Clinical Anesthesia Practice

Clinical Anesthesia Practice

ROBERT R. KIRBY, M.D.
Professor of Anesthesiology
Department of Anesthesiology
University of Florida College of Medicine
Gainesville, Florida

NIKOLAUS GRAVENSTEIN, M.D.
Professor and Executive Associate Chairman
Department of Anesthesiology, and
Professor of Neurosurgery
Department of Neurosurgery
University of Florida College of Medicine
Gainesville, Florida

W.B. SAUNDERS COMPANY
A Division of Harcourt Brace & Company
Philadelphia   London   Toronto   Montreal   Sydney   Tokyo

W.B. SAUNDERS COMPANY
A Division of
Harcourt Brace & Company

The Curtis Center
Independence Square West
Philadelphia, Pennsylvania 19106

Library of Congress Cataloging-in-Publication Data

Clinical anesthesia practice / [edited by] Robert R. Kirby, Nikolaus Gravenstein.

    p.   cm.

ISBN 0–7216–3328–5

1. Anesthesiology.   I. Kirby, Robert R.   II. Gravenstein, Nikolaus.

[DNLM: 1. Anesthesia. WO 200 C6412 1994]

RD81.C584 1994

617.9′6—dc20

DNLM/DLC   93–41602

Clinical Anesthesia Practice   ISBN 0–7216–3328–5

Printed in the United States of America

Last digit is the print number: 9   8   7   6   5   4   3   2   1

Contributors

R. DENNIS BASTRON, M.D.

Professor of Anesthesiology, Texas A&M University Health Science Center, College of Medicine, College Station, TX; Anesthesiologist, Scott and White Clinic, Temple, TX
Nephrology Consultation

JERRY J. BERGER, M.D.

Associate Professor of Anesthesiology, and Director of Pain Management, University of Florida College of Medicine; Staff Member, Shands Hospital at the University of Florida, Gainesville, FL
Genitourinary Surgery

DAVID R. BEVAN, M.B., M.R.C.P., F.F.A.R.C.S.

Professor and Head, Department of Anaesthesia, Faculty of Medicine, The University of British Columbia; Head, Department of Anaesthesia, Vancouver General Hospital, Vancouver, British Columbia, Canada
Acid-Base

SUSAN BLACK, M.D.

Associate Professor, Department of Anesthesiology, University of Florida College of Medicine, Gainesville, FL
Abnormal Intracranial Pressure

ROBERT BLACKSHEAR, M.D.

Clinical Assistant Professor of Anesthesiology, University of Florida College of Medicine, Gainesville, FL; and University of Utah College of Medicine, Salt Lake City, UT
Positioning the Surgical Patient

PHILIP G. BOYSEN, M.D., F.A.C.P., F.C.C.P.

Professor, Anesthesiology and Medicine, University of Florida College of Medicine; Chief, Anesthesia Services, and Co-Director, Surgical Intensive Care Unit, Veterans Administration Medical Center, Gainesville, FL
Pulmonary Consultation; Anesthetic Considerations for Thoracic Surgery

DAVID L. BROWN, M.D.

Associate Professor, Department of Anesthesiology, Mayo Medical School, and Consultant, Mayo Clinic and Foundation, Rochester, MN
Risk and Outcome Analysis: Myths and Truths; Regional Anesthesia

ROY D. CANE, M.B., B.Ch., F.F.A.(S.A.)

Professor of Anesthesiology, Department of Anesthesiology, University of South Florida College of Medicine; Director, Critical Care Medicine, Department of Anesthesiology, Tampa General Hospital, Tampa, FL
Hypoxemia; Abnormal Ventilation

DONALD CATON, M.D.

Professor of Anesthesiology and Obstetrics and Gynecology, and Graduate Research Faculty, University of Florida College of Medicine; Chief, Obstetrical Anesthesia Service, J. Hillis Miller Health Center, Shands Hospital at the University of Florida, Gainesville, FL
The Obstetric Patient

WILLIAM T. CEFALU, M.D.

Assistant Professor of Medicine, Bowman Gray School of Medicine of Wake Forest University; Staff Member, North Carolina Baptist Hospital, Inc., Winston-Salem, NC
Endocrine Consultation

JESSE L. CHAI, M.D.

Resident in Radiology, Department of Radiology, Duke University Medical Center, Durham, NC
Radiology Consultation

JERRY A. COHEN, M.D.

Associate Professor of Anesthesiology, Department of Anesthesiology, University of Florida College of Medicine; Associate Chief of Staff for Quality Management; Chairman, Patient Care Evaluation Committee; Chairman, Medical Staff Evaluation Committee; and Chairman, Medical Records Committee, Shands Hospital at the University of Florida, Gainesville, FL
Quality Assurance in Anesthesiology

RANDALL C. CORK, M.D., Ph.D.

Professor of Anesthesiology, Louisiana State University; Professor, Department of Anesthesiology, Louisiana State University Medical Center, New Orleans, LA
Temperature Monitoring

EDWARD T. CROSBY, B.Sc., M.D., F.R.C.P.C.

Assistant Professor, Department of Anesthesia, University of Ottawa; Consultant Staff Member, Ottawa General Hospital, Ottawa, Ontario, Canada
The Spine

ROY CUCCHIARA, M.D.

Professor and Chairman of Anesthesiology, Department of Anesthesiology, University of Florida School of Medicine, Gainesville, FL
Abnormal Intracranial Pressure

CHRISTINE A. CZEPIZAK, M.S., P.A.-C.

Physician Assistant, Department of Critical Care Medicine, Memorial Medical Center, Jacksonville, FL
Vascular System Anatomy; Vascular Access

LAURIE K. DAVIES, M.D.

Associate Professor of Anesthesiology, Department of Anesthesiology, University of Florida College of Medicine; Staff Physician, Shands Hospital at the University of Florida; Staff Physician, Department of Veterans Affairs Medical Center, Gainesville, FL
Anesthesia for Pediatric Cardiovascular Surgery

DONN M. DENNIS, M.D.

Assistant Professor of Anesthesiology and Pharmacology and Experimental Therapeutics, University of Florida College of Medicine; Staff Member, Shands Hospital at the University of Florida, Gainesville, FL
Anesthesia for Aortic Vascular Surgery

STEPHEN F. DIERDORF, M.D.

Professor of Anesthesia, Indiana University School of Medicine; Director, Anesthesia Section, Richard L. Roudebush Veterans Affairs Medical Center, Indianapolis, IN
Anesthesia for Patients with Chronic Obstructive Pulmonary Disease; Anesthesia for Patients with Bronchial Asthma

CHERYL L. DIXON, M.D.

Assistant Professor of Anesthesiology, Department of Anesthesiology, University of Florida College of Medicine; Associate Director, Pain Management Clinic, and Director, Acute Pain Service, Shands Hospital at the University of Florida, Gainesville, FL
Pain Management Consultation in Adult Patients

ERAN DOLEV, M.D.

Associate Professor of Internal Medicine, Sackler School of Medicine, Tel Aviv University, Tel Aviv; Head, Department of Internal Medicine "E", Wolfson Hospital, Holon, Israel
Battlefield Surgery and Anesthesia

THOMAS J. EBERT, M.D.

Associate Professor of Anesthesiology, and Adjunct Professor of Physiology, The Medical College of Wisconsin and Affiliated Hospitals, Milwaukee, WI
Autonomic Nervous System

JAMES ECKHART, ESQ.

Carey, Dwyer, Eckhart, Mason, and Spring P.A.; Lead Counsel, Anesthesiologists' Professional Assurance Company, Miami, FL
Medicolegal Issues and Concerns

JAY S. ELLIS, M.D., Lt. Col., U.S.A.F., M.C.

Arthur B. Tarrow Chairman, Department of Anesthesiology, Wilford Hall United States Air Force Medical Center/59th Medical Wing, Lackland Air Force Base, Lackland, TX; Clinical Assistant Professor, Department of Anesthesiology, University of Texas Health Science Center, San Antonio, TX; Clinical Assistant Professor, Department of Anesthesiology, Uniformed Services University of the Health Sciences, F. Edward Hebert School of Medicine, Bethesda, MD
Local Anesthetics; Battlefield Surgery and Anesthesia

F. KAYSER ENNEKING, M.D.

Assistant Professor, Department of Anesthesiology, University of Florida College of Medicine; Staff Anesthesiologist, Shands Teaching Hospital at the University of Florida, Gainesville, FL
Anesthesia for Orthopedic Surgery

BURTON S. EPSTEIN, M.D.

Seymour Alpert Professor of Anesthesiology, The George Washington University School of Medicine; Attending Physician in Anesthesia, The George Washington University Hospital, Washington, DC
Outpatient Surgery

MICHAEL J. FEFFER, M.D.

Assistant Professor of Anesthesiology, State University of New York Health Science Center at Brooklyn, Brooklyn, NY
Otolaryngologic and Maxillofacial Surgery

JEFFREY M. FELDMAN, M.D., M.S.E.

Assistant Professor of Anesthesiology, Temple University School of Medicine; Director of Anesthesia Research, Albert Einstein Medical Center, Philadelphia, PA
The Anesthetic Record

ORLANDO G. FLORETE, Jr., M.D.

Clinical Assistant Professor, University of Florida Health Science Center.
Airway Devices and Their Application

H. JERREL FONTENOT, M.D., Ph.D.

Vice Chairman, Department of Anesthesiology; Associate Professor of Anesthesiology and Pharmacology, Department of Anesthesiology; Medical Director, Operating Room and Clinical Services, University of Arkansas for Medical Sciences, Little Rock, AR
Neuromuscular Junction Monitoring and Nerve Stimulation

PHILLIP GAUKROGER, M.D., F.F.A.R.A.C.S.

Clinical Lecturer, University of Adelaide; Senior Consultant in Anaesthesia, Department of Anaesthesia, Women's and Children's Hospital, North Adelaide, South Australia, Australia
Pain Management Consultation in Pediatric Patients

PETER GERNER, M.D.

Research Fellow, Department of Anesthesiology, University of Arkansas for Medical Sciences, Little Rock, AR
Neuromuscular Junction Monitoring and Nerve Stimulation

HUGH C. GILBERT, M.D.

Assistant Clinical Professor, Division of Anesthesia, Northwestern University Medical School; Staff Member, The Evanston Hospital, Evanston, IL
Cardiovascular Monitoring

JULIAN M. GOLDMAN, M.D.

Assistant Professor of Anesthesiology, and Director of Anesthesia Research, University of Colorado School of Medicine; Staff Anesthesiologist, University Hospital; Staff Anesthesiologist, Veterans Affairs Medical Center, Denver, CO

Respiratory Monitoring

MICHAEL L. GOOD, M.D.

Associate Professor of Anesthesiology, Department of Anesthesiology, University of Florida College of Medicine, Gainesville, FL

The Anesthesia Machine, Anesthesia Ventilator, Breathing Circuit, and Scavenging System

SALVATORE R. GOODWIN, M.D.

Associate Professor of Anesthesiology and Pediatrics, University of Florida College of Medicine; Medical Director, Pediatric Intensive Care Unit, Shands Hospital at the University of Florida, Gainesville, FL

Drug Interactions

ALEXANDER W. GOTTA, M.D.

Professor of Clinical Anesthesiology, State University of New York Health Science Center at Brooklyn; Chief of Service—Anesthesia, Kings County Hospital Center, Brooklyn, NY

Otolaryngologic and Maxillofacial Surgery

J. S. GRAVENSTEIN, M.D.

Graduate Research Professor, Department of Anesthesiology, University of Florida College of Medicine, Gainesville, FL

Introduction to Monitoring: Clinical Monitoring; General Anesthesia: Induction, Maintenance, and Emergence

NIKOLAUS GRAVENSTEIN, M.D.

Professor, Department of Anesthesiology, and Professor of Neurosurgery, Department of Neurosurgery, University of Florida College of Medicine, Gainesville, FL

Positioning the Surgical Patient

SERGIO GREGORETTI, M.D.

Assistant Professor, Department of Anesthesiology, University of Alabama School of Medicine, University of Alabama at Birmingham, Birmingham, AL

Abdominal Surgery

GREGORY M. GULLAHORN, M.D., L.C.D.R., M.C., U.S.N.R.

Clinical Instructor, Director of Neuroanesthesiology, and Co-Director of Critical Care Anesthesiology, Naval Medical Center San Diego; Clinical Instructor, University of California at San Diego; Staff Member, Departments of Anesthesiology and Critical Care Medicine, and Hyperbaric Medicine, Naval Medical Center San Diego; Department of Anesthesiology, Mercy Hospital and Medical Center San Diego; Departments of Anesthesiology, Critical Care, and Hyperbarics, University of California at San Diego, San Diego, CA

Monitoring During Patient Transport

RAAFAT S. HANNALLAH, M.D.

Professor of Anesthesiology and Pediatrics, The George Washington University Medical Center; Vice Chairman of Anesthesiology, Childrens National Medical Center, Washington, DC

Outpatient Surgery

MAXIMILIAN W. B. HARTMANNSGRUBER, M.D.

Scientific Assistant, Department of Anesthesiology, Ludwig-Maximilians-Universität; Staff Member, Klinikum Grossbaden, Munich, Germany

Thermal Injuries: Pathophysiology and Anesthetic Considerations

STEPHEN O. HEARD, M.D.

Associate Professor of Anesthesiology and Surgery, and Co-Director, Surgical Intensive Care Units, University of Massachusetts Medical Center; Staff Member, University of Massachusetts Medical Center, Worcester, MA

Preanesthetic Evaluation

JAN C. HORROW, M.D.

Professor and Deputy Chair, Department of Anesthesiology, Hahnemann University; Director, Cardiothoracic Anesthesia, Hahnemann University Hospital, Philadelphia, PA

Electrical Safety

MICHAEL D. INGRAM, M.D.

Assistant Professor of Anesthesiology, Medical College of Pennsylvania, Philadelphia, PA; Associate Attending Staff, Division of Anesthesiology, Allegheny General Hospital, Pittsburgh, PA

Shock

CHRISTOPHER F. JAMES, M.D.

Associate Professor of Anesthesiology, Department of Anesthesiology, University of Florida College of Medicine; Staff Anesthesiologist, Shands Hospital at the University of Florida; Veterans Administration Medical Center, Gainesville, FL

Nonobstetric Surgery in the Pregnant Patient

KENNETH M. JANIS, M.D.

Associate Professor, Department of Anesthesiology, University of New Mexico; Assistant Chief of Anesthesiology, Veterans Administration Hospital, Albuquerque, NM

The Geriatric Patient

VINCENT G. JOHNSON, D.O.

Medical Director, Surgicenter of Kansas City; Staff Member, Baptist Medical Center, Kansas City, MO

The Pediatric Patient

ROBERT KETTLER, M.D.

Associate Professor of Anesthesiology, Medical College of Wisconsin; Attending Physician, Milwaukee County Medical Complex, Froedtert Memorial Lutheran Hospital, Veterans Administration Medical Center, Milwaukee, WI

Autonomic Nervous System

ROBERT R. KIRBY, M.D.

Professor of Anesthesiology, Department of Anesthesiology, University of Florida College of Medicine; Staff Anesthesiologist and Medical Director, Respiratory Care, Shands Hospital at the University of Florida, Gainesville, FL

General Anesthesia: Induction, Maintenance, and Emergence; Fluids and Electrolytes; Cardiopulmonary Resuscitation; Battlefield Surgery and Anesthesia

A. JAY KOSKA, M.D., Ph.D.

Assistant Professor, Departments of Anesthesiology and Pediatrics, University of Florida College of Medicine; Staff Member, Shands Hospital at the University of Florida, Gainesville, FL

Intravenous Agents

A. JOSEPH LAYON, M.D., F.A.C.P.

Associate Professor, Departments of Anesthesiology and Medicine, University of Florida College of Medicine; Director, Preoperative Evaluation Clinic, Shands Hospital at the University of Florida, Gainesville, FL

Thermal Injuries: Pathophysiology and Anesthetic Considerations; Occupational Hazards in the Operating Room

THOMAS W. LEBERT, II, M.D.

Staff Attending Anesthesiologist, St. Joseph's Hospital of Atlanta, Atlanta, GA

Nonobstetric Surgery in the Pregnant Patient

JERROLD H. LEVY, M.D.

Associate Professor of Anesthesiology, Department of Anesthesiology, Emory University School of Medicine; Staff Member, Division of Cardiothoracic Anesthesia and Critical Care, The Emory Clinic, Atlanta, GA

Allergy and Immunology

MONTE LICHTIGER, M.D.

Professor of Clinical Anesthesiology, University of Miami School of Medicine; Vice Chairman, Department of Anesthesiology, Mt. Sinai Medical Center of Greater Miami; Medical Director, Gumenick Ambulatory Surgical Facility, Mt. Sinai Medical Center of Greater Miami, Miami, FL

Medicolegal Issues and Concerns

RICHARD B. LILLY, Jr., M.D.

Assistant Director, Department of Anesthesiology, and Director of Ambulatory Surgery, Hartford Hospital, Hartford CT; Senior Staff Anesthesiologist, Newington Childrens Hospital, Newington, CT

Temperature Fluctuations

MARIAN C. LIMACHER, M.D.

Associate Professor of Medicine, and Director of Preventive Cardiology, Division of Cardiovascular Medicine, University of Florida College of Medicine; Associate Chief of Cardiology, and Director, Cardiology Non-Invasive Laboratory, Veterans Administration Medical Center; Attending Cardiologist, Shands Hospital at the University of Florida, Gainesville, FL

Cardiology Consultation

MARTIN J. LONDON, M.D.

Associate Professor of Anesthesiology, University of Colorado Health Sciences Center; Chief, Anesthesia Service, Veterans Affairs Medical Center, Denver, CO

Myocardial Ischemia and Dysfunction

SALVATORE LoPALO, C.R.N.A., M.S. Ed., M.A.

Associate in Anesthesiology, Department of Anesthesiology, University of Florida College of Medicine; Staff Member, Shands Hospital at the University of Florida, Gainesville, FL

Occupational Hazards in the Operating Room; Battlefield Surgery and Anesthesia

ANNE C. P. LUI, M.Sc., M.D., F.R.C.P.C.

Lecturer, Department of Anaesthesiology, University of Ottawa; Active Attending Staff Member, Ottawa Civic Hospital, Ottawa, Ontario, Canada

The Spine

MICHAEL E. MAHLA, M.D.

Associate Professor of Anesthesiology and Neurosurgery, and Chief, Division of Neuroanesthesia, University of Florida College of Medicine; Director of Neuroanesthesia, and Director of Neurologic Monitoring Laboratory, Shands Hospital at the University of Florida, Gainesville, FL

Monitoring the Nervous System; Neurologic Surgery

VINOD MALHOTRA, M.D.

Associate Professor, Department of Anesthesiology, Cornell University Medical College; Attending Anesthesiologist, The New York Hospital; Director, Post Graduate Training, Department of Anesthesiology, The New York Hospital–Cornell University Medical Center, New York, NY

Extracorporeal Shock Wave Lithotripsy

J. R. MARSHALL, M.D.

Clinical Professor of Anesthesiology, University of Miami; Director, Anesthesiology Training Program, Mt. Sinai Medical Center; Staff Member, Mt. Sinai Medical Center, Miami, FL

Cardiopulmonary Resuscitation

THOMAS J. MARTIN, M.D.

Attending Anesthesiologist, Hartford Hospital, Hartford, CT

Cardiopulmonary Bypass; Anesthesia for Adult Cardiovascular Surgery

TIMOTHY W. MARTIN, M.D.

Assistant Professor of Anesthesiology, University of Arkansas for Medical Sciences; Staff Anesthesiologist, Arkansas Children's Hospital, Little Rock, AR

The Neonate; The Pediatric Patient

EDWARD K. McGOUGH, M.D.

Staff Anesthesiologist, Memorial Medical Center of Jacksonville, Jacksonville, FL

Fluids and Electrolytes

ROGER S. MECCA, M.D.

Chairman, Department of Anesthesiology, Danbury Hospital, Danbury, CT; Clinical Associate Professor, Department of Anesthesiology, Yale–New Haven Hospital, New Haven, CT

Postanesthesia Recovery; Management of the Difficult Airway

RICHARD J. MELKER, M.D., PH.D.

Associate Professor of Anesthesiology, Surgery, and Pediatrics, University of Florida College of Medicine, Gainesville, FL

Cardiopulmonary Resuscitation

W. JERRY MERRELL, M.D.

Clinical Associate Professor, Departments of Anesthesiology and Pharmacology and Therapeutics, University of Florida College of

Medicine, Gainesville, FL; Staff Anesthesiologist, Florida Hospital, Orlando, FL

Basic Pharmacologic Applications in Anesthesia; Intravenous Agents

EDWARD D. MILLER, Jr., M.D.

E. M. Papper Professor of Anesthesiology and Chairman, Department of Anesthesiology, College of Physicians and Surgeons, Columbia University; Director, Anesthesiology Service, Presbyterian Hospital, New York, NY

Surgery of the Endocrine System

MARK C. MONROE, M.D.

Staff Anesthesiologist, Memorial Medical Center of Jacksonville, Jacksonville, FL

Anesthetic Management for Heart Transplantation

S. S. MOORTHY, M.D.

Professor of Anesthesia and Respiratory Care, Indiana University School of Medicine; Staff Member, Indiana University Medical Center; Richard L. Roudebush Veterans Affairs Medical Center, Indianapolis, IN

Anesthesia for Patients with Bronchial Asthma; Anesthesia for Patients with Chronic Obstructive Pulmonary Disease

THOMAS C. MORT, M.D.

Associate Professor of Surgery, University of Connecticut School of Medicine, Farmington, CT; Clinical Assistant of Anesthesiology; Associate Director, Surgical Intensive Care Unit; and Medical Director, Postanesthesia Care Unit, Hartford Hospital, Hartford, CT

Temperature Fluctuations

MARY BETH MYERS, R.N., M.S.

Clinical Adjunct Faculty, Illinois Wesleyan University; and University of Illinois College of Medicine, Chicago, IL; Trauma Coordinator, Carle Foundation Hospital, Urbana, IL

Trauma

SCOTT H. NORWOOD, M.D.

Director, Trauma Services, East Texas Medical Center/Mother Frances Hospital, Tyler, TX

Trauma

K. PATRICK OBER, M.D.

Associate Professor of Internal Medicine (Endocrinology and Metabolism), Bowman Gray School of Medicine of Wake Forest University; Staff Member, North Carolina Baptist Hospital, Winston-Salem, NC

Endocrine Consultation

JAMES M. O'CALLAGHAN, P.A.-C., B.M.Sc.

Physician's Assistant to the Director of Critical Care, Memorial Medical Center of Jacksonville, Jacksonville, FL

Vascular System Anatomy; Vascular Access

ANNETTE G. PASHAYAN, M.D.

Associate Professor of Anesthesiology and Neurosurgery, University of Florida College of Medicine; Staff Anesthesiologist, Shands Hospital at the University of Florida, Gainesville, FL

Lasers and Laser Safety

DAVID A. PAULUS, M.D.

Professor of Anesthesiology and Mechanical Engineering, University of Florida College of Medicine; Cardiovascular Anesthesiologist, Shands Hospital at the University of Florida; Medical Director, Shands HomeCare at Shands Hospital, Gainesville, FL

Medicine and Anesthesia: Financial and Other Costs

AZRIEL PEREL, M.D.

Associate Professor of Anesthesiology and Intensive Care, Sackler School of Medicine, Tel Aviv University, Tel Aviv; Chairman, Department of Anesthesiology and Intensive Care, Sheba Medical Center, Tel Hashomer, Israel

Battlefield Surgery and Anesthesia; Pulmonary Edema

JUKKA RÄSÄNEN, M.D.

Associate Professor of Anesthesiology, Department of Anesthesiology, University of South Florida College of Medicine; Staff Anesthesiologist, Department of Anesthesiology, Tampa General Hospital, Tampa, FL

Hypoxemia; Abnormal Ventilation

CARL E. RAVIN, M.D.

Professor of Radiology, Department of Radiology, and Chairman of Radiology, Duke University Medical Center, Durham, NC

Radiology Consultation

WILLIAM C. ROBBINS, M.D.

Interventional Cardiology Fellow, University of Florida College of Medicine, Gainesville, FL

Cardiology Consultation

MARK E. ROMANOFF, M.D.

Staff Anesthesiologist, Carolinas Medical Center, Charlotte, NC

Radiologic Procedures, Computed Tomography Scans, Magnetic Resonance Imaging, and Radiation Therapy

MARK T. SCARBOROUGH, M.D.

Assistant Professor, Department of Orthopaedic Surgery, University of Florida College of Medicine, Gainesville, FL

Anesthesia for Orthopedic Surgery

ERAN SEGAL, M.D.

Instructor in Anesthesiology, Sackler School of Medicine, Tel Aviv University, Tel Aviv; Attending Anesthesiologist, Department of Anesthesiology and Intensive Care, Sheba Medical Center, Tel Hashomer, Israel

Pulmonary Edema

AVNER SIDI, M.D.

Associate Professor of Anesthesiology, Department of Anesthesiology, University of Florida College of Medicine; Staff Anesthesiologist, Shands Hospital at the University of Florida, Gainesville, FL

Orthotopic Liver Transplantation; Renal Transplantation

DALE E. SOLOMON, M.D.

Assistant Professor, Department of Anesthesiology, University of Texas Health Science Center at San Antonio; Staff Anesthesiologist,

Audie L. Murphy Memorial Veterans Hospital Medical Center; Director of the Post-Anesthesia Care Unit, San Antonio Regional Hospital, San Antonio, TX

Neurologic Consultation

DIANE H. SOLOMON, M.D.

Assistant Professor, Department of Medicine, Division of Neurology, University of Texas Health Science Center at San Antonio; Staff Neurologist, Audie L. Murphy Memorial Veterans Hospital Medical Center, San Antonio, TX

Neurologic Consultation

JENNIFER SOUDERS, M.D.

Acting Instructor, Department of Anesthesiology, University of Washington School of Medicine; Staff Physician, University of Washington Medical Center, and Harborview Medical Center, Seattle, WA

Respiratory Monitoring

DONALD S. STEVENS, M.D.

Assistant Professor of Anesthesiology, and Staff Member, University of Massachusetts Medical Center, Worcester, MA

Preanesthetic Evaluation

WENDELL C. STEVENS, M.D.

Professor of Anesthesiology, Oregon Health Sciences University; Attending Anesthesiologist, Oregon Health Sciences University Hospital, and Veterans Affairs Medical Center, Portland, OR

Inhalation Agents

COLLEEN A. SULLIVAN, M.B., Ch.B.

Clinical Professor of Anesthesiology, State University of New York Health Science Center at Brooklyn; Medical Director, Ambulatory Surgery, Kings County Hospital Center, Brooklyn, NY

Otolaryngologic and Maxillofacial Surgery

JERRY J. TOMASOVIC, M.D.

Clinical Associate Professor of Pediatrics, University of Texas Health Science Center at San Antonio; Staff Physician, Southwest Texas Methodist Hospital, Santa Rosa Children's Hospital, Laurel Ridge Hospital, and Baptist Memorial Hospital System, San Antonio, TX

Neurologic Consultation

DAVID J. TORPEY, Jr., M.D.

Professor and Chairman, Department of Anesthesiology, Allegheny Campus, Medical College of Pennsylvania; Senior Attending Staff, and Director, Division of Anesthesiology, Allegheny General Hospital, Pittsburgh, PA

Shock

LEROY D. VANDAM, Ph.B., M.D., M.A.

Professor of Anaesthesia, Emeritus, Harvard Medical School; Anesthetist, Brigham and Women's Hospital, Boston, MA

Functional Anatomy of the Airway

MARK VEERMAN, Pharm.D.

Clinical Associate Professor, Department of Pharmacy Practice, University of Florida College of Pharmacy; Clinical Pharmacy Specialist, Pediatrics, Shands Hospital at the University of Florida, Gainesville, FL

Drug Interactions

JEFFERY S. VENDER, M.D., F.C.C.M.

Associate Professor of Anesthesiology, Northwestern University Medical School, Chicago, IL; Chief of Anesthesia and Director, Medical-Surgical Intensive Care, Evanston Hospital, Evanston, IL

Cardiovascular Monitoring

BAHMAN VENUS, M.D., F.C.C.P., F.C.C.M.

Chairman and Director, Critical Care Medicine, Memorial Medical Center, Jacksonville, FL

Vascular System Anatomy; Vascular Access

SNO E. WHITE, M.D.

Assistant Professor of Anesthesiology, Department of Anesthesiology, University of Florida College of Medicine; Staff Member, Shands Hospital at the University of Florida, and the Veterans Administration Medical Center, Gainesville, FL

The Preoperative Visit and Premedication

GARY P. ZALOGA, M.D., F.A.C.P., F.C.C.M.

Professor of Anesthesia and Medicine (Endocrinology), Bowman Gray School of Medicine of Wake Forest University; Head, Section on Critical Care, Department of Anesthesia, North Carolina Baptist Hospital, Winston-Salem, NC

Endocrine Consultation

Preface

In the 1960s, when one of us (RRK) received his training, the number of anesthesiology textbooks was limited. Authors such as Wylie, Churchill-Davidson, Dripps, Eckenhoff, Vandam, Adriani, Cullen, Moore, Lee, and Collins were well known to practicing anesthesiologists and residents alike. By the early 1980s, when NG was in training, an explosion in anesthesia publishing was already underway. New names—Miller, Stoelting, Gregory, Orkin, Cooperman, Cousins, Blitt, Martin, Shnider, Barash, Benumof, Kaplan, and others too numerous to mention—became as well known as their predecessors. Their books were comprehensive, informative, and, in many cases, encyclopedic. More texts already were available than most practitioners could hope to read and assimilate in a lifetime.

Why then, in the face of apparent plenty, should this textbook have been conceived, yet alone published? We are convinced that an approach to clinical anesthesia that differs in several ways from that presented in available texts can be of practical use. Specifically, our goal has been to incorporate the clinical practice of anesthesia, equivalent to two volumes, under a single cover. To do so, we have divided the text roughly as follows. The first nine sections (54 chapters) deal with fundamental concepts with which everyone who practices or is learning about anesthesia should be familiar. The subject matter is generic in the sense that the information is applicable to almost any case. Rather than to make these discussions all-encompassing, we asked the contributors to focus their discussions on what they consider to be the *clinically relevant* and, to the reader, *clinically applicable* features of the particular concepts being considered.

In order to provide up-to-date, expert treatments with a fresh outlook, we chose many contributors who have published or lectured on their topics but have not written on the same topics in one of the major anesthesiology texts. This arrangement allows the reader to obtain a different perspective in areas where opinions and approaches are divergent; conversely, it may confirm that an approach to a case is standard when it mirrors information that is available in other writings.

The 10th section (comprising 26 chapters) arises out of our observation that, when preparing for a type of case we have not done recently (or may never have done before), we are often frustrated by having to piece together the relevant facts from numerous sources. For that reason, we asked the contributors to include the relevant anatomy, physiology, pharmacology, and surgical procedure/anesthetic interactions in their approach to clinical management. Specifically, they were requested to organize their discussions as if they were describing their approach to a colleague who had not dealt with a particular problem for some time. In all cases, they were requested to provide "tips" or "pearls" that they have found useful in their practice and that are of practical use even if they are not validated scientifically.

We also requested that contributors don their soothsayer caps whenever possible and project what future major advances or changes appear likely in their specialties and subspecialties. The reader exposed to such prognostication may thus be stimulated to peruse a scientific article on a subject with no apparent current clinical relevance, but which he or she recognizes as having the potential to become a "hot" topic in the next few years.

We attempted to render each of the chapters similar one to another with respect to style but without altering the flavor of each individual author's contributions. Usually, a reference text is perused to answer a question. Therefore, we have introduced each major topic with a question, and this question is followed by the information that provides the answer. The discerning reader will note duplication of some subject matter and even of a few illustrations in some chapters. This approach was deliberate on our part and is based on our annoyance when we must break our trains-of-thought while reading intently and are referred to another part of a book for a figure, table, or related discussion. Although we have not resolved this problem completely, we have tried to make chapters stand on their own merit as much as possible.

Our sincere thanks go to Lew Reines, President and Chief Executive Officer of W.B. Saunders Company, who finally convinced us (we think!) that this effort was worthwhile. The editors also commend the work of the copy editor, Frank Messina, who achieved the miraculous with late entries and revisions and whose gracious cooperation was indispensable in maintaining the high standards set forth for this book. Finally, the editors thank Hope Olivo, our assistant editor, who, as so often in the past, made it all possible!

We wish to dedicate this textbook to T.W. Andersen, M.D., Professor of Anesthesiology, who has been a mentor, teacher, friend, and role model for faculty and residents alike at the University of Florida for over 30 years.

ROBERT R. KIRBY, M.D.
NIKOLAUS GRAVENSTEIN, M.D.

Contents

SECTION I

Toward a Safer Practice 1

Chapter 1

Preanesthetic Evaluation 1
STEPHEN O. HEARD, M.D.
DONALD S. STEVENS, M.D.

Purposes 1
Procedures 1
Historical Information 2
Medications 5
Allergic Responses 9
Social History 9
Physical Examination 9
Laboratory Testing 11
Special Testing 12
Consultations 14
Preoperative Medication 15
Nil Per Os Status 15

Chapter 2

The Anesthetic Record 21
JEFFREY M. FELDMAN, M.D., M.S.E.

Purposes of the Record 21
Creating the Record 24
The Automated Anesthesia Record 28
Postanesthesia Documentation 29
Conclusions 29

Chapter 3

Quality Assurance in Anesthesiology 31
JERRY A. COHEN, M.D.

Historical Considerations 31
Peer Review Organizations 32
Current Quality Assurance 33
Current Ground Rules and Implementation 38
Joint Commission on Accreditation of Healthcare
    Organizations Survey 40

Quality Assurance in Anesthesia Practice 41
Appendix I Abstract of 1992 JCAHO Accreditation Manual
    for Hospitals 49
Appendix II Selection of Quality Assurance Database
    Software 51

Chapter 4

Medicolegal Issues and Concerns 53
MONTE LICHTIGER, M.D.
JAMES ECKHART, ESQ.

Introduction 53
The Malpractice Insurance Crisis 53
Current Status 54
Negligence 55
Future Problems 56
Adverse Events 57
Defense 57
Types of Liability 59
The Anesthesiologist As an Expert Witness ... 59
Malpractice Insurance 60

Chapter 5

Risk and Outcome Analysis: Myths and Truths 62
DAVID L. BROWN, M.D.

Risk Stratification 62
Outcome Measurement 63
Preoperative Risk Assessment 64
Functional Physiologic Risk Factors 64
Anesthetic Prescription 67
Postoperative Analgesia 70

Chapter 6

Postanesthesia Recovery 73
ROGER S. MECCA, M.D.

General Concerns 73
Pain Control 76
Postoperative Oxygenation 77

Postoperative Ventilation 81
Pulmonary Aspiration Syndrome 85
Postoperative Hypotension 88
Postoperative Hypertension 91
Postoperative Electrocardiographic Abnormalities 92
Postoperative Renal Problems 94
Central Nervous System Function 95
Postoperative Nausea and Vomiting 99
Postoperative Hypothermia 100
Postoperative Hyperthermia 101
Postoperative Acid-Base Problems 101
Postoperative Glucose and Electrolyte Abnormalities 102
Miscellaneous Postoperative Complications 103

Chapter 7

Medicine and Anesthesia: Financial and Other Costs 109

DAVID A. PAULUS, M.D.

Alternatives to the Present Health Care System in the
    United States 109
The Future 110
The Environment 114
Hospital Waste 114
Monitoring 116
Funding of Equipment Costs 118
Conclusion 120

SECTION II

Perioperative Consultations 125

Chapter 8

Cardiology Consultation 125

MARIAN C. LIMACHER, M.D.
WILLIAM C. ROBBINS, M.D.

Cardiac Risk Factors 126
Assessment: The Cardiologist's Role 135
Postoperative Consultation 138

Chapter 9

Pulmonary Consultation 143

PHILIP G. BOYSEN, M.D., F.A.C.P., F.C.C.P.

General Considerations 143
Specific Measures 144
Intraoperative Consultation 145
Postoperative Care 146

Chapter 10

Neurologic Consultation 152

DALE E. SOLOMON, M.D.
DIANE H. SOLOMON, M.D.
JERRY J. TOMASOVIC, M.D.

The Perioperative Neurologic Consult 152
Myasthenia Gravis 153
Parkinson's Disease 154
Stroke 154
Multiple Sclerosis 155
Muscular Dystrophy 156
Guillain-Barré Syndrome 156
Huntington's Disease 157
Pseudotumor Cerebri 157
Pre-Eclampsia/Eclampsia 157
Neuroleptic Malignant Syndrome 158
Known Seizure Disorders 159
Obstructive Sleep Apnea 161
Peripheral Nerve Injury 161
Neurologic Complications After Spinal or
    Epidural Anesthesia 163
Postanesthetic Neurologic Examination 163
Postoperative Delirium 165
Postischemic/Hypoxic Brain Injury 166
Postoperative Headache 167
Status Epilepticus 167
Conclusion 168

Chapter 11

Nephrology Consultation 170

R. DENNIS BASTRON, M.D.

Purpose of the Consultation 170
Hypertension 170
Fluid Therapy 171
Sodium 172
Potassium 173
Calcium 175
Magnesium 176
Phosphorus 177
Renal Function Tests 178
Compromised Renal Function 179
Renal Toxicity 182
Dialysis Patients 183

Chapter 12

Endocrine Consultation 185

GARY P. ZALOGA, M.D., F.A.C.P., F.C.C.M.
K. PATRICK OBER, M.D.
WILLIAM T. CEFALU, M.D.

Pituitary Disease 185
Adrenal Disease 189
Thyroid Disease 196
Parathyroid Disease 202
Diabetes Mellitus 205

Chapter 13

Radiology Consultation 211

JESSE L. CHAI, M.D.
CARL E. RAVIN, M.D.

The Thorax 211
The Neck 223
The Abdomen 226

Chapter 14

Pain Management Consultation in Adult Patients 233
CHERYL L. DIXON, M.D.

The Adult Pain Management Consultation 233
Management Techniques 239
Controversies 250
Regional Anesthetic Techniques 253
Neurolytic Blocks 254
Neuroaugmentation 254
Physical Therapy 255
Psychologic Therapy 256

Chapter 15

Pain Management Consultation in Pediatric Patients 261
PHILLIP GAUKROGER, M.D., F.F.A.R.A.C.S.

Pediatric Pain Management 261
Spectrum of Pediatric Pain 262
Assessment and Measurement of Pain in Children 263
Postoperative Pain Management 263
Techniques of Analgesic Administration 265
Regional Blockade 267
Procedural Pain in Children 270
Analgesia for Burns 271
Cancer Pain 271
Chronic Noncancer Pain 272
Pediatric Pain Management Services 273

SECTION III

Tools of the Trade and Their Applications 276

Chapter 16

The Anesthesia Machine, Anesthesia Ventilator, Breathing Circuit, and Scavenging System 276
MICHAEL L. GOOD, M.D.

Basic Concepts 276
High-Pressure System 276
Low-Pressure System 281
Breathing System 285
Waste Gas Scavenging Systems 288
Troubleshooting the Gas Delivery System 291
Monitoring the Anesthesia Machine 294
Standards and Changes in Anesthesia Machine Design ... 296
Future Developments 296

Chapter 17

Airway Devices and Their Application ... 298
ORLANDO G. FLORETE, Jr., M.D.

Oral and Nasal Airways 298

Esophageal, Pharyngeal, and Laryngeal Tubes 299
Facemask/Bag-Valve Ventilation 301
Laryngoscopes 302
Bronchoscopes 305
Fiberoptic Laryngoscopes 306
Single-Lumen Endotracheal Tubes 307
Double-Lumen Endotracheal Tubes 312
Ancillary Equipment 315
Alternative Management Techniques 316

Chapter 18

Cardiopulmonary Bypass 320
THOMAS J. MARTIN, M.D.

Bypass Circuits 320
Myocardial Protection 323
Reperfusion Injury 325
Pathophysiology of Cardiopulmonary Bypass 326

SECTION IV

Monitors and Their Applications 333

Chapter 19

Introduction to Monitoring: Clinical Monitoring 333
J. S. GRAVENSTEIN, M.D.

Underlying Concepts 333
Basic Monitoring Without Instruments
     (Other than a Stethoscope) 334
Basic Monitoring Instrumentation 337

Chapter 20

Respiratory Monitoring 341
JULIAN M. GOLDMAN, M.D.
JENNIFER SOUDERS, M.D.

Arterial Blood Gas Analysis 341
Oxygen Monitoring 343
Airway Pressure Monitoring 344
Tidal Volume Monitoring 345
Agent Monitoring 348
Carbon Dioxide Monitoring 350
Pulse Oximetry 354
Carbon Dioxide Absorption 356
Conclusion 358

Chapter 21

Cardiovascular Monitoring 360
HUGH C. GILBERT, M.D.
JEFFREY S. VENDER, M.D., F.C.C.M.

The Electrocardiogram 360
Arterial Blood Pressure 367
Central Venous Pressure 373
Pulmonary Artery Pressure 375
Cardiac Output 378
Transesophageal Echocardiography 380
Urine Output 384

Chapter 22

Monitoring the Nervous System 389
MICHAEL E. MAHLA, M.D.

Implications for Intraoperative Management 389
The Clinical Neurologic Examination 390
Cerebral Blood Flow Monitoring During
  General Anesthesia 392
Direct Measurement of Cerebral Blood Flow 395
Balance of Cerebral Oxygen Supply and Demand:
  Jugular Bulb Saturation 398
Cerebral Oxygen Supply/Demand Balance:
  The Electroencephalogram 398
Cerebral Oxygen Supply and Demand:
  Evoked Potentials 402
Facial Nerve Monitoring 408
Conclusions 409

Chapter 23

**Neuromuscular Junction Monitoring
and Nerve Stimulation** 412
H. JERREL FONTENOT, M.D., Ph.D.
PETER GERNER, M.D.

Practical Considerations 412
Technique 413
Interpretation of Stimulus Frequency Data 416
Other Methods to Assess Neuromuscular Blockade 419

Chapter 24

Monitoring During Patient Transport 421
GREGORY M. GULLAHORN, M.D., L.C.D.R., M.C., U.S.N.R.

Basic Considerations 421
A Rational Approach 423
Selection of Monitors 425

Chapter 25

Temperature Monitoring 429
RANDALL C. CORK, M.D., Ph.D.

Temperature Probes 429
Anatomic Sites for Monitoring 430
Intraoperative Hypothermia 433

SECTION V

Clinically Relevant Anatomy 439

Chapter 26

Functional Anatomy of the Airway 439
LEROY D. VANDAM, Ph.B., M.D., M.A.

Phylogenetic Considerations 439
Topical Anatomy of the Airway 439
The Trachea 442
The Larynx 444
Tracheal Intubation 450

Chapter 27

The Spine 458
EDWARD T. CROSBY, B.Sc., M.D., F.R.C.P.C.
ANNE C. P. LUI, M.Sc., M.D., F.R.C.P.C.

Embryologic Development 458
Vertebral Anatomy 458
The Cervical Spine 460
The Thoracic Spine 468
The Lumbar Spine 471
The Sacral Spine 478

Chapter 28

Autonomic Nervous System 482
THOMAS J. EBERT, M.D.
ROBERT KETTLER, M.D.

Anatomic and Functional Characteristics 482
Sympathetic Nerve Block 485
Autonomic Dysfunction: Dysreflexia 492

Chapter 29

Vascular System Anatomy 496
JAMES M. O'CALLAGHAN, P.A.-C., B.M.Sc.
CHRISTINE A. CZEPIZAK, M.S., P.A.-C.
BAHMAN VENUS, M.D., F.C.C.P., F.C.C.M.

Arterial Cannulation 496
Peripheral Venous Cannulation 498
Central Venous Cannulation 500

SECTION VI

Techniques and Procedures 503

Chapter 30

Positioning the Surgical Patient 503
ROBERT BLACKSHEAR, M.D.
NIKOLAUS GRAVENSTEIN, M.D.

Special Considerations 503
Avoidance of Position-Related Injuries 504
Documentation of Measures 505
Incidence of Potentially Position-Related Complications ... 505
Specific Considerations 505
Peripheral Nerve Injury 511
The Patient with a Neck Injury 512
Rheumatoid Disorders 512

Chapter 31

Regional Anesthesia 514
DAVID L. BROWN, M.D.

Philosophy of Regional Anesthesia 514
Making It Work 515
Centroneuraxis Blockade: Spinal Anesthesia 516
Centroneuraxis Blockade: Epidural Anesthesia 520

Centroneuraxis Blockade: Caudal Anesthesia 523
Upper Extremity Blocks 524
Lower Extremity Blocks 531
Truncal Blocks 534
Complications 536

Chapter 32

Vascular Access 542

CHRISTINE A. CZEPIZAK, M.S., P.A.-C.
JAMES M. O'CALLAGHAN, P.A.-C., B.M.Sc.
BAHMAN VENUS, M.D., F.C.C.P., F.C.C.M.
NIKOLAUS GRAVENSTEIN, M.D.

Equipment 542
Preparation 543
Venous Catheterization 544
Arterial Catheter Placement 545
Pulmonary Artery Catheterization 545
Techniques of Peripheral Venous Catheterization 546
Arterial Catheterization Techniques 547
Techniques of Central Venous Catheterization 550
Pulmonary Artery Catheterization Techniques 557

SECTION VII

Pharmacologic Considerations and Anesthetic Administration **561**

Chapter 33

Basic Pharmacologic Applications in Anesthesia 561

W. JERRY MERRELL, M.D.

Drug Disposition: Pharmacokinetics 561
Membrane Transport 565
Drug Removal 566
Dosing Regimens 567
Perioperative Concerns 567
Drug Accumulation 568
The Response to Anesthesia 569
Characteristics of Drug Response 569
Anesthetic Agents 570
Anesthetic Induction 571
Anesthetic Drug Selection 571

Chapter 34

The Preoperative Visit and Premedication 576

SNO E. WHITE, M.D.

Psychologic Preparation 576
Pharmacologic Evaluation 578
Benzodiazepines 579
Modification of Gastric Contents 581
Miscellaneous Drugs 583
Summary 583

Chapter 35

General Anesthesia: Induction, Maintenance, and Emergence 585

J. S. GRAVENSTEIN, M.D.
ROBERT R. KIRBY, M.D.

Preliminary Concerns 585
Preoxygenation 586
Induction of Anesthesia 588
Maintenance of Anesthesia 591
Emergence and Extubation 594

Chapter 36

Intravenous Agents 597

A. JAY KOSKA, M.D., Ph.D.

Pharmacokinetic Properties of Intravenous Agents 597
Intravenous Anesthetic Agents 601

Chapter 37

Inhalation Agents 606

WENDELL C. STEVENS, M.D.

The History of Inhaled Anesthetics 606
Pharmacokinetics and Pharmacodynamics:
   Clinical Implications 607
Considerations in Patients with Central Nervous
   System Diseases 608
Management of Breathing 610
Management of the Circulation 612
Neurohumoral Response to Surgery 613
Renal Function 613
The Liver and Inhaled Agents 614
Endocrine Effects 614
Obesity 614
Muscle Relaxation 615
Bone Marrow Transplantation 615
Trauma 615
Prolonged Anesthesia 616
Pregnancy and the Puerperium 616
Ambulatory Surgery 617
Conclusion 617

Chapter 38

Local Anesthetics 621

JAY S. ELLIS, M.D., Lt. Col., U.S.A.F., M.C.

Mechanisms of Action 621
Clinical Applications 625
Toxicity 631

Chapter 39

Drug Interactions 640

SALVATORE R. GOODWIN, M.D.
MARK VEERMAN, Pharm.D.

Drug Compatibility 640

Pharmacokinetic Drug Interactions 641
Pharmacodynamic Interactions 650
Summary 659

SECTION VIII

Physiologic Aberrations and Their Control 663

Chapter 40

Shock 663
DAVID J. TORPEY, Jr., M.D.
MICHAEL D. INGRAM, M.D.

Hypotension 663
Vascular Endothelium 664
Pharmacologic Treatment 665
Oxygen Delivery and Oxygen Consumption 666
Prehospital Resuscitation 666
Fluid Resuscitation 667
Hemoglobin and Hematocrit 668
Myocardial Oxygen Consumption 668
Cardiogenic Shock 672
Mechanical Complications of Acute
    Myocardial Infarction 677
Right Ventricular Infarction 678
Other Causes of Acute Right Ventricular Dysfunction 679
Monitoring in Shock 679
Anaphylactic Shock 680
Spinal Cord Shock 682
Septic Shock 686
Intraoperative Management of Shock 688
Intraoperative Hemodynamic Stabilization 689
Pulmonary Dysfunction 692
Hypothermia 693
Organ Responses to Shock 694

Chapter 41

Thermal Injuries: Pathophysiology and Anesthetic Considerations 699
MAXIMILIAN W. B. HARTMANNSGRUBER, M.D.
A. JOSEPH LAYON, M.D.

Pathology 699
Classification 700
Pathophysiology 701
Pulmonary Injury 704
Initial Therapy 704
Definitive Therapy 705
Anesthetic Management 708
The Chronic Phase 711

Chapter 42

Fluids and Electrolytes 714
EDWARD K. McGOUGH, M.D.
ROBERT R. KIRBY, M.D.

Fluid Compartments 714
Origins of Therapeutic Misconceptions 715
Fluid Balance During Surgery 715
Intraoperative and Postoperative Fluid Therapy 716
Hypertonic Solutions 720
Blood Substitutes 721
Indications for Glucose in Water 721
Estimation of Fluid Requirements 722
Perioperative Electrolyte and Glucose Management 723
Fluid Therapy and Coagulation 727
Complications of Fluid Therapy 728
Transurethral Resection of the Prostate 729
Sepsis 730
Liver Failure 730
Neurosurgery 730
Pediatric Patients 730
Burn Patients 731

Chapter 43

Acid-Base 732
DAVID R. BEVAN, M.B., M.R.C.P., F.F.A.R.C.S.

Physiology 732
Ventilation and Acid-Base Status 734
Renal Responses to Acid-Base Disturbance 735
The Liver and Acid-Base Regulation 736
Acid-Base Disturbances 737
Effects of Acid-Base Disturbances 740
Conclusion 741

Chapter 44

Allergy and Immunology 743
JERROLD H. LEVY, M.D.

Antigens and Antibodies 743
Anaphylaxis 744
Nonimmunologic Release of Histamine 746
Perioperative Anaphylaxis 748
Summary 750

Chapter 45

Myocardial Ischemia and Dysfunction ... 752
MARTIN J. LONDON, M.D.

Perioperative Myocardial Ischemia 752
Anesthesia and Intraoperative Ischemia 756
Myocardial Dysfunction 757
Intraoperative Ischemia 760
Postoperative Myocardial Infarction 761
Treatment of Perioperative Myocardial Dysfunction 764
Preoperative ''Optimization'' of Patients with
    Myocardial Dysfunction 767

Chapter 46

Abnormal Intracranial Pressure 769
SUSAN BLACK, M.D.
ROY CUCCHIARA, M.D.

Determinants of Intracranial Pressure 769
Intracranial Pressure and Anesthesia 774
Summary 781

Chapter 47

Hypoxemia 782
ROY D. CANE, M.B., B.Ch., F.F.A.(S.A.)
JUKKA RÄSÄNEN, M.D.

Hypoxemia, Arterial Oxyhemoglobin Saturation,
and Oxygen Content 782
Assessment of Hypoxemia 786

Chapter 48

Abnormal Ventilation 799
JUKKA RÄSÄNEN, M.D.
ROY D. CANE, M.B., B.Ch., F.F.A.(S.A.)

Ventilatory Work 799
Alveolar Hypoventilation 800
Alveolar Hyperventilation 807
Ventilatory Work 809
''Abnormal'' Ventilatory Therapy 814

Chapter 49

Temperature Fluctuations 817
RICHARD B. LILLY, Jr., M.D.
THOMAS C. MORT, M.D.

Thermoregulatory Responses in Anesthetized Patients 817
Heat Loss 818
Pathophysiology of Hypothermia 819
Special Postoperative Problems 820
Prevention and Treatment of Hypothermia 822
Hyperthermia 823
Malignant Hyperthermia 826

Chapter 50

Cardiopulmonary Resuscitation 835
RICHARD J. MELKER, M.D., Ph.D.
ROBERT R. KIRBY, M.D.
J. R. MARSHALL, M.D.

Airway 835
Breathing 836
Circulation 840
Pharmacologic Therapy 843
Drugs to Improve Cardiac Output and Blood Pressure 849
Life-Threatening Dysrhythmias 850

SECTION IX

Hazardous Environments 853

Chapter 51

**Occupational Hazards in the
Operating Room** 853
SALVATORE LoPALO, C.R.N.A., M.S. Ed., M.A.
A. JOSEPH LAYON, M.D., F.A.C.P.

HIV Infection 853
HIV-Negative CD4⁺ Lymphopenia 858

Hepatitis 858
Herpetic Whitlow 862
Chicken Pox/Herpes Zoster 862
Cytomegalovirus Infection 864
Tuberculosis 865
Drug Abuse 865
Fatigue 868
Trace Gas Exposure 868

Chapter 52

Battlefield Surgery and Anesthesia 874
AZRIEL PEREL, M.D.
ERAN DOLEV, M.D.
JAY S. ELLIS, M.D., Major, U.S.A.F., M.C.
ROBERT R. KIRBY, M.D.
SALVATORE LoPALO, C.R.N.A., M.S. Ed., M.A.

Wartime Surgery 874
The Mission 875
Urban Warfare 876
Multitrauma 877
Terrorism 877
Anesthesia Practice 877
Future Considerations 881
Summary 883

Chapter 53

Electrical Safety 885
JAN C. HORROW, M.D.

Historical Considerations 885
Electrocution 885
The Operating Room 890
Electrosurgery 891
Living with Pacemakers 893
How to Think Electrically 895
Summary 896

Chapter 54

**Radiologic Procedures, Computed
Tomography Scans, Magnetic Resonance
Imaging, and Radiation Therapy** 897
MARK E. ROMANOFF, M.D.

Environmental Hostility 897
Anesthetic Concerns 900
Reactions to Contrast Agents 901
Diagnostic Radiologic Procedures 905
Therapeutic Vascular Interventions 905
Therapeutic Nonvascular Interventions 906
Computed Tomography Scans 909
Magnetic Resonance Imaging 911
Radiation Therapy 916

SECTION X

**Anesthetic Considerations, Special
Problems, Approaches, and
Problem-Solving** 921

Chapter 55

Management of the Difficult Airway 921
ROGER S. MECCA, M.D.

General Principles 921
Facemask Ventilation 922
Difficult Intubation 928
Nasal Intubation 933
Potentially Difficult Intubation 934
Intubation After Anesthetic Induction 938
Tube Placement 943
Esophageal Intubation 944
Difficult Ventilation and Oxygenation 945
Problems After Extubation 949

Chapter 56

Anesthesia for Patients with Bronchial Asthma 955
S. S. MOORTHY, M.D.
STEPHEN F. DIERDORF, M.D.

Pathophysiology 955
Characteristics 956
Treatment 957
Perioperative Management 958
Anesthetic Management 959
Intraoperative Bronchospasm 960
Postoperative Care 961

Chapter 57

Anesthesia for Patients with Chronic Obstructive Pulmonary Disease 963
S. S. MOORTHY, M.D.
STEPHEN F. DIERDORF, M.D.

Pathophysiology 963
Signs and Symptoms 964
Treatment 965
Perioperative Management 965
Anesthetic Management 966
Postoperative Management 967

Chapter 58

Pulmonary Edema 969
ERAN SEGAL, M.D.
AZRIEL PEREL, M.D.

Pathogenesis 969
Pathophysiology 969
Clinical Implications 971
Preoperative Treatment 973
Intraoperative Pulmonary Edema 976
Postoperative Pulmonary Edema 978
Miscellaneous Causes 979

Chapter 59

Trauma 982
SCOTT H. NORWOOD, M.D.
MARY BETH MYERS, R.N., M.S.

Epidemiology 982
Assessment of Injury Severity 984
Emergency Department Logistics and Operating
    Room Preparation 985
Initial Patient Assessment and Resuscitation Strategy 990
Alcohol and Drug Intoxication 999
The Full Stomach 1000
Cervical Spine Injury 1001
Retroperitoneal Injuries 1001
Head Injuries 1001
Pregnant Trauma Victims 1002
Pediatric Trauma Victims 1003
An Approach to Victims of Multiple Trauma 1005
Postoperative Complications 1006

Chapter 60

The Neonate 1013
TIMOTHY W. MARTIN, M.D.

Pain and Its Perception 1013
The Respiratory System 1014
The Cardiovascular System 1015
The Kidneys 1016
Heat Loss 1017
Pre-Existing Medical Problems 1017
Retinopathy of Prematurity 1020
Anesthetic Problems of Former Premature Infants 1021
Preoperative Fasting Guidelines 1021
Premedication 1022
Airway Management 1022
Intraoperative Ventilation 1023
Vascular Access 1024
Fluid Administration 1024
Intraoperative Monitoring 1025
Pyloric Stenosis 1026
Congenital Abdominal Wall Defects 1027
Necrotizing Enterocolitis 1028
Patent Ductus Arteriosus 1029
Tracheoesophageal Fistula 1030
Congenital Diaphragmatic Hernia 1031
Neonatal Resuscitation 1033

Chapter 61

The Pediatric Patient 1038
TIMOTHY W. MARTIN, M.D.
VINCENT G. JOHNSON, D.O.

Preanesthetic Assessment: General Considerations 1038
Upper Respiratory Tract Infection 1041
Asthma 1042
Congenital Heart Disease 1043
Malignant Hyperthermia 1044
Premedication 1046
Anesthetic Induction 1049
Anesthetic Maintenance 1054
Fluid Therapy and Blood Transfusion 1056
Monitoring 1059
Regional Anesthesia 1060
Postanesthetic Problems 1061
Common Anesthetic Procedures 1062

Chapter 62

The Geriatric Patient 1067
KENNETH M. JANIS, M.D.

Demographics 1067
Life Span and Longevity 1067
Perioperative Mortality 1068
Common Surgical Procedures in the Elderly 1069
Changes That Affect Anesthetic Management 1070
Monitoring 1073
General Anesthetic Drugs 1074
Muscle Relaxants and Reversal Agents 1076
Regional Anesthetic Drugs 1076
Postoperative Pain Relief 1077
Drug Interactions 1078
Alzheimer's Disease 1079
Postoperative Cerebral Dysfunction 1079
Outpatient Anesthesia 1079
Preoperative Do-Not-Resuscitate Orders 1080
Summary and Conclusions 1080

Chapter 63

The Obstetric Patient 1082
DONALD CATON, M.D.

Normal Changes in Pregnancy 1082
Labor Analgesia: General Considerations 1085
Epidural Analgesia 1087
Inhalation Analgesia 1089
Cesarean Section: General Considerations 1089
General Anesthesia 1091
Regional Anesthesia 1092
Maternal Complications of Cesarean Section 1093
Coexisting Medical or Surgical Problems 1093
Fetal Monitoring 1095
Neonatal Resuscitation 1097

Chapter 64

Nonobstetric Surgery in the Pregnant Patient 1099
CHRISTOPHER F. JAMES, M.D.
THOMAS W. LEBERT, II, M.D.

Anesthetic Considerations 1099
Fetal Risks 1101
Preparing the Pregnant Patient for Surgery 1104
Anesthetic Administration 1105
Summary 1107

Chapter 65

Abdominal Surgery 1109
SERGIO GREGORETTI, M.D.

The Abdominal Wall 1109
General Anesthesia 1109
Muscle Relaxants 1110
Spinal and Epidural Anesthesia 1113
Hypotension Related to Surgical Maneuvers 1114
Nitrous Oxide and Bowel Distention 1115
Narcotic Administration and Biliary Spasm 1116
Nasogastric Tubes 1117

Rapid-Sequence Induction in Emergency Abdominal Surgery 1118
Intraoperative Fluid Management 1119
Useful Rules of Thumb 1120
Acute Gastrointestinal Bleeding 1121
Splenectomy 1122
Obstructive Jaundice 1122
Hepatic Resection 1123
Patients with Ascites 1124
Peritoneovenous Shunting 1125
Portosystemic Shunts 1126
Effects of Abdominal Surgery on Pulmonary Function 1130
Pulmonary Complications 1132
Postoperative Intestinal Motility 1133
Surgery of the Abdominal Wall and Abdominal Wall Hernias 1133

Chapter 66

Anesthesia for Pediatric Cardiovascular Surgery 1138
LAURIE K. DAVIES, M.D.

Major Congenital Heart Lesions 1138
Physiologic Considerations 1139
Preoperative Assessment 1141
Equipment and Infusions 1144
Anesthetic Induction and Maintenance 1145
Monitoring 1148
Cardiopulmonary Bypass 1150
Postbypass Issues 1154

Chapter 67

Anesthesia for Adult Cardiovascular Surgery 1157
THOMAS J. MARTIN, M.D.

Preoperative Evaluation 1157
The Preoperative Period 1163
Anesthetic Management Before Cardiopulmonary Bypass 1169
Anesthetic Techniques 1173
Management of Surgical Events in Cardiac Surgery 1176
Weaning and Separating from Cardiopulmonary Bypass ... 1179
Problems After Bypass 1181
Anesthesia for Thoracic Aortic Procedures 1190
Procedures Not Requiring Cardiopulmonary Bypass: Pacemaker Implantation 1191
Automatic Internal Cardioverter-Defibrillator Implantation 1193
Pericardiotomy 1195

Chapter 68

Anesthetic Considerations for Thoracic Surgery 1200
PHILIP G. BOYSEN, M.D., F.A.C.P., F.C.C.P.

Pulmonary Function Testing 1200
Intraoperative Anesthetic Management 1202
Mediastinal Lesions 1207
Postoperative Pain Management 1207

Chapter 69

Anesthesia for Aortic Vascular Surgery .. 1210
DONN M. DENNIS, M.D.

Aortic Disease 1210
Anatomic Considerations 1215
Anesthesia for Central Aortic Surgery 1217
Anesthetic Induction and Maintenance 1222
Conclusion 1230

Chapter 70

Genitourinary Surgery 1234
JERRY J. BERGER, M.D.

Anatomic Considerations 1234
Interpleural Anesthesia 1237
Prostatic Surgery 1237
The TURP Syndrome 1240
Nephrectomy 1242
Cystectomy 1242
Nonchromaffin Paragangliomas 1243
Laser Surgery 1243
Noninvasive Urologic Surgery 1244

Chapter 71

Anesthesia for Orthopedic Surgery 1246
F. KAYSER ENNEKING, M.D.
MARK T. SCARBOROUGH, M.D.

Orthopedic Trauma 1246
Total Joint Replacement 1248
Rheumatoid Arthritis 1250
Orthopedic Oncology 1251
Scoliosis 1252
Amputations and Phantom Limb Pain 1254
Ambulatory Orthopedic Surgery 1254
Regional Anesthesia 1255
Antibiotics 1258
Blood Loss 1259
Positioning 1260
Tourniquets 1261
Splinting 1263
Venous Thromboembolism 1263
Pain Control 1264

Chapter 72

Otolaryngologic and Maxillofacial Surgery 1268
ALEXANDER W. GOTTA, M.D.
MICHAEL J. FEFFER, M.D.
COLLEEN A. SULLIVAN, M.B., Ch.B.

Myringotomy 1268
Adenotonsillectomy 1269
Middle Ear Surgery 1271
Otologic and Parotid Surgery 1271
Cleft Lip and Palate 1272
Caldwell-Luc Procedure 1272

Pharyngeal Abscess 1273
Ludwig's Angina 1273
Airway Neoplasia 1274
Radical Head and Neck Surgery 1274
Airway Edema 1275
Dental Repairs in Retarded and Uncooperative Patients 1275
Craniofacial Trauma 1276
Awake Tracheal Intubation 1279
Alternative Techniques to Secure the Airway 1280

Chapter 73

Neurologic Surgery 1283
MICHAEL E. MAHLA, M.D.

Neurophysiology and Neuropharmacology 1283
Positioning 1286
Impact of Neurologic Disease on
    Anesthetic Management 1286
Neurovascular Surgery 1288
Spinal Column and Spinal Cord Surgery 1295
Intracranial Neoplasm 1302
Conclusions 1309

Chapter 74

Surgery of the Endocrine System 1312
EDWARD D. MILLER, Jr., M.D.

Pituitary Gland 1312
Parathyroid Glands 1313
Thyroid Gland 1314
Insulinoma 1316
Adrenal Glands 1317

Chapter 75

Anesthesic Management for Heart Transplantation 1321
MARK C. MONROE, M.D.

Selection Criteria 1321
End-Stage Heart Disease 1322
Preanesthetic Management 1322
Preinduction Period 1324
Anesthetic Induction 1325
Anesthetic Maintenance 1325
The Anesthesiologist's Responsibilities During
    Cardiopulmonary Bypass 1326
The Operative Procedure 1326
Denervated Heart Function 1326
Weaning from Cardiopulmonary Bypass 1327
Anesthesia After Cardiac Transplantation 1329

Chapter 76

Orthotopic Liver Transplantation 1333
AVNER SIDI, M.D.

General Considerations 1333
Preanesthetic Evaluation 1335

Anesthetic Induction 1342
Anesthetic Management 1343
Surgical Stages in Orthotopic Liver Transplantation 1345
Specialized Equipment 1352
Pediatric Orthotopic Liver Transplantation 1355
Recovery After Orthotopic Liver Transplantation 1356
Anesthesia for Retransplantation 1356
Associated Procedures Immediately After Orthotopic
    Liver Transplantation 1356

Chapter **77**

Renal Transplantation 1358
AVNER SIDI, M.D.

General Considerations 1358
Preoperative Concerns 1358
Anesthetic Induction 1362
Anesthetic Maintenance 1364
Postoperative Care 1365
Cadaveric Donor Harvesting 1366
Living-Related Donor Harvesting 1366

Chapter **78**

Lasers and Laser Safety 1370
ANNETTE G. PASHAYAN, M.D.

Basic Principles 1370
Medical Applications 1371
Special Concerns During Laryngeal Laser Operations 1374
Special Concerns Regarding the Lower Respiratory
    Tract During Laser Surgery 1378
Management of Airway Fire 1378

Chapter **79**

Extracorporeal Shock Wave Lithotripsy 1380
VINOD MALHOTRA, M.D.

Technical Aspects 1380
Preoperative Considerations 1380
Physiologic Effects of Immersion 1383
Patient Safety 1384
Stone Movement 1385
Anesthetic Technique 1385
Miscellaneous Considerations 1387
Summary 1387

Chapter **80**

Outpatient Surgery 1389
BURTON S. EPSTEIN, M.D.
RAAFAT S. HANNALLAH, M.D.

Screening 1389
Procedures 1393
The Perioperative Period 1394
The Preinduction Period 1395
General Anesthesia 1396
Airway Management 1398
Intravenous Infusions 1399
Regional Anesthesia 1400
Monitored Anesthesia Care 1400
The Recovery Period 1401
Unplanned Hospitalization 1402
Morbidity and Mortality 1404
Quality Improvement Programs 1405

Index 1407

Toward a Safer Practice

CHAPTER 1

Preanesthetic Evaluation

STEPHEN O. HEARD, M.D.

DONALD S. STEVENS, M.D.

First impressions often have lasting effects. The preanesthetic evaluation is likely to be the first time a patient interacts with a member of an anesthesia department. Although the evaluation encounter usually is brief, it is very important. This chapter examines the first encounter between a patient and the anesthesiologist and gives practical suggestions to the anesthesiologist on how to improve the skills needed to perform the preanesthetic evaluation.

PURPOSES

What Are the Purposes of the Preoperative Evaluation?

Meeting the Patient

The preoperative evaluation is important for three main reasons.[1] First, the anesthesiologist is able to meet the patient. Although busy clinicians may downplay this interaction, many studies have shown that the preoperative interview is very effective in reducing a patient's anxiety.[2–4] In light of current practice, it is assumed (but unclear) that this effect is continued after the patient is evaluated by a member of an anesthesia department to when he or she is provided intraoperative care by a member of another department.

Delineating the Problem

Second, the anesthesiologist is able to delineate the current problem through the history, physical examination, and use of laboratory studies. Coexisting problems are also determined and evaluated.

Obtaining Informed Consent

Third, the anesthesiologist is able to obtain the patient's informed consent for anesthesia procedures.[1]

PROCEDURES

How Is Information Obtained?

Much of the preoperative evaluation can be done by reviewing the patient's medical record. However, examining, counseling, and reassuring the patient are still essential aspects of the preoperative assessment.

Communicating Information

Because of changes in medical and surgical practice that have occurred over the last decade, the preoperative evaluation has become more difficult to complete. Large percentages of patients now have surgery in the ambulatory setting or are admitted to the hospital on the day of surgery instead of on the night before surgery. One consequence of this practice is that the anesthesiologist sometimes must interview and examine the patient in the preoperative holding area. Frequently, the anesthesiologist who evaluated the patient preoperatively is not the one who will perform the anesthesia administration. Unless a good system exists for communication between these anesthesiologists, delays or cancellation of procedures may result. Also, the "new" anesthesiologist must take the time and effort necessary to familiarize himself or herself with the patient. If the new anesthesiologist does not do this, the patient's anxiety may actually increase rather than decrease.

Computerized Questionaires

Ideally, a personal interview is part of the initial preoperative evaluation. Several computerized questionnaires have been developed to assist in obtaining the medical history of the patient.[5] Although one might expect patient responses to such questionnaires to be incomplete, one study has indicated that they are as accurate and helpful in obtaining the medical history as is the interview.[5] It is important to emphasize that the purpose of these questionnaires is not to replace the personal interview but to assist the physician in obtaining the history and to suggest what laboratory tests should be ordered. Using these questionnaires can make the personal interview much more efficient.

HISTORICAL INFORMATION

What Can Be Learned from the History of the Present Illness?

Knowledge of the current surgical problem is obviously crucial. The anesthetic management depends on the type of surgery to be performed. The disease state being treated may also have implications for anesthetic management or may suggest other underlying medical conditions. For example, pneumoencephaly after skull fracture would be a contraindication to the use of nitrous oxide. A craniotomy in the sitting position for a posterior fossa tumor would place the patient at risk for venous air emboli. This possibility would prompt insertion of a central venous catheter, use of precordial Doppler ultrasound, and monitoring of end-tidal carbon dioxide. A parathyroidectomy for hypercalcemia should alert the anesthesiologist to the possibility of an undiagnosed multiple endocrine neoplasia syndrome.

Specifics regarding organ system involvement by the primary process undergoing surgical treatment are considered later.

Why Is the Previous Surgical and Anesthetic History Important?

Previous surgery may affect the anesthetic plan. For instance, the patient with limited neck motion after a cervical fusion may be managed differently than a patient with a normal airway. Presence of an arteriovenous dialysis fistula would contraindicate placement of an intravenous catheter or blood pressure cuff on the involved extremity.

Adverse Drug Reactions

Important information is obtained from prior anesthetic experience. Adverse reactions to particular anesthetic agents in the past would presumably preclude their use for the impending anesthetic procedure. In particular, the interviewer should determine whether the patient has ever had a prolonged episode of paralysis following succinylcholine administration or whether the patient has ever been thought to have malignant hyperthermia.

Questions To Be Asked

Such information can be obtained easily by asking the patient such questions as, Have you had any operations before? What kind of anesthesia did you have? Did you have any problems with the anesthesia? Unexpected specific answers, such as "I'm allergic to Anectine," have been obtained by such questioning. Most commonly, nausea and vomiting are reported as problems. If such side effects are almost always

present postoperatively, then use of a technique aimed at limiting this complication (e.g., a regional or propofol-based anesthetic, and early antiemetic therapy) might be helpful.

What Can Be Learned from the Medical History?

As complete a medical history as possible should be obtained before anesthetizing the patient. Many different approaches can be used, but regardless of which one is chosen, the anesthesiologist should be sure that all relevant information is obtained. Our approach is based on a *review of systems,* and is as follows:

Cardiovascular System

Questions concerning the cardiovascular system should focus on a history of hypertension, valvular or ischemic heart disease, and peripheral vascular insufficiency. Presence of dysrhythmias (commonly called "arrhythmias") as well as presence of a pacemaker also needs to be determined.

Hypertension

If the patient has a history of hypertension, the anesthesiologist should inquire about the duration of the disease and the duration and adequacy of treatment. Patients with untreated or inadequately treated hypertension may have a greater risk of perioperative hemodynamic fluctuations, resulting in increased morbidity.[6-9]

Valvular Disease

The patient should be questioned about his or her history of rheumatic fever or heart murmurs, especially if a history of syncope is elicited. Syncope is associated with mitral valve prolapse and hypertrophic cardiomyopathy.

Coronary Artery Disease

Patients of appropriate age should be asked about a history of angina, previous myocardial infarction (MI), or congestive heart failure. Reports suggest that the prevalence of perioperative morbidity and mortality associated with surgery in patients who have suffered an MI less than 6 months before surgery ("recent MI") is much lower at the time of this writing than that reported in the 1960s and 1970s.[10-13] The prevalence of morbidity and mortality for those patients with an MI 6 months or more prior to surgery ("remote MI") is also lower compared with that reported in earlier studies. However, there are not enough data in the most recent studies to demonstrate whether there are differences in morbidity and mortality between those patients with a recent MI and those with a remote MI who are undergoing noncardiac surgery[14] (Fig. 1–1).

A recent MI still dictates that elective surgery be delayed or, if surgery is urgent, that invasive hemodynamic monitoring be used during and after the procedure. Angina of new onset or a change in a previous anginal pattern should be a warning that the patient be evaluated more thoroughly before surgery. In many cases, a cardiologist should assist with this evaluation.

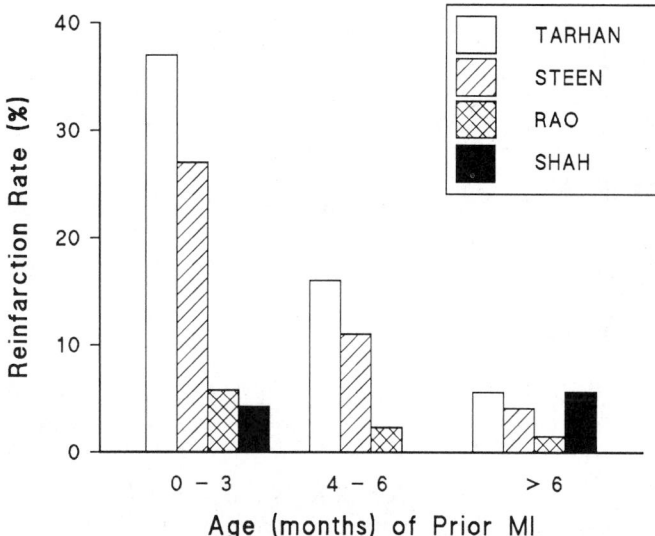

FIGURE 1–1. Reinfarction rates from several studies in patients who have had prior myocardial infarction. (Adapted from McCulloch HA, Sprague DH: Myths in vascular anesthesia. Probl Anesth 1991; 5:453–467.)

Symptomatic Dysrhythmias

Symptomatic dysrhythmias can also be important. Palpitations often indicate premature ventricular contractions that may require treatment before elective surgery. A history of a rapid heart beat can indicate paroxysmal supraventricular tachycardia, which may arise during surgery. Several types of dysrhythmias are associated with increased perioperative cardiac risk and include a rhythm other than sinus, premature atrial contractions, and five or more premature ventricular contractions per minute.[15]

Pacemakers

Inquiries as to the presence, type, and location of a pacemaker should be made. Since electrocautery can interfere with pacemaker function, reprogramming the pacemaker to an asynchronous mode prior to surgery may be indicated. Moreover, the older practice of using a magnet to convert a demand pacemaker to an asynchronous pacemaker[16] may not work well with newer pacing devices. Reports of patients whose pacemakers have been reprogrammed to unwanted rates by the use of a magnet are found in the literature.[17, 18] Use of the appropriate type of reprogramming device, with the assistance of a cardiologist, may be the safest course.[19, 20]

Identifying the pacemaker's location allows intraoperative placement of the electrocautery grounding pad in a location where the current flow from the electrocautery at the surgical site is least likely to pass through or near the pacemaker.

Pulmonary System

Questions related to the pulmonary system should focus on a history of emphysema, bronchitis, asthma, recent upper respiratory tract infection, productive or nonproductive cough, or sinusitis. The patient's exercise capacity should be elicited by asking such questions as, Can you climb up one flight of stairs? and Are you out of breath at the top? Remember that dyspnea may also be the presenting symptom for cardiovascular problems.

Chronic Obstructive Lung Disease

In patients with chronic obstructive lung disease (COLD), the amount of sputum that is expectorated per day should be determined. A change in the amount or color of the sputum from its usual quality may indicate an acute upper respiratory tract infection. Elective surgery in the presence of a current or recent upper respiratory tract infection is controversial.[21, 22] At our institution, elective surgery is delayed until 2 weeks after the resolution of the infection.

Miscellaneous Conditions

The anesthesiologist should remember that a nonproductive cough may be the sole manifestation of asthma or silent regurgitation and aspiration of stomach contents.[23, 24] Nasotracheal intubation may be contraindicated in patients with a history of sinusitis or nasal polyposis.

Gastrointestinal System

Aspiration of Gastric Contents

One of the most feared anesthetic complications is pulmonary aspiration of gastric contents. The anesthesiologist must determine whether the patient is at risk for the development of aspiration pneumonitis should regurgitation and aspiration occur during anesthesia and surgery. Pain, recent injury, insufficient duration of fasting, diabetes mellitus, obesity, pregnancy, and use of narcotics, β-adrenergic agents, and anticholinergic agents can delay gastric emptying or alter lower esophageal sphincter tone, thus theoretically increasing the risk of aspiration.[25, 26] A hiatal hernia is believed to increase the risk for aspiration, but reflux symptoms (i.e., heartburn), rather than the hiatal hernia itself, probably identify the patient at risk[27] (Fig. 1–2).

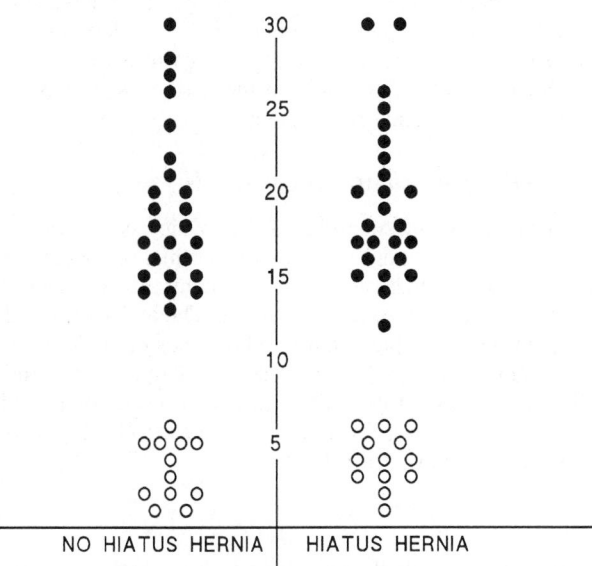

FIGURE 1–2. Resting lower esophageal sphincter (LES) pressure (in mm Hg) in patients with or without a hiatal hernia and with *(open circles)* or without *(filled circles)* the symptoms of reflux. LES pressures were higher in patients without symptoms of reflux irrespective of the presence of a hiatal hernia. (Reprinted from Cohen S, Harris LD: Does hiatus hernia affect competence of the gastroesophageal sphincter? N Engl J Med 1971; 284:1053, by permission of the New England Journal of Medicine.)

Liver Disease

A history of blood transfusions or hepatitis, hematemesis, or hematochezia should also be elicited. When indicated, questions concerning chronic liver disease (e.g., cirrhosis and hypoalbuminemia) need to be asked, since the pharmacokinetics and pharmacodynamics of various drugs often will be altered in such disease. Coagulation studies may also be abnormal in patients with altered liver function.

Genitourinary System

Renal Insufficiency

Renal insufficiency may be a manifestation of diseases of organ systems other than the genitourinary system. Thus, the patient with diabetes mellitus, connective tissue disease, hypertension, or peripheral vascular disease should be carefully questioned about signs and symptoms of renal insufficiency. In patients with chronic renal failure, the anesthesiologist should be sure to establish the time of the patient's last dialysis procedure, as significant changes in blood volume and serum potassium level may occur before and after dialysis.

Urinary Tract Infection

Inquiries into recent or chronic urinary tract infections should also be made.

Pregnancy

In the female of childbearing age, the possibility of pregnancy should be considered, and appropriate inquiries should be made.

Endocrine System

Diabetes Mellitus

All patients should be asked whether they have diabetes mellitus. Diabetic patients are at risk for silent myocardial ischemia, autonomic neuropathy, and gastroparesis. Attention should be carefully focused on the cardiovascular system as well as on other end organ systems.

Adrenal Suppression/Corticosteroids

In those patients with diseases in which corticosteroid use is common (e.g., asthma, ulcerative colitis, or rheumatoid arthritis), the anesthesiologist should inquire as to the dose and the time of last use of corticosteroids. The incidence of adrenal suppression is not predictable and depends on the potency and frequency of steroid dose and on the length of steroid therapy. Suppression can occur with cumulative doses of prednisone <0.4 g and can last for as long as 1 year following cessation of steroid therapy[28] (Fig. 1–3).

Thyroid Disease

In patients with thyroid disease, the adequacy of thyroid hormone replacement therapy (for hypothyroidism) or antithyroidal treatment (for hyperthyroidism) should be established. Although recent retrospective data suggest that elective anesthesia and surgery can be performed on patients with stable hypothyroidism,[29] delay of elective operations is prudent so as to allow for adequate thyroid replacement.[30]

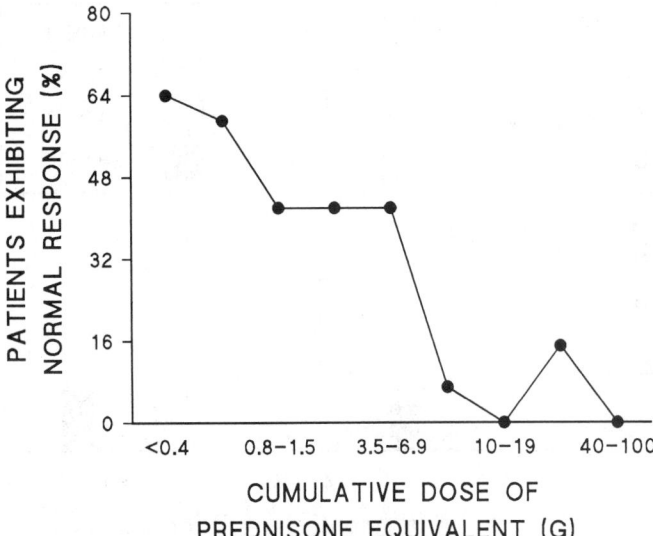

FIGURE 1–3. Relationship between the cumulative dose of glucocorticoid and the adrenal response to exogenous corticotropin-releasing hormone (CRH). A normal response was a 1.5-fold increase in the plasma cortisol level to at least a level of 276 nmol · L^{-1} or a peak cortisol level of 552 nmol · L^{-1}. A blunted response was a plasma cortisol level between 83 and 276 nmol · L^{-1} after CRH administration or an increase of less than 1.5 times the basal level if the basal level was greater than 179 nmol · L^{-1}. No response was defined as basal and stimulated cortisol levels of less than 83 nmol · L^{-1}. (Adapted from information appearing in Schlaghecke R, Kornely E, Santen RT, et al: The effect of long-term glucocorticoid therapy on pituitary-adrenal responses to exogenous corticotropin-releasing hormone. N Engl J Med 1992; 326:226, by permission of the New England Journal of Medicine.)

Miscellaneous

Other endocrine disease, such as primary hyperparathyroidism, may suggest the existence of an underlying multiple endocrine neoplasia syndrome. Further evaluation may be needed to rule out endocrine abnormalities, such as pheochromocytoma or medullary carcinoma of the thyroid gland.

Neurologic System

The anesthesiologist should ask the patient whether he or she has a history of central and peripheral nervous system problems.

Intracranial Pressure

If the patient has an intracranial lesion, symptoms of intracranial hypertension should be sought. Pituitary lesions may cause endocrine abnormalities that must be carefully managed in the perioperative period. A history of recent transient ischemic attack, with signs and symptoms of less than 24 hours' duration; reversible ischemic neurologic deficits, with signs and symptoms of less than 72 hours' duration; or cerebrovascular accidents ("completed strokes") suggests that careful neurologic evaluation be undertaken before proceeding with surgery.

Seizures

The anesthesiologist should ask the patient about a history of seizures, particularly regarding their type, frequency, and last occurrence as well as the anticonvulsants the patient is receiving.

Spinal Cord Injuries

In patients with spinal cord injury, the level of the neurologic deficit must be determined. Episodes of autonomic hyperreflexia can occur with cutaneous stimulation or distention of a hollow viscus with deficits above T-7.[31] Recent spinal cord lesions preclude the use of succinylcholine because of the massive release of intracellular potassium caused by this drug.[32]

Musculoskeletal System

A history of rheumatoid arthritis may indicate several problems that need to be evaluated[33] (Fig. 1–4). Airway management can be more difficult owing to altered laryngeal anatomy (see Fig. 1–4) and decreased range of joint motion. Cervical spine instability may also exist at the atlantoaxial joint, requiring that special precautions be taken during intubation. Because of the reduced range of motion in arthritic joints, positioning can be difficult after anesthetic induction.

The presence of a muscular disorder, such as a muscular dystrophy, should also be ascertained. Specific anesthetic agents, such as succinylcholine, may be contraindicated in patients with such a disorder.

Integumentary System

Recent burns contraindicate the use of depolarizing muscle relaxants because of the danger of hyperkalemia.[32] If emergent surgery is required, careful airway evaluation and assessment of the adequacy of fluid resuscitation also are essential.[34]

Hematologic System

Asking about previous bleeding problems and about the need for blood transfusions almost always identifies the patient who may develop perioperative hemorrhage.[35] In addition, if the preoperative assessment is performed sufficiently early, the anesthesiologist can identify a patient who is suitable for preoperative autologous blood donation. This procedure should be used more frequently.[36, 37] Use of recombinant erythropoietin also can increase the efficiency of preoperative autologous blood donation (Fig. 1–5).[38]

MEDICATIONS

What Medications Should Be Continued or Stopped Prior to Surgery?

Antihypertensives

In general, antihypertensive agents other than diuretics should be continued up to the time of surgery. Many studies have documented the adverse hemodynamic effects of discontinuing β-adrenergic blockers or clonidine in the perioperative period.[39, 40]

Diuretics

Use of diuretics is usually stopped prior to surgery. Patients taking thiazide diuretics have frequent hypokalemia regardless of potassium supplementation or the use of potassium-sparing agents.[41] Serum potassium concentrations <3.5 mEq $\cdot$ L^{-1} occur in 15% of patients, and concentrations <3.0 mEq $\cdot$ L^{-1} occur in 10%.

The perioperative consequences of a low serum potassium level may not be as severe as once was believed.[42, 43] Delay of surgery probably is not justified for patients at low risk for perioperative cardiac complications whose preoperative serum potassium concentration is in the range of 3 to 3.5 mEq $\cdot$ L^{-1}.[44] However, for patients thought to be at higher risk, the potassium concentration should be >3.5 mEq $\cdot$ L^{-1}. The incidence of ventricular dysrhythmias is twofold greater when serum potassium concentration is <3.0 mEq $\cdot$ L^{-1} than when it is >3.0 mEq $\cdot$ L^{-1} (Fig. 1–6).[41]

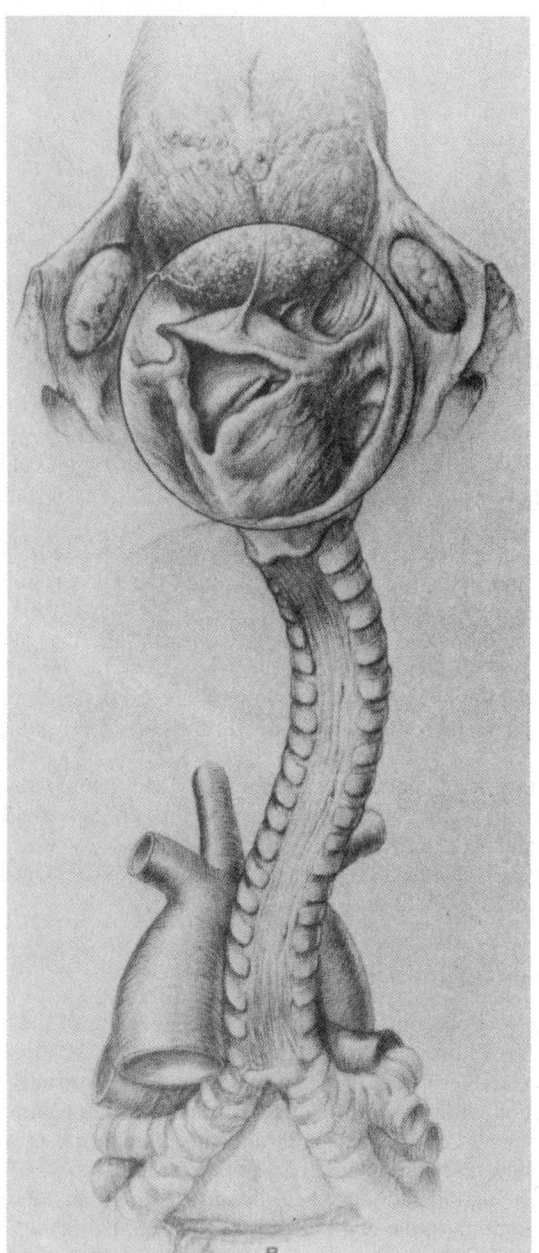

FIGURE 1–4. The effect of severe erosive polyarticular arthritis on the anatomy of the larynx and trachea. The larynx is rotated, deviated, and tilted forward; the trachea becomes redundant. (From Keenan MA, Stiles CM, Kaufman RL: Acquired laryngeal deviation associated with cervical spine disease in erosive polyarticular arthritis. Anesthesiology 1983; 58:441.)

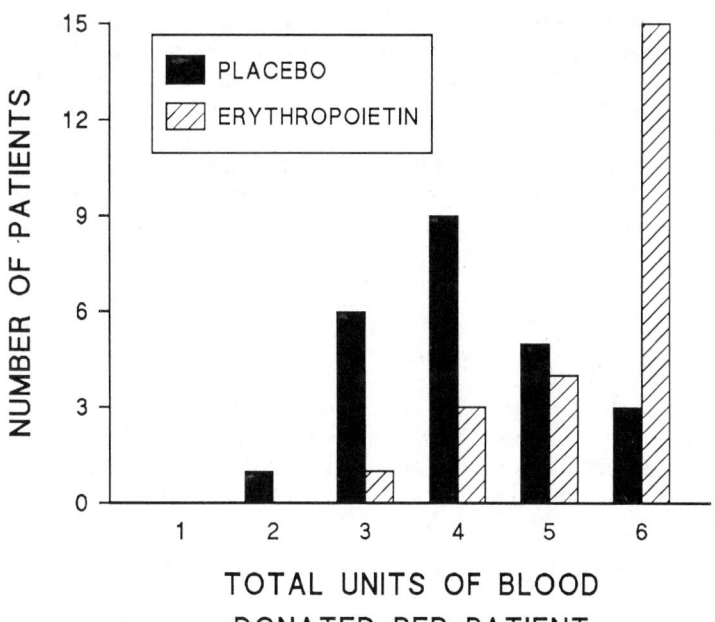

FIGURE 1–5. Efficiency of preoperative autologous blood donation in patients receiving erythropoietin compared with those given a placebo. Erythropoietin-treated patients were able to donate a significantly greater number of units of blood than were placebo-treated patients. (Adapted from Goodnough LT, Rudnick S, Price TH, et al: Increased preoperative collection of autologous blood with recombinant human erythropoietin therapy. N Engl J Med 1989; 321:1163, by permission of the New England Journal of Medicine.)

Digitalis Glycosides

Digoxin use should be continued in the perioperative period. It is efficacious in patients with congestive heart failure in classes III or IV (New York Heart classification).[45, 46] However, recent data suggest that its utility in atrial fibrillation is limited.[47, 48]

Antianginal Medication

Use of all medications used to treat angina pectoris, including nitrates, calcium channel blockers, and β-adrenergic receptor blockers should be continued up to the time of surgery.[40, 49]

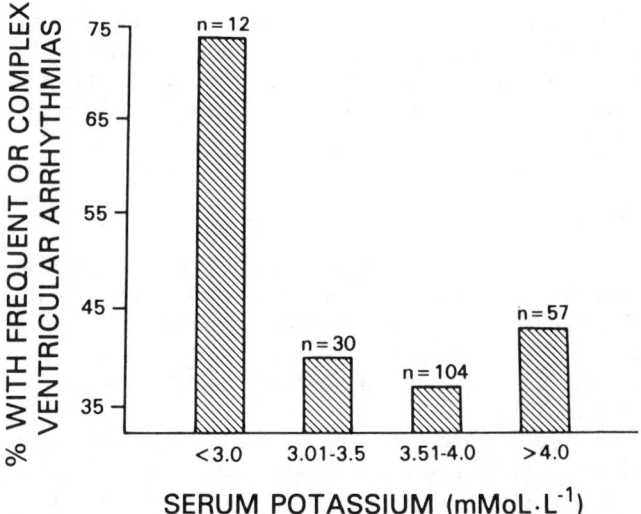

FIGURE 1–6. Incidence of frequent or complex ventricular dysrhythmias as a function of serum potassium levels in hypertensive men taking thiazide diuretics. Those patients with a serum potassium level of less than or equal to 3 mmol · L⁻¹ had a significantly higher incidence of dysrhythmias compared to those with patients with potassium levels greater than 3 mmol · L⁻¹. (Redrawn from Siegel D, Hulley SB, Black DM, et al: Diuretics, serum and intracellular electrolyte levels, and ventricular arrhythmias in men. JAMA 1992; 267:1083–1089. Copyright 1992, American Medical Association.)

If taken orally, they should be given at their usual dosing interval. If required, they can be given during surgery as well.

Antidysrhythmic Agents

Depending on their original indication, antidysrhythmic medications should be continued in the perioperative period. However, several of these drugs can have significant side effects relevant to anesthesia. The administration of quinidine to patients with stable digoxin blood levels causes a decrease in the clearance of digoxin and may result in toxicity.[50] Both quinidine and procainamide can cause the QT prolongation syndrome.

Disopyramide is a myocardial depressant and may increase the cardiac depression observed with volatile anesthetics. Amiodarone has been associated with altered thyroid function, particularly thyrotoxicosis, and with hypersensitivity pneumonitis.[51, 52]

Intravenous lidocaine is a commonly used antidysrhythmic agent. It should be remembered that this drug decreases the minimum alveolar concentration for volatile anesthetic agents and has been used as an adjunct to intravenous anesthetic techniques in the past.[53]

Bronchodilators

The role of aminophylline in the management of the patient with bronchospastic disease is controversial.[54] Although it is an effective bronchodilator, it does not add significantly to the bronchodilating effects of inhaled β-adrenergic or anticholinergic agents.[55] Besides inhibiting phosphodiesterase, aminophylline causes the release of norepinephrine.

Since halothane sensitizes the myocardium to circulating catecholamines, the combined use of aminophylline and halothane may result in ventricular dysrhythmias.[56] In addition, toxic serum concentrations of aminophylline may occur in the perioperative period due to alterations in drug metabolism by the liver that have been induced by changes in parenteral nutritional content.[57]

Our practice is to give aminophylline only if a patient is receiving a stable dose preoperatively. Otherwise, we avoid aminophylline and instead use aerosolized bronchodilators and corticosteroids for bronchospasm secondary to reactive airway disease. If a patient uses aerosolized medications routinely, we administer them 30 to 60 minutes preoperatively.

Insulin and Oral Hypoglycemic Agents

Insulin

The optimal management of blood glucose levels in the diabetic patient remains controversial; "tight" and "loose" control regimens have been proposed.[58] Those who favor tight control argue that better management of perioperative blood glucose level results in decreased postoperative morbidity, including fewer wound infections and enhanced wound healing.[59]

Those who favor loose control believe that sound data supporting the notion that tight control reduces perioperative morbidity is lacking, the resources needed for tight control are too expensive, and that without these resources, the danger of hypoglycemia is significant.[60]

We favor loose control. If the patient has adult-onset insulin-dependent diabetes mellitus, one half the usual dose of insulin is administered on the morning of surgery after an intravenous infusion of a dextrose-containing crystalloid solution has been begun.[60]

Oral Hypoglycemics

Oral hypoglycemic agents should not be administered on the day of surgery, particularly those agents with a long duration of action, such as chlorpropamide, glipizide, and glyburide. They bind ionically to serum albumin and may be displaced from their binding sites by drugs used in the perioperative period.[61] Asymptomatic hypoglycemia can occur in the somnolent postoperative patient who has been taking long-acting oral hypoglycemic drugs.

Corticosteroids

The patient who is taking corticosteroids or adrenocorticotropic hormone (ACTH) should receive appropriate perioperative corticosteroid replacement[62] (Table 1-1). For the patient who is taking a corticosteroid with a potency of >300 mg of hydrocortisone per day, hydrocortisone use is not substituted for the perioperative steroid treatment; the routine dose of steroid can be administered. For example, if a patient is taking 3 mg of dexamethasone every 6 hours, this daily dose meets the stress dose requirements of surgery. The patient will be protected from adrenal insufficiency if this drug and dosing regimen is continued perioperatively.

Thyroid Medication

Because of its long half-life (1.4–10 days), thyroxine does not have to be given on the day of surgery. Antithyroid medications include methimazole and propylthiouracil. These agents should be given on the morning of surgery.

Anticonvulsant Medications

The use of these medications should be continued up to the time of surgery. Many anticonvulsants induce the hepatic mi-

TABLE 1–1. Suggested Steroid Coverage for Preoperative Patients with Adrenocortical Insufficiency or Suppression

	Hydrocortisone Sodium Succinate or Equivalent
Preoperative Day 1	25 mg at 6:00 PM and 12:00 AM, IV or IM
Day of Operation	100 mg IV during surgery
Postoperative Day 1	100 mg IV q.8h times 24h
	50 mg IV q.8h times 24h
	25 mg IV q.8h times 24h

(From Chin R: Corticosteroids. *In* The Pharmacologic Approach to the Critically Ill Patient. 2nd ed. Chernow B (ed). Baltimore, Williams & Wilkins, 1988, pp 559–583.)
Abbreviation: IV = intravenously; IM = intramuscularly; q.8h = every 8 hours.

crosomal enzyme system and may cause alterations of the pharmacokinetics of other perioperative medications, particularly the barbiturates.

However, recent treatment with anticonvulsants may *not* have the desired effect. The prophylactic value of phenytoin in reducing the incidence of seizures in patients who have suffered closed head injuries is only effective during the first week of therapy; thus, the anesthesiologist still should be wary of seizures perioperatively despite prophylactic "preventive therapy."[63]

Antipsychotics and Antidepressants

These medications are usually administered up to the time of the surgical procedure. However, several special situations deserve consideration.

Monoamine Oxidase Inhibitors

Use of monoamine oxidase inhibitors (MAOIs) is generally discontinued 2 weeks before surgery. They have been implicated in a number of adverse reactions in the perioperative period, including cardiac dysrhythmias and death. However, several reports note patients taking MAOIs who had uneventful anesthetic procedures. The risk of administering anesthetics to these patients must be weighed against the possible psychiatric complications associated with preoperative cessation of the drug.[64, 65]

Lithium

Lithium carbonate, used in the treatment of manic depression, can potentiate the effect of muscle relaxants and may decrease anesthetic requirements.

Tricyclic Antidepressants

The tricyclic antidepressants (TCAs) block the reuptake of norepinephrine and deplete the terminal nerve stores of this neurotransmitter. Although animal studies suggest an interaction of TCAs with pancuronium and halothane, resulting in the development of fatal ventricular dysrhythmias, there are no published clinical reports suggesting such an interaction in humans.[66]

Anti-inflammatory Drugs

Anti-inflammatory agents affect coagulation owing to their effect on platelets. Acetylsalicylic acid (aspirin) irreversibly acetylates the platelet enzyme cyclooxygenase, resulting in decreased platelet aggregation for the life of the platelet (7–10 days).[67]

Other nonsteroidal anti-inflammatory drugs (NSAIDs) appear to inhibit the same enzyme but do so reversibly, with effects lasting at most 2 days after a single NSAID dose.[68] Whether aspirin or other NSAIDs increase bleeding during and after surgery is controversial,[69] but "minor hemorrhagic complications" of epidural anesthesia appear to be increased.[70] This effect is also important in surgeries in which small amounts of bleeding may be detrimental, such as in intracranial procedures.

We recommend that aspirin be stopped at least 7 days prior to elective surgery, that the use of other NSAIDs be stopped at least 48 hours prior to surgery, and that a bleeding time be checked prior to performing a major regional nerve block if such medications have been continued until the time of surgery.

Anticoagulants

In general, use of anticoagulants should be discontinued before a surgical procedure. In some cases, their effects may require reversal before surgery can proceed. If the patient is receiving warfarin and surgery is urgent, fresh frozen plasma should be given for quick reversal of the anticoagulant effect. If surgery is elective, an oral dose of 5 mg of phytonadione (vitamin K_1) should cause the prothrombin time to normalize within 24 hours.[71] Use of vitamin K_1, however, makes anticoagulation following surgery more difficult.

If a heparin infusion is used, it may be stopped 3 to 4 hours before surgery, allowing sufficient time for the return of normal values for coagulation parameters. If reversal is urgently needed, protamine sulfate can be used. We do not stop heparin therapy in patients with unstable angina or recent MI who are undergoing coronary artery bypass grafting because of the risk of intracoronary thrombosis before the institution of cardiopulmonary bypass.

Antineoplastic Agents

Cancer patients should be asked about the chemotherapeutic agents used in their treatment. The anesthesiologist should determine what agents were given and how long ago they were administered. In addition, an assessment of bone marrow recovery should be made.

Doxorubicin

Specific problems also exist apart from bone marrow suppression. Adverse effects of doxorubicin on the heart have been well described.[72] The anesthesiologist needs to determine the total dose given to the patient.[72] Although myocardial damage can be detected by subendocardial biopsies after doses of 250 mg $\cdot$ M$^{2-1}$, clinically significant congestive heart failure is rare with doses <500 mg $\cdot$ M$^{2-1}$.[72] Concurrent administration of cyclophosphamide and doxorubicin increases the risk of cardiac toxicity. If the patient reports symptoms suggestive of congestive heart failure, an assessment of cardiac function should be undertaken preoperatively.

Bleomycin

Bleomycin can cause interstitial pulmonary fibrosis and may sensitize the lungs to damage from inspired oxygen concentrations >28%.[73] If a history of bleomycin use is obtained, particularly if the dose is >500 mg, it is probably wise to limit the perioperative inspired oxygen concentration to <30% while carefully monitoring the patient's arterial hemoglobin oxygen saturation using pulse oximetry. Administration of corticosteroids preoperatively may be of benefit in preventing perioperative respiratory failure in patients with a history of bleomycin treatment.[74]

Antiglaucoma Agents

Use of antiglaucoma agents is routinely continued in the perioperative period. Two important medications in this class are the cholinesterase inhibitors echothiophate and isoflurophate. They irreversibly inhibit plasma cholinesterase, which prolongs the duration of action of succinylcholine.[75]

Systemic absorption of ophthalmic medication may also occur in those patients who use ophthalmic β-blockers. The cardiovascular reserve to stress may be blunted in such patients[76] (Fig. 1–7).

Antibiotics

Many antibiotics, particularly the aminoglycosides, potentiate neuromuscular blockade. This effect can present difficulties in the reversal of neuromuscular relaxation at the end of surgery or in the presence of a respiratory acidosis. A partial list is presented in Table 1–2.[77]

Opioids and Benzodiazepines

Opioids and benzodiazepines are frequently withheld after midnight the night before surgery. However, this course of action leaves a patient's preoperative pain untreated or may

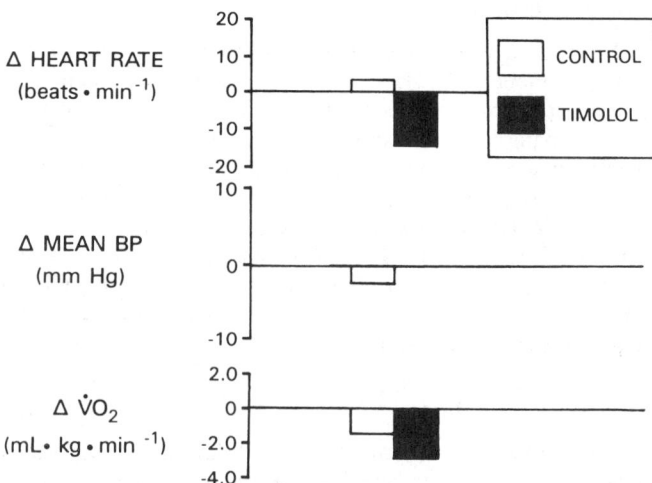

FIGURE 1–7. Cardiovascular responses to exercise following 4 weeks of therapy with 0.5% ophthalmic timolol maleate or artificial tears in healthy volunteers. The responses to exercise represent changes from baseline exercise periods performed at the beginning of the 4-week therapy. Exercise capacity (heart rate and oxygen consumption [$\dot{V}O_2$]) was significantly reduced in those volunteers who were treated with timolol. (Reproduced with permission from Leier CV, Baker D, Weber PA: Cardiovascular effects of timolol. Ann Intern Med 1986; 104:197.)

TABLE 1–2. Interaction Among Antibiotics, Muscle Relaxants, Neostigmine, and Calcium*

Antibiotic	dTc	Succinylcholine	Neostigmine	Calcium
Neomycin	Yes	Yes	Usually	Usually
Streptomycin	Yes	Yes	Usually	Usually
Gentamicin	Yes	†	Sometimes	Usually
Kanamycin	Yes	Yes	Sometimes	Sometimes
Paromomycin	Yes	†	Yes	Yes
Viomycin	Yes	†	Yes	Yes
Polymyxin A	Yes	†	No	No
Polymyxin B	Yes	Yes	No‡	No
Colistin	Yes	Yes	No	Sometimes
Tetracycline	Yes	No	Partially	Partially
Lincomycin	Yes	†	Partially	Partially
Clindamycin	Yes	†	Partially	Partially

(From Miller RD, Savarese JJ: Pharmacology of muscle relaxants and their antagonists. *In* Anesthesia. 3rd ed. Miller RD (ed). New York, Churchill Livingstone, 1990, pp 389–435.)
*Increase in neuromuscular block from antibiotic.
†Not studied.
‡Block is augmented by neostigmine.
Abbreviation: dTc = d-tubocurarine–like drugs, which include other nondepolarizing muscle relaxants.

precipitate panic attacks or withdrawal symptoms. These drugs should be continued until the time of surgery. If the use of oral medications is deemed unwise, parenteral therapy can be instituted instead.

ALLERGIC RESPONSES

What Specific Information Is Important?

Allergic Responses Versus Side Effects

Any allergies to medications must be documented, and the exact nature of the allergic responses should be determined and included in the record. This documentation is important because patients may confuse side effects with allergic responses. For example, codeine may cause nausea (a side effect) or a pruritic rash (an allergic response), but either may be interpreted as an "allergy" by the patient. Also, tachycardia due to epinephrine mixed with lidocaine given for dental procedures may lead the patient to say that he or she is allergic to local anesthetics.

True Allergies

True allergies do exist. A 10% to 15% rate of allergic cross-reaction exists between penicillins and cephalosporins. In patients with a history of an immediate hypersensitivity reaction to penicillin (e.g., anaphylactic shock, angioedema, and hives) a cephalosporin should not be used as a substitute antibiotic. Cephalosporins may be used if a history of a delayed type of allergic reaction to penicillins *only* is elicited.

Allergies to iodine-containing compounds preclude the use of anesthetic agents that contain iodine (e.g., metocurine or gallamine). If intravenous radiographic contrast agents are absolutely required, pretreatment with corticosteroids and antihistamines can be used to decrease or eliminate the allergic response.[78]

Anesthetic Agents

True allergy to anesthetic agents is extremely rare. Allergy to ester-based local anesthetic agents may be to *para*-amino-

benzoic acid, a metabolite of that group of compounds. True allergy to the amide local anesthetics has been reported but is even more rare than that observed with ester anesthetics. Intradermal challenge testing for true allergy to local anesthetics can be done prior to elective surgery or elective nerve block through consultation with an allergist.[79] Similar testing can also be used for other medications.[79]

SOCIAL HISTORY

Why Is the Social History Important?

Smoking and Alcohol

Questions concerning tobacco and alcohol use need to be asked, including those addressing the amount and duration of consumption. Cigarette smoke has several adverse effects, including alteration of mucus secretion and clearance and decrease of small airway caliber. It also may alter the immune response. The chronic smoker should be encouraged to abstain from smoking for at least 2 months prior to the operation,[80] but stopping smoking for even <24 hours may produce benefits in cardiovascular physiology.[81]

Illicit Drug Use

Inquiries into illicit or "recreational" drug use or behavior that would place a patient into a high-risk group for infection with the human immunodeficiency virus also need to be made. Once drug use is identified (whether it is prescribed or illicit), strategies for the prevention or treatment of withdrawal syndromes in the perioperative period can be formulated.

The patient who is suffering from a withdrawal syndrome should not undergo anesthesia and surgery unless the surgery is urgent. Also, an increased requirement for opioids should be expected both intraoperatively and postoperatively in patients that have a preoperative history of medicinal opioid use or opioid abuse.

Questions concerning anabolic steroid use should be asked of athletes, as these drugs can have significant side effects on the liver.[82] Cholestatic jaundice can occur as a result of the use of anabolic steroids.[83]

PHYSICAL EXAMINATION

What Should Be Checked?

General Assessment

A quick *general assessment* of the patient frequently provides important information. For example, cyanosis may be observed; if it is present, a careful examination of the cardiovascular and pulmonary systems should be performed. A pulse oximeter–determined baseline arterial oxygen saturation value confirms or refutes the clinical impression of cyanosis. The chronically ill–appearing patient with anasarca has an altered volume of distribution for most of the drugs that are used in the perioperative period.

Vital Signs

Vital signs, including weight (in kilograms), should be documented. In patients with peripheral vascular disease, blood pressure is measured in both arms. Up to 21% of such patients present with a pressure disparity of greater than 20 mm Hg between the two extremities that is presumably due to atherosclerosis[84] (Fig. 1–8). Such differences in pressure require a change in the location of a radial artery catheter, because the arm with the higher blood pressure reflects the central arterial pressure more accurately.[84]

If available, a preoperative baseline measure of hemoglobin saturation (SpO_2) is also of value, as it not only identifies a respiratory abnormality but also establishes a realistic goal for postoperative saturation before the patient is discharged from the postanesthesia recovery area. The need for supplemental oxygen is also assessed. In many institutions, SpO_2 is becoming the fifth vital sign.

Airway

An accurate assessment of the airway must be made and includes examination of cervical spine mobility, temporomandibular joint function, and dentition. Problems with orotracheal intubation should be expected in those patients who are unable to open their mouth greater than 4 cm, whose distance from the thyroid notch to the mandible is less than three fingerbreadths, who have a high, arched palate, or who demonstrate decreased cervical spine mobility.[85]

A simple clinical examination has been proposed to predict a difficult tracheal intubation.[86] In those patients whose faucial pillars, soft palate, and uvula were visible (class I), adequate exposure of the glottis during direct laryngoscopy was achieved.

If the faucial pillars and soft palate were visible but the uvula was masked by the base of the tongue (class II), adequate exposure of the glottis was achieved in only approximately 66% of cases.

If only the soft palate could be visualized (class III), adequate visualization of the glottis was achieved by direct laryngoscopy in fewer than 7% of patients[86] (Fig. 1–9).

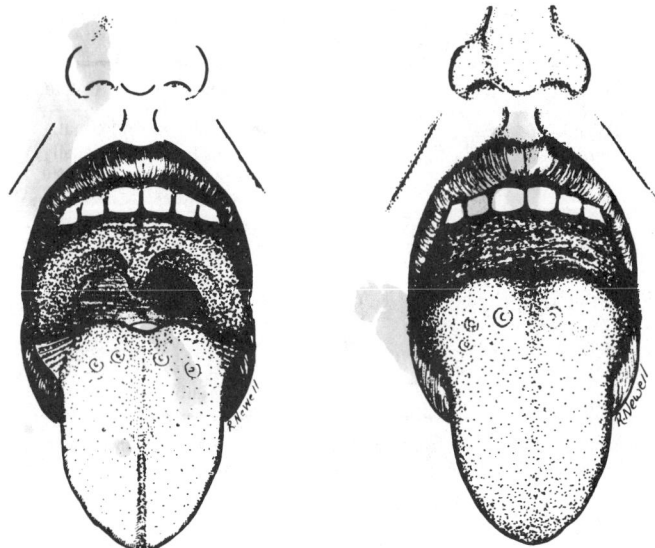

FIGURE 1–9. Examples of Mallampati class I ([*left*] faucial pillars; soft palate and uvula are visible) and class III ([*right*] no pharyngeal structures are seen) airways. Difficulty may be encountered when intubating the patient with the class III airway. (From Mallampati SR, Gugino LD, Desai SP, et al: A clinical sign to predict difficult tracheal intubation: a prospective study. Can Anaesth Soc J 1985; 32:429.)

Dentition

Examination of dentition is important as well. The presence of chipped or otherwise damaged teeth should be noted on the medical record. Teeth that are in imminent danger of falling out should be pulled before the administration of anesthesia to avoid aspiration. This procedure, of course, must be done with the patient's consent.

Neck

Examination of the neck should be performed in addition to the airway examination just described. A carotid bruit indicates the presence of peripheral vascular disease and may be an indication for further evaluation but does not necessarily reflect an increased risk for a perioperative stroke.[87, 88] Palpation of the thyroid gland can also be performed quickly and easily.

Lungs

Auscultation of the lungs may reveal evidence of disease in otherwise asymptomatic individuals and may indicate that further evaluation is needed. Bronchospasm in an asthmatic patient who has been "cleared" for surgery indicates that the patient has not been prepared optimally. Similarly, evidence of rales or wheezing in a patient with a history of congestive heart failure may be suggestive of subclinical congestive heart failure. Diaphragmatic excursion should be checked if an interscalene block is planned, since ipsilateral phrenic nerve paralysis occurs regularly with this technique.[89]

Heart

Examination of the heart should include an assessment of the heart rate and rhythm (regular, irregular, presence of extrasystolic beats) and determination as to whether murmurs or

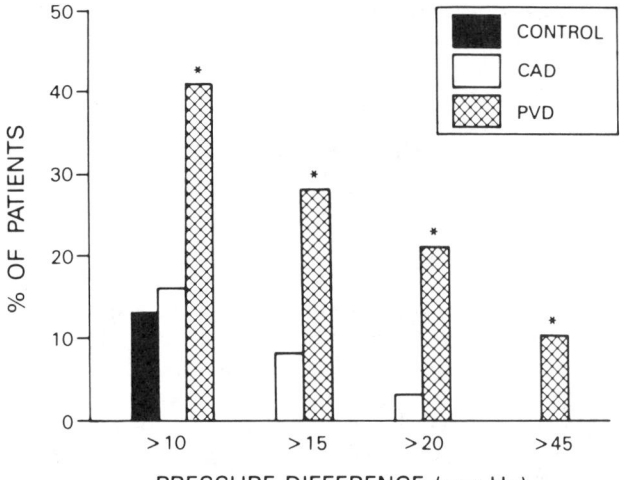

FIGURE 1–8. Systolic blood pressure differences between the right and left arm in three groups of patients: control patients without atherosclerotic disease, patients with coronary artery disease (CAD), and patients with peripheral vascular disease (PVD). There is a significantly greater number of patients with PVD who have systolic pressure differences between the two arms compared with the other two groups. (Adapted from Frank SM, Norris EJ, Christopherson R, et al: Right- and left-arm discrepancies in vascular surgery patients. Anesthesiology 1991; 75:457.)

TABLE 1–3. Useful Bedside Maneuvers to Determine the Type of Cardiac Murmur

Type of Murmur	Müller's Maneuver	Valsalva's Maneuver	Squatting	Standing	Amyl Nitrate
Right-sided heart murmurs	↑		Should ↑		
Hypertrophic cardiomyopathy		↑	↓	↑	↑
Aortic stenosis	↓	↓	Should ↑	↓	↑
Mitral regurgitation			Should ↑	↓	↓
Mitral valve prolapse		±		↑	±
Aortic insufficiency			↑		↓
Pulmonic stenosis					↑
Tricuspid regurgitation				↓	↑
Pulmonic regurgitation					↑

(Reproduced with permission, from Rothman A, Goldberger AL: Aids to cardiac auscultation. Ann Intern Med 1983; 99:346.)

extra heart sounds (e.g., a third heart sound) or jugular venous distention is present. Determination of the type of murmur may be assisted by the use of amyl nitrate and several bedside maneuvers[90] (Table 1–3).

Extremities and Back

The extremities and back should also be examined. If use of a regional anesthetic is contemplated, examination of the site is important to identify that it is clear of lesions and that the appropriate landmarks are present to determine the feasibility of the technique.

A modification of Allen's test (Table 1–4)[91] is usually performed to provide some assessment of the adequacy of ulnar collateral flow if cannulation of the radial artery is considered. However, the utility of this test in patients without peripheral vascular disease has been called into question.[92]

Neurologic Function

If a regional anesthetic technique is planned, the anesthesiologist should document the neurologic function in the area to be anesthetized. Likewise, if the patient is to be operated on in an unusual position, the anesthesiologist should determine the neurologic function of areas that could be affected by the position. A corollary to this approach is to have the patient assume the anticipated intraoperative position to determine whether it is easily tolerated.

Pre-existing Deficits

Documentation of pre-existing neurologic deficits is important, especially considering that 15% of closed malpractice

TABLE 1–4. Modified Allen's Test

Both radial and ulnar arteries are compressed
The patient clenches and unclenches the fist repeatedly until the palm develops pallor
One of the arteries is released
The amount of time required for blushing of the palm is noted
The procedure is repeated for the other artery
Normal palmar blushing should be evident within 7 s
An equivocal test is 8–14 s
An abnormal test is present if it takes 15 s or longer for the palm to blush
A pulse oximeter may also be helpful to determine the time to return of flow

(From Seneff M: Arterial line placement and care. *In* Intensive Care Medicine. 2nd ed. Rippe JM, Irwin RS, Alpert JS, et al (eds). Boston, Little, Brown & Co, 1991, pp 37–47.)

claims made against anesthesiologists involved peripheral nerve injury after anesthesia.[93] If a neurologic deficit is present, succinylcholine may be contraindicated owing to increased muscle membrane chemosensitivity and resultant hyperkalemia.[32]

LABORATORY TESTING

What Tests Are Appropriate?

Extensive literature has been published over the past decade regarding routine preoperative blood tests. The most important screening "test" to detect disease processes is still a thorough history and physical examination.

Routine Testing

Much data exist supporting the concept that routine laboratory screening tests are not cost-effective in the asymptomatic patient.[1] Tests are often inefficient and do not always identify symptomatic disease.[94] Notable to consider is that since a "normal" laboratory test result is usually defined as the mean value for the test plus or minus 2 standard deviations, an "abnormal" test result appears in 5% of the healthy population[95] and increases with the number of tests performed. The probability of healthy individuals having a completely normal 12-test biochemical profile is only 54%.[95]

In addition to the inefficiency of routine testing, abnormalities that are discovered frequently do not have a measurable effect on perioperative anesthetic management or on patient outcome; furthermore, an abnormal test result may cause the ordering of other tests, which increases risk to the patient.[1, 96]

For the apparently healthy, asymptomatic male who is younger than 40 years of age and who is undergoing surgery with minimal expected blood loss, no preoperative blood testing is necessary.[1, 96] Those patients with underlying disease as detected by history and physical examination should undergo preoperative testing.[1, 96]

Electrocardiogram

The utility of routine electrocardiograms is also questionable. Abnormal electrocardiographic findings are common in surgical patients and their prevalence increases with age (Fig. 1–10)[97]; such findings usually do not alter perioperative medical management.[97, 98] The significance of the abnormalities

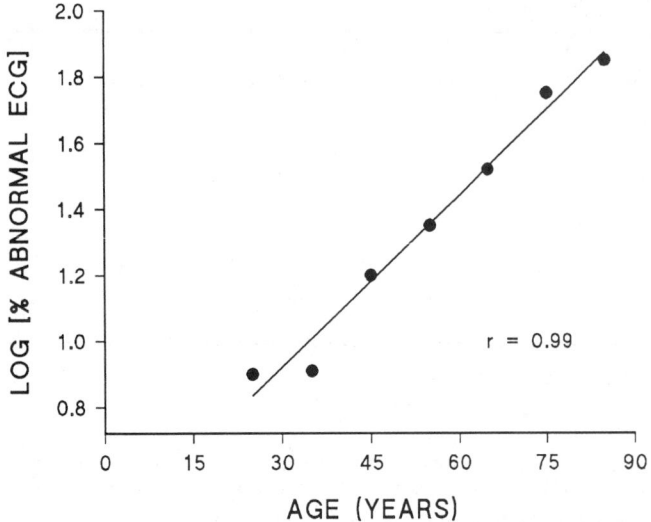

FIGURE 1–10. Prevalence of electrocardiographic (ECG) abnormalities as a function of age. The ECG abnormalities increase exponentially with age. (Reproduced with permission, from Goldberger AL, O'Konski M: Utility of the routine electrocardiogram before surgery and on general hospital admission: a critical review and new guidelines. Ann Intern Med 1986; 105:552.)

depends in part on the prevalence of the disease state. In young, healthy patients, Q waves or ST-T wave changes usually are not due to ischemic heart disease.[97]

The probability of detecting cardiac disease based on the admission electrocardiogram and not during the taking of the patient history or physical examination is low irrespective of age, but it increases in patients over 44 years of age or in those who also have a history of a cardiac abnormality.[97]

Although no consensus states when a routine preoperative electrocardiogram should be obtained,[97] it is reasonable to request one for patients older than 40 to 45 years of age, particularly if a history of cardiac disease is suggested.[95, 97, 98]

Previous Tests

If a patient has a normal complete blood count, sodium, potassium, and creatinine levels, prothrombin time, and partial thromboplastin times within 1 year prior to surgery, the likelihood that a current preoperative value is abnormal is less than 0.5%.[99] Up to 20% of preoperative tests results will be abnormal if a previous test result is also abnormal.[99]

Despite specific criteria for preoperative tests, recent data suggest that a large number of unnecessary tests are still ordered and that indicated testing is often not performed.[100] Table 1–5 presents proposed guidelines for the minimal amount of preoperative testing in the *healthy* patient. Of note is that routine urinalysis is of no apparent value.

SPECIAL TESTING

What Special Preoperative Tests Are Available?

Cardiac Disease

Each year, approximately 7 to 8 million noncardiac surgical patients are at risk for cardiac morbidity and mortality.[101] A significant number of these patients have *undetected* coronary

artery disease. Identification of this high-risk group preoperatively is important. Several useful cardiac risk indices have been developed in the last 15 years. A "low risk" does *not* exclude a patient from suffering a perioperative cardiac event but merely indicates a low probability of its occurrence.[102, 103] The use of a Bayesian approach (i.e., determination of the likelihood that a patient has a disease given a certain test result) to assess cardiac risk may be of further benefit.[104]

Clinical findings such as uncontrolled congestive heart failure or an MI within 6 months indicates that elective surgery should be delayed. In those cases that are urgent but not true emergencies, application of medical decision-making algorithms may be helpful in deciding on the appropriate timing of surgery.[105]

Coronary Artery Disease

Significant advances in the diagnostic evaluation of patients with known or suspected coronary artery disease have occurred.

Dipyridamole-thallium Imaging. One test in particular—dipyridamole-thallium imaging—has received widespread attention. Dipyridamole is a potent coronary artery vasodilator and diverts coronary blood flow from areas with fixed arterial lesions. Thallium 201 (^{201}Tl) is taken up by normal myocytes and is detected by scintigraphy. The thallium is administered after dipyridamole has been infused. Areas of the myocardium that do not take up thallium during and after dipyridamole-induced vasodilation are considered areas of infarct. Areas of the myocardium that do not take up thallium during vasodilation but do so afterward (reperfusion defect) are considered at risk for ischemia and infarction (Fig. 1–11).

Dipyridamole-thallium imaging is also helpful in detecting significant coronary artery disease in high-risk patients who cannot be tested using other methods (i.e., patients with peripheral vascular disease who cannot perform treadmill testing). If the reperfusion defect is sufficiently severe, the patient may be referred for coronary angiography and possible angioplasty or revascularization instead of undergoing the scheduled elective procedure. Even if the proposed procedure is urgent enough to postpone coronary revascularization, the knowledge that a particular patient is at high risk for perioperative ische-

TABLE 1–5. Suggested Minimal Preoperative Test Requirements

Age (y)	Test Required
<40	None
40–59	Electrocardiography; measurement of creatinine and glucose
≥60	Complete blood cell count; electrocardiography; chest roentgenography; measurement of creatinine and glucose

Guidelines	

A complete blood cell count is indicated in all patients who undergo blood typing and who are screened or cross-matched

Measurement of potassium is indicated in patients taking diuretics or undergoing bowel preparation

Chest roentgenography is indicated in patients with a history of cardiac or pulmonary disease or with recent respiratory symptoms

A history of cigarette smoking in patients older than 40 y of age who are scheduled for an upper abdominal or thoracic surgical procedure may be an indication for spirometry (determination of forced vital capacity)

(From Narr BJ, Hansen TR, Warner MA: Preoperative laboratory screening in healthy Mayo patients: cost-effective elimination of test and unchanged outcomes. Mayo Clin Proc 1991; 66:155–159, by permission.)

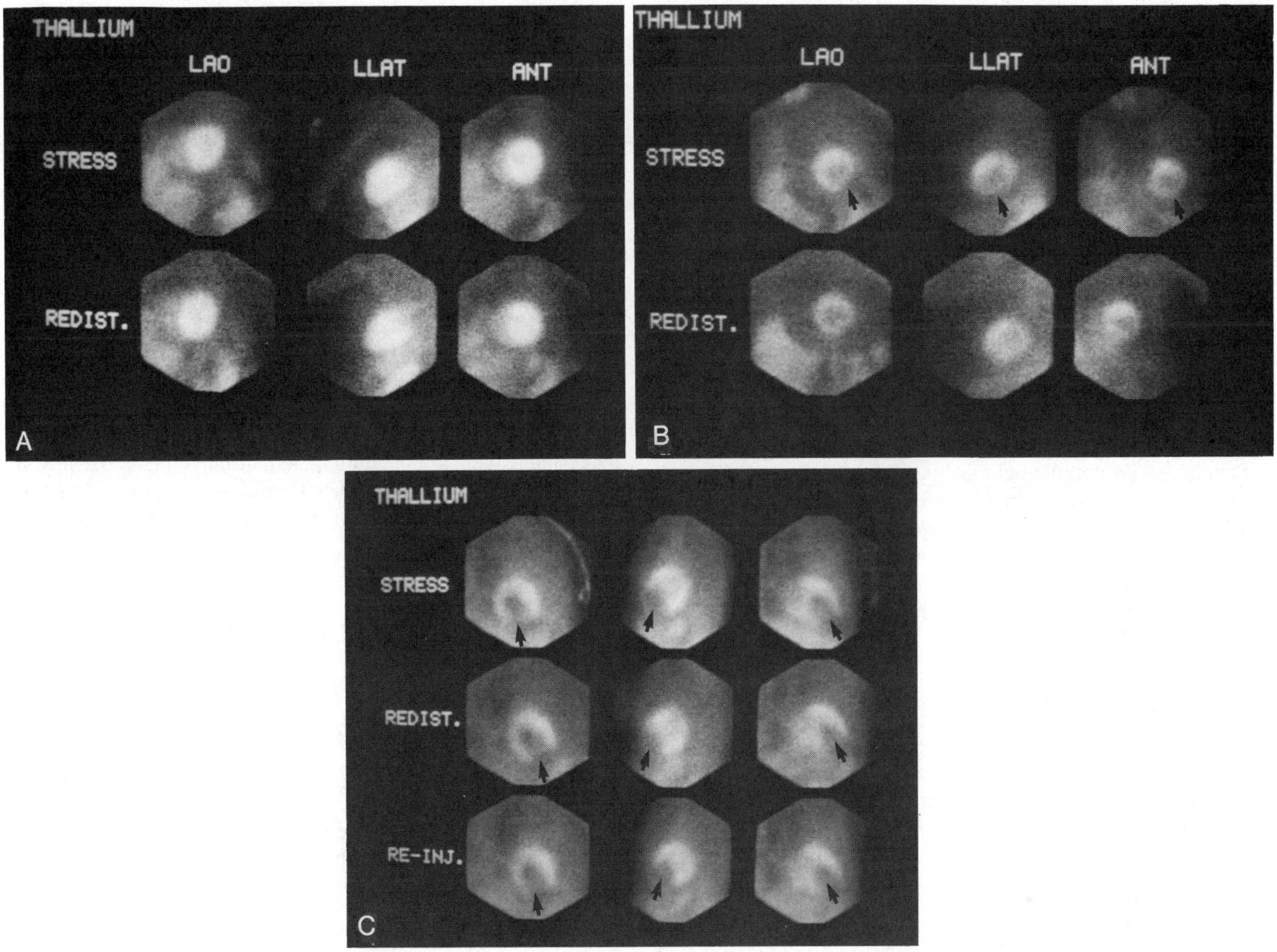

FIGURE 1–11. Dipyridamole-thallium images from patients with normal coronary arteries *(A)*, coronary artery disease (as evidenced by a reperfusion defect [*B*]), and a previous myocardial infarction (persistent defect [*C*]). See text for details. (Images provided by Jeffrey Leppo, M.D. and Seth Dahlberg, M.D.)

mia or infarction is still highly useful information, as monitoring or anesthetic techniques might change.[106, 107]

Although dipyridamole-thallium scanning is very sensitive in detecting coronary artery disease, the presence of a reperfusion defect does *not* specifically mean that a perioperative cardiac event will occur.[107] Therefore, it is not absolutely clear which patients should undergo preoperative dipyridamole-thallium testing. Some data suggest that patients scheduled for peripheral vascular surgery who meet certain clinical criteria may benefit from preoperative thallium-dipyridamole testing[108, 109] (Fig. 1–12).

Other Tests. Preoperative ischemia detected by *Holter monitoring* may identify vascular surgery patients at risk for perioperative cardiac events.[110] *Echocardiography* and *gated radionuclide angiography* can be useful ancillary tests in those patients with a history of cardiac dysfunction, because such tests can assess the degree and location of cardiac wall motion abnormalities.

Pulmonary Function

Spirometry

For those patients undergoing nonthoracic surgery, few studies exist that validate the clinical usefulness of routine pulmonary function testing in the preoperative period.[111] Spirometry is no better than a careful history and physical examination in predicting postoperative pulmonary complications following upper abdominal surgery.[112, 113] In addition, no single

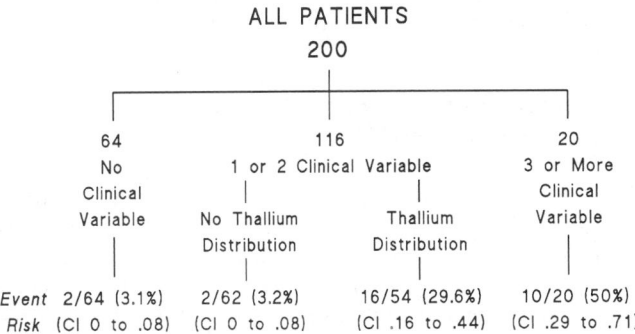

FIGURE 1–12. Algorithm combining clinical variables (Q wave on electrocardiogram, age >70 years, history of angina, history of ventricular ectopic activity requiring therapy, and diabetes mellitus requiring treatment) and the results of dipyridamole-thallium imaging to stratify cardiac risk in 200 patients undergoing major vascular surgery. An ''event'' refers to postoperative unstable angina, ischemic pulmonary edema, myocardial infarction, or cardiac death. CI = confidence intervals. (Adapted from Eagle KA, Singer DE, Brewster DC, et al: Dipyridamole-thallium scanning in patients undergoing vascular surgery: optimizing preoperative evaluation of cardiac risk. JAMA 1987; 257:2185. Copyright 1987, American Medical Association.)

TABLE 1–6. Indicators That Predict Postoperative Pulmonary Complications

ASA physical status category greater than II
Upper abdominal surgery
Residual intra-abdominal sepsis
Age greater than 59 y
Obesity
Preoperative stay >4 d
Colorectal or gastroduodenal surgery
Cardiac surgery with pleurotomy
Preoperative $PaCO_2$ >45

abnormal finding on standard pulmonary function testing contraindicates surgery. Patients with a forced expiratory volume in 1 second (FEV_1) as low as 0.45 L have tolerated surgery.[112]

Several easily obtained clinical parameters are predictive of postoperative pulmonary complications after laparotomy (Table 1–6).[114] In those patients in whom a pneumonectomy is contemplated, more extensive testing that includes split pulmonary function testing, exercise studies, and right-sided heart catheterization with pulmonary artery pressure measurements is generally indicated.[112–114]

Arterial Blood Gas Analysis

Besides a careful clinical evaluation, the most important and easily obtained test relating to pulmonary function is the arterial blood gas measurement.[113] In the absence of neuromuscular disease or drug-induced alveolar hypoventilation, an arterial carbon dioxide tension ($PaCO_2$) >45 mm Hg reliably predicts pulmonary complications.[112, 113]

Which Medication Levels Should Be Determined Preoperatively?

Not all patients who are taking medications that are monitored by assaying serum concentrations need to have repeat assays before a surgical procedure. If a medication has been taken chronically and the patient has been clinically stable, no additional testing need be done.[115] However, recent changes in dosing or in the clinical condition make determination of the serum concentration of the medication in question prudent.

When Should Preoperative Invasive Monitoring Be Used?

In many institutions, selected patients are admitted routinely to the surgical intensive care unit preoperatively for invasive hemodynamic monitoring so that cardiovascular hemodynamics can be optimized before the scheduled operation. Uncontrolled studies suggest that such a practice identifies high-risk patients and that correction of abnormal hemodynamic variables preoperatively decreases morbidity and mortality.[116]

A recent prospective, randomized trial in patients undergoing peripheral vascular surgery showed that preoperative pulmonary artery catheterization and correction of abnormal hemodynamic variables resulted in fewer adverse intraoperative events (tachycardia, dysrhythmias, and hypotension) and reduced perioperative morbidity (mainly graft thrombosis) compared with a control group that received no invasive monitor-

ing.[117] However, no differences in mortality, length of stay, or hospital costs between control and study groups were noted.

Although this study suggests that preoperative pulmonary artery catheterization may be beneficial in this patient population, these data should be considered preliminary. The results should be verified before *routine* preoperative invasive monitoring is advocated for patients undergoing peripheral vascular surgery.

The number of patients occupying the intensive care units in many hospitals is too great to allow *routine* preoperative invasive monitoring. We believe that high-risk patients can be identified preoperatively by history and physical examination and by performing tests such as echocardiography or dipyridamole-thallium scanning. Appropriate invasive catheters can be inserted on the day of surgery, and abnormal hemodynamic variables can be corrected at that time. If postoperative surgical intensive care is anticipated, arrangements should be made preoperatively. Surgery should not begin on patients requiring such care until a bed is available in the surgical intensive care unit.

CONSULTATIONS

When Is Preoperative Consultation Appropriate?

After the history and physical examination are completed and the laboratory data have been reviewed, additional testing or treatment may be indicated. Assistance from other medical specialists is appropriate to help in better preparing the patient for surgery or to perform additional diagnostic tests (see Chapters 9 to 16).

When requesting the services of a consultant, the anesthesiologist should ask a specific question rather than request "preoperative clearance." Without such specific direction, the consultant, who may lack an understanding of intraoperative practice, often suggests methods of intraoperative monitoring, medication use, or anesthetic techniques that are inappropriate or condescending.[118]

Some medical centers have developed preoperative anesthesia consultation clinics where anesthesiologists direct the evaluation of patients deemed at high risk for anesthesia and surgery.[119] The interviewing anesthesiologist should contact the consultant directly by telephone to discuss the specifics of the situation and to expedite the consultation. This approach helps to prevent delays in elective surgical cases (see Chapters 9 to 16).

How Is the Risk of Anesthesia Estimated?

The overall risk of death from anesthesia in several reports ranges from 0.01% to 0.0005%.[120] This range is for primary anesthetic mortality only and not for anesthetic-associated deaths from iatrogenic causes. A preoperative grading system that evaluates patients according to their general state of health and the severity of their underlying diseases was first published by Saklad.[121] This system was later revised by Dripps and coworkers into the American Society of Anesthesiologists (ASA) Physical Status Scale[122] (Table 1–7).

Although interobserver variations in score assignment and vagueness in the definitions have been noted,[123] several studies

TABLE 1–7. ASA Physical Status

Category	Description
I	Healthy patient
II	Mild systemic disease; no functional limitation
III	Severe systemic disease; definite functional limitation
IV	Severe systemic disease that is a constant threat to life
V	Moribund patient who is unlikely to survive 24 h with or without operation

showed the ASA physical status scale to be a good predictor of noncardiac deaths when it is applied to total operative mortality.[102, 103] The scale is much less sensitive when it is used as a means to predict anesthesia-related deaths[124] (see Chapter 5).

PREOPERATIVE MEDICATIONS

What Medications Should Be Given Preoperatively?

As discussed previously, the most important medications should be continued on the day of surgery. Preoperative medications, including sedative/hypnotics and analgesics, are discussed in Chapter 80. Other specific medication needs to be mentioned.

Antibiotics

If the patient is at risk for the development of infective endocarditis, appropriate antibiotic prophylaxis should be instituted. Table 1–8 provides the most recent American Heart Association guidelines for perioperative endocarditis prophylaxis.[125]

Many patients receive preoperative prophylactic antibiotics to reduce the incidence of wound or prosthetic device–related infections. Such antibiotics must be given 2 hours or less before incision; otherwise, their effectiveness is reduced[126] (Fig. 1–13).

Aspiration Prophylaxis

Those patients at risk for vomiting and aspiration of gastric contents should receive prophylaxis with nonparticulate antacids or histamine$_2$ blockers with or without metoclopramide.[127] Recent data suggest that proton pump inhibitors such as omeprazole are also effective in keeping gastric pH above 2.5.[128]

Prophylaxis For Venous Thrombosis

Some patients are at high risk for the development of venous thrombophlebitis in the perioperative period (Table 1–9). Prophylactic measures should be used. Various methods include the use of low-dose heparin, intermittent calf compression, warfarin (particularly in total hip replacements), or dextran.[129, 130] Regrettably, recent studies indicate methods to prevent venous thromboembolism are underutilized.[131]

NIL PER OS STATUS

How Long Should a Patient Be Kept Nil Per Os?

The duration of preoperative fasting has come under scrutiny since the late 1980s. The stomach empties clear liquids in 1 to 2 hours but takes longer than 3 hours to clear solids.[132] Recent studies indicate that in both children and adults (ASA I or II), gastric volume and pH are unchanged after

TABLE 1–8. Bacterial Endocarditis Prophylaxis

A. Conditions for Which Prophylaxis Is Recommended
1. Prosthetic heart valves, including bioprosthetic and homograft valves
2. Previous bacterial endocarditis
3. Most congenital cardiac malformations
4. Rheumatic and other acquired valvular dysfunction
5. Hypertrophic cardiomyopathy
6. Mitral valve prolapse with valvular regurgitation

B. Surgical Procedures for Which Prophylaxis Is Recommended
1. Dental procedures known to induce gingival or mucosal bleeding
2. Tonsillectomy and/or adenoidectomy
3. Surgical procedures that involve intestinal or respiratory mucosa
4. Bronchoscopy with a rigid bronchoscope
5. Sclerotherapy for esophageal varices
6. Esophageal dilatation
7. Gallbladder surgery
8. Cystoscopy
9. Urethral dilatation
10. Urethral catheterization if urinary tract infection is present
11. Prostatic surgery
12. Incision and drainage of infected tissue
13. Vaginal hysterectomy
14. Vaginal delivery in the presence of infection

C. Standard Prophylactic Regimen for Patients at Risk

Drug	Dosing Regimen
Amoxicillin	3.0 g orally 1 h before procedure, then 1.5 g at 6 h after initial dose

Amoxicillin/Penicillin–Allergic Patients

Erythromycin *or*	Erythromycin ethylsuccinate, 800 mg, or erythromycin stearate, 1.0 g, orally 2 h before procedure, then one-half this dose 6 h later
Clindamycin	300 mg orally 1 h before procedure, then 150 mg at 6 h after initial dose

Patients Unable to Take Oral Medications

Ampicillin	IV or IM administration of ampicillin, 2.0 g, 30 min before procedure, then IV or IM administration of ampicillin, 1.0 g at 6 h after initial dose

Ampicillin/Amoxicillin/Penicillin–Allergic Patients Unable to Take Oral Medications

Clindamycin	IV administration of clindamycin, 300 mg, 30 min before procedure and an IV or oral administration of 150 mg at 6 h after initial dose

Patients Considered High-Risk and Not Candidates for Standard Regimen

Ampicillin	IV or IM administration of ampicillin, 2.0 g, and gentamicin, 1.5 mg · kg^{-1} (not to exceed 80 mg), 30 min before procedure, followed by amoxicillin, 1.5 g, orally at 6 h after initial dose; alternatively, the parenteral regimen may be repeated 8 h after initial dose

Ampicillin/Amoxicillin/Penicillin–Allergic Patients Considered High-Risk

Vancomycin	IV administration of 1.0 g over 1 h, starting 1 h before procedure; no repeat dose necessary

Alternative Low-Risk Patient Regimen

Amoxicillin	3.0 g orally 1 h before procedure, then 1.5 g at 6 h after initial dose

(Modified from Dajani AS, Bisno AL, Chung KJ, et al: Prevention of bacterial endocarditis. Recommendations by the American Heart Association. JAMA 1990; 264:2919. Copyright 1990, American Medical Association.)

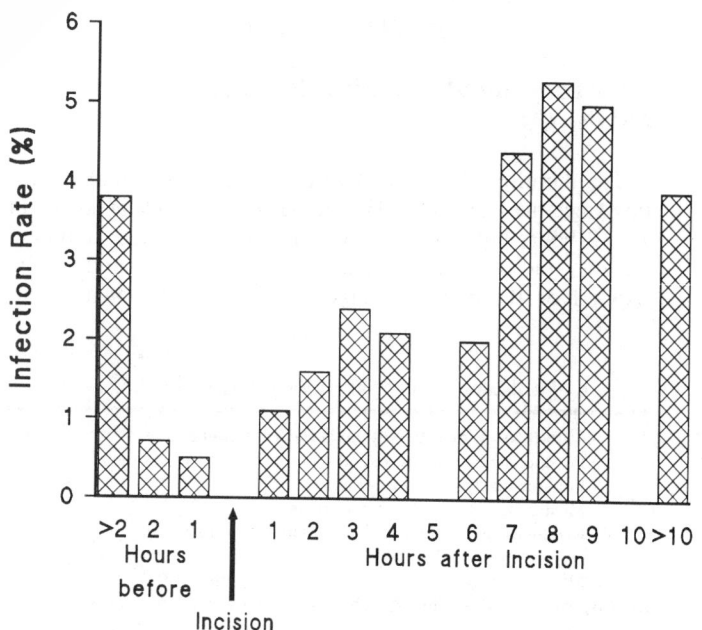

FIGURE 1-13. Surgical wound infection rates as a function of the time of initial perioperative antibiotic dose. There is a significant trend toward higher infection rates for each hour that antibiotic administration was delayed following surgical incision. (Reprinted from Classen DC, Evans S, Pestotnik SL, et al: The timing of prophylactic administration of antibiotics and the risk of surgical-wound infection. N Engl J Med 1992; 326:281, by permission of the New England Journal of Medicine.)

TABLE 1-9. Risk Groups for Venous Thromboembolism

Patient Group	Incidence of Venous Thrombosis (%)	Site of Thrombosis	Incidence of Fatal Pulmonary Embolus (%)	Prophylaxis
Hip fracture	40–70	Thigh and calf	7–10	Any of the following: dextran, adjusted-dose heparin, low-dose warfarin, pneumatic compression
Total hip replacement	40–70	Thigh and calf	4–7	See hip fracture
Total knee replacement	40–70	Thigh and calf	3–7	See hip fracture
Urologic surgery	15–20	Calf	<5	Pneumatic compression
General gynecologic surgery	15–20	Calf	1	Low-dose heparin
Neurologic surgery	15–20	Calf	<1	Pneumatic compression
Medical patients	<15	Calf	<1	Low-dose heparin

(From Hyers TM, Hull RD, Weg JC: Antithrombotic therapy for venous thromboembolic disease. Chest 1986; 89 (Suppl): 26S–35S.)

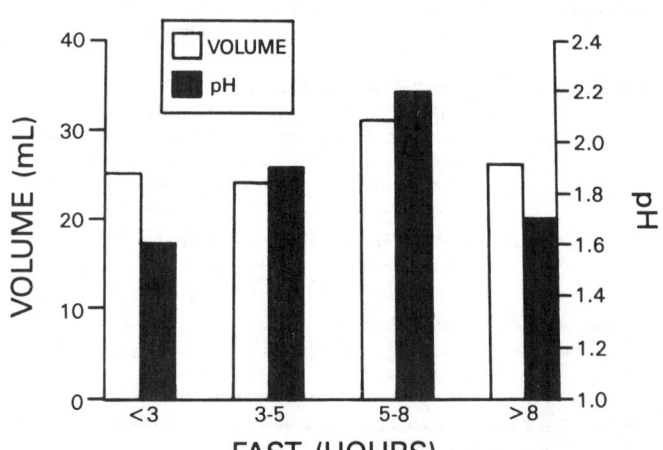

FIGURE 1-14. Gastric volume and pH as a function of preoperative duration of fast for liquids. There are no significant differences among groups. (Data from Scarr M, Maltby JR, Jani K, et al: Volume and acidity of residual gastric fluid after oral fluid ingestion before elective ambulatory surgery. Can Med Assoc J 1989; 141:1151.)

TABLE 1–10. Suggested Fasting Guidelines for Elective Surgical Patients

---

No ingestion of solid food on the day of surgery
Unrestricted clear fluids are permitted until 3 h before the scheduled time of surgery
Oral medications with 30 mL of water are allowed up to 60 min before surgery
In those patients at risk for regurgitation and aspiration of gastric contents, the administration of a clear antacid or H_2-receptor blocker should be considered

---

(Goresky GV, Maltby JR: Fasting guidelines for elective surgical patients. Can J Anaesth 1990; 37:493.)

ingestion of 2 to 3 mL · kg^{-1} of clear liquids (e.g., tea, coffee, fruit juice, and water) 2 to 3 hours before the scheduled start of surgery compared with those of the gastric contents of patients who fasted for more than 6 hours[133–136] (Fig. 1–14). Many hospitals have begun to relax fasting guidelines for preoperative patients[137] (Table 1–10; see also Chapter 80).

How Should the "Do-Not-Resuscitate" Patient Be Treated?

Approximately 15% of patients with do-not-resuscitate orders undergo a surgical procedure.[138] These patients present a special problem to the anesthesiologist: should the do-not-resuscitate orders be suspended during anesthesia and surgery?

Because the administration of anesthesia involves the use of potent cardiovascular depressants and often requires some degree of resuscitation (whether it be with fluids or inotropes and vasopressors), some anesthesiologists recommend that do-not-resuscitate orders be suspended in the perioperative period.[138–141] However, in the preoperative evaluation, the patient's do-not-resuscitate status should be clarified. If the goals of surgery and anesthesia are consistent with that clarification and if the patient and health care team agree, the operation can proceed. Appropriate resuscitative and supportive measures can then be undertaken should hemodynamic instability or arrest occur in the perioperative period as a result of the anesthesia or surgery.

If the cause of the arrest is the patient's underlying condition or is believed to be irreversible, resuscitative efforts do not have to be instituted.[139] The most important point that needs to be emphasized is that good preoperative communication and agreement must be present among physicians, the patient, and the members of the patient's family.[138, 139]

References

1. Roizen MF: Preoperative evaluation. *In* Anesthesia. 3rd ed. Miller RD (ed). New York, Churchill-Livingstone, 1990, pp 743–772.
2. Egbert LD, Battit GE, Turndorf H, et al: The value of the preoperative visit by the anesthetist. JAMA 1963; 185:553.
3. Egbert LD: Preoperative anxiety: the adult patient. Int Anesthesiol Clin 1986; 24:17.
4. Leigh JM, Walker J, Jananaganathan P: Effect of preoperative anaesthetic visit on anxiety. Br Med J 1977; 2:987.
5. Lutner RE, Roizen MF, Stocking CB, et al: The automated interview versus the personal interview: do patient responses to preoperative health questions differ? Anesthesiology 1991; 75:394.
6. Prys-Roberts C, Meloche R, Foex P: Studies of anesthesia in relation to hypertension. I: Cardiovascular responses of treated and untreated patients. Br J Anaesth 1971; 43:122.
7. Goldman L, Caldera DL: Risks of general anesthesia and elective operation in the hypertensive patient. Anesthesiology 1979; 50:285.
8. Bedford RF, Feinstein B: Hospital admission blood pressure: a predictor for hypertension following endotracheal intubation. Anesth Analg 1980; 59:367.
9. Asiddao CB, Donegan JH, Whitesell RC, et al: Factors associated with perioperative complications during carotid endarterectomy. Anesth Analg 1982; 61:631.
10. Tarhan S, Moffitt EA, Taylor WF, et al: Myocardial infarction after general anesthesia. JAMA 1972; 220:1451.
11. Steen PA, Tinker JH, Tarhan S: Myocardial reinfarction after anesthesia and surgery. JAMA 1978; 239:2566.
12. Rao TL, Jacobs KH, El-Etr AA: Reinfarction following anesthesia in patients with myocardial infarction. Anesthesiology 1983; 59:499.
13. Shah KB, Kleinman BS, Sami H, et al: Reevaluation of perioperative myocardial infarction in patients with prior myocardial infarction undergoing noncardiac operations. Anesth Analg 1990; 71:231.
14. McCulloch HA, Sprague DH: Myths in vascular anesthesia. Probl Anesthesiol 1991; 5:453–467.
15. Goldman L, Caldera DL, Nussbaum SR, et al: Multifactorial index of cardiac risks in noncardiac surgery patients. N Engl J Med 1977; 297:845.
16. Simon AB: Perioperative management of the pacemaker patient. Anesthesiology 1977; 46:127.
17. Domino KB, Smith TC: Electrocautery-induced reprogramming of a pacemaker using a precordial magnet. Anesth Analg 1983; 62:609.
18. Shapiro WA, Roizen MF, Singleton MA, et al: Intraoperative pacemaker complications. Anesthesiology 1985; 63:319.
19. Atlee JL: Pacemakers and cardioversion. *In* Cardiac Anesthesia. 2nd ed. Kaplan JA (ed). Philadelphia, WB Saunders, 1987, pp 855–879.
20. Bloomfield P, Bowler GMR: Anaesthetic management of the patient with a permanent pacemaker. Anaesthesia 1989; 44:42.
21. Cohen MM, Cameron CB: Should you cancel the operation when the child has an upper respiratory infection? Anesth Analg 1991; 72:282.
22. DeSoto H, Patel RI, Soliman IE, et al: Changes in oxygen saturation following general anesthesia in children with upper respiratory infection signs and symptoms undergoing otolaryngological procedures. Anesthesiology 1988; 68:276.
23. Corrao WM, Braman SS, Irwin RS: Chronic cough as the sole presenting manifestation of bronchial asthma. N Engl J Med 1979; 300:633.
24. Irwin RS, Corrao WM, Pratter MR: Chronic persistent cough in the adult: the spectrum and frequency of causes and successful outcome of specific therapy. Am Rev Respir Dis 1981; 123:413.
25. Olsson GL, Hallen B, Hambraeus-Jonzon K: Aspiration during anaesthesia: a computer-aided study of 185,358 anesthetics. Acta Anaesthesiol Scand 1986; 30:84.
26. Knieriem K, Stehling L: Aspiration pneumonitis. Semin Anesth 1990; 9:54.
27. Cohen S, Harris LD: Does hiatus hernia affect competence of the gastroesophageal sphincter? N Engl J Med 1971; 284:1053.
28. Schlaghecke R, Kornely E, Santen RT, et al: The effect of long-term glucocorticoid therapy on pituitary-adrenal responses to exogenous corticotropin-releasing hormone. N Engl J Med 1992; 326:226.
29. Weinberg AD, Brennan MD, Gorman CA, et al: Outcome of anesthesia and surgery in hypothyroid patients. Arch Intern Med 1983; 143:893.
30. Litt L, Roizen MF: Anesthetic and surgical risk in hypothyroidism. Arch Intern Med 1984; 144:657.
31. Schonwald G, Fish KJ, Perkash I: Cardiovascular complications during anesthesia in chronic spinal cord injured patients. Anesthesiology 1981; 55:550.
32. Gronert GA, Theye RA: Pathophysiology of hyperkalemia induced by succinylcholine. Anesthesiology 1975; 43:89.
33. Keenan MA, Stiles CM, Kaufman RL: Acquired laryngeal deviation associated with cervical spine disease in erosive polyarticular arthritis. Anesthesiology 1983; 58:441.
34. Vassalo SA, Martyn JAJ: Pathophysiology and anesthetic management of burn injury. Semin Anesth 1989; 8:275.
35. Rapaport SI: Preoperative hemostatic evaluation: which tests, if any? Blood 1983; 61:229.
36. The National Blood Resource Education Program Expert Panel: The use of autologous blood. JAMA 1990; 263:414.
37. Owings DV, Kruskall MS, Thurer RL, et al: Autologous blood donations prior to elective cardiac surgery: safety and efficacy of subsequent blood use. JAMA 1989; 262:1963.
38. Goodnough LT, Rudnick S, Price TH, et al: Increased preoperative collection of autologous blood with recombinant human erythropoietin therapy. N Engl J Med 1989; 321:1163.

39. Kaplan JA, Dunbar RW, Bland JW Jr, et al: Propranolol and cardiac surgery: a problem for the anesthesiologist? Anesth Analg 1975; 54:571.

40. Goldman L: Noncardiac surgery in patients receiving propranolol: case reports and a recommended approach. Arch Intern Med 1981; 141:193.

41. Siegel D, Hulley SB, Black DM, et al: Diuretics, serum and intracellular electrolyte levels, and ventricular arrhythmias in men. JAMA 1992; 267:1083.

42. Vitez TS, Soper LE, Wong KC, et al: Chronic hypokalemia and intraoperative dysrhythmias. Anesthesiology 1985; 63:127.

43. Hirsch IA, Tomlinson DL, Slogoff S, et al: The overstated risk of preoperative hypokalemia. Anesthesiology 1988; 67:131.

44. McGovern B: Hypokalemia and cardiac arrhythmias. Anesthesiology 1985; 63:127.

45. Lewis RP: Digitalis: a drug that refuses to die. Crit Care Med 1990; 18:S5–S13.

46. Kulick DL, Rahimtoola SH: Current role of digitalis therapy in patients with congestive heart failure. JAMA 1991; 265:2995.

47. Falk RH, Knowlton AA, Bernard SA, et al: Digoxin for converting recent-onset atrial fibrillation to sinus rhythm: a randomized, double-blinded trial. Ann Intern Med 1987; 106:503.

48. Falk RH, Leavitt JI: Digoxin for atrial fibrillation: a drug whose time has gone? Ann Intern Med 1991; 114:573.

49. Kates RA: Antianginal drug therapy. *In* Cardiac Anesthesia. 2nd ed. Kaplan JA (ed). Philadelphia, WB Saunders, 1987, pp 451–518.

50. Mungall DR, Robichaux RP, Perry W, et al: Efficacy of quinidine on serum digoxin concentration: a prospective study. Ann Intern Med 1980; 93:689.

51. Stoelting RK: Pharmacology and physiology in anesthetic practice. Philadelphia, JB Lippincott, 1987, pp 322–334.

52. Kennedy JI, Myers JL, Plumb VJ, et al: Amiodarone pulmonary toxicity: clinical, radiologic, and pathologic correlations. Arch Intern Med 1987; 147:50.

53. Steinhaus JE, Howland DE: Intravenously administered lidocaine as a supplement to nitrous oxide–thiobarbiturate anesthesia. Anesth Analg 1958; 37:40.

54. Rossing TH: Methylxanthines in 1989. Ann Intern Med 1989; 110:502.

55. Lam A, Newhouse MT: Management of asthma and chronic airflow limitation: are methylxanthines obsolete? Chest 1990; 98:44.

56. Roizen MF, Stevens WC: Multiform ventricular tachycardia due to interaction of aminophylline and halothane. Anesth Analg 1978; 57:738.

57. Pantuck EJ, Pantuck CB, Weissman C, et al: Effects of parenteral nutritional regimens on oxidative drug metabolism. Anesthesiology 1984; 60:534.

58. Roizen MF: Anesthetic implications of concurrent disease. *In* Anesthesia. 3rd ed. Miller RD (ed). New York, Churchill Livingstone, 1990, pp 798–799.

59. Palumbo PJ: Blood glucose control during surgery. Anesthesiology 1981; 55:94.

60. Roizen MF: Is tight perioperative control of diabetes warranted? Anesthesiology 1982; 56:242.

61. Stoelting RK: Pharmacology and physiology in anesthetic practice. Philadelphia, JB Lippincott, 1987, pp 415–422.

62. Chin R: Corticosteroids. *In* The Pharmacologic Approach to the Critically Ill Patient. 2nd ed. Chernow B (ed). Baltimore, Williams & Wilkins, 1988, pp 559–583.

63. Temkin NR, Dikmen SS, Wilensky AJ, et al: A randomized, double-blind study of phenytoin for the prevention of post-traumatic seizures. N Engl J Med 1990; 323:497.

64. Wong KC: Preoperative discontinuation of monoamine oxidase inhibitor therapy: an old wives' tale? Semin Anesth 1986; 5:145.

65. Bready LL, Solomon DE: Preparation for surgery. Probl Anesth 5:386–400.

66. Edwards RE, Miller RD, Roizen MF, et al: Cardiac effects of imipramine and pancuronium during halothane anesthesia and enflurane anesthesia. Anesthesiology 1979; 50:421.

67. Macdonald R: Aspirin and extradural blocks. Br J Anaesth 1991; 66:1.

68. Cronberg S, Wallmark E, Soderberg I: Effect on platelet aggregation of oral administration of 10 non-steroidal analgesics to humans. Scand J Haematol 1984; 33:155.

69. Dahl JB, Kehlet H: Non-steroidal anti-inflammatory drugs: rationale for use in severe postoperative pain. Br J Anaesth 1991; 66:703.

70. Horlocker TT, Wedel DJ, Offord KP: Does preoperative antiplatelet therapy increase the risk of hemorrhagic complications associated with regional anesthesia? Anesth Analg 1990; 70:631.

71. O'Reilly RA: Anticoagulant, antithrombotic, and thrombolytic drugs. *In* Goodman and Gilman's The Pharmacologic Basis of Therapeutics. 7th ed. Gilman AG, Goodman LS, Rall TW, Murid F (eds). New York, MacMillan Publishing Co, 1985, pp 1338–1359.

72. Calabresi P, Parks RE Jr: Antiproliferative agents and drugs used for immunosuppression. *In* Goodman and Gilman's The Pharmacological Basis of Therapeutics. 7th ed. Gilman AG, Goodman LS, Rall TW, Murid F (eds). New York, MacMillan Publishing Co, 1985, pp 1247–1306.

73. Waid-Jones MI, Coursin DB: Perioperative considerations for patients treated with bleomycin. Chest 1991; 99:992.

74. Ingrassia TS 3d, Ryu JH, Trastek VF, Rosenow EC 3d: Oxygen-exacerbated bleomycin pulmonary toxicity. Mayo Clin Proc 1991; 66:173.

75. Cavallaro RJ, Krumperman LW, Kugler F: Effect of echothiophate therapy on the metabolism of succinylcholine in man. Anesth Analg 1968; 47:570.

76. Leier CV, Baker D, Weber PA: Cardiovascular effects of timolol. Ann Intern Med 1986; 104:197.

77. Miller RD, Savarese JJ: Pharmacology of muscle relaxants and their antagonists. *In* Anesthesia. 3rd ed. Miller RD (ed). New York, Churchill Livingstone, 1990, pp 389–435.

78. Lasser EC, Berry CC, Talner LB, et al: Pretreatment with corticosteroids to alleviate reactions to intravenous contrast material. N Engl J Med 1987; 317:845.

79. Levy JH: Anaphylactic Reactions in Anesthesia and Intensive Care. 2nd ed. Boston, Butterworths-Heinemann, 1992.

80. Warner MA, Offord KP, Warner ME, et al: Role of preoperative cessation of smoking and other factors in postoperative pulmonary complications: a blinded prospective study of coronary artery bypass patients. Mayo Clin Proc 1989; 64:609.

81. Pierce AC, Jones RM: Smoking and anesthesia: preoperative abstinence and perioperative mortality. Anesthesiology 1984; 61:576.

82. Murad F, Haynes RC Jr: Androgens. *In* Goodman and Gilman's The Pharmacological Basis of Therapeutics. New York, Macmillan Publishing Co, 1985, pp 1440–1458.

83. Brown BB: Anesthesia in Hepatic and Biliary Tract Disease. Philadelphia, FA Davis, 1988.

84. Frank SM, Norris EJ, Christopherson R, et al: Right- and left-arm discrepancies in vascular surgery patients. Anesthesiology 1991; 75:457.

85. Stone DJ, Gal TJ: Airway management. *In* Anesthesia. 3rd ed. Miller RD (ed). New York, Churchill Livingstone, 1990, pp 1265–1292.

86. Mallampati SR, Gugino LD, Desai SP, et al: A clinical sign to predict difficult tracheal intubation: a prospective study. Can Anaesth Soc J 1985; 32:429.

87. Heyman A, Wilkinson WE, Heyden S, et al: Risk of stroke in asymptomatic persons with carotid arterial bruits: a population study in Evans County, Georgia. N Engl J Med 1980; 302:838.

88. Ropper AH, Wechsler LR, Wilson LS: Carotid bruit and the risk of stroke in elective surgery. N Engl J Med 1982; 307:1388.

89. Urmey WF, Talts KH, Sharrock NE: One hundred percent incidence of hemidiaphragmatic paresis associated with interscalene brachial plexus block anesthesia as diagnosed by ultrasonography. Anesth Analg 1991; 72:498.

90. Rothman A, Goldberger AL: Aids to cardiac auscultation. Ann Intern Med 1983; 99:346.

91. Seneff M: Arterial line placement and care. *In* Intensive Care Medicine. 2nd ed. Rippe JM, Irwin RS, Alpert JS, et al (eds). Boston, Little, Brown & Co, 1991, pp 37–47.

92. Slogoff S, Keats AS, Arlund C: On the safety of radial artery cannulation. Anesthesiology 1983; 59:42.

93. Kroll DA, Caplan RA, Posner K, et al: Nerve injury associated with anesthesia. Anesthesiology 1990; 73:202.

94. Pauker SG, Kopelman RI: Trapped by an incidental finding. New Engl J Med 1992; 326:40.

95. Cebul RD, Beck JR: Biochemical profiles: applications in ambulatory screening and preadmission testing of adults. Ann Intern Med 1987; 106:403.

96. Narr BJ, Hansen TR, Warner MA: Preoperative laboratory screening in healthy Mayo patients: cost-effective elimination of test and unchanged outcomes. Mayo Clin Proc 1991; 66:155.

97. Goldberger AL, O'Konski M: Utility of the routine electrocardiogram before surgery and on general hospital admission: a critical review and new guidelines. Ann Intern Med 1986; 105:552.

98. Turnbull JM, Buck C: The value of preoperative screening investigations in otherwise healthy individuals. Arch Intern Med 1987; 147:1101.

99. Macpherson DS, Snow R, Lofgren RP: Preoperative screening: value of previous tests. Ann Intern Med 1990; 113:969.

100. Blery C, Charpak Y, Szatan M, et al: Evaluation of a protocol for selective ordering of preoperative tests. Lancet 1986; 1:139.

101. Mangano DT: Perioperative cardiac morbidity. Anesthesiology 1990; 72:153.
102. Goldman L: Cardiac risks and complications of noncardiac surgery. Ann Intern Med 1983; 98:504.
103. Freeman WK, Gibbons RJ, Shub C: Preoperative assessment of cardiac patients undergoing noncardiac surgical procedures. Mayo Clin Proc 1989; 64:1105.
104. Detsky AS, Abrams HB, Forbath N, et al: Cardiac assessment for patients undergoing noncardiac surgery: a multifactorial clinical risk index. Arch Intern Med 1986; 146:2131.
105. Eckman MH, McNutt RA, Parkinson DR, et al: The timing of radical cystectomy after recent myocardial infarction: waiting for Godot. Med Decis Making 1987; 7:52.
106. Boucher CA, Brewster DC, Darling RC, et al: Determination of cardiac risk by dipyridamole-thallium imaging before peripheral vascular surgery. N Engl J Med 1985; 312:389.
107. Leppo J, Plaja J, Gionet M, et al: Noninvasive evaluation of cardiac risk before elective vascular surgery. J Am Coll Cardiol 1987; 9:269.
108. Eagle KA, Singer DE, Brewster DC, et al: Dipyridamole-thallium scanning in patients undergoing vascular surgery: optimizing preoperative evaluation of cardiac risk. JAMA 1987; 257:2185.
109. Eagle KA, Coley CM, Newell JB, et al: Combining clinical and thallium data optimizes preoperative assessment of cardiac risk before major vascular surgery. Ann Intern Med 1989; 110:859.
110. Raby KE, Goldman L, Creager MA, et al: Correlation between preoperative ischemia and major cardiac events after peripheral vascular surgery. N Engl J Med 1989; 321:1296.
111. American College of Physicians: Preoperative pulmonary function testing. Ann Intern Med 1990; 112:793.
112. Gass GD, Olsen GN: Preoperative pulmonary function testing to predict postoperative morbidity and mortality. Chest 1986; 89:127.
113. Zibrak JD, O'Donnell CR, Marton K: Indications for pulmonary function testing. Ann Intern Med 1990; 112:763.
114. Hall JC, Tarala RA, Hall JL, et al: A multivariate analysis of the risk of pulmonary complications after laparotomy. Chest 1991; 99:923.
115. Troupin AS: The measurement of anticonvulsant agent levels. Ann Intern Med 1984; 100:854.
116. Del Guercio LRM, Cohn JD: Monitoring operative risk in the elderly. JAMA 1980; 243:1350.
117. Berlauk JF, Abrams JH, Gilmour IJ, et al: Preoperative optimization of cardiovascular hemodynamics improves outcome in peripheral vascular surgery. Ann Surg 1991; 214:289.
118. Choi JJ: An anesthesiologist's philosophy on ''medical clearance'' for surgical patients. Arch Intern Med 1987; 147:2090.
119. Berger JJ: The patient for outpatient surgery. Part I: Preoperative evaluation. Probl Anesth 1991; 5:613–626.
120. Ross AF, Tinker JH: Anesthesia and risk. *In* Anesthesia. 3rd ed. Miller RD (ed). New York, Churchill Livingstone, 1990, pp 743–772.
121. Saklad M: Grading of patients for surgical procedures. Anesthesiology 1941; 2:281.
122. American Society of Anesthesiologists: New classification of physical status. Anesthesiology 1963; 24:111.
123. Christou NV: Evaluation of operative risk. *In* Care of the Surgical Patient. Perioperative Management and Techniques. Vol. 2. Sec. 5. Wilmore DW, Brennan MF, Harken AH, et al (eds). New York, Scientific American, 1988, pp 3–15.
124. Ross AF, Tinker JH: Risk and anesthesia. *In* Perioperative Management. Breslow MJ, Miller CF, Rogers MC (eds). St Louis, CV Mosby, 1990, pp 13–21.
125. Dajani AS, Bisno AL, Chung KJ, et al: Prevention of bacterial endocarditis: recommendations by the American Heart Association. JAMA 1990; 264:2919.
126. Classen DC, Evans S, Pestotnik SL, et al: The timing of prophylactic administration of antibiotics and the risk of surgical-wound infection. N Engl J Med 1992; 326:281.
127. Davies JM, Davison JS, Nimmo WS, et al: The stomach: factors of importance to the anaesthetic. Can J Anaesth 1990; 37:896.
128. Moore J, Flynn RJ, Sampaio M, et al: Effect of single-dose omeprazole on intragastric acidity and volume during obstetric anaesthesia. Anaesthesia 1989; 44:559.
129. National Institutes of Health Consensus Conference: Prevention of venous thrombosis and pulmonary embolism. JAMA 1986; 256:744.
130. Hyers TM, Hull RD, Weg JC: Antithrombotic therapy for venous thromboembolic disease. Chest 1986; 89(Suppl):26S–35S.
131. Anderson FA, Wheeler HB, Goldberg RJ, et al: Physician practices in the prevention of venous thromboembolism. Ann Intern Med 1991; 115:591.
132. Minani H, McCallum RW: The physiology and pathophysiology of gastric emptying in humans. Gastroenterology 1984; 86:1592.
133. Crawford M, Lerman J, Christensen S, et al: Effects of duration of fasting on gastric fluid pH and volume in healthy children. Anesth Analg 1990; 71:400.
134. Shevde K, Trivedi N: Effects of clear liquids on gastric volume and pH in healthy volunteers. Anesth Analg 1991; 72:528.
135. Hutchinson A, Maltby JR, Reid CRG: Gastric fluid volume and pH in elective inpatients. Part I: coffee or orange juice versus overnight fast. Can J Anaesth 1988; 35:12.
136. Scarr M, Maltby JR, Jani K, et al: Volume and acidity of residual gastric fluid after oral fluid ingestion before elective ambulatory surgery. Can Med Assoc J 1989; 141:1151.
137. Goresky GV, Maltby JR: Fasting guidelines for elective surgical patients. Can J Anaesth 1990; 37:493.
138. Truog RD: ''Do-not-resuscitate'' orders during anesthesia and surgery. Anesthesiology 1991; 74:606.
139. Cohen CB, Cohen PJ: Do-not-resuscitate orders in the operating room. N Engl J Med 1991; 325:1879.
140. Couper C: DNR in the OR (Letter). JAMA 1992; 267:1465 .
141. Franklin C, Rothenberg DM: DNR in the OR (Letter). JAMA 1992; 267:1465.

CHAPTER 2

The Anesthetic Record

JEFFREY M. FELDMAN, M.D., M.S.E.

The year is 1894, and E. A. Codman, a surgical house officer at the Massachusetts General Hospital, is about to create the first anesthesia record.[1] Listen, if you will, to the quiet of the surgical suite. The anesthetist drops ether while the surgeon busies himself with the surgical procedure at hand, the silence broken only by the occasional clang of a metal instrument and some quiet conversation. Picture Codman, with pen in hand, scribbling heart and respiratory rates every 5 minutes (Fig. 2–1).

Today, most anesthesiologists are still scribbling heart and respiratory rates as part of the anesthesia record, although the rhythm of the operating room is anything but quiet, with monitors beeping, lights blinking, pagers buzzing, phones ringing, and a host of operating room sounds in the background. Even though the amount of information documented in the record has certainly increased, what has changed most dramatically is the significance of the anesthesia record for those who provide anesthesia. Little did Codman know that what began as an academic exercise would become a fundamental—and controversial—part of anesthesia practice.

One of the first skills taught to new trainees in anesthesia is how to create an anesthetic record. New trainees learn that preparation of a quality anesthesia record requires careful attention to detail. The record should be legible, complete, and accurate. Once an appreciation is gained of the many functions of the record, the diligent clinician endeavors to create a useful document.

Underlying the meticulous creation of the record is concern about liability exposure. Given the rather aggressive medicolegal climate in the United States, such concern is reasonable and appropriate. No doubt the ultimate form of the record is influenced by the manner in which each individual who has contributed to its preparation reacts to liability potential. Some anesthesiologists feel that the most detailed, high-quality record possible is the best defense. Others may not include details of every physiologic change, arguing that fluctuations in vital signs typical during anesthesia may be misinterpreted as potentially harmful by a lay reviewer.

These emotions and concerns about the record have led to a great deal of controversy regarding how the anesthesia record

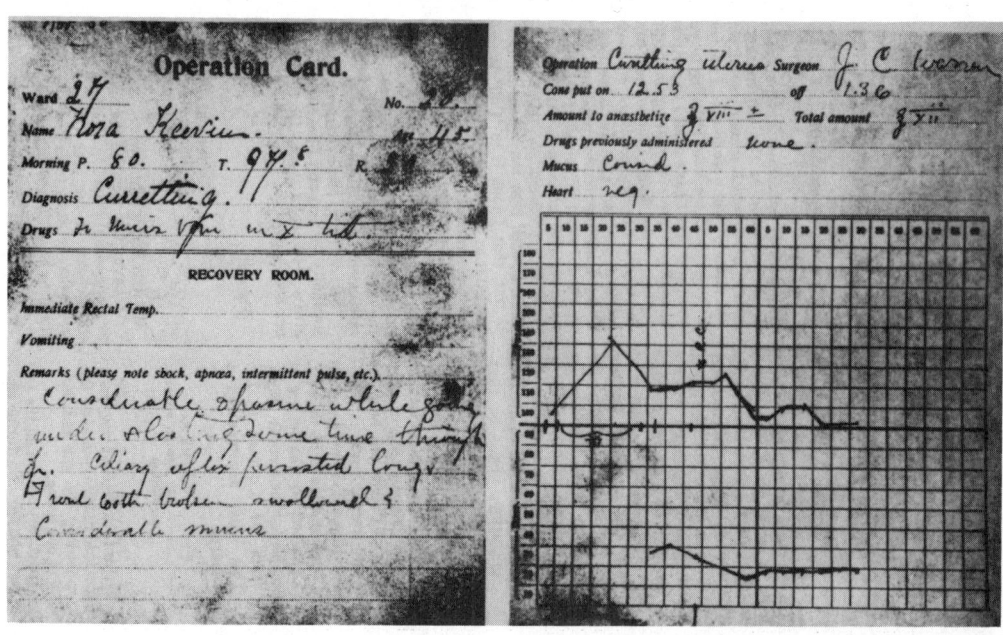

FIGURE 2–1. An early anesthesia record created by EA Codman. (From Beecher HK: The first anesthesia records. Surg Gynecol Obstet 1940; 71:689–693. By permission of Surgery, Gynecology, & Obstetrics.)

TABLE 2–1. Individual Users of the Record

Patient Care Delivery (Providers)	Patient Care Management and Support
Chaplains	Administrators
Dental hygienists	Financial managers and accountants
Dentists	Quality assurance managers
Laboratory technologists	Records professionals
Nurses	Risk managers
Occupational therapists	Unit clerks
Optometrists	Utilization review managers
Pharmacists	
Physical therapists	**Patient Care Reimbursement**
Physicians	Benefit managers
Physician assistants	Insurers (federal, state, and private)
Podiatrists	
Psychologists	**Other**
Radiology technologists	
Respiratory therapists	Accreditors
Social workers	Government policymakers and legislators
Patient Care Delivery (Consumers)	Lawyers
	Health care researchers and clinical investigators
Patients	
Families	Health sciences journalists and editors

(Reprinted with permission from The Computer-Based Patient Record: An Essential Technology for Health Care. Copyright 1991 by the National Academy of Sciences. Courtesy of the National Academy Press, Washington, DC.)

TABLE 2–2. Primary Uses of Patient Records

Patient Care Delivery (Patient)	Patient Care Management
Document services received	Document case mix in institutions and practice
Constitute proof of identity	Analyze severity of illness
Self-manage care	Formulate practice guidelines
Verify billing	Manage risk
Patient Care Delivery (Provider)	Characterize the use of services
	Provide the basis for utilization review
Foster continuity of care (i.e., serve as a communication tool)	Perform quality assurance
Describe diseases and causes (i.e., support diagnostic work)	**Patient Care Support**
Support decision-making about diagnosis and treatment of patients	Allocate resources
Assess and manage risk for individual patients	Analyze trends and develop forecasts
Facilitate care in accordance with clinical practice guidelines	Assess workload
Document patient risk factors	Communicate between departments
Assess and document patient expectations and patient satisfaction	**Billing and Reimbursement**
Generate care plans	Document services for payments
Determine preventive advice or health maintenance information	Bill for services
Remind clinicians (e.g., screens, age-related reminders)	Submit insurance claims
Support nursing care	Adjudicate insurance claims
Document services provided (e.g., drugs, therapies)	Determine disabilities (e.g., workmen's compensation)
	Manage costs
	Report costs
	Perform actuarial analysis

(Reprinted with permission from The Computer-Based Patient Record: An Essential Technology for Health Care. Copyright 1991 by the National Academy of Sciences. Courtesy of the National Academy Press, Washington, DC.)

should be kept. The demands on the clinician in the operating room have made quality handwritten recordkeeping increasingly difficult. Emerging technology to perform automated recordkeeping offers the potential to improve the recordkeeping process but has met with a very mixed response.

The intent of this chapter is to explore the issues important to quality recordkeeping and the suitability of both handwritten and automated anesthesia records to that task.

PURPOSES OF THE RECORD

The purpose of the first anesthesia record is subject to debate.[1] *Cushing has written that a wager between Codman and himself concerning who was the best "etherizer" was the motivation for the first anesthesia records. Codman, noting Cushing's flair for the dramatic, explained that F. B. Harrington, Codman's chief when he was a house officer, suggested that anesthesia records be kept to document the anesthetic course. However, it is certain that there were probably very few individuals other than Dr. Codman and his colleagues who took an interest in their content.*

Current handwritten records are subjected to much more intense scrutiny. Not only is the primary care provider interested in the content of the record, but other physicians and nurses, the anesthesiologists who will care for the patient in the future, administrators, accountants, peer review organizations, researchers, and attorneys also will require access to it[2] (Table 2–1). Although the modern anesthesia record serves many masters and contains more information than did the first record, the basic approach to recordkeeping has changed very little.

How Is It Used?

A recent study of the computer-based patient record conducted by the Institute of Medicine of the National Academy

of Sciences highlights its many different uses. Four categories of use were identified: direct patient care, administration and management, reimbursement, and research (Table 2–2). These uses are considered primary if they are associated with the provision of patient care (i.e., with the provision, management, or reimbursement of care services) and secondary if they do not influence the encounter between provider and patient directly but rather the environment in which care is provided.[3] To emphasize issues important to anesthesia practice, the following uses of the anesthesia record are considered: patient care, administration (including reimbursement), research and education, and medicolegal purposes.

Patient Care

As an instrument for patient care, the anesthesia record serves both intraoperative and postoperative functions. For the intraoperative anesthesia care provider, the anesthesia record functions as both a log book and a clinical management tool.[4]

Log Book

The clinician uses the anesthesia record as a log book to record information about the patient that should be readily available. For example, preoperative data, patient medications, patient weight, allergies, and perhaps a succinct list of medical problems are included. This information is typically transcribed from the medical record into the record or preoperative evaluation note, since otherwise it may not be easily found when needed. It provides a useful summary for other anesthetists that become involved with the patient.

Documentation of the anesthetic care is the most obvious

role of the record as a log book. This documentation should include operating room location, time of the operation, identification numbers for the anesthesia machine, notes on airway management and other procedures, a list of the drugs administered, and a record of vital signs. All practicing clinicians are familiar with this aspect of the record and with the difficulty of maintaining a quality record when occupied with patient care.

Clinical Management Tool. As the record evolves, a trend plot is created that may indicate a change that is not apparent from observing individual values on the monitor. When multiple parameters are plotted together, the relationship between these parameters (e.g., heart rate and blood pressure) can indicate subtle but important physiologic changes (e.g., progressive hypovolemia). The relationship between drug doses and physiologic response demonstrates the dose-response relationship for the individual patient. For the clinician who assumes responsibility for anesthesia care from another individual, the carefully constructed record can be invaluable for developing and continuing an appropriate anesthetic plan.

Postoperative users include the physicians and nurses who care for the patient in the postanesthesia care unit, on the postoperative surgical ward, or in the intensive care unit. These physicians and nurses consult the anesthesia record for information such as intraoperative blood loss, fluids and drugs administered, and overall physiologic stability. The other postoperative beneficiaries of a quality record are the anesthesiologists and anesthetists who consult the record when preparing to administer a subsequent anesthetic to the same patient.

Administration

Whereas the primary purpose of the record traditionally has been to facilitate the management of patient care, its administrative uses are becoming fundamental to the delivery of health care. Since anesthesiology is a hospital-based practice, two aspects of the administrative use of the record are identifiable:

1. The anesthesiologist or anesthesiologists responsible for the administration of the department must make decisions about such aspects as the quality of care, patient outcome, implications of practice patterns, and the utilization of manpower. The information in the anesthesia record constitutes the documentation necessary for making and supporting these decisions.
2. Hospital administrators also rely on the information in the anesthesia record to make decisions regarding utilization of hospital facilities and allocation of personnel, equipment, and supplies.

    Reimbursement for anesthesia services has become an increasingly complex undertaking given the number of third-party payers and the regulations applied to reimbursement for anesthesia services. The anesthesia record is the document that confirms the billing information and, conversely, provides the data on which the bill is based. Auditors seek to confirm entries on the anesthesia record by comparing them with information in other documentation, such as nurse's notes and the surgeon's dictation. All documents must be in agreement if questions about billing practices are to be avoided.

    Quality assurance and peer review auditors examine the anesthesia record to fulfill their responsibilities. Accreditation agencies insist upon ongoing quality assurance pro-

grams and carefully audit records for this information. As managed care becomes more prevalent, quality assurance activities will utilize the anesthetic record as a means to compare the services rendered by different providers.

Research and Education

Educational activities are served whenever a record is reviewed with the goal of improving care. Conferences that focus on discussion of a difficult case utilize the record as the primary documentation of events. Research activities are also facilitated by an accurate record. Despite the limitations of retrospective chart review, a careful review of records can help to identify undesirable practice patterns.

Medicolegal Purposes

As any practicing anesthesiologist knows, the importance of the anesthesia record as a medicolegal document cannot be understated. During anesthesia-related legal proceedings, the anesthesia record undergoes intense scrutiny. Verbal testimony regarding the quality of care has little credibility if the anesthesia record does not corroborate the testimony. The attorney for a plaintiff often asserts that if "it isn't charted, it didn't happen."

Since most clinicians are consumed with patient care activities during anesthetic induction, emergence, and emergencies, little information is recorded on the anesthesia record during these time periods. However, it is during these periods when physiologic changes are typically most dramatic and the greatest potential for serious problems exists.[5]

What Constitutes a Meaningful Record?

The anesthesia record serves many users, but the responsibility for creating the record lies only with the anesthesiologist. How can the individual clinician develop a record that serves the purposes of all its potential users? What information should be included? How should the information be organized and presented?

A meaningful record should be a complete rendition of events that anyone can review to understand what has transpired. Furthermore, sufficient detail should be included to identify the cause or causes of intraoperative and postoperative events. This description of the meaningful record is easier to state than it is to achieve in practice. The clinician may not always appreciate the wide range of information of interest to all potential users of the record. The most diligent clinician may simply not have enough time (or space) while caring for the patient during surgery to include all the pertinent data. Finally, the record may not present information in a manner conducive to interpretation. Both the information content and the manner in which the information are presented are important aspects of a meaningful record.

What Information Should the Record Contain?

The American Society of Anesthesiologists (ASA) has developed a sample anesthetic record as a model for clinicians (Fig. 2–2). This record exemplifies both the range of informa-

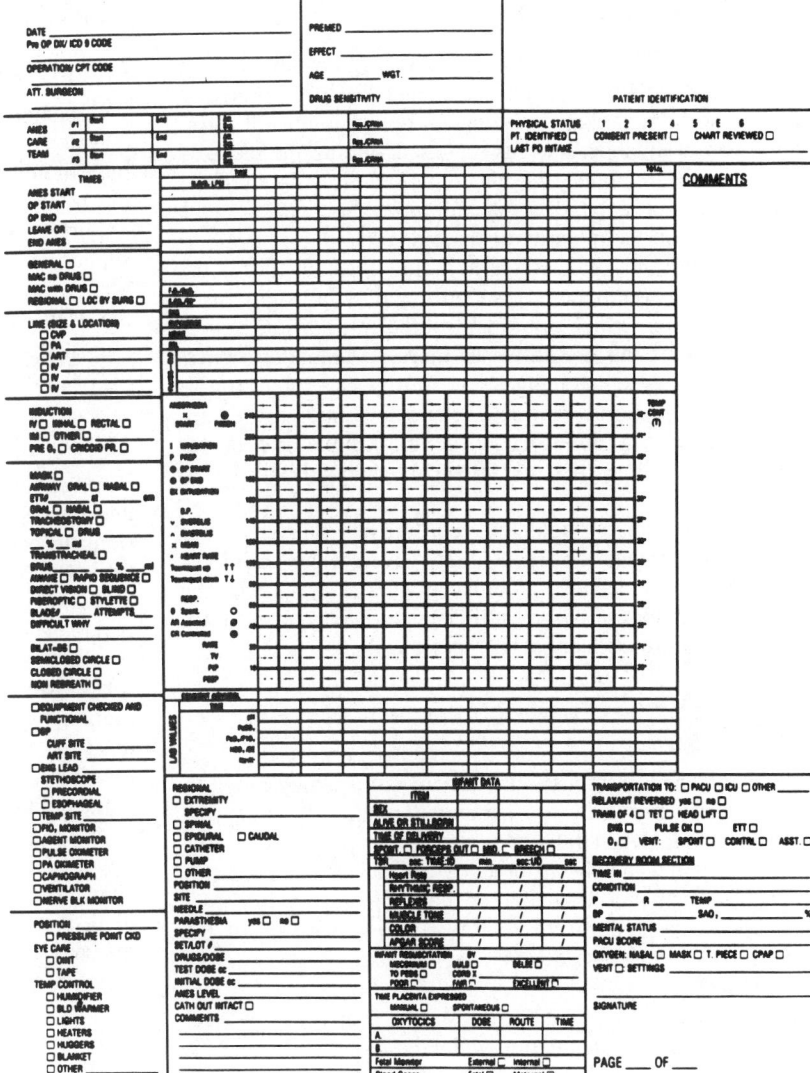

FIGURE 2–2. Sample anesthetic record proposed by the American Society of Anesthesiologists. (From American Society of Anesthesiologists, Park Ridge, IL.)

tion that should be included as well as the difficulty in portraying this information in a usable format. One glance at this record and one is immediately struck by the density of the print. The appearance is due to the need to represent an extensive amount of information on an 8½ × 11-inch piece of paper. The limitations of this format notwithstanding, if this record is completed faithfully, much useful information will be recorded.

Equipment Checks and Airway Management

The ASA record incorporates details that are applicable to every anesthetic procedure: confirmation that equipment is checked, details of the monitors used, a record of the catheters inserted, airway management notes, and emergence (postanesthesia care unit) transfer notes. Of these details, confirmation that equipment is checked should be indicated clearly to avoid citation by accreditation auditors. Notes on management of the airway should be explicit and legible, especially when airway management is not straightforward. No patient should be resubjected to the risks of an airway problem simply because the previous occurrence was poorly documented.

Investigation of Postoperative Problems

Information that will facilitate investigation of postoperative problems is difficult to define prospectively, since the wide range of potential problems is not always anticipated. One area—the documentation of lot numbers for the drugs and materials used—stands out as an example of a detail that might serve that purpose. Ideally, all lot numbers should be recorded; however, as indicated on the ASA record, the lot number is usually recorded only for regional anesthesia sets.

Limited Applicability Data

Much information indicated in the ASA record is not applicable to the majority of anesthetic procedures. Large spaces are dedicated to obstetric and regional anesthesia notes, even though these are used in the minority of anesthetic procedures. The obstetric anesthesia note space accommodates triplet delivery, which occurs rarely even with the increasing application of in vitro fertilization. Space for blood gas analysis results, central venous pressure, and pulmonary artery occlusion pressure measurements is also unlikely to be used in the majority of anesthetic procedures.

Limitations of Inclusiveness

Although a valiant effort is made to be inclusive in the ASA record, the detail that can be documented is incorporated at the expense of vital sign recording. Only 90 minutes of information can be included on this record, assuming the use of a 5-minute recording interval. This limitation results in multiple-page records for a large number of procedures, with much wasted space on the majority of these records.

More important than concerns about wasted space, the ASA format perpetuates the recording of vital signs at 5-minute intervals, which, although rooted in tradition, serves the purposes of the recordkeeper more so than the record. Important physiologic changes are in no way related to a 5-minute interval. Some require intervention much more rapidly than every 5 minutes. Therefore, a 5-minute interval for vital sign recording does not reflect true physiologic variation.

When the patient is stable, the recording of vital signs every 5 minutes is perhaps too frequent. However, when an important event occurs, accurate recordkeeping is essential; yet, the current format does not allow sufficient resolution or space for a very meaningful reflection of what transpired.

Billing Data

As mentioned previously, the record is inspected by auditors to verify that bills are generated accurately. Accurate billing practice is a vital function, since it provides for the viability of the anesthesia practice and can ensure against accusations of fraud. Inclusion of the preoperative diagnosis and surgical procedure are central to the generation of the patient's bill, but these details are only part of the required information.

Efforts to reduce health care costs for anesthesia services have focused on documentation of the duration of care and the manner in which care is supervised. The ASA record incorporates an important feature to document the individuals involved with providing anesthesia care and the time during which the care was provided. For complete accuracy, even temporary relief should be recorded in this fashion. The total anesthesia time is also documented (along with surgical times) to confirm the ongoing anesthesia care prior to and following the surgical procedure.

Penalties for Inaccuracy

The consequences of record inaccuracies that lead to conviction of fraudulent Medicare billing practices can be significant economic and professional penalties. The civil monetary penalties law (CMPL 42 U.S.C. §1320a-7a) authorizes the Secretary of Health and Human Services to penalize any health care provider who presents a claim that is ''for a medical service that the person knows, or should have known, was not provided as claimed.'' The penalties include a $2000 fine for each such item, assessment for up to twice the amount claimed, and exclusion from Medicare and Medicaid programs. Legal precedent exists to consider ''unartful'' description on the record of services rendered to be a description of services that were not provided as claimed.[6] Accurate description on the anesthetic record of billable services is therefore essential.

How Should the Information Be Presented?

Interpretation

Although a great deal of thought has been applied to the question of what information to include in the record, very little thought has been directed to its presentation. Legibility is the basic requirement of a well-presented record, but, more important, information should be presented in a manner that supports interpretation. Current anesthesia records do little to present information in a manner conducive to interpretation by the users. The sample ASA record is so crowded with space allocated for infrequently used information that important details are not emphasized.

Trend Plotting

The clinician can use the current record as a trend plotter, and it serves this function well in many instances. The relationship between heart rate, blood pressure, and the administration of drugs is relatively well shown if the record is legible and complete. However, if one wants to examine the various parameters that impact on respiratory function, the current record format does not allow the ready identification of the relationships among pertinent history, hemoglobin oxygen saturation (SpO_2), fresh gas flow, ventilator settings, blood gas analysis, end-tidal carbon dioxide, surgical position, fluids administered, and so on. To assess these parameters, one must extract the data from the record and attempt to relate the values in a meaningful fashion. Presenting the data appropriately might identify the change in tidal volume that accompanies a change in fresh gas flow, or the alveolar-arterial oxygen gradient that is inappropriately large for the current fraction of inspired oxygen. Such a presentation of information may draw attention to a problem rather than allow a diagnosis only after the problem occurs.

Auditing

The presentation of information on the record can also be tailored to the needs of many different users. The Medicare auditor who must shuffle through a large number of barely legible, poorly organized records is more likely to find fault simply owing to an inability to locate appropriate information. If the important information is clearly displayed for that individual, it becomes more difficult to find fault where none exists.

The ASA-proposed record is one example of the type of information and detail necessary to develop a meaningful record. However, the conventional format has important limitations, especially with regard to the manner in which information is presented. As the number of the record's users and uses increases, their needs cannot be ignored. We must divorce ourselves from conventional notions about the anesthesia record and consider new methods of recordkeeping that better serve the needs of anesthesiologists and others who use it. Not only the form and content of the record must be examined, but also the ability of the handwritten record to satisfy recordkeeping needs now and in the future.

CREATING THE RECORD

The foregoing discussion created a perspective on the essential elements of a quality anesthetic record. Whereas the record traditionally has been created by hand, technology for creating it automatically is proliferating. Given the importance of the record, the means by which it is created merits close inspection. Clearly, the handwritten record may not be an adequate document. Unfortunately, *automated anesthesia recordkeepers* (AARKs) may not be the indispensable tools their proponents would have us believe.

What Are the Handwritten Record's Strengths?

The handwritten anesthesia record has many strengths. It is portable, can be used at the bedside, and is easily integrated into the crowded anesthesia workspace. All clinicians possess the skills to create a record. "Soft" data, such as the subjective descriptions of managing an airway or performing a procedure, are easily recorded.[7] These are obvious strengths and the primary reasons why the use of the handwritten anesthesia record has become so entrenched in clinical practice.

However, the handwritten record must satisfy other requirements in which its strengths are not as obvious. The clinician must have the time available to create the record. The record must also be accurate, complete, and legible. The process of recordkeeping must not interfere with patient care.

The literature contains numerous studies that compare handwritten recordkeeping to AARKs. A critical review of these studies highlights the strengths and limitations of each method of recordkeeping.

How Much Time Is Spent Recordkeeping?

Time demands in the operating room are significant. The clinician not only must manage the patient and facilitate the surgical procedure but also must communicate with the laboratory, manage infusion pumps, insert monitoring devices, and troubleshoot equipment. Therefore, the time required to maintain the record has increased significantly and often exceeds the time available for contemporaneous handwritten entry.

AARK Versus Handwritten Recordkeeping

The time spent in recordkeeping during coronary artery bypass[8] and general surgical procedures[9] has been studied by means of videotape examination of these procedures. Meijler compared the studies by equating the tasks studied and by plotting the results on the same graph[10] (Fig. 2–3). The task of logging data on the chart consumed 6% of the anesthesiologists' time during general surgery and 12% of their time during coronary artery bypass surgery.

Proponents of automated recordkeeping contend that with its application the anesthetist could spend less time keeping a record and, therefore, have additional time to better manage the anesthetic procedure. For this contention to be true, less time should be required to keep a record using an AARK than is needed for handwritten recordkeeping. Since an AARK records monitored data automatically, the user should be spared the time usually required to transcribe data from the monitors. However, time savings may be offset by the increased time spent entering notations into the AARK. This task may be more awkward than is handwritten notation.

Although the overall percentage of available time devoted to recordkeeping during anesthesia is of interest, it does not reflect those situations in which 100% of the anesthetist's attention is directed to the patient and, thus, no time for recordkeeping is available. An AARK faithfully records monitored information with a resolution that reflects true physiologic change. Reflecting this detail in recordkeeping is not possible for a human, particularly when intensive patient care demands are present. Every practitioner has experienced the frustration that occurs after management of a serious adverse

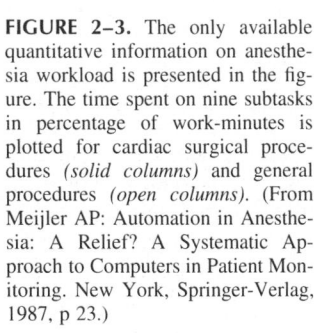

FIGURE 2–3. The only available quantitative information on anesthesia workload is presented in the figure. The time spent on nine subtasks in percentage of work-minutes is plotted for cardiac surgical procedures *(solid columns)* and general procedures *(open columns)*. (From Meijler AP: Automation in Anesthesia: A Relief? A Systematic Approach to Computers in Patient Monitoring. New York, Springer-Verlag, 1987, p 23.)

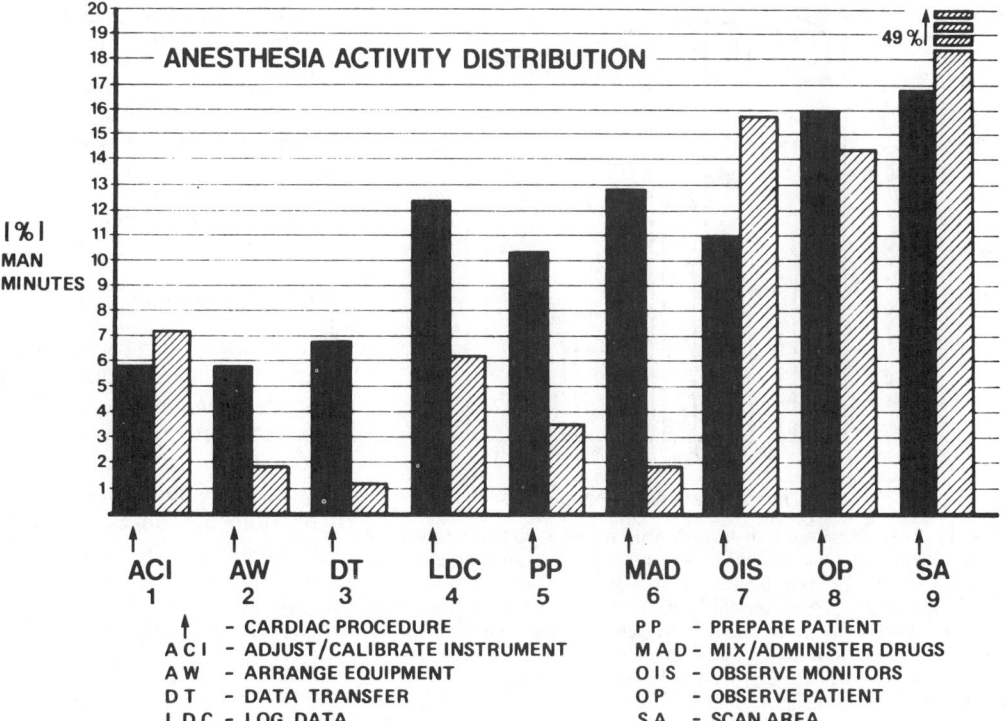

event in the operating room when it is virtually impossible to create an accurate and complete rendition of what took place. It is during such an event that an accurate recording is most needed.

How Accurate Is the Typical Record?

The accuracy of handwritten records has been examined by comparing them with those produced by an AARK. Studies have identified major discrepancies between manually recorded and computer-recorded values.[11, 12] These discrepancies were found to occur often during induction of and emergence from anesthesia, when the clinician was occupied with clinical

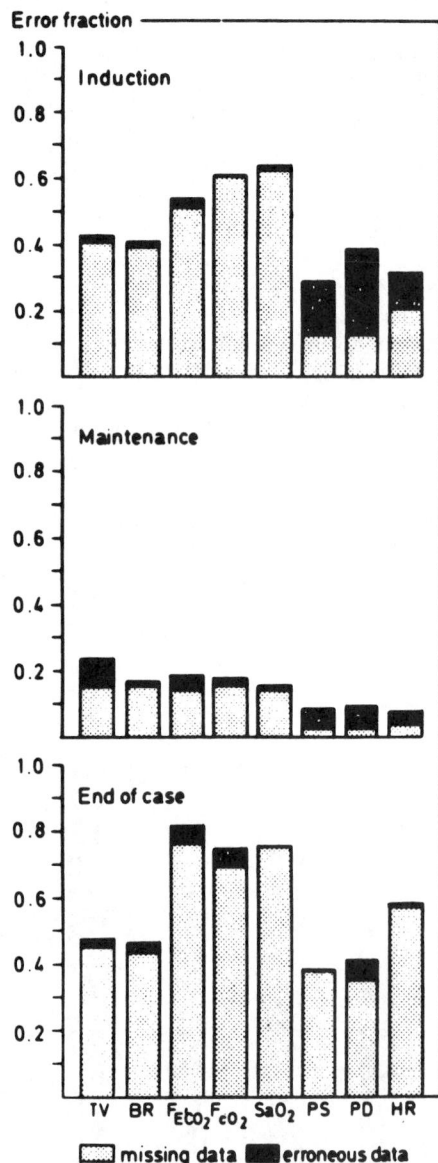

FIGURE 2–4. The amount of missing and erroneous data on handwritten records is shown for the three major periods of anesthesia: induction (first 15 minutes), end of case (last 10 minutes), and maintenance (period in between). TV = tidal volume; BR = breathing rate; F_{ETCO_2} = end-tidal CO_2; F_{CO_2} = oxygen fraction in the circuit; S_{aO_2} = oxygen saturation by pulse oximetry; PS = systolic blood pressure; PD = diastolic blood pressure; HR = heart rate. (From Lerou JGC, et al: Automated charting of physiological variables in anaesthesia: a quantitative comparison of handwritten versus automated records. J Clin Monit 1988; 4:37–47.)

care and, therefore, had to make retrospective entries on the record from memory (Fig. 2–4).

Blood Pressure Comparisons

The accuracy of recording blood pressure measurements has been examined, and interesting discrepancies have been found between handwritten values and those recorded automatically.[13] Fifty patients undergoing a variety of surgical procedures were studied. In the handwritten recording of blood pressure values, the investigators found a tendency toward the elimination of extreme values. The highest and lowest blood pressure values measured did not appear on the record. Although 33 instances of automatically recorded diastolic blood pressure greater than 110 mm Hg occurred, no handwritten record contained a diastolic blood pressure measurement >110 mm Hg. Since extremes in blood pressure may be construed by some to represent suboptimal anesthetic management, these findings likely represent a bias toward the recording of less controversial values.

Three conclusions can be drawn from these studies: (1) the clinician is often occupied, especially during induction and emergence, and unable to make timely notations on the record; (2) entries made from memory are often inaccurate; and (3) a bias, whether it be conscious or unconscious, is likely present during the creation of the handwritten record.

Automated Anesthesia Recordkeeper Artifacts

The handwritten record may be inaccurate for a number of reasons, but the automated record may also be flawed. An AARK records exactly what is displayed on the monitor whether or not it is artifactual.[14, 15] Studies of the incidence of artifact recorded by AARKs demonstrate that a small percentage of data—between 0.1% and 6%, depending on the parameter of interest—is artifactual. Of perhaps greater interest, however, is that both studies demonstrated that the incidence of artifact decreased as AARK technology matured.

Artifactual data usually appear on the record as markedly different from the other values recorded. As such, artifact is unlikely to be regarded as a manifestation of poor anesthetic management.

How Complete Is the Record?

AARKs seem to create a more accurate rendition of monitored parameters than does the clinician. Can the AARK facilitate the creation of a more complete record as well?

Entry Frequency

An anesthetic record can be incomplete because data are not entered or are not entered at the desired resolution. For most handwritten records, data is recorded every 5 minutes for the most frequently recorded information and every 15 minutes for other parameters, such as SpO_2. As noted earlier, this frequency, although well accepted, is not indicative of important physiologic changes. Significant heart rate and blood pressure alterations can occur within seconds. This interval is not practical for a human data recorder, but AARKs with modern computer technology can acquire data well within the frequency of physiologic changes. One approach to avoid storing large amounts of normal data is to program the automated record to eliminate high-resolution normal data but to retain a high resolution during periods of interest.

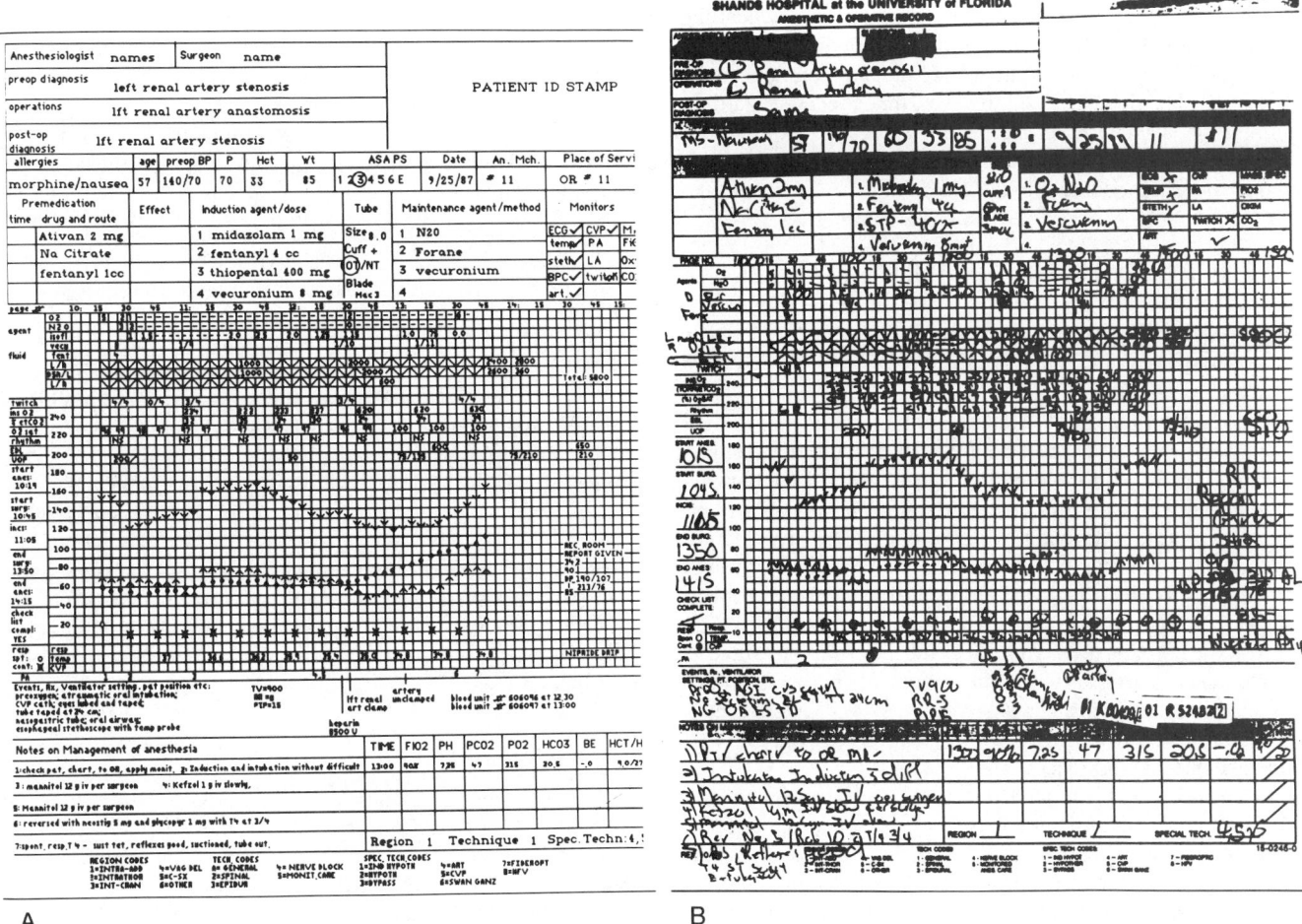

FIGURE 2–5. *A*, Representative automated anesthetic record. *B*, The same record shown as it would be handwritten. (From Gravenstein JS: The uses of the anesthesia record. J Clin Monit 1989; 5:251–255.)

Printed Versus Magnetic Records

The printed record generated by an AARK typically displays data at the intervals customary on handwritten records. AARK systems that record data to magnetic disk actually do so more frequently than is printed on the handwritten record. If these "magnetic records" are retained, events can be reviewed in much greater detail than that provided by either the printed or handwritten records.

Messages, Checklists, and Automated Prompts

AARKs can also be programmed to determine whether the information entered onto the record is complete. Messages, checklists, or automated prompts can be programmed into an AARK as reminders to the user to be sure that essential items are included. For example, before the record is considered complete, the AARK can check to ensure that billing information or any other required details are complete. It can then prompt the user for additional information as it is needed.

Is the Record Legible?

The light-hearted comment often made to someone with illegible handwriting that he or she would make a good physician has an unfortunate ring of truth. In fact, many health care professionals either have poor handwriting or the legibility of their handwriting deteriorates when they attempt to record rapidly changing events. Figure 2–5 shows examples of a typical automated record *(A)* and a representative handwritten record *(B)*. The automated record is clearly the more legible of the two.

Why is legibility important? Obviously, an illegible record fails to serve the function for which it was created, that is, the documentation of the course of an anesthetic procedure. Furthermore, an illegible anesthetic record may have serious medicolegal implications. A jury may interpret a sloppy record as an indication of a sloppy approach to patient care. If important data are missing from the record, it may prove difficult to alter the jury's interpretation.

Do AARKs Interfere with Vigilance?

One purported advantage of the handwritten record is that the physical act of entering data on the record makes the clinician aware of physiologic trends. Does the clinician using an AARK suffer a decrement in vigilance by having monitored data charted automatically? Unfortunately, little objective data assess the impact of an AARK on vigilance.

One study suggests that vigilance may not be as well maintained with the use of an AARK.[16] The investigators found that clinicians who used an AARK were less likely to know the values of current monitored parameters than when the same clinicians kept the record by hand. Whether this difference translates into less optimal patient care remains to be determined. The data suggest, however, that concern regarding the impact of an AARK on vigilance may be justified. Perhaps clinicians who use an AARK need to modify their practice patterns to ensure continued vigilance.

THE AUTOMATED ANESTHESIA RECORD

Unnecessary Technology or an Indispensable Tool?

We have seen that the AARK offers many advantages over the handwritten record. The true utility of the AARK is a topic of heated debate, and the technology has yet to be embraced by more than a handful of clinicians. AARK proponents assert that this technology provides a better-quality and more complete, accurate, and legible record than handwritten recording. Detractors of AARKs feel that reduced vigilance is a problem and that recording of artifactual data may open the possibility of medicolegal exposure. The foregoing information suggests that elements of truth are present in both of these assertions. How can these opposing views be resolved? Will AARK technology ultimately fade away, or will it become an integral part of the anesthesia workplace?

In order to gain acceptance into routine clinical practice, a new device must satisfy one or more of the following criteria: it must (1) improve patient care, (2) reduce physician workload, (3) decrease cost, (4) be medicolegally compelling, or (5) perform one or more important tasks that would otherwise not be done.[17] Does AARK technology satisfy any of these criteria?

Can an AARK Improve Patient Care?

No data are available to document that AARKs improve patient care. Further, a study is unlikely to collect such data, given the low incidence of patient injury due to anesthesia and the multitude of factors that potentially contribute to such injury. AARKs may improve care by increasing the amount of time available to observe the patient, or they may be detrimental by reducing the awareness of monitored data. Given the paucity of objective information, each user must make a personal judgment about the potential impact on patient care. In any event, AARKs are unlikely to gain acceptance based on the criteria of improved patient care.

Do AARKs Reduce the Physician's Workload?

Clearly, AARKs reduce the work associated with entering physiologic data on the record, since these data are recorded automatically. The clinician using an AARK, however, is not freed from all recordkeeping activities, since demographic, procedural, and drug information must still be entered manually. Current AARK technology does not provide a method for entering information that can be more conveniently entered by hand.

Of the data-entry devices that have been tried, including bar code readers,[18] voice recognition systems,[19] and touch screens,[20] none has replaced the keyboard. Since many clinicians do not have typing skills, manual annotation remains awkward. Prerecorded annotations can reduce the amount of manual entry required but do not eliminate it entirely. The workload advantages of the AARK are apparent during those situations when all attention must be directed to the patient; however, such situations likely do not occur frequently enough to drive acceptance of the technology.

Is an AARK Cost-Effective?

Whether AARKs will decrease the cost of care remains to be determined. With medical costs soaring, the cost of any new technology will be a factor in its acceptance. At first glance, it appears that AARKs are excessively expensive, and this is likely a major factor in their rather slow acceptance. The only costs associated with the handwritten record are those incurred by printing forms and buying pens. The cost of one AARK (which can function only in one location) approaches the cost of an integrated physiologic monitor. The decision to purchase an AARK must, therefore, involve a cost/benefit analysis.

Billing and Collection

The cost savings associated with AARKs have yet to be documented, but AARKs may in fact pay for themselves. If one accepts the premise that the quality documentation provided by an AARK might decrease malpractice liability, the cost is clearly minimal. Since the AARK is used to record information necessary for billing purposes, it may help to improve collections. In the future, AARKs will be linked electronically to billing services, thereby eliminating clerical processing of billing information. Thus, bills will be generated more quickly and with fewer errors. The Workgroup for Electronic Data Interchange of the U.S. Department of Health and Human Services estimates that automating the flow of information between insurers and health care providers could reduce health care costs by between 4 and 10 billion dollars.[21]

Quality Assurance

AARKs can also facilitate tasks that now consume both clerical and physician time in an anesthesia practice. Quality assurance analysis is required of all anesthesia practices and is increasingly scrutinized by hospital-accrediting agencies. A busy anesthesia practice generates a large amount of quality assurance information that must be processed and analyzed. The AARK stores a large amount of the information that is necessary to support quality assurance. That information can be transferred automatically to quality assurance software to generate the appropriate reports, thus reducing clerical and physician time devoted to updating quality assurance records. In addition, because the AARK data are more complete and accurate than those obtained from the handwritten record, quality assurance should be better when the data has been collected using an AARK.

Although no one to date has evaluated the cost-effectiveness of AARKs, some potential major advantages can translate into significant cost savings and offset the cost of the devices. As AARK technology matures, its costs may decrease, and

AARKs will become incorporated into sophisticated data management systems that improve the quality and efficiency of not only recordkeeping but also billing and quality assurance.

Does an AARK Increase or Decrease Liability Exposure?

When viewed from a medicolegal perspective, AARK technology is highly controversial. It is striking, however, that professionals who defend physicians overwhelmingly support the use of automated records. The consensus of these individuals is that the "poor or incomplete anesthesia record" is the greatest obstacle to successful defense against a malpractice claim.[22] Crawford Morris, an attorney experienced at defending physicians in malpractice litigation, writes about AARKs:

"With the use of such devices, each side is going to lose some malpractice cases it might have won with poorly decipherable records, and vice versa, but on balance, the presentation of actual facts should not only promote justice but also lead to more reasonable settlements."[23]

To date, no malpractice claims have been won or lost because of the use of an AARK. As their application proliferates, malpractice litigation will ultimately involve data collected by AARKs. The role of the AARK in litigation almost certainly will have a major impact on acceptance of the technology.

Can an AARK Facilitate New Tasks?

AARKs have the potential to perform information management functions that are not currently possible. This potential will ultimately drive their acceptance. In the 1990s, an increasing demand is being placed on the anesthesia record for information. Following is the foremost recommendation of an Institute of Medicine study on the computer-based patient record:

"Health care professionals and organizations should adopt the computer-based patient record (CPR) as the standard for medical and all other records related to patient care."[24]

The basis for this recommendation is the recognition that the computer-based patient record, of which the AARK is one element, will facilitate the access to information in ways that are not possible with current approaches to recordkeeping.

Access to Medical Records

Merely obtaining an old medical record can be a frustratingly slow process, whereas the pressure to care for more patients in less time is increasing. Patients are often poor historians and do not relate significant past complications that could be readily gleaned from their old charts if they were available. The AARK offers the potential to archive patient records and make them immediately accessible when needed.

Research Activities

Any number of research activities can be supported if accurate information is entered into the record. Retrospective chart reviews can provide useful information but are hampered by the difficulty involved in locating information and by the inconsistency of information entered onto the record.

In the future, studies will be facilitated by AARK technology. Data that are collected in the operating theater will be more easily categorized and analyzed. Prospective studies involving more than one institution will be quite feasible, since data formats will be standardized and readily exchangeable.

POSTANESTHESIA DOCUMENTATION

What Is Important?

Postanesthesia documentation is required at the time of discharge from the recovery room and at one or more days after the anesthetic procedure, particularly if a complication occurs. With the increase in same day surgery, documentation of discharge readiness has become an important issue. Whenever a patient is allowed to leave a postanesthesia care unit (PACU), some assessment of physiologic stability should be documented.

For the patient returning home, this documentation should include not only that the patient is awake but also that he or she is able to take fluid by mouth, void, and ambulate. Although the inpatient need not ambulate, physiologic stability and some assessment of pain control should be documented. Furthermore, if a problem had occurred in the PACU, the effect of treatment of that problem should be noted.

The postanesthesia documentation that occurs after discharge from the PACU should indicate that a postoperative visit occurred and should identify problems that relate to the rendering of anesthetic care. Patients who suffer an adverse consequence related to anesthesia are typically comforted by explanation. Time should be spent addressing the issue with the patient, and the amount of time spent should be clearly documented in the record.

The extension of anesthesia quality assurance into the postoperative period has not been extensively pursued but is potentially of great value. If we are to measure practice patterns in terms of outcome, recording of data throughout the postoperative period is essential.

CONCLUSIONS

The anesthetic record is the final arbiter of the manner in which patient care is rendered. The record no longer exists solely for the benefit of its creator. As viewed by other users, it is a reflection of the person caring for the patient. To create an effective record, anesthetists must think of the manner in which they would like each user of the records to view the care they provide.

It is becoming increasingly difficult for the handwritten anesthetic record to satisfy all the demands now being placed on the record. In addition, a clear mandate is emerging to move to computer-based patient records. In order for the anesthesia community to satisfy this mandate, AARK technology needs to be closely examined. AARKs have the potential to improve patient care in a multitude of ways. Not only can information be presented in a fashion that aids clinical decision making but also the accessibility and quality of data will be improved.

Outcomes research, which requires extensive data collection procedures, often by many institutions, will be enhanced through the definition of uniform information formats. Costs will be contained through improved efficiency and better data for accounting procedures. If we continue to think of the AARK only as an alternative means to reproduce the existing anesthesia record, acceptance will remain slow and the rewards limited. We must think beyond existing misconceptions about what the record is to what it might become if we were to utilize the technologic power available to us.

References

1. Beecher HK: The First Anesthesia Records. Surg Gynecol Obstet 1940; 71:689.
2. Gravenstein JS: The uses of the anesthesia record. J Clin Monit 1989; 5:256.
3. The computer-based patient record: Meeting health care needs. *In* The Computer-Based Patient Record: An Essential Technology for Health Care. Dick RS, Steen EB (eds). Washington DC, National Academy Press, 1991, pp 34–35.
4. Gravenstein JS: The automated anesthesia record. Int J Clin Monit Comput 1986; 3:131.
5. Whitcher C: Advantages of automated record keeping. *In* The Automated Anesthesia Record and Alarm Systems. Gravenstein JS, Newbower RA, Ream AK, et al (eds). Boston, Butterworths, 1987.
6. Anesthesiologists Affiliated versus Sullivan. 941 F2d 678 [8th Cir 1991].
7. Introduction. *In* The Computer-Based Patient Record: An Essential Technology for Health Care. Dick RS, Steen EB (eds). Washington DC, National Academy Press, 1991, p 14.
8. Kennedy PJ, Feingold A, Wiener EL, et al: Analysis of tasks and human factors in anesthesia for coronary artery bypass. Anesth Analg 1976; 55:374.
9. Boquet G, Bushman JA, Davenport HT: The anaesthetic machine, a study of function and design. Br J Anaesth 1980; 52:61.
10. Meijler AP: Automation in Anesthesia: A Relief? A Systematic Approach to Computers in Patient Monitoring. New York, Springer-Verlag, 1987, p 23.
11. Zollinger RM, Kreul JF, Schneider AJL: Man-made versus computer-generated anesthesia records. J Surg Res 1977; 22:419.
12. Lerou JGC, Dirksen R, van Daele M, et al: Automated charting of physiological variables in anesthesia: a quantitative comparison of automated versus handwritten anesthesia records. J Clin Monit 1988; 4:37.
13. Cook RI, McDonald JD, Nunziata E: Differences between handwritten and automatic blood pressure records. Anesthesiology 1989; 71:385.
14. Edsall DW: Analysis and frequency of artifacts generated by anesthesia information management systems. Anesthesiology 1990; 73:A481.
15. Stanley TE, Smith LR, White WD, et al: Incidence of vital sign artifact in automated anesthesia records. Anesthesiology 1990; 73:A483.
16. Yablock DO: Comparison of vigilance using automated versus handwritten records. Anesthesiology 1990; 73:A416.
17. Gravenstein N, Feldman JM: Anesthesia records and automation. Semin Anesth 1989; 8:119.
18. Block FE, Burton LW, Rafal MD, et al: Two computer-based anesthetic monitors: the DUKE automatic monitoring equipment (DAME) system and the microdame. J Clin Monit 1985; 1:30.
19. Brien RA, Smith NT, Quinn ML, et al: The accuracy of voice recognition in the operating room. Anesthesiology 1988; 69:A331.
20. Klocke H, Inform D, Trispel S, et al: An anesthesia information system for monitoring and recordkeeping during surgical anesthesia. J Clin Monit 1986; 2:246.
21. McIlrath S: Panel wants most paper claims to go the way of the dinosaur. Am Med News, August 10, 1992, p 1.
22. Gibbs RF: The present and future medicolegal importance of recordkeeping in anesthesia and intensive care: the case for automation. J Clin Monit 1989; 5:251.
23. Morris C: Legal aspects of monitoring. *In* The Automated Anesthesia Record and Alarm Systems. Gravenstein JS, Newbower RS, Ream AK, et al (eds). Boston, Butterworths, 1987, pp 270–271.
24. Summary. *In* The Computer-Based Patient Record: An Essential Technology for Healthcare. Dick RS, Steen EB (eds). Washington DC, National Academy Press, 1991, p 6.

CHAPTER 3

Quality Assurance in Anesthesiology

JERRY A. COHEN, M.D.

"Those who fail to remember the past are condemned to repeat it."

GEORGE SANTAYANA

In the broad sense, quality assurance (QA) increases the likelihood that medical intervention will improve patient outcome and reduces the probability that it will precipitate a bad outcome.[1] When QA works effectively, it provides a systematic mechanism by which problems are detected and corrected, efficiency is improved, and care is rendered in a manner convenient for patients and health care providers. When it fails, usually from superficiality or disuse, the history of practice problems is repeated.

In October 1988, at the American Society of Anesthesiologists' (ASA) Workshop on Quality Assurance held at the annual meeting in San Francisco,[2] the question was asked, "How many people are here because they are interested in passing the Joint Commission on Accreditation of Healthcare Organizations (JCAHO) audit, and how many people are here because they would like to learn more about how to evaluate and improve quality?" Approximately 99% of the attendees indicated that their major motivation was passing the JCAHO audit, and only 1% were interested in using QA techniques to improve their practice.

Three years later, in June 1991, at another ASA workshop for QA and risk management, the same question was asked.[3] This time the answers were reversed; 99% of the attendees indicated that they wanted to improve the quality of their practice and reduce their perceived quality problems, and only 1% were primarily concerned about passing the next JCAHO audit.

Interest in quality improvement has become a hot topic in the literature of corporate management, in the popular press, and in medicine. Provision of the best possible quality of care is now perceived as more efficient, more economical, more profitable, and less of a liability than the alternative.

HISTORICAL CONSIDERATIONS

How Did the "Quality" Concept Enter Medical Practice?

The Agricultural Experience

Medical QA derives from the same scientific foundations as those principles originally designed to improve the outcome in agriculture, an area affected by numerous uncontrolled variables, such as rainfall, soil conditions, and temperature. Early controlled studies were designed to identify the ideal mixture of factors that were controllable. Statisticians plotted out large areas of land and divided them into squares, varying the nutrients, soil, irrigation, and other factors. They observed great variation in productivity, depending on the combination of these factors. The concept of controlling the process of a previously uncontrollable enterprise, farming, developed into a science that made America the breadbasket of the world.

Major concepts of statistical quality control were derived to a great extent from agriculture. Contributors such as E. A. Fisher, who applied the science of mathematic statistics to agricultural problems, eventually developed statistical methods by which complex interactions could be analyzed. Two individuals who contributed greatly to the concept of analysis of variance were W. Edwards Deming and W. A. Shewhart. Their understanding of the relationship of inherent variation in processes, control limits, and outcome subsequently led to the notion that complex undertakings, such as medical performance and outcome, also can be expected to perform within limits determined by the underlying structure and process of medical practice.[4]

Although Deming's original writings were highly technical and difficult to read, even when they were intended for the public, the methodology used and its impact on the rise of Japanese industry were captured in a very accessible, well-written book by Mary Walton.[5] Today we use Deming's principles of statistical quality control to improve practices that work and to eliminate those that do not. At the same time, we attempt to improve the efficiency and economy of medical practice.

What Was the Stimulus for Early Quality Assurance Development?

Because of the poor quality of American hospitals at the beginning of the 20th century, a major effort to improve the standards of care developed. The Flexner Report,[6] Codman Survey,[7] and early work by the American College of Surgeons coalesced into the Hospital Standardization Program. This program eventually became highly effective. In the initial report of 1917, 87% of the hospitals surveyed failed the audit; later, only 6% of hospitals failed a much more rigorous audit.

Because the program had expanded and required more resources than the American College of Surgeons could provide, the Joint Commission on Accreditation of Hospitals (JCAH) was established in 1951. This commission was composed of the American Hospital Association, the American Medical Association, the American Dental Association, the American College of Physicians, and the American College of Surgeons.

From its beginning to the present time, hospital accreditation has dwelt largely on the area of quality and the observance of quality standards. Seventy-eight per cent of the average JCAHO audit and more than 60% of the contingencies have dealt with QA in recent years. Although the current JCAHO audit is, in theory, voluntary, successful passage is required for Medicare reimbursement. This fact alone has made the JCAHO the most influential purveyor of QA concepts in American medicine.

Who Was E. A. Codman?

E. A. Codman developed a concept of outcome analysis. When he identified areas of poor outcome, he designed his surgical program to improve them. He realized that a number of factors affected outcome, including the skill of the surgeon, the nursing personnel, anesthesia, equipment, and the patients' disease.[7] In a speech in 1914, he said, in essence:

"I am called an eccentric for saying in public that hospitals:

Must find out what their results are
Must analyze these results to find out their strong and weak points
Must compare their results with those of other hospitals
Must care for the cases they can care for well and avoid attempting to care for the cases that they are not qualified to care for
Must welcome publicity not only for their successes but also for their errors **so that the public will give them help when it is needed** [emphasis added]
Must promote members of the staff on the basis [of] . . . what they can accomplish for their patients

Such opinions will not be eccentric in a few years."

Clearly, Codman was nearly three-quarters of a century early in his pronouncements. His concepts, although extremely well developed, were left to twist idly in the wind and had to be rediscovered later by people such as Avedis Donabedian.[8]

The public has come to expect predictable good outcome within rather narrow acceptable limits. Although patients and physicians alike at one time were willing to accept the concept that "all anesthetics are dangerous . . .," this hundred-year-old expectation is as foreign to modern anesthesia as it is to modern aviation, with which it still shares many of the opportunities for excitement as well as terror. Contemporary journalism exploits the public's desire for excellence in medicine. The annual survey of America's best hospitals by *U.S. News and World Report* gives people the bottom-line message that not too many hospitals are desirable places in which patients would like to find themselves.

Despite the role of the JCAHO in improving medical practice, its seal of approval has come under fire in recent years. On October 12, 1988, the *Wall Street Journal* published a chilling article including a list of dozens of accredited hospitals that had failed state inspections between 1986 and 1988.[9]

As a result of this and other pressures, the JCAHO responded with the so-called Agenda for Change,[10] which introduced practice parameters as part of the concept that standards of practice could improve outcome. The JCAHO also outlined a system for ongoing quality analysis and assessment and by 1992 had begun to foster the notion of continuous quality improvement.[11]

PEER REVIEW ORGANIZATIONS

What Were the Legislative Initiatives?

To a great extent, the battle between cost and quality has been spearheaded by a series of legislative initiatives. The Social Security Act of 1965 established Medicare and with it the requirement for JCAH accreditation. Utilization review soon followed in the Social Security Act of 1967. In order to review the quality and appropriateness of care and to establish some form of ongoing review, the Peer Standards Review Organization (PSRO) was enacted into law in 1972. A decade of profound disinterest in the PSRO followed, because physicians saw it more as an intrusion than a help.

Subsequently, as part of the Tax, Equity, and Fiscal Responsibility Act in 1982, the Peer Review Improvement Act (PRIA) was passed. The PRIA replaced the PSRO with the Professional Review Organization (PRO). Some critics commented that the PRO was merely the PSRO without standards. The next year, 1983, saw the implementation of Diagnosis-Related Groups as part of the Social Security Act. This act mandated the prospective payment system (PPS) and had almost no QA measures. The deficit soon was remedied by the Comprehensive Omnibus Budget Reconciliation Act of 1985, in which QA and discharge planning were mandated.

The flurry of legislative activity culminated in 1986 in the Health Care Quality Improvement Act (HCQIA), which mandated a federal data bank for reporting QA issues. The items to be reported included any restriction of privileges for more than a 30-day period, liability settlements, professional society restrictions, and restrictions of a practitioner's medical license.

What Is the Role of the Peer Review Organization?

Mark Holoweiko, writing in *Medical Economics*,[12] quoted William Roper, then head of the Health Care Financing Administration (HCFA) and later Deputy Assistant to the President for Domestic Policy: "The time has come for the federal government to become intricately involved in the writing of medical-practice standards." Roper anticipated that the PRO would be the government's agent in this effort. Although this statement did not mark the beginning of the federal government's interest in controlling the quality of care for which it paid, it was a major cannon ball delivered across the bow of organized medicine. It represents the continuing contest between the cost and quality of care, characterized by the PRO's third contract cycle.

The PRO was largely responsible for administrating the HCFA's quality intervention plan, which included sanctions for quality deficiencies. The legitimacy of quality review provided by the PRO rested to a large extent on the validity of the governmental assumption that health care providers will render poor care because of the combination of financial incentives and disincentives introduced by the PPS.

The adversarial nature of the PRO with respect to medical practice included its punitive measures, bureaucratic orientation, negative rather than positive incentives, and overconcentration on case outliers, all of which have been a continuing annoyance to physicians. This irksome set of characteristics was not helped by the lack of demonstrated effect on outcome. Consequently, the National Academy of Sciences Institute of Medicine recommended that Congress totally redesign the PRO to oversee Medicare quality in a manner to reflect realistic and meaningful standards and to improve outcome.[13]

What Is the Impact of Malpractice Legislation and Tort Law?

The courts have established some general guidelines regarding the relationship of hospitals and the physicians to whom they extend privileges.[14, 15] In these corporate negligence cases, the responsibility of hospitals to guarantee the extension of clinical privileges only to physicians who are well qualified was established as a matter of law.

As a consequence of these decisions and the actions of the PRO, hospitals have an interest in evaluating the quality of care, not only with respect to the hospital as a corporate entity but also with respect to the individual providers of care. This concept parallels the shift in emphasis by the JCAHO from focused studies of problems, which were typical in the early 1980s, to the trending of quality indicators and providers, which became *de rigueur* by the end of the 1980s.

Malpractice legislation also has a major impact on quality of care evaluation and risk management. As an example, the Florida Comprehensive Medical Malpractice Reform Act of 1985 mandated the disclosure of (1) a series of defined severe adverse outcomes to be reported to a hospital (institutional)-based risk manager; (2) an annual report to the state of the frequency of adverse outcomes, their cause, and the providers involved; (3) the malpractice claims against a provider and the institution; (4) any modification of clinical privileges made by the hospital for a provider; and (5) all deaths and neurologic damage–related problems.

Three years later, the Medical Incident Recovery Act was enacted. It created a Division of Medical Quality Assurance within the Department of Professional Regulation. This act also extended immunity to all persons reporting on quality issues, including protection from antitrust actions. The state realized that the potential for exposure of QA documentation would greatly chill the entire process; it therefore extended legal protection to all QA documentation, making it nondiscoverable for any purpose other than quality improvement (i.e., data reported to the DPR were protected from use in medical malpractice suits).

Protection of Peer Reviewers

What protection is afforded peer reviewers with respect to the liability for their actions? As was mentioned, legislation such as that in Florida has been passed by many individual states.

Title 19

Defects in the law of the state of Oregon, demonstrated in the continuing case of *Patrick v Burger*,[16] were instrumental in the genesis of protective federal legislation. In this suit, brought by a physician who was deprived of his right to practice by the peer review committee of his hospital, the committee was held liable under the antitrust laws for improper restraint of trade. Further, confidential documents involving the review process were exposed to public scrutiny.

This frightening precedent was promptly dealt with on the federal level. The HCQIA extended protection via Title 19 of the Social Security Act to peer reviewers. Under the provisions of this act, peer reviewers who act on a reasonable belief that they are improving the quality of care, who make a reasonable effort to obtain the appropriate and relevant facts in the case, who provide appropriate notice to physicians being reviewed, who give them an opportunity to rebut the charges, and who base their decisions on the facts of the case are immune to prosecution or suit under the Federal Antitrust Laws.

The act further protects the peer review/QA documents from exposure in medical malpractice cases and specifically provides for up to 6 months imprisonment or a $1000 fine or both for persons who expose these documents improperly through any publication, distribution, or factual description outside of the peer review process.

Regardless of legislative initiatives, the real solution to liability and exposure is the observance of scrupulously fair procedures for peer review, including written criteria for review that are made part of the hospital bylaws.

CURRENT QUALITY ASSURANCE

What Are Its Common Problems?

The difficulties in developing a productive QA program are numerous. The QA infrastructure sometimes develops in a manner that is overly complex and inefficient. The database produced by that system may not be sufficiently robust or accurate to describe the quality of each service's activities in a meaningful fashion. As such, it cannot form the foundation for significant action. Several internal and external problems reduce the productivity of a QA program.

Reactionary Evolution

QA evolved as a reaction to JCAHO demands, which have been advanced in a manner that has often lacked detail and consistency. Although the JCAHO has been our greatest stimulus to develop quality assessment and improvement techniques, its leadership has straddled the fence on the specifics of implementation, causing great confusion to those who are attempting to comply. Its recent pilot studies on quality indicators revealed a simplistic approach that contrasts markedly with the detailed pilot study of severe morbidity and mortality performed by Battelle and the ASA.[17] The JCAHO methodology was characterized by the development of a few indicators of severe morbidity and mortality that pertain to a small minority of patients. They serve poorly to reflect the overall quality of the hospital and the concerns of most patients.[18] A robust meaningful database probably is not much more expensive than the abbreviated one advocated by the JCAHO; the latter organization, however, chose a simple system in order to make it more palatable.

Herein lies one of the principal paradigms for failure in QA: adoption of an overly simple system in order to obtain acceptance. This approach fails because it does not produce meaningful assessment and action in a predictable fashion. It fails in particular institutions because many hours are spent by the medical staff to produce reports (the necessary paperwork) but little real improvement in quality is derived from the effort. This produces frustration and cynicism.

Gathering of Data

The indicators used by the medical staff to reflect quality of care may be gathered in a manner that produces statistical inaccuracy. The QA staff can help individual specialties by analyzing the medical record post hoc to determine the occurrence of indicators. Because data are gathered by nonphysicians who are unfamiliar with the patients and long after the problem occurred, they often are incomplete.

An informal study made with the QA staff of my hospital several years ago demonstrated that they were unable to determine accurately which patients suffered from various common perioperative problems, including hypertension, hypotension, airway obstruction, hypoxemia, and so forth. The failure was attributable to their understandably limited ability to make medical judgments.

This hypothesis has been reinforced by the sporadic nature of reports of quality indicators, such as hypotension and nausea, referred to the department of anesthesiology by the QA staff, in contrast to the much more frequent incidence of these problems detected by our physician-based departmental QA tracking system.

Applicability of Indicators

The indicators used to reflect quality may apply to a minority of patients. Because most systems are driven by regulators, we tend to direct our efforts toward assessment of the worst possible problems. In fact, few patients suffer the extremes in poor quality of care, but many have minor and frequent problems that are annoying, prolong their hospital stay, and reduce profitability.

Method of Assessment

The way in which recognized problems in care are assessed may prevent systematic action. Assessments should be clear and forthright. Labeling problems as "expected," "unexpected," and "possibly outside the standards of care" does not express the true preventability or severity of the problems being addressed. These categories do not even exist along the same continuum and, at best, are ambiguous and perhaps disingenuous.

The tendency of hospitals to adopt obscure assessment categories derives in part from legal concerns that labeling such

as "preventable/nonpreventable," treated "properly/improperly," and leading to "short-term/permanent damage" or escalation of care could have adverse tort claim effects. However, because federal statutes limit the discovery of QA data, this specter has not materialized.

To be useful, any assessment system should reflect the medical, ethical, and legal severity of the problems observed. We must differentiate between trivial problems and those that lead to escalation of care, severe morbidity, or even death. The system should account for the preventability of the event. (Is it unrelated to our process, or is it something we can improve?) Finally, it should form the basis for effective action.

Accuracy of Aggregate Data

Methodology may be inadequate to obtain consistently accurate aggregate data that serve to inform practitioners and the hospital administration of the quality of care. Many institutions use a mixture of normalized data (the frequency of events per patient at risk or per other meaningful cohort grouping) and non-normalized data (total number of events without reference to a denominator). Also, when the data are gathered by nonphysician QA workers rather than concurrently with patient care, the number of problems detected may represent only a fraction of the total. Therefore, the data that are obtained cannot serve as a barometer of the current status, nor can they be the basis for meaningful improvement. A well-structured, robust system is less expensive to operate and more productive in terms of improving quality of care, public image, and profitability.

In order to be useful, data should include relevant measurements of how well the structure, process (including practice parameters generally accepted as leading to good outcome), and outcome of current medical practices are functioning (i.e., how often a good or bad outcome occurs per patient at risk). Compilation of statistics that are not related to risk or cost of care are largely noncontributory and wasteful of resources.

Much of the information needed for computing frequency statistics is available on existing hospital databases, especially those that form the cohort denominators. Rekeying of these data is wasteful. The relevant data should be centralized as much as possible and distributed in a common electronic form for QA review and use. This method provides a cost-effective uniform standard for calculating frequency statistics.

Quality of Definitions

Quality and the purpose of QA may be poorly defined. A well-understood concept of what constitutes quality should lead to the development of meaningful indicators based on the scope of care, including all services; therapeutic modalities; their desired outcome; and their associated risks. Problem/outcome indicators must be designed by the individual specialties in terms meaningful to their practice. Some of these indicators may require long-term follow-up of neurologic dysfunction, efficacy of pain therapies, or headache secondary to lumbar puncture, for example.

A two-tiered system of quality assessment bookkeeping—one for the JCAHO and one that we report in our specialty journals or talk about in the lounge—must be eliminated by devising a scientifically meaningful database and using it to guide change. This approach should have a positive impact on the economics of care and could also lead to sustained demonstrable improvements in outcome.

Academic Organization

Academic institutions often have an organizational structure that parallels that of the affiliated medical school, which time and tradition have made virtually unchangeable. Although several layers of this system could be eliminated, most academic hospitals choose to retain the departmental organizational skeleton. The strengths of departmental organization and current technology can be used in these institutions to help facilitate individual departmental QA programs. Departments should retain the role of developing meaningful quality indicators and of providing the QA system with realistic definitions of quality.

The hospital QA service can provide basic support for the medical staff to collect data for problems related to individual patients. Physicians have more confidence in data they collect as a matter of course than in distantly post hoc data gathered by others.

Existing data can be provided in electronically usable form. Hospital computer resources can help to customize existing software, resulting in uniformity, standardization, and a marked reduction in personnel requirements. The departmental QA officer can then review only the outliers of quality instead of screening chart after chart; time saved allows review of the ''big picture'' and formulation of meaningful action.

Paperwork

Many practitioners believe that filling out forms to please the JCAHO is QA. This statement is an exaggeration, but not much of one. We need to re-educate ourselves concerning the utility of quality management/improvement systems. We need to convince our colleagues that such systems are in their best interest and that they reduce medical and legal risks and make medicine more rewarding. We probably cannot wholly separate out the credentialing aspects of QA, but we can promote the idea that it can detect the problems that individual practitioners are having before their credentials are at risk.

Regulators

Some problems in dealing with our regulators are not of our making. To resolve these problems, we must continue to work with them to establish firmly what the ground rules are, although we must not make them the centerpiece of our QA program. Although the specifics in the JCAHO accreditation manual[11] (see Appendix I at the end of this chapter) are not exquisitely detailed, their intent is clear. The JCAHO wants physicians to develop a system for monitoring quality that has some meaning with respect to outcome (although they do not describe exactly how to do it). One suspects that they will not relate precisely how to implement the system in the Accreditation Manual for Hospitals (AMH) but will give examples through their other publications. Of course, they will tell individual departments at the time of inspection whether or not they succeeded.

What Is the Theoretic Basis of Medical Quality Assurance?

Some of the concepts of industrial QA were translated into medical terms by Avedis Donabedian.[8, 19] The overall goal of his unified quality assessment theory was to advance simple but powerful principles that would expose the sources of variation in medical management, then reduce them by making the outcomes of care more predictable.

To achieve this goal, the quality assessment process is divided into three functionally related categories: structure, process, and outcome. A quality indicator may fall into one or more of these divisions. Donabedian postulated that the structures and processes of medical care result in the observed outcomes.

Structure

Quality indicators that are primarily structural are derived from the institutional elements that support care. These include elements relating to the physical plant, including the anesthetic gas delivery system, the anesthesia machine and its components, disposable equipment, the logistic means by which items are supplied to the anesthesiologist, and the patient-monitoring systems. Also included are the means of deploying personnel, established operating room safety procedures, and well-accepted management algorithms, such as basic cardiac life support or the Harvard anesthesia practice standards.[20, 21]

Process

Process elements are derived from the generally accepted techniques, methodologies, and judgment processes that contribute to patient care. These include the indications for anesthetics, blood components, drugs, invasive monitoring, and pain management.

Outcome

Changes in structure and process are generally systematic and should lead to improvement in outcome by reducing the frequency of problem events related to these elements. To be useful, structure and process review requires specific criteria defining the problem area to be improved, the goals of improvement stated in terms of enhanced outcome and performance, and a description of the changes in process that are to be used to effect the improvement. If the problems, goals, or methodologies are poorly defined, improvement is unlikely.

Similarly, if the structural and process elements of practice are not reviewed continuously over time, improvement may be ephemeral. For example, if a QA program detected a large number of hypotensive episodes attributable to rapid vancomycin infusions (i.e., ''red man syndrome''),[22] improving the structures and processes involved should lead to improved outcome. This goal might be accomplished by pretreating patients with an antihistamine, by using only infusion pumps to deliver the drug over a 1-hour period, or by infusing the drug even more slowly over an 8-hour period before surgery.

Such changes in the structure and process of vancomycin administration should reduce the number of reactions to rapid administration virtually to zero. In this case, the goal, the methods to achieve that goal, and the resulting outcome are clear and achievable. Continued monitoring of the problem ensures that the improvement is sustained.

Problems of Analysis

Outcome cannot be improved directly, except by time travelers and other miracle workers; rather, it improves as a consequence of improved structure, process, or a change in the overall severity of patients' illness. Review of outcome is useful principally to determine the consequences that the structure and process elements have on care. Outcome elements include mortality and morbidity rates, overuse or underuse of blood products and monitoring techniques, cost of care, length of stay, and patients' satisfaction. To the extent that outcome reflects the impact that antecedent structures and processes have on care, it is a useful measurement, but it should not be used alone as a quality indicator. It can serve best as a gross confirmation of the success or failure of changes to improve defined end points of care.

Confounding Variables

Outcome assessment is limited by several factors. In medicine, unlike industry, many uncontrollable variables in patients' physiology and behavior conspire to limit the effectiveness of the health care system. Hence, poor outcome does not always indicate substandard care.[23]

The relationship of process and structure to outcome may be obscured by confounding offsetting variables. Outcome can best be understood in relationship to the severity of pre-existing illness, but even MedisGroups admission severity groups fail to give unbiased estimates of outcome.[24] This limitation severely reduces our ability to compare the standard expected outcome, weighted for severity of illness, with the actual outcome. It also compromises efforts by the JCAHO and the PROs to set simple normative standards for outcome.

Adverse outcome may be delayed, thereby obscuring problems in care. Such is the case with hepatitis or human immunodeficiency virus disease. The effect of knowing the severity of outcome biases the review of process.[25] Reviewers regularly judge care to be substandard when they are told that permanent injury or death occurred.

The consequence of overzealous reliance on outcome assessment may be an inappropriate reduction manipulation of case mix. Both individuals and institutions may improve their outcome statistics by reducing the number of high-risk admissions.[26] For all of these reasons, change in outcome resulting from systemwide changes in process and structure are useful measurements of the effectiveness of change. However, outcome is not, in itself, an independent indicator of quality.

What Is the Approach to Quality Assurance of the Joint Commission on Accreditation of Healthcare Organizations?

More than any other body, the JCAHO has the greatest single influence on medical QA because of its roots and its quasi-regulatory status. The JCAHO sets forth its theory and regulations in the annual AMH. Building on the concepts of structure, process, and outcome, the JCAHO has transformed QA from an almost useless bureaucratic waste of paper into a reasonably scientific approach to quality assessment and improvement (QA/I). Some of this transformation, as noted previously, occurred in response to external criticism.[9]

Statistical Quality Control

In developing its concepts of QA/I, the JCAHO borrowed heavily from the theories of statistical quality control, especially those of Deming.[4] It has at times developed its methodology before its theory, such as when it mandated the development of indicators of care before clearly explaining their basis in the service/risk profile (Fig. 3–1). On balance, the history of QA, under the aegis of the JCAHO, has been a gradual evolution from procedure/diagnosis spot checks to the use of aggregate data gathered concurrently with patient care, divided into relevant cohort groupings, and stated in terms of frequency of occurrence.

Retrospective Review

In the 1970s and early 1980s, the JCAHO promoted retrospective review in the form of the problem-oriented medical audit, also espoused by Brown.[27] Essential elements of quality assessment were promulgated: identification of the problem, determination that it was a real problem affecting outcome, investigation of its exact cause (structure and process), and implementation of corrective action.

Without the concept of a logical set of indicators and an aggregate database, the case audit method did not evaluate medical practice comprehensively. It depended on the episodic identification of problems, from various sources (e.g., incident reports, mortality and morbidity conferences), but without prioritization in terms of the source or the level of the problem. The audits were conducted often enough to please the JCAHO. However, long-term systematic follow-up was inadequate.

Departmental Quality Assurance

The requirement for case audits was eventually extended to individual departments. Departments appointed a QA officer who was tasked to perform a monthly or quarterly audit of a problem. The problems of random selection of the subject of the audit, the lack of a foundation for systematic screening, and the assumption that once solved, the problem was gone forever were now reproduced on the departmental level. Time was wasted; little changed.

Freestanding Review Committees

The need for systematic identification of ongoing problems eventually gave rise to freestanding review committees: surgical tissue, blood use, medical records, infection control, and pharmacy and therapeutics. These committees met monthly to evaluate specific problems in their area of concern. They began to compile data and to trace the occurrence of problems with the goal of making systematic changes to reduce their frequency.

Quality Screening/Concurrent Monitoring

Paradoxically, the means by which to interpret the data, the structure-process-outcome relationship, preceded the introduction of concurrent monitoring, by which the data were acquired. In 1984, the JCAHO introduced the quality screening concept,[28] thereby providing the basis for developing a statistically credible quality assessment database.

The foundation of concurrent monitoring is the set of defined quality indicators. These indicators are based on the scope of care and are derived from the service/risk profile that describes the services offered by a specialty and their associated risks (see Fig. 3–1).[29] Quality indicators are based on the

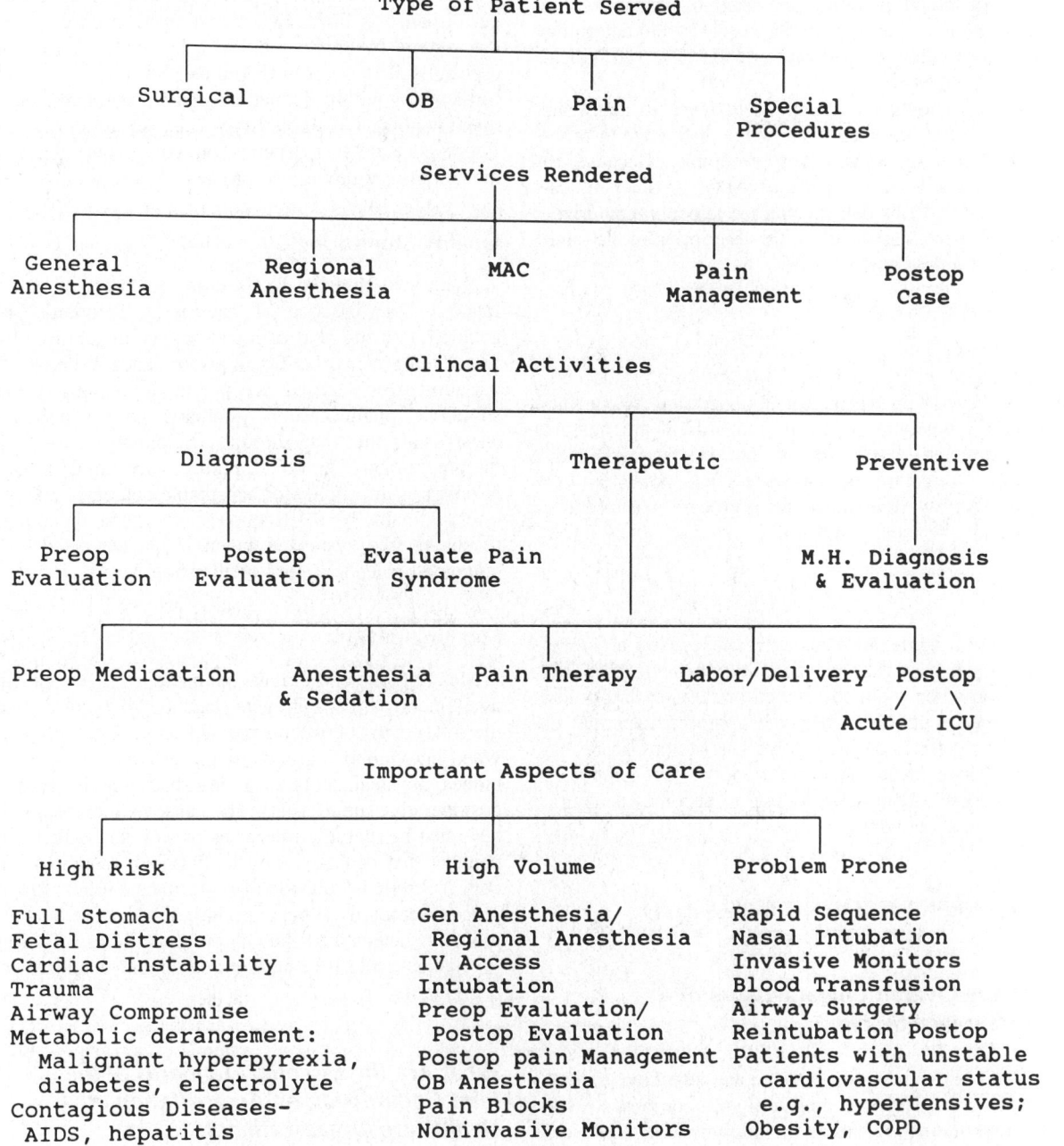

FIGURE 3–1. Risk Service Profile (After Cohen JA: Quality assurance and risk management. *In* Manual of Complications in Anesthesia. Gravenstein N (ed). JB Lippincott, 1991, pp 1–44.)

risks, as well as demographic and administrative cohort groupings (Fig. 3–2).[29] Each patient is screened for the occurrence of the defined indicators according to predefined criteria.[30]

Quality indicators are usually adverse patient outcomes (APOs), but they may also be positive occurrences. Generic indicators include cohort groupings such as anesthetic type or ASA physical status. The criteria (e.g., acceptable upper and lower limits of blood pressure) are used to determine the occurrence of an indicator. Other criteria are used to determine the severity, preventability, and cause of the observed indicator.

Data for each patient are combined to form an aggregate database that can be tabulated to show the difference in problems between corresponding cohort groupings. Because all patients are screened, the incidence of APOs or other indicators can be trended. If the data are entered into a computerized database, a powerful, statistically valid description of the quality indicators of a department results.

Limitations

The usefulness of this database is limited only by the definition of the criteria on which it is founded and by the fact that it is largely outcome driven. If standards of practice are used to develop indicators, process can also be tracked directly. However, direct tracking of process indicators is limited in medicine by the various outcomes a process may produce in a heterogeneous patient population.

Advantages

Ultimately, the aggregate database can be used to assess quality in a statistically valid manner and to provide a rational basis for action when problems exceed predefined thresholds. Further, action can be directed at the appropriate patient or provider cohort. Effectiveness of corrective action can be detected as a change in the incidence of those problems (i.e., improved outcome). Long-term follow-up becomes a natural result of continuous trending.

CURRENT GROUND RULES AND IMPLEMENTATION

What Are the Overall Characteristics of a Quality Assurance System?

QA activities must primarily evaluate and affect the practice of anesthesiologists. They can do so only if a consensus exists among the practitioners regarding the appropriateness of techniques, standards of practice, and expected outcomes. They must be structured broadly enough to detect most of the objectives and problems generic to the practice of anesthesiology. To achieve this goal, QA must continuously assess readily verifiable indicators of care relating to daily practice. This assessment should be reasonable and relate to accepted definitions of appropriate practice. The assessment of the frequency of problems, their degree of preventability and appropriateness of treatment, and their distribution among cohorts (e.g., patient, provider, location) should lead to actions that improve outcome. Improved outcome should be evident from subsequent QA data.

Industrial Quality Control Methodology

Most of the objectives of QA/I in medicine parallel those in industrial quality control. The industrial model of statistical quality control discussed previously is largely applicable.[4] In industry, variation is an expected part of all processes. It results from the way in which the system is defined and taught and how and which support equipment is used. Individual performance is limited by variation engendered primarily by the system, by chance, and to a lesser extent by individuals, especially if they are well trained. So long as individual performance is within defined acceptable standards, outcome remains within predictable limits (i.e., the system is in control). Improved outcome depends on continuous small improvements in the structure and process of the system.

Quality Monitoring

Quality monitoring focuses on indicators of outcome that relate to the practice of anesthesia. Standards should be adopted with the goal of improving predictability of outcome by reducing the variability in performance. When performance variation goes beyond acceptable limits, improvement first should be sought through systematic changes in the process of anesthesia rather than through disciplinary actions directed at the practitioners. To do so, performance limits must be stated in terms of thresholds for acceptable outcome. This process is often definable by the frequency of adverse outcomes. Action to change the system is taken if the frequency of adverse outcomes exceeds agreed-on threshold levels.

Meaningful Data

Meaningful action must be based on a statistically valid assessment of the aggregate database. It requires analysis of the differences between expected and actual outcome, subdivided into cohort groups (e.g., providers, anesthetic techniques, physical status, locations, discharge destinations, acute postoperative monitoring). The cause of the observed disparities must be identified in terms of structure and process components that can be changed. Provider behavior is modified only if it remains outside of performance limits. The modified process/standards should produce a reduction in preventable problems detected by the QA program. The monitoring-analysis-change cycle is continual and should result in steady improvement.

What Are the Essential Standards of the Joint Commission on Accreditation of Healthcare Organizations?

The principles promulgated by the JCAHO for focusing on priority issues have been outlined in the last several AMHs. They are similar to those principles described earlier (Table 3–1) and were later expanded into the so-called 10-step process (Table 3–2). A specific person, usually the departmental chairman, is responsible for monitoring and evaluation of quality.

The QA process is based on an understanding of the scope of care and those important aspects from which specific quality indicators are developed. Action is taken when established thresholds are exceeded in order to correct the systematically identified problems. The quality indicator data-gathering proc-

```
CLINICAL QUALITY ASSURANCE PEER REVIEW AUDIT
(Return form with anesthesia record to OR desk.
Do not make copies.  Do not attach to patient record.)


Date        _____          Pre op:  [ ] Complete
OR#         _____                   [ ] Completed in OR (e.g., labs)
Operation   _____                   [ ] Incomplete (explain below)
ASA Class   _____                   [ ] Made by another anesthetist
                                        [ ] Plan changed (explain below)

Anesthetic [ ] General    [ ] Regional    [ ] MAC
Anesthesiologist _____   Anesthesiology Resident _____
Surgeon _____     Surgery Resident _____
Recovery Room Nurse _____     Discharge:[ ] ONR [ ] ICU [ ] Ward [ ] Home


[ ] NO UNTOWARD EVENTS               [ ] UNTOWARD EVENTS (check below)


OR RR      Airway                  OR RR      Respiratory
_ _  Chipped tooth/loosened tooth  _ _  Post op ventilatory assistance
_ _  Stridor, Laryngospasm, Obstruction         (unplanned)
_ _  Failed rapid sequence induction _ _  Significant Hypoxemia/hypercapnia
_ _  Nose bleed or other trauma of airway _ _  Pneumothorax
_ _  Inability to intubate by route _ _  Inappropriate bronchial
        originally planned                      intubation
_ _  Esophageal intubation         _ _  Aspiration-respiratory
_ _  Lip trauma                             distress syndrome
_ _  Accidental extubation         _ _  Reintubation (other than accidental
                                            extubation)
            CV                     _ _  Bronchospasm
_ _  Death
_ _  Cardiac arrest                         Miscellaneous
_ _  Significant Hypertension (sustained  _ _  Other (describe below)
        >30% above preop systolic)  _ _  Hyperpyrexia >38 C
_ _  Significant Hypotension (sustained  _ _  Hypothermia <34 C (uninduced)
        <30% below preop diastolic)  _ _  Wrong medication/dose given
_ _  Significant Bradycardia (30% below         (describe below)
        preop or that associated with  _ _  Drug reaction (allergic/adverse)
        hypotension)                _ _  Intravascular line problem
_ _  Significant Tachycardia (30% above  _ _  Delayed or erroneous lab report/other
        preop or that associated with  _ _  Nausea and vomiting
        hypertension)               _ _  Equipment failure (explain below)
_ _  Myocardial ischemia/MI suspected  _ _  Pain medication delayed/inadequate
_ _  Congestive heart failure/pulmonary edema
_ _  Dysrhythmia associated with one or  Regional (including pain therapy)
        more of above              _ _  Pain unresponsive to block
                                   _ _  Failed block, inadequate block
        Discharge planning         _ _  Toxic reaction
_  Unplanned outpatient admission  _ _  Excessive block (high spinal)
_  Unplanned transfer to ICU       _ _  Wet tap (epidural)
_  Unplanned return to OR
_  Unscheduled ONR                         Neurological
_  > 3 hr. stay in RR              _ _  Prolonged neuromuscular block
_  Delayed waiting for M.D. to evaluate  _ _  Prolonged sedation
_  Delayed waiting for X-ray       _ _  Peripheral nerve injury
_  Delayed waiting for Room        _ _  Stroke
_  Delayed for medical reasons     _ _  Recall
_  Other delay (explain below)     _ _  Seizure
                                   _ _  Other damage (explain below)

For each of the above, describe briefly on back:

Event location   [ ] OR        [ ] RR

A)  Cause of Event
B)  Treatment of Event
C)  Result of Treatment
```

FIGURE 3–2. Example of a QA report form. (After Cohen JA: Quality assurance and risk management. *In* Manual of Complications in Anesthesia. Gravenstein N (ed). JB Lippincott, 1991, pp 1–44.)

TABLE 3–1. The Joint Commission on Accreditation of Healthcare Organizations Method for Focusing on Priority Issues

Identification of important aspects of care
Measurable indicators to monitor these care aspects
Evaluation of care when thresholds are reached
Action taken to correct problems
Assessment of effectiveness of actions
Systematic, ongoing, routine collection of data
    For each patient
    For each provider

ess is ongoing and is used to assess the effectiveness of changes. All providers are regularly informed of the findings and actions of the QA program.

During the past decade, the JCAHO has incorporated vast amounts of QA theory into its accreditation manual. Appendix I abstracts the portions of that manual[11] currently applicable to anesthesiology departments; the wording in the AMH is followed closely. The elements of structure, process, and outcome described by Donabedian[11, 19] and the notion of performance limits and quality improvement described by Deming[4, 5] have led to a gradual refinement of the JCAHO theories regarding QA and the rules by which those theories are to be implemented.

The term *quality assurance* has become a liability to the JCAHO, which changed it to *quality assessment* and added *quality improvement.* Interestingly, *quality assessment* was a term in use more than a decade ago by the JCAH and does have the advantage of being value neutral. The QA concept became infused with the notion that it is a method for removing the ''bad apples'' from medicine, with the dubious expectation that medical practice will, therefore, improve.

New Directions

Beginning with the 1992 AMH,[11] the JCAHO initiated a major effort to encourage the application of the principle of continuous quality improvement, a part of the Agenda for Change.[10] The concept of indicators of care and a database derived from the services and risks presented to patients by various services, methods of monitoring, and trending remain largely the same.

Most important in the current AMH is a decrease in the total number of standards and a transfer of some of the standards previously under surgery and anesthesia to the medical

TABLE 3–2. Joint Commission on Accreditation of Healthcare Organizations 10-Step Process

- Assign responsibility for monitoring and evaluation.
- Delineate scope of care provided.
- Identify important aspects of care.
- Identify clinical care indicators.
- Establish thresholds that trigger evaluation.
- Monitor each indicator by collecting ongoing data.
- Evaluate care when thresholds are reached.
- Take actions to correct identified problems.
- Assess effectiveness of actions.
    Improved outcome
    Decreased incidence of problems
    Increased productivity
- Communicate results.

staff and QA sections. Standards affecting anesthesia include the general staff standards for review of surgical and other invasive procedures and blood or blood product use.

Emphasis on continuous improvement rather than solving of isolated nonsystemic problems continues to evolve but appears to be more a philosophic reorientation than a change in methodology. The JCAHO is now emphasizing the problems resulting from the overall process of care and service rather than the performance of individual physicians. The purpose is to provide a means by which continuous quality improvement is possible even when problems are not clearly above threshold levels. Rather than being purely department based, contemporary quality review requires cross-departmental attention to problems that involve patients whose care depends on many different hospital services.

Trending of individual performance is expected to demonstrate quality problems resulting more from flaws in the existing systems rather than individual flaws. However, evaluation of individual performance will remain a secondary objective. Specific requirements are abstracted in Appendix I. (Note: In 1994, significant changes in JCAHO guidelines are anticipated; these changes represent an attempt to integrate hospital-based health care more comprehensively than in the past.)

JOINT COMMISSION ON ACCREDITATION OF HEALTHCARE SURVEY

What Preparations Should Be Made?

The JCAHO survey is voluntary and is paid for by the institution under review. Although passing the JCAHO survey is desirable and prestigious and certifies the institution for Medicare reimbursement, it is not essential and it does not replace state-mandated audits. Some hospitals choose not to endure the rigors of a JCAHO audit to qualify for Medicare, opting instead for a direct audit by the HCFA. The latter organization does not charge for the audit, and the process is somewhat simpler.

Passing the JCAHO survey requires a thorough understanding of the principles applied to the institution/department under review (Table 3–3). Specific examples of how the department interprets and implements the 10-step process are essential. The service risk profile should be available in writing (see Fig. 3–1), as should the indicators derived from it (see Fig. 3–2). The indicators should embrace all of the important aspects of care, including high-risk, high-volume, and problem-prone activities. Thresholds for triggering further review of rate-based indicators and evidence of review of sentinel events should be documented. Specific issues identified and corrected using the QA process should be presented.

The hospital's chief of staff and QA/UR (utilization review) director should be available at the time of the departmental interview. Their presence is supportive and is essential for documenting the interaction of the departmental and hospital QA activities.

The JCAHO survey differs from those conducted by HCFA or the PRO. The JCAHO audit surveys the QA process but does not specifically look at outcome, whereas the PRO/HCFA audits are more intensely focused on outcome. JCAHO audits are voluntary, but the HCFA (Medicare) audit is required if JCAHO accreditation is not obtained.

TABLE 3–3. Joint Commission on Accreditation of Healthcare Organizations Accreditation Survey

Understand the JCAHO Principles
• The 10-step process
• The relation of structure, process, and outcome
• The terminology: APO, generic screen, concurrent monitoring, etc.
• Concept of continuous quality improvement
• Scoring guidelines for specialty—review the AMH
• How your own QA program fulfills JCAHO guidelines
General Guidelines and Nomenclature—Be Ready to Discuss:
• Scope of service
    Risk/service profile (including locations of service)
    Important aspects of care: high-risk, high-volume, problem-prone activities
• Indicators of care/standards for case review
    Sentinel events: always reviewed, e.g., deaths, myocardial infarctions
    Rate-based indicators: reviewed when they exceed pre-established threshold
• Identification of problem issue: a problem with care that you have identified by monitoring
• Actions taken to correct problems in care
• Effective follow-up on corrective actions
• Assistance of chief of staff, QA and UR (utilization review) supervisors
• Regard the surveyor as consultant as well as examiner
Who Does the Review?
• Physicians, nurses, ambulatory care expert, administrator
What Do They Look at in a Nutshell?
• Compliance with the process published in the AMH
• Not a review of outcome per se
What Does the Exit Interview Mean?
• A chance for the chief executive officer to give overall conclusions, list specific issues for possible contingencies
• Open session for staff—educational
How Does JCAHO Differ from PRO/Medicare/HCFA Review?
• Outcome versus process-based review
    Medicare/PRO reviews are based on outcomes
    JCAHO review is based on compliance with QA process
• Voluntary versus mandatory
    JCAHO voluntary
    Medicare audit mandatory for payment if no JCAHO certification obtained
• Reviewers
    JCAHO: physician review
    HCFA/PRO: nurse screening
• Objectives
    JCAHO: institution-oriented quality improvement
    PRO: institutional/practitioner penalties, denial of payment

Abbreviations: APO = adverse patient outcome; AMH = Accreditation Manual for Hospitals; QA = quality assurance; JCAHO = Joint Commission on Accreditation of Healthcare Organizations; PRO = Professional Review Organization; HCFA = Health Care Financing Administration.

QUALITY ASSURANCE IN ANESTHESIA PRACTICE

How Can It Work Efficiently?

The principles discussed in this chapter are more easily implemented in anesthesiology than in many other areas of medicine. The data-driven nature of anesthesiology, coupled with an organized way of recording that data, facilitates the maintenance of an aggregate database. The highly focused scope of care and well-defined expectations easily translate into standards of practice and an accepted set of quality indicators. In a way, QA programs in anesthesiology are prototypical of what is likely to develop in other areas of medicine as their activities become more precisely defined.

Ongoing Measurement

At the foundation of improvement is an ongoing measurement of the state of affairs. A summary of the steps used in our institution is outlined in Table 3–4. Quality indicators should be collected on all patients and combined to form an aggregate database. This can be done most easily by attaching an indicator form to the anesthesia record (see Fig. 3–2). The form can be completed by the anesthesia provider during the case and passed on to the postanesthesia care unit staff for their additions. A short summary of the cause, treatment, and result of treatment facilitates the assessment of problem cases without the need to perform a detailed chart review. The finished forms should be deposited in a central location for collection. Other forms can facilitate postoperative follow-up (Fig. 3–3).

Computerized Data Entry

After being checked for completeness, the information can be entered into a computerized database. This process is not absolutely necessary, but cross-tabulation of data, division of data into cohort groupings, and frequency calculations can be automated with appropriate software. Hand calculation is not only time-consuming but also requires marked constriction of the data analysis to be affordable. By contrast, software is consistently accurate, does not receive a salary, takes no coffee breaks, and has no personal agenda.

TABLE 3–4. Guide to Data Collection and Entry

1. Use a QA report form such as that in Figure 3–2 to document basic demographic data and adverse events.
2. Make sure that the providers know how to fill out the form and that they understand how to fill out the description of events section. These descriptions enable the QA review officer to assess and code events without reviewing each medical record.
3. Attach the QA report form to the anesthesia record or billing form so that the providers do not have to look for it separately. This maximizes ease of compliance.
4. Provide a single central location for the QA forms. Keeping them with the billing form or the department's copy of the anesthesia record works quite well. If you collect the operative data, you need to designate a location for postoperative evaluation forms.
5. Make sure that a QA form is filled out for each case.
   Cross-check the QA forms against the OR log daily and make sure that missing data are obtained promptly.
6. Enter the data into the database or import it from another source, such as the billing database.
7. Code incomplete entries. Use the database to summarize incomplete QA reports to track incomplete forms. Recode incomplete to complete when the record is corrected (completed).
8. Separate the QA forms without adverse events from the others. Give the forms with events to the QA officer for assessment (coding and narrative summary) of each of the events. The QA officer should number and code each event, indicate if further audit is necessary, and write a brief narrative summary. For efficiency, you may restrict the narratives to the records with at least one code-2 event.
9. Collect the coded forms and enter the assessment codes and narrative comments on the database. Code the audits as pending (P) on the database. This allows you to use the database to produce the summary of audited cases. Use this report to help you when ordering medical records for auditing.
10. Submit the medical records for further audit to the QA officer when available and type in the case review audit reports.
11. Transcribe the case review audits and enter any resulting changes in the database. Change the audit code from pending (P) to audited (A).
12. Use the database software to generate the reports.

Abbreviations: QA = quality assurance; OR = operating room.

DEPARTMENT OF ANESTHESIOLOGY   NAME:

FORM TYPE 1
POST-OP ANESTHESIA EVALUATION   MEDICAL RECORD NUMBER:

Postoperative Diagnosis: Post op day: #

Operation: surgery:	Anesthetic:	Anesthesiologist: [G] [R] [M]	Resident:	Date of

Postoperative Notes:

	Y	N	COMMENTS
Sore Throat			
Drug Reaction			
Nausea/Vomiting			
Muscle Pain			
Respiratory Distress			
Nerve Injury			
Stroke			
Headache			
Recall			
CV Instability			
Cardiac Arrest			
M. I.			
Death			
Organ Failure			
Escalation of Care			
Other			

RECOMMENDATIONS:

Physicians signature:

Date:_____ Time:_____

FIGURE 3–3. Example of a postoperative report form.

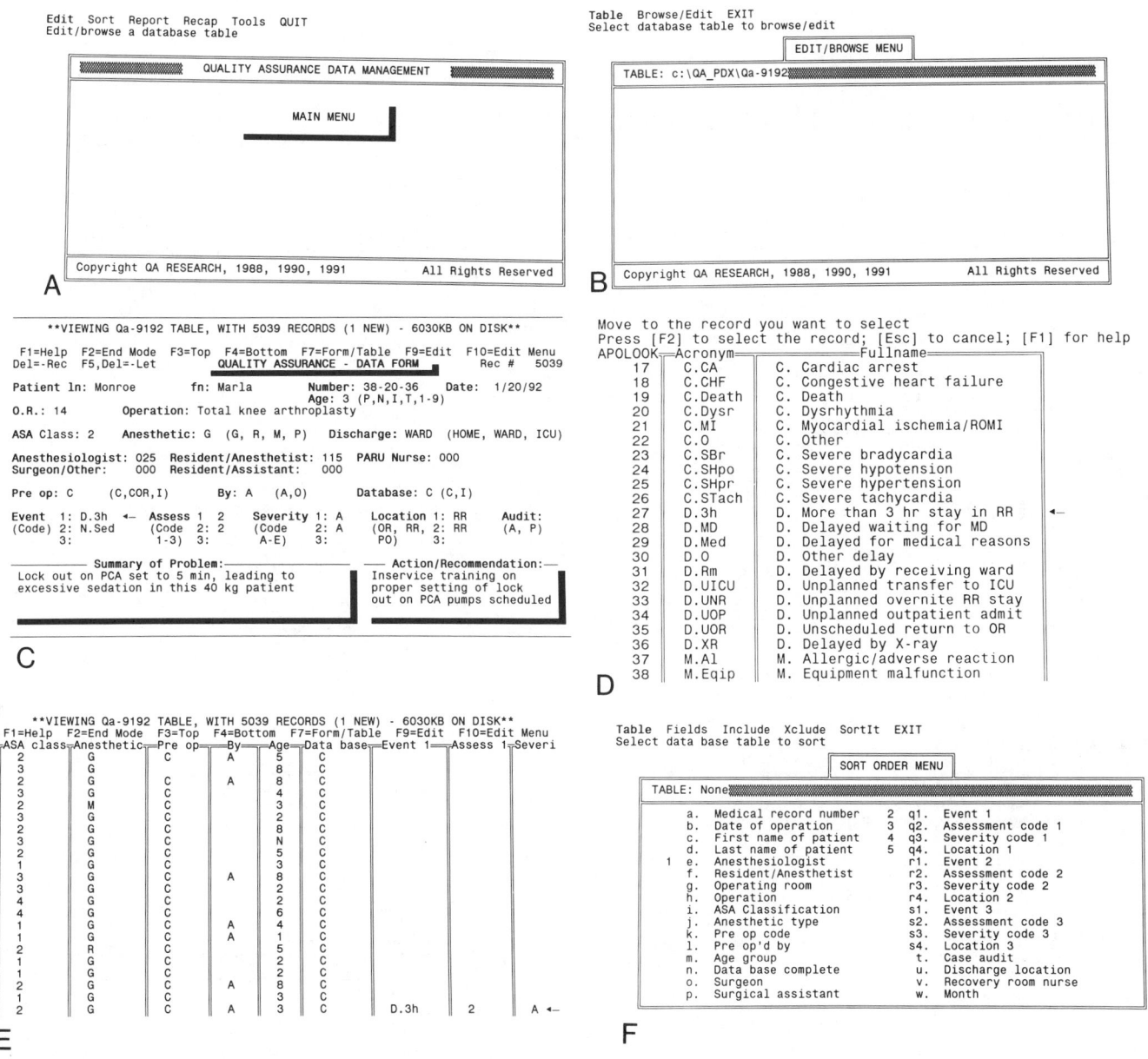

FIGURE 3–4. Examples of the appearance of a computerized database (Courtesy of QA RESEARCH, Gainesville, FL.)

A, The MAIN MENU provides access to all of the system menus. These menus are listed on the top line of the display. Pressing the Enter key selects the highlighted selection. An explanation of the highlighted selection appears on the second line. **Q**UIT causes the system to exit properly to DOS.

B, The EDIT/BROWSE MENU provides access to QA database tables and to the system's data entry and editing functions. **B**rowse/edit displays the data entry form for the data table chosen with **T**able.

C, Data are entered on the form to the left. The first line of the form displays the database table name, size, number of new records added, and the remaining memory on the current directory's disk. The second line displays frequently used functions. The third line displays, to the far left, the purpose of the **D**el key when in the Edit mode (this area is otherwise blank) and, to the far right, the current record number. Data are entered onto the body of the form. Narrative comments may be entered into the two fields at the bottom of the form.

D, Pressing the **F**1 key in the edit mode while the cursor is in one of the "Event" fields displays the lookup table (to the right) containing all of the adverse event acronyms and their full names. Pressing **F**2 copies the acronym from the line on which the cursor is located.

E, The **F**7 key toggles the display between the form and table views. The table view displays more records but fewer fields at any given time. Data can be viewed from the table view but neither entered nor edited. The table columns can be rearranged using the column rotate (Ctrl R) function. The **F**10 key terminates editing or viewing and displays the EDIT/BROWSE MENU. The **F**3/**F**4 keys toggle between the comment field and other fields.

F, The SORT ORDER MENU provides access to the functions used to select a database table and re-sort the display. **T**able selects the database to be sorted, and **F**ields displays prompts for setting the sort order. **I**nclude or **X**clude can be used to restrict sorting to a subset of the database. **S**ort initiates the sort and displays the sorted data in the same manner as the EDIT/BROWSE MENU functions, except that the sorted table may be printed. **E**xit saves all settings and returns the display to the MAIN MENU.

Illustration continued on following page

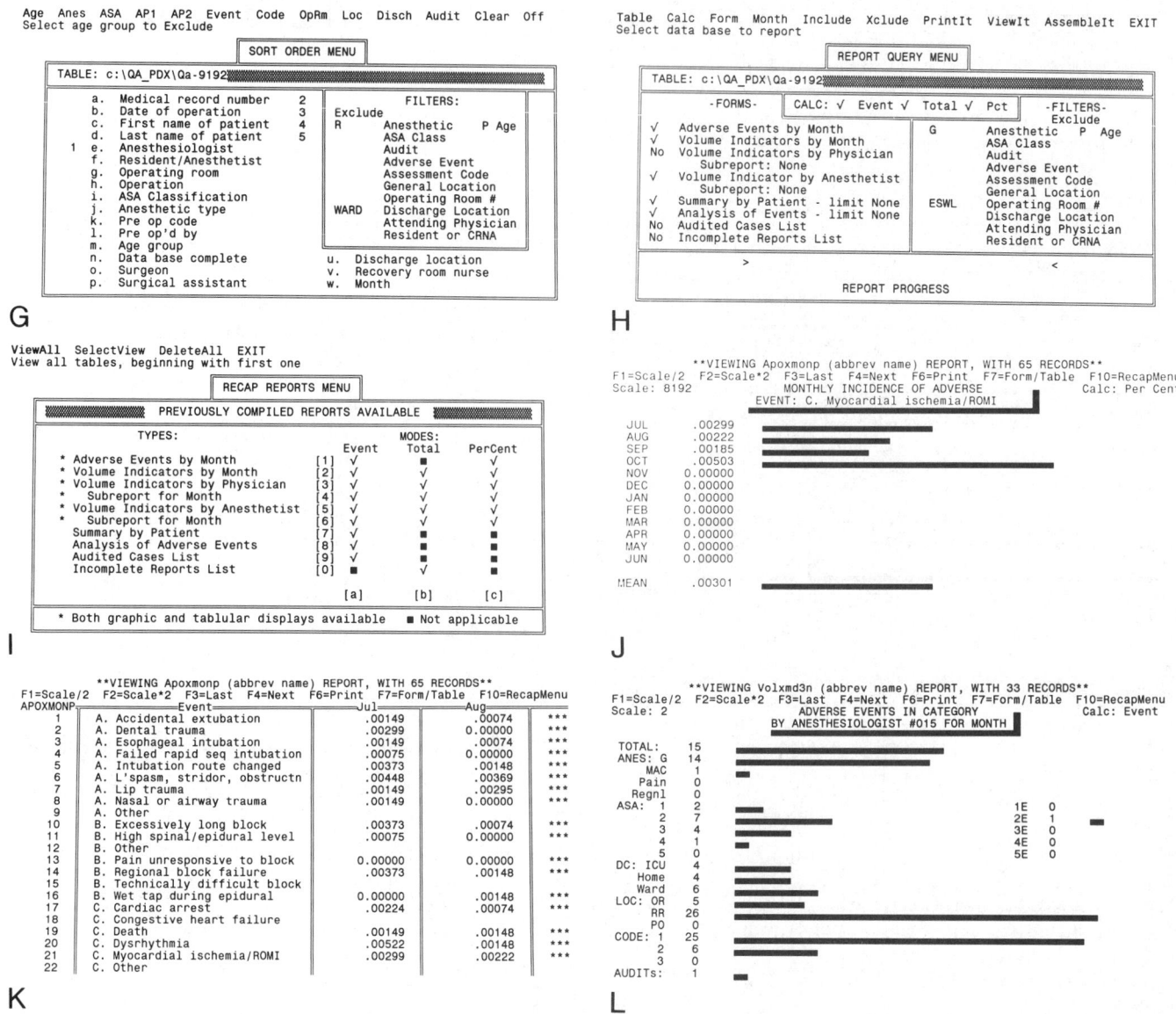

FIGURE 3–4 *Continued G*, Pressing **I**nclude or **X**clude displays the filters listed on the first line of the display. The filters selected are displayed in the drop down window. Filters can be turned **O**ff without loosing the settings. As with sorting, **I**nclude and **X**clude may be used to restrict a report's data to a subset of the database.

H, The REPORT QUERY MENU provides access to the systems's report functions. The primary menu choices, which are displayed on the first line to the left, provide access to the submenus (capitalized in the boxes of the menu) that are used to configure and select reports. **E**xit saves all settings and returns the display to the MAIN MENU.

I, The RECAP REPORTS MENU provides access to previously compiled reports. Any or all reports may be viewed: **S**elect**V**iew displays the selected report (1a–0c), whereas **V**iew**A**ll places all of the existing reports in memory. The existing reports are indicated by the checkmarks. The system replaces an old report each time one is compiled, resulting in a set of reports that can differ in age. **D**elete**A**ll clears *all* old reports. **E**xit returns the display to the MAIN MENU.

J, A recap of a report, located in position ''1c'' on the RECAP REPORTS MENU, is shown to the left. The principal display controls are displayed on the second line. The display consists of a window (middle of third line) that shows the event displayed. The data are presented numerically and in the form of bar graphs by column item. PgUp and PgDn toggle between column items. **F**1 and **F**2 adjust the relative scale of the bar graph. The scale selected is shown on the third line at the far left. The calculation mode is shown on the third line at the far right.

K, **F**7 toggles the view between the graphic form and the tabular display. As with the other tabular displays, the columns may be rearranged. The report may be reprinted, as shown below in the Example Reports section, by pressing **F**6.

L, A recap of a report appears to the left. As with the other recap displays, a description of the report and the row (in the printed report) that is displayed is shown in the window in the middle of the third and fourth lines. The report (printed) column labels are displayed along the right margin, with the data and graphic display to the right.

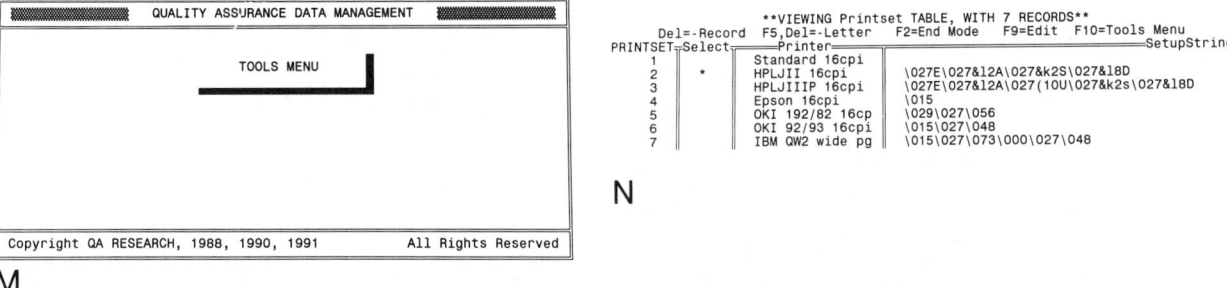

```
New  Copy  Del  Merge  Rename  Import  LookupEdit  Printer  SetPath  Pak  EXIT
Create a new data table in directory c:\QA_PDX\
```

FIGURE 3–4 *Continued M*, The TOOLS MENU provides access to the file, lookup table, data import, and printer management functions shown on the top line of the display. Further instructions are given after a particular tool is selected. **E**xit returns the display to the MAIN MENU.

N, Selecting **P**rinter from the main menu displays the screen shown to the left. Entering an asterisk in the "Select" column selects the printer. Printers may be added as needed by entering their names and setup stings. **F**10 saves the settings and returns to the TOOLS MENU. The current settings are displayed each time the system starts.

The computerized database shown in the examples (Fig. 3–4) can import data from other computer databases; trend volume and quality indicators by month or provider; trend adverse event indicators by month; filter and sort the data; display reports graphically or print tabular reports; and provide various summary reports including adverse event assessments and recommendations (Fig. 3–5). It can calculate indicators for the entire patient population, those with events, or the percentage of patients with events. Database software like this are commercially available and range in price from $2000, such as the one illustrated, to $15,000. A guide to selecting QA software appears in Appendix II at the end of this chapter.

Responsive Action

The trended data form the basis for actions taken to reduce the observed incidence of problems. Other data contribute to the decision to take action, such as the evaluation of sentinel events or referrals from other departments or the hospital QA committee or other quality-monitoring committees, such as pharmacy, blood use, or infection control. The relevant findings should be reviewed monthly and summarized in a report or minutes (Fig. 3–6). Effective actions should produce a decrease in the observed problem indicators.

How Important Are Normalized Data?

Use of normalized data to compute QA statistics is essential for valid inferences. The probability that the analysis of QA data will lead to actions that improve the quality of care is critically dependent on the quality of the data. Conclusions may be erroneous if the problems and cohort groupings of the patients with adverse events (numerator) are evaluated without respect to the total population at risk. However, when problems in the numerator are divided by the total population in the corresponding denominator, the relative distribution of the data, hence the conclusions, may change. The relationship of incidence of adverse events to total number of adverse events within cohorts is often poor.[31]

Use of non-normalized data to point to the source of problems among providers is inaccurate because of the wide disparities in case load. The distribution of totals grossly distorts the apparent relative occurrence of common events. Providers who have a heavy case load often have a higher total number but much lower incidence of adverse events than those who perform fewer anesthetics.

The apparent increase in gross problem rates associated with increasing ASA physical status ranking among patients undergoing regional anesthesia is apparent only from the incidence statistics alone, not from the enumeration of totals. The influence of physical status on the gross adverse event rate is similarly obscured by evaluating the numerator alone. Thus, the numerators of care (total numbers of events) must always be analyzed in relationship to the denominators of care that provide the context in which these events occur. Otherwise, meaningless statistics may lead to spurious efforts to improve quality.

What Are the Pitfalls?

The major pitfall in any QA program is consistent reporting of data. Until fully automated methods that acquire data directly from monitoring systems[32] become common and cost less than $20,000 per operating room, provider-generated reports will still be essential. To avoid resistance engendered by the additional time needed to fill out a quality audit, a succinct check-off form should be used. Demographic data can be imported from existing databases to avoid unnecessarily encumbering anesthetists.

To avoid inaccuracies caused by fear of self-reporting, providers must participate in the development of the QA program, including the standards of practice, development of indicators, and ground rules for assessment of data. Confidentiality of data must be absolute. Appropriate resources, such as a personal computer and one part-time clerk must be provided.

At least one department member must take charge of the system and be willing to spend 3 to 4 hours a week evaluating the data and occasionally reviewing cases that represent severe problems. Finally, meaningful improvements in the structure and process of practice must result in improved outcome, or the entire QA system will degenerate into a meaningless pantomime.

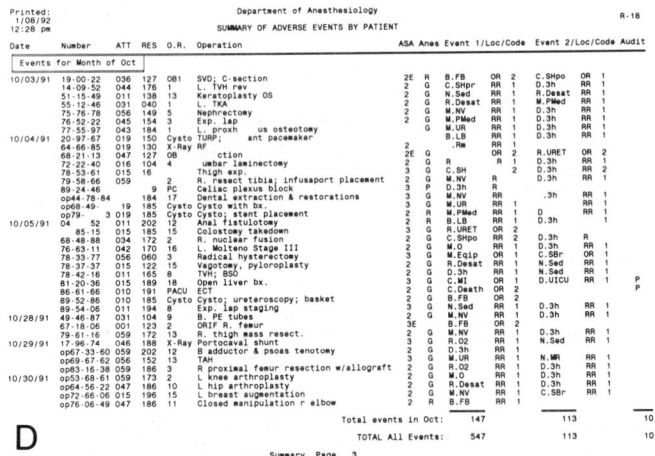

FIGURE 3–5. Examples of printouts of various reports. Note that the data used to illustrate the appearance of the reports do not represent actual findings. *A*, Sample printout of incidence of events trended by month. *B*, Sample printout of incidence of volume indicators trended by month. *C*, Sample printout of incidence of indicators trended by anesthesiologist. *D*, Sample printout of event summary. *E*, Sample printout of event analysis.

REPORTING PERIOD: *month, year*
DEPARTMENT: *Anesthesiology*

Minutes
Quality Assurance Committee
DEPARTMENT OF ANESTHESIOLOGY

Meeting Date:

Meeting Called to Order at:

Meeting Place:

Those who were required to be **present** and were (listed alphabetically):

Those who were required to be present but were **absent** (listed alphabetically):

Old Business:

Follow up on referrals/issues from the following:

Medical Staff Monitors (concurrent generic monitors):

Blood Utilization (transfusion practice):

Medical Records:

Surgical Case Review:

Unscheduled Ambulatory Admissions:

Pharmacy and Therapeutics:

Infection Control:

Other referrals:

A   Other:

FIGURE 3–6. Example of QA report/minutes.

Illustration continued on following page

<u>New Business</u>:

<u>Medical Staff Monitors and referrals for the month of</u>:

    1. Volume: Total cases __. See also Volume Indicator Reports

    2. Quality Review:

        a. General Summary:

            1) General Review/Analysis - See also Analysis of Adverse Events Report

            2) Generic trends by month and provider - See also Adverse Event by Month Reports

        b. Case Reviews - internal and external referrals (next pages)

<u>Utilization Review Referrals</u>:

<u>Blood Utilization (transfusion practice)</u>:

<u>Medical Records</u>:

<u>Surgical Case Review</u>:

<u>Unscheduled Ambulatory Admissions</u>:

<u>Pharmacy and Therapeutics</u>:

<u>Infection Control</u>:

<u>Other referrals</u>:

<u>Other</u>:

Meeting adjourned at:

B   _____   _____
       Chairman, Quality Assurance Committee   Chairman, Department of
           Department of Anesthesiology   Anesthesiology

FIGURE 3–6 *Continued*

References

1. Cohen JA: Quality assurance initiatives. Probl Anest 1991; 5:277.
2. American Society of Anesthesiologists: Workshop on quality assurance, San Francisco. Park Ridge, IL, ASA, 1988.
3. American Society of Anesthesiologists: Workshop on quality assurance, Milwaukee. Park Ridge, IL, ASA, 1991.
4. Deming W: Out of the Crisis. Cambridge, Massachusetts Institute for Advanced Engineering Studies, 1986, pp 484–485.
5. Walton M: The Deming Management Method. Chicago, Putnam, 1986.
6. Anonymous: What is the safest anesthetic? JAMA 1887; 8:520.
7. Codman EA: A Study in Hospital Efficiency. Boston, Thomas Todd, 1918.
8. Donabedian A: The quality of medical care: methods for assessing and monitoring the quality of care for research and quality assurance programs. Science 1978; 200:856.
9. Bogdanich W: Small comfort: Prized by hospitals, accreditation hides perils patients face. Wall Street Journal 212(12):A1,A12, October 12, 1988.
10. Joint Commission on the Accreditation of Health Organizations: Task forces lay groundwork for new survey process. *In* Agenda for Change Update. Vol. 1, No. 1. Chicago, JCAHO, 1987, pp 1–6.
11. Joint Commission on Accreditation of Healthcare Organizations: Accreditation Manual for Hospitals. Chicago, JCAHO, 1992.
12. Holoweiko M: What cookbook medicine will mean for you. Medical Economics 1989; 66:118.
13. Lohr KN: Institute of Medicine (IOM) study urges a major shift in QA strategy. QA Review 1990; 2:1.
14. Darling vs. Charleston Community Hospital, 1965.
15. Johnson vs. Misericordia Community Hospital, 1981.
16. Patrick vs. Burger, 800 F2d 1498 [9th Cir.] [1986].
17. Battelle Human Affairs Research Center: Study Coordinators Manual—ASA/CDC Anesthesia Mortality and Morbidity Study. Washington, DC, Battelle, 1988.
18. Eichhorn JW: Quality Assurance in Anesthesiology in International Anesthesia Research Society 1989 Review Course Lectures. Lake Buena Vista, March, 1989, pp 36–42.
19. Donabedian A: Evaluating the quality of medical care. Milbank Mem Fund Q 1966; 44:166.
20. Eichhorn JH, Cooper JB, Cullen DJ, et al: Anesthesia practice standards at Harvard: a review. J Clin Anesth 1988; 1:55.
21. Eichhorn JH, Cooper JB, Cullen DJ: Standards for patient monitoring during anesthesia at the Harvard medical school. JAMA 1986; 256:1017.
22. Polk RE, Healy DP, Schwartz LB, et al: Vancomycin and the red-man syndrome: pharmacodynamics of histamine release. J Infect Dis 1988; 157:502.
23. Schroeder SA, Kabcenall AI: Do bad outcomes mean substandard care? (Editorial). JAMA 1991; 265:1995.
24. Blumberg MS: Biased estimates of expected acute myocardial infarction mortality using MedisGroups admission severity groups. JAMA 1991; 265:2965.
25. Caplan RA, Posner KL, Cheney FW: Effect of outcome on physician judgements of appropriateness of care. JAMA 1991; 265:1957.
26. Ferrante J: What can medical sociologists say about clinical outcome measurements? Am J Public Health 1978; 77:1155.
27. Brown E: Quality assurance in anesthesiology—the problem-oriented audit. Anesth Analg 1984; 63:611.
28. Joint Commission on Accreditation of Healthcare Organizations: Accreditation Manual for Hospitals. Chicago, JCAHO, 1984.
29. Cohen JA: Quality assurance and risk management. *In* Manual of Complications in Anesthesia. Gravenstein N (ed). Philadelphia, JB Lippincott, 1991, pp 1–44.
30. Roberts JS, Walczak RM: Toward effective quality assurance: the evolution and current status of the JCAH standard. QRB Qual Rev Bull 8:11, 1984.
31. Cohen JA: Normalizing data improves quality assurance inference. Anesthesiology 1992; 77:A1099.
32. Edsall DW: Quality assessment with a computerized anesthesia information management system (AIMS). Qual Rev Q 1991; June:182.

Appendix I
Abstract of 1992 JCAHO Accreditation Manual for Hospitals

The relevant portions of the 1992 AMH[11] are abstracted below. Significant changes to these portions are anticipated in 1994. The wording, when relevant, and intent are preserved as closely as possible.

Section MS—Medical Staff. Of interest, clinical privileges referred to in this section are defined as "permission to provide medical or other patient care services in the granting institution, within well-defined limits based on the individual's professional license and his or her experience, competence, and judgment." This wording implies that the granting of clinical privileges includes the right to use the facility but does not specifically say so, but it does note that the medical staff is to be governed by specific written bylaws, rules, and regulations of the medical staff and of the hospital. In this system, each clinical department is responsible for developing its own criteria for recommending specialty privileges. Whatever the mechanism is for granting privileges, they are related to the individuals' experience in categories of treatment or procedures, the results of treatment, and the conclusions drawn from quality assessment and improvement activities, when available. Board certification is considered to be a benchmark but not essential. **Section MS.5** delineates the responsibilities of the medical staff for continuous quality improvement. This section is very similar to that previously noted in the AMH. Specifically, important problems in patient care are to be identified and resolved, and areas that can be improved are to be improved. A review of all invasive procedures is conducted monthly, the purpose being to improve the appropriateness and effectiveness of these procedures.

Procedures that require review are most importantly those that are performed very commonly, have high risk, or are suspected or known to be problem prone. This is an old concept, now applied specifically to invasive procedures. This type of review is to be made in a systematic manner and with a view to helping improve the performance of individuals who are having problems.

The exact intent of applying this to invasive procedure and anesthesia is not spelled out in the AMH. Specific areas of evaluation of patient care with respect to invasive procedures include (1) selection of the appropriate procedure, (2) preparation of patients for the procedure, (3) performance of the procedure and monitoring of patients during the procedure, and (4) post-procedure care.

Drug use evaluation is specifically spelled out in the current AMH and is aimed at an ongoing criteria-based process designed to improve the effectiveness of drug use. Included are (1) evaluation of the appropriateness of medications prescribed, (2) appropriate preparation dispensing of medication, (3) appropriate administration, and (4) monitoring of medication effects.

Similarly, review of blood and blood component administration is mandated in order to make sure that (1) appropriate blood components are ordered, (2) their distribution and dispensing are appropriate, (3) they are given in an appropriate manner, and (4) the effects of blood and blood component administration are appropriately monitored. Specific criteria for the administration of blood are conspicuously absent. Review is limited to components that are used in high volume, pose a substantial risk, and are known or thought to be potentially problematic. As is the JCAHO tradition, specifics are absent.

Section QA—Quality Assessment and Improvement. Quality is now defined as that which increases the probability of a desired outcome. Emphasis is now more patient based than physician or service based. The overall thrust of this change is to try to deal with the multiple inter-related problems within an institution instead of attributing them to individual physicians. In order to implement these changes, the JCAHO now requires the administrative organizational leaders to undergo specific education in quality improvement.

Monitoring of the quality of care is done on a department-by-department basis and includes the identification, as usual, of the important aspects of care. The most important aspects of care are considered to be those that occur frequently and affect large numbers of patients who are hospitalized where care is not properly provided or is provided when not properly indicated. In-depth evaluation of particular care problems is indicated when important single events or a pattern of problems exists. This requirement is not a departure from previous JCAHO guidelines. New is the encouragement to initiate improvement or changes in policy to improve overall performance.

The current guidelines mandate peer review when analysis of care provided by an individual practitioner is being considered. Conspicuously absent is the use of the JCAHO 10-step process. This process has been incorporated but not identified, as such, into the current guidelines. The concept that someone in the department must be in charge of quality review, that a systematic means of using indicators to assess quality must be in place, and of taking action when possible has not changed. The need to monitor the effectiveness of action and the need to document the success of the actions are also unchanged.

SA—Surgical and Anesthesia Services. This section is abstracted in somewhat greater detail than those preceding.

SA1.2. The care of patients who receive surgical and anesthesia services is the responsibility of *licensed independent practitioners with appropriate clinical privileges.*

SA1.3.1.2.1. Except in extreme emergencies, surgery is to be performed only after an appropriate history, physical examination, and any indicated laboratory and x-ray examinations have been completed.

SA1.4. Organized anesthesia services are directed by a physician member of the medical staff with appropriate clinical and administrative experience. This individual makes recommendations regarding clinical privileges of all licensed independent practitioners and personally provides or provides through his or her designee(s) the formulation of mechanisms

and material to help provide uniform quality of anesthesia services throughout the hospital. These mechanisms include means to ensure that anesthesia services are consistent with patients' needs and the current standards of practice, the type and amount of physical resources necessary for administering anesthesia and providing resuscitative measures, and approaches to monitor and evaluate effectively the quality of anesthesia care provided by individuals in *any* department, including ambulatory care, dental, emergency, obstetric, psychiatric, special care, and special procedures units within a hospital.

Guidelines must be developed to include those for administering general anesthesia with an anesthesia machine, the use of safety devices including but not limited to oxygen analyzers, pressure and disconnect alarms, PIN index safety systems, gas-scavenging systems, and oxygen pressure interlock systems.

It also appears that the chief of anesthesia services is responsible for not only policies related to the giving of anesthetics by an anesthesiologist but also the administration of anesthesia in other departments as well as the hospital's cardiopulmonary resuscitation program (SA1.4.1.2.6.3).

A preanesthetic evaluation is mandated for every patient for whom anesthesia is contemplated (note the language). It includes gathering sufficient information to formulate an anesthetic plan intelligently. Objective diagnostic data, an interview with the patient, and a discussion of his or her medical, anesthetic, and drug history, as well as a review of his or her physical status, are required. It also includes a determination that the patient is an appropriate candidate for the anesthetic planned. Before the induction of anesthesia, this determination must be made by a licensed independent practitioner with appropriate clinical privileges.

Immediately before the induction of anesthesia, patients must be re-evaluated, and equipment, drugs, and gas supplies checked. Patients must be appropriately monitored during anesthesia. Documentation is required for monitoring, dosage of all drugs and agents used, the type and amounts of fluids administered including blood and blood products, the technique or techniques used, unusual events during the anesthetic period, and the status of patients at the conclusion of anesthesia.

A patient's postoperative status is evaluated on admission to and from the postanesthesia recovery room (PARR). Documentation includes vital signs and level of consciousness, intravenous fluid and drugs administered, unusual events or postoperative complications, and the management of those events. Discharge from the PARR is the responsibility of a licensed independent practitioner with appropriate clinical privileges. If this person is not physically present, his or her name must be recorded in the patient's medical record along with the relevant criteria applied to determine the readiness for discharge. These criteria must have been previously approved by the medical staff.

SA.2. Patients with the same health status and condition must receive comparable levels of quality of surgery and anesthesia care throughout the hospital. This section addresses the need for uniformity between different areas of the hospital, in particular the need for the standards in ambulatory surgery to be identical to those for inpatient surgery and the need to provide outpatients with a means of obtaining assistance in the event of postoperative complications. The standards specifically mandate that patients who receive other than local anesthesia on an ambulatory basis be accompanied at discharge by a designated and responsible person who is responsible for the patient.

AMH Appendix D. The JCAHO previously devised basic indicators during the past 3 years, which they submitted for field testing. The following indicators are to be used in monitoring and evaluating the quality of anesthesia:

AN-1. Patients developing a central nervous system (CNS) complication during or within two postprocedural days of a procedure involving anesthesia subcategorized by ASA physical status, age, central nervous system (CNS) versus non-CNS–related procedures.

AN-2. Patients developing a peripheral neurologic deficit during or within 2 days of a procedure involving anesthesia administration.

AN-3. Patients developing an acute myocardial infarction during or within two postprocedural days of a procedure involving anesthesia administration subcategorized by ASA physical status, age, cardiac versus noncardiac procedure.

AN-4. Patients suffering cardiac arrest during or within one postprocedural day of procedures involving anesthesia administration, excluding patients with required intraoperative cardiac arrest, subcategorized by ASA physical status, age, and cardiac versus noncardiac procedures.

AN-5. Patients with unplanned respiratory arrest during or within one postprocedural day of procedures involving anesthesia.

AN-6. Death of patients within two postprocedural days of procedures involving anesthesia administration, subcategorized by ASA physical status and a patient's age.

AN-7. Unplanned admission of a patient to the hospital within one postprocedural day after outpatient procedures involving anesthesia.

AN-8. Unplanned admission of patients to an intensive care unit (ICU) within one postprocedural day for procedures involving anesthesia and with ICU stay >1 day.

Additional indicators not retained after β-testing included patients with fulminant pulmonary edema during or within 1 day of anesthesia, patients with aspiration pneumonia, patients developing postural headache after spinal anesthesia or epidural anesthesia, patients experiencing dental injury, and patients experiencing ocular injury involving anesthesia care.

As can be noted from these indicators, they are the most severe problems, not the most common, most annoying, or most expensive problems on the basis of the total numbers of patients seen. Therefore, they are unlikely to pass JCAHO muster as embracing all of the quality problems attributable to anesthesia. Further, they require subcategorization and the calculation of frequencies not specifically mentioned in the JCAHO manual but mentioned in other JCAHO publications.

Postoperative follow-up is required for 1 to 2 days postoperatively. Calculations of frequency and cohort subgroupings require careful systematic and massive manipulation of data, making QA a process that will increasingly require outside consultation for its design. The patient care committee can be very useful to the membership in helping with setting up QA programs for individual departments.

Appendix II
Selection of Quality Assurance Database Software

System Overview. A database system can simplify handling of even large amounts of data. It requires organization, beginning with a logical series of menus that guide you in using the system. A well-organized top-level menu should branch no more than two or three times before reaching any essential function. All of the basic functions of the system should be accessible from the main menu. Use of the functions is guided by a series of on-line instructions and tables. Validity checks can detect mistakes immediately and prompt appropriate corrections. Such a system should provide an easy-to-use but robust capacity to enter data, manage data files, alter lookup tables, add users, maintain security, sort the database, and generate and review past reports graphically or on paper. A system consistent with the characteristics outlined in this appendix appears in the illustrations in Figure 3–4.

Data Entry and Browsing. The computer entry form should serve as a visual metaphor for the paper audit form. The name of the data table, its size, number of new entries, and remaining disk space should appear on the display, as should the meaning of frequently used special function keys. The system should use validity checks to permit only plausible data to be entered. Lookup tables for hard-to-remember acronyms should be available by pressing a help key. Codes for

providers, entered in separate lookup tables, should remain in the background and translate the initials of the providers into code numbers to keep the data and reports confidential.

The default entry for the current field should be enterable by pressing a single key, such as the space bar. The system should have data entry and error prevention methods to protect against data loss and corruption. Memo fields should be included on the form to enter assessments and actions. For rapid browsing, it is helpful if the data can also be viewed in a spreadsheet format. The system should be able to easily locate the occurrence of any field entry or one like it.

Reporting Data. A QA database system should provide various useful reports. The reports should be available by filling out a simple report query menu. Available reports should include records of the number of untoward events in a category for common volume indicators and adverse occurrences for providers. Generation of reports should be possible for the entire patient database or for events on a percentage basis. Statistical and database filtering functions should be provided to help enhance and tailor reports.

Means and standard deviation calculations help to put an individual provider's statistics into perspective. Filters can be set to include or exclude specific data from reports. Special summary reports can enable support staff to monitor cases that require further auditing, summarize all or part of the database, produce a report of the analysis of specific problems sorted by type of problem, and follow up on incomplete reports.

Reviewing Reports Graphically. The database system should save a copy of all of your printed reports, to be reviewed using a recap function available from another check-off style menu. Reports should be viewable either as bar-type graphs or in tabular form. A graph-resizing function should be included to adjust the size of the graph. This feature is useful when dealing with outliers that might be too large or too small to be displayed otherwise. Cursor controls to move between fields and reports should be easy to use.

Sorting Data. Sorting provides a way to examine the database in a manner not readily provided by the preconfigured reports. Sorted data can be filtered using the same functions available with the report functions. Sorted data should be displayed on a screen like the data entry screen, which also may be toggled to show a tabular view of the data. Tables should be able to be sorted repeatedly without affecting the source database. A report of the sorted data should be available.

General Characteristics. When designing or selecting an existing system for managing QA data, several general characteristics are desirable. In addition to a user-friendly interface and robust data manipulation capabilities, the following should also be present:

Color—The system makes judicious but not excessive use of color, just enough to separate prompts, field labels, data entries, system messages, and headings.

Installation—The system runs on available equipment without having to purchase add-ons. Installation should be simple and fast. It should not require major changes in your computer's configuration.

Memory—The data management system should be able to use all available hard disk space available to store and manipulate data. It should not limit the size of the database to the

size of the computer's random access memory (RAM). It should be able to use all available RAM, not just the conventional 600 or so kilobytes. To enhance speed, it should be able to run by swapping blocks of code into and out of memory as needed, leaving the maximum amount of RAM for data manipulation.

Compatibility—The system program code should be compatible with DOS, other shells such as Windows (Microsoft), and TSRs such as a spell checker.

Error prevention—The program should have parameter checks and lookup tables that supervise your work. It should format all data files uniformly. It should automatically join all associated files that you need at the time each database is created, copied, merged, or renamed. It should check the media before writing to it to make sure there is adequate space and advise you if there is not before copying.

Messages—Help messages should appear generously, as needed. When a violation is committed, the program should instruct the user in how to correct the error rather than ejecting to the DOS prompt. This feature includes checking to make sure that the printer or disk drive is ready, multiple times during an operation if necessary. Unless the disk drive is turned off or the disk is removed in the middle of an operation, the program should be able to recover from virtually any error as long as the computer or disk does not run out of memory.

Data security—Although an encryption process should be available, the physical records in the database do not always need protection. The encryption process should be optional. Encrypting schemes often slow down processing, make exporting data unduly complex, and may provide a false sense of security. Entry to the program and the confidential look-up tables should be password protected.

Tools—File management tools should allow the user to create, move, delete, rename, import, and merge files and maintain the lookup and printer tables.

CHAPTER 4

Medicolegal Issues and Concerns

MONTE LICHTIGER, M.D.

JAMES ECKHART, ESQ.

INTRODUCTION

What Is the Scope of the Medicolegal Problem?

In the past 50 years, the incidence of personal injury suits against physicians has increased tremendously. General practice physicians in the 1940s and 1950s lacked the scientific armamentarium and the technologic advances that we have today. However, they made up for this deficiency with the rapport they developed with their patients. These patients knew their doctors well, thought of them as benefactors of society, and realized that they had limitations.

The Impact of Specialization

With increasing emphasis on specialization, medical science advanced so rapidly that one individual could not keep abreast of all the advances in the many specialties and subspecialties. However, physicians could truly cure or effectively treat many of the ailments that humans were prone to develop. New devices capable of diagnosing diseases in their early stages were introduced. Better therapeutic modalities were commonplace. Indeed, life expectancy itself increased rapidly, and the geriatric age group became an increasingly large percentage of the total population.

Patients now came to their physicians with great expectations. They saw these doctors as all-knowing individuals who could take care of almost all their illnesses. Excellent results were not merely hoped for; they were expected. Should problems occur, someone must, therefore, presumably be at fault. Consequently, physicians were sued not only for negligence but also for the unexpected, poor result.

Interpersonal Relationships

The age of specialization brought great medical advances, but often lost was the personal relationship patients had with their physicians. The greater abilities of physicians to cure disease led to their spending less time with patients to provide emotional support. Patients had difficulties relating to their doctors, and doctors were thought of as impersonal. Therefore, patients had no qualms about suing them if they were unhappy with the results of their therapy.

Public Perception

Compounding this state of affairs was the fact that the "old country doctor," who was paid with poultry and produce, no longer existed. Physicians were not viewed as benefactors of humankind. To the contrary, they had an exceptionally high income and were perceived as individuals earning their "fortune" from the ills of humanity. This image was, of course, aided by the increased cost of this better medical care and the fact that many physicians adorned themselves with the external accoutrements of success to impress their patients.

The Effect of Malpractice Insurance

Patients also became aware of the fact that doctors carried professional liability insurance. Consequently, should they have any positive feelings toward the physician against whom they wished to bring suit, they could rationalize these feelings with the knowledge that it was the insurance carrier, not the doctor, who would compensate them. "It's just business, not personal."

The Contribution of Plaintiff Attorneys

The change in medical science, the change in attitudes of physicians in developing rapport with their patients, the increase in the cost of health care, and the knowledge of the existence of malpractice insurance led to what has been called the "malpractice crisis." To be complete, another factor must be mentioned—the increased number of attorneys in this country who viewed doctors with their malpractice insurance as legitimate targets. Some of these plaintiff-oriented attorneys, unfortunately, seemed to care little about whether negligence had occurred. If a poor result was associated with a sympathy factor that would sway a jury, they were eager to institute a suit.

THE MALPRACTICE INSURANCE CRISIS

How Did It Arise?

In many cases, the previously mentioned circumstances led juries with little medical or economic knowledge to award millions of dollars to the "victims" of medical malpractice. This upward spiral in awards eventually led to escalating insurance premiums, as well as the financial failure of many insurance carriers in a number of states, and became what doctors refer to as the "malpractice insurance crisis."

How Did Anesthesiologists Fare?

Anesthesiologists, in particular, were singled out as very high-risk physicians. They were doctors who spent most of their time in a very high-risk environment (i.e., the operating room, the emergency room, the intensive care unit). They also had little time (or inclination) to develop rapport with their patients. In fact, patients rarely knew their anesthesiologist. He or she simply was that doctor who put them to sleep. They had little or no knowledge of what this physician had to do while they were anesthetized. Indeed, many patients felt that after the anesthesiologists gave them an injection to put them to sleep, they left the operating room.

This patient perception, coupled with the lack of rapport between the patient and the anesthesiologist, contributed to the malpractice problem in anesthesiology. Malpractice insurance premiums rose precipitously as insurance carriers had large verdicts returned against anesthesiologists. The incidence of anesthetic problems was very low, but their severity was extremely high.[1] Hypoxia or anoxia led to brain damage. Medication and technical errors when performing central nervous system blocks led to paralysis.

CURRENT STATUS

Is the Situation Getting Worse?

The previously referred to medical advances, of course, also took place in anesthesiology. In the past 10 years, we have witnessed the advent of new monitoring techniques and seen the expansion of our pharmacologic armamentarium. These new drugs and monitors enhance patients' safety and can prevent poor results. In essence, the techniques of the physiology laboratory have been brought into the operating room. Not uncommonly, patients are monitored with central venous, arterial, and pulmonary artery catheters to determine a number of directly measured variables and various calculated derivatives (Table 4–1).

The American Society of Anesthesiologists (ASA) has also published rather specific standards regarding intraoperative and perioperative monitoring.[2] Most notable inclusions are the routine use of pulse oximetry in the operating room and recovery room and identification of carbon dioxide in the expired gas of any patient in whom an endotracheal tube is inserted.

What Is the Impact of Technologic Advances on Malpractice Actions?

These advances in anesthesiology have improved patients' safety and seem to have decreased the number of anesthetic mishaps,[3] although this point is debated.[4] This fact should decrease our medicolegal problems, and our experience is that this is, in fact, the case. One of the major problems leading to large judgments against anesthesiologists was brain damage secondary to unrecognized esophageal intubation.[5] This prob-

TABLE 4–1. American Society of Anesthesiologists' Statement on Invasive Monitoring in Anesthesiology*

A major contribution to the current practice of medicine is made by the galaxy of monitoring equipment and techniques developed in the past two decades. They have had a vital role in improving our ability to prevent, recognize, and treat many conditions that previously contributed to morbidity and mortality.

These techniques, particularly those involving insertion of central venous pressure (CVP) monitoring lines, intra-arterial catheters (A-lines), and Swan-Ganz catheters (PA lines), all carry with their application some varying degree of risk to a patient. This statement attempts to minimize such risk by outlining our position on the provision of such procedures in the delivery of anesthesia care by anesthesia care team personnel.

- The decision to use invasive monitoring is a medical judgment and should therefore be made only by a qualified physician.
- Invasive monitoring techniques should be prescribed by a physician. Depending on its risk, each should be applied only by a competent and trained physician or under the personal and immediate medical direction of such a competent and responsible physician.
- Training and credentialing of nonphysician members of the anesthesia care team who may perform invasive monitoring techniques should be approved at the local medical staff level by the anesthesia department and the active medical staff.
- Some of the invasive monitoring tasks, namely the insertion of CVP lines placed via the upper extremity and of arterial lines (A-lines), may be delegated to properly trained and credentialed members of an anesthesia care team. Performance, however, should be under the immediate and personal medical direction of the leader of the team, preferably an anesthesiologist.
- Insertion of pulmonary artery catheters is a relatively hazardous procedure and should only be done by a properly trained physician.

(Excerpted from the American Society of Anesthesiologists' Statement on Invasive Monitoring in Anesthesiology, 1984, of the American Society of Anesthesiologists. A copy of the full text can be obtained from ASA, 520 N. Northwest Highway, Park Ridge, Illinois, 60068–2573.)

lem seldom arises now. However, it has been replaced in part by brain damage secondary to the inability to establish an airway. Thus, better monitoring permits us to diagnose the malintubation but does not secure the airway for us. The bottom line, however, is that early diagnosis frequently leads to correction. Therefore, it is probable that anesthetic complications are declining.

Are Anesthetic Medicolegal Problems Decreasing?

A decrease in anesthetic problems should reduce anesthetic medicolegal problems, which in turn should be reflected by reduced premiums for malpractice insurance. If this sequence is correct, we can conclude that our medicolegal problems, indeed, are declining. In the past 5 years, these premiums have decreased about 40% for anesthesiologists. We have even witnessed a reclassification of anesthesiologists by many insurance carriers from insurance rate or risk classification 5 to 3 on a scale of 1 to 7. Category 1 represents the benchmark—for example, a physician not engaged in invasive procedures. Now we are placed in lower-risk groups, whereas less than a decade ago we were considered among the highest of insurance risks.

The Texas Health Policy Task Force Study

The improvement in anesthetic risk classification may reflect overall improvement in the malpractice situation in general. Plaintiff attorneys and defendant physicians and hospitals have traditionally been adversarial in and out of the courtroom.

Inflammatory rhetoric has obscured the facts concerning how serious the problem of malpractice is and how much it costs.

One published study was funded jointly by the Texas Hospital Association, Texas Medical Association, and Texas Trial Lawyers' Association.[6] Apart from the uniqueness reflected by the cooperation of these often contentious groups, the findings were remarkable and included the following:

1. Few claimants received multimillion dollar payments.
2. Overall caps tend to shift, rather than reduce overall costs.
3. Few cases are resolved by jury judgments.
4. Noneconomic damages do not appear to be a major factor in payments to claimants.

Of perhaps more interest to physicians was the finding that the economic impact of medical malpractice to total health care expenditures in Texas was 0.62% (approximately 260 million dollars). This figure was very close to national findings of 0.74% reported to Congress in March 1992 by the Congressional Budget Office.[7] Presumably, these findings are applicable to anesthesiologists. Although these dollar amounts are significant, they seem less than generally have been assumed. Perhaps the malpractice crisis is abating.

NEGLIGENCE

Where Do Our Problems Arise?

Anesthetic Induction

Years ago, we would answer this question by stating that most of our problems occurred during anesthetic induction, although this perception was disputed as early as 1976.[8] Many problems were related to improper intubation (i.e., esophageal intubation). As was already stated, undiagnosed malintubation now is rare. However, the esophagus is still intubated on occasion, and injury may result. Esophageal perforation or tearing still occurs. We also have alluded to the fact that the inability to establish or maintain an airway is a significant cause of hypoxic damage.[8, 9] Despite our better monitoring techniques, we still have major problems associated with induction and airway maintenance, even when regional techniques are used.[10]

Negligence

Legally, negligence is the failure to use reasonable care, which is that level of care, skill, and treatment that, in light of all relevant circumstances, is recognized as acceptable and appropriate by reasonably careful physicians in the same field. As a practical matter, negligence is whatever a plaintiff's expert witness says is a deviation from that reasonable care and which a jury believes.

Is the inability to intubate a patient negligence? Many expert witnesses are willing to state, under oath, that it is. However, a responsible and honest expert witness will admit that some patients have anatomy that misleads an anesthesiologist; they appear to have a feasible airway yet are difficult or impossible

to intubate by the conventional approach. A physician is negligent only if he or she does not have and use a plan (e.g., algorithm) to manage these patients. Every anesthesiology department should have such a plan that is consistent with the equipment and expertise available to it. For example, fiberoptic intubation techniques should not be included in a department's scheme if a fiberoptic bronchoscope is unavailable.

Also, members of a department must be familiar with that department's policies and procedures. If, for example, the policies and procedures state that patients in whom muscle relaxants are used must be monitored with a nerve stimulator, then this policy must be followed; to do otherwise constitutes negligence. As policies and procedures vary from department to department and are periodically updated, it is important to familiarize yourself with them.

Aspiration of gastric contents may also occur during induction, especially in a patient with a "full stomach." This problem is a known complication of anesthesia, but lawsuits for death or brain damage secondary to aspiration continue to appear. Anesthesiologists must document all the steps taken to prevent this complication. Their best defense rests with their demonstrating awareness of the potential problem and a complete record showing that their management was aimed at avoiding it (e.g., antacid prophylaxis and induction with cricoid pressure).

The largest awards for negligence against anesthesiologists have been for incidents resulting in brain damage. Most of these are related to hypoxic or anoxic encephalopathy secondary to failure to establish an airway. Attempts to intubate a patient with a difficult airway can be traumatic. Bleeding with possible blood aspiration, avulsion of laryngeal cartilages, vocal cord damage, and perforation of the trachea, esophagus, or pyriform sinuses may result. The latter problems may lead to pneumothorax, pneumomediastinum, and subcutaneous emphysema. Although problems can arise at any time during an anesthetic,[9] the most costly ones do so during induction.

Emergence

Emergence from anesthesia can be fraught with problems. Again, the most severe cases relate to death and brain damage. One of the most important incidents leading to severe problems is premature extubation of the trachea, for example, in a patient with Ludwig's angina. If the patient was intubated successfully, an anesthesiologist may be comfortable with extubation once the patient awakens and is able to follow commands. All too often, however, delayed respiratory obstruction occurs, after which the patient may be more difficult to intubate than before surgery. The ensuing hypoxia may lead to death or brain damage.

Other respiratory problems that may occur during emergence include aspiration pneumonitis, laryngeal spasm, and noncardiogenic pulmonary edema. The latter problem may be related to respiratory obstruction, aspiration, and central nervous system hypoxia. The results of a traumatic intubation may not be noted until after the patient has emerged from anesthesia and has been extubated, even though it occurred during induction. Documentation in the record that a patient is able to follow simple commands and has no evidence of residual neuromuscular blockade is strong evidence that a conservative approach was taken regarding timing of extubation. It also decreases the impact of a negligence accusation.

How Do Postanesthesia Care Unit Problems Impact on Anesthesiologists?

An anesthesiologist's responsibility for care does not end with a patient's arrival in the postanesthesia care unit (PACU). Indeed, in most institutions, the PACU is under the direction of the anesthesiology department. Many legal precedents hold anesthesiologists responsible for the caliber of care rendered by a hospital's PACU employees. If a patient in a PACU suffers an adverse outcome as a result of a nurse's negligence, the anesthesiologist often is named in the suit. If not named as a defendant because he or she left the patient in the PACU in an unsafe condition (e.g., still anesthetized so that airway obstruction was possible), the anesthesiologist is often designated as the physician who has the responsibility for care given by the nurse. Record of a formal transfer of patient care responsibility from the anesthesiologist to the PACU nurse by a note to that effect in the record; acceptable vital signs; and a PACU recovery score document that the transfer of responsibility took place, was organized, and was appropriate.

Within the past few years, we have witnessed an increased number of cases of severe outcome in the PACU. As intraoperative monitoring has improved, we have noted fewer cases of hypoxic brain damage in the operating room and more in the PACU. This observation has prompted insurance carriers to require improved PACU monitoring as a condition for coverage. We can anticipate that better PACU monitoring (e.g., pulse oximetry) will decrease morbidity and mortality in this area.

If an emergency occurs in the PACU, ideally an anesthesiologist should respond. However, if all the anesthesiologists are busy with patients in the operating rooms, a plan must be available to the PACU nurses so they know who to call for the emergency.[2] The plan may include coverage of an operating room case by a Certified Registered Nurse Anesthetist to free up an anesthesiologist for the PACU. Alternatively, an intensivist, an emergency room physician, or an emergency team in the institution must be designated so that help is available in the PACU. Whatever plan is formulated must be designed to provide expedient and appropriate care.

Such a plan, if accepted at the institution, ameliorates an anesthesiologist's liability for any alleged negligence in the PACU. The specifics of the plan differ from hospital to hospital. However, it must be a workable approach to emergencies occurring in the PACU, and it must be accepted by all parties involved.

FUTURE PROBLEMS

How Can They Be Avoided?

Vigilance

Vigilance is one of the most important characteristics that anesthesiologists can bring to bear. Close monitoring with an awareness of the pitfalls of monitoring devices is essential. However, with the increased importance that monitoring has assumed in our practices, we must still remember to pay close

attention to our patients. Not uncommonly, cases arise in which too much attention was given to the monitors and too little to the patient.

As an example, a patient suffered a cardiac arrest with resultant brain damage secondary to an obstructed endotracheal tube, even though a pulse oximeter was in use. The physician, who was alerted to the problem by the oximeter's alarm, spent a great deal of time readjusting the transducer and checking the monitor while his patient was hypoxic. We must first assume that the monitor is correct and check the patient.[4] The monitors should be checked *only* after we have satisfied ourselves that the patient is all right. Do not shoot the messenger!

Patient Rapport

Good patient rapport is another important aspect of care that must be pursued to avoid future problems. Lawsuits are easier to initiate against someone with whom one does not have a positive relationship. Conversely, a patient may be reluctant to pursue legal action against a doctor who has taken a great deal of time to explain the anticipated procedures, who has answered questions, and who has generally attempted to make the upcoming surgery and anesthesia as comfortable as possible. This concept was espoused by an anesthesiologist who wrote a letter to the editor encouraging other anesthesiologists to ensure that our role in patient care is properly presented to the media. He felt that this would enhance our stature with the public.[12] The response follows:

"One thing we learned after the expenditure of huge sums of money on public relations consultants was the fact that 'we have met the enemy, and they is us.' Failure to carry out meaningful preoperative and postoperative interviews with patients was determined to be a glaring deficit shared by a majority of anesthesiologists."

We must spend some time with our patients and show that we are both informed and caring individuals. Doctors are human, and humans sometimes make mistakes. It is surprising how forgiving patients can be if we demonstrate humanity when dealing with them.

The Hospital Record and Anesthesia

We must also have thorough records and record events appropriately. Write legibly and use ink when charting. Make all entries promptly and use only acceptable abbreviations. Date, time, and sign each entry. On the anesthesia record, timing and dating are routine, but anesthesiologists often are less compulsive in this regard when writing preoperative notes. Another useful practice is to cosign with date and time the anesthesia preoperative evaluation if it was performed by another member of your department. This measure confirms in the record that you are informed about the patient before caring for him or her. Cross out all errors in charting with a single line, and initial and date these corrections. To a jury, a sloppy record designates a sloppy doctor.

The anesthetic record should tell a complete story of what occurred in the operating room. The plaintiff always argues that if it wasn't charted, it wasn't done; thus, details regarding positioning changes and any notable occurrences are important to record. The record is a medicolegal document that can, if complete, represent the anesthesiologist as well as an attorney, if not better. Finally, the medical record is not an editorial forum, and one must resist making editorial comments in it about a patient's care by yourself or others.

ADVERSE EVENTS

What Should Be Done If One Occurs?

An adverse event should be reported promptly to your insurance carrier and risk manager. This process is not only important for your ultimate defense but may also be required so that your insurance policy covers any potential expenses that arise out of the adverse event. It also alerts your carrier to hidden cases and allows him or her to review and collect facts, settle, assume hospital bills, or prepare a defense. You should also write down your own recollection of the events involved while they are fresh in your mind. Keep this narrative in a safe place where you can retrieve it in the future. Some plaintiff attorneys may wait to file suit in the hope that the defendant will have forgotten many of the facts of the case.

Remember to preserve any evidence that relates to the problem, including equipment that may have malfunctioned and medications.[13] This action may be a great help to you and may also protect other patients in your institution.

How Should You Interact with the Patient and Family?

Maintain good rapport with the patient and the patient's family. You must present yourself as a concerned physician. As stated previously, people can be very forgiving if they are treated with care and regard. Explain the problem in terms that they can understand. A logical explanation of the complication may help the patient and family accept the outcome.

What Should Not Be Done?

Above all, do not attempt to cover up the incident either in the medical records or in talking to the patient. When this action is discovered, as it almost always is, you will be confronted by an angry patient and his or her attorney. Hiding a problem can also result in punitive charges being brought against you. An award for punitive damages usually is not covered by your insurance carrier.

Alteration of Records

Some physicians have tried to conceal their liability by altering medical records. To do so is unethical and dishonest. This approach should never even be considered. Handwriting experts may be called on to examine these records and are almost always able to detect these changes. When they testify at trial, you will lose all credibility.

Examination of medical records has become very scientific. An expert in this field is able to discern if the record was altered some time after it was initially entered. One of the ways in which this determination is made is by ink analysis. Ink manufacturers change certain fluorescent components in their inks on a yearly basis at the direction of the Internal Revenue Service to enable them to detect recent changes in

records made by taxpayers. Chromatographic studies can also be performed on the ink in the records. A needle is used to punch out a sample from the chart, and the ink is separated from the paper by a solvent. Chromatographic studies on this dissolved ink can then establish the manufacturer of the ink as well as the year it was made.

Other examinations routinely used include infrared reflectance and infrared luminescence photography, which demonstrate differences in writing instruments. Precision typewriter grids are also available and can show where additions have been made when the records are reinserted into the typewriter.

One of the most interesting new instruments, designed to detect interlineation and substitution of pages, is an electrostatic detection apparatus (ESDA), which makes a permanent record of indentations appearing on the surface of a sheet of paper. One can actually read the writing that was present before the changes were made. These are just some of the modern technology methods that are now available to detect record changes.

If an addition or alteration is made, it should be as with any other record change (i.e., a single line through the deleted comment with your initials and date in such a way that the original comment is still legible). For late additions, identify them as such, time, date, and sign. In general, little is gained by late entries or deletions, even when they are made according to the appropriate protocol.

Contact with the Plaintiff's Attorney

You should avoid all contact with the plaintiff's attorney. Do not discuss the case with anyone except your attorney or a representative of your insurance company. Be careful not to make any derogatory remarks or loose comments about patients or colleagues. Be in control at all times while speaking about the adverse incident. Furthermore, do not mention anything about a report you may have written, either for yourself or your insurance company. And remember, do not admit liability that has yet to be determined.

DEFENSE

How Does One Prepare?

Assuming you obtained informed consent and have not done anything to cover up the incident, you are now ready to prepare for your defense. Some steps can be taken to assist in your defense before reporting the incident to your carrier and before an attorney is assigned to represent you. These steps are often the key to a successful outcome of your case, whether you are appearing before an institutional review panel, a state regulatory body, or a jury (Table 4–2).

TABLE 4–2. How to Prepare for a Possible Lawsuit

Obtain complete copies of all records.
Make written verbatim copies of records.
Do not discuss the case or make written reports unless such activities are
　protected from later discovery.
If served with suit papers, do not discuss anything with the patient, family,
　or opposing attorney.
Obtain supporting medical literature and read it.
Be active in your defense.

Copies of Pertinent Records

Obtain complete copies of all pertinent hospital records as quickly as possible. By getting your copies early, you protect yourself from the hospital's "locking up" the chart, which could prevent you from reviewing these records. By copying the records soon after the incident, you obtain excellent evidence to demonstrate late entries, changes, or attempts to alter the records by others involved in the case. Remember that even minor changes or attempts at altering the records can destroy the credibility of the person making them. Should another physician or nurse make such alterations, your defense is solidified.

Prepare a legible verbatim copy of your records and a narrative summary of events. Aside from the embarrassment of not being able to read your own chart entries, a thought or idea that was in your mind at the time of the incident is very often lost because a word or phrase cannot be read. At times, the emergent nature of an incident precludes a contemporaneous entry in the medical records.

Certainly even the most compulsive physician will not be able to chart everything as accurately as desired. However, by preparing a summary immediately after the incident (no matter how time-consuming or unpleasant), events can be kept in perspective for questions that will almost certainly arise. Furthermore, this summary allows you to detail what actually occurred better than the chart entries alone. The combination of the two can greatly assist you in whatever defense is ultimately presented.

Discussion of the Case

Do not discuss the incident with anyone who may be on the other side. Resist the temptation to discuss the case with the other physicians or personnel involved. Any such discussions that are not in the context of a quality assurance or attorney/client discussion, especially if reduced to writing, are discoverable and can become evidence against you. Decline to meet with the hospital's risk manager unless you are certain that your conversation is legally protected from discovery. You must also be aware of the fact that the hospital may become your adversary in court.

Never talk to the patient, the patient's family, or the patient's attorney if served with suit papers or a preliminary presuit screening notice. Whatever you say (or write) at that point can and will be used against you. It will not change their decision to proceed with the suit.

Review of Medical Literature

Obtain medical literature that supports your diagnosis and treatment. If possible, do so early while the facts of the case are still fresh in your mind. Such action will help in your defense later when your insurance carrier and your attorney become involved. It will also assist you by suggesting potential expert witnesses for your defense.

This supporting literature gives you a psychologic advantage, as well. It demonstrates to your attorney and your insurance carrier that what you did is an accepted practice. It helps to educate your attorney and to plan for your defense. This approach provides everyone involved in your defense with a positive outlook. It certainly is preferable to just telling your defense team that you followed an accepted practice. Without supporting medical literature, they may be skeptical about your

actions until an expert is retained to verify your position. This action also demonstrates your concern and interest in assisting with the defense.

How Active Should Your Participation Be?

Become actively involved in your defense. All defense attorneys appreciate a client who is willing to spend the time to become involved in the defense of a claim. Anesthesiologists too often assume that their attorney will take care of everything. They fail to spend the necessary time to educate the attorney in the medical issues of a case. This educational process helps the anesthesiologist and lawyer to gain confidence in each other and creates a team concept. They can feel comfortable enough to discuss the weaknesses of the case and to analyze them rationally when preparing the defense. The anesthesiologist will also feel more secure in questioning his or her lawyer about how things are proceeding and what can be expected in the future.

Proper preparation is the key to a successful defense. It includes explaining (1) the facts and circumstances, (2) how the medical literature supports your actions, and (3) any deviations from accepted standards. Do not assume that the case will go away or avoid addressing any mistakes on your part (no matter how painful). If you fail to do these things during your preparation, you will be even more uncomfortable explaining your actions at a deposition or a hearing; by then, it may be too late.

Once you have taken a position on the record under oath, it is almost impossible to change without losing credibility. Ask your counsel to discuss all the ramifications of the case with you so that you are fully prepared and have no surprises when you give your testimony. Follow the advice of your attorney and ask questions about the legal sequence of events if you do not understand what is going to happen. This action helps to eliminate the fear and uncertainty surrounding litigation. Remember that you know more medicine than the plaintiff's attorney. You really have the upper hand if you use your head and stay in control. A good defense counsel will be able to prepare you for your deposition and for any trick questions you may be asked.

What Do the Plaintiff and Defense Look for in a Record?

States differ in terms of what information is admissible and what is discoverable at the time of trial. Generally speaking, physicians should recognize that a good attorney, whether plaintiff or defendant, will look at the documents summarized in Table 4–3. Once these records are obtained, the attorney will ascertain the defendant's education, training, and qualifications.

The extent of independent recollection of events in the case must be learned during the discovery period to prevent sudden "convenient" recall testimony at the time of trial. The records will be scrutinized to develop a sequence of events that will be covered in detail during the testimony of all involved parties. Everything from first visit or contact through history, physical examination, diagnostic tests, and findings and the medical significance of all of these items will be covered.

Conversations with the plaintiff will also be explored, as

TABLE 4–3. Documents of Particular Interest to Plaintiff Attorneys

A complete set of hospital records, including those from the emergency room, postanesthesia care unit, intensive care unit, labor and delivery areas, obstetric logs, and so forth, as well as an autopsy report (if available). Nurses' notes are heavily scrutinized because they are often much more detailed and detached than those of physicians.
Complete sets of records from all physicians who provided treatment.
Health care provider certificates or applications for state licensure and hospital staff privileges.
Corporate information on your professional group.
Medical staff bylaws and the rules and regulations of the departments involved in the case.
Incident reports if discoverable in your state.

will the treatment given and any communication with other doctors and medical personnel involved in the plaintiff's care. The anesthetic given and the thought processes behind your decisions will also be considered. Alternative methods of care will be discussed, including your reasons for adopting or rejecting them. Any possible conflicts in the records and testimony will be explored thoroughly.

Evidence of Finger Pointing

In particular, the opposing attorney will look for inconsistencies and "finger pointing." Again, the hospital record should not be used for airing grievances or editorializing; however, this practice sometimes occurs despite all instructions to avoid it. The defendant anesthesiologist should be aware of other physicians' notes that suggest his or her culpability. He or she should also look for any nursing notes that are incomplete or that conflict with the doctors' notes or with his or her recollection of the facts. The anesthesiologist must pay particular attention to notes made in the PACU.

Attorneys will also examine the original records to determine if anything has been rewritten or changed. Of course, a record that is too neat also arouses suspicion. Remember that almost without exception, every negligence case changes in theory as the case develops and discovery proceeds. This fact of life results from the witnesses' interpretation of the records and testimony, which often depends on what is in their own best interest.

TYPES OF LIABILITY

How Do They Differ?

Individual Liability

Most states have statutes or case decisions defining or interpreting what is meant by this aspect of fault determination. If you are the only one sued, individual liability is apparent. The problem occurs when many parties are potentially responsible.

Joint and Several Liability

Under the doctrine of joint and several liability, a plaintiff who recovers a judgment against only one defendant can recover against that defendant or any other defendants for any reason he or she chooses. Consequently, a defendant found to be only 1% at fault may pay the entire judgment, allowing another more responsible defendant to escape payment entirely. Clearly, this distribution of blame is inequitable.

Comparative Negligence

Most state jurisdictions now have elected to use a comparative negligence system, in which the percentage of fault is equated with the percentage of liability. However, as with most things in law, the manner in which this doctrine is applied to defendants varies. Some states have adopted the principle of pro rata contribution among defendants, in which one's percentage of fault is one's percentage of the judgment recoverable. Other states have a sliding scale of fault. An example of this system is a state in which a defendant found to be 20% or more at fault would be in a situation where joint and several liability was applicable. However, if his or her percentage of fault was determined to be less than 20%, pro rata contribution would apply. One must be aware of the law in effect in his or her state to understand how the theory of joint and several liability impacts his or her practice.

THE ANESTHESIOLOGIST AS AN EXPERT WITNESS

What Is the Desired Role?

The role of expert witnesses in a medical malpractice case is crucial in determining the outcome of the case. Expert witnesses provide testimony about whether a breach in the standard of care occurred and whether that breach was the proximate cause of the injury sustained. The suggestion has been made that an expert witness should render an honest opinion based on scientific principles and facts. The ASA suggests that at a minimum, expert witnesses should be qualified for their role and should follow a clear and consistent set of ethical guidelines (Table 4–4). In theory, either side, plaintiff or defendant, should be able to use the testimony regardless of who retained the expert.

Unfortunately, in the real world, this idealistic approach is rarely the case. Perhaps it should not be. A completely bland recitation of facts and principles by an uninspired witness is unlikely to be comprehensible and may well be soporific. Both plaintiff and defendant want an expert who testifies enthusiastically and favorably for their side. This need has led to shopping for experts to provide the desired testimony. Certainly, the proliferation of expert witness services and brokering agencies attests to this situation. Also, some itinerant medical testifiers constantly solicit attorneys, thus demeaning both the legal and medical professions.

How Is Accountability Determined?

Irresponsible medical experts (so-called hired guns) can testify to anything they wish. They may be devious, partisan, and uninformed physicians who can present to a jury outrageous testimony that is completely unfounded and without merit. In our present system, they usually need not fear accountability for their testimony. Without such accountability, hired guns can provide their often ludicrous opinions for many years. The only problem they may encounter is a well-prepared attorney on the other side who is aware of this expert's prior testimony. The hired gun can then be exposed during cross-examination.

Are Expert Witnesses Qualified?

Part of the reason for this problem relates to the lack of precise qualifications that an expert witness should possess before being allowed to testify. The various state legislatures have been reluctant to define such qualifications. Consequently, individual courts have wide latitude in allowing testimony from expert witnesses. In fact, most courts permit almost any type of medical testimony to be presented, as long as it assists the jury to understand the evidence or to determine a fact at issue. The response to an opposing attorney's objections is that the weight to be given to the testimony is for the jury to decide.

Without an irresponsible medical expert, a plaintiff will not get very far with many cases. Very few medical malpractice cases can be successfully tried without a medical expert. Fortunately, the defense bar has started some clearing-house organizations to gather information on these hired gun experts. This information results in a more effective cross-examination, enabling attorneys to eliminate many of these physicians who constantly testify in a manner adverse to the medical profession.

What Is Being Done by Professional Medical Organizations?

Similar efforts are now taking place in some medical specialty organizations. The American Medical Association and numerous medical specialty organizations are in the process of creating guidelines for expert witnesses' qualifications. They are also seeking ways of providing some means of accountability for their testimony. Until this goal is accomplished, *true* medical experts should be objective, render honest and scientifically valid opinions, and present what the standard of care was at the time of the occurrence, not what it is today if standards have changed. They should also recognize the wide range of acceptable medical approaches when presenting their expert opinion. To do otherwise is irresponsible and is a disservice to the medical profession.

MALPRACTICE INSURANCE

What Types Are Available?

Space does not allow an exhaustive discussion of the many types of insurance policies available. However, two basic types of insurance can be purchased by physicians.

Occurrence

The first is the traditional occurrence policy (almost nonexistent nowadays), which insures for damage that occurs during the policy period, regardless of when the claim is made. The occurrence determines whether or not coverage is applicable.

Claims-Made

The more common form of insurance is the claims-made policy. Generally speaking, this policy covers only those claims made during the policy period. Unfortunately, there are many variations of claims-made policies. Each particular pol-

TABLE 4–4. American Society of Anesthesiologists' Guidelines for Expert Witness Qualifications and Testimony*

The integrity of the civil litigation process in the United States depends in part on the honest, unbiased testimony of expert witnesses. Such testimony serves to clarify and explain technical concepts and to articulate professional standards of care. The American Society of Anesthesiologists supports the concept that such expert testimony by anesthesiologists should be readily available, objective, and unbiased. To limit uninformed and possibly misleading testimony, experts should be qualified for their role and should follow a clear and consistent set of ethical guidelines.

Expert Witness Qualifications
1. The physician (expert witness) should have a current valid and unrestricted state license to practice medicine.
2. The physician should be board certified in anesthesiology or hold an equivalent specialist qualification as recognized by the American Board of Anesthesiology.
3. The physician should be familiar with the clinical practice of anesthesiology at the time of the occurrence and should have been actively involved in clinical practice at the time of the event.

Guidelines for Expert Testimony
1. The physician's review of the medical facts should be thorough and impartial and should not exclude any relevant information to create a view favoring either the plaintiff or the defendant. The ultimate test for accuracy and impartiality is willingness to prepare testimony that could be presented unchanged for use by either the plaintiff or defendant.
2. The physician's testimony should reflect an evaluation of performance in light of generally accepted standards, neither condemning performance that clearly falls within generally accepted practice standards nor endorsing or condoning performance that clearly falls outside accepted medical practice.
3. The physician should make a clear distinction between medical malpractice and adverse outcomes not necessarily related to negligent practice.
4. The physician should make every effort to assess the relationship of the alleged substandard practice to the patient's outcome. Deviation from a practice standard is not always causally related to a poor outcome.
5. Fees for expert testimony should relate to the time spent and in no circumstances should be contingent on outcome of the claim.
6. The physician should be willing to submit such testimony for peer review.

(Excerpted from the American Society of Anesthesiologists' Guidelines for Expert Witness Qualifications and Testimony, 1990, of the American Society of Anesthesiologists. A copy of the full text can be obtained from ASA, 520 N. Northwest Highway, Park Ridge, Illinois, 60068–2573.)

icy should be carefully read before you purchase the insurance to assure yourself that you are getting the coverage you desire. Some, for example, may require both the occurrence and the claim to take place during the policy period. Others may require that both the claim and report of the occurrence be made during the policy period. In other words, some claims-made policies are more limited than others in the coverage they provide.

Some companies, however, cover the insured anesthesiologist forever on any case for which an incident report was filed with the company during the policy period (e.g., Anesthesiologists' Professional Assurance Company, Miami, FL). In essence, this policy becomes an occurrence policy for those claims for which an incident report was filed during the policy period.

Tail Coverage

To further protect yourself when insured with a claims-made policy, it is advisable to purchase extended reported or tail coverage. Then, if you have not reported a potential claim to your prior carrier to activate coverage, your tail coverage should provide coverage with your current carrier.

Self-Insurance

Self-insurance is another alternative to the traditional insurance company policies. Two general forms of self-insurance are available. The first requires the individual to join a group or association of licensed individuals in the same profession, who then establish a trust fund to provide coverage. This type of insurance is strictly regulated by statutes in the states where it is allowed.

The second form is self-insurance in the literal sense, with the individual physician meeting the financial responsibility required by state statutes. In general, some type of bond is purchased from a licensed surety, or an escrow account is established with the required money. Of course, if a judgment is rendered in excess of the amount of the bond or escrow account required, the physician can be personally liable. This fact should be considered before deciding on any self-insurance program. Furthermore, if involved in one of these programs, physicians obviously should take the necessary steps to try to make themselves judgmentproof.

Going Bare

Finally, physicians may elect to practice while uninsured (''going bare''). In this case, they are banking on an injured party's looking to others for his or her damages. This is an extremely risky position to take because of the personal asset exposure plus the need to pay for legal defense, which can be quite costly.

How Much Malpractice Insurance Should One Have?

For those physicians practicing in states having a state insurance fund to protect them, they need only secure the limits required by that state. Other doctors must decide on coverage with which they are comfortable. Frequently, hospital attorneys or risk managers may be in a position to suggest appropriate insurance limits based on their experience with jury verdicts in that community.

We recognize that finances may dictate the amount of coverage that an individual physician can purchase. Notwithstanding that fact, limits of 1 million dollars are almost always sufficient to resolve a case and to protect the assets of the individual physician.

References

1. Brunner EA: The national association of insurance commissioners closed claim study. Int Anesthesiol Clin 1984; 22:21.
2. American Society of Anesthesiologists: 1992 Directory of Members, pp 675–701.
3. Eichorn JH: Prevention of intraoperative anesthesia accidents and related injury through safety monitoring. Anesthesiology 1989; 70:572.
4. Orkin FK: Practice standards. The Midas touch or the emperor's new clothes. Anesthesiology 1989; 70:567.
5. Caplan RA, Posner KL, Ward RJ, et al: Adverse respiratory events in anesthesia: a closed claims analysis. Anesthesiology 1990; 72:828.
6. Medical and Hospital Professional Liability: A report prepared for the Texas Health Policy Task Force (Tonn and Associates). July, 1992.
7. Rerschauer R: Congressional Budget Office Testimony, Ways and Means, U.S. House of Representatives, March 4, 1992.
8. Taylor G, Larson CP Jr, Prestwich R: Unexpected cardiac arrest during anesthesia and surgery. JAMA 1976; 236:2758.
9. Cheney FW, Posner KL, Caplan RA: Adverse respiratory events infrequently leading to malpractice suits. A closed claims analysis. Anesthesiology 1991; 75:932.
10. Caplan RA, Ward RJ, Posner K, et al: Unexpected cardiac arrest during spinal anesthesia: a closed claims analysis of predisposing factors. Anesthesiology 1988; 68:5.
11. Davis DA: An analysis of anesthetic mishaps from medical liability claims. Int Anesthesiol Clin 1984; 22:31.
12. Cheney F: ASA Newsletter 1990; 54:4.
13. Spooner RB, Kirby RR: Equipment-related anesthetic incidents. Int Anesthesiol Clin 1984; 22:133.

CHAPTER 5

Risk and Outcome Analysis: Myths and Truths

DAVID L. BROWN, M.D.

Since the introduction of effective inhalational anesthetics approximately 100 years ago, the term *anesthetic risk* has often been used interchangeably with anesthetic mortality. Perhaps this fundamental confusion in conceptualizing anesthetic risks has to do with a somewhat unique aspect of anesthesia. Intraoperative anesthesia care, except in rare circumstances, is not therapeutic. The best we can hope for as anesthesiologists is that patients emerge from their anesthetics in no worse physiologic state than when anesthesia was induced.

This problem has become accentuated during the past 50 years with the ever increasing narrow focus on specialization and subspecialization in medical practice. This factor allows patients to receive care predicated on the latest advances in a specialty; however, it often prevents a single physician from being in a position to weigh all risk and benefit decisions impacting our surgical patients comprehensively. Because it is easier to understand perioperative death than it is the more elusive term *anesthetic risks,* many take the less rigorous approach and accept death due to anesthesia as the essence of anesthetic risks.

RISK STRATIFICATION

What Is the Risk of Anesthetic Mortality?

It has been suggested that the overall risk of anesthetic-related mortality is approximately 1 death per 10,000 anesthetic procedures. Nevertheless, this-easy-to-conceptualize incidence blurs many subtleties. For instance, the collaborative confidential inquiry into perioperative death (CEPOD) conducted in England in the mid-1980s showed that unequivocal anesthetic mortality occurred at a rate of 1 in approximately 185,000 anesthetics.[1] Natof, in a survey of ambulatory surgical centers spanning the years 1975 to 1980, reported a rate of anesthetic mortality of 1 in approximately 450,000 anesthetics.[2] Eichhorn and colleagues evaluated anesthetic-related deaths and severe central nervous system (CNS) injury in patients classified as American Society of Anesthesiologists (ASA) physical status 1 and 2 in the Harvard-affiliated hospitals during the years 1976 to 1988. They found a rate of

anesthetic death or significant CNS injury of 1 per 112,000 anesthetics.[3]

How Should the Data Be Interpreted?

What do these data mean? For ASA status 1 or 2 patients undergoing non–life-threatening surgery, it is likely that the incidence of anesthetic mortality is on the favorable side of 1 per 100,000 anesthetics. In our higher-risk patients, those with more physiologic dysfunction or undergoing life-threatening procedures, the anesthetic-related mortality rate is likely higher. The difficulty in these more critically ill patients is that the specific cause of death is often blurred between a patient's disease, the surgical procedure, and the anesthetic care. Because anesthetic mortality in our "healthy" patients occurs so infrequently, it seems important for us to begin to understand and define the more frequently occurring nonmortal anesthetic complications.

How Should We Define and Assess Anesthetic Complications?

One of the difficulties in understanding anesthetic complications is the confusion that exists between complications and physiologic side effects related to our anesthetics. The most evident example of this confusion has to do with blood pressure decreases related to anesthetics. The anesthetic literature is replete with references to hypotension as a complication of various anesthetic techniques; nevertheless, many of these are likely simply physiologic responses to vasodilatation accompanying both general and regional anesthetics.

This imprecision in language should be one of the principal focuses of ongoing anesthesia outcome analyses. I believe the term *complication* should be reserved for those situations in which a morbidity measure reaches a predetermined threshold of severity. This approach certainly makes outcome analyses more complex; however, over time, it also increases the precision of our language and deepens our understanding of anesthetic complications.

OUTCOME MEASUREMENT

Are Morbidity and Mortality Suitable Indicators?

Morbidity and mortality are certainly the most useful measures of anesthetic outcome. The difficulty arises in agreeing on their definitions. For example, when defining anesthetic mortality, should a death occurring 7 days after operation be considered a mortality but that occurring 8 days after an anesthetic be excluded? This question has practical implications, because our critical care units have become increasingly skilled at prolonging the lives of our most at-risk and critically ill patients.

How Should Mortality Be Defined?

Mortality is a suitable measure of outcome, and the focus of our research should be to agree on suitable time-linked mortality measures. Moving the time limit for mortality toward operation improves its specificity but clearly decreases its sensitivity.

How Is Morbidity Defined?

The question of morbidity as an appropriate measure of outcome is even more complex, since most morbid events do not have a uniformly agreed-on definition, such as a mortality end point. It is in this area of anesthetic outcome analysis that imprecision in language most often confuses morbidity and side effects.

To measure anesthetic morbidity accurately, the morbid event should require either additional therapy, prolongation of the patient's stay, or a patient's dissatisfaction. If one of these three requirements was fulfilled before determining that morbidity occurred, practical precision in our outcome language would be increased.

Despite this belief, circumstances exist in which intermediate variables, such as myocardial ischemia, may be practical measures of anesthetic outcome. Slogoff and Keats have shown that an intermediate variable (myocardial ischemia) is linked to the development of perioperative myocardial infarctions.[4] There are likely other intermediate variables that can be linked to adverse outcomes and may be appropriately included in outcome analysis once that link is established.

When and By Whom Should Anesthetic Outcome Be Measured?

The measurement of anesthetic outcome is inevitably time linked. The length of outcome observation is necessarily shorter for our outpatients than it is for critically ill inpatients. Once again, the length of time needs to be determined by multiple factors, including the magnitude and urgency of the operation, a patient's age, ASA physical status assessment, and others appropriate for given surgical and anesthetic techniques.

Is Peer Assessment Appropriate?

Another aspect of outcome measurement that needs to be considered when undertaking outcome studies is the reliability of peer assessments of anesthetic outcome. Goldman showed that in peer assessment, physicians' agreement regarding the quality of care is only slightly better than the level expected by chance.[5] Likewise, Caplan and colleagues have shown that knowledge of the severity of outcome of an injury related to anesthetic care influences a reviewer's judgment on the appropriateness of that care.[6] These studies highlight that retrospective outcome analyses can be significantly influenced by reviewer bias, and they suggest that reviewers of medicolegal situations are likely influenced by the severity of outcome when determining the appropriateness of care.

Can the Process Be Improved?

An extension of this observation is that to accumulate data in an objective fashion, the data collection should be "unhooked" from those providing clinical anesthetic care. Cohen and Duncan took this approach in their study of anesthetic outcome in Winnipeg. Their study design template is likely an effective method of data collection.[7] However, it is more expensive for an independent observer to categorize morbidity and mortality in anesthetic practice than is self-reporting by practitioners.

What Is the Role of Patient Satisfaction?

Another aspect of outcome analysis receiving increasing attention is the linking of patient satisfaction with anesthetic care and outcome measurements. In this age of consumerism, not surprisingly, quality anesthetic practice may be tied to patients' satisfaction with the care provided. Today, there are few data to substantiate this concept as a valid measure of anesthetic outcome or quality anesthetic practice, but it will likely and appropriately be studied as a measure of outcome during the next decade.

How Is the Statistical Problem of Rare Events Addressed?

Anesthetic care has become increasingly safe through the years, a positive development. However, when events occur infrequently, statistical analysis is problematic.

What Are the Pitfalls?

Statistical analysis is the means by which the effects of random variation are estimated. When we use inferential statistics to formulate conclusions about a larger group from a selected number of individuals (a sample), we take risks. As an example, during a multi-institutional English report involving 108,878 patients and 2391 deaths, the author stated: "Although we examined more than 100,000 operations, the numbers were still too small to allow analysis of the risk of the preoperative conditions for specific operations or even separately for males and females."[8]

Data Dredging

Further, as computerization of clinical databases has become commonplace, one of the statistical problems in outcome studies has been the problem of multiple comparisons. As investigators attempt to generate hypotheses from many of these databases, the problem of "data dredging" can occur. That is, any time they compare 20 outcome measures from the database, one of the observations of $P < 0.05$ is likely to be erroneous because the commonly accepted statistical handling of a type I error sets the alpha at 1 per 20 observations (or ≤ 0.05).

To highlight the issues involved in studying rare events, consider the estimated cost of more than one million dollars to study general anesthetic agents and outcome in a multi-institutional prospective evaluation of 17,000 patients.[9]

Default Mode of Anesthetic Prescription

The final difficulty in understanding anesthetic risk and outcome is the implicit bias that technique comparisons use a general anesthetic as the benchmark of measure. Most anesthesiologists' default mode of anesthetic prescription is general anesthesia.

As previously outlined, when morbid or mortal events occur infrequently, it is difficult and expensive to document an improvement in outcome related to anesthetic technique, especially in this era of relative anesthetic safety. We should be willing to state, in order to be "scientifically" honest, that in particular patient situations, neither general nor regional anesthesia has been shown to be safer. Detailed risk-benefit analysis demands that we be honest in this regard, both for our patients and for our legal colleagues, who frequently become involved in patient care after adverse outcomes.

PREOPERATIVE RISK ASSESSMENT

Because anesthetic care is not therapeutic, the focus of most of our preoperative risk management efforts has been to ensure that patients are physiologically "optimized" when they arrive in the operating theater.

Which Perioperative Risk Factors Are Not Modifiable?

Anesthesiologists know that perioperative risk variables fall into two broad classes. Some, such as a patient's age, intended operation, urgency of operation, personnel experience, and the institution in which the procedure is to be performed, are impossible (or nearly so) to change preoperatively. Conversely, a number of patient variables may be amenable to optimization before operation—that is, organ system physiologic function. These issues are next addressed sequentially.

What Is the Impact of Advanced Age?

The most striking example in this category is a patient's age. Most clinicians assume that as patients age, perioperative and mortality risks increase. However, many investigations suggest that age is primarily a marker of an increasing number of concurrent diseases or physiologic derangements.[10] The CE-POD study showed that approximately 80% of perioperative deaths occurred in patients older than 65 years.

An additional relationship of age to perioperative risks is the life expectancy remaining for elderly patients undergoing operation. Decisions to operate or not to operate are often affected by a misunderstanding of the extent of life remaining for 85- to 90-year-old patients[11] (Table 5–1). Many more years are predicted actuarially for elderly patients than physicians weighing risk-benefit decisions realize.

What Are the Effects of the Personnel and Institution?

Other nonmodifiable risk factors are the personnel and institution involved. Slogoff and Keats showed that the incidence of myocardial ischemia accompanying coronary artery bypass grafting procedures may vary depending on the individual performing the anesthetic.[4] This concept has been strengthened by data from Merry and colleagues, who also showed that specific anesthesiologists impact perioperative outcome.[12] Although the concept is speculative, specific surgical colleagues probably can also be linked to changes in perioperative outcome.

Once a decision has been made to operate, the institution in which the operation is to be performed is most often not alterable. For specific operations, a frequency-dependent minimum exists, below which perioperative outcomes are less desirable.[13] Additionally, for what are thought to be similar types of institutions, such as academic centers performing coronary artery bypass grafting procedures, even in age- and disease-matched patients, a 21-fold variation in perioperative mortality can result.[14]

When Is the Type of Surgery a Factor?

Other factors that impact perioperative risk relate to the surgical procedure itself. Superficial operations, such as repair of fractures of the extremities, are associated with a lower risk of adverse outcomes than are intrathoracic, major intra-abdominal, or intracranial procedures.[15, 16]

An additional feature having a major influence over adverse perioperative outcome is the elective or emergent nature of operation. Although elective and emergent procedures may never be quite "the same operation," for a similar operation, emergent conditions increase the risk of adverse outcome by a factor of three- to sixfold.[17–19]

FUNCTIONAL PHYSIOLOGIC RISK FACTORS

Which Cardiovascular Functions Are Important?

Hypertension

Treatment of even mild hypertension prolongs life.[20] Between 10% and 50% of an anesthesiologist's patients, de-

TABLE 5–1. Geriatric Life Expectancy

Current Age (Years)	Years of Life Remaining	
	Men	*Women*
65	14	18
67	12	16
70	11	14
75	9	11
80	7	9
85	5	7

(Modified from Eiseman B: What Are My Chances? Philadelphia, WB Saunders, 1980, p 15.)

pending on the type of practice, may have hypertension. Thus, this risk factor must be analyzed. Some studies suggest that mild to moderate hypertension is not associated with adverse perioperative outcome.

Improved vasoactive drugs have led some investigators to believe that uncontrolled hypertension should not postpone a scheduled surgical procedure.[21] This study of approximately 1000 patients with hypertension must be placed in perspective. The patients all received a general anesthetic. Whether their data can be applied to patients receiving regional anesthesia must remain speculative. Additionally, only a limited number of patients with severe hypertension were included in their investigation, thus making a type II (false-negative) statistical error possible.

Coronary Artery Disease

Patients with coronary artery disease are widely variable, ranging from those only experiencing angina to others with documented myocardial infarction. Prior myocardial infarction has a time-linked relationship to adverse perioperative myocardial events. The link of angina to adverse outcomes is less clear.[22]

Anesthesiologists have interpreted Rao and colleagues' data to suggest that the well-established truism that surgical procedures should be postponed for 6 months after a myocardial infarction when possible may no longer be valid.[23] Nevertheless, a preponderance of evidence, even in Rao's study, shows that performing a surgical procedure within 6 months of prior myocardial infarction significantly increases the perioperative risk of subsequent myocardial events.[22]

Why recent myocardial infarction markedly increases surgical risk is not clear, nor is the reason why an interval of 6 months affords risk reduction. One may speculate that this interval is necessary for healing or for scarring of the myocardium to mature. Likewise, this time may be necessary for the development of sufficient collateral circulation to protect areas of myocardium at risk in the perimeter around prior infarcts.

Congestive Heart Failure

Congestive heart failure is associated with significant morbidity and mortality in the perioperative period. In Goldman's study, patients who were older than 40 years and who developed congestive heart failure had a 57% incidence of perioperative mortality.[24] The best preoperative predictors of postoperative heart failure are jugular venous distention and third heart sounds or a prior history of congestive heart failure.[25] Important valvular heart disease, particularly aortic stenosis, is also reported to cause new or worsening heart failure in 20% of those so affected.[23]

Complicating analyses of the impact congestive heart failure has on adverse perioperative outcomes are the different and often clinically imprecise criteria used to diagnose the condition. Postoperative myocardial reinfarction occurs at a higher rate in patients with preoperative congestive heart failure.[25] Mangano and colleagues found that a history of congestive heart failure was a univariant predictor of adverse postoperative cardiac outcome.[26]

Is an Admission Electrocardiogram Useful?

An admission electrocardiogram (ECG) usually is obtained for patients older than some predetermined age. The usefulness of this practice continues to be debated. Moorman and colleagues[27] evaluated ECGs in 1410 general medical patients and found the admission ECG provided new information in only 1% of cases of patients with no cardiac problems suggested by history or physical examination. In patients suspected of having cardiac problems, admission ECGs provided additional information in 6.9% of cases.[27]

Indications

Some have suggested that Moorman's findings indicate that a preoperative ECG is unnecessary in patients with no evidence of cardiac disease. However, in Moorman's patients, 75% of the 1410 admission ECGs were abnormal. Because these patients were scheduled for surgery, it remains speculative whether obtaining a preoperative ECG would allow alteration of anesthetic management to lower the risk of adverse cardiac outcomes.

Despite the scarcity of outcome data, a preoperative ECG to evaluate cardiovascular risk factors probably is reasonable in men aged 40 years or older; in patients with hypertension, peripheral vascular disease, or diabetes; in patients at risk for electrolyte abnormalities; in patients undergoing intrathoracic, intraperitoneal, aortic, major neurologic, or emergency surgery; and in patients with a history of physical findings suggestive of heart disease, including dysrhythmias.

What Other Tests Are Meaningful?

Technologic advances in noninvasive cardiac function assessment provide a number of options in preoperative cardiac assessment. The difficulties anesthesiologists experience in understanding the optimum use of these tests include the fact that traditional lower-cost tests are not discarded as new (and expensive) noninvasive tests become practical. The most important risk management decision for anesthesiologists, I believe, is to voice concerns to our cardiologist colleagues. By the time an individual patient is evaluated, a multitude of tests have often already been performed. A practical discussion may better focus the preoperative evaluation.

Echocardiography

Patients often undergo an echocardiographic study before their surgical procedure; this study is an excellent means to assess valvular and overall ventricular functions. A significantly decreased ejection fraction, in the 25% to 35% range, likely identifies a high-risk group.[28] Remember, however, that preoperative ejection fraction measurements assess only function. A normal ejection fraction does not rule out the presence of significant coronary artery disease.[29]

Radionuclide Studies

A patient who has a history suggestive of myocardial ischemia and who has not undergone a thallium radionuclide-type study is unusual today. Thallium acts like potassium and follows myocardial perfusion. In a normal patient, an image of homogeneous myocardial perfusion results. A scar in the myocardium, similar to that found after a myocardial infarction, is identified as a cold spot.

To fully understand the use of thallium imaging, one must

be familiar with stress thallium scans. Exercise or dipyridamole is used to produce coronary vasodilatation during a thallium scan. An immediate image is obtained, followed by another after a 2- to 3-hour delay. If homogeneous perfusion is shown on the initial and delayed scans, the study is interpreted as normal. However, if a defect is noted on the initial scan and is not observed on the delayed scan, a diagnosis of viable myocardium at risk is made. If the initial scan shows a defect that persists to the delayed scan, a fixed defect, such as myocardial infarction, is diagnosed.

Clinical Application

Boucher and colleagues in 1985 published a widely discussed study suggesting that preoperative dipyridamole-thallium imaging could predict adverse cardiac outcomes in patients undergoing peripheral vascular surgery.[30] Several permutations of this work have been developed since that time. Overall thallium redistribution does indicate a high incidence of adverse cardiac outcomes; however, a normal dipyridamole-thallium scan does not ensure an uneventful postoperative course.[31]

Exercise Studies

Further confounding the appropriate use of nuclear medicine studies are reports by Gerson and coworkers[32, 33] in which bicycle exercise testing was a better predictor of perioperative pulmonary, cardiac, and combined cardiopulmonary complications than were nuclear medicine studies. An inability to perform 2 minutes of supine bicycle exercise sufficient to raise the heart rate above 99 beats per minute was the best predictor of adverse cardiac events in patients undergoing elective noncardiac surgery. Elderly patients who were able to perform this bicycle exercise had a five- to sixfold reduction in major perioperative pulmonary, cardiac, and combined cardiopulmonary complications.

How Important Are Pulmonary Risk Factors?

The ASA closed-claims project shows that at least one third of all claims against anesthesiologists are related to respiratory events.[34] European data also suggest that the majority of adverse outcomes are related to cardiopulmonary complications following operation.[15] The difficulty for a clinical anesthesiologist is highlighted by the data presented by Caplan and colleagues showing that even patients with normal lung function may experience postoperative pulmonary complications.[34]

In patients with abnormal pulmonary function, no single test accurately predicts postoperative complications.

Operative Site

The incidence of postoperative pulmonary complications increases if the operative site involves the upper abdomen and diaphragm.[35] Thoracic and upper abdominal operations are associated with the highest incidence of postoperative pulmonary complications. Provision of adequate analgesia is one means of limiting the adverse effects of such operations. However, despite using adequate analgesia, Ford and associates showed that after these procedures, a shift from abdominal to rib cage breathing still occurs.[36] These data suggest that either

direct diaphragmatic irritation or initiation of a neural reflex becomes established and inhibits diaphragmatic function.

Chronic Obstructive Lung Disease

Another well-established perioperative risk factor for pulmonary complications is chronic obstructive lung disease (COLD). Because postoperative pulmonary changes are primarily restrictive in character, a patient with underlying COLD may be especially compromised.

A number of studies indicate that a combination of pulmonary function tests, such as forced vital capacity, forced expiratory volume in 1 second (FEV_1), and maximal voluntary ventilation, are the best predictors of postoperative respiratory dysfunction.[37–40]

Similar to the suggestion for dialogue with cardiology colleagues about the optimal preoperative evaluation, a discussion with our pulmonary colleagues about the ideal method of evaluating patients with significantly compromised pulmonary function should occur in advance of the need for such evaluations. Despite increased risk, patients with a FEV_1 as low as 0.45 L may survive the perioperative period.[40]

Asthma

Asthmatic patients, or those with reversible airflow obstruction, also are at increased perioperative risk. Common dictum suggests that avoidance of a general anesthetic and tracheal tube minimizes asthmatic exacerbations.[41] Shnider and Papper studied 687 asthmatic patients in a group of more than 55,000 patients (1.2% prevalence of asthma) requiring anesthesia.[42] In those asthmatic patients whose wheezing was quiescent preoperatively, 6.5% wheezed intraoperatively (40% on induction and 60% during anesthetic maintenance). In these patients, increasing age increased the incidence of exacerbation. Contrary to traditional teaching, patients undergoing regional anesthetics had the same incidence of intraoperative wheezing as nonintubated patients receiving general anesthesia.

Gold and Helrich reviewed the perioperative course of approximately 200 asthmatic patients and documented that the site of surgical procedure is an important predictor in the asthma exacerbation equation.[43] They found the highest incidence of pulmonary complications occurred during upper abdominal procedures.

To minimize risks, asthmatic patients should be established to be in their optimum condition, and an anesthetic approach tailored for the specific patient should be developed. Postoperative analgesia requirements should be considered before formulating an intraoperative anesthetic plan.

Should Routine Chest Radiographs Be Obtained?

The question of obtaining a routine chest radiograph before surgical procedures has been better defined over time. Roizen suggests the risks of chest radiography probably exceed its benefits if a patient is asymptomatic and younger than 60 years. He emphasizes that this assumption is predicated on maximizing the benefit to society in general rather than to individual patients.[44]

What Is the Impact of Neurologic Dysfunction?

Preoperative neurologic dysfunction often influences anesthetic selection. However, little information suggests that well-conducted general or regional anesthetics significantly alter the incidence of adverse neurologic outcome. Preoperative concern over patients with cerebrovascular disease has been prevalent for years. I believe that the primary benefit of identifying cerebrovascular disease preoperatively is that it highlights a patient's risk of adverse cardiovascular outcome, such as myocardial infarction.[45]

Blood Pressure Control

A generally accepted dictum is that blood pressure in patients with cerebrovascular disease needs to be maintained at a higher level perioperatively than in patients without a history of cerebrovascular disease. However, data gathered from patients who were resuscitated after cardiac arrest and who died from 1 day to several weeks later suggest that the risk of precipitating brain infarcts by lowering blood pressure is not much greater in atherosclerotic than in nonatherosclerotic individuals.[46]

Carotid Bruits

In patients older than 45 years, between 4% and 5% have asymptomatic carotid bruits.[47] When patients who are older than 55 years and are undergoing elective surgery are considered, the incidence increases to 14%.[48] The presence of a carotid bruit suggests that a patient has a higher risk of atherosclerosis involving other blood vessels. Myocardial infarction occurs 2.5 times more commonly in patients with asymptomatic bruits than in age-matched controls.[47]

Progressive Neurologic Disease

Another situation in which neurologic dysfunction often impacts anesthetic prescription occurs in patients with progressive neurologic diseases. In many cases, anesthesiologists alter their usual prescription of a regional anesthetic in favor of a general anesthetic for fear that the regional technique might be implicated in further deterioration of neurologic function. No data show that a well-conducted regional anesthetic places a patient at higher risk than a well-conducted general anesthetic in patients with conditions such as diabetes mellitus or other peripheral neuropathies. Nevertheless, a thorough discussion with a patient before the surgical procedure is indicated if one believes a regional anesthetic has advantages.

ANESTHETIC PRESCRIPTION

What Is the Proper Role of Monitoring?

One of the first decisions required when considering anesthetic prescription is which monitoring devices to use. Risk management in this area has been affected by the ASA'S basic intraoperative monitoring standards, the latest revision of which became effective in January of 1992 (Table 5–2).

Since anesthesiologists began monitoring patients with a finger on the pulse many years ago, new monitoring devices have been resisted by many. One early report suggesting that ECG was useful as an intraoperative monitor documented an 80% incidence of dysrhythmias during surgical procedures.[49] A reviewer questioned whether this high incidence was clinically significant and whether the advances in operating room monitoring were justified. He stated, "It seems to me that the question is not whether irregularities occur or what causes them particularly, but whether the patient gets through the operation."[49]

This same tone has been taken by many anesthesiologists as additions have been made to what is considered basic intraoperative monitoring (Table 5–3).

Does Monitoring Reduce Anesthetic Risk?

One of the difficulties in assessing whether added monitoring decreases the risks of operation is that most devices have been included in the monitoring schema before randomized studies documenting their usefulness. One of the most-discussed additions during the past decade is pulse oximetry as a continuous monitor during all anesthetics. No randomized prospective study documents its value, and in fact, one large prospective study of 20,802 patients could not show that pulse oximetry affected early postanesthesia outcome.[50] However, Eichhorn presented retrospective data suggesting a lowered incidence of perioperative complications since its introduction.[3]

The ASA closed-claims database has been analyzed to determine if negative outcomes could have been prevented by the proper use of additional monitoring devices. More than 1000 cases were reviewed, and more than 30% of the negative outcomes were believed to have been preventable by the application of additional monitors, chiefly pulse oximetry plus capnometry.[51] When Caplan and colleagues looked at the ASA closed-claims database and assessed adverse outcomes related to respiratory events, they stated that 72% of the adverse outcomes could have been prevented by better monitoring.[34]

Does Monitoring Introduce Additional Problems?

A report by Kestin and colleagues highlights one of the increasing difficulties of intraoperative monitoring. In a pediatric population, they assessed the significance of auditory alarms that sounded during routine anesthetics. Seventy-five per cent of all auditory alarms did not originate from changes in the physiologic variables for which the monitor was designed, and only 3% presented any patient risk.[52] Although many industrial suppliers are addressing this issue, nonintegrated and nonhierarchic alarms remain one of the unsolved problems of risk management in patient monitoring.

When Is Patient Risk Increased?

When anesthesiologists become concerned about higher levels of risk in surgical patients, they often escalate the monitoring schema to include invasive hemodynamic devices. Many believe this continuous assessment of arterial or pulmonary arterial blood pressure creates a margin of safety.

Some operations, such as cardiac surgery, carotid endarterectomy, and aortic aneurysm repair, would be very difficult to conduct without continuous invasive monitors. Nevertheless,

TABLE 5–2. American Society of Anesthesiologists' Standards for Basic Intraoperative Monitoring

These standards apply to all anesthesia care, although in emergency circumstances, appropriate life support measures take precedence. These standards may be exceeded at any time based on the judgment of the responsible anesthesiologist. They are intended to encourage high-quality patient care, but observing them cannot guarantee any specific patient outcome. They are subject to revision from time to time, as warranted by the evolution of technology and practice. This set of standards addresses only the issue of basic intraoperative monitoring, which is one component of anesthesia care. *In certain rare or unusual circumstances, (1) some of these methods of monitoring may be clinically impractical and (2) appropriate use of the described monitoring methods may fail to detect untoward clinical developments. Brief interruptions of continual† monitoring may be unavoidable. Under extenuating circumstances, the responsible anesthesiologist may waive the requirements marked with (‡); it is recommended that when this is done, it be so stated (including the reasons) in a note in the patient's medical record.* These standards are not intended for application to the care of obstetric patients in labor or in the conduct of pain management.

Standard I

Qualified anesthesia personnel shall be present in the room throughout the conduct of all general anesthetics, regional anesthetics, and monitored anesthesia care.

Objective

Because of the rapid changes in patient status during anesthesia, qualified anesthesia personnel shall be continuously present to monitor the patient and provide anesthesia care. In the event that a direct known hazard (e.g., radiation) to the anesthesia personnel might require intermittent remote observation of the patient, some provision for monitoring the patient must be made. In the event that an emergency requires the temporary absence of the person primarily responsible for the anesthetic, the best judgment of the anesthesiologist will be exercised in selection of the person left responsible for the anesthetic during the temporary absence.

Standard II

During all anesthetics, the patient's oxygenation, ventilation, circulation, and temperature shall be continually evaluated.

Oxygenation

Objective

To ensure adequate oxygen concentration in the inspired gas and the blood during all anesthetics.

Methods

1. Inspired gas: During every administration of general anesthesia using an anesthesia machine, the concentration of oxygen in the patient breathing system shall be measured by an oxygen analyzer with a low oxygen concentration limit alarm in use. ‡
2. Blood oxygenation: During all anesthetics, a quantitative method of assessing oxygenation such as pulse oximetry shall be used. ‡ Adequate illumination and exposure of the patient are necessary to assess color.

Ventilation

Objective

To ensure adequate ventilation of the patient during all anesthetics.

Methods

1. Every patient receiving general anesthesia shall have the adequacy of ventilation continually evaluated. While qualitative clinical signs such as chest excursion, observation of the reservoir breathing bag, and auscultation of breath sounds may be adequate, quantitative monitoring of the CO_2 content or volume of expired gas is encouraged.
2. When an endotracheal tube is inserted, its correct positioning in the trachea must be verified by clinical assessment and by identification of CO_2 in the expired gas. † End-tidal CO_2 analysis, in use from the time of endotracheal tube placement, is strongly encouraged.
3. When ventilation is controlled by a mechanical ventilator, there shall be in continuous use a device that is capable of detecting disconnection of components of the breathing system. The device must give an audible signal when its alarm threshold is exceeded.
4. During regional anesthesia and monitored anesthesia care, the adequacy of ventilation shall be evaluated, at least, by continual observation of qualitative clinical signs.

Circulation

Objective

To ensure the adequacy of the patient's circulatory function during all anesthetics.

Methods

1. Every patient receiving anesthesia shall have the electrocardiogram continuously displayed from the beginning of anesthesia until preparing to leave the anesthetizing location.‡
2. Every patient receiving anesthesia shall have arterial blood pressure and heart rate determined and evaluated at least every 5 minutes.‡
3. Every patient receiving general anesthesia shall have, in addition to the above, circulatory function continually evaluated by at least one of the following: palpation of a pulse, auscultation of heart sounds, monitoring of a tracing of intra-arterial pressure, ultrasound peripheral pulse monitoring, or pulse plethysmography or oximetry.

Body Temperature

Objective

To aid in the maintenance of appropriate body temperature during all anesthetics.

Methods

There shall be readily available a means to measure continuously the patient's temperature. When changes in body temperature are intended, anticipated, or suspected, the temperature shall be measured.

(Excerpted from the American Society of Anesthesiologists' Standards for Basic Monitoring, 1992, of the American Society of Anesthesiologists. A copy of the full text can be obtained from ASA, 520 N. Northwest Highway, Park Ridge, Illinois, 60068–2573.)
†Note that *continual* is defined as "repeated regularly and frequently in steady rapid succession" whereas *continuous* means "prolonged without any interruption at any time."
‡Requirements that may be waived by the anesthesiologist under certain circumstances.

TABLE 5–3. Basic Intraoperative Monitors, Circa 1994

Automated blood pressure
Electrocardiograph
Pulse oximeter
Capnometer
Precordial/esophageal stethoscope
Circuit oxygen analyzer
Airway pressure (high/low)
Temperature probe

few data suggest that invasive hemodynamic monitors have lowered perioperative risks.

Additional advantages of direct over noninvasive blood pressure monitoring include reduced intraoperative workload, immediate detection of the hemodynamic effects of cardiac dysrhythmias or surgical manipulation of vascular structures, and better assessment of lower blood pressures.[53]

Direct Arterial Pressure Monitoring

In any risk-benefit analysis, the benefits of a technique (monitor) must be weighed against the risks of the device itself. One of the factors encouraging widespread use of direct systemic arterial blood pressure monitoring is the minimal risk attendant to its use. Superficial skin infections occur in approximately 4% of patients,[54, 55] and radial artery occlusion may occur in up to 40% of patients.[56, 57] Nevertheless, compromise of hand or digits is rare and does not appear to result in the absence of concurrent vasopressor therapy, multiple particulate emboli from the heart, or prolonged periods of low cardiac output.

Central Venous and Pulmonary Artery Pressure Monitoring

Central pressure monitoring, including central venous pressure (CVP) and pulmonary artery pressure (PAP), have increased during the past 20 years, partly because of their widespread application in cardiovascular surgical patients. Once again, randomized trials do not document their effectiveness. It seems unlikely that such trials will ever be performed effectively.

Complications. Unlike direct systemic arterial blood pressure monitoring, the risks associated with both CVP and PAP monitoring must be seriously considered in risk-benefit analyses. Carotid artery puncture, infection, thrombosis of central veins, and pulmonary artery rupture (including death) occur with these techniques. Despite these problems, the pulmonary artery catheter has made available tremendous amounts of information to anesthesiologists, allowing classification of many perioperative disease states into understandable terms and treatment regimens.

Application. The prescription of invasive central monitoring for an individual patient must be predicated on many of the factors already discussed. Shoemaker and colleagues proposed that the use of a pulmonary artery catheter to direct "supraphysiologic cardiovascular function" lowered perioperative deaths in high-risk general surgical patients.[58] The final choice about using pulmonary artery and central venous catheters needs to be based on your particular institution and practice style. I believe that CVP monitoring alone to direct hemodynamic therapy is misguided in many situations. The risks

of adverse outcomes are lower with CVP catheters than with pulmonary artery catheters; however, useful hemodynamic information is less frequently obtained from the former devices.

What Advantages Accrue to Regional Anesthesia?

Advantages of regional anesthesia over general anesthesia are difficult to confirm in most circumstances. In certain clinical situations, however, regional techniques are clearly advantageous. A decreased incidence of deep venous thrombosis follows centroneuraxis blocks during hip repair and prostatectomy.[59] Fewer episodes of congestive heart failure occur during low spinal anesthesia.[60] Organ function also appears better preserved, and decreased morbidity and possibly reduced mortality are noted in critically ill patients for whom prolonged epidural analgesia is used in the intensive care unit.[61, 62]

A long-quoted criticism of regional anesthesia is that it "takes too long," an accurate assessment if such techniques are infrequently used.[63] Because many anesthesia trainees have limited access to comprehensive regional anesthesia experience, the development of efficient regional anesthesia skills may be difficult.[64] Conversely, if regional anesthesia is conducted in a comprehensive manner using induction rooms and appropriate levels of sedation, skilled anesthesiologists can keep turnover time to a minimum and provide efficient anesthetic care.

Postoperative Analgesia

If a stand-alone regional anesthetic is used before surgical incision or as part of a general anesthetic technique, postoperative pain may be lessened for a period of time even after the local anesthetic effect has resolved. Tverskoy and colleagues showed that regional anesthesia during herniorrhaphy is associated with less postoperative pain than are general anesthesia and routine opioids for postoperative analgesia in similar patients.[65] My belief is that the advantages of regional anesthesia, in most circumstances, are related to prolonged postoperative analgesia.

What Advantages Accrue to General Anesthesia?

A recurring theme during preoperative discussion with many surgical patients is their desire to be "asleep." If anesthesiologists interpret this to mean a patient wishes a general anesthetic, appropriate prescription can be difficult. From the times of Crile and Lundy,[66, 67] it has been clear that most patients prefer to be amnestic for their operative experience. With the addition of anesthetic agents such as midazolam, propofol, and fentanyl and its congeners, amnesia for the operative experience does not preclude a regional anesthetic. Conversely, as noted earlier, in only a few situations is it clear that regional anesthesia has advantages over general anesthesia. Therefore, administration of a general anesthetic for almost any operative procedure may be easily justified.

Which Considerations Are Important?

General anesthetic techniques can be provided with quite different methods. Primarily inhalational anesthesia, using the

TABLE 5–4. Severe Adverse Anesthetic Outcome in General Anesthesia

Anesthetic	Tachycardia	Hypertension	Ventricular Dysrhythmia
Halothane	0.7%	0.5%	8.6%*
Isoflurane	1.5%*	0.8%	0.8%
Fentanyl	1.0%	2.4%*	1.3%

(From Forrest JB, Rehder K, Cahalan MK, et al: Multicenter study of general anesthesia. III. Predictors of severe perioperative adverse outcomes. Anesthesiology 1992; 76:3.)
*Significantly different from other anesthetics.

lungs as the route of anesthetic uptake, or high-dose opioid techniques, using intravenous administration, can be applied with equal facility. However, when high-dose opioid techniques are used, that consideration must include the need for postoperative mechanical ventilation.

Familiarity

Despite the concept that one should administer whatever general anesthetic technique with which one has had the most experience, recent data from the multi-institutional general anesthetic study by Forrest and colleagues document that statistically different incidences of adverse outcomes depend on the general anesthetic technique chosen (Table 5–4).[16] Thus, hypertension is more common with fentanyl, ventricular dysrhythmias are more common with halothane anesthesia, and tachycardia is more common when isoflurane is used as a primary anesthetic agent.[16]

Data Interpretation

Additional information about differences in general anesthetic prescription comes from a contrary interpretation of the data of Yeager and colleagues.[61] They showed that prolonged epidural analgesia in high-risk patients lowered their risk of morbidity and mortality, compared with patients receiving a moderate- to high-dose fentanyl general anesthetic. The striking differences perhaps would not have been as large if the patients receiving general anesthesia had received a lower dose of opioid or an inhalational-based anesthetic.

As a result of the moderate- to high-dose opioid technique chosen in the general anesthetic group, patients required on average more than 80 hours of tracheal intubation and mechanical ventilation, compared with approximately 7 hours in the patients having regional anesthesia. Perhaps what really was shown in this study was that prolonged postoperative mechanical ventilation is not as risk free as many anesthesiologists believed. This alternative interpretation must remain speculative, because it was not designed as part of the original study.

TABLE 5–5. Major Risks Associated with Analgesia Techniques

Analgesia Technique	Complication	Incidence
Peridural opioid	Severe respiratory depression	1:500–1:1100[70, 71]
Parenteral opioid (intravenous, subcutaneous, intramuscular)	Respiratory depression	1:100[72]
Intercostal nerve block	Symptomatic pneumothorax	1:1100[73]

Additional data highlight the differences between general anesthetic techniques. Anand and Hickey found that infants anesthetized for the repair of complex congenital heart lesions had lower perioperative mortality when administered a high-dose sufentanil opioid anesthetic that was continued into the postoperative period, compared with a similar group receiving a traditional halothane technique.[68] This study is sound in design and, coupled with data from Forrest and colleagues,[16] suggests that anesthesiologists using primarily general anesthetic techniques must be willing to alter their anesthetic prescription to specific patient requirements.

POSTOPERATIVE ANALGESIA

Interest in postoperative analgesia care for surgical patients has humanitarian as well as practical implications. The benefit of anesthesia is that patients are able to undergo a surgical procedure without the ''mortal pain'' that accompanied surgical care before the 1840s.

Although most anesthesiologists are supportive of the advances made in postoperative analgesia, some suggest that acute postoperative pain services are not in their best interests. This concept smacks of those mid-1840s days when some physicians criticized the introduction of effective general anesthetics.[69] Because anesthesia practice is based on the basic concept of pain relief, it seems important to me for anesthesiologists to continue to advance patient care in that area.

What Are the Advantages?

On the practical side, increasing evidence suggests that the nervous system and its pain recognition components are not the ''hard-wired'' structures that many of us learned in medical school. Rather, prevention of pain through the use of more effective regional analgesic or parenteral techniques may affect the degree of pain a patient experiences at a time remote from the anesthetic and analgesic intervention.[70]

Yeager and coworkers[61] and Tuman and colleagues[62] demonstrated that epidural analgesia carried into the postoperative period of high-risk surgical patients can reduce the mortality and morbidity associated with these surgical procedures. Tverskoy and colleagues found that a common surgical procedure, inguinal herniorrhaphy, is associated with less postoperative pain if a regional anesthetic technique is used as part of the anesthetic.[65]

What Are the Risks?

If analgesia was prescribed and carried out without any associated increased morbidity, this discussion would be moot. However, almost all analgesia is associated with small but measurable risks (Table 5–5). Epidural opioid analgesia provides excellent analgesia for major intra-abdominal procedures,[61, 62] but it may lead to respiratory depression. Should this potential problem prevent anesthesiologists from prescribing the technique? Probably not. The often forgotten part of the risk-benefit equation is that respiratory depression accompanies routine parenteral opioid analgesia.

What Are the Costs?

Yeager and colleagues included data about physician and hospital costs associated with random assignment to traditional or epidural analgesia techniques.[61] Although their study was small, including only 53 patients, the costs associated with epidural analgesia were significantly less overall than those associated with traditional analgesia.

Because physicians and hospital administrators are most comfortable in thinking of medical costs in an unbundled fashion, many fail to recognize that money spent for analgesia may, in the long run, may save money during the period of an entire hospitalization. If techniques allow patients to return to their jobs sooner because of improved analgesia, further decreases in incremental costs may accrue.

References

1. The lessons of CEPOD (Editorial). Br J Anaesth 1988; 60:753.
2. Natof HE: Complications. *In* Anesthesia for Ambulatory Surgery. Wetchler BV (ed). Philadelphia, JB Lippincott, 1985, p 349.
3. Eichhorn JH: Prevention of intraoperative anesthesia accidents and related severe injury through safety monitoring. Anesthesiology 1989; 70:572.
4. Slogoff S, Keats AS: Does perioperative myocardial ischemia lead to postoperative myocardial infarction? Anesthesiology 1985; 62:107.
5. Goldman RL: The reliability of peer assessments of quality of care. JAMA 1992; 267:958.
6. Caplan RA, Posner KL, Cheney FW: Effect of outcome on physician judgments of appropriateness of care. JAMA 1991; 265:1957.
7. Cohen MM, Duncan PG, Pope WDB, et al: A survey of 112,000 anaesthetics at one teaching hospital (1975–83). Can Anaesth Soc J 1986; 33:22.
8. Fowkes FGR, Lunn JN, Farrow SC, et al: Epidemiology in anaesthesia III: mortality risk in patients with coexisting physical disease. Br J Anaesth 1982; 54:819.
9. JB Forrest: Personal communications, 1986.
10. Cohen MM, Duncan PG, Tate RB: Does anaesthesia contribute to operative mortality? JAMA 1988; 260:2859.
11. Eiseman B: What Are My Chances? Philadelphia, WB Saunders, 1980, p 15.
12. Merry AF, Ramage MC, Whitlock RML, et al: First-time coronary artery bypass grafting: the anaesthetist as a risk factor. Br J Anaesth 1992; 68:6.
13. Luft HS, Bunker JP, Einthoven AC: Should operations be regionalized? The empirical relation between surgical volume and mortality. N Engl J Med 1979; 301:1364.
14. Kennedy JW, Kaiser GC, Fischer LD, et al: Clinical and angiographic predictors of operative mortality from the collaborative study in coronary artery surgery (CASS). Circulation 1981; 63:793.
15. Pedersen T, Eliasen K, Henriksen E: A prospective study of risk factors and cardiopulmonary complications associated with anaesthesia and surgery: risk indicators of cardiopulmonary morbidity. Acta Anaesthesiol Scand 1990; 34:144.
16. Forrest JB, Rehder K, Cahalan MK, et al: Multicenter study of general anesthesia. III. Predictors of severe perioperative adverse outcomes. Anesthesiology 1992; 76:3.
17. Practice Standards: The Midas Touch or The Emperor's New Clothes? (Editorial). Anesthesiology 1989; 70:567
18. Tiret L, Desmonts JM, Hatton F, et al: Complications associated with anaesthesia—a prospective survey in France. Can Anaesth Soc J 1986; 33:336.
19. Tiret L, Hatton F, Desmonts JM, et al: Prediction of outcome anaesthesia in patients over 40 years: a multifactorial risk index. Stat Med 1988; 7:947.
20. The Hypertension Detection and Follow-Up Program: The effect of treatment on mortality in ''mild'' hypertension: results of the hypertension detection and follow-up program. N Engl J Med 1982; 307:976.
21. Goldman L, Caldera DL: Risks of general anesthesia and elective operation in the hypertensive patient. Anesthesiology 1979; 50:285.
22. Ross AF, Tinker JH: Cardiovascular disease. *In* Risk and Outcome in Anesthesia. Brown DL (ed). Philadelphia, JB Lippincott, 1992, pp 39–76.
23. Rao TLK, Jacobs KH, El-Etr AA: Reinfarction following anesthesia in patients with myocardial infarction. Anesthesiology 1983; 59:499.
24. Goldman L, Caldera DL, Southwick FS, et al: Cardiac risk factors and complications in noncardiac surgery. Medicine 1978; 57:357.
25. Goldman L: Cardiac risks and complications of noncardiac surgery. Ann Surg 1983; 198:780.
26. Mangano DT, Browner WS, Hollenberger M, et al: Association of perioperative myocardial ischemia with cardiac morbidity and mortality in men undergoing noncardiac surgery. N Engl J Med 1990; 323:1781.
27. Moorman JR, Hlatky MA, Eddy DM, et al: The yield of the routine admission electrocardiogram—a study in a general medical service. Ann Intern Med 1985; 103:590.
28. Pasternack PF, Imparato AM, Bear G, et al: The value of radionuclide angiography as a predictor of perioperative myocardial infarction in patients undergoing abdominal aortic aneurysm resection. J Vasc Surg 1984; 1:320.
29. Moraski RE, Russell RO, Smith M, et al: Left ventricular function in patients with and without myocardial infarction and one, two, or three vessel coronary artery disease. Am J Cardiol 1975; 35:1.
30. Boucher CA, Brewster DC, Darling RC, et al: Determination of cardiac risk by dipyridamole-thallium imaging before peripheral vascular surgery. N Engl J Med 1985; 312:389.
31. Eagle KA, Boucher CA: Cardiac risk of noncardiac surgery. N Engl J Med 1989; 321:1300.
32. Gerson MC, Hurst JM, Hertzberg VS, et al: Cardiac prognosis in noncardiac geriatric surgery. Ann Intern Med 1985; 103:832.
33. Gerson MC, Hurst JM, Hertzberg VS, et al: Prediction of cardiac and pulmonary complications related to elective abdominal and noncardiac thoracic surgery in geriatric patients. Am J Med 1990; 88:101.
34. Caplan RA, Posner KL, Ward RJ, et al: Adverse respiratory events in anesthesia: a closed claims analysis. Anesthesiology 1990; 72:828.
35. Meneely GR, Ferguson JL: Pulmonary evaluation and risk in patient preparation for anesthesia and surgery. JAMA 1961; 175:1074.
36. Ford GT, Whitelaw WA, Rosenal TW, et al: Diaphragm function after upper abdominal surgery in humans. Am Rev Respir Dis 1983; 127:431.
37. Latimer RC, Dickman M, Day WC, et al: Ventilatory patterns and pulmonary complications after upper abdominal surgery determined by preoperative and postoperative computerized spirometry and blood gas analysis. Am J Surg 1971; 122:622.
38. Gracey DR, Divertie MB, Didier EP: Preoperative pulmonary preparation of patients with chronic obstructive pulmonary disease. Chest 1979; 76:123.
39. William CD, Brenowitz JB: Prohibitive lung function and major surgical procedures. Am J Surg 1976; 132:763.
40. Milledge JS, Nunn FJ: Criteria for fitness for anesthesia in patients with chronic obstructive lung disease. Br Med J 1975; 3:670.
41. Kingston HGG, Hirschman CA: Perioperative management of the patient with asthma. Anesth Analg 1984; 63:844.
42. Shnider SM, Papper EM: Anesthesia for the asthmatic patient. Anesthesiology 1961; 22:886.
43. Gold MI, Helrich M: A study of complications related to anesthesia in asthmatic patients. Anesth Analg 1963; 42:283.
44. Roizen MF: Preoperative evaluation. *In* Anesthesia. Miller RD (ed). New York, Churchill Livingstone, 1990, p 753.
45. Dexter DD, Whisnant JP, Connolly DC, et al: The association of stroke and coronary heart disease: a population study. Mayo Clin Proc 1987; 62:1077.
46. Torvik A, Skullerud K: How often are brain infarcts caused by hypotensive episodes? Stroke 1976; 7:255.
47. Wolf PA, Kannel WB, Sorlie P, et al: Asymptomatic carotid bruit and risk of stroke: the Framingham study. JAMA 1981; 245:1442.
48. Ropper AH, Wechsler LR, Wilson LS: Carotid bruit and the risk of stroke in elective surgery. N Engl J Med 1982; 307:1388.
49. Kurtz CM, Bennett JH, Shapiro HH: Electrocardiographic studies during surgical anesthesia. JAMA 1936; 106:434.
50. Moller JT, Pedersen T, Rasmussen L, et al: Randomized evaluation of pulse oximetry in 20,802 patients (I and II). Anesthesiology 1993; 78:436, 445.
51. Tinker JH, Dull DL, Caplan RA, et al: Role of monitoring devices in prevention of anesthetic mishaps: a closed claims analysis. Anesthesiology 1989; 71:541.
52. Kestin IG, Miller BR, Lockhart CH: Auditory alarms during anesthesia monitoring. Anesthesiology 1988; 69:106.
53. Wagner DL: Hemodynamic monitoring. *In* Risk and Outcome in Anesthesia. 2nd ed. Brown DL (ed). Philadelphia, JB Lippincott, 1992, pp 283–312.
54. Pinilla JC, Ross DF, Martin T, et al: Study of the incidence of intravascular catheter infection and associated septicemia in critically ill patients. Crit Care Med 1983; 11:21.
55. Gardner RM, Schwartz R, Wong HC: Percutaneous indwelling radial artery catheters for monitoring cardiovascular function. Prospective study of the risk of thrombosis and infection. N Engl J Med 1974; 290:1227.

56. Slogoff S, Keats AS, Arlund C: On the safety of radial artery cannulation. Anesthesiology 1983; 59:42.
57. Bedford RF, Wollman H: Complications of percutaneous radial artery cannulation: an objective prospective study in man. Anesthesiology 1973; 38:228.
58. Shoemaker WC, Appel PL, Kram HB, et al: Prospective trial of supranormal values of survivors as therapeutic goals in high-risk surgical patients. Chest 1988; 94:1176.
59. Brown DL: Anesthetic choice. *In* Risk and Outcome in Anesthesia. Brown DL (ed). Philadelphia, JB Lippincott, 1992, pp 193–234.
60. Greene NM: Physiology of Spinal Anesthesia. Baltimore, Williams & Wilkins, 1981, p 93.
61. Yeager MP, Glass DD, Neff RK, et al: Epidural anesthesia and analgesia in high-risk surgical patients. Anesthesiology 1987; 66:729.
62. Tuman KJ, McCarthy RJ, March RJ, et al: Effects of epidural anesthesia and analgesia on coagulation and outcome after major vascular surgery. Anesth Analg 1991; 73:696.
63. Bonica JJ: Regional anesthesia in private practice. Anesthesiology 1960; 21:554.
64. Bridenbaugh LD: Are anesthesia resident programs failing regional anesthesia? Reg Anesth 1982; 7:26.
65. Tverskoy M, Cozacov C, Ayache M, et al: Postoperative pain after inguinal herniorrhaphy with different types of anesthesia. Anesth Analg 1990; 70:29.
66. Crile GW: Nitrous oxide anaesthesia and a note on anociassociation, a new principle in operative surgery. Surg Gynecol Obstet 1911; 13:170.
67. Lundy JS: Balanced anesthesia. Minn Med 1926; 9:399.
68. Anand KJS, Hickey PR: Halothane-morphine compared with high-dose sufentanil for anesthesia and postoperative analgesia in neonatal cardiac surgery. N Engl J Med 1992; 326:1.
69. Brown DL: Anesthesia risk: a historical perspective. *In* Risk and Outcome in Anesthesia. Brown DL (ed). Philadelphia, JB Lippincott, 1992, pp 1–35.
70. Dickenson AH, Sullivan AF: Subcutaneous formalin-induced activity of the dorsal horn neurons in the rat: differential response to an intrathecal opiate administered pre or post formalin. Pain 1987; 30:349.
71. Ready LB, Loper KA, Nessly M, et al: Postoperative epidural morphine is safe on surgical wards. Anesthesiology 1991; 75:452.
72. Rawal N, Arner S, Gustafsson LL, et al: Present state of extradural and intrathecal opioid analgesia in Sweden. Br J Anaesth 1987; 59:791.
73. Miller RR, Greenblatt DG (eds): Drug Effects in Hospitalized Patients: Experiences of the Boston Collaborative Drug Surveillance Program, 1966–75. New York, John Wiley & Sons, 1976.
74. Moore DC, Bridenbaugh LD: Intercostal nerve block in 4,333 patients. Anesth Analg 1962; 41:1.

CHAPTER **6**

Postanesthesia Recovery

ROGER S. MECCA, M.D.

An organized clinical environment that enhances one's ability to perform individualized, problem-oriented patient assessment and care is essential to ensure optimal postoperative recovery with minimum risk, inconvenience, and expense. Facility design, staffing, and equipment requirements for a postanesthesia care unit (PACU) are reviewed elsewhere.[1, 2] The standards for postanesthesia care described in the American Society of Anesthesiologists (ASA) Directory of Members are listed in Table 6–1.

GENERAL CONCERNS

The administrative structure of a PACU service can have dramatic impact on the quality of clinical care offered and liability exposure for physicians, PACU nurses, and hospitals. Clear lines of authority for patient care and disposition must be established and observed to avoid any confusion about which physician is responsible when clinical decisions are necessary or when problems arise.

What Are the Minimal Administrative Considerations?

Patient Coverage

Policies governing patient coverage by PACU nurses should address the method of assignment and minimum staff-to-patient ratios. A primary PACU nurse should be assigned to each patient on admission, and a PACU nurse should not be responsible for more than two patients at a time. Depending on patient acuity, one-to-one coverage is often appropriate. It is also important to have and be aware of the policy for ensuring the availability of a physician capable of managing complications in the PACU if an anesthesiologist is not available.

Performance Evaluation

Compulsive staff development, interdisciplinary medical education, and performance evaluation are required to ensure that every patient can be cared for by a nurse with sufficient skill and judgment to recognize and process evolving problems of airway management, pulmonary function, and cardiovascular dynamics.

Policies and Procedures

A comprehensive policy and procedure manual must be created to ensure that all aspects of clinical care in the PACU are optimal. Medical directors should be cautious about creating policies that are unrealistic or cannot be followed because the inevitable lack of compliance can make appropriate clinical activity appear to fall below an unachievable local standard of care. Finally, an aggressive program of interdisciplinary quality assurance and risk management is essential to ensure that care available in the PACU remains safe, appropriate, and up to date.

Does Every Patient Need to Go Through the Postanesthesia Care Unit?

The level of postoperative care that a patient requires varies with the underlying illness, duration and complexity of anesthesia and surgery, and risk of postoperative complications. Straightforward patients receiving local infiltration, digital blocks, or field blocks can often be transferred from the operating room to less intensive discharge settings, even after moderate sedation. Patients should always be admitted to a PACU if there is any concern about their ability to recover safely in an unmonitored setting. It is clear that the PACU has an important role in the acute postoperative management of patients; this is evident in Figure 6–1, which shows the frequency of various complications encountered in this setting from a prospective study of more than 18,000 patients.[3]

What Are the Initial Steps on Admission?

Monitoring

When patients are admitted to a PACU, their heart rate, systemic blood pressure, and ventilatory rate should be recorded initially and at least every 5 minutes for the first 15 minutes, and thereafter every 15 minutes. Their temperature should be documented at least on admission and discharge and

TABLE 6–1. Standards for Postanesthesia Care*

These standards apply to postanesthesia care in all locations. These standards may be exceeded based on the judgment of the responsible anesthesiologist. They are intended to encourage high-quality patient care but cannot guarantee any specific patient outcome. They are subject to revision from time to time as warranted by the evolution of technology and practice. Under extenuating circumstances, the responsible anesthesiologist may waive the requirements marked with an asterisk (*); it is recommended that when this is done, it should be so stated (including the reasons) in a note in the patient's medical record.

Standard I:

All patients who have received general anesthesia, regional anesthesia, or monitored anesthesia care shall receive appropriate postanesthesia management.

1. A postanesthesia care unit (PACU) or an area that provides equivalent postanesthesia care shall be available to receive patients after surgery and anesthesia. All patients who receive anesthesia shall be admitted to the PACU except by specific order of the anesthesiologist responsible for the patient's care.
2. The medical aspects of care in the PACU shall be governed by policies and procedures that have been reviewed and approved by the Department of Anesthesiology.
3. The design, equipment, and staffing of the PACU shall meet requirements of the facility's accrediting and licensing bodies.
4. The nursing standards of practice shall be consistent with those approved in 1986 by the American Society of Post Anesthesia Nurses (ASPAN).

Standard II:

A patient transported to the PACU shall be accompanied by a member of the anesthesia care team who is knowledgeable about the patient's condition. The patient shall be continually evaluated and treated during transport with monitoring and support appropriate to the patient's condition.

Standard III:

On arrival in the PACU, the patient shall be re-evaluated and a verbal report provided to the responsible PACU nurse by the member of the anesthesia care team who accompanies the patient.

1. The patient's status on arrival in the PACU shall be documented.
2. Information concerning the preoperative condition and the surgical/anesthetic course shall be transmitted to the PACU nurse.
3. The member of the anesthesia care team shall remain in the PACU until the PACU nurse accepts responsibility for the nursing care of the patient.

Standard IV:

The patient's condition shall be evaluated continually in the PACU.

1. The patient shall be observed and monitored by methods appropriate to the patient's medical condition. Particular attention should be given to monitoring oxygenation, ventilation, and circulation. During recovery from all anesthetics, a quantitative method of assessing oxygenation such as pulse oximetry shall be used in the initial phase of recovery.*† This is not intended for application during the recovery of obstetric patients in whom regional anesthesia was used for labor and delivery.
2. An accurate written report of the PACU period shall be maintained. Use of an appropriate PACU scoring system is encouraged for each patient on admission, at appropriate intervals before discharge, and at the time of discharge.
3. General medical supervision and coordination of patient care in the PACU should be the responsibility of an anesthesiologist.
4. There shall be a policy to ensure the availability in the facility of a physician capable of managing complications and providing cardiopulmonary resuscitation for patients in the PACU.

Standard V:

A physician will be responsible for the discharge of the patient from the postanesthesia care unit.

1. When discharge criteria are used, they must be approved by the Department of Anesthesiology and the medical staff. They may vary depending on whether the patient is discharged to a hospital room, to the intensive care unit, to a short-stay unit, or to home.
2. In the absence of the physician responsible for the discharge, the PACU nurse shall determine that the patient meets the discharge criteria. The name of the physician accepting responsibility for discharge shall be noted on the record.

(From 1993 ASA Directory of Members. Park Ridge, IL, American Society of Anesthesiologists, 1993.)
*Approved by the House of Delegates on October 12, 1988, and last amended on October 21, 1992.
†To become effective as soon as feasible but no later than January 1, 1992.

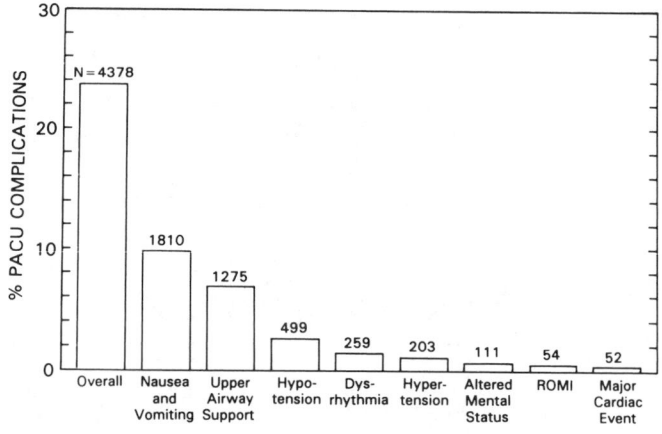

FIGURE 6–1. Major PACU complications by percentage of occurrence and number of patients (*above the bars*) experiencing each complication. Nausea and vomiting were the most frequently observed PACU complications, occurring in 1810 patients (9.8%). (From Hines R, Barash PG, Watrous G, et al: Complications occurring in the postanesthesia care unit: a survey. Anesth Analg 1992; 74:503.)

more frequently if appropriate. Axillary or oral routes are usually acceptable, although rectal, tympanic, or esophageal determination is necessary if an assessment of core temperature is important.

Documentation of the level of consciousness, skin color, character of ventilation, and airway patency is important. Every patient in a PACU should be monitored with a pulse oximeter and single-lead continuous electrocardiography (ECG). Continuous capnographic monitoring is not essential for all patients but should be used when mechanical ventilation is required or when a patient is at risk for compromised ventilation. Signals from invasive devices such as arterial, central venous, and pulmonary artery catheters should be transduced and recorded.

Transfer to the Postanesthesia Care Unit Staff

Before anesthesiology personnel transfer responsibility for a patient's care, the PACU staff should have ample opportunity to ascertain admission vital signs and to record a succinct clinical report (Table 6–2), which facilitates rapid evaluation and intervention if sudden postoperative complications arise. A standardized format printed on the PACU record is useful.

Location of a responsible anesthesiologist must be clearly identified, and orders for required laboratory evaluations or therapeutic interventions should be thoroughly reviewed. A patient should never be left with PACU personnel if airway patency, ventilation, or hemodynamic stability is uncertain. A final check of intravenous catheters and monitoring devices should be completed. Appropriate reporting and careful, legible documentation not only decrease clinical risks but also reduce potential liability exposure for claims of negligence or abandonment should complications occur during the PACU interval.[4]

Routine Laboratory Tests

Routine postoperative laboratory testing should be avoided. Tests such as hematocrit and electrolyte determinations, arterial blood gas (ABG) measurements, ECG, and chest radiography should be ordered individually based on each patient's requirements.[5]

TABLE 6–2. Postanesthesia Care Unit Admission Report

Pertinent History

Significant medical illnesses	Chronic medications, last dose
Pertient previous surgery	Medication allergies and sensitivities

Preoperative Status

Acute conditions (ischemia, dehydration)	Premedication and preoperative meds
Traumatic injuries	NPO status

Intraoperative Factors

Surgeon and anesthesiologist	Surgical procedure
Amount and time of narcotic administration	Type of anesthetic and specific agents
Relaxant and reversal status	Amount and type of intravenous
Urine output	fluids
Intraoperative vital sign ranges	Estimated blood loss and
Unexpected surgical and anesthetic events	replacement
	Other medications (steroids, diuretics, antibiotics)
	Intraoperative laboratory findings

Status on Admission to PACU*

Systemic pressure	Heart rate and rhythm
Level of consciousness	Airway patency and ventilatory
Size and location of intravenous catheters	adequacy
	Intravascular volume status
Endotracheal tube position	Function and readings, invasive
Overall assessment of status	monitors
	Overall assessment of status
	Anesthetic equipment (epidural catheters)

Postoperative Instructions

Acceptable urine output and blood loss	Acceptable vital sign ranges
	Anticipated cardiovascular problems
Anticipated airway and ventilatory status	Diagnostic tests to be secured
	Orders for therapeutic interventions
Therapeutic goals and end points	
Surgical instructions (positioning, wound care)	
Location of the responsible anesthesiologist	

*Clinical judgment should supersede guidelines, because not every patient will meet all criteria. If any doubt exists about a patient's viability beyond the PACU, discharge should be delayed.

When Is a Patient Ready to Leave the Postanesthesia Care Unit?

Assessment

A decision to release a patient from a PACU is usually based on both objective and subjective criteria. Use of only fixed discharge criteria introduces an element of additional risk, because interpatient variability is significant. Scoring systems that quantify physical status are useful to facilitate assessment[6, 7] but should not replace individual evaluation. Vital signs should be stable, and pulse oximetry should verify adequate oxygenation. These indices and any laboratory results should always be interpreted in the context of a patient's clinical condition.

In an ideal setting, every patient should be discharged by an anesthesiologist using consistent criteria after thorough evaluation of the anesthetic, PACU course, and the patient's condition (Table 6–3). The level of care available at a patient's destination must also be considered, especially for ambulatory patients who will be leaving the medical facility.

Mental and Physical Status

Before discharge, patients should be able to evaluate their physical condition, communicate perceived problems, and summon assistance. Airway protective reflexes must be sufficiently recovered to prevent aspiration, and pulmonary function should be adequate to overcome potential minor deterioration in ventilation and oxygenation. Systemic blood pressure and heart rate need to be relatively constant for at least 1/2 hour before discharge from the PACU.

Complete rewarming to normal body temperature is not absolutely necessary in many patients, but shivering and discomfort should be resolved. Intravascular volume and peripheral perfusion must be stable. The evolution of potentially adverse surgical sequelae or complications of pre-existing conditions like coronary artery disease, diabetes, or bronchospastic diseases should be evaluated.

Late Interventions

Be sure to assess the peak impact of late therapeutic interventions before discharge. After discontinuation of supplemental oxygen (O_2) therapy, staff must watch for 15 to 20 minutes to detect unexpected hypoxemia with room air ventilation. Patients should be observed for at least 20 to 30 minutes after administration of any medication with potential cardiovascular or ventilatory side effects (i.e., narcotics and sedatives, antihypertensives, calcium channel or β-adrenergic blockers, and antidysrhythmics). A sufficient period of observation is also necessary after reinforcement of regional anesthetic tech-

TABLE 6–3. Criteria for Discharge from a Postanesthesia Care Unit*

General

Oriented to time, place, and surgical procedure
Follows simple instructions
Adequate strength and mobility for minimal self-sufficiency (?)
Suitable control of nausea and vomiting
Appropriate appearance without cyanosis or splotches
Control of acute surgical complications (bleeding, edema, diminished pulses)
Status appropriate for destination
Ambulates without dizziness, hypotension, or support (ambulatory patients)
Suitable control of motion related to nausea and vomiting (ambulatory patients)
Ability to drink or eat if appropriate (ambulatory patients)

Airway Maintenance

Adequate level of consciousness
Protective reflexes (swallow, gag) intact
Absence of stridor, retraction, or other signs of obstruction
Assistance not needed for airway support

Ventilation and Oxygenation

Spontaneous ventilatory rate >10, <30
Forced vital capacity approximately twice tidal volume
Adequate ability to cough and clear secretions
Qualitatively acceptable work of breathing

Systemic Blood Pressure: Heart Rate and Rhythm

Within ±20% resting preoperative value
Relatively constant for at least 30 min
Acceptable intravascular volume status
Resolution or clearance of any new dysrhythmia
Suspicion of myocardial ischemia clarified

Renal Function

Urine output >30 mL · hr^{-1}
Appropriate color and appearance of urine, notation of hematuria
Follow-up orders if spontaneous voiding has not occurred
Acceptable hematocrit for hydration, blood loss, and potential future loss
Appropriate blood glucose and electrolyte status
Chest radiograph electrocardiogram, and other tests reviewed

*Clinical judgment should supersede guidelines, because not every patient will meet all criteria. If any doubt exists about a patient's viability beyond the PACU, discharge should be delayed.

niques. Results of postoperative diagnostic tests should be reviewed.

Postponement of Discharge

If any doubt remains about a patient's stability outside the PACU, the discharge can be postponed or the patient transferred to a specialized unit for extended definitive care and monitoring. Remember that the level and quality of care are decreased if a patient is discharged to any area of the hospital except a special care unit.

PAIN CONTROL

What Is an Acceptable Approach to Postoperative Pain Management?

Narcotics

The clinical end point for postoperative analgesic therapy is relief of surgical pain without undesired side effects. Surgical pain can be effectively treated with intermittent intravenous opiate administration. Long-acting agents such as morphine or meperidine are useful, although shorter-acting narcotics are more appropriate in ambulatory settings. Very large doses of narcotics are acceptable when required by tolerant patients who take analgesics chronically or who abuse opioids or alcohol.

Intravenous narcotic administration permits expeditious titration to a safe, appropriate level of analgesia with minimal risk of respiratory or cardiovascular depression. Such "loading" in the PACU is a first step in the transition to postoperative patient-controlled analgesia (PCA). The physician responsible for regulating postoperative PCA must be familiar with patients' intraoperative and PACU narcotic regimens.

Alternate Routes of Administration

Administration of postoperative analgesics by the intramuscular route is less desirable because of delayed onset, unpredictable uptake in hypothermic patients, requirement for larger doses, and the fact that most intramuscular injections ($\leq 85\%$) are actually subcutaneous. Selected pediatric patients may benefit from rectal administration of analgesics. Oral and transdermal routes are usually ineffective during immediate postoperative recovery.

Non-Narcotic Analgesics

Non-narcotic analgesics generally offer little advantage over narcotics for PACU applications. However, supplementation of narcotic analgesia with agents like ketorolac or clonidine can significantly reduce narcotic analgesic requirements and side effects. Be aware that hypotension can occur after their administration.[8-11]

Hypotension Following Pain Relief

Relief of pain decreases sympathetic nervous system (SNS) activity, reducing postoperative hypertension, tachycardia, and agitation. Analgesia, in conjunction with vasodilation secondary to decreased venous adrenergic tone or narcotic-induced histamine release, can precipitate hypotension. Hypovolemic patients who rely on SNS activity to support cardiovascular function are at especially high risk of hypotension with a reduction of postoperative pain. Any normotensive or hypotensive patient with signs and symptoms of severe postoperative pain is most likely hypovolemic, especially if tachycardia is also present.

Fear and Anxiety

Removal of offending stimuli through repositioning, extubation of the trachea, or Foley catheter removal decreases the level of postoperative discomfort. If fear, anxiety, or agitation accentuates the reaction to postoperative pain during emergence from general anesthesia, titration of intravenous diazepam or midazolam often decreases these psychogenic components.

Be sure to differentiate between analgesic and sedative requirements. Opiates are relatively ineffective sedatives, whereas benzodiazepines and other sedatives do not provide analgesia. Choice of the wrong drug type only increases the risk of unnecessary side effects. A calm and reassuring manner shown by the anesthesiologist and PACU personnel is as important as the drugs given.

How Should the Intensity and Severity of Pain Be Assessed?

The intensity of postoperative pain after a given surgical procedure is affected by surgical skill, anesthetic techniques, and an individual patient's pain tolerance. A poor correlation is often found between cognitive perception of postoperative pain and the SNS response, which is probably caused by cultural, psychologic, and cardiovascular variations. Some patients exhibit hypertension, tachycardia, and ectopic cardiac complexes on the ECG with minimal complaint of discomfort, whereas others perceive severe pain without evidence of unusual autonomic nervous system tone.

Appropriateness of Pain

Before medicating a patient, make sure that the nature and degree of pain being treated are consistent with the operative procedure and anesthetic technique.[12] This step helps to avoid inadvertent masking of signs of an evolving surgical complication or unrelated condition. In addition, central nervous system (CNS) manifestations of hypoxemia, respiratory acidemia, or cerebral hypoperfusion often mimic signs of postoperative pain, especially after general anesthesia.

Hypoventilation or hypotension can be acutely exacerbated by parenteral analgesic or sedative administration, leading to cardiorespiratory collapse. Careful assessment of arousal and orientation, as well as systemic perfusion pressure and minute ventilation, usually identifies these patients.

What Alternative Techniques Are Useful?

Alternative modalities are available to provide analgesia through and beyond the PACU stay.

Epidural and Subarachnoid Narcotics

Epidural or subarachnoid narcotics administered during surgery can yield prolonged postoperative analgesia in selected patients.[13, 14] However, both immediate and delayed ventilatory depression may occur secondary to vascular uptake and rostral cerebrospinal fluid (CSF) spread. Hence, epidural or intrathecal narcotics use mandates careful ventilatory monitoring.[15]

Nausea and pruritus are bothersome side effects of both PCA and spinal narcotic administration. Addition of local anesthetics to continuous-infusion epidural narcotic regimens augments postoperative analgesia but adds to the risk of unwanted motor blockade or inadvertent subarachnoid injection. After major abdominal surgery, epidural techniques are particularly useful to facilitate weaning patients with morbid obesity or severe chronic obstructive lung disease (COLD) from mechanical ventilation.[16] Clonidine enhances analgesia and decreases the intensity of side effects from epidural opiates.[8, 17, 18]

Regional Blocks

Long-acting regional blocks effectively reduce postoperative pain, improve postoperative ventilatory function, and control SNS activity in selected patients. An interscalene block almost completely relieves pain after shoulder and upper extremity procedures and causes minimal motor impairment. Caudal analgesia is effective in pediatric patients after inguinal or genital procedures, as is a penile block after circumcision. Intraoperative local anesthetic infiltration of joints or incisions also decreases the intensity of postoperative pain.

Percutaneous intercostal blocks decrease analgesic requirements after thoracic or high abdominal procedures such as thoracotomy, cholecystectomy, chest tube placement, or gastrostomy, although their effects on pulmonary function are still debated.[19–20]

"Nonconventional" Techniques

Positive auditory input during surgery might influence analgesic requirements and recovery course.[21, 22] More innovative analgesic modalities such as acupuncture, hypnosis, transcutaneous nerve stimulation, or auditory overstimulation have limited use in the immediate postoperative period.

Summary

When PCA, continuous-infusion epidural opiates, or sustained postoperative regional analgesia is used, careful planning of a therapeutic course and assessment of potential risks are essential. Implementation of an extended postoperative analgesic regimen should commence before induction of surgical anesthesia and continue through the anesthetic and PACU course. If an extended modality fails, caution should be used before switching to a second therapy in order to minimize the complexity of management and the risk after discharge from the PACU.

POSTOPERATIVE OXYGENATION

Mechanical, hemodynamic, and pharmacologic factors related to surgery and anesthesia can profoundly affect postoperative pulmonary function.[23, 24] Arterial oxygenation, pulmonary ventilation, maintenance of airway patency, and protection of the airway can be considered separately to categorize these factors' impact and to assist in selecting appropriate therapy.

How Is It Assessed?

The most reliable indicator of O_2 transfer from alveolar gas to pulmonary venous blood is the systemic arterial partial pressure of O_2 (PaO_2). Analysis of arterial hemoglobin O_2 saturation using pulse oximetry (SpO_2) indicates the adequacy of arterial oxygenation but yields little information on alveolar-arterial gradients. Pulse oximetry is also affected by changes in hemoglobin structure (i.e., methemoglobin).

Mixed venous O_2 content, venous hemoglobin saturation, and metabolic acidemia are most useful to assess peripheral O_2 delivery and use. Even though PaO_2 may be adequate, arterial perfusion pressure, cardiac output, and distribution of systemic blood flow might not be sufficient to maintain tissue oxygenation. Marked tissue ischemia can also occur with normal PaO_2 secondary to peripheral shunting in sepsis, anemia, hemoglobin dissociation abnormalities, and poisoning with carbon monoxide, arsenic, or cyanide.

Acceptable Limits

In the PACU, an acceptable lower limit for PaO_2 at a given fraction of inspired O_2 (FIO_2) must be established for each patient. This limit, for example, can be based on the baseline preoperative SpO_2. Reduction of PaO_2 to <60 mm Hg can cause significant arterial hemoglobin desaturation, although tissue O_2 delivery may still be adequate. However, the risk of interventions necessary to maintain PaO_2 must also be considered. Maintaining the PaO_2 between 80 and 100 mm Hg (saturation >93–95%) ensures adequate peripheral oxygenation and usually requires minimal intervention.

Increasing the PaO_2 to >100 to 110 mm Hg offers little benefit because hemoglobin saturation is little increased and the additional O_2 dissolved in serum is negligible. During routine postoperative mechanical ventilation, if the PaO_2 exceeds 80 mm Hg (SpO_2 >93%) with a 0.4 FIO_2 and 5 cm H_2O positive end-expiratory pressure (PEEP) or continuous positive airway pressure (CPAP), patients usually sustain adequate peripheral oxygenation after tracheal extubation.

What Postoperative Factors Cause Decreased Alveolar Oxygen Tension?

Many factors reduce arterial O_2 saturation after surgery (Table 6–4). A global reduction of the alveolar partial pressure of oxygen (PAO_2) causes severe hypoxemia, especially if due to a decrease of fresh gas delivery to alveoli.

Respiratory Depression

Whenever uptake of O_2 from the alveoli exceeds delivery, the PAO_2 and arterial oxygenation fall precipitously. If hypoventilation is caused by respiratory center depression from excessive opioid administration, hypoxemia usually evolves more gradually.

Arterial desaturation also results from periodic apnea or

TABLE 6–4. Causes of Hypoxemia in the
Postanesthesia Care Unit

Reduced P_{AO_2}	Severe hypoventilation
	Decreased hypoxic ventilatory drive
	Airway obstruction
$\dot{V}/\dot{Q}$ mismatching: distribution of ventilation	Atelectasis secondary to reduced functional residual capacity
	Hydrostatic pulmonary edema increased lung water
	Postobstructive pulmonary edema
	Mucus plugging/airway obstruction
	Mainstem intubation/lobar bronchus occlusion
	Aspiration
$\dot{V}/\dot{Q}$ mismatching: distribution of perfusion	Variations in pulmonary artery pressure
	Gravitational effects secondary to positioning
	Pulmonary arteriolar dilation from drugs, sepsis, cirrhosis
	Decreased hypoxic pulmonary vasoconstriction
	Varying airway pressure
Reduced mixed venous P_{O_2}	Accentuates impact of $\dot{V}/\dot{Q}$ mismatching

airway obstruction.[25] Hypoxemia is accentuated when opiates and residual anesthetic levels suppress the hypoxic respiratory drive. If obesity or other factors reduce the functional residual capacity (FRC), the decreased volume of O_2 available in the lungs accelerates hypoxemia.[26]

Suppression of Hypoxic Drive

Although rare, apnea resulting from the administration of supplemental O_2 to patients with severe COLD represents another example of hypoventilation-related hypoxemia.

Airway Obstruction

Complete airway obstruction caused by soft tissue swelling or laryngospasm fosters rapid depletion of alveolar O_2 as does a marked increase in airway resistance that prevents effective ventilation. Partial upper airway obstruction or moderate increases in airway resistance reduce ventilation enough to affect P_{AO_2}, especially when supplemental O_2 is not being administered.

Should Oxygen Be Administered Postoperatively?

Increasing O_2 content in the FRC safeguards against hypoxemia from transient hypoventilation and airway obstruction and is the main indication for supplemental O_2 in the postoperative period. Hypoventilation must be severe for hypoxemia to appear; thus, in the PACU, a patient who has moderate hypoventilation and is receiving supplemental O_2 usually presents with respiratory acidemia, not hypoxemia.

The risk of hypoxemia in the immediate postoperative period has been interpreted to mandate that all patients, including those given regional anesthetics, receive supplemental O_2 during transfer and in the initial recovery period.[27–30] Supplemental O_2 administered in the PACU does not guarantee that hypoxemia will not develop[31]; thus, pulse oximetry monitoring is essential during and especially after supplemental O_2 admin-

istration. Careful clinical observation and assessment of cognitive function do not accurately detect hypoxemia.[32–34] Hypoxemia also occurs in children, especially if perioperative upper respiratory infections or chronic adenotonsillar hypertrophy are present.[35–39]

Supplemental O_2 often improves the P_{aO_2}, although the effectiveness of a given F_{IO_2} is variable. The actual F_{IO_2} is difficult to predict with face masks, tents, or nasal prongs because ambient air is entrained with each inspiration.[40] If hypoxemia is caused by "shunting," supplemental O_2 does not significantly increase P_{aO_2} because the shunted blood is not exposed to the increased F_{IO_2}, whereas blood passing ventilated alveoli is already fully saturated. Hypoxemia caused by low ventilation/perfusion ($\dot{V}/\dot{Q}$) units improves when the increased F_{IO_2} augments O_2 delivery to marginally ventilated air spaces.

Resorption Atelectasis/Pulmonary Oxygen Toxicity

At an $F_{IO_2} > 0.8$, replacement of inert nitrogen with O_2 in poorly ventilated alveoli may cause resorption atelectasis. Inspiration of 100% O_2 for 24 to 36 hours might generate the early stages of pulmonary O_2 toxicity, which can progress to alveolar epithelial degeneration and capillary leak pulmonary edema.[41] O_2 toxicity is increased in patients undergoing hyperbaric O_2 therapy but probably is minimal during or after bleomycin therapy.[42–44] Nevertheless, the P_{aO_2} probably should be maintained as low as possible, consistent with adequate arterial saturation. The routine use of humidified O_2 yields little additional benefit unless tracheal intubation or tracheotomy inhibits its natural humidification.

Some clinicians, however, choose to administer supplemental O_2 only as necessary rather than routinely. This practice allows hypoventilating patients to be identified because of the attendant decrease in SpO_2, provoked by the increase in P_{aCO_2}, as predicted by the alveolar gas equation:

$$P_{AO_2} = P_{IO_2} - \frac{P_{aCO_2}}{R}$$

R, the respiratory exchange ratio, normally is 0.8.

The rationale is that patients who require extra attention in the PACU can be identified. It does not distinguish patients who have a decreased SpO_2 from other causes. An additional benefit is that it also saves the expense associated with O_2 administration in those patients who do not require it.

Diffusion Hypoxia

At the end of a general anesthetic, a very rapid outpouring of relatively insoluble nitrous oxide from pulmonary arterial blood into the alveoli can cause volume displacement of alveolar gas. The P_{AO_2} can be lowered to dangerous levels, especially if a patient is breathing ambient air or is hypoventilating.[45] The risk of hypoxemia is minimized by administration of 100% O_2 to dilute the alveolar nitrous oxide and to maintain P_{AO_2}. This problem usually is manifested in the operating room but rarely may present in the PACU, particularly when a patient hypoventilates.

Why Does Ventilation/Perfusion Maldistribution Cause Postoperative Hypoxemia?

The most common cause of hypoxemia in the PACU is $\dot{V}/\dot{Q}$ mismatch resulting from loss of volume in dependent lung areas. Reduction of the FRC decreases radial traction in small airways, causing airway collapse and distal atelectasis. A $\dot{V}/\dot{Q}$ mismatch can progressively worsen for 24 to 36 hours after surgery. Hypoventilation of dependent lung areas is particularly damaging to $\dot{V}/\dot{Q}$ matching because gravity disproportionately directs pulmonary blood flow to these same areas.[46, 47]

Reduction of Functional Residual Capacity

Age and Chronic Lung Disease

Older patients and those with COLD are at increased risk for reduction of the FRC during and after surgery, because they normally suffer loss of airway traction and some airway closure at end-expiration.[48]

Obesity and Increased Intra-Abdominal Pressure

Limitation of diaphragmatic excursion and lung expansion due to obesity or increased intra-abdominal pressure decreases lung volume as does decreased pulmonary compliance caused by increased lung water, atelectasis, pleural effusions, or restrictive disorders. During upper abdominal surgery, retraction, packing, and external abdominal compression by leaning surgical assistants also contribute. Prone, lithotomy, or Trendelenburg's positions are disadvantageous in obese patients.

Thoracic Operations

Reduction of FRC and profound $\dot{V}/\dot{Q}$ mismatching frequently occur during thoracic surgery, especially with one-lung anesthesia. Direct surgical compression, the weight of unsupported mediastinal contents, and displacement of the paralyzed dependent diaphragm into the chest cavity preferentially reduce dependent lung volume.[49, 50] Gravity and lymphatic obstruction lead to the accumulation of interstitial fluid, which accentuates $\dot{V}/\dot{Q}$ mismatching and causes a ''down lung syndrome'' that appears as unilateral pulmonary edema on a postoperative chest radiograph. Increased blood flow through the dependent lung worsens intrapulmonary shunting, especially when volatile anesthetic agents that interfere with hypoxic pulmonary vasoconstriction (HPV) are used.[51]

Pulmonary Edema

Acute postoperative pulmonary edema caused by overhydration, ventricular dysfunction, or increased capillary permeability interferes with O_2 diffusion and $\dot{V}/\dot{Q}$ matching.[52] Edema and loss of lung volume also occur with strong inspiratory efforts against an obstructed airway (negative-pressure pulmonary edema).[53]

Miscellaneous Causes

Pneumothorax or hemothorax, pulmonary contusion, and intrapulmonary hemorrhage also alter $\dot{V}/\dot{Q}$ matching and promote hypoxemia. Mucus plugging or severe bronchospasm promotes hypoventilation of distal air spaces as does obstruction of larger airways by mainstem bronchial intubation, foreign body aspiration, or external compression. Partial right mainstem intubation is a frequently overlooked cause of right upper lobe collapse and significant postoperative hypoxemia.

What Treatment Is Indicated?

Conservative measures to restore lung volume in the PACU often produce significant improvement in arterial oxygenation. Deep tidal ventilation, vigorous cough, and chest physiotherapy mobilize secretions, increase FRC, and acclimate a patient to the incisional discomfort associated with deep inspiration. Incentive spirometry may be helpful to maintain FRC. Intermittent positive-pressure breathing techniques are probably less effective,[54, 55] but CPAP is a valuable adjunct and may be applied with a mask or nasal prongs. Obese patients should recover in a semi-sitting position, if possible, to reduce the pressure of abdominal contents on the diaphragms.

Analgesia

Adequate postoperative analgesia is vital, especially after upper abdominal or thoracic surgery. Pain with ventilation encourages rapid, shallow breathing, which provides adequate minute ventilation but fails to restore and maintain lung volume. Effective analgesia can be provided with the previously discussed techniques. Continuous regional analgesia is helpful in weaning patients with limited pulmonary reserve from ventilatory support.[56]

Continuous Positive Airway Pressure or Positive End-Expiratory Pressure

CPAP is effective for restoring and maintaining FRC. It can be delivered at low levels by face or nasal mask for several hours to maintain the Pao_2 until the loss of lung volume resolves.[57] However, persistent arterial hypoxemia may necessitate tracheal intubation for delivery of CPAP.

Positive-pressure ventilation should be added only if the $Paco_2$, the arterial pH, and the work of breathing indicate ventilatory insufficiency.[58] Usually, 5 to 10 cm of CPAP or PEEP supports Pao_2 without causing hypotension or increased intracranial pressure.[59]

If the Pao_2 does not improve with 5 to 10 cm H_2O of positive pressure, the cause of hypoxemia should be re-evaluated. Higher positive pressure is seldom effective unless significant pulmonary pathology, such as the adult respiratory distress syndrome (ARDS), is present. Pressures >10 to 15 cm H_2O cause greater cardiovascular compromise and may be associated with an increased incidence of barotrauma.[60-62] High airway pressure may actually worsen $\dot{V}/\dot{Q}$ matching by increasing vascular resistance in compliant regions of the lung and by diverting blood flow into poorly ventilated areas.

Intubation

In general, intubated patients should exhale against some positive pressure. Tracheal intubation eliminates so-called physiologic PEEP, which presumably helps to maintain lung volume during spontaneous ventilation. Exposing an intubated patient to ambient airway pressure can lead to gradual, progressive reduction of the FRC and arterial hypoxemia. Young, slender patients, however, can tolerate up to an hour of ambient pressure and are able to restore the FRC easily after extubation. The routine use of PEEP/CPAP in otherwise healthy, intubated patients has been questioned.

Is Postoperative Oxygenation Affected by Pulmonary Perfusion?

The distribution of pulmonary blood flow is determined primarily by pulmonary arterial and venous pressures and by arteriolar and capillary resistance. These factors, in turn, are affected by airway pressure, gravity, lung volume, and cardiovascular dynamics. Blood flow distribution is also modulated by HPV, which diverts flow away from poorly ventilated air spaces with low P_{AO_2}. Inappropriate distribution of pulmonary perfusion interferes with $\dot{V}/\dot{Q}$ matching and causes hypoxemia.

Increased Pulmonary Artery Pressure

In the PACU, increased adrenergic tone caused by pain, hypoxemia, or acidemia can increase cardiac output and pulmonary vascular resistance, thus elevating pulmonary artery pressure. Increased pulmonary artery pressure can increase blood flow to nondependent lung areas, through the bronchial circulation, and through pulmonary arteriovenous anastomoses, thereby interfering with $\dot{V}/\dot{Q}$ matching. Recruitment of pulmonary vessels reduces the effectiveness of HPV in regulating the localized distribution of blood flow.[63]

Reduced Pulmonary Artery Pressure

A reduction of pulmonary artery pressure may also interfere with $\dot{V}/\dot{Q}$ matching. If perfusion to the uppermost parenchyma is compromised by decreased pulmonary artery pressure while atelectasis in dependent lung areas simultaneously redistributes fresh ventilation to nondependent lung areas, regional $\dot{V}/\dot{Q}$ mismatch results. A low pulmonary artery pressure also reduces the differences in flow resistance among various areas of the vascular bed, thereby also reducing the effectiveness of HPV. Hypoxic pulmonary vasoconstriction actually varies with pulmonary artery pressure in a bimodal fashion.[64]

Position Changes

Position changes affect oxygenation if gravity augments flow to areas with reduced ventilation. Placing a patient with a unilateral ventilatory abnormality such as pneumonia or a mainstem intubation in a lateral position with the poorly ventilated lung dependent can seriously reduce P_{aO_2}; conversely, placing the poorly ventilated lung in a nondependent position can improve arterial oxygenation. However, a diseased lung in a nondependent position increases the risk of drainage of purulent or obstructing material to the unaffected, dependent lung.

Changes in Airway Pressure

Pulmonary blood flow distribution can also be affected by airway pressure.[65] Positive-pressure lung inflation may increase resistance in both intra-alveolar and extra-alveolar vessels, whereas spontaneous "negative-pressure" inspiration

probably decreases extra-alveolar vascular resistance. A decrease in capillary transmural pressure gradients caused by reduction of dependent lung volume may promote an increase in dependent vascular resistance, improving $\dot{V}/\dot{Q}$ matching by diverting blood from poorly ventilated areas. Redistribution of flow to nondependent lung regions can also worsen matching. The net impact of lung volume changes on $\dot{V}/\dot{Q}$ matching is difficult to predict.

Drug and Humoral Effects

$\dot{V}/\dot{Q}$ matching is also affected by inhalation anesthetics or sympathomimetics, which alter pulmonary arterial and venous pressures.[66] Nitrous oxide and ketamine cause direct pulmonary vascular constriction, whereas nitroglycerin/phentolamine and sodium nitroprusside cause pulmonary vasodilation. Inhalation anesthetics and vasodilators also impair HPV,[67] perhaps contributing to an increased alveolar-arterial O_2 gradient during general anesthesia. The effects of anesthetics on HPV persist well into the recovery period.

Antihypertensives and β-mimetic drugs probably interfere with $\dot{V}/\dot{Q}$ matching and oxygenation. Circulating humoral substances related to inadequate hepatic metabolism seem to cause poor $\dot{V}/\dot{Q}$ matching and hypoxemia in patients with cirrhosis of the liver.[68] Endotoxin impairs HPV, contributing to hypoxemia in patients with systemic sepsis.[69]

Therapy

In routine clinical settings, $\dot{V}/\dot{Q}$ abnormalities are more easily resolved by improving the distribution of ventilation than by manipulating pulmonary blood flow. Maintenance of a relatively normal pulmonary artery pressure probably optimizes $\dot{V}/\dot{Q}$ matching. Avoidance of dependent placement of severely underventilated lung regions improves oxygenation. Weaning from β-mimetic or vasodilatory medications, if possible, may also improve P_{aO_2}, but the therapeutic benefits of the medication usually require that they be continued until the problem for which they were ordered is resolved.

Why Does Desaturation of Mixed Venous Blood Contribute to Arterial Hypoxemia?

The mixed venous partial pressure of O_2 ($P_{\bar{v}O_2}$) varies with cardiac output, arterial O_2 content, tissue O_2 extraction, and the proportional contributions of different tissue beds to mixed venous blood. If P_{aO_2} decreases or global tissue extraction increases, the $P_{\bar{v}O_2}$ may fall.

A reduction of $P_{\bar{v}O_2}$ amplifies the impact of $\dot{V}/\dot{Q}$ mismatch on P_{aO_2}, because blood with low $P_{\bar{v}O_2}$ that is distributed to low $\dot{V}/\dot{Q}$ units causes a larger proportional reduction of P_{aO_2} after equilibration in the pulmonary veins. Reduced $P_{\bar{v}O_2}$ also increases the extraction of O_2 from alveolar gas, accelerating a decline in P_{AO_2} when hypoventilation or airway obstruction reduces fresh gas delivery to the alveoli. The impact of low $P_{\bar{v}O_2}$ can be attenuated with supplemental O_2.

Shivering, infection, or hypermetabolism lowers $P_{\bar{v}O_2}$ by decreasing tissue O_2 delivery, increasing O_2 consumption, or both.

POSTOPERATIVE VENTILATION

Effective alveolar ventilation delivers fresh gas to perfused alveoli and washes out a sufficient volume of carbon dioxide (CO_2) to match peripheral CO_2 production. Dead space ventilation (i.e., airways and nonperfused alveoli) does not participate in gas exchange. Pa_{CO_2} rises when control mechanisms or physiologic observations prevent an adequate ventilatory response.

What Are the Normal Control Mechanisms?

Ventilation is regulated primarily by medullary center receptors sensitive to pericellular pH in CSF. When hypercarbia causes CSF acidosis, neural output increases the ventilatory rate and tidal volume, augmenting both total minute ventilation and effective alveolar ventilation and reducing Pa_{CO_2}. Consequent resolution of CSF acidosis creates a negative feedback loop that keeps Pa_{CO_2} relatively constant.

Minute ventilation can also increase in response to peripheral chemoreceptors, which monitor carotid Pa_{O_2} and guard against hypoxemia secondary to hypoventilation. Respiratory rate, depth, and pattern are further modulated by neural elements such as chest wall mechanoreceptors, slow adapting parenchymal stretch receptors, and J-receptors. Subconscious and conscious cortical input can override these physiologic regulating mechanisms.[70, 71]

What Factors Reduce Ventilatory Drive?

A number of factors increase Pa_{CO_2} during the immediate postoperative period (Table 6–5). Residual effects of intravenous or inhalational anesthetics blunt the ventilatory sensitivity to hypercarbia and hypoxemia.[71–75] Medullary centers that regulate autonomic activity are also affected. Blunting of SNS response to acidemia and hypoxemia by agitation, tachycardia, and hypertension often conceals inadequate ventilation.

Drug-Induced Respiratory Depression

Mild respiratory acidemia is expected in postoperative patients, but a cautious balance must be struck between a safe degree of postoperative ventilatory depression and an acceptable level of pain or agitation. Serious hypoventilation and hypercarbia often begin insidiously during transfer to the PACU.[27]

Intravenous narcotics administered toward the end of surgery frequently exert their peak ventilatory depression effect in the PACU, and certain neuroleptic or opiate anesthetic techniques may generate delayed respiratory depression.[76, 77] Sedatives depress ventilation through synergistic actions with opiates and anesthetics, direct depression of ventilatory drives, and blunting of the conscious will to ventilate.[78–80] The time, amount, and route of all respiratory depressant medications given to patients must be clearly documented.

Reversal

Careful titration of intravenous naloxone[81] can reverse respiratory depression from narcotics without affecting analgesia, whereas flumazenil often counteracts depression from

TABLE 6–5. Causes of Postoperative Hypoventilation and Hypercarbia

Decreased ventilatory drive	Depression of pH drive by anesthetics/narcotics/sedatives
	Suppression of hypoxic drive
	Abrupt withdrawal of noxious stimuli
	Sedation with decreased volitional will to ventilate
	Emergence of chronic drive problems (sleep apnea)
	Chronic carbon dioxide retention
	Intracranial pathology
Increased work of breathing	Increased upper or small airway resistance
	Decreased lung compliance
	Decreased chest cavity compliance
	Increased intra-abdominal pressure/gastric distention
Decreased mechanical capacity	Ventilatory muscle fatigue
	Neuromuscular paralysis
	Splinting against a painful incision
	Phrenic nerve paresis or anesthesia
	Chronic obstructive changes
	Recurrence of chronic neuromuscular weakness
Increased dead space	Pulmonary air or thromboembolism
	Airway expansion secondary to continuous positive pressure
	Gas trapping secondary to airway resistance/high ventilation rates
	Adult respiratory distress syndrome with microvascular destruction
Increased carbon dioxide production	Reversal of neuromuscular relaxant/warming
	Increased work of breathing
	Shivering
	Fever/sepsis
	Hyperalimentation
	Malignant hyperthermia

benzodiazepines.[82, 83] Doxapram, a central respiratory stimulant, can also be administered to improve ventilation in postoperative patients,[84] although its routine use is probably not advisable.

Noxious Stimuli

Other factors interfere with postoperative ventilatory drive. Abrupt diminution of a noxious stimulus by extubation of the trachea or administration of a postoperative regional analgesic block reduces excitation from stimuli that counteracts medication-induced respiratory depression. Hypoventilation or airway obstruction may result.

Patients suffering from abnormal CO_2/pH responses associated with morbid obesity, chronic upper airway obstruction, chronic CO_2 retention, or sleep apnea disorders are often uniquely sensitive to respiratory depressants. They are at increased risk of inadequate postoperative ventilation, especially when their hypoxic drive is suppressed by medications or if they are chronic CO_2 retainers using a hypoxic respiratory drive that is suppressed by excess supplemental O_2.

Apnea of Prematurity

After anesthesia, the risk of apnea in preterm infants varies with their postconceptional age[85, 86] and preoperative hematocrit.[87] Although the type of anesthetic administered may influence the incidence of postoperative apnea and bradycardia, all preterm infants <60 weeks total age (gestational and postnatal) should be monitored for at least 12 hours after surgery and perhaps admitted overnight.[88]

Neurologic Sequelae

Hypoventilation or apnea can be the presenting symptom of intracranial hemorrhage or edema after posterior fossa craniotomy.[89] Damage to the carotid bodies after bilateral carotid endarterectomy sometimes ablates peripheral hypoxic drive.[90, 91]

What Is the Effect of Increased Upper Airway Resistance?

High airways resistance to gas flow increases the work of breathing and thereby also CO_2 production. If the inspiratory muscles are unable to sustain a sufficient pressure gradient to overcome airway resistance and maintain effective alveolar ventilation, progressive respiratory acidemia occurs. A number of factors predispose to this problem (Table 6–6).

Soft Tissue Obstruction

In the PACU, increased airways resistance to gas flow is commonly caused by pharyngeal obstruction from posterior tongue displacement or soft tissue collapse. Immediate relief of airway obstruction is essential. Simple airway maneuvers such as jaw lift, mandible elevation, lateral positioning, or placement of an oropharyngeal or nasopharyngeal airway usually relieve pharyngeal obstruction. Improving the level of consciousness can be equally useful.

Laryngeal Obstruction

Acute extrinsic upper airway compression from an expanding neck hematoma should be decompressed as soon as possible. Obstruction can also occur at the laryngeal level from laryngospasm or laryngeal edema. Assuming that an airway is clear of vomitus or foreign bodies, most episodes of laryngospasm resolve spontaneously or with application of gentle positive pressure in the oropharynx using 100% O_2. For prolonged laryngospasm, a small dose of succinylcholine (e.g., 0.1 mg · kg^{-1}) yields sufficient relaxation to restore airway patency.

Edema of the vocal cords, glottis, or tracheal mucosa sometimes reduces upper airway caliber after extubation of the trachea, bronchoscopy, or airway surgery. This problem is especially common in children. Complete obstruction from edema is rare, and airway compromise can often be ameliorated with nebulized racemic epinephrine inhaled in O_2.

TABLE 6–6. Causes of Increased Airways Resistance

Soft tissue necrosis	Tongue, tonsils, adenoids, hematoma, edema
Laryngeal obstruction	Laryngospasm, vocal cord edema, foreign body, vomitus
Fixed obstruction	Epiglottitis, retropharyngeal abscess, Ludwig's angina, tracheal stenosis, extrinsic compression, kinked endotracheal tube
Bronchospasm	Suctioning, aspiration, tracheal intubation, allergic reactions, pulmonary embolization
Airway edema	Asthma, smoking
Loss of radial traction	Chronic obstructive lung disease

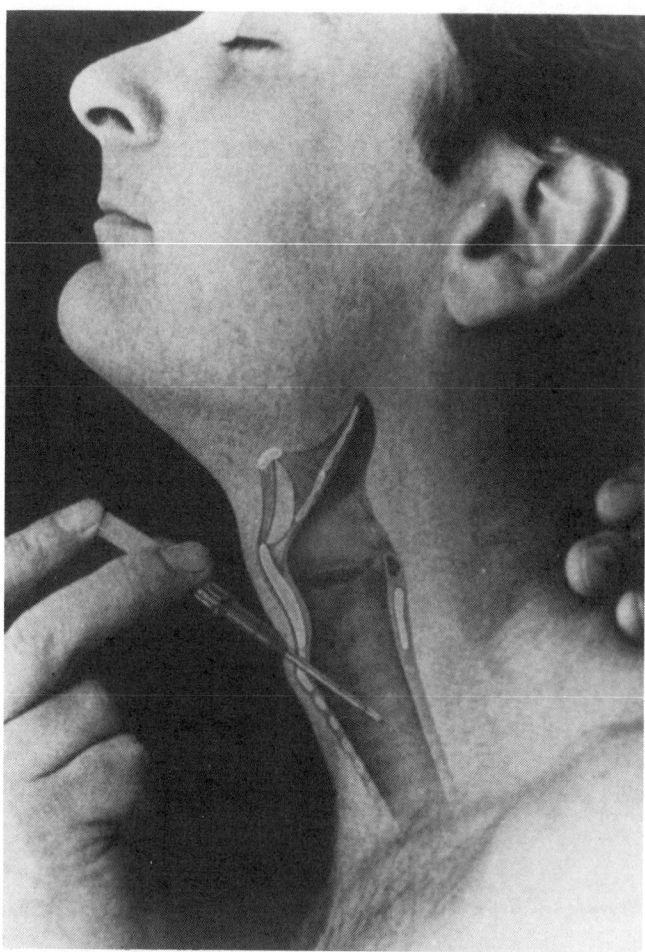

FIGURE 6–2. Cricothyroidotomy using large-bore (12- to 14-gauge) intravenous catheter. (From Benumof JF: Clinical Procedures in Anesthesia and Intensive Care. Philadelphia, JB Lippincott, 1992, p 199.)

Emergency Treatment

If tracheal intubation and face mask ventilation prove impossible after paralysis, one is faced with a life-threatening situation, most likely proximal airway obstruction that is refractory to standard therapy. Given these risks, equipment and personnel necessary for emergency cricothyroidotomy or tracheotomy should be readily available. Cricothyroidotomy using a 14-gauge intravenous catheter attached to a high-pressure O_2 source permits oxygenation and marginal ventilation until the airway can be definitely secured[92] (Figs. 6–2 and 6–3). This subject is covered in more detail in Chapters 50 and 55. More distal large airway obstruction from extrinsic compression or tracheal stenosis is unusual.

What Is the Role of Distal Airway Resistance?

Because resistance varies inversely with the fourth power of airway radius during laminar airflow, reduction of the cross-sectional area, particularly in small airways, causes a significant increase in overall airway resistance. Pharyngeal or tracheal stimulation from secretions, suctioning, aspiration, or intubation elicits reflex constriction of bronchial smooth muscle, especially after the bronchodilatory effects of inhalation

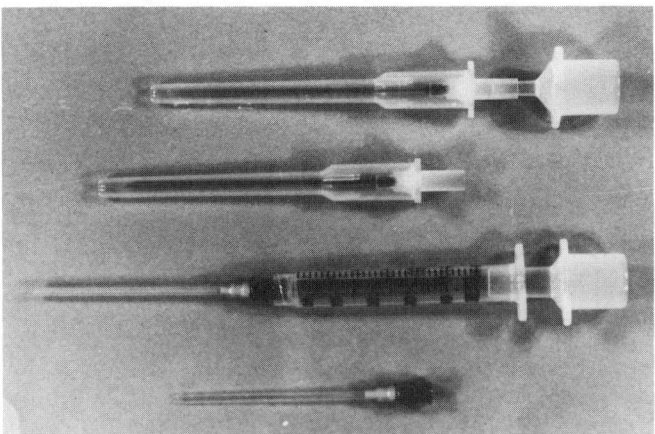

FIGURE 6–3. Devices for attaching a cricothyroidotomy catheter to a positive pressure source for ventilation. An adapter from a 3.0-mm-ID pediatric tracheal tube fits directly into the Luer lock on the catheter. An adapter from a 7.0-mm-ID endotracheal tube fits into the barrel of a 3-mL syringe, which in turn engages the Luer lock on the catheter.

anesthetics wane. Histamine release secondary to medication or allergic reactions can also cause bronchospasm.

Decreased airway caliber is worsened by airway wall edema in asthmatic patients or in smokers with reactive airway disease. Reduction of lung volume and radial airway traction can also decrease airway cross-sectional area in patients exhibiting COLD, obesity, excess lung water, or hypoexpansion caused by incisional pain.

If ventilatory requirements are increased by shivering, hyperthermia, or increased work of breathing, high flow rates convert normal laminar flow to chaotic turbulent flow and increase flow resistance. (Flow resistance during turbulent airflow varies inversely with the fifth power of the radius.)

Diagnosis

A forced vital capacity expiration often reveals high airway resistance in spontaneously ventilating patients. Resistance is higher during expiration because positive intrathoracic pressure compresses intermediate diameter airways.

Signs of increased small airways resistance mimic those of decreased pulmonary compliance. Spontaneously breathing patients have increased work of breathing, accessory muscle recruitment, and labored ventilation with either condition, whereas mechanically ventilated patients exhibit elevated peak inspiratory pressure. Increased airways resistance does not always cause audible turbulent airflow (wheezing), because ventilation may be so restricted that no sound is produced.

Treatment

Bronchospasm

Postoperative bronchospasm usually resolves after the administration of isoetharine or metaproterenol nebulized in O_2. Intramuscular or sublingual terbutaline can be added. Patients whose bronchospasm is resistant to β_2-sympathomimetic medications may occasionally respond to a parasympatholytic medication such as atropine.[93]

An aminophylline loading dose and maintenance infusion or epinephrine infusion can be administered if effective ventilation is still compromised. Treatment of high resistance in small airways should always include an attempt to eliminate the offending laryngeal or tracheal stimulus.

Mechanical Factors

Increased small airways resistance caused by mechanical factors such as loss of lung volume or pulmonary edema is usually refractory to bronchodilators. Incentive spirometry or deep tidal ventilation can restore lung volume and increases external radial traction on small airways, thereby decreasing flow resistance.

If high airway resistance is caused by increased lung water, reduction of left ventricular filling pressures is beneficial. Airway wall edema and interstitial fluid accumulation require time to resolve. An acute exacerbation of chronic bronchospasm sometimes seems resistant to bronchodilators because prolonged contraction of airway smooth muscle causes venous and lymphatic obstruction in airway walls, which persists even after smooth muscle relaxation occurs.

How Does Reduction of Pulmonary Compliance Interfere?

Factors that reduce pulmonary compliance, the change in lung/chest wall volume per unit change in transthoracic pressure, increase work of breathing (Table 6–7). Very low compliance causes ventilatory muscle fatigue, which leads to hypoventilation and respiratory acidemia, and decreased lung volume, which leads to $\dot{V}/\dot{Q}$ mismatching and hypoxemia.[94, 95]

Preoperative Factors

Pulmonary compliance in the postoperative period depends in part on preoperative status. Obesity reduces compliance, especially if adipose tissues compress the thoracic cage in the supine or lateral positions.[96, 97]

Increased intra-abdominal pressure due to obesity, pregnancy, tumors, ascites, or bowel obstruction impedes diaphragmatic excursion, reduces FRC, and promotes airway closure and atelectasis.[98] Re-expansion of atelectatic parenchyma and airways requires increased energy expenditure.

Pulmonary contusion, consolidation, or hemorrhage secondary to trauma interferes with lung expansion and accentuates the work of breathing. Restrictive lung diseases, musculoskeletal abnormalities, intrathoracic tumors or aneurysms, and massive cardiomegaly also reduce pulmonary compliance.[99] Increased pulmonary fluid and blood volume secondary to hydrostatic or high-permeability pulmonary edema increase

TABLE 6–7. Causes of Reduced Pulmonary Compliance

Preoperative	Obesity
	Increased intra-abdominal pressure (pregnancy, ascites, tumor, bowel obstruction)
	Pulmonary parenchymal problems (contusion, tumors, edema, restrictive disease)
Intraoperative	Mainstem intubation
	Abdominal manipulation
	Hemothorax, pneumothorax
	Unusual positions (lateral, decubitus, prone without adequate chest roll placement)
	Restrictive dressings

the weight and inertia of the lungs, whereas accumulation of air space fluid interferes with the modulation of surface tension by pulmonary surfactant.

Intraoperative Factors

Numerous intraoperative factors promote atelectasis and reduce compliance, including gastric or bowel distention, intra-abdominal manipulation or fluid accumulation, mainstem tracheal intubation, excessive airway suctioning, and hemothorax or pneumothorax. Mediastinal compression and interstitial fluid accumulation lower compliance in the dependent lung after prolonged lateral positioning. Tight chest or abdominal dressings are also contributory.

Treatment

In the PACU, allowing patients to recover in a semi-sitting position (60° inclination) rather than supine or full sitting improves diaphragmatic excursion and decreases work of breathing.[100, 101] Chest physiotherapy, incentive spirometry, PEEP, and CPAP are useful to restore inflation.[102, 103] However, in patients with COLD, positive airway pressure must be applied cautiously because it can overdistend the highly compliant lungs past the equilibrium point of the chest cavity, paradoxically increasing the muscular effort required to breathe.

What Neuromuscular Problems Interfere?

Inadequate Muscle Relaxant Reversal

Incomplete reversal of neuromuscular relaxation is a serious potential cause of postoperative hypoventilation. Almost total paralysis may be preferable to partial reversal. It is difficult to overlook an agitated, discoordinate patient with severe airway obstruction. In contrast, a somnolent patient with marginal neuromuscular function exhibiting mild stridor and partial obstruction is more easily missed. Insidious respiratory acidemia or regurgitation and aspiration may occur well after admission to the PACU, when observation is often less intense.

Neuromuscular Disease States

Administration of muscle relaxants to patients with neuromuscular deficiencies such as myasthenia gravis, Eaton-Lambert syndrome, periodic paralysis, or muscular dystrophies often results in prolonged paralysis. These patients may suffer postoperative ventilatory insufficiency, even when relaxants are omitted as well, and therefore deserve especially careful observation and monitoring.[104]

Neuromuscular relaxation can be inadvertently potentiated by antibiotics, furosemide, and propranolol, as well as by hypocalcemia or hypermagnesemia.[105] Patients with atypical pseudocholinesterase have a dramatic increase in the duration of succinylcholine-induced paralysis.

Diaphragmatic and Intercostal Muscle Function Compromise

Strength and coordination of diaphragmatic contraction are probably compromised in certain postoperative patients, reducing their ability to deal with decreased compliance or increased ventilatory demands.[106] Postoperative diaphragmatic fatigue may improve with aminophylline infusion.[107] Residual thoracic spinal or epidural blockade impedes external intercostal muscle function and can reduce ventilatory ability, especially in patients with COLD. Morphine also may compromise intercostal function, further compounding ventilatory inadequacy.[108]

Phrenic Nerve Impairment

Phrenic nerve impairment due to trauma, thoracic and neck surgery, or interscalene anesthesia immobilizes the ipsilateral hemidiaphragm. Though adequate ventilation can normally be maintained with one hemidiaphragm and marginal ventilation with only the external intercostal muscles, increased work of breathing or ventilatory demands usually precipitate ventilatory failure.[109] Patients with Guillain-Barré syndrome, cervical spinal cord trauma, and severe kyphosis or scoliosis are at risk for postoperative ventilatory insufficiency.[110]

Flail Chest

Paradoxical inspiratory chest wall collapse secondary to flail chest impedes thoracic cavity expansion so that ventilatory failure occurs. Loss of compliance from an underlying pulmonary contusion undoubtedly is of greater significance with respect to ventilatory impairment than is the flail.[111]

How Is the Ability to Ventilate Assessed?

Simple bedside tests can assess the mechanical ability to ventilate. A forced vital capacity >10 to 12 mL $\cdot$ kg^{-1} and inspiratory pressure more negative than -25 cm H_2O usually indicate adequate ventilatory muscle strength, although many patients with chronic lung diseases cannot meet these criteria preoperatively. The ability to sustain head elevation for ≥ 5 seconds in a supine position is a rough index of muscular recovery that ensures functional airway protective reflexes.[112] Hand grip, pedal flexion, and other maneuvers are less reliable indicators.

Clinical Appearance

A clinical impression of postoperative ventilatory insufficiency occasionally occurs with adequate minute ventilation. Splinting inspiration against a painful incision can present as a rapid, shallow breathing pattern characteristic of inadequate ventilation. However, incisional pain seldom causes respiratory acidemia, and the labored ventilatory pattern usually disappears with analgesia.

Prolonged ventilation with small tidal volumes caused by thoracic restriction or reduced compliance often leads to dyspnea, labored breathing, and accessory muscle recruitment despite appropriate minute ventilation. This problem also occurs during mechanical ventilation with low inspired volumes. Providing patients with a large, "satisfying" lung expansion often decreases the afferent input from pulmonary stretch receptors and relieves these symptoms. Hyperventilation to compensate for metabolic acidemia may generate a breathing pattern of tachypnea and labored ventilation. When assessing potential ventilatory insufficiency and any questions that remain, always evaluate the Pa_{CO_2} and pH.

TABLE 6–8. Factors Causing Changes in Dead Space

Decrease	Tracheal intubation, tracheotomy
Increase	Circuit valve reversal
	Prolonged inspiration-to-expiration ratios during mechanical ventilation
	Positive end-expiratory pressure/continuous positive airway pressure
	Increased airways resistance
	Embolic phenomena (air, fat, thromboembolism)
	Shock, pulmonary hypotension
	Adult respiratory distress syndrome

How Does Increased Dead Space Interfere?

Ventilation of air spaces that are not perfused (e.g., dead space ventilation) does not contribute to CO_2 excretion, whereas ventilation of alveoli with high $\dot{V}/\dot{Q}$ ratios is less effective in removing CO_2. If dead space volume increases while tidal volume remains constant, the fraction of each inspiration wasted in dead space VDS/VT increases. A decreased tidal volume also increases VDS/VT.

High dead space necessitates a proportionally larger increase in total minute ventilation to meet increased ventilatory demands. Patients with high VDS/VT, therefore, are at greater risk for postoperative ventilatory failure. A VDS/VT between 0.55 and 0.60 (normal 0.30) usually necessitates mechanical assistance to maintain adequate ventilation and CO_2 excretion. A ratio >0.60 to 0.65 often precludes adequate ventilation with even conventional positive-pressure ventilation techniques. High-frequency ventilation may facilitate CO_2 removal at higher VDS/VT.

Changes in Dead Space

A number of factors decrease or increase dead space (Table 6–8).

Mechanical

Tracheal intubation or tracheotomy reduces upper airway dead space by approximately 75%. However, valve reversal in breathing circuits or incorrect connection of tubing increases circuit dead space and forces rebreathing of exhaled gas rich in CO_2. Increased airway volume with PEEP or CPAP increases anatomic dead space, if pulmonary compliance is high. Interruption of expiration by a subsequent inspiration forces spent alveolar gas back into exchanging air spaces, mimicking an increase in dead space.

Gas trapping and CO_2 retention also occur when high airway resistance lengthens the time required for complete exhalation. Improper (prolonged) inspiratory-to-expiratory time ratios or excessive ventilatory rates during mechanical ventilation lead to the same problems.

Embolic Phenomena

Pulmonary embolization with air, thrombus, cellular debris, or foreign matter generates an increase in physiologic dead space. The impact of high $\dot{V}/\dot{Q}$ units on CO_2 excretion is often masked by increased minute ventilation mediated by reflex responses to emboli or ventilatory response to hypercarbia.[113] Evaluation of end-expired PCO_2 trends or comparison with $PaCO_2$ is useful to detect embolization.

Other Causes

Pulmonary hypotension increases VDS/VT.[114] If a pathologic process disrupts or destroys pulmonary microvasculature, an irreversible increase in dead space occurs. ARDS related to sepsis, massive transfusion, trauma, or hypoxemia progressively increases VDS/VT.

When Does Increased Carbon Dioxide Production Lead To Postoperative Ventilatory Failure?

CO_2 production varies directly with metabolic rate, body temperature, and substrate availability. General anesthesia reduces CO_2 production by 20% to 40% as hypothermia lowers metabolic activity and neuromuscular relaxation reduces baseline muscle tone. Postoperative warming restores metabolic rate, O_2 consumption, and CO_2 production toward normal.

Causes

Shivering, increased work of breathing, SNS activity, and carbohydrate metabolism during hyperalimentation accelerate CO_2 production.[115] Even small increases in postoperative CO_2 production can precipitate respiratory acidemia if ventilatory reserve is compromised. An episode of malignant hyperthermia dramatically increases CO_2 production, which rapidly exceeds normal ventilatory capacity, causing severe respiratory acidemia.

Treatment

Control of CO_2 production in the PACU most commonly revolves around controlling shivering. This can be accomplished by warming using lights, blankets, forced warm-air systems, or in extreme cases by chemical paralysis. Administration of small amounts (10–20 mg) of meperidine has also been shown efficacious.[116] The need to adjust hyperalimentation or treat malignant hyperthermia is rare. If dead space is so high that optimal mechanical ventilation can no longer control the $PaCO_2$, paralysis and deliberate hypothermia may reduce CO_2 production and decrease those VDS/VT components that are reversible.

PULMONARY ASPIRATION SYNDROME

Pulmonary aspiration during or after anesthesia is responsible for postoperative morbidity of varying severity, depending on the type or volume of aspirate. Aspiration of acidic gastric contents is most widely feared, although other aspiration syndromes may occur in the perioperative period (Table 6–9).

TABLE 6–9. Aspiration Syndromes

Acid
Clear oral (saliva)
Blood
Solid foreign matter (e.g., food, coins, buttons, teeth)

What Problems Occur With Other Types of Aspiration?

Clear Oral Secretions

Aspiration of clear oral secretions during face mask ventilation following extubation of the trachea or during emergence from anesthesia is both common and usually insignificant, although repeated aspiration of large volumes might promote small airway obstruction or infection. Transient cough or laryngospasm frequently is the only clinical sequela.

Blood

Blood aspiration secondary to trauma, epistaxis, or surgical bleeding in the airway is cleared from air spaces by resorption and phagocytotic processes. The impact of blood aspiration on pulmonary function generally is minimal, although the radiographic presentation is often dramatic. Secondary infection can occur, especially if bits of tissue or purulent matter are also aspirated. Massive blood aspiration interferes with gas exchange and may lead to subsequent pulmonary hemochromatosis. Residual fibrinous deposits also increase pulmonary morbidity.

Solid Foreign Matter

Aspiration of solid foreign matter such as unswallowed food, small objects, teeth, or pieces of dental appliances usually causes persistent cough and diffuse reflex bronchospasm. Obstruction of the trachea or mainstem bronchi can predispose to life-threatening interferences with ventilation and oxygenation. Complications secondary to obstruction of smaller airways, such as distal atelectasis and infection, are often localized and treatable with antibiotics and conservative pulmonary care once the foreign matter is expelled or removed via bronchoscopy.

What Problems Result from Aspiration of Acidic Gastric Contents?

Aspiration of acidic gastric contents initially causes diffuse bronchospasm, hypoxemia, and atelectasis. Subsequent chemical pneumonitis involves airway epithelial degeneration, interstitial and alveolar edema, and air space hemorrhage. A fulminating ARDS with high-permeability pulmonary edema, $\dot{V}/\dot{Q}$ mismatch, and marked reduction in compliance often follows.

Destruction of type I and II pneumocytes greatly reduces surfactant activity. Damage to the pulmonary microvasculature increases pulmonary vascular resistance, pulmonary arterial pressure, and V_{DS}/V_T. If a patient survives, later sequelae include accumulation of fibrinous deposits, hyaline membrane formation, and emphysematous changes caused by parenchymal destruction.

Severity

Severity and eventual resolution probably depend on the volume and pH of the aspirate. Morbidity sharply increases when the pH is <2.0 to 2.5. Aspiration of fluid with pH >2.5 is less damaging but still interferes with surfactant activity and disrupts pulmonary function.[117] Morbidity also increases as the volume of aspirate increases.

Pneumonitis is more severe if partially digested food is aspirated as well. Food particles obstruct small airways and promote secondary bacterial infection. Aspirated vegetable matter causes a chronic granulomatous reaction resembling that caused by miliary tuberculosis.[118]

How Is the Risk of Aspiration Increased?

Loss of Protective Airway Reflexes

The risk of aspiration is particularly high when protective airway reflexes are suppressed by muscle relaxants and depressant medications such as inhalation anesthetics, barbiturates, and opiates.[119] The ability to sustain spontaneous ventilation does not guarantee that sufficient neuromuscular recovery has occurred to maintain airway protection. Trauma or anesthesia of the airway or laryngeal and pharyngeal muscle innervation seriously compromises airway reflexes.

Interference with Gastric Emptying

The risk also is increased when patients requiring emergency surgery present with large volumes of intragastric food and fluid. Many factors interfere with gastric emptying, including bowel obstruction, pain, anxiety, narcotics, salt depletion, and peristaltic abnormalities. Pregnancy or morbid obesity results in increased gastric volume and hyperacidity, and the associated mechanical displacement of the gastroesophageal junction interferes with sphincter integrity.[120] Abnormalities that affect gastroesophageal tone or swallowing, such as achalasia, hiatal hernia, esophageal diverticuli or tumors, and amyotrophic lateral sclerosis, also increase the risk of regurgitation and aspiration.

What Steps Should Be Taken to Prevent Aspiration?

Nil Per Os Status

Prevention of aspiration is critical, because therapy is limited. Traditionally, a nil per os (NPO) status was believed to be necessary for at least 8 to 12 hours before induction of anesthesia to allow gastric emptying, even when a regional anesthetic technique was planned. Despite ongoing revision of the guidelines for preoperative fasting (shorter NPO period), the vigilance for potential regurgitation and aspiration in any patients with a history of recent ingestion should not be reduced.

Nonparticulate Antacids

Nonparticulate antacids such as sodium citrate increase the pH of gastric fluid without excessively increasing volume, but particulate antacids should be avoided because subsequent aspiration of these medications can cause chronic granulomatous reactions.[121]

Histamine Blockers and Metoclopramide

Histamine$_2$-receptor blockers such as cimetidine or ranitidine decrease the production and increase the pH of gastric fluid, whereas metoclopramide improves gastroesophageal sphincter tone and accelerates gastric emptying.[122, 123]

Nasogastric Suction

Decompression with a nasogastric tube before an anesthetic induction interferes with gastroesophageal sphincter integrity and is often ineffective to remove particulate matter. However, gastric contents should be emptied as much as possible after induction.

What Is the Risk of Aspiration in the Postanesthesia Care Unit?

Protective reflex function is often marginal during emergence from general anesthesia, and postoperative nausea and vomiting are still a significant problem, especially if gas has accumulated in the stomach. The effects of intraoperative interventions to reduce airway irritability such as topical local anesthetics or laryngeal nerve blocks can persist, decreasing a patient's airway protection. Residual neuromuscular paralysis reduces protective laryngospasm or cough, whereas hypotension, hypoxemia, or acidemia increases the risk of aspiration by causing both emesis and obtundation.

Anatomic distortion caused by mandibular fractures or stabilization or soft tissue trauma interferes with airway protection. Mandibular fixation impedes expulsion of vomitus, blood, or secretions from the mouth. Instruments necessary to release the fixation apparatus should be immediately available in the PACU.

How Long Should Patients Remain Intubated?

Patients at high risk of aspiration should remain intubated until restoration of airway reflexes is complete. An endotracheal tube does not preclude aspiration past a nonsealing cuff.[124] Appropriate pharyngeal suctioning reduces the incidence of silent aspiration. Unnecessary tracheal tube cuff deflation increases the risk of aspiration because the rigid tube prevents laryngeal closure.

During extubation, the pharynx must be completely suctioned. Cuff deflation and extubation should be performed at end-inspiration, preferably with positive airway pressure, to promote vigorous expulsion of material trapped below the vocal cords but above the inflated cuff. After tracheal extubation, airway reflexes can be temporarily impaired; thus, patients should be carefully monitored.

What Should Be Done When Vomiting or Regurgitation Occurs?

The appearance of gastric secretions in the pharynx mandates immediate lateral head positioning, pharyngeal suctioning, and perhaps tracheal intubation if airway reflexes are compromised. Great care must be taken when clearing the airway of a patient with a cervical spine injury.

Positioning

Trendelenburg positioning may promote regurgitation, but it also aids in clearing vomitus once regurgitation has occurred. Head elevation should be avoided if airway reflexes are marginal, because establishing a gravitational gradient from pharynx to lungs promotes aspiration.

Airway Management

If tracheal intubation is performed in a patient who has regurgitated, the trachea should be suctioned through the tube before instituting positive-pressure ventilation. This action avoids further dissemination of aspirated material into distal airways. Instillation of saline or alkalizing solutions into the tracheal tube is contraindicated. Determining tracheal aspirate pH is of little value because buffering is almost immediate. Assessment of pH in a pharyngeal aspirate is more reliable but of little practical value.

Postoperative Assessment

If intraoperative or postoperative aspiration is suspected, the patient should be observed carefully for 24 to 48 hours. Serial temperature checks, differential white blood cell counts, blood gas determinations, and pulmonary function testing can be helpful. Infiltrates can appear on repeated chest radiographs anytime within 24 to 36 hours, and hypoxemia may evolve insidiously as lung pathology progresses.

Therapy

Aggressive chest physiotherapy and incentive spirometry are thought by some to minimize atelectasis and $\dot{V}/\dot{Q}$ mismatching. Medications for pre-existing chronic pulmonary conditions such as asthma should be reinstituted. Should the likelihood of significant aspiration be small, outpatients can be discharged (with planned follow-up) if hypoxemia, wheezing, cough, or chest radiographic abnormalities do not appear within 4 to 6 hours.[125] Patients must be instructed to contact a medical facility if fever, cough, chest pain, or other symptoms of pneumonitis appear.

What Should Be Done When Aspiration Is Documented?

If significant aspiration causes hypoxemia, increased airway resistance, or pulmonary edema, mechanical ventilation, supplemental O_2, and PEEP or CPAP are usually necessary. The therapeutic approach is similar to that used for ARDS. High-permeability pulmonary edema should not be treated with diuretics unless high ventricular filling pressures are present. Hypovolemia from vascular to pulmonary fluid translocation after aspiration often necessitates aggressive fluid administration.

High-dose steroids do not yield improvement in long-term outcome after aspiration. Prophylactic antibiotic administration promotes colonization by resistant organisms. If secondary bacterial infection appears, specific antibiotic therapy should be instituted based on sputum culture results. If culture results are equivocal, broad-spectrum antibiotics should be chosen with coverage for gram-negative rods and anaerobes including *Bacteroides fragilis*.[126, 127]

Causes of Postoperative Hypotension

Relative hypovolemia	Inappropriately large blood pressure cuff
	Improperly zeroed arterial catheter
	Damped arterial catheter trace
	Inadequate replacement of preoperative deficits, third space losses, and intraoperative blood loss
	Occult or continued hemorrhage in postanesthesia care unit
	Increased venous capacity with rewarming
	Sympathectomy secondary to regional anesthetics
	Orthostasis
	Sudden decrease in α-adrenergic venous tone
	Direct venodilation by medications (furosemide, morphine, nitrates)
	Venodilation secondary to α-adrenergic blockade (droperidol, chlorpromazine)
	Venodilation secondary to histamine release (barbiturates, relaxants, morphine)
	Allergic or anaphylactoid reactions, anaphylaxis
	Interference with venous return (caval compression, high airway pressure, tension pneumothorax)
	Interference with ventricular filling (pericardial tamponade)
Ventricular dysfunction	Acute ischemic myocardiopathy
	Overhydration, ventricular dilation, and nonischemic failure
	Reduced endogenous sympathetic nervous system activity
	Beta-receptor or calcium channel blockade
	Severe acidemia/alkalemia
	Decreased ionized calcium, acute steroid deficiency
	Acute valvular dysfunction, air embolism, thromboembolism
Dysrhythmia	Bradycardia (sinus or heart block) with decreased cardiac output
	Tachydysrhythmia with decreased ventricular filling
	Tachycardia with underlying valvular lesions
	Life-threatening ventricular tachycardia, fibrillation, or asystole
Decreased systemic vascular resistance	Sympathectomy from major regional anesthesia
	Direct arterial dilating medications (hydralazine, nitroprusside)
	Alpha-adrenergic blockade (droperidol, chlorpromazine)
	Decreased endogenous sympathetic nervous system tone
	Blunted baroreceptor function, intracranial pathology
	Severe hypoxemia or acidemia
	Arteriolar dilation secondary to sepsis, blood components
	Acute steroid deficiency

POSTOPERATIVE HYPOTENSION

Hypotension in the immediate postoperative period is a common problem with various causes (Table 6–10). Systemic hypotension can lead to hypoperfusion of vital organs. Inadequate O_2 delivery causes tissue hypoxia, inefficient aerobic metabolism, and lactic acid accumulation. In response, the SNS diverts perfusion to the brain, heart, and kidneys, where autoregulatory vascular dilation helps to preserve blood flow. If symptoms of hypotension such as nausea, disorientation, loss of consciousness, angina, or oliguria suggest hypoperfu-sion of these vital systems, the compensatory reserve already has been used.

What Are the Complications?

Complications of hypotension include myocardial, cerebral, and renal ischemia or infarction. Viability of the spinal cord and bowel can be jeopardized, and the risk of deep vein thrombosis may be increased at low venous flow velocities. Decreased hepatic O_2 delivery may trigger alternate pathways for drug metabolism and lead to hepatic damage from the accumulation of toxic metabolites. The minimum acceptable systemic blood pressure is higher in patients with chronic hypertension, arteriosclerotic disease, fixed stenotic vascular lesions, increased intracranial pressure, or conditions that interfere with autoregulation.[128]

Is the Measurement Valid?

Ensuring that a low blood pressure reading is accurate avoids the risk of serious iatrogenic hypertension resulting from inappropriate treatment. Blood pressure cuff width should equal approximately two thirds of arm circumference. Inappropriately large cuffs yield artificially low values.

If an arterial catheter transducer system is improperly zeroed or damped by air bubbles or catheter obstruction, readings can be erroneously low. Intra-arterial readings from radial or even brachial insertions can be reduced below the true central pressure by arterial constriction in hypothermic patients or those receiving α-adrenergic agonist medications.

What Is Absolute Hypovolemia?

Absolute hypovolemia implies that the circulating intravascular volume is insufficient to support ventricular filling and cardiac output. SNS responses mediated by baroreceptor reflexes usually can maintain systemic pressure despite a 15% to 20% loss of intravascular volume. Greater deficits overcome the salutary compensation from tachycardia, increased systemic vascular resistance (SVR), and venoconstriction; as a result, systemic blood pressure falls. Several factors may be responsible.

Inadequate Blood and Fluid Replacement

Postoperative hypovolemia is frequently caused by inadequate replacement of preoperative fluid deficits, evaporative losses during surgery, and blood loss. In the PACU, additional hemorrhage, insensible fluid loss, and exudation of fluid into tissues exacerbate hypovolemia. Muscle hemorrhage after trauma or orthopedic procedures, diffuse oozing related to acute coagulopathy, and retroperitoneal bleeding are difficult to recognize.[129]

Third Space Losses

Third space losses continue for 24 to 48 hours postoperatively and can lead to profound hypovolemia through the accumulation of ascites, pulmonary edema, or anasarca.

Hypothermia and Rewarming

Hypothermia often masks hypovolemia on admission to the PACU through arterial and venous constriction. On rewarming, venous capacitance increases, afterload decreases, and hypovolemia with hypotension is revealed.[130]

What Is Relative Hypovolemia?

Relative hypovolemia is implied when an otherwise normal intravascular volume is inadequate to maintain blood pressure. A number of causes are known.

Sympathectomy

Increased venous capacitance due to sympathectomy after spinal or epidural anesthesia decreases ventricular filling pressures and prevents venoconstriction in response to hemorrhage or position changes.

Decreased Sympathetic Nervous System Activity

After general anesthesia, vasovagal responses, extubation of the trachea, or relief of pain can cause a sudden reduction in SNS activity and increased venous capacity. Medications with α-adrenergic blocking properties such as droperidol and chlorpromazine increase venous capacity, as do those that dilate veins, such as nitrates or furosemide.

Histamine Release

After allergic responses or administration of medications such as barbiturates or morphine, histamine may cause significant venous pooling. Blood products or low-molecular-weight dextrans sometimes cause venodilation, which probably is secondary to histamine release.

Impedance to Venous Return

Factors that impede venous return to the right atrium, such as compression of thoracic veins by positive-pressure ventilation or tension pneumothorax, and inferior vena caval compression due to a gravid uterus or increased intra-abdominal pressure cause relative hypovolemia. Acute pericardial tamponade also impedes ventricular filling.

How Is Volume Status Assessed?

On admission to the PACU, a patient's preoperative fluid status, estimated blood loss, and intraoperative fluid loss and replacement should be reviewed and a qualitative assessment of current intravascular volume and hemostasis completed. The variation of systolic blood pressure during positive-pressure ventilation provides a qualitative warning of reduced intravascular volume.[131] This can be identified by inspection of either an arterial catheter or pulse oximeter–derived pulse waveform (Fig. 6–4). A quick assessment is also possible by lifting a patient's legs to increase venous return. A sustained increase in mean arterial pressure confirms the diagnosis of hypovolemia.

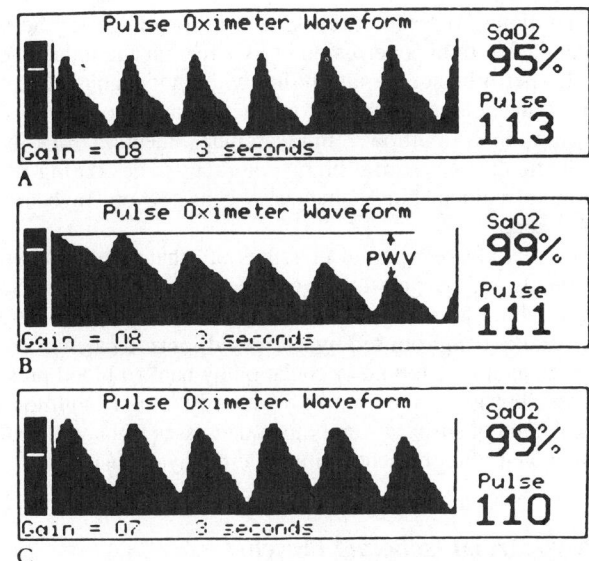

FIGURE 6–4. Pulse oximeter waveform representation. *A,* When the patient arrived in the operating room, central venous pressure (CVP) was 8 mm Hg. Little variation was seen in the waveform with positive-pressure ventilation. *B,* After third space translocation and blood loss, CVP was 4 to 5 mm Hg. The pulse waveform varied with respiration. The method for measuring pulse waveform variation (PWV) is shown. *C,* After fluid resuscitation, CVP was 8 mm Hg. The pulse waveform no longer shows significant variation with respiration. (From Partridge BL: Use of pulse oximetry as a noninvasive indicator of intravascular volume status. J Clin Monit 1987; 3:263.)

Urine output is a potentially misleading index of intravascular volume in the PACU because surgery and anesthesia interfere with renal concentrating ability. Also, unrecognized hyperglycemia promotes glycosuria and osmotic diuresis, which overcomes normal renal fluid retention mechanisms during hypovolemia.

Insertion of a central venous or pulmonary arterial catheter may be indicated to assess right or left ventricular filling pressures, respectively, if intravascular volume status is uncertain.

Is Ventricular Dysfunction Present?

Hypotension from postoperative ventricular dysfunction usually occurs in patients who have impaired baseline ventricular contractility and who require elevated left ventricular end-diastolic pressure (LVEDP) and intense SNS activity to maintain cardiac output and is therefore uncommon.

Overhydration

Overhydration causes ventricular dilation, decreased cardiac output, hydrostatic pulmonary edema, and hypotension in such patients. Excessive fluid administration initially may be concealed in patients recovering from spinal or epidural anesthesia because sympathectomy dramatically increases venous capacity. When SNS blockade resolves, a characteristically high level of SNS outflow causes venoconstriction and an acute increase of central vascular volume.

Drug Treatment

Patients who have severe ventricular dysfunction and rely on maximal SNS activity may exhibit hypotension after administration of β-receptor blocking drugs or analgesics. Severe acidemia due to hypoperfusion or hypercarbia can reduce ventricular performance by interfering with endogenous or exogenous catecholamine-receptor interaction and by directly depressing SNS outflow. Intravascular injection of local anesthetic or uptake from highly vascular tissues during postoperative regional blocks may also cause severe myocardial depression.

Residual alveolar partial pressures of inhalation anesthetics marginally reduce ventricular contractility and decrease SNS outflow, limiting cardiac output increase. Ventricular contractility also is compromised by decreased ionized calcium from acute alkalemia, dilution, or chelation by banked blood preservatives; however, the impact is usually minor. Pulmonary thromboembolism or air embolism decreases right ventricular outflow and often presents with systemic hypotension.

Is Myocardial Ischemia Present?

Intraoperative hypotension and reduced diastolic filling during tachycardia may be precipitating events for postoperative myocardial ischemia or infarction in patients with coronary artery disease.[132] In the PACU, inadequate aortic diastolic blood pressure reduces myocardial perfusion, as does tachycardia in response to hypotension, pain, acidemia, anxiety, or medications. Myocardial O_2 consumption increases during shivering or if ventricular wall tension is increased by high SVR or overhydration. Hypoxemia caused by hypoventilation, airway obstruction, or $\dot{V}/\dot{Q}$ mismatching can generate myocardial ischemia despite adequate coronary perfusion.

Recognition

Postoperative ischemia is often difficult to recognize.[133] Most cases are truly silent. Analgesia from residual anesthetics or narcotics treats anginal as well as incisional pain. Chest pain can also be overshadowed by discomfort from upper abdominal incisions, esophageal reflux, vomiting, or gastric distention. Routine ECG monitoring is relatively inadequate for evaluation of ischemic changes but remains the standard. In patients considered to be at increased risk for ischemic monitoring, lead V5 is most efficacious. A high incidence of benign postoperative dysrhythmias makes differentiation of ischemia-induced dysrhythmias difficult.

Ischemia accompanied by hypotension secondary to ischemic ventricular dysfunction can progress to irreversible infarction. Close evaluation of hemodynamic responses to fluid challenge, ST segment and T wave morphology on 12-lead ECG, and assessment of cardiovascular dynamics may uncover ischemia before hypotension occurs. Careful control of precipitating factors and timely therapy are important to decrease morbidity.[134, 135]

What Is the Effect of Decreased Systemic Vascular Resistance?

Decreased SVR is an important cause of postoperative hypotension associated with regional anesthesia, vasoactive blood components, and warming, although venous dilation also has a role. Severe systemic acidemia reduces SVR by a direct vasodilatory effect and by interfering with catecholamine actions on α-receptors. Hydralazine and nitroprusside reduce SVR and blood pressure by dilating muscular arterioles, whereas α-receptor and ganglionic blocking drugs interfere with peripheral SNS effects.

Hypotension due to systemic sepsis is often related to a decrease in SVR caused by endotoxin, although myocardial depression is usually superimposed in end-stage sepsis. Decreased SVR can also be caused by blunted baroreceptor function,[90, 136] by intracranial pathology,[89] or by acute steroid deficiency if prior exogenous steroid administration has suppressed the pituitary-adrenal axis. The latter problem is often preceded by lethargy, fever, or nausea and accompanied by hyperkalemia, hyponatremia, and hypoglycemia. Response to supplemental steroids is often dramatic.

Which Dysrhythmias Reduce Blood Pressure?

Postoperative hypotension caused by a cardiac dysrhythmia is more common in patients with a history of myocardial disease or rhythm disturbances. Sinus or nodal bradycardia decreases cardiac output and blood pressure, as do slow ventricular rhythms associated with complete heart block.

Paroxysmal atrial tachycardia (PAT), atrial fibrillation or flutter, and fast ventricular tachycardia that generate rates >140 to 150 beats per minute often do not provide adequate diastolic intervals for ventricular filling. Stroke volume, cardiac output, and systemic blood pressure all decrease. Needless to say, ventricular fibrillation, asystole, or electromechanical dissociation causes lethal reduction in cardiac output.

Why Are Valvular Abnormalities Particularly Dangerous?

The effects of SNS tone on cardiac performance can precipitate hypotension in patients with valvular abnormalities. Tachycardia in a patient with mitral stenosis interferes with left ventricular filling, increases left atrial pressure, and decreases cardiac output and systemic pressure.

With mitral regurgitation, high SVR increases the regurgitant fraction and compromises cardiac output. Tachycardia in a patient with aortic stenosis reduces systolic ejection time and increases LVEDP, promoting decreased cardiac output, hypotension, and ventricular dilation. Increased contractility or heart rate causes similar problems with hypertrophic subaortic stenosis.

What Treatment Is Indicated?

A 20% to 30% reduction of systemic arterial systolic pressure below chronic preoperative levels usually is an indication for therapy, as is the appearance of symptoms referable to vital organ hypoperfusion. If a high risk for hypotensive complications is present, acceptable limits for pressure and heart rate should be defined when a patient is admitted to the PACU.

Before treatment for significant hypotension is initiated, the pressure determination should be quickly validated. Palpation of carotid or femoral pulses and auscultation of heart sounds are useful qualitative indicators of central blood pressure. Cardiac rate and rhythm, breath sounds, and O_2 saturation should be checked immediately. Tracheal intubation and cardiopulmonary resuscitation must be instituted immediately if ventilation or pulses are absent. Depending on the circumstances, a 12-lead ECG, an ABG sample, or a chest radiograph may be ordered.

Trendelenburg positioning is controversial, but every patient should receive supplemental O_2. Infusions that might cause vasodilation should be discontinued, and recent drug administration should be noted. Simple maneuvers such as lateral uterine displacement in pregnant patients or supine positioning and elevating the legs of patients with orthostatic changes should be used if appropriate.

Initial Therapy

Definitive therapy should be directed toward the specific problem responsible for reducing systemic blood pressure. An etiologic diagnosis should be confirmed repeatedly based on the response to interventions. Because hypovolemia is by far the most common cause of postoperative hypotension, the intravenous infusion rate initially should be increased to maximum. Crystalloids are usually sufficient, although plasma expanders or blood facilitates more rapid volume expansion. Only small amounts of unnecessary fluid are infused while spurious hypotension or hypotension caused by ischemia is evaluated. Tension pneumothorax must be immediately evacuated.

Vasopressors

Although vasopressors are not appropriate therapy for absolute hypovolemia, judicious administration of sympathomimetic agents that increase SVR and venous return can help maintain systemic pressure until sufficient volume is infused. Relative hypovolemia caused by increased venous capacity or obstruction to venous return can be appropriately treated with an α-adrenergic drug such as phenylephrine to supplement fluid therapy. Ephedrine is less desirable because an increase in heart rate and contractility is usually unnecessary. However, its ready availability makes it a popular choice.

Myocardial Dysfunction

If 300 to 500 mL of fluid does not improve blood pressure, myocardial dysfunction should be considered as a possible cause. When hypotension is caused by myocardial ischemia, resolution of ischemia usually restores baseline myocardial function. Therapy of acute ischemia is dependent on the circumstances.

In the presence of significant hypotension associated with myocardial ischemia, support of aortic diastolic pressure with an α-adrenergic agonist such as phenylephrine and reduction of LVEDP with nitroglycerin are useful to maximize the coronary artery perfusion pressure.[137]

Control of heart rate with analgesics, sedatives, or β-receptor blockers is essential. If dysfunction is not related to ischemia, drugs that augment contractility such as calcium chloride, ephedrine, or dopamine, in conjunction with carefully titrated systemic vasodilators, often restore cardiac output and systemic pressure.

Because therapy for ischemia can acutely worsen hypovolemia-induced hypotension, decreased SVR, or nonischemic ventricular dysfunction, it is critical that the diagnosis of ischemia be accurate. Suspicion that hypotension is caused by ventricular dysfunction represents an indication for echocardiography or pulmonary artery catheterization to measure cardiac output and pulmonary artery occlusion.

Dysrhythmias

Tachycardia. PAT often responds to alteration of cardiac conduction rates by vagal maneuvers or medication, whereas digitalization or calcium channel blockade reduces the ventricular rate during atrial fibrillation. Low-energy (50 J) direct-current cardioversion can be used if hypotension due to a tachydysrhythmia is life threatening.

Bradycardia. Atropine, glycopyrrolate, or ephedrine resolves hypotension secondary to sinus bradycardia unrelated to hypoxemia. Refractory bradycardia caused by sinus node disease or complete heart block usually requires intravenous administration of epinephrine or isoproterenol or cardiac pacing.

Decreased SVR

Low SVR with high cardiac output sometimes can be resolved with phenylephrine, although with advanced sepsis or catecholamine depletion, norepinephrine infusion may be required.

POSTOPERATIVE HYPERTENSION

Moderate elevation of systemic blood pressure is acceptable in the PACU, but significant hypertension increases morbidity and should be aggressively evaluated and treated.[138] Hypertension increases postoperative hemorrhage and third space losses.

Ventricular dilation or myocardial fiber stretch secondary to high LVEDP can cause cardiac dysrhythmias, whereas an increase in myocardial wall tension may precipitate ischemia. Hypertension also exacerbates increased intracranial pressure, cerebral edema, intracranial hemorrhage, and elevated intraocular pressure. Disruption of major vascular suture lines can also occur.

If a blood pressure cuff is inappropriately small, it yields erroneously high readings. This is a particular problem in the evaluation of obese patients. An improperly zeroed or calibrated transducer or an excessive amount of resonance and electronic "overshoot" can lead to overestimation of systolic pressure. Overshoot usually does not significantly change the mean arterial pressure value.

What Is the Role of Sympathetic Nervous System Activity?

Hypertension due to increased SNS activity after surgery usually reflects an appropriate response to noxious stimuli or adverse physiologic conditions (Table 6–11).

Increased α-Adrenergic Stimulation

Enhanced α-adrenergic receptor stimulation causes arteriolar and venous constriction, increasing SVR and venous return, respectively. Increased $β_1$-receptor stimulation increases heart

TABLE 6–11. Factors That Increase Postoperative Sympathetic Activity

Increased sympathetic activity	Noxious stimuli:	Surgical pain, discomfort, anxiety, full bladder, endotracheal intubation, carinal stimulation
	Adverse physiologic conditions:	Hypercarbia/acidemia; hypoxemia, hypotension, hypoglycemia, congestive heart failure, myocardial ischemia, increased intracranial pressure, pulmonary hypoexpansion, pulmonary embolism
	Medications:	Pressors (ephedrine, isoproterenol, epinephrine, dopamine, dobutamine)
		Bronchodilators (terbutaline, albuterol, aminophylline)
		Antihypertensives (hydralazine, nitroprusside)
		Anesthetics (ketamine, isoflurane)
Decreased parasympathetic activity	Parasympatholytic medications:	Atropine, glycopyrrolate, pancuronium, gallamine

rate and ventricular contractility. Patients with pre-existing hypertension often exhibit noncompliant arteriosclerotic vasculature and elevated peripheral vascular tone mediated by the renin-angiotensin system. Each of these factors causes exaggerated blood pressure responses to stimuli in the PACU.

Precipitating Causes

Increased SNS activity can occur as a baseline condition or can be caused by exogenous sympathomimetics or very rarely by monoamine oxidase inhibition or pheochromocytoma. Intravascular volume expansion increases cardiac output and blood pressure despite compensatory decreases in SVR and heart rate, especially in hypothermic, vasoconstricted patients. After carotid endarterectomy, abnormal baroreceptor sensitivity can produce significant hypertension.[139] Central SNS regulation can be disrupted by cerebral vascular accidents, hypoxic encephalopathy, increased intracranial pressure, or osmotic changes, causing severe hypertension.[89]

How Should It Be Treated?

Treatment of postoperative hypertension is usually indicated when systolic or diastolic pressure exceeds 120% to 130% of resting pressure or when signs of complications such as headache, bleeding, visual changes, angina, or ST segment depression occur.

Patients with increased intracranial pressure, open eye injury, mitral regurgitation, or intracardiac shunts are at increased risk of morbidity and should be treated more aggressively. To avoid hypoperfusion of vital organs in patients with chronic hypertensive disease, pressure should not be reduced below preoperative baseline levels.

Drug Therapy

Elimination of increased SNS activity by administration of analgesics for pain or sedatives for anxiety, correction of acidemia or hypoxemia, or bladder decompression often suffice. Intravenous labetalol,[140] esmolol,[141] or nicardipine[142] in small incremental doses is useful for short-term pressure control, as is a combination of intravenous hydralazine and propranolol. Alpha-methyldopa yields longer lasting control that can easily be switched to an oral regimen. Potent intravenous vasodilators such as sodium nitroprusside, nitroglycerin, or trimethaphan should be reserved for severe or refractory hypertension.

POSTOPERATIVE ELECTROCARDIOGRAPHIC ABNORMALITIES

After general anesthesia, ECG changes that often appear suggest abnormal myocardial physiology and yet are unrelated to clinical signs or symptoms of actual cardiac pathology.[143] These findings most likely are caused by a combination of autonomic nervous system imbalance, the electrophysiologic effects of inhalation anesthetics, electrolyte imbalance, and hypothermia.[144]

Transient alterations in axis, intraventricular conduction, P and T wave morphology, and ST segments almost always resolve spontaneously within 3 to 6 hours. Repeat ECG recording and perhaps CK-MB enzyme determinations are in order if sufficient question remains about the origin of such changes.

Where Do Premature Complexes Originate?

Atrial

An aberrant impulse from the atrium, atrioventricular (AV) node, or upper bundle of His usually generates an atrial premature contraction (APC), which is followed by an early but otherwise normal QRS complex. In postoperative patients, they usually result from increased SNS activity and seldom lead to hemodynamic compromise. Control of SNS activity (pain management, sedation) is usually sufficient to eliminate APCs.

Ventricular

Origination of an impulse peripherally in ventricular conducting tissue generates a ventricular premature complex (VPC). Peculiar QRS complexes on ECG are often categorically assumed to be VPCs, although the majority are caused by other benign electrophysiologic mechanisms.[145] Ventricular premature impulses usually occur at varying intervals from previous normal QRS complexes. Also, the interval between previous and subsequent normal QRS complexes is often twice the normal interval between sinus complexes (compensatory pause) (Fig. 6–5).

Spontaneous ventricular depolarization is often associated with increased parasympathetic nervous system (PNS) or SNS activity. Excess PNS influence reduces the rate of supraventricular pacemakers, allowing the emergence of ventricular escape beats. Treatment using vagolytic or sympathomimetic medications accelerates supraventricular pacemaker rates.

Excess SNS activity accelerates spontaneous ventricular de-

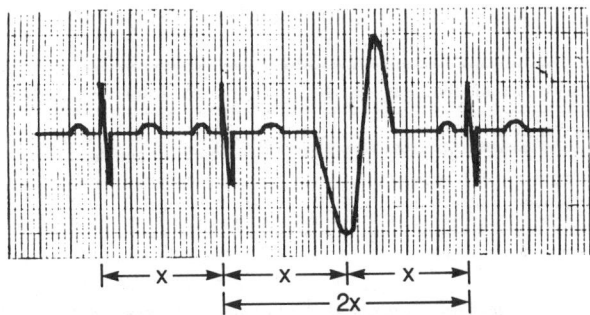

FIGURE 6–5. Ventricular premature contraction. Note wide, high-amplitude configuration, reverse initial deflection, and compensatory pause between previous and subsequent normal QRS complexes. x = normal RR interval; 2x = full compensatory pause. (From Mecca RS: Postanesthesia recovery. *In* Clinical Anesthesia. Barash PG, Cullen BF, Stoelting RK (eds). Philadelphia, JB Lippincott, 1989, p 1405.)

polarization rates or fosters the emergence of parasystolic foci. Myocardial fiber stretch, digitalis toxicity, electrolyte disturbances, and mechanical stimulation from central catheters also cause ventricular depolarization. Elimination of autonomic nervous system imbalance usually resolves the dysrhythmia; β-receptor blockade is also effective. Mechanical stimulation-induced arrhythmias are best and most predictably treated by withdrawing the catheter out of the ventricle or atrium.

Refractory ventricular depolarizations suggest that myocardial ischemia is causing nonphysioloic depolarization.[146] Intravenous antidysrhythmics such as lidocaine, bretylium, or procainamide can be useful to control ischemic ventricular automaticity.

Supraventricular Premature Impulses with Aberrant Conduction

If an aberrantly conducted atrial premature depolarization enters the ventricular conduction system before complete recovery of excitability, asynchronous ventricular depolarization generates wide, high-amplitude ECG complexes that are similar to PVCs (Fig. 6–6). Aberrantly conducted premature supraventricular depolarizations often resemble normal complexes in general shape and are sometimes preceded by a P wave that

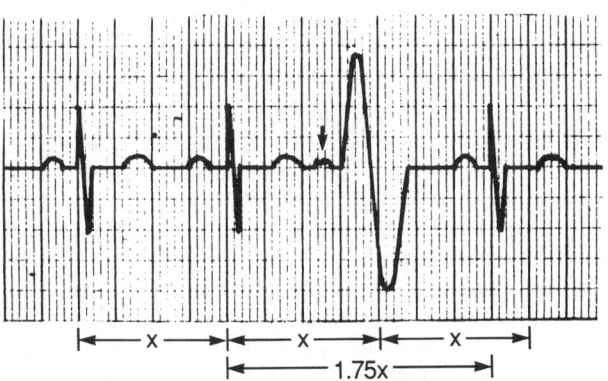

FIGURE 6–6. Aberrantly conducted atrial premature depolarization. Note initial deflection and general configuration similar to normal QRS complex, presence of abnormal preceding P wave *(arrow)*, and noncompensatory pause between previous and subsequent normal QRS complexes. x = normal RR interval; 2x = full compensatory pause; 1.75x = noncompensatory pause. (From Mecca RS: Postanesthesia recovery. *In* Clinical Anesthesia. Barash PG, Cullen BF, Stoelting RK (eds). Philadelphia, JB Lippincott, 1989, p 1405.)

may be different from the normal P waves. The interval between a previous and subsequent normal QRS is usually less than twice the normal interval (noncompensatory pause).

Increased SNS activity is the usual cause of premature supraventricular impulses with aberrant conduction, but delayed recovery of conducting tissues caused by chronic disease, general anesthetics, or electrolyte abnormalities also favors aberrant conduction. If the frequency of aberrantly conducted impulses compromises cardiac output, control of SNS activity usually restores regular rhythm.

Re-Entrant Depolarization

If a sinus impulse is delayed in a ventricular conduction pathway long enough to encounter tissue that has recovered excitability, the impulse causes a second, re-entrant depolarization that spreads throughout the heart.[147] Re-entrant depolarizations generate wide, high-amplitude complexes that also resemble VPCs but are uniform in configuration, manifest full compensatory pauses, follow a preceding normal complex by a constant interval (fixed coupling), and often appear in a bigeminal pattern (Fig. 6–7).

Postoperative re-entry also is often related to increased SNS activity, especially after inhalation anesthesia. Control of SNS tone and elimination of factors that cause conduction delay or nonuniform recovery of excitability usually suppress re-entry dysrhythmias.

Most abnormal ventricular complexes seen on PACU monitors are caused by re-entrant dysrhythmias or aberrantly conducted supraventricular complexes. Differentiation from actual ventricular ectopy is important, because re-entry and aberrant conduction seldom require treatment. Frequent ventricular ectopy may also be benign, particularly if it was evident preoperatively, or may reflect a serious underlying abnormality that could cause degeneration into a more serious dysrhythmia.

When Is Tachycardia Significant?

Sinus Tachycardia

Sinus tachycardia, the most common dysrhythmia encountered in the PACU, is usually harmless. It seldom interferes with ventricular filling but can exacerbate hypertension or reduce cardiac output in patients with stenotic valvular lesions. Decreased diastolic filling time may precipitate acute myocardial ischemia in patients with coronary artery disease.[133]

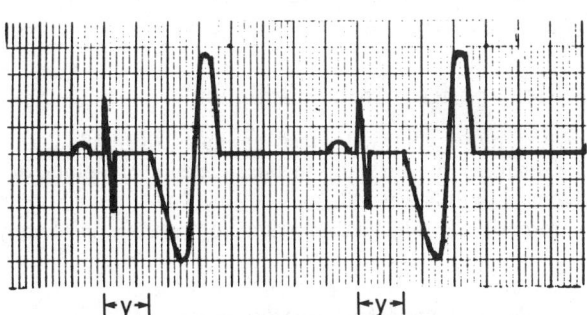

FIGURE 6–7. Re-entry with fixed coupling. Note uniform configuration of abnormal QRS complex, and fixed interval (y) between preceding normal QRS complex and abnormal complex. (From Mecca RS: Postanesthesia recovery. *In* Clinical Anesthesia. Barash PG, Cullen BF, Stoelting RK (eds). Philadelphia, JB Lippincott, 1989, p 1405.)

Because tachycardia might be caused by serious conditions such as acidemia, hypoxemia, or malignant hyperthermia, it is important to identify and treat an underlying cause. Intravenous fluids to counteract hypovolemia, analgesics to treat postoperative pain, or sedatives to calm anxiety usually suffice. Relief of bladder distention by catheterization often slows the rate. When tachycardia presents a medical risk or the underlying cause is beyond control, β-blockade with esmolol is useful. Digoxin is ineffective unless ventricular failure is the underlying cause.

Atrial Fibrillation

Untreated atrial fibrillation can generate ventricular rates in excess of 150 beats per minute. At this high a rate, it often appears as a nearly regular supraventricular tachycardia on ECG. Patients recovering from thoracic surgical procedures exhibit a higher incidence of postoperative atrial fibrillation, as do patients with mitral valvular disease or pulmonary embolism.

A fast ventricular rate often causes significant hypotension or myocardial ischemia, so treatment involves decreasing the number of impulses that can traverse the AV node per minute with digoxin or calcium channel blockers. Direct-current cardioversion might be indicated in urgent circumstances.

Atrial Flutter

Atrial flutter is rare in postoperative patients. It usually presents with a rapid, regular ventricular rate at some fraction of the atrial rate. Decreasing the ventricular rate and regulating atrial electrical activity are the major goals of therapy.

Paroxysmal Atrial Tachycardia

PAT is usually caused by circus re-entry in conduction tissue, although a small percentage result from discrete, rapidly firing groups of pacemaker cells. When PAT emerges, the resulting excessive ventricular rate interferes with ventricular filling and reduces cardiac output.

Treatment of PAT involves slowing cardiac conduction velocity to interrupt re-entrant synchrony. This approach allows a dominant pacemaker to recapture the heart at a slower rate. Depression of conduction by residual anesthetic levels may contribute to the relative rarity of PAT in the PACU setting. Increasing PNS influence on the heart (Table 6–12) resolves PAT. Digoxin or calcium channel blockers can also be useful. PAT caused by a rapidly firing atrial pacemaker may slow with β-blockade.

Ventricular Tachycardia/Fibrillation

Postoperative ventricular tachycardia or fibrillation usually reflects severe myocardial ischemia, systemic acidemia, or hypoxemia. Controlled ventilation and oxygenation, cardiopulmonary resuscitation, and cardioversion are mainstays of therapy.

When Is Postoperative Bradycardia Significant?

A decrease in SNS activity or an increase in PNS activity slows down spontaneous depolarization in supraventricular

TABLE 6–12. Factors That Increase Postoperative Parasympathetic Influence

Increased Parasympathetic Activity	Decreased Sympathetic Activity
Vagal Reflexes	
Carotid sinus massage, gagging, Valsalva's maneuver, rectal examination, increased ocular pressure, bladder distention, pharyngeal stimulation	T1–T4 spinal or epidural sympathectomy Decreased stimulus (extubation, analgesia) Emptying bladder Severe acidemia/hypoxemia
Parasympathomimetic Medications	*Sympatholytic Medications*
Cholinesterase inhibitors (neostigmine, edrophonium) Alpha-adrenergics (phenylephrine hydrochloride [Neo-Synephrine], norepinephrine) Narcotics (morphine, fentanyl) Succinylcholine	Beta-blockers (propranolol, esmolol) Narcotics/sedatives/general anesthetics Ganglionic blockers Local anesthetics

pacemakers, leading to sinus bradycardia. The sinus rate also falls with sick sinus syndrome, sinus nodal ischemia, or severe hypoxemia. Hypotension usually does not result until the rate falls below 40 to 45 beats per minute.

Therapy involves elimination of autonomic nervous system imbalance or restoration of SNS or PNS tone. Excess PNS activity usually responds to muscarinic blocking drugs such as atropine or glycopyrrolate, whereas decreased SNS activity is usually resolved with a β-mimetic drug such as ephedrine.

Nodal Rhythm

The sinus node sometimes is more sensitive to increased PNS activity than are other supraventricular pacemakers; thus, autonomic imbalance can promote emergence of a pacemaker in the lower AV node or bundle of His. If sinus node impulses are prevented from reaching the ventricle by sinus nodal exit block or AV nodal block, a nodal rhythm can also emerge.

When the ventricular rate is sufficient to maintain cardiac output and blood pressure, nodal rhythm usually does not require treatment. However, lack of coordinated atrial contraction can decrease cardiac output by 10% to 15%, especially in patients with noncompliant ventricles. If hypotension occurs, atropine or β-mimetic medications may restore the sinus node as the dominant pacemaker; occasionally, however, they serve only to increase the nodal rate. Blood pressure support may be necessary until spontaneous resolution of the rhythm occurs.

Idioventricular Bradycardia

Idioventricular bradycardia almost always indicates third-degree heart block, hypoxemia, acidemia, or myocardial ischemia. A slow idioventricular rhythm usually does not generate adequate blood pressure. If acute third-degree AV nodal block is secondary to digitalis toxicity or ischemia, atropine sometimes marginally improves AV nodal conduction and allows supraventricular impulses to reach the ventricles.

Should acceleration of the ventricular rate be necessary, epinephrine, isoproterenol, or cardiac pacing is used. Vagolytic medications do not increase the depolarization rates of ventricular pacemakers.

POSTOPERATIVE RENAL PROBLEMS

Opiates and the parasympathomimetic side effects of regional anesthetics accentuate urinary sphincter tone and can lead to difficulty with micturition. If a patient cannot spontaneously void, extended observation after discharge from the PACU is necessary to avoid urinary retention. Patients with indwelling catheters should have urine output recorded hourly.

How Is Renal Function Assessed?

Assessment of postoperative urine output as the sole index of renal function can be misleading, because osmotic diuresis or the effects of surgery and anesthesia interfere with renal regulatory mechanisms. Urine color is a poor predictor of renal concentrating ability but can suggest pyuria or hematuria.

A urine sodium concentration far below serum concentration indicates renal tubular viability, as does a urine potassium concentration above serum. Urine osmolarity better reflects tubular function than does specific gravity. An osmolarity >450 mOsm $\cdot$ L^{-1} implies intact tubular concentrating ability.[148]

Acidification or alkalization of urine requires intact tubular function; thus, urine pH reflects tubular viability. Electrolyte osmolarity and pH values close to those in serum can be normal or might signify acute tubular necrosis.

What Is the Significance of Polyuria?

A number of conditions lead to polyuria (Table 6–13). Profuse postoperative urine output usually reflects the excretion of generous intraoperative fluids. However, sustained polyuria (>4–5 mL $\cdot$ kg^{-1} $\cdot$ hr^{-1}) that compromises intravascular volume and systemic blood pressure sometimes denotes abnormal regulation of free water clearance. Polyuria also can reflect the persistent effects of intraoperatively administered diuretics. High-output renal failure should also be considered.

Osmotic Diuresis

Osmotic diuresis secondary to hyperglycemia and glycosuria can generate massive urine output, especially if glucose-containing crystalloid solutions are used to replace urinary losses. Once urine and serum glucose determinations reveal the problem, glucose restriction usually is the only therapy required for this self-limited process.

Diabetes Insipidus

Polyuria caused by diabetes insipidus can occur after intracranial surgery, pituitary ablation, or head trauma. Increased intracranial pressure or inadvertent omission of preoperative vasopressin also interferes with free water reabsorption. Comparison of electrolytes and osmolarity between urine and serum is diagnostic, and the administration of vasopressin is therapeutic.[89]

TABLE 6–13. Causes of Postoperative Polyuria

Liberal intraoperative fluid administration
Diuretics
High-output renal failure
Osmotic diuresis (glucose, mannitol)
Diabetes insipidus (central or nephrogenic)

TABLE 6–14. Causes of Postoperative Oliguria

Inadequate intraoperative fluid administration
Hypotension
Elevated antidiuretic hormone secretion (pain, anxiety, stress)
Hyponatremia
Acute renal insufficiency (acute tubular necrosis)
Ureteral ligation
Catheter occlusion
Renal vascular occlusion
Narcotic administration
Residual effects of spinal, epidural, caudal anesthesia

What Is the Significance of Oliguria?

Urine volume of <0.5 mL $\cdot$ kg $\cdot$ hr^{-1} usually reflects an appropriate kidney response to hypovolemia, elevated antidiuretic hormone levels, or systemic hypotension but can indicate abnormal renal function and other problems (Table 6–14). Oliguria should always be evaluated, especially after procedures involving aortic cross-clamping, possible ureteral ligature, severe hypotension, or massive transfusion.

Urinary catheter patency should be checked because obstruction by blood clots or debris mimics oliguria, as does positioning that forces the catheter tip above the urine level in the bladder. For patients without urinary catheters, assessment of bladder fullness, the urge to void, and the interval since last voiding helps to differentiate between urinary retention and oliguria.

Hypovolemia

To assess whether oliguria represents an appropriate response to hypovolemia, a 300- to 500-mL intravenous crystalloid bolus should be given after urine samples for electrolyte and osmolarity testing are obtained. If output does not improve, a larger fluid bolus or a diagnostic trial of 5 mg of furosemide is appropriate. Furosemide increases urine output if oliguria is caused by increased tubular reabsorption.

Hypoperfusion due to systemic hypotension can reduce urine output. The systemic blood pressure that provides minimally adequate renal perfusion varies, depending on the usual preoperative pressure.

What Should Be Done If Oliguria Persists?

If oliguria persists despite adequate perfusion pressure, hydration, and a small furosemide challenge, the possibilities of ureteral obstruction, acute tubular necrosis, renal artery or vein occlusion, or inappropriate antidiuretic hormone secretion must be evaluated. Intravenous pyelography, angiography, or radioisotope imaging helps to clarify current renal status, whereas pulmonary artery catheterization can determine the adequacy of cardiovascular function. Osmotic or loop diuretics and low-dose dopamine or dobutamine probably are useful to attenuate renal damage.[149, 150] Perioperative administration of desmopressin usually has minimal effect on postoperative urinary output.

CENTRAL NERVOUS SYSTEM FUNCTION

When the reasons for prolonged unconsciousness are sought, preoperative responsiveness must be taken into consideration to rule out unrecognized chronic mental dysfunction or drug or alcohol intoxication (Table 6–15). All depressant medications administered before and during surgery should be noted.

Pupillary size and response are unreliable as diagnostic indices because many drugs affect pupillary signs. However, the rate and character of spontaneous ventilation can serve to identify residual anesthetic. Systemic blood pressure and heart rate suggest the adequacy of cerebral perfusion and the prevailing level of autonomic tone. A firm tactile stimulus is often more effective than verbal stimulation to elicit arousal.

Are Residual Drug Effects Present?

Residual depression from intraoperative sedative medications frequently causes somnolence.[151] Inhalation anesthetics are more likely to prolong unconsciousness after long surgical procedures, especially in obese patients. Continuing high inspired concentrations of such agents through the end of surgery to facilitate deep extubation often leave patients unresponsive in the PACU.

Intraoperatively administered narcotics or sedatives generally cause dose-related sedation, although perioperative administration of long-acting sedatives such as lorazepam, scopolamine, pentobarbital, hydroxyzine, or promethazine significantly prolong emergence.

Narcotics

If unconsciousness persists beyond 60 to 90 minutes, low-dose intravenous naloxone in 40-μg increments every 2 minutes should reverse the sedative effects and respiratory depression due to intraoperative narcotics without precipitating dangerous reversal of analgesia. A maximum dose of 200 to 400 μg should increase ventilatory rate and arousal unless the patient has been massively overdosed with narcotics.

Sedative Drugs

Flumazenil, a new competitive benzodiazepine antagonist, is useful to identify and reverse sedation from benzodiazepines,[152–154] although residual sedative effects of the benzodiazepines may recur after flumazenil's 1-hour duration of action. Intravenous physostigmine, 1.25 mg, sometimes nonspecifically counteracts sedation from residual inhalation anesthetics, anticholinergics, tricyclic antidepressants, and other sedatives.[155] Lack of response to adequate doses of naloxone, flumazenil, or physostigmine does not categorically preclude unrecognized preoperative or intraoperative overdose with sedative medications as a possible cause.

Neuromuscular Paralysis

Profound residual neuromuscular paralysis can mimic unconsciousness and may be a factor in patients with unrecognized neuromuscular disease, phase II blockade caused by excessive succinylcholine administration, or pseudocholinesterase deficiency. Purposeful motion, spontaneous ventilation, reflex activity, or other evidence of neuromuscular function eliminates residual paralysis as an explanation for unresponsiveness.

Which Less Common Etiologies Should Be Considered?

Preoperative exhaustion often delays emergence from an anesthetic, especially if sleep patterns are interrupted in children undergoing emergency surgery at night. Caffeine withdrawal is an uncommon cause but should be considered. A family member can usually provide a history of significant chronic caffeine ingestion (e.g., >10 cups per day) if this is the case.

Intravenous caffeine promptly reverses this cause of delayed emergence. On occasion, a patient feigns unresponsiveness. If hypoglycemia is suspected, an immediate empiric trial of intra-

---

TABLE 6–15. Differential Diagnosis of Persistent Unconsciousness

Routine Cases	
Residual depression from general anesthetics	Usually resolves within 60–90 min
Excessive narcotic administration	Identify and treat with naloxone titration
Prolonged effect of long-acting sedative premedication	Either medical drugs or substance abuse. If benzodiazepines given, treat with flumazenil titration.
Preoperative exhaustion	Causes deep sleep, arousable with stimulus
Preoperative decreased level of consciousness	Intoxication, chronic low level of arousal
Global Physiologic Disorders	
Profound residual neuromuscular paralysis	Precluded if any motor responses noted
Systemic hypotension	Severe if hypoperfusion causes unconsciousness
Profound hypoxemia	Caused by airway obstruction, hypoventilation
Marked hypercarbia	High carbon dioxide acts as sedative; often with hypoxemia
Severe hypoglycemia	Suspicion indicates 50% dextrose trial
Hypothermia	Below 30°C, unusual cause or deep sedation
Severe hyperglycemia/hyperosmolarity	Unusual, treated with insulin/potassium
Hyponatremia/hypo-osmolarity	Treated with furosemide to waste free water
Central Nervous System Dysfunction	
Seizure activity	Seizure or postictal phase decreases responses
Intraoperative cerebral anoxia	Hypotension, disconnection, dysrhythmia
Unrecognized subarachnoid injection of local anesthetic	Can occur during "general-regional" techniques
Undiagnosed preoperative high intracranial pressure/subdural hematoma	Multiple trauma with unrecognized head injury
Cerebral embolism	Fibrillation, air embolism, invasive neck catheters
Stroke/increased intracranial pressure	Mostly after carotid or cardiac/neurosurgery

venous 50% dextrose should be administered while serum glucose determination is pending.

Hypo-osmolarity secondary to acute hyponatremia can affect consciousness, so serum electrolyte concentrations and osmolarity should be checked. Serum sodium level <125 mEq $\cdot$ L^{-1} is cause for concern, as is a serum osmolarity <260 mOsm $\cdot$ L^{-1}. Glucose and electrolyte determinations also reveal severe hyperglycemia or hypernatremia causing acute hyperosmolar coma.

Hypothermia <33 °C can impair consciousness or accentuate the depressant effects of some medications. Fixed pupillary dilation, areflexia, and coma can occur at core temperatures <30 °C. ABG analysis assesses whether unrecognized hypoxemia or marked hypercarbia with CO_2 narcosis is contributory.

What Should Be Done If the Cause Is Indeterminate?

A thorough, carefully documented neurologic evaluation in consultation with a neurologist should be carried out if the diagnosis is still unclear. Subclinical seizures secondary to delirium tremens or an underlying seizure disorder can present as unresponsiveness in the PACU, as can CNS depression due to intravenous local anesthetic toxicity or inadvertent subarachnoid injections during analgesic blocks.[156]

Central Nervous System Pathology

Unrecognized intraoperative cerebral hypoxia secondary to severe hypotension, dysrhythmias, or hypoxemia must be considered. In trauma victims, covert head trauma or increased intracranial pressure should be sought. Increased intracranial pressure due to bleeding or edema also causes unconsciousness after intracranial surgery.

Cerebral embolism is another possible etiology following vascular surgery[157] or after the insertion of internal jugular, subclavian, or intra-arterial catheters. A history of atrial fibrillation, carotid disease, or hypercoagulability increases the risk of thromboembolism.[158] Air embolism through a right-to-left intracardiac shunt and intracerebral hemorrhage secondary to hypertension also cause postoperative coma.[159]

Cerebrovascular accidents are rare in lower risk patients and usually occur later in the postoperative course.[160]

Why Does Altered Sensorium Occur?

Inappropriate mental reactions ranging from lethargy and confusion to extreme disorientation and physical combativeness can occur in the PACU (Table 6–16). These reactions are disturbing to staff and other patients and pose substantial risks, including contusion or fracture due to contact with equipment or bed side rails, corneal abrasion due to dislodged O_2 apparatus, and sprains due to violent struggling.

Combative, thrashing patients jeopardize suture lines, vascular grafts, and orthopedic fixation and dislodge drains, tracheal tubes, or vascular catheters. High SNS activity in agitated patients causes tachycardia and hypertension and the potential for serious medical complications. The risk of injury to the PACU staff struggling to contain a combative patient is also significant.

Patients at Risk

Although difficult to predict, extreme emergence reactions are more prevalent in children and young adults, whereas the elderly may recover cognitive function more slowly.[161] Parental separation increases anxiety in young children. Preoperative aberrations often complicate the emergence of individuals with mental retardation, clinically evident psychiatric disorders, organic brain dysfunctions, or hostile affect.

Psychologic, ethnic, and cultural differences have some role,[162, 163] especially if a language barrier interferes with reassurance by the PACU staff. Oral fixation or tracheal intubation interferes with communication and generates frustration or fear. The incidence of stormy emergence is probably higher after procedures such as breast or testicular biopsies, which are associated with unusual anxiety or emotion.

Reversible Factors

Failure to Process Sensory Input

For a short period during emergence from general anesthesia, the ability to process and react to sensory input can be

TABLE 6–16. Differential Diagnosis of Altered Sensorium During Emergence

General Causes	Effects
Disorientation during emergence	Poor integration of sensory input, 10 min
Postoperative surgical pain	Treat with analgesia if pain clearly from procedure
Nonsurgical discomfort	Full bladder, nausea, gastric distention, positioning
Postoperative anxiety/fear	Separation from parents, emotional diagnoses, death
Inability to move/poor positioning	Escalating combativeness against restraint
Individual variation	Affected by intelligence, culture, gender, retardation
Unrecognized preparation intoxication	Marked combativeness, disorientation
Scopolamine/ketamine/etomidate	Occasional postoperative dysphoria
Atropine/meperidine	Rare anticholinergic-induced postoperative delirium
Serious Underlying Abnormalities	
Pulmonary dysfunction	↑ Work of breathing/poor expansion/vascular distention
Hypoxemia	Clouding of sensorium, disorientation, mild agitation
Hypercarbia/acidemia	Marked agitation, disorientation, dyspnea, tachypnea
Hypotension	Cerebral hypoperfusion, confusion, nausea, somnolence
Hypoglycemia	Agitation/confusion/disorientation, sympathetic nervous system activity
Hyponatremia/hypo-osmolarity	Confusion/visual disturbances/seizures
Residual paralysis	Terrifying, flopping motions, mimic agitation

impaired. Lack of integration may present as gradually clearing somnolence, disorientation, and sluggish mental responsiveness or as wide emotional swings with uncontrollable weeping. An occasional patient exhibits escalating combativeness against positioning and restraint.

Sedatives and Psychiatric Drugs

Preoperative administration of long-acting sedatives or psychogenic medications can cloud the sensorium and cause disorientation in the PACU. Preoperative alcohol or drug abuse often generates bizarre emergence behavior secondary to intoxication or withdrawal.

Disorientation, paranoia, and combativeness after parenteral scopolamine administration can be treated with intravenous physostigmine. Prolonged preoperative meperidine therapy or atropine premedication can also cause anticholinergic-induced postoperative delirium.[164, 165] Etomidate induction may be associated with increased postoperative restlessness.[166] Postoperative dysphoria and hallucination secondary to acute ketamine reactions are rare.

Pain and Discomfort

Pain or discomfort amplifies confusion, agitation, and aggressive behavior during emergence, so adequate postoperative analgesia is essential early in the PACU course. Urinary bladder or gastric distention generates marked discomfort and agitation in emerging patients. Tracheal or nasogastric tubes, urinary catheters, infiltrated vascular catheters, tight dressings, or painful phlebotomy can also be troublesome.

Unusual sources of pain such as corneal abrasion, entrapment of sensitive body parts, or small pieces of equipment left beneath a patient occasionally are responsible. Nausea and dizziness are very distressing, as is severe pruritus caused by medication reactions.

Position and Restraint

Obese patients or those with gastroesophgeal reflux or pulmonary congestion sometimes struggle vigorously to move from a supine into a semi-sitting position. Patients often fight vigorously against physical restraint until the restraint is relaxed. Partial neuromuscular relaxation causes severe agitation during emergence, even if ventilation is adequate, and can elicit violent, uncoordinated motion that might be mistaken for disorientation or combativeness.

Respiratory Dysfunction

Confusion, delirium, or combativeness after anesthesia sometimes indicates serious respiratory dysfunction. Hypoxemia is associated with disorientation, clouded mentation, or agitation that is similar to that caused by pain. Respiratory acidemia also elicits profound agitation, although if hypercarbia is caused by respiratory center suppression, the visible responses may be reduced by coincident depression of higher CNS functions. Hypercarbia without acidemia is often asymptomatic unless CO_2 narcosis causes somnolence and disorientation.

Increased work of breathing from high airway resistance or partial upper airway obstruction causes marked agitation, as does the inability to cough or clear secretions. Pulmonary vascular engorgement or early interstitial pulmonary edema causes symptoms of chest fullness and air hunger well before airway flooding occurs.

Restriction of inspiratory volume by tight dressings, gastric distention, splinting, or inappropriately low tidal volume settings during mechanical ventilation cause vague manifestations similar to air hunger. This phenomenon is probably mediated by stretch receptors that monitor lung volume. Agitation caused by problems with the mechanics of ventilation can be profound, even though ventilation and oxygenation are adequate.

Abnormal Perfusion

Lactic acidemia caused by poor peripheral perfusion results in anxiety and mild disorientation. Cerebral hypoperfusion is associated with lethargy, disorientation, agitation, or combativeness. Sedatives or analgesics administered to quell anxiety or pain may lead to cardiopulmonary collapse.

Metabolic Changes

Metabolic abnormalities can interfere with lucidity. Acute hyponatremia and hypo-osmolarity after transurethral prostatic resection markedly cloud the sensorium, although glycine toxicity may also play a part. Cerebral fluid shifts occur after dialysis, acute repletion of severe dehydration, or massive fluid infusion. Moderate hypoglycemia results in significant agitation or diminished responsiveness, whereas acute hyperglycemia due to excess glucose infusion or insufficient insulin can alter consciousness.

Primary Neurologic Problems

A primary neurologic problem must be considered once reversible causes of delirium or agitation are eliminated. Seizure activity in patients with epilepsy, head trauma, chronic alcohol abuse, or cocaine intoxication can mimic agitation and combativeness and can generate disorientation and somnolence during the postictal phase. Cerebral embolism, hemorrhage, or infarct sometimes presents with disorientation, inability to vocalize, or a reduced level of consciousness.[167]

What Therapy Is Appropriate?

Therapy for altered mental status in the PACU is generally supportive. Most emergence reactions disappear as residual anesthesia resolves, although unpleasant sequelae can persist.[168] Reassuring patients that they are doing well can be invaluable, especially if a patient's and surgeon's name are frequently used and time and location are emphasized. Allowing patients to determine their own position can be helpful.

A small amount of sedative is sometimes necessary to reduce fear or anxiety. Of course, adequate analgesia is essential. Identifying whether a patient is reacting to pain or to anxiety before treatment is important, for narcotics are relatively poor sedatives and benzodiazepines or barbiturates are ineffective analgesics.

Physical restraint should be used when a patient's physical safety is in jeopardy (e.g., intubated, agitated). Altered mental status caused by a physiologic abnormality such as hypoxemia, acidemia, hypoglycemia, or hypotension should be treated by resolving the underlying problem.

POSTOPERATIVE NAUSEA AND VOMITING

The incidence of nausea and vomiting varies with age, surgical procedure, and anesthetic technique.[169–172] Postoperative vomiting often delays PACU discharge or necessitates admission of ambulatory patients, reducing efficiency and overall satisfaction with the procedure. Vomiting is unpleasant for patients and staff and poses genuine medical risks for aspiration of gastric contents, especially if airway reflexes are marginal or postoperative oral fixation interferes with airway clearance.

Increased intra-abdominal pressure can jeopardize abdominal or inguinal closures, and increased central venous pressure may increase morbidity after ocular, tympanic, or intracranial procedures. The SNS responses to vomiting and pain due to increased movement elevate heart rate and systemic blood pressure, increasing the risk of myocardial ischemia and dysrhythmias. Gagging and retching can also elicit a parasympathetic response with bradycardia and hypotension.

What Are the Risk Factors?

A history of preoperative emesis or motion sickness has some predictive value. A general anesthetic near menses increases the incidence of vomiting in women,[173] perhaps related to an increase in circulating E2 estrogen levels.[174] The risk of nausea is higher after procedures involving extraocular muscles or middle ear manipulation, peritoneal or intestinal irritation, and testicular traction.[175, 176]

Anesthetic Contribution

Anesthetic effects on chemotactic centers, autonomic imbalance, starvation, and postoperative pain probably increase the risk.[177] Swallowed blood or tissue promotes postoperative vomiting, as does accumulation of gas in the stomach. Regional anesthesia probably generates less immediate postoperative vomiting than does general, although vomiting frequently occurs when parenteral narcotics are required after a regional block has resolved.

Inhalational Agents

Exclusion of nitrous oxide from an anesthetic might reduce the incidence of postoperative vomiting,[178, 179] although this finding is controversial.[180–183] The incidence of nausea does not appear to differ whether halothane, enflurane, or isoflurane is used.[184]

Intravenous Agents

Barbiturate induction seems less offensive than ketamine or etomidate; propofol induction may have the lowest incidence.[184] Narcotic analgesics probably increase postoperative nausea when compared with "pure" inhalation techniques, especially in ambulatory surgical patients.[185] Meperidine might generate a higher incidence of postoperative nausea than morphine.

Non-narcotic analgesics such as ketorolac, in conjunction with small doses of narcotics, may reduce the severity of emesis. Neostigmine administered during reversal of neuro-

muscular relaxants or physostigmine given to counteract sedation also increases the incidence of postoperative nausea.[186, 187]

How Is Nausea Prevented?

Several interventions help to prevent postoperative nausea. Adequate postoperative analgesia is important, as is limiting postoperative vestibular stimulation by minimizing brisk head motion. Avoiding gastric distention by evacuation of stomach contents with an orogastric tube is of questionable utility.[188, 189]

Drug Therapy

Droperidol

The antiemetic effect of intravenous droperidol has been extensively evaluated.[176, 190–193] Perioperative administration of intravenous droperidol decreases the incidence and severity of postoperative nausea, although the efficacy varies among procedures and individual patients. A dose <1 to 2 $\mu g \cdot kg^{-1}$ or 1.25 mg total in adults should not cause excessive sedation.

Additional intravenous droperidol helps treat breakthrough nausea in the PACU, although the resultant sedation may delay discharge. The α-adrenergic blocking properties of droperidol can precipitate hypotension in hypovolemic patients. Transient extrapyramidal side effects are infrequent and usually inconsequential.[194]

Metoclopramide

Intravenous metoclopramide, alone or with droperidol, probably decreases the incidence of postoperative vomiting.[192, 195–197] Whether metoclopramide merely reduces gastric volume or has an additional central antiemetic action is unclear. Rarely it causes dysphoria.[198]

Histamine₂ Blockers

Cimetidine or ranitidine helps to decrease gastric volume. Dimenhydrinate or thiethylperazine may also be effective to treat nausea.[199, 200]

Scopolamine

Intravenous scopolamine causes unacceptable psychogenic reactions when used as an antiemetic. Low efficacy and a tendency to cause visual disturbances make transdermal scopolamine a poor substitute for other agents.[201–203]

Ephedrine

Ephedrine might be effective for postoperative nausea related to ambulation or motion, but its efficacy is unclear.[204–207]

Ondansetron

Ondansetron, a new serotonin receptor blocker, may prove to be a useful antiemetic for postoperative nausea, but its effectiveness compared with droperidol or metoclopramide still needs to be established. Its cost may be prohibitive.[208–211]

Acupuncture stimulation and acupressure are alleged to reduce the incidence of postoperative vomiting.[212] Before instituting treatment, it is always important to evaluate more serious causes of nausea and emesis such as hypotension, increased intracranial pressure, hypoxemia, hypoglycemia, or gastric bleeding.

POSTOPERATIVE HYPOTHERMIA

Many patients exhibit hypothermia after surgery. The level at which the body actively begins to regulate temperature (i.e., the thermoregulatory threshold) is decreased by approximately 2.5 °C during general anesthesia.[213]

Why Does It Occur?

Heat is lost through evaporation during skin preparation, by the humidification of dry gases, and through radiation and convection from the skin and surgical wound. A reduction in core temperature is accelerated by low ambient temperatures and cold intravenous fluids.

The ability to maintain temperature is severely compromised even after temperature reaches the reset thermoregulatory threshold. Paralysis and anesthesia impair shivering, and nonshivering thermogenesis is relatively ineffective in adults.[214] Peripheral thermoregulatory vasoconstriction decreases heat loss but is less effective in anesthetized patients.[215] It is associated with decreased reliability of pulse oximetry, intra-arterial pressure monitoring, and peripheral nerve stimulation.

Heat loss is approximately the same during general and regional anesthetics, but rewarming is slower after regional anesthetics because residual vasodilation and paralysis interfere with heat generation and retention. Infants are at increased risk because their body mass is relatively low compared with surface area. Cachectic, traumatized, or burned patients are prone to more serious temperature reduction.

What Are the Adverse Effects?

The adverse effects of hypothermia are many and varied (Table 6–17). Hypothermia increases postoperative morbidity because it increases SNS activity, elevates peripheral vascular resistance, and decreases venous capacitance.[216] Hypoperfusion of peripheral tissues promotes hypoxia and metabolic acidemia, jeopardizing the viability of marginal tissue grafts. Increased avidity of hemoglobin for O_2 further compromises oxygenation in hypothermic tissues. Decreased biotransforma-

TABLE 6–17. Adverse Effects of Hypothermia

Increased systemic vascular resistance
Decreased venous capacitance
Hypoperfusion
Increased oxyhemoglobin affinity
Decreased metabolic biotransfusion
Increased sedation
Hyperglycemia
Platelet sequestration
Decreased renal function
Cardiac dysrhythmias
Shivering

tion and reduced perfusion may increase the duration of sedation and neuromuscular relaxation.

The minimal alveolar concentration of inhalation anesthetics decreases 5% to 7% per 1 °C reduction in core temperature, accentuating sedation from residual alveolar partial pressures. Moderate hyperglycemia occurs, and visceral sequestration of platelets, decreased platelet function, and reduced activity of clotting factors may cause mild coagulopathy.

Severe hypothermia interferes with cardiac rhythm generation and impulse conduction, lengthening PR, QRS, or QT intervals and generating J waves on ECG. The risk of dysrhythmia after mechanical stimulation of the myocardium is increased, and spontaneous ventricular fibrillation can occur at temperatures <28 °C.

Why Is Shivering Detrimental?

During emergence from general anesthesia, hypothalamic regulation steps up metabolic activity and generates shivering to increase endogenous heat production. Postoperative shivering increases the risk of incidental trauma and makes routine postoperative care more difficult. Shivering increases O_2 consumption and CO_2 production by 200% to 800%. The associated increase in cardiac output and minute ventilation may precipitate myocardial ischemia or ventilatory failure in patients with coronary artery disease or limited ventilatory reserve.

The intensity of postoperative shivering is sometimes accentuated by inhalation anesthetic–related tremor, which manifests both clonic and tonic components.[217] The former may be triggered by hypothermia but seems related to decreased cortical influence on spinal cord reflexes.[218]

Treatment

Morphine, meperidine, droperidol, butorphanol, chlorpromazine, magnesium sulfate, and methylphenidate all have been advocated to suppress shivering.[219–222] Withholding the reversal of neuromuscular relaxants in intubated, ventilated, sedated patients attenuates shivering but increases rewarming time. Additional relaxant administration to eliminate shivering in patients with limited cardiac reserve in the PACU is an option but usually is not indicated.

How Is Hypothermia Decreased or Prevented?

During surgery, covering exposed body and head surfaces[223] and warming of ambient air, intravenous fluids, and irrigating solutions are useful to counteract temperature loss. Surface or radiant warmers and heated humidification of inspired gases also help. Reduction of core temperature is <2 to 3 °C in most patients, so spontaneous rewarming during routine recovery is usually sufficient, although moderate shivering often occurs.

Patients undergoing prolonged major surgical procedures with significant fluid replacement can suffer more profound hypothermia. All hypothermic patients should receive supplemental O_2 in the PACU. Core temperature <35 °C is an indication for assisted rewarming using heating blankets, reflective coverings, radiant lighting, or forced air.[224–226] As body temperature rises, hypotension caused by increasing venous capacitance can occur.

POSTOPERATIVE HYPERTHERMIA

What Is the Impact?

Fever is less common in the PACU than hypothermia. Self-limited hyperthermia is occasionally caused by close draping and aggressive heat preservation in the operating room. Acute postoperative fever may be caused by atelectasis or respiratory infection secondary to intraoperative loss of lung volume or retention of secretions but is usually not detected in the PACU. Unrecognized intraoperative aspiration sometimes causes fever.

Exacerbation of an existing infection during resection of infected tonsils or appendix, abscess drainage, and urinary tract manipulation are other frequent causes. Emergence of a previously asymptomatic condition such as influenza, sinusitis, otitis, or upper respiratory infection can also cause postoperative fever.

Increased body temperature is a presenting sign of a drug or transfusion reaction. Muscarinic blocking agents like atropine interfere with cutaneous cooling and can contribute to postoperative fever. Fever occurs during malignant hyperthermia, but other signs such as tachycardia, muscle rigidity, acidemia, and increased CO_2 production generally precede it. Rare causes of hypermetabolism like thyroid storm must be considered.

How Is It Treated?

Therapy for fever is generally supportive. Aggressive chest physiotherapy, incentive spirometry, and appropriate administration of antipyretics are usually sufficient. If a drug or transfusion reaction is suspected, the offending medication or blood product should be withheld. The physician responsible for long-term care should be notified to observe for a serious underlying complication.

POSTOPERATIVE ACID-BASE PROBLEMS

Why Does Respiratory Acidemia Occur?

Respiratory acidemia frequently occurs in the PACU because inhalation anesthetics, narcotics, and sedative medications promote hypoventilation. Hypercarbia and acidemia are usually mild in awake, spontaneously breathing patients in the PACU. However, some patients are unable to sustain adequate ventilation. Residual neuromuscular paralysis, increased airway resistance, or decreased pulmonary compliance can impede ventilation and generate progressive respiratory acidemia despite appropriate CNS drive to breathe. Elevated CO_2 production caused by shivering, fever, hyperalimentation, or malignant hyperthermia amplifies the problem, as does increased dead space.[115, 116]

Effects

Respiratory acidemia causes agitation, confusion, dyspnea, and tachypnea, as well as hypertension, tachycardia, and dysrhythmias due to increased SNS activity. When caused by CNS depression, it produces less intense SNS activity because central autonomic responses are also depressed. Cerebral blood flow is increased and intracranial pressure rises in patients with head injury, intracranial tumor, or cerebral edema. At very low pH, heart rate and blood pressure can decrease precipitously.

Treatment

Compensation for acute respiratory acidemia is limited and requires hours to days before renal conservation of bicarbonate is fully effective. Therapy involves correction of the imbalance between effective alveolar ventilation and CO_2 production. Reversal of narcotics or neuromuscular relaxants, relief of airway obstruction, or improvement of ventilatory mechanics may be all that is necessary. If CO_2 elimination cannot be maintained with spontaneous ventilation, tracheal intubation and mechanical ventilation are required. Control of CO_2 production by decreasing fever, shivering, and work of breathing may be helpful, but extreme measures such as core cooling or paralysis are seldom appropriate.

Why Does Metabolic Acidemia Occur?

Postoperative metabolic acidemia sometimes indicates ketoacidosis in severely diabetic patients. Elevated serum glucose levels and urinary or blood ketones are diagnostic. Patients suffering from renal failure, renal tubular acidosis, or small bowel drainage are usually identified by history and often exhibit preoperative metabolic acidemia. Overdose with phenformin, aspirin, or methanol rarely causes postoperative metabolic acidemia.

Once ketoacidosis or a pre-existing metabolic problem is ruled out, postoperative metabolic acidemia is almost always caused by lactic acid accumulation secondary to insufficient delivery or use of tissue O_2. Peripheral hypoperfusion is often caused by low cardiac output due to hypovolemia, cardiac failure, or dysrhythmia.

Hypotension due to decreased SVR during sepsis, catecholamine depletion, or sympathectomy also causes lactic acidemia. Intense arteriolar constriction reduces tissue perfusion, as does inappropriate distribution of blood flow. Hypoxemia, decreased O_2-carrying capacity of blood, interference with release of O_2 from hemoglobin, or inability to use O_2 in the mitochondria also generates lactic acidemia.

Effects

A spontaneously ventilating patient should generate a respiratory compensation to offset metabolic acidemia, but anesthetic agents and narcotics interfere with the ventilatory response.[227] The sympathetic response to acute metabolic acidemia usually is less than that to respiratory acidemia because hydrogen and bicarbonate ions cross the blood-brain barrier with more difficulty than CO_2.

Treatment

Therapy is aimed at resolving the condition causing accumulation of metabolic acid. Fluids and intravenous insulin, potassium, and glucose are used to treat ketoacidosis. Mild lactic acidemia resolves spontaneously through acid metabolism and renal excretion of hydrogen ions once cardiac output and systemic blood pressure are improved. Rewarming also improves perfusion. Intravenous sodium bicarbonate or a suitable substitute is useful to maintain pH near normal when acidemia is severe or progressive despite other therapy.

Why Does Respiratory Alkalemia Occur?

Pain or anxiety during emergence commonly causes spontaneous hyperventilation and acute respiratory alkalemia. Pathologic causes of spontaneous hyperventilation include cerebrovascular accident, sepsis, or paradoxical CNS acidosis. Pain due to clumsy blood sampling sometimes generates a spurious alkalemia.

Excessive mechanical ventilation frequently causes postoperative respiratory alkalemia, especially when hypothermia or paralysis has reduced CO_2 production.

Effects

Acute respiratory alkalemia causes confusion or dizziness, atrial dysrhythmias, and mild cardiac conduction abnormalities. Alkalemia decreases cerebral blood flow and may lead to hypoperfusion and cerebral ischemia in patients with cerebrovascular disease. More severe alkalemia precipitates muscle fasciculation or tetany resulting from reduction of serum ionized calcium. Very high pH levels directly depress cardiovascular and CNS function and interfere with catecholamine-receptor function.

Treatment

Large renal time constants for bicarbonate excretion limit metabolic compensation for acute respiratory alkalemia. Correction of respiratory alkalemia necessitates reduction of effective alveolar ventilation, usually through the administration of analgesics and sedatives to control pain and anxiety. Rebreathing of exhaled CO_2 or addition of CO_2 to inspired gases is not useful.

Why Does Metabolic Alkalemia Occur?

New metabolic alkalemia is unusual in patients in the PACU. Preoperative vomiting, gastric suctioning, dehydration, or potassium wasting frequently generates alkalemia that persists through surgery. Metabolism of excess sodium lactate or citrate in blood products usually requires 24 hours to generate significant postoperative alkalemia. However, excessive intraoperative bicarbonate administration may cause postoperative metabolic alkalemia.

Effects

Retention of CO_2 to compensate for metabolic alkalemia is rapid but somewhat limited because hypoventilation causes hypoxemia at some point.

Treatment

Hydration and correction of hypochloremia and hypokalemia are important for the kidneys to excrete bicarbonate. Hy-

drochloric acid infusion through a central venous catheter is seldom necessary but is effective to treat severe life-threatening metabolic alkalemia. Acetazolamide, 250 to 500 mg intravenously given once or twice in a 4-hour period, works well if hypochloremia has been corrected.

POSTOPERATIVE GLUCOSE AND ELECTROLYTE ABNORMALITIES

Why Does Postoperative Hyperglycemia Occur?

Glucose infusions and stress response commonly elevate serum glucose levels in patients recovering from surgery, but hyperglycemia may indicate severe insulin deficiency and evolving ketoacidosis in diabetic patients.[228]

Effects

Moderate hyperglycemia ($200-300$ mg $\cdot$ dL^{-1}) probably has little significant effect on wound healing and usually resolves spontaneously. Higher glucose levels cause glycosuria and osmotic diuresis and reduce the accuracy of serum electrolyte determinations. Severe hyperglycemia can increase serum osmolarity and generate cerebral disequilibrium and hyperosmolar coma.

Treatment

Treatment of severe hyperglycemia includes titration of intravenous regular insulin by small incremental bolus or continuous infusion. Potassium replacement and monitoring of serial blood glucose levels are essential.

Why Does Hypoglycemia Occur?

Hypoglycemia in the PACU can be caused by inadvertent or excessive insulin administration or by endogenous insulin secretion. Sedation or excessive SNS activity may mask signs and symptoms of hypoglycemia during recovery. Serious postoperative hypoglycemia is rare and easily treated by intravenous administration of 50% dextrose followed by glucose infusion.

Why Does Hyponatremia Occur?

Postoperative hyponatremia occurs if excess free water is infused or absorbed during surgery. Uptake of sodium-free irrigating solution via prostatic venous sinuses during transurethral prostatic resection is a classic example, although the effects of serum glycine or its metabolite, ammonia, exacerbate the signs.[229–231] Inappropriate secretion of antidiuretic hormone, prolonged labor induction with oxytocin, and respiratory uptake of nebulized water droplets can also result in free water retention.

Effects

Symptoms of moderate hyponatremia include nausea, agitation, disorientation, and visual disturbances. More severe dilution causes decreased effectiveness of airway reflexes, unconsciousness, and grand mal seizures.

Treatment

Therapy of acute hyponatremia incorporates water restriction in mild cases; infusion of normal saline and intravenous furosemide in moderate to severe cases; and, in particularly severe instances, the infusion of hypertonic saline with careful monitoring of serum sodium concentration and osmolarity.

Why Does Hypokalemia Occur?

A potassium deficit caused by chronic diuretic administration, prolonged nasogastric suctioning, or vomiting usually underlies postoperative hypokalemia.[232] In surgery, dilution during volume replacement, urinary and hemorrhagic losses, or insulin therapy often exacerbates potassium deficits. A shift of potassium into cells during β-adrenergic therapy or acute respiratory alkalemia acutely exacerbates hypokalemia in the PACU.

Effects

Hypokalemic patients should be closely observed during infusion of calcium, insulin, or β-mimetic medications and during periods of increased SNS activity.[233] Postoperative hypokalemia is usually inconsequential but occasionally can generate serious dysrhythmia, especially in patients taking digitalis preparations.

Treatment

Addition of supplemental potassium to routine intravenous fluids usually restores an acceptable serum concentration, but infusion of concentrated solutions through a central catheter may be necessary. Correction of serum concentration does not imply repletion of the total body deficit.

Why Does Hyperkalemia Occur?

Postoperative hyperkalemia can result from excessive potassium administration, chronic renal failure, or malignant hyperthermia.[232] Acute acidemia exacerbates postoperative hyperkalemia.[234] Succinylcholine may increase serum potassium to dangerous levels in patients with burns or old neurologic injuries or during reperfusion of severely ischemic tissue.

Effects

Cardiac dysrhythmia culminating in cardiac arrest at levels >7.5 to $8 \text{ mEq} \cdot \text{dL}^{-1}$ are the major complications of hyperkalemia.

Treatment

Intravenous insulin and glucose are efficacious to acutely lower serum potassium level, whereas intravenous calcium transiently counters myocardial effects. Whenever an unusually high serum potassium level appears with no apparent cause, one should suspect spurious hyperkalemia caused by a hemolyzed specimen or sampling near an intravenous infusion containing potassium or banked blood.

Why Does Hypocalcemia Occur?

Hypocalcemia is rarely a problem in the PACU. Massive fluid replacement or underlying parathyroid disease reduces total body calcium, although symptomatic hypocalcemia seldom occurs. Transfusion of blood-containing chelating agents also rarely causes symptomatic hypocalcemia.

Effects

Hypocalcemia secondary to surgical parathyroidectomy usually takes several hours to cause clinical symptoms but can present with acute laryngospasm within 3 hours of excision. Further reduction of the critical ionized fraction by metabolic or respiratory alkalemia may cause myocardial conduction and contractility abnormalities, decreased vascular tone, or tetany.

Treatment

Administration of calcium chloride to hypocalcemic patients can improve cardiovascular dynamics and response to intravenous fluid administration. Calcium salts are no longer recommended during cardiopulmonary resuscitation unless hypocalcemia is known to be present.

MISCELLANEOUS POSTOPERATIVE COMPLICATIONS

Anesthetized patients may suffer incidental trauma from equipment, positioning, and nonsurgical manipulations.

What Are the Causes of Corneal Injury?

Corneal injury due to drying or inadvertent eye contact during airway manipulation causes pain, photophobia, tearing, and decreased visual acuity. Abrasions usually heal spontaneously within 72 hours, but severe injury can lead to cataract formation and impaired vision. Fluorescein staining is useful for diagnosis, whereas treatment with artificial tears and eye closure is primarily symptomatic.[235]

Why Does Soft Tissue Trauma Occur?

Soft tissue mouth trauma frequently results from laryngoscopy, indwelling airways, or biting. Lip, tongue, or gum abrasions require only an ice pack for treatment, but penetrating injuries caused by entrapment of tissue between the teeth and laryngoscope blade or airway may benefit from topical antibiotic application.

Upper airway edema or hematoma due to traumatic or difficult tracheal intubation must be considered before extubation. Nebulized racemic epinephrine may improve stridor and edema. A dental consultation should be obtained if teeth or dental appliances are loosened or broken, and the patient should be monitored for signs of foreign body aspiration.

Airway Effects

Adults

Tracheal intubation causes sore throat and hoarseness in 20% to 50% of patients. Symptoms vary with the degree of trauma during laryngoscopy and oropharyngeal suctioning, the duration of tracheal intubation, and the type of tube.[236–239] Mucosal irritation often presents as unquenchable dryness in the mouth and throat. Anesthetic ointments used to lubricate endotracheal tubes probably do little to decrease the incidence and may cause additional irritation to the tracheal mucosa.[240] Sore throat can also be caused by breathing unhumidified gases or trauma resulting from oral airways and suctioning.[241]

Children

The severity of postintubation laryngeal edema or tracheitis in pediatric patients depends on age, intubation trauma, duration of intubation, and degree of movement with the tracheal tube in place.[242] Cool mist therapy is usually sufficient, although racemic epinephrine often improves the signs of upper airway obstruction.

Other traumatic complications of laryngoscopy and intubation include desquamation of mucosa, vocal cord avulsion, airway wall ulceration, tracheal perforation, and hypoglossal, lingual, or recurrent laryngeal nerve damage.[243, 244]

What Factors Predispose to Peripheral Nerve Injury?

Peripheral nerve compression against hard surfaces during general or regional anesthesia sometimes causes permanent sensory and motor deficits, as do stretch injuries resulting from inadvertent hyperextension of an extremity.[245–247] Any complaint of pain, numbness, or weakness should be evaluated. Whenever pressure-related bruising or skin breakdown is noted, underlying nerve damage must be considered. Occlusion of retinal perfusion by ocular compression can generate postoperative visual disturbances ranging from loss of acuity to permanent blindness.

What Problems Are Associated with Positioning?

Ischemia and necrosis of soft tissue can occur during long surgical procedures, especially if pressure points are not properly padded. Entrapment of breasts, genitalia, ears, and skin folds may cause necrosis, especially in the lateral or prone positions. Scalp pressure may cause localized alopecia. Regional ischemia secondary to arterial inflow occlusion is possible although rare. Joint or muscle hyperexpansion can cause postoperative pain, stiffness, back ache, and even joint instability.[248]

Which Injuries Occur in the Postanesthesia Care Unit?

Incidental injury also occurs in the PACU, especially with thrashing during emergence. Bruising resulting from contact with stretcher rails, damage to dental appliances from biting on rigid airways, and corneal injury caused by rigid disposable face masks are relatively common. Dislocation or infiltration of vascular catheters can lead to hematoma formation or extravasation of caustic medications. Discovery of a complication in the PACU requires careful documentation, notification of primary physicians, consultation of appropriate subspecialists, and assiduous follow-up.

What Are the Causes of Postoperative Skeletal Muscle Pain?

Postoperative muscle pain undoubtedly is caused by various intraoperative factors. Prolonged immobility and excessive muscle stretch during positioning often contribute to stiffness and aching after surgery. Symptoms referable to joint hyperextension also lead to postoperative complaints.

Fasciculation during depolarizing blockade with succinylcholine has been implicated as a cause of postoperative myalgias.[249–250] A subparalyzing dose of nondepolarizing relaxant may reduce the incidence or severity,[251] although this approach is controversial. Acute myalgia occurs less frequently after the administration of other relaxants; it also occurs in patients receiving no relaxant whatsoever. Delayed-onset muscle fatigue that appears days after surgery usually resolves spontaneously.

References

1. Finch JS: Equipment and monitoring. *In* Recovery Room Care. Israel JS, DeKornfeld TJ (eds). Chicago, Year Book Medical Publishers, 1987, p 25.
2. DeFranco M: Planning the physical structure of the PACU. *In* Post Anesthesia Care Unit. Frost EAM (ed). St Louis, CV Mosby, 1990, p 187.
3. Hines R, Barash PG, Watrous G, et al: Complications occurring in the postanesthesia care unit: a survey. Anesth Analg 1992; 74:503.
4. DeKornfeld TJ: Medico-legal considerations in the recovery room. Curr Rev Nurs Anesth 1992; 14:166.
5. Cooper MH, Primrose JN: The value of postoperative chest radiology after major abdominal surgery. Anaesthesia 1989; 44:306.
6. Aldrete JA, Kroulik D: A postanesthetic recovery score. Anesth Analg 1970; 49:924.
7. Steward DJ: A simplified scoring system for the postoperative recovery room. Can Anaesth Soc J 1975; 22:111.
8. Bonnet F, Boico O, Rostaing S, et al: Clonidine-induced analgesia in postoperative patients: epidural versus intramuscular administration. Anesthesiology 1990; 72:423.
9. Segal IS, Jarvis DA, Duncan SR, et al: Perioperative use of transdermal clonidine as an adjunctive agent. Anesth Analg 1989; 68:S79.
10. Bernard JM, Lechevalier T, Pinaud M, et al: Postoperative analgesia by IV clonidine. Anesthesiology 1989; 71:A154.
11. Bailey PL, Sperry RJ, Johnson GK, et al: Respiratory effects of clonidine alone and combined with morphine in humans. Anesthesiology 1991; 74:43–48.
12. Henderson JJ, Parbrook GD: Influence of anaesthetic technique on postoperative pain. Br J Anaesth 1976; 48:587.
13. Cuschieri RJ, Morran CG, Howie JC, et al: Postoperative pain and pulmonary complications: comparison of three analgesic regimens. Br J Surg 1985; 72:495.
14. Cousins MJ, Mather LE: Intrathecal and epidural administration of opioids. Anesthesiology 1984; 61:276.
15. Palmer CM: Early respiratory depression following intrathecal-fentanyl-morphine combination. Anesthesiology 1991; 74:1153.
16. Pflug AE, Murphy TM, Butler SH: The effects of postoperative peridural analgesia in pulmonary therapy and pulmonary complications. Anesthesiology 1974; 41:8.
17. Motsch J, Graber E, Ludwig K: Addition of clonidine enhances postop-

erative analgesia from epidural morphine: a double-blind study. Anesthesiology 1990; 73:1067.

18. Mendez R, Eisenbach JC, Kashtan K: Epidural clonidine analgesia after cesarean section. Anesthesiology 1990; 73:848.

19. Ross WB, Tweedle JH, Leong YP, et al: Intercostal blockade and pulmonary function after cholecystectomy. Surgery 1989; 105:166.

20. Miguel R, Hubbell D: Postoperative pain management and pulmonary function after thoracotomy: a prospective randomized study. Anesthesiology 1990; 73:A777.

21. Evans C, Richardson PH: Improved recovery and reduced postoperative stay after therapeutic suggestions during general anaesthesia. Lancet 1988; 4:491.

22. Boeke S, Bonke B, Bouwhuis-Hoogerwerf ML, et al: Effects of sounds presented during general anaesthesia on postoperative course. Br J Anaesth 1988; 60:697.

23. Beard K, Jick H, Walker AM: Adverse respiratory events occurring in the recovery room after general anesthesia. Anesthesiology 1986; 64:269.

24. Hewlett AM, Branthwaite MA: Postoperative pulmonary function. Br J Anaesth 1975; 47:102.

25. Catley DM, Thornton C, Jordan C, et al: Pronounced episodic oxygen desaturation in the postoperative period: its association with ventilatory pattern and analgesic regimen. Anesthesiology 1985; 63:20.

26. Jensen HG, Dubin SA, Silverstein PI, et al: Effect of obesity on safe duration of apnea in anesthetized humans. Anesth Analg 1991; 72:89.

27. Sybert DA, Block FE, McDonald JS: Oxygenation and ventilation during transport to recovery room. Anesthesiology 1989; 71:A442.

28. Hudes ET, Marans HJ, Hirano GM, et al: Recovery room oxygenation: a comparison of nasal catheters and 40 percent oxygen masks. Can J Anaesth 1989; 36:20.

29. Zvara MJ, Labaille T, Benlabed M, et al: Does significant postoperative arterial desaturation occur with regional anesthesia? Anesthesiology 1989; 71:A898.

30. Tait AR, Kyff JV, Crider B, et al: Postoperative arterial oxygen saturation—up in a puff of smoke? Anesth Analg 1989; 86:284.

31. Moller JT, Wittrup M, Johansen SH: Hypoxemia in the postanesthesia care unit: an observer study. Anesthesiology 1990; 73:890.

32. Russell GB, Graybeal JM: Persistent occurrence of postoperative arterial oxygen desaturations despite oxygen therapy. Anesthesiology 1990; 73:A540.

33. Kimovec MA, Grutsch JF, Napcil JA: Incidence of postoperative hypoxemia prior to recovery room discharge. Anesthesiology 1989; 71:A373.

34. Daley MD, Colmenares ME, Sandler AN, et al: Continuous pulse oximetry in the post anesthesia care unit. Anesth Analg 1990; 70:S77.

35. McGowan FX, Kenna MA, Kleinman CS, et al: Hypoxemia and pulmonary hypertension in children with adenotonsillar hypertrophy. Anesthesiology 1989; 71:A1010.

36. Pulleritis J, Burrows FA, Roy WL: Arterial desaturation in healthy children during transfer to the recovery room. Can J Anaesth 1987; 34:470.

37. Tomkins DP, Gaukroger PB, Bentley MW: Hypoxia in children following general anaesthesia. Anaesth Intensive Care 1988; 16:177.

38. Kataria BK, Harnik EV, Mitchard R, et al: Postoperative arterial oxygen saturation in the pediatric population during transportation. Anesth Analg 1988; 67:280.

39. Pandit UA, Levy L, Randel GI, et al: Perioperative respiratory complications in children with upper respiratory infection. Anesthesiology 1989; 71:A1011.

40. Gibson RL, Comer PB, Beckman RW: Actual tracheal oxygen concentrations with commonly used oxygen equipment. Anesthesiology 1976; 44:71.

41. Klein J: Normobaric pulmonary oxygen toxicity. Anesth Analg 1990; 70:195.

42. Blom-Muilwijk MC, Vriesendorp R, Veninga TS, et al: Pulmonary toxicity after treatment with bleomycin or in combination with hyperoxia: studies in the rat. Br J Anaesth 1988; 60:91.

43. LaMantia KR, Glick JH, Marshall BE: Supplemental oxygen does not cause respiratory failure in bleomycin treated patients. Anesthesiology 1984; 60:65.

44. Goldiner PG, Carlon GC, Cvifkovic E: Factors influencing postoperative morbidity and mortality in patients treated with bleomycin. Br J Med 1978; 1:1664.

45. Fink BR, Carpenter SL, Holaday DA: Diffusion anoxia during recovery from nitrous oxide/oxygen anesthesia. Fed Proc 1954; 13:354.

46. Craig DB: Postoperative recovery of pulmonary function. Anesth Analg 1981; 60:46.

47. Tokics L, Hedenstierna G, Strandberg A, et al: Lung collapse and gas exchange during general anesthesia: effects of spontaneous breathing, muscle paralysis, and positive end-expiratory pressure. Anesthesiology 1987; 66:157.

48. Rehder K, Marsh HM, Rodarte JR: Airway closure. Anesthesiology 1977; 47:40.

49. Larsson A, Malmkvist G, Werner O: Variations in lung volume and compliance during pulmonary surgery. Br J Anaesth 1987; 59:585.

50. Kerr JH, Crampton Smith AC, Prys-Roberts C: Observations during endobronchial anaesthesia, II: oxygenation. Br J Anaesth 1974; 46:84.

51. Benumof JL: One-lung ventilation and hypoxic pulmonary vasoconstriction. Anesth Analg 1985; 64:821.

52. Warner MA, Wever BA, Warner ME: Etiologies and incidence of acute pulmonary edema in the immediate postoperative period. Anesth Analg 1990; 70:S421.

53. Jackson FN, Rowland V, Corssen G: Laryngospasm induced pulmonary edema. Chest 1980; 78:819.

54. Inverson LIG, Ecker RR, Fox HE, et al: A comparative study of IPPB, the incentive spirometer, and blow bottles: the prevention of atelectasis following cardiac surgery. Ann Thorac Surg 1978; 25:197.

55. Craven JL, Evans GA, Davenport PJ, et al: The evaluation of the incentive spirometer in the management of postoperative pulmonary complications. Br J Surg 1974; 61:793.

56. Spence AA, Smith G: Postoperative analgesia and lung function: a comparison of morphine with extradural block. Br J Anaesth 1971; 43:144.

57. Greenbaum DM, Millen JE, Eross B: Continuous positive airway pressure without tracheal intubation in spontaneously breathing patients. Chest 1976; 69:615.

58. Jardin F, Delorme G, Hardy A, et al: Reevaluation of hemodynamic consequences of positive pressure ventilation: emphasis on cyclic right ventricular afterloading by mechanical lung inflation. Anesthesiology 1990; 72:966.

59. Qvist J, Pontoppidan H, Wilson R: Hemodynamic responses to PEEP. Anesthesiology 1975; 42:45.

60. Haake R, Schlichtig R, Ulstad DR, et al: Barotrauma: pathophysiology, risk factors, and prevention. Chest 1987; 91:608.

61. Huseby JS, Pavlin EG, Butler J: Effect of PEEP on intracranial pressure. J Appl Physiol 1978; 44:225.

62. Cullen DJ, Caldera DL: The incidence of ventilator-induced pulmonary barotrauma in critically ill patients. Anesthesiology 1979; 50:185.

63. Benumof JL, Wahrenbrock EH: Blunted hypoxic pulmonary vasoconstriction by increasing lung vascular pressure. J Appl Physiol 1975; 38:846.

64. Marshall C, Kim SD, Marshall BE: The influence of vascular pressure on hypoxic pulmonary vasoconstriction. Anesthesiology 1990; 73:A1139.

65. Roos A, Thomas LJ, Nagel EL: Pulmonary vascular resistance as determined by lung inflation and vascular pressures. J Appl Physiol 1961; 16:77.

66. Mathers J, Benumof JL, Wahrenrock EA: General anesthetics and regional hypoxic pulmonary vasoconstriction. Anesthesiology 1977; 46:111.

67. Benumof JL: Hypoxic pulmonary vasoconstriction and sodium nitroprusside perfusion. Anesthesiology 1979; 50:481.

68. Daoud FS, Reeves JT, Schaefer JW: Failure of hypoxic pulmonary vasoconstriction in patients with liver cirrhosis. J Clin Invest 1972; 51:1076.

69. Reeves JT, Grover RF: Blockade of acute hypoxic pulmonary hypertension by endotoxin. J Appl Physiol 1974; 36:328.

70. Shea SA, Walter J, Pelley K, et al: The effect of visual and auditory stimuli upon resting ventilation in man. Respir Physiol 1987; 68:345.

71. Mitchell RA, Berger AJ: Neural regulation of respiration. Am Rev Respir Dis 1975; 111:206.

72. Hudson HE, Harber PI, Smith TC: Respiratory depression from alkalosis and opioid interaction in man. Anesthesiology 1974; 40:543.

73. Harper MH, Hickey RF, Cromwell TH: The magnitude and duration of respiratory depression produced by fentanyl and fentanyl plus droperidol in man. J Pharmacol Exp Ther 1976; 199:464.

74. Jordan C: Assessment of the effects of drugs on respiration. Br J Anaesth 1982; 54:763.

75. Knill RL, Gelb AW: Ventilatory responses to hypoxia and hypercarbia during halothane sedation and anesthesia in man. Anesthesiology 1978; 49:244.

76. Krane BD, Kreutz JM, Johnson DL, et al: Alfentanil and delayed respiratory depression: case studies and review. Anesth Analg 1990; 70:557.

77. Clark NJ, Meuleman T, Liu WS, et al: Comparison of sufentanil-N_2O in patients without cardiac disease undergoing general surgery. Anesthesiology 1987; 66:130.

78. Bailey PL, Pace NL, Ashburn MA: Frequent hypoxemia and sedation with midazolam and fentanyl. Anesthesiology 1990; 73:826.

79. Alexander CM, Gross JB: Sedative doses of midazolam depress hypoxic ventilatory responses in humans. Anesth Analg 1988; 67:377.

80. Fink BR: Influence of cerebral activity in wakefulness on regulation of breathing. J Appl Physiol 1961; 16:15.

81. Radvanyi T, Marin F, Bikhazi GB, et al: Antagonism of the postoperative respiratory depression caused by large doses of morphine. Anesthesiology 1990; 73:A1173.

82. Gross JB, Weller RS, Conard P, et al: Flumazenil antagonism of midazolam-induced ventilatory depression. Anesthesiology 1991; 75:179.

83. Geller E, Halpern P, Chernilas J, et al: Cardiorespiratory effects of antagonism of diazepam sedation with flumazenil in patients with cardiac disease. Anesth Analg 1991; 72:207.

84. Gupta PK, Dundee JW: Postoperative pain relief with morphine combined with doxapram and naloxone. Anaesthesia 1974; 29:33.

85. Kurth CD, LeBard SE, Downes JJ: Association of airway obstruction, hypoxemia, and postoperative apnea in preterm infants. Anesthesiology 1990; 73:A1131.

86. Kurth CD, Spitzer AR, Broennle AM, et al: Postoperative apnea in preterm infants. Anesthesiology 1987; 66:483.

87. Welborn LG, Hannallah RS, Higgins T, et al: Does anemia increase the risk of postoperative apnea in former preterm infants? Anesthesiology 1990; 73:A1091.

88. Welborn LG, Rice LJ, Hannallah RS, et al: Postoperative apnea in former preterm infants: prospective comparison of spinal and general anesthetics. Anesthesiology 1990; 72:838.

89. Marsh ML, Marshall LF, Shapiro HM: Neurosurgical intensive care. Anesthesiology 1977; 47:149.

90. Wade JG, Larson CP Jr, Hickey RF: Effect of carotid endarterectomy on carotid chemoreceptor and baroreceptor function in man. N Engl J Med 1977; 282:823.

91. Lugliani R, Whipp BJ, Seard C: Effect of bilateral carotid body resection on ventilatory control at rest and during exercise in man. N Engl J Med 1971; 285:1105.

92. Slutsky AS, Watson J, Leith DE, et al: Tracheal insufflation of oxygen (TRIO) at low flow rates sustains life for several hours. Anesthesiology 1985; 63:278.

93. Ingram RA, Wellman JS, McFadden ER: Relative contributions of large and small airways to flow limitation in normal subjects before and after atropine and isoproterenol. J Clin Invest 1977; 59:696.

94. Aldrich TK: Respiratory muscle fatigue. Clin Chest Med 1988; 9:225.

95. Aubier M, Banzett RB, Bellamare F, et al: Respiratory muscle fatigue: report of the respiratory muscle fatigue workshop group. Am Rev Respir Dis 1990; 142:474.

96. Paul DR, Hoyt JL, Boutros AR: Cardiovascular and respiratory changes in response to change of posture in the very obese. Anesthesiology 1976; 45:73.

97. Hedenstierna G, Santesson J: Breathing mechanics, deadspace, and gas exchange in the extremely obese. Acta Anaesthesiol Scand 1976; 20:248.

98. Weinberg JSE, Weiss ST, Cohen WR, et al: Pregnancy and the lung. Am Rev Respir Dis 1980; 121:559.

99. Bergofsky EH: Respiratory failure in disorders of the thoracic cage. Can Med Assoc J 1979; 119:643.

100. Crosbie WJ, Sim DT: The effect of postural modification on some aspects of pulmonary function following surgery of the upper abdomen. Physiotherapy 1988; 72:487.

101. Melendez JA, Alagesan R, Weissman C, et al: Effect of postural changes on post thoracotomy respiratory muscle mechanics during incentive spirometry. Anesthesiology 1990; 73:A1176.

102. Chuter TAM, Weissman C, Matthews DM, et al: Abdominal breathing maneuvers increase diaphragmatic motion after surgery. Anesthesiology 1989; 71:A1114.

103. Katz JA, Marks JD: Inspiratory work with and without continuous positive airway pressure in patients with acute respiratory failure. Anesthesiology 1985; 63:598.

104. d'Empaire G, Hoaglin DC, Perlo VP, et al: Effect of prethymectomy plasma exchange on postoperative respiratory function in myasthenia gravis. J Thorac Cardiovasc Surg 1985; 89:592.

105. Burkett L, Bikhazi GB, Thomas KC: Mutual potentiation of the neuromuscular effects of antibiotics and relaxants. Anesth Analg 1976; 58:107.

106. Ford GT, Whitelaw WA, Rosenal TW, et al: Diaphragm function after upper abdominal surgery in humans. Am Rev Respir Dis 1983; 127:43.

107. Dureuil B, Desmonts JM, Mankikian B, et al: Effects of aminophylline on diaphragmatic dysfunction after upper abdominal surgery. Anesthesiology 1985; 62:242.

108. Rigg RA, Rondi P: Changes in rib cage and diaphragm contribution in ventilation after morphine. Anesthesiology 1981; 55:507.

109. Loh L, Hughes JMB, Newson Davis J: The regional distribution of ventilation and perfusion in paralysis of the diaphragm. Am Rev Respir Dis 1979; 119:121.

110. Troyer AD, Heilporn A: Respiratory mechanics in quadriplegia: the respiratory function of the intercostal muscles. Am Rev Respir Dis 1980; 122:591.

111. Richardson JD, Adams L, Flint LM: Selective management of flail chest and pulmonary contusion. Ann Surg 1982; 128:481.

112. Pavlin EG, Holle RH, Schoene RB: Recovery of airway protection compared with ventilation in humans after paralysis with curare. Anesthesiology 1989; 70:381.

113. Moser KM: Pulmonary embolism. Am Rev Respir Dis 1977; 115:829.

114. Khambatta HJ, Stone JG, Matteo RS: Effect of sodium nitroprusside induced hypotension on pulmonary deadspace. Br J Anaesth 1982; 54:1197.

115. Askanazi J, Mordenstraum J, Rosenbaum SH, et al: Nutrition for the patient with respiratory failure. Anesthesiology 1981; 54:373.

116. Claybon LE, Hirsh RA: Meperidine arrests postanesthesia shivering. Anesthesiology 1980; 63:S180, 1980.

117. Schwartz DJ, Wynne JW, Gibbs CP: The pulmonary consequences of aspiration of gastric contents at pH values greater than 2.5. Am Rev Respir Dis 1980; 121:119.

118. Vidyarthi SC: Diffuse miliary granulomatosis of the lungs due to aspirated vegetable cells. Arch Pathol 1967; 83:215.

119. Laxmaiah M, Colliver JA, Marrero TC, et al: Assessment of age related acid aspiration risk factors in pediatric, adult, and geriatric patients. Anesth Analg 1985; 64:11.

120. James CF, Gibbs CP, Banner T: Postpartum perioperative risk of aspiration pneumonia. Anesthesiology 1984; 61:756.

121. Gibbs CP, Schwartz DJ, Wynne JW: Antacid pulmonary aspiration in the dog. Anesthesiology 1979; 51:380.

122. Manchikanti L, Colliver J, Marrero T, et al: Ranitidine and metoclopramide for prophylaxis of aspiration pneumonitis in elective surgery. Anesth Analg 1984; 63:903.

123. Solanki DR, Suresh M, Ethridge HC: The effects of intravenous cimetidine and metoclopramide on gastric volume and pH. Anesth Analg 1984; 63:599.

124. Petring OU, Adelhoj B, Jensen BN, et al: Prevention of silent aspiration due to leaks around cuffs of endotracheal tubes. Anesth Analg 1986; 65:777.

125. Wever JG, Warner MA, Warner ME: Perioperative pulmonary aspiration: incidence of risk factors. Anesthesiology 1990; 73:A1017.

126. Bynum LJ, Pierce AK: Pulmonary aspiration of gastric contents. Am Rev Respir Dis 1976; 114:1129.

127. Bartlett JG, Gorbach SL, Finegold S: The bacteriology of aspiration pneumonia. Am J Med 1974; 56:202.

128. Lindrop MJ: Complications and morbidity of controlled hypotension. Br J Anesth 1975; 47:799.

129. Ellison N: Diagnosis and management of bleeding disorders. Anesthesiology 1977; 47:171.

130. Ivanov J, Weisel RD, Mickelborough LL, et al: Rewarming hypovolemia after aortocoronary bypass surgery. Crit Care Med 1984; 12:1049.

131. Partridge BL: Use of pulse oximetry as a noninvasive indicator of intravascular volume status. J Clin Monit 1987; 3:263.

132. Mangano DT: Perioperative cardiac morbidity. Anesthesiology 1990; 72:153.

133. Wong MG, Wellington MS, London MJ, et al: Prolonged postoperative myocardial ischemia in high risk patients undergoing noncardiac surgery. Anesthesiology 1988; 69:A57.

134. Becker RC, Underwood DA: Myocardial infarction in patients undergoing noncardiac surgery. Cleve Clin J Med 1987; 54:25.

135. Slogoff S, Keats AS: Does perioperative myocardial ischemia lead to postoperative myocardial infarction? Anesthesiology 1985; 62:107.

136. Bove EL, Fry WJ, Gross WS, et al: Hypotension and hypertension as consequences of baroreceptor dysfunction following carotid endarterectomy. Surgery 1979; 86:633.

137. Myers RW: Effects of nitroglycerin and nitroglycerin-methoxamine during acute myocardial ischemia in dogs with preexisting multivessel coronary occlusive disease. Circulation 1975; 51:632.

138. Gal TJ, Cooperman LH: Hypertension in the immediate postoperative period. Br J Anesth 1975; 47:70.

139. Satiani B, Vasko JS, Zarins CK: Hypertension following carotid endarterectomy. Arch Surg 1982; 1117:1073.

140. Leslie JB, Kalayjian RW, Sirgo MA, et al: Intravenous labetalol for treatment of postoperative hypertension. Anesthesiology 1987; 67:413.

141. Kataria BK, Bubois MY, Gadde PL, et al: Evaluation of intravenous esmolol for treatment of postoperative hypertension. Anesth Analg 1990; 70:S192.

142. IV Nicardipine Safety Group: Efficacy and safety of intravenous nicardipine in the control of postoperative hypertension. Chest 1991; 99:393.

143. Breslow MJ, Miller CF, Parker SD, et al: Changes in T-wave morphology following anesthesia and surgery: a common recovery room phenomenon. Anesthesiology 1986; 64:398.

144. Atlee JL, Bosnjak ZJ: Mechanisms for cardiac dysrhythmias during anesthesia. Anesthesiology 1990; 72:347.

145. Pratila MG, Pratila V: Anesthetic agents and cardiac electromechanical activity. Anesthesiology 1978; 49:338.

146. Cranefield PF, Wit AL, Hoffman BF: Genesis of cardia arrhythmias. Circulation 1973; 47:408.

147. Wit AL, Rosen MR, Hofman BF: Electrophysiology and pharmacology of cardiac arrhythmias, II: relationship of normal and abnormal electrical activity of cardiac fibers to genesis of arrhythmias. B: Reentry. Am Heart J 1974; 88:664.

148. Berns AS, Linas SL, Miller TR: Urinary diagnostic indices in acute renal failure. Kidney Int 1976; 10:495.

149. Hilberman M, Maseda J, Stinson EB, et al: The diuretic properties of dopamine in patients after open heart operation. Anesthesiology 1984; 61:489.

150. Levinsky NG, Bernard DB, Johnson TA: Mannitol and loop diuretics in acute renal failure. *In* Acute Renal Failure. Brenner BM, Lazarus JM (eds). Philadelphia, WB Saunders, 1983, p 462.

151. Denlinger JK: Prolonged emergence and failure to regain consciousness. *In* Complications in Anesthesiology. Orkin FK, Cooperman LH (eds). Philadelphia, JB Lippincott, 1983, p 368.

152. Fragen RJ, Katz JA, Dunn KL: Flumazenil reversal of midazolam sedation in the elderly. Anesth Analg 1990; 70:S113.

153. Ghoneim MM, Dembo JB, Block RI: Time course of antagonism of sedative and amnesic effects of diazepam by flumazenil. Anesthesiology 1989; 70:899.

154. Jensen S, Knudsen L, Kirkegaard L, et al: Flumazenil used for antagonizing the central effects of midazolam and diazepam in outpatients. Acta Anaesthesiol Scand 1989; 33:26.

155. Bourke DL, Rosenberg M, Allen PD: Physostigmine: effectiveness as an antagonist of respiratory depression and psychomotor effects caused by morphine or diazepam. Anesthesiology 1984; 1:523.

156. Douglass JH, Ross JD, Bruce DL: Delayed awakening due to lidocaine overdose. J Clin Anesth 1989; 2:126.

157. Skillman JJ: Neurologic complications of cardiovascular surgery, I: procedures involving the carotid arteries and abdominal aorta. *In* Neurological and Psychological Complications of Surgery and Anesthesia. Hidman BJ (ed). Boston, Little, Brown & Co, 1986, p 135.

158. Gutierrez IZ, Barone DL, Makula PA, et al: The risk of perioperative stroke in patients with asymptomatic carotid bruits undergoing peripheral vascular surgery. Am Surg 1987; 53:487.

159. Hindman BJ: Perioperative stroke: the noncardiac surgical patient. *In* Neurological and Psychological Complications of Surgery and Anesthesia. Hindman BJ (ed). Boston, Little, Brown & Co, 1986, p 101.

160. Larsen SF, Zaric D, Boysen G: Postoperative cerebrovascular accidents in general surgery. Acta Anaesthesiol Scand 1988; 32:698.

161. Chung F, Seyone C, Dyck B, et al: Age-related cognitive recovery after general anesthesia. Anesth Analg 1990; 71:217.

162. Jamison RN, Parris WC, Maxson WS: Psychological factors influencing recovery from outpatient surgery. Behav Res Ther 1987; 25:31.

163. Taenzer P, Melzack R, Jeans ME: Influence of psychological factors in postoperative pain, mood, and analgesic requirements. Pain 1986; 24:331.

164. Hammon K, Demartino BK: Postoperative delirium secondary to atropine premedication. Anesth Prog 1985; 32:107.

165. Eisenrath SJ, Goldman B, Douglas J, et al: Meperidine induced delirium. Am J Psychiatry 1987; 144:1062.

166. Heath PJ, Kennedy DJ, Ogg TW, et al: Which intravenous induction agent for day surgery? A comparison of propofol, thiopentone, methohexitone, and etomidate. Anaesthesia 1988; 43:365.

167. Oliver SB, Cucchiara RF, Warner MA, et al: Unexpected focal neurologic deficit on emergence from anesthesia: a report of three cases. Anesthesiology 1987; 67:823.

168. Suresh D: Nightmares and recovery from anesthesia. Anesth Analg 1991; 72:404.

169. Hines RL, Barash PG, Dubow H, et al: Ambulatory surgical complications in the postoperative period: we can't just walk away. Anesth Analg 1989; 86:S122.

170. Palazo MG, Strunin L: Anesthesia and emesis, II: prevention and management. Can Anaesth Soc J 1984; 31:407.

171. Palazzo MG, Strunin L: Anesthesia and emesis, I: Etiology. Can Anaesth Soc J 1984; 31:178.

172. Patel RI, Hannallah RS: Anesthetic complications following pediatric ambulatory surgery: a three year study. Anesthesiology 1988; 69:1009.

173. Lindblad T, Beattie WS, Buckley DN, et al: Menstruation increases risk of postoperative emesis. Anesthesiology 1990; 73:A17.

174. Beattie WS, Forrest JB, Buckley DN, et al: Nausea and vomiting correlates with estrogen levels and liter dose response for droperidol. Anesthesiology 1989; 71:A957.

175. Caldamone AA, Rabinowitz R: Outpatient orchiopexy. J Urol 1982; 127:286.

176. Lerman J, Eustis S, Smith DR: Effect of droperidol pretreatment on postanesthetic vomiting in children undergoing strabismus surgery. Anesthesiology 1986; 65:322.

177. Anderson R, Crohg K: Pain as a major cause of postoperative nausea. Can Anaesth Soc J 1976; 23:366.

178. Melnick BM, Johnson LS: Effects of eliminating nitrous oxide in outpatient anesthesia. Anesthesiology 1987; 67:982.

179. Lonie DS, Harper NJN: Nitrous oxide anaesthesia and vomiting. Anaesthesia 1986; 41:703.

180. Hovorka J, Korttila K, Erkola O: Nitrous oxide does not increase nausea and vomiting following gynaecological laparoscopy. Can J Anaesth 1989; 36:145.

181. Sengupta P, Plantevin OM: Nitrous oxide and day-case laparoscopy: effects on nausea, vomiting, and return to normal activity. Br J Anaesth 1988; 60:570.

182. Muir JJ, Warner MA, Offord KP, et al: Role of nitrous oxide and other factors in postoperative nausea and vomiting: a randomized and blinded prospective study. Anesthesiology 1987; 66:513.

183. Carter JA, Dye AM, Cooper GM: Recovery after day-case anaesthesia: the effect of different inhalational anaesthetic agents. Anaesthesia 1985; 40:545.

184. Marais ML, Maher MW, Wetchler BV, et al: Reduced demands on recovery room resources with propofol (Diprivan) compared to thiopental-isoflurane. Anesthesiol Rev 1989; 16:29.

185. Hunt TM, Plantevin OM, Gilbert JR: Morbidity in gynaecological day-case surgery: a comparison of two anaesthetic techniques. Br J Anaesth 1979; 51:785.

186. Toro-Matos A, Rendon-Platas AM, Avil-Valez E, et al: Physostigmine antagonizes ketamine. Anesth Analg 1980; 59:644.

187. King MJ, Milazkiewicz R, Carli F, et al: Influence of neostigmine on postoperative vomiting. Br J Anaesth 1988; 61:403.

188. Kraynack BJ, Bates MF, Gintautas J, et al: Antiemetic efficacy of ranitidine, metoclopramide, and gastric suctioning in outpatient laparoscopy. Anesth Analg 1990; 70:S218.

189. McCarroll SM, Mori S, Bras PJ, et al: The effect of gastric intubation and removal of gastric contents on the incidence of postoperative nausea and vomiting. Anesth Analg 1990; 70:S262.

190. Morgensen NH, Coyle JP: Effect of intravenous droperidol upon nausea and vomiting using alfentanil anesthesia. Anesth Analg 1989; 68:S139.

191. Williams JJ, Goldbert ME, Boerner TF, et al: A comparison of three methods to reduce nausea and vomiting after alfentanil anesthesia in outpatients. Anesth Analg 1989; 68:S311.

192. Pandit SK, Kothary SP, Pandit UA, et al: Dose-response study of droperidol and metoclopramide as antiemetics for outpatient anesthesia. Anesth Analg 1989; 68:798.

193. Eustis S, Lerman J, Smith D: Droperidol pretreatment in children undergoing strabismus repair: the minimal effective dose. Can Anaesth Soc J 1986; 33:S115.

194. Melnick BM: Extrapyramidal reactions to low-dose droperidol. Anesthesiology 1988; 69:424.

195. Broadman LM, Ceruzzi W, Patane PS: Metoclopramide reduces the incidence of vomiting following strabismus surgery in children. Anesthesiology 1990; 72:245.

196. Doze VA, Shafer A, White PF: Nausea and vomiting after outpatient anesthesia: effectiveness of droperidol alone and in combination with metoclopramide. Anesth Analg 1987; 66:S41.

197. Cohen SE, Woods WA, Wyner J: Antiemetic efficacy of droperidol and metoclopramide. Anesthesiology 1984; 60:67.

198. Horton BF, Chadwick D: Metoclopramide may cause dysphoria. Anesthesiology 1990; 73:A38.

199. Bidwai AV, Meulman T, Thatte WP, et al: Prevention of postoperative nausea with dimenhydrinate (Dramamine) and droperidol (Inapsine). Anesth Analg 1990; 68:S25.

200. Jacobs BR, O'Connor TZ: Controlled comparison of the antiemetic efficacy of thiethylperazine and droperidol in outpatient surgery. Anesth Analg 1991; 72:S122.

201. Uppington J, Dunnet J, Blogg CE: Transdermal hyoscine and postoperative nausea and vomiting. Anaesthesia 1986; 41:16.

202. Bailey PL, Streisand JB, Pace NL, et al: Transdermal scopolamine reduces nausea and vomiting after outpatient laparoscopy. Anesthesiology 1989; 72:977.

203. Tigerstedt I, Salmela L, Aroma U: Double-blind comparison of transdermal scopolamine, droperidol, and placebo against postoperative nausea and vomiting. Acta Anesthesiol Scand 1988; 32:454.

204. Poler SM, White PF: Does ephedrine decrease nausea and vomiting after outpatient anesthesia? Anesthesiology 1989; 71:A995.

205. Rothenberg DM, Parnass SM, Litwack K, et al: Efficacy of ephedrine in the prevention of postoperative nausea and vomiting. Anesth Analg 1991; 72:58.

206. Rothenberg D, Parnass S, Newman L, et al: Ephedrine minimizes postoperative nausea and vomiting in outpatients. Anesthesiology 1989; 71:A322.

207. Sung YF, Tillette T: Placebo, ephedrine, and antiemetics in postoperative nausea and vomiting in ambulatory surgery patient. Anesth Analg 1991; 72:S285.

208. Wetchler BV, Sung YF, Duncalf D, et al: Odansetron decreases emetic symptoms following outpatient laparoscopy. Anesthesiology 1990; 73:A36.

209. Bodner M, Poler SM, White PF: Initial evaluation of odansetron—a novel antiemetic. Anesthesiology 1990; 73:A328.

210. Rosenblum F, Azad SS, Bartkowski R, et al: Odansetron: a new, effective antiemetic prevents postoperative nausea and vomiting. Anesth Analg 1991; 72:S230.

211. Leeser J, Lip H: Prevention of postoperative nausea and vomiting using odansetron, a new selective, 5-HT3 receptor antagonist. Anesth Analg 1991; 72:751.

212. Dundee JW, Ghaly RG, McKinney MS: P6 acupuncture antiemesis comparison of invasive and noninvasive techniques. Anesthesiology 1989; 71:A310.

213. Sessler DI, Olofsson CI, Rubinstein EH, et al: The thermoregulatory threshold in humans during halothane anesthesia. Anesthesiology 1988; 68:836.

214. Hynson JM, Sessler DI, Moayeri A, et al: Absence of nonshivering thermogenesis in anesthetized adults. Anesth Analg 1991; 72:S119.

215. Sessler DI, Moayeri A, Stoen R, et al: Thermoregulatory vasoconstriction decreases cutaneous heat loss. Anesthesiology 1990; 73:656.

216. Slotman GJ, Jed EH, Burchard KW: Adverse effects of hypothermia in postoperative patients. Am J Surg 1985; 149:495.

217. Sessler DI, Israel D, Pozos RS, et al: Spontaneous post-anesthetic tremor does not resemble thermoregulatory shivering. Anesthesiology 1988; 68:843.

218. Sessler DI, Rubinstein EH: Hypothermia triggers spontaneous postanesthetic tremor. Anesthesiology 1990; 73:A173.

219. MacIntyre PE, Pavin EG, Dwersteg JF: Effect of meperidine on oxygen consumption, carbon dioxide production, and respiratory gas exchange in post anesthesia shivering. Anesth Analg 1987; 66:751.

220. Rodriguez JL, Weissman JC, Damask MC, et al: Physiologic requirements during rewarming: suppression of the shivering response. Crit Care Med 1983; 11:490.

221. Claybon LE, Hirsch RA: Meperidine arrests postanesthetic shivering. Anesthesiology 1983; 59:S180.

222. Vogelsang J, Hayes SR: The differential effects of butorphanol, meperidine, and morphine treatment of postanesthesia shaking. Anesth Analg 1991; 72:S310.

223. MacDonald LE, Franklin C, Wiseman E: Using a head covering of T-727 thermal fabric to conserve core body temperature during anesthesia. Anesth Analg 1991; 72:S166.

224. Saunders PR, McCarroll SM, Harris J: Does heated humidified oxygen in the recovery room aid warming of the hypothermic patient? Anesthesiology 1989; 71:A185.

225. Lennon RL, Hosking MP, Conover MA, et al: Evaluation of a forced air system for warming hypothermic postoperative patients. Anesth Analg 1990; 70:424.

226. Lipton JM, Schroeder T, Banish P, et al: Control of postanesthetic shivering by localized regulated radiant heat. Anesth Analg 1990; 70:S243.

227. Knill RL, Clement JL: Ventilatory responses to acute metabolic acidemia in humans awake, sedated, and anesthetized with halothane. Anesthesiology 1985; 62:745.

228. Doze VA, White PF: Effects of fluid therapy on serum glucose levels in fasted outpatients. Anesthesiology 1987; 66:223.

229. Alexander JP, Polland A, Gillespie IA: Glycine and transurethral resection. Anesthesia 1986; 41:1189.

230. Wang JM-L, Creel DJ, Wong KC: Transurethral resection of the prostate, serum glycine levels, and ocular evoked potentials. Anesthesiology 1989; 70:36.

231. Roesch RP, Stoelting RK, Lingeman JE: Ammonia toxicity resulting from glycine absorption during a transurethral resection of the prostate. Anesthesiology 1983; 58:577.

232. Kliger AS, Hayslett JB: Disorders of potassium balance. *In* Acid Base and Potassium Homeostasis. Brenner BM, Stein JH (eds). New York, Churchill Livingstone, 1978, p 168.

233. Brown MJ, Brown DC, Murphy MB: Hypokalemia from beta-2 receptor stimulation by circulating epinephrine. N Engl J Med 1983; 309:1414.

234. Scribner BH, Fremont-Smith K, Burnell JM: The effect of respiratory acidosis on the internal equilibrium of potassium. J Clin Invest 1975; 34:1278.

235. Batra KY, Bali ML: Corneal abrasion during general anesthesia. Anesth Analg 1977; 56:363.

236. Stout DM, Bishop MJ, Dwersteg JF, et al: Correlation of endotracheal tube size with sore throat and hoarseness following general anesthesia. Anesthesiology 1987; 67:419.

237. Loeser EA, Stanley TH, Jordan W, et al: Postoperative sore throat: influence of tracheal tube lubrication versus cuff design. Can Anaesth Soc J 1980; 27:156.

238. Jensen PJ: Sore throat after operation: influence of tracheal intubation, intracuff pressure, and type of cuff. Br J Anaesth 1982; 54:453.

239. Monroe MC, Gravenstein N, Saga-Rumley SA: Postoperative sore throat: effect of oropharyngeal airway. Anesthesiology 1989; 71:A951.

240. Stock MC, Downs JB: Lubrication of tracheal tubes to prevent sore throat from intubation. Anesthesiology 1982; 57:418.

241. Bogetz MS, Tupper BJ, Vigil AC: Too much of a good thing: uvular trauma caused by overzealous suctioning. Anesth Analg 1991; 72:125.

242. Koka BV, Jeon IS, Andre JM, et al: Postintubation croup in children. Anesth Analg 1977; 56:501.

243. Keane WM, Denneny JC, Rowe LD, et al: Complications of intubation. Ann Otol Rhinol Laryngol 1982; 91:584.

244. Friedman M, Toriumi DM: Esophageal stethoscope: another possible cause of vocal cord paralysis. Arch Otolaryngol Head Neck Surg 1989; 115:95.

245. Kroll DA, Caplan RA, Ward RJ, et al: Perioperative nerve injuries. Anesthesiology 1989; 71:A929.

246. Alvine FG, Schurrer ME: Postoperative ulnar nerve palsy: are there predisposing factors? J Bone Joint Surg 1987; 69:A255.

247. Dornete WHL: Compression neuropathies: medial aspects and legal implications. *In* Neurological and Psychological Complications of Surgery and Anesthesia. Hindman BJ (ed). Boston, Little, Brown & Co, 1986, p 201.

248. Trepanier CA, Brousseau C, Lacerte L: Myalgia in outpatient surgery: a comparison of atracurium and succinylcholine. Can J Anaesth 1988; 35:255.

249. Manchikanti L, Grow JB, Colliver JA, et al: Atracurium pretreatment for succinylcholine induced fasciculations and postoperative myalgia. Anesth Analg 1985; 64:1010.

250. O'Sullivan EP, Williams NE, Calvey TN: Differential effects of neuromuscular blocking agents on suxamethonium induced fasciculations and myalgia. Br J Anaesth 1988; 60:367.

251. Pace NL: Prevention of succinylcholine myalgias: a meta analysis. Anesth Analg 1990; 70:477.

CHAPTER 7

Medicine and Anesthesia: Financial and Other Costs

DAVID A. PAULUS, M.D.

The cost of anesthesia services is a small part of the total cost of health care in the United States. To place the former into perspective, one must start with a more comprehensive, overall view. Concern over national health costs and coverage has resulted in a growing debate. The opportunity to cure disease or to ameliorate its effects is brought about by new developments. Marwick writes that the rate of growth of health care costs in the United States is probably unsustainable.[1] Since the early 1960s, health care costs have risen from 6% to about 12% of the gross national product. By the year 2000 they may be 17%, and by the year 2030 they could approach 37%. Corporations are feeling the pressure, and Marwick further writes that spending by employers for health care benefits has exceeded 50% of pretax corporate profits.[2] Corporations, in their negotiations with labor unions, are pressing this point as they seek to have larger copayments made by employees.

At present, Americans spend 650 billion dollars each year on health care. The number of uninsured persons is estimated to be >33 million.[3] In 1988, 10% of the population in Massachusetts was uninsured, whereas in Louisiana, Texas, and New Mexico, the per cent of uninsured was >25%.[4] Strikingly, 85% of the uninsured were workers or family members of workers. Many small businesses find that they cannot obtain health care insurance for their workers. Frequently, service-oriented organizations do not insure many of their full-time workers and, often, none of their part-time workers.

Those of us who provide health care usually find that it does not significantly stress our personnel resources. Our mandate as care providers is to contribute leadership to our nation in solving what our citizens view as a significant problem and what society increasingly views as a right. In addition, we should keep in mind that what we and other health care providers do in our everyday work generates costs that are not only financial. Increasingly, we must also be concerned about the environmental impact of our specialty in particular and of medicine in general.

ALTERNATIVES TO THE PRESENT HEALTH CARE SYSTEM IN THE UNITED STATES

What Is the Canadian System?

Owing to Canada's geographic location and its similarity to the United States with respect to language and culture, the Canadian health care system is probably the most popular alternative to the current health care system in the United States. The Canadian-funded health care system consists of 10 province-based plans that share common elements for all medically necessary hospital and physician services. The provincial governments are the single payors for both hospitals and physicians, and they make key decisions on financing. This arrangement enables them to establish budgets for hospital and physician fees and, at the same time, to regulate access to new equipment.

The system has no deductibles or copayments for covered services. Therefore, the patient is not responsible for payment. Covered services do not include adult dental care, cosmetic surgery, or hospital room amenities. Since there is a single payor in each province, administrative costs are much reduced from those of the United States. If United States health care administration were as efficient as that in Canada, the administrative cost difference possibly would pay the health insurance costs for Americans who are currently uninsured and reduce, or possibly eliminate, copayments and deductibles. By mandating the health care cost environment, Canadians are able to dictate or constrain growth, thereby molding the system to each province's will.

In Canada, the percentage of generalists is much higher than in the United States. They are the gatekeepers to the system. Since no costs accrue to the patient, health care service use is higher in Canada than in the United States. In 1989, Canada spent $670 less per person than did the United States, primarily because of savings in administrative costs (one-fifth those of the United States). Reimbursement to physicians in Canada is one-third less per capita than in the United States, and the per capita cost of beds is 18% less.

Physician professional expenses in the United States average 48% of gross income, whereas in Canada they are 36%. Additionally, Canadian malpractice premiums are about 10% of those in the United States. In 1971, when Canada had fully implemented the system, both countries spent approximately the same share of their gross national products on health care. In 1989, the United States' share became 11.6%, whereas Canada's was 8.9%. The difference reflects lower Canadian spending on insurance administration and physician and hospital reimbursement, despite the fact that Canadians have a longer average hospital stay than do Americans.

How Do Germans Pay for Health Care?

The German system is more similar to the American system than to the Canadian. This system is based on insurance for which the employees and employers each pay one-half. Unemployed or retired persons are cared for through a retirement or unemployment fund. Health insurance is compulsory for all those who earn under a certain salary level. Hence, over 90% of the population in Germany is covered by such insurance. Only the very wealthy are exempt from this mandate.

In Germany, as in the United States, many funds finance health care (over 1100 insurance funds exist). The system focuses on interlocking obligations by the participants in the health care sector. Included is the obligation of health care providers, including physicians in hospitals, to provide necessary care for all patients. Common knowledge that patients who receive small and moderate salaries cannot pay for medical care out of their own pockets led to their obligation to procure health insurance, one-half the cost of which is borne by the employer. These interlocking obligations often include a retirement fund that is used to provide assistance in the purchase of insurance.

Since everyone is obligated to purchase insurance, insurers, in turn, are obligated to insure everyone. This process eliminates problems attendant to obtaining such insurance in the United States, including pre-existing health conditions, requirements for small business employers, and restrictions for those employed in certain industrial occupations. Health insurance trust funds are nonprofit organizations, just as private sector organizations regulated as public utilities are in the United States. Fees and budgets are established through regional and national organizations. The fees for budgets and rates are set for all providers. Once again, the interlocking obligations between hospitals, physicians, labor unions, employers, sickness funds, and retirement funds result in a self-regulated system.

Ambulatory care physicians are the gatekeepers in this system. They control all referrals to hospitals and to hospital-based physicians. On the other hand, patients can choose their own physician. Hospital-based physicians are obligated to return the patient to the ambulatory care physician upon discharge. The former group is paid by the hospital; a relative value scale is used to allocate the fee-for-service basis for ambulatory care. Some structural features of the systems of Germany (and the Netherlands) are shown in Figure 7–1. In Germany and the Netherlands, the private sector, not the government, is responsible for providing universal coverage. The systems are not supported by progressive income taxes but rather by income-based premiums. Health care costs in both Germany and the Netherlands are lower than they are in the United States. Furthermore, the obligation to take care of all patients is fundamental in the German system. Table 7–1 shows cost data comparing health care systems of the United States, the Netherlands, and Germany.

THE FUTURE

What Does It Hold for the United States?

Kirkman-Liff suggests several lessons for the United States system[6]:

1. Public discussions about underlying values are important if a strategy is to be obtained for health insurance. The employee and employer must contribute. For the employee, cost awareness in the sense of shared ownership is brought about by contributing 50% of the income base to the premium for family coverage.

2. Mandated employee-employer coverage is essential to achieve universal coverage. No worker should ever be without health insurance, and this insurance should be transferable from one place of employment to another. National and regional negotiations are essential to develop fees and budgets that compensate all providers while ensuring that costs are controlled. In these instances, the training and qualifications of physicians in Canada, the United States, Germany, and the Netherlands are reasonably equal.

What Is the Resource-Based, Relative-Value Scale?

In 1988, Hsiao and coworkers presented an alternative to the system of payment based on charges.[7] They proposed a resource-based, relative-value scale known by its initials as RBRVS. This scale caused numerous controversies.

Basic Premises

The authors recognized that three resources are required to provide medical services and procedures: (1) the total work input by the physician; (2) funds for practice costs, including malpractice premiums; and (3) the opportunity for physicians to acquire postgraduate training to become qualified. They also argued that a purely competitive health care market does not exist because the conditions are not favorable to a competitive environment. Patients are not very price-sensitive because most are insured; price does not much influence physician choice; patients do not have many choices as to therapy; and the medical profession has monopolistic powers over prescription writing and hospital admission. Hsiao and coworkers proposed the use of resource input cost as the basis for reimbursement. Expressed mathematically, the RBRVS is as follows:

$$RBRVS = (TW)(1 + RPC)(1 + AST)$$

where TW is the total work input by the physician, RPC is an index of relative specialty-practice costs, and AST is an index of amortized value for the opportunity cost of specialized training.

After dividing the total effort into preservice, intraservice,

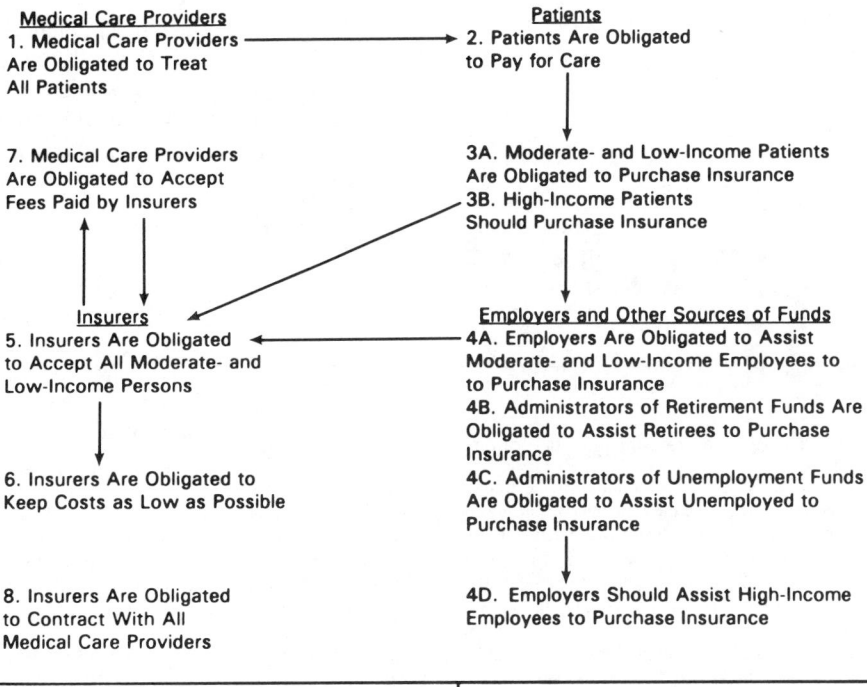

FIGURE 7–1. Structure of obligations in the Dutch and German health care systems. (From Kirkman-Liff BL: Health insurance values and implementation in the Netherlands and the Federal Republic of Germany: an alternative path to universal coverage. JAMA 1991; 265:2496–2505. Copyright 1991, American Medical Association.)

and postservice work, they applied the *Physician's Current Procedural Terminology, Fourth Edition* (CPT-4) to measure relative physician work input. To account for the variation in the complexity and severity of patient condition, they enlisted the help of consulting physicians. Two of the questions that the authors attempted to answer were, What is the physician's work input for each service performed? and, Can work be measured in a reliable and valid manner? They concentrated on the intraservice work and considered the preservice and postservice work in addition to the RPC and AST. Anesthesiology work estimates varied, on an arbitrary scale, from 68 (anesthesia for dilation and curettage of the cervix and uterus) to 518 (anesthesia for repair of abdominal aortic aneurysm). By comparison, the general surgeons rated uncomplicated indirect inguinal hernia repair at 100 and lower anterior resection for rectal carcinoma at 445.

The underlying assumption is that physician work input into services can be defined. It is assumed that it consists of "time, mental effort and judgement [sic], technical skill and physical effort, and stress."[8] The ratings of work did not vary much among physicians, so "it is feasible to quantify systematically the relative resource-input costs of physician's services in each specialty."[8]

This report established the validity of resource-based relative values for physician compensations. The results and policy implications of RBRVSs were then studied.[9] Maintaining a "budget neutral" assumption, the impact of RBRVS-based fee schedules was applied to 1986 Medicare payments (Fig. 7–2).[9] A comparison with Ontario was made that showed a strong similarity between what would be paid through RBRVSs and what was paid in Ontario. The approaches were quite different, but the results were similar.

Criticisms

The criticisms of a relative value approach to compensation are many. No accommodation for variation in patient condition exists within a CPT-4 code, nor is a difference in quality assumed. Furthermore, the benefits of a service are not quan-

TABLE 7–1. Health Care Costs in the Netherlands, Germany, and the United States

Indicator	Netherlands	Germany	United States
GNP for health care (%)			
1975	7.7	7.8	8.4
1987	8.5	8.1	11.1
% Change	9.7	2.9	33.5
Per capita health costs			
1975	$428	$409	$614
1987	$1038	$1072	$2051
% Change	142	162	234
1987 Health expenditures (%)			
Inpatient care	57	39	47
Ambulatory care	26	29	31
Pharmaceutical	10	22	7
Other health costs	7	10	15
1987 Filled inpatient care beds per 1000 population	11.8	11.0	5.3
1987 Inpatient care costs per occupied bed	$50,500	$38,300	$182,700
1987 Practicing physicians per 1000 population	2.4	2.8	2.3
1987 Ambulatory care costs per physician	$114,500	$108,900	$275,300

(From Health Insurance Values and Implementation in the Netherlands and the Federal Republic of Germany. JAMA 1991; 265:2496–2505. Copyright 1991, American Medical Association.)
Abbreviation: GNP = gross national product.

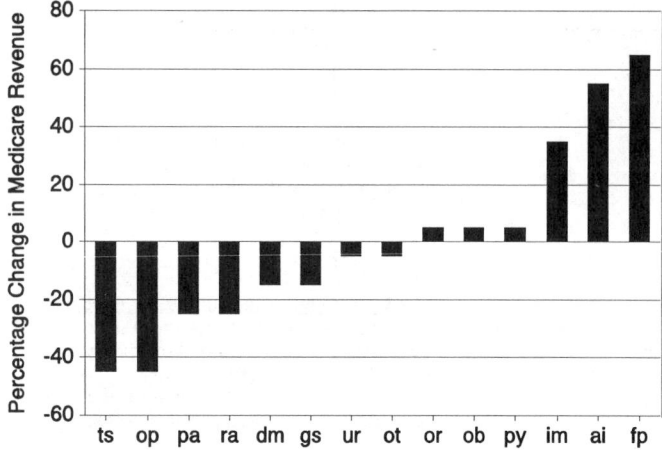

FIGURE 7–2. Results of simulation of the impact of an RBRVS-based fee schedule on 1986 Medicare payments according to specialty. Total Medicare payments in each specialty were calculated from the RBRVS, service volume, and a monetary conversion factor. ts = Thoracic and cardiovascular surgery; op = ophthalmology; pa = pathology; ra = radiology; dm = dermatology; gs = general surgery; ur = urology; ot = otolaryngology or orthopedic surgery; ob = obstetrics/gynecology; py = psychiatry; im = internal medicine; ai = allergy and immunology; fp = family practice. (Reprinted from Hsiao WC, Braun P, Dunn D: Special report—Results and policy implications of the resource-based relative-value study. N Engl J Med 1988; 319:881, by permission of the New England Journal of Medicine.)

tified. For the anesthesiologist, the time variable is not specifically addressed. In spite of these problems, the system is being used for Medicare reimbursement and will be used in other compensation schemes.

How Will Costs Be Minimized?

Containing health care costs in the United States has been on the minds of many in government and in medicine. Rice suggests several cost containment strategies.[10]

Users

The first strategy is aimed at users. By encouraging patient copayments as in Germany, use of health care will be discouraged. Patients will be asked to be released from hospitals earlier and presumably will seek physician care only when it is needed. By taxing the employer's health insurance contribution, the employer would be even more anxious to reduce costs.

Holmer suggests that some elasticity is present in health care costs.[11] For example, the sum of copayments and deductibles was no greater than $1000 annually or, up to this amount, 25% of costs; consumers spent an average of $630 on medical care per year compared with $777 for patients who received free care. Thus, the copayment requirement reduced costs by almost 20%. If tax deductibility of employer contributions for health insurance were to be eliminated, demand for services would be reduced from about 5%.[12]

Einthoven and Kronick have written provocatively about restructuring the way in which health care is financed in the United States.[13, 14] They suggest that the incentive for consumers and providers in the United States' system is rather perverse and predict that competitive forces would make the health care system more efficient and less costly. Furthermore,

health care plans could compete for consumers by offering the most competitive package premiums. For individuals, the employer would be required to sponsor coverage, and the employee could choose from among various plans. Incentives to be more frugal would be stronger, and utilization management would be improved.

Providers

The strategies just mentioned appeal to the users. One could try to appeal to both users and providers. Insurance providers can control the price paid for each unit of service, and they can control the quantity of service through utilization review. Presently, five common utilization management activities are performed:

1. High-cost case management, in which the insurer coordinates and explicitly monitors the care of individuals who are undergoing extensive diagnostic or health care exercises.
2. Preadmission certification, in which prior approval must be obtained in order for the charges to be covered.
3. Concurrent review.
4. Retrospective review.
5. Mandatory second opinion, typically applied to surgery.

Studies to determine the effectiveness of these attempts at cost control and reduction are relatively few. Although preadmission certification initially reduced hospital days and health care costs, savings obtained immediately after implementation have not continued.[15] As to second opinion, not much evidence exists that a review is helpful in terms of reducing costs.[16] However, a study of patients urged to undergo coronary angiography revealed that 80% were judged not to require angiography as a result of the second opinion process. The national implications are enormous.[17]

Health Maintenance Organizations

Another strategy aimed at both users and providers is to alter the organization through which patients receive and physicians provide care. The Health Maintenance Organization (HMO) is probably the oldest such organization. HMO groups have increased in popularity; more than 32 million people belong to them. They are attractive to both employers and employees because of their emphasis on prevention and their relatively low premiums. However, they are closed systems, requiring that patients receive care from a contracted provider to ensure coverage.[18] Patients sacrifice some freedom of choice in order to receive the "nearly free" care. The primary care physician is the gatekeeper. Interestingly, two-thirds of the HMOs in this country pay the preferred care physician on a capitative basis.

How do HMOs reduce costs? The answer is not clear. Initially, savings on the order of 30% were realized, but these seem to have been a one-time occurrence. Hospitalization rates are decreased, but cost inflation is not; HMOs are not insulated from the underlying causes of health care cost inflation.[19] Compared with fee-for-service medicine, in which no patient cost sharing is required, HMOs probably provide substantial savings; however, when cost-sharing is required, the patients participate in reducing the costs.[20]

HMOs probably can control costs if they can garner an increase in market share. However, patients want to have a role in choosing their physician. Three-quarters of Americans generally prefer some sort of national health plan, but if limits are placed on their choice of physician, the approval rate drops to 30%.[21] People who join HMOs probably are less sick than those in the general population. This group of people is attracted to HMOs because they are already interested in preventive medicine. The cost of HMOs to the government for certain risk contracts is up to 74% higher in HMOs than if patients had been cared for in a fee-for-service program.[22]

Preferred Provider Organizations

In response to some of the reluctance to join HMOs, preferred provider organizations (PPOs) have arisen. The PPO agrees to provide service to a certain group of individuals at a discounted rate, providing an incentive for the patient. This system may conserve some medical resources and preserves patient choice. The PPO can choose among hospitals that bid to provide services. It can conduct utilization reviews and can attempt to reduce expenses. Of course, the discounts that the hospitals give may represent cost-shifting. Studies do not indicate that PPOs have been successful in reducing costs.

Practice Guidelines

Practice guidelines are being developed to define appropriate medical care. Many medical organizations have groups to define practice parameters. The latter include guidelines, standards, and other patient management strategies. These guidelines are recommendations for patient management, and the standards are generally accepted principles for patient management.[23] The development of practice parameters began in the 1930s, when only one physician organization was developing them. In 1992, over 32 organizations were involved in their development.

The American Society of Anesthesiologists (ASA) joined the trend by initiating practice parameter development in two areas: (1) management of a difficult airway, and (2) use of the pulmonary artery catheter. The impetus for the development of practice parameters probably comes mainly out of the fear of other organizations impressing their views upon a group such as anesthesiologists and out of the recognition that such parameters might help to improve quality of care. Practice parameters do not appear to increase professional liability and may have a moderating effect. State-of-the-art treatment may be enhanced by the use of practice parameters. The ASA parameters on standards for intraoperative monitoring were published in 1986 and strengthened in 1990 and 1991.[24] Much debate about the standards has taken place. Do they improve care? Intuition and the reduction in malpractice premiums allow us to infer that they do; however, the proof is not convincing.

Anesthesiologists have been very fortunate in reducing the risk of anesthesia. As malpractice premiums rose dramatically, the increase for anesthesiologists was less rampant and, in some cases, it was reduced. Nevertheless, medical practices do change as physicians practice "defensive medicine." An investigation in New York State through a physician payment review commission found that only 10% of patients who received injuries during hospitalization filed a malpractice claim.[25] Limitations on malpractice suits may reduce awards as well. Some states have reduced the amount of recovery for injury and suffering through legislation. Rates have decreased dramatically as a result.

Several strategies aimed at providers have been employed in an attempt to reduce costs. Hospitals and physicians have become targets in this effort.

Certificate of Need

The certificate of need strategy was developed in an attempt to reduce costs. It is designed according to Roemer's law, which states that "a bed built is a bed occupied."[26] The purpose of the certificate of need is "to eliminate the unnecessary investment and expansion of capacity and to halt offerings of new services that are or were deemed to duplicate the existing ones."[27]

Certificate of need programs are ineffective in controlling hospital expenditures.[28] One possible reason is that the makeup of boards issuing certificates of need may include representatives who view the expansion of a community hospital as positive for their locale. Another possible explanation is that the health planning boards do not bear the risk of being wrong; thus, no financial incentive exists. If the health care board were responsible for health care expenses, it might put more vigor in the certificate of need process; such is the case in Canada, where the provinces bear full fiscal responsibility and thus have an inherent obligation to control facility expenditures. The American populace is not as enthusiastic about the idea of limiting availability. Support for national health insurance plummets when patients perceive the need to wait to receive care.[29]

Technology Control

Technology control is quite effective in reducing expenditures for new technology. Whether the quality of care is affected is unclear. For example, when key comparisons between the United States and Canada were made, it was found that there are (1) nearly eight times more magnetic resonance imaging (MRI) scanners and radiation therapy units per capita in the United States; (2) over six times more lithotripsy centers per capita in the United States; (3) roughly three times more cardiac catheterization and open heart surgery units per capita in the United States; and (4) slightly greater availability of organ transplant units per capita in the United States.[30]

Hospital Rate Setting

Hospital rate setting is another measure that appears to be successful in reducing cost pressures. However, one must be careful to recognize that rate setting for one group often means cost-shifting to another. The Medicare system in the United States adopted the diagnosis-related groups as a strategy to reduce hospital expenditures. Hospital admissions between 1983 and 1989 decreased by 11%, even though the number of eligible patients increased by 13%.[31] A plateau has been placed on length of hospital stay. Concurrently, however, expenditures for prehospitalization and posthospitalization care have increased markedly. Some of these shifts probably were appropriate; others may not have been. The morbidity rate of patients discharged from the hospital has declined slowly; however, inappropriate discharge of patients is a concern. I am unaware of any study that discusses this problem relative to discharge from the postanesthesia care unit.

Another way of saving funds affects global hospital budgets. Canada has a lower cost per day, but has not reduced the length of hospital stay as has the United States. However, staffing levels per hospital bed are much higher in the United States. It is not clear that the mortality rate is higher in Canada than it is in the United States.[32]

Physician Fees

Physician fees have come under attack at various times since the early 1970s. The Health Care Financing Administration (HCFA) has been vigorous in trying to create a revised way of reimbursing physicians. An emphasis has been placed on reducing the level of payment to specialists in certain areas, including anesthesiologists, while at the same time increasing the level for generalists. The HCFA quotes "relative value scales for physician services."[33] It assumes that for every 1% reduction in payment to physicians, physicians increase volume and intensity of service by 0.5%. In Canadian provinces with strict fee controls, volume did increase but not enough to offset the savings derived from fee control. Certain provinces, however, capped expenditures so that volume could not increase by very much. In the United States, this approach may not work because physicians may bias their work towards another payor.

Physician Supply

The question of supply leading to concerns about costs recently has come to the fore. The most aggressive example of restricting the supply of physicians has taken place in British Columbia.[34] Here, billing numbers were restricted not unlike taxicab licenses are restricted in New York City. Unless a physician has a billing number, he or she cannot get paid. Whether restricting physician supply influences health care costs is unclear. Over 50% of Canadian physicians are general or family practitioners.

In 1990, Canada had 388 anesthesiologists, 522 pediatricians, 1392 family medicine physicians, and 1194 internists in training; and a ratio of 8 pediatric, internal medicine, or family medicine postgraduate trainees for each anesthesiologist in training.[35] In 1992, 6233 pediatricians, 18,662 internists, 5610 family practice physicians, and 5213 anesthesiology residents were in training in the United States. This ratio of primary care physicians to anesthesia residents in training was 6:1.[36] Increased pressure has developed to raise the number of general and family practice physicians in the United States. Only 15% of physicians are in this category in the United States compared with over 50% in Canada.[37]

THE ENVIRONMENT

What Are the Nonmedical Effects of Anesthesia?

Personnel

In the 1960s, several studies reported an increased incidence of spontaneous abortion, cancer, congenital anomalies, and deaths among operating room personnel.[38, 39] However, Tannenbaum and Goldberg analyzed the studies and concluded that they were flawed.[40] They suggested that no correlation existed between the presence of waste anesthetic gases and the previously reported adverse effects. Spence and Hemminiki and associates reported similar findings.[41, 42] The use of nitrous

oxide during dental procedures may, however, be another matter.[43] The fertility rate among women employed as dental assistants who are exposed to high levels of nitrous oxide was lower than for women not exposed or exposed only to low levels of nitrous oxide.

Ozone Depletion

Chlorofluorocarbons

Although the inhaled anesthetic agents do not appear to have an adverse health effect on operating room personnel, the possibility that these chlorofluorocarbons may adversely influence the concentration of ozone in the atmosphere is another consideration. Ozone is produced continuously in the stratosphere when solar radiation at wavelengths less than 242 nm dissociates molecular oxygen into atoms that attach themselves to oxygen. Destruction of ozone appears to be proceeding more rapidly than its production. In the stratosphere, ozone destruction is primarily caused by the catalytic reaction of nitrogen, hydrogen, chlorine, and oxides.[44] The effects of chlorine from chlorofluorocarbons were predicted by Molina and Roland.[45] Ozone depletion by chlorofluorocarbons has been implicated as a factor that increases our risk of skin cancer and cataracts.

Hydrochlorofluorocarbons

Hydrochlorofluorocarbons in volatile anesthetic agents persist in the atmosphere for only 3 to 5 years, whereas chlorofluorocarbons last 40 to 150 years; this allows time for their circulation above the ozone layer. The volatile anesthetics are chlorofluorocarbons that combine with carbon hydrogen bonds when exposed to hydroxyl radicals in the atmosphere, producing hydrochloric acid, hydrobromic acid, and carbon dioxide. They return to earth in rain; only a minimal amount of the hydrochlorofluorocarbons reaches the ozone layer, that is, only 1% of halothane ever reaches the ozone layer.[46]

Production of chlorofluorocarbons is approximately 630,000 tons per year, whereas that of hydrochlorofluorocarbons is approximately 6400 tons per year.[47] However, anesthetic agents are not included in the United Nations' list of substances harmful to the ozone layer.[48]

Nitrous Oxide and the Greenhouse Effect

Nitrous oxide contributes to the greenhouse effect by combining with oxygen to produce nitric oxide.[49] The tropospheric concentration of nitrous oxide is increasing at a rate of 0.25% per year, primarily as a result of agricultural nitrate breakdown by microbes. Some investigators believe that agricultural products and nitrous oxide contribute to the problem of global warming.[50]

HOSPITAL WASTE

How Important Is It?

In 1987, several beaches in the United States experienced washups of medical waste and as a result were closed. As unpleasant as these episodes were, no incidences of public illness were reported to have been caused by such exposures.

Subsequent studies pointed out that medical waste could not be traced to illegal dumping or to specific sources such as hospitals.[51–55] The Environmental Protection Agency reported that of the medical waste that washed ashore in 1988, 65% was syringe-related and came from home health care and illegal intravenous drug use.[56] Insulin or cocaine was found in 60% of the syringes.[57] Despite the failure to reveal the illegal dumping of medical waste or any evidence that any person has ever been infected outside of a health care facility, the Medical Waste Tracking Act was signed into law on November 1, 1988.[58]

What Waste Merits Special Handling?

The Centers for Disease Control have made recommendations for the prevention of human immunodeficiency virus transmission in health care settings:

There is no epidemiologic evidence to suggest that most hospital waste is any more infective than residential waste. Moreover, there is no epidemiologic evidence that hospital waste has caused disease in the community as the result of improper disposal. Therefore, identifying waste for which special precautions are indicated is largely a matter of judgement [sic] about the relative risk of disease transmission.

The most practical approach to the management of infectious waste is to identify that waste with the potential for causing infection during handling and disposal and for which some precautions appear prudent. Hospital waste for which special precautions appear prudent include microbiologic laboratory waste, pathology waste, and blood specimens or blood products. While any item that is in contact with blood, exudates, or secretions may be potentially infective, it is not usually considered practical or necessary to treat all such waste as infective. Infective waste, in general, should be either incinerated or should be autoclaved before disposal in a sanitary landfill. Bulk blood, suctioned fluid, excretions, and secretions may be carefully poured down a drain connected to a sanitary sewer. Sanitary sewers may also be used to dispose of other infectious waste capable of being ground and flushed into the sewer.[59]

Inconsistencies

Some internal inconsistencies appear to be present in the guidelines of the Centers for Disease Control, and definitions of terms are problematic. Rutala and colleagues provided the following suggestions:[60]

1. *Hospital* or *solid waste* refers to all waste, biologic or nonbiologic, that is discarded and not intended for further use.
2. *Medical waste* refers to materials that were generated as a result of diagnosis, treatment, or immunization of human beings or animals.
3. *Infectious waste* refers to that portion of the medical waste that could transmit an infectious disease.

The United States Congress and the Environmental Protection Agency use the term ''regulated medical waste'' rather than ''infectious waste'' out of concern for the remote possibility of disease transmission. Medical waste is a subset of hospital waste; regulated medical waste is synonymous with infectious waste and is a subset of medical waste.

What Is the Medical Waste Tracking Act?

The Medical Waste Tracking Act of 1988 was signed by President Ronald Reagan just prior to the November election. The Environmental Protection Agency was directed to implement a 2-year pilot program for the disposal of infectious waste. The program insisted that waste leaving the institution be accompanied by a tracking manifesto. The Environmental Protection Agency should be notified through the tracking system whenever the waste does not reach its intended destination. The program is designed primarily for hospitals but also includes nursing homes, laboratories, and physician's offices. Home waste, which is considered by other definitions to be infectious, is exempt.[58]

What Is Hospital Waste?

Hospital waste in the United States constitutes 1% of the 158 million tons of municipal solid waste produced annually; this amounts to approximately 15 lb of waste per patient per day.[60] Shands Hospital, with which I am affiliated, generates 20 lb of ''red bag'' waste and 18 lb of ''regular'' waste per patient per day. Nationally, approximately 15% of total hospital waste is classified as infectious.

Most surgical waste is classified as infectious. At present, it costs us $0.02 per pound for disposal of noninfectious waste and $0.16 per pound to dispose of infectious waste.[61] Tieszen and Gruenberg studied 27 surgical cases that produced 610 lb of waste, which occupied 171 cu ft.[61] Disposable linens accounted for 39% of the weight, paper—7%, plastic—26%, and miscellaneous items—27%. The authors estimate that the annual surgical waste associated with the examined procedures (back, heart, abdomen, hip, knee, and herniorrhaphy) is 50 million pounds and 14 million cu ft. An estimated reduction of 73% in weight and 30% in volume is possible. Nationwide, manufacturers of disposable draping materials capture 80% of the market share.[62] Reusable operating room materials are equal in performance and should be considered. Of course, there are concerns relative to the need to increase laundry services.

How Can Hospital Waste Be Reduced?

Total rubbish output in the United States presently is 220,000,000 tons per year,[63] and United States hospital waste output is 32,000,000 tons per year.[64] The overall contribution of medicine is only 0.25% of total refuse deposited in landfills throughout the United States. The biggest components are household, yard, and organic material.[65] Of the 5500 landfills in the United States, 90% will be full within the next decade. In order to reduce both costs and the size of the waste stream, several approaches have been tried.

The first approach addressed is the recovery and resterilization of unused surgical supplies.[66] During an 11-month trial, 1713 kg of material with an estimated value of $158,854 was recovered and distributed to established charitable organizations for medical material relief work. In the United States, recovery and resterilization of disposable products can be problematic because in donating supplies, hospitals need to limit their liability and avoid any inference of an implied warranty.[67] The University of Florida College of Medicine's insurance trust fund recommends against the reuse of single-use items. However, in Canada, resterilization and reuse of disposable devices is routine.[68] Open but unused drapes that have been resterilized pose no problem.[69] The issue of the use of disposables versus reusables calls for weighing of the costs of each system.[70] Many hospitals are now adding the cost of disposal to the cost of material. Many also have inadequate laundry facilities should disposable items be completely replaced.

Treatment of biomedical waste has generated a number of approaches. Local landfills are often reluctant to process such waste. The natural life cycle of items that are disposable is actually longer than that of reusable items. For example, a cloth diaper lasts approximately 6 months in a landfill, whereas the ''disposable'' diaper may last 30 years. Options for disposal include incineration, deposition in a landfill, carting, irradiation, and acid reduction.

Incineration can be problematic in that the volume of waste may exceed the capacity of the local incinerator. Also, incinerators must meet environmental standards. Once incineration takes place, items still must be disposed. The advantage, of course, is that heat sterilizes the products of incineration.

MONITORING

What Are Clinical Monitoring Standards?

In 1850, Snow advocated the measuring of pulse and respiration when chloroform anesthesia was administered. However, monitoring standards did not exist until 1986, when the ASA took an unprecedented step by defining minimal standards for the monitoring of anesthetized patients.[71] Although these standards leave room for discretion in some instances, the fact of their publication carries much weight.

How Have These Standards Evolved?

Initially, in the standards promulgated by the ASA, the use of capnographs and pulse oximeters was ''encouraged.'' Such encouragement made it nearly impossible for the individual practitioner to ignore them unless the most persuasive arguments against their benefit could be advanced. Experience has brought several changes in the standards. The evolution of clinical practice mandated the changes and contributes to their being dynamic and reflective of changing environments.

Current Form

The standards for basic intraoperative monitoring that were approved by the ASA House of Delegates on October 21, 1986 and were last amended on October 21, 1992 are listed in the Appendix to this chapter. Not included is the use of a nerve stimulator to check neuromuscular junction integrity. Yet, the manufacturers of both atracurium and vecuronium mention the desirability of monitoring neuromuscular activity with a nerve stimulator in patients receiving either drug. Recommendations in the inserts that pharmaceutical companies prepare for their drugs are checked and approved by the Food and Drug Administration. This is another example of a recommendation that can be ignored by the practitioner, but that may receive a rather exhaustive examination should a malpractice suit result and neuromuscular function be of importance in the etiology of whatever difficulty the plaintiff/patient developed.

The anesthesia machine is not addressed in the monitoring standards, but clearly it is very important. Furthermore, one may choose to procure an anesthesia machine with an integral monitoring system. Whether one chooses totally integrated systems or separate machines and monitors is a matter of choice, past experience, and prediction of problems inherent in either approach.

My monitors for a routine anesthetic procedure generally include the following:

- oscillometric sphygmomanometer
- electrocardiogram
- stethoscope (pretracheal, precordial, or esophageal)
- airway gas analysis (oxygen, carbon dioxide, anesthetic agents)
- thermometer
- nerve stimulator
- pulse oximeter
- spirometer in expiratory limb of anesthesia circuit

For patients with complex problems, additional monitors may include a second electrocardiogram lead, two or perhaps three channels with which to measure blood pressures invasively (arterial, central venous, pulmonary artery). Devices are commonly used to determine cardiac output; to assess the state of coagulability of a patient's blood; to determine arterial blood gas partial pressures, electrolytes, and blood glucose; to perform esophageal echocardiography and electroencephalography; to monitor evoked potentials; and to collect and measure the volume of urine.

Presently, a basic monitoring system costs from $15,000 to $20,000; a more advanced system may cost as much as $50,000.

How Are Monitoring Device Costs Evaluated?

In the analysis of cost, the life expectancy of the monitor has a significant role. A unit that serves for only 3 years costs twice as much per year as one that lasts for 6 years. All other factors being equal, device cost generally is based on 7 years of useful life of the instrument. Obsolescence, maintenance, and incompatibility are three factors that affect the duration of a unit's service.

Obsolescence

When a new and markedly improved device becomes available, an institution may decide to replace an older monitor with it, not because the older unit fails to function but rather because the newer unit offers significant advantages. Although a replacement of this type immediately increases the cost of the unit that has been discarded (fewer years for amortization), the still serviceable monitors often are transferred to other clinical units (for instance, postanesthesia recovery unit or the intensive care unit) or to research laboratories where the requirements may not be quite as demanding as those in an operating room.

Although this process may save the hospital or other institution money, the administrative entity (e.g., the anesthesia department or the operating room) responsible for the purchase of a new monitoring device usually shows the entire cost of the purchase. No benefit is gained from offsetting the recovery or salvage value of the replaced machine that has been handed over to other users.

Maintenance

An electronic device may not last 7 years and may, therefore, have to be replaced because repairs become too expensive or because the functioning of the unit is too unreliable. Maintenance costs can become excessive, and the purchase of a new monitor may be more cost-effective. Additionally, the use of unreliable monitors is not risk-free. Such risks may translate into enormous liability costs.

Incompatibility

New devices may have been designed to work in conjunction with existing equipment. However, existing equipment may no longer be compatible with new equipment. The old device may, therefore, require costly modifications to be of service with the add-on new equipment. These considerations, each with its own unpredictable aspects, show why the listing of a purchase price amortized over 7 years presents at best an estimate subject to many modifications.

How Are Maintenance and Repair Costs Assessed?

One of the factors most difficult to assess is the cost of maintenance and repairs. Maintenance can be obtained through service contracts with vendors or manufacturers or through hospital engineering personnel. A biomedical engineering department in larger institutions is quite costly in its own right. As an example, the Shands Hospital administration (the 550-bed teaching hospital associated with the University of Florida College of Medicine) estimates that it spends $531,081 annually in maintaining the biomedical engineering department overall and that approximately 15%, or almost $80,000, is attributed to anesthesiology. We have an additional separate maintenance contract covering 30 anesthesia machines that currently costs the hospital almost $21,000.[72] With 30 anesthetizing locations and 15,000 cases per year, the average annual cost per anesthetizing location is $3880, or $7 per case. Although the biomedical technicians service other equipment, we estimate that 75% of their time is spent on electronic devices related to monitoring.

To complicate matters further, some expensive systems save money in unexpected ways. For instance, a service contract for the maintenance and calibration of vaporizers (for halothane, enflurane, isoflurane, and desflurane) annually costs $285 per vaporizer. For 30 anesthetizing locations, each with 3 vaporizers, the total cost is $25,650 per year. Newer vaporizers do not need yearly maintenance. Since we have airway gas monitoring systems with agent identification, we monitor the accuracy of the vaporizers daily. Thus, a service contract for our vaporizers is unnecessary. As a result, considerable expense is avoided. In actuality, the savings is probably less than $25,000, since occasionally a vaporizer must be sent out for repair.

What Is the Cost of Consumable Supplies?

Consumable supplies are costly and frequently ignored items in the monitoring budget. Prices vary widely, depending on the contract the hospital can negotiate with a vendor. A reasonable cost estimate for five disposable electrocardiogram electrodes is $1.25; for a disposable esophageal stethoscope, it is $3.50; and for a disposable finger probe for pulse oximetry, it is $10. Two stick-on skin electrodes for the nerve stimulator add another $0.50.

For an invasive arterial pressure measurement setup, the estimates for disposable items are shown in Table 7–2. In addition, we must include the cost of the extra time required to apply monitors and the cost of the time that may be saved by their use in the short or long run (i.e., in the operating room and the postanesthesia recovery unit, or the intensive care unit, respectively). Preparation of a pressure monitoring system, together with insertion and securing of an arterial catheter, consumes physician and nurse time and can extend the amount of time the patient spends in the operating room. If we assume that this activity represents 10 minutes of the physician's time and operating room time simultaneously, the cost for the anesthesiologist might be $25 (based on a point system in which a 10-minute time unit is valued at $25) and the cost for the operating room might be $150 (assuming a rate of $900 per hour). Alternative methods of monitoring arterial pressure continuously and noninvasively require little or no time for preparation and application and are very attractive by comparison.

Monitoring can save money when information on inspired and expired anesthetic gases and repeated assessment of neuromuscular blockade allow accurate control of anesthetic depth and rapid emergence at the end of the procedure. Thus, the expenses associated with prolonged recovery and drug use in excess of that required can be avoided.

How Can the Cost of Monitoring Be Placed in Perspective?

The price one pays for monitoring must be balanced against its tangible and intangible benefits; these benefits are not easily measured. Morbidity and mortality statistics, for example, are difficult to obtain (and even impossible to collect for a single department). Yet, the bulk of the evidence points to increased safety for patients under anesthesia when capnography and pulse oximetry are used routinely.[73, 74] Quoted benefits also include reduced insurance premiums when comprehensive monitoring is applied as well as steeply increased premiums if a lawsuit results and monitoring is found to have fallen below standards.[74] For a teaching institution, other benefits accrue, namely those of exposing future practitioners to modern methods (some of which may well become common) and perhaps a reduction in educational requirements in the future. For all available monitors, justifications for their use can be developed.

TABLE 7–2. Disposable Items for Invasive Arterial Pressure Measurements

Item	Cost
Disposable transducer	$10.00
Heparin	$0.03
Bag with normal saline	$0.05
Catheter	$1.00
Alcohol sponge or material for sterilization of the skin	$0.01
Sponges	$0.02
Adhesive tape	$0.01

Nevertheless, extensive monitoring is expensive. We estimate the cost of a basic monitoring package as follows: electrocardiogram, oscillometric automated blood pressure, pulse oximetry, and capnography—$20,000; precordial or esophageal auscultation and temperature measurement—$1 to $4; and neuromuscular junction monitoring—$100 to $500. These costs represent about $4 to $10 for the monitors and $15 to $20 for disposable items per patient, if we assume that all instruments will work for 7 years; that their annual maintenance equals 10% of their purchase price; that disposable items are limited to electrodes, esophageal stethoscope, and a disposable finger probe for the pulse oximeter; and that all monitors are used in 750 patients per year.

Clearly, the greatest savings can be realized by a most parsimonious use of disposables, careful negotiations of service contracts, and thrift in the arrangements for maintenance without jeopardizing the reliability of the monitors. When viewed as a percentage of the overall cost of anesthesia or operating room fees and the professional fees charged by surgeons and anesthesiologists, the additional $20 to $30 per anesthetic procedure for safety is a bargain no one is likely to ignore. Comprehensive, noninvasive monitoring probably costs less than 1% of the sum of all hospital and medical charges for the hours the patient spends in the operating room.

FUNDING OF EQUIPMENT COSTS

How Can We Obtain the Equipment We Need?

Present anesthesia practice is much more quantitative and instrument-oriented than it was in the past. Not too many years ago, the operating room was equipped with a monitor and a very simple anesthesia machine, both of which lasted for years. New technology has presented to the clinician a wide variety of instruments, some of which are coveted as we seek to improve quality of care and reduce risk. The time between our first desire to obtain new instruments and the time that they finally are obtained can span months or even years, much of which generates frustration. It is the frustration we wish to reduce by suggesting ways to obtain instruments more efficiently, as no budget is ever adequate to acquire everything on our wish list.

Identification of the Problem Set

The first step is to develop a set of the clinical problems to be solved or avoided; then, to the greatest extent possible, this set should be agreed upon within the practice group. The larger the proportion in the group that agrees, the better. Prioritizing the problems becomes a necessity in most cases. To develop a set of problems that are to be solved or partially solved by capital equipment purchases, we must first be certain that the applicable standards (state, federal, and societal) are met.

The department of anesthesiology may wish to adopt standards (e.g., the practice standards suggested by the ASA) as a starting point. Monitoring standards may be included using other sources, such as those published by Harvard University, the University of Arizona, and Stanford University. Others are sure to follow, and many will necessitate additional equipment purchases.

Unique problems in each practice may require or invite

solutions. For example, if laser therapy is to be used in the intubated patient, an anesthesia machine capable of delivering helium as well as an airway gas monitor that is not affected by helium *may* be desirable. If surgical patients are at risk for air embolus (e.g., as in sitting position craniotomy), a precordial Doppler ultrasound instrument is added to the instrument armamentarium.

Of concern also are changes in the anesthesia/monitoring needs predicted for the next fiscal year. Is the hospital considering lithotripsy, organ transplantation, or cardiac surgery that might require additional anesthesia-related equipment? Since hospitals tend to think in terms of fiscal years for purchasing, early identification of perceived needs is helpful.

Loss Minimization

Identification of areas in your practice in which improved or new equipment might reduce patient risk helps to prioritize efforts. Data come from published sources and local experience. For example, Cooper and associates suggest that vigilance for disconnections of all kinds is particularly problematic in patients who had "near misses" or had come to grief in the perioperative period.[75] Management of the airway contributed mightily to the near misses. They recommend particular emphasis be placed on this aspect of care, on airway monitoring, and on training.

Locally, a review of perioperative near misses or morbidity can be quite helpful. Over the past several years, have patients had bad outcomes owing to airway mismanagement that a capnograph might have helped to prevent? Did an esophageal intubation in a patient undergoing a cesarean section lead to preventable morbidity? How much did each occurrence cost? If the cost of an accident multiplied by the probability of its occurrence exceeds the cost of the occurrence, we are negligent for not spending enough to avoid the accident. For example, if an unrecognized esophageal intubation costs $1,000,000 and the occurrence of that or a similar accident is once every 5 years, we are obligated, according to this reasoning, to spend up to $200,000 per year if the accident can be avoided for that sum of money.

The ASA Closed Claims study suggests that prevention of accidents is cost-effective.[76] The total cost of preventable injury or death and the total cost of nonpreventable injury or death were not calculated because the non-normal distribution potentially would bias the results. However, the authors noted, "The median payment for cases deemed preventable by additional monitoring was $250,000, whereas the median payment for cases not deemed preventable was $22,500."[76]

Justification

To justify, identify, and prioritize equipment purchases is one matter; turning the justification into hardware requires more than passively saying, "The hospital never buys us anything" or aggressively marching into the administrator's office saying, "Patients are going to die unless you buy this." Both approaches will fail.

Success depends on familiarization with the hospital budgetary process, since the hospital usually funds capital equipment purchases. Knowing the deadlines for requests is not enough. Usually, the hospital requires a written justification and a deadline for its submission. This task, viewed by some as onerous, is necessary for the proper understanding of what the equipment is meant to do. The administrator will be concerned as to how the equipment contributes to the "bottom line." Will it generate revenue or reduce costs? The answer can be considered from both a macroeconomic and a microeconomic sense.

Whitcher and colleagues[77] calculated that by using the standard monitoring equipment described previously (Fig. 7–3), the reduction in cost is $14,000 per operating room per year with an associated 50% reduction in claims. How does that analysis relate to my hospital? you might ask. Review your experience over the past several years to identify cases that cost, or could have cost, the institution much more. Frequently, the administrator only needs to be reminded of an incident and a method to prevent its recurrence to consider funding a request. Similarly, if you feel that an outlying area is underequipped, you need only remind the administrator that both the Joint Commission on the Accreditation of Healthcare Organizations and ASA standards state that all patients must receive a similar level of care no matter where in the hospital their care is provided.

Enlistment of Support

Once you have enlisted the aid of the department of anesthesiology, seek broader support (surgeons and other physicians). To do so costs them little. Next, identify other support groups within the hospital. If the nursing, respiratory therapy, or other departments see the utility, support may come in many ways. Written support is direct and helpful, but do not minimize the support your request may receive at staff meetings. Those departments may need your help in some of their efforts; this is an opportunity to work together.

Other resources include loss prevention or risk management

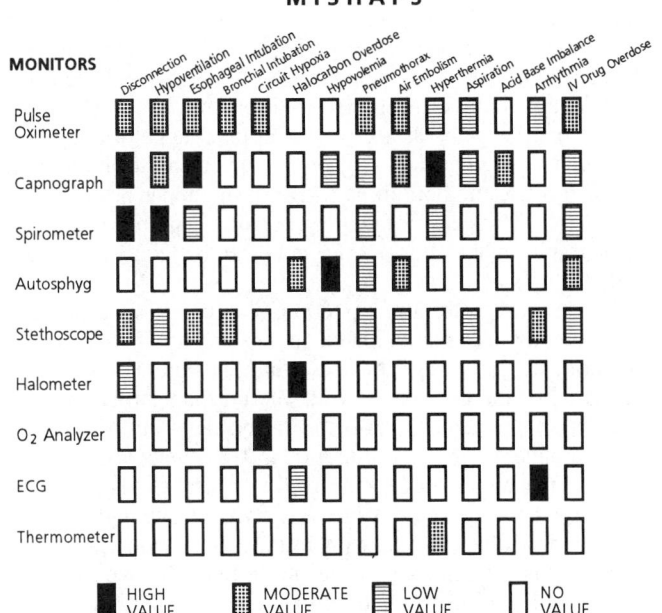

MISHAPS

FIGURE 7–3. Matrix of monitoring equipment versus type of mishap. This matrix represents the authors' estimate of the relative value of each monitoring modality. IV = Intravenous; Autosphyg = automatic noninvasive sphygmomanometer; O₂ Analyzer = breathing circuit oxygen analyzer; ECG = monitor of cardiac electrical activity. (From Whitcher C, Ream AK, Parsons D, et al: Anesthetic mishaps and the cost of monitoring: a proposed standard for monitoring equipment. J Clin Monit 1988; 4:5–15.)

personnel and insurance carriers. Defense attorneys can also lend a sympathetic voice or letter. These supporters may recognize additional reasons for the capital equipment you did not appreciate.

Fund Allocation

Today's hospital administrators face very difficult tasks in managing their resources. Physicians requesting capital equipment must understand what priorities face the administrator in allocating funds. It is a time-consuming task that inevitably requires funding cuts on some requests or only partial funding of others. Reduced to its essence, it is a cost/risk benefit calculation that requires a combination of inputs to arrive at the most efficacious allocation of resources.

Prioritization

Familiarity with hospital funding priorities is essential to understand funding decisions. You will need to make some effort to do this, but diligence in this area can bear fruit. A hospital priority list might look something like this:

1. New Programs/Personnel

The hospital administrator will try to support new programs that directly or indirectly contribute to the hospital as a whole. For example, if a heart transplant program or cardiac surgical unit is planned, that program will get first priority. Anesthesiologists must carefully analyze what they will have to do to support that program and to make associated capital equipment needs known. Since equipment bought for one program frequently can be used in more than one location, thinking in terms of broader applications is helpful. If an additional anesthesia machine is required, consider the most flexible arrangement. If pediatric patients are treated in your hospital, configure the system to handle them even though the primary use would be for adults. If a magnetic resonance imaging system is contemplated, an anesthesia setup compatible with this technology is needed. Justification of an extra $10,000 attached to a $500,000 project is much easier than is an individual $10,000 effort.

2. Compliance with Standards

The hospital will attempt to meet all relevant standards. If the anesthesia department standards are reasonable but not met with the existing equipment, a significant justification is that, "without this equipment, we do not meet standards." Insurance carriers, the Joint Commission on the Accreditation of Healthcare Organizations and the ASA are helpful references.

3. Attractive Technologies

Although everything new is not what is desired in any hospital, employing new technologies is attractive to hospitals even if only for positive public relations. Of course, hospitals need more justification than this. However, if a new magnetic resonance imaging scanner is purchased, the amount of specialized anesthesia care may increase, necessitating additional monitoring for an anticipated larger patient load.

4. Safety

As disappointing as it may seem, patient safety may not be the highest priority. In the absence of studies showing a decrease in morbidity and mortality, the safety argument may well fall on deaf ears; after all, everybody makes such an argument.

Funding Sources

Although we usually think of the hospital as the sole fund provider, in special circumstances, other sources may be available. First, we should look to ourselves. If it is believed that a piece of equipment will be helpful, we should buy the first one ourselves, thus proving the value and the strength of our commitment to others. As an alternative to outright purchase, leasing or renting can also be considered. If a monitoring charge can be assessed, a method of payment can be arranged.

A frequently ignored source of funds is the hospital volunteer groups. Equipment to be purchased for children or parturients often is particularly attractive to these groups. Service organizations may also help. Lastly, in return for an evaluation, vendors may donate equipment. During product development, clinical evaluation can be interesting for you and useful to a firm.

CONCLUSION

These steps discussed earlier will prove helpful in understanding how to obtain adequate support to meet equipment and monitoring needs. Although the national and international considerations about health care costs and access should concern us all, it is in our own workplaces—hospitals, outpatient centers, and pain clinics—that we in anesthesiology can directly affect charges and costs. Professional medical societies, government, health care organizations, and trade organizations are clamoring for us to reduce our charges. We resent the implication that we are not worth what we are charging. We resent the various plans to reduce physician reimbursement. However, we have perhaps not done a very effective job at convincing the public that we deserve what we bill.

An opportunity exists to save payers their money. It depends, in large part, on how efficiently we work, squeezing the most out of available resources. Our obligation is to do so; certainly the patient cannot control costs once he or she is under our care. As Johnstone and Martines point out, "Quantifying the benefits of anesthesia is possible but must be approached with an economic perspective in that the utility of anesthetic benefits must incorporate the feasibility of selecting anesthetic plans. The feasibility of an anesthetic plan will, in turn, depend on valuing the costs of anesthesia and its determinations and components."[78] Patients deserve the most efficiency and the best of care, regardless of the amount we are being paid. How can this goal be achieved? Let us consider a few ways.

Drug Costs

A substantial portion of anesthesia supply charges is the cost of drugs. At Shands Hospital, pharmaceuticals constitute one-third to one-half of the total anesthesia supply budget. What is our justification for using the drugs we use? Is the newest drug the best? Can an expensive inhalation agent, an expensive muscle relaxant, or an expensive hypnotic be justified only because it is new? Saidman writes, "Is desflurane sufficiently better than currently available inhaled anesthetics, especially isoflurane, to warrant widespread incorporation into widespread practice?"[79]

Antebi[80] suggests a simple way to calculate the costs of inhalational anesthetics using the following equation:

$$C = 3Fc$$

where C is the consumption in $mL \cdot h^{-1}$, F is the fresh gas flow rate in $L \cdot h^{-1}$, and c is the delivered per cent concentration of the anesthetic. Whitcher and coworkers[77] calculated that at minimum alveolar concentration, their hospital costs for a 1-hour procedure are $15.18 with isoflurane, $15.12 with enflurane, and less than $1 with halothane.

Lampotang and associates[81] calculate that by decreasing anesthetic flow rate uniformly from $5 L \cdot min^{-1}$ to $2.5 L \cdot min^{-1}$, $225 million could be saved annually worldwide. This figure translates to $8300 annual savings per operating room.

Whitcher and coworkers further note that at their institution, 1 mg of doxacurium costs $5.94; 1 mg of pipecuronium—$3.50; and 1 mg of pancuronium—$0.18. For 30 minutes of muscle relaxation in a 70-kg patient, succinylcholine (Anectine Flow-Pack, Burroughs-Wellcome, Research Triangle Park, NC) costs $9.50; succinylcholine (Quelicine vials, Abbott Laboratories, Abbott Park, IL) costs $2.94; vecuronium costs $12.32; atracurium costs $14.70; and mivacurium costs $10.80. To reverse muscle relaxation, neostigmine costs $0.80 for 4 mg, and edrophonium costs $4.50 for 70 mg. One should ask whether the substantial increases of cost in some cases can be justified.

A good knowledge of both pharmacology and the patient should lead us to appropriate patient care and economic decisions. Some suggest that the problem is a bit more complex and that other factors should be considered. Marias and colleagues suggest that there are reduced demands on postanesthesia care unit resources when propofol is used.[82] Less emesis and earlier tolerance of fluids by mouth are strong considerations in patient management, and the agent selected can make a difference.

In Shands Hospital, we have audited fresh gas flows to verify that they are $\leq 2.5 L \cdot min^{-1}$ compared with the traditional use of a $5 L \cdot min^{-1}$ flow rate, which made copper kettle concentration calculations easier. We also have altered our soda lime canister exchange protocol. Where previously we changed both cartridges when a color change was noted, we now do not remove the upper canister until the bottom one begins to show signs of use (e.g., a color change or a temperature that is warmer than that of the upper one to the touch). We then rotate the bottom cartridge to the upper position and put a new cartridge in the bottom position. The routine use of capnography makes this a safe and effective economy measure.

We discourage the use of propofol infusions as a primary technique for cases anticipated to last longer than 2 hours; similarly, we discourage the use of intermediate-acting muscle relaxants for these cases as well. We no longer routinely administer supplemental oxygen in the postanesthesia care unit unless a patient's oxygen saturation is >2% below baseline, is <92%, or is anticipated to fall below this level.[84] This modification has reduced our oxygen use by over one-half and is a cost-saving, safe measure with routine continuous pulse oximetry monitoring in the postanesthesia care unit. We routinely use reusable pulse oximeter probes in the operating room, reserving disposable probes for those patients in whom a reusable probe cannot be applied.

References

1. Marwick C: Groups survey health care costs, charges. JAMA 1991; 265:2454.

2. Cantor JC, Barrand NL, Desonia RA, et al: Data watch: business leaders' views on American health care. Health Aff (Millwood) 1991; 10:98–105.

3. Wilensky GR: From the Health Care Financing Administration. JAMA 1991; 265:2461.

4. Friedman E: The uninsured: from dilemma to crisis. JAMA 1991; 265:2491.

5. General Accounting Office (GAOHRD-91-90 Canadian Health Insurance Lessons for the United States).

6. Kirkman-Liff BL: Health insurance values and implementation in the Netherlands and the Federal Republic of Germany: an alternative path to universal coverage. JAMA 1991; 265:2496.

7. Hsiao WC, Braun P, Yutema D, et al: Estimating physicians work for a resource-based relative-value scale. N Engl J Med 1988; 319:835.

8. Hsiao WC, Braun P, Becker ER, et al: The resource-based relative value scale: toward the development of an alternative physician payment system. JAMA 1987; 258:799.

9. Hsiao WC, Braun P, Dunn D, et al: Results and policy implications of the resource-based relative-value scale. N Engl J Med 1988; 319:881.

10. Rice T: Containing health care costs. US Med Care Rev 1992; 49:19.

11. Holmer M: Tax policy and the demand for health insurance. Health Econ 1989; 3:203.

12. Manning WG, Newhouse JP, Duane N, et al: Health insurance and demand for medical care: evidence from a randomized experiment. Med Econ Rev 1987; 77:251.

13. Einthoven AC, Kronick R: A consumer choice health plan for the 1990s. N Engl J Med 1989; 320:31.

14. Einthoven AC: Consumer choice health plan. N Engl J Med 1978; 298:650, 709.

15. Wickizier TM, Wheeler RJC, Feldstein PJ: Does utilization review reduce the necessary hospital care and contain cost? Med Care 1989; 28:632.

16. Lindsey PA, Newhouse JP: The cost and value of second surgical opinion programs: the critical review of the literature. J Health Polit Policy Law 1990; 15:543.

17. Graboys TB, Biegelsen B, Lampert S, et al: Results of a second opinion trial among patients recommended for coronary angiography. JAMA 1992; 268:2537.

18. Ossorio RC, Alper MH: Fee-for-service medicine, preferred provider organizations, and health maintenance organizations. In The Business of Medicine. Gitnick J, Rothenberg F, Weiner J (eds). New York, Elsevier, 1991, p 24.

19. Newhouse JP: Is competition the answer? J Health Econ 1982; 1:110.

20. Jones SB: Multiple choice health insurance: the lessons and challenge to private insurers. Inquiry 1990; 27:161.

21. Blendon RJ, Donelan K: The public and the emerging debate over national health insurance. N Engl J Med 1990; 323:208.

22. Langwell KM, Hadley JP: Evaluation of the Medicare competition demonstrations. Health Care Financ Rev 1989; 11:65.

23. Arens JF: A practice parameters overview. Anesthesiology 1993; 78:229.

24. ASA Standards for Intraoperative Monitoring. Park Ridge, IL, American Society of Anesthesiologists, 1992.

25. Physician Payment Review Commission Annual Report to Congress. Washington, DC, Physician Payment Review Commission, 1990.

26. Shain M, Roemer MI: Hospital costs relate to the supply of beds. Mod Hosp 1959; 168:71.

27. Rice TW: Health services planning and regulation. In Introduction to Health Services. Williams SG, Torrence PR (eds). New York, Wiley, 1988, p 393.

28. Steinwall B, Sloan FA: Regulatory Approaches to Hospital Cost Containment: A Synthesis of the Empirical Evidence and a New Approach to the Economics of Health Care. Olsen M (ed). Washington, DC, The American Enterprise Institute for Public Policy Research, 1981.

29. Blendon RJ, Donelan K: The public and the emerging debate over National Health Insurance. N Engl J Med 1990; 323:208.

30. Rublee D: Medical technology in Canada, Germany, and the United States. Health Aff (Millwood) 1989; 8:181.

31. Wilensky GR: Medicare at 25: Better value and better care. American Medical Association #264. Chicago, American Medical Association, 1990, pp 1996–1997.

32. Roos LL, Fisher ES, Sharp SM, et al: Post surgical mortality in Manitoba and New England. JAMA 1990; 263:2453.

33. Health Care Financing Administration: Relative value scales for physician services. In Medicare Physician Payment. Washington, DC, Health Care Financing Administration, October 1989.

34. Baier ML: Regulating physician supply, the evolution of British Columbia's bill 41. J Health Polit Policy Law 1988; 13:1.

35. Medical Schools in Canada. (Provided by Eva Ryten, Info Service, Association of Canadian Medical Colleges.) Appendix 1B, Table 5. JAMA 1992; 268:1167.

36. Graduate Medical Education. Appendix 2. JAMA 1992; 268:1170.

37. United States Public Health Service DHHS Publication No. DHS89-1232, Rockville, MD, March 1989.

38. Bruce DL, Eide KA, Linde HW, et al: Causes of death among anesthesiologists: a 20-year survey. Anesthesiology 1968; 29:565.

39. Vaisman AL: Work in surgical theaters and its influence on the health of anesthesiologists. Eksp Khir Anesteziol 1967; 3:44.

40. Tannenbaum TN, Goldberg RJ: Exposure to anesthetic gases and reproductive outcome: a review of the epidemiologic literature. J Occup Med 1985; 27:669.

41. Spence AA: Environmental pollution by inhalation anesthetics. Br J Anaesth 1987; 59:96.

42. Hemminiki K, Kyyronen P, Lindbohn ML: Spontaneous abortion and malformations in the offspring of nurses exposed to anesthetic gases, cytostatic drugs, and other potential hazards in hospitals based on registered information of outcome. J Epidemiol Community Health 1985; 39:141.

43. Rowland AS, Baird DD, Weinberg CR, et al: Reduced fertility among women employed as dental assistants exposed to high levels of nitrous oxide. N Engl J Med 1992; 327:993.

44. Stolarski R, Bojkov R, Bishop L, et al: Measured transient stratospheric ozone. Science 1992; 256:342.

45. Molina MJ, Roland FS: Stratospheric sink for chlorofluromethanes: chlorine atom–catalysed destruction of ozone. Nature 1974; 249:810.

46. Logan M, Farmer JG: Anesthesia and the ozone layer (Editorial). Br J Anaesth 1989; 63:645.

47. Hammitt JK: Future emission scenarios for chemicals that may deplete the stratospheric ozone. Nature 1987; 330:711.

48. Johnston K: First steps in ozone protection agreed. Nature 1987; 329:189.

49. Logan MF, Farmer JT: Anesthesia and the ozone layer (Editorial). Br J Anaesth 1989; 63:645.

50. Kole TE: Environmental and occupational hazards of the anesthesia workplace (Editorial). J Assoc Nurse Anesthetists 1990; 58:327.

51. Investigation: Sources of beach washups in 1988. Albany, NY, New York State Department of Environmental Conservation, 1988.

52. US Environmental Protection Agency: Inventory of medical waste beach washups. June-October 1988. Fairfax, VA, ICF Incorporated, 1989.

53. O'Hara KJ: Center for Marine Conservation: Trash on America's beaches: a national assessment. Washington, DC, Center for Marine Conservation, 1989.

54. Debenham P, Younger LK: Center for Marine Conservation: Cleaning North America's beaches, 1990 Beach Cleanup Results. Washington, DC, Center for Marine Conservation, 1991.

55. Rutala WA, Mayhall G: Medical waste. Infect Control Hosp Epidemiol 1992; 13:38.

56. US Environmental Protection Agency: Standards for the tracking and management of medical waste; intra-panel report rule and request for comment. Fed Reg 1989; 54:12326–12395.

57. US Environmental Protection Agency: Medical Waste Management in the United States: Second Interim Report to Congress. EPA/530-SW-90-087A; 1990.

58. Farber BF: The disposal of medical waste: The New York experience under the Medical Tracking Act. Infection Control Hosp Epidemiol 1991; 12:251.

59. Centers for Disease Control: Recommendations for prevention of HIV transmission in health care settings. MMWR Morb Mortal Wkly Rep 1988; 36:125.

60. Rutala WA, Odette RL, Samsa GP: Management of infectious waste by U.S. hospitals. JAMA 1989; 262:1635.

61. Tieszen ME, Gruenberg JC: A quantitative, qualitative, and critical assessment of surgical waste. JAMA 1992; 267:2765.

62. Wagner M: Environment, cost concerns spur new interest in reusables. Mod Health Care 1990; 20:46.

63. Grossman D, Shulman S: Down in the dumps. Discover 1990; 11:36.

64. Council on Scientific Affairs, American Medical Association: Infectious medical waste. JAMA 1989; 262:1669.

65. Rathje WL: Once and future landfills. National Geographic 1991; 179:117–134.

66. Rosenblatt WH, Silverman DG: Recovery, resterilization, and donation of unused surgical supplies. JAMA 1992; 268:1441.

67. Decker R: Hospitals need to limit their liability when selling used and surplus equipment. Hosp Materials Manage 1989; 14:20.

68. Campbell BA, Wells GA, Palmer WN, et al: Reuse of disposal medical devices in Canadian hospitals. Am J Infect Control 1987; 15:196.

69. Mayhall CG: Types of disposable medical devices reused in hospitals. Infect Control 1986; 7:491.

70. Bruning LM: Disposables vs. reusables in OR practice: Part II. Weighing costs, risks, and wastes. Nurs Management 1992; 23:72I–72P.

71. Eichhorn JH, Cooper JB, Cullen DJ, et al: Standards for patient monitoring during anesthesia at Harvard Medical School. JAMA 1986; 256:1017.

72. Sembroski G: Shands Hospital at the University of Florida. Personal communication, March 1987.

73. Wood MD: Monitoring equipment and loss reduction: an insurer's view. *In* Gravenstein JS, Holzer JF (eds). Anesthesia Safety and Cost Containment. Stoneham, Butterworths, 1988, pp 47–54.

74. Whitcher C, Parsons D, Ream AK, et al: Anesthetic safety and cost effective monitoring. Scientific exhibit, ASA Annual Meeting, Las Vegas, October 19–21, 1986.

75. Cooper JB, Newbower RS, Long CD, et al: Preventable anesthetic mishap: a study of human factors. Anesthesiology 1978; 49:399.

76. Tinker JH, Dull DL, Caplan RA, et al: Role of monitoring devices in prevention of anesthetic mishaps: a closed claims analysis. Anesthesiology 1989; 71:547.

77. Whitcher C, Ream AK, Parsons D, et al: Anesthetic mishaps and the cost of monitoring: a proposed standard for monitoring equipment. J Clin Monit 1988; 4:5.

78. Johnstone RE, Martines CL: Costs of anesthesia. Anesth Analg 1993; 76:840.

79. Saidman LJ: The role of desflurane in the practice of anesthesia. Anesthesiology 1991; 74:399.

80. Antebi ME, Patel AJ: Cost containment in anesthesia. Scientific exhibit, ASA Annual Meeting, Las Vegas, October 19–23, 1990.

81. Lampotang S, Nyland ME, Gravenstein N: The cost of wasted anesthetic gases. Anesth Analg 1991; 71:S151.

82. Marias ML, Maher MW, Wetchler BV, et al: Reduced demands on recovery room resources with propofol (Diprivan) compared to thiopental-isoflurane. Anesth Rev 1989; 16:29.

83. Korttila K, Ostman P, Faure E, et al: Randomized comparison of recovery after propofol-nitrous oxide versus thiopentone-isoflurane-nitrous oxide anesthesia in patients undergoing ambulatory surgery. Acta Anaesthesiol Scand 1990; 34:400.

84. Dibenedetto R, Graves SA, Gravenstein N, et al: O$_2$ as needed based on pulse oximetry in the postanesthesia recovery unit: a way to save (Abstract). Anesthesiology 1992; 77:A1127.

APPENDIX

Standards for Basic Intraoperative Monitoring (Approved by House of Delegates on October 21, 1986 and last amended on October 21, 1992)

These standards apply to all anesthesia care although, in emergency circumstances, appropriate life support measures take precedence. These standards may be exceeded at any time based on the judgement of the responsible anesthesiologist. They are intended to encourage quality patient care, but observing them cannot guarantee any specific patient outcome. They are subject to revision from time to time, as warranted by the evolution of technology and practice. This set of standards addresses only the issue of basic intraoperative monitoring, which is one component of anesthesia care. In certain rare or unusual circumstances, (1) some of these methods of monitoring may be clinically impractical, and (2) appropriate use of the described monitoring methods may fail to detect untoward clinical developments. Brief interruptions of continual† monitoring may be unavoidable. *Under extenuating circumstances, the responsible anesthesiologist may waive the requirements marked with an asterisk (*); it is recommended that when this is done, it should be so stated (including the reasons) in a note in the patient's medical record.* These standards are not intended for application to the care of the obstetrical patient in labor or in the conduct of pain management.

†Note that "continual" is defined as "repeated regularly and frequently in steady rapid succession," whereas "continuous" means "prolonged without any interruption at any time."

STANDARD I

Qualified anesthesia personnel shall be present in the room throughout the conduct of all general anesthetics, regional anesthetics, and monitored anesthesia care.

Objective

Because of the rapid changes in patient status during anesthesia, qualified anesthesia personnel shall be continuously present to monitor the patient and provide anesthesia care. In the event there is a direct known hazard, e.g., radiation, to the anesthesia personnel which might require intermittent remote observation of the patient, some provision for monitoring the patient must be made. In the event that an emergency requires the temporary absence of the person primarily responsible for the anesthetic, the best judgement of the anesthesiologist will be exercised in comparing the emergency with the anesthetized patient's condition and in the selection of the person left responsible for the anesthetic during the temporary absence.

STANDARD II

During all anesthetics, the patient's oxygenation, ventilation, circulation, and temperature shall be continually evaluated.

Oxygenation

Objective

To ensure adequate oxygen concentration in the inspired gas and the blood during all anesthetics.

Methods

1. Inspired gas: During every administration of general anesthesia using an anesthesia machine, the concentration of oxygen in the patient breathing system shall be measured by an oxygen analyzer with a low oxygen concentration limit alarm in use.*
2. Blood oxygenation: During all anesthetics, a quantitative method of assessing oxygenation such as pulse oximetry shall be employed.* Adequate illumination and exposure of the patient is necessary to assess color.*

Ventilation

Objective

To ensure adequate ventilation of the patient during all anesthetics.

Methods

1. Every patient receiving general anesthesia shall have the adequacy of ventilation continually evaluated. While qualitative clinical signs such as chest excursion, observation of the reservoir breathing bag, and auscultation of breath sounds may be adequate, quantitative monitoring of the CO$_2$ content and/or volume of expired gas is encouraged.

2. When an endotracheal tube is inserted, its correct positioning in the trachea must be verified by clinical assessment and by identification of carbon dioxide in the expired gas.* End-tidal CO_2 analysis, in use from the time of endotracheal tube placement, is strongly encouraged.
3. When ventilation is controlled by a mechanical ventilator, there shall be in continuous use a device that is capable of detecting disconnection of components of the breathing system. The device must give an audible signal when its alarm threshold is exceeded.
4. During regional anesthesia and monitored anesthesia care, the adequacy of ventilation shall be evaluated, at least, by continual observation of qualitative clinical signs.

Circulation

Objective

To ensure the adequacy of the patient's circulatory function during all anesthetics.

Methods

1. Every patient receiving anesthesia shall have the electrocardiogram continuously displayed from the beginning of anesthesia until preparing to leave the anesthetizing location.*
2. Every patient receiving anesthesia shall have arterial blood pressure and heart rate determined and evaluated at least every 5 minutes.*
3. Every patient receiving general anesthesia shall have, in addition to the above, circulatory function continually evaluated by at least one of the following: palpation of a pulse, auscultation of heart sounds, monitoring of a tracing of intra-arterial pressure, ultrasound peripheral pulse monitoring, or pulse plethysmography or oximetry.

Body Temperature

Objective

To aid in the maintenance of appropriate body temperature during all anesthetics.

Methods

There shall be readily available a means to continuously measure the patient's temperature. When changes in body temperature are intended, anticipated or suspected, the temperature shall be measured.

(Excerpted from 1993 Directory of Members. 58th ed., of the American Society of Anesthesiologists. A copy of the full text can be obtained from ASA, 520 N. Northwest Highway, Park Ridge, Illinois 60068-2573.)

Perioperative Consultations

CHAPTER 8

Cardiology Consultation

MARIAN C. LIMACHER, M.D.

WILLIAM C. ROBBINS, M.D.

The referral of a patient for a consultation with a cardiologist is frequent prior to surgery. Most surgical procedures are performed in adults who are, by virtue of their age and other prevalent factors, at risk for cardiac disease at the time of surgery (Fig. 8–1).[1] Management of cardiac conditions, therefore, represents a significant portion of the medical care of the surgical patient. Yet, many consultations result in no meaningful alterations in management and ultimately appear to have been unnecessary. Are these consultations unwarranted, or does good practice indicate that subspecialists should closely follow patients at risk in order to intervene in the event of an untoward development? When should an anesthesiologist or surgeon consult with a cardiologist?

This chapter outlines the information that can be provided

by a cardiac assessment and, specifically, by the cardiologist. Information pertaining to preoperative risk assessment and perioperative cardiac management is reviewed. Guidelines for appropriate utilization of the cardiology consultant are also developed. In our opinion, no consultant can "clear" a patient for surgery. The decision to undergo a surgical procedure is made by the patient and the surgeon. The risks and benefits of surgery already will have been weighed before a consultant is called in. The cardiologist asked to evaluate a surgical patient may provide a variety of services, but applying a "stamp of approval" (i.e., clearance) that the patient (or the patient's heart) will safely endure the proposed procedure is not one of them. As is detailed subsequently, a cardiologist may clarify the extent of disease, make recommendations for additional

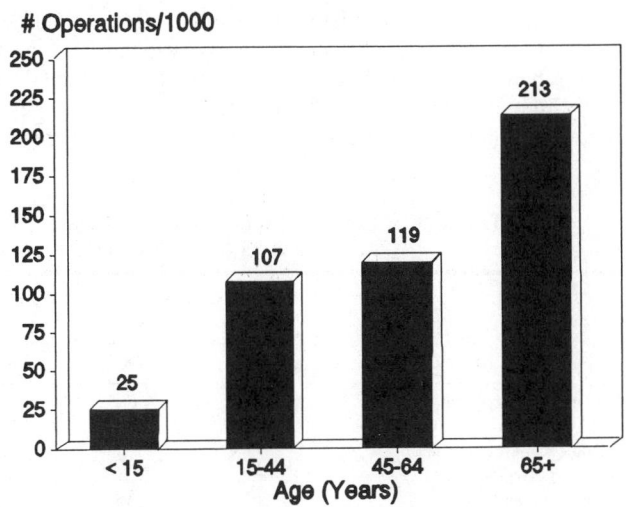

FIGURE 8–1. Prevalence of coronary artery disease (CAD) in four age groups in 1988 *(left panel)*, and the number of surgical operations performed in 1988 *(right panel)*. (From Mangano DT: Perioperative cardiac morbidity. Anesthesiology 1990; 72:155, 157.)

evaluation, assist in the management of known disease to optimize a patient's condition before, during, and following a surgical procedure, or assist in the evaluation and management of an acute problem. At all phases, open communication, preferably by direct discussion and in addition to review of complete chart notes, is the best policy for ensuring optimal patient care.

CARDIAC RISK FACTORS

How Are They Categorized?

Perioperative Myocardial Infarction Mortality

An extensive experience of over 30,000 patients undergoing general anesthesia for noncardiac surgery at the Mayo Clinic in 1967 and 1968 was reported by Tarhan and coworkers.[2] They also found that 6.6% of patients with evidence of previous myocardial infarction (MI) developed reinfarction compared with only 0.13% of patients without prior infarction. The death rate for patients developing a postoperative MI was 62% and was not higher among those with previous MI. Two other important observations emerged from this landmark study: (1) MIs were most prevalent on the third postoperative day; and (2) patients operated on within 3 months of preceding MI had the highest reinfarction rate (37%) compared with a reinfarction rate of 16% if the operation was within 3 to 6 months, and 4% to 5% if it was >6 months previously.[2]

A follow-up series of patients undergoing surgery a decade later (1974 and 1975) was reported by the same group and demonstrated a reduction in incidence of postoperative MI to 6.1% in patients who had previous MI.[3] The death rate from suffering postoperative reinfarction, however, remained high at 69%. Yet, the reinfarction incidence if the operation was within 3 months of previous infarction had declined to 27%, and was 11% if the previous infarction had occurred between 3 and 6 months. The report of Rao and associates from 1983 confirmed both a marked increase in risk of reinfarction with previous MI and a high mortality due to perioperative MI.[4]

Noncardiac Vascular Surgery

Among surgical procedures, noncardiac vascular surgery has been demonstrated to produce an exceptional risk for cardiac ischemic events and death. Early experience at the Cleveland Clinic determined that 45% of deaths after elective repair of an abdominal aortic aneurysm were due to MI, as were 67% of deaths after lower extremity revascularization utilizing the aorta. Early mortality was 2.9% for patients with no clinical indication of coronary artery disease but 9.5% for those with documented symptoms or events.[5] Hertzer and colleagues determined that only 8% of patients referred for noncardiac vascular surgery have normal coronary arteries as demonstrated by angiography (Table 8–1).[5] At the time of this assessment, 25% of patients studied were found to have severe, correctable coronary artery disease and were referred for coronary artery bypass surgery. No patients in this study were treated with coronary angioplasty. Higher percentages of severe coronary artery disease were noted in patients with clinically suspected disease, in patients over age 70 years, and in men (for operable disease only).

A more recent report from the Aneurysm Study Group of the Canadian Society for Vascular Surgery defined the overall mortality rate for repair of nonruptured abdominal aortic aneurysms to be 4.8%. The mortality rate for patients with no history or clinical evidence of coronary disease (not all patients underwent cardiac catheterization) was 0.8% compared with 6.2% in those with a history of MI, angina, congestive heart failure, or electrocardiogram (ECG) evidence of infarction or ischemia. Likewise, cardiac morbidity, including postoperative MI, congestive heart failure (CHF), dysrhythmia, or cardiac death, or any combination of these, occurred in 12.1% of patients without and in 26.6% of patients with clinical coronary artery disease.[6]

For this group of patients at high risk for cardiac events, MI within 6 months, remote history of CHF, and an increase in the Canadian Cardiovascular Association Classification were associated with increased risk of mortality. However, the traditional cardiac risk factors of smoking, hypertension, diabetes, and obesity were not statistically related to increased operative mortality.[6] In the same cohort of 666 patients, the mortality rate for MI occurring after abdominal aneurysm repair was 50%. Infarction was more likely in patients of advanced age, in those with a previous history of angina, or in those with a prolonged aortic cross-clamp time.[7]

How Can Cardiac Risk Be Assessed?

Cooperman's Equation

A number of strategies have been developed to attempt to quantify preoperatively an individual patient's cardiac risk for the planned surgical procedure. Cooperman and colleagues developed an equation for use in peripheral vascular patients

TABLE 8–1. Extent of Coronary Artery Disease, According to Type of Primary Peripheral Vascular Diagnosis in 1000 Patients Undergoing Routine Preoperative Catheterization

Coronary Artery Disease	Abdominal Aortic Aneurysm		Lower Extremity Ischemia		Cerebrovascular Disease		Other		Total	
	No.	%	No.	%	No.	%	No.	%	No.	%
None; normal coronary arteries	16	6	38	10	27	9	4	7	85	8
Mild to moderate (<70% stenosis)	77	29	125	33	94	32	21	34	317	32
Advanced "compensated"*	77	29	111	29	80	27	21	34	289	29
Severe, correctable	81	31	79	21	77	26	14	23	251	25
Severe, inoperable†	12	5	28	7	17	6	1	2	58	6

(Modified from Hertzer NR, Beven EG, Young JR, et al: Coronary artery disease in peripheral vascular patients. Ann Surg 1984; 199:227.)
*"Compensated" = >70% stenosis of at least one vessel, but myocardium supplied by collaterals or myocardium already scarred.
†Inoperable = diffuse, distal diseases, or generalized ventricular impairment.

based on preoperative risk factors.[8] Angina, dysrhythmias, carotid bruits, prior stroke, serum cholesterol level >300 mg · dL^{-1}, triglyceride level >150 mg · dL^{-1}, fasting glucose level >110 mg · dL^{-1}, 2-hour postprandial glucose level >120 mg · dL^{-1}, hypertension, previous MI, CHF, smoking, syphilis, and transient ischemic attacks were analyzed for significance by chi-squared testing. Only CHF, MI, cerebral vascular accident (CVA), ECG abnormalities, angina, and dysrhythmia were significantly associated with outcome and were then included in the following probability equation:

$$\text{Cooperman equation: } P_{complication} = \\ \text{antilog}_2 (c_1x_1 + c_1x_2 + \ldots + c)$$

where x_1 = angina, c_1 = 0.46, x_2 = CHF, c_2 = 1.02, x_3 = dysrhythmia, c_3 = 0.62, x_4 = MI, c_4 = 0.64, x_5 = CVA, c_5 = 1.15, x_6 = abnormal ECG, c_6 = 1.25, and c = −3.81.[8]

For example, a patient with CHF (controlled), prior CVA, abnormal ECG, and no previous MI, angina, or dysrhythmia would have a probability of 68% of experiencing a postoperative cardiac event. When applied retrospectively to a group of 450 patients with 37 postoperative deaths, 23 of which were due to cardiovascular complications, the equation accurately predicted complications throughout the range of risk and reliably separated very-high- and very-low-risk patients.[8]

American Society of Anesthesiologists Physical Status Classification

Several other careful risk assessments have been performed. The earliest classification attempt is the physical status scale developed by Dripps as a modification of the American Society of Anesthesiologists (ASA) physical status scale. In a study designed to assess the role of spinal or general anesthesia in surgical death, the number of deaths were related directly to worsening physical status (modified 1 through 5 scale). No deaths occurred in Physical Status Classification 1 patients, 4 of 87 (5%), whereas mortality was 5% in class 5.[9] The Classification of Physical Status was later revised by the ASA in 1963 into the current format (Table 8–2).[10] Vacanti and coworkers subsequently validated the predictive capability of the Physical Status scale in 58,078 surgical procedures.[11]

Goldman's Cardiac Risk Index

The most widely known of the preoperative cardiovascular risk assessments is the scale developed by Goldman and associates.[12] In a retrospective analysis of 1001 patients, several

factors correlated with postoperative cardiac death in multivariate analysis: MI in the previous 6 months; a third heart sound; jugular venous distention in the immediately preoperative period; >5 premature ventricular beats per minute documented at any time preoperatively; rhythm other than sinus, or premature atrial contractions on preoperative ECG; age >70 years; significant valvular aortic stenosis (assessed clinically); emergency operation; and a ≥33% fall in systolic blood pressure for >10 minutes intraoperatively. They also noted no association of mortality with traditional cardiac risk factors (smoking, glucose intolerance, hyperlipidemia, peripheral vascular disease, angina, and distant MI). A "Cardiac Risk Index" was developed from the multivariate predictors; the Index assigns a maximum of 53 points for the 9 independent risk factors previously identified (Tables 8–3 and 8–4).[13]

The Goldman Cardiac Risk Index has been validated in a prospective study of over 1100 patients by Zeldin.[14] Zeldin found that the risk of complications was markedly increased between classes 3 and 4 compared with that in classes 1 and 2. Patients in class 4 had an 8-fold higher risk of life-threatening cardiac events and a 20-fold increased risk of cardiac death; 43% of cardiac deaths occurred in class 4 patients.[14]

TABLE 8–3. Goldman's Multifactorial Cardiac Risk Index

		Points
History	Myocardial infarction within 6 mo	10
	Age over 70 y	5
Physical examination	S3 gallop or jugular venous distention	11
	Important aortic stenosis	3
Electrocardiogram	Rhythm other than sinus or sinus plus APBs* on last preoperative electrocardiogram	7
	More than 5 premature ventricular beats per minute at any time preoperatively	7
Poor general medical status	Pao$_2$ <60 mm Hg, Paco$_2$ >50 mm Hg, K$^+$ <3.0 mEq · L^{-1}, HCO$_3^-$ <20 mEq · L^{-1}, BUN >50 mg · dL^{-1} (18 mmol · L^{-1}), Creatinine >3 mg · dL^{-1} (260 mmol · L^{-1}), abnormal SGOT, signs of chronic liver disease, patient bedridden from noncardiac causes	3
Intraperitoneal, intrathoracic, or aortic surgery		3
Emergency operation		4
	Total:	53

(Reprinted from Goldman L, Caldera D, Nussbaum SR, et al: Multifactorial index of cardiac risk in non-cardiac surgical procedures. N Engl J Med 1977; 197:848, by permission of the New England Journal of Medicine.)
*APB = atrial premature beat.

TABLE 8–2. Classification of Physical Status*

Class	Description
1	A normal healthy patient
2	A patient with mild systemic disease
3	A patient with a severe systemic disease that limits activity but is not incapacitating
4	A patient with an incapacitating systemic disease that is a constant threat to life
5	A moribund patient not expected to survive 24 h with or without operation

(From American Society of Anesthesiologists, Inc: New Classification of Physical Status. Anesthesiology 1963; 24:111.)
*In the event of an emergency operation, precede the number with the letter "E."

TABLE 8–4. Prediction of Perioperative Cardiac Complications by Points in the Goldman Index

	Point Total	Cardiac Death (%)	Other Life-Threatening Complications* (%)
Class I	0–5	0.2	0.7
Class II	6–12	2.0	5.0
Class III	13–25	2.0	11.0
Class IV	≥26	56.0	22.0

(Reprinted from Goldman L, Caldera D, Nussbaum SR, et al: Multifactorial index of cardiac risk in non-cardiac surgical procedures. N Engl J Med 1977; 197:848, by permission of the New England Journal of Medicine.)
*Nonfatal MI, CHF, and ventricular tachycardia.

TABLE 8–5. Detsky's Multifactorial Index

Coronary artery disease	MI within 6 mo	10
	MI more than 6 mo previously	5
	Canadian Cardiovascular Society Angina:	
	Class III	10
	Class IV	20
Alveolar pulmonary edema	Within 1 wk	10
	Ever	5
Valvular disease	Suspected critical aortic stenosis	20
Arrhythmias	Rhythm other than sinus or sinus plus APBs on last preoperative electrocardiogram; more than 5 premature ventricular contractions at any time prior to surgery	5
Poor general medical status*		5
Age over 70 y		5
Emergency operation		10

(From Detsky AS, Abrams HB, McLaughlin JR, et al: Predicting cardiac complications in patients undergoing non-cardiac surgery. J Gen Intern Med 1986; 1:213.)
*Pao_2 <60 mm Hg, $Paco_2$ >50 mm Hg, K^+ <3.0 mEq · L^{-1}, HCO_3^- <20 mEq · L^{-1}, BUN >50 mg · dL^{-1} (18 mmol · L^{-1}), creatinine >3 mg · dL^{-1} (260 mmol · L^{-1}), abnormal SGOT, signs of chronic liver disease, patient bedridden from noncardiac causes.

Jeffrey and colleagues also carried out a prospective evaluation of the Goldman Cardiac Risk Index but in a much smaller number of patients undergoing abdominal aortic surgery.[15] They found that patients in classes 2 and 3 did have a higher incidence of cardiac complications, but that even patients in class 1 undergoing elective aortic surgery experienced a 7% incidence of cardiac events, including MI, pulmonary edema, ventricular tachycardia, and death.

Detsky's Multifactorial Index

Detsky and colleagues developed a modified cardiac risk index stratified by the type of planned surgery (Table 8–5).[16] Their modification takes into account the impact of a specific surgical procedure on the increase in perioperative cardiac complications. The likelihood ratios presented in Table 8–6 convert a given pretest probability of complications rate for patients undergoing a particular surgical procedure into the post-test probability, or change in risk based on the points assigned by the Detsky Index. Thus, although it does not represent a simple percentage of events experienced by patients in a given risk class, a likelihood ratio of >1 denotes an incremental increase in risk over the pretest probability that a high point score imparts to a given procedure.[16] Freeman and associates have illustrated the Bayesian analysis of risk utilizing the data presented by Detsky (Fig. 8–2).[17]

TABLE 8–6. Likelihood Ratios of Perioperative Cardiac Complications* by Points in the Detsky Index

Class (Points)	Major Surgery	Minor Surgery	All Surgery
I (0–15)	0.42	0.39	0.43
II (15–30)	3.58	2.75	3.38
III (>30)	14.93	12.20	10.60

(From Detsky AS, Abrams HB, McLaughlin JR, et al: Predicting cardiac complications in patients undergoing non-cardiac surgery. J Gen Intern Med 1986; 1:217.)
*Defined as MI pulmonary edema, ventricular tachycardia or fibrillation, new or worsening CHF, and coronary insufficiency.

What Are the Shortcomings of Cardiac Risk Assessment?

These frequently utilized indices of cardiac risk assessment appear to be most reliable in identifying those at highest risk. However, a low score does not guarantee that a patient will be free from cardiac events but merely that he or she is at lower risk. Also, the outcome for specific surgical procedures in one's own institution and differences in one's patient population must be considered in determining the applicability of a risk assessment score for an individual patient.

The reliability of each of these indices must be considered in assigning a score. The Goldman and Detsky scales utilize physical examination as the only tool for determining left ventricular function. Aortic stenosis was estimated without echocardiographic or Doppler ultrasound assessment. Auscultation of a third heart sound or observation of jugular venous distention can be missed by even experienced examiners. Quantification of left ventricular ejection fraction, especially in the presence of an abnormal ECG or chest radiograph, is a much more accurate technique for stratifying cardiac function. Left ventricular ejection fraction has been shown to accurately predict overall outcome in patients with coronary artery disease.[18, 19]

Measured ejection fraction has not been included as an independent component in multifactorial risk indices. However, evidence suggests that the degree of left ventricular dysfunction predicts outcome in noncardiac surgery. Patients enrolled in the Coronary Artery Surgery Study (CASS) Registry who underwent noncardiac procedures during the follow-up period were grouped according to their coronary disease status: group 1 had no significant coronary artery disease based on angiography; group 2 had coronary disease and had undergone coronary artery bypass surgery; and group 3 had significant coronary artery disease but had not had previous bypass surgery. Although patients were not randomly assigned to surgery in the CASS Registry, those in group 3 were found to have a higher death rate and more postoperative chest pain than did patients in the other two groups. Left ventricular wall motion scores (a higher value indicating more severe impairment) were strong indicators of operative morbidity and mortality by both univariate and multivariate analyses.[20]

The cardiac risk indices remain imperfect but useful tools for determining perioperative risk for cardiac events. Additional cardiac tests are routinely employed in determining a patient's current risk status even if the test results cannot be applied to one of the published risk scores.

Of What Value Is the Patient History?

The first and arguably most important assessment tool is the patient history. The surgeon and anesthesiologist must have a complete medical history. Occasionally, a cardiologist is able to facilitate documentation of information and to interpret a patient's current status, especially if he or she is also the primary physician. The patient's complete symptom and event record should be investigated. Cardiac symptoms, especially indicators of myocardial ischemia and CHF, should be documented as to their onset, frequency, severity, and current treatment.

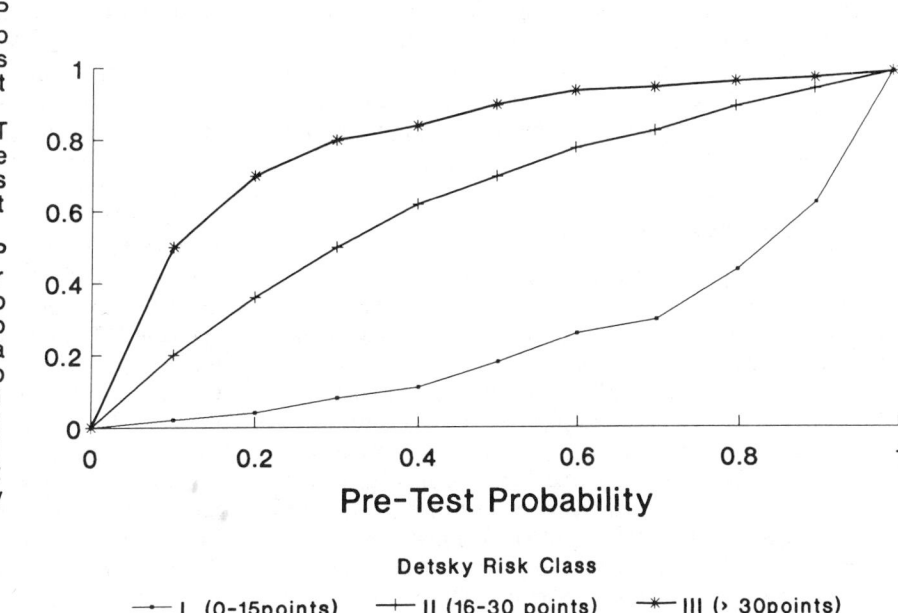

FIGURE 8–2. Bayesian analysis of perioperative cardiac risk of noncardiac surgery. Curves represent classification by the risk index of Detsky and coworkers.[16] (From Freeman WK, Gibbons RJ, Shub C: Preoperative assessment of cardiac patients undergoing noncardiac surgical procedures. Mayo Clin Proc 1989; 64:1109.)

Documentation

Prior hospitalizations, prolonged episodes of symptoms, previous diagnostic evaluations, and preceding interventions must be elicited and documented. Although patients and their families may be able to provide this information, documentation of MI in particular must be objective; many patients consider that chest pain necessitating hospitalization represents a "heart attack." Patients who relate having had five or more heart attacks most likely had episodes of unstable angina without myocardial damage.

Admittedly, documentation of previous medical history may require considerable effort. In the current age of population mobility, hospital and physican records are rarely located in one facility. Phone calls, express mail, and facsimile transmissions aid the thorough investigator. Determining that a patient has had a cardiac catheterization or two previous MIs is critical to the complete preoperative assessment. Likewise, documentation of normal coronary arteries or a negative result on a recent stress test is also very important.

Positive Historical Features

The actual contribution of positive historical features of cardiac disease is debated in the literature. In the more than 35-year period of investigation represented by the previously discussed investigations, a number of differences in practice and study methodology have evolved that explain some of their discrepant conclusions. Studies may be observational, retrospective, randomized, large-scale, utilize comparable assessment items or techniques, or use comparable statistical methods; all of these possibilities contribute to the difficulty in comparing multiple studies.[1] Although most studies confirmed that documented MI within 6 months predicts increased risk,[2, 5, 12, 21, 22] some did not.[4, 20] MI occurring earlier than 6 months previously seems to impart less risk, with an average 6% cardiac event rate.[1, 12] However, some authors have not demonstrated a significant decreased risk for perioperative infarction[12] or operating morbidity and mortality[20] after 6 months.

Clinical Prevalence

The description of typical exertional angina in middle-aged men and older women is highly predictive of coronary artery stenosis in at least one vessel.[23] However, its value as a preoperative risk factor is debatable. In fact, Goldman and associates reported that stable angina was a "conspicuously insignificant" predictor of perioperative risk.[13] Inability to quantitate severity of coronary disease from a subjective report of even typical angina may explain some of the difficulty in determining the impact of this intuitively important risk factor. It should also be pointed out that an assessment of the severity or instability of angina pattern has yet to be thoroughly studied as a predictor of operative outcome.

Is the Preoperative Electrocardiogram Valuable?

Performance of routine 12-lead ECGs in an ambulatory, healthy population is of little value in medical decision-making.[24] The proportion of patients with abnormal resting ECGs depends on age, presence of hypertension, underlying cardiac disease, and other medical conditions. In a large-scale epidemiologic study of men and women aged 18 to 65 years, 55% had completely normal tracings, but 20% of women and 9% of men had ST depression.[25] In a hypertensive population, only 41.1% had normal ECGs, whereas signs of left ventricular hypertrophy were present in 21.3% of males and 14.6% of females. Again, ischemic ST-T changes were found more frequently in females (18.1% compared with 5.7% in men).[26]

In the setting of a general hospital, routine preoperative ECG results were positive in 7.4% of patients over age 40 years and in only 4.5% under age 40 years. When ECGs were performed in the context of an abnormal physical finding or positive history, 31% were abnormal.[27] McCleane and McCoy also reported that routine preoperative ECGs were more likely to be abnormal with increasing age and with class 2 or higher ASA Physical Status Classification. In a population of 877 patients, 45% of ECGs were abnormal.[28] Despite a 42.7%

incidence of abnormal ECGs in another study of 751 preoperative ambulatory surgery patients, only 12 adverse cardiac events occurred perioperatively (1.6%).[29] The authors felt that the preoperative ECG was not predictive of cardiac complications and was rarely of clinical value in patients appropriate for ambulatory surgery.[29]

Findings That Predict Morbidity

The bulk of reported evidence and the majority of clinical experience substantiate the lack of utility of the routine preoperative ECG. Yet, abnormal rhythm[8, 12, 13, 20] and other findings, such as bundle branch block, Q wave infarctions, ST shifts, and left axis deviation,[30, 31] predict cardiovascular morbidity and mortality. Questions that remain unanswered and prevent development and implementation of widespread guidelines for obtaining ECGs are, (1) Will management be altered after identifying an ECG abnormality? (2) Does any altered management based on an ECG abnormality reduce the risk of perioperative morbidity and mortality? and (3) Does selected ordering of ECGs reduce the unnecessary testing without sacrificing risk stratification information?

Without large-scale randomized clinical trials to answer these questions, prudence indicates identification of populations within individual medical centers in whom preoperative ECGs will be performed. These might include patients undergoing major abdominal, thoracic, or aortic procedures; patients over age 40 years who have not had a previous baseline ECG; patients with known or suspected cardiac disease; and patients with abnormal physical findings, such as irregular heart beats. The healthy, active, younger patient undergoing low-risk procedures has a low likelihood of having an abnormal ECG and an even lower probability of having an underlying cardiac condition that is both diagnosable by ECG and serious enough to alter perioperative management.

Facsimile-Transmitted Electrocardiograms

The quality of an electrocardiographic tracing is occasionally called into question, especially when outlying surgical centers utilize facsimile transmission of data and ECGs. In our experience, a facsimile tracing is usually of adequate quality to permit accurate interpretation. This general perception may not hold in the event of a dysrhythmia, in which P wave assessment may be difficult with a poor-quality tracing. A questionably abnormal ECG that requires review by a cardiologist can be repeated or the original tracing examined.

Are Routine Preoperative Chest Radiographs Valuable?

The rationale for performing routine preoperative chest radiographs has more basis in intuition than in documentation. Observational studies have demonstrated that preoperative radiographs have little impact on patient management or outcome, whether they are obtained in high-risk vascular patients[32] or in younger patients undergoing elective surgery.[33] In addition, misleading radiographic findings can lead to additional diagnostic studies, delays in surgery, and even inappropriate treatments, such as the beginning of therapy for tuberculosis because of unexplained parenchymal findings.[32]

In 1979, a large study based in England found that there exists no rational approach to the ordering of preoperative chest films.[34] Guidelines suggested from that study subsequently were evaluated in a prospective study of 3883 patients undergoing general, orthopedic, plastic, gynecologic, and obstetric surgical procedures.[35] Only 9% of abnormal findings were felt to have an impact on surgical and anesthetic plans when outcomes were carefully evaluated. The major cardiac abnormality detected on routine radiographs is cardiac enlargement that is seen increasingly with older age (Fig. 8–3). However, this finding occurred most commonly in patients with known cardiac or hypertensive disease and did not alter management.[35] The series of Foster and coworkers found that cardiomegaly predicts perioperative complications,[20] whereas that of Goldman and associates did not.[12] Parenthetically, and worthy of note, no lung cancers were detected in the study of Charpak and colleagues.[35]

Based on available information, selective rather than routine preoperative chest radiographic screening is recommended. The criteria established by Charpak and colleagues (Table 8–7)[35] are recommended by some.[33] McKee and Scott recommend the study in patients who are older than 60 years of age who are to undergo major surgery.[36]

Is Exercise Testing Useful?

Preoperative exercise ECG testing has been utilized with some success as a screening tool for coronary artery disease. Cutler and coworkers demonstrated that vascular surgery patients with a positive study had a 37% incidence of postoperative MI.[37] Patients at highest risk were those who achieved less than 75% of predicted maximum heart rate and had ST segment depression >1 mm at peak exercise. Conversely, patients who were able to exercise to over 75% of their predicted maximum heart rate and also had no exercise-induced ECG changes had no mortality.[37]

In a population including patients other than those needing vascular procedures, Carliner and associates found that ECG findings, but not exercise stress test results, predicted postoperative cardiac complications by multivariate analysis.[31] However, patients unable to exercise beyond 5 METs (one metabolic [MET] unit = 3.5 mL of oxygen uptake $\cdot$ kg^{-1} $\cdot$ min^{-1}) or those found to have an abnormal exercise ECG were more likely to have postoperative cardiac complications.

McPhail and coworkers reported that during exercise treadmill testing, failure to obtain 85% of the predicted maximum heart rate identified patients who had a cardiac complication rate that was four times greater than that of patients achieving adequate exercise heart rates (24.3% versus 6.6%).[38] A significant relationship was demonstrated between either maximum heart rate or METs at peak exercise and the probability of developing a postoperative cardiac complication (Fig. 8–4).[39] Unfortunately, 70% of the 101 patients in the study were unable to achieve 70% of maximum predicted heart rate. Although ECG stress testing can be useful in patients undergoing high-risk vascular surgery, it has limited applicability in the patients at highest risk because these patients are not able to achieve adequate levels of exercise.

When Is Stress Testing Indicated?

Thallium Scintigraphy

When used for the diagnosis of coronary artery disease, exercise testing with thallium scintigraphy generally improves

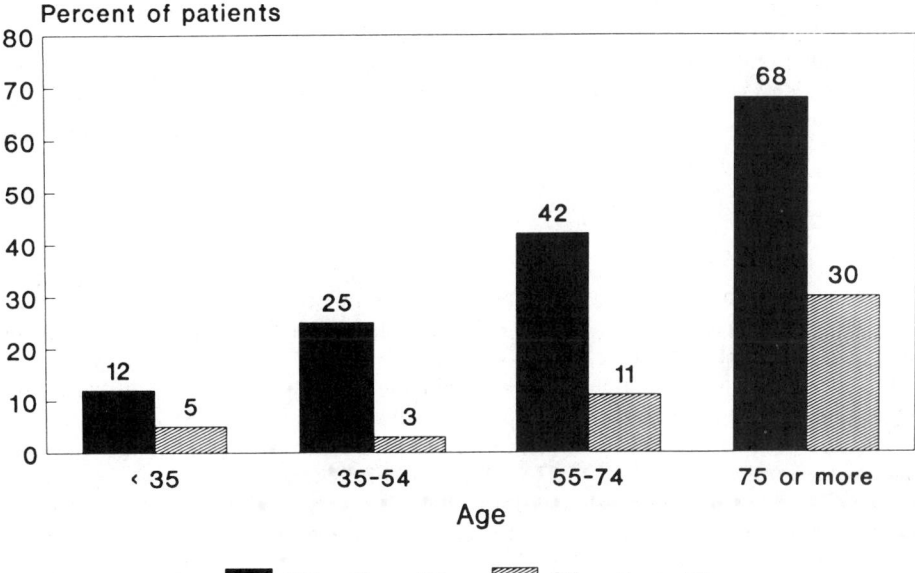

FIGURE 8–3. Frequency of finding cardiac enlargement on preoperative chest x-rays in patients grouped by age. (Data from Charpak Y, Blery C, Chastang C, et al: Prospective assessment of a protocol for selective ordering of preoperative chest x-rays. Can J Anaesth 1988; 35:262.)

sensitivity and specificity compared with exercise ECG testing alone. In one review, the average reported sensitivity for exercise thallium scintigraphy was 84%, and the specificity was 87%.[39] When an exercise test is believed to be indicated and the patient has an abnormal resting ECG, or when information regarding the probability of viability of apparently infarcted myocardial regions is needed, thallium scanning clearly is the preferred technique.[40] However, thallium scintigraphy has not been combined routinely with exercise testing preoperatively, undoubtedly because of the emergence of nonexercise, pharmacologic methods of inducing myocardial ischemia with agents such as dipyridamole, dobutamine, and adenosine.

Pharmacologic Methods

The first major report of preoperative thallium imaging and intravenous dipyridamole to induce maximum coronary vasodilation (thus enhancing the relative lack of blood flow in stenotic arteries) included 54 patients with suspected coronary artery disease. Eight of 48 patients (17%) who underwent elective peripheral vascular surgery without preoperative coronary angiography suffered ischemic cardiac complications. The finding of a redistribution abnormality was highly predictive of a postoperative cardiac ischemic event (all patients who had complications were noted to have redistribution perfusion defects).[41] No ischemic events occurred in patients with persistent defects only on the preoperative scan. This finding is consistent with prior MI but no inducible ischemia.

TABLE 8–7. Recommendations for Preoperative Chest X-Ray

Lung disease
Cardiovascular disease
Known malignant disease
Major surgical emergencies
Current smoking history in patients over age 50 y
Immunodepression (malnutrition, steroid treatment, chemotherapy)
Lack of prior health examination in immigrants

(From Charpak Y, Blery C, Chastang C, et al: Prospective assessment of a protocol for selective ordering of preoperative chest x-rays. Can J Anaesth 1988; 35:259.)

Lette and coworkers found a significant correlation between indices of severity and the extent of coronary artery disease found by intravenous dipyridamole thallium testing and the occurrence of postoperative events, even in patients undergoing nonvascular surgery.[42] However, they found no statistical association between clinical features, the Dripps-ASA class, or the Goldman Cardiac Risk Index and postoperative cardiac events.[42]

Oral administration of dipyridamole was found to be effec-

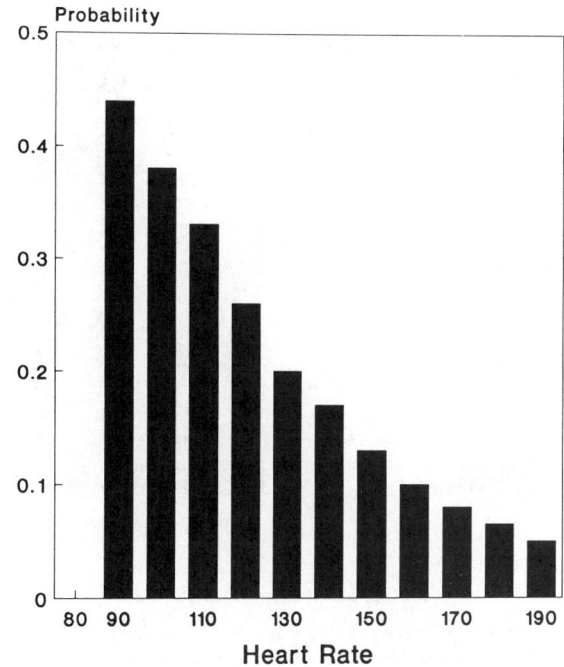

FIGURE 8–4. Relationship, by logistic regression, of maximum heart rate obtained by exercise testing to the probability of postoperative cardiac complications (defined as acute myocardial infarction, acute congestive heart failure, ventricular tachycardia or fibrillation, or cardiac death.) (Modified from McPhail N, Calvin JE, Shariatmadar A, et al: The use of preoperative exercise testing to predict cardiac complications after arterial reconstruction. J Vasc Surg 1988; 7:63.)

tive in inducing perfusion defects and to correlate with angiographically detected coronary artery disease.[43] At least one report found oral dipyridamole testing to be accurate in identifying patients at high risk for cardiac complications after vascular surgery.[44]

Relative Merits

In a comparison of pharmacologic stress and thallium scanning with exercise testing, McPhail and coworkers showed that exercise treadmill testing alone had a poor sensitivity (23%) in predicting cardiac complications; thallium scanning had much greater sensitivity (86%).[45] Despite reports that thallium imaging is superior to clinical predictors, Eagle and associates suggested that the combination of ECG Q waves, a history of ventricular ectopy, diabetes mellitus, age >70 years, or angina with the thallium results was most sensitive for the prediction of cardiac risk in vascular surgery patients.[46] They advise first identifying the pertinent clinical risk indicators. If none are present, no further testing is recommended. If one or two clinical variables are present, dipyridamole thallium redistribution identifies a high-risk patient subset (Fig. 8–5). The risk of MI or cardiac death in patients with three or more clinical features was 50%; thallium scanning did not distinguish further risk.[46]

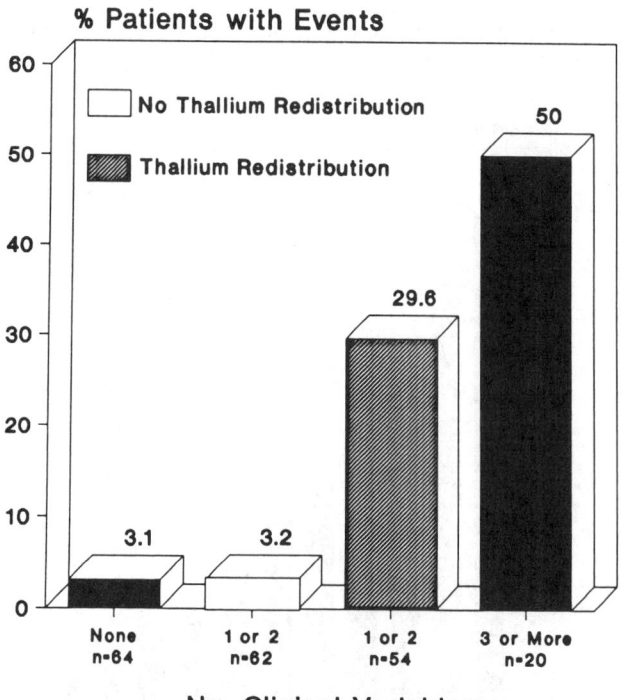

% Patients with Events

☐ No Thallium Redistribution
▨ Thallium Redistribution

	None n=64	1 or 2 n=62	1 or 2 n=54	3 or More n=20
value	3.1	3.2	29.6	50

No. Clinical Variables

FIGURE 8–5. Risk of postoperative cardiac events (defined as cardiac death, acute nonfatal myocardial infarction, unstable angina pectoris, and acute ischemia-related pulmonary edema) as assessed by clinical variables (Q wave on ECG, age >70 years, history of angina, history of ventricular ectopic activity requiring treatment, and diabetes mellitus requiring treatment). Results of dipyridamole thallium imaging is displayed only for patients with one or two clinical variables. (Data from Eagle KA, Coley CM, Newel JB, et al: Combining clinical and thallium data optimizes preoperative assessment of cardiac risk before major vascular surgery. Ann Intern Med 1989; 110:863.)

How Is the Vascular Surgery Patient Assessed?

The strategy of complete clinical assessment guiding additional myocardial testing in the vascular patient has been further refined by Wong and Detsky.[47] Like Eagle and associates, Wong and Detsky recommend thallium testing for patients at intermediate risk for postoperative cardiac events (Fig. 8–6). Intermediate risk is defined as the presence of one or two of Eagle and associates' clinical markers[46] or as the patient's inability to walk two blocks without developing angina. Patients falling into either low-risk or high-risk categories by clinical assessment could proceed with surgery or undergo catheterization without thallium scanning. This algorithm, including decisions based on ability to walk and the recommendations for invasive monitoring, has not been validated.[47] Nonetheless, the practical application of clinical risk assessment in combination with selected additional testing serves as a logical guideline for approaching the vascular surgical patient. Whether additional myocardial testing, including pharmacologic stress testing, should be undertaken in patients undergoing nonvascular procedures has not been addressed widely. However, Younis and associates studied a group of 131 patients, 20 of whom underwent nonvascular surgery.[48] Reversible dipyridamole thallium scanning defects were the strongest predictors of late (24-month) cardiac complications in addition to those that occurred in the immediate perioperative course.[48]

Contrary to the report of a composite sensitivity of 85% and specificity of 91% for coronary artery disease using dipyridamole scintigraphy,[49] Mangano and colleagues found that thallium redistribution did not predict adverse cardiac events in 7 of 13 patients undergoing elective vascular surgery.[50] When continuous 12-lead ECG and transesophageal echocardiographic monitoring of wall motion were used to detect ischemia, no correlation between thallium redistribution defects and ischemia was found.[50] Thus, thallium imaging may not be as potent a predictor of risk as was hoped. The relatively small sample size of most studies undoubtedly predisposes to discrepant findings. Likewise, differences in the definition of end points and imaging techniques contribute to the difficulty in comparing findings across study populations.[51]

What Is the Role for Echocardiography?

Thallium scintigraphy is not the only noninvasive method for assessing stress-induced myocardial dysfunction. Echocardiography is a reliable method for assessing left ventricular wall motion and has been used with exercise[52, 53] to demonstrate changes in wall motion that are indicative of myocardial ischemia. Dipyridamole has also been successfully employed as a pharmacologic stressor for the echocardiographic detection of wall motion changes in patients with suspected coronary artery disease.[53] As with thallium scanning, the improved sensitivity achieved with cardiac imaging makes echocardiography an attractive addition to the preoperative evaluation of the high-risk patient.

Tischler and coworkers demonstrated that the appearance of a new regional wall motion abnormality or worsening of pre-existing wall motion abnormalities successfully predicted major postoperative cardiac events. Seven of 9 patients with new or worsening wall motion defects had MIs, unstable angina,

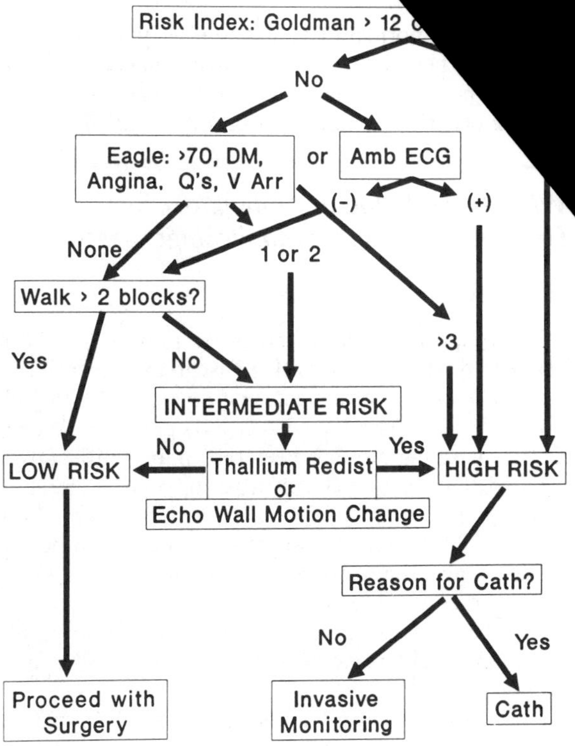

Risk Index: Goldman > 12

FIGURE 8–6. Suggested algorithm for stratifying cardiac risk before surgery. DM = Diabetes mellitus requiring treatment; Q = Q waves on ECG; V Arr = ventricular ectopic activity requiring treatment; Amb = ambulatory; Redist = redistribution defect; cath = cardiac catheterization and coronary angiography. (Modified with permission from Wong T, Detsky AS: Preoperative cardiac risk assessment for patients having peripheral vascular surgery. Ann Intern Med 1992; 116:751.)

pulmonary edema, or died. Only one such event occurred in 100 patients without positive echocardiographic findings.[54]

Recently, dobutamine also was shown to be a useful pharmacologic stress agent for detecting myocardial ischemia with echocardiography.[55, 56] Lalka and associates found that patients demonstrating new or worsening wall motion abnormalities with intravenous dobutamine infusion (to a peak dose of 50 $\mu g \cdot kg^1 \cdot min^{-1}$) had a 29% incidence of postoperative cardiac events in contrast with only a 4.6% incidence in patients without an abnormal test result.[57]

How Is the "Right" Test Chosen?

The choice of noninvasive preoperative myocardial testing should be made after consideration of the availability and expertise for given techniques in one's individual institution. Thallium imaging, although more often available, also is more expensive than echocardiography. However, more experience is needed for performing stress imaging studies than is commonly available in many echocardiography laboratories.

The type of stress, likewise, will be an individual choice for each institution. Intravenous dipyridamole only recently has been released for noninvestigative use. Adenosine is being used in some laboratories,[58] and dobutamine may have advantages of more closely simulating the myocardial workload produced by exercise. Unfortunately, no comprehensive comparison studies that assess the relative merits and disadvantages of each technique have been performed.

How Is Left Ventricular Function Assessed?

Gated Nuclide Ventriculography

Resting ventricular ejection fraction is a powerful predictor of prognosis in patients surviving MI.[59, 60] Left ventricular

ejection fraction obtained by gated radionuclide ventriculography (multigated angiographic [MUGA] scans) correlates directly with the perioperative infarction rate. Pasternack and coworkers reported an increased risk of perioperative MI in vascular patients (predominantly undergoing nonaortic surgery) if the preoperative ejection fraction was <35%.[61] In addition, patients with ejection fractions >55% were at very low risk, experiencing no MIs or postoperative deaths.[61] Kazmers and associates also demonstrated reduced survival in patients with low ejection fractions.[62] However, a subsequent report found no statistical difference in the incidence of postoperative cardiac events between patients with normal ejection fractions compared with those with low ejection fractions. Still, the incidence of CHF was higher in patients with lower ejection fractions.[63]

Comparison of Methods

A preliminary report compared the prognostic value of resting echocardiography, dipyridamole thallium scanning, and clinical indices for perioperative cardiac events in patients undergoing nonvascular surgery. Cardiac events were predicted only by the presence of left ventricular dysfunction found on the resting echocardiogram and by a redistribution defect on the dipyridamole thallium scan. Death, MI, unstable angina, or CHF occurred in 23% of patients. Thallium redistribution abnormalities were found in 29%, and resting global or segmental abnormalities, or both, were demonstrated by echocardiography in 48%.[64] Although the experience is varied in different centers, assessment of left ventricular dysfunction can aid in assessing operative risk. Although most studies use MUGA scans, echocardiographic assessment of ejection fraction is also reliable.[65–67] In patients who have undergone cardiac catheterization with left ventricular angiography, an additional test for ejection fraction is not necessary. Whether a

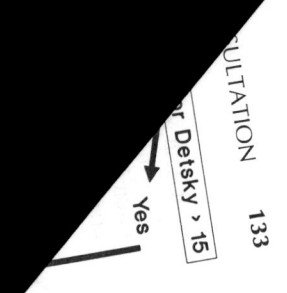

...d no history for previous cardiac ...e assessment of left ventricular ...group already is at low risk for ...perative period.

...latory ...oring?

The frequency of detectable preoperative ischemic episodes, defined by the presence of ST segment depression, ranges from 18% to 42% of patients, with up to 94% being clinically silent.[68–70] Silent ischemia detected by preoperative ambulatory ECG monitoring also has been shown to significantly increase the risk for development of a perioperative cardiac event in patients undergoing peripheral vascular surgery. In 176 patients, 12 of 32 with preoperative ischemia had postoperative events. Only 1 adverse event occurred in the 144 patients without preoperative ischemia.[71] The sensitivity of preoperative ischemia was 92%, specificity 88%, positive predictive value 38%, and negative predictive value 99% for adverse events.

These findings were replicated in another study that included both 67 vascular and 79 nonvascular surgical patients.[72] Preoperative demonstration of silent ischemia had a predictive value of 38% for postoperative cardiac events in both groups. However, absence of preoperative silent ischemia predicted an excellent outcome in nonvascular patients (99%). The negative predictive value for vascular patients was somewhat reduced but still substantial at 86%.[73]

Correlation with Postoperative Cardiac Events

Pasternack and colleagues studied 200 patients undergoing peripheral vascular surgery preoperatively (mean monitoring time = 21.2 hours), intraoperatively (mean monitoring time = 5.4 hours), and postoperatively (mean monitoring time = 38.6 hours).[73] Nearly 40% of these patients experienced intraoperative ischemia, and 50% of them had postoperative ischemia. In these patients, only preoperative ischemia and angina at rest were found to be significant predictors of perioperative MI.

Mangano and coworkers similarly monitored 474 patients preoperatively, intraoperatively, and postoperatively but found that in the 41% of patients with detectable postoperative ischemia, a 2.8-fold increase in the likelihood of a postoperative cardiac event (defined here as ischemic events, CHF, or ventricular tachycardia) was present.[74] That postoperative ischemia can lead to additional adverse cardiac events might be predicted by the known increased stresses in the immediate postoperative period.[75] Pain, changes in intravascular volume, temperature, and ventilatory status may alter the balance between myocardial oxygen supply and demand.[76] Tarhan and coworkers previously had documented the increased rate of MI by the third postoperative day.[2] Indeed, the heart rates were significantly higher in the postoperative period (90 beats per minute versus 74 and 72 beats per minute preoperatively and intraoperatively, respectively).[74]

Although these reports have identified the presence of myocardial ischemia as a predictor of perioperative cardiac risk, the definition of events and the comparative value of preoperative or postoperative ischemia detection differed. In addition, extensive, continuous ECG monitoring in patients undergoing coronary artery bypass surgery demonstrated that 52% had preoperative ST changes and 48% had postoperative ischemia. Yet, no patients with postoperative ischemia had an adverse cardiac outcome, an observation that raises questions about the clinical utility of ischemia detection.[76]

Current Role

Because of its relatively high sensitivity and low cost, continuous ECG monitoring has appeal as a cost-effective modality for assessing cardiac perioperative risks. Its use may also be limited in many evaluation proceedings because of time constraints. At present, continuous ECG monitoring should not be routinely applied for preoperative risk screening. There is not yet sufficient evidence that it can add discriminating risk stratification compared with exercise or stress testing and clinical variables. In addition, reduction in perioperative risk by reducing or eliminating ECG evidence for myocardial ischemia, either medically or by revascularization, has not been demonstrated. Clearly, additional research is needed.

When Should Cardiac Catheterization Be Performed?

Coronary angiography remains the "gold standard" for defining the anatomy of the coronary circulation; as such, it should be applied when knowledge of the extent and severity of coronary artery disease will alter planned management.[77] In most instances, cardiac catheterization is in the second tier of testing to further evaluate findings of severe ischemia by other noninvasive tests (see Fig. 8–6). Detection of regions of redistribution with stress by thallium scanning, wall motion abnormalities by stress echocardiography, prolonged episodes of ST segment depression by continuous ECG monitoring, or symptoms consistent with significant myocardial ischemia should lead to a recommendation of coronary angiography *only if coronary revascularization is anticipated.*

Not all patients are candidates for revascularization, especially through coronary artery bypass surgery. The urgency of the surgical condition may preclude such intervention, or the risk of revascularization may be felt to be unacceptably high, in which case patients may be referred for surgery with intensified perioperative monitoring. Effective risk stratification tools make routine catheterization, which had been previously advised,[78] no longer widely recommended.

When Is "Preoperative" Coronary Revascularization Indicated?

Reduction in cardiac mortality has been reported following successful coronary bypass surgery prior to major vascular or thoracic procedures.[20, 79, 80] However, the studies that gave rise to these reports have not reflected randomized, controlled trials. In addition, the morbidity and mortality of the revascularization procedure must be taken into account before it is recommended that it be performed pre-emptively to reduce the risk of the original procedure.

Coronary angioplasty is a common nonsurgical revascularization technique applied to selected stenotic coronary artery lesions in symptomatic patients.[81, 82] There has been one report that angioplasty in patients with significant anginal symptoms undergoing noncardiac surgery results in lower cardiac morbidity and mortality than had been previously reported for nonrevascularized patients.[83] However, this study was retrospective, nonrandomized, and subject to selection bias. Until an appropriate randomized clinical trial can be performed to answer whether revascularization should be performed prior to noncardiac surgery, the decision to recommend angioplasty or coronary artery bypass surgery for an individual patient can be made only after the risks and benefits of each procedure and of combined procedures have been carefully assessed.

In practice, a patient with unstable angina, defined as frequent, prolonged angina with minimal exertion or at rest despite medical therapy, should undergo cardiac catheterization, even if noncardiac surgery is not being planned. If severe multivessel or left main disease is identified, and if the patient is otherwise an acceptable candidate, coronary artery bypass surgery will be recommended if he or she has documented ischemia (as determined by ECG or imaging techniques). If single or multivessel disease is discovered and the vessels are of suitable morphology to anticipate both a high success of reducing the degree of stenosis and a low risk of morbidity and mortality, angioplasty should be performed. If significant ischemia is determined to be present by preoperative risk assessment but the patient does not have symptoms of angina, it is our practice to recommend revascularization only if significant ischemia can be demonstrated by low-level exercise or by pharmacologic stress in the region perfused by a vessel amenable to angioplasty. High-risk surgery, especially that involving the aorta (thoracic or abdominal) tends to influence the decision toward rather than against a preoperative revascularization procedure when significant coronary artery lesions are identified. This strategy is purely subjective and has not been rigorously tested, but it does reflect a practical approach to a common problem.

ASSESSMENT: THE CARDIOLOGIST'S ROLE

The patient who requires surgical intervention must be evaluated carefully by the surgeon and anesthesiologist. A complete history and physical examination combined with the review of past medical records does not usually require interpretation by a subspecialist. However, if the patient has documented cardiac disease, he or she also very likely will be under the current care of a physician who is familiar with the condition. Only if the primary physician is unaware of the planned surgical procedure, if a change in the patient's condition has occurred, or if a new question or condition has developed should specific additional consultation be requested.

The patient referred by an internist or a cardiologist who is quite stable and has already undergone previous bypass surgery but who now requires elective cholecystectomy very likely does not need and would not benefit from an additional consultation at the time of planned surgery. However, communication *is* necessary at every stage of planning and execution. If the patient does not have adequate available medical records or a recent evaluation by a medical physician, or if he or she presents for medical attention initially because of the surgical procedure, specific consultation may well be indicated. In this context, the cardiologist's role is defined in Table 8–8. The major concern is the impact of coronary artery dis-

TABLE 8–8. Role of the Cardiologist

To assess the extent and severity of any cardiac disease
To direct the diagnostic investigation
To recognize problems that may be correctable or modifiable before surgery
To identify the patient for whom the cardiac risks are so high that the benefits of the planned procedure may be outweighed
To identify the patient who might benefit from specific monitoring and management

ease on outcome; the bulk of risk assessment and management is directed toward this most prevalent condition.

How Is a Murmur Evaluated?

A cardiologist may be asked to assess the significance of a murmur or other abnormal physical finding. The patient will be approached as for any other evaluation—that is, primarily through history and physical examination. There are no universally accepted criteria for what constitutes a "significant" murmur. However, if the examining physician identifies a murmur that has not been previously diagnosed, further evaluation is probably indicated. Findings that should be referred include a systolic murmur associated with other features of significant aortic stenosis (delayed or reduced carotid upstroke, diminished aortic component of the second heart sound, palpable systolic thrill over the aortic area, radiation of the murmur to the carotids), any diagnostic murmur, and a loud holosystolic murmur, which is especially associated with a third heart sound gallop or with findings of CHF. Patients with such significant abnormal heart sounds and murmurs are best evaluated by transthoracic echocardiography. If the transthoracic echocardiogram identifies a moderately severe or severe valvular lesion, a cardiologist is required to direct further investigations, including transesophageal echocardiography, cardiac catheterization, and interventions.

Although a complete cardiologic assessment may be desired by the noncardiologist, such a request may constitute a desire for reassurance more than a true need for intervention prior to any planned surgery. We recommend that patients be evaluated by a cardiologist *after* a clinical risk assessment places the patient at intermediate or high risk by the scheme outlined in Figure 8–6 or by echocardiographic findings. Other appropriate considerations best evaluated by a cardiologist are outlined in Table 8–9.

How Is Hemodynamic Assessment Performed?

The incidence of perioperative morbidity and mortality related to ischemic heart disease is higher in the patient with known coronary artery disease, particularly in those with a previous MI. Recent reported experience suggests that aggressive monitoring and hemodynamic management of these patients may decrease the perioperative event rate. Berlauk and coworkers conducted a careful, randomized trial of hemodynamic monitoring and intervention for patients undergoing peripheral vascular reconstruction.[84] Utilizing an algorithm similar to that outlined in Figure 8–7, they found that patients successfully achieving the predetermined hemodynamic parameters as determined by pulmonary artery catheter measure-

TABLE 8–9. Patient Features Supporting Need for Cardiac Consultation

- Previously documented MI or revascularization (angioplasty or bypass surgery) without recent evaluation
- Presence of current typical angina pectoris (defined by patient description of pressure or squeezing-type precordial chest pain with exertion that radiates to the arms or neck, is relieved by rest or nitroglycerin, and is associated with sweating, nausea, or shortness of breath)
- Chest pain that has some features of angina but which may be somewhat atypical; for example, pain that is sharp but brought on by exertion; and neck or arm discomfort without any chest symptoms that is brought on by exertional or emotional stress
- History or examination consistent with CHF; in particular, evidence of recent paroxysmal nocturnal dyspnea, orthopnea, edema (with or without chest pain), physical examination evidence of pulmonary râles, gallop rhythm, hepatomegaly, jugular venous distention, or peripheral edema
- Finding of significant undiagnosed valvular disease (presence of [loud] grade 3/6 systolic murmur, any diastolic murmur, or abnormal echocardiogram), or presence of significant valvular disease or previous valve surgery
- History of rheumatic fever* (positive Jones criteria) if accompanied by a significant murmur or with abnormal echocardiogram
- History of episodic paroxysmal dysrhythmias (including unexplained syncope, supraventricular arrhythmias, or uncomfortable palpitations)
- Suspicion of congenital heart disease either based on patient history or physical examination, including evidence for right ventricular failure with parasternal heave, right-sided murmur, hepatomegaly, cyanosis, or edema
- Any patient currently taking obvious cardiac medications (e.g., long-acting nitrates, ACE inhibitors for nonhypertension indications, and digoxin) if the patient is not actively followed by a medical specialist

Jones Criteria

Major	Carditis
	Polyarthritis
	Sydenham's chorea
	Erythema marginatum
	Subcutaneous nodules
Minor	Fever
	Arthralgia
	Previous rheumatic fever* or rheumatic heart disease
	Elevated acute-phase reactants (C-reactive protein, erythrocyte sedimentation rate)
	Prolonged PR interval on electrocardiogram

(Jones Criteria from Special Writing Group of the Committee on Rheumatic Fever, Endocarditis, and Kawasaki Disease of the Council on Cardiovascular Disease in the Young of the American Heart Association: Guidelines for the diagnosis of rheumatic fever: Jones criteria, 1992 update. JAMA 1992; 268:2069. Copyright 1992, American Medical Association.)

*Diagnosis of rheumatic fever requires presence of two major or one major and two minor criteria as well as supporting evidence for preceding streptococcal infection (history of recent scarlet fever, positive throat culture for group A streptococcus, increased ASO titer or other streptococcal antibodies).

ments had fewer adverse intraoperative events, fewer cardiac complications, and less early graft thrombosis than did the patients in the control group. A trend toward fewer deaths was noted. However, no difference in outcome could be related to the duration of hemodynamic management (12 hours versus fewer than 3 hours prior to surgery).[84]

What Is the Value of Transesophageal Echocardiography?

Transesophageal echocardiography (TEE) has been applied as a myocardial monitoring tool and is particularly effective for detecting changes in regional wall motion during surgery.[85] When evaluated in conjunction with pulmonary artery occlusion pressure readings in a series of coronary artery bypass surgery patients, wall motion abnormalities were readily detected in 14 of 98 patients before or after induction of anesthe-

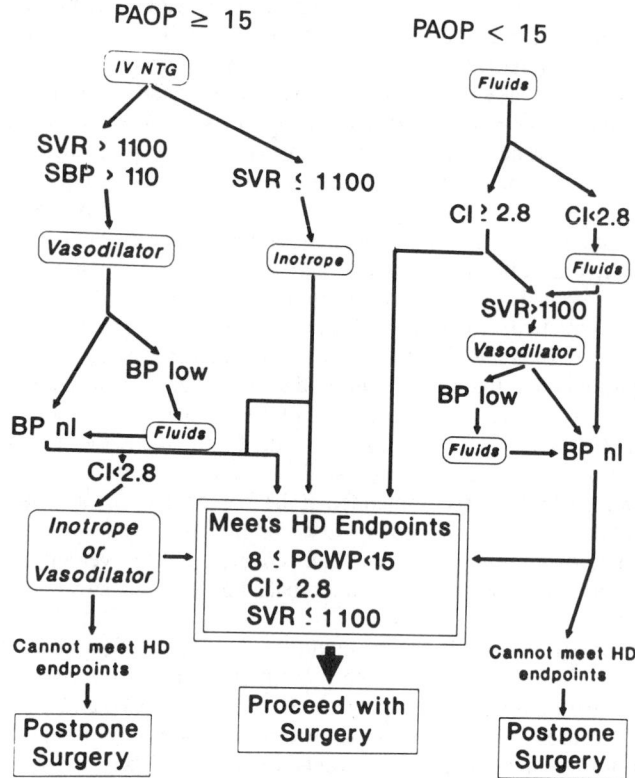

FIGURE 8–7. Algorithm for invasive preoperative cardiovascular assessment and management. Measurements are repeated after each intervention. PAOP = Pulmonary artery occlusion pressure; IV NTG = intravenous nitroglycerin; SVR = systemic vascular resistance; SBP = systolic blood pressure; CI = cardiac index; inotrope = dobutamine or dopamine; HD = hemodynamic; nl = normal. Units are mm Hg for pressure, dyne-s cm⁻⁵ for SVR, and L · min⁻¹ · m²⁻¹ for CI. Vasodilators are nitroglycerin or nitroprusside. (Modified from Berlauk JF, Abrams JH, Gilmour IJ, et al: Preoperative optimization of cardiovascular hemodynamics improves outcome in peripheral vascular surgery: a prospective, randomized clinical trial. Ann Surg 1991; 214:290.)

sia. Associated ST segment depressions were noted in 10 of these 14 patients. The pulmonary artery occlusion pressure increased by a mean of 3.5 mm Hg during ischemia, but an increase was predictive of ischemia in only 15% of patients.[86]

Although TEE has been advocated for the monitoring of high-risk surgical patients, a recent comparison between continuous ECG and TEE monitoring demonstrated a lack of concordance in ischemia detection.[87] Only a minor contribution to prediction of perioperative outcome was made with TEE compared with clinical assessment. The lack of adequate clinical trials with outcome measurements makes the routine utilization of intensive intraoperative monitoring techniques ill-advised. However, TEE is the best monitoring technique when information regarding volume status, ventricular contractility, and valvular competence is required. The more experienced the anesthesiologist, the more useful are the findings provided by any technology. Close collaboration with a cardiology expert in TEE enhances the value of myocardial assessment.

What Is the Value of Intravenous Nitroglycerin?

Intravenous nitroglycerin has been tested as an agent to reduce the consequences of perioperative myocardial ischemia.

In a small group of high-risk patients, high-dose nitroglycerin administration (≤ 1 μg · kg^{-1} · min^{-1}, mean dose = 0.91 μg · kg^{-1} · min^{-1}) resulted in few episodes of intraoperative myocardial ischemia.[88] However, other investigators could not demonstrate a benefit with lower doses of nitroglycerin.[89] Thus, convincing evidence that routine application of anti-ischemic medication clearly provides benefit to even high-risk surgical patients is lacking. Nonetheless, careful assessment of defined parameters, as developed by Berlauk and coworkers,[84] provides logical direction for guided intervention to control factors likely to produce ischemia.

How Should Patients with Suspected Valvular Heart Disease Be Managed?

The finding of a murmur suggestive of valvular heart disease during the preoperative evaluation is not unusual. However, patients with proven moderate valvular heart disease who are well compensated at rest and who have only mild limitations of activity are at very low risk of cardiac complications with surgery. In these patients, all that is needed is endocarditis prophylaxis following the American Heart Association guidelines (Tables 8–10 and 8–11).[90] However, patients with severe aortic or mitral stenosis are at increased risk of perioperative complications.

Aortic Stenosis

The clinical assessment for severe aortic stenosis is not difficult because it reveals a history of syncope, new onset of CHF, dyspnea on exertion, or angina in conjunction with the physical examination finding of a typical systolic murmur. These findings identify a patient who requires further investigation prior to surgery. The peak instantaneous valvular gradient is accurately obtained by continuous wave Doppler echocardiography using the modified Bernoulli equation[91, 92]:

TABLE 8–10. Cardiac Conditions* for Which Endocarditis Prophylaxis Recommended or Not Recommended

Recommended	Prosthetic cardiac valves, including bioprosthetic and homograft valves
	Previous bacterial endocarditis, even in the absence of heart disease
	Most congenital cardiac malformations
	Rheumatic and other acquired valvular dysfunction, even after valvular surgery
	Hypertrophic cardiomyopathy
	Mitral valve prolapse with valvular regurgitation
Not recommended	Isolated secundum atrial septal defect
	Surgical repair without residual >6 mo ago for secundum atrial septal defect, ventricular septal defect, or patent ductus arteriosus
	Previous coronary artery bypass graft surgery
	Mitral valve prolapse without valvular regurgitation†
	Physiologic, functional, or innocent heart murmurs
	Previous Kawasaki disease without valvular dysfunction
	Previous rheumatic fever without valvular dysfunction
	Cardiac pacemakers and implanted defibrillators

(From Dajani AS, Bisno AL, Chung KJ, et al: Prevention of bacterial endocarditis: recommendations by the American Heart Association. JAMA 1990; 264:2920. Copyright 1990, American Medical Association.)
*This table lists selected conditions, and is not meant to be all-inclusive.
†Individuals who have a mitral valve prolapse associated with thickening or redundancy of the valve leaflets may be at increased risk for bacterial endocarditis (particularly men 45 y of age and older).

TABLE 8–11. Dental or Surgical Procedures* for Which Endocarditis Prophylaxis Is Recommended or Not Recommended

Recommended	Dental procedures known to induce gingival or mucosal bleeding, including professional cleaning
	Tonsillectomy or adenoidectomy, or both
	Surgical operations that involve intestinal or respiratory mucosa
	Bronchoscopy with a rigid bronchoscope
	Sclerotherapy for esophageal varices
	Esophageal dilation
	Gallbladder surgery
	Cystoscopy
	Urethral dilation
	Urethral catheterization if urinary tract infection is present†
	Urinary tract surgery if urinary tract infection is present†
	Prostatic surgery
	Incision and drainage of infected tissue†
	Vaginal hysterectomy
	Vaginal delivery in presence of infection†
Not recommended‡	Dental procedures not likely to induce gingival bleeding, such as simple adjustment of orthodontic appliances or fillings above the gum line
	Injection of local intraoral anesthetic (except intraligamentary injections)
	Shedding of primary teeth
	Tympanostomy tube insertion
	Endotracheal intubation
	Bronchoscopy with inflexible bronchoscope, with or without biopsy
	Cardiac catheterization
	Endoscopy with or without gastrointestinal biopsy
	Cesarean section
	In the absence of infection: urethral catheterization, dilation and curettage, uncomplicated vaginal delivery, therapeutic abortion, sterilization procedures, or insertion or removal of intrauterine devices

(From Dajani AS, Bisno AL, Chung KJ, et al: Prevention of bacterial endocarditis: recommendations by the American Heart Association. JAMA 1990; 264:2920. Copyright 1990, American Medical Association.)
*This table lists selected procedures, and is not meant to be all-inclusive.
†In addition to prophylactic regimen for genitourinary procedures, antibiotic therapy should be directed against the most likely bacterial pathogen.
‡In patients who have prosthetic heart valves, a previous history of endocarditis, or surgically constructed systemic-pulmonary shunts or conduits, physicians may choose to administer prophylactic antibiotics, even for low-risk procedures that involve the lower respiratory, genitourinary, or gastrointestinal tracts.

$$\Delta P = 4 \, V_{max}^2$$

Although the peak instantaneous Doppler gradient is usually larger than the traditional peak-to-peak gradient recorded at the time of cardiac catheterization, simultaneous Doppler echocardiographic and catheterization studies show that the mean gradient across a stenotic aortic valve is accurately measured by both techniques.[93]

The aortic valve area also may be assessed using the continuity equation, which states that systolic flow in the left ventricular outflow tract must equal flow in the ascending aorta. Since the area in the outflow tract can be measured echocardiographically and because the velocity of flow can be measured in the outflow tract and in the aorta, the stenotic valve area can be calculated with a reported correlation coefficient of 0.95 and a standard error of the estimate of 0.15 cm^2.[94]

Patients with severe aortic stenosis tolerate tachycardia or hypotension poorly because of a relatively fixed stroke volume secondary to the stenotic valve orifice. Perfusion of the hypertrophic myocardium is also a potential problem with severe aortic stenosis when the aortic diastolic pressure is low and the left ventricular end-diastolic pressure is high. This combination of increased wall stress and concomitant increased oxygen consumption can induce cardiac ischemia.

A review by O'Keefe and associates at the Mayo Clinic showed that with careful monitoring during anesthesia, even patients with severe aortic stenosis can undergo a noncardiac operation with minimal risk of major cardiac complications.[95] For patients with severe aortic stenosis in whom aortic valve replacement is not possible, palliative percutaneous balloon valvuloplasty occasionally has been used with success by some investigators.[96, 97]

Mitral Stenosis

For patients with moderate to severe mitral stenosis, tachycardia—whatever its origin—is poorly tolerated because of the decreased diastolic filling time. Careful monitoring of rate and hemodynamic control are the keys to avoiding CHF and concomitant hypotension. Balloon mitral valvuloplasty has emerged as effective treatment for selected patients.[98, 99] For patients needing noncardiac surgery, such therapy can be considered prior to surgery. Although preoperative balloon valvuloplasty has not been reported extensively, the analogous situation in pregnancy is well described as a safe and effective treatment option.[100, 101]

Aortic and Mitral Regurgitation

The impact of valvular regurgitation on surgical morbidity and mortality has not received a great deal of attention. A complete preoperative evaluation that includes Doppler echocardiography can reliably determine the severity of regurgitant lesions. If intervention is not warranted but the lesion is of more than trivial severity, careful hemodynamic monitoring may be indicated. Afterload reduction for both mitral[102] and aortic regurgitation[103] has proved beneficial. In addition, endocarditis prophylaxis may be required (see Tables 8–10 and 8–11).[90]

Hypertrophic Obstructive Cardiomyopathy

In patients with hypertrophic obstructive cardiomyopathy, left ventricular obstruction results from excessive narrowing of the left outflow tract from the hypertrophied subaortic muscle and systolic displacement of the anterior leaflet of the mitral valve. Situations that increase cardiac contractility (e.g., sympathetic stimulation) or decrease preload (e.g., hypovolemia) increase the degree of left ventricular outflow obstruction.

Halothane, which has myocardial depressant activity and causes only a slight change in systemic vascular resistance, historically has been recommended as the primary anesthetic. The treatment of choice for hypotension is administration of phenylephrine and fluid.[104, 105] Pretreatment of these patients with β-blockers or calcium channel antagonists is now standard therapy.

In a large series of patients with hypertrophic cardiomyopathy undergoing surgery, 56 procedures were performed with no deaths and only 1 episode of perioperative CHF.[106] Therefore, the risk of operating on patients with hypertrophic cardiomyopathy appears to be very low when proper preoperative preparation and anesthetic management is undertaken.

How Is the Anticoagulated Patient with a Prosthetic Valve Managed?

The predominant question that arises in the management of patients with a prosthetic heart valve is the timing of discontinuation of anticoagulant use preoperatively. Tinker and colleagues followed 159 patients with prosthetic valves undergoing 180 noncardiac surgeries.[107] They observed no thromboembolic events when anticoagulant use was discontinued 3 days preoperatively and subsequently restarted an average of 2.5 days postoperatively.[107]

One analysis has reinforced the concept that the length of hospital stay not be increased to stop or restart anticoagulation, since the risk of thromboembolism is very low.[108] However, patients whose prosthetic valves are associated with a relatively high risk of thrombosis (Björk-Shiley mitral valves) should be hospitalized, warfarin use should be discontinued, and heparin therapy should be begun and continued until 8 hours prior to surgery. Heparin and warfarin use can then be restarted 24 hours after surgery.

POSTOPERATIVE CONSULTATION

Most major complications of cardiac morbidity and mortality arise postoperatively. MI occurring either early (within the first 24 hours) or late (3–5 days postoperatively), CHF, dysrhythmias, and hypertension are the postoperative complications most commonly requiring consultation by the cardiologist.

How Is the Diagnosis of Myocardial Infarction Made?

Strategies for diagnosing postoperative MI vary considerably. Charlson and associates systematically followed over 260 patients after noncardiac surgery to determine the most sensitive and specific approach.[109] Their recommendation is to follow all patients with preoperative abnormal resting ECGs, and those with a Goldman risk classification of 2 or 3 with both serial enzyme analysis and serial ECGs. Creatinine kinase MB enzyme analysis alone was nonspecific and was found to be confusing among asymptomatic patients with normal ECGs in whom the likelihood of ischemic coronary artery disease was extremely low. Their data also suggested that the most frequent period of MI occurrence was within the first 48 hours (non–Q wave infarctions). Classic Q wave infarctions peaked more commonly at 48 to 72 hours.[109]

How Is Congestive Heart Failure Manifested?

The majority of patients develop postoperative CHF within the first 3 days after surgery. Most are not acutely ischemic or infarctive in origin; rather, they involve relative fluid overload. Simple fluid diuresis without the addition of a cardiac inotrope is adequate therapy unless left ventricular function is compromised (i.e., left ventricular ejection fraction is <40%).

The differentiation between cardiogenic and noncardiogenic sources of pulmonary edema can be made with pulmonary artery occlusion pressure measurements and echocardiographic assessment of left ventricular function. For patients without an adequate transthoracic window for echocardiographic imaging—for example, those with chronic obstructive lung disease and lung interposition between the chest wall and thoracic structures—TEE can provide appraisal of left ventricular function.[110, 111]

How Are Postoperative Dysrhythmias Managed?

Sinus Tachycardia

The most common postoperative dysrhythmia is sinus tachycardia. Its prevalence is not in itself abnormal but rather reflects an underlying disorder such as pain, anemia, CHF, ischemia, infection, hypovolemia, hypoxia, fever, or other metabolic derangement. Therefore, pharmacologic treatment directed toward slowing the heart rate usually is not appropriate until the underlying condition is correctly diagnosed and treated. An exception to this general guideline is the patient who is tachycardic and manifesting signs of myocardial ischemia; in such a case, concomitant titration of β-blockers is a reasonable option.

Atrial Fibrillation

Atrial fibrillation can be seen in the same setting as sinus tachycardia, especially in patients with atrial dilation with associated valvular or myocardial dysfunction. Treatment of atrial fibrillation first requires control of ventricular rate with digoxin, calcium channel antagonists, or β-blockers. Many patients then undergo spontaneous conversion to sinus rhythm without further intervention. If fibrillation persists and an underlying etiology cannot be found, anticoagulation and cardioversion should be considered.[112]

Supraventricular dysrhythmias, especially atrial fibrillation and flutter, occur very commonly after coronary bypass surgery. A recent meta-analysis of treatment trials to prevent supraventricular dysrhythmias concluded that β-blockade alone was effective in preventing the dysrhythmia.[113] Digoxin, verapamil, and β-blockers were able to reduce ventricular rate in patients who developed the dysrhythmia.[113]

Another analysis concluded that the combination of digoxin and a β-blocker significantly reduced the incidence of postoperative supraventricular dysrhythmias.[114] Many clinicians do not routinely begin prophylactic medications but continue use of previously prescribed digoxin, calcium channel blockers, or β-blockers. However, consensus may be developing to begin routine prophylactic β-receptor blockade in patients with preserved left ventricular function (ejection fraction > 30%) who undergo bypass surgery.

Atrial Flutter

Atrial flutter is another common supraventricular rhythm with similar predisposing etiologies as those discussed for sinus tachycardia and atrial fibrillation. Atrial flutter may be particularly difficult to control, although treatment with digoxin, calcium channel blockers, or β-blockers effectively lowers the ventricular rate. If medical treatment fails and identifiable precipitating factors are eliminated, atrial flutter usu-

ally converts with low-energy (5–40 joules) synchronized DC cardioversion. Anticoagulation is not needed for atrial flutter without intermittent atrial fibrillation.

Premature Ventricular Contractions

Frequent ventricular ectopy or ventricular tachycardia may be a marker for ischemic heart disease. Prompt recognition and therapy to decrease potential cardiac ischemia along with evaluation for evolving MI are warranted. Recommendations for such an evaluation are shown in Table 8–12.

The appearance of such dysrhythmias necessitates an urgent investigation for metabolic factors (hypoxia, acidosis, electrolyte imbalances) or mechanical factors (central venous or pulmonary artery catheters, or pacing wires) that may precipitate them. If no other treatable factors can be identified, antidysrhythmic therapy with a type I-B agent (lidocaine) may be used. Lidocaine may also be considered for prophylactic use in the patient with a history of sustained ventricular dysrhythmias or cardiac arrest.[115]

Conduction Blocks

Patients with ECG evidence of conduction blocks, including bundle branch block or bifascicular block, do not require prophylactic pacing.[116, 117]

Should Preoperative Medications Be Altered?

Concerns about the use of some antihypertensive agents throughout surgery are largely unfounded. General guidelines suggest that current antihypertensive regimens be continued through the day of surgery and be resumed as rapidly as possible following the procedure.[118] This approach is especially important for the patient taking a preoperative β-blocker or clonidine. Beta-blockade should not be withdrawn because of concerns that myocardial ischemia may be precipitated.[119] For the patient taking preoperative clonidine in the ideal circumstances, use of this drug should either be continued according to the usual dosage schedule, or transition to nil per os status can be accommodated by switching the patient to a clonidine patch regimen. Despite the dramatically described case reports of acute rebound hypertension associated with acute clonidine withdrawal, it is a relatively rare syndrome but has also been reported in patients making the transition from oral to patch clonidine.[120, 121]

One exception to this rule is the use of angiotensin-converting enzyme inhibitors, especially enalapril. Significant hypotension following induction of anesthesia is more prevalent if use of this medication is continued through the morning of surgery.[122] Perioperative hypertension can be controlled with rapidly-acting intravenous preparations, which may include

TABLE 8–12. Initial Ventricular Arrhythmia Work-up

Electrolytes (K^+, Mg^+)
12-lead electrocardiogram
Arterial blood gas (Pao_2, $Paco_2$, pH)
Medication history
Mechanical source

ultrashort-acting esmolol or nitroprusside, depending on the clinical setting.

References

1. Mangano DT: Perioperative cardiac morbidity. Anesthesiology 1990; 72:153.
2. Tarhan S, Moffitt EA, Taylor WF, et al: Myocardial infarction after general anesthesia. JAMA 1972; 220:1451.
3. Steen PA, Tinker JH, Tarhan S: Myocardial reinfarction after anesthesia and surgery. JAMA 1978; 239:2566.
4. Rao TLK, Jacobs KH, El-Etr AA: Reinfarction following anesthesia in patients with myocardial infarction. Anesthesiology 1982; 59:499.
5. Hertzer NR, Beven EG, Young JR, et al: Coronary artery disease in peripheral vascular patients. Ann Surg 1984; 199:223.
6. Johnston KW, Scobie TK: Multicenter prospective study of nonruptured abdominal aortic aneurysms: I. Population and operative management. J Vasc Surg 1988; 7:69.
7. Johnston KW: Multicenter prospective study of nonruptured abdominal aortic aneurysms: Part II. Variables predicting morbidity and mortality. J Vasc Surg 1989; 9:437.
8. Cooperman M, Pflug B, Martin EW Jr, et al: Cardiovascular risk factors in patients with peripheral vascular disease. Surgery 1978; 84:505.
9. Dripps RD, Lamont A, Eckenhoff JE: The role of anesthesia in surgical mortality. JAMA 1961; 178:261.
10. American Society of Anesthesiologists, Inc: New classification of physical status. Anesthesiology 1963; 24:111.
11. Vacanti CJ, VanHouten RJ, Hill RC: Physical status and postop mortality. Anesth Analg 1970; 49:564.
12. Goldman L, Caldera DL, Southwick FS, et al: Cardiac risk factors and complications in non-cardiac surgery. Medicine 1978; 57:357.
13. Goldman L, Caldera D, Nussbaum SR, et al: Multifactorial index of cardiac risk in non-cardiac surgical procedures. N Engl J Med 1977; 197:845.
14. Zeldin RA: Assessing cardiac risk in patients who undergo noncardiac surgical procedures. Can J Surg 1984; 27:402.
15. Jeffrey CC, Kunsman J, Cullen DJ, et al: A prospective evaluation of cardiac risk index. Anesthesiology 1983; 58:462.
16. Detsky AS, Abrams HB, McLaughlin JR, et al: Predicting cardiac complications in patients undergoing non-cardiac surgery. J Gen Intern Med 1986; 1:211.
17. Freeman WK, Gibbons RJ, Shub C: Preoperative assessment of cardiac patients undergoing noncardiac surgical procedures. Mayo Con Proc 1989; 64:1105.
18. Mock MB, Ringqvist I, Fisher LD, et al: Survival of medically treated patients in coronary artery surgery study (CASS) registry. Circulation 1982; 66:562.
19. The Multicenter Postinfarction Research Group: Risk stratification and survival after myocardial infarction. N Engl J Med 1983; 309:331.
20. Foster ED, Davis KB, Carpenter JA, et al: Risk of noncardiac operation in patients with defined coronary disease: the coronary artery surgery study (CASS) registry experience. Ann Thorac Surg 1986; 41:42.
21. Schoeppel LS, Wilkinson C, Waters J, et al: Effects of myocardial infarction on perioperative cardiac complications. Anesth Analg 1983; 62:493.
22. Larsen SF, Oleson KH, Jacobsen E, et al: Prediction of cardiac risk in noncardiac surgery. Eur Heart J 1987; 8:179.
23. Diamond GA, Forrester JS: Analysis of probability as an aid in the clinical diagnosis of coronary artery disease. N Engl J Med 1979; 300:1350.
24. Nissan R, Encarnacion M: Clinical value of the electrocardiogram in ambulatory care. J Fam Pract 1987; 24:361.
25. Jonsson B, Astrand I: Electrocardiographic findings in men and women aged 18–65. Scand J Soc Med 1977; 5:41.
26. Zamboni S, Ambrosio BG, Bertoldero G, et al: Electrocardiograms in hypertensive subjects from a population random sample: basic characteristics and correlations with some biological variables. G Ital Cardiol 1985; 15:375.
27. Sommerville TE, Murray WB: Information yield from routine preoperative chest radiography and electrocardiography. S Afr Med J 1992; 81:190.
28. McCleane GJ, McCoy E: Routine preoperative electrocardiography. Br J Clin Pract 1990; 44:92.
29. Gold BS, Young ML, Kinman JL, et al: The utility of preoperative electrocardiograms in the ambulatory surgical patient. Arch Intern Med 1992; 152:301.
30. Rettke SR, Shub C, Naessena JM, et al: Significance of mildly elevated creatine kinase (myocardial band) activity after elective abdominal aortic aneurysmectomy. J Cardiothorac Vasc Anesth 1991; 5:425.
31. Carliner NH, Fisher ML, Plotnick GD, et al: Routine preoperative exercise testing in patients undergoing major noncardiac surgery. Am J Cardiol 1985; 56:51.
32. Tape TG, Mushlin AI: How useful are routine chest x-rays of preoperative patients at risk for postoperative chest disease? J Gen Intern Med 1988; 3:15.
33. Gagner M, Chiasson A: Preoperative chest x-ray films in elective surgery: a valid screening tool. Can J Surg 1990; 33:271.
34. National study by the Royal College of Radiologists: Preoperative chest radiology. Lancet 1979; ii:83.
35. Charpak Y, Blery C, Chastang C, et al: Prospective assessment of a protocol for selective ordering of preoperative chest x-rays. Can J Anaesth 1988; 35:259.
36. McKee RF, Scott EM: The value of routine preoperative investigations. Ann R Coll Surg Engl 1987; 69:160.
37. Cutler BS, Wheeler HT, Paraskos JA, et al: Applicability and interpretation of electrocardiographic stress testing in patients with peripheral vascular disease. Am J Surg 1981; 141:501.
38. McPhail N, Calvin JE, Shariatmadar A, et al: The use of preoperative exercise testing to predict cardiac complications after arterial reconstruction. J Vasc Surg 1988; 7:60.
39. Kotler TS, Diamond GA: Exercise thallium-201 scintigraphy in the diagnosis and prognosis of coronary artery disease. Ann Intern Med 1990; 113:684.
40. American College of Physicians Position Paper: Efficacy of exercise thallium-201 scintigraphy in the diagnosis and prognosis of coronary artery disease. Ann Intern Med 1990; 113:703.
41. Boucher CA, Brewster CD, Darling RC, et al: Determination of cardiac risk by dipyridamole-thallium imaging before peripheral vascular surgery. N Engl J Med 1985; 312:389.
42. Lette J, Waters D, Lapointe J, et al: Usefulness of the severity and extent of reversible perfusion defects during thallium-dipyridamole imaging for cardiac risk assessment before noncardiac surgery. Am J Cardiol 1989; 64:276.
43. Homma S, Callahan RJ, Ameer B, et al: Usefulness of oral dipyridamole suspension for stress thallium imaging without exercise in the detection of coronary artery disease. Am J Cardiol 1986; 57:503.
44. Makaroun MS, Shuman-Jackson N, Rippey A, et al: Cardiac risk in vascular surgery: the oral dipyridamole-thallium stress test. Arch Surg 1990; 125:1610.
45. McPhail NV, Ruddy TD, Calvin JE, et al: A comparison of dipyridamole-thallium imaging and exercise testing in the prediction of postoperative cardiac complications in patients requiring arterial reconstruction. J Vasc Surg 1989; 10:51.
46. Eagle KA, Coley CM, Newel JB, et al: Combining clinical and thallium data optimizes preoperative assessment of cardiac risk before major vascular surgery. Ann Intern Med 1989; 110:859.
47. Wong T, Detsky AS: Preoperative cardiac risk assessment for patients having peripheral vascular surgery. Ann Intern Med 1992; 116:743.
48. Younis LT, Aguirre F, Byers S, et al: Perioperative and long-term prognostic value of intravenous dipyridamole thallium scintigraphy in patients with peripheral vascular disease. Am Heart J 1990; 119:1287.
49. Beller GA: Pharmacologic stress imaging. JAMA 1991; 265:633.
50. Mangano DT, London MJ, Tubau JF, et al: Dipyridamole thallium-201 scintigraphy as a preoperative screening test: a reexamination of its predictive potential. Study of Perioperative Ischemia Research Group. Circulation 1991; 84:493.
51. Pohost GM: Dipyridamole thallium test: is it useful for predicting coronary events after vascular surgery? Circulation 1991; 84:931.
52. Limacher MC, Quinones MA, Poliner LP, et al: Detection of coronary artery disease with exercise two-dimensional echocardiography: description of a clinically applicable method and comparison with radionuclide ventriculography. Circulation 1983; 67:121.
53. Picano E, Lattanzi F, Masini M, et al: High dose dipyridamole echocardiography test in effort angina pectoris. J Am Coll Cardiol 1986; 8:848.
54. Tischler MD, Lee TH, Hirsch AT, et al: Prediction of major cardiac events after peripheral vascular surgery using dipyridamole echocardiography. Am J Cardiol 1991; 68:593.
55. Segar DS, Brown SE, Sawada SG, et al: Dobutamine stress echocardiography: correlation with coronary lesions severity as determined by quantitative angiography. J Am Coll Cardiol 1992; 19:1197.
56. Mazeika PK, Nadazdin A, Oakley CM: Dobutamine stress echocardiography for detection and assessment of coronary artery disease. J Am Coll Cardiol 1992; 19:1203.
57. Lalka SG, Sawada SG, Dalsing MC, et al: Dobutamine stress echocar-

diography as a predictor of cardiac events associated with aortic surgery. J Vasc Surg 1992; 15:831.

58. Zoghbi W, Cheirif J, Kleiman NS, et al: Diagnosis of ischemic heart disease with adenosine echocardiography. J Am Coll Cardiol 1991; 18:1271.

59. Mock MB, Ringqvist I, Fisher LD, et al: Survival of medically treated patients in the Coronary Artery Surgery Study (CASS) Registry. Circulation 1982; 66:562.

60. The Multicenter Postinfarction Research Group: Risk stratification and survival after myocardial infarction. N Engl J Med 1983; 309:331.

61. Pasternack PF, Imparato AM, Riles TS, et al: The value of the radionuclide angiogram in the prediction of perioperative myocardial infarction in patients undergoing lower extremity revascularization procedures. Circulation 1985; 72(Suppl 2):II11.

62. Kazmers A, Cerqueira MD, Zierler RE: The role of preoperative radionuclide ejection fraction in direct abdominal aortic aneurysm repair. J Vasc Surg 1988; 8:128.

63. Franco CD, Goldsmith H, Veith FJ, et al: Resting gated pool ejection fraction: a poor predictor of perioperative myocardial infarction in patients undergoing vascular surgery for infrainguinal bypass grafting. J Vasc Surg 1989; 10:656.

64. Takase B, Younis LT, Labovitz AJ, et al: Comparative prognostic value of rest two-dimensional echocardiography, dipyridamole stress thallium myocardial imaging and clinical indices for perioperative cardiac events in major nonvascular surgery patients (Abstract). JACC 1992; 19:101A.

65. Wyatt H, Heng MK, Meerbaum S, et al: Cross-sectional echocardiography: II. Analyses of mathematical models for quantifying volume of formalin-fixed left ventricle. Circulation 1980; 61:1119.

66. Folland ED, Parisi AF, Moynihan PF, et al: Assessment of left ventricular ejection fraction and volumes by real-time two-dimensional echocardiography. Circulation 1979; 60:760.

67. Starling MR, Crawford MH, Sorensen SG, et al: Comparative accuracy of apical biplane cross-sectional echocardiography and gated equilibrium radionuclide angiography for estimating left ventricular size and performance. Circulation 1981; 63:1075.

68. Knight AA, Hollenberg M, London MJ, et al: Perioperative myocardial ischemia: importance of the preoperative ischemic pattern. Anesthesiology 1988; 68:681.

69. Muir AD, Reeder MK, Foex P, et al: Preoperative silent myocardial ischaemia: incidence and predictors in a general surgical population. Br J Anaesth 1991; 67:373.

70. Mangano DT, Hollenberg M, Fegert G, et al: Perioperative myocardial ischemia in patients undergoing noncardiac surgery: I. Incidence and severity during the 4 day perioperative period. The Study of Perioperative Ischemia (SPI) Research Group. JACC 1991; 17:843.

71. Raby K, Goldman L, Creager MA, et al: Correlation between preoperative ischemia and major cardiac events after peripheral vascular surgery. N Engl J Med 1989; 321:1296.

72. Fleisher LA, Rosenbaum SH, Nelson AH, et al: The predictive value of preoperative silent ischemia for postoperative ischemic cardiac events in vascular and nonvascular surgery patients. Am Heart J 1991; 122:980.

73. Pasternack PF, Grossi EA, Baumann FG, et al: The value of silent myocardial ischemia monitoring in the prediction of perioperative myocardial infarction in patients undergoing peripheral vascular surgery. J Vasc Surg 1989; 10:617.

74. Mangano DT, Browner WS, Hollenberg M, et al: Association of perioperative myocardial ischemia with cardiac morbidity and mortality in men undergoing noncardiac surgery. N Engl J Med 1990; 323:1781.

75. Mangano DT, London MJ, Hollenberg M, et al: Predicting cardiac morbidity in surgical patients. Prim Cardiol 1992; 18:27.

76. Smith RC, Leung JM, Mangano DT: SPI Research Group: postoperative myocardial ischemia in patients undergoing coronary artery bypass graft surgery. Anesthesiology 1991; 74:464.

77. Ross J, Brandenburg RO, Dinsmore RE, et al: Guidelines for coronary angiography: a report of the ACC/AHA Task Force on Assessment of Diagnostic and Therapeutic Cardiovascular Procedures. J Am Coll Cardiol 1987; 10:935.

78. Hertzer NR, Young JR, Kramer JR, et al: Routine coronary angiography prior to elective aortic reconstruction: results of selective myocardial revascularization in patients with peripheral vascular disease. Arch Surg 1979; 114:1336.

79. Crawford ES, Morris GC Jr, Howell JF, et al: Operative risk in patients with previous coronary artery bypass. Ann Thorac Surg 1978; 26:215.

80. Mahar LJ, Steen PA, Tinker JH, et al: Perioperative myocardial infarction in patients with coronary artery disease with and without aortocoronary artery bypass grafts. J Thorac Cardiovasc Surg 1978; 76:533.

81. Ryan TJ, Faxon DP, Gunnar RM, et al: ACC/AHA Task Force Report: guidelines for a percutaneous transluminal coronary angioplasty: a report of the American College of Cardiology/American Heart Association Task Force on Assessment of Diagnostic and Therapeutic Cardiovascular Procedures (Subcommittee on Percutaneous Transluminal Coronary Angioplasty). J Am Coll Cardiol 1988; 12:529.

82. Ryan TJ: Revised ACC/AHA Task Force Guidelines for percutaneous transluminal angioplasty. J Am Coll Cardiol 1993; (in press).

83. Huber KC, Evans MA, Bresnahan JF, et al: Outcome of noncardiac operations in patients with severe coronary artery disease successfully treated preoperatively with coronary angioplasty. Mayo Clin Proc 1992; 67:15.

84. Berlauk JF, Abrams JH, Gilmour IJ, et al: Preoperative optimization of cardiovascular hemodynamics improves outcome in peripheral vascular surgery: a prospective, randomized clinical trial. Ann Surg 1991; 214:289.

85. Clemens FM, de Bruijn NP: Perioperative evaluation of regional wall motion by transesophageal two-dimensional echocardiography. Anesth Analg 1987; 66:249.

86. Van Daele ME, Sutherland GR, Mitchell MM, et al: Do changes in pulmonary capillary wedge pressure adequately reflect myocardial ischemia during anesthesia: a correlative preoperative hemodynamic, electrocardiographic, and transesophageal echocardiographic study. Circulation 1990; 81:865.

87. Eisenberg MJ, London MJ, Leung JM, et al: Monitoring for myocardial ischemia during noncardiac surgery: a technology assessment of transesophageal echocardiography and 12-lead electrocardiography. JAMA 1992; 268:210.

88. Fusciardi J, Daloz M, Coriat P, et al: Prevention of myocardial ischemia by nitroglycerin in patients with severe coronary artery disease undergoing noncardiac surgery (Abstract). Anesthesiology 1980; 53:S80.

89. Thomson IR, Mutch WAX, Culligan JD: Failure of intravenous nitroglycerin to prevent intraoperative myocardial ischemia during fentanyl-pancuronium anesthesia. Anesthesiology 1984; 61:385.

90. Dajani AS, Bisno AL, Chung KJ, et al: Prevention of bacterial endocarditis: recommendations by the American Heart Association. JAMA 1990; 264:2919.

91. Stamm RB, Martin RP: Quantification of pressure gradients across stenotic valves by Doppler ultrasound. J Am Coll Cardiol 1983; 2:707.

92. Berger M, Berdoff RL, Gallerstein PE, et al: Evaluation of aortic stenosis by continuous wave Doppler ultrasound. J Am Coll Cardiol 1984; 3:150.

93. Currie PJ, Seward JB, Reeder GS, et al: Continuous-wave Doppler echocardiography assessment of severity of calcific aortic stenosis: a simultaneous Doppler-catheter correlative study in 100 adult patients. Circulation 1985; 71:1162.

94. Zoghbi WA, Farmer KL, Soto JG, et al: Accurate noninvasive quantification of stenotic aortic valve area by Doppler echocardiography. Circulation 1986; 73:452.

95. O'Keefe JH, Shub C, Rettke SR: Risk of noncardiac surgical procedures in patients with aortic stenosis. Mayo Clin Proc 1989; 64:400.

96. Hayes SN, Holmes DR, Nishimura RA, et al: Palliative percutaneous aortic balloon valvuloplasty before noncardiac operations and invasive diagnostic procedures. Mayo Clin Proc 1989; 64:753.

97. Roth RB, Palacios IF, Block PC: Percutaneous aortic balloon valvuloplasty: its role in the management of patients with aortic stenosis requiring major noncardiac surgery. J Am Coll Cardiol 1989; 13:1039.

98. Vahanian A, Pichel PL, Cormoier B, et al: Results of percutaneous mitral commissurotomy in 200 patients. Am J Cardiol 1989; 63:847.

99. The NHLBI Balloon Valvuloplasty Registry Participants: Multicenter experience with balloon mitral commissurotomy: NHLBI Balloon Valvuloplasty Registry report on immediate and 30-day followup results. Circulation 1992; 85:448.

100. Esteves CA, Ramos AI, Braga SL, et al: Effectiveness of percutaneous balloon mitral valvotomy during pregnancy. Am J Cardiol 1991; 68:930.

101. Gangbar EW, Watson KR, Howard RJ, et al: Mitral balloon valvuloplasty in pregnancy: advantages of a unique balloon. Cathet Cardiovasc Diagn 1992; 25:313.

102. Chatterjee K, Parmley WW, Swan HJC, et al: Beneficial effects of vasodilator agents in severe mitral regurgitation due to dysfunction of subvalvular apparatus. Circulation 1973; 48:684.

103. Miller RR, Vismara LA, DeMaria AN, et al: Afterload reduction therapy in severe aortic regurgitation: improved cardiac performance and reduced regurgitant volume. Am J Cardiol 1976; 38:564.

104. Chambers DA: Acquired valvular heart disease. In Cardiac Anesthesia. Kaplan JA (ed). New York, Grune & Stratton, 1979; pp 197–240.

105. Reitan JA, Wright RG: The use of halothane in a patient with asymmetrical septal hypertrophy: a case report. Can Anaesth Soc J 1982; 29:154.

106. Thompson RC, Liberthson RR, Lowenstein E: Perioperative anesthetic risk of noncardiac surgery in hypertrophic obstructive cardiomyopathy. JAMA 1985; 254:2419.

107. Tinker JH, Tarhan S: Discontinuing anticoagulant therapy in surgical patients with cardiac valve prostheses. JAMA 1978; 239:738.

108. Eckman MH, Beshansky JR, Durand-Zalesky I: Anticoagulation for noncardiac procedures in patients with prosthetic heart valves. JAMA 1990; 263:1513.

109. Charlson ME, MacKenzie CR, Ales KL, et al: The postoperative electro-cardiogram and creatine kinase: implications for diagnosis of myocardial infarction after noncardiac surgery. J Clin Epidemiol 1989; 42:25.

110. Oh JK, Seward JB, Khandheria BK, et al: Transesophageal echocardi-ography in critically ill patients. Am J Cardiol 1990; 66:1492.

111. Pearson AC, Castello R, Labovitz AJ: Safety and utility of transesopha-geal echocardiography in the critically ill patient. Am Heart J 1990; 119:1083.

112. Pritchett ELC: Management of atrial fibrillation. N Engl J Med 1992; 326:1264.

113. Andrews TC, Reimold SC, Berlin JA, et al: Prevention of supraventric-ular arrhythmias after coronary artery bypass surgery: a meta-analysis of randomized control trials. Circulation 1991; 84(Suppl 5):III–236.

114. Kowey PR, Taylor JE, Rilas SJ, et al: Meta-analysis of the effectiveness of prophylactic drug therapy in preventing supraventricular arrhythmia early after coronary artery bypass grafting. Am J Cardiol 1992; 69:963.

115. Goldman L: Assessment and management of the cardiac patient before, during, and after noncardiac surgery. *In* Cardiology. Vol. 2. Parmley WW, Chatterjee K (eds). Philadelphia, JB Lippincott Co, 1988, pp 1–15.

116. Pastore JO, Yurchak PM, Janis KM, et al: The risk of advanced heart block in surgical patients with right bundle branch block and left axis deviation. Circulation 1978; 57:677.

117. Frye RL, Collins JJ, DeSanctis RW, et al: Guidelines for permanent cardiac pacemaker implantation, May 1984: A report of the Joint Amer-ican College of Cardiology/American Heart Association Task Force on Assessment of Cardiovascular Procedures (Subcommittee on Pacemaker Implantation). Circulation 1984; 70:331A.

118. Goldman L, Wolf MA, Braunwald E: General anesthesia and noncardiac surgery in patients with heart disease. *In* Heart Disease: A Textbook of Cardiovascular Medicine. 3rd ed. Braunwald E (ed). Philadelphia, WB Saunders, 1988, pp 1693–1705.

119. Goldman L: Noncardiac surgery in patients receiving propranolol: case reports and a recommended approach. Arch Intern Med 1981; 141:193.

120. Brenner WI, Lieberman AN: Acute clonidine withdrawal syndrome fol-lowing open-heart operation. Ann Thorac Surg 1977; 24:80.

121. Stewart M, Burris JF: Rebound hypertension during initiation of trans-dermal clonidine. Drug Intell Clin Pharm 1988; 22:573.

122. Coriat P, Douraki T, Contani E, et al: Chronic treatment with converting enzyme inhibitors. Anesthesiology 1992; 77:A77.

CHAPTER 9

Pulmonary Consultation

PHILIP G. BOYSEN, M.D.

The incidence of postoperative pulmonary complications ranges from 2% to 70%, depending on the criteria used to identify them.[1] Preoperative evaluation of pulmonary function and consultation with a pulmonary specialist can be helpful for several reasons. Assessment of chronic pulmonary disease is useful in designing the preoperative regimen, altering intraoperative management, and planning for postoperative respiratory care. In addition, documentation of changes in pulmonary function can be useful in assessing risk and, in combination with the pulmonary consultation, in better advising patients of the benefits, risk, and outcome of the surgical procedure. Alteration in organ function may be so severe that therapeutic management of the chronic disease has been undertaken. A pulmonary consultant can help to assess the benefits of that therapy, the effect on organ function, and the need to alter therapy before undergoing surgery. Particular risk factors suggesting that consultation will be beneficial are listed in Table 9–1.

GENERAL CONSIDERATIONS

Who Benefits from Preoperative Pulmonary Consultation?

As pulmonary function testing has become more widely available, the patients who are candidates for assessment of preoperative pulmonary function and possible evaluation by a pulmonary consultant have increased in number.

Thoracic and Upper Abdominal Surgery

Routine performance of pulmonary function testing for all patients who are scheduled for thoracic surgery generally is

TABLE 9–1. Factors Increasing the Risk of Postoperative Pulmonary Complications

Thoracic and upper abdominal surgery
Age >70 y
Morbid obesity
Smoking
Pre-existing pulmonary disease

considered reasonable, especially if its intention is to resect functional lung tissue.[2] Patients about to undergo upper abdominal surgical procedures should also have a preoperative evaluation of pulmonary function. The cost of such testing must be balanced against the likelihood of gaining useful information. Therefore, if the preoperative history and physical examination suggest some reason to suspect compromised pulmonary function, further testing and evaluation are in order.

In thoracic or upper abdominal surgery, a major element of postoperative pulmonary function abnormalities concerns diaphragmatic muscle dysfunction. This phenomenon may be transient but relatively severe in the early postoperative period, particularly in patients whose pulmonary function is already compromised.

Smokers

Patients with a history of heavy smoking and cough may also benefit from preoperative pulmonary function testing as a means of documenting dysfunction. A pulmonary consultation may be necessary to design a preoperative regimen of bronchopulmonary toilet.

Obese Patients

Obese patients may have severe restrictive lung disease, as well as chronic obstructive lung disease (COLD) if they smoke. Such individuals are particularly affected shortly after the operation.

Patients With Pre-existing Pulmonary Disease

Patients with other types of pulmonary disease associated with restrictive or obstructive pathophysiology also are candidates for pulmonary function testing and preoperative consultation.

Older Patients

In the past, a pulmonary evaluation was recommended for all patients older than 70 years. Advanced age might or might not necessitate pulmonary function testing. Patients in this age group are probably at increased risk because they have lost elastic recoil as a result of aging of lung tissue and are, therefore, more prone to postoperative pulmonary complications.

When Is a Pulmonary Consultation Superfluous?

If the intent of preoperative pulmonary function testing and pulmonary consultation is to maximize function before the surgical procedure and administration of an anesthetic, such testing and consultation are superfluous if the recommendations are not followed and the goals are not met. In the event that chronic organ dysfunction has been previously identified and perhaps documented by pulmonary function testing and lung function has been maximized by therapy, additional consultation has little to offer. Obviously, selection of the anesthetic technique, procedure, and monitoring is within the purview of the anesthesiologist, not the pulmonary consultant. The consultant, however, may be in a very good position to make recommendations for further therapy, especially if he or she had prior involvement in the management of the patient's chronic lung disease.

SPECIFIC MEASURES

What Is the Role of Bronchodilators?

Several issues must be addressed preoperatively for patients with chronic pulmonary disease. First is documentation of the degree of pulmonary dysfunction. Second is an attempt to maximize pulmonary function before the operative procedure is begun. Along these lines, control of bronchospasm and infections is of utmost importance.

A bronchospastic patient's response to bronchodilator therapy may range from minimal to very impressive. Evaluation of pulmonary function by the pulmonary consultant and the objective response to bronchodilation are very important in this regard. Currently, intermittent use of nebulized β_2-agonists by metered-dose inhaler (MDI) is the most popular means of achieving maximum bronchodilation (Table 9–2). These drugs and this form of delivery are usually effective, well tolerated, associated with minimal side effects, and easy to use if patients are properly instructed.[3] Relative to other drugs and considering their minimal side effects, the cost of MDIs is not exorbitant.

Administration

In preparation for surgery, maximal bronchodilation can usually be accomplished by coaching patients and by adequate instruction and administration of the metered dose during deep inspiration. Use of a chambered collection device, which maintains the vapor in the proximity of the patient's airway and facilitates introduction of the volatilized agent to the alveoli by minimizing loss of drug through deposition on the posterior pharynx, may be most beneficial. Although popular in the past, administration of these drugs through intermittent positive-pressure ventilation is no longer routinely recommended. However, some patients who are unable to breathe deeply spontaneously are best able to tolerate and administer the nebulized bronchodilator by this technique.

Assessment

Improvement in airflow after nebulized bronchodilator therapy may indicate a more favorable postoperative prognosis. Some patients with minimal improvement in midflow measurements (i.e., forced expired volume between 25% and 75% of the exhaled volume [$FEV_{25\%-75\%}$]) respond to intensive use of bronchodilators, hydration, antibiotics, and cessation of smoking. For those whose $FEV_{25\%-75\%}$ or maximum voluntary ventilation (MVV) does not improve, a higher incidence of postoperative pulmonary complications is to be anticipated.

How Important Is Infection Control?

Control of infection is important because of the tendency for patients who have bacterial colonization to develop bronchitis and pneumonia in the postoperative state. Antibacterial agents and facilitation of the clearance of secretions are important in alleviating such postoperative complications. Bronchodilation is usually effective in allowing an effective cough after a deep breath and facilitates clearance of secretions. Adequate attention to hydration is also beneficial, whereas the use of other agents administered into the airway is not generally efficacious.

Diagnosis and Treatment

When administering antibiotics, remember that many species of organisms colonize the upper airways and trachea. If a patient has been in the hospital or has received other medical attention, these organisms are often gram-negative types. The cost and efficacy of culturing them have been debated. Antibiotic therapy administered preoperatively seems prudent, assuming that the surgical procedure is elective, without incurring the cost and delay of first culturing secretions from the airway.

Ampicillin, tetracycline, trimethoprim/sulfamethoxazole, and other broad-spectrum antibiotics have been recommended as the most reasonable therapeutic agents.[4] The appearance of purulent sputum is enough of an indication to begin such therapy. It is also reasonable to expect that the sputum will clear and the amount will decrease if appropriate antibiotic therapy has been instituted. This change should, in turn, improve the postoperative outcome.

Education

Patient education is also an important part of the preoperative evaluation and should be emphasized by the pulmonary consultant to ensure postoperative compliance in the performance of deep breathing and coughing maneuvers. If incentive spirometry has been ordered as a means of achieving postoperative lung inflation, patients should be coached and observed to comply with the intent and purpose of the device.

Are Cessation of Smoking and Loss of Weight Helpful?

Smoking

If adequate time exists before surgery is performed, smoking cessation is often recommended. However, the ability to

TABLE 9–2. Metered-Dose Bronchodilators

Drug	Trade Name	Manufacturer	Concentration/Puff
Terbutaline	Brethaire	Geigy	200 μg
Albuterol	Proventil	Schering	90 μg
	Ventolin	Glaxo	
Metaproterenol	Alupent	Boehringer Ingelheim	650 μg
	Metaprel	Dorsey	
Isoetharine	Bronkometer	Winthrop-Breon	340 μg
Bitolterol	Tornalate	Winthrop-Breon	370 μg
Isoproterenol	Isuprel Mistometer	Winthrop-Breon	130 μg
	Medihaler-Iso	Riker	75 μg
Isoproterenol and phenylephrine	Duo-Medihaler	Riker	160 μg 240 μg Phenyl
Epinephrine*	Asthmahler	Norcliff Thayer	160 μg
	Bronitin Mist	Whitehall	
	Bronkaid Mist	Winthrop-Breon	
	Medihaler-Epi	Riker	
	Primatene Mist	Whitehall	
Ipratropium	Atrovent	Boehringer Ingelheim	18 μg

(From: Gold ML, Marcial E: An anesthetic adaptor for all metered dose inhalers [Letter to the editor]. Anesthesiology 1988; 68:965.)
*Other concentrations available: 200 μg, 270 μg.

affect outcome by discontinuation of smoking is somewhat controversial.[5–7] Recovery from the effects of cigarettes is a long and slow process, but mucociliary escalation begins to improve almost immediately. This change should ensure more effective and complete removal of airway secretions. Clearly, however, cessation of smoking is of more benefit and is an issue better addressed as a long-term goal to maintain pulmonary function than to alter postoperative management and immediate postoperative outcome.[5]

Weight Loss

Similarly, weight reduction may be appropriate. If a patient undergoes a surgical procedure after considerable weight loss, particularly if he or she is morbidly obese, outcome is improved. In either case, prolonged periods before the operation are necessary to achieve the desired improvement.

INTRAOPERATIVE CONSULTATION

What Is the Role?

Continuous monitoring and examination of the patient are necessary to achieve maintenance of lung function and improvement of postoperative outcome. The reduction in anesthesia time is of importance but is closely linked to the ongoing surgical procedure; thus, it often is not under control of the anesthesiologist or the pulmonary consultant. Once a surgical procedure extends beyond 3 hours and the patient is continuously in the same position, the tendency toward accumulation of secretions and the incidence of postoperative pulmonary complications and infections rises.[8]

Intraoperative control of secretions is essential. Adventitious sounds in the airways are an indication for intermittent suction to maintain clearance of secretions; a more aggressive approach may necessitate direct observation and suctioning via fiberoptic bronchoscopy.

Aspiration of Gastric Contents

A patient with pulmonary compromise is at tremendous risk for postoperative morbidity and mortality should gastric contents be aspirated into the tracheobronchial tree. Every effort should be made, beginning with anesthetic induction, to avoid such occurrences (rapid-sequence induction with a Sellick maneuver, proper positioning, techniques to minimize or neutralize gastric secretions, awake intubation of the trachea when necessary).

Bronchodilator Therapy

Bronchodilatation that has begun before the operation should be maintained intraoperatively. Many techniques are available; most depend mainly on inhaled bronchodilators. An MDI can be used to introduce the drug into the anesthesia circuit just proximal to the endotracheal tube, or continuous nebulization into the anesthesia circuit can be performed.[9] Because significant "rain out" of these agents into the ventilator tubing occurs, continued therapy may be necessary for a long time to obtain the desired clinical response. Because anesthetized patients cannot undergo spirometric testing, end points include assessments of lung compliance, airways resistance, slope of the capnographic tracing, end-tidal carbon dioxide (CO_2) pressure ($P_{ET}CO_2$), pulse oximetric oxygen (O_2) saturation (SpO_2), and so forth.

Parasympatholysis

If optimal bronchodilatation is not obtained by the inhalation of β_2-agonists, the next choice is an agent capable of achieving some degree of parasympatholysis. Inhaled atropine has been used for many years; atropine analogues such as ipratropium bromide are now commonly used. These drugs are particularly worth considering in patients who are about to undergo a general anesthetic and who have a tendency toward exacerbation or bronchospasm.

This response to manipulation or intubation has been described as a vagally mediated alteration in bronchomotor tone.

Parasympatholysis specifically blocks this response and therefore should be extremely useful in intubated patients or patients undergoing general anesthesia with a volatile agent. Such agents can also be administered into the anesthetic circuit, either by a MDI or by nebulization of the drug through a system introduced into the anesthesia circuit between the Y-piece and the endotracheal tube.[9] If a β_2-agonist and a parasympatholytic agent have been instituted preoperatively, they should be used intraoperatively at the same time intervals to maintain optimal response to drug therapy.

Theophylline

Maintenance of intravenous theophylline therapy is a third choice when assessing bronchodilators, and use of this drug and other agents is considered subsequently. For patients who have not received theophylline previously, an initial dose of 6 to 7.5 mg $\cdot$ kg^{-1} of aminophylline over 15 to 30 minutes is indicated, depending on the severity of the attack.[10] A continuous infusion of 0.7 mg $\cdot$ kg^{-1} $\cdot$ h^{-1} should follow. After the loading dose, a serum level of 12 to 15 μg $\cdot$ mL^{-1} usually results.

If patients previously have been receiving theophylline, a serum level should be ascertained and half the loading dose given if longer-acting oral preparations were taken. Although theophylline is inferior to β_2-agonists, it may be indicated for patients with status asthmaticus or those who are refractory to the latter agents. Its nonbronchodilator effects (diaphragmatic strengthening, inotropism, respiratory stimulation), although limited, may be useful.

Volatile Agents

All of the volatile anesthetics currently in use are powerful bronchodilators. Halothane has long enjoyed the reputation of being the most potent, but enflurane, isoflurane, and desflurane are probably equally useful. Deepening the anesthetic in bronchospastic patients may be efficacious and can provide an essentially wheeze-free state during the course and conduct of the anesthetic. However, such patients often again wheeze when the volatile agent is withdrawn; therefore, anesthetic maintenance with the volatile anesthetic is prudent, while bronchodilator therapy is provided at the same time by inhaled techniques in anticipation of anesthetic emergence.

How Should Mechanical Ventilation Be Provided?

During anesthesia, mechanical ventilation should be provided with an 8 to 10 mL $\cdot$ kg^{-1} tidal volume at a rate sufficient to maintain a normal CO_2 partial pressure (PaCO_2). The rate and inspiratory-to-expiratory time ratio should be altered to allow complete exhalation in bronchospastic patients and to avoid or minimize hyperinflation and gas trapping. This approach is assessed by observing that the expiratory valve settles before the next inspiration or by noting that the spirometer turbine stops before the subsequent inhalation begins. If not, the expiratory time is lengthened or additional bronchodilator therapy as described earlier is instituted. Ventilatory therapy can be guided by the PETCO$_2$ and the capnographic slope. However, in some patients, measurement of the PaCO_2 may be necessary to assess intraoperative events.

POSTOPERATIVE CARE

How Is Lung Volume Maintained?

The main feature of postoperative care emphasizes continuation of pre- and intraoperative therapeutic regimens with particular attention to lung inflation. This goal may be achieved by encouraging deep-breathing exercises, by passive lung inflation with intermittent positive pressure breathing (IPPB) machines, continuous positive airway pressure (CPAP), or sustained maximum inspiration (incentive spirometry).[11] The key element is postoperative pulmonary function maintenance, recovery of the functional residual capacity (FRC), and clearance of secretions. Because coughing is often painful and, when not associated with a deep inspiration, may be counterproductive (i.e., decreases lung volume and collapses small airways), patients should be coached to take a maximum inspiration and to hold it as long as possible. This maneuver creates the highest, longest duration of subambient intrapleural pressure and, therefore, best restores the FRC. The tendency to cough after exhalation, with further expulsion of air at end-tidal volumes, actually accentuates airway collapse.

The exhalation phase, whether forced or otherwise, moves secretions proximally. If a patient is instructed to do so several times an hour (e.g., each time a commercial appears on television) and is able to comply, incentive spirometry devices become almost superfluous. Mobilization of secretions and early ambulation are necessary to maximize bronchopulmonary toilet. Bronchodilatation by previously described techniques is aggressively maintained in the early postoperative period.

How Is Pain Relief Provided?

Of major importance to anesthesiologists is the provision of adequate analgesia in the early postoperative period. Whether for emotional or physiologic reasons, patients who are undergoing a painful postoperative course are more prone to bronchospasm. Adequate analgesia can be provided in a number of ways.

Intramuscular and Intravenous Narcotics

The classic approach uses intramuscular or intravenous drug therapy. Such therapy is problematic because of the tendency to have very high plasma levels of narcotics, resulting in suppression of ventilatory drive, versus a later period of subtherapeutic blood levels and return to the painful state.[12] Low-dose infusion of narcotics has been helpful in this regard.

Patient-Controlled Analgesia

Some patients benefit from a patient-controlled analgesia (PCA) technique with or without a baseline infusion of narcotic. Intermittent on-demand boluses of very low doses of narcotic have a psychotherapeutic benefit because of the control exerted by the patient on his or her environment. A lower overall dose of narcotic is required to achieve adequate pain relief. Other patients, however, cannot or will not cooperate with such devices. Other mechanisms of pain relief may be useful in this type of patient and in many others. These include local anesthetic infiltration, regional block therapy, or cryoanalgesia.

Epidural Narcotics

Of major benefit to many compromised, elderly, postoperative patients is postoperative administration of epidural narcotics.[13, 14] Nociception is altered at spinal narcotic receptor sites that are occupied by the introduction of these agents into the epidural space. Some absorption of the narcotic agents obviously occurs, but to a much lesser degree than with intravenous or intramuscular administration of the same drug.

Although morphine migrates rostrally, with a biphasic tendency toward suppression of ventilation, this complication is extremely uncommon unless parenteral narcotics have been used intraoperatively. Epidural analgesia leaves patients wide awake and alert but with minimal perception of pain. Morphine, meperidine, fentanyl, and sufentanil have been used to achieve this effect.

Effects on Pulmonary Function

Adequate pain management has an additional benefit that has been underemphasized. Both PCA and epidural narcotics seem to have a salutary effect on pulmonary function.[15] In particular, with epidural narcotics, the breathing pattern is slowed, the tidal volume is increased, and patients are more cooperative in trying to achieve deep lung inflation. Similarly, PCA is associated with increased FRC and vital capacity and improved outcome.

These changes may simply be due to alleviation of pain and the ability of the patient to inspire deeply without splinting, even if the incision is in the upper abdomen or the thorax. Additionally, some neurogenic inhibitory reflex mediated at the spinal cord appears to alter diaphragmatic function postoperatively. Epidural narcotics occupying receptor sites along the spinal cord may interrupt this inhibitory reflex so that improved diaphragmatic function is achieved in the early postoperative period.[15, 16] Whatever the reason, adequate pain management, combined with physical examination and assessment of a patient's breathing rate, tidal volume, and capacity for deep inspiration, is a useful means to achieve and assess therapeutic goals in the early postoperative time frame.

In Whom Should Delay of Elective Surgery Be Considered?

Thoracic Surgery

No single test predicts postoperative pulmonary function or outcome. Instead, a combination of tests is usually necessary, and the pattern demonstrated by a particular patient gives an indication of the postoperative course (Fig. 9–1). For thoracotomy patients, the parameters listed in Table 9–3 indicate the ability to withstand the incision and give some indication of the remaining lung function should resection up to and including a pneumonectomy be performed. In my experience, the most useful parameters are the forced expired volume in 1 second (FEV_1), which should exceed 2.0 L, and the MVV, which should exceed 50 L $\cdot$ min^{-1}, or 50% of the predicted value. These data are also useful when combined with ventilation or perfusion radionuclide scanning in predicting the ultimate remaining lung function after resection.

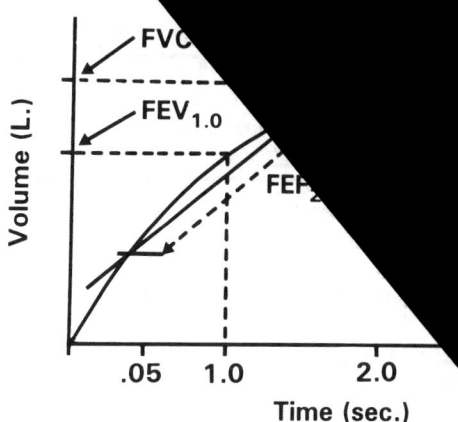

FIGURE 9–1. Normal spirogram with the relevant componen

In those patients being assessed for thoracotomy, se restriction of pulmonary function indicates that no lung tiss can be resected without severely compromising the patient and possibly causing his or her demise. In some studies, even an incision to obtain a biopsy without resection of functional lung tissue has resulted in disastrous consequences.

Even in the event that only a partial resection is performed on one lung, the remaining lung may be severely edematous in the early postoperative period and may take several months to achieve its ultimate function.[17, 18] During this time, adequate attention to physical therapy, removal of secretions, antibiotics, and so forth are essential to maximize function for that particular lung. Carefully titrated positive end-expiratory pressure (PEEP)/CPAP may be useful in conjunction with positive-pressure ventilation.

Upper Abdominal Surgery

For patients undergoing upper abdominal surgery, parameters that define patients at moderate risk, should the incision be close to the diaphragm, are listed in Table 9–4. Close attention to detail, particularly preoperative, intraoperative, and postoperative bronchopulmonary toilet, are especially important. Maximizing function, as indicated by improved spirometric values, during this period, has been associated with a lesser tendency for patients to develop postoperative pneumonia and therefore to have an improved outcome.

The parameters listed in Table 9–5 define a severe degree of risk. In these individuals, postoperative mechanical ventilation should be maintained for a period of 24 to 48 hours in an intensive care unit (ICU) so that continuous monitoring and therapeutic intervention are possible. Such planning does not preclude a trial at extubation should the patient look better than expected, but don't plan on it!

A clinically useful approach to assessment of risk that in-

TABLE 9–3. Increased Risk of Pulmonary Complications Following Pneumonectomy

Forced vital capacity	<50% predicted or <1.75–2 L
Forced expired volume in 1 s	>2 L, mortality = 10%
	<2 L, mortality = 20–45%
	<0.8 L, nonoperable
Maximum voluntary ventilation	<50–60% predicted, mortality = 5–32%

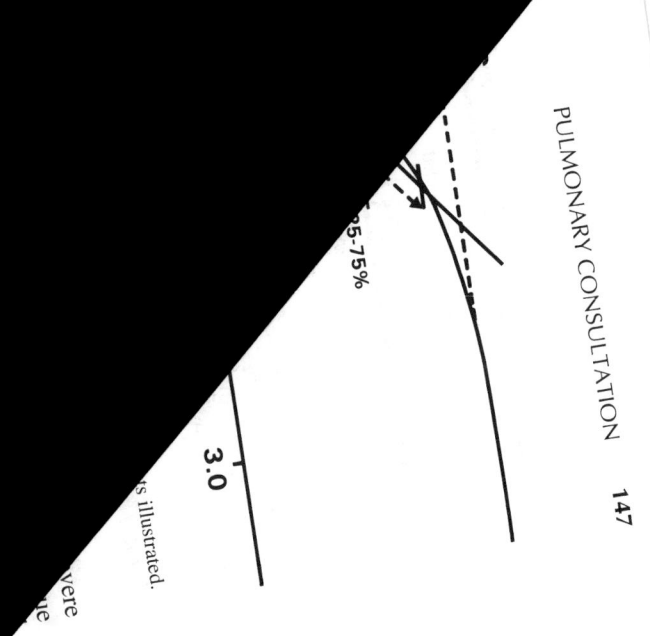

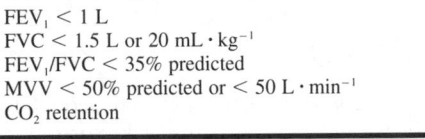

TABLE 9–5. Abdominal Surgery: High Risk

$FEV_1 < 1$ L
$FVC < 1.5$ L or 20 mL · kg^{-1}
$FEV_1/FVC < 35\%$ predicted
MVV $< 50\%$ predicted or < 50 L · min^{-1}
CO_2 retention

Abbreviations: FEV_1 = forced expired volume in 1 s; FVC = forced vital capacity; MVV = maximum voluntary ventilation; $FEV_{25\%-75\%}$ = forced expired volume between 25% and 75% of the exhaled volume.

be supported through) the most severe period of respiratory compromise.

Careful assessment of breathing patterns is essential in the event that patients are allowed to trigger the ventilator or are supported by intermittent or synchronized intermittent mandatory ventilation (IMV and SIMV).[20] Pressure support ventilation may be particularly advantageous, because it allows patients to control respiratory rate, respiratory flow rate, and tidal volume during spontaneous breathing with mechanical ventilation. This support can be varied from maximum (PSV MAX),[21] in which almost total support is provided (i.e., a tidal volume of 10–12 mL · kg^{-1}), through lesser amounts designed to overcome only the imposed work from the ventilator circuit and endotracheal tube.[22]

What Are the Principal Goals of Mechanical Ventilation?

No one best way can be advocated to ventilate patients with pulmonary disease. A major therapeutic goal is to reduce the O_2 cost of breathing and to minimize energy expenditure, achieving deep lung inflation and delivering adequate fraction of inspired O_2 (FIO_2) at a frequency sufficient to result in the desired arterial blood gas values.

Adequate attention to control of pain is essential, and it is hoped that subsequent withdrawal of ventilatory therapy can be accomplished within 48 to 72 hours. The frequency with which patients who have been extubated successfully are

This loss of lung ..... or pulmonary secretions and results in a ...ght-to-left intrapulmonary shunt and subsequent hypoxemia.

For this reason, therapy is specifically focused on achieving deep lung inflation and reclaiming lung volumes. This approach should minimize the intrapulmonary shunt. The nadir of these changes usually occurs within the first 24 hours; therefore, during this period, not only intensive respiratory care but also mechanical ventilation may be necessary.

Reduction of Work of Breathing

Reduction in lung volume and alteration in breathing patterns are associated with a severe increase in the mechanical work of breathing. Compromised patients may be unable to assume this extra ventilatory workload, and respiratory failure can ensue. By assuming the respiratory muscle work and maintaining lung inflation with mechanical ventilation and some form of PEEP or CPAP, patients can often overcome (or

TABLE 9–6. Classification System for Risk of Pulmonary Complications Following Thoracic and Abdominal Procedures

	Assessment	Points*
Expiratory spirogram	Normal: % FVC + % FEV$_1$/FVC > 150	0
	% FVC + % FEV$_1$/FVC = 100–150	1
	% FVC + % FEV$_1$/FVC < 100	2
	Preoperative FVC < 20 mL · kg^{-1}	3
	Postbronchodilator FEV$_1$/FVC < 50%	3
Cardiovascular system	Normal	0
	Controlled hypertension, myocardial infarction without sequelae for more than 2 y	0
	Dyspnea on exertion, orthopnea, paroxysmal nocturnal dyspnea, dependent edema, congestive heart failure, angina	1
Nervous system	Normal	0
	Confusion, obtundation, agitation, spasticity, discoordination, bulbar malfunction	1
	Significant muscle weakness	1
Arterial blood gas values	Acceptable	0
	PaCO$_2$ > 50 mm Hg or PaO$_2$ < 60 mm Hg with room air	1
	pH > 7.5 or < 7.3	1
Recovery	Ambulation (at minimum, sitting at bedside) expected within 36 h	0
	Complete bed confinement expected for at least 36 h	1

(Modified from Clinical Application of Respiratory Care. 4th ed. Shapiro BA, Kacmarek RM, Cane RD, et al (eds). Chicago, Mosby-Year Book Medical Publishers, 1989.)
*0 points = low risk; 1–2 points = moderate risk; >3 points = high risk.
Abbreviations: FVC = forced vital capacity; FEV = forced expiratory volume; FEV$_1$ = forced expiratory volume in 1 s; PaCO$_2$ = arterial partial pressure of carbon dioxide; PaO$_2$ = arterial partial pressure of oxygen.

TABLE 9–7. Postoperative Pathophysiologic Pulmonary Changes Following Abdominal Surgery

Decreased	Forced vital capacity
	Lung volumes, especially functional residual capacity and total lung capacity
	Tidal volume
	Lung compliance
	↓ PaO_2
	↓ $PaCO_2$

TABLE 9–8. Criteria for Weaning and Tracheal Extubation

Respiratory muscle strength	PNP >20–30 cm H_2O
Ventilatory mechanics	VC >10–15 mL · kg^{-1}
	V_T >5 mL · kg^{-1}
	C_{ST} >30 mL · cm H_2O
Ventilatory reserve	MVV >2 × $\dot{V}_E$ and normal (for patient) $PaCO_2$ and pHa
Minute ventilation	$\dot{V}_E$ with normal $PaCO_2$ and pHa
	<10 L · min^{-1}
	<180 mL · kg^{-1} · min^{-1}
Dead space	V_D/V_T <0.6

Abbreviations: PNP = peak negative pressure; VC = vital capacity; V_T = tidal volume; C_{ST} = static compliance; $\dot{V}_E$ = minute ventilation; V_D/V_T = dead space to tidal volume ratio; $PaCO_2$ = arterial partial pressure of carbon dioxide; pHa = arterial pH; MVV = maximum voluntary ventilation.

readmitted to the ICU on the second or third postoperative day because of inadequate pain management is impressive. Elderly and obese patients are particularly problematic in this regard.

Thus, documentation of organ function by pulmonary function testing is essential to assess the degree of compromise and the response to therapy. In such cases, extubation criteria such as those listed in Table 9–8 may be used. Remember, however, that the values listed are only guidelines that must be modified by clinical assessment.

What Patterns of Pulmonary Function Tests Are Seen?

Obstructive Disease

Patients with moderate compromise can achieve nearly normal vital capacity. However, because exhaled flows are diminished throughout the forced vital capacity (FVC) maneuver, the FEV at ½ second, 1 second, 2 seconds, and 3 seconds is usually reduced (Fig. 9–2). The hallmark of obstructive lung disease is a reduction in the FEV_1/FVC. Maximum midexpiratory flow rates are also measured as a means of assessing damage or compromise to the smaller airways. This particular test is very useful in the event that maximum bronchodilator therapy improves this limitation.

Restrictive Disease

A restrictive ventilatory defect (RVD) results in limitation of inspiration and, therefore, a reduction in the vital capacity (see Fig. 9–2). Exhaled flow is usually normal. Thus, the FEV_1, as a percentage of the FVC, is also normal; in fact, it may be very high because the ventilatory restriction can result in rapid reduction of lung volume after deep inspiration.

Clinical Implications

Chronic Obstructive Lung Disease

In either obstructive disease or restrictive disease, further testing will delineate the type of abnormalities that are encountered. Emphysematous patients, for example, have a loss of effective surface area for gas transfer and a reduction in diffusing capacity. As the tethering effect of the pulmonary parenchyma is lost, a tendency toward gas trapping and hyperinflation occurs. Increases in the FRC and residual volume (RV) follow. In particular, the RV/TLC and FRC/TLC are greatly affected. In contrast, patients with chronic bronchitis may have nearly normal lung volumes unless they are undergoing an exacerbation of bronchospasm.

Emphysematous patients respond little or not at all to ad-

ministration of nebulized or inhaled bronchodilators, whereas chronic bronchitic patients may show a dramatic response of 10% or more in all affected parameters above baseline values. Asthmatic patients, who are usually younger and have episodic bronchospasm, have an even greater response (up to 25% above baseline) to bronchodilators given immediately during testing.

Restrictive Ventilatory Defects

Patients with a RVD also have alterations in lung volumes and diffusing capacity. With intrinsic RVD, the diffusing capacity is usually reduced and a concentric reduction in all lung volumes is present. Thus, the RV, FRC, and TLC are reduced by approximately the same percentage.

Patients with an extrinsic ventilatory defect (ascites, paralyzed diaphragm, pulmonary edema, and pleural effusion) have a significant reduction in TLC but a lesser reduction in FRC and RV. Therefore, the reduction in lung volumes is not concentric. In addition, these patients usually have a normal surface area for gas transfer and a normal diffusing capacity.

What Changes Are Expected in Arterial Blood Gas Values?

Given the pathophysiology described, patients with COLD are categorized as "pink puffers" or "blue bloaters." Emphy-

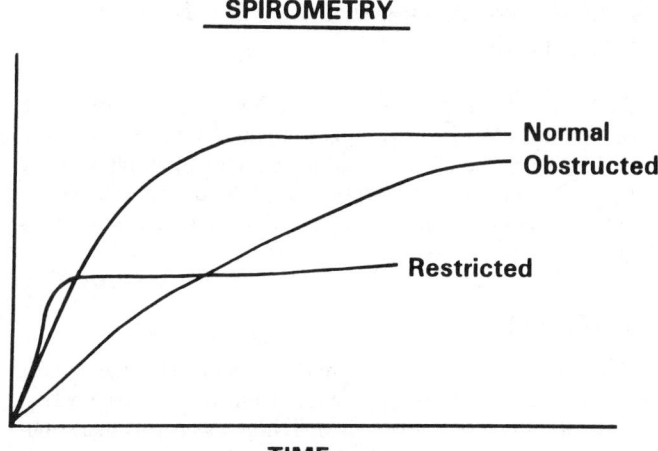

SPIROMETRY

Normal
Obstructed
Restricted

TIME

FIGURE 9–2. Alteration of spirometric tracings in obstructive and restrictive lung disease. Plot of expiratory volume versus time.

sematous patients are dubbed pink puffers because of the previously mentioned changes and the tendency for arterial blood gas values to be very close to normal. In other words, patients are not hypoxemic, nor do they have a tendency to retain CO_2. Minimal or no bronchospasm is present, there is little tendency to retain secretions or sputum, and bacterial colonization and airway infection are uncommon.

Blue bloaters with chronic bronchitis are often hypoxemic and retain CO_2. They have multiple episodes of bronchospasm and a tendency toward right heart failure, concomitant with hypoxemia. Sputum is usually copious and colonized, and tracheal bronchitis and pneumonia are frequent. The response to bronchodilators is often dramatic, resulting not only in improved airflow but also a markedly improved ability to clear secretions and maintain bronchopulmonary hygiene.

Postoperative Management Goals

Assessment of a patient's status is enhanced by arterial blood gas analysis before surgery. In combination with pulmonary function testing and the history and physical examination, it leads to better categorization of a patient in terms of diagnosis and outcome. In addition, baseline values help to tailor postoperative therapy. A patient who normally has a SpO_2 of 90% and arterial O_2 partial pressure (PaO_2) of 60 mm Hg will not be greatly improved after surgery. These values are the best that can be hoped for as postoperative goals during breathing of room air.

The inability of a patient to maintain a PaO_2 that is consistent with good SpO_2 and O_2 delivery may indicate the necessity to administer O_2 postoperatively, often for long periods. In particular, patients with COLD, whose clinical pattern suggests chronic bronchitis, often benefit greatly from low-flow O_2 therapy. Conversely, a $SpO_2 \geq 94\%$ precludes both hypoxemia and hypercarbia if the patient is breathing room air.

As long as the PaO_2 is approximately 60 mm Hg and the SpO_2 can be maintained at 90%, a patient will have nearly maximum O_2 delivery for a specific cardiac output and hemoglobin level with no tendency to aggravate hypoventilation and CO_2 accumulation (Fig. 9–3). Further increases in saturation above 90% not only offer little therapeutic benefit but may actually be deleterious to a patient's eventual outcome through ventilatory suppression.

When Should Preoperative Drug Levels Be Measured?

Most bronchodilators exert their effect topically on the mucosa of the airway. The β_2-agonists and the atropine or atropine-like drugs therefore should have a maximum physiologic effect with minimum absorption. For these drugs, measurement of function is superior to measurement of a specific drug level.

Theophylline

Theophylline poses a different problem. The therapeutic plasma level for theophylline ranges from 10 to 20 $\mu g \cdot mL^{-1}$. Below this suggested level, theophylline has a less than optimal therapeutic effect, and above this level, a considerable increase in the incidence of side effects occurs. At approximately 20 $\mu g \cdot mL^{-1}$, gastrointestinal side effects (primarily manifested as nausea and vomiting) predominate. If a blood level of 40 $\mu g \cdot mL^{-1}$ is reached, cardiovascular side effects, premature ventricular contractions, or runs of ventricular tachycardia predominate. When the blood level exceeds 60 $\mu g \cdot mL^{-1}$, seizures that are poorly responsive to therapy tend to occur and often result in a patient's death.[10]

If a patient has received chronic theophylline therapy, obtain a blood sample to determine the presumably steady-state blood level. Augmentation of blood levels can be accomplished by small intravenous boluses of the drug. In general, a dose of 1 mg $\cdot$ kg^{-1} increases the serum level approximately 2 $\mu g \cdot mL^{-1}$, although marked variability in response occurs.[10] When an adequate therapeutic range has been established, oral dosing of theophylline up to and including the time of surgery is usually recommended.

Halothane, when combined with theophylline, causes an increase in cardiac toxicity.[23] Although this volatile anesthetic agent was recommended for many years because of its bronchodilator capacity, it should be avoided altogether in patients to whom theophylline has been administered. Isoflurane has adequate bronchodilator properties and no such adverse interaction.

What Other Drugs Are Problematic?

Corticosteroids

Corticosteroids and β-blockers present potential problems. When corticosteroid therapy has been initiated before surgery, especially within the past 6 months, adequate dosing should be administered perioperatively to offset potential adrenal suppression. These drugs have little effect in the treatment of acute bronchospasm, requiring hours to days for the optimal therapeutic effect to occur.

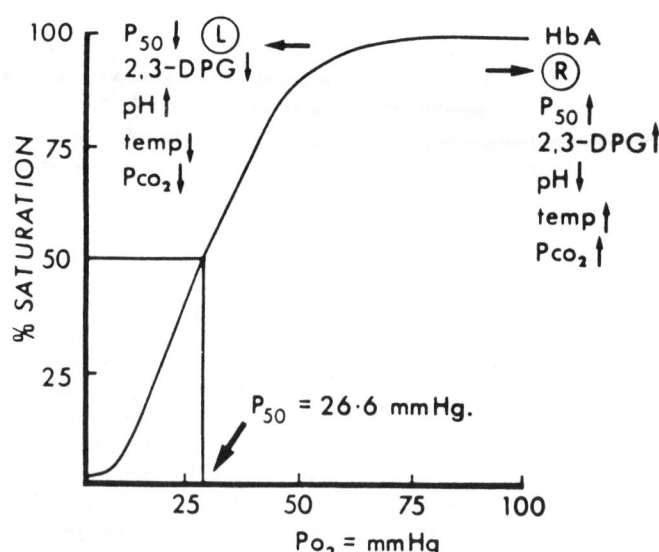

FIGURE 9–3. The oxyhemoglobin dissociation curve. Oxygen saturation of hemoglobin is 90% at a PaO_2 approximately 60 mm Hg. Other factors that may alter the position of the curve are illustrated for the sake of completeness.

β-Blockers

When tachycardia or hypertension is problematic, β-blockers often are administered intravenously. Drugs such as propranolol, which block both the β$_1$- and the β$_2$-receptor sites, tend to cause acute bronchospasm. The search for specific β$_1$-blockers has led to the concept that receptor sites can be selectively blocked to control heart rate without any effect on those receptors that cause bronchodilatation. Beta-blockers such as esmolol are particularly useful for this purpose because of their short duration of action, their rapid elimination, their specificity for β$_1$-receptor sites, and because they do not induce bronchospasm.[24] Unfortunately, the response to β-blockade in these patients is not easily predicted.

In patients undergoing maximum bronchodilator therapy, small doses of propranolol can be very effective in controlling heart rate and blood pressure without causing bronchospasm. If bronchospasm occurs, it can be treated with isoproterenol. Other methods to control blood pressure (e.g., clonidine) should also be considered to avoid β-blockade altogether. Labetalol, which is a selective α$_1$-antagonist and nonselective β$_1$- and β$_2$-antagonist, appears less likely to induce bronchospasm than other nonselective β-adrenergic antagonists.[25]

Narcotics

Narcotics can be used to control intraoperative hemodynamics but may cause reduction in central ventilatory drive in the early postoperative period. Because sophisticated testing of the response to CO_2 and hypoxia is usually not performed preoperatively, the ability to administer these drugs without consequence is generally unknown until such time as they are needed. Small incremental dosing and careful assessment are essential to provide the desired therapeutic effect without invoking unwanted or untoward side effects.[16, 18]

CONCLUSIONS

In summary, patients with COLD or RVD pose a challenging problem for clinicians about to administer an anesthetic. The status of organ dysfunction, the effects of therapy, and the proposed therapeutic regimen must be carefully assessed, sometimes in conjunction with a formal pulmonary consultation. Maintenance of such regimens preoperatively, intraoperatively, and postoperatively is necessary to achieve the desired outcome. In those patients with severe pulmonary compromise, administration of an anesthetic is fraught with difficulties that often are more problematic than the surgical procedure for which the anesthetic is to be provided.

References

1. Latimer RG, Dickman M, Day WC, et al: Ventilatory patterns and pulmonary complications after upper abdominal surgery determined by preoperative and postoperative computerized spirometry and blood gas analysis. Am J Surg 1971; 122:622.
2. Tisi GM: Preoperative evaluation of pulmonary function: validity, indications, and benefits. Am Rev Respir Dis 1979; 119:293.
3. Myers DL: Pharmacologic therapy of respiratory failure. *In* Respiratory Failure. Kirby RR, Taylor RW (eds). Chicago, Year Book Medical Publishers, 1986, pp 482–484.
4. Cicale MJ, Block AJ: Acute respiratory failure in chronic obstructive pulmonary disease. *In* Critical Care. 2nd ed. Civetta JM, Taylor RW, Kirby RR (eds). Philadelphia, JB Lippincott, 1992, pp 1313–1323.
5. Ashley K, Kannel WB, Sorlie PD, et al: Pulmonary function: relation to aging, cigarette habit, and mortality. Ann Intern Med 1975; 82:739.
6. Chodoff P, Margand PMS, Knowles CL: Short term abstinence from smoking: its place in preoperative preparation. Crit Care Med 1975; 3:131.
7. Wheatley IC, Hardy KJ, Barter CE: An evaluation of preoperative methods of preventing postoperative pulmonary complications. Anaesth Intensive Care 1977; 5:56.
8. Dripps RD, Deming MV: Postoperative atelectasis and pneumonia. Ann Surg 1946; 124:94.
9. Gold MI, Marcial E: An anesthetic adaptor for all metered dose inhalers (Letter to the editor). Anesthesiology 1988; 68:965.
10. Dellinger RP: Life-threatening bronchospasm in the asthmatic. *In* Critical Care. 2nd ed. Civetta JM, Taylor RW, Kirby RR (eds). Philadelphia, JB Lippincott, 1992, pp 1331–1332.
11. Stock MC, Downs JB, Gauer PK, et al: Prevention of postoperative pulmonary complications with CPAP, incentive spirometry, and conservative therapy. Chest 1985; 87:151.
12. Austin KL, Stapleton JV, Mather LE: Relationship between blood meperidine concentrations and analgesic response: a preliminary report. Anesthesiology 1980; 53:460.
13. Ready LB: Acute peridural narcotic therapy. *In* Perioperative Analgesia. Problems in Anesthesia. Brown DL (ed). Philadelphia, JB Lippincott, 1988, pp 327–338.
14. Cousins MJ, Mather LE: Intrathecal and epidural administration of opioids. Anesthesiology 1984; 61:276.
15. Boysen PG: Postoperative respiratory dysfunction. *In* Critical Care. 2nd ed. Civetta JM, Taylor RW, Kirby RR (eds). Philadelphia, JB Lippincott, 1992, pp 607, 608.
16. Brown DL, Flynn JF, Owens BD: Pain control. *In* Critical Care. 2nd ed. Civetta JM, Taylor RW, Kirby RR (eds). Philadelphia, JB Lippincott, 1992, pp 220, 221.
17. Ali MK, Mountain CF, Ewer MS, et al: Predicting loss of pulmonary function after pulmonary resection for bronchogenic carcinoma. Chest 1980; 77:337.
18. Boysen PG: Pulmonary resection and postoperative pulmonary function (Editorial). Chest 1980; 77:718.
19. Shapiro BA, Kacmarek RM, Cane RD, et al: Clinical Application of Blood Gases. 4th ed. Chicago, Mosby-Year Book Medical Publishers, 1989.
20. MacIntyre NR, Stock MC: Weaning mechanical ventilatory support. *In* Clinical Application of Ventilatory Support. Kirby RR, Banner MJ, Downs JB (eds). New York, Churchill Livingstone, 1990, pp 263–276.
21. MacIntyre NR: Respiratory function during pressure support ventilation. Chest 1986; 89:677.
22. Banner MJ, Blanch PB, Kirby RR, et al: Decreasing imposed work of the breathing apparatus to zero using pressure support ventilation. Crit Care Med 1993; 21:1333.
23. Stoelting RK: Pharmacology and Physiology in Anesthetic Practice. Philadelphia, JB Lippincott, 1987, p 267.
24. Gold MR, Dee GW, Cocca-Spofford D, et al: Esmolol and ventilatory function in cardiac patients with COPD. Chest 1991; 100:1215.
25. Stoelting RK: Pharmacology and Physiology in Anesthetic Practice. Philadelphia, JB Lippincott, 1987, p 303.

CHAPTER 10

Neurologic Consultation

DALE E. SOLOMON, M.D.

DIANE H. SOLOMON, M.D.

JERRY J. TOMASOVIC, M.D.

Patients with neurologic disease present unique challenges to anesthesiologists in the perioperative period. Many neurologic diseases are rare and are even more rarely encountered in the operating room, yet they have associated manifestations that require specific knowledge for optimal perioperative management. A neurologist as consultant can provide assistance in the perioperative period by (1) preoperatively identifying and optimizing medical management of neurologic disorders, (2) providing advice about perioperative management of patients with specific neurologic diseases, (3) performing intraoperative electrophysiologic assessments, and (4) diagnosing and treating postoperative sequelae and complications. The intent of this chapter is to provide answers to questions that anesthesiologists might commonly ask a neurologist and to share with neurologists the unique challenges that an anesthesiologist encounters while caring for patients with neurologic disease.

THE PERIOPERATIVE NEUROLOGIC CONSULT

What Are the Components of an Effective Consultation?

An effective neurologic consultation (Table 10–1) begins with a clear communication of the questions to be addressed by the consultant. When the question is ill defined or nebulous, the resultant assessment and recommendations are also likely to be vague. Even when the cause of the problem is unknown, a directed question can be formulated. For example, "Does this patient have a reversible neurologic condition?" is a better

TABLE 10–1. Effective Consultation Requirements

Direct contact between the consulting and consultant physicians
Limited number of recommendations
Emphasis on high-priority recommendations
Specification of drug, dosage, route, and duration
Continued follow-up and repeated offering of recommendations

consult request than "Please see postoperative patient in coma."

Next, the degree of urgency must be adequately communicated to the consultant. Thus, a patient in status epilepticus represents a more urgent problem than does a work-up of a perioperative nerve injury.

The consultant then gathers data (history, physical examination, diagnostic tests) to formulate an opinion. Ideally, data gathering and interpretation of findings by the consultant are performed independently to remove the bias of previous examinations and assessments. A neurologist's skill in taking detailed histories and performing expert neurologic examinations is extremely important at this point.

Finally, the consultant communicates his or her assessment and recommendations to the physician requesting the consult. Ideally, this communication is brief, specific to the question, diplomatic, and timely. The recommendations should include contingency plans for courses that the disease process are likely to take as well as subsequent tests that might be needed during the perioperative period. Follow-up by the consultant can ensure that potential new problems are adequately addressed.[1]

The spectrum of circumstances for which a neurologic consultation might be requested are summarized in Table 10–2.

What Should a Routine Preoperative Neurologic Evaluation Comprise?

Pre-Existing Disease

First, the presence of known pre-existing disease should be well documented, with particular attention to the duration of the disease, the current manifestations, the drug therapy, the physical examination findings, and the laboratory data that substantiate the diagnosis. Whenever inconsistencies are noted between the current findings and the presumed diagnosis, further investigation is needed. In addition, careful testing of disabilities immediately preoperatively allows more accurate postanesthetic assessment of neurologic dysfunction.

TABLE 10–2. Indications for Neurologic Consultation

Preoperative diagnosis of neurologic signs or symptoms	Headache Spells Transient or chronic focal symptoms Weakness Movement disorder Altered mental status
Preoperative assessment of chronic disease	Poorly controlled seizures Myasthenia gravis Pseudotumor cerebri Parkinson's disease Multiple sclerosis Muscular dystrophy Symptomatic carotid disease
Intraoperative monitoring of neurologic function	Electroencephalography or evoked responses for cerebral ischemia Somatosensory evoked responses for spine surgery Brainstem auditory evoked responses for posterior fossa surgery Electromyography and nerve conduction velocity for cranial or peripheral nerve monitoring
Postoperative complications	Failure to awaken, coma Delirium, encephalopathy New focal neurologic sign or nerve injury Headache Seizure Brain death determination

Absence of Known Disease

History

For patients without known neurologic diseases, a screening history and physical examination detect most neurologic diseases that have important anesthetic consequences. Every patient should be specifically questioned about a history of headache, loss of consciousness, weakness, and focal neurologic symptoms such as transient monocular blindness, diplopia, numbness, and dysphagia. Headache may denote tumor or other mass lesions, increased intracranial pressure (ICP), hydrocephalus, intracranial aneurysm, or arteriovenous malformation.

Loss of consciousness, described as fainting or blackouts, may indicate cardiovascular disease or a seizure disorder. Weakness, when diffuse, may suggest the presence of neuromuscular diseases (e.g., muscular dystrophy, myasthenia gravis, or a polyneuropathy) or endocrine or metabolic disorders. Unilateral episodes of weakness are most often associated with stroke, transient ischemic attack (TIA) (now also referred to as *reversible ischemic neurologic deficit*), or spinal root pathology.

Finally, focal neurologic symptoms may be due to various central and peripheral neurologic diseases and may indicate that further neurologic evaluation is necessary.

Physical Findings

Patients with identified and unstable disease or new symptoms or who are undergoing procedures that place them at risk for postoperative neurologic dysfunction should undergo more in-depth evaluation, perhaps by a neurologist.

MYASTHENIA GRAVIS

What Factors Are Important in Preoperative Evaluation?

Myasthenia gravis is due to loss of postjunctional acetylcholine receptors, resulting in weakness and easy fatigability. All muscles can be affected, but those of most concern to an anesthesiologist are the pharyngeal/laryngeal muscles protecting the airway and the muscles of respiration. These muscles must be assessed by testing the gag reflex, the ability to handle secretions, and the force of cough. Most patients should undergo pulmonary function studies to help anticipate the need for postoperative ventilatory assistance.

Drug Therapy

Accurate documentation of baseline strength is important. If a patient is weak, therapy should be maximized before elective surgery. Anticholinesterase drugs are used to prevent metabolism of acetylcholine at the neuromuscular junction. Most frequently used is pyridostigmine (Mestinon) at doses averaging 60 mg orally every 4 to 6 hours. If the disease is not controlled with pyridostigmine, steroids are usually added. However, approximately 8% of cases of myasthenia gravis transiently worsen when steroid therapy is initiated.

Immunosuppressive agents are used in severe myasthenia or if the response to steroids is inadequate. A full response to steroids or chemotherapeutic agents may take weeks to months. Plasmapheresis may provide the most rapid improvement in poorly controlled cases. When pheresis was provided 1 to 4 times at 2 to 13 days before thymectomy in patients with severe myasthenia, the need for postoperative mechanical ventilation, time to extubation, and length of stay in the intensive care unit (ICU) all decreased.[2]

Associated Diseases

A search for frequently associated diseases including thyroid disease, rheumatoid arthritis, systemic lupus erythematosus, and pernicious anemia should be made. Predictors of the need for postoperative mechanical ventilation include a duration of the disease >6 years, a history of chronic respiratory disease, pyridostigmine dose >750 mg · d^{-1} and vital capacity <2.9 L.[3]

How Is the Patient Managed Perioperatively?

Preoperative sedation is avoided because narcotics and benzodiazepines can affect respiratory and neuromuscular function. Most antibiotics except penicillins and cephalosporins can exacerbate weakness. Preoperative anticholinesterase medications are continued until the day of surgery. Patients treated with steroids should receive perioperative coverage.

Awake intubation or rapid-sequence induction with cricoid pressure is used in patients with bulbar involvement. Use of succinylcholine is avoided because of its potential for phase II blockade and prolonged action due to anticholinesterase therapy. In most cases, tracheal intubation can be performed without pharmacologically induced muscle relaxation, often with deep inhalation anesthesia alone.

Drugs (e.g., magnesium, local anesthetics, cardiac antidysrhythmics) and other factors (hypothermia, respiratory acidosis) that can potentiate nondepolarizing muscle relaxants should be avoided. Patients may be extremely sensitive to nondepolarizing muscle relaxants. When further muscle relaxation is needed, very small doses of nondepolarizing relaxants can be titrated with monitoring of neuromuscular blockade. Atracurium appears to be the relaxant of choice.[4]

Reversal of nondepolarizing muscle relaxants is performed in a titrated fashion with 1 to 2 mg of neostigmine every 5 minutes to avoid anticholinergic overdose, resultant cholinergic crisis, and an increase in weakness.

What Are the Postoperative Concerns?

If a patient is unable to resume oral pyridostigmine, it can be given intravenously at approximately 1/30 of the oral dose.[5] In the past, a Tensilon test was frequently performed in the postoperative period to distinguish cholinergic toxicity from worsening primary myasthenic weakness. Edrophonium (Tensilon) is a short- and rapid-acting anticholinesterase that improves weakness in myasthenic patients except in cases of excessive anticholinesterase medication. In the latter circumstance, the cholinergic effect of edrophonium causes increased weakness.

Because most neurologists no longer use very large doses of pyridostigmine and anesthesiologists limit their use of cholinergic drugs, cholinergic crisis is now uncommon as a cause of worsening weakness. Unless large doses of neostigmine are given as a muscle relaxant reversal, the Tensilon test is usually unnecessary. If patients are difficult to wean after restarting anticholinesterase therapy, plasmapheresis is begun. Protocols vary, but most begin with daily single plasma volume exchanges for 2 to 3 days, followed by alternate-day exchanges, depending on the clinical response.

PARKINSON'S DISEASE

Which Organ Systems Can Be Affected?

Depletion of dopamine in the striatonigral pathways of the basal ganglia causes the neurologic manifestations of Parkinson's disease: tremor, rigidity, bradykinesia, and impairment of postural and righting reflexes. Autonomic dysfunction results in orthostatic hypotension, impaired thermoregulation, and labile hemodynamics during anesthesia. There is a tendency toward dementia, delirium, and psychosis.

Pharyngeal and laryngeal muscle dysfunction may place patients with Parkinson's disease at an increased risk for aspiration. In addition, difficulty in eating and swallowing may affect the blood volume and nutritional status. Restrictive pulmonary disease results from rigidity and bradykinesia of the respiratory muscles and spinal kyphosis. Preoperative pulmonary function studies, arterial blood gas analysis, and pulmonary teaching are often recommended. Carbidopa-levodopa (Sinemet), the drug most frequently used to treat Parkinson's disease, can sensitize the myocardium to dysrhythmias and cause hypotension or hypertension.

What Are the Anesthetic Considerations?

Carbidopa-levodopa and other antiparkinsonian medications should be continued until the day of surgery. When the pharyngeal/laryngeal musculature is affected, rapid-sequence induction with cricoid pressure is used. Moderated doses of cardiodepressant anesthetics are used because of altered homeostatic adrenergic responses to hypotension. Succinylcholine has been reported in one case to cause hyperkalemia.[6] Normal responses to nondepolarizing muscle relaxants have been reported.

Use of antidopaminergic drugs such as metoclopramide, droperidol, and thorazine should be avoided. Regional anesthetic techniques can be used, but positioning may be difficult. Patients should be awake, and special attention should be given to verification of intact or at least baseline pharyngeal/laryngeal reflexes and adequate pulmonary function before extubation.

Withdrawal of carbidopa-levodopa in the postoperative period can cause severe exacerbation of symptoms. Therapy should be restarted as soon as possible to prevent irreversible rigidity and bradykinesia. In patients who are unable to take medications orally or by gastric tube, parenterally administered anticholinergic drugs such as trihexyphenidyl, benztropine, or diphenhydramine can be administered.

Other postoperative care is centered on pulmonary toilet and prevention of thromboses and, most importantly, early physical therapy and ambulation. Postoperative delirium is not uncommon and may be due to pre-existing dysfunction, intravenous anticholinergics, or medication withdrawal.

STROKE

What Is the Risk?

Perioperative stroke risk depends on the type of surgery. Cumulative data indicate that stroke incidence ranges from as low as 0.2% for patients undergoing general surgery to 4% in patients having cardiac or carotid surgery (Table 10–3). If patients with a prior history of cerebrovascular disease are excluded, the risk of stroke in adults undergoing general surgery decreases by more than half. Additional risk predictors include peripheral vascular disease, hypertension, atrial fibrillation, and possibly age >70 years[7, 8] (Table 10–4).

What Preventive Strategies May Be Used?

Preoperative

Treatment of coronary artery disease, atrial fibrillation, and hypertension should be optimized before surgery. New atrial

TABLE 10–3. Perioperative Stroke Risk

Surgery	Incidence	Range
General	0.2%	0.1–0.4%
Peripheral vascular	1.5%	1–2%
Cardiac	4%	1–6%
Carotid artery	4%	1–8%

(Data from Lee T, Goldman L: Role of the consultant. *In* Perioperative Management. Breslow M, Miller C, Rogers M (eds). St Louis, CV Mosby, 1990, p 49, *and* Landercasper J, Merz BJ, Cogbill TH, et al: Perioperative stroke risk in 173 consecutive patients with a past history of stroke. Arch·Surg 1990; 125:986.)

TABLE 10–4. Predictors of Perioperative Stroke

Predictor	Relative Risk
Prior stroke/transient ischemic attack	× 20
Peripheral vascular surgery	× 8
Atrial fibrillation	× 4
Advanced age	× ?

(Data from Larsen SF, Zaric D, Boysen G: Postoperative cerebrovascular accidents in general surgery. Acta Anaesthesiol Scand 1988; 32:698, *and* Hart RG, Easton JD: Management of cervical bruits and carotid stenosis in preoperative patients. Stroke 1983; 14:290.)

fibrillation should be converted to normal sinus rhythm, if possible, or the ventricular rate should be well controlled in chronic atrial fibrillation. Asymptomatic atrial fibrillation is treated prophylactically with aspirin or coumadin,[9] but these medications are discontinued before most operative procedures.

The cause of past strokes and TIAs should be determined. This work-up includes a computed tomographic (CT) scan of the brain to rule out intracerebral hemorrhage or subdural hematoma, carotid screening with carotid ultrasonography/Doppler, and angiography in selected cases. Preventive therapy is directed by the stroke's cause. Because angiographically determined stenosis of >70% on the symptomatic side of stroke or TIA has been identified as an indication for carotid endarterectomy (CEA), angiography should probably be performed before elective surgery.[10] Noncardioembolic strokes without significant carotid disease are primarily treated with aspirin. Patients who are intolerant of aspirin or who have stroke symptoms despite aspirin therapy may now be treated with ticlopidine (Ticlid), a platelet inhibitor.[11] However, ticlopidine is associated with a 1% risk of neutropenia and requires biweekly complete blood counts with differentiation for at least 3 months.

If a patient has a history of coronary artery disease, valvular heart disease, or cardiac dysrhythmias, echocardiography and possibly 24-hour ambulatory electrographic monitoring are warranted. In patients with known atrial fibrillation or those considered at high risk for emboli of cardiac origin (large left atrial size, stroke in posterior cerebral artery territory), a transesophageal echocardiogram should be considered if a transthoracic echocardiogram is nonrevealing.[12] Unlike transesophageal echocardiography, transthoracic echocardiography does not easily visualize the left atrium, and clots often are missed. If a cardiac thrombus is identified, sodium warfarin is usually given for a minimum of 3 months and then as indicated by repeat echocardiogram.

Intraoperative

Intraoperatively, stroke prevention involves blood pressure control and optimal oxygen transport. Most strokes occur postoperatively and are not a result of intraoperative hypotension even in the presence of carotid occlusive disease. An exception to this observation is that intraoperative hypotension may have a role in stroke during aortic surgery. These patients have a high likelihood of carotid disease, and transient acute hypotension is common at the time of vessel clamp release, thus increasing the risk of stroke on this basis.[7]

It is commonly recommended that mean perfusion pressure be maintained at >50 mm Hg in patients with significant occlusive carotid disease. However, no controlled prospective studies address this issue. A transcranial Doppler study showed that when mean arterial pressure was kept >60 mm Hg, blood flow velocity was maintained despite severe unilateral stenosis.[13] However, Brusino and colleagues[14] found no difference in cerebral blood flow in a patient with >80% bilateral carotid stenosis with mean arterial pressures at 35 mm Hg versus 85 mm Hg. Cerebral autoregulation appears to remain intact over a wide range of pressures despite old age and severe cerebrovascular disease if a vasoconstrictor is used to increase the mean arterial pressure and thereby the cerebral perfusion pressure.

When Are Antiplatelet Agents and Anticoagulants Stopped Before Surgery?

Guidelines for discontinuing aspirin depend on the vascularity of the surgical site and the "comfort" of the surgeon. For most operations, aspirin is stopped 5 to 10 days before surgery and restarted 48 to 72 hours postoperatively. Aspirin is not usually stopped before CEA and is continued immediately afterward. One study suggests expeditiously resuming aspirin is especially important to prevent myocardial infarction in post-CEA patients.[15] Ticlopidine is similar to aspirin in terms of its effect on bleeding time, and similar guidelines are appropriate.

Substituting heparin for sodium warfarin (Coumadin) 3 to 4 days before surgery allows avoidance of the use of vitamin K for reversal because when vitamin K is used, reanticoagulation with sodium warfarin may be difficult. Sodium warfarin is restarted 12 to 24 hours postoperatively in patients with mitral valve prosthesis and 24 to 48 hours postoperatively in most other conditions.

When Is It Safe to Operate After a Stroke?

By convention, anesthesia and surgery are delayed 4 to 6 weeks after acute stroke. This practice is based on our knowledge of loss of autoregulation in the ischemic penumbra surrounding the infarct. Neuronal perfusion is directly related to systemic blood pressure when autoregulation is absent. This relationship puts the susceptible peri-infarct tissue at high risk for irreversible damage from relatively mild hypotension.

How Long Should the Use of Succinylcholine Be Avoided After a Hemiparetic Stroke?

Unless a compelling reason necessitates the use of succinylcholine, it should probably be avoided for the remainder of the patient's life. However, a hyperkalemic response to succinylcholine has not been reported later than 6 months after stroke.[16]

MULTIPLE SCLEROSIS

What Elements Are Necessary in the Preoperative Evaluation?

Clinical Findings

White matter degeneration in the brain of patients with multiple sclerosis can cause diverse clinical findings. Sensory, motor, autonomic, optic, and integrative pathways all may be affected. Respiratory function may be affected by demyelinating lesions of the cervical spinal cord or medullary respiratory centers. Pulmonary function studies and arterial blood gas analysis should be obtained to evaluate the respiratory reserve. Pharyngeal and laryngeal muscle dysfunction places some patients at increased risk for aspiration of gastric contents. Patients with paraplegia or quadriplegia may be prone to autonomic hyper-reflexia. Symptoms or signs of this syndrome should be sought.

Medications

Medications used to treat associated spasticity have anesthetic implications.[16] Propantheline can potentiate nondepolarizing neuromuscular relaxants, delay gastric emptying, and cause autonomic blockade. Baclofen and dantrolene may potentiate nondepolarizing muscle relaxants. Diazepam potentiates the sedative effects of anesthetic drugs. A history of recent (within 1 year) steroid therapy should be solicited. Exacerbations are sometimes treated with steroids, and stress coverage for surgery often is necessary.

What Are the Anesthetic Considerations?

Spinal and epidural anesthesia have been reported to cause exacerbations of the disease, but may be used when other patient factors argue against general anesthesia.[17, 18] When general anesthesia is chosen, rapid-sequence induction is indicated if pharyngeal/laryngeal muscle involvement is present. Invasive hemodynamic monitoring is warranted in the presence of autonomic insufficiency.[19]

Succinylcholine may cause significant potassium release with multiple sclerosis (Table 10–5). Close monitoring of neuromuscular function is needed when nondepolarizing muscle relaxants are used because they may have an exaggerated or prolonged effect. Hyperthermia should be avoided because exacerbation of multiple sclerosis weakness can occur as a consequence of fever. Patients with multiple sclerosis present one of the few noncardiac surgery situations in which we actively strive to keep patients cool. The disease may be worsened by the stress of anesthesia and surgery.

TABLE 10–5. Neurologic Diseases in Which Succinylcholine May Cause an Exaggerated Potassium Release

Neurologic Disease	Period of Vulnerability
Hemiplegia (stroke)	7 d–6 mo
Parkinson's disease	? if any
Multiple sclerosis	not reported
Encephalitis	not reported
Head injury	not reported
Subarachnoid hemorrhage	not reported
Tetanus	not reported
Paraplegia (traumatic)	3 wk–3 mo
Anterior horn disease (amyotrophic lateral sclerosis)	not reported
Muscle denervation	3 wk–3 mo
Myotonia*	always
Muscular dystrophy*	always

(Modified from Azar I: The response of patients with neuromuscular disorders to muscle relaxants: a review. Anesthesiology 1984; 61:173.)
*Increased susceptibility to succinylcholine-induced malignant hyperthermia.

MUSCULAR DYSTROPHY

Which Organ Systems Are Affected?

Of most interest to anesthesiologists is the fact that muscular dystrophy may affect the muscles of the pharynx and glottis, the respiratory system, and the cardiovascular system. Delayed gastric emptying, difficulty with swallowing, and inability to handle secretions place patients at risk for perioperative aspiration. In addition, glottic muscle weakness may restrict expiratory airflow.

Respiratory muscle dysfunction often manifests as tachypnea, smaller tidal volumes, and paradoxical breathing with use of accessory muscles of respiration. Many times, baseline respiratory function appears normal but reserve is severely limited. In addition, the ventilatory response to hypercapnia and hypoxemia may be depressed.

Myocardial function can be severely compromised in myotonic dystrophy, Duchenne's muscular dystrophy, Becker's muscular dystrophy, limb-girdle dystrophy, and fascioscapulohumeral muscular dystrophy.[20] Cardiac conduction abnormalities are common. Preoperative testing, including electrocardiography (ECG) and some measure of myocardial contractility (echocardiogram or multigated angiogram), should be performed.

What Are the Anesthetic Considerations?

Intraoperatively, patients with muscular dystrophy most often require assisted or controlled ventilation to compensate for the negative effects of anesthetics on muscle function and ventilatory response to elevated carbon dioxide tension ($PaCO_2$). ECG and frequent blood pressure monitoring are important to assess the effect of anesthesia on cardiac function. When cardiac reserve is compromised preoperatively, invasive hemodynamic monitoring is indicated. Postoperatively, the trachea is extubated when patients are awake and have return of baseline motor function, and when weaning criteria are met (i.e., peak negative pressure at least -20 to -30 cm H_2O and vital capacity at least 15 mL $\cdot$ kg^{-1} with acceptable arterial blood gas values and pH).

GUILLAIN-BARRÉ SYNDROME

How Is the Nervous System Affected?

Guillain-Barré syndrome presents most often after an otherwise inconsequential viral infection, but has been reported in postoperative patients without evidence of antecedent viral infection.[20] It consists of a symmetric ascending weakness evolving over several days and caused by demyelination of peripheral nerves.

In one half of cases, cranial nerve involvement compromises respiratory and bulbar function. Sensory deficits can occur. Autonomic dysfunction is common, resulting in hemodynamic instability. Nerve conduction studies reveal slowed conduction velocities early on and denervation potentials late in the course of the disease. Other polyneuropathies may mimic the disease.

What Are the Anesthetic Implications?

With regard to muscle weakness, attention to airway management and respiratory support is similar to that with muscular dystrophy. Succinylcholine may cause massive potassium release in chronically denervated muscles (see Table 10–5). Close hemodynamic monitoring, including continuous ECG and intra-arterial blood pressure monitoring, are indicated because of the instability of the cardiovascular system with resultant lability of heart rate and blood pressure. Central venous or pulmonary artery catheter monitoring may be useful to ensure euvolemia, because with autonomic insufficiency, heart rate and blood pressure are unreliable indicators of the volume status.

HUNTINGTON'S DISEASE

What Are the Anesthetic Considerations?

Huntington's disease is a genetically transmitted condition associated with neuronal destruction in the caudate nucleus and putamen. Patients manifest progressive chorea, dementia, and depression. They may have prolonged sedation with normal doses of induction drugs. Also, prolonged paralysis with succinylcholine has been suggested, although it has not been confirmed in other reports.[21] Anticholinergic drugs may exacerbate the choreiform movements.[22] Because of involvement of the pharyngeal musculature, an increased risk of aspiration may be present in the perioperative period.

Haloperidol, a butyrophenone, is most commonly used to treat the choreiform movements. The α-adrenergic blocking properties of this agent may potentiate hypotension during induction or maintenance of anesthesia, whereas the sedative properties potentiate the hypnotic and respiratory depressant effect of anesthetic drugs.

PSEUDOTUMOR CEREBRI

What Is It?

Pseudotumor cerebri (also called *benign intracranial hypertension*) is a syndrome that causes elevated ICP without an intracranial mass. It occurs four to eight times more frequently in women than in men[23] and is associated with headache, papilledema, visual disturbances, and cranial nerve dysfunction (usually VI).[24] The etiology is most often idiopathic but can include abnormalities of cerebral venous drainage, cerebrospinal fluid (CSF) secretion/outflow, or endocrine, metabolic, and immunologic diseases. The lumbar CSF pressure is elevated to >200 mm H_2O. Lumbar CSF drainage is often beneficial in treating symptoms of headache, but should be done only after a mass lesion has been ruled out with contrast CT scanning or magnetic resonance imaging.[25] Hydrocephalus is not present; in fact, the ventricles are normal or small.

How Is Anesthesia Managed?

Preoperative Management

Careful preoperative documentation of the current visual abnormalities is important to assess postoperative dysfunction adequately. Patients undergoing spinal or epidural anesthesia may benefit from a CT scan of the head to rule out impending herniation syndromes. When the condition has been stable for months or years, anesthesia and surgery can proceed. However, recent deterioration in visual acuity or cranial nerve function necessitates further assessment and therapy before surgery. Perioperative steroid coverage is required for patients who have recently been treated with steroids.

Regional Anesthesia

Spinal anesthesia is safe in the great majority of cases and in fact has been advocated because CSF drainage, which constitutes part of the normal therapy for this condition, may be instituted immediately before injection of the spinal anesthetic in many patients.[26] Epidural anesthesia would be a less desirable choice because injection of fluid into the epidural space increases the ICP.

General Anesthesia

When general anesthesia is necessary, drugs and techniques that actually decrease or prevent increases in ICP are used. Abnormal responses to muscle relaxants have not been reported, nor do these patients appear more sensitive to sedative-hypnotics. Because a majority of patients with pseudotumor cerebri are obese, standard techniques for induction, emergence, and extubation of obese patients should be instituted.

PRE-ECLAMPSIA/ECLAMPSIA

What Further Neurologic Evaluation Is Necessary?

The typical pre-eclamptic patient has arterial hypertension, peripheral edema, proteinuria, and onset of the disease between 20 weeks' gestation and 48 hours post partum. Many of these patients complain of headache, photophobia, and visual difficulty and may have altered mental status and nausea and vomiting. Patients with these symptoms who do not have other typical findings of pre-eclampsia need further neurologic evaluation.

In patients who have pre-eclampsia/eclampsia and evidence of focality on neurologic examination or who are comatose, CT scan of the head may rule out processes that require surgical intervention such as intracerebral hemorrhage with mass effect or hydrocephalus due to posterior fossa edema and CSF pathway obstruction.[27]

Comatose patients with diffuse cerebral edema and papilledema should receive therapy for increased ICP similar to that used for other conditions that cause elevated ICP. Although radiologic evaluation is recommended for patients with focality or in coma, CT scans of the head are usually not necessary in patients with "typical" eclampsia.[28]

How Are Eclamptic Seizures Best Treated?

Eclampsia is defined as the occurrence of seizures during pregnancy or in the postpartum period in a patient with pre-eclampsia. Eclampsia rarely occurs before 20 weeks' gestation or later than 48 hours post partum. Of course, any pregnant patient, including those with pre-eclampsia, can have seizures secondary to disease processes that cause seizures in the general population.

Several signs and symptoms in pre-eclamptic patients can portend the onset of seizures. These include severe and persistent headache, blurred vision, photophobia, vomiting, and hyperactive deep tendon reflexes with clonus.[29]

General Considerations

The initial considerations during eclamptic convulsion are to ensure adequate oxygenation and ventilation, to minimize the risk of pulmonary aspiration of gastric contents, and to prevent injury during the convulsion.

Magnesium Sulfate

Use of magnesium sulfate remains the standard of care in the United States for treatment of eclamptic seizures by obstetricians,[30] but its use for that purpose is coming under increasing scrutiny by neurologists. It is administered as an intravenous bolus of 4 to 6 g, followed by an intravenous infusion of 1 to 2 g · h^{-1}. If convulsions recur, another 2 to 4 g is given over 5 minutes.[31]

Many neurologists argue that drug treatment for eclamptic seizures should be no different than that for seizures due to other causes. This opinion is based on the premise that magnesium sulfate is not a proven anticonvulsant; that its use in eclampsia has been based on historical rather than clinical research data; that many patients have seizures despite adequate serum magnesium concentrations; and that established anticonvulsive drugs are effective in treating eclamptic seizures with minimal side effects.[32, 33] Thus, use of an intravenous benzodiazepine (lorazepam, 1–2 mg; diazepam, 5–10 mg; or midazolam, 2–5 mg) titrated to stop the seizure, followed by intravenous phenytoin administration (10 mg · kg^{-1} given at a rate <25 mg · min^{-1}) may be an alternative to stop eclamptic seizures. Blood pressure and ECG monitoring are required during phenytoin loading.

Intramuscular midazolam, 10 mg, has been used to stop seizures when intravenous access cannot be obtained.[34] After the seizure has been controlled and adequate oxygenation, ventilation, and blood pressure are ensured, further care is administered, including control of blood pressure and delivery of the fetus.[35]

NEUROLEPTIC MALIGNANT SYNDROME

What Is It?

Neuroleptic malignant syndrome (NMS) is an idiosyncratic reaction that occurs in one of two pharmacologic settings:

1. After administration of drugs that block central dopaminergic pathways. These drugs include chlorpromazine, droperidol, metoclopramide, prochlorperazine, and many other neuroleptics used primarily in psychiatry, including butyrophenones, phenothiazines, and thioxanthines.
2. During withdrawal of dopaminergic agonists used for treatment of parkinsonism.[36]

Dopamine is an integral neurotransmitter in thermoregulatory neural and striatal motor pathways. Interference with dopaminergic activity can lead to impairment of temperature regulation and drug-induced parkinsonism. Fever results from altered thermoregulation in the presence of increased thermogenesis due to exaggerated muscle activity. Thus, NMS should be suspected in the proper pharmacologic setting when parkinsonism, manifested as tremor and rigidity, or other movement disorders such as dystonia are associated with fever in the absence of infection. In addition, autonomic instability, altered mental status, and elevations in creatine kinase levels may be present.

What Is the Incidence and Associated Mortality?

NMS occurs in about 1 in 100 to 1 in 1000 patients treated with neuroleptic medications. The overall mortality has been about 10% since 1984. Excess mortality occurs when the syndrome is associated with myoglobinemia and renal failure.[37] The use of dopamine agonists (bromocriptine, amantadine) and dantrolene does not appear to decrease mortality.

What Is the Differential Diagnosis of Fever and Movement Disorder?

These signs can occur with encephalitis, meningitis, idiopathic or drug-induced Parkinson's disease with ongoing infection, heat stroke, malignant hyperthermia, alcohol or benzodiazepine withdrawal, and lethal catatonia, a mental disorder that results in continuous uncontrollable motor activity and fever.

What Is the Treatment?

Initial treatment is supportive. Neuroleptic medication is stopped. Adequate oxygenation and ventilation are ensured, with muscle relaxants if necessary. Nondepolarizing agents provide muscle relaxation in NMS. Hyperpyrexia is treated with cooling blankets, alcohol-water baths, and antipyretics. Cardiovascular stability is achieved with fluid and inotropes in hypotensive patients and with vasodilators or α-blockers when severe hypertension is present.

Dantrolene can decrease the muscle rigidity and aid in lowering the fever, but an improvement in mortality has not been demonstrated with its use.[37] The dopamine agonists carbidopa-levodopa, amantadine, and bromocriptine can shorten the duration of the illness.[38, 39] When myoglobinuria is present, vigorous fluid therapy and diuresis are required to prevent renal failure.

Are Agents that Trigger Malignant Hyperthermia Safe in Patients with Neuroleptic Malignant Syndrome?

Succinylcholine has been used safely many times in patients with NMS, although a case report describes a hyperkalemic response.[40] Nevertheless, use of nondepolarizing muscle relaxants seems warranted when their relatively long duration will not complicate the procedure.[41] Patients have been safely anesthetized with volatile anesthetics, a fact that emphasizes the differences in pathophysiology between NMS and malignant hyperthermia.

KNOWN SEIZURE DISORDERS

What Is Important in the Preoperative Evaluation?

In patients who have a known seizure disorder and are being treated with anticonvulsants, the type of seizures, their frequency, and drug therapy and serum concentration should be known. In patients whose seizure disorder is well controlled or who suffer only from absence seizures, surgery can proceed without adjustment of their usual anticonvulsant regimen. Patients who have experienced an increasing frequency of seizures or who have frequent generalized tonic-clonic seizures should be evaluated for potential causes of exacerbation of seizures.

Common contributors include medication noncompliance, alcohol, and illness. Electrolyte, creatinine, and albumin determinations, a complete blood count with differential, and urinalysis are performed. If the anticonvulsant level is subtherapeutic, the patient is given a loading dose of the applicable agent. However, elective surgery should be delayed until the patient's seizure control is stabilized, because an intraoperative seizure would likely remain unnoticed and therefore untreated in a patient undergoing general anesthesia with neuromuscular blockade. However, therapy for complications related to seizures, such as dehiscence of a surgical wound or loss of airway access, often requires muscle relaxant use.

How Are Anticonvulsants Handled Perioperatively?

Table 10–6 lists commonly used anticonvulsants. Most patients maintain acceptable blood levels of drug by taking the usual oral dose of medication with sips of water during the nil per os (NPO) preoperative period. For patients who remain in NPO status postoperatively, the oral medications can be given via nasogastric tube; alternatively, a change to intravenous phenytoin or phenobarbital can be made.

When poor oral absorption can be anticipated in elective surgery, a switch to phenytoin or phenobarbital several weeks before surgery allows attainment of steady-state levels and avoidance of an intravenous loading dose.

Valproic acid given rectally to children has good absorption.[42] A preceding cleansing enema is required for predictable absorption. Rectal absorption of carbamazepine is unreliable.

The relatively long half-life of these drugs means that by doubling the last oral dose before surgery, one can maintain therapeutic blood levels throughout the day of surgery despite the omission of one or two doses.

How Is Anesthesia Managed for Patients with Seizures?

Regional Anesthesia

Although toxic doses of local anesthetics can cause seizures, no evidence shows that the serum concentrations associated with routine epidural or brachial plexus anesthesia are unsafe in patients with a seizure disorder. Nevertheless, when regional anesthesia is chosen, it would seem prudent, when possible, to use spinal anesthesia, with its much lower local anesthetic dose.

General Anesthesia

Many of the intravenous and inhaled anesthetics in common use can enhance or suppress seizure activity, depending on the dose administered and the clinical situation. Ketamine (especially when combined with theophylline) and methohexital have been reported to be epileptogenic in patients with a seizure disorder.[43]

Enflurane, at high doses ($\geq 2.5\%$) with hyperventilation ($Pa_{CO_2} \leq 25$ mm Hg), produces electroencephalographic (EEG) evidence of seizure activity. Avoidance of enflurane use is recommended as is maintenance of normocarbia in the perioperative period. Halothane may be metabolized to a greater extent because of the up-regulation of hepatic microsomal enzymes, resulting in a potentially increased incidence of hepatotoxicity. Isoflurane is a potent anticonvulsant.[44]

Awareness of the sedative side effects of this group of drugs and their effect on hepatic metabolism and protein binding of concurrently administered drugs is important. In addition, chronic phenytoin and carbamazepine therapy have been associated with resistance to nondepolarizing neuromuscular relaxants.

What Intraoperative Monitoring Is Indicated?

Electroencephalography

EEG measures the summation of spontaneous brain electrical activity immediately adjacent to recording electrodes placed on the scalp or on brain tissue itself. The raw EEG can

TABLE 10–6. Commonly Used Anticonvulsant Medications

Drug	Serum Half-Life (Hours)	Therapeutic Blood Level (μg/mL)	Dose-Related Side Effects
Phenytoin	24 ± 12	10–20	Nystagmus, ataxia, lethargy
Phenobarbital	96 ± 12	15–40	Lethargy, nystagmus, ataxia
Carbamazepine	12 ± 3	28–12	Lethargy, diplopia, blurred vision
Primidone	12 ± 6	5–12	Lethargy, nystagmus, ataxia
Ethosuximide	30 ± 6	40–100	Hiccups, headache, drowsiness, N & V
Valproic acid	12 ± 6	50–100	N & V, drowsiness, increasing absences
Clonazepam	22–32	5–50	Sedation, tolerance, behavior problems

Abbreviations: N & V = nausea and vomiting.

record voltage changes with time over a large percentage of the brain using a 16-channel montage. By noting the frequency of the resultant electrical waveform (in hertz) and its amplitude and symmetry, inferences can be made about the degree of activation and metabolic state of underlying brain (Table 10–7). For example, increasing frequency of the waveform is associated with seizure activity and with use of low-dose barbiturates and ketamine. Low-frequency high-amplitude waveforms are associated with narcotic anesthesia and deeper levels of inhalational anesthesia. Low-frequency low-amplitude activity may occur with hypoxia, ischemia, and higher dose barbiturates. Finally, an isoelectric EEG is found with brain death, severe hypothermia, profound hypoperfusion, barbiturate-induced coma, and twice minimal alveolar concentration levels of isoflurane.

Computer Processing

Computer processing of the raw EEG transforms the data into power (amplitude squared) versus frequency and can display the data in a graphically simplistic manner. For example, the compressed spectral array (CSA) monitor plots power versus frequency over time in a three-dimensional plot, often with a display of the spectral edge frequency—that is, the frequency below which 97% of the power is occurring (Fig. 10–1). Processed EEG monitors are primarily used to detect global cerebral ischemia and miss episodes of focal ischemia that can be detected by a 16-channel raw EEG.

Evoked Potentials

Evoked potentials (often also referred to as *evoked responses*) measure the electrical response in the central nervous system to a stimulus applied to a more peripheral nerve. The clinical use of evoked potentials requires that (1) an intact neural pathway be accessible for stimulation distally and monitoring proximally and that (2) this neural pathway be anatomically proximate or physiologically similar to the neural elements at risk during surgery. By signal averaging and electronic filtering, the low-amplitude evoked potentials can be recorded and analyzed for their latency (time from stimulation to generation of an electrical signal) and amplitude. In addition, near-field (close to the recording electrode, e.g., the cerebral cortex) and far-field potentials (recording deeper transmission through deeper brain structures, e.g., brainstem) can be recorded.

Current evoked potential modalities include (1) somatosensory evoked potentials (SSEPs), elicited by stimulating a peripheral nerve in the arm or leg and recording the nerve impulse at the scalp, over the spine, at an interspinous ligament, or in an epidural space; (2) brainstem auditory evoked potentials (BAEPs), in which cranial nerve VIII is stimulated with an audible click and recording of the generated potentials in the brainstem occurs over the posterior scalp; and (3) visual evoked potentials, in which cranial nerve II is stimulated with flashes of light and potentials are recorded over the anterior cranial fossa.

Electromyography and Nerve Conduction Velocity

In addition, electromyography (EMG) and nerve conduction velocity monitoring can be used by surgeons to assess the

TABLE 10–7. Electroencephalographic Waveform: Characteristics and Interpretation

Rhythm	Frequency (Hz)	State of Arousal
Delta	0–4	Coma, hypoxia/ischemia, deep anesthesia
Theta	4–8	Sleep, surgical anesthesia
Alpha	8–13	Relaxed, eyes closed, light anesthesia
Beta	13–30	Awake, alert, low-dose barbiturate

integrity of motor and cranial nerve pathways during dissection of proximate tissue.

Indications for Electrophysiologic Monitoring

The Therapeutics and Technology Assessment Subcommittee of the American Academy of Neurology has published an assessment of intraoperative electrophysiologic monitoring.[45]

Carotid Endarterectomy

For CEA and other procedures in which cerebral ischemia is a risk, the order of preference for cerebral monitoring is (1) a 16-channel EEG, (2) 4-channel EEG monitoring with electrodes placed over the anterior and posterior regions of both hemispheres, or (3) SSEPs.

Resection of Abnormal Brain Tissue

Electrocorticography from surgically exposed cortex can help to define the optimal limits of surgical resection of abnormal brain tissue, either for biopsy or resection, such as during surgery for epilepsy.

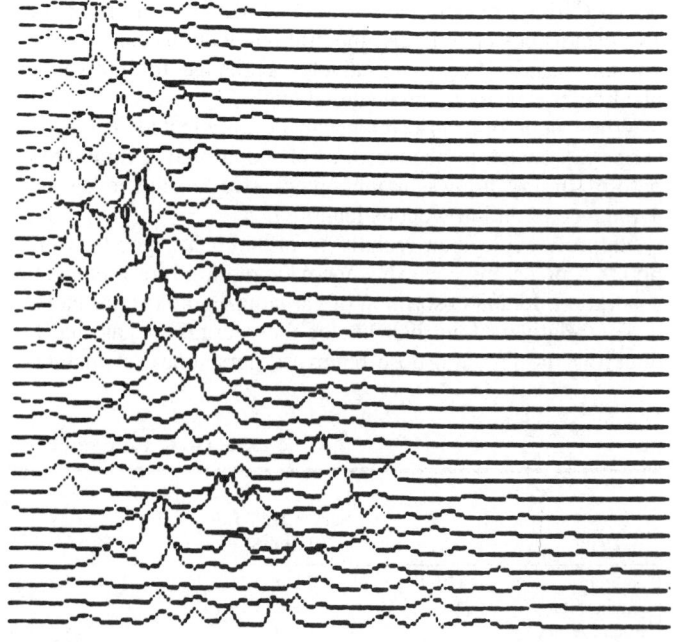

FIGURE 10–1. Compressed spectral array plotting of power and frequency against time. This frequency domain display allows easy recognition of frequency concentration shifts over long periods of time. However, the large amplitude of some traces can obscure activity in others. (From Kirby RR: Monitoring of neurologic function. *In* Critical Care. 1st ed. Civetta JM, Taylor RW, Kirby RR (eds). Philadelphia, JB Lippincott, 1988, p 353.)

Posterior Fossa Surgery

During posterior fossa surgery, BAEPs and facial nerve (VII) monitoring by nerve stimulation with EMG are indicated to identify cranial nerve impairment caused by compression, retraction, or ischemia.

Spine Surgery

SSEP monitoring is indicated during orthopedic spine surgery, especially scoliosis surgery and neurosurgical spinal cord surgery, and when the thoracic aorta is cross-clamped.

Peripheral Nerve Grafting/Dissection

EMG and nerve conduction velocity measurements are indicated for identifying peripheral nerves that are damaged and need grafting, for identifying nerve pathways and monitoring their function during surgical dissection, and for monitoring nerve function during intraoperative procedures (traction, compression, limb positioning) that may damage nerves.

The subcommittee cautions that intraoperative monitors not be used in clinical situations where the risk of nervous system damage is low. When the risk is high, electrophysiologic monitoring is probably safe and efficacious.

In addition to these published recommendations, many anesthesiologists are using the EEG and SSEPs to monitor depth of anesthesia, to ensure adequate brain and spinal cord perfusion during induced hypotension, and to achieve an isoelectric EEG pattern when the brain is at risk for ischemic events.

Anesthetics For Evoked Potential Monitoring

Most intravenous and inhalational anesthetics affect the SSEPs to a variable and inconsistent degree, with cortical SSEPs recorded from the scalp being more greatly affected than subcortical SSEPs or BAEPs. Barbiturates cause a small increase in the latency and decrease the amplitude but do not abolish the SSEP even when the cortical EEG is isoelectric. The volatile anesthetics and nitrous oxide have the greatest effect on cortical SSEPs by increasing the latency and decreasing the amplitude of the recorded potential.[46] Opiates tend to decrease the amplitude and increase the latency of recorded potentials, but clinically useful SSEPs can be obtained even with high-dose narcotic anesthesia. Etomidate, ketamine, and propofol may actually potentiate SSEPs.[47]

The most common technique for maintenance of anesthesia during SSEP monitoring is with narcotic, usually fentanyl, supplemented with $\leq60\%$ nitrous oxide or $\leq1\%$ isoflurane. General anesthesia appears to have little effect on either peripheral (e.g., cervical SSEPs) or short-latency auditory evoked potentials.[48]

The most important anesthetic factor in producing an easily interpretable recording is that the depth of anesthesia be maintained at a stable level during baseline and subsequent monitoring and that the individual interpreting the evoked potentials be made aware when clinical circumstances dictate a change in the anesthetic technique. Other physiologic variables must be maintained constant, such as body temperature, acid-base status, hematocrit, and blood pressure.

OBSTRUCTIVE SLEEP APNEA

Obese patients with obstructive sleep apnea remain at maximum risk for postoperative complications related to preoperative sedation, general anesthetics, or both. Reduced lung volumes contribute to airway compromise. Maintenance of a patent upper airway may also be compromised by analgesics and decreased muscle tone. Finally, blunting of the normal ventilatory drive responses to increased $PaCO_2$ is frequently present and may be worsened by airway edema associated with surgical procedures such as a uvulopalatopharyngoplasty.

Surprisingly, many cases of obstructive sleep apnea remain undiagnosed. If an obese patient or a family member provides a history of excessive daytime somnolence, a consultation by a pulmonary or neurology specialist in sleep disorders should be obtained to identify the extent of this problem before initiating perioperative management. Pulmonary function tests and arterial blood gas analysis are important for comprehensive evaluation. An elevated resting $PaCO_2$ is particularly worrisome and is associated with a significantly increased risk of postoperative pulmonary complications. Careful evaluation for any evidence of early cor pulmonale is essential; morbidity and mortality are significantly increased if it is present.

PERIPHERAL NERVE INJURY

How Common Is It?

Historical data indicate that nerve injury occurs in about 0.1% of anesthetized patients.[49] Surgery for myocardial revascularization carries an incidence of nerve injury of 2.6% to 13%.[50, 51] Surgical positions other than level supine probably increase the risk of nerve injuries.[52] The use of muscle relaxants, which allow abnormal stretching of limbs, has been suggested as a risk factor for nerve injury.[53]

What Are the Mechanisms?

Nerves may be injured by various mechanisms. Ischemia due to mechanical pressure can be caused by external compression, traction, or stretching. Other causes include interruption of blood flow or inadequate oxygen supply due to vascular disease, anemia, or hypotension. Direct trauma may result from surgical misadventure, needle trauma, and intraneural injection.

The incidence of nerve injury is increased when paresthesias are sought during performance of a nerve block.[54] Neurotoxicity due to high perineural concentration of local anesthetics can occur. Various chemical compounds when injected into the subarachnoid space or around peripheral nerves are potentially toxic. These compounds include local anesthetics at high concentration, antibiotics, electrolyte solutions, and bactericidal and chemotherapy agents.

Which Nerves Are Most Likely to Be Injured?

An examination of the database of the American Society of Anesthesiologists' (ASA) Closed Claim Study reveals that nerve injury accounted for 15% of the malpractice claims reviewed, and was the second most common cause of claims.[55] Of those, 34% involved injury to the ulnar nerve, 23% to the brachial plexus, and 16% to the lumbosacral nerve roots. The remaining 28% of claims were nearly equally divided between the spinal cord, sciatic nerve, median nerve, radial nerve, femoral nerve, and other peripheral and cranial nerves. Overall, nerve injuries were equally divided between men and women, although a 3:1 male predominance was noted in ulnar nerve injury, similar to a 5:1 predominance cited in another study.[56]

How Does Nerve Injury Present?

Of the 22 cases in the ASA Closed Claims Study in which the time of onset of symptoms was described, only 8 were noted on the first postoperative day. The remainder were first detected as long as 1 month after surgery. The presenting symptoms may include paresthesia, dysesthesia, weakness, clumsiness, or pain in the affected nerve distribution. Many nerve injuries may be subtle or not appreciated by a patient, for example, Horner's syndrome (after cervical sympathetic chain injury) or a unilateral phrenic nerve palsy. A postanesthetic nerve assessment directed by the intraoperative position has been advocated.[57] Table 10–8 lists nerves at particular risk with different intraoperative positions.

What Should Be Done After a Potential Nerve Injury Is Discovered?

First, reversible causes of nerve dysfunction should be sought and rectified. This process may include release of orthopedic casts and traction devices, correction of anemia, or surgical decompression of nerves compressed by edema, hematoma, or surgical devices.

History and Physical Findings

A detailed history and neurologic examination most often reveal which nerves are affected and why. First, the nature of the nerve deficit (sensory, motor, both, unilateral, bilateral) should be determined. Next, whether the suspected lesion can be explained on an anatomic basis (peripheral nerve, nerve root, or spinal cord lesion) or on a physiologic basis—for example, residual local anesthetic or neuromuscular blockade, electrolyte abnormality, or coexisting nerve-muscle disease—should be established. Finally, whether surgical trespass or positioning could have caused the lesion is determined.[58] Examples include lithotomy position (affecting the peroneal nerve) and inguinal exploration (affecting the femoral nerve). When a spinal or epidural hematoma is suspected, immediate

TABLE 10–8. Relationship Between Positioning and Potential Nerve Injury

Position	Nerves at Risk
Supine	Ulnar, suprascapular
Fracture table (vertical perineal post)	Obturator, pudendal, common peroneal
Lithotomy	Obturator, peroneal, femoral, saphenous
Sitting	Ulnar, sciatic, cervical spinal cord
Trendelenburg's (shoulder braces)	Brachial plexus, long thoracic
Lateral decubitus	Brachial plexus, peroneal, cervical sympathetic chain, facial nerve
Prone	Brachial plexus, ulnar, lateral femoral cutaneous, facial, optic

myelography, computed tomography, or magnetic resonance imaging is indicated.

Electrophysiologic Studies

Electrophysiologic measurements may help to localize the nerve lesion and determine whether loss of axonal continuity has occurred. EMG signs of muscle denervation (fibrillation potentials and positive sharp waves) do not become evident until 2 to 3 weeks after the nerve injury and even then are not 100% sensitive or specific for axonal loss. This is a critically important feature because an EMG in the immediate postoperative period can implicate the presence of pre-existing pathology and serve as a baseline for later studies when pathologic changes attributable to the perioperative period should become evident. Nerve conduction studies can localize the area along the course of the nerve that has become injured. Later, motor and sensory evoked responses may indicate when regeneration is occurring.[59]

What Is the Prognosis After Nerve Injury?

The prognosis depends on the mechanism of injury. Neuropraxia is an injury in which a portion of the nerve fibers becomes demyelinated but the continuity of the nerve and the endoneural sheath is preserved. Remyelinization allows recovery of function in 6 to 8 weeks.

Axonotmesis occurs when complete disruption of axons takes place within an intact epineural and perineural sheath. In this type of lesion, recovery depends on regeneration of neurons within endoneural tubes, and spontaneous recovery can occur, with a favorable prognosis after months to years. A rule of thumb is that the nerve regenerates at a rate of $1 \text{ mm} \cdot \text{d}^{-1}$. Thus, a proximal injury requires longer to recover than does a distal one.

Neurotmesis is complete transection of the axon and myelin sheath. With the fascicular anatomy disrupted, connective tissue proliferation and scarring occur within the nerve, preventing spontaneous generation down the nerve tract. These injuries are sometimes amenable to surgical repair.[60]

What Therapy Is Available After Nerve Injury Has Occurred?

Little can be done to aid nerve regeneration after traumatic nerve injuries. If nerve transection has occurred, reapproximation of the nerve ends may allow some regeneration to occur. A clean laceration caused by a slip of the scalpel in the operating room should be immediately repaired. If the injury is less well demarcated, nerve repair should be delayed 3 to 6 weeks. The determination must be made in the immediate postoperative period that the nerve dysfunction is not due to extrinsic compression that can be relieved surgically.

Control of metabolic factors, such as diabetes and uremia, and nutritional supplementation in patients suffering from hypovitaminosis caused by alcoholism or nutritional diseases may speed recovery. Anti-inflammatory medications may lessen the extent of the injury. Carbamazepine and phenytoin have been used to treat painful dysesthesia. Finally, sympathectomy may be needed to treat causalgia.[60, 61]

What Nerve Injuries Are Common in Pregnancy?

Neurologic complications are common in parturients who do not receive an anesthetic, occurring perhaps in 1 of 3000 deliveries.[62, 63] Thus, polyneuropathies and mononeuropathies should be identified in the preanesthetic period so that anesthetic procedures can be eliminated in the differential diagnosis of a neuropathy that is discovered post partum.

Many mononeuropathies that in nonpregnant patients would be attributed to the anesthetic or positioning can be caused by pregnancy and childbirth. For example, brachial plexus and lateral femoral cutaneous nerve injury can be caused by weight gain and changes in spinal curvature. A median neuropathy at the wrist is very common.[64] Peripartum ulnar neuropathy has been described.

Vaginal delivery may injure the femoral nerve, the obturator nerve, and the lumbosacral plexus.[65] Surgical procedures, vaginal instruments, and stirrups can injure the femoral nerve, lumbosacral trunk, and peroneal nerves, respectively. The weight of a term fetus and the effects of pregnancy can injure the sciatic nerve and cause radiculopathies. Radiculopathies may present at any time in the peripartum period with severe weakness. Bladder dysfunction is not uncommon after delivery. Backache occurs in about 40% of parturients not receiving an epidural anesthetic.[66]

In evaluating parturients for postanesthetic nerve injury, remember that repeated injection of long-acting local anesthetics (as would occur with labor analgesia) can produce a very long-lasting effect as a result of the partition coefficient of the anesthetic, in which it is in effect concentrated within the neural tissue.[67, 68] The duration and difficulty of labor, the use of instruments and retractors, and local anesthetics injected by the obstetrician are also important in determining the etiology of nerve lesions.

NEUROLOGIC COMPLICATIONS AFTER SPINAL OR EPIDURAL ANESTHESIA

Why Do They Occur?

Although nerve lesions associated with spinal or epidural anesthesia are exceedingly rare and probably occur no more frequently than with general anesthesia, permanent nerve damage can occur.[69, 70] Lumbosacral nerve injury has been reported and seems to be associated with paresthesia or pain on advancing the needle or during local anesthetic injection. Needle trauma to the spinal cord is unreported in the literature.[71] The toxic effects of local anesthetics, their preservatives, or both have been thought to cause neural deficits,[72, 73] cauda equina syndrome,[74] and backache.[75] Meningitis—bacterial or aseptic—can result from subarachnoid or epidural injection.[76–80] Several case reports describe spinal epidural abscesses after needle instrumentation.[81, 82]

Epidural hematomas can occur whether or not a patient is undergoing anticoagulation.[83] Unintentional injection of toxic substances into the subarachnoid space may cause adhesive arachnoiditis, and a technique has been described for "washing out" toxic substances.[84] Dural puncture can cause headache and has been associated with postoperative hearing loss and cranial nerve abnormalities.[85, 86]

Spinal anesthesia has been implicated in exacerbation of multiple sclerosis. Back pain occurs with a frequency of a few per cent after spinal or epidural anesthesia but may be just as frequent after general anesthesia. Preservative-free 2-chloroprocaine has been implicated as a cause of back pain.[87] Finally, paraplegia has occurred after epidural anesthesia without the presence of abscess or hematoma. Arterial hypotension and body positioning were thought to have contributed to spinal cord ischemia.[88]

POSTANESTHETIC NEUROLOGIC EXAMINATION

Many physical findings that are considered pathologic in healthy patients are commonly found in patients emerging from anesthesia. It is not unusual to find sustained ankle clonus, muscle spasticity, an up-going plantar response (positive Babinski's sign), and nonreactive pupils as long as 40 minutes after anesthesia.[89, 90] However, all abnormal findings should be symmetric, and a new unilateral finding of weakness, pathologic reflexes, or cranial nerve dysfunction requires immediate investigation.

A patient with a prior stroke or other intracranial process occasionally manifests lateralizing neurologic signs on awakening from general anesthesia. If the signs resolve within 30 minutes, they may be attributed to "differential awakening."[91] This is distinct from a procedure-related neurologic deficit, which recovers more slowly if at all. Theories that explain the phenomenon of differential awakening speculate that injured tissue is more sensitive to low concentrations of anesthetic, that injured tissue is less well perfused and therefore requires a longer time for drug elimination, or that compensatory pathways that evolve during recovery of the injured tissue only function when the patient is in the completely awake state.[91]

When Should the Anesthesiologist Become Concerned About Delayed Awakening?

Drug Effects

Impaired cerebral functioning in the postoperative period is a normal consequence of the pharmacologically induced anesthetic state. Lingering effects of anesthetic drugs are expected to depress mental function for a variable period of time after the end of surgery. In addition, antiemetics, analgesics, and the psychologic response to pain may alter the postoperative mental status.

Clearly, most cerebral dysfunction is due to the effects of administered drugs. For example, after anesthesia with isoflurane—the most quickly eliminated volatile anesthetic currently available—cerebral dysfunction can persist for days.[92] This effect may be due to the prolonged half-life of inhaled anesthetics in brain tissue.[93] Natural sleep patterns are disturbed for several days after surgery.[94] Even small antiemetic doses of droperidol can cause prolonged sedation in patients after ambulatory surgery.[95] The concept that most postoperative cerebral dysfunction is drug induced is reinforced by the knowledge that although prolonged postanesthetic sedation is frequently encountered, new neurologic events occur with an incidence of less than 1 in 2500 general anesthetics.[96]

No guidelines state at what point postoperative sedation has become prolonged, and clinical experience remains the most important factor in deciding when emergence has become excessively delayed. Expectations of emergence from anesthesia are strongly influenced by the type, route, and total dose of administered drug and must take into account patient characteristics that influence the pharmacodynamics and pharmacokinetics of those drugs. Even in patients who are susceptible to prolonged sedation, awakening should be expected to occur by 60 to 90 minutes after arrival in the postanesthesia care unit.[97] When emergence from anesthesia seems abnormal or prolonged compared with the clinician's expectations, further neurologic evaluation should be carried out.

Evaluation

When emergence from anesthesia has taken longer than expected, a systematic work-up is required. The differential is not unlike that of any patient with coma or excessive somnolence, and diagnosis should first rule out reversible conditions that can cause permanent neurologic injury. Afterward, less threatening yet common causes of prolonged sedation or coma are sought based on the patient's medical history, drug history, and perioperative course. Finally, less common etiologies are considered.

Most importantly, the airway, ventilation, and circulation are assessed and supported if necessary. Adequate blood oxygenation, ventilation, and perfusion are verified by arterial blood gas analysis, blood pressure measurement, and determination of hematocrit. Hypoglycemia is ruled out by serum glucose measurement. The presence of ongoing seizure activity is carefully sought, by EEG examination if necessary, because status epilepticus can cause permanent dysfunction if untreated.

Intracranial pathology, which may require immediate intervention, includes subarachnoid or intracerebral hemorrhage, tumor edema, or cerebral ischemia after cerebrovascular surgery. In most cases, neurosurgical emergencies present with lateralizing neurologic signs such as asymmetric motor activity, reflexes, or pupillary findings. Cyanide toxicity should be considered in patients who have received sodium nitroprusside.

After these problems are addressed, a careful search of the medical record, a more complete neurologic examination, and further laboratory studies are carried out in a search for the most likely cause of neurologic dysfunction.

The medical record must be examined for pre-existing medical conditions that predispose to metabolic abnormalities. Table 10–9 lists medical conditions that may delay emergence from anesthesia. Laboratory studies are carried out according to the likelihood of causative factors based on the medical history. The medication list is carefully searched for drugs with sedative side effects such as clonidine, methyldopa, lithium, lidocaine, and antihistamines. Anesthetic and other perioperative drugs are surveyed to ascertain that they were given in an amount appropriate for the patient.

Narcotics, benzodiazepines, inhaled anesthetics, anticholinergics, droperidol, and muscle relaxants all may cause failure to arouse. Narcotic overdose is indicated by slow deep respirations and miotic pupils, whereas patients with residual volatile anesthetic have faster, shallow respirations and pupils that are not small. Patients who are unarousable because of muscle paralysis demonstrate minimal to no response to electrical nerve stimulation.

Drug Overdose

When drug overdose is either relative (e.g., patient sensitivity or synergistic drug interaction) or absolute (e.g., administration error or unanticipated short procedure), specific antag-

TABLE 10–9. Conditions That May Delay Emergence

Diabetes mellitus	Hypoglycemia, ketoacidosis, nonketotic hyperosmolar coma, hyponatremia, stroke
Hepatic disease	Hepatic encephalopathy, altered drug pharmacokinetics, hypoglycemia, intracranial hemorrhage, cerebral edema, acidosis
Renal failure	Uremia, acidosis, hyponatremia, hypocalcemia, hypermagnesemia, hypoglycemia, cerebral edema, altered drug pharmacokinetics, postdialysis syndrome
Hypothyroidism	Hypothermia, increased sensitivity to anesthetics, hyponatremia, hypoglycemia
Hyperparathyroidism	Hypercalcemia
Seizure disorder	Ongoing seizure activity, postictal state, toxic anticonvulsant levels
Alcoholism	Acute ethanol intoxication, Wernicke's encephalopathy, Korsakoff's psychosis, subdural hematoma, hypoglycemia
Adrenal insufficiency	Altered pharmacodynamics and pharmacokinetics, hyponatremia, hypoglycemia
Malignant hyperthermia	Acidosis, hypoxemia, electrolyte abnormalities
Sepsis	Impaired cerebral metabolism, anemia, hypotension, acidosis
Fat embolism	Impaired cerebral metabolism
Porphyria	Altered porphyrin metabolism
Pre-eclampsia, eclampsia	Hypermagnesemia, seizure, cerebral edema, intracranial hemorrhage, venous sinus thrombosis
Substance abuse	Drug interactions, acute intoxication
Cancer	Hypercalcemia, hyponatremia, brain tumor edema
Malnutrition	Altered pharmacokinetics, hypoglycemia

onists should be administered to rule out neurologic injury. Naloxone, administered intravenously in titrated doses of 20 to 40 μg, reverses the sedation and respiratory depression of narcotics without causing severe pain, hypertension, and tachycardia. Flumazenil given in 0.2-mg increments promptly reverses benzodiazepine-induced sedation. It should be used very cautiously in patients receiving continuous benzodiazepine or tricyclic therapy. Physostigmine, 1 to 2 mg intravenously, can reverse the sedation of anticholinergic drugs, droperidol, and inhaled anesthetics. Finally, neostigmine or edrophonium is used to reverse neuromuscular blockade.

Surgical Procedures

Certain surgical procedures are commonly associated with neurologic dysfunction. After transurethral resection of the prostate, hyponatremia is a common cause of mental dysfunction, and glycine absorption can cause blindness. Stroke is more common after carotid and open heart surgery than after general surgery. Hypocalcemia is relatively more common after thyroid or parathyroid surgery. Vasospasm may cause coma after surgery for cerebral aneurysm when subarachnoid hemorrhage has occurred. The anesthesia record is carefully surveyed for evidence of hypotension/hypoxemia, which may be causing postischemic/hypoxic encephalopathy. Hypothermia may cause coma, in addition to potentiating anesthetic drugs and muscle relaxant effect.

Assessment should carefully rule out lateralizing signs in motor function and reflexes or pupillary findings that indicate focal cerebral pathology. When suspected, immediate cranial imaging is necessary.

TABLE 10–10. Assessment of Postoperative Coma, Sedation, Delirium

Immediately
1. Ensure adequate airway, oxygenation, ventilation: verify with arterial blood gas
2. Ensure adequate cerebral perfusion and energy utilization: check blood pressure, glucose; rule out seizures and cyanide toxicity
3. Check for lateralizing signs that may indicate an intracranial mass lesion and impending herniation

Further Testing
(Directed by History and Neurologic Examination)

Medical/Surgical	Drug Effect	New Neurologic Deficit
History: Electrolytes, blood urea nitrogen, magnesium, calcium, ammonia, thyroid function, alcohol level, temperature	Specific reversal agents: naloxone, flumazenil, physostigmine	CT or MRI of head, lumbar puncture, evoked potentials, angiogram
CT scan or MRI, angiogram, electroencephalogram	Check serum level: lidocaine, phenobarbital, phenytoin, magnesium	
	Check neuromuscular function with nerve stimulator	

Abbreviations: CT = computed tomography; MRI = magnetic resonance imaging.

Rare Events

Finally, rare events must be considered. Cardioembolic stroke may occur in patients with cardiac dysrhythmias or congestive heart failure. Echocardiography may detect intracardiac thrombi. Paradoxical air embolism through a patent foramen ovale can occur after procedures in which the surgical incision is higher than the central venous pressure level, and paradoxical CO_2 embolism after abdominal CO_2 insufflation has been reported. Embolic events should evidence lateralizing signs on neurologic examination but do not necessarily show immediate changes with cranial imaging techniques.

Pneumocephalus can occur after neurosurgical procedures that drain CSF. Unrecognized seizure activity during the intraoperative period may cause a postictal state that manifests as difficulty in arousal. Preoperative illicit drug use should be considered. If a spinal or epidural anesthetic was administered, total spinal anesthesia may have occurred.

Finally, the presence of meningitis and encephalitis should be ruled out by lumbar puncture in patients with fever and depressed mental function, especially in the presence of a stiff neck and when other causes of cerebral dysfunction have been eliminated. Table 10–10 presents an algorithm for assessing patients with postoperative coma.

POSTOPERATIVE DELIRIUM

What Are the Causes?

Some patterns of emergence from anesthesia are clearly abnormal. Delirium—a confusional state involving altered sensorium that is often associated with agitation, restlessness, and combativeness—is probably the most common abnormal postanesthetic condition. As with delayed emergence, various external factors influenced by psychologic and physiologic patient characteristics can cause postoperative delirium.

Differential Diagnosis

The differential diagnosis of postoperative delirium is similar to causative factors for encephalopathy in the general population. In addition, many of the conditions, which in a more severe form cause coma or delayed emergence, in a less severe form present as delirium.

Cerebral Oxygenation

Of greatest importance is the quick ruling out of disturbances in cerebral oxygen delivery and utilization, pulmonary ventilation, and arterial circulation. Thus, the initial evaluation includes the determination of arterial blood gases and oxyhemoglobin saturation, hematocrit, blood pressure, and blood glucose levels. A partially obstructed airway or ventilator dyssynchrony can cause severe agitation.

New or Pre-existing Medical Problems

After airway, breathing, and circulation problems are ruled out, other diagnoses are entertained. Pre-existing medical or psychiatric conditions, new neurologic conditions, drug side effects, intraoperative complications, and metabolic and endocrine abnormalities are sought. Table 10–9 lists medical conditions that can result in coma; however, delirium may also be the initial presentation.

The use of glucose-containing solutions in malnourished alcoholic patients can result in Wernicke's disease and Korsakoff's psychosis. Patients with organic brain syndromes, mental retardation, personality disorders, and psychiatric illness are more prone to postoperative delirium or agitation. Patients at the extremes of age have a higher incidence of stormy emergence and postoperative delirium. Those with acute psychosis may appear to be suffering from delirium.

Metabolic/Endocrine

Metabolic and endocrine factors may be causative, including electrolyte abnormalities, uremia, hepatic dysfunction, hypothyroidism and hyperthyroidism, and adrenal disease. Also, sepsis, fat embolism, encephalitis, meningitis, malignant hyperthermia, and NMS may result in delirium.

Brain Injury

Brain injury after ischemic/hypoxic events may also present as encephalopathy. Neurologic examination should be especially tuned to lateralizing signs indicating the presence of stroke, hemorrhage, or other intracranial mass lesion.

Drugs

Delirium is most commonly caused by the side effects or sequelae of preoperatively or intraoperatively administered drugs. Commonly implicated drugs are ketamine, atropine, scopolamine, droperidol, lidocaine, and cimetidine. Probably every drug administered by anesthesiologists, including antibiotics, has been blamed for causing delirium.

Pain

Some patients react to severe pain with restlessness, agitation, and confusion. Occult causes of discomfort may be present, such as tight surgical dressings, bladder or gastric distention, intravenous infiltration, and nausea.

Restraint/Partial Paralysis

Physical restraint in some patients may cause extreme agitation that can present as delirium. Finally, patients who are partially paralyzed may be restless and unable to speak as they attempt to breathe. Fortunately, in most cases, delirium is due simply to a loss of higher integrative functions because of residual anesthesia and resolves as the anesthetic state abates.

POSTISCHEMIC/HYPOXIC BRAIN INJURY

What Can Be Done?

General Measures

In most cases, patients with this type of brain injury—for example, that caused by cardiac arrest, arterial hypoxemia, or both—should receive primarily supportive care. Strict attention to hemodynamics and maintenance of at least normal and perhaps supranormal blood pressures may ensure perfusion of areas of brain at risk during the postinjury phase.[98, 99] Vasopressors may be needed to maintain blood pressure after euvolemia is attained with dextrose-free intravenous fluids. Cerebral metabolism should be minimized when possible. Induced hypothermia has been advocated; certainly, hyperthermia is to be avoided.[100] Small doses of intravenous thorazine (1–2 mg) to inhibit normal temperature regulation may be helpful in this regard as long as hypotension is avoided.

Seizures

Evidence of seizure activity should be quickly abated with sodium thiopental, phenytoin, or a benzodiazepine titrated as needed. Sedative drugs, however, alter the results of prognostic neurologic examinations.

Pharmacologic Agents

Various pharmacologic agents, including steroids,[101] barbiturates,[102] and calcium channel blockers,[103, 104] have been administered to comatose survivors of cardiac arrest without evidence of benefit in clinical trials. The 30° head-up position may help maintain cerebral perfusion pressure by enhancing jugular venous drainage.

Ventilatory Support

Controlled ventilation is maintained for several hours or until normal pulmonary function and adequate mental status are ensured. The use of hyperventilation is controversial.[105] Straining, bucking on the ventilator, and excessive muscle activity are controlled with muscle relaxants if needed.

Miscellaneous Support

Severe hyperglycemia is avoided, the hematocrit is kept in the 30% range, and the serum osmolality is kept between normal and 320 mOsm · L^{-1}. ICP is not normally elevated after global brain ischemia, but imaging or physical examination evidence of elevated ICP warrants ICP monitoring. When ICP is found to be elevated, normal protocols involving hyperventilation, osmotic/loop diuretics, barbiturates, and hypothermia can be followed.

In the future, other therapies, including free radical scavengers and blockers of excitatory neuroreceptors,[106, 107] other regulators of humorally mediated responses,[108] or hypothermic cardiopulmonary bypass,[109] may be used.

Can Outcome Be Predicted After Cardiac Arrest?

A multitude of patient characteristics at the time of cardiac arrest influence the eventual outcome. These factors include age, concurrent drug therapy, hematocrit, serum glucose level, body temperature, reperfusion pattern, acid-base status, serum osmolality, and premorbid conditions of the brain. Levy and colleagues observed physical signs that predicted the eventual level of recovery after 1 year (Table 10–11).[110] For example, patients who on initial examination (within 6 h of injury) had intact pupillary reflexes, flexor or extensor motor responses, and at least roving conjugate eye movements went on to independent function the great majority of the time. Unfortunately, no clinical or laboratory test is 100% predictive of eventual neurologic outcome.[111]

How Is Brain Death Diagnosed?

The diagnosis of brain death is made when signs of brain activity are absent and the patient is comatose in the absence of drug intoxication, hypothermia, or reversible metabolic, electrolyte, or endocrine disturbances. Spontaneous respiratory activity does not occur despite elevations in $Paco_2$ >50 to 60 mm Hg and evidence that peripheral neuromuscular function is intact. Electrical nerve stimulation or the presence of spinal reflexes demonstrates that apnea is not due to chemical paralysis.

Absence of brainstem reflexes, including the pupillary response to light, the corneal reflex, and the vestibulo-ocular reflex (ice-water calorics), must be demonstrated. Spinal reflexes to somatic stimulation may be present, but cranial nerve responses and decorticate/decerebrate posturing are absent. EEG, cerebral angiography, and positron emission tomography can verify the diagnosis of brain death but are not essential.[112]

TABLE 10–11. Predicting Outcome After Cardiac Arrest

Time	Good Prognosis	Poor Prognosis
Initial examination	Roving conjugate (or better) eye movements	Absent pupillary reflexes
	Extensor or flexor motor response	No motor response
3 days	Orienting eye movements, withdrawal or purposeful motor responses	Extensor or flexor motor response
1 week	Obeys commands	Spontaneous eye opening only

(From Levy DE, Caronna J, Singer B, et al: Predicting outcome from hypoxic-ischemic coma. JAMA 1985; 253:1420. Copyright 1985, American Medical Association.)

TABLE 10–12. Differential Diagnosis of Postanesthetic Headache

Mass lesion
    Tumor, aneurysm
    Hematoma, arteriovenous malformation
Increased intracranial pressure
    Cerebral edema, venous sinus thrombosis
    Hydrocephalus
    Malignant hypertension
Cerebrovascular insufficiency
Hypercapnia
Meningitis/encephalitis
Pneumocephalus
Postdural puncture
Post-traumatic (concussion, closed head injury)
Pre-eclampsia
Hypoglycemia
Referred pain
    Sinusitis
    Degenerative spine disease
    Carotid dissection
    Increased intraocular pressure
Migraine headache
Cluster headache
Tension headache
Caffeine withdrawal
Anemia/polycythemia
Vasodilator: nitroglycerin, nitroprusside
Vasoconstrictor: phenylephrine

POSTOPERATIVE HEADACHE

What Diagnostic Work-up Is Reasonable?

Headache is a frequent complaint in the general population and has a reported incidence of 13% to 80% after general anesthesia.[113, 114] Bromide, a by-product of halothane metabolism, can cause headache in up to 60% of patients anesthetized with halothane.[115] However, one survey of more than 18,000 patients admitted to the postanesthesia care unit did not list headache as a complication.[116] Thus, patients complaining of headache deserve further evaluation (Table 10–12).

History

The preanesthetic case history should be reviewed to determine whether a long-standing syndrome is present (e.g., migraine or cluster headaches) and whether risk factors are present for conditions that might cause headache. For example, patients with coagulopathy would be at higher risk for a subdural hematoma, hypertensive patients for intracerebral bleeds, patients with collagen vascular diseases for vasculitic headaches, and febrile patients for meningitis.

Coffee drinkers who abstain from caffeine intake on the day of surgery may be at increased risk for withdrawal headache.[117] The medication record should be reviewed because vasodilators, such as nitroglycerin, can also cause headache.

Examination

Malignant hypertension should be ruled out by blood pressure determination. A careful neurologic and fundoscopic examination should be performed to rule out the presence of mass lesions and elevated ICP. Laboratory studies should include hematocrit, white blood cell count, and blood glucose determination. When a mass lesion is suspected, CT scanning of the head is indicated.

Spinal Anesthesia

Patients who had spinal anesthesia are at risk for postdural puncture headache. This problem occurs more frequently in young females and pregnant patients, when larger needles are used, when the needle bevel is oriented perpendicular to the spine, and perhaps when the needle passes through povidone-iodine solution.[118]

The onset of a postdural puncture headache is within a few days after dural puncture or when a patient first assumes an upright position. The headache is most often described as being frontal, radiating toward the occiput, dull or throbbing, and almost invariably relieved by a horizontal body position. Visual and auditory disturbances are common, and nausea and vomiting are a frequent accompaniment. Cranial nerve abnormalities, especially diplopia (VI) and hyperacusis (VIII), may be encountered.

If a headache that resembles a postdural puncture headache does not respond to conservative measures such as hydration or administration of analgesics or caffeine or if it continues after epidural blood patch, further diagnostic endeavors must be undertaken. Postpartum patients present additional diagnostic dilemmas because the incidence of postpartum headache without anesthesia has been estimated at 30% to 40%[119] and because these patients are at risk for unusual causes of headaches such as venous sinus thrombosis, cerebral edema due to hypertensive disease of pregnancy,[120] subarachnoid hemorrhage, pituitary tumors, and cerebral choriocarcinoma.[121]

STATUS EPILEPTICUS

When seizures are so frequent that recovery of function does not occur between them, status epilepticus is present. Immediate and aggressive treatment is necessary to prevent permanent neurologic damage associated with this entity. Table 10–13 presents a protocol for treatment.

TABLE 10–13. Treatment of Generalized Tonic-Clonic Status Epilepticus

Immediate Intervention (first 10 min)
1. Support circulation
2. Support respiration; most, if not all, patients should be intubated
3. Draw blood for anticonvulsant levels, glucose, electrolytes, complete blood count, calcium
4. Measure arterial blood gas values
5. Administer 50 mL of 50% glucose intravenously
6. Administer 100 mg thiamine intramuscularly

Intermediate Intervention (2nd 10 min)
1. Diazepam, 10 mg (lorazepam 4 mg) intravenously at 2–4 mg · min^{-1} until seizure stops or to a total of 30 mg (lorazepam 12 mg). For children, diazepam 0.1 mg · kg^{-1}, up to 0.3 mg · kg^{-1}, is given over 5 to 30 min
2. Slow intravenous infusion (<50 mg · min^{-1}) of phenytoin to a total of 20 mg · kg^{-1}
3. Perform general and neurologic examination with attention to evidence of primary or secondary trauma, pupils, fundi, extremity movements, pathologic reflexes

Further Intervention (next 40–60 min) (if seizures persist)
1. Phenobarbital intravenously at 50 mg · min^{-1} to a total of 20 mg · kg^{-1}
2. Thiopental drip (1 g · 500 mL^{-1}) or general anesthesia to obtain EEG burst suppression *or*
3. 4% paraldehyde solution in normal saline

CONCLUSION

Working together, anesthesiologists and neurologists can effect optimal perioperative care of patients with chronic or acute neurologic disease. Neurologists have specific and detailed knowledge about the diagnosis, pathophysiology, and therapy of unique disease processes, whereas the knowledge and skills of anesthesiologists are required to support patients through various pharmacologic, hemodynamic, and respiratory challenges.

References

1. Lee T, Goldman L: Role of the consultant. *In* Perioperative Management. Breslow M, Miller C, Rogers M (eds). St Louis, CV Mosby, 1990, p 49.
2. d'Empaire G, Hoaglin D, Perlo V, et al: Effect of prethymectomy plasma exchange on postoperative respiratory function in myasthenia gravis. J Thorac Cardiovasc Surg 1985; 89:592.
3. Leventhal S, Orkin F, Hirsh R: Prediction of the need for postoperative mechanical ventilation in myasthenia gravis. Anesthesiology 1980; 53:26.
4. Brown T, Gebert R, Meretoja O, et al: Myasthenia gravis in children and its anaesthetic complications. Anaesth Intensive Care 1990; 18:466.
5. Merli G, Bell R: Preoperative management of the surgical patient with neurologic disease. Med Clin North Am 1987; 71:511.
6. Gravlee GP: Succinylcholine-induced hyperkalemia in a patient with Parkinson's disease. Anesth Analg 1980; 59:444.
7. Hart RG, Hindman B: Mechanisms of perioperative cerebral infarction. Stroke 1982; 13:766.
8. Larsen SF, Zaric D, Boysen G: Postoperative cerebrovascular accidents in general surgery. Acta Anaesthesiol Scand 1988; 32:698.
9. Stroke prevention in atrial fibrillation investigators: Stroke prevention in atrial fibrillation study, final results. Circulation 1991; 84:527.
10. North American symptomatic carotid endarterectomy trial collaborators: Beneficial effect of carotid endarterectomy in symptomatic patients with high-grade carotid stenosis. N Engl J Med 1991; 325:445.
11. Hass WK, Easton JD, Adams HP Jr, et al: Ticlopidine aspirin stroke study group: a randomized trial comparing ticlopidine hydrochloride with aspirin for the prevention of stroke in high-risk patients. N Engl J Med 1989; 321:501.
12. Hart RG: Cardiogenic embolism to the brain. Lancet 1992; 339:589.
13. Von Reutern GM, Hetzel A, Bernbaum D, et al: Transcranial Doppler ultrasonography during cardiopulmonary bypass in patients with severe carotid stenosis or occlusion. Stroke 1988; 19:674.
14. Brusino FG, Reves JG, Smith LR, et al: The effect of age on cerebral blood flow during hypothermic cardiopulmonary bypass. J Thorac Cardiovasc Surg 1989; 97:541.
15. Mayo asymptomatic carotid endarterectomy study group: Results of a randomized controlled trial of carotid endarterectomy for asymptomatic carotid stenosis. Mayo Clin Proc 1992; 67:513.
16. Kearse L: Neurologic disorders and spinal cord injuries. *In* Manual of Anesthesia and the Medically Compromised Patient. Cheng EY, Kay J (eds). Philadelphia, JB Lippincott, 1990, pp 317–341.
17. Warren T, Datta S, Ostheimer G: Lumbar epidural anesthesia in a patient with multiple sclerosis. Anesth Analg 1982; 61:1022.
18. Bader AM, Hunt Co, Datta A, et al: Anesthesia for the obstetric patient with multiple sclerosis. J Clin Anesth 1988; 1:21.
19. Jones RM, Healy T: Anaesthesia and demyelinating disease. Anaesthesia 1980; 35:879.
20. Borel C: Neuromuscular disease. *In* Perioperative Management. Breslow M, Miller C, Rogers M (eds). St Louis, CV Mosby, 1990, pp 417–426.
21. Browne MG, Cross R: Huntington's chorea. Br J Anaesth 1981; 53:136.
22. Stewart JT: Huntington's disease. Am Fam Physician 1988; 37:105.
23. Durcan FJ, Corbett J, Wall M: The incidence of pseudotumor cerebri. Arch Neurol 1988; 45:875.
24. Baker RS, Bauman RJ, Buncic JR: Idiopathic intracranial hypertension (pseudotumor cerebri) in pediatric patients. Pediatr Neurol 1989; 5:5.
25. Corbett JJ, Mehta M: Cerebrospinal fluid pressure in normal obese subjects and patients with pseudotumor cerebri. Neurology 1983; 33:1386.
26. Abouleish E, Ali V, Tang R: Benign intracranial hypertension and anesthesia for cesarean section. Anesthesiology 1985; 63:705.
27. Devitt J, Noseworthy T, Shustack A, et al: Acute hydrocephalus and eclampsia. Can Med Assoc J 1986; 134:370.
28. Brown CE, Purdy P, Cunningham FG: Head computed tomographic scans in women with eclampsia. Am J Obstet Gynecol 1988; 159:915.
29. Barton J, Sibai B: Cerebral pathology in eclampsia. Clin Perinatol 1991; 18:891.
30. Dinsdale HB: Does magnesium sulfate treat eclamptic seizures? Yes. Arch Neurol 1988; 45:1360.
31. Sibai BM: Magnesium is the ideal anticonvulsant in preeclampsia-eclampsia. Am J Obstet Gynecol 1990; 162:1141.
32. Kaplan P, Lesser RP, Fisher RS, et al: No, magnesium sulfate should not be used in treating eclamptic seizures. Arch Neurol 1988; 45:1361.
33. Kaplan PW, Lesser RP, Fisher RS, et al: A continuing controversy: magnesium sulfate in the treatment of eclamptic seizures. Arch Neurol 1990; 47:1031.
34. Mayhue F: IM midazolam for status epilepticus in the emergency department. Ann Emerg Med 1988; 17:643.
35. Pritchard J: Magnesium sulfate in the treatment of eclampsia. Arch Neurol 1989; 46:947.
36. Granner MA, Wooten GF: Neuroleptic malignant syndrome or parkinsonism hyperpyrexia syndrome. Semin Neurol 1991; 11:228.
37. Shalev A, Hermesh H, Munitz H: Mortality from neuroleptic malignant syndrome. J Clin Psychiatry 1989; 50:18.
38. Dickey W: The neuroleptic malignant syndrome. Prog Neurobiol 1991; 36:425.
39. Ebadi M, Pfeiffer RF, Murrin LC: Pathogenesis and treatment of neuroleptic malignant syndrome. Gen Pharmacol 1990; 21:367.
40. George A, Wood C: Succinylcholine-induced hyperkalemia complicating the neurologic malignant syndrome. Ann Intern Med 1987; 106:172.
41. Geiduschek J, Cohen S, Khan A, et al: Repeated anesthesia for a patient with neuroleptic malignant syndrome. Anesthesiology 1988; 68:134.
42. Woody R, Grollady E, Fiedorek S: Rectal anticonvulsants in seizure patients undergoing gastrointestinal surgery. J Pediatr Surg 1989; 24:474.
43. Modica PA, Tempelhoff R, White PF: Pro- and anticonvulsant effects of anesthetics. Anesth Analg 1990; 70(pt 1):433.
44. Modica PA, Tempelhoff R, White PF: Pro- and anticonvulsant effects of anesthetics. Anesth Analg 1990; 70(pt 2):303.
45. Therapeutics and Technology Assessment Subcommittee of the American Academy of Neurology: Assessment: intraoperative neurophysiology. Neurology 1990; 40:1644.
46. Goodrich JT: Electrophysiologic measurements: intraoperative evoked potential monitoring. Anesthesiol Clin North Am 1987; 5:477.
47. Gugino V, Chabot R: Somatosensory evoked potentials. Int Anesthesiol Clin 1990; 28:154.
48. Levine R: Short-latency auditory evoked potentials: intraoperative applications. Int Anesthesiol Clin 1990; 28:147.
49. Thompson GE, Lui A: Perioperative nerve injury. *In* Anesthesia and Perioperative Complications. Benumof JL, Saidman, LJ (eds). St Louis, Mosby-Year Book, 1992, pp 160–172.
50. Lederman R, Breuer A, Hanson M, et al: Peripheral nervous system complications of coronary artery bypass graft surgery. Ann Neurol 1982; 12:297.
51. Keates J, Innocenti D, Ross D: Mononeuritis multiplex, a complication of open-heart surgery. J Thorac Cardiovasc Surg 1975; 69:820.
52. McAlpine FS, Seckel BR: The peripheral nervous system. *In* Positioning in Anesthesia and Surgery. 2nd ed. Martin JT (ed). Philadelphia, WB Saunders, 1987, pp 303–328.
53. Parks B: Postoperative peripheral neuropathies. Surgery 1973; 74:348.
54. Selander D, Edshage S, Wolff T: Paresthesiae or no parasthesiae? Nerve lesions after axillary blocks. Acta Anaesthesiol Scand 1979; 23:27.
55. Kroll DA, Caplan RA, Posner K, et al: Nerve injury associated with anesthesia. Anesthesiology 1990; 73:202.
56. Cameron M, Stewart O: Ulnar nerve injury associated with anesthesia. Can Anaesth Soc J 1975; 22:253.
57. Aldrete J: Recovery room assessment. *In* Positioning in Anesthesia and Surgery. Martin J (ed). Philadelphia, WB Saunders, 1987, pp 329–335.
58. Chadwick HS, Ross BK: Causes and consequences of maternal-fetal perianesthetic complications. *In* Anesthesia and Perioperative Complications. Benumof JL, Saidman LJ (eds). St Louis, Mosby-Year Book, 1992, pp 520–547.
59. Dawson DM, Krarup C: Perioperative nerve lesions. Arch Neurol 1989; 46:1355.
60. Ducker T: Management of peripheral nerve injuries. *In* Neurologic Emergencies Recognition and Management. 2nd ed. Salcman E (ed). New York, Raven Press, 1990, pp 221–233.
61. Massey EW, Cefalo RC: Managing the carpal tunnel syndrome of pregnancy. Contemp Obstet Gynecol 1977; 9:39.

62. Massey EW: Mononeuropathies in pregnancy. Semin Neurol 1988; 8:193.

63. Hill EC: Maternal obstetric paralysis. Am J Obstet Gynecol 1962; 83:1452.

64. Berry PR, Wallis WE: Venepuncture nerve injuries. Lancet 1977; 1:1236.

65. Adelman J, Goldberg G, Puckett J: Postpartum bilateral femoral neuropathy. Obstet Gynecol 1973; 42:845.

66. Grove LH: Backache, headache and bladder dysfunction after delivery. Br J Anaesth 1973; 45:147.

67. Pathy G, Rosen M: Prolonged block with recovery after extradural analgesia for labour. Br J Anaesth 1975; 47:520.

68. Cuerdan C, Buley R, Downing JW: Delayed recovery after epidural analgesia for labour. Anaesthesia 1977; 32:773.

69. Kane R: Neurologic deficits following epidural or spinal anesthesia. Anesth Analg 1981; 60:150.

70. Vandam L, Dripps R: A long-term follow-up of 10,098 spinal anesthetics. Surgery 1955; 38:463.

71. Murphy TM, O'Keeffe D: Complications of spinal, epidural and caudal anesthesia. In Anesthesia and Perioperative Complications. Benumof JL, Saidman LJ (eds). St Louis, Mosby-Year Book, 1992, pp 38–51.

72. Wang BC, Hillman DE, Spielholz NI, et al: Chronic neurological deficits and nesacaine-CE: an effect of the anesthetic, 2-chloroprocaine, or the antioxidant, sodium bisulfite? Anesth Analg 1984; 63:445.

73. Reisner L, Hochman B, Plumer M: Persistent neurologic deficit and adhesive arachnoiditis following intrathecal 2-chloroprocaine injection. Anesth Analg 1980; 59:452.

74. Rigler M, Drasner R, Krejcie T, et al: Cauda equina syndrome after continuous spinal anesthesia. Anesth Analg 191; 72:275.

75. Fibuch E, Opper S: Back pain following epidurally administered nesacaine-MPF. Anesth Analg 1989; 69:113.

76. Ready LB, Helfer D: Bacterial meningitis in parturients after epidural anesthesia. Anesthesiology 1989; 71:988.

77. Goldman WW, Sanford JP: An ''epidemic'' of chemical meningitis. Am J Med 1960; 29:94.

78. Berga S, Trierweiler MW: Bacterial meningitis following epidural anesthesia for vaginal delivery: a case report. Obstet Gynecol 1989; 74:437.

79. McHale S, Clark MM: Meningitis after spinal anaesthesia. Anaesthesia 1990; 45:987.

80. DiGiovanni AJ, Galbert MW, Phillips JN: ''Chemical meningitis'' tied to cleaning fluid bacteria. JAMA 1970; 214:2129.

81. Goucke CR, Graziotti P: Extradural abscess following local anaesthetic and steroid injection for chronic low back pain. Br J Anaesth 1990; 65:427.

82. Baker A, Ojemann R, Swartz M, et al: Spinal epidural abscess. N Engl J Med 1975; 293:463.

83. Owens E, Kasten G, Hessel E: Spinal subarachnoid hematoma after lumbar puncture and heparinization: a case report, review of the literature and discussion of anesthetic implications. Anesth Analg 1986; 65:1201.

84. Tartiere J, Gerard JL, Peny J, et al: Acute treatment after accidental intrathecal injection of hypertonic contrast media. Anesthesiology 1989; 71:169.

85. Fog J, Wang L, Sundberg A, et al: Hearing loss after spinal anesthesia is related to needle size. Anesth Analg 1990; 70:517.

86. Robles R: Cranial nerve paralysis after spinal anesthesia. Northwest Medicine 1968; 67:845.

87. Fibuch E, Opper S: Back pain following epidurally administered nesacaine-MPF. Anesth Analg 1989; 69:113.

88. Bromage P: ''Paraplegia following epidural analgesia'': a misnomer. Anaesthesia 1976; 31:947.

89. Rosenberg H, Clofine R, Bialik O: Neurologic changes during awakening from anesthesia. Anesthesiology 1981; 54:125.

90. Cucchiara RF: Differential awakening (Letter to the editor). Anesth Analg 1992; 75:467.

91. McCulloch PR, Milne B: Neurological phenomena during emergence from enflurane or isoflurane anesthesia. Can J Anaesth 1990; 37:739.

92. Davison L, Steinhelber J, Eger E, et al: Psychological effects of halothane and isoflurane anesthesia. Anesthesiology 1975; 43:313.

93. Mills P, Sessler D, Moseley M, et al: An in vivo ^{19}F nuclear magnetic resonance study of isoflurane elimination from the rabbit brain. Anesthesiology 1987; 67:169.

94. Knill R, Moote C, Skinner M, et al: Anesthesia with abdominal surgery leads to intense REM sleep during the first postoperative week. Anesthesiology 1990; 73:52.

95. Melnick B, Sawyer R, Karambelkar D, et al: Delayed side effects of droperidol after ambulatory general anesthesia. Anesth Analg 1989; 69:748.

96. Crosby G: Impaired central nervous system function. In Anesthesia and Perioperative Complications. Benumof JL, Saidman LJ (eds). St Louis, Mosby-Year Book, 1992, pp 356–377.

97. Mecca RS: Complications during recovery. Int Anesthesiol Clin 1991; 29:37.

98. Safar P: Cerebral resuscitation after cardiac arrest: a review. Circulation 1986; 74(suppl 4):IV-138.

99. Sterz F, Leonov Y, Safar P, et al: Hypertension with or without hemodilution after cardiac arrest in dogs. Stroke 1990; 21:1178.

100. Sterz F, Safar P, Tisherman S, et al: Mild hypothermic cardiopulmonary resuscitation improves outcome after prolonged cardiac arrest in dogs. Crit Care Med 1991; 19:379.

101. Jastremski M, Sutton-Tyrrell K, Vaagenes P, et al: Glucocorticoid treatment does not improve neurological recovery following cardiac arrest. JAMA 1989; 262:3427.

102. Brain resuscitation clinical trial I study group: A randomized clinical study of thiopental loading in comatose survivors of cardiac arrest. N Engl J Med 1986; 314:397.

103. Brain resuscitation clinical trial II study group: A randomized clinical study of a calcium-entry blocker (lidoflazine) in the treatment of comatose survivors of cardiac arrest. N Engl J Med 1991; 324:1225.

104. Roine R, Kaste M, Kinnunen A, et al: Nimodipine after resuscitation from out of hospital ventricular fibrillation. JAMA 1990; 264:3171.

105. Loughhead MG: Brain resuscitation and protection. Med J Aust 1988; 148:458.

106. Rogers MC, Kirsch JR: Current concepts in brain resuscitation. JAMA 1989; 261:3143.

107. Safar P: resuscitation from clinical death: Pathophysiologic limits and therapeutic potentials. Crit Care Med 1988; 16:923.

108. Rochanek PM: Novel pharmacologic approaches to brain resuscitation after cardiorespiratory arrest in the pediatric patient. Crit Care Clin 1988; 4:661.

109. Sterz F, Safar P, Tisherman S, et al: Mild hypothermic cardiopulmonary resuscitation improves outcome after prolonged cardiac arrest in dogs. Crit Care Med 1991; 19:379.

110. Levy DE, Caronna J, Singer B, et al: Predicting outcome from hypoxic-ischemic coma. JAMA 1985; 253:1420.

111. Reinmuth O, Vaagnes P, Abramson N, et al: Predicting outcome after resuscitation from clinical death. Crit Care Med 1988; 16:1043.

112. Critchley E: Neurological Emergencies. Philadelphia, WB Saunders, 1988, pp 88–93.

113. Fennelly M, Galletly DC, Purdie GI: Is caffeine withdrawal the mechanism of postoperative headache? Anesth Analg 1991; 72:449.

114. Cosh PH: Headache after general anesthesia. Anaesthesia 1988; 43:889.

115. Tyrrell M, Feldman S: Headache following halothane anesthesia. Br J Anaesth 1968; 40:99.

116. Hines R, Barash P, Watrous G, et al: Complications occurring in the postanesthesia care unit. Anesth Analg 1992; 74:503.

117. Fennelly M, Galletly DC, Purdie GI: Is caffeine withdrawal the mechanism of postoperative headache? Anesth Analg 1991, 72:449.

118. Gurmarnik S: Skin preparation and spinal headache. Anaesthesia 1988; 43:1057.

119. Stein G, Morton J, Marsh A, et al: Headaches after childbirth. Acta Neurol Scand 1984; 69:74.

120. Reik L: Headaches in pregnancy. Semin Neurol 1988; 8:187.

121. Fox M, Harms R, Davis D: Selected neurologic complications of pregnancy. Mayo Clin Proc 1990; 65:1595.

122. Landercasper J, Merz BJ, Cogbill TH, et al: Perioperative stroke risk in 173 consecutive patients with a past history of stroke. Arch Surg 1990; 125:986.

123. Hart RG, Easton JD: Management of cervical bruits and carotid stenosis in preoperative patients. Stroke 1983; 14:290.

124. Azar I: The response of patients with neuromuscular disorders to muscle relaxants: a review. Anesthesiology 1984; 61:173.

CHAPTER 11

Nephrology Consultation

R. DENNIS BASTRON, M.D.

Identification of an electrolyte abnormality often results in a nephrology consult. A range outside of which a laboratory value signifies severe electrolyte imbalance is somewhat meaningless because each patient responds differently to electrolyte changes. For example, a patient with slowly developing hyponatremia may be asymptomatic with a serum sodium level of 120 mEq $\cdot$ L^{-1}, whereas another patient with acute hyponatremia may have major symptoms at a level of 130 mEq $\cdot$ L^{-1}. In this chapter, severe electrolyte imbalance is defined as a disorder that causes signs or symptoms or is outside of the range that a patient's current physicians feel confident about treating.

Similarly, chronic renal disease is characterized by slow, irreversible, progressive loss of some nephrons and is accompanied by compensatory changes in the remaining nephrons. Patients pass through several stages before they develop uremia and require dialysis. Each stage has anesthetic implications, but a preoperative nephrology consultation usually is not necessary until the patient requires dialysis. In contrast, patients with acute renal failure (ARF) should have a nephrologist involved in their care as soon as practical.

PURPOSE OF THE CONSULTATION

A nephrology consultation should answer these questions:

1. What is the patient's diagnosis and pathophysiology?
2. Is the patient in optimum condition for anesthesia and surgery?
3. If not, what must be done to make the patient's condition optimum?

This information is valuable to help plan the timing of nonemergency surgery. Specifically, a nephrologist can help with perioperative fluid management, antihypertensive therapy, selection and dosage of certain drugs, and dialysis should it be necessary.

When Is a Consultation Superfluous?

A consultation is superfluous when a patient's problems do not lie outside the confidence zone of the treating physicians, when the consultation indicates something that is already known ("monitor the patient and keep the patient well oxygenated"), or when the advice is outside the consultant's area of expertise ("general anesthesia is contraindicated").

HYPERTENSION

About 10% of Americans are hypertensive, and nearly 12 million develop renal disease annually.[1] The size of the patient population that is anesthetized determines the frequency of nephrology consultations that are requested, but this number is probably small.

How Is the Efficacy of Antihypertensive Therapy Assessed?

Five to 10 years ago, patients were admitted to the hospital a day or two before surgery, and several recorded blood pressure measurements usually were available to evaluate control of a patient's hypertension. Today, the odds are that your first contact with a patient will be in the preoperative holding area, and perhaps one blood pressure measurement will be recorded in the chart. It may be recorded in several places by different people, but it is uncanny how the numbers are the same. This blood pressure value probably was measured just as the patient had been told that the risks of surgery and anesthesia might include death, coma, and permanent neurologic damage. This measurement often is higher than usual, and it is on this insufficient information that a judgment must be made about whether the antihypertensive therapy is adequate.

What Are Allowable Blood Pressure Limits?

If the blood pressure is <160 mm Hg systolic and 90 mm Hg diastolic, there probably is no problem. If it is 190/100 mm Hg, the anesthetist should be concerned but can medicate the patient to see if decreasing anxiety or pain decreases the blood pressure. If the diastolic blood pressure exceeds 110 mm Hg, it is not controlled by the current therapy.[2]

To assess the effectiveness of treatment, the patient's usual blood pressure (many hypertensive patients know this value) must be known. Whether the patient is adequately treated, has a rare pathologic process (thyrotoxicosis, pheochromocytoma), or has some temporary and reversible cause of hypertension (severe pain, distended bladder) must then be determined. Also of concern is the possibility of a drug reaction (e.g., Neo-Synephrine eye or nose drops), withdrawal (missed morning dose), or interaction (meperidine and monoamine oxidase inhibitor).

When Should Surgery Be Delayed?

Surgery should not be delayed for a patient whose diastolic pressure is <110 mm Hg. When the diastolic pressure exceeds 110 mm Hg, several determinations should be made while you try therapeutic maneuvers. These include catheterization of the bladder or administration of sedatives, tranquilizers, narcotics, vasodilators, β-blockers, or calcium channel blockers (Table 11–1). After the pressure decreases to a tolerable range (and it almost always does), proceed with anesthesia. Careful blood pressure control intraoperatively and, perhaps more importantly, postoperatively is essential.[3–6] When the inevitable peaks and valleys of blood pressure occur, react appropriately but do not over-react.

Delay surgery only in the following rare circumstances:

1. The diastolic blood pressure cannot be controlled (i.e., it is >110 mm Hg).
2. You suspect thyrotoxicosis or pheochromocytoma.
3. The patient has myocardial ischemia or congestive heart failure.
4. Signs and symptoms of end-organ failure (renal, central nervous system) are present.

Is Perioperative Medication Change Indicated?

Changing a patient's medication in the perioperative period may cause an unsteady state that can be more of a problem than if the medication were not changed. The medication schedule should usually be maintained right up to the time of surgery. Any doses scheduled after the nil per os (NPO) time period can safely be taken with a sip of water.

Is Clonidine a Problem?

Rebound hypertension may occur after withdrawal of clonidine. It is more common at doses >0.6 mg daily and can be treated with direct vasodilators (especially α-methyldopa [Aldomet], which is also centrally active), adrenergic antagonists, or calcium channel blockers. When the parenteral clonidine preparations used in Europe become available in the United States, this issue will become moot. Until then, clonidine patches can be used to replace the oral clonidine. Because these patches require a 2- to 3-day absorption period, one approach is to apply a clonidine patch in the morning of day 1 and give the usual oral dose. Then, on day 2, the blood pressure is checked: if it is elevated, half the usual oral dose is given; if not, the dose remains unchanged. On the third day, the blood pressure is checked again to verify that the patch is effective.

FLUID THERAPY

How Are Intravenous Fluids Chosen?

This discussion is limited to routine surgery and does not address the colloid/crystalloid debate or blood component replacement for patients in shock (see Chapter 42). Surgical patients need salt.[7, 8] The practice of giving 5% dextrose in water (D_5W) as the only intravenous fluid for intraoperative and postoperative patients has been abandoned. The questions of importance are which salt solution to use and whether the solution should contain dextrose.

What Fluids Are Useful?

The most common salt solutions available in surgical suites are 0.9% sodium chloride (NS) and lactated Ringer's solution (LR).[9, 10] The use of LR is generally safe despite theoretic considerations about the presence of lactate. On the other hand, NS is a perfectly acceptable solution for intraoperative use as well, despite the excess chloride. With very few exceptions—primarily patients with severe electrolyte imbalance—it really does not make any difference whether NS or LR is used. Sometimes the best solution is whatever is warm.

Is Dextrose a Problem?

The dextrose question is a little more complicated (Table 11–2). Historically, intravenous glucose was administered to surgical patients for several reasons. Glucose protected the liver from the toxic effects of chloroform. In the era when salt was not given to patients in the perioperative period, D_5W was the primary alternative. Moreover, with long preoperative fast-

TABLE 11–1. Useful Drugs for Treating Perioperative Hypertension

Drug	Dose	Route	Action
Hydralazine*	5 mg every 5 min	Intravenous	Direct vasodilator
Labetalol	5–20 mg	Intravenous	Alpha/beta-blocker
Nifedipine	10 mg	Sublingual	Calcium channel blocker
Diazepam	2–10 mg	Intravenous	Tranquilizer
Midazolam	1–2 mg	Intravenous	Tranquilizer
Fentanyl	50–100 μg	Intravenous	Narcotic
Morphine	2–10 mg	Intravenous	Narcotic

*Current production has been halted by manufacturer (July, 1993).

TABLE 11–2. To Sweeten or Not to Sweeten— That Is the Question

No Sugar	Sugar
Parturient	Diabetic who received insulin
Global central nervous system ischemia related to:	Prolonged fast
Neurosurgery	
Spinal column surgery	
Carotid artery surgery	
Cardiopulmonary bypass	
Diabetic with elevated blood sugar	Starvation
	Morbid obesity

ing periods, physicians feared that some patients might become symptomatically hypoglycemic.

In the early days of surgical treatment of morbid obesity, several deaths were caused by embolic phenomena. These were thought to be a result of elevated levels of free fatty acids, which are suppressed by administering dextrose.

Maternal administration of dextrose during labor has been shown to cause severe hypoglycemia in the newborn. Administration of intravenous glucose can increase the damage caused by experimentally induced brain ischemia. Moreover, many patients who receive more than 1 L of D₅LR develop significant hyperglycemia. On the basis of this information, many anesthesiologists have abandoned the use of dextrose-containing solutions in the operating room.

When Can Dextrose Be Administered?

Opponents of dextrose solutions intraoperatively take the approach that no one really needs glucose, that it is harmful in a parturient, and that it may be harmful in certain patients, including those undergoing cardiac surgery, carotid artery surgery, and neurosurgery, and in those suffering cardiac arrest.

I take the opposite approach and use dextrose solutions in patients in whom they are not specifically contraindicated. Some patients who are maintained NPO for long periods before surgery, who are malnourished, or who are morbidly obese receive some benefit from dextrose. Each patient is not treated as though a perioperative cardiac arrest will occur. Certainly a diabetic patient who has received insulin should have some dextrose if the NPO period is prolonged.

Except for reasonably clear-cut cases, 1 L of D₅LR can be given to most patients. If all patients had clear liquids by mouth up until 3 or 4 hours before anesthesia, I would be more inclined to abandon dextrose solutions. However, many patients, including young children, arrive in the operating room having been in NPO status for 12 to 16 hours. The decision whether to use dextrose in most patients is based on something other than hard data.

SODIUM

Sodium is the major solute in extracellular fluid and is the major determinant of extracellular fluid volume and osmolality.[11] Glucose and urea contribute lesser amounts to osmolality. Sodium concentration (140 ± 5 mEq $\cdot$ L^{-1}), osmolality (287 ± 7 mOsm $\cdot$ kg^{-1}), and extracellular fluid volume, especially the circulating blood volume, are regulated closely by the body. Plasma osmolality (Posm) can be estimated as follows:

$$Posm = 2[Na^+] + \frac{glucose\ (mg \cdot dL^{-1})}{18} + \frac{BUN\ (mg \cdot dL^{-1})}{2.4}$$

Equation 1

A measured osmolality >9 mOsm $\cdot$ kg^{-1} from that calculated indicates the presence of exogenous molecules such as mannitol or radiographic dyes.

Alterations in sodium concentration result when a disproportionate change in either sodium or water occurs. These changes may be associated with normal or abnormal physiologic mechanisms, normal or abnormal osmolality, and normal or abnormal total body water. To evaluate patients with sodium imbalance, the general fluid status (volume, osmolality) as well as the renal response (urine volume, osmolality, and sodium excretion) should be known. A carefully taken history and a physical examination reveal the cause of sodium imbalance in most patients.

What Is the Significance of Hyponatremia?

Hyponatremia can be caused by water intoxication, rarely because of polydipsia. More often, it is caused by decreased glomerular filtration rate (GFR), decreased obligatory solute excretion, or chemical interference with the diluting mechanism, especially by thiazide diuretics. It may be encountered with stress, decreased thyroid or adrenal function, diuretic administration, or the syndrome of inappropriate release of antidiuretic hormone.[11]

Manifestations

Serum sodium concentration and signs or symptoms often are poorly correlated. Patients are more likely to become symptomatic with rapid or extreme changes. The signs and symptoms of hyponatremia (Table 11–3) usually begin with anorexia, confusion, headaches, and muscle cramps, progressing to nausea, vomiting, and personality changes and finally to convulsions, coma, and death. Acute symptomatic hyponatremia is associated with significant morbidity and mortality. Chronic symptomatic hyponatremia has a lower mortality rate, and chronic asymptomatic hyponatremia is associated with a very low mortality rate. Nevertheless, relatively low levels of

TABLE 11–3. Signs and Symptoms of Hyponatremia

Anorexia
Confusion
Disorientation
Apathy
Headache
Muscle cramps
Lethargy
Nausea
Vomiting
Stupor
Seizures
↓ Deep tendon reflexes
Coma

hyponatremia, especially in young females, may result in death or permanent neurologic sequelae.

Treatment

A good rule of thumb in treatment is to treat rapidly if hyponatremia occurred rapidly and to treat slowly if it evolved slowly. Asymptomatic to mild hyponatremia is treated by restricting water intake to <1 L $\cdot$ d^{-1}. Excess fluid can be calculated as follows:

$$\text{Water excess (kg)} = \text{wt (kg)} \times 0.6 \times \frac{140 - [Na^+]}{140} \qquad \text{Equation 2}$$

Example: A 70-kg patient has a serum sodium of 126 mEq $\cdot$ L^{-1}:

$$[70 \times 0.6] \times \frac{140 - 126}{140}$$

$$42 \times 0.1 = 4.2 \text{ kg (L) excess fluid}$$

Patients with acute neurologic symptoms are treated more aggressively.

$$\text{Sodium deficit (mEq)} = \text{wt (kg)} \times 0.6 \times (140 - [Na^+]) \qquad \text{Equation 3}$$

A useful rule of thumb is that an infusion of 1 mEq $\cdot$ kg^{-1} of sodium per hour raises the serum sodium level 2 to 3 mEq $\cdot$ L^{-1}. Another method for rapid correction of symptomatic hyponatremia is to administer furosemide (1 mg $\cdot$ kg^{-1}), measure the hourly sodium excretion, and replace it with 3% sodium chloride (sodium concentration of 513 mEq $\cdot$ L^{-1}). The goal is to increase serum sodium concentration 1 to 2 mEq $\cdot$ L $\cdot$ h^{-1}. Stop aggressive treatment when relief of symptoms occurs and a sodium level between 120 and 130 mEq $\cdot$ L^{-1} is achieved. More rapid correction or overcorrection may cause fluid overload or potentially fatal central nervous system complications (i.e., central pontine myelinolysis). Intravenous sodium bicarbonate, 2 mL $\cdot$ kg^{-1} over several minutes, increases serum sodium by about 6 mEq $\cdot$ L^{-1} in infants and small children.

What Is the Significance of Hypernatremia?

Hypernatremia rarely is caused by excessive sodium intake (e.g., saltwater near-drowning, accidental substitution of salt for sugar in infant formula, problems during hypertonic saline abortions). More often the cause is limited access to water or inability to ingest water to replace renal or extrarenal water loss (diabetes insipidus [central or nephrogenic], osmotic diuresis, excessive sweating, diarrhea). A carefully taken history is helpful in diagnosing the cause of hypernatremia.

Manifestations

Acutely increased serum osmolality initially causes intracellular dehydration of the brain, with restlessness, lethargy, and headache. This complex may progress to confusion, seizures,

TABLE 11–4. Signs and Symptoms of Hypernatremia

Restlessness
Lethargy
Headache
Disorientation
Confusion
↑ Deep tendon reflexes
Seizures
↑ Muscle tone
Stupor
Coma

coma, and death (Table 11–4). The brain responds to this dehydration by forming intracellular solutes (idiogenic osmoles) with partial restoration of intracellular volume. This process begins within 4 to 6 hours and takes several days to reach equilibrium. The presence of idiogenic osmoles in chronic hypernatremia makes rapid correction dangerous because of a resulting predisposition to cerebral edema.

Treatment

Calculate total water deficit by the following formula:

$$\text{Water deficit (kg)} = (\text{wt (kg)} \times 0.6) \times \frac{([Na^+] - 140)}{140} \qquad \text{Equation 4}$$

The treatment of hypernatremia is to control shock, if present, with crystalloids or colloids to stabilize the cardiovascular system. Treat accompanying acidosis with sodium bicarbonate only if the pH is <7.20. Alternatively, carbicarb or dichloroacetate can be used to avoid further sodium load. Replace the calculated fluid deficit slowly with hypotonic fluid (0.25 or 0.5 NS). The goal is to decrease plasma osmolality by no more than 2 mOsm $\cdot$ kg^{-1} $\cdot$ h^{-1}. Measure plasma sodium and osmolality every 2 hours.

While treating either hyponatremia or hypernatremia, always remember to consider and treat the underlying disease.

POTASSIUM

Potassium is the second most abundant cation within the body and the major intracellular cation. The intracellular concentration of potassium is about 150 mEq $\cdot$ L^{-1}. About 2% of total body potassium is extracellular, with a concentration of 3.5 to 4.5 mEq $\cdot$ L^{-1}.[11, 12]

What Is the Significance of Hypokalemia?

Hypokalemia can occur without a change in total body content when extracellular potassium moves to the intracellular space (internal shift). A decrease in total body potassium results because of inadequate intake or excessive loss of potassium.

Shifts of potassium into cells occur with metabolic or respiratory alkalosis, endogenous or exogenous catecholamines (especially β-adrenergic agonists), and elevated insulin levels. Alkalosis predictably decreases serum potassium about 0.5 mEq $\cdot$ L^{-1} for each 0.1 increase in pH (10 mm Hg decrease in $Paco_2$).

Inadequate intake of potassium as a cause of hypokalemia is relatively unusual because the kidneys can decrease obligatory potassium losses to around 10 to 30 mEq $\cdot$ d^{-1}. It may occur in starvation and anorexia nervosa, as well as in elderly and alcoholic patients. Excessive potassium loss usually causes the hypokalemia. These losses may be through the skin (excessive sweating), gastrointestinal tract (vomiting, diarrhea), or kidneys (diuretics, hyperaldosteronism).[12]

Manifestations

Because the ratio of intracellular to extracellular potassium determines cell membrane potential, most of the signs and symptoms of hypokalemia are related to cells that depolarize (Table 11–5). With moderate hypokalemia, patients may develop muscle weakness, cramps, fatigue, and decreased gastrointestinal motility with constipation or ileus. More severe hypokalemia (usually <2.5 mEq $\cdot$ L^{-1}) may cause paralysis (including respiratory), rhabdomyolysis, and decreased vascular resistance. Electrocardiographic (ECG) changes include flattening of the T waves, depressed ST segments, and U waves. Susceptibility to atrial and ventricular dysrhythmias is increased, especially in the presence of digitalis.

Critical Limits

The old rule of canceling surgery for patients with potassium levels <3 or even 3.5 mEq $\cdot$ L^{-1} is not valid. Surgery should not be canceled for asymptomatic, chronically moderately hypokalemic, nondigitalized patients without ECG changes. Most patients with potassium levels <2.7 mEq $\cdot$ L^{-1} have ECG changes. Hypokalemia in digitalized patients and patients with ischemic heart disease or cardiomyopathy is of greater concern because they may be more susceptible to dysrhythmias.

When anesthetizing a hypokalemic patient, maneuvers such as hyperventilation and administration of sodium bicarbonate, glucose, insulin, or catecholamines should be avoided as they further decrease the serum potassium level. Techniques or drugs associated with a higher incidence of dysrhythmias (e.g., halothane, atropine) should also not be used. Hypokalemia is worsened by epinephrine administration and lowers the threshold for epinephrine-induced dysrhythmias. Hypokalemia may increase the effectiveness of nondepolarizing muscle relaxants and may increase the requirement for reversal agents for the neuromuscular blocking drugs.

Treatment

The primary treatment of asymptomatic hypokalemia is to address the cause. Each 1 mEq $\cdot$ L^{-1} decrease in serum potassium approximates a 200 to 400 mEq total body deficit.

TABLE 11–5. Signs and Symptoms of Hypokalemia

Digitalis toxicity
Electrocardiogram changes (flattened T waves, depressed ST segments, prolonged PR interval, U waves)
Muscle weakness
Constipation
Ileus
Orthostatic hypertension
Vasodilation
Rhabdomyolysis
Dysrhythmias
Paralysis

Oral

The deficit should be replaced slowly, preferably by mouth, over several days while monitoring both serum levels and urinary excretion. Rapid intravenous replacement may be hazardous because of rapid changes in the intracellular-to-extracellular ratio and, therefore, the cell membrane potential.

Intravenous

Treat symptomatic hypokalemia with intravenous potassium using ECG monitoring. The maximum recommended rate of replacement is 0.5 to 0.7 mEq $\cdot$ kg^{-1} $\cdot$ h^{-1} given in a maximum concentration of 80 to 120 mEq $\cdot$ L^{-1}. Hyperkalemia is possible with rapid intravenous potassium administration, especially in insulin-dependent diabetic patients and patients receiving nonselective β-blockers.

What Is the Significance of Hyperkalemia?

Shifts of potassium from intracellular to extracellular fluid or an increase in total body potassium from excessive load or diminished excretion of potassium can cause hyperkalemia.[12]

Significant internal shifts (i.e., intracellular to extracellular) can be caused by respiratory or metabolic acidosis. Acute hyperosmolality of extracellular fluid (hyperglycemia, mannitol, radiocontrast media) increases serum potassium by 0.3 to 0.5 mEq $\cdot$ L^{-1} for each 10 mOsm $\cdot$ kg^{-1} increase in plasma osmolality. Anesthesiologists are familiar with the rise in plasma potassium following succinylcholine administration and associated with malignant hyperthermia. Deficiencies in insulin (diabetes), catecholamines (e.g., with β-blockers), and aldosterone decrease cellular potassium uptake. When these deficiencies occur in combination (severe diabetes) and in the presence of an increased potassium load (e.g., vigorous exercise in a β-blocked person) or decreased excretory ability (ARF or chronic renal failure, use of ''potassium-sparing'' diuretics), clinically significant and even fatal hyperkalemia can occur.

Increased potassium loads result from exogenous or endogenous sources. Exogenous potassium loads are usually iatrogenic, in the form of potassium salts administered orally or intravenously for potassium replacement, or incidentally (e.g., large doses of potassium penicillin). Endogenous sources include cell lysis, trauma, rhabdomyolysis, hypercatabolic states (e.g., malignant hyperthermia), and hemolysis (gastrointestinal tract hemorrhage, resolution of massive hematomas). Excessive loads are rarely a problem without diminished cellular uptake or renal excretion of potassium.

Severely decreased GFR, hypoaldosteronism, and aldosterone-blocking agents (spironolactone, triamterine amiloride) cause decreased renal potassium excretion.

Manifestations

Signs and symptoms of hyperkalemia usually are absent or insignificant with plasma levels <6 mEq $\cdot$ L^{-1} and are frequent and severe with levels >8 mEq $\cdot$ L^{-1} (Table 11–6). ECG changes begin with peaked T waves and prolongation of the PR interval, progressing to disappearance of P waves, widening of the QRS complex to a sine wave configuration, and finally ventricular fibrillation or asystolic cardiac arrest.

TABLE 11–6. Signs and Symptoms of Hyperkalemia

Electrocardiogram changes (peaked T waves, prolonged
  PR intervals, bradycardia, absent P waves, widened
  QRS complex, sine wave pattern)
Paresthesias
Dysrhythmias
Vasodilation
Hypotension
Paralysis

These ECG abnormalities are accentuated by concomitant hyponatremia, hypocalcemia, and acidosis. Vasodilation and hypotension may occur, along with paresthesias, weakness, and eventually paralysis of extremity and respiratory muscles.

Critical Limits

The adage about canceling elective surgery if the potassium level exceeds 5.5 mEq $\cdot$ L^{-1} needs re-evaluation. The most common cause of hyperkalemia in surgical patients is chronic renal failure. Many patients with chronic renal failure tolerate high levels of potassium without signs or symptoms. Consider dialysis of patients who often exceed this level several times a week.

Without ECG changes, I proceed with anesthesia regardless of the potassium level. Elective surgery should be delayed if the process is acute, if the cause is unknown, or if the patient has heart disease (especially conduction defects) that may predispose to dysrhythmias. Finally, if a patient is diabetic, is taking β-blockers, or has symptoms suggestive of hyperkalemia (including ECG changes), delay is also recommended.

When anesthesia is conducted in a hyperkalemic patient, certain drugs (succinylcholine) and techniques that lead to acidosis (hypoventilation) are avoided, intravenous glucose is infused, and hyperventilation is used.

Treatment

Asymptomatic Patients

Asymptomatic patients are treated by correcting or treating the cause of hyperkalemia. Patients with normal muscle tone and peaked T waves but no other ECG changes can be managed by decreasing oral potassium intake, by administering loop diuretics to increase potassium excretion, and, if indicated, by using ion exchange resin (Kayexalate) or dialysis. The dose of Kayexalate is 15 to 30 g in 20% sorbitol orally or 50 g rectally; this regimen removes 0.5 to 1 mEq of potassium per gram of resin.

Symptomatic Patients

Any patient with muscle weakness or ECG changes more severe than peaked T waves constitutes a medical emergency. Treatment must counteract the membrane effects of hyperkalemia (Ca^{2+} and hypertonic saline) to cause internal shifts of potassium into cells (bicarbonate, glucose, insulin). These regimens have a relatively rapid onset (within minutes) and short duration (15 to 60 min).

Administration of calcium (1–2 g of calcium chloride or 30–60 mL of calcium gluconate) should be assessed with constant ECG monitoring and stopped when the abnormal ECG changes reverse. Calcium is used with caution in digitalized patients to avoid digitalis toxicity. It must never be mixed with bicarbonate or it precipitates. A convenient way to make hypertonic saline is to add 2 ampules of sodium bicarbonate to 1 L of 0.9% saline, giving a final sodium concentration of 216 mEq $\cdot$ L^{-1}.

Ten per cent glucose (with or without insulin), sodium bicarbonate, and hyperventilation cause internal shifts of potassium. These modalities have a somewhat slower onset and longer duration of action. Because none actually lowers total body potassium, begin ion exchange therapy or dialysis as soon as practical.

CALCIUM

Bone contains more than 99% of the total body calcium; about 0.6% is intracellular, and 0.1% is in the extracellular fluid. Most intracellular calcium is in various membrane structures. The free, ionized intracellular calcium is 100 to 200 nmol $\cdot$ L^{-1}. Ionized calcium serves many second-messenger functions and regulates several enzyme systems.[13]

Extracellular calcium exists in three phases:

1. Ionized (about 50%)
2. Complexed to various anions (about 10%)
3. Bound to plasma proteins, mostly albumin (40%)

Ionized calcium is physiologically active and should be measured. Many laboratories still measure total calcium.

Changes in ionized and total calcium are not always proportionate. As examples, hypoalbuminemia decreases total extracellular calcium without affecting ionized calcium; alkalosis increases protein binding and decreases ionized calcium without changing total calcium concentration; and hyponatremia also increases protein binding but to a lesser extent. Normal levels of total serum calcium are 8.5 to 10.5 mg $\cdot$ dL^{-1} (2.0–2.5 mEq $\cdot$ L^{-1}).

What Is the Significance of Hypocalcemia?

Hypocalcemia (ionized calcium <2 mg $\cdot$ dL^{-1} or total calcium <8.5 mg $\cdot$ dL^{-1}) can occur because of increased sequestration of calcium (hyperphosphatemia, chelation with citrate of ethylenediaminetetra-acetic acid, acute pancreatitis, rhabdomyolysis, bone deposition from osteoblastic metastases, or severe osteitis fibrosa cystica). Significant hypocalcemia due to citrate intoxication associated with blood transfusion is extremely rare and very transient when it does occur. Other causes include hypoparathyroidism, hypomagnesemia, vitamin D deficiency, phenytoin, and mithramycin.

Manifestations

The symptoms of hypocalcemia are primarily neuromuscular and cardiovascular (Table 11–7).

Central Nervous System

Central nervous system symptoms begin with lethargy and depression and may progress to psychosis, dementia, and sei-

TABLE 11–7. Signs and Symptoms of Hypocalcemia

Paresthesias
Muscle cramps
Chvostek's sign
Trousseau's sign
Lethargy
Seizures
Fractures
Bone pain
Depression
Dementia
Tetany
Hypotension
Dysrhythmias*

*Especially heart block and ventricular fibrillation.

zures. Neuromuscular excitability begins with paresthesias and hyper-reflexia. Positive Chvostek's sign (facial twitching when the facial nerve is tapped) and Trousseau's sign (carpal spasm after 3 min of arm ischemia) may occur. With progression, patients develop muscle cramps and finally tetany and laryngeal stridor.

Cardiovascular

Cardiovascular signs and symptoms include prolonged QT interval, heart block, hypotension, heart failure, and ventricular fibrillation. The response to digitalis is decreased. All of these symptoms may be exacerbated by concurrent hypomagnesemia, alkalosis, or hyperkalemia.

Treatment

Asymptomatic Patients

Hypocalcemia should be treated to avoid progression to potentially fatal symptoms. If a patient is asymptomatic, give oral calcium, vitamin D supplements, and perhaps a thiazide diuretic to reduce urinary calcium loss. Treat hyperphosphatemia, if present, before calcium is supplemented. Calcium supplementation should proceed cautiously in digitalized patients to avoid digitalis toxicity.

Symptomatic Patients

Treat severe, symptomatic hypocalcemia urgently with an initial bolus of intravenous calcium followed by an infusion. Monitor replacement by frequent determinations of ionized calcium. Administer calcium in a dose just sufficient to reverse the symptoms and normalize the plasma concentration. Begin oral calcium and vitamin D supplements as soon as possible.

The intravenous preparations are calcium gluconate 10% and calcium chloride 10%. Calcium gluconate produces less venous irritation. A bolus dose of 10 to 30 mL over 10 to 15 minutes is followed by an infusion of 10 to 15 mg of calcium per kilogram of body weight in 1 L D_5W over 4 to 6 hours. Each 10 mL of calcium gluconate contains 93 mg (4.7 mEq) of calcium. Calcium chloride (273 mg, 14 mEq $\cdot$ 10 mL^{-1}) is given through a central venous catheter in the same doses (about one third the volume) as calcium gluconate.

What Is the Significance of Hypercalcemia?

Hypercalcemia occurs when calcium enters the extracellular fluid faster than regulatory hormones (parathyroid hormone and vitamin D) or renal excretory mechanisms can respond or when disorders of the hormones are present. More than one mechanism is usually involved. Increased intestinal absorption, increased bone release, and decreased renal excretion usually occur together in significant hypercalcemia. The most common causes of hypercalcemia are hyperparathyroidism, vitamin D intoxication, certain malignancies, chronic renal failure, milk-alkali syndrome, and iatrogenic causes.

Manifestations

Signs and symptoms (Table 11–8) include depression, lethargy, confusion, coma, muscle weakness, and decreased deep tendon reflexes. Hypertension is common, and dysrhythmias and digitalis toxicity may occur. ECG changes include shortening of the QT interval. Gastrointestinal symptoms include nausea, vomiting, and constipation. Metastatic calcification may cause pruritus, band keratopathy, and conjunctivitis.

Treatment

Most cases of hypercalcemia should be treated. Treatment of the causative disorder usually suffices in asymptomatic patients. The main treatment of acute symptomatic hypercalcemia is a brisk saline diuresis (5–10 L $\cdot$ d^{-1}) induced by rapid administration of intravenous saline. This approach must proceed cautiously in patients with significant heart disease.

Once the diuresis is established, it can be enhanced by the administration of furosemide, 20 to 40 mg intravenously every 2 to 3 hours. Urinary losses of sodium, potassium, and magnesium should be measured and replaced. Hemodialysis may be necessary in patients with very low GFR.

MAGNESIUM

How Is Magnesium Imbalance Managed?

Like calcium, magnesium is primarily an intracellular ion, only 1% to 2% being extracellular. Of the extracellular magnesium, about 60% is free, 15% is complexed to anions, and 25% is protein bound. Magnesium is an essential cofactor in more than 300 enzymatic reactions.

TABLE 11–8. Signs and Symptoms of Hypercalcemia

Nausea
Vomiting
↓ Deep tendon reflexes
Shortened QT interval
Constipation
Lethargy
Muscle weakness
Depression
Hypertension
Digitalis toxicity
Peptic ulcer
Dysrhythmias
Coma

What Is the Significance of Hypomagnesemia?

Normal plasma magnesium concentrations are between 1.7 and 2.7 mg · dL^{-1} (1.4–2.3 mEq · L^{-1}). Internal shifts are rarely a cause of hypomagnesemia. The most common causes are decreased intestinal absorption (starvation, alcoholism, malabsorption, diarrhea) or increased renal excretion (diuresis). Urine excretion is usually appropriately low <10 mg · d^{-1}, if the cause is intestinal and >10 mg · d^{-1} if the cause of the hypomagnesemia is renal.

Manifestations

Hypomagnesemia is common in postoperative patients in an intensive care unit. It may be accompanied by hypocalcemia and hypokalemia, which exacerbate the signs and symptoms. Symptoms very similar to those of hypokalemia include apathy, nausea, positive Chvostek's, and Trousseau's signs, muscle spasticity, increased deep tendon reflexes, tetany, and seizures. Ventricular dysrhythmias may occur, especially in digitalized patients (Table 11–9). Hypomagnesemia may hamper treatment of hypokalemia because it interferes with establishing the normal transcellular gradient for potassium and often must be corrected in order to correct the potassium deficit.

Treatment

Patients with seizures, tetany, or dysrhythmias should receive 100 to 200 mg (8–16 mEq) of magnesium intravenously over 10 to 15 minutes. With less severe symptoms, the infusion can proceed intravenously at a rate of 12 mg · kg^{-1} · d^{-1}. Deep tendon reflexes should be checked frequently and the infusion stopped if they decrease. Asymptomatic hypomagnesemia is treated with oral supplementation.

What Is the Significance of Hypermagnesemia?

Hypermagnesemia is almost always iatrogenic (from treatment of pre-eclampsia) or due to uncontrolled magnesium intake (in antacids, cathartics) in patients with severe reductions in GFR.

Manifestations

Signs and symptoms (Table 11–10) include lethargy, confusion, nausea, hypotension, muscle weakness, decreased deep tendon reflexes, dysrhythmias, respiratory paralysis, and coma.

TABLE 11–9. Signs and Symptoms of Hypomagnesemia

↑ Deep tendon reflexes
Chvostek's sign
Trousseau's sign
Muscle spasticity
Nausea
Apathy
Tetany
Dysrhythmias

TABLE 11–10. Signs and Symptoms of Hypermagnesemia

Muscle weakness
↓ Deep tendon reflexes
Nausea
Lethargy
Confusion
Hypotension
Coma
Dysrhythmias

Hypermagnesemia increases the effectiveness of both depolarizing and nondepolarizing neuromuscular blocking agents.

Treatment

Mild, asymptomatic hypermagnesemia does not need treatment other than to limit magnesium intake. If the plasma magnesium level is >10 mg · dL^{-1}, or if a patient is symptomatic, administer calcium intravenously to provide 15 mg · kg^{-1} over a 4-hour period. If renal function permits, establish a diuresis by volume expansion and loop diuretics. Otherwise, dialysis may be necessary.

PHOSPHORUS

How Is Phosphorus Imbalance Managed?

Only about 0.03% of total body phosphorus is in plasma; the remainder exists in bone (85%) and cells (14%). Intracellular phosphorus is critically important in most cell functions. Plasma inorganic phosphate is primarily dibasic (HPO$_4^{-2}$) and monobasic phosphate (H$_2$PO$_4^-$). Changes in albumin concentration do not influence plasma phosphorus levels.

Normal plasma inorganic phosphorus concentrations are 2.5 to 4.5 mg · dL^{-1} in adults and 3.5 to 6.0 mg · dL^{-1} in children. Significant internal redistribution occurs with respiratory alkalosis but not metabolic alkalosis or glucose/insulin administration. Hypophosphatemia secondary to respiratory alkalosis is asymptomatic.

What Is the Significance of Hypophosphatemia?

Hypophosphatemia can result from decreased absorption (starvation, alcoholism, phosphate binders, vitamin D deficiency) and from excessive renal loss (hyperparathyroidism, carbonic anhydrase inhibitors).

Manifestations

Symptoms of hypophosphatemia are largely attributable to decreased intracellular adenosine triphosphate and impaired oxygen delivery secondary to decreased red blood cell 2, 3-diphosphoglycerate (Table 11–11). These include irritability, confusion, stupor, coma, seizures, paresthesias, muscle weakness, hemolysis, rhabdomyolysis, and decreased cardiac output. There is poor correlation between plasma and total body phosphorus. Symptoms usually do not occur until the total body deficit exceeds 10 g.

TABLE 11–11. Signs and Symptoms of Hypophosphatemia

Paresthesias
Muscle weakness
Confusion
Irritability
Stupor
Seizures
Hemolysis
Rhabdomyolysis
Decreased cardiac output
Coma

Treatment

Hypophosphatemia is treated by increasing oral phosphorus intake. If the plasma phosphorus is <1.5 mg $\cdot$ dL^{-1} or if a patient is symptomatic, give intravenous phosphorus, 2.0 to 7.5 mg $\cdot$ kg^{-1}, three to four times daily until the plasma concentration exceeds 2.0 mg $\cdot$ dL^{-1} (Table 11–12). Do not give parenteral phosphorus in the presence of hypocalcemia. Give phosphorus cautiously if the GFR is reduced. Metastatic calcification can occur if the phosphorus and calcium product exceeds 60.

What Is the Significance of Hyperphosphatemia?

Hyperphosphatemia may result from internal shifts (hemolysis, rhabdomyolysis, tumor lysis), excessive exogenous load (phosphorus-containing antacids, enemas, laxatives), or diminished excretion (decreased GFR). Renal dysfunction is almost always a factor.

Manifestations

Symptoms are generally attributed to secondary changes in calcium concentration and ectopic tissue deposition with calcium. A phosphorus and calcium concentration product of 60 or greater must be aggressively treated.

Treatment

In the presence of adequate renal function, the treatment consists of volume expansion to increase the GFR. Once accomplished, a carbonic anhydrase inhibitor (acetazolamide) is administered. The alternative is hemodialysis. Less severe or asymptomatic hyperphosphatemia is treated by decreasing phosphorus intake and the cautious use of phosphorus binders such as oral antacids containing aluminum, magnesium, or calcium (see Tables 11–12 and 11–13).

RENAL FUNCTION TESTS

Clinically available methods for evaluating renal function include urinalysis and measurement of urine output, blood urea nitrogen (BUN), serum creatinine (Scr), and rarely creatinine clearance (Ccr).[14] All have significant limitations that should be considered when interpreting results.

TABLE 11–12. Electrolyte Solutions Useful in Treating Electrolyte Imbalance*

3% NaCl: 513 mEq $\cdot$ L^{-1} Na$^+$
Calcium gluconate: 10% = 93 mg (4.7 mEq) Ca^{2+} $\cdot$ 10 mL^{-1}
Calcium chloride: 10% = 273 mg (14 mEq) Ca^{2+} $\cdot$ 10 mL^{-1}
Magnesium sulfate:
  50% = 50 mg (4 mEq) Mg^{2+} $\cdot$ mL^{-1}
  25% = 25 mg (2 mEq) Mg^{2+} $\cdot$ mL^{-1}
  10% = 10 mg (1 mEq) Mg^{2+} $\cdot$ mL^{-1}
Sodium phosphate = 93 mg PO$_4^-$ $\cdot$ mL^{-1} (4 mEq $\cdot$ mL^{-1} Na$^+$)
Potassium phosphate = 93 mg PO$_4^-$ $\cdot$ mL^{-1} (4 mEq $\cdot$ mL^{-1} K$^+$)

*See text for doses and indications.

When Is Urinalysis Useful?

Urinalysis is one of the most common laboratory tests ordered for preoperative patients. It is more useful to establish a diagnosis of urinary tract disease than to evaluate renal function. The presence of protein, sugar, and abnormal sediment tells little about kidney function. In most cases, urine concentration and pH cannot be interpreted meaningfully. Extremely concentrated or dilute urine (specific gravity ≥ 1.025 or ≤ 1.005) indicates that the renal concentrating or diluting mechanisms are functioning. They may also give an idea of the patient's fluid status at the time the specimen was collected.

Of What Significance Is the Urine Volume?

Urine volume is a nonspecific indicator of renal function because many factors influence urine output, including protein and fluid intake, nonrenal fluid loss, stress, pain, drugs, and cardiovascular status. Therefore, a great deal must be known about a patient to judge the appropriateness of the urine output. Normal urine output is in the range of 0.7 to 1.5 mL $\cdot$ kg^{-1} $\cdot$ h^{-1}. Under unusual circumstances, it may be lower or higher. Despite the limitations of urine output as a measure of renal function, it is the most routinely available if not the best test in the operating room.

What Does Blood Urea Nitrogen Indicate?

Urea nitrogen is an end product of hepatic protein metabolism. Ingestion of large amounts of protein, catabolic states, anabolic steroids, and blood in the gut all increase urea nitrogen production. Urea nitrogen is freely filterable by the kid-

TABLE 11–13. Summary of Signs and Symptoms of Electrolyte Imbalance

	↓Na	↑Na	↓K	↑K	↓Ca	↑Ca	↓Mg	↑Mg	↓PO₄
Lethargy	+	+			+	+	+		
Coma	+	+				+		+	+
Seizures	+				+		+		+
↑ Deep tendon reflexes		+					+		
↓ Deep tendon reflexes	+					+		+	
Muscle weakness			+	+		+		+	
Positive (+) Trousseau's sign				+	+				
Positive (+) Chvostek's sign				+	+				
Electrocardiogram changes			+	+	+	+	+	+	
Rhabdomyolysis		+							+

neys and is both secreted and reabsorbed by the tubules. The amount reabsorbed increases as urine flow decreases.

If all factors are constant, an inverse relationship between GFR and BUN exists (Fig. 11–1). Oliguria, hypercatabolism, and blood in the gut may increase the BUN without a decrease in GFR.

With complete cessation of glomerular filtration, the BUN rises about 10 to 20 mg $\cdot$ dL^{-1} $\cdot$ d^{-1}. After massive trauma, sepsis, or other problems associated with hypercatabolic states, the BUN may rise as much as 100 mg $\cdot$ dL^{-1} $\cdot$ d^{-1}. Elevation of the BUN:Scr ratio, which is normally 10:1, may mean that extracellular fluid depletion is causing the azotemia. Severe liver disease, decreased protein intake, and extracellular volume expansion decrease the BUN.

When Is Serum Creatinine Measurement Useful?

Scr level is also inversely proportional to GFR (see Fig. 11–1). Creatinine is produced by muscle, and its rates of production and release are related to the muscle mass. Creatinine is freely filtered by the glomeruli; very little is secreted or reabsorbed by the tubules. Scr $\times$ GFR is a constant. If GFR is halved, Scr doubles. This relationship holds only when a steady state exists.

If GFR ceases, the Scr rises about 0.5 to 1.0 mg $\cdot$ dL $\cdot$ d^{-1} (Fig. 11–2). This increase may be much greater with severe trauma or rhabdomyolysis. Because creatinine production is related to muscle mass, loss of muscle tissue with renal failure may result in a deceptively low Scr level. Neither BUN nor Scr values accurately reflect acute changes in GFR.

A more accurate method for determining GFR uses Ccr, which can be calculated as follows:

$$Ccr = Ucr \times V/Pcr \qquad \text{Equation 5}$$

where Ucr is the urine creatinine concentration, V is urine volume during a given period of time, and Pcr is the plasma creatinine concentration sampled during the urine collection period.

This test is fraught with collection errors and is rarely available (or appropriate) in the acute situation usually found in the operating room. It is, however, useful in patients with chronic renal dysfunction and some patients in the ICU. Like Scr determination, Ccr is not an accurate estimate of GFR unless a steady state exists.

COMPROMISED RENAL FUNCTION

The kidneys are the primary organs for maintaining homeostasis of the internal milieu. This function is accomplished by glomerular filtration and by tubular secretion and absorption. When the ability to maintain homeostasis is interfered with by physiologic, pathologic, or pharmacologic means, renal dysfunction exists. Changes can be gradual (aging, chronic renal disease) or abrupt (renal artery thrombosis, diuretics, acute tubular necrosis).

Are the Changes Acute or Chronic?

When we think of compromised renal function, we are usually concerned with ARF or chronic renal failure. ARF can be oliguric (urine output <400 mL $\cdot$ day^{-1}) or nonoliguric (urine output >400 mL $\cdot$ d^{-1}). Inadequately treated functional renal failure may eventuate in acute tubular necrosis.[15]

What Are the Hallmarks of Chronic Failure?

Patients with chronic renal failure may pass through several stages (Fig. 11–3).

FIGURE 11–1. Theoretical relationship among BUN, Scr, and GFR. (Reprinted from Kassirer JP: Clinical evaluation of kidney function: glomerular function. N Engl J Med 1971; 285:385, by permission of the New England Journal of Medicine.)

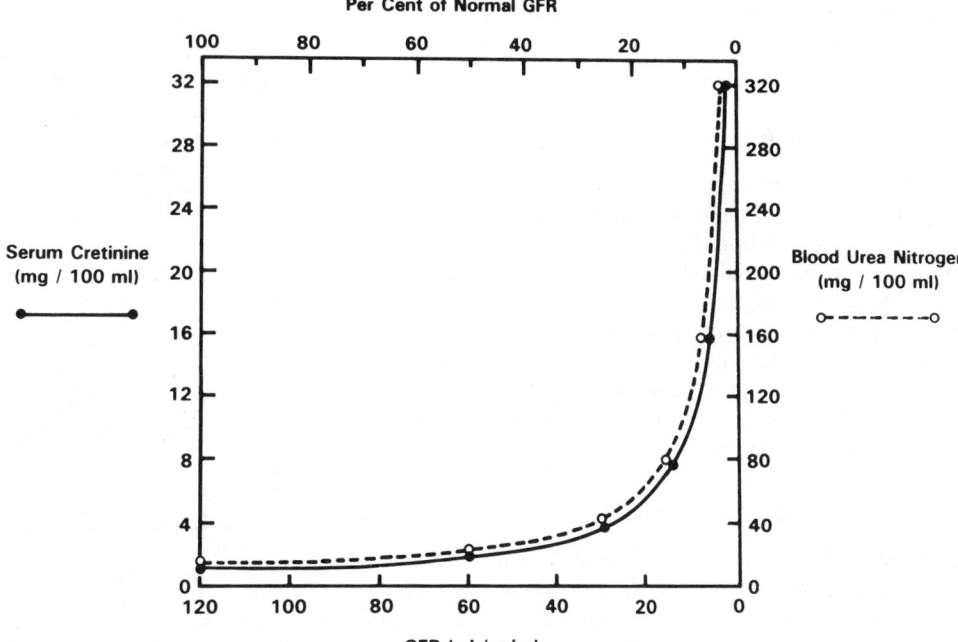

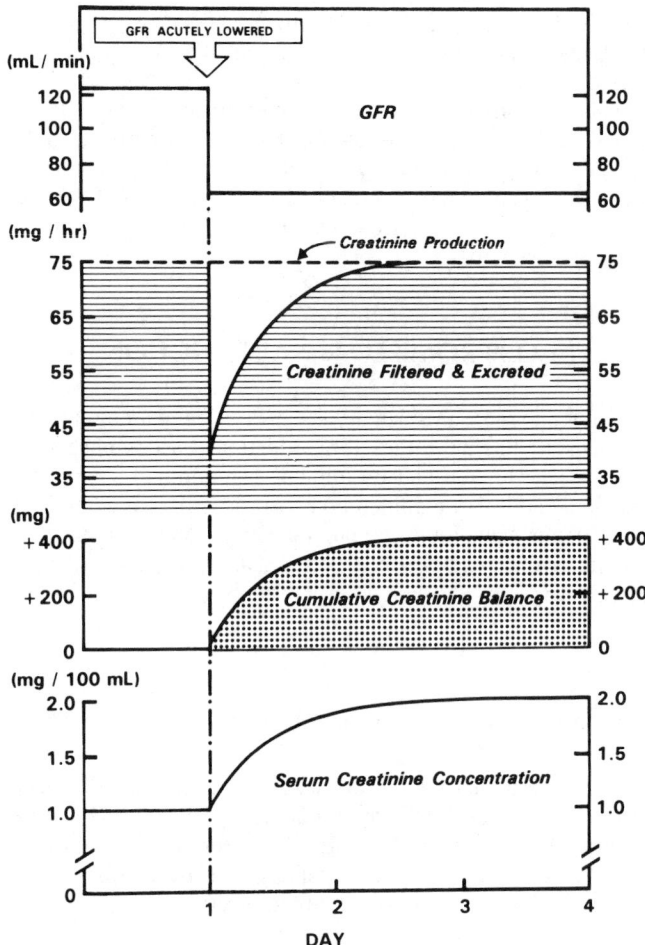

FIGURE 11–2. Effects of an acute decrease in GFR on creatinine balance, excretion, and serum concentration. (Reprinted from Kassirer JP: Clinical evaluation of kidney function. N Engl J Med 1971; 285:385, by permission of the New England Journal of Medicine.)

Decreased Renal Reserve

Until about 60% of nephron mass is lost, patients are in a stage of decreased renal reserve. They generally have no signs or symptoms of renal dysfunction and present no special problems for an anesthesiologist.

Early Renal Insufficiency

Subsequently, they enter the stage of renal insufficiency and may develop mild degrees of azotemia, anemia, and acidosis; decreased concentrating ability; and nocturia. Any decrease in effective circulating blood volume in these individuals can cause devastating further deterioration of renal function. The implications of even a small decrease in GFR are illustrated in Figure 11–4. The main anesthetic implications of renal insufficiency are, therefore, careful attention to fluid replacement and renal perfusion. With this in mind, these patients can surely undergo major surgery.

Advanced Renal Insufficiency

As renal disease evolves, azotemia, anemia, and acidosis become more severe. Isosthenuria, polyuria, nocturia, hyperchloremia, hyperphosphatemia, hyponatremia, and hypocalcemia are common. Infection is a constant threat. The major

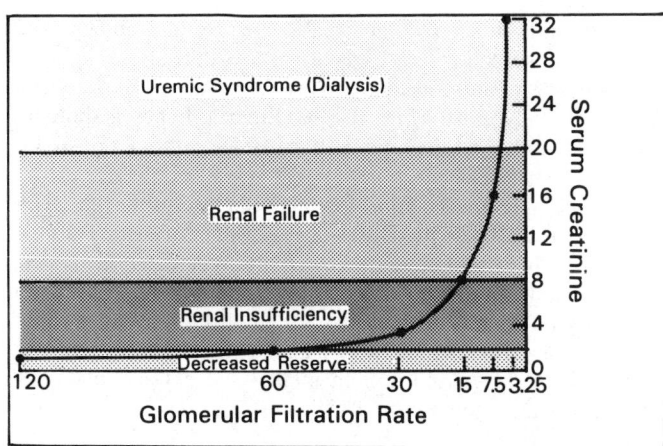

FIGURE 11–3. Changes in glomerular filtration rate and serum creatinine in chronic renal failure. (Modified from Bastron RD: Chronic renal failure, clinical implications. In Current Reviews in Clinical Anesthesia, 1982. Lesson 8. Vol. 3. Miami, FL, Current Reviews in Clinical Anesthesia, 1982, p 60.)

anesthetic problems in patients with renal failure are drug elimination, fluid balance, and sepsis (Fig. 11–5).

Decompensation

With further progression, decompensation occurs. Uremia and all the manifestations of renal disease become overt. Significant anesthesia implications of uremia are discussed later in this chapter.

When Should Urine Output Be Monitored?

No hard and fast rules are available to determine when to measure urine output. Certain perioperative risk factors (Table 11–14), high-risk procedures (Table 11–15), and nephrotoxins (Table 11–16) are associated with higher incidences of ARF.

Some factors such as shock, massive blood transfusion, aortic cross-clamping, hemolysis, rhabdomyolysis, and major trauma are strong indications for monitoring urine output. Others are relative indicators for such monitoring. As an example, measurement of urine output in a patient with pre-existing renal dysfunction having major bowel surgery is advisable but is unnecessary during less extensive surgery such as hernia repair, cataract extraction, or median nerve decompression. This decision is a clinical one, and common sense serves as a guide.

Note that indications for monitoring urine output are not the

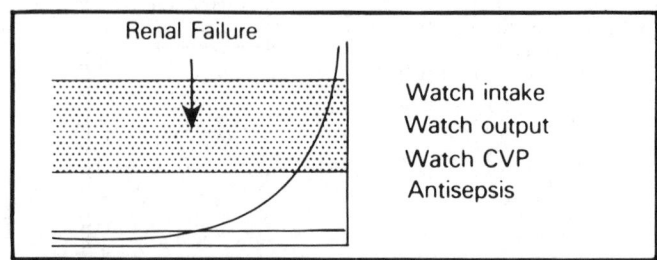

FIGURE 11–4. The patient with renal failure requires strict attention to fluid balance and aseptic technique. (Modified from Bastron RD: Chronic renal failure, clinical implications. In Current Reviews in Clinical Anesthesia, 1982. Lesson 8. Vol. 3. Miami, FL, Current Reviews in Clinical Anesthesia, 1982, p 63.)

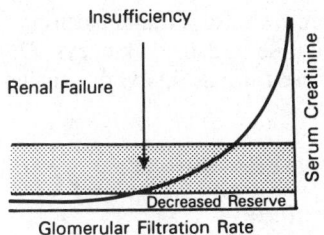

FIGURE 11–5. The primary concern in renal insufficiency is meticulous fluid replacement. (Modified from Bastron RD: Chronic renal failure, clinical implications. *In* Current Reviews in Clinical Anesthesia, 1982. Lesson 8. Vol. 3. Miami, FL, Current Reviews in Clinical Anesthesia, 1982, p 63.)

same as indications for inserting a urethral catheter. The latter may be useful in a young, healthy person undergoing a long otolaryngologic procedure in order to drain the bladder, but not to measure hourly urine flow. Like any other test, false-positive or negative results can be misleading, and decisions based on those results can be incorrect.

What Are Oliguria and Polyuria?

When the kidneys sense abnormalities in extracellular fluid volume or osmolarity, they respond by either increasing or decreasing the amount of urine excreted. The standard definition of oliguria in an adult is urine output <400 mL · d^{-1}.[16] This is the amount of maximally concentrated urine required to excrete the normal daily nitrogenous waste produced by the body's metabolism.

In the operating room, anesthesiologists generally deal with patients for hours rather than days and consider a urine output of <0.5 mL · kg^{-1} · h^{-1} to represent oliguria. Using this definition, oliguria may represent normal renal function to conserve water and electrolytes in response to decreased intake, excessive extrarenal loss, stress, pain, positive-pressure ventilation, or anesthesia. On the other hand, oliguria may represent a pathologic response of the kidneys such as prerenal failure, acute tubular necrosis, or postrenal failure.

Similarly, polyuria may result from excessive fluid intake (polydipsia, intravenous fluids), a high osmotic load (glycosuria), or the use of diuretic agents. It also may be a pathologic response caused by central or renal diabetes insipidus, severe hypokalemia, or high-output renal failure. The diagnosis can be made on the basis of a carefully taken history, physical examination, and laboratory tests.

Why Is Oliguria Present?

The cause of normally occurring oliguria (long-term NPO status, stress, pain, or anesthesia) is usually apparent. The main

TABLE 11–14. Perioperative Risk Factors for Renal Failure

Advanced age
Pre-existing renal dysfunction (serum creatinine >2 mg · dL^{-1})
Vasomotor nephropathy (sepsis, congestive heart failure, liver failure)
Obstructive jaundice (bilirubin >8 mg · dL^{-1})
Rhabdomyolysis, myoglobinemia
Shock (hypovolemic, cardiogenic, septic)
Massive blood transfusion

(Modified from Sladen RN: Perioperative renal protection. *In* ASA 1991 Annual Refresher Course Lectures. Park Ridge, IL, 1991, pp 1–7. A copy of the full text can be obtained from ASA, 520 N. Northwest Highway, Park Ridge, Illinois, 60068-2573.)

problem is oliguria in patients with the previously mentioned risk factors. High-risk patients with oliguria should be evaluated systematically to rule out or to prevent ARF. One such approach is discussed next.

Likely Causes

The main causes of renal failure in surgical patients are:

1. Prerenal (hypovolemia, pump failure)
2. Intrinsic—acute tubular necrosis (vascular, toxic)
3. Postrenal (obstruction, extravasation)

Assessment

The first step in the evaluation of oliguric patients is to be certain that urine being formed can get to the collection receptacle. Insert a urethral catheter or irrigate a catheter that is already in place. Be sure that all collection tubing is properly connected and patent. Males with pelvic trauma should have an injection urethrogram before insertion of a urethral catheter. Anuria is a hallmark of postrenal failure, although oliguria or intermittent anuria is more common.

The second and most important step is to be certain that perfusion is optimum. Correction of preload (effective circulating blood volume); cardiac rate, rhythm, and contractility; and afterload (peripheral vascular resistance) is critical.[17] The approach may be as simple as a fluid challenge or may entail the use of the most sophisticated cardiac monitoring devices and the infusion of potent drugs, depending on the clinical situation. Remember that many critically ill patients need to be hyperdynamic—that is, they require a higher than normal filling pressure and cardiac index.

Indications for Diuretics

Most of the time, these steps are sufficient both to evaluate and treat oliguric patients. If the cause of oliguria is prerenal, it should be reversed by providing optimum perfusion. If a patient remains oliguric despite optimum perfusion, diuretics may be helpful.[18]

Mannitol, 12.5 to 25 g, or furosemide, 1 to 2 mg, can be administered intravenously. Mannitol increases blood volume and should be used with caution in patients with heart disease. If a low dose of furosemide is not effective, a second dose of up to 1 mg · kg^{-1} may be given. If oliguria persists, assume that the patient has acute tubular necrosis. Should urine output increase, carefully monitor and maintain the patient's volume and electrolyte status. Consider a nephrology consultation for any patient who requires this latter step.

Diuretics may be indicated in well-hydrated patients in several circumstances.[19] These include cardiopulmonary bypass, aortic cross-clamp, or kidney transplantation. They may be

TABLE 11–15. High-Risk Procedures

Cardiac surgery
Aortic cross-clamp
Biliary tract surgery (sepsis, obstructive jaundice)
Complicated obstetrics
Major trauma

TABLE 11–16. Nephrotoxins

Endogenous nephrotoxins:	Myoglobin
	Hemoglobin
	Conjugated bilirubin
	Uric acid
Exogenous nephrotoxins:	Volatile anesthetic agents with fluoride metabolites
	Chemotherapeutic agents (aminoglycosides, amphotericin B)
	Immunosuppressives (cyclosporin, *cis*-platinum)
	Contrast dyes (especially in dehydrated, elderly, hypertensive, diabetic patients)
	Low-molecular-weight dextrans

(Modified from Sladen RN: Perioperative renal protection. ASA 1991 Annual Refresher Course Lectures. Park Ridge, IL, 1991, pp 1–7. A copy of the full text can be obtained from ASA, 520 N. Northwest Highway, Park Ridge, Illinois, 60068-2573.)

requested by a surgeon to increase urine flow (e.g., to make the ureteral orifices easier to identify during cystoscopy) or by a neurosurgeon or ophthalmologist to decrease intracranial or intraocular pressure, respectively. The only contraindication to diuretics is volume depletion, which may be aggravated by the diuretic administration.

Occasionally, a lung-versus-kidney or heart-versus-kidney situation is encountered with respect to therapy. With careful monitoring of renal, pulmonary, and cardiac function, this dilemma should not occur often. When it does, erring in favor of the kidneys is recommended. There are countless therapies for congestive heart failure but none for acute tubular necrosis. Pulmonologists and cardiologists do not always agree with this approach. When it is necessary to choose among these vital organs, the decision is made on a case-by-case basis.

Is Sophisticated Testing Necessary?

The fractional excretion of sodium, the renal failure index, and other urinary indices for differentiating prerenal failure from acute tubular necrosis are of limited clinical value for an anesthesiologist. I have never seen them used in the operating room and only rarely in the ICU when an aggressive approach to oliguria, such as outlined earlier, is used. If the reader believes these indices to be necessary, a nephrology consultation is additionally required. If you anticipate using any of them, be sure to collect the urine and plasma samples for analysis before giving any diuretic agents.

RENAL TOXICITY

What Are the Causative Factors?

A wide variety of compounds, including heavy metals, organic solvents, analgesics, antibiotics, radiocontrast dyes, and anesthetics, can be nephrotoxic. Of most interest to anesthesiologists are antibiotics, radiocontrast dyes, and anesthetics. The prototypical nephrotoxic antibiotic is gentamicin. Gentamicin nephrotoxicity can be limited by measuring peak and trough levels, keeping them below toxic levels, and monitoring Scr values for signs of decreased renal function. This speaks in favor of giving gentamicin in the operating room via slow infusion rather than as a bolus.

Nephrotoxicity due to radiocontrast dyes can be minimized by avoiding dehydration. Prolonged use of enflurane can produce sufficient free inorganic fluoride to damage kidneys. Enflurane should probably not be used in patients with existing renal dysfunction.

How Are the Kidneys Protected?

Duration of insult is probably the most important factor causing renal dysfunction during and after high-risk procedures. Anesthesiologists have little or no control over a procedure's duration. The best one can do is to ensure adequate cardiac output and circulating blood volume to minimize vasoconstriction and to maximize renal perfusion.

Hypotension associated with vasoconstriction (low cardiac output or circulating blood volume) is associated with a higher incidence of postoperative dysfunction than is hypotension caused by vasodilators. Diuretics and possibly low-dose dopamine, given before the insult, may be helpful to protect the kidneys as well. Use monitoring techniques appropriate for the patient, surgeon, and surgical procedure.

What Intravenous Fluids Are Best?

Intraoperative fluid therapy is aimed at replacing fluids lost by normal body functions that are not replaced during the NPO period, as well as blood and third space losses caused by the surgical procedure. The main concern is to maintain adequate circulating blood volume and extracellular fluid volume. This goal is best achieved with salt solutions, either isotonic NS or nearly isotonic LR.

The main argument against balanced salt solutions is that they contain potassium, and patients with renal failure may be hyperkalemic. Realistically, the 4 mEq · L^{-1} of potassium in the balanced salt solutions does no harm. NS may be selected for use if a patient is significantly hyperkalemic or will be receiving large volumes of banked blood, which will provide a large potassium load. Otherwise, it makes no difference which fluid is chosen.

How Does Renal Failure Affect Drug Choice and Dosage?

Patients with uremic syndrome may have unusual responses to drugs for several reasons.[18, 19] Protein binding is abnormal, and drugs such as sodium thiopental, which are highly protein bound, may cause exaggerated or prolonged effects. Pseudocholinesterase levels may be diminished but rarely enough to cause clinically significant prolongation of succinylcholine-induced blockade (and presumably that of mivacurium).

Electrolyte imbalance, especially hypokalemia and hypermagnesemia, may potentiate the neuromuscular blocking agents. Drugs such as gallamine, which are totally dependent on renal excretion, should be used with caution if at all. Other drugs depend on renal excretion of active metabolites (e.g., meperidine). Most drugs that are partially dependent on renal excretion require smaller than usual doses or longer intervals between doses.

Preoperative Blood Levels

Renal dysfunction per se is not an indication to measure any drug level. The usual indication for monitoring drug levels is to confirm a clinical impression that drug levels are subtherapeutic, therapeutic, or toxic. This same indication should be used for patients with renal failure.

DIALYSIS PATIENTS

In addition to the usual concerns for any preoperative patient, the main consideration in preoperative patients on dialysis is to assess the adequacy of dialysis. Dialysis replaces the kidneys to maintain homeostasis of the internal milieu as well as possible. It should correct water and electrolyte imbalance (Table 11–17) as well as several other abnormalities associated with the uremic syndrome.

Why Is Timing Important?

Determine the time of the last dialysis, which ideally should be within 24 hours. Serum electrolytes measured the day of surgery should be within normal limits if dialysis is adequate. Verifying the absence of hypertension and comparison of predialysis and postdialysis weight are the best clinical methods for determining the status of the water balance. Patients usually know their dry weight and the amount of fluctuation in weight that they experience with each dialysis cycle.

Nephrologists often remove more water than usual in preoperative patients to allow the anesthesiologist to give more intravenous salt solutions during the procedure.

Is a Tilt Test Advisable?

Although theoretically attractive, a tilt test to determine adequacy of autonomic nervous system function is not necessary. A patient's response to anesthesia and blood loss is determined primarily by the effective circulating blood volume and is treated accordingly, regardless of the results of a tilt test.

What Blood Studies Are Important?

Be aware of the degree of anemia and how well it is tolerated. If a patient is inadequately dialyzed or has just recently

TABLE 11–17. Water and Electrolyte Imbalance in Uremia

↑ Intake
Hypervolemia
Peripheral edema
Pulmonary edema
Ejection murmurs
Hypertension
Encephalopathy
↓ Intake, extrarenal loss
Hypovolemia
Hypotension
Shock
↑ H^+, PO_4^{2-}, Mg^{2+}, K^+
↓ Na^+, Ca^{2+}

(Modified from Bastron RD: Chronic renal failure, clinical implications. *In* Current Reviews in Clinical Anesthesia, Lesson 8. Vol. 3. Miami, Current Reviews in Clinical Anesthesia, 1982.)

TABLE 11–18. Abnormalities Caused by Dialysis

Rebound heparinization
Disequilibrium syndrome
Encephalopathy
Hepatitis/human immunodeficiency virus
Ascites, pericardial effusion
Hypersplenism

(Modified from Bastron RD: Chronic renal failure, clinical implications. *In* Current Reviews in Clinical Anesthesia, Lesson 8. Vol. 3. Miami, Current Reviews in Clinical Anesthesia, 1982.)

been dialyzed, check for clotting abnormalities. Inadequately dialyzed patients may have abnormal platelet function; the best test for this situation is determination of bleeding time. Recently dialyzed patients may still be heparinized or develop rebound heparinization (Table 11–18), which can be ruled out by an activated clotting time. Because most of these patients will have received multiple transfusions, they should be considered at increased risk for hepatitis or human immunodeficiency virus infection.

If a patient is confused or nauseated and has been dialyzed in the immediate preoperative period, the disequilibrium syndrome may be to blame. This results from cerebral edema subsequent to a decrease in plasma osmolality relative to cerebral osmolality. It requires up to 24 hours to resolve. This situation suggests that it is appropriate to treat such patients as though they had increased intracranial pressure if postponement of the procedure is not an option.

How Should Arteriovenous Fistulas or Other Dialysis Sites Be Managed?

Dialysis sites are the lifeline of these patients and must be protected carefully. Do not measure blood pressure or start intravenous infusions on the arm with an arteriovenous fistula; carefully protect the fistula from external pressure, kinking, or obstruction due to arm flexion; and when feasible, do not place intravenous infusion catheters in veins that may be needed later for arteriovenous fistulas. Document on the anesthesia record that the fistula was protected and functioning.

Why Is the Postoperative Period Critical?

Postoperatively, these patients may develop a hypercoagulable state. This problem may explain why arteriovenous fis-

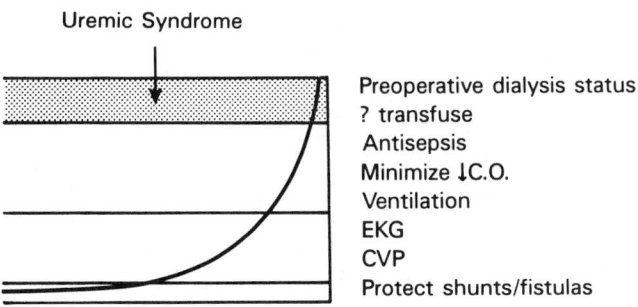

FIGURE 11–6. Anesthetic implications of uremia and dialysis. (Modified from Bastron RD: Chronic renal failure, clinical implications. *In* Current Reviews in Clinical Anesthesia, 1982. Lesson 8. Vol. 3. Miami, FL, Current Reviews in Clinical Anesthesia, 1982, p 63.)

tulas clot at this time. Therefore, fistulas must be carefully protected in the postoperative period as well. The lumina of temporary dialysis catheters may be filled with a solution containing 10,000 U of heparin per milliliter. If one of these lumina must be used for intravenous access, aspirate to clear it of heparin before injecting anything through the catheter.

What Are the Anesthetic Implications?

The importance of preoperative dialysis cannot be overemphasized (Fig. 11–6). Adequate dialysis corrects the problems caused by fluid and electrolyte imbalance. Evaluate and treat anemia according to your hospital's current guidelines. Compensation for severe anemia involves increased cardiac output, which reduces available cardiac reserve, and increased red blood cell 2,3-diphosphoglycerate, which shifts the oxygen dissociation curve to the right (more favorable for tissue oxygenation). Therefore, avoid or minimize reductions in cardiac output and increases in pH during anesthesia. Blood gas partition coefficients may be reduced by as much as 20% in patients with severe anemia, affecting induction and recovery times from inhaled anesthetics.

Monitor the ECG with particular attention to electrolyte-related changes. Poorly prepared patients may have hyperkalemic metabolic acidosis with compensatory hyperventilation. Failure to maintain hyperventilation may result in more severe acidosis and a catastrophic rise in serum potassium levels.

Immunosuppressive drugs used in transplant recipients potentiate a natural susceptibility to infections. Therefore, special attention to aseptic technique is important when performing any invasive procedure. Hepatitis is endemic in the dialyzed population, and appropriate precautions including vaccination should be followed.

All types of anesthetic techniques and agents have been successfully used in dialyzed patients and transplant recipients. No single agent or technique is always appropriate.[20–22] A choice is made on the basis of the principles discussed, a patient's psychologic and physiologic state, and the requirements of the surgical procedure.

References

1. Roberts SL, Tinker JH: Cardiovascular disease. *In* Risk and Outcome in Anesthesia. Brown DL (ed). Philadelphia, JB Lippincott, 1988, pp 34–36.
2. Brown DL, Thompson GE: Anesthetic choice. *In* Risk and Outcome in Anesthesia. Brown DL (ed). Philadelphia, JB Lippincott, 1988, pp 166–168.
3. Prys-Roberts C: Anesthetic management of the hypertensive patient. Acta Anaesthesiol Belg 1988; 39(Suppl 2):9–12.
4. Miller ED Jr: Anesthesia and the hypertensive patient. 1987 Review Course Lectures. International Anesthesia Research Society, 1987, pp 6–10.
5. Miller ED Jr: Perioperative hypertension: An overview. ASA Forty-Second Annual Refresher Course Lectures and Clinical Update Program. 1991.
6. Longnecker DE: The case for perioperative blood pressure control. ASA 1991 Annual Review Course Lectures. 1991, pp 62–64.
7. Berry FA: Anesthetic Management of Difficult and Routine Pediatric Patients. 2nd ed. New York, Churchill Livingstone, 1990, pp 89–120.
8. Cheung AT, Chernow B: Perioperative electrolyte disorders. *In* Anesthesia and Perioperative Complications. Benumof JL, Saidman LJ (eds). St Louis, Mosby-Year Book, 1992, pp 466–506.
9. Gravenstein JS: Fluid and electrolytes and acid-base balance. *In* Manual of Complications During Anesthesia. Gravenstein N (ed). Philadelphia, JB Lippincott, 1991, pp 353–382.
10. Cogan MG: Fluid and Electrolytes: Physiology and Pathophysiology. Norwalk, Appleton & Lange, 1991.
11. Kokko JP, Tannel RL: Fluids and Electrolytes. 2nd ed. Philadelphia, WB Saunders, 1990.
12. Solomon RJ, Katz JD: Disturbances of potassium homeostasis. *In* Advances in Anesthesia. Vol. 3. Stoelting RK, Barash PG, Gallagher TJ (eds). Chicago, Year Book Medical Publishers, 1986, pp 169–194.
13. Prielipp R, Zaloga GP: Calcium action and general anesthesia. *In* Advances in Anesthesia. Vol. 8. Stoelting RK, Barash PG, Gallagher TJ (eds). St Louis, Mosby-Year Book, 1991, pp 241–278.
14. Kaufman BS, Contreras J: Preanesthetic assessment of the patient with renal disease. Anesthesiol Clin North Am 1990; 8:677–695.
15. Takala J, Ruokonen E, Kari A: Acute renal failure. Anesthesiol Clin North Am 1988; 6:173–184.
16. Prough DS: Oliguria: Significance and management. International Anesthesia Research Society 1987 Review Course Lectures. 1987, pp 112–119.
17. Prough DS, Zaloga G: Hypovolemia and renal dysfunction. *In* Anesthesia and Perioperative Complications. Benumof JL, Saidman LJ (eds). St Louis, Mosby-Year Book, 1992, pp 434–465.
18. Sladen RN: Perioperative renal protection. ASA Forty-Second Annual Refresher Course Lectures, #255. Park Ridge, IL, 1991.
19. Prough DS: Perioperative management of acute renal failure. *In* Advances in Anesthesia. Vol. 5. Stoelting RK, Barash PG, Gallagher TJ (eds). Chicago, Year Book Medical Publishers, 1988, p 192.
20. Barr L, Miller ED Jr: Preserving renal function. Anesthesiology Report 1989; 1:290–294.
21. Gelman S: Preserving renal function during surgery. International Anesthesia Research Society 1991 Review Course Lectures. 1992, pp 88–92.
22. Borland LM, Cook DR: Anesthesia for organ transplantation. *In* Advances in Anesthesia. Vol. 3. Stoelting RK, Barash PG, Gallagher TJ (eds). Chicago, Year Book Medical Publishers, 1986, pp 12–17.

CHAPTER **12**

Endocrine Consultation

GARY P. ZALOGA, M.D., F.A.C.P., F.C.C.M.
K. PATRICK OBER, M.D.
WILLIAM T. CEFALU, M.D.

Anesthesiologists frequently encounter patients who have underlying endocrine disease and are about to undergo surgery. Surgery may be unrelated to the endocrine disease or may be part of the treatment for the disease. It is important to understand the metabolic alterations that result from the underlying endocrine abnormality and be knowledgeable about their treatment. This chapter addresses six common endocrine diseases: pituitary disease, adrenal disease, pheochromocytoma, thyroid disease, parathyroid diseases, and diabetes mellitus. It summarizes the pathophysiology and metabolic alterations that occur with the various diseases and outlines the important factors to consider in the preoperative evaluation and perioperative treatment of such patients. Some diseases, such as diabetes mellitus, are common and seldom require consultative services unless a problem such as diabetic ketoacidosis (DKA) arises. Others are uncommon or rare. Such cases (e.g., uncontrolled hypertension due to pheochromocytoma) should prompt a consultation as soon as is possible.

PITUITARY DISEASE

What Is Acromegaly?

Acromegaly is a chronic debilitating disorder caused by excessive growth hormone production.[1–7] Morbidity due to the disease is caused by the multiple metabolic actions of growth hormone and growth hormone–dependent growth factors (in particular, insulin-like growth factor I [IGF-I] or somatomedin C). Most cases of acromegaly are associated with a growth hormone–secreting pituitary tumor; some patients have problems related to the local effects of the intracranial mass.

Clinical Features

Clinical features develop slowly and gradually, and the disease is usually present for many years before the diagnosis is made.[1–3] Soft tissue changes are prominent. Facial features are coarsened, skin tags are frequently seen, and an increased risk of colon polyps and carcinoma has been reported. Stimulation of cartilage and bone also occurs, resulting in osteoarthritis (which may be severe and disabling), frontal bossing, prognathism, and dental malocclusion. The hands, feet, and tongue are typically enlarged.

Visceromegaly is commonly reported at autopsy but may not be apparent clinically. It is characterized by enlargement of the heart, kidneys, liver, and spleen. Entrapment neuropathies, especially carpal tunnel syndrome, are frequent accompaniments. Insulin resistance is a common metabolic consequence of growth hormone excess, although clinical diabetes mellitus is present in only 10% to 20% of acromegalic patients.

The mass effect due to the pituitary tumor may cause visual field defects by compression of the optic nerves and chiasm. Compression or destruction of normal pituitary tissue by the tumor may lead to hypopituitarism, with a resultant need for thyroid hormone, adrenal steroids, and sex hormone replacement therapy. Downward tumor growth can penetrate the sphenoid sinus and cause cerebrospinal fluid (CSF) rhinorrhea and risk of central nervous system (CNS) infection.

How Is Acromegaly Diagnosed?

The diagnosis of acromegaly is made on the basis of biochemical criteria, including elevation of basal growth hormone, failure to suppress growth hormone by oral administration of glucose, and elevation of IGF-I. In most cases, a pituitary adenoma can be visualized by computed tomography (CT) or magnetic resonance imaging (MRI). In rare instances, acromegaly is caused by ectopic production of growth hormone–releasing hormone (GHRH) rather than by a pituitary adenoma.

How Is Acromegaly Treated?

The preferred therapy is selective transsphenoidal resection of the pituitary adenoma.[4, 5] Radiation therapy may also be effective but is very slow to have an effect, usually taking many years, and frequently produces hypopituitarism. Radiation therapy is usually used as an adjunct if surgery has not been totally successful.

Medical therapy is also used as an adjunct to surgery or radiation. Bromocriptine (a dopamine agonist) may lower growth hormone levels in some patients, and the somatostatin analogue, octreotide, may cause tumor shrinkage in addition to biochemical and clinical improvement.[6, 7] However, the effects of these drugs are not consistent in all patients, and the expense and potential side effects of these treatments are problematic.

Perioperative Management

Thoughtful perioperative assessment and management of acromegalic patients are essential (Table 12–1). Unrecognized pituitary insufficiency, which can be precipitated by general anesthesia and surgical stress, is a potentially life-threatening complication of the pituitary tumor.

Associated Endocrinopathies

Documentation of normal thyroid function preoperatively is crucial. Measurement of thyroid-stimulating hormone (TSH) is not the best means of assessing thyroid status in patients with large pituitary tumors because a low-normal value is impossible to interpret. Documentation of a normal free thyroxine index (FTI) is the preferred method of confirming euthyroid status.

Adrenal Function

Because of the risk of secondary hypoadrenalism in these patients, stress level glucocorticoid therapy should be administered in the perioperative period if adrenal insufficiency cannot be ruled out. Diabetes insipidus is rare in acromegaly, but the increased risk of diabetes mellitus mandates careful monitoring of serum glucose and electrolyte values. Hypopituitarism may develop after transsphenoidal resection of pituitary adenomas. Careful postoperative evaluation of adrenal and thyroid status is mandatory. Diabetes insipidus may also occur.

Cardiac Disease

Although the existence of a specific acromegaly-associated cardiac disorder (i.e., cardiomyopathy) is controversial, a careful cardiac evaluation is warranted because of the frequent occurrence of hypertension, left ventricular hypertrophy, and abnormalities in left ventricular function.

Respiratory Dysfunction

Respiratory problems are of particular concern in the perioperative treatment of acromegalic patients. Enlargement of

TABLE 12–1. Potential Disease Complications of Acromegaly

Deficiency	Management
Hypopituitarism	Thyroid hormone (hypothyroidism)
	Glucocorticoid coverage (adrenal insufficiency)
Diabetes mellitus	Measure serum glucose level; administer insulin
Diabetes insipidus	Measure serum electrolytes, intake and output; administer vasopressin
End-organ dysfunction	Cardiac evaluation
	Airway/respiratory tract evaluation

the tongue, soft tissue swelling, and growth in the upper airway may lead to difficulties with application of a face mask, assisted manual ventilation, airway obstruction, and tracheal intubation. Upper respiratory tract infections can exacerbate the obstruction, leading to the acute onset of dyspnea and inspiratory stridor.

Sleep apnea is also a common problem in acromegaly. Airway obstruction (macroglossia and inspiratory collapse of the hypopharynx) has been implicated in some cases, although the incidence of central sleep apnea is also increased. A history of snoring suggests that apnea is likely to be a problem postoperatively, particularly because the nose is occluded by the surgical dressing.

What Is Diabetes Insipidus?

Diabetes insipidus results from inadequate antidiuretic hormone (ADH, also known as *vasopressin*) secretion or action.[8-11] It is manifested by an inability to conserve water, resulting in polyuria and polydipsia. Polyuria is defined as urine volumes >30 mL $\cdot$ kg $\cdot$ d^{-1}; most patients become aware of symptoms when urine volumes exceed 3 to 4 L $\cdot$ d^{-1}. Serum hypertonicity may also be a feature. This condition is usually manifested as the laboratory finding of hypernatremia during blood chemistry testing. However, hypernatremia is not essential for the diagnosis. An alert patient with an intact thirst mechanism and ready access to water is able to compensate for the increased renal excretion of dilute urine by increased intake of fluid.

Classic

Classic diabetes insipidus, which is often referred to as *central* or *neurogenic* diabetes insipidus, is caused by inadequate secretion of ADH. Head trauma, CNS tumors (primary or metastatic), and neurosurgical procedures are among the most common causes. Other causes include infiltrative hypothalamic disorders such as sarcoidosis, histoplasmosis, Wegner's granulomatosis, and Langerhan's cell histiocytosis (histiocytosis X).

Postoperative/Post-Traumatic

Three patterns of postoperative or post-traumatic diabetes insipidus have been described. *Transient diabetes insipidus* accounts for 50% to 60% of cases of postsurgical diabetes insipidus. It usually occurs after transsphenoidal resection of pituitary adenomas and typically resolves in 3 to 5 days. *Permanent diabetes insipidus,* frequently noted after transfrontal resection of large masses with suprasellar extension, occurs in 30% to 40% of cases of postoperative diabetes insipidus. *Triphasic diabetes insipidus,* often occurring after complete pituitary stalk section, is the least common form. In this pattern, acute onset of diabetes insipidus is followed by an antidiuretic interval lasting 2 to 14 days. During this time, excessive fluid therapy and ADH administration are particularly treacherous because of the risk of inducing profound hyponatremia. Subsequently, permanent diabetes insipidus develops.

How Is Diabetes Insipidus Diagnosed?

The extent of evaluation (Table 12–2) required depends on the clinical setting. In a postoperative neurosurgical patient

TABLE 12–2. Diabetes Insipidus: Diagnosis and Management Strategies

Establish the diagnosis	Rule out osmotic diuresis
	Rule out excessive intravenous fluid administration
	Document hypotonic polyuria in clinical setting of hypernatremia/serum hypertonicity
Therapy	Monitor electrolytes, intake and output
	Ensure availability of water to alert patients
	Replace water loss with intravenous fluid replacement as needed; avoid saline solutions
	Cautious use of desamino-8-D-arginine vasopressin (DDAVP), 1–4 μg subcutaneously every 12 h

with an elevated serum sodium concentration and low urine osmolality (<200 mOsm $\cdot$ kg^{-1}), the diagnosis can be considered to be established, and a positive therapeutic response to ADH is confirmatory.

In situations not involving neurosurgery before the diagnosis is established, other causes of polyuria must be precluded.[12]

Osmotic Diuresis

The possibility of an osmotic diuresis should always be considered. This process can be triggered by pharmacologic solutes such as mannitol, which may be used to treat cerebral edema. Physiologic solutes such as glucose can also be responsible. Diabetes mellitus can be induced by the high doses of glucocorticoids used to treat neurosurgical patients, as can urea in postobstructive diuresis. The normal renal threshold for glucosuria is approximately 180 mg $\cdot$ dL^{-1}.

Excessive Fluid Administration

Administration of large volumes of intravenous fluid in the operative and postoperative period may also lead to large urine volumes, which can be incorrectly diagnosed as diabetes insipidus. Recovery from or mobilization of intraoperative fluid administration should be considered in polyuric postoperative patients with a normal or low serum sodium level. A decrease in urine volume, increase in urine concentration, and maintenance of a normal serum sodium value after a decrease in the rate of fluid infusion confirm the diagnosis of iatrogenic volume overload. Continued excretion of large volumes of dilute urine, as the serum sodium rises above normal, establishes the diagnosis of diabetes insipidus.

Dehydration Test/Response to Vasopressin

In nonsurgical patients who have normal electrolytes and in whom the diagnosis of diabetes insipidus is considered, a more formalized evaluation may include a dehydration test aimed at producing hypertonicity of the serum, followed by assessment of a patient's response to ADH administration. This approach is aimed at establishing the diagnosis of diabetes insipidus, differentiating diabetes insipidus from other causes of hypotonic polyuria such as "psychogenic water drinking," and distinguishing between central diabetes insipidus (ADH deficiency) and nephrogenic diabetes insipidus (ADH resistance).

Diagnostic criteria[12] are not always clear-cut because of difficulties in interpreting the results. Consultation with an endocrinologist or nephrologist is advised if such testing is believed to be warranted. It should be emphasized that the dehydration test is *unnecessary* and *dangerous* in patients who are already hypertonic or hypovolemic.

How is Diabetes Insipidus Treated?

Fluids

Appropriate fluid replacement is the cornerstone of diabetes insipidus therapy (see Table 12–2). Alert patients with an intact thirst mechanism can usually maintain appropriate volume intake if given free access to water. Treatment is more difficult in patients with decreased mental status or impaired recognition of thirst. Intravenous fluid replacement is essential in such cases, with careful and frequent monitoring of body weight, serum electrolytes, and fluid intake and output. Fluid replacement should be almost exclusively in the form of dextrose-containing water solutions. The primary fluid lost is free water, and infusion of saline solutions, perhaps the most common error made in diabetes insipidus management, leads to a continuing solute load that increases renal water loss.

Antidiuretic Agents

Antidiuretic agents (ADH or its analogues) should be used only when the diagnosis of diabetes insipidus is firmly established. Risks of excessive or inappropriate therapy include hyponatremia with cerebral edema, confusion, seizures, or coma. Desamino-8-D-arginine vasopressin (DDAVP) is the preferred agent because of its rapid onset of action (within 1 h), reasonable duration of action (6–24 h), and absence of clinical pressor effects.[8, 9, 13, 14] DDAVP administered subcutaneously at doses of 1 to 4 μg every 12 hours usually controls diabetes insipidus adequately; "breakthrough" polyuria may occur at the lower dose limit, and hyponatremia can occur at the higher dose limit. This drug may also be administered intravenously or intranasally.

Anterior Pituitary Dysfunction

The possibility of anterior pituitary dysfunction should always be considered in patients with postoperative diabetes insipidus. Corticosteroid supplementation should be provided until anterior pituitary function can be formally assessed. Acute problems with hypothyroidism are less likely because of the long half-life (1 wk) of thyroxine. However, hypothyroidism should be ruled out in these patients.

What Is the Syndrome of Inappropriate Antidiuretic Hormone Secretion?

The syndrome of inappropriate antidiuretic hormone (SIADH) secretion is initially suggested by the finding of a low serum sodium level (<130 mEq $\cdot$ L^{-1}). Hyponatremia is a common laboratory disorder in hospitalized patients, and SIADH represents only one of several different causes.[15–18]

How Is the Syndrome of Inappropriate Antidiuretic Hormone Secretion Diagnosed?

Factitious Hyponatremia

Evaluation of hyponatremic patients (Table 12–3) should begin by ruling out factitious hyponatremia. In patients with

TABLE 12–3. Syndrome of Inappropriate Secretion of Antidiuretic Hormone: Diagnosis and Management Strategies

Establish the diagnosis	Rule out "factitious" hyponatremia Rule out hypervolemia or hypovolemia Rule out hypothyroidism or cortisol deficiency Confirm the diagnosis by documenting low serum osmolality with inappropriate elevations of urine Na⁺ and urine osmolality
Seek an underlying disorder	Infection, malignancy, drug, surgery
Therapy	Treat the underlying disease Free water restriction Loop diuretic Monitor fluid and electrolyte balance Demeclocycline for chronic, refractory syndrome of inappropriate secretion of antidiuretic hormone Aggressive normal saline or hypertonic saline *only* when hyponatremia is of acute onset and associated with neurologic impairment (*risk:* central pontine myelinolysis with overly rapid correction of chronic hyponatremia in asymptomatic patient)

substantial elevations of plasma proteins (e.g., multiple myeloma or Waldenstrom's macroglobulinemia) or lipids (e.g., hypertriglyceridemia), the sodium-containing serum water is displaced by protein or lipid, leading to an artifactual underestimation of sodium level. A low serum sodium value can also occur with any osmotically induced shift of water into the intravascular space (e.g., mannitol administration or hyperglycemia).

Factitious hyponatremia should be suspected when a normal serum osmolality is found in the setting of a low serum sodium value. Some patients may develop hyperosmolar hyponatremia as a result of the presence of a circulating nonsodium solute such as glucose, mannitol, or ethyl alcohol. Patients with a nonsodium, nonglucose solute have an osmolar gap (i.e., the difference between measured and calculated osmolality exceeds 10). The measured osmolality can be determined by the clinical laboratory, and calculated osmolality is derived from the following formula:

$$\text{Osmolality (mOsm} \cdot \text{kg}^{-1}) = 2 \times [\text{Na}^+] + [\text{glucose}]/18 + [\text{BUN}]/2.4$$

Volume Status

Clinical assessment of a patient's volume status is a major component of the evaluation of hyponatremia.

Hypervolemia

Hyponatremia can occur in patients with *hypervolemia* (e.g., congestive heart failure, cirrhosis, nephrotic syndrome). The ineffective circulating volume caused by the underlying disorder leads to aldosterone-mediated sodium retention and ADH-mediated water retention. These patients frequently have edema and other clinical features of volume excess. In the absence of renal disease, they have hyponatremia with concentrated urine (due to ADH) and low urine sodium concentration (secondary to elevated aldosterone). Therapy includes restriction of sodium and fluid intake, in addition to treatment specifically targeted at the underlying disease (i.e., improving cardiac output).

Hypovolemia

Hyponatremia can also occur concomitantly with *hypovolemia,* which may be caused by gastrointestinal fluid loss, renal dysfunction, diuretics, or aldosterone deficiency. Similar to the situation in hypervolemic patients, hyponatremia in hypovolemic patients is secondary to water retention, which is stimulated by increased ADH secretion that is triggered by volume depletion. Hypovolemic patients may have orthostatic hypotension, dry mucous membranes, poor skin turgor, and laboratory features of prerenal azotemia. Fluid and sodium administration is a major component of the therapy of volume-contracted hyponatremic patients. Other patients with hyponatremia appear to have normal volume status. SIADH is the chief consideration in euvolemic hyponatremia.

Laboratory Studies

Helpful laboratory studies include measurements of blood urea nitrogen (BUN) and uric acid, which are usually decreased in patients with SIADH (when glomerular filtration is preserved) and elevated in patients whose hyponatremia is due to other causes. In addition, urinary sodium level is frequently increased in SIADH because of increased ADH and suppressed aldosterone, whereas decreased levels of urinary sodium are encountered in both hypervolemic and hypovolemic hyponatremia. This finding reflects the action of the increased aldosterone secretion on renal sodium conservation in these settings.[19] Urinary sodium measurement is not a foolproof diagnostic test. Levels may be increased in patients who are volume depleted because of diuretics, salt-wasting nephropathies, and aldosterone deficiency. Patients with SIADH may have low urinary sodium levels if salt and water intake have been restricted. In patients with euvolemic hyponatremia, measurement of urine osmolality is the most reliable diagnostic test. A value >200 mOsm $\cdot$ kg⁻¹ in a euvolemic, hyponatremic patient is highly suggestive of SIADH.

What Are the Causes of the Syndrome of Inappropriate Antidiuretic Hormone Secretion?

When the diagnosis of SIADH has been made, identification of the underlying cause is necessary. SIADH can be a manifestation of pain, nausea, malignancy, CNS pathology, pulmonary disease, or drug effect. Consultation with an endocrinologist or nephrologist should be considered if the cause is not apparent. Particularly important is ruling out hypothyroidism or cortisol deficiency in euvolemic hyponatremic patients who fulfill the criteria for SIADH but have no obvious underlying cause. These diagnoses are usually missed unless they are specifically sought.

How Is the Syndrome of Inappropriate Secretion of Antidiuretic Hormone Managed?

Treatment of SIADH must be individualized (see Table 12–3).[15–22] Therapy of the underlying disorder (e.g., drainage of a subdural hematoma or antibiotics for pulmonary tuberculosis) is obviously important. The specifics of fluid and electrolyte management are more controversial, because severe complications can ensue from either aggressive or excessively conservative therapy of hyponatremia.[20, 21]

The rate of development of hyponatremia (acute versus chronic) and the presence or absence of neurologic symptoms are more important than the absolute sodium concentration. Acute development of hyponatremia over an interval of 2 to 3 days, with a decline in sodium of 0.5 mEq · L · h^{-1} or faster, is frequently associated with neurologic symptoms. Therapy consists of normal or hypertonic (3%) saline combined with furosemide aimed at increasing serum sodium by approximately 1 mEq · L · h^{-1}. Furosemide is usually added to the saline to diminish the ability of the renal tubules to produce free water.

If the hyponatremia is chronic and the patient has few symptoms, aggressive sodium replacement can lead to central pontine myelinolysis with permanent neurologic impairment or death. The sodium in these patients should be corrected more slowly, at approximately 0.5 mEq · L · h^{-1} (12 mEq · L · d^{-1}).

Hypertonic Saline

Hypertonic saline should be given slowly (0.1 mL · kg^{-1} · min^{-1}) until the sodium is at a "safe" asymptomatic level (usually 120–125 mEq · L^{-1}).

Fluid Restriction

In patients who have SIADH and in whom aggressive correction is not necessary, restriction of free water to 500 to 800 mL · d^{-1} should lead to gradual improvement of hyponatremia.

Demeclocycline

For those who have chronic SIADH and in whom the underlying disease, such as with some malignancies, is refractory to therapy, therapy with demeclocycline (600–1200 mg daily in divided doses) causes nephrogenic diabetes insipidus and counteracts the effect of the high ADH levels.[22]

ADRENAL DISEASE

The adrenal glands are composed of the adrenal cortex and adrenal medulla. The cortex contains the zona glomerulosa (aldosterone synthesis), zona fasciculata (glucocorticoid synthesis), and zona reticularis (androgen and glucocorticoid synthesis). Glucocorticoid synthesis is regulated via the hypothalamic-pituitary-adrenal (HPA) axis. Corticotropin-releasing hormone (CRH) secreted by the hypothalamus stimulates the secretion of adrenocorticotropic hormone (ACTH) from the pituitary, in turn increasing cortisol production by the adrenal cortex. Cortisol feedback inhibits CRH and ACTH synthesis in a negative-feedback fashion. Mineralocorticoid production is regulated primarily by the renin-angiotensin system, extracellular potassium level, and blood pressure.

What Are the Effects of Corticosteroids?

Glucocorticoids affect global cellular metabolism. They are essential for energy production; for glucose, protein, and fat metabolism; for immune and cardiovascular function; for

membrane integrity; and for many other activities. Mineralocorticoids regulate sodium, potassium, and hydrogen balance. In the kidneys, aldosterone stimulates sodium reabsorption, kaliuresis, and hydrogen ion secretion.

What Is Cushing's Syndrome?

Excess circulating levels of glucocorticoids result in Cushing's syndrome. This syndrome may result from exogenous use of glucocorticoids, excess hypothalamic production of CRH, excess production of ACTH by the pituitary (e.g., pituitary adenoma) or "ectopic" tissue, or excess production of glucocorticoids by hyperplastic or adenomatous adrenal glands.[23–26]

What Is Addison's Disease?

A deficiency of glucocorticoid production results in adrenal insufficiency, or Addison's disease.[27–37] Adrenal insufficiency[27–37] may result from adrenal gland failure (i.e., primary adrenal insufficiency) or failure of hypothalamic-pituitary secretion of CRH or ACTH (i.e., secondary adrenal insufficiency).

Primary Adrenal Failure

Primary glandular failure may occur secondary to infection (e.g., human immunodeficiency virus [HIV], cytomegalovirus [CMV], tuberculosis, fungi, meningococcemia, *Pseudomonas* septicemia); tumor destruction; hemorrhagic necrosis (i.e., stressed patients receiving anticoagulants; disseminated intravascular coagulopathy); autoimmunity; or drugs that block adrenal steroid synthesis (i.e., ketoconazole, etomidate, aminoglutethimide). Primary adrenal insufficiency usually results in loss of both glucocorticoid and mineralocorticoid secretion.

Secondary Adrenal Failure

Secondary adrenal insufficiency may occur as a result of acute withdrawal of exogenous glucocorticoids; HIV infection; pituitary or hypothalamic tumors; and pituitary necrosis, hemorrhage, infarction, trauma, or pituitary removal. These patients maintain normal secretion of mineralocorticoids. When patients with adrenal disorders are evaluated, the specific cause must be determined and appropriate therapy for the underlying disease instituted.

How Is Cushing's Syndrome Managed Preoperatively?

A high index of suspicion is required for the diagnosis of adrenal disorders. Cushing's syndrome should be suspected when clinical features are consistent with excess glucocorticoid effects (Table 12–4). Untreated Cushing's syndrome results in higher perioperative morbidity and mortality. Patients lose protein mass. Wound healing, immune function, muscle strength, and the response to stress are impaired. Bone loss is common and predisposes to fractures. Many patients develop hypertension and hyperglycemia.

TABLE 12–4. Clinical Features of Adrenal Dysfunction

Excess Glucocorticoids (Cushing's)	Adrenal Insufficiency (Addison's)
Central obesity	Glucocorticoid deficiency
Weakness/proximal myopathy	Weight loss
Muscle atrophy	Hypoglycemia
Hypertension	Asthenia, fatigue
Skin changes	Impaired cardiac contractility
Thin skin/bruising	Hypotension
Acne, greasy skin	Diminished plasma volume
Hirsutism	Syncope
Plethora	Vomiting, nausea
Abdominal striae	Impaired gut absorption
Infection (e.g., tinea)	Diarrhea
Pigmentation	Hyponatremia, syndrome of inappropriate secretion of
Impaired wound healing	antidiuretic hormone
Psychiatric changes (e.g., psychosis)	Myalgia, arthralgia
Pseudotumor cerebri	Amelioration of diabetes insipidus
Oligo/amenorrhea	Muscle weakness
Impotence	Anemia
Osteoporosis	Eosinophilia
Aseptic necrosis of bone	Neutropenia
Pathologic fracture	Hypercalcemia
Thirst, polyuria	Mental slowing
Glucose intolerance/hyperglycemia	Electrocardiogram: Low voltage, ST and T wave flattening
Peripheral edema	Diminished glomerular filtration rate and renal plasma flow
Renal calculi	Hyperprolactinemia
Exophthalmos	Skin pigmentation
Headache	Mineralocorticoid deficiency
Abdominal pain	Renal salt wasting
Peptic ulcers	Hypotension, volume depletion
Pancreatitis	Hyperkalemia
Impaired immune function	Metabolic acidosis
Hypokalemic alkalosis	Impaired cardiac contractility
Glaucoma, cataracts	Decreased pressor response to norepinephrine

Diagnosis

Cushing's syndrome is diagnosed by the demonstration of sustained and excessive secretion of cortisol and the lack of response to normal physiologic manipulations.[23–26] Patients with Cushing's syndrome have increased cortisol levels, nonsuppression of cortisol levels with dexamethasone, and loss of circadian variation of cortisol and ACTH, and they fail to increase cortisol in response to hypoglycemia. Patients with endogenous depression may demonstrate increased cortisol levels, nonsuppression with dexamethasone, and loss of circadian variation of cortisol and ACTH. However, these patients demonstrate a plasma cortisol response to hypoglycemia.

The differential diagnosis of Cushing's syndrome depends on the presence or absence of circulating ACTH and differentiating between ACTH-dependent and ACTH-independent hypersecretion of cortisol. ACTH dependence is demonstrated by showing measurable circulating ACTH at a time when a patient is hypercortisolemic.

Corticotropin-Releasing Hormone

The CRH test is useful in the differential diagnosis of Cushing's syndrome.[38] It can distinguish most cases of ACTH-dependent Cushing's syndrome (ACTH-secreting pituitary adenomas and ectopic ACTH-secreting tumors) from ACTH-independent forms of the disease (adrenal adenoma, adrenal carcinoma, exogenous glucocorticoids). In the presence of documented Cushing's syndrome, undetectable plasma ACTH is also suggestive of an adrenal tumor. Adrenal CT scan can confirm the diagnosis and localize the lesion, and it frequently distinguishes adenoma from carcinoma.

Pituitary Versus Ectopic Adrenocorticotropic Hormone Production

The differentiation of pituitary versus ectopic ACTH production as the cause of Cushing's syndrome is more difficult, particularly if the ectopic source is small. Patients with ectopic ACTH production, such as due to carcinoids or malignant tumors, are frequently hypokalemic and have an associated alkalosis.[25] Most patients with Cushing's disease (pituitary ACTH) show suppression of urinary hydroxycorticosteroids, plasma cortisol, and ACTH after high-dose dexamethasone administration (2 mg orally every 6 h for 48 h). The test is not specific, however; 10% to 15% of patients with ectopic ACTH may also show suppression, and 10% to 20% of patients with Cushing's disease may not.

The CRH test also may be useful to differentiate pituitary from ectopic ACTH production. Most patients with pituitary ACTH secretion demonstrate an increase in ACTH after CRH administration, whereas most patients with ectopic ACTH secretion fail to respond.[38] The positive predictive value of the test is 90%, but the predictive value of a negative test (i.e., failure to respond to CRH) is only 63%. Techniques for localizing tissue producing ACTH include venous sampling and CT scanning.

Treatment

Appropriate treatment for Cushing's syndrome depends on the specific diagnosis. Cushing's disease, with a pituitary source of ACTH, is usually treated surgically. Most patients can have their tumors removed by transsphenoidal surgery. Pituitary irradiation may also be effective in controlling the disease. Patients who fail to respond to these therapies respond to bilateral adrenalectomy.

Medical

Medical therapy may occasionally be necessary to lower serum cortisol levels if, for example, a patient suffers from cortisol-induced psychosis or harbors a cortisol-producing malignancy. Metyrapone (an inhibitor of cortisol synthesis), mitotane (o,p'-DDD, an adrenolytic drug), aminoglutethimide, ketoconazole, bromocriptine, and cyproheptadine (an antiserotoninergic agent) have demonstrated clinical efficacy.

Surgical

Ectopic Vasopressin Secretion. The key to the treatment of ectopic ACTH secretion is finding the source of the ACTH. Most ectopic ACTH-secreting tumors are found in the chest. Other tumors secreting ACTH include medullary carcinoma of the thyroid, islet cell tumors, and pheochromocytomas. Surgical resection is the treatment of choice. If surgical cure is impossible, medical adrenalectomy (ketoconazole) is indicated.

Adrenal Tumors. Adrenal carcinoma and adenomas are treated by surgical ablation. Adrenal carcinomas are inefficient producers of hydrocortisone and are usually large at the time of diagnosis. The adrenolytic agent o,p'-DDD is used when surgery fails to control the disease. The drug dose is increased to toxicity (i.e., neurologic side effects including ataxic gait, nausea, diarrhea). If time permits, patients should undergo pituitary testing to assess the adequacy of other hormonal systems (i.e., thyroid).

How Is Addison's Disease Managed Preoperatively?

Adrenal insufficiency should be suspected after glucocorticoid use. It should also be considered in patients with acquired immunodeficiency, CMV infection, tuberculosis, fungal infection, and meningococcemia and in those receiving drugs that interfere with glucocorticoid synthesis. Many of the effects of glucocorticoid deficiency are nonspecific (see Table 12–4), and the diagnosis can easily be overlooked.

Adrenal insufficiency should be considered in patients with circulatory collapse, hypoglycemia, hyponatremia, weight loss, nausea and vomiting, dehydration, hypothyroidism, and hyperpigmentation. At times, however, only a vague history of malaise, low-grade fever, nausea, arthralgias, or other nonspecific complaints may be elicited. In humans, sudden complete glucocorticoid deficiency can be fatal in 7 to 10 days. Mineralocorticoid deficiency may result in salt-losing nephropathy, hyperkalemia, hyponatremia, and metabolic acidosis. These disturbances should raise the question of adrenal insufficiency.

Diagnosis

In most situations, a single measurement of plasma cortisol does not permit a reliable appraisal of pituitary-adrenal function. Thus, provocative tests are usually required to identify patients with inadequate adrenal cortisol production.

Cortisol Response

Adrenal insufficiency is best diagnosed by demonstrating an impaired serum cortisol response to induced stress (i.e., insulin-induced hypoglycemia) or metyrapone (suppresses cortisol feedback).[28] A normal response to symptomatic hypoglycemia (i.e., glucose <35 mg $\cdot$ dL^{-1}) is a peak plasma cortisol level >20 μg $\cdot$ dL^{-1} (60–90 min after insulin). Administration of glucose after induced hypoglycemia does not alter the cortisol response.

Metyrapone Test

The metyrapone test may be extremely dangerous in patients with adrenal insufficiency because it inhibits cortisol synthesis. It is best reserved for evaluating the cause of Cushing's syndrome. The response to stress assesses the integrity of the entire CNS-HPA axis.

Adrenocorticotropic Hormone Stimulation

The short ACTH stimulation (i.e., Cortrosyn) test assesses the integrity of the adrenal glands.[28, 31] A plasma cortisol level ≥20 μg $\cdot$ dL^{-1} 30 to 60 minutes after ACTH (250 μg) administration is a normal response. Severe endogenous ACTH deficiency results in adrenal atrophy and an impaired response to exogenous ACTH. On the other hand, patients who secrete small amounts of endogenous ACTH may respond normally to exogenous ACTH. Secretion of ACTH may be inadequate in stimulating adrenal cortisol production under stress. This phenomenon has been described in patients with pituitary tumors.

Dynamic Pituitary Testing

Because basal ACTH and cortisol measurements often do not discriminate between patients with mild secondary adrenal insufficiency and normal individuals, we recommend dynamic pituitary testing (i.e., insulin tolerance tests). The CRH stimulation test has also been shown to be reliable for predicting the cortisol response to stress in patients with primary and secondary adrenal insufficiency.[33, 34] If urgent therapy is required, dexamethasone can be given while the short ACTH or CRH test is being performed. Dexamethasone immediately suppresses the HPA axis and does not significantly affect the measurement of plasma cortisol.

Serum Cortisol Determination

If a patient is already stressed (i.e., severe pain, hypotension, postsurgery, hypoglycemia, sepsis), serum cortisol testing alone is sufficient to rule out adrenal insufficiency. A level >20 μg $\cdot$ dL^{-1} after stress, ACTH, or CRH indicates adequate adrenal glucocorticoid secretion. If cortisol insufficiency is confirmed, investigation is required to determine the exact cause and the possibility of associated endocrine abnormalities. Inappropriately elevated ACTH levels with a simultaneous low plasma cortisol level suggest primary adrenal insufficiency.[31] Failure of the adrenal glands to respond to prolonged ACTH stimulation also suggests primary glandular failure.

Renin and Aldosterone Levels

Measurement of plasma renin (PRA) and aldosterone (ALDO) levels is helpful in separating primary from secondary adrenal insufficiency. PRA/ALDO ratios are high in primary adrenal insufficiency and low in secondary adrenal insufficiency.[31]

Diagnostic Imaging

Diagnostic imaging may be helpful in determining the cause of adrenal gland failure. Bilaterally enlarged adrenal glands demonstrated by CT scan suggest adrenal hemorrhage, neoplastic disease, fungal infection, or tuberculosis. Small adrenal glands suggest atrophy due to autoimmune disease or lack of ACTH.

Individual Susceptibility to Suppression by Steroids

Individual susceptibility to HPA axis suppression by steroids is variable. Anatomic evidence of a steroid effect on the hypothalamus, anterior pituitary, and adrenal cortex appears within 5 days of steroid initiation. Patients receiving supraphysiologic doses of corticosteroids (i.e., hydrocortisone >20 to 30 mg $\cdot$ d^{-1}) for longer than 3 to 4 weeks should be considered to have clinically significant adrenal insufficiency. Those who receive 12.5 mg or more of prednisone per day for 1 month to 8 years show HPA suppression.[32] On the other hand, those receiving 4 mg or less per day do not. Variable responses are found in the dose range of 4 to 12.5 mg of prednisone per day. Withdrawal of exogenous steroids may leave patients with adrenal insufficiency.[32]

Short-acting steroids produce less HPA axis suppression than long-acting steroids, and single daily or every-other-day doses produces less suppression than multiple daily doses (Table 12–5). Once suppressed, the HPA axis can take as long as a year to recover.[39, 40]

The long-held belief that large daily doses of corticosteroids and prolonged treatment dependably predict HPA axis suppression has been questioned. Schlaghecke and colleagues[33] evaluated the response to CRH and hypoglycemia in patients treated with glucocorticoids. A poor correlation was found between the cortisol response to CRH and dose or duration of therapy. Of the 279 patients receiving glucocorticoid therapy, 103 had normal responses to CRH, 133 had blunted responses, and 43 had no response. Basal plasma cortisol values were poor indicators of HPA function in these patients.

TABLE 12–5. Adrenal Replacement Therapy

Agent	Daily Dose (mg)	Mineralo-corticoid Potency	Gluco-corticoid Potency	Duration of Action (h)
Dexamethasone	0.75	0	25	72
Methylprednisolone	4.0	0.5	5	36
Prednisolone	5.0	0.8	4	24
Prednisone	5.0	0.8	4	24
Cortisol	20.0	1.0	1.0	8
Hydrocortisone	25.0	1.0	1.0	8
Cortisone	25.0	1.0	0.8	8
Fludrocortisone	0.1	125	10	20

Response to Stress

How test results of HPA axis function correlate with cardiovascular and other responses to acute stress remains unclear.[34] Some patients with normal findings on HPA axis function tests may not withstand stress without corticosteroid supplementation.[35] On the other hand, those with blunted HPA axis function tolerate stress without difficulty. Jasani and colleagues compared plasma cortisol concentrations after four provocative tests (i.e., corticotropin, ADH, metyrapone, and insulin-induced hypoglycemia) with concentrations during surgery (synovectomy) in corticosteroid-treated patients.[36] The response to corticotropin correlated best with levels during surgery. However, many patients lacking an increase in plasma cortisol levels during surgery fared well. Intuitively, this makes sense because the goal of many anesthetic techniques is just that—namely, to block the stress response to surgery. These investigators concluded that hypotension during surgery in patients with relative hypoadrenalism is the exception rather than the rule.

Kehlet and Binder studied corticosteroid-treated patients undergoing surgery without steroid supplementation.[37] Hypotension was observed in 18 of 74 patients undergoing major surgery and responded to volume infusion. In 11 of these, the reduction in blood pressure was caused by bleeding, infection, or an anaphylactic response. Adrenocortical function was normal in eight and slightly impaired in three patients. That hypotension was caused by adrenocortical insufficiency seemed unlikely because it reversed without glucocorticoid administration. Hypotension occurred in some patients with appropriate plasma cortisol values, whereas other patients with suppressed adrenal function fared well. Which patients will develop clinical adrenal insufficiency is difficult to predict, and we are not sure which tests of adrenal function best predict a patient's clinical response to stress. Indeed, factors other than HPA axis adequacy are involved in the stress response.

Conclusions

Based on the available data, a number of conclusions appear justified: (1) Plasma cortisol alone is an insufficient index of HPA function (except under severe stress). (2) Provocative tests are a better measure of HPA axis adequacy. (3) Insulin-induced hypoglycemia and the CRH test appear best to assess the response of the HPA axis to acute stress. (4) The response to provocative testing of the HPA axis may not correlate with a patient's response to severe illness or surgery. (5) Short-term corticosteroid therapy is safe and may prevent steroid withdrawal syndromes. Thus, when a question of adrenal insufficiency arises during an emergency, we advocate short-term supplemental corticosteroids until adrenal integrity can be assessed.

How Is Addison's Disease Treated Preoperatively?

Mineralocorticoid deficiency is treated with fluid and electrolyte administration (i.e., high sodium, low potassium). The abnormalities can frequently be corrected without the addition of exogenous mineralocorticoids. Fludrocortisone may occasionally be required.

Glucocorticoid deficiency impairs the function of all cells and is best treated with glucocorticoid replacement. Normal adult replacement doses are 20 to 30 mg of hydrocortisone equivalent per day (see Table 12–5). Two thirds is usually given in the morning and one third in the evening to approximate normal diurnal variation. Higher doses are required during stress (see How Is Addison's Disease Managed Perioperatively, later).

How Is Cushing's Syndrome Managed Perioperatively?

Corticosteroid Supplementation

Patients undergoing removal of their pituitary gland or adrenal glands for treatment of Cushing's syndrome should be considered to have postoperative adrenal insufficiency. Preoperative hypercortisolemia suppresses ACTH secretion from nontumorous pituitary tissue. We recommend "stress" doses (discussed later) of glucocorticoids in the immediate postoperative period (i.e., 24–48 h). If patients are stable, exogenous glucocorticoids should be slowly tapered until maintenance doses are reached. Remember that these patients are accustomed to high circulating levels of cortisol.

A glucocorticoid withdrawal syndrome may develop if exogenous glucocorticoids are tapered rapidly. We prefer to administer hydrocortisone to these patients. At high doses (i.e., $>150 \text{ mg} \cdot \text{d}^{-1}$) hydrocortisone possesses adequate glucocorticoid and mineralocorticoid activity. However, as the dose approaches maintenance levels (i.e., $20–30 \text{ mg} \cdot \text{d}^{-1}$), addition of a mineralocorticoid may be necessary. Mineralocorticoid replacement is required if hyperkalemia, salt loss, or hypotension (especially orthostatic) becomes problematic.

Other Hormonal Systems

After pituitary surgery, diabetes insipidus is common in the immediate postoperative period and may require treatment with DDAVP. Suppression of TSH, gonadotropin, and growth hormone secretion may also occur. Failure of recovery may indicate thyroid hormone deficiency.

How Is Addison's Disease Managed Perioperatively?

Adrenal insufficiency is managed with glucocorticoid/mineralocorticoid replacement (see Table 12–5). Traditionally, patients undergoing stress (i.e., surgery, sepsis, shock) have received large doses of glucocorticoids (for "stress coverage"). However, the requisite quantity of exogenous glucocorticoid during stress has never been adequately studied. Many patients with adrenal insufficiency following pituitary surgery or after withdrawal of exogenous glucocorticoids tolerate stress well and do not require glucocorticoid therapy. One strategy of caring for these patients is to wait and watch. If they demonstrate features of adrenal insufficiency such as cardiovascular instability, only then is treatment initiated. This approach is beneficial when high-dose glucocorticoids may be harmful (i.e., impaired wound healing after lung transplant).

Minor Illnesses/Surgery

For minor surgical procedures, no extra steroid is needed in patients with adrenal insufficiency. The same is true of minor illnesses such as viral gastroenteritis, influenza, and pharyngitis. For these minor illnesses, it is important that patients continue their steroid dose, not stop it.

Major Stress

For major stress (i.e., major surgery, trauma, major illness), however, we prefer to treat with exogenous glucocorticoids. Patients who have received prolonged therapy with supraphysiologic doses of glucocorticoids and who have been withdrawn from these regimens are assumed to be at risk of adrenal insufficiency for 1 year after withdrawal. High-dose glucocorticoids are usually well tolerated by most patients for short durations.

Patients under severe stress rarely secrete $>200 \text{ mg} \cdot \text{d}^{-1}$ of cortisol. Thus, stress doses of glucocorticoids consist of 200 to 300 mg of cortisol equivalent per day (i.e., hydrocortisone, 100 mg intravenously every 8 h). Dosage frequency is dictated by the half-life of the drug administered (see Table 12–5). We prefer to administer glucocorticoid by the intravenous route in the immediate postoperative period. High-dose glucocorticoids are tapered to maintenance levels (i.e., 20–30 mg of hydrocortisone per day) over 5 to 7 days, provided a patient continues to improve.

Mineralocorticoids

In patients with primary adrenal insufficiency, mineralocorticoids are usually unnecessary when large doses of glucocorticoids are administered (i.e., $>150 \text{ mg}$ of hydrocortisone per day). However, as the dose is lowered, mineralocorticoid therapy may become necessary to control salt loss and hyperkalemia. Intravenous saline should also be administered, because patients usually suffer from intravascular volume depletion. Blood glucose levels should be monitored and treated accordingly.

Preoperative Evaluation

Preoperative evaluation includes an assessment of hydration, metabolic status (i.e., serum levels of sodium, potassium, glucose, calcium, urea nitrogen, creatinine; blood cell counts; acid-base status), cardiovascular function (blood pressure, heart rate) and fluid balance. Postural changes in blood pressure and heart rate can help to evaluate the adequacy of intravascular volume.

On the day of surgery, patients are given hydrocortisone, 100 mg intravenously before surgery and every 8 hours after surgery. Intraoperatively, the anesthesiologist should periodically monitor electrolyte and glucose levels. Stress doses of steroids are continued postoperatively until recovery is under way and then tapered back to maintenance levels.

What Are the Perioperative Complications in Cushing's Syndrome?

Complications in patients with Cushing's syndrome primarily result from the long-term effects of elevated circulating cortisol levels. These include poor skin integrity, impaired wound healing, diminished protein reserves, impaired muscle function, decreased immunity, and diminished bone mass.

After pituitary or adrenal surgery, complications may occur

as a result of adrenal insufficiency. After pituitary surgery, patients may also develop features of other endocrine deficiency states (i.e., hypothyroidism, diabetes insipidus), leak of CSF, injury to the carotid artery or cranial nerves (i.e., II, IV, VI), local hemorrhage, or meningitis.

Long-standing complications related to hypertension, including hypertensive cardiomyopathy or hyperglycemia (i.e., cardiac, renal, vascular disease), can be problematic. After total adrenalectomy, pituitary macroadenomas associated with very high ACTH levels and skin pigmentation (Nelson's syndrome) can occur.

What Are the Perioperative Complications in Addison's Disease?

Complications of adrenal insufficiency result from under- or over-replacement of glucocorticoids and mineralocorticoids. Inadequate replacement of glucocorticoids can impair the response to stress and may manifest as cardiovascular insufficiency. However, the most common manifestations of adrenal insufficiency are weakness, lassitude, fatigue, mental depression, and hypotension. Inadequate replacement of mineralocorticoids can result in hyperkalemia, salt-losing nephropathy, hyponatremia, dehydration, hypoperfusion, and hypotension.

Excess Corticosteroid Replacement

Excess glucocorticoid replacement is generally benign for short periods. Long periods of supraphysiologic glucocorticoid therapy result in iatrogenic Cushing's syndrome (see Table 12–4).[40] Excess mineralocorticoid replacement may result in salt retention, weight gain, peripheral and pulmonary edema, congestive heart failure, and hypertension.

Steroids should be tapered or discontinued as soon as possible to minimize complications. They can be abruptly discontinued or tapered to maintenance doses if treatment has been limited to <6 days. The activity of the precipitating condition dictates the rate of tapering. Gradual withdrawal may be required to avoid recurrent disease.

Hypothyroidism slows the metabolic clearance of cortisol, and thyroxine may consume the small amount of residual cortisol in patients with adrenal insufficiency. Thyroxine should not be given to patients with adrenal insufficiency until glucocorticoid replacement is initiated. Sudden restoration of free water clearance with glucocorticoids can unmask diabetes insipidus and result in dehydration and hypernatremia. These patients respond well to DDAVP therapy. Glucocorticoid replacement can also unmask diabetes mellitus or increase insulin requirements.

Corticosteroid Interactions with Other Agents

Barbiturates, phenytoin, and rifampin reduce the effectiveness of corticosteroids by inducing hepatic microsomal enzymes. Raising the dose of steroid may be necessary. Estrogens enhance the anti-inflammatory and gluconeogenic actions of glucocorticoids by delaying their inactivation. Corticosteroids blunt the action of antidiabetic drugs. They augment diuretic-induced potassium loss and act synergistically with nonsteroidal anti-inflammatory agents in causing gastric ulceration.

Corticosteroid Metabolism

Corticosteroid metabolism is slowed with advanced age. Although children metabolize corticosteroids similarly to adults, these agents markedly inhibit growth. The liver is the principal site of corticosteroid metabolism, and diseases of the liver (e.g., cirrhosis, hepatitis) impair metabolism of glucocorticoids. Prednisolone may be preferable to prednisone in patients with major liver disease owing to defective inactivation of prednisone.

Alternate-day steroids spare the HPA axis from glucocorticoid suppression and can reduce the complications of hypercortisolism. A short-acting corticosteroid is preferred because the long-acting agents do not allow for a period of nonexposure.

What Is Pheochromocytoma?

Pheochromocytomas are adrenomedullary tumors that secrete dopamine, epinephrine, or norepinephrine.[41–47] Nonadrenal tumors arising from the sympathetic nervous system are designated extra-adrenal pheochromocytomas or functioning paragangliomas. The most common locations are within the abdomen (i.e., Zuckerkandl's organ, aortic bifurcation, bladder wall), chest, and neck (i.e., carotid and glomus jugulare bodies). Although rare, occurring in 1 to 2 per 100,000 adults, pheochromocytomas can occur in patients of any age.

Clinical Features

The clinical features of these tumors result from the catecholamines that they secrete. $Alpha_1$-adrenergic receptor activation causes vasoconstriction; α_2-adrenergic activation decreases insulin secretion; β_1-adrenergic activation results in cardiac inotropy and chronotropy; β_2-adrenergic activation causes vasodilation and bronchodilation; and dopamine-1 receptor activation results in renal and mesenteric vasodilation.

Most patients present with hypertension (0.1–0.5% of hypertensives), headache, pallor, diaphoresis, anxiety, palpitations, tachycardia, angina, hyperglycemia, and weight loss. Hypertension may be paroxysmal or persistent. A pressor response to histamine, glucagon, droperidol, tyramine, metoclopramide, saralasin, tricyclics, and phenothiazines should also suggest the possibility of this tumor. Definitive therapy for pheochromocytoma is surgical excision.

How Is Pheochromocytoma Assessed Preoperatively?

Proper diagnosis, localization, and control of the underlying disease are essential in the preoperative period. Biochemical diagnosis is accomplished by determining plasma and urinary catecholamine levels or urinary catechol metabolites (i.e., vanillylmandelic acid, metanephrines). Rarely are suppressive tests (i.e., clonidine suppression test) or provocative tests (i.e., glucagon) required.

Stimulation of endogenous catecholamines by surgery or stroke, exogenous catecholamines, and various drugs such as α_2-agonists, methyldopa, converting enzyme inhibitors, monoamine oxidase inhibitors, phenothiazines, and tricyclic antidepressants interfere with measurements of plasma and urinary catecholamines.

After biochemical confirmation of excess catecholamine production, tumors are localized using various scanning techniques such as metacodobenzylguanidine, CT, or MRI or venous blood sampling for catecholamines. Arteriography is rarely used because it may precipitate hypertensive crisis.

Pheochromocytoma may be accompanied by other endocrine tumors (i.e., thyroid, parathyroid, ganglioneuromas). Many patients may also have end-organ dysfunction, including cardiomyopathy and renal disease, due to long-standing hypertensive disease. Diabetes mellitus may also be present. All patients should be evaluated for other disease processes and organ dysfunction.

How Is Pheochromocytoma Managed Preoperatively?

Proper preoperative management is the most important factor determining a successful surgical outcome. The goals of preoperative medical therapy are to control blood pressure, attain adequate blood volume status, and treat tachydysrhythmias, heart failure, and glucose intolerance.

Blood Pressure

Alpha-adrenergic blockade is the basis of preoperative pharmacologic management of hypertension (Table 12–6). Patients are usually treated for 1 to 2 weeks with oral phenoxybenzamine. Prazosin and labetalol have also been used successfully. Alpha-blockade is tapered to produce a 10 to 15 mm Hg orthostatic decrease in blood pressure. A 1- to 2-week course allows replenishment of intravascular volume that had been diminished by excess circulating catecholamines. Tachycardia may result from unopposed β-adrenergic receptor activation. Reflex tachycardia is less with prazosin and labetalol than it is with phenoxybenzamine.

Alpha-methylparatyrosine may be used to control blood pressure in patients who cannot tolerate α-adrenergic blockade (i.e., postural hypotension). Phenoxybenzamine and α-methylparatyrosine are a reasonable combination. Effective control of hypertension can be obtained with lower doses of phenoxybenzamine using this combination, thereby reducing the adverse effects of α-blockade. Postoperative hypotension and tachycardia are also less common.

Tachycardia

If tachycardia is present, a β-adrenergic blocker should be added. We usually give a β-blocker when the heart rate exceeds 110 beats per minute. Many patients do not require β-blocker therapy. Propranolol, atenolol, and labetalol all have been used successfully. Beta-antagonists should not, however, be administered before the institution of α-adrenergic blockade. Elimination of the vasodilatory effects of β-receptors results in unopposed α-adrenergic vasoconstriction and may provoke a hypertensive crisis. In addition, the negative inotropic effects of β-blockade may precipitate heart failure in the presence of hypertension.

Reduction of Catecholamine Levels

Alpha-methylparatyrosine inhibits tyrosine hydroxylase, the rate-limiting enzyme in catecholamine synthesis. This drug reduces catecholamine levels and is useful in treating pheochromocytomas when other agents are not effective (i.e., heart failure). Alpha-adrenergic blockers may result in hypotension, β-adrenergic blockers may impair cardiac contraction, and diuretics may further reduce intravascular volume in patients with heart failure.

Dysrhythmias

Patients with dysrhythmias are treated with standard antidysrhythmic agents. However, we usually add a β-adrenergic blocker. Adequate blood should be available for transfusion in the perioperative period, because pheochromocytomas are vascular tumors and frequently bleed.

Cardiomyopathy and Heart Failure

Excessive levels of catecholamines are toxic to the myocardium, and heart failure, as a result of long-standing hypertension or cardiomyopathy, may occur. Phenoxybenzamine may be beneficial by reducing systemic vascular resistance. However, α-blockers must be used cautiously because hypotension may result when cardiac reserve is insufficient to overcome the decrease in vascular resistance.

Diuretics should be used sparingly because intravascular volume is already constricted by catecholamines. On the other hand, administration of excessive amounts of fluids can worsen heart failure. Alpha-methylparatyrosine is useful in treating catecholamine-induced cardiomyopathy. The drug allows gradual repletion of intravascular volume, and postoperative hypotension is decreased because α-receptors are not blocked.

Hyperglycemia

Hyperglycemia may result from the gluconeogenic and anti-insulin effects of catecholamines. The hyperglycemia responds to reduction in circulating catecholamines (i.e., α-methylparatyrosine) and insulin. Hypoglycemia may occur after tumor removal.

How Is Pheochromocytoma Managed Perioperatively?

Intraoperative management goals are to balance hypertension and arrhythmias due to catecholamine release against hypotension and bradycardia due to blood loss, hypovolemia, and a sudden fall in catecholamines after tumor removal. Pre-

TABLE 12–6. Preoperative Pharmacologic Management of Pheochromocytoma

Alpha-adrenergic blockade (titrate to 10–15 mm Hg orthostatic drop in blood pressure)	Phenoxybenzamine (10–50 mg twice daily) Prazosin, 1–4 mg every 8 h (increase to 10 mg every 8 h) Labetalol, 100 mg every 6 h (increase to 200 mg every 6 h)
Beta-adrenergic blockade (for heart rate >110/min)	Propranolol, 20–60 mg PO every hour Atenolol, 50–100 mg PO every 12–24 h Labetalol, 100 mg every 6 h (increase to 200 mg every 6 h)
Alpha-methylparatyrosine	250 mg 4 times daily (increase to 1000 mg 4 times daily)

operatively, hypovolemia should be corrected with α-adrenergic blockade and the associated intravascular volume expansion. Drugs that cause catecholamine release or that potentiate catecholamine action should be avoided.

Basic monitoring includes a continuous electrocardiogram (ECG), intra-arterial catheter, Foley catheter, pulse oximeter, central venous or pulmonary artery catheter, temperature sensor, and periodic blood glucose determinations. In general, short-acting drugs are preferable to long-acting ones. Premedication is frequently accomplished with a benzodiazepine. Morphine is usually avoided because of histamine-induced catecholamine release. Droperidol and phenothiazines generally should also be avoided because of catecholamine interactions in that they block catecholamine uptake. Atropine may cause significant tachycardia and aggravate catecholamine-induced hypertension and myocardial ischemia.

Anesthetic Choice

The optimal anesthetic for surgery has not been fully defined. Thiopental, fentanyl/alfentanil, and etomidate all have been used with good results. Many consider vecuronium the muscle relaxant of choice. This agent has no autonomic effects and does not stimulate the release of catecholamines. Tubocurarine and atracurium may cause histamine release, and pancuronium may increase catecholamines. Succinylcholine may result in sympathetic stimulation, hypertension, and tachycardia. Nitrous oxide, isoflurane, and enflurane are frequently used to supplement a balanced narcotic technique.

Rapid changes in cardiovascular parameters may develop in response to changes in catecholamines during surgical manipulation of a tumor. Decreases in blood pressure occur after isolation of the venous drainage. Intraoperative hypertension is treated with phentolamine (2–5 mg boluses), titrated nitroprusside infusion, or labetalol. Tachycardia is usually treated with esmolol, propranolol, or labetalol. Dysrhythmias frequently respond to esmolol and lidocaine.

Hypotension

Hypotension is common after tumor removal. Causes include a decrease in circulating catecholamines, constricted vascular volume, operative blood loss, receptor down-regulation, α-adrenergic antagonists, and β-adrenergic blockade. Pheochromocytomas are vascular tumors and frequently originate adjacent to major vessels. Significant hemorrhage is a potential hazard. Hypotension usually responds to fluid administration. Vasopressor (phenylephrine) administration may occasionally be needed.

Glucose

Blood glucose levels should be monitored. Hypoglycemia is common after tumor removal as a consequence of loss of catecholamine-induced hyperglycemia. Glucocorticoids or mineralocorticoids or both are required for patients undergoing bilateral adrenalectomies.

Postoperative Considerations

Postoperatively, the goals are to control blood pressure, maintain volume status, monitor glucose, prevent dysrhythmias, and treat heart failure if it is present. Hypovolemia is managed with fluid/blood administration. Recurrent hypertension should suggest the possibility of residual tumor.

THYROID DISEASE

Thyroid hormone is essential for normal metabolic function of all cells. On binding to its DNA receptor, triiodothyronine (T_3) initiates biochemical and physiologic responses that affect cardiovascular, respiratory, gastrointestinal, neuromuscular, and other organ systems. It is required for the synthesis of contractile proteins and adrenergic receptors. Excess thyroid hormone causes hyperthyroidism or thyrotoxicosis.[48–51] Thyroid hormone deficiency results in hypothyroidism or myxedema.[52, 53]

Thyroid hormone secretion is controlled by the hypothalamus, which secretes thyrotropin-releasing hormone (TRH). The latter stimulates pituitary secretion of TSH. TSH causes the thyroid to secrete thyroxine (T_4) and smaller amounts of T_3. T_3 is the active form of thyroid hormone. Most T_3 is produced from monodeiodination of circulating T_4 in peripheral organs. T_4 and T_3 circulate bound to serum proteins; however, it is the free T_4 (FT_4) and free T_3 (FT_3) fractions that are metabolically active. T_3 inhibits the pituitary production of TSH via negative feedback.

How Is Thyroid Dysfunction Diagnosed?

The diagnosis of thyroid dysfunction relies on serum levels of thyroid hormones and TSH (Table 12–7).[54] The most commonly measured hormones are T_4 and T_3. These hormones circulate bound to serum proteins; alterations in these proteins may increase or decrease the serum level of total T_4 and T_3 without altering the biologically active free hormone concentrations. Thus, FT_4 levels better reflect thyroid performance.

If FT_4 is not available, it can be estimated using the FTI, which is calculated by multiplying total T_4 by T_3 resin uptake (T_3RU), a measure of binding. TSH reflects pituitary function and pituitary tissue sensitivity to thyroid hormone.

TABLE 12–7. Effect of Thyroid Disease or Illness on Thyroid Hormone Levels

	Hypothyroidism	Hyperthyroidism	Euthyroid-Sick
Thyroxine (T_4)	N, ↓	↑	N, ↓
Free thyroxine (FT_4)	↓	↑	↓
Triiodothyronine (T_3)	N, ↓	↑	↓
Free triiodothyronine (FT_3)	↓	↑	↓
Thyroid-secreting hormone (TSH)	↑	↓	N
Free triiodothyronine (T_3RU)	↓	↑	↑
Reverse T_3 (rT_3)	↓	↑	↑

Ratio of Thyroid-Stimulating Hormone to Thyroxine

New immunometric TSH assays can detect very low levels of TSH and are sensitive to levels as low as 0.01 mU/L. A strong inverse relationship exists between free T_4 and TSH. A 2-fold change in FT_4 produces a 160-fold change in TSH. Each patient has an individual, genetically determined set-point for the TSH/T_4 relationship. Hyperthyroidism is characterized by a decreasing TSH/T_4 relationship. TSH becomes subnormal while T_4 levels are still within normal limits. Hypothyroidism is characterized by a rising TSH/T_4 ratio. TSH is elevated while T_4 is still within normal limits (increasing TSH compensates for falling T_4 levels). During subclinical disease, the TSH/T_4 ratio changes relative to a patient's set-point.

The TSH/T_4 ratio is only valid when hypothalamic-pituitary function is intact. Serum T_3 determination is a poor indicator of thyroid function except in hyperthyroid states. Most T_3 is produced outside the thyroid gland. As the thyroid fails, the serum T_4 level falls and a compensatory increase in T_3 production occurs, maintaining serum T_3 levels close to normal until T_4 deficiency is significant. On the other hand, serum T_3 increases early in hyperthyroid states. T_4 is metabolized to T_3 and reverse T_3 (rT_3). Reverse T_3 increases in hyperthyroid states and decreases in hypothyroid states.

Nonthyroidal Illness

Many patients with nonthyroidal illnesses (e.g., surgery, infection, pneumonia, renal failure) demonstrate changes in thyroid hormone and TSH measurements.[55] A decrease in total T_3 and FT_3 occurs early and results from inhibition of $5'$-deiodinase, the enzyme that converts T_4 to T_3. T_4 is metabolized to rT_3, resulting in an elevation in rT_3 levels. As the severity of illness increases, total T_4 and FT_4 also decrease. Most ill patients have normal TSH values. Therefore, a normal TSH level usually precludes significant hypothyroidism or hyperthyroidism during nonthyroidal illnesses. Patients with mild hypothyroidism may have their slightly elevated TSH levels suppressed into normal ranges by nonthyroidal illness. Binding of thyroid hormones is decreased, resulting in an elevation in T_3RU.

Increase in serum T_4 concentrations, without thyrotoxicosis, may occur in various conditions and is referred to as *euthyroid hyperthyroxinemia*.[56] These include liver disease, pregnancy, and acute psychiatric illness. Serum TSH and FT_4 are the most useful tests for diagnosing thyroid disease (see Table 12–7). If direct measurement of FT_4 is not available, it may be estimated (i.e., FTI).

How Is Hypothyroidism Assessed Preoperatively?

Thyroid testing is not recommended in sick hospitalized patients unless clinically significant thyroid disease is suspected. Clinical features suggestive of thyroid disease are listed in Table 12–8. Mild subclinical hyperthyroidism and hypothyroidism are usually well tolerated and do not appear to increase operative mortality. On the other hand, overt disease alters organ function and increases operative complications and mortality.

A diagnosis of hypothyroidism or hyperthyroidism is confirmed by measuring TSH and FT_4 (or FTI) (see Table 12–7).

The most common cause of hypothyroidism is Hashimoto's thyroiditis (an autoimmune disease). Subclinical hypothyroidism is present in about 5% of the population and overt primary hypothyroidism in 1% of the population and is more common in women. Other causes of hypothyroidism include surgical removal of the gland, radioiodine treatment, hypopituitarism (e.g., pituitary infarction or tumors), and drugs (e.g., lithium, amiodarone). Findings suggestive of hypothyroidism include a goiter, previous neck surgery, and treatment for hyperthyroidism (e.g., surgery, radioactive iodine).

Clinical Features

The most common clinical features of hypothyroidism relate to depressed CNS, cardiovascular, respiratory, and gastrointestinal function (see Table 12–8). Patients with hypothyroidism frequently have underlying coronary artery disease, impaired cardiac contractility, impaired ventilation, hyperlipidemia, anemia, electrolyte disturbances, free water retention, impaired renal function, and diabetes mellitus.

How Is Hypothyroidism Managed Preoperatively?

Patients with hypothyroidism require supportive care and thyroid hormone. Maintenance of body temperature, correction of hypovolemia, support of cardiovascular and respiratory function, assessment of electrolyte status, monitoring of glucose and renal function, maintenance of adequate nutrition, treatment of underlying illness (e.g., sepsis), and assessment of hypothalamic-pituitary status (e.g., adrenal function) are important.

Replacement Therapy

Five thyroid hormone preparations are available: L-thyroxine (T_4), L-triiodothyronine (T_3), liotrix (T_4 and T_3), desiccated thyroid, and thyroglobulin.

Synthetic Thyroxine

The majority of patients are treated with synthetic L-thyroxine (i.e., Synthroid, Levothroid) or desiccated thyroid. L-Thyroxine is well absorbed from the small intestine (50–90%). It has a 7-day half-life, which permits single daily dosing. Because of its long half-life, L-thyroxine requires 3 to 4 weeks to reach steady-state levels. Increasing the dose before reaching steady state may result in production of a hyperthyroid state.

The average L-thyroxine replacement dose in patients with hypothyroidism ranges from 0.075 to 0.10 mg daily. Replacement dose is lower in the elderly. Thyroid hormone replacement can be initiated with a full dose (0.075–0.1 mg of L-thyroxine) in healthy patients.

When therapy is initiated in patients with symptomatic long-standing hypothyroidism, the elderly, or patients with underlying ischemic heart disease, it is started with small doses of L-thyroxine (12.5–25 $\mu g \cdot d^{-1}$). L-Thyroxine can precipitate or worsen ischemic heart disease. Dose increases should be small (12.5–25 $\mu g \cdot d^{-1}$ every 4 to 6 wk). Before each change in dose, patients should be questioned about chest pain and TSH/T_4 concentrations measured. Cardiac symptoms

TABLE 12–8. Clinical Features of Thyroid Disease

Hyperthyroidism	Hypothyroidism
Cardiovascular	*Cardiovascular*
Tachycardia	Bradycardia
Tachydysrhythmias (supraventricular tachycardia, atrial fibrillation)	Depressed contractility
Ventricular dysrhythmias	Decreased cardiac output
Increased cardiac output, increased contractility	Hypertension, high systemic vascular resistance
Reduced systemic vascular resistance	Pericardial effusion
Cardiomyopathy, heart failure	Atherosclerosis
Angina pectoris	Elevated creatine phosphokinase
Myocardial infarction	*Decreased oxygen consumption*
Increased oxygen consumption	*Respiratory*
Respiratory	Airway obstruction, enlarged tongue
Tachypnea	Impaired ventilation
Decreased lung compliance	Impaired response to hypoxia and hypercapnia
Increased response to hypoxia/hypercapnia	Muscle weakness
Nervous system	*Nervous system*
Nervousness, tremors	Fatigue
Short attention span	Diminished reflexes
Seizures, chorea	*Other common features*
Coma	Diminished mental status
Diminished mental status	Cold intolerance
Hyper-reflexia	Hyperlipidemia
Other	Anemia
Muscle weakness, myopathies	Glucose intolerance
Periodic paralysis	Gastroparesis
Increased appetite	Hyponatremia
Heat intolerance, diaphoresis	
Diarrhea	
Weight loss	
Abdominal pain	
Hypercalcemia	
Osteopenia	
Glucose intolerance	
Malnutrition	

should prompt a reduction in dose and evaluation for possible coronary artery bypass surgery. Many patients with hypothyroidism and angina cannot tolerate full replacement therapy.

Desiccated Thyroid

Desiccated thyroid contains both T_4 and T_3. These preparations have variable potency. Because T_3 is more rapidly and completely absorbed and has a shorter serum half-life than T_4, serum T_3 levels transiently rise and may cause symptoms (i.e., cardiac). One grain (60 mg) of desiccated thyroid is approximately equivalent to 0.1 mg of L-thyroxine.

Optimal Dosage

The optimal dose of thyroid hormone in patients with primary hypothyroidism is one that normalizes the serum TSH level. However, TSH may be an unreliable indicator of the adequacy of thyroid hormone replacement in some situations. Levels may be suppressed in patients receiving dopamine or glucocorticoids, during acute psychiatric illness, with severe nonthyroidal illness, and during pregnancy. Under these circumstances, an FTI or FT_4 in the mid to high normal range suggests adequate replacement. Overtreatment with thyroid hormone may adversely increase metabolism in the heart, kidneys, bone, and liver. A T_4 level in the midnormal range is a reasonable treatment end point in patients with secondary hypothyroidism.

Associated Endocrinopathies

Hypothyroidism resulting from pituitary or hypothalamic disease requires a full evaluation of pituitary function. If adrenal insufficiency is present, glucocorticoid therapy must precede thyroxine replacement to avoid an increase in metabolic rate and precipitation of adrenal crisis.

Euthyroid Sick Syndrome

Hypothyroidism may at times be difficult to distinguish from the euthyroid sick syndrome. Both states are characterized by low serum T_4 levels.[28] An increased serum TSH concentration suggests primary hypothyroidism. In some instances, however, increased TSH may be suppressed into the normal range by the acute illness and use of certain drugs (i.e., glucocorticoids, dopamine). TSH may also be decreased in secondary hypothyroidism. Reverse T_3, T_3RU, and FT_4 can help distinguish between the two states. To date, studies have failed to find an advantage to administering thyroid hormone to euthyroid sick patients.[57, 58]

Myxedema Coma

If myxedema coma is suspected, we recommend treating the patient empirically with thyroid hormone even before results of laboratory tests are available. Delay in treatment is believed to increase morbidity and mortality. Although some patients may receive treatment unnecessarily, therapy is unlikely to cause harm.

How Is Hyperthyroidism Assessed Preoperatively?

The major causes of hyperthyroidism are Graves' disease, toxic multimodular goiter, toxic adenoma, exogenous thyroid hormone, thyroiditis, and syndromes of excess TSH secretion. Determination of serum T_4 and TSH levels, a thyroid scan, and radioactive iodine uptake (RAIU) are helpful in establishing a specific diagnosis (see Table 12–7). RAIU is elevated in Graves' disease, toxic multimodular goiter, toxic adenoma, and syndromes of excess TSH production. It is low in thyroiditis, exogenous thyroid hormone excess, and ectopic thyroid hormone production.

Clinical Features

The major goals of preoperative assessment of hyperthyroidism are to control hypermetabolism and associated cardiovascular effects (Tables 12–8 and 12–9) and to prevent severe thyrotoxicosis. Thyroid hormone increases cardiac contractility and heart rate. The increased oxygen demand of the myocardium may cause ischemia in patients with coronary artery disease as well as cardiomyopathy, congestive heart failure, and dysrhythmias.

CNS abnormalities include nervousness, tremors, seizures, depressed mental status, and coma. Muscle weakness and myopathy are also common.

Thyrotoxic crisis (thyroid storm) represents a life-threatening complication of hyperthyroidism characterized by multiorgan decompensation. It is frequently precipitated by illness (i.e., infection, surgery, labor/delivery, stroke, trauma) in patients with untreated hyperthyroidism.

How Is Hyperthyroidism Managed Preoperatively?

Selection of optimal therapy for hyperthyroidism requires knowledge of the specific cause and assessment of clinical status. The objective of therapy is to reverse the hypermetabolic state and normalize tissue levels of thyroid hormone. General measures include treatment of fever, hydration, maintenance of adequate nutrition, electrolyte replacement, and maintenance of cardiorespiratory function. Acetaminophen is preferred to salicylates, because the latter decrease binding of T_4 and T_3 to binding proteins. A precipitating event (e.g., infection, pancreatitis) should be identified and treated.

Normalization of Thyroid Hormone

Normalization of thyroid hormone may be accomplished with antithyroid drugs, radioactive iodine, or surgery (see Table 12–9). Propylthiouracil (PTU) and methimazole are the principal antithyroid drugs. They block the synthesis of new hormone. A high rate of recurrence of hyperthyroidism occurs after drug withdrawal.

Radioactive iodine requires 4 to 6 months to have an effect. Undertreatment may lead to recurrence of hyperthyroidism, and overtreatment may result in hypothyroidism. In addition, a high proportion of patients in whom a euthyroid state follows radioiodine therapy ultimately suffer hypothyroidism during the ensuing years.

Subtotal thyroidectomy may also result in post-therapy hypothyroidism or persistent hyperthyroidism (depending on the extent of resection). Thus, patients previously treated for hyperthyroidism should have their thyroid status assessed before surgery.

Blockade of Thyroid Hormone Synthesis

Our initial approach to hyperthyroidism is to block the synthesis of thyroid hormone with a thionamide drug (see Table 12–9), gradually reversing the hypermetabolic state. These drugs inhibit new hormone synthesis but have no effect on the release of stored thyroid hormone. We prefer PTU because it has the added effect of inhibiting peripheral conversion of T_4 to T_3. In general, 1 to 2 weeks is required for a significant clinical effect, and euthyroidism is not attained for 6 to 8 weeks. The adrenergic hyperactivity associated with thyroid hormone can be reduced with β-adrenergic antagonists (see Table 12–9). Hypermetabolism may also be decreased by blocking the peripheral conversion of T_4 to T_3 with PTU, β-adrenergic antagonists, or glucocorticoids.

Unlike PTU, steroids penetrate the CNS and may prevent T_3 production centrally. PTU crosses the placenta less than methimazole and is preferred during pregnancy. It also penetrates breast milk less than methimazole and is the drug of choice for treating hyperthyroidism in breast-feeding mothers. Iodides acutely inhibit T_4 release. They should be given after initiation of antithyroid therapy so that the large iodide load will not provide additional substrate for new thyroid hormone synthesis (e.g., 1–2 h).

Radioiodine and Surgery

Radioiodine is the preferred therapy for definitive treatment of hyperthyroidism in most patients. However, surgery may be the treatment of choice for young patients, pregnant patients, patients with large goiters, and patients with "cold" nodules. Before surgery, patients should be rendered euthyroid with antithyroid drugs.

TABLE 12–9. Treatment of Hyperthyroidism

Antithyroid therapy	Antithyroid drugs (thionamides):
	• Propylthiouracil (200–400 PO/NG q 6 h)
	• Methimazole (20–40 mg rectally q 6 h)
	Radioactive iodine
	Surgery
Agents blocking T_4 to T_3 conversion	Propylthiouracil (200–400 mg PO q 6 h)
	Beta-adrenergic antagonists (propranolol)
	Glucocorticoids (dexamethasone, 2 mg q 6 h)
	Ipodate (0.5–1.0 g · d^{-1} PO)
Agents antagonizing hyperadrenergic activity	Beta-adrenergic antagonists (i.e., propranolol, 1–5 mg IV prn; 40–120 mg PO q 6 h)
	Catecholamine depleters (i.e., reserpine, guanethidine)
Inhibit T_4 release	Iodides:
	• SSKI (5 drops q 6 h PO)
	• NaI (1–2 g IV q 8–12 h)
	Ipodate (0.5–1 g · d^{-1} PO)
	Lithium (300–900 mg · d^{-1})
General measures	Antipyresis (i.e., acetaminophen)
	Hydration
	Nutrition
	Cardiovascular support

Abbreviations: q = every; PO = orally; NG = nasogastric; IV = intravenously, prn = as needed; SSKI = saturated solution of potassium iodide; NaI = sodium iodide.

Beta-Blockade

Thyroid crisis may develop during labor or in untreated hyperthyroid patients who require emergency surgery. These patients should be treated. Beta-blockade alone has been effective. However, we also advocate administration of antithyroid drugs.

How Is Hypothyroidism Managed Perioperatively?

Symptomatic hypothyroidism and myxedema coma may be precipitated by acute illness, anesthesia, surgery, and infection in patients with unrecognized hypothyroidism. Myxedema coma has a mortality rate as high as 80%. It should be considered in stuporous or comatose patients, particularly when hypothermia is present and when a reason for the diminished level of consciousness is not clear. Early treatment of myxedema coma can reduce mortality.

Therapy for hypothyroid states includes ventilation, volume expanders, thyroxine, glucocorticoids, passive warming, and treatment of precipitating causes such as infection, sedatives, narcotics, gastrointestinal bleeding, myocardial infarction, and stroke. Because laboratory confirmation of myxedema may be delayed, therapy should begin when the diagnosis is seriously suspected. Short-term administration of thyroxine is well tolerated in euthyroid patients and can be life saving in hypothyroid individuals.

Thyroid Hormone

As soon as a patient is stabilized with adequate oxygenation and perfusion, thyroid hormone should be administered. Severe hypothyroidism in the absence of coma is treated by administering small doses of thyroid hormone and waiting for the effects to be fully developed before increasing the dose (i.e., 12.5–25 $\mu g \cdot d^{-1}$ for 2 to 3 weeks, increasing by 12.5–25 μg daily at 2- to 3-wk intervals).

Myxedema coma, however, appears to be associated with an improved outcome with early use of large doses of intravenous T_4. Although large doses predispose to cardiac dysrhythmias, the cost/benefit ratio is still favorable. We recommend administering 200 to 300 μg of L-thyroxine as an intravenous bolus, followed by 50 to 100 μg of L-thyroxine per day. The serum total T_4 is measured on the second day of treatment. If levels are <5 $\mu g \cdot dL^{-1}$, a second bolus of 200 to 300 μg of L-thyroxine may be administered if the patient remains stuporous or comatose.

Respiratory Problems

Maintenance of normal organ functions is important in the care of hypothyroid patients. Ventilation is commonly impaired, and respiratory failure may occur. Increased sensitivity to drugs that depress respiration is common. The tongue is frequently enlarged and may contribute to airway obstruction. Respiratory muscles may be weak, and respiratory drive impaired. Mechanical ventilation may be needed to maintain oxygenation. Weaning from the ventilator may be impaired because of respiratory insufficiency and slow metabolism of sedatives. Hypotonia of the gut is common and results in constipation, ileus, and megacolon. Gastroparesis predisposes

to aspiration and sometimes requires postpyloric administration of nutrients.

Cardiovascular Problems

Hypothyroid patients are insensitive to the β-adrenergic agents. They are predisposed to hypotension and cardiac insufficiency. Patients usually have peripheral vasoconstriction, and plasma volume is diminished. Fluids are preferred over α-adrenergic agents for treating hypotension. Dysrhythmias may occur, especially during initiation of thyroid hormone. Hypothyroid patients may have bradycardia and low QRS voltage on the ECG. Pericardial effusions can occur but rarely impair cardiac function. Creatine kinase (including MB bands) level may be elevated and is not necessarily indicative of myocardial injury.

Hypothermia

Patients may become hypothermic as a result of lowered metabolic rate. Warming may be necessary. Passive warming with a blanket is preferred to active warming. A rise in body temperature is usually evident within 24 hours of starting thyroid hormone therapy.

Adrenal Insufficiency

Because adrenal insufficiency may coexist with primary hypothyroidism, patients are usually treated with cortisol equivalent, 50 to 100 mg intravenously every 8 hours. The serum cortisol level should be determined from a blood sample obtained before beginning steroid therapy. If the results are subsequently found to be appropriately elevated, consistent with stress, the dose of hydrocortisone can be quickly tapered and discontinued.

Fluids

Intravenous fluids should be administered cautiously. Hypothyroid patients frequently have hyponatremia and impaired free water excretion. Hypotonic fluids may exacerbate free water retention. If hypoglycemia is present, dextrose-containing fluid should be given. Drug metabolism is decreased in hypothyroidism. Drugs with a narrow therapeutic/toxic ratio must therefore be monitored particularly closely.

How Is Hyperthyroidism Managed Perioperatively?

Hyperthyroid patients require close monitoring in the perioperative period to avoid thyrotoxic crisis. Elective surgery should be postponed in thyrotoxic patients until hyperthyroidism is controlled. If surgery is emergent, patients should be treated with a combination of antithyroid drugs, a β-adrenergic blocker, and agents that decrease T_4-to-T_3 conversion (see Table 12–9). We prefer the combination of PTU, propranolol, iodine, and glucocorticoids. Although β-adrenergic blockade alone has been used to prepare patients with uncomplicated hyperthyroidism for thyroidectomy, preparation of hyperthyroid patients for thyroidectomy usually involves antithyroid drugs and iodine.

Thionamides

Thionamides inhibit the synthesis of thyroid hormone and reduce thyroid hormone stores. These agents reduce perioperative morbidity and mortality. After inhibition of thyroid hormone synthesis, a 10-day preoperative course of inorganic iodine leads to involution and decreased vascularity of the thyroid gland, facilitating its removal. Thionamide therapy must be continued during iodine administration to prevent accumulation of iodine within the thyroid (and aggravation of thyrotoxicosis).

Ipodate Sodium

Ipodate sodium has also been used successfully to treat hyperthyroidism, particularly in patients allergic to thionamides. In doses of 0.5 to 1.0 g daily, it inhibits peripheral T_4-to-T_3 conversion. Released inorganic iodine blocks release of hormone from the thyroid gland and causes involution of the gland.

Cardiovascular Problems

Heart failure and atrial fibrillation are usually treated with digoxin. Increased metabolism necessitates an increased dose of the drug. Muscarinic antagonists (atropine, scopolamine) should be avoided in uncontrolled hyperthyroidism because they may cause even more rapid heart rates. Tachycardia and atrial fibrillation have responded to diltiazem.

Beta-adrenergic antagonists attenuate the hyperadrenergic manifestations of hyperthyroidism. These agents are useful for reducing tachycardia, hypermetabolism, and cardiac toxicity, as well as anxiety.

Airway Obstruction

Patients with large goiters may develop respiratory tract obstruction. Distortion of the airway and larynx or compression of the tracheal lumen is frequent. Tracheomalacia may also occur, especially after thyroidectomy.

Fever

Reduction of fever is important because fever increases metabolic demands and the percentage of T_4. Acetaminophen is the drug of choice because salicylates decrease thyroid hormone binding, thereby elevating free levels. Large volumes of fluid are frequently needed to replace insensible losses. Patients are catabolic and have increased nutritional requirements for vitamins, glucose, protein, and electrolytes.

What Are the Perioperative Complications of Hypothyroidism?

Hypothyroidism diminishes body metabolism and organ function. Mild hypothyroidism is usually well tolerated. On the other hand, moderate to severe hypothyroidism impairs physiologic responses and increases complications and mortality. These patients demonstrate respiratory muscle weakness, impaired responses to hypoxia/hypercarbia, impaired sympathetic responses, diminished drug metabolism, and impaired nervous system function (see Table 12–8). Metabolism of drugs used during anesthesia is slowed, and weaning from the ventilator may be prolonged. Respiratory failure is a major cause of death.

Airway Obstruction

The thyroid normally resides in the anterior portion of the neck. Some individuals may have thyroid tissue extending substernally and intrathoracically. Enlargement of the thyroid (goiter) may cause upper airway obstruction.[59] Flow volume loops are believed to be the most sensitive and reliable tests for detecting airway obstruction.[60] After removal of a goiter, tracheomalacia may develop. Other postoperative causes of airway distress include wound hematoma, laryngeal edema, and vocal cord paralysis due to recurrent laryngeal nerve injury.

Surgical Outcome

Several studies have evaluated the effect of hypothyroidism on surgical outcome. Weinberg and colleagues found that hypothyroidism did not affect the duration of anesthesia, the lowest intraoperative blood pressure, the need for vasopressors, the frequency of dysrhythmias, fluid/electrolyte imbalance, or the duration of hospital stay.[61] However, hypothyroid patients had longer duration of intubation and more bleeding complications.

Ladenson and associates reported that hypothyroidism had no effect on the difficulty of tracheal intubation, the frequency of perioperative infarctions, dysrhythmias, pulmonary complications, tissue integrity and wound healing, infection, blood loss, hyponatremia, hypothermia, intensive care unit/hospital stay, or death.[62] However, intraoperative hypotension and postoperative gut dysfunction were noted to be more common in the hypothyroid patients they studied.

Of 559 patients undergoing cardiopulmonary bypass surgery, 13 were found to have unrecognized mild to moderate hypothyroidism.[55, 63] Hypothyroidism was not associated with an increased complication rate.

Patients with severe coronary artery disease and hypothyroidism may have an exacerbation of their ischemic disease if thyroid hormone is administered before coronary artery bypass surgery. These patients are best treated by initiating thyroid hormone therapy after surgery.[64]

Treatment With L-Thyroxine

When adrenal insufficiency coexists with hypothyroidism, glucocorticoids should be given first before increasing metabolism with L-thyroxine. Thyroid hormone accelerates the clearance of endogenous glucocorticoids and exacerbates adrenal insufficiency.

Treatment of hypothyroidism with L-thyroxine is remarkably safe. Major complications result from overtreatment and the development of iatrogenic hyperthyroidism. Manifestations include anxiety, nervousness, tremor, tachycardia, palpitations, headaches, insomnia, sweating, and weight loss. Overtreatment may precipitate angina pectoris, cardiac dysrhythmias, myocardial infarction, and heart failure. Cardiac symptoms are more common in the elderly and in patients with ischemic heart disease.

What Are the Perioperative Complications of Hyperthyroidism?

Medical

Complications of thionamide therapy for the treatment of hyperthyroidism include pruritus, rash, agranulocytosis, hepatotoxicity, arthralgias, and arthritis. Radioactive iodine produces an intense radiation thyroiditis followed by fibrosis and atrophy of the thyroid gland. The thyroiditis, which peaks 10 to 14 days after radioiodine therapy, may release large quantities of stored thyroid hormone and result in adverse cardiovascular effects. Therefore, a course of thionamide therapy is desirable before radioiodine therapy. Beta-adrenergic antagonists are also helpful in blocking hyperadrenergic effects.

Surgical

Complications of thyroidectomy include damage to the recurrent laryngeal nerves resulting in vocal cord paralysis, hypoparathyroidism, wound hematoma, and tracheomalacia.

PARATHYROID DISEASE

Calcium is essential for maintenance of excitation-contraction coupling in muscle, secretion, neurotransmission, cell division, blood coagulation, and many other functions. It is a major intracellular messenger, coupling cell surface events (i.e., β- and α-adrenergic receptor activation) to intracellular events (i.e., contraction, secretion). Calcium is also important for activation of many intracellular enzymes (e.g., proteases, lipases) and for proper function of the coagulation cascade. In general, cellular processes that require movement involve calcium.

Because of its importance in cellular physiology, the blood calcium level is maintained within narrow limits (ionized calcium 1.0–1.3 mmol $\cdot$ L^{-1}) via the coordinated effects of parathyroid hormone (PTH) and vitamin D.[65–72] PTH increases the release of calcium from bone, stimulates calcium absorption from the gut via vitamin D–dependent processes, and stimulates calcium reabsorption from renal tubules. Its secretion is stimulated by ionized hypocalcemia and mild hypomagnesemia, and is inhibited by ionized hypercalcemia, severe hypomagnesemia, hypermagnesemia, and 1,25-dihydroxyvitamin D.

What Are Hypoparathyroidism and Hyperparathyroidism?

PTH deficiency (hypoparathyroidism) presents with ionized hypocalcemia, whereas PTH excess (hyperparathyroidism) presents with ionized hypercalcemia. Hypoparathyroidism is usually acquired and may result from hypomagnesemia, sepsis, burns, pancreatitis, rhabdomyolysis, and surgical removal of the parathyroid glands (Table 12–10). Primary hypoparathyroidism is rare and of autoimmune etiology.

Hyperparathyroidism is primary or secondary (ectopic PTH) (see Table 12–10). Primary hyperparathyroidism can result from a parathyroid adenoma, hyperplasia of multiple glands, or parathyroid cancer. A state of transient hyperparathyroidism with ionized hypercalcemia may also occur after a period of

TABLE 12–10. Causes of Hypoparathyroidism and Hyperparathyroidism

Hypoparathyroidism	Primary	Autoimmune
	Secondary	Severe hypomagnesemia
		Hypermagnesemia
		Suppression during systemic inflammatory diseases
		Sepsis
		Pancreatitis
		Burns
		Rhabdomyolysis
		Trauma
		Surgery
		Neck trauma
Hyperparathyroidism	Primary	Adenoma
		Hyperplasia
		Carcinoma
	Secondary (ectopic)	Carcinoma
	Transient	Posthypocalcemia

ionized hypocalcemia. Hyperplasia of the parathyroid glands and increased PTH secretion continue after resolution of the hypocalcemia. This type of hyperparathyroidism typically corrects itself in 1 to 2 weeks.

How Is Parathyroid Function Assessed Preoperatively?

The clinical manifestations of hypocalcemia and hypercalcemia are listed in Table 12–11. These manifestations should prompt an investigation of parathyroid function as well as other causes of the calcium abnormality.[65–72] However, while parathyroid gland function is being evaluated, treatment of hypocalcemia or hypercalcemia is frequently necessary.

Ionized Calcium

Parathyroid gland function is evaluated by measuring the level of circulating ionized calcium. Total circulating calcium is composed of a protein-bound fraction, a chelated fraction, and an ionized fraction. The ionized fraction is the physiologically active and homeostatically regulated fraction.[65, 66, 68, 72]

Total blood calcium levels are altered by albumin binding, acid-base status, and free fatty acid levels. Although levels are decreased in patients with hypoalbuminemia, the magnitude of the decrease is variable and cannot be used to predict true ionized calcium concentrations accurately in critically ill patients.[73, 74]

Parathyroid Hormone

If the ionized calcium level is abnormal, PTH can be measured to assess parathyroid gland secretory status. We recommend measuring either an intact or N-terminal PTH fragment, because these fragments are not renally cleared and better reflect secretory status in sick patients. The measured PTH level should be interpreted with regard to the ionized calcium value. A low PTH value in the presence of ionized hypocalcemia denotes hypoparathyroidism. A normal or elevated PTH concentration in the presence of ionized hypercalcemia implies hyperparathyroidism.

TABLE 12–11. Clinical Features of Hypocalcemia and Hypercalcemia

Hypocalcemia		Hypercalcemia	
Cardiovascular	Hypotension	General	Fatigue
	Cardiac failure		Lethargy
	Bradycardia		Depression
	Dysrhythmia		Anorexia
	Cardiac arrest		Polydipsia
	Digitalis insensitivity		Dehydration
	ECG: QT and ST prolongation,	Cardiovascular	Hypertension
	T wave inversion		Dysrhythmia
Respiratory	Weakness		Digitalis sensitivity
	Laryngeal spasm		Epinephrine resistance
	Bronchospasm		ECG: QT shortening
Neuromuscular	Tetany	Psychiatric	Mental dullness
	Chvostek's or Trousseau's sign		Confusion, disorientation
	Muscle spasm		Coma
	Paresthesias		Depression
	Seizures		Anxiety
			Dementia
	Weakness		Psychosis
	Extrapyramidal signs		Seizures
Psychiatric	Anxiety	Neuromuscular	Aches and pains
	Dementia		Weakness
	Depression	Gastrointestinal	Abdominal pain
	Irritability		Constipation
	Psychosis		Peptic ulcer disease
	Confusion		Pancreatitis
			Nausea/vomiting
		Renal	Stones
			Nephrocalcinosis
			Renal failure
			Polyuria/nocturia
			Tubular dysfunction
			Interstitial nephritis
		Skeletal	Osteopenia
			Osteitis fibrosa
			Fractures
			Painful bones
			Arthralgias
			Gout

Abbreviations: ECG = electrocardiogram.

Other Causes of Hypocalcemia and Hypercalcemia

Hypocalcemia and hypercalcemia may result from causes other than parathyroid disease.[65–72] Hypocalcemia occurs in vitamin D deficiency and in the presence of circulating chelators such as the citrate found in stored blood. These diseases are characterized by ionized hypocalcemia and an elevated PTH concentration.

Hypercalcemia may result from malignancy, granulomatous disease (e.g., sarcoidosis, tuberculosis), immobilization, and exogenous calcium administration. These conditions are characterized by hypercalcemia and low PTH values, which are compatible with nonparathyroid hypercalcemia.

The specific cause of hypocalcemia or hypercalcemia should be determined before surgery, because the underlying disease may alter the response and indications for surgery. Clearly, a specific diagnosis of hyperparathyroidism should be made before parathyroid gland removal for hypercalcemia. Treatment of infectious diseases such as tuberculosis and histoplasmosis should be initiated before surgery. Patients with hyperparathyroidism should be evaluated for multiple endocrine neoplasia syndromes, which involve tumors of the pituitary, thyroid, parathyroids, pancreas, and adrenal glands (pheochromocytoma). Associated diseases may require specific treatment before surgery.

Metabolic Evaluation

A complete metabolic evaluation to assess disease activity and associated disorders is essential. Serum magnesium and phosphorus levels should be measured and normalized. Magnesium-related parathyroid disease responds poorly to therapy aimed at correcting circulating calcium but does respond to normalization of magnesium concentrations. Correction of hyperphosphatemia may improve hypocalcemia. On the other hand, administration of calcium to hyperphosphatemic patients can result in calcium precipitation and organ damage. The level of circulating calcium must be assessed. Although mild hypocalcemia and hypercalcemia are well tolerated, severe alterations should be treated.

How Is Severe Preoperative Hypocalcemia Treated?

Hypocalcemia is usually treated with calcium or vitamin D administration. Vitamin D derivatives have various physiologic durations of action, and this property should be taken into consideration when prescribing treatment. Serum calcium levels may fluctuate in patients receiving oral calcium and vitamin D supplements for treatment of hypoparathyroidism (i.e., hypocalcemia). Fluctuations result from intermittent dosing, variation in absorption, and variation in bioavailability among different calcium preparations.

For patients undergoing major surgery, we prefer preoperative stabilization with an intravenous calcium infusion given via a central venous catheter to avoid the irritating and sclerosing effect on peripheral veins. An endocrinologist can adjust and regulate the infusion to maintain circulating calcium in the perioperative period. Therapy must be individualized and closely monitored.

How Is Preoperative Severe Hypercalcemia Treated?

Severe hypercalcemia should be treated before surgery. Initial treatment consists of hydration to expand intravascular volume and maintain organ perfusion. Hypercalcemia causes nephrogenic diabetes insipidus, and these patients are frequently dehydrated. Further dehydration may result in calcium precipitation and organ damage. Hydration with isotonic saline expands intravascular volume, dilutes circulating calcium, and improves organ perfusion.

Sodium competes with calcium for reabsorption in the renal tubules, resulting in calcium diuresis. Once intravascular volume is restored, addition of furosemide assists in maintaining calcium diuresis. Renal function must be evaluated and monitored in hypercalcemic patients because hypercalcemia can cause permanent renal damage. Calcium can be removed from the circulation by dialysis in patients with renal failure.

Pre-Existing Therapy

Patients with severe hypercalcemia may be receiving various treatments, depending on the etiology, for control of their hypercalcemia.[65, 66, 68, 69, 72] These agents decrease calcium mobilization from bone (e.g., diphosphonates, mithramycin) or chelate calcium (i.e., phosphates). The pharmacokinetics of the specific agents must be understood. Diphosphonates and mithramycin have effects lasting from days to a few weeks. Phosphates, in contrast, are short acting, with an effect that is measured in hours.

Changes in drug effects can result in rebound hypercalcemia. Long-acting agents can impair recovery from hypocalcemia, which may occur during surgery.

Some patients may be receiving glucocorticoids or chemotherapy agents for treatment of their disease. Failure to administer glucocorticoids in the perioperative period may result in exacerbation of hypercalcemia and adrenal insufficiency.

Bone Involvement

Many causes of hypercalcemia and their treatments result in osteopenia and pathologic fractures. Preoperative assessment of the degree of bony involvement can help minimize skeletal damage during the perioperative period.

Summary

Preoperative assessment of patients with parathyroid disease is aimed at determining disease activity by ionized calcium and PTH measurements, normalizing circulating ionized calcium concentrations, correcting associated electrolyte abnormalities (i.e., magnesium, phosphorus), replacing intravascular

volume, and assessing underlying organ function, particularly that of the kidneys and heart.

How Is Parathyroid Disease Managed Perioperatively?

The essence of perioperative parathyroid disease management is close monitoring of serum ionized calcium and correction of electrolyte and fluid abnormalities. Alterations in serum proteins, acid-base status, circulating lipid levels, serum osmolality, and other factors in the postoperative period distort the total serum calcium value, irrespective of ionized calcium levels. Total serum calcium does not accurately reflect ionized calcium concentrations.

Ionized Calcium

Calcium is important for normal cardiovascular and neuromuscular function. Ionized hypocalcemia predisposes to bradycardia, impaired cardiac contractility, hypotension, muscle weakness, muscular irritability, and tetany (including seizures) (see Table 12–11). The ECG may demonstrate ST-T wave changes and QT interval prolongation. However, life-threatening hypocalcemia can occur without ECG alterations. Circulating calcium levels may change rapidly depending on urine output, considering that diuresis increases calcium losses, and administration of chelating agents such as citrate in blood or phosphates.

Hypoparathyroidism can be controlled by maintaining circulating ionized calcium within normal levels. This goal is best accomplished with an intravenous infusion through a central venous catheter.

Emergency Treatment of Hypocalcemia

For emergency treatment of hypocalcemia, we recommend 10 ml of 10% calcium gluconate (93 mg of elemental calcium) over 10 minutes ("rule of 10s"). Note that calcium gluconate can be administered via a peripheral vein but calcium chloride cannot. For children, we recommend 2 mg·kg^{-1} elemental calcium. Most adult patients require 0.5 to 2 mg of elemental calcium per kilogram per hour to maintain normal levels. Dosages vary greatly, however, and less calcium is required in patients with renal insufficiency. Symptoms of hypocalcemia resolve promptly after normalization of the ionized calcium level.

Hyperparathyroidism

Perioperative management of hyperparathyroidism can be divided into two major categories: parathyroid surgery and nonparathyroid surgery. Attempts to lower ionized calcium into the normal to slightly hypercalcemic range should be made before surgery. Treatment usually consists of hydration and diuresis. Organ dysfunction may be precipitated in patients with severe hypercalcemia. Mildly hypercalcemic hyperparathyroid patients tolerate nonparathyroid surgery in the same way as their eucalcemic counterparts.

Parathyroid Surgery

Response to parathyroid surgery depends on the underlying cause of the hyperparathyroidism. Most patients have a single parathyroid adenoma. The remaining parathyroid glands are normal and suppressed by the hypercalcemia. These patients are hypercalcemic before parathyroid gland removal but develop acute hypocalcemia afterward. The degree of hypocalcemia depends on the preoperative level of hypercalcemia (gland suppression) and underlying bone disease.

Severe Hypercalcemia. Patients with severe preoperative hypercalcemia and extensive bone disease develop severe postoperative hypocalcemia as a result of parathyroid gland suppression and bone uptake of calcium. This has been termed the *hungry bone syndrome.* Hypocalcemia develops within a few hours after surgery. The frequency of ionized calcium measurement is dictated by the degree of underlying disease. We recommend that ionized calcium levels be monitored every 30 to 60 minutes in the immediate postoperative period until a trend is apparent. These patients often require postoperative calcium replacement to prevent cardiovascular and neuromuscular compromise.

Mild to Moderate Hypercalcemia. Patients with less severe disease are more commonly encountered today, and most may be treated without exogenous calcium. Mild hypocalcemia develops after surgery, but eucalcemia usually is restored within 24 to 48 hours as the remaining parathyroid glands recover. We recommend monitoring ionized calcium levels every 4 to 6 hours until eucalcemia is restored. Do not over-replace calcium in the early postoperative period, because elevated ionized calcium levels impair recovery of the suppressed glands.

Glandular Hyperplasia. Patients may also develop hyperparathyroidism as a result of glandular hyperplasia. This process involves all the parathyroid glands. Hypocalcemia is unusual unless all parathyroid tissue is removed. Less than half of one parathyroid gland is needed to maintain normal circulating calcium levels. Surgery in these patients usually involves removal of three and one half of the four glands.

Some patients have all glands removed and have some of the removed tissue transplanted to another site such as the arm. Failure of calcium levels to normalize in the postoperative period suggests either the presence of more than four glands (some patients have as many as six to eight glands), failure to remove enough glandular tissue, or the presence of metastatic parathyroid carcinoma.

What Are the Perioperative Complications?

Anatomic

Complications of surgery for hyperparathyroidism relate to anatomic and metabolic alterations. Anatomic complications include bleeding, infection, and pain. Edema and bleeding in the neck can result in acute airway compromise. Damage to the recurrent laryngeal nerve may also result in airway compromise.

Metabolic

Metabolic complications result primarily from alterations in the circulating calcium level. Hypocalcemia commonly causes cardiovascular (i.e., hypotension, bradydysrhythmias) and neuromuscular symptoms (i.e., weakness, seizures, laryngeal spasm, tetany) (see Table 12–11). Hypercalcemia commonly results in CNS depression, hypertension, polyuria, and organ dysfunction (see Table 12–11). Organ dysfunction includes

renal tubular dysfunction, nephrocalcinosis, nephrolithiasis, renal insufficiency, gastrointestinal dysfunction, and psychiatric abnormalities.

Drug Interactions

A number of drugs have important interactions with calcium. Thiazide diuretics enhance renal tubular calcium reabsorption and may precipitate hypercalcemia. In contrast, loop diuretics increase calcium excretion and may cause hypocalcemia in patients with hypoparathyroidism. Glucocorticoids antagonize the actions of vitamin D on the gut and reduce calcium absorption. Drugs like phenytoin and others that induce hepatic microsomal oxidases increase metabolism of vitamin D. Aluminum and magnesium hydroxide antacids precipitate calcium in the gut and limit its absorption. Cholestyramine binds vitamin D and prevents its gut absorption.

DIABETES MELLITUS

How Is Blood Glucose Regulated?

Diabetes mellitus represents abnormal regulation of blood glucose due to either an absolute or relative deficiency of insulin or relative resistance to the action of insulin. The blood glucose level is dependent on the interplay between glucose production and glucose use. Glucose production in the fasting state results from metabolic processes in the liver, fat, and muscle.[75] During states of fasting, blood glucose is maintained within normal ranges by the breakdown of preformed glycogen in tissues and gluconeogenesis from amino acids. Peripheral mobilization of amino acids depends on low levels of insulin and increases (acting as counter-regulatory hormones) in glucagon, cortisol, growth hormone, and epinephrine.[76, 77] During acute illness and surgery, other factors come into play as well (Fig. 12–1).

Insulin Deficiency

Relative insulin deficiency also allows mobilization of free fatty acids from adipose tissue, shifting the body's energy consumption to that of lipids. Blood glucose is conserved for tissues, such as the brain, that cannot use fatty acids.[78, 79] The fatty acids released can be taken up by the liver, converted to ketones, and oxidized by nonhepatic tissues such as the brain to provide back-up substrate for the CNS should hepatic glucose production fail.[80] These changes characterize the fasting or postprandial state. They end at the next meal, and no significant ketosis or acidosis develops.

When the postprandial state is extended and an individual does not eat for a prolonged period, ketone concentrations increase to the range of 2 to 4 $mmol \cdot L^{-1}$. Higher ketone levels do not occur because ketones stimulate insulin release.[81] This release of insulin prevents a further increase in rate of adipose tissue breakdown, thereby fixing ketosis in a relatively safe range by limiting substrate production.[81]

Diabetic Ketoacidosis

DKA results from a lack of insulin or from stress-induced counter-regulatory hormone release that overrides the amount of insulin. As a result, the concentrations of ketone bodies and

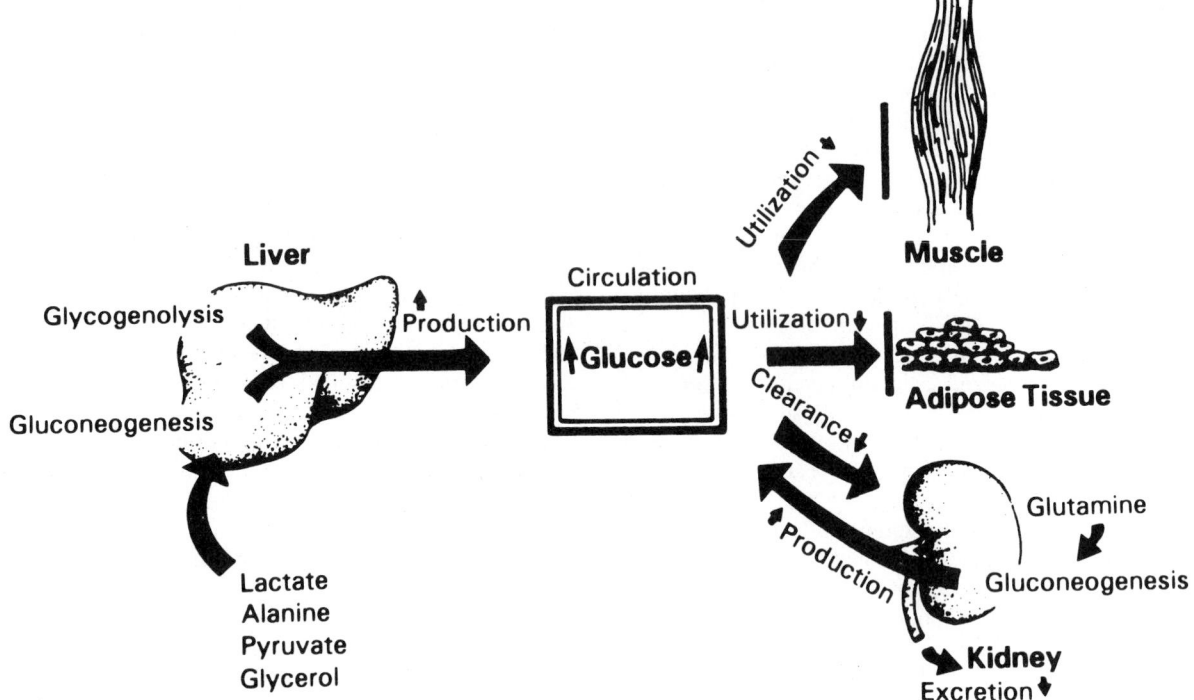

FIGURE 12–1. Factors raising the blood glucose concentration during acute illness and surgery. Increased production is secondary to enhanced glycogenolysis and gluconeogenesis in the liver and to renal gluconeogenesis during fasting. Clearance of glucose from the circulation is decreased as relative insulin deficiency inhibits entry of glucose into both muscle and fat tissue. If dehydration is severe, renal excretion of glucose also decreases. (Adapted with permission from Schade DS: Surgery and diabetes. Med Clin North Am 1988; 72:1531.)

free fatty acids rise uncontrollably and produce the marked acidosis that characterizes the DKA state.

Summary

During states of fasting, glucose remains in the normal range as a result of increased hepatic glucose production. After a meal, blood glucose is maintained from exogenous sources. The rise in blood glucose stimulates the β-cells of the pancreas to produce insulin, and the increase in insulin level peripherally reduces or inhibits fat mobilization and muscle breakdown. The body shifts to an anabolic state in which fuel such as glucose and fat is stored. Thus, normal glucose homeostasis requires adequate production of glucose from the liver, adequate stores of both fat and muscle, and adequate reserve of insulin from the pancreas.

What is Diabetes Mellitus?

Diabetes mellitus can be categorized into two major types.[82, 83]

Type I

Type I diabetes mellitus is characterized by an absolute destruction of the pancreatic β-cells. It is believed to be autoimmune in origin, and islet cell antibodies are demonstrable.

Clinically, these patients have their disease onset at a younger age than in type II, and the diagnosis is made acutely, either in the form of severe weight loss and the demonstration of hyperglycemia or by the presentation of DKA.[82, 83] Treatment consists of lifelong insulin administration combined with a diet and exercise program.

Type II

Type II diabetes mellitus is associated with diminished insulin action or insulin resistance. A deficiency in the timing of insulin release is also present. Generally, these patients are obese and older at onset (i.e., >40 years).[82, 83] However, the disease may also present at younger ages.

Characteristics

Patients with type I diabetes mellitus usually present with severe hyperglycemia because of ketosis and the absolute or relative deficiency of insulin. These patients are placed on insulin at the time of diagnosis.

Type II diabetes mellitus may be treated with diet and exercise only, with oral agents, or with insulin. The diagnosis may have been made when a patient was asymptomatic or complained of fatigue or weakness of many months' duration. These cases are diagnosed when an elevated fasting blood sugar >140 mg · dL^{-1} is found on two occasions but ketosis is not identified in the blood. They may have elevated basal or postprandial insulin levels at diagnosis, reflecting an insulin-resistant state. Patients with type II diabetes mellitus often describe a history of being treated with diet and exercise for several months, followed by the initiation of oral agents, and then, after failing control by oral agents, the initiation of insulin therapy.

Regardless of the diabetic state, both type I and type II diabetic patients frequently develop complications resulting from tissue injury. A thorough history should be taken and a review of systems carried out on all patients before surgery. Specific questions relevant to the diabetic state should be asked.

Visual Disturbances

Transient decrease in vision after meals may reflect osmotic changes in the lens of the eye due to poor metabolic control. Patients may complain of a gradual decrease in vision over years, reflecting an underlying retinopathy. An ophthalmologic consult may be important for detecting and treating active bleeding in the eyes, cataracts, and retinopathy.

Gastrointestinal Problems

Patients may complain of nausea and vomiting or postprandial fullness due to gastroparesis secondary to autonomic neuropathy. This finding increases their risk for aspiration during induction of anesthesia. Intermittent episodes of diarrhea may reflect bacterial overgrowth resulting from decreased intestinal motility.

Genitourinary Problems

Urinary incontinence or frequent urinary tract infections may indicate genitourinary involvement. Rarely is gross hematuria related to the diabetic condition. Males may complain of failure to obtain an erection, secondary to either vascular or neuropathic conditions.

Peripheral Neuropathy

Patients may report a long history of paresthesias or numbness in the hands and feet as a result of peripheral neuropathy.

Cardiovascular Symptoms

Finally, conditions such as shortness of breath, dizziness on exertion, and chest pain should be sought in every diabetic patient, because these may reflect underlying cardiovascular disease that could alter the type of anesthesia and timing of surgery. Significantly, many of these patients suffer from silent myocardial ischemia; therefore, absence of cardiac symptoms should not be construed to rule out significant coronary artery disease.

What Assessment Should Be Made?

Physical Examination

A physical examination should be performed to assess diabetic complications. If a change in the vision is suspected, the eyes should be checked for evidence of hemorrhages or exudates. Irregularities in the pulse or orthostatic blood pressure changes may denote autonomic neuropathy. In addition, the physical examination should test proprioceptive and vibratory sense in the upper and lower extremities to assess for evidence of peripheral neuropathy. Cardiac, pulmonary, and extremity examinations may reveal evidence of cardiac failure, and the extremities should be evaluated for vascular insufficiency.

Blood Glucose Control

Blood glucose should be measured to assess diabetic control. Review of home blood glucose measurements also aids in the assessment of antecedent diabetic control. An objective way to determine antecedent control if a patient is unable to provide a reliable history is to measure glycosylated hemoglobin, which reflects average blood glucose during the 2 to 3 months before surgery.[84, 85]

Renal Function

Renal function should be evaluated by measuring BUN and serum creatinine levels. Comparison with previous values aids in determining progressive renal disease. Creatinine clearance and protein excretion values are also helpful. Adjustment of medications for renal insufficiency may be in order. Other valuable laboratory tests include serum electrolyte determinations (especially potassium), blood cell counts, and assessment of acid-base status.

How Is Diabetes Managed Perioperatively?

No consensus has been reached on a single treatment regimen for perioperative management of diabetes. Many successful approaches have been described.[86–92] The reason for diversity resides in the fact that diabetic patients are a heterogeneous group, encompassing patients with relatively well-preserved insulin secretory function to those with absolute deficiency of endogenous insulin production. In addition, they exhibit various degrees of insulin resistance, obesity, and complications (eyes, heart, kidneys, and neuropathic syndromes). The surgery to be performed also needs to be considered; one standard perioperative protocol may not be appropriate for all types of surgery. For these reasons, an individualized approach to perioperative care is recommended.

Complication Assessment

Based on review of the history, physical examination, laboratory test results, and consultation with the primary care physician, one should have a good understanding of a patient's condition and potential problems to be encountered. Of primary concern are those complications that may require special consideration in the perioperative period, such as pre-existing hypertension, cardiac conduction disturbances, atherosclerotic cardiovascular disease, renal insufficiency, and autonomic neuropathy.

Glucose Monitoring

Bedside capillary blood glucose monitoring is strongly encouraged during the perioperative period. Patients should be checked frequently, and insulin adjustments made. Stabilization of the blood glucose level before surgery is important. The average blood glucose goal should be 200 to 250 mg · dL^{-1}. This value should minimize the chances of hypoglycemia and preventing severe hyperglycemia.

Insulin Therapy

Insulin administration should be considered in every diabetic patient anticipating surgery. Insulin needs increase after the stress of surgery owing to the production of counter-regulatory hormones. Insulin is of primary importance in preventing hyperglycemia and inhibiting fat mobilization, which may precipitate and worsen ketone production. Therefore, with the exception of patients with diet-controlled type II diabetes, all other diabetic patients anticipating surgery usually require insulin administration.[93]

Route of Administration

The route of administration of insulin (i.e., subcutaneous, intravenous, or intramuscular) should be based on each individual case and the preference of the anesthesiologist. An individual who is well controlled by oral agents and is anticipating a short surgical procedure may be an appropriate candidate for subcutaneous or intramuscular insulin. However, a brittle type I diabetic patient undergoing a more extensive procedure benefits most from a continuous intravenous insulin infusion managed by an intensivist or endocrinologist and frequent monitoring of blood glucose levels. A consideration of the type and duration of surgery is the major determining factor in deciding on appropriate insulin dosing during surgery (Table 12–12).

Several regimens have been advocated for managing diabetes during surgery.[86–92] Insulin stimulates intracellular glucose, potassium, phosphorus, and magnesium entry. Thus, it is essential that one also monitor levels of these electrolytes.

TABLE 12–12. Intravenous Insulin Infusion for Maintenance of Glucose Homeostasis in Insulin-Dependent Patients

A	B
• Thin	• Obese
• Minimum illness, minimum surgery	• Severe illness, major surgery
• Usual insulin requirement <50 U/day	• Usual insulin requirement >50 U/day
• Infusion fluid: 1 L sodium chloride (0.45 mol · L^{-1}) plus 20 mEq · L^{-1} potassium chloride plus 500 U heparin plus 50 U rapid-acting insulin	• Infusion fluid: 1 L sodium chloride (0.45 mol · L^{-1}) plus 20 mEq · L^{-1} potassium chloride plus 500 U heparin plus 100 U rapid-acting insulin

Blood Glucose Concentration (mg · dL^{-1})	Infusion Rate (mL · h^{-1})	A Insulin (U · h^{-1})	B Insulin (U · h^{-1})
0–50	5	0.25	0.50
5–100	10	0.50	1.00
100–150	15	0.75	1.50
150–200	20	1.00	2.00
200–250	25	1.25	2.50
250–300	30	1.50	3.00
300–350	35	1.75	3.50
350–400	40	2.00	4.00
>400	50	3.00	6.00

(Adapted from Schade DS: Surgery and diabetes. Med Clin North Am 1988; 72:1531.)

Changes in potassium occur the fastest and can precipitate lethal dysrhythmias. Note that potassium is included in both of the intravenous insulin infusion regimens shown in Table 12–12.

Same-Day Surgery

Patients anticipating same-day surgery for minor procedures are usually not allowed intake of food or drink after midnight. A patient's evening NPH or Lente insulin should be reduced by 10% to 20% to decrease the possibility of morning hypoglycemia.[93]

Once a patient arrives at the hospital, blood glucose is measured and a 5% dextrose solution infusion is begun at 100 mL · h^{-1}. We then recommend giving two thirds of the customary morning NPH or Lente insulin dose subcutaneously, plus regular insulin as sliding scale coverage.[93] A suggested sliding scale consists of 3 to 5 units of regular insulin for every 50 mg · dL^{-1} of measured glucose above the presurgical goal of 200 mg · dL^{-1}.[93] Blood glucose is measured at 3- to 4-hour intervals, and regular insulin administered accordingly.

After surgery and recovery from anesthesia, the lunch meal may be served, the dextrose discontinued, and the patient discharged provided that the blood glucose level is believed to be stable at <250 mg · dL^{-1}.[93] Frequent blood glucose checks by patients are recommended, and a regular routine is encouraged.

Major Surgery/Uncontrolled Blood Glucose

Major surgical procedures or surgery in a diabetic patient with uncontrolled blood glucose should be performed using continuous intravenous infusion of glucose and insulin. Frequent monitoring of blood glucose levels is essential. One regimen for administering insulin is listed in Table 12–12. An alternate regimen is to mix 100 units of regular insulin in 200 ml of normal saline.[93] Twenty-five milliliters of solution is rapidly discarded through the intravenous tubing to coat the plastic because it absorbs insulin. The insulin infusion rate is started at 0.03 to 0.05 units · kg · h^{-1}. Blood glucose level is checked hourly, and the infusion rate increased or decreased to achieve a target blood glucose level of 200 to 250 mg · dL^{-1}.

Oral Agents

For those type II diabetic patients taking oral agents, consideration of the half-life is important. For example, if a patient is taking chlorpropamide, which has a long half-life, the dose should be halved the day before surgery and omitted completely on the day of surgery.[93] Other first- and second-generation shorter acting sulfonylureas may be discontinued the morning of surgery and restarted after resuming oral intake.

References

1. Baumann G: Acromegaly. Endocrinol Metab Clin North Am 1987; 16:685–703.
2. Molitch ME: Clinical manifestations of acromegaly. Endocrinol Metab Clin North Am 1992; 21:597–614.
3. Chang-DeMoranville BM, Jackson IMD: Diagnosis and endocrine testing in acromegaly. Endocrinol Metab Clin North Am 1992; 21:649–668.
4. Laws ER Jr: Pituitary surgery. Endocrinol Metab Clin North Am 1987; 16:647–665.

5. Fahlbusch R, Honegger J, Buchfelder M: Surgical management of acromegaly. Endocrinol Metab Clin North Am 1992; 21:669–692.

6. Jaffe CA, Barkan AL: Treatment of acromegaly with dopamine agonists. Endocrinol Metab Clin North Am 1992; 21:713–735.

7. Lamberts SWJ, Reubi JC, Krenning EP: Somatostatin analogs in the treatment of acromegaly. Endocrinol Metab Clin North Am 1992; 21:737–752.

8. Hall J, Robertson G: Diabetes insipidus. Problems in Critical Care 1990; 4:342–354.

9. Ober KP: Endocrine crises. Diabetes insipidus. Crit Care Clin 1991; 7:109–125.

10. Blevins LS Jr., Wand GS: Diabetes insipidus. Crit Care Med 1992; 20:69–79.

11. Miller M, Dalakos T, Moses AM, et al: Recognition of partial defects in antidiuretic hormone secretion. Ann Intern Med 1970; 73:721–729.

12. Zaloga GP: Hyperosmolar states. In Critical Care. 2nd ed. Civetta JM, Taylor RW, Kirby RR (eds). Philadelphia, JB Lippincott, 1992, pp 447–456.

13. Chanson P, Jedynak CP, Czernichow P: Management of early postoperative diabetes insipidus with parenteral desmopressin. Acta Endocrinol 1988; 117:513–516.

14. Robinson AG: DDAVP and the treatment of central diabetes insipidus. N Engl J Med 1976; 294:507–511.

15. Zaloga GP: Electrolyte disorders. In Critical Care. 2nd ed. Civetta JM, Taylor RW, Kirby RR (eds). Philadelphia, JB Lippincott, 1992, pp 481–505.

16. Sterns RH: The management of hyponatremic emergencies. Crit Care Clin 1991; 7:127–142.

17. Anderson RJ, Chung HM, Kluge R, et al: Hyponatremia: a prospective analysis of its epidemiology and the pathogenetic role of vasopressin. Ann Intern Med 1985; 102:164–168.

18. Chung HM, Kluge R, Schrier RW, et al: Postoperative hyponatremia. A prospective study. Arch Intern Med 1986; 146:333–336.

19. Zaloga GP, Hughes SS: Oliguria in patients with normal renal function. Anesthesiology 1990; 72:598–602.

20. Berl T: Treating hyponatremia: what is all the controversy about? Ann Intern Med 1990; 113:417–419.

21. Sterns RH: Severe hyponatremia: the case for conservative management. Crit Care Med 1992; 20:534–539.

22. Forrest JN Jr, Cox M, Hong C, et al: Superiority of demeclocycline over lithium in the treatment of chronic syndrome of inappropriate secretion of antidiuretic hormone. N Engl J Med 1978; 298:173–177.

23. Nelson DH: Cushing's syndrome. In Endocrinology. 2nd ed. Vol. 2. DeGroot LJ, Besser GM, Cahill GF et al (eds). Philadelphia, WB Saunders, 1989, pp 1660–1675.

24. Loriaux DL: The treatment of Cushing's syndrome and adrenal cancer. Endocrinol Metab Clin North Am 1991; 20:767–771.

25. Howlett TA, Rees LH, Besser GM: Cushing's syndrome. Clin Endocrinol Metab 1985; 14:911–945.

26. Gomez MT, Chrousos GP: Cushing's syndrome. In Current Therapy in Endocrinology and Metabolism. Bardin CW (ed). Philadelphia, BC Decker, 1991, pp 134–137.

27. Bethune JE: The diagnosis and treatment of adrenal insufficiency. In Endocrinology. 2nd ed. Vol. 2. DeGroot LJ, Besser GM, Cahill GF, et al (eds). Philadelphia, WB Saunders, 1989, pp 1647–1659.

28. Burke CW: Adrenocortical insufficiency. Clin Endocrinol Metab 1985; 14:947–976.

29. Muir A, Maclaren NK: Adrenocortical insufficiency. In Current Therapy in Endocrinology and Metabolism. Bardin CW (ed). Philadelphia, BC Decker, 1991, pp 124–129.

30. Chin R: Adrenal crisis. Crit Care Clin 1991; 7:23–42.

31. Oelkers W, Diederich S, Bahr V: Diagnosis and therapy surveillance in Addison's disease: rapid adrenocorticotropin (ACTH) test and measurement of plasma ACTH, renin activity, and aldosterone. J Clin Endocrinol Metab 1992; 75:259–264.

32. Christy NP: Corticosteroid withdrawal. In Current Therapy in Endocrinology and Metabolism. Bardin CW (ed). Philadelphia, BC Decker, 1991, pp 116–124.

33. Schlaghecke R, Kronely E, Santen RT, et al: The effect of long-term glucocorticoid therapy on pituitary-adrenal responses to exogenous corticotropin-releasing hormone. N Engl J Med 1992; 326:226–230.

34. Christy NP: Pituitary-adrenal function during corticosteroid therapy. Learning to live with uncertainty. N Engl J Med 1992; 326:266–267.

35. Amatruda TT Jr, Hurst MM, D'Esopo ND: Certain endocrine and metabolic facets of the steroid withdrawal syndrome. J Clin Endocrinol Metab 1965; 25:1207–1217.

36. Jasani MK, Freeman PA, Boyle JA, et al: Studies of the rise in plasma 11-hydroxycorticosteroids (11-OHCS) in corticosteroid-treated patients with rheumatoid arthritis during surgery: correlations with the functional integrity of the hypothalamo-pituitary-adrenal axis. Q J Med 1968; 37:407–421.

37. Kehlet H, Binder C: Adrenocortical function and clinical course during and after surgery in unsupplemented glucocorticoid-treated patients. Br J Anaesth 1973; 45:1043–1048.

38. Loriaux DL, Nieman L: Corticotropin-releasing hormone testing in pituitary disease. Endocrinol Metab Clin North Am 1991; 20:363–369.

39. Graber AL, Ney RI, Nicholson WE, et al: Natural history of pituitary-adrenal recovery following long-term suppression with corticosteroids. J Clin Endocrinol Metab 1965; 25:11–16.

40. Christy NP: Principles of systemic corticosteroid therapy in nonendocrine disease. In Current Therapy in Endocrinology and Metabolism. Bardin CW (ed). Philadelphia, BC Decker, 1991, pp 109–116.

41. Raum WJ: Pheochromocytoma. In Current Therapy in Endocrinology and Metabolism. 4th ed. Bardin CW (ed). Philadelphia, BC Decker, 1991, pp 152–158.

42. Hull CJ: Phaeochromocytoma. Diagnosis, preoperative preparation and anesthetic management. BR J Anaesth 1986; 58:1453–1468.

43. Shapiro B, Fig LM: Management of pheochromocytoma. Endocrinol Metab Clin North Am 1989; 18:443–481.

44. Bravo EL, Gifford RW Jr: Current concepts. Pheochromocytoma: diagnosis, localization and management. N Engl J Med 1984; 311:1298–1303.

45. Sheps SG, Jiang NS, Klee GG, et al: Recent developments in the diagnosis and treatment of pheochromocytoma. Mayo Clin Proc 1990; 65:88–95.

46. Mueller GL: Pheochromocytoma. Problems in Critical Care 1990; 4:372–381.

47. Shapiro B, Gross MD: Endocrine crises. Pheochromocytoma. Crit Care Clin 1991; 7:1–21.

48. Smallridge RC: Metabolic and anatomic thyroid emergencies: a review. Crit Care Med 1992; 20:276–291.

49. Burch HB, Wartofsky L: Hyperthyroidism. In Current Therapy in Endocrinology and Metabolism. 4th ed. Bardin CW (ed). Philadelphia, BC Decker, 1991, pp 58–64.

50. Benua RS, Becker DV: Thyroid storm. In Current Therapy in Endocrinology and Metabolism 4th ed. Bardin CW (ed). Philadelphia, BC Decker, 1991, pp 68–70.

51. Klein I, Ojamaa K: Clinical review 36: cardiovascular manifestations of endocrine disease. J Clin Endocrinol Metab 1992; 75:339–342.

52. Gaitan E, Cooper DS: Primary hypothyroidism. In Current Therapy in Endocrinology and Metabolism. 4th ed. Bardin CW (ed). Philadelphia, BC Decker, 1991, pp 75–78.

53. Rapoport B: Myxedema coma. In Current Therapy in Endocrinology and Metabolism. 4th ed. Bardin CW (ed). Philadelphia, BC Decker, 1991, pp 79–82.

54. Zaloga GP, Smallridge RC: Thyroidal alterations in acute illness. Semin Respir Med 1985; 7:95–107.

55. Zaloga GP, Chernow B, Smallridge RC, et al: A longitudinal evaluation of thyroid function in critically ill surgical patients. Ann Surg 1985; 201:456–464.

56. Borst GC, Eil C, Burman KD: Euthyroid hyperthyroxinemia. Ann Intern Med 1983; 98:366–378.

57. Becker RA, Vaughan GM, Ziegler MG, et al: Hypermetabolic low triiodothyronine syndrome of burn injury. Crit Care Med 1982; 10:870–875.

58. Brent GA, Hershman JM: Thyroxine therapy in patients with nonthyroidal illnesses and low serum thyroxine concentration. J Clin Endocrinol Metab 1986; 63:1–8.

59. Alfonso A, Christoudias G, Amaruddin Q, et al: Tracheal or esophageal compression due to benign thyroid disease. Am J Surg 1981; 142:350–354.

60. Miller MR, Pincock AC, Oates GD, et al: Upper airway obstruction due to goiter: detection, prevalence and results of surgical management. Q J Med 1990; 74:177–188.

61. Weinberg AD, Brennan MD, Gorman CA, et al: Outcome of anesthesia and surgery in hypothyroid patients. Arch Intern Med 1983; 143:893–897.

62. Ladenson PW, Levin AA, Ridgway EC, et al: Complications of surgery in hypothyroid patients. Am J Med 1984; 77:261–266.

63. Drucker DJ, Burrow GN: Cardiovascular surgery in the hypothyroid patient. Arch Intern Med 1985; 145:1585–1587.

64. Becker C: Hypothyroidism and atherosclerotic heart disease: pathogenesis, medical management, and the role of coronary artery bypass surgery. Endocr Rev 1985; 6:432–440.

65. Zaloga GP: Electrolyte disorders. In Critical Care. 2nd ed. Civetta JM, Taylor RW, Kirby RR (eds). Philadelphia, JB Lippincott, 1992, pp 481–505.

66. Zaloga GP: Hypocalcemic crisis. Crit Care Clin 1991; 7:191–200.

67. Davis KD, Attie MF: Management of severe hypercalcemia. Crit Care Clin 1991; 7:175–190.

68. Zaloga GP: Calcium disorders. Problems in Critical Care 1990; 4:382–401.

69. Mundy GR: Calcium Homeostasis—Hypercalcemia and Hypocalcemia. London, England, Martin Dunitz, 1989, pp 1–240.

70. Downs RW Jr: Hypocalcemia and hypoparathyroidism. *In* Current Therapy in Endocrinology and Metabolism. 4th ed. Bardin CW (ed). Philadelphia, BC Decker, 1991, pp 440–444.

71. Bilezikian JP: Primary hyperparathyroidism. *In* Current Therapy in Endocrinology and Metabolism. 4th ed. Bardin CW (ed). Philadelphia, BC Decker, 1991, pp 448–452.

72. Zaloga GP, Chernow B: Divalent ions: calcium, magnesium, and phosphorus. *In* The Pharmacologic Approach to the Critically Ill Patient. 3rd ed. Chernow B, Holaday JW, Zaloga GP, Zaritsky AL (eds). Baltimore, William & Wilkins, in press.

73. Zaloga GP, Chernow B, Cook D, et al: Assessment of calcium homeostasis in the critically ill patient. The diagnostic pitfalls of the McLean Hastings nomogram. Ann Surg 1985; 202:587–594.

74. Ladenson JH, Lewis JW, Boyd JC: Failure of total calcium corrected for protein, albumin, and pH to correctly assess free calcium status. J Clin Endocrinol Metab 1978; 46:986–993.

75. Foster DW, McGarry JD: Intermediary metabolism of carbohydrates, lipids, and proteins. *In* Harrison's Principles of Internal Medicine. 10th ed. Petersdorf RG, Adams RD, Braunwald E, et al (eds). New York, McGraw-Hill, 1983, pp 490–495.

76. McGarry JD, Foster DW: Hormonal control of ketogenesis. Biochemical considerations. Arch Intern Med 1977; 137:495–501.

77. Unger RH, Orci L: Glucagon and the A cell: physiology and pathophysiology. N Engl J Med 1981; 304:1518–1524, 1574–1580.

78. Ruderman NB, Aoki TT, Cohill GF Jr: Gluconeogenesis and its disorders in man. *In* Gluconeogenesis: Its Regulation in Mammalian Species. Hanson RW, Mehlman MA (eds). New York, John Wiley & Sons, 1976, pp 515–532.

79. Cahill GF Jr: Starvation in man. N Engl J Med 1970; 282: 668–675.

80. Drenick EJ, Alvarez LC, Tamasi GC, et al: Resistance to symptomatic insulin reactions after fasting. J Clin Invest 1972; 51:2757–2762.

81. Foster DW, McGarry JD: Acute complications of diabetes: ketoacidosis, hyperosmolar coma, lactic acidosis. *In* Endocrinology. 2nd ed. Vol. 2. DeGroot LJ, Besser GM, Cahill GF, et al (eds). Philadelphia, WB Saunders 1989, pp 1439–1453.

82. National Diabetes Data Group: Classification and diagnosis of diabetes mellitus and other categories of glucose intolerance. Diabetes 1979; 28:1039–1057.

83. Genuth S: Classification and diagnosis of diabetes mellitus. Clinical Diabetes 1983; 1:1–20.

84. Gabbay KH, Hasty K, Breslow JL, et al: Glycosylated hemoglobins and long-term blood glucose control in diabetes mellitus. J Clin Endocrinol Metab 1977; 44:859–864.

85. Gonen B, Rubenstein A, Rochman H, et al: Haemoglobin A_1: an indicator of metabolic control of diabetic patients. Lancet 1977; 2:734–737.

86. Shuman CR: Surgery and diabetes. *In* Diabetes Mellitus: Diagnosis and Treatment. Ellenberg M, Rifkin H (eds). New Hyde Park, NY, Medical Examination Publishers, Inc., 1983, pp 679–687.

87. Alberti KG, Gill GV, Elliot MJ: Insulin delivery during surgery in the diabetic patient. Diabetes Care 1982; 5:65–77.

88. Fetchick DA, Fischer JS: Perioperative management of the patient with diabetes mellitus undergoing outpatient or elective surgery. Clin Podiatr Med Surg 1987; 4:439–443.

89. Fletcher J, Langman MJS, Kellock TD: Effect of surgery on blood-sugar levels in diabetes mellitus. Lancet 1965; 2:52–54.

90. Gallina DL, Mordes JP, Rossini AA: Surgery in the diabetic patient. Compr Ther 1983; 9:8–16.

91. Galloway JA, Shuman CR: Diabetes and surgery. A study of 667 cases. Am J Med 1963; 34:177–191.

92. Schade DS: Surgery and diabetes. Med Clin North Am 1988; 72:1531–1543.

93. Kreines K: Diabetes management during same-day surgery or procedures. Clinical Diabetes 1992; 10:52–54.

CHAPTER 13

Radiology Consultation

JESSE L. CHAI, M.D.
CARL E. RAVIN, M.D.

The purpose of this chapter is to demonstrate normal plain film anatomy of the thorax, neck, and abdomen and to illustrate pathologic processes in these regions that are of clinical concern to an anesthesiologist.

THE THORAX

What Factors Affect Chest Radiograph Assessment?

Initial review of a chest radiograph should include assessment of the radiographic technique, patient positioning, and lung volumes. Understanding the factors that vary from radiograph to radiograph enables an observer to discriminate more easily between technical variation, true pathology, and normal anatomy.

Position of X-Ray Film

Most preoperative chest films are taken with a patient standing at a 6-foot focal-film distance (from the x-ray tube to the x-ray film) and are exposed at full inspiration. Almost all normal radiographic measurements of structures in the thorax are defined only for the standard erect posteroanterior (PA) chest film.

However, most films of critically ill patients, such as those in intensive care units, are performed in an anteroposterior (AP) projection with a patient supine and a focal-film distance of 40 to 48 inches. Because of the physics involved, this alteration in technique results in significant magnification of many intrathoracic structures, particularly those located more anteriorly in the chest, such as the heart. In addition, the change in position from erect to supine often results in increased venous volume, causing additional enlargement of venous structures. Finally, low lung volumes may result in distortion of underlying lung parenchyma and apparent increase in heart size.

Patient Position

Interpreting radiographs of ill patients may be difficult. Rotation of a patient's body can confound findings. Not infre-

quently a patient is radiographed in a semierect position, which is particularly confusing, because the actual position can vary from almost supine to almost erect. Lung volumes are often low. Assessing patient positioning (generally indicated on the film by the technologist) is especially important when looking for pneumothoraces or pleural fluid because air and fluid move freely in the pleural space in the absence of adhesions. Thus, a pneumothorax would be visible in the apex of the chest with a patient in the erect position; with a patient supine, a pneumothorax would be anterior and medial and would be more difficult to see. Fluid would be posterior and basal with a patient in the erect position, and posterior and medial with a patient supine. In some cases, fluid actually is better seen in a lateral view if a patient must remain supine.

Radiographic Techniques

Moreover, radiographic technique can vary greatly from film to film, depending on the experience of the technologists. For the most part, any judgment regarding edema, pulmonary vascularity, and heart size should be made cautiously on low lung volume films. In addition, edema can appear worse with "light" underexposed films or appear improved with larger lung volumes or on "dark" overexposed films. A dark film should always be viewed over a bright light in addition to the standard "view box."

What Is the Normal Anatomy on the Chest Radiograph?

Chest radiography is invaluable in assessing placement of endotracheal tubes, central venous and pulmonary artery catheters, monitoring devices, or pacemakers. Understanding normal anatomy aids in identifying the location of these devices.

Figure 13–1 demonstrates the normal anatomy of a PA and lateral chest radiograph.[1-3]

Venous Structures

The subclavian vein is the continuation of the axillary vein and courses along the inner surface of the clavicle. It joins the

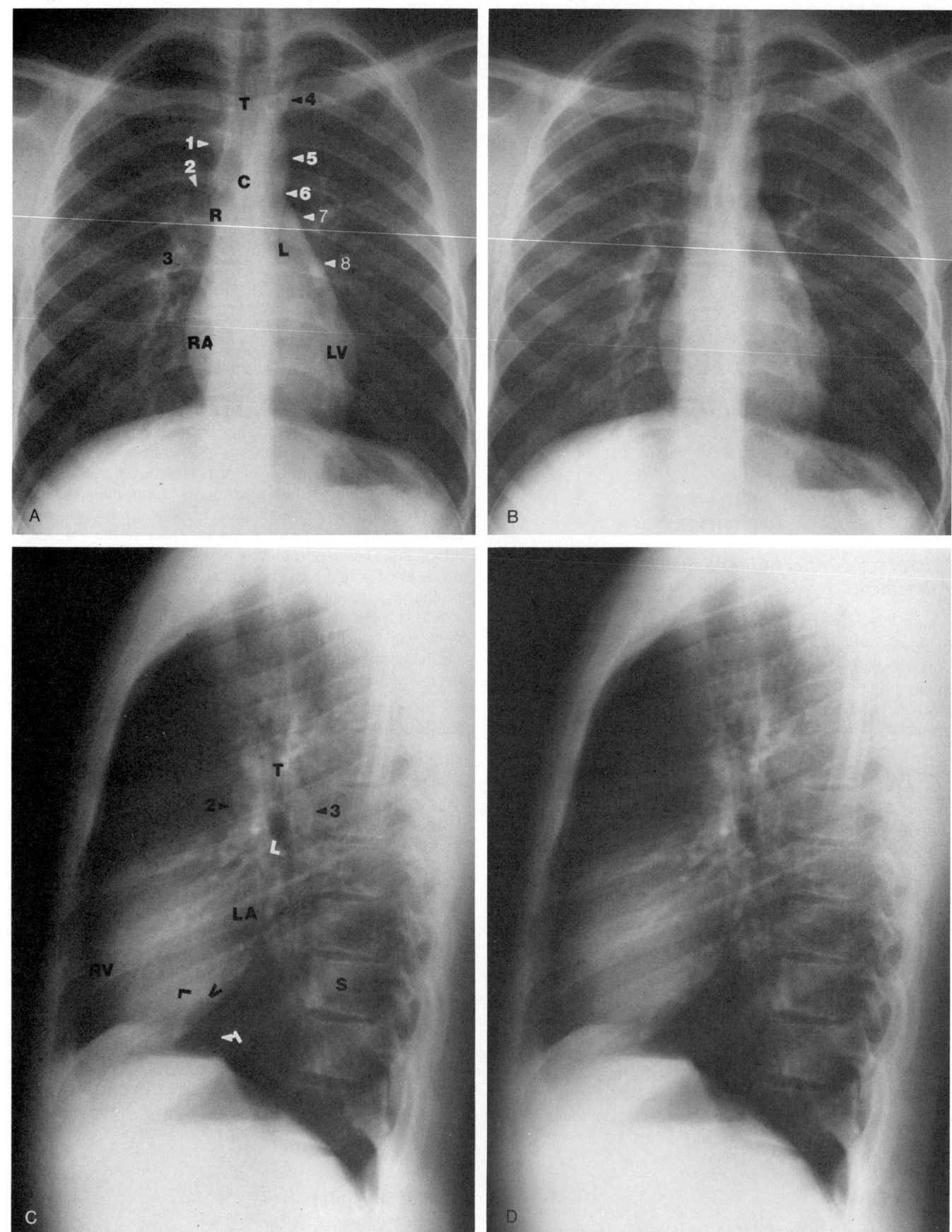

FIGURE 13–1. Normal chest film. *A,* PA view. T = trachea; C = carina; R = right mainstem bronchus; L = left mainstem bronchus; RA = right atrium; LV = left ventricle; 1 = superior vena cava; 2 = azygos vein; 3 = right interlobar pulmonary artery; 4 = left subclavian artery; 5 = aortic arch; 6 = pleural reflection from aorta onto main pulmonary artery; 7 = main pulmonary artery; 8 = left atrial appendage. *B,* Same PA view without labels. *C,* Lateral view. T = trachea; L = distal left mainstem bronchus; LA = left atrium; LV = left ventricle; RV = right ventricle; S = spine; 1 = inferior vena cava; 2 = right pulmonary artery; 3 = left pulmonary artery. The right upper lobe bronchus is not visualized on this film. *D,* Same lateral view without labels.

internal jugular vein to form the brachiocephalic vein behind the sternoclavicular joint. The left brachiocephalic vein courses obliquely downward and to the right; the right brachiocephalic vein passes directly downward behind the manubrium. The union of the brachiocephalic veins forms the superior vena cava (SVC), which then enters the right atrium. The right atrium is a border-forming structure of the normal cardiac silhouette on a frontal chest film. A normal-sized right ventricle is not seen on a frontal chest radiograph.

At about the level of T-4, the azygos vein arches forward over the right mainstem bronchus to empty into the back wall of the superior vena cava (Fig. 13–2). Enlargement of the azygos vein is seen in disease states that result in either elevated right heart end-diastolic pressures, tricuspid insufficiency, or increased venous return such as right-sided heart failure or inferior vena cava obstruction. A diameter of the azygos vein as seen en face of ≤10 mm on a standard PA chest radiograph is considered normal. A measurement >10 mm is considered pathologic except in pregnant women.[4]

Cardiomediastinal Silhouette

The left border of the cardiomediastinal silhouette is formed (superiorly to inferiorly) by the left subclavian artery, the aortic arch, the pleural reflection from the aorta onto the main pulmonary artery, the left border of the main pulmonary artery, the left atrial appendage, and the left ventricle.

On the lateral view, the right ventricle is the most anterior border-forming structure of the heart and normally abuts the sternum; it generally occupies no more than a third of the distance from the anterior costophrenic angle to the sternomanubrial joint.

The left ventricle is the chamber that most frequently enlarges in adults and tends to enlarge more posteriorly than laterally. An often quoted sign of left ventricular enlargement is the Hoffman-Rigler sign (Fig. 13–3).

Heart Size

The normal heart size on a standard PA chest radiograph ranges from 11.5 to 15.5 cm. The widely used 50% rule for describing the upper limits of normal for the cardiothoracic ratio should be used with caution because at least 10% of normal patients exceed this ratio. In addition, patients with a small heart that subsequently enlarges pathologically sometimes do not approach this 50% ratio.[5]

Airway and Pulmonary Arteries

On the frontal view, the trachea divides at the carina into the right and left mainstem bronchi at approximately the level of T-5. On the lateral view, the trachea ends in a rounded radiolucent structure that represents the distal left mainstem/left upper lobe bronchus (see Fig. 13–1C). Above the left mainstem bronchus, another rounded lucent structure representing the right upper lobe bronchus can occasionally be seen. The left pulmonary artery arches over the left mainstem bronchus. Projected anterior to the left mainstem bronchus is the right pulmonary artery.

Pulmonary Vasculature

Appreciation of normal pulmonary vascularity is best learned through experience. The normal pulmonary vasculature radiates from the hilum and branches toward the periphery of the lung. On an erect chest radiograph, the upper lung vessels are smaller and less numerous than those in the lower lungs because of differences in blood flow related to hydrostatic pressure differences. This discrepancy tends to disappear on a supine chest radiograph as the hydrostatic pressure differences between upper and lower lungs are eliminated.

What Are the Radiographic Findings in Emphysema?

The role of chest radiography in diagnosing emphysema has been the subject of contentious debate. Most radiologists are uncomfortable with the term *chronic obstructive pulmonary disease* because it describes function (or malfunction) and is therefore a clinical diagnosis. Emphysema, on the other hand, is defined structurally as "enlargement of air spaces distal to the terminal respiratory bronchiole accompanied by destruction of the alveolar walls."[6] Although some experts believe that emphysema is a pathologic diagnosis rather than a radiologic one, we are comfortable diagnosing emphysema because radiographs reflect structure. However, in general, when the disease is evident radiographically, clinical and physiologic clues to the diagnosis are also evident.

Hyperinflation

Various criteria have been proposed for diagnosing emphysema radiographically. Those relating to hyperinflation appear to be the most reproducible and reliable whereas those reflecting tissue destruction are subject to more intraobserver and interobserver variation.

Signs of hyperinflation include the following:

1. Depression and flattening of the hemidiaphragms with blunting of the costophrenic angles on the PA or lateral view. The contour of the hemidiaphragms is more important than the actual level. If the highest level of a hemidiaphragm is <1.5 cm above a line drawn from the costophrenic angle to the vertebrophrenic junction, then the diaphragm can be regarded as flat (Fig. 13–4).

2. Increased retrosternal space on the lateral view. Radiolucency measuring 2.5 cm or more from the sternum to the most anterior margin of the ascending aorta is considered abnormal.[7, 8]

Tissue Destruction

Discerning tissue destruction can be difficult. However, alterations of the normal dichotomous branching pattern of pulmonary vascularity with displacement of vessels around areas of pulmonary destruction is a reliable radiograhic sign. Increased lucency within the lungs corresponds to abnormal enlargement of air spaces associated with alveolar destruction. The lucencies may be focal or diffuse. Focal lucencies may reflect bullae, which are thin-walled air-filled spaces >1 cm (Fig. 13–5). They appear radiographically as well-demarcated avascular spaces. Blebs, another finding in emphysema, are collections of air within the layers of the visceral pleura.[9]

Pulmonary Artery Enlargement

Complications of emphysema or any other long-standing pulmonary disease include pulmonary arterial hypertension. A

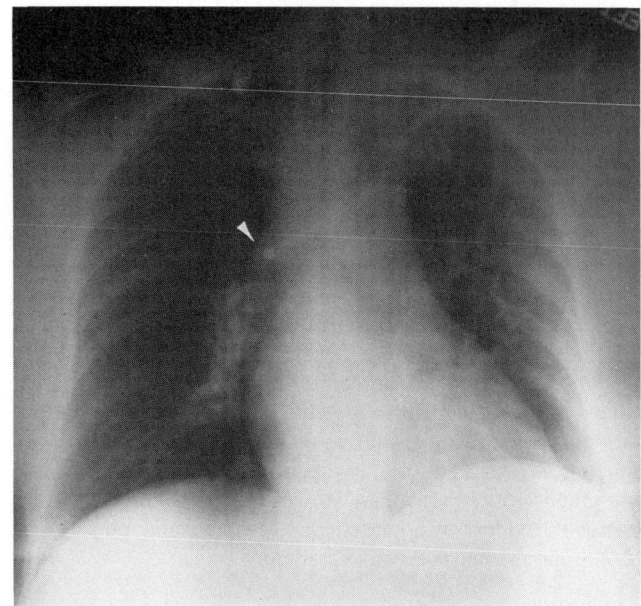

FIGURE 13–2. The course of the azygos vein is more clearly delineated on this film because of inadvertent placement of a catheter into the azygos vein. This left subclavian catheter traverses the left brachiocephalic vein and the superior vena cava and then courses posteriorly into the azygos vein. The distal 5 cm of the catheter is in the azygos vein *(arrowhead).* (Courtesy of James Chen, M.D.)

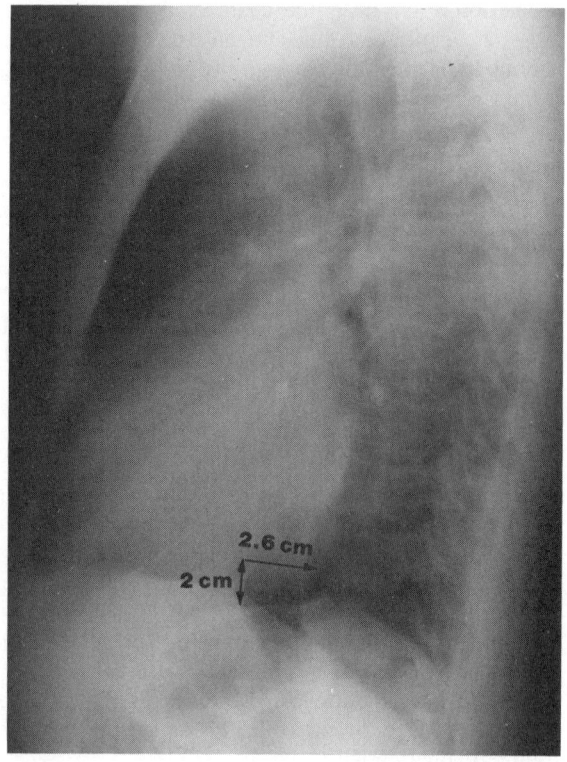

FIGURE 13–3. Hoffman-Rigler sign. On the lateral view, a measurement of >1.7 cm at a point 2 cm cephalad from the crossing of the inferior vena cava with the left ventricle indicates left ventricular enlargement. The measurement should be made on a plane parallel to the endplates of the vertebral bodies of the spine. This sign is not specific in the presence of a pectus excavatum deformity and right ventricular hypertrophy, since both of these processes tend to displace the left ventricle posteriorly even in the absence of left ventricular enlargement. Also, a true lateral film is required for utilization of this sign, since the left ventricle can be positioned more posteriorly on a rotated film. This 42-year-old male has marked left ventricular enlargement secondary to mitral valvular insufficiency. The measurement of 2.6 cm greatly exceeds the upper limits of normal.

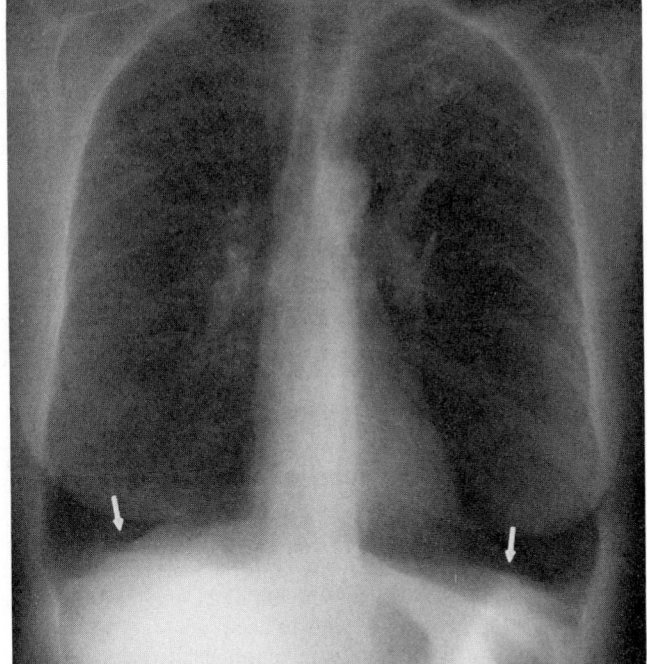

FIGURE 13–4. This 52-year-old female has emphysema from α_1-antitrypsin deficiency (A1AD) and is a candidate for lung transplantation. Note the marked flattening of the hemidiaphragms *(arrows)*. Also, the lower lungs are more lucent than the upper lungs and have fewer vascular markings. The emphysematous changes in α_1-antitrypsin deficiency are typically more prominent in the bases of the lungs.

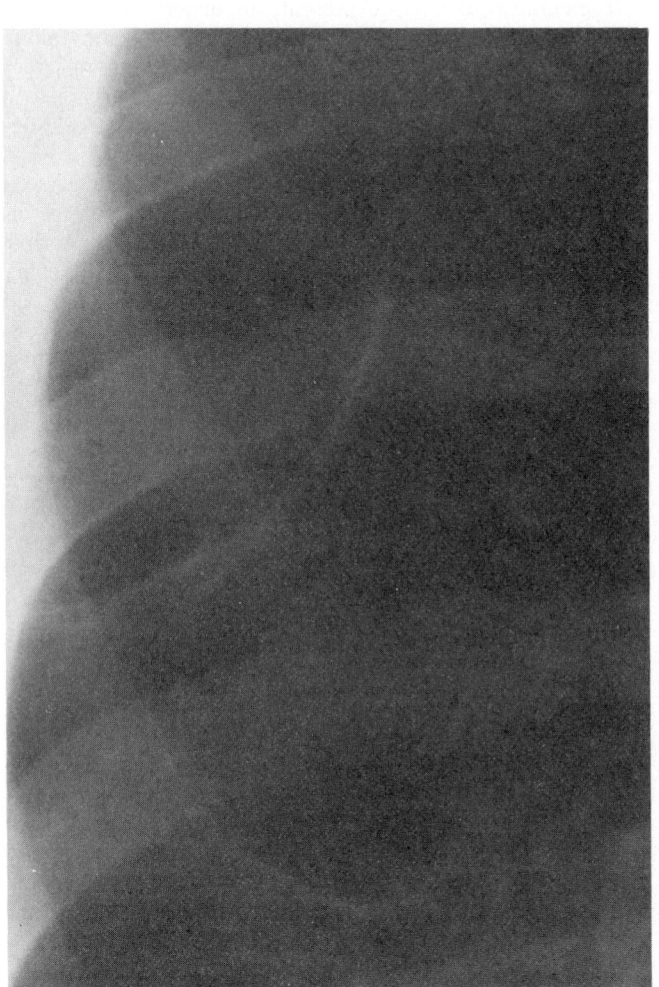

FIGURE 13–5. Bullae are seen radiographically as thin curvilinear lines demarcating avascular spaces.

characteristic finding is enlargement of the central pulmonary arteries (Fig. 13–6). Increase in diameter of the right descending (interlobar) pulmonary artery (>16 mm in males and >15 mm in females) has been shown to correlate well with the diagnosis of pulmonary arterial hypertension.[10]

Right Ventricular Hypertrophy

Long-standing pulmonary arterial hypertension can lead to right ventricular hypertrophy or cor pulmonale (Fig. 13–7). Roentgenologically, right ventricular hypertrophy may be difficult to detect, especially in emphysematous patients with generous lung volumes. Comparison with prior films is helpful to determine interval increase in size of the right ventricle.

What Are the Radiographic Findings of Pulmonary Edema?

When pulmonary capillary pressure is markedly increased or when the permeability of the capillary wall is increased above normal, excess fluid tends to accumulate in the interstitial space. When the quantity increases such that it fills the interstitial compartment, fluid then floods the alveoli.

Pulmonary Vasculature

Pulmonary edema most commonly results from elevated pulmonary venous pressure secondary to left-sided heart failure. Detecting early interstitial edema can be difficult and is subject to considerable interobserver variability. One of the earliest radiographic signs is loss of the normal sharp definition of the pulmonary vessels. With increasing venous pressure, vasoconstriction occurs in the lower lungs, and blood flow is redistributed from the lower to the upper lungs.

Later, septal lines may be present. The most common form, most often referred to as *Kerley B lines,* are short (<2 cm), straight, thin lines oriented perpendicular to the pleural surface and are most clearly seen along the lateral border of the lower lungs or in the retrosternal region (Fig. 13–8). Peribronchial thickening may be appreciated in the perihilar regions. Subpleural edema, which is manifested as thickened interlobar fissures, may also be noted.[11]

Cardiogenic Pulmonary Edema

Interstitial edema precedes alveolar edema. In cardiogenic alveolar edema, opacities are usually bilateral and symmetric but can be asymmetric and rarely unilateral. Typically, the opacities are irregular, ill defined, and scattered and are more confluent in the medial third of the lungs. The "butterfly" or "bat wing" pattern describes a distribution of alveolar edema in which the "medulla" of the lungs is consolidated with relative sparing of the "cortex," the peripheral 2 to 3 cm of the lungs. This pattern was initially described in and is more common with uremia but may also be seen in congestive heart failure.[12, 13]

Congestive Heart Failure

In congestive heart failure, the heart size is usually enlarged and pleural effusions are generally present. The left ventricle is the chamber that most commonly enlarges (Fig. 13–9). A normal heart size associated with cardiogenic edema is noted in acute myocardial infarctions or dysrhythmias (Fig. 13–10). Resolution of the edema generally begins peripherally and ends medially. The radiographic findings may lag behind the clinical findings but generally clear rapidly once therapy is instituted.

Noncardiogenic Pulmonary Edema

The pulmonary opacities of noncardiogenic pulmonary edema resemble those of cardiogenic edema. However, heart size is generally normal. Common causes include acute increase in intracranial pressure, inhalation of noxious substances, anaphylaxis, and drug reaction.

Adult Respiratory Distress Syndrome

The pulmonary edema of adult respiratory distress syndrome is generally associated with altered permeability of the pulmonary capillaries. The most common precipitating events include sepsis, hypotensive or hypovolemic shock, trauma, and pancreatitis. There is generally a delay of up to 12 hours between the clinical onset of respiratory failure and radiographic abnormality.

At 12 to 24 hours, patchy irregular opacities appear bilaterally and resemble those of cardiogenic edema. However, cardiomegaly, pleural effusions, and cephalization of the pulmonary vessels are generally absent unless these abnormalities were pre-existent.

If pleural effusions are present, an underlying infection, pulmonary infarction, or superimposed cardiogenic failure should be ruled out. At 24 to 48 hours, the patchy opacities coalesce into homogeneous consolidated regions. By 5 to 7 days, the consolidation often becomes inhomogeneous, suggesting improved aeration.

As aeration improves, a coarse reticular pattern is seen and corresponds pathologically to fibrin deposition on the alveolar walls. The radiographic findings may revert to normal in 2 to 3 weeks (Fig. 13–11) or may progress to pulmonary fibrosis.[11, 14, 15]

Mechanical ventilation improves lung expansion and consequently often improves the radiographic picture of diffuse pulmonary parenchymal disease even if clinical findings do not suggest improvement. Conversely, when mechanical support is discontinued, radiographic findings associated with hypoaerated lungs may falsely suggest worsening of the parenchymal process despite an improving clinical picture.[16]

What Are the Radiographic Findings of Pulmonary Barotrauma?

Pulmonary Interstitial Emphysema

When intra-alveolar pressure rises and an alveolus ruptures, air dissects along the bronchovascular bundle. Air in the interstitium is termed *pulmonary interstitial emphysema* (PIE). When positive-pressure ventilation is a cause of this complication, the bronchovascular sheaths dilate and become filled with air. Radiographically, these dilated structures resemble tortuous bubbles, 2 to 3 mm in diameter, which radiate outward from the hilum (Fig. 13–12). Inspiratory and expiratory films demonstrate that these structures do not decompress.

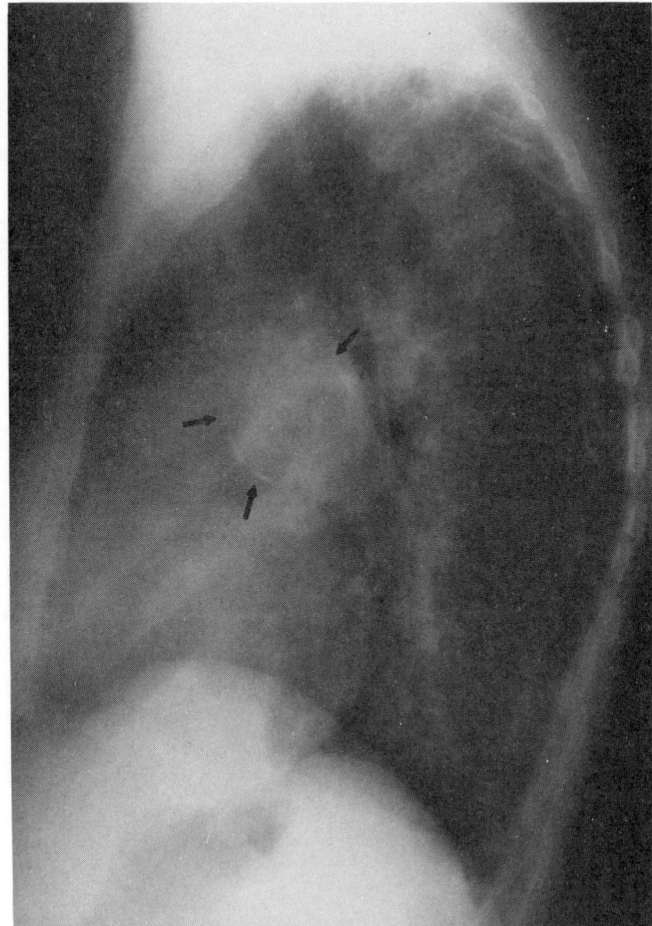

FIGURE 13–6. This 67-year-old woman has long-standing pulmonary arterial hypertension from an atrial septal defect. On the lateral view, the right pulmonary artery *(arrows)* is markedly enlarged and calcified. (Courtesy of Edward Patz, M.D.)

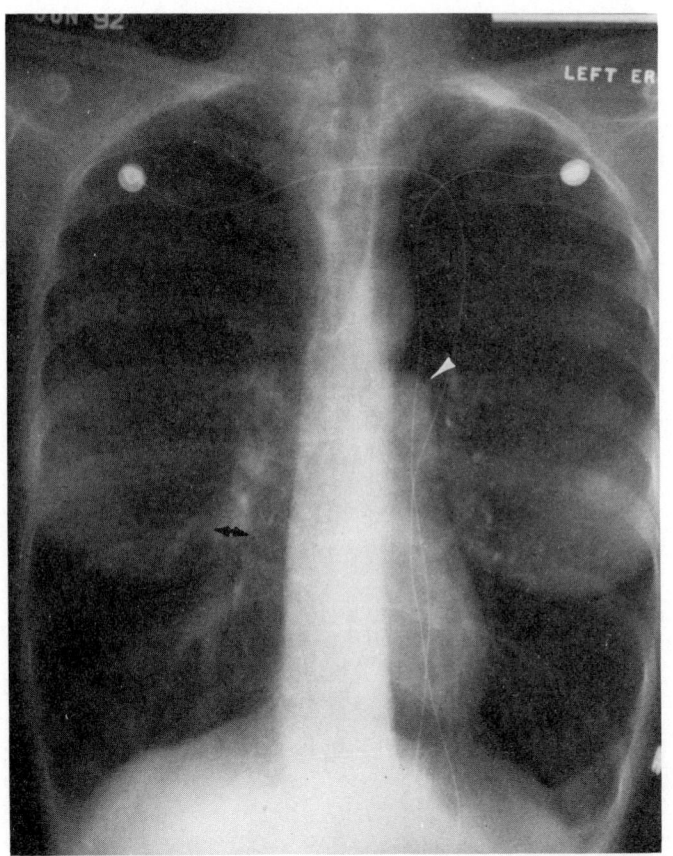

FIGURE 13–7. This 43-year-old woman has severe emphysema, pulmonary arterial hypertension, and cor pulmonale. Note the marked flattening of the hemidiaphragms. The main pulmonary artery *(white arrowhead)* is enlarged, the right interlobar pulmonary artery *(double-headed arrow)* measures 17 mm, and the right ventricle is enlarged.

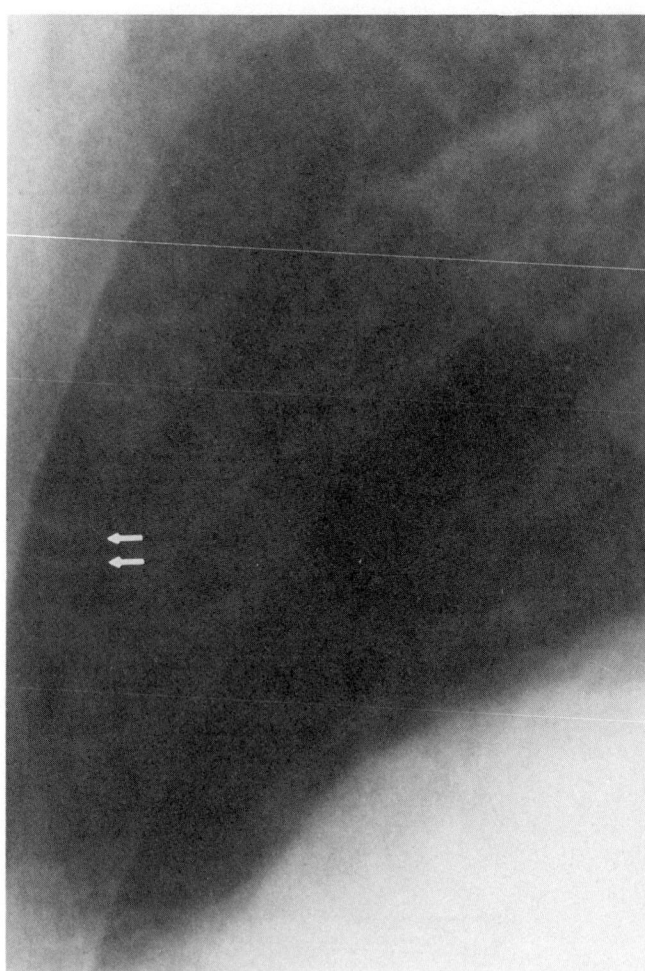

FIGURE 13–8. Septal lines *(arrows)* are best seen along the lateral borders of the lower lungs (as in this case) and in the retrosternal space.

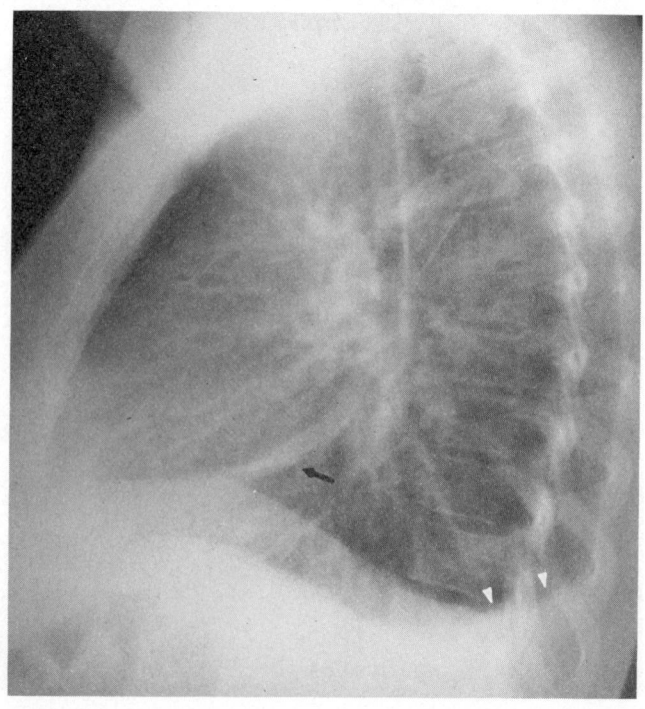

FIGURE 13–9. This 34-year-old woman developed postpartum congestive heart failure. Interstitial edema is demonstrated by interstitial thickening and septal lines *(black arrowhead)*. Small bilateral pleural effusions *(white arrowheads)* are present. Fluid is also present in the right major fissure *(arrow)*. The heart is mildly enlarged.

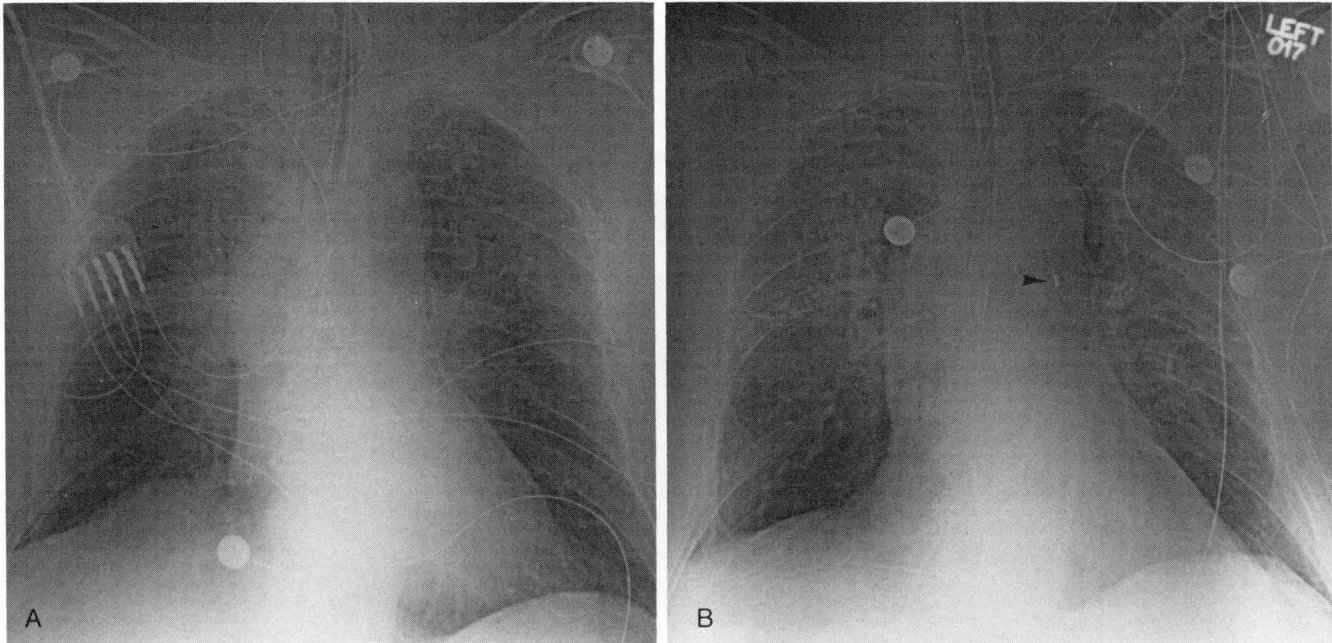

FIGURE 13–10. This 74-year-old man suffered an acute myocardial infarction. *A,* Initial chest radiograph reveals bilateral hazy perihilar opacities consistent with cardiogenic pulmonary edema. The heart size is normal; this can be seen in the setting of acute myocardial infarction. The endotracheal tube is in satisfactory position. *B,* The bilateral perihilar opacities are improved after diuretic therapy and placement of an intra-aortic balloon pump *(arrowhead).* There has been interval placement of a pulmonary artery catheter via a femoral vein.

With continued positive-pressure ventilation, these structures dilate even more and can enlarge into large cysts.

PIE is more commonly encountered in children than adults and usually resolves when positive-pressure ventilation is stopped.[17] If the air decompresses by bursting through the visceral pleura into the pleural space, pneumothorax results. If the air decompresses into the mediastinum, pneumomediastinum results.

Pneumothorax

The radiographic diagnosis of pneumothorax is established when the visceral pleural line is visualized. In an erect patient, air in the pleural space normally rises to the apex of the hemithorax and causes local compression of the lung (Fig. 13–13). In a supine patient, air rises to the most superior portion of the hemithorax, which in this position is located in the region of the hemidiaphragm in the anteromedial and subpulmonic recesses. A deep costophrenic sulcus may be seen, and the upper quadrant of the abdomen may be relatively lucent (Fig. 13–14).[18, 19]

If a pneumothorax is suspected clinically but not demonstrated radiographically, a lateral decubitus view often establishes the diagnosis because the pleural line is more easily seen along the lateral chest wall, where there are fewer confounding shadows. An expiratory film may also be used.

"Tension" pneumothorax is a clinical diagnosis, not a radiologic one. Shift of the mediastinum toward the contralateral side does not necessarily indicate increased pressure from the pneumothorax.[11] A pneumothorax that develops in a mechanically ventilated patient is very likely to become a tension pneumothorax if not treated appropriately.

Pneumomediastinum

Pneumomediastinum is manifested radiographically as lateral displacement of the mediastinal pleural line or linear ver-

tically oriented collections of air in the mediastinum. The line is usually more evident on the left, and a longitudinal line can be seen paralleling the heart and sometimes the aorta (Fig. 13–15).

Pneumothorax is a common complication of pneumomediastinum and results from rupture of the mediastinal pleura. Air in the mediastinal space can also decompress into the soft tissues of the neck and thorax and into the retroperitoneum.

The presence of subcutaneous emphysema on a radiograph may be one of the first signs of barotrauma, and a developing pneumothorax or pneumomediastinum should be suspected if this is observed.

What Are the Common Radiographic Findings in Catheter and Tube Placement?

Endotracheal Tubes

Most endotracheal tubes are marked by a radiodense stripe that extends to the tip. The tip of a single-lumen endotracheal tube is ideally placed in the region of the thoracic inlet and should be no more distal than 2 cm from the carina.[20] Intubating a mainstem bronchus results in atelectasis or collapse of the contralateral lung and may result in barotrauma of the portion of the lung that is selectively aerated. In contrast, a proximal intubation predisposes to inadvertent extubation and laryngeal or tracheal stenosis. (The vocal cords are located at the level of approximately C5–6.)

Chest Tubes

The correct position for chest tubes depends on the reason for placement. Pleural fluid drainage tubes should be placed posteriorly for a supine patient and posteriorly and inferiorly for an ambulatory patient. A tube used to evacuate pleural air

Text continued on page 223

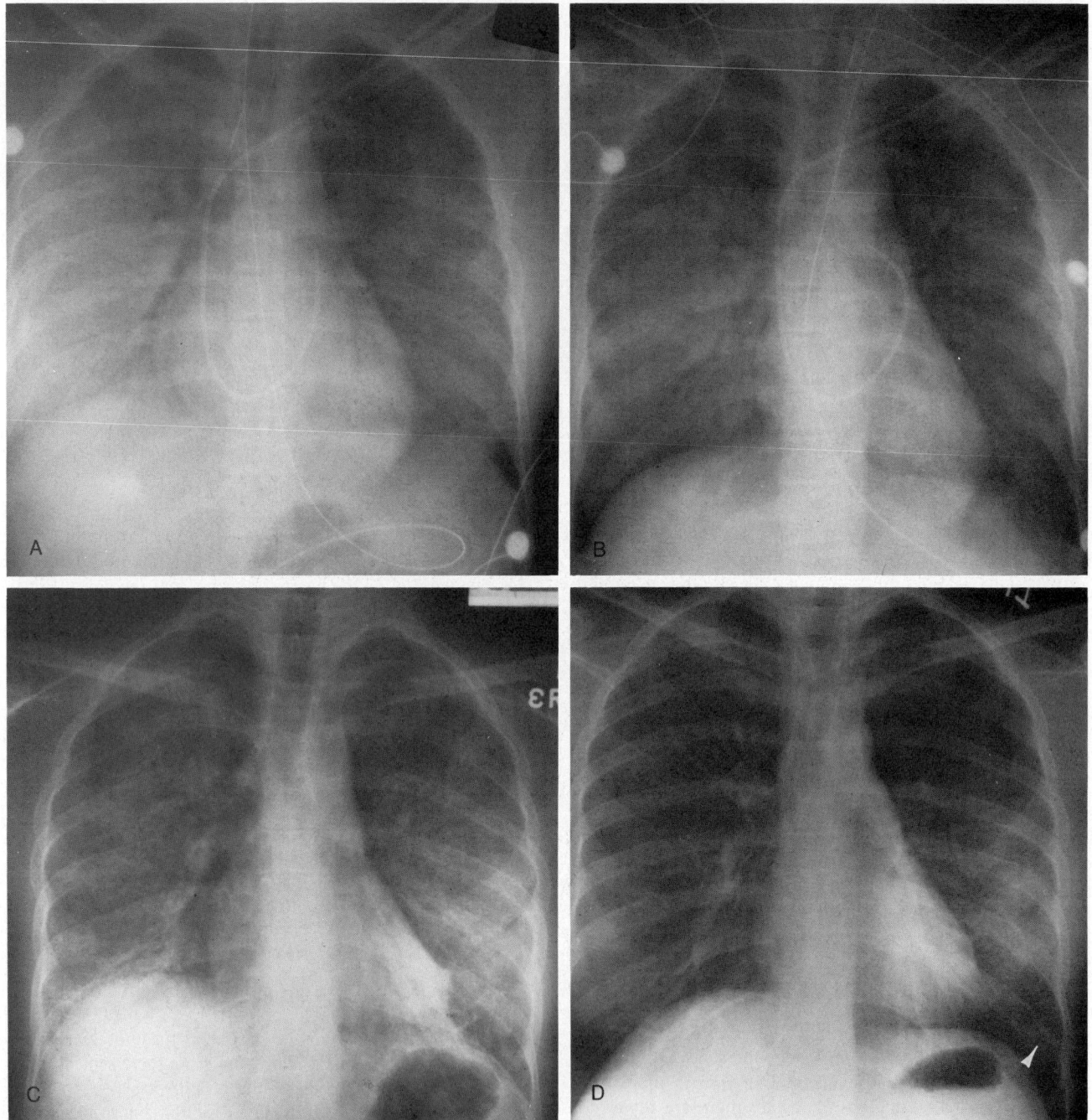

FIGURE 13–11. This 16-year-old young woman was brought comatose and hypotensive into the emergency room following an overdose of ethchlorvynol (Placidyl). The patient subsequently developed adult respiratory distress syndrome. *A,* Chest radiograph 4 hours after admission reveals bilateral dense alveolar opacities. The endotracheal tube is in satisfactory position with the tip 2 cm above the carina. The Swan-Ganz catheter terminates in the right ventricular outflow tract and needs to be advanced. *B,* Chest radiograph 2 days later demonstrates slight interval clearing of the alveolar opacities. The endotracheal tube tip is now 2 cm above the thoracic inlet, and the Swan-Ganz catheter tip is now in the proximal right pulmonary artery. *C,* Three weeks later, interstitial opacities remain. *D,* Chest radiograph taken 3 months later reveals resolution of the opacities except for minimal scarring *(arrowhead)* at the left lung base.

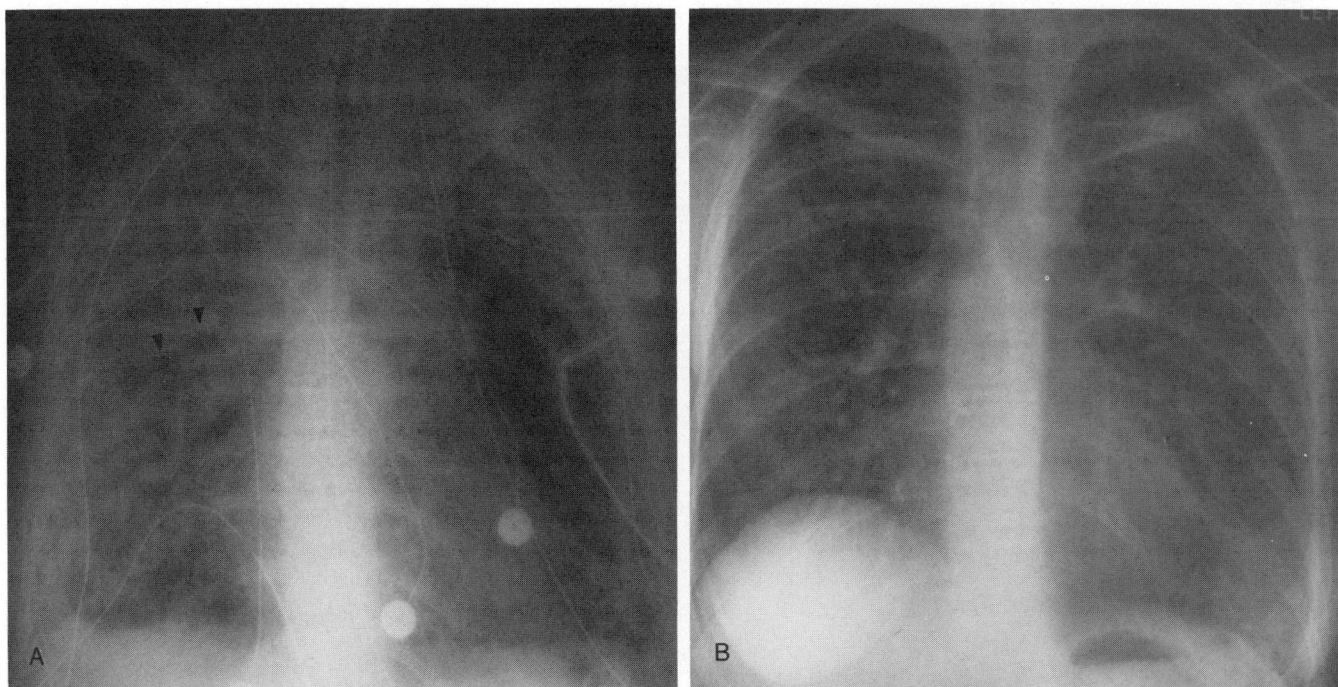

FIGURE 13–12. This 19-year-old woman had a prolonged course in an intensive care unit secondary to meningococcemia and adult respiratory distress syndrome. *A*, Multiple tortuous radiolucencies *(arrowheads)* represent air within the bronchovascular sheaths, a finding of pulmonary interstitial emphysema. *B*, Three months later, coarse interstitial opacities reflect pulmonary fibrosis, a complication of adult respiratory distress syndrome and oxygen toxicity.

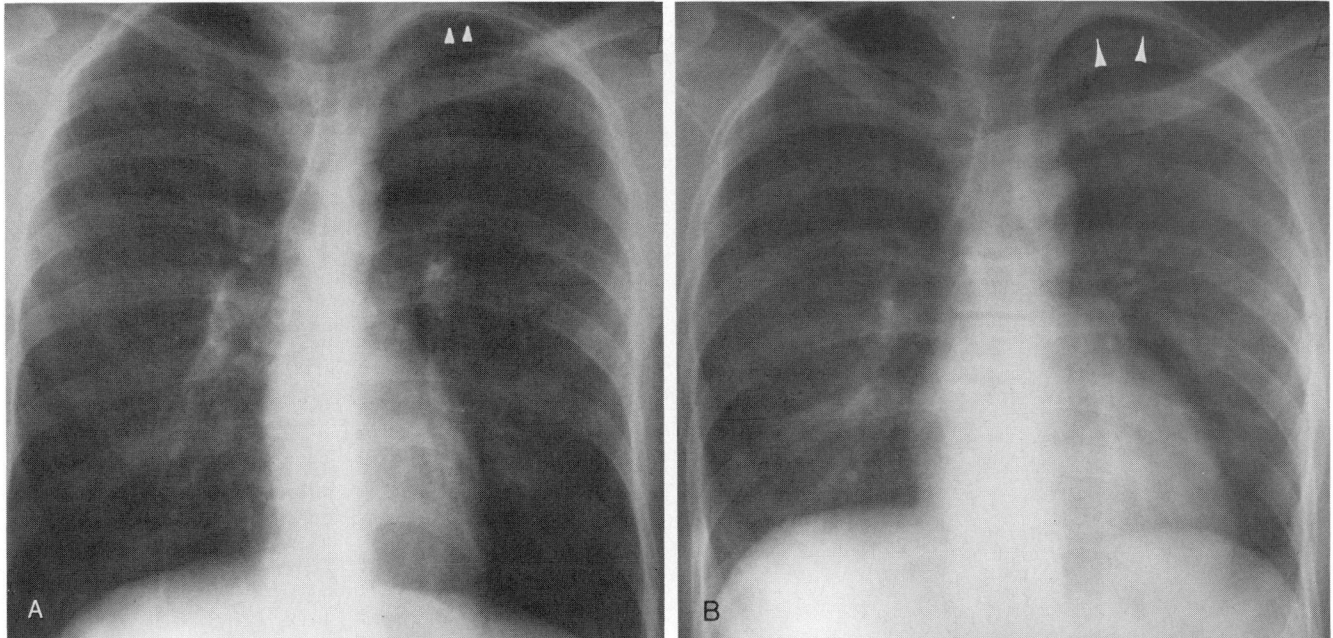

FIGURE 13–13. *A*, On this upright inspiratory film, a left apical pneumothorax is demonstrated by visualization of the visceral pleural line *(arrowheads)*. *B*, The visceral pleural line *(arrowheads)* is more easily seen on the expiratory film.

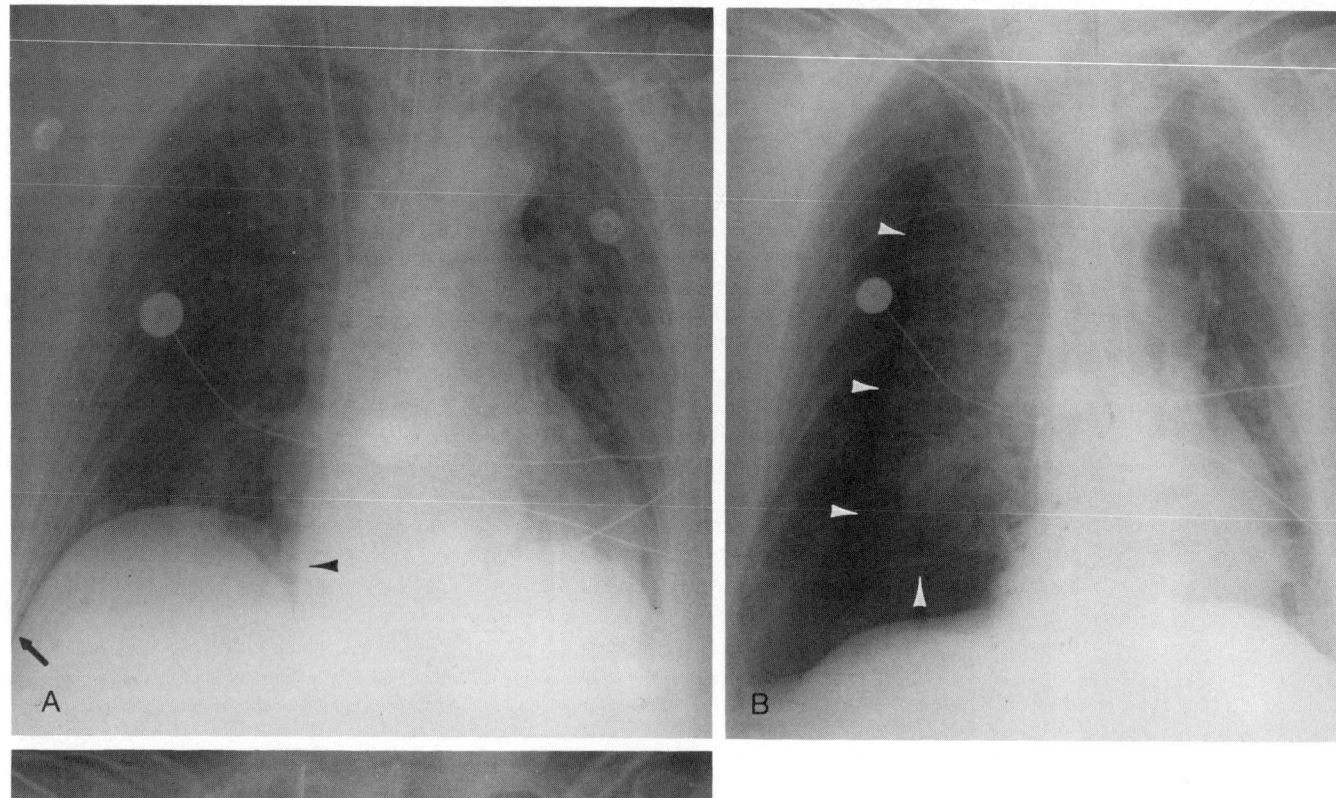

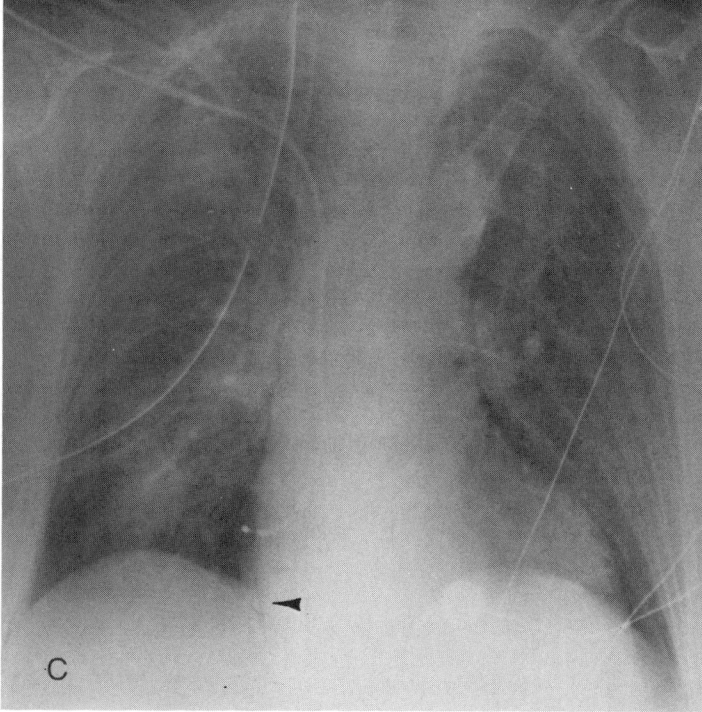

FIGURE 13–14. *A,* On a supine film, the findings of a pneumothorax can be subtle. A deep costophrenic sulcus *(arrow)* and air in the antero-medial recess *(arrowhead)* indicate that there is air in the pleural space. Also, the right upper quadrant of the abdomen is relatively more lucent than the left. *B,* Three hours later, a large right pneumothorax develops. The visceral pleural line *(arrowheads)* is easily seen. *C,* The pneumothorax is markedly decreased in size after placement of a chest tube. A tiny amount of residual air remains in the anteromedial recess *(arrowhead).*

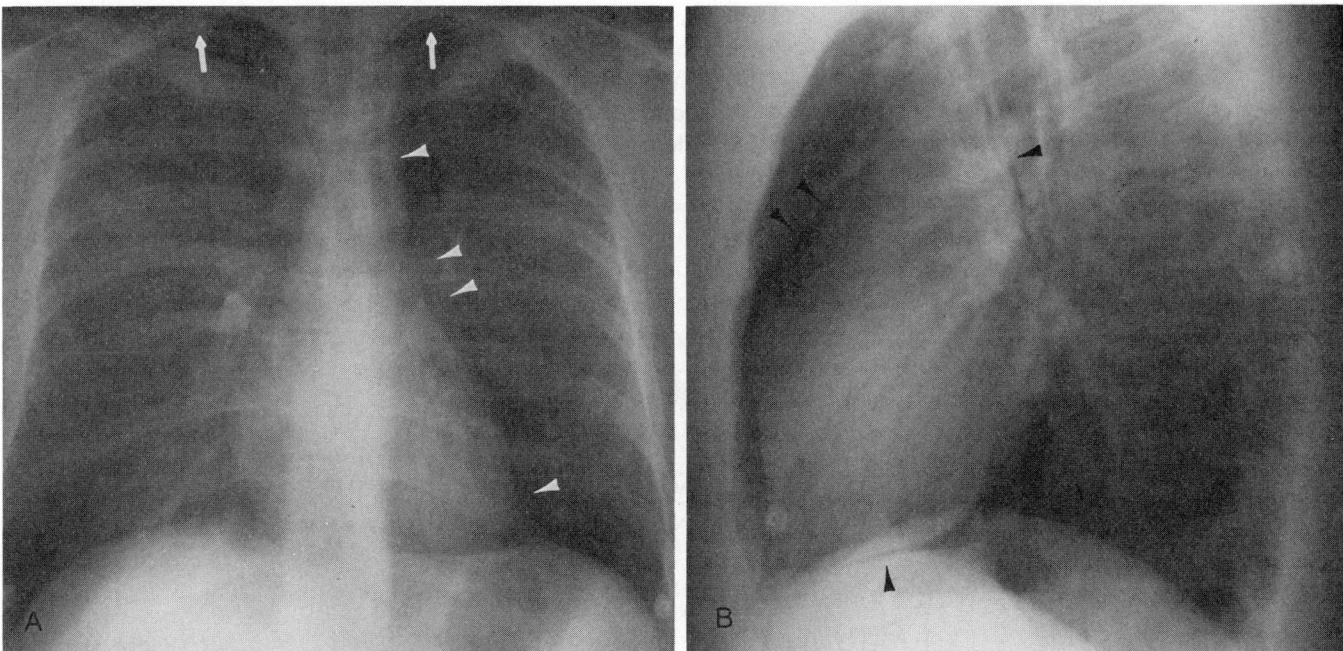

FIGURE 13–15. This 20-year-old man developed chest pain following cocaine use. *A,* Pneumomediastinum is demonstrated by visualization of a line *(arrowheads)* paralleling the heart and aortic arch. Small biapical pneumothoraces *(arrows)* are present. Subcutaneous air is seen as streaky radiolucencies projecting over the upper mediastinum. *B,* Air in the mediastinal space *(arrowheads)* is easily seen on the lateral film.

should be placed anteriorly in a supine patient and superiorly in an ambulatory patient.

Central Venous Catheters

Because as many as one third of central venous catheters are initially malpositioned, placement should be checked radiographically. The distal tip of the catheter should be located in the SVC, proximal to but not in the right atrium. Extension into the right atrium or beyond predisposes to perforation of the heart by the catheter tip.[21] Extension into the region of the tricuspid valve can cause valvular insufficiency as well as ectopy. Overinsertion of the catheter into the right ventricle also predisposes to ectopy and perforation of the heart.[22] The ideal catheter tip position zone is proximal to the right atrium within the SVC above the pericardial reflection, with the catheter tip parallel to the SVC (Fig. 13–16). In addition, to minimize the chance of SVC perforation, the catheter tip should not have an impingement angle with the SVC of >40°.[22] Because of the close anatomic relationship between the subclavian vein and the underlying lung, pneumothorax is a common complication following subclavian line placement and should also be ruled out.

Pulmonary Artery Catheters

Pulmonary artery catheters are typically radiodense. The tip should be placed in either the right or left pulmonary artery or in a main descending branch. The catheter tip should be no more than 2 cm lateral to the hilum; otherwise, pulmonary infarction or perforation may result.

Central venous and pulmonary artery catheters may knot or break, with subsequent migration of the free fragment. Such fragments may often be retrieved using interventional radiographic techniques obviating surgery.

Intra-Aortic Balloon Pump Catheters

An intra-aortic balloon pump (IABP) measures about 26 cm in length and has a radiodense marker at the tip, which is inserted proximally. The proximal end of the IABP should be placed just distal to the aortic arch so that the left subclavian artery or left common carotid artery is not occluded. Distally, the balloon should be above the origins of the renal and celiac arteries to avoid obstruction of these arteries when the balloon inflates during diastole.[21]

THE NECK

Regardless of etiology, diseases of the upper airway often lead to obstruction. Any insult to the larynx and trachea can result in airway compromise that may require the emergent attention of an anesthesiologist. Children are especially susceptible because of the smaller caliber of their airways. Frontal and lateral radiographs of the neck are useful for detecting pathology. The lateral view demonstrates the majority of abnormalities.

What Are the Radiographic Findings of Acute Laryngeal Pathology?

The anatomy of the soft tissues of the larynx in a normal adult is illustrated in Figure 13–17. The anatomy is similar in children older than 3 years.

The vallecular recess is an air-containing structure between the base of the tongue and the epiglottis. The epiglottis has a smooth anterior surface and a pointed superior tip. The aryepiglottic folds arise from the tip of the epiglottis and continue posteriorly and inferiorly to end in the arytenoid area.

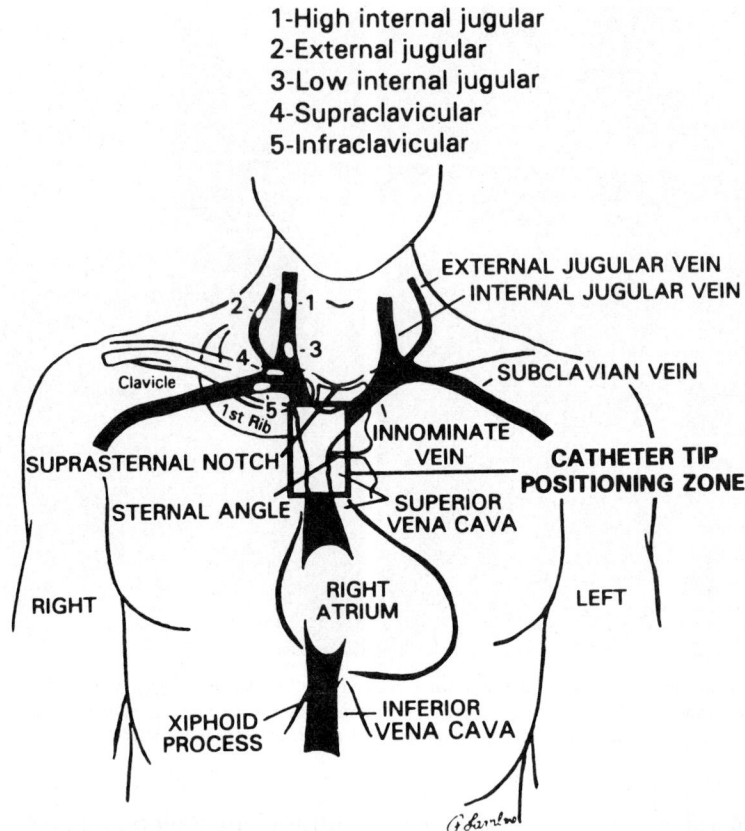

1-High internal jugular
2-External jugular
3-Low internal jugular
4-Supraclavicular
5-Infraclavicular

EXTERNAL JUGULAR VEIN
INTERNAL JUGULAR VEIN

SUBCLAVIAN VEIN

INNOMINATE VEIN

CATHETER TIP POSITIONING ZONE

Clavicle

1st Rib

SUPRASTERNAL NOTCH

STERNAL ANGLE

SUPERIOR VENA CAVA

RIGHT

RIGHT ATRIUM

LEFT

XIPHOID PROCESS

INFERIOR VENA CAVA

FIGURE 13–16. Central venous access sites and catheter tip positioning zone. (From package insert for triple lumen central venous catheter manufactured by Cook Critical Care, a division of Look, Inc., Bloomingdale, IN, 1986.)

Epiglottitis

Swelling of the epiglottis or aryepiglottic folds can be life threatening. The most common cause is epiglottitis, which occurs in all age groups but more commonly in children. Epiglottitis is manifested radiographically as enlargement of the epiglottis so that it becomes a thumblike mass rather than a thin, pointed one. The aryepiglottic folds become thickened, and the vallecular recess is obliterated (Fig. 13–18). Ingestion of caustic substances may also result in swelling of the epiglottis and may create a radiographic picture similar to epiglottitis.[21]

Foreign Bodies

Aspiration of a foreign body can also lead to airway compromise. Metallic and radiodense foreign bodies are easily visualized radiographically. Substances such as plastic, wood, or food are more difficult to detect.

Prevertebral Soft Tissues

The width of the prevertebral soft tissues anterior to C-3 normally does not exceed 4 to 5 mm with the neck in neutral position, and the width of the retrotracheal tissues anterior to C-6 normally does not exceed 22 mm in adults and 14 mm in children. The prevertebral soft tissues enlarge in the presence of infection (retropharyngeal abscess), trauma, neoplasia, and angioneurotic edema. Prevertebral soft tissue swelling associ-

ated with anterior displacement and narrowing of the airway suggests airway compromise.

What Are the Radiographic Findings of Atlantoaxial Subluxation?

Manipulation of the head and neck in the presence of an unstable cervical spine can lead to injury to the spinal cord, resulting in paralysis or death. Most cervical spine injuries secondary to trauma are known or suspected by an anesthesiologist before intubation. Atlantoaxial subluxation, however, can be overlooked. High-risk patients should be screened so that they can be appropriately managed in the operating room.

Causes

The transverse atlantal ligament holds the dens adjacent to the anterior arch of C-1. Disruption or laxity of this ligament leads to abnormal movement of C-1 on C-2, which can impinge on the spinal cord. Inflammatory causes are common and include rheumatoid arthritis, juvenile rheumatoid arthritis, ankylosing spondylitis, and pharyngitis. Ligamentous laxity secondary to hyperemia from adjacent inflammation is thought to be the pathogenesis. The incidence of atlantoaxial subluxation in rheumatoid patients is estimated to be 20% to 25%.[23–25]

Atlantoaxial instability is also encountered in patients with Down's syndrome and is presumed to be secondary to inherent

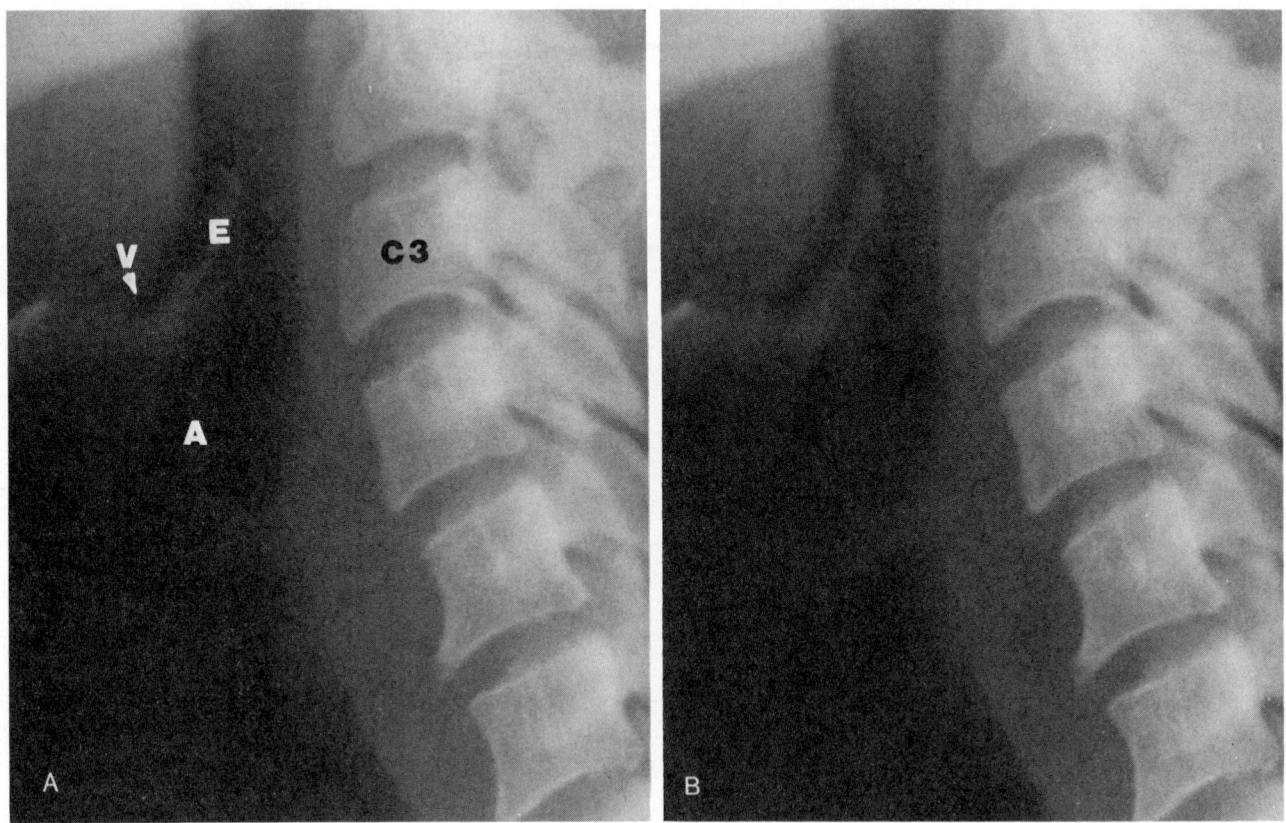

FIGURE 13–17. *A*, The normal soft tissues of the neck in an adult. V = vallecular recess; E = epiglottis; A = aryepiglottic folds. The prevertebral soft tissues are normal anterior to the C3 vertebral body. *B*, Same lateral view of the neck without labels.

FIGURE 13–18. Epiglottitis in an adult. The epiglottis *(arrows)* is enlarged and blunted, and the aryepiglottic folds *(arrowheads)* are markedly thickened. The vallecular recess is obliterated. (Courtesy of Phyllis Kornguth, M.D.)

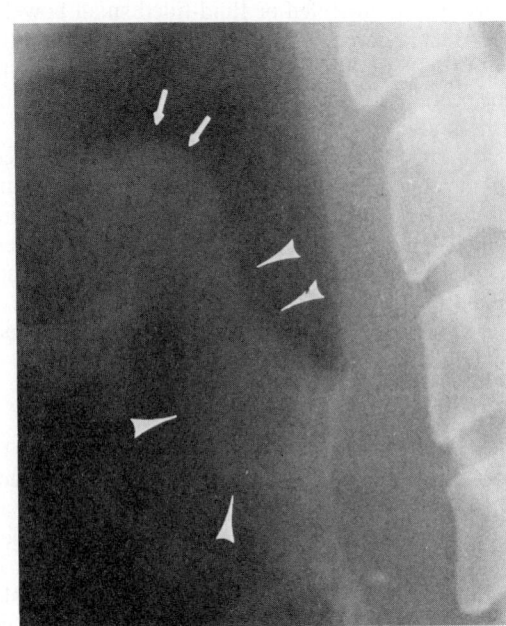

ligamentous laxity. Traumatic causes are rare and are often accompanied by fractures of the odontoid process.

In adults, the distance between the posterior surface of the anterior arch of the atlas and the anterior surface of the dens does not normally exceed 2.5 mm on neutral, flexion, or extension positions. The normal distance in children is 3.5 to 4.5 mm. When these measurements are exceeded on carefully monitored flexion and extension series, atlantoaxial instability is present (Figs. 13–19 and 13–20). Flexion/extension views are contraindicated when a dens fracture is suspected or when a patient is insensitive to pain.

THE ABDOMEN

Abdominal distention is a common finding in critically ill patients. Radiographic monitoring is necessary to rule out significant acute abdominal pathology. For the most part, gaseous distention is not disconcerting unless bowel loops are dilated or perforation has occurred.

Colonic gas is normally located in the periphery of the abdomen. The colon has haustral indentations that are irregularly spaced, indent the surface of the colon, and do not typically extend across the whole lumen. Gas in the small bowel is located more centrally in the abdomen. Small bowel loops have thin, closely spaced lines that extend across the whole lumen; these lines represent the valvulae conniventes. The normal small bowel loop is generally no more than 3 cm in diameter.

What Are the Radiographic Manifestations of Bowel Obstruction?

Seventy-five per cent of small bowel obstructions are caused by adhesions. Other causes include hernia, gallstone ileus, volvulus, intussusception, and neoplasm. In small bowel obstruction, air-filled or fluid-filled small bowel loops are dilated and relatively little gas or stool is seen in the colon (Fig. 13–21). Upright or decubitus films may demonstrate a "string of pearls" sign (Fig. 13–22), which represents multiple small air-fluid levels in the small bowel.

In large bowel obstruction, the colon is dilated to the level of obstruction (Fig. 13–23). The sigmoid, cecum, and transverse colon are affected, in decreasing order of frequency. The small bowel may or may not be dilated, depending on the competency of the ileocecal valve. Carcinomas account for the majority of colonic obstructions. Diverticulitis and volvulus are frequently encountered but are less common causes of colonic obstruction.

Ileus

Adynamic ileus is characterized by generalized dilatation of the stomach, small bowel, and colon without an underlying mechanical obstruction. *Colonic ileus* refers to generalized dilatation of the colon without obstruction. Ileus is a common finding following surgery and trauma and is also associated with sepsis, electrolyte imbalances, and drugs such as narcotics. Differentiating between a low colonic obstruction and ileus can be difficult. Prone or left lateral decubitus views may rule out a low colonic obstruction by demonstrating air rising into the rectum (Fig. 13–24).[26]

A subclassification of colonic ileus is cecal ileus, in which the cecum is dilated out of proportion to the remainder of the colon. The major risk of cecal ileus is perforation, especially when the cecum is mobile and rotates anteromedially. Risk of perforation correlates more with the duration of dilatation than with actual cecal size. Aggressive decompression measures should be considered when the cecum is dilated >10 cm for more than 2 to 3 days.[27]

What Are the Radiographic Findings of Pneumoperitoneum?

A plain film of the abdomen is performed with a patient supine, and the radiographic findings of pneumoperitoneum on a supine film can be quite subtle. Radiographic findings (Figs. 13–25 and 13–26) include the following:

1. Outlining of the bowel wall by air inside and outside the lumen (Rigler's sign)
2. Outlining of the falciform ligament by air
3. Lucency in the right upper quadrant, indicating air anterior to the liver
4. Subhepatic air
5. Triangular extraluminal lucencies between bowel loops

When pneumoperitoneum is suspected but not readily detected on a supine abdominal film, a left lateral decubitus or an upright film often simplifies diagnosis.[26, 28] Pneumoperitoneum is an expected finding in patients who have recently undergone abdominal surgery or who are on peritoneal dialysis.

What Is the Correct Gastric or Enteric Tube Position?

Nasogastric

Nasogastric tubes are used to relieve gastric distention. Most nasogastric tubes have radiopaque linear markers that are continuous except in the region of the side ports. The side port should be located in the stomach and specifically should not be positioned in the distal esophagus. Positioning of a side port in the distal esophagus or at the gastroesophageal junction predisposes to aspiration. A nasogastric tube can also be inadvertently placed in a mainstem bronchus or can be coiled in a hiatal hernia.

Nasoenteric

The course of nasoenteric tubes is more difficult to visualize radiographically; most have radiodense tips. The position of a nasoenteric feeding tube should be checked radiographically before starting tube feedings.

Complications of these tubes are related to malpositioning and include mainstem bronchus intubation, pneumothorax, and perforation of a mediastinal structure. Many clinicians place these tubes fluoroscopically to avoid these complications. The tip should be located in the third or fourth portion of the duodenum to avoid aspiration of tube feedings (Fig. 13–27). However, no study has confirmed that intragastric feeding is less safe in the absence of gastroesophageal reflux, gastroparesis, or gastric outlet obstruction.[29]

Text continued on page 232

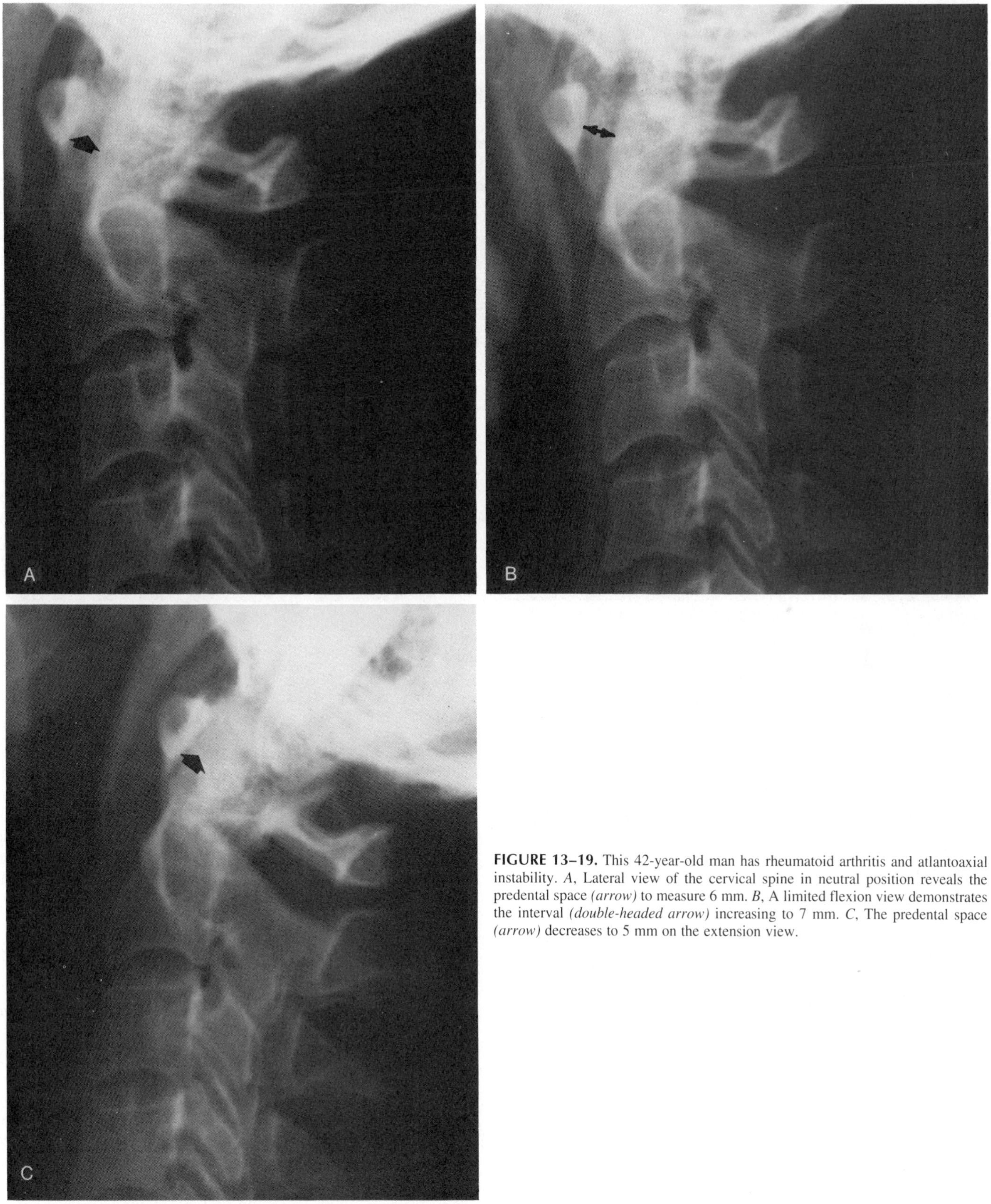

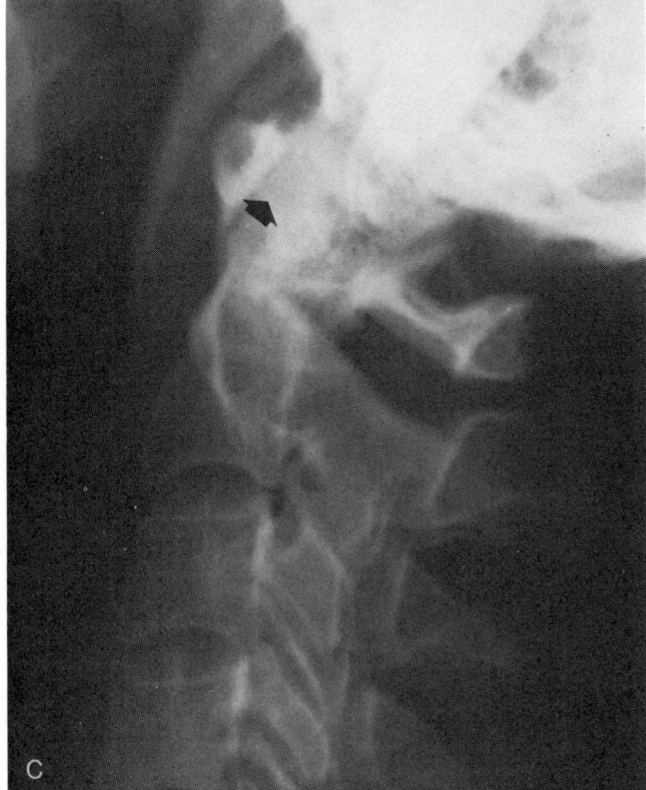

FIGURE 13–19. This 42-year-old man has rheumatoid arthritis and atlantoaxial instability. *A*, Lateral view of the cervical spine in neutral position reveals the predental space *(arrow)* to measure 6 mm. *B*, A limited flexion view demonstrates the interval *(double-headed arrow)* increasing to 7 mm. *C*, The predental space *(arrow)* decreases to 5 mm on the extension view.

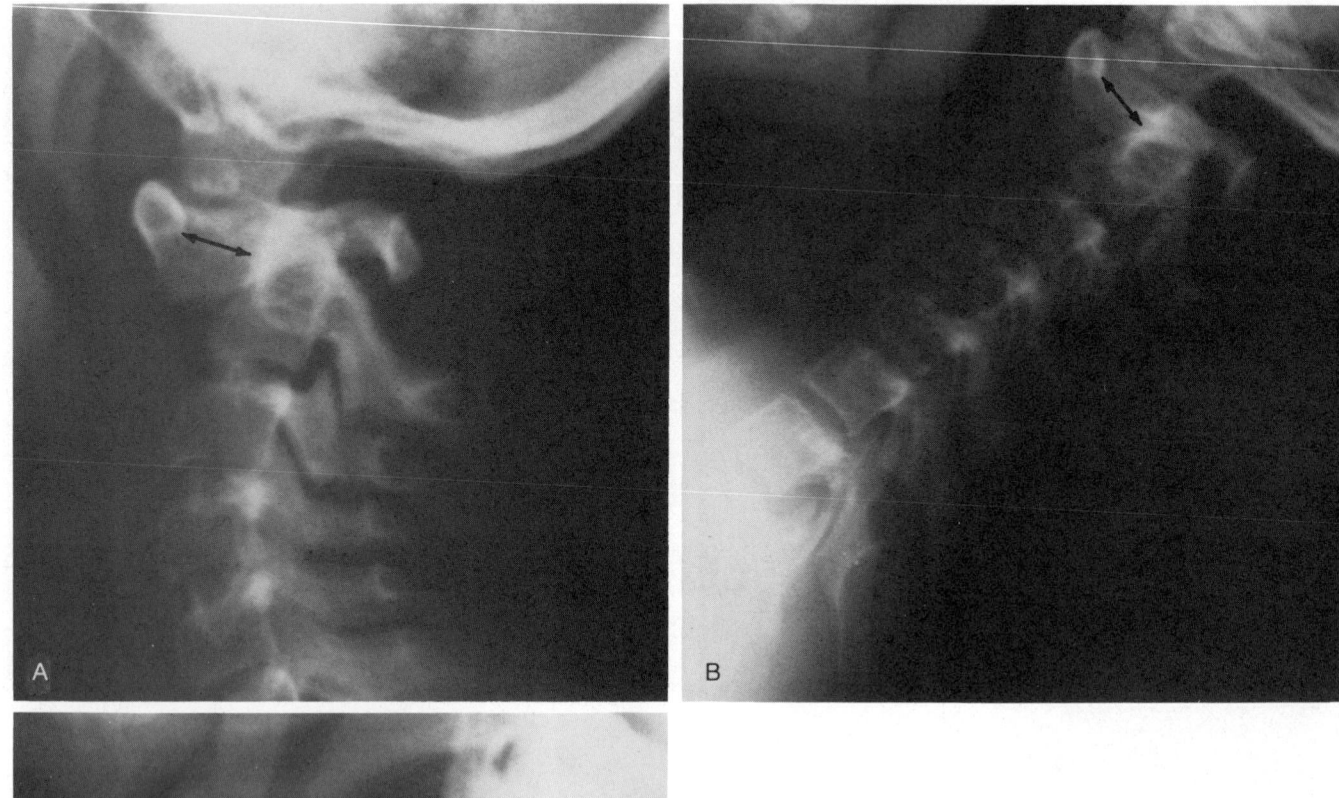

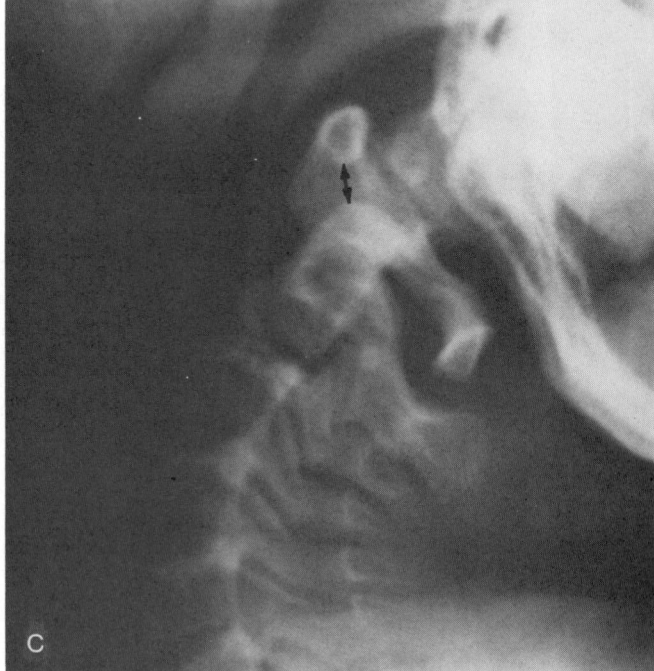

FIGURE 13–20. This 16-year-old boy with Down's syndrome also has atlan-toaxial instability. *A*, The predental space *(double-headed arrow)* measures 11 mm on the neutral view. *B*, This interval *(double-headed arrow)* is unchanged on the limited flexion view. *C*, Extension view demonstrates the predental space *(double-headed arrow)* decreasing to 5 mm.

FIGURE 13–21. This 60-year-old man developed abdominal distention several days after repair of an abdominal aortic aneurysm. Supine film of the abdomen reveals multiple dilated small bowel loops with relatively little air in the colon *(arrows)*. The radiographic findings are consistent with an early or partial small bowel obstruction. Note the closely spaced, thin, parallel lines of the valvulae conniventes *(arrowheads)*, indicating small bowel loops.

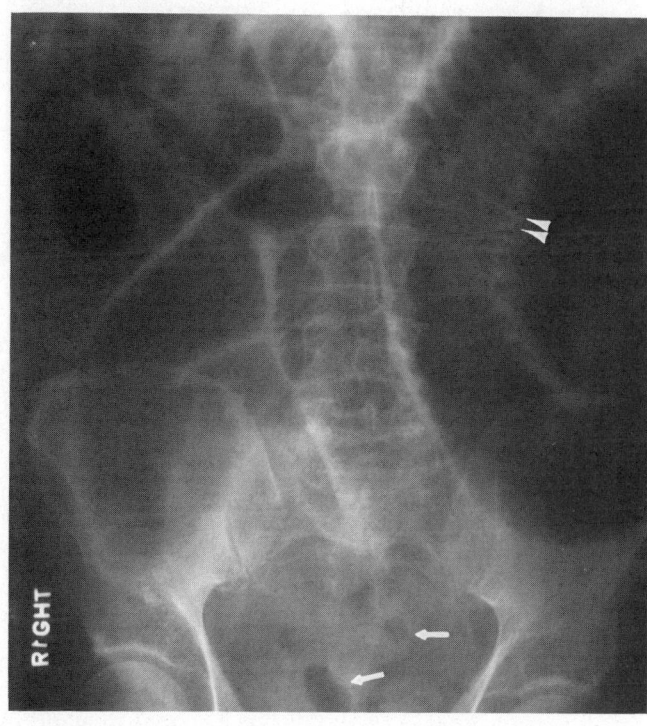

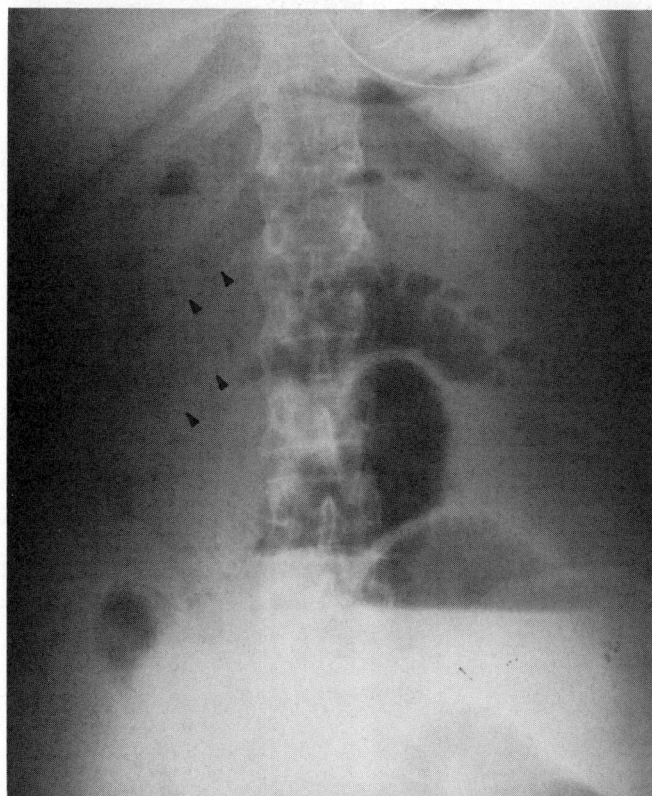

FIGURE 13–22. Upright abdominal film of a 62-year-old woman demonstrates the "string of pearls" sign *(arrowheads)* of small bowel obstruction. (Courtesy of Reed P. Rice, M.D.)

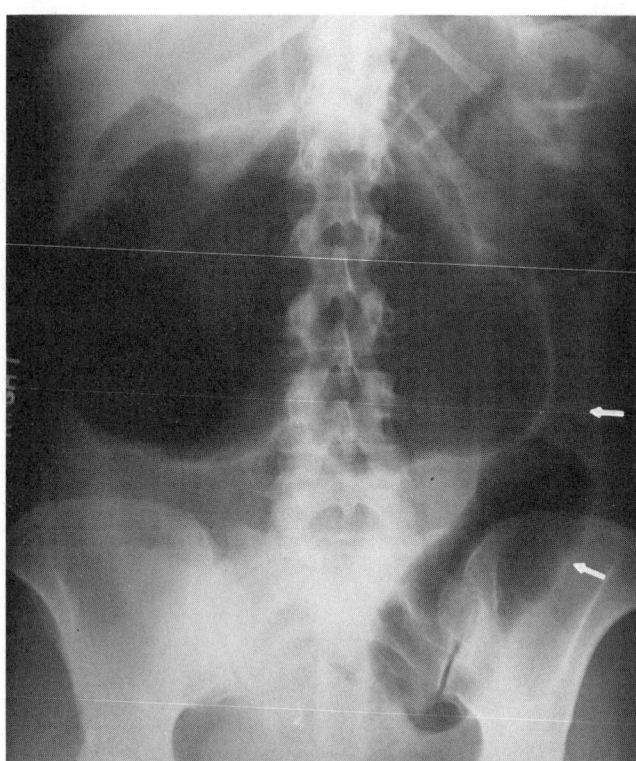

FIGURE 13–23. This 31-year-old woman developed colonic obstruction from serosal metastases. Supine film of the abdomen reveals dilated colonic loops to the level of obstruction, which, in this instance, is the distal segment of the sigmoid colon. The haustra *(arrows)* are seen as irregularly spaced lines that in general do not traverse the entire lumen.

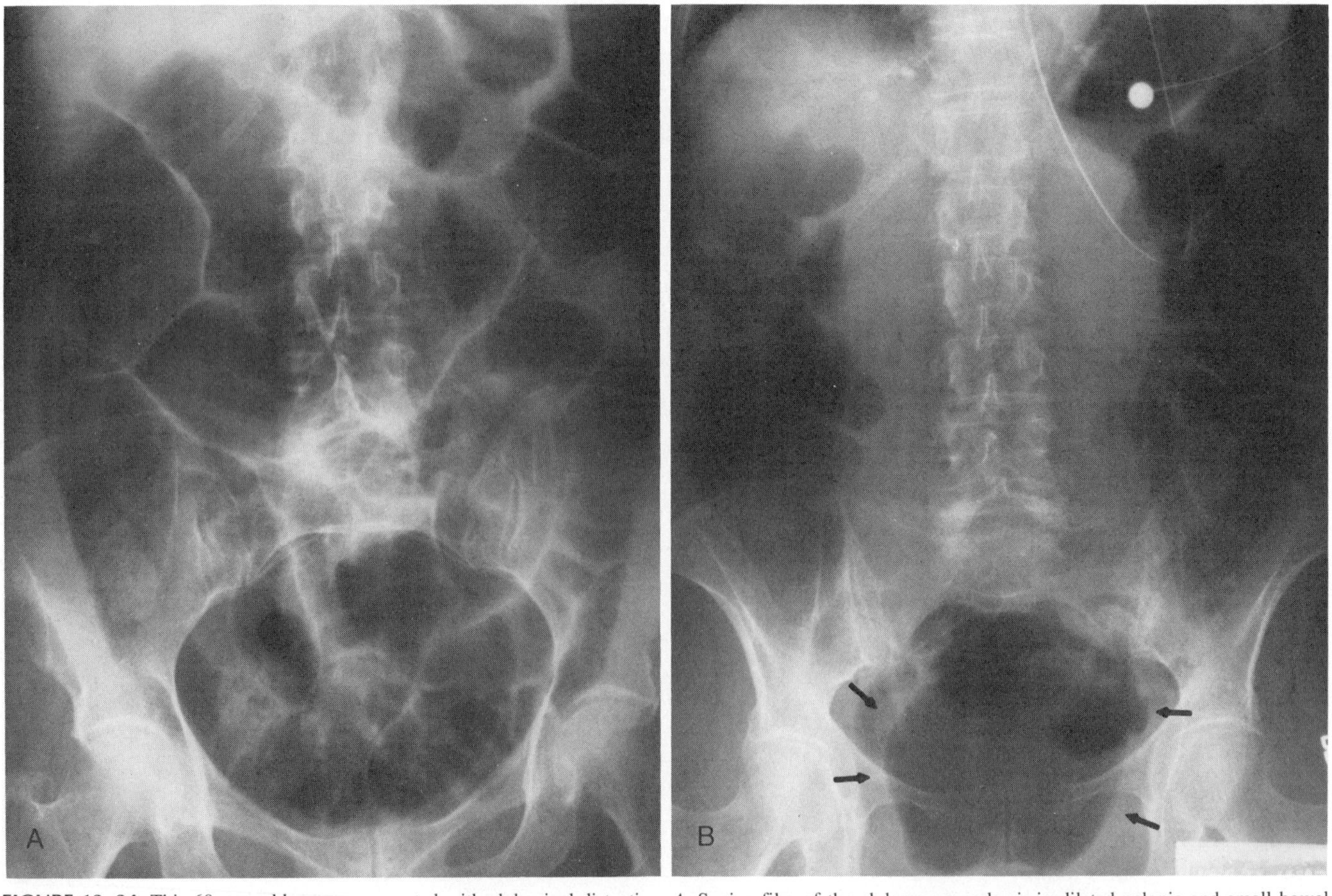

FIGURE 13–24. This 60-year-old woman presented with abdominal distention. *A,* Supine film of the abdomen reveals air in dilated colonic and small bowel loops. These findings do not distinguish between adynamic ileus and large bowel obstruction with an incompetent ileocecal valve. *B,* Prone film demonstrates air rising into the rectum *(arrows),* a finding seen in adynamic ileus. (Courtesy of Reed P. Rice, M.D.)

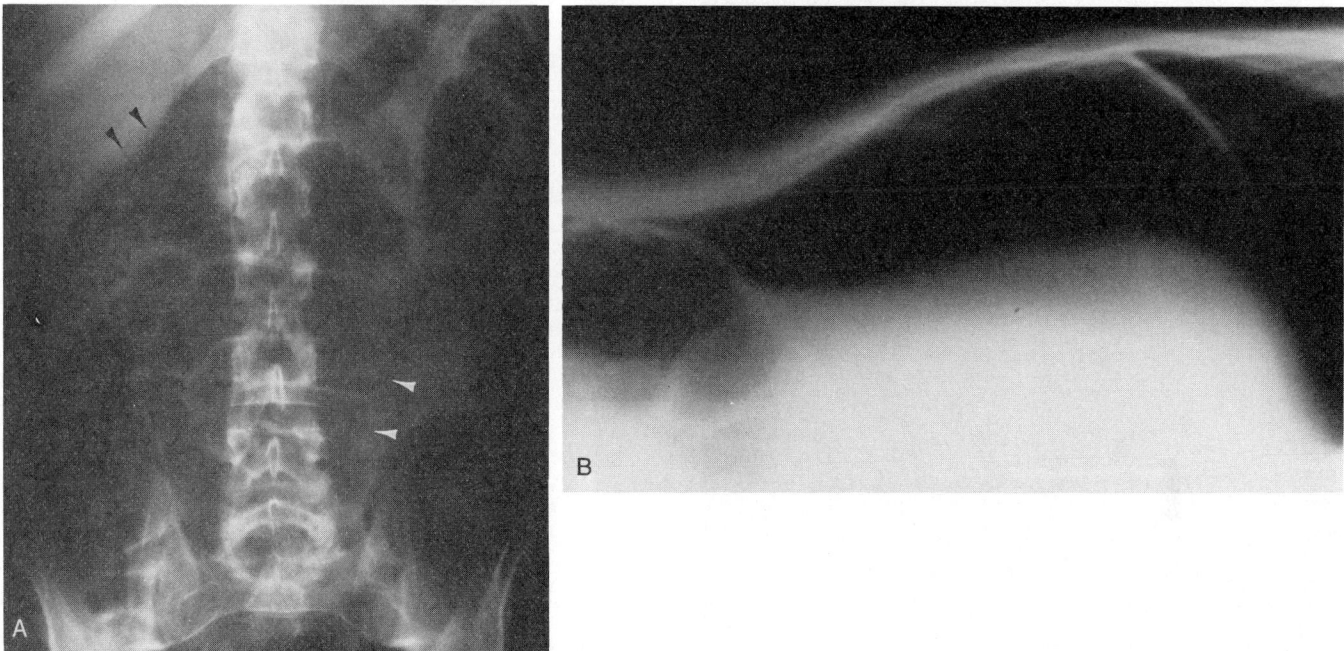

FIGURE 13–25. This 22-year-old man presented with abdominal pain. *A,* Supine film of the abdomen reveals a large amount of extraluminal subhepatic air *(black arrowheads)* and air outlining the bowel walls *(white arrowheads). B,* Left lateral decubitus film confirms the findings of pneumoperitoneum. (Courtesy of Reed P. Rice, M.D.)

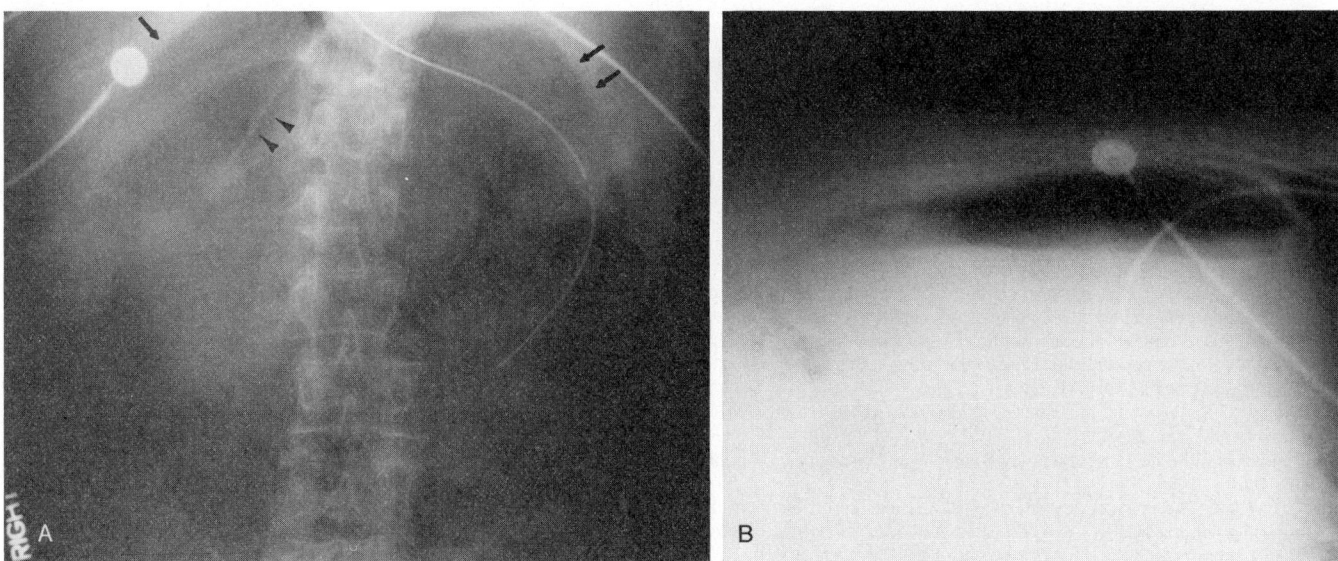

FIGURE 13–26. *A,* Pneumoperitoneum on this supine film is demonstrated by the outlining of the falciform ligament *(arrowheads)* by air and relative radiolucency *(arrows)* in the upper abdomen. *B,* Left lateral decubitus view reveals air rising superior to the liver.

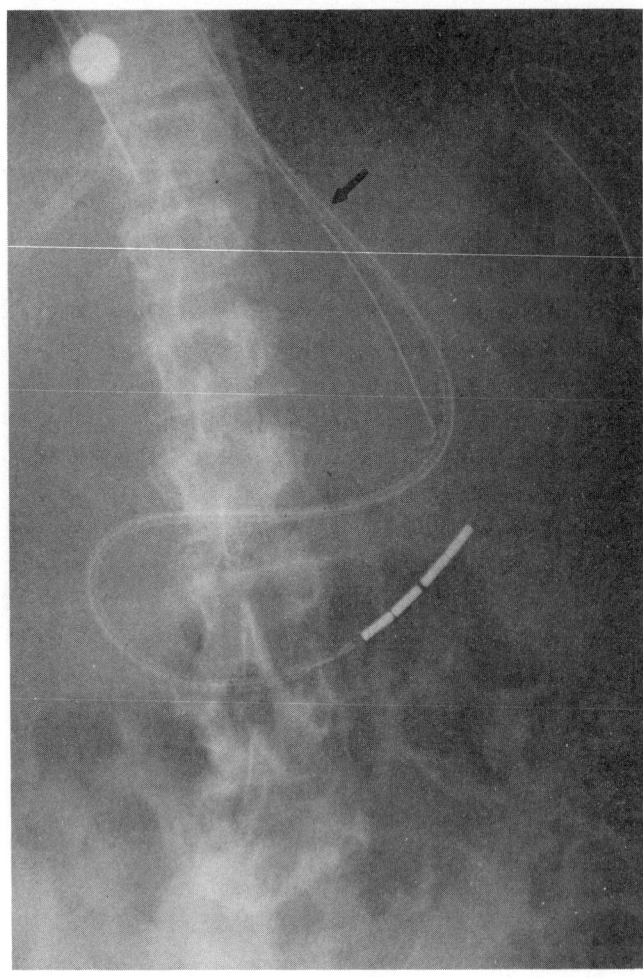

FIGURE 13–27. The Dobhoff tube is in satisfactory position with the tip in the region of the ligament of Treitz. The nasogastric tube is also in good position, with the sideport *(arrow)* in the body of the stomach.

References

1. Godwin JD, Chen JTT: Thoracic venous anatomy. AJR 1986; 147:674.
2. Ravin CE: Introduction to chest radiography. *In* Textbook of Diagnostic Imaging. Putman CE, Ravin CE (eds). Philadelphia, WB Saunders, 1988, pp 413–425.
3. Heitzman ER: The Mediastinum: Radiologic Correlations with Anatomy and Pathology. 2nd ed. Berlin, Springer-Verlag, 1988.
4. Felson B: Chest Roentgenology. Philadelphia, WB Saunders, 1973.
5. Simon G: Principle of Chest X-ray Diagnosis. 3rd ed. London, Butterworth, 1971.
6. American Thoracic Society: Chronic bronchitis, asthma, and pulmonary emphysema: statement by the committee on diagnostic standards for nontuberculous respiratory disease. Am Rev Respir Dis 1962; 85:762–768.
7. Pratt PC: Role of conventional chest radiography in diagnosis and exclusion of emphysema. Am J Med 1987; 82:998.
8. Pratt PC: Radiographic appearance of the chest in emphysema. Invest Radiol 1987; 22:927.
9. Heitzman ER: The Lung: Radiologic-Pathologic Correlations. St Louis, CV Mosby, 1984.
10. Chang CH: The normal roentgenographic measurement of the right descending pulmonary artery in 1,085 cases. AJR 1962; 87:929.
11. Pare JA, Fraser RG: Synopsis of Diseases of the Chest. Philadelphia, WB Saunders, 1983.
12. Nessa CG, Rigler LG: The roentgenological manifestations of pulmonary edema. Radiology 1941; 37:35.
13. Hodson CJ: Pulmonary oedema and the ''bat's wing'' shadow. J Fac Radiol 1950; 1:176.
14. Joffe N: Roentgenologic findings in post-shock and postoperative pulmonary insufficiency. Radiology 1970; 94:369.
15. Ostendorf P, Birzle H, Vogel W, et al: Pulmonary radiographic abnormalities in shock. Radiology 1975; 115:257.
16. Johnson TH, Altman AR, McCaffree RD: Radiologic considerations in the adult respiratory distress syndrome treated with positive and expiratory pressure (PEEP). Clin Chest Med 1982; 3:89.
17. Swischuk LE: Respiratory system. *In* Imaging of the Newborn, Infant, and Young Child. 3rd ed. Swischuk LE (ed). Baltimore, Williams & Wilkins, 1989, pp 1–206.
18. Rhea JT, vanSonnenberg E, McLoud TC: Basilar pneumothorax in the supine adult. Radiology 1979; 133:593.
19. Tocino IM, Miller MH, Fairfax WR: Distribution of pneumothorax in the supine and semirecumbent critically ill adult. AJR 1985; 144:901.
20. Goodman LR, Putman CE: Critical Care Imaging. Philadelphia, WB Saunders, 1992.
21. Ellis L, Vogel S, Copeland E: Central venous catheter vascular erosions. Diagnosis and clinical course. Ann Surg 1989; 209:475.
22. Blackshear RH, Gravenstein N: Critical angle of incidence for delayed vessel perforation by central venous catheter: a study of in vivo data (Abstracted). Ann Emerg Med 1992; 21:659.
23. Conlon PW, Isdale IC, Rose BS: Rheumatoid arthritis of the cervical spine: an analysis of 333 cases. Ann Rheum Dis 1966; 25:120.
24. Resnick D, Niwayama G: Diagnosis of Bone and Joint Disorders. 2nd ed. Philadelphia, WB Saunders, 1988.
25. Mathews JA: Atlanto-axial subluxation in rheumatoid arthritis. Ann Rheum Dis 1969; 28:260.
26. Rice RP: The plain film of the abdomen. *In* Radiology: Diagnosis—Imaging—Intervention. Vol. 4. Tavaras JM, Ferrucci JT (eds). Philadelphia, JB Lippincott, 1990, pp 1–21.
27. Johnson CD, Rice RP, Kelvin FM, et al: The radiologic evaluation of gross cecal distension: emphasis on cecal ileus. AJR 1985; 145:1211–1217.
28. Laufer B.: The left lateral view in the plain film assessment of abdominal distention. Radiology 1976; 119:265.
29. Gutierrez ED, Balfe DM: Fluoroscopically guided nasoenteric feeding tube placement: results of a 1-year study. Radiology 1991; 178:759.

CHAPTER 14

Pain Management Consultation in Adult Patients

Cheryl L. Dixon, M.D.

The role of the anesthesiologist as a pain management consultant is changing rapidly. Pain management has evolved into a legitimate subspecialty, in and of itself, and is no longer a "black art." Our understanding of the anatomic and physiologic mechanisms of pain is expanding almost daily. As basic scientists discover more and more pieces to the pain puzzle, our pharmacologic and therapeutic options expand as well. The goal of this chapter is to delineate a clinical approach to the adult patient that will elicit the correct pain diagnosis and allow full consideration and implementation of all therapeutic options.

THE ADULT PAIN MANAGEMENT CONSULTATION

What Is the Best Approach?

On the first day of the "pain rotation," an anesthesiology resident must experience the same feelings of inadequacy that medical students feel as they try to complete their first history and physical examination, differential diagnosis, and treatment plan. The principles of medical diagnosis are applicable to the pain patient, regardless of the nature and duration of the problem.

Initial Assessment

Portenoy outlined an approach to pain diagnosis in cancer patients that can be modified to apply to the evaluation and assessment of all patients with pain (Fig. 14–1).[1] With this problem-solving strategy in mind, even the beginning pain management consultant can be successful both in diagnosing and treating pain.

Several basic components to the evaluation process must be thoroughly examined (Table 14–1). The consultant must assess key elements of a pain-related history; understand the impact that psychologic, psychiatric, and social factors have on the problem; and know when to ask for further evaluation. This approach is basic to all pain consultations, aids in the classification of pain, and expedites the eventual diagnosis. A basic

medical history is imperative to pain diagnosis, therapeutic strategy, and prediction of outcome. A generalized physical examination and detailed examination of the targeted area should also be performed.

Laboratory Assessment

Based on the information obtained, the consultant next employs laboratory testing to aid in the differential diagnosis. The most common tests (selectively applied based on the previously obtained information) include spine radiography, computed tomography (CT), magnetic resonance imaging (MRI),

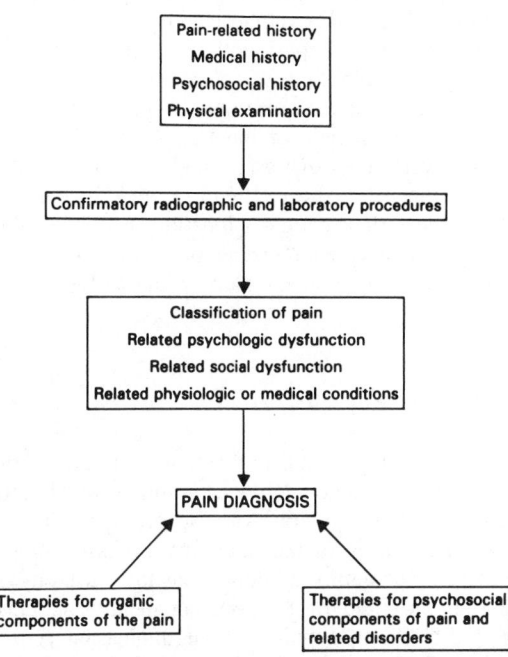

FIGURE 14–1. The pain diagnosis incorporates the multifactorial nature of pain and its associated symptoms and signs and is a guide to targeting interventions appropriately and efficiently. See text for the various classifications of pain. (From Portenoy RK: Diagnosis of cancer pain syndromes. *In* Pain Syndromes in Neurologic Practices. Field H (ed). New York, Butterworth Publishing Company, 1990, p 240.)

TABLE 14–1. Key Points in Obtaining a Thorough Pain History

Definition of the pain problem (acute, chronic, or cancer-related; nociceptive or neuropathic)
Course of the pain problem from the onset
Characteristics of the pain intensity (quality, duration, periodicity, location, and distribution)
Exacerbating factors
Associated factors (stress, depression, sleep disturbances)
Current therapeutic modalities
Results of all diagnostic and therapeutic procedures

electromyography (EMG), nerve conduction studies, bone scanning, and determination of complete blood count, erythrocyte sedimentation rate, and vitamin B_{12} and folate levels.

Diagnosis

Once this information is gathered, the pain and associated medical and psychosocial conditions can be classified and a pain diagnosis established. Not until this problem-solving approach has been performed thoroughly can the patient be adequately treated with an expected good outcome. The methodology used distinguishes a "block" clinic from a "pain" clinic. Therapeutic options specific to the classification of pain as well as to the individual patient can then be recommended.

Treatment

Treatment options to be discussed in greater detail later include pharmacologic approaches via all routes (oral to neuraxial); regional anesthetic techniques (single injection to neurolytic blockade); neuroaugmentation, including transcutaneous electrical nerve stimulation (TENS) and spinal cord stimulation (SCS); and psychiatric and psychologic therapy.

Patients experiencing pain with an expected short duration and a limited etiology (e.g., postoperative pain in young healthy adults) usually require only a simple therapeutic modality. Patients with pain of long duration and no chance of medical recovery (e.g., that associated with metastatic prostate cancer) require the most attention and inventive strategies. Regardless of a patient's location in this spectrum, the pain management consultant can offer something that is of help, often with tremendous success and to the patient's delight.

What Are the Key Historical Elements?

Before discussing a pain problem with a patient, the anesthesiologist should have an understanding of the definitions of pain, since treatment options vary accordingly. The Subcommittee on Taxonomy of the International Association for the Study of Pain has published definitions to be used by all those working in the field of pain management. The universally accepted definition of pain is "an unpleasant sensory and emotional experience associated with actual or potential tissue damage, or described in terms of such damage."[2]

Chronicity

Bonica takes this definition one step further by differentiating acute from chronic pain.[3] This modifier is vitally important

because the etiology, pathophysiology, symptomatology, diagnosis, and therapy of both are potentially different.

Acute Pain

Acute pain, as defined by Bonica, "is a complex constellation of unpleasant sensory, perceptual, and emotional experiences and certain autonomic, psychologic, emotional, and behavioral responses."[3] Acute pain patients lack psychopathology as a primary cause of their problem. Their pain is self-limiting in nature and usually resolves within days to weeks.

Chronic Pain

Chronic pain is "pain that persists a month beyond the usual course of an acute disease or a reasonable time for an injury to heal, or that is associated with a chronic pathologic process that causes continuous pain, or the pain recurs at intervals for months or years."[3] It may well have associated psychopathology, either as a cause or result, and may have irreversible pathophysiology if not recognized and treated in a timely fashion. Chronic pain may be caused by cancer, in which case additional pathophysiology is introduced and variations in treatment modalities are employed.

The term *chronic, benign pain* describes nonmalignant pain; nothing is "benign" about chronic pain, which can be devastating to both patients and associates. Bonica recommends that the term "chronic pain" be reserved for nonmalignant pain and that "cancer pain" be used for those pain problems that are related to a malignant process. Finally, adding to the complexity of the problem is the well-known fact that patients with malignancies can have acute and chronic pain.

Mechanisms

Another way to define pain uses a mechanistic approach that removes the emotional aspect of pain and suffering but is helpful in determining the best medical approach to the underlying problem. Portenoy proposed three general mechanisms of chronic pain that might be helpful in classification. These include nociceptive, neuropathic, and psychogenic pain (Fig. 14–2).[4]

Nociceptive pain is pain that occurs under normal conditions and is related to ongoing activation of nociceptive pathways of somatic or visceral origin. *Neuropathic pain* is related to the pathologic effects of an injury to a nerve, a nerve plexus, or the central nervous system (CNS).

Psychogenic pain historically was termed *idiopathic pain*. It is applied to patients whose pain is associated with no evidence of an organic lesion or to those with pain in excess of the extent of the organic lesion.

This definition presents some difficulties, since many chronic pain patients appear to have pain in excess of the inciting lesion owing to both the chronicity of the problem, often without successful treatment, and to the confounding anxiety and depression. We have much to learn about the pathophysiology of pain and its mechanisms within the CNS. I am reluctant to label a patient as having psychogenic pain until all other possibilities have been exhausted and multiple pain experts have been involved in evaluation and treatment.

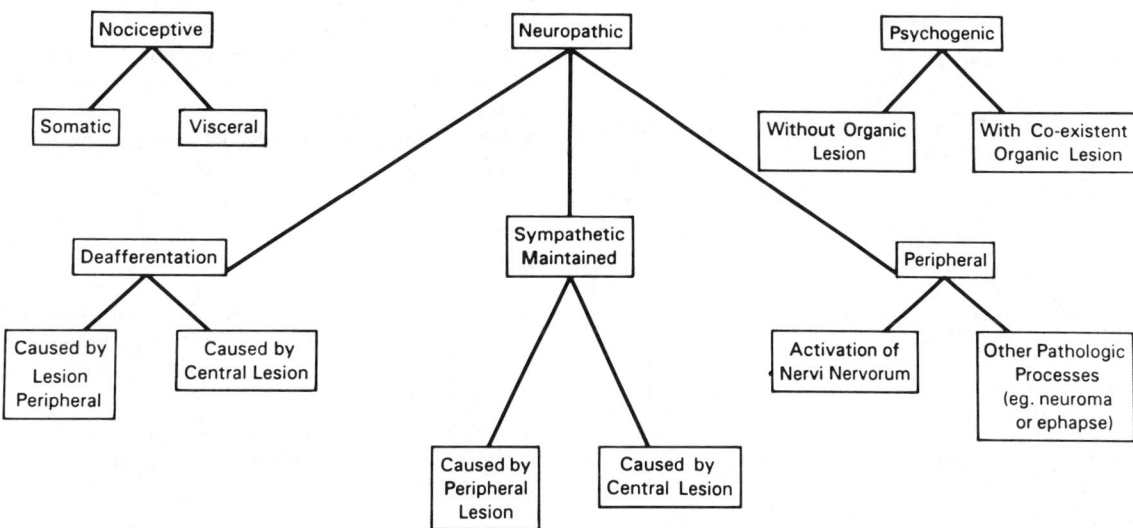

FIGURE 14–2. Proposed taxonomy of chronic pain based on presumed pathophysiologic distinctions. (From Portenoy RK: Mechanisms of clinical pain, observations and speculations. Neurol Clin 1989; 7:207.)

Intensity

Scales and Percentages

Once the chronicity of the pain problem has been established, the intensity must be evaluated. Multiple tools have been utilized to assess this aspect, but the visual analogue scale is the most popular and has been used for many years both in the clinical arena and in research. It is a reliable and a valid tool.[5]

In the traditional use of the visual analogue scale, the patient is shown a 10-cm line with endpoint descriptors of "NO PAIN" on the left and "THE WORST PAIN IMAGINABLE" on the right. The patient is then asked to place a mark at the position that represents his or her current level of pain (Fig. 14–3).[6] Some patients find it easier to use if the numerical scale is already present on the line (see Fig. 14–3). Others are only able to use words to describe their pain level (see Fig. 14–3).

Another method of evaluation that is very useful in elderly patients involves the use of percentages. Many will be able to tell you what "percentage" of pain they experience out of 100% or what "percentage" decrease in pain they achieve in response to your treatment but have tremendous difficulty in using a 0-to-10 scale. The key is to find the method of pain assessment that works for each patient and then use it consistently.

Individual Perception

One major point that must be understood when pain is assessed is the belief that the most reliable indicator of pain is the patient's reporting.[7] Loeser developed a model of the components of pain that well illustrates this point (Fig. 14–4).[8] It incorporates the physiologic processing of pain (nociception); the perceptions (pain) and emotional responses to the pain (suffering); and the only assessable part (pain behavior). The anesthesiologist must constantly remind himself or herself that pain behavior—that is, what the patient does or does not say or do—is the *only* measurable component. In so doing, one quickly discards any temptation to second guess this evaluation process.

Physical Signs

The pain management novice is tempted to rely on objective measures such as heart rate, blood pressure, and facial expressions when assessing pain or pain management techniques. Although these signs should be included in the evaluation

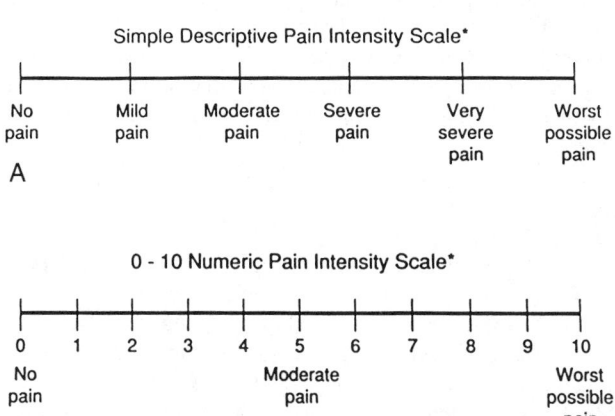

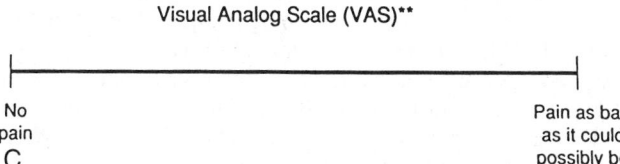

FIGURE 14–3. Examples of pain intensity and pain distress scales. *A*, Descriptive pain intensity scale. *B*, Numeric pain intensity scale (from 1 to 10). *C*, Visual analogue scale (VAS). (From Acute Pain Management Guideline Panel: Acute Pain Management: Operative or Medical Procedures and Trauma. Clinical Practice Guideline. AHCPR, Pub. No. 92-0032. Rockville, MD: Agency for Health Care Policy and Research, Public Health Service; 1992. US Department of Health and Human Services publication AHCPR 92-0032, p 116.)

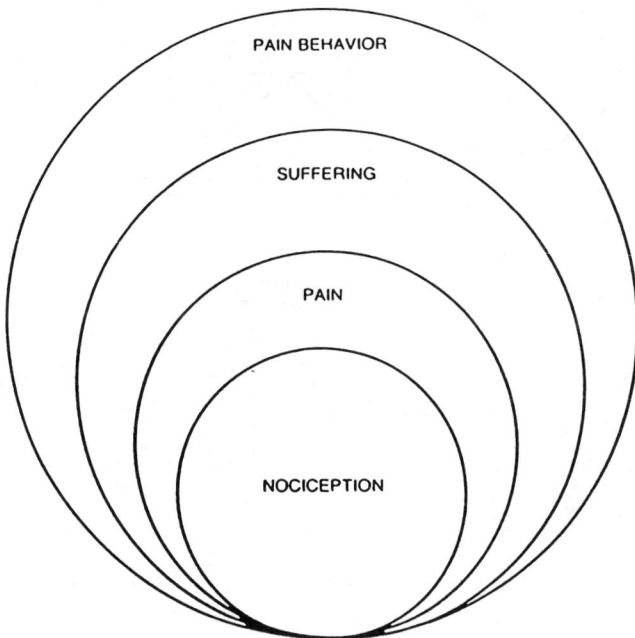

FIGURE 14–4. A multifaceted model of the components of pain. (From Loeser JD: Concepts of pain. *In* Chronic Low Back Pain. Staton-Hicks M, Boas R (eds). New York, Raven Press, 1982, p 146.)

process, they are not as reliable as the patients' self-report.[9] An example familiar to anesthesiologists is the patient in the postanesthesia care unit (PACU) who sleeps intermittently yet complains of pain when awake. This scenario is easy to understand when the intraoperative drug history is reviewed. As long as centrally-acting drugs influence the patient's level of consciousness, he or she may legitimately feel pain when awake yet intermittently fall asleep until the blood level of the sedative/hypnotic/analgesic combination deteriorates. Withholding appropriate pain medications at that point only delays a satisfactory degree of pain management as well as the PACU discharge.

Quality

The quality of pain can be a clue to its etiology. Examples of differentiating pain descriptors include cutaneous (sharp, pricking, burning, throbbing, stabbing); deep somatic (dull, aching, diffuse); visceral (vague, poorly localized, diffuse dull, aching); and sympathetic (burning, aching, throbbing).

Similarities between deep somatic (i.e., in muscles, tendons, joints, and bones) and visceral pain have been noted. The characteristics are similar, but significant differences involve the pain pathways and the embryologic origin of the structures involved. Although sensory innervation involves A delta and C fibers, those fibers traveling from the viscera run in association with the sympathetic fibers. Also, the structures involved in deep somatic pain are of mesodermal origin, whereas those of the viscera are of endodermic origin.[10]

Duration and Periodicity

The duration and periodicity of pain are also characteristics that are helpful in a differential diagnosis. Lewis described many well-known pains using a time-intensity curve that in-

corporates the length of time between episodes, the way pain starts, and the rate of rise, frequency, and rate of decline of the curve (Fig. 14–5).[11] Questions to elicit this information address whether the pain is intermittent or continuous, or pulsatile or wavelike. The relationship in time to injuries, changes in weather, stressful life events, and medical problems can all be helpful as well.

Location

The location of pain also is a key to its diagnosis. This fact must be tempered with the realization that only cutaneous pain is well localized. Deep somatic pain and visceral pain may be very difficult to locate because of the amount of referred pain involved. Furthermore, sympathetically mediated pain does not follow classic dermatome distributions.

Course

Be sure to determine exacerbating factors and relieving maneuvers, particularly if the pain is chronic or cancer-related. For all pain problems except the most acute, the previously discussed characteristics must be analyzed from the onset of the pain to the time of evaluation. Has the pain intensity worsened or improved? Is the pain now intermittent or constant? Does it have any association with physical or emotional stress? Has the location changed?

Also be sure to obtain the results of previous diagnostic and therapeutic procedures. This information is best sought from the referring physician, as the patient will have a very difficult time remembering results, especially if pain relief from a therapeutic procedure was only short-lived.

Current therapeutic modalities must also be elicited. Many patients have cognitive deficits associated with centrally-acting medications that are used to treat the problem, the chronic nature of their pain, and its potential association with depression. This problem may lead to long-term sleep disturbances, thus adding to their cognitive dysfunction. Be prepared to involve all health care providers and family members familiar with the patient to develop a complete pain history.

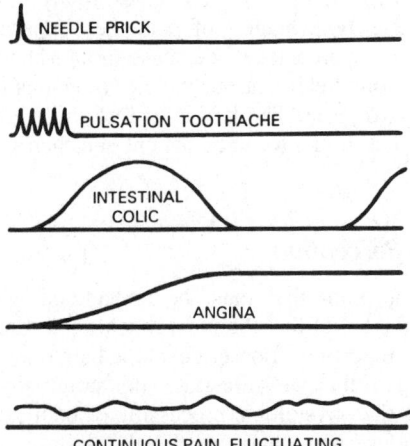

FIGURE 14–5. A diagram illustrating time-intensity curves of various well-known pains, namely, needle prick, pulsating toothache, intestinal colic, angina, and continuous fluctuating pain. (From Lewis T: Pain. New York, MacMillan Publishing Co, 1942, p 173.)

Is the Concurrent Medical Condition a Factor?

The next step in the development of a pain diagnosis involves obtaining a separate medical history (see Fig. 14–1). The young, healthy patient with an easily diagnosed and treatable pain problem does not present a dilemma; the elderly patient with multiple organ system dysfunctions is more challenging and difficult. These patients are problematic regardless of whether their pain is acute, chronic, or cancer-related. The major problem involves potential adverse effects associated with both pharmacologic and nonpharmacologic treatment options.

Pharmacologic Interactions

Drug interactions and pharmacokinetics must be considered when treatment is recommended. Regardless of the route used, opiates can potentially produce clinically significant adverse interactions with any other class of centrally-acting drugs (all CNS depressants, anticonvulsants, alcohol, and some drugs with a primary site of action outside the CNS).

Tricyclic Antidepressants and Narcotics

Adjuvant tricyclic antidepressant use can be problematic in cancer patients who are not obtaining satisfactory pain relief with opiates alone. Even a low dose of amitriptyline can cause delirium and major management problems.[12] This drug interaction may take hours to days to resolve once the source of the problem has been identified owing to the long half-life of the tricyclic antidepressant. Obviously, dose titration is crucial in these and similar patients and requires very close observation and gradual increase in the antidepressant dose while all other drug doses are maintained at a stable level.

Steroids

Treatment for several types of low back pain involves the placement of steroids in the epidural space. Although the depot form is used, gradual uptake occurs with the potential for systemic effects. A common problem in patients with diabetes mellitus is an increase in the insulin or oral hypoglycemic requirements and the need for stricter diet control. Thus, a plan for close monitoring of blood glucose must be in place prior to administration of depot steroid to a diabetic patient.

Steroids administered by any route may cause serious gastrointestinal bleeding problems in patients who are taking aspirin or nonsteroidal anti-inflammatory drugs (NSAIDs). Both of these drug therapies may be overlooked by the patient during the medical and drug history unless questions are specifically asked.

Finally, the rare but serious potential for an epidural hematoma if an epidural steroid injection is performed must be considered in patients who are taking aspirin or NSAIDs. Although controversy abounds regarding the validity of bleeding time measurements as prognosticators of this problem, the conservative approach is to obtain the test before attempting an epidural steroid injection.

Calcium Channel Blockers

The administration of calcium channel blockers for the treatment of reflex sympathetic dystrophy, although potentially useful for the pain problem, may become very problematic in the patient with hypertension or coronary artery disease currently treated with other medications. A complicated pain patient focuses pain and often makes light of other controlled medical problems, not realizing the potential complicating factors.

Pharmacokinetic Alterations

The pharmacokinetics of medications used in the treatment of pain may be altered by hepatic, renal, or cardiac disease. Cirrhosis and liver failure can result in decreases in drug clearance; decreases in enzymatic biotransformation; and a greater potential for drug sensitivity and toxicity. The reduction in plasma proteins results in a greater delivery of larger amounts of free drug to target organs.[13]

Renal dysfunction can lead to an increase in plasma drug levels or in their active metabolites because of decreased clearance or uremia-induced hypoalbuminemia.[14]

Cardiac dysfunction, particularly congestive heart failure, results in decreased blood flow to both the liver and the kidneys, further impairing hepatic clearance, biotransformation, and renal elimination.[15] Obviously, the prescription of medications to pain patients with major systemic disease, those taking other medications, or both, must be done with great caution, reductions in dose, and close communication with the patient's primary physician.

Nonpharmacologic Interactions

Nonpharmacologic treatment options might also be problematic in patients with significant medical problems. Such individuals most likely have difficulty participating in active exercise programs that are often imperative in the recovery process of a myofascial pain problem. The primary physician can help to determine the acceptable level of physical activity.

What Is the Impact of Psychologic/ Psychiatric Dysfunction?

Psychologic and psychiatric factors may play important roles in the perception and response to pain. Pain becomes a problem once it can no longer be ignored. At this point, the emotional or *affective* aspects of the pain become increasingly important (Table 14–2).[16]

The Minnesota Multiphasic Personality Inventory reveals that chronic pain patients have higher scores in hysteria, depression, and hypochondriasis.[17] Such patients have reduced scores once their pain is treated successfully.[18]

TABLE 14–2. Psychologic Effects of Pain

Depressed mood
Sleep disturbance
Somatic preoccupation
Reduced activity
Reduced libido
Irritable
Anxiety

(From Pelz M, Merskey H: A description of the psychological effects of chronic painful lesions. Pain 1982; 14:293.)

Emotional Disorders

Emotional disorders often predispose to increased susceptibility or decreased tolerance for pain. Such problems include major depression, dysthymia, somatization, conversion disorders, hypochondriasis, and psychogenic pain.[19] Depression impairs the patient's ability to cope with the pain, whereas somatization disorder and hypochondriasis result in a persistent search for the "etiology" of the pain problem, often involving invasive tests and surgery. Obviously, when such a problem might exist, a screening evaluation by a trained psychiatrist is needed.

Environmental Factors

Environmental factors also can influence a patient's response to pain. The consequences of one's pain behavior are at the heart of this relationship. Behavior may be rewarded or punished, depending on environmental factors. The learning model of pain holds that reinforcement of pain behavior sustains it even in the absence of the noxious somatic stimulus that initially elicited the pain.[20]

The issue of disability payments is a common problem seen in chronic pain patients. Financial compensation for pain and injury is a positive reinforcer to continue the pain and to stay away from work. Inactivity is another commonly seen problem. Initially, avoiding activity lessens the pain; eventually, the inability to be active is reinforced by the avoidance of unpleasant tasks or the attention of family members, or both. Physicians often contribute to this problem in their attempts to identify the organic cause of the pain without evaluating the other possible psychosocial etiologies.

Preliminary questions that need be asked to screen for these features are listed in Table 14–3.

How Should the Physical Examination Be Approached?

The physical examination is crucial to the differential pain diagnosis. It includes a general examination as well as a thorough evaluation of the painful region. Height, weight, blood pressure, heart rate, respiratory rate, and temperature are essential as screening data. A complete cardiopulmonary examina-

TABLE 14–3. Screening Questions to Detect Psychologic, Psychiatric, Emotional, and Environmental Problems

Have you felt sad, blue, depressed, hopeless, down in the dumps lately?
Have you noticed a decrease in your appetite or weight loss?
Are you able to sleep at night?
Have you lost interest in your usual pleasurable activities?
Have you noticed a loss of energy or the onset of fatigue?
Are you able to concentrate in your usual fashion?
Have you had recurrent thoughts of death or suicide?
Have you at any time had psychiatric or psychologic treatment for any condition?
Has anyone in your family been diagnosed with a psychiatric problem?
Do others consider you a sickly person?
If your present pain condition was caused on or by your job, do you feel that your employer has treated you fairly?
Have you received compensation for your injury?
Are you bringing suit because of your pain?
Do you expect to sue or are you thinking about suing?
When you are in pain, what does your spouse do?

tion is also mandatory as is a screening neurologic examination that includes assessment of cranial nerve function, spinal nerve function (sensory and motor), coordination, and cerebral function. The anesthesiologist should explain to the patient that this initial examination process is for screening purposes to assure the physician that nothing is missed. Otherwise, a patient will be confused and possibly resentful when the initial examination involves nonpainful areas. Examination of the most painful area should be performed last so as not to interfere with the rest of the process.

The Painful Area

Inspection

Inspection gives further evidence that is needed to make the correct pain diagnosis. When pain is secondary to chronic reflex sympathetic dystrophy, the skin in the involved area is mottled, often sweaty, and sustains hair loss; ridging of the nails is common. Patients with myofascial pain may exhibit observable muscle asymmetry in the area of muscle spasm, or they may experience limited range of motion. Denervation hypersensitivity can be observed in skin supplied by damaged nerve roots when cool air provokes the pilomotor reflex.[21] This response may be short-lived, occurring at the time of undressing and possibly resolving shortly thereafter, but it can be reproduced by stroking or scratching the affected area.

Palpation

Palpation adds more information on which to base the pain diagnosis. If the history and qualitative description of the pain are suggestive of reflex sympathetic dystrophy of 6 months' duration or greater, the skin will feel cold to the touch. Since the first stage of reflex sympathetic dystrophy can last from 6 weeks to 6 months, the area may feel warm during this period.[22]

In myofascial pain, tender muscle areas are palpable as nodules or bands; palpation reproduces the patient's pain. The patient may jump or withdraw when relatively light pressure is applied to these tender areas. The muscle itself may even twitch under the palpating finger (jump sign), further supporting the diagnosis.[23]

In some neuropathic pain problems, sensation is diminished in the dermatomal distribution of the affected nerve or nerves, whereas the surrounding areas may reveal hyperesthesia, dysesthesia, allodynia, or hyperalgesia. These findings are elicited by gently stroking the contralateral mirror-image region followed by the affected area. If the affected area is more sensitive than the normal region, the patient is said to have hyperesthesia; dysesthesia is an unpleasant sensation, and allodynia is a painful sensation.[2] Also seen with neuropathic pain is an increased response to a painful stimulus that is termed *hyperalgesia.*[2] It can be elicited by pinprick testing that compares normal and painful areas. Palpation over a neuroma, also classified as neuropathic by some, reproduces the sharp, shooting pain that is the patient's major complaint.

What Laboratory Or Radiographic Data Are Necessary to Make a Pain Diagnosis?

Although pain management experts rely heavily on physical examination, they also find certain tests to be of value (Table

TABLE 14–4. Useful Laboratory and Radiographic Tests in Pain Evaluation

Plain radiography
CT scan
EMG
Contrast radiography
Nuclear medicine
Laboratory tests (other than blood tests)
CBC
Thermography
Electroencephalography
Electrocardiography

(From Rudy TE, Turk DC, Brena SF: Differential utility of medical procedures in the assessment of chronic pain patients. Pain 1988; 34:167.)

14–4).[24] Usually, patients coming to a chronic pain clinic or center will have had these studies performed in the recent past. The pain management consultant must interpret these tests appropriately and know when to order further tests.

Radiographic Studies

Radiographic studies are useful in evaluation of a number of musculoskeletal pain problems, including arthritis, bone tumors (primary and metastatic), and fractures.

Computed Tomography Scans

CT scans are commonly used to evaluate the spine. The spinal cord and any extrinsic defects in the canal may be visualized as can facet joint disease and spinal stenosis. The CT scan is noninvasive and thus preferable to myelography, which carries potential significant risks.

Myelography

Myelography is helpful to determine whether a patient has a surgically correctable disease and, if so, to localize the lesion prior to surgery. Over 90% of lumbar herniated disks are diagnosed by CT scanning alone; the myelogram is reserved for those cases in which CT scanning fails to find an abnormality.[25]

Magnetic Resonance Imaging

MRI is noninvasive and visualizes the spinal anatomy in much the same way as contrast myelography but without the associated risks. The MRI scan is superior for the evaluation of intervertebral disk disease and is the examination of choice for many spinal conditions.

Electromyography

EMG is useful in the diagnosis of nerve trauma, plexopathies or nerve root lesions, diffuse polyneuropathies, and primary muscle diseases.

Screening Laboratory Studies

The causes of painful neuropathies are extensive; laboratory screening studies include determination of complete blood counts, erythrocyte sedimentation rate, and muscle enzyme levels; serum protein electrophoresis; immunoglobulin measurement; LE cell preparation; antinuclear antibodies; glucose tolerance testing; vitamin B_{12}, folate, and niacin determination; and serologic assay for syphilis.

Thermography

Thermography has been used to diagnose many pain syndromes. However, since the test measures surface temperature, it yields positive results in many situations and cannot necessarily be used as a specific diagnostic tool. It is useful in the following situations: soft tissue injury, nerve root compression or irritation, bone and joint disorders, myofascial pain syndromes, neurovascular compression, sprains, infections, and sympathetic mediated pain.

MANAGEMENT TECHNIQUES

Once the history, physical examination data, and laboratory results have been obtained and a pain diagnosis determined, a treatment plan is generated. Treatment should provide the most benefit with the least side effects. Unfortunately, the diagnosis is not always readily apparent on the first visit, and the patient may require several trials, a combination of treatments, or both. Combination therapy often minimizes side effects and maximizes pain relief by blocking pain pathways at multiple sites within the peripheral and central nervous system.

What Is the Basis of Pharmacologic Approaches?

Table 14–5 lists the major classes of drugs that are available for consideration. Some are not indicated for every patient. A long-acting opiate such as morphine sulfate is not the drug of choice in a patient with postoperative pain in whom the problem is expected to be short-lived. Similarly, a short-acting drug that must be administered in multiple doses each day is less than desirable for the management of a long-term, chronic pain problem.

Classification of Pain and Associated Drug Therapy

Drug therapies are often selected in accordance with the classification of pain the patient is experiencing. Primary drugs

TABLE 14–5. Major Drug Classifications Utilized in Pain Management

Nonopiate analgesics
Opiate analgesics
Local anesthetics
Antidepressants
Anticonvulsants
Muscle relaxants
Sympatholytics
Corticosteroids
Analeptics
Neuroleptics
Antihistamines
Benzodiazepines
Miscellaneous (e.g., baclofen, clonidine)

utilized for acute pain include nonopiate and opiate analgesics and occasionally a benzodiazepine (Tables 14–6 to 14–8).[26] Chronic pain patients present a different therapeutic dilemma by the nature of the chronicity of the disease and the potential for psychologic involvement. With these facts in mind, the most common drug therapies include use of nonopiate analgesics, antidepressants, oral local anesthetics (e.g., mexiletine), anticonvulsants, neuroleptics, sympatholytics, and miscellaneous drugs such as baclofen (Tables 14–9 and 14–10).[27]

One principle to follow in the prescription of ''pain'' medication to chronic pain patients is to avoid the long-term use of medications known to produce tolerance and physical dependence until all other options have undergone adequate trials (including a multidiscipline inpatient program, when appropriate). Occasionally, such medications may be necessary in the beginning (e.g., use of a muscle relaxant such as cyclobenzaprine [Flexeril] for myofascial pain). The pain consultant should be certain to prescribe a short course of any such medication and to follow these patients closely until they no longer require medications to control their problem.

Opioids and Nonmalignant Pain

A growing body of literature concerns opioid therapy for the treatment of chronic (nonmalignant) pain. Significant controversy surrounds this issue.[28–30] Some topics for discussion include analgesic efficacy, tolerance, goals, risk of adverse pharmacologic outcomes, toxicity, side effects, drug dependence, and drug addiction.[28] Many experts believe that a subset of chronic pain patients obtains improved pain relief without significant toxicity or addiction. One should be aware of the recommendations for opioid therapy (Table 14–11).[28]

Cancer Pain

Cancer pain patients present a different set of problems owing to the nature of the disease and the impact it has on the patient and the family.[31–33] Such patients can experience a combination of acute and chronic pain and often have a limited life expectancy. Therefore, they have even more medication needs as well as some unique problems specific to their group.

The World Health Organization (WHO) has developed a three-step analgesic ladder that is applicable to all cancer pain patients both in developed and undeveloped countries (Fig. 14–6).[31] In addition, use of corticosteroids, analeptics, neuroleptics, antihistamines, and miscellaneous drugs such as antiemetics and anticonstipation agents must be considered early (Tables 14–12 to 14–15).[33]

Known Efficacy

Appropriate pharmacotherapy may be chosen based on drug groups that are known to be efficacious in the treatment of a specific pain syndrome or problem. The simplest mechanistic approach, after determining if the pain is acute, chronic, or cancer-related, is to classify the pain as nociceptive or neuropathic.

Physicians of all specialties know the utility of nonopiate

TABLE 14–6. Nonopioid Analgesics for the Treatment of Acute Pain

Agent	Adult Dose (mg per os)	Interval (h)	Maximum Dose per Day (mg)	Comments
Salicylates				
Aspirin	500–1000	4–6	6000	1. Gastrointestinal upset and bleeding 2. Irreversible decrease in platelet aggregation
Diflunisal (Dolobid)*	1000 initial 500 subsequent	8–12	1500	No antiplatelet effect at lower doses
Choline magnesium trisalicylate (Trilisate)	1000–1500	12	4000	No antiplatelet effect
Acetaminophen	500–1000	4–6	4000	Hepatotoxic with sustained high doses
NSAIDs				
Ibuprofen	200–400	4–6	3200	All NSAIDS: 1. Reversible decrease in platelet aggregation 2. Can produce gastrointestinal effects 3. Can cause renal insufficiency 4. Can cause CNS impairment
Naproxen*	500 initial 250 subsequent	12	1250	
Fenoprofen (Nalfon)	300–600	6–8	3000	
Indomethacin*	25	8–12	150	
Sulindac (Clinoril)	150–200	12	400	
Mefenamic acid (Ponstel)	500 initial 250 subsequent	6	1000	Do not use longer than 7 days
Meclofenamate (Meclomen)	50	6	400	
Tolmetin (Tolectin)	400	8	2000	
Piroxicam (Feldene)*	10	12	30	
Ketoprogen*	50	6–8	300	
Diclofenac*	50–100	6–12	200	
Benzidamine*	50	?	?	
Metamizol/Dypirone*	500	?	?	
Ketorolac (Toradol)*	30–60	6	150	
Tenoxicam†	20	24	20	

(From Task Force on Acute Pain: Management of Acute Pain: A Practical Guide. Ready BH, Edwards WT (eds). Seattle, IASP Publications, 1992, pp 11–21.)
*Injectable form is available in some countries.
†Intramuscular or intravenous route only.

TABLE 14–7. Systemic Opioids for the Treatment of Acute Pain

	Drug	Route of Administration (mg · kg^{-1})	Front Load*† (mg · kg^{-1})	Maintenance Dose‡ (mg · kg^{-1})	Frequency§ (h)
Agonists	Codeine	PO	1.5	0.75	3–4
		SC, IM	1.0	0.5	3–4
	Hydrocodone‖ (Vicodin)	PO	0.15	0.07–0.15	4–6
	Oxycodone (Percodan)	PO	0.15	0.07–0.15	3–4
	Morphine	PO	0.5–1.0	0.5–1.0	4
		Slow-release	1.0	1.0–2.0	12
		PO¶	0.15	0.1–0.2	3–4
		SC, IM	0.15	0.01–0.04 per h	Continuous
		IV			
	Meperidine (Pethidine)	PO	2.5–3.5	1.5–3.0	3–4
		SC, IM	1.5–2.0	1.0–1.5	3–4
		IV	1.5–2.0	0.3–0.6 per h	Continuous
	Omnopon (Pantopon)	SC, IM	0.3	0.1–0.2	4
	Hydromorphone	PO	0.04–0.08	0.04–0.08	3
	(Dilaudid)	SC, IM	0.02–0.04	0.03–0.06	3
		IV	0.02	0.01 per h	Continuous
	Nicomorphine††	SC, IM	0.15	0.1–0.2	3–4
		IV	0.15	0.01–0.04 per h	Continuous
	Diamorphine†† (Heroin)	SC, IM	0.03–0.07	0.01–0.04	2
		IV	0.03–0.07	0.01–0.04 per h	2
	Oxymorphone	SC, IM	0.15	0.1–0.2	3–4
	Methadone	PO	0.2–0.4	0.1–0.4	**, ‡‡
		SC, IM	0.14	0.1–0.2	**, ‡‡
		IV	0.15	§§	
	Levorphanol	PO	0.02–0.04	0.02–0.04	**, ‡‡
		SC, IM	0.02	0.01	**, ‡‡
		IV	0.02	§§	
	Fentanyl	IV‖‖	0.0008–0.0016	0.0003–0.0016 per h	Continuous
		Transdermal			
	Sufentanil	IV‖‖	0.001–0.0003	Not established	—
	Alfentanil	IV‖‖	0.03–0.05	0.06–0.09 per h	Continuous
Mixed Agonist-antagonists	Pentazocine¶¶ (Talwin)	PO	1.5–2.5	1.0–1.5	6
		SC, IM	1.0	0.7–1.0	6
		IV	1.0	0.7–1.0 per h	6
	Nalbuphine (Nubain)	SC, IM	0.05–0.01	0.05–0.1	3–4
		IV	0.05–0.01	0.05–0.1 per h	3–4
	Butorphanol¶¶ (Stadol)	SC, IM	0.03	0.02–0.04	3
		IV	0.03	0.02–0.04	3
		Intranasal			
Partial Agonist	Buprenorphine	Sublingual	0.006	0.004	6–8
	(Buprenex)	SC, IM	0.004	0.002	6
		IV	0.004	0.002 per h	6

(From Task Force on Acute Pain: Management of Acute Pain: A Practical Guide. Ready BH, Edwards WT (eds). Seattle, IASP Publications, 1992, pp 11–21.)
*IV front-loading dose should be titrated slowly to reduce risk of overdose.
†Except in pediatric patients, body weight is not an accurate predictor of effective opioid dose. Titration to desired effect for each patient is necessary.
‡If pain breakthrough occurs before administration of scheduled maintenance dose, give one additional maintenance dose and continue schedule.
§Maintenance dose is usually approximately one-half the effective loading dose.
‖Available only in combination with aspirin or acetaminophen in the United States.
¶Nearest dosage increment must be chosen; if tablets are broken, immediate release can occur.
**Metabolic normeperidine accumulates; CNS stimulation can lead to seizures; higher doses or prolonged infusions are not recommended.
††Not available in the United States.
‡‡Watch for accumulation, especially after 48 h of administration.
§§Long duration of action renders drug unsuitable for continuous infusion.
‖‖Short duration of action makes IV infusion the only practical route of administration.
¶¶Can precipitate withdrawal in opioid-dependent patients.
Abbreviations: PO = oral; IV = intravenous; IM = intramuscular; SC = subcutaneous.

TABLE 14–8. Benzodiazepines as Adjuncts in the Treatment of Acute Pain

	Half-Life of Drug or Metabolites (h)	Route	Adult Dose (mg)	Interval (h)	Comments
Diazepam (Valium)	30–60	Oral	2–10	6	1. Injection is painful
		IV	2–5	3–4	2. Long-acting active metabolite
Chlordiazepoxide (Librium)	5–15	Oral	10–25	8–12	
		IMV, IV	5–25	6–8	
Flurazepam (Dalmane)	50–100	Oral	10–30	12–24	Hypnotic
Lorazepam (Ativan)	10–20	Oral	0.5–3	6–12	May accumulate in elderly patients
		IM, IV	0.5–2	6–12	
Oxazepam (Serax)	5–10	Oral	10–20	6–8	
Triazolam (Halcion)	1.3–3	Oral	0.125–0.5	8–12	Hypnotic
Midazolam (Versed)	1.2–12	IM	1–3	2–4	1. Amnesia is pronounced
		IV	0.5–2	0.3–3	2. Well suited to IV infusion (0.5–5 mg · h^{-1})

(From Task Force on Acute Pain: Management of Acute Pain: A Practical Guide. Ready BH, Edwards WT (eds). Seattle, IASP Publications, 1992, pp 11–21.)

TABLE 14–9. Dosages and Effects of Antidepressants Used in Pain Management

	Drug	Initial Dosage*	Maintenance Dosage*	Efficacy in Depression	Adverse and Side Effects	
					Orthostatic Hypotension	*Sedation*
Heterocyclics	Tricyclics					
	Amitriptyline	10–300	10–150	+ + + +	+ +	+ + +
	Clomipramine	20–200	20–150	+ + + +	+ +	+ +
	Desipramine	75–300	75–100	+ + + +	+ +	−
	Doxepin	30–300	30–200	+ + + +	+ +	+ + + +
	Imipramine	20–300	20–150	+ + + +	+ + +	+
	Nortriptyline	50–150	50–150	+ + + +	+	+
	Trimipramine	50–225	75–150	+ + + +	+ +	+ + +
	Second-generation drugs					
	Maprotiline	75–300	75–125	+ + + +	+	+ +
	Trazodone	50–600	100–300	+ + +?	+ +	+ + +
Monoamine Oxidase Inhibitor	Phenelzine	45–90	45–75	+ +	+ + +	−

(From Monks R: Psychotropic drugs. *In* The Management of Pain. Bonica JJ (ed). Philadelphia, Lea & Febiger, 1990, pp 1676–1689.)
*Antidepressant dose reflects material from the clinical literature cited in this chapter and the author's personal experience.
Value of effects: + + + + = marked; + + + = moderate; + + = mild; + = minimal; − = absent; ? = questionable (data inadequate). Only values in vertical columns should be compared.

TABLE 14–10. Dosages and Side Effects of Neuroleptics Used for Pain Management

	Drug	Initial Dosage* (mg · d^{-1} PO)	Maintenance Dosage† (mg · d^{-1} PO)	Side and Adverse Effects‡	
				Anticholinergic	*Autonomic (Hypotension)*
Phenothiazines	Chlorpromazine	75–500	25–150	+ + +	+ + +
	Fluphenazine	1–10	1–3	+	+
	Methotrimeprazine	5–100	15–50	+ + +	+ + +
	Pericyazine	5–200	5–100	+ + +	+ + +
	Perphenazine	8–64	4–16	+ +	+ +
	Thioridazine	10–200	25–75	+ + +	+ + +
	Trifluoperazine	3–20	3–10	+	+
Thioxanthenes	Chlorprothixene	50–200	50–150	+ + +	+ + +
	Flupenthixol	0.5–2	0.5–1	+	−
Miscellaneous	Haloperidol	0.5–30	0.5–10	+	+

(From Monks R: Psychotropic Drugs. *In* The Management of Pain. Bonica JJ (ed). Philadelphia, Lea & Febiger, 1990, pp 1676–1689.)
*Neuroleptic doses reflect data from the clinical material cited in this chapter and from the author's personal experience.
†Modified from Baldessarini RJ: Drugs and the treatment of psychiatric disorders. *In* The Pharmacological Basis of Therapeutics. 7th ed. Goodman L, Gilman AG (eds). New York, Macmillan Publishing Co, 1985.
‡Value of effects: + + + = moderate; + + = mild; + = minimal; − = absent. Only values in vertical columns should be compared.

TABLE 14–11. Proposed Guidelines in the Management of Opioid Maintenance Therapy for Nonmalignant Pain

1. Should be considered only after all other reasonable attempts at analgesia have failed
2. A history of substance abuse should be viewed as a relative contraindication
3. A single practitioner should take primary responsibility for treatment
4. Patients should give informed consent before the start of therapy; points to be covered include recognition of the low risk of psychologic dependence as an outcome, potential for cognitive impairment with the drug alone and in combination with sedative/hypnotics, and understanding by female patients that children born when the mother is on opioid maintenance therapy will likely be physically dependent at birth
5. After drug selection, doses should be given on an around-the-clock basis; several weeks should be agreed upon as the period of initial dose titration, and although improvement in function should be continually stressed, all should agree to at least partial analgesia as the appropriate goal of therapy
6. Failure to achieve at least a partial analgesia at relatively low initial doses in the nontolerant patient raises questions about the potential treatability of the pain syndrome with opioids
7. Emphasis should be given to attempts to capitalize on improved analgesia by gains in physical and social function
8. In addition to the daily dose determined initially, patients should be permitted to escalate dose transiently on days of increased pain; two methods are acceptable: (1) prescription of an additional four to six ''rescue doses'' to be taken as needed during the month; and (2) instruction that one or two extra doses may be taken on any day, but they must be followed by an equal reduction of dose on subsequent days
9. Most patients should be seen and drugs prescribed at least monthly. Patients should be assessed for the efficacy of treatment, adverse drug effects, and the appearance of either misuse or abuse of the drugs during each visit. The results of the assessment should be clearly documented in the medical record
10. Exacerbations of pain not effectively treated by transient, small increases in dose are best managed in the hospital, where dose escalation, if appropriate, can be observed closely, and return to baseline doses can be accomplished in a controlled environment
11. Evidence of drug hoarding, acquisition of drugs from other physicians, uncontrolled dose escalation, or other aberrant behaviors should be followed by tapering and discontinuation of opioid maintenance therapy

(Reprinted by permission of Elsevier Science Publishing Co., Inc., from Chronic opioid therapy in non-malignant pain, by Portenoy RK. Journal of Pain and Symptom Management, Vol. 5(Suppl), p. 546. Copyright 1990 by the U.S. Cancer Pain Relief Committee.)

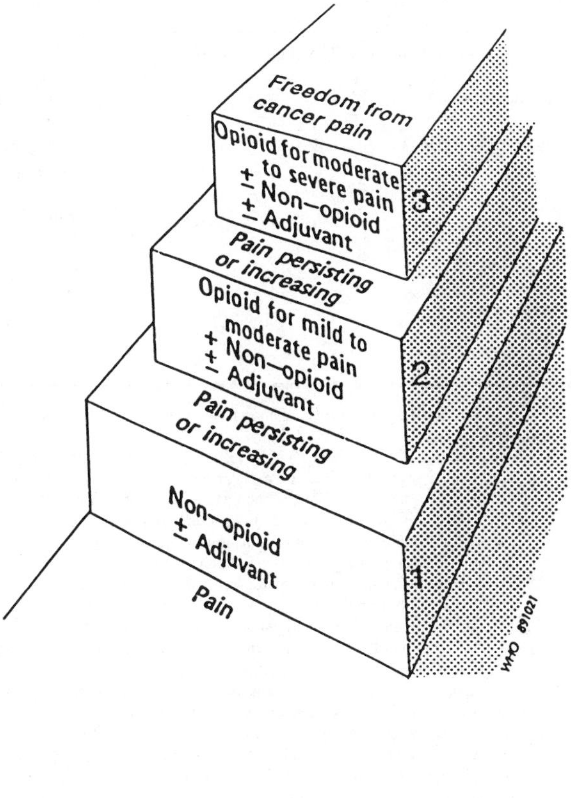

FIGURE 14–6. The WHO three-step analgesic ladder. (Reproduced, by permission, from Cancer pain relief and palliative care. Report of a WHO Expert Committee. Geneva, World Health Organization, 1990, WHO Technical Report Series No. 804, p 9.)

TABLE 14–12. Steroid Therapy for Cancer Pain

Dose	Dexamethasone*	Pain
Low	2–4 mg PO 2 or 3 times per day	Soft tissue infiltration
Moderate	4–8 mg PO 2 to 3 times per day	Nerve compression; visceral distention; lymphedema
High	4–12 mg PO 3 to 4 times per day	Increased intracranial pressure

(From Patt RB, Szalados JE, Wu CL: Pharmacotherapeutic guidelines. *In* Cancer Pain. Patt RB (ed). Philadelphia, JB Lippincott, 1993, p 574.)

and mild opiate analgesics for the treatment of nociceptive pain related to injury, particularly musculoskeletal-type injuries. However, once the problem outlives the usual course of healing, such therapies often cease to be effective. At this point, antidepressants that are efficacious in both nociceptive and neuropathic pain problems should be considered.[34]

For neuropathic pain problems not controllable with antidepressants, oral local anesthetics, sympatholytics, anticonvulsants, neuroleptics, and baclofen use should be considered.[35–40] The order in which the drugs are chosen is based on the degree of pain, the potential for side effects, and the known efficacy of the drug for a particular pain syndrome. The consultant must have a thorough understanding of the pharmacology of the chosen drug and of the pathophysiology and proven treatment modalities for each pain problem before instituting a treatment plan.

When Is the Intravenous Route Appropriate?

Opiates

Although intravenous opiates have long been used for acute pain problems, only recently have anesthesiologists successfully managed acute pain with inventive, invasive techniques. Intravenous opiate delivery, whether by intermittent bolus, by continuous infusion, or by a combination of the two, is appropriate for any patient experiencing acute pain that is uncontrollable with oral opiates or other analgesics or who is unable to take medications by mouth (Table 14–16; see also Table 14–7).[26] Included are postoperative patients, cancer pain patients with an acute exacerbation, obstetric patients, patients with burns, intensive care unit patients, and chronic pain patients in the acute phase of their disease (e.g., those with cardiac pain, herpes zoster, or sickle cell crisis).

Regardless of whether the pain problem is acute, chronic, or cancer-related, the oral route should be utilized as soon as

TABLE 14–13. Miscellaneous Drugs With Analgesic Potential

	Generic Name	Trade Name	Dose Range	Comments
Oral local anesthetics/sodium channel blockers	Mexiletene	Mexitil	600–900 mg · d^{-1}	1
	Tocainide	Tonocard	200–400 mg 3 times a day	2
Psychostimulants	Dextroamphetamine	Dexedrine	5–20 mg every 6–12 h	3
	Methylphenidate	Ritalin	5–20 mg 2 times a day	3
Major tranquilizers	Methotrimeprazine	Levoprome	10–50 mg per 4–8 h	4
	Phenothiazines	—	—	5
Anxiolytic/antihistamines	Hydroxyzine	Vistaril, Atarax	50–100 mg per 4–6 h	6
	Antihistamines			7
	Benzodiazepines			8
Miscellaneous	Baclofen	Lioresal	20–120 mg · d^{-1}	9
	Nifedipine	Procardia	10–60 mg · d^{-1}	10
	Phenoxybenzamine	Dibenzyline	10–120 mg · d^{-1}	11
	Clonidine	Catapres		12
	Tetrahydrocannibinol	Marinol	5–15 mg · m$^{2-1}$	13

(From Patt RB, Szalados JE, Wu CL: Pharmacotherapeutic guidelines. *In* Cancer Pain. Patt RB (ed). Philadelphia, JB Lippincott, 1993, p 574.)

Comments

1. Frequently considered for management of neuropathic pain in patients who have failed trials of antidepressants, anticonvulsants, or both. Potential adverse effects include cardiac dysrhythmia, confusion, dysarthria, nystagmus, tremor, nausea, vomiting, and constipation.
2. Considered as a third line drug for neuropathic pain for patients who have failed trials of antidepressants, anticonvulsants, and mexiletine. Side effect profile similar to but more severe than that of mexiletine. In addition, administration has been associated with rare incidences of pneumonitis, hepatitis, and immunologic, allergic, and psychotic reactions.
3. Primary indication is as a psychostimulant to enhance alertness in patients with opioid-induced sedation. Analgesic effect has been demonstrated with some reliability, although pain per se is not a primary indication. Although not indicated as an analgesic, its analgesic effect, together with its rapid antidepressant activity, are beneficial side effects.
4. Phenothiazine. Available only in parenteral (IM) form, although there is anecdotal support for safe IV use. Equianalgesic with morphine (15 mg methotrimeprazine = 10 mg MSO4). Use is associated with sedation, making it a good choice in anxious patients with advanced illness who have not responded to more conventional analgesics or who are unable to take opioids. Potent antiemetic. Use may be associated with the appearance of extrapyramidal signs (see text for details).
5. With the exception of methotrimeprazine, generally regarded as not possessing intrinsic analgesic activity, although sedative and antiemetic properties make these agents useful in the treatment of agitation, nausea and vomiting.
6. Antihistamine. Only drug of this class with demonstrated analgesic activity. Often coadministered with an opioid for acute pain and anxiety. IM injection may be painful. Not recommended in the management of chronic cancer pain.
7. With the exception of hydroxyzine, generally regarded as not possessing intrinsic analgesic activity, although sedative and antipruritic actions may be useful.
8. Direct analgesic/coanalgesic activities have not been demonstrated. Well-established role in treatment of insomnia and anxiety. May have an indirect role in managing pain when complaints are presumed to stem in large part from anxiety or sleep deprivation. Should not be used as a substitute for analgesics.
9. Antispasmodic agent (γ-aminobutyric acid analogue). Has not been studied in cancer patients but may be useful as an adjunctive pharmacologic agent in the treatment of neuropathic pain.
10. Calcium channel blocker. Has not been studied in patients with cancer pain. Anecdotal support for use as a systemic vasodilator in the presence of sympathetically maintained pain. Common adverse effects include orthostatic hypotension, headache, and peripheral edema.
11. Alpha-adrenergic antagonist. Has not been studied in patients with cancer pain. Anecdotal support for use as a systemic vasodilator in the presence of sympathetically maintained pain. Common adverse effects include orthostatic hypotension, headache, and peripheral edema.
12. Centrally-acting antihypertensive. Has not been studied in cancer pain. Indications for use still unclear. Analgesic by intraspinal routes; available as transdermal patch; used as an adjunct in the management of opioid and nicotine withdrawal.
13. Cannabinoid/psychotropic. Capacity to relieve pain is controversial. Use is associated with psychomimetic effects that many patients find undesirable. Indication is mainly as an antiemetic and, more recently, an appetite stimulant.

TABLE 14–14. Recommended Prophylactic Antiemetics

Prochlorperazine (Compazine), 5 mg PO every 4 h (range: 5 mg every 6 h to 20 mg every 4 h)	
If the above is too sedating or ineffective:	Haloperidol (Haldol), 0.5 mg PO every 8 h (range: 0.5 mg every 12 h to 1.0 mg every 4 h)
If sedation is desired in an agitated, nauseated patient:	Chlorpromazine (Thorazine), 10 mg PO every 4 h (range: 10 mg every 6 h to 25 mg every 4 h)
If gastric outlet obstruction is a problem, switch to or add to above:	Metoclopramide (Reglan), 10 mg PO every 8 h (range: 10 mg every 8 h to 20 mg every 6 h)

(From Patt RB, Szalados JE, Wu CL: Pharmacotherapeutic guidelines. *In* Cancer Pain. Patt RB (ed). Philadelphia, JB Lippincott, 1993, p 574.)

possible. Conversion from parenteral to oral opiates should take into consideration the previous 24-hour needs that produced adequate analgesia as well as the length of time opiate therapy has been required (Table 14–17).[41] If such therapy has been of short duration, a 1:6 intramuscular-to-oral ratio is utilized; if the patient has required opiate therapy for some time, a 1:2 to a 1:3 ratio is more appropriate.[42]

Lidocaine and Mexiletine

Intravenous lidocaine is utilized successfully for many neuropathic pain problems.[43] Although this approach was reported

TABLE 14–15. Bowel Preparation Protocol

Begin with a stool softener and gentle laxative:
- Diocytil sodium sulfosuccinate, 100 mg, plus casanthranol, 30 mg (Peri-Colace), 1 capsule PO 3 times a day (range: 1 capsule once per day to 2 capsules 3 times per day)
- Docusate calcium, 60 mg, plus Danthron, 50 mg (Doxidan), 1 capsule twice per day (range: 1 capsule once per day to 2 capsules 3 times per day)
- Docusate sodium, 50 mg, plus senna, 187 mg (Senokot S), 1 tablet orally 3 times per day (range: 1 tablet once per day to 4 tablets 3 times per day)

If no bowel movement in any 48-hour period, add one of the following:
- Senna (Senokot), 187 mg, 2 to 3 tablets PO HS (range: 2 tablets HS to 4 tablets 3 times per day)
- Bisacodyl (Dulcolax), 10–15 mg PO HS (range: 5 mg PO HS to 15 mg 3 times per day)
- Milk of magnesia, 30–60 mL PO HS (range: once to twice per day)
- Haley's M-O, 30–60 mL PO HS (range: once to twice per day)
- Lactulose (Chronulac: 10 g per 15 mL), 30–45 mL PO HS (range: 15–60 mL HS, twice per day)

If no bowel movement by 72 hours, perform rectal examination to rule out impaction:
- If not impacted, try one of the following:
  Bisacodyl (Dulcolax) suppository, 10 mg
  Magnesium citrate, 8 oz PO
  Senna extract (X-Prep liquid), 2.5 oz PO
  Mineral oil, 30–60 mL PO
  Fleet enema
- If impacted:
  Manually disimpact if stool is soft enough (consider pretreatment of patient with analgesic or tranquilizer)
  Soften with glycerin suppository or olive oil retention enema, then disempact manually
  Follow-up with enema or enemas of choice (e.g., tap water, soap suds) until clear and then increase intensity of daily bowel preparation

(From Patt RB, Szalados JE, Wu CL: Pharmacotherapeutic guidelines. *In* Cancer Pain. Patt RB (ed). Philadelphia, JB Lippincott, 1993, p 574.)

TABLE 14–16. Guidelines for Patient-Controlled Intravenous Opioid Administration*

Drug (Concentration)	Size of Bolus (mg)	Lockout Interval (min)
Morphine (1 mg · mL^{-1})	0.5–2.5	5–10
Meperidine (10 mg · mL^{-1})	5–25	5–10
Hydromorphone (0.2 mg · mL^{-1})	0.05–0.25	5–10
Methadone (1 mg · mL^{-1})	0.5–2.5	8–20
Oxymorphone (0.25 mg · mL^{-1})	0.2–0.4	8–10
Fentanyl (0.01 mg · mL^{-1})	0.010–0.020	3–10
Sufentanil (0.002 mg · mL^{-1})	0.002–0.005	3–10
Alfentanil (0.1 mg · mL^{-1})	0.1–0.2	5–8
Pentazocine (10 mg · mL^{-1})	5–30	5–15
Nalbuphine (1 mg · mL^{-1})	1–5	5–15
Buprenorphine (0.03 mg · mL^{-1})	0.03–0.1	8–20

(From Task Force on Acute Pain: Management of Acute Pain: A Practical Guide. Ready BH, Edwards WT (eds). Seattle, IASP Publications, 1992, pp 11–21.)
*Individual patient requirements vary widely. Small doses should be used initially for elderly or very sick patients.

previously,[44–46] renewed interest developed with the introduction of mexiletine, an oral analogue to parenteral local anesthetics.[47]

The first studies of this approach involved diabetic patients with neuropathy.[48] Following a 1 mg · kg^{-1} lidocaine bolus given over 2 to 3 minutes, an infusion was instituted with 4 mg · kg^{-1} over 30 minutes. A significant number of these patients experienced improvement in pain that lasted days to weeks. A follow-up study showed the utility of mexiletine in long-term treatment when the intravenous therapeutic result was short-lived.[49] Subsequently, this therapy has been found to be useful in patients with burn pain,[50] postherpetic neuralgia,[51] and neuropathic pain in a variety of other syndromes.[47]

Since mexiletine takes several days to have an effect, acute pain is best treated with intravenous lidocaine initially; if this drug is effective, mexiletine is started at 5 to 10 mg · kg^{-1} · d^{-1} in divided doses.[49]

The most common side effects of mexiletine use are nausea, tremor, and dizziness; therefore, dose titration is imperative in patients with a predisposition to any of these side effects. The gastrointestinal side effects can be minimized if the medication is taken with food.

TABLE 14–17. Oral-to-Parenteral Dose Ratios and Equianalgesic Doses for Various Opioids (Reference Dose: 10 mg Morphine Intramuscularly to Treat Severe Pain)

Drug	Oral Dose	Oral-to-Parenteral Dose Ratio	Parenteral Dose
Morphine			
Single dose	60 mg	6:1	10 mg
Repeated dose	30 mg	3:1	10 mg
Hydromorphone	8 mg	5:1	1.6 mg
Methadone hydrochloride	20 mg	2:1	10 mg
Levorphanol	2 mg	1:1 (approximate)	2 mg
Meperidine hydrochloride	300 mg	4:1	75 mg
Codeine	200 mg	1.5:1	130 mg

(From Hill CS: Oral opioid analgesics. *In* Cancer Pain. Patt RB (ed). Philadelphia, JB Lippincott, 1993, p 137.)

What Is the Value of Peridural Analgesics In Acute Pain?

As has been mentioned in previous sections, the type of pain experienced is a primary determinant of the appropriateness of therapy. Peridural opiates have different indications in acute, chronic, and cancer-related pain.

Most literature has focused on the use of peridural opiates in the acute pain setting. Bonica summarized the clinical responses to acute pain in relationship to each level affected in the CNS (Fig. 14–7).[52]

Pulmonary Changes

The pulmonary system is the most affected and most important organ system in relation to potential postoperative complications. Following upper abdominal surgery, up to 70% of patients may develop atelectasis, pneumonia, and arterial hypoxemia.[53] These complications are related to reductions in vital capacity, functional residual capacity, tidal volume, and the forced expired volume in 1 second. The ability to cough and clear secretions is reduced as is chest wall compliance.[53-56] The changes in respiratory mechanics are greatest following thoracic and upper abdominal procedures and are least following extra-abdominal and nonthoracic procedures.[54, 57, 58] Pain from peripheral surgical procedures, such as major orthopedic surgery, can produce pulmonary dysfunction as well.[59]

Cardiovascular Function

The cardiovascular system is also affected. Pain activates the sympathetic nervous system and the neuroendocrine system, producing multiple responses that impact on myocardial oxygen supply and demand. The addition of these stress responses to a patient with known cardiovascular disease increases the potential for ischemia and cardiac failure.[60, 61] In addition, pain affects the development of deep venous thrombosis by way of platelet-fibrinogen activation and impairs a patient's ability to ambulate, with resulting decreased venous flow.[62-64]

Gastrointestinal Problems

The gastrointestinal system becomes problematic with the development of postoperative ileus, which is thought to occur in response to spinal reflexes triggered by pain and the stress of the surgical procedure.[65, 66] If these expected postoperative responses to surgery and pain are superimposed on pre-existing cardiopulmonary illness or morbid obesity, the outcome is questionable without good pain control.

Outcome Studies

Studies have been completed in an attempt to determine whether peridural analgesia can alter the impact that acute pain has on the pathophysiologic changes discussed earlier. The neuroendocrine response is decreased to a greater extent when pain is adequately controlled with epidural opiates than when it is managed with intravenous opiates alone.[67-70] Epidural morphine also improves postoperative immune function and nitrogen balance.[71] Postoperative epidural opiate analgesia is said to improve pulmonary function and reduce morbidity when it is compared with patient-controlled analgesia with morphine.[72]

A decreased incidence in pulmonary complications follows upper abdominal[71, 73, 74] or thoracic[55, 75, 76] procedures when postoperative epidural analgesia is utilized. These same observations apply to patients with morbid obesity. Epidural morphine compared with intramuscular morphine in obese patients results in less sedation, earlier ambulation, return of bowel function, and fewer pulmonary complications.[74]

Epidural or intrathecal opiates given for postoperative pain management may improve cardiac outcome.[77, 78] Finally, epidural analgesia may reduce morbidity and mortality in high-risk patients.[79]

What Is the Effect of Added Local Anesthetics?

The combination of peridurally administered local anesthetics and opiates more completely blunts the neuroendocrine response than the use of opiates alone[63, 67, 69, 80] and improves

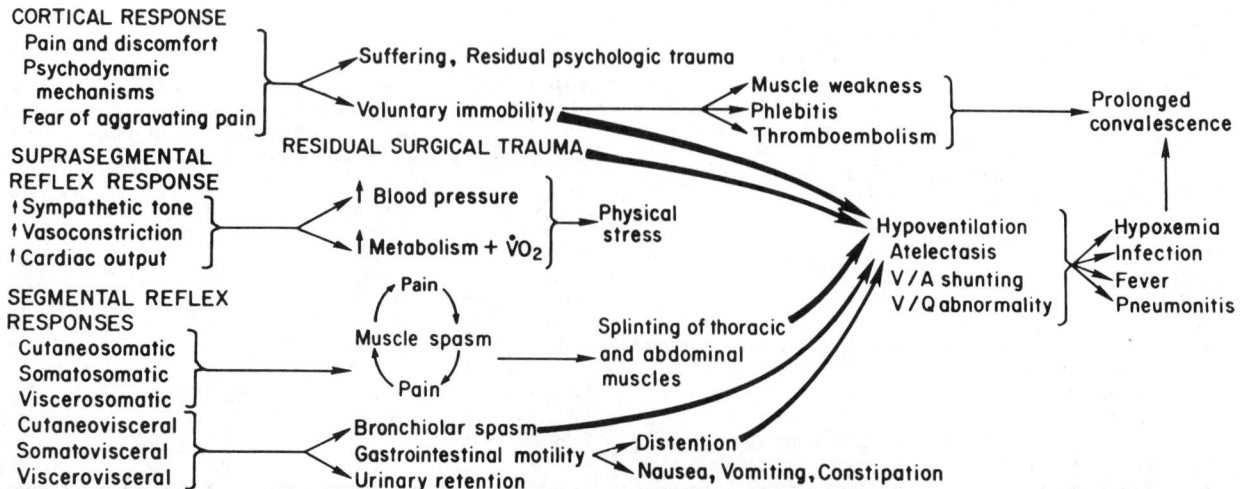

FIGURE 14–7. Schematic depiction of the pathophysiology of postoperative pain. (From Bonica JJ: Postoperative pain. *In* The Management of Pain. Bonica JJ (ed). Philadelphia, Lea & Febiger, 1990, p 466.)

TABLE 14–18. Situations in Which Peridural Opiates, Local Anesthetics, or Both, Might Be Beneficial

Surgical considerations	Thoracoabdominal procedures, major vascular procedures, major orthopedic procedures, urologic procedures, cesarean sections
	Increased risk associated with ileus, risk of the development of chronic pain
Medical considerations	Cardiovascular disease, pulmonary disease, obesity, multisystem disease, high-risk patients, elderly
Patient-related factors	History of a good past experience with epidural analgesia, desire for health care professionals to manage their pain control
	No patient preference but the procedure or the underlying medical problem suggests benefit of epidural analgesia
	Desire for regional anesthesia

pain relief better than the use of local anesthetics alone.[81] However, no difference in postoperative pulmonary morbidity or mortality results. Local anesthetics administered through thoracic epidural catheters significantly decrease hospital stays following major abdominal or hip operations compared with intramuscularly administered morphine.[83]

Vascular Surgery

Outcome after major vascular surgery improves with use of combined general/epidural anesthesia followed by epidural administration of fentanyl/bupivacaine for postoperative pain control compared with balanced general anesthesia followed by postoperative parenteral administration of opiates.[84] The general anesthesia/parenteral analgesia group experienced a greater incidence of cardiovascular and infectious complications, multisystem complications, and vascular graft thrombosis.

Hip Arthroplasties

Epidural anesthesia followed by use of epidural local anesthetics for postoperative pain relief can reduce the incidence of lower extremity thrombosis and pulmonary embolism in patients undergoing total hip arthroplasties.[64] Local anesthetics perhaps increase fibrinolytic activity and inhibit platelet aggregation.[85, 86]

Gastrointestinal Motility

Several studies show an improvement in postoperative gastrointestinal motility with peridural local anesthesia or analgesia that is not seen with epidural opiate administration.[87] In fact, both epidural and parenteral use of opiates delay return of bowel function, although this effect is more pronounced with parenteral administration.[74, 88, 89] A significant reduction in hospital stay follows use of epidural opiates or local anesthetics for perioperative pain relief.[83, 90–92]

Chronic Pain Syndromes

In addition to blunting the responses to acute pain, local anesthetics administered by multiple routes prevent chronic pain syndromes related to surgical procedures. The best examples include prevention of acute and chronic pain associated with iliac crest bone donor sites by local anesthetic infusions through iliac crest catheters[93] and of phantom limb pain with peridural local anesthetics and opiates.[94, 95] This renewed idea of "pre-emptive analgesia" dates back to the early 1900s. Postoperative mortality was thought to be significantly reduced if the transmission of the response to the surgical procedure (pain/stress) could be blocked prior to the incision.[96] More recent studies have verified this observation; patients require significantly less postoperative analgesia when local anesthetic blockade is provided before the surgical incision.[97–99]

Factors to consider when deciding whether peridural opiates, local anesthetics, or both, might be beneficial to the acute pain patient are summarized in Table 14–18.

How Is the Dose of Peridural Opiates and Local Anesthetics Determined?

Opiates

The majority of clinicians initially utilized morphine as the drug of choice for peridural postoperative pain management. Table 14–19 is an excellent guide for determining the dose of epidural morphine, taking into consideration the patient's age, site of the surgical incision, and site of the epidural catheter.[26] More recently, morphine has been administered successfully by constant infusions in an attempt to minimize the periods of pain experienced with intermittent bolus injections (Table 14–20).[100] Again, the dose is based on the site of incision and, to a lesser extent, on the site of catheter insertion. Table 14–21 summarizes the dosing intervals of all the commonly used opiates for both intrathecal and epidural administration.[26]

Bupivacaine

Many practitioners add local anesthetics in analgesic doses to gain their previously described benefits and to minimize the side effects of opiates. Bupivacaine at concentrations of 0.0625% to 0.25% is most frequently utilized. Patient-controlled epidural analgesia has become increasingly popular. One technique is outlined in Table 14–22.[101] Following these guidelines, a self-administered dose of morphine can reach 1.2 mg · h^{-1} as well as the superimposed background infusion of 0.4 mg · h^{-1}. This total is a significant dose for an elderly patient or one with any degree of opiate sensitivity. A lower

TABLE 14–19. Initial Dose (mg) of Epidural Morphine for Incisional Pain*

Patient Age (y)	Nonthoracic Surgery (Lumbar or Caudal Catheter)	Thoracic Surgery	
		Thoracic Catheter	*Lumbar Catheter*
15–44	4	4	5
45–65	3	3	4
66–75	2	2	3
76+	1	1	2

(From Task Force on Acute Pain: Management of Acute Pain: A Practical Guide: Ready BH, Edwards WT (eds). Seattle, IASP Publications, 1992, pp 11–21.)
*These doses should only be considered as guidelines. They are based on the use of undiluted 0.1% preservative-free morphine. Safe and effective doses for individual patients may vary considerably.

TABLE 14–20. Recommended Epidural Morphine Doses for Various Surgical Procedures

Operation	$(mg \cdot h^{-1})$	$(mL \cdot h^{-1})$
Total hip arthroplasty	0.2–0.5	2–5
Prostatectomy	0.3–0.8	3–8
Total abdominal hysterectomy*	0.4–1.0	4–10
Colectomy	0.4–1.0	4–10
Hepatic resection	0.5–1.0	5–10
Cholecystectomy	0.6–1.0	6–10
Total knee arthroplasty	0.5–1.5	5–15
Thoracotomy		
Lumbar	0.8–1.5	8–15
Thoracic	0.3–0.6	3–6

(From Benson JP: Organization of a postoperative pain service. *In* Anesthesia Update #6, Supplement to Anesthesia. 3rd ed. Miller RD (ed). New York, Churchill Livingstone, 1992, pp 137–153.)
*Rates given are for lumbar catheters unless otherwise specified.

dose or a longer lockout interval may be appropriate in such patients.

Why and How Should Patients Be Monitored?

Problems that require special monitoring include sedation and respiratory depression. Sedation may result from the direct central effects of the opiate secondary to the hypercarbia associated with opiate-induced respiratory depression or from the additive effects of other adjuvant medications. It should be thought of as a sign of respiratory depression until proven otherwise.

Respiratory Depression

Peridural opiate–related respiratory depression occurs in two phases.

Early

Early respiratory depression is caused by systemic absorption of the opiate through the epidural veins. This effect is

TABLE 14–21. Intraspinal Opioids for the Treatment of Acute Pain

	Drug	Single Dose* (mg)	Infusion Rate† $(mg \cdot h^{-1})$	Onset (min)	Duration of Single Dose‡ (h)
Epidural	Morphine	1–6	0.1–1.0	30	6–24
	Meperidine	20–150	5–20	5	4–8
	Methadone	1–10	0.3–0.5	10	6–10
	Hydromorphone	1–2	0.1–0.2	15	10–16
	Diamorphine	4–6	?	5	12
	Fentanyl	0.025–0.1	0.025–0.10	5	2–4
	Sufentanil	0.01–0.06	0.01–0.05	5	2–4
	Alfentanil	0.5–1	0.2	15	1–3
Subarachnoid	Morphine	0.1–0.3		15	8–24*
	Meperidine	10–30		?	10–24*
	Diamorphine	1–2		?	20
	Fentanyl	0.005–0.025		5	3–6

(From Task Force on Acute Pain: Management of Acute Pain: A Practical Guide. Ready BH, Edwards WT (eds). Seattle, IASP Publications, 1992, pp 11–21.)
*Low doses may be effective when administered to the elderly or when injected in the cervical or thoracic region.
†If combining with a local anesthetic, consider using 0.0625% bupivacaine.
‡Duration of analgesia varies widely; higher doses produce longer duration.

TABLE 14–22. Usual Parameters of Epidural Infusion Patient-Controlled Analgesia Employed (Plain Morphine 0.2 mg $\cdot$ mL^{-1} or with Additional 0.1% to 0.125% Bupivacaine)

Parameter	Amount
Load	2–3 mg of morphine
Infusion	0.4 mg $\cdot$ h^{-1}
Patient-controlled dose	0.2 mg
Lockout	10 min

(From Walmsley PNH: Patient-controlled epidural analgesia. *In* Acute Pain: Mechanisms & Management. Sinatra RS, Hord AH, Ginsberg B, et al (eds). St Louis, Mosby–Year Book, 1992, pp 312–325.)

more likely to be of concern with the use of potent lipophilic agents, such as fentanyl and sufentanil, and occurs within the first 1 to 2 hours after administration. The degree of respiratory depression is similar to that seen with an equivalent dose of parenterally administered opiate.[102]

Late

The late phase of respiratory depression occurs primarily with hydrophilic opiates, such as morphine, that tend to accumulate in the cerebrospinal fluid and spread rostrally to the brainstem respiratory centers. This problem is noted between 8 and 12 hours after the opiate administration.[103]

Nursing Care

The best monitor to ensure patient safety is a well-trained, vigilant nurse. One of the contraindications to peridural opiate analgesia is inadequate nursing education.[104] Standard orders must accompany the institution of peridural opiate therapy and should include the monitoring procedures that are expected to occur. Figure 14–8 is an example of the epidural order form utilized at the Shands Hospital at the University of Florida in Gainesville.

Techniques

Standard monitoring procedures include frequent checks of respiratory rate and the level of sedation (Table 14–23).[105] Ready suggests the use of a respiratory monitor for patients with the following risk factors: age ≥50 years; ASA physical status 3, 4, or 5; thoracic or upper abdominal incisions; surgical procedures lasting >4 hours; concomitant use of long-acting anesthetics, opiates, or other CNS depressants either before or during surgery; and epidural morphine dose of ≥6 mg or intrathecal morphine dose of ≥0.5 mg.[106] High-risk patients should be monitored more extensively in intensive care units or in intermediate care units where the nurse-to-patient ratio is greater than on a medical-surgical floor.

Peridural Local Anesthetics

Patients receiving local anesthetics through an epidural catheter may develop hypotension related to the sympathetic blockade, extensive sensory blockade, and muscle weakness if an excessive dose or inappropriately placed catheter is utilized. Vital signs should be taken according to protocol as ordered, but in the case of local anesthetics, additional orthostatic blood

PHYSICIAN'S ORDERS
SHANDS HOSPITAL
at the
UNIVERSITY OF FLORIDA

ADDRESSOGRAPH:

Generic equivalent permitted unless this square
initialed by physician.

DATE/TIME	**EPIDURAL NARCOTIC** **DOCTOR'S ORDERS**	
	1) This patient is receiving epidural narcotics. Notify APS on arrival. Label head of	
	bed, front of chart, infusion bag, and infusion tubing.	
	2) Epidural bolus of duramorph _____ mg @ _____ AM/PM.	
	3) Epidural infusion of: a) 5 mcg/ml/fentanyl a) 1/16% BUPIVICAINE	
	(Circle desired solution) b) 7.5 mcg/ml/fentanyl b) 1/32% BUPIVICAINE	
	c) 4 mcg/ml/fentanyl	
	d) _____	
	in ____ ml PFNS. Bolus ____ ml and begin basal infusion @ ____ ml/hr.	
	4) Program BARD® pump as follows: Vol. limit ____ ml, Concentration _ø_ , Dose _ø_ ,	
	Basal ____ ml/hr, Bolus _ø_ .	
	5) Give no additional narcotics, anti-emetics, or sedatives without clearance from APS	
	6) Continuous pulse oximetry monitoring with low sat alarm @ 90%.	
	7) Monitor and record: O_2 SAT, RR, LOC Q 15 min x 2, then Q one hour x 4, then Q	
	2H for duration of infusion. Repeat Q 15 min and Q 1H sequence for subsequent	
	boluses or rate increases.	
	8) Resume routine unit monitoring 2 hours after D/C fentanyl infusion or 12 hours after	
	D/C duramorph.	
	9) Maintain venous access until routine monitoring resumed.	
	10) Naloxone 400 mcg/cc @ bedside, attached to epidural pump with syringe and needle.	
	11) If patient is receiving epidural bupivicaine assess sensation changes and motor	
	strength BLE prior to getting patient OOB. May ambulate with assistance only.	
	12) Managing side effects:	
	a) Itching: Naloxone (400 mcg/cc) .1 - .2cc IV.	
	Then place remainder of vial in > 500cc maintenance IV fluids, run @	
	maintenance rate. Call APS for itching unrelieved by above.	
	b) Nausea: Reglan 10mg IV in 50cc NS x one dose. Call APS if ineffective.	
	c) Urinary retention > 8°: Notify APS.	
	d) Resp. rate < 12/min or O_2 SAT < 90%: Notify APS.	
	e) Resp. rate < 8/min or pt. unresponsive:	
	1. Notify APS, STAT. (Beeper # 2482)	
	2. Turn off epidural infusion.	
	3. Give naloxone (400 mcg/cc) .5cc IV, repeat until responsive or RR > 12/min.	
	f) Sedation > 1: Notify APS.	

CHART COPY

FIGURE 14–8. Physician order sheet. (Courtesy of Shands Hospital at the University of Florida, Gainesville, FL.)

TABLE 14–23. Example of Bedside Sedation Scale

Sedation	Description
0 (None)	Alert
1 (Mild)	Occasionally drowsy; easy to arouse
2 (Moderate)	Frequently drowsy; easy to arouse
3 (Severe)	Somnolent; difficult to arouse
S (Sleeping)	Normal sleep; easy to arouse

(From Ready LB, Loper KA, Nessly M, et al: Postoperative epidural morphine is safe on surgical wards. Anesthesiology 1991; 75:452.)

pressure checks may be necessary as well. Nursing assessment should also include testing for sensation and strength in the lower extremities before ambulation and with each routine pain assessment. This level of nursing assessment, coupled with that of the pain consultant (Fig. 14–9), minimizes the attendant risks.

Pulse Oximetry

Pulse oximetry is an alternative monitoring technique on the ward that best identifies respiratory depression if a patient is not receiving supplemental oxygen. Periodic end-tidal carbon dioxide checks are also useful in the high-risk patient. The risk of respiratory depression from peridural opiate therapy is 0.2% to 0.4%.[105, 107]

When Should Cancer Patients Receive Peridural Analgesia?

Indications

The majority of physicians who work with cancer pain patients believe that 80% of their patients' pain can be controlled with oral analgesics, following the WHO three-step program.[108] However, 60% to 80% of terminally ill cancer patients have significant pain.[109] Patients most likely to need invasive delivery systems for analgesic therapy include those receiving around-the-clock strong opiates in adequate doses but without adequate pain relief; those with intolerable side effects from systemic opiates; and those without a tumor in the epidural space or thecal sac.[110]

A therapeutic trial of peridural opiate therapy, usually with morphine, is utilized to ensure that the patient will experience adequate pain relief. The dose to be used for the trial is based on the patient's previous 24-hour morphine requirement.

Changeover to Peridural Administration

A conversion schema should include[111] the 24-hour oral morphine requirement change to parenteral morphine (see Table 14–17), the 24-hour nonmorphine requirement change to parenteral morphine, and administration of one-half of this calculated dose (owing to incomplete cross-tolerance). The epidural morphine dose is equal to the 24-hour parenteral morphine dose divided by 10; the intrathecal morphine dose is equal to the epidural dose divided by 10.

Concern about opiate withdrawal during the changeover to the peridural route of administration is justified. Withdrawal can be avoided if the initial 24-hour opiate dose reduction is no more than 50% and if further reductions are limited to 20%

of the original need per day. A positive response to this therapeutic trial is found when the patient reports a 50% reduction in pain, a 50% reduction in the 24-hour opiate requirement, or both.[111]

Delivery System

Once a positive therapeutic trial has been established, the appropriate delivery system must be chosen. A commonly held practice is to utilize an entirely implantable system for any patient with a life expectancy >3 months; patients with an anticipated life expectancy <3 months are candidates for a tunneled epidural catheter with an external pump for continuous infusion or utilization of intermittent injections (Fig. 14–10).[111]

Other issues to be considered include patient preference, physician preference, cost, drug/dose requirements, and location and type of pain. The issues of surgical complications (bleeding, infection, pump pocket seroma, cerebrospinal fluid leaks, and postspinal headache), mechanical complications, and pharmacologic management via the chosen delivery system must be well considered ahead of time. The patient and his or her family members should be aware of the potential problems and solutions.

When Should Chronic Pain Patients Receive Peridural Analgesia?

Considerable controversy surrounds peridural opioids in this patient population. Concerns about stable opiate use and efficacy, addiction, tolerance, and dependence, whether founded or not, are widespread. These individuals normally do not have a limited life expectancy. Chronic pain patients can be helped with this therapy. Successful case reports describe implantable infusion systems.[112] The reversible nature of the procedure, even though it initially involves surgical implantation at a significant cost, makes it more desirable and less risky than irreversible neuroablative procedures.

The patient selection criteria proposed by Krames seem reasonable, taking into account that the long-term effects of intraspinal infusional therapy are unknown (Table 14–24).[111] These criteria state that the chronic pain patient should have tried all nonopiate and opiate medications as well as all the other pain management treatment modalities prior to the institution of invasive infusional opiate therapy.

CONTROVERSIES

How Should Patients with Opiate Dependence Be Managed?

Opiate dependence must be evaluated for its cause, which may be:

1. The appropriate use of opiates without psychologic dependence or drug seeking behavior, as in cancer patients;

2. The appropriate use of opiates, with psychosocial and physiologic reinforcers, as in chronic pain patients;

3. Drug tolerance, physical dependence, and psychologic dependence from the use of illegal drugs or alcohol; and

4. The potential for psychologic dependence, but current

SHANDS HOSPITAL
at the University of Florida
Gainesville, Florida 32610

History

Physical Examination

Progress Notes

Patient Name: _____   MR#: _____

Anesthesiology Pain Service

Date: _____   Time: _____   POD: _____   Catheter Day: _____

Patient report: _____

Pain location: _____   VAS: rest _____ move _____ /10

Side effects: *Sedation _____   **Nausea _____   Pruritus _____   Urinary retention _____

Current therapy: _____

SaO2: _____ RA ____ O2 ____ Tx: ____ L/min   RR: ____ /min   Incentive spirometer _____ cc

O2 saturation trend last 8 hrs.: _____

B/P: _____ Tmax: _____ Wt.: _____ kg

Motor exam: _____   Sensory exam: _____

Site: L ____ T ____ : Clean/dry _____   Other: _____

Assessment: _____

Plan: _____

☐ Continue current therapy.

☐ Change analgesics as follows: _____

☐ Treat side effects as follows: _____

☐ Discontinue therapy today. Further analgesic orders per primary service. _____

_____
_____
_____
_____
_____
_____
_____
_____
_____

/APS

**0 = none   1 = no tx required   2 = tx with relief   3 = tx without relief

*Sedation: 0 = None   1 = arouses to voice   2 = requires physical stimulation

3 = Unarousable   5 = Normal sleep

Rev 9 92   PS3079099215C

FIGURE 14–9. University of Florida daily assessment form. (Courtesy of Shands Hospital at the University of Florida, Gainesville, FL.)

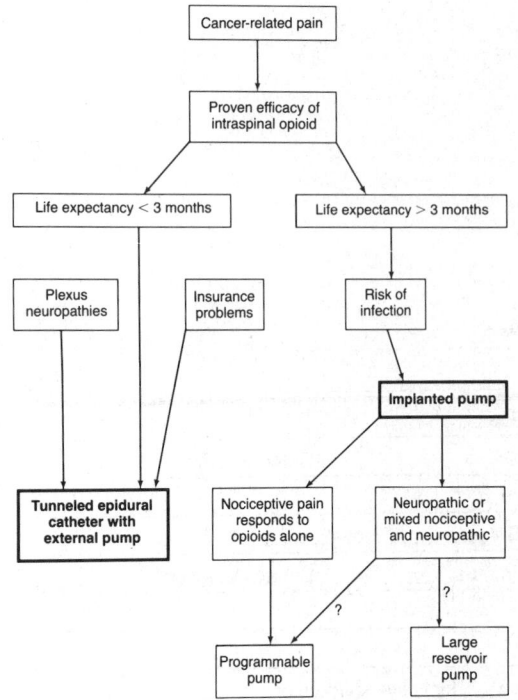

FIGURE 14–10. Algorithm for choosing the appropriate peridural opiate delivery system in cancer pain patients. (Reprinted by permission of Elsevier Science Publishing Co., Inc. from Intrathecal infusional therapies for intractable pain: patient management guidelines, by ES Krames, Journal of Pain and Symptom Management, Vol. 8, p. 36. Copyright 1993 by the U.S. Cancer Pain Relief Committee.)

TABLE 14–24. Selection Criteria for Opioid Infusional Therapy for Patients With Noncancer-Related Pain

Therapy of last resort
Baseline neurologic examination
Psychologic report unequivocally stating nonfunctional pain state

(Reprinted by permission of Elsevier Science Publishing Co., Inc. from Intrathecal infusional therapies for intractable pain: patient management guidelines, by Krames ES. Journal of Pain and Symptom Management, Vol. 8, p. 36. Copyright 1993 by the U.S. Cancer Pain Relief Committee.)

useful in the opiate-tolerant patient without psychologic dependence as long as an equivalent dose is prescribed to avoid withdrawal. Select the dose of epidural opiate based on the previous opiate use as follows:

1. Convert the average daily preoperative opiate use to its intravenous morphine equivalent;

2. Divide this dose by 24 to obtain the hourly intravenous morphine equivalent;

3. Divide by 4 to obtain the hourly epidural morphine equivalent.[113]

Psychologic Dependence

Patients with psychologic opiate dependence do not do well with epidural opiate analgesia as they do not experience the central effect they normally obtain. They demand much higher doses than the physician feels comfortable prescribing and do better with an equivalent dose of intravenous opiate. Local anesthetics administered by peripherally placed catheters or epidural catheters are useful to reduce postoperative pain and opiate needs. The equivalent dose of preoperatively used opiate should be prescribed by way of intravenous patient-controlled analgesia to prevent opiate withdrawal.

Benzodiazepines

Benzodiazepines are useful in allaying anxiety but should be avoided in opiate-dependent patients who are naive to this class of drugs.[113] They must be used in larger doses than normal in those patients who are also dependent on them. Most other adjuvant drugs do not have a role in the treatment of acute pain.

Specific Abuse Behavior

Specific abuse behavior should be recognized and dealt with firmly and consistently by all health care providers. Limits must be set to avoid ongoing and excessive negotiations regarding drug use for pain management. Utilize other consultants early in difficult cases. Psychologists, psychiatrists, substance abuse experts, and neurologists can be most helpful.

Who Is at Risk of a Peridural Hematoma?

Patients Receiving Subcutaneous Heparin

Patients with a pre-existing major coagulopathy are at risk and should not be considered for regional anesthesia.[115, 116] Controversy exists when a regional anesthetic technique is considered for a patient who is receiving subcutaneous heparin therapy, for one who will be anticoagulated during the procedure, or for one who will remain anticoagulated afterwards. With regard to subcutaneous heparin prophylaxis, several concerns must be taken into account. Wide variations in heparin levels follow this administration.[117] A retrospective review of 136 patients indicated this is not a problem,[117] yet individual

lack of tolerance or dependence, as in the recovering alcoholic or substance abuser.[113]

General Principles

Several general principles of management deserve attention. The expected result of the operation and the reason for preoperative opiate use will determine the therapeutic plan for postoperative pain management.[113] If the preoperative pain problem is expected to be cured by the surgical procedure, the opiates can be quickly and easily weaned postoperatively. But if the reason for the use of preoperative opiates will not be eliminated, the need will continue. This is not the time to begin an opiate taper. In fact, every effort should be made to control postoperative pain. Confidence in the patient-physician relationship will increase, thus allowing the potential for successful dependency treatment once the acute pain problem has resolved. The patient and all involved health care providers should be well informed as to the plan for both short-term and long-term management.

Specific Methods

Specific management includes all of the techniques discussed previously. Some caveats include a preferred avoidance of opiate use in recovering addicts and the fear of loss of control by others. Intravenous patient-controlled analgesia is very useful in the second group of patients, since it does not carry the risk of renewed or worsening dependence.[114] In addition, this technique prevents withdrawal as long as opiate agonist-antagonists are not used. Epidural opiate analgesia is

case reports still appear, at times without resolution of the neurologic deficit.[119]

Although many of us feel comfortable placing epidural catheters atraumatically just prior to the next dose of heparin, the recommendations of Cousins and Bridenbaugh should be kept in mind:[120]

1. If the benefits of the heparin are minimal and the anesthetic technique of choice is epidural blockade, heparin therapy should be omitted.

2. If heparin prophylaxis is strongly indicated and is practical for the proposed surgery, a single-shot epidural technique may be used before starting the heparin therapy.

3. If heparin therapy must be started before the patient is taken to the operating room, do not use an epidural block in any form.

4. The epidural catheter can be placed the night before surgery; this is followed by preoperative heparin administration if it is needed.

Patients Who Are Anticoagulated Intraoperatively and Postoperatively

The literature is a bit more thorough concerning the issue of epidural catheter placement in patients who are to receive anticoagulation intraoperatively, postoperatively, or both. Odoom and Sih reported no side effects related to hemorrhage or hematoma in 950 patients receiving preoperative oral anticoagulants and intraoperative intra-arterial heparin infusions at a rate of 250 to 300 $\mu g \cdot min^{-1}$.[121] They placed epidural catheters after induction of general anesthesia and left them in place for 48 hours.

Baron and coworkers also reported no untoward neurologic events attributable to an epidural hematoma in 912 patients. Patients in this group were anticoagulated transiently with heparin, 75 $U \cdot kg^{-1}$; this elevated their activated partial thromboplastin time to 100 seconds or more.[122]

Rao and El-Etr prospectively reviewed the results of 3164 patients who received epidural anesthesia and 847 patients who received spinal anesthesia for vascular surgery.[123] The patients were given 500 units of heparin every 3 minutes intraoperatively to maintain an ACT level twice baseline. The catheters were removed 24 hours postoperatively just before the next dose of heparin. The only untoward events were complaints of postoperative paresthesias (4 patients with epidural anesthesia, 1 patient with spinal anesthesia) that resolved spontaneously and of low back pain (9 patients with epidural anesthesia, and 6 patients with spinal anesthesia) that resolved with analgesia therapy.

As expected, case reports describe epidural and subdural hematomas with anticoagulation, with and without regional anesthesia.[124–126] Recommendations based on the preceding information follow[126]:

1. Avoid lumbar puncture in a patient who is receiving anticoagulants or who has known coagulopathy or significant thrombocytopenia, except in extraordinary circumstances.

2. Discuss the risks and benefits of regional anesthesia with a patient and document the discussion if this approach is chosen in the face of anticoagulation.

3. Use an atraumatic midline approach to the peridural space.

4. Monitor anticoagulation activity and minimize heparin doses.

5. Use short-acting local anesthetics intraoperatively to allow immediate assessment of motor and sensory function.

6. Remove catheters when the heparin levels are low, as determined by appropriate laboratory studies.

7. Continue to monitor the patient's neurologic status closely during the hospital stay and at the follow-up visit.

8. Evaluate the spine radiologically if prolonged, severe low back pain occurs with or without neurologic signs, local tenderness, fever, or leukocytosis.

Utilize opioid analgesia postoperatively without local anesthetics to ensure complete assessment of the neurologic status.

REGIONAL ANESTHETIC TECHNIQUES

Regional anesthesia and pain management represent different areas of anesthetic practice; however, considerable overlap between these two areas occurs. Most important is knowing *when* to apply the regional techniques in pain management. Such techniques are used diagnostically, prognostically, prophylactically, and therapeutically. With the exception of peridural analgesia, no concise recommendations for regional anesthetic techniques exists in pain management. Nevertheless, some principles that help with everyday decision making can be followed[127]:

1. Utilize data from the history, physical, laboratory, and radiologic examinations to determine both the classification and the location of the pain problem.

2. Utilize the least invasive and lowest risk procedure possible (e.g., administer a trigger point injection first when trying to differentiate between low back pain of myofascial origin and nerve root irritation).

3. Use diagnostic nerve blocks *only* when alternative therapy that will then be as successful and as longlasting is available (Note: Short-term pain relief is almost always possible with some type of regional anesthetic technique, but this relief may give the patient with chronic benign pain a false sense of hope, and the patient may be devastated once the block wears off).

4. Know the literature with regard to the etiology of the pain problem you are attempting to treat and familiarize yourself with the treatments that have been most successful in the past. A wealth of knowledge that dates back many decades is still valid in this subspecialty. Your patients deserve the benefit of both the historical and current literature when deciding on the best course of action.

5. Combine other modalities of pain management, such as physical therapy or psychologic therapy, to gain the best result possible. Rarely will nerve block alone cure a pain problem of a magnitude that would prompt a patient to seek the help of a pain management expert.

A more extensive set of principles is available for review if these techniques are to become a part of your pain management practice.[128]

What Techniques Are Applicable?

Continuous Catheter Infusions for Acute Pain

Repeated injections into nerves or nerve plexi are less than desirable from the standpoint of patient comfort and manpower requirements. Placement of a catheter into the nerve sheath or plexus sheath permits a continuous infusion, thus eliminating those problems. Catheters have been used, among other locations, in the wound, in nerve sheaths after amputation, in the brachial plexus, and in the sciatic nerve sheath.[129–132] Lower extremity catheters are indicated when only one extremity is involved or when a patient's medical status dictates a minimum of hemodynamic change.

Cancer Pain

Once oral analgesics are no longer controlling the pain, are causing intolerable side effects, or both, and once the pain is well localized, well characterized, somatic or visceral in origin, and does not comprise a component of a pain syndrome characterized by multifocal aches and pains, regional techniques may be considered.[133] They should always be utilized prognostically before neurolytic or ablative procedures to predict efficacy and to allow the patient to experience the expected loss of sensation.

Specific somatic blocks, trigger point injections, and sympathetic nerve blocks are also useful in the treatment of cancer pain related to reflex sympathetic dystrophy, some neuropathic conditions, and acute and chronic herpes zoster.[134] Lastly, regional techniques can be used as an alternative to opioid analgesics in crisis management due to intractable pain. This approach allows the reversal of tolerance that would otherwise occur, especially as the tumor process progresses.

Chronic Pain

The chronic benign pain patient can also benefit from regional anesthetic techniques in some of the same situations as the cancer pain patient.

Epidural Steroid Injection

Epidural steroid injections are a mainstay of treatment for both acute herniated disks and in chronic low back pain due to nerve root irritation, postsurgical lumbalgia, degenerative joint disease, osteoarthritis, or radicular pain related to metastatic infiltration of nerve roots.[135]

The following are guidelines for epidural steroid injections.

1. Place the patient in the lateral decubitus position with the affected side down because the steroid becomes hyperbaric when it is mixed with saline or local anesthetic.

2. Once the epidural space is located, mix the steroid with 2 to 4 mL of saline or local anesthetic. The patient may experience transient radicular pain with the injection.

3. Clear the steroid from the needle prior to its removal from the epidural space.

4. Keep the patient in position with the affected side down for at least 10 minutes to ensure that the steroid has had time to bathe the affected nerve root.

5. If local anesthetic has been used, test for correct placement of the drug by having the patient perform a straight leg test; performance should be improved compared with that of the preinjection period.

6. Warn the patient that the local anesthetic effect (if used) wears off in a number of hours and that the full steroid effect may not be apparent for 5 to 6 days.

Neuroma Injection

Another commonly used technique involves the injection of local anesthetics and steroids into the area of a neuroma. Nerves can be trapped in scar tissue after surgery or other injury and can be treated effectively in this manner. Corticosteroids suppress spontaneous ectopic discharges from entrapped nerves, stabilizing the nerve membrane for 2 weeks or longer.[136] The injection of a combination of local anesthetic and depot corticosteroid is useful in the treatment of myofascial pain with trigger points, arthritic joint pain, and facet joint pain.[137–140]

NEUROLYTIC BLOCKS

When and How Are They Used?

A neurolytic block involves the application of a chemical agent onto or into a nerve, the epidural space, the subdural space, or the subarachnoid space to destroy the axon or the cell bodies of somatic nerves, sympathetic nerves, or both. The agents most frequently used are phenol, alcohol, or glycerol. Although many clinicians perform neurolytic blocks for chronic benign pain, the risk of a severe neuralgia during nerve regeneration has led experts in the field of pain management to state that ". . . with few special exceptions, neurolytic block of somatic spinal nerves should not be done in patients with nonmalignant chronic pain."[141] On the other hand, if a series of prognostic blocks with local anesthetic relieves cancer pain in a patient with limited life expectancy, the neurolytic block is indicated.

The principles of neurolytic block application, combined with the general principles of regional anesthetic techniques used for pain management, are as follows[141]:

1. Only physicians with extensive experience, skill, and knowledge of the procedures and the management of chronic pain should perform neurolytic blocks.

2. Neurolytic blocks should be used in conjunction with all other appropriate pain management techniques, since they do not necessarily relieve all pain and eventually lose effectiveness.

3. Careful patient selection should be combined with the least invasive technique that has the least side effects and the best potential for pain relief.

4. The patient and the patient's family must be informed regarding the details of the procedure, the expected outcome, and the potential side effects and complications.

5. The neurolytic block must be preceded by two or three diagnostic or prognostic blocks with local anesthetic.

6. Assessment of the results of the block necessitates close observation by the physician, nurses, and the patient's family members and must take into consideration that many factors can influence a patient's report of pain relief or lack thereof.

7. Pain relief in a patient previously requiring large doses of opiate analgesics carries the risk of causing respiratory depression (as the respiratory stimulus [pain] is removed) and withdrawal symptoms (if the opiate is stopped too quickly).

NEUROAUGMENTATION

How Does a Transcutaneous Electrical Nerve Stimulator Work?

Two basic mechanisms are thought to explain the effective pain relief found with TENS and SCS.

Gate Control

The first involves an understanding of the gate control theory of pain, which was first described by Melzack and Wall in 1965.[142] A delta and C fibers are responsible for the transmission of pain to the spinal cord. Once they synapse on interneurons in the substantia gelatinosa, the "gate" is opened, reducing presynaptic inhibition and allowing the painful stimulus to continue up the central neuraxis.

When transmission from large-diameter, myelinated A fibers occurs (carrying sensations of light touch and pressure), the gate closes, facilitating presynaptic inhibition of the gelatinosa cells and blocking the flow of painful information. Neurostimulation is thought to involve stimulation of the large-diameter A fibers, thus blocking the transmission of pain via the C fibers to the brain.

Release of Endogenous Opioids

Electrical stimulation also may release endogenous opioid-like substances that act at the opiate receptors in the CNS to mediate the pain response. Beta-endorphin levels are elevated in the plasma[143] and in the cerebrospinal fluid[144] regardless of which mode of stimulation is used. However, other investigators have found no difference in endorphin levels before, during, or after TENS therapy.[144]

Who Is a Candidate for a Transcutaneous Electrical Nerve Stimulator Unit?

Acute Pain

The majority of research evaluating the effectiveness of a TENS has been done in the area of acute pain. Ordog found a TENS to be useful for sprains, lacerations, fractures, hematomas, and contusions and as effective as acetaminophen with codeine.[146] It is also useful for postoperative pain, dental pain, and the pain of labor and delivery.[147–149]

Chronic Pain

A TENS is reported to be effective in the treatment of chronic low back pain, peripheral neuropathies, postherpetic neuralgia, reflex sympathetic dystrophy, phantom limb pain, arthritis, and pain associated with malignancies.[150–154] Although a decline in use occurs with time, Johnson and associates reported that 58% of patients surveyed found that the efficacy remained unchanged with long-term use (mean duration of 4 years).[155] As can be seen from the preceding list of indications, the majority of successfully treated pain problems are of neuropathic origin. Those of nociceptive origin are less likely to respond to TENS.[156]

When Is a Spinal Cord Stimulator Considered?

Generally, patients who benefit from a TENS also benefit from a SCS. Therefore, the same indications hold true. Consider using a SCS when the degree of pain relief from a TENS is insufficient. This therapy has been in use for over 20 years with reported variable responses. Initial enthusiasm after the first trials in the 1970s subsided over time when long-term

TABLE 14–25. Neurogenic, Neuropathic, Deafferentation, and Other Pain Syndromes Likely to Respond to Dorsal Column Stimulators

Peripheral Nerve and Root Lesions	Post-traumatic neuropathy: Trauma due to injuries, surgery, entrapment, or incisional scar Causalgia and reflex sympathetic dystrophy Postamputation pain (stump and phantom) Coccygodynia Diabetic neuropathy Plexus lesions induced by trauma, malignancy, and radiation* Rhizopathy Postherpetic neuralgia Cervical syndrome Low back pain (particularly radicular pain due to arachnoiditis and epidural fibrosis)
Spinal Cord Lesions	Postcordotomy dysesthesia Multiple sclerosis Paraplegia (radicular pain at level of lesion and pain below level of lesion with preservation of sensibility)
Peripheral Vascular Disease	

(From Meyerson BA: Electrical stimulation of the spinal cord and brain. *In* The Management of Pain. Bonica JJ (ed). Philadelphia, Lea & Febiger, 1990, pp 1862–1877.)
*Plexus avulsion pain is not likely to respond to DCS.

relief was not always as good as anticipated. This finding possibly was a result of "uncritical overuse" of this reversible and extremely safe surgical treatment.[155]

In the 1970s, percutaneous dorsal column stimulators (DCSs) were also introduced with the same level of enthusiasm owing to their ease of insertion and decreased invasiveness. Similarly, however, the number of late failures caused significant reevaluation of the use and indications for the DCSs and the SCS. A review of over 500 patients treated with DCSs up to 1978 showed a long-term satisfactory outcome of between 30% and 40%.[157] Successful results after 4 years were only 26%.[157] With the percutaneous approach, the short-term success rate reportedly is ≤80%; long-term success is ≤50%.[158] A list of indications is presented in Table 14–25.[159]

PHYSICAL THERAPY

Rehabilitation and physical therapy have been used for the treatment of acute injuries for many years and with great success. Problems develop when patients have pain that is out of proportion to their injury and that prevents completion of therapy to aid recovery. In many cases, physical therapists can decrease acute, subacute, and chronic pain problems. Cancer pain patients also should have the benefit of the physical therapy during all phases of their disease, including the terminal stage, when the risk of pain is highest.

Three goals of physical therapy used specifically for pain control are described by Yeh and colleagues:[160]

1. Determination of the most effective means of decreasing pain.
2. Correction of the identified dysfunction or dysfunctions.
3. Restoration of a patient's confidence in his or her ability to move and to enjoy physical activity by reducing the fear of further injury or pain.

When Should Physical Therapy Be Prescribed?

Therapeutic Exercise

In acute pain states, active exercise may be contraindicated owing to the potential for further injury or problems with healing. The advice of an orthopedist or a psychiatrist should be sought in this circumstance. In the healing phase, passive range of motion exercises are indicated to maintain muscle and joint mobility.

Once healing has occurred and chronic pain is the main problem, the patient must be encouraged to increase activity, first with the aid of analgesics and injections when appropriate. Eventually, with improved pain control, minimal to no need for any other management technique will occur. When a specific chronic pain problem such as reflex sympathetic dystrophy or radicular pain is treated, physical therapy should be prescribed immediately following a regional anesthetic technique if one is employed initially.

The goals of physical therapy in cancer pain initially are the same as for acute and chronic pain. In advanced stages, the specific needs of the cancer patient population come into play, including respiratory management to allow free and effective breathing, encouragement of independence in daily living (e.g., the ability to transfer himself or herself from bed to wheelchair), and relaxation therapy (both peripheral and general).[160, 161]

Other Options

Besides therapeutic exercise, the physical therapist has many other options for pain management. Techniques to consider include thermotherapy (Table 14–26),[162] cryotherapy (cold packs, vapo-coolant sprays), electrotherapy (iontophoresis, TENS), and passive mechanotherapies (massage, manipulation, traction). Since these interventions are applied without *active* patient participation, some experts question their utility in the treatment of chronic pain. Although the final goal is independent, pain-free activity without analgesics, the initial treatment phase is a time for building trust between the patient and health care provider. Very few patients will be successful if they are asked to begin a vigorous exercise program that involves a painful extremity without the application of analgesic techniques.

TABLE 14–26. Therapeutic Heating Modalities

Primary Mode of Heat Transfer	Modality	Depth
Conduction	Hot packs	Superficial heat
	Paraffin bath	Superficial heat
Convection	Hydrotherapy	Superficial heat
	Fluidotherapy	Superficial heat
Conversion	Infrared	Superficial heat
	Shortwaves	Deep heat
	Microwaves	Deep heat
	Ultrasound	Deep heat

(From Lee MHM, Itoh M, Yang G-FW, et al: Physical therapy and rehabilitation medicine. *In* The Management of Pain. 2nd ed. Bonica JJ (ed). Philadelphia, Lea & Febiger, 1990, pp 1769–1788.)

PSYCHOLOGIC THERAPY

When Should a Psychologist or Psychiatrist Become Involved?

After thorough evaluation and assessment of psychosocial dysfunction, the appropriate psychologic intervention can be applied. Psychiatrists and psychologists are trained in many of the techniques utilized. Choosing the appropriate specialist is based on that individual's level of interest and expertise in the interventional therapy requested.

Suicide Precautions

You must have access to psychiatrists who are willing to evaluate and treat severely depressed patients who are suicidal. The psychologist often uncovers the suicidal intention during the initial assessment. The psychiatrist is then consulted to confirm the diagnosis and to admit the patient to the psychiatric unit, if needed. This task can be very emotional and difficult, not only for the patient but also for his or her family and health care providers. All involved must understand that the decision for psychiatric admission is made with the patient's best interest in mind and to allow further therapy to help alleviate depression and pain.

Chronic Pain Evaluation

Aside from this rare but very important need for psychiatric support, a psychiatrist or a psychologist can and should evaluate all chronic pain patients as part of the multidisciplinary approach to chronic pain management. The interventions used are adjuvants to the medical treatments discussed earlier. The objective of such therapy is to change the perception of pain by altering the meaning of the pain experience or the effect associated with it, by changing the pain behavior and expression, or both. Many times, an accurate medical diagnosis and treatment plan fails without this additional psychologic treatment. Family members or loved ones also must be incorporated into the treatment plan to ensure a successful therapeutic trial. Acute pain patients also can benefit from many of these same therapies, particularly if a history of chronic pain is present. Cancer pain patients have the additional psychologic problems associated with death and dying that can be tempered with many of the same techniques.

What Are Appropriate Cognitive and Behavioral Interventions?

No psychologic technique is appropriate for all pain patients. Each situation requires careful evaluation, possibly over many return visits, to determine the best approach. Several techniques are potentially useful, including cognitive-behavioral therapy, biofeedback therapy, hypnosis, and psychotherapy.

Cognitive-Behavioral Therapy

The idea behind the application of cognitive-behavioral treatment strategies (Table 14–27)[162] is that a patient can learn to change the negative impact of pain, thus decreasing suffering and pain behavior (see Fig. 14–4) increasing control over

TABLE 14–27. Major Types of Cognitive-Behavioral Therapies for Pain

Cognitive Restructuring	Patients are taught to monitor and evaluate negative thoughts and to generate more accurate and adaptive cognitions. *Example:* A chronic pain patient who responds to increased pain by thinking, ''I can't take this anymore'' is taught to examine such thoughts and develop more accurate and adaptive ones; for example, ''Is it really true that I can't deal with this? No. It may be difficult, but I've done it before and can do it again.''
Coping Skills Training	Patients are provided a rationale for the use of techniques and then taught various skills for managing pain and stress.
Relaxation	*Example:* Physical or mental relaxation methods
Imagery	*Example:* Imagining pleasant scenes
Coping self-statements	*Examples:* ''Relax.'' ''I can cope.'' ''Focus on what you have to do.''

(From Turner JA, Romano JM: Cognitive-Behavioral therapy. *In* The Management of Pain. 2nd ed. Bonica JJ (ed). Philadelphia, Lea & Febiger, 1990, pp 1711–1721.)

the pain. These techniques have been found to be useful in a variety of pain problems.

Biofeedback

Biofeedback is a very different approach that utilizes an electronic device to detect and amplify biologic responses and convert them into information that patients can utilize to change their response to the pain. This technique has been found to be successful in the treatment of tension or migraine headaches, myofascial pain, and temporomandibular joint syndrome.

Hypnosis

Hypnosis has been successful in reducing or eliminating a variety of clinical pain problems, including acute and chronic pain syndromes.

Psychotherapy

Lastly, psychotherapy is defined as any form of treatment for mental illness, behavioral maladaptation, and other problems assumed to be of an emotional nature. The therapist deliberately establishes a professional relationship with a patient for the purpose of modifying, removing, or retarding existing symptoms, attenuating or reversing disturbed patterns of behavior, and promoting positive personality growth and development.[164] This type of therapy must be chosen carefully and is appropriate when[165]:

1. Much or all of the problem seems to follow from a psychologic disorder without a major physical contribution;

2. Emotional changes have developed in response to suffering related to a prolonged and severe illness without evidence of premorbid predisposition to psychologic illness;

3. The aim of treatment is to change subjective distress related to relationships, conflicts, and the sense of self.

The major types of psychotherapy used in the treatment of chronic pain patients include supportive, dynamic, family, and group therapies.

References

1. Portenoy RK: Diagnosis of cancer pain syndromes. *In* Pain Syndromes in Neurologic Practices. Field H (ed). New York, Butterworth Publishing Co, 1990, pp 237–255.
2. Mersky H (ed): Classification of chronic pain: description of chronic pain syndromes and definition of pain terms. Pain 1986; S1(Suppl. 3):217.
3. Bonica JJ: Definitions and taxonomy of pain. *In* The Management of Pain. Bonica JJ (ed). Philadelphia, Lea & Febiger, 1990, pp 18–27.
4. Portenoy RK: Mechanisms of clinical pain, observations and speculations. Neurol Clin 1989; 7:205.
5. Revill SI, Robinson JO, Rosen M, et al: The reliability of a linear analogue for evaluating pain. Anaesthesia 1976; 31:1991.
6. Acute Pain Management Guideline Panel: Acute Pain Management: Operative or Medical Procedures and Trauma. Clinical Practice guideline. Rockville, MD: Agency for Health Care Policy and Research, Public Health Service; 1992. US Department of Health and Human Services publication AHCPR 92-0032, p 116.
7. National Institutes of Health Consensus Panel: The integrated approach to the management of pain. J Pain Symptom Manage 1987; 2:35.
8. Loeser JD: Concepts of pain. *In* Chronic Low Back Pain. Staton-Hicks M, Boas R (eds). New York, Raven Press, 1982, pp 145–148.
9. Beyer JE, McGrath PJ, Berde CN: Discordance between self-report and behavior pain measures in children age 3–7 years after surgery. J Pain Symptom Manage 1990; 5:350.
10. Cervero F: Deep and visceral pain. *In* Pain and Society. Kosterlitz HW, Terenius LY (eds). Chemie, Weinheim Verlag GmbH, 1980, pp 263–282.
11. Lewis T: Pain. New York, MacMillan Publishing Co, 1942, pp 173–180.
12. Bruera E, Ripamonti C: Adjuvants to opioid analgesics. *In* Pratt RB (ed). Cancer Pain. Philadelphia, JB Lippincott, 1993, pp 143–159.
13. Stoelting RK: Pharmacokinetics and pharmacodynamics of injected and inhaled drugs. *In* Pharmacology and Physiology in Anesthetic Practice. Stoelting RK (ed). Philadelphia, JB Lippincott, 1987, pp 2–34.
14. Reidenberg MM: Effect of disease states on plasma protein binding of drugs. Med Clin North Am 1974; 58:1103.
15. Hudson RJ: Basic principles of pharmacology. *In* Clinical Anesthesia. Barash PG, Cullen BF, Stoelting RK (eds). Philadelphia, JB Lippincott, 1989, pp 137–164.
16. Pelz M, Merskey H: A description of the psychological effects of chronic painful lesions. Pain 1982; 14:293.
17. Sternbach RA, Wolf SR, Murphy RW, Akeson WH: Traits of pain patients: the low-back ''loser.'' Psychosomatics 1973; 14:226.
18. Sternbach RA, Timmermans G: Personality changes associated with reduction of pain. Pain 1975; 1:177.
19. Fields HL: The psychology of pain. *In* Pain. Fields HL (ed). New York, McGraw-Hill, 1987, pp 171–203.
20. Fordyce WE: The acquisition of operant pain. *In* Behavioral Methods for Chronic Pain and Illness. Fordyce WE (ed). St Louis, Mosby, 1976, pp 41–73.
21. Gunn CC, Milbrandt E: Early and subtle signs of low back pain. Spine 1978; 3:267.
22. Bonica JJ: Causalgia and other reflex sympathetic dystrophies. *In* The Management of Pain. Bonica JJ (ed). Philadelphia, Lea & Febiger, 1990, pp 220–243.
23. Travell J: Myofascial trigger points: clinical view. *In* Advances in Pain Research and Therapy, 1. Bonica JJ, Albe-Fessard D (eds). New York, Raven Press, 1976, pp 919–926.
24. Rudy TE, Turk DC, Brena SF: Differential utility of medical procedures in the assessment of chronic pain patients. Pain 1988; 34:167.
25. Schipper J, Kardaun JWPF, Braakman R, et al: Lumbar disk herniation: diagnosis with CT or myelography? Radiology 1987; 165:227.
26. Task Force on Acute Pain: Management of Acute Pain: A Practical Guide. Ready BH, Edwards WT (eds). Seattle, IASP Publications, 1992, pp 11–21.
27. Monks R: Psychotropic Drugs. *In* The Management of Pain. Bonica JJ (ed). Philadelphia, Lea & Febiger, 1990, pp 1676–1689.
28. Portenoy RK: Chronic opioid therapy in non-malignant pain. J Pain Symptom Manage 1990; 5(Suppl.):S46.
29. Fishbain DA, Rosomoff HL, Rosomoff RS: Review article: drug abuse, dependence, and addiction in chronic pain patients. Clin J Pain 1992; 8:77.
30. Portenoy RK, Foley KM: Chronic use of opioid analgesics in nonmalignant pain: report of 38 cases. Pain 1986; 25:171.
31. World Health Organization: Cancer Pain Relief and Palliative Care. WHO Technical Report Series 804. Geneva, Switzerland, 1990, p 9.

32. Levy MH: Pain management in advanced cancer. Semin Oncol 1985; 12:394.

33. Patt RB, Szalados JE, Wu CL: Pharmacotherapeutic guidelines. *In* Cancer Pain. Patt RB (ed). Philadelphia, JB Lippincott, 1993, p 574.

34. Onghena P, Van Houdenhove B: Antidepressant-induced analgesia in chronic nonmalignant pain: a meta-analysis of 39 placebo-controlled studies. Pain 1992; 49:205.

35. Tanelian DL, Brosse WG: Neuropathic pain can be relieved by drugs that are use-dependent sodium channel blockers: Lidocaine, Carbamazepine, and Mexilitene. Anesthesiology 1991; 74:949.

36. Davis KD, Treede RD, Raja SN, et al: Topical application of clonidine relieves hyperalgesia in patients with sympathetically maintained pain. Pain 1991; 47:309.

37. Raskin NH, Levinson SA, Hoffman PM, et al: Post-sympathectomy neuralgia: amelioration with diphenylhydantoin and carbamazepine. Am J Surg 1974; 128:75.

38. Kocher R: Use of psychotropic drugs for the treatment of chronic severe pain. *In* Advances in Pain Research and Therapy. Vol. 1. Bonica JJ, Albe-Fessard D (eds). New York, Raven Press, 1976, pp 579–582.

39. Fromm GH, Terrence CF, Chattha AS: Baclofen in the treatment of trigeminal neuralgia: double-blind study and long-term follow-up. Ann Neurol 1984; 15:240.

40. Ghostine SY, Comair YG, Turner DM, et al: Phenoxybenzamine in the treatment of causalgia. J Neurosurg 1984; 60:1263.

41. Hill CS: Oral opioid analgesics. *In* Cancer Pain. Patt RB (ed). Philadelphia, JB Lippincott, 1993, p 137.

42. Patt RB, Szalados JE, Wu CL: Pharmacotherapeutic guidelines. *In* Cancer Pain. Patt RB (ed). Philadelphia, JB Lippincott, 1993, pp 565–575.

43. Marchettini P, Lacerenza M, Marangoni C, et al: Lidocaine test in neuralgia. Pain 1992; 48:377.

44. Graubard DJ, Robertazzi RW, Peterson MC: One year's experience with intravenous procaine. Anesth Analg 1948; 27:222.

45. Boas RA, Covino BG, Shahnarian A: Analgesic responses to IV lignocaine. Br J Anaesth 1982; 54:501.

46. Edwards WT, Habib F, Burney RG, et al: Intravenous lidocaine in the management of various chronic pain states: a review of 211 cases. Reg Anesth 1983; Jan-March:1.

47. Glazer S, Portenoy RK: Review article: systemic local anesthetics in pain control. J Pain Symptom Manage 1991; 6:30.

48. Kastrup J, Peterson P, Dejgard R, et al: Intravenous lidocaine infusion: a new treatment of chronic painful diabetic neuropathy? Pain 1987; 28:69.

49. Dejgard A, Peterson P, Kastrup J: Mexilitine for treatment of chronic painful diabetic neuropathy. Lancet 1988; i:9.

50. Jönsson A, Cassuto J, Hanson B: Inhibition of burn pain by intravenous lignocaine infusion. Lancet 1991; 338:151.

51. Dixon CL, Berger JJ: Intravenous lidocaine in the treatment of postherpetic neuralgia (Abstract). Reg Anesth 1992; 17(Suppl):61.

52. Bonica JJ: Postoperative pain. *In* The Management of Pain. Bonica JJ (ed). Philadelphia, Lea & Febiger, 1990, p 466.

53. Brown DL, Carpenter RL: Perioperative analgesia: a review of risks and benefits. J Cardiothorac Anesth 1990; 4:363.

54. Ali J, Weisel RD, Layug AB, et al: Consequences of postoperative alterations in respiratory mechanics. Am J Surg 1974; 128:376.

55. Buckley DN, MacIntosh J, Beattie WS: Epidural analgesia prevents loss of lung volume (Abstract). Anesthesiology 1990; 73(Suppl):A764.

56. Zimmerman M: Peripheral and central nervous system mechanisms of nociception, pain and pain therapy: facts and hypothesis. *In* Advances in Pain Research and Therapy. Bonica JJ, Liebeskind JC, Albe Fessard DC (eds). New York, Raven Press, 1979, pp 3–32.

57. Craig DG: Postoperative recovery of pulmonary function. Anesth Analg 1981; 60:46.

58. Mankikian B, Cantineau JP, Bertrand M, et al: Improvement of diaphragmatic function by a thoracic extradural block after upper abdominal surgery. Anesthesiology 1988; 68:379.

59. Modig J: Respiration and circulation after total hip replacement surgery: a comparison between parenteral analgesics and continuous lumbar epidural block. Acta Anaesth Scand 1976; 20:225.

60. Christopherson R, Rock P, Parker S, et al: Tachycardia occurs more frequently postoperatively than intraoperatively in patients at risk for perioperative myocardial ischemia. Anesthesiology 1989; 71:A950.

61. Ellis JE, Busse JR, Foss JF, et al: Postoperative management of myocardial ischemia. Anesth Clin 1991; 9:609.

62. Breslow MJ: Neuroendocrine responses to surgery. *In* Perioperative Management. Breslow MJ, Miller CF, Rogers MC (eds). St Louis, Mosby–Year Book, 1990, pp 180–193.

63. Cousins MJ: Acute pain and the injury response: immediate and prolonged effects. Reg Anesth 1989; 16:162.

64. Modig J, Borg T, Karlström G, et al: Thrombo-embolism after total hip replacement: role of epidural and general anesthesia. Anesth Analg 1983; 62:174.

65. Bing HI: Viscerocutaneous and cutaneovisceral thoracic reflexes. Acta Med Scand 1936; 89:57.

66. Nimmo WS: Effect of anaesthesia on gastric motility and emptying. Br J Anaesth 1984; 56:29.

67. Philbin DM, Rosow CE, Schneider RC, et al: Fentanyl and sufentanil anesthesia revisited: how much is enough? Anesthesiology 1990; 73:5.

68. Suchner U, Rothkopf MM: Metabolic effects of the neuroendocrine stress response. Anesth Clin North Am 1988; 6:1.

69. Ruthberg H, Hakanson E, Anderberg B, et al: Effect of extradural administration of morphine or bupivacaine on the endocrine response to upper abdominal surgery. Anaesthesia 1985; 40:748.

70. Traynor C, Paterson JL, Ward ID, et al: Effects of extradural analgesia and vagal blockade on the metabolic and endocrine response to upper abdominal surgery. Br J Anaesth 1982; 54:319.

71. Kehlet H: Modification of responses to surgery by neural blockade: clinical implications. *In* Neural Blockade in Clinical Anesthesia and Management in Pain. 2nd ed. Cousins MJ, Bridenbaugh PO (eds). Philadelphia, JB Lippincott, 1988, pp 145–188.

72. Bell SD: The correlation between pulmonary function and resting and dynamic pain scores in post-aortic surgery patients. Anesth Analg 1991; 72:S18.

73. Hendolin H, Lahtinen J, Lärsimies E, et al: The effect of thoracic epidural analgesia on respiratory function after cholecystectomy. Acta Anaesth Scand 1987; 31:645.

74. Rawal N, Sjöstrand U, Christoffersson E, et al: Comparison of intramuscular and epidural morphine for postoperative analgesia in the grossly obese: influence of postoperative ambulation and pulmonary function. Anesth Analg 1984; 63:583.

75. Hasenbos M, van Egmond J, Gielen M, et al: Post-operative analgesia by high thoracic epidural versus intramuscular nicomorphine after thoracotomy. Part III: The effect of pre- and post-operative analgesia on morbidity. Acta Anaesth Scand 1987; 31:645.

76. Shulman M, Sandler AN, Bradley JW, et al: Post-thoracotomy pain and pulmonary function following epidural and systemic morphine. Anesthesiology 1984; 61:569.

77. El-Baz N, Goldin M: Continuous epidural infusion of morphine for pain relief after cardiac operations. J Thorac Cardiovasc Surg 1987; 93:878.

78. Vanstrum GS, Bjornson KM, Ilko R: Postoperative effects of intrathecal morphine in coronary artery bypass surgery. Anesth Analg 1988; 67:261.

79. Yeager MP, Glass DD, Neff RK, et al: Epidural anesthesia and analgesia in high risk surgical patients. Anesthesiology 1987; 66:729.

80. Waskinck J, Hurford W, Gelb C, et al: Epidural opioid analgesia does not alter the neuro-endocrine response to thoracotomy. Anesth Analg 1990; 70:S422.

81. Scott NB, Mogensen T, Bigler D, et al: Continuous thoracic extradural 0.5% bupivacaine with or without morphine: effect on quality of blockade, lung function and surgical stress response. Br J Anaesth 1989; 62:252.

82. Bonnet F, Blery C, Zatan M, et al: Effect of epidural morphine on postoperative pulmonary function. Acta Anaesth Scand 1984; 28:147.

83. Pflug AE, Murphy TM, Butler SH, et al: The effects of postoperative peridural analgesia on pulmonary therapy and pulmonary complications. Anesthesiology 1974; 41:8.

84. Tuman KJ, McCarthy RJ, March R, et al: Epidural anesthesia—analgesia improves outcome after major vascular surgery: a hypothesis reconfirmed (Abstract). Anesth Analg 1991; 72(Suppl):S302.

85. Borg T, Modig J: Potential antithrombotic effect of local anesthetics due to their inhibition of platelet aggregation. Acta Anaesthesiol Scand 1985; 29:739.

86. Modig J, Borg T, Bagge L, et al: Role of epidural and of general anesthesia in fibrinolysis and coagulation after total hip replacement. Br J Anaesth 1983; 55:625.

87. Ahn H, Bronge A, Johansson K, et al: Effect of continuous postoperative epidural analgesia on intestinal motility. Br J Surg 1988; 75:1176.

88. England DW, Davis JJ, Timmins AE, et al: Gastric emptying: a study to compare the effects of intrathecal morphine and i.m. papaveretum analgesia. Br J Anaesth 1987; 59:1403.

89. Scheinin B, Asantila R, Orko R: The effect of bupivacaine and morphine on pain and bowel function after colonic surgery. Acta Anaesthesiol Scand 1987; 31:161.

90. Grass JA, Sakina NT: Epidural anesthesia and analgesia results in shorter hospital stay after total abdominal hysterectomy (Abstract). Reg Anesth 1992; 17(Suppl):77.

91. Bellamy CD, McDonnell FJ, Colclough GW: Postoperative epidural pain management results in shorter hospital stay than IV PCA morphine: a

comparison in anterior cruciate ligament repair (Abstract). Anesthesiology 1989; 71(Suppl):A685.

92. Dixon CL, Sefton W, Gravenstein N: Epidural analgesia after donor nephrectomy decreases duration of hospitalization (Abstract). Reg Anesth 1992; 17(Suppl):75.

93. Brull SJ, Lieponis JV, Murphy MJ, et al: Acute and long-term benefits of iliac crest donor site perfusion with local anesthetics. Anesth Analg 1992; 74:145.

94. Jacobson L, Chabal C: Prolonged relief of acute post-amputation phantom limb pain with intrathecal fentanyl and epidural morphine. Anesthesiology 1989; 71:984.

95. Bach S, Noreng MF, Tjellden NU: Phantom limb pain in amputees during the first 12 months following limb amputation, after preoperative lumbar epidural blockade. Pain 1988; 33:297.

96. Crile GW, Lower WE: Anoci-association. Philadelphia, WB Saunders, 1914.

97. Tverskoy M, Cozacov C, Ayache M, et al: Postoperative pain after inguinal herniorrhaphy with different types of anesthesia. Anesth Analg 1990; 70:29.

98. McQuay HJ, Carroll D, Moore RA: Postoperative orthopedic pain: the effect of opiate premedication and local anesthetic blocks. Pain 1988; 33:291.

99. Jebeles JA, Reilly JS, Gutierrez JF, et al: The effect of pre-incisional infiltration of tonsils with bupivacaine on the pain following tonsillectomy under general anesthesia. Pain 1991; 47:305.

100. Benson JP: Organization of a postoperative pain service. In Anesthesia Update #6: Supplement to Anesthesia. 3rd ed. Miller RD (ed). New York, Churchill Livingstone, 1992, pp 137–153.

101. Walmsley PNH: Patient-controlled epidural analgesia. In Acute Pain: Mechanisms & Management. Sinatra RS, Hord AH, Ginsberg B, et al (eds). St Louis, Mosby–Year Book, 1992, pp 312–325.

102. Sinatra RS: Pharmacokinetics and pharmacodynamics of spinal opioids. In Acute Pain: Mechanisms & Management. Sinatra RS, Hord AH, Ginsberg B, et al (eds). St Louis, Mosby–Year Book, 1992, pp 102–111.

103. Kafer ER, Brown JT, Scott DD, et al: Biphasic depression of ventilatory responses to CO_2 following epidural morphine. Anesthesiology 1983; 58:418.

104. Ready LB, Oden R, Chadwick HS, et al: Development of an anesthesiology-based postoperative pain management service. Anesthesiology 1988; 68:100.

105. Ready LB, Loper KA, Nessly M, et al: Postoperative epidural morphine is safe on surgical wards. Anesthesiology 1991; 75:452.

106. Ready LB: Regional analgesia with intraspinal opioids. In The Management of Pain. 2nd ed. Bonica JJ (ed). Philadelphia, Lea & Febiger, 1990, pp 1967–1979.

107. Rawal N, Arner S, Gustafsson LL, et al: Present state of extradural and intrathecal opioid analgesia in Sweden. Br J Anaesth 1987; 59:791.

108. Ventafridda V, Tamburini M, Caraceni A, et al: A validation study of the WHO method for cancer pain relief. Cancer 1987; 59:851.

109. Foley KM: Treatment of cancer pain. N Engl J Med 1985; 313:84.

110. Krames ES, Gershow J, Glassberg A, et al: Continuous infusion of spinally administered narcotics for the relief of pain due to malignant disorders. Cancer 1985; 56:696.

111. Krames ES: Intrathecal infusional therapies for intractable pain: patient management guidelines. J Pain Symptom Manage 1993; 8:36.

112. Plummer JL, Cherry DA, Cousins MJ, et al: Long-term spinal administration of morphine in cancer and non-cancer pain: a retrospective study. Pain 1991; 44:215.

113. Hord AH: Postoperative analgesia in the opioid-dependent patient. In Acute Pain: Mechanisms & Management. Sinatra RS, Hord AH, Ginsberg B, et al (eds). St Louis, Mosby–Year Book, 1992, pp 390–398.

114. Stacey BR, Brody MC, Burke DF: Patients with a substance abuse history can effectively use PCA (Abstract). Anesthesiology 1990; 73(Suppl):A759.

115. Eichhorn JH: Spinal anesthesia and anticoagulant therapy: questions and answers. JAMA 1989; 262:411.

116. Bromage PR: Epidural Anesthesia. Philadelphia, WB Saunders, 1978, pp 283–346.

117. Cook ED, Lloyd MJ, Bowcock SA, et al: Monitoring during low dose heparin prophylaxis. N Engl J Med 1976; 294:1066.

118. Lowson SM, Goodchild CS: Low-dose heparin therapy and spinal anaesthesia. Anaesthesia 1989; 44:67.

119. Darnat S, Guggiari M, Grob R, et al: Un cas d'hematome extradural rachidien au cours de la mise en place d'un catheter peridural. Ann Fr Anesth Reanim 1986; 5:550.

120. Cousins MJ, Bridenbaugh PO: Epidural neural blockade. In Neural Blockade in Clinical Anesthesia and Management of Pain. 2nd ed. Cousins MJ, Bridenbaugh PO (eds). Philadelphia, JB Lippincott, 1988, pp 253–360.

121. Odoom JA, Sih IL: Epidural analgesia and anticoagulant therapy. Anaesthesia 1983; 38:254.

122. Baron HC, LaRaja RD, Rossi G, et al: Continuous epidural analgesia in the heparinized vascular surgical patient: a retrospective review of 912 patients. J Vasc Surg 1987; 6:144.

123. Rao TLK, El-Etr AA: Anticoagulation following placement of epidural and subarachnoid catheters: an evaluation of neurologic sequelae. Anesthesiology 1981; 55:618.

124. Owens EL, Kasten GW, Hessel EA: Spinal subarachnoid hematoma: a case report, review of the literature, and discussion of anesthetic implications. Anesth Analg 1986; 65:1201.

125. Helperin SW, Cohen DD: Hematoma following epidural anesthesia: report of a case. Anesthesiology 1971; 35:641.

126. DeAngelis J: Hazards of subdural and epidural anesthesia during anticoagulant therapy: a case report and review. Anesth Analg 1972; 51:676.

127. Dixon, CL: Preoperative assessment for regional anesthesia. Probl Anesth 1991; 5:591.

128. Bonica JJ, Buckley FP: Regional analgesia with local anesthetics. In The Management of Pain. Bonica JJ (ed). Philadelphia, Lea & Febiger, 1990, pp 1883–1966.

129. Levack SP, Holmes JD, Robertson JS: Abdominal wound perfusion for the relief of postoperative pain. Br J Anaesth 1986; 58:615.

130. Malawer MM, Buck R, Khurana JS, et al: Postoperative infusional continuous regional analgesia. Clin Orthop 1991; 266:227.

131. Rosenblatt R, Pepitone-Rockwell R, McKillop RJ: Continuous axillary analgesia for traumatic hand injury. Anesthesiology 1979; 51:565.

132. Smith BD: Continuous sciatic nerve block. Anaesthesia 1984; 39:155.

133. Patt RB, Jain S: Therapeutic decision-making for invasive procedures. In Cancer Pain. Patt RB (ed). Philadelphia, JB Lippincott, 1992, pp 275–283.

134. Ferrer-Brechner T: Anesthetic techniques for the management of cancer pain. Cancer 1989; 63:2343.

135. Rowlingson JC, Chalkley J: Common pain syndromes: diagnosis and management. Semin Anesth 1985; 4:223.

136. Devor M, Govrin-Lippimann R, Raber P: Corticosteroids suppress ectopic neural discharge originating in experimental neuromas. Pain 1985; 22:127.

137. Simons DG: Myofascial pain syndromes of head, neck and low back. In Pain Research and Clinical Management. Vol. 3. Proceedings of the Fifth World Congress on Pain. Dubner R, Gehhart GF, Bond MR (eds). New York, Elsevier, 1988, pp 186–200.

138. Pybus PK: Control of pain and stiffness in osteoarthritis of the hand. S Afr Med J 1981; 59:514.

139. Dory MA: Arthrography of the cervical facet joints. Radiology 1983; 148:379.

140. Wedel DJ, Wilson PR: Cervical facet arthrography. Reg Anesth 1985; 10:7.

141. Bonica JJ, Buckley FP, Moricca G, et al: Neurolytic blockade and hypophysectomy. In The Management of Pain. Bonica JJ (ed). Philadelphia, Lea & Febiger, 1990, pp 1980–2039.

142. Melzack R, Wall PD: Pain mechanisms: a new theory. Science 1965; 150:971.

143. Hughes GS, Lichstein PR: Response of plasma beta-endorphins to TENS in healthy subjects. Phys Ther 1984; 64:1062.

144. Facchinetti F, Sforza G: Central and peripheral beta-endorphin response to TENS. NIDA Res Monogr 1986; 75:555.

145. O'Brien WJ, Rutan FM: Effect of TENS on human blood beta-endorphin levels. Phys Ther 1984; 64:1367.

146. Ordog GJ: TENS vs oral analgesic: a randomized double-blind controlled study in acute traumatic pain. J Emerg Med 1987; 5:6.

147. Schomberg FL, Carter-Baker SA: Transcutaneous electrical nerve stimulation for postlaparotomy pain. Phys Ther 1983; 63:188.

148. Solomon FA, Vierstein MC: Reduction of postoperative pain and narcotic use by TENS. Surgery 1980; 87:142.

149. Warfield CA: Physical therapy for pain relief. Hosp Pract 1984; 19:84E.

150. Gersh MR, Wolf SL: Applications of transcutaneous electrical stimulation in the management of patients with pain. Phys Ther 1985; 65:314.

151. Melzack R: TENS for low back pain: a comparison of TENS with massage for pain and range of motion. Phys Ther 1983; 63:489.

152. Carabelli RA, Kellerman WC: Phantom limb pain: relief by application of TENS to contralateral extremity. Arch Phys Med Rehab 1985; 66:466.

153. Robaina FJ, Rodriguez JL: TENS and spinal cord stimulation for pain relief in reflex sympathetic dystrophy. Stereotact Funct Neurosurg 1989; 52:53.

154. Wolf SL, Gersh MR: Examination of electrode placements and stimulating parameters in treating chronic pain with conventional TENS. Pain 1981; 11:37.

155. Johnson MI, Ashton CH, Thompson JW: An in-depth study of long-

term users of transcutaneous electrical nerve stimulation (TENS). Implications for clinical use of TENS. Pain 1991; 44:221.

156. Meyerson BA: Electrostimulation procedures: effects, presumed rationale, and possible mechanisms. *In* Advances in Pain Research and Therapy. Vol. 5. Bonica JJ (ed). New York, Raven Press, 1983, pp 495–533.

157. Sedan R, Lazorthes Y: La neurostimulation electrique therapeutique. Neurochirurgia 1978; 24(Suppl 1):1.

158. Urban BJ, Nashold BS: Percutaneous epidural stimulation of the spinal cord for relief of pain. Neurosurgery 1978; 48:323.

159. Meyerson BA: Electrical stimulation of the spinal cord and brain. *In* The Management of Pain. Bonica JJ (ed). Philadelphia, Lea & Febiger, 1990, pp 1862–1877.

160. Yeh C, Gonyea MB, Lemke J, et al: Physical therapy: evaluation and treatment of chronic pain. *In* Evaluation and Treatment of Chronic Pain. Aronoff GM (ed). Baltimore, Urban & Schwarzenberg, 1985, pp 251–261.

161. Marcant D, Rapien C-H: Role of the physiotherapist in palliative care. J Pain Symptom Manage 1993; 8:68.

162. Lee MHM, Itoh M, Yang G-FW, et al: Physical therapy and rehabilitation medicine. *In* The Management of Pain. 2nd ed. Bonica JJ (ed). Philadelphia, Lea & Febiger, 1990, pp 1769–1788.

163. Turner JA, Romano JM: Cognitive-Behavioral therapy. *In* The Management of Pain. 2nd ed. Bonica JJ (ed). Philadelphia, Lea & Febiger, 1990, pp 1711–1721.

164. OHIP Schedule of Benefits. Physician's Services: Ontario, Ministry of Health, 1984.

165. Tunks ER, Merskey H: Psychotherapy in the management of chronic pain. *In* The Management of Pain. 2nd ed. Bonica JJ (ed). Philadelphia, Lea & Febiger, 1990, pp 1751–1756.

CHAPTER **15**

Pain Management Consultation in Pediatric Patients

PHILLIP GAUKROGER, M.D., F.F.A.R.A.C.S.

The past 10 years have seen an escalation of interest in the management of all forms of pain in children. This interest stemmed from the publication of several significant studies. Mather and Mackie[1] investigated the incidence of postoperative pain in 170 Australian children and found fundamental problems in the way analgesia was prescribed and delivered. They found that the incidence of severe pain was 13% on the day of surgery and 17% on the first postoperative day. Analgesia was not ordered for 16% of children, and there was a marked reluctance to administer narcotic analgesics to children. Prescribing habits were poor, and in many cases the doses of medication were too small and too infrequent. "As needed" was interpreted to mean "as little as possible." Children expressed a fear of "the needle" and preferred to put up with pain rather than have a shot. The researchers concluded that there was considerable scope for improving pediatric pain relief.

Beyer and colleagues[2] surveyed analgesic prescription in 50 adults and 50 children after cardiac surgery. They found that adults received 70% of the analgesic doses and children received 30%. Young children were less likely to be prescribed narcotic analgesics. Six children were the only patients in the study to receive no analgesia at all.

A review of the literature at the time reveals that very little was known about pediatric pain relief. The pharmacology of analgesics in children was unknown, and the common methods and doses of drugs for analgesics were merely scaled-down adult regimens that often did not consider special pediatric needs.

In 1987, Anand and Hickey demonstrated that infants who undergo surgery with little or no analgesia mount a significant stress response, as measured by the release of catecholamines, growth hormone, glucagon, and corticosteroids and the suppression of insulin release.[3] This work provided evidence that neonates feel pain, and subsequent studies showed that outcome can be improved by providing adequate anesthesia and analgesia.[4–6] It increased the awareness that neonatal analgesia was poorly managed and stimulated considerable debate, including at least five editorials in 1987.[7–11]

Deficiencies in pediatric pain relief were demonstrated not only in the perioperative period but also in burn units in the United States. Perry and Heidrich found that children were four times less likely to receive narcotic analgesia than adults, despite the fact that respondents felt that the degree of pain experienced by children and adults was the same.[12]

Procedural pain also was studied. In 1985, Hockenberry and Bologna-Vaugh reported that only 12% of institutions routinely premedicated children before bone marrow biopsies and lumbar punctures.[13] These procedures often create intense fear and anxiety in pediatric oncology patients.

PEDIATRIC PAIN MANAGEMENT

Why Was It Ignored?

Commonly Accepted Myths

Table 15–1 summarizes the reasons for ignorance about pediatric pain. Clearly, many myths were promulgated for years and tended to be handed down as gospel. Several deserve special comment.

The myth that children and infants feel no pain probably

TABLE 15–1. Reasons for Undertreatment of Pediatric Pain

Myths	Children don't feel pain
	Children don't remember pain
	Children will become addicted to narcotics
Attitudes	Pain builds character
	"It is not a painful operation"
	Children are powerless
Research difficulties	Measuring pediatric pain
	Technical (e.g., blood sampling in small children)
	Ethical
Poor education	Medical
	Nursing
	Allied health professions
	Child and parent
Poor clinical application	Unsuitable methods (e.g., intramuscular injections)
	Drugs not approved for children
	Poor prescribing practices
	Acute pain management poorly developed in adult practice
Economic	Difficult to demonstrate cost effectiveness of pain management in children

arose from arguments that myelination of nerves is incomplete at birth. The immaturity of nervous tissue, however, does not affect pain perception, and Anand's studies clearly have put to rest that myth.[3-6]

The myth that pain is not remembered by children is often argued for infants undergoing neonatal circumcision. However, behavioral changes persist in infants who have undergone surgery without pain relief or who undergo many painful procedures in neonatal intensive care units.[14] Furthermore, addiction has never been documented to be a problem in the management of acute pain,[12, 15] and this observation is especially so for children.

A common attitude is that pain is a normal part of growing up and that it ''builds character,'' yet recurrent procedures in children are usually detrimental to a child's self-development. Also, many hospital staff subconsciously underestimate distress and pain in children as a way of coping with their role as causers of pain.

Research and Education

The lack of pediatric pain research is in part due to difficulties that are peculiar to childhood. Assessment and measurement of pain in such a wide range of ages and developmental stages is clearly difficult. Pharmacokinetic studies have been hindered by difficulties in collecting sufficient quantities of blood. Ethical issues such as consent are more complex in children.

The deficiencies of education of medical, nursing, and allied health professionals is clearly illustrated by examining past syllabuses and textbooks that paid little or no attention to pediatric pain. Fortunately, this situation is rapidly improving. Pain relief tended not to be discussed in the past, but it is clear now that both children and parents benefit from knowledge about pain relief methods.

Clinical issues are relevant. Methods of drug delivery designed specifically for children were uncommon until recent times. Also, many drugs are restricted or not approved for use in children.

Financial Incentives

Finally, we always have to consider the economic reasons. A strong financial impetus encourages improved chronic pain management in adults. The costs of third-party claims, workers' compensation injuries, and sickness benefits were considerable, enabling adult pain management services to put forward very strong arguments that their therapies were cost effective in that they allowed many patients to return to work. For obvious reasons, this type of argument is difficult to advance in children. Pediatric pain is most commonly acute pain, and acute pain has been equally neglected in adults.

Is the Management Changing?

Response to the considerable problems of providing pain relief to children has been relatively quick. We are optimistic that a progressive reduction in the number of children unnecessarily experiencing pain will occur.[16] Promising signs include the increasing number of textbooks dealing specifically with this topic; the setting up of both acute and chronic pain management services and pain interest groups for children; the

development of special interest groups such as the Pain in Childhood group formed through the International Association for the Study of Pain (IASP); the inclusion of pain management topics in undergraduate curricula; and the development of better techniques of managing acute pain in children.

SPECTRUM OF PEDIATRIC PAIN

Clear differences are demonstrated in the spectrum of pain experienced by children and adults (Table 15–2). Because of these differences, many adult pain relief therapies and experience are inappropriate when applied to pediatric pain.

What Types of Pain Do Children Experience?

Acute

The majority of childhood pain is acute. This situation is different in adults, in whom chronic noncancer and cancer pain are very common. Postoperative pain management is of obvious relevance to anesthetists and is an area in which the benefits of improved pain management are readily seen.

Other forms of acute pain are particularly important in children. Procedural pain causes considerably more distress, especially if recurrent procedures are required. The difficulty in explaining the benefits of blood tests, lumbar punctures, and intravenous insertions to small children is obvious. Burns and trauma are major pain management problems and may require ongoing pain therapy for periods of weeks to months.

Cancer

Cancer pain is vastly different in children, a fact that is often not perceived by workers in adult oncology and palliative care teams. Pediatric cancers are uncommon, constituting only 1% of malignancies. Hematologic malignancies predominate and have much higher cure rates than do adult cancers. Therapy is thus much more aggressive in children, and therapy-related pain is more common. On the other hand, adult cancer pain usually occurs during the terminal phase of the illness and is most commonly due to tumor spread.

TABLE 15–2. Spectrum of Pediatric and Adult Pain

Type of Pain	Pediatric	Adult
Acute pain (common)	Postoperative	Postoperative
	Procedural	Trauma
	Trauma	Burns
	Burns	
Cancer pain	Therapy-related pain predominates	Tumor-related pain predominates
Chronic noncancer pain	Juvenile chronic arthritis	Low back pain
	Headache	Cervical spine pain
	Recurrent abdominal pain	Postherpetic neuralgia
	Sickle cell disease	Phantom limb pain
	Hemophilia	Workers' compensation injuries
	Sympathetically maintained pain	Sympathetically maintained pain
	Progressively debilitating diseases	Neuralgias
	Miscellaneous	Miscellaneous

Noncancer

Chronic noncancer pain is relatively common in both adults and children but is much less likely to be debilitating in children. As can be seen from Table 15–2, the diseases causing chronic pain in children are vastly different from those in adults.

ASSESSMENT AND MEASUREMENT OF PAIN IN CHILDREN

Poor assessment of pain in children was a major factor inhibiting early research. Considerable effort has recently been expended in the development of suitable pain measurement and assessment tools.[17, 18] Although numerous methods now are available, none has been universally accepted and none is truly applicable to all age groups.

What Methods Are Clinically Useful?

In clinical practice, routine recording of pain as a nursing observation is to be encouraged because it increases awareness, allows more rational decisions about therapy, and gives a more accurate picture of how a patient has progressed. In my experience, simple verbal rating scales for pain and side effects such as sedation, nausea, and vomiting are easy to understand and have been a useful first step toward better recording of these important observations.[19] However, for the purposes of research, validated methods are required.

Self-Reporting

Because pain is a subjective phenomenon, self-report methods such as the 10-cm visual analogue scale (VAS) have become universally accepted for use by adults. The use of a VAS in children is limited by a child's cognitive development. The standard 10-cm VAS can be used reliably by most children as young as 6 to 7 years.

Most children older than 3 years can communicate "pain" or "hurt." Self-report measures can be applied, but methods that are easily understood by a child are more likely to be successful. The use of happy and sad faces is the most common modification to the VAS (Fig. 15–1).[17, 18, 20] Children must be made aware that the faces communicate their feelings about pain and not other emotions.

Behavioral Methods

Behavioral methods are necessary for measuring pain in smaller children and infants. Behavioral changes associated with pain can be classified as simple motor responses, crying, facial expression, and other more complex patterns. The major limitations are that some have been designed to measure responses to a specific procedure (e.g., heel lance) and some can only be applied to a limited age group.

Physiologic Measures

Physiologic variables such as pulse rate and blood pressure, transcutaneous oxygenation, palmar sweating, and hormonal changes occur with painful experiences, but no physiologic responses directly reflect a child's perception of pain.[21]

POSTOPERATIVE PAIN MANAGEMENT

Postoperative pain is the most common type treated by pediatric anesthesiologists. It is also an area that is undergoing considerable improvement with the introduction of newer techniques.

What Are the General Considerations?

The following principles are important if postoperative pain techniques are to be effective and properly applied. It is preferable to prevent pain than to treat it.[22] With respect to postoperative pain, a child is better off arriving in the recovery room with adequate analgesia from a loading dose of opiate or local anesthetic. If children are allowed to wake up in severe pain, more opiate will be required to settle them down. Opiates given in the recovery room should be titrated intravenously for rapid onset of effect.

Preanesthetic Assessment

The anesthesiologist should discuss postoperative analgesia during the preoperative visit. Not only will the child, parent, and ward staff benefit from this knowledge, but the anesthesiologist can plan for rational use of analgesic drugs. Unfortunately, healthy children commonly receive a short-acting opiate (e.g., fentanyl, alfentanil) in the operating room and arrive in the recovery room with severe pain. Titration with a different opiate for postoperative analgesia then follows. Whenever possible, the same drug should be used throughout for intraoperative and postoperative analgesia.

Psychologic Needs

The psychologic needs of children must be considered. Parental presence and comforting help most children experiencing pain; thus, it is common and appropriate that parents are allowed to be with their children during the postanesthesia recovery period.

Children benefit from an honest explanation of how much pain they are likely to experience and how it will be relieved. They are then able to prepare themselves psychologically, and clinically they appear to cope with painful surgery much better. Many school-aged children wish to know more about postoperative pain and prefer an honest explanation of how much pain they are likely to experience.

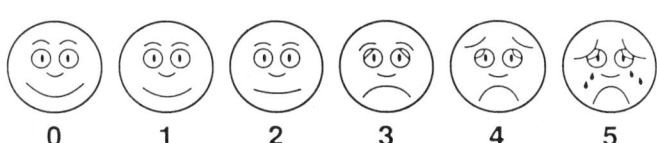

FIGURE 15–1. Face 0 = Very happy, has no hurt; face 1 = still happy, but not quite as happy as "0"; face 2 = is not very happy or sad, is kind of "in between," hurts just a little bit; face 3 = sad, hurts a little more; face 4 = even more sad and hurts a whole lot; face 5 = is very, very sad; hurts as bad as it can be. (Courtesy of Perdue Frederick Co., Norwalk, CT.)

Staff Education

Education and support for ward nursing and medical staff are essential to implement new techniques and to improve the way other techniques are managed. The greatest benefits in postoperative pain management are achieved in the general wards rather than in the high-care areas; hence, the general wards should not be ignored when new techniques are introduced. Commonly used drugs are listed in Table 15–3.

How Should Acetaminophen Be Used?

Acetaminophen is a useful analgesic and antipyretic drug that is very well tolerated by children. It is most often used for minor procedures, for day case surgery, and to supplement regional blockade. The principal questions are, "How much should I give?" and "When should I give it?"

Manufacturer's recommendations are often quoted for antipyresis, not analgesia, and usually underestimate the latter required dose considerably. For postoperative pain, oral doses of 15 to 20 mg · kg^{-1} every 4 hours and rectal doses of 20 to 30 mg · kg^{-1} every 6 hours are required.

Oral doses take approximately 30 minutes and rectal doses approximately 60 minutes for effect. Thus, premedication with 20 mg · kg^{-1} of acetaminophen orally, 30 to 60 minutes before the operation, is sensible, especially for ear, nose, and throat, ophthalmologic, dental, and minor general surgical procedures that are short. A commonly used alternative is to give 25 to 30 mg · kg^{-1} rectally immediately after induction of anesthesia. Both methods are preferable to attempting to administer acetaminophen in the recovery room or on return to the ward.

What Is the Value of Nonsteroidal Anti-Inflammatory Drugs?

Nonsteroidal anti-inflammatory drugs (NSAIDs) remain a controversial area of pediatric anesthetic practice. Aspirin fell from favor in pediatric practice when the potential association with Reye's syndrome was described.[23] For this reason and because of the well-documented side effects of gastric irritation and platelet dysfunction, aspirin is not used for pediatric postoperative pain management. Other NSAIDs such as ibuprofen, diclofenac, and naproxen are available in pediatric formulations and are commonly used for children in many countries. Pediatric suppository formulations do not exist in most countries.

These drugs provide equal or better analgesia than acetaminophen, do not sedate, and do not predispose to as much nausea and vomiting as opiates. However, the problem of platelet dysfunction prevents their more widespread use. In most institutions, NSAIDs are not administered routinely but are considered when opiate side effects such as sedation and nausea become troublesome. Because NSAIDs are also antipyretic, if concern about masking a fever is an issue, an opiate analgesic is preferred. The parenteral NSAID ketorolac[24] is still being evaluated but may overcome some of the logistic problems of trying to administer oral or rectal NSAIDs to children in the perioperative period. I give 1 mg · kg^{-1} either intramuscularly or intravenously as a loading dose and repeat 0.5 mg · kg^{-1} every 6 hours for up to 20 doses.

When Are Opioids Indicated?

When pain is not adequately ameliorated by simple analgesics or local anesthesia, opiate analgesics remain the drugs of choice. Healthy children 3 months of age and older absorb, metabolize, and excrete opiates similarly to healthy young adults. Studies by Hertzka and colleagues suggest that children older than 6 months have no more respiratory depression than adults.[25] Premature and term newborns, on the other hand, have reduced clearance of most opioids[26] and possibly increased blood-brain permeability. Along with their immature responses to hypoxia and hypercarbia, they are rendered more susceptible to the respiratory depressant effects.

Morphine

Morphine remains the opioid of choice for postoperative pain, although meperidine and other synthetic agents such as

---

TABLE 15–3. Pediatric Analgesic Dosage Guidelines

Drug	Prescription	Comments
Simple Analgesics		
Acetaminophen	15–20 mg · kg^{-1} PO q 4 h	Minor procedures
	20–30 mg · kg^{-1} PR q 6 h	Local anesthetic infiltration
Nonsteroidal anti-inflammatory drugs		Nonsedating; inhibit platelet function, antipyretic
Naproxen	5–7 mg · kg^{-1} PO q 12 h	Available in syrup, tablets, suppositories
Ibuprofen	4–8 mg · kg^{-1} PO q 6 h	Syrup, tablets, over the counter
Ketorolac	1 mg · kg^{-1} loading dose, then 0.5 mg · kg^{-1} q 6 h IM or IV	Parenteral nonsteroidal anti-inflammatory drugs
Opiate Analgesics		
Codeine	0.5–1 mg · kg^{-1} q 4 h	Partial agonist
Morphine	IV bolus: 0.05 mg · kg^{-1} q 1–2 h prn	Most commonly used
	IV infusion: 0–50 μg · kg^{-1} · h^{-1} or IV PCA: bolus 15–20 μg · kg^{-1}, background 15 μg · kg^{-1} · h^{-1}	
Meperidine	Multiply morphine doses by 10	Not for prolonged use (normeperidine toxicity)
Methadone	0.2 mg · kg^{-1} IV bolus	Intraoperative single dose
	0.2 mg · kg^{-1} PO q 12 h	Oral starting dose for prolonged pain
Fentanyl	1–3 μg · kg^{-1} · h^{-1} infusion	Short-acting drug

Abbreviations: PCA = patient-controlled analgesia; PO = orally; PR = rectally; q = every; IM = intramuscular(ly); IV = intravenous(ly).

fentanyl and sufentanil are common alternatives. Considerable clinical experience, economy, and the lack of superior alternatives favor morphine. However, side effects such as nausea and vomiting, sedation, and pruritus are common and may limit the extent of analgesia achievable.

Meperidine

Meperidine produces similar analgesic effects and side effects. It is more lipid soluble and has a slightly more rapid onset of analgesia but a shorter half-life than morphine.

Meperidine has a potentially toxic metabolite, normeperidine, which can cause agitation and seizures in susceptible individuals. For this reason, it is not recommended for longer-term analgesia or for analgesia in patients with impaired renal function.

Fentanyl and Sufentanil

Fentanyl and sufentanil are more lipid-soluble drugs that, because of rapid redistribution, have a relatively short duration of action. They cause little histamine release, an attribute that is especially useful in patients troubled by opiate-induced pruritus or rash. Disadvantages include skeletal muscle rigidity at higher doses and considerably greater expense. They are best administered as continuous infusions because of their short duration of effect.

Methadone

Methadone has been considered for postoperative pain but has a long half-life of approximately 19 hours, making it slightly difficult to titrate. However, a loading dose of 0.2 mg $\cdot$ kg^{-1} at the start of anesthesia may provide postoperative analgesia for most of the first day.[27] If overdose occurs, side effects will also be long lasting. Most anesthesiologists prefer a more titrable drug for postoperative analgesia.

Codeine

Codeine is a partial agonist opioid still in common use for pediatric analgesia. Clinically, it seems to have fewer side effects than the full agonist drugs, but it also appears to have a ceiling effect on analgesia. Codeine is commonly used when postoperative pain is not severe and sedation is to be avoided, as in neurosurgery. One of every 10 to 20 patients lacks the ability to metabolize codeine to its active metabolite, morphine. In these patients, it is ineffective.

Other Drugs

Other opioids are available, but none offers any significant advantage over those discussed earlier. Drugs commonly used for postoperative pain have not changed in recent years. For pediatric patients, the method of administration is more important than the choice of drug; the greatest advances in pediatric postoperative pain management have been made in this area.

TECHNIQUES OF ANALGESIC ADMINISTRATION

In recent years, a bewildering array of methods to administer opioids to children has been devised, including oral, rectal, intravenous, subcutaneous, oral transmucosal, nasal transmucosal, transdermal, and inhalational routes.[28] How does one sift through this array to decide what is the most appropriate method for pediatric patients?

Is the Intramuscular Route Outmoded?

Considerations include the advantages and disadvantages of each method (Table 15–4), the age and cognitive development of the child, and the interest of staff in considering the use of alternative methods.

Intramuscular opiate administration was the mainstay of analgesia for decades in both adults and children. However, such injections should never be used routinely in children. The most common fear children have of hospitals is needles. Children are quick to discover that the expression of pain after surgery is frequently followed by an intramuscular injection. It does not take long before a child denies pain in order to avoid further injections. In children requiring frequent hospitalization, this fear becomes a major management problem. Clearly, pain-free methods of analgesic administration in children are essential.

Intravenous and oral routes of administration are the most useful methods currently used. Various options are available for intravenous opiates. Most pediatric institutions offer three methods of administration: intermittent intravenous boluses as

TABLE 15–4. Methods of Opiate Delivery in Children

Method	Advantages	Disadvantages
Oral	Simple Acceptable to children	Difficult if child vomiting Variable effect and speed of onset
Rectal	Simple Effective in vomiting child No special equipment needed	May be disliked by child May be socially unacceptable
Intramuscular	No special equipment needed	Children hate injections Variable effect Encourages pain cycle
Intravenous		
Boluses	Avoids painful injections Quick onset	Frequent doses required Time-consuming method
Infusion	Continuous analgesia Avoids injections	Needs close observation Incident pain difficult to control
Patient-controlled analgesia	Patient in control Allows for variability High patient satisfaction Safety Reduced nursing staff workload	Expensive equipment Needs staff training
Subcutaneous	Relatively simple Continuous analgesia	Variability in responses Slow onset Needle site discomfort
Epidural	Good quality analgesia Often less sedation	Invasive technique Urinary retention more common Pruritus more common
Transmucosal	Simple administration Bypasses first-pass metabolism Avoids needles	Taste may be deterrent Needs cooperation
Transdermal	Simple Acceptable to children	Slow onset, slow offset Incident pain difficult to control

necessary, continuous infusions, and patient-controlled analgesia (PCA).

How Should Intermittent Intravenous Boluses Be Used?

This technique involves the injection of boluses of morphine, 0.05 mg · kg^{-1}, or meperidine, 0.5 mg · kg^{-1}, directly into the side port of the intravenous infusion over a 5-minute period. Alternatively, these doses can be infused over 20 minutes via a burette.

This technique is advantageous because it is painless, and intravenous boluses work more quickly than intramuscular or subcutaneous injections. However, it should only be used after minor procedures, when the administration of opiates is unlikely to be needed after the first postoperative day, or when a clinician is unsure about whether opiates will be required at all.

The disadvantages of intravenous boluses are that in smaller children, very small increments of drug have to be calculated and drawn up, increasing the possibility of administration errors. Also, if pain is more severe, doses have to be given at 1- to 2-hour intervals, a process that is very time consuming for ward nurses. In this situation, continuous intravenous infusions or PCA is more suitable.

How Are Intravenous Infusions Administered?

This method was described in children in the early 1980s[29, 30] and was a considerable advance over intramuscular administration. The argument for continuous administration is that it provides smooth, consistent analgesia by maintaining a constant blood level of the drug. Intravenous infusions have become one of the most commonly accepted methods of pediatric postoperative pain relief.

Infusions are most commonly used when moderate to severe pain is expected, usually in preschool children and those unsuitable for PCA. Infusions are, in effect, scheduled rather than administered on an as-needed basis. Hence, they require closer observation to allow titration lest drug accumulation and attendant side effects occur.

Syringe pumps are commonly used for intravenous infusions. A simple regimen is to add 0.5 mg · kg^{-1} of morphine or 5 mg · kg^{-1} of meperidine to a 50-mL syringe and dilute to 50 mL with normal saline or 5% dextrose (D$_5$W). The infusion is then run at 0 to 5 mL · h^{-1} (equals 0–50 μg · kg · h^{-1} of morphine). Most institutions allow and encourage ward nurses to use their discretion in titrating this infusion rate within the prescribed limits.

Background Versus Incident Pain

The theory behind infusion therapy is a bit erroneous in that postoperative pain is not constant. We must consider control of both background pain (pain that occurs when a patient lies still in bed) and incident pain (pain on movement or with procedures). Background pain is well managed with intravenous infusions; incident pain is more difficult to control. To help overcome this problem, supplementary boluses of 3 to 4 mL of the solution (30–40 μg · kg^{-1} morphine) can be administered as required, either in anticipation of incident pain (e.g., before getting out of bed, removing drains, physiotherapy) or to settle a patient when background pain is not well controlled.

For infants younger than 3 months, we use a modified regimen with the same concentration of morphine but a reduced infusion rate of 0 to 2 mL · h^{-1} (0–20 μg · kg · h^{-1}). These infants require closer observation than is usually possible on most general wards. Apnea monitoring, continuous pulse oximetry, and a high level of nursing care are highly desirable.

For meperidine, the foregoing regimens may be used, but doses need to be multiplied by 10. Morphine infusions can also be delivered through a normal intravenous set and burette. In this situation, add 0.5 mg · kg^{-1} morphine (or 5 mg · kg^{-1} meperidine) to 500 mL of normal saline or D$_5$W and run as a continuous infusion at up to 50 mL · h^{-1}. The burette prevents the contents of the entire bag from being inadvertently emptied into the patient.

How Is Patient-Controlled Analgesia Used?

PCA is becoming the standard of care for acute pain management with opioids. Its use in children was described in the late 1980s[31, 32] Initial fears regarding the ability of children to administer their own pain relief were unfounded; the technique has been used in children as young as 4 years.[33, 34]

The fundamental difference between PCA and staff-administered techniques is the issue of control. The psychologic benefits of "control" in children and adolescents, in particular, should not be underestimated. Commonly recognized benefits are individualization of a patient's opiate requirements, better control of incident pain, high patient and parental satisfaction, and safety.

Some practical applications must be considered when PCA is prescribed for children.

Management

Many hospitals prefer not to set a lower age limit but offer PCA to all children who can understand the simple concept of pressing a button when they hurt.[35] With this factor in mind, the majority of children age 7 years and older have no trouble with PCA. Children between 4 and 6 years often require extra time to understand the concept and to benefit from being shown the machine. Ask a child to tell you in his or her own words what the machine is for, so that you are satisfied that he or she comprehends.

PCA is also better managed if the parents are able to reinforce this concept before and after surgery. However, they are not allowed to press the button, because to do so removes the fundamental safeguard with PCA—that is, that the patient has to be awake and able to press a button to receive morphine.

All children benefit from the explanation that analgesics do not completely take the pain away but merely reduce it to a level that is well tolerated. Setting honest and realistic goals is important.

Prescribing

The settings need to vary with the size of the child; therefore, most regimens are related to body weight. Common settings for morphine are as follows:

1. Bolus dose: 15 to 20 $\mu g \cdot kg^{-1}$
2. Lockout interval: 5 minutes
3. Background infusion: 15 $\mu g \cdot kg \cdot h^{-1}$

In PCA pumps using 60-mL syringes, we use a concentration of 1 $mg \cdot kg^{-1}$ of morphine in 60 mL (maximum 60 mg). A bolus dose of 1 mL (16 $\mu g \cdot kg^{-1}$) and a background infusion of 1 $mL \cdot h^{-1}$ (16 $\mu g \cdot kg \cdot h^{-1}$) are then easily programmed.

Similar concentrations can be used for PCA pumps using different-sized syringes or cartridges. Care must be taken with most systems to ensure that the bolus dose size remains above 0.5 mL.[36]

Background Infusion

The use of a background infusion remains controversial in adult practice[37] but has been shown to be advantageous in children. Berde and colleagues demonstrated the increased efficacy of PCA over intramuscular analgesics in children and also studied the effect of adding a 15 $\mu g \cdot kg \cdot h^{-1}$ background infusion to PCA.[38] In children undergoing orthopedic surgery, they found that adding a background infusion reduced episodes of severe pain and did not affect morphine requirements or the incidence of side effects. A background infusion provides children with better sleep and better pain control after surgery. The background infusion may be discontinued after 24 to 48 hours when requirements decrease or if a child is experiencing opiate side effects.

Long-term PCA for children with prolonged acute pain episodes due to burns, cancer, and sickle cell disease is a promising technique.[34, 39, 40] Giving these children control of their pain medication for longer periods of time is of psychologic as well as pharmacologic benefit.

The PCA concept extended to oral medications has been described in adolescents.[41]

REGIONAL BLOCKADE

The swing toward greater use of regional analgesia in children has been well justified. Advantages and disadvantages are listed in Table 15–5. The benefits of most importance clinically are the ability of local anesthetics to produce complete analgesia without sedation, without opiate side effects, and with a quicker recovery. However, because of dislike of needles and reduced cooperation in smaller children, regional blockade is rarely the sole anesthetic technique; it is more often used to provide intraoperative and postoperative analgesia.[42–45]

TABLE 15–5. Regional Analgesia in Children

Advantages	Disadvantages
Total pain relief is possible	Technical expertise required
No sedation	Usually requires general anesthesia
Quick recovery	Risk of local anesthetic toxicity
Control of muscle spasm, bladder spasm, etc.	May mask pressure necrosis or compartment syndrome
Usually fewer side effects	Technical problems with catheter techniques
	Other side effects (e.g., motor block, urinary retention)

TABLE 15–6. Suggested Maximum Local Anesthetic Doses in Children

Lidocaine	7 $mg \cdot kg^{-1}$
Lidocaine with adrenaline	10 $mg \cdot kg^{-1}$
Prilocaine	8 $mg \cdot kg^{-1}$ (not in neonates)
Bupivacaine	3 $mg \cdot kg^{-1}$
Bupivacaine with adrenaline	5 $mg \cdot kg^{-1}$
Etidocaine	4 $mg \cdot kg^{-1}$
Tetracaine	2 $mg \cdot kg^{-1}$

When Is It Contraindicated?

Absolute contraindications are similar to those for adults. The presence of infection near the site of the block, coagulopathy, and the lack of consent are obvious contraindications. Relative contraindications include ongoing degenerative axonal disease, meningomyelocele or uncorrected hypovolemia for central neuraxis blocks, and the possibility of compartment syndromes in patients with plaster casts. In these situations, the benefits need to be weighed against the disadvantages and discussed with the parents and surgeon before proceeding with the block.

How Does Local Anesthetic Pharmacology Differ in Children?

Differences in children relate mainly to neonates and infants. Older children handle local anesthetics in a manner similar to young adults. Esters such as tetracaine are metabolized by plasma cholinesterase, and infants younger than 6 months have reduced levels of this enzyme.[46] However, no evidence suggests that this difference is of clinical importance.

With amides, plasma protein binding and hepatic clearance need to be considered. Neonates may be at increased risk of local anesthetic toxicity because of reduced levels of albumin and α_1-acid glycoproteins,[47] which allow higher levels of free drug in the plasma. Immature hepatic enzyme systems compound this problem by also increasing free drug levels. These observations are clearly important for bupivacaine, which is highly plasma protein bound. On the other hand, the greater volume of distribution in neonates may confer some protection against local anesthetic toxicity.

Is Local Anesthetic Toxicity a Problem?

Cardiovascular and central nervous system (CNS) toxicity from local anesthetics are uncommonly reported in children.[43] The most likely explanations are that general anesthesia masks signs of CNS toxicity, and the large volume of distribution results in lower blood levels after the initial dose. Also, children older than 6 months have outgrown their immaturity, have a relatively large liver and excellent renal function, and appear to eliminate these drugs more quickly than adults.

Suggested maximum doses of local anesthetics are listed in Table 15–6. Plasma bupivacaine levels following caudal blockade with 3 $mg \cdot kg^{-1}$ have been reported to be within safe limits[48] and may be lower than in adults. These recommendations assume that the local anesthetic has not been injected intravenously or intra-arterially, in which case toxic effects occur at much lower doses.

What Are the Common Local Anesthetic Techniques?

Many procedures performed on children are suitable for the application of regional techniques. Benefits are particularly evident in children undergoing day surgery, when rapid return to normal function is important.

Infiltration

This is the simplest and one of the most reliable applications of local anesthesia. Wound infiltration of up to 3 mg $\cdot$ kg^{-1} (1.2 mL $\cdot$ kg^{-1}) of plain 0.25% bupivacaine at the end of minor general and plastic surgical procedures prevents a child from waking up in significant pain. This approach is particularly suitable in neonates and infants undergoing inguinal herniorrhaphy or pyloromyotomy.

Bear in mind that other forms of analgesia (e.g., acetaminophen) may be required after the local anesthetic effect dissipates. Counsel the parents about what dose to administer to the child after leaving the hospital and about timing it so that drug effect is present before the local anesthetic wears off.

Lower Limb Blocks

Femoral nerve blocks are commonly used in children presenting with femoral shaft fractures. They not only provide analgesia for the application of traction but also prevent painful muscle spasm. Continuous femoral blockade via a 19-gauge epidural catheter may prolong the benefits of this technique. Combined femoral nerve and lateral cutaneous nerve blocks of the thigh may be useful in providing analgesia for skin graft donor sites.[49, 50]

Sciatic nerve blockade has been used for procedures on the foot in children; posterior, anterior, and lateral approaches have been described.[51–53] Other nerve blocks around the knee are sometimes useful.[54] The main limitations to peripheral blocks is the concern, particularly by orthopedic surgeons, that compartment syndromes and pressure necrosis will not be recognized in patients with plaster casts. Many anesthesiologists do not have sufficient technical expertise to perform certain blocks reliably, in which case some other form of analgesia is used. Again, we must recognize the need for alternative analgesia when the block wears off.

Brachial Plexus Blocks

Brachial plexus blockade is easily performed in children using the commonly described approaches for adults. These blocks are uncommon, however, because of the need for general anesthesia or heavy sedation to perform the blocks, thus negating some of their advantages.

Penile Blocks

Penile blocks are often used as an alternative to caudal analgesia after circumcision[55] because they are easy to perform. In the hands of many pediatric anesthesiologists, caudal blockade is more reliable.

Ilioinguinal and Iliohypogastric Blocks

Ilioinguinal and iliohypogastric nerve blocks[56] can be simply inserted during inguinal surgery, either under direct vision by the surgeon or percutaneously by the anesthesiologist. Wound infiltration is usually performed as well to cover the skin incision. The femoral nerve occasionally is blocked, in which case the child will be unable to ambulate until the block recedes.

Intercostal Block

Intercostal nerve blocks may be used to supplement analgesia following thoracotomy and in patients with rib fractures. Interpleural analgesia has been described in children[57] but has limited application, because unilateral subcostal incisions are uncommon in pediatric surgery.

Sympathetic Block

Sympathetic blockade may be indicated in children with peripheral ischemia, for accidental intra-arterial injections, or for the treatment of sympathetically maintained pain. Stellate ganglion block[58] and lumbar sympathetic block can be performed in children using techniques similar to those used in adults. Neurolytic blockade is rarely performed in children.

If prolonged sympathetic blockade is required, continuous catheter administration of bupivacaine for the lower extremity and axillary catheter or interpleural administration of bupivacaine for the upper limb are useful. Surgical sympathectomy may be indicated if a good response is obtained after the block. Details about how to perform these blocks can be found in several reviews.[42, 43, 59, 60]

What Is the Role of Epidural Techniques?

Epidural techniques have been used widely in adults and are gaining general acceptance in children.[61–62] No method of providing epidural analgesia is universally accepted. Options for the anesthesiologist are to decide whether to use a single-shot or continuous technique, whether the caudal or lumbar approach is appropriate, and which drug or drug combination should be used.

Indications

The type of surgery is the major determinant of whether an epidural technique is suitable. Table 15–7 provides suggested guidelines for the applicability. Urologic surgery is particularly suitable.

Circumcision

Children undergoing circumcision with general anesthesia are usually given 0.5 mL $\cdot$ kg^{-1} of 0.25% bupivacaine into the caudal space. Intraoperative and postoperative analgesia usually lasts 4 to 6 hours. The child awakens clearheaded, with no pain, and can usually eat and drink more quickly than after opiate analgesia. A single-shot technique is used because these children are treated as same-day discharge patients. As with infiltration techniques, parents should be advised concerning appropriate analgesia (e.g., acetaminophen, 15–20 mg $\cdot$ kg^{-1} orally every 4 hours) after the caudal block wears off.

Hypospadias Repair

Hypospadias repair can be particularly distressing to children of all age groups, especially for those who return for

TABLE 15–7. Indications for Epidural Analgesia in Children

Single-shot caudal	Circumcision
	Rectal prolapse
	Imperforate anus procedures
	Hypospadias
	Lower limb procedures
	Inguinal surgery (hernia, hydrocele, orchidopexy)
Continuous caudal catheter	Hypospadias
	Epispadias
	Perineal surgery for ambiguous genitalia
Continuous lumbar epidural	Lower abdominal urology
	Pyeloplasty
	Abdominal tumor surgery
	Spinal surgery
Continuous thoracic epidural	Thoracotomy
	Major upper abdominal surgery
	Chest trauma (less common in children)
Comments	Lumbar and thoracic catheters may be placed via caudal route
	Continuous methods used when children already have a urinary catheter
	Single-shot caudals need to be followed by other suitable analgesic techniques
	Single-shot caudals are mostly bupivacaine alone
	Continuous techniques are mostly low-dose bupivacaine/fentanyl mixtures
	Single-shot and intermittent epidural morphine used in some centers

repeat procedures or second-stage repairs. In the past, common practice was to administer a single-shot caudal, followed by management with intermittent acetaminophen or intravenous opiates. However, in our experience, continuous epidural infusions via caudally placed epidural catheters have been spectacularly successful.

Lower Abdominal Surgery

Lower abdominal operations such as ureteral reimplantation, other bladder operations, and loin operations such as pyeloplasty are also suitable for continuous epidural techniques. These children all have urinary catheters as part of their surgery, thus removing the worry of urinary retention as a complication. Reduction of bladder spasm is often quoted as offering an advantage over systemically administered opiates. Catheters for these procedures are usually placed via a lumbar approach, although in children it is very easy to feed epidural catheters up to a lumbar or even thoracic level from the caudal canal.[63, 64]

Differences in Children

Caudal catheters are easily placed because the sacral hiatus is almost always accessible in children (Fig. 15–2). Catheters placed via 18- or 19-gauge Tuohys or Crawford's needles are fed several centimeters into the epidural space. Those supplied with 18-gauge sets are less likely to kink, block, or cause syringe pump occlusion and can be used in children as young as 2 years. In children younger than 2 years, 19-gauge sets are preferable.

The most difficult part of the procedure is to provide a comfortable, secure dressing. Transparent plastic adhesive dressing achieves this better than traditional tapes and prevents

soiling of the site. Syringe pumps are the most accurate way of infusing the small volumes of drug required in children.

Management of Continuous Epidural Mixtures

An epidural mixture can easily be prepared by adding 20 mL of 0.25% bupivacaine, 2 mL (100 μg) of fentanyl, and 28 mL of saline to a 50-mL syringe. The final concentration is 0.1% bupivacaine, 1 mg · mL^{-1}, and fentanyl, 2 μg · mL^{-1}. Many other combinations are possible, but the mixture must be balanced between local anesthetic effects and opioid effects. Low concentrations of bupivacaine have the advantage of not causing leg weakness, which may be otherwise distressing for children and limit early mobilization.

Low-dose epidural mixtures provide complete pain relief after procedures such as hypospadias repair and almost complete relief after lower abdominal urologic procedures. Required infusion rates vary with the type of procedures and the site of the catheter. Generally speaking, for lower abdominal surgery (and also thoracic surgery), the previously described mixture can be infused at rates of up to 0.2 mL · kg · h^{-1}. For a continuous sacral block, 0.1 mL · kg · h^{-1} usually provides excellent analgesia.

Although continuous epidural analgesia can provide pain relief for orthopedic procedures and other abdominal operations, the frequent need for urinary catheterization mitigates

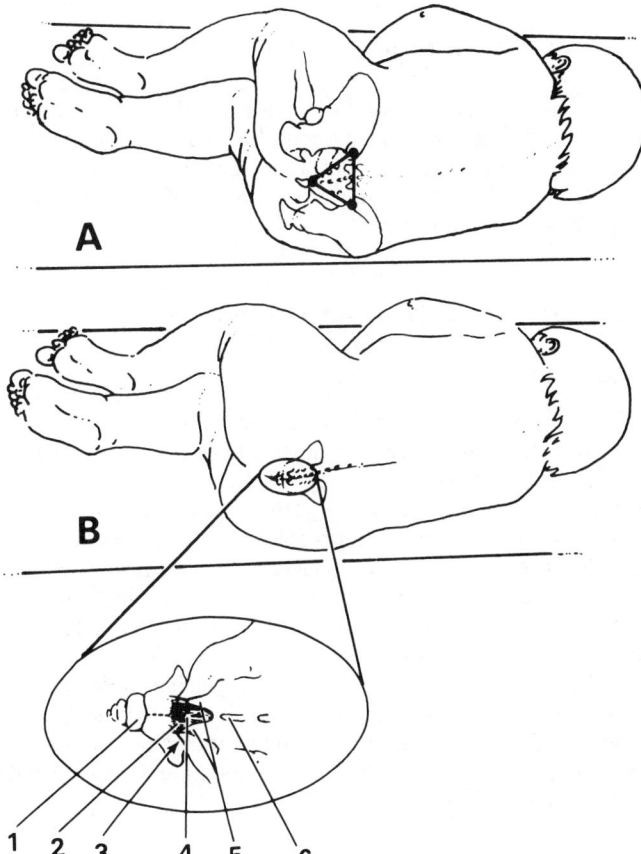

FIGURE 15–2. Localization of the sacral hiatus in children. *A,* Landmarks: the equilateral triangle. *B,* The sacrococcygeal membrane. 1 = Coccyx; 2 = sacrococcygeal membrane; 3 = sacrococcygeal joint; 4 = site of puncture; 5 = sacral cornua; 6 = spinous process of L5. (Reproduced with permission from Pediatric Regional Anesthesia. Dalens BJ (ed). Boca Raton, FL, CRC Press, 1990, p 361. Copyright CRC Press, Boca Raton, FL.)

against its general use and favors, instead, well-administered systemic opiates.

Epidural Opioids As Sole Agents

Epidural opioids are less commonly used as sole agents in children. Epidural morphine in a single dose of 0.05 to 0.1 mg · kg^{-1} provides analgesia lasting 10 to 12 hours.[65–67] Delayed respiratory depression is uncommon in children but has been described[68] and necessitates a higher degree of respiratory monitoring. Side effects such as nausea, vomiting, urinary retention, and itching may be troublesome.

For these reasons, many anesthesiologists prefer to use more lipophilic agents such as fentanyl via infusion or PCA. Epidural opioids alone in children provide no additional benefits over well-administered systemic opioids.

PROCEDURAL PAIN IN CHILDREN

Procedural pain is a common problem in pediatric hospitals and presents major difficulties in management. Painful dressing changes, suturing, intravenous cannulation, blood taking, lumbar punctures, and bone marrow aspirations strike fear into many children and constitute some of the main reasons why children are scared of hospitals. Various options are available to reduce these fears.

When Is Nitrous Oxide Useful?

The analgesic effects of nitrous oxide have been well known since the 19th century. Quick onset of action and quick recovery make it one of the best potent analgesics for short procedures in children.[28, 69] Optimal concentration for venous cannulation in children is 50%.[70]

How Are Topical Local Anesthetics Applied?

Intact Skin

Eutectic mixture of local anesthetics (EMLA) cream has been popular in European countries for several years and is now available in North America. EMLA cream is a eutectic mixture of 5% lidocaine and 5% prilocaine that penetrates the relatively impermeable barrier provided by skin. Most experience has been with venous cannulation,[72–74] but EMLA cream is also useful before lumbar puncture, for superficial skin procedures, and for other needle procedures such as accessing implanted access ports.

EMLA cream is applied under an occlusive dressing and needs to be present for at least 1 hour before the procedure. Methemoglobinemia can result from the prilocaine component when used in small infants,[75] but the mixture is considered safe in infants older than 3 months.[76]

Wound Analgesia and Suturing

EMLA cream is not recommended for use in wounds and on broken skin. To overcome this problem and to provide analgesia for wound suturing, a topical anesthetic solution containing tetracaine 0.5%, adrenaline 1:2000, and cocaine 11.8% (TAC) has been developed.[77–79] This solution is instilled into the wound and then onto a gauze in the wound for 10 to 20 minutes. When it is removed, painless suturing is possible, although supplementary lidocaine infiltration is occasionally required. Because TAC solution is a potent vasoconstrictor, it should not be used in areas supplied by an end artery. Clinical signs of cocaine toxicity are rare.[80]

Is Conscious Sedation an Option?

The use of short-acting analgesics and sedatives (commonly fentanyl and midazolam) for short painful procedures, usually in pediatric oncology patients, is referred to as *conscious sedation*. The report of the Consensus Conference on the Management of Pain in Childhood Cancer[81] provided suitable guidelines for the management of procedural pain in these children.

Fentanyl

Fentanyl, 1 to 2 μg · kg^{-1} intravenously, can be given concurrently for analgesia. Intravenous sedation must be undertaken in a room with appropriate resuscitation facilities and should be administered by well-trained medical staff. Continuous monitoring with pulse oximetry is essential.

Midazolam

Midazolam is useful not only for anxiolysis but also for amnesia. Children who are sleepy from midazolam rarely have any recall of painful procedures. This drug is especially useful for children who undergo frequent burn and oncologic procedures. Midazolam is titrated to effect intravenously with 0.05 mg · kg^{-1} increments or given orally, 0.5 to 1 mg · kg^{-1}, 45 minutes before the procedure.

Is Transmucosal Drug Administration of Value?

Both fentanyl and midazolam are highly lipid-soluble drugs that are well absorbed across the oral mucosa, making them suitable for transmucosal premedication before procedures or induction of anesthesia. The benefits of transmucosal administration are rapid onset and absence of first-pass metabolism. The disadvantage is that the drug needs to be supplied in a form that has an acceptable taste for children.

Fentanyl

Oral transmucosal fentanyl citrate (OTFC) has been evaluated both as an anesthetic premedicant[82–84] and as an analgesic before painful procedures.[85] It is presented in the form of a "lollipop" that is sucked (not eaten) 10 to 30 minutes before the painful procedure. Nausea, vomiting, and facial pruritus may occur.

Midazolam

Transmucosal application of intravenous midazolam has been described via both intranasal and sublingual routes.[86] Not surprisingly, most children find the transnasal route unacceptable; it offers no advantage over the sublingual route. A commonly used dose is 0.2 mg · kg^{-1}.

Are Nonpharmacologic Techniques Useful?

Children are excellent subjects for behavioral method techniques, particularly for oncology and burn therapy.[87–89] Hypnotherapy and other strategies such as distraction and relaxation should be considered as part of the overall management of procedural pain and should complement pharmacologic management.

ANALGESIA FOR BURNS

Pain management in children with burns presents considerable difficulty because of the need to perform frequent painful procedures and the often lengthy rehabilitation. These problems are compounded by the devastating cosmetic and social effects of a burn injury, not only on the child but also on the family.

Pain results from the initial injury, daily or twice daily dressing changes, surgical debridement, and skin grafting procedures. Several weeks or, in severe cases, several months may elapse before skin coverage is complete.

What Pharmacologic Techniques Are Useful?

Most children with >10% burn surface area require intravenous access. In this situation, I manage initially with an intravenous morphine infusion.

PCA has been used in children with burns for periods as long as 131 days.[34] In this series of 11 children, PCA was started at the time of first debridement, usually 7 to 10 days after the burn. A perceived benefit of PCA was that the children were given control over their pain, a positive psychologic effect. There was considerable variability in morphine requirements. Three children developed tolerance to morphine, but it was easily managed by increasing doses. All children weaned themselves from opiates when skin closure was complete and painful procedures were no longer required.

Various techniques are available to ameliorate the pain of dressing changes. If intravenous access is available, titration with midazolam and fentanyl (see *Procedural Pain in Children,* earlier) is commonly used. If not, inhalational analgesia with nitrous oxide is a useful patient-controlled method for school-aged children. A protocol must be at hand to avoid bone marrow toxicity. Oral premedication with midazolam, 0.5 to 1.0 mg · kg^{-1}, has a reliable amnesic and anxiolytic effect. These therapies should be used from the outset instead of waiting for pain management difficulties to develop.

Longer-term analgesia may also be achieved with oral slow-release morphine preparations or oral methadone. Additional analgesia is still required to ease the acute pain of dressing changes.

CANCER PAIN

Pain is common in children with cancer,[90] and the importance of adequately managing it cannot be overestimated.

TABLE 15–8. Differences Between Pediatric and Adult Cancer

	Children	Adults
Incidence	Uncommon (1%)	Common (99%)
Tumors	Many hematologic	Mostly solid tumors
Outcome	Mostly curable	Mostly incurable
Treatment	Very aggressive	Less aggressive
Pain problems	Therapy-related pain common	Tumor-related pain common
Palliative care	Usually short (weeks)	Often months to years
Bony metastases	Less common	More common
Managed by	Pediatric oncology team	Various specialties

How Does Pediatric Cancer Pain Differ?

Fundamental differences must be considered in the types of cancer pain experienced by children (Table 15–8). For this reason, extrapolation of adult cancer pain management practices to pediatric patients is difficult.

Pediatric cancers are relatively uncommon. Only 1% of cancers occur in children. Many general practitioners have no experience with pediatric cancer, the treatment for which is largely confined to larger pediatric institutions. Types of cancers experienced by children are listed in Table 15–9. Almost half of pediatric malignancies are hematologic; carcinomas are very rare. Bony metastases, which are the most common cause of cancer pain in adults, are rare in children.

Survival rates from pediatric cancers are increasing because of improvements in aggressive chemotherapy, radiotherapy, and surgery. However, such therapy causes many pain management problems. Bone marrow aspirations, lumbar punctures, intravenous therapy, and surgery are frequent, and children may develop painful complications such as oral mucositis and infections. Therapy-related pain, therefore, predominates in children.

Pediatric palliative care is a poorly developed specialty because most communities have too few cases. Most children and their parents prefer for palliative care to be provided in the home environment, where children are happy with their surroundings and usually have parents and siblings to provide care.

How Is Therapy-Related Pain Managed?

Various options are available. Placement of long-term central venous catheters reduces problems of intravenous access and blood taking and simplifies administration of intravenous sedation or general anesthesia.

General Anesthesia

Bone marrow biopsies and lumbar punctures remain a major pain management problem. In some countries, general anesthe-

TABLE 15–9. Pediatric Malignancies

Leukemias	30%
Cerebral tumors	18%
Lymphoma	13%
Neuroblastoma	11%
Wilms' tumor	10%
Bone tumors	5%
Miscellaneous	13%

sia is routinely used. The procedures are then painless, and intravenous therapy or blood taking can also be performed while the child is anesthetized. Although some children dislike general anesthesia, it is close to ideal for the majority.

Conscious Sedation

In hospitals where general anesthesia is not feasible, conscious sedation, often with midazolam and fentanyl, is used. Nitrous oxide is a suitable alternative. These methods are considerably more reliable and acceptable than is intramuscular opioid analgesia.

Opioids and Local Anesthetics

Oral mucositis is a painful ulceration of the upper alimentary tract frequently encountered after bone marrow transplantation. Patients usually are unable to swallow and often experience extreme discomfort. Systemic opioids (often using PCA), transdermal fentanyl patch therapy, topical local anesthetics, and mouth washes are the mainstays of providing comfort.

Behavioral Intervention

In addition to pharmacologic approaches, behavioral and psychologic intervention are important, especially in children whose treatments may take several years. Hypnosis, distraction, and relaxation are commonly used in children.

How Is Pediatric Palliative Care Pain Managed?

Making the decision to administer palliative care is stressful for children, parents, and hospital and community staff. The decision to discontinue treatment is often made after considerable time and effort with aggressive therapies, and it is difficult for parents to accept that their child is not curable.

The likelihood of pain depends on the type of neoplasia. Leukemias usually produce generalized bone pain during the terminal stages. Medulloblastomas may spread caudally from the posterior fossa and cause spinal pain. Bone tumors may cause pain from local spread or metastases. Neuroblastomas often cause abdominal and chest pain due to tumor spread and may give rise to neuropathic pain from nerve compression.

An analgesic ladder similar to the one proposed by the World Health Organization is worthwhile, but many of the medications used are different in children. Therapy must be individualized to the needs of each child.[91, 92]

Acetaminophen and Codeine

Mild pain is often treated with simple analgesics such as intermittent acetaminophen and codeine. Syrup, tablet, or rectal formulations are used according to a child's preference.

Nonsteroidal Anti-Inflammatory Drugs

NSAIDs are a useful next step, especially if bone pain is present. The platelet dysfunction caused by NSAIDs can occasionally lead to problems such as nosebleeds in children who are thrombocytopenic, but the benefits in terms of quality of pain relief often outweigh this disadvantage in the palliative care situation. Drugs such as naproxen need to be administered only twice daily and are available in tablet, syrup, and suppository formulations.

Opioids

Opioids are often required in combination with NSAIDs, and longer-acting preparations are useful for the majority of children with cancer pain. Slow-release morphine tablets, methadone syrup, and oxycodone suppositories are three commonly used drugs, depending on which route of administration is suitable for an individual child. Vomiting may prevent reliable use of the oral route, necessitating rectal administration.

Intravenous and subcutaneous infusions[93] are often not required until a child is no longer ambulant. Epidural opiates are rarely required for children when the other routes are used in an appropriate manner. Many children develop progressive tolerance to opioids and require escalating doses. Side effects such as nausea, constipation, and pruritus need to be anticipated and treated before they become severe. If drowsiness and reduced ambulation are not a major consideration, midazolam administered orally, rectally, or parenterally is useful to reduce distress.

Other Drugs

Other adjuvants may be required. Amitriptyline syrup or tablets may help to promote sleep and is particularly useful if neuropathic pain is present. Carbamazepine or phenytoin is usually required for neuropathic pain; plasma levels should approximate the lower end of the anticonvulsant range.

CHRONIC NONCANCER PAIN

The spectrum of chronic noncancer pain problems is children is vastly different from adults (see Table 15–2). Although many of these problems are common in children (headaches occur in 75%), they are rarely debilitating. Most are managed by pediatricians, pediatric neurologists, rheumatologists, psychiatrists, and psychologists and rarely require the services of a pediatric anesthesiologist. However, as with adult pain management, a multidisciplinary approach is very useful for difficult chronic pain problems.

What Treatments Are Required?

Headache

Headache is common in children and adolescents, and efforts are initially focused on ruling out serious causes. Tension headaches and migraines are the most common and, if mild, are treated conservatively with simple measures such as rest, simple analgesics, simple physical measures such as massage, and psychologic strategies such as relaxation and biofeedback training.[94, 95] More difficult cases may require aggressive drug therapy in addition to these measures.

Abdominal Pain

Recurrent abdominal pain is another relatively common pediatric problem (15% of school children); to find a clear-cut organic cause for this problem is uncommon.[95] If recurrent abdominal pain is troublesome, these children are most often referred to a pediatrician, pediatric gastroenterologist, or pediatric surgeon for investigation and treatment.

Reflex Sympathetic Dystrophy

Sympathetically maintained pain (or reflex sympathetic dystrophy syndrome) was poorly recognized in children until recently. Female adolescents are more likely to develop the syndrome (male-to-female ratio approximately 1:6).[96] No uniform method of management is available, although a combination of physical therapies, psychologic assessment and therapy, and sympathetic blockade may offer the best approach for more difficult cases. A comprehensive treatment approach based on experience at The Childrens Hospital, Boston, is outlined by Berde and colleagues.[94]

Sickle Cell Crisis

Sickle cell crisis causes episodic pain due to occlusion of small blood vessels and distal infarction. Painful episodes may be mild and respond to simple analgesics such as codeine, acetaminophen, or ibuprofen. When pain is severe, parenteral opioids may may be required. They should not be withheld because of fear of addiction. The harmful effects of uncontrolled pain outweigh this fear in most cases. PCA is useful, because children and adolescents react positively to being able to control this aspect of their care.[97, 98]

PEDIATRIC PAIN MANAGEMENT SERVICES

Pediatric pain management services have been described only recently.[99] However, during the past 5 years there has been a considerable increase in the number of hospitals providing pediatric pain management facilities, particularly in North America. This trend is likely to continue into the future; however, cost constraints in many countries have inhibited such growth.

How Are Anesthesiology Departments Involved?

Many anesthesiology departments, particularly in pediatric hospitals, provide acute pain management facilities for children and respond to requests for PCA and epidural techniques. The question of expanding this ''informal'' therapy to include services for pediatric cancer pain and palliative care, burns, procedural pain, and the wide range of chronic noncancer pains in children must be answered by individual departments.

Acute Pain Management

An acute pain management service[100–102] is the most common first option because it requires fewer resources than does a full multidisciplinary pain management service. The pain management problems encountered are relevant to anesthetic practice. Good working relationships with surgical colleagues and nursing staff are essential for the smooth running of such a service.

Extended Acute Pain Management

My experience at the Adelaide Childrens Hospital (ACH) encompasses an extended acute pain management service that is involved with cancer pain, burns, and procedural pain, all of which are experienced on the hospital campus. A small amount of community palliative care work is also provided.

The involvement in all areas is to facilitate and coordinate pain management methods within the hospital and to provide hospital protocols, prescription guidelines, education, and maintenance of pain management equipment. Individual surgeons are encouraged to participate in managing the common techniques including PCA, although prescribing, machine programming, and overall supervision of such techniques remain with anesthetic personnel. There is no outpatient service.

Chronic pain problems continue to be managed by appropriate pediatric specialties and, if severe, may be referred to adult pain management services. The advantage of this approach at the ACH was implementation at minimal cost. Surgeons do not believe that this aspect of their postoperative care has been taken away from them, and we are involved in the majority of pediatric pain problems.

This approach suits the nature of practice at the ACH. Pediatric pain services must always be individualized to meet demands of the clinical workload in a particular institution. The opinions and needs of clinicians within the anesthesiology department and other clinical services must be respected.

Comprehensive Multidisciplinary Pain Management

The third option is to provide maximum care in the form of a comprehensive multidisciplinary pain management service.[103] This service needs input from specialists in anesthesia, pediatric surgery, orthopedics, neurosurgery, pediatric medicine, psychiatry, psychology, nursing, social work, pharmacy, and rheumatology who have a dedicated interest in pediatric pain management. Several key individuals should coordinate the service, which needs to receive patients from an extensive referral base. Although this approach is ideal for major pediatric referral centers, cost constraints and recruiting sufficiently interested individuals are commonly encountered difficulties.

Many comprehensive clinics (i.e., oncology, burn) already have a weekly multidisciplinary group meeting to discuss patient management problems. This group usually consists of doctors, ward nurses, ward play leader, hospital school teacher, community nurse representative, clinical psychologist, social worker, and sometimes research staff. The addition of an acute pain management specialist such as an anesthesiologist is valuable.

Pain Interest Groups

Another simple option is to set up a pain interest group. These groups have regular meetings to discuss pain management problems within an institution and to assist in coordinating the way pain is managed. They can offer advice and opinion concerning individual cases. Such a group requires interested individuals from anesthesia, surgery, medicine, psychiatry, nursing, social work, and allied specialties and should be open to any interested individuals within the hospital.

References

1. Mather L, Mackie J: The incidence of postoperative pain in children. Pain 1983; 15:271.
2. Beyer JE, DeGood DE, Ashley LC, et al: Patterns of postoperative analgesic use with adults and children following cardiac surgery. Pain 1983; 17:71.
3. Anand KJS, Hickey PR: Pain and its effects in the human neonate and fetus. N Engl J Med 1987; 317:1321.
4. Anand KJS, Sippell WG, Aynsley-Green A: Randomised trial of fentanyl anaesthesia in preterm babies undergoing surgery: effects on the stress response. Lancet 1987; 1:243.
5. Anand KJS, Sippell WG, Schofield NM, et al: Does halothane anaesthesia decrease the metabolic and endocrine stress responses of newborn infants undergoing operation? Br Med J 1988; 296:668.
6. Anand KJS, Hickey PR: Halothane-morphine compared with high-dose sufentanil for anesthesia and postoperative analgesia in neonatal cardiac surgery. N Engl J Med 1992; 326:1.
7. Fletcher AB: Pain in the neonate. N Engl J Med 1987; 317:1347.
8. Hatch DJ: Analgesia in the neonate. Br Med J 1987; 294:920.
9. Pain, anaesthesia, and babies (Editorial). Lancet 1987; 2:543.
10. Yaster M: Analgesia and anesthesia in neonates. J Pediatr 1987; 111:394.
11. Gauntlett IS: Analgesia in the neonate. Br J Hosp Med 1987; 37:518.
12. Perry S, Heidrich G: Management of pain during debridement: a survey of U.S. burn units. Pain 1982; 13:267.
13. Hockenberry MN, Bologna-Vaugh S: Preparation for intrusive procedures using non-invasive techniques in children with cancer. Cancer Nursing 1985; 8:97.
14. Marshall RE, Stratton WC, Moore JA, et al: Circumcision: effects on newborn behavior. Infant Behav Dev 1980; 3:1.
15. Porter J, Jick H: Addiction rare in patients treated with narcotics (Letter to the editor). N Engl J Med 1980; 302:123.
16. McGrath PJ: Pediatric pain: a good start. Pain 1990; 41:253.
17. McGrath PA: Pain assessment in infants and children. In Pain in Children—Nature, Assessment and Treatment. McGrath PA (ed). New York, Guildford Press, 1990, pp 41–87.
18. Beyer JE, Wells N: The Assessment of Pain in Children. Pediatr Clin North Am 1989; 36:837.
19. Gaukroger PB: Pediatric analgesia—which drug? which dose? Drugs 1991; 41:52.
20. Bieri D, Reeve RA, Champion GD, et al: The Faces Pain Scale for the self-assessment of the severity of pain experienced in children: development, initial validation, and preliminary investigation for ratio scale properties. Pain 1990; 41:139.
21. McGrath PA: An assessment of children's pain: a review of behavioral, physiological and direct scaling techniques. Pain 1987; 31:147.
22. Cousins MJ: Prevention of postoperative pain. In Proceedings of the VIth World Congress on Pain. Bond MR, Charlton JE, Woolf CJ (eds). New York, Elsevier, 1991, pp 41–52.
23. Barrett MJ, Hurwitz ES, Schonberger LB, et al: Changing epidemiology of Reye syndrome in the United States. Pediatrics 1986; 77:598.
24. Maunuksela E-L, Olkkola KT, Kokki H: Pharmacokinetics of intravenous ketorolac and its efficacy in relieving postoperative pain in children (Abstract). J Pain Symptom Manage 1991; 6:143.
25. Hertzka RE, Gauntlett IS, Fisher DM, et al: Fentanyl-induced respiratory depression: effects of age. Anesthesiology 1989; 70:213.
26. Koren G, Butt W, Chinyanga H, et al: Postoperative morphine infusion in newborn infants: assessment of disposition characteristics and safety. J Pediatr 1985; 107:963.
27. Berde CB, Beyer JE, Bournaki M-C, et al: Comparison of morphine and methadone for prevention of postoperative pain in 3-to 7-year-old children. J Pediatr 1991; 119:135.
28. Gaukroger PB: Novel techniques of analgesic delivery. In Pain Management in Children and Adolescents. Schechter N, Berde CB, Yaster M (eds). Baltimore, Williams & Wilkins (in press).
29. Bray RJ: Postoperative analgesia provided by morphine infusion in children. Anaesthesia 1983; 38:1075.
30. Dilworth NM, MacKellar A: Pain relief for the pediatric surgical patient. J Pediatr Surg 1987; 22:264.
31. Rodgers BM, Webb CJ, Stergios D, et al: Patient-controlled analgesia in pediatric surgery. J Pediatr Surg 1988; 23:259.
32. Gaukroger PB, Tomkins DP, Van der Walt JH: Patient-controlled analgesia in children. Anaesth Intensive Care 1989; 17:264.
33. Gaukroger PB: Patient-controlled analgesia in children. In Pain Management in Children and Adolescents. Schechter N, Berde CB, Yaster M (eds). Baltimore, Williams & Wilkins (in press).
34. Gaukroger PB, Chapman MJ, Davey RB: Pain control in pediatric burns—the use of patient-controlled analgesia (PCA). Burns 1991; 17:396.
35. Gaukroger PB, Tomkins DP, van der Walt JH: Letter to the editor. J Pediatr Surg 1988; 23:1227.
36. Patient-controlled analgesic infusion pumps. Health Devices 1988; 17:137.
37. Gaukroger PB, Tomkins DP, van der Walt JH: Background infusions with PCA (Letter to the editor). Anaesth Intensive Care 1991; 19:134.
38. Berde CB, Lehn BM, Yee JD, et al: Patient-controlled analgesia in children and adolescents: a randomised, prospective comparison with intramuscular administration of morphine for postoperative analgesia. J Pediatr 1991; 118:460.
39. Mowbray MJ, Gaukroger PB: The use of long-term patient-controlled analgesia in children. Anaesthesia 1990; 45:941.
40. Shapiro B, Cohen D, Howe C: Use of patient-controlled analgesia for patients with sickle cell disease (Abstract). J Pain Symptom Manage 1991; 6:176.
41. Litman RS, Shapiro BS: Oral patient-controlled analgesia in adolescents. J Pain Symptom Manage 1992; 7:78.
42. Brown TCK, Schulte-Steinberg O: Neural blockade for pediatric surgery. In Neural Blockade in Clinical Anesthesia and Management of Pain. 2nd ed. Cousins MJ, Bridenbaugh PO (eds). Philadelphia, JB Lippincott, 1988, pp 669–692.
43. Arthur DS, McNicol LR: Local anaesthetic techniques in paediatric surgery. Br J Anaesth 1986; 58:760.
44. Dalens B: Regional anesthesia in children. Anesth Analg 1989; 68:654.
45. Yaster M, Maxwell LG: Pediatric regional anesthesia. Anesthesiology 1989; 70:324.
46. Zsigmond EK, Downs JR: Plasma cholinesterase activity in newborns and infants. Can Anaesth Soc J 1971; 18:278.
47. Wood M, Wood AJJ: Changes in plasma drug binding and alpha-1 acid glycoprotein in mother and newborn infant. Clin Pharmacol Ther 1979; 19:426.
48. Eyres RL, Bishop W, Oppenheim RC, et al: Plasma bupivacaine concentrations in children during caudal epidural anaesthesia. Anesth Intensive Care 1983; 11:20.
49. McNicol LR: Lower limb blocks for children—lateral cutaneous and femoral nerve blocks for postoperative pain relief in paediatric practice. Anaesthesia 1986; 41:27.
50. Brown TCK, Dickens DRV: A new approach to lateral cutaneous nerve of thigh block. Anaesth Intensive Care 1986; 14:126.
51. Dalens B, Tanguy A, Vanneuville G: Sciatic nerve blocks in children: comparison of the posterior, anterior, and lateral approaches in 180 pediatric patients. Anesth Analg 1990; 70:131.
52. McNicol LR: Sciatic nerve block for children—sciatic nerve block by the anterior approach for postoperative pain relief. Anaesthesia 1985; 40:410.
53. Guardini R, Waldron BA, Wallace WA: Sciatic nerve block: a new lateral approach. Acta Anaesthesiol Scand 1985; 29:515.
54. Kempthorne PM, Brown TCK: Nerve blocks around the knee in children. Anaesth Intensive Care 1984; 12:14.
55. Bacon AK: An alternative block for post circumcision analgesia. Anaesth Intensive Care 1977; 5:63.
56. Casey WF, Rice LJ, Hannallah RS, et al: A comparison between bupivacaine instillation versus ilioinguinal iliohypogastric nerve block for postoperative analgesia following inguinal herniorrhaphy in children. Anesthesiology 1990; 72:637.
57. McIlvaine WB, Chang JHT, Jones M: The effective use of intrapleural bupivacaine for analgesia after thoracic and subcostal incisions in children. J Pediatr Surg 1988; 23:1184.
58. Parris WC, Reddy BC, White HW, et al: Stellate ganglion blocks in pediatric patients. Anesth Analg 1991; 72:552.
59. Dalens B (ed): Pediatric Regional Anesthesia. Boca Raton, CRC Press, 1991.
60. Saint-Maurice C, Schulte-Steinberg O: Regional Anesthesia in Children. Norwalk, Appleton & Lange/Mediglobe, 1990.
61. Dalens B, Chrysostome Y: Intervertebral epidural anesthesia in pediatric surgery: success rate and adverse effects in 650 consecutive procedures. Pediatr Anesth 1991; 1:107.
62. Sethna N, Strafford M, Berde CB: Experience with 852 epidural infusions in a childrens hospital (Abstract). J Pain Symptom Manage 1991; 6:164.
63. Bosenberg AT, Bland BAR, Schulte-Steinberg O, et al: Thoracic epidural anesthesia via caudal route in infants. Anesthesiology 1988; 69:265.
64. Rasch DK, Webster DE, Pollard TG, et al: Lumbar and thoracic epidural analgesia via the caudal approach for postoperative pain relief in infants and children. Can J Anaesth 1990; 37:359.

65. Tyler DC, Krane EJ: Epidural Opioids in Children. J Pediatr Surg 1989; 24:469.
66. Krane EJ, Jacobson LE, Tyler DC: Caudal epidural morphine in children: a comparison of three doses. Anesthesiology 1988; 69:3A, A763.
67. Glenski JA, Warner MA, Dawson B, et al: Postoperative use of epidurally administered morphine in children and adolescents. Mayo Clin Proc 1984; 59:530.
68. Krane EJ: Delayed respiratory depression in a child after caudal epidural morphine. Anesth Analg 1988; 67:79.
69. Miser AW, Ayesh D, Broda E, et al: Use of a patient-controlled device for nitrous oxide administration to control procedure-related pain in children and young adults with cancer. Clin J Pain 1988; 4:5.
70. Henderson JM, Spence DG, Komocar LM, et al: Administration of nitrous oxide to pediatric patients provides analgesia for venous cannulation. Anesthesiology 1990; 72:269.
71. Amos RJ, Amess JAL, Nancekievill DG, et al: Prevention of nitrous oxide-induced megaloblastic changes in bone marrow using folinic acid. Br J Anaesth 1984; 56:103.
72. Mauneksela E-L, Korpela R: Double-blind evaluation of a lignocaine-prilocaine cream (EMLA) in children. Br J Anaesth 1986; 58:1242.
73. Hallen B, Olsson GL, Uppfeldt A: Pain-free venipuncture. Effect of timing of application of local anaesthetic cream. Anaesthesia 1984; 39:969.
74. Hallen B, Uppfeldt A: Does lidocaine-prilocaine cream permit painfree insertion of IV catheters in children? Anesthesiology 1982; 57:340.
75. Frayling IM, Addison GM, Chattergee K, et al: Methaemoglobinaemia in children treated with prilocaine-lignocaine cream. Br Med J 1990; 301:153.
76. Selbst SM: Managing pain in the pediatric emergency department. Pediatr Emerg Care 1989; 5:56.
77. Pryor GJ, Kilpatrick WR, Opp AR: Local anesthesia in minor lacerations: topical TAC versus lidocaine infiltration. Ann Emerg Med 1990; 9:568.
78. Bonadio WA: TAC: a review. Pediatr Emerg Care 1989; 5:128.
79. Bonadio WA, Wagner V: Efficacy of tetracaine-adrenaline-cocaine topical anesthetic without tetracaine for facial laceration repair in children. Pediatrics 1990; 86:856.
80. Fitzmaurice LS, Wasserman GS, Knapp JF, et al: TAC use and absorption of cocaine in a pediatric emergency department. Ann Emerg Med 1990; 19:515.
81. Zeltzer LK, Altman A, Cohen D, et al: Report of the subcommittee on the management of pain associated with procedures in children with cancer. Pediatrics 1990; 86:826.
82. Nelson PS, Streisand JB, Mulder SM, et al: Comparison of oral transmucosal fentanyl citrate and an oral solution of meperidine, diazepam, and atropine for premedication in children. Anesthesiology 1989; 70:616.
83. Streisand JB, Stanley TH, Hague B, et al: Oral transmucosal fentanyl citrate premedication in children. Anesth Analg 1989; 69:28.
84. Ashburn MA, Streisand JB, Tarver S, et al: Oral transmucosal fentanyl citrate for premedication in pediatric outpatients. Can J Anaesth 1990; 37:857.
85. Schechter NL, Weisman SJ, Rosenblum, et al: Oral transmucosal fentanyl citrate for pediatric procedures: a randomised clinical trial. J Pain Symptom Manage 1991; 6:178.
86. Karl HW, Larach MG, Ruffle JM: Transmucosal midazolam for preinduction of anesthesia in pediatric patients: comparison of intranasal and sublingual routes (Abstract), Anesthesiology 1991; 75:A922.
87. Zeltzer LK, Jay SM, Fisher DM: Management of pain associated with pediatric procedures. Pediatr Clin North Am 1989; 36:941.
88. Osgood PF, Szyflbein SK: Management of burns pain in children. Pediatr Clin North Am 1989; 36:1001.
89. Maron M, Bush JP: Burn injury treatment pain. *In* Children in Pain: Clinical and Research Issues From a Developmental Perspective. Bush JP, Harkins SW (eds). New York, Springer-Verlag, 1991, pp 275–295.
90. Miser AW, Dothage JA, Wesley RA, et al: The prevalence of pain in a pediatric and young adult cancer population. Pain 1987; 29:73.
91. Berde C, Ablin A, Glazer J, et al: Report of the subcommittee on disease-related pain in childhood cancer. Pediatrics 1990; 86:818.
92. Miser AW, Miser JS: The treatment of cancer pain in children. Pediatr Clin North Am 1989; 36:979.
93. Miser AW, Moore L, Greene R, et al: Prospective study of continuous intravenous and subcutaneous morphine infusions for therapy-related or cancer-related pain in children and young adults with cancer. Clin J Pain 1986; 2:101.
94. Berde CB, Anand KJS, Sethna NF: Pediatric pain management. *In* Pediatric Anesthesia 2nd ed. Gregory GA (ed). New York, Churchill Livingstone, 1989, pp 679–727.
95. McGrath PA: Recurrent pain syndromes. *In* Pain in Children—Nature, Assessment and Treatment. New York, Guilford Press, 1990, pp 251–308.
96. Wilder RT, Berde CB, Wolohan M, et al: Reflex sympathetic dystrophy in children: follow-up of 70 patients (Abstract). Anesthesiology 1991; 75:A693.
97. Shapiro BS: The management of pain in sickle cell disease. Pediatr Clin North Am 1989; 36:1029.
98. Shapiro B, Cohen D, Howe C: Use of patient-controlled analgesia for patients with sickle cell disease (Abstract). J Pain Symptom Manage 1991; 6:176.
99. Berde CB, Sethna NF, Masek B, et al: Pediatric pain clinics: recommendations for their development. Pediatrician 1989; 16:94.
100. Ready LB, Oden R, Chadwick HS, et al: Development of an anesthesiology-based postoperative pain management service. Anesthesiology 1988; 68:100.
101. Ready LB: Acute pain services: an academic asset. Clin J Pain 1989; 5(Suppl 1):S28.
102. Gaukroger PB: An acute pain management service for children. Pain 1990; (Suppl 5):S6.
103. Berde CB, Lacouture PG, Masek BJ, et al: Initial experience with a pediatric pain treatment service. Pain 1987; 4(Suppl):S99.

Tools of the Trade and Their Applications

CHAPTER **16**

The Anesthesia Machine, Anesthesia Ventilator, Breathing Circuit, and Scavenging System

MICHAEL L. GOOD, M.D.

The eloquent simplicity of early anesthesia "systems" such as the Morton inhaler demanded few technical skills but great clinical acumen from the anesthesiologist. With the early systems, a "dose" of anesthetic was administered; this was followed by close observation of the patient's clinical response to determine whether the next dose should be increased or decreased relative to the first. Today, oxygen (O_2) and anesthetic gases are precisely metered, mixed, measured, and delivered into the lungs of an anesthetized patient. The patient's pulmonary ventilation is assessed with a spirometer and capnograph and is automatically controlled by a mechanical ventilator.

The "cost" of this enhanced precision in gas delivery and pulmonary ventilation is a proportional increase in the complexity of anesthesia gas delivery systems. Today's anesthesiologist can no longer just "look" at an anesthesia machine and deduce intuitively how it is supposed to work. Contemporary anesthesia machines are indeed complex, contain hundreds of functionally distinct components, and have dozens of controls that need to be adjusted, numerous gauges and displays that must be watched, and a multitude of possible failure modes.

This complexity is overwhelming for many anesthesiologists. Yet, patients expect their anesthesiologists to protect them from injury should the anesthesia and life support equipment malfunction. Thus, anesthesiologists must understand how an anesthesia machine works, be able to detect machine malfunctions, and know when and how to take corrective action to prevent patient injury.

BASIC CONCEPTS

The anesthesia gas delivery system has three primary functions: (1) to provide O_2, (2) to blend and deliver an anesthetic gas mixture, and (3) to support ventilation of the patient's lungs.

What Are the Four Component Subsystems?

A better understanding of the anesthesia gas machine is achieved by functionally dividing it into four component subsystems (Fig. 16–1). Pipeline and cylinder gas supplies (e.g., O_2, nitrous oxide [N_2O], and helium) are connected to the *high-pressure system*. Concealed within the anesthesia machine, the high pressure system connects to the *low pressure system*, in which an O_2 and anesthetic gas mixture (often called the "fresh gas mixture") is blended according to the control settings. The fresh gas mixture passes through the fresh gas hose into the *breathing system*, which includes the mechanical ventilator. Excess gas from the breathing system is collected by the *scavenging system* and transported into the waste gas evacuation system.

Monitoring Instruments

Note that this classification scheme does not include monitoring instruments (e.g., O_2 analyzer, capnograph, and pulse oximeter) as a component subsystem of the anesthesia machine. Although they play an important role in monitoring anesthesia machine performance,[1] monitors may or may not be built-in features of an anesthesia gas delivery system. Descriptive and technical aspects of monitoring instruments, as well as their vital role in monitoring a patient's physiologic status, are discussed in separate chapters of this textbook.

HIGH-PRESSURE SYSTEM

What Are the Structural Components?

Gas Sources

The structures and safety features of the high-pressure system are listed in Table 16–1 and illustrated graphically in

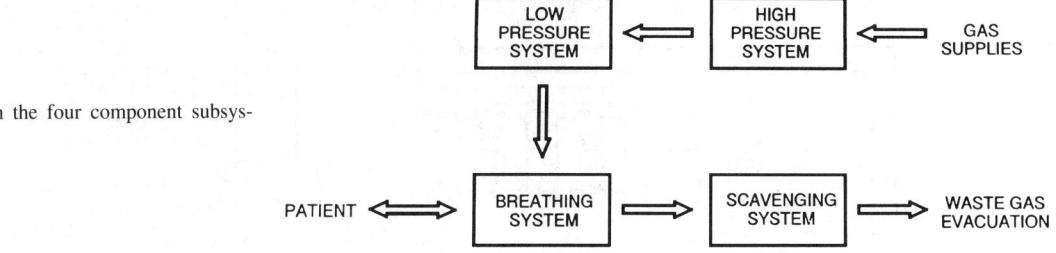

FIGURE 16–1. Gas flow through the four component subsystems of an anesthesia machine.

Figure 16–2. The pipeline gas inlets (see Fig. 16–2.1) provide connection sites for high-pressure gas hoses (see Fig. 16–2.2) that are connected to the hospital's pipeline gas supply (see Fig. 16–2.3). Hanger yokes allow cylinders of compressed gas to be securely attached to the anesthesia machine. When a gas cylinder is connected to the yoke and the stem valve on the cylinder is opened, gas can flow through the cylinder gas inlet (see Fig. 16–2.4) into the anesthesia machine. Check valves (see Fig. 16–2.5) are located on the machine side of both the pipeline and the cylinder inlets and prevent gas from leaking retrograde through the back of the anesthesia machine. On machines that accommodate more than one cylinder of each gas, the cylinder inlet check valves also prevent gas from a cylinder with higher pressure from transfilling a second cylinder with lower pressure.

Pressure Regulation

Pressure gauges (see Fig. 16–2.6), which are typically located on the front or side of the anesthesia machine, indicate the gas pressure in the hospital pipeline and in an *open* gas cylinder. The pressure in a cylinder of medical gas is related to the volume of compressed gas in the cylinder and to the physical characteristics of the contained gas—specifically, to whether the gas enters the liquid phase when compressed.

Regardless of the pressure in the cylinder (which may be as high as 2000 psig [gauge pressure in pounds per square inch]), the cylinder pressure regulator (see Fig. 16–2.7) reduces this pressure to approximately 45 psig, which is below the 50- to 55-psig operating pressure of the hospital pipeline gas supply. This pressure differential (pipeline gas at 50 psig; cylinder gas at 45 psig) allows the pipeline gas to be used preferentially if the anesthesia machine is connected to the hospital pipeline gas supply and if a reserve gas cylinder is simultaneously (and inadvertently) opened.

TABLE 16–1. Structures and Safety Features in the High-Pressure System

Structures	Pipeline gas inlets and check valves
	Cylinder gas inlets and check valves
	Cylinder hanger yokes
	Cylinder pressure regulator
	Gas supply pressure gauges
	O_2 (ventilator) power outlet
	O_2 flush valve
	Second-stage O_2 pressure regulator
Safety features	Diameter index safety system
	Pin index safety system
	Low O_2 supply pressure alarm
	O_2 pressure failure safety mechanism ("fail-safe")

Oxygen

The O_2 portion of the high-pressure system also includes an O_2 power outlet (see Fig. 16–2.8) (which is typically connected to a pneumatically driven mechanical ventilator) and the O_2 flush valve (see Fig. 16–2.9). On Ohmeda/Ohio (Madison, WI) anesthesia machines, the O_2 in the high-pressure system is reduced from 50 psig to approximately 16 psig by the second-stage pressure regulator (see Fig. 16–2.10). This arrangement minimizes movement ("bobbing") of the O_2 flow meter float that is caused by variations in O_2 pressure (such as that which accompanies cycling of the mechanical ventilator) and ensures that a decreasing O_2 supply pressure triggers the low O_2 supply pressure alarm before affecting the O_2 flow to the patient.

Safety Features

A number of safety features are built into the high-pressure system. All are designed to prevent the anesthesia machine from delivering hypoxic gas.

Diameter Index Safety System Connections

The Diameter Index Safety System (DISS; see Fig. 16–2.11) is designed to prevent the misconnection of a gas supply hose to the wrong pipeline gas inlet (e.g., N_2O supply hose connected to the O_2 pipeline inlet). The DISS standard specifies nut, nipple, and thread combinations (Fig. 16–3) that preclude such incorrect interconnections.

Quick Connectors

Many hospital pipeline systems use so-called "quick connectors" (Fig. 16–4) that allow faster connection of gas supply hoses to the pipeline outlets than do the DISS connectors, which must be slowly screwed on and off. The quick connector systems are also specifically designed to prevent misconnections.

Pin Index Safety System Connections

Analogous to the DISS is the Pin Index Safety System (PISS; see Fig. 16–2.12), which uses unique pin and receptacle combinations (Fig. 16–5) on cylinder hanger yokes to prevent the misconnection of a gas cylinder to the wrong cylinder inlet. The PISS system can be inappropriately defeated by pulling out the pins or by placing extra washers between the hanger yoke and the cylinder stem.

Low Oxygen Supply Pressure Alarm

The low O_2 supply pressure alarm (see Fig. 16–2.13) is designed to warn the anesthesiologist when the O_2 pressure

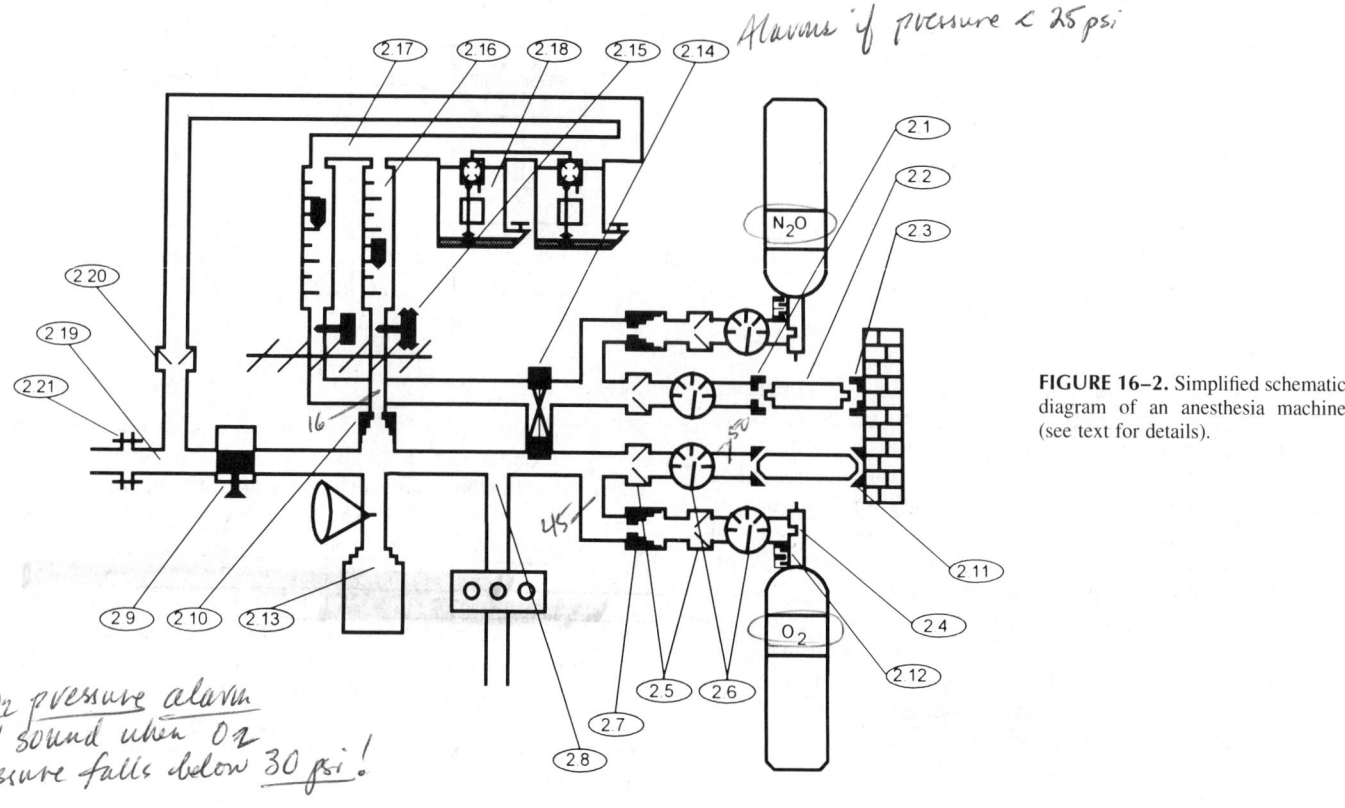

Alarms if pressure < 25 psi

FIGURE 16–2. Simplified schematic diagram of an anesthesia machine (see text for details).

low O_2 pressure alarm will sound when O_2 pressure falls below 30 psi!

falls below approximately 30 psig. Machine performance standards recommend that the alarm sound for at least 7 seconds if the O_2 pressure decreases below the threshold level.[2]

One anesthesia machine manufacturer implements this device mechanically using a pressure reservoir and a reed connected to the O_2 high-pressure line (Fig. 16–6). When the anesthesia machine is first connected to a high-pressure O_2 source (pipeline or cylinder) and is turned on, gas flows from the high-pressure line into the pressure reservoir, causing the reed to ''sound'' an alarm.

This feature explains why the low O_2 supply pressure alarm is activated when the anesthesia machine is first turned on. Once the pressure in the reservoir equilibrates with the high-pressure O_2 line, gas stops flowing across the reed, and the alarm is silent. Should the O_2 supply pressure decrease below a preset threshold, usually 30 psig, gas begins to flow from the pressure reservoir into the O_2 high-pressure line, once again causing the alarm to sound.

Oxygen Pressure Failure Safety Mechanisms

Perhaps the most inappropriately named safety feature of the high-pressure system is the O_2 pressure failure safety mechanism (see Fig. 16–2.14). This device often is referred to only as the ''fail-safe,'' implying that it eliminates the possibility of the anesthesia machine delivering hypoxic gas. The O_2 pressure failure safety mechanism arrests (Ohmeda/Ohio machines) or proportionally reduces (North American Dräger machines [Telford, PA]) the flow of non-O_2 gases when the pressure in the O_2 pipeline decreases to ≤25 psig (Fig. 16–7).

Continued flow of N_2O, helium, or other non-O_2 gases in the absence of O_2 quickly causes the gas mixture inspired by the patient to become hypoxic. Note, however, that if the O_2 pipeline or cylinder is pressurized with a gas other than O_2 (e.g., argon), the ''fail-safe'' does not activate. As long as the O_2 line in the high-pressure system is pressurized by *any* gas,

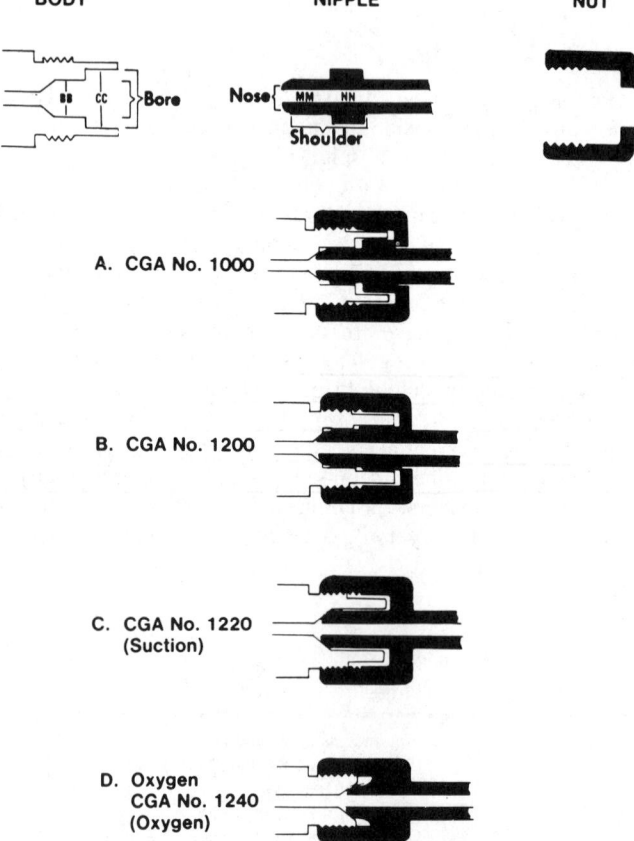

FIGURE 16–3. Diameter Index Safety System (1000 Series). With increasing Compressed Gas Association (CGA) number, the small shoulder of the nipple becomes larger and the large diameter becomes smaller. Noninterchangeability of connections is assured, since either MM will be too large for BB or NN will be too large for CC if assembly of a nonmating body and nipple is attempted. (From Dorsch JA, Dorsch SE: Understanding Anesthesia Equipment. 2nd ed. Baltimore, Williams & Wilkins, 1984, p 25.)

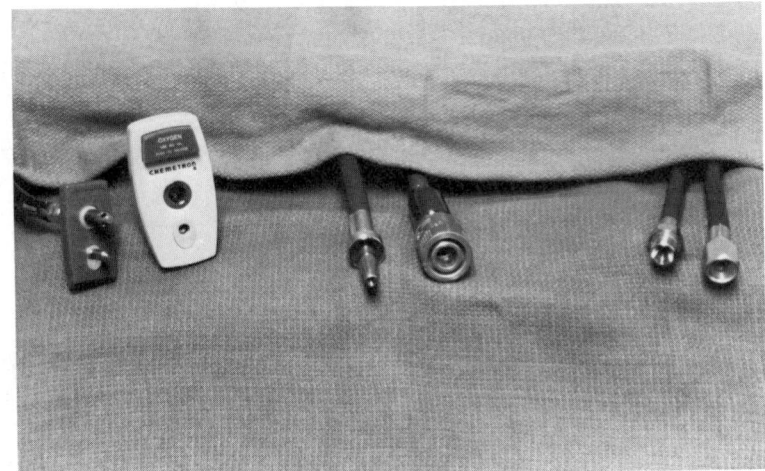

FIGURE 16–4. Examples of quick connectors, which, like DISS connectors, prevent misconnections of high-pressure gas hoses. The quick coupler and the attached hose should be color-coded for the specific gas.

the fail-safe continues to let all gases flow, even hypoxic mixtures.

When Should the Pressure Gauges Be Checked?

Pipeline

The pipeline pressure gauge for each gas should be included in the daily pre-use check of the anesthesia machine. An appropriate pressure reading verifies that the anesthesia machine is connected to each pipeline gas, that the pipeline is charged with gas, and that the operating pressure is correct. Each gauge should be checked periodically during the anesthetic procedure to verify that the correct pressure is maintained. Occasionally, pipeline pressure is lost or may change dramatically (e.g.,

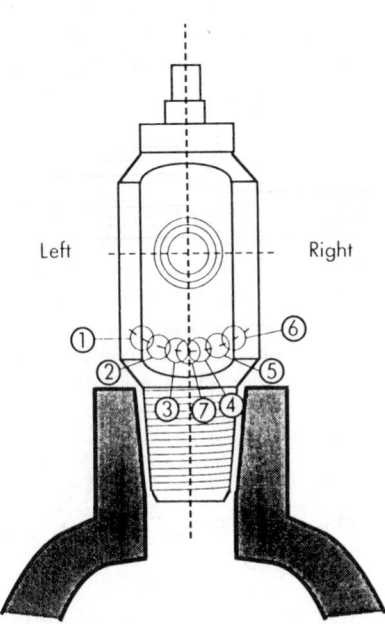

FIGURE 16–5. Pin Index Safety System pin location. Perspective shown looking at the placement of holes in the tank. Pins are placed precisely complementary in the tank yoke. Two pins are used to identify each type of gas. (From Eichhorn JH, Ehrenwerth J: Medical gases: storage and supply. *In* Anesthesia Equipment: Principles and Applications. Ehrenwerth J, Eisenkraft JB (eds). St Louis, Mosby–Year Book, 1993.)

decrease to 25 psig). Unexpected and confusing changes in machine performance (e.g., switching from pipeline to cylinder gas source) may result if the anesthesiologist is unaware of the change in the gas supply pressure.

Cylinder

The cylinder pressure gauge shows the gas pressure within the cylinder only if the cylinder stem valve is open. Pressure in the O_2 cylinders should be checked each day as part of the pre-use machine check. Pressure in other gas cylinders (N_2O, air, helium) need to be checked only according to periodic maintenance schedules, depending on local usage and practice. After checking the pressure in the gas cylinders, be sure to close the stem valve to prevent undesired leakage or inadvertent use of the cylinder gas.

What Is the Normal Pipeline Operating Pressure?

Operating pressure for the central hospital pipeline should be 50 ± 5 psig.[3] During mechanical ventilation or when the O_2 flush valve is opened, small pressure fluctuations can be observed on the pipeline pressure gauge. These fluctuations are caused by the momentary high demand for O_2 flow, which causes a corresponding decrease in the high-pressure system.

Such fluctuations should be small, typically <5 psig.[3] If they exceed this value, the anesthesia machine is "having difficulty" responding to the momentary demand for increased O_2 flow. Possible causes include a failure within the hospital pipeline system, a kinked supply hose (e.g., caused by a machine wheel resting on top of the hose), or an otherwise defective connection between the anesthesia machine and the pipeline wall outlet. Failures in the hospital pipeline system should simultaneously affect multiple anesthetizing locations and anesthesia machines, whereas problems with supply hoses affect only one site.

What Are Full E-Cylinder Pressures?

Oxygen

A full E-cylinder contains 660 L of O_2 and has a pressure of 1900 psig.[4] Oxygen remains in the gaseous phase when

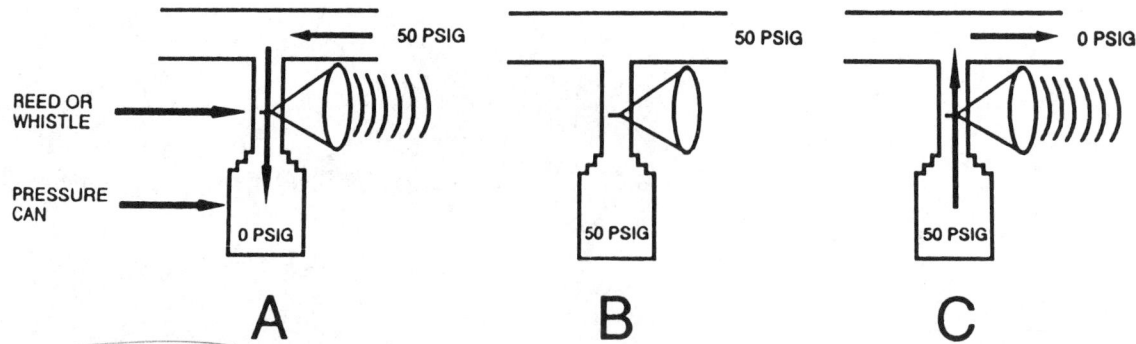

FIGURE 16–6. Low oxygen supply pressure alarm. *A,* When the anesthesia machine is connected to the oxygen supply and is turned on, oxygen at approximately 50 psig rushes by a reed or whistle as it passes into the pressure can. *B,* When oxygen pressure remains above a manufacturer's preset threshold (e.g., 30 psig), the can remains pressurized and the reed or whistle is silent. *C,* If the oxygen supply pressure drops below the manufacturer's preset threshold, gas rushes from the pressure can into the depressurized oxygen supply and causes the reed or whistle to sound the low oxygen supply pressure alarm. (From Good ML, Cooper JB: Monitoring the anesthesia machine. *In* Monitoring in Anesthesia. 3rd ed. Saidman LJ, Smith NY (eds). Boston, Butterworth-Heinemann, 1993.)

compressed at room temperature. Thus, the amount of gas remaining in an E-cylinder is directly proportional to its pressure (Fig. 16–8*A*). In other words, the volume of O_2 remaining in the cylinder is equal to the cylinder pressure (psig) multiplied by 660 L and divided by 1900 psig. At 950 psig, 330 L of O_2 remain compressed in the cylinder, and at 475 psig, 165 L of O_2 remain.

Nitrous Oxide

A full E-cylinder of N_2O contains 1600 L and has a pressure of approximately 750 psig. Nitrous oxide enters the liquid phase when it is compressed at room temperature. As long as any of the N_2O in the E-cylinder is in the liquid phase, the pressure remains 750 psig (Fig. 16–8*B*). When the volume of N_2O remaining in the cylinder reaches approximately 255 L (one-sixth of its initial value), all of the N_2O in the cylinder is in the gaseous phase.[5] From this point on, pressure correlates directly with the volume remaining, just as with O_2. Thus, a N_2O E-cylinder with a pressure of 750 psig may contain as little as 255 L or as much as 1600 L of gaseous N_2O. Only by

weighing the cylinder can one ascertain the exact amount of gas remaining. At a pressure of 375 psig, 128 L of N_2O remain within the cylinder; at 187 psig, 64 L remain.

Practical Applications

These relationships are used to determine how long an anesthesia machine can function on the reserve E-cylinder gas supplies. For example, suppose general anesthesia is needed in a remote site that is not supplied with pipeline gas. An E-cylinder of O_2 has a pressure of 1000 psig, and an E-cylinder of N_2O has a pressure of 745 psig. Assuming fresh gas flows of 5 L · min^{-1} each for O_2 and N_2O, how long can anesthesia be provided? Using the previously described relationships, 1000 psig corresponds to 347 L of O_2 (1000/1900 × 660 = 347), which will last longer than 1 hour at a flow rate of 5 L · min^{-1}. At a pressure of 745 psig, the N_2O E-cylinder contains any value between 255 and 1600 L, which, in a worst case scenario, provides a 5 L · min^{-1} flow for 51 minutes.

For spontaneous respiration or manual positive-pressure ventilation administered with the breathing bag, these calculations are sufficient. However, if an O_2-powered mechanical ventilator is used, you must also account for the extra usage. Oxygen usage by mechanical ventilators varies widely, ranging from 5 to 28 L · min^{-1}. This additional usage is at least equal to the patient's minute ventilation.[6] Thus, if minute ventilation is 5 L, total O_2 usage per minute is at least 10 L. Since only 347 L of O_2 are left in the E-cylinder, anesthesia and mechanical ventilation with the O_2-powered ventilator can be provided for just over 30 minutes.

When using E-cylinders as the sole gas source, it is practical to obtain an anesthesia machine that has two O_2 hangar yokes and inlet ports. This setup allows one O_2 cylinder to be used while the other is being exchanged.

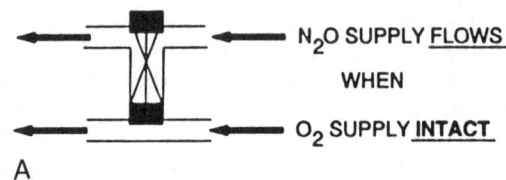

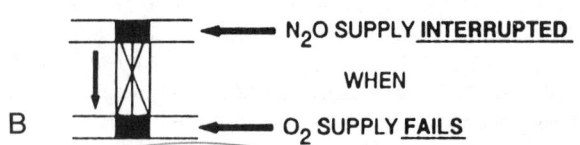

FIGURE 16–7. Oxygen pressure failure safety mechanism (fail-safe). *A,* When the oxygen system is pressurized, the fail-safe mechanism allows nitrous oxide to flow through the anesthesia machine. *B,* If the oxygen supply pressure decreases below the manufacturer's preset threshold (e.g., 25 psig), the fail-safe mechanism shifts to interrupt the flow of nitrous oxide, either completely or in proportion to the decrease in oxygen pressure. (From Good ML, Cooper JB: Monitoring the anesthesia machine. *In* Monitoring in Anesthesia. 3rd ed. Saidman LJ, Smith NY (eds). Boston, Butterworth-Heinemann, 1993.)

What Is the Flow Rate When the Oxygen Flush Valve Is Pressed?

Note that the O_2 flush valve provides a direct connection between O_2 at 50 psig in the high-pressure system and the breathing system, which is in continuity with the patient's lungs (see Fig. 16–2.9). When the O_2 flush valve is depressed, the breathing system is flooded with 35 to 75 L · min^{-1} of O_2.

If the adjustable pressure-limiting (APL, or "pop-off")

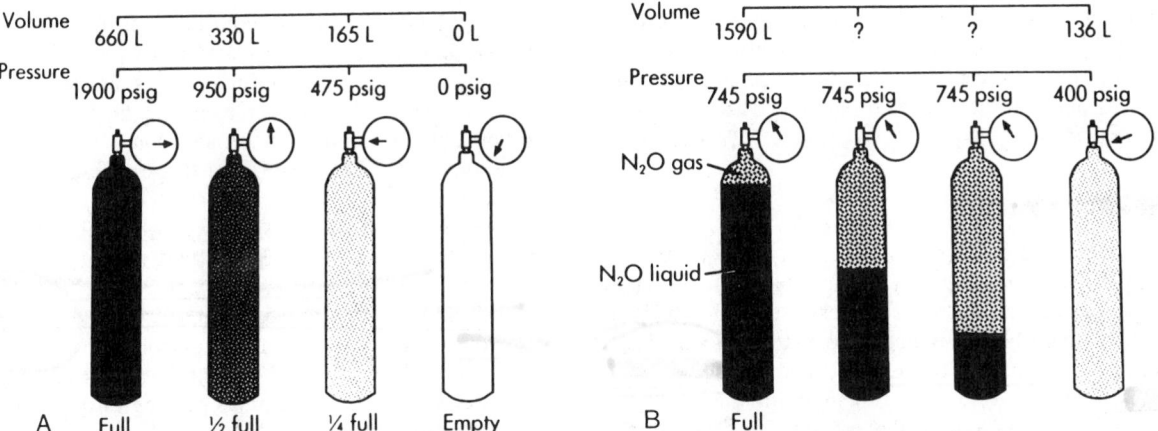

FIGURE 16–8. *A,* Oxygen remains a gas under high pressure. The pressure falls linearly as the gas flows from the cylinder; thus, in contrast to nitrous oxide, the oxygen pressure remaining always reflects the amount of gas remaining in the cylinder. *B,* At ambient temperature (20 °C), nitrous oxide liquefies under high pressure, and the pressure of the gas above the liquid remains constant *independently* of how much liquid remains in the cylinder. Only when all the liquid has evaporated does the pressure start to fall; as the residual gas flows from the cylinder, the pressure falls rapidly. (From Eichhorn JH, Ehrenwerth J: Medical gases: storage and supply. *In* Anesthesia Equipment: Principles and Applications. Ehrenwerth J, Eisenkraft JB (eds). St Louis, Mosby–Year Book, 1993, p 5.)

valve is partially or completely closed during spontaneous ventilation or if the pressure relief valve in the mechanical ventilator is closed during mechanical inspiration, this high flow may cause pressure to increase rapidly in the breathing system, potentially leading to cardiovascular compromise and pulmonary barotrauma.

To help guard against this complication, push the O_2 flush valve in short, intermittent bursts while observing the patient's chest or the airway pressure gauge. Never hold the flush valve open during the inspiratory phase of mechanical ventilation.[7]

How Can a Hypoxic Gas Mixture Be Delivered with a Fail-Safe Mechanism?

The fail-safe designation is misleading because it implies that the anesthesia machine cannot deliver a hypoxic gas mixture. Unfortunately, the device protects against only the continued flow of N_2O or other non-O_2 gas (e.g., helium) following a loss of O_2 supply pressure. As was already discussed, if any other pressurized gas source is attached inadvertently to the O_2 source, the fail-safe will be defeated.

Several other mechanisms also can cause a hypoxic gas mixture, including a contaminated O_2 pipeline or cylinder supply, inadequate O_2 flow, hypoxic N_2O-O_2 fresh gas flows, and leaks in the low-pressure system.[8] Although devices such as the fail-safe decrease the likelihood of hypoxic gas delivery, they do not eliminate it. Anesthesiologists must use calibrated O_2 analyzers with an audible alarm to ensure that a rare but often lethal hypoxic inspired gas mixture is rapidly detected.

LOW-PRESSURE SYSTEM

What Are the Structural Components?

Flow Control Valves

The components and safety features in the low-pressure system are listed in Table 16–2 and illustrated graphically in Figure 16–2. The high-pressure system is separated from the low-pressure system by the flow control valves (see Fig. 16–

2.15). As gas passes through the small orifice of the flow control valve, its pressure drops substantially. The flow control valves are simple but relatively precise variable-orifice needle valves. The anesthetic gas mixture is blended by turning the flow control valves to adjust the flow of O_2, N_2O, air, or other gases (e.g., helium, CO_2) that may be installed in a particular anesthesia machine.

Flow Meters

As gas emerges from the flow control valve, it passes immediately into a flow meter (see Fig. 16–2.16). (Many anesthesiologists incorrectly state that they ''adjust the flow meter.'' Technically speaking, one adjusts the flow control *valve* and observes the resulting flow on the flow *meter*.) Most anesthesia machines use a float or bobbin within a tapered, calibrated flow tube to measure the flow of gas emerging from the flow control valve. The greater the flow, the higher the float is lifted in the flow tube. Floats and flow tubes are calibrated as a pair for a specific gas. Use a flow meter only with the gas for which it was calibrated; if either the float or the tube is damaged, both must be replaced or gas flow will be measured incorrectly.

Manifold

Anesthesia machines usually have at least two, often three, and sometimes four or more separate gas sources, each with

TABLE 16–2. Structures and Safety Features in the Low-Pressure System

Structures	Flow control valves
	Flow meters (flow tubes)
	Manifold
	Calibrated vaporizers
	Common gas outlet check valve
	Common gas outlet
Safety features	Touch-sensitive O_2 flow control knob
	Hypoxic guard (link or proportioned)
	Minimum O_2 flow
	Vaporizer interlock/exclusion system

its own flow control valve and flow meter. Since the purpose of the low-pressure system is to blend a gas mixture, the gas emerging from each flow meter must be joined together; this junction takes place in the manifold (see Fig. 16–2.17) of the low-pressure system.

Calibrated Vaporizers

As the gas mixture emerges from the flow meters and travels through the low-pressure system manifold, it may detour through one of the calibrated vaporizers (see Fig. 16–2.18) attached to the manifold. Contemporary anesthesia vaporizers usually are of the variable bypass type and are temperature compensated. The new volatile anesthetic desflurane has physical characteristics that require the special Tec 6 desflurane vaporizer (Ohmeda, Madison, WI).

Common Gas Outlet

The low-pressure system arbitrarily ends with the common gas outlet (see Fig. 16–2.19). Some Ohmeda/Ohio anesthesia machines position a common gas outlet check valve (see Fig. 16–2.20) just proximal to the outlet. The check valve is designed to prevent retrograde flow from the flush valve or breathing system into the low-pressure system. Newer anesthesia machines use special antidisconnect connectors (see Fig. 16–2.21) to help prevent accidental disconnection of the fresh gas hose from the common gas outlet.

Is the Arrangement of the Gas Flow Meters Important?

Yes! The O_2 flow meter should connect to the manifold at the point closest to the common gas outlet.[9] This arrangement is safest should a leak occur in one of the flow tubes or in the manifold. For example, let us assume that a two-gas anesthesia machine with N_2O and O_2 each flowing at $1 \text{ L} \cdot \text{min}^{-1}$ has a $1.5\text{-L} \cdot \text{min}^{-1}$ leak in one of the flow tubes (Fig. 16–9). If the O_2 flow meter is positioned farther from the common gas outlet than the N_2O flow meter (see Fig. 16–9A and B), approximately $1 \text{ L} \cdot \text{min}^{-1}$ of O_2 and $0.5 \text{ L} \cdot \text{min}^{-1}$ of N_2O escape through the leak; $0.5 \text{ L} \cdot \text{min}^{-1}$ of pure N_2O flows through the common gas outlet to the patient; and a hypoxic gas mixture rapidly develops in the breathing system.

Consider the same situation, but switch the order of the O_2 and N_2O flow meters such that the O_2 flow meter is closest to the common gas outlet (see Fig. 16–9C and D). In this configuration, $1 \text{ L} \cdot \text{min}^{-1}$ of N_2O and $0.5 \text{ L} \cdot \text{min}^{-1}$ of O_2 escape through the leak in the manifold, whereas $0.5 \text{ L} \cdot \text{min}^{-1}$ of O_2 flows to the common gas outlet. Although the patient does not receive the intended 50:50 N_2O-O_2 gas mixture, the inspired gas is not hypoxic.

How Do Variable-Bypass Vaporizers Meter Anesthetic Vapor?

The functional components of a variable-bypass vaporizer (Fig. 16–10) include the gas inlet (see Fig. 16–10.1), bypass channel, vaporizing chamber (see Fig. 16–10.5), concentration control (see Fig. 16–10.2), temperature compensator (see Fig. 16–10.3 and 16–10.6), fluctuating back pressure compensator

(see Fig. 16–10.4), bypass control valve (see Fig. 16–10.8), and gas outlet (see Fig. 16–10.7). When the concentration control is in the "off" position, the inlet and outlet port valves close, isolating the vaporizer from the fresh gas flow. When the concentration control is turned "on," the vaporizer inlet and outlet port valves open, and the fresh gas mixture flows into the vaporizer.

From this point, the fresh gas flow is divided; part flows through the bypass channel, and part through the vaporizing chamber. The portion that travels along each route depends on the concentration control setting and on the temperature compensator. As the concentration control setting increases, the proportion of gas directed into the vaporizing chamber increases (see Fig. 16–10.10). Gas passing through the chamber becomes fully saturated with anesthetic vapor; as it emerges, it rejoins the gas passing through the bypass channel and exits through the vaporizer outlet port.

Do Contemporary Vaporizers Compensate for Ambient Pressure? _Temperature?_

Contemporary anesthetic vaporizers are temperature compensated. The temperature-compensating mechanism includes a sensing component (see Fig. 16–10.6) and a valve (see Fig. 16–10.3). As the liquid anesthetic cools, the temperature-compensating valve directs more gas into the vaporizing chamber, and vice versa. Thus, the vaporizer automatically compensates for changes in the vaporization of liquid anesthetic at different temperatures.

Do Contemporary Vaporizers Compensate for Barometric Pressure?

Although the concentration (i.e., volume/volume%) of anesthetic vapor emerging from a vaporizer is dependent on barometric pressure, compensation for changes in barometric pressure do not occur within contemporary vaporizers. Remember that the partial pressure (i.e., mm Hg) and not the concentration (i.e., per cent) of anesthetic agent correlates with depth of anesthesia. Thus, although a vaporizer set to deliver 1% isoflurane at sea level delivers approximately 0.5% when the barometric pressure is decreased to 380 mm Hg, the gas mixture has an isoflurane partial pressure of approximately 7 mm Hg, the same as it would at sea level. Anesthetic potency is unchanged.

If the barometric pressure were increased to 1520 mm Hg, the 1% vaporizer setting actually would deliver 2%. Again, however, the partial pressure of isoflurane is 7 mm Hg. Thus, even though the vaporizer does not possess a formal barometric "pressure compensator," and although changes in barometric pressure alter concentration of the anesthetic output, the applicable physical principles of anesthetic vaporization enable the vaporizer to perform in a satisfactory manner.

Do Contemporary Vaporizers Compensate for Fluctuating Back Pressure?

Intermittently fluctuating pressure in the breathing system, such as that generated by positive-pressure ventilation or by intermittent pressing and releasing of the O_2 flush valve,

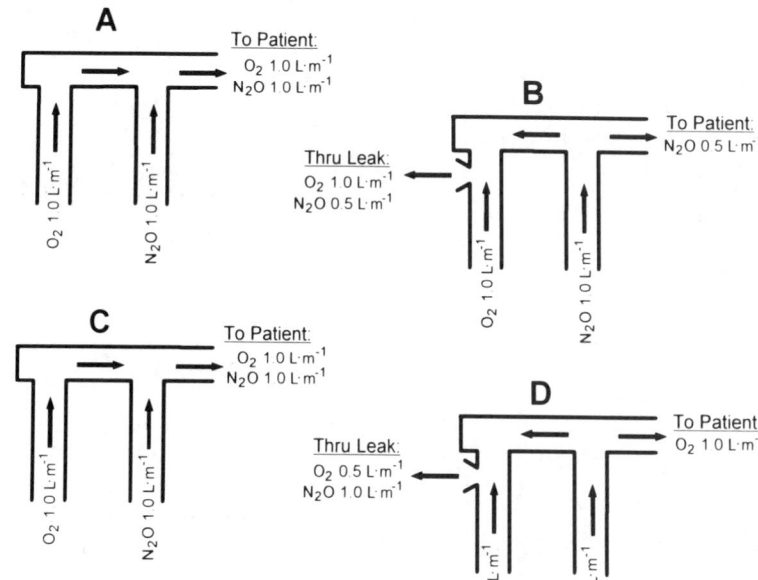

FIGURE 16–9. Optimal arrangement of flow meters in low pressure system (see text for explanation).

causes fluctuating back pressure to be transmitted into the low-pressure system. Earlier vaporizer designs were susceptible to this pumping effect.[10, 11] If breathing system pressure was increased sufficiently, the pressure and, therefore, the volume of gas in both the vaporizing chamber and the bypass channel also increased. When the pressure was released, gas in the vaporizing chamber was able to flow retrograde into the bypass channel as it decompressed. The result of this pumping effect was an increased concentration of anesthetic delivered. New anesthetic vaporizers (Tec 4, Tec 5, and Dräger 19.1) incorporate mechanisms that decrease the size of the vaporizing chamber relative to the bypass channel and increase the volume of the inflow channel. Accordingly, vapor-saturated gas cannot make its way back into the bypass channel, and thus the pumping effect is prevented.

Are Contemporary Vaporizers Accurate at Very Low Fresh Gas Flow Rates?

Some clinicians erroneously claim that vaporizer output is inaccurate at low fresh gas flow rates. During low flow anes-

thesia, the anesthetic agent concentration measured in the breathing system differs greatly from that set on the vaporizer concentration control. However, constant flow performance data clearly demonstrate that anesthetic vaporizers are very accurate, even when the fresh gas flow is only 500 mL · min⁻¹ (Fig. 16–11).

The discrepancy observed between vaporizer setting and measured anesthetic concentration in the breathing circuit is due to the low flow, not to inaccuracy of the vaporizers. At low fresh gas flows, even though a specific concentration of anesthetic agent emerges from the fresh gas hose, the volume of anesthetic emerging is low compared with the volume at high fresh gas flows. Hence, at low flow rates, patient uptake and dilution into the volume of the breathing circuit significantly reduce the breathing system concentration.

What Happens If the Wrong Agent Is Added to a Vaporizer?

The concentration of anesthetic that emerges from the vaporizer depends on the vaporization characteristics of the

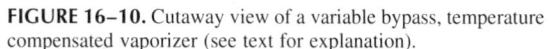
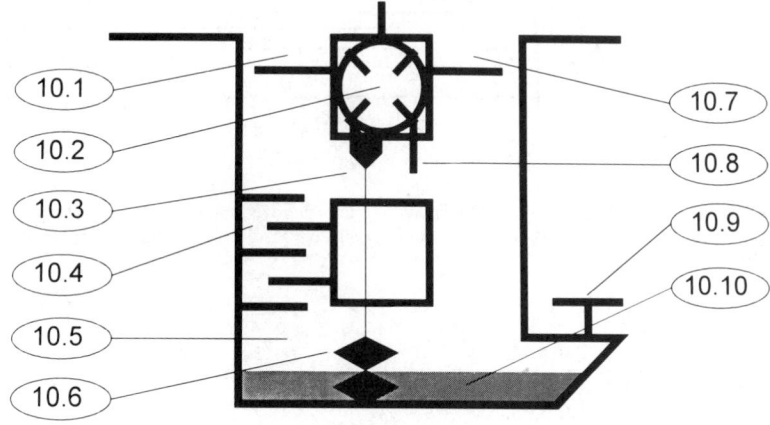

FIGURE 16–10. Cutaway view of a variable bypass, temperature compensated vaporizer (see text for explanation).

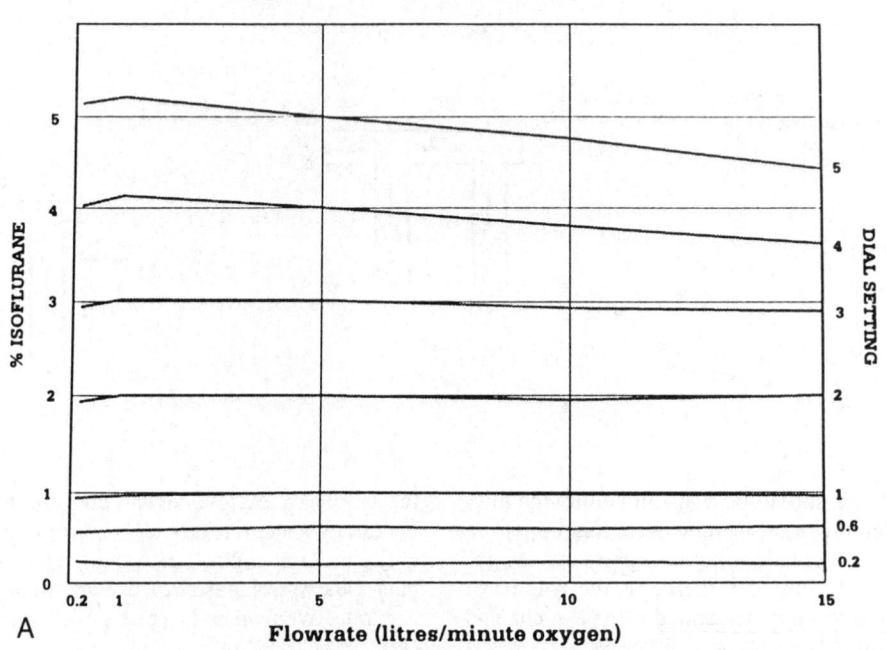

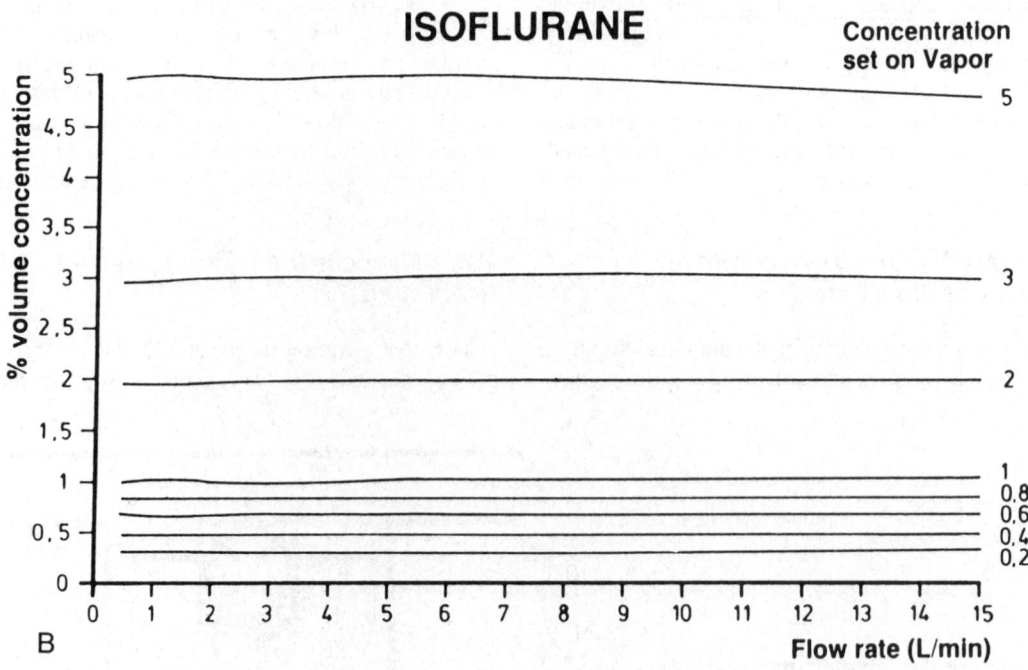

FIGURE 16–11. Performance graphs comparing the vaporizer control (''dial'') setting and the measured vaporized output as a function of fresh gas flow. (*A* from Tec 5 Operation and Maintenance Manual. Ohmeda, Madison, WI, 1989. *B* from Dräger-Vapor 19.1, Operating Instructions. Drägerwerk, Lübeck, Germany, 1987.)

TABLE 16–3. Effect of Misfilling Vaporizer

| Anesthetic Agent | Vapor Pressure at 20° C (mm Hg) | Vaporizer Type (Set at 1 MAC) | | |
		Enflurane	*Isoflurane*	*Halothane*
Enflurane	184	1 MAC	<1 MAC	<1 MAC
Isoflurane	239	>1 MAC	1 MAC	<1 MAC
Halothane	243	>1 MAC	>1 MAC	1 MAC

(From Good ML, Paulus DA: Equipment. *In* Manual of Complications During Anesthesia. Gravenstein N (ed). Philadelphia, JB Lippincott, 1991, p 107.)

agent. Isoflurane and halothane have nearly identical vaporization constants; thus, the concentration of anesthetic emerging from the vaporizer should be similar even if misfilling occurs. However, halothane is more potent than isoflurane. Therefore, the patient receives a relative overdose when an isoflurane vaporizer is filled with halothane.

Calculations are somewhat more complicated when a halothane or isoflurane vaporizer is filled with enflurane or when an enflurane vaporizer is filled with either halothane or isoflurane. In general, the difference in anesthetic potency (i.e., the minimum alveolar concentration [MAC]) is of greater significance than differences in vapor pressure. Thus, an enflurane vaporizer filled with either isoflurane (MAC = 1.1%) or halothane (MAC = 0.75%) also delivers a relative overdose. The effects of misfilling combinations are shown in Table 16–3.

BREATHING SYSTEM

What Are the Structural Components?

Structures and safety features in the breathing system are listed in Table 16–4 and illustrated in Figure 16–12. The anesthetic gas mixture blended in the low-pressure system is delivered through the fresh gas hose (see Fig. 16–12.1), which connects to the breathing system at the fresh gas inlet (see Fig. 16–12.2) on the carbon dioxide [CO_2]–absorbent canister (see Fig. 16–12.3).

The circle anesthesia breathing system includes the inspiratory (see Fig. 16–12.4) and expiratory (see Fig. 16–12.5) unidirectional valves, breathing hoses (see Fig. 16–12.6), and Y-piece (see Fig. 16–12.7). Located on the CO_2-absorbent

TABLE 16–4. Structures and Safety Features in the Breathing System

Structures	Fresh gas hose
	Fresh gas inlet
	Inspiratory unidirectional valve
	Expiratory unidirectional valve
	Breathing hoses
	Y-piece
	APL or ''pop-off'' valve
	CO_2-absorbent canister
	''Airway'' (breathing system) pressure gauge
	Return tube
	Breathing bag
	Bag/ventilator selector switch
	Ventilator hose
	Mechanical ventilator control unit
	Ventilator bellows
	Ventilator pressure relief (''spill'') valve
Safety features	Antidisconnect fresh gas hose connectors
	Ventilator low airway pressure alarm

canister are the APL or pop-off valve (see Fig. 16–12.8), ''airway'' or, more precisely, breathing system pressure gauge (see Fig. 16–12.9), return tube (see Fig. 16–12.10), breathing bag (see Fig. 16–12.11), and the bag/ventilator selector switch (see Fig. 16–12.12).

Also included are the mechanical ventilator and associated components, specifically the ventilator hose (see Fig. 16–12.13), mechanical ventilator control unit (see Fig. 16–12.14), ventilator bellows (see Fig. 16–12.15), and ventilator pressure relief (''spill'') valve (see Fig. 16–12.16).

Safety Features

Although many equipment-related injuries are caused by problems in the breathing system, relatively few safety features are found in this portion of the anesthesia machine. Newer anesthesia machines have antidisconnect fresh gas hose connectors (see Fig. 16–12.17) on both the machine and circuit side of the fresh gas hose rather than the older friction-slip-fit–type connectors. Also, contemporary anesthesia ventilators include a ventilator low airway pressure alarm that is designed to warn the clinician in the event of a partial or complete disconnection.

When Is Carbon Dioxide Removed from the Respiratory Gas?

Despite its deceiving simplicity, tracing the flow of gas through a circle anesthesia breathing system is more difficult than might seem to be the case. To better understand this gas flow, one can divide the respiratory cycle into three phases: mechanical inspiration, active exhalation, and the expiratory pause. Gas flow patterns for each phase are graphically illustrated in Figure 16–13, summarized in Table 16–5, and described in detail in the following sections.

Mechanical Inspiration

The control unit of the mechanical ventilator can be thought of as a timer and flow controller. When it initiates a mechanical breath, a high flow of gas (usually O_2 or an O_2-air mixture from the O_2 high-pressure system and entrained air) passes into the outer drive chamber of the mechanical ventilator (see Fig. 16–13A). The duration of this high flow state (''mechanical inspiration'') and the volume of gas delivered to the outer chamber are determined by the tidal volume and inspiratory flow or inspiratory-to-expiratory (I:E) ratio settings on the control unit.

Pressurization within the drive chamber compresses the bellows and ''pushes'' gas, under positive pressure, into the ventilator hose and the breathing circuit. Pressure against the ma-

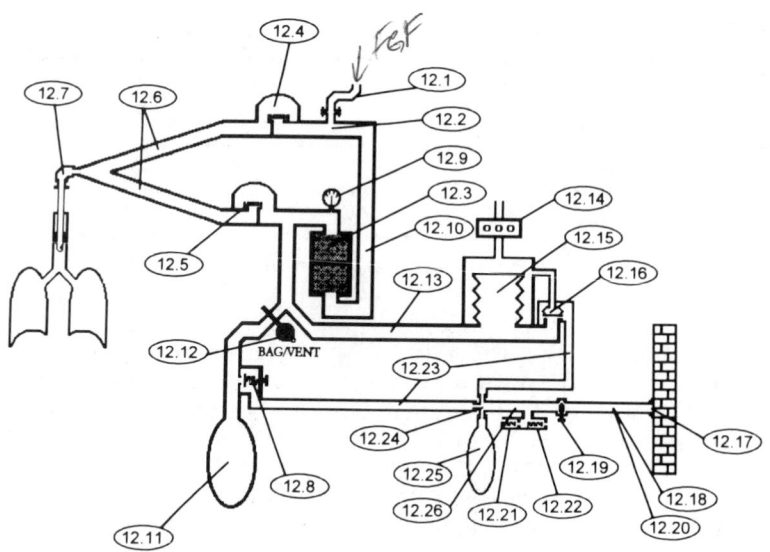

FIGURE 16–12. Simplified schematic diagram of the breathing and scavenging systems (see text for explanation).

chine side of the expiratory unidirectional valve causes it to close, preventing gas from entering the expiratory limb of the circuit. Thus, the gas moves down through the CO_2-absorbent canister and up the return tube that is concealed within. At the top of the CO_2 canister, the positive-pressure breath from the ventilator is augmented by the continuously flowing fresh gas mixture. The combined gas volume moves through the inspiratory unidirectional valve, down the inspiratory limb, through the Y-piece and endotracheal tube, and into the patient's lungs.

Active Exhalation

This phase of the respiratory cycle commences as soon as the ventilator control unit ends the inspiratory phase and depressurizes the outer drive chamber of the mechanical ventilator. Elastic recoil of the patient's lungs pushes gas through the airway and Y-piece and into the expiratory limb.

As the exhaled gas passes into the canister, it is joined by the continuously flowing fresh gas mixture (see Fig. 16–13B). When the inspiratory unidirectional valve closes at the beginning of active exhalation, the fresh gas flow can no longer continue its course into the patient; instead, the path of least resistance is now retrograde, down the return tube, and back through the CO_2-absorbent canister, where it joins the exhaled gas from the patient's lungs. This gas mixture (exhaled and fresh gas) then passes through the bag/ventilator selector switch, ventilator hose, and into the ventilator bellows, which re-expands to its initial position.

When the ventilator bellows reaches this position, pressure momentarily begins to increase in the breathing system. However, as soon as the pressure reaches approximately 2 cm H_2O, the ventilator pressure relief valve opens to allow the remaining exhaled gas to enter the waste gas scavenging system.

Expiratory Pause

The time between the end of active exhalation and the start of the next mechanical inspiration is designated as the *expiratory pause*. No gas movement occurs in or out of the patient's lungs nor in the inspiratory and expiratory limbs of the breathing system. However, fresh gas continues to flow into the

absorbent canister (Fig. 16–13C). The path of least resistance for this gas also is down the return tube, up in a retrograde fashion through the CO_2-absorbent canister, through the bag/ventilator selector switch and ventilator hose, into the ventilator bellows, and out the ventilator pressure relief valve. The fresh gas flow during this phase begins to purge the CO_2-containing gas from the ventilator hose and ventilator. The degree to which purging occurs is dependent on the fresh gas flow rate and on the duration of the expiratory pause. Thus, at high fresh gas flows (e.g., >12 L $\cdot$ min^{-1}), the circle system can be used as a nonrebreathing system, and it allows adequate ventilation, even without CO_2 absorbent.

What Is the Effect of an Incompetent Unidirectional Valve?

The flow of gas during the three phases of respiration can be re-examined in the case of an incompetent inspiratory valve and an incompetent expiratory valve.

Inspiratory Valve

With an incompetent inspiratory valve, mechanical inspiration proceeds normally, since the inspiratory valve is supposed to be open at this time. During active exhalation, however, the inspiratory valve fails to close, and part of the exhaled gas enters the inspiratory limb. If the volume of the exhaled gas entering the inspiratory limb exceeds the volume of the inspiratory hose, the excess gas passes down the return tube, enters the absorbent canister, and CO_2 is removed. During the expiratory pause, fresh gas flows retrograde through the return tube, flushing the CO_2-containing gas into the CO_2 absorber.

With the next mechanical inspiration, previously exhaled gas in the inspiratory limb is pushed back into the patient's lungs, causing CO_2 rebreathing. Because the volume of most standard breathing hoses is 300 to 600 mL, and since the tidal volume for adults exceeds the volume of the breathing hose, some fresh gas eventually reaches the patient's lungs. Thus, an incompetent inspiratory valve causes partial rebreathing,

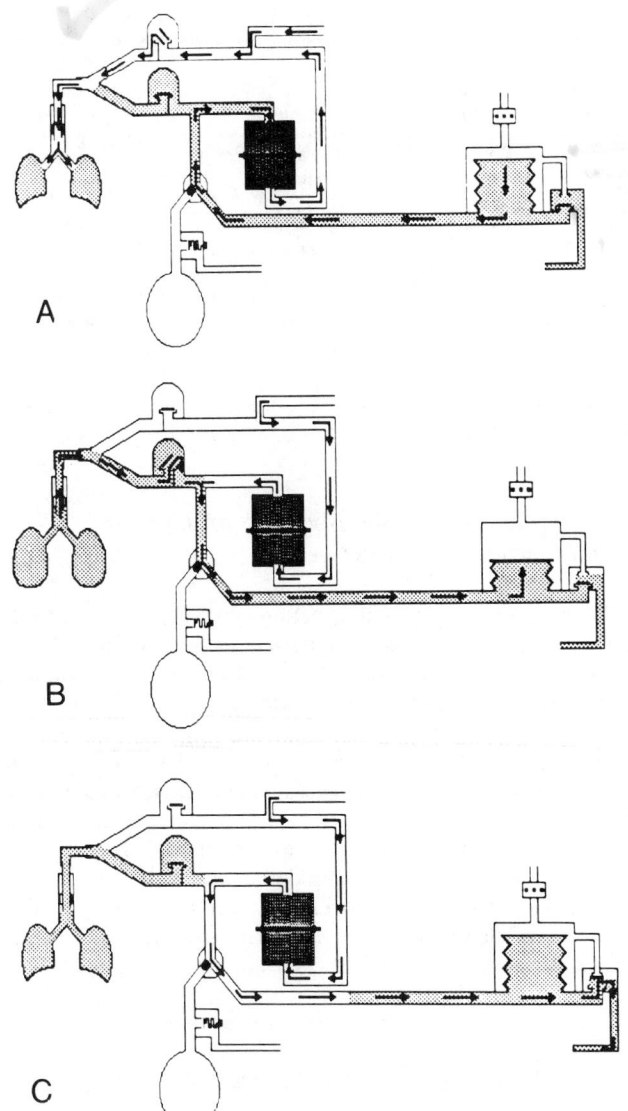

FIGURE 16–13. Gas flow through the circle anesthesia breathing system during the three phases of mechanical ventilation. *A,* Mechanical inspiration. *B,* Expiration. *C,* Expiratory pause. (See text for explanation.)

the amount of which is determined primarily by the volume of the inspiratory hose relative to the tidal volume.

Expiratory Valve

When the expiratory valve is incompetent, active exhalation proceeds normally, since the expiratory valve is supposed to be open at this time. During mechanical inspiration, however, the expiratory valve fails to close. A portion of the inspiratory gas from the ventilator bellows is thus directed to the patient through the expiratory limb, and rebreathing of CO_2 results. In this case, the abnormal reservoir for CO_2 includes not only the expiratory limb but also the gas in the ventilator hose and ventilator bellows (2 L or more). Thus, an incompetent expiratory valve causes significantly more CO_2 rebreathing than does an incompetent inspiratory valve.

What Is the Compliance of the Breathing Hoses?

The "compliance" of anesthesia breathing hoses varies greatly, depending on the type and manufacturer (Table 16–6). Most anesthesiologists use the term *compliance* to include collectively the distensibility of the breathing hose and volume of gas that can be compressed within it. This information is important to determine the volume of gas trapped in the breathing system that does not reach the patient's lungs. It is calculated as the plateau inspiratory pressure (Pplat) multiplied by the breathing circuit compliance. If the Pplat is 20 cm H_2O and the circuit compliance is 7 mL · cm H_2O^{-1}, the volume of gas compressed within the hoses during mechanical inspiration is 140 mL. For an adult with an 800-mL tidal volume, this loss is not clinically significant. However, for a small child with a 300-mL tidal volume, it represents almost a 50% decrease.

Gas compressed within and distending the breathing hoses during mechanical inspiration does not enter the patient's lungs. During active exhalation, the breathing hoses decompress, and the trapped gas exits with gas from the patient's lungs through the expiratory hose. Thus, a spirometer located on the expiratory limb includes both gas components (patient-ventilated and compressed gas) and may mislead the anesthesiologist into thinking that the patient's tidal volume is appropriate when it really is low. The compliance of a breathing circuit can be estimated by occluding the Y-piece, pressurizing the circuit by cycling the ventilator, and observing the exhaled volume measured by a spirometer adjacent to the expiratory valve. The compliance (expressed as milliliters per centimeter of H_2O) is determined from this value and the measured circuit pressure.

How Is Carbon Dioxide Removed from the Respiratory Gas?

Chemical Absorbent

During inspiration, the gas from the previous exhalation is directed through the CO_2-absorbent canister that contains a chemical CO_2 absorbent. Such absorbents, most commonly soda lime or Baralyme, chemically remove CO_2 from the gas. The chemical reactions require water and produce heat (Table 16–7).

Dye Indicator

The CO_2 absorbent includes a dye indicator designed to turn the normally white absorbent to a purple color when it is exhausted and no longer capable of removing CO_2. Normally, the dye indicator performs as it should. However, the color change is not permanent and may fade over time. Fluorescent lights also adversely affect absorbent performance.[13] Capnography serves as an additional and perhaps more reliable means to detect exhausted CO_2 absorbent, which is indicated by an elevated inspiratory baseline.

In certain instances, respiratory gas may channel through the inner core of the absorbent-filled canister and exhaust this portion. The outer rim of absorbent remains white, concealing

TABLE 16–5. Summary of Gas Flow Characteristics During Mechanical Ventilation Through a Circle Anesthesia Breathing System

Respiratory Phase	Ventilator Control Unit	Ventilator Bellows	Gas and Flow in CO_2 Absorbent	Flow in Return Tube	Fresh Gas Flow	Ventilator Pressure Relief Valve
Mechanical inspiration	Pressurizes drive chamber	Compresses	Exhaled gas with CO_2 flows top to bottom	Bottom to top	Toward inspiratory limb	Closed
Active exhalation	Depressurizes drive chamber	Re-expands to initial position	Fresh gas flows bottom to top	Top to bottom	Into return tube and absorbent canister	Closed
Expiratory pause	Inactive	Stationary at initial position	Fresh gas flows bottom to top	Top to bottom	Into return tube and absorbent canister	Open

the purple, exhausted absorbent. In this situation, the dye indicator change is not seen by the anesthesiologist; however, the capnograph detects the problem.

Why Doesn't Positive End-Expiratory Pressure Register on the Breathing Pressure Gauge?

The airway pressure gauge (which, as noted before, is more correctly called the "breathing system pressure gauge") is typically positioned within the CO_2-absorbent canister on older machines (see Fig. 16–12.9). In this position, it is a long distance from the patient's airway and separated from it by the inspiratory and expiratory unidirectional valves. When positive end-expiratory pressure is added to the breathing circuit, typically through the placement of a valve on the expiratory port of the absorbent canister, the end-expiratory pressure is maintained on the patient side of the unidirectional valves but is not transmitted into the absorbent canister. Thus, the pressure gauge indicates only peak inspiratory pressure and returns to zero during exhalation.

On newer anesthesia machines, the gauge remains on the absorbent canister, but the pressure sensor is tunnelled through the canister to measure the pressure on the patient side of the unidirectional valve (Fig. 16–14). In this position, it is closer to the patient's airway, more accurately reflects the pressure there, and registers positive end-expiratory pressure.

What Is the Difference Between an Upright and a Hanging Bellows?

An ascending ("upright") bellows ascends during exhalation and descends during inspiration. A descending ("hanging") bellows descends during exhalation and ascends during inspiration. Hence, the terms "ascending" or "descending" refer to the motion of the bellows during exhalation. The important difference between the two is that the ascending bellows requires that the patient's exhaled gas fill it, whereas the descending bellows refills on its own because gravity pulls it back to its initial position. In the event of a disconnection within the breathing system, the descending bellows ventilator continues to refill and to cycle. By contrast, the ascending bellows ventilator collapses, triggering the ventilator's low airway pressure alarm and alerting the anesthesiologist that a problem exists (Fig. 16–15).

WASTE GAS SCAVENGING SYSTEMS

How Are They Classified?

Gas scavenging systems are classified (Table 16–8) as active or passive and as valved ("closed") or valveless ("open"). A vacuum source (see Fig. 16–12.17), vacuum hose (see Fig. 16–12.18), and vacuum control (see Fig. 16–12.19) distinguish an active scavenging system, whereas a waste gas evacuation hose (see Fig. 16–12.20) replaces these components in a passive scavenging system.

The negative pressure source of the active scavenging system, usually a component of the hospital pipeline system, actively "pulls" the excess gas from the anesthesia machine, transports it through the hospital gas disposal system, and typically releases it from the roof. Passive scavenging systems

TABLE 16–6. Compression Volume Versus Pressure*

	Peak Inflation Pressure (cm H_2O)				
Circuit	10	20	30	40	50
Mapleson D Circuits					
Bain (H)	20	60	100	120	167
Piggy back (H)	27	67	127	147	180
Our own (H)	27	53	94	120	160
Circle Circuits					
Adult rubber	127	240	353	487	600
Adult rubber (H)	147	267	380	547	687
Adult plastic	74	147	220	294	347
Adult plastic (H)	100	187	274	360	447
Adult wire	53	127	187	240	294
Adult wire (H)	74	147	220	280	353
Pediatric rubber	53	107	167	207	260
Pediatric rubber (H)	67	133	200	267	320
Pediatric plastic	53	113	174	233	267
Pediatric plastic (H)	67	140	200	274	333

*This table presents the mean volume of compressed oxygen (in milliliters) of six determinations at each peak inflation pressure (in centimeters of H_2O). The letter H indicates that the study was carried out with a heated humidifier (see text for details). (From Coté CJ, Petkau AJ, Ryan JF, et al: Wasted ventilation measured in vitro with eight anesthetic circuits with and without inline humidification. Anesthesiology 1983; 59:442.)

TABLE 16–7. Chemical Reactions of Carbon Dioxide with Soda-Lime (Top) and Baralyme (Bottom)

$$CO_2 + H_2O \rightleftharpoons H_2CO_3$$
$$H_2O + 2NaOH(KOH) \rightleftharpoons Na_2CO_3(K_2CO_3) + Heat$$
$$Na_2CO_3(K_2CO_3) + Ca(OH)_2 \rightleftharpoons CaCO_3 + 2NaOH(KOH)$$

$$Ba(OH)_2 + 8H_2O + CO_2 \rightleftharpoons BaCO_3 + 9H_2O + Heat$$
$$9H_2O + 9CO_2 \rightleftharpoons 9H_2CO_3$$
$$9H_2CO_3 + 9Ca(OH)_2 \rightleftharpoons 9CaCO_3 + 18H_2O + Heat$$

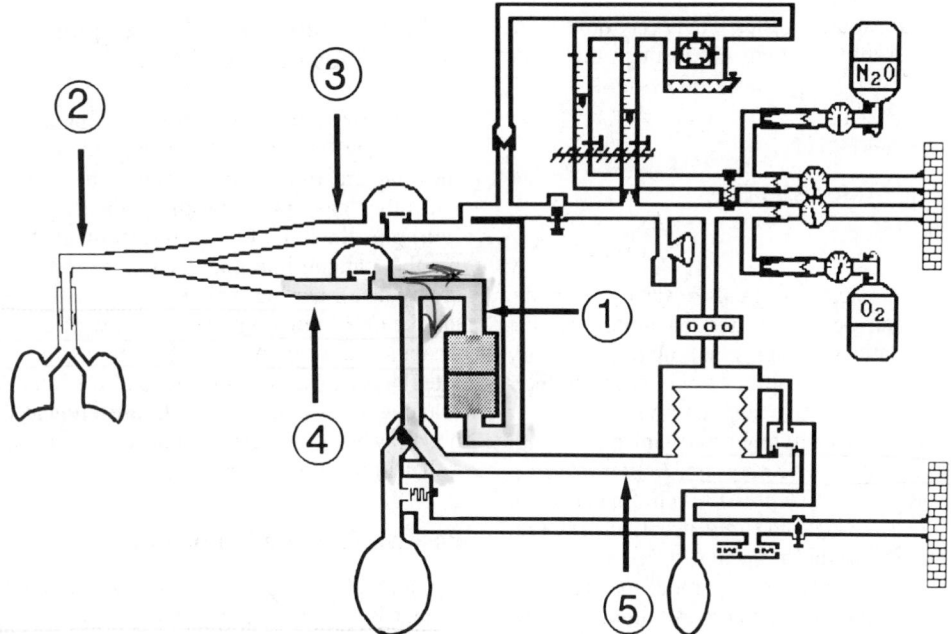

FIGURE 16–14. Breathing system pressure sensor sites. (1) In older breathing systems, pressure is sensed within the absorber canister. PEEP, which is constrained to the patient side of the unidirectional valves, does not register when breathing system pressure is sensed in this location. (2) If breathing system pressure is measured close to the patient's airway, it more accurately reflects pressure in the patient's lungs. However, pressure sensors that are connected at this site tend to promote displacement of endotracheal tubes, are sometimes bulky, and increase the number of potential disconnection sites. (3) and (4) Breathing system pressure sensors placed on the patient side of unidirectional valves correctly register PEEP when present. Site 4 is preferred to site 3, because at site 3, pressure fluctuations are registered (and prevent low pressure alarms from sounding) with a disconnection if a partial obstruction occurs between the pressure sensor and the patient's airway. (5) Breathing system pressure should never be measured in the ventilator portion of the breathing system. Again, breathing system pressure fluctuations may register even though a complete disconnection has occurred further downstream. (Modified from Good ML, Cooper JB: Monitoring the anesthesia machine. *In* Monitoring in Anesthesia. 3rd ed. Saidman LJ, Smith NT (eds). Boston, Butterworth-Heinemann, 1993, p 387.)

FIGURE 16–15. Comparison of an upright (ascending) and hanging (descending) bellows mechanical ventilator during disconnection. The upright bellows ventilator cycles normally when the breathing system is intact *(A)* but collapses during disconnection *(B)* because the patient's exhaled gas no longer lifts the bellows to its initial position. The hanging bellows ventilator cycles normally when the breathing system is intact *(C);* it continues to cycle up and down despite a disconnection *(D)* because the bellows is pulled by gravity to its initial position. (From Good ML, Cooper JB: Monitoring the anesthesia machine. *In* Monitoring in Anesthesia. 3rd ed. Saidman LJ, Smith NT (eds). Boston, Butterworth-Heinemann, 1993, p 386.)

SYSTEM INTACT   DISCONNECTION

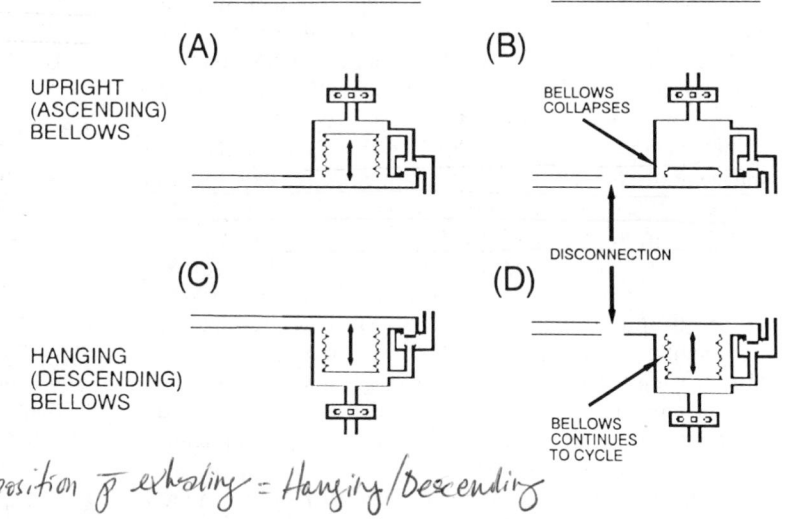

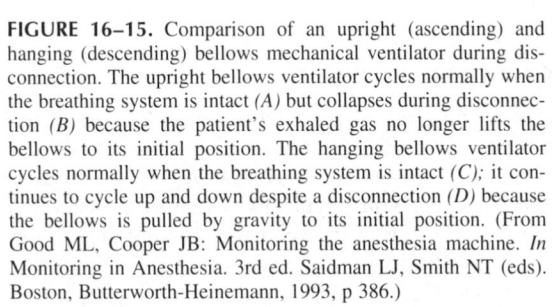

TABLE 16–8. Classification of Gas Scavenging Systems

Manufacturer	Model	Active	Passive	Valved*	Valveless†
Ohmeda/Ohio	Waste gas scavenging interface valve	×‡	×‡	×	
North American Dräger	Scavenger interface for air conditioning systems		×	×	
	Scavenger interface for suction systems	×		×	
	Open reservoir scavenger	×			×

*Also referred to as "closed."
†Also referred to as "open."
‡This scavenging system can be used in either an active or a passive configuration.

do not require the vacuum source; instead, they rely on a slight positive pressure to push the waste gas out through the waste gas evacuation hose and into the gas disposal system.

Can Gas Scavenging Systems Injure Anesthetized Patients?

If excessive positive or negative pressure develops in the scavenging system, it can be transmitted back through the breathing system to the patient's lungs, resulting in pulmonary barotrauma and cardiovascular collapse. To minimize the likelihood of these events, both active and passive scavenging systems include a positive-pressure relief mechanism (see Fig. 16–12.21) to vent undesired positive pressure. Active scavenging systems also include a negative-pressure relief mechanism (see Fig. 16–12.22) to dissipate undesired negative pressure. Some systems use gravity-driven or spring-loaded valves for the positive-pressure and negative-pressure relief mechanisms. Other systems accomplish the same objectives without valves.

What Are the Structural Components?

The structures and safety features of the waste gas scavenging system are listed in Table 16–9 and illustrated in Figure 16–12. Excess anesthetic gas must be collected from the APL and ventilator pressure relief valves (see Fig. 16–12.8 and 16–12.16). A scavenging system collecting hose (see Fig. 16–12.23) connects each of these to the scavenging system intake ports (see Fig. 16–12.24). The scavenging system may have just one intake port that must be divided to allow both collecting hoses to be connected. If more than two intake ports are present, those not in use should be capped off to ensure proper function of the scavenging system.

The vacuum control (see Fig. 16–12.19) typically is an adjustable needle valve that controls the flow rate of gas from the scavenging system into the hospital gas disposal system. A gas reservoir (see Fig. 16–12.25) is also required for an active scavenging system. The vacuum hose, vacuum control, intake ports, and reservoir bag are joined together by the scavenging system manifold (see Fig. 16–12.26), which is also called the "scavenging system interface" because it interfaces the anesthesia machine and the hospital gas disposal system. The passive scavenging system has a waste gas evacuation hose (see Fig. 16–12.20). This hose connects the scavenging manifold with the environment into which the waste gas will be delivered (e.g., an air conditioning intake duct or an open window).

TABLE 16–9. Structures and Safety Features of the Gas Scavenging System

Structures	Collecting hoses (19-mm connectors)
	Inlet ports
	Reservoir
	Manifold
	Vacuum port and control (active)
	Exhaust port and evacuation hose (passive)
Safety features	19-mm connectors
	Positive-pressure relief mechanism
	Negative-pressure relief mechanisms

Why Does an Active Scavenging System Need a Gas Reservoir?

The flow rate of gas from the breathing system into the scavenging system can be calculated as the total fresh gas flow into the breathing system minus the rate of O_2 consumption and other gas uptake by the patient (e.g., N_2O during induction) plus the rate of CO_2 production and other gas elimination by the patient into the breathing system (e.g., N_2O during emergence). During maintenance anesthesia, with minimal gas uptake or elimination, the total flow of gas into the scavenging system is approximately the same as the total fresh gas flow rate. Unfortunately, knowledge of the total flow of gas into the scavenging system is of little use clinically because gas does not flow into the scavenging system at a continuous rate but rather in discrete "boluses."

Positive-Pressure Ventilation

Table 16–5 and Figure 16–13 demonstrate that when the patient is receiving controlled mechanical ventilation, gas enters the scavenging system through the ventilator pressure relief valve only during late exhalation and the expiratory pause after the ventilator bellows has returned to its initial position. When the anesthesiologist delivers positive-pressure breaths manually with the breathing bag, gas enters the scavenging system when the breathing system pressure exceeds the opening pressure of the APL valve.

Spontaneous Breathing

When the patient breathes spontaneously, gas enters the scavenging system through the APL valve only during late expiration and the expiratory pause after the breathing bag is fully distended.

Reservoir Function

Regardless of the mode of ventilation, gas delivery to the scavenging manifold is discontinuous. Gas flow out of the scavenging system, however, is continuous and constant. Therefore, the gas reservoir—typically a bag or canister—is needed to provide buffering between the discontinuous flow into and continuous flow out of the scavenging system. Without a reservoir (see Fig. 16–12.25), excessively high vacuum would be required to capture all the waste gas; more likely, inadequate vacuum flows would result in spillage of waste anesthetic gas into the operating room environment.

Vacuum Control

From the preceding discussion, one deduces that if the volume of the gas reservoir is adequate, the vacuum flow rate should be set slightly greater than the total fresh gas flow rate. In clinical practice, however, this precise an adjustment is difficult. With one open reservoir system, the vacuum flow is adjusted using a flow meter.[14] For systems that use an anesthesia bag as the reservoir, the vacuum flow is adjusted until the reservoir bag is neither fully collapsed nor fully distended.

Recall, however, that each time the rate of fresh gas flow into the breathing system changes, the rate of gas flow out of the breathing system and into the scavenging system also changes. The rate of fresh gas flow changes many times during a typical anesthetic procedure, since very high flow rates of O_2 (e.g., 6–12 L · min^{-1}) are provided during denitrogenation and mask ventilation prior to intubation; high flows (e.g., 5 L · min^{-1}) of O_2 and N_2O or air occur during the rapid uptake phases; low or very low flows (e.g., 0.5–2 L · min^{-1}) are provided during maintenance anesthesia; periodic increases to higher flow (3–5 L · min^{-1}) are used to quickly increase or decrease the concentration of volatile agent in the breathing system; and a return to high flows (e.g., 5 L · min^{-1}) occurs just prior to emergence to hasten elimination of anesthetic gases from the breathing system. To prevent the reservoir bag from overdistending or collapsing, each change in fresh gas flow would need to be accompanied by a concomitant change in the vacuum control knob.

Practical Considerations

Because this approach is not clinically practical, we must choose the "lesser of two evils": (1) having the reservoir bag fully distended and venting anesthetic gas into the room, with a risk of excessively high airway pressures if the positive pressure relief mechanism fails; or (2) allowing the reservoir bag to be fully collapsed and room air to be entrained, with the risk of subatmospheric pressures if the negative pressure relief mechanism fails.

In my opinion, the fully collapsed bag is a more attractive option. During pre-use check of the anesthesia machine, I follow the advice of a colleague: I completely close the vacuum control knob and then open it one-half turn (personal communication, David G. Bjoraker, M.D.). This technique results in a collapsed reservoir bag at low fresh gas flow rates and in a partially distended reservoir bag at high flow rates. The one-half turn may have to be adjusted in each practitioner's institution, depending on the strength of the vacuum.

Can Scavenging and Breathing Circuit Hoses Be Used Interchangeably?

Scavenging and breathing system hoses are very similar in appearance. For safety reasons, however, scavenging collecting hoses are fitted with 19-mm connectors and breathing hoses that have 22-mm connectors. The 19-mm connectors are often color-coded with yellow tape or molded from yellow plastic to distinguish them clearly from breathing hoses, which have black or clear plastic connectors.

Misconnection of scavenging hoses to the breathing system or vice versa can have disastrous consequences. A particularly hazardous situation develops with the inadvertent attachment of the scavenging hose from the ventilator to the mount for the breathing bag. This misconnection prevents any gas exit from the mechanical ventilator and quickly increases airway pressures; pulmonary barotrauma is a possible outcome.

What Happens If the Ventilator Scavenging Hose Becomes Obstructed?

Obstruction of either gas collecting hose is dangerous because it prevents gas from exiting the breathing system. Because fresh gas continues to flow in, breathing system and airway pressures increase dramatically and rapidly, and again barotrauma can occur.

During manual positive-pressure ventilation, the anesthesiologist usually recognizes that a problem exists because the breathing bag "gets stiff" and continues to distend even though the APL valve is fully opened. With mechanical ventilation, however, this important clinical sign is not available because the bag is not held in the hand. A distended ventilator bellows, abnormal ventilator sounds, or elevated airway pressures may be the first clues.

Precautions to prevent patient injury include keeping collecting hoses as short as possible so that they are not run over and obstructed by the wheels of the anesthesia machine. Never use adhesive tape to incorrectly mate a 22-mm breathing hose connector to a 19-mm mount. The tape can work itself free and obstruct the lumen of the collecting hose, and this obstruction will not be visible. Patency of the scavenging collecting hoses should be assessed during the pre-use check of the anesthesia machine.

TROUBLESHOOTING THE GAS DELIVERY SYSTEM

Anesthesiologists must apply their technical knowledge of the anesthesia machine by (1) conducting a pre-use check each day prior to first use; (2) monitoring the performance of the machine during an anesthetic procedure; and (3) troubleshooting the machine to identify and correct malfunctions when they occur.

What Needs to Be Checked?

Equipment malfunction is an infrequent but recurrent cause of iatrogenic patient injury. Numerous case reports describing patient injuries and "near misses" resulting from equipment malfunction fill the anesthesia literature. Nearly every component of the anesthesia gas delivery system has been implicated. In one large study of untoward outcomes in anesthesia, patient injury from equipment malfunction (including breathing system disconnection) accounted for approximately 14% of all critical incidents.[15]

Patients usually are not directly injured by an equipment failure. Instead, the equipment malfunction compounds and worsens an evolving crisis in which the primary causative factor is a nonequipment problem (most often human error).[16] In large surveys of critical anesthesia incidents, "failure to check" is one of the most frequently cited "associated factors."[15]

A Critical Example

Suppose that a syringe of succinylcholine is mislabeled as fentanyl. During monitored anesthesia care, the patient receives 100 μg (2 mL) of "fentanyl," promptly "has a seizure," and becomes apneic. Anticipating a spontaneously breathing patient, the anesthesiologist failed to check the anesthesia machine prior to beginning the anesthetic procedure. Now, a malfunctioning bag/ventilator selector switch prevents the patient from receiving positive-pressure ventilation by either the breathing bag or the mechanical ventilator. The backup self-inflating resuscitation bag is missing from the anesthesia cart. The patient suffers several minutes of hypoxemia before a Mapleson circuit and E-cylinder of O_2 are brought to the operating room, assembled, connected, and used to restore ventilation. The primary problem was human error—specifically, the mislabelling of a syringe. However, the patient would have done well if the anesthesia machine and the backup ventilation equipment had been present and properly checked before the case began.

How Well Are Systems Checked?

Can anesthesia practitioners properly check an anesthesia gas machine? In the early 1980s, Buffington and coworkers studied the ability of anesthesia personnel to detect anesthesia machine malfunctions.[17] Anesthesia machines were preconfigured with five machine faults: (1) removal of inspiratory and expiratory unidirectional check valves; (2) removal of the PISS, which allowed interchange of N_2O and O_2 reserve E-cylinders; (3) malfunction of the fail-safe mechanism; (4) interchange of O_2 and cyclopropane flow tubes; and (5) misfilling of the halothane vaporizer with methoxyflurane.

Anesthesiologists were asked to examine the anesthesia machines and determine what was wrong. On average, only 2.2 of the five faults were identified. No faults were detected by 7.3% of participants, and only 3.4% detected all five faults. Participants with more than 10 years of clinical anesthesia practice identified more faults (2.46) then did those with less experience (2.04). No correlation was found between professional background (physician, nurse, technician, dentist, designer, manufacturer, or service personnel) and the number of faults detected.

Are Pre-Use Check Protocols Useful?

Because "failure to check" is a frequent associated factor in the iatrogenic injury of anesthetized patients, manufacturers of anesthesia machines, the American Society of Anesthesiologists (ASA), the Anesthesia Patient Safety Foundation, and the Food and Drug Administration (FDA) support the use of pre-use check protocols to help anesthesia practitioners ensure that their anesthesia machine is properly functioning and fit for patient use. The FDA designed a generic protocol, entitled *Anesthesia Apparatus Checkout Recommendations,* that was first published in 1986[18] and has since been widely disseminated.[19, 20]

The effectiveness of the FDA protocol was subsequently evaluated in the early 1990s.[21] Residents in training and private practitioners attending continuing medical education meetings were challenged to identify one set of four machine faults using their own check methods, then a different set of four machine faults using the FDA protocol. The specific machine faults included a malfunctioning O_2/N_2O ratio protection system, malfunctioning fail-safe mechanism, malfunctioning O_2 analyzer, leak in the low-pressure system, leak in the mechanical ventilator, leak in the vaporizer, incompetent unidirectional valve, and a leak in the high-pressure system.

Participants detected an average of only 1.03 of four faults (25.8%) using their own check methods and only 1.20 of four faults (29.9%) using the FDA check protocol. Only the malfunctioning O_2/N_2O ratio protection system was detected more frequently using the FDA check protocol than the participants' own methods. Anesthesiology residents detected more faults (2.46 of eight total, or 30.8%) than did practicing clinicians

(1.98 of eight total, or 23.9%). The investigators concluded that " . . . mere introduction of the FDA checklist did not improve the ability of anesthesiologists to detect anesthesia machine faults."[21]

Why Do Pre-Use Protocols Fail?

Two important considerations help us to understand why detailed pre-use check protocols by themselves fail to improve the ability to detect anesthesia machine malfunctions.

Understanding

The written protocol provides specific instruction for completing the pre-use check, but it does not help one to understand the anesthesia machine. In some instances, the anesthesia practitioner is able to complete each step of the protocol but does not understand its purpose or what specific malfunctions are being sought.

In a pilot study, the FDA confirmed this hypothesis by providing a group of resident anesthesiologists with the pre-use check protocol; written and didactic educational materials designed to help the residents understand their anesthesia machine; and the rationale for each step in the check protocol. Subjects who completed the educational program were able to identify 4 of the 8 preconfigured machine faults. This score was statistically different from that obtained in previous studies that did not include the accompanying educational curriculum.

Length of the Precheck List

A second factor contributing to poor acceptance and understanding of the pre-use machine check is its length. Existing protocols often include 70 or more individual tasks and may take 10 minutes or more to complete. They include checking machine components that fail infrequently and that do not immediately jeopardize the patient when they do fail. Basically, these protocols are too long and too verbose to anticipate high compliance by a majority of anesthesia practitioners.

What Is the Revised Food and Drug Administration Pre-Use Check Protocol?

Recognizing these deficiencies, the ASA Committee on Equipment and Facilities met with representatives from the FDA and the anesthesia machine manufacturers in 1992 to develop a revised pre-use check protocol. Table 16–10 shows the 1993 draft of this document.

The objective in designing this revised protocol was to emphasize checking components that "fail" frequently or that quickly and severely jeopardize the safety of the anesthetized patient when they do fail. Anesthesia machine components that fail infrequently and those that do not jeopardize patient safety if they do fail were eliminated from the daily pre-use check protocol and relegated to periodic maintenance.

For example, the O_2 supply pressure fail-safe mechanism is a durable mechanical device that rarely fails. Even if it should fail, it does not injure the anesthetized patient except with a simultaneous loss of the O_2 supply pressure. Even in this "worst case" scenario, the low O_2 supply pressure alarm on

TABLE 16–10. Anesthesia Apparatus Checkout Recommendations (1993)

Emergency Ventilation Equipment
*1. Verify that backup ventilation equipment is available and functioning.

High-Pressure System
*2. Check O_2 cylinder supply.
    a. Open O_2 cylinder and verify that it is at least half-full (about 1000 psi).
    b. Close cylinder.
*3. Check central pipeline supplies.
    a. Check that hoses are connected and that pipeline gauges read about 50 psi.

Low-Pressure System
*4. Check initial status of low-pressure system.
    a. Close flow control valves and turn vaporizers off.
    b. Check fill level and tighten vaporizers' filler caps.
*5. Perform leak check of machine low-pressure system.
    a. Verify that the machine's master switch and flow control valves are off.
    b. Attach "suction bulb" to common (fresh) gas outlet.
    c. Squeeze bulb repeatedly until fully collapsed.
    d. Verify that bulb stays *fully* collapsed for at least 10 s.
    e. Open one vaporizer at a time and repeat steps c and d above.
    f. Remove suction bulb and reconnect fresh gas hose.
*6. Turn on machine's master switch and all other necessary electrical equipment.
*7. Test flow meters.
    a. Adjust flow of all gases through their full range, checking for smooth operation of floats and undamaged flow tubes.
    b. Attempt to create a hypoxic O_2-N_2O mixture and verify correct changes in flow and alarm operation.

Scavenging System
*8. Adjust and check scavenging system.
    a. Ensure proper connections between the scavenging system and both APL (pop-off) valve and ventilator relief valve.
    b. Adjust waste gas vacuum (if possible).
    c. Fully open APL valve and occlude Y-piece.
    d. With minimum O_2 flow, allow scavenging reservoir bag to collapse completely and verify that absorber pressure gauge reads about zero.
    e. With the O_2 flush activated, allow the scavenger reservoir bag to distend fully, and then verify that absorber pressure gauge reads <10 cm H_2O.

Breathing System
*9. Calibrate O_2 monitor.
    a. Ensure that monitor reads 21% in room air.
    b. Verify that low O_2 alarm is enabled and functioning.
    c. Reinstall sensor in circuit and flush breathing system with O_2.
    d. Verify that monitor now reads >90%.
10. Check initial status of breathing system.
    a. Set selector switch to bag mode.
    b. Check that breathing circuit is complete, undamaged, and unobstructed.
    c. Verify that CO_2 absorbent is adequate.
    d. Install breathing circuit accessory equipment (e.g., humidifier, positive end-expiratory pressure valve) to be used during the case.
11. Perform leak check of the breathing system.
    a. Set all gas flows to zero (or minimum).
    b. Close APL (pop-off) valve and occlude Y-piece.
    c. Pressurize breathing system to about 30 cm H_2O with O_2 flush.
    d. Ensure that pressure remains fixed for at least 10 s.
    e. Open APL (pop-off) valve and ensure that pressure decreases.

Manual and Automatic Ventilation Systems
12. Test ventilation systems and unidirectional valves.
    a. Place a second breathing bag on Y-piece.
    b. Set appropriate ventilator parameters for next patient.
    c. Switch to automatic ventilation (ventilator) mode.
    d. Turn ventilator on and fill bellows and breathing bag with O_2 flush.
    e. Set O_2 flow to minimum, other gas flows to zero.
    f. Verify that during inspiration bellows delivers appropriate tidal volume and that during expiration bellows fills completely.
    g. Set fresh gas flow to about 5 L · min⁻¹.
    h. Verify that the ventilator bellows and simulated lungs fill *and empty appropriately* without sustained pressure at end-expiration.
    i. *Check for proper action of unidirectional valves.*
    j. Exercise breathing circuit accessories to ensure proper function.
    k. Turn ventilator off and switch to manual ventilation (bag/APL) mode.
    l. Ventilate manually and ensure inflation and deflation of artificial lungs and appropriate feel of system resistance and compliance.
    m. Remove second breathing bag from Y-piece.

Monitors
13. Check, calibrate, or set alarm limits of all monitors (capnometer, pulse oximeter, oxygen analyzer, respiratory volume monitor (spirometer), pressure monitor with high and low airway pressure alarms).

Final Position
14. Check final status of machine; make sure that:
    a. Vaporizers are off.
    b. APL valve is open.
    c. Selector switch is moved to bag mode.
    d. All flow meters read zero (or minimum).
    e. Patient suction level is adequate.
    f. Breathing system is ready to use.

*If an anesthesia provider uses the same machine in successive cases, these steps need not be repeated or may be abbreviated after the initial checkout.

the anesthesia machine, the low O_2 supply pressure alarm on the mechanical ventilator, the O_2 analyzer, and eventually the pulse oximeter alarm should warn of a developing hypoxic gas mixture in sufficient time for corrective action to be taken.

The revised FDA pre-use check protocol can be completed in 5 minutes or less. After its final revision, editing, and publication, additional studies will be needed to determine its effectiveness.

MONITORING THE ANESTHESIA MACHINE

How Do Anesthesia Gas Machines Injure Patients?

The primary purposes of an anesthesia gas machine are (1) to provide O_2; (2) to blend an anesthetic gas mixture; and (3) to facilitate spontaneous, assisted, or controlled ventilation of the patient's lungs. Accordingly, anesthesia gas machines injure patients when they (1) cause the patient to respire a hypoxic gas mixture; (2) deliver an incorrect anesthetic dose; and (3) inappropriately ventilate the patient's lungs.

What Are the Consequences of Inspiring a Hypoxic Gas?

Inspiring a hypoxic gas mixture (one that contains <21% O_2) rapidly causes oxyhemoglobin desaturation. In general, irreversible hypoxic injury of the central nervous system is thought to begin after approximately 4 minutes of arterial desaturation. Surprisingly, small or even no changes in hemodynamic variables are initially observed even when arterial hypoxemia is severe.

Must All Anesthesia Gas Delivery Systems Provide Supplemental Oxygen?

Theoretically no, but from a practical standpoint, yes. Anesthesia gases can be delivered to the patient's lungs using room air—in other words, without providing supplemental O_2. For example, a drawover vaporizer system,[22] which is often used for providing anesthesia in a military environment, in Third World countries, and in other locations without compressed O_2 supplies, can deliver anesthesia gases to the patient using room air. However, all but the healthiest of patients require supplemental O_2 administration to maintain arterial O_2 saturation during mechanical ventilation.[23] Thus, to be of use in contemporary civilian anesthesia practice, the anesthesia machine must provide O_2 and a control system to meter its release into the inspired gas mixture.

What Malfunctions Cause Respiration of Hypoxic Gas?

Malfunctions that allow the anesthesia machine to create a hypoxic gas mixture are shown in Table 16–11. The entire list of problems may or may not be applicable to a specific make and model of anesthesia machine. For example, the loss of O_2

TABLE 16–11. Malfunctions That Result in Hypoxic Gas

Obstructed fresh gas hose
Hypoxic fresh gas flow ratios
Inaccurate flow meters
Inadequate O_2 flow
Leak in the low-pressure system
Loss of O_2 supply pressure
Contaminated O_2 supply

supply pressure should not lead to a hypoxic gas mixture if the anesthesia machine is equipped with a functioning O_2 supply pressure fail-safe mechanism. Similarly, the hypoxic guard mechanism should prevent the user from setting a hypoxic O_2/N_2O flow ratio. However, certain malfunctions can cause hypoxic gas to flow from even the newest of anesthesia machines.

As an example, if the O_2 pipeline or cylinder is misfilled with a gas other than O_2, the anesthesia machine will deliver hypoxic gas. This type of malfunction, whether due to a pipeline cross-over or a direct misfilling, can be detected only with a functioning O_2 analyzer. Leaks in the low-pressure system of the anesthesia machine may also cause a hypoxic gas mixture if O_2 is preferentially lost through the leak (see Fig. 16–9).

An inadequate flow rate of O_2 may also lead to a hypoxic gas mixture. Consider fresh gas flow rates of 300 mL · min^{-1} for both O_2 and N_2O. The O_2 concentration emerging from the fresh gas hose is 50%. However, a typical adult patient consumes approximately 250 mL of O_2 each minute. Thus, the net delivery of O_2 to the breathing system is 50 mL · min^{-1}, whereas that of N_2O (assuming minimal uptake or elimination) is 300 mL · min^{-1}. Over time, the O_2 concentration approaches 16%, eventually causing oxyhemoglobin desaturation.

Can the Anesthesia Machine Provide Oxygen Through a Nasal Cannula?

Because supplemental O_2 is often administered to nonintubated, spontaneously breathing patients through a nasal cannula during regional or monitored anesthesia care, an attractive feature of some anesthesia machines is a separate flow control and flow meter for metering O_2.

Without this secondary system, the anesthesiologist who desires to administer O_2 through a nasal cannula must attach that cannula to the common gas outlet on the anesthesia machine or connect it to the Y-piece of the breathing system. The first option requires temporary disassembly of the machine. In the event of complications requiring emergent transition to general anesthesia, the nasal cannula must be disconnected from the common gas outlet and the fresh gas hose reconnected.

The second option is fraught with several problems. First, because the resistance of the nasal cannula tubing is high, a significant amount of pressure is required to push O_2 flow through it; therefore, if the APL valve is not fully closed, an indeterminate amount of O_2 escapes into the scavenging system and is not delivered to the patient. Even if the pop-off valve is closed, because of the relative compliance of the breathing system and breathing bag, a limited (usually about 3 L · min^{-1}) and indeterminate amount of O_2 is delivered through the nasal cannula.

What Are the Consequences of an Inappropriate Anesthetic Dose?

Anesthetic overdose or underdose may injure the patient. An underdose may lead to awareness and recall and, in some patients, to sympathetic stimulation that results in tachycardia and hypertension. Depending on the underlying medical problems, this sympathetic stimulation may have adverse sequelae (e.g., myocardial ischemia). An anesthetic overdose results in hypotension, may cause bradycardia, and, if severe enough, eventually leads to cardiovascular collapse.[24]

What Malfunctions Cause an Inappropriate Anesthetic Dose?

Anesthetic underdose and overdose are most often related to titration "errors" by the anesthesiologist. However, faults within the machine may also cause problems. A leak in the low-pressure system allows anesthetic gas to escape into the operating room and not be delivered to the breathing system. A vaporizer that is filled with the wrong anesthetic agent may also cause an anesthetic underdose or overdose, depending on the specific type of vaporizer and the anesthetic with which it is filled (see Table 16–4). Spillage of liquid anesthetic into the breathing system also may cause an inadvertent overdose.

What Are the Consequences of Inappropriate Ventilation?

Inadequate ventilation leads initially to hypercapnia and eventually to hypoxemia. Hypercapnia increases pulmonary vascular resistance and causes changes in acid-base regulation, serum potassium concentration, cerebral blood flow, and sympathetic stimulation, whereas prolonged hypoxemia leads to irreversible central nervous system damage.

What Should Be Done If a Machine Malfunction Is Suspected?

The course of action taken when an anesthesia machine malfunction is discovered or suspected depends on the specific clinical circumstances. The anesthesiologist should have a systematic, organized, and rehearsed plan for responding to equipment malfunction.

Hypoxic Gas Mixture

If the O_2 analyzer indicates a hypoxic gas mixture, I recommend immediate disconnection of the patient from the anesthesia machine. If the patient is not breathing spontaneously, ventilation can be supported using a self-inflating resuscitation bag. A Mapleson breathing circuit is not an ideal backup ventilation system unless it is accompanied by a separate E-cylinder of O_2 and a pressure regulator. An O_2 pressure source is necessary with the Mapleson circuit; if the anesthesia machine is suspected of delivering hypoxic gas, one does not want to connect it to the Mapleson circuit. Conversely, the self-inflating resuscitation bag can be used with or without an O_2 supply.

Inappropriate Anesthetic Dose

Underdose

If an anesthetic underdose is suspected, the concentration on the vaporizer is increased in an attempt to deliver additional anesthetic. At some point, the concentration set on the vaporizer will seem inappropriately high; at this time, a vaporizer or machine malfunction will be suspected.

The liquid fill level on the vaporizer should be checked to ensure that the vaporizer is filled with liquid anesthetic. Also, check the filler cap (see Fig. 16–10.9) and drain port to ensure that they are closed tightly. Small leaks in this portion of the anesthesia machine can result in the loss of all or nearly all of the anesthetic vapor. If these maneuvers do not improve the situation, use another vaporizer or intravenous anesthetics. Appropriate service personnel should be contacted to verify vaporizer performance and to check the contents of the vaporizer.

Overdose

If an anesthetic overdose is suspected, first turn off the vaporizer and turn on high fresh gas flows to wash the volatile agent from the breathing system. If an overdose continues to be suspected, smell the gas emerging from the fresh gas hose; minimal volatile odor should be present with the vaporizer turned off. Finally, disconnect the patient from the machine to guarantee that a volatile anesthetic agent is not being inhaled.

Anesthetic Agent Analysis

The clinical utility of an anesthetic agent monitor is readily apparent when one considers machine malfunctions that cause these problems. Without such a monitor, the anesthesiologist must make decisions with an incomplete data set; differentiation of patient variation and errors in titration from anesthesia equipment malfunction is difficult and sometimes impossible. Anesthetic agent analyzers eliminate this uncertainty.

Inappropriate Ventilation

If inadequate ventilation is suspected or if data from the spirometer and capnograph indicate such a condition, the cause must be sought. Leaks are suggested by low inspiratory pressure, whereas high inspiratory pressure suggests obstruction. When searching for the location of a breathing system leak, I divide the anesthesia machine into three components: (1) the ventilator, (2) the breathing system, and (3) the endotracheal tube and patient.

Ventilator

Ventilator-associated problems are easily eliminated by switching to the breathing bag and manually inflating the patient's lungs. If the leak disappears, its location is pin-pointed to the ventilator portion of the breathing system.

Breathing System

If the leak persists, disconnect the patient from the breathing system, occlude the Y-piece, and perform the standard positive-pressure leak check of the breathing system. If it fails to hold pressure, the site of the leak is in the breathing system.

Endotracheal Tube

If the breathing system is leak-free, the leak most likely involves the endotracheal tube cuff or a misplaced endotracheal tube. A leak around the endotracheal tube cuff is easily confirmed by placing a stethoscope over the larynx and auscultating during sustained application of positive pressure in the breathing system; if a leak is present, a rush of gas occurs.

STANDARDS AND CHANGES IN ANESTHESIA MACHINE DESIGN

What Are They?

Anesthesia gas delivery systems are durable and dependable pieces of equipment. Historically, anesthesia machine manufacturers followed the guidelines of the American National Standards Institute, which published standards for anesthesia machines in the Z-79 document.[25] Subsequently, for legal and other reasons, the American Safety and Testing Materials Society (ASTM) took over. Voluntary anesthesia machine performance guidelines are published in the ASTM F1161 document.[26]

Integration of Monitoring Instruments

Notable recent changes include the integration of monitoring instruments into the anesthesia machine. This feature ensures that the monitoring instruments are turned on with the anesthesia machine (an F1161 requirement for O_2 analyzer). Such integration also enables all data, on both patient and machine, to be available on a common data bus, which lends itself to automated anesthesia recordkeeping.

Elimination of the Ventilator Hose

Elimination of the ventilator hose represents an attractive design improvement, since critical incident studies indicated that ventilator-hose disconnection was a frequent problem. This configuration prevents disconnection of the ventilator hose from either its canister attachment or its attachment to the ventilator bellows because no ventilator hose is present to disconnect.

Isolation of the Adjustable Pressure-Limiting Valve

Similarly, isolation of the APL valve from the breathing system during mechanical ventilation is another important improvement. In this position, even if the valve is inadvertently left open during mechanical ventilation, the entire ventilator breath will be delivered to the patient; no gases will leak out of the open APL valve.

Measurement of Breathing System Pressure

Finally, newer anesthesia machines measure the breathing system pressure on the patient side of the inspiratory unidirectional valve. This previously discussed design improvement allows the airway pressure gauge, which is still physically located on the absorbent canister, to identify and measure PEEP.

FUTURE DEVELOPMENTS

What Changes Are Anticipated?

The newest feature for anesthesia machines will be the desflurane vaporizer. Also in the future, look for servo-control options to appear. One possibility is a mechanical ventilator that adjusts minute ventilation so as to maintain a user-specific expired concentration of CO_2. Similarly, automatic vaporizers will meter volatile anesthetic agents to achieve a specific inspired or expired concentration of anesthetic.

When Is an Anesthesia Machine Obsolete?

Exactly when an anesthesia gas machine becomes obsolete is difficult to determine. Intuition suggests that the design and safety features of contemporary anesthesia machines should decrease the incidence of patient injuries attributable to equipment malfunction and that older anesthesia machines without these features should no longer be used. However, solid scientific data addressing this issue are lacking. The suggestion has been advanced that more harm than good may result when a practitioner with years of experience who uses a particular "outdated" anesthesia gas machine is forced to replace it with a new, "safer" anesthesia machine with which he or she is much less familiar.

Yet, certain types of equipment-related patient injuries seem to be recurrent problems. For example, the copper kettle and vernitrol vaporizers frequently caused anesthetic overdoses in the past. They are no longer commercially available, and service contracts for them are no longer available; thus, in effect, they have been declared obsolete.

Following a panel discussion at the 1989 annual meeting, the ASA Committee on Equipment and Standards proposed the following *Policy for Assessing Obsolescence*, which was subsequently approved by the ASA Board of Directors[27]:

The age of an anesthesia machine has not been demonstrated to be a factor in anesthetic mishaps. An anesthesia gas machine, however, which no longer functions as designed and is not modified to meet acceptable levels of performance and monitoring should not be used.

Each anesthesia department should establish a protocol to assure that all anesthesia staff members are qualified in the operation of each type of gas machine, ventilator, and monitor in use.

The Anesthesia Patient Safety Foundation (APSF) Committee on Technology recently prepared a report that addresses obsolescence as it relates to anesthesia equipment.[28] Like the ASA policy statement, this document also notes that "age alone does not create obsolescence . . . neither does the failure to continue in widespread use." Modularity is viewed as an attractive feature that prevents obsolescence because " . . . failure of a module does not render the entire system obsolete."

Specific definitions of obsolescence are provided with regard to the maintenance (e.g., cost required to keep device working is too great), reliability (e.g., the device is not as "fail-safe" as newer devices), ergonomics (e.g., avoidable injuries occur owing to "user errors"), and function (e.g., higher morbidity than with newer alternatives) of anesthesia equipment.

The committee report goes on to note that " . . . the use of time threshold to define obsolescence introduces problems." Specific examples are given:

1. Time alone does not adequately characterize changes in function.

2. Failure with wear can be reversed with repair or replacement. A time threshold removes the option of repair.

3. Innovation does not occur at a constant rate. A time threshold can therefore trigger unnecessary replacement or delay necessary replacement.

4. A time threshold increases the probability of inadequate maintenance of older equipment (i.e., older equipment is not serviced if it is expected to be replaced by newer equipment).

5. A time threshold implies economic stability for manufacturers, even if they do not innovate, and thus reduces the incentive to innovate.

6. A time threshold causes economic expense for users, whether or not it is required for patient safety.

In the end, every practitioner must decide whether his or her anesthesia machine or any other piece of anesthesia equipment is obsolete. As should be evident from the aforementioned ASA and APSF documents, functionality and safety features, not age, are the characteristics on which this determination should be based. Anesthesia machine standards such as ASTM F1161 as well as texts such as this are designed to help each practitioner make an educated decision.

References

1. Good ML, Cooper JB: Monitoring the anesthesia machine. *In* Monitoring in Anesthesia. Saidman LJ, Smith NT (eds). Boston, Butterworth-Heinemann, 1993.
2. Anesthetic machines for use with humans. International Standards Organization Document 5358.
3. Health Care Facilities: NFPA 99. Quincy, MA, National Fire Protection Association, 1990, pp 59–63.
4. Characteristics and safe handling of medical gases: Publication P-2. 7th ed. Arlington, VA, Compressed Gas Association, 1989.
5. Eisenkraft JB: The anesthesia delivery system: Part one. Progr Anesth 1989; 3:1–9.
6. Raessler KL, Kretzman WE, Gravenstein N: Oxygen consumption by anesthesia ventilators. Anesthesiology 1988; 69:A271.
7. Andrews JJ: Understanding your anesthesia machine and ventilator: 1989 Review Course Lectures. Cleveland, International Anesthesia Research Society. 1989.
8. Good ML, Paulus DA: Complications during Anesthesia. *In* Equipment. Gravenstein N (ed). Philadelphia, JB Lippincott, 1991.
9. Eger EI, Hylton RR, Irwin RH, Guadagni N: Anesthetic flow meter sequence: a cause for hypoxia. Anesthesiology 1963; 24:396–397.
10. Hill DW, Lowe HJ: Comparison of concentration of halothane in closed and semiclosed circuits during controlled ventilation. Anesthesiology 1962; 23:291–298.
11. Hill DW: The design and calibration of vaporizors for volatile anaesthetic agents. Br J Anaesth 1968; 40:648–659.
12. Cooper JB, Newbower RS, Kitts RJ: An analysis of major errors and equipment failures in anesthesia management: consideration for prevention and detection. Anesthesiology 1984; 60:34–42.
13. Andrews JJ, Johnston RV, Bee DE, Arens JF: Photodeactivation of ethyl violet: a potential hazard of Sodasorb. Anesthesiology 1990; 72:59–64.
14. North American Dräger Operator Instruction Manual: Open reservoir scavenger. Telford, PA, North American Dräger, 1986.
15. Cooper JB, Newbower RS, Kitz RJ: An analysis of major errors and equipment failures in anesthesia management: considerations for prevention and detection. Anesthesiology 1984; 60:34.
16. Gaba DM, Maxwell M, DeAnda A: Anesthetic mishaps: breaking the chain of accident evolution. Anesthesiology 1987; 66:670.
17. Buffington CW, Ramanathan S, Turndorf H: Detection of anesthesia machine faults. Anesth Analg 1984; 63:79.
18. United States Food and Drug Administration: Anesthesia apparatus checkout recommendations. Rockville, MD, Federal Register, February 1987.
19. Carstensen P: FDA Issues Pre-Use Checkout. Anesthesia Patient Safety Foundation Newsletter. 1986; 1:13.
20. American Society of Anesthesiologists Newsletter. American Society of Anesthesiologists, October 1986, pp 5–6.
21. March MG, Crowley JJ: An evaluation of anesthesiologist's present checkout methods and the validity of the FDA checklist. Anesthesiology 1991; 75:724.
22. Mackie A: Drawover anaesthetic systems. Anaesthesia 1987; 42:299.
23. Borland CW, Herbert P, Pereira NH, et al: Evaluation of a new range of air drawover vaporizers: the PAC series—laboratory and field studies. Anaesthesia 1983; 38:852.
24. Keenan RL, Boyan CP: Cardiac arrest due to anesthesia: a study of incidence and causes. JAMA 1985; 253:2373.
25. Minimum performance and safety requirements for components and systems of continuous flow anesthesia machines for human use: ANSI Z79.8-1979. New York, American National Standards Institute, 1979.
26. Standard specification for minimum performance and safety requirements for components and systems of anesthesia gas machines: F1161-88. Philadelphia, American Society for Testing and Materials, 1989.
27. Lees DE: Older anesthesia equipment target of study, panel; ASA policy recommended. Anesthesia Patient Safety Foundation Newsletter 1989; 4:13.
28. Critical issues relating standards for technology to patient safety: a report by the Committee on Technology of the Anesthesia Patient Safety Foundation. April 1992.

CHAPTER 17

Airway Devices and Their Application

ORLANDO G. FLORETE, JR., M.D.

Establishment of a patent airway is essential to the practice of anesthesiology. Indeed, anesthesiologists must be procedural experts for quality airway management. To this end, familiarity with airway equipment is mandatory. Airway devices can be divided into two broad categories: (1) those that are essential and must be available, regardless of the anesthetic technique (facemasks, oral and nasal airways, laryngoscopes, and endotracheal tubes); and (2) those that are ancillary or adjunctive and used to facilitate airway control as dictated by the patient's peculiar anatomic characteristics and pathologic problem or by the surgical procedure (fiberoptic bronchoscopes, lightwands, specialized or modified laryngoscopes, tube changers, and other related devices).

In the operating room (OR), airway management may be performed simply with basic devices for oxygen (O_2) delivery such as a nasal cannula or facemask. Complete airway control is achieved by tracheal intubation and manual or mechanical ventilation. During emergencies, cricothyroidotomy or tracheotomy may be employed. Various resources are used to facilitate airway access, successful airway control, and adequate ventilation and oxygenation. This chapter addresses the different types of airway devices and their indications, contraindications, complications, techniques of utilization, maintenance, and care.

ORAL AND NASAL AIRWAYS

What Are Their Clinical Applications?

During anesthetic induction or emergence, patients often manifest signs and symptoms of airway obstruction. The most common cause is the falling back of the tongue into the oropharynx. Displacement of the mandible anteriorly and backward head tilt (Jackson's position) usually relieve the obstruction. Failure to correct the problem necessitates the use of an oral or nasal airway, which provides an artificial passage to airflow by separating the tongue from the posterior pharyngeal wall.[1, 2]

An oral airway is preferred to a nasal airway during induction owing to its ease of insertion and lesser likelihood of causing trauma and bleeding. During emergence, a nasal airway is much better tolerated as it reduces gagging, vomiting, and laryngeal spasm. An oral airway may also be inserted after

orotracheal intubation to prevent the patient from biting the endotracheal tube. The oral airway facilitates insertion of an esophageal stethoscope and nasogastric tube and allows suctioning of the mouth and oropharynx as necessary.

A nasal tube may be particularly useful in patients who develop masseter spasm or trismus. If the nares are partially blocked or if pharyngeal obstruction is only partially relieved by a nasal airway, an oral airway is preferable; however, it should be avoided in conscious or uncooperative patients. Nasal airways are contraindicated in the presence of coagulopathy, basal skull fracture, and nasopharyngeal infection or anatomic deformity.

How Are They Inserted?

Oral

Oral airways are metallic, black rubber, or, most commonly, plastic devices in the shape of an S or semicircular curve. They are available in various sizes, ranging from those suitable for neonates to those for adults. An appropriate size is one that holds the tongue in the normal anatomic position and follows its natural curvature. Adult sizes range from 80 to 100 mm (also labeled as numbers 3, 4, and 5). Sizes for children range from 50 to 70 mm (numbers 0, 1, and 2). Smaller airways are also available for premature and newborn infants.

Most commonly used are the S-shaped Guedel and Berman airways (Fig. 17–1). The Guedel design has a large flange, reinforced bite area, and a large tubular lumen for increased air exchange and insertion of a suction catheter. A specially designed metal airway (Patil-Syracuse endoscopic airway) is available for use during fiberoptic tracheal intubation. This device has a central groove to hold the endoscope in the midline. A slit is provided distally to direct it into the larynx. Lateral channels are also provided for suctioning.

The Williams airway intubator (round hole airway) is cylindric on its proximal half and open on the distal half of the lingual surface (see Fig. 17–1). It serves as an oropharyngeal airway, a means of intubating the trachea, and a guide for fiberoptic laryngoscope placement.

Insertion of an oral airway is enhanced with a tongue blade that depresses the tongue and moves it laterally. The oral airway is inserted by turning the curved side up, then by

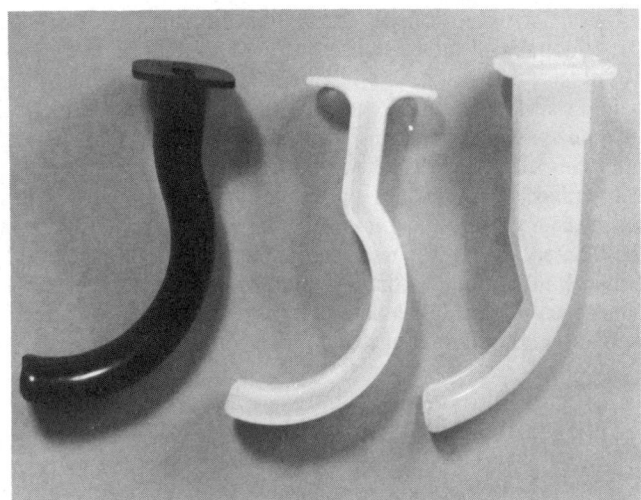

FIGURE 17–1. The Guedel oral airway (*left*) is commonly made of black rubber and is provided with a tubular lumen that facilitates airway exchange and insertion of suction catheters. The Berman oral airway (*center*) is a plastic device similar to shape to the Guedel airway but is not provided with an air channel. The Williams airway intubator (*right*) is made of plastic and is cylindrical on its proximal half and open on the distal half of the tongue surface. It has a central opening to allow passage of fiberoptic airway devices, endotracheal tubes, and suction catheters.

advancing it toward the posterior end of the tongue while rotating it 90° downward into the position of function. Alternatively, it may be inserted upside down and rotated 180° into the proper position.

Problems

Problems associated with oral airway insertion are uncommon. The gag reflex may be elicited in conscious or lightly anesthetized patients as may coughing, vomiting, laryngospasm, and bronchospasm. Therefore, they should only be used in unconscious, well-anesthetized, or comatose patients. Improper placement may push the tongue against the pharynx and aggravate airway obstruction. Malposition can also traumatize the teeth, tongue, and pharynx. Placement should be checked periodically, especially in long procedures.

If the patient's mouth cannot be pried open, and if time permits, one useful approach is to insert two tongue blades, one on top of the other, between the molars and then to place additional tongue blades between them until an adequate mouth opening is achieved.

Nasal

A nasal airway is a soft rubber or pliable plastic, uncuffed tube approximately 15 cm in length. It is useful for short-term airway management and is inserted via the naris into the posterior pharynx. It is better tolerated in conscious patients, in those with sensitive gag reflexes, or in instances when the oral route is inaccessible because of oral or lower facial trauma. Measurement of the tube size is based on its outer diameter and circumference and expressed in French sizes 28 to 30 for women and 32 to 34 for men. Smaller nasal airways for pediatric patients are also available. Most commonly used are the straight red rubber Rusch airway, the neoprene rubber Bardex airway, and the soft, pliable plastic modified Saklad nasal airway (Fig. 17–2). A binasal airway can also be used and is

provided with an adaptor that may be connected to the anesthesia machine.

Several important points should be remembered during insertion. First, the more patent naris should be selected. In patients with septal deviation, the airway should be inserted in the side with the smaller external orifice, since the ipsilateral nasal chamber is usually larger. Second, the nasal tube should be adequately lubricated with lidocaine jelly to facilitate insertion. A local vasoconstrictor like phenylephrine or 4% cocaine should be applied prior to insertion to minimize bleeding. Third, the length of the nasal tube to be inserted can roughly be estimated by measuring the distance from the nasal tip to the external auditory meatus. The tip of the nasal airway should be directed perpendicular to the face, not toward the cribriform plate. Insertion should be done smoothly and slowly; any resistance requires that the tube be gently rotated until no obstruction is felt. The tip of the airway should be at a point just above the epiglottis.

Problems

Complications associated with nasal airway insertion include epistaxis and nasopharyngeal trauma. Aspiration into the lower airway may occur. A large safety pin inserted off center at the top prevents this problem. A nasal airway should not be used in any patient with suspected or proven basilar skull fracture; otherwise it may be passed into the cranium.

ESOPHAGEAL, PHARYNGEAL, AND LARYNGEAL TUBES

How Are They Used?

Other devices for maintenance of a patent airway are available, but their role in the OR is undefined. They are confined

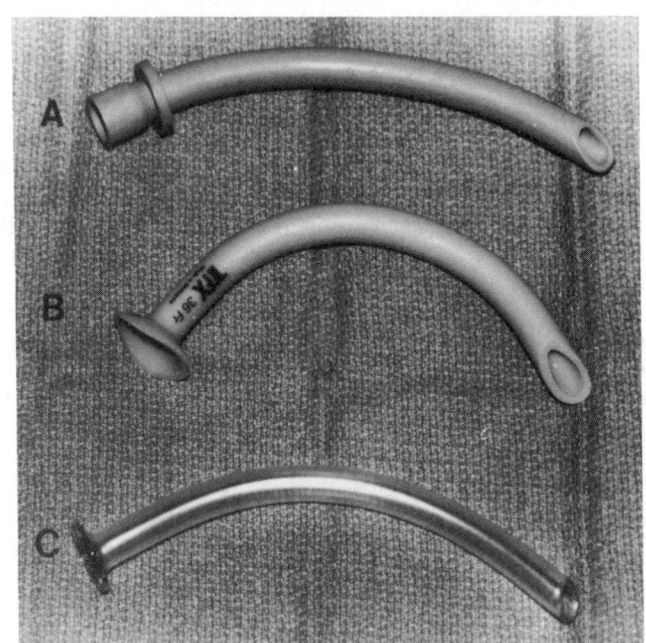

FIGURE 17–2. Nasal airways. *A,* The Rusch nasal airway is a soft, red rubber device with a firm, adjustable flange at the nasal end and a bevel at the pharyngeal end. *B,* The Bardex airway is a soft rubber nasal airway with a large flange at the nasal end and a bevel at the pharyngeal end. *C,* The modified Saklad-type nasal airway is made of plastic and has a small flange at the nasal end and a blunted bevel at the pharyngeal end.

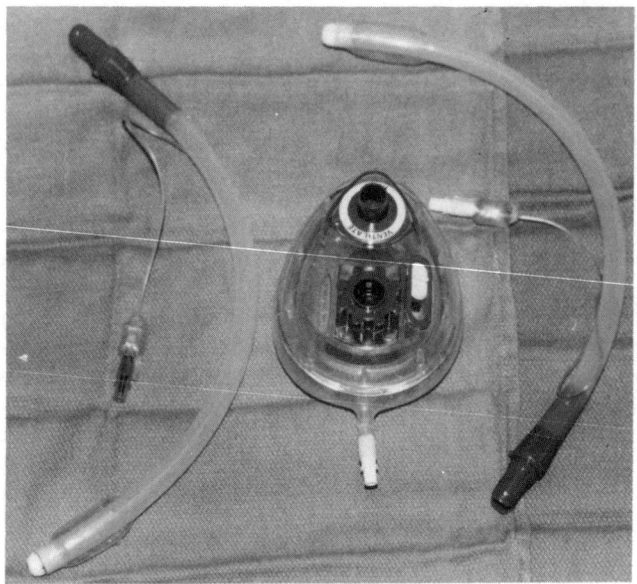

FIGURE 17–3. The esophageal obturator airway.

mainly to emergency situations and out-of-hospital resuscitation and include the esophageal obturator airway (EOA), the pharyngeal tracheal lumen airway (PTLA), and the esophageal tracheal combitude (ETC). Conversely, the binasal pharyngeal airway (BNPA) and laryngeal mask airway (LMA) have been used with variable success in the operating room.

Esophageal Obturator Airway

The EOA is a plastic tube 34 cm in length with a balloon at its distal end designed to be inflated in the esophagus (Fig. 17–3).[3] Sixteen holes 3 mm in diameter are present in the upper third of the tube and allow for the passage of air during ventilation. The EOA is attached to a self-sealing facemask and is inserted into the esophagus at a level just distal to the carina. Insertion does not require visualization and is facilitated by grasping the mandible between the thumb and the index finger and lifting it forward while the tube is inserted into the esophagus with the other hand. The balloon is inflated with 30 mL of air once the tube is in place, and the mask is fitted to the face. Air is blown into the tube through the small holes in the upper part of the tube into the airways. Inflation of the balloon prevents gas passage into the stomach.

Unfortunately, no convincing evidence of EOA effectiveness exists for clinical situations in which it has been used, (e.g., during cardiopulmonary resuscitation in prehospital cardiac arrest).[4–6] Complications, some of which are fatal, include esophageal rupture, inadvertent tracheal intubation and occlusion, massive gastric distention, vomiting, and aspiration.[7–9]

Pharyngeal Tracheal Lumen Airway

The PTLA is a modification of the EOA. This device consists of two tubes, an endotracheal tube and a shorter tube that is designed to terminate in the hypopharynx.[10] A large, 150- to 200-mL cuff is attached proximal to the port of the pharyngeal tube; inflation prevents oral and nasal secretions from entering the airway and prevents oral escape of air delivered via the pharyngeal tube.[11] A smaller, 30-mL distal cuff is attached to the endotracheal tube.

The PTLA also is inserted blindly, allowing placement of the endotracheal tube component into the trachea or esophagus. Once the airway is in position, air is injected into the balloon port, inflating both the oropharyngeal and endotracheal tube cuffs. Air is then blown into the pharyngeal tube. If lung inflation occurs, a resuscitator bag is attached to the tube, and ventilation is continued. If lung inflation does not occur when the pharyngeal tube is ventilated, the endotracheal tube is in the trachea. The resuscitator bag is then attached to the endotracheal tube and ventilation initiated, following which the pharyngeal balloon is deflated. Unlike with the EOA, the facemask is not required to maintain an effective seal.

Esophageal Tracheal Combitude

The ETC is a variant of the PTLA. Its proximal cuff is smaller than that of the PTLA and is placed between the base of the tongue and the hard palate.[12] It is inserted in the same manner as the PTLA. Ventilation is similar to that of the EOA except for the absence of a facemask.

Binasal Pharyngeal Airway

The BNPA is made up of two soft nasopharyngeal tubes connected to a suitable 15-mm male adaptor (Fig. 17–4).[13] It is inserted in both nares in a similar manner to that for a single nasal airway. This airway has been successfully used to ventilate patients in the operating room.[14] Gastric dilatation is unlikely because excess air escapes through the mouth. The BNPA is contraindicated in patients with full stomachs and specifically recommended only during difficult intubation when skilled personnel or more sophisticated equipment is not available.

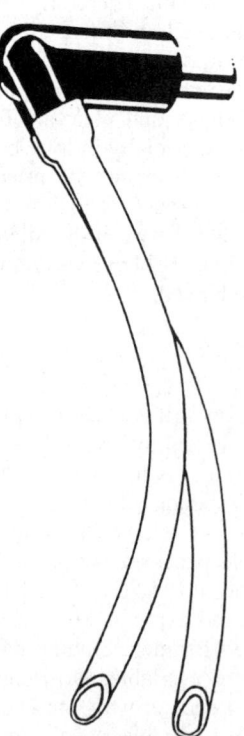

FIGURE 17–4. Binasal pharyngeal airway.

Laryngeal Mask Airway

The LMA consists of a shortened endotracheal tube attached to a cuff of a shallow facemask (Fig. 17–5).[14] It conforms to the shape of the laryngeal inlet and can be inserted without direct visualization. The tube is inserted facing backwards and is rotated 180° as it is passed downward into the larynx. Inflation of the cuff holds the device in place over the larynx, and the position of the mask is adjusted if a good seal is not obtained. This device does not require a laryngoscope for insertion. It is expensive but can be autoclaved and is reusable. It is widely used in the United Kingdom for airway management during general anesthesia[15] and is gaining some popularity in the United States. The LMA is available in various sizes (sizes 1, 2, 2½, 3, and 4) for neonates, infants, children, and adults.

Advantages

Smith and White found the LMA to be associated with fewer episodes of desaturation, less difficulty in maintenance of a patent airway, and decreased arm and hand fatigue when compared with a conventional facemask.[16] It can serve as an emergency airway during difficult intubation or when ventilation is not possible with a standard facemask and bag.[17–19] It can also serve as an airway conduit for an intubating tracheal stylet or fiberoptic bronchoscope, through which an endotracheal tube may be passed when airway management or intubation is difficult.[20–22] Fiberoptic diagnostic visualization of the airway and fiberoptic laser ablation of tracheobronchial tree tumors are facilitated as is management of patients with facial burns and those who need multiple anesthetics in a short period of time.[22–25] Finally, it may be useful in patients with unstable cervical spines, since its insertion does not require neck manipulation.[26]

Problems

The most common problem during insertion is failure to achieve correct placement as a result of inadequate anesthesia or inadequate relaxation; with failure to negotiate the 90° turn from the posterior pharynx to the hypopharynx; and with the selection of the wrong LMA size.[20] The device is difficult to insert in patients with small mouths, large tongues or tonsils, or a posteriorly displaced pharynx. The esophagus may be exposed to positive pressure, resulting in gastric dilatation and regurgitation. Failed insertion occurs in as many as 5% of attempts.

Contraindications

The LMA is contraindicated in patients with pharyngeal or laryngeal pathology; in patients who are at risk of regurgitation or aspiration or who have blood present in the upper airway; or when >25 cm H$_2$O peak inflation pressure is required to ventilate the lungs. It is relatively contraindicated for situations in which tracheal intubation cannot be performed immediately, for example, in a patient in the prone position or when the operating table is away from the anesthesiologist's field.[27]

FACEMASK/BAG-VALVE VENTILATION

Prior to tracheal intubation, and sometimes throughout surgery, oxygenation is achieved by ventilating the patient through a facemask. Currently available facemasks are made of black rubber or of colorless, clear plastic. An ideal facemask should be large enough to fit snugly over the patient's mouth and nose. It should have a soft, pliable rim to create an effective seal with the cheeks. A clear mask is preferred because it provides direct visualization of the mouth, lips, nose, emesis, or secretions. An airtight seal is necessary to allow adequate ventilation and avoids escape of the anesthetic agent during induction.

Various mask sizes are available for children and adults (Fig. 17–6). Some version of the Cornell anatomic mask is most commonly used in adults, whereas the Rendell-Baker-Soucek mask is commonly used in children because it is relatively flat, conforms well to a child's face, and has minimal dead space. The Patil-Syracuse endoscope facemask may be used during fiberoptic tracheal intubation. It has a port for the bronchoscope and permits endotracheal tube insertion.

How Should a Facemask Be Applied?

Facemask placement can be achieved by single-handed or double-handed technique. With the former method, the anes-

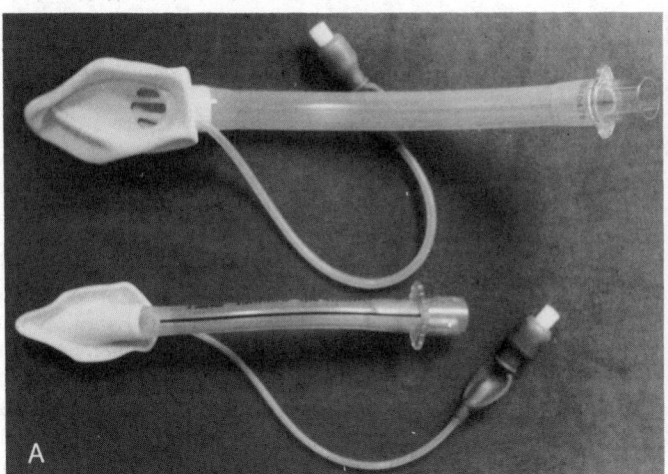 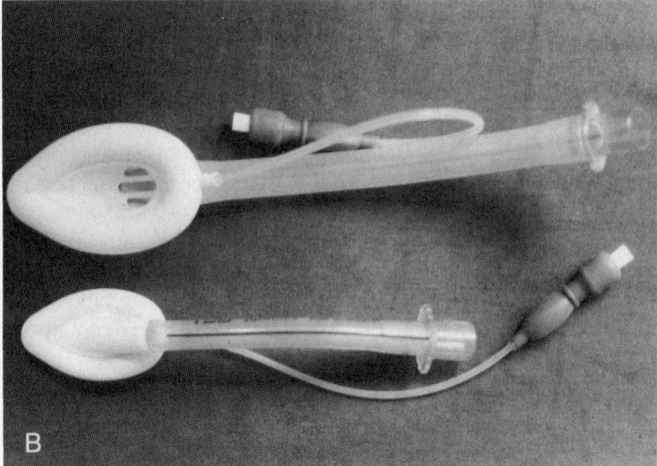

FIGURE 17–5. The laryngeal mask airway (LMA). *A,* A correctly deflated LMA that forms a smooth, flat wedge shape structure, allowing easy passage around the back of the tongue and behind the epiglottis. *B,* Properly inflating a LMA with the correct volume of air allows proper positioning of the device and provides a seal around the laryngeal aperture.

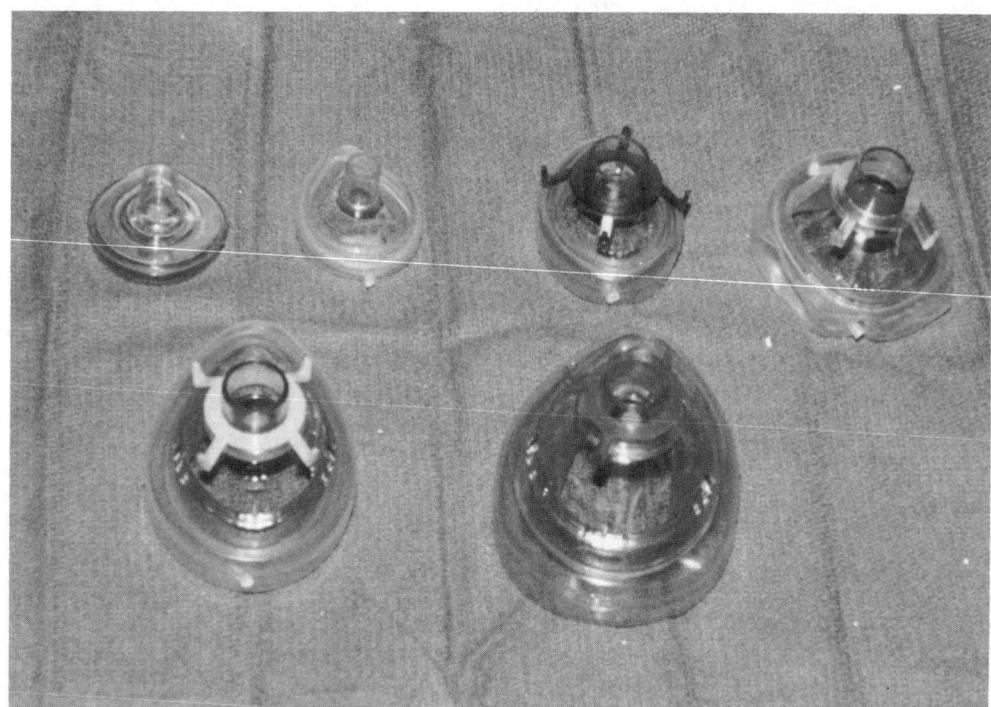

FIGURE 17–6. The most commonly used facemask is made of clear, colorless plastic with a soft pliable rim. It is available in various sizes for children and adults.

thesiologist fits the mask snugly on the patient's face, using the thumb and the index finger in a pincer grip while simultaneously displacing the mandible upward and lifting the chin with the other three fingers. The middle finger is placed on the anterior mandible, the ring finger is midway between the mandibular angle and the chin, and the little finger rests on the angle of the jaw. Pressure on the soft tissues should be avoided because it can raise the base of the tongue and can cause airway obstruction. It is also uncomfortable and sometimes painful to the awake patient.

On occasion, ventilation may be inadequate or airway obstruction may be unrelieved with the single-handed technique. If an oral or nasopharyngeal airway does not relieve the obstruction, the mask can be held by both hands. The fingers are placed as with the single-handed technique but on both sides of the face. The chin is lifted, and the mandible is pulled upward. An assistant is necessary to provide manual ventilation if the patient is not breathing spontaneously.

What Problems May Occur?

Problems associated with mask ventilation include inability to ventilate, pressure damage to soft tissues and the eyes, gastric distention, and pulmonary aspiration of gastric contents. If a tight mask strap is left in place over the facial nerve for a prolonged period, a facial nerve palsy may result. Cricoid pressure (Sellick's maneuver) may be applied during prolonged mask ventilation to avoid regurgitation of gastric contents. Decompressing the stomach with a nasogastric tube may reduce gastric distention but does not guarantee an empty stomach.

Is a Manual Resuscitator Bag Necessary in the Operating Room?

Although mask ventilation is readily achieved by connecting the facemask to the anesthesia machine circuit, in the rare instance of machine or breathing circuit failure, a manual resuscitator bag is mandatory. A manual bag also may be necessary or desirable during transport to the postanesthesia or intensive care unit. Various designs are available, but a self-inflating, manual resuscitation bag is preferable because it allows ventilation even if the O_2 supply is cut off (Fig. 17–7).

The standard parts should include a delivery port with a 15-mm inside diameter and a 22-mm outside diameter that can be connected to an endotracheal tube or to a facemask. The self-inflating system must allow delivery of an O_2-rich mixture. It should have a valve that allows both spontaneous and controlled positive-pressure ventilation. A positive end-expiratory pressure valve can also be incorporated. Pediatric manual resuscitation bags are usually provided with a 25- to 30-cm H_2O pop-off valve to avoid excessive positive airway pressure. Because the bag is usually reusable and is dismantled during cleaning, proper functioning and especially appropriate valve component reassembly must be assured before any attempt to use it is made.

LARYNGOSCOPES

What Are the Components?

Handles

The basic rigid laryngoscope incorporates a handle that allows attachment of various blade types. The power source is provided by batteries (C cells for adult handles and AA cells for pediatric handles). The handle surface is roughened to allow a better grip. The top has a crossbar to which the blade adaptor locks. When the blade is snapped into the position of use, current flows between electrical contacts at its base and the handle, and the bulb is illuminated. To ensure proper contact, the electrical contacts should be clean. The blade should be detached from the handle or folded when it is not in use. Failure of the bulb to illuminate indicates low battery power, bulb failure, improper blade positioning, or use of a wrong blade (e.g., the handle for fiberoptic blades cannot be used for standard blades with replaceable light bulbs because the contact points differ). The light source of a standard rigid laryngoscope is the light bulb; that for the fiberoptic bundle is in the handle.

Blades

The laryngoscope blade has four main parts: the light source, the flange, the spatula, and the blade tip. The light source allows illumination and visualization of the airway while the flange helps to guide the endotracheal tube. The spatula provides the means to compress and manipulate the tongue and soft tissue while the blade tip presses on the vallecula (curved blade) or supports the epiglottis (straight blade) for vocal cord exposure.

How Are Blades Shaped?

Curved

The MacIntosh (MAC) curved blade is designed to elevate the epiglottis when its tip is pressed into the vallecula. It provides increased space during intubation, reduces trauma to the teeth and epiglottis, and purportedly is associated with a reduced incidence of laryngospasm, since it does not touch the lower surface of the epiglottis. The MAC 1 (87 mm in length) is used for infants, whereas the MAC 2 (108 mm in length) is used for children. The MAC 3 (130 mm in length) is most frequently employed in adults, although a MAC 4 (158 mm in length) can be useful in large adults. The curved blade has a ridge that prevents the tongue from intruding into the path of vision. However, the ridge may also provide a fulcrum for leverage against the upper teeth when improper techniques are employed. The light source is located one-third of the blade length from the tip.

Straight

Straight blades commonly have a straight tip (the Jackson-Wisconsin blade) or a curved tip (the Miller blade [MIL]). The

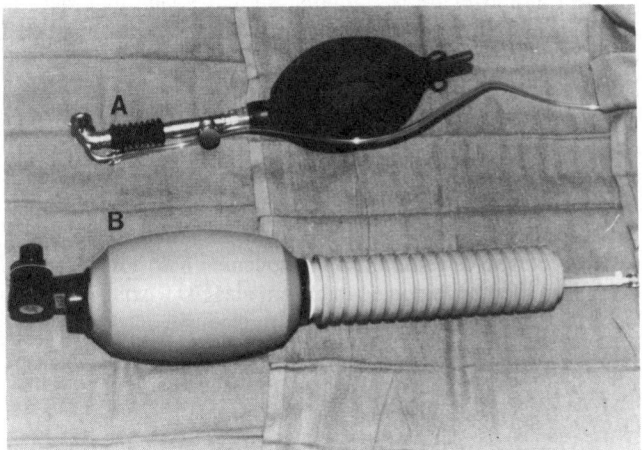

FIGURE 17–7. Commonly available manual resuscitation bags. *A,* The Mapleson bag is not self-inflating and requires a continuous oxygen source for proper functioning. *B,* A self-inflating manual resuscitator allows ventilation even if the oxygen supply is cut off.

blade is designed to be placed directly behind the epiglottis, which is then elevated directly to expose the vocal cords. It is the preferred blade for small children and is advantageous when the mouth opening is small or when the larynx is "anterior." It also has a left-sided ridge that protects the visual pathway from obstruction by the tongue. Its light source is located just behind the blade tip on the right side of the MIL and on the left side of the Wisconsin-Jackson blade.

The MIL is the most popular of the straight blades and is available in various sizes, depending on patient age. The MIL 0 is intended for premature infants and newborns, the MIL 1—for infants and toddlers, the MIL 2—for older children and average adults, and the MIL 3—for large adults. An MIL 4 is also available. Jackson-Wisconsin blades come in three sizes. A modification of this blade, the Wisconsin-Hippe blade, is especially designed for infants (aged 9 months to 2 years). Figure 17–8 shows the two most commonly used laryngoscope blades.

What Modifications Are Available?

Curved Blades

Siker

This blade allows visualization of an anterior larynx through a stainless steel, mirrored surface that reflects an inverted image of the cords.[28] This feature makes the blade difficult to use without practice, especially if the patient has a small mouth.[28, 29]

Huffman

A prism clipped to the base of the blade allows one to see the blade's tip without inversion of the image.[20, 29, 30] It is useful during difficult intubation when the larynx cannot be readily visualized with standard blades.

Bizarri-Guiffrida

This is a modified MAC blade with the left ridge removed and a light bulb placed in the blade's midportion.[31] It allows easy insertion in a patient with a small oral opening, short thick neck, or an extremely anterior larynx.

Fink

The Fink blade is a modified curved blade with the left ridge reduced in size at the hook, a wider spatula, and an increased curvature at the tip. Unlike with the Bizarri-Guiffrida blade, the light source is closer to the tip.

Polio

The angle formed by the blade and the handle is more obtuse (Fig. 17–9),[31, 33, 34] allowing easier insertion into the mouth. It is useful in patients with increased anteroposterior chest wall diameter that impedes handle rotation and blade insertion.

Blechman

The Blechman blade has an angled tip to further elevate the glottis in a patient with a short neck. Viewing is enhanced by removal of part of the flange near the lock of the blade.

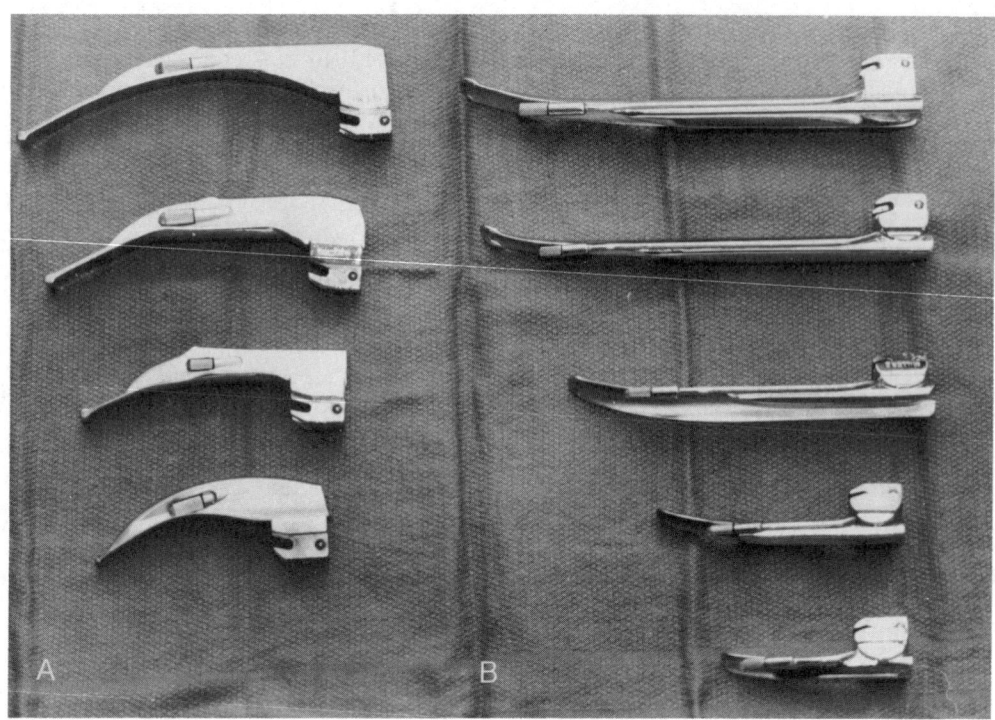

FIGURE 17–8. Laryngoscope blades. *A,* Curved (Macintosh) blades. *B,* Straight (Miller) blades.

Straight Blades

Guedel

The angle between the handle and the blade is 72° instead of 90°. The light bulb is located just behind the slightly curved tip.

Flagg

This blade has a C-shaped flange. An angle of 90° is formed between the blade and handle, and the light bulb is located just behind the tip.

Whitehead

This blade has a smaller left-sided ridge. It allows easy insertion in a patient with a small mouth opening and reduces pressure against the upper teeth.

Bennett

A reduced left-sided ridge (as with the Whitehead blade) is present, and the angle formed between the handle and the blade is 72° when in a position of function (as with the Guedel blade).

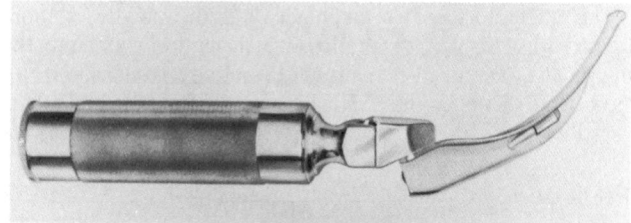

FIGURE 17–9. The polio laryngoscope. (From Dorsch JA, Dorsch SE: Understanding Anesthesia Equipment. 1st ed. Baltimore, Williams & Wilkins, 1975, p 236.)

Snow

This blade has a reduced left-sided flange and a raised tip.

Eversole

The C-shaped ridge is reduced over the distal half of the blade.

Bellhouse

The Bellhouse blade is modified by a forward angulation of 115° at the midpoint.[35] The spatula has vertical and horizontal components that are significantly lower than in the MAC blade. The light bulb is located near the tip. Alternatively, a prism can be added for a better view of the larynx.

Bainton

The Bainton blade is a tubular straight blade that can displace tissues circumferentially, permitting rapid viewing of the larynx when the pharyngeal space is limited. A tube 7 cm in length is present in the distal portion, and an intraluminal light source is protected from tissues that might otherwise cover and obstruct it.

Mathews

This blade is designed for difficult nasopharyngeal intubation. It has a unique petalloid configuration that allows the tip of the endotracheal tube to be guided between the vocal cords. Its peculiar shape also allows better visualization of the hypopharynx and the supraglottic area.

Handles

The Stunted Handle

This handle has a reduced height to facilitate blade insertion. It is particularly useful in patients with increased anteroposterior chest wall diameter, in pregnant patients, in patients with large breasts, or in morbidly obese patients whose body habitus causes the standard handle to press on the chest wall during insertion. The stunted handle has largely replaced the polio blade in this respect.

The Howland Adapter Handle

The handle is modified to allow changes in the angle between the handle and the blade.[29, 36] It decreases the angle and the axis that the blade makes with the horizontal axis of the patient and brings the handle forward, thus improving exposure. It may, however, be more difficult to use in patients with increased anteroposterior chest wall diameter.

The Seward Laryngoscope

This modified laryngoscope has a narrow handle and a small straight blade. It facilitates intubation of neonates and infants by improving access into the mouth and exposure of the larynx.

Other modifications incorporate adjustable double-angle or multiple-angle adapters that are useful in a patient with a receding mandible, anterior larynx, protruding teeth, bullneck, facial fractures, and decreased jaw mobility.[37–39]

BRONCHOSCOPES

Bronchoscopic devices allow easy and direct visualization of the airway and can be used as a means to pass an endotracheal tube. They permit verification of tube position and evaluation of the airway in patients with diffuse parenchymal lung disease, atelectasis, hemoptysis, and blunt chest trauma. Aspirates and tissue samples can be obtained for microbiologic, cytologic, or chemical analysis, and foreign bodies, excessive secretions, and blood clots can be removed from the airway.[40] Effective use of a bronchoscope requires skill and experience and should not be relegated to the newcomer.

What Types Are Available?

Available types include diagnostic (Negus and Storz), rigid intubating (Magill), rigid Venturi (Sanders injector), and flexible fiberoptic bronchoscopes.[41]

Diagnostic Bronchoscopes

Diagnostic bronchoscopes are rigid instruments inserted via the mouth to examine the trachea and the major bronchi. They allow extraction of foreign bodies and endobronchial resection of granulomatous tissue following prolonged or traumatic intubation. They can be fitted with a fiberoptic light source. The Storz bronchoscope can be used to ventilate a patient, using either the Sanders injector or via connection to a standard breathing circuit.

Rigid Intubating Bronchoscope

The rigid Venturi bronchoscope has a jet ventilator attachment.[42] It allows continuous ventilation and extends bronchoscopy time. However, the fraction of inspired O_2 available to the patient at the distal end of the bronchoscope is unpredictable as a result of air entrainment by the O_2 jet. Lung ventilation may be inadequate, especially if airway resistance is increased.

Flexible Fiberoptic Bronchoscope

The flexible fiberoptic bronchoscope is inserted via the nose or mouth and allows direct visualization up to the fifth bronchial branching. It is frequently utilized for preoperative assessment and management of a potentially difficult airway; as a conduit for the endotracheal tube during intubation; to verify correct single-lumen or double-lumen tracheal tube position; and to facilitate intubation in awake patients and bronchial toilet.[43–47] It is relatively easy to use, is associated with few complications, allows excellent exposure of the tracheobronchial tree, and does not require general anesthesia during induction.

What Should an Anesthesiologist Know About Fiberoptic Bronchoscopes?

Components

The standard flexible fiberoptic bronchoscope has three basic components: the light source, the elongated flexible portion, and the handle with the control section. The elongated flexible portion is marked in centimeters throughout most of its length and is provided with a distal bending section. The upward or downward movement of the tip can be controlled by manipulating the knob on the handle.

A channel or side port at the control section is provided, allowing O_2, local anesthetic, and irrigation fluid administration; attachment to a vacuum source permits the suctioning of secretions. It also provides access for a guidewire over which an endotracheal tube can be passed. A wire basket can be placed for the removal of foreign bodies from the airway, and a biopsy forceps or cytologic brush can be used to sample tissue for cytopathologic studies.

The handle has an adjustable proximal eyepiece and a control knob for upward and downward manipulation of the distal end. Pediatric and adult-sized bronchoscopes are available. A 4.5-mm endotracheal tube is the smallest tube that passes over current commercially available fiberoptic bronchoscopes. A teaching head may be fitted over the control section to allow others to see the airway as the operator manipulates the instrument. If the bronchoscope is inserted orally in an awake patient, a specially designed hollow, oral airway (oral airway intubator) should be used to protect the instrument against damage from patient biting.[48, 49]

Maintenance

The fiberoptic bronchoscope is an expensive and delicate instrument. To ensure that it ''survives'' and functions properly, appropriate handling and storage are mandatory. Prior to use, a clear, water-soluble lubricant should be applied to the elongated flexible portion of the endotracheal tube.[29, 36] Propylene glycol–containing ointments should be avoided, since they may damage the covering. An antifogging substance can be applied to the lens.

The distal end should be dipped in warm water for 30

seconds to minimize fogging, and suction should be applied to extricate any secretion remaining in the instrument. Avoid unnecessary bending of the flexible portion to prevent breaking the fiberoptic bundles. Fracture or break of individual fibers results in small black dots in the field of view.

After use, dip the distal end of the scope in soap and water and apply suction to remove any secretions. Sterilization may be done by soaking the flexible portion in a 30% ethanol solution or by gas sterilization. An anesthesia technician should be familiar with the care and cleaning of the instrument according to the individual manufacturer's specific recommendations.

Potential Problems

Hypoxemia

A number of complications are associated with fiberoptic bronchoscopy, which has an overall complication rate of 6.5% to 8.1% and an associated mortality of 0.01% to 0.04%.[50–53] Minor complications include bleeding, nausea, vomiting, vasovagal reaction, and fever. The patient may become hypoxic owing to prolonged suctioning, endotracheal instillation of lidocaine or irrigant, or respiratory depression secondary to sedative use. Hypoxemia-induced catecholamine release can predispose a patient to myocardial ischemia, cardiac dysrhythmia, hypotension, and, in rare instances, cardiac arrest. The incidence of bronchoscopy-induced hypoxemia is decreased by delivery of 100% O_2 either via facemask with a bronchoscope adapter or with a suction port throughout the procedure; by shortening the bronchoscopy time; by suctioning secretions intermittently for 10 seconds at a time or less; and by carefully titrating sedatives.

Laryngospasm/Bronchospasm

Laryngospasm or bronchospasm is seen in 0.1% to 0.4% of patients. It is more common in patients with reactive airway disease. Bronchodilator therapy before the procedure reduces the incidence of this problem.

Trauma

Damage to laryngeal, tracheal, and bronchial mucosa may occur; pneumothorax rarely has been observed. Epistaxis and severe hemorrhage may occur during nasal insertion of the bronchoscope. Other reported problems include allergic reaction to the premedications or local anesthetic, aphonia, pneumonia, mechanical trauma, subglottic edema, and upper airway obstruction on passage of the bronchoscope through an area of tracheal stenosis.

Failure to Intubate

Failure to thread the endotracheal tube over the bronchoscope after it has been inserted into the trachea is occasionally encountered.[54] The point of obstruction during oral bronchoscopy is commonly caused by the catching of the bevel at the distal end of the endotracheal tube by the right arytenoid cartilage, thus hindering smooth advancement into the trachea. Rotation of the endotracheal tube's radiopaque stripe to the patient's right places the Murphy tip under and slightly anterior to the epiglottis and corrects the problem. Similarly, during nasal fiberoptic intubation, obstruction may result owing to catching of the Murphy tip on the epiglottis. Rotation of the endotracheal tube (positioning the strip to the patient's left, which places the tip posteriorly) usually facilitates passage.

Miscellaneous Considerations

Certain conditions are associated with increased risks of complications. Bronchoscopy should not be performed when an experienced bronchoscopist is not available or when a patient is uncooperative. Patients with an unstable cardiac history, bleeding diathesis, untreated asthma, chronic obstructive lung disease, active untreated tuberculosis, advanced malignancy, persistent hypoxemia with supplemental O_2 and persistent hyperbaric pulmonary hypertension are poor candidates.

FIBEROPTIC LARYNGOSCOPES

What Types Are Available?

Newer devices with fiber-guided light paths for airway visualization and illumination are available.[36] They include flexible, malleable, and specialized rigid types.

Flexible Fiberoptic Laryngoscope

The flexible fiberoptic laryngoscope is similar to the bronchoscope. It is useful for oral and nasal intubation and has a laryngoscopic handle, optic bundle, and a port for suctioning or administration of O_2, local anesthetics, and irrigants. Its light source may be supplied by portable batteries within the handle; alternatively, a separate, high-intensity source may provide light through a fiberoptic cable. The eyepiece is adjustable, and a control knob can be manipulated to move the tip of the bundle upward or downward.

Malleable Fiberoptic Laryngoscope

The malleable fiberoptic laryngoscope is designed primarily for oral and nasotracheal intubation. It is most useful for patients with neck injury. A malleable fiberoptic stylet can be molded to the shape of the patient's oropharyngeal anatomy without the need to move the neck. The light source also is powered by portable batteries within the handle or supplied via a fiberoptic cable attached to a high-intensity lamp. Unlike the flexible fiberoptic laryngoscope, it does not have a channel for suctioning or drug administration.

The Rigid Storz Fiberoptic Laryngoscope

The rigid Storz laryngoscope is similar to a rigid bronchoscope and has excellent optical characteristics. The rigid stylet has a narrow diameter, which allows the endotracheal tube to be placed over it. Because of its rigidity, patient conformation to the configuration of the laryngoscope through neck extension may be necessary. It is, therefore, contraindicated in patients with suspected cervical injury. A fiberoptic cable attached to a high-intensity source provides illumination.

The Rigid Bullard Fiberoptic Laryngoscope

The Bullard laryngoscope is used primarily for indirect oral laryngoscopy.[55–59] Because of its shape and low blade profile, it requires minimal manipulation of the head and neck. It is useful in patients with abnormal or difficult airways and is available in adult and pediatric sizes.

Components include a handle, a blade that angulates 90° from the handle, and a halogen bulb that is powered by 2 C cells or a light post that accepts a fiberoptic cable from a light source. It has a fixed focus eyepiece with an optional snap-on diopter corrector. A teaching attachment provides an additional eyepiece.

Two working ports are between the handle and the viewing arm. The smaller one has a female Luer lock and may be used to administer O_2, local anesthetics, or irrigant solution, or to suction. A larger working port is used for insertion of an intubation forceps or a dedicated stylet. This port can be plugged by a rubber stopper if the smaller port is being used for suctioning or the administration of drugs or O_2. The pediatric Bullard laryngoscope is provided with a shorter blade and is recommended for use in patients up to 10 years of age (Fig. 17–10).[56]

Insertion

The instrument may be inserted orally in a manner similar to that used for an oral airway. Several techniques of tracheal intubation have been described.[52] A dedicated grasping forceps can be inserted through a channel in the scope to hold the endotracheal tube in place at the Murphy eye. The scope and the endotracheal tube are then inserted together into the oropharynx. Once the larynx is identified, the endotracheal tube is advanced by applying pressure on the thumb lever at the proximal end of the forceps. Additional pressure on the lever

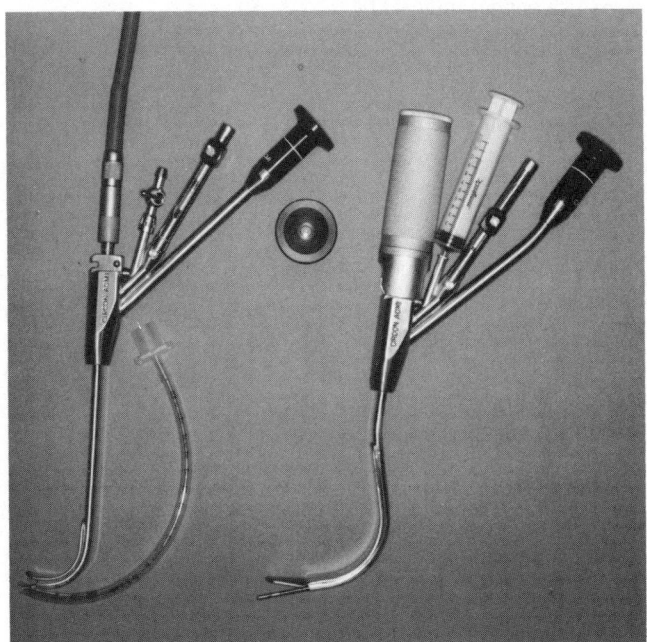

FIGURE 17–10. The Bullard laryngoscope. The pediatric Bullard laryngoscope (*left*) has a fiberoptic cable attachment. Note that the blade is smaller and that a pediatric endotracheal tube is held in place by a grasping forceps at the Murphy eye. The adult Bullard laryngoscope (*right*) is shown with a laryngoscope handle as the light source. The smaller working part has a syringe attachment to show the site to administer drugs, oxygen, or emergent solutions. The larger working part is used for insertion of the intubation forceps or a dedicated stylet. (From Bjoraker DG: The Bullard intubating laryngoscope. Anesthesiology Rev 1990; 17:64.)

releases the endotracheal tube, which is then inserted to its proper depth in the trachea.

The instrument also functions as a regular laryngoscope. A dedicated stylet may be attached at the same site as the forceps, thus maintaining the tube closely applied to the underside of the blade. The entire apparatus is introduced into the pharynx. Once the larynx is visualized, the tube is advanced into its proper position using the right hand. It allows minimal displacement of the tongue or epiglottis for visualization of the vocal cords, making awake intubation more comfortable than conventional laryngoscopy. It is safe for patients with an unstable neck and avoids the complications associated with nasal intubation.

Problems

Problems encountered with this instrument include inadvertent laceration of the endotracheal tube cuff by the forceps teeth during insertion and failure to intubate adults with longer necks owing to inadequate blade length. Complications associated with standard oral laryngoscopy may also be encountered.

The instrument is expensive. Maintenance and cleaning require proper training. It has several potential mechanical problems, and considerable training and familiarization are required before it can be used, especially in patients with difficult airways.

SINGLE-LUMEN ENDOTRACHEAL TUBES

How Are They Constructed?

Materials

Endotracheal tube design has progressed hand-in-hand with the development of anesthesia. Present-day endotracheal tubes are made of polyvinyl chloride, medical-grade silicone rubber, red rubber, nylon, or Teflon plastic.[60] Polyvinyl chloride is most commonly used. In its pure form, polyvinyl chloride is brittle, hard, inflexible, translucent, and degrades easily when exposed to heat. Chemicals are added during the manufacturing process to increase its flexibility (plasticizers) and stability (stabilizers).

Medical-grade silicone rubbers are opaque and very flexible. They bend easily, a quality that sometimes interferes with insertion unless a stylet is used. Red rubber is a natural product that has a variable composition. Such tubes are reusable and therefore less expensive to use than tubes made of different materials. However, certain chemical additives in the rubber may be harmful to the trachea; accordingly, red rubber largely has been supplanted by plastic.

Nylon tubes are rigid, lightweight, and reusable. Their chemical composition is variable, but they are nontoxic to tissues and can be sterilized by autoclaving. Teflon tubes are hard, rigid, reusable plastic tubes that can be boiled, steam autoclaved, or chemically sterilized.

Because of the many chemicals used in the manufacture of endotracheal tubes, extensive testing has been done to ensure patient safety. Most tubes are stamped ''I.T.'' (Implant Tested) or ''Z-79'' (Z-79 Committee of the American National Standards Institute) to indicate that they have been tissue-tested and are free of toxicity or irritant properties.

Components

Standard endotracheal tubes have several important parts: (1) the *bevel* is the distal, stented end of the tube; (2) the *cuff* is the inflatable sleeve around the distal end of the endotracheal tube that is inflated to provide an effective seal between the tube and the trachea; (3) the *machine* or proximal portion projects from the patient and is attached to the breathing circuit via a 15-mm adaptor; (4) the *pilot balloon* connects to the cuff and gives some indication of the cuff inflation pressure; in such instances, pressure is controlled through a pressure-regulating valve incorporated within the pilot balloon; (5) the *inflating pilot tube* connects the pilot balloon to the cuff; and (6) the *Murphy eye* is a side port near the distal end of the tube that allows ventilation when the main port is occluded by secretions, blood clot, or tracheal wall. Not all endotracheal tubes have a Murphy eye.

Calibration and Dimensions

Endotracheal tubes are calibrated in internal and external diameter (millimeters) as well as in length (centimeters). Oral and nasal tubes have a radius of curvature of 14 cm ± 10%. The bevel angle of oral and nasal tubes is 45° and 30°, respectively, in relation to their long axis except for smaller nasal tubes (<6 mm ID), which have a similar bevel angle as the oral tube. The bevel opening faces left in oral tubes; nasal tube bevels face in either direction.

The cuff length is generally 2 to 4 cm, and the maximum length of the cemented end is 1.0 cm. The distance between the cemented end of the cuff and the tip of the endotracheal tube is usually <13 mm except in tubes with an ID ≤4.5 mm, in which the distance is 5 to 6 mm. Cuff sizes vary with tube size.

Pediatric endotracheal tubes have single and double black marks located 2 and 3 cm from the tip of the tube, respectively. Endotracheal tubes are also provided with a stripe of radiographically opaque material along the wall to facilitate confirmation of tube position. Uncuffed tubes are generally used for children younger than 6 years of age. Since the smallest portion of the pediatric airway is at the level of the cricoid cartilage, which is circumferential, an appropriately selected uncuffed tube provides an adequate seal.

Special Modifications

Single-lumen tubes are most commonly used and can be inserted orally or nasally. They may be cuffed or uncuffed and vary in size from 2.5 to 11.0 mm ID. Preformed or RAE tubes are also available in oral and nasal forms. The portions that emerge from the nose or mouth are angulated to direct their proximal path away from the surgical field. They are useful in oromaxillofacial surgery.

Armored, anode, or wire-reinforced tubes have a spiral metal wire or nylon filament embedded in their wall that provides resistance to kinking or collapse. Their flexibility necessitates the use of a stylet during insertion. Owing to their flexibility and kink resistance, they may also be inserted through a tracheotomy or laryngectomy stoma and fastened to the skin.

The guidable tube (Endotrol) has a built-in stylet system and is useful for blind nasal or difficult oral intubation. A ring or trigger at the machine (proximal) end of the tube is provided with a thread that runs through a channel in the inner curvature of the tube wall up to its distal end. Traction on the ring decreases the radius of the tube's distal end, causing the curvature to increase and facilitating its guidance into the larynx.

Other single-lumen tubes are designed specifically for laser surgery.[61] Double-cuffed, silicone-coated metal tubes decrease the risk of fire associated with airway laser use but are expensive. Protected endotracheal tubes (wrapped with metallic tapes) also reduce the fire hazard. When properly wrapped with metallic tape or copper foil, red rubber tubes are more flame-resistant than are polyvinyl chloride, stainless steel laser-flex, and other commercially available laser-resistant tubes; however, the cuff still remains unprotected.

How Are Tube Size and Length Chosen?

Adults

Oral intubation generally requires an 8.0- to 9.0-mm-ID endotracheal tube for adult males and a 7.0- to 8.0-mm-ID tube for adult females. Tubes that are 1 mm less in size are used for nasal intubation. The tube's length from the alveolar ridge to the tip is usually 20 to 22 cm for females and 22 to 24 cm for males. For nasotracheal intubation, 2 to 3 cm is added to the length from the naris to the tube tip.

Children

For children, the internal diameter of the endotracheal tube is selected on the basis of age and size (Table 17–1). A tracheal tube one size above and below the calculated size should be immediately available to allow proper selection after visualization of the glottic opening. The following formulas can be used to calculate uncuffed tube sizes for children 6 years or younger in age:

$$\text{Size (mm ID)} = 4.0 + \frac{\text{age in years}}{4}$$

Equation 1

Alternatively, this formula can be used:

$$\text{Size (mm ID)} = \frac{16 \text{ to } 18 + \text{age}}{4}$$

Equation 2

An ideally sized tube allows a leak at 20 to 25 cm H_2O of airway pressure. If the leak occurs at ≤10 cm H_2O, the tube should be replaced with the next larger size (e.g., from 4.0 to 4.5).

TABLE 17–1. Recommended Sizes for Pediatric Endotracheal Tubes

Age of Patient	Internal Diameter of Tube (mm)*
Newborn	3.0
6 mo	3.5
18 mo	4.0
3 y	4.5
5 y	5.0
6 y	5.5
8 y	6.0
12 y	6.5
16 y	7.0

(Modified from Florete OG: Airway management. *In* Critical Care. 2nd ed. Civetta JM, Taylor RW, Kirby RR (eds). Philadelphia, JB Lippincott, 1991, p 1427.)
*One size larger or one size smaller should be allowed for individual intra-age variations.

The depth to which the tube should be inserted may also be calculated using a formula based on the child's age:

$$\text{(Oral) Tube length (cm)} = 12 + \frac{\text{age}}{2} \qquad \text{Equation 3}$$

$$\text{(Nasal) Tube length (cm)} = 15 + \frac{\text{age}}{2} \qquad \text{Equation 4}$$

These values estimate the distance of the tracheal tube from the alveolar ridge or naris to the tip positioned in the midtrachea.

Why Is the Correct Size Important?

Cuff Inflation

Appropriate endotracheal tube size and length are important, especially in children. Too large a tube may cause laryngotracheal trauma or failure to intubate. A higher incidence of postoperative sore throat, laryngeal damage, and tracheal stenosis also occurs when a tube that is too large is used. An inappropriately small tube may result in gas leakage, especially if it is uncuffed; conversely, with a cuffed tube, the cuff may have to be excessively inflated to maintain a seal, thereby creating a high-pressure cuff.

Resistance

Work of breathing and airway resistance vary inversely with tube size. For 1-mm decrease in the internal diameter of the endotracheal tube, the work of breathing increases by 34% to 154%, and the airway resistance increases by 25% to 100%.[62] This factor also emphasizes the importance of not using a tube that is too small.

Positioning

In adults, the correct position of the tracheal tube tip is approximately 5 cm above the carina. Neck extension moves the tip an average of 1.9 cm away from the carina toward the pharynx, whereas flexion moves it toward the carina. Lateral rotation moves the tube 0.7 cm away from the carina.[63] In children, the length of the trachea varies with age. The vocal cord–to–carina distance in newborns is about 4 cm.

Since the tube tip moves with head movement, the best approach is to verify position by auscultation with the neck flexed and extended after intubation to identify a tube that is positioned too deeply (potential mainstem intubation) or not deeply enough (potential extubation).

How Is Intubation Performed?

Orotracheal

Orotracheal intubation is most commonly employed because it permits direct airway visualization. It is fast and easy to perform in awake, sedated, or fully anesthetized and paralyzed patients. Awake intubation requires patient cooperation. It may be advantageous because airway reflexes are maintained with minimal depression of the cardiovascular, respiratory, and ner-

vous systems. However, gagging and vomiting may be induced. General anesthesia ensures patient "cooperation," removes language barriers, provides amnesia, and promotes muscle relaxation. However, airway reflexes are lost, inability to intubate may occur, and adverse drug reactions, although rare, may result.

Initial Steps

Administration of 100% O_2 for at least 1 minute (preferably 3–5 minutes) before intubation promotes denitrogenation, corrects underlying hypoxemia, and provides a buffer against developing hypoxia. The patient's head is placed in a sniffing position, aligning the axial plane of the mouth, pharynx, and trachea. A pillow or blanket elevates the head 10 cm above the shoulders and helps to align the pharyngeal and laryngeal axes.

Positioning

The anesthesiologist stands behind the patient, with the bed height adjusted so that the patient's head is at the level of the xiphoid. He or she holds the laryngoscope with the left hand so that the blade is below the hypothenar eminence. The right hand tilts the patient's head back, automatically opening the patient's mouth. Occasionally, the right hand may be placed inside the patient's mouth to open the jaw using the crossed-finger or scissors maneuver, which depresses the lower teeth with the thumb and raises the upper teeth with the index finger.

Blade Insertion

The laryngoscope blade is inserted at the right side of the mouth along the groove between the tongue and alveolar ridge; the tongue is swept to the left side by the flange of the blade as it is gently and deliberately advanced. A key concept to ensure optimal visualization is not to allow any part of the tongue to appear on the right side of the blade. A curved blade follows the base of the tongue anterior to the epiglottis, with the tip in the vallecula. Gentle pressure on the vallecula opens the epiglottis and exposes the vocal cords. A straight blade tip is used to lift the epiglottis. Once the blade is inserted, the handle is pulled forward; in this way, wrist flexion is avoided. This movement allows elevation of the tongue and visualization of the vocal cords. It also avoids injury to the teeth and maintains the larynx within sight.

Tube Insertion

Once the vocal cords are seen, the endotracheal tube is inserted at the right side of the mouth just lateral to the laryngoscope. An assistant may retract the right corner of the mouth to facilitate tube insertion. The tube is gently advanced between the vocal cords. A stylet may be used to guide the endotracheal tube into the larynx, but it should be removed as soon as the tube tip passes the cords. The tube is advanced 2 to 4 cm beyond the glottic opening in a child and several centimeters beyond disappearance of the cuff from view in an adult. The laryngoscope blade is then removed, and the proximal end of the tube is attached to the breathing circuit.

Cuff Inflation

The tube cuff is inflated with sufficient air to create a seal while positive-pressure breaths are delivered. Chest movement

TABLE 17–2. Common Errors During Intubation

Step	Error	Correction
Position	Axes not aligned	Put patient in ''sniffing'' position
Mouth opening	Mouth not wide open	Tilt back head or open mouth using crossed-finger technique
Blade insertion	Wrong size or wrong blade	Change blade
	Blade not inserted on right side of tongue	Withdraw blade and reinsert on the right side
Vocal cord exposure	Leverage rather than traction	Keep wrist rigid and pull handle upward and apply traction
Tube introduction	Obscuring line of vision of tube	Reinsert tube along right side of mouth lateral to path of blade
	Failure to maintain natural curve of tube	Use a stylet
	Angulation of trachea due to excessive traction	Release traction
Tube position	Endobronchial intubation/esophageal intubation	Auscultate for breath sounds; check chest radiograph
	Inadvertent extubation	Secure and tape tube in place

(Adapted from information appearing in the New England Journal of Medicine by Salem MR, Mathrubhutham M, Bennett EJ: Difficult intubation. N Engl J Med 1976; 295:879.)

is observed. Bilateral auscultation of the chest in the axillary area and over the epigastrium helps to confirm tube position. Table 17–2 lists the common errors that occur during intubation and the means to correct them.[64]

Nasotracheal

Although most patients are intubated orally, certain clinical situations require nasotracheal intubation. Patients with an unstable cervical spine who are conscious, those with a fractured mandible, neck abnormalities, temporomandibular problems, oropharyngeal infection, and those scheduled for oral or facial surgery may be candidates for nasotracheal intubation.

This technique is more difficult to perform, takes longer, and is more traumatic than oral intubation and often causes epistaxis. It may be performed blindly or under direct visualization with conventional laryngoscopy or fiberoptic bronchoscopy. Nasotracheal intubation is avoided in patients with basal skull fractures or bleeding diathesis, those receiving anticoagulant therapy, those with nasal obstruction or nasal fractures, or those at risk for bacteremia (i.e., patients with heart prosthesis or valvular disease). Details are provided in Chapter 55.

Problems/Considerations

Problems may occur any time during intubation, after placement, during extubation, and after extubation (Table 17–3).[64]

What Problems Are Associated with Cuff Inflation?

Endotracheal tubes for adults and children older than 6 years of age are provided with inflatable cuffs at the distal end. The cuff serves two purposes. Once inflated, it creates a seal against the underlying tracheal mucosa, making aspiration of pharyngeal or gastric contents into the trachea less likely. It also helps to prevent air leak, thereby facilitating positive-pressure ventilation.

High-Pressure, Low-Volume Cuffs

Cuffs are classified as either high-pressure or low-pressure. High-pressure cuffs have low volume and compliance and can exert as much as 180 to 250 mm Hg of pressure on the tracheal mucosa before creating an effective seal. When inflated, these cuffs are spherical and narrow and have a small area of tracheal contact. They expand the trachea until the normal C-shaped tracheal contour is lost, at which point the trachea is forced to assume the cuff's shape.[65]

High cuff pressure transmission exceeds the capillary perfusion pressure (normally 25–35 mm Hg), and ischemia results. Persistent ischemia leads to tracheal necrosis, stricture, or tracheoesophageal fistula formation. The mechanism of high pressure–induced tracheal injury is illustrated in Figure 17–11.[66] Low compliance cuffs may also expand asymmetrically, deforming the trachea and producing tracheal dilatation. When tracheal injury occurs, the rigid, nonyielding tracheal

TABLE 17–3. Risks of Tracheal Intubation/Extubation

Time	Tissue Injury	Mechanical Problems	Other
Tube placement	Corneal abrasion; nasal polyp dislodgment; bruise/laceration of lips/tongue; tooth extraction; retropharyngeal perforation; vocal cord tear; cervical spine subluxation or fracture; hemorrhage; turbinate bone avulsion	Esophageal/endobronchial intubation; delay in cardiopulmonary resuscitation	Dysrhythmia; pulmonary aspiration; hypertension; hypotension
Tube in place	Tear/abrasion of larynx, trachea, bronchi	Airway obstruction; migration of tube; ignition of tube during laser surgery	Bacterial infection (secondary); pulmonary aspiration; paranasal sinusitis; problems related to mechanical ventilation (e.g., pulmonary barotrauma)
Extubation	Damage to vocal cords (failure to deflate cuff)	Difficult extubation; airway obstruction from blood; foreign bodies, dentures, or throat packs	Pulmonary aspiration; laryngeal edema; laryngospasm; tracheomalacia

(Modified from Florete OG: Airway management. *In* Critical Care. 2nd ed. Civetta JM, Taylor RW, Kirby RR (eds). Philadelphia, JB Lippincott, 1991, p 1427.)

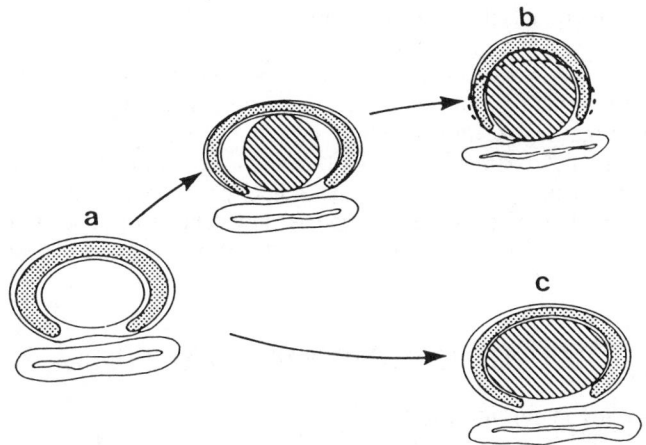

FIGURE 17–11. Mechanism of tracheal injury by high-pressure cuff inflation. A high-pressure cuff produces a narrow, spherically shaped structure with a small area of tracheal contact. It expands the trachea until the normal C-shape of the tracheal form is lost and the trachea assumes the cuff's shape. Pressure on the tracheal wall exceeds capillary perfusion pressure, resulting in mucosal ischemia, inflammation, hemorrhage, and ulceration. This ultimately leads to tracheal dilatation, granuloma formation, tracheomalacia, tracheal stenosis, and, in some instances, erosion into the innominate artery. (From Cooper JD, Grillo HC: The evolution of tracheal injury due to ventilatory assistance through cuffed tubes: a pathologic study. Ann Surg 1969; 169:334.)

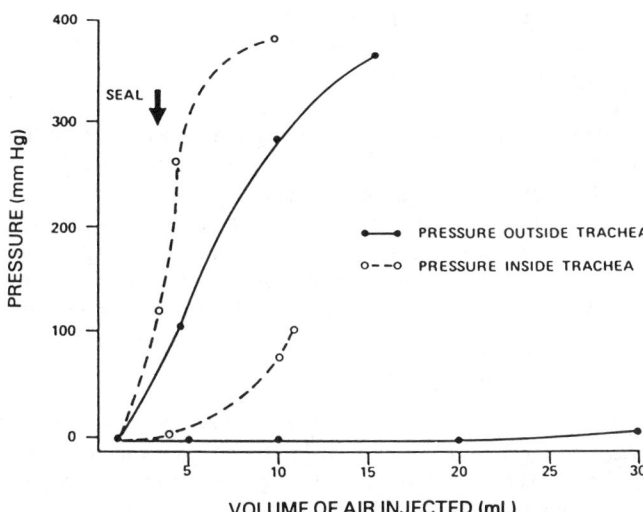

FIGURE 17–12. Difference in volume and pressure curves of low-pressure and high-pressure endotracheal tube cuffs. *Solid* and *dotted lines* show the volume and pressure curves of low-pressure and high-pressure cuffs, respectively. (From Dunn CR, Dunn DL, Moser KH: Determinants of tracheal injury by cuffed tracheostomy tubes. Chest 1974; 65:128.)

wall suffers more extensive damage than does the posterior membranous portion.[66–68]

Low-Pressure, High-Volume Cuffs

Low-pressure, high-volume cuffs adapt to the tracheal contour without deforming its shape. When used correctly, they inflate symmetrically and provide a seal with the trachea at relatively low intraluminal cuff pressures. Their sausage-like shape allows the pressure to be transferred to the trachea over a wide area, causing a lower tracheal wall pressure at any given point. The lower pressure causes less obstruction to mucosal blood flow than occurs with high-pressure cuffs.[69–71] Pressures >25 mm Hg cause at least partial obstruction to tracheal mucosal perfusion.[72–75]

Remember that even at low cuff pressures, normal tracheal mucosal architecture may be disrupted. Superficial histologic damage and ciliary denudation have been observed at the cuff site when pressure was <25 mm Hg.[72, 76] Figure 17–12 shows the comparison of the pressure volume curves of high-pressure and low-pressure cuffs before and after placement in the trachea, clearly illustrating the significant difference in intracuff pressure necessary to create a seal.[77]

Cuff Size

Although available modern endotracheal tubes are classified as low-pressure and high-volume, not all behave the same way under different clinical settings.[78] Cuffs of nearly identical diameter (internal diameters one and one-half times that of the trachea) but of different lengths provide an equal and adequate tracheal seal at peak inflation pressures <25 mm Hg. When lung compliance is reduced and peak inflation pressure is increased to 80 cm H₂O, shorter cuffs need an inflation pressure of nearly 50 mm Hg compared with one of only 30 mm Hg in longer ones. The difference in performance is attributed to the length of their tracheal contact. The distal ends of both cuffs

collapse when the peak airway pressure is increased, whereas the proximal end bulges outward, changing the cuff shape from cylindric to conical (Fig. 17–13).[78]

Inflation Volume and Pressure

Ideally, the cuff should be inflated to a point that allows a seal without jeopardizing tracheal mucosal blood flow. Careful monitoring and control of cuff pressure is necessary to prevent significant changes. Patients with poor lung compliance or high airway resistance may require higher pressure to seal, thus limiting the protection afforded by low-pressure, high-volume cuffs.[78] During general anesthesia with nitrous oxide, intracuff pressure increases because of nitrous oxide diffusion into the cuff.[79–81] This can be prevented by inflating the cuff with gas from the breathing circuit rather than with air.[82, 83]

Following prolonged intubation, cuff pressures have been observed to decrease with time, although the magnitude of decrease and time were not correlated.[84] This reduction is believed to be due to diffusion of gas and to slow movement (creeping) of plastic in the cuff. Intermittent increases occur during positive-pressure ventilation if the airway pressure exceeds that in the cuff. Transient large increases are seen during coughing, chest physiotherapy, and when a patient struggles with the ventilator.[85]

Measurement of Pressure and Volume

Measurement and monitoring of intracuff volume and pressure are necessary during prolonged periods of tracheal intubation. The equipment is simple and composed of a sphygmomanometer and a syringe attached to the female port of a three-way stopcock.[60] The male element of the stopcock is attached to the pilot balloon in the closed position to prevent air escape from the pilot line. After suctioning the pharynx free of secretions, the stopcock is opened, and the entire air volume is aspirated and measured. The air is then reinjected back into the cuff, and the stopcock is again turned to the off position. The stopcock is then rotated to the second orifice to allow cuff pressure to be measured by the sphygomanometer. It is then rotated once again to allow air from the cuff to be aspirated into the syringe.

The volume obtained at this point is lower than the original volume because some of the air filling the pressure measuring system previously was in the cuff. Additional air is reinjected into the cuff to compensate for that lost to the manometer tube, and the stopcock is again rotated to the position that allows pressure to be read from the manometer. This pressure is higher than the initial reading and is the true intracuff pressure, compensated for the volume of air in the manometer.

Minimal Leak Cuff Inflation

To minimize the possibility of an excessively high intracuff pressure, the minimal leak inflation technique is increasingly preferred. The cuff is inflated during positive-pressure ventilation until total occlusion occurs between the cuff and the tracheal wall. Air is then gradually aspirated until a minimal air leak is heard at peak inspiratory pressure. The tidal volume is then adjusted to compensate for the minimal loss through the leak in this system. This approach minimizes tracheal damage at low to moderate peak inflation pressure but not when very high ventilatory pressure is necessary.

No Leak Cuff Inflation

In some clinical situations, the minimal leak technique may not be helpful, and total occlusion is desirable, particularly for patients who aspirate repeatedly, have poor lung compliance, or require high levels of positive end-expiratory pressure to maintain adequate ventilation and oxygenation. In these instances, a "no leak" technique with minimal occluding volume is used to inflate the cuff. This approach requires fre-

quent, round-the-clock monitoring of intracuff pressure and volume.

To assure that minimum pressure and volume are used, the cuff is inflated and deflated in a similar manner as for the minimal leak technique. Once a minimal leak is observed, an additional volume of air is slowly injected until no leak is appreciated. This process is periodically repeated. This technique of cuff pressure inflation is prevalent in the operating room to avoid contamination of the room with anesthetic gases.

DOUBLE-LUMEN ENDOTRACHEAL TUBES

What Is Their Role?

Double-lumen tubes (DLTs) are primarily utilized for one-lung ventilation.[86] These devices functionally consist of two tubes attached together, side by side, with one side longer than the other and with the tip curved to the longer side. They are available with a left-sided or right-sided orientation. The former allows placement of the left catheter into the left mainstem bronchus and the right catheter into the trachea. The latter functions in opposite fashion.

Regardless of the type or manufacturer, DLTs have common characteristics, as shown in Figure 17–14.[87] Two pilot balloons are provided, one of which leads to the tracheal cuff and the other to the bronchial cuff (as indicated by a capital "T" [trachea] or "B" [bronchial] label). The distal portion of the tube has two lumens. Currently, left-sided endobronchial tubes are preferred because of their ease of placement and margins of safety.

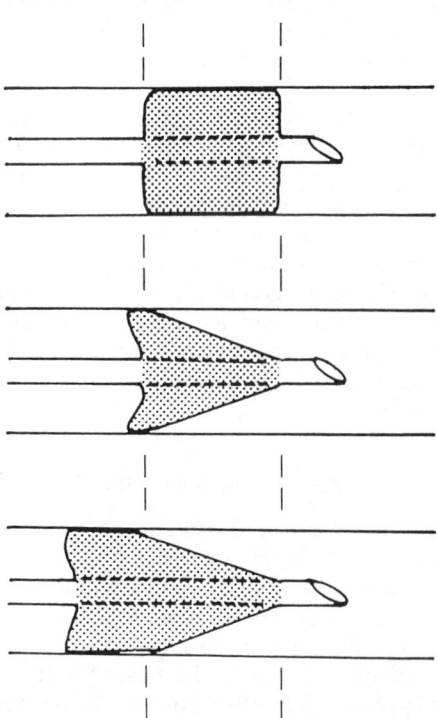

FIGURE 17–13. Effect of increased peak airway pressure on an endotracheal tube cuff's shape (see text for explanation). (From Guyton DC: Endotracheal and tracheotomy tube cuff design: influence on tracheal damage. Crit Care Updates 1990; 1:1.)

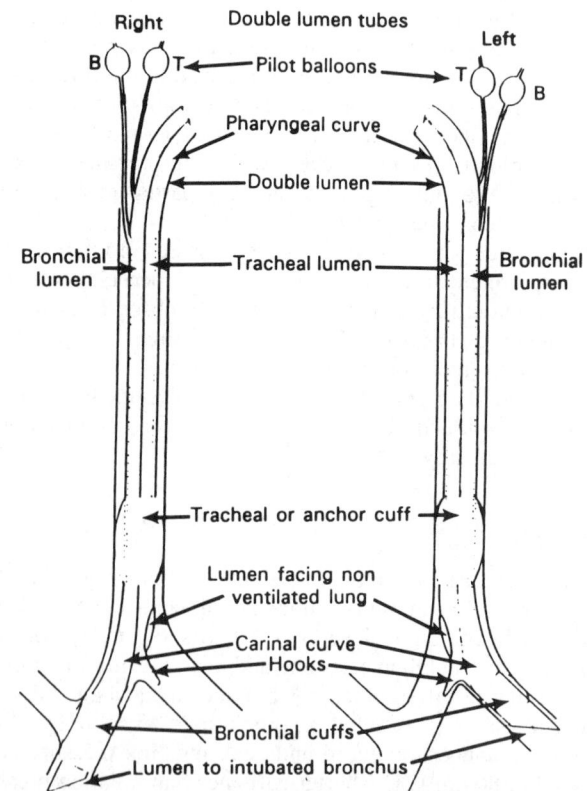

FIGURE 17–14. Parts of right-sided and left-sided double-lumen tubes. (From Vaughan RS: Endobronchial intubation. *In* Difficulties in Tracheal Intubation. Latto IP, Rosen M (eds). London, Bailliere Tindall, 1983, p 158.)

What Types Are Available?

The Carlens Tube

The Carlens DLT was the first such tube used in anesthesia. It is left-sided and made of soft rubber or plastic and has tracheal and bronchial cuffs, two pilot balloons, and a carinal hook to facilitate tube placement and to avoid distal tube movement. Occasionally, the carinal hook may be amputated during or after intubation and may make intubation difficult. It may also cause laryngeal trauma, tube malposition, or physical interference during surgery.[88] Four sizes are available: 35, 37, 39, and 41 French (with internal diameters of 5.0, 5.5, 6.0, and 6.5 mm, respectively).

The White Tube

The White tube is essentially a right-sided Carlens tube.[89] It has a slotted cuff on its right side, thus permitting right upper lobe ventilation.

The Bryce Smith Tube

The Bryce Smith tube has right-sided and left-sided versions. It lacks a carinal hook, and the right-sided version has a slotted cuff that promotes right upper lobe ventilation.

The Robertshaw Tube

The Robertshaw tube has an enlarged lumen to decrease resistance to airflow and facilitate suctioning of secretions.[90] The original design was made of reusable red rubber, but this has been replaced by a modern version made of disposable, clear, nontoxic tissue-implantable plastic.[91] It does not have a carinal hook; this facilitates tube insertion and permits ligation of a mainstem bronchus close to the carina for pneumonectomy.[92] Left-sided or right-sided tubes are available. The right-sided version has a slotted tip in the endobronchial cuff, permitting right upper lobe ventilation. The left-sided model has a beveled bronchial lumen with restricted bronchial cuff inflation on the medial side. This design reduces interference with right lung ventilation.

Tube sizes are 28, 35, 37, 39, and 41 French (with internal diameters for each lumen of 4.5, 5.0, 5.5, 6.0, 6.5 mm, respectively). Only a left-sided tube is available in the 28 French size. Both cuffs are low-pressure and high-volume. The bronchial cuff is colored bright blue, allowing easy recognition during fiberoptic bronchoscopy. The tube also has a black radiopaque line at the end of both lumens that is used as a radiographic marker. Malleable stylets and nonadhering suction catheters are usually provided in the package of the disposable Robertshaw tube.

What Are the Indications?

For thoracotomies requiring ventilation of the left lung and collapse of the right, a left-sided DLT should be utilized. For left thoracotomies, either a left-sided or right-sided tube may be used. If a right-sided tube is selected, the ventilation slot in the endobronchial cuff should be closely opposed to the right upper lobe orifice to permit unobstructed right upper lobe ventilation. The best way to achieve this precise positioning of the ventilation slot is to position it using the flexible fiberoptic bronchoscope. Otherwise, because of wide anatomic variation in the exact position of the right upper lobe opening and in the length of the right mainstem bronchus, the slot of the endobronchial cuff may not be in proper position, resulting in the risk of inadequate right upper lobe ventilation. This problem accounts for the popularity of the left-sided tube even during left lung surgery.[93, 94] If the left mainstem bronchus needs to be clamped, the DLT can be pulled back into the trachea and used as a single-lumen tracheal tube to ventilate the right lung.

What Are the Contraindications?

The presence of strictures, tumors, tracheobronchial disruption, extraluminal compression of the airway (e.g., aortic arch aneurysm) or any lesion along the double tube's pathway contraindicates DLT use. Such tubes are relatively contraindicated in patients with full stomachs or at high risk of aspiration; critically ill patients with a single-lumen endotracheal tube in place who cannot tolerate even a short period of removal from mechanical ventilation; and instances in which it is difficult or impossible to perform conventional, direct vision intubation.[86] Tenting of the left mainstem bronchus with a take-off angulation from the trachea of 90° or greater may make insertion of the left endobronchial tube extremely difficult and hazards left mainstem bronchus injury.

How Are They Inserted?

Insertion of the DLT may be performed using conventional laryngoscopy or fiberoptic bronchoscopy. If conventional laryngoscopy is selected, a MAC blade is preferable because it approximates the tube's curvature. Once the vocal cords are visualized, the tube is inserted into the mouth with the concave side up; it is then rotated 90°. As the tube tip passes the larynx, the stylet is removed, and the tube is rotated 90° back to the original position in order to advance the bronchial portion into the appropriate bronchus. Turning the head and neck to the opposite side may facilitate insertion. Advancement continues until the proximal end of the double-lumen binder mold is near or at the level of the teeth, or when mild resistance to further advancement is encountered, indicating that the tube tip is positioned endobronchially. The tracheal and bronchial cuffs are then inflated. Generally, less than 3 mL of air is required to inflate the bronchial cuff.

Verification of Placement

Bilateral ventilation is checked by delivering several positive-pressure breaths, auscultating breath sounds, and observing the chest. If only one side of the chest moves and unilateral breath sounds are appreciated, both lumens may have entered a single mainstem bronchus. The cuffs should be deflated and the tube withdrawn 1 to 2 cm at a time. The cuffs are reinflated, the chest is observed for movement, the lungs are auscultated until bilateral chest movement is seen, and breath sounds are heard equally in both lung fields.

If the tube is in its proper place, clamping of one connecting tube results in disappearance of breath sounds on the ipsilateral side. Only the contralateral side of the chest rises and falls with ventilation, giving it a rocking-boat motion. Tube con-

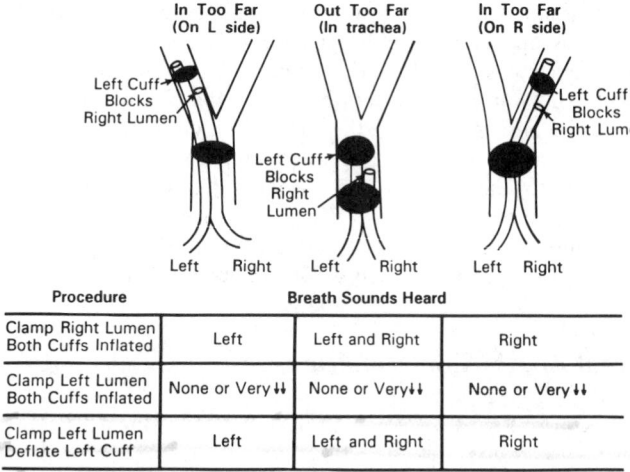

Procedure	Breath Sounds Heard		
Clamp Right Lumen Both Cuffs Inflated	Left	Left and Right	Right
Clamp Left Lumen Both Cuffs Inflated	None or Very ↓↓	None or Very↓↓	None or Very ↓↓
Clamp Left Lumen Deflate Left Cuff	Left	Left and Right	Right

FIGURE 17–15. Different types of double lumen tube malpositioning. (From Benumof JL: Anesthesia for thoracic surgery. International Anesthesia Research Society, 1988 Review Course Lectures, p 120.)

densation is only observed on exhalation from the ventilated side. The ventilated lung should feel reasonably compliant and easy to ventilate.

Breath sounds should be equally appreciated at the basal, medial, and apical portions. If right-sided apical breath sounds are not audible, the upper lobe on that side may not be ventilated. Pulling the tube back 1 cm at a time until apical breath sounds are heard corrects the problem. If the lumen cap is opened proximal to the clamp, no air leakage should be noted to indicate adequate seal by the bronchial cuff. Once the clamp is removed and the lumen cap is replaced, bilateral breath sounds and chest movement should be observed. Further confirmation of tube placement must be done by chest radiography or fiberoptic visualization.

Malpositioning

If the patient is moved and repositioned, tube position should again be reconfirmed; head flexion may advance the tracheal tube into the mainstem bronchus or cut off right upper lobe ventilation. Head extension may cause the bronchial cuff to move out of the mainstem bronchus.[95, 96]

Three major malpositions of the DLT have been described following blind insertion (Fig. 17–15).[96] They can be ascertained by chest auscultation combined with unilateral clamping and by endobronchial cuff inflation-deflation. When the left cuff is inflated and the left lumen is clamped, ventilation occurs only through the right lumen. In all three malpositions, this maneuver results in blockage of the right lumen, and breath sounds are either absent or diminished. When the left cuff is deflated, breath sounds are heard only on the left if the tube is too far into the left bronchus; bilateral breath sounds are heard if the tube is out too far in the trachea; and only right breath sounds are appreciated if the tube is too far into the right bronchus.

If the patient has pre-existing lung disease, breath sounds may not be a good indicator of proper tube positioning, and fiberoptic bronchoscopy should be used to confirm position. The tube may only be slightly malpositioned and thus difficult to diagnose. Also, surgical manipulation, head movement, or patient turning during the procedure may change the position of the tube. In all cases, ready access to and use of fiberoptic bronchoscopy is considered by many to be essential to avoid complications of malpositioning.

Fiberoptic Bronchoscopic Examination

The blind method of DLT insertion is associated with a high failure rate and malposition (25–48%), even when clinical signs indicate proper tube position.[97, 98] Fiberoptic bronchoscopy is associated with a more accurate placement.[93, 98–100] Some argue, however, that routine use of fiberoptic bronchoscopy to position a DLT is unnecessary, expensive, and time consuming and discourages the use of such tubes.[101, 102] Furthermore, movement of the tube is likely to occur several times during surgery as a result of the patient's positioning, surgical procedure, or head movement, making the use of fiberoptic bronchoscopy impractical.

Nevertheless, most anesthesiologists use a fiberoptic bronchoscope to confirm tube position. It may be passed through the tracheal lumen to check the position of both the bronchial cuff and the tracheal lumen opening relative to the mainstem bronchus that leads to the other lung. Insertion of the instrument into the tracheal lumen should provide a clear view of the carina, the endobronchial tube going into the appropriate bronchus, and the upper surface of the blue bronchial balloon visible just below the carina. Fiberoptic bronchoscopy readily detects gross malposition and excessive bronchial cuff inflation pressure that results in cuff herniation, carinal deviation, and excessive left lumen constriction. Additionally, it localizes the right upper lobe ventilation slot of the right-sided DLT and its relation to the right upper lobe orifice.

A pediatric fiberoptic bronchoscope is preferred for insertion and confirmation of tube position because it can pass down the lumens of all commercially available DLTs. Once the tube is in the trachea, positive-pressure ventilation may be continued during bronchoscopy by inserting the bronchoscope through a self-sealing diaphragm in the elbow connector to the bronchial lumen.

What Are the Potential Complications?

Ventilation/Perfusion Mismatch

Several complications of DLTs have been reported. The most common is arterial hypoxemia following induction and insertion of the tube.[103] Arterial desaturation may result from obstruction of the right upper lobe bronchus or increased shunt secondary to ventilation/perfusion mismatch during one-lung ventilation. It may also result from excessive intra-alveolar pressure when the tidal volume delivered to one lung remains the same as it was originally for both lungs. To minimize this problem, the fraction of inspired O_2 may be increased to 1.0, the tidal volume appropriately reduced, and the respiratory rate increased to maintain the same minute ventilation.

Use of volatile anesthetics that increase the shunt through pulmonary vasodilatation may have to be discontinued and intravenous agents substituted. If hypoxemia persists, the steps listed in Table 17–4 should be followed. Persistent hypoxemia is unusual if the ventilated lung receives a fraction of inspired O_2 of 1.0 and the nonventilated lung is inflated with O_2 and 5 cm positive end-expiratory pressure.

TABLE 17–4. Approaches to Independent Lung Ventilation in Lateral Decubitus Position

"Up" Lung	"Dependent" Lung
CPAP (5–10 cm H$_2$O) (apneic oxygenation)	Ventilate
Constant CPAP, apneic oxygenation, periodic ventilation	Ventilate
No ventilation	Ventilate with CPAP (5–10 cm H$_2$O)
High-frequency ventilation	Ventilate with or without CPAP

Abbreviation: CPAP = continuous positive airway pressure.

Tube Malposition

The most common cause of malposition is selection of a tube that is inappropriately long, allowing its placement too far into the bronchus.[103, 104] Malposition may result in airway obstruction, atelectasis, inability to isolate and collapse the lung, and O$_2$ desaturation. If the DLT is too large, it may be difficult to position into the appropriate bronchus. Proper tube selection and fiberoptic bronchoscopy obviate this problem.

Tracheobronchial Rupture

A dreaded complication of DLT insertion is tracheobronchial rupture.[105–107] Risk factors include insertion by inexperienced operators, use of intubating stylets, multiple vigorous attempts at intubation, presence of tracheobronchial abnormalities, overdistention of the tracheal or bronchial cuff, and advanced patient age.[108–111] Diagnosis can be difficult, and clinical signs such as hemorrhage, cyanosis, subcutaneous emphysema, pneumothorax, or compliance changes may be absent or slow to develop.

To prevent this problem, the bronchial cuff should not be inflated with more than 2 to 3 mL of air and should be deflated before the patient is moved. The integrity of the intubated bronchus can be checked with the bronchial cuff deflated at the time of testing of the resected bronchus for air leak.

Miscellaneous Problems

Other reported complications include traumatic laryngitis,[88] cardiac arrest due to pulmonary outflow tract obstruction,[112] and suture of a pulmonary vessel to the DLT.[113] Trauma during extubation may also occur and includes slight bleeding and ecchymosis of mucous membranes, arytenoid dislocation, laryngeal and vocal cord damage, and accidental tooth extraction.

ANCILLARY EQUIPMENT

Several ancillary devices facilitate intubation. These include specialized forceps, flexible lumen finders, tube changers, laryngotracheal anesthesia kits, malleable stylets, lighted stylets, and lightwands.

How Are Intubating Forceps Utilized?

The forceps is used during direct laryngoscopy to direct the tip of the endotracheal tube into the glottic inlet. The Magill forceps has a handle angle relative to its length of about 50°. The Rovenstein forceps has a 90° handle angulation and a deeper tip with which to grasp the endotracheal tube. The Aillon forceps is provided with a spring-loaded handle and is used to grasp and bend the endotracheal tube's tip to align it with the laryngeal axis. The forceps is generally held in the right hand and is used to grasp the endotracheal tube distally above the point of attachment of the cuff. The tube is advanced by an assistant while the operator directs it to the glottic opening with the aid of the forceps.[114, 115]

Is a Stylet Helpful?

A stylet is an elongated, malleable introducer made from a variety of materials, including copper wire, coat hanger wire, brass rods, flexible stainless steel, or disposable plastic rods.[116–118] When inserted into an endotracheal tube, it permits customizing of the tube's shape to facilitate intubation. The stylet is lubricated and passed into the endotracheal tube, and the distal end is bent gradually in a J or "hockey stick" shape. The tube is inserted with the curvature directed towards the coronal plane (glottic opening).

A stylet should not protrude through the Murphy eye or the tip of the endotracheal tube, nor should it be used to force entry into the trachea. Instead, its tip should lie at least 2 cm from the tube's end to avoid trauma and possible perforation of the larynx, trachea, or esophagus. Its proximal end should be bent over the rim of the 15-mm adaptor to avoid accidental advancement beyond the tube tip during intubation. It should be withdrawn once the tube is seen to pass the vocal cords.

Since most intubations can be performed rapidly and safely without a stylet, I do not recommend that a stylet be used routinely; it should be reserved for rapid sequence induction or emergency intubation, when a difficult airway is anticipated, or if an armored tube is used. Although a stylet is utilized primarily for oral intubation, it may be employed for nasotracheal intubation.[116] Reported complications of stylet use include bleeding, hematoma formation, submucosal dissection, tracheobronchial rupture, esophageal perforation, pneumomediastinum, and pneumothorax.

What Is a Lightwand?

A flexible, battery-operated stylet (lightwand) with a smooth tip and a bulb at its distal end for illumination is available.[119–124] The lightwand is lubricated and placed inside the endotracheal tube, and the distal end is preformed to the anticipated path of entry to the glottic opening. The stylet is inserted orally and transilluminates the neck when it passes through the vocal cords. A bright cherry red glow is appreciated at the region of the cricothyroid membrane, indicating proper positioning of the stylet. If the stylet is somewhere else, the light is noted laterally or not at all. The transillumination is most easily observed in a dark room. Once the characteristic glow is noted, the tube is passed over the lightwand into the trachea.

Insertion

This technique of insertion does not require direct laryngoscopy and can be performed safely in adults and children.[122–124] It has been utilized for routine and difficult intubation in awake as well as in anesthetized patients. Its greatest value is in patients whose glottic opening cannot be completely visualized by direct laryngoscopy. Minimal movement of the neck is required; thus, it may also be useful in patients with suspected neck injury.

Potential Problems

Blood and secretions in the oropharynx do not interfere with its use as they might with direct laryngoscopy or fiberoptic intubation. The lightwand cannot be used in children younger than 5 years of age or in those requiring an endotracheal tube <5.5 mm ID because of the bulb size. Problems associated with its use are uncommon and include hoarseness, postoperative sore throat, and cricoarytenoid subluxation. Complications associated with the use of the lightwand are similar to those occasionally seen with a malleable stylet.

What Is a Flexible Lumen Finder?

Another modification of the stylet is a flexible lumen finder and intubation guide.[125] It has a proximal control handle, trigger, inner rod, and notched outer tube that allows the operator's right hand to maneuver the distal tip with the proximal trigger. The smooth, flexible tip can be directed anteriorly, posteriorly, or laterally. The distal 5 cm should be well lubricated before the endotracheal tube is inserted through it. Direct laryngoscopy is performed, and the stylet tip is maneuvered towards the glottic inlet. Once the distal tip of the finder enters the trachea, the tracheal tube is advanced, and the lumen finder is removed.

How Does the Laryngotracheal Anesthesia "Stylet" Function?

Although a laryngotracheal anesthesia kit is generally used to spray topical anesthesia into the larynx and trachea, it may also function as a stylet. The distal end is inserted into the Murphy eye of the endotracheal tube. Following direct laryngoscopy, the tip is directed into the rima glottidis.[126] The endotracheal tube is then advanced over the elongated portion. The tube often hangs up on the laryngeal inlet when it is advanced over the stylet. This problem is usually resolved by rotating the endotracheal tube 90° to 180°.

What Is a Tube Changer?

A tube changer is a hollow or solid elongated plastic tube that can be used to exchange a malfunctioning endotracheal tube or that can be used as an introducer during initial intubation in a patient with a difficult airway. To change the tube, the tube changer is first lubricated and inserted into the trachea through the in situ endotracheal tube, which is then pulled out while the position of the tube changer is maintained. A new endotracheal tube is then inserted over the tube changer into proper position. The tube changer is withdrawn, and the tube is secured.

Hollow tube changers can be connected to a high-pressure O_2 source, and oxygenation can be achieved with either O_2 insufflation or ventilation using a Sanders-type injector. Suc-

tion catheters may function as tube changers but are a less secure option because they are too flexible and often of insufficient length. Complications associated with tube changer manipulation are similar to those encountered with stylets. An additional reported complication is bronchial rupture caused by a tube changer that has advanced beyond the carina.

ALTERNATIVE MANAGEMENT TECHNIQUES

The incidence of failed tracheal intubation ranges from 5 to 35 per 10,000 patients.[127–130] Inability to mask ventilate and intubate patients ranges from 0.01 to 2.0 per 10,000 patients.[132, 133] Failure to oxygenate and ventilate patients is responsible for 50% to 75% of cardiac arrests during general anesthesia.[133–135] Hence, alternative methods of securing the airway must be available. These include needle cricothyroidotomy with transtracheal jet ventilation[136–139]; percutaneous cricothyroidotomy[140–144]; surgical cricothyroidotomy or tracheotomy[145–147]; and retrograde tracheal intubation. Percutaneous cricothyroidotomy is easier and safer than emergency tracheotomy.[145–149]

When Is Retrograde Catheter Placement Useful?

Retrograde tracheal intubation is indicated when translaryngeal intubation fails and the glottic inlet is not totally obstructed.[150–158] The procedure can be done in an awake, sedated, or anesthetized patient, and the endotracheal tube can be passed orally or nasally. It involves puncture of the cricothyroid membrane with a hollow needle, followed by passage of a wire or small catheter through the membrane and upward into the pharynx. The posterior pharynx is visualized, and the catheter is grasped with a forceps and directed toward the mouth or nose. It is then used as a guide to insert the endotracheal tube into the airway. Once the endotracheal tube is seen to pass through the cords, the catheter is gently removed, and the tube is secured in place. Clinical signs as previously described should be observed for proper tube placement.

Although its success rate is high, the technique is time-consuming and sometimes difficult to perform. It is not popular among anesthesiologists and serves only as a last resort when other easier methods, such as fiberoptic intubation or percutaneous cricothyroidotomy, fail to secure the airway. Complications include inability to secure the airway, minor bleeding at the puncture site or nose, hematoma formation, and barotrauma. Potential complications observed during percutaneous cricothyroidotomy and standard translaryngeal intubation may occur.

When Is Tracheotomy Performed?

Emergency tracheotomy should only be performed by a trained surgeon. Indications include rare instances of laryngeal trauma and emergency airway control in infants.[156] Elective tracheotomy is indicated for relief of upper airway obstruction, to improve suctioning, to reduce work of breathing, to improve airway access for prolonged mechanical ventilation, to assist in weaning mechanically ventilated patients with marginal pulmonary function, to reduce dead space, and to relieve patient discomfort. It should generally not be done in patients with fresh sternotomies because of the danger of the spread of infection from the stoma to the surgical site. It should also be avoided in most cases of emergency airway access because of a high morbidity and mortality rate.[157, 158] Emergent tracheotomy has a reported complication rate of as high as 42%; mortality is 2% to 5% even in elective cases.[157, 159–162]

Tube Types

"Standard" tubes consist of an inner and outer cannula, an obturator, a flange, and a cuff. The inner cannula has a 15-mm universal adapter that can be connected to a self-inflating bag or to the anesthesia machine breathing circuit. The cannula is made of metal or plastic and is shorter, wider, and less curved than a standard endotracheal tube. Only implant-tested tubes should be used, and a low-pressure, high-volume cuff is preferable. A tracheotomy button is available to maintain a tracheostomy stoma after decannulation when one has doubts about whether a patient can chronically maintain a patent airway without the tracheotomy tube. A fenestrated tracheotomy tube allows breathing through the upper respiratory tract, permitting phonation and humidification of the inspired gas.

Early Complications

Early complications include pneumothorax, subcutaneous emphysema, bleeding, aspiration, and aerophagia. The most important and potentially lethal complication is tube displacement following initial insertion. Blind attempts to reinsert the tube may cause tracheal compression and upper airway obstruction. If the tube is displaced and the path to the trachea is not clear, translaryngeal intubation should be attempted to secure the airway. If necessary, a pediatric laryngoscope can be used to visualize the trachea directly through the stoma, and careful cannulation can be performed with a small, cuffless endotracheal tube. Once the patient is stable, the tracheotomy tube can be reinserted.

Late Complications

Late complications include lower respiratory tract infection, which is observed in more than 50% of patients,[162] stricture, tracheal stenosis, erosion of the brachiocephalic artery with tracheobrachiocephalic fistula formation, and tracheal hemorrhage.[162] Tracheal necrosis and tracheoesophageal fistula may be caused by excessive intracuff pressure or by a poorly fitting tracheotomy tube.[163] Other chronic problems include swallowing dysfunction, tube obstruction, aspiration, stomal infection, and unsightly scar formation.

References

1. Applebaum EL, Bruce DL: A short history of tracheal intubation. *In* Tracheal Intubation. Applebaum EL, Bruce DL (eds). Philadelphia, WB Saunders, 1976, p 1.
2. Welch GW, Rippe JW: Airway management and endotracheal intubation. Intensive Care Medicine. *In* Rippe JM, Irwin RS, Alpert JS, et al (eds). Boston, Little, Brown & Co, 1985, p 1.
3. Smith JP, Bodai BI, Seifkin A, et al: The esophageal obturator airway: a review. JAMA 1983; 250:1081.
4. Meislin HW: The esophageal obturator airway: a study of respiratory effectiveness. Ann Emerg Med 1980; 9:54.
5. Schofferman J, Oill P, Lewis AD: The esophageal obturator airway: a clinical evaluation. Chest 1984; 69:63.
6. Smith JP, Bodai BI, Aubourg R, et al: A field evaluation of the esophageal obturator airway. J Trauma 1983; 23:317.
7. Harrison EE, Ward HJ, Bleman RW: Esophageal perforation following use of the esophageal obturator airway. Ann Emerg Med 1980; 9:21.
8. Jancey W, Wear SR, Kamajian G: Unrecognized tracheal intubation: a complication of the esophageal obturator airway. Ann Emerg Med 1980; 9:18.
9. Key GK: Use of the esophageal obturator airway with a report of an unusual complication. Postgrad Med 1980; 67:189.
10. Niemann JT, Rosborough JP, Myers R, et al: The pharyngeo-tracheal lumen airway: preliminary investigation of a new adjunct. Ann Emerg Med 1984; 13:591.
11. Bartlett RL, Martin SD: The pharyngeo-tracheal lumen airway: an assessment of airway control in the setting of upper airway hemorrhage. Ann Emerg Med 1987; 16:343.
12. Frass M, Frenzer R, Zdrahl F, et al: The esophageal tracheal combitude: preliminary results with a new airway for CPR. Ann Emerg Med 1987; 16:768.
13. Elam JO, Titel JH, Feingold A, et al: Simplified airway management during anaesthesia or resuscitation: a binasal pharyngeal system. Anesth Analg 1969; 48:407.
14. Brain AIJ: The laryngeal mask: a new concept in airway management. Br J Anaesth 1983; 55:801.
15. Leach AB, Alexander CA: The laryngeal mask: an overview. Eur J Anaesthesiol Suppl 1991; 4:19.
16. Smith I, White PF: Use of the laryngeal mask airway as an alternative to a face mask during outpatient arthroscopy. Anesthesiology 1992; 77:850.
17. Brain AIJ: The laryngeal mask: a new concept in airway management. Br J Anaesth 1983; 55:801.
18. Calder I, Ordman AJ, Jackowski A, et al: The brain laryngeal mask airway: an alternative to emergency tracheal intubation (case report). Anaesthesia 1990; 45:137.
19. Riley RH, Swan HD: Value of the laryngeal mask during thoracotomy (Letter). Anesthesiology 1992; 77:1051.
20. Benumof JL: Laryngeal mask airway. Indications and contraindications. Anesthesiology 1992; 77:843.
21. Benumof JL: Management of the difficult airway: with special emphasis on the awake tracheal intubation. Anesthesiology 1991; 75:1087.
22. Brimacombe J: The laryngeal mask airway and flexible bronchoscopy (Letter). Thorax 1991; 46:591.
23. Walker RWM, Murrel D: Yet another use for the laryngeal mask airway. Anaesthesia 1991; 46:591.
24. Tanigawa K, Inoue Y, Iwata S: Protection of recurrent laryngeal nerve during neck surgery: a new combination of neutracer, laryngeal mask airway, and fiberoptic bronchoscope (Letter). Anesthesiology 1991; 74:918.
25. Grebenik CR, Ferguson C, White A: The laryngeal mask airway in pediatric radiotherapy. Anesthesiology 1990; 72:474.
26. Logan AS: Use of the laryngeal mask in a patient with an unstable fracture on the cervical spine (Letter). Anesthesia 1991; 46:987.
27. Fisher JS, Ananthanarayan C, Edelist G: Role of the laryngeal mask in airway management. Can J Anaesth 1992; 39:1.
28. Siker ES: A mirror laryngoscope. Anesthesiology 1956; 17:38.
29. Finucane BT, Santora A: Difficult intubation. *In* Principles of Airway Management. Philadelphia, FA Davis, 1988, p 146.
30. Huffman JP, Elam JO: Prisms and fiberoptics for laryngoscopy. Anesth Analg 1971; 50:64.
31. Dorsch JA, Dorsch SE (eds). Understanding Anesthesia Equipment. 1st ed. Baltimore, Williams & Wilkins, 1975, p 232.
32. Huffman JP: The development of optical prism instruments to view and study the human larynx. J Am Assoc Nurse Anesth 1970; 38:197.
33. Weeks DB: A new use for an old blade. Anesthesiology 1974; 40:200.
34. Kessell J: A laryngoscope for obstetrical use. Anaesth Intensive Care 1977; 5:265.
35. Bellhouse CP: An angulated laryngoscope for routine and difficult tracheal intubation. Anesthesiology 1988; 69:126.
36. Roberts JT: Fundamentals of Tracheal Intubation. New York, Grune & Stratton, 1983.
37. Patil VU, Stehling LC, Zander HL: An adjustable laryngoscope handle for difficult intubation. Anesthesiology 1984; 60:609.
38. Dhara SS, Cheong TW: An adjustable multiple angle laryngoscope adaptor. Anaesth Intensive Care 1991; 19:243.
39. Nunn G: A new laryngoscope. Anaesthesia 1987; 42:877.
40. Corwin RW, Irwin RS: Bronchoscopy. *In* Intensive Care Medicine. Rippe JM, Irwin RS, Alpert JS et al (eds). Boston, Little, Brown & Co, 1985, p 73.
41. Vaughan RS: Endobronchial intubation. In Difficulties in Tracheal Intubation. Latto IP, Rosen M (eds). London, Bailliere Tindall, 1983, p 162.

42. Sanders R: Two ventilating attachments for bronchoscopes. Del Med J 1968; 39:170.
43. Landa JF: Indications for bronchoscopy. Chest 1978; 73(Suppl):686.
44. Sackner MA: State of the art: bronchofiberoscopy. Ann Rev Respir Dis 1975; 111:62.
45. Udaya BS, Prakash MD, Stubbs SE: Bronchoscopy: indications and technique. Semin Respir Med 1981; 3:17.
46. Fulkerson WJ: Current concepts: fiberoptic bronchoscopy. N Engl J Med 1984; 311:511.
47. Dellinger DP: Fiberoptic bronchoscopy in adult airway management. Crit Care Med 1990; 18:882.
48. Williams RT, Maltabey JR: Airway intubator. Anesth Analg 1982; 61:309.
49. Hogan K, Harpier MH, Pollard BJ: Use of a pharyngeal guide to aid intubation with the fiberoptic laryngoscope. Anaesth Intensive Care 1984; 12:18.
50. Pereira W Jr, Kounet DM, Snider GL: A prospective cooperative study of complications following flexible fiberoptic bronchoscopy. Chest 1978; 73:813.
51. Suratt PM, Smiddy JF, Gruber B: Deaths and complications associated with fiberoptic bronchoscopy. Chest 1976; 69:747.
52. Credle WF, Smiddy JF, Elliott RC: Complications of fiberoptic bronchoscopy. Am Rev Respir Dis 1974; 109:67.
53. Simpson FB, Arnold AG, Purvis A, et al: Postal survey of bronchoscopic practice by physicians in the United Kingdom. Thorax 1986; 41:311.
54. Katsnelson T, Frost EA, Farcon E, et al: When the endotracheal tube will not pass over flexible fiberoptic bronchoscope. Anesthesiology 1992; 76:151.
55. Saunders PR, Geisecke AH: Clinical assessment of the adult Bullard laryngoscope. Can Anaesth Soc J 1989; 36:S118.
56. Bjoraker DG: The Bullard intubating laryngoscopes. Anesthesiology Rev 1990; 17:64.
57. Gorback MS: Management of the challenging airway with the Bullard laryngoscope. J Clin Anaesth 1991; 3:473.
58. Borland LM, Caselbrant M: The Bullard laryngoscope: a new indirect oral laryngoscope (pediatric version). Anesth Analg 1990; 70:105.
59. Dyson A, Harris J, Bhatia K: Rapidity and accuracy of tracheal intubation in a mannequin: comparison of the fiberoptic with the Bullard laryngoscope. Br J Anaesth 1990; 65:268.
60. Caldwell SL, Sullivan KN: Artificial airways. In Respiratory Care. A Guide to Clinical Practice. Burton GG, Hodgin JF (eds). Philadelphia, JB Lippincott, 1984, p 493.
61. Sosis MB: What is the safest endotracheal tube for Nd-YAG laser surgery? A comparative study. Anesth Analg 1989; 69:802.
62. Bolder PM, Healey TEJ, Bolder AR: The extra work of breathing through adult endotracheal tubes. Anesth Analg 1986; 65:853.
63. Conrardy PA, Goodman LR, Lainge F, et al: Alteration of endotracheal tube position: flexion and extension of the neck. Crit Care Med 1976; 4:8.
64. Florete OG Jr: Airway management. In Critical Care. Civetta JM, Taylor RW, Kirby RR (eds). Philadelphia, JB Lippincott, 1992, p 1419.
65. Cooper JD, Grillo HC: Analysis of problems related to cuffs on endotracheal tubes. Chest 1972; 62:24S.
66. Cooper JD, Grillo HC: The evolution of tracheal injury due to ventilatory assistance through cuffed tubes: a pathologic study. Ann Surg 1969; 169:334.
67. Cooper JD, Grillo HC: Experimental production and prevention of injury due to cuffed tracheal tubes. Surg Gynecol Obstet 1969; 129:1235.
68. Grillo HC, Cooper JD, Geffin B, et al: A low pressure cuff for tracheostomy tubes to minimize tracheal injury. J Thorac Cardiovasc Surg 1971; 62:898.
69. Ching NP, Nealon TB Jr: Clinical experience with new low-pressure, high-volume tracheostomy cuffs: importance of limiting intracuff pressure. NY State J Med 1974; 74:2379.
70. Dobrin P, Canfield T: Cuffed endotracheal tubes: mucosal pressure and tracheal wall blood flow. Am J Surg 1977; 133:562.
71. Leigh JM, Maynard JP: Pressure on the tracheal mucosa from cuffed tubes. Br Med J 1979; 1:1173.
72. Nordin U: The tracheal and cuff-induced tracheal injury. Acta Otolaryngol Suppl (Stockh) 1977; 345:1.
73. Bjorkund S, Ekedahl C, Hansson PG, et al: Experimental tracheal wall injury. Acta Otolaryngol 1973; 75:387.
74. Dobrin P, Canfield T: Cuff endotracheal tubes: mucosal pressures and tracheal wall blood flow. Am J Surg 1972; 133:562.
75. Nordin U, Lindholm CE, Wolfgast M: Blood flow in the rabbit tracheal mucosa under normal conditions and under the influence of tracheal intubation. Acta Anaesth Scand 1977; 21:8.
76. Klainer AS, Turndorf H, Wen-Hsien WV, et al: Surface alterations due to endotracheal intubation. Am J Med 1975; 58:674.
77. Dunn CR, Dunn DL, Moser KM: Determinants of tracheal injury by cuffed tracheostomy tubes. Chest 1974; 65:128.
78. Guyton DC: Endotracheal and tracheotomy tube cuff design: influence on tracheal damage. Crit Care Updates 1990; 1:1.
79. Stanley TH, Kawamura R, Graves C: Effects of nitrous oxide on volume and pressure of endotracheal tube cuffs. Anesthesiology 1974; 41:256.
80. Stanley TH: Effects of anesthetic gases on endotracheal tube cuff gas volumes. Anesth Analg 1974; 53:480.
81. Stanley TH: Nitrous oxide and pressures and volumes of high and low pressure endotracheal tube cuffs in intubated patients. Anesthesiology 1975; 42:637.
82. Stanley TH, Liu WS: Tracheostomy and endotracheal tube cuff volume and pressure changes during thoracic operations. Ann Thorac Surg 1975; 20:144.
83. Ravenas B, Lindholm CE: Pressure and volume changes in tracheal tube cuffs during anesthesia. Acta Anaesthesiol Scand 1976; 20:321.
84. Jacobsen L, Greenbaum R: A study of intracuff pressure measurements, trends and behaviour in patients during prolonged periods of tracheal intubation. Br J Anaesth 1981; 53:97.
85. Mackenzie CF, Klose S, Browne DRG: A study of inflatable cuffs on endotracheal tubes. Br J Anaesth 1976; 48:105.
86. Benumof JL: Anesthesia for Thoracic Surgery. Philadelphia, WB Saunders, 1987.
87. Vaughan RS: Endobronchial intubation. In Difficulties in Tracheal Intubation. Latto IP, Rosen M (eds). London, Bailliere Tindall, 1983, p 156.
88. Newman RW, Finer GE, Downs JE: Routine use of the Carlens double-lumen endobronchial catheter: an experimental and clinical study. J Thorac Cardiovasc Surg 1961; 42:326.
89. White G: A new double lumen tube. Br J Anaesth 1960; 32:232.
90. Robertshaw F: Low resistance, double-lumen endobronchial tubes. Br J Anaesth 1962; 34:576.
91. Clapham MC, Vaughan RS: Bronchial intubation: a comparison between polyvinyl chloride and red rubber double lumen tubes. Anaesthesia 1985; 40:1111.
92. Zeitlin GL, Short DH, Ryder GH: An assessment of the Robertshaw double-lumen tube. Br J Anaesth 1965; 57:858.
93. Benumof JL, Partridge BL, Salvatierra C, et al: Margin of safety in positioning double-lumen endotracheal tubes. Anesthesiology 1987; 67:729.
94. Black AMS, Harrison GA: Difficulties with positioning Robertshaw double lumen tubes. Anaesth Intensive Care 1975; 3:299.
95. Saito S, Dohi S, Naito H: Alteration of double-lumen endobronchial tube position by flexion and extension of the neck. Anesthesiology 1985; 62:696.
96. Benumof JL: Anesthesia for thoracic surgery. International Anesthesia Research Society 1988 Review Course Lectures, 1988, p 120.
97. Read NC, Friday CD, Eason CN: Prospective study of the Robertshaw endobronchial catheter in thoracic surgery. Ann Thorac Surg 1977; 24:156.
98. Smith GB, Hirsch NP, Ehrenwerth J: Sight and sound: can double-lumen endotracheal tubes be placed accurately without fiberoptic bronchoscopy? Anesth Analg 1986; 65:S1.
99. Ovassapian A, Braunschweig R, Joshi CW: Endobronchial intubation using a flexible fiberoptic bronchoscope. Anesthesiology 1983; 59:501.
100. Shinnick JP, Freedman AP: Bronchofiberscopic placement of a double-lumen endotracheal tube. Crit Care Med 1982; 10:544.
101. Burk WJ: Should a fiberoptic bronchoscope be routinely used to position a double-lumen tube? Anesthesiology 1988; 68:826.
102. Grum D, Porembka D: Misconceptions regarding double tubes and bronchoscopy. Anesthesiology 1988; 68:826.
103. Wilson RS: Endobronchial intubation. In Thoracic Anesthesia. Kaplan JA (ed). New York, Churchill Livingstone, 1983, p 389.
104. Brodsky JB, Shulman MS, Mark JB: Malposition of left-sided double lumen endotracheal tubes. Anesthesiology 1985; 62:667.
105. Wagner DL, Gammage GW, Wong ML: Tracheal rupture following the insertion of a disposable double lumen endotracheal tube. Anesthesiology 1985; 63:698.
106. Heiser M, Steinberg JJ, MacVaugh H III, et al: Bronchial rupture, a complication of use of the Robertshaw double-lumen tube. Anesthesiology 1979; 51:88.
107. Foster JNG, Lau OJ, Alimo EB: Ruptured bronchus following endobronchial intubation. Br J Anaesth 1983; 55:687.
108. Hood RM, Sloan HE: Injuries of the trachea and major bronchi. J Thorac Cardiovasc Surg 1959; 18:458.
109. Tornvall SS, Jackson KH, Oyanedel ET: Tracheal rupture: complication of cuffed endotracheal tube. Chest 1971; 69:237.
110. Blanc FV, Trembal NAG: Complications of tracheal intubation: a new classification and a review of the literature. Anesth Analg 1976; 53:202.

111. Thompson DS, Reed RC: Rupture of the trachea following endotracheal intubation. JAMA 1968; 204:995.

112. Wells DG, Zelcer J, Podolakin W, et al: Cardiac arrest from pulmonary outflow tract obstruction due to a double lumen tube. Anesthesiology 1987; 66:422.

113. Dryden GE: Circulatory collapse after pneumonectomy (an unusual complication from the use of a Carlens catheter): a case report. Anesth Analg 1977; 56:451.

114. Bearman AJ: Device for nasotracheal intubation. Anesthesiology 1962; 23:130.

115. Munson ES, Cullen SC: Endotracheal intubation in a patient with ankylosing spondylitis of the cervical spine. Anesthesiology 1965; 26:365.

116. Cass NM, James NR, Lines V: Difficult direct laryngoscopy complicating intubation for anaesthesia. Br Med J 1956; ii:488.

117. Bowen RA: An introducer for difficult intubation. Anaesthesia 1967; 22:150.

118. Brechner VL: Unusual problems in the management of airways; flexion extension mobility of the cervical vertebrae. Anesth Analg Curr Res 1968; 47:362.

119. Ducrow M: Throwing light on blind intubation. Anaesthesia 1978; 33:827.

120. Elis DG, Jackymec A, Kaplan RE, et al: Guided orotracheal intubation in the operating room using a lighted stylet: a comparison with direct laryngoscopic technique. Anesthesiology 1986; 64:823.

121. Weis FR, Hatton MN: Intubation by the use of the light wand: experience in 253 patients. J Oral Maxillofac Surg 1989; 47:577.

122. Rayburn RL: Light wand intubation (Letter). Anaesthesia 1979; 34:677.

123. Holzman RS, Nargozian CD, Florence B: Lightwand intubation in children with abnormal airways. Anesthesiology 1988; 69:784.

124. Fox DJ, Matson MD: Management of the difficult pediatric airway in an austere environment using the lightwand. J Clin Anesth 1990; 2:123.

125. Rao TLK, Mathru M, Gorski DW, et al: Experience with a new intubation guide for difficult tracheal intubation. Crit Care Med 1982; 10:882.

126. Rosenberg MB: Use of the LTA kit as a guide for endotracheal intubation. Anesth Analg 1977; 56:287.

127. Samsoon GLT, Young JRB: Difficult tracheal intubation: a retrospective study. Anaesthesia 1987; 42:487.

128. Lyons G: Failed intubation. Anaesthesia 1985; 40:759.

129. Cormack RS, Lehane J: Difficult tracheal intubation in obstetrics. Anaesthesia 1984; 39:1105.

130. Glassenburg R, Vaisrub N, Albright G: The incidence of failed intubation in obstetrics: is there an irreducible minimum? (Abstract). Anesthesiology 1990; 73:A1061.

131. Bellhouse CP, Dore C: Criteria for estimating likelihood of difficulty of endotracheal intubation with MacIntosh laryngoscope. Anaesth Intensive Care 1988; 16:329.

132. Tunstall ME: Failed intubation in the parturient (Editorial). Can J Anaesth 1989; 36:611.

133. Keenan RL, Boyan CP: Cardiac arrest due to anesthesia. JAMA 1985; 253:2373.

134. Holland R: Anesthesia-related mortality in Australia. Int Anesthesiol Clin 1984; 22:61.

135. Tiret L, Desmonts JM, Hatton F, et al: Complications associated with anaesthesia: a prospective survey in France. Can Anaesth Soc J 1986; 33:336.

136. Benumof JL, Scheller MS: The importance of transtracheal jet ventilation in the management of the difficult airway. Anesthesiology 1989; 71:769.

137. Griggs WM, Worthley LIG, Gillegan GE, et al: A simple percutaneous tracheostomy technique. Surg Gynecol Obstet 1990; 170: 543.

138. Toye FJ, Weinstein JD: Clinical experience with percutaneous tracheostomy and cricothyroidotomy in 100 patients. J Trauma 1988; 26:1034.

139. Wain JC, Wilson DJ, Mathisen DJ: Clinical experience with mini-tracheostomy. Ann Thorac Surg 1990; 49:881.

140. Walls RM: Cricothyroidotomy. Emerg Med Clin North Am 1988; 6:725.

141. Mace SE: Cricothyrotomy. J Emerg Med 1988; 6:309.

142. Roven AN, Clapham MC: Cricothyroidotomy. Ear Nose Throat J 1983; 62:68.

143. Corke C, Cranswick P: A Seldinger technique for mini-tracheostomy insertion. Anesth Intensive Care 1988; 16:206.

144. Melker RJ, Banner MJ: Work imposed by breathing through cricothyrotomy tube. 6th World Congress on Emergency and Disaster Medicine, Hong Kong, September 1989.

145. Boyd AD, Romita MC, Conlan AA, et al: A clinical evaluation of cricothyrotomy. Surg Gynecol Obstet 1979; 149:365.

146. Essess BA, Jafek BW: Cricothyroidotomy: a decade of experience in Denver. Ann Otol Rhinol Laryngol 1987; 96:519.

147. O'Connor JV, Reddy K, Ergin MA, et al: Cricothyroidotomy for prolonged ventilatory support after cardiac operations. Ann Thorac Surg 1988; 39:353.

148. Sise MJ, Shaelford SR, Cruickshank JC, et al: Cricothyroidotomy for long term tracheal access. Ann Surg 1984; 200:13.

149. Kress TD, Balasbramanian S: Cricothyroidotomy. Ann Emerg Med 1982; 11:197.

150. Waters DJ: Guided blind endotracheal intubation. Anaesthesia 1963; 18:158.

151. Powell WF, Ozdil T: A translaryngeal guide for tracheal intubation. Anesth Analg 1967; 46:231.

152. Bourke D, Levesque PR: Modification of retrograde guide for endotracheal intubation. Anesth Analg 1974; 53:1013.

153. Harmaer M, Vaughan RS: Guided blind oral intubation. Anaesthesia 1980; 35:921.

154. Robert KW: New use for Swan-Ganz introducer wire. Anesth Analg 1981; 60:67.

155. Borland LM, Swan DM, Leff S: Difficult pediatric intubation: a new approach to the retrograde technique. Anesthesiology 1981; 55:577.

156. Piotrowskii JJ, Moore EE: Emergency department tracheostomy. Emerg Med Clin North Am 1988; 6:737.

157. Heffner JE, Miller KS, Sahn SA: Tracheostomy in the intensive care unit: Part I. Indications, technique, and management. Chest 1986; 90:269.

158. Heffner JE, Sahn SA: The technique of tracheostomy and cricothyroidotomy. J Crit Care Illness 1987; 2:79.

159. Meade JW: Tracheotomy: its complications and their management. N Engl J Med 1961; 264:587.

160. Heffner JE, Miller KS, Sahn SA: Tracheostomy in the ICU: Part 2. Complications. Chest 1986; 90:430.

161. Selecky PA: Tracheostomy: a review of present-day indications, complications, and care. Heart Lung 1974; 3:272.

162. Cross AS, Roup B: Role of respiratory assistance devices on endemic nosocomial pneumonia. Am J Med 1981; 70:681.

163. Thomas AN: The diagnosis and treatment of tracheoesophageal fistula caused by cuffed tracheal tubes. J Thorac Cardiovasc Surg 1973; 65:612.

CHAPTER 18

Cardiopulmonary Bypass

THOMAS J. MARTIN, M.D.

One of the most significant contributions in medicine was the development of cardiopulmonary bypass (CPB). The ability to take over cardiac and pulmonary function by mechanical means enabled cardiac surgery to be carried out with improved operating conditions and relative safety. CPB remains an evolving technology as we learn more about its "pathophysiology," for it involves an extremely abnormal set of physiologic circumstances for a patient. How best to construct a CPB circuit and to conduct CPB continues to be defined. This chapter focuses on the basic components of the circuit, techniques of myocardial preservation, the pathologic effects of CPB, and patient management as we attempt to limit the adverse effects.

BYPASS CIRCUITS

What Are the Typical Components?

The function of CPB is to drain venous blood from the patient, deliver oxygen (O_2) to the blood and remove carbon dioxide (CO_2) from it, warm or cool it, and return it to the patient's arterial circulation. The components are listed in Table 18–1. A typical CPB circuit is diagrammed in Figure 18–1.

Venous Cannula

Venous blood is siphoned by gravity through a venous cannula, usually placed in either the right atrium (to drain the superior vena cava [SVC] and inferior vena cava [IVC]) or a femoral vein (to drain the IVC). Drainage via the right atrium may be accomplished through the use of a single two-stage cannula, which drains both the SVC and IVC, or two separate cannulas in the SVC and IVC. Two cannulas are used during procedures requiring access to the mitral valve, tricuspid valve, and right atrium. Venous blood flows into a reservoir. The flow of venous blood to the CPB pump is commonly referred to as *venous return.*

Because flow is dependent on gravity, it is determined by the height of the operating table, the patient's intravascular volume, and the size and position of the venous cannula. The venous cannula and its tubing should be relatively free of air,

because if enough air enters the venous line, an air lock may result, preventing venous return. If this problem occurs, it must be corrected immediately by raising the tubing and "milking" the air toward the reservoir. Without adequate venous return, the reservoir quickly empties, and the perfusionist is unable to deliver blood to the arterial circulation. If the venous return is excessive and causes the right atrium to collapse and re-expand intermittently, the surgical procedure becomes more difficult. This problem can be corrected by asking the perfusionist to partially occlude the venous return between the patient and the oxygenator.

Cardiotomy Sucker

Blood also may pass from the patient to the reservoir through two or more suction lines, with suction generated by roller pumps. The cardiotomy sucker is used by the surgeon to scavenge shed blood at the operative site from the time the patient is heparinized until the administration of protamine after CPB.

The surgeon must be careful not to use the cardiotomy sucker to aspirate dilute fluids, such as cardioplegia solution or iced saline used for topical cooling of the heart, into the CPB reservoir, or excessive hemodilution results. Such dilute fluids should be aspirated into disposable suction canisters or an intraoperative blood salvage device.

Cardiotomy suction is most efficacious when the sucker can be submerged in blood. Aspiration of small amounts of blood maximizes the blood-air interface, which is one of the most significant sources of trauma to red blood cells and platelets. It also may increase the risk of microscopic air emboli, if suction is allowed to run continuously.

TABLE 18–1. Components of a Typical Cardiopulmonary Bypass

Venous drainage line
Cardiotomy sucker
Left ventricular vent
Venous and arterial filters
Oxygenator (bubble or membrane)
Heat exchanger
Main pump (roller or centrifugal)
Cardioplegia devices (antegrade arterial or retrograde venous)

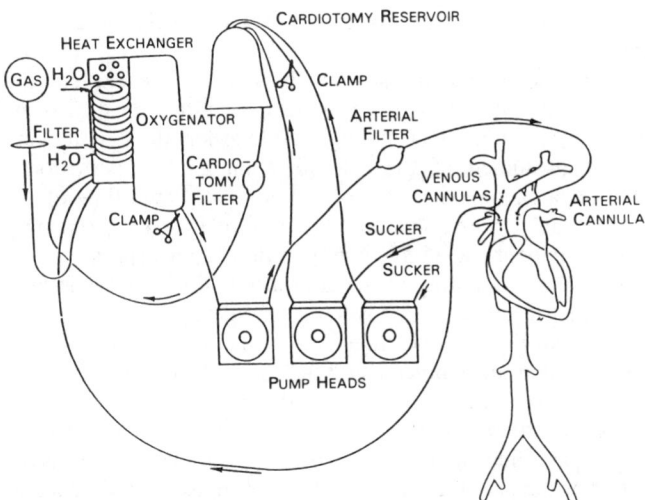

FIGURE 18-1. The components of a typical CPB circuit. Venous blood flows by gravity through a venous cannula or cannulas to the pump. Pump heads generate suction to aspirate shed blood from the surgical field and to vent the left ventricle. Blood passes through an oxygenator (either a bubble- or membrane-type) and a heat exchanger before being pumped back to the patient through an arterial cannula. Both venous and arterial blood may be filtered. (From Lake CL, Schwartz AJ, Campbell FW: Extracorporeal circulation. *In* Pediatric Cardiac Anesthesia. 1st ed. Lake CL (ed). Norwalk, Appleton & Lange, 1988, pp 155–179.)

Left Ventricular Vent

Another suction line commonly used during CPB is the left ventricular (LV) vent or sump. The LV vent is a tube attached to suction and placed in the left ventricle, usually via the right superior pulmonary vein, through the left atrium, and across the mitral valve. It may also be placed directly into the apex of the left ventricle, the left atrium, or the aortic root.

The purpose of the vent is to decompress the left ventricle, thereby decreasing wall tension and myocardial O_2 consumption ($M\dot{V}O_2$), as well as providing a bloodless field during aortic or mitral valve procedures. Without a LV vent, the ventricle may fill with blood as a result of aortic insufficiency and thebesian and bronchial venous return to the left side of the heart.

Filters

Blood from the venous cannulas, the cardiotomy suction, and the LV vent is usually passed through a 40-μm filter built into the CPB reservoir or added in-line to the CPB circuit. Filtered venous blood then travels to either the oxygenator or the pump, depending on which type of oxygenator is used. When a bubble oxygenator is used, it is usually placed before the pump. When a membrane oxygenator is used, it is usually placed after the pump. The greater resistance to flow across a membrane oxygenator necessitates a higher driving pressure. Another filter is placed in the arterial line between the arterial pump head and the patient (see Fig. 18–1).

Oxygenators

The oxygenator is responsible for adding O_2 to the blood (oxygenation) and removing CO_2 (ventilation). A water-mediated heat exchanger is incorporated into the oxygenator to facilitate warming and cooling of the perfusate. Two types are commonly used.

Bubble

Bubble oxygenators maximize contact between blood and O_2 by creating a foam of tiny O_2 bubbles in the blood. Oxygenation is determined by the blood-O_2 surface area, which is greater with small bubbles than with large bubbles. Excessively small bubbles, however, limit CO_2 elimination, and the bubbles may be difficult to remove. Ventilation is increased with increased gas flow (O_2 or a mixture of O_2 and CO_2) through the oxygenator. Blood foam passes through a defoaming device, consisting of a silicone polymer bonded to a polypropylene or polyurethane mesh. Most of the foam is removed, and oxygenated ("arterial") blood then enters a reservoir compartment. Any residual foam remains on top, and oxygenated blood exits through an outlet at the bottom of the reservoir.

Membrane

The direct blood-O_2 interface in bubble oxygenators produces blood trauma, resulting in hemolysis and protein denaturation. Membrane oxygenators were developed to reduce these effects by separating O_2 and blood with a thin gas-permeable membrane. This type of oxygenator more closely simulates the exchange of O_2 and CO_2 across the alveolar-capillary membranes of the lungs.

Gas transfer depends on the permeability of the membrane, the diffusion distance of the gas in blood, and the driving pressure of gas across the membrane. Differential control of oxygenation and ventilation is more easily achieved with a membrane oxygenator than with a bubble oxygenator. The O_2 partial pressure (Po_2) can be controlled by the use of an air-O_2 blender. CO_2 partial pressure (Pco_2) is controlled by the rate of gas flow. The perfusionist adjusts the air-O_2 blender and gas flow rate based on serial arterial blood gas determinations after CPB is initiated.

Pumps

Two types of pumps are currently used: the nonocclusive roller pump and the centrifugal pump.

Roller

The action of a roller pump causes blood to flow by compression of plastic tubing between the roller head and a horseshoe-shaped back plate as the roller turns within a stationary raceway (Fig. 18–2). The rotation of the roller pump is not affected by distal pressure, so it is said to be "resistance independent." Although this property is advantageous in ensuring the flow rate set by the perfusionist, it can also lead to disastrous rupture or disconnection of tubing if excessive pressures are generated. Pressures in excess of 300 mm Hg are worrisome.

The roller pump can be set to deliver pulsatile flow by adjusting the instantaneous rate of rotation of the pump head. Although roller pumps have been implicated as a source of hemolysis, large-diameter rollers, large-diameter tubing, and a low occlusion setting minimize blood trauma.[1] Other factors, particularly the cardiotomy sucker, type of oxygenator, and duration of CPB, appear to be more important in determining the degree of hemolysis during CPB.

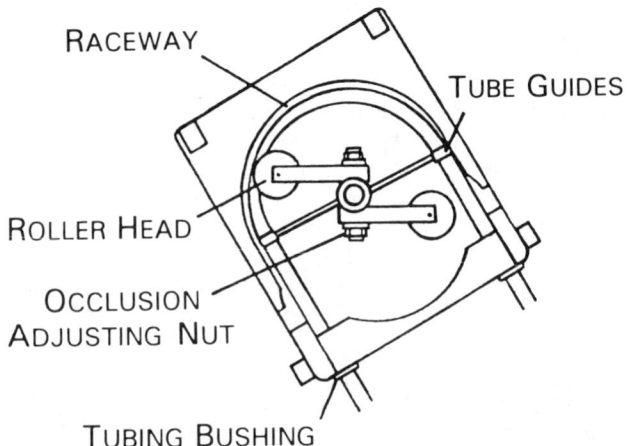

FIGURE 18–2. The nonocclusive roller pump. Blood flow within the tubing is generated by compression of the tubing between the roller heads and the backplate of the raceway. The amount of occlusion by the roller head is varied by the occlusion-adjusting nut on the pump head. Flow is determined by the volume of tubing compressed by the roller head and the number of revolutions per minute. (From High KM, Williams DR, Kurusz M: CPB circuits and design. *In* The Practice of Cardiac Anesthesia. 1st ed. Hensley FA Jr., Martin DE (eds). Boston, Little, Brown & Co, 1990, pp 583–601.)

Centrifugal

The centrifugal pump produces flow by the rotation of a series of cones within a clear plastic housing (Fig. 18–3). This action causes circular motion of blood with the development of flow and pressure by centrifugal force. The centrifugal pump is resistance dependent. Hence, the pump output varies with distal pressure and resistance. This property adds to its safety by preventing rupture or separation of the tubing if a sudden increase in pressure occurs. However, because flow does not necessarily correspond to pump speed, a flowmeter must be placed in the arterial line to allow CPB flow rate to be monitored.

A large bolus of air is much less likely to be delivered to the patient with a centrifugal pump than with a roller pump, because the centrifugal pump does not function if it becomes filled with air. However, if a centrifugal pump stops owing to loss of electrical power or pump failure, the aortic pressure exceeds pump pressure; air then may be entrained into the aorta and arterial line through the aortic cannulation or aortic root cardioplegia cannula sites. A centrifugal pump with rotating fins, manufactured by Sarns (3M Health Care, Ann Arbor, MI), is capable of delivering pulsatile flow; the Bio-pump (Bio-Medicus, Eden Prairie, MN) with rotating cones is not.

Arterial Cannula

Blood returns to the patient through the arterial cannula, which usually is placed in the ascending aorta. It may also be placed in a femoral artery. A pressure gauge on the arterial line is important. Pressure measured before initiation of CPB should be pulsatile and should be nearly equal to the patient's pressure measured with an intra-arterial catheter. If it is lower, the discrepancy may indicate improper zeroing or placement of the transducer, placement of the arterial cannula within the false lumen of a pre-existing or iatrogenic dissection, or connection of the arterial line to a venous cannula. Conversely, a pressure that reads higher in the arterial cannula than the radial artery implies a zeroing or reference level discrepancy, the cannula tip against the aortic wall, or central aortic-radial ar-

tery blood discrepancy suggestive of a subclavian atherosclerotic plaque.

During CPB, the pressure in the arterial line exceeds the patient's pressure because of the resistance that must be overcome in pumping blood through the long length of tubing and the small lumen of the arterial cannula. The perfusionist chooses a cannula size that provides a calculated flow of 2.4 $L \cdot min \cdot m^{2-1}$ with a gradient of 100 mm Hg or less, assuming that the patient's anatomic configuration can accept it.

Pressure monitoring in the arterial line during CPB is very important in detecting inadvertent clamping or kinking of the tubing. An arterial line filter is also included to trap debris, thrombi, and air bubbles (see Fig. 18–1). It usually has a 40-μm pore size. A bypass line around the filter remains clamped unless the filter becomes obstructed. If this problem occurs, the bypass line is opened to permit continuous CPB flow. Whether the use of an arterial line filter makes a difference in neurologic outcome after CPB remains controversial.

Temperature is monitored in both the venous and arterial lines. It is particularly important during cooling and rewarming to determine the temperature gradient between the patient (venous line) and the CPB circuit (arterial line).

Anesthesia Vaporizer

An anesthesia vaporizer is often placed in the fresh gas line to deliver volatile anesthetics via the oxygenator. Administration of anesthesia during CPB is discussed later. The vaporizer should be rigidly mounted to minimize the possibility of accidental spills of volatile anesthetic agents on the plastic components of the CPB circuit during filling. Spilled vapor can cause anything from cracking and softening of the plastic housing to complete shattering.[2, 3]

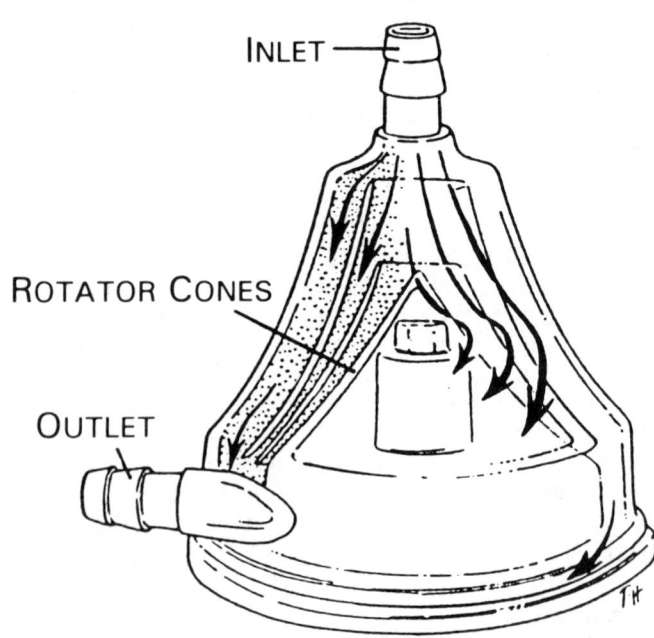

FIGURE 18–3. The centrifugal pump manufactured by Bio-Medicus (Eden Prairie, MN). Blood enters through an inlet at the axis of the pump. An impeller of spinning cones causes centrifugal acceleration of blood; blood exits through an outlet at the periphery of the pump. (From Reed CC, Stafford TB: Cardiopulmonary Bypass. 2nd ed. Houston, Texas Medical Publications, 1985, p 378.)

Cardioplegia Apparatus

The cardioplegia apparatus consists of a separate roller pump at the opposite end of the pump that is used to deliver a cardioplegia solution that is hyperkalemic, iso-osmolar or slightly hyperosmolar, crystalloid or blood based, oxygenated, and usually cooled to 4 °C to 12 °C. It may be delivered antegrade through an aortic root or coronary ostia cardioplegia cannula, retrograde through the coronary sinus, or by both routes.

MYOCARDIAL PROTECTION

Perioperative myocardial infarction can limit the success of a technically flawless cardiac repair. The extent of perioperative myocardial necrosis as determined by creatine kinase (CK) MB isoenzyme activity is inversely related to postoperative cardiac index, postoperative need for pharmacologic and mechanical support, and ultimately survival rate (Fig. 18–4). Thus, myocardial protection is an extremely important part of CPB and cardiac surgery.

What Are the Important Elements?

Prevention and treatment of myocardial ischemia during cardiac surgery is an important part of the anesthesiologist's role. However, despite careful hemodynamic control, perioperative ischemia not associated with hemodynamic aberrations still occurs.[4, 5] Sensitive detection of ischemia with the electrocardiogram (ECG), pulmonary artery and pulmonary artery occlusion pressure monitoring, and transesophageal echocardiography is extremely important. Ischemic myocardial damage is most likely to occur during CPB.[6, 7]

Myocardial Oxygen Consumption

After the initiation of CPB, the empty heart continues to beat and the myocardium is still perfused by native coronary blood flow until the aortic cross-clamp is applied. Until cooling begins, a coronary perfusion pressure of 60 to 70 mm Hg seems reasonable to prevent myocardial and cerebral ischemia. Hemodilution with the CPB prime reduces the hemoglobin concentration, but a concentration of 7 g · dL^{-1} or more probably provides adequate myocardial O_2 delivery.

Tachycardia may develop after the initiation of CPB and can markedly increase $M\dot{V}O_2$. Administration of a β-adrenergic blocker, such as esmolol, may prevent tachycardia-associated increases in $M\dot{V}O_2$ and may even lessen the detrimental effects of myocardial ischemia after aortic cross-clamping.[8, 9] If systemic hypothermia is induced with initiation of CPB, bradycardia is more commonly encountered.

Pharmacologic arrest of the heart by instillations of cardioplegia solution is accomplished immediately after aortic cross-clamping, usually with simultaneous cooling. Diastolic arrest of the heart is the single most important factor to reduce $M\dot{V}O_2$. In an animal study of empty beating hearts, fibrillating hearts, and arrested hearts at 37 °C, 32 °C, 28 °C, and 22 °C, the $M\dot{V}O_2$ of arrested hearts was lower at each temperature by 70% to 80% than empty beating or fibrillating hearts[10] (Table 18–2). Myocardial wall tension increased with lower temperatures in the empty beating and fibrillating hearts.

Pharmacologic arrest chemically depolarizes the cell membrane and places the heart in sustained diastole.[11] Arrest should be induced rapidly, because cellular adenosine triphosphate stores can be significantly depleted during an intervening period of ventricular fibrillation.[12]

Metabolic Requirements

When the heart is arrested during CPB, little energy production is needed to meet basal myocardial metabolic requirements. However, the only energy production that is ongoing at that time is derived from anaerobic metabolism of glycogen and glucose. Hence, another important role of cardioplegia infusion is to wash away accumulated anaerobic metabolites. Hypothermia reduces basal metabolic requirements beyond the effect of electromechanical arrest alone, so it is commonly used in conjunction (i.e., iced cardioplegic solution and topical application of iced saline). Interest recently has been renewed in continuous normothermic blood cardioplegia, which may offer some advantages over hypothermic cardioplegia. This subject is discussed later.

How Is Hypothermia Induced?

Three methods of hypothermia, in the order they are introduced after initiation of CPB, are systemic cooling, topical myocardial cooling, and hypothermic cardioplegia.

Systemic Cooling

With the initiation of CPB or shortly thereafter, temperature of the CPB perfusate is reduced, usually until the patient's temperature reaches 25 °C to 28 °C. O_2 consumption and basal metabolic activity of the heart, brain, and other organs are thereby reduced >50%. Rewarming of the heart after it has been cooled by other methods is also decreased by limiting the transfer of heat from surrounding tissues by placing an insulating pad or iced sponge behind the heart. If a transesophageal echocardiography probe is in place, it is turned off dur-

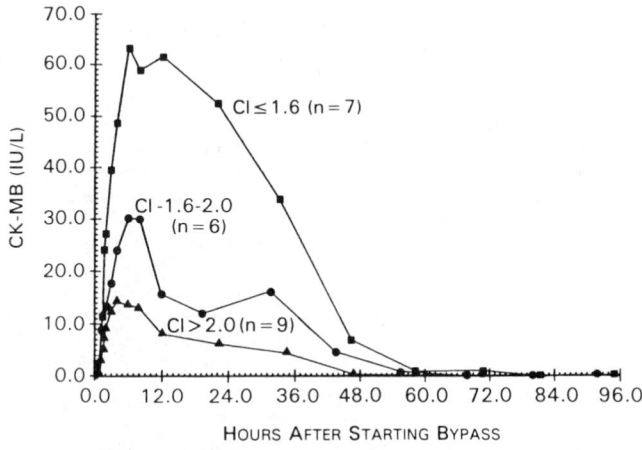

FIGURE 18–4. Inadequate myocardial protection leads to poor outcome after cardiac surgery. Blood creatine phosphokinase MB isoenzyme levels (CK-MB) were inversely related to cardiac index (CI) in the hours after starting cardiopulmonary bypass. Patients underwent mitral valve replacement in 1975 with simple cold ischemic arrest. (From Kirklin JW, Barratt-Boyes BG: Cardiac Surgery. New York, Churchill Livingstone, 1986, p 87.)

TABLE 18–2. Myocardial Metabolism During Hypothermia*

	37 °C	32 °C	28 °C	22 °C
Heart rate (bpm) (n = 12)	164 ± 10	118 ± 10	77 ± 7	31 ± 3
M$\dot{v}o_2$/beat (mL/100 g/min) (n = 12)	0.033 ± 0.003	0.041 ± 0.005	0.051 ± 0.005	0.086 ± 0.12
M$\dot{v}o_2$/min (mL/100 g/min)				
Beating empty (n = 12)	5.59 ± 1.95	4.93 ± 1.80	3.93 ± 1.10	2.87 ± 0.90
Fibrillating (n = 14)	6.50 ± 1.60	3.84 ± 0.51	2.93 ± 1.02	1.95 ± 0.86
Arrest (n = 7)	1.10 ± 0.41	0.83 ± 0.23	0.59 ± 0.30	0.31 ± 0.12

(From Buckberg GD, Brazier JR, Nelson RL, et al: Studies of the effects of hypothermia on regional myocardial blood flow and metabolism during cardiopulmonary bypass. I. The adequately perfused beating, fibrillating, and arrested heart. J Thorac Cardiovasc Surg 1977; 73:88.)
*n = number of observations. Values are mean ± ISD.
Abbreviations: M$\dot{v}o_2$ = left ventricular myocardial oxygen consumption.

ing the period of aortic cross-clamping to eliminate it as a heat source.

Topical Myocardial Cooling

Topical methods assist in myocardial cooling and produce a more homogeneous temperature than that obtained by hypothermic cardioplegia alone.[13] A cold crystalloid solution such as normal saline or lactated Ringer's is generally used. A saline slush may also be used, but this approach may be associated with transient postoperative phrenic nerve paresis.[14, 15]

Hypothermic Cardioplegia

Antegrade Arterial

Antegrade administration of hypothermic cardioplegia solution, usually at 4 °C to 12 °C, via the coronary arteries efficiently cools the myocardium. However, the distribution of cardioplegic solution, and thus cooling, may be nonuniform in the presence of coronary stenoses or ventricular hypertrophy. Monitoring of myocardial temperature for a target temperature of 10 °C to 15 °C may identify areas of inadequate protection. Cardioplegia solution is usually infused at an aortic root pressure of 80 to 100 mm Hg. It is reinfused when myocardial temperature exceeds 15 °C or every 20 minutes.

Retrograde Venous

Topical cooling[13] and retrograde cardioplegia via the coronary sinus[16] often overcome the problem of antegrade arterial maldistribution. The coronary venous system is not affected by atherosclerosis, so retrograde coronary sinus perfusion provides homogeneous distribution of cardioplegia solution regardless of the severity of coronary artery disease. The surgeon inserts a catheter into the coronary sinus under direct vision through an atriotomy or by blind transatrial intubation.[17]

Indications for retrograde cardioplegia are not completely defined, but its use is increasingly common. Examples of situations in which it may be beneficial include (1) severe coronary stenoses, occlusions, or poor collaterals such that antegrade cardioplegia distribution is likely to be very poor,[18] (2) aortic insufficiency, (3) aortic valve surgery, and (4) reoperation with patent saphenous vein grafts or internal mammary artery graft. Advantages and disadvantages of retrograde cardioplegia are listed in Table 18–3.

Problems of slower induction of arrest and poor distribution of cardioplegia to the right ventricle may be overcome by combined antegrade cardioplegia to arrest the heart and retro-

grade cardioplegia for maintenance.[19] Coronary sinus injury is avoided if the balloon on the catheter is gently inflated without an excessively tight fit; if the catheter is positioned in the terminal portion of the coronary sinus, partially within the atrium; and if the infusion rate and coronary sinus pressure are limited to 100 mL · min^{-1} and 40 mm Hg, respectively.[20]

What Is the Composition of Cardioplegia Solutions?

The exact composition of cardioplegia solutions differs among institutions and individual surgeons. Most solutions contain potassium chloride in a concentration of 15 to 30 mEq · L^{-1}. Diastolic arrest of the heart results from raising extracellular potassium concentration and lowering the resting membrane potential of myocardial cells to cause depolarization.

Hypothermia reduces the potassium concentration necessary to cause depolarization and helps to maintain asystole. Magnesium is frequently included in cardioplegia solutions to limit intracellular calcium influx. Even though calcium entry should be limited during ischemia, a small amount of calcium is added to cardioplegia solutions because reperfusion injury is worsened if myocardial cells are exposed to a calcium-containing solution (i.e., blood) after the use of calcium-free cardioplegia.[21]

Cardioplegia solutions can be oxygenated by adding oxygenated blood, bubbling O_2 through crystalloid solution, or adding a perfluorocarbon. Other components and their presumed roles are listed in Table 18–4.

TABLE 18–3. Retrograde Cardioplegia

Advantages	Improved flow to areas supplied by an occluded coronary artery
	Avoidance of ostial cannulation-associated coronary artery injuries
	Continuous cardioplegia infusion rather than intermittent infusion with interruption of surgery
	Elimination of coronary artery cannulas that obscure the surgical field during aortic valve surgery
Disadvantages	Slower induction of cardiac arrest compared with antegrade cardioplegia via the aortic root
	Coronary sinus injury with improper cannula insertion or improper balloon inflation
	Poor cardioplegia distribution to the right ventricle
	The need for bicaval cannulation if an atriotomy is used
	The need for left ventricular venting

TABLE 18–4. Components of Cardioplegia Solutions

Component	Purpose
Potassium chloride	Maintains asystole
Blood oxygenated crystalloid	Provides oxygen delivery to myocardium
Albumin, mannitol	Make solution iso-osmolar or slightly hyperosmolar
Sodium bicarbonate, phosphates, tris(hydroxymethyl)aminomethane histidine	Buffers to prevent metabolic acidosis
Calcium (in very low concentration)	Prevents calcium paradox
Magnesium	Antagonizes calcium entry into cells
Calcium channel blockers	Antagonize calcium entry into cells
β-Adrenergic blockers	Reduce myocardial metabolism
Procaine, lidocaine	Membrane stabilization, prevention of fibrillation during rewarming
Glucose	Substrate (may worsen acidosis if metabolites are not washed out by intermittent reperfusion)
Glutamate, aspartate	Replenish Krebs' cycle intermediates
Allopurinol, coenzyme Q	Free radical scavenging
Nitroglycerin	Vasodilator
Adenosine	Vasodilator, enhances repletion of adenosine triphosphate

Is Blood-Based Cardioplegia Superior to Crystalloid Cardioplegia?

The rationale for adding blood to cardioplegia solutions includes a higher O_2 content than that of crystalloid cardioplegia owing to the presence of both dissolved and hemoglobin-bound O_2, superior buffering capacity, the presence of plasma proteins to provide oncotic support, and the avoidance of the cost necessary to make a crystalloid solution with comparable qualities.[22]

Temperature

At normothermia, blood cardioplegia delivers O_2 to the myocardium more effectively than oxygenated crystalloid cardioplegia solutions. As temperature is reduced, however, the hemoglobin-O_2 dissociation curve is shifted to the left, and O_2 is less readily released to the myocardium. The mild myocardial metabolic acidosis that develops during cardioplegic arrest only partially opposes this shift in the curve. Below 20 °C, the advantage of blood cardioplegia, containing both dissolved and bound O_2, compared with crystalloid cardioplegia, which contains only dissolved O_2, is lost.

Buffering

The superiority of blood cardioplegia in providing buffering capacity and oncotic support due to the presence of plasma proteins is somewhat diminished by dilutional changes. In addition to the approximately 30% dilution of blood and plasma proteins due to the CPB prime, blood cardioplegia is usually prepared as a 4:1 dilution (four parts blood and one part crystalloid). Hemoglobin, the histidine component of plasma proteins, and carbonic anhydrase all are effective buffering systems found in blood.

Free Radical Scavenging

Theoretically, blood cardioplegia may be better at free radical scavenging than crystalloid cardioplegia because of the presence of plasma proteins, ascorbate, vitamin E, urate, catalase, superoxide dismutase, and glutathione. However, this potential benefit is unproven.

Summary

Clinical studies have not shown the clear superiority of blood or crystalloid cardioplegia. In terms of O_2 delivery during hypothermia, the dissolved O_2 in either type is most important. In this respect, crystalloid cardioplegia is equally efficacious.

Is Continuous Warm Cardioplegia Safe?

The safety of continuous warm blood cardioplegia is based on the notion that an electromechanically arrested, blood-perfused heart allows aerobic metabolism and represents the optimal state during CPB. Because the major determinant of $M\dot{V}O_2$ is electromechanical work, aerobic metabolism may provide sufficient energy to the arrested heart, making additional hypothermia-induced decreases in $M\dot{V}O_2$ unnecessary. This approach also avoids the potentially detrimental effects of hypothermic arrest. Favorable results have been reported with continuous antegrade cardioplegia via the aortic root and with antegrade arrest followed by continuous retrograde cardioplegia via the coronary sinus.[23–25]

Reported advantages include a decreased need for defibrillation after reperfusion, good post-CPB ventricular function, and a low incidence of perioperative myocardial infarction. In addition, very long cross-clamp times are tolerated, because cross-clamp time is not truly ischemic time. No difference has been noted in anesthetic dose requirement, management of anticoagulation, or postoperative care compared with patients undergoing surgery with hypothermic CPB.[26]

REPERFUSION INJURY

What Is It and How Can It Be Limited?

After a period of ischemia without infarction, reperfusion of myocardium restores the delivery of O_2 and nutrients and allows preservation of contractile function. However, the introduction of calcium, O_2, and neutrophils into myocardium recovering from ischemia may initiate a deleterious cascade of cellular events referred to as *reperfusion injury*.[26, 27]

Oxygen-Free Radicals and Hydrogen Peroxide

The reintroduction of O_2 to cells that are hypoxic appears to promote the production of the free radical superoxide anion (O_2^-), hydrogen peroxide (H_2O_2), and the hydroxyl radical (·OH). Normal cellular antioxidant systems may be relatively inactive during ischemia, limiting the availability of superoxide dismutase, glutathione peroxidase, glutathione reductase, and catalase. Free radicals are then able to interact with cellular constituents, such as lipids, to form species that damage cells. Inclusion of free radical scavengers in cardioplegia solution is intended to limit these effects, but clinical outcome data have not demonstrated consistent benefit.

Neutrophils

Neutrophil adherence to endothelial cells is increased by ischemia and hypoxia. Neutrophil activation produces an inflammatory response that leads to increased phospholipase activity and products of arachidonic acid. Leukotrienes cause increased vasoconstriction, potentiate platelet aggregation, increase endothelial permeability, and release proteolytic enzymes. Endothelial damage results, and capillaries may become plugged with neutrophils. This sequence further decreases blood flow to myocytes (the "no reflow" phenomenon) and may lead to cell death.

Is Effective Therapy Possible?

Calcium seems to have a role in the release of toxic substances, including proteolytic enzymes and free radicals, from activated neutrophils. Inhibitors of neutrophil function are being studied. Adenosine may counteract the vasoconstriction and platelet aggregation and therefore may prove to be a useful adjunct to cardioplegia solutions.[28] Calcium channel blockers and β-blockers may provide benefit if administered before or during the ischemic injury, but not during the reperfusion period.[29] The indications for administration of calcium salts after CPB should be carefully considered (see Chapter 67).

PATHOPHYSIOLOGY OF CARDIOPULMONARY BYPASS

CPB induces an abnormal physiologic state that affects multiple organ systems. Some of the effects can be directly attributed to certain components of the CPB circuit. Others may relate to the manner in which bypass is conducted, in terms of the pressure and flow rate of perfusion, management of acid-base status, delivery of anesthesia, and so forth. Bypass methodology is filled with controversial issues. The effects of CPB on the coagulation system and the management of post-CPB coagulation problems are discussed in Chapter 67. This section focuses on the effects of CPB on metabolism, central nervous system (CNS) function, and renal function.

What Is the Physiologic Stress Response to Cardiopulmonary Bypass?

The stress response to surgery involves the release of hormones and vasoactive substances from various organs. This response is especially pronounced during CPB. Consider the abnormal conditions the body encounters: hypothermia, nonpulsatile blood flow, hemodilution, changes in blood pressure and volume status, alteration in tissue perfusion, and perhaps relative ischemia of some organs including the heart (Fig. 18–5).

Catecholamines

The most notable hormonal response to CPB involves the adrenergic system. A ninefold increase in epinephrine concentration has been demonstrated, with a peak during rewarming near the time of aortic cross-clamp release.[30] Norepinephrine concentration increases to a lesser degree. Catecholamine concentrations may remain elevated during CPB because of isolation of the lungs from the circulation. The lungs are normally responsible for a significant amount of catecholamine metabolism. Both opioids and inhalational anesthetics alter the stress response to CPB, including the adrenergic component, and the depth of anesthesia appears to determine the degree of attenuation.

What Are the Effects of Cardiopulmonary Bypass on Neurologic Outcome?

Numerous studies of neurologic outcome after cardiac surgery have demonstrated a 3% to 6% incidence of stroke[31–33] and a 13% to 79% incidence of more subtle neuropsychologic dysfunction.[32, 34] The etiology of CNS injury associated with cardiac surgery and CPB is probably multifactorial.

Mechanisms of Injury

Three categories of injury have been suggested (Table 18–5). Whether the safety of CPB depends on perfusion pressure, duration of CPB, type of oxygenator, use of an arterial line filter, technique of acid-base management, control of blood glucose, or various other characteristics has been the source of considerable debate.

Embolization

The higher incidence of focal neurologic deficits after open ventricle procedures (valve replacement, aneurysmectomy), in

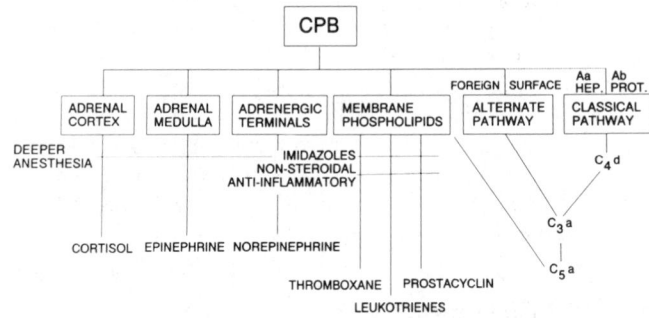

FIGURE 18–5. Various organs and tissues release mediators in the stress response to CPB. Release of cortisol and catecholamines may be reduced by deeper levels of anesthesia. Release of prostaglandins may be reduced by treatment with anti-inflammatory drugs. (From Reves JG, Croughwell N, Jacobs JR, Greeley W: Anesthesia during cardiopulmonary bypass: Does it matter? *In* Cardiopulmonary Bypass: Current Concepts and Controversies. Tinker JH (ed). Philadelphia, WB Saunders, 1989, pp 69–97.)

TABLE 18–5. Suggested Mechanisms of Central Nervous System Injury Following Cardiac Surgery

Microembolization	Macroembolization	Reduced Cerebral Perfusion
Air	Air	Decreased blood flow
Atherosclerotic plaque	Atherosclerotic plaque	Low perfusion pressure
Cellular aggregates	Calcium deposit	Cerebrovascular disease
	Intracardiac thrombus	Technical problems with aortic cannula placement
		Inadequate drainage of superior vena cava

which air and particulate matter would be more likely to enter the circulation, suggests that an embolic cause is more common than is reduced cerebral blood flow (CBF).[32] Transcranial Doppler ultrasonography has demonstrated a high incidence of microemboli in the middle cerebral artery associated with CPB, particularly with insertion of the aortic cannula.[35]

Cerebral Hypoperfusion

Global neuropsychologic deficits may be related more to cerebral hypoperfusion on the basis of hemodynamic instability than factors related to the conduct of CPB. Analysis of multiple risk factors and variables in one study showed that only the use of post-CPB pressors and placement of an intra-aortic balloon pump were associated with the incidence of post-CPB encephalopathy.[36]

What Perfusion Pressure Is Necessary for Adequate Cerebral Blood Flow?

In order to determine the relation between perfusion pressure and neurologic outcome, Stockard and colleagues examined continuous arterial pressure, intermittent electroencephalographic (EEG) monitoring, and preoperative and postoperative neurologic testing in 25 patients undergoing CPB.[37] Flow was maintained at $2.2 \ L \cdot min \cdot m^{2-1}$ at all times. The depth and duration of perfusion pressure below 50 mm Hg were determined from the pressure tracing as [50 − MAP] dt (MAP = mean arterial pressure), expressed in the units millimeters of mercury per minute of perfusion <50 mm Hg, or tm^{50}. *Trends of greater incidence of intraoperative EEG abnormalities and*

postoperative neurologic dysfunction with increasing tm^{50} were demonstrated (Fig. 18–6). No patients with tm^{50} <100 had intraoperative EEG changes or postoperative neurologic dysfunction.

Although these findings probably have contributed to a reluctance among surgeons, anesthesiologists, and perfusionists to maintain CPB perfusion pressure at <50 mm Hg, numerous subsequent studies have failed to confirm the relationship of low perfusion pressure and post-CPB neurologic dysfunction.[31, 32, 38] Low-flow low-pressure perfusion has been shown to be safe, even with very large tm^{50} values.[31] CBF and cerebral metabolism decrease during hypothermic CPB, and cerebral autoregulation appears to be maintained to a pressure as low as 30 mm Hg.[39] Hemodilution during CPB probably promotes cerebral perfusion by improving the flow characteristics of blood.

Advantages of Low Perfusion Pressure

Low perfusion pressure during CPB offers other potential advantages (Table 18–6).[40] Although the lower limit of safe perfusion pressure has not been clearly defined in terms of neurologic outcome, a pressure between 40 and 50 mm Hg is probably safe during hypothermia. A slightly higher pressure, perhaps 60 to 70 mm Hg, during normothermic CPB is advised because of greater cerebral metabolism. Higher pressures may be necessary in subsets of patients with cerebrovascular disease or diabetes, as discussed subsequently.

How Should Acid-Base Status Be Managed?

The choice of acid-base management involves the controversy about whether blood gas values should be temperature corrected and whether CO_2 should be added to a patient's blood during CPB. As temperature is lowered, the solubility of CO_2 in blood increases, the P_{CO_2} decreases, and the pH increases. When blood gas partial pressures are measured during hypothermic CPB, the sample is warmed in the blood gas machine to 37 °C. The results can be reported for a temperature of 37 °C or may be "temperature corrected" down to the patient's temperature through the use of a nomogram to determine the values at the perfusion temperature.

pH-Stat

The pH-stat method of acid-base management strives to keep a patient's P_{CO_2} at 40 mm Hg and pH at 7.40 no matter

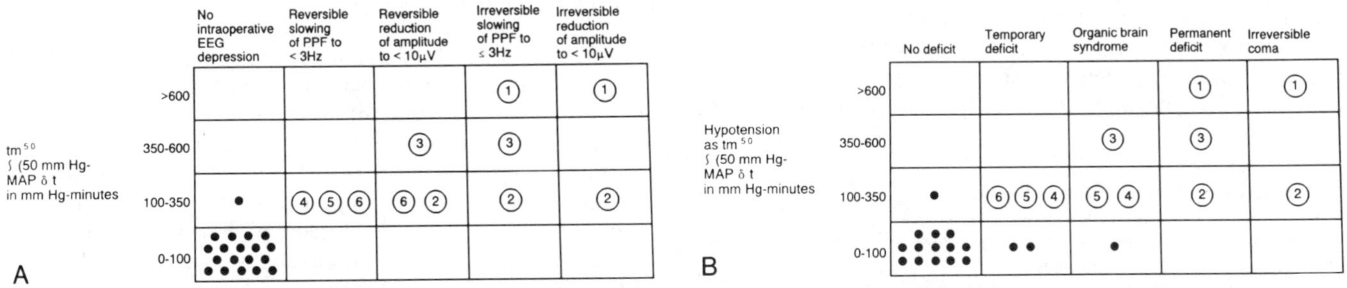

FIGURE 18–6. Postoperative neurologic complications were correlated with depth and duration of hypotension *(A)* and electroencephalographic changes *(B)* during cardiopulmonary bypass in 23 patients. The units of hypotension are mm Hg–minutes of perfusion below 50 mm Hg (tm^{50}). The *circled numbers* represent the 6 patients who had hypotension >100 mm Hg–minutes, EEG changes, and postoperative neurologic deficits. The *solid circles* represent the other 17 patients. Several more recent studies have failed to confirm this correlation of neurologic deficits with depth and duration of hypotension during CPB. (From Stockard JJ, Bickford RG, Schauble JF: Pressure-dependent cerebral ischemia during cardiopulmonary bypass. Neurology 1973, 23:521.)

what the temperature. This goal is accomplished by adding CO_2 to the CPB circuit.

α-Stat

The α-stat method maintains the P_{CO_2} at 40 mm Hg and pH at 7.40 in a blood sample measured at 37 °C. Blood gas values and pH are thus temperature corrected, and CO_2 is not added to the CPB circuit. Because P_{CO_2} and pH are allowed to change with temperature, intracellular electrochemical neutrality rather than pH is maintained constant.

The "α" refers to the α-imidazole ring on the histidine amino acid residue in various cellular proteins, the most important charged species determining intracellular electrochemical charge. A theoretic benefit of α-stat acid-base management is that normal protein structure and function, particularly enzyme function, are maintained in an electrochemically neutral environment.[41]

Practical Applications

CBF reactivity to varying P_{CO_2} is maintained during hypothermic CPB.[39, 42] Thus, CBF tends to be greater during pH-stat management because of a greater degree of cerebral vasodilation. However, cerebral autoregulation and flow/metabolism coupling are lost during pH-stat management, whereas they are maintained during α-stat management.[43]

Although CBF in excess of metabolic requirements occurs with pH-stat management, whether this "luxury perfusion" is an advantage or a disadvantage remains unclear. If CNS dysfunction after CPB is most commonly related to embolic events, increasing CBF through pH-stat management may, in theory, lead to more frequent delivery of embolic materials to the cerebral vasculature.

When phenylephrine is used to increase perfusion pressure, CBF does not increase in patients managed with the α-stat technique (i.e., autoregulation is preserved). When phenylephrine is administered to a patient undergoing CPB with pH-stat acid-base management, CBF increases linearly with the increase in perfusion pressure (i.e., autoregulation is not preserved).[44]

Conclusions

Maintenance of intracellular electrochemical neutrality, preservation of cerebral pressure-flow autoregulation, and preservation of flow-metabolism coupling all make α-stat management attractive. However, a randomized study of patients undergoing cardiac surgery with CPB using either pH-stat or α-stat management, moderate hypothermia (28 °C to 32 °C), and perfusion pressure within a range of 60 to 80 mm Hg failed to show any differences in neuropsychologic or cardiac outcome.[45] Despite what appear to be very significant effects

TABLE 18–6. Potential Advantages of Low Cardiopulmonary Bypass Perfusion Pressure

---

Reduced trauma to blood elements
Less stress on pump tubing and connections
Decreased trauma to aortic cannulation and cross-clamp sites
Less bleeding into the operative field
Decreased heart warming through noncoronary collateral vessels
Smaller venous and arterial cannula size

---

on CBF, the choice of acid-base management during CPB does not appear to be a critical factor in determining the occurrence of neurologic dysfunction.

What Other Factors Affect Central Nervous System Outcome?

Oxygenator

The direct contact of blood with air in a bubble oxygenator increases the delivery of microemboli to a patient over that with a membrane oxygenator.[35] Greater numbers of circulating platelet microaggregates are present when a bubble oxygenator is used.[46] However, postoperative neurologic dysfunction has not been shown to be worse after use of a bubble oxygenator than after a membrane oxygenator.

Arterial Line Filter

Although an arterial line filter should prevent cellular aggregates and debris larger than 20 or 40 μm (depending on the filter pore size used) from traveling from the CPB circuit to the patient, studies have not demonstrated improved neurologic outcome.[33, 47]

Duration of Cardiopulmonary Bypass

Some studies have shown an increase in postoperative neurologic dysfunction with increasing CPB duration, but others have not. Correlation of neurologic dysfunction with the duration of CPB may be more related to the complexity of the surgery and perhaps hemodynamic compromise after CPB than a problem inherent in the duration of CPB.

Miscellaneous Considerations

Although several aspects of CPB taken together may affect neurologic outcome, the attribution of neurologic dysfunction to any single characteristic is difficult. Other factors, such as a patient's preoperative cerebrovascular and neurologic status, complexity of the surgical procedure, and hemodynamic stability, all may be more important.

Do Barbiturates Confer Cerebral Protection?

Open Chamber Heart Surgery

In light of several animal studies that suggested improved neurologic outcome after incomplete cerebral ischemia, a randomized prospective trial of barbiturate administration was carried out in patients undergoing cardiac surgery that involved opening a chamber of the heart.[48] Sodium thiopental was infused in the study group of patients, at a rate sufficient to produce and maintain an isoelectric EEG, from 10 minutes before aortic cannulation until the discontinuation of CPB.

A significantly lower incidence of neuropsychiatric complications was found in the thiopental group on the 10th postoperative day. A rather large dose of thiopental (mean = 39.5 mg · kg^{-1}) was administered, however, leading to more frequent need for inotropic support, delayed awakening (by 2.5

hours), and prolonged tracheal intubation (by 5 hours) compared with the control group.

This study was criticized for several technical aspects of CPB that differed from common practice at other institutions (normothermic CPB, use of a bubble oxygenator, absence of an arterial line filter, and loose control of perfusion pressure). As noted previously, these differences in practice may be less important in the production of CNS dysfunction than previously thought.[47] Nevertheless, the use of thiopental for cerebral protection is not common except in selected situations (i.e., deep hypothermia and circulatory arrest).

Coronary Artery Bypass Grafting

Thiopental use in patients undergoing coronary artery bypass grafting (CABG) also has been investigated.[49] Hypothermic CPB was used with a membrane oxygenator, arterial line filter, and perfusion pressure >50 mm Hg. No significant difference was noted in the incidence of neurologic complications between thiopental and control groups. The doses of thiopental were comparable to those required in the open chamber heart study.[48] Similar delays in awakening and extubation and an increased need for inotropic support were also demonstrated.

Summary

Thiopental may offer potential benefit in some high-risk patients, but routine use does not appear justified. Its administration in patients undergoing cardiac surgery in the doses described is not benign, as demonstrated by the tendency for myocardial depression and prolonged times to awakening and extubation.

Is Control of Blood Glucose Concentration Important?

Blood glucose concentration commonly increases during CPB. This increase is most likely due to the increased concentrations of catecholamines, cortisol, and glucagon that occur during the stress response. The release of insulin is also inhibited during hypothermic CPB.

In nonsurgical patients, evidence suggests that cerebral ischemia (i.e., cardiac arrest, stroke) with hyperglycemia is associated with worse neurologic outcome than when it occurs in a normoglycemic patient.[50-52] Whether a causal relationship exists between blood glucose concentration and neurologic dysfunction after cerebral ischemia is uncertain. Large increases in blood glucose may also be a marker of difficult and prolonged resuscitation, which is associated with worse neurologic outcomes.[51, 53]

Children undergoing cardiac surgery with deep hypothermia and circulatory arrest have a greater incidence of neurologic deficits if hyperglycemia is present.[54] This indirect evidence suggests that tight glucose control during CPB is important to lessen the risk of post-CPB neurologic dysfunction.

Neuropsychiatric Dysfunction

Elevations of blood glucose concentration during CPB have not been shown to correlate with postoperative neuropsychiatric dysfunction.[55] Perhaps blood glucose concentration is more important in determining outcome after global cerebral ischemia than after focal events. Its importance may also differ between nondiabetic and diabetic patients. Diabetic patients may be at greater risk of postoperative neurologic deficits for reasons other than hyperglycemia (Table 18-7).[56-59]

Tight Glucose Control

Tight control of blood glucose concentration has not been compared prospectively with less aggressive glucose management as a determinant of postoperative neurologic outcome. The use of a glucose-containing priming solution may produce very high glucose concentrations during CPB,[60] but this effect is not associated with any worsening of neurologic outcome.[61]

Although it has been suggested that the blood glucose concentration should be maintained below 200 mg · dL^{-1} whenever a risk of brain ischemia is present,[62] currently available data do not provide a conclusive answer about whether tight control is beneficial during CPB that does not involve circulatory arrest. Prompt treatment of hyperglycemia after CPB may add stability to postoperative metabolic and electrolyte status.

How Can Perfusion Pressure Be Controlled?

When systemic vascular resistance (SVR) and perfusion pressure become excessively elevated during CPB, one may choose to administer an inhalational anesthetic to the CPB circuit or an intravenous agent such as sodium nitroprusside (SNP) or nitroglycerin (NTG). All of these agents have rapid onset, can be titrated, and are of short duration.

Of the inhalational anesthetics, isoflurane is the most logical choice because it is an effective vasodilator and may offer benefit in terms of cerebral protection. Similar to thiopental, 1% isoflurane produces EEG burst suppression and reduces the cerebral metabolic rate for O_2 (CMRo$_2$) during hypothermic CPB.[63] Its advantages over thiopental are that it is readily eliminated at the end of CPB, and it does not have persistent detrimental effects on myocardial function.

Inhalational anesthetics prevent increases in catecholamine and cortisol concentrations at least as effectively as opioids during CPB.[64, 65] One approach is to use isoflurane when necessary to decrease perfusion pressure during most of the course of CPB and then to convert to SNP or NTG or both if needed near the end of CPB.

Are Patients with Carotid Disease at Increased Risk of Neurologic Deficits?

Patients with symptomatic, hemodynamically significant carotid artery stenoses commonly undergo carotid endarterec-

TABLE 18-7. Risk Factors for Postoperative Neurologic Dysfunction in Diabetes

Chronically impaired cerebral autoregulation
Increased blood viscosity
Reduced red blood cell deformability
Hypercoagulability due to reduced antithrombin III activity
Increased platelet adhesion
Increased platelet aggregation

tomy before or combined with cardiac surgery. Patients with asymptomatic carotid stenoses for elective cardiac surgery and patients with symptomatic carotid disease undergoing emergency cardiac surgery present interesting management considerations during CPB. One may choose to monitor the EEG intraoperatively and to administer thiopental to decrease $CMRo_2$.

Perfusion Pressure

Anesthesiologists and perfusionists commonly maintain perfusion pressure higher than in patients without known carotid disease, usually choosing an arbitrary lower limit of acceptable pressure somewhere between 50 and 70 mm Hg. The rationale is that a higher driving pressure across stenotic lesions preserves downstream flow. Pressure is maintained by increased pump flow or α-adrenergic agonists such as phenylephrine. CBF was measured using ^{133}Xe clearance in a single patient with significant bilateral carotid stenoses and was found to be equal at perfusion pressures of 30 and 80 mm Hg.

Because the most common cause of post-CPB neurologic dysfunction is probably an embolic event,[32] carotid stenosis and the perfusion pressure during CPB may be of secondary importance. Further study of this patient population, including patients with severe carotid stenosis and patients with symptomatic disease, is warranted to determine whether maintaining an elevated perfusion pressure is beneficial.

How Are Renal Blood Flow and Renal Function Affected?

Nonpulsatile Cardiopulmonary Bypass

Even though mean arterial pressure and overall renal blood flow may be maintained during nonpulsatile CPB, a progressive reduction of flow to the outer cortex and relative increase in flow to the inner cortex occur.[66] Simultaneously, an increase in renin release is noted and may be responsible for the redistribution of renal cortical blood flow rather than a result of it.

Perfusion Pressure

The renal perfusion pressure during CPB is important in determining the transglomerular filtration pressure and, therefore, the glomerular filtration rate (GFR). Maintenance of a higher perfusion pressure with phenylephrine (>70 mm Hg) during CPB increases GFR and creatinine clearance compared with values at lower pressures. However, raising perfusion pressure to optimize these measures of renal function intraoperatively is probably of little overall importance and has not been shown to improve postoperative renal function.[67]

Pulsatile Cardiopulmonary Bypass

Pulsatile CPB has been suggested to provide some advantages in patients at risk for postoperative renal dysfunction. Studies have suggested that pulsatile perfusion is superior to nonpulsatile perfusion in preservation of renal function, maintenance of normal renal metabolism, reduction in renin release, preservation of outer cortical flow, and prevention of histologic evidence of ischemia.[68] Data from other studies have been inconsistent and contradictory.

Analysis of perioperative variables to predict postoperative renal dysfunction has not implicated the flow and pressure characteristics of CPB as important contributors. Preoperative renal dysfunction and perioperative hemodynamic instability, especially when severe enough to require vasopressors, intra-aortic balloon counterpulsation, large blood transfusions, and reoperation, are most important in determining postoperative renal dysfunction.[69]

Postoperative Renal Failure

The incidence of postoperative renal failure after cardiac surgery has been reported to vary from 2.5% to 31%.[70, 71] Mortality has been reported to be as high as 89%.[72] For this reason, anything that can be done to prevent worsening of preoperative renal dysfunction should be considered. The CPB prime usually contains mannitol to induce diuresis. Assuming adequate intravascular volume and CPB flow, additional doses of mannitol or other diuretics should be considered when urine output is low. Low-dose dopamine (2 to 3 $\mu g \cdot kg^{-1} \cdot min^{-1}$) may also improve renal blood flow. Pulsatile CPB may also provide some benefit, although the existing data are not conclusive.

What Are the Other Potential Advantages of Pulsatile over Nonpulsatile Cardiopulmonary Bypass?

Pulsatile flow appears to offer physiologic advantages to several organ systems, but clinical evidence of improved outcome has been difficult to demonstrate. The inconsistent findings reported for pulsatile CPB may reflect differences in the perfusion systems used and the interaction of such systems with the arterial system of a patient. The waveform of pulsatile flow depends on both the system and the patient's vascular impedance. If a pulsatile perfusion system is unable to deliver pulsatile waveform flow to the various organ beds, it is no different from a nonpulsatile system.

Pulsatile flow has been provided in the past by several devices including an intra-aortic balloon pump. Most commonly today it is achieved by a standard roller pump with instantaneous variation of the rate of pump head rotation. It can also be generated by the previously mentioned Sarns centrifugal pump.

Blood Pressure and Systemic Vascular Resistance

Pulsatile CPB appears to be associated with smaller increases in concentrations of epinephrine, norepinephrine, and vasopressin than nonpulsatile CPB.[73, 74] Perhaps as a consequence, mean arterial pressure and SVR tend to be higher during nonpulsatile CPB.[74] Also, smaller increases in catecholamines may favor better perfusion of vascular beds. Variable results have been reported concerning the effects of pulsatile CPB on microcirculatory perfusion and tissue metabolism.

Cerebral Blood Flow

CBF has received little study during pulsatile CPB. A higher cerebrospinal fluid Po_2 and lower jugular venous lactate concentration occur during pulsatile than nonpulsatile CPB.[75, 76]

Otherwise, no convincing evidence shows that pulsatile perfusion is more favorable for cerebral metabolism. Whether pulsatile CPB improves CBF in patients with cerebrovascular disease is unknown.

Miscellaneous Effects

Pulsatile CPB may provide better perfusion to the pancreas, thereby preventing ischemic injury and preserving metabolic function.[77] Some forms of pulsatile CPB have been shown to be less damaging to red blood cells and platelets, but others have produced more damage. Cannula sizes and shapes, connections, and the type of pump are probably important factors.

References

1. Noon GP, Kane LE, Feldman L, et al: Reduction of blood trauma in roller pumps for long-term perfusion. World J Surg 1985; 9:65.
2. Maltry DE, Eggers GWN: Isoflurane-induced failure of the Bentley-10 oxygenator. Anesthesiology 1987; 66:100.
3. Cooper S, Levin R: Near catastrophic oxygenator failure. Anesthesiology 1987; 66:101.
4. Slogoff S, Keats AS: Does perioperative myocardial ischemia lead to postoperative myocardial infarction? Anesthesiology 1985; 62:107.
5. Slogoff S, Keats AS: Further observations on perioperative myocardial ischemia. Anesthesiology 1986; 65:539.
6. Delva E, Maille J-G, Solymoss BC, et al: Evaluation of myocardial damage during coronary artery grafting with serial determinations of CPK MB isoenzymes. J Thorac Cardiovasc Surg 1978; 75:467.
7. Jalonen J, Heikkila H, Arola M, et al: Myocardial oxygen balance and cardiopulmonary bypass in patients undergoing coronary artery bypass grafting. J Cardiothorac Anesth 1989; 3:311.
8. Magee PG, Gardner ATJ, Flaherty JT, et al: Improved myocardial protection with propranolol during induced ischemia. Circulation 1980; 62(Suppl):I–49.
9. Rao PS, Brock FE, Cleary K, et al: Effect of intraoperative propranolol on serum creatine kinase MB release in patients having elective cardiac operations. J Thorac Cardiovasc Surg 1984; 88:562.
10. Buckberg GD, Brazier JR, Nelson RL, et al: Studies of the effects of hypothermia on regional myocardial blood flow and metabolism during cardiopulmonary bypass. I. The adequately perfused beating, fibrillating, and arrested heart. J Thorac Cardiovasc Surg 1977; 73:87.
11. Buckberg GD: A proposed "solution" to the cardioplegic controversy. J Thorac Cardiovasc Surg 1979; 77:803.
12. Wright RN, Levitsky S, Holland C, et al: Beneficial effects of potassium cardioplegia during intermittent aortic cross-clamping and reperfusion. J Surg Res 1978; 24:201.
13. Landymore RW, Tice D, Trehan N, et al: Importance of topical hypothermia to ensure uniform myocardial cooling during coronary artery bypass. J Thorac Cardiovasc Surg 1981; 82:832.
14. Rousou JA, Parker T, Engelman RM, et al: Phrenic nerve paresis associated with the use of iced slush and the cooling jacket for topical hypothermia. J Thorac Cardiovasc Surg 1985; 89:921.
15. Marco JD, Hahn JW, Barner HB: Topical cardiac hypothermia and phrenic nerve injury. Ann Thorac Surg 1977; 23:235.
16. Gundry SR, Kirsh MM: A comparison of retrograde cardioplegia versus antegrade cardioplegia in the presence of coronary artery occlusion. Ann Thorac Surg 1984; 38:124.
17. Chitwood WR Jr: Retrograde cardioplegia: Current methods. Ann Thorac Surg 1992; 53:352.
18. Partington MT, Acar C, Buckberg GD, et al: Studies of retrograde cardioplegia. I. Capillary blood flow distribution to myocardium supplied by open and occluded arteries. J Thorac Cardiovasc Surg 1989; 97:605.
19. Partington MT, Acar C, Buckberg GD, et al: Studies of retrograde cardioplegia. II. Advantages of antegrade/retrograde cardioplegia to optimize distribution in jeopardized myocardium. J Thorac Cardiovasc Surg 1989; 97:613.
20. Menasche P, Subayi J-B, Piwicna A: Retrograde coronary sinus cardioplegia for aortic valve operations: a clinical report on 500 patients. Ann Thorac Surg 1990; 49:556.
21. Zimmerman ANE, Daems W, Hulsmann WC, et al: Morphological changes of heart muscle caused by successive perfusion with calcium-free and calcium-containing solutions (calcium paradox). Cardiovasc Res 1967; 1:201.
22. Barner HB: Blood cardioplegia: a review and comparison with crystalloid cardioplegia. Ann Thorac Surg 1991; 52:1354.
23. Lichtenstein SV, Ashe KA, Dalati HE, et al: Warm heart surgery. J Thorac Cardiovasc Surg 1991; 101:269.
24. Lichtenstein SV, Abel JG, Panos A, et al: Warm heart surgery: experience with long cross-clamp times. Ann Thorac Surg 1991; 52:1009.
25. Salerno TA, Christakis AGT, Abel J, et al: Technique and pitfalls of retrograde continuous warm blood cardioplegia. Ann Thorac Surg 1991; 51:1023.
26. Kavanagh BP, Mazer CD, Panos A, et al: Effect of warm heart surgery on perioperative management of patients undergoing urgent cardiac surgery. J Cardiothorac Vasc Anesth 1992; 6:127.
27. Forman MB, Virmani R, Puett DW: Mechanisms and therapy of reperfusion injury. Circulation 1990; 81(Suppl):IV–69.
28. Bolling SF, Bies LE, Gallagher KP, et al: Enhanced myocardial protection with adenosine. Ann Thorac Surg 1989; 47:809.
29. Opie LH: Reperfusion injury and its pharmacologic modification. Circulation 1989; 80:1049.
30. Reves JG, Karp RB, Buttner EE, et al: Neuronal and adrenomedullary catecholamine release in response to cardiopulmonary bypass in man. Circulation 1980; 66:49.
31. Kolkka R, Hilberman M: Neurologic dysfunction following cardiac operation with low-flow, low-pressure cardiopulmonary bypass. J Thorac Cardiovasc Surg 1980; 79:432.
32. Slogoff S, Girgis KZ, Keats AS: Etiologic factors in neuropsychiatric complications associated with cardiopulmonary bypass. Anesth Analg 1982; 61:903.
33. Aris A, Solanes H, Camara ML, et al: Arterial line filtration during cardiopulmonary bypass: neurologic, neuropsychologic, and hematologic studies. J Thorac Cardiovasc Surg 1986; 91:526.
34. Shaw PJ, Bates D, Cartlidge NEF, et al: Neurologic and neuropsychological morbidity following major surgery: comparison of coronary artery bypass and peripheral vascular surgery. Stroke 1987; 18:700.
35. Padayachee TS, Parsons S, Theobold R, et al: The detection of microemboli in the middle cerebral artery during cardiopulmonary bypass: a transcranial Doppler ultrasound investigation using membrane and bubble oxygenators. Ann Thorac Surg 1987; 44:298.
36. Breuer AC, Furlan AJ, Hanson MR, et al: Central nervous system complications of coronary artery bypass graft surgery: prospective analysis of 421 patients. Stroke 1983; 14:682.
37. Stockard JJ, Bickford RG, Schauble JF: Pressure-dependent cerebral ischemia during cardiopulmonary bypass. Neurology 1973; 23:521.
38. Sotaniemi KA: Brain damage and neurological outcome after open-heart surgery. J Neurol Neurosurg Psychiatry 1980; 43:127.
39. Govier AV, Reves JG, McKay ARD, et al: Factors and their influence on regional cerebral blood flow during nonpulsatile cardiopulmonary bypass. Ann Thorac Surg 1984; 38:592.
40. Garman JK: Optimal pressures and flows during cardiopulmonary bypass. Pro: a low-flow, low-pressure technique is acceptable. J Cardiothorac Vasc Anesth 1991; 5:399.
41. Hickey PR, Hansen DD: Temperature and blood gases: the clinical dilemma of acid-base management for hypothermic cardiopulmonary bypass. In Cardiopulmonary Bypass: Current Concepts and Controversies. Tinker JH (ed). Philadelphia, WB Saunders, 1989, pp 1–20.
42. Prough DS, Stump DA, Roy RC, et al: Response of cerebral blood flow to changes in carbon dioxide tension during hypothermic cardiopulmonary bypass. Anesthesiology 1986; 64:576.
43. Murkin JM, Farrar JK, Tweed WA, et al: Cerebral autoregulation and flow/metabolism coupling during cardiopulmonary bypass: the influence of $Paco_2$. Anesth Analg 1987; 66:825.
44. Rogers AT, Stump DA, Gravlee GP, et al: Response of cerebral blood flow to phenylephrine infusion during hypothermic cardiopulmonary bypass: influence of $Paco_2$ management. Anesthesiology 1988; 69:547.
45. Bashein G, Townes BD, Nessly ML, et al: A randomized study of carbon dioxide management during hypothermic cardiopulmonary bypass. Anesthesiology 1990; 72:7.
46. Dutton RC, Edmunds LH, Hutchinson JC, et al: Platelet aggregate emboli produced in patients during cardiopulmonary bypass with membrane and bubble oxygenators and blood filters. J Thorac Cardiovasc Surg 1974; 67:258.
47. Nussmeier NA, Fish KJ: Neuropsychological dysfunction after cardiopulmonary bypass: a comparison of two institutions. J Cardiothorac Vasc Anesth 1991; 5:584.
48. Nussmeier NA, Arlund C, Slogoff S: Neuropsychiatric complications after cardiopulmonary bypass: cerebral protection by a barbiturate. Anesthesiology 1986; 64:165.
49. Zaidan JR, Klochany A, Martin WM, et al: Effect of thiopental on neurologic outcome following coronary artery bypass grafting. Anesthesiology 1991; 74:406.

50. Longstreth WT Jr, Inui TS: High blood glucose level on hospital admission and poor neurological recovery after cardiac arrest. Ann Neurol 1984; 15:59.

51. Longstreth WT Jr, Diehr P, Cobb LA, et al: Neurologic outcome and blood glucose levels during out-of-hospital cardiopulmonary resuscitation. Neurology 1986; 36:1186.

52. Candelise L, Landi G, Orazio EN, et al: Prognostic significance of hyperglycemia in acute stroke. Arch Neurol 1985; 42:661.

53. Hallstrom AP, Cobb LA, Swain M, et al: Predictors of hospital mortality after out-of-hospital CPR. Crit Care Med 1985; 13:927.

54. Steward DJ, Da Silva CA, Flegel T: Elevated blood glucose levels may increase the danger of neurological deficit following profoundly hypothermic cardiac arrest (Letter to the editor). Anesthesiology 1988; 68:653.

55. Frasco P, Croughwell N, Blumenthal J, et al: Association between blood glucose level during cardiopulmonary bypass and neuropsychiatric outcome (Abstract). Anesthesiology 1991; 75:A55.

56. Bentsen N, Larsen B, Lassen NA: Chronically impaired autoregulation of cerebral blood flow in long term diabetes. Stroke 1975; 6:497.

57. Barnes AJ, Locke P, Scudder PR, et al: Is hyperviscosity a treatable component of diabetic microcirculatory disease? Lancet 1977; 2:789.

58. Ceriello A: Heparin preserves antithrombin III biological activity from hyperglycemia induced alteration in insulin dependent diabetes. Haemostasis 1986; 16:458.

59. Colwell JA, Nair RMG, Halushka PV, et al: Platelet adhesion and aggregation in diabetes mellitus. Metabolism 1979; 28:394.

60. McKnight CK, Elliot MJ, Pearson DT, et al: The effects of four different crystalloid bypass pump-priming fluids upon the metabolic response to cardiac operation. J Thorac Cardiovasc Surg 1985; 90:97.

61. Metz S, Keats AS: Benefits of a glucose-containing priming solution for cardiopulmonary bypass. Anesth Analg 1991; 72:427.

62. Sieber FE, Smith DS, Traystmann RJ, et al: Glucose: a reevaluation of its intraoperative use. Anesthesiology 1987; 67:72.

63. Woodcock TE, Murkin JM, Farrar JK, et al: Pharmacologic EEG suppression during cardiopulmonary bypass: cerebral hemodynamic and metabolic effects of thiopental or isoflurane during hypothermia and normothermia. Anesthesiology 1987; 67:218.

64. Samuelson PN, Reves JG, Kirklin JK, et al: Comparison of sufentanil and enflurane-nitrous oxide anesthesia for myocardial revascularization. Anesth Analg 1986; 65:217.

65. Fiezzani P, Croughwell N, McIntyre RW, et al: Isoflurane decreases the cortisol response to cardiopulmonary bypass. Anesth Analg 1986; 65:1117.

66. Goodman TA, Gerard DF, Bernstein EF, et al: The effects of pulseless perfusion on the distribution of renal cortical blood flow and on renin release. Surgery 1976; 80:31.

67. Urzua J, Troncoso S, Bugedo G, et al: Renal function and cardiopulmonary bypass: effect of perfusion pressure. J Cardiothorac Vasc Anesth 1992; 6:299.

68. Hickey PR, Buckley MJ, Philbin DM: Pulsatile and nonpulsatile cardiopulmonary bypass: review of a counterproductive controversy. Ann Thorac Surg 1983; 36:720.

69. Slogoff S, Reul GJ, Keats AS, et al: Role of perfusion pressure and flow in major organ dysfunction after cardiopulmonary bypass. Ann Thorac Surg 1990; 50:911.

70. Hilberman M, Myers BD, Carrie BJ, et al: Acute renal failure following cardiac surgery. J Thorac Cardiovasc Surg 1979; 77:880.

71. Bhat JG, Gluck MC, Lowenstein J, et al: Renal failure after open heart surgery. Ann Intern Med 1976; 84:677.

72. Abel RM, Buckley MJ, Austen WG, et al: Etiology, incidence, and prognosis of renal failure following cardiac operations: results of a prospective analysis of 500 consecutive patients. J Thorac Cardiovasc Surg 1976; 71:323.

73. Philbin DM, Levine FH, Kono K, et al: Attenuation of the stress response to cardiopulmonary bypass by the addition of pulsatile flow. Circulation 1981; 64:808.

74. Minami K, Korner MM, Vyska K, et al: Effects of pulsatile perfusion on plasma catecholamine levels and hemodynamics during and after cardiac operations with cardiopulmonary bypass. J Thorac Cardiovasc Surg 1990; 99:82.

75. Geha AS, Salaymeh MT, Abe T, et al: Effect of pulsatile cardiopulmonary bypass on cerebral metabolism. J Surg Res 1972; 12:381.

76. Geha AS, Malt SH, Nara Y, et al: Effect of cardiopulmonary bypass on cerebral metabolism. J Thorac Cardiovasc Surg 1971; 61:200.

77. Nagaoka H, Innami R, Watanabe M, et al: Preservation of pancreatic beta cell function with pulsatile cardiopulmonary bypass. Ann Thorac Surg 1989; 48:798.

Monitors and Their Applications

CHAPTER **19**

Introduction to Monitoring: Clinical Monitoring

J. S. GRAVENSTEIN, M.D.

The pioneers in anesthesia had no monitors and, in fact, knew little about what they should monitor. Through the years, a routine evolved for monitoring ventilation and circulation without instruments. Then, one by one, monitoring instruments were developed, not to replace the largely qualitative clinical judgment but to add quantitative assessments.

UNDERLYING CONCEPTS

What Are the Principal Objectives Served by Monitoring?

Titration

We titrate the effects of anesthetic and adjuvant drugs, such as a muscle relaxant, or adjust the ventilator to a desired end point. If patients' responses were predictable, titration would not be necessary.

Safety

We must discover unexpected perturbations of vital functions before a patient suffers harm—for example, from hypotension when the surgeon compresses the vena cava.

Equipment Function

We must monitor equipment function because malfunction can cause injury—for example, from an occluded scavenger system.

How Is Monitoring Applied?

Today, as was the case a century ago, all monitoring starts with inspection, auscultation, and palpation—that is, with the assessment of clinical signs. For two reasons, this routine continues to come first. (1) Some clinical signs are subtle, and no instruments yet exist to take their place. (2) Instruments may fail or cannot be applied, for example, in a patient suffering severe burns.

Even without instruments, clinicians must be capable of caring for their patients as safely as possible. Indeed, experienced clinicians appear to have a sixth sense for perceiving trouble. They may identify a problem well before it becomes obvious. That sixth sense deserves continual cultivation. Monitoring instruments cannot replace it, but they amplify and quantify the information we collect clinically.

In What Order Should We Sample Monitored Data?

Monitoring can be pursued according to a geographic or a conceptual approach. Both have proponents.

The Geographic Approach

The geographic approach calls for scanning of all variables in a predetermined sequence—for example, starting with a patient's left hand, which might carry a pulse oximeter probe; working up the arm and checking the intravenous site; auscultating across the chest for breath and heart sounds; progressing to the other arm to measure blood pressure; and moving down to the wrist of the right hand to the nerve stimulator. An alternative geographic sequence would call for scanning the instruments from one side to the other, regardless of their physiologic relationship.

TABLE 19–1. Monitoring Variables*

Ventilation	Circulation
Gas supply	Patient's color (perfusion)
	Skin
	Mucous membranes/wound
Gas flow rates	Appearance of skin (moist/dry)
Inspired gas concentrations	Heart sounds
Oxygen	
Carbon dioxide (system OK?)	
Anesthetic vapors	
Peak inspiratory pressures	Arterial pressure
End-expiratory pressures	Venous pressure
	Neck veins
	Other veins
Bellows or bag excursions	Electrocardiogram (rate and rhythm)
Tidal volume	Pulse oximeter saturation (plethysmogram)
Respiratory rate	Capnogram (pulmonary circulation)
Expired gas concentrations	Urine output
Patient's color	Cerebral perfusion
	Conscious > orientation
	Unconscious
	Pupils
	Electroencephalogram, evoked potentials
Chest excursion	
Patterns of breathing	
Breath sounds	
Pulse oximeter saturation	

*Grouped according to the conceptual approach and combined clinical observation and use of instruments.

The Conceptual Approach

The conceptual approach, in contradistinction, calls for assessment of variables according to physiologic systems. One may start with ventilation, which in most patients under general anesthesia includes the system that brings gases to the patient, and then the circulation (Table 19–1). Other systems can be added—for example, neuromuscular integrity (the feel of the bag or the peak inspiratory pressure; how relaxed the muscles are in the surgical field; and the response to nerve stimulation) or metabolic variables such as control of blood sugar or regulation of electrolytes and pH.

The conceptual system has intellectual appeal because a clinician thinks in terms of concepts and systems rather than individual variables. Ideally, the geographic and the conceptual system should merge—that is, monitoring instruments should be arranged according to concepts rather than by dint of their size and their ability to fit in this or that empty hole on the anesthesia machine. The following discussion adopts the conceptual approach.

BASIC MONITORING WITHOUT INSTRUMENTS (OTHER THAN A STETHOSCOPE)

First we address the basics: monitoring without instruments, which is essential and continuous yet is the least expensive of all monitoring approaches.[1] According to the *Oxford English Dictionary* (Clarenden Press, Oxford, 1989), both *continual* and *continuous* have been used to mean "incessant, perpetual, without intermission." However, the word *continual* is some-

times used to describe actions that are repeated with brief intermissions. The American Society of Anesthesiologists has embraced the latter definition of *continual* (see Appendix) and reserves the word *continuous* for actions without interruption.

How Should Conscious Patients Be Managed?

Good medical care requires that an anesthesiologist maintain contact with conscious patients. This contact should be frequent, should be verbal, and should include touching a patient to feel the pulse, to mop a brow, or to adjust a gown, drape, or blanket. Patients are justifiably anxious. Concern shown by the anesthesiologist and the human touch go a long way toward lessening anxiety.

Next we elaborate on a system-by-system assessment by inspection, auscultation, and palpation.

Ventilation

Is a patient breathing adequately? We check color and breathing. Remember that even in white patients, cyanosis is a late and unreliable sign of deoxygenation.[1] Table 19–2 includes data from an old study that is still valid.

The Pattern of Breathing

During normal sleep, healthy people breathe so quietly that one can barely discern inspiration and expiration. Any deviation from a peaceful, smooth pattern of breathing must give rise to questions. Such deviations typically occur in a progression, from the most subtle signs in patients minimally affected by disease or weakness to grossly obvious manifestations of severe respiratory impairment. The following signs of breathing, discussed next, are ranked from subtle to obvious. One should make it a habit to check for abnormal signs. If none is detected, so much the better.

Respiratory Rate. You may have to put your hand on the patient's epigastrium to count respirations. Fewer than 12 breaths per minute in an adult should raise questions.

Abdominal Motion. With quiet ventilation in a healthy subject, abdominal motion is barely noticeable. In distressed patients, the abdomen may rise during inspiration. During expiration, the muscles of the abdomen may tighten. That pattern is typically observed in patients with obstructive pulmonary disease. Because of their obstruction and the loss of elastic recoil of the lungs, these patients must exhale actively using accessory muscles of respiration.

TABLE 19–2. Per Cent of Observers Who Detected Cyanosis in White Men

Pao_2	No Cyanosis	Slight Cyanosis	Definite Cyanosis
100–96	68	26	6
95–91	43	40	17
90–86	32	37	31
85–81	14	37	49
80–76	10	40	50
75–71	3	22	75

(From Comroe JH Jr, Botelho S: The unreliability of cyanosis in the recognition of arterial anoxemia. Am J Med Sci 1947; 214:1.)
Abbreviation: Pao_2 = arterial oxygen pressure.

One can easily imagine what happens when such a patient's abdominal muscles are paralyzed, such as during spinal or epidural anesthesia. Active expiration is impossible, and a patient is unable to exhale fully. The functional residual capacity is likely to increase. A desperate situation can arise in asthmatic patients, in whom a high epidural or spinal block paralyzes the sympathetic innervation of the lungs without inhibiting the vagus innervation, resulting in even greater constriction of the bronchial tree.

Chest Motion. Healthy patients, breathing quietly, show little motion of the chest. During inspiration, the chest may rise slightly and symmetrically. Tightening of the intercostal muscles during inspiration cannot be seen. However, when the intercostal muscles are paralyzed and a patient is inhaling forcefully, the intercostal spaces may retract, together with the jugular area just above the sternum.

In spontaneously breathing patients who have upper airway obstruction or are weakened by neuromuscular disease, the chest may show a paradoxical motion, the so-called rocking of the boat. The upper anterior chest sinks instead of rising during inspiration, while the abdomen rises.

The Sounds of Breathing

That we can and will listen to the breath sounds goes without saying. These sounds should be of equal quality on the left and right. In children, breath sounds are easy to hear, regardless of where we apply the stethoscope. In adults, the loudest sounds are heard over the trachea in the suprasternal notch, where air passes by with great velocity during each breath. There, we can also hear if a patient swallows, gags, or retches and if, once he or she is intubated and mechanically ventilated, the cuff on the endotracheal tube leaks. We care for many patients with a history of wheezing. Make sure wheezing does not worsen after the administration of drugs such as antibiotics and morphine, which may release histamine.

Circulation

Perfusion

The brain is the critical organ. If patients are awake, oriented to person, time, and place, and can answer questions, their brains are adequately perfused and oxygenated. Talking with conscious patients is the very best monitor. It reassures patients and it represents good clinical practice. As long as the brain receives adequate blood and oxygen (O_2), we may assume that other organs are adequately perfused and that blood pressure is satisfactory.

I like to inspect a patient's palpebral conjunctiva. My impression is that it turns pale early in hypovolemia and anemia and that it is less likely to be blanched by vasoconstriction than are the nail beds. Check it before starting anesthesia and whenever questions about hypovolemia or anemia arise.

Arterial Blood Pressure

It is difficult to estimate arterial pressure by palpation, but the extremes of hypotension (thready or absent pulse) or hypertension (a taut, hard vessel) can usually be detected. When counting heart rate in a hypotensive patient, some clinicians recommend feeling one's own pulse at the same time to avoid confusing it with that of the patient.

Cardiac Function

Auscultation of breath sounds with a precordial stethoscope has become so routine that some consider it negligent to omit this inexpensive device during regional anesthesia. We can monitor the quality of heart sounds without interruption, beat by beat, and do so for pennies per anesthetic.

The first heart sound is produced by the vibration of the taut atrioventricular valves, the second by the vibration of the semilunar valves. In addition, vibrations of the ventricular wall and, for the second sound, the walls of the aorta and pulmonary artery contribute to the heart sounds. Thus, whenever the contractile force of the heart decreases and blood pressure falls, the vibrations diminish and the heart sounds become muffled.

Of course, in addition to characterizing the heart sounds, auscultation gives continuous information about heart rate and, to a degree, rhythm. Explore with the stethoscope chest piece where the heart sounds are heard best. Sometimes, in obese and emphysematous patients, the suprasternal notch transmits heart sounds more clearly than does the precordium.

How Should Anesthetized Patients Be Managed?

Ventilation

Is a patient getting O_2? If a patient turns blue, it makes little sense to start fretting over ventilation, shunts, alveolar dead space, and the like when the problem all along is the supply of O_2. Therefore, first make sure that O_2 is available to the patient. Your checklist (you could be modern and call it an algorithm) should be O_2 flow meter > inspired O_2 concentration > ventilation. That inspection should require less than 30 seconds; then proceed.

Inspection and Palpation

The Tracheal Tug. During normal ventilation in healthy people, the larynx does not move. With beginning emphysema, in patients with muscle weakness, with mild respiratory obstruction, or with processes that interfere with normal gas exchange, such as pneumonia, the larynx moves down a little with every inspiration. If the reader is young and healthy, he or she should now put a hand over his or her larynx and observe the lack of motion with normal ventilation. Now take a rapid, deep breath and feel how the larynx moves down during inspiration; that is a tracheal tug.

Check your patient before starting anesthesia. If no tracheal tug is felt, the patient should not have one after recovery from anesthesia. If one develops, search for an explanation. The most common causes are muscle relaxant ''hangover,'' with weakening of the respiratory muscles; obstruction of the upper airway; and atelectasis.

Tracheal tugs can be so subtle that one cannot discern them by inspection, particularly in obese patients with a short neck. Put your hand over the larynx or place three fingers along the larynx and trachea and feel for the tug. Do this before starting anesthesia and again before leaving a patient in the postanesthesia care unit.

The more severe the problem with ventilation, the more pronounced is the tracheal tug. First, only the larynx moves a few millimeters, then, with graver respiratory problems, even the floor of the mouth tightens with every inspiration. With very severe respiratory distress, the nares may flare and the mouth may open with every inspiratory gasp.

Where Is the Tube?

Check the Chest. Listen over the anterior chest and in the axillary line before induction of anesthesia to obtain baseline impressions. After intubation, do two things:

1. Listen for breath sounds over the left and right chest, in front, and in the axillary lines. Remember that it is not always easy to determine whether the endotracheal tube has slipped into a mainstem bronchus. The tip may have been located just over the carina; on flexion of the patient's head, it may have descended into a bronchus, most often but not invariably to the right.

2. Feel for the endotracheal tube cuff. It should be palpable just under the larynx. I gently increase and decrease the volume in the cuff by pushing and releasing the plunger of the inflating syringe while I palpate the trachea between larynx and jugular. In most adult patients, one can confirm the position of the cuff: If you can feel it, the tip of the tube cannot be in a mainstem bronchus. Some press on the trachea and feel for the transmitted pulsation in the partially compressed pilot balloon; others squeeze the pilot balloon and feel over the trachea.

Fastening the tube to the skin of the cheek and lip prevents it from being pushed in all the way or coming out all together. However, the skin, lip, and cheek are quite loose; they give the tube enough slack to get where it is not supposed to go—namely, into a mainstem bronchus or, particularly in babies, out of the larynx.

Check the Trachea. The breath sounds heard over the trachea are loud and serve well to monitor breathing (and the absence of a disconnection), particularly during mechanical ventilation. It is also useful to listen there while applying a little positive inspiratory pressure in order to discover leaks around the endotracheal tube. If the cuff of the tube is not adequately inflated, the leak causes a noise at the end of inspiration. Usually, however, the cuff is overinflated, exerting >15 mm Hg pressure on the mucous membrane of the trachea. In hypotensive patients, such pressure jeopardizes perfusion of the fine ciliary epithelium.

Because the cuff swells during nitrous oxide anesthesia (Fig. 19–1), I recommend deflating it about every half hour until a leak can be heard and then inflating it just enough to make the leak disappear. An alternative is to fill the cuff with nitrous oxide and O_2 from the breathing bag, which eliminates the gradient of nitrous oxide pressure across the membrane of the cuff.

Check the Breathing Hose. Some surgical procedures preclude application of the stethoscope to the chest or the suprasternal notch. Remember that you can clearly hear breath sounds after putting the stethoscope over the expiratory tube or, even better, bringing the breathing tube to your ear. Try it. Breath sounds over the breathing tubes tend to be harsher in mechanically ventilated patients than in those breathing spontaneously.

Circulation

Our principal concern is perfusion of the vital organs—the brain and heart. If a patient is anesthetized, the adequacy of

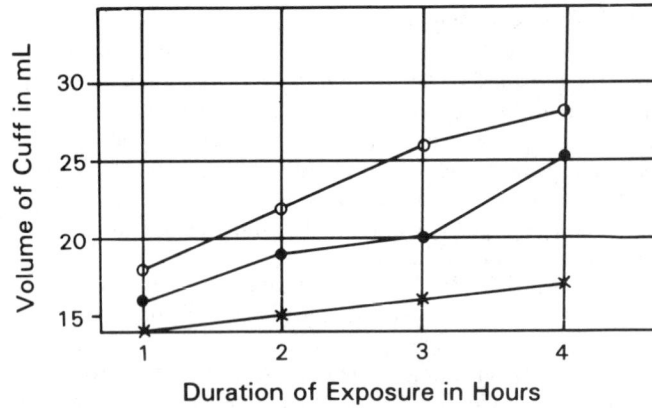

FIGURE 19–1. Volume of 10-mL cuff of a 34 French latex rubber endotracheal tube exposed to nitrous oxide. (From Stanley TH, Kawamura R, Graves C: Effects of nitrous oxide on volume and pressure of endotracheal tube cuffs. Anesthesiology 1974; 41:256.)

cerebral circulation is difficult to judge. Here are a few clinical signs that can prove useful.

Inspection

A patient's mucous membranes should be pink in areas well above the heart. Remember that blood pools in dependent areas, which appear to be pink. They blanch with pressure and then refill, even in severe hypotension, although perhaps not as briskly as normal.

Also look at the eyes. I recommend taping patients' eyes *only* when there is danger of damaging them. At all other times, we should not deprive ourselves of the advantage of checking pupil size; they should be constricted when all is well, and the palpebral conjunctiva should be well perfused and pink.

Look at the veins. In the areas hydrostatically below the right atrium, the veins should be dilated if blood volume is adequate and if the patient's sympathetic system is not working overtime. Use a patient's hand veins for a quick and rough estimate of right atrial pressure. Lift the hand until it is at the same height as the right atrium.

One can perform the same maneuver by using a simple U-tube concept: Open a stopcock of the intravenous infusion tubing to air, hold the open stopcock at heart level, and slowly lift it, watching where the meniscus of water begins to recede into the tubing. You can also put tubing on the stopcock and watch the water level (Fig. 19–2). The smaller the intravenous catheter, the more time it takes for the system to equalize its pressure.

Palpation

Pulse. Feel the pulse. Before the introduction of the precordial or esophageal stethoscope, it was customary to hold a finger over the external maxillary, temporal, or preauricular artery. I do not recommend keeping a finger on the carotid artery because compression of that vessel may not be tolerated well by patients with easily compromised carotid blood flow.

Heart rate can reveal a great deal. Tachycardia does not invariably signal hypovolemia, and hypovolemia is not invariably accompanied by tachycardia. Nevertheless, hemorrhage

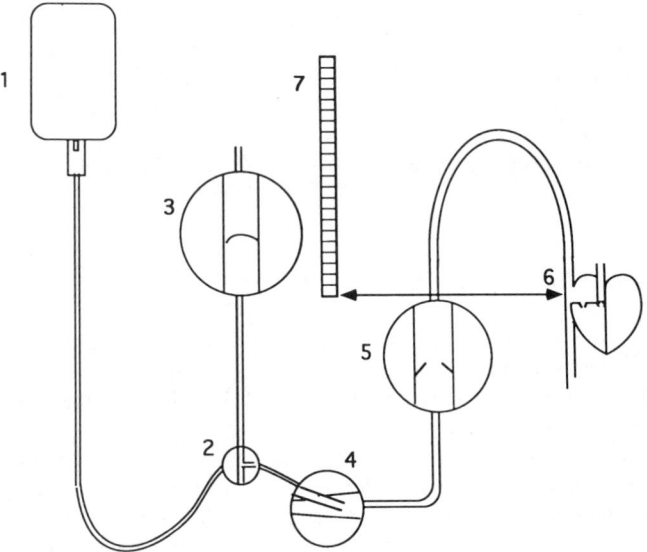

FIGURE 19–2. A simple, clinical estimation of central venous pressure. 1 = intravenous solution bag; 2 = three-way stopcock connecting vein to open-ended tubing; 3 = meniscus of fluid in open-ended tubing; 4 = catheter or needle in peripheral vein; 5 = valve in vein; 6 = superior vena cava; 7 = measuring stick.

When estimating central venous pressure, fill the open-ended tubing with intravenous fluid and hold the end of the tubing well above the level of the right atrium. Turn the stopcock to allow fluid to drain into the vein. The fluid will stop flowing when the pressure in the system and the central venous pressure equalize. Since there are valves in peripheral veins, it is important to let the fluid drain into the vein rather than to wait for blood to return from the vein into the tubing. Watch for respiratory fluctuations if the patient's lungs are being mechanically ventilated. Instead of attaching the tubing to watch the meniscus, the open stopcock can simply be lifted until a meniscus forms.

must be ruled out when the heart rate accelerates (Table 19–3).

A simple rule of thumb calls for feeling the radial artery pulse. If it is palpable, the pressure is presumably acceptable (perhaps 90 mm Hg systolic or higher); if it is absent, feel for the carotid artery pulse. If it is palpable but the radial pulse is not, the pressure may be around 60 mm Hg systolic.

Capillary Refill. Momentarily blanch the skin or a nail bed to look for capillary refill. It should occur promptly, in no more than about a second. Raise the patient's hand or pick the point highest above the heart when checking capillary refill.

Auscultation

Listening to the heart sounds in an anesthetized patient is more important than in an awake patient, in whom you can monitor the adequacy of cerebral perfusion by nothing more than a conversation. Listen for muffled heart sounds and for dysrhythmias.

If a patient had a carotid bruit before induction of anesthesia, listen for the bruit. The quality of its sound should not change. If it does, blood flow through the stricture has decreased, and cerebral perfusion may be jeopardized.

Autonomic Nervous System

We monitor the autonomic nervous system by inspection, even though we frequently do not think of it as a separate system; instead, we infer the depth of anesthesia from its activity. The three most important variables assessed by in-

spection are the size of the pupils (worry when they are dilated), tearing (the patient is inadequately anesthetized), and sweating (also a sign of light anesthesia). Arterial pressure and heart rate, also under control of the autonomic system, were discussed previously. High heart rates and systolic pressure are taken as evidence of light anesthesia.

BASIC MONITORING INSTRUMENTATION

What Should Be Done First?

Blood Pressure Cuff Application

As a general principle, establish baseline data before starting anesthesia. These data include arterial blood pressure. Ask patients about the comfort or discomfort of the cuff during blood pressure measurement. Use a cuff of appropriate size. Cuffs should be 20% wider than the circumference of the arm; if they are smaller, they report falsely high systolic pressures and they hurt more than cuffs of appropriate size.

A skin fold caught under the cuff is quite painful. Pressure of the tubing exerted on the ulnar or radial nerve close to the elbow can damage the nerve during a long anesthetic.[2] Therefore, apply the cuff so that the tubing from the cuff emerges proximally rather than distally. For long anesthetics, apply the cuff after wrapping cast padding around the arm. This procedure strikingly reduces the incidence of skin lesions.

Traditionally, the cuff is applied to the upper arm, leaving the elbow joint free for access to the brachial artery, where the stethoscope is applied. With the oscillometric technique, the cuff can also be wrapped around the forearm or the leg. The forearm is suitable if that extremity is needed for venous cannulation, which can then be obtained proximally. If the cuff is applied to the leg, place it just above the ankle, where it hurts less than higher up. Avoid the thigh whenever possible.

Blood Pressure Variation

Normally, small differences in systolic and diastolic pressure are noted, depending on where the pressure is measured, even if the sites of cuff application are all at the same (heart) level. Systolic pressure tends to be highest in the lower extremity. Because mean pressure must decrease with the distance from the heart, the pressure waveform changes in peripheral arterial vascular beds. Hence, the systolic pressure may be

TABLE 19–3. Questions Raised When Two Commonly Monitored Variables Change*

Heart Rate	↑	Blood Pressure	↓
↑	Early hypoxemia? Hyperpyrexia? Hypercapnia? Hyperthyroid? Light anesthesia?		Hemorrhage? Obstruction of venous return? Septicemia?
↓	High intracranial pressure? Baroreceptor hypertension due to vasopressors?		Severe hypoxemia? Cardiovascular collapse Myocardial failure? Toxins? Vagal reflex?

*The entries are ranked in terms of concern, not frequency. That is to say, rising heart rate and blood pressure are usually signs of light anesthesia, but it is more important quickly to rule out far more troublesome possible causes, such as hypoxemia.

higher in the calf than in the aorta. The preinduction blood pressure should be close to the values recorded preoperatively. If not, check for an explanation (mechanical, e.g., a cuff too small for the patient; or a variation in the patient's anatomy or physiology).

Pulse Oximetry

Record the pulse oximeter saturation (SpO_2) while the patient is breathing room air. Again, make sure the probe is comfortable. Some reusable probes can be pushed too far onto the finger and can cause sloughing of the finger tip.

Electrocardiographic Monitoring

Run an electrocardiogram (ECG) strip before inducing anesthesia. Obtain at least a V_5 tracing in adults to record whether this patient did or did not have dysrhythmias, flipped T waves, or ST segment depression. Even with a three-lead ECG, one can get a useful, if modified, lead V_5 tracing (Fig. 19–3).

Once anesthesia is under way, proceed system by system, using all electronically or mechanically monitored variables *in addition* to the clinical assessment without instruments.

How Is Ventilation Assessed?

Start with the supply of O_2; check the pressure gauge, flowmeters, and fraction of inspired O_2 (FiO_2); proceed to check gas exchange with tidal volume and end-tidal Pco_2 (around 35 mm Hg, or 4%). Also make sure that end-tidal O_2 concentration (if available) is reasonable—that is 3% to 6% (approximately 40 mm Hg) below the inspired O_2 concentration.

There should be no carbon dioxide (CO_2) in the inspired gas. If there is, your instrument may be sluggish (damped waveform) or noisy (artifact), or a little rebreathing may be occurring. If the $Pico_2$ is <4 mm Hg, the patient will not be harmed, but your system deserves an examination to detect the imperfection.

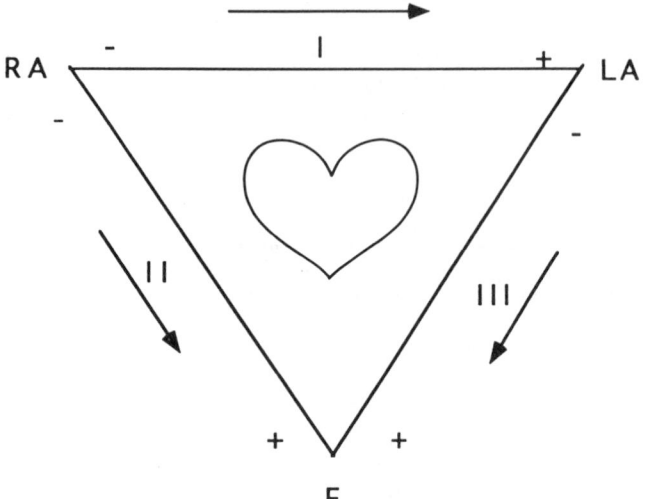

FIGURE 19–3. The traditional Einthoven' triangle shows the classical limb leads. Remember that the exploring electrode is always positive. For a modified VC_5, place the F (left leg) over the anterior axillary line in the 5th intercostal space, move the right arm electrode close to the manubrium, and run lead II.

Capnography has now assumed an important place in monitoring for safety.[3] The two completely preventable causes of major disasters in anesthesia can be detected by capnography: esophageal intubation and disconnection (see also Chapter 22). Check SpO_2.

Remember the advantages of observing the patient, as described earlier.

How Is Circulation Assessed?

Start by measuring blood pressure. It might decrease with injection of intravenous induction agents, increase with intubation, and settle down to steady, slightly reduced values during anesthesia maintenance. If you use an automated noninvasive method for blood pressure measurement—for example, an oscillometric device—let it cycle once a minute during induction but do not forget to reset it to a lower cycling frequency (i.e., once every 3 min) for the balance of the anesthetic. Even at that frequency, many patients develop petechial hemorrhages under the cuff, usually longitudinal, where folds of the cuff press into the skin or where skin folds are compressed by the cuff.

Remember also that our blood vessels are alive and reactive. It is quite possible to have constricted vessels (and low pressures) in the periphery (e.g., radial and digital arteries) and high pressures in the aorta. Monitor lead V_5 (best for detecting ST segment depression) and lead II (best for P wave monitoring), if you can look at two leads at once.

Remember the advantages of observing a patient, as described earlier. In addition to listening to the precordial stethoscope, insert an esophageal stethoscope if a patient is intubated. Advance it to optimize the auscultation of heart sounds.

How Is Temperature Assessed?

Feel a patient's forehead, even though you cannot determine his or her temperature to the exact degree. If a patient feels hot or cold but a temperature probe reports differently, get another probe or check the temperature the old-fashioned way, with a system used by nurses (electronic or mercury). Put the probe under the tongue or in the axilla. It will not give you a continuous reading, but it will tell whether you need to worry about your patient.

During general anesthesia, temperature is most conveniently measured in the esophagus, even though numerous other sites are available: the nose, the rectum, the forehead (with a strip that changes color and numbers), the tympanic membrane or the ear canal, the bladder or the pulmonary artery, and finally the axilla. Any of these sites is preferable to not measuring temperature at all. All have their drawbacks.

For routine monitoring, you really need not worry about accuracy or about how closely the temperature you measure reflects core temperature. You need to know whether your patient is getting a fever or is getting too cold. In either case, you need to act (see Chapter 55).

How Is Muscle Relaxation Assessed?

Once a patient is paralyzed, it becomes difficult to gauge the degree of relaxation by means other than a nerve stimulator, affectionately known as a twitch monitor. Apply the electrodes close to the wrist over the ulnar nerve, so that their current stimulates nerve rather than muscle. The nerve stimulator delivers a direct current; however, if you put the electrodes close together (i.e., a couple of centimeters apart), you need not worry about which is the anode and which the cathode. Optimally, you should increase the stimulating current until you obtain a maximum response, then set the stimulator to 10% above that maximum value. However, do not do that until a patient is asleep, because the current is painful.

Practical Applications

Many nerve stimulators offer the option of delivering single shocks, single shocks repeated every second, a train-of-four, train-of-four shocks repeated every 10 seconds, or tetany. There is a science to nerve stimulation and the interpretation of the responses (see Chapter 25). A simple clinical approach calls for turning the stimulator on as soon as the anesthetic is induced, selecting the optimal power setting, and setting it to single stimuli to be repeated every second while the first dose of the muscle-relaxing drug takes effect. Once the response to stimulation is absent, intubation is appropriate, provided the patient is adequately anesthetized. After that, switch to a train-of-four stimulation and test periodically to monitor the degree of relaxation.

How Often Should Vital Signs Be Checked?

Ideally, patients should be monitored continuously. Although we can and should inspect without interruption and listen to the precordial or esophageal stethoscope continuously, many variables cannot be monitored without interruption. A simple formula lets clinicians determine the minimal monitoring intervals[4]:

$$TT_{max} = \frac{delta_{max}}{slope_{max}}$$

where TT_{max} is the maximum interval between determinations, $delta_{max}$ is the maximum difference the clinician is willing to ascribe to acceptable physiologic variability, and $slope_{max}$ is the maximum rate of change the clinician foresees for this variable in this particular patient.

For example, $delta_{max}$ for blood pressure might be set at 50 mm Hg; this would mean that a change of that magnitude would require attention. Blood pressure $slope_{max}$ might be set as a 50 mm Hg change in 60 seconds. That is to say, one postulates that short of a cardiac arrest, the pressure is not likely to change faster than that. The monitoring interval, therefore, would be set at once a minute, as suggested during induction of anesthesia. With invasive monitoring, of course, continuous readings are available.

How Should Alarms on Monitoring Devices Be Set?

Today, many monitors have automatic alarms that are useless or harmful if not properly used. Do not treat them non-chalantly. Numerous disasters and lost lawsuits have resulted when anesthesiologists have disabled or turned off an alarm and forgotten to turn it back on or ignored it.

Important points are as follows:

1. Use the alarms. *Do not disable them.* If you must disable them, do so temporarily; make a positive identification of the alarm and its origin, take the necessary action, and turn it back on as soon as possible.

2. Set alarm limits with a little forethought. For variables that are not likely to change greatly, set the limits close to the values you expect to achieve. For example, it makes no sense to set the F_{IO_2} alarm at 0.21 if you are administering 50% O_2 or to set the alarm on the tidal volume meter at 300 mL if you are ventilating a patient with a tidal volume of 800 mL.

3. Set alarms for blood pressure and heart rate with wide margins, because these variables are likely to change greatly during anesthesia. Alarms for these variables are often disabled because they are improperly set and sound too often, for example, during intubation.

4. Adapt the alarm to the clinical circumstance. Set it with wider margins at the beginning and at the end of anesthesia than during the maintenance phase.

Are Monitoring Standards Useful?

Many countries have adopted minimal monitoring standards. An international version, showing different levels appropriate to the resources of individual countries, was presented at the meeting of the World Federation of Anesthesia Societies in 1992. Standards published by the American Society of Anesthesiologists as of 1993 are presented in the Appendix at the end of this chapter.

Many questions must be raised about standards. Are they helpful? The answer depends not only on how they affect outcome (not known) but also on how they affect the practice of the specialty (also not known). Can we drop standards that require expensive systems? Should instruments that are now available or likely to become available be incorporated into existing standards? Would practice standards (or guidelines), rather than or in addition to equipment standards, be useful? Anesthesiology has made a dramatic step in adopting a first set of standards. The clock will not be turned back. How our experience with the first steps will influence the next steps remains to be seen.

References

1. Comroe JH Jr, Botelho S: The unreliability of cyanosis in the recognition of arterial anoxemia. Am J Med Sci 1947; 214:1.
2. Gravenstein JS, Paulus DA: Clinical Monitoring Practice. 2nd ed. Philadelphia, JB Lippincott, 1987, p 62.
3. Gravenstein JS, Paulus DA, Hayes TJ: Capnography in Clinical Practice. 2nd ed. Stoneham, MA, Butterworths, 1992.
4. Gravenstein JS, DeVries A, Beneken JEW: Sampling intervals for clinical monitoring of variables during anesthesia. J Clin Monit 1989; 5:17.

Appendix

STANDARDS FOR BASIC INTRAOPERATIVE MONITORING
(Approved by House of Delegates on October 21, 1986, and last amended on October 23, 1990, placed in effect January 1, 1991)

These standards apply to all anesthesia care, although in emergency circumstances, appropriate life support measures take precedence. These standards may be exceeded at any time based on the judgment of the responsible anesthesiologist. They are intended to encourage high-quality patient care, but observing them cannot guarantee any specific patient outcome. They are subject to revision from time to time, as warranted by the evolution of technology and practice. This set of standards addresses only the issue of basic intraoperative monitoring, which is one component of anesthesia care. In certain rare or unusual circumstances, (1) some of these methods of monitoring may be clinically impractical and (2) appropriate use of the described methods may fail to detect untoward clinical developments. Brief interruptions of continual* monitoring may be unavoidable. *Under extenuating circumstances, the responsible anesthesiologist may waive the requirements marked with a dagger* (†). It is recommended that when this is done, it should be so stated (including the reasons) in a note in the patient's medical record. These standards are not intended for application to the care of obstetric patients in labor or in the conduct of pain management.

STANDARD I

Qualified anesthesia personnel shall be present in the room throughout the conduct of all general anesthetics, regional anesthetics, and monitored anesthesia care.

OBJECTIVE

Because of the rapid changes in a patient's status during anesthesia, qualified anesthesia personnel shall be continuously present to monitor the patient and provide anesthesia care. If a direct known hazard (e.g., radiation) to the anesthesia personnel might require intermittent remote observation of the patient, some provision for monitoring the patient must be made. In the event that an emergency requires the temporary absence of the person primarily responsible for the anesthetic, the best judgment of the anesthesiologist will be exercised in comparing the emergency with the anesthetized patient's condition and in the selection of the person left responsible for the anesthetic during the temporary absence.

STANDARD II

During all anesthetics, the patient's oxygenation, ventilation, circulation, and temperature shall be continually evaluated.

OXYGENATION

OBJECTIVE

To ensure adequate oxygen concentration in the inspired gas and the blood during all anesthetics.

METHODS

1. Inspired gas: During every administration of general anesthesia using an anesthesia machine, the concentration of oxygen in the patient's breathing system shall be measured by an oxygen analyzer with a low oxygen concentration limit alarm in use.†
2. Blood oxygenation: During all anesthetics, a quantitative method of assessing oxygenation such as pulse oximetry shall be used.† Adequate illumination and exposure of the patient are necessary to assess color.†

VENTILATION

OBJECTIVE

To ensure adequate ventilation of the patient during all anesthetics.

METHODS

1. Every patient receiving general anesthesia shall have the adequacy of ventilation continually evaluated. Although qualitative clinical signs such as chest excursion, observation of the reservoir breathing bag, and auscultation of breath sounds may be adequate, quantitative monitoring of the carbon dioxide content and/or volume of expired gas is encouraged.
2. When an endotracheal tube is inserted, its correct positioning in the trachea must be verified by clinical assessment and by identification of carbon dioxide in the expired gas.† End-tidal carbon dioxide analysis, in use from the time of endotracheal tube placement, is encouraged.
3. When ventilation is controlled by a mechanical ventilator, there shall be in continuous use a device that is capable of detecting disconnection of components of the breathing system. The device must give an audible signal when its alarm threshold is exceeded.
4. During regional anesthesia and monitored anesthesia care, the adequacy of ventilation shall be evaluated, at least, by continual observation of qualitative clinical signs.

CIRCULATION

OBJECTIVE

To ensure the adequacy of the patient's circulatory function during all anesthetics.

METHODS

1. Every patient receiving anesthesia shall have the electrocardiogram continuously displayed from the beginning of anesthesia until preparing to leave the anesthetizing location.†
2. Every patient receiving anesthesia shall have arterial blood pressure and heart rate determined and evaluated at least every 5 minutes.†
3. Every patient receiving general anesthesia shall have, in addition to the above, circulatory function continually evaluated by at least one of the following: palpation of a pulse, auscultation of breath sounds, monitoring of a tracing of intra-arterial pressure, ultrasound peripheral pulse monitoring, or pulse plethysmography or oximetry.

BODY TEMPERATURE

OBJECTIVE

To aid in the maintenance of appropriate body temperature during all anesthetics.

METHODS

There shall be readily available a means to measure the patient's temperature continuously. When changes in body temperature are intended, anticipated, or suspected, the temperature shall be measured.

---

*Note that *continual* is defined as "repeated regularly and frequently in steady rapid succession," whereas *continuous* means "prolonged without any interruption at any time."

CHAPTER 20

Respiratory Monitoring

JULIAN M. GOLDMAN, M.D.

JENNIFER S. STROM, M.D.

It is said that our raison d'être as anesthesiologists is to preserve a patient's oxygenation and ventilation. Modern practitioners rely on numerous technically complex devices to monitor respiratory status and the functioning of ventilatory equipment in order to enhance therapeutic intervention. Without sound knowledge of the function, strengths, and shortcomings of this equipment, we may be misled by erroneous data. A thorough understanding of our monitoring equipment is essential in order to maximize its diagnostic utility while minimizing misdirected therapeutic actions that are based on incorrect data. Perhaps these should be the guiding principles of monitoring: If the data are suspect, confirm them by other means if possible; and when treating a patient, err on the side of enhancing the margin of safety. We must always remember that an instrument ultimately derives its value through critical analysis by a human expert—the anesthesiologist.

ARTERIAL BLOOD GAS ANALYSIS

Despite advances in new, sophisticated, noninvasive monitoring techniques, the analysis of arterial blood gas (ABG) partial pressures and pH remains essential for a thorough evaluation of respiratory and overall physiologic function in anesthetized patients.

Why Are the Measurements Important?

Verify the Normal

Certain physiologic parameters must be within a narrow range for homeostasis. In fact, we *treat these numbers* (normally we treat the patient) for the following reasons:

1. Arterial pH is corrected to ensure an optimum milieu for the functioning of enzymes and drugs.
2. Arterial oxygen partial pressure (Pa_{O_2}) is normalized to permit cellular aerobic metabolism.
3. Arterial carbon dioxide partial pressure (Pa_{CO_2}) is regulated to maintain normal organ perfusion; because of its pervasive interaction via the sympathetic nervous system; and as

a therapeutic intervention (e.g., control of intracranial hypertension).

Identify the Abnormal

In addition to the previously cited reasons, ABG analysis is used to indicate the presence of abnormal physiologic states. Once they are identified, diagnosis and treatment of the underlying problem can proceed. (In this case, we treat the problem that has caused the abnormal ABG, not the number.)

1. Abnormal pH may indicate organ or endocrine dysfunction (e.g., organ hypoperfusion, renal tubular acidosis, or ketoacidosis).
2. Abnormal Pa_{O_2} may indicate pulmonary dysfunction or abnormal O_2 delivery.
3. Abnormal Pa_{CO_2} may indicate ventilatory dysfunction or abnormal CO_2 production (e.g., malignant hyperthermia).

ABG monitoring will increase in utility as continuous intra-arterial blood gas monitors are introduced into clinical practice. These monitors use an ultrathin fiberoptic bundle that is passed through an arterial catheter to continuously measure the pH, Pa_{CO_2}, and Pa_{O_2}. The tips of the fibers are coated with fluorescent dyes that alter their optical properties as the concentrations of specific interactive substances change.[1, 2] New monitoring applications surely will be developed as a consequence of the introduction of these devices.

What Is Measured and What Is Calculated?

Clinical blood gas machines use three electrodes: one each for Pa_{CO_2}, Pa_{O_2}, and pH. These variables are directly measured and may be temperature corrected before display (more about temperature correction later). In contrast, bicarbonate (HCO_3^-), base excess, and percent saturation of hemoglobin by O_2 (Sa_{O_2}) are *calculated* from the directly measured variables. (Sa_{O_2} can be directly *measured* with a spectrophotometric automatic hemoglobin analyzer, or co-oximeter.)

Units of Measurement

The newest measurement system, Système Internationale (SI), is in use in many countries but has not yet achieved popularity in the United States. These values are based on meter-kilogram-second units and do not include gravity-based units such as the millimeter of mercury. The kilopascal (kPa) is the appropriate SI unit for the description of clinical pressure measurement. One kilopascal is equal to 7.50 mm Hg or 10.2 cm H_2O. Although kilopascals were introduced a number of years ago, their acceptance as the clinical unit of measure of fluid pressures has been delayed for reasons described by Nunn as ''. . . an entirely specious attachment to the mercury or water manometer.''[3] Kilopascals are probably here to stay.

How Quickly Must a Blood Sample Be Analyzed?

Most clinicians accept the observation that if a sample is stored in a plastic syringe at room temperature, no significant abnormalities will be induced by waiting up to 20 minutes before analysis.[4] Exceptions to this rule of thumb are blood samples from patients who are polycythemic or who have leukocytosis and a higher total metabolic rate of the white blood cells. However, some investigators recommend a more conservative time limit of 10 minutes if the sample is not stored on crushed ice (i.e., at 0 °C).[5] Regardless of philosophy, no harm results from analyzing it even sooner or, conversely, putting it on ice if you are uncertain about how much time will elapse before analysis. Note that when whole blood samples for ABG analysis are stored on crushed ice, glass syringes may confer more stability than plastic syringes.[6]

Be careful to avoid producing foam when aspirating arterial blood and to eliminate all air bubbles. Residual air in the sample syringe will begin to equilibrate with the blood sample and alter the PaO_2 and $PaCO_2$ within 2 minutes.[7]

Should Temperature-Corrected or Noncorrected Values Be Used?

Blood gas machines are warmed and perform their measurements with the blood sample brought to exactly 37 °C. If a patient's temperature is less, as the blood sample is warmed to 37 °C in the blood gas machine, the partial pressure of the gases in solution will increase and the pH will decrease. Blood gas results may be reported *uncorrected*—that is, at the new partial pressure and pH that resulted from this temperature change. Conversely, they may be mathematically *temperature corrected* to report the partial pressures that exist in a patient at the *patient's body temperature*.

Although temperature correction is a complex and controversial topic, the following generalization can be made: Correct the temperature of the blood gas sample if you want to accurately assess the relationship of blood gas partial pressures to inspired or alveolar gas partial pressures. Alternatively, the ABG can be left uncorrected, and the alveolar gas sample partial pressure could be reported as if it were measured at 37 °C.

What Are α-Stat and pH-Stat Methods?

α-Stat

Failure to correct for temperature of the blood gas sample yields a pH and $PaCO_2$ that differ from those in the in vivo state. Despite the appearance of introducing artifact, the practice of maintaining uncorrected ABG values in a normal range has a sound physiologic basis and is called α-stat. The premise of α-stat is to maintain intracellular electrochemical neutrality, in which the *ratio* of hydrogen [H^+] to hydroxyl [OH^-] ions is kept constant during changes in temperature. As temperature decreases, the degree of H^+-OH^- dissociation decreases and the concentrations of both H^+ and OH^- are reduced.

Because the concentration of H^+ decreases and because pH is defined as the negative log of the hydrogen ion *concentration,* pH increases. H^+ concentration, *not* ratio, determines pH. Therefore, in a closed system, as temperature falls, pH rises. Applying the α-stat method during hypothermic cardiopulmonary bypass entails regulating ventilation so that the pH and $PaCO_2$ are within normal limits after the blood sample is warmed to 37 °C in the blood gas analyzer. This approach is in contrast to the assumption that the pH should always be 7.40 once it is corrected for a patient's body temperature.[8–10]

An important element in the concept of maintaining a constant ratio of H^+ and OH^- is the maintenance of the milieu of the α-amino group of the imidazole-histidine residues of intracellular proteins—hence the term α-stat (think of a thermostat, which maintains a constant temperature). (See Chapters 18 and 67 for further discussion.)

pH-Stat

An alternative method for managing ABGs is pH-stat. With pH-stat, the ABG is temperature corrected during hypothermia (i.e., the lower $PaCO_2$ that exists in vivo is calculated and ventilation is decreased or CO_2 is added in order to maintain normal temperature-corrected values for pH and $PaCO_2$). See Chapters 18 and 67 for additional discussion.

If I Know the Fraction of Inspired Oxygen, How Can I Calculate the Predicted PaO_2?

Several methods predict what the PaO_2 should be when a given fraction of inspired O_2 (FIO_2) is breathed. For a normal adult breathing room air at sea level, the PaO_2 can be estimated by the following equation[3]:

$$PaO_2 \text{ in mm Hg} = 102 - (age/3)$$
$$PaO_2 \text{ in kPa} = 13.6 - 0.044 \text{ (age)}$$

If a patient with lung disease breathes supplemental O_2, an accurate estimate of PaO_2 can be obtained by measuring the FIO_2, calculating the pulmonary shunt fraction, and using the iso-shunt diagram to diagram plots of FIO_2 against PaO_2 for a range of calculated shunt values[11] (Fig. 20–1).

In contrast to estimating PaO_2, calculating the alveolar PO_2 (PAO_2) is considerably simpler, as long as we do not require great accuracy. For *clinical* purposes, the following form of the alveolar air equation can be used:

$$PAO_2 = PIO_2 - PaCO_2/R$$

where R is the respiratory exchange ratio (equal to pulmonary CO_2 elimination/O_2 consumption) and PIO_2 is the inspired partial pressure of O_2.

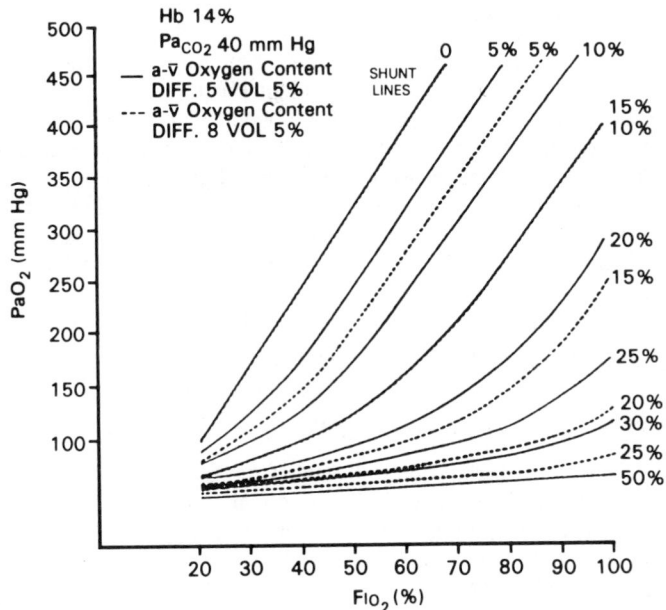

FIGURE 20–1. Theoretic relationships between Pao$_2$ and Fio$_2$ for different values of shunt at two different values of arterial/mixed venous O$_2$ content difference. Note that the curves are displaced but that their pattern is unaltered. (From Benatar SR, Hewlett AM, Nunn JF: The use of iso-shunt lines for control of oxygen therapy. Br J Anaesth 1973; 45:713.)

This equation is appropriate for a calculation performed intraoperatively, when a simple and easy estimate of the alveolar-arterial oxygen gradient (P[A − a]o$_2$) is necessary and less accuracy is acceptable. This form of the alveolar air equation does not account for differences in the volume of inspired and expired gas due to the respiratory exchange ratio or due to the exchange of inert gases.[3] Despite these shortcomings, this estimate of the Pao$_2$ can be used to evaluate a patient's pulmonary function (as reflected by the P[A-a]o$_2$ gradient); even patients with normal lungs have a gradient of about 15 mm Hg (2 kPa).[3]

How Are Respiratory and Metabolic Disturbances Differentiated?

A systematic approach to ABG interpretation simplifies intraoperative diagnosis and treatment of acid-base derangements that inevitably arise during anesthesia. We suggest first examining the pH value to determine whether acidemia or alkalemia is present. This initial assessment is followed by evaluation of the Paco$_2$, which is elevated in the presence of respiratory acidosis and decreased in the presence of respiratory alkalosis. Finally, the values for bicarbonate and base excess are examined; a low bicarbonate and negative base excess indicate a metabolic acidosis, whereas an elevated bicarbonate and base excess are associated with metabolic alkalosis. Obviously, different combinations of acid-base derangements can be present simultaneously and can infrequently produce an overall normal pH (see Chapter 43 for additional discussion).

An important fact to consider when interpreting ABGs is that the values for both bicarbonate and base excess are calculated by the blood gas analyzer; hence, they are derived values that vary based on the algorithm used by the machine. This is one reason why evaluation of the directly measured

values of pH and Paco$_2$ first is important before treating a patient for a presumptive metabolic disturbance. However, although they are derived values, they are useful to many clinicians because they simplify assigning the metabolic contribution of pH derangements.

OXYGEN MONITORING

Monitoring the Fio$_2$ delivered to a patient has been advocated as an intraoperative monitoring standard by the American Society of Anesthesiologists (ASA) since 1986. The O$_2$ monitor, when it incorporates an activated low-concentration alarm, provides an easy and inexpensive way to avoid the catastrophic consequences of hypoxic gas mixture delivery from the anesthesia machine.

O$_2$ concentration is usually measured by a relatively slowly responding sensor placed in the inspiratory limb of the circle breathing circuit. It indicates what the *circuit is delivering* to the patient but does not necessarily indicate the concentration of the fresh gas delivered to the circuit from the anesthesia machine, nor does it reveal anything about the expired O$_2$ concentration. This monitoring technology has obvious limitations.

How Can the Oxygen Sensor Mislead Us?

Calibration

O$_2$ analyzers can produce incorrect values as a result of faulty initial calibration. Therefore, we recommend that the analyzer be calibrated at least once daily, usually during the initial anesthesia machine check, and that it be calibrated with room air as opposed to 100% O$_2$ in order to maximize its accuracy in the low concentration range and to facilitate the detection of a hazardously low concentration. In addition to faulty calibration, some of the commonly used older polarographic or galvanic O$_2$ sensors have been reported to be sensitive to nitrous oxide (N$_2$O), particularly as the battery power for the sensor fails.[12]

Sensor Position

The O$_2$ sensor's position in the breathing circuit influences its ability to provide accurate information about the Fio$_2$. Because the sensor is typically placed in the inspiratory limb of the breathing circuit near the inspiratory valve, it cannot measure a change in O$_2$ concentration resulting from air entrainment in the circuit at a site distal to it. Therefore, a spontaneously breathing patient could be inspiring room air around a deflated endotracheal tube (ETT) cuff or through a partially disconnected or leaking circuit that would escape detection by an inspiratory limb O$_2$ sensor.

Supply/Demand Balance

Finally, the O$_2$ analyzer sensing the fresh gas flow (FGF) detects only whether the set Fio$_2$ is delivered from the anesthesia machine. If a patient's O$_2$ requirements exceed the amount of O$_2$ delivered, a standard sensor that does not display the circuit or, even better, the expired O$_2$ concentration will not identify the relative O$_2$ deficiency. In this case, the problem will be detectable only through the use of ABG analysis or pulse oximetry to assess hemoglobin saturation (SpO_2).

Can the Oxygen Sensor's Diagnostic Utility Be Improved?

One method is to place the sensor in the expiratory limb, which facilitates the detection of leaks or disconnections. However, moisture condensation on the sensor can damage it and render it useless.[13] Moving the location of the O_2 sensor is not even an option in many newer anesthesia machines, because they have incorporated their O_2 analyzers into the soda lime canister. Perhaps for reasons of durability and reducing liability, manufacturers want to prove that their machines *deliver* a sufficient O_2 concentration, although we would prefer to know that a patient *receives* sufficient O_2. Hence, enthusiasm has surrounded the development and use of "fast" airway O_2 sensors that actually create an O_2 waveform or oxygram.

What Is Fast Oxygen Monitoring?

Fast O_2 monitoring refers to the use of rapidly responding O_2 analyzers to measure inspired and expired O_2 at the mouth or ETT.[14] Current technologies capable of fast O_2 analysis include mass spectroscopy, Raman spectroscopy, and paramagnetic O_2 analysis. (Mass spectroscopy and Raman spectroscopy are described further in the section *Agent Monitoring*.)

Paramagnetic Sensors

Paramagnetic O_2 sensors take advantage of the fact that O_2 is one of only a few molecules that has two electrons in unpaired orbits, allowing it to exhibit a magnetic property. The paramagnetic sensor uses an alternating magnetic field to generate a pressure in the presence of O_2 molecules. The difference in pressure between a reference cell and a sample cell is proportional to the difference in O_2 partial pressures. When used with a sufficiently small sample cell, the paramagnetic sensor provides a fast response time that gives breath-by-breath measurements of inspired and expired oxygen.[15]

Oxygraphy

Oxygraphy, which is the continuous waveform display of these breath-by-breath O_2 time-concentration waveform measurements, may detect ventilatory abnormalities such as circuit disconnections and leaks in a fashion similar to that for capnography (the CO_2 time-concentration waveform).

Oxygen Delivery and Uptake

The difference between the inspired and expired O_2 concentrations (ΔO_2) can be measured. This value provides a noninvasive estimate of the relationship between alveolar O_2 delivery (a function of FiO_2 and alveolar ventilation) and alveolar O_2 uptake (primarily affected by cardiac output and mixed venous O_2). Hence, inadequate O_2 delivery for a given O_2 consumption can be detected. An increase in the ΔO_2 has been demonstrated to be a more sensitive indicator of alveolar hypoventilation than a change in SpO_2.[16]

Denitrogenation

Another useful application of oxygraphy involves examining the decrease in ΔO_2 as a patient breathes 100% O_2, in order to provide an estimate of the adequacy of preinduction denitrogenation (preoxygenation). As demonstrated in Figure 20–2, the decrease in alveolar nitrogen (N_2) concentration is accompanied by a complementary increase in the alveolar O_2 concentration. Figure 20–2 illustrates that alveolar N_2 can be rapidly exchanged for O_2 in a healthy patient who takes big breaths. In contrast, during quiet breathing, N_2 washout requires between 2 and 3.5 minutes in a healthy patient and 10 to 12 minutes in a patient with emphysema.[17]

Detection of Circuit Valve Leaks

We have compared the efficacy of oxygraphy with that of capnography for the detection of circle-circuit valve leaks and spontaneous respiratory efforts during mechanical ventilation. In our experiments, performed with a mechanical lung and mass spectrometer, oxygraphy was not as useful as capnography for detecting an expiratory valve leak (Fig. 20–3).

AIRWAY PRESSURE MONITORING

What Is the Value of Intraoperative Measurement?

Many benefits accrue to continuous intraoperative airway pressure monitoring, particularly when high- and low-pressure alarms and a graphic pressure-time display are used. The likelihood of barotrauma can be reduced by adjusting the ventilator's tidal volume (V_T) and inspiratory flow rate to optimize peak and mean airway pressures. In addition, some newer anesthesia ventilators can be set to terminate inspiration at a predetermined "safe" peak airway pressure. A loss of pressure, as occurs with a disconnection, similarly can be detected. Compliance changes, including those caused by ETT obstruction, bronchospasm, or pneumothorax, may be reflected as changes in the airway pressure. Finally, an airway pressure monitor allows a rough evaluation of a patient's respiratory mechanics before extubation through measurement of the negative inspiratory and positive expiratory pressures.

Does a Manometer Accurately Measure Intratracheal and Circuit Pressure?

Not always! It overestimates intratracheal pressure during mechanical ventilation and underestimates it during spontaneous breathing. The error is a function of inspiratory flow and ETT size (Fig. 20–4). The gradient across a small pediatric ETT can easily exceed 20 cm H_2O. When knowledge of the precise intratracheal pressure is important, application of an end-inspiratory hold or plateau (i.e., a period of no flow, therefore no resistance) allows the circuit and intratracheal pressures to equilibrate.

Sensor Location

The location of the pressure sensor may also influence accuracy. Positioning the pressure sensor within the CO_2 ab-

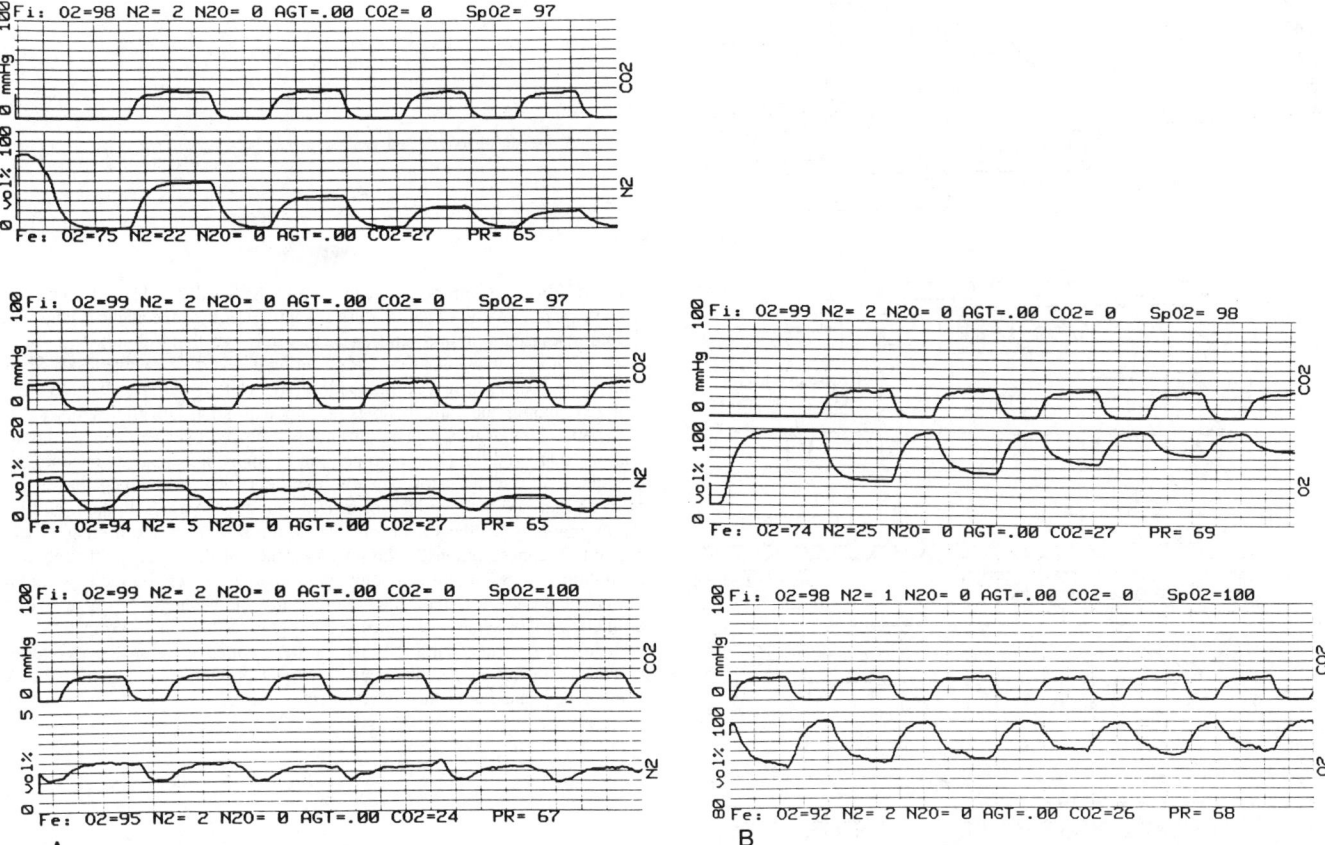

FIGURE 20–2. *A*, Preinduction denitrogenation (commonly called "preoxygenation"). Breathing pure O_2 exchanges N_2 for O_2 in the patient's pulmonary functional residual capacity. The capnogram and N_2 curve from this patient breathing O_2 by face mask illustrate the rapid decline in expired N_2 concentration. Nitrogen washout in this healthy adult patient is almost complete after four large breaths. (Note that the N_2 scale is different on each printout. Gas analyzed by Ohmeda Rascal II Raman spectroscopic analyzer.) *B*, Preinduction denitrogenation oxygram. Simultaneous oxygram and capnogram from same patient and under same conditions as in *A*. The end-tidal O_2 concentration rises as N_2 washout occurs. (Note that the O_2 scale is different on each printout.)

sorber canister, as is the case in older anesthesia machines, produces an incorrect positive end-expiratory pressure (PEEP) measurement owing to isolation of the sensor by the inspiratory valve (Fig. 20–5). PEEP devices usually are added between the expiratory limb and the expiratory valve. Therefore, the PEEP-induced circuit pressure increase occurs only in that portion of the circuit bounded by the inspiratory valve and the PEEP valve. To detect PEEP, the measurement must take place anywhere in the patient segment of the circuit between the two valves. The old Ohio Anesthesia Absorber incorporated a pressure gauge in the canister. Although this measured intracanister pressure, it did not measure pressure produced with a typical PEEP valve. It would detect inadvertent PEEP produced by other factors, such as a scavenger valve defect. (See Chapter 16 for additional discussion.)

TIDAL VOLUME MONITORING

Why Does the End-Tidal Carbon Dioxide Decrease When I Increase the Fresh Gas Flow?

Change in Tidal Volume

The V_T delivered to the breathing circuit comes from two parallel sources: the ventilator bellows excursion and the FGF.

FGF is added continuously to the circuit gas; because the circuit pop-off is closed during the inspiratory phase of mechanical ventilation, FGF contributes to the inspired V_T during mechanical inspiration (Fig. 20–6). The resultant increase is a function of the inspiratory time and the FGF.

For example, with a ventilator-delivered V_T of 600 mL at a respiratory rate of 10 breaths per minute and an inspiratory-to-expiratory (I:E) ratio of 1:2, inspiratory time is 2 seconds. If the FGF is 6 L · min^{-1}, 200 mL will be added to each 600-mL breath that is delivered by the ventilator bellows. The patient actually receives 800 mL per breath, producing a discrepancy between the set V_T (noted on the ventilator control panel or the ventilator bellows excursion) and the measured V_T.

If the FGF is decreased to 2 L · min^{-1}, only 66 mL is added to each 600-mL breath. The effect of changes in FGF on delivered V_T may be particularly important for children, immediately after induction of general anesthesia when FGF is reduced from a very high to a lower value, and just before emergence when a low FGF is increased to a higher one. An analogous effect on V_T occurs when the I:E ratio is reduced (i.e., the longer the inspiratory [I] time, the longer the V_T).

Spirometer Design

Several other factors influence the discrepancy between the set and delivered V_T measured by an in-circuit spirometer.

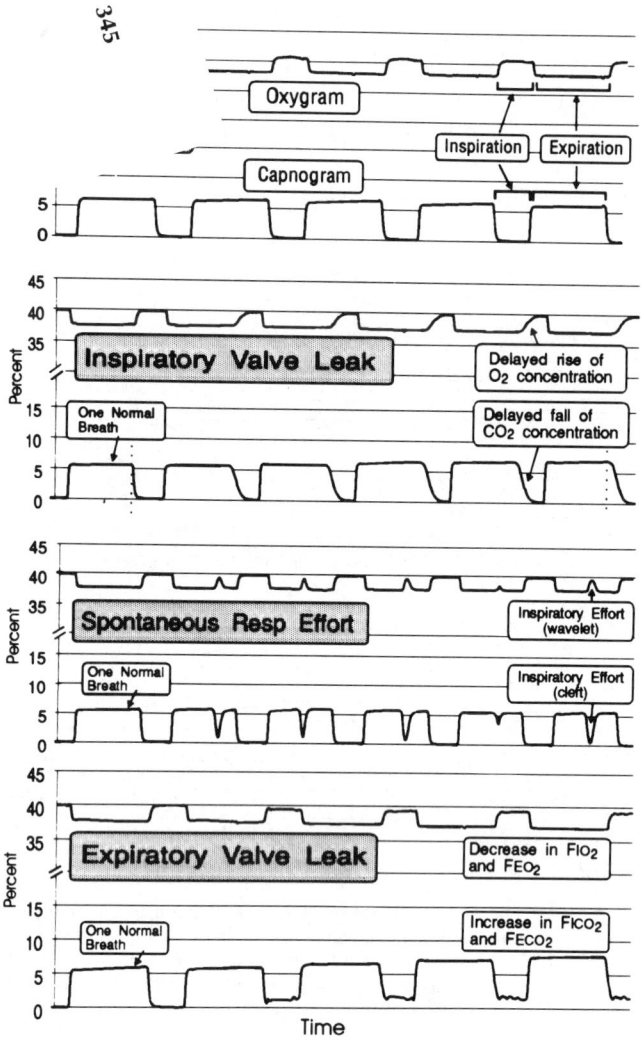

FIGURE 20–3. Oxygrams and capnograms with valve defects. Comparison of the capnogram and oxygram during ventilation by a mechanical lung with a volume-cycled ventilator and an adult circle breathing circuit. Inspiratory and expiratory valve leaks were produced by elevating the valve disks. Spontaneous inspiratory efforts during expiration ("cleft") were produced by manually expanding the lung bellows during expiration. In all examples, the oxygram is similar to a capnogram that is "flipped over vertically." Abnormalities that produce clear morphologic changes are apparent on both gas concentration tracings. However, the expiratory gas rebreathing that results from an expiratory valve leak primarily changes the concentration, and not the morphology, of the waveforms. Thus, the slow decrease in inspired and expired O_2 concentrations is the only evidence of the defect. Although concentration changes are also the only abnormalities evident on the capnogram, the baseline change is more obvious because the capnogram rises above its normally zero baseline. In contrast, the oxygram's "baseline" normally varies with inspired O_2 concentration. The *vertical dotted lines* on the inspiratory valve leak tracing indicate the beginning of inspiration (see Figure 20–9 for a complete explanation of this valve defect).

Different spirometer designs are affected by various breathing circuit conditions and flow patterns.

Turbine

A rotating mechanical (turbine) spirometer's accuracy may be reduced at low flow rates because of the inertia of the turbine element. If moisture condenses on the turbine, its mass may increase so that very low gas flows do not initiate turbine rotation, falsely indicating absence of gas flow.

Pneumotachograph

A pneumotachograph calculates flow by measuring the pressure drop across a flow resistor (e.g., fine-mesh screen) located in the circuit. The resultant pressure drop is a function of the flow. The Datex Capnomac Ultima uses a unique implementation of pneumotachography to measure flow at the ETT and to produce flow-volume and pressure-volume loops. Correct interpretation of the flow-induced pressure drop depends on careful calibration of the pneumotachograph with a specific ETT size.

A change in placement of the pneumotachograph (e.g., from the proximal side to the distal side of an elbow connector) also may necessitate recalibration. Gas composition changes during an anesthetic procedure are analyzed by the Ultima, which automatically compensates the pneumotachograph's calibra-

tion to maintain accuracy in the presence of gas density changes. A pneumotachograph offers the benefits of potentially high accuracy, but it may incorrectly measure circuit flow if not used with careful attention to detail.

Does A V_T Setting Change Produce a Corresponding Patient V_T Change?

Circuit Compression and Expansion

Anesthesia ventilators compress the bellows with O_2 to drive circuit gas into a patient's lungs. The set V_T is the volume that would be delivered by the ventilator into a chamber at ambient pressure. However, for the volume to be delivered into a patient's lungs and the anesthesia circuit, it must be pressurized; this pressure increase compresses some gas within the ventilator bellows, ventilator hose, CO_2 absorber, and breathing circuit. The actual volume delivered to a patient's lungs reflects the set V_T minus the resultant volume of gas compressed during inspiration. Additional V_T loss occurs as a result of expansion of the breathing circuit tubing. The longer and more compliant the breathing circuit, the greater is the latter.

Subtle differences between the methods of operation of the Ohmeda and North American Dräger anesthesia machine ven-

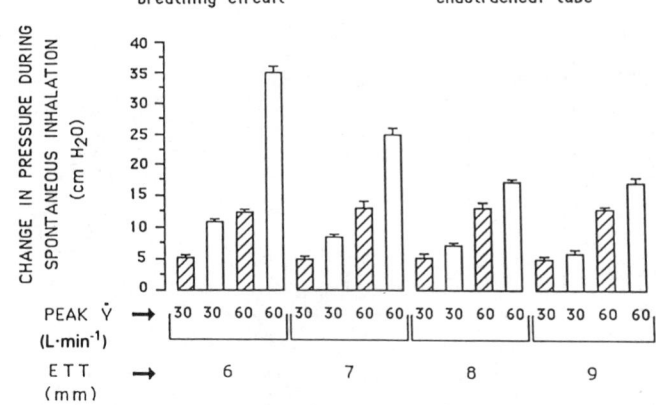

FIGURE 20-4. Comparison of pressure changes measured at the Y-piece of the breathing circuit tubing and at the tracheal (or carinal) end of the endotracheal tube (ETT) during spontaneous inhalation at different peak sinusoidal inspiratory flow rate demands ($\dot{V}$) with four different endotracheal tube sizes (6.0, 7.0, 8.0, and 9.0). Note that the narrower the internal diameter of the ETT and the greater the peak inspiratory flow rate demand, the greater the discrepancy between pressures measured at the Y-piece and at the tracheal end of the ETT. Measuring pressure at the Y-piece results in significant underestimations of pressure changes, especially when the ETT has a small internal diameter and the peak inspiratory flow rate demand is high.

tilators influence the effect of pulmonary compliance on apparent delivered volume.

Ohmeda Ventilator

The Ohmeda ventilator bellows always fills to its capacity (about 1600 mL). It then partially empties when a volume of gas equal to the set V_T is introduced into the bellows housing, compresses the bellows, and forces circuit gas into the patient. Because the bellows is emptying against the resistance imposed by an increasing circuit pressure, the driving gas introduced around the bellows will be compressed, resulting in a smaller bellows volume change (as indicated by a reduction in bellows excursion) than would be expected. In other words, the bellows may descend only to the 650-mL mark on the bellows housing, despite a V_T setting at 800 mL. If the exhaled V_T is measured after a return to ambient pressure, the volume will re-expand to a value close to the set V_T. In contrast, the patient's lung volume increases only by a volume equal to the compressed breath (650 mL in this example). This effect can be partially offset by increasing the set V_T until the bellows descends the desired amount.

Dräger Ventilator

The Dräger ventilator uses an adjustable stop to limit bellows capacity. Ventilator inspiratory flow is adjusted to ensure complete emptying of the bellows. If the bellows capacity is adjusted to 800 mL, this volume, measured at ambient pressure, is delivered. However, it is variably compressed during inspiration, depending on the peak inspiratory pressure. The reduction in actual lung volume change that results from V_T compression is similar to that which occurs with the Ohmeda ventilator. However, with the Dräger ventilator, no objective indication shows that this volume compression is occurring.

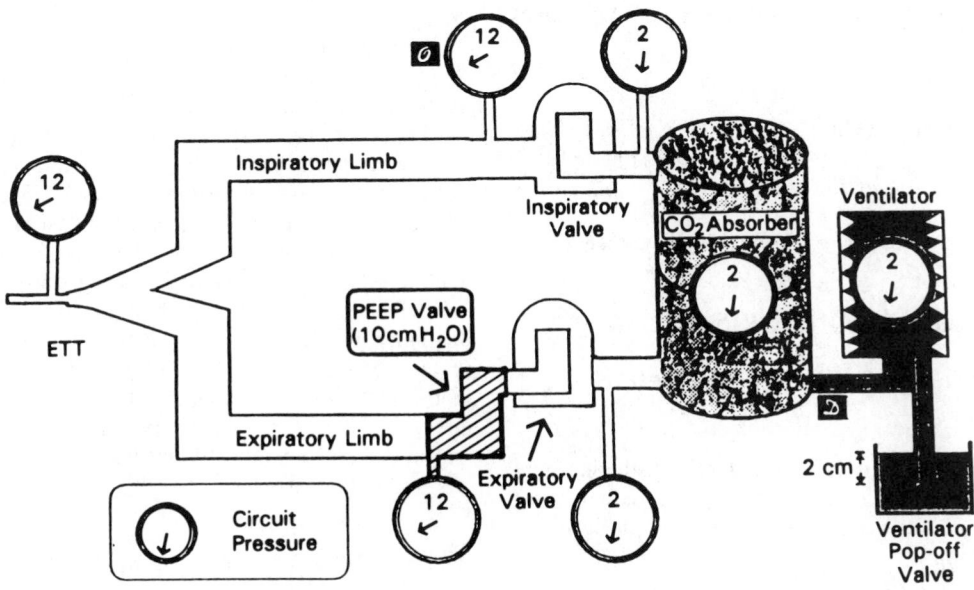

FIGURE 20-5. Breathing circuit pressure distribution. Schematic diagram of circle breathing circuit (during expiration) with a PEEP valve added to the expiratory limb. Ventilator bellows, which rise on expiration, incorporate a low pressure pop-off valve to maintain positive pressure within the bellows during expiration (depicted here by a water column "valve"). Note that with the PEEP valve placed at the expiratory valve, the pressures on the circuit side are different from those on the canister side of the inspiratory and expiratory valves. Currently, both North American Dräger (Telford, PA) and Ohmeda (Madison, WI) supply anesthesia machines that incorporate adjustable PEEP valves into the absorber head in locations that differ from those shown on this figure (and from each other). The Ohmeda machine measures circuit pressure at O in the figure, and the Dräger machine incorporates the PEEP valve and measures circuit pressure at D. Both machines correctly measure circuit pressure on the patient side of the PEEP valves. (See text for discussion.)

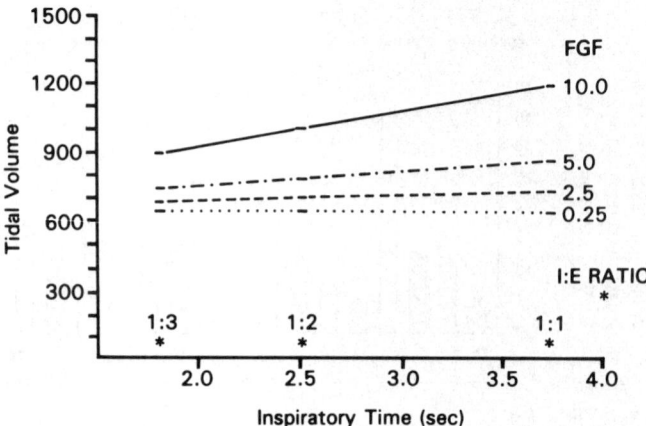

FIGURE 20–6. The effect of the ratio of inspiratory time to expiratory time (I:E) and FGF on the delivered V_T as determined with a test lung. The ventilator was set for a V_T of 600 mL by observing the bellows excursion at 8 breaths per minute. I:E was 1:3, 1:2, and 1:1 at the corresponding inspiratory times indicated by asterisks. Data are means ± SD. (From Gravenstein N, Banner MJ: Tidal volume changes due to the interaction of anesthesia machine and anesthesia ventilator. J Clin Monit 1987; 3:187.)

Summary

The brand of ventilator may also affect V_T delivery. Additional circuit volume increases circuit compliance. With a set V_T of 600 mL, the residual volume of the Ohmeda bellows is 1 L more than the Dräger bellows. Hence, a larger total volume is present in the Ohmeda system than in the Dräger system, even if the patient circuit, soda lime canister, and ventilator hose volumes are the same.

The breathing circuit spirometer measures only that gas that flows by it in the expiratory limb (gas exhaled by a patient and gas that distends the circuit or is compressed within it during inspiration). It does not include the portion of the V_T that is sequestered in the ventilator, ventilator hose, and soda lime canister. Only when the FGF is sufficient to make up this lost volume will the set and measured exhaled V_T values match.

Hence:

$$V_T \text{ delivered to patient} = \text{bellows excursion} + \text{FGF} \times T_I \\ - \text{ gas lost to compression and} \\ \text{circuit compliance}$$

where FGF = $mL \cdot s^{-1}$ and T_I = inspiratory time (seconds).

AGENT MONITORING

What Is the Value of Monitoring Anesthetic Concentration?

To argue that continuous monitoring of anesthetic agent concentration is essential for the conduct of a safe general anesthetic is difficult. However, clear benefits are derived and include the following:

1. Detection of an inadvertent agent overdose due to either vaporizer malfunction or human error
2. "Precision timing" of reaching MAC-awake and achievement of a desired or target end-tidal concentration[18, 19]
3. Detection of vaporizer filling errors through agent-specific monitoring

4. Observation of inhalation kinetic principles
5. Assurance that the desired concentration is actually delivered, particularly when low flows cause equilibrium to be reached very slowly and produce a large discrepancy between the vaporizer dial setting and inspired agent concentration

Modern agent analyzers use one of several technologies. See Table 20–1 for a comparison of these devices.

What Are the Potential Sources of Error?

Ethanol has an infrared (IR) absorption peak within the wavelengths used by an IR analyzer to detect anesthetic agents. Therefore, exhaled ethanol acts to elevate falsely the reported values of exhaled anesthetics. If you are using an IR analyzer without automatic agent identification capability and the monitor is set to read enflurane or isoflurane, ethanol vapor will have minimal effects. In contrast, if halothane is selected, ethanol can artifactually increase the halothane reading by 3.5 times the blood alcohol per cent concentration. We can apply this phenomenon to our clinical practice by selecting halothane during preoxygenation in order to detect potential interference by ethanol. This effect could also be anticipated in the presence of other organic hydrocarbons that have similar IR absorption (ketones, methanol, or isopropyl alcohol).[20]

"Unusual" Gases

Ethanol, which could constitute only a small fraction of the gas mixture, would affect the mass spectrometer minimally. However, other unusual gases may have a more profound effect. The mass spectrometer reports each detected gas as a fraction of all the detectable gases. Because those used in anesthesiology usually do not detect nonanesthetic gases, their presence is ignored. Thus, the mass spectrometer may report falsely elevated levels of anesthetic agents in the presence of nondetectable gases such as helium or other organic hydrocarbons.

If we administer 20% helium, the isoflurane concentration is read according to its fraction in the remaining 80% of the respiratory gas that the mass spectrometer "sees"; a 1% dial setting on the vaporizer is associated with a 1.25% reading on the mass spectrometer. (Explained another way, if a patient inspires a mixture of helium 33%, O_2 33%, and N_2 33%, a clinical mass spectrometer that is not designed to detect helium would report concentrations of O_2 50% and N_2 50%.) If a metered-dose inhaler is used during mass spectroscopy, the propellant, a chlorofluorocarbon like the volatile agents, artifactually increases the reported anesthetic concentration.

In contrast to mass spectroscopy, Raman spectroscopy reports the measured concentration of each detectable gas present. Thus, the Raman spectrometer should continue to provide accurate values for anesthetics even in the presence of unidentifiable gases.

Water Vapor

All agent analyzers are affected by water vapor. IR analyzers are subject to interference by water vapor, particularly in the CO_2 absorption wavelengths. A wet sample cell causes an increase in the baseline and end-tidal values.

Mass spectrometers and Raman analyzers are subject to mechanical failure as a result of water condensate in the sam-

TABLE 20–1. Comparison of Methods Used for Anesthetic Agent Analysis*

Technology	Principle of Operation	Benefits	Weaknesses	Notes
Infrared (IR) spectroscopy	Anesthetic agents absorb certain IR wavelengths. Concentration is determined by the absorption difference between the sample cell (which contains the gas to be analyzed) and reference cell (a sealed cell containing a known gas concentration).	Newer analyzers with automated agent detection ("agent ID") detect incorrect agent in vaporizer and obviate manual agent identification.[47]	In most analyzers, the user must select the specific agent to be analyzed. Mistakenly selecting the wrong agent results in an inaccurate value. Cannot detect O_2, N_2, argon, or other nonpolar molecules.	Older monitors are being replaced by IR monitors that can identify specific anesthetic agents automatically.
Piezoelectric crystal adsorption	Measurement is performed by two quartz crystals, one of which is coated with a synthetic oil that adsorbs agents, the other of which serves as a reference. Adsorption of agent molecules (or water) on the crystal's surface decreases the crystal's vibrational frequency as a function of agent concentration.	Although the agent must be selected, the displayed error due to incorrect agent selection (with halothane, enflurane, and isoflurane) is minimal. (Error with desflurane may be higher.) Infrequent calibration requirements.	Agent to be measured must be selected manually. Cannot be used for measurement of CO_2 or other respiratory gases.	Developed in 1982, but not in widespread use.
Raman spectroscopy	Raman scattering describes the phenomenon in which sample gas illuminated by light (usually a laser beam) re-emits a small portion of the light at a different wavelength. Analysis of the resultant Raman spectrum identifies and quantifies the sampled gases.	Reports the measured concentration of each gas detected (in contrast to mass spectroscopy). Therefore, the presence of undetectable gases does not influence the measured concentration of the identified gases. Measures all gases.	Like mass spectroscopy, requires frequent calibration. Laser light source has a limited life span.	Improvements in solid-state laser technology may permit further miniaturization.
Mass spectroscopy	Sampled gases are ionized, and the resultant particles are deflected by a magnetic field in a vacuum chamber. The particles are separated by their mass/charge ratios. Each gas produces particles with an identifiable pattern of mass/charge ratios.	Potentially long delay time if long sample tubing is used in a multiplexed (shared) installation.	It reports each detected gas as a fraction of all detected gases. Therefore, it gives incorrect results if an undetected gas (e.g., helium) dilutes the other gases (see text for elaboration).	Single-user monitors are becoming available but remain expensive.

*In order of increasing list price of a representative monitor of each technology.

ple cell. In addition, mass spectrometers yield errors in measurement if the analyzed gas is not dried, for the same reasons that they yield errors when nonstandard gases are present. Raman spectrometers have a separate scattering peak for water that is far removed from the peaks for other respiratory gases.

Piezoelectric crystal adsorption monitors are sensitive to water molecules deposited on the measuring crystal's surface. The water is misidentified as anesthetic agent and produces an artifactual increase in agent concentration.

Eliminating Water from Sampling Lines

In order to have dry gas for analysis, many agent monitors use in-line hydrophobic filters and frequently combine them with Nafion tubing. Nafion is a copolymer of tetrafluoroethylene and a fluorosulfonyl monomer that selectively adsorbs water without affecting the other respiratory gases present in the sample. After water vapor is adsorbed to the inner surface of Nafion tubing, it passes through the wall and evaporates.

Because Nafion is ineffective in eliminating water droplets, it is most efficacious when used at the airway, where the water is still vaporized, rather than near the analyzer, at which point it has condensed. The unique properties of Nafion also allow selective removal of alcohols, ketones, and some ethers, thus decreasing interference from these compounds.

Simpler solutions include positioning the sampling site such that it is in a nondependent position. If an "artificial nose" is used, place it between the patient and sampling site, thereby eliminating most of the water vapor before it reaches the sample line.

Calibration, Leaks, Machine Faults

Three other reasons for apparent gas analysis errors should be considered if the displayed concentrations seem inaccurate:

1. The gas monitor requires calibration.
2. The gas monitor is not sampling what you think it is (the sampling catheter may have a leak).
3. The anesthesia machine is not delivering the gas mixture that you think it is.

Calibration

Begin your evaluation with two simple tests: First let the monitor sample room air; then exhale into the sampling catheter. Room air provides known concentrations of CO_2 (0%), O_2 (21%), and N_2 (79%). If these values are not displayed, the monitor requires calibration (or perhaps servicing). If room air is measured correctly, your exhaled gas provides CO_2 at about 33 to 38 mm Hg. If room air values were correct but your breath was not, try repeating the test with a new gas-sampling catheter. The monitor may be aspirating room air through a

pling catheter, resulting in dilution of
...e.

...ery

...ese tests, it should be performing
...purposes; you then should consider the
...uat the anesthesia machine is delivering an incorrect gas mixture. For example, a vaporizer may require calibration, or the FIO_2 may be decreased because N_2 is accumulating
in the circuit during a low-flow or closed-circuit anesthetic.

Sampling Line Leak

Inspection of the capnogram (the respiratory CO_2 concentration-time tracing) may provide a clue about the equipment
problem. Figure 20–7 shows CO_2 and N_2 waveforms collected
during and after correction of small and large gas monitor
sampling catheter leaks. In the top print-out, a small sampling
catheter leak produced a small rise in the terminal portion of
the capnogram's alveolar plateau.

The capnogram abnormality associated with a sampling line
leak is subtle and may not arouse suspicion by itself. However,
the concentration of N_2 and its waveform are also abnormal.
Because the patient was breathing a mixture of O_2, N_2O, and
isoflurane, we should not detect more than a small amount of
(residual) N_2. Inspection of the N_2 waveform (Fig. 20–7A)
reveals that the N_2 concentration varied from 1% to 12%
during the respiratory cycle and that its concentration decreased as the capnogram's alveolar plateau suddenly increased.

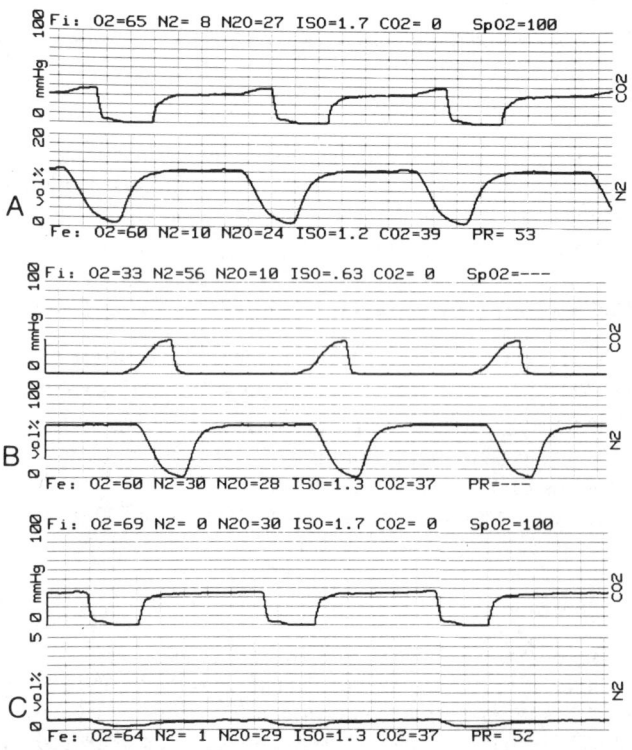

FIGURE 20–7. Large, small, and corrected respiratory gas monitor sampling
catheter leak. Nitrogen and CO_2 concentration-time curves aspirated from a
circle-circuit Y-piece during intermittent positive-pressure ventilation of an
anesthetized adult patient. *A,* Small leak in gas monitor sampling catheter. *B,*
Large sampling catheter leak. *C,* Leak eliminated. Note that the N_2 scale is
different on each printout. (See text for discussion.)

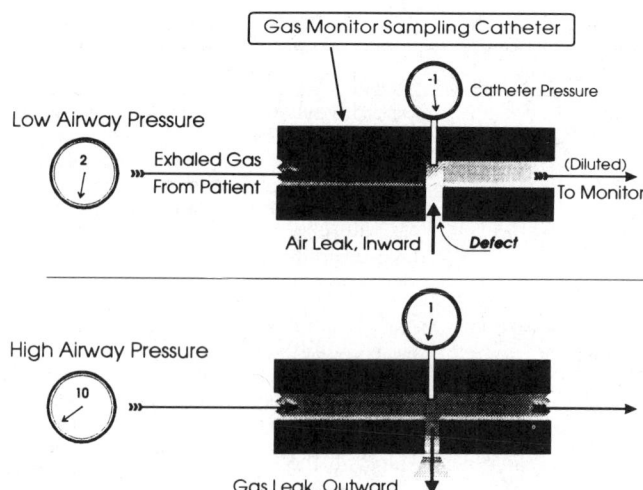

FIGURE 20–8. Respiratory gas monitor sampling catheter leak. Variable
respiratory gas sample dilution occurs when a leak is present in the gas
monitor's sampling catheter. The monitor continuously aspirates sample gas;
this generates a negative pressure (compared with ambient pressure), which
causes entrainment of room air into the gas sample. When circuit pressure
rises (during intermittent positive pressure ventilation), the sample catheter
pressure rises (and usually becomes greater than ambient pressure). Room air
is no longer entrained, and the gas sample may be accurately measured
(although the capnogram is distorted). (Figure 20–7 shows resultant CO_2 and
N_2 waveforms.)

Figure 20–8 is a schematic representation of a segment of
gas-sampling catheter and helps to explain this phenomenon.
During the early part of expiration, the gas monitor samples
respiratory gas that has been diluted by the aspiration of room
air through a leak in the sampling catheter. When the ventilator
cycles and pressurizes the breathing circuit and gas-sampling
catheter, room air entrainment stops and an undiluted sample
is aspirated by the gas monitor. The point of pressurization of
the breathing circuit is evident on the N_2 tracing; note that N_2
concentration falls toward zero as room air entrainment stops.

Circuit Leaks and Air Embolization

Analysis of the sampling catheter leak underscores the value
of a monitor that can detect N_2. The same principle, that of
observing an unexpectedly high concentration of N_2, applies
to detecting breathing circuit discontinuities that entrain room
air. Similarly, entrainment of air into the venous system (venous air embolization), with subsequent elimination of atmospheric N_2 by the lungs, can be detected by noting a sudden
increase in concentration of expired N_2.[21]

CARBON DIOXIDE MONITORING

What Is Meant by "End-Tidal Carbon Dioxide"?

The $PETCO_2$ is the partial pressure of exhaled CO_2 obtained
at the end of a tidal breath. It is measured by selecting the
highest concentration of CO_2 achieved in a single breath and
is usually indicated by the terminal portion of the alveolar
plateau of the capnogram (Fig. 20–9). Respiratory CO_2 concentration may be measured by a capnometer, which displays
only the CO_2 concentration (peak or instantaneous), or by a
capnograph, which displays the CO_2 concentration-time waveform.

The key principle underlying the significance of PETCO₂ is that it is an end-tidal gas sample composed primarily of alveolar gas. The concentration of CO_2 in alveolar gas is, in turn, used to estimate PaCO₂ noninvasively. When PETCO₂ differs from PaCO₂, we can glean clinically relevant information from P(a − ET)CO₂ gradient.

Of course, the process really is not that straightforward. Because of the complex nature of pulmonary gas exchange and the effects of mixing expired gas and ventilatory gas at the sampling site, whether we are truly sampling alveolar gas may be difficult to ascertain. Therefore, a capnometer, which only indicates the CO_2 concentration (e.g., with a bar graph or digital display) but does not have a graphic display, may lead to errors in measuring and interpreting the PETCO₂.[22] Even when using a capnograph, we must be suspicious that a PETCO₂ value that was not measured at the terminal portion of a capnogram with a normal alveolar plateau may substantially underestimate the PaCO₂.

As an example, the capnogram with the steep plateau in Figure 20–9 could have been measured from a patient with severe obstructive lung disease. The steep plateau may indicate that expiration was not complete before the ventilator produced the next inspiration and returned the capnogram to baseline. Had expiration been permitted to continue, the capnogram would have continued to rise and may have finally measured a sample of undiluted alveolar gas. It is also possible that the PETCO₂ measured with a steep alveolar plateau is *greater* than PaCO₂, but this finding is unusual.[23]

Another example of a potential difficulty in determining alveolar CO_2 occurs when capnography is applied to nonintubated patients. Sampling of expiratory gas can be performed by modifying nasal cannulas or by inserting a sampling catheter in the naris, among other methods.[24] A reliable alveolar sample that reflects PaCO₂ may be obtained, but only from a capnogram with a normal alveolar plateau.[25, 26]

What Is the Relationship Between PETCO₂ and PaCO₂?

PETCO₂ may be greater than, equal to, or less than PaCO₂. This variable relationship is influenced by the sampling technique, equipment, and a patient's (patho)physiology (Fig. 20–10). In healthy patients, the P(a − ET)CO₂ gradient is about 5 mm Hg,[27] but it varies during the course of an anesthetic.[28]

In order to consider the relationship between PETCO₂ and PaCO₂, we must first consider the factors that impede acquisition of an alveolar gas sample. Obstruction to expiratory gas flow, as in asthma or with a partially occluded ETT, produces an artifactually low PETCO₂ because a true end-exhaled sample is not obtained. Sampling from a loose-fitting or large dead space face mask causes dilution of the alveolar sample with fresh gas. The presence of a leak in the sampling catheter permits aspiration of room air by the gas monitor, again producing an artifactually low PETCO₂.

In patients with severe pulmonary ventilation-perfusion ($\dot{V}/\dot{Q}$) abnormalities, such as may be induced by pulmonary

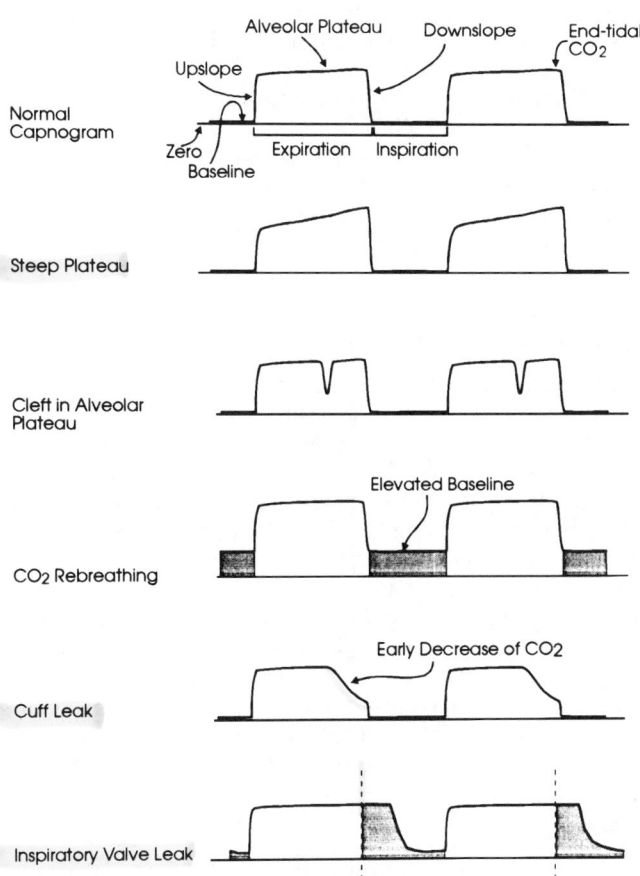

FIGURE 20–9. Archetypical capnograms. Note that *baseline, upslope,* and *alveolar plateau* correspond approximately to phase I, phase II, and phase III, respectively, of the classic physiologic description of a single breath analysis of CO_2.[23] These capnograms may be seen with a circle breathing circuit and mechanically ventilated patient. *Shaded areas* indicate duration and concentration of rebreathed CO_2. *Dotted lines* of inspiratory valve leak tracing indicate the point at which inspiration commenced and at which the capnogram should be returning to baseline. (This phenomenon is explained in detail in Figure 20–12.)

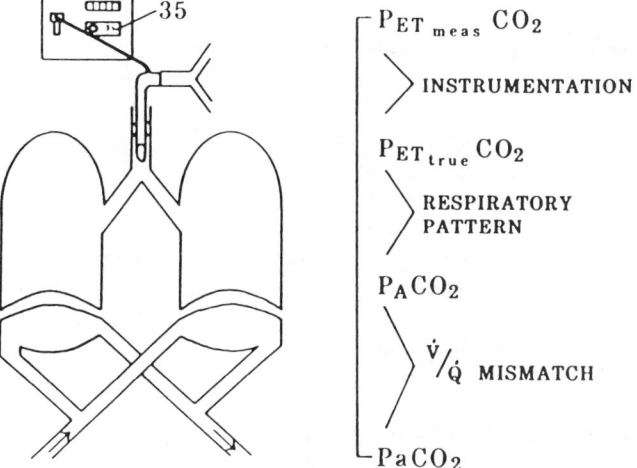

FIGURE 20–10. The difference between PaCO₂ and PETCO₂ can be divided into three components. The first component is the difference between PaCO₂ and PACO₂. Ventilation/perfusion mismatching causes this component of the PaO₂–PETCO₂ difference to increase. The second component is the difference between PACO₂ and true PETCO₂ (PET$_{true}$CO₂). Respiratory patterns that do not deliver mixed alveolar gas to the upper airway (e.g., rapid shallow breathing) increase this component of the PaCO₂–PETCO₂ difference. The third component is the difference between PET$_{true}$CO₂ and measured PETCO₂ (PET$_{meas}$CO₂). This component of the PaCO₂–PETCO₂ difference increases in the presence of problems related to instrumentation (e.g., miscalibrated CO_2 analyzer, sampling line leak). (From Good ML: Capnography: uses, interpretation, and pitfalls. *In* Refresher Courses in Anesthesiology. Vol. 18. Park Ridge, IL, American Society of Anesthesiologists, 1990, p 185.)

hypotension or a pulmonary embolus, alveoli with little or no pulmonary blood flow (high $\dot{V}/\dot{Q}$) contribute their gas (which has not acquired CO_2) to gas from normally perfused alveoli. If these groups of alveoli empty in parallel, the average exhaled CO_2 is lower than the concentration in the normally perfused alveoli, and $PETCO_2$ is lower than "true" alveolar CO_2. The resulting alveolar dead space decreases $PETCO_2$ without necessarily producing an abnormal alveolar plateau.[23]

If Conditions Are Perfect, Will P_{ETCO_2} Equal P_{ACO_2}?

Although clinicians expect $PETCO_2$ to be close to $PaCO_2$, let's ask a different question: What does the $PETCO_2$ value actually represent? In the ideal setting (assuming absent pathology), the end-expiratory gas contains alveolar gas from the terminal portion of expiration (the last gas to leave the alveoli remains in the conducting airways and cannot be measured). Alveolar PCO_2 varies throughout the respiratory cycle.

At the start of inspiration, alveolar gas that had remained behind from the previous breath is nearly in equilibrium with mixed venous blood and has a $PACO_2$ of about 44 mm Hg. As fresh gas floods the alveoli, $PACO_2$ decreases to about 39 mm Hg.[4] During expiration, the $PACO_2$ rises to a value greater than $PaCO_2$ as mixed venous blood continues to deliver CO_2 to the alveoli. If this alveolar gas, undiluted by respiratory dead space gas, is then sampled, $PETCO_2$ may be greater than $PaCO_2$.

The key point is that $PaCO_2$ represents the average of the phasic changes in $PACO_2$, whereas $PETCO_2$ represents the highest $PACO_2$ that can be sampled. Conditions that favor obtaining a sample of alveolar gas with a $PETCO_2$ greater than $PaCO_2$ include healthy lungs, minimal alveolar dead space, low respiratory rate, and large VT.[29] These conditions promote equilibration of end-expiratory gas with mixed venous gas.

Why Is the Relationship Between P_{ETCO_2} and P_{ACO_2} Emphasized?

This relationship is emphasized for several reasons. The parameter that we wish to know is $PaCO_2$; effort is thus placed on assessing its relationship to $PETCO_2$ under varying clinical conditions. Also, $PETCO_2$ represents the physiologic, integrated value of $PACO_2$ throughout the lung,[30] and by convention, it is equal to "ideal alveolar" CO_2.[4] In addition, an arterial blood sample usually is easier to acquire than a mixed venous one for studying these relationships.

What Are the Consequences of Drying Respiratory Gases Before Analysis?

Concentration Versus Partial Pressures

Removal of water vapor increases the concentration of each gas in the gas mixture. However, before investigating this phenomenon, we must understand that gas monitors are calibrated with gases of known fractional percentages (e.g., 5% CO_2). Calibrating the monitor to a fractional gas concentration instead of partial pressure is important for practical reasons. For example, we can calibrate a monitor with 5% CO_2 from a pressurized tank, irrespective of the barometric pressure. When

released from the tank, the gas expands until it equals atmospheric pressure. The concentration of CO_2 remains 5% regardless of whether calibration is performed in Seattle at an ambient pressure of 760 mm Hg or in Denver at an ambient pressure of 630 mm Hg. The measured gas per cent concentration is converted to a partial pressure value by multiplying the percentage by the barometric pressure (e.g., 0.05×760 mm Hg = 38 mm Hg). Therefore, the partial pressure of CO_2 is 38 mm Hg in Seattle (5% of 760 mm Hg) and 31.5 mm Hg in Denver (5% of 630 mm Hg).

Practical Implications

The implication of calibrating a monitor with dry gas and then measuring water vapor–saturated exhaled gas is that if the $PETCO_2$ is 38 mm Hg, the equivalent fraction of CO_2 in saturated alveolar gas is 5% (38 mm Hg/760 mm Hg). Because we know that saturated water vapor exerts a constant partial pressure of 47 mm Hg at body temperature, we can also calculate the concentration of water vapor: 47 mm Hg/760 mm Hg = 6.2%.

Let us assume that O_2 is the only other gas present and that its concentration is 88.8% (675 mm Hg/760 mm Hg). If water vapor were removed from the alveolar gas sample, the remaining O_2 and CO_2 would increase in concentration but their relative proportions would remain unchanged. Therefore, the new concentration of CO_2 would be its old concentration (5%) divided by the sum of CO_2 and O_2, or 5%/(5% + 88.8%) = 5.3%. Similarly, the new concentration of O_2 would be 94.6% (88.8%/[5% + 88.8%]).

A more common and mathematically equivalent way of calculating the expected concentration change that results from removal of water vapor is to divide the partial pressure by $(760 - 47)$ mm Hg. For example, the new concentration of CO_2 would be 38 mm Hg/$(760 - 47)$ mm Hg = 5.3%.

Open and Closed Systems

If we had sealed these gases in a box (closed system) before removing the water vapor, the number of molecules of CO_2 and O_2 could not change, and by definition, the partial pressures of the CO_2 and O_2 would be unchanged despite an increase in each gas's concentration. However, drying of the gas sample is occurring within the monitor or Nafion gas-sampling line, which is an open system, so that additional gas can replace the water vapor as it is removed. Therefore, the number of molecules of CO_2 and O_2 increases in proportion to the increase in concentration of these gases as water vapor is removed. The new partial pressures of these gases can be calculated by multiplying the new concentrations by 760 mm Hg. From our previous example, the new partial pressure of CO_2 is 5.3% of 760 mm Hg, or 0.053×760 = 40.3 mm Hg.

Summary

In summary, the gas monitor analyzes the dried sample gas and measures 5.3% CO_2. If the monitor displays a gas concentration as a partial pressure, it may calculate 5.3% of 760 mm Hg and report $PETCO_2$ as 40.5 mm Hg, or it may adjust the partial pressure value to reflect saturated alveolar conditions by calculating 5.3% of $(760 - 47)$ mm Hg and report $PETCO_2$ as 38 mm Hg.

Respiratory physiology nomenclature conventions recommend displaying the fractional percentage unchanged (e.g.,

5.3% CO_2) while displaying the partial pressure (P_{ETCO_2}) adjusted to saturated conditions.[31] Unfortunately, not all monitors correct their partial pressure measurement to water vapor–saturated conditions, and whether a specific monitor is displaying dry or water vapor–saturated gas partial pressure is not readily apparent.

Another confounding problem is that only partial drying of the gas sample may occur before analysis. An interesting consequence of this artifactual increase in P_{ETCO_2} is a reduction in the apparent gradient between Pa_{CO_2} and P_{ETCO_2}.

What Is the Difference Between Capnographs and Chemical Carbon Dioxide Detectors?

A mainstream analyzer uses a cuvette attached to the ETT to measure CO_2. The IR optics are located in the cuvette itself, so that analysis of the gas sample is very rapid. In contrast, a sidestream analyzer must aspirate the gas sample through a sampling catheter. Therefore, the sidestream analyzer imposes an additional delay in sampling and modest alteration of the waveform due to the transit of the gas sample in the sampling catheter.[32]

The advantage of the mainstream analyzer is the high fidelity of the resultant capnograms. Disadvantages include the cost and fragility of some brands of cuvettes. In addition, the cuvette adds apparatus dead space to the breathing circuit, is relatively heavy, and is awkward and bulky.

We prefer sidestream analyzers because the lightweight and inexpensive disposable sampling catheter permits flexibility in selecting a gas-sampling location. Unfortunately, these monitors aspirate sufficient gas (about 200 mL $\cdot$ min^{-1}) from the breathing circuit that they require special consideration during low-flow or closed-circuit anesthesia for pediatric applications.

A third technology for P_{ETCO_2} monitoring is the chemical detector. The chemical reaction $CO_2 + CO_3^- + H_2O \rightleftarrows 2HCO_3^-$ drives a pH reaction to one of six color zones. These devices are disposable and semi-quantitative, add 38 mL of apparatus dead space, and are not recommended for more than 10 minutes' use. This technology should be considered a backup rather than a primary technique in the operating room (Table 20–2). However, it is useful in remote locations to confirm ETT placement and the effectiveness of cardiopulmonary resuscitation.

What Can We Learn by Examining Capnogram Morphology?

We can learn a great deal about patients and equipment by examining a capnogram. Figure 20–9 shows capnogram nomenclature and several classic capnogram abnormalities that may be observed with a circle breathing circuit attached to a mechanically ventilated patient. The normal capnogram is labeled to explain the various parts of the waveform. Note that the baseline of the capnogram should be zero; if it is not, rebreathing of CO_2 is probably occurring. Here are examples of conditions that could produce the capnograms illustrated in Figure 20–9.

Steep Plateau

A steep plateau may occur in a patient with bronchoconstriction or during ventilation at a slow respiratory rate and large V_T. Typically, in a patient with bronchospasm, the peak CO_2 concentration achieved during expiration is abnormally less than the Pa_{CO_2}. This change is due, in part, to providing inadequate time for completion of expiration, so that an adequate alveolar gas sample is not obtained before initiation of the next inspiration. Therefore, as illustrated in Figure 20–11, we can improve the estimation of Pa_{CO_2} in these patients by permitting expiration to continue for 10 to 20 seconds and noting the peak CO_2 concentration.

Alveolar Plateau Cleft

A cleft in the alveolar plateau results from CO_2-free gas passing from the inspiratory limb and back toward the patient (and CO_2 sampling site) during expiration. This transient reversal of gas flow briefly decreases the concentration of CO_2, until expiration recommences. The cleft sometimes results from the sudden release of a surgeon's elbow pressure from a patient's chest. It often heralds a patient's recovery of neuromuscular function and the return of (weak) spontaneous respirations. In a normally functioning circle breathing circuit, the regular, repetitive appearance of a cleft is a sensitive indicator of spontaneous inspiratory efforts.

Elevated Baseline

Rebreathing of CO_2 is evident from the elevated capnogram baseline. This capnogram may occur when a circle-circuit ex-

TABLE 20–2. Comparison of Chemical and Electronic Carbon Dioxide Monitors

Characteristic	Chemical Devices	Sidestream Electronic Devices	Mainstream Electronic Devices
Breath-by-breath	+	+	+
Increased dead space	+ +	−	±
Quantitative	−	+	+
Long-term use	−	+	+
Requires calibration gas	−	+	−
Respiratory rate	−	+	+
Alarm	−	+	+
Diagnose hypercapnia	−	+	+
Power requirement	−	+	+

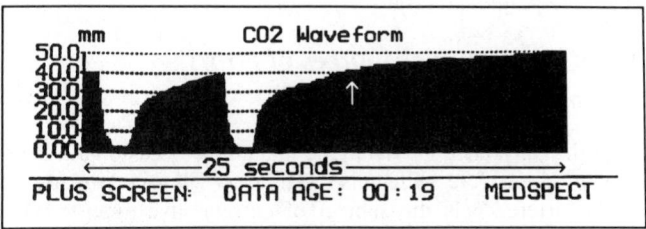

FIGURE 20–11. Steep alveolar plateau. In this adult patient with severe obstructive pulmonary disease, the apparent P_{ETCO_2} on the capnogram misrepresents alveolar pCO_2. The first capnogram demonstrates an abnormally steep alveolar plateau. It appears that P_{ETCO_2} is 39 mm Hg. When expiration was permitted to continue uninterrupted for about 18 seconds, expired CO_2 concentration increased to 50 mm Hg as alveolar CO_2 finally reached the ETT sampling site. Arterial pCO_2 was 55 mm Hg. (The *vertical white arrow* indicates the point at which inspiration would have commenced had mechanical ventilation not been interrupted.)

piratory valve becomes incompetent and permits bidirectional flow or with exhausted soda lime. In either case, during inspiration, CO_2-laden expired gas mixes with fresh gas from the inspiratory limb and is inspired with it. If the expiratory valve is absent, no recognizable undulations may occur in the capnogram.

Early Decrease of Carbon Dioxide

A leaking ETT cuff may permit the escape of ventilating gas past the cuff and into the upper airway during inspiration and expiration. The leak during late expiration permits fresh circuit gas to enter the ETT, pass the CO_2 sampling site, and decrease the measured CO_2 concentration. The greater the leak and the greater the FGF, the greater the distortion of the capnogram.

Inspiratory Valve Leak

A leaking inspiratory valve causes CO_2 rebreathing that is detectable on a capnogram by identifying the prolonged alveolar plateau and abnormal downslope. This abnormality is shown in Figure 20–9 and is illustrated in detail in Figure 20–12.

PULSE OXIMETRY

What Does a Pulse Oximeter Really Measure?

Pulse oximetry computes arterial O_2 saturation by using variations in the absorption of light in the red and IR wavelengths caused by the pulsation of arterial blood.[33] Arterial O_2 saturation determined by a pulse oximeter is designated as SpO_2 (Fig. 20–13). Increased arterial blood flow during systole expands tissue beds by delivering additional blood with each pulse. These arterial pulsations alter the amount of transmitted light. By working only with the pulsatile light, the pulse oximeter can ignore light absorption by nonpulsatile elements in the light transmission pathway (e.g., tissue, bone, or pigmented skin).[34] The technology just described is called *transmission oximetry* and uses light at wavelengths of 660 nm (red light, primarily absorbed by reduced hemoglobin) and 910 or 940 nm (IR light, primarily absorbed by oxyhemoglobin). A newer technology is *reflectance oximetry,* which monitors SpO_2 by measuring light reflected from perfused tissues. This approach is advantageous for monitoring at nontransilluminable sites (e.g., the pulmonary artery).

What Are Potential Sources of Error?

Nail Polish

Both nail polish and synthetic nails have occasionally been shown to interfere with pulse oximetry. The exact nature of this interference is the subject of current investigation. Obviously, opaque nail polish diminishes the intensity of transmitted light and may result in decreased signal strength.[35] Nail polish that incorporates a blue pigment similarly has been shown to cause an artifactual lowering of the reported SpO_2 value. Options are to remove nail polish on one digit or to select another probe site, a reasonable option for a patient who has an expensive manicure and is undergoing outpatient surgery. Alternatively, you can also verify that the baseline SpO_2

is normal; therefore, the nail polish is not altering the monitor's ability to accurately reflect SpO_2.

Insufficient Signal Strength

Insufficient signal strength may be caused by incorrect probe:sensor-detector alignment or placement and typically results in either a falsely low saturation, if the probe is extending too far off the finger tip, or lack of signal detection. The former is obviously the more bothersome problem and is thought to result from incorporation of venous pulsations, thus contaminating what is presumed to be a purely arterial signal.[36] Patients who are warm and peripherally vasodilated are most prone to this phenomenon, termed the *penumbra effect.*[36] Placing the sensing site more proximal (i.e., over larger arterial or capillary vessels) resolves the problem.

In contrast, patients who are vasoconstricted from cold, shock, vasculitis, or drugs can have reduced blood flow through the finger tips. When the probe is not optimally positioned, no signal is detected. This problem can be remedied by a digital nerve block with a local anesthetic or the application of topical nitroglycerin.[37]

Other causes of low perfusion such as arm elevation, arterial compression, and hypotension can cause similar effects; in fact, the pulse oximeter probe can be positioned specifically to aid in detecting arterial pulsations.

Noisy Signals

Noisy signals are commonly caused by ambient light (especially IR warming lights), motion, and stray electromagnetic energy from the electrosurgical unit (ESU) or magnetic resonance imaging (MRI). ESUs and ambient light can cause either falsely high or falsely low saturations and heart rates. The entry of ambient light may be reduced with a close-fitting probe and may be blocked with an opaque probe cover. MRI interferes with pulse oximetry (and vice versa) and can cause abrupt changes in SpO_2 with the start of imaging.

Probe motion may cause absent or incorrect readings. The readings usually decrease to a "default" SpO_2 value of 85%, which implies a red-to-IR light transmission ratio of one (corresponding to a SpO_2 of 85%). Extensive effort has been put into developing probes that are less sensitive to motion, including coupling of the electrocardiogram signal to the oximeter. An additional source of error occurs when a large dicrotic notch is detected as a separate heartbeat, causing the displayed pulse rate to be twice the actual pulse rate.[37]

Dyes and Abnormal Hemoglobins

Another source of pulse oximetry error that deserves mention is the interference caused by dyes and abnormal hemoglobins. Methylene blue, indocyanine green, and indigo carmine cause transient, apparent desaturation when administered intravenously. Methylene blue has the most profound and complex effects on SpO_2. It both produces and clears methemoglobin, causes a transient increase in cardiac output followed by cardiac depression, and has an absorbance peak at 668 nm that interferes with the oximeter's detection of red absorbance and indicates desaturation.[34]

Methemoglobin can cause falsely high or low SpO_2 readings, depending on the relative amounts of oxyhemoglobin and reduced hemoglobin. However, as the methemoglobin

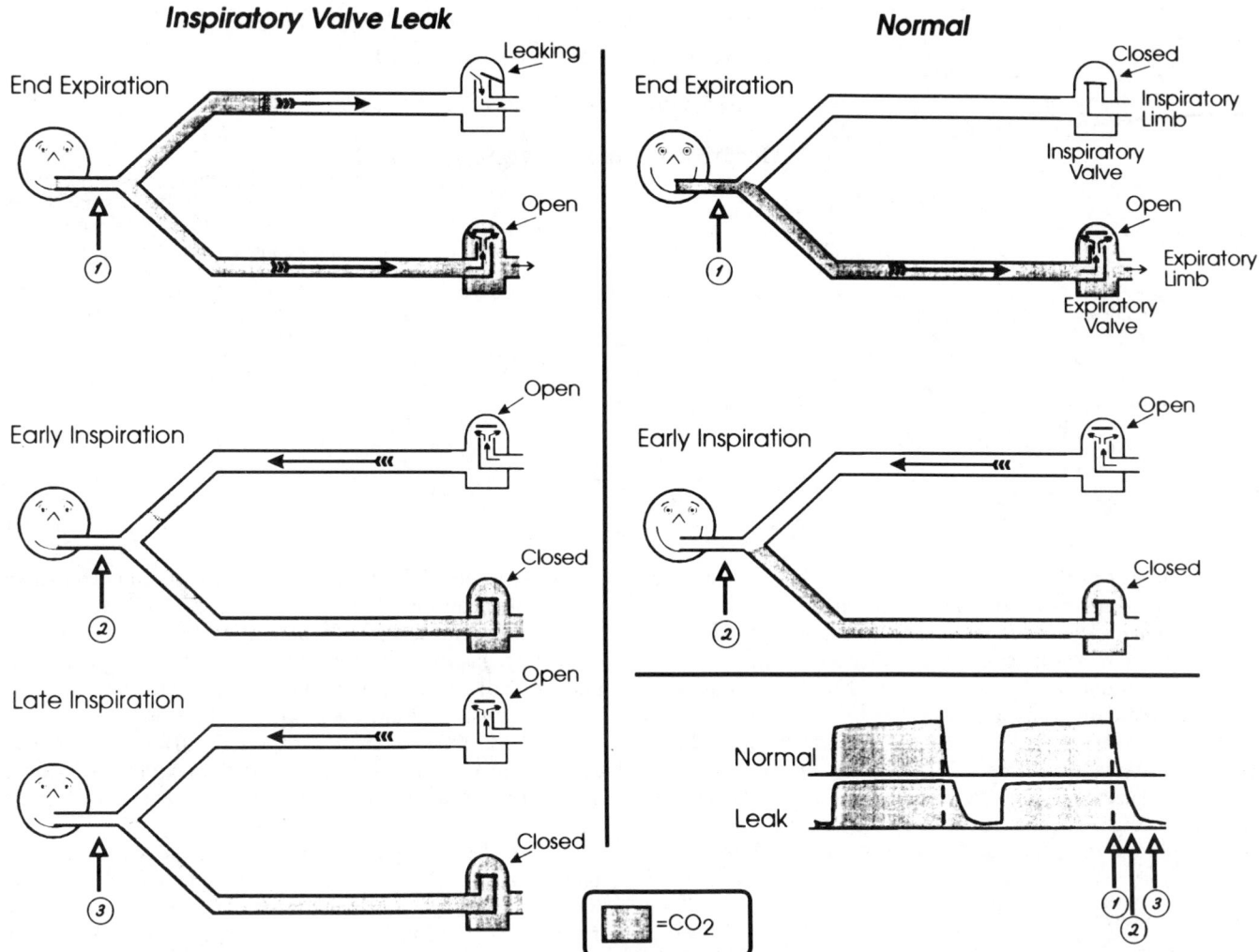

FIGURE 20–12. Pattern of gas flow with a leaking inspiratory valve. Diagram of CO_2 flow in a circle breathing circuit with a leaking inspiratory valve and under normal conditions. Normally during expiration, CO_2-laden expiratory gas flows only through the expiratory limb and is measured by the capnograph (1). Then, as inspiration begins, fresh gas (devoid of CO_2) flows through the inspiratory limb and is sampled by the capnograph (2). This results in the rapid downslope of the capnogram during inspiration.

If the inspiratory valve leaks and permits bidirectional gas flow, expired gas will flow through both the expiratory and inspiratory limbs of the circuit during expiration. Then, as inspiration begins, the capnogram will demonstrate the continued presence of CO_2 at the endotracheal tube (2). As inspiration progresses, the inspired limb CO_2 may completely wash into the patient, or a residual amount may still remain at the end of inspiration (3). The gradual washout of CO_2 from the inspiratory limb produces a capnogram with a prolonged plateau and an abnormal downslope. The severity of CO_2 rebreathing depends on the amount of reverse flow in the inspiratory limb. The capnogram may return to baseline during inspiration if the tidal volume is large relative to the volume of gas that flows backward into the inspiratory limb.

level increases, the SpO_2 decreases to 80%–85% and then remains constant.

Carboxyhemoglobin is read as approximately 90% saturated by pulse oximeters. Therefore, it can cause falsely elevated SpO_2 readings in heavy smokers or in those with carbon monoxide poisoning if they have "true" low SaO_2 levels with elevated carboxyhemoglobin levels. Fetal hemoglobin has no clinically significant effect on pulse oximetry.[38]

What Other Applications Are Useful?

Remote Areas/Transport

Pulse oximetry has become a standard of care in the postanesthesia care unit that parallels that in the operating room. Not surprisingly, its introduction into the postanesthesia care unit has revealed a high incidence of postanesthetic hypox-

emia.[39] In areas where parenteral sedation is given (e.g., dental offices, angiography suites, or endoscopy units), pulse oximetry should be standard as well.

We use pulse oximetry to monitor critically ill (and especially ventilator-dependent) patients during transport to and from the intensive care unit. Critically ill patients are frequently monitored with continuous pulse oximetry as a noninvasive and inexpensive method for assessing O_2 requirements. However, poor perfusion and movement artifact may reduce its reliability in this group of patients.

Circulatory Assessment

The plethysmographic display capability of the pulse oximeter has been proposed as a means of monitoring the circulation. Although studies have used this display to estimate intravascular volume status, the technique has limited clinical applicability.[40] The problem stems from the pulse oximeter's

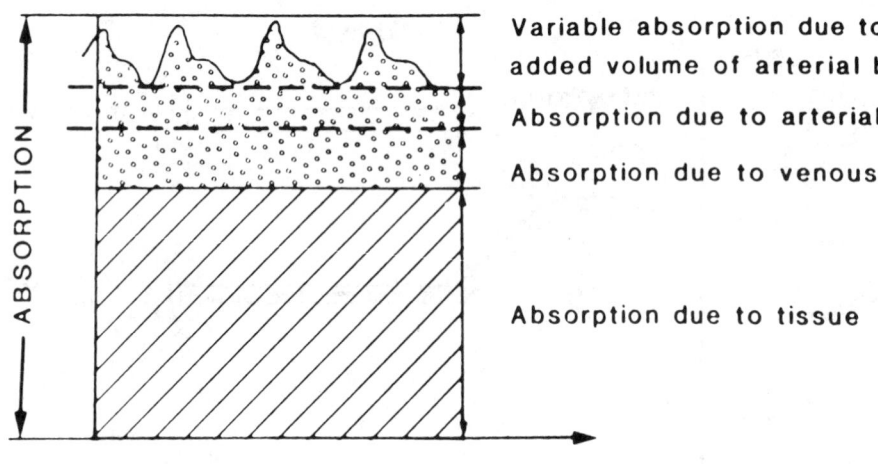

Variable absorption due to pulse-added volume of arterial blood

Absorption due to arterial blood

Absorption due to venous blood

Absorption due to tissue

ABSORPTION

TIME

FIGURE 20–13. Tissue composite showing dynamic and static components that affect light absorption during pulse oximetry. (Adapted from Ohmeda 3700, Pulse Oximeter Users Manual. Madison, WI, Ohmeda, 1989, p 22. Provided by Ohmeda, Inc., The BOC Group.)

scaling of the plethysmographic display to compensate for alterations in amplitude that are unrelated to perfusion. For instance, changes in saturation change plethysmographic amplitude. Some newer pulse oximeters display an index of perfusion that is unrelated to saturation and may overcome the limitations of current instruments.

Pulse oximetry also has been used to assess the palmar collateral circulation before arterial cannulation. However, its ability to detect even minute pulsations (i.e., <10% of the normal blood flow) can be a problem because such pulsations may be present in the absence of adequate collateral flow.[41–43]

Blood Pressure

The disappearance of the plethysmographic waveform during slow blood pressure cuff inflation can provide an estimate of systolic blood pressure.[44] We have found this to be an effective technique for measuring blood pressure in pediatric patients undergoing general anesthesia for MRI. Note that this technique of blood pressure determination occurs during *inflation*. Systolic pressure corresponds to the *loss* of the plethysmographic signal. During deflation of the cuff signal, reacquisition of the pulse signal is sufficiently slow that this end point predictably underestimates systolic pressure.

CARBON DIOXIDE ABSORPTION

How Much Carbon Dioxide Can Soda Lime Absorb?

Soda lime is a CO_2 absorbent composed mainly of calcium hydroxide [$Ca(OH)_2$] and smaller amounts of sodium hydroxide or potassium hydroxide as a dry mixture bound to inert silicate.[45] A related product uses a combination of barium hydroxide (as an octahydrate compound) and sodium hydroxide as the absorbent (Baralyme). Barium hydroxide is heavier than calcium hydroxide. Therefore, under ideal conditions, 100 g of soda lime absorbs 23 L of CO_2, whereas 100 g of barium hydroxide absorbs only 18 L. A typical canister contains about 1200 g.

During closed-circuit anesthesia, when we require that all CO_2 produced by a patient be absorbed, the amount of time to exhaustion of the CO_2 absorber can be calculated if you know its absorbing capacity. In a properly packed canister, 100 g of soda lime should absorb a minimum of 15 L of CO_2 before the exiting gas exceeds 1% CO_2. The average to maximum production of CO_2 in healthy adult males under general anesthesia is between 12 and 18 $L \cdot h^{-1}$.[45] Therefore, about 100 g of fresh soda lime is required to absorb all of the CO_2 produced during each hour of general anesthesia; for added safety, the usual estimate is 1 kg of soda lime for every 8 hours of use.

Because the average CO_2 absorber holds two soda lime containers, each of 1 to 1.5 kg capacity, a total of 16 hours of CO_2-absorbing capacity should be possible with a new canister of soda lime. In semi-closed anesthesia systems, a portion of the CO_2 is vented to the scavenging system; hence the CO_2 absorbent lasts longer. The higher the fresh gas flow, the longer the absorbent lasts (Fig. 20–14).

Calcium hydroxide is consumed during the process of CO_2 absorption, which occurs in three steps as follows:

$$2CO_2 + 2H_2O \rightarrow 2H_2CO_3$$

$$2H_2CO_3 + 2NaOH + 2KOH \rightarrow Na_2CO_3 + K_2CO_3 + 4H_2O$$

$$Na_2CO_3 + K_2CO_3 + 2Ca(OH)_2 \rightarrow 2CaCO_3 + 2NaOH + 2KOH$$

What Factors Govern the Efficiency of Absorption?

The efficiency of CO_2 absorption can be influenced by the physical characteristics of the soda lime and the method of packing the soda lime into the canister.

Shape

Soda lime granules have irregular shapes to increase the surface area for CO_2 absorption.

Size

Limitation of granule size to 4 to 8 mesh optimizes the surface area without increasing the resistance to breathing.

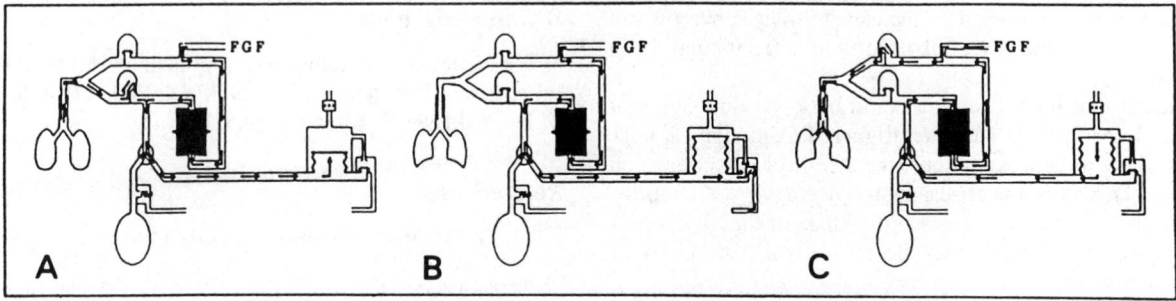

FIGURE 20–14. Mechanism by which the rate of fresh gas flow affects the CO_2 absorbent. (FGF = fresh gas flow; CO_2-containing gases are represented by the *blacked-in portions* of the circuit). *A,* Carbon dioxide–containing gases from the patient pass through the ventilator hose into the ventilator bellows during exhalation. *B,* Carbon dioxide–containing gases pass through the ventilator hose, into the ventilator bellows, and out of the spill valve during the respiratory pause. *C,* Gases flow retrograde through the absorbent during inspiration. (From Öhrn M, Gravenstein N, Good ML: Duration of carbon dioxide absorption by soda lime at low rates of fresh gas flow. J Clin Anesth 1991; 3:104. Reproduced by permission of Butterworth-Heinemann.)

(Mesh is a measure of the screen size through which the granules pass; the greater the mesh, the smaller the granule size.)

Hardness

Granules must have a specific minimum hardness to prevent the formation of caustic dust particles.

Packing

Granules must be firmly packed to prevent *channeling,* which is the formation of vertical pathways with very low resistance to gas flow. Channeled gases contact only a small portion of the absorbent granules, thus allowing CO_2-containing gas to pass through the absorber canister and be rebreathed.

When Is the Soda Lime Nearly Exhausted?

In order to facilitate recognition of soda lime's loss of CO_2-absorbing capacity, manufacturers incorporate an indicator dye in the granules. This indicator, ethyl violet, has a critical pH of 10.3. As calcium hydroxide is consumed and the pH in the canister falls, the indicator dye turns purple. The color change becomes more prominent as the absorbing capacity is progressively exhausted.

The manufacturer of Sodasorb recommends that the upper canister be replaced when the majority of visible granules just begin to show a change in color.[45] The lower canister, which is generally spared by the CO_2-containing gas flow, is then switched to the upper location. Another option is to compare the temperature of the two canisters by touching them with the back of your hand. The reaction sequence described is exothermic. When the lower canister is warmer, the upper canister is depleted.

North American Dräger and Ohmeda recommend changing soda lime when any visible color change is present. We cannot find any evidence to support this wasteful approach. Our practice is to remove the upper canister and replace it with the lower as soon as a color change is noted in the lower canister (proof that CO_2 is passing through the upper canister).

Routine use of capnography identifies rebreathing, which may occur if either channeling through or exhaustion of the lower canister's absorbing ability occurs. This problem is readily remedied by increasing the FGF, thereby turning the system into a nonrebreathing one (see Fig. 20–14).

Is a Carbon Dioxide Absorber Without Purple Discoloration Fresh?

Maybe not! The indicator dye is helpful only when the anesthesia machine is in use. If the machine has been allowed to stand idle for more than 30 minutes with no exposure to CO_2, the soda lime may regenerate a small amount of absorptive capacity, increasing the pH sufficiently to cause the indicator to revert to a colorless state. In this instance, the absence of a color change belies the presence of nearly exhausted absorbent with limited remaining capacity. "It is thus evident that white Sodasorb always has absorptive capacity, but its whiteness is not a quantitative indication. Sodasorb which is purple, however, is always at or very near the point of clinical—not chemical—exhaustion."[45]

Photoreactivation of ethyl violet caused by exposure to fluorescent light can also cause inability to detect absorbent exhaustion. A significant dose-response relationship is present between the duration of light exposure and the amount by which the ethyl violet concentration declines. In addition, ethyl violet decays with time after a container of soda lime has been opened, even if it is stored in the dark.[46]

Finally, unknown to you, your absorbent may be of a type that lacks an indicator, in which case the color change that you are expecting will never occur. Without capnography, you would not know that CO_2 rebreathing was occurring until abnormal physical or vital signs aroused your suspicion and prompted you to perform an ABG analysis. If CO_2 rebreathing is documented by the appearance of inspired CO_2 on the capnogram, exhausted CO_2 absorbent can be differentiated from a leaking expiratory valve by increasing the FGF to exceed the minute ventilation. This process converts the circle system into a nonrebreathing circuit and should return the capnogram to normal if the CO_2 absorbent is exhausted (see Fig. 20–14).

Why Is the Soda Lime Canister Warm?

The chemical reaction of CO_2 with a strong base is exothermic; therefore, a warm canister indicates that CO_2 absorption is occurring. The temperature is not proportional to the remaining absorptive capacity and may not decrease as the absorber is nearing exhaustion.[45] The canister may remain warm for considerable time after all absorbing capacity has been exhausted.

A canister that feels quite hot could be a warning sign that malignant hyperthermia has been triggered. Although capnography is likely to be a more sensitive means of detecting such a reaction, the heat of the absorbent is a useful way of confirming fears that the capnogram is provoking. In the absence of capnography, this change may be one of the first clues of impending disaster.

Is Carbon Monoxide Poisoning a Risk?

Intraoperative carbon monoxide poisoning has been described during both closed-circuit and semi–closed-circuit anesthesia. The levels of carboxyhemoglobin were, in many instances, too high to be the result of smoking and high enough to cause poisoning. One study noted that the cases of unexplained poisoning were also the first anesthetic cases on Monday morning. The hypothesis was advanced that when fluorinated anesthetics are permitted to incubate with the absorbent, carbon monoxide may be produced.[47] Further investigation may ultimately support the practice of flushing the absorber with fresh gas after an idle period. However, the small number of reported cases of carbon monoxide contamination should not discourage the use of a CO_2 absorbent.

CONCLUSION

We are reminded of a fascinating analysis, that performed by J. F. Nunn, that we believe emphasizes the importance of monitoring respiratory function.[3] He reviewed the situations that could most rapidly produce the ultimate physiologic insult—cerebral anoxia. Nunn summarized these situations as follows:

1. Circulatory arrest produces loss of cerebral circulation and results in loss of consciousness in about 10 seconds.
2. Exposure to an ambient pressure of 47 mm Hg (6.3 kPa) causes body fluids to boil. Water vapor replaces alveolar gas, and consciousness is lost in one circulation time (about 15 s).
3. Hyperventilation with pure N_2 washes out alveolar O_2 and produces cerebral anoxia in about 30 seconds.
4. Inhalation of pure N_2O produces loss of consciousness more slowly than inhalation of N_2 (unspecified time). The difference in speed of action occurs because N_2O is more soluble than N_2, so that removal of N_2O from the lungs by pulmonary blood flow decreases the rate of rise of alveolar N_2O, and hence the resultant fall in PaO_2 is slowed.
5. Apnea ultimately leads to loss of consciousness, but the time to development of cerebral anoxia is dependent on the rate of O_2 consumption and alveolar O_2 stores. Loss of consciousness could occur within 90 seconds of apnea (after breathing room air).

Respiratory monitoring permits immediate detection of four of these five causes of cerebral anoxia. An altimeter detects the remaining one. Although these scenarios represent the extremes of untoward events, they do underscore the value of such respiratory monitoring.

Acknowledgments

We express our gratitude to our colleagues for their thoughtful comments: Robert W. Phelps, M.D., Ph.D., Paul S. Nelson, M.D., and Lyle E. Kirson, D.D.S.

References

1. Shapiro BA: In-vivo monitoring of arterial blood gases and pH. Respiratory Care 1992; 37:165.
2. Greenblott G, Barker SJ, Tremper KK, et al: Detection of venous air embolism by continuous intraarterial oxygen monitoring. J Clin Monit 1990; 6:53.
3. Nunn JF: Applied Respiratory Physiology. 3rd ed. Boston, Butterworths, 1987.
4. Nanji AA, Whitlow KJ: Is it necessary to transport arterial blood samples on ice for pH and gas analysis? Can Anaesth Soc J 1984; 31:568.
5. Lenfant C, Aucutt C: Oxygen uptake and change in carbon dioxide tension in human blood stored at 37°C. J Appl Physiol 1965; 20:503.
6. Mahoney JJ, Harvey JA, Wong RJ, et al: Changes in oxygen measurements when whole blood is stored in iced plastic or glass syringes. Clin Chem 1991; 37:1244.
7. Biswas CK, Ramos JM, Agroyannis B, et al: Blood gas analysis: effect of air bubbles in syringe and delay in estimation. Br Med J (Clin Res Ed) 1982; 284:923.
8. Reeves RB: An imidazole alphastat hypothesis for vertebrate acid-base regulation: tissue carbon dioxide content and body temperature in bullfrogs. Respir Physiol 1972; 14:219.
9. Ream RK, Reitz BA, Silverberg G: Temperature correction of PCO_2 and pH in estimating acid-base status. Anesthesiology 1982; 56:41.
10. Nattie EE: The alphastat hypothesis in respiratory control and acid-base balance. J Appl Physiol 1990; 69:1201.
11. Benatar SR, Hewlett AM, Nunn JF: The use of iso-shunt lines for control of oxygen therapy. Br J Anaesth 1973; 45:711.
12. Piernan S, Roizen MF, Severinghaus JW: Oxygen analyzer dangerous—senses nitrous oxide as battery fails. Anesthesiology 1979; 50:146.
13. Westenskow DR, Jordan WS, Jordan R, et al: Evaluation of oxygen monitors for use during anesthesia. Anesth Analg 1981; 60:53.
14. Linko K, Paloheimo M: Inspiratory end-tidal oxygen content difference: a sensitive indicator of hypoventilation. Crit Care Med 1989; 17:345.
15. Merilainen PT: A differential paramagnetic sensor for breath-by-breath oximetry. J Clin Monit 1990; 6:65.
16. Linko K, Paloheimo M: Monitoring of the inspired and end-tidal oxygen, carbon dioxide, and nitrous oxide concentrations: clinical applications during anesthesia and recovery. J Clin Monit 1989; 5:149.
17. Boothby WM, Lundin G, Helmholz HF Jr: Gaseous nitrogen elimination test to determine pulmonary efficiency. Proc Soc Exp Biol Med 1948; 67:558.
18. Gaumann DM, Mustaki JP, Tassonyi E: MAC-awake of isoflurane, enflurane and halothane evaluated by slow and fast alveolar washout. Br J Anaesth 1992; 68:81.
19. Stoelting RK, Longnecker DE, Eger E II: Minimum alveolar concentrations in man on awakening from methoxyflurane, halothane, ether and fluroxene anesthesia: MAC awake. Anesthesiology 1970; 33:5.
20. Guyton DC, Gravenstein N: Infrared analysis of volatile anesthetics: impact of monitor agent setting, volatile mixtures, and alcohol. J Clin Monit 1990; 6:203.
21. Matjasko J, Petrozza P, Mackenzie CF: Sensitivity of end-tidal nitrogen in venous air embolism detection in dogs. Anesthesiology 1985; 63:418.
22. Block FE Jr: A carbon dioxide monitor that does not show the waveform is worthless. J Clin Monit 1988; 4:213.
23. Fletcher R, Jonson B, Cumming G, et al: The concept of deadspace with special reference to the single breath test for carbon dioxide. Br J Anaesth 1981; 53:77.
24. Goldman JM: A simple, easy, and inexpensive method for monitoring $ETCO_2$ through nasal cannulae (Letter to the editor). Anesthesiology 1987; 67:606.
25. Bowe EA, Boysen PG, Broome JA, et al: Accurate determination of end-tidal carbon dioxide during administration of oxygen by nasal cannulae. J Clin Monit 1989; 5:105.
26. McNulty SE, Roy J, Torjman M, et al: Relationship between arterial carbon dioxide and end-tidal carbon dioxide when a nasal sampling port is used. J Clin Monit 1990; 6:93.
27. Nunn JF, Hill DW: Respiratory dead space and arterial to end-tidal CO_2 tension difference in anesthetized man. J Appl Physiol 1960; 15:383.
28. Raemer DB, Francis D, Philip JH, et al: Variation in PCO_2 between

arterial blood and peak expired gas during anesthesia. Anesth Analg 1983; 62:1065.

29. Bhavani Shankar K, Maseley H, Vemula V, et al: Physiological dead space during general anaesthesia for caesarean section. Can J Anaesth 1987; 34:373.

30. Riley RL, Lilienthal JL Jr, Proemmel DD, et al: On the determination of the physiologically effective pressures of oxygen and carbon dioxide in alveolar air. Am J Physiol 1946; 147:191.

31. Severinghaus JW: Water vapor calibration errors in some capnometers: respiratory conventions misunderstood by manufacturers? Anesthesiology 1989; 70:996.

32. Gravenstein JS, Paulus DA, Hayes TJ: Capnography in Clinical Practice. Stoneham, MA, Butterworths, 1989.

33. Severinghaus JW, Honda Y: History of blood gas analysis. VII. Pulse oximetry. J Clin Monit 1987; 3:135.

34. Kelleher JF: Pulse oximetry. J Clin Monit 1989; 5:37.

35. Coté CJ, Goldstein EA, Fuchsman WH, et al: The effect of nail polish on pulse oximetry. Anesth Analg 1988; 67:683.

36. Kelleher JF, Ruff RH: The penumbra effect: vasomotion-dependent pulse oximeter artifact due to probe malposition. Anesthesiology 1989; 71:787.

37. Severinghaus JW, Kelleher JF: Recent developments in pulse oximetry. Anesthesiology 1992; 76:1018.

38. Pologe JA, Raley DM: Effects of fetal hemoglobin on pulse oximetry. J Perinatol 1987; 7:324.

39. Canet J, Ricos M, Vidal F: Early postoperative arterial desaturation: determining factors and response to oxygen therapy. Anesth Analg 1989; 69:207.

40. Partridge BL: Use of pulse oximetry as a noninvasive indicator of intravascular volume status. J Clin Monit 1987; 3:263.

41. Lawson D, Norley I, Korbon G, et al: Blood flow limits and pulse oximeter signal detection. Anesthesiology 1987; 67:599.

42. Cheng EY, Lauer KK, Stommel KA, et al: Evaluation of the palmar circulation by pulse oximetry. J Clin Monit 1989; 5:1.

43. Glavin RJ, Jones HM: Assessing collateral circulation in the hand—four methods compared. Anaesthesia 1989; 44:594.

44. Wallace CT, Baker JD III, Alpert CC, et al: Comparison of blood pressure measurement by Doppler and by pulse oximetry techniques. Anesth Analg 1987; 66:1018.

45. The Sodasorb Manual of Carbon Dioxide Absorption. WR Grace & Co, Dewey and Almy Chemical Division, 1962.

46. Andrews JJ, Johnston RV Jr, Bee DE, et al: Photodeactivation of ethyl violet: a potential hazard of Sodasorb. Anesthesiology 1990; 72:59.

47. Moon RE, Ingram C, Brunner EA, et al: Spontaneous generation of carbon monoxide within anesthetic circuits (Abstract). Anesthesiology 1991; 75:A873.

CHAPTER 21

Cardiovascular Monitoring

HUGH C. GILBERT, M.D.
JEFFREY S. VENDER, M.D.

Cardiovascular monitoring is an essential component of intraoperative anesthesia care. The cardiovascular system frequently is influenced not only by anesthetic drug therapy but also by dynamic changes related to surgical intervention. Historically, anesthesiologists relied on their senses to assess anesthetic depth and patients' well-being. By observing patterns of ventilation, muscle tone, pupillary size, movement, and skin color, they monitored the effects of anesthetics in order to reduce the prospect of anesthetic overdose and the potential for anesthetic-induced mortality.

Cardiovascular monitoring uses instrumentation to assess current cardiovascular status; to manipulate, maintain, or restore cardiovascular homeostasis; and to detect or eliminate preventable untoward events. Ensuring the adequacy of circulatory function during anesthesia care is an essential component of basic intraoperative monitoring. This chapter examines key elements and specific techniques necessary to monitor the adequacy of circulatory function. Electronic signal processing, computer data acquisition, and new transducers have revolutionized the potential for assessment. Nevertheless, clinical judgment remains an essential aspect of monitoring. Sophisticated instrumentation cannot serve anesthetized patients unless knowledgeable clinicians integrate monitored data with judgment and experience.

THE ELECTROCARDIOGRAM

The electrocardiogram (ECG) was the first electronic monitor to be used intraoperatively.[1] Described principally as a means of detecting intraoperative dysrhythmias, continuous display of the ECG has been incorporated into routine intraoperative monitoring.[2]

What Is the Value of Electrocardiographic Monitoring?

Studies have demonstrated a high incidence of dysrhythmias associated with the administration of anesthesia.[3, 4] Although the majority are of no clinical consequence, the potential for a dysrhythmia that requires alteration of the anesthetic management plan, addition of specific drug therapy, or even cardioversion is always present. Table 21-1 lists the most commonly associated factors. Patients with pre-existing heart disease are more prone to perioperative dysrhythmias.[5] Because intraoperative dysrhythmias occur frequently, anesthesiologists must be skillful in monitoring and interpreting ECG changes. The prevalence of coronary artery disease also has focused attention on the potential use of ECG criteria to diagnose and treat intraoperative ischemia or infarction.

What Does the Electrocardiogram Represent?

Electrocardiography is based on the recording and interpretation of alterations in electrical potentials that result from the electrically active cells of the heart. Although the electrical gradients resulting from the depolarization and repolarization potentials of the atria and ventricles are very small, impulse conduction recording is easily performed.

A multitude of electrode arrays and instrumentation are available. Central to ECG interpretation is the concept that a spatial vector can describe the cumulative current flow associated with myocardial depolarization and repolarization. Spatial vectors define the magnitude and direction of electrical events measured by a set of electrodes (bipolar leads). Intraoperatively, interest is focused on alterations of atrial and ventricular depolarization and ventricular repolarization.

TABLE 21-1. Factors That May Contribute to Intraoperative Dysrhythmias

Factor	Mechanism
Inhalational anesthetic agents	Re-entry, sensitization
Hyperventilation	Hypokalemia, alkalosis
Electrolyte imbalance	Re-entry, automaticity
Endotracheal intubation	Autonomic activation
Pre-existing cardiac disease	Myocardial ischemia; conduction defects
Catheter insertions	Irritation of myocardium
Drug interaction	Sensitization

What Factors Determine Electrocardiographic Deflection?

When bipolar leads are used, a current vector in the direction of the positive electrode results in an upward deflection. A downward deflection occurs when the current flow is reversed. If the electrode pair is perpendicular to the current flow, no deflection occurs. If the electrode pair is parallel to the current flow, the deflection is maximum.

An infinite number of surface bipolar leads and vectors are possible. Electrocardiologists have devised 12 standardized lead positions to optimize the clinical applicability of ECG recordings. The electrical signals obtained from surface electrodes require amplification in order to be displayed. Computerization of ECG monitors facilitates the processing of these signals, permitting real-time analysis.

What Leads Are Used?

Intraoperative ECG, by convention, is based on information obtained from placing three or five surface leads. Three leads placed on both arms and the left leg can be used to monitor the standard limb leads (I, II, III) or any modified bipolar lead. A fourth lead, the right leg lead, is necessary to establish a reference ground for the augmented leads (aVR, aVL, aVF). Many microprocessor-based intraoperative monitors require application of the right leg (green) lead to reduce interference and to permit dysrhythmia processing.

Color Coding

Color coding the standard leads permits quick identification of the proper electrode pairs. In the United States, the white lead is applied to the right arm, the black lead is placed on the left arm, the green lead is applied to the right leg, and the red lead is applied to the left leg. The brown chest lead is used to monitor unipolar V leads. An easy mnemonic to remember is to consider the patient as the driver of a car. The left leg operates the brake (red), the right leg the gas pedal (green), the left arm hangs out the window and gets suntanned (black), while the right arm is pale (white). The remaining chest lead is brown.

Limb Leads

The standard limb leads record potential differences in accordance with Einthoven's triangle, in which lead I detects the potential difference from the right arm to the left arm; lead II detects the potential difference from the right arm to the left leg; and lead III detects the potential difference from the left arm to the left leg.[7]

Augmented and Precordial Leads

The augmented leads (aVR, aVL, and aVF) use a "zero" potential indifferent electrode by connecting the three limb leads to 5000-ohm resistors. This indifferent central terminal serves as a common negative electrode. The positive, exploring electrode for the augmented leads can be switched from the right arm, left arm, or left leg, representing the positive electrodes for the aVR, aVL, and aVF leads, respectively.[8] The precordial leads (V_1–V_6) constitute the unipolar leads recorded during a standard 12-lead ECG.

Five-Cable Systems

A five-electrode cable enables display of a precordial lead by placement of one electrode on each extremity and the remaining electrode (brown lead) over the precordium. During anesthesia, this unipolar lead is usually positioned along the left anterior axillary line in the fifth intercostal space (V_5). Therefore, a five-lead cable permits intraoperative monitoring of 7 of the 12 standard leads (I through aVF) as well as a precordial lead of choice. When a precordial unipolar lead is monitored, all of the limb leads serve as the indifferent central terminal (negative).

Three-Cable Systems

Table 21–2 depicts commonly used lead placements for intraoperative monitoring with a three-cable ECG system. If the shoulders, precordium, and left leg are available, electrodes placed in MV_5 array (white, right arm; black, V_5; red, left leg) permit monitoring of a modified V_5 lead when the selector switch is turned to "lead I" and of the standard lead II when the selector is turned to "lead II." Modified V_5 and lead II monitoring affords excellent capability to detect inferior and anterior myocardial ischemia and to track P waves.

What Characteristics Are of Interest to Anesthesiologists?

Monitored waveforms are dependent on the following six "electrical linkages": heart → skin → electrode → lead → cable → ECG amplifier → display.

TABLE 21–2. Electrocardiogram Electrode Placement Options for Three-Lead Cables

Limb Leads	White	Black	Red	Switch	Benefit
Lead I	Right arm (−)	Left arm (+)	Ground	Lead I	Lateral ischemia
Lead II	Right arm (−)	Ground	Left leg (+)	Lead II	Dysrhythmias, inferior ischemia
Lead III	Ground	Left arm (−)	Left leg (+)	Lead III	Inferior ischemia
		Modified Bipolar Leads—Infinite Varieties			
MV_5	Right arm (−)	V_5 (+)	Ground	Lead I	Anterior ischemia
CS_5	Subclavicular (−)	V_5 (+)	Ground	Lead I	As above
CB_5	Scapula (−)	V_5 (+)	Ground	Lead I	Like true V_5
MCL1	Ground	Subclavicular (−)	V_1 (+)	Lead III	Dysrhythmias

Abbreviations: M = modified; C or CL = central; S = subclavicular; B = back; V_n = precordial positions; (+) = positive electrode; (−) = negative electrode.

Atrial Depolarization

Normal cardiac electrophysiology results in a progression of events commencing with the spontaneous depolarization of the sinoatrial (SA) node, followed by right and left atrial depolarization. Atrial depolarization is evident by the development of the P wave (Fig. 21–1). The size and shape of the P wave depend on the vector relationship between atrial depolarization and the displayed monitoring lead. In sinus rhythm, the P wave is normally upright in I and II and inverted in aVR. After the depolarization of both atria, a delay in the conduction of the depolarization potential (PR interval) is associated with ejection of blood into the ventricles.

Ventricular Depolarization

After conduction through the atrioventricular (AV) node, the electrical impulse is transmitted through the bundle of His to the left and right bundle branches, Purkinje's fibers, and both ventricles. Like its atrial counterpart, the size and protection of the depolarization vector of the ventricles vary, depending on the spatial relationships of the monitoring lead and the propagation of ventricular depolarization. The ventricular depolarization ECG wave is termed the *QRS complex* (see Fig. 21–1). Numerous variations can be observed. By definition, the first positive deflection is called an *R wave*. Secondary positive deflections are labeled *R'*.

Repolarization

Unlike depolarization, which is propagated throughout the heart from cell to cell, repolarization is an energy-dependent process that occurs at a specific rate in each myocardial cell. Although the summation of repolarization is manifested on the ECG by the T wave (see Fig. 21–1), its orientation is complex and also includes the preceding ST segment interval and occasionally a following U wave. With a limb lead, V_5 or MV_5 monitoring, the ST segment is usually isoelectric, and the T wave vector is usually positive.

Signal Fidelity

Figure 21–2 and Table 21–3 summarize common features that reduce the fidelity of the ECG monitor display and depict important aspects of ECG trouble-shooting. Any decrease in fidelity or addition of artifact interferes with the user's ability

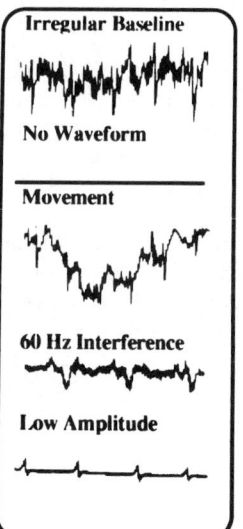

Monitor Waveforms	Summary of Causes
Irregular Baseline	**Patient Factors:**
No Waveform	• **Electrodes over muscles**
Movement	• **Electrodes Loose**
	• **Skin Hairy**
	• **Skin resistence high**
	• **Excessive Shivering**
60 Hz Interference	**Equipment Factors:**
	• **"Dried-out" Electrodes**
Low Amplitude	• **Corroded Connectors**
	• **Ungrounded Equipment**
	• **Leadwire Strain**
	• **Broken Connection**

Corrective Action

Skin Preparation
Reapply Electrodes
New Cables
Remove Faulty Equipment

FIGURE 21–2. Factors that reduce ECG waveform fidelity.

to identify abnormalities or respond with appropriate intervention.

What Information Is Derived?

In healthy patients, the ECG helps to assess heart rate, rhythm disturbances, and electrolyte abnormalities. In critically ill patients or patients with cardiovascular disease, it provides data to assess ischemia, acute myocardial infarction, conduction disturbances, dysrhythmias, acute pulmonary hypertension, or pulmonary emboli and other diseases with profound influences on myocardial function (Table 21–4).

A strip-chart ECG recording is valuable to evaluate the size, shape, and character of the ECG waves and to determine ST and T wave changes. Comparisons between the preoperative ECG tracing, preferably a strip-chart recording from the operating room monitor before induction, and intraoperative recording are valuable in determining alterations and the need for therapy.

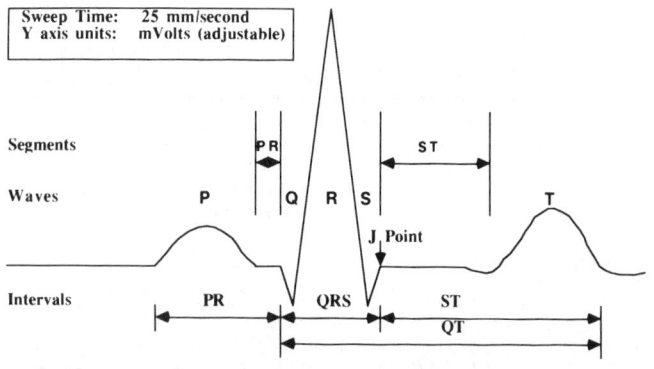

FIGURE 21–1. The ECG waves and intervals. (From Thys DM: The normal ECG. *In* The ECG in Anesthesia and Critical Care. Thys DM, Kaplan JA (eds). New York, Churchill Livingstone, 1987, p 14.)

TABLE 21–3. Trouble-shooting Reduction in Fidelity of the Electrocardiogram Monitor Display

Summary of causes	*Patient factors:*
	Electrodes over muscles
	Loose electrodes
	Hairy skin
	High skin resistance
	Excessive shivering
	Equipment factors:
	"Dried-out" electrodes
	Corroded connectors
	Ungrounded equipment
	Lead wire strain
	Broken connection
	Interference from adjacent electrical cables
Corrective action	Prepare skin
	Reapply electrodes
	Replace cables
	Remove faulty equipment
	Reposition cables

TABLE 21–4. Alterations of Electrocardiographic Waves and Intervals

Alteration in PR Interval	Abnormality	Associated Condition(s)
Shortened PR interval		Pre-excitation due to Wolff-Parkinson-White syndrome or junctional rhythm
Prolonged PR interval	1st-degree block	Normal athletes; digitalis; heart disease, vagotonia
	2nd-degree block (Mobitz I)	Digitalis; heart disease; inferior myocardial infarction; mitral valve disease; aortic valve disease; atrial septal defect; vagotonia
	2nd-degree block (Mobitz II)	Anterior MI; valvular heart disease
Advanced	3rd degree	Inferior MI
P wave morphology	Peaked	Cor pulmonale
	Notched	Mitral valvular disease
	Absent	Junctional block; atrial fibrillation
Q waves		MI; idiopathic hypertrophic subaortic stenosis
QRS complex	Prolonged blocks	
	Left bundle branch	MI; IHD
	Right bundle branch	MI; IHD
QT interval	Prolonged	IHD; hypocalcemia; hypomagnesemia; MI
	Shortened	Hypercalcemia
ST segment	Depression	IHD; MI; ventricular hypertrophy; digitalis; intraventricular conduction defects
	Elevation	Myocardial injury; IHD; Prinzmetal's angina; acute pericarditis; ventricular aneurysms; left bundle branch block; left ventricular hypertrophy
T wave	Tall peaked	Hyperkalemia; IHD
	Inverted	MI; IHD; ventricular hypertrophy; subendocardial infarction; pericarditis; subarachnoid hemorrhage; nonspecific
U wave	Increased	Hypokalemia; hypercalcemia; thyrotoxicosis
	Inverted	Left ventricular strain; IHD; intracranial hemorrhage

Abbreviations: MI = myocardial infarction; IHD = ischemic heart disease.

How Does an Electrocardiogram Help to Identify Ischemia?

During periods of coronary insufficiency, repolarization of ischemic myocardial cells is delayed and electrical events in the region of ischemia are manifested as changes in the ST segment and the T wave. Although the ECG changes during ischemia, injury, and infarction are specific when recorded from epicardial electrodes, detection from surface electrodes may be confusing because of technical aspects of electrode placement and the frequency response of the recording system used. Instrumentation and practice standards for ECG monitoring in special care units have been formulated.[9]

Classic Changes

The following discussion summarizes the classic changes associated with ischemia using an *epicardial* electrode. (For a more complete explanation, refer to Schamroth L: *The ECG of Coronary Artery Disease.* Oxford, Blackwell, 1984.)

During periods of subendocardial ischemia, an unopposed increase in the repolarization vector results in tall, upright T waves. If the ischemia becomes transmural, the direction of repolarization travels from the epicardium to the endocardium, producing an inverted T wave. Figure 21–3 demonstrates ST and T wave changes recorded from the region of ischemia. Ischemic changes are best observed in leads parallel to the T wave vector.

ST and T wave changes also result from conduction defects, left ventricular hypertrophy, electrolyte disorders, and drug effects. Data from exercise stress testing suggest that simultaneous monitoring of leads II and V5 detect approximately 96% of all ECG-detectable ischemic events.[10] However, London and colleagues, using continuous intraoperative 12-lead ECG,

found that monitoring leads II and V5 had a sensitivity of only 80%; monitoring of leads II, V4, and V5 was necessary to detect 96% of intraoperative ischemic events.[11]

Monitoring Criteria

Criteria for the detection of intraoperative ischemia require ST segment displacement of at least 1 mm 60 milliseconds after the J point (see Fig. 21–1). A more inclusive set of criteria to determine the incidence of intraoperative myocardial ischemia with continuous 12-lead ECG includes[11]:

1. New ST depression ≥1 mm (0.1 mV) in a horizontal or downsloping ST segment measured 60 milliseconds after the J point

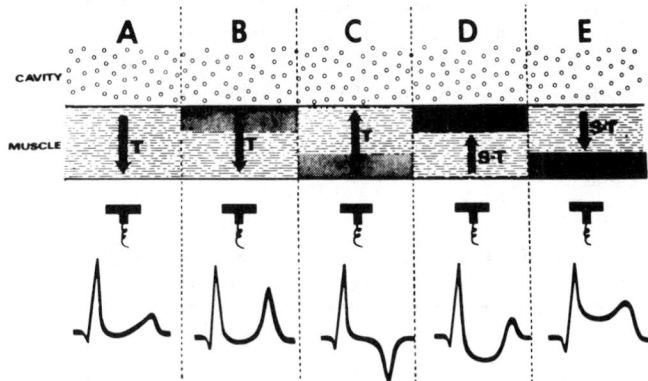

FIGURE 21–3. The T wave vector during ischemia and injury recorded from the area of ischemia. A = normal; B = subendocardial ischemia; C = subepicardial ischemia; D = subendocardial infarction; E = subepicardial infarcton. (From Schamroth L: The ECG of Coronary Artery Disease. Oxford, Blackwell, 1984.)

2. ST segment depression ≥1.5 mm in a slowly upsloping ST segment

3. ST segment elevation ≥1.5 mm from baseline in a non-Q wave lead

4. ST segment elevation ≥1.0 mm if associated with a simultaneous ST elevation of ≥1.5 mm of another ECG lead

ST segment changes occurring with dysrhythmias do not always indicate ischemia. Displacement that meets inclusion criteria must be interpreted cautiously when it is observed in populations that are not at risk for myocardial ischemia or when it is detected by ECG monitoring systems in which the characteristics of electronic filtering are unknown.[12]

New-Onset ST Segment Displacement

Studies of patients undergoing coronary artery bypass grafting or major vascular surgery have demonstrated a high incidence of new-onset ST segment displacement.[6, 13, 14] When it occurs in high-risk patients, it should be regarded as an important indicator for development of intraoperative myocardial ischemia, even if the changes are not accompanied by hypertension and tachycardia.

Silent Ischemia

Silent ischemia occurs in patients with asymptomatic coronary artery disease as well as in those recovering from myocardial infarction.[15] Most of these events are unrelated to major alterations in heart rate or blood pressure. Although ECG monitoring is not as sensitive as wall motion abnormalities in assessing intraoperative ischemia, its ubiquity makes it the most accessible intraoperative ischemia monitor.

Clinical Applications: Computer Analysis

Little information is available regarding the diagnostic precision of clinicians in assessing intraoperative ECG ST segment changes. London and colleagues suggest that a clinical display and three- or five-lead cables may elicit a sensitivity of 75%.[11] Intraoperative ST segment evaluation lends itself to computer analysis, and several reports suggest that this technology enhances both sensitivity and specificity.[16, 17]

Intraoperative ST segment changes suggesting myocardial ischemia require clinical correlation. Because perioperative myocardial ischemia in patients with coronary artery disease may lead to postoperative myocardial infarction, the need for improved intraoperative ST surveillance remains an area of increasing interest. ST segment analysis programs are often incorporated into intraoperative ECG monitors. Although the exact algorithms are proprietary, several factors must be addressed when this technology is used in an acute care setting (Table 21–5).

TABLE 21–5. Factors Necessary for Computerized ST Segment Detection

Dysrhythmia detection algorithm	Detects ectopic or bundle branch blocks
Timing algorithm	Identifies onset and offset of QRS complex and J point
Artifact rejection algorithm	Detects artifacts, movement, and electrical interference
Signal processing	Proper filtering and amplification

The ST segment is measured as the vertical difference between the T-P isoelectric point (reference) and the ST point (60 milliseconds after the J point). ST segment measurements are stored in memory with graphic programs for display on the monitor screen. Alarm limits can be set to warn when ischemia develops. Representative samples of the average digitized signals are available for evaluation. An artificial pacemaker or abnormal conduction pathways circumvent many P-QRS-T algorithms.

What Are the Characteristics of Myocardial Injury and Infarction?

Injury

Early ischemia results in a current of injury, which theoretically accounts for ST and T wave changes. If conditions causing subendocardial injury currents are reversed, the ST segment changes resolve. If the area of ischemia increases to include the epicardium, an endocardial-to-epicardial injury current is established. The result is ST-T wave elevation in leads "facing" the current vector and ST-T wave depression in opposite leads.[18] Figure 21–4 illustrates ST-T wave changes involving the anterior, inferior, and posterior walls monitored from an epicardial electrode. If conditions responsible for injury currents are not reversed, myocardial infarction results.

Infarction

Myocardium that has undergone *transmural* necrosis is no longer electrically active (depolarization does not occur), and Q waves are recorded from leads facing the infarct. Abnormal Q waves (Q wave > 0.04 s) are the classic finding following transmural necrosis. Unfortunately, localization of infarction by ECG patterns of necrosis is imprecise, particularly when conduction disturbances exist. Furthermore, the pathologic correlation between transmural infarction and the presence of Q waves is incomplete. Table 21–6 lists ECG findings that are expected after myocardial infractions associated with Q waves. Non-Q wave infarction also is a well-recognized clinical entity.

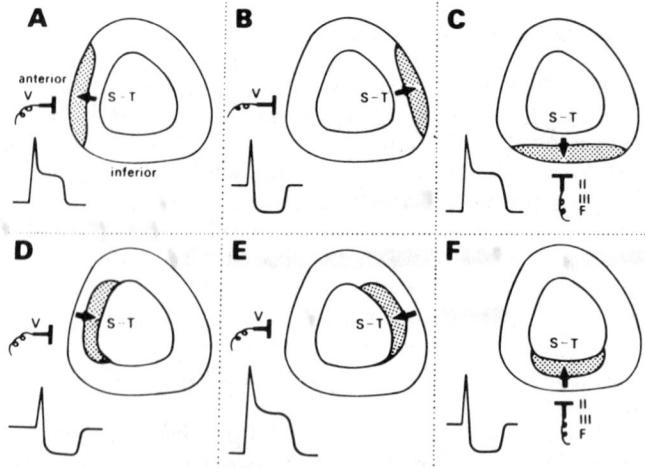

FIGURE 21–4. Injury patterns. *A–C,* The theoretic ECG during epicardial injury of the anterior, posterior, and inferior walls. *D–F,* Subendocardial injury of corresponding areas of myocardium. (From Schamroth L: The ECG of Coronary Artery Disease. Oxford, Blackwell Scientific, 1984.)

TABLE 21–6. Electrocardiogram Findings Associated with Q Wave Myocardial Infarction

Left ventricular infarctions	
Anteroseptal	Abnormal Q: V_1, V_2, V_3
Anterior	Abnormal Q: V_2, V_3, V_4
Anterolateral	Abnormal Q: V_1 or V_2; V_3, V_4
Inferior	Abnormal Q: II, III, aVF
Posterolateral	Abnormal Q: I, V_6
Posterior	Abnormal tall and wide R wave: V_1 and V_2
Right ventricular infarctions	Abnormal Q: II, III, aVF, inferior posterior leads with ST segment elevation right precordium (V_{3R-6R})

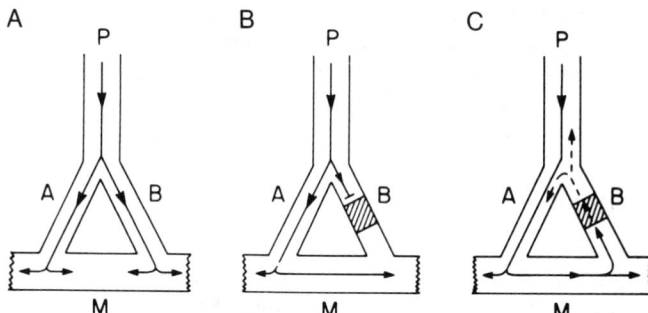

FIGURE 21–5. Re-entry. *A,* Normal conduction. *B,* Area of impaired conduction in B. *C,* Impulse from A activates B following the recovery of the area of impaired conduction. M = myocardium. (From Chou Te-C: Electrocardiography in Clinical Practice. Philadelphia, WB Saunders, 1991.)

How Do Dysrhythmias Originate?

For simplicity, dysrhythmias are described as resulting from abnormalities of impulse formation, impulse conduction, or combinations thereof. Electrophysiologic studies have identified four phases that describe the transmembranous potential changes in electrically active cells of the heart. If the resting potential of these cells is reduced or the Na^+ or Ca^{2+} ion currents are appreciably altered, abnormal automaticity or irritability results.

Spontaneous diastolic depolarization (phase 4 of the action potential) usually occurs in the SA node. In a normal heart, automaticity (spontaneous diastolic depolarization) is a characteristic of the heart's conducting system. Ectopic beats or abnormal rhythms can be expected if the SA node is suppressed, if the conduction pathways are altered, or if the automaticity of other cardiac cells of the conduction system is enhanced.

Genesis

The genesis and propagation of dysrhythmias are complex. Dominant pacemaker function may shift from the SA node to an ectopic site (subsidiary pacemakers). Local cellular changes occurring in the atria, AV node, or ventricles may induce spontaneous diastolic depolarization, which, if conducted, is displayed on the ECG as an ectopic beat. The refractory period for cardiac fibers is long. Therefore, a normal or ectopic impulse must remain active somewhere in the heart in order to re-excite a portion of heart.

Re-entry

Re-entry, precipitated by slow conduction and unidirectional conduction block, explains the genesis of some dysrhythmias. Figure 21–5 depicts the genesis of a ventricular dysrhythmia by re-entry, resulting from slow conduction and a unidirectional conduction block in Purkinje's fibers. This mechanism has been implicated in the genesis of lethal dysrhythmias accompanying myocardial infarction.[19]

Automaticity

All currently administered potent inhalational agents affect automaticity.[20] The effects are complex, involving the entire conduction cascade, and may influence impulse formation and impulse conduction. Drug effects, sympathetic stimulation, electrolyte imbalance, and metabolic factors have an important role in the genesis of intraoperative dysrhythmias. "Cardiac" and antidysrhythmic drugs potentially alter the membrane permeability of ions responsible for normal conduction. Confounding variables such as digitalis, hyperkalemia, and preexisting first-degree heart block often make it difficult to define the etiologic events that lead to intraoperative dysrhythmias. Table 21–7 lists many of the dysrhythmias that may occur during anesthesia care.

What Are the Characteristics of Atrial Dysrhythmias?

Although the mechanism for the genesis of intraoperative dysrhythmias is always important (e.g., pulling the viscera during subarachnoid block, causing sinus bradycardia), the *hemodynamic consequences* require prompt recognition and treatment. This section highlights the ECG diagnosis and intraoperative significance of dysrhythmias starting from the SA node.

Sinus Dysrhythmia

Intraoperative sinus dysrhythmia is common in healthy patients. It most often is related to inspiration and probably arises

TABLE 21–7. Intraoperative Dysrhythmias

Mechanism	Location	Electrocardiogram Finding
Enhanced automaticity	SA node	Sinus tachycardia
Sympathetic stimulation	Atria,* AV node	Supraventricular tachycardia
Drugs, electrolyte disturbances	Atria*	PAC
Metabolic diseases, hyperthermia	Ventricle*	PVC
Reduced automaticity	SA node	Bradycardia, PAC
Parasympathetic stimulation	Atria*	Junctional rhythm
Drugs, electrolyte disturbances	His, AV node	
Re-entry	Atria*	Atrial flutter, fibrillation
Diseases	Purkinje's fibers	Ventricular tachycardia
Electrolyte disturbances	Ventricle*	Ventricular tachycardia, ventricular fibrillation

*Indicates cardiac tissues that normally do not demonstrate spontaneous diastolic depolarization.

Abbreviations: SA = sinoatrial; AV = atrioventricular; PAC = premature atrial contraction; PVC = premature ventricular contraction.

from reflex changes in vagal tone. Parasympathomimetic drugs may also be responsible. The ECG diagnosis is evident when the P wave morphology remains constant but the PP interval varies, usually at slow sinus rates. Sinus dysrhythmia occurs frequently in children.

Sinus Bradycardia

In adults, sinus bradycardia is defined as a heart rate <60 beats per minute (bpm). The intraoperative ECG has a normal P wave and normal PR interval. Sinus bradycardia may be prevalent in healthy athletic adults and in patients taking β-blockers or calcium channel blockers. Hypothyroidism or hypothermia can depress SA function. Sinus bradycardia is commonly associated with acute myocardial infarction.[21] It may occur intraoperatively as a vagal response to traction of the mesentery, as a result of the stretching of extraocular muscles in children, or after the second intravenous administration of succinylcholine. New-onset bradycardia associated with hypotension, ventricular dysrhythmia, or signs of diminished perfusion requires prompt evaluation and treatment. Myocardial ischemia must be ruled out.

Sinus Tachycardia

In adults, a sinus heart rate >100 bpm defines sinus tachycardia. The ECG monitor displays normal P waves, but the PR interval may shorten. ST segment depression is occasionally associated with fast rates, and the QT interval is shortened. Differentiation of pure sinus tachycardia from other supraventricular tachycardias is often difficult when the heart rate is >150 bpm. Finding P waves cements the diagnosis and may require changing monitor leads (e.g., from V_5 to II). Sinus tachycardia can occur under various clinical situations. The underlying disorder (e.g., hypovolemia, hypoxemia, hyperthermia, sympathetic response, pain, drug effects) warrants treatment depending on the etiology. Patients with ischemic heart disease are at risk for ischemia.

Sick Sinus Syndrome

The ECG characteristics of sick sinus syndrome are bradycardia, sinus arrest, bradycardia-tachycardia, and absence of rhythm. Many causes are known.[22] Patients with sick sinus syndrome have a diminished response to intravenous atropine.[23] The condition most often is observed in patients with ischemic cardiomyopathies or hypertensive heart disease. Intraoperative treatment may require β-agonists or pacing.

Paroxysmal Atrial Tachycardia

Paroxysmal atrial tachycardia (PAT) is an uncommon intraoperative dysrhythmia that is often initiated and sustained by re-entrant or ectopic atrial foci. In healthy patients, PAT is usually short-lived and has no significant hemodynamic effects. Atrial rates of 100 to 250 bpm are followed by normal-appearing QRS complexes. Secondary ST segment and T wave changes may suggest ischemia. P waves may be difficult to identify. Digitalis toxicity is a common cause of PAT with associated heart block. Sustained PAT (unlike paroxysmal supraventricular tachycardia) usually indicates organic heart disease. Under anesthesia, PAT may predispose to severe hemodynamic deterioration.[24]

Atrial Flutter

Atrial flutter results from circus movement. Saw-tooth flutter (F) waves of constant timing and morphology distinguish atrial flutter (240–350 bpm) from atrial fibrillation (AF), which has fibrillatory (f) waves of irregular timing and morphology at rates >350 bpm. ST segment tracking during atrial flutter is difficult. Most patients with atrial flutter have organic heart disease. Other causes include pulmonary disease, hyperthyroidism, and pericarditis.

Atrial Fibrillation

As with atrial flutter, AF results from an induced circus movement. However, the chaotic depolarizations in the atria are conducted through the AV junction at random intervals. In AF, P waves are absent and the atrial rate is very rapid (350–700 bpm). The RR intervals are usually irregular. Fibrillatory waves often are identifiable in right precordial leads. The most common causes include coronary artery disease, valvular heart disease, hypertensive heart disease, congestive heart failure (CHF), chronic obstructive lung disease, and pulmonary embolism.

What Are the Characteristics of Atrioventricular Dysrhythmias?

The atrioventricular junction (AVJ) retards conduction from the atria to the ventricles. AVJ cells are capable of spontaneous phase 4 depolarization. Under anesthesia, the AVJ may become the dominant pacemaker if SA node automaticity is slowed or fails. The ECG monitor usually displays a rate of 40 to 60 bpm and a normal-appearing Q wave. P waves may precede, coincide with, or follow the QRS complex, depending on the location of the junctional pacemaker and the relative velocity of conduction to the atria and ventricles. Intraoperative junctional rhythms are commonly associated with decreases in blood pressure.[25]

If the SA node or the atria lose their automaticity, the AVJ normally assumes pacemaker function. Re-entrant and automatic junctional mechanisms have been described to occur at the AVJ. Premature junctional beats or junctional tachycardias may occur under anesthesia. The effect of potent inhalational agents on AV nodal function remains obscure. Enhancement of impulse formation occasionally occurs in the AV node, producing accelerated AV junctional rhythms.

What Are the Characteristics of Atrioventricular Block?

AV dissociation is defined by independent atrial and ventricular rates. It is always a secondary phenomenon that develops from other disturbances in cardiac rhythm (e.g., heart block, default of the primary pacemaker with escape of a subsidiary pacemaker, or usurpation by a faster pacemaker).[26]

Complete

Serious reductions in cardiac output often result when AV conduction is blocked. If a complete disruption occurs, the atria beat at the rate set by the SA node and the ventricular rate is determined by a slower "pacemaker" situated in the AV node, bundle of His, or within the ventricular muscle. During complete disruption (third-degree AV block), the ECG displays P and QRS-T waves that may have normal morphology but are asynchronous. New-onset third-degree block often requires drug therapy or pacing.

Incomplete

Incomplete disruptions of AV conduction may also be of clinical importance. Disruption can occur after acute myocardial infarction. Gradually increasing PR intervals followed by nonconducted P waves (Wenckebach's phenomenon) is the ECG hallmark of a Mobitz type I block. Mobitz I block usually results from an abnormality of the AV node, and Mobitz II blocks usually occur in the bundle of His or the bundle branches. First-degree AV block (PR interval > 0.20 s) is common and usually does not influence anesthesia care.

What Are the Characteristics of Ventricular Dysrhythmias?

Premature Ventricular Contractions

Premature ventricular contractions (PVCs) alter the sequence of coordinated ventricular contraction. The QRS complex is abnormal and prolonged; ST-T wave changes are expected because ventricular repolarization is also abnormal. P waves are not associated with PVCs, but retrograde depolarization or blocked sinus beats may add confusing appearances to the complexes. (Premature atrial contractions [PACs] with aberrant ventricular conduction may mimic the wide and bizarre QRS complexes that result from ventricular ectopy. They may or may not reset the sinus rhythm and are not hemodynamically significant.)

PVCs commonly are observed in patients with pre-existing cardiac disease. They also may be observed in healthy patients during periods associated with sympathetic stimulation. New-onset PVCs may be ominous signs of impending life-threatening dysrhythmias, myocardial infarction, ongoing myocardial ischemia, digitalis toxicity with hypokalemia, or hypoxemia due to any cause. Therefore, the occurrence of PVCs during anesthesia requires prompt identification of any clinical aberrations that may be corrected.

Intraoperative PVCs are significant when they are frequent ($>6 \cdot min^{-1}$), multifocal, occur early in the normal cardiac cycle (R on T), or occur in patients with recent myocardial infarction. Continuation of PVCs may lead to the development of ventricular tachycardia (VT) and ventricular fibrillation (VF).

Ventricular Tachycardia

Intraoperative VT is not commonly observed other than in cardiac surgery. It occurs when three or more PVCs take place in a row.[27] The conduction pattern is aberrant, and AV dissociation frequently is present. The rhythm is usually regular, with a heart rate of 100 to 250 bpm. Recognition of VT is important, because its acute onset is hemodynamically significant, may be life threatening, and requires immediate treatment.

Ventricular Fibrillation

VF is characterized by rapid, disorganized depolarization of the ventricles. The ECG displays irregular complexes. Discrete QRS-T waves are not present. During VF, cardiovascular collapse can be expected, because the rhythm does not permit ventricular ejection. The causes of intraoperative VF include ongoing hypoxia, severe myocardial ischemia, electric shock, hyperkalemia, hypothermia, and malignant hyperpyrexia.

What Electrocardiographic Changes Occur with Electrolyte Disturbances?

An ECG may be useful in identifying intraoperative electrolyte disturbances, especially significant changes in potassium and calcium. Unfortunately, the observed changes may also be caused by drugs, intrinsic cardiac disease, and even extracardiac pathologic states. Once the diagnosis of a specific electrolyte abnormality is documented, monitoring the ECG provides a convenient, noninvasive guide to therapy (Table 21–8).

ARTERIAL BLOOD PRESSURE

Measurement of arterial blood pressure has been an essential element of anesthesia care since 1855. The relationship between left ventricular ejection and blood pressure is complex. Estimates of the arterial blood pressure to a great degree depend on the generation and propagation of the arterial pressure wave.

What Are the Characteristics of the Arterial Pressure Wave?

Immediately after ejection, a fluid wave begins in the central aorta and propagates throughout the arterial tree. As the peripheral vasculature divides, the contour, size, and character of the arterial pressure wave vary. Factors contributing to the propagation and character of the pressure pulse include the energy content imparted by ventricular systole (1–600 W), contour transformation by the vascular tree, and reflective waves produced at the periphery (Table 21–9).

Wave Reflection and Propagation

Wave reflection and propagation vary with physiologic and pathologic conditions. In most species, the systolic pressure component of the arterial pulse wave is artifactually augmented as the wave passes from the central aorta into the peripheral vessels. Similarly, the diastolic component is lowered. Peripheral augmentation can exceed central aortic pressure measurements by 20% to 30%. Figure 21–6 demonstrates the changes in size and shape of the pressure wave observed at various sites.[28] The pulse contour can be influenced by occlusive vascular disease, dynamically changing peripheral vascular resistance, and physical constraints of the measuring system.

TABLE 21–8. Electrocardiographic Changes Associated with Electrolyte Abnormalities

Hyperkalemia	T wave changes: tall, peaked, narrow ST segment elevation; QRS prolongation	AV conduction defects; tachydysrhythmias (VT, VF); ventricular arrest

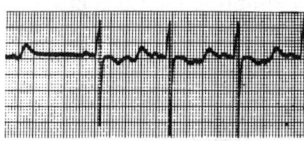

$K^+ = 7.4$ mEq $\cdot$ L^{-1}

Hypokalemia	T wave changes: small prominent U wave; ST segment depression; minimal DQRS prolongation; QT-U prolongation	PAT 1st- and 2nd-degree heart block; VT; VF; torsades de pointes

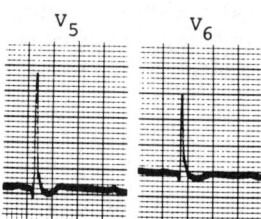

$K^+ = 1.6$ mEq $\cdot$ dL^{-1}

Hypercalcemia	Decrease in QTc interval; prolongation of PR interval	Rare: 1st- and 2nd-degree heart block

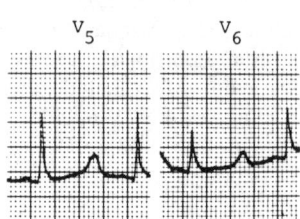

$Ca^{2+} = 17.4$ mg $\cdot$ dL^{-1}

Hypocalcemia	Prolongation of QTc interval; increased duration of ST segment	Uncommon

$Ca^{2+} = 5.6$ mg $\cdot$ L^{-1}

Hypermagnesemia	Increase in PR interval; prolonged QRS	SA block; AV block
Hypomagnesemia	Peaked T waves; normal QTc	Variable effects; torsades de pointes

(Electrocardiograms from Chou TC: Electrocardiography in Clinical Practice. Philadelphia, WB Saunders, 1991.)
Abbreviations: AV = atrioventricular; VT ventricular tachycardia; VF = ventricular fibrillation; PAT = paroxysmal atrial tachycardia; SA = sinoatrial.

TABLE 21–9. Factors Influencing the Characteristics of the Arterial Pulse Wave

Dynamics of pulsatile flow
Acceleration and deceleration of blood
Elasticity of the large conducting arteries
Modulated impedance controlling regional blood flow (systemic vascular resistance)

How Is Blood Pressure Measured Noninvasively?

Manual (Nonautomated) Techniques

Anesthesiologists have used palpatory or auscultatory techniques to measure blood pressure. These traditional methods require placement of an appropriately sized blood pressure cuff around an extremity. Inflation of the cuff above systolic pressure flattens the underlying regional artery. With gradual deflation, the pressure at which arterial flow resumes can be determined if the encircling cuff is attached to a calibrated manometer.

Resumption of Arterial Blood Flow

The end point for arterial flow can be determined using several methods. Palpation of distal pulses during slow deflation of a blood pressure cuff provides a reasonable estimate of systolic blood pressure. Palpatory techniques are a valuable back-up when primary monitoring techniques fail or estimates of blood pressure require verification. Sophisticated modifications are possible when photoplethysmographic finger probes (oximetry probes), indwelling arterial catheters, or Doppler ultrasound transducers are used to determine the point at which distal arterial flow resumes.

Auscultation of Korotkoff's Sounds

Auscultation of Korotkoff's sounds permits estimation of systolic and diastolic blood pressure. Mean arterial pressure (MAP) can be calculated using an estimating equation:

$$MAP = \text{diastolic pressure} + 1/3 \ (\text{systolic} - \text{diastolic}) \ \text{pressure}$$

Korotkoff's sounds result from turbulent flow within an artery in response to the mechanical deformation from the blood pressure cuff (Fig. 21–7). Systolic blood pressure is signaled by the appearance of the first Korotkoff's sound. Disappearance of the sounds or a muffled tone signals the diastolic blood pressure. The detection of sound changes is subjective and prone to errors based on deficiencies in sound transmission or poor hearing. Cuff deflation rate also influences accuracy. Quick deflations ($>3 \ mm \ Hg \cdot s^{-1}$) underestimate blood flow and are unreliable during conditions of low flow.[29]

Nonautomated blood pressure measurements are reasonably accurate when aneroid gauges are within calibration, the encircling cuff is appropriately positioned, the inflation is greater than the true systolic pressure, and Korotkoff's sounds or pulse is properly identified. Nevertheless, palpatory and auscultatory techniques have for the most part been replaced by automated devices that free the anesthesiologist from the hands-on tasks needed to determine repeated blood pressure measurements.

The accuracy of a blood pressure estimate is, to a great extent, dependent on the proper use of the encircling blood pressure cuff. Simpson and colleagues demonstrated that too small a cuff or one applied too loosely results in blood pressure estimates that are high.[30] A larger than necessary cuff does not affect accuracy as long as the pressure of the cuff is transmitted to the underlying artery and compresses it. Geddes suggests that the optimal width of a blood pressure cuff is 40% of the circumference of the arm.[31]

Doppler Sphygmomanometry

Doppler sphygmomanometry detects the Doppler shift ultrasound signal after the restoration of blood flow on deflation of a blood pressure cuff. Studies have shown excellent correlation

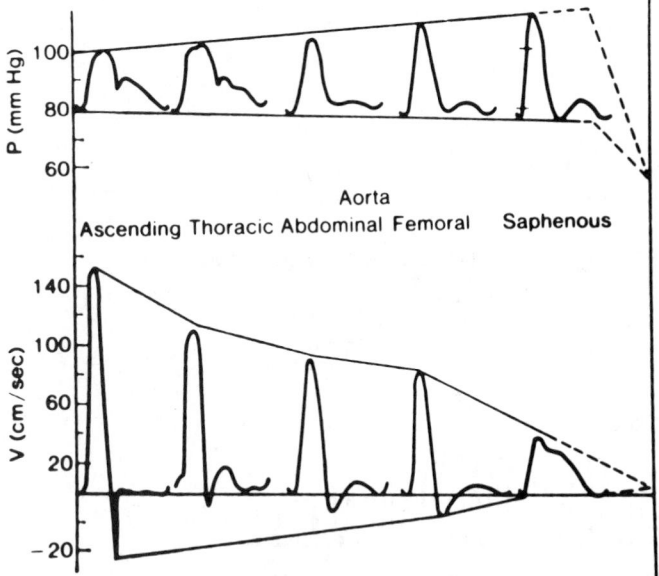

FIGURE 21–6. Pressure-velocity measurements from the aorta and its branches in the dog. Amplification of the pressure wave by reflected waves is demonstrated. (Modified from Milnor WR: Hemodynamics. Baltimore, Williams & Wilkins, 1989.)

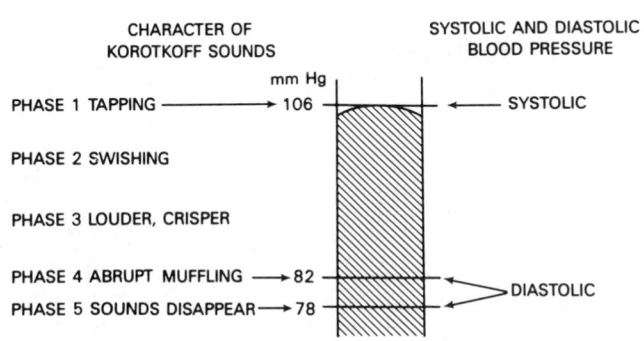

FIGURE 21–7. Graphic representation of the relationship of the Korotkoff sounds to blood pressure measurement. (From Whelton PK, Russell RP: The Principles and Practice of Medicine. 21st ed. Harvey AM, Johns RJ, Mckusik VA, et al (eds). Norwalk, CT, Appleton-Century-Crofts, 1984, p 279.)

with direct arterial measurements.[32, 33] Compact battery-powered Doppler devices are helpful in clinical situations in which detection of the systolic arterial blood pressure is difficult owing to low flow. The Doppler shift signal is best identified over the compressed arterial wall using a coupling gel to enhance the transmittance of the sound waves. Automated Doppler-based devices have been used to estimate blood pressure during induced hypotension.[33]

Automated Devices

Since 1976, microprocessor-controlled oscillotonometers (MCOs) largely have replaced auscultatory and palpatory techniques for routine intraoperative blood pressure monitoring. Advantages of these devices are listed in Table 21–10. Oscillometry measures mean blood pressure by sensing the point of maximal fluctuations produced while a blood pressure cuff is deflated.

Methodology

Modern MCOs (e.g., Dinamap, Critikon, Inc., Tampa, FL) measure systolic, diastolic, and mean pressures by sampling oscillations in the cuff and determining parameter identification points (PIPs) for each respective measurement.[34] Substantial differences exist among the many MCOs.

A "generic" MCO senses cuff pressure with a transducer, and the output is digitized for processing. After the cuff is inflated by an air pump, pressure is held constant while oscillations are sampled. If no oscillations are detected, the cuff pressure is greater than arterial blood pressure; the computer then opens a deflation valve for sampling at the next lower level. MCOs assign the systolic pressure to the point of appearance of pressure oscillations in the cuff; MAP is the pressure at which maximal oscillations occur; and diastolic pressure is the point of maximal oscillatory decline.

Artifact-rejection algorithms are implemented by the stepwise deflation-PIPs cycle. Important to recognize is the fact that MCOs compare the amplitude of oscillation pairs and numerically display their estimates. This technique requires that a patient be relatively still. A dysrhythmia such as AF, in which the amplitude of successive pulses varies widely, renders accurate measurements problematic. Figure 21–8 graphically depicts the responses of a Dinamap. During this inflation cycle, respiratory variation, a PVC, and cuff movement are demonstrated.

Accuracy

Automated oscillometry correlates well with direct intra-arterial measurement of mean and diastolic blood pressures.[35] Underestimation of systolic blood pressure may occur, with mean errors reported from −6.9 to −8.6 mm Hg compared with direct radial artery pressures.[36] The Association for the Advancement of Medical Instrumentation (AAMI) recommends that MCOs have a mean error of <5 mm Hg compared with a centrally placed arterial catheter.[34]

Oscillometry requires the careful evaluation of several cardiac cycles at each increment of deflation in order to smoothe out pronounced respiratory variations or motion artifacts. Cuff movement or erratic pulse transmission influences the accuracy of all MCOs. The time necessary to display the measured MAP and the estimates of systolic and diastolic pressures vary,

TABLE 21–10. Benefits of Microprocessor-Controlled Oscillotonometers

Hands-free operation
Programmable time cycle
Adaptable to all age groups
Measures mean, systolic, and diastolic pressures
Functions on all extremities
Programmable alarms
Digitized output for computerized records
Acceptable accuracy in wide range of patients

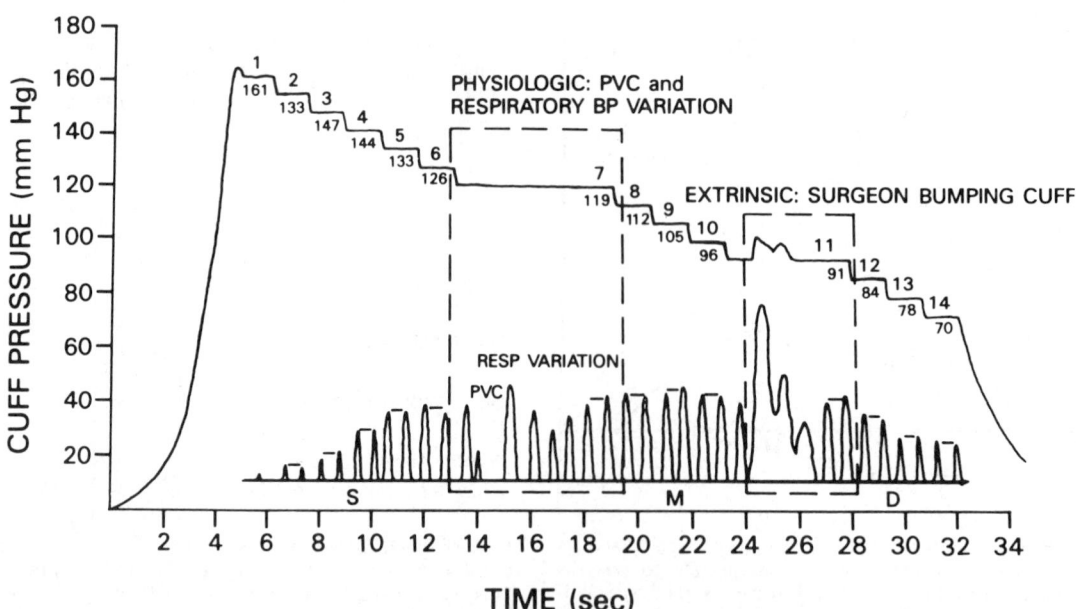

FIGURE 21–8. Diagram illustrates motion artifact, premature ventricular contraction, and respiratory artifact recorded using a Dinamap MCO. PVC = Pressure-volume curve; BP = blood pressure. (From Ramsey M: Blood pressure monitoring: automated oscillometric devices. J Clin Monit 1991; 7:56.)

depending on the proprietary software that integrates the inflation-deflation cycle and the analysis of the amplitude of oscillations. Many MCOs operate in a "STAT mode," in which the inflation-deflation cycle is shortened.

In anesthetized patients, automated oscillometry is usually accurate and versatile. Although upper arm cuff placement is most commonly used, other locations are acceptable, including the thigh, calf, ankle, or forearm (as long as the cuff size is appropriate to the site of measurement). Difficulties can be expected when shock or low pressure reduces the oscillations. Shivering produces motion artifacts that degrade MCO performance. In these circumstances, many MCOs display only estimates of mean pressure.

Benefits and Risks

MCOs have simplified the task of obtaining accurate blood pressure measurements. However, improper cuff deflation has the potential to promote venous congestion. Placement of an automated blood pressure cuff on the same extremity in which venous access has been established may influence the rate of fluid administration and the response to administered drugs. This problem is particularly annoying during a rapid-sequence induction. The potential for direct compression of superficial peripheral nerves is minimized by careful cuff application.[37]

Photoplethysmography

Peñaz described a method that holds the size of the digital arteries of a finger constant and alters the pressure within a finger cuff.[38] The device uses infrared light and detects oscillations within the finger cuff. A very fast servo mechanism and pump adjust the pressure in the finger cuff during each cardiac cycle, preventing the digital arteries from expanding (loading) during systole and shrinking (unloading) during diastole.

This technique permits the measurement and display of a beat-to-beat pressure pulse wave that *simulates* the arterial blood pressure tracing. Clinical trials in healthy patients undergoing routine surgical procedures suggest that it correlates with direct arterial blood pressure measurements. Arterial spasm following cardiopulmonary bypass or the administration of phenylephrine affected the reliability of early prototypes.[39] The device is also susceptible to hydrostatic errors resulting from changing the position of the transducer-servo mechanism.

Pulse Wave Velocity

Another unique approach for continuous noninvasive blood pressure monitoring involves measurement of the pulse wave velocity using photoplethysmography. A linear relationship between the pulse wave velocity and changes in mean arterial blood pressure has been described.[40] ARTRAC estimates arterial blood pressure by measuring the pulse wave velocity and changes in blood volume with two photometric sensors placed on the forehead and a digit. The technique requires calibration from a built-in MOC.

Because this technique uses the AC signal of two reflectance oximeter probes, the computer can also calculate oxygen (O_2) saturation. Clinical trials have demonstrated that ARTRAC detects beat-to-beat changes in arterial blood pressure and compares favorably with intra-arterial measurements.

Arterial Tonometry

Satisfactory estimates of the blood pressure waveform and measurement of systolic, mean, and diastolic pressures can be obtained using arterial tonometry (AT) (N-CAT, Nellcor, Hayward, CA). AT uses an array of 15 piezoelectric pressure transducers placed on the wrist over the radial artery. The transducer assembly contains an air chamber that places sufficient pressure on the skin to flatten the wall of the artery, at which time the intra-arterial blood pressure is transmitted through the subcutaneous tissues and is sensed at the skin.

The accuracy of AT requires tension exerted on the artery to be perpendicular to the sensor. Clinical tonometry incorporates a computer analysis of the multiple sensors in order to determine which transducer elements faithfully monitor the flattened arterial wall. Kemmotsu and associates have found close correlation between AT and intra-arterial blood pressure.[41]

How Is Blood Pressure Measured Invasively?

Direct invasive arterial blood pressure monitoring is often used. Indications are limited primarily to high-risk patients necessitating beat-to-beat blood pressure measurements, arterial blood gas analysis, or frequent blood sampling.

Components

All intravascular pressure measurements require placement of a catheter into a vessel and attachment to a rigid fluid-filled tubing. The tubing links the pressure wave to a transducer that converts pressure (force per unit area) into an electrical signal that is amplified and filtered electronically. This processed electrical signal is displayed as the monitored arterial pressure tracing.

Cardiovascular pressure waves have unique shapes that are often characterized as complex periodic sine waves. High-fidelity recordings and analysis of the arterial pressure tracing (Fourier's series of power spectrum analysis) indicate that the arterial pressure wave (input) contains frequencies from 1 to 30 Hz (1 Hz = 60 cycles per second). Most of the frequency components are <10 Hz.

The behavior of transducers, fluid couplings, signal amplification, and display can be described by a second-order differential equation in which the mass, elasticity, and resistance of the transducing system are related to input. Solution of the equation predicts the output (transduced arterial pressure trace) and characterizes the system's performance. Table 21–11 lists the properties of a fluid-coupled transducing system.

TABLE 21–11. Properties of Fluid-Coupled Transducing Systems

Feature	Definition
Frequency response	How faithfully input = output. Ideally, fluid-coupled transducing systems should have a flat frequency response up to 20 Hz.
Natural frequency—Fo (resonant frequency)	The frequency at which the system resonates. As the input frequencies approach Fo, amplification and distortion of output result.
Damping coefficient (ζ)	The expression describing the tendency for fluid to extinguish motion.

Fidelity

The fidelity of any fluid-coupled transducing system is constrained by two properties: damping (ζ) and natural frequency (Fo). Therefore, the fidelity of the transduced pressure depends on optimizing ζ and Fo, thus permitting to-and-fro movement of the coupling fluid and transducer to faithfully reproduce the range of frequencies contained in the arterial pressure wave (the system's bandwidth).

Natural Frequency

Fo describes the tendency for the measuring system to resonate. Conventional disposable transducers, coupled with 60 inches of pressure tubing, have a Fo of approximately 20 to 40 Hz. Should the Fo approach the frequencies found in the arterial pressure wave (<10 Hz), estimates of the systolic blood pressure increase because the fluid-filled coupling system resonates.

Damping Coefficient

The damping coefficient describes the tendency for fluid in the measuring system to extinguish motion. Damping lowers the effective bandwidth. If the system is underdamped ($\zeta = 0.2$), the effective bandwidth is reduced by approximately two thirds of the Fo. Figure 21–9 demonstrates the effect of damping on the character of an arterial pressure trace. Fidelity is optimized when catheters and tubings are very stiff, the mass of the fluid is small, the number of stopcocks is limited, and the connecting tubing is as short as possible. Air bubbles lower the Fo of catheter-transducer systems.[42, 43]

In clinical practice, underdamped catheter-transducer systems tend to overestimate systolic pressure by 15 to 30 mm Hg and to amplify artifact (catheter whip). Overdamping reduces the fidelity of the system, underestimates the systolic pressure, and overestimates the diastolic pressure. The MAP wave is most resistant to inadequate frequency response or damping characteristics. Dynamic calibration can determine the fidelity of the pressure-recording system.

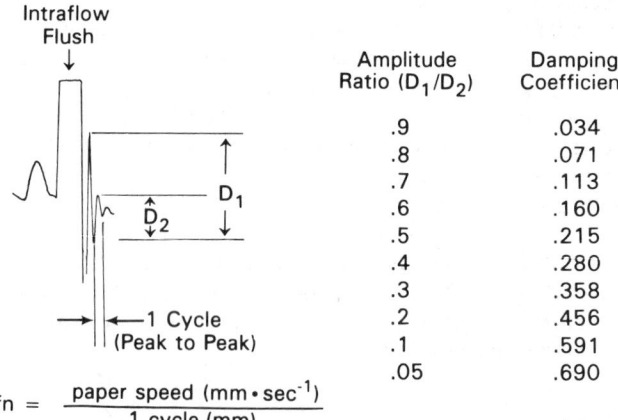

$$fn = \frac{paper\ speed\ (mm \cdot sec^{-1})}{1\ cycle\ (mm)}$$

FIGURE 21–10. Example of the fast flush test. (From Bedford H: Invasive blood pressure monitoring. *In* Monitoring in Anesthesia and Critical Care Medicine. Blitt CD (ed). New York, Churchill Livingstone, 1985, p 59.)

Clinical Applications

Damping and Fo can be estimated when a strip-chart recorder is part of the transducer-monitor system. After arterial cannulation and zeroing, a rapid high-pressure flush is initiated while the system's output is recorded. Fluid-coupled transducer systems show a square wave followed by oscillations during the "fast flush." Fo is estimated by dividing the paper speed by the distance measured between two consecutive oscillations. Damping is estimated by the ratio of the amplitude of the first and second oscillations. Figure 21–10 demonstrates the calculation of Fo and ζ using the fast flush test.

If a pen recorder is not present, observation of the display during a fast flush test identifies systems that oscillate. Systems with damping coefficients of 0.4 to 0.6 perform ideally (they are optimally damped). For the most part, transducer systems used in clinical anesthesia are underdamped ($\zeta = 0.2$ to 0.36). Resonance elimination devices enhance the performance of underdamped systems by increasing ζ and improve the accuracy of systolic blood pressure measurements.[43]

Monitor manufacturers filter the transducer signal, removing the higher frequencies carried in the electrical signal, thereby reducing the fidelity of the monitoring system. However, filtering (electrical damping) is beneficial in reducing noise from electrocautery and may improve overall performance.

Arterial Cannulation

The radial artery is most commonly used. Alternative cannulation sites are listed in Table 21–12.

Complications and Their Prevention

Abnormal radial artery blood flow following the removal of arterial catheters occurs frequently. Studies suggest that blood flow normalizes in 3 to 70 days.[44, 45] Radial artery thrombosis can be minimized by using nontapered 20- to 22-gauge catheters constructed of Teflon and reducing the duration of arterial cannulation.[45–47] Using a catheter smaller than 20 gauge when the wrist circumference is <15 cm may also decrease the risk of thrombosis. The potential for thromboembolism possibly is

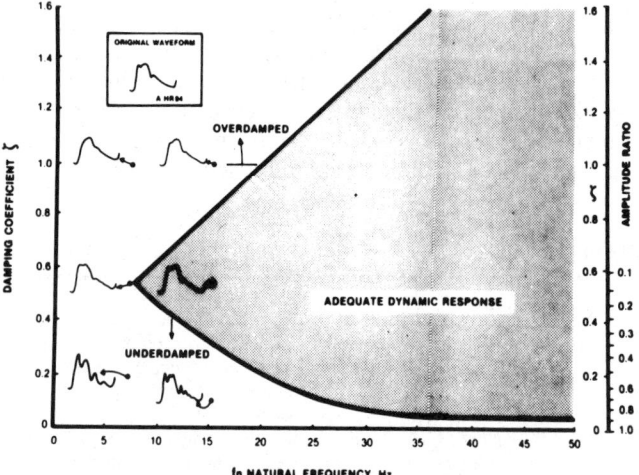

FIGURE 21–9. Ranges of damping coefficients and natural frequencies. The *shaded area* represents the regions of best fidelity. (From Gardner RM: Blood pressure: dynamic response needs. Anesthesiology 1981; 54:227.)

TABLE 21–12. Alternate Arterial Cannulation Sites

Ulnar	Complications similar to radial, ulnar nerve adjacent. Primary source of hand blood flow.
Brachial	Insertion site medial to biceps tendon. Median nerve damage is potential hazard. Can accommodate 18-gauge cannula.
Axillary	Insertion site at junction of pectoralis major and deltoid muscles. Specialized catheter kit available.
Femoral	Easy access in low-flow states. Potential for local and retroperitoneal hemorrhage. Longer catheters preferred. Access for intra-aortic balloon.
Dorsalis pedis	Adequate collateral flow needs verification.

(From Gilbert HC, Vender JS: Monitoring the anesthetized patient. *In* Clinical Anesthesia. 2nd ed. Barash PG, Cullen BF (eds). Philadelphia, JB Lippincott, 1992, p 748.)

diminished by compressing the proximal and distal artery while aspirating the cannula during withdrawal.[48]

Ischemia following radial artery cannulation resulting from thrombosis, proximal or distal embolization, and prolonged shock has been described.[49, 50] Contributing factors include severe atherosclerosis, diabetes mellitus, low cardiac output, intense peripheral vasoconstriction, or use of vasoconstrictors. Ischemia, hemorrhage, thrombosis, embolism, cerebral air embolism, aneurysm formation, arteriovenous fistula formation, and infection have occurred as the result of arterial cannulation, arterial blood sampling, or pressure flushing.

Continuous-flush devices are incorporated into disposable transducer kits and infuse fluid at 3 to 6 mL · h^{-1}. In neonates, even this low an infusion volume may contribute to fluid overload. Continuous-flush devices have little effect on the blood pressure measurement. However, pressurized flush devices may serve as a source of air embolism. Removing air from the pressure bag, stopcocks, and tubings minimizes the potential for air embolism and reduces damping.

CENTRAL VENOUS PRESSURE

Where Are Catheters Placed?

Central venous pressure (CVP) cannulas are important portals for intraoperative vascular access. Table 21–13 lists several clinical indications for intraoperative CVP cannula placement. The right internal jugular vein is the preferred site of cannulation by anesthesiologists because it is accessible from the head of the operating table, has a predictable anatomy, and is associated with a high success rate in both adults and children.[51]

Left-sided internal jugular cannulation can also be used but should be considered a second choice. It is less desirable

TABLE 21–13. Indications for Intraoperative Central Venous Cannulation

Vascular access: rapid infusion of fluids; parenteral alimentation; central drug administration (especially caustic drugs)
Monitoring central venous pressure
Access route for insertion of pulmonary artery catheter; transvenous pacemaker
Therapeutic uses: Treatment of venous air embolism

because of the potential for damage of the thoracic duct, puncture of the apex of the left lung, and difficulty in maneuvering and positioning catheters through the left jugular–left subclavian vein junction. The potential for accidental puncture of the left carotid artery and embolization to the left dominant cerebral hemisphere is often cited as an additional reason to avoid this site.

Alternatively, right and left external jugular and subclavian veins can be used. A J-tipped guidewire increases the success of central line placement through the external jugular veins. The success and safety of central venous cannulation require knowledge of regional anatomy and attention to detail (see Chapter 32).

What Are the Normal Pressure Waves?

CVP monitoring measures and displays a waveform that is essentially equivalent to right atrial pressure (RAP). Conditions affecting RAP are reflected by changes in the CVP. The normal CVP waveform is depicted in Figure 21–11.

a Wave

The a wave reflects the pressure change associated with atrial contraction following the P wave of the ECG. It occurs at the end of ventricular diastole and provides the "atrial kick" that primes the right ventricle.

c Wave

As the right atrium relaxes, the right ventricle contracts. The resulting upward motion of the tricuspid valve is reflected by a transient increase in pressure—the c wave. Because it occurs in early systole (ventricular), it follows the QRS complex.

x Descent

As ventricular systole continues, the relaxed right atrium is pulled down. This motion is reflected by a decrease in RAP that is termed the x descent.

v Wave

The last positive wave, the v wave, results when venous filling of the atrium occurs (atrial diastole).

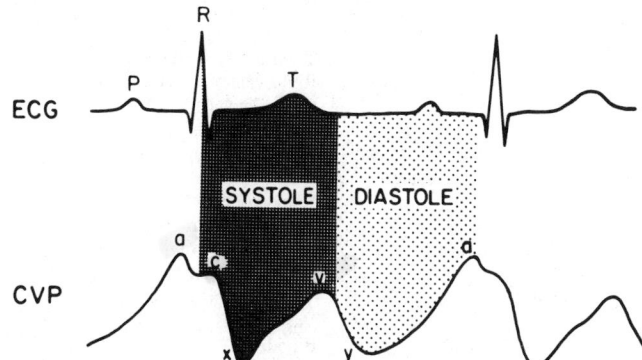

FIGURE 21–11. The relationship of normal CVP waves to ventricular systole and diastole. (From Mark JB: Central venous pressure monitoring: clinical insights beyond the numbers. J Cardiothorac Vasc Anesth 1991; 5:163.)

y Descent

The y descent is ascribed to the opening of the tricuspid valve, which rapidly empties blood from the right atrium into the right ventricle.[52]

What Conditions Are of Particular Interest to Anesthesiologists?

Many factors influence the character of the CVP tracing and often have diagnostic significance (Table 21–14). Table 21–15 lists features of particular interest to anesthesiologists. Right ventricular ischemia is often difficult to diagnose; a prominent v wave in the CVP tracing is suggestive of right ventricular papillary muscle ischemia and tricuspid regurgitation.[53] The CVP waveform in patients with diminished right ventricular compliance often demonstrates elevated pressures with prominent a and v waves that create an M or W configuration.[52]

CVP monitoring is helpful in the diagnosis and treatment of pericardial tamponade. As the CVP tracing becomes monophasic, the y descent is lost. Equalization of CVP, right ventricular and pulmonary artery diastolic pressures, and pulmonary artery occlusion pressure (PAOP) is characteristic of hemodynamically significant pericardial constriction and tamponade.[54] After treatment, a dramatic drop in filling pressures, restoration of systemic blood pressure, and normalization of the CVP waveform should occur.

What Conditions Warrant Central Venous Catheter Placement?

Central venous access is indicated in patients with hypovolemia, multiple trauma, or shock and whenever surgical procedures may be associated with large fluid shifts. For patients in shock, a subclavian approach may be preferred, because the subclavian vein has a constant size because of fascial attachments regardless of intravascular volume status. In contrast, the caliber and ease of cannulation of the jugular vein are completely pressure dependent. Monitoring is indicated in car-

TABLE 21–15. Central Venous Pressure Morphology in Conditions of Interest to Anesthesiologists

Clinical Condition	Changes in Morphology
Sinus tachycardia	Fusion of a and c waves
Atrial fibrillation	Absent a waves
Impaired right atrial emptying	Large a waves
Tricuspid stenosis	
Right ventricular hypertrophy	
Acute lung injury	
Chronic obstructive lung disease	
Pulmonary hypertension	
Tricuspid regurgitation	Giant v waves
Constrictive pericarditis	Large a, v waves; prominent x, y descents
Pericardial tamponade	Rapid x, blunted y descents

diac procedures (CVP or CVP port of a pulmonary artery catheter) and in patients with pre-existing cardiovascular disease.

Table 21–16 focuses attention on the difficulty in interpreting the clinical relevance of "mean CVP numbers." Changes in the numbers during anesthesia care are often helpful in monitoring fluid resuscitation and assessing the need for a pulmonary artery catheter. At higher CVP values, however, intraoperative fluid management is best guided by monitoring pulmonary artery pressures.

What Are the Complications?

Carotid Puncture

Potentially serious complications have been described for virtually every vascular access location. Table 21–17 lists complications of CVP placement that are common to all central venous access sites. Use of either carotid artery palpation or a Doppler pencil probe makes carotid artery puncture less likely.

Dysrhythmias

Dysrhythmias are most commonly associated with mechanical irritation of the myocardium by the guidewire. The guidewire is normally twice as long as the catheter; limiting its insertion distance to <20 cm avoids most dysrhythmias. Prevention of improper catheter position-related injuries is predicated on review of the follow-up chest radiograph to identify

TABLE 21–14. Factors That Influence Central Venous Pressure Tracing

Cardiac	Heart rate
	Heart rhythm
	Conduction disturbances
	Tricuspid valve function
	Right ventricular compliance
	Cor pulmonale
	Constrictive pericarditis
	Pericardial tamponade
Intrathoracic pressure	Pneumothorax
	Hemothorax
	Mechanical ventilation
Blood volume	Intravascular volume
	Rate of fluid administration
Drug therapy	Vasopressors
	Vasodilators
Pulmonary emboli	Blood
	Fat
	Air
Artifacts	Misdirected catheters
	Kinks

TABLE 21–16. Central Venous Pressure: The Numbers Game

Clinical Situations	Ventilation	Range of Values
Healthy patients	Spontaneous	−2 to +6 cm H_2O
	Mechanical	+4 to +12 cm H_2O
Surgical patients (mild hypovolemia)	Spontaneous	−4 to +2 cm H_2O
	Mechanical	0 to +3 cm H_2O
Critically ill patients (severe hypovolemia)	Mechanical + positive end-expiratory pressure	−4 to +1 cm H_2O
(fluid resuscitation)		+10 to 15 cm H_2O

TABLE 21–17. Complications Common to All Central Venous Cannula Placement Techniques

Accidental arterial puncture
    Hematoma
    False aneurysm
    Arteriovenous fistula
Poor positioning of catheter during placement
    Dysrhythmias
    Wall perforation
Injury to surrounding structures
Clot and fibrinous sleeve formation
Thrombosis of the vein
Catheter-related infections
Guidewire embolus
Bleeding

that the catheter tip is within the superior vena cava, not the right atrium, and that the angle between the catheter tip and the superior vena cava is <40°.

Miscellaneous Insertion Problems

Additional complications inherent to internal jugular and subclavian access include (1) pneumothorax from puncture of pleura or lung, (2) arterial puncture leading to hemothorax or hemomediastinum, (3) puncture of the lymphatic ducts leading to chylothorax or chylomediastinum, (4) pleural effusion, and (5) brachial plexus injury.

Infection

Central venous catheters are identified as important sources of nosocomial infections and sepsis. Catheter contamination may occur during insertion (poor technique), as a result of colonization from a distant infected site (hematogenous spread), or as a consequence of skin contamination at the insertion site. Both local and systemic infections have been reported. Overall risk of central venous catheter infections is approximately 4%.[55]

The practice of using transparent polyurethane dressings is associated with an increased risk of bacterial infections and suggests that a sterile gauze dressing is preferred.[56] Anesthesiologists are often responsible for inserting CVP catheters or vascular sheaths in surgical patients and should perform these procedures aseptically. Prevention of catheter-related infections requires knowledge of and adherence to institutional guidelines for dressing and tubing changes.

PULMONARY ARTERY PRESSURE

Flow-directed balloon flotation pulmonary artery catheters advanced the concept of clinical hemodynamic monitoring and are an important tool in the quantitative assessment of cardiopulmonary function. Right heart pressures often provide unreliable estimates of left ventricular filling pressures. This disparity is particularly true of patients who are elderly or have pre-existing cardiopulmonary disease.[57, 58]

What Are the Indications?

Pulmonary artery pressure monitoring originally was used to aid in the management of complicated myocardial infarction.[59] Indications are broadly defined. If one views the pulmonary artery catheter as a physiologic monitor, insertion should be guided by the need for information to diagnose and treat the underlying condition. Such monitoring provides anesthesiologists the unique opportunity to assess (1) intracardiac pressures, (2) thermodilution cardiac output, (3) mixed venous oxygenation, and (4) derived hemodynamic indices (e.g., systemic vascular resistance [SVR] and left ventricular stroke work index [LVSWI]). This information can help to define clinical problems, monitor the progression of hemodynamic dysfunctions, and guide the adequacy of and response to therapy.[60]

Clinical Applications

The measurement of intracardiac pressures is helpful to assess left ventricular preload, pulmonary hypertension, and cardiac or noncardiac causes of pulmonary edema. Analysis of the CVP and pulmonary artery port pressure waveforms provides diagnostic insights regarding the functional characteristics of rapid and reproducible ($\pm 10\%$) measurements of thermodilution-derived cardiac output. Cardiac output measurements are helpful to assess cardiac function, calculate O_2 delivery ($\dot{D}O_2$) (cardiac output $\times$ arterial O_2 content [CaO_2]), and evaluate alterations in cardiac performance. Mixed venous blood samples (or measurement of O_2 saturation by reflectance oximetry) are necessary to calculate intrapulmonary and intracardiac shunts.

Hemodynamic Assessment

Hemodynamic management is often predicated on the manipulation of preload, afterload, and contractility. Several of the derived indices of hemodynamic function necessitate cardiac output measurement (more later). Table 21–18 lists derived hemodynamic variables that require pulmonary artery catheter insertion. The pulmonary artery catheter is used to measure intracardiac pressure, in particular the PAOP. The latter value is used to assess left ventricular preload (left ventricular end-diastolic volume [LVEDV]) by reflecting changes in left ventricular end-diastolic pressure (LVEDP).

The clinical value of the PAOP is based on the assumption that an open conduit from the catheter tip to the left ventricle results when the pulmonary artery catheter is in the "wedged" position. During end-diastole, cessation of forward blood flow

TABLE 21–18. Derived Hemodynamic Variables

Name	Abbreviation	Calculation
Cardiac index	CI	CO/body surface area
Systemic vascular resistance	SVR	(MAP − CVP/CO) × 80
Pulmonary vascular resistance	PVR	(MPAP − PWP/CO) × 80
Stroke index	SI	CI/heart rate
Left ventricular stroke work index	LVSWI	SI × (MAP − PWP) × 0.0136
Right ventricular stroke work index	RVSWI	SI × (MAP − CVP) × 0.0136

(From Gilbert HC, Vender JS: Monitoring the anesthetized patient. *In* Clinical Anesthesia. 2nd ed. Philadelphia, JB Lippincott, 1992, p 752.)
Abbreviations: CO = cardiac output; MAP = mean arterial pressure; CVP = central venous pressure; MPAP = mean pulmonary artery pressure; PWP = pulmonary wedge pressure.

occurs, and a static fluid column is presumed to exist from the left ventricle to the pulmonary artery catheter tip. Ideally, changes in LVEDP are reflected by all proximal pressures (i.e., pulmonary artery end-diastolic pressure [PAEDP], PAOP, pulmonary venous pressure [PVP], and left atrial pressure [LAP]).

What Factors Affect Data Validity?

Pulmonary Vascular Resistance

Normally, pulmonary vascular resistance (PVR) and the impedance to pulmonary blood flow are minimal. Any significant increase in PVR alters the relationship between PAOP and PAEDP. Acute or chronic parenchymal pulmonary disease, pulmonary emboli, alveolar hypoxia, acidosis, hypoxemia, and many vasoactive drugs may increase PVR. Tachycardia shortens ventricular diastole, reducing distal runoff of pulmonary blood flow and increasing PVR.[61] When these situations exist, the PAEDP cannot be assumed to reflect distal diastolic pressures, including the PAOP.

Pulmonary Artery Catheter Tip Placement

Accurate measurement of PAOP can also be affected by the position of the catheter tip in the pulmonary artery and by changes in intrathoracic pressure. West and colleagues described a gravity-dependent difference between ventilation and perfusion in the lung.[62] Only in zone III do pulmonary artery and venous pressures consistently exceed alveolar pressure. Therefore, only zone III locations meet the requirement for uninterrupted blood flow and continuous communication with distal intracardiac pressures.[63]

Increase in alveolar pressure, decrease in perfusion (e.g., hypovolemia, hypotension, reduced cardiac output), or changes in posture may convert areas of zone III to either zone I or II. Accurate measurement necessitates a pulmonary artery catheter tip to be placed in zone III. Because pulmonary artery catheters are flow directed, they usually advance to areas of highest blood flow. Catheter position can be confirmed by a lateral chest radiograph to ascertain that the catheter tip is below the level of the left atrium.

Several characteristics suggest that the catheter tip is not in zone III: (1) a PAOP greater than the PAEDP, (2) nonphasic PAOP tracing, (3) an increase in PAOP >50% of the increased alveolar pressure (positive end-expiratory pressure [PEEP] therapy), and (4) the inability to aspirate blood from the distal port when the catheter is wedged. Factors that influence the accuracy and validity of the PAOP are listed in Table 21–19.

Waveform Characteristics

When the pulmonary artery balloon is inflated, the pressure tracing looks like the CVP or atrial trace. Pulmonary artery v waves are present at the end of ventricular systole when the left atrium is maximally filled. The size of the v wave is most often associated with changes in left atrial compliance rather than regurgitant volume.

Decreases in left ventricular compliance, aortic regurgitation, and premature closure of the mitral valve may reverse the normal pressure gradient so that the LVEDP is greater than LAP.[64, 65] Therefore, the accuracy of the measured pulmonary pressures and their correlation with LVEDP does not always ensure a valid reflection of left ventricular preload.

TABLE 21–19. Factors Affecting the Accuracy of Pulmonary Artery Occlusion Pressure

Cause	Potential Effect
Increases in pulmonary vascular resistance (e.g., acidosis, alveolar hypoxia, hypoxemia, chronic pulmonary disease)	PAD > PAOP
Increases in airway pressure (e.g., PEEP therapy, positive-pressure ventilation)	PAOP > LAP
Mitral stenosis Left atrial myxoma	LAP > LVEDP
Abnormal ventricular compliance	LVEDP > LVEDV

Abbreviations: PAD = pulmonary artery diastolic pressure; PAOP = pulmonary artery occlusion pressure; LAP = left atrial pressure; LVEDP = left ventricular end-diastolic pressure; LVEDV = left ventricular end-diastolic volume.

Ventricular Compliance

The relationship between LVEDP and LVEDV is not linear. Changes in ventricular compliance result from inherent alterations in ventricular stiffness.[64–66] Ventricular compliance is a dynamic factor that can be influenced by many physiologic and pathologic variables. Factors that affect ventricular compliance are shown in Table 21–20. Appropriate use of pulmonary artery catheters necessitates an appreciation and understanding of these pitfalls and limitations.[61, 66, 67]

What Do the Numbers Mean?

The preceding discussion emphasizes many factors that affect the character of the pulmonary artery tracing as well as the absolute numbers. Pulmonary artery catheters, by virtue of their multiple ports, provide simultaneous measurements of CVP and PAOP. These numbers, along with information obtained from thermodilution cardiac output measurement, enhance our capabilities to assess fluid status and cardiac performance. However, use of the numbers sometimes is difficult.

Consider the example of a failing left ventricle versus new-onset left ventricular ischemia. In both situations, the LVEDP may have the same absolute value. However, the intraventricular volumes are likely to be different, because the conditions may be associated with dissimilar changes in ventricular compliance. To assume that abnormal values by themselves mandate specific therapeutic interventions is unwise.

Recognition of artifacts, understanding of clinical circumstances in which pulmonary artery catheter data may be misleading or difficult to obtain, and knowledge of the interaction of pathophysiologic states and diseases common to surgical

TABLE 21–20. Factors That Influence Ventricular Compliance

Decreased Left Ventricular Compliance	
Myocardial ischemia	Cardiac tamponade
Restrictive myopathies	Myocardial fibrosis
Right-to-left intraventricular shunts	Inotropic drugs
Aortic stenosis	Hypertension

Increased Ventricular Compliance	
Vasodilator therapy	Congestive myopathies
Mitral regurgitation	Aortic regurgitation

(From Gilbert HC, Vender JS: Monitoring the anesthetized patient. *In* Clinical Anesthesia 2nd ed. Baresh PG, Cullen BF (eds). Philadelphia, JB Lippincott, 1992, p 755.)

patients define the cognitive skill of clinicians who use these catheters.

For many years, anesthesiologists have debated the worth of pulmonary artery monitoring, particularly with respect to its value as a sensitive indicator of new-onset ischemia.[68] Many cardiac anesthesiologists do not routinely insert pulmonary artery catheters. Patients with poor left ventricular function (ejection fraction <0.4), documented left ventricular wall motion abnormality, recent myocardial infarction, significant angina, or documented left main or left main equivalent stenosis are considered for pulmonary artery monitoring on an individual basis. Such monitoring requires a knowledgeable anesthesia care team in order to minimize complications and to maximize the clinical value.[69]

What Are the Complications?

Pulmonary artery catheters are associated with numerous complications.[70] Factors that appear to reduce complications include experience, supervision, and attention to details. One large study suggests a low incidence of morbidity and mortality,[71] but others suggest significant comorbidity[72] and even comortality,[73] referable to pulmonary artery catheter use. The majority of complications can be categorized into three groups: (1) insertion risks, (2) catheter passage risks (advancement and removal), and (3) risk associated with use (maintenance).

Insertion

Insertion risks are identical to those described for CVP cannulation.

Advancement and Removal

Complications of advancement and removal are related to problems associated with cardiac performance or structure. Dysrhythmias are the most common complication of catheter passage.[72] Right bundle branch block and even complete heart block have been reported. Intravenous lidocaine can be administered either therapeutically or prophylactically, but its utility is unpredictable.[74] If complete heart block is a concern, as in patients who have a pre-existing left bundle branch block and in whom a superimposed right bundle branch block would result in complete heart block, a catheter with pacing capabilities may be used.

Table 21–21 lists some of the complications that have been associated with catheter advancement and removal. Difficult insertions can be anticipated in patients having right ventricular enlargement, low-flow states, or tricuspid valvular disease.

TABLE 21–21. Complications of Pulmonary Artery Catheter Passage

Dysrhythmias
Knotting
Valvular damage
Perforation of the atrium, ventricle, or pulmonary artery
Heart block
Kinking or coiling

(From Gilbert HC, Vender JS: Monitoring the anesthetized patient. *In* Clinical Anesthesia. 2nd ed. Baresh PG, Cullen BF (eds). Philadelphia, JB Lippincott, 1992, p 755.)

TABLE 21–22. Complications of Pulmonary Artery Catheter Maintenance

Thrombosis
Pulmonary artery rupture
Sepsis
Endocarditis
Balloon rupture
Pulmonary infarction
Thrombocytopenia
Valvular damage
Thrombocytopenia
Dysrhythmias

In these situations, patient positioning (head up, right side down),[75] deep breathing, or fluoroscopic guidance may be necessary.

Maintenance

Numerous complications have been associated with the continued use of pulmonary artery catheters (Table 21–22).[60, 76] The most dramatic and potentially catastrophic complication is pulmonary artery perforation and hemorrhage.[77] Predisposing risk factors include hypothermia, pulmonary hypertension, advanced age, female gender, and poor insertion/use technique. Perforations and subsequent hemorrhage can be avoided by restricting overwedging through rigorous monitoring of the pulmonary artery tracing during gradual balloon inflation, continuously monitoring the pulmonary artery pressure tracing to recognize spontaneous wedging, and minimizing the number of balloon inflations (inflate only as necessary rather than according to an arbitrary schedule). Serious pulmonary hemorrhage from pulmonary artery perforation is associated with hemoptysis and may require single-lung ventilation and surgical intervention.

Catheter-related infections (sepsis or endocarditis) are well recognized causes of morbidity that can be minimized when infection control protocols are implemented.[75, 78]

How Is Pulmonary Artery Catheter Use Enhanced?

Several modifications enhance pulmonary artery catheter monitoring capabilities. The first significant improvement was the incorporation of a thermistor at the tip, enabling cardiac output measurement by thermodilution technique. Other features have been introduced for clinical use or are undergoing clinical evaluation. These include measurement of mixed venous oximetry, right ventricular ejection fraction, and continuous cardiac output. Additionally, some pulmonary artery catheters have cardiac pacemaker capabilities. Right ventricular ejection fraction (RVEF) and continuous cardiac output monitoring are discussed later.

Mixed Venous Oximetry

Advances in fiberoptic technology led to the development of pulmonary artery catheters that can continuously monitor mixed venous O_2 saturation ($S\bar{v}O_2$). The accuracy of these in vivo measurements has been confirmed by comparison studies with co-oximetry. Continuous $S\bar{v}O_2$ monitoring provides a minute-to-minute reflection of total tissue O_2 balance (i.e., the relationship between $\dot{D}O_2$ and O_2 consumption [$\dot{V}O_2$]).

Oxygen Delivery, Demand, and Consumption

Understanding the value of continuous $S\bar{v}O_2$ monitoring necessitates a review of the factors influencing $\dot{D}O_2$, O_2 demand, and $\dot{V}O_2$. $\dot{D}O_2$ (mL · min^{-1}) equals CaO_2 (mL · L^{-1}) times cardiac output (L · min^{-1}). $\dot{D}O_2$ = hemoglobin × 13.8 × cardiac output. The constant 13.8 represents the volume of O_2 carried by hemoglobin (g · L^{-1}). This equation does not include the dissolved O_2 content, which in most cases is insignificant. $\dot{V}O_2$ is determined by the difference between arterial and venous O_2 content times cardiac output. The relationship between $S\bar{v}O_2$, $\dot{V}O_2$, and cardiac output is demonstrated in the following equation:

$$S\bar{v}O_2 = SaO_2 - \frac{\dot{V}O_2}{(\text{hemoglobin} \times 13.8)} \times \text{cardiac output}$$

where SaO_2 represents the percent saturation of hemoglobin by O_2.

Clinical Implications

Increases in O_2 extraction are reflected by a decrease in $S\bar{v}O_2$. At critical $\dot{D}O_2$ levels, the $S\bar{v}O_2$ plateaus because the $\dot{V}O_2$ is maximum.[79] When the $S\bar{v}O_2$ is <30%, tissue O_2 balance is compromised and anaerobic metabolism ensues. $S\bar{v}O_2$ is determined by the previously mentioned variables and, therefore, is not exclusively a reflection of changes in cardiac output. A normal $S\bar{v}O_2$ does not ensure a normal metabolic state but suggests that O_2 kinetics are either normal or compensated.

Figure 21–12 demonstrates the $S\bar{v}O_2$ recording of a patient recovering from cardiac surgery. In this example, a decrease in $S\bar{v}O_2$ was observed despite marked increases in cardiac output, suggesting an imbalance between $\dot{D}O_2$ and $\dot{V}O_2$. A reduction in $\dot{V}O_2$ (reduced shivering) restored the balance between $\dot{V}O_2$ and $\dot{D}O_2$, reflected by a step-up of the $S\bar{v}O_2$ despite a decrease in cardiac output.

Mixed venous oximetry is a powerful tool for both diagnos-

TABLE 21–23. Conditions Associated with Normal or High $S\bar{v}O_2$

Sepsis
Peripheral shunts
Left-to-right intracardiac shunts
Hemoglobinopathies
Arteriovenous fistulas
Cirrhosis
Paget's disease
Cyanide poisoning
Unintentional pulmonary artery catheter wedging
Cyanide toxicity

tic and therapeutic assessments of critically ill patients. The combination of continuous SaO_2 and $S\bar{v}O_2$ monitoring (dual oximetry) provides continuous information regarding the cardiopulmonary effects of PEEP.[80]

As with all monitoring, technologic and physiologic limitations affect clinical utility.[60, 61] Although low $S\bar{v}O_2$ often is considered ominous, normal or high $S\bar{v}O_2$ does not always indicate adequate tissue O_2 balance. $S\bar{v}O_2$ is a global measurement. Normal $S\bar{v}O_2$ does not ensure the adequacy of regional (specific vital organs) tissue O_2 balance. Table 21–23 lists some of the pathophysiologic conditions that may be associated with normal or high $S\bar{v}O_2$.

Other Modifications

Table 21–24 lists other adaptations that have been engineered into flow-directed pulmonary artery catheters. Monitoring of RVEF requires a rapid-response thermistor, allowing quantification of the beat-to-beat variations in pulmonary artery temperature. Ejection fraction estimates are reasonably accurate as long as regurgitant flow or cardiac dysrhythmias are not present.[81, 82] However, the value of and appropriate clinical situation for monitoring RVEF during anesthesia care have not been fully explored.

CARDIAC OUTPUT

Cardiac output and hemodynamic variables derived from estimates of blood pressure and flow are important indices of myocardial performance and the status of the circulatory system. Estimates of cardiac output, although not a routine measurement during anesthesia, are of great importance when managing critically ill patients or patients with documented or newly acquired cardiac dysfunction.

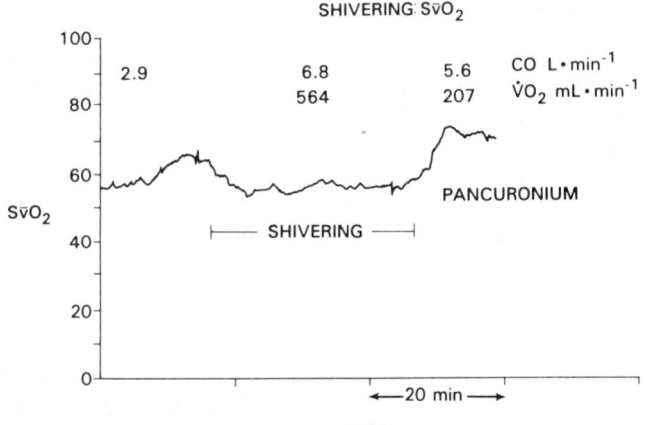

FIGURE 21–12. Effects of shivering (increased $\dot{V}O_2$) on the balance of $\dot{D}O_2$ and $\dot{V}O_2$ as reflected by changes in $S\bar{v}O_2$ and cardiac output.

TABLE 21–24. Pulmonary Artery Catheter Modifications

Modification	Utility
Pacing wires/leads	Atrial and ventricular pacing
Electrocardiography	Dysrhythmia diagnosis
Ventricular ports	Access for placing Chandler's wire
Infusion port	Central drug infusion
Fast thermistors	Monitoring right ventricular ejection
Heating elements	Continuous cardiac output
Piezoelectric crystals	Continuous cardiac output
Fiberoptic cables	Monitoring oxygen saturation

How Is It Measured Invasively?

The earliest technique for cardiac output measurement was proposed by Adolph Fick in 1870. Modern invasive techniques, to a great extent, are based on adaptations of this principle. Fick found that the size of a fluid stream can be calculated by instilling an indicator into the stream and measuring the concentration difference over time between the inflow and outflow. Traditionally, O_2 has been used as the indicator substance, and cardiac output is determined by measuring the $\dot{V}O_2$ and dividing it by the arterial-venous O_2 content difference $C(a - \bar{v})O_2$.

The direct Fick cardiac output measurement technique is the standard by which other methods are judged. Implicit in its use is the assumption that a steady state exists with respect to O_2 saturation, $\dot{V}O_2$, and cardiac output during the period of data collection. Values are inaccurate if cardiac, pulmonary, or hepatic shunts are present.[83] The traditional Fick cardiac output determination has been superseded by the thermodilution technique that was introduced into clinical practice in 1971.[84] Direct Fick cardiac output measurement in the operating room is cumbersome because of the requirement to measure $\dot{V}O_2$. However, intraoperative mass spectrometry and spirometry can be adapted to estimate $\dot{V}O_2$.

Indicator-Dilution Techniques

Indocyanine Green Dye

Indicator dilution determinations of cardiac output are based on a concept proposed by Stewart and tested by Hamilton and colleagues.[85] A known amount of indicator (usually indocyanine green dye) is injected into a CVP catheter, arterial blood is withdrawn at a constant rate, and assay is performed by an in-line photodensitometer. The output of the photodensitometer is graphed as a concentration-time curve. Today computers calculate the average concentration over time. In adults, 50 mL of blood is withdrawn during each calculation. In children, 4 to 5 mL can be used without sacrificing accuracy.[86] This technique is not often used in clinical practice and has been replaced by thermodilution cardiac output determinations.

Thermodilution

Thermodilution cardiac output determination (TCO) is the most widely used adaptation of the indicator dilution principle. This technique was first described by Fegler in 1954.[87] Today, 5% dextrose or 0.9% saline is injected into the central venous port of a thermodilution pulmonary artery catheter. A thermistor at the catheter tip records the decrease in temperature as blood, cooled by the injectate, passes through the pulmonary artery. Computers contend with the complexity of the thermodilution cardiac output equation, which, although similar to that for dye dilution, includes the following factors: specific heat and gravity of blood and indicator, volume of the injectate, catheter size, and the area of the blood temperature curve.

Accuracy. Unlike dye dilution, the small amount of injected indicator in TCO does not recirculate. Comparison studies suggest that either room temperature or iced injectate can be used with equal accuracy for clinical measurements of TCO when a 10-mL injectate volume is used.[88] Iced injectate produces more accurate results in children or adults when 5 mL

TABLE 21–25. Factors That Affect Thermodilution Accuracy and Precision

Theoretic concerns	Cardiac output is constant during measurement
	Blood volume is constant
Sources of errors	Intracardiac shunts
	Computer algorithm catheter computation constant mismatch
	Thermistor drift
	Variable rate of injectate administration
	Coadministration of intravenous fluids at a changing rate
	Respiratory cycle variation
Factors that enhance accuracy and precision	Measure at peak inspiration or end expiration
	Injectate rate = 2–4 s
	Constant, precise injectate volume
	Delay repetition of injections 60–90 s
	Observation of the temperature decay curve
	Proper sample handling
	Accurate injectate temperature

injectate is used. Properly performed, TCO correlates very well with both direct Fick and dye dilution determinations.[89,90] In clinical practice, triplicate determinations are averaged to increase precision. Differences in values of 12% to 15% are not of clinical significance. Factors that influence the accuracy and precision of TCO determinations are listed in Table 21–25.

Sources of Error. Observation of the thermal curve is helpful in assessing the accuracy of TCO determinations. Low-amplitude curves result when (1) cardiac output is very high or injectate volume is too small, (2) the temperature differential between injectate and the patient is small, or (3) the thermistor is improperly positioned.[90] Tricuspid or pulmonic regurgitation and intracardiac shunts may produce recirculation errors.[89] A diminished height of the concentration-time (thermodilution) curve can also occur from incomplete filling of the syringe, from loss of injectate through leaks, or from a thrombus insulating the pulmonary artery thermistor. Each of these conditions results in a falsely high cardiac output measurement.

Intravenous infusions can influence cardiac output determinations. Rapid infusions should be maintained at a constant rate or discontinued before measurement.[91] Irregularities in the thermal curve should be evaluated before initiation of therapy based on possibly erroneous cardiac output determination. Stetz and colleagues[92] found disparities were greatest when single measurement comparisons were studied rather than those performed in triplicate (13% versus 23%, respectively). This finding is of importance when considering alternative methods for estimating cardiac output.

Continuous Cardiac Output Techniques

Continuous-wave and pulsed Doppler techniques have been incorporated into specialized pulmonary artery catheters that can estimate cardiac output by determining the average velocity of blood flow and multiplying it by the estimate of the pulmonary artery diameter. Clinical studies suggest that the Doppler pulmonary artery catheter permits monitoring of instantaneous as well as mean cardiac output. Cardiac output estimates compare with triplicate thermodilution measurements.[93]

Critical to the accuracy of this technique is positioning the Doppler piezoelectric crystals so that accurate estimates of the pulmonary artery diameter are obtained. In patients undergoing cardiac catheterization, Doppler catheter-determined cardiac output measurements modestly underestimate Fick cardiac values.[94] Clinical use of this technique in anesthetized patients has been limited.

Another adaptation of the pulmonary artery catheter places a heating filament proximal to the thermistor. Heat from the filament is used as the indicator.[95] Clinical studies evaluating the accuracy, precision, and physiologic benefits are ongoing and appear quite promising.

How Is It Measured Noninvasively?

The quest for technically simple, noninvasive methods to estimate cardiac output has a long history. Two methods are currently available for clinical use.

Impedance Plethysmography

Impedance plethysmography (IP) is based on measurement of the pulsatile change in resistance during the cardiac cycle. Four electrodes are applied to the neck and thorax. Impedance measurements are made in two pairs while a continuous small electric current is applied across the thorax. The maximum rate of impedance change during systole (max dZ/dT) is proportional to the stroke volume and the ventricular ejection time.[96]

Cardiac output monitors based on IP are commercially available (Biomed Medical Instruments, Irving, CA). Electrode placement is an important source of error.[97] Other factors that influence bioimpedance include intrathoracic fluid shifts and changes in hematocrit. Although IP has not gained wide use, the technique offers clinicians a quick method for determining cardiac output with minimum risk to patients.

Continuous- or Pulsed-Wave Doppler Ultrasonography

Continuous-wave or pulsed-wave Doppler ultrasonography can measure the velocity of blood in the ascending aorta. Cardiac output is calculated by multiplying the time-weighted average velocity of blood flow by an estimate of aortic cross-sectional area. Aortic area can be measured or predicted from a nomogram.

The accuracy and precision of Doppler-based cardiac output estimates are dependent on the reliability of the estimate of aortic diameter and the alignment of the Doppler probe to the blood flow jet in the aorta. Velocity measurements are most accurate when the Doppler beam and flow are parallel. In clinical practice, velocity measurements become unreliable when the angle exceeds 25°.

Suprasternal and transesophageal probes have been designed for determining cardiac output *noninvasively* using continuous-wave Doppler ultrasonography. A pulsed-wave transtracheal device that measures aortic diameter and blood flow has been introduced. Comparison studies continue to question the precision and accuracy of cardiac output determinations using suprasternal, transesophageal, and transtracheal Doppler techniques.[98–101]

TRANSESOPHAGEAL ECHOCARDIOGRAPHY

Transesophageal echocardiography (TEE) adds a new dimension to intraoperative monitoring because it creates beat-to-beat cardiac imaging with the capability of measuring intracardiac blood flow. This approach offers clinicians information that complements data obtained from surface ECGs, invasive hemodynamic monitoring, and clinical signs. In experienced hands, TEE may provide information about the onset of myocardial ischemia, valvular competency, graphic representations of blood flow during diastole and systole, estimates of chamber volumes, quantification of cardiac output, and estimates of regional myocardial function.

What Are the Clinical Applications?

Despite the potential for esophageal damage or irritation, TEE has an excellent record of safety with few reports of complications.[102] As anesthesiologists learn to use TEE, its application for intraoperative clinical decision making expands to include estimation of preload and measurement of stroke volume,[103] tracking of changes in left ventricular filling during noncardiac surgery,[104] assessment of intraoperative inotropy following cardiopulmonary bypass,[105] and determination of the incidence and location of intracardiac air.[106] Enhancements in instrumentation and computer software have improved the quality of images and expanded the utility of TEE. Unfortunately, the equipment is expensive and user *un*friendly, and the learning curve for clinical interpretation requires considerable hands-on training.

How Does It Work?

Methodology

Modern intraoperative TEE uses Doppler-shifted ultrasound to penetrate intracardiac structures. The TEE processes reflected sound waves using complex instrumentation to depict graphically the size and shape of the heart chambers during filling and ejection. Direction of blood flow across valves, intracardiac chambers, coronary and pulmonary arteries, and pulmonary veins can be determined. Valvular motion can be depicted, and the presence or absence of intracardiac masses or septal defects can be defined.

Sound is transmitted through matter (water, tissue) as ripples (sine waves) that are depicted when the amplitude of the sound energy is plotted against time. When sound waves enter a homogeneous medium, the velocity of the wave is constant and equals the product of the cycle length and frequency:

$$V = f(\lambda)$$

The ability of ultrasound to discern structures depends on the distance between the structures, the interface between the object(s) of interest, the frequency of the probing wave, and attenuation of this frequency by intervening tissues.

Transesophageal Versus Transthoracic Techniques

Modern TEE uses high-frequency ultrasound (5–7.5 MHz) to probe the heart through the thin-walled esophagus. Although the ultrasonic beams are weakened as they penetrate tissues, the beating heart is ideal for ultrasonic probing because strong reflections termed *specular echos* are produced at the blood-tissue interfaces. TEE is more sensitive than transthoracic techniques because penetration of the chest wall is avoided, the lungs do not interfere with imaging, and higher frequencies may be used.

What Are the Types of Echocardiograms?

The display produced by ultrasonic probing is called an *echocardiogram.* Transesophageal equipment can produce echocardiograms using various formats. A complete TEE evaluation includes M-mode, two-dimensional (2D) imaging, and Doppler flow studies.

M-Mode Studies

M-mode echocardiograms (time-motion displays) are produced when an ultrasonic beam is aimed at oscillating cardiac structures, and the reflected beam is displayed as wavy lines (due to oscillations of intervening heart tissues). Distance away from the transducer is displayed on the vertical axis, and time is displayed on the horizontal axis. M-mode echocardiograms are valuable because M-mode transducers can track rapidly moving structures such as valve leaflets.

Two-Dimensional

Two-dimensional echocardiograms result when the TEE collects a series of B-mode (brightness mode) scans and aligns them in their appropriate anatomic orientation. Four approaches have been engineered to acquire the B-mode scan lines that create 2D echocardiograms. Many crystals or a rap-

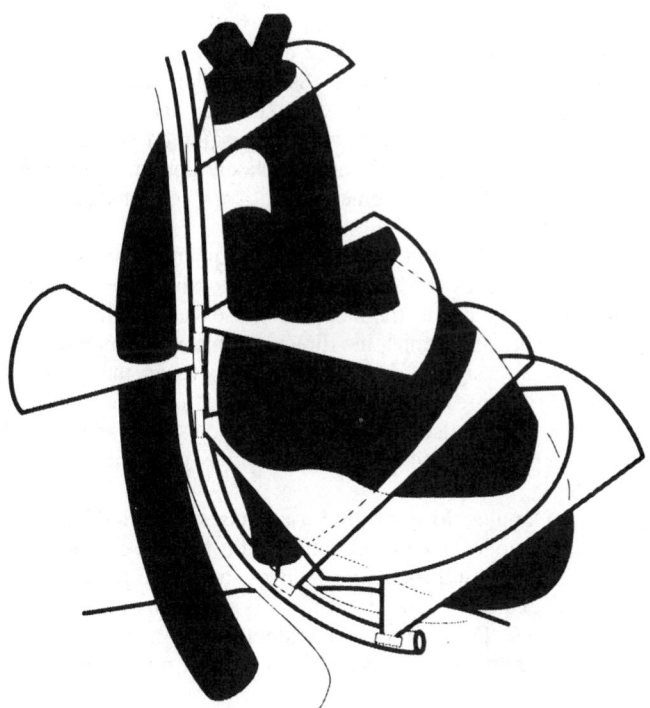

FIGURE 21–14. Positioning of the TEE probe to obtain views of areas of interest. (Redrawn from Sutherland GR, Roelandt JPTC: Transesophageal echocardiography. *In* Clinical Practice. London, Gower Medical Publishing, 1991.)

idly moving single crystal create multiple views of cardiac structures that can be graphically reconstructed and collated into a 2D image. Today, most TEE probes use phased-array technology to provide the input for imaging processing. Figure 21–13 depicts how a phased-array probe acquires a series of B-mode scans to display the cardiac structures graphically.

Two-dimensional echocardiograms display cardiac structures with amazing clarity. The imaging process is minimally invasive, and no adverse effects of ultrasound have been demonstrated after its use. Two-dimensional scans depend on the reflected waves that are perpendicular to the ultrasonic beam. Esophageal probes (modified gastroscopes) can be positioned to optimize the spatial resolution of the scans. Figure 21–14 depicts the positioning of the TEE esophageal probe during a complete examination. At each level, structures of interest are present, and the operator must be skilled in orienting the esophageal probe to produce the best images.[107] Definition in two dimensions provides an enormous advantage to new users, because the image is intuitively more obvious in terms of how it defines anatomic structures. Two-dimensional imaging does not provide direct imaging of blood flow.

Doppler Flow

Color imaging is based on the principle of Doppler-shifted ultrasound and uses sophisticated processing of the reflected echo waves to estimate flow characteristics. Because the velocity of the wave (pulsed or continuous) through the tissues is nearly constant, the distance between interfacing tissues can be determined by timing the reflected wave at the probe site. The shift of the frequency and amplitude of the reflected waves can be processed to provide color flow enhancement. Flow in the direction of the transducer is depicted in one color

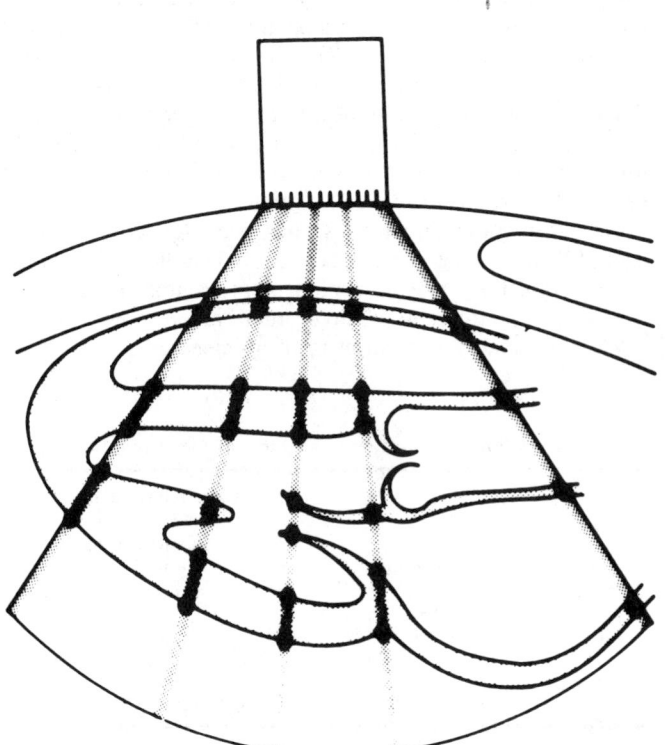

FIGURE 21–13. Depiction of transthoracic phased-array B-mode scanning of cardiac structures.

(e.g., red), and that away from the transducer is shown in another (e.g., blue). Increasing velocity in either direction is depicted by increases in the intensity of color shading.

These studies are useful to verify cardiac anatomy, identify intracardiac shunts, assess valvular regurgitation, and evaluate myocardial perfusion.[108] Contrast echocardiograms are made by enhancing the echo characteristic of blood using saline "microbubbles."

Pulsed Doppler studies may provide quantitative estimates of flow as long as the sampling frequency is higher than the velocities measured. If the Doppler shift exceeds half the sampling rate (Nyquist limit), the direction of flow is ambiguously presented as a signal of the highest velocity in the opposite direction (aliasing). Aliasing can be used to define areas of increased flow. Pulsed Doppler flow studies are range gated and susceptible to aliasing when blood is examined at high velocities.

Color Doppler flow imaging uses pulsed Doppler information and encodes mean velocities with 16 to 32 shades of colors. Color flow processing reduces the frame refresh rate, density of scan lines, the frequency of resolution, and depth of simultaneous 2D scanning.[109] Intraoperative color flow studies have been found to be sensitive indicators of mitral regurgitation.[110]

What Are the Clinical Uses?

Intraoperative Monitoring

With the introduction of phased-array esophageal transducers in 1982, the potential for intraoperative TEE monitoring became a reality.[111] Before the design of practical TEE probes, anesthesiologists, cardiologists, and cardiac surgeons depended on transthoracic and epicardial echocardiography for intraoperative cardiac imaging. These techniques, although helpful, were cumbersome to perform and had limited resolution.

Intraoperative TEE, unlike other cardiovascular monitors, provides almost real-time beat-to-beat information about valvular function, cardiac filling and ejection, and the presence of air embolism. The clinical interpretation of wall motion abnormalities is helpful to diagnose intraoperative ischemia. Electronic processing of echocardiographic signals can assist clinicians in monitoring myocardial performance in a minimally invasive manner. Although most of the experience has been gained in patients undergoing cardiac surgery, the role of TEE as an intraoperative monitor in noncardiac surgery and critical care is constantly expanding.

Detection of Myocardial Infarction

For many years, graded reductions in myocardial perfusion pressure have been known to be associated with quantifiable alterations in wall motion.[112] During cardiac catheterization, cardiologists grade regional wall motion by assessing systolic ventriculographic patterns. Similarly, TEE images can be used to detect segmental wall motion abnormalities (SWMA). Two-dimensional imaging and cineangiography show excellent correlation.[113] Acute myocardial ischemia can be assessed by evaluating SWMA and wall thickening with intraoperative TEE.

Most intraoperative reports use four quadrants to describe

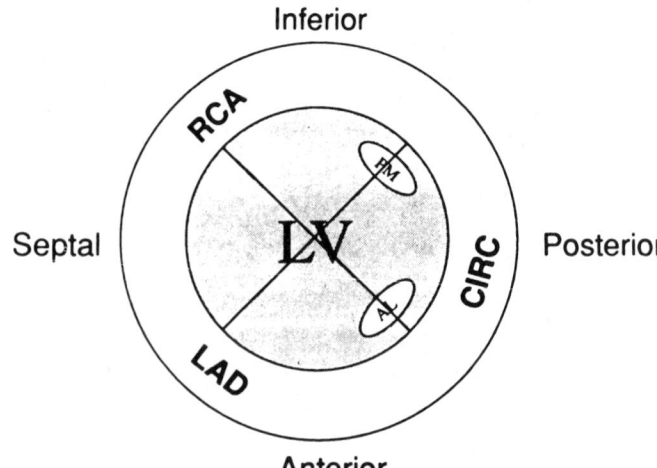

FIGURE 21–15. Transgastric, short axis TEE view of the left ventricle. RCA = right coronary artery; LAD = left anterior descending coronary artery; CIRC = circumflex coronary artery; PM = posteromedian; AL = anterolateral. (From Calahan MK: Transesophageal echocardiography. ASA Refresher Courses in Anesthesiology. American Society of Anesthesiologists, 1990.)

left ventricular wall motion using a short-axis 2D image at the level of the papillary muscles (transgastric view). Figure 21–15 depicts this short-axis view of the left ventricle. Table 21–26 lists the criteria used to grade SWMA.

Comparison with Electrocardiographic Monitoring

Monitoring for SWMA has been found to be more sensitive than intraoperative ECG monitoring for early detection of intraoperative ischemia.[114, 115] Leung and colleagues evaluated the prognostic value of intraoperative TEE and compared SWMA with two-channel ECG monitoring.[116] An "echo episode" suggesting ischemia was defined as a worsening of SWMA of two or more grades, lasting longer than 1 minute. TEE was more sensitive than the ECG and was particularly useful in detecting ischemic changes occurring in the posterior or lateral quadrants of the left ventricle.

No other pathologic process has been found to produce acute SWMA to the same degree as myocardial ischemia resulting from the acute disruption of myocardial blood flow. Conversely, correction of myocardial blood flow reverses SWMA associated with coronary insufficiency.[117]

TABLE 21–26. Grading Wall Motion Abnormalities

Grade	Features	Criterion (Radial Shortening and Thickening During Systole)
1	Normal	>30%
2	Mild hypokinesis	10–30%
3	Severe hypokinesis	<10%
4	Akinesis	None
5	Dyskinesia	Bulging out and thinning

(Modified from Calahan MK: Transesophageal echocardiography: Should I be using it? *In* ASA Annual Refresher Course Series. Vol. 18. Park Ridge, IL.)

Future Applications

The pioneering studies of TEE have confirmed its sensitivity as a qualitative monitor of ischemia when analyzed off line. For the technique to become popular as an intraoperative monitor, it must be determined that SWMA can be detected with confidence in all patients at risk for myocardial ischemia and that SWMA can be detected on line in the operating room by practicing anesthesiologists. Of note is that SWMA outside of the literally paper-thin plane being observed will go unnoticed. Thus, TEE supplements but does not replace ECG monitoring. To that end, biplane probes, split-screen displays, and enhanced computer graphics may facilitate intraoperative detection. Quantitative computer analysis of SWMA is currently undergoing investigation and offers anesthesiologists the potential for continuous evaluation of wall motion (smaller segments) without the need for constant observation of TEE images.

Analysis of Valvular Function

TEE has advantages over precordial echocardiographic imaging techniques in assessing the structure and function of AV valves. Higher-quality images are provided without compromising the sterility of the surgical field. Analysis of mitral regurgitation is often dramatic when color flow studies are performed. Color flow mapping is helpful in ascertaining diastolic and systolic flow within the atria, across the valves, and in the pulmonary veins.

The clinical performance of prosthetic heart valves and complicating factors such as perforation of leaflets and intracardiac fistulas can be evaluated before and after surgical correction. With increasing degrees of mitral regurgitation, antegrade systolic flow in the pulmonary veins becomes abnormal. Experienced echocardiographers can also help cardiac surgeons to identify potential problems during rewarming before cessation of cardiopulmonary bypass.

Effects of Anesthesia

Several investigations have focused attention on the use of echocardiography to assess the effect of anesthesia on ventricular function. Most studies used transthoracic techniques. Narcotic techniques appear to have very little effect on ventricular function.[104, 118] Potent inhalational agents vary in their effects. Table 21–27 annotates the application of echocardiography in assessing the effects of anesthesia on myocardial performance. Clinical assessment of myocardial performance using echocardiographic indices requires careful consideration of loading conditions, heart rate, and differences in blood/gas and tissue/blood partition coefficients of potent inhalational agents.

TABLE 21–27. Echocardiography Assessment of Myocardial Performance: Anesthetic Effects (Healthy Patients)

Agent	Findings
Halothane	26% reduction in ejection fraction*
	36% reduction in Vcf
	Significant decrease in Fs
Enflurane	Insignificant
Isoflurane	Insignificant*

Abbreviations: Vcf = circumferential fiber shortening; FS = fractional shortening.
*Studies in children.

Miscellaneous Additional Applications

Aortic Dissection

TEE is a valuable tool for assessing aortic dissections. Comparison studies have demonstrated equivalent sensitivity and specificity with angiography and computed tomographic scanning.[118] Intraoperative monitoring permits assessment of aortic valve function, estimation of luminal thrombus, delineation of aortic size and the extent of dissection, the presence of pericardial fluid, involvement of the coronary ostia, and quantification of flow in the false lumen.[119]

Embolic Events

The technique is of great value in monitoring intraoperative embolic events. Unlike conventional monitoring for air embolus, TEE offers capabilities to monitor and diagnose systemic as well as venous embolic events.[106] Although TEE has been demonstrated to be very sensitive in detecting venous air embolism, its utility as a technique to check for residual intracardiac air after heart surgery has been questioned.[120]

Congenital Lesions

Intraoperative TEE has been advocated for assessing the surgical repair of a wide spectrum of congenital lesions.[121] Single-plane miniaturized TEE probes permit the monitoring of shunt and regurgitant and obstructive lesions in patients as small as 3 kg.[122, 123]

What Problems Must Be Addressed?

Although wide applications for intraoperative TEE monitoring are possible, its availability is limited because of its expense and complexity. Although the use of TEE as a diagnostic tool for defining cardiac morphology in patients of all ages is well established, its role as an integral intraoperative monitor is still emerging. Nevertheless, anesthesiologists involved in the care of patients with heart disease clearly benefit from such TEE imaging.

Evaluations with TEE often influence the conduct of anesthesia. The equipment is cumbersome and requires attention; therefore, many institutions use a team approach when studies are performed intraoperatively. During rewarming, after hypothermic cardiopulmonary bypass, esophageal temperatures often exceed manufacturer's set-points, requiring manual override for imaging.

Despite the potential for esophageal injury, continued observation of anesthetized patients has not revealed increased risks for esophageal damage. Pharyngeal and especially esophageal injury during placement, as well as laryngeal trauma following prolonged TEE, have been described. The size of TEE probes (6–11 mm) makes esophageal passage difficult in some patients.

A complete history of esophageal problems should be taken in all patients for whom TEE is planned. Esophageal tumor or stricture contraindicates TEE evaluation. Esophageal varices have been cited as a contraindication as well, but TEE use during liver transplantation is common and without reported sequelae. Thus, esophageal varices probably should not preclude TEE monitoring if the benefits are thought to outweigh the risks.

URINE OUTPUT

The composition and production of urine offer anesthesiologists insights into the adequacy of the circulation and intraoperative renal function. The kidneys, more than any other organ, have a central role in the regulation of blood volume, extracellular fluid volume, osmolality of body fluids, concentration of ions, acidity, and excretion of drugs and metabolic by-products. Thus, their function is a reflection of overall cardiovascular performance and stability. For this reason, monitoring the quality and quantity of urine output is included in this chapter. The indications for bladder catheterization are listed in Table 21–28.

What Factors Determine Urine Output?

Urine homeostasis results from two variables, glomerular filtration and tubular reabsorption. Additionally, unwanted substances can be cleared by tubular secretion. In healthy kidneys, the glomerular filtration rate (GFR) is autoregulated by pressure inside the glomerular capillaries, pressure outside Bowman's capsule, and the colloid oncotic pressure (COP).

Autoregulation of Glomerular Filtration and Renal Blood Flow

The mechanisms for autoregulation of glomerular filtration and renal blood flow (RBF) are complex. When glomerular filtration falls, a decrease in the concentration of sodium at the macula densa results. The reduction of sodium and chloride ions at the macula densa initiates two responses. The afferent arterioles dilate, and the juxtaglomerular cells release renin, causing the formation of angiotensin II. Angiotensin II induces efferent arterioles to constrict, favoring the reabsorption of water and electrolytes by reducing peritubular pressure and increasing the COP of the peritubular capillaries. Feedback mechanisms that enhance tubular reabsorption of water and salt reduce the quantity of urine production.

Healthy kidneys maintain (autoregulate) RBF and GFR as long as the MAP is sustained between 80 and 180 mm Hg.[123] The precise mechanism for autoregulation is not fully understood. Apart from autoregulation, renal function is controlled by the interaction of complex neurohumoral systems that are influenced by trauma, surgical stress, and drug therapy to various degrees (Fig. 21–16).

TABLE 21–28. Indications for Bladder Catheterization and Monitoring of Urine Output

During procedures anticipated to last longer than 4 h
During pelvic surgery (potential damage to ureters)
When the potential for large blood losses, excessive fluid losses, or replacement is anticipated
During deliberate hypotensive anesthesia
When diuretic therapy is anticipated
In all major vascular procedures requiring aortic cross-clamp
In most intracranial neurosurgical procedures
In all procedures using cardiopulmonary bypass
In all procedures performed after major trauma or burns
Any time monitoring hourly urine output is deemed helpful during anesthesia care

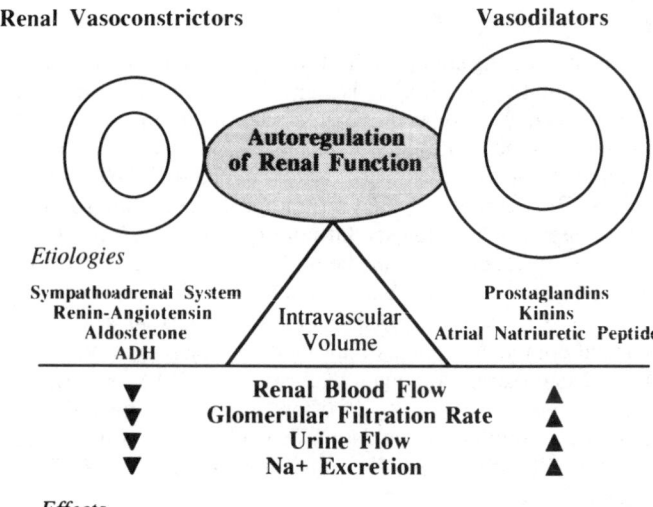

FIGURE 21–16. Factors affecting renal function during anesthesia.

What Factors Promote Vasoconstriction and Salt Retention?

Each day, 160 to 180 L of water is filtered by the kidneys. This ultrafiltrate of plasma contains 300 mOsm of solute per liter. Nephrologists define *oliguria* as a reduction of urine output to <0.3 mL $\cdot$ kg^{-1} $\cdot$ h^{-1}. Anesthesiologists become concerned when intraoperative urine output falls to <0.5 to 1 mL $\cdot$ kg^{-1} $\cdot$ h^{-1}. Studies suggest that the effects of anesthetic agents and techniques on renal function are mediated by extrarenal circulatory changes rather than by direct action on kidney function.[124] Surgical wounds (stress stimulation) have been suggested to promote the stimulation of systems that foster vasoconstriction and salt retention.

Catecholamines

The release of norepinephrine from autonomic nerve fibers and stimulation of the adrenal medulla diminish GFR and RBF. Slight α-adrenergic stimulation is not associated with significant changes. However, high-level α-adrenergic stimulation promotes afferent arteriolar vasoconstriction, decreasing RBF and GFR. Beta-adrenergic stimulation is associated with the release of renin from the juxtamedullary apparatus. Therefore, increases in adrenergic tone associated with intraoperative events may promote vasoconstriction and sodium retention.

Renin-Angiotensin-Aldosterone

The renin-angiotensin-aldosterone complex (RAAC) is important in regulating GFR, vasoconstriction, and salt homeostasis. Renin release is controlled by several factors. Baroreceptors in the renal afferent arterioles are primary modulators of the RAAC. Beta-adrenergic receptors in the vicinity of the juxtaglomerular cells also influence the release of renin. In addition to its vascular and renal effects, angiotensin II activation promotes the secretion of aldosterone from the zona glomerulosa of the adrenal cortex. Aldosterone increases sodium and water absorption from the distal convoluted tubules.

Antidiuretic Hormone

Antidiuretic hormone (ADH) secretion normally is stimulated by changes in osmolality, blood volume, and blood pressure; however, it is also influenced by surgical stimulation. Inappropriate ADH secretion following major surgery may result in fluid retention, hypo-osmolality, and hyponatremia.[125]

Positive-Pressure Ventilation

When controlled ventilation, with or without PEEP, is used postoperatively, urine production often diminishes. This effect results from a contraction of the central circulation (decreased venous return) that concomitantly reduces RBF. Sympathetic, ADH, and renin-angiotensin modulations are the responses that maintain central arterial circulation. For a more extensive review of the effects of positive-pressure ventilation on renal function and the enigmatic associated hormonal interactions, refer to the reports by Berry,[126] Sladen and colleagues,[127] and Hemmer and associates.[128]

What Factors Promote Vasodilatation and Salt Excretion?

A protective role has been defined for the production of intrarenal prostaglandins.[129] During periods of hypotension or ischemia or after catecholamine or angiotensin II stimulation, local prostaglandin production is increased. Prostaglandins produce renal vasodilatation, maintain intrarenal hemodynamics, and block sodium reabsorption within the distal convoluted tubules. Renal prostaglandins modulate renin secretion.[130] Intrarenal kinins also have prominent roles in producing vasodilatation and enhancing the actions of prostaglandins.[131]

A series of peptides that have been extracted from atrial tissues promote natriuresis and interact with the renin-aldosterone axis.[132] If hypotension and hypovolemia ensue during anesthesia, release of renin and atrial natriuretic hormone is triggered. Atrial natriuretic hormone inhibits the release of renin, blocks angiotensin-induced vasoconstriction, and blocks aldosterone release, thereby promoting vasodilatation and salt-losing urine production.

Why Does Oliguria Occur?

Oliguria is common postoperatively. Intraoperative oliguria usually is associated with decreases in circulating blood volume because of inadequate fluid replacement or hidden fluid losses. If severe and persistent hypotension occurs, the potential for oliguric renal failure must be considered in the early postoperative period.

Differential Diagnosis

Urinary diagnostic tests are helpful to distinguish the cause of acute oliguria. Laboratory evaluation of renal function is based on examination of the urine formed elements and blood and urine chemistry studies. Creatinine, urea, and sodium in plasma and urine are central to differentiating prerenal and renal causes of oliguria. Urinalysis may help to differentiate

TABLE 21–29. Diagnostic Tests for Oliguria

Test	Prerenal	Renal
Urinary Na^+ (mEq $\cdot$ L^{-1})	<20	>40
Urine osmolarity (mOsm $\cdot$ L^{-1})	>500	<350
Urine/plasma osmolality	>1.3	<1.1
Urine/plasma urea ratio	>8	<3
Urine/plasma creatinine ratio	>40	<20
Fractional excretion of Na^+ (%)	<1	>2

(Modified from Bauman LA, Prough DS: Acute perioperative renal dysfunction. *In* Post Anesthesia Care. Vender JS, Spies BD (eds). Philadelphia, WB Saunders, 1992, p 147.)

renal from tubular obstruction by assessing the presence or absence of granular casts, epithelial cells, or urine histiocytes.

Table 21–29 lists laboratory values that help to distinguish prerenal and renal oliguria. Urine osmolarity and urine sodium values are readily available intraoperatively. Urea, creatinine, and the fractional excretion of sodium can be measured in the early postoperative period. Potential causes of postoperative oliguria are multifactorial (Table 21–30).

Why Does Polyruia Occur?

A number of physiologic and pathologic processes may result in an increase in urine production. If the kidneys' ability to concentrate or dilute is impaired, urine production can be affected. Intraoperative polyuria requires evaluation.

Fluid Drug Therapy

If hypotonic fluids are administered preoperatively, one should anticipate ADH secretion in response to decreases in

TABLE 21–30. Causes of Perioperative Oliguria

Postrenal etiologies	Catheter obstruction	Kink
	Ureteral obstruction	Calculi
		Prostatism
		Surgical accidents
	Extravasation	Rupture of bladder
		Ureteral disruption
		Catheter disconnection
Prerenal etiologies	Hypovolemia	Hypotension
		Hemorrhage
		Fluid sequestration
		Diuretic dependence
	Cardiovascular failure	Hypotension
		Sepsis
		Myocardial ischemia
	Vascular obstructions	Renal artery
		Thrombosis/embolus
		Renal vein thrombosis
Renal etiologies	Intravascular hemolysis	Transfusion reactions
	Rhabdomyolysis/ myoglobinuria	Malignant hyperpyrexia
		Trauma
		Exotic muscle disease
	Nephrotoxins	Eclampsia (pregnancy related)
		Drug reactions
		Immune complexes

(Modified from Dooley JR, Mazze RI: Oliguria. *In* Complications in Anesthesia. Orkin FR, Cooperman LH (eds.). Philadelphia, JB Lippincott, 1983, p 406.)

serum osmolarity. Glucose-containing fluids often produce an osmotic diuresis, because the glucose load may exceed the renal threshold for reabsorption. Reducing glucose administration to 50 to 100 g during surgery diminishes the incidence of intraoperative polyuria.

Diuretics

Perioperative diuretic therapy may also account for increased urine production. Diuretics are often administered to neurosurgical or ophthalmologic patients. Mannitol is an important component of cardiopulmonary bypass primes and cardioplegia solutions.

Diabetes Insipidus

The potential for surgically induced diabetes insipidus should be entertained after neurosurgical procedures near the supraopticohypophyseal axis. In most instances, adequate stores of ADH are present to maintain water conservation for 12 hours.

Anesthetic Agents

Most anesthetic agents and techniques lower GFR and RBF so that urine output is diminished compared with the awake state.[133] These effects are related to changes in renal hemodynamics and are readily reversible.

A syndrome of polyuric renal failure, characterized by loss of concentrating ability and progressive azotemia, sometimes occurs after the administration of methoxyflurane. Studies of rats[134] and humans[135] show that inorganic fluoride (Fi) is responsible for this reversible renal tubular dysfunction. Fi is a metabolite of methoxyflurane and enflurane. Isoflurane and halothane produce negligible amounts of Fi. In most instances, the threshold for Fi-induced polyuric renal failure approaches 100 to 150 μmol $\cdot$ L^{-1}. Toxicity may be enhanced by the concomitant administration of aminoglycosides or by prolonged anesthetic exposure in patients with previous renal dysfunction.

References

1. Kurtz CM, Bennett JH, Shapiro H: Electrocardiographic studies during surgical anesthesia. JAMA 1936; 106:434.
2. American Society of Anesthesiologists: Standards for Basic Intraoperative Monitoring (effective January 1, 1994). Park Ridge, IL, American Society of Anesthesiologists, 1994.
3. Bertrand CA, Steiner NV, Jameson AG, et al: Disturbances of cardiac rhythm during anesthesia and surgery. JAMA 1971; 216:1615.
4. Katz RL, Bigger JT: Cardiac arrhythmias during anesthesia and operation. Anesthesiology 1970; 33:193.
5. Angelini L, Feldman MI, Lufschonoski R, et al: Cardiac arrhythmias before and after heart surgery: diagnosis and management. Prog Cardiovasc Dis 1974; 16:469.
6. Slogoff S, Keats AS: Does perioperative myocardial ischemia lead to postoperative myocardial infarction? Anesthesiology 1985; 62:107.
7. Einthoven W, Fahr G, de Waart A: On the direction and manifest size of the variations of potential in the human heart and the influence of the position of the heart on the form of the electrocardiogram. Am Heart J 1950; 40:163.
8. Wilson FN, Kossman CE, Burch GE, et al: Recommendations for standardization of electrocardiography. Circulation 1954; 10:564.
9. Mirvis DM, Berson AS, Goldberger AL, et al: Instrumentation and practice standards for electrocardiographic monitoring in special care units. Circulation 1989; 79:464.
10. Blackburn H, Katigbak R: What ECG lead to take after exercise? Am Heart J 1964; 67:184.
11. London MJ, Hollenberg M, Wong MG, et al: Intraoperative myocardial ischemia: localization by continuous 12-lead electrocardiography. Anesthesiology 1988; 69:232.
12. Palmer CM, Norris MC, Giudici MC, et al: Incidence of electrocardiographic changes during cesarean delivery under regional anesthesia. Anesth Analg 1990; 70:36.
13. Slogoff S, Keats AS, David Y, et al: Incidence of perioperative myocardial ischemia detected by different electrocardiographic systems. Anesthesiology 1990; 73:1074.
14. Haggmark S, Hobner P, Ostman M, et al: Comparison of hemodynamic, electrocardiographic, mechanical, and metabolic indicators of intraoperative myocardial ischemia in vascular patients with coronary artery disease. Anesthesiology 1989; 70:19.
15. Epstein SE, Quyyumi AA, Bonow RD: Current concepts: myocardial ischemia—silent or symptomatic? N Engl J Med 1988; 318:1038.
16. Kotter GS, Bernstein JS, Kotrly KJ, et al: ECG changes detect coronary artery bypass graft occlusion without hemodynamic instability. Anesth Analg 1984; 63:1133.
17. Kotrly KJ, Kotter GVS, Mortara D, et al: Intraoperative detection of myocardial ischemia with an ST segment trend monitoring system. Anesth Analg 1984; 63:343.
18. Gunnar RM, Pietras RJ, Blackaller J, et al: Correlation of vectorcardiographic criteria for myocardial infarction with autopsy findings. Circulation 1967; 35:158.
19. Wit AL, Bigger JT: Possible electrophysiological mechanisms for lethal arrhythmias accompanying myocardial ischemia and infarction. Circulation 1975; 51(Suppl) and 52:III–96.
20. Basnijak ZJ, Kampine JP: Effects of halothane, enflurane, and isoflurane on the SA node. Anesthesiology 1983; 58:314.
21. Meltzer LE, Kitchell JB: The incidence of arrhythmias associated with acute myocardial infarction. Prog Cardiovasc Dis 1966; 9:50.
22. Rubeinstein JJ, Schulman CL, Yurchak PM, et al: Clinical spectrum of the sick sinus syndrome. Circulation 1972; 46:5.
23. Rosen KM, Loeb HS, Sinno MZ, et al: Cardiac conduction in patients with symptomatic sinus node disease. Circulation 1971; 43:836.
24. Sprague DH, Mandel SD: Paroxysmal supraventricular tachycardia during anesthesia. Anesthesiology 1977; 46:75.
25. Haldemann G, Schoer H: Haemodynamic effect of transient atrioventricular dissociation in general anesthesia. Br J Anaesth 1972; 44:159.
26. Chou TE-C: Electrocardiography in Clinical Practice. Philadelphia, WB Saunders, 1991.
27. Kastor JA, Horowitz LN, Harken AH, et al: Clinical electrophysiology of ventricular tachycardia. N Engl J Med 1981; 304:1004.
28. MacDonald DA: Blood Flow in Arteries. London, Edward Arnold, 1974.
29. Cohn JN: Blood pressure measurement in shock. JAMA 1967; 199:118.
30. Simpson JA, Jamieson G, Dickhaus DW, et al: Effect of size of cuff bladder on accuracy of measurement of indirect blood pressure. Am Heart J 1965; 70:206.
31. Geddes LA: The Direct and Indirect Measurement of Blood Pressure. Chicago, Year Book Medical Publishers, 1970.
32. Stegall HF, Kardon MB, Kemmerer WT: Indirect measurement of arterial blood pressure by Doppler ultrasonic sphygmomanometry. J Appl Physiol 1968; 25:793.
33. Poppers PJ, Epstein RM, Donham RT: Automatic ultrasound monitoring of blood pressure during induced hypotension. Anesthesiology 1972; 35:431.
34. Ramsey M: Blood pressure monitoring: automated oscillometric devices. J Clin Monit 1991; 7:56.
35. Ramsey M: Noninvasive automatic determination of mean arterial blood pressure. Med Biol Eng Comput 1979; 17:11.
36. Epstein RH, Huffnagle S, Barkowski RR: Comparative accuracies of a finger blood pressure monitor and an oscillometric blood pressure monitor. J Clin Monit 1991; 7:161.
37. Sy WP: Ulnar nerve palsy possibly related to use of automatically cycled blood pressure cuff. Anesth Analg 1981; 60:687.
38. Peñaz J: Photoelectric measurement of blood pressure volume and flow in the finger. Digest, 10th International Conference of Medical Biological Engineers, 1973, p 104.
39. Kurki T, Smith NT, Head N, et al: Noninvasive continuous blood pressure measurement from the finger: optimal measurement conditions and factors affecting reliability. J Clin Monit 1987; 3:6.
40. Branwell JC, Hill AV: The velocity of the pulse wave in man. Proc Soc Lond [Biol] 1922; 93:298.
41. Kemmotsu O, Ueda M, Otsuka MU, et al: Evaluation of arterial tonometry for noninvasive, continuous blood pressure monitoring during anesthesia. Anesthesiology 1990; 71:A406.
42. Gardner RM: Blood pressure—dynamic response needs. Anesthesiology 1981; 54:227.

43. Hipkins SF, Rutten AJ, Runciman WB: Experimental analysis of catheter-manometer systems in vitro and in vivo. Anesthesiology 1989; 71:893.

44. Slogoff S, Keats AS, Arlund C: On the safety of radial artery cannulation. Anesthesiology 1980; 59:42.

45. Bedford RF, Wollman H: Complications of percutaneous radial artery cannulation: an objective prospective study in man. Anesthesiology 1973; 38:232.

46. Davis FM, Steward JM: Radial artery cannulation. Br J Anaesth 1980; 52:674.

47. Downs JB, Rackstein AD, Klein EF, et al: Hazards of radial artery catheterization. Anesthesiology 1973; 38:283.

48. Bedford RF: Removal of radial artery thrombi following percutaneous cannulation for monitoring. Anesthesiology 1977; 46:430.

49. Vender JS, Watts RD: Differential diagnosis of hand ischemia in the presence of an arterial cannula. Anesth Analg 1982; 61:465.

50. Wilkins RG: Radial artery cannulation and ischaemic damage: a review. Anaesthesia 1985; 40:896.

51. Sanford TJ: Internal jugular vein cannulation versus subclavian cannulation: an anesthesiologist's view: the right internal jugular vein. J Clin Monit 1985; 1:58.

52. Mark JB: Central venous pressure monitoring: clinical insights beyond the numbers. J Cardiothorac Vasc Anesth 1991; 5:163.

53. Trager MA, Feinberg BI, Kaplan JA: Right ventricular ischemia diagnosed by an esophageal electrocardiogram and right atrial pressure tracing. J Cardiothorac Anesth 1987; 1:123.

54. Sharkey SW: Beyond the wedge: clinical physiology and the Swan-Ganz catheter. Am J Med 1987; 83:111.

55. Maki DG: Infections associated with intravascular lines. In Current Topics in Clinical Infectious Disease. Swartz M, Remington J (eds). New York, McGraw-Hill, 1982, pp 309–363.

56. Hoffman KK, Weber DJ, Gregory P, et al: Transparent polyurethane film as an intravenous catheter dressing. JAMA 1992; 276:2072.

57. Civetta JM, Gabel JC: Flow-directed pulmonary artery catheterization. Indications and modification of technique. Ann Surg 1972; 176:753.

58. Samii K, Counseiller C, Viars P: Central venous pressure and pulmonary wedge pressure. Arch Surg 1976; 111:1122.

59. Swan HJC, Ganz W, Forrester JS, et al: Catheterization of the heart in man with the use of flow-directed balloon-tipped catheters. N Engl J Med 1970; 283:447.

60. Vender J: Pulmonary artery catheter monitoring. Anesth Clin North Am 1988; 6:743.

61. Tuman KJ, Carroll GC, Ivankovich AD: Pitfalls of interpretations of pulmonary artery catheter data. J Cardiovasc Anesth 1989; 3:625.

62. West JB, Dollery CT, Naimark A: Distribution of blood flow in isolated lung: relation to vascular and alveolar pressures. J Appl Physiol 1984; 19:713.

63. Marini JJ: Obtaining meaningful data from the Swan-Ganz catheter. Crit Care Clin 1988; 2:572.

64. Carlile PV: Pitfalls in the interpretation of hemodynamic data. Prog Crit Care Med 1985; 2:69.

65. Jardin F, Farcot JC, Boisante L, et al: Influence of positive end-expiratory pressure on left ventricular performance. N Engl J Med 1981; 305:387.

66. Weber KT, Janiold JS, Shroff S, et al: Contractile mechanics and interaction of the right and left ventricles. Am J Cardiol 1981; 47:686.

67. Marini JJ: Hemodynamic monitoring with the pulmonary artery catheter. Crit Care Clin 1986; 2:551.

68. Kaplan JA, Wells PH: Early diagnosis of myocardial ischemia using the pulmonary arterial catheter. Anesth Analg 1981; 60:792.

69. Iberti TJ, Fischer EP, Leibowitz AB, et al: A multicenter study of physicians knowledge of the pulmonary artery catheter. Pulmonary artery study group. JAMA 1990; 264:2928.

70. Puri VK, Carlson RW, Bander JT, et al: Complications of vascular catheterization in the critically ill. Crit Care Med 1980; 8:495.

71. Shah KB, Rao TLK, Laughlin S, et al: A review of pulmonary artery catheterization in 6,245 patients. Anesthesiology 1984; 61:27.

72. Voukydis PC, Cohen SI: Catheter-induced arrhythmias. Am Heart J 1974; 88:588.

73. Robin ED: Death by pulmonary artery flow-directed catheter. Time for a moratorium (Editorial). Chest 1987; 94:727.

74. Salmenpera M, Peltola K, Rosenberg P: Does prophylactic lidocaine control cardiac arrhythmias associated with pulmonary artery catheterization? Anesthesiology 1982; 56:210.

75. Keusch DJ, Winters S, Thys DM: The patient's position influences the incidence of dysrhythmias during pulmonary artery catheterization. Anesthesiology 1989; 70:582.

76. Band JD, Maki DG: Infections caused by arterial catheters used for hemodynamic monitoring. Am J Med 1979; 67:735.

77. Barash PG, Nardi D, Hammond G, et al: Catheter-induced pulmonary artery perforation, mechanisms, and management and modifications. J Thorac Cardiovasc Surg 1981; 82:5.

78. Heard SO, Davis LF, She&vertz RJ, et al: Influence of sterile protective sleeves on the sterility of pulmonary artery catheters. Crit Care Med 1987; 15:499.

79. Mohsinifar Z, Goldbach P, Tachkin DP, et al: Relationship between O_2 delivery and O_2 consumption in the adult respiratory distress syndrome. Chest 1983; 84:267.

80. Räsänen J, Downs JB: Titration of continuous positive airway pressure by real-time dual oximetry. Crit Care Med 1987; 15(a):395.

81. Kay H, Afshari M, Barash PG, et al: Measurement of ejection fraction by thermal dilution techniques. J Surg Res 1983; 34:337.

82. Urban P, Scheidegger D, Gabathular J, et al: Thermodilution determination of right ventricular volume and ejection fraction: a comparison with biplane angiography. Crit Care Med 1987; 15:652.

83. Taylar SH, Silke B: Is the measurement of cardiac output useful in clinical practice? Br J Anaesth 1988; 60:90S.

84. Ganz W, Donoso R, Marcus HS, et al: A new technique for measurement of cardiac output by thermodilution in man. Am J Cardiol 1971; 27:392.

85. Hamilton WF, Moore JW, Kinsman JM, et al: Studies on the circulation IV: further analysis of the injection method and of changes in hemodynamics under physiologic and pathologic condition. Am J Physiol 1932; 99:534.

86. Truccone NJ, Spontnitz HM, Gersony WM, et al: Cardiac output in infants and children after open-heart surgery. J Thorac Cardiovasc Surg 1976; 71:410.

87. Fegler G: Measurement of cardiac output in anesthetized animals by thermodilution method. Q J Exp Physiol 1954; 39:153.

88. Shellock FG, Riedinger MS, Bateman TM, et al: Thermodilution cardiac output determination in hypothermic postcardiac surgery patients: room vs. iced temperature injectate. Crit Care Med 1983; 11:668.

89. Fischer AP, Benis AM, Jurado RA, et al: Analysis of errors in measurement of cardiac output by simultaneous dye and thermal dilution in cardiothoracic surgical patients. Cardiovasc Res 1978; 12:190.

90. Levitt JM, Replogle RL: Thermodilution cardiac output: a critical analysis and review of the literature. J Surg Res 1979; 27:392.

91. Wetzel RC, Latson TW: Major errors in thermodilution cardiac output measurement during rapid volume infusion. Anesthesiology 1985; 62:684.

92. Stetz CW, Miller RG, Kelly CE, et al: Reliability of the thermodilution method in the determination of cardiac output in clinical practice. Am Rev Respir Dis 1982; 126:1002.

93. Segal J, Gaudiani V, Nishimura T: Continuous determination of cardiac output using a flow-directed Doppler pulmonary artery catheter. J Cardiothorac Vasc Anesth 1991; 5:309.

94. Segal J, Nassi M, Ford AJ, et al: Instantaneous and continuous cardiac output in humans obtained with a Doppler pulmonary artery catheter. J Am Coll Cardiol 1990; 16:1398.

95. Yelderman M: Continuous measurement of cardiac output with the use of stochastic system identification techniques. J Clin Monit 1990; 6:322.

96. Kubicek WG, Karnegis JN, Patterson RP, et al: Development and evaluation of an impedance cardiac output system. Aerospace Med 1966; 37:1208.

97. Bernstein DP: A new stroke volume equation for thoracic electrical bioimpedance: theory and rationale. Crit Care Med 1986; 14:902.

98. Kamal GD, Symreng T, Starr J: Inconsistent esophageal Doppler cardiac output during acute blood loss. Anesthesiology 1990; 72:95.

99. Siegel LC, Pearl RG: Noninvasive cardiac output measurement: troubled technologies and troubled studies. Anesth Analg 1992; 74:790.

100. Siegel LC, Shafer SL, Martinez GM, et al: Simultaneous measurements of cardiac output by thermodilution, esophageal Doppler, and electrical impedance in anesthetized patients. J Cardiothorac Anesth 1988; 2:590.

101. Abrams JH, Weber RE, Holman KD: Continuous cardiac output determination using transtracheal Doppler: initial results in humans. Anesthesiology 1989; 71:11.

102. Urbanowitz JH, Kernoff RE, Oppenheim G, et al: Transesophageal echocardiography and its potential for esophageal damage. Anesthesiology 1990; 72:40.

103. Martin RW, Bashein G: Measurement of stroke volume with three-dimensional transesophageal ultrasonic scanning. Comparison with thermodilution measurement. Anesthesiology 1989; 70:470.

104. Roizen MF, Beaupre PN, Alpert RA, et al: Monitoring with two-dimensional transesophageal echocardiography; comparison of myocardial

function in patients undergoing supraceliac, suprarenal-infrarenal or infrarenal aortic occlusion. J Vasc Surg 1984; 1:300.

105. Topol EJ, Humphrey LS, Blanck TJJ, et al: Characterization of postcardiopulmonary bypass hypotension with intraoperative transesophageal echocardiography (Abstract). Anesthesiology 1983; 59:2a.

106. Cucchiara RF, Seward JB, Nishmura RA, et al: Identification of patent foramen ovale during sitting position craniotomy by transesophageal echocardiography with positive airway pressure. Anesthesiology 1985; 63:107.

107. Powis RL, Powis W: A Thinker's Guide to Ultrasonic Imaging. Baltimore, Urban & Schwarzenberg, 1984.

108. Lang RM, Feinstein SB, Feldman T, et al: Contrast echocardiography for evaluation of myocardial perfusion: effects of coronary angioplasty. J Am Coll Cardiol 1986; 8:232.

109. Kisso J, Adams DB, Belkin RN: Doppler color flow imaging. New York, Churchill Livingstone, 1988.

110. Czer LSC, Maurer G, Bolger AF, et al: Intraoperative evaluation of mitral regurgitation by Doppler color flow mapping. Circulation 1987; 76(Suppl 3):III.

111. Schlüter M, Langenstein BA, Polster J, et al: Transesophageal cross-sectional echocardiography with a phased array transducer system. Techniques and initial clinical results. Br Heart J 1982; 48:67.

112. Forrester JS, Wyatt HL, Paluz PL, et al: Functional significance of regional ischemic contraction abnormalities. Circulation 1976; 54:64.

113. Kisslo J, Robertson D, Gilbert B, et al: A comparison of real-time, two-dimensional echocardiography and cineangiography in detecting left ventricular asynergy. Circulation 1977; 55:134.

114. Smith JS, Cahalan MK, Benefiel DJ, et al: Intraoperative detection of myocardial ischemia in high risk patients: electrocardiography versus two-dimensional transesophageal echocardiography. Circulation 1985; 72:1015.

115. von Daele M, Sutherland GR, Mitchell MM, et al: Do changes in pulmonary capillary wedge pressure adequately reflect myocardial ischemia during anesthesia? Circulation 1990; 81:865.

116. Leung JM, O'Kelly B, Browner WS, et al: Prognostic importance of postbypass regional wall motion abnormalities in patients undergoing coronary artery bypass graft surgery. Anesthesiology 1989; 71:16.

117. Koolen JJ, Visser CA, Van Wezel WB, et al: Influence of coronary artery bypass surgery on regional left ventricular wall motion: an intraoperative two-dimensional transesophageal echocardiography study. J Cardiothorac Anesth 1987; 1:276.

118. Schieber M, Stiller R, Cook R: Cardiovascular and pharmacodynamic effects of high-dose fentanyl in newborn piglets. Anesthesiology 1985; 63:166.

119. Erbel R, Engberding R, Daniel W, et al: Echocardiography in diagnosis of aortic dissection. Lancet 1989; i:457.

120. Topol EJ, Humphrey LS, Borkon AM, et al: Value of intraoperative left ventricular microbubbles detected by transesophageal two-dimensional echocardiography in predicting neurologic outcome after cardiac operations. Am J Cardiol 1985; 56:773.

121. Muhiudeen IA, Roberson DA, Silverman NH, et al: Intraoperative echocardiography for evaluation of congenital heart defects in infants and children. Anesthesiology 1992; 76:165.

122. Ritter SB: Transesophageal real-time echocardiography in infants and children with congenital heart disease. J Am Coll Cardiol 1991; 18:1991.

123. Shipley RE, Study RS: Changes in renal blood flow, extraction of insulin, glomerular filtration rate, tissue pressure and urine flow with acute alterations of renal artery pressure. Am J Physiol 1951; 197:676.

124. Sladen RN: Effect of anesthesia and surgery on renal function. Crit Care Clin 1987; 3:373.

125. Bartter FC, Schwartz WB: The syndrome of inappropriate secretion of antidiuretic hormone. Am J Med 1967; 42:790.

126. Berry A: Respiratory support and renal function. Anesthesiology 1981; 55:655.

127. Sladen A, Laver MB, Pontoppidan H: Pulmonary complications and water retention in prolonged mechanical ventilation. N Engl J Med 1968; 279:448.

128. Hemmer M, Viguerat CE, Suter PM, et al: Urinary antidiuretic hormone excretion during mechanical ventilation and weaning in man. Anesthesiology 1980; 52:399.

129. Anggard E, Oliw E: Formation and metabolism of prostaglandins in the kidney. Kidney Int 1981; 19:771.

130. Gerber JG, Olsen RD, Nies AS: Interrelationship between prostaglandins and renin release. Kidney Int 1981; 19:816.

131. Nasjletti A, Malik KU: Renal kinin-prostaglandin relationship: implications for renal function. Kidney Int 1981; 19:860.

132. Laragh JH: Atrial natriuretic hormone, the renin-aldosterone axis, and blood pressure-electrolyte homeostasis. N Engl J Med 1985; 313:1330.

133. Priano LLO: Effects of anesthetic agents on renal function. *In* Refresher Courses in Anesthesiology. Vol. 13. Barash PG (ed). Philadelphia, JB Lippincott, 1985, p 143.

134. Cousins MJ, Mazze RI, Kosek JC: The etiology of methoxyflurane nephrotoxicity. J Pharmacol Exp Ther 1974; 190:523.

135. Cousins MJ, Mazze RI: Methoxyflurane nephrotoxicity: a study of dose response in man. JAMA 1973; 225:1611.

22

Monitoring the Nervous System

MICHAEL E. MAHLA, M.D.

The central and peripheral nervous systems can be readily examined in an awake patient to determine whether they are functioning normally. This examination may consist of a neurological physical examination and laboratory tests such as an electroencephalogram (EEG) or a magnetic resonance imaging (MRI) study, or both. Abnormalities of the central nervous system (CNS) (e.g., aneurysms, tumors), its supporting structures (e.g., spondylitic myelopathy, scoliosis), or its blood supply (e.g., carotid artery arteriosclerosis, thoracoabdominal aortic or intracranial aneurysms) may require surgery for correction. When surgery is required, the patient must be prevented from experiencing the pain associated with operation.

Some operations may be performed under local or regional anesthesia with the patient awake. The parts of the patient's nervous system not anesthetized may then be examined while surgery is being performed. However, local or regional anesthesia is inadequate for many operations, and general anesthesia must be used. When general anesthesia is used, the nervous system can no longer be assessed by neurologic examination unless the patient is awakened during the operation. Over the past several decades, clinicians have begun to use tests previously used only in the diagnostic laboratory as continuous intraoperative "monitors" for various portions of the central and peripheral nervous systems.

Nervous system monitors may be divided into those that assess nervous system blood flow and those that assess nervous system function (Table 22–1). This chapter provides an overview and clinical examples of how different diagnostic tests have been adapted for such monitoring during surgery. Common surgical procedures in which such monitors have been found useful are presented in Table 22–2.

IMPLICATIONS FOR INTRAOPERATIVE MANAGEMENT

For a monitor of the nervous system to have maximum utility, it must meet the requirements set forth in Table 22–3. Monitors measure function only at the time they are being used. No monitor in the operating room has been shown to change or reliably predict outcome. The electrocardiogram (ECG) used in the operating room can detect only a small fraction of the number of instances of myocardial ischemia that occurs during surgery, even if it is watched continuously (and it is not!). Certainly, patients with intraoperative ischemia detected by ECG have a higher likelihood of perioperative myocardial infarction, but ECG detection of intraoperative ischemia does not reliably predict myocardial infarction, nor does its absence guarantee that myocardial infarction will not occur postoperatively.

No studies demonstrate that monitoring of the ECG during surgery reduces the likelihood of perioperative myocardial infarction or even of ischemia, yet ECG monitoring is a standard of care according to the American Society of Anesthesiolo-

TABLE 22–1. Monitors of the Nervous System

Monitors of blood flow	Blood pressure
	Intracranial pressure
	Jugular venous po_2
	Radioactive (^{133}Xe) washout
	Transcranial Doppler blood flow velocity
Monitors of function	
Neurologic examination	Discontinuous: wake-up test
	Continuous: local or regional technique
EEG	Scalp recordings (unprocessed, processed)
	Direct cortical recordings
Evoked potentials	*Somatosensory*
	Cortical: scalp recordings; cortical recordings
	Subcortical: surface recordings; direct recordings
	Peripheral: surface recordings; direct nerve recordings
	Auditory
	Brainstem (BAEPs)
	Middle latency cortical (MLAEPs)
	Visual (VEPs)
	Cortical
	Direct nerve recordings
	Motor (MEPs)
	Electrical or magnetic cortical stimulation
	Electrical or magnetic spinal cord stimulation
	Electromyography
	Peripheral muscle recordings
	Facial nerve monitoring: active and passive
	Other cranial nerve monitoring

TABLE 22–2. Surgical Procedures in Which Electrophysiologic Monitoring Is Used Successfully

Operation	Monitor
Carotid endarterectomy	Awake patient, EEG, SSEP, TCD, rCBF
Thoracoabdominal aneurysm repair, coarctation of aorta repair	SSEP, MEP
Posterior spinal fusion, anterior cervical fusion, vertebral body resection	SSEP, MEP, wake-up test
Intracranial aneurysm clipping	SSEP, VEP, BAEP, EEG, TCD, rCBF
Resection of intracranial or spinal cord tumor	SSEP, BAEP, VEP, EEG, EMG, MEP
Selective dorsal rhizotomy	EMG, SSEP
Induced hypotension (during many different operations)	EEG, SSEP, BAEP
Microvascular decompression of cranial nerve V or VII	BAEP, EMG

Abbreviations: SSEP = somatosensory evoked potential; MEP = motor evoked potential; BAEP = brainstem auditory evoked potential; EMG = electromyogram; TCD = transcranial Doppler; rCBF = regional cerebral blood flow (using ^{133}Xe).

gists. Most clinicians who routinely utilize neurologic monitoring have become convinced of its utility, not because scientific studies have demonstrated its usefulness, but rather because cases in which major changes in therapy guided by monitoring have resulted in good outcome. These clinicians would be totally unwilling at this point in time to participate in prospective studies designed to test the utility of neurologic monitoring, just as many anesthesiologists would be uncomfortable with testing the utility of pulse oximetry, capnometry, and blood pressure monitoring.

How Well Do Monitors of Neurologic Function Predict Outcome?

Numerous retrospective studies have addressed this question. Most utilized either EEG, somatosensory evoked potentials (SSEPs), or brainstem auditory evoked potentials (BAEPs) as monitors of neurologic function, and their results were very impressive. In a series of >1000 patients undergoing carotid endarterectomy at the Mayo Clinic, no patient awakened with a new neurologic deficit that was not detected by EEG.[1] Monitoring of evoked potentials has a similar accuracy record for scoliosis surgery.[2-6] However, a few cases have been reported in which neurologic monitoring was used and bad neurologic outcome occurred, even though there was no

TABLE 22–3. Requirements for a Nervous System Monitor

- The monitor must reflect the function of the part of the nervous system at risk from either surgery or compromise of blood supply
- The operator must understand the anatomic pathways assessed by the monitor and the pathophysiologic mechanisms of injury that might occur during surgery
- The monitor should be used continuously, if possible, particularly during periods of risk
- The number of other factors affecting the monitor must be kept to a minimum
- Strict quality control must be observed to avoid technical problems with recordings

change in the monitored parameters (i.e., false-negative results).[7, 8] Indeed, it would be extremely surprising if such cases were not reported.

Even if all of the reported false-negative results were valid (most were not), the number of such events is exceedingly small compared with the total number of patients monitored.[9] Many of these results were generated by an inappropriate use of the monitor—for example, the monitored pathway did not correspond to the part of the nervous system at risk from the operation, or inadequate quality control resulted in technical problems with the recordings. However, some of the reports of unacceptable outcomes have improved our understanding of how well the function of the monitored pathway predicts the function of adjacent areas of the brain and spinal cord. As a result, we are better able to define the monitor's limitations.[8, 10]

Cases in which a perceived or real failure of a monitor occurred must be kept in perspective. When used carefully and appropriately, intraoperative neurologic monitoring appears to be useful for the early detection of a change in the monitored function and for the initiation of therapeutic interventions to prevent permanent neurologic injury.

THE CLINICAL NEUROLOGIC EXAMINATION

Why Is Preoperative Assessment Important?

If the clinical neurologic examination is to be used as a monitor of function during surgery (or after emergence from anesthesia), the clinician must know the level of baseline function. A patient who cannot perform a task preoperatively cannot be expected to perform this task during surgery or postoperatively. For example, if a wake-up test is planned during scoliosis surgery, one should ensure that the necessary commands (e.g., "move your toes," and "squeeze my hand") can be followed preoperatively. A patient with a pre-existing motor weakness from a stroke does not function immediately following carotid endarterectomy. On the contrary, pre-existing neurologic deficits may be transiently aggravated by general anesthesia. A patient with a preoperative mild residual left hemiparesis, for example, may experience a more dense motor weakness for a few hours postoperatively.

How Can the Examination Be Used Intraoperatively?

The Wake-Up Test

The neurologic examination may be used intraoperatively either intermittently (the wake-up test) or continuously (during local or regional anesthesia). The wake-up test is used to test neurologic function following a *reversible* surgical manipulation that has the potential to cause neurologic damage. Nothing is gained by awakening a patient to assess neurologic function if nothing can be done to correct a problem that is detected.

The wake-up test can be used safely only when movement will not cause damage. As an example, waking a patient following clipping of an aneurysm to assess function is extremely hazardous. Movement of a patient secured in a pin head holder may cause cervical spine injury as well as severe scalp lacerations. In addition, coughing, straining, and hypertension associated with wake-up may cause cerebral swelling. The test is most commonly used following distraction of the spinal column during surgery for correction of kyphoscoliosis.

Techniques

Table 22–4 shows one of the many effective techniques for applying the wake-up test. The hypnotic (but not the analgesic) component of the anesthetic is reversed for a brief period, and the patient is asked to follow simple commands with both the upper extremities (not at risk from surgery) and the lower extremities (at risk from surgery). The patient must follow a command voluntarily. Interruption of the blood supply to the corticospinal tracts in the thoracic spinal cord results in complete failure of voluntary lower extremity movement. Reflex movement in response to pain, however, will still be intact as long as blood supply to the lumbar cord is intact and the patient is not experiencing ''spinal shock.'' Thus, grasping the leg and applying a painful stimulus may evoke movement of the leg via spinal reflex and is not an appropriate method of applying the wake-up test.

Validity

The wake-up test has been considered for many years to be the gold standard for assessment of spinal cord function during scoliosis surgery. However, its sensitivity is open to question. The test is applied only intermittently. Long periods occur in which nervous system function is unknown. Thus, the effects of induced hypotension, which potentially places spinal cord function at risk, particularly when distraction is applied to the spinal column, are not assessed except during the test performance.

The appropriate time or times to apply the wake-up test are not clear. Both the spinal cord and brain have gray and white

TABLE 22–5. Some Procedures During Which the Clinical Neurologic Examination Has Been Applied, and Anesthetic Techniques That May Be Used in Them

Procedure	Anesthetic Technique or Techniques
Carotid endarterectomy	Local infiltration, cervical plexus block interscalene block, ± sedation
Electrocorticography and resection of seizure focus	Local infiltration, multiple nerve blocks, ± sedation
Resection of brain tumor from eloquent area of the cortex	Local infiltration, multiple nerve blocks, ± sedation
Non-neurologic surgery on patient with head or neck injury following trauma or otherwise unstable CNS function	Local infiltration, nerve blocks, epidural or spinal anesthesia, ± sedation

matter. Gray matter has a higher metabolic need for oxygen (O_2) and stops functioning within seconds after a complete interruption in blood supply. White matter, which consumes much less O_2, may continue to function for many minutes after a complete interruption. Partial interruption of blood supply to white matter may take much longer (even hours) to manifest loss of function. Thus, a wake-up test applied immediately after spinal column distraction may fail to detect loss of blood flow to white matter pathways in the midthoracic spinal cord (the area at highest risk for ischemia) and cannot reliably detect partial loss of blood flow that may later become critical.

In summary, the wake-up test can evaluate both motor and sensory function at the time it is applied. It cannot assess function at other times during the procedure. Despite these shortcomings, results of the wake-up test seem to correlate well with neurologic outcome (in only one reported case and in one case in my personal experience did a patient demonstrate a neurologic deficit postoperatively that was not detected by an intraoperative wake-up test).[11, 12]

Potential Complications

The wake-up test is potentially dangerous, since the patient may become agitated and dislodge monitoring, life-support, and surgical instrumentation. Ideally, the test is applied in conjunction with other less dangerous and more continuous forms of neurologic function monitoring. In this way, it can be used as a confirmatory test when the results of other monitoring are uninterpretable or when such monitoring suggests a potential problem.

Continuous Clinical Monitoring

Table 22–5 lists operations in which local or regional anesthesia has been used successfully for continuous clinical CNS assessment. The level of sedation and airway accessibility are two special considerations during these operations (Table 22–6).

Continuous assessment of the awake patient is extremely useful in any situation in which unstable CNS function may occur. Patients under local or regional anesthesia who have an unstable neck (e.g., in rheumatoid arthritis, or in cervical myelopathy secondary to degenerative arthritis) may be positioned while they are awake, and neurologic examination can be conducted during surgery. A patient with compromised

TABLE 22–4. How May the Wake-Up Test Be Performed?

Prior to surgery	Document level of preoperative neuologic function. Can the patient understand and perform the necessary commands? Discuss the test to prepare the patient psychologically and to reduce intraoperative panic.
Anesthetic technique	Narcotic infusion with potent inhalation agent, ± nitrous oxide, partial neuromuscular blockade
Prior to wake-up	Document at least two of four twitches with blockade monitor, and partially reverse relaxant if needed (not usually necessary).
Wake-up	1. Discontinue administration of potent inhalation agent and nitrous oxide. 2. Continue narcotic infusion. 3. Begin calling patient by name until he or she responds. 4. Ask the patient to squeeze your hand and then to let go. Asking the patient to let go differentiates a voluntary response from a spinal reflex grasp. 5. After the patient voluntarily follows an upper extremity command, ask the patient to move toes and feet. For completeness, strength in each leg should be compared with that in the arms. Having the patient move the leg in response to pain is not a valid wake-up test! Movement following painful stimulus is a reflex and tests only lumbar cord function. 6. Sensation to a pinprick may be tested in a similar fashion, beginning with the upper extremities and continuing with the lower extremities.

TABLE 22–6. Special Considerations For Monitoring of the Central Nervous System in the Awake Patient

Sedation	Overuse of sedation makes this type of monitoring useless. Recommended drugs: Narcotics: fentanyl, sufentanil, alfentanil Hypnotics: propofol, midazolam,* droperidol Amnestics: midazolam*
Airway	If the surgery itself limits airway access, consider risk/benefit ratio for sedation carefully.

*Avoid use during electrocorticography for location of seizure focus, as this drug or any in its class may depress any seizure activity.

blood supply to the head (severe carotid stenosis) may be assessed continuously to make certain that his or her cerebral perfusion pressure (CPP) is adequate to supply the brain's needs. Neurologic function may be monitored similarly in carotid surgery during application of a carotid cross-clamp.

The clinical neurologic examination also is particularly useful during non-CNS surgery following trauma that produces a closed head injury or cervical spine injury. If regional or local anesthesia is feasible and not contraindicated for other reasons (e.g., the presence of coagulopathy, or lack of cooperation or combativeness on the part of the patient), continuous awake neurologic assessment enables the anesthesiologist to detect neurologic deterioration associated with cerebral edema or delayed intracranial hematoma formation, particularly if intracranial pressure monitoring is not available.

In the case of a neck injury and an unstable cervical spine, the neurologic examination can be followed closely during and following positioning for surgery to ensure that the position has not compromised spinal cord function.

Surgery to Control Seizures

Patients have surgery to control seizures because medical control has proved unsuccessful or because medical treatment produces significant side effects. The location of the seizure focus may be determined by several methods, including preoperative EEG scalp recording, continuous EEG monitoring, recording from depth EEG electrodes or subdural grid electrodes placed in the operating room, and intraoperative direct cortical EEG mapping.

If the location of the focus involves brain tissue that controls important neurologic function such as speech or motor activity, resection might produce an unacceptable neurologic injury. In the awake patient, the function of the area of the brain that is the source of the seizure activity may be tested. An electric current is applied directly to the applicable portion of the cortex. This current causes the patient to experience sensation or movement of a particular portion of the body or temporarily results in the cessation of function of that area of the brain. If application of the electric current to an area of active epileptic activity causes the patient to stop talking until the current is removed, resection of that area of the cortex will likely produce postoperative aphasia. The surgeon can then assess the cost/benefit ratio of resection.

Candidates

Patients who undergo awake monitoring for either neurologic or non-neurologic surgery must be chosen carefully. Those who are very anxious or who cannot understand what

is happening may require so much sedation to tolerate the procedure that an adequate clinical examination cannot be carried out.

When the planned surgical procedure is conducted near or on the head and neck and limits access to the airway, patients frequently feel claustrophobic. Special care with positioning and surgical draping is needed to provide an open space around the face, to allow free breathing, and to permit the patient to maintain visual contact with the surroundings. If neurologic deterioration that results in compromised ventilation occurs, quick access to the airway is necessary. This factor must be considered when determining the advisability of awake CNS monitoring.

Sedation/Analgesia

Awake neurologic monitoring may be difficult during lengthy procedures. A 3-hour limit is probably expedient. Patients often become uncomfortable after lying in the same position for a prolonged period; they may require analgesics and sedation to tolerate the procedure. At some point, such therapy may decrease the sensitivity and specificity of the neurologic examination to detect injury.

Some investigators recommend propofol infusion for "unconscious sedation" during longer procedures that require only limited patient cooperation. For example, during craniotomy for electrocorticography and cortical mapping, the patient may be maintained with propofol during the relatively painful opening portion of the operation.[13] Propofol may then be discontinued, and the patient returns rapidly to baseline neurologic function for the testing period.

This technique has three drawbacks. First, neurologic monitoring is no longer continuous; therefore, it is not helpful during operations such as carotid endarterectomy in which continuous CNS assessment is desirable. Second, oversedation with loss of airway patency and aspiration may occur. Third, some drug effect will persist into the testing period, and the results of neurologic testing, particularly during EEG monitoring, will be affected.[14]

CEREBRAL BLOOD FLOW MONITORING DURING GENERAL ANESTHESIA

During general anesthesia, the clinical neurologic examination, except during the wake-up test, is unavailable. Thus, complete functional monitoring is impossible. However, two other techniques can be readily performed: cerebral blood flow (CBF) monitoring (direct and indirect) and partial functional monitoring (EEG, SSEP and BAEP, motor evoked potential [MEP], and electromyography [EMG]).

Why Is Cerebral Blood Flow Monitoring Important?

The brain has a high metabolic O_2 requirement. When blood flow falls below a level sufficient to meet the cerebral metabolic requirements for O_2 ($CMRo_2$), cerebral function fails before cellular integrity is lost (resulting in permanent damage). Thus, if CBF is restored in a timely fashion, function is also restored without permanent damage. If CBF falls further,

TABLE 22–7. Brain and Spinal Cord Blood Flow Monitors

Monitor Type	Method of Assessment	Location of Blood Flow
Monitors that measure blood flow indirectly	Blood pressure	B, SC
	Intracranial pressure	B, SC
Monitors that measure blood flow directly	Radioactive ^{133}Xe washout	B
	Transcranial Doppler blood flow velocity	B
Monitor that measures balance between O_2 supply and demand directly	Jugular venous pO_2	B
Monitors that measure balance between supply and demand functionally	EEG	B
	SSEPs	B, SC
	MEPs	B, SC

Abbreviations: B = brain; SC = spinal cord.

however, insufficient O_2 is available to supply energy for cell maintenance, and brain cells die. Flow may be monitored indirectly, directly, or by measuring the balance between cerebral O_2 supply and demand (Table 22–7).

How Is Indirect Assessment Performed?

The most commonly monitored parameter that gives information about the adequacy of the blood supply to the brain is blood pressure. Normally, the relationship between blood pressure and CBF is described by the cerebral autoregulation curve (Fig. 22–1). CPP is defined as the mean arterial pressure (MAP) minus the intracranial pressure (ICP) or central venous pressure (CVP), whichever is higher:

$$CPP = MAP - ICP \text{ (or CVP)}$$

CBF is normal and constant over perfusion pressures that range from 50 to 150 mm Hg (see Fig. 22–1). If cerebral autoregulation is intact and ICP is known and constant, blood pressure may be used to indirectly monitor the adequacy of CBF. Blood pressure that maintains CPP between 50 mm Hg and 150 mm Hg provides adequate CBF in normal patients.

What Are the Limitations?

The most important limitation to blood pressure monitoring of CBF is uncertainty regarding the limits of cerebral autoreg-

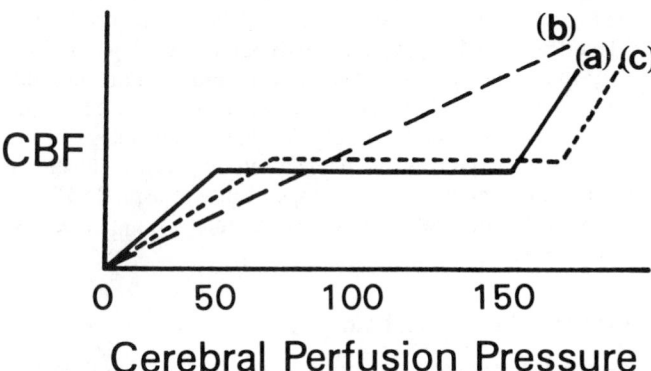

FIGURE 22–1. Relationship between CBF and cerebral perfusion pressure. a = Normal; b = failure of autoregulation; c = hypertensive patient.

ulation and whether autoregulation is intact in the individual patient. Patients with poorly controlled hypertension generally have higher limits for cerebral autoregulation. This effect is reflected by a rightward shift of the curve in Figure 22–1. These limits return to normal with control of blood pressure.[15, 16] The actual limits for autoregulation in an individual patient are not known unless CBF is actually measured.

Autoregulation is impaired in many patients with intracranial pathology; in such patients, knowledge of CBF may be critically important (Table 22–8). The actual relationship between blood pressure and blood flow in these patients is unknown without some measurement of CBF or cerebral function. Blood pressures within the normal range may be inadequate to maintain sufficient CBF. Anesthetic drugs may also impair cerebral autoregulation and change the relationship between blood pressure and CBF even when autoregulation is intact.

Decreased Cerebral Perfusion Pressure

If CPP decreases to <50 mm Hg, blood flow decreases linearly with blood pressure. The blood pressure at which CBF becomes inadequate depends on the mechanism of blood pressure reduction and, again, cannot be known for certain without some measurement of cerebral function (level of consciousness, EEG, or evoked potentials). I have observed unexpectedly normal evoked potentials during aneurysm clipping performed with sustained, severe sodium nitroprusside–induced hypotension (MAP = 30 mm Hg). CBF was maintained at acceptable levels despite the low perfusion pressure because of the cerebral vasodilating effects of nitroprusside.

Increased Cerebral Perfusion Pressure

In normotensive patients with increases in CPP to >150 mm Hg, blood flow varies directly with blood pressure. As CBF increases, cerebral edema, intracranial hemorrhage, or both become more likely. Until either of these events occurs, however, function remains normal.

Clinical Implications

Blood pressure is not a very sensitive monitor of CBF when CPP is outside the limits of autoregulation. The likelihood of blood flow abnormalities that will produce functional damage to the brain probably increases with the duration and magnitude of CPP variance from the autoregulatory limits.

The discussion thus far has ignored changes in ICP. Many patients have a constant, normal ICP during surgery; changes in CBF are related to changes in blood pressure alone. However, ICP may be variable in patients with different types of CNS pathology. Unless ICP is measured, CPP is unknown.

TABLE 22–8. Some Conditions in Which Autoregulation May Fail

Head trauma
Subarachnoid hemorrhage
Brain tumor
Hypoxemia
Hypercarbia
High concentration of volatile anesthetic

Summary

Because blood pressure measurement is noninvasive and very easy to perform, it is the most frequently used monitor of CBF. In normal patients (ICP ≤ 10 mm Hg), blood pressure relates directly to CPP and is a reasonably good indicator of CBF. In patients with intracranial pathology or with altered autoregulation secondary to hypertension or drug administration, blood pressure at best crudely estimates CBF and may be misleading. Generally, blood pressure should be kept within the awake range throughout which function is documented. If it must be adjusted outside this range for surgical or medical reasons, some form of functional monitoring is needed.

How Does Intracranial Pressure Relate to Cerebral Blood Flow?

The relationship between ICP and CBF in normal patients is also described by the cerebral autoregulation curve (see Fig. 22–1). If blood pressure is constant, as ICP rises, CPP falls. Changes in blood flow will not occur until the limits for autoregulation are exceeded. However, in patients with impaired autoregulation (see Table 22–8 and Fig. 22–1*B*), CBF, as noted previously, varies directly with CPP (i.e., the curve is "straightened"). In these patients, as ICP rises, CBF falls, unless blood pressure increases by the same amount.

ICP commonly refers to supratentorial pressure that is subarachnoid on the surface, subdural, epidural, or intraventricular. However, ICP reflects complex interactions within the craniospinal system, and pressure may be quite different in the various intracranial and intraspinal compartments.

How Is Intracranial Pressure Measured?

ICP can be measured using any of the techniques shown in Table 22–9.

Ventricular Catheter

Fluid-coupled intracranial pressure measurement is perhaps the least controversial method when it is performed with a ventricular catheter (Fig. 22–2). A small burr hole is made in the head, and a needle is passed through the dura and the substance of the brain into the lateral ventricle. A catheter is passed over the needle, and the needle is removed. The catheter is connected to a fluid-filled system and attached to a pressure transducer that is zeroed at the level of the foramen of Monro, which corresponds roughly to the surface landmarks of the nasion, the inion, or the external auditory meatus. *Note: This transducer system should not be attached to a flush sys-*

TABLE 22–9. Methods of Intracranial Pressure Assessment

Lumbar cerebrospinal fluid pressure
Fluid-coupled transducer systems
Ventriculostomy
Subdural bolt (the Richmond screw)
Implanted intracranial transducer
Optical methods
Pressure transducer
Neuroradiologic studies

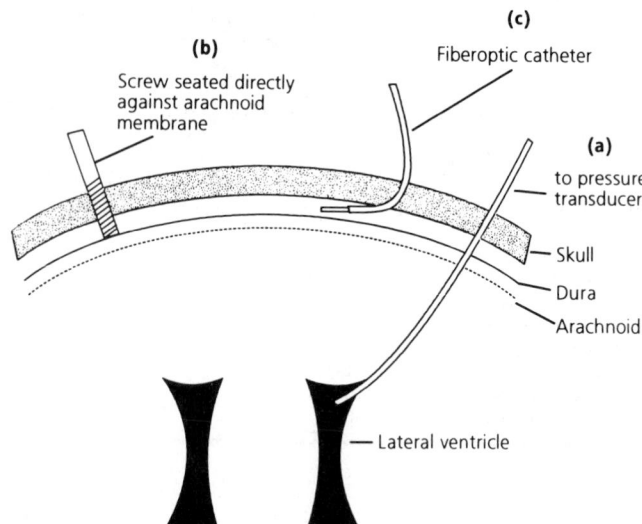

FIGURE 22–2. Schematics of intracranial pressure monitors. a = Ventriculostomy; b = Richmond screw; c = fiberoptic intracranial pressure transducer.

tem of any sort. If it is, infusion of fluid into the ventricle will occur, resulting in potentially disastrous elevations in ICP. Since this system does not involve blood, the catheter is very unlikely to become occluded, and flush systems are not needed.

A ventricular catheter is felt by many to provide the most accurate monitor of ICP. A major advantage of this system is that it can be both diagnostic and therapeutic, since cerebrospinal fluid (CSF) may be removed during treatment for elevated ICP. Complications associated with insertion and use include an approximately 1% risk of bleeding[17] and an infection rate as high as 6.3% if the device is left in place for more than a few days.

Subdural Bolt

The second fluid-coupled ICP measurement device is the subdural bolt or Richmond screw (see Fig. 22–2). A small incision is made in the scalp, and a ¼-inch twist drill hole is made in the skull. The dura is opened, and a hollow bolt is screwed through the skull so that the open end protrudes 1 to 2 mm below the inner table and rests directly against the brain surface. The hole in the skull is sealed. The hollow bolt is filled with fluid and connected through fluid-filled tubing to a pressure transducer. *Again, no flush device should be attached.* The transducer is zeroed at the level of the foramen of Monro.

The Richmond screw reportedly gives readings that are lower than those for simultaneously recorded intraventricular pressure. Some feel that this discrepancy is caused by the leaking of fluid around the bolt. A major disadvantage of this system when compared with the ventriculostomy catheter is that the bolt cannot be used therapeutically to aspirate CSF. It is also easily occluded with debris and thus requires frequent, careful irrigation.

Intracranial Pressure Transducers

Several ICP transducers do not require fluid coupling (see Fig. 22–2). They do not share the potential risk of inadvertent attachment of heparin flush to the transducer. The level at which these transducers are zeroed is not important because they are intracranial. The major drawback of these systems, again, is their inability to be used therapeutically for CSF withdrawal. The sensing catheters also are quite expensive and are not designed for multiple patient use.

Lumbar Cerebrospinal Fluid Catheters

Lumbar CSF pressure may be measured easily by inserting a small, fluid-filled catheter designed for epidural use into the subarachnoid space through a Tuohy needle. This catheter is attached to a transducer without a flushing device. Lumbar CSF pressure correlates well with ICP, provided that the transducer is zeroed at the level of the foramen of Monro and that the lumbar CSF space communicates with the lateral ventricles.

Any blockage of CSF circulation may prevent this communication. Hence, lumbar CSF pressure may be substantially lower than supratentorial ICP. Such a blockage makes insertion of a lumbar catheter dangerous as well; leakage of CSF from the lumbar space increases the pressure gradient between the supratentorial and lumbar compartments and may cause downward herniation of the intracranial contents.

Scanning Techniques

Computed tomography (CT) and MRI scans of the head can give information about increased ICP. However, both studies are intermittent and their results can be very misleading, thus they should not be considered as monitors. Evidence of increased ICP on CT or MRI scans is by no means quantitative and does not substitute for pressure measurements (Table 22–10).

TABLE 22–10. Computed Tomography and Magnetic Resonance Imaging Indicators of Elevated Intracranial Pressure

Shift of structures
Small or absent ventricles
Loss of cortical folds
Loss of cerebrospinal fluid in prepontine and mesencephalic cisterns
Cerebral edema (white matter)
Tumor with hydrocephalus
Tumor ≥ 3 cm with edema

DIRECT MEASUREMENT OF CEREBRAL BLOOD FLOW

How Is Regional Blood Flow Assessed?

Direct measurements of regional CBF are not commonly used. The only "practical" intraoperative measurement involves injection of a radioactive isotope of xenon into the carotid artery, followed by measurement of the radioactivity washout with a gamma detector placed over a specific area of the brain (Fig. 22–3). This method cannot measure CBF over other areas of the brain and cannot distinguish flow at different depths (gray and white matter). Rather, regional CBF measurements reflect average gray/white matter flow. The technique is not continuous; therefore, during most of the operation, CBF is unknown. Indirect measurements, in contradistinction, can be used continuously. Despite its shortcomings, this method has been used in combination with other continuous infusional monitoring, particularly during carotid endarterectomy surgery.[1]

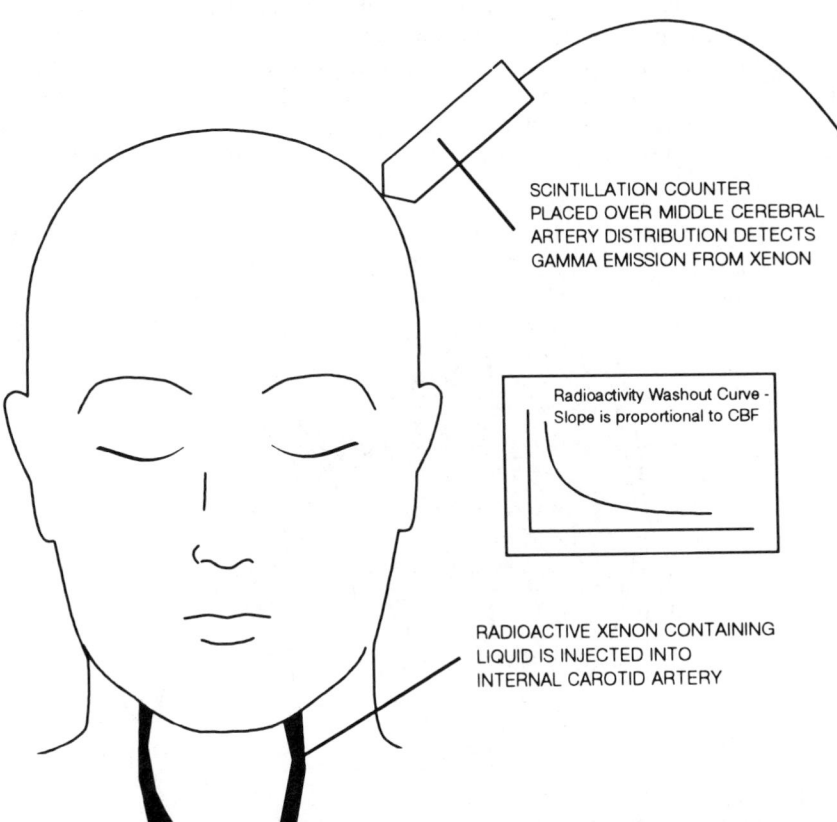

FIGURE 22–3. Schematic representation of radioactive xenon CBF measurement.

SCINTILLATION COUNTER PLACED OVER MIDDLE CEREBRAL ARTERY DISTRIBUTION DETECTS GAMMA EMISSION FROM XENON

Radioactivity Washout Curve - Slope is proportional to CBF

RADIOACTIVE XENON CONTAINING LIQUID IS INJECTED INTO INTERNAL CAROTID ARTERY

How Is Transcranial Doppler Ultrasound Utilized?

An easy-to-apply, direct, continuous, and noninvasive monitor of CBF employs transcranial Doppler (TCD) ultrasound. It has found increasing application as a monitor in the operating room and intensive care unit.

Methodology

Ultrasound waves are used to measure the velocity of blood flow in the basal arteries of the brain. These waves are transmitted through the relatively thin temporal bone (Fig. 22–4). When they contact moving red blood cells, they are reflected at a changed frequency through the brain and skull back to a detector. The change in frequency as blood cells move toward or away from the ultrasound transmitter and detector is an example of Doppler-shifted ultrasound that is related to the velocity and direction of flow. Velocity increases during systole and decreases during diastole; blood in the center of the lumen moves faster than does that near the vessel wall, producing a spectrum of flow velocities. This spectrum resembles the shape of the waveform produced by an intra-arterial pressure transducer (Fig. 22–5).

TCD flow velocity measurements are most commonly and easily made in the middle cerebral and internal carotid arteries but are also possible in other vessels, including the anterior cerebral, anterior communicating, posterior cerebral, posterior communicating, and basilar arteries.

Flow Velocity and Cerebral Blood Flow Relationships

Two assumptions must be made in order for TCD-measured blood flow velocity to have a direct relationship with CBF. First, flow and flow velocity are directly related only if the diameter of the artery at the point of flow velocity measurement and the measurement angle of the Doppler probe (angle of insonation) remain constant (Fig. 22–6). The angle of insonation may be kept constant by rigidly mounting the TCD probe on the patient's head with a headset. Second, the blood flow

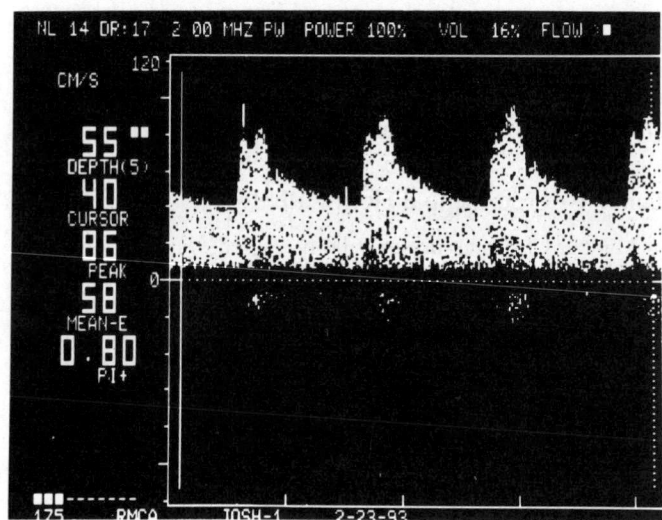

FIGURE 22–5. Typical TCD waveform showing middle cerebral artery blood flow velocity spectrum.

in the basal arteries of the brain must be directly related to cortical CBF.

Neither of these assumptions has been proved. TCD technology has not been adequately validated in a large series of intraoperative cases against established monitors of CBF such as the EEG or against direct cortical CBF measurements.

Clinical Applications

Carotid Endarterectomy

The major reported intraoperative use of TCD ultrasound involves testing CBF adequacy while the carotid artery is cross-clamped during carotid endarterectomy. Studies that compare gamma detector–measured CBF with TCD ultrasound–derived middle cerebral artery flow have not shown a particularly good correlation.[18] In addition, the period of carotid cross-clamping is only a small portion of the time that

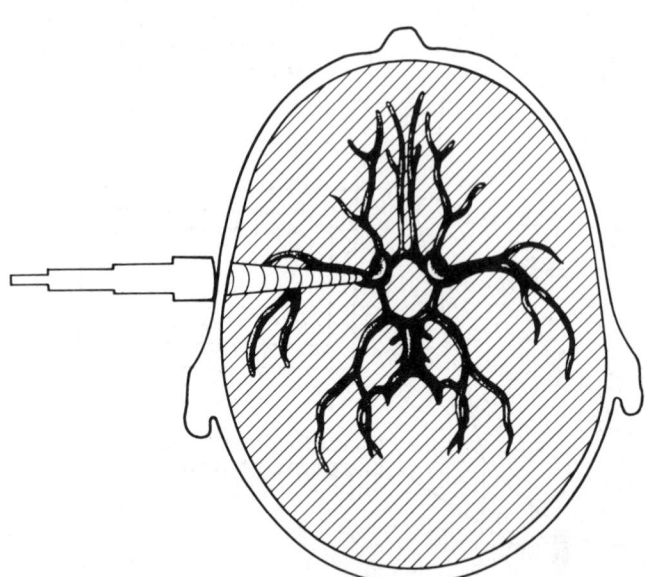

FIGURE 22–4. Schematic representation of TCD. (From Mahla ME: Update on anesthesia for intracranial aneurysm surgery. Adv Anesth 1993; 10:103.)

$$\text{FLOW VELOCITY} = 60\,\text{cm} \cdot \text{s}^{-1}$$

$$\text{FLOW} = 100\,\text{mL} \cdot \text{min}^{-1}$$

$$\text{FLOW VELOCITY} = 30\,\text{cm} \cdot \text{s}^{-1}$$

$$\text{FLOW} = 100\,\text{mL} \cdot \text{min}^{-1}$$

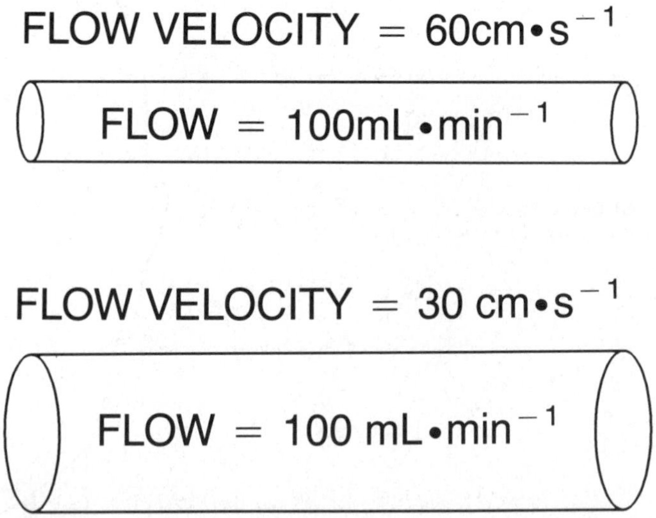

FIGURE 22–6. Schematic representation of changes in blood flow velocity that occur with constant blood flow and a change in artery diameter. (From Mahla ME: Update on anesthesia for intracranial aneurysm surgery. Adv Anesth 1993; 10:103.)

the patient with carotid disease is at risk for ischemia; most strokes occur at other times during or after surgery. Few data are available about the nature and degree of acceptable TCD changes during the remainder of the operation.

Normal variations in blood flow velocities during surgery in patients without cerebrovascular disease appear to be large.[19] Thus, in 1994, recommending TCD ultrasound as the optimal monitor of CBF during carotid surgery probably is premature. Electroencephalographic and SSEP monitoring appears to be more sensitive and specific, although TCD ultrasound technology may have a supplementary role, particularly when it is used for detection of emboli following endarterectomy.[20]

Cardiopulmonary Bypass

These measurements also have been made during cardiopulmonary bypass to assess CBF[21] and to detect emboli.[22] Based on a limited number of studies involving a small number of patients, correlation between CBF and TCD ultrasound measurements appears to be reasonably good as long as the management of arterial carbon dioxide partial pressure ($PaCO_2$) is based on temperature-uncorrected blood gas measurements. Emboli are readily detected, but studies to determine whether the incidence and severity of TCD ultrasound–detected emboli correlate with neurologic outcome have not yet been completed.

Detection of Vasospasm

Measurements of CBF have had much greater and more successful application in the intensive care unit. Detection and documentation of the severity of vasospasm following subarachnoid hemorrhage are possible.[23, 24] As the diameter of the arterial lumen decreases with vasospasm, the velocity of blood flowing through the narrowed vessel must increase if flow is to be maintained (Figs. 22–7 and 22–8). If studies involving greater numbers of patients confirm reasonable sensitivity and specificity, TCD ultrasound measurement will facilitate the detection of vasospasm in patients who are still asymptomatic. Early detection allows prophylactic treatment and close monitoring. In addition, preoperative evidence of vasospasm in asymptomatic patients with subarachnoid hemorrhage can alert

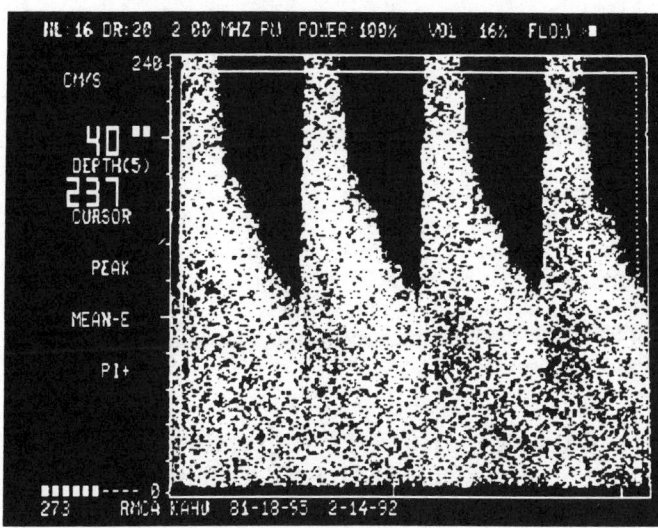

FIGURE 22–8. Typical TCD waveform in a patient after the development of cerebral vasospasm following subarachnoid hemorrhage. Note greatly increased flow velocity compared with that in Figure 22–7.

the anesthesiologist to the patient who may be at greater risk for ischemia during hypotension if hypotension is needed for aneurysm clipping.

Confirmation of Brain Death

Studies have demonstrated a characteristic blood flow velocity pattern in patients who are clinically brain dead (Fig. 22–9).[25] Measurements are easily performed at the bedside, and in a few centers the TCD ultrasound method is used to determine whether definitive studies to document brain death need to be performed. For example, if TCD ultrasound does *not* show the flow velocity pattern characteristic of brain death, angiographic or radioactive xenon blood flow studies are *unlikely* to show absent cortical CBF. Transport of these critically ill patients for CBF studies is thus unnecessary.

On the other hand, if a TCD ultrasound study does show the pattern characteristic of brain death (see Fig. 22–9), the patient can be transported for definitive blood flow studies without further delay or expenditure of resources. Further stud-

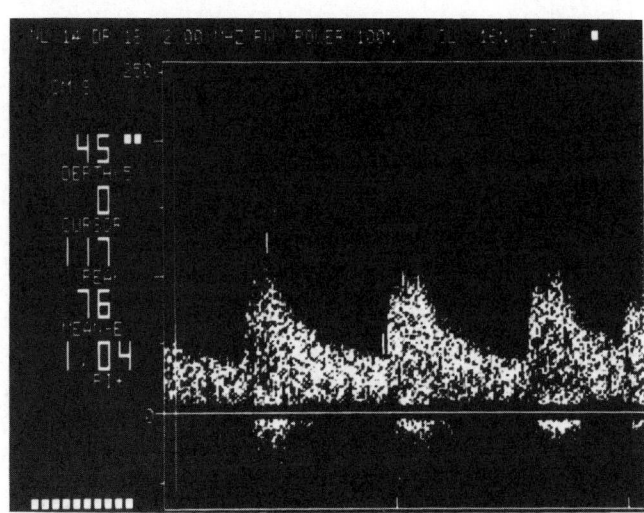

FIGURE 22–7. Typical TCD waveform in a patient prior to the development of cerebral vasospasm following subarachnoid hemorrhage.

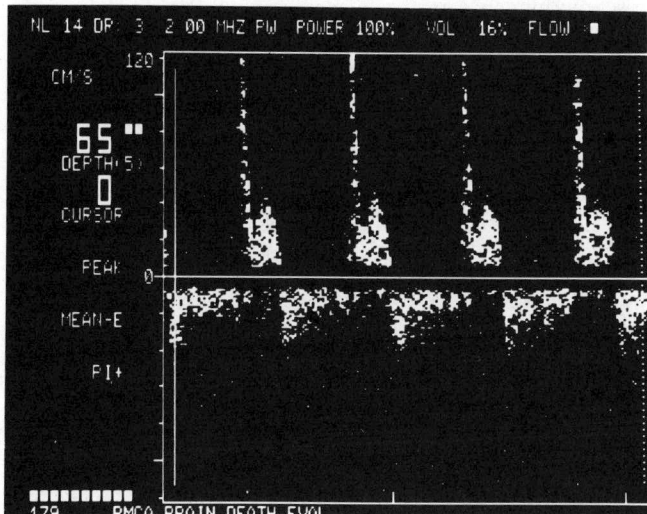

FIGURE 22–9. TCD waveform in a patient with intracranial circulatory arrest. Note reversal of blood flow direction during diastole.

ies documenting the sensitivity and specificity of this test in the diagnosis of brain death are needed before this test can be used alone to confirm brain death.

Summary

Technically satisfactory recordings cannot be obtained in some patients (particularly elderly females), thus rendering TCD ultrasound diagnosis or monitoring useless. When recordings can be made, TCD ultrasound is very attractive because it is a continuous method and is easy to use. It clearly is of benefit in the laboratory evaluation of patients with cerebrovascular disease.

BALANCE OF CEREBRAL OXYGEN SUPPLY AND DEMAND: JUGULAR BULB SATURATION

Cerebral O_2 demand (requirement) varies with changing CNS conditions. Reduction of brain temperature by 5 °C may reduce O_2 needs by $\geq 35\%$. CBF may be adequate for cerebral function and cellular integrity at 32 °C but inadequate at 37 °C. Cerebral O_2 delivery varies with CBF and O_2 content. Cerebral function is determined by the *balance* between cerebral O_2 demand and supply. Thus, numerical values of CBF, taken alone, do not guarantee either preservation or loss of function; they must be interpreted with regard to O_2 demand and supply.

Clinically applicable direct measurements of O_2 demand are not available at this time. The EEG can be used to assess O_2 demand indirectly. Generation of spontaneous electrical activity uses roughly 50% of the total O_2 consumed by the brain. As a corollary, if drugs are given to totally suppress spontaneous electrical activity, the O_2 demand will be reduced by about 50%.

How Is Jugular Bulb Saturation Utilized?

Measurements that reflect the balance between O_2 supply and demand, however, can be made directly or by measuring the O_2 saturation in the jugular venous blood (SvO_2) returning from the brain. A catheter is advanced retrograde under fluoroscopic guidance in the jugular vein until its tip lies in the jugular bulb. Blood can then be aspirated and saturation measured. When cerebral O_2 delivery falls (as a result of decreased blood O_2 content, decreased CBF, or both), cerebral O_2 extraction increases. This change results in decreased SvO_2 of venous blood returning from the brain. Measurement also can be made continuously using a small fiberoptic catheter similar to that used to measure mixed venous oxygen saturation in the pulmonary artery.

Jugular SvO_2 monitoring has been used primarily in head trauma patients who require control of increased ICP with hyperventilation or barbiturates, or both.[26] Hyperventilation decreases CBF; too much can produce cerebral ischemia. Several clinical series have described knowledge of jugular SvO_2 as helpful in detecting excessive hyperventilation.[26] Although hyperventilation was found to lower ICP, the accompanying decrease in CBF caused O_2 delivery to fall below demand. These data suggested that another technique to control ICP (e.g., barbiturate coma, ventriculostomy, or CSF drainage) might be safer.

Several problems occur with this technique. Blood in a single jugular bulb comes from sources on both sides of the brain (70% ipsilateral, 30% contralateral). This measurement technique evaluates the *global* balance between cerebral O_2 supply and demand. Inadequate CBF to a small area of cortex may be masked by blood that has a higher SvO_2 from areas of adequately perfused brain in either hemisphere. Thus, a high saturation can be falsely reassuring. More importantly, placement of a catheter in the jugular vein may block jugular outflow or cause thrombosis after prolonged use. Even unilateral placement sometimes impedes jugular outflow sufficiently to raise ICP in patients with decreased intracranial compliance. These problems have prevented widespread use of such monitoring.

CEREBRAL OXYGEN SUPPLY/DEMAND BALANCE: THE ELECTROENCEPHALOGRAM

When O_2 delivery falls below a level sufficient to meet the $CMRo_2$, function fails. Since function is disrupted before cellular integrity is lost, monitors of function provide early warning of inadequate O_2 supply and provide opportunity to correct this problem before irreversible damage occurs. Such monitors can be used to guide therapy when CNS O_2 supply may be compromised during surgery and to detect surgically induced structural damage that produces changes in function.

The function of some motor and sensory pathways, as well as the spontaneous electrical activity of the cerebral cortex, is easily monitored during general anesthesia. These pathways and spontaneous electrical activity of the cerebral cortex reflect only a portion of the entire nervous system. Changes in one monitored parameter may *imply* damage to other nearby areas of the nervous system; however, damage to unmonitored portions of the nervous system may occur without detection. Thus, when areas of the nervous system that cannot be monitored are at risk during surgery, false-negative monitoring patterns should be expected.

What Is the Electroencephalogram?

The EEG recorded from the scalp is a summation of excitatory and inhibitory postsynaptic potentials produced in the pyramidal layer of the cerebral cortex. These electrical signals range in amplitude from <10 μV to around 100 μV.

Recording

As with recording of the ECG, EEG electrodes are placed in a standardized fashion so that tracings from one individual may be compared either with later tracings from the same individual or with those of other individuals. The International Ten-Twenty Electrode System[27] (Fig. 22–10) places EEG electrodes or electrodes for recording evoked potentials over specific areas of the cerebral cortex and is based on measurements made between pairs of specific sites on the patient's head. Each recording point is designated with a letter and a number and can often be associated with underlying CNS structures; for example, C_3, C_z, and C_4 are all associated with the motor cortex. By convention, recording electrodes placed over the

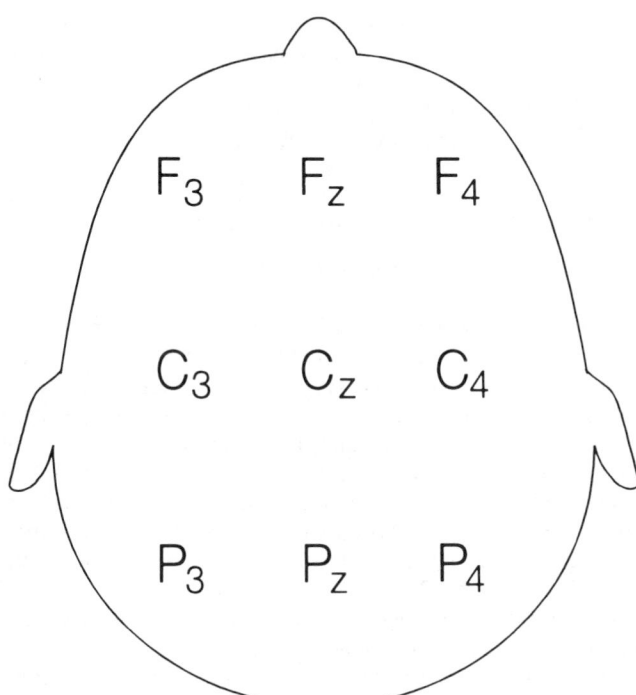

FIGURE 22–10. Schematic representation of the ten-twenty system of electrode placement.

SCHEMATIC OF THE 10-20 SYSTEM

right hemisphere are even-numbered, and those placed over the left hemisphere are odd-numbered. Midline electrodes are designated by a ''z.''

These electrodes are connected in pairs to an amplification system and their recordings are displayed, just as with the ECG, as a plot of voltage versus time. Each EEG channel represents the electrical activity of one electrode pair. The recording of multiple EEG channels simultaneously on paper at speeds of up to $3 \ cm \cdot s^{-1}$ creates a large amount of on-line data; a technician or neurologist must monitor the EEG output constantly for maximum utility.

Alternative Displays

Reduction in the number of channels or simplification and suitable formatting of data enable personnel such as anesthesiologists, who also have other intraoperative tasks, to use the EEG for intraoperative monitoring. The display can be simplified through signal processing techniques, which include power spectrum analysis, frequency analysis, filtering, and rectification. Data are displayed in time-compressed formats such as compressed spectral array and density spectral array (Fig. 22–11). Of extreme importance, however, is the retention of

FIGURE 22–11. Processed EEG. The two most common types of EEG processing are density spectral array (top) and compressed spectral array (bottom).

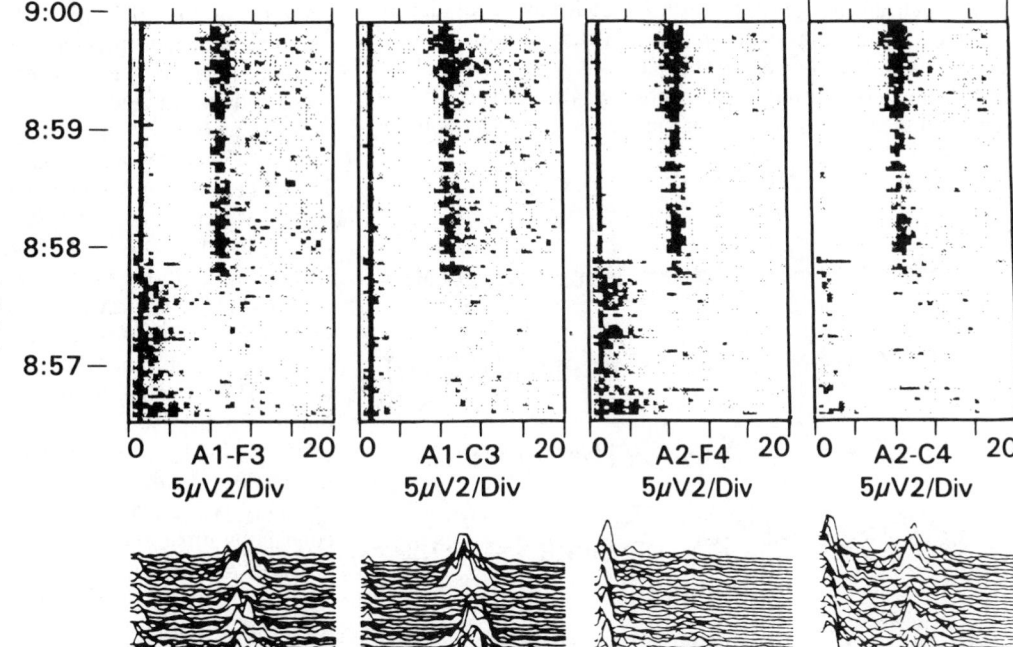

access to the real-time, unprocessed EEG. Except for gross artifact rejection by voltage criteria, these simplified monitors do not yet have the ability to distinguish brain activity from other biologic signals (e.g., ECG) or noise. Noise is processed as if it were electrical brain activity.

Number of Leads for Meaningful Data

The largest clinical series that examined the usefulness of EEG monitoring during carotid surgery used 16 channels of acquired data for analysis.[1] Although no carefully performed studies have compared lesser numbers of channels systematically to the 16-channel unprocessed recordings, data suggest that fewer numbers of channels may be very useful. One study compared 2-channel, computer-processed EEGs interpreted by an inexperienced observer with 16-channel hard copy EEGs monitored by a trained technician and a neurologist. The inexperienced observer was able to identify 75% of the significant EEG changes seen on the 16-channel EEG.[28] This study suggests that even 2-channel EEGs (one channel examining each cerebral hemisphere) are very useful for monitoring a carotid endarterectomy. One channel on each hemisphere helps to differentiate EEG changes that are caused by global factors (e.g., anesthetic drugs) from those changes that are caused by more regional factors (e.g., carotid cross-clamping).

What Is the Significance of Electroencephalogram Frequency and Amplitude?

For pattern recognition in the EEG, the complex waveforms are described in terms of frequency (cycles $\cdot$ s^{-1} = hertz = Hz) and amplitude (voltage). Four basic EEG rhythms or frequency patterns are analyzed (Fig. 22–12): delta (0–4 Hz); theta (4–8 Hz); alpha (8–13 Hz); and beta (>13 Hz).

Delta rhythm occurs during deep sleep and deep anesthesia and in many pathologic states such as ischemia, drug overdose, and severe metabolic derangements. Theta rhythm is commonly seen during general anesthesia and may occur during the same pathologic states in which delta rhythm is seen. Alpha rhythm can be recorded, mainly over the occipital region, in an alert, relaxed patient whose eyes are closed. During lighter surgical planes of anesthesia, this 8- to 13-Hz activity

can be recorded over much of the cortex but especially in the anterior leads.

Beta rhythm accompanies mental concentration or may be induced with low doses of many sedative and hypnotic drugs such as barbiturates or benzodiazepines. Deep anesthesia, ischemia, or other pathologic states abolish both alpha and beta frequencies, after which slower frequencies predominate.

Changes in EEG amplitude normally result from synchronization or desynchronization of cortical electrical activity. Larger EEG amplitude is seen during sleep or surgical anesthesia. However, very deep levels of anesthesia cause a loss in EEG amplitude secondary to direct depression of cortical neuronal activity. Awakening usually produces a decrease in amplitude and the appearance of higher frequency patterns such as beta rhythm. An extremely strong stimulus under anesthesia may cause the appearance of an alerting pattern that consists of high-voltage delta and theta frequency patterns.

How Is the Electroencephalogram Useful to the Anesthesiologist?

Relationship to Brain Function

Electroencephalographic activity—that is, cortical electrical activity—requires roughly 50% of the total O_2 consumed by the brain; the remaining 50% is needed to maintain cellular integrity. When O_2 delivery is compromised by either hypoxemia or decreased blood supply, O_2 that ordinarily would be used to produce electrical activity is instead diverted to maintain cellular integrity. Depression of EEG activity thus reflects decreased O_2 delivery.

Practical Considerations

The first step in using an unfamiliar monitor is to define it in terms of a monitor that is familiar. Electrocardiography is routinely used by anesthesiologists, who have learned the various normal and abnormal ECG patterns that may occur during surgical operations. For example, ST segment depression immediately causes concern about myocardial ischemia. Interpretation of CNS monitoring also involves pattern recognition. Slowing of the EEG (Fig. 22–13) may be associated with cerebral ischemia. Interventions based on recognition of these patterns may be made in much the same fashion in which interventions are made after recognition of ECG changes.

The most important intraoperative use for the EEG is to monitor O_2 supply and demand balance in the cerebral cortex. In a large series of patients undergoing carotid endarterectomy at the Mayo Clinic,[1] the EEG was compared with regional CBF using the ^{133}Xe washout method. This study validated the EEG as an indicator of the adequacy of regional CBF.

Normal CBF in gray and white matter averages 50 mL $\cdot$ 100 g^{-1} $\cdot$ min^{-1}. With most anesthetic techniques, the EEG begins to become abnormal when CBF falls to 20 mL $\cdot$ 100 g^{-1} $\cdot$ min^{-1}. However the threshold for EEG changes appears to be much lower (8–10 mL $\cdot$ 100 g^{-1} $\cdot$ min^{-1} when isoflurane is used.[29] Cellular survival is not threatened until CBF falls to 12 mL $\cdot$ 100 g^{-1} min^{-1} (lower with isoflurane). Thus, a margin of safety is present between the time at which the EEG becomes abnormal and that at which cellular damage begins to occur. Severe anemia and decreases in O_2 saturation also decrease O_2 delivery. The EEG activity becomes abnormal once increased blood flow cannot compensate for decreased arterial oxygen content.

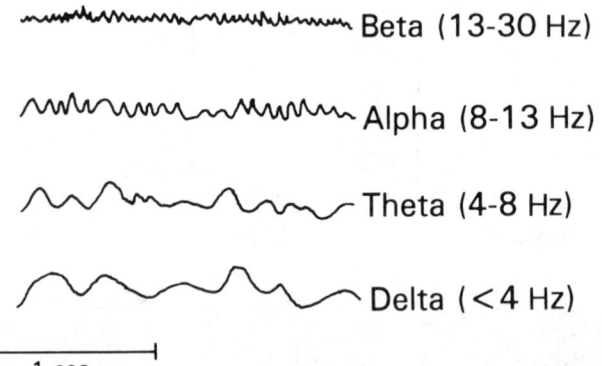

FIGURE 22–12. EEG frequency patterns in order of declining frequency.

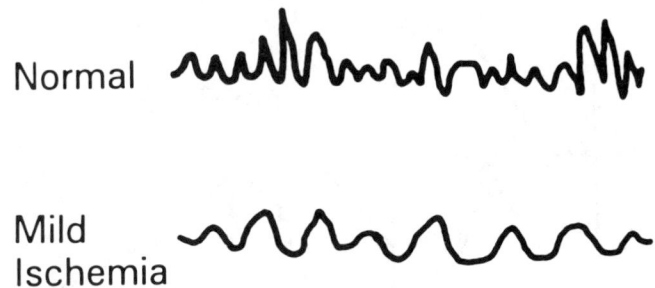

Normal

Mild
Ischemia

Severe
Ischemia

FIGURE 22–13. Schematic of EEG changes during ischemia.

Why Is the Electroencephalogram Useful During Carotid Surgery?

Determination of Inadequate Oxygen Delivery

Serious intraoperative reduction in cerebral O_2 supply may result from surgical factors (e.g., carotid cross-clamping) that are usually beyond the anesthesiologist's control and from factors that the anesthesiologist can correct. Reduction in CBF produced by hyperventilation, hypotension, or temporary occlusion of major blood vessels sometimes is corrected by reducing ventilation, by restoring normal blood pressure, or, in the case of temporary vessel occlusion, by increasing blood pressure above normal. Since the EEG correlates with CBF adequacy, it serves as a monitor of the effectiveness of therapy instituted to correct ischemia.

Ideally, EEG use is continuous; yet, it has been described most frequently as a spot check to determine the need for shunt placement after carotid cross-clamping in anesthetized patients. However, this short-term use detects only a small portion of the neurologic injuries that can occur during and after carotid surgery. Critical carotid luminal narrowing risks cerebral hypoperfusion during hypotension or positioning. These problems will be missed if the EEG is not monitored continuously.

Shunt Placement

If monitoring of the EEG could be proved scientifically to reduce the incidence of stroke, the question introducing this section would require no discussion. Data demonstrating this, however, do not exist. What information is available is less than satisfactory. In a large series of patients undergoing carotid endarterectomy with selective shunting who were monitored with 16-channel unprocessed EEG, no patient awakened with a new neurologic deficit that was not predicted by EEG.[1] Transient, correctable EEG changes were not associated with stroke. Persistent changes were associated with stroke.

Based on laboratory data, the ischemic tolerance of neural tissue is directly related to both the severity of CBF reduction and the duration of the insult.[30] Since the EEG detects reductions in CBF that would not otherwise be apparent in unmonitored patients and thus permits intervention that may correct

the problem (usually placement of a shunt), EEG monitoring should be useful in reducing the incidence of stroke when selective shunting is used.

More difficult to prove is that EEG monitoring is useful when all patients are shunted during carotid clamping. Such monitoring has detected correctable shunt malfunction, and investigators have described hypotension-related EEG changes in patients with critical stenoses and poor collateral circulation.[31, 32]

Finally, a recent multicenter study of 1495 carotid endarterectomies provides convincing data that shunting of patients without evidence of decreased cerebral perfusion actually increases the incidence of stroke more than six-fold.[33]

Hypotension

Without EEG monitoring, blood pressure decreases that occur during surgery are treated empirically. Elevation of blood pressure with a vasopressor is known to increase the likelihood of myocardial ischemia. Monitoring of the EEG helps to determine whether hypotension actually produces a reduction in CBF that requires treatment and helps to determine the risk/benefit ratio for treating hypotension.

How Else Can the Electroencephalogram Be Used?

Barbiturate Suppression of the CMR_{O_2}

The EEG may be used to monitor cerebral O_2 demand. Barbiturates administered to lower ICP do so by depressing cortical electrical activity and, thus, by lowering the CMR_{O_2}. In response to decreased O_2 requirement, CBF and blood volume decrease; this, in turn, decreases ICP.

Since barbiturates and other drugs that depress cerebral metabolism are almost without exception cardiovascular depressants, the minimum dose of drug necessary for the intended effect on CMR_{O_2} should be given. Once cortical electrical activity is abolished, barbiturates cannot further reduce CMR_{O_2}, CBF, or ICP. Hence, the EEG may be used to determine the minimum dose of drug necessary to obtain the maximum effect (i.e., near total EEG suppression).

Induced Hypotension

Monitoring cerebral cortical function during induced hypotension or cardiopulmonary bypass is a logical extension of EEG use in carotid surgery. Carefully controlled studies appearing in the literature describe the use of EEG for these purposes, but the monitoring methods and EEG changes used to guide therapy vary widely from institution to institution, and little standardization of intraoperative techniques exists.

What Effects Do Anesthetic Drugs Have on the Electroencephalogram?

Low doses of potent inhalation agents with nitrous oxide produce an active EEG with alpha and beta frequencies present. Steady-state anesthesia, regardless of the agent used, usually produces a stable EEG pattern. Be aware that deep anesthesia and ischemia produce similar EEG changes. In both cases, fast activity is replaced by slower, larger EEG waveforms. As anesthesia is further deepened or as ischemia worsens, additional slowing occurs, and the EEG amplitude decreases and ultimately becomes flat (isoelectric).

Boluses of anesthetic drugs may produce large EEG changes that are indistinguishable from those seen during ischemia; such changes in the anesthetic regimen should be avoided during surgery when ischemia is a risk. In addition, monitoring of areas that are not at risk for ischemia during surgery may help to distinguish anesthetic effect, which should be global, from surgically induced decreases in blood flow, which may be only regional.

What Information Is Not Provided by Electroencephalogram Monitoring?

Electroencephalographic monitoring provides information about the overall electrical functioning of the cerebral cortex but not much information about the subcortical brain, spinal cord, or cranial and peripheral nerves. The functioning of CNS sensory or motor pathways that may be at risk during surgical procedures is monitored using SSEPs and MEPs.

CEREBRAL OXYGEN SUPPLY AND DEMAND: EVOKED POTENTIALS

The EEG records *spontaneous* electrical activity produced by the CNS. Sensory evoked potentials (EPs) consist of CNS electrical activity that is evoked by sensory stimuli (electrical [most common], auditory, or visual [least common]). Sensory EPs are of three types: (1) peripheral or cranial nerve, (2) subcortical, and (3) cortical.

From Where Are Evoked Potentials Recorded?

EPs from peripheral nerves that are generated by propagated action potentials usually are recorded directly over the nerve or plexus and are very large. Subcortical EPs are produced by synaptic activity generated in subcortical groups of nerve cells and action potentials traveling on connecting nerve pathways. They cannot usually be recorded near the cells or pathways that produce the EPs and therefore have small amplitude. Instead, they are recorded over the spinal cord and brainstem.

Cortical EPs, as with the EEG, are produced by the summation of postsynaptic potentials in the pyramidal layer of the cerebral cortex and also have a small amplitude. These EPs are recorded over the cerebral cortex. The amplitude of spontaneous background EEG activity is generally much larger than that of either subcortical or cortical EPs and easily obscures these smaller signals. This problem is solved through the application of filtering and signal averaging techniques.

How Do Evoked Potentials Appear, and How Are They Described?

EPs are described in terms of latency and amplitude (Fig. 22–14). Latency is the time measured from the application of the stimulus to the point of maximum amplitude of the EP.

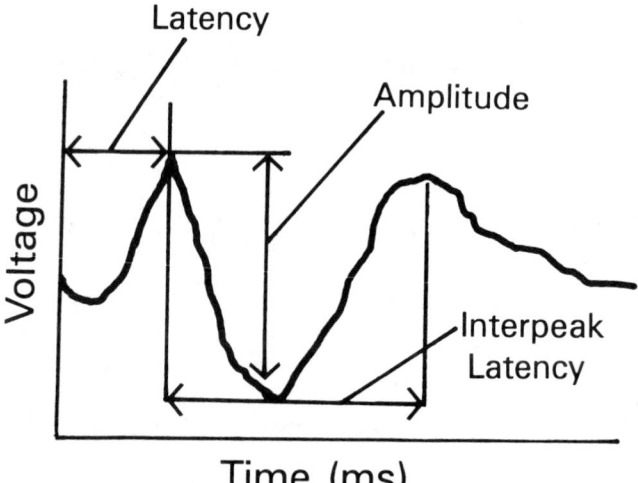

FIGURE 22–14. Evoked potentials are described in terms of time after stimulus (latency) and size (amplitude).

Some types of EPs have more than one peak. Latency measured between EP peaks (interpeak latency) is often important clinically. Amplitude is defined as the voltage difference between two peaks of opposite polarity or between an EP peak and a reference level that represents zero potential.

What Are Somatosensory Evoked Potentials?

SSEPs monitor the function of the somesthetic sensory system that extends throughout the peripheral and central nervous systems. Thus, peripheral nerve, spinal cord, subcortical, and cortical structures in the brain may be monitored. The somesthetic system carries sensory information, including that concerning vibration, proprioception, and light touch. An SSEP is generated when repetitive electrical stimuli are applied to a peripheral nerve, and many single responses are averaged to record the evoked response. Responses may be recorded over the peripheral nerve, nerve plexus, spinal cord, brainstem, and cerebral cortex (Fig. 22–15). Recording sites are related directly to the somesthetic pathway. As with the EEG, cortical recording electrode locations are based on the International Ten-Twenty System of electrode placement.

Recording Channels

The number of recording channels varies with the type of case being monitored. In an ideal situation, recordings should be made over each peripheral nerve being stimulated, the spinal cord rostral to the nerve's entry, the second cervical vertebra, and the opposite cerebral cortex. In addition, if possible, a portion of the somatosensory system not at risk from surgery should be monitored as well to help differentiate the previously mentioned changes in SSEPs produced by global factors such as anesthetic drugs. Thus, during a right carotid endarterectomy, cortical responses to both left and right median nerve stimulation should be recorded. During surgery for correction of thoracolumbar scoliosis, responses from both posterior tibial nerves as well as from at least one median nerve are desirable. Generally, these requirements translate into at least four channels of data.

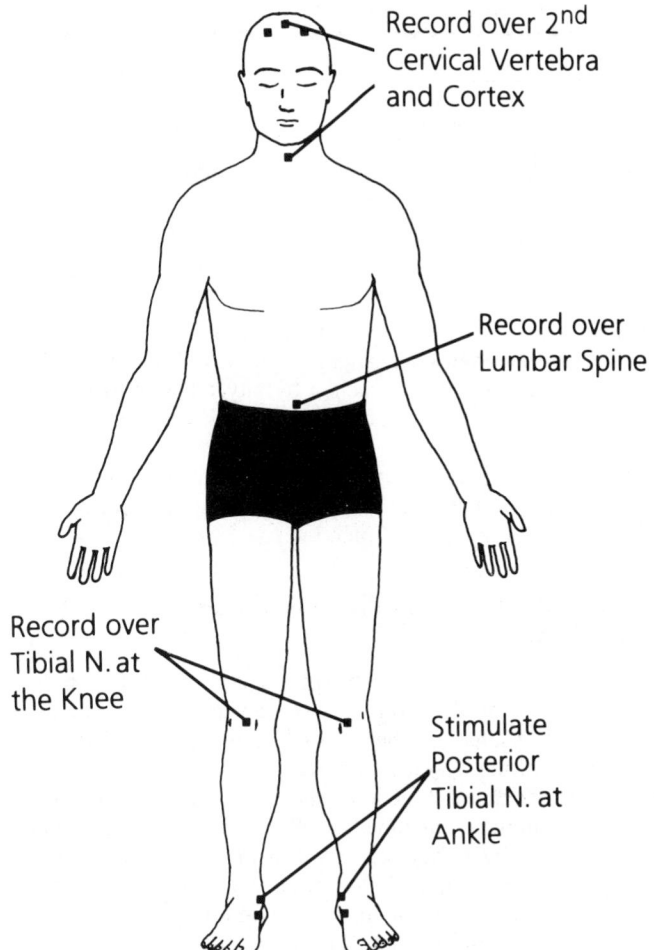

Record over 2nd Cervical Vertebra and Cortex

Record over Lumbar Spine

Record over Tibial N. at the Knee

Stimulate Posterior Tibial N. at Ankle

FIGURE 22–15. Schematic representation of spinal cord monitoring showing sites of recording electrode placement.

Usefulness of Peripheral and Spinal Cord Recordings

Adequacy of Stimulus

The most important use of peripheral nerve recordings is to make certain that a stimulus is actually reaching the CNS. If the SSEP disappears during a surgical procedure, one must ensure that the cause is not failure to stimulate adequately. A peripheral nerve response rules out this technical failure.

Peripheral Nerve Injuries

Recordings over the peripheral nerves and plexuses also have been useful during surgical explorations of peripheral nerve injuries and may help to direct the most appropriate treatment of these lesions (i.e., lesion resection and nerve grafting versus leaving the nerve intact with lysis of scar and adhesions).[34] If SSEPs can be recorded on both sides of a peripheral nerve lesion, neurolysis usually suffices to improve function. If proximal recording cannot be obtained, resection of the lesion and nerve grafting is needed.

Technical Failure, and Choice of Anesthetic

Recordings over the spinal cord also ensure against technical failure. In addition, they monitor spinal cord function be-

low the level of electrode placement. In the case of operations on the spinal cord or on the spinal column, if recordings over the spinal cord rostral to the operative site can be made, cortical recordings become less important. Recordings made over the spinal cord are much less sensitive to the effects of anesthetic drugs than are recordings made over the cortex (Fig. 22–16). Reliance on spinal recordings allows the anesthesiologist much greater freedom in drug choice. Spinal recordings, however, give little information about cortical function and show only that a stimulus has reached the CNS.

Significant Changes

Since factors other than surgery may alter the SSEP signal, the clinician must be able to decide when a change is significant and requires treatment. On the basis of many clinical series (not studies) and of studies addressing the effects of different anesthetic agents on the SSEP (Table 22–11), many experts quote a 50% decrease in amplitude or a 10% increase in latency as the degree of change that should provoke concern. Amplitude changes are considered the more important factor.

In an environment where factors known to influence the SSEP (e.g., anesthetic drugs, temperature, or $Paco_2$) cannot be controlled, these guidelines may be appropriate. If tight control of these factors can be maintained (Table 22–12), any amount of *event-related change* in the SSEP should be considered significant. In the absence of any observable event occurring around the time of an SSEP change, the aforementioned latency and amplitude criteria should be used to help decide when a change needs to be investigated urgently.

How Are Somatosensory Evoked Potentials Used Intraoperatively?

Spinal Operations

Spinal cord monitoring is the most widely applied intraoperative use of SSEPs, particularly during spinal instrumentation for the treatment of kyphoscoliosis. It has been used to a lesser

Stimulate Lt. Posterior Tibial Nerve

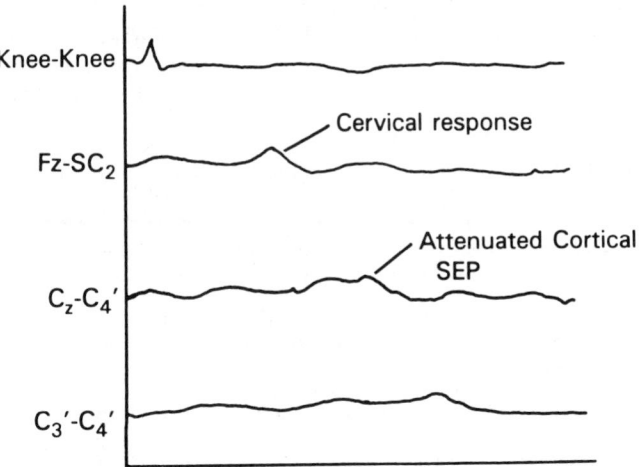

Knee-Knee

Fz-SC$_2$ — Cervical response

C$_z$-C$_4$' — Attenuated Cortical SEP

C$_3$'-C$_4$'

FIGURE 22–16. Cervical responses are not affected by high concentrations of potent inhalation agents.

TABLE 22–11. Anesthetic Susceptibility of Evoked Potential Responses

	Somatosensory	Auditory	Motor	Visual
Resistant	Peripheral nerve Lumbar/thoracic potentials Subcortical potential at C$_2$	Brainstem	Spinal cord Peripheral nerve	None
Moderate	Primary cortical response	Middle latency responses	None	None
Severe	Long latency responses	Long latency responses	All responses recorded from muscle (EMG)	Primary cortical response

extent during other operations on the spinal cord and its supporting structures, such as resection of spinal cord tumors or vascular malformations, diskectomies, and stabilization procedures for trauma or degenerative disease.

The incidence of postoperative paraplegia following posterior spinal fusion for scoliosis ranges from approximately 1% to 10%, depending on the type of instrumentation used. The highest incidence occurs when sublaminar wires are used, as in the Luque fusion. Before intraoperative SSEPs came into common use, the wake-up test was used to assess lower extremity motor function intraoperatively. This test has the advantage of being simple and inexpensive. However, as was discussed previously, it has numerous disadvantages. Also, it is only an intermittent monitor of spinal cord function.

In contrast, SSEP monitoring may be performed continuously, and trauma associated with intraoperative wake-up is avoided. In most centers, clinicians now omit the wake-up test if SSEPs are monitored and remain unchanged. If clear changes occur, the wake-up test may be performed; distraction is removed or reduced if motor deficits are detected. Alternatively, in the case of clear SSEP changes associated with distraction, the distraction may be removed or reduced without the performance of a wake-up test. The wake-up test is also used when changes in SSEP are equivocal.

Anterior Spinal Cord Monitoring

The SSEP generated from lower extremity nerve stimulation is carried in the spinal cord primarily by the posterior columns but also by the anterior spinothalamic tract and the ventral spinocerebellar tract. The SSEP, therefore, does not primarily reflect motor function. Interestingly, however, SSEP monitoring during posterior spinal fusion has correlated very well with postoperative sensory and motor neurologic outcome.[2–5] In some previously discussed case reports, however, SSEPs did not change during surgery, and the patients awakened with motor deficits (false-negative results).[7, 8] These cases are ex-

tremely rare, and most are controversial. Even if the data are correct, the reported false-negative rate is still much less than 1%, a frequency not approached by any other intraoperative monitor. MEPs may be useful in overcoming this limitation of SSEPs.

Occasionally, technically satisfactory waveforms cannot be obtained. In this case, the wake-up test must be used, if feasible, to monitor spinal cord function.

Operations That Jeopardize Spinal Cord Blood Flow

SSEPs have been used to monitor spinal cord function during operations on the thoracic aorta (aneurysm or coarctation correction); results have been variable. A normal SSEP at the conclusion of the operation clearly does not guarantee normal postoperative motor function. The most important factor in predicting ultimate outcome with SSEP monitoring is the *duration* of time over which the SSEP is lost during aortic cross-clamping.[35–39] Restoration of a normal SSEP after aortic cross-clamping release does not ensure a good outcome if the SSEP was lost for >14 minutes during cross-clamping. Loss of SSEPs for <14 minutes, with subsequent return to normal, is associated with good outcome during coarctation repair.[35]

Changes in the SSEP during surgery may be corrected by a trial of clamp reposition, shunting, induced hypertension, spinal fluid drainage, or intercostal reimplantation in an attempt to re-establish adequate spinal cord blood flow. Well-documented reports indicate that if normal SSEPs are continuously monitored and remain unchanged throughout surgery, major new neurologic deficits will not occur.

Are Somatosensory Evoked Potentials Useful for Monitoring Cerebral Cortical Function?

Cortical structures can also be monitored by SSEPs. Inadequate perfusion of the somatosensory cortex eliminates the cortical but not the subcortical components. The reduction in CBF necessary to suppress the SSEP appears slightly greater than that needed to suppress the EEG; thus, SSEPs may not be as sensitive as the EEG.[40] Such monitoring is successful during procedures that may compromise blood flow, including carotid endarterectomy, cerebral aneurysm clipping (Fig. 22–17), induced hypotension prior to aneurysm clipping, and arteriovenous malformation resection.

Correlation of SSEP recordings with neurologic outcome is strong, particularly when the middle and anterior cerebral circulations are involved. Irreversible loss of the SSEP nearly always predicts postoperative sensory and motor deficits. Preservation of cortical SSEPs is associated with an unchanged neurologic examination in the vast majority of patients.[41–43]

TABLE 22–12. Techniques to Minimize Influence of Anesthetics on Interpretation of Evoked Potentials

No changes in anesthetic technique should be made during critical periods of monitoring (e.g., induced hypotension, carotid cross-clamping, aneurysm clipping).

An area of the brain or spinal cord not at risk from the surgical procedure should also be monitored using the same evoked potential modality (see Fig. 22–23).

If SSEPs are being monitored, use cervical responses (see Fig. 22–22) whenever possible, since they are not influenced significantly by anesthetic agents.

If cervical responses cannot be recorded or if evoked potentials susceptible to anesthetics must be monitored, use favorable anesthetic techniques.

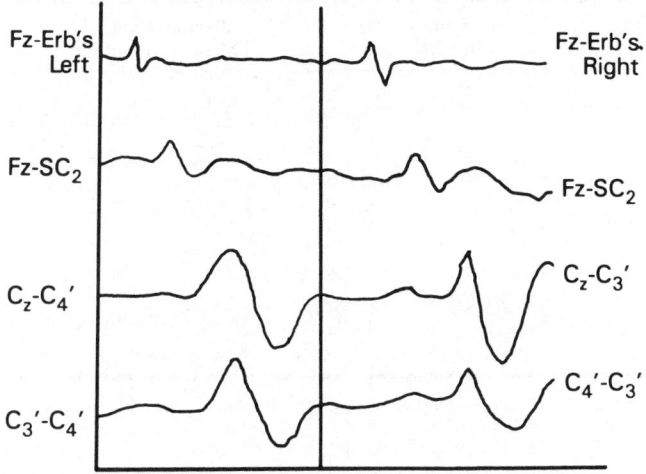

Stimulate Lt. Median N.   Stimulate Rt. Median N.

Fz-Erb's Left   Fz-Erb's Right

Fz-SC$_2$ Fz-SC$_2$

C$_z$-C$_4'$ C$_z$-C$_3'$

C$_3'$-C$_4'$ C$_4'$-C$_3'$

FIGURE 22–17. Changes in the cortical SSEP ipsilateral to the aneurysm is likely caused by the surgery. Bilateral changes are likely caused by anesthesia. Monitoring a part of the CNS not at risk for surgical manipulation allows this differentiation. In this figure, both hemispheres are monitored by sequential stimulation of the median nerve.

False-negative monitoring patterns usually occur during neurovascular procedures that involve the basilar and posterior cerebral circulations. Large portions of the brainstem may become ischemic or suffer infarction with no effect on the somatosensory pathway or the SSEP.[44]

Are Somatosensory Evoked Potentials Helpful in Preventing Neurologic Injury?

As with other monitors, no carefully controlled studies prove that SSEP monitoring improves outcome following neurologic surgery. The absence of such outcome studies, however, should not prevent clinicians from utilizing this monitoring modality. It has an excellent overall correlation with neurologic outcome. Feedback to the surgeon is rapid; this, in turn, enables rapid intervention, either surgical or anesthetic, to prevent permanent neurologic deficit. In Figure 22–18, note that the cortical SSEP disappeared following middle cerebral artery aneurysm clipping after removal of retraction from the frontal and temporal lobes. The brain then shifted, causing the clip to kink the middle cerebral artery. Retractors were again placed, and the clip position was adjusted so that no further problems occurred. Prompt feedback prevented a major neurologic injury.

Provided that other factors affecting SSEPs are kept constant, increases in latency and decreases in amplitude are ominous signs; surgical causes should be sought and corrected rapidly, if possible. Changes in SSEPs usually reflect damage to motor pathways as well. However, because motor and sensory pathways are located in different parts of the brain and spinal cord and because in some places they have a different blood supply, the SSEP will not always reflect motor function. Such monitoring is most effective when a large area of brain or spinal cord or its blood supply is threatened during surgery.

FIGURE 22–18. SSEP change caused by kinking of the middle cerebral artery after removal of frontal and temporal lobe retraction following the placement of an aneurysm clip. (From Mahla ME: Update on anesthesia for intracranial aneurysm surgery. Adv Anesth 1993; 10:113.)

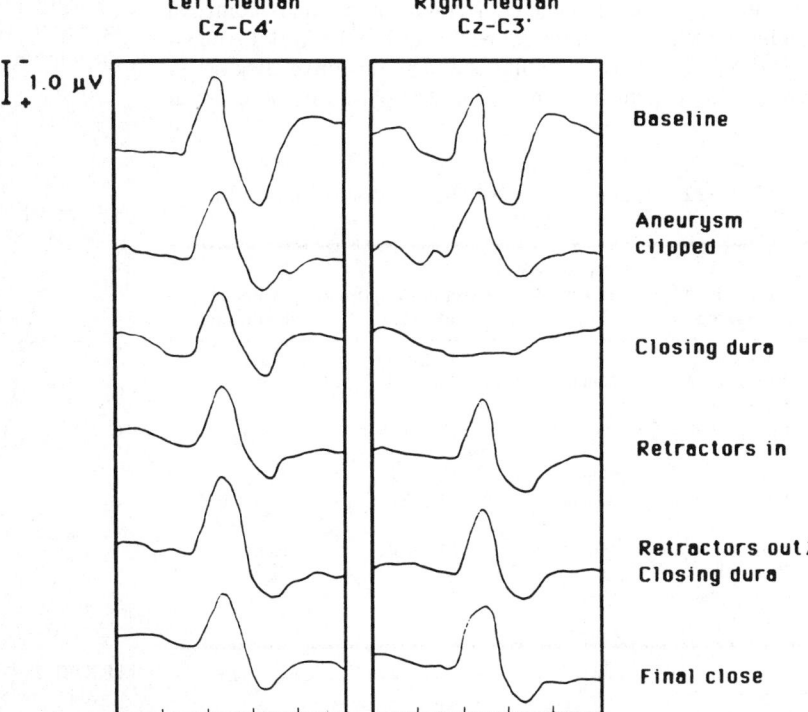

Sequential Median Nerve SEP

Left MCA Aneurysm Surgery

Left Median Cz-C4'   Right Median Cz-C3'

1.0 µV

Baseline

Aneurysm clipped

Closing dura

Retractors in

Retractors out; Closing dura

Final close

0ms   50ms   0ms   50ms

TABLE 22–13. Effects of Anesthetics on Somatosensory Evoked Potentials[45–52]

Anesthetic Drug	Effect on Peripheral Nerve Potential	Effect on Subcortical Potential	Effect on Cortical Potential Latency	Effect on Cortical Potential Amplitude
Barbiturates	None	None	1 to 2+ D	1 to 3− D
Nitrous oxide	None	None	1+	1 to 2− D
Halothane Enflurane Isoflurane	None	None	1 to 4+ D	1 to 4− D
Narcotics	None	None	+/−	+/−
Benzodiazepines	None	None	1+	1 to 2−
Etomidate	None	None	1+	2 to 4+ D
Ketamine	None	None	1+	1 to 2+
Propofol	None	None	1 to 2+ D	1 to 2− D
Muscle relaxants	May clarify if EMG noise is a problem	May clarify if EMG noise is a problem	None; may clarify if EMG noise is present	None; may clarify if EMG noise is present

Key: 1+ = >10% increase; 2+ = >20% increase; 3+ = >50% increase; 4+ = ≥100% increase; 1− = >10% decrease; 2− = >20% decrease; 3− = >50% decrease; 4− = incompatible with monitoring; D = dose-related.

What Factors Other Than Surgical Damage Change the Somatosensory Evoked Potentials?

Intraoperative depression of SSEPs can be caused by decreased body temperature, cold irrigation to the surgical field, hypoxemia, variations in $Paco_2$, and anesthetic agents. Of these, changes in anesthetic drug dose are the most important (Table 22–13).[45–52] Most of these factors can be kept constant during SSEP monitoring.

What Do Brainstem Auditory Evoked Potentials Monitor?

The BAEP is a monitor of auditory system function, which begins with the eighth cranial nerve and extends up through the medulla and pons to the temporal lobe.[53–55] BAEPs are the subcortical components of the auditory evoked response and monitor function of the eighth cranial nerve and brainstem auditory pathway up through the nucleus of the lateral lemniscus (Fig. 22–19). The stimulus is a loud, repetitive click delivered to the patient by small ear inserts placed in the external auditory canal. Since recording electrodes cannot be placed close to the brainstem, the BAEP is recorded from the scalp quite far from the generating structures. It is thus very small, and as many as 2000 repetitions may be required to produce a good averaged response.

Use During Surgery

Intraoperative monitoring of BAEPs has been used most frequently for monitoring eighth nerve and brainstem function during surgical procedures in the posterior fossa. This monitoring has been used successfully by surgeons attempting to preserve hearing during resection of acoustic neuromas.[56] Preservation of an unchanged BAEP is associated with functional hearing postoperatively. Loss of all components of the BAEP predicts deafness.

During microvascular decompression of the fifth or seventh cranial nerve in the posterior fossa (the Jannetta procedure), retractor placement may damage the eighth nerve and cause postoperative deafness (Fig. 22–20). Detection of ischemia of the eighth nerve allows retractors to be repositioned before

TABLE 22–14. Effects of Anesthetics on Brainstem Auditory Evoked Potentials[45, 53–55]

Anesthetic Drug	Effect on I-V Interpeak Latency	Effect on Amplitude of Wave V	Clinical Significance*
Barbiturates	Increases	Decreases	None
Nitrous oxide	Minimal	Minimal	None
Halothane Enflurane Isoflurane	Increases	Decreases	Minimal
Narcotics	None	None	None
Benzodiazepines	Minimal	Minimal	Minimal
Etomidate Ketamine Propofol	Minimal	Minimal	None
Muscle relaxants (all types)	None	None	None

*Clinical significance is based on criteria for significant changes at the University of Florida.

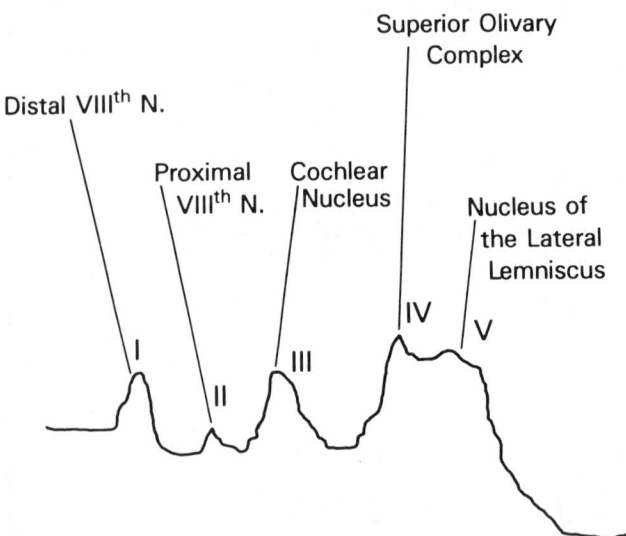

FIGURE 22–19. Brainstem auditory evoked potential. The generator of each wave is shown.

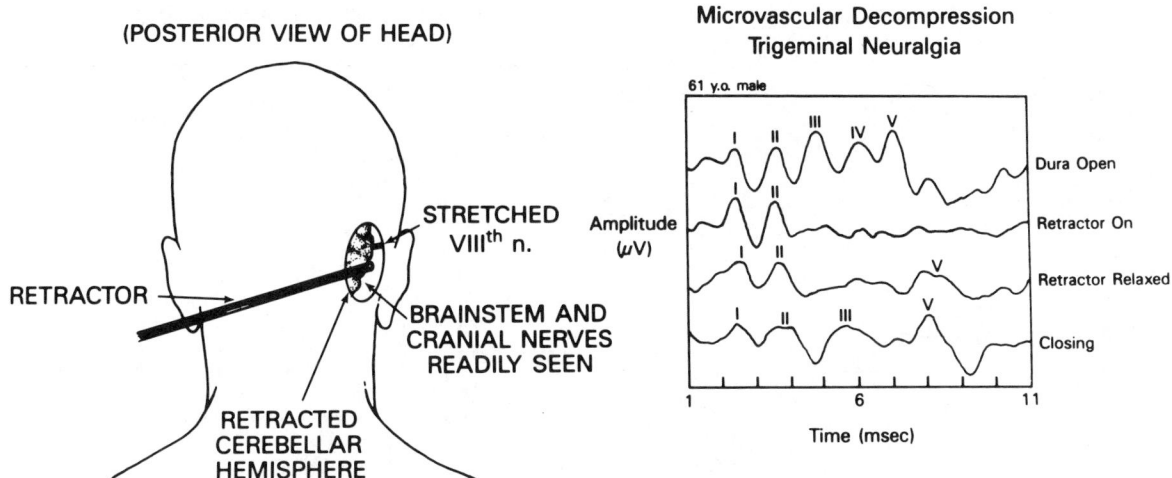

(POSTERIOR VIEW OF HEAD)

RETRACTOR

STRETCHED VIIIth n.

BRAINSTEM AND CRANIAL NERVES READILY SEEN

RETRACTED CEREBELLAR HEMISPHERE

Microvascular Decompression
Trigeminal Neuralgia

61 y.o. male

Amplitude (µV)

Dura Open

Retractor On

Retractor Relaxed

Closing

Time (msec)

FIGURE 22–20. Cerebellar retraction during the Janetta procedure stretches the eighth nerve.

irreversible damage occurs. Monitoring BAEPs has made possible a reduction of the incidence of deafness associated with the Jannetta procedure.[57]

Brainstem function during surgery involving the posterior cerebral circulation (basilar artery and its branches) also can be assessed with BAEP monitoring. As with SSEPs, however, false-negative monitoring patterns may occur. Combined monitoring of SSEPs and BAEPs evaluates the function of a larger portion of the brainstem and may be more useful than isolated monitoring of either during vascular surgery in this region.

Factors Other Than Surgical Damage That Change the Brainstem Auditory Evoked Potentials

Resistance to nonsurgical factors such as hypothermia and anesthetic drugs is greater with BAEPs than with other EPs. They may be recorded successfully during any anesthetic technique. In contrast with SSEP monitoring, changes in anesthetic technique (Table 22–14) are unlikely to produce a change in the BAEP waveform that will be mistaken for a surgically induced change.

What Do Visual Evoked Potentials Monitor?

Visual evoked potentials (VEPs) reflect the function of the visual pathway, which extends from the optic nerve through the chiasm to the visual cortex. The VEP is generated primarily by the visual cortex. Intraoperatively, the stimulus is usually applied by goggles that deliver a repetitive bright flash through closed eyelids. Contact lenses containing light-emitting diodes also have been applied directly to the cornea. This arrangement takes up less space and is less likely to interfere with surgical exposure; also, when contact lenses are used, a closed eyelid does not interfere with delivery of the stimulus as it does when goggles are used. Recordings are from scalp electrodes placed over the calcarine cortex.

Use During Surgery

VEPs are not widely used during surgery. They have been used for visual function monitoring in operations near the optic

nerve and chiasm (most commonly during pituitary surgery). They can also be monitored during resection of intracranial tumors such as meningiomas that involve or compress the optic nerve.

Correlation between changes in VEPs and outcome has not been evaluated in a large series of patients. Which VEP changes during manipulation of the optic nerve and chiasm are normal and which are ominous have not been identified. The major reasons for this lack of data are difficulties with stimulus application and the exquisite sensitivity of the VEP to anesthetic agents. Some investigators believe that VEPs are too variable intraoperatively to be of any clinical use.[58, 59]

What Are Motor Evoked Potentials?

MEP monitoring was developed specifically to assess the function of motor pathways; thus, it overcomes one of the major limitations of SSEP monitoring. Many variants exist. The most common involves placement of stimulating electrodes on the scalp over the motor cortex; an electrical current is passed through the motor cortex transcranially to provide stimulation. An experimental new method of stimulating the motor cortex also has been used. A powerful magnetic stimulator is placed on the scalp over the motor cortex. Brief repetitive applications of a strong magnetic field induce current in the motor cortex and produce an MEP. Both methods also probably activate surrounding cortical structures as well as subcortical white matter pathways (sensory and motor) (Fig. 22–21).

Propagation of the stimulus is blocked by synapses in all of the ascending (sensory) pathways, but the stimulus is propagated easily via descending pathways. The evoked responses may be recorded over the spinal cord, the peripheral nerve, and the involved muscle (EMG) (see Fig. 22–21). To enhance, the MEP, these responses may be averaged in the same manner as for sensory EPs; however, averaging often is unnecessary.

A third method to produce the MEP involves electrical stimulation of the spinal cord above the area at risk during surgery. Responses are recorded over the peripheral nerve and muscle.

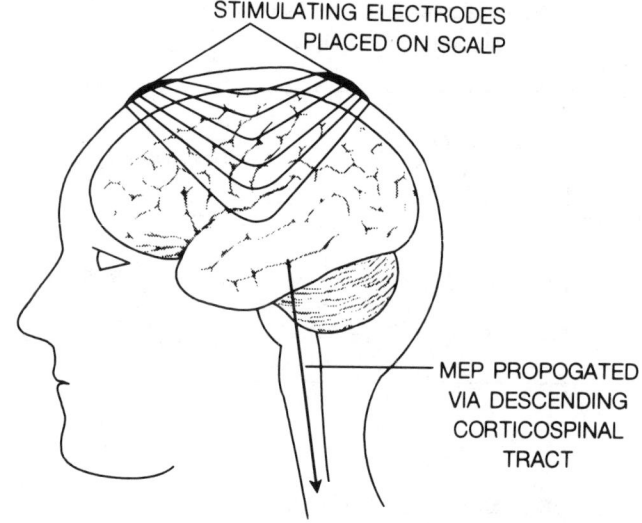

STIMULATING ELECTRODES PLACED ON SCALP

MEP PROPOGATED VIA DESCENDING CORTICOSPINAL TRACT

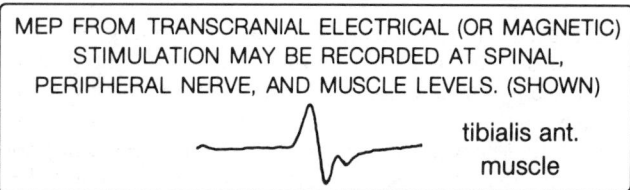

MEP FROM TRANSCRANIAL ELECTRICAL (OR MAGNETIC) STIMULATION MAY BE RECORDED AT SPINAL, PERIPHERAL NERVE, AND MUSCLE LEVELS. (SHOWN)

tibialis ant. muscle

FIGURE 22–21. Schematic representation of transcranial motor evoked potential for magnetic stimulation. Electrodes are replaced by a magnetic coil that is positioned over the motor strip.

Clinical Applications

This monitoring modality, although promising in some aspects, has many problems that remain to be solved. The exact pathways involved have not been completely determined. Intraoperative experience is relatively limited. Anecdotal reports suggest that MEP monitoring during surgery on the spine or its blood supply may be very useful.[60, 61] Whether this monitor can be used to guide management and predict postoperative neurologic function in a large series of patients is unknown. Some recent data suggest that MEPs may be no more effective in predicting motor function following major aortic surgery than are SSEPs. Responses recorded over the lumbar cord are insensitive indicators of motor function following aortic cross-clamping in several animal models.[62, 63]

Anesthetic Effects

Anesthetic agent effects are surprisingly profound, particularly on EMG recordings of the MEP produced by either transcranial electrical or magnetic stimulation (Table 22–15).[64–69] Recordings produced by stimulation of the spinal cord are less sensitive to anesthetic agents.

Safety

Limited data are available regarding the short-term or long-term safety of magnetic or electrical transcranial stimulation of the cortex. Neither stimulation method is approved for use in humans; at this time, MEP monitoring should still be considered experimental.

TABLE 22–15. Effects of Anesthetics on Motor Evoked Potentials: Transcranial Magnetic and Electrical[64–69]

Anesthetic Drug	Muscle Potential (EMG)
Barbiturate	P
Nitrous oxide	P (D)
Halothane	P
Enflurane	
Isoflurane	
Narcotics	A
Benzodiazepines	P
Ketamine	A
Etomidate	A
Propofol	?P*
Muscle relaxant	A†

*Conflicting data in literature
†Provided that 1–2 twitches are maintained.
Abbreviations: A = acceptable; P = prohibitive in clinically used concentrations <1 maximum alveolar concentration.

FACIAL NERVE MONITORING

Why Is It Important?

Some operations in the posterior fossa, particularly those involving resection of acoustic neuromas and the base of the skull, may result in damage to the facial nerve (cranial nerve VII). Postoperative weakness or paralysis of the facial nerve produces serious morbidity. First, eye closure may be incomplete, producing corneal drying and damage; second, muscles of facial expression can fail to function, with resulting serious disfigurement.

How Can It Be Monitored During Surgery?

Direct Observation

The simplest method involves direct observation of the face while the surgeon uses a nerve stimulator to locate the facial nerve in the surgical field. This method is limited for several reasons. First, the facial nerve is not assessed except when the surgeon attempts to locate it with a nerve stimulator. Serious damage that will not be detected can occur at other times during surgery (e.g., during exposure of an acoustic tumor over which the facial nerve has been stretched). Second, the face may not be readily visible for direct observation. For example, during procedures conducted in the three-quarter prone position, which is commonly used for posterior fossa explorations, the face cannot be seen unless the clinician crawls under the table and shines a light on it.

Electromyography

For facial nerve monitoring, EMG recording needles are placed in the orbicularis oculi and orbicularis oris muscles (Fig. 22–22). To locate the facial nerve, a repetitive electrical stimulus is applied, and EMG activity is recorded from these muscles (Fig. 22–23). The EMG response is displayed on a screen and converted to an audio signal that gives immediate, direct feedback to the surgeon.

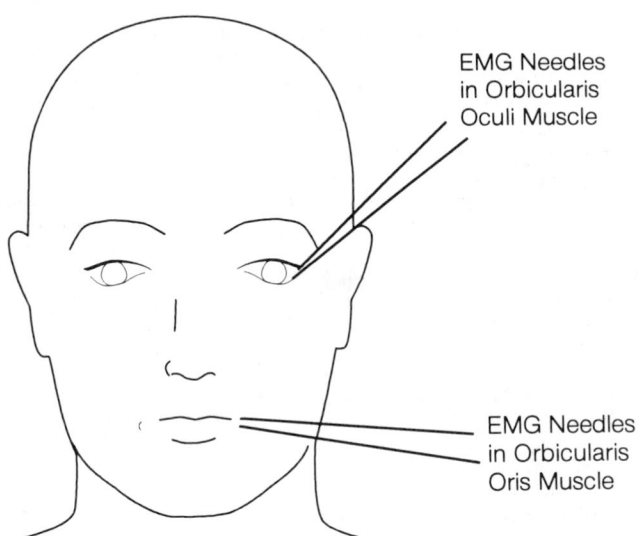

FIGURE 22–22. Schematic representation of facial nerve monitor.

Passive Monitoring

The facial nerve may also be passively monitored. Whenever surgical manipulation involves touching of or retraction on the facial nerve, spontaneous electrical activity increases, and the audio signal, which sounds like static on a radio, immediately alerts the surgeon to the proximity of the nerve.

Summary

These techniques are much more reliable than mere observation for facial twitching. Facial nerve monitoring leads to improved facial nerve function following acoustic tumor removal.[70] The EMG is also safer than facial observation because the anesthesiologist does not have to disturb the arrangement of equipment, personnel, or drapes to see the face. Motor cranial nerves III, IV, VI, X, XI, and XII also can be monitored in a similar fashion to detect surgical trauma in the posterior fossa.

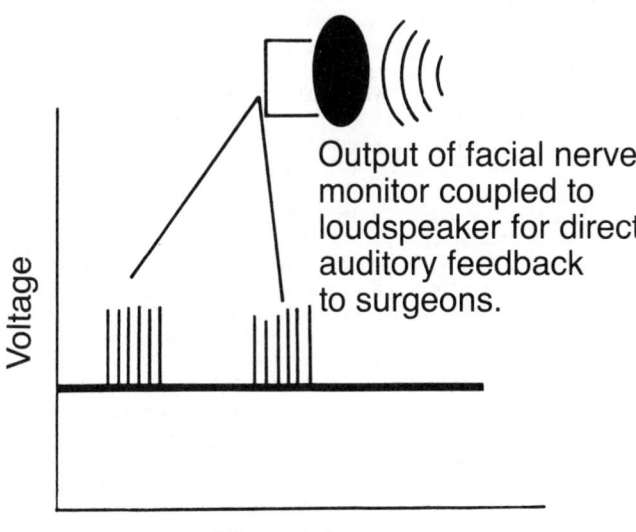

FIGURE 22–23. Active monitoring of the facial nerve.

Can Neuromuscular Blocking Agents Be Used?

For EMG monitoring to be successful, the patient cannot be completely paralyzed. A recent study demonstrated that partial paralysis (twitch height 50% of control) is compatible with successful location of the facial nerve.[71] Whether such paralysis affects the sensitivity of passive facial nerve monitoring is unclear. Many experts involved in seventh nerve monitoring still recommend complete avoidance of neuromuscular blockade during the time at which the facial nerve is considered at risk. Higher concentrations of potent inhalation agents, with or without nitrous oxide, facilitate patient immobility in the absence of neuromuscular blocking agents.

CONCLUSIONS

A large portion of the anesthesiologist's job is to assess organ function during surgery. Advances such as the pulmonary artery catheter, mixed venous oximetry, transesophageal echocardiography, capnography, and pulse oximetry have been mastered by most anesthesiologists involved in the care of critically ill patients. Similar advances have been made in the monitoring of neurologic function.

The nervous system can be placed at risk during surgery by a reduction in O_2 supply or by structural damage from positioning or surgical manipulation. Monitoring gives information about blood flow or neurologic function that would not otherwise be available. The surgeon can alter the procedure, and the anesthesiologist may intervene to increase blood pressure, change patient position, increase the amount of inspired O_2, or administer drugs to decrease O_2 demand, thus restoring blood flow or CNS function to normal levels. Anesthesiologists should embrace CNS monitoring as a part of their practice when they provide perioperative care for patients at risk for neurologic damage.

References

1. Sundt TM Jr, Sharbrough FW, Piepgras DG, et al: Correlation of cerebral blood flow and electroencephalographic changes during carotid endarterectomy: with results of surgery and hemodynamics of cerebral ischemia. Mayo Clin Proc 1981; 56:533.
2. Nash CL, Lorig RA, Schatzinger LA, et al: Spinal cord monitoring during operative treatment of the spine. Clin Orthop 1977; 126:100.
3. Dinner DS, Lüders H, Lesser RP, et al: Intraoperative spinal somatosensory evoked potential monitoring. J Neurosurg 1986; 65:807.
4. York DH, Chabot RJ, Gaines RW: Response variability of somatosensory evoked potentials during scoliosis surgery. Spine 1987; 12:864.
5. Bieber E, Tolo V, Uematsu S: Spinal cord monitoring during posterior spinal instrumentation and fusion. Clin Orthop 1988; 229:121.
6. Grundy BL, Nash CL, Brown RH: Arterial pressure manipulation alters spinal cord function during correction of scoliosis. Anesthesiology 1981; 54:249.
7. Ginsburg HH, Shetter AG, Raudzens PA: Postoperative paraplegia with preserved intraoperative somatosensory evoked potentials: a case report. J Neurosurg 1985; 63:296.
8. Lesser RP, Raudzens PA, Lüders H, et al: Postoperative neurological deficits may occur despite unchanged somatosensory evoked potentials. Ann Neurol 1986; 19:22.
9. Friedman WA, Grundy BL: Monitoring of sensory evoked potentials is highly reliable and helpful in the operating room. J Clin Monit 1987; 3:38.
10. Little JR, Lesser RP, Lüders H: Electrophysiologic monitoring during basilar aneurysm operation. Neurosurgery 1987; 20:421.
11. Hall JE, Levine CR, Sudhir KG: Intraoperative awakening to monitor spinal cord function during Harrington instrumentation and spine fusion. J Bone Joint Surg 1978; 60A:533.

12. Ben DB, Taylor PD, Haller GS: Posterior spinal fusion complicated by posterior column injury: a case report of a false-negative wake-up test. Spine 1987; 12:540.

13. Silbergeld DL, Mueller WM, Colley PS, et al: Use of propofol (Diprivan) for awake craniotomies: technical note. Surg Neurol 1992; 38:271.

14. Oei-Lim VL, Kalkman CJ, Bouvy-Berends EC, et al: A comparison of the effects of propofol and nitrous oxide on the electroencephalogram in epileptic patients during conscious sedation for dental procedures. Anesth Analg 1992; 75:708.

15. Hoffman WE, Miletich DJ, Albrecht RF: The influence of antihypertensive therapy on cerebral autoregulation in aged hypertensive rats. Stroke 1982; 13:701.

16. Paulson OB, Strandgaard S, Edvinsson LTI: Cerebral autoregulation. Cerebrovasc Brain Metab Rev 1990; 2:161.

17. Sundbarg G, Nordstrom CH, Soderstrom S: Complications due to prolonged ventricular fluid pressure recording. Br J Neurosurg 1988; 4:485.

18. Halsey JH, McDowell HA, Gelmon S, et al: Blood velocity in the middle cerebral artery and regional cerebral blood flow during carotid endarterectomy. Stroke 1989; 20:53.

19. Pashayan AG, Mahla ME: Unpublished data.

20. Spencer MP, Thomas GI, Nicholls SC, Sauvage LR: Detection of middle cerebral artery emboli during carotid endarterectomy using transcranial Doppler ultrasonography. Stroke 1990; 21:415.

21. van der Linden J, Wessler O, Tyder H, et al: Transcranial Doppler versus thermodilution measurements of cerebral blood flow during cardiac surgery. J Cardiothorac Anesth 1989; 3:68.

22. van der Linden J, Casimir-Ahn H: When do cerebral emboli occur during open heart operations? A transcranial Doppler study. Ann Thorac Surg 1991; 51:237.

23. Sloan MA, Haley EC Jr, Kassell NF, et al: Sensitivity and specificity of transcranial Doppler ultrasonography in the diagnosis of vasospasm following subarachnoid hemorrhage. Neurology 1989; 39:1514.

24. Grosset DG, Straiton J, du Trevou M, et al: Prediction of symptomatic vasospasm after subarachnoid hemorrhage by rapidly increasing transcranial Doppler velocity and cerebral blood flow changes. Stroke 1992; 23:674.

25. Petty GW, Mohr JP, Pedley TA, et al: The role of transcranial Doppler in confirming brain death. Neurology 1990; 40:300.

26. Sheinberg M, Kanter MJ, Robertson CS, et al: Continuous monitoring of jugular venous oxygen saturation in head-injured patients. J Neurosurg 1992; 76:212.

27. Jasper HH: The ten-twenty electrode system of the International Federation. Electroencephalogr Clin Neurophysiol 1958; 10:371.

28. Spackman TN, Faust RJ, Cucchiara RF, et al: A comparison of aperiodic analysis of the EEG with standard EEG and cerebral blood flow for the detection of ischemia. Anesthesiology 1987; 66:229.

29. Messick JM Jr, Casement B, Sharbrough FW, et al: Correlation of regional cerebral blood flow (rCBF) with EEG changes during isoflurane anesthesia for carotid endarterectomy: critical rCBF. Anesthesiology 1987; 66:344.

30. Sundt TM Jr, Michenfelder JD: Focal transient ischemia in the squirrel monkey: effect on brain adenosine triphosphate and lactate levels with electrocorticographic and pathologic correlation. Circ Res 1972; 30:703.

31. Silbert BS, Koumoundouros E, Davies MJ, et al: Comparison of the processed electroencephalogram and awake neurologic assessment during carotid endarterectomy. Anaesth Intensive Care 1989; 17:298.

32. Whittemore AD, Kauffman JL, Kohler TR, et al: Routine electroencephalographic (EEG) monitoring during carotid endarterectomy. Ann Surg 1983; 193:707.

33. Halsey JH Jr: Risks and benefits of shunting in carotid endarterectomy. the international transcranial Doppler collaborators. Stroke 1992; 23:1583.

34. Landi A, Copeland SA, Wynn-Parry CB, et al: The role of somatosensory evoked potentials and nerve conduction studies in the surgical management of brachial plexus injuries. J Bone Joint Surg 1980; 4:492.

35. Kaplan BJ, Friedman WA, Alexander JA, Hampson SR: Somatosensory evoked potential monitoring of spinal cord ischemia during aortic operations. Neurosurgery 1986; 19:82.

36. Crawford ES, Mizrahi EM, Hess KR, et al: The impact of distal aortic perfusion and somatosensory evoked potential monitoring on prevention of paraplegia after aortic aneurysm operation. J Thorac Cardiovasc Surg 1988; 95:357.

37. Maeda S, Miyamoto T, Murata H, et al: Prevention of spinal cord ischemia by monitoring spinal cord perfusion pressure and somatosensory evoked potentials. J Cardiovasc Surg 1989; 30:565.

38. Laschinger JC, Cunningham JN, Cooper MM, et al: Monitoring of somatosensory evoked potentials during surgical procedures on the thoracoabdominal aorta: I. Relationship of aortic cross-clamp duration, changes in somatosensory evoked potentials, and incidence of neurologic dysfunction. J Thorac Cardiovasc Surg 1987; 94:260.

39. Cunningham JN, Laschinger JC, Spencer FC: Monitoring of somatosensory evoked potentials during surgical procedures on the thoracoabdominal aorta: IV. Clinical observations and results. J Thorac Cardiovasc Surg 1987; 94:275.

40. Branston NM, Symon L, Crockard HA, et al: Relationship between the cortical evoked potential and local cortical blood flow following acute middle cerebral artery occlusion in the baboon. Exp Neurol 1974; 45:195.

41. Friedman WA, Chadwick GM, Verhoeven FJS, et al: Monitoring of somatosensory evoked potentials during surgery for middle cerebral artery aneurysms. Neurosurgery 1991; 29:83.

42. Schramm J, Koht A, Schmidt G, et al: Surgical and electrophysiologic observations during clipping of 134 aneurysms with evoked potential monitoring. Neurosurgery 1990; 26:61.

43. Mooij JJA, Buchthal A, Belopavlovic M: Somatosensory evoked potential monitoring of temporary middle cerebral artery occlusion during aneurysm operation. Neurosurgery 1987; 21:492.

44. Little JR, Lesser RP, Lüders H: Electrophysiological monitoring during basilar aneurysm operation. Neurosurgery 1987; 20:421.

45. Sebel PS, Ingram DA, Flynn PJ, et al: Evoked potentials during isoflurane anaesthesia. Br J Anaesth 1986; 58:580.

46. Drummond JC, Todd MM, U HS: The effect of high dose sodium thiopental on brainstem auditory and median nerve somatosensory evoked responses in humans. Anesthesiology 1985; 63:249.

47. McPherson RW, Sell B, Traystman RJ: Effects of thiopental, fentanyl and etomidate on upper extremity somatosensory evoked potentials in humans. Anesthesiology 1986; 62:626.

48. McPherson RW, Mahla ME, Johnson R, et al: Effects of enflurane, isoflurane and nitrous oxide on somatosensory evoked potentials during fentanyl anesthesia. Anesthesiology 1985; 62:626.

49. Schubert A, Drummond JC, Peterson DO, et al: The effect of high-dose fentanyl on human median nerve somatosensory-evoked responses. Can J Anaesth 1987; 34:35.

50. Sloan TB, Ronai AK, Toleikis JR, et al: Improvement of intraoperative somatosensory evoked potentials by etomidate. Anesth Analg 1988; 67:582.

51. Koht A, Schütz W, Schmidt G, et al: Effects of etomidate, midazolam, and thiopental on median nerve somatosensory evoked potentials and the additive effects of fentanyl and nitrous oxide. Anesth Analg 1988; 67:435.

52. Maurette P, Simeon F, Castagnera L, et al: Propofol anaesthesia alters somatosensory evoked cortical potentials. Anaesthesia 1988; 43(Suppl):44.

53. Drummond JC, Todd MM, Schubert A, et al: Effect of the acute administration of high dose pentobarbital on human brainstem auditory and median nerve somatosensory evoked responses. Neurosurgery 1987; 20:830.

54. DuBois MY, Sato S, Chassy J, et al: Effects of enflurane on brainstem auditory evoked responses in humans. Anesth Analg 1982; 61:898.

55. Manninen PH, Lam AM, Nicholas JF: The effects of isoflurane and isoflurane–nitrous oxide anesthesia on brainstem auditory evoked potentials in humans. Anesth Analg 1985; 64:43.

56. Watanabe E, Schramm J, Strauss C, et al: Neurophysiologic monitoring in posterior fossa surgery: II. BAEP-waves I and V and preservation of hearing. Acta Neurochir (Wien) 1989; 98:118.

57. Moeller AR, Moeller MB: Does intraoperative monitoring of auditory evoked potentials reduce incidence of hearing loss as a complication of microvascular decompression of cranial nerves? Neurosurgery 1989; 24:257.

58. Raudzens PA: Intraoperative monitoring of evoked potentials. Ann N Y Acad Sci 1982; 388:308.

59. Grundy BL: Monitoring of sensory evoked potentials during neurosurgical operations: methods and applications. Neurosurgery 1982; 11:556.

60. Edmonds HL Jr, Paloheimo MP, Backman MH, et al: Transcranial magnetic motor evoked potentials for functional montoring of motor pathways during scoliosis surgery. Spine 1989; 14:683.

61. Owen JH, Bridwell KH, Grubb R, et al: The clinical application of neurogenic motor evoked potentials to monitor spinal cord function during surgery. Spine 1991; 16(8 Suppl):S385.

62. Elmore JR, Gloviczki P, Harper CM, et al: Spinal cord injury in experimental thoracic aortic occlusion: investigation of combined methods of protection. J Vasc Surg 1992; 15:789.

63. Elmore JR, Gloviczki P, Harper CM, et al: Failure of motor evoked potentials to predict neurologic outcome in experimental thoracic aortic occlusion. J Vasc Surg 1991; 14:131.

64. Zentner J, Albrecht T, Heuser D: Influence of halothane, enflurane, and isoflurane on motor evoked potentials. Neurosurgery 1992; 31:298.

65. Jellinek D, Platt M, Jewkes D, et al: Effects of nitrous oxide on motor evoked potentials under total anesthesia with intravenously administered propofol. Neurosurgery 1991; 29:558.

66. Ghaly RF, Stone JL, Levy WJ, et al: The effect of etomidate on motor evoked potentials induced by transcranial magnetic stimulation in the monkey. Neurosurgery 1990; 27:936.

67. Zentner J, Kiss I, Ebner A: Influence of anesthetics—nitrous oxide in particular—on electromyographic response evoked by transcranial electrical stimulation of the cortex. Neurosurgery 1989; 24:253.

68. Kalkman CJ, Drummond JC, Ribberink AA, et al: Effects of propofol, etomidate, midazolam, and fentanyl on motor evoked responses to trans-cranial electrical or magnetic stimulation in humans. Anesthesiology 1992; 76:502.

69. Kalkman CJ, Drummond JC, Kennelly NA, et al: Intraoperative monitoring of tibialis anterior muscle motor evoked responses to transcranial electrical stimulation during partial neuromuscular blockade. Anesth Analg 1992; 75:584.

70. Harner SG, Daube JR, Ebersold MJ, et al: Improved preservation of facial nerve function with use of electrical monitoring during removal of acoustic neuromas. Mayo Clin Proc 1987; 62:92.

71. Lennon RL, Hosking MP, Daube JR, et al: Effect of partial neuromuscular blockade on intraoperative electromyography in patients undergoing resection of acoustic neuromas. Anesth Analg 1992; 75:729.

CHAPTER 23

Neuromuscular Junction Monitoring and Nerve Stimulation

H. JERREL FONTENOT, M.D., Ph.D.

PETER GERNER, M.D.

More than 3 decades have passed since the initial account of the use of nerve stimulators in the objective assessment of neuromuscular function during anesthesia was published. For many years, few anesthetists used nerve stimulators routinely; instead, the degree of neuromuscular blockade during and after anesthesia was evaluated using clinical criteria alone (Table 23–1). Since the early 1970s, increasing awareness of the problems of postoperative residual neuromuscular blockade has been documented.[1, 2] The present medicolegal practice setting and the quest for objective measurement in such a setting have advanced peripheral nerve stimulation monitoring during and after muscle relaxant administration. The value of this equipment for routine monitoring of neuromuscular blockade is now widely applied and appreciated.[3, 4]

PRACTICAL CONSIDERATIONS

In awake patients, muscle force can be evaluated with tests of voluntary muscle strength; however, this approach is not practical during either general anesthesia or during the initial recovery from anesthesia. Instead, the clinician uses clinical assessment to directly assess muscle power and to indirectly estimate neuromuscular function (muscle tone, the feel of the anesthesia bag, tidal volume, and inspiratory pressure). Unfortunately, all of these clinical parameters are influenced by factors other than the degree of neuromuscular blockade. Therefore, whenever more precise information regarding the status of neuromuscular functioning is necessary, objective assessment using a neuromuscular stimulator is essential.

Why Monitor?

Presently available and prospective neuromuscular blocking agents have been designed to optimize control of neuromuscular blockade. Limiting factors include our understanding of their pharmacology and, potentially, our ability to assess accurately the magnitude of blockade. The latter problem can be handled by observation of the muscle response to nerve stimulation. By so doing, we overcome the possible clinical assessment deficiencies related to interpatient pharmacokinetic and pharmacodynamic variability. The information derived helps to identify the optimal time to intubate and extubate the trachea; the precise dose of drug necessary to produce neuromuscular blockade; the optimal time to reverse the blockade; and whether reversal of neuromuscular blockade is adequate. Documentation of neuromuscular function on the anesthesia record is especially warranted if a clinician elects not to use a reversal agent following the administration of a nondepolarizing blocking agent.

Many variables impact on the physiology of the neuromuscular junction; many drugs modify that physiology. Therefore, predictability of individual patient response in other than the crudest of fashions is likely to be inaccurate following neuromuscular blocking drug administration. This response is even more uncertain in pathologic conditions that directly or indirectly involve the neuromuscular junction. The acquisition of relevant data contributes to a more predictable and rational approach to the use of neuromuscular blocking agents and, consequently, to better patient care.

How Is Neuromuscular Blockade Assessed Clinically?

Muscle Control and Strength

The basic clinical approach is to observe provoked or spontaneous clinical signs such as the eye opening, tongue protru-

TABLE 23–1. Clinical Assessment of Neuromuscular Function

Eye opening
Tongue protrusion
Swallow
Grip strength
Head lift
Tidal volume
Vital capacity
Peak negative pressure

sion, swallowing, hand grip strength, and head lift. The most definitive indicator of significant residual neuromuscular blockade is the failed head lift (i.e., the inability of a supine patient to lift his or her head off the bed for at least 5 seconds).

Respiratory Variables

In addition, some anesthesiologists also assess specific respiratory variables such as tidal volume, vital capacity, inspiratory force (peak negative pressure), and expiratory force (pressure) to indicate the presence or absence of any residual weakness secondary to neuromuscular block.[3] Obviously, measurement of voluntary movement cannot be carried out in unconscious patients, and involuntary movements may be depressed by the central actions of analgesics and anesthetics rather than by peripherally acting neuromuscular blocking agents. Some patients may also be inhibited from performing a head lift or other clinical test by pain, bandages, or residual sedation. Attempts to judge recovery from the effects of muscle relaxants on clinical criteria (patient movement, tidal volume, vital capacity) without the aid of a peripheral nerve stimulator (i.e., an evoked response to peripheral nerve stimulation) may result in failure to appreciate significant residual neuromuscular blockade (Table 23–2).[5]

Respiratory Depression

The supposition that relaxants are responsible for respiratory depression after emergence from anesthesia can only be determined when impairment of neuromuscular function is confirmed. Pavlin and coworkers demonstrated that adequate ventilation in unanesthetized volunteers did not guarantee the ability to adequately protect the airway (Fig. 23–1).[6] Only when individuals were able to lift their heads for 5 seconds could they perform all maneuvers "guaranteed" to maintain a functionally intact airway.

Because this study was performed with unanesthetized volunteers, the implication for patients who are exposed to a variety of drugs and drug interactions is that even stricter criteria are appropriate. A study in awake volunteers receiving vecuronium again placed serious doubt on the reliability of clinical assessment in the determination of "complete rever-

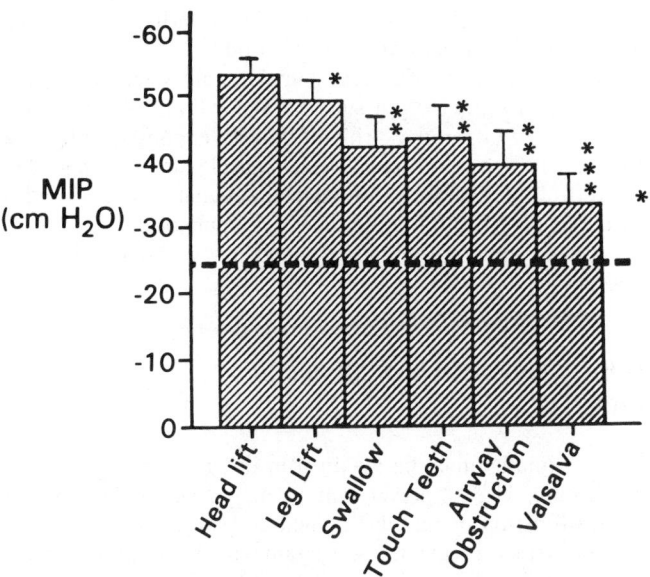

FIGURE 23–1. Levels of neuromuscular blockade in awake volunteers with d-tubocurarine (dTc) indicated by maximum inspiratory pressure (MIP ± SE) below which the indicated clinical maneuvers could not be accomplished. Head lift and straight leg raising are the most sensitive indicators of neuromuscular blockade with dTc. No maneuvers indicating airway protection could be accomplished by any of the subjects at a MIP of -25 cm H_2O. * = $P < .001$ compared with MIP = -25 cm H_2O; ** = $P < .2$ compared with MIP = -25 cm H_2O; *** = $P < .05$ compared with MIP = -25 cm H_2O. (From Pavlin EG, Holle RH, Schoene RB: Recovery of airway protection compared with ventilation in humans after paralysis with curare. Anesthesiology 1989; 70:383.)

sal."[7] A significant decrease in response to hypoxia was noted despite a train-of-four ratio (T_4/T_1) of 0.7 that indicated normal recovery. It also suggested an effect of vecuronium on carotid body chemosensitivity (i.e., depression of the hypoxic ventilatory response).

The most reliable method of monitoring neuromuscular function is stimulation of an accessible peripheral motor nerve and measurement of the evoked response of the skeletal muscle innervated by that nerve. In contrast to voluntary movement, evoked responses do not require patient cooperation and, if applied with a supramaximal stimulus, ensure full activation of all nerve and muscle fibers.

TECHNIQUE

What Is the Proper Stimulus Pattern?

The response of the whole muscle to a stimulus depends on the number of muscle fibers activated. The single muscle fiber responds in a quantal fashion—that is, it either responds or does not (no graded response occurs). If a nerve is stimulated with sufficient intensity, all muscle fibers supplied by the nerve contract, and the response is maximal.

Following the administration of a neuromuscular blocking drug, the response of the whole muscle decreases in parallel with the number of fibers blocked. The reduction in response during constant stimulation reflects the degree of neuromuscular blockade. A nerve stimulator should deliver a square-wave stimulus of sufficient intensity to depolarize the nerve

TABLE 23–2. Assessment of Neuromuscular Function

Test	Per Cent of Receptors Occupied Before Abnormal	Disadvantages
Tidal volume	75–80	Insensitive, significantly altered by anesthetic agents
Twitch height	75–80	Insensitive, uncomfortable
Tetanic stimulation (30 Hz)	75–80	Insensitive, uncomfortable
Vital capacity	75–80	Insensitive, patient cooperation required
Train-of-four	75–80	Requires <50% T_4/T_1 to be visible
Tetanic stimulation	50	Painful
Head lift/hand grip	33	Patient cooperation

fibers; duration of stimulus should be less than that of the neuromuscular junction refractory period.[8-10]

Desirable features of a nerve stimulator are detailed in Table 23–3. Stimuli that are not square-wave and are of long duration can cause repetitive firing of the nerve; consequently, the patient will appear to have greater muscle strength than that which truly exists. Most commercial stimulators deliver pulse durations of 0.1 to 0.3 milliseconds. Stimulator characteristics are usually quite specifically detailed in the product description.

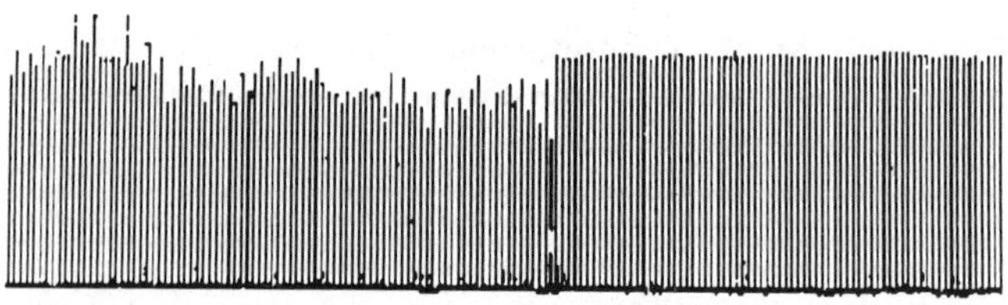

FIGURE 23–2. Submaximum versus supramaximum stimulation. The left half of the twitch recording represents the variety of responses to a control situation with submaximum stimulation, whereas the right half demonstrates the very uniform response to supramaximum stimuli.

Why Is Supramaximal Stimulation Preferred?

The stimulus must be maximal in order to ensure accurate monitoring. Use of lower current may result in an overall underestimation of muscle strength and an overestimation of neuromuscular blockade. A supramaximal stimulus ensures that all nerve fibers are stimulated each time, even though current output or skin impedance may have changed.

Desired Level

The optimal supramaximal electrical stimulus is usually at least 20% to 25% above that necessary for a maximal response. Increasing the stimulus to a supramaximal level does not obtain a higher response but does ensure a maximal response and one that is reproducible, reliable, and useful (Fig. 23–2).

Current Requirement

In 75% of patients, when surface electrodes (not needles) are used over the ulnar nerve at the wrist, the supramaximal current is in the range of 15 to 40 mA (obese patients may require 50–60 mA).

What Are Desirable Nerve Stimulator Characteristics?

The nerve stimulator should be able to generate 60 to 70 mA, but not more than 100 mA (see Table 23–3).[11] Most com-

mercially available stimulators deliver only 25 to 50 mA and a constant current only when skin resistance is below 2500 Ω. This limitation becomes a significant clinical problem during cooling, when skin resistance may increase to approximately 5000 Ω. As a result, the current delivered may fall below the supramaximal level, leading to a decrease in the stimulatory response.

In general practice, you are best served by a stimulator with a current level display that alerts the user when the current selected is not being delivered because of resistance changes or decreased battery life. Some modern stimulators supply a constant current of ≤ 80 mA that is unaffected by changes in skin impedance.

Stimulators that provide multiple patterns are desirable as they have more versatile and clinically useful applications. The availability of high and low output sockets is important if the nerve stimulator is attached to a block needle for nerve identification during regional anesthetia.

How Should Electrodes Be Placed and Used?

Pregelled, adhesive electrocardiographic electrodes are most commonly used, although special electrodes and needles for neuromuscular monitoring are manufactured. The actual gelled electrode surface must not be too large, otherwise current density is reduced and a supramaximal stimulus may not be delivered. Ideally, the skin should be cleansed properly and rubbed with an abrasive before application of the electrodes. When supramaximal response cannot be obtained by using surface electrodes, another site should be tried or needle electrodes should be placed. Assess for supramaximal stimulus by increasing the output of the nerve stimulator incrementally and observing the evoked twitch. Once the maximum twitch has been observed, the output of the monitor is increased another 20% to ensure that it is supramaximal.

In general, any superficially located peripheral motor nerve can be used in the monitoring of neuromuscular function. In clinical anesthesia, the ulnar nerve is the most popular site; the median, posterior tibial, common peroneal, and facial nerves are also used. The ulnar nerve offers several advantages, including ease of electrode application, decreased potential for direct muscle stimulation of the adductor muscle of the thumb, and a sensitivity index between that of laryngeal muscles and the diaphragm.

Ulnar Nerve

For stimulation of the ulnar nerve, the electrodes are best applied at the volar side of the wrist (Fig. 23–3). The distal

TABLE 23–3. Desirable Features of a Nerve Stimulator

Essential	Square-wave impulse, <0.5-ms duration
	Ability to maintain selected current for duration of impulse (i.e., constant current, variable voltage)
	Battery power
	Multiple patterns of stimulation; single-twitch, train-of-four, double-burst, tetanus, post-tetanic count
Optional	Rheostat for adjustable current output
	Polarity output indicator
	Ability to calculate and display fade ratio and/or per cent depression of single-twitch amplitude from control value
	High-output (≤80–100 mA) and low-output (<5 mA) sockets
	Audible signal with each stimulus delivered
	Alarm for excessive impedance, lead disconnect, and low battery
	Battery charge indicator

(From Brull SJ, Silverman DG: Neuromuscular block monitoring. *In* Anesthesia Equipment Principles and Applications. Ehrenworth J, Eisenkraft JB (eds). St Louis, CV Mosby, 1993, p 300.)

electrode should be placed about 1 cm proximal to the point where the proximal flexion crease of the wrist crosses the radial side of the tendon to the ulnar flexor muscle of the wrist. The proximal electrode preferably should be within 3 cm of the distal electrode. Placement of the electrode any more proximally frequently results in direct muscle stimulation of the flexor muscles of the forearm, especially if the proximal electrode is negative. The closer the electrode is to the wrist, the more circumscribed the effect is to the ulnar nerve–innervated hand muscles.

Correct placement of electrodes over the ulnar nerve and adequate stimulation produce only finger flexion and thumb adduction. If the proximal electrode is placed over the ulnar groove at the elbow, thumb adduction often appears more pronounced because of the stimulation of the ulnar flexor muscle of the wrist (see Fig. 23–3). In children, placement at the ulnar groove may be preferable (because of the size of the stimulating electrodes); in this case, the active negative electrode should be at the wrist to ensure a maximal response.[12, 13]

Facial Nerve

Stimulation of either the facial nerve or one of its major trunks can be accomplished by placing electrodes lateral to the

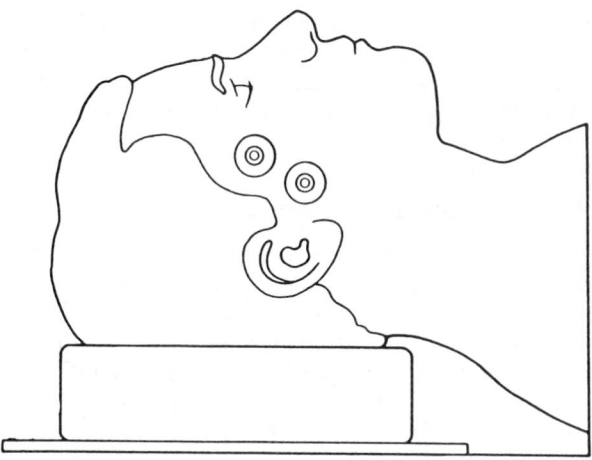

FIGURE 23–4. Positioning of stimulating electrodes over nerve. The electrode nearest the eye is negative. (Modified from Caffrey RR, Warren ML, Becker KE Jr: Neuromuscular blockade monitoring comparing the orbicularis oculi and adductor pollicis muscles. Anesthesiology 1986; 65:96.)

eye and anterior to the ear (the negative electrode should be placed distally over the course of the nerve) (Fig. 23–4). Generally, visual assessment is more difficult because the target muscles are not available for tactile or mechanical assessment. Response of the facial nerve–innervated musculature (orbicular muscle of the eye, orbicular muscle of the mouth) precedes that of ulnar nerve stimulation; this presents the danger of underestimating the degree of blockade or of overestimating the degree of recovery.[14] The recovery to both one and four twitches occurs almost twice as fast at the face compared with at the ulnar nerve at the wrist.[14]

The Larynx

Although we are not able to place a twitch monitor on the larynx, we are interested in how the laryngeal muscle response to muscle relaxants compares with that of the adductor muscle of the thumb. Multiple studies confirm that one and one-half times the dose of nondepolarizing relaxant necessary to obtain twitch ablation of the adductor muscle of the thumb is required to suppress laryngeal response to stimulation.[15] Curiously, depolarizing relaxants (i.e., succinylcholine) are more effective at the larynx than at the adductor muscle of the thumb.

The Leg

Other options include stimulation of the common peroneal nerve as it courses around the head of the fibula or the posterior tibial nerve just behind the medial malleolus. Stimulation of the common peroneal nerve results in ankle flexion, whereas stimulation of the posterior tibial nerve causes plantar flexion.

What Alternate Electrodes Can Be Used?

Needles

Needle electrodes may be placed subcutaneously, overlying the nerve. The only major advantage of needle electrodes is the elimination of major resistance (due to the skin, oils, and moisture) and the subsequent reduction in optimal current flow

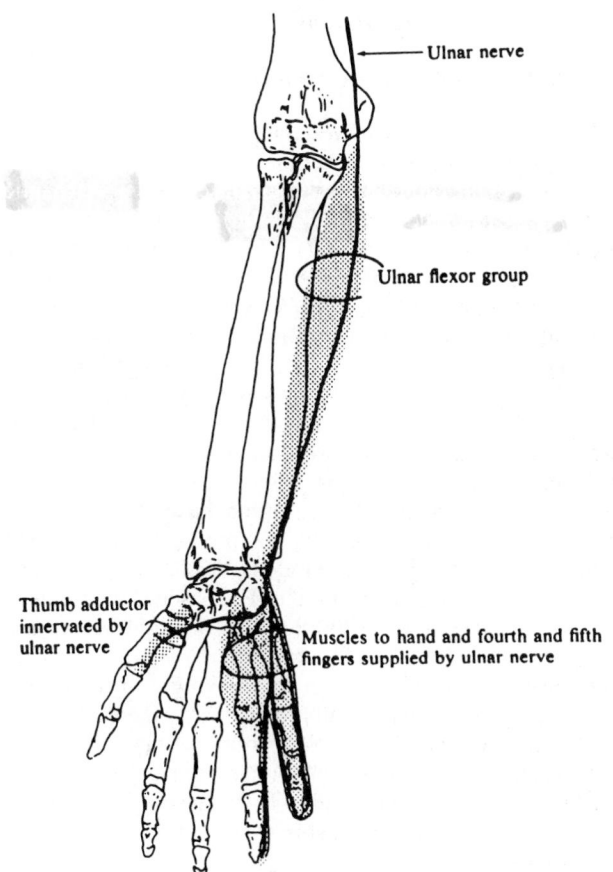

FIGURE 23–3. Semidiagrammatic picture of muscles supplied by the ulnar nerve. The ulnar nerve supplies, in the forearm, a group of muscles that produce flexion of the wrist and fingers. It is not desirable to stimulate these. Therefore, the negative electrode should not be placed over the ulnar nerve at the elbow. The ulnar nerve also supplies the muscles of the hand, the fourth and fifth fingers, and the thumb. Stimulating the ulnar nerve at the wrist causes these muscles to contract. (From Gravenstein JS, Paulus DA: Clinical Monitoring Practice. Philadelphia, JB Lippincott, 1987, p 217.)

Labels in Figure 23–3: Ulnar nerve; Ulnar flexor group; Thumb adductor innervated by ulnar nerve; Muscles to hand and fourth and fifth fingers supplied by ulnar nerve

(supramaximal current) necessary for accurate monitoring. The needle must not be inserted into the nerve. The potential for needle stick injury is real and should not be discounted. Needles may be useful in trauma patients and in the obese or burned patient.

Built-In Stimulating Electrodes

Hand-held stimulators with protruding rounded tip or ball electrodes are often used. However, the positioning of the electrodes over the nerve is critical. Because of the sensitivity to stimulation current requirement as related to electrode placement, even minor movement in electrode position may prevent accurate or useful comparison of previous or subsequent muscle responses.

Negative Versus Positive Electrode

An electrode placed directly over a nerve is termed the *active electrode*. The electrode placed at a distance is the *inactive* or *indifferent electrode*. If the active electrode is negative for a given, preset current, the force of muscle contraction is greater than that observed if the active electrode is positive.[12] If, however, both electrodes are close together over the nerve, the difference is clinically insignificant. In general, the negative electrode should be placed over the more distal portion of the nerve. If the polarity of a nerve stimulator is in doubt, place the electrodes adjacent to each other or reverse the polarity to see which pairing gives the most discreet thumb adduction response.

Rationale

The optimal use of neuromuscular blocking agents in all clinical settings (e.g., operating room, intensive care unit) requires titration of these drugs to a desired response. A peripheral nerve stimulator permits titration of muscle relaxant doses to produce optimal skeletal muscle relaxation in association with a $\geq 90\%$ depression of twitch response. This level correlates with adequate skeletal muscle relaxation for intubation of the trachea or performance of intra-abdominal surgery (in the presence of adequate concentrations of anesthetic drugs).[16]

On the other hand, surgical planes of neuromuscular blockade may not be necessary to optimize ventilator parameters in the intensive care unit. Ventilator mechanics may improve and adverse side effects may decrease with only minimal neuromuscular blockade (e.g., 25% depression of twitch response).

We use nerve stimulators routinely whenever an intermediate or long-acting neuromuscular blocking drug is given. The response is by observation and touch. Only in selected cases are the responses monitored by means of a strip recorder.

Specific Indications

The benefits dramatically outweigh the minor inconvenience and expense of monitoring. Some clinical situations arise that make monitoring difficult or impossible; however, such monitoring should be considered mandatory in the following situations:

1. When pathologic states cause significant changes in the effect of the drug at the neuromuscular junction (e.g., in neuromuscular diseases such as myasthenia gravis and myasthenic syndrome, and in Eaton-Lambert syndrome).

2. When one wishes to avoid the use of anticholinesterases for reversal of neuromuscular blockade (e.g., in symptomatic bronchial asthma).

3. When postoperative muscle strength should be maximal or when clinical evaluation suggests marginal respiratory reserve (e.g., severe pulmonary disease or marked obesity).

In most instances, tactile evaluation of the response to nerve stimulation is sufficient. One must remain cognizant of the well-documented observations that describe our inability to record precisely small changes in twitch response by tactile evaluation.[17] Personnel could not perceive a significant difference in twitch response until a $\geq 60\%$ decrease in recorded T_4 versus T_1 twitch height occurred. This observation is noteworthy because adequate recovery of neuromuscular function is not considered to have occurred until a $<30\%$ difference between the first and fourth twitch of a train-of-four stimulation is present.

A general tendency to underestimate neuromuscular blockade—and, thus, overestimate recovery—exists when clinicians rely solely on observation or palpation of the twitch response. The investigators conclude that "postoperative absence" of visual and manual face in the train-of-four response does not exclude neuromuscular blockade.[17]

INTERPRETATION OF STIMULUS FREQUENCY DATA

Presynaptic Versus Postsynaptic

With repetitive stimulation (tetanus, train-of-four, and double-burst), two aspects of neuromuscular function are observed: (1) depression of initial response (i.e., postsynaptic); and (2) degree of fade (i.e., presynaptic). When the presynaptic fade response has resolved ($T_4/T_1 > 0.7$), clinicians generally consider that the neuromuscular blockade has worn off sufficiently for the patient to be discharged from the postanesthesia care unit. However, absence of fade is an indication of full recovery only if the two effects (depression of initial amplitude and fade) are representative of the same physiologic action.

Basic science data suggest that depression of initial amplitude occurs mainly because of postjunctional receptor blockade, whereas fade arises from a separate mechanism that is dependent on prejunctional receptor blockade. Alpha-bungarotoxin blocks postjunctional but not prejunctional receptors; when it depresses twitch amplitude by 90%, T_4/T_1 remains at 1.0 (100%) with no fade. Consequently, absence of fade is not always characteristic of restored normal neuromuscular function.

Fortunately, the neuromuscular-blocking drugs currently used, although not identical, all produce fade when a decreased twitch amplitude is present. Furthermore, with all currently used agents, the "fade effect" is more persistent than is depression of twitch amplitude. Thus, absence of fade, although not perfect, is a reasonably good indication of recovery from blockade.

How Are Stimulation Patterns Assessed?

Single Twitch

Single-twitch stimuli usually are of 200-millisecond duration, and square-wave impulses are applied every 10 seconds

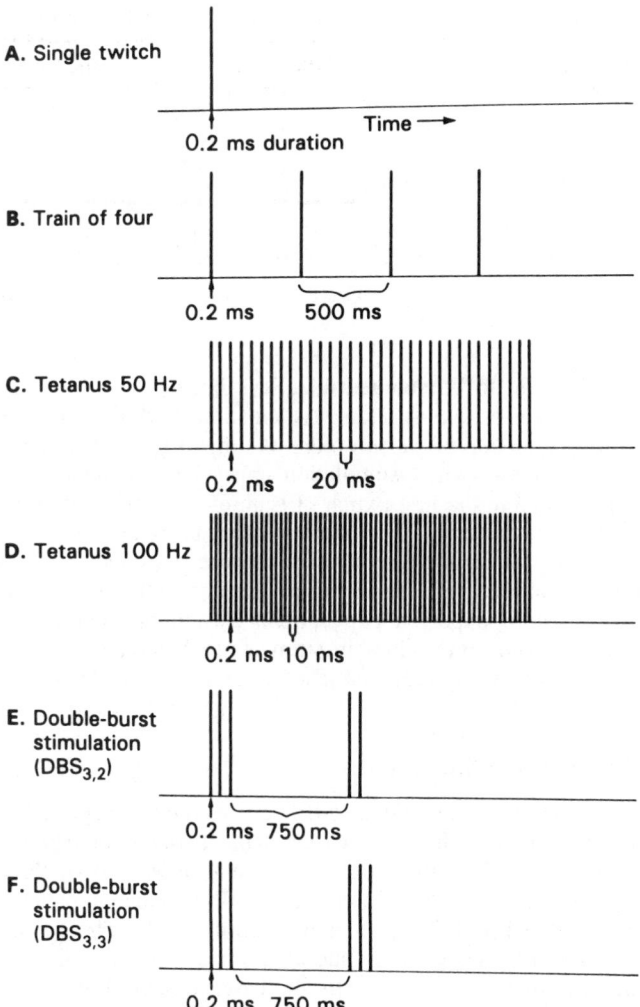

FIGURE 23–5. Peripheral nerve stimulators create various patterns of electrical impulses. See text for details. (From Morgan GE, Mikhail MS: Clinical Anesthesiology. 1st ed. Norwalk, CT, Appleton & Lange, 1992, p 97.)

75% to 80% of cholinergic receptors at the neuromuscular junction are blocked (see Table 23–2), whereas it disappears when 90% of receptors are blocked.

Train-of-Four

The train-of-four pattern of nerve stimulation is two 200-millisecond stimuli per second (2 Hz) for a period of 2 seconds (i.e., four equal supramaximal stimuli at half-second intervals) (Fig. 23–6; see also Fig. 23–5). Individual trains-of-four are usually repeated no more often than every 10 seconds. Division of the amplitude of the fourth response by the amplitude of the first response provides the train-of-four ratio. In the control period (the response obtained before administration of muscle relaxant), all four responses ideally are the same (i.e., the ratio is 1.0).

Each stimulus in the train causes the muscle to contract and "fade." The appearance of the contraction sequence also depends on the type of block (see Fig. 23–6). During a partial nondepolarizing block, the ratio decreases and is inversely proportional to the degree of blockade. During a partial depolarizing block (succinylcholine), the twitch height decreases evenly in four responses, but no fade occurs. Fade of the response (which makes it appear like a nondepolarizing block) after injection of a depolarizing agent signifies the development of a phase II block.

The value of train-of-four stimulation is best appreciated during nondepolarizing blockade because the degree of block can be read directly from the response, even though a control value is absent. With the onset of neuromuscular block, the fourth response is eliminated at approximately 75% depression of the first twitch; the third and fourth responses are abolished at 80% suppression of the first twitch; and the second twitch vanishes at about 90% block of the first twitch depression.[20–22] These observations provide the scientific basis for the clinical practice of counting the number of twitches in the train-of-four response; this makes it possible to quantify the dose of relaxant needed to achieve relaxation.

Neuromuscular blockade ranging from 75% to 95% twitch

(0.1 Hz) to every second (1 Hz) (Fig. 23–5). The muscle response to single-twitch stimulation depends on the frequency of the stimuli. More specifically, if the rate of delivery is increased to >0.15 Hz, the evoked response gradually decreases and settles at a lower level of twitch tension.[18] Therefore, a frequency of 0.1 to 0.15 Hz is usually used for assessment of single twitch. Higher frequencies (1.0 Hz) are useful to quickly establish supramaximal stimulation during induction of anesthesia. Once the supramaximal stimulus has been established, lower frequencies of stimulation are recommended to preserve optimal monitoring conditions. Intraoperative data can only be accurately compared if they are collected at identical stimulation frequencies. Thus, 1-Hz single-twitch, 0.1-Hz single-twitch, and 2-Hz (train-of-four) muscle responses cannot be directly compared.[19]

Changing the stimulus frequency from 0.1 Hz to 1.0 Hz can decrease the ED_{95} (the effective dose for 95% twitch suppression of thumb adduction) for d-tubocurarine by a factor of three or more.[18] The ED_{95} of d-tubocurarine at 0.1 Hz is approximately 0.5 mg·kg^{-1}, compared with 0.16 mg·kg^{-1} at 1.0 Hz. The onset time and the duration of action of the relaxant accordingly appear to differ when the stimulation frequency is varied.

Finally, a single-twitch response may not be reduced until

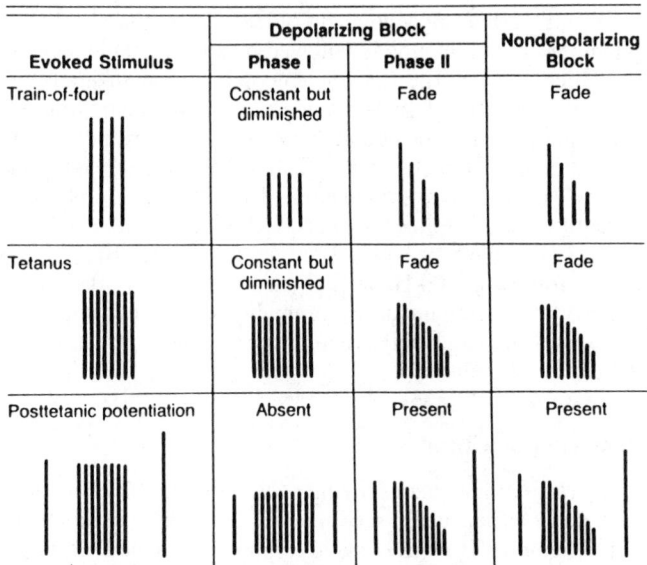

FIGURE 23–6. Evoked responses during depolarizing (phase I and phase II) and nondepolarizing block. (From Morgan GE, Mikhail MS: Clinical Anesthesiology. 1st ed. Norwalk, CT, Appleton & Lange, 1992, p 137.)

inhibition provides satisfactory clinical relaxation during nitrous oxide narcotic anesthesia. During anesthesia provided by potent inhalation agents, lesser degrees of twitch suppression are often adequate. This quantal assessment is appropriate for tactile determination of neuromuscular blockade; however, it should not be confused with the train-of-four ratio, which compares only the first and fourth twitch response. Clinically, a ratio of 75% (four full twitches) is thought to reflect adequate recovery of neuromuscular function.[23–28] Unlike tetanic stimulation, train-of-four stimulation does not affect subsequent monitoring.

Tetanic Stimulation

Tetanic stimulation consists of rapid electrical stimuli at 50 or 100 Hz. The 100-Hz stimuli are administered every 10 milliseconds, whereas the 50-Hz stimulation pattern is presented every 20 milliseconds. The most commonly used pattern in clinical practice is 50-Hz stimulation for 5 seconds. Depolarizing neuromuscular blocking agents allow a sustained muscle response to 50-Hz tetanic stimulation (see Fig. 23–6). During a nondepolarizing block (and a phase II depolarizing block), the response is not sustained, and obvious fade occurs before the 5-second 50-Hz stimulation is completed.

Tetanic stimulation is commonly used to evaluate residual neuromuscular blockade. In simplified terms, it stresses neuromuscular function, demonstrating the ability of the presynaptic nerve terminal to mobilize and release enough acetylcholine to maintain a favorable concentration gradient. However, except in connection with the technique of post-tetanic count, tetanic stimulation has very little role in everyday clinical anesthesia. If the response to nerve stimulation is recorded, all of the information required can be obtained from the response to train-of-four nerve stimulation. If, on the other hand, the response to nerve stimulation is evaluated only by feel or by observation, even experienced observers cannot judge the response of tetanic stimulation with sufficient certainty to exclude residual neuromuscular blockade.

Post-Tetanic Facilitation

During partial nondepolarizing blockade or phase II block, tetanic nerve stimulation is followed by a post-tetanic increase in twitch tension (i.e., post-tetanic facilitation of transmission).[29] The clinical implication is that subsequent train-of-four, single-twitch, or double-burst stimulation responses are stronger; single-twitch height is increased; and decreased fade follows double-burst stimulation. This facilitated response, thought to be due to increased acetylcholine release, is proportional to the depth of block. The duration of the effect is also longer following 100-Hz tetanus than it is after a 50-Hz tetanus with vecuronium and presumably other neuromuscular blockers. This facilitated twitch effect is gone 2 minutes after the tetanic stimulus.

Post-Tetanic Count

Injection of a nondepolarizing neuromuscular blocking drug in a dose sufficient for very intense blockade causes single-twitch, train-of-four, and tetanic responses to be undetectable. If a 50-Hz tetanic stimulus is applied for 5 seconds and followed after a pause of 3 seconds by stimulation at 1 Hz, the number of post-tetanic twitches due to post-tetanic facilitation

TABLE 23–4. Minutes Until Detectable Twitch Response*

Post-Tetanic Counts	Atracurium	Pancuronium
2	7	30
4	4	20
6	2	10
8	0–2	5

(From Brull SJ, Silverman DG: Neuromuscular block monitoring. *In* Anesthesia Equipment Principles and Applications. Ehrenworth J, Eisenkraft JB (eds). Mosby, 1993, p 304.)
*Number of responses to single-twitch stimuli at 1 Hz following 50-Hz tetanus for 5 s.

may be able to be counted. The less intense the block, the more responses to post-tetanic twitch stimulation appear.

After injection of pancuronium, 0.1 mg · kg^{-1}, the response to post-tetanic twitch stimulation appears approximately 37 minutes before the first twitch of train-of-four stimulation becomes noticeable.[31, 32] This method of ensuring or monitoring the degree of paralysis is useful to ensure profound paralysis for ophthalmologic or airway procedures as well as to indicate how soon to expect a conventional twitch or train-of-four response. Thus, it provides an estimate of when the patient can be expected to respond to anticholinesterase (Table 23–4).

Double-Burst Stimulation

Double-burst stimulation (DBS) is a method of nerve stimulation, similar to the train-of-four, that consists of three pulses at 50 Hz, a 750-millisecond pause, and either two or three additional pulses at 50 Hz.[33–35] These DBS stimulation patterns are identified as DBS$_{3,3}$ and DBS$_{3,2}$ respectively. The advantages of DBS over train-of-four monitoring is that if no recording is available, as is typically the case, it is much easier to identify residual blockade; the response is larger, and it is easier to differentiate between the two twitches of DBS than between the first and fourth twitches of train-of-four, which are, of course, separated by the second and third twitches (Fig. 23–7).

The train-of-four ratio is numerically close to the DBS ratio when recordings are compared, but the strength of contractions with DBS is almost three times greater. DBS fade is detected when the train-of-four ratio is judged to be 0.7 to 0.8 by most observers, even by those without prior experience with this pattern of stimulation. These advantages of DBS make it an

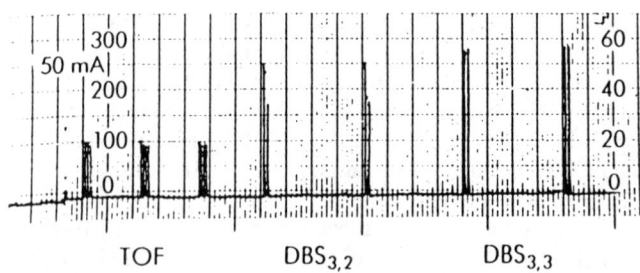

FIGURE 23–7. Evoked responses of train-of-four (TOF; every 12 seconds), DBS$_{3,2}$ and DBS$_{3,3}$ (every 20 seconds) in an unmedicated volunteer. Although the magnitude of the individual responses is greater for DBS, the T$_4$/T$_1$ ratio of TOF and the D$_2$/D$_1$ ratio of DBS$_{3,3}$ are virtually equivalent; the D$_2$/D$_1$ ratio of DBS$_{3,2}$ is lower because its second burst has a shorter duration than does its first burst. (From Brull SJ, Silverman DG: Neuromuscular block monitoring. *In* Anesthesia Equipment Principles and Applications. Ehrenworth J, Eisenkraft JB (eds). St Louis, CV Mosby, 1993, p 307.)

appealing technique and a likely replacement for clinical monitoring of the neuromuscular junction in the future.

When Is Neuromuscular Blockade Reversible?

The question frequently arises as to whether dense neuromuscular blockade can safely be reversed in a patient. For reversal of a nondepolarizing neuromuscular blocking agent, the concept should be related to the basic physiology of the neuromuscular junction; that is, reversal is a competitive process. If the administration of small quantities of anticholinesterase result in a measurable response, the concentration gradient is surmountable.

Data indicate that the dose response curves for the anticholinesterases are relatively steep (i.e., addition of small quantities of drug results in a significant change in response); therefore, if any response is elicited by a small dose, complete reversal is likely with the administration of a full reversal dose.

Clinically, this pharmacologic challenge should only be applied to the short and intermediate acting agents because of the differences in the elimination characteristics of the longer-acting agents compared with those of the reversal agents. If the patient does not develop a palpable twitch after administration of <10% of total reversal dose, the appropriate clinical course is to maintain a secure airway and institute (or continue) manual or mechanical ventilation.

OTHER METHODS TO ASSESS NEUROMUSCULAR BLOCKADE

Several other techniques can be used to supplement twitch monitoring.

What Is Electromyography?

Electromyography displays the compound muscle action potential in response to nerve stimulation. It is most often obtained using muscles innervated by the ulnar or median nerves. Stimulating electrodes are placed over the appropriate nerve as with twitch monitoring, whereas recording electrodes are placed over the thenar, hypothenar, or first dorsal interosseous muscle of the hand. The monitor displays the measured response as either a per cent of control or as a train-of-four ratio. The electromyogram recording is very sensitive to electrode placement. Proper placement is difficult to verify unless the monitor also provides a display of the electromyogram.

What Is Mechanomyography?

Mechanomyography is the traditional ''gold standard'' for measuring muscle response to electrical stimulation. The mechanomyograph uses a force displacement transducer that is attached via a ring to the thumb and to a rigid armboard. Because the adductor muscle of the thumb is the only muscle in the thumb innervated by the ulnar nerve, it is the one used in mechanomyography. In order to obtain correct and reproducible measurements, the forces generated are isometric; therefore, a constant preload is required. This preload is usu-

ally 100 to 300 g. In addition to constant preload, the device also requires that the axis of contraction and the axis of the transducer are the same. Once these requirements are met, monitoring can begin, with the caveat that the reaction to control supramaximal stimulation increases for up to 12 minutes after commencement of stimulation. This device can then be used for very precise train-of-four or other stimulation pattern recording.

What Is Accelerometry?

The newest approach to evoked muscle response monitoring is accelerometry, which is thought to be equivalent to mechanomyography.[36] This method uses a piezoelectric motion transducer that is attached to the thumb. It is a dynamic method that does not require a set preload or rigid fixation of the hand. One difference between accelerometry and other tests is that it is *not* useful for assessing the response to a tetanic stimulation, since the tetanic stimulation test has a nondynamic component. Although the accelerometer is easier to use than the mechanomyograph, its ultimate role in clinical monitoring has yet to be determined.

References

1. Viby-Mogensen J, Chraemmer-Jorgensen B, Ording H: Residual curarization in the recovery room. Anesthesiology 1979; 50:539.
2. Lennmarken C, Lofstrom JB: Partial curarization in the postoperative period. Acta Anesthesiol Scand 1984; 28:260.
3. Ali HH, Savarese JJ: Monitoring of neuromuscular function. Anesthesiology 1976; 45:216.
4. Ali HH: Mechanomyography and electromyography. *In* Muscle Relaxation. Buzello W (ed). New York, Georg Thieme Verlag Stuttgart, 1981, pp 82–88.
5. Bevan DR, Smith CE, Donati F: Postoperative neuromuscular blockade: a comparison between atracurium, vecuronium, and pancuronium. Anesthesiology 1988; 69:272.
6. Pavlin EG, Holle RH, Schoene RB: Recovery of airway protection compared with ventilation in humans after paralysis with curare. Anesthesiology 1989; 70:381.
7. Eriksson LI, Sata M, Severinghaus JW: Effect of a vecuronium-induced partial neuromuscular block on hypoxic ventilatory response. Anesthesiology 1993; 78:693.
8. Viby-Mogensen J: Clinical assessment of neuromuscular transmission. Br J Anaesth 1982; 54:209.
9. Epstein RA, Wyte SR, Jackson SH, et al: The electromechanical response to stimulation by the Block Aid Monitor. Anesthesiology 1969; 30:43.
10. Epstein RA, Jackson SH: Repetitive muscle depolarization from single indirect stimulation in anesthetized man. J Appl Physiol 1970; 28:407.
11. Kopman AF, Lawson D: Milliamperage requirements for supramaximal stimulation of the ulnar nerve with surface electrodes. Anesthesiology 1984; 61:83.
12. Berger JJ, Gravenstein JS, Munson ES: Electrode polarity and peripheral nerve stimulation. Anesthesiology 1982; 56:402.
13. Rosenberg H, Greenhow DE: Peripheral nerve stimulator performance: the influence of output polarity and electrode placement. Can Anaesth Soc J 1978; 25:424.
14. Caffrey RR, Warren ML, Becker KE, Jr: Neuromuscular blockade monitoring comparing the orbicularis oculi and adductor pollicis muscles. Anesthesiology 1986; 65:95.
15. Donati F, Plaud B, Meistelman C: Vecuronium neuromuscular blockade at the adductor muscles of the larynx and adductor pollicis. Anesthesiology 1991; 74:827.
16. Meistelman C, Plaud B, Donati F: Neuromuscular effects of succinylcholine on the vocal cords and adductor pollicis muscle. Anesth Analg 1991; 73:278.
17. Viby-Mogensen J, Jensen NH, Engbaek J, et al: Tactile and visual evaluation of the response to train-of-four nerve stimulation. Anesthesiology 1985; 63:440.

18. Ali HH, Savarese JJ: Stimulus frequency and dose-response curve to d-tubocurarine in man. Anesthesiology 1980; 52:36.

19. Curran MJ, Donati F, Bevan DR: Onset and recovery of atracurium and suxamethonium-induced neuromuscular blockade with simultaneous train-of-four and single twitch stimulation. Br J Anaesth 1987; 59:989.

20. Lee C-M: Train-of-four quantitation of competitive neuromuscular block. Anesth Analg 1975; 54:649.

21. Gibson FM, Mirakhur RK, Clarke RSJ, et al: Quantification of train-of-four responses during recovery of block from nondepolarizing muscle relaxants. Acta Anaesthesiol Scand 1987; 31:655.

22. O'Hara DA, Fragen RJ, Shanks CA: Comparison of visual and measured train-of-four recovery after vecuronium-induced neuromuscular blockade using two anaesthetic techniques. Br J Anaesth 1986; 58:1300.

23. Ali HH, Utting JE, Gray TC: Quantitative assessment of residual antidepolarizing block. Br J Anaesth 1971; 43:478.

24. Ali HH, Wilson RS, Savarese JJ, et al: The effect of tubocurarine on indirectly elicited train-of-four muscle response and respiratory measurements in humans. Br J Anaesth 1975; 47:570.

25. Ali HH, Utting JE, Gray TC: Quantitative assessment of residual antidepolarizing block (Part I). Br J Anaesth 1971; 43:473.

26. Brand JB, Cullen DJ, Wilson NE, et al: Spontaneous recovery from nondepolarizing neuromuscular blockade: correlation between clinical and evoked responses. Anesth Analg 1977; 56:55.

27. Jones RM, Pearce AC, Williams JP: Recovery characteristics following antagonism of atracurium with neostigmine or edrophonium. Br J Anaesth 1984; 56:453.

28. Engbaek J, Ostergaard D, Viby-Mogensen J: Clinical recovery and train-of-four ratio measured mechanically and electromyographically following atracurium. Anesthesiology 1989; 71:391.

29. Brull SJ, Connelly NR, O'Connor TZ, et al: Effect of tetanus on subsequent neuromuscular monitoring in patients receiving vecuronium. Anesthesiology 1991; 74:64.

30. Viby-Mogensen J, Howardy-Hansen P, Chraemmer-Jorgensen B, et al: Posttetanic count (PTC): a new method of evaluating an intense nondepolarizing neuromuscular blockade. Anesthesiology 1981; 55:458.

31. Bonsu AK, Viby-Mogensen J, Fernando PUE, et al: Relationship of posttetanic count and train-of-four response during intense neuromuscular blockade caused by atracurium. Br J Anaesth 1987; 59:1089.

32. Mucchal KK, Viby-Mogensen J, Fernando PUE, et al: Evaluation of intense neuromuscular blockade caused by vecuronium using posttetanic count (PTC). Anesthesiology 1987; 66:846.

33. Engbaek J, Ostergaard D, Viby-Mogensen J: Double burst stimulation (DBS): a new pattern of nerve stimulation to identify residual curarization (Abstract). Acta Anaesth Scand 1987; 31:A198.

34. Engbaek J, Ostergaard D, Viby-Mogensen J: Double burst stimulation (DBS): a new pattern of nerve stimulation to identify residual neuromuscular block. Br J Anaesth 1989; 62:274.

35. Brull SJ, Connelly NR, Silverman DG: Correlation of train-of-four and double burst stimulation ratios at varying amperes. Anesth Analg 1990; 71:489.

36. May O, Kirkegqaard-Nielson H, Werner MV: The acceleration transducer: an assessment of its precision in comparison with a force displacement transducer. Acta Anaesth Scand 1988; 32:239.

CHAPTER 24

Monitoring During Patient Transport

GREGORY M. GULLAHORN, M.D., L.C.D.R., M.C., U.S.N.R.

Anesthesiologists use a vast array of monitors to assess physiologic status and the functioning of the anesthesia machine, ventilator, and other life support equipment. Such monitoring is applied not only in the operating room (OR) and intensive care unit (ICU) but also in the postanesthesia care unit (PACU) and emergency room, where anesthesiologists may routinely be involved in patients' care. We feel uncomfortable managing critically ill or anesthetized patients without monitoring in such settings; yet what parameters should be monitored while transporting patients between these locations or to other diagnostic and therapeutic areas within the hospital is less clear. A number of questions must be addressed.

BASIC CONSIDERATIONS

Why Monitor?

Patients who have serious illnesses or injuries or who are anesthetized may have altered organ system function and abnormal responses to stress.[1, 2] We use our senses—and monitors as an extension of these senses—to identify trends or problems that require intervention and then to assess the effects of therapy. Monitors that check functions on which our treatment may have an impact are clearly the most efficacious (i.e., pulse oximeters to evaluate the adequacy of oxygenation in anesthetized or sedated patients).

In the OR and the ICU, these monitors are well established (see also Chapters 21–23 and 25). In all settings, simple inspection is the most basic and least invasive form of monitoring. Precordial or esophageal stethoscopes, pulse oximetry, electrocardiography, blood pressure (invasive or noninvasive) measurement, and capnography now represent standards of care in the OR. Temperature monitoring and assessment of neuromuscular activity are indicated by a patient's status and the surgery.

Anesthesiologists would be hesitant to administer a full induction dose of sodium thiopental to a pale, diaphoretic trauma victim and would pause before performing laryngoscopy and intubation on a patient with an intracranial aneurysm without measuring blood pressure. At the end of surgery, however, less concern may be directed to a patient who is making a trip from the OR to the PACU or the ICU. Realistically, however,

is the potential for fluctuations in blood pressure, changes in heart rate or rhythm, problems with oxygenation or unplanned extubation any less during this transport process, and are these considerations less important because of the hopefully limited time frame?

Cardiovascular Changes

Insel and colleagues examined cardiovascular changes occurring during transport from the OR to the ICU after major general or vascular surgery, carotid endarterectomy, or coronary artery bypass. In the first three groups, significant increases in blood pressure and pulse and initial lability were noted. In the major vascular/general surgery group, 20% of patients required vigorous fluid resuscitation for hypotension on arrival in the ICU, and 36% required either nitroglycerin or sodium nitroprusside for control of hypertension.[3]

Hypoxemia

Hypoxemia may also be common. Tyler and associates reported a 35% incidence of decreased oxyhemoglobin saturation (SaO_2) to <90% during the transport of adults from the OR to the PACU; 12% fell to <85%.[4] Healthy pediatric patients appear to be equally at risk. Kataria and coworkers found that even with 3 minutes of 100% O_2 administration after surgery, a significant age-related reduction in SaO_2 occurred during a 120- to 180-second transfer to the PACU. The mean SaO_2 was 88% in children younger than 6 months.[5]

Tomkins and colleagues examined children with the American Society of Anesthesiologists physical status I or II and found that 24% had a SaO_2 <90% during the first 10 minutes after anesthesia. Clinical signs such as cyanosis or upper airway obstruction correlated poorly with measured hypoxemia.[6] "Modest" desaturation was also demonstrated in adult patients during transfer from an anesthesia induction room to the OR. Despite an average transfer time of only 51 seconds, 21 of 25 patients had a decline in SaO_2. In two patients, a decrease to 90% occurred. All patients were either apneic or breathing room air.[7]

Although the risk of hypoxemia in most postsurgical patients during a brief transfer from the OR to the PACU is minimized by routine administration of supplemental O_2, the potential for mishaps probably increases with prolonged transit times en route to an ICU and in patients with pre-existing or new-onset pulmonary disease.

What Does Intrahospital Transport Entail?

Many experienced anesthesiologists correctly assume that the potential for clinically significant problems during transfer from the OR is fairly remote except in specific population groups; the challenge is to identify those at risk. The possibility of adverse events may be just as pronounced in other types of intrahospital transport. Venkataraman and Orr defined four common scenarios for intrahospital transport (Table 24–1).[8]

Conceptual Differences

Vigilance is the cornerstone of anesthesiology and is vital in all transport scenarios. However, differences do exist. When patients leave a critical care setting, their physiologic status should be stable, with continued normalization expected. They no longer need as intensive monitoring as they had in the operating room or ICU. Major risks involve airway problems or changing level of consciousness.

Individuals being taken to a critical care area, however, present different problems. Examples include trauma victims transported to the OR after initial resuscitation in the emergency room or septic patients who have deteriorated on the ward and are now being transferred to the ICU. In these settings, the baseline requirements for monitoring are increasing as the potential for significant physiologic changes grows.

Secondary Insults

In head-injured patients, "secondary insults" such as hypoxia, hypotension, and intracranial hypertension clearly worsen outcome.[9] Andrews and colleagues found secondary insults during transport in 47% of patients being transferred from the emergency department. Eighty per cent of these patients suffer secondary injuries within 4 hours of their transfer.[10] Significantly, Gentlemen and Jennet reported airway compromise in 43 of 164 head-injured patients on arrival at a neurosurgical unit; 15% to 22% of patients were hypoxic.[9] Better monitoring of these patients might have a profound impact on outcome, if problems leading to secondary injury can be identified and corrected.

Critical Care Transport

Modern critical care units provide extensive monitoring of physiologic functions and multiple life support modalities. The

TABLE 24–1. Common Intrahospital Transport Scenarios

Movement from critical care areas	OR to PACU
	OR to ward
	ICU to ward
One-way transfer to critical care areas	
Round-trip transport between critical care and noncritical care areas	ICU to radiology and back
	ICU to cardiac catheterization laboratory and back
Transfer between critical care areas	ICU to OR
	OR to ICU

Abbreviations: OR = operating room; PACU = postanesthesia care unit; ICU = intensive care unit.

ICU concentrates equipment and personnel who are experienced in managing severely ill or injured patients, as well as the complications they may develop. For those of us involved in critical care, transporting patients from the ICU to other parts of the hospital and back is sure to evoke anxiety. Any anesthesiologist may be called on to assist in this process, however. The provision of sedation or anesthesia for unstable or combative patients who must undergo computed tomographic (CT) scans, angiography, other invasive radiologic procedures, or even radiation therapy is increasingly common.

Transport of Anesthetized Patients

Movement of anesthetized patients to and from these ancillary areas presents special logistic and clinical challenges; the decision to proceed with such moves must carefully weigh the potential benefits of the planned procedure or test against the potential for misadventure. Venkataraman and Orr divide adverse events during transport into physiologic changes and equipment mishaps.[8] Small changes in heart rate or blood pressure may be of no consequence, whereas unplanned extubation or the loss of intravenous access in a patient requiring multiple pressors for hemodynamic support can be lethal. Clearly, early detection of such changes is critically important for definitive intervention.

Mortality

In the 1970s, Wadell reported a 5-month study of both critically ill ICU patients and postoperative patients who had undergone at least one intrahospital transport. Among the critically ill patients, one per month suffered cardiac arrest or died of causes attributed to the transport process.[11]

Mechanically Ventilated Patients

Many patients in an ICU require ventilatory support and are prone to transport complications related to inadvertent changes in tidal volume, minute ventilation, continuous positive airway pressure, or ventilatory mode. These changes may adversely impact the cardiovascular system or intracranial pressure (ICP).

Braman and colleagues prospectively studied changes in arterial blood gas partial pressures and hemodynamic parameters in 36 ventilator-dependent patients who required procedures outside the ICU.[12] Two groups were examined: The first were ventilated manually during transport, and the second via a portable, volume-limited ventilator (with settings matched to the bedside ventilator). Several patients in both groups had significant (>10 mm Hg) changes in arterial carbon dioxide pressure (P_{CO_2}) and pH, as well as hypotension; however, the incidence was considerably greater in the manually ventilated group (75% versus 44%), and two developed new cardiac dysrhythmias. Hypotension and dysrhythmias were strongly correlated with blood gas deterioration.

Gervais and associates found that both manual ventilation without volume monitoring and portable mechanical ventilation with preset but unmonitored volumes resulted in significant decreases in P_{CO_2} and increases in pH.[13] These changes were not noted when tidal volume was controlled using a spirometer during manual ventilation.

Adverse Effects of Positive Airway Pressure

Changes in airway pressure may have profound impact on venous return, blood pressure, and intracranial elastance. Unrecognized changes in arterial O_2 pressure (Po_2), Pco_2, pH, and blood pressure are potentially deleterious for patients with coronary or cerebrovascular disease, particularly those with head injuries. Such patients are of particular concern because they are likely to undergo multiple transports to CT or nuclear magnetic resonance (NMR) scanning facilities, the OR, or the angiography suite.

In Gentleman's review, more than a third of deaths in patients referred to a neurosurgical unit had avoidable contributing factors.[9] Andrews's series showed that during transport of head-injured patients from the ICU, pretransfer insults (e.g., episodes of hypotension, hypoxia, or intracranial hypertension) were predictive of increased ICP during transport and the likelihood of further insults during the first 4 hours after return to the ICU.[10] This observation supports the admonition that adequate resuscitation and stabilization are vital before transport.

Complications

Smith and colleagues reviewed 125 intrahospital transports from the ICU to identify factors related to mishaps.[14] The latter were defined as events having a detrimental effect on a patient's stability (e.g., monitor failure, intravenous catheter infiltration or disconnect, vasoactive drug infusion disconnect, ventilator disconnects, extubation, invasive monitor or line-related mishaps). More than one third of transports involved at least one mishap, and 11% involved multiple events. On return to the ICU, 24% of patients were judged to be less stable.

Intensive Care Unit to Computed Tomography Scanner

Several interesting factors were apparent in this series. Mishaps were more common during transport to the CT scanner than to any other location, especially when a wait occurred at the destination. Transfer of a patient from the bed to the scanner and physical isolation during scanning were believed to be important contributors. Overall, 75% of mishaps occurred at the study site. Surprisingly, no correlation was noted between the number of catheters and monitors and the likelihood of mishaps, nor was an increased incidence of mishaps noted during emergent transports, perhaps reflecting increased vigilance in these settings.

Critical Care to Critical Care

When a patient is transferred between critical care areas (from the OR to ICU or from the ICU to OR), isolation in remote areas of the hospital with limited resources is unlikely. Nevertheless, issues involving the transport process are still relevant. Just as Insel and associates showed significant hemodynamic changes in adults during transfer from the OR to the ICU,[3] Venkataraman and colleagues demonstrated major cardiorespiratory changes in children going from the OR to the ICU, many of which required interventions such as ventilator changes or vasoactive infusions to stabilize.[8] Petre and coworkers noted that patients with complex cardiothoracic problems may leave the OR with multiple inotropic or vasoactive infusions, invasive monitors, and at times pacemakers and intra-aortic balloon pumps, all requiring monitoring and adjustment during the transport process.[15] They found that patients frequently arrived in the ICU in unstable condition.

We frequently are asked to maintain tight control of moderate induced hypotension in awake patients immediately after complex neurovascular procedures, during emergence from anesthesia, transport to the ICU, and transfer to the critical care team. This approach is vital after resection of high-flow arteriovenous malformations to prevent hemorrhage and edema and requires close and constant monitoring. The same potential for physiologic deterioration certainly is present when patients are transferred from the ICU to the OR; in this setting, the added factor of an emergent situation is often present.

A RATIONAL APPROACH

What Factors Determine Monitoring Requirements?

Cost-benefit relationships have been demonstrated with monitors and monitoring.[1, 2] The costs may be economic (related to the equipment), physical (iatrogenic injury to the patient), or a combination of the two (increased time or personnel requirements). Benefits are related to improved patient care, reduced complications, shorter ICU or hospital stays, and, hopefully, better outcomes.

Risk Analysis

Risks and costs increase with progression from simple clinical observation, to noninvasive equipment-assisted monitoring, to invasive monitors; clearly not all monitors are needed for all patients. A decision about what monitors should be used during transport must be based on an individual patient's physiologic status and the stress imposed by injury, disease process, surgery, anesthesia, and medications. These needs are modified by the length and type of transport. General guidelines can be developed for the previously mentioned scenarios described by Venkataraman and colleagues.[8]

Patients should be stabilized as much as possible before any movement.[8–12, 14, 16, 17] In healthy patients after elective surgery, a regular heart rate and rhythm, adequate airway with regular respirations, and acceptable blood pressure before transfer usually are all that is required.

How Is a Patient Prepared for Transport?

In critically ill patients, transport should be broken down into the *preparatory phase, transfer phase,* and *post-transport stabilization.*[8] The first phase should start with the carefully weighed decision to transport made by the primary members of the critical care, trauma, or surgical team (including the anesthesiologist). Once this decision is made, adequate and appropriate personnel should be gathered, and a careful systems review of the patient should be made to determine if any further interventions can optimize stabilization of the patient.

If a patient is receiving vasoactive infusions, they should be steady state, not in a continuous state of flux.[16] In patients with shock due to trauma, volume resuscitation should be well under way or complete before movement, and all necessary vascular catheters should be in place. If blood pressure cannot be stabilized, surgical exploration and control of bleeding must take precedence over *any* further diagnostic procedures.[9, 10]

A ventriculostomy catheter can be placed in the OR in hypotensive trauma victims with severe head injury during other surgical exploration, and an air ventriculogram used to lateralize a mass lesion if the ICP is increased. Control of the airway and some level of adequate oxygenation and ventilation should be achieved. In a neurologically injured or impaired patient (or any patient with a depressed level of consciousness) who is not intubated, careful consideration should be given to securing the airway electively before transport.

Equipment Needs

Parameters to be monitored during transport must be transferred to portable monitors. Dedicated transport beds with built-in monitors may seem attractive; however, the risk of dislodging catheters and an endotracheal tube or of inducing changes in ICP with a patient's movement suggests that patients should be transported in their ICU beds if possible. Self-contained critical care transport carts may be attached or detached quickly from the ICU bed. These are set up with appropriate monitors, compressed gas cylinders, transport or ICU ventilators, infusion pumps, and battery power sources.[18-21] During monitor transfer, brief periods of blackout for the parameter(s) being transferred often are needed to permit rezeroing of transducers.

The TRAM System

The transport team must be familiar with the operation and function of the additional equipment. One concept that has been developed to ease this problem is the transport remote acquisition monitor (TRAM) system. The TRAM is designed around a self-contained data acquisition and processing module, to which ECG leads, invasive or noninvasive pressure transducers, pulse oximeter probes, temperature probes, and other monitoring modalities may be attached. This module may be plugged into a permanent (fixed) operating room or bedside monitor; before disconnection from the primary monitor, it is linked to the portable TRAM LCD display screen. When a patient is moved, the module is simply removed from the fixed monitor and ''follows'' the patient without the need to detach any of the monitoring lines.[22]

An alternative approach to avoid gaps is to duplicate monitoring between the bedside and transport systems. This process involves placing a separate set of ECG pads and leads for the transport monitor, if cardiac rhythm is a concern, and measuring blood pressure noninvasively while invasive lines are transferred. The real utility of the TRAM system is evident when multiple invasive monitors are to be followed or a patient must be transported to an intermediate location (e.g., CT scans or angiography) en route between the OR and ICU.

Management of Tubing

Not only must monitoring be transferred in preparation for transport, but care must be taken to ensure that the various infusion tubings and cables are organized and identifiable. Patient safety necessitates that lines and infusions not be confused. An inadvertent fluid bolus through an infusion tubing filled with a vasoactive medication obviously can have serious consequences. Our approach has been to try to simplify things as much as possible. At least one route for intravenous administration should be maintained in all patients, but other access

ports may be flushed and capped off if they are not required during transport. Bundling of lines and cables, along with adequate labeling, may be helpful.

The Intensive Care Unit Bed

The Cleveland Clinic has developed a rather elegant system to increase safety and efficiency during transfer of patients undergoing cardiothoracic surgery. Their concept centers around the ICU bed as the primary transport device, with which they interface other equipment (Fig. 24–1). Monitoring is based on the TRAM system, in the OR, during transport, and in the ICU. At the head of the bed is a bracket designed to hold all the patient-monitoring transducers and the TRAM display. The TRAM module is placed in a receptacle under the bed. An infusion rack is used for all intravenous infusion fluids and medications and incorporates intravenous hooks, an adjustable intravenous pole, and volumetric pumps. This rack is suspended from an overhead mount in the OR, then attached to the side of the ICU bed for transport, and then again suspended from a ceiling mount in the ICU. Thus, the monitoring system and infusion/medication systems follow the patient as a unit.

Although the hardware for this system cost more than $1000 per bed in 1988, it was believed to be cost effective because of an estimated 50% time savings in the transport process and increased ability of transport personnel to focus on a patient rather than on movement of equipment.[15, 23] Even if this particular system is too complex for some institutions, the concept of maintaining uninterrupted monitoring and moving infusions as a unit is worth noting.

Nursing and Respiratory Care

Nursing care is vital to patient care in the ICU and is mandatory during transport to ensure that vasoactive infusions are adjusted, medications are administered, and accurate records are maintained. When a patient is unstable or is at risk for airway problems, a physician who is familiar with the patient and is skilled in managing tracheal intubation and other potential complications should be present.[16, 17, 24] A respiratory therapist or perfusionist may be required for specific problems. Resuscitative and scheduled medications, appropriate intravenous fluids or blood products, a portable defibrillator, and airway supplies should be available. Access to the head of the bed for airway management and to the chest, should cardiopulmonary resuscitation be required, is mandatory.

Transport Route

The final part of the preparatory phase is to make sure that everyone knows the route of the transport, elevators are standing by, and diagnostic facilities are ready to accept the patient. Similarly, before a patient is moved from the OR to the ICU, report should be given so that the ICU team can prepare. Notice should be called when the patient is actually ready to leave the OR.

How Is the Transport Phase Managed?

During the transport phase, the goal is to provide the same level of care as the patient had in the OR or ICU: (1) Maintain

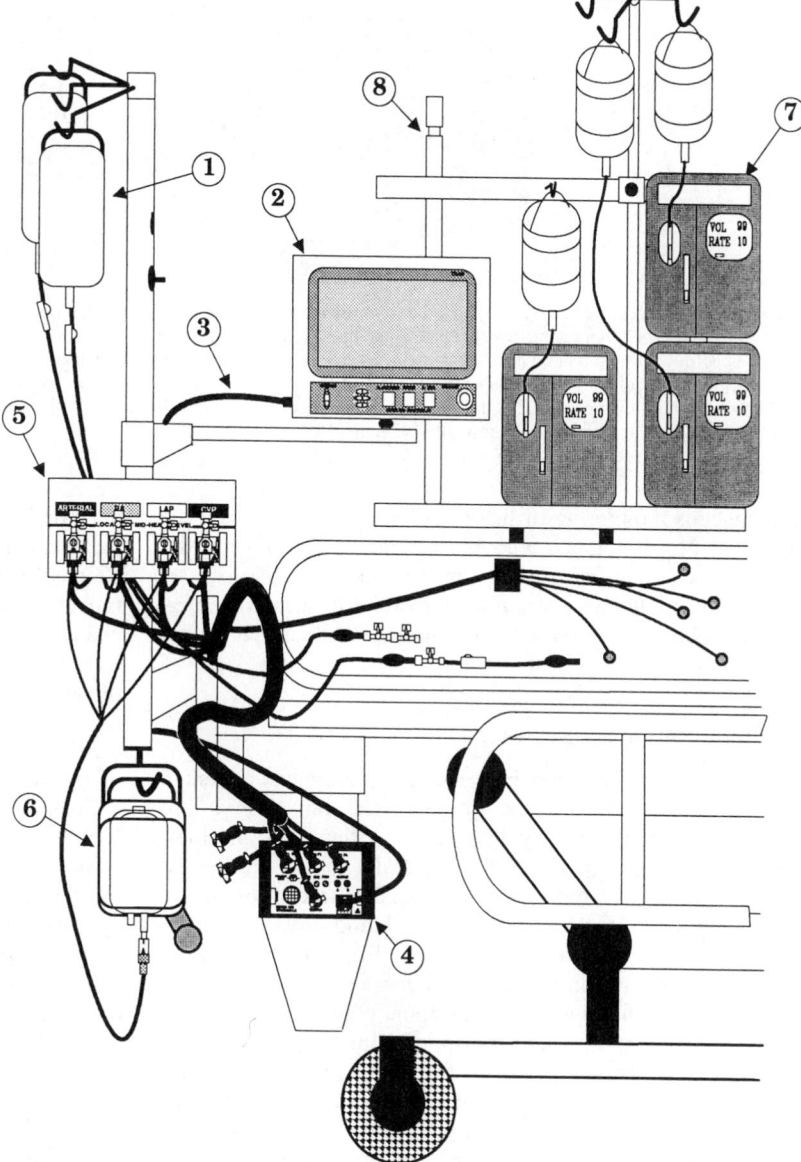

FIGURE 24–1. Integrated transport system. Support pole at head (1) holds pressure transducer mount (5) and pressurized flush solution (6) as well as hooks for intravenous solutions. The TRAM display screen (2) is mounted on the pole via a moveable sidearm and is connected to the TRAM module (4) by an electrical cord (3). The infusion bracket (8) is mounted on the side of the bed, and can support multiple intravenous solutions and up to six infusion pumps (7). (From Hendren W, Higgins T: Immediate postoperative care of the cardiac surgical patient. Semin Thorac Cardiovasc Surg 1991; 3:6).

stability of the patient through monitoring, (2) continue the present ongoing management, and (3) avoid iatrogenic mishaps.[8] Every attempt should be made to return monitoring and care to the ICU level during the diagnostic or therapeutic procedure. Parameters such as pulmonary artery pressure, which may be difficult to measure in a moving patient, can be monitored in a stationary location. Close adherence to the principles of adequate preparation and minimization of time spent during the transport phase should decrease the potential for complications.

What Problems Occur in the Post-Transport Stabilization Phase?

On arrival at or return to the ICU, no less attention should be paid to the post-transport stabilization phase.[3, 9, 14] Additional issues arise, and communication is essential. The primary surgical team may be unaware of problems that began in the operating room. The anesthesiologist must review these issues with the critical care team, particularly in the case of

trauma victims who may be treated by physicians from several disciplines.[24]

SELECTION OF MONITORS

What Factors Should Be Considered?

Hypoxemia

The evidence for hypoxemia following general anesthesia in all age groups is now quite convincing; thus, the routine use of supplemental O_2 during transport to the PACU is justifiable. When underlying pulmonary disease or the nature of the surgical procedure suggests that a patient may not be able to maintain adequate oxygenation with simple face mask or blow-by O_2, observation, including pulse oximetry, should take place in the OR, using the transport mode of supplemental O_2. One can assess the rate and depth of respirations by feeling exhalations on the palm of the hand while helping to support the airway (Fig. 24–2). The precordial stethoscope permits

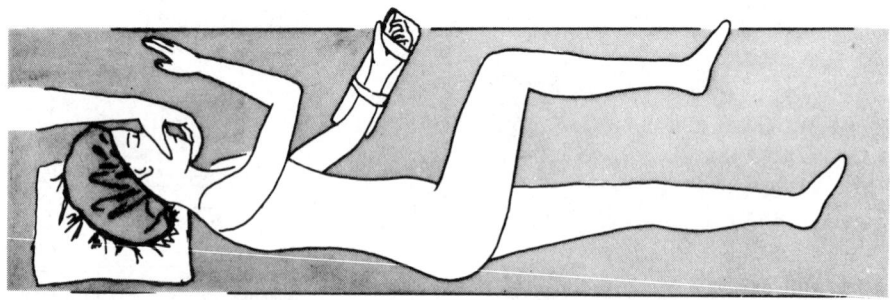

FIGURE 24–2. The optimal position of an unconscious patient during transport from the operating room to the PACU. The patient is placed on his or her side. If the patient had been in a lateral position during the operation, he or she is to be positioned with the side with the incision down. Straighten the lower leg and flex the upper leg 90° at hip and knee. This provides stability to the hip. Bring both arms and hands forward to stabilize the shoulder girdle. Support the head by placing a pillow or folded blanket under the occiput so that the face is turned slightly downward; this causes the jaw and tongue to fall forward, preventing obstruction while allowing saliva, gastric juice, or vomitus to drain from the mouth rather than pool in the hypopharynx. (From Gravenstein J, Paulus D: Monitoring Practice in Clinical Anesthesia. Philadelphia, JB Lippincott, 1982, p 33.)

simultaneous monitoring of heart rate and rhythm (as well as tone) and breath sounds, with the patient on his or her side and the occiput cushioned. In this position, soft tissues are pulled forward and away from the airway, decreasing obstruction and allowing secretions (or emesis, should it occur) to drain out of the corner of the mouth.[1]

Cardiopulmonary Assessment

Additional monitors may be desirable in individual patients, even during the brief transfer to the PACU, but observation and a stethoscope generally suffice. If a patient was anesthetized in a location other than the OR and a longer transfer is required, a pulse oximeter is advisable. Electrocardiographic monitoring and automated noninvasive blood pressure monitoring are desirable if a potential exists for volume shifts or bleeding during transport. Such occurrences may be noted after invasive radiologic or angiographic procedures. Various lightweight battery-operated transport monitors follow these parameters and also allow vascular pressures to be transduced.

During transfer from the ICU or PACU to the ward, clinical observation should form the base of monitoring. Unless a patient is moved to a "step-down" unit or a telemetry ward, electrocardiographic and blood pressure measurement is not required. If a patient has been receiving supplemental O_2, however, and may continue to need it on the ward, O_2 should be administered during transport.

Ventilator-Dependent Patients

Ventilator-dependent patients are clearly at risk for deterioration during critical care transport. How ventilation should be

accomplished and what additional monitors should be used are pertinent questions during transport. Gervais and colleagues showed that manual ventilation with spirometry measurement prevents alterations in arterial blood gas and hemodynamic changes that accompany unmonitored manual ventilation or use of a transport ventilator.[13] Weg and Haas found that stable hemodynamic and respiratory status for most patients could be maintained by a trained respiratory therapist using manual ventilation matched to the inspired O_2 and minute ventilation of the bedside ventilator.[25] Other investigators have reported similar findings, although a tendency toward hyperventilation with bag inflation compared with that of a transport ventilator is noteworthy (Table 24–2).[26] My experience suggests that most ventilator-dependent patients can be satisfactorily managed using a Mapleson D circuit with a gauge attached to monitor airway pressures. This combination allows some control over positive end-expiratory pressure (PEEP) and prevents overdistention and barotrauma.[16] Available transport ventilators and their characteristics are summarized in Table 24–3.[26]

Choice of Ventilator

Critically ill patients may require high levels of continuous positive airway pressure (CPAP) or complex ventilatory modes such as pressure control ventilation with inverse inspiration-to-expiration ratios to maintain oxygenation. In these patients, manual ventilation is likely to be ineffective, and a transport ventilator must be used. Unfortunately, the modes of an ICU ventilator (intermittent mandatory ventilation, pressure support ventilation, CPAP/PEEP, pressure control ventilation, and so on) may be different or impossible to match with these devices. The safest approach whenever possible in such cases

TABLE 24–2. Comparing Self-Inflating Bag and Transport Ventilator

	Conventional Ventilation Before Transport	Self-Inflating Bag Used During Transport	Transport Ventilator Used During Transport
pHa	7.39 ± 0.3	7.51 ± 0.2*	7.40 ± 0.3
$Paco_2$ (mm Hg)	39 ± 4	30 ± 3*	39 ± 3
Pao_2 (mm Hg)	116 ± 17	109 ± 24	117 ± 20
Heart rate (beats per minute)	106 ± 23	115 ± 19	109 ± 25
Systolic pressure (mm Hg)	130 ± 36	112 ± 24	136 ± 31
Diastolic pressure (mm Hg)	86 ± 12	73 ± 10	81 ± 20

(From Branson RD, McGough EK: Transport ventilators. Probl Crit Care 1990; 4:261.)
*$P < .05$ compared with conventional ventilation.
Average transport time = 9 ± 3 min during manual ventilation with a self-inflating bag; 8 ± 3 min during ventilation with a transport ventilator.

TABLE 24–3. Ventilatory and Monitoring Characteristics of Transport Ventilators

Ventilator	Cycling Variables	Modes	Rate (breaths per minute)	Tidal Volume (mL)	Minute Volume (L/min)*	I:E Ratio (Minimum)	Peak Flow Rate (L/min)	Fio₂	PEEP (cm H₂O)†	Alarms	Monitoring	Demand-Flow Valve	Manual Breath
Hamilton MAX	Time	IMV, CMV	2–30	50–1500	45.0	1:1	90	1.0	No	Low inlet pressure and low battery (audible and visual). High airway pressure (audible)	Airway pressure	Yes	Yes
Biomed IC2A	Time	CMV, IMV, CPAP	1–66	130–2500	37.5	4:1	75	1.0	0–25	None	Airway pressure	No‡	Yes
Healthdyne 105	Time	IMV, CPAP, CMV	1–150	10–4000	20.0	4:1	60	0.21–1.0	0–20	Audible/visual; low/high pressure, low inlet pressure, system interrupt, insufficient expiratory time, reverse I:E, power loss, disconnect	Airway pressure	No, continuous flow only	Yes
Impact Universal	Time	CMV	14, 20, 30 child; 12, 18 adult	10–1250	22.5	1:2	90	1.0	No	Visual low battery; audible high pressure	None	No	Yes
Life support products Auto Vent 2000	Time	IMV, CMV	8–20	400–1200	24.0	1:1	48	1.0	No	High pressure audible	None	Yes	No
Life support products Auto Vent 3000	Time	IMV, CMV	9–27 child; 8–20 adult	200–600 child; 400–1200 adult	24.0 adult; 16.0 child	1:1	48	1.0	No	High pressure audible	None	Yes	No
Newport E100i	Time or pressure	IMV, CMV, A/C, CPAP	1–80	100–3600	36.0	1:1	72	0.21–1.0	0–25	Visual/audible high/low pressure, inspiration time too long	Airway pressure	No, continuous flow only	Yes
Ohmeda Logic 07	Time	CMV	10–40	100–2000	20.0	1:2	65	0.5 or 1.0	No	Audible high pressure	Airway pressure	No	No
Penlon 350	Time	CMV	10–85	10–300 neonate/child; 50–2000 adult	0.1–9.0 neonate/child; 1.0–3.0 adult	2:1	60	1.0	No	Audible high pressure	Airway pressure	No	No
Pneupac Model 2-R	Time	CMV	11, 12, 13, 14, 16, 19, and 21	340–1450	16.0	1:1.5	40	0.45 or 1.0	No	Audible high pressure	None	No	No
Stein-Gates	Time	CMV	1–150	30–3000	20.0	2:1	45	1.0	No	None	None	No	No
Bird Space Technologies Mini-TXP	Time	CMV	4–15	50–2500	30.0	1:2	120	0.45–0.8	No	None	None	No	Yes

(From Branson RD, McCough EK: Transport ventilators. *In* Banner M (ed). Problems in Critical Care. Philadelphia, JB Lippincott, 1990, p 264.)

*Maximum available minute volume with an I:E of 1:1.

†PEEP can be provided in all ventilators with an external PEEP valve.

‡During spontaneous inhalation, the ventilator cycles "on," but the exhalation valve remains depressurized to allow venting of gas to the atmosphere. Depending on the inspiratory flow rate and time settings, gas flow rate for a specific duration of time is available for spontaneous breathing. The system does not function as a demand-flow valve.

Abbreviations: I:E = inspiration-to-expiration; Fio₂ = fraction of inspired oxygen; PEEP = positive end-expiratory pressure; IMV = intermittent mandatory ventilation; CMV = controlled mechanical ventilation; CPAP = continuous positive airway pressure.

may be to use the ICU ventilator for transport and, if necessary, for any surgical procedure in the OR.[16] The ventilator may be moved independently, with compressed gas tanks, or more ideally as part of a transport cart.[20]

In addition to pulse oximetry, ventilated patients should have airway pressure monitored during transport. A spirometer is helpful to ensure adequate and consistent tidal volumes. At the minimum, a colorimetric carbon dioxide (CO_2) detector should be available. Critically ill patients or those with reduced intracranial elastance should have continuous end-tidal CO_2 monitoring.[20, 27]

Head Injury Cases

Patients with a neurologic injury present special challenges. Clinical examination remains the best monitor of neurologic status, both during transport and in the ICU. Unfortunately, the need to pursue diagnostic studies in an uncooperative patient or to perform surgical procedures may necessitate sedation or other medications that can obscure the neurologic findings. Sedation and intubation in a relatively controlled setting, before transport to the CT scanner or other areas of the hospital, is often advisable. Short-acting sedatives, especially propofol, are useful, allowing rapid emergence so that patients may be clinically assessed at the end of the transport or procedure.

Patients with severe head injuries or other causes of increased ICP are likely to have ICP monitors in place. They are intubated and hyperventilated and are likely to be in a 20° to 30° head-up position. Newer modalities include somatosensory evoked potential monitoring and jugular bulb oximetry. These patients are at high risk of secondary insults yet are also quite likely to require transport for radiologic studies or to the OR.

Although jugular bulb oximetry and evoked potential monitoring are unnecessary during transport, oxygenation, blood pressure, and end-tidal CO_2 should be maintained as constant as possible. The head-up position should be continued. Because ICP changes are common during transport, ICP monitoring should be continued. This assessment is easily accomplished with the newer fiberoptic devices but may require careful attention to transducer height and monitor function if a ventriculostomy catheter or Richmond's bolt is being used.

Spinal Cord Injury Patients

Spinal cord–injured patients present special logistic concerns related to the traction and stabilization devices that may be used. Any movement or transport should be performed with a member of the neurosurgical team. Airway protection in spinal cord injury must also take into consideration the potential for progressive ventilatory muscle insufficiency. Although this problem is unlikely to occur rapidly, it must be addressed before any prolonged transport.

Hemodynamically Unstable Patients

Optimal preparation is crucial to the safe transport of hemodynamically unstable patients. Resuscitation fluids should be available with blood (if appropriate), together with a plentiful supply of any infusions or medications. Consideration should be given to having at least one individual available for the sole purpose of fluid/blood administration and to ensuring that the nurse or other designated individual will have uninterrupted access to vasoactive infusions.

References

1. Gravenstein J, Paulus D: Monitoring Practice in Clinical Anesthesia. Philadelphia, JB Lippincott, 1982.
2. Blitt C: A philosophy of monitoring. *In* Monitoring in Anesthesia and Critical Care Medicine. Blitt C (ed). New York, Churchill Livingstone, 1985, pp 1–4.
3. Insel J, Weissman C, Kemper M, et al: Cardiovascular changes during transport of critically ill and postoperative patients. Crit Care Med 1986; 14:539.
4. Tyler I, Tatisara B, Winter P, Moloyana E: Continuous monitoring of arterial oxygen saturation with pulse oximetry during transfer to the recovery room. Anesth Analg 1985; 64:1108.
5. Kataria B, Harnik E, Mitchard R, et al: Postoperative arterial oxygen saturation in the pediatric population during transportation. Anesth Analg 1988; 67:280.
6. Tomkins D, Gaukroger P, Bentley M: Hypoxia in children following general anesthesia. Anaesth Intensive Care 1988; 16:177.
7. Riley R, Davis N, Finucane K, Christmas P: Arterial oxygen saturation in anaesthetised patients during transfer from induction room to operating room. Anaesth Intensive Care 1988; 16:182.
8. Venkataraman S, Orr R: Intrahospital transport of critically ill patients. Crit Care Clin 1992; 8:525.
9. Gentleman D, Jennet B: Audit of transfer of unconscious head-injured patients to a neurosurgical unit. Lancet 1990; 335:330.
10. Andrews P, Piper I, Dearded N, Miller J: Secondary insults during intrahospital transport of head-injured patients. Lancet 1990; 335:327.
11. Waddel G: Movement of critically ill patients within hospital. Br Med J 1975; 2:417.
12. Braman S, Dunn S, Amico C, Millman R: Complications of intrahospital transport in critically ill patients. Ann Intern Med 1987; 107:469.
13. Gervais H, Eberle B, Konietzke D, et al: Comparison of blood gases of ventilated patients during transport. Crit Care Med 1987; 15:761.
14. Smith I, Fleming S, Cernaianu A: Mishaps during transport from the intensive care unit. Crit Care Med 1990; 18:278.
15. Petre J, Bazaral M, Estafanous F: Patient transport: an organized method with direct clinical benefits. Biomed Instrum Technol 1989; 23:100.
16. Melker R, Gallagher TJ: Transport of the critically ill/injured patient. *In* Critical Care. 2nd ed. Civetta J, Taylor R, Kirby R (eds). Philadelphia, JB Lippincott, 1992, pp 1797–1808.
17. Fromm R, Dellinger R: Transport of critically ill patients. J Intensive Care Med 1992; 7:223.
18. Kondo K, Herman S, O'Reilly P, Simeonidis S: Transport system for critically ill patients. Crit Care Med 1985; 13:1081.
19. Vandermeersch E, Muller E, Mulier J, et al: A new mobile artificial respiration and monitoring system for transporting critically ill (emergency) patients. Anasth, Intensivther, Notfallmed 1988; 23:276.
20. Link J, Krause H, Wagner W, Papadopoulos G: Intrahospital transport of critically ill patients. Crit Care Med 1990; 18:1427.
21. Schirmer U, Heinrich H, Siebeneich H, Vandermeersch E: Safe intraclinical transfer of intensive care patients—a concept to avoid monitoring and treatment gaps. Anasthesiol Intensivmed Notfallmed Schmerzther 1991; 26:112.
22. Weinfurt P: TRAM: a new concept in transport monitoring. Int J Clin Monit Comput 1987; 4:149.
23. Hendren W, Higgins T: Immediate postoperative care of the cardiac surgical patient. Semin Thorac Cardiovasc Surg 1991; 3:3.
24. Watson C, Norfleet E: Anesthesia for trauma. Crit Care Clin 1986; 2:717.
25. Weg J, Haas C: Safe intrahospital transport of critically ill ventilator-dependent patients. Chest 1989; 96:631.
26. Branson RD, McGough EK: Transport ventilators. Prob Crit Care 1990; 4:254–274.
27. End-tidal carbon dioxide measurement in emergency medicine and patient transport. Health Devices 1991; 20:35.

CHAPTER 25

Temperature Monitoring

RANDALL C. CORK M.D., Ph.D.

The physiology of temperature regulation is discussed in Chapter 49, as is the way in which the body temperature drops during anesthesia. Intraoperative hypothermia as a significant problem is best illustrated by the significant problem of hypothermia in the postanesthesia care unit (PACU).[1] Better monitoring and, thereby, management of patients' temperature during surgery diminish the problem of abnormal temperature postoperatively.

How temperature should be monitored during anesthesia involves two variables: (1) temperature probe selection and (2) temperature monitoring site selection. When one realizes the various sites and probes used, the availability of a probe for every orifice is apparent. Orifices tend to be the best sites, because access is thereby gained to core rather than surface temperature. Before examining alternative sites, let us first review the various probes available.

TEMPERATURE PROBES

What Are Contact Probes?

With the exception of infrared and special tympanic membrane probes, all others are contact probes—that is, they must contact the tissue that is to be monitored for temperature. The prototype, of course, is the somewhat fragile glass mercury thermometer, which has an equalization period of 3 to 5 minutes. Use of mercury now is ecologically unsound and represents a hazardous waste disposal problem. The main physiologic conduit for mercury intoxication is via inhalation, and mercury vaporizes at room temperature. Concentrations can be unusually high in a confined space, such as an incubator.

Thermocouples and Thermistors

Thermocouples and thermistors provide newer ways to measure temperature without toxic hassles. Thermistors are electrical resistors that vary as a function of temperature. Thermocouples are two metals in proximity that produce different electrical current as a function of temperature. Thermistors were available first, but the introduction of thermocouples provided low-cost disposability, a key advantage in our ecologically unconcerned, throw-away culture. However, at pres-

ent, both are fast (20- to 30-s equilibration period), and both are disposable.

Liquid Crystal

The latest craze in temperature probes is liquid crystal temperature indicators. The color of liquid crystal probes changes as a function of temperature; thus liquid crystal tape affixed to the skin can identify the temperature of the skin surface just by its color. Advantages include no equipment expenditures and no maintenance costs. The problem with liquid crystal thermometry is not the technology, which works well, but the site of measurement. Liquid crystal probes measure only skin temperature, and skin temperature does not necessarily reflect core temperature.

As a concession to this shortcoming, virtually all liquid crystal temperature indicators have a button measurement offset that is intended to make the displayed temperature more representative of core temperature (Table 25–1). Note the wide range of offsets. Interestingly, most manufacturers do not include the offset in the product literature.

What happens during anesthesia may be visualized as relaxation of a total body temperature "sphincter," as depicted in Figure 25–1. Heat redistributes during anesthesia, and peripheral temperature may even increase as core temperature decreases. As patients warm up again in the PACU, liquid crystal temperature readings diverge widely from core temperature.[2] This fact, together with the use of temperature offsets in most of these devices, limits the utility of liquid crystal temperature measurement in the operating room to that of trend monitoring alone.

When an accurate core temperature is desired or required, another method should be used. Forehead temperature measured by liquid crystal thermometers has been shown to correlate with esophageal temperature during rapid rewarming after cardiopulmonary bypass.[3] This situation is not representative of most anesthetic procedures, because patients coming off bypass are undergoing rewarming by retransfusion of warmed blood from the bypass pump, resulting in vasodilatation of the cutaneous vessels of the head.

Needle

The ultimate probe is a needle, which can be placed in any tissue at any depth. However, the risks of puncturing holes in

TABLE 25–1. Offset Between Displayed and Actual Temperatures for Different Types of Liquid Crystal Temperature Indicators

Type of Liquid Crystal Temperature Indicator	Temperature (°F)		
	Claimed Accuracy	Offset	
		Mean*	Range
Stat Temp II†	± 0.42	5.3	3.0–8.7
Stat Temp II WR†	± 0.42	6.2	3.4–9.0
RediTemp, oval‡	± 0.04	4.5	3.2–5.2
RediTemp, strip‡	± 0.04	3.1	2.6–4.0
TriTemp§	± 0.05	3.5	3.0–4.2
Temp-a-Strip§	—	0.6	0.2–1.0
Protect§	± 0.5	3.2	2.8–4.0
Crystalline§	± 0.5	4.9	4.5–5.0
EZ Temp‖	—	1.7	0.0–2.5
Omni Combo¶	± 0.5	3.5	2.7–3.6
Omni II¶	± 0.5	5.0	3.8–5.8
Omni OR¶	± 0.5	5.3	4.4–6.6
Omni Wide Range¶	± 0.5	4.7	2.0–6.6
Anesthesia Monitor**	—	2.3	0.0–5.4

(From Shomaker TS, Bjoraker DG: Measurement offset with liquid crystal temperature indicators. Anesthesiology 1990; 73:A425.)
*Mean offset was based on eight readings; displayed temperature was always greater than actual temperature.
†Trademark Medical Corp.
‡Medical Products of America
§Sharn, Inc.
‖Seven Cs, Inc.
¶Omnitherm, Inc.
**Clinitemp, Inc.

people generally outweigh the benefit. The needle temperature probe has found appropriate specific applications in two areas: cardiac surgery and isolated hyperthermia as a treatment for cancer. The temperature of the heart during cold cardioplegia is a direct predictor of protection from myocardial ischemia; the temperature to which different tissues in an isolated, perfused limb are heated is a key factor in monitoring hyperthermia treatment for cancer. In the heart, the interventricular septum is the usual location for placement of the needle probe (Fig. 25–2).

Which probe one uses depends on a number of considerations. Some of the factors commonly considered in selecting a temperature probe are time savings, ease of use, accuracy, precision, hospital area, calibration, service, and durability.

How Are Infrared Detectors Used?

All objects in the universe that are not *black bodies* (a term used in physics to describe heat sinks) emit infrared radiation; this radiation is a function of the surface temperature. At first glance, one might suppose that infrared detectors suffer from the same problem as liquid crystal thermometers, because the temperature at the surface is not the temperature of the core. However, infrared detectors have found application at a specific temperature site, the tympanic membrane, which provides our best index of brain temperature.[2]

An infrared detector, which looks like an otoscope (Fig. 25–3) or a gun to shoot into a patient's ear, has become widely accepted. Its response time is less than 5 seconds. Disposable plastic film covers the sensor to reduce the risk of cross-contamination and prevent build-up of cerumen on the probe.

Advantages of the infrared probe are better infection control because no mucous membrane is contacted, the need for fewer special handling procedures, and less tissue damage risk. Disadvantages are that only intermittent measurements are made and the device must be accurately aimed at the tympanic membrane because the temperature of the ear canal is lower.

ANATOMIC SITES FOR MONITORING

Many anatomic locations, mainly orifices, are used to monitor temperature. During one of our studies at the University of Arizona, the residents frequently commented, "Show us an orifice, and we'll show you a probe for it." Not far from the truth! Figure 25–4 diagrams the sites most commonly used during anesthesia.

What Are the Characteristics at Each Site?

Oral

The classic oral location for a temperature probe is sublingual. The probe is placed on either side of the frenulum, but temperature of tissue just lateral to this position may be significantly different. Sublingual temperature is subject to a number of external factors, such as mouth breathing, crying, and recent ingestion of hot or cold liquids. Oral temperatures can be measured in a cooperative patient in the preanesthetic holding

The Total Body Temperature "Sphincter"

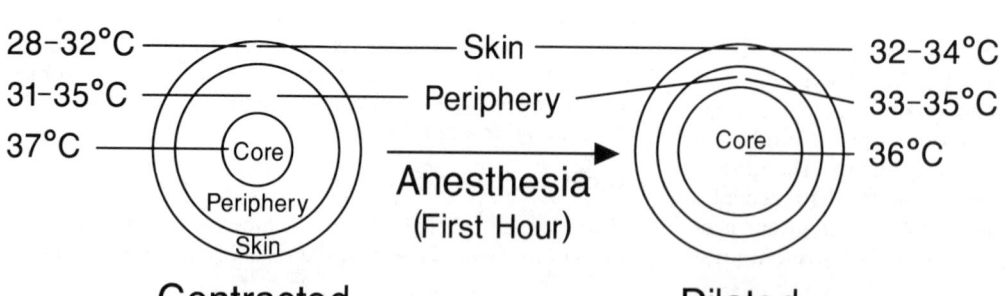

FIGURE 25–1. The total body temperature "sphincter" is relaxed under anesthesia, so temperature from the core is redistributed to the periphery.

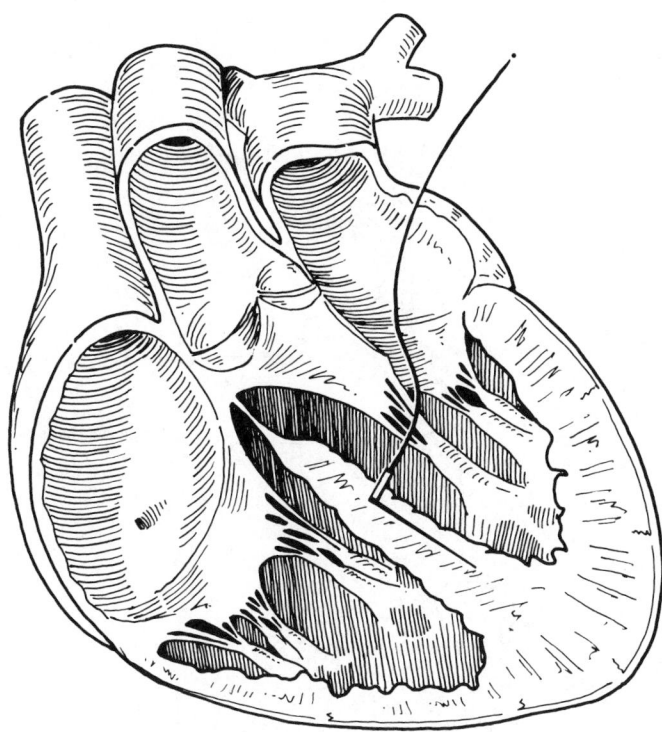

FIGURE 25–2. Placement of a needle probe into the interventricular septum to monitor myocardial temperature during cardiopulmonary bypass.

area and in the PACU; however, they are not conveniently monitored during an anesthetic.

Tympanic Membrane

The temperature of the tympanic membrane approximates brain temperature better than any other site. The blood supply

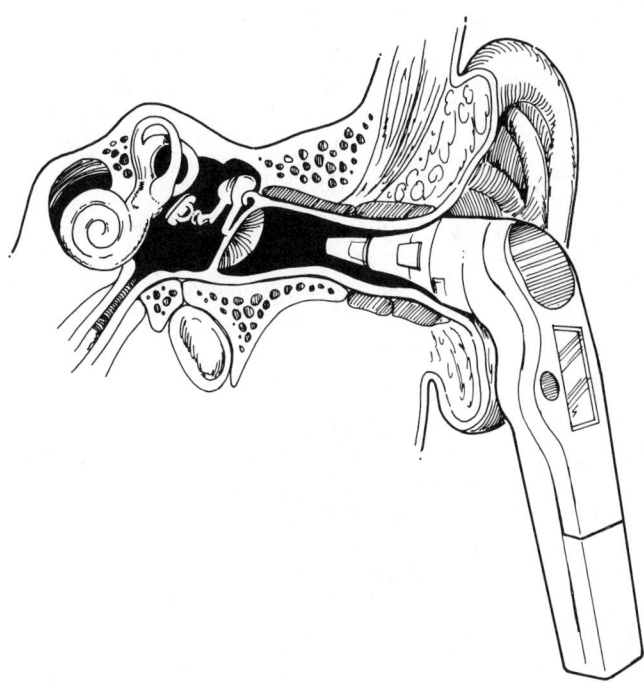

FIGURE 25–3. An infrared detector of tympanic membrane temperature. It is excellent for making single determinations, especially during recovery, but not for use as a continuous monitor. The detector must be accurately aimed at the tympanic membrane rather than at the wall of the ear canal.

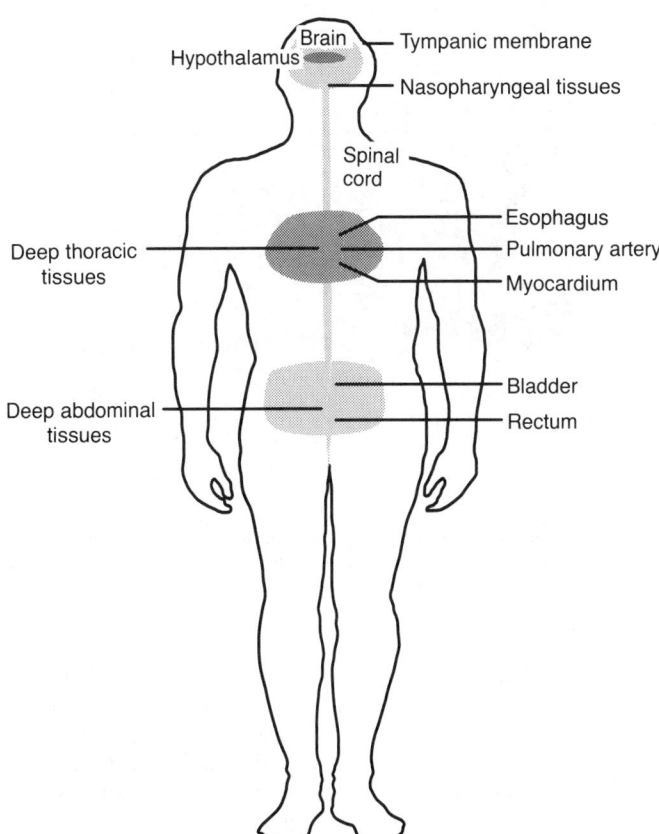

FIGURE 25–4. Anatomic sites frequently used for monitoring temperature under anesthesia.

to the tympanic membrane is via the internal carotid artery, which also supplies the hypothalamus, where the central thermostat is located.[4]

Tympanic probes have lateral stabilizers, which give them the appearance of badminton shuttlecocks (Fig. 25–5). In anesthetized patients particularly, perforation of the tympanic membrane is a risk.[5] These probes should be placed after an otoscopic examination and while patients are awake and alert. Noncontact tympanic membrane probes have been designed,[6] and the infrared temperature detectors discussed previously need no tissue contact. Because the tympanic membrane shares the same vascular supply as the brain, hyperventilation-associated vasoconstriction decreases blood flow to the tympanic membrane and causes a decrease in temperature.[7]

Pulmonary Artery

Pulmonary artery catheters have a probe to monitor blood temperature. This feature is necessary to determine cardiac output by thermodilution, but it provides a useful monitor of intrathoracic temperature as well. Keep in mind that any type of thoracic surgery may affect this monitor, especially cardiac surgery involving cold cardioplegia. A cardiac output monitor that provides a continuous display of pulmonary artery temperature is preferable to one that requires pushing a button each time the temperature is to be checked.

Nasopharynx

The nasopharyngeal temperature probe (Fig. 25–6) should be inserted via a nostril to a depth equal to the distance from

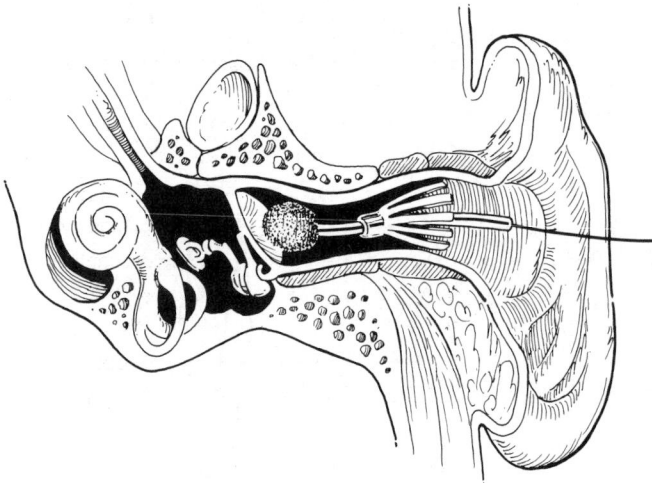

FIGURE 25–5. Probe designed for monitoring of tympanic membrane temperature. It should only be placed in the awake patient prior to anesthesia in order to minimize risk of tympanic membrane injury.

the tragus of the ear to the ala nasi; when inserted too far, it becomes an oropharyngeal or esophageal probe. The temperature of the nasopharynx also is a close approximation of brain temperature.[8] Proper positioning puts the probe in contact with tissue close to the internal carotid artery. Measurement can be adversely affected by gas flow from ventilation, resulting in lower temperatures with higher flows.[9] The danger of causing epistaxis is a consideration, especially in heparinized patients.

Esophagus

The esophagus is close to the great vessels and the heart; hence, the function of an esophageal probe can be combined with that of an esophageal stethoscope (Fig. 25–7). A temper-

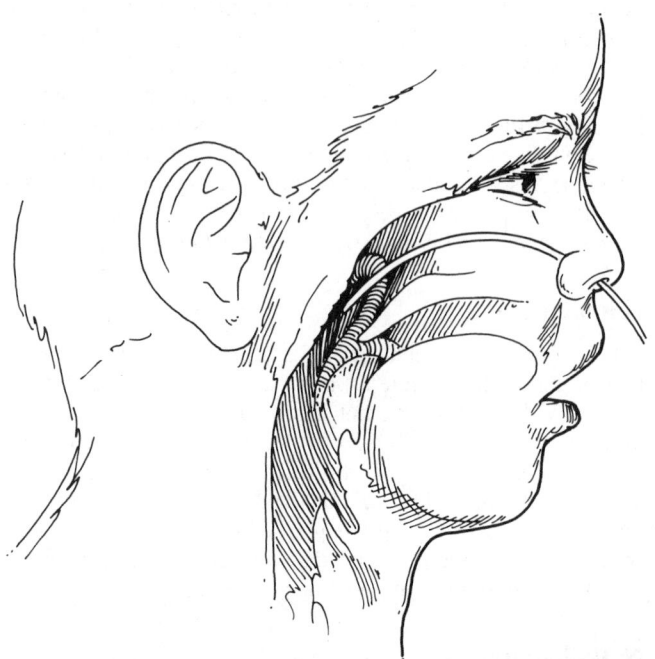

FIGURE 25–6. The nasopharyngeal probe should be inserted only as far as the posterior nasopharynx. This is about the same distance as from the tragus of the ear to the ala nasi.

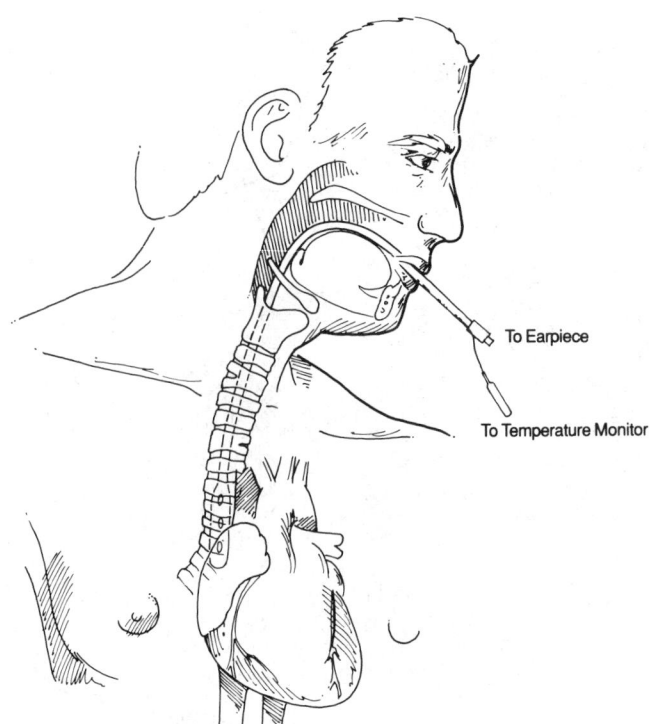

FIGURE 25–7. The esophageal temperature probe can be combined with the esophageal stethoscope. It is best placed where the heart sounds are loudest.

ature gradient is noted along the length of the esophagus. The proximal two thirds is affected by airway temperature; the distal one third offers a true estimate of core temperature.

A combined device may aid in placement of the temperature probe, because it is best located where heart sounds are the loudest.[10] However, esophageal probes are typically inserted only into the middle third of the esophagus, where both heart and breath sounds can be heard effectively. This point usually is between the left atrium and the aorta, about 24 cm below the larynx, or about 37 cm from the incisors in an adult patient. Measurements here are affected by artifactual cooling or heating of respiratory gases in the trachea. Even when an esophageal probe is properly located, temperature measurement can be affected by thoracic surgery, just as with a pulmonary artery temperature probe.

If precise temperature measurement is important, insert the probe to the hilt to ensure that it is in the distal esophagus, or 12 to 16 cm beyond the site of best combined heart and breath sounds.[10]

Bladder

To reinforce the idea that for every orifice there is a probe, thermocouples have been incorporated into the Foley catheter (Fig. 25–8) to measure bladder temperature.[11] This idea is sound because bladder temperature is a reliable index of core temperature.[8] Bladder temperature is more accurate and precise than rectal temperature and not as messy to monitor. Lower abdominal procedures and irrigation artifactually lower the measured temperature.

Rectum

Rectal temperature is a traditional measure of core temperature, but a poor one.[8] Feces tend to act as an insulator. Rectal

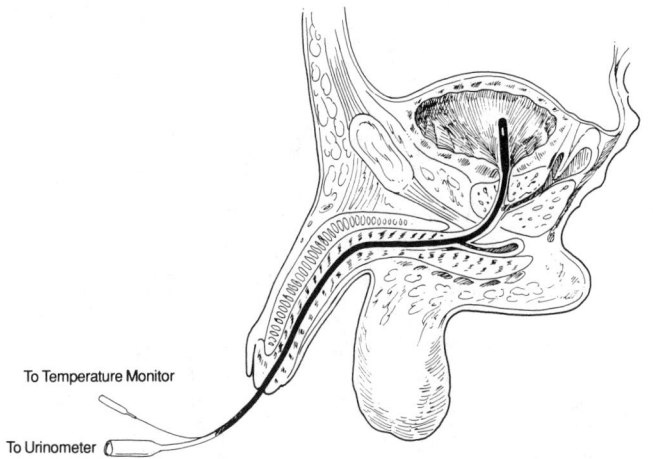

To Temperature Monitor

To Urinometer

FIGURE 25–8. The bladder temperature probe is combined with the Foley catheter. It is especially helpful during major surgery and in the intensive care unit, since it provides an accurate, precise, and continuous measurement of core temperature.

temperature reflects core temperature better in infants than it does in adults. Measurement of rectal temperature is generally fraught with problems in execution, patient discomfort, and safety. Infection control is a real problem, as is nosocomial cross-contamination. As with bladder temperature, surgical procedures involving peritoneal lavage or cystoscopy decrease the utility of this anatomic site for temperature monitoring.

Skin

Heat is radiated from the skin to the environment. More than 90% of heat loss is through the skin. The amount of heat loss is a function of the amount of skin exposed.[12] In fact, the ''rule of nines,'' commonly used for assessing the percentage of burned skin in burned victims,[13] can also be used to roughly assess the percentage of potential heat loss in a partially covered patient. For instance, a savings of 9% of potential heat loss is realized by insulating the head.

Skin temperature is not a reliable index of core temperature, because the degree of vasoconstriction or vasodilation can significantly affect the measurements obtained (see Fig. 25–1). For instance, no skin surface probe at any anatomic site serves as a reliable warning of malignant hyperthermia because of the associated cutaneous vasoconstriction.

Forehead

The forehead has received a lot of attention as an anatomic site for temperature monitoring because of the introduction of liquid crystal temperature-sensitive adhesive strips. Several Canadian studies investigating protection against accidental hypothermia[14, 15] are frequently cited by the proponents of liquid crystal forehead temperature monitoring to illustrate the importance of the forehead in heat loss. Indeed, these studies did show that heat lost via the forehead at low temperatures can account for up to 50% of total heat production. However, this fact was demonstrated at very low temperatures (below freezing) in subjects with heavy thermal insulation over all of their bodies except the forehead. At normal operating room temperatures, heat lost from the forehead is no more or less than heat lost from any other part of the body with the same surface area exposed.

Axilla

The key advantage of axillary temperature measurement is accessibility in awake patients, particularly in the PACU, where axillary temperatures are most commonly measured. The probe is placed over the pulse from the axillary artery, but the reading may take as long as 15 minutes to equilibrate.

Axillary temperature is not an accurate index of core temperature[8] because of hair, a patient's movement, blood pressure cuff inflation, and ipsilateral intravenous infusions. Infrared monitoring of tympanic membrane temperature is rapidly replacing the axillary probe as the preferred method of temperature measurement in the PACU.

Toe

The toe as an anatomic site for temperature monitoring was suggested by cardiac surgeons who noticed during their postoperative rounds that those patients with higher cardiac output had warmer feet than those with lower cardiac output.[16] The investigators conducted a small descriptive study, which showed a close correlation between cardiac output and toe temperature in postoperative patients.

Peripheral temperatures of the hands, fingers, and toes are frequently measured to assess adequacy of sympathetic blockade (Fig. 25–9); the better the block, the warmer the peripheral temperature.[17] We included the toes as an anticipated least-reliable site in our analysis of the accuracy and precision of various anatomic sites as indicators of core temperature.[8] We did so expecting to find no association at all but found that the longer the anesthetic lasted, the more accurate and precise measurement of toe temperature became—an excellent example of how anesthesia tends to make homeothermic poikilotherms of us all.

How Do the Various Sites Compare As Indices of Core Temperature?

Temperature sites can be compared in terms of accuracy and precision. In the previously mentioned study, accuracy was defined as absolute deviation from the gold standard of tympanic membrane temperature; precision was defined as the tracking ability at the various sites to that same standard. A study by Stone and colleagues[18] demonstrates the close association between tympanic membrane temperature and direct measurements of brain temperature. We found esophageal, nasopharyngeal, and bladder temperatures to be more reliable indices of core temperature (i.e., tympanic membrane temperature) than forehead, axillary, rectal, and, of course, toe temperatures (Figs. 25–10 and 25–11).

INTRAOPERATIVE HYPOTHERMIA

How Can It Be Prevented or Treated?

Figure 25–12 illustrates a number of potential options available to anesthesiologists to maintain temperature of anesthetized and recovering patients.

Room Temperature

The first place to start is with room temperature regulation. Two early studies demonstrated that if the operating room temperature is kept at >21 °C, more patients maintain core temperature above 36 °C after 2 hours of surgery.[19, 20]

Surgeons tend to complain of temperature discomfort at room temperatures >17 °C. A compromise that has been proposed involves preheating the room to between 22 °C and 24 °C before a patient arrives to minimize radiant and convective heat loss before draping, followed by lowering of room temperature to 17 °C afterward.

In apparent conflict with these studies are the findings by Roizen and colleagues,[21] who showed no difference in the incidence of hypothermia at room temperatures of 17 °C to 20 °C versus 21 °C to 23 °C. However, in this study, other methods were used to preserve heat, such as heating mattresses set to 38 °C, fluid warmers, and cotton blankets over as much surface as possible. Thus, temperature maintenance during anesthesia and surgery is a multivariate endeavor, with room temperature an important variable but certainly not a solitary one.

Heating and Humidifying of Inspired Gases

Aside from the damage caused by drying of respiratory epithelium, approximately 10% of hourly heat production is lost via the airway during ventilation with unheated dry gases. Heating and humidifying gases to 35 °C to 37 °C and 100% relative humidity has been shown to be effective in preventing intraoperative heat loss during major surgical procedures.[22, 23] In addition, this process decreases the incidence of postoperative shivering.[24]

Some considerations must be taken into account in the numerator of the risk-benefit ratio. These include the potential for bacterial contamination, condensation, and tracheal injury. Bacterial contamination is avoided with close attention to antimicrobial technique. Single-use cartridge systems are available with some of the current heating and humidification systems.

"Rain out" in the anesthetic circuit is not a benign meteorologic observation; it can accumulate to such a degree that it causes circuit valve failure or tubing obstruction. Condensation must be monitored and treated with periodic tube emptying. Inadvertent tracheal injury, known as "hot pot tracheitis," can occur if the heated and humidified gases are too hot.[25] Use temperatures <41 °C.

Artificial Noses

Although not as effective as active systems, passive heat and humidity retention systems, also known as *artificial noses,* retain heat and moisture of the exhaled gases and release it to the inhaled gases.[26] In addition to reducing the rate of intraoperative heat loss, some also serve as disposable bacterial filters. Efficiency increases with lower fresh gas flow rates. Patients with artificial noses demonstrated a reduced rate of cooling with room temperatures of 20 °C to 21 °C and gas flows of 3 L · min⁻¹.[27] Other benefits of artificial noses include prevention of drying of the respiratory mucosa and preservation of respiratory epithelium ciliary function and pulmonary mechanics.[28] However, they increase airway resistance significantly as they become "soaked," a factor that may be of some concern in spontaneously breathing patients.

Passive heat retention with artificial noses is about 50% as effective at temperature maintenance as active heating and humidification. Both are more effective in infants and children than adults. In fact, a real risk of inadvertent hyperthermia is

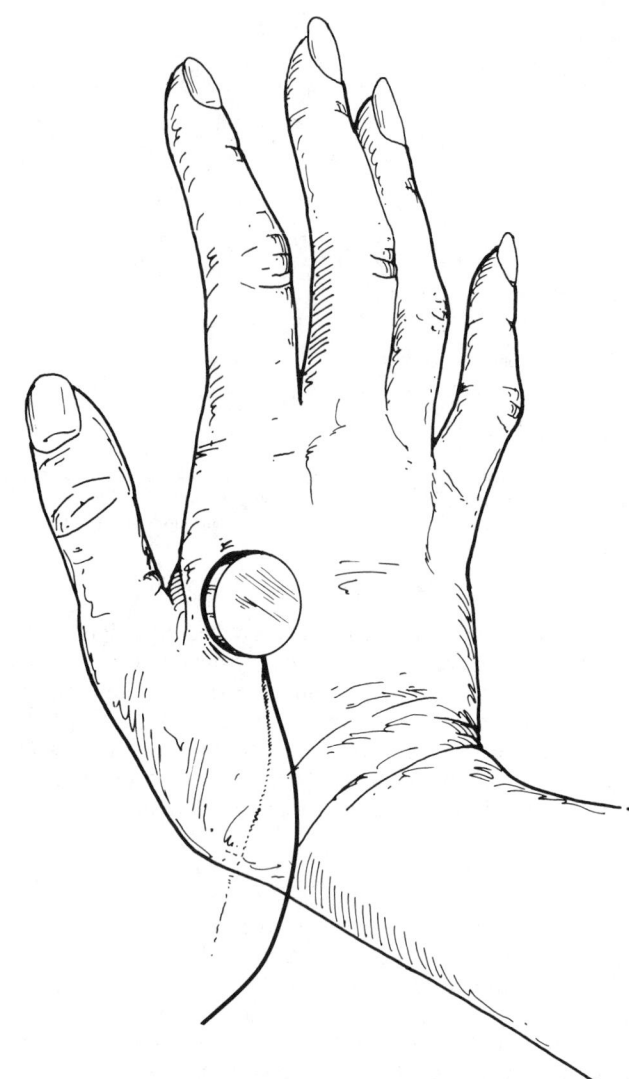

FIGURE 25–9. An adhesive skin probe can be used to measure the temperature of the hands, fingers, and toes in order to monitor sympathetic blockade. Also, temperatures of the forehead and axillae have been used as indices of core temperature.

present in infants and children during active heating and humidification. In combination with limb tourniquets, active heating and humidification significantly increases core temperature (1.7 ± 0.6 °C) in children.[29]

Covers

Covers placed over a patient decrease heat loss from radiation and convection and help to maintain temperature. Various materials have been used: cotton, plastic, paper, and permeable Mylar with reflective metal, such as aluminum foil. Reflective blankets alone have been shown to be ineffective in preventing hypothermia in the operating room unless 60% or more of the body surface area can be covered.[30] All materials reduce heat loss approximately 30% in fully covered patients. As noted in the previous discussion of skin surface temperature, heat loss reduction is proportional to the amount of body surface area covered.

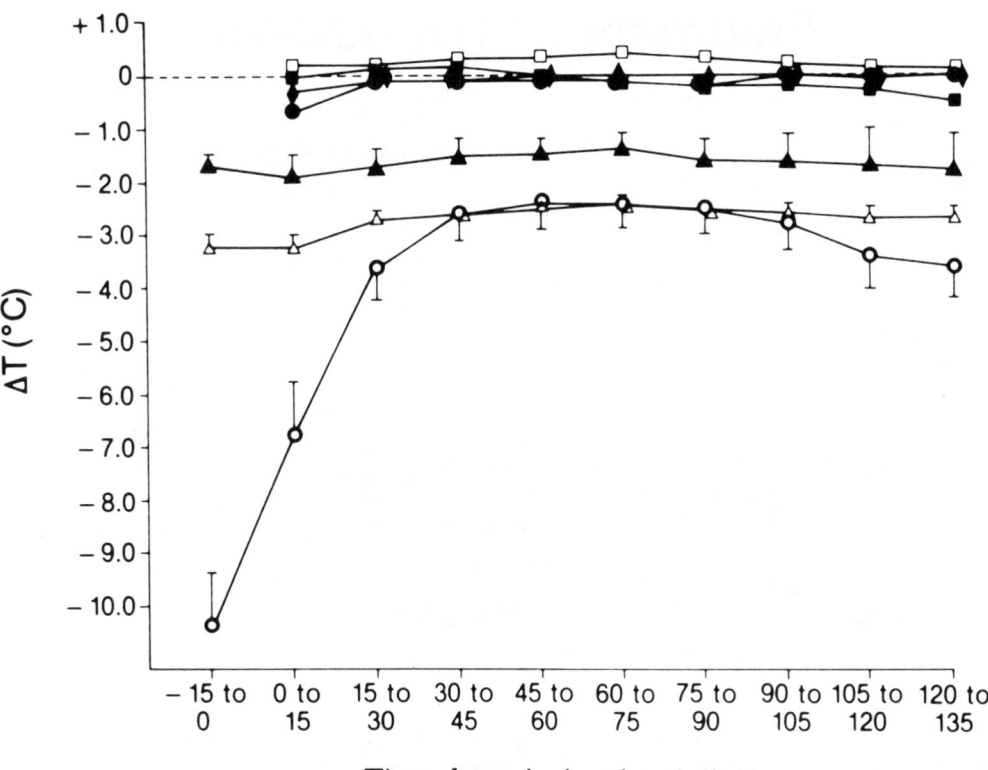

FIGURE 25–10. Accuracy of temperature measurement at various sites compared with the accuracy of temperature measurement at the tympanic membrane (TM). Rectal (□), bladder (■), esophageal (♦), and nasopharyngeal (●) measurements are the most accurate, with mean axillary (▲) temperatures 1.5 to 1.9 °C below mean TM temperature and with mean forehead (△) temperature 2.4 to 3.2 °C below mean TM temperature. Great toe (○) temperature averages 10.4 °C below mean TM temperature at the beginning of anesthesia, but measurement becomes more accurate as the anesthesia progresses. (From Cork RC, Vaughan RW, Humphrey LS: Precision and accuracy of intraoperative temperature monitoring. Anesth Analg 1983; 62:212. Reproduced with permission of the author.)

Active Skin Surface Warming

If blankets can be considered to prevent heat loss passively, a number of methods are available for active skin surface warming. These methods include various types of radiant heaters and heating blankets that use heated water or forced air convection.

Radiant Heaters

Radiant heaters use infrared radiation and are best employed for heat maintenance during skin preparation and draping of patients before surgery or for treatment of hypothermia during emergence in the PACU. Attempts at intraoperative use of radiant heaters interfere with the surgeon and may dry exposed viscera. Although portable infrared lamps are usually used, thermal ceilings have been installed in many PACUs, because the incidence of intraoperative hypothermia (60%) is so common.[1] In the PACU, radiant heat has been shown to decrease postanesthetic shivering without affecting core temperature.[31]

Heating Blankets

Heating blankets set at 38 °C to 40 °C provide heat transfer of up to 8 to 10 Kcal · h⁻¹ during surgery. However, at least

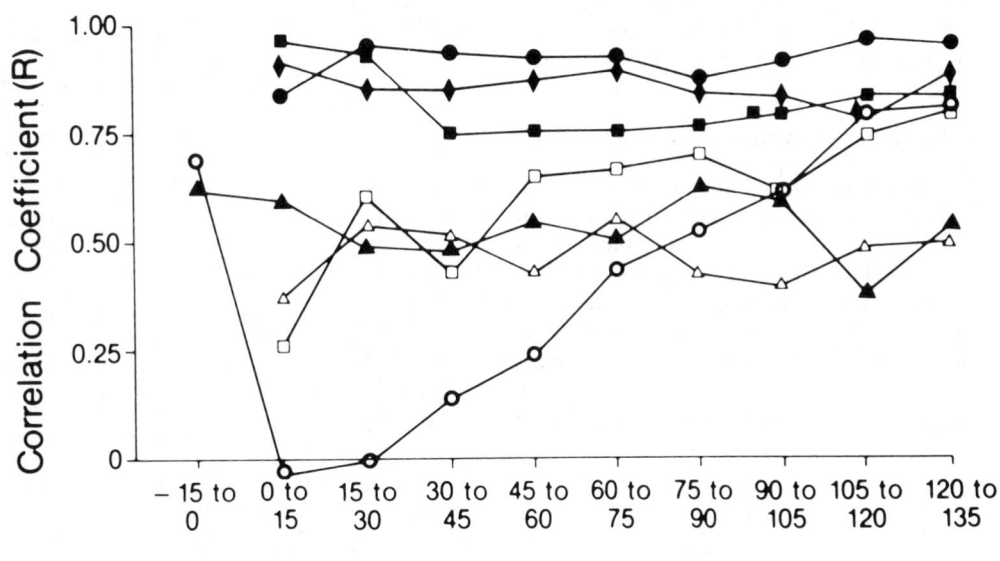

FIGURE 25–11. Precision of bladder (■), esophageal (▲), nasopharyngeal (●), forehead (△), rectal (□), axillary (▲), and great toe (○) temperature measurements as correlated with tympanic membrane temperature measurements. Precision is quantitated by correlation coefficients. Precision of rectal temperature measurement gradually improves from a correlation coefficient of 0.26 at 0 to 15 min, to 0.81 at 120 to 135 min. Marked improvement in precision during anesthesia is exhibited when great toe temperature is measured (improving from a correlation with TM temperature of −0.04 at the beginning of anesthesia to 0.82 after 2 h of anesthesia). (From Cork RC, Vaughan RW, Humphrey LS: Precision and accuracy of intraoperative temperature monitoring. Anesth Analg 1983; 62:213. Reproduced with permission of the author.)

Treatment of Hypothermia

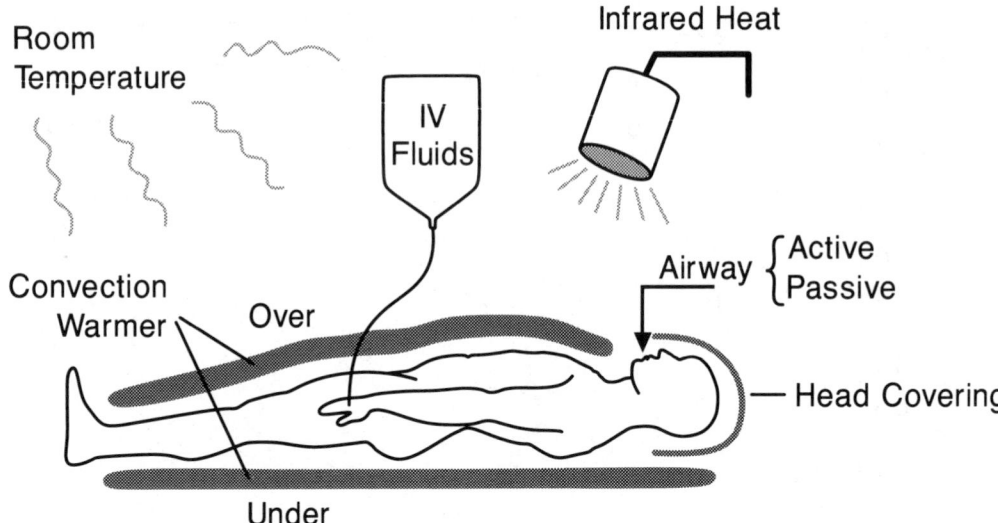

FIGURE 25–12. A number of options are available to help control or maintain patient temperature during anesthesia.

one study has shown that when used as the sole warming technique in a cold operating room (<21 °C), heating blankets are ineffective in preventing hypothermia.[32] This study serves to reinforce the idea that prevention of hypothermia is multivariate. When combined with a heated humidifier and warm room temperatures, heating blankets are very effective at preventing hypothermia.[33] The most important caveat, especially in long operations, is the risk of contact burns with any heating blanket.

Types of Thermal Insulation

A comparison of the different types of thermal insulation reveals little difference in maintenance of a patient's temperature during the first hour of anesthesia.[34] This observation is consistent with the period of redistribution of body heat, which is unpreventable. However, prewarming with a convection blanket before anesthesia does attenuate the drop in temperature associated with the previously mentioned redistribution of body heat during the first hour of anesthesia.[35]

Warming of Intravenous Fluids and Blood

In addition to warming the outside of the patient, the anesthesiologist has the opportunity to warm the inside by heating the intravenous fluids. Warming of intravenous fluids prevents approximately 0.2 °C temperature loss per liter of fluid infused attributable to the administration of intravenous fluid at room temperature. Two units of packed red blood cells at 4 °C lowers core temperature by 0.5 °C, equivalent to a loss of 16 Kcal. Infusion of 1 L of crystalloid at room temperature results in the same 16 Kcal lost. An anesthetized adult generates only 50 to 60 Kcal $\cdot$ h^{-1}, so a 16-Kcal loss is significant.

References

1. Vaughan MS, Vaughan RW, Cork RC: Postoperative hypothermia. Am J Nurs 1981; 81:1198.

2. Vaughan MS, Cork RD, Vaughan RW: Inaccuracy of liquid crystal thermometry to identify core temperature trends in postoperative adults. Anesth Analg 1982; 61:284.

3. Allen G, Horrow JC, Rosenberg H: Does forehead liquid crystal temperature accurately reflect "core" temperature? Can J Anaesth 1990; 37:659.

4. Benzinger TH: Heat regulation: homeostasis of central temperature in man. Physiol Rev 1969; 49:671.

5. Wallace CT, Marks WE, Adkins WY, et al: Perforation of the tympanic membrane, a complication of tympanic thermometry during anesthesia. Anesthesiology 1974; 41:290.

6. Moore JW, Newbower RS: Noncontact tympanic thermometer. Med Biol Eng Comput 1978; 36:580.

7. Romanelli VA, Hiesstand DC, Howie MB, et al: The effect of hyperventilation on tympanic membrane temperature as measured by infrared scanning (Abstract). Anesthesiology 1991; 75:A482.

8. Cork RC, Vaughan RW, Humphrey LS: Precision and accuracy of intraoperative temperature monitoring. Anesth Analg 1983; 62:211.

9. Hendricks HHL, Trahey GE: Paradoxical inhibition of decreases in body temperature by use of heated and humidified gases (Letter to the editor). Anesth Analg 1982; 61:393.

10. Kaufman RD: Relationship between esophageal temperature gradient and heart and lung sounds heard by esophageal stethoscope. Anesth Analg 1987; 66:1946.

11. Lilly JK, Boland JP, Zekan S: Urinary bladder temperature monitoring: a new index of body core temperature. Crit Care Med 1980; 8:742.

12. Sessler DI, Moayeri A: Skin-surface warming: heat flux and central temperature. Anesthesiology 1990; 73:218.

13. Knaysi GA, Crikelair GF, Cosman B: The rule of nines: its history and accuracy. Plast Reconstruct Surg 1968; 41:560.

14. Burton AC, Froese G: Heat losses from the human head. J Appl Physiol 1957; 10:235.

15. Edwards M, Burton A: Temperature distribution over the human head, especially in the cold. J Appl Physiol 1960; 15:209.

16. Joly HR, Weil MH: Temperature of the great toe as an indicator of the severity of shock. Circulation 1969; 39:131.

17. Löfström JB, Lloyd JW, Cousins MJ: Sympathetic neural blockade of the upper and lower extremity. In Neural Blockade in Clinical Anesthesia and Management of Pain. Cousins MJ, Bridenbaugh PO (eds). Philadelphia, JB Lippincott, 1980, pp 355–382.

18. Stone JG, Yong WL, Smith CR, et al: Do temperatures recorded at standard monitoring sites reflect actual brain temperature during deep hypothermia? (Abstract) Anesthesiology 1991; 75:A483.

19. Morris RH: Influence of ambient temperature on patient temperature during intraabdominal surgery. Ann Surg 1971; 173:230.

20. Morris RH, Wilkey BR: The effects of ambient temperature on patient temperature during surgery not involving body cavities. Anesthesiology 1970; 32:102.

21. Roizen MF, Sohn YJ, L'Hommedieu CS, et al: Operating room tempera-

ture prior to surgical draping: effect on patient temperature in recovery room. Anesth Analg (Cleve) 1980; 59:852.

22. Stone DR, Downs JB, Paul WL, et al: Adult body temperature and heated humidification of anesthetic gases during general anesthesia. Anesth Analg (Cleve) 1981; 60:736.

23. Tausk HC, Miller R, Roberts RB: Maintenance of body temperature by heated humidification. Anesth Analg 1976; 55:719.

24. Pflug AE, Aasheim GM, Foster C, et al: Prevention of post-anesthesia shivering. Can Anaesth Soc J 1973; 25:43.

25. Klein EF, Graves SA: "Hot pot" tracheitis. Chest 1974; 65:225.

26. Chalon J, Markham JP, Ali MM, et al: The Pall Ultipor breathing circuit filter: an efficient heat and moisture exchanger. Anesth Analg 1984; 63:566.

27. Haslam KR, Nielsen CH: Do passive heat and moisture exchangers keep the patient warm? Anesthesiology 1986; 64:379.

28. Weeks DB, Ramsey FM: Laboratory investigation of six artificial noses for use during endotracheal anesthesia. Anesth Analg 1983; 62:758.

29. Blach EC, Ginsberg B, Binner RA, et al: Limb tourniquets and central temperature in anesthetized children. Anesth Analg 1992; 74:486.

30. Bourke DL, Wurm H, Rosenberg M, et al: Intraoperative heat conservation using a reflective blanket. Anesthesiology 1984; 60:151.

31. Murphy MT, Lipton JM, Loughran MB, et al: Postanesthetic shivering in primates: inhibition by peripheral heating and by taurine. Anesthesiology 1985; 63:161.

32. Morris RH, Kumar A: The effect of warming blankets on maintenance of body temperature of the anesthetized, paralyzed adult patient. Anesthesiology 1972; 36:408.

33. Tollusfrud SG, Gunderson Y, Anderson R: Perioperative hypothermia. Acta Anaesthesiol Scand 1984; 28:511.

34. Sessler DI, McGuire J, Sessler AM: Perioperative thermal insulation. Anesthesiology 1991; 74:875.

35. Moayeri A, Hynsen JM, Sessler DI, et al: Preinduction skin-surface warming prevents redistribution hypothermia (Abstract). Anesthesiology 1991; 75:A1004.

Clinically Relevant Anatomy

CHAPTER 26

Functional Anatomy of the Airway

LEROY D. VANDAM, Ph.B., M.D., M.A.

Perhaps it is superfluous to state that maintenance of the airway is one of two essentials of anesthetic management, the other being circulatory homeostasis. In support of this tenet are those reports originating from closed-claim analysis of medicolegal actions in which respiratory events involving hypoxia formed the single largest class of adverse anesthetic events, 762 of 2046 cases.[1] Relatively infrequent were airway trauma, pneumothorax, subcutaneous emphysema, aspiration of gastric contents into the lungs, barotrauma, and bronchospasm.

In the conscious state, exchange of oxygen and carbon dioxide (CO_2) at the lungs is vital to survival. During anesthesia, any difficulty that might have existed beforehand is surely magnified by the use of sedatives, the central depressant effects of general anesthetics, the use of neuromuscular blocking agents, the supine position with relaxation of the jaw, or any of the many unusual body positions required for surgical procedures.

Despite these findings, and nearly 150 years after the introduction of anesthesia, airway management continues to bedevil anesthesiologists, as demonstrated by a spate of articles, symposia, and monographs on the subject. Perhaps this publicity is a manifestation of increasing technology in anesthesia so that clinicians are no longer the observant physicians they once were.

In their respective fields, medical specialists, particularly radiologists and surgeons, are obliged to be experts on the anatomic basis for their diagnoses and operations. Nevertheless, I am unaware of any sustained effort on the part of anesthesiologists to return consistently to the dissecting room to learn the essentials about how the airway is related to the maneuvers they must perform. Because recall of the details once learned in medical school is hardly possible, we must rely instead on textbook illustrations, radiographs, or observations made during surgery for the necessary information—hardly substitutes for the three-dimensional views, relationship of structures, and tissue textures of the anatomy we should have in mind.

PHYLOGENETIC CONSIDERATIONS

Humans' problems with the airway are of evolutionary origin, dating back to distant times when oxygen transport became necessary for survival: the development of gills in fish, the emergence of aquatic creatures from the sea, and the development of the extremities for locomotion and finally bipedalism.[2] These phylogenetic matters are emphasized in the subsequent discussion on laryngeal anatomy.

What Are the Effects of the Erect Position?

Anthropologists have advanced several theories for the change from four-footed locomotion to two footed: the need to use one pair of extremities for foraging, for climbing, for defense, or for travel at a distance in the search for food while carrying the young in arms.[3]

Despite these advantages that distinguish the anthropoids from other mammalian species, the erect position has its tradeoffs.[4] The cranium became set at a right angle to the vertebral column, thus detouring and adding resistance to airflow in respiration; the eyes became centered for vision, with loss of part of the lateral visual fields; and the more mobile cervical spine became susceptible to degenerative changes with aging, as well as the liability of injury and trauma to the spinal cord. Further, the utility of only two extremities in locomotion and running and the inability to gallop have placed obligate two-footed species at a disadvantage with the felines, hounds, and horses in the matter of speed.

TOPICAL ANATOMY OF THE AIRWAY

Since the introduction of artificial airways to improve gas exchange—initially simple oropharyngeal or nasopharyngeal devices and tracheotomy in an emergency, later tracheal intubation—the need to examine the existing features of the airway beforehand has been emphasized. The vast majority of misadventures can be avoided by this appraisal alone.

With a patient's head at a right angle to the spine, some of the probable difficulties encountered in airway establishment are notable (Table 26–1). Nevertheless, despite attempts to predict difficulty in airway placement, one is occasionally taken aback by some unforeseen problems; therefore, one must be ready for any contingency.

How Should the Oral Cavity Be Examined?

Kaban[5] has described the manner in which the airway should be examined before contemplating induction of anesthesia. In addition to other obligatory elements of the physical examination, this approach impresses patients with the seriousness of the anesthetic experience and the role of the professional in this endeavor.

The Face and Jaw

One should inspect the structure of the face and jaws with regard to mask fit during induction. A large protruding nose, a receding jaw, a wide mouth, or a heavy beard in a man can defeat the tight mask fit required for assisted ventilation and oxygenation. As clues to temporomandibular joint dysfunction and the accompanying pain that often presents as neuralgia or headache, one should look for hypomobility or the possibility of dislocation of the jaw during intubation by listening for clicking sounds, as well as remain alert for elicitation of pain.

The Mouth and Oropharynx

The mucous membranes of the mouth and tongue and their coloration may offer clues to underlying disease: anemia, leukoplakia, or early epidermoid carcinoma. The soft palate and uvula should be observed as a patient says ''ah,'' to discover cranial nerve dysfunction and deviation of the tongue (Fig. 26–1), and the tongue should be examined to see if it is excessively large as it is protruded.

With the use of a wooden tongue depressor, the oropharynx is examined for any pathologic changes in the faucial pillars and tonsils while watching for secretions from the salivary ducts. For example, clear saliva should issue from Stensen's duct adjacent to the second molar maxillary teeth.

The Teeth and Dental Appliances

Look at tooth structure, and examine for the presence of periodontal infection, caries, looseness, and the general state of dental hygiene, as well as edentia and prostheses.

TABLE 26–1. Examination of the Airway: Clues to Problems

Inability to open the mouth widely
Temporomandibular joint problems: pain, masseter spasms, trismus
Protruding upper incisors
Agnathia
Nasal obstruction: old fractures, posterior choanal atresia
Hypertrophied tonsils and adenoids
Ankylosis of the cervical spine; dislocation, fractures
Short, thick, muscular neck; ''turkey'' neck; scarring from burns
Congenital malformations
Endocrine disease; acromegaly, goiter, exophthalmos

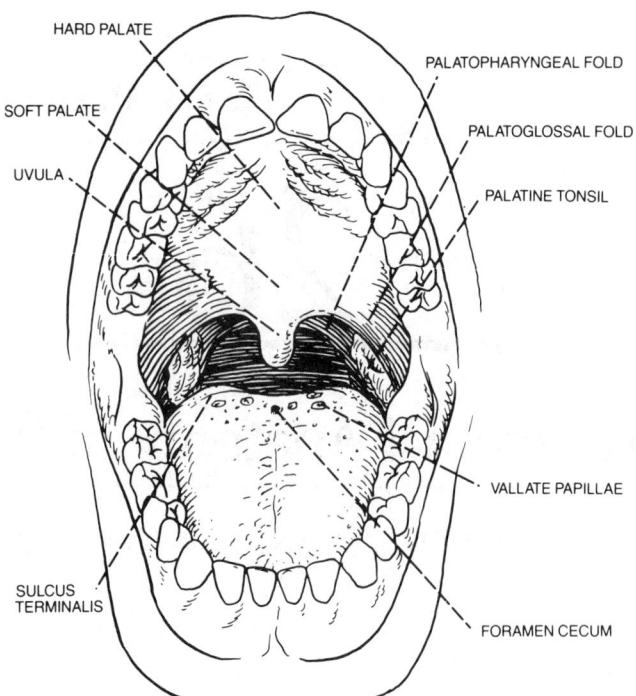

FIGURE 26–1. The open mouth showing the base of the tongue, uvula, and faucal pillars. (From Snell RS, Katz J: Clinical anatomy for anesthesiologists. Norwalk, Appleton & Lange, 1988.)

Although removable bridgework should be taken out before induction of anesthesia, a mask fit is more easily obtained if complete dental plates are retained. A risk here is the possible loss of these important appliances if removed and misplaced during the course of anesthesia. Any abnormalities detected should be noted in a patient's chart along with advice to the patient that injury may occur during anesthesia. Before intubation, when there is concern, the teeth can be protected against damage by means of a malleable mold.

What Anatomic Considerations Are Important to Intubation?

The airway extends from the nostrils to the pulmonary alveoli, but for intubation purposes, the distance to the tracheal bifurcation is more pertinent. Proctor[6] defines the upper airway as consisting of the area for airflow between nasal passages and larynx, the former from the nostrils to the posterior termination of the nasal septum; the nasopharynx from the end of the septum to the lower border of the soft palate; and the pharynx from the soft palate to the larynx. Under some circumstances, the mouth must also be included as part of the airway.

The Nose and Nasopharynx

The nasal passage is a double airway with a complex shape. The nasopharynx is the region where closure can separate the nasal passage from the pharynx; the pharynx is an airway common to both nasal and oronasal breathing and, along with the larynx, more or less forms a bottleneck.

The tip of the nose with its nostrils is fairly mobile and prone to necrosis of the skin if a tracheal tube is allowed to exert pressure on it. This mobile area of the nose consists of several hyaline cartilages, which articulate with the nasal bones laterally and the maxillary and frontal bones superiorly (Fig. 26–2). Cartilages can be injured or even fractured as a result of rough treatment.

The nares, or external choanae, are larger in diameter than the posterior choanae, which lead to the nasopharynx. Both dilation and stabilization of the nares are afforded by the dilator nares muscles. In humans, dilation of the nostrils can be seen during respiratory distress (air hunger) and commonly occurs in animals running at high speed.

Functions

As pointed out by Courtiss and colleagues,[7] the nose provides several basic functions: air conditioner, air cleanser, airway, olfaction, phonation, and reflex responder. Flow of air is both laminar and turbulent, with the main flow passing through the middle meatus; that flow, in turn, is influenced by mucus, ciliary action, and vasoconstriction or vasodilation.

Warming and Humidification. During inspiration, air is warmed nearly to body temperature before reaching the larynx, a conditioning process requiring from 75 to 100 calories of energy expenditure per day. Approximately 90% humidification is achieved before air reaches the lungs, consuming about 1 L of water per day.

Air Cleansing. Air cleansing, an essential protective measure, includes impingement of gross particles suspended in air, with the larger particles caught in the vibrissae of the nostrils and electrostatic changes causing the adhesion of others. The cilia of the upper airway, with their covering mobile blanket of mucus, constantly propel foreign particles toward the exterior, and coughing is the main means by which larger foreign bodies are expelled.

Airway. In adults, the nasal airway is approximately 10 to 14 cm long, divided into two parts by the septum and convo-

luted by the scroll-like structure of the turbinate cartilages (the superior, middle, and inferior conchae attached to the lateral wall) (see Fig. 26–2). The entrance to the nose forms a funnel-shaped vestibule. The entry initially points upward, so the nostrils should be lifted to form a straight passage when inserting an airway. Beyond the vestibule, the passage becomes horizontal but slopes backward, widens at the nasopharynx, and then makes a 90° curve downward toward the larynx.

The roof of the nose is formed by the olfactory plate. For some obscure reason, anosmia has been reported as a complication of general anesthesia. In the supine position, the nasal cavity slopes downward, and the greater space for airway placement lies below the inferior turbinate (see Fig. 26–2).

Epistaxis

Because of the air-conditioning function of the nasal passages, the mucous membranes are highly vascular and erectile. Thus, epistaxis readily occurs with rough manipulation, suggesting the advisability of local application of vasoconstrictors with any intranasal procedures.

The blood supply derives mainly from branches of the maxillary artery, and a common bleeding site is anterior (Kiesselbach's plexus), where the sphenopalatine branch of the maxillary artery anastomoses with the septal branch of the superior labial artery. If anticoagulants have been given, the nasal cavity should not be intubated with nasal airways, nasogastric tubes, or tracheal tubes. Hemorrhage can be intractable, and one should know how to apply nasal packs to stem the bleeding.

Sinusitis

Note that the nasolacrimal ducts and the several cranial sinuses open into the nasal cavity. The sinuses occasionally are infected or occluded by polyps in the allergic state, and postnasal intubation sinusitis may occur. Equalization of air pressure between the middle ear and pharynx is provided by the eustachian tubes and may be obstructed by a nasotracheal tube on that side.

Topical Anesthesia

The nose inside and out is innervated by the superior, medial, and inferior branches of the trigeminal nerve. The terminal nerve endings are superficial in the mucosa, rendering them susceptible to topical anesthesia. Rhinoplasty and other surgical procedures performed on the nose are readily accomplished under regional anesthesia. Injection at the exiting foramina of the infratrochlear and external nasal extensions of the maxillary divisions of the trigeminal nerves is easily accomplished.

What Pharyngeal Factors Are Important for Intubation?

The shape of the pharynx is like a flattened cylinder, constantly changing contour by constriction or relaxation of the pharyngeal muscles and positioning of the soft palate, uvula, and tongue (see Fig. 26–1). During examination, the tongue can be drawn forward to widen the oropharyngeal cavity, in order to visualize the structures more clearly and to apply topical anesthesia. Although indirect laryngoscopy has become

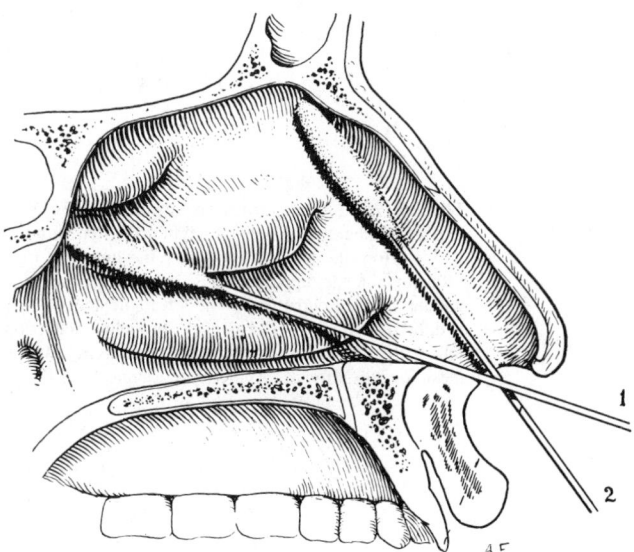

FIGURE 26–2. The lateral wall of the nasal cavity showing the vestibule-like entry, the turbinates, the hard and soft palates, and the adjacent sinuses. The swabs (*1* and *2*) illustrate how topical anesthesia may be applied to the mucous membranes. Notice the space below the inferior turbinate, where there is more room for the passage of air. (From Labat G: Regional Anesthesia: Its Technical and Clinical Application. 2nd ed. Philadelphia, WB Saunders, 1928.)

a lost art among most physicians,[8] the anesthesiologist, using head and laryngeal mirrors, with reflected light, should be proficient in examining the larynx to detect pathologic changes and to observe movement of the vocal cords.

Potential Difficulty of Intubation

As a simple means of detecting possible difficulty in tracheal intubation, Mallampati and colleagues[9] have shown that the size of the tongue at its base is a major factor (see Fig. 26–1). If the base of the tongue when protruded is sufficiently large and the faucial pillars and uvula are concealed during laryngoscopy, the larynx will be overshadowed and its visualization made difficult.

In a prospective study, the degree of obscuration by the tongue of the faucial pillars and uvula was graded and matched with subsequent ability to expose the glottis fully (see Chapter 1, Fig. 1–9). Grades I and II were compatible with adequate exposure, and grades III and IV were predictive of inadequate exposure, the findings having statistical significance.

Another means of predicting possible difficult intubation is by using ultrasound scanning, a noninvasive means of visualizing the vocal cords and larynx.

Anticipated Problems

Proctor[6] points out that the pharynx and larynx comprise, in essence, a bottleneck of the airway. This observation is most evident in neonates and younger children, in whom the presence of infection, mucosal swelling, inspissated secretions, enlarged adenoids and tonsils, and various degrees of choanal atresia can virtually obstruct the airway. The consequent increase in airway resistance may set off a vicious circle, with development of negative pressure causing the tongue and epiglottis to fall backward into the air passages; emergency treatment—laryngeal intubation and occasionally tracheotomy—may be required.

In adults, virulent infection can also lead to airway difficulty in the presence of epiglottitis. Further, sleep apnea can cause major physiologic changes. The cause of sleep apnea has not been established, but many studies implicate a discordant action of the glossal and pharyngeal muscles.

THE TRACHEA

Which Anatomical Considerations Are Important?

The trachea, about 15 cm long in adults, extends from the cricoid cartilage of the larynx to the bronchial bifurcation approximately at the level of the fifth thoracic vertebra and the manubrium sterni (Fig. 26–3). Hyaline cartilaginous rings, about three to five of which are palpable in the neck, encircle the trachea, keeping its patency. Tracheotomy or tracheostomy is preferably performed below the level of the first cartilage to avoid development of chondritis of the cricoid ring.

The cartilages are incomplete posteriorly and are joined by fibroelastic tissue and highly reactive smooth muscle, the Reis-

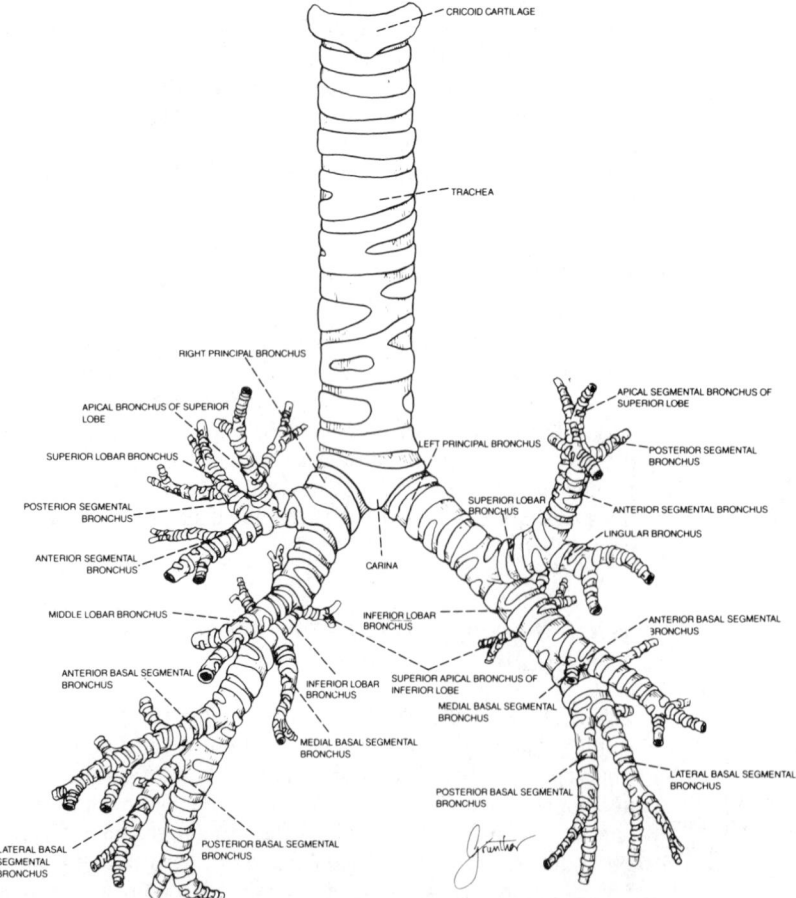

FIGURE 26–3. The trachea and its bifurcation. Notice the lesser angle at which the right mainstem bronchus derives from the trachea as well as the high exit of the bronchus of the upper lobe. Conversely, observe the greater angle of departure of the left main stem bronchus and the relatively lower exits of the bronchus to the upper lobe. (From Snell RS, Karz J: Clinical anatomy for anesthesiologists. Norwalk, Appleton & Lange, 1988.)

seisen's muscle (Fig. 26–4), which receives the same autonomic innervation as does the gut. Thus, the trachea dilates during inspiration and narrows during expiration, almost completely closing during cough to enhance development of positive intrathoracic pressure. The epithelial lining is composed of stratified ciliated columnar epithelium and mucus-secreting goblet cells (Fig. 26–5). The mucus covering under ciliary action propels microparticles in an oral direction.

Mainstem Intubation

Because the right lung consists of three lobes, the right mainstem bronchus is larger in diameter than the left, diverging from the trachea at a lesser angle to the midline (see Fig. 26–3). Consequently, foreign bodies preferentially lodge there, and inadvertent bronchial intubation usually occurs on that side. In children, this difference is less pronounced, and thus the right-sided prevalence of foreign bodies is less obvious. Further, the bronchus to the right upper lobe arises a mere 2 cm below the bifurcation, whereas the left upper lobe bronchus originates about 5 cm below the bifurcation. As a result, inflation of the cuff on an ordinary or double-lumen tracheal tube

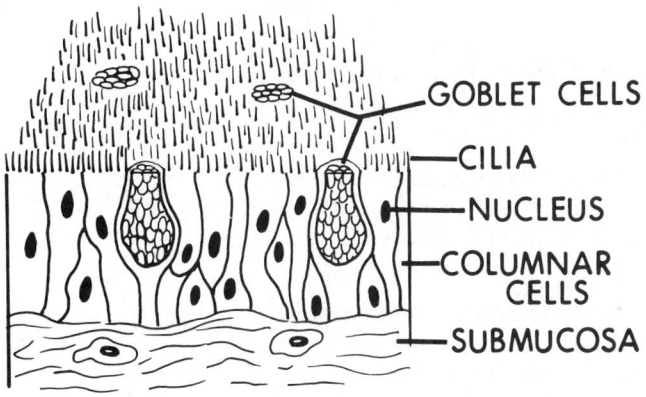

FIGURE 26–5. Mucosal lining of the trachea.

may easily occlude the right upper lobe bronchus. In any case, the operator should listen with a stethoscope over the lobes of both lungs to be sure of proper tube positioning as well as to detect esophageal intubation.

Bronchial Suctioning

Because of the difference in the angles of the right and left mainstem bronchi, Kubota and colleagues[10] found that catheters for suctioning of secretions or treatment of atelectasis entered the right bronchus in about 85% of insertions and the left bronchus in about 11% and coiled up in the upper airway in the remaining 4%.

In order to circumvent this haphazard approach to selective bronchial suctioning, Kubota's group developed a curved-tip catheter with a guide mark at the proximal end to indicate the direction of the curve on its rotation (Fig. 26–6). With this method, they had a success rate ranging from 89% to 97% for left bronchial catheterization. Later, and with equal success, they used a J-shaped catheter tip to aspirate the upper lobe bronchi on either side.

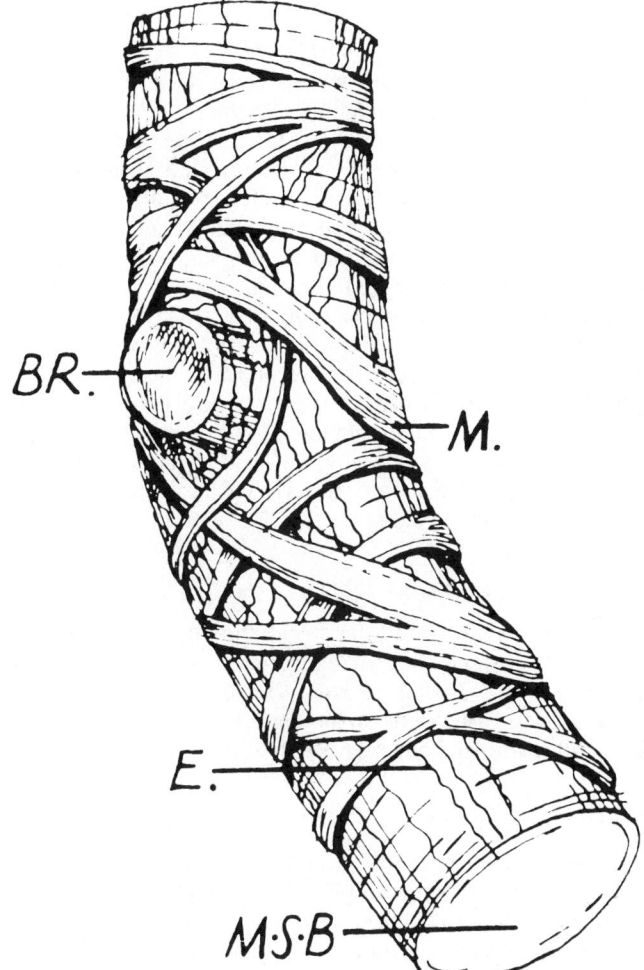

FIGURE 26–4. Smooth muscle (M) and elastic fibers (E) of the trachea at a place where a branch (BR) departs from the mainstem bronchus (MSB) of the lung. By contracting and relaxing, the smooth muscle (Reisseisen) with its spiral arrangement can cause marked changes in both length and caliber of the trachea and bronchi. (From Vandam LD: The functional anatomy of the lung. Anesthesiology 1952; 13:130.)

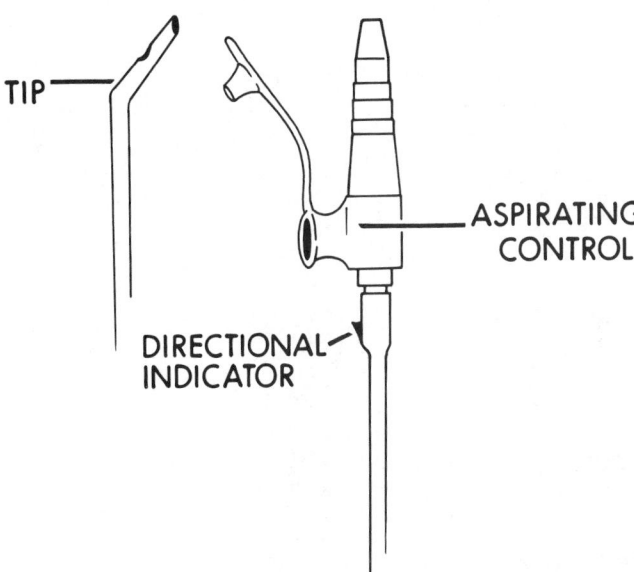

FIGURE 26–6. Curved-tip suctioning catheter with directional indicator.

THE LARYNX

What Are Its Functions?

Phonation

To paraphrase Negus,[2] an eminent British laryngologist who studied the comparative anatomy of the larynx by dissecting the larynges of hundreds of species stored in the museum of the Royal College of Surgeons:

"Much has been written about the larynx, its anatomical structure, its physiology and the diseases which affect it. And yet, this small organ performs its work enshrouded in mystery. It is generally known as the organ of voice, and yet it takes but a moment's reflection to observe that thousands of species which have a larynx never (or practically never) make use of voice. In the human, voice is a poor thing—the individual speaks in a monotone—the range is limited—few are able to execute elaborate songs. Those who can sing through a wide range are hard to find."

Control of Entry to the Respiratory Tract

According to Negus's monograph,[2] elements of a larynx first began to appear in those species that emerged from the sea to take up an amphibious existence (Fig. 26–7). When the lung buds developed as an outpouching of the foregut, a sphincter mechanism was required to prevent inundation of the lungs on re-entry to the aqueous milieu. As a consequence, it is worth noting that the pharmacologic reactions of tracheal smooth muscle present in mammals are the same as those of the intestinal tract, based presumably on their similar autonomic innervation.

A primitive sphincter is present at the aditus to the lungs in the lungfish (Kamongo of East Africa), then elaborated in the evolutionary ascent through the amphibians, avians, and mammals. Thus, from the human standpoint, even though voice seems to be the dominant function, the larynx must be viewed as a valvular mechanism controlling entrance to the respiratory tract.

Valves of any kind, whether physiologic (as in living crea-

tures) or elements of machinery (anesthetic apparatus), consist of a housing within which the moving parts perform their function. In that context, the human larynx is described here.

What Are the Laryngeal Cartilages?

Because of their subcutaneous location in the anterior triangles of the neck, most of the structures of the larynx are easily palpable and serve as topographic landmarks for performance of such maneuvers as tracheal intubation, regional anesthesia, and resuscitation as in cricothyroidotomy or tracheostomy. In preparation for tracheal intubation, these structures should always be examined beforehand.

The Thyroid Cartilage

There are nine cartilages in the larynx (Fig. 26–8), of which the largest and most evident is the hyaline thyroid cartilage, so called because it is shaped like a shield. The broad laminae of this cartilage meet anteriorly at an acute angle to form a prominence (Adam's apple) in men that is less acute in women. Masculinizing tumors in women cause male-type morphologic changes, as well as deepening of the voice.

Attachments

The broad plates of the cartilage serve as attachments for the sternothyroid, sternohyoid, cricothyroid, and strap muscles in the neck (Fig. 26–9), which act to tether the larynx during such functions as swallowing, sneezing, vomiting, and coughing. Innervation of these muscles comes from the ansa hypoglossi, with elements contributed by the hypoglossal nerves and branches of the cervical plexus, thus suggesting the interactive complexity of laryngeal function.

Superiorly, the thyroid cartilage is attached to the hyoid bone via the thyrohyoid membrane. The muscles of the tongue are attached to the hyoid and secondarily therefore to the mandible and other structures of the neck. The intubationist should understand that intubation of the larynx, no matter which laryngoscopic blade is used, involves both suspension and elevation of the larynx because the beak of a blade is always beneath the hyoid bone.

The Cricoid Cartilage

A second large hyaline laryngeal cartilage is the cricoid, shaped like a signet ring, with the signet facing posteriorly (see Fig. 26–8). This is the only complete cartilage of the airway, a narrowing point or bottleneck, thus accounting for the fact that foreign bodies usually lodge at this junction.

Attachments

As part of the larynx, the cricoid is attached to the thyroid cartilage by the cricothyroid membrane, which is immediately subcutaneous, easily palpated, and readily incised in the midline for large needle insertion or incision during resuscitation.

Invagination of the membrane contributes to formation of the true and false vocal cords internally. Further, the cricoid lies at the level of the sixth cervical vertebra, serving as a landmark when stellate ganglion nerve block is performed and the injecting needle strikes the prominent Chassaignac's tubercle of the sixth vertebra.

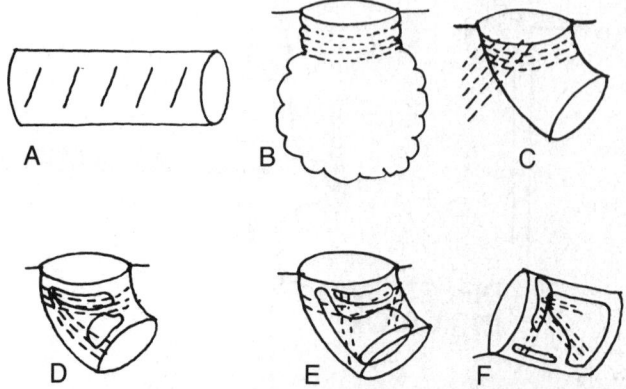

FIGURE 26–7. Evolution of the larynx. *A,* Pharynx of fish with gill slits. *B,* Pulmonary outgrowth from the floor of the pharynx with sphincter mechanism. *C,* In the mudfish, the trachea turns toward the thorax; constrictor and dilator fibers are seen. *D,* The newt shows early cartilaginous formation. *E and F,* Cartilaginous formation is further elaborated in the bird and mammal. (From Negus VE: The Comparative Anatomy and Physiology of the Larynx. New York, Grune & Stratton, 1949.)

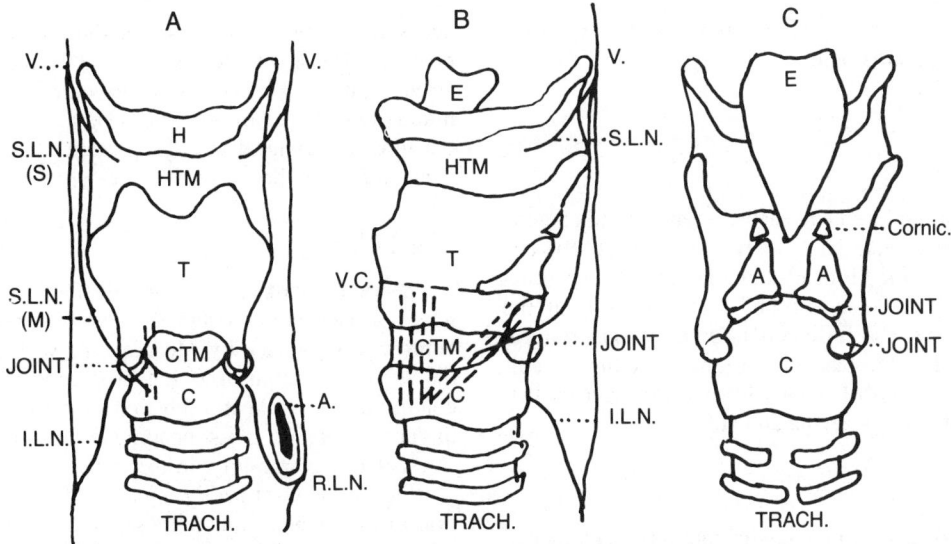

FIGURE 26–8. The cartilage of the larynx and the nerve supply in anterior *(A)*, lateral *(B)*, and posterior *(C)* views. The thyroid (T), cricoid (C), and arytenoid (A) cartilages are the essential elements. Epiglottis (E), corniculate cartilages (Cornic.), and cuneiform cartilages (not shown) are of little functional importance. Note the presence of synovial membrane–lined joints between arytenoid and cricoid cartilages, and between cricoid and thyroid cartilages. These joints permit movement owing to action of the intrinsic muscles in the former case and to contraction of the cricothyroid muscle (shown as *dotted lines*) in the latter . The hyoid bone (H), the hyothyroid membrane (HTM), and the cricothyroid membrane (CTM) are important landmarks both for regional anesthesia and for resuscitation. The vagus (V) departs from the superior laryngeal nerve (SLN) and provides sensory function (S) to the upper portion of the larynx and motor function (M) to the only intrinsic muscle, the cricothyroid muscle. Contraction of the latter rotates the cricoid cartilage and tenses the vocal cords. The inferior laryngeal nerves (ILNs) are also mixed nerves, providing sensory function to the lower larynx and motor function to all of the intrinsic muscles. (From Vandam LD: Functional anatomy of the larynx. Weekly Anesth Update 1977; 1:2.)

The cricoid cartilage also articulates with the thyroid cartilage bilaterally by way of diarthrodial joints, permitting a rocking motion of the former in an anterior-posterior direction under the action of the external cricothyroid muscles. As noted later, this motion serves to tense the vocal cords.

The Arytenoid Cartilages

The remaining cartilages of functional significance are the paired arytenoids (ladle shaped), which sit atop the signet portion of the cricoid posteriorly.

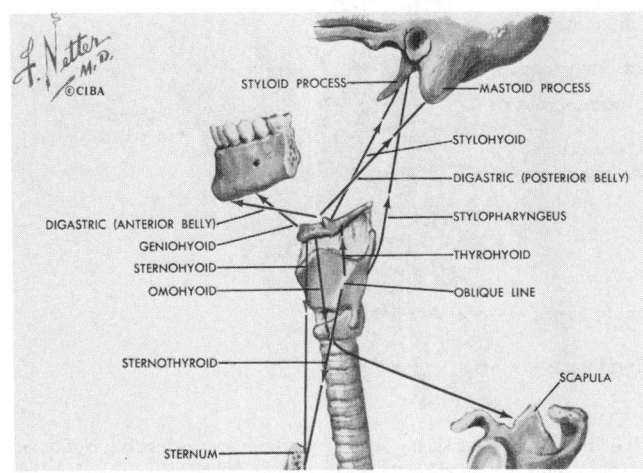

FIGURE 26–9. The extrinsic muscles of the larynx and their action. Notice the direction of action of these muscles, their attachment to the hyoid bone, the sternum, the mandible, the mastoid and styloid processes of the temporal bone, the scapula, and the thyroid cartilage. During a variety of physiologic functions (e.g., voice production, swallowing, coughing, sneezing, use of the shoulder girdle), these muscles act jointly to tether the larynx. (From Saunders WH: The larynx. Clinical Symposia (CIBA) 1964; 16:75.)

Attachments

All of the intrinsic muscles of the larynx, both abductor and adductor, are attached to the arytenoid cartilages. Motion of these cartilages is again facilitated by the presence of synovially lined diarthrodial joints located between the cricoid and arytenoids. Thus, the arytenoids can move anteriorly, posteriorly, or laterally according to actions of the intrinsic muscles.

Rheumatoid Arthritis

These cricoarytenoid joints, as well as the cricothyroid joints, may be affected by rheumatoid arthritis along with others in the body. Consequently, the glottis may be narrowed while movements of the vocal cords, both true and false, are limited. In severely arthritic patients, this affliction is often revealed by a high-pitched weak voice accompanied by a fixed lordotic cervical spine and ankylosis of the temporomandibular joints. Tracheal intubation becomes difficult, and for these reasons, a tracheal tube of smaller diameter than usual should be selected, particularly in nasotracheal intubation, which may be the approach of choice in the presence of an arthritic spine.

Airway Obstruction

Although the cricoid cartilage in adults is cylindrically shaped, that of infants is in the form of an inverted cone, narrow at its apex.[11] Even moderate degrees of mucosal inflammation at that level may cause croup (often in association with epiglottitis) and respiratory difficulty, calling for early tracheal intubation and use of both antibiotics and adrenocortical steroids to diminish the swelling.

A second related phenomenon in infants is the development of subglottic edema and obstruction following extubation of the trachea when a large-diameter tube had been in place. On laryngoscopy, one can clearly see the glottis and vocal cords with the obstructing edema below.

The Epiglottis

Attachments

The remainder of the laryngeal cartilages are of little significance and are mostly vestigial elements (see Fig. 26–8). The largest of this group is the fibrocartilaginous epiglottis (petiolepetal), the stem of which is attached to the interior of the thyroid cartilage above the false cords. On the oropharyngeal side, it is connected to the base of the tongue by the hyoepiglottic ligament, vestigial of a muscle in lower species that apposed the epiglottis to the uvula and soft palate.

Function

In running animals and in infants, the epiglottis is elongated so that its approximation to the palate effectively separates the nasopharyngeal and oropharyngeal cavities. This arrangement permits a running predatory animal with its long snout to maintain a streamlined airway to the glottis and trachea while retaining access of air to the olfactory plate for scenting prey.

Occasionally, in humans, inflammation can result in epiglottitis and edema,[12] which may obstruct the airway. Contrary to popular opinion, the epiglottis does not serve as a cover on a box to close the glottis. Rather, during swallowing and in other functions in which the airway must close, the larynx is apposed to the base of the tongue by action of the extralaryngeal muscles noted previously.[13]

From the standpoint of topical anesthesia, the oral surface of the epiglottis receives its innervation from the glossopharyngeal nerve, and the laryngeal surface from the sensory division of the superior laryngeal branch of the vagus.

The Corniculate and Cuneiform Cartilages

The paired corniculates (horn shaped) and the cuneiforms (wedge shaped) are mainly of evolutionary interest (see Fig. 26–8). The corniculates can be seen as translucent structures during laryngoscopy or can be palpated in anatomic specimens as horn-shaped objects at the tips of the arytenoids, where they once functioned as attachments or davits for the cricopharyngeal sphincter muscles.

Functions

In lower species and in the developmental stages of humans, the wedge-shaped cuneiform cartilages are present in the aryepiglottic folds, perhaps adding to their stiffness (as in a starched collar) and width and possibly protecting the glottis against aspiration of liquids and foreign bodies.

Because human fetuses and infants recapitulate phylogeny, these paired cartilages and the aryepiglottic folds, as well as the epiglottis, are quite prominent to be reckoned with during laryngoscopy, and they are of some physiologic significance.[11]

Why Is Nerve Block of the Larynx Performed?

Before proceeding to discuss the actions of the intrinsic muscles of the larynx, a description of their innervation is

necessary. Topical anesthesia of the airway is easily accomplished because of the submucosal location of the sensory nerve endings. The larynx, in its entirety, both sensory and motor, is supplied by the vagus nerve, although elements of the glossopharyngeal may be present via the 10th nerve nucleus in the hindbrain (see Fig. 26–8).

Vagal Block

The vagi enter and exit from the skull in company with the glossopharyngeal and spinal accessory nerves and jugular veins. As introduced by Mushin,[14] nerve block of the vagi at the jugular foramina (no longer practiced) provided superb conditions for tracheal intubation in awake patients, although the accompanying glossopharyngeal and spinal accessory paralysis led to respiratory obstruction.

When vocal cord paralysis is found in any patient, in addition to the more common causes, the anesthesiologist should consider the possible presence of a brainstem lesion and search for accompanying paralysis of the glossopharyngeal and spinal accessory nerves.

Superior Laryngeal Nerves

One branch of the vagus, the mixed motor and sensory superior laryngeal nerve, leaves the parent nerve at the site of the nodose ganglion at the skull base. (A ganglion always implies the presence of sensory neuronal bodies.) An internal

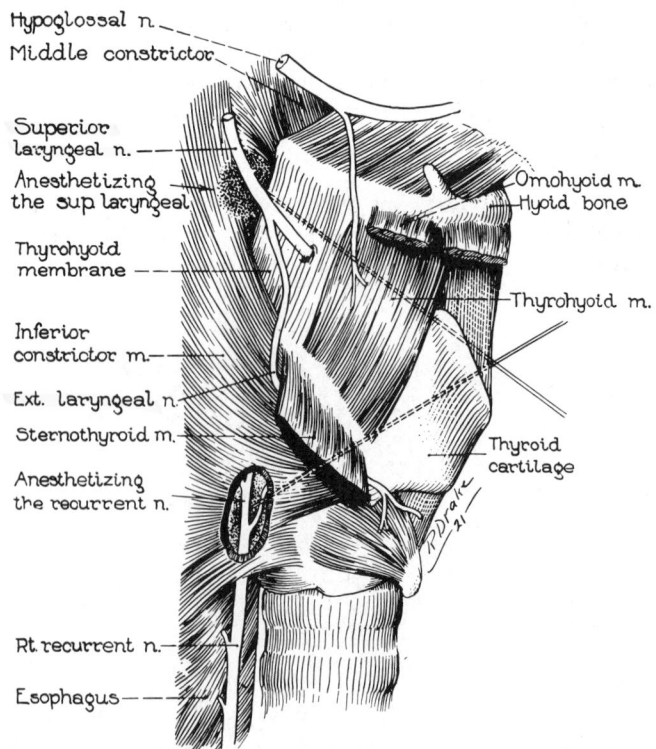

FIGURE 26–10. Nerve supply to the larynx from the vagus nerve. Notice the internal branch (sensory) of the superior laryngeal nerve as it pierces the thyrohyoid membrane and the external branch (motor) (external laryngeal nerve), which supplies the cricothyroid muscle. Also shown below is the recurrent branch of the vagus as it ascends toward the larynx. *Dotted lines* show the needle pathway for injection of the superior and inferior laryngeal nerves via the thyroid notch. (From Labat G: Regional Anesthesia: Its Technical and Clinical Application. 2nd ed. Philadelphia, WB Saunders, 1928, p 143.)

branch pierces the hyothyroid membrane to provide sensation to the larynx and part of the pharynx (glossopharyngeal plexus) above the level of the vocal cords (Figs. 26–10 and 26–11).

Motor Activity

The motor branch of the superior laryngeal supplies the only extrinsic muscle of the larynx, the cricothyroid (see Figs. 26–8, 26–10, and 26–11). Because of both vertical and diagonal fiber direction and because of the cricothyroid joint, contraction of the cricothyroid muscles causes a rocking motion of the cricoid in the sagittal plane, thus tensing the vocal cords as noted earlier. This action occurs because the arytenoids move with the cricoid, and the internal thyroarytenoid muscle or musculus vocalis is thereby stretched.

Effects of Nerve Block

Nerve block of the superior laryngeal nerve at its entry to the hyothyroid membrane, along with performance of pharyngeal and transtracheal topical anesthesia, provides excellent conditions for tracheal intubation in awake patients. Sensory anesthesia of the larynx and trachea results, and the vocal cords are relaxed. Superior laryngeal nerve block is also helpful for treatment of laryngeal pain, as might be present in tuberculous ulceration or infiltrating carcinoma.

Technique

The nerve is anesthetized by fanning the needle after insertion anterior to a finger tip placed between the cornu of the hyoid bone and superior cornu of the thyroid cartilage. Paresthesias are referred to the external auditory canal, which receives some of its sensory innervation from the vagus nerve.

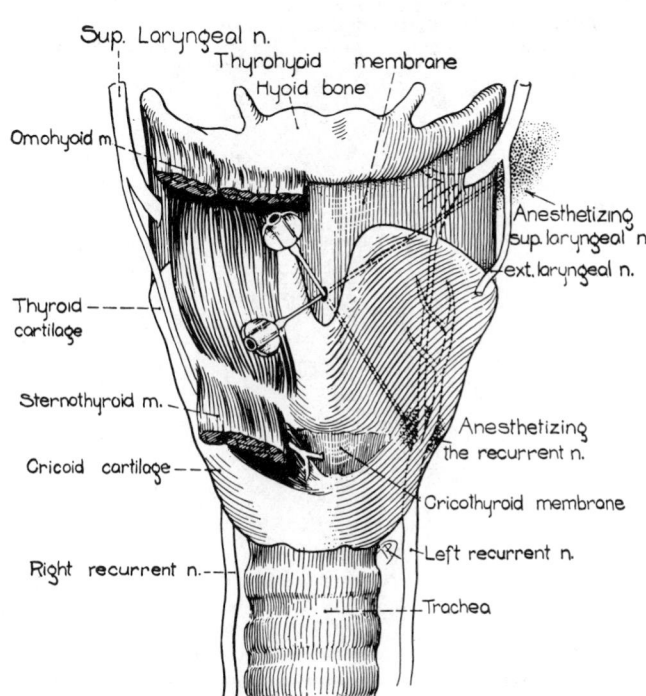

FIGURE 26–11. Approach to local anesthetic injection of the superior laryngeal nerve. (From Labat G: Regional Anesthesia: Its Technical and Clinical Application. 2nd ed. Philadelphia, WB Saunders, 1928, p 143.)

Alternatively, as described by Labat,[15] superior laryngeal nerve block may be accomplished by inserting the needle at the thyroid notch and directing it upward and backward toward the thyrohyoid membrane (see Fig. 26–11).

Inferior Laryngeal Nerves

The inferior laryngeal or recurrent nerves pass toward the larynx from below, upward to provide sensation to the trachea below the level of the vocal cords (see Figs. 26–10 and 26–11). Furthermore, all of the intrinsic muscles of the larynx are supplied by the inferior laryngeal nerve.

Anatomic Relationships

On the left, the inferior laryngeal nerve is truly recurrent as it encircles the arch of the aorta close to the ligamentum arteriosum (the obliterated ductus arteriosus). Thus, the left or recurrent nerve is more subject to injury, not only during thyroidectomy but also during ligation of a patent ductus arteriosus, because of pressure from an expanding aortic aneurysm and rarely because of atrial enlargement in mitral stenosis.

Technique

The inferior nerve can be anesthetized close to the inferior cornu of the thyroid. Anesthetization of the superior and inferior nerves along with superficial cervical plexus block permits performance of laryngectomy purely under regional anesthesia.

What Should Be Known About Laryngeal Blood Supply?

The blood supply to the larynx derives from the inferior laryngeal branch of the thyrocervical trunk of the first portion of the subclavian artery and the superior laryngeal artery (the first branch of the external carotid). Because the inferior laryngeal artery lies close to the recurrent laryngeal nerve, injury to the nerve may occur in attempts to control bleeding during thyroidectomy, the most common cause of vocal cord paralysis.

Because the nerves may already have divided into their branches at that point, vocal cord paralysis may be partial or complete, depending on the number of branches injured and, incidentally, accounting for the variable positions of the cords found in paralysis.

What Are the Intrinsic Muscle Activities?

As noted, all of the muscles of the larynx are supplied by the recurrent laryngeal nerves, and they may be grouped according to dilator (abductor) or constrictor (adductor) action. The muscles extend between the muscular processes of the arytenoid cartilages at the one end to the cricoid or thyroid cartilage at the other. In evolutionary development, the constrictors dominate, for only one set of dilators is present. Figures 26–12 and 26–13 give a view of the glottis as seen on laryngoscopy. One can envision how the muscles act during adduction or abduction of either the true or false vocal cords (ventricular bands).

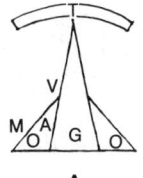 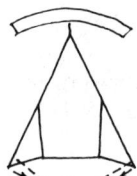 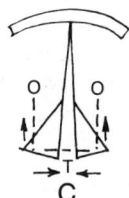 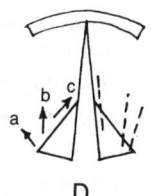

FIGURE 26–12. The glottis (G) and movement (M) of the arytenoid (A) cartilages. *A,* The vocal cords (V) are shown attached to the thyroid cartilage anteriorly and to the vocal process of the arytenoid cartilages posteriorly. Note that the posterior third of the glottis is bounded by the arytenoid cartilages, which are covered with squamous epithelium. *B,* The action of the posterior cricoarytenoid muscles is shown, attached to the posterior face of the arytenoid cartilages, thus opening the glottis. *C,* The glottis is nearly closed owing to the action of the transverse interarytenoid (T) and oblique interarytenoid (O) muscles. *D,* The remainder of the adductors are shown, indicating action of the lateral cricoarytenoid muscles (a), action of the external thyroarytenoid muscles (b), and action of the internal thyroarytenoid or vocalis muscles (c). (From Vandam LD: Functional anatomy of the larynx. Weekly Anesth Update 1977; 1:95.)

Laryngeal Dilators

The posterior, paired cricoarytenoid muscles connect the posterior aspect of the vocal processes of the arytenoids to the broad posterior plate of the cricothyroid cartilage, thus rotating the arytenoids laterally to abduct the cords. These are the only dilator muscles. Consequently, when the cords are found in adduction after nerve injury, paralysis is usually said to be the cause (see Figs. 26–12 and 26–13).

Laryngeal Constrictors

Several muscles form a complete sphincter for the larynx (see Figs. 26–12 and 26–13).

Interarytenoids

The interarytenoids, transverse and oblique in direction, bring the arytenoids together. The transverse elements ascend in the aryepiglottic folds as the aryepiglottic muscles.

Lateral Cricoarytenoids

The paired lateral cricoarytenoids extend from the anterior surface of the muscular processes of the arytenoids to the interior of the cricoid ring, thus rotating the cartilages inward.

Internal Thyroarytenoids

The paired internal thyroarytenoid or vocal muscles extend from the vocal processes of the arytenoids to the inner surface of the thyroid cartilage. As vocal muscles, they both close the glottis and tense the cords (as do the extrinsic cricothyroid muscles).

The vocal cords are covered by stratified squamous epithelium, the source of epidermoid carcinoma. Vocal cord polyps are more likely to develop at the posterior third of the glottis, where a tracheal tube rests against the underlying vocal processes of the arytenoids.

Movement of the larynx in light planes of anesthesia (swallowing, cough) may abrade the epithelium. During healing of the ulceration, fibrous organization results in polyp formation with continued cord movement. Postintubation polyp formation, not a rare complication, is suggested by chronic hoarseness. An unusual complication of prolonged intubation, in addition to tracheal erosion and stenosis, is arytenoid cartilage dislocation.

External Thyroarytenoids

The paired external thyroarytenoid muscles extend from the vocal processes of the arytenoids to a higher level of the interior of the thyroid cartilage, thus forming the ventricular bands (see Figs. 26–12 and 26–13). An evagination of the larynx between the true and false cords forms the laryngeal ventricles and Morgagni's vestigial saccules.

Why Is Intubation Sometimes Difficult?

Anesthetists should realize that the larynx is of considerable depth, extending from the level of the third cervical to the sixth cervical vertebra (Fig. 26–14). In difficult intubations, the problem is not so much that the larynx is "too anterior," as often stated, for it is always anterior in the neck, but that it is relatively high in a short, thick-necked individual. Visualization of the glottis is difficult because of the correspondingly more acute angle between oropharynx and pharynx; hence the need for a tracheal tube stylet, curved blade, or fiberoptic laryngoscope becomes obvious.

What Are the Sphincter Functions of the Larynx?

In addition to its function in vocalization, the larynx also serves as a true valve of the respiratory tract.

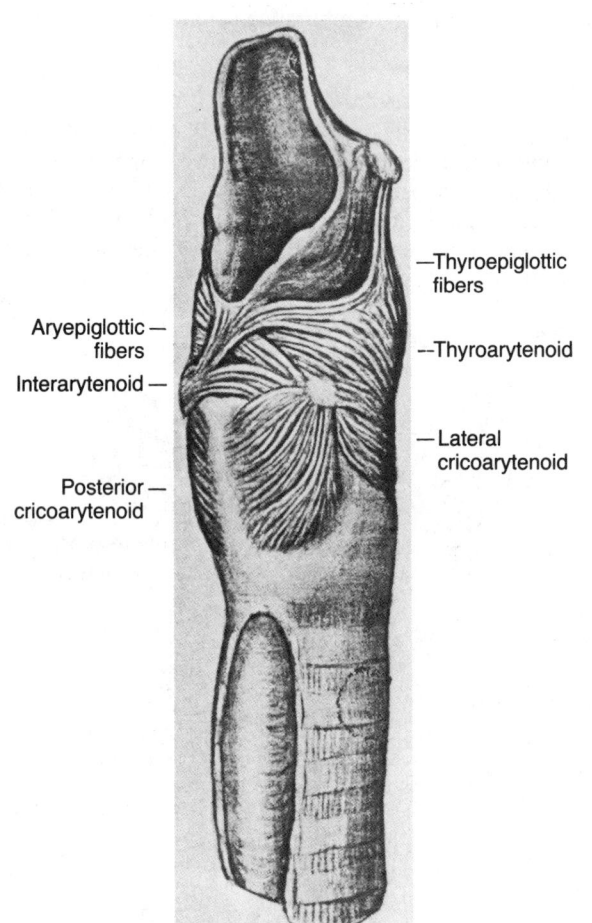

FIGURE 26–13. The dilator muscles of the larynx (posterior cricoarytenoid) and the components of the sphincteric group. Note how the latter form a complete sphincter from the larynx. Note also the height of the larynx from the cricoid cartilage below to the tip of the epiglottis. (From Negus VE: The Comparative Anatomy and Physiology of the Larynx. New York, Grune & Stratton, 1949.)

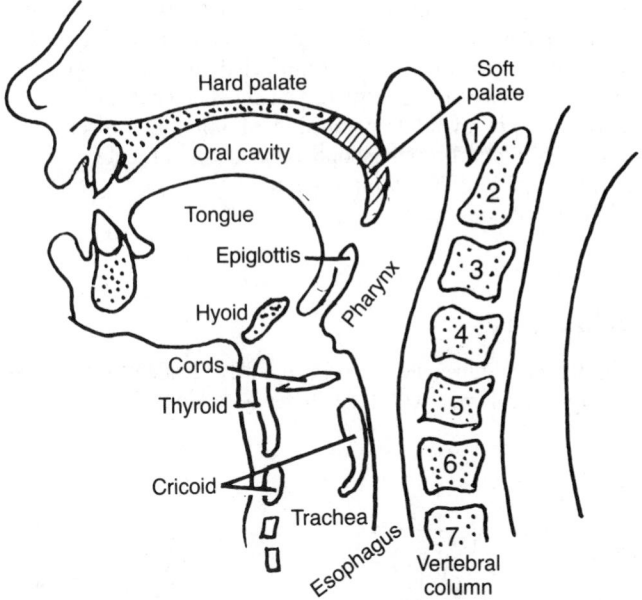

FIGURE 26–14. Sagittal section through the upper airway. Note that the larynx, from the tip of the epiglottis to the cricoid cartilage below, corresponds to a span of four cervical vertebrae (C-3 through C-6). If an intubation is difficult to perform, it is not because the larynx lies anteriorly (it always does) but because it is relatively high on the cervical column in the short-necked person. The angle between oral cavity and pharynx is acute and it is not easily negotiated on intubation. (From Vandam LD: Functional anatomy of the larynx. Weekly Anesth Update 1977; 1:95.)

Increase of Intrathoracic Pressure

In order to increase intrathoracic pressure with Valsalva's maneuver and during coughing or sneezing, the larynx must close before thoracic pressure can be raised.

Increase of Intra-abdominal Pressure

Similarly, to increase intra-abdominal pressure, the diaphragm must be stabilized by laryngeal closure before the abdominal muscles can contract effectively during urination, defecation, or bearing down in labor (Fig. 26–15). Further, when the upper extremities are used for lifting or for chinning on a bar, the shoulder girdle muscles attached to the chest can only function effectively with a stable thorax as provided by laryngeal closure.

Improved Efficiency of Alveolar Ventilation

Finally, the larynx serves to improve the efficiency of alveolar ventilation, because both the glottis and tracheobronchial tree dilate during inspiration to permit laminar airflow, and constrict during exhalation, with reflux of dead space air into the alveoli.[16]

Because of the sphincter actions of the larynx, patients with a tracheostomy cannot cough effectively and cannot expel secretions efficiently. Although anatomic dead space is decreased after tracheostomy, alveolar ventilation is not as efficient: Respiratory rate increases, and a minor degree of respiratory alkalosis develops.

Reflex Airway Closure

Laryngospasm and bronchospasm are manifestations of the reflex defensive system of the lungs.

Laryngospasm

Muscle spasm in response to mechanical or chemical stimuli intrinsically or painful stimuli extrinsically involves all of the intrinsic muscles of the larynx, as well as the smooth muscles of the tracheobronchial tree and the extrinsic muscles of the larynx and chest wall. The resulting complete closure of the airway is stubbornly resistive to positive airway pressure and does not respond to atropine injection for obvious reasons. However, because the muscles of the larynx are of the special visceral kind, thus permitting both voluntary and involuntary action, they are readily subject to temporary paralysis by neuromuscular blocking agents.

Standard treatment consists of elimination of the offending stimulus, manual forward and upward thrust of the jaw, intravenous administration of succinylcholine, and oxygen given by positive-pressure ventilation.

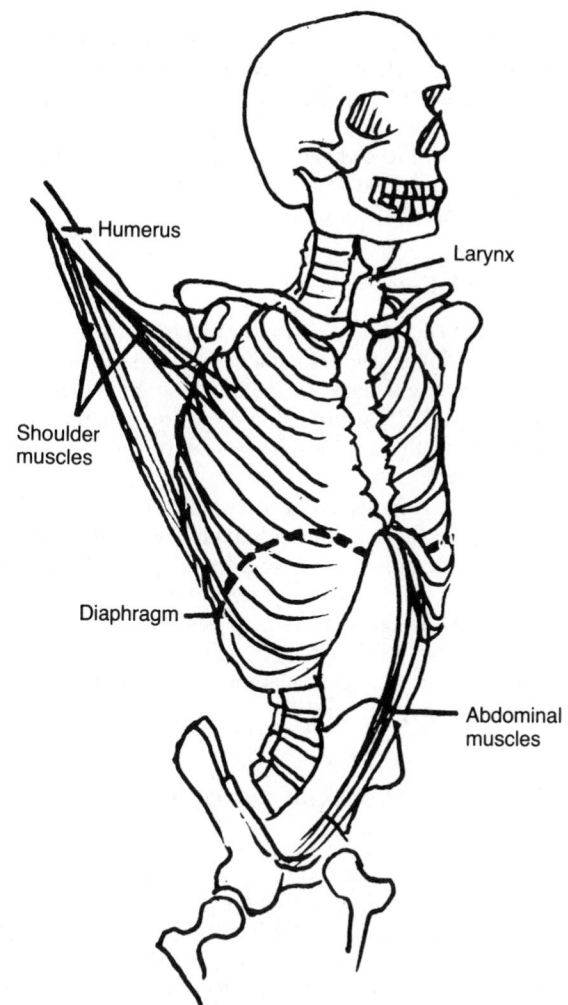

FIGURE 26–15. Sphincter mechanism of the larynx. Closure of the larynx stabilizes the volume of air within the thorax and fixes the diaphragm *(dotted line)*. This permits the abdominal muscles to contract effectively and increase intra-abdominal pressure for such purposes as urination, defecation, and bearing down during labor. Similarly, closure of the laryngeal sphincter allows the development of positive pressure within the thorax for the purpose of coughing or sneezing. Lastly, in order to use the shoulder girdle muscles effectively, the muscles must act from a fixed thorax, with the diaphragm stabilized. In all of these situations, the Valsalva maneuver is employed. (From Vandam LD: Functional anatomy of the larynx. Weekly Anesth Update 1977; 1:95.)

Bronchospasm

Bronchospasm is a complex phenomenon caused by one or more of the following: parasympathetic activity, allergens and drugs, histamine, prostaglandins, and slow-reacting substance of anaphylaxis. Narrowing of the airway is also affected by body temperature, extrinsic bronchial pressure, congestive heart failure, pulmonary edema, and pulmonary embolism.

Standard therapy consists of elimination of the stimulus and one or several of the following: positive airway pressure with oxygen, use of β-sympathetic agonists, anticholinergic therapy, administration of hydrocortisone, occasionally also intravenous aminophylline, and elimination of any chest wall spasm with a neuromuscular blocker.

TRACHEAL INTUBATION

What Are the Advantages?

Patency of the airway is reasonably assured. Secretions can be removed from the tracheobronchial tree with relative ease. Positive pressure can be applied to the airway without distention of the stomach; a patient can be placed in any position during surgery, with less chance of compromising the airway; and the anesthetist can be seated at a distance from the patient while still maintaining control of respiration.

Assisted Ventilation

Intubation is necessary to assist ventilation in patients with ventilatory insufficiency and to protect the lungs when reflexes of the larynx are inadequate. Tracheal intubation is mandatory in patients at high risk for aspiration of gastric contents and in operations such as thoracotomy when positive-pressure ventilation is necessary.

Intubation is also indicated in the prone, sitting, lateral, or Trendelenburg's positions, in which maintenance of an airway by mask and application of positive-pressure ventilation would be unreliable, and it is necessary in operations on patients who already have a compromised airway.[17] Appropriate equipment is shown in Figure 26–16. Some, such as the hemostat, Y-adaptor, and universal metal adaptors, are seldom required with modern circuitry and tubes.

What Equipment Should Be Available?

Laryngoscopes

A laryngoscope is used to expose the glottis. The instrument is made of metal and consists of a handle, a blade, and a light source. The handle contains batteries to provide current for a light bulb that is fitted into the tip of the blade, the latter with a hook-on attachment to the handle. The C-shaped blade, in cross section, displaces the tongue to the left away from the path of vision, which is kept open to the right for passage of a tracheal tube (Fig. 26–17).

Blades

Laryngoscope blades are of two principal kinds, curved and straight, varying in size for use in infants, children, or adults

(see Fig. 26–16). Many varieties of both the curved and straight blades have been designed to facilitate passage of a tracheal tube. However, an accomplished anesthesiologist can manage with two or three blades at most. Disposable blades are available to avoid transmission of infectious disease. A flexible fiberoptic bronchoscope is used for intubation under difficult conditions (for a more detailed discussion, see Chapter 17).

Tracheal Tubes

Most tracheal tubes are disposable and are made of clear, pliable, polyvinylchloride, with little tendency to kink. They are steri-

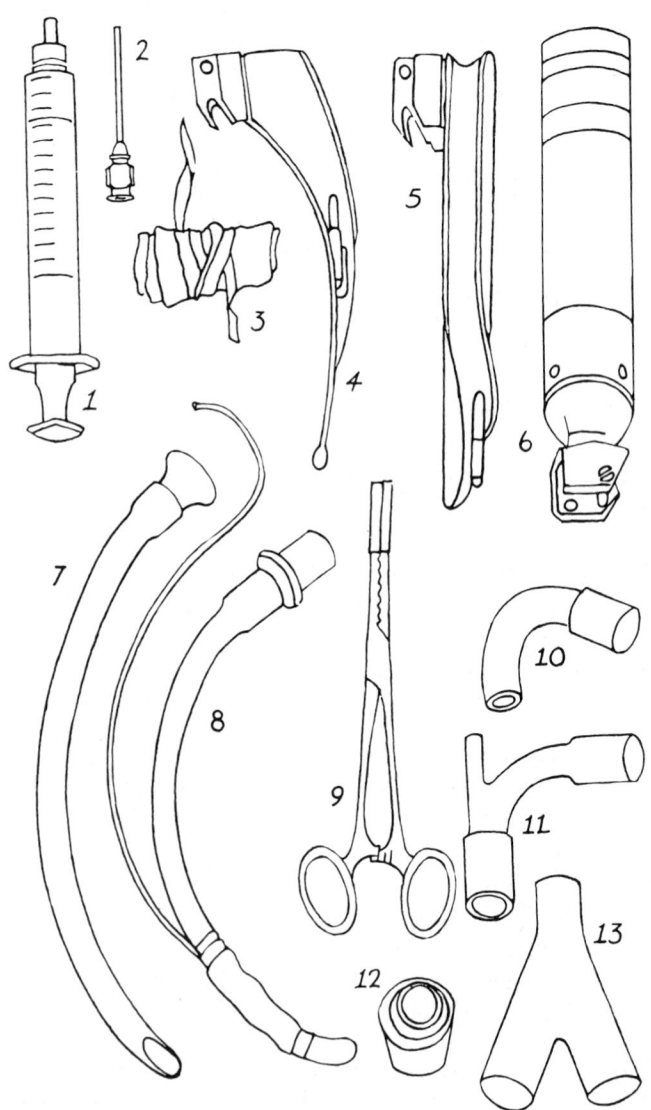

FIGURE 26–16. Endotracheal equipment. 1 = Syringe and 2 = blunt-tipped needle to inflate cuff on endotracheal tube; 3 = bite block; 4 = curved laryngoscope blade; 5 = straight laryngoscope blade; 6 = laryngoscope handle and battery holder; 7 = nasotracheal tube with funnel; 8 = cuffed endotracheal tube with straight slip joint; 9 = hemostat to maintain cuff inflation; 10 = curved endotracheal tube connector; 11 = curved endotracheal tube connector with suction tube nipple; 12 = universal metal adapter; 13 = catheter Y-adapter. (From Dripps RD, Eckenhoff JE, Vandam LD: Introduction to Anesthesia: The Principles of Safe Practice. 1st ed. Philadelphia, WB Saunders, 1957.)

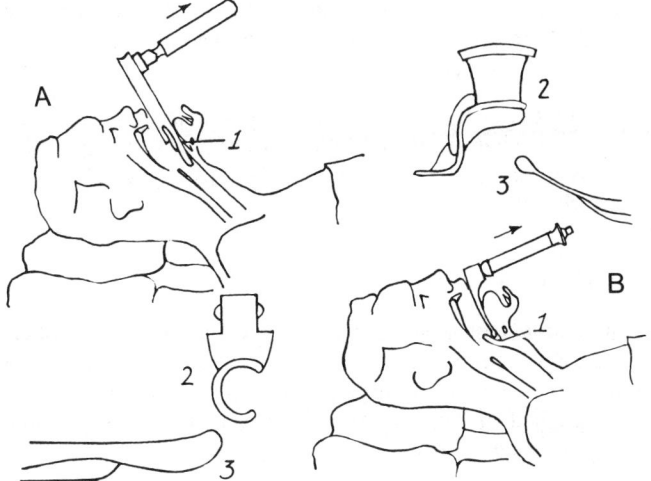

FIGURE 26–17. Upward lift of laryngoscopy at 45° angle to expose the glottis. *A*, Straight blade beneath the (1) epiglottis. 2 = End view of the straight blade with semicircular construction to keep tongue to the left; 3 = tip of the straight blade to lift the hyoid bone when placed beneath the epiglottis. *B*, Curved blade proximal to (1) the epiglottis. 2 = End view of curved blade with right-angle construction to keep the tongue to the left; the flange lifts the tongue. (From Dripps RD, Eckenhoff JE, Vandam LD: Introduction to anesthesia: The Principles of Safe Practice. 1st ed. Philadelphia, WB Saunders, 1957.)

lized by the manufacturer with ethylene oxide and thoroughly vented before use. At body temperature, the tubes mold to the contour of the upper airway and present a smooth interior for easy passage of suction catheters or a flexible bronchoscope.

Construction

Tracheal tubes are of measured length, marked in 0.5-cm increments according to diameter, with inflatable cuffs optional above 5 mm, and with a Magill's or Murphy's tip. The latter has an opening opposite the bevel. They are usually longer than necessary when received from the manufacturer and benefit from shortening to lessen the possibility of bronchial intubation or to prevent kinking at the nose or mouth. After the proximal end of the tube is cut, the connector should be reinserted firmly.

Cuffs

Built-in cuffs are used in adults and older children; when inflated, the cuff ensures a closed system, permitting easy control of ventilation and minimizing the possibility of aspiration of vomitus or blood.

Cuffs may be of the high- or low-pressure volume variety, depending on the volume of air required for their inflation. When inflated, a high-pressure cuff has a short length; thus, a small surface is in contact with the tracheal wall and a high internal cuff pressure is required to seal the trachea. Low-pressure cuffs offer both a larger volume and diameter plus a broad contact with the tracheal wall.

If a cuff is overinflated, regardless of whether it is a high-pressure–low-volume or low-volume–high-pressure cuff, pressure on the tracheal wall may cause mucosal ischemia; therefore, the cuff is inflated with only enough air to obtain a seal. Esophageal temperature probes and nasogastric tubes may readily pass into the tracheal beside a low-pressure cuff.

Cuffed tracheal tubes usually incorporate a pilot balloon with a self-sealing valve at the inflation site. Moreover, the cuffs are permeable to nitrous oxide and over time increase in volume and pressure; thus, during a prolonged anesthetic, the volume should be readjusted to prevent excessive pressure.

Special Purpose Tracheal Tubes

1. Armored or anode tubes are reinforced with coiled wire to prevent occlusion as a result of external pressure or kinking. Noncollapsible tubes are useful in patients with a tracheostomy and in operations performed with a patient in the sitting or face-down position when the head is sharply flexed. Magill's forceps or a stylet is needed for insertion.

2. Preformed tubes have molded angles placed at the point of emergence from mouth or nose; the molded curve minimizes kinking and obstruction.

3. Pediatric tubes are small, <5.0 mm in diameter, and generally without a cuff.

4. Laser-shield tubes (various types) have been made of silicone impregnated with metal particles covering the main shaft and cuff to withstand laser-induced heat and ignition. Nitrous oxide should not be used during anesthesia, and the cuff should be inflated with sterile saline.

5. Double-lumen tubes are used for selective ventilation or airway protection.

Additional discussion is found in Chapter 17.

Accessory Intubating Instruments

Stylets

A stylet made of malleable metal or plastic is inserted in a tracheal tube to improve the curvature and add stiffness to it. The stylet is lubricated to aid in its withdrawal and should not protrude beyond the tip.

Intubating Forceps

Magill's intubating forceps are used to assist in passage of flaccid or regular tracheal tubes, to aid in passage of a nasogastric tube, or to insert pharyngeal packing. Damage to the cuff may occur if it is handled with forceps.

Which Techniques Are Preferred?

The method of intubation is predicated not only on the site of operation but also on the projected need for postoperative ventilation.

Orotracheal Intubation

Before induction of anesthesia, all necessary equipment should be tested and readied for use. A tube of appropriate diameter and length should be selected—in women, 7.5 mm inside diameter and in a man, 8 to 9 mm. The tube should be cut to size before intubation, examined for patency, and the cuff inflated to detect air leak. The adapter placed in the proximal end should fit snugly, lying at the level of the teeth; otherwise, its projection may lead to kinking or to downward displacement into a bronchus. The tube is kept in its sterile wrapper and not handled until ready for insertion.

After preoxygenation and induction of anesthesia, relaxation is usually achieved with a neuromuscular blocker, and the lungs are oxygenated by positive-pressure ventilation before attempted intubation. In teaching, an instructor should set a limit of 45 seconds for placement of the tube, followed by a second period of ventilation with oxygen.

Curved Blade Technique

The maneuvers are as follows:

1. The height of the operating table is adjusted so that the table is at the level of the anesthesiologist's iliac crest. This position allows laryngeal suspension with the left arm flexed and elbow held against the body at the level of the crest.
2. The patient's head, resting on a pillow or pad, is brought into the "sniffing" position to align the axes of the trachea, pharynx, and mouth. The head is extended at the atlanto-occipital joint, and the cervical spine is flexed (Fig. 26–18). This position was earlier proposed by Bannister and Macbeth in 1944.[18]
3. The fingers of the anesthetist's gloved right hand open the jaws widely, the thumb on the lower molars, with the second and third fingers on the upper teeth, thus spreading the lips to prevent bruising. Gentleness and avoidance of pressure on teeth or gums are essential. A protective shield or plastic mold placed over the upper incisors can prevent damage.
4. Held in the left hand, the moistened or lubricated laryngoscope blade is introduced at the right side of the mouth and advanced in the midline, displacing the tongue to the left. The epiglottis is then seen at the base of the tongue, the tip of the blade fitting into the vallecula (see Fig. 26–17). The wrist is held rigid to avoid using the upper teeth as a fulcrum for the laryngoscope blade. A forward and upward lift of the laryngoscope and blade stretches the hypoepiglottic ligament, thus folding the epiglottis upward and further exposing the glottis. As a result, the larynx is suspended on the tip of the blade via the hyoid bone.
5. The tracheal tube, with cuff deflated and concavity di-rected anterolaterally, is passed to the right of the laryngoscope through the glottis into the trachea until the cuff passes 2 to 3 cm beyond the vocal cords.

The glottis occasionally is not fully visible, but intubation is possible when only the arytenoid cartilages and posterior commissure are seen. A curved stylet helps to direct the tube anteriorly.

Straight Blade Technique

Intubation with a straight blade (see Fig. 26–17) involves the same maneuvers but with one major difference. The blade is slipped *beneath* the epiglottis, and exposure of the larynx is accomplished by an upward and forward lift at a 45° angle. Again, leverage must not be applied.

Comparison of Straight and Curved Blade Techniques

Theoretically, the advantages of the curved blade relate to the sensory innervation of the laryngeal or inferior surface of the epiglottis, where sensation is derived from the superior laryngeal branch of the vagus: Stimulation by a straight blade placed beneath the epiglottis is said to predispose more to laryngospasm and cough.

The pharyngeal or superior surface is innervated by the glossopharyngeal nerve, stimulation of which is less likely to cause spasm. Further, the curved blade allows more room for passage of the tracheal tube between the teeth than does a straight blade. Occasionally, however, exposure of the glottis is not as good as that obtained with the straight blade, so a stylet may be required to improve the curvature of the tube.

When a patient's mouth cannot be opened widely, as when the teeth protrude or are in poor condition or in stout-necked individuals, a curved blade is more useful. If the glottis is not easily exposed, depression of the cricoid cartilage (Sellick's maneuver) by an assistant may help, although suspension of the larynx is counteracted. This maneuver commonly is used to prevent regurgitation of stomach contents during induction of anesthesia.[19] An extra pillow or pad placed beneath the head may also prove of value.

Failure to Intubate

With either technique, the common causes of failure to intubate are as follow: inadequate position of the head; misplacement of the laryngoscope blade; inadequate muscle relaxation; insufficient depth of general anesthesia; allowing the tongue to obscure the glottis; and lack of familiarity with the anatomy, especially where there are pathologic changes.

Inserting a laryngoscope blade too deeply results in lifting of the entire larynx and esophagus if the tip of the blade is not placed in the vallecula.

Nasotracheal Intubation

Nasotracheal intubation is commonly used in oral and maxillofacial operations and in emergency situations outside the operating room. Although nasotracheal intubation is indicated in a patient with trismus or a fractured jaw, it is avoided in patients with a basilar skull fracture, a fractured nose, or nasal

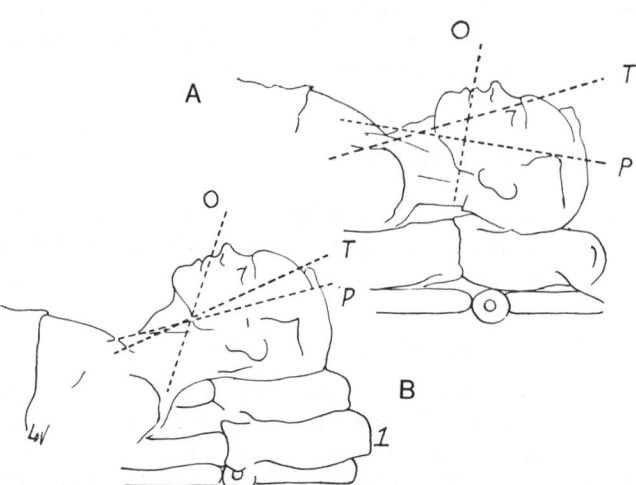

FIGURE 26–18. Position of the head for laryngoscopy and intubation of the trachea. *A*, Ordinary position. T = Axis of the trachea; P = axis of the pharynx; O = axis of the oral cavity. *B*, Modified position achieved with an extra head rest. Flexion of the cervical spine and extension at the atlanto-occipital joint bring the three axes more nearly into line. (From Dripps RD, Eckenhoff JE, Vandam LD: Introduction to Anesthesia: The Principles of Safe Practice. 7th ed. Philadelphia, WB Saunders, 1988.)

obstruction. It is also contraindicated in the presence of acute sinusitis or mastoiditis, because the infection may spread to the rest of the airway.

The technique may be applied either with a patient awake and well sedated or after induction of general anesthesia and use of a neuromuscular blocker. Nasal intubation may be performed blindly or under direct vision using a laryngoscope or flexible fiberoptic bronchoscope.

Blind

1. The patient's occiput rests on a firm pillow, somewhat higher than that used for oral intubation, with the chin further elevated. Prior topical application of cocaine, 5%, or lidocaine, 4% with phenylephrine, 0.25%, in 2- to 4-mL amounts is used to shrink mucous membranes. Gentle exploration should be carried out with cotton swabs to detect nasal obstruction, particularly at the posterior choanae.

2. A tube, smaller in diameter than required for oral intubation, should be soft and pliable to avoid injuring the nasal mucosa or turbinates but should also be of a consistency to resist compression and to maintain a reasonable curvature. These conditions can be met by warming the plastic tube in hot water just before intubation.

3. The tube, well lubricated, is introduced with its concavity forward, bevel directed laterally; advancement is slow and gentle, with rotation when resistance is encountered. Rough maneuvers, large-bore rigid tubes, poor lubrication, and use of force against obstruction easily induce epistaxis.

Guides to ultimate success during intubation include the following:

1. Watching the neck for the bulging produced by the tip of the tube in the hypopharynx
2. Increase or decrease in breath sounds heard by listening at the proximal end of the tube in spontaneously breathing patients
3. Resistance to passage

Rotation of the tube and manual depression or elevation of the larynx may be required in order to succeed. Voluntary hyperpnea helps if the patient is awake, as well as hyperpnea produced by hypercapnia, because maximal abduction of the cords is present during inspiration. Entry into the trachea is signified by consistent breath sounds transmitted via the tube and inability to speak if the patient is breathing, as well as by lack of resistance, often accompanied by cough. One can then feel the inflation of the tracheal cuff below the larynx, followed by connecting the tube to the rebreathing system and expanding the lungs.

Direct Vision

Nasotracheal intubation under direct vision is accomplished during laryngoscopy with or without the help of Magill's forceps. The tube is inserted through one nostril into the oropharynx, with the bevel pointing laterally. The vocal cords are then exposed, and the tube advanced under direct vision into the trachea. If it does not progress, Magill's forceps are used to direct the tip toward the glottis, with an assistant then advancing the tube. Magill's forceps may also be useful during conscious nasotracheal intubation under direct vision.

Advantages of nasotracheal over oral intubation are as follow:

1. The tube is easily secured, with less tendency for accidental extubation.
2. It is more comfortable for awake patients and eliminates the possibility of occlusion by their biting on the tube.
3. Oral feeding is possible during long-term nasotracheal intubation.

The following are disadvantages:

1. Damage to nasal tissues (epistaxis, dislodgement of adenoidal tissue) is possible.
2. Infection can be transmitted from nose to trachea and lungs.
3. The need for smaller tubes results in increased resistance to breathing.
4. Secretions are more difficult to suction.

Why Is Tracheal Intubation Performed in Conscious Patients?

An anesthesiologist should be able to intubate the trachea with a patient awake when induction of general anesthesia is considered unsafe, as in the absence of an assured airway. Indications for ''awake'' intubation are listed in Table 26–2. Preanesthetic preparation should include a detailed explanation of the procedure to ensure maximum cooperation by patients.

Requirements
Sedation

Intubation of conscious patients can be performed either orally or nasally. Patients require sedation for relaxation and to minimize unpleasant recollections. Sedation is best achieved with incremental intravenous doses of sedatives or opioids such as diazepam, midazolam, and fentanyl. Topical anesthesia of the airway is also necessary.

Topical Anesthesia

Topical anesthesia of the upper airway can be accomplished by means of nebulizer, application of cotton swabs, superior laryngeal nerve block, transtracheal injection of local anesthetic via the cricothyroid membrane, or spraying with a topical anesthetic under direct vision with a laryngoscope. The structures are anesthetized in the following order: oropharynx, base of tongue, epiglottis, pyriform fossae, vocal cords, and finally the larynx and upper trachea by instillation of 2 mL of local anesthetic through the glottis.

For nasotracheal intubation, the mucosa should also be thoroughly anesthetized. A minimal amount of anesthetic is used to prevent untoward reactions, not more than 4 mL of 4% lidocaine or 5% cocaine, using ''wrung out'' swabs.

TABLE 26–2. Indications for Intubation in a Conscious Patient

Threat of aspiration of gastric contents during induction of general anesthesia
Intubation of the trachea or mask ventilation after induction of anesthesia is anticipated to be difficult or impossible because of pathologic changes in the pharynx, larynx, neck, or mediastinum
Inflammatory swelling encroaching on the mouth or pharynx
Malformation of the jaws
Scar tissue resulting from burns or operations about the head and neck
Congenital abnormalities of the upper airway
Morbid obesity

Risk of Aspiration

The use of topical anesthesia and heavy sedation for tracheal tube placement is controversial in patients with a full stomach. Sedation, opioids, and topical anesthesia may result in an incompetent larynx and thus risk of aspiration should regurgitation or vomiting occur. Sellick's maneuver is usually used. Awake tracheal intubation is generally less traumatic and more often successful if performed with a flexible fiberoptic bronchoscope.

What Care Is Necessary After Intubation?

The first steps after intubation include

1. Cuff inflation using the minimum leak method to seal off the trachea and to avoid excessive cuff pressure
2. Observation of chest movement as the lungs are inflated with oxygen
3. Observing the repetitive presence of exhaled CO_2 and listening for breath sounds bilaterally high in the axillae and over the epigastrium to make certain that the trachea, not the esophagus or a bronchus, has been entered

As noted, a tube more easily enters the right mainstem bronchus than the left because of their relative angles at the bifurcation. Failure of one side of the chest to move with ventilation and absence of breath sounds suggest bronchial intubation, in which case the tube should be withdrawn several centimeters beyond where breath sounds are bilaterally and equally audible.

Tube Stabilization and Fixation

After orotracheal intubation, an oropharyngeal airway or soft bite block is typically placed between the teeth to prevent biting on the tube. The tube is secured with adhesive or umbilical tape tied around the neck; suturing to the teeth or gums may be required during maxillofacial operations.

When secretions are excessive, as in the face-down position, or when solutions used to prepare the operative field may loosen adhesive, preparation of the skin with tincture of benzoin before taping is useful. Nasotracheal tubes should also be fixed securely, with the connector at the level of the nares, not deforming the nasal cartilages.

Why Does Coughing Occur, and How Is it Treated?

Cough after intubation frequently occurs when topical anesthesia is inadequate, during light planes of general anesthesia, and when the tube touches the carina. If cough is mild, only transient hypertension and tachycardia result. In the more severe response, thoracic muscle spasm and bronchospasm may be difficult to overcome and ventilation is impaired, resulting in hypoxia. If the tube touches the carina, it should be withdrawn slightly. If coughing persists, intravenous injection of a small amount of lidocaine or neuromuscular blocker followed by controlled ventilation usually relieves chest wall spasm.

What Factors Affect Tube Movement?

When a patient's position on the operating table is subsequently changed, the position of the tube must again be verified. Flexion of the head, shortening the distance from teeth to carina, and steep Trendelenburg's position, causing the abdominal contents to elevate the hila of the lungs and carina, may direct a tube into a mainstem bronchus.

How Is Esophageal Intubation Detected?

Clinical Signs

A tracheal tube inadvertently placed in the esophagus is suggested by absence of clear breath sounds and exhaled CO_2, progressive distention of the stomach with attempted ventilation, deterioration in saturation as seen on pulse oximetry, and development of cyanosis. While listening over the stomach with a stethoscope, the anesthetist may detect air entry as the reservoir bag is compressed.

When in doubt, one should immediately remove the tracheal tube and ventilate the lungs with a face mask. Then, after tracheal intubation has been accomplished, the stomach should be emptied of gas by orogastric or nasogastric suctioning.

Capnography is essential in detecting esophageal intubation, because absence of CO_2 in exhaled air is diagnostic and minimizes the time for corrective action. Unrecognized esophageal intubation is one of the common causes of anoxia and not an infrequent factor leading to medicolegal action.

How Is Extubation Performed?

Preparation

Before extubation, the oropharynx is suctioned, neuromuscular blockade is reversed, and the adequacy of spontaneous ventilation is ensured. Routine tracheal suctioning is unnecessary; however, when it is indicated, a sterile suction catheter should be used. Although it is essential to rid the trachea or pharynx of secretions before extubation, one should not persist if coughing is protracted and cyanosis develops.

Oxygen Administration

Before and after tracheal suctioning, oxygen is administered. Tape or other fixation devices are removed, the cuff is deflated, and the tube withdrawn as the lungs are inflated with oxygen. A tube should not be removed with the aspirating catheter in place, because this technique depletes the lungs of oxygen, nor is this maneuver effective in preventing aspiration. Should the catheter brush against the vocal cords, bleeding or laryngospasm can result.

Technique

After the tube is removed, the patient is given oxygen by mask; if necessary, the oropharynx is again suctioned. Should laryngospasm develop, it is now less threatening because the lungs have been inflated with oxygen before extubation. To avoid laryngospasm, extubation can be carried out at a relatively deep plane of anesthesia during spontaneous ventilation or when a patient has reacted sufficiently to have regained airway control. Laryngospasm and cough may be minimized by injection of lidocaine, 50 to 100 mg intravenously, a minute or two before extubation.

Why Is Extubation Sometimes Difficult?

Removal of a tracheal tube is occasionally difficult or impossible. The common causes are failure to deflate the cuff or unintentional suturing of a nasotracheal tube to the tissues during maxillofacial surgery. Also, a patient may have bitten down on the tube.

What Precautions Are Necessary?

A tracheal tube should not be removed in the presence of oxygen desaturation and cyanosis, when respiratory exchange is inadequate or uncontrollable with mask and bag, or when the operation has compromised the airway.

In patients with a full stomach, a tube is left in place until the patient is fully awake and extubation then accomplished with the patient in the lateral decubitus position.

When maxillofacial operations result in a compromised airway, elective tracheostomy may be necessary before extubation. Should respiratory exchange be inadequate, the tube is left in place, the patient transported to the recovery room with assisted breathing, and ventilation continued mechanically until adequate.

What Are the Complications of Tracheal Intubation?

Complications related to tracheal intubation are many, so they must be carefully weighted against the benefits gained (Table 26–3; Fig. 26–19).

TABLE 26–3. Untoward Sequelae of Tracheal Intubation

Immediate
　Esophageal or bronchial intubation
　Kinking of the tube
　Occlusion due to distended cuff
　Bevel against the tracheal wall
　Sympathetic response
Delayed and postextubation
　Overdistention of the cuff (nitrous oxide)
　Accidental extubation of bronchial entrance
　Secretions
　Laryngospasm
　Inadequate oxygenation
　Full stomach
　Postoperative compromised airway
Trauma
　Dental damage
　Lacerations
　Mediastinal emphysema
　Aspiration of gastric contents
　Vocal cord paralysis
　Polyp formation
　Laryngeal edema and tracheitis

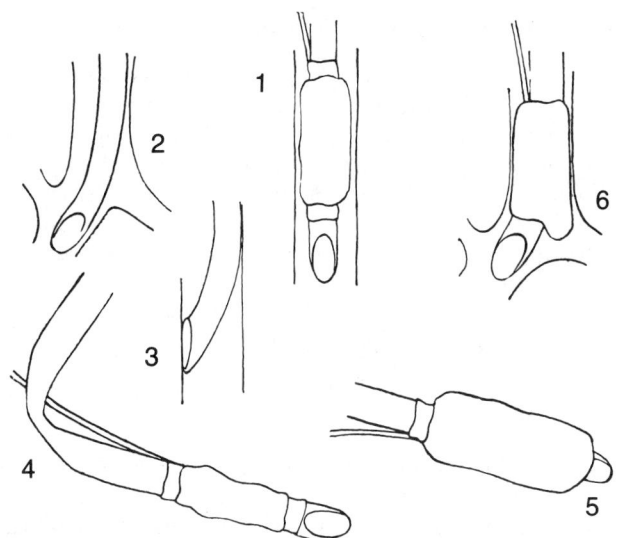

FIGURE 26–19. Accidents with tracheal intubation. 1 = Normal position of the tube; 2 = intubation of the right main bronchus; 3 = tube opening against side of trachea, resulting in one-way valve effect; 4 = kinked tube; 5 = endotracheal cuff inflated with partial occlusion of opening; 6 = inflated cuff partially occluding left main bronchus. (From Dripps RD, Eckenhoff JE, Vandam LD: Introduction to Anesthesia: The Principles of Safe Practice. 1st ed. Philadelphia, WB Saunders, 1957.)

Immediate

Trauma

Intubation may result in lacerated or bruised lips and tongue; chipped, loosened, or dislodged teeth; laceration of the pharyngeal wall; dislodged adenoidal tissue; and epistaxis. Rupture of the hypopharynx, esophagus, or trachea may result in mediastinal or subcutaneous emphysema and pneumothorax, perhaps more often encountered when a stylet has been used. Pneumothorax requires immediate diagnosis, insertion of chest tubes, and re-expansion of the lungs.

Cardiovascular Responses

Hypertension and tachycardia almost always accompany laryngoscopy and tracheal intubation, the so-called stress response. Dysrhythmias may also be precipitated. Perhaps a shorter time during laryngoscopy may minimize the magnitude and duration of these changes.

In patients with coronary artery disease, hypertension and tachycardia may cause myocardial ischemia and infarction. Dysrhythmias such as polymorphic ventricular tachycardia and premature ventricular beats more often occur with those agents (halothane) that sensitize the myocardium to the action of catecholamines. Deepening anesthesia and hyperventilation usually eliminate the dysrhythmias. Additional drug therapy may be necessary.

Lidocaine. Laryngotracheal spray with 4% lidocaine immediately preceding placement of a tracheal tube often does not prevent the circulatory reaction. Lidocaine, $1 \text{ mg} \cdot \text{kg}^{-1}$, given intravenously 1 minute before laryngoscopy may modify the response by depressing airway reflexes and by deepening the level of anesthesia, but a significant cardiovascular response may still occur.

Narcotics and β-Adrenergic Blockers. Intravenous injection of one of the ultrapotent opioids or a short-acting β-adrenergic blocker may be the treatment of choice.

Spinal Cord and Vertebral Column Injury

Patients with cervical spinal fractures and dislocations, osteoporosis, osteolytic lesions, and congenital malformations of the spine are susceptible to spinal cord and cervical vertebral injury during laryngoscopy and attempted tracheal intubation. Both flexion and hyperextension of the neck, as usually practiced during laryngoscopy with a rigid laryngoscope, should be avoided. Alternate techniques, such as fiberoptic or "blind" nasotracheal intubation, should be considered. In most of these patients, fiberoptic intubation can easily be accomplished without manipulating the neck.

Esophageal Intubation

Esophageal intubation is a more common complication than realized; recognition must be prompt to avoid hypoxia. It is easily detected under most circumstances, but in occasional patients even an experienced anesthetist may have difficulty in immediately recognizing the problem. Signs of hypoxia, desaturation on the pulse oximeter, and electrocardiographic changes may be delayed if the lungs have been preoxygenated. Monitoring end-tidal CO_2 is the key element in detection.

Aspiration of Gastric Contents

Special precautions should be taken in patients at high risk for aspiration. Awake tracheal intubation or rapid-sequence induction and intubation, with Sellick's maneuver, are the two most commonly used techniques. Fiberoptic tracheal intubation may be of value in awake patients.

Partial airway obstruction, distention of the stomach during mask anesthesia, or spontaneous breathing against an obstructed airway facilitates regurgitation and aspiration. Extubation before protective reflexes return increases the risk during emergence from anesthesia.

Laryngospasm

Painful stimulation of the patient during anesthesia, attempts at tracheal intubation with inadequate anesthesia or without a neuromuscular blocker, and the presence of blood or secretions in the airway after extubation can result in laryngeal spasm.

Bronchial Intubation

Bronchial intubation may take place during intubation or subsequent positioning when flexing the neck or when a steep Trendelenburg's position is used.

Delayed

Vocal Cord Paralysis

The mechanism of vocal cord paralysis following intubation is unknown.[20] Paralysis may be unilateral, presenting as hoarseness, or bilateral, causing inspiratory obstruction because the relaxed cords are drawn to the midline. Pressure exerted by an overinflated cuff on branches of the recurrent laryngeal nerve has been implicated as a cause, as have poorly aerated tubes after ethylene oxide sterilization. Most often the occurrence is unexplained. The paralysis is usually transient.

Laryngeal Edema and Tracheitis

Subglottic edema, the gravest of the laryngeal edemas, occurs mostly in children younger than 3 years; onset is apparent within 1 to 2 hours after extubation. Treatment includes inhalation of humidified oxygen and humidification. Dexamethasone is helpful, as is nebulized racemic epinephrine, to reduce vascular engorgement. Reintubation or tracheotomy may be necessary in refractory cases.

Infection

Maxillary sinusitis and retropharyngeal abscess may follow nasotracheal intubation. Bacteremia has been shown to be more common after nasotracheal than after oral intubation.

Sore Throat

Sore throat is the most frequent sequel of tracheal intubation. It is sometimes severe, and the incidence is high after head and neck operations. Laryngitis, as manifested by hoarseness and a sore throat, appears in a small percentage of patients but is transient. Recovery is usual, and special treatment is not needed.

Failed Intubation

Inability to obtain a secure airway often results in disaster. To minimize the consequences, the emergency must be detected early and prearranged maneuvers immediately applied. For such emergencies outside the operating suite, an emergency cart stocked with necessary equipment and supplies should be available.

References

1. Caplan RA, Posner KL, Ward RJ, et al: Adverse respiratory events in anesthesia: a closed claims analysis. Anesthesiology 1990; 72:828.
2. Negus VE: The Comparative Anatomy and Physiology of the Larynx. New York, Grune & Stratton, 1949.
3. Bramble DM, Carrier DM: Running and breathing in mammals. Science 1983; 219:25.
4. Lewin R: Four legs bad, two legs good. Science 1987; 235:969.
5. Kaban LB: Dental and oral problems. In To Make The Patient Ready for Anesthesia. 2nd ed. Vandam LD (ed). Menlo Park CA, Addison-Wesley, 1984, pp 208–233.
6. Proctor DF: Form and function of the upper airways and larynx. In Handbook of Physiology, Section 3. The Respiratory System. Vol. III. Mechanics of Breathing. Part I. Bethesda, MD, American Physiological Society, 1982.
7. Courtiss EH, Gorgon TJ, Courtiss GB: Nasal physiology. Ann Plast Surg 1984; 13:214.
8. Klein HC: Why can't physicians examine the larynx? JAMA 1982; 247:2111.
9. Mallampati SR, Gugino LD, Desai SP, et al: A clinical sign to predict difficult tracheal intubation: a prospective study. Can Anaesth Soc J 1985; 32:429.
10. Kubota Y, Magaribuchi T, Toyoda Y, et al: Selective bronchial suctioning in the adult using a curve-tipped catheter with a guide mark. Crit Care Med 1982; 10:767.
11. Eckenhoff JE: Some anatomic considerations of the infant larynx influencing endotracheal anesthesia. Anesthesiology 1951; 12:401.
12. Warner JA, Finlay WEI: Fulminating epiglottitis in adults: report of three cases and review of the literature. Anaesthesia 1985; 40:348.
13. Fink BR: The etiology and treatment of laryngeal spasm. Anesthesiology 1956; 17:569.
14. Mushin WW: Bilateral vagus nerve block. Proc R Soc Med 1944; 38:308.
15. Labat G: Regional Anesthesia. Its Technical and Clinical Application. 2nd ed. Philadelphia, WB Saunders, 1928, p 143.

16. Bartlett D Jr: Respiratory functions of the larynx. Physiol Rev 1989; 69:33.

17. Dripps RD, Eckenhoff JE, Vandam LD: Introduction to Anesthesia: The Principles of Safe Practice. 7th ed. Philadelphia, WB Saunders, 1988.

18. Bannister FB, Macbeth RG: Direct laryngoscopy and tracheal intubation. Lancet 1944; 2:651.

19. Sellick BA: Cricoid pressure to control regurgitation of stomach contents during induction of anaesthesia. Lancet 1961; 2:404.

20. Halley HS, Gildea JE: Vocal cord paralysis after tracheal intubation. JAMA 1971; 215:281.

General Reading

Benumof JL: Management of the difficult airway. Anesthesiology 1991; 75:1087.

Fink BR, Demaret RJ: Laryngeal biomechanics. Cambridge, Harvard University Press, 1978.

Finucaine BT, Santura AH: Principles of airway management. Philadelphia, FA Davis, 1988.

Negus VE: The comparative anatomy and physiology of the larynx. New York, Grune & Stratton, 1949.

Snell RS, Katz J: Clinical anatomy for anesthesiologists. Norwalk, CT, Appleton & Lange, 1988.

Vandam LD: Functional anatomy of the larynx. Weekly Anesthesia Update 1977; 1:95.

CHAPTER 27

The Spine

EDWARD T. CROSBY, B.Sc., M.D., F.R.C.P.C.
ANNE C. P. LUI, M.Sc., M.D., F.R.C.P.C.

The ability to assess spinal function and to appreciate the impact of altered anatomy and biomechanical function on anesthetic techniques should be part of every anesthesiologist's clinical repertoire. This review is intended to help the reader gain such an appreciation by highlighting important aspects of the anatomy and function of the spine and noting the implications of both congenital and acquired processes. For the purposes of the discussion, the spine is divided into cervical, thoracic, lumbar, and caudal portions. The clinical focus of the discussion of the cervical spine is on tracheal intubation and airway maneuvers; that of the thoracic spine, on the effects of thoracic spinal deformity on anesthesia; and that of the lumbosacral spine, on regional anesthesia.

EMBRYOLOGIC DEVELOPMENT

Beginning at about 3 weeks' gestational age, mesodermal somites begin to appear along each side of the neural groove. Each somite differentiates into a dorsolateral myotome (muscle plate) and a ventromedial sclerotome (vertebral plate). Growth of the sclerotomes occurs in three directions: medially to surround the notochord and establish the vertebral body, dorsally to enclose the neural tube and produce the vertebral arch and spinous process, and laterally to give rise to the transverse processes. Chondrification centers arise in the arch rudiments and in the primitive body. In the third month of gestation, ossification centers replace the chondrogenous centers.

At birth, each hemiarch and its corresponding body is separated by cartilaginous plates. Hemiarches unite dorsally during the first postnatal year, and the completed arches join the vertebral bodies during the third to sixth years of life. Absence of an ossification center in the vertebral body may result in formation of a hemivertebra. Failure of closure of the neural arch results in spina bifida. Finally, failure of the arch to fuse with the ossified vertebral body results in spondylolysis.

VERTEBRAL ANATOMY

What Are the Common Characteristics?

The spine is composed of 33 vertebrae (7 cervical, 12 thoracic, 5 lumbar, 5 fused sacral, and 4 coccygeal) and describes four curves (Fig. 27–1). The cervical and lumbar curves are convex anteriorly (lordotic), and the thoracic and sacral curves are convex posteriorly (kyphotic).

A typical vertebra (C-3 to L-5) consists of a body anteriorly and a neural arch posteriorly (Fig. 27–2).

The Body

The heavy body resembles a short, long bone, and its principal function is to support weight. The bodies of the vertebrae

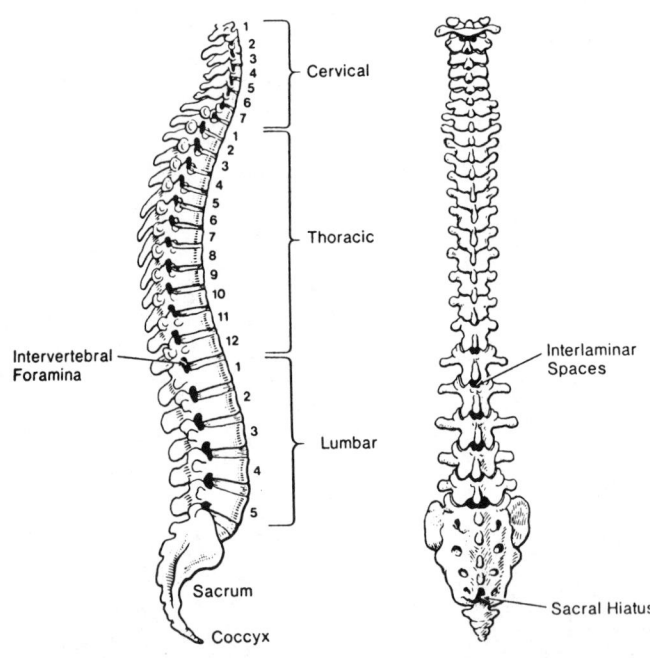

FIGURE 27–1. The vertebral column. Lateral and posterior views.

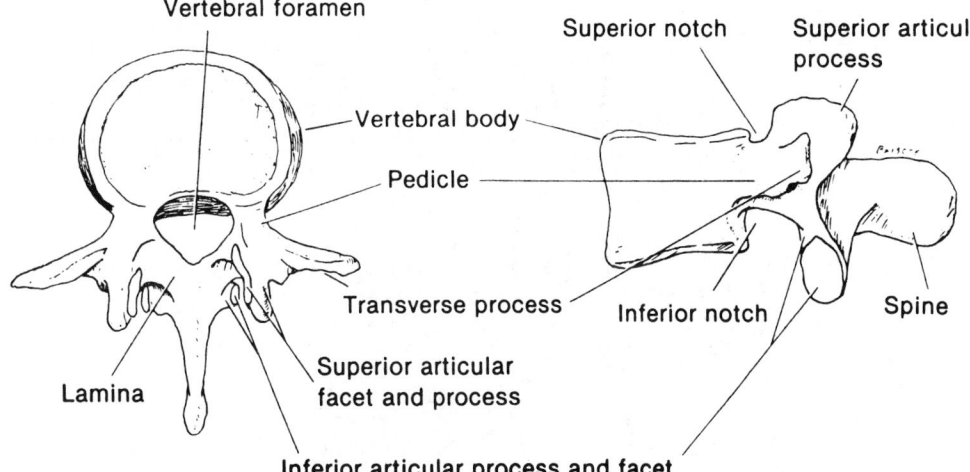

FIGURE 27–2. Typical vertebral body. (From Levinson G: Spinal anesthesia. *In* Clinical Procedures in Anesthesia and Intensive Care. Benumof JL (ed). Philadelphia, JB Lippincott, 1992, p 646.)

from C-3 to L-5 become progressively larger in order to bear incrementally greater weight.

Neural Arch

The dorsal neural arch serves to shelter and protect the neural elements. It is formed by two pedicles rising from the vertebral body to constitute the side walls of the arch, which is closed superiorly by the laminae.

Articular Processes

Four articular processes (two superior and two inferior), two laterally placed transverse processes, and a dorsal spinous process arise from the neural arch. The pedicles are notched both inferiorly and superiorly. When two vertebrae are in articulation, the large inferior notch of the more cephalic vertebra is adjacent to the smaller superior notch of the caudal vertebra to form the intervertebral foramen. These foramina contain the dorsal root ganglia and conduct the spinal nerves.

What Are the Major Joints?

The vertebrae from C-2 to S-1 articulate with each other through three joints: one anterior nonsynovial joint, the intervertebral disk; and two posterior synovial joints, the zygapophyseal or facet joints.

Intervertebral Disks

The intervertebral disks account for about 25% of total spinal length. They are composed of peripheral fibrous tissue and fibrocartilage arranged in concentric rings (the annulus fibrosus), surrounding a soft central core (the nucleus pulposus). They adhere above and below to hyaline cartilage, which covers the articular surfaces of the vertebral bodies.

Facet Joints

The facet joints are true synovial joints. Their articular surfaces are covered with hyaline cartilage, and each joint is surrounded by an articular capsule. These capsules are longer and looser in the cervical region than in the subcervical spine, allowing for greater range of joint motion.

What Are the Important Ligamentous Structures?

The spinal column is bound together, through its length, by several ligaments, which give it stability and elasticity (Fig. 27–3).

Supraspinous Ligament

The supraspinous ligament is a strong fibrous cord that connects the apices of the spinous processes from the sacrum to C-7, above which it continues to the external occipital protuberance as the ligamentum nuchae.

Interspinous Ligament

The interspinous ligament is a thinner, more membranous structure that connects the spinous processes, blending ventrally with the ligamentum flavum and dorsally with the supraspinous ligament.

Ligamentum Flavum

The ligamentum flavum lies deep to the interspinous ligament and connects the laminae of adjacent vertebrae. It covers the interlaminar space and forms the roof of the epidural space.

Longitudinal Ligaments

The anterior and posterior longitudinal ligaments bind the vertebral bodies together. The anterior ligament inserts on the intervertebral disks and adjacent vertebrae and ascends along the anterior surface of the spine. The posterior longitudinal ligament courses upward along the dorsal surface of the vertebral bodies, forming the floor of the neural canal.

Intertransverse Ligament

The intertransverse ligaments connect adjacent transverse processes and are insignificant membranous ligaments.

Anterior   **Posterior**

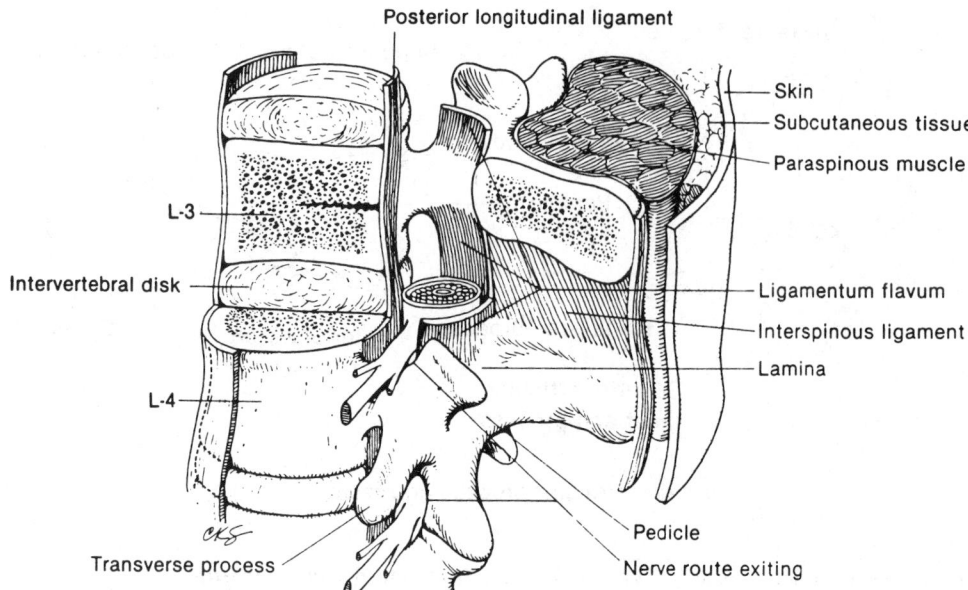

FIGURE 27-3. Ligaments of the spine. (From Reisner LS, Ellis J: Epidural and caudal puncture. *In* Clinical Procedures in Anesthesia and Intensive Care. Benumof JL (ed). Philadelphia, JB Lippincott, 1992, p 663.)

What Are the Subdivisions Within the Neural Canal?

The Epidural Space

The epidural space is the outermost division of the neural canal. It extends from the foramen magnum, where the dura is fused to the base of the skull to the sacral hiatus, where it is covered by the sacrococcygeal ligament. Its boundaries are the posterior longitudinal ligament anteriorly, the pedicles laterally, and the anterior surfaces of the lamina and the ligamentum flavum posteriorly.

The anterior epidural space is very narrow because of the close proximity of the dura to the posterior longitudinal ligament. Trabeculations between the dura and the posterior ligament are common, rendering this space discontinuous across the midline. Hogan has demonstrated the existence of a membranous lateral extension of the posterior longitudinal ligament, isolating the anterior epidural space.[1] These previously described trabeculations and newly described membranes may provide a barrier to the circumferential spread of solutions deposited in the anterior epidural space.

The epidural space is widest in its sagittal plane posteriorly and varies with the vertebral level, ranging from 1 to 1.5 mm at C-5; 2.5 to 3.0 mm at T-6; and, at its widest point, 5 to 6 mm at L-2. In addition to the nerve roots that cross it, the contents of the epidural space include fat, areolar tissue, lymphatics, arteries, and an extensive internal vertebral venous plexus.

The Subdural Space

The subdural space is a potential space, bounded by the dura externally and the pia-arachnoid membranes internally, and containing a small amount of serous fluid.[2] It extends laterally over the nerve roots and ganglia and is greater in its posterior aspects. It has been written that one cannot pierce the dura without penetrating the arachnoid membrane as well—that is, one cannot perform a subdural injection. This is

not the case; both intentional and accidental subdural injections have been reported.[3–6] Injections into the subdural space tend to localize primarily in its posterior aspects; a predominantly sensory (dorsal root) blockade results.

The Subarachnoid Space

The subarachnoid space is bound internally by the pia and externally by the arachnoid and is filled by the cerebrospinal fluid, brain, spinal cord, and nerve roots. It has three divisions; cranial, spinal and nerve root, all of which are in free communication with one another.

THE CERVICAL SPINE

What Are the Relevant Anatomic Features?

The Atlas

The first cervical vertebra, the atlas, has thick anterior and posterior arches that blend laterally into large masses (Fig. 27–4). The occipital condyles of the skull articulate with large kidney-shaped depressions on the superior aspects of these lateral masses. The flatter inferior surfaces of the lateral masses transmit the weight of the skull onto the superior facet joints of the axis, the second cervical vertebra (Fig. 27–5). On the inner aspects of the anterior arch of the atlas, arising bilaterally and projecting inward, two bony tubercles give rise to the transverse ligament.

The Axis

Laterally placed on the superior surface of the axis (C-2) are circular facets that articulate with the lateral masses of the atlas (see Fig. 27–5). The centrum or body of the axis extends upward to form the odontoid process. The narrowed waist of the odontoid process is compressed by the transverse ligament of the atlas. Alar and apical ligaments fan upward from the

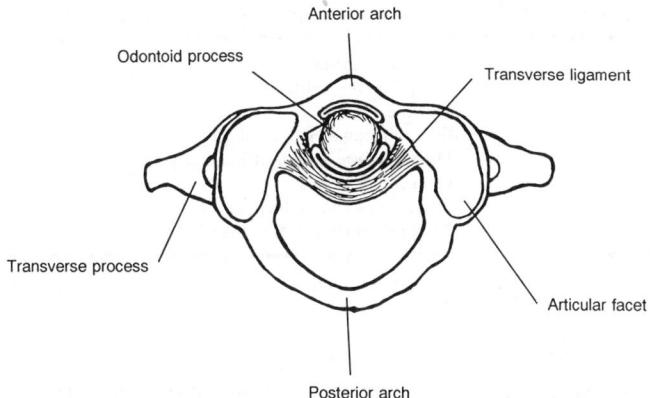

FIGURE 27–4. The atlas. Superior view of the atlantoaxial articulation (skull removed) detailing superior surface anatomy of the atlas. (From Crosby ET, Lui A: The adult cervical spine: implications for airway management. Can J Anaesth 1990; 37:77.)

odontoid process to insert on the anterior margins of the foramen magnum (Fig. 27–6). The spinous process of the axis is large and heavy, allowing muscle and ligamentous insertion.

The Lower Cervical Vertebrae

The lower five cervical vertebrae are anatomically more typical. The transverse processes are the unique features, with laterally projecting costal processes and the foramen transversarium, transmitting the vertebral artery through most of the cervical spine. The arches of the second to seventh cervical vertebrae articulate via horizontally oriented facet joints. There is an intervertebral disk between C-2 and C-3 and each subjacent pair of vertebrae.

The Longitudinal Ligaments

Anterior and posterior longitudinal ligaments extend the length of the cervical spine. The anterior ligament terminates over the anterior arch of the atlas, forming the anterior atlantooccipital ligament, which inserts on the base of the skull (see Fig. 27–6). The posterior ligament courses upward along the dorsal surface of the vertebral bodies, fans over the body of the axis and the odontoid process, and terminates as the tectorial membrane, which inserts into the basiocciput.

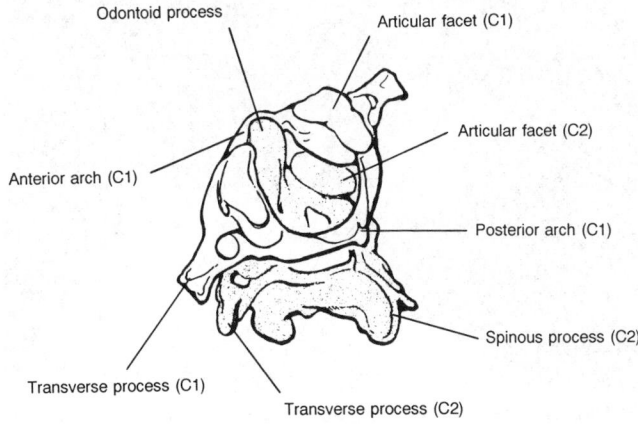

FIGURE 27–5. The atlantoaxial joint. Details of the articulating surfaces of the atlantoaxial joint.

TABLE 27–1. Bony Anomalies Involving the Cervical Spine

Cranio-occipital anomalies	Occipitalization of vertebrae
	Occipital dysplasia
	Condylar hypoplasia
	Assimilation of the atlas
	Arnold-Chiari malformation
	Foramen magnum stenosis (achondroplasia)
Anomalies of the atlas and axis	Arch aplasias—atlas
	Odontoid anomalies
	Aplasia
	Hypoplasia
	Os odontoideum
	Ossiculum terminale
Anomalies below C-2	Failure of segmentation (Klippel-Feil syndrome)
	Failure of fusion (spina bifida; spondylolisthesis)
	Cervical ribs

How Does Cervical Spinal Anatomy Differ in the Pediatric Age Group?

Many of the anatomic differences in the pediatric cervical spine relative to that of an adult result from variances in the ossification centers, unfused synchondroses, and laxity of the ligamentous structures.[7]

Anterior wedging of the incompletely ossified vertebral body in young children can produce the appearance of a compression fracture. Anterior pseudosubluxation, especially at or above C-3, as well as an increase in the atlas-dens interval (ADI), are due to laxity of the spinal ligaments and are normal anatomic variants in young children.

Finally, with puberty, secondary ossification centers appear at the superior and inferior borders of the vertebral bodies and may not close until into the third decade. These secondary centers may be confused with chip fractures of the vertebral body.

What Are Common Congenital Anomalies?

A large number of bony anomalies involve the cervical spine (Table 27–1).

The Odontoid

The odontoid process of the axis is formed from paired centers that appear in the fifth gestational month. An additional center appears above the cleft tip of the odontoid. Between the third and sixth years of life, the separate components of the axis meet and fuse, and ossification is completed during puberty. Failure of the ossification centers in the odontoid process results in an aplastic or hypoplastic process (Fig. 27–7).

Hypoplasia

If the paired centers fail to fuse, a bifid odontoid process results. If these centers fail to fuse to the body of the axis, an os odontoideum develops. Hypoplasia of the odontoid process is encountered in a number of syndromes and may occur as an isolated anomaly[8] (Table 27–2). Both odontoid hypoplasia and os odontoideum result in loss of the buttressing action of the dens during extension of the head and neck. The atlas subluxes anteriorly on the axis, reducing the space available for the cord and resulting in compression of the neural elements. Patients with both Morquio's syndrome and disproportionate dwarfism

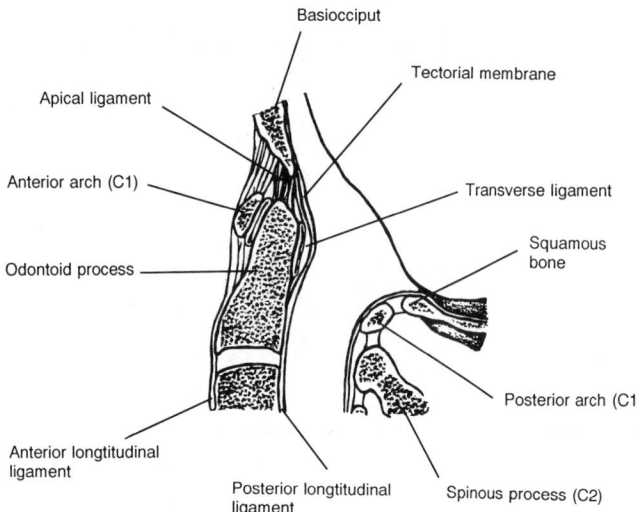

Basiocciput
Tectorial membrane
Apical ligament
Anterior arch (C1)
Transverse ligament
Odontoid process
Squamous bone
Posterior arch (C1)
Anterior longtitudinal ligament
Posterior longtitudinal ligament
Spinous process (C2)

FIGURE 27–6. The occipitoatlantoaxial articulation. Lateral view, sagittal section. (From Crosby ET, Lui ACP. The cervical spine: fundamental considerations. *In* Anesthesia and Musculoskeletal Disorders. Crosby ET, Lui ACP (eds). Probl Anesth 1991; 5:1.)

are at risk for odontoid hypoplasia, with resulting atlantoaxial subluxation (AAS) and decreased joint stability; spinal cord injury may result after even minor trauma.[9–11]

Down's Syndrome

Laxity of the transverse ligament and atlantoaxial instability are encountered in 14% to 22% of children with Down's syndrome.[12–14] Extension of the head may sublux the atlas anteriorly on the axis, with resultant compression of the cord by the odontoid process. Case reports in the anesthesiology literature have documented both rotatory subluxation of the atlantoaxial joint and posterior subluxation of the axis as new postoperative findings.[13, 14]

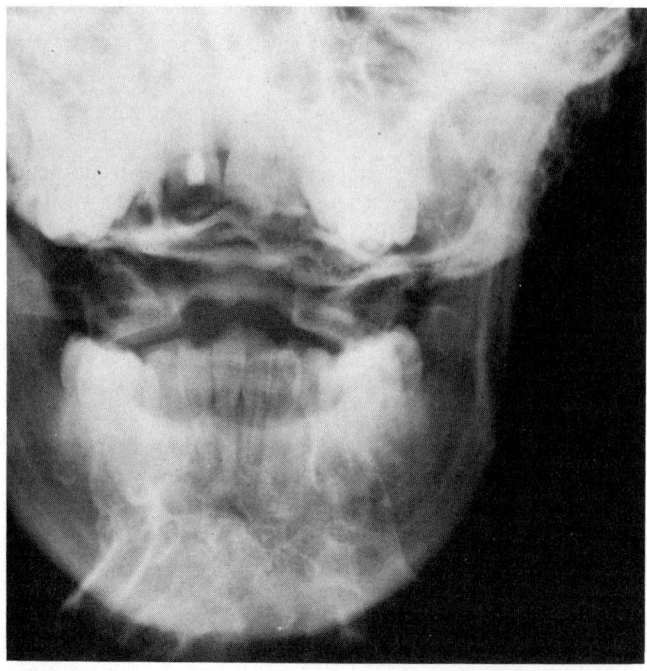

FIGURE 27–7. Aplasia of the odontoid process. Anteroposterior view of the atlantoaxial joint. The odontoid process is absent.

TABLE 27–2. Syndromes Associated with Odontoid Hypoplasia

Morquio's syndrome
Klippel-Feil syndrome
Down's syndrome
Spondyloepiphyseal dysplasia
Disproportionate dwarfism
Congenital scoliosis
Osteogenesis imperfecta
Neurofibromatosis

(From Crosby ET, Lui A: The adult cervical spine: implications for airway management. Can J Anaesth 1990; 37:77.)

Excessive laxity of other joints correlates well with the presence of AAS in Down's syndrome. It is thought that such patients have an intrinsic defect of the collagen fibers that form their ligamentous structures.[15] Other cervical spine abnormalities noted in Down's syndrome include spina bifida of the atlas, vertebral occipitalization, os odontoideum, and Klippel-Feil syndrome.[8]

Klippel-Feil Syndrome

Klippel-Feil syndrome is characterized by ankylosis of the cervical spine and has also been noted in trisomy 18, Turner's syndrome, and other less common syndromes, as well as being described as an isolated anomaly[16] (Fig. 27–8). Fusion of several cervical vertebrae into an osseous mass is encountered, as are abnormalities of the occipitoatlantoaxial complex.[17] In severely affected individuals, a single slender block vertebra

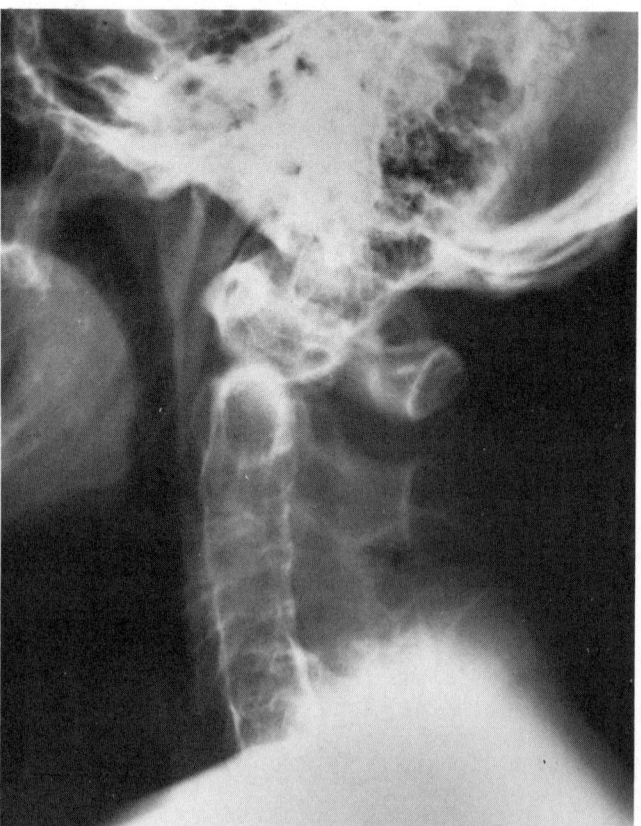

FIGURE 27–8. Klippel-Feil syndrome. Lateral view of the cervical spine. The cervical spine is fused into a single block of vertebrae. Also of note is the absence of the odontoid process (see also Fig. 27–7).

replaces the lower cervical spine. Neck movements are severely limited in all planes. Neurologic symptoms are variable and are predicted by associated anomalies rather than by the fusion itself.[16]

Clinical Significance

The clinical significance of an anomaly in the cervical spine is related to its effect on the stability of the spine and joint articulation. Important anomalies are usually a result of failed fusion of bone structures, laxity of ligamentous structures, or excess ossification in the spine.

Many congenital abnormalities of the cervical spine result in an actual or potential reduction in the lumen of the spinal canal. Thus, the space available for the cord is reduced, and the neural elements are at risk. A dynamic component to the luminal reduction may be present, as in AAS, with symptoms precipitated in some patients only by movement. Other congenital anomalies, such as odontoid hypoplasia, often reduce the threshold tolerance for traumatic injury and spinal instability; cord damage may result from seemingly trivial trauma.

Preanesthetic Evaluation

Patients with Down's syndrome and other congenital syndromes known to be associated with important cervical spinal anomaly should have clinical and radiographic evaluation of the cervical spine before receiving an anesthetic. Adequate assessment includes a review of the lateral cervical spine radiographs in the neutral, flexed, and extended positions for evidence of AAS. Measurements of the space available for the spinal cord (SAC) rather than the ADI may be of greater clinical relevance in an abnormal cervical spine. A difficult intubation should be anticipated in those patients with ankylosis and decreased neck mobility. Postoperatively, neck symptoms or altered neurologic status should be assessed. If present, they should prompt an urgent clinical and radiographic evaluation.

Asymptomatic patients with Down's syndrome do not routinely require radiographic evaluation of the cervical spine before anesthesia. However, preoperative radiographic assessment is recommended when endotracheal intubation is expected to be difficult, possibly requiring neck positioning at the extremes of the ranges of motion, or when the surgical procedure involves unusual head positioning or repeated manipulations of the head and neck.

The costal elements of the seventh cervical vertebra occasionally persist as cervical ribs. The brachial plexus may be compressed by the cervical rib as the plexus passes through the triangle formed by the musculus scalenus anticus and medius and the first rib, giving rise to the scalenus anticus syndrome. Additionally, a fibrous band in the musculus scalenus medius between the costotransverse elements of the C-7 vertebra and the first rib may compress the lower trunk of the brachial plexus and result in the scalenus medius syndrome. These syndromes are characterized by vague shoulder and upper extremity pain marked by positional exacerbation.

What Important Anatomic Changes Occur with Advancing Age?•

Degeneration of the cervical spinal joints and disk spaces is radiologically demonstrable in 80% to 90% of the population by age 40 years and is the result of normal aging. The radiologic changes of cervical spondylosis are listed in Table 27–3.[18] These changes are thought to result from the accumulated effects of years of weight bearing on the joints and desiccation of the disk. An age-associated reduction in normal lordosis, loss of joint cartilage and intervertebral disk height, and increased new bone formation in the cervical spine occur. These changes are common throughout the aging population, although in some patients they become apparent at an earlier age and follow a more rapidly progressive course.

Osteophyte formation is common, and new bone may encroach on spinal foramina or the canal, giving rise to root or cord compression, respectively. These changes usually do not interfere with tracheal intubation, although Lee reported difficulties related to hypertrophic bony changes on the anterior aspects of the C-5 to C-7 vertebral bodies.[19] Rotation and displacement of the trachea and difficulty achieving intubation were noted.

Ossification of the Posterior Longitudinal Ligament

Ossification of the posterior longitudinal ligament is a condition of unknown etiology,[20] usually occurring in the midcervical spine. The ligament is evident on a lateral radiograph as an ossified plaque of variable thickness, along the posterior margins of the vertebral bodies and disks. The ossified ligament may encroach on the spinal canal, producing cord or root lesions. Associated anterior osteophyte formation is common.

Diffuse Idiopathic Skeletal Hyperostosis

Diffuse idiopathic skeletal hyperostosis (DISH, ankylosing hyperostosis, Forestier's disease) is an ossifying diathesis in elderly patients that leads to spinal and extraspinal new bone formation as well as ligament calcification and ossification[21] (Fig. 27–9). Isolated or predominant cervical spine involvement has been reported, but thoracic and lumbar segments are more typically involved.

Abnormalities are more common in the lower cervical region and begin with cortical hyperostosis along the anterior surface of the vertebral body. Bony outgrowths eventually extend across the anterior intervertebral disk. Apophyseal joint narrowing is common, as is ossification of the ligamentum nuchae. Skip areas of involvement along the anterior spine are frequent; the posterior aspects of the vertebral bodies and the intervertebral disks are usually spared.

The more limited bony bridging of DISH causes less loss of motion and allows greater spinal flexibility than does ankylosing spondylitis.[22] Therefore, tracheal intubation is not likely to be rendered more difficult in patients with cervical spinal DISH. However, large anterior osteophytes may result in distortion of the airway and interfere with intubation.

TABLE 27–3. Radiologic Changes of Cervical Spondylosis

Narrowing of the disk space
Osteophyte formation at the anterior and posterior margins
  of the vertebral bodies
Vertebral endplate sclerosis
Osteoarthritic changes of the synovial joints
Ossification of the longitudinal ligaments
Narrowing of the sagittal diameter of the spinal canal

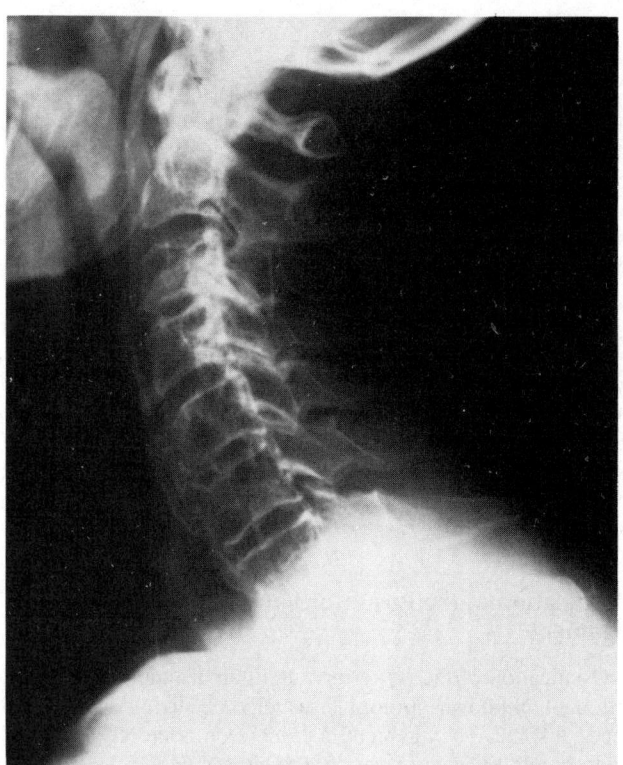

FIGURE 27–9. Diffuse idiopathic skeletal hyperostosis. Lateral view of the cervical spine. There is a large anterior osteophyte at C4 as well bridging osteophytes at C5-6 and C6-7. There is anterior bowing of the trachea over the osteophytes at the C5 to C7 levels.

What Factors Control Cervical Spinal Movement?

Flexion-extension occurs in the upper cervical spine at both the atlanto-occipital and atlantoaxial articulations; a combined 35° of motion may be achieved.[23] Flexion is limited by contact between the odontoid process and the anterior border of the foramen magnum at the atlanto-occipital articulation and by the tectorial membrane and posterior elements at the C-1 to C-2 level. Extension is limited by the contact of the posterior arch of the atlas with the occiput superiorly and with the arch of the axis inferiorly. A further 66° of flexion-extension may be achieved in the lower cervical spine, with the C-5 to C-7 segments contributing the largest component.[23]

Implications for Tracheal Intubation

The distance from the posterior arch of the atlas to the occiput is termed the *atlanto-occipital gap* (AOG); a narrow AOG has been cited as a common cause of difficult intubation.[20, 24] With the head in the sniffing position, the lower cervical spine is relatively straight. Curvature increases from C-4 to C-2, and the atlantoaxial complex is at or near full extension.

Attempts to extend the head farther in patients with a narrow AOG result in anterior bowing of the cervical spine, forward displacement of the larynx, and difficulty visualizing the larynx during laryngoscopy.[24] If difficulty in laryngeal visualization is encountered, additional neck flexion may facilitate intubation. A short interspace between the posterior

arches of the atlas and the axis may result in the same phenomenon, although to a lesser degree.[20]

Clinical Evaluation

Bedside evaluation of atlanto-occipital extension may be performed by having the patient sit straight and face directly to the front, with the head held erect. In this position, the occlusal surface of the upper teeth is horizontal and parallel to the ground. The patient extends the atlanto-occipital joint as much as possible, and the examiner estimates the angle traversed by the occlusal surface of the upper teeth. Any reduction in extension can be expressed as a fraction of normal (35°). This information may be used, in conjunction with other clinical information, to predict the probability of difficulty in both obtaining a line of vision during laryngoscopy and achieving endotracheal intubation.[25]

How Is Cervical Spinal Movement Affected by Advancing Age?

As age increases, cervical mobility decreases. Hayashi compared three groups of healthy volunteers ages 20 to 40, 40 to 60, and 60 to 82 years.[26] A 25% reduction in maximum flexion-extension occurred in the 60- to 82-year group compared with the 20- to 40-year group. Much of the lost range of motion occurs in the lower cervical spine and is not likely to result in difficult intubation. However, calcification of the anterior longitudinal ligament resulting in limitation of spinal movement has been reported as a rare cause of difficult intubation in elderly patients.[27]

How Do Inflammatory Arthropathies Alter Cervical Spine and Airway Anatomy?

The cervical spine is commonly involved in both adult- and juvenile-onset rheumatoid arthritis, with 43% to 70% of patients having symptoms referable to the neck and 17% to 86% demonstrating radiologic evidence of neck involvement.[28, 29]

Rheumatoid Arthritis

Atlantoaxial Subluxation

AAS is the most common radiographic finding in rheumatoid arthritis, occurring in 25% of patients. It results from attenuation or disruption of the transverse ligament, allowing for anterior movement of C-1 on C-2 during neck flexion. Radiographically, AAS is marked by an increase in the ADI. This change is best demonstrated on a lateral cervical spine radiograph with the neck flexed (Fig. 27–10).

Odontoid Subluxation

Vertical subluxation of the odontoid process through the foramen magnum and into the posterior fossa may occur in 4% to 35% of patients with rheumatoid arthritis, is far more common in elderly patients with severe and long-standing disease, and usually occurs in conjunction with anterior AAS.[30] As the odontoid process migrates superiorly and posteriorly, a

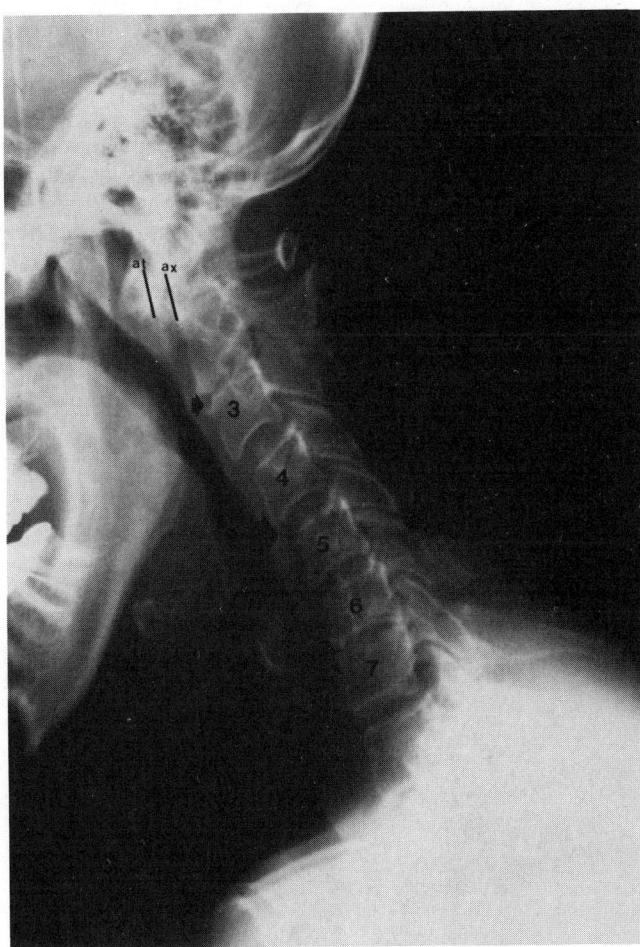

FIGURE 27–10. Rheumatoid arthritis. Lateral view of the cervical spine. There is generalized osteoporosis. Six millimeters of atlantoaxial subluxation is measured from the posterior aspects of the anterior arch of the atlas (at) and the anterior aspects of the odontoid process of the axis (ax). A subaxial subluxation is at C4-5, and vertebral endplate erosions are at C2-3 and C6-7.

larynx relative to the sternal notch is noted, resulting in difficult intubation (Fig. 27–13).

What Anatomic Structures Determine Cervical Spine Stability?

Stability is the property of the spine that, under conditions of physiologic loading, maintains vertebral relationships and prevents damage of the neural structures contained within the spinal column.[34] With instability, head and neck movement causes patterns of vertebral displacement that jeopardize the spinal cord or nerve roots.

severe reduction in the lumen of the spinal canal results (Fig. 27–11). Consequently, 10% to 50% of patients with the combined subluxation develop cord compression.[30, 31]

Ankylosing Spondylitis

Ankylosing spondylitis is an inflammatory arthropathy marked by increasing calcification and ankylosis of the axial skeleton.[32] Complete ankylosis of the cervical spine, characteristically in the flexed position, is the end result (Fig. 27–12).

Clinical Implications

Many patients with inflammatory arthropathies manifest a decrease in the safe range of neck motion, and spinal cord compromise can result from inappropriate neck manipulation. In addition, the mandibular space may be reduced by temporomandibular joint involvement, resulting in relative anterior positioning of the larynx and difficulty obtaining a line of vision for intubation.

A scoliotic deformity of the trachea and larynx secondary to neck shortening from vertical subluxation has been reported in patients with long-standing rheumatoid arthritis.[33] Laryngeal deviation may result, and a rotational malalignment of the

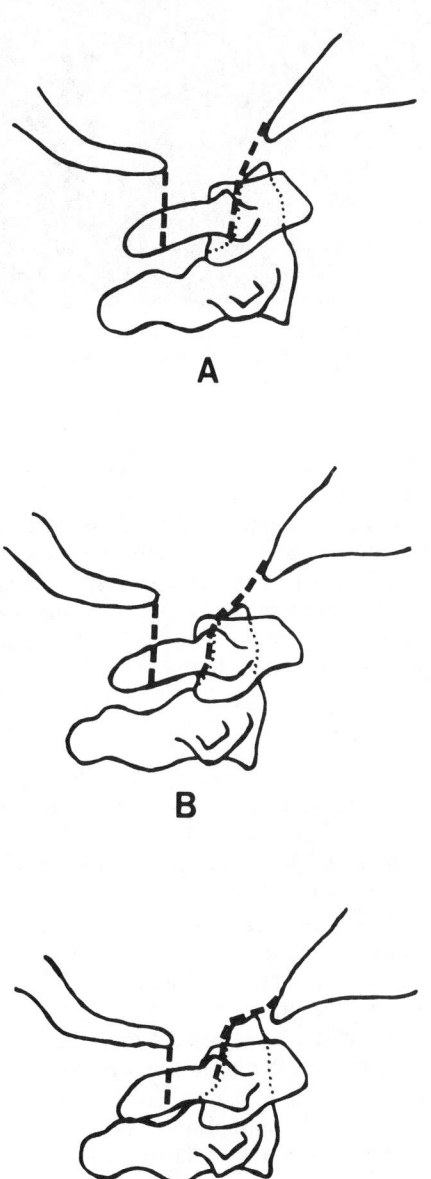

FIGURE 27–11. Atlantoaxial subluxation. Lateral views, occipitoatlantoaxial complex. The space available for the cord (SAC) is outlined by the *bold, dashed line.* The odontoid process is outlined by the *smaller dashed line. A,* Normal complex. *B,* Anterior subluxation. The SAC is decreased in the anteroposterior plane. *C,* Combined anterior and vertical subluxation. The SAC is severely reduced, with the potential for brainstem compression by the odontoid process. (From Crosby ET, Lui A: The adult cervical spine: implications for airway management. Can J Anaesth 1990; 37:77.)

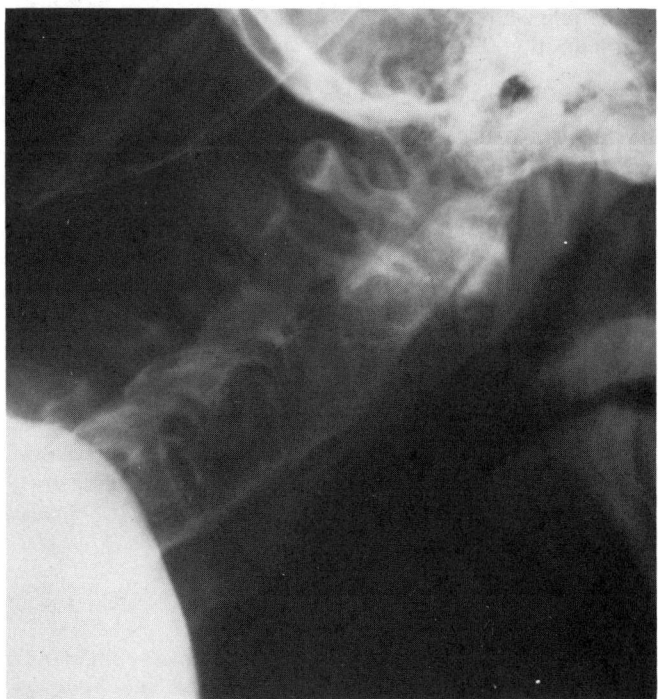

FIGURE 27–12. Ankylosing spondylitis. Lateral view of the cervical spine. There is fusion of the cervical spine as well as marked and generalized osteoporosis.

Although the neck muscles exert some stabilizing forces, the high incidence of secondary neurologic injury in trauma victims not initially recognized to be at risk for a spinal injury suggests that this muscle splint is insignificant. Conversely, the role of the ligamentous structures, intervertebral disks, and osseous articulations in determining stability has been demonstrated repeatedly. Conditions associated with instability of the cervical spine are listed in Table 27–4.

Upper Cervical Spine

Contributing to stability of the upper cervical spine complex are the transverse, apical, and alar ligaments and the superior terminations of the anterior and posterior longitudinal ligaments.[35] In adults, the transverse ligament normally allows no more than 3 mm of ADI anteroposterior translation. If the transverse ligament is disrupted but the alar and apical ligaments remain intact, as much as 5 mm of movement may be seen.[35] If all the ligaments are disrupted, 10 mm or more of displacement may result.

Significant posterior displacement of the dens reduces the SAC in the vertebral column. In a normal spine, the SAC at C-1 is approximately 20 mm. Cord compressions do not occur when the SAC is >18 mm but may occur if it is <14 mm.[36] Steel defined a rule of thirds.[37] The area of the vertebral canal at C-1 may be divided into one-third odontoid, one-third cord, and one-third "space." The one-third space allows some encroachment of the spinal lumen without cord compromise. However, once this margin of safety is compromised, compression of neural elements occurs.

Lower Cervical Spine

In the lower cervical spine, structures contributing to stability include, from anterior to posterior, the anterior longitudinal ligament, the intervertebral disks, the posterior longitudinal ligament, the facet joints with their capsular ligaments and the intertransverse ligaments, the interspinous ligament, and the supraspinous ligaments.[34, 38]

The posterior longitudinal ligament and the structures anterior to it are grouped as the anterior elements or anterior column. The posterior elements or posterior column comprises those elements behind the posterior ligament. The anterior column contributes more to the stability of the spine in extension, and the posterior column exerts its major forces in flexion.[38]

One element in an injured column must be preserved to achieve spinal stability. If a single column is disrupted, a small amount of movement in the opposite column is permissible, but none in the disrupted column. If both columns are likely to have been disrupted, no movement is permissible.

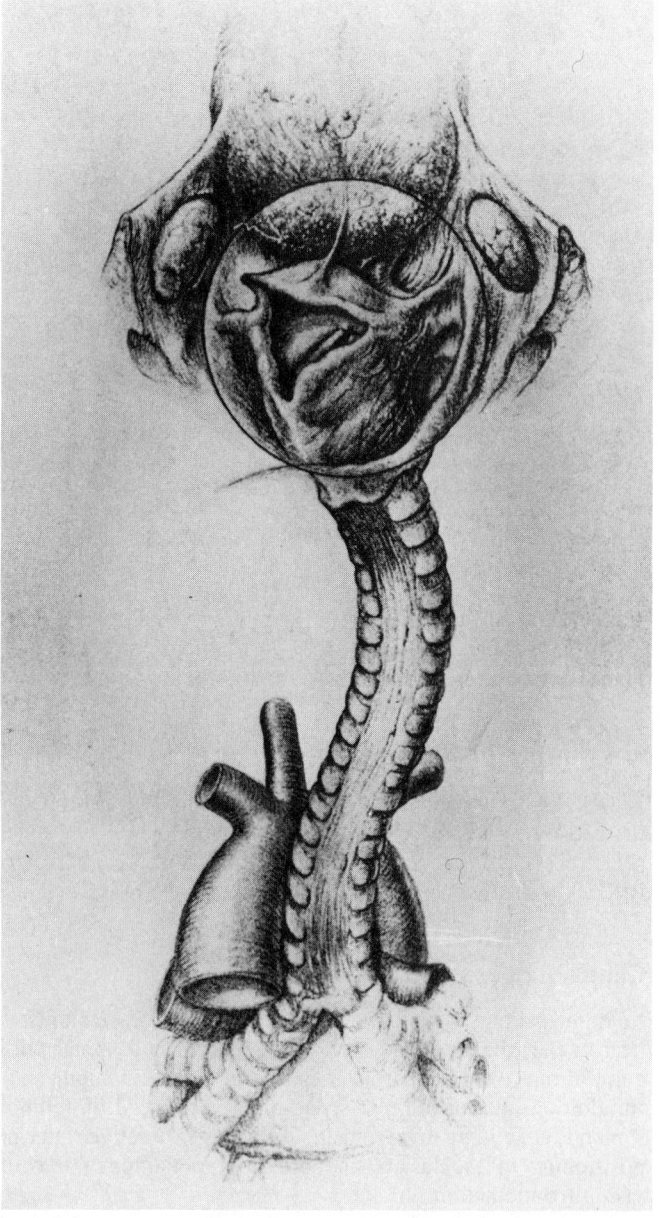

FIGURE 27–13. The airway in severe cervical spinal arthritis. The larynx is displaced anterolaterally, tilted forward and rotated. (From Keenan MA, Stiles CM, Kaufman RL: Acquired laryngeal deviation associated with cervical spine disease in erosive polyarticular arthritis. Anesthesiology 1983; 58:441.)

TABLE 27-4. Conditions Associated with Cervical Spinal Instability

Congenital	Isolated bony malformations
	Klippel-Feil syndrome
	Chromosomal anomalies
	Transverse ligament laxity
Inflammatory	Rheumatoid arthritis
	Juvenile rheumatoid arthritis
	Seronegative arthritides
	Ankylosing spondylitis
Infectious	Tuberculosis
	Osteomyelitis
	Grisel's syndrome
Neoplastic, benign	Bone cysts
	Histiocytosis X
	Osteoid osteoma
	Osteoblastoma
	Giant cell tumors
Neoplastic, malignant	Multiple myeloma
	Sarcomas
	Chordomas
Neoplastic, metastatic	Lung
	Breast
	Prostate
	Kidney
	Thyroid
Degenerative disorders	Cervical spondylosis
	Diffuse idiopathic skeletal hyperostosis (DISH)
	Ossification of the posterior longitudinal ligament
Trauma	

How Is the Cervical Spine Rendered Unstable by Injury?

Spinal injuries may be classified according to the mechanism of injury (Table 27-5; Fig. 27-14).

Flexion

Flexion injuries usually result from blows to the back of the head or forceful decelerations; they cause compression of the anterior column and distraction of the posterior column. Pure flexion trauma may result in wedge fracture of the vertebral body without ligamentous injuries. These injuries are stable and are rarely associated with neurologic injuries. With more extreme trauma, elements of the posterior column are disrupted as well, and bilateral facet joint dislocation may result. These injuries are unstable and are associated with a high incidence of cord damage.

Flexion-Rotation

Flexion-rotation injuries disrupt the posterior ligamentous complex and may produce unilateral facet joint dislocation. They tend to be stable and are not usually associated with spinal cord injury. However, cervical root injury is common.

Hyperextension

Hyperextension injuries result from a blow to the anterior part of the head or from an acceleration (whiplash) injury and cause compression of the posterior column and distraction of the anterior column. Hyperextension combined with compressive forces (e.g., diving injury) may result in injury to the lateral vertebral masses, pedicles, and laminae. Because both anterior and posterior columns are disrupted, this injury is unstable and is associated with a high incidence of cord dysfunction.

Violent hyperextension, with fracture of the pedicles of C-2 and forward movement of C-2 on C-3, produces a traumatic spondylolisthesis of the axis, or "hangman's fracture." The fracture is unstable, but the degree of neurologic compromise is highly variable, because the bilateral pedicular fractures serve to decompress the spinal cord at the site of injury.

Burst Fractures

Burst fractures are caused by compressive loading of the vertex of the skull in the neutral position and are not as common as flexion-extension injuries. Compressive forces in the lower cervical spine result in the explosion of compressed disk material into the vertebral body. Depending on the magnitude of the compression loading and associated angulating forces, the resulting injury ranges from loss of vertebral body height with relatively intact margins, to complete disruption of the vertebral body. Posterior displacement (retropulsion) of comminuted fragments may result, producing cord injury. Despite cord injury, the spine is usually stable.

What Are the Characteristics of Pediatric Cervical Spine Injury?

Cervical spine injury is a rare occurrence in the pediatric population.[7] Sixty per cent to 70% of pediatric spinal injuries occur in children older than 12 years, result largely from the same traumatic events that lead to adult injuries, and have a similar distribution. In children younger than 8 years, injuries are primarily restricted to the upper cervical spine. Children age 8 to 12 years have a distribution of injuries in transition from that of young children to that of adults.

An unusual pattern of cord injury in the pediatric population is that of spinal cord injury without radiographic abnormalities (SCIWORA).[7] It is most common in children younger than 8 years and is thought to result from mechanisms that lead to a disruption in the microvascular blood supply of the spinal

TABLE 27-5. Classification of Spinal Injuries by Mechanism of Injury

Hyperflexion	Anterior subluxation
	Bilateral interfacetal dislocation
	Wedge compression fracture
	Flexion teardrop fracture
Hyperflexion and rotation	Unilateral interfacetal dislocation
Hyperextension	Hyperextension fracture-dislocation
	Fracture of posterior arch of atlas
	Traumatic spondylolisthesis (hangman's fracture)
	Laminar fracture
Vertical compression	Wedge compression fracture
	Burst fracture
	Jefferson's burst fracture (C1)
Mixed mechanism	Atlanto-occipital dislocation
	Odontoid fractures
	Total ligamentous disruption

(From Crosby ET, Lui A: The adult cervical spine: implications for airway management. Can J Anaesth 1990; 37:77.)

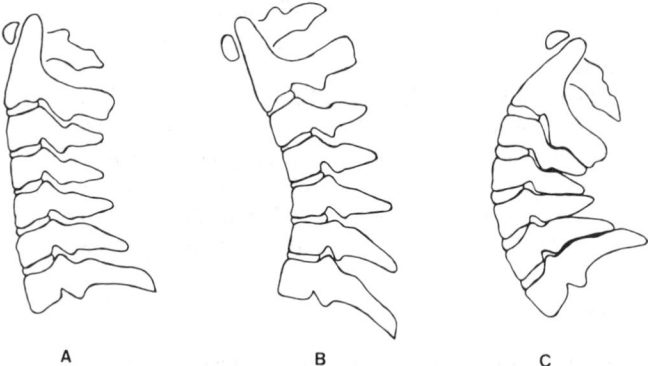

A   B   C

FIGURE 27–14. Mechanisms of injury. Lateral view, cervical spine. *A,* Normal. *B,* Hyperflexion with compression of the anterior elements and distraction in the posterior column. *C,* Hyperextension with compression of the posterior elements and distraction in the anterior column. (From Crosby ET, Lui A: The adult cervical spine: implications for airway management. Can J Anaesth 1990; 37:77.)

cord. Ligamentous laxity in an immature cervical spine may allow longitudinal distraction and flexion-compression of the spinal cord and has been cited as a possible explanation for SCIWORA.

Assessment

Interpretation of pediatric cervical spine radiographs may be perplexing. A number of normal variants that mimic spinal injury result from incomplete ossification and ligamentous laxity. Anterior wedging sometimes is seen in adjacent vertebrae in younger children and may represent incompletely ossified vertebrae. Pseudosubluxations are common in very young children. An ADI of up to 5 mm may be seen in normal individuals owing to normal laxity of the transverse ligament.[7] Finally, the indirect signs of injury, including loss of lordosis and increased retropharyngeal and retrotracheal soft tissue spaces, are even less specific in children than they are in adults.

What Are the Effects of Airway Maneuvers on the Injured Neck?

After surgical disruption of the anterior and most of the posterior column in a human cadaver, the effects of airway maneuvers were studied with lateral cervical spine radiographs.[39] Basic maneuvers included chin lift, jaw thrust, head tilt, and placement of oral and esophageal airways. Advanced maneuvers included placement of an esophageal obturator airway, insertion of an orotracheal tube using both straight and curved laryngoscope blades, and blind placement of a nasotracheal tube.

Chin lift and jaw thrust resulted in expansion of the disk space more than 5 mm at the site of injury. When blind nasotracheal intubation was effected with anterior pressure to stabilize the airway, 5 mm of posterior subluxation occurred at the site of injury. The other advanced airway maneuvers produced 3 to 4 mm of disk space enlargement. Maneuvers were then repeated after the application of soft and semi-rigid cervical collars. Neither type immobilized the neck effectively and consistently.

In-Line Traction

Bivins and colleagues studied the effects of in-line traction in deceased victims of blunt trauma.[40] In those cadavers without injury to the spinal column, in-line traction resulted in lengthening of the spinal column. When unstable spinal injuries were present, traction resulted in average distraction at the fracture site of 7.75 mm, with up to 4 mm of posterior subluxation. Traction during intubation produced less subluxation than occurred during intubation without traction, but the benefit was negated by the increased distraction at the injury site.

Of note is the fact that 21.8 kg of traction was applied across the neck using a head halter device. This amount is far in excess of what would be applied during conventional manual in-line stabilization during intubation.

THE THORACIC SPINE

What Are the Relevant Anatomic Characteristics?

Spinous Processes

The spinous processes of the 12 thoracic vertebrae are long and directed caudally. From T-1 to T-4, they are bladelike and project backward at an angle of about 40° from the perpendicular. The middle four spinous processes are longer and directed at an angle of 60°, with the spines completely overlapping the subjacent vertebrae. The spines of the four most inferior thoracic vertebrae resemble the first four in direction and shape.

Flexion and Extension

Rib attachments to the upper segments of the thoracic spine limit flexion-extension of this area; these movements become freer in the lower thoracic segments. Flexion increases the interlaminar distance, allowing easier access to the intraspinal space. A slight cephalad displacement of the termination of the spinal cord occurs with flexion, allowing safe insertion of a spinal needle even at the level of L-2 to L-3.

Spinal Cord

The spinal cord is enlarged in two regions of the thoracic spine.[41] The cervical enlargement includes the C-3 to T-2 cord segments and is found at the corresponding vertebral levels. The lumbar enlargement is composed of the L-1 to S-3 cord segments and extends from the body of T-11 to that of L-1. The spinal cord is widest in the upper thorax (9 mm), narrows through the midthorax (6.5–8 mm), and is expanded again in the lower thorax (7–9 mm) before terminating in the conus medullaris in the upper lumbar spine.[42]

Epidural Space

The dorsal epidural space is narrowest in its midsagittal dimension in the upper thorax (3–4 mm), increases through the midthorax (3–5 mm), and is largest at the thoracolumbar junction (4–6 mm).

Based on these considerations, the optimum site for performing a thoracic epidural anesthetic is in the midthoracic spine; here the narrowest portion of the spinal cord is associated with a relatively wide epidural space. However, this is the site of the most extreme angulation of the spinous processes, and the midline approach may be difficult.

How Is Epidural Puncture Achieved?

Midline Approach

When approaching the thoracic epidural space, consider both the size of the spinal cord and the orientation of the spinous processes at the different spinal levels. At T-1, the spinous process is almost horizontal, and the epidural space is easily reached by the midline approach.

In the midthorax, between T-4 and T-8, the midline approach is feasible only with the needle directed at an angle of 60° or more from the perpendicular (Fig. 27–15). The needle may enter the epidural space at 7 cm or more from the skin.

The advantage of the midline approach for an anesthesiologist experienced with lumbar epidural blocks is that it provides the security and ''feel'' associated with traversing the usual

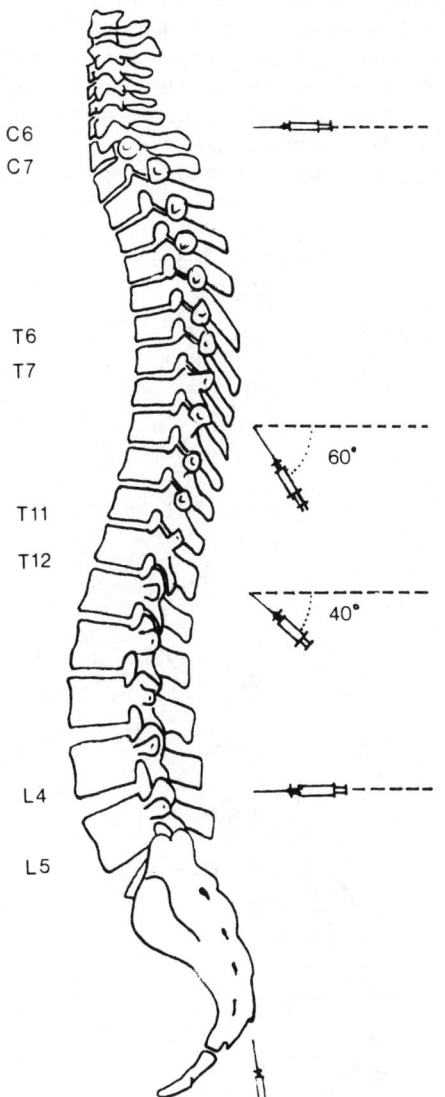

FIGURE 27–15. Lateral aspect of the vertebral column illustrating the angle of needle entry required with the midline approach to access the intraspinal space.

TABLE 27–6. Etiologic Classification of Scoliosis

Idiopathic
Neuromuscular
Congenital
Neurofibromatosis
Mesenchymal disorders
Rheumatoid disease
Trauma
Osteochondrodystrophies
Metabolic disorders
Tumors

ligamentous structures. The midline approach becomes more straightforward below T-8, where the spines are shorter and less acutely angulated and the vertebral segment can be flexed to optimize access to the interlaminar space (see Fig. 27–15).

Paramedian Approach

The paramedian approach avoids the sharp angulations approach in the midthorax and the longer distance to the epidural space. This technique may provide the only access to the epidural space when the bony elements deter midline access. A key to success in using the paramedian approach is to enter immediately beside the spinous process. This method avoids being so far lateral that the needle never encounters the ligamentum flavum and reduces the likelihood of entering the epidural space in its narrow lateral aspects. The risk of a failed epidural block or accidental dural puncture may be reduced.

How Are Abnormal Curvatures of the Spine Described?

The terms *scoliosis, kyphosis, lordosis,* and combinations of *kyphoscoliosis* or *lordoscoliosis* are often encountered. *Scoliosis* (derived from the Greek word *skoliosis,* meaning ''crookedness'') refers to a lateral curvature of the spine. *Kyphosis,* meaning ''humpback,'' describes a backward convexity of the spine, and *lordosis* describes a forward convexity of the spine. For the purpose of this discussion, only the classification of scoliosis is presented, because it is representative of spinal deformity in general and covers most of the etiologies (Table 27–6).

Congenital abnormalities of the subcervical spine are the result of defects in formation or segmentation (Fig. 27–16). Failure to form the lateral aspects of the vertebral body results in formation of a hemivertebra, manifested clinically as scoliosis. Pure defects in the formation of the anterior vertebral body result in kyphosis. Mixed defects are common and result in kyphoscoliosis and lordoscoliosis.[43] Symmetric defects of segmentation result in ''block'' vertebrae, whereas asymmetric defects result in an unsegmented bar, the location and lesion determining the curvature of the spine.

What Problems Are Associated with Scoliosis?

Scoliotic curves can be subdivided into structural and nonstructural variants. Nonstructural curves are those seen in postural scoliosis or related to sciatica or leg length discrepancies;

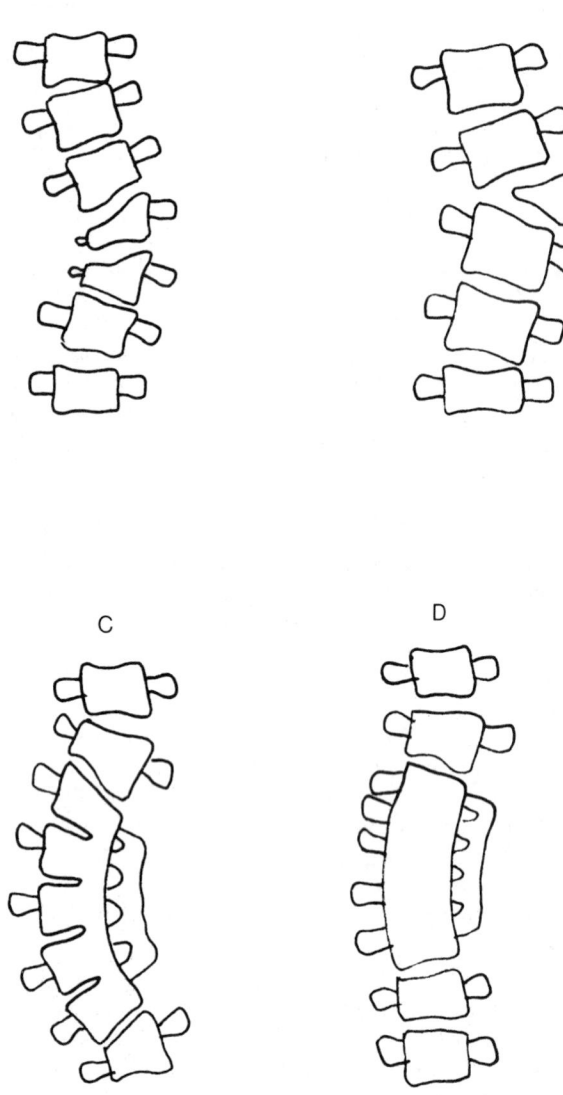

FIGURE 27–16. Congenital deformities of the spine, mechanisms for failed development. *A*, Partial unilateral failure of formation. *B*, Complete unilateral failure of formation. *C*, Unilateral failure of segmentation. *D*, Bilateral failure of segmentation.

they are nonprogressive. The spine appears completely normal on clinical and radiographic examination.

Structural curves are associated with spinal rotation as well as lateral curvature. The direction of rotation is into the convexity of the curvature, such that the spinous processes point toward the concavity (Fig. 27–17). This observation is of obvious consequence when one performs an epidural block. The majority of structural curves are idiopathic. The remaining cases are associated with syndromes or diseases that pose unique anesthetic challenges (Table 27–7) in addition to those considerations relating to the spinal deformity.

Cardiopulmonary Dysfunction

Growth and Development of the Lungs

Although the incidence of respiratory failure in scoliosis is unknown, the deterioration in pulmonary function correlates with the severity of the curvature.[44, 45] Scoliosis interferes with

the formation, growth, and development of the lungs. Because the number of alveoli increases by a factor of 10 between birth and age 8 years, the occurrence of scoliosis before lung maturity may reduce the number of alveoli formed. The pulmonary vasculature forms in parallel with the alveoli and is likewise affected, resulting in increased pulmonary resistance and, in severe cases, right heart failure.

Ventricular Perfusion Abnormalities

The most common blood gas abnormality is an increased alveolar-to-arterial oxygen partial pressure gradient. The reduction in arterial oxygen content coupled with normal levels of carbon dioxide suggests ventilation/perfusion mismatch with venoarterial shunting and altered regional perfusion.

Mechanical Function

The pulmonary pathophysiology of scoliosis also includes the effects of the vertebral and rib cage deformity on the mechanical function of the lungs. The most common pulmonary function abnormality is a restrictive pattern with reduction in vital capacity, total lung capacity, and lung compliance. This pattern is encountered in all patients with thoracic curves >65°. The rotation of the spine and thoracic cage puts the lungs at a mechanical disadvantage, and the work of breathing may increase to five times normal.[46]

Other factors that may impair lung function in patients with

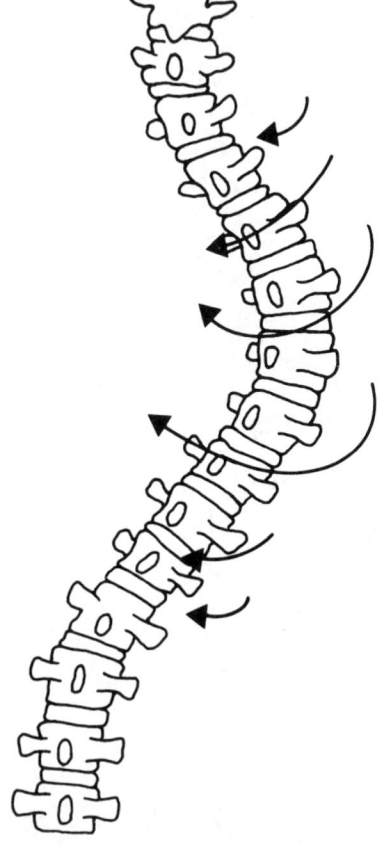

FIGURE 27–17. Idiopathic scoliosis. Both lateral curvature and rotation of the spine occur. The direction of the rotation is such that the spinous processes rotate into the concavity of the lateral curve.

TABLE 27–7. Anesthetic Considerations in Patients with Scoliosis

Syndrome	Anesthetic Considerations
Idiopathic scoliosis (>65°)	Mitral valve prolapse, pulmonary hypertension, right ventricular hypertrophy, restrictive respiratory defect
Neuropathic disorders (cerebral palsy)	Recurrent pneumonia, upper airway obstruction, malnutrition, difficult vascular access, positioning difficulties
Myopathic disorders (muscular dystrophy, myotonia, central core disease)	Cardiomyopathy, mitral valve prolapse, arrhythmias, respiratory failure, upper airway obstruction, altered responses to neuromuscular blockers, hyperkalemia with succinylcholine, malignant hyperthermia
Neurofibromatosis	Pulmonary valvular stenosis, fibrosing alveolitis, airway obstruction, pheochromocytoma
Mesenchymal disorders (Marfan's syndrome)	Aortic dissection and incompetence
Rheumatoid disease (rheumatoid arthritis)	Pericarditis, valvular involvement, pulmonary fibrosis, pleural effusions, atlantoaxial subluxation, Felty's syndrome, positioning difficulties
Osteochondrodystrophies (Morquio's syndrome)	Aortic valvular incompetency, heart failure, atlantoaxial instability
Metabolic disorders (osteogenesis imperfecta)	Aortic valvular incompetence, abnormal platelets, positioning difficulties

scoliosis include associated lordosis, poor muscle function, and reduced distensibility of the lungs.

Associated Cardiac Abnormalities

Roth and colleagues suggested that scoliosis and cardiac anomalies have common embryogenic etiology.[47] In adolescent scoliosis, the incidence of mitral valve prolapse exceeds 25%.[48] Children with congenital heart disease have an increased incidence of scoliosis. A high incidence of right ventricular hypertrophy and hypertensive pulmonary vascular changes is found at autopsy in patients with thoracic scoliosis. A wide variety of disease processes, ranging from neuromuscular disorders to inborn errors of metabolism, are associated with scoliosis. With each disease or syndrome, associated cardiovascular abnormalities also may be present.[49]

What Are the Mechanisms of Injury to the Thoracolumbar Spine?

The 17 vertebrae that form the thoracolumbar spine are designed to support the body in an erect position and to allow limited motion of the trunk. In the thoracic region, the rib cage restricts motion to a minimum degree of flexion, as experienced during normal respiration. Below T-8, the costal attachments are less rigid, permitting increased mobility in forward flexion, lateral flexion, extension, and some rotatory motion.

The basic mechanisms of injury to the thoracolumbar spine are flexion, extension, rotation, and shear. Flexion accounts for almost 85% of injuries. Because the natural curvature of the thoracic spine is predominantly one of flexion, a vertical force acting on the spine increases the flexion. The resultant injury is a wedge fracture of the vertebral body. As the vertical compressive force is increased, the likelihood of a comminution injury to the vertebral body is presented. Retropulsion of a comminuted fragment into the canal may result in cord injury.

When Is the Thoracic Spine Unstable?

As with the cervical spine, stability of the thoracic column depends on the integrity of not only the skeletal components but also the ligaments, intervertebral disks, and facet joints.

Thoracic instability is defined by Denis's three-column concept of the spine.[50] The anterior column extends from the anterior longitudinal ligament to a vertical line drawn through the middle and posterior third of the vertebral body. The middle zone extends from this line to the posterior longitudinal ligament. The posterior zone extends from the posterior longitudinal ligament to the supraspinous ligament. Instability occurs when injury disrupts the middle zone.

THE LUMBAR SPINE

What Are the Relevant Anatomic Characteristics?

In the lumbar spine, the spinous processes are oriented more horizontally. When the spine is flexed, access to the spinal canal through the interlaminar space becomes relatively easy (Fig. 27–18). The neural canal becomes more triangular in the lumbar region, and the epidural space is increased to 5 to 6 mm in its anterior-posterior dimension.

Plicae Mediana Dorsalis and Posterior Dural Fold

Dissection and injection studies have demonstrated a midline connective tissue membrane (plicae mediana dorsalis) as well as a posterior dural fold in the lumbar epidural space.[51, 53] Both the plicae and the median dural fold tend to be consistent through several successive lumbar vertebral levels and have the effect of dividing the posterior lumbar epidural space into two dorsolateral compartments. These structures have been cited as the etiologic factors responsible for unilateral epidural blockade[51, 53, 54] (Fig. 27–19).

Posterior Epidural Fat Pad

Hogan, using cryomicrotome technology, was unable to demonstrate the posterior midline epidural septa but did describe the consistent presence of a posterior epidural fat pad and a midline pedicle for the pad.[1] It is likely that these structures represent the same structure labeled the plicae mediana dorsalis.[52, 53]

EXTENSION

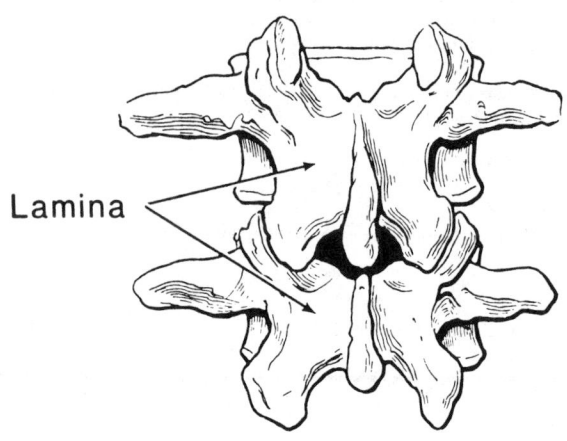

Lamina

FLEXION

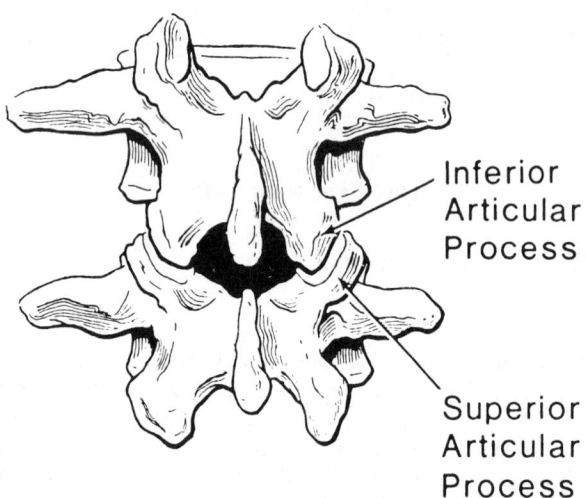

Inferior
Articular
Process

Superior
Articular
Process

FIGURE 27–18. Interlaminar space, lumbar region, in flexion and extension. In extension, the boundaries are the roots of spinous processes and the laminae. With flexion, the space is widened in both dimensions, and the new lateral boundaries are the articular processes. (From Cousins MJ: Epidural neural blockade. *In* Neural Blockade in Clinical Anesthesia and Management of Pain. Cousins MJ, Bridenbaugh PO (eds). Philadelphia, JB Lippincott, 1980, p 192.)

Anterior Epidural Space

A consistent feature that may be responsible for unilateral blockade is the small and discontinuous anterior epidural space. When the tip of the catheter is positioned in the anterolateral aspects of the epidural space, inadequate block may result as the injected local anesthetic solution spreads predominantly ipsilaterally[55] (Fig. 27–20). Bilateral blockade is dependent on retrograde flow around the dura in the posterior epidural space. Large volumes of local anesthetic solution that approach or exceed the recommended safe dose may be required for some patients. A technique to salvage inadequate epidural blockade uses large volumes of the relatively nontoxic local anesthetic chloroprocaine.[56]

What Are the Common Congenital Anomalies of the Lumbar Spine?

Spina Bifida

Spina bifida refers to the condition of failed closure of the neural arch. Spina bifida cystica is marked by herniation of the meninges (meningocele) or the meninges and neural elements (myelomeningocele) through the vertebral defect. These conditions are relatively uncommon, occurring in 1 to 3 in 1000 births.[57] Neurologic deficits involving the lower extremities and sphincters are common. Although regional anesthesia has been reported in patients with spina bifida cystica, experience is limited.[58, 59]

Spina bifida occulta is the failed fusion of the neural arch without herniation of meninges or neural elements and is much more common, occurring in about 5% to 36% of the population.[60, 61] Superficial signs of a lesion include a tuft of hair, cutaneous angioma, lipoma, or skin dimple, but they are not invariable. Unlike the cystica syndrome, patients with spina bifida occulta usually do not have symptoms related to their anomaly.

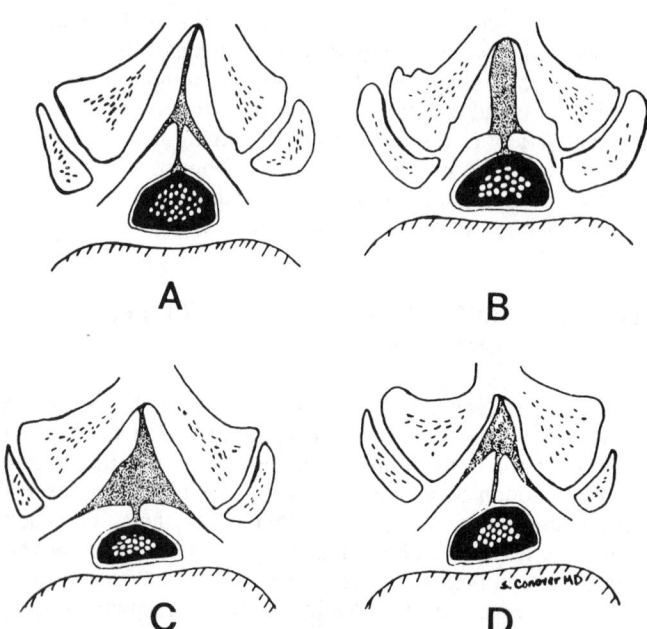

A   B

C   D

FIGURE 27–19. The plicae mediana dorsalis. The anatomic configuration of both the plicae and the posterior epidural space approximates one of the four general patterns determined by the amount and location of fatty material deposited between the membranes. *A*, Seven of 40 patients showed thin linear membranes with minimal fatty content. *B*, Two of 40 patients showed a somewhat thicker configuration of the plica but still retained a linear orientation. *C*, Eighteen of 40 patients showed a large triangular junction of membranes, with copious fat contributing to the extra bulk of the midline structure. Such a configuration might impede or deflect an epidural catheter or, perhaps, even receive injection of solutions within the midline structure itself. *D*, Thirteen of 40 patients demonstrated a smaller triangular membrane junction located posteriorly on the plica. The junction produced less bulk but, by virtue of its location, could possibly interfere with catheter introduction through a Tuohy needle. (From Savolaine ER, Pandya JB, Greenblatt SH, et al: Anatomy of the human lumbar epidural space: new insights using CT-epidurography. Anesthesiology 1988; 68:217.)

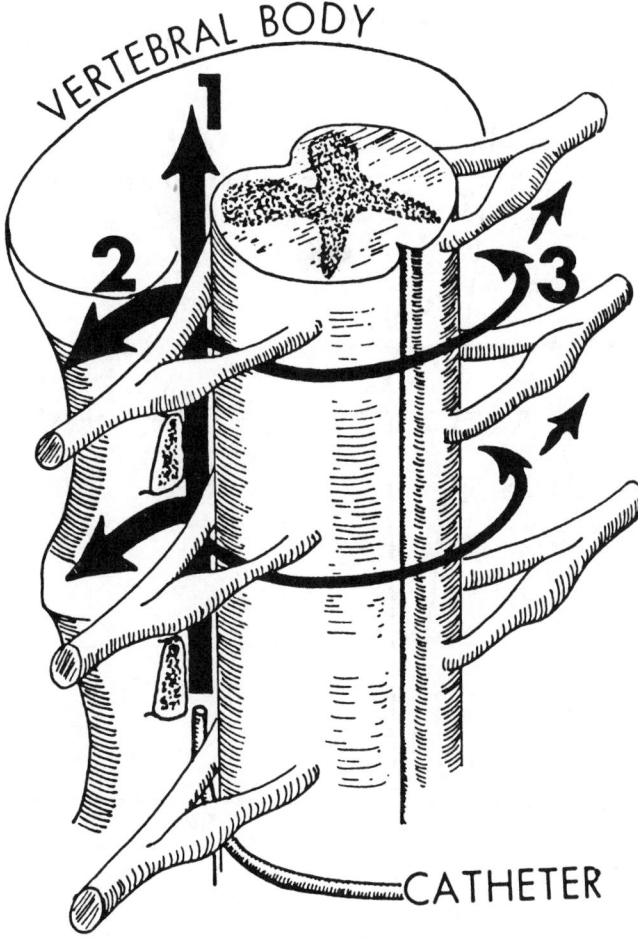

FIGURE 27–20. With the tip of the catheter in the anterior or anterolateral epidural space, longitudinal (1) and ipsilateral transverse (2) spread of the local anesthetic solution predominates. The magnitude of the circumferential spread around the dura (3) determines the quality of contralateral blockade. (From Usubiaga JE, Dos Reis A, Usubiaga LE: Epidural misplacement of catheters and mechanisms of unilateral blockade. Anesthesiology 1970; 32:158.)

Epidural Blockade

Because of the absent lamina and variable formation of the ligamentum flavum at the site, the epidural space may be incompletely formed, discontinuous, or even absent across the level of the lesion. Attempted epidural block performed over an occulta lesion is unpredictable and likely to result in dural puncture. Successful epidural analgesia has been reported with the catheter situated within the zone of the lesion.[57] It is possible that flow of anesthetic solutions through the lateral and anterolateral epidural spaces may be sufficient to extend a block beyond the level of the lesion.

Despite its common occurrence in the population, spina bifida occulta is rarely a clinical problem in regional anesthesia. This observation is likely accounted for by two factors. First, the lesions most commonly occur at the L-5 to S-1 levels, below the levels at which the majority of major regional blocks are performed.[59, 61] Second, the most common anomaly is a simple midline split in the lamina; it is unlikely to interfere with either the performance or development of an epidural block. Although more extensive occulta lesions involving multiple vertebral segments have been reported, they are not as common as the more limited lesions.[61]

Tethered Cord

The spinal cord may be attached (tethered) to a congenitally abnormal structure in the lumbar spine in patients with spina bifida.[61, 62] This condition is marked by a low-lying (L2–3) conus medullaris anchored by a thick filum terminale.[63] Magnetic resonance imaging studies show that tethering is present in virtually all patients with myelomeningocele. What percentage of patients with spina bifida occulta have a tethered cord is unclear, but the incidence is low. The implication of the tethered cord for regional anesthesia is that the terminal portion of the spinal cord lies at a lower than normal vertebral level, and care must be taken to identify the lowermost cord level before attempting intraspinal block.

Scoliosis

Scoliosis is a lateral deviation in the vertical axis of the spine, encountered most commonly in females. Minor thoracolumbar curves are common, whereas uncorrected major curves are less frequently seen. A rotatory component is associated with the scoliotic curve, as was noted earlier, and the axial rotation of the vertebral body is always into the convexity of the lateral curve so that the spinous process rotates back into the concavity[64] (see Fig. 27–17). Hence, the midline of the epidural space is deviated toward the convexity of the curve relative to the spinous process palpable at the skin level.

The needle should enter the selected interspace and be directed toward the convexity of the curve. An experienced individual can track the resistance and feel both the interspinous ligament and the ligamentum flavum to maintain a true course into the epidural space. Minor functional curves, such as those commonly seen in term pregnant women, rarely result in any significant rotatory deviation of the vertebrae. Little if any accommodation in technique is required for successful needle or catheter placement.

What Age-Related Changes Occur in the Lumbar Spine?

With advancing age, desiccation of the intervertebral disks and loss of disk height occur. Osteoporosis, occurring especially in women, leads to compression fractures that are common to the weight-bearing vertebrae of the lumbar spine. Both processes tend to diminish separation of the posterior elements of the lumbar spine and result in smaller interlaminar spaces. In addition, osteophyte formation and ligamentous ossification result in encroachment of foramina and interspaces and may, as well, result in smaller interlaminar spaces. The net result is greater difficulty as attempts are made to pass a needle into either the epidural or subarachnoid spaces.

How Deep Is the Epidural Space?

In the majority of adults, the epidural space lies 4 to 6 cm below the skin.[65–69] The depth increases from L2-3 to L4-5, but the difference is not great.[65, 67] Increasing weight and body mass index correlate with increasing depth, but maternal height reportedly does not.[65, 66] This difference is likely an artifact of small study population size, with few patients at the extremes of height being assessed; depth probably does correlate with height at the extremes of height. In support of this hypothesis is Mieklejohn's observation that women of Asian races with smaller stature had epidural spaces that were less distant from the skin than taller European females.[69]

In very few adults is the epidural space <3 cm from the skin.[65-69] Thus a perceived loss of resistance at 3 cm or less from the skin rarely identifies the epidural space. A depth of >7 cm is also relatively uncommon.[65-69] Narang and Linter reported that as the depth of the space increased, so did the incidence of unsatisfactory blocks.[68] It was suggested that the greater distance traveled was associated with an increased likelihood that the epidural space was entered in its lateral aspects, with obvious implications for both local anesthetic distribution and the resultant block (Fig. 27–21). Although Narang and Linter reported that only 2.8% of patients have a space 6 cm or more from the skin, others have noted incidences of such depth from 13% to 20%.[65-67, 69]

Finally, Harrison observed that the distance to the space increases as the needle is angled off the perpendicular.[67] However, the error introduced is relatively small and is likely to increase the depth of the space by only 0.2 to 0.3 cm.

What Changes Occur with Pregnancy?

Back Pain

An increase in the lumbar lordotic curve occurs during pregnancy as the pelvis rotates forward. This alteration exaggerates the normal loads borne by the posterior aspects of the intervertebral disks and the zygapophyseal joints. Back pain is common, occurring in about half of all parturients at some point during their pregnancy.[70] The pain is usually related to softening of the sacroiliac and pubic ligaments, with resultant mechanical instability in these joints. True pathology (i.e., herniated disk) related to pregnancy is uncommon; it should be recognized and distinguished from the more benign forms of gestational back problems.[71, 72]

Spinal Canal And Epidural Venous Plexus

As a result of caval obstruction caused by a gravid uterus, enhanced blood flow occurs through the vertebral venous plexus, with engorgement of the epidural venous plexus (Fig. 27–22). The result is a decrease of the cerebrospinal fluid volume, smaller relative spinal canal volume, and lower volume requirements for local anesthetics during major regional blockade.[73] Additionally, an increased risk of epidural vascular trauma occurs in parturients, compared with nonpregnant patients. This risk may be reduced by using softer catheters and perhaps by injecting a volume of saline or local anesthetic through the epidural needle before attempting to pass the catheter.[74, 75]

How Deep Is the Epidural Space Via the Paramedian Approach?

Blomberg compared the median and paramedian approaches to the epidural space using fiberoptic epiduroscopy[76] (Fig. 27–23). In the 14 subjects studied, the epidural space was an average 9.3 mm farther from the skin with the paramedian approach than with the median approach. Once loss of resis-

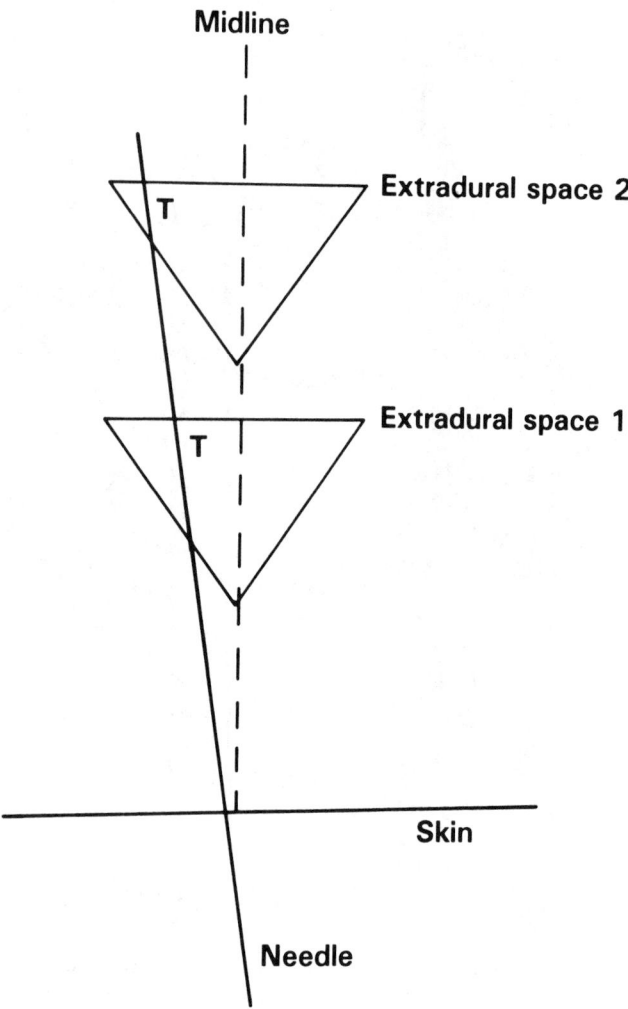

FIGURE 27–21. Diagram showing increasing lateral displacement of the tip of the needle (T) as the skin–to–extradural space distance increases from extradural space 1 to epidural space 2. (From Narang VPS, Linter SPK: Failure of extradural blockade in obstetrics. Br J Anaesth 1988; 60:402.)

tance to air was recognized, the needle could travel another 3.9 mm until dural contact with the median approach, compared with 7.6 mm with the paramedian approach. On this basis, accidental dural puncture was concluded to be more likely with the median approach.

With the midline technique, the catheter entered the space at right angles, and the catheter caused tenting of the dura in all subjects. By comparison, with the paramedian approach, the catheter entered the space at 120° to 135° to the dura and did not cause dural tenting. It was concluded that the risk of dural puncture by the catheter was greater with the median technique.

The catheter moved in a cephalad direction in all cases in the paramedian trial but in only 29% of the median attempts. It moved laterally in the epidural space in 64% of the median insertions, theoretically increasing the risk for blood vessel trauma with the median technique.

This study appears to confirm the advantages cited for the paramedian approach: a lower incidence of accidental dural puncture, blood vessel cannulation, and paresthesia and a straighter, predictable course for the catheter in the epidural space. However, comparisons of the techniques do not dem-

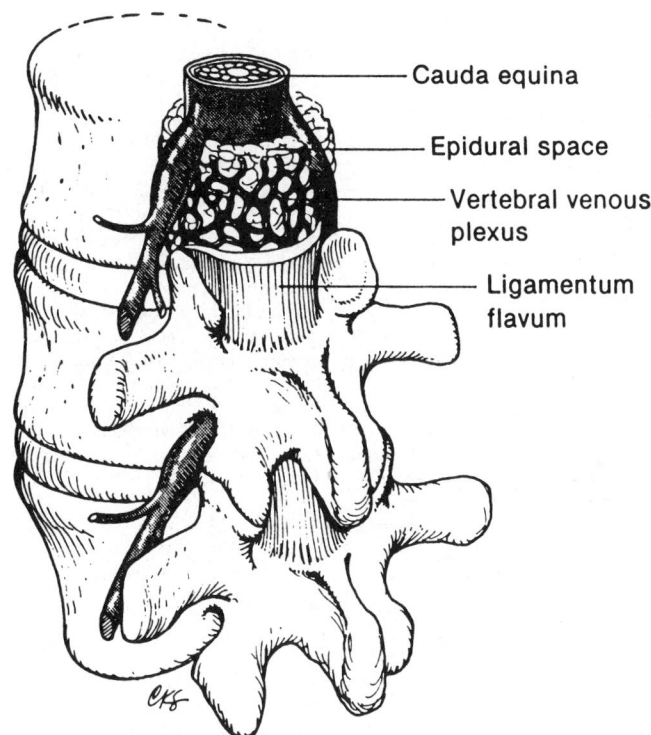

Cauda equina

Epidural space

Vertebral venous plexus

Ligamentum flavum

FIGURE 27–22. Epidural venous plexus. The large epidural venous plexus may become engorged with increased intra-abdominal pressure and during pregnancy. (From Reisner LS, Ellis J: Epidural and caudal puncture. *In* Clinical Procedures in Anesthesia and Intensive Care. Benumof JL (ed). Philadelphia, JB Lippincott, 1992, p 663.)

onstrate a consistent, clinically important advantage for the paramedian technique.[77, 78]

Is a Paramedian Approach Really More Difficult?

Blomberg and colleagues reported a higher incidence of difficult insertions and difficulty encountered in identifying the epidural space, as well as catheter-related problems with the median approach.[79] However, their reported incidence of difficulties with the median approach is much higher than that reported by others, thus skewing their comparison.

Jaucot, reporting more than 1000 epidurals, described no important differences between median and paramedian techniques.[77] A slightly increased incidence of paresthesias, blood vessel puncture, and inability to pass the catheters was recorded in the midline approach group, but the overall incidences of these events were small. The success rate on the first attempt was 94.5% with the median approach and 98% with the paramedian approach, not an important difference.

Finally, Griffin and Scott reported similar success with catheter placement, difficulty locating the space, analgesia on the first attempt, the incidence of passing the catheter, and blood vessel cannulation.[78] A higher incidence of pain was observed with the paramedian approach but was attributed to the small volumes of local anesthetic used to provide anesthesia.

Why Does Low Back Pain Occur?

Pain may arise from three distinct anatomic areas in the spinal column, each of which gives rise to a characteristic pain syndrome[80] (Fig. 27–24).

Type A Pain

Type A pain originates in the motion segments and associated ligamentous and muscular structures and is most common. It is a dull, deep, aching pain, poorly localized, and it is not associated with neurologic findings.

Type B Pain

Type B pain arises in the superficial structures of the vertebral column and is usually well localized to the area of injury.

Type C Pain

Type C pain is caused by involvement of nerve trunks associated with the vertebral column. It is a sharp radiating pain that is often referred and is associated with neurologic findings.

Spinal pain may originate from one anatomic structure, but because injuries may not be so limited, various degrees of overlap of pain type do occur. The majority of instances of acute low back pain are types A and B or combinations thereof and represent minor self-limited injuries to the motion segments and adjacent structures. The pain of these acute injuries may be reproduced by injection of hypertonic saline into supraspinous, interspinous, and longitudinal ligaments, ligamenta flava, and the facet joint capsules.[81, 82]

In about 1% of these cases, prolapse of the nucleus pulposus occurs with compression of neural elements, resulting in type C pain (sciatica). This injury most commonly occurs in the L-4 to L-5 or L-5 to S-1 motion segments in patients 20 to 50 years of age.[83]

What Makes Back Pain Chronic?

Three months after an episode of acute low back pain, only about 5% of patients have persistent symptoms and chronic low back pain. A number of conditions are associated with chronic low back pain[84] (Table 27–8). Anatomic features common to many of these conditions are hypertrophic bony changes and disk degeneration. The bony changes may reduce the lumen of the spinal or nerve root canal and result in chronic compression of neural elements and pain.

When the disk degenerates, changes occur throughout the motion segment, any or all of which may result in pain. Load bearing of the facet joints is increased, distribution of stress concentration is altered in the endplates and the subchondral bone of the vertebrae, and encroachment on the nerve root canal occurs. Finally, an increased demand is placed on intersegmental muscles and ligaments to stabilize the motion segments.[85]

The association between abnormal anatomy and pain is not entirely clear, because these pathologic conditions, including disk degenerations and herniations, are found in many asymptomatic patients.[83] In a significant proportion of patients with chronic low back pain, no anatomic pathology is demonstrable.

What Are the Effects of Spinal Injury and Surgery on the Epidural Space?

Intervertebral Disk Abnormalities

Benzon and colleagues reported that the onset of epidural anesthesia was delayed in patients with back pain or sciatica,

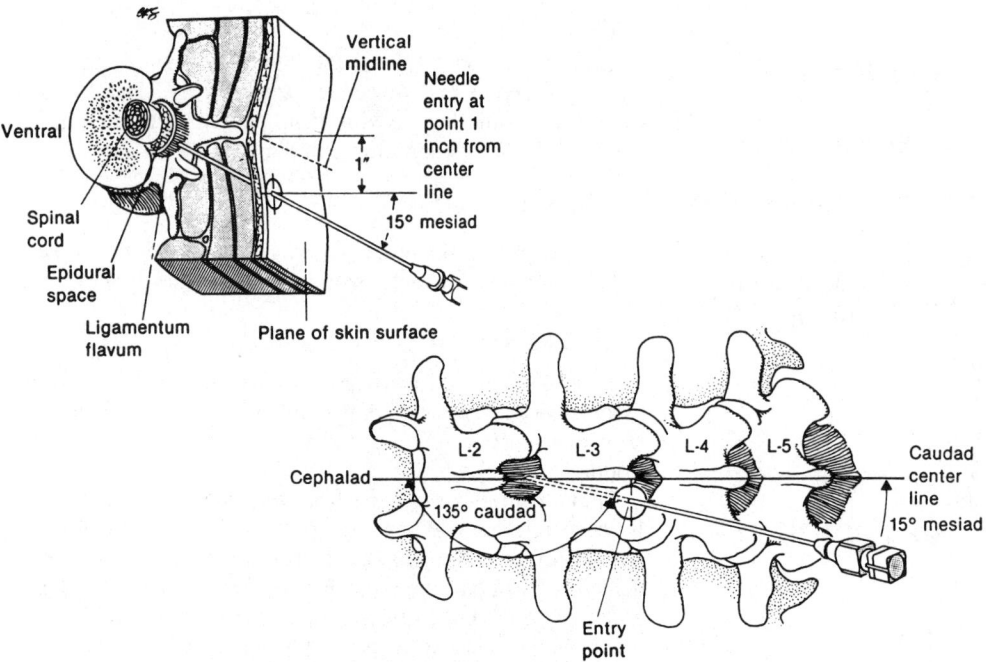

FIGURE 27–23. Epidural puncture: paramedian approach. The paramedian approach avoids the overlap of spinous processes but is not characterized by the same feel as the midline approach because the supraspinous and interspinous ligaments are avoided. (From Reisner LS, Ellis J: Epidural and caudal puncture. *In* Clinical Procedures in Anesthesia and Intensive Care. Benumof JL (ed). Philadelphia, JB Lippincott, 1992, p 663.)

the affected roots being blocked 10 to 70 minutes later than contralateral roots at the same level.[86] Central disk herniations resulted in delayed onset of the block beyond the level of the lesion. Delay in block onset was suggested to result from the inability of local anaesthetic to diffuse into the area of the injured root.

Luyendijk and Van Voorthuisen analyzed 600 epidurograms and confirmed that contrast material failed to reach the nerve root in 33% of patients with uncomplicated disk prolapse and did not move beyond the affected disk space in 4.9% of cases.[52] Schachner and Abram confirmed that contrast material failed to diffuse upward past bulging disks and tended to

escape the epidural space via the foramina below the affected level.[87]

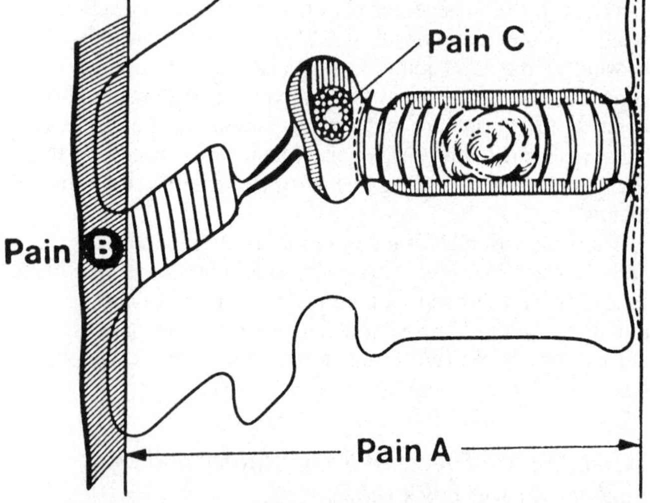

Prolapse of the intervertebral disk thus may result in relative or total obstruction to local anaesthetic flow within the epidural space. The unblocked area includes the affected segment but may also include all segments distal to the affected level in an ipsilateral or bilateral distribution. Either a double catheter technique or, more reliably, a subarachnoid injection of local anaesthetic could be used to manage the unblocked segments.

Postsurgical Epidural Blocks

Some distinction should be made between the more limited decompressions and fusions undertaken in the lumbar area for disk disease and the more extensive fusions involving the thoracolumbar spine used in corrective surgery for scoliosis (Table 27–9). Patients with more limited spinal operations have been reported to have high rates (91.2%) of successful epidural anaesthesia when the block was performed by experienced clinicians.[88] However, the success rate was lower than that experienced by the same clinicians in a population not previously subjected to back surgery (98.7%). The investigators attributed the increased rate of failures to the distortion of

FIGURE 27–24. Low back pain. Back pain may arise from three distinct anatomic areas in the spinal column, each area giving rise to a characteristic pain syndrome (see text). (From O'Brien JP: Mechanisms of spinal pain. *In* Textbook of Pain. Wall PD, Melzack R (eds). New York, Churchill Livingstone, 1984, p 240.)

TABLE 27–8. Anatomic Irregularities Correlating with Chronic Low Back Pain

Likely causes	Spondylolisthesis (moderate to severe)
	Spinal stenosis
	Multiple narrowed disk spaces
	Diffuse idiopathic skeletal hyperostosis
	Inflammatory spondyloarthropathies
	Congenital kyphosis
	Scoliosis (severe)
Questionable causes	Spondylolisthesis (mild)
	Scoliosis (mild to moderate)
	Retrolisthesis of vertebral body
	Lumbar scoliosis
	Single level disk space narrowing

TABLE 27–9. Technical Considerations in Postsurgical Epidural Blocks

- Reliable surface landmarks may be absent
- Epidural needle insertion may not be possible through the mass of osseous graft material
- False loss of resistance is common
- Degenerative changes occur in the spine below the lower level of the fusion at a greater rate in nonscoliotic patients. Both retrolisthesis and spondylolisthesis are increased.
- The ligamentum flavum may be injured during surgery, resulting in adhesions in the epidural space and partial or total obliteration of the epidural space; this may interfere with local anesthetic spread.
- Obliteration of the epidural space may make accidental dural puncture inevitable. It may not be possible to perform an epidural blood patch if a significant postdural puncture headache results.

surface anatomy and the tethering of the dura to the ligamentum flavum by scar formation, rendering the epidural space discontinuous.

Laminectomy Membranes

Support for this latter hypothesis of block failure was provided by LaRocca and Macnab's description of the laminectomy membrane.[89] They noted after laminectomy the formation of an organized fibrous tissue surrounding the dura and, at times, binding the nerves to the posterior aspects of the disk and adjacent vertebral body. The fibrous response was proportional to the extent of the surgical trauma, being more marked with wider operative exposures. Peridural fibrosis extended beyond the laminectomy defect in the more extensive exposures, obliterating the epidural space at that level.

Sharrock and colleagues recommended that epidural anesthesia should be attempted one to two interspaces above the operated segment(s) to improve the likelihood of successful block.[88]

Spinal Fusion

Lumbar epidural anaesthesia also has been reported in patients who have undergone extensive spinal fusion for kyphoscoliosis or after traumatic spinal injury.[90–93] The major factor determining successful outcome appears to be the persistence of lumbar interspaces not involved in the fusion. When the fusion terminates in the upper lumbar spine, successful outcome is likely. Some difficulties may be experienced, including multiple attempts before successful catheter placement, catheter-induced blood vessel trauma, difficulties defining the epidural space, and patchy or ineffective blocks.[90, 92, 93]

About 20% of fusions include L-4 and below; in these patients, lower success rates are reported (Fig. 27–25). Hubbert noted an 80% rate of successful epidural blockade in obstetric patients with fusions ending above L-4 and sparing the lower lumbar interspaces but only a 41% success rate in patients with fusions involving the entire lumbar spine.[93]

Caudal and subarachnoid blocks may be used in situations in which it has proved impossible to obtain an effective epidural block.

What Are the Etiologic Factors Implicated in Postoperative or Postpartum Back Ache?

Time

Back ache is common after anesthesia and surgery or labor and delivery.[94–98] The incidence of back ache after surgery appears to be unrelated to position during surgery, but it does increase with increasing duration of surgery.[94, 98] This observation suggests that anesthesia may permit prolongation of surgery beyond the limits of postural tolerance.

Anatomic Support

Lumbar supports and the lawn chair (contoured supine) position have been advocated to reduce the incidence of post-

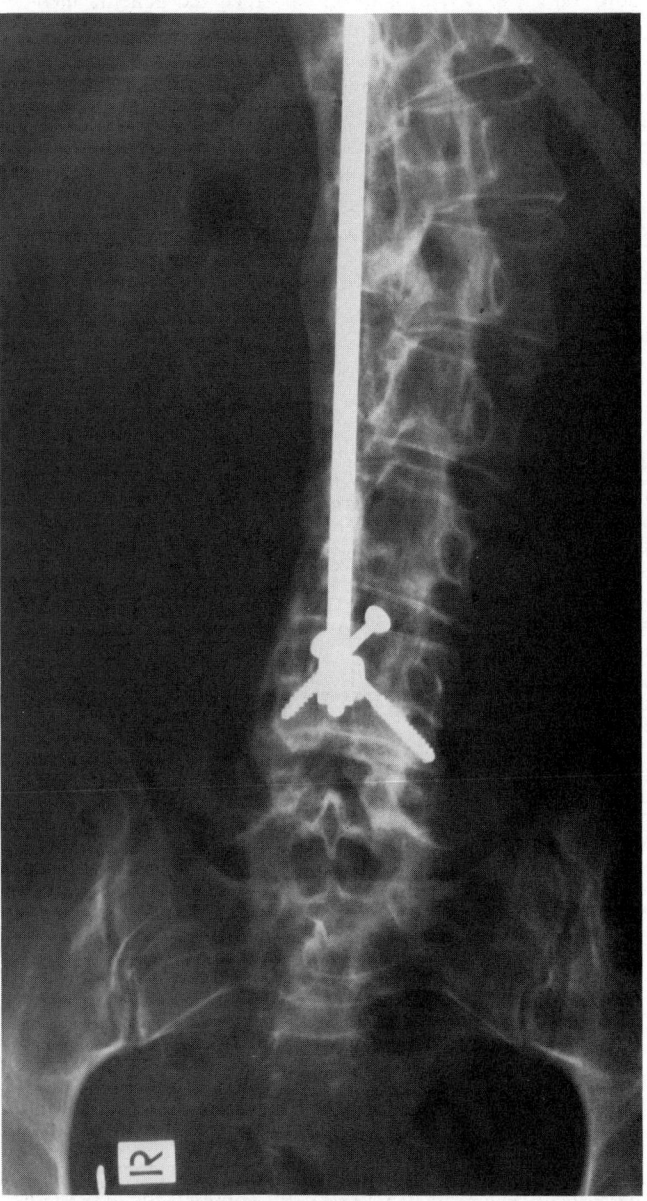

FIGURE 27–25. Spinal fusion for scoliosis. Anteroposterior view of the thoracolumbar junction and lumbar spine demonstrating fusion that involves the entire lumbar spine. There is rotation of the lumbar spinous processes into the concavity of the lateral curve, and the transverse processes are seen in the midline of the midlumbar vertebrae.

operative back ache. These techniques may be effective in maintaining lumbar lordosis, thus providing back ache prophylaxis, but no data attest to their effectiveness. Careful positioning of patients in the lithotomy position, taking care to raise and lower both legs simultaneously, is recommended to prevent a tension injury to the ligamentous structures of the lumbar spine.[99]

Anesthetic Technique

Back pain after surgery had been reported to be unrelated to the type of anesthesia.[94, 98] However, studies have reported an increased incidence of postoperative back ache in patients who received epidural or subarachnoid anesthesia compared with patients who had general anesthesia.[100, 101]

Postoperative back ache occurred in 26% of patients receiving subarachnoid block (26-gauge needle) for knee arthroscopy but in only 4% of those who received general anesthesia.[100] The back aches were characterized as mild and lasted an average of 2 days. In 22% of patients, multiple attempts were required for dural puncture, a factor that may have had some influence on the incidence. Back ache was reported in 9.34% of 682 patients who received epidural anesthesia for day care surgery.[101] Again, the back ache was characterized by a short, 2-day duration and a benign course. Patients' satisfaction with the anesthetics was not diminished by its occurrence.[100, 101]

Parturition

Postpartum back ache (PPB) is a common complaint. Previous back pain, including symptoms during the pregnancy, appears to confer the highest risk for PPB.[96] Epidural anesthesia increases the risk in multiparas without previous back ache but not in primiparous patients. Factors associated with PPB are local pain at the time of needle insertion and the occurrence of unilateral block. Presumably, these factors reflect the degree of local tissue trauma and perhaps lateral passage of the needle.

Paramedian approaches to the spinal spaces have been reported to result in greater discomfort at the time of the procedure compared with midline approaches.[78] Although a field block before lumbar puncture has been reported to reduce the incidence of postdural puncture back ache, this finding has not been consistent after labor lumbar epidural analgesia.[102, 103]

THE SACRAL SPINE

What Are the Relevant Anatomic Considerations?

The sacrum is a large triangular wedge-shaped bone, usually composed of five fused vertebrae. In some patients, the first sacral vertebra is not fused to the sacrum; this variant is termed *lumbarization*. Sacralization of the fifth lumbar vertebra occurs in a similar proportion of the population. These conditions have been related to low back pain, although this association has been disputed.[84] The spinous processes of the upper sacral vertebrae are fused to form the median sacral crest. This crest ends at the sacral hiatus as an upside down V and is covered by the thick, fibrous sacrococcygeal ligament.

The Sacral Hiatus

The sacral cornua are found on either side of the hiatus and provide useful landmarks to identify it during the performance of a caudal block. The hiatus varies widely in size and shape, ranging from longitudinal to horizontal slits, and is absent in up to 7.7% of the population.[104] The apex of the hiatus is usually below the lower third of S-4 but can be higher; complete sacral spina bifida is found in about 1% of specimens.

The fused sacral transverse processes form the lateral sacral crest. They can form a sufficient bump to be confused with the sacral cornua, creating a "decoy" hiatus. Injection into a decoy hiatus covered by ligament is usually met with resistance.

The Sacral Canal

The variable volume (12–65 mL) of the sacral canal and the range in size and patency of the sacral foramina, which deter-

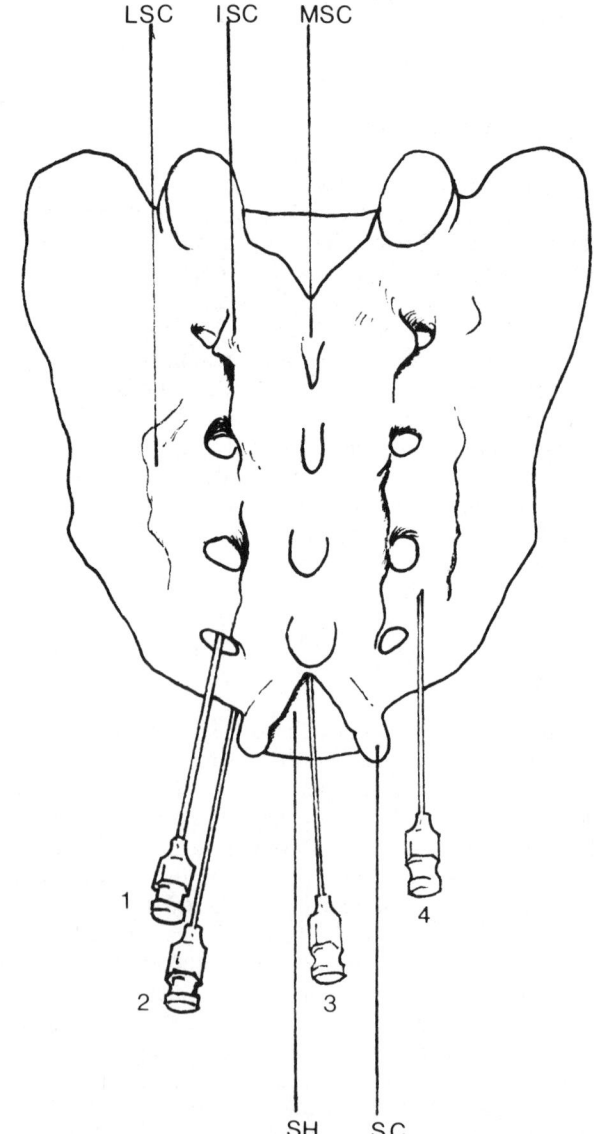

FIGURE 27–26. The sacrum and misplacements of attempted caudal blocks. 1 = Entry into the S-4 foramen; 2 = entry into the presacral area; 3 = correct needle placement for caudal block; 4 = entry into "decoy" hiatus; LSC = lateral sacral crest; ISC = intermediate sacral crest; MSC = median sacral crest; SH = sacral hiatus; SC = sacral cornua.

mine the amount of extravasation out of the sacral canal, make the volume of local anesthetic necessary for effective caudal analgesia unpredictable.[105]

How Likely Is Dural Puncture During Caudal Anesthesia?

The risk of dural puncture during a caudal block is very real, because the distance between the bottom of the dural sac and the top of the sacral hiatus can vary between 16 and 75 mm (average 45 mm).[106] In 5% of the population, the antero-posterior diameter of the sacral canal may be <2 mm, barely wide enough to admit a 21-gauge needle.

Where Do Misplaced Injections Go?

The needle can be easily misplaced during attempts to perform caudal epidural block (Fig. 27–26). Lateral needle placement can result in injection into the S-4 foramen. Subcutaneous injections occur, particularly in obese patients, in whom palpable landmarks may be difficult to appreciate. Injections into the presacral soft tissues are also possible, and injection into the fetal scalp has been reported during caudal blockade for labor analgesia.[107] Entry into the thin cortical bone overlying the anterior wall of the sacral canal can have a similar feel to traversing the sacrococcygeal ligament but results in injection into the bone marrow.

What Sacral Abnormalities Are Significant?

Sacral agenesis, congenital absence of the sacrum, is rare and is associated with maternal diabetes.[108–10] Other anomalies in the remainder of the spine are often associated with the agenesis and include scoliosis, spina bifida, vertebral fusion, tethered cord, lipoma, dermoid cyst, and diastematomyelia. A low-lying tethered cord may be associated with a more caudal termination of the subarachnoid space.[111] Sacral agenesis also is often associated with important anomalies of the digestive and genitourinary tracts as well as other musculoskeletal malformations.[108, 109, 112]

Congenital lumbosacral spinal anomalies do not represent an absolute contraindication to epidural anesthesia. However, preoperative evaluation of the lumbosacral spine in order to delineate the anatomy and an awareness of the implications of these anomalies for major regional anesthesia are necessary to ensure safe performance.

References

1. Hogan QH: Lumbar epidural anatomy: a new look by cryomicrotome technology. Anesthesiology 1991; 75:767.
2. Blomberg RG: The lumbar subdural extraarachnoid space of humans. An anatomical study using spinaloscopy in autopsy cases. Anesth Analg 1987; 66:177.
3. Crosby ET, Halpern SH: Failure of a lidocaine test dose to identify subdural placement of an epidural catheter. Can J Anaesth 1989; 36:445.
4. Reynolds F, Speedy HM: The subdural space: the third place to go astray. Anaesthesia 1990; 45:120.
5. Lubenow T, Keh-Wong E, Kristof K, et al: Inadvertent subdural injection: a complication of an epidural block. Anesth Analg 1988; 67:175.
6. Morgan B: Unexpectedly extensive conduction blocks in obstetric epidural analgesia. Anaesthesia 1990; 45:148.
7. Fesmire FM, Luten RC: The pediatric cervical spine: developmental anatomy and clinical aspects. J Emerg Med 1989; 7:133.
8. Poznanski AK: Congenital anomalies of the cervical spine. In The Cervical Spine. Bailey RW (ed). Philadelphia, Lea & Febiger, 1974, p 47.
9. Lipson SJ: Dysplasia of the odontoid process in Morquio's syndrome causing quadriparesis. J Bone Joint Surg 1977; 59-A:340.
10. Herrick IA, Rhine EJ: The mucopolysaccharidoses and anaesthesia: a report of clinical experience. Can J Anaesth 1988; 35:67.
11. Walts LF, Finerman G, Wyatt GM: Anaesthesia for dwarfs and other patients of pathological small stature. Can Anaesth Soc J 1975; 22:703.
12. Pueschel SM, Scola FH: Atlantoaxial instability in individuals with Down's syndrome: epidemiologic, radiographic and clinical studies. Pediatrics 1987; 80:555.
13. Moore RA, McNicholas KW, Warran SP: Atlantoaxial subluxation with symptomatic spinal cord compression in a child with Down's syndrome. Anesth Analg 1987; 66:89.
14. Williams JP, Somerville GM, Miner ME, et al: Atlantoaxial subluxation and trisomy-21: another perioperative complication. Anesthesiology 1987; 67:253.
15. Kobel M, Creighton RE, Steward DJ: Anaesthetic considerations in Down's syndrome: experience with 100 patients and a review of the literature. Can Anaesth Soc J 1982; 29:593.
16. Pizzutillo PD: Klippel-Feil syndrome. In The Cervical Spine. 2nd ed. Cervical Spine Research Society, Editorial Committee. Philadelphia, JB Lippincott, 1989, pp 258–271.
17. Naguib M, Farag H, Ibrahim AEW: Anaesthetic considerations in Klippel-Feil Syndrome. Can Anaesth Soc J 1986; 33:66.
18. Jeffreys E: Cervical spondylosis. In Disorders of the Cervical Spine. Jeffreys E (ed). London, Butterworths, 1980, pp 90–105.
19. Lee HC, Andree RA: Cervical spondylosis and difficult intubation. Anesth Analg 1979; 58:434.
20. White A, Kander PL: Anatomical factors in difficult direct laryngoscopy. Br J Anaesth 1975; 47:468.
21. Resnick D: Hyperostosis and ossification in the cervical spine. Arthritis Rheum 1984; 27:564.
22. Houk RW, Hendrix RW, Lee C, et al: Cervical fracture and paraplegia complicating diffuse idiopathic skeletal hyperostosis. Arthritis Rheum 1984; 27:472.
23. Jofe MH, White AA, Panjabi MM: Clinically relevant kinematics of the cervical spine. In The Cervical Spine. 2nd ed. Cervical Spine Research Society, Editorial Committee. Philadelphia, JB Lippincott, 1989, pp 57–69.
24. Nichol HC, Zuck D: Difficult laryngoscopy—the "anterior" larynx and the atlanto-occipital gap. Br J Anaesth 1983; 55:141.
25. Bellhouse CP, Dore C: Criteria for estimating likelihood of difficulty of endotracheal intubation with the Macintosh laryngoscope. Anaesth Intensive Care 1988; 16:329.
26. Hayashi H, Okada K, Hamada M, et al: Etiologic factors of myelopathy. A radiographic evaluation of the aging changes in the cervical spine. Clin Orthop 1987; 214:200.
27. Brechner VL: Unusual problems in the management of airways: flexion-extension mobility of the cervical spine. Anesth Analg 1968; 47:362.
28. Komusi T, Munro T, Harth M: Radiologic review: the rheumatoid cervical spine. Semin Arthritis Rheum 1985; 14:187.
29. Grantham SA: Rheumatoid arthritis and other noninfectious inflammatory diseases: Atlantoaxial instability. In The Cervical Spine. 2nd ed. The Cervical Spine Research Society, Editorial Committee. Philadelphia, JB Lippincott, 1989, pp 564–598.
30. Weissman BNW, Aliabadi P, Weinfeld MS, et al: Prognostic features of atlantoaxial subluxation in rheumatoid arthritis patients. Radiology 1982; 114:745.
31. Pellicci PM, Ranawat CS, Tsairis P, et al: A prospective study of the progression of rheumatoid arthritis of the cervical spine. J Bone Joint Surg 1981; 63-A:342.
32. Sinclair JR, Mason RA: Ankylosing spondylitis, the case for awake intubation. Anaesthesia 1984; 39:3.
33. Keenan MA, Stiles CM, Kaufman RL: Acquired laryngeal deviation associated with cervical spine disease in erosive polyarticular arthritis. Anesthesiology 1983; 58:441.
34. White AA, Southwick WO, Panjabi MM: Clinical instability in the lower cervical spine. Spine 1976; 1:15.
35. Johnson RM, Wolf JW: Stability. In The Cervical Spine. Cervical Spine Research Society, Editorial Subcommittee. Philadelphia, JB Lippincott, 1983, pp 35–53.
36. Hensinger RN: Congenital anomalies of the atlantoaxial joint. In The

Cervical Spine. 2nd ed. Cervical Spine Research Society, Editorial Committee. Philadelphia, JB Lippincott, 1989, pp 236–243.

37. Steel HH: Anatomical and mechanical considerations of the atlantoaxial articulations. J Bone Joint Surg 1968; 50:14.

38. White AA, Johnson RM, Panjabi MM, et al: Biomechanical analysis of clinical stability in the cervical spine. Clin Orthop 1975; 109:85.

39. Aprahamian C, Thompson BM, Finger WA, et al: Experimental cervical spine injury model: examination of airway management and splinting techniques. Ann Emerg Med 1984; 13:584.

40. Bivins HG, Ford S, Bezmalinovic Z, et al: The effect of axial traction during orotracheal intubation of the trauma victim with an unstable cervical spine. Ann Emerg Med 1988; 17:25.

41. Moore KL: The back. In Clinically Oriented Anatomy. Baltimore, Williams & Wilkins, 1980, pp 605–673.

42. Wagner F: Thoracic epidural anesthesia. In Regional Anesthesia. Zenz M, Panhans C, Niesel H, et al (eds). Chicago, Year Book, 1988, pp 117–125.

43. Bradford DS, Moe JH, Winter RB: Scoliosis and kyphosis. In The Spine. 2nd ed. Simeone FA (ed). Philadelphia, WB Saunders, 1982, p 316.

44. Kafer ER: Respiratory and cardiovascular functions in scoliosis and the principles of anesthetic management. Anesthesiology 1980; 52:339.

45. Shannon DC, Riseborough EJ, Valenca LM, et al: The distribution of abnormal lung function in kyphoscoliosis. J Bone Joint Surg 1968; 50:466.

46. Bergofsky EH: Respiratory failure in disorders of the thoracic cage. Am Rev Respir Dis 1979; 119:643.

47. Roth A, Rosenthal A, Hall JE, et al: Scoliosis and congenital heart disease. Clin Orthop 1973; 93:95.

48. Hirschfeld SS, Ruder C, Nasch CL, et al: The incidence of mitral valve prolapse in adolescent scoliosis and thoracic hypokyphosis. Pediatrics 1982; 40:451.

49. Sullivan PJ, Miller DR, Wynands JE: Cardiovascular manifestations of musculoskeletal diseases. In Anesthesia and Musculoskeletal Disorders. Lui ACP, Crosby ET (eds). Problems in Anesthesia 1991; 5:107.

50. Denis F: Spinal instability as defined by the three column spine concept in acute spinal trauma. Clin Orthop 1984; 189:65.

51. Husemeyer RP, White DC: Topography of the lumbar epidural space. Anaesthesia 1980; 35:7.

52. Luyendijk W, Van Voorthuisen AE: Contrast examination of the spinal epidural space. Acta Radiol 1966; 5:1051.

53. Savolaine ER, Pandya JB, Greenblatt SH, et al: Anatomy of the lumbar epidural space: new insights using CT-epidurography. Anesthesiology 1988; 68:217.

54. Boezaart AP: Computerized axial tomo-epidurographic and radiographic documentation of unilateral epidural analgesia. Can J Anaesth 1989; 36:697.

55. Usubiaga JE, DosReis A Jr, Usubiaga LE: Epidural misplacement of catheters and mechanisms of unilateral blockade. Anesthesiology 1970; 32:158.

56. Crosby E, Reid D: Salvaging inadequate epidural anaesthetics: the chloroprocaine save. Can J Anaesth 1991; 38:136.

57. McGrady EM, Davis AG: Spina bifida occulta and epidural anaesthesia. Anaesthesia 1988; 43:867.

58. Cooper MG, Sethna NF: Epidural analgesia in patients with congenital lumbosacral spinal anomalies. Anesthesiology 1991; 75:370.

59. Vaagenes P, Fjaerestad I: Epidural block during labor in a patient with spina bifida cystica. Anaesthesia 1981; 36:299.

60. Rothman RH, Simeone FA: The spine. 2nd ed. Philadelphia, WB Saunders, 1978, p 241.

61. McAllister VL: Plain spine x-ray. In Spina Bifida Occulta. James CCM, Lassman LP (eds): London, Academic Press, 1981, pp 60–78.

62. Rekate HL: Neurosurgical management of the child with spina bifida. In Comprehensive Management of Spina Bifida. Rekate HL (ed). Boca Raton, CRC Press, 1991, pp 93–111.

63. James CCM, Lassman LP: Tight filum terminale and tethered cord syndromes. In Spina Bifida Occulta. James CCM, Lassman LP (eds). London, Academic Press, 1981, pp 202–209.

64. White AA III, Panjabi MM: Practical biomechanics of scoliosis and kyphosis. In Clinical Biomechanics of the Spine. 2nd ed. White AA III, Panjabi MM (eds). Philadelphia, JB Lippincott, 1990, p 127.

65. Crosby ET: Epidural catheter migration during labor: a hypothesis for inadequate analgesia. Can J Anaesth 1990; 37:789.

66. Palmer SK, Abram SE, Maitra AM, et al: Distance from the skin to the lumbar epidural space in an obstetric population. Anesth Analg 1983; 62:944.

67. Harrison GR, Clowes NWB: The depth of the lumbar space from the skin. Anaesthesia 1985; 40:685.

68. Narang VPS, Linter SPK: A failure of extradural blockade in obstetrics. Br J Anaesth 1988; 60:402.

69. Meiklejohn BH: Distance from skin to the epidural space in an obstetric population. Reg Anesth 1990; 15:134.

70. Ostgaard HC, Anderson GBJ, Karlsson K: Prevalence of back pain in pregnancy. Spine 1991; 16:549.

71. Artal R, Friedman MJ, McNitt-Gray JL: Orthopedic problems in pregnancy. Physician Sportsmed 1990; 18:93.

72. Laban MM, Perrin JCS, Latimer FR: Pregnancy and the herniated lumbar disc. Arch Phys Med Rehabil 1983; 64:319.

73. Albright GA: Lumbar epidural anesthesia. In Anesthesia in Obstetrics: Maternal, Fetal and Neonatal Aspects. Albright GA, Ferguson JE II, Joyce TH III, et al (eds). Boston, Butterworths, 1986, pp 278–309.

74. Rolbin SH, Hew E, Ogilvie G: A comparison of two types of epidural catheters. Can J Anaesth 1987; 34:459.

75. Verniquet AJW: Vessel puncture with epidural catheters. Anaesthesia 1980; 35:660.

76. Blomberg RG: Technical advantages of the paramedian approach for lumbar epidural puncture and catheter introduction. Anaesthesia 1988; 43:837.

77. Jaucot J: Paramedian approach of the peridural space in obstetrics. Acta Anaesthesiol Belg 1986; 37:187.

78. Griffin RM, Scott RPF: A comparison between the midline and paramedian approaches to the extradural space. Anaesthesia 1984; 39:584.

79. Blomberg RG, Jaanivald A, Walther S: Advantages of the paramedian approach for lumbar epidural analgesia with catheter technique: a clinical comparison between midline and paramedian approaches. Anaesthesia 1989; 44:742.

80. O'Brien JP: Mechanisms of spinal pain. In Textbook of Pain. Wall PD, Melzack R (eds). New York, Churchill Livingstone, 1984, pp 240–251.

81. McCall IW, Park WM, O'Brien JP: Induced pain referral from posterior lumbar elements in normal subjects. Spine 1979; 4:441.

82. Hirsch C, Ongelmark B-E, Miller M: The anatomical basis for low back pain: studies on the presence of sensory nerve endings in ligamentous, capsular and intervertebral disc structures in the human lumbar spine. Acta Orthop Scand 1963; 33:1.

83. Frymoyer JW: Back pain and sciatica. N Engl J Med 1988; 318:291.

84. White AA III, Panjabi MM: The clinical biomechanics of spine pain. In Clinical Biomechanics of the Spine. 2nd ed. White AA III, Panjabi MM (eds). Philadelphia, JB Lippincott, 1990, pp 379–474.

85. Nachemson AL: Advances in low back pain. Clin Orthop 1985; 200:266.

86. Benzon HT, Braunschweig R, Molloy RE: Delayed onset of epidural anesthesia in patients with back pain. Anesth Analg 1981; 60:874.

87. Schachner SM, Abram SE: Use of two epidural catheters to provide analgesia of unblocked segments in a patient with lumbar disc disease. Anesthesiology 1982; 56:150.

88. Sharrock ME, Urqhart B, Mineo R: Extradural anaesthesia in patients with previous lumbar spine surgery. Br J Anaesth 1990; 65:237.

89. LaRocca H, Macnab I: The laminectomy membrane. Studies in its evolution, effects and prophylaxis in dogs. J Bone Joint Surg 1974; 56:545.

90. Crosby ET, Halpern SH: Obstetric epidural anaesthesia in patients with Harrington instrumentation. Can J Anaesth 1989; 36:693.

91. Feldstein G, Ramanathan S: Obstetrical lumbar epidural anesthesia in patients with previous posterior spinal fusion for kyphoscoliosis. Anesth Analg 1985; 64:83.

92. Daley MD, Morningstar BA, Rolbin SH, et al: Epidural anesthesia for obstetrics after spinal surgery. Reg Anesth 1990; 15:280.

93. Hubbert CH: Epidural anesthesia in patients with spinal fusion. Anesth Analg 1985; 64:843.

94. Brown EM, Elman DS: Postoperative backache. Anesth Analg 1961; 40:683.

95. Moir DD, Davidson S: Postpartum complications of forceps delivery performed under epidural and pudendal nerve block. Br J Anaesth 1972; 44:1197.

96. Lecog G, Hamza J, Narchi P, et al: Risk factors associated with postpartum backache in obstetric patients (Abstract). Anesthesiology 1990; 73:A966.

97. Benlabed M, Hamza J, Jullien P, et al: Risk factors for postpartum backache associated with epidural anesthesia (Abstract). Anesthesiology 1990; 73:A996.

98. Middleton MJ, Bell CR: Postoperative backache: attempts to reduce the incidence. Anesth Analg 1965; 44:446.

99. Welborn SG: The lithotomy position. Anesthesiologic considerations. In Positioning in Anesthesia and Surgery. 2nd ed. Martin JT (ed). Philadelphia, WB Saunders, 1987, pp 57–69.

100. Dahl JB, Schultz P, Anker-Moller E, et al: Spinal anaesthesia in young patients using a 29-gauge needle: technical considerations and an eval-

uation of postoperative complaints compared with general anaesthesia. Br J Anaesth 1990; 64:178.

101. Sarma VJ, Lundstrom J: Epidural anaesthesia for day care surgery: a retrospective study. Anaesthesia 1989; 44:683.

102. Peng ATC, Behar S, Blancato LS: Reduction of postlumbar puncture backache by the use of field block anesthesia prior to lumbar puncture. Anesthesiology 1985; 63:227.

103. Halpern S, Huh C, Djordjevic V: The use of a spinal field block before epidural analgesia for labour. Annual Meeting of the Society of Obstetrical Anesthesia and Perinatology, Boston, May 1991.

104. Black MG: Anatomic reasons for caudal anesthesia failure. Anesth Analg 1949; 28:33.

105. Bromage PR: Epidural Analgesia. Philadelphia, WB Saunders, 1978, pp 258–282.

106. Trotter M: Variations of the sacral canal: their significance in the administration of caudal analgesia. Anesth Analg 1947; 26:192.

107. Finster M, Poppers PJ, Sinclair JC, et al: Accidental intoxication of the fetus with local anesthetic drug during caudal anesthesia. Am J Obstet Gynecol 1965; 92:922.

108. Andrish J, Kalamachi A, MacEwen GD: Sacral agenesis: a clinical evaluation of its management, heredity and associated anomalies. Clin Orthop 1979; 139:52.

109. Cooper MG, Sethna NF: Epidural analgesia in patients with congenital lumbosacral spinal anomalies. Anesthesiology 1991; 75:370.

110. Denton JR: The association of congenital spinal anomalies with imperforate anus. Clin Orthop 1982; 162:91.

111. Brooks SB, El Gammal T, Hartlage P, et al: Myelography of sacral agenesis. AJNR 1981; 2:319.

112. Craigmile TK: Congenital anomalies of the spine. *In* Spinal Disorders: Diagnosis and Treatment. Ruge D, Wiltse LL (eds). Philadelphia, Lea & Febiger, 1977, pp 223–245.

CHAPTER 28

Autonomic Nervous System

THOMAS J. EBERT, M.D.

ROBERT KETTLER, M.D.

The autonomic nervous system (ANS) consists of a network of neural connections that maintains body homeostasis by regulating tissue and organ function. Autonomic outflow arises in the medullary vasomotor centers and is modulated by ascending input from peripheral sensors and by descending signals from higher brain centers. The ANS is segmental and, to some degree, parallels the somatic distribution to skeletal muscle. Sympathetic control is from thoracolumbar segments, and parasympathetic control is from the cranial and sacral segments (Fig. 28–1). The ANS is primarily an effector system that is tonically active and maintains visceral organs in a state of intermediate function. This activity permits central control and peripheral reflex mechanisms to augment or diminish autonomic outflow in order to adjust blood flow and visceral organ function in response to environmental changes.

ANATOMIC AND FUNCTIONAL CHARACTERISTICS

What Factors Distinguish the Autonomic and Somatic Nervous Systems?

Synapses

The ANS is sometimes referred to as the *visceral* motor system, in contrast to the *somatic* motor system. Two characteristics distinguish it from the somatic nervous system. First, the ANS essentially is under involuntary control (i.e., it is automatic). Second, the majority of somatic motor neurons are located within the central nervous system (CNS), and their efferent pathway to skeletal muscle is monosynaptic. In contrast, all autonomic motor neurons are peripherally located within ganglia that lie outside the CNS (postganglionic neurons). Preganglionic neurons that originate in the brainstem and the spinal cord synapse with these peripheral ganglia and activate postganglionic neural fibers. Thus, the ANS is a disynaptic system.

Nerve Fibers

The autonomic nerves are composed of small myelinated and unmyelinated fibers. Preganglionic B fibers are generally myelinated, have diameters of <3 μm, and conduct impulses at a speed of 2 to 14 $m \cdot s^{-1}$. Postganglionic C fibers are largely unmyelinated, have a diameter that ranges from 0.3 to 1.3 μm, and conduct impulses at <2 $m \cdot s^{-1}$.

Sympathetic

The sympathetic divisions of the ANS consist of preganglionic fibers that exit the spinal cord from the first thoracic to the third lumbar vertebral levels. Most of these fibers make synaptic connections in the lateral sympathetic chain, but some extend to peripheral ganglia before synapsing. In addition, preganglionic fibers make direct connections with the adrenal medulla (Fig. 28–2).

Parasympathetic

In the parasympathetic system, preganglionic fibers terminate in ganglia close to or within specific organs. Very short postganglionic fibers extend into the organ tissue. No interconnections are present between the cranial and sacral components. Furthermore, the parasympathetic system innervates only selected smooth muscle, tissue, and visceral organs (see Fig. 28–1).

Enteric

A third division is the enteric system, which is composed of local sensory neurons that respond to alterations in the tension and chemical environment of gut walls in order to regulate gastrointestinal, pancreatic, and gallbladder activity. The enteric system can function autonomously, although its activity normally is regulated by CNS reflexes.

Activity

The sympathetic nervous system is the ''fight or flight'' division, whereas the parasympathetic system functions to ''rest and digest.'' Activation of the sympathetic nervous system under stress (e.g., in the presence of blood loss, temperature change, or exercise) increases sympathetic neural activity to the heart and other viscera, peripheral vasculature, sweat glands, ocular muscles, and piloerector muscles. The results are increases in cardiac output, blood glucose, pupillary dilation, and body temperature. In contrast, activation of the parasympathetic system slows heart rate, respiration, digestion, and metabolism.

How Is Sympathetic Control Regulated?

A useful principle to facilitate an understanding of the pertinent neuroanatomy of the sympathetic nervous system is that it "disseminates" and "amplifies" information related to maintenance of body homeostasis[1-3] (Fig. 28–3).

Preganglionic Fibers

The preganglionic sympathetic neurons lie in the intermediolateral cell columns of the spinal cord gray matter, extending from T-1 to L-2. Axons of the sympathetic neurons are small and myelinated. They leave the spinal cord in the ventral spinal roots along with somatic alpha motor neurons and gamma motor neurons; they then branch off into the white (myelinated) rami communicantes and enter the paravertebral ganglia. These ganglia are arranged as a bilateral vertical chain running the length of the spinal column and located anterolateral to the vertebral bodies.[3] Prevertebral, intermediate, and terminal ganglia also are present.

The preganglionic fiber can synapse with one or more sympathetic neurons in the ganglion that it has entered; can ascend or descend in the paravertebral chain (with or without synapsing with a neuron in the entry level ganglion); or synapse with neurons at other levels. After traveling up or down the paravertebral chain, the preganglionic fiber may leave the paravertebral chain via a ramus communicans griseus. It can then join a somatic nerve and travel to an effector site (e.g., the blood vessels), synapse with an intermediate ganglion cell, or synapse with a prevertebral ganglion cell.

Although preganglionic fibers are present in the various sympathetic ganglia, and, in fact, sometimes exit from them, they are so named because they have not yet synapsed with a

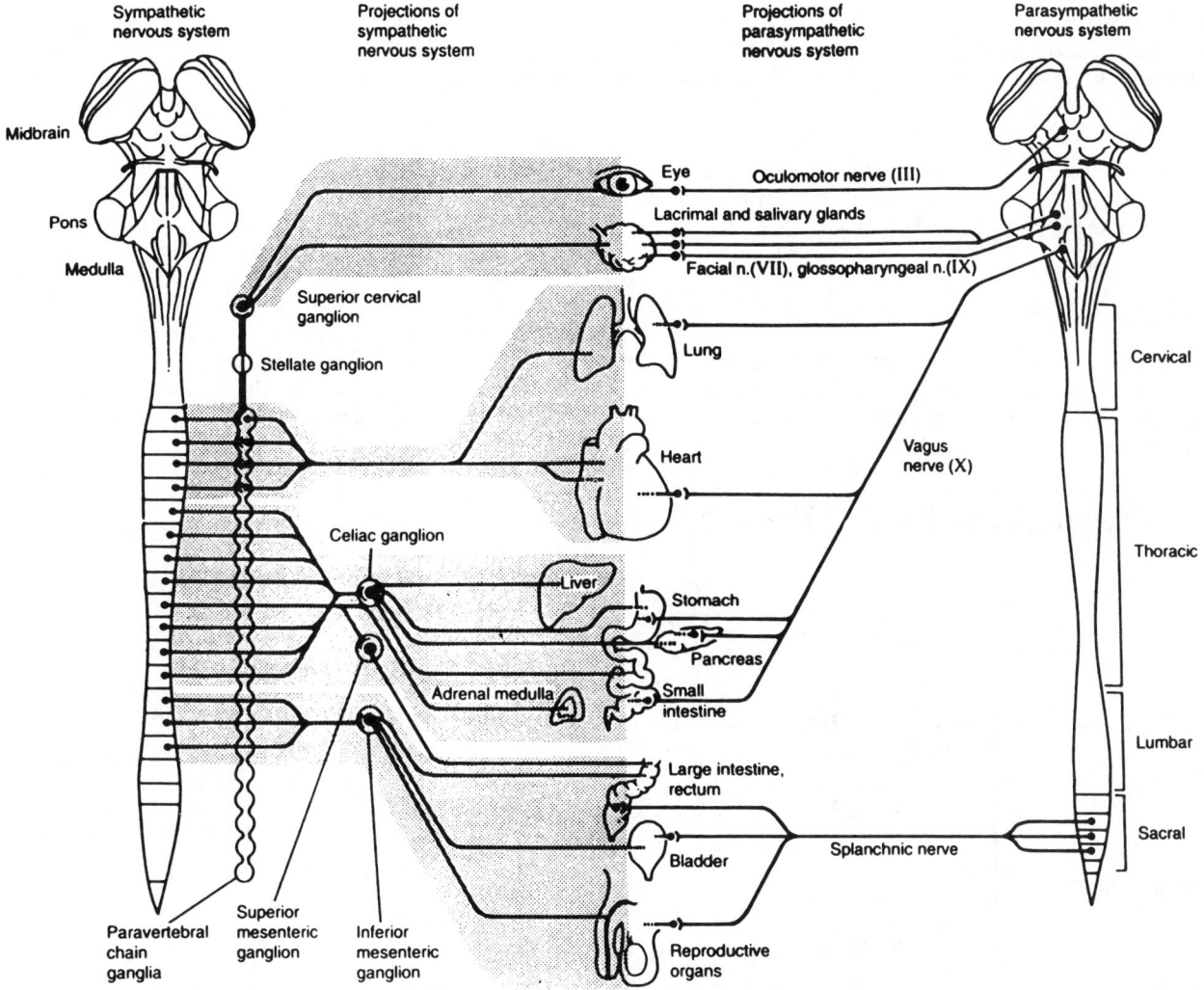

FIGURE 28–1. Sympathetic and parasympathetic divisions of the autonomic nervous system. Preganglionic neurons of the sympathetic division extend from the first thoracic spinal segment to lower lumbar segments. Parasympathetic ganglionic neurons are located within the brainstem and from segments S-2 to S-4 of the spinal cord. This figure also illustrates the coordinate innervation of a subset of targets by these two divisions of the autonomic nervous system. (From Dodd J, Role LW: The autonomic nervous system. *In* Principles in Neural Science. 3rd ed. Kandel ER, Schwartz JH, Jessell TM (eds). New York, Elsevier Scientific Publishing Co, 1991, p 763.)

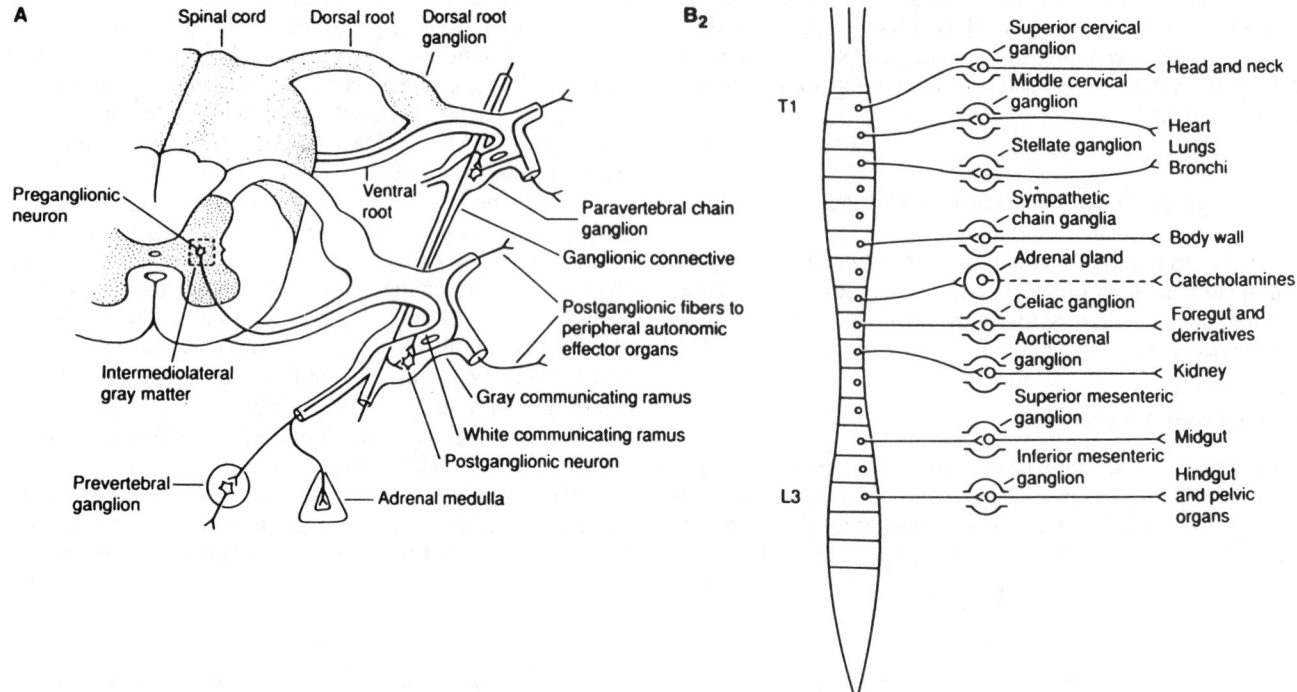

FIGURE 28–2. Schematic representation of the sympathetic system. (From Dodd J, Role LW: The autonomic nervous system. *In* Principles in Neural Science. 3rd ed. Kandel ER, Schwartz JH, Jessell TM (eds). New York, Elsevier Scientific Publishing Co, 1991, p 764.)

ganglion cell. Likewise, postganglionic fibers are so named because they are the terminal fibers of a ganglion cell and synapse with the appropriate end-organ.

Intermediate Ganglia

The intermediate ganglia are small structures, occasionally microscopic, that are located near the paravertebral chain. Their significance for the anesthesiologist is unclear.

Prevertebral Ganglia

Prevertebral ganglia are composed of a network of preganglionic and postganglionic sympathetic fibers, parasympathetic fibers, and ganglion cell bodies. Those of most significance to an anesthesiologist performing autonomic nerve blocks are the celiac ganglia and, possibly, the superior hypogastric (mesenteric) ganglia. Other prevertebral ganglia include the superior and middle cervical ganglia, the stellate ganglion, the first thoracic ganglia, the aortorenal ganglion, and the inferior mes-

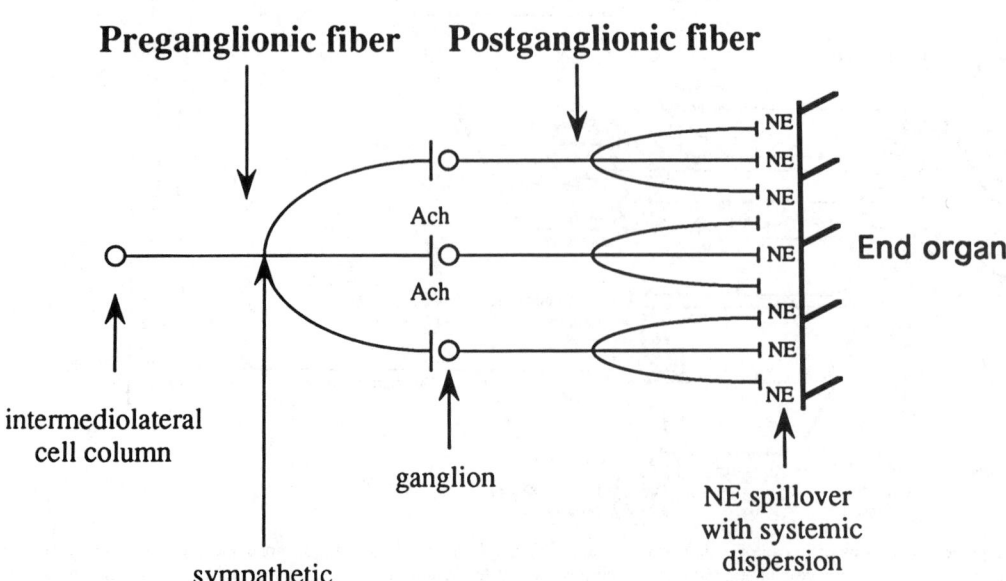

FIGURE 28–3. Schematic drawing of the organization of the sympathetic nervous system that results in dispersion and amplification of efferent signals. Ach = acetylcholine; NE = norepinephrine.

enteric ganglion (see Fig. 28–2). The terminal ganglia lie in close proximity to their end-organs (e.g., the urinary bladder and the rectum).

Postganglionic Fibers

The postganglionic sympathetic fibers are not myelinated. Like preganglionic fibers, one postganglionic fiber can synapse with a number of effector cells; however, a postganglionic fiber synapses with only one type of end-organ. For example, one postganglionic fiber might synapse with several vascular smooth muscle cells but would not simultaneously synapse with a sweat gland and a piloerector muscle. The important end-organs include the eye, the secretory structures (including the sweat glands), the heart, the blood vessels, the adrenal medulla, the abdominal and pelvic viscera, and the piloerector muscles.

Dispersion and Amplification

The sympathetic nervous system has evolved so that its efferent outflow is dispersed and amplified. This process is accomplished by preganglionic and postganglionic fibers that synapse with multiple effector cells. With a great burst of sympathetic activity, the release of the postganglionic neurotransmitter norepinephrine may exceed the capacity of the local uptake system and enzymatic breakdown that terminates its action. This excess norepinephrine (or overflow) can be dispersed by the circulatory system and result in widespread effects (see Fig. 28–3).

SYMPATHETIC BLOCKADE

What Are the Indications?

Sympathetic blockade can benefit surgical anesthesia through its vasodilating effects or its ability to reduce postoperative sympathetically induced pain.[4–6] However, some practitioners believe that sympathetic blockade is not beneficial and suggest that anesthetic and surgical outcome may actually be worsened when it is used.[7,8] Their discussions usually focus on the beneficial or harmful effects of the resultant hypotension. However, hypotension from a sympathetic block can be significantly reduced with the use of selective techniques.

Sympathetic blockade also has been recommended for the treatment of sympathetically maintained pain,[9] acute herpes zoster (shingles),[10] vascular insufficiency,[11] neuropathic pain,[12] and a number of miscellaneous conditions.[13–17] Celiac plexus blockade has been used in the management of pain due to upper abdominal malignancy[18] and chronic pancreatitis.[19] Likewise, superior hypogastric plexus blockade has been suggested for pain from pelvic malignancy.[20]

Much of the rationale for sympathetic blockade has resulted from extrapolation of what is known of the neurophysiology of the sympathetic nervous system. However, many practitioners question the benefit of blocks carried out for traditional indications,[21–24] partly because of a lack of randomized clinical trials that are needed to establish efficacy and outcome in surgical or pain patients undergoing such treatment. Despite the lack of convincing clinical studies, many of the blocks have become a traditional component of the solution for various pain management problems[21–24] (Table 28–1).

TABLE 28–1. Indications for Sympathetic Blocks

Vasodilation	Vascular surgery
	Replantation surgery
	Rest pain of lower extremities
	Intra-arterial injection of caustic substances (e.g., thiopental)
Pain management	Sympathetically maintained pain
	Shingles
	Neuropathic pain
	Intractable visceral pain
Prognostic	Before surgical sympathectomy

What Agents and Techniques Are Applicable?

Parenteral Drugs

Blockade of the ANS can be performed with parenteral agents that block the parasympathetic muscarinic receptor (e.g., atropine); that inhibit sympathetic outflow by central mechanisms (e.g., clonidine); or that inhibit sympathetic end-organ responses (e.g., α- and β-blockers). In addition, sympathetic ganglia can be blocked with intravenous agents such as hexamethonium.

Regional Block

Regional anesthetic techniques that use local anesthetics and neurolytic agents can also be employed. Central neuraxial anesthetic techniques, such as spinal or epidural anesthesia, provide sympathetic block of the preganglionic fibers; these techniques and their pertinent anatomy are discussed in Chapter 31. Note, however, that epidural anesthesia commonly results in incomplete block of the sympathetic nerves.

Selective regional sympathetic blockade can also be performed by injecting pharmacologic agents in proximity to the paravertebral and prevertebral ganglia. Such techniques provide a postganglionic block. Finally, intravenous regional approaches have been used to perform sympathetic blocks at an end-organ level.

Local Agents

Lidocaine, 1% to 2%, bupivacaine, 0.25% to 0.5%, and chloroprocaine, 2% to 3%, are frequently used. Bretylium, reserpine, and guanethidine have been used for intravenous regional anesthesia to interrupt synaptic nerve function. With many sympathetic blocks, the duration of local anesthetic action is not important; rather, the goal is to perform a series of blocks in an effort to achieve progressive improvement in pain through transient interruptions of sympathetic nervous system activity.

Neurolytic Drugs

Various neurolytic agents have been used to provide long-lasting sympathetic block; the most common are ethanol and phenol. Both agents work by disruption of myelin and precipitation of protein elements. They do not always provide a permanent block because neural fibers can regenerate; however, if the neural cell bodies in the ganglion are destroyed, permanent loss of neural function can be achieved.

Controversy exists regarding the exact role of neurolytic agents in sympathetically mediated pain. However, a neurolytic celiac plexus block for treatment of pain secondary to upper abdominal malignancy is accepted therapy; the patient's life expectancy is often less than the time required for neural regrowth. The techniques of neurolytic blockade and the pharmacology of ethanol, phenol, and other neurolytic agents are covered in a number of pain management texts.[25–27]

What Preparation Is Needed?

The practitioner must assess each situation in terms of the patient's general condition, the expected ease of intravenous catheter placement, and the likelihood of a complication. Preparation for a sympathetic block can be largely inferred from the information contained in the discussion of complications. The operating room table provides a useful surface for performing the block, since it can be used to place the patient in the Trendelenburg position and provides a firm surface for cardiopulmonary resuscitation, if needed. Suction equipment to clear an obstructed airway, a system to provide oxygen and positive-pressure ventilation, and an assortment of airway equipment (e.g., laryngoscopes, endotracheal tubes, and pharyngeal airways) must be immediately available.

In addition to monitoring equipment for assessment of the block, an electrocardiograph and sphygmomanometer are commonly employed. Intravenous access should be available to administer anxiolytic agents and emergency drugs, even though specific recommendations to this effect are absent in the literature. Resuscitative drugs include thiopental sodium, benzodiazepines, succinylcholine, epinephrine, atropine, lidocaine, and bretylium.

How Is a Block Evaluated?

The success of a block is assessed similarly in most procedures: symptoms are elicited, a physical examination is performed, and data from special studies are evaluated. For example, after stellate ganglion block, the patient can be queried about nasal congestion, a warm sensation in the extremity, or relief of pain. Signs of Horner's syndrome or increased temperature of the extremity can be noted. Postblock change in the patient's pain is commonly evaluated with a visual analogue pain scale.[28] Pain relief alone is not an indicator of sympathetic blockade but is an important part of the assessment. A number of special studies can be performed.[29]

Physical Characteristics

The obvious findings present on physical examination can be predicted based on one's knowledge of ANS neuroanatomy. Several end-organs have special significance.

Skin

A careful skin examination should reveal that the skin has become smooth and dry because of piloerector muscle and sweat gland inactivation.

Vascular Bed

Venous dilation may be obvious because of anesthetic denervation of the venular smooth muscle. This sign may be present even when the arteriolar system is too diseased to respond to sympathetic blockade (e.g., in patients with peripheral vascular disease). When arteriolar dilatation is present, the pressure at the arteriolar side of the capillary circulation is decreased; with simultaneous venous dilatation and facilitated drainage, the pressure on the venous side is reduced. This combination results in an increased blood flow in the capillary bed, which is apparent as a rapid filling time after blanching beneath a fingernail.

Horner's Syndrome

Probably the most striking set of physical findings are those of Horner's syndrome produced by a stellate ganglion block. The classic triad consists of ptosis, miosis, and anhidrosis. These are apparent on the side of the face ipsilateral to the block.

Temperature

Following a sympathetic block, the volume of blood in the capillaries increases, bringing skin surface temperature closer to core body temperature. This increase in temperature can be measured by placement of a temperature probe on the skin in the anatomic distribution of the block. Bilateral temperature probes can be used to compare the blocked and unblocked sides.

Plethysmographic Waveforms

The waveform obtained from a photoplethysmograph can also be used to evaluate a successful sympathetic block. In its simplest application, a pulse oximeter is placed on a digit of the extremity to be blocked. Because most pulse oximeters incorporate an automatic gain control to create a prominent waveform, unless the gain setting can be fixed, this approach can be misleading. A control pulse tracing should be compared with the postblock tracing. A successful sympathetic block results in an increase of amplitude and area beneath the pulse waveform.

Successful blockade also can be evaluated by a cold pressor test (typically the immersion of an unblocked extremity in ice water for 60 seconds). This preblock maneuver causes a reduction in the pulse amplitude. When a sympathetic block has been successfully performed, the waveform, which has increased in size owing to the block, should not change during the cold stimulus.

Sympathogalvanic Reflex

In patients with severe peripheral vascular disease, the aforementioned tests may not be positive despite the presence of successful blockade. In this situation, the sympathogalvanic reflex is useful. A two-lead electrocardiographic monitoring system is employed. The positive and negative leads are placed on the patient's skin in the area to be blocked; a ground electrode is placed elsewhere. The waveform displayed is a representation of cutaneous electrical current.

When sympathetic activity to the skin increases (e.g., in

response to a noxious stimulus, such as loud noise, skin pinch, or startle response), a positive deflection of the waveform occurs in response to the increased sympathetic discharge. After a successful sympathetic block, the increase in cutaneous conductance during a noxious stimulus is absent, and the waveform deflection is not apparent (Fig. 28–4).

Sweat Tests

Finally, tests of sweat gland function can assess sympathetic activity. In the Ninhydrin, cobalt blue, and starch iodide tests, color changes in certain dyes occur with increased skin surface moisture (sweat). Successful block eliminates sweating in the affected areas. These tests are used infrequently because they are less convenient and are messy compared with those previously mentioned.

Critique

The utility of any of the tests mentioned, including the subjective sensation of pain relief, has proponents and critics. Individual tests and combinations of tests have been used in numerous studies of sympathetic blockade.[17, 30–33] However, none of the commonly used methods to evaluate end-organ function has been rigorously studied for utility (specificity and sensitivity). A thorough evaluation of these tests should include the variability inherent in each, the variability of results in normal subjects, the establishment of a "gold standard" with which the tests can be compared, and determination of each test's diagnostic discrimination.[34, 35] Perhaps the best approach is to combine physical assessment, a practical test for the given clinical setting, and a therapeutic goal.[36]

What Should You Know About Paravertebral Block?

Anatomic Features

Stellate ganglion and lumbar sympathetic blocks are performed fairly frequently. The thoracic sympathetic chain is

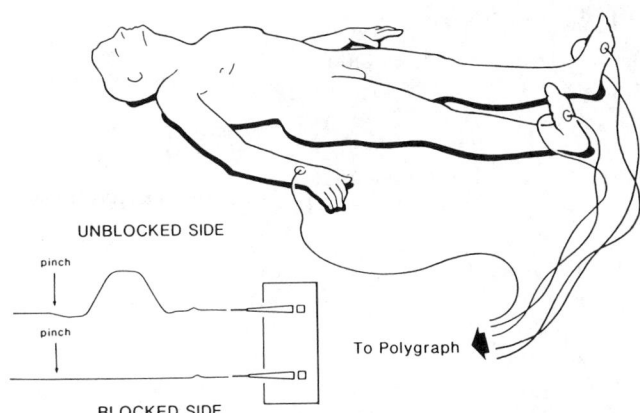

FIGURE 28–4. Sympathogalvanic response. Electrodes are placed on the front and back of hands or feet, and a ground electrode is placed elsewhere on the body. Changes in baseline level on an electrocardiographic recorder indicate changes in sweat gland activity. (From Lofstrom JB, Cousins MJ: Sympathetic neural blockade of upper and lower extremity. *In* Neural Blockade. Cousins MJ, Bridenbaugh PO (eds). Philadelphia, JB Lippincott, 1988, p 475.)

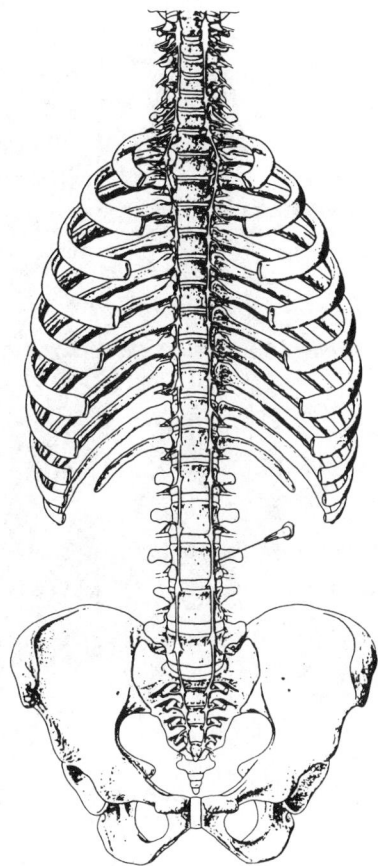

FIGURE 28–5. Anatomic location of the thoracic sympathetic ganglia increases the likelihood of a pneumothorax when a block in this region is attempted. The lumbar sympathetic chain is more easily accessed and with fewer complications. (From Scott DB: Techniques of Regional Anaesthesia. Norwalk, CT, Appleton & Lange, 1989, p 205.)

less commonly blocked. In the neck, the paravertebral ganglia lie against the vertebral transverse processes; they are more anterior in the thorax, lying in front of the heads of the rib insertions. The lumbar paravertebral chain lies along the anterolateral aspect of the lumbar vertebral bodies. In the pelvis, the sympathetic chains are anterior to the sacrum and terminate as a single ganglion located anterior to the coccyx (Fig. 28–5).

Potential Complications

The location of the thoracic sympathetic ganglia means that a pneumothorax is a potential complication of an attempt to block this portion of the paravertebral chain; a thoracic epidural or intercostal nerve block is an alternative, although each technique has associated potential complications as well.

The paravertebral chain in the neck also lies in close proximity to a number of structures that, when pierced, can give rise to complications. These include the dural sleeves that invest the cervical nerve roots, the vertebral artery, and the dome of the pleura. Other nearby structures are the phrenic and vagus nerves, carotid artery, jugular vein, esophagus, trachea, and cervical disks. Lumbar sympathetic chains are also close to structures of importance, including the kidneys, lumbar nerve roots and their associated dural sleeves, genitofemoral nerves, and major blood vessels (Figs. 28–6 and 28–7).

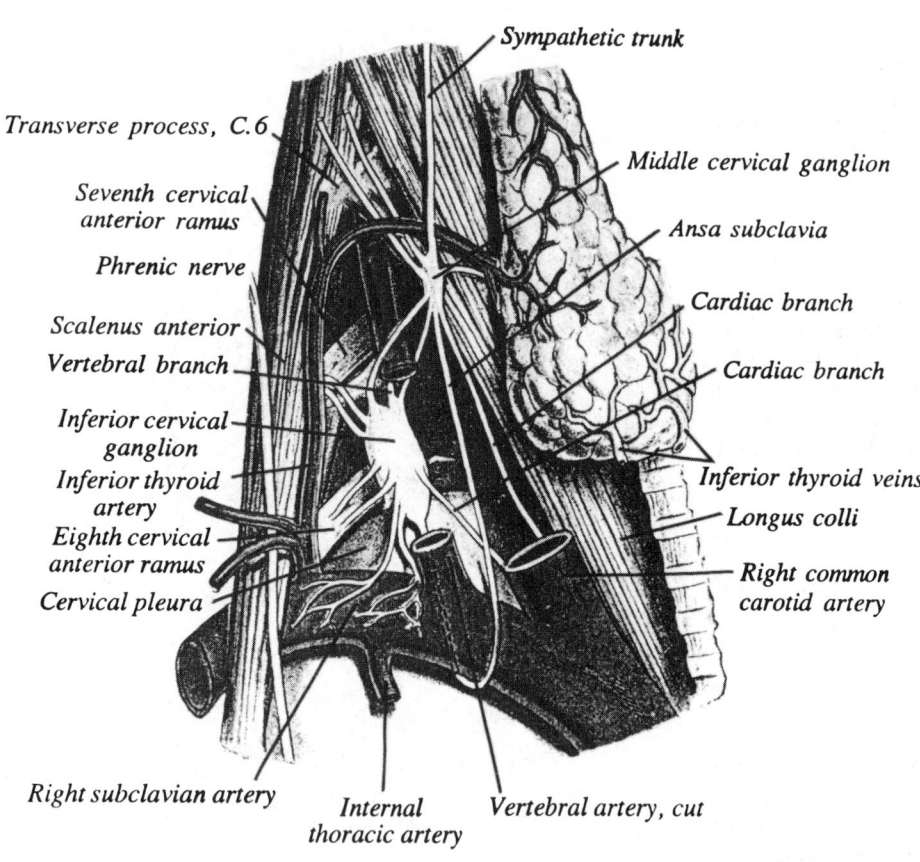

Sympathetic trunk

Transverse process, C.6

Seventh cervical
anterior ramus

Phrenic nerve

Scalenus anterior

Vertebral branch

Inferior cervical
ganglion

Inferior thyroid
artery

Eighth cervical
anterior ramus

Cervical pleura

Middle cervical ganglion

Ansa subclavia

Cardiac branch

Cardiac branch

Inferior thyroid veins

Longus colli

Right common
carotid artery

Right subclavian artery

Internal
thoracic artery

Vertebral artery, cut

FIGURE 28–6. Anterior view of the inferior cervical (or stellate) ganglion. Part of the vertebral artery has been excised to show the inferior cervical ganglion. Surrounding structures could be inadvertently penetrated during needle placement. (From Williams PL, Warwick R, Dyson M, et al (eds): Gray's Anatomy. 37th ed. New York, Churchill Livingstone, 1989, p 1161.)

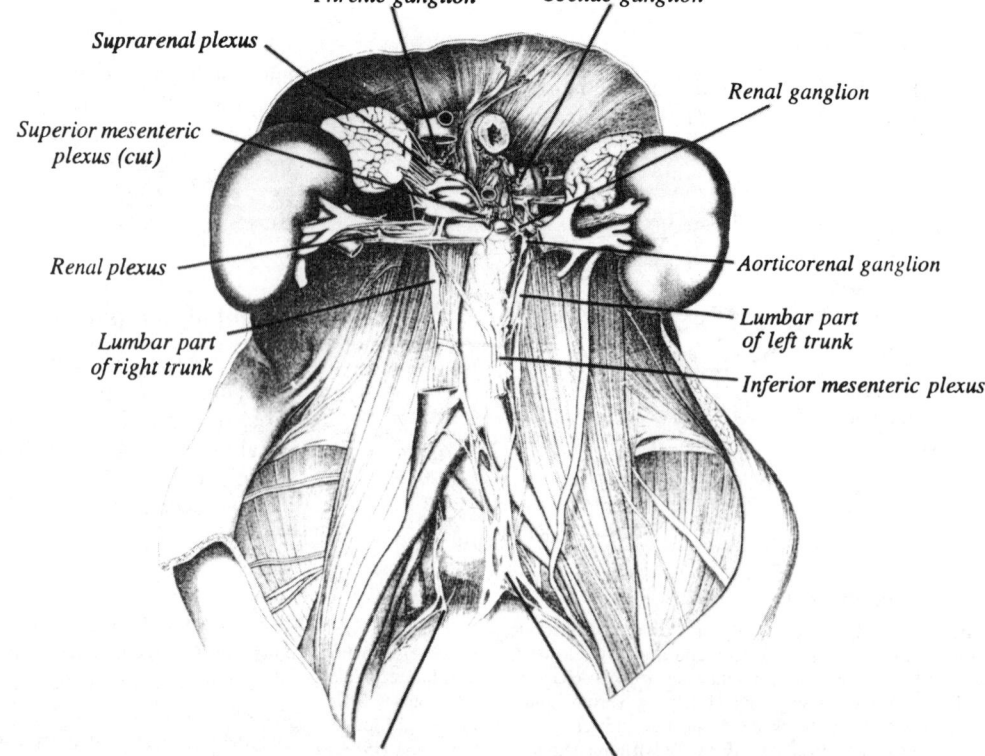

Phrenic ganglion

Coeliac ganglion

Suprarenal plexus

Renal ganglion

Superior mesenteric
plexus (cut)

Renal plexus

Aorticorenal ganglion

Lumbar part
of left trunk

Lumbar part
of right trunk

Inferior mesenteric plexus

Pelvic part of right trunk

Superior hypogastric plexus

FIGURE 28–7. The abdominal part of the sympathetic system. Structures adjacent to the ganglia could be penetrated during needle placement. (From Williams PL, Warwick R, Dyson M, et al (eds): Gray's Anatomy. 37th ed. New York, Churchill Livingstone, 1989, p 1163.)

TABLE 28–2. Common Sympathetic Blocks

Neuraxial	Spinal
	Epidural
Paravertebral	Cervicothoracic (stellate ganglion)
	Lumbar sympathetic
Prevertebral	Celiac plexus
	Hypogastric plexus

Despite the potential for complications owing to needle puncture or injection of local anesthetics into nearby structures along the paravertebral chain, the cervical and lumbar portions of the chain are more safely approached and thus more frequently blocked than are the thoracic elements (Table 28–2).

What Should You Know About Ganglionic Block?

Celiac Plexus

Celiac plexus blocks are the most common of the prevertebral blocks. These procedures are typically called ''plexus blocks'' because they involve a relatively large area that contains ganglia and several types of nerve fibers.

Anatomic Relationships

The celiac plexus is located at the level of the T-12 and L-1 vertebral bodies. It is anterior to the aorta and surrounds the celiac artery and the root of the superior mesenteric artery. The adrenal glands form the lateral border. Preganglionic fibers penetrate the crura of the diaphragm and synapse in the plexus. The greater splanchnic nerve (T5-10), the lesser splanchnic nerve (T9-11), and the least splanchnic nerve (T-12) are the preganglionic nerves that join with branches of the vagus and phrenic nerves and with postganglionic fibers to form the neural network of the plexus. Also contained in the plexus are the celiac ganglia and the aorticorenal ganglia.

Interestingly, the target of a local anesthetic or neurolytic block of the celiac plexus is the visceral afferent fibers, which carry nociceptive information from the abdominal viscera. These fibers do not synapse in the preaortic ganglia and, in fact, are not part of the sympathetic nervous system. They are like other primary nociceptive afferents in that their cell bodies are in the dorsal root ganglion, and they synapse in the dorsal horn of the spinal cord gray matter.

Superior Hypogastric Plexus

The superior hypogastric plexus is located in a more caudal direction by several lumbar levels.[26] It is composed of branches of the aortic plexus, the third and fourth lumbar splanchnic nerves, and the superior hypogastric ganglia. The plexus is anterior to the aortic bifurcation, from the body of L-5 to the sacral promontory, and between the iliac arteries. It is continuous with the inferior hypogastric plexus in a more caudal direction.

Because the pelvic viscera have a dual afferent innervation that consists of nociceptive fibers traveling with both the sympathetic fibers and the sacral parasympathetic fibers, a superior hypogastric plexus block may not provide complete pelvic analgesia.

How Are Sympathetic Blocks Performed?

Intravenous Regional

A capped intravenous catheter is placed in the distal portion of the extremity to be blocked with a tourniquet positioned on the proximal limb. The extremity is exsanguinated by elevation and an Esmarch wrap, and the arterial inflow is occluded by inflation of the tourniquet above systolic pressure. A sympatholytic agent (e.g., guanethidine, reserpine, or bretylium, usually with 0.5% lidocaine) is slowly injected through the intravenous catheter. After a minimum of 20 minutes, the tourniquet can be released in a staged fashion.[30]

Stellate Ganglion

The patient is placed in a supine position. The cricoid cartilage is identified by palpation. A 22-gauge, short-bevel needle is inserted just lateral to the cricoid cartilage in a slight medial direction but otherwise toward the surface on which the patient is lying. When the transverse process of C-6 is contacted by the needle tip, the needle is withdrawn slightly. Aspiration to check for intravascular or subarachnoid placement is performed. If the aspiration is negative, 5 to 10 mL of local anesthetic is slowly injected with repeated attempts at aspiration after every few milliliters of injection.[29]

An alternative technique is to perform the block at the level of the C-7 transverse process. The insertion site is located two fingerbreadths lateral and cephalic to the suprasternal notch. Again, the needle is inserted until the transverse process is contacted and is then withdrawn slightly.

The approach at C-6 has several anatomic advantages.[3]

1. The needle is more distant from the dome of the pleura, which lowers the risk of pneumothorax.

2. At the C-6 level, the vertebral artery passes through the transverse process (in contrast to its superficial location at C-7).

3. The bifid transverse process of C-6 protects the roots of the brachial plexus, whereas the transverse process of C-7 does not.

Lumbar Sympathetic

The patient is placed with a pillow beneath the hips to flex the lumbar spine. The spinous process of L-2 is identified by palpation, and a point 8 to 12 cm lateral to its cephalic position is marked. The variability in distance from the midline depends on the body habitus. In general, the insertion site is just lateral to the border of the paraspinous muscle.

A 12-cm, 20-gauge needle is inserted toward the vertebral body at a 45° angle to the horizontal plane of the patient's back (the cephalic tip of the spinous process usually corresponds to a midpoint level of the vertebral body). When the vertebral body is contacted, the needle is withdrawn, and its angle is increased to about 60° (from the horizontal toward the perpendicular); it is then advanced again. The tip of the needle should slide off the anterolateral portion of the vertebral body and lie in proximity to the lumbar sympathetic chain. After a negative aspiration, 10 to 20 mL of local anesthetic is slowly injected with frequent aspiration[29] (Fig. 28–8).

Celiac Plexus

The technique of celiac plexus blockade is a modification of the lumbar sympathetic block technique except that bilateral

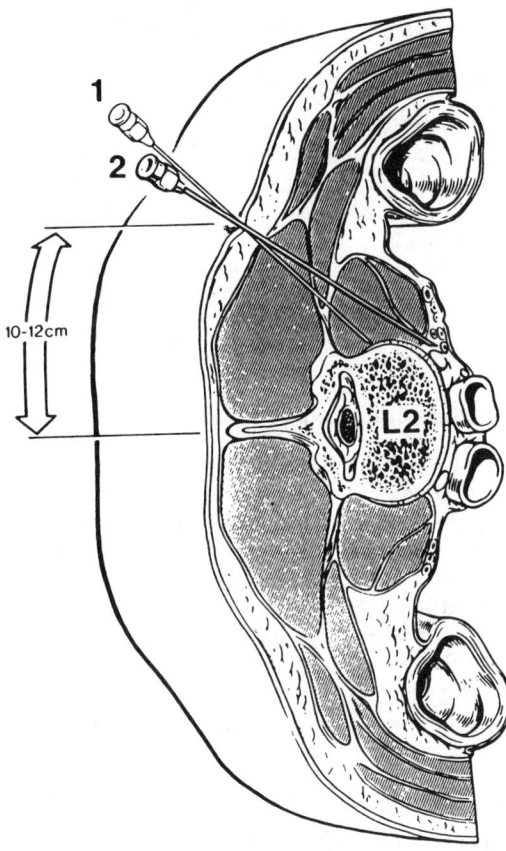

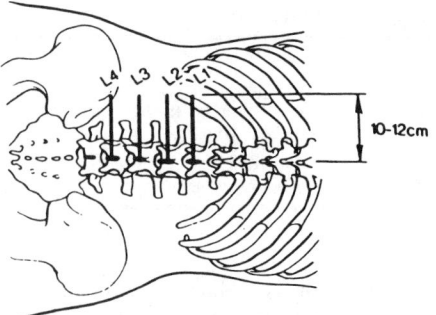

FIGURE 28–8. Technique of lumbar sympathetic block. Note location of skin marks for L-1 and L-5 spinous processes; these marks permit identification of L-2 and L-3. A line is drawn through the center of the spinous processes. Needle insertion is at the lateral margin of the erector spinae muscle (approximately 10–12 cm from midline). If the depth of the transverse process is to be checked, the needle must be angled cephalad. Otherwise, the needle is inserted at approximately 45° toward the vertebral body until this structure is located. The needle is then angled more steeply until it slips just past the vertebral body and through the psoas fascia (2). A single needle can be used instead of 2 or 3 needles; however, with a single needle, an increased volume must be injected. (From Lofstrom JB, Cousins MJ: Sympathetic neural blockade of upper and lower extremity. *In* Neural Blockade in Clinical Anesthesia and Management of Pain. Cousins MJ, Bridenbaugh PO (eds). Philadelphia, JB Lippincott, 1988, p 487.)

needles are placed.[37] Because of marked vasodilation, intravascular volume expansion is important before the block. A point 8 to 10 cm lateral to the spinous process of L-1 is located on both flanks. Again, the paraspinous muscles are a useful landmark; the intersection of the lateral border of these muscles and the caudad edge of the 12th rib usually marks the insertion site. This site should lie at the level of the caudal edge of the L-1 spinous process. The caudal portion of T-12 is palpated and marked. Be sure to form a ''mind's eye'' picture of a point anterior to the vertebral column that should locate the celiac plexus.

A 12-cm, 20-gauge needle is advanced to this point, initially with an angle of 45° to a horizontal plane. Once the vertebral body is contacted, the needle is withdrawn and redirected to a steeper angle (more perpendicular); it is then inserted until it lies along the anterolateral aspect of the vertebral body.

Some practitioners prefer to insert the left needle first. This needle is advanced slowly until pulsations of the aorta are noted at the needle hub. The needle is then withdrawn slightly, and the right-sided needle placed in a similar direction and to a similar depth.

After aspiration and use of a test dose to check for intravascular and subarachnoid placement, 20 to 25 mL of local anesthetic or neurolytic agent is slowly injected through each needle. If only a single, left-sided needle is used, 40 to 50 mL of anesthetic are injected slowly. Most practitioners prefer to use fluoroscopy or computed tomography to guide needle

placement, particularly when a neurolytic celiac plexus block is contemplated.

Superior Hypogastric Plexus

This technique has been described for the management of pelvic pain.[20] The patient is placed in the prone position with a pillow beneath the hips. Like celiac plexus blockade, bilateral needles are employed. The needle insertion sites are located at the level of the L4-5 interspace, 5 to 7 cm from the midline. They are directed in a medial and caudal direction. The medial direction should be at a 45° angle to the sagittal plane. The caudal direction should be at a 30° angle to a horizontal plane on the patient's back. The needles are positioned so that the tips lie at the anterolateral aspect of the L5-S1 interspace.

What Does Radiologic Assistance Contribute?

Radiologic techniques can be used to assist or confirm needle placement in any of the blocks just described. Various radiologic imaging procedures have added to our knowledge of the pertinent anatomy but have generated controversy about the proper needle placement. Considerable discussion has focused on whether radiologic techniques help to reduce complications.[38–48]

Our opinion is that good outcome from these procedures is based on a combination of anatomic knowledge, experience, and the use of test doses. If the patient's body habitus makes palpation of landmarks difficult, radiologic imaging can facilitate needle placement. When a neurolytic procedure is performed, radiographic visualization of needle placement may reduce the likelihood of serious neurologic complications. However, controlled studies that employ rigorous methodology and compare the success of "blinded" techniques to those performed with imaging techniques have not been done.

What Are the Complications?

The potential complications are of two general types: (1) complications related to needle trauma; and (2) those related to the substance injected. Trauma to neural structures is possible with any regional anesthetic technique. However, a review of the literature does not reveal the frequency with which this problem occurs in clinical practice. Trauma to proximate structures is also possible; most can be surmised from a review of the regional anatomy pertinent to each ganglion.

During a stellate ganglion block, the following structures are at risk of needle trauma: the vertebral artery, the cervical nerve roots (and the accompanying dural sleeve), the pleura, the trachea, and the esophagus. With celiac plexus and lumbar sympathetic blocks, nerve roots and dural sleeves, the major abdominal vessels, the kidneys, the bowel, and the pleura (celiac plexus block) are at risk (see Table 28–3).

How Are These Complications Managed?

Puncture of Abdominal Viscera

Some of the potential complications are not of great clinical significance, and routine follow-up may be all that is necessary. If bowel perforation occurs with an anterior celiac plexus block using a 22-gauge or smaller needle, adverse outcome is rare.[49, 50] The technique of lumbar sympathetic block has been modified to reduce the likelihood of renal puncture. Patients should be alerted to the possibility that hematuria may develop if it occurs. Hematuria is usually transient and of little clinical consequence. If the patient develops flank pain with a mass, persistent or heavy hematuria, or hypertension, urologic con-

sultation should be ordered. Many of the complications are self-limited and do not require further anesthesia or surgical management.[51]

Vascular Trauma and Bleeding

Needle-induced vascular trauma also seems to be a relatively rare serious event. In fact, the lumbar approach for aortography is similar to that used for lumbar sympathetic block and celiac plexus block. Serious hemorrhage is rare with both blocks if small-gauge needles are used and if the patient has a normal blood coagulation profile. Whether neuraxial blocks should be performed in patients with a pathologic or therapeutic coagulopathy[52] or in those receiving nonsteroidal anti-inflammatory drugs is debated.[53] Probably the most prudent approach is to weigh the benefits to be gained from the block against the risk of hemorrhage (unquantified) and to observe the patient carefully for signs or symptoms of hematoma formation or other signs of hemorrhage.

Pneumothorax

Puncture of the pleura can result in a pneumothorax; this complication occurs with celiac plexus block or stellate ganglion block (especially if performed at C-7). Chest pain, dyspnea, cyanosis, loss of fremitus over the chest wall, hyperresonance of the ipsilateral hemithorax, and loss of breath sounds are pertinent findings.[54] Inspiratory and expiratory chest radiographs facilitate the diagnosis. A thoracic surgery consult for chest tube placement should be considered if the pneumothorax is greater than 20%. If a pneumothorax results in rapid deterioration, a large-bore intravenous catheter (14- to 16-gauge) can be inserted in the second intercostal space in the midclavicular lines.

Esophageal Perforation

Puncture of the esophagus with a subsequent osteitis of the transverse process or mediastinitis is a potential but apparently very rare complication.[10]

Neural Injury

The incidence of neural injury from needle trauma during sympathetic blockade has not been studied. Appropriate management should include careful documentation of symptoms and neurologic deficit (if present) and careful follow-up to ensure resolution of the problem. Most symptoms gradually diminish over several months. Often, nonsteroidal anti-inflammatory drugs help to alleviate symptoms.

Intravascular Injection

Unrecognized injection of local anesthetics into a blood vessel can result in local anesthetic toxicity. The likelihood of a seizure depends on the quantity and rapidity of local anesthetic delivered to the brain. During an attempted lumbar sympathetic block, 20 mL of 0.5% lidocaine (100 mg) could be injected into the inferior vena cava with a relatively low risk of toxicity. However, during an attempted stellate ganglion block, less than 1 mL of local anesthetic injected into the vertebral artery likely will result in a seizure because of direct delivery to the brain.

TABLE 28–3. Complications of Sympathetic Blockade

Needle trauma	Nerves and dura
	Blood vessels
	Viscera (kidney, bowel)
	Pleura
Effect of injected substance	Local anesthetic toxicity
	Extensive sympathetic blockade (hypotension)
	Extensive spread of neurolytic solution, causing somatic nerve injury or bowel or bladder dysfunction
Miscellaneous	Infection (very rare)
	Vasovagal response
	Allergic reaction to contrast dye or local anesthetic

Prior to injection, perform careful aspiration to identify improper intravascular positioning. All injections should be made in small (2- to 5-mL) increments. The patients must be observed for signs of local anesthetic toxicity (tinnitus, perioral numbness, blurred vision, slurred speech, seizure) during and after injection.

If a seizure occurs, a patent airway, adequate ventilation, and circulatory stability need to be maintained. Hyperventilation with 100% oxygen is always indicated. Administration of a benzodiazepine or other CNS depressant (e.g., thiopental) to terminate the seizure and a muscle relaxant to facilitate airway management may be necessary. The decision to use these agents must be based on the practitioner's assessment of each situation.

Subarachnoid Injection

The accidental injection of anesthetic solution into the subarachnoid space can result in extensive sympathetic blockade, respiratory arrest, and, if untreated, cardiovascular collapse. Profound hypotension secondary to arterial vasodilation, impaired venous return, and cardiac sympathectomy (T1-T4) with reduced cardiac rate and contractile function often occur. Reduced venous return can also result from celiac plexus or lumbar sympathetic block owing to sequestration of venous blood in the viscera or lower extremities. Appropriate management of this problem is the immediate restoration of venous return by leg elevation, rapid infusion of intravenous fluids, and administration of temporizing drugs such as ephedrine, atropine, or phenylephrine.[56]

Neurolytic Agent Spread

Unexpected extensive spread of neurolytic agents can lead to neurologic damage of a prolonged nature. The best management of this problem is prevention. In all cases, an analysis of risk versus benefit is in order. The procedures must be done with care; a test dose of local anesthetic and radiographic confirmation of needle placement are indicated.

AUTONOMIC DYSFUNCTION: DYSREFLEXIA

Patients with spinal cord injury are frequently seen in the operating room for plastic reconstruction and for orthopedic, genitourinary, and neurologic surgery. For each patient, the degree of derangement of sympathetic control systems is a function of the level, completeness, and duration of the spinal cord injury.

Acute spinal cord trauma is a medical emergency. The major cause of morbidity and mortality is impaired respiratory function. Patients may be unable to protect their airway and clear bronchial secretions; therefore, prevention of aspiration of gastric contents is a recurring concern. Pulmonary edema and bronchopneumonia frequently occur.

In addition, these patients are functionally hypovolemic and frequently require intravenous fluids and vasopressors to support blood pressure. This relative hypovolemia stage is due to a low systemic vascular resistance that is caused by disruption of sympathetic vasoconstrictor mechanisms. The vasodilated state of the acute spinal cord injury patient also leads to significant heat loss and a predisposition to hypothermia.

Autonomic dysreflexia (AD) is a hypertensive crisis that occurs in paraplegic and quadriplegic patients. It is due to massive sympathetic vasoconstriction that is initiated below the segmental level of the spinal cord lesion (Fig. 28–9).

What Patients Are at Risk?

Two to 3 weeks following acute spinal cord trauma, sweating and the appearance of reflex flexor activity in the legs coincide with the return of autonomic responsiveness below the cord lesion. From this point forward, many spinal cord injured patients are at risk for AD. About 65% to 85% of spinal cord injury patients with lesions at or above the T-7 level have hypertensive episodes in their daily activities.[57] Patients with lesions between T-5 and T-10 may have only mild elevations in blood pressure during AD-triggering episodes. With cord lesions below T-10, the occurrence rate is relatively low (<10%).[58] In patients with an infarcted spinal cord or a cord that has otherwise been damaged, a minimal risk of AD episodes is present, since spinal reflexes are generally abolished.

Why Does It Occur?

The gradation of hypertensive responses relative to the level of spinal cord lesion is due to neurophysiologic mechanisms. Most commonly, visceral stimuli (e.g., bowel and bladder distension) and, less commonly, somatic and cutaneous stimuli can trigger AD (Fig. 28–10). Afferent signals are believed to travel to the spinal cord through sacral routes via the pudendal (somatic, S2-4) and pelvic (parasympathetic, S2-4) nerves. They proceed up the spinal cord via the spinothalamic tracks and dorsal columns.[58, 59] These signals can trigger both ipsilateral and contralateral increases in sympathetic outflow at each spinal level below the cord lesion.[60]

In normal individuals, this outflow is inhibited by descending signals from higher CNS centers. This descending inhibition is interrupted in the spinal cord injury patient. If splanchnic sympathetic outflow is included in the sympathetic response (cord lesions at or above T-7), the ensuing vasoconstriction can precipitate large increases in blood pressure that cannot be adequately compensated for by baroreflex-mediated cardiac slowing and sympathoinhibition to vascular sites above the lesion. The neurally intact adrenal medulla can also participate in the response. In addition, the denervated blood vessels of spinal cord injury patients appear to be hypersensitive to sympathetic stimulation and to catecholamines.[59]

Spinal cord transection does not interfere with afferent neural connections from the carotid and aortic arch baroreceptors (cranial nerves IX and X) to the brainstem. These receptors are activated by systemic hypertension during an AD episode. They promote reflex slowing of the heart through an intact vagus and reduced sympathetic activity to the vasculature above the level of the cord lesion. In patients with low cord injuries (T-10 or below), reflex inhibition of sympathetic outflow to the splanchnic circulation can also participate in the compensatory response to an AD episode. In this situation, blood pressure may increase only moderately, despite large increases in regional sympathetic outflow below the cord lesion.

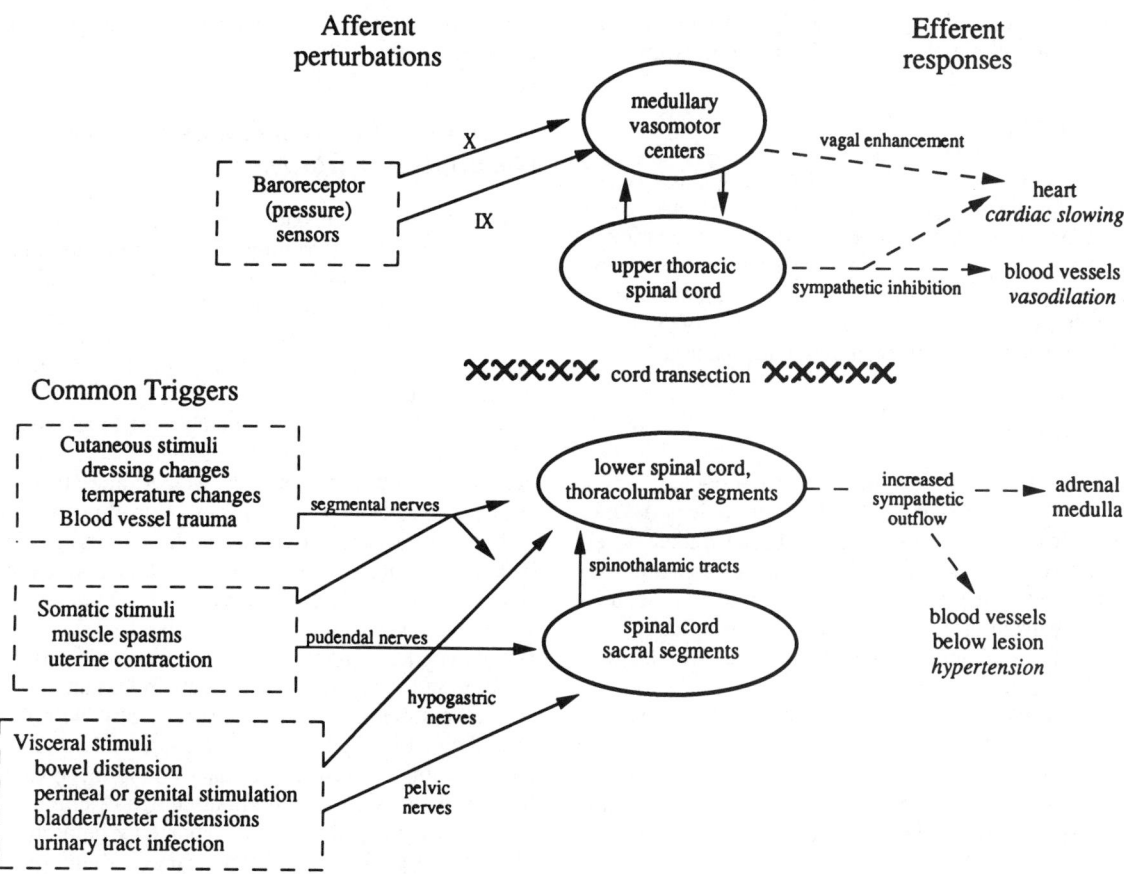

FIGURE 28–9. Autonomic dysreflexia. Neural pathways involved in autonomic dysreflexia. Triggering stimuli below the lesion leads to increased sympathetic outflow and hypertension. The baroreceptors sense the pressure elevation and elicit increases in vagal (parasympathetic) outflow and decreases in sympathetic outflow.

What Are the Stimuli, Signs, and Symptoms?

Many of the common visceral triggers for an AD episode have been mentioned. Others include dressing changes over decubiti, urinary tract infections, uterine contractions during labor, skeletal muscle spasms, and hypotension during orthostatic stress. Patients who experience an episode may report sensations of facial tingling, nasal stuffiness, headache, shortness of breath, nausea, or blurred vision. Associated signs include cutaneous vasodilation above and vasoconstriction below the lesion, sweating, cutis anserina (''goose flesh''), hypertension, bradycardia, and, on occasion, dysrhythmias. Severe episodes can be associated with seizure, loss of consciousness, and retinal, cerebral, or subarachnoid hemorrhage.[57–59]

Who Needs Preventive Treatment?

Should spinal cord injury patients with lesions below T-7 and no previous history of AD receive preventive therapy during surgical procedures below the lesions (where sensations are absent)? Because of the potential morbidity of an unablated episode, the answer probably is ''Yes.''

An important consideration is that autonomic responses are proportional to the strength of the stimulus. In daily activities, the strength and duration of potential triggering stimuli for AD may be much less than those of the stimuli that occur during surgical procedures. Thus, a patient with a low spinal cord transection and a negative history for AD might still have a major episode during a stimulating surgical procedure.

An additional consideration is that during an AD episode, reflex compensatory responses above the level of the cord lesion are dependent on intact baroreceptor mechanisms. Aging, hypertension, and various systemic diseases and medications can impair baroreceptor reflex function.[61] Thus, many spinal cord injury patients with low lesions are still at significant risk for uncontrolled hypertension due to pathologic or iatrogenic impairment of reflex buffering mechanisms.

What Therapeutic Modalities Are Useful?

The most common preventive strategy is to block the neural pathways with a general or regional anesthetic.[61–65]

Regional Anesthesia

Although spinal anesthesia is commonly employed, it may be difficult to perform or difficult to control, may be incomplete, or may lead to hypotension. The majority of these concerns have not been substantiated in recent studies.[4, 65] However, 7% to 27% of at-risk spinal cord injury patients given spinal anesthesia still have episodes of AD during surgery. The local anesthetic chosen should be sufficient to last throughout the planned surgical procedure. Epidural analgesia may result in inadequate block of L-5 or S-1 dermatomes. An inadvertent intrathecal injection may be difficult to ascertain.

General Anesthesia

Many anesthesiologists choose inhalation anesthetics. However, these agents do not always prevent AD because deep levels of anesthesia are needed to obtund sympathetic reflexes sufficiently.[65] An adequate plane of anesthesia without substantial hypotension in the spinal cord injury patient may be difficult to achieve. Moreover, a 23% incidence of AD has been reported in patients undergoing general anesthesia.[65]

Vasoactive Drugs

Other techniques that inhibit sympathetic outflow have been employed to treat AD episodes.[57, 58, 66] Ganglionic blocking agents such as trimethaphan are excellent because their onset of action is relatively quick and the magnitude of the response is fairly well titrable. Alpha-adrenergic antagonists (phentolamine, phenoxybenzamine) and direct-acting vasodilators (nitroprusside, calcium channel antagonists, and hydralazine) have been employed effectively.

Beta-adrenergic blockers are not indicated, since tachycardia is not a problem. Clonidine has been used prophylactically and has been reported to reduce hypertension during bladder stimulation.[67] This effect has been attributed to its ability to act either on spinal preganglionic neurons or on peripheral

presynaptic α_2-adrenoceptors. Clonidine may also reduce skeletal muscle spasms.[59]

What Special Considerations Apply to the Quadriplegic Parturient?

The uterus has a capacity to contract normally during labor despite complete interruption of its efferent neural regulation.[68] When the spinal cord is completely severed, labor is painless but can be associated with AD. Recurring episodes of AD may, in fact, be the only indication of the onset of labor.[68–70] In this situation, the nociceptive stimulus originates from the contracting uterus.

Epidural opioids have been employed to attenuate AD activity owing to their ability to modulate nociceptive transmission at the posterior horn cells. Meperidine (100 mg) has also been reported to be successful in controlling AD in the quadriplegic parturient.[69] However, epidural fentanyl (75-μg bolus; 10-μg · h^{-1} infusion) has failed in this application, perhaps owing to incomplete suppression of cord transmission of neural signals and to the use of such a low dose.[70] Meperidine may have been more effective because it has both opioid receptor and local anesthetic effects in humans.

Higher doses of other opioids may also be effective; however, they carry the usual risk of opioid side effects, including nausea, vomiting, pruritus, urinary retention, sedation, and respiratory depression. The optimal choice of epidural anesthetic for the quadriplegic patient in labor may be a combination of a low dose ($\leq$0.125%) of bupivacaine and an opioid.

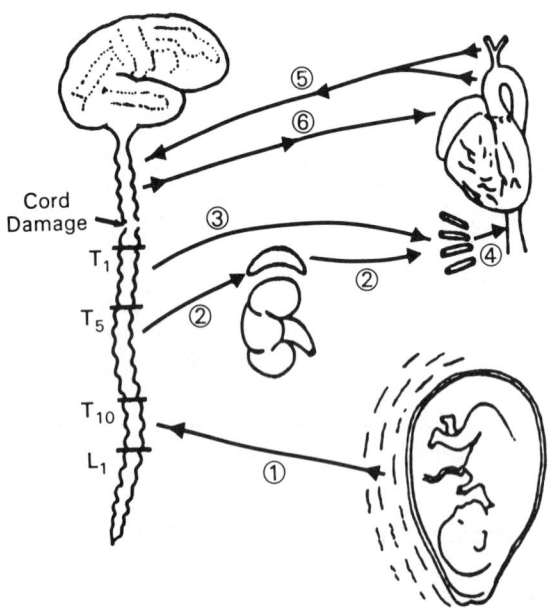

FIGURE 28–10. Mechanism of cardiovascular changes in autonomic hyperreflexia. Afferent impulses from contracting uterus to spinal cord segments T-10 through L-1. *2,* Efferent impulses from segments T-5 to T-9 to adrenal medulla causing discharge of catecholamines. Efferent impulses from sympathetic centers T-1 through L-1 directly to vascular bed causing vasoconstriction. *4,* Increase in arterial blood measure as a result of stimuli by *2* and *3. 5,* Afferent impulses from carotid sinus and aortic arch to cardiac centers in medulla oblongata. *6,* Efferent impulses through vagus nerves to heart causing bradycardia. (From Abouleish EI, Hanley ES, Palmer SM: Can epidural fentanyl control autonomic hyperreflexia in a quadriplegic parturient? Anesth Analg 1989; 68:523–526.)

References

1. Lykowitz RJ, Hoffman BB, Taylor P: Neurohumoral transmission: The autonomic and somatic motor nervous system. *In* Goodman and Gilman's The Pharmacological Basis of Therapeutics. 8th ed. Gilman AG, Rall TW, Nies AS, et al (eds). New York, Pergammon Press, 1990, pp 84–121.
2. Livingston RB: Visceral control mechanisms. *In* Best and Taylor's Physiological Basis of Medical Practice. 12th ed. West JB (ed). Baltimore, Williams & Wilkins, 1991, pp 1053–1067.
3. Williams PL, Warwick R, Dyron M, et al (eds): Gray's Anatomy. 37th ed. Edinburgh, Churchill Livingstone, 1989, pp 1154–1169.
4. Shanahan PT: Replantation of extremities. Anesth Clin North Am 1989; 7:675.
5. Hobelmann CF Jr, Delon AL: Use of prolonged sympathetic blockade as an adjunct to surgery in the patient with sympathetic-maintained pain. Microsurgery 1989; 10:151.
6. Ladd AL, DeHaven KE, Thanik J, et al: Reflex sympathetic imbalance: response to epidural blockade. Am J Sports Med 1989; 17:660.
7. Gamulin Z, Forster A, Simonet F, et al: Effects of renal sympathetic blockade on renal hemodynamics in patients undergoing major aortic abdominal surgery. Anesthesiology 1986; 65:688.
8. VanTwisk R, Gielen JM, Pavlov PW, et al: Is additional epidural sympathetic block in microvascular surgery contraindicated? A preliminary report. Br J Plast Surg 1988; 41:37.
9. Bonica JJ: Causalgia and other reflex sympathetic dystrophies. *In* The Management of Pain. 2nd ed. Bonica JJ (ed). Philadelphia, Lea & Febiger, 1990, pp 220–243.
10. Colding A: The effect of regional sympathetic blocks in the treatment of herpes zoster. Acta Anaesthesiol Scand 1969; 13:133.
11. Bonica JJ: Pain due to vascular disease. *In* The Management of Pain. 2nd ed. Bonica JJ (ed). Philadelphia, Lea & Febiger, 1990, pp 502–537.
12. Tasker RR, Dostrovsky JO: Deafferentation and central pain. *In* Textbook of Pain. Wall PD, Melzak R (eds). Edinburgh, Churchill Livingstone, 1989, pp 154–180.
13. Bengsston A, Bengsston M: Regional sympathetic blockade in primary fibromyalgia. Pain 1988; 33:161.

14. DeWitt RFE, Remme JJ: A report on the efficacy of regional intravenous sympathetic blocks (RIS-blocks) with guanethidine (Ismelin) in long-standing and complicated leg ulcers. Arch Dermatol Res 1989; 281:206.

15. Dyson A, Henderson AM: Continuous axillary brachial plexus blockade following intra-arterial injection of nicotinic acid. Anesth Intensive Care 1987; 15:462.

16. Floyd JB: Traumatic cerebral edema relieved by stellate ganglion anesthesia. South Med J 1987; 80:1328.

17. Sanchez V, Segedin ER, Moses M, et al: Role of lumbar sympathectomy in the pediatric intensive care unit. Anesth Analg 1988; 67:794.

18. Bonica JJ, Ventafridda V, Twyerors RG: Cancer pain. *In* The Management of Pain. 2nd ed. Bonica JJ (ed). Philadelphia, Lea & Febiger, 1990, pp 400–460.

19. Bell S, Cole R, Robert-Thompson IC: Coeliac plexus block for control of pain in chronic pancreatitis. Br Med J 1980; 281:1604.

20. Plancarte R, Amescua C, Patt RB, et al: Superior hypogastric plexus block for pelvic cancer pain. Anesthesiology 1990; 73:236.

21. Leung JWC, Bowen-Wright M, Aveling W, et al: Coeliac plexus block for pain in pancreatic cancer and chronic pancreatitis. Br J Surg 1983; 70:730.

22. Nurmikko T, Wells C, Bowsher D: Pain and allodynia in postherpetic neuralgia: role of somatic and sympathetic nervous systems. Acta Neurol Scand 1991; 84:146.

23. Sharfman WH, Walsh TD: Has the analgesic efficacy of neurolytic celiac plexus block been demonstrated in pancreatic cancer pain? Pain 1990; 41:267.

24. Yanagida H, Suwa K, Corssen G: No prophylactic effect of early sympathetic blockade on postherpetic neuralgia. Anesthesiology 1987; 66:73.

25. Bonica JJ, Buckley FP, Moricca G, et al: Neurolytic blockade and hypophysectomy. *In* The Management of Pain. 2nd ed. Bonica JJ (ed). Philadelphia, Lea & Febiger, 1990, pp 1980–2039.

26. Verrill P: Sympathetic ganglion lesions. *In* Textbook of Pain. 2nd ed. Wall PD, Melzak R (eds). Edinburgh, Churchill Livingstone, 1989, pp 773–783.

27. Wood KM: Peripheral nerve and root chemical lesions. *In* Textbook of Pain. 2nd ed. Wall PD, Melzak R (eds). Edinburgh, Churchill Livingstone, 1989, pp 768–772.

28. Reading AE: Testing pain mechanisms in persons in pain. *In* Textbook of Pain. 2nd ed. Wall PD, Melzak R (eds). Edinburgh, Churchill Livingstone, 1989, pp 269–280.

29. Lofstrom JB, Cousins MJ: Sympathetic blockade of upper and lower extremity. *In* Neural Blockade in Clinical Anesthesia and Management of Pain. 2nd ed. Cousins MJ, Bridenbaugh PO (eds). Philadelphia, JB Lippincott, 1988, pp 461–500.

30. Benzon HT, Cheng SC, Avram MJ, et al: Sign of complete sympathetic blockade: sweat test or sympathogalvanic response? Anesth Analg 1985; 64:415.

31. Diaz P: Use of liquid crystal thermography to evaluate sympathetic blocks. Anaesthesia 1976; 44:443.

32. Higa K, Dan K, Manabe H, et al: Factors influencing the duration of treatment of acute herpetic pain with sympathetic nerve block: importance of severity of herpes zoster assessed by the maximum antibody titers to varicella-zoster virus in otherwise healthy patients. Pain 1988; 32:147.

33. Malmquist L-A, Tryggvasm B, Bengtsson M: Sympathetic blockade during extradural analgesia with mepivacaine or bupivacaine. Acta Anaesthesiol Scand 1989; 33:444.

34. Riegelman RK, Hirsch RP: Studying a Study and Testing a Test: How To Read The Medical Literature. 2nd ed. Boston, Little, Brown & Co, 1989, pp 127–183.

35. Haynes RB: How to read clinical journals: II. To learn about a diagnostic test. Can Med Assoc J 1981; 124:703.

36. Hannington-Keff JG: Pharmacological target blocks in painful dystrophic limbs. *In* Textbook of Pain. 2nd ed. Wall PD, Melzak R (eds). Edinburgh, Churchill Livingstone, 1989, pp 754–766.

37. Thompson GE, Moore GC: Celiac plexus, intercostal, and minor peripheral blockade. *In* Neural Blockade in Clinical Anesthesia and Management of Pain. 2nd ed. Cousins MJ, Bridenbaugh PO (eds). Philadelphia, JB Lippincott, 1988, pp 503–530.

38. Brown DL, Bulley CK, Quiel EL: Neurolytic celiac plexus block for pancreatic cancer pain. Anesth Analg 1987; 66:869.

39. Brown EM, Kunjappen V: Single needle lateral approach for lumbar sympathetic block. Anesth Analg 1975; 54:725.

40. Fujita Y, Takaori M: Pleural effusion after CT-guided alcohol celiac plexus block. Anesth Analg 1987; 66:911.

41. Hardy PAJ, Wells JDC: Coeliac plexus block and cephalic spread of injectate. Ann R Coll Surg Engl 1989; 71:48.

42. Hogan QH, Erickson SJ, Haddox JD, et al: The spread of solutions during stellate ganglion block. Reg Anaesth 1992; 17:78.

43. Kirvela O, Svedstrom E, Lundblom N: Ultrasonic guidance of lumbar sympathetic and celiac plexus block: a new technique. Reg Anaesth 1992; 17:43.

44. Lieberman RP, Waldman SD: Celiac plexus neurolysis with the modified transaortic approach. Radiology 1990; 175:274.

45. Moore DC, Bush WH, Burnett LL: Celiac plexus block: a roentgenographic anatomic study of technique and spread of solution in patients and corpses. Anesth Analg 1981; 60:369.

46. Moore DC, Bush WH, Burnett LL: An improved technique for celiac plexus block may be more theoretical than real. Anesthesiology 1982; 57:347.

47. Singler RC: An improved technique for alcohol neurolysis of the celiac plexus. Anesthesiology 1982; 56:137.

48. Sprague RS, Ramamurthy S: Identification of the anterior psoas sheath as a landmark for lumbar sympathetic block. Reg Anaesth 1990; 15:253.

49. Lieberman RP, Nance PN, Cuka DJ: Anterior approach to celiac plexus block during interventional biliary procedures. Radiology 1988; 167:562.

50. Matamala AM, Lopez FV, Sanchez JLA, et al: Percutaneous anterior approach to the coeliac plexus using ultrasound. Br J Anaesth 1989; 62:637.

51. Wheatly JK, Motamedi F, Hammonds WD: Page kidney resulting from massive subcapsular hematoma: complication of lumbar sympathetic nerve block. Urology 1984; 24:361.

52. Owens EL, Kasten GW, Hersel EA: Spinal hematoma after lumbar puncture and heparinizaton. Anesth Analg 1986; 65:1201.

53. Horlocker TT, Wedel DJ, Offord KP: Does preoperative antiplatelet therapy increase the risk of hemorrhagic complications associated with regional anesthesia? Anesth Analg 1990; 70:631.

54. DeGowin RL: DeGowin and DeGowin's Bedside Diagnostic Examination. 5th ed. New York, Macmillan Publishing Co, 1987, p 948.

55. Lofstran B: Stellate ganglion block. *In* Illustrated Handbook in Local Anesthesia. 2nd ed. Copenhagen, I. Chr. Sorenson & Co, A/S, 1979, p 143.

56. Greene NM: Physiology of Spinal Anesthesia. 3rd ed. Baltimore, Williams & Wilkins, 1981, pp 63–146.

57. Schonwald G, Fish KJ, Perkash I: Cardiovascular complications during anesthesia in chronic spinal cord injured patients. Anesthesiology 1981; 55:550.

58. Johnson B, Thomason R, Pallares V, et al: Autonomic hyperreflexia: a review. Mil Med 1975; 140:345.

59. Mathias CJ, Frankel HL: Cardiovascular control in spinal man. Ann Rev Physiol 1988; 50:577.

60. Fagius J, Karhuvaara S: Sympathetic activity and blood pressure increases with bladder distension in humans. Hypertension 1989; 14:511.

61. Ebert TJ, Stowe DF: Peripheral circulation: recent insights into autonomic nervous control and endothelial factors relevant to cardiovascular disease and anesthesia. Curr Opin Anaesth 1991, pp 3–11.

62. Lambert DH, Deane RS, Mazuzan JE: Anesthesia and the control of blood pressure in patients with spinal cord injury. Anesth Analg 1982; 61:344.

63. Broecker BH, Hranowski N, Hackler RH: Low spinal anesthesia for the prevention of autonomic dysreflexia in the spinal cord injury patient. J Urol 1979; 122:366.

64. Katz RL, Thorp JM, Cefalo RC: Epidural analgesia and autonomic hyperreflexia: a case report. Am J Obstet Gynecol 1990; 162:471.

65. Stowe DF, Bernstein JS, Madsen KE, et al: Autonomic hyperreflexia in spinal cord injured patients during extracorporeal shock wave lithotripsy. Anesth Analg 1989; 68:788.

66. Dykstra DD, Sidi AA, Anderson LC: The effect of nifedipine on cytoscopy-induced autonomic hyperreflexia in patients with high spinal cord injuries. J Urol 1987; 138:1155.

67. Mathias CJ, Frankel HL: Autonomic failure in tetraplegia. *In* Autonomic Failure. 2nd ed. Banister R (ed). Oxford, Oxford University Press, 1988, pp 453–488.

68. Robertson DNS: Pregnancy and labor in the paraplegic. Paraplegia 1972; 10:209.

69. Baraka A: Epidural meperidine for control of autonomic hyperreflexia in a paraplegic parturient. Anesthesiology 1985; 62:688.

70. Abouleish EI, Hanley ES, Palmer SM: Can epidural fentanyl control autonomic hyperreflexia in a quadriplegic parturient? Anesth Analg 1989; 68:523.

CHAPTER 29

Vascular System Anatomy

JAMES M. O'CALLAGHAN, P.A.-C., B.M.Sc.
CHRISTINE A. CZEPIZAK, M.S., P.A.-C.
BAHMAN VENUS, M.D., F.C.C.M., F.C.C.P.

Vascular access is an important part of many diagnostic procedures and clinical monitoring. Rapid, safe access can be achieved with practice and solid knowledge of the anatomy of the vascular system.

Arterial cannulation is desirable for invasive blood pressure monitoring, for sampling in arterial blood gas analysis, and for providing access for invasive diagnostic procedures such as arteriography. Occasionally, it is indicated for patients who require frequent blood sampling but have poor peripheral veins.

Venous cannulation provides a direct route for the delivery of drugs, fluids, electrolytes, and nutrients. The type of therapy, duration of catheterization, and condition of the patient may determine whether intravenous access is located peripherally or centrally, or both.

ARTERIAL CANNULATION

The most common sites for arterial cannulation are the radial and femoral arteries because of their superficial location and low complication rates.[1]

Where Is the Radial Artery?

The radial artery is a branch of the brachial artery, which in 90% of patients bifurcates just below the elbow (Fig. 29–1). Proximally, the radial artery is overlapped by the brachioradial muscle. Distally, it resides between the brachioradial and the radial flexor muscle of the wrist. It passes over the distal part of the radius, making the pulse easily palpable at this point. Collateral arterial blood flow to the hand is supplied via the ulnar artery as well as via the dorsal arch in the back of the hand. Cannulation of the radial artery is preferable at the wrist because it is more superficial and because the radial nerve is separate from the artery at this location.

The left radial artery is generally cannulated in preference to the right because it originates from the left subclavian artery. Thus, a retrograde embolus introduced into the systemic

circulation during irrigation of an arterial catheter will likely go to the descending aorta; in contrast, one entering via the right radial and subclavian arteries must first traverse the origins of arterial inflow to the cerebral vessels, making a central nervous system complication more likely.

In patients with peripheral vascular disease, a discrepancy in blood pressure between the right and left brachial arteries (and, thus, both radial arteries) is frequently present. This difference is attributed to proximal atherosclerotic stenosis. Hence, one should compare blood pressures in both arms. If a ≥10-mm Hg difference exists, the side with the higher blood pressure is cannulated.

Where Is the Femoral Artery?

The femoral artery lies together with the femoral vein in a fibrous sleeve called the *femoral sheath* (Fig. 29–2). It begins distal to the inguinal ligament and continues along the medial and anterior aspects of the thigh. The artery lies superficially within the femoral triangle, and the pulse generally can be located midway on an imaginary line between the symphysis pubis and the anterior superior spine of the ilium. Note that the proximity of the femoral nerve makes it vulnerable to block and thus, to weakness of the quadriceps muscle of the thigh when local anesthetic is infiltrated into this area. Collateral flow is via the anastomoses between several branches originating off of the femoral artery distally. The femoral vein lies just medial to the artery within the femoral sheath. The femoral artery commonly has atherosclerotic lesions. These may break off and embolize or interfere with cannulation.

What Alternate Sites Can Be Used?

Axillary Artery

The axillary artery is the continuation of the subclavian artery as it crosses beneath the first rib (see Fig. 29–1). It becomes the brachial artery at the distal border of the tendon

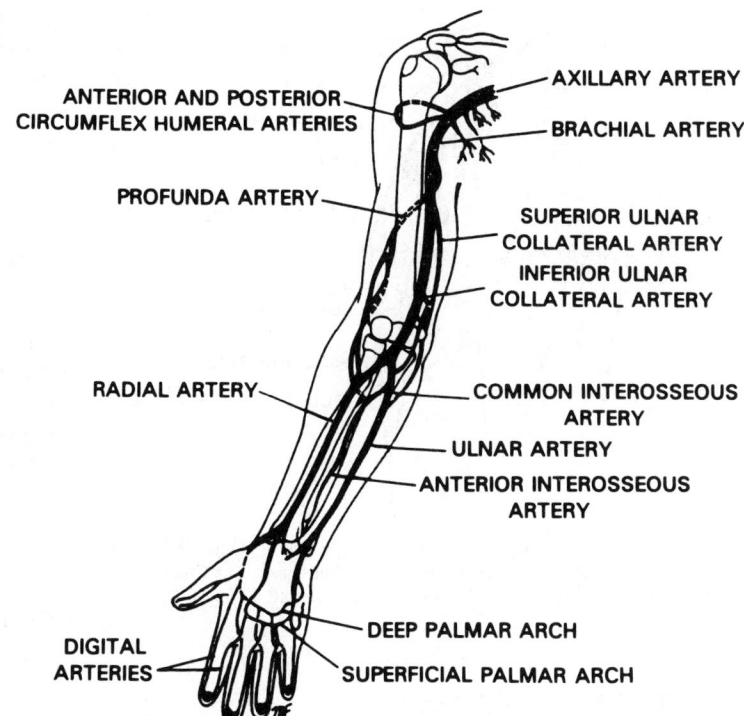

FIGURE 29–1. Axillary, brachial, and radial artery relationships at the upper arm and elbow. Note important anastomoses at the elbow. (From Snell RS, Katz J: Clinical Anatomy for Anesthesiologists. Norwalk, CT, Appleton & Lange, 1988, p 88.)

of the teres major muscle. This segment is superficial and can be cannulated. The artery can be palpated as it is compressed against the shaft of the humerus along the lower border of the pectoralis major muscle. Lateral to it is the coracobrachial muscle, and on its medial border lies the axillary vein. In close proximity and within the enshrouding neurovascular sheath are the branches of the brachial plexus. Collateral flow to this segment of the axillary artery is via its subscapular, posterior humeral circumflex and anterior humeral circumflex branches.

To expose this artery, the patient is positioned with the hand on the side to be cannulated under his or her head. If the artery is difficult to palpate, the arm can be slightly adducted from this position. The vessel can also be located by pencil-probe Doppler ultrasound or by applying a pulse oximeter probe to the hand and finding the point where compression of the axilla causes the pulse oximeter signal to disappear. Even more so than with the more distally located radial or brachial arterial sites, the left side is preferred because of a lower incidence of retrograde embolic stroke.

Brachial Artery

The brachial artery begins where the axillary artery terminates at the distal margin of the tendon of the teres major muscle (see Fig. 29–1). It runs down the arm medial to the humerus until it approaches the bend of the elbow, where it lies anterior and midway between the two epicondyles. The artery is relatively superficial throughout its course and is covered by several layers of fascia. It can be palpated in the antecubital fossa of the extended arm.

Collateral circulation is via the deep brachial nutrient artery of the humerus and the superior ulnar collateral, inferior ulnar collateral, and muscular arteries. This collateral blood source is often considered insufficient should thrombi form after cannulation of the brachial artery.[1] Hence, the brachial artery is not a first choice for this purpose. Since it runs medial and adjacent to the median nerve at the elbow, care should be exercised not to injure this nerve during cannulation.

Dorsalis Pedis Artery

The dorsalis pedis artery is the continuation of the anterior tibial artery. It lies anterior on the ankle joint and passes to the medial side of the dorsum of the foot (Fig. 29–3). On its tibial side is the tendon of the long extensor muscle of the great toe, and along its fibular side lies the first tendon of the long extensor muscle of the toes. It is a superficial artery palpable along its course.

Collateral flow is to the foot via the posterior tibial artery and the perforating branch of the peroneal artery. The dorsalis pedis artery is not commonly a first choice for cannulation. Its anatomy and size are less predictable, and its distal location results in systolic overshoot and diastolic underestimation of central aortic pressures. Mean arterial pressure is, however, representative of central pressures in the supine patient who does not have peripheral vascular disease. It is absent or too small to cannulate in 12% of individuals.

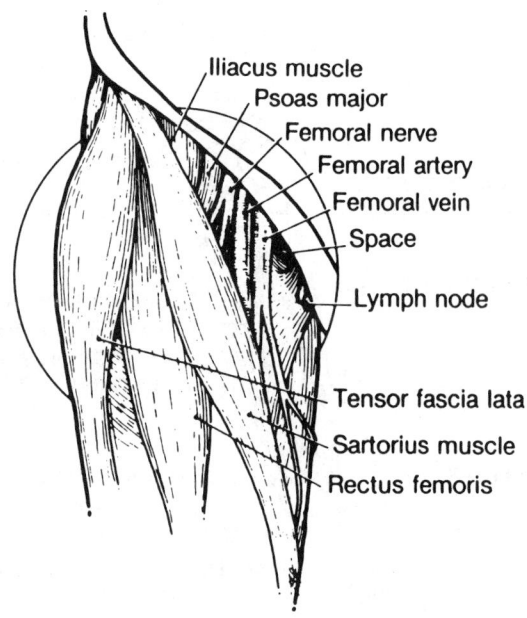

FIGURE 29–2. Anatomy of the right femoral region. (From Otto CW: Central venous pressure monitoring. *In* Monitoring in Anesthesia and Critical Care Medicine. 2nd ed. Blitt CD (ed). New York, Churchill Livingstone, 1990, p 205.)

Superficial Temporal Artery

The superficial temporal artery is used for cannulation in children and infants. It is one of two terminal branches of the external carotid artery. This artery originates in the parotid gland, crosses the posterior segment of the zygomatic process of the temporal bone, and then divides into two branches above the zygoma. It can be palpated just anterior to the auricle of the ear. It is an extremely small and tortuous artery; thus, a cannula that is 22 gauge or smaller is commonly inserted.

Because of its small volume (<1 mL) and origin off the carotid artery, air or particulate emboli may travel to the brain.[2] Thus, it is used only if attempts at other sites are unsuccessful or if other sites are inappropriate. It was a more commonly utilized site prior to the advent of pulse oximetry because it served as another site for collecting preductal blood specimens and for monitoring in newborns when other preductal arteries could not be cannulated.

PERIPHERAL VENOUS CANNULATION

Which Peripheral Veins Are Easiest to Access?

In adults, the most common veins used, in order of accessibility, are: the metacarpal veins, the branches of the basilic and cephalic veins, and the superficial pedal veins. Use of the pedal veins is not highly recommended, since they have a propensity for thrombosis as well as blood backflow from extremity dependence.[3] Generally, they are chosen in an acute setting as a temporizing measure.

Metacarpal Veins

The metacarpal veins are usually the first to consider.[4, 5] They lie on the dorsal aspect of the hand and run between the metacarpal bones. This site is ideal in that the veins usually are easily seen, palpated, or both. Even if they are not visible, their location is relatively constant, and they can often be cannulated by trial and error. The metacarpal bones provide stability, but if the tip of the cannula crosses the wrist joint, the wrist should be stabilized with an "arm board." This technique decreases mechanical damage to the intima by decreasing catheter movement within the vein.

Basilic Vein Branches

The basilic and cephalic veins are fairly large and have adequate subcutaneous tissue to provide stability during cannulation (Fig. 29–4). The basilic vein begins on the anterior, ulnar aspect of the forearm. As the vein ascends the forearm, it crosses the antecubital fossa, runs deep through the subcutaneous fascia, and eventually joins other deep veins of the upper arm to become the axillary vein. From the basilic vein, a fairly long and straight branch, the median antebrachial vein, travels laterally across the brachial muscle. It curves distally and then runs straight along the posterior aspect of the forearm.[4, 6–9] This vein may be difficult to locate in some patients.

Cephalic Vein Branches

Below the antecubital fossa, a straight branch of the cephalic vein, the accessory cephalic vein, is the most commonly used tributary on the forearm. The cephalic vein begins along the dorsal, radial aspect of the lower forearm and ascends the lateral side of the arm. It becomes anterior at the antecubital fossa, while passing over the brachial artery and median nerve. Instead of running deep, it continues superficially across the biceps muscle before entering the subcutaneous tissue.

Median Cubital Vein

The median cubital vein connects the basilic and cephalic veins within the antecubital fossa (see Fig. 29–4). This vein is

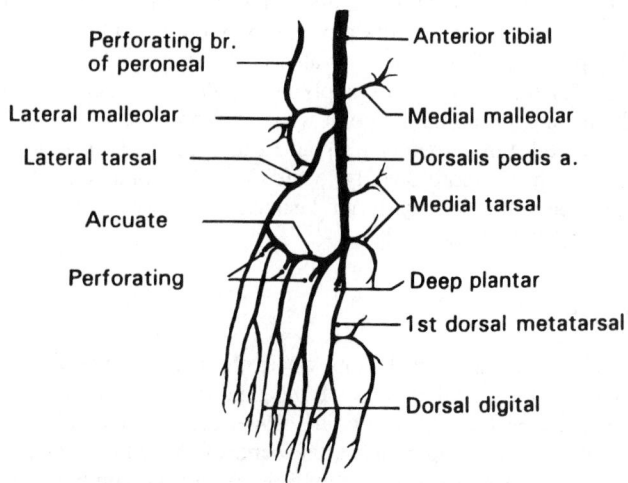

FIGURE 29–3. Arteries of the dorsum of the foot.

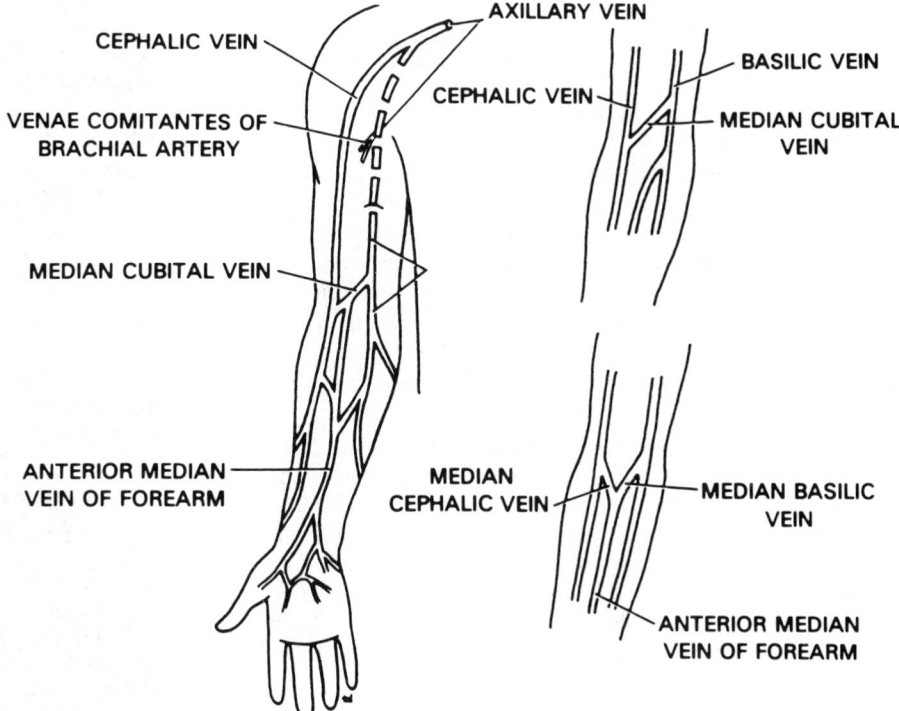

FIGURE 29–4. Superficial veins of the upper limb. The common variations seen in the region of the elbow are also shown. (From Snell RS, Katz J: Clinical Anatomy for Anesthesiologists. Norwalk, CT, Appleton & Lange, 1988, p 101.)

Labels in figure: CEPHALIC VEIN, VENAE COMITANTES OF BRACHIAL ARTERY, MEDIAN CUBITAL VEIN, ANTERIOR MEDIAN VEIN OF FOREARM, AXILLARY VEIN, CEPHALIC VEIN, BASILIC VEIN, MEDIAN CUBITAL VEIN, MEDIAN CEPHALIC VEIN, MEDIAN BASILIC VEIN, ANTERIOR MEDIAN VEIN OF FOREARM

rarely covered by fat, and many of its tributaries are readily visible or palpable. Use of these veins at the level of the antecubital fossa in nonurgent situations is discouraged because flexion of the forearm poses an increased risk for cannula occlusion, thrombosis, and patient discomfort.[10] However, in an emergent situation, or for a long procedure in which the arm is straight, these veins make excellent choices for peripheral intravenous access because of their large caliber and relatively straight course.[3, 5, 11]

Summary

When choosing a vein for venipuncture, one should avoid areas that include valves. They commonly occur at points of bifurcation and may present as obstructions as the catheter is advanced.[7] Once a vein has been chosen, the order of the sites for cannulation attempts is from distal to proximal to allow maximum availability in the event that further access is required or if the initial cannulation attempt is unsuccessful.

What Alternate Sites Can Be Used?

In the nonemergent setting, other sites can be considered for peripheral cannulation. They include digital veins lying along the dorsolateral aspect of the fingers[5]; deep dorsal hand veins, which form an arch and are one-third of the distance proximal to the metacarpal-phalangeal joints[6]; pedal veins, including the median and lateral margin veins of the foot; and the long saphenous vein.[4, 8, 11] The last of these is recommended for use only in infants and small nonambulatory children.[12]

Intraosseous Sites

In adults, the sternum or ribs may be used for intraosseous infusions. The body of the sternum, just above the xiphoid process, is the sternal site of choice. Its thin cortex makes insertion easy; however, the close proximity of the underlying great vessels and pleura increase the risk of serious complications. Alternatively, the lateral aspect of the sixth through ninth ribs may be cannulated. Again, care must be taken to avoid puncturing the pleural cavity. The medial (tibial) malleolus is a safer and easily accessible site in both pediatric and adult patients. The special needle is introduced approximately 2 cm above the distal process of the tibial tubercle.

Corpora Cavernosa and Dorsal Vein of the Penis

Use of the corpora cavernosa of the penis as a route for fluid administration in emergent situations has been suggested.[13] The corpora cavernosa have a rich venous drainage system with many communications between the superficial dorsal vein and the deep veins of the penis. Subcutaneous hematoma formation is a possible complication.[14]

Theoretically, direct cannulation of the superficial dorsal

vein is possible in emergent situations requiring intravenous access. The safety and efficacy of using the penis for fluid and or drug administration have not been formally evaluated.

Other Peripheral Sites in Children

In the newborn, superficial veins may tend to be more visible than in adults; however, as the child develops, the formation of subcutaneous tissue and fat make access much like that in the adult.[15] Veins of the scalp are often utilized in neonates.[12] They include the frontal, superficial temporal, posterior auricular, supraorbital, occipital, and posterior facial veins. These superficial veins are thin, small, and course caudally and laterally until they drain into the external jugular vein at the angle of the mandible. Veins on the ventral surface of the wrist may also be used. The foot and long saphenous veins of the medial lower limb are also available.

Intraosseous Sites

Intraosseous sites may be used in emergency situations to infuse fluids or drugs. The spacious venous sinusoids in the marrow function as a rich venous drainage route. In children and infants, the proximal tibia and distal humerus are locations of choice. Infusion needles may be inserted 2 to 3 cm below the tibial tubercle along the flat anterior surface or 3 cm above the external condyle of the femur in the anterior midline. Care must be taken to avoid the epiphyseal plates of the long bones in children.

CENTRAL VENOUS CANNULATION

The most commonly used central veins are the internal jugular vein (IJV), the subclavian vein (SCV), and the femoral vein. The external jugular vein can be used for either peripheral or central venous access.

Where Is the Internal Jugular Vein?

The IJV lies beneath the sternocleidomastoid muscle. This vein exits the skull via the jugular foramen posterior to the internal carotid artery near the angle of the mandible and enters a sheath that surrounds the IJV and common carotid artery. As it courses distally toward the SCV, its relationship changes such that it is anterolateral to the carotid artery at the level of the cricoid cartilage. The IJV is medial to the sternocleidomastoid at its most cephalad portion. It becomes posterior to the triangle formed by the two heads of this muscle in the middle and finally is posterior and lateral to the sternal head at its caudal portion (Fig. 29–5).

The IJV is smallest at its origin and increases in diameter until it terminates at the SCV. On the right, the IJV joins the SCV to form the short brachiocephalic vein, which is 1 to 2 cm in length. On the left, the IJV joins the SCV at an acute angle posterior to the medial head of the clavicle, forming a more pronounced and longer (3- to 5-cm) brachiocephalic vein.[3, 8, 9, 16] The IJV on the right is generally larger than the one on the left. This difference is thought to reflect the greater amount of blood entering it from the superior sagittal sinus via the sigmoid sinus.[17]

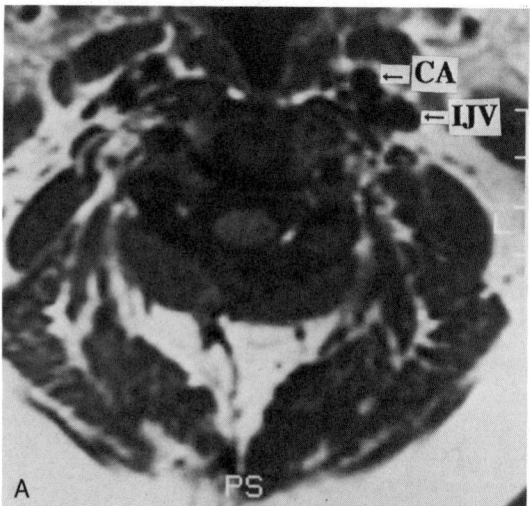

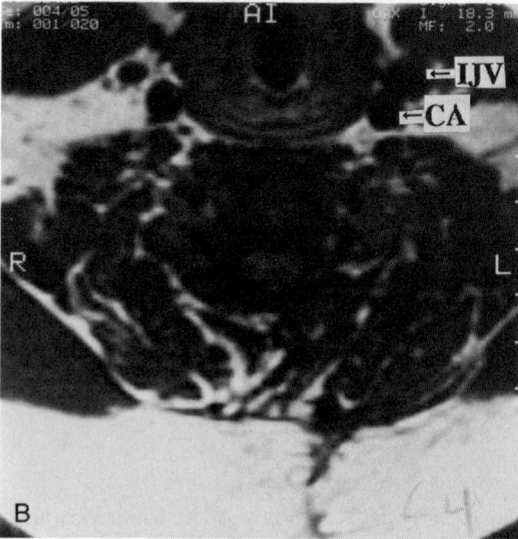

FIGURE 29–5. *A,* Magnetic resonance image of the neck at the level of the carotid bifurcation. Note that the internal jugular vein is posterolateral to the carotid artery. *B,* At the level of C-4, the rotation has resulted in an anterolateral jugular vein position. IJV = internal jugular vein; CA = carotid artery.

Adjacent Structures

Carotid Artery, Vagus and Phrenic Nerves, and Stellate Ganglion

The carotid artery is usually palpated medial and posterior to the IJV. Posterior to the carotid artery lies the stellate ganglion and cervical sympathetic trunk. Important nerves include the phrenic nerve, which runs lateral to the vascular bundle and medial to the attachment of the anterior scalene muscle. The vagus nerve is located outside the sheath posterior to and between the carotid artery and the IJV. The thyroid gland is medial and in the same plane as the IJV. This gland, lateral to the cricoid cartilage, is easily palpated and avoided. The platysma, superficial aponeurosis, and the epidermis are the outer remaining structures.

Vertebral and Thyroid Arteries

The vertebral and thyroid arteries lie underneath the anterior triangle of the neck. The branches of the inferior thyroid and ascending cervical arteries pass in front of the anterior scalene muscle and behind the internal jugular vein. The vertebral artery runs through the transverse foramina of C-6 to C-1. Of note is that low in the neck, at the level of C-7, the vertebral artery is not protected by a bone canal and is thus even more vulnerable to needle injury. The vertebral artery lies posterior to the common and then to the internal carotid artery as it ascends in the neck.

Thoracic Duct

Another noteworthy adjacent structure is the thoracic duct. This lymphatic drainage channel is present on both sides of the neck but is much larger on the left side. It courses up and out of the thorax adjacent to the esophagus. It then loops just posterior to the carotid sheath behind the carotid artery and vein at the base of the neck and then empties posteriorly into the junction of the internal jugular and subclavian veins.

Cupola of the Lung

The inner chest wall is covered by the parietal pleura. The apex of each hemithorax is called the ''cupola.'' The cupola can extend up to 3 cm superior to the middle third of the clavicle posterior to the sternocleidomastoid muscle and brachial plexus. Because the pleural cupola is dome-shaped, it does not extend as far superior at the medial or lateral margins of the clavicle. Although some anatomists note that the cupola is lower on the right side than on the left, this opinion is not uniformly held.

Precautions

The IJV has been shown to be typically rhomboid in shape, and it becomes more circular as the head is rotated. This maneuver increases its lumenal cross-sectional area.[18] The relationship between the sternocleidomastoid and IJV changes with head position. By rotating the head 30° to 45° toward the contralateral side, the sternocleidomastoid muscle stretches, making it both more visible and palpable. Once the head is rotated beyond 45°, the medial portion of the muscle begins to overlie the IJV, making it more difficult to locate.[18] Head rotation also tends to rotate the vein, which in the anterior triangle of the neck is predominately anterior and lateral in the sheath over the carotid artery.[19]

Head rotation beyond 45° predisposes to carotid puncture when the vein overlies the artery and the needle passes through the back wall of the vein during cannulation. Another consideration is that the angle between the IJV and SCV becomes smaller as the head is rotated away from the side of cannulation (i.e., the veins become more aligned). This relationship predisposes to entry of the guidewire and catheter into the ipsilateral SCV rather than into the brachiocephalic vein and superior vena cava. The vein is 1.5 to 2.5 cm deep to the skin at the level of the cricoid cartilage. This depth remains fairly constant with changes in head positioning.

Where Is the Subclavian Vein?

The SCV originates from the axillary vein at the outer aspect of the first rib just below the middle third of the clavicle (Fig. 29–6). It is 1 to 2 cm in diameter and 3 to 4 cm in length. Its orientation is medial and superior to the first rib. After crossing the rib, the SCV continues medially until it is separated from the subclavian artery by the anterior scalene muscle at its attachment to the first rib. On the left side, the SCV and IJV join to form the brachiocephalic vein located behind the superior lateral border of the manubrium. This vein is longer on the left side and curves downward behind the manubrium, where it joins the short, right brachiocephalic vein to form the superior vena cava–brachiocephalic junction.[20, 21] The size of the subclavian vein is not influenced by intravascular volume or central venous pressure as it is held open by its investing fascia. This feature is of consequence because it

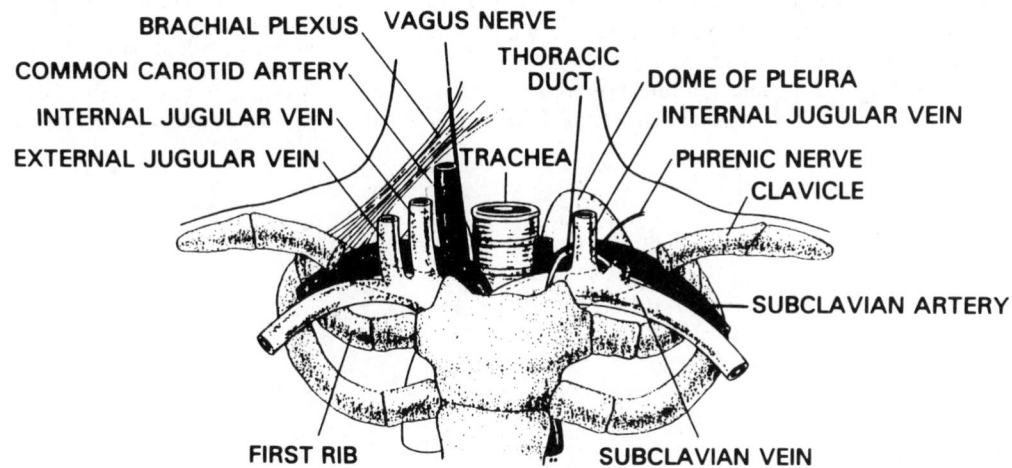

FIGURE 29–6. Anatomic relationships of vascular and associated structures. Note the close proximity of arterial and venous structures, the prominent thoracic duct and higher pleural cupola on the left, and the perpendicular entry of the left IJV into the left SCV. The right IJV and the SCV-IJV junction are on a straight path to the SCV. The left SCV courses in a less angulated orientation than the right. Venipunctures in the lateral region of the clavicle are more prone to arterial puncture, brachial plexus injury, and pneumothorax. (From Novak R, Venus B: Clavicular approaches for central vein cannulation, ''Vascular cannulation.'' Probl Crit Care 1988; 2:244.)

BRACHIAL PLEXUS VAGUS NERVE
COMMON CAROTID ARTERY THORACIC DUCT DOME OF PLEURA
INTERNAL JUGULAR VEIN INTERNAL JUGULAR VEIN
EXTERNAL JUGULAR VEIN TRACHEA PHRENIC NERVE
CLAVICLE
SUBCLAVIAN ARTERY
FIRST RIB SUBCLAVIAN VEIN

predisposes the patient to venous air embolism; however, it is more easily cannulated than the IJV during shock or low flow states.

Adjacent Structures

Important surrounding structures are the clavicular notch at the level of the SCV-IJV junction, the right and left thoracic ducts that enter the SCV at its superior margin just lateral to the SCV-IJV junction, and the subclavius muscle that lies anterior along the length of the SCV.

Other structures closer to the junction of the IJV and SCV may vary according to their position on the left or right side. The pleural dome is located just posterior to the IJV-SCV junction and brachiocephalic vein. The apical aspect on both sides potentially may be higher in thin individuals or in those with chronic obstructive lung disease.[16, 21]

Where Is the External Jugular Vein?

The external jugular vein begins at the bifurcation of the anterior facial and posterior auricular veins just anterior to the ear lobe and behind the angle of the mandible. It runs at an oblique angle superficially across the anterior aspect of the body of the sternocleidomastoid muscle, continues distally, then turns inward at the middle third of the clavicle, and terminates at the SCV lateral to the insertion of the IJV.[6, 8, 18]

Valsalva's maneuver, fluid bolus, Trendelenburg's position, or finger compression on the skin just above the clavicle to obstruct its drainage can assist in defining the vein's course. In younger individuals, valves are prominent, especially at the terminal site, and may make cannulation difficult.

The acute angle of entry of the external jugular vein into the SCV can make catheter passage into the brachiocephalic vein and superior vena cava difficult. A flexible tip guidewire is important to avoid perforation of the inferior wall of the SCV as the wire is advanced.

Where Is the Femoral Vein?

The femoral vein is relatively superficial and a direct continuation of the popliteal vein in the lower thigh. Below the inguinal ligament, the vein travels cephalad within a femoral sheath, always medial to the femoral artery (see Fig. 29–2). Above the inguinal ligament, it runs posteriorly to become the external iliac vein. The femoral vein can be located below the inguinal ligament by palpating the artery in the femoral triangle. It is 1 to 2 cm medial to the artery. A useful mnemonic to remember that the vein is located medial to the femoral artery is NAVL (Nerve, Artery, Vein, Lymphatic vessels, from lateral to medial).

References

1. Seneff M: Arterial line placement and care. *In* Intensive Care Medicine. Rippe JM, Irwin RS, Fink MP (eds). Boston, Little, Brown & Co, 1991, pp 37–47.
2. Prian GW, Wright GB, Runack CM, et al: Apparent cerebral embolizations after temporal artery cannulation. J Pediatr 1978; 93:113.
3. Intravenous nursing standards of practice. National Intravenous Therapy Association, 1980; 4:8.
4. Kaye W, Dubin H: Vascular cannulation. *In* Critical Care. Civetta JM, Taylor RW, Kirby RR (eds). Philadelphia, JB Lippincott, 1988, pp 211–225.
5. Vicari M, Swecker M: Care of vascular cannulas, "Vascular cannulation." Probl Crit Care 1988; 2:214.
6. Grant JC: Grant's Atlas of Anatomy. 6th ed. Baltimore, Williams & Wilkins, 1972.
7. Hardaway L: An overview of vascular access devices inserted via the antecubital area. J Intraven Nurs 1990; 13:297.
8. Tortora G, Anagnostakos N: Principles of Anatomy and Physiology. 2nd ed. New York, Canfield Press, 1978, p 480.
9. Otto CW: Central venous pressure monitoring. *In* Monitoring in Anaesthesia and Critical Care Medicine. 2nd ed. Blitt C (ed). New York, Churchill Livingstone, 1985, pp 142–161.
10. Plumer AL, Casentina F: Principles and Practice of Intravenous Therapy. 7th ed. Boston, Little, Brown & Co, 1987.
11. Wax F, Talan D: Advances in cutdown techniques. Emerg Med Clin North Am 1989; 7:65.
12. O'Biran R: Starting intravenous lines in children. J Emerg Nurs 1991; 17:225.
13. Godec CJ, Cass AS: The penis: a possible alternative emergency venous access for males? Ann Emerg Med 1982; 11:266.
14. Venus B, Mallory DL: Vascular cannulation. *In* Critical Care. 2nd ed. Civetta JM, Taylor RW, Kirby RR (eds). Philadelphia, JB Lippincott, 1992, pp 149–169.
15. Murdock L, Bingham R: Venous cannulation in infants and small children. Br J Hosp Med 1990; 44:405.
16. Parsa MH, Tabora F, Al-Saurwaf M, et al: Vascular access techniques. *In* Textbook of Critical Care. 2nd ed. Shoemaker W (ed). Philadelphia, WB Saunders, 1990, pp 122–126.
17. Moore KL, Keith L: Clinical Oriented Anatomy. 2nd ed. Baltimore, Williams & Wilkins, 1985, p 1014.
18. Mallory DL, Shawtzer T, Evans RG, et al: Effects of clinical maneuvers on sonographically determined internal jugular vein size during venous cannulation. Crit Care Med 1990; 18:1269.
19. Sulek CA, Weiss L, Gravenstein N: Influence of head position on relationship between internal jugular vein and carotid artery. Crit Care Med 1993; 21:S218.
20. McGee WT, Mallory D: Cannulation of the internal and external jugular veins, "Vascular cannulation." Probl Crit Care 1988; 2:217–242.
21. Novak R, Venus B: Clavicular approaches for central vein cannulation, "Vascular cannulation." Probl Crit Care 1988; 2:242–246.

Techniques and Procedures

CHAPTER 30

Positioning the Surgical Patient

ROBERT BLACKSHEAR, M.D

NIKOLAUS GRAVENSTEIN, M.D.

Positioning the patient for surgery is an important but sometimes underappreciated aspect of patient care in anesthesiology. Closed claims review indicates that 15% of closed malpractice claims related to anesthesia care are filed for peripheral nerve injuries.[1] These injuries usually are directly or indirectly attributed to the patients' positioning for surgery. Correct positioning is a necessary consideration if the incidence of intraoperative nerve injury is to decrease.

In positioning a patient, a number of goals are promoted. Important to the surgeon is that the patient's position facilitate the surgery without injury, whether it be to nerves or skin or secondary to physiologic alterations caused by the particular position. Another goal is to optimize access to the anatomic target to facilitate the surgical process. A more efficiently completed procedure decreases the incidence of injury secondary to positioning. A third goal is to preserve the anesthesiologist's access to the patient so that he or she can maintain the airway, monitoring devices, and intravascular catheters.

Ultimately, the responsibility for positioning to minimize nerve injury or patient discomfort lies with the anesthesiologist, the surgeon, and the circulating nurse, who together must act as a team. At one extreme, assignment of primary responsibility is to the individual who renders the patient unable to respond to pain. Some consider the anesthesiologist generally to be responsible for positioning and position-related injuries to the upper half of the body and the surgeon and nurse to be accountable for injuries to the lower half. A hybrid view considers that the anesthesiologist is responsible for the upper half of the body, since that is where he or she works, monitors, and has access, as well as for those parts of the lower half of the body that are readily visible. Regardless of one's personal philosophy, a patient expects to leave the hospital without a nerve injury, and likely will attempt to hold all who provided care responsible if such injury does occur.

SPECIAL CONSIDERATIONS

How Should the Patient Be Moved and Positioned?

A number of inherent problems are confronted when a patient is anesthetized. The first is how he or she is to be transferred from one place to another. Whenever possible, the patient should position himself or herself by moving unassisted to the operating room table from the stretcher and then should assume the position for the surgical procedure while he or she is still awake. Any elements of the positioning that may compromise patient comfort can thus be detected. If the position required for the procedure is not assumed until after induction of anesthesia, the anesthesiologist should verify before induction that the patient can lie on the applicable side. If the arms are to be abducted, request that the patient assume the necessary position before induction, and ensure that the abducted position can be accomplished without pain or discomfort. Sometimes these goals can be accomplished by questioning the patient or by having him or her try the position during the preanesthetic interview.

What Is the Effect of Pre-Existing Medical Problems?

Pre-existing anatomic or medical conditions should also be considered. Exposure of the operative site may be compromised by a painful spine, excessive bulk, or skeletal deformity. Conditions such as congestive heart failure or increased intracranial pressure should also be considered, as they too can affect what positioning is best. In patients with either of these conditions, an elevated head position would be expected to have a beneficial effect, whereas a supine or lowered head position might aggravate the condition.

Why Does Postoperative Back Ache Occur?

Postoperative back ache is often attributed to positioning, but this problem is more commonly a function of the duration of surgery, the use of muscle relaxants, the associated loss of the normal lumbar lordosis, and the stretching of intervertebral ligaments.[2] The incidence of postoperative back ache ranges from 12% to 37%.[2, 3] Other than slightly flexing the hips and knees, placing a pillow under the knees, using a semi-reclining beach chair position, or inserting a small lumbar support, we know of no definitive preventive measures.

How Does Cardiorespiratory Compromise Occur?

Potential compromise of cardiorespiratory function is a well-recognized effect of positioning. Positions that minimize respiratory compromise (e.g., the head elevated position) may aggravate circulatory insufficiency, and vice versa. Some positions with a kidney rest (e.g., the prone and lateral decubitus positions) interfere with venous return from the lower body and decrease lung-thorax compliance and functional residual capacity.

When Is Neurovascular Compromise a Problem?

Neurovascular compromise can lead to peripheral nerve injury (from compression or stretching of the intraneural vasa nervorum, or both), resulting in nerve ischemia.[4] This complication most likely occurs when a nerve or plexus has a long and a superficial course between two points of fixation (Fig. 30–1). Another mechanism involves compression of a nerve between internal structures (e.g., bone) and external structures (e.g., operating room table, stirrups). The most detrimental circumstances occur when stretching and compression are combined; a stretched nerve is exquisitely vulnerable to ischemic compression.[5]

Compression of tissue is more likely to produce nerve injury when it occurs in a small area. Impacting on this form of injury is the duration of the compression.[5] As a general rule, at least 20 minutes of ischemic compression are required for a nerve injury to occur. For example, consider how long your arm or leg takes to become numb when the nerve supply to either is compressed. A stretch injury, in contrast, can occur instantaneously (e.g., brachial plexus avulsion).

The most common cause of nerve injury is likely a combination of stretch and compression, since neither alone would be sufficient to cause such an injury. The anesthetized patient is unable to move or change position independently and is unable to identify pain or paresthesia associated with position-induced neurovascular compromise. Thus, the risk of injury is *always* present.

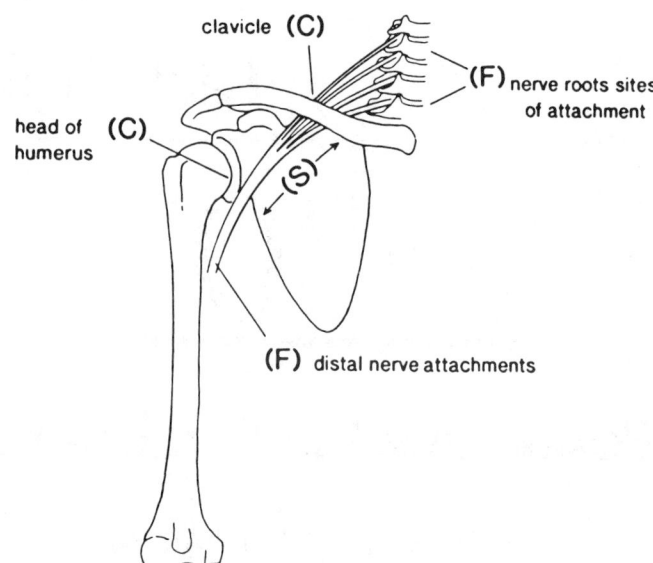

FIGURE 30–1. Schematic diagram of brachial plexus injury. Positioning may stretch (S) the plexus between points of fixation (F), increasing the likelihood of compression injury at several sites (C). (From Mahla ME: Nervous system. *In* Manual of Complications During Anesthesia. Gravenstein N (ed). Philadelphia, JB Lippincott, 1991, p 384.)

AVOIDANCE OF POSITION-RELATED INJURIES

Awake positioning, as was mentioned in the introductory remarks, is the best method to detect and to prevent potential injury. This approach is possible in the vast majority of cases.

How Are Pressure Points Managed?

Pressure points and nerve stretch should also be considered as causes of nerve injury. Careful padding of pressure points and devoting strict attention to the patient's position or to a change in this position during the surgical process are also important. Pressure points vary with patient position (Table 30–1). The operating room table mattress is adequate to support the scapulae, hips, and sacrum in all short procedures. Areas of special concern are the occiput, elbows, and heels, all of which require extra padding. The occiput and heels are particularly problematic because of the considerable weight that is distributed over their small areas. Weight distribution and the very superficial course of the ulnar nerve cause potential difficulties at the elbows.

Why Do Stretch Injuries Occur?

Avoiding stretch injuries is best accomplished by considering the course and fixation points of superficial nerves (Figs.

TABLE 30–1. Pressure Points

Supine	Prone	Decubitus
Occiput	Forehead	Ear
Scapula	Eyes	Axilla
Elbows	Chest	Hip
Hips	Elbows	Knee (peroneal nerve)
Sacrum	Iliac crests	Ankle
Heels	Knees	

30–2 and 30–3). Gentle flexion of the hips and knees; abduction of the arms to <90° extension (in or forward of the plane of the body); and conformance of the cervical spine to the neutral or ''sniffing'' position ensures absence of nerve stretch. We emphasize that the absence of pain and the use of muscle relaxants allow placement of a patient into an otherwise intolerable position. Prolongation of surgery beyond the limits of what the patient would otherwise tolerate contributes to injury that may occur.

DOCUMENTATION OF PROTECTIVE MEASURES

Patient positioning should be documented in the anesthesia record in order to demonstrate that it was duly considered and carefully determined. The patient's response to the position should be indicated on the chart if he or she is awake during the procedure or just prior to induction. A description of the padding should also be included. A comment such as ''pressure points padded and checked'' on the chart, although common on anesthesia records, does not provide much information. We have adopted the practice of teaching residents to draw a stick figure of the patient on which the position and associated padding can be shown. Figure 30–4 is an example of such a drawing for a supine patient. Note the identification of specific padding and arm abduction, which is clearly <90°.

INCIDENCE OF POTENTIALLY POSITION-RELATED COMPLICATIONS

According to Kroll and coworkers, of the 1541 claims reviewed up to 1990 and recorded in the American Society of

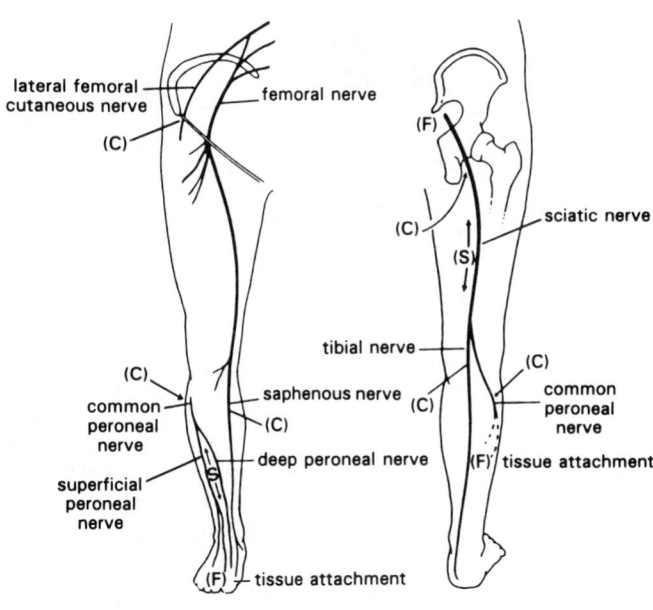

FIGURE 30–3. Schematic diagram of selected lower extremity nerve injuries. *A,* Anterior view. The lateral femoral cutaneous nerve may be compressed (C) between an external appliance and the iliac spine. The common peroneal nerve may be compressed (C) between the head of the fibula and an external appliance. Pressure against the medial aspect of upper one-third of tibia may compress (C) the saphenous nerve. The superficial and deep peroneal nerves may be stretched (S) if the foot is plantar flexed. *B,* Posterior view. The sciatic nerve may be stretched (S) between its fixation points by flexion of the hip without flexion at the knee. It may also be compressed (C) at the ischial tuberosity. The tibial nerve is susceptible to compression (C) at the popliteal fossa. (From Mahla ME: Nervous system. *In* Manual of Complications During Anesthesia. Gravenstein N (ed). Philadelphia, JB Lippincott, 1991, p 388.)

Anesthesiologists' (ASA) closed claims study database, 227 were for anesthesia-related nerve injury.[1] The most frequent claimed injury was ulnar neuropathy, which represented 34% of all nerve injuries. Less frequent were brachial plexus (23%) and lumbosacral (16%) injuries.

Of interest were the authors' conclusions that although nerve damage is a significant source of anesthesia-related claims, most often it cannot be explained. In particular, ulnar nerve injuries seem to occur without any identifiable mechanism.[1, 6] Body habitus may also be an important variable. For example, in the closed claims analysis, 61% of the ulnar nerve damage claims were made by men, even though the overall gender distribution of claims was equal.[1]

SPECIFIC CONSIDERATIONS

What Problems Are Associated with the Supine Position?

Padding

When the patient is placed in a supine position, the weight is borne by the occiput, scapulae, elbows, sacrum, calves, and heels (see Table 30–1). Appropriate padding must be placed at each pressure point to prevent pressure injuries, especially in older patients undergoing prolonged procedures (Fig. 30–5). The use of soft foam or gel-filled padding is advocated.

We pad the sacrum in adults undergoing cardiopulmonary bypass owing to the associated lower perfusion pressures and

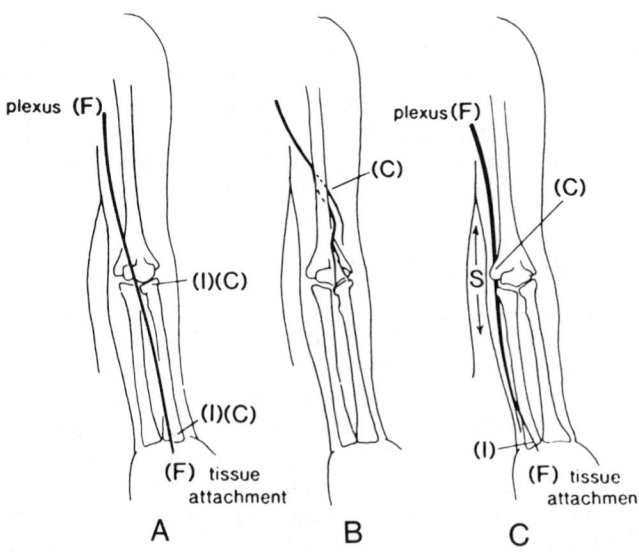

FIGURE 30–2. Schematic diagram of selected upper extremity nerve injuries. *A,* Median nerve. Injuries may occur by direct damage from intravenous catheter insertion (I) or intravenous filtration with resultant compression (C). Stretching may occur between points of fixation (F) by dorsiflexion of the wrist. *B,* The radial nerve is susceptible to compression against the posterior surface of the humerus (C), usually by an external appliance or by the operating table. *C,* The ulnar nerve is susceptible to stretching (S) between fixation points (F) by elbow flexion. In addition, it is vulnerable to compression at the elbow (C). (From Mahla ME: Nervous system. *In* Manual of Complications During Anesthesia. Gravenstein N (ed). Philadelphia, JB Lippincott, 1991, p 387.)

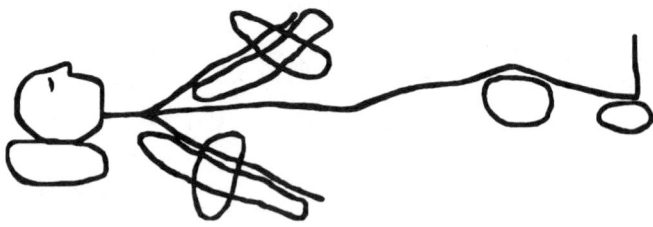

FIGURE 30–4. Schematic representation of position and pressure point documentation of a patient in the supine position.

long case duration. An often neglected pressure point is the occiput; a number of cases describe pressure alopecia secondary to poor occipital circulation that causes an obliterative vasculitis when inadequate padding is placed beneath the head.[3] Although the scalp is vascular, the occiput is still vulnerable because of the head's weight and the small area that is in contact with the bed or table. Padding serves not only to soften the contact point but also to enlarge it by allowing the weight to be distributed over a greater area.

Additional means to protect against positioning trauma in the supine position include the placement of pillows under the knees to prevent hyperextension and resultant tibial and peroneal nerve stretch, and the positioning of the safety belt above the knees and below the hips to avoid compressing the peroneal and lateral femoral cutaneous nerves, respectively.

Positioning of the Arms

Flexed and Wedged

How to position the patient's arms (i.e., whether they should be tucked at the patient's side, extended on an armboard, or flexed and wedged) is an additional consideration. The literature is contradictory with respect to the incidence of brachial nerve injury and ulnar neuropathy when the arms are tucked, abducted to an angle of <90°, or flexed and wedged over the head.[7, 8] Similarly, the relative advantages of having the forearms supinated, prone, or in an in-between position are un-

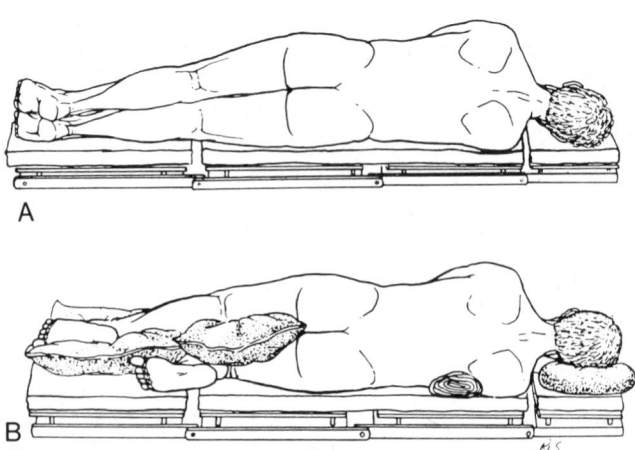

FIGURE 30–5. The standard right lateral decubitus position. *A,* Improper head position and inadequate padding. *B,* Proper padding is present over bone prominences, a chest roll is placed to protect the axilla, and the cervical spine is properly aligned. A flexed lower leg stabilizes the torso and relaxes the lower extremity. (From Lawson NW: The lateral decubitus position. *In* Positioning in Anesthesia. Martin JT (ed). Philadelphia, WB Saunders, 1987, p 156.)

clear. Our practice is to place soft wedges under each arm and to place the arms above the head. This position is analogous to the touching of the ears with the upper arms abducted 30° in front of the plane of the body.

Abducted

If a patient's arms are positioned out and to the sides on armboards, close attention must be given that they maintain an angle of <90° with the plane of the body. Make sure that the brachial plexus is not being stretched by feeling the degree of tension placed on the pectoral muscle in the axilla. Also be careful that the height of the armboard padding is matched to that of the mattress so that the humerus does not lie behind the plane of the body. Should this occur, the head of the humerus moves anteriorly and results in pressure and stretch on the axillary portion of the brachial plexus. Conversely, if the armboard padding is higher than the mattress, the radial nerve may be compressed by the edge of the armboard pad as it courses around the posterior surface of the humerus.

Tucked

If the patient's arms are tucked at the side, they should be padded and secured. A shield or *toboggan* placed under the mattress prevents the arm from falling off the table and protects it from being leaned against by workers in the operating room. If a shield is used, it too should be padded. An alternative approach is to secure the arms to the bed by encircling them with the draw sheet, which is then tucked underneath the patient (not under the table!).

Regardless of which position is selected, the ulnar nerve—or at least the ulnar groove—should be palpated to ensure that it is not being compressed. Theoretically, supination of the forearm moves the cubital tunnel away from the surface of the bed and, thus, protects the ulnar nerve; however, no data have shown this position to be efficacious. Therefore, routine internal or external rotation of the arm cannot be recommended. Choose the position that feels best to the patient and avoids ulnar nerve compression. A final consideration is to verify that the patient's fingers are away from the hinge in the bed so that they are not injured if the foot/leg portion of the bed is raised.

Contoured Supine Position

The contoured supine position is also called the "lawnchair position." (Fig. 30–6) The back of the bed is elevated 10° to 20°, and the table is contoured so that the hips and knees are slightly flexed. A conscious patient lying supine and motionless can usually maintain normal distribution of tissue perfusion for about 1 hour before he or she notices increasing discomfort that necessitates moving. This "lying-at-attention" position, also known as the "rigid supine position," results in significant discomfort to the patient who is awake while undergoing a protracted procedure.

In contrast, the lawnchair position adds to patient comfort by more uniformly distributing his or her weight and by providing support along the full length of the dorsal body surface. It also permits gentle flexion of the hips and knees, which helps to put these joints into more anatomically neutral positions.

The lawnchair position is advantageous for patients in shock because it allows the head and both lower extremities to be

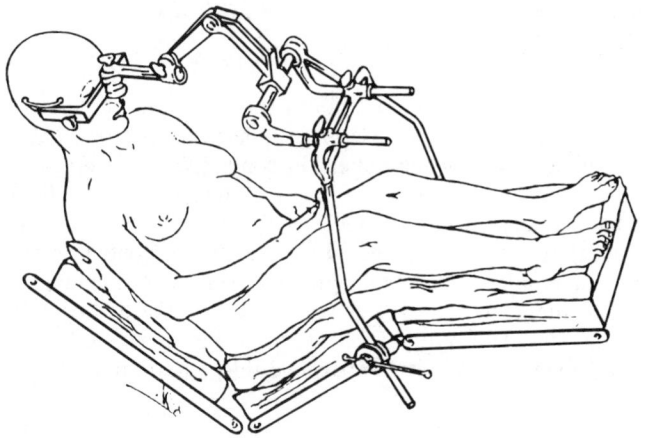

FIGURE 30–6. Patient in position using a three-pin clamp. (Reproduced with permission from Anderton JM, Keen RI, Neave R (eds). Positioning the Surgical Patient. London, Butterworth-Heinemann, Ltd., 1988, p 68.)

raised above the level of the heart. Venous drainage into the superior and inferior vena cava augments central blood volume. Elevation of the head above the level of the heart also lessens cerebral venous pressure and minimizes the chances for producing or increasing cerebral edema.

Because the horizontal axis of the trunk is not changed, pulmonary blood volume is usually not redistributed; thus, venous congestion in the poorly ventilated pulmonary apices, as would typically occur in a patient in the Trendelenburg position, is avoided.

What Problems Are Associated with the Prone Position?

The prone position (or the ventral decubitus position) is useful for operations involving the rectum, the spine, or the dorsum of the body (Fig. 30–7). When this position is used, attention is focused primarily on cardiorespiratory effects. Potential respiratory problems mainly involve restriction of the diaphragm during inspiration by abdominal contents or by the weight of the patient against the thorax. Both problems create a restrictive defect, compromise chest expansion, and increase work of breathing in the spontaneously ventilating patient. Positive-pressure ventilation is effective in overcoming the decreased lung-thorax compliance. However, the cardiovascular system is affected by compression of the abdomen, which obstructs flow in the inferior vena cava and decreases preload to the right ventricle.

Moving Supine to Prone

Technique

An effective way to place the patient in the prone position after induction of anesthesia is to align the patient's torso (with the arms at his or her sides) with the padding on the frame that is to be used. The anesthesiologist is responsible for the head and neck and a second person for the feet and legs. A third person rolls the patient into the arms of a fourth who is leaning across the padding or support frame. This "catcher" secures the patient's arms while the stretcher is moved out of the way. The patient's torso is centered over the frame, and

the arms are positioned and padded, either at the sides or adjacent to the head on armboards. In the latter situation, the arms are abducted with the elbows flexed and padded so that the hands are near the head in front of the plane of the body. A sufficient number of people must be available if injury—not only to the patient but also to the personnel helping in the lifting process—is to be avoided. Again, we stress that when an anesthetized patient is to be placed on the operating room table, all accessories (e.g., armboards, pillows, support for the patient's head) should already be prepositioned at their appropriate locations.

Precautions

If a patient is placed in the prone or three-quarter prone position for a neurosurgical technique in which the head is to be supported by pins, the anesthesiologist should be directly involved. It should be verified that no undue flexion or extension of the neck occurs, that the pinning apparatus is well attached to the table, and that the endotracheal tube is adequately secured once the new position is achieved. We affirm that at least two fingerbreadths of space are present between the chin and sternum to avoid excessive flexion.

Head

Positioning of the head in the prone position is done with strict attention devoted to the eyes as well as to the cervical spine, the ears, and the endotracheal tube. Pressure on the eyes can result in retinal artery thrombosis and postoperative blindness. Pressure can fold the ear when the head is turned to the side and thus cause cartilaginous damage.[3]

Endotracheal Tube

Endotracheal tube management in the prone patient is problematic because we are unable to assess tube position or identify possible kinking or secretions that cause loss of tape adherence. Administration of an antisialagogue to minimize secretions is recommended for any prone patient.

In our experience, use of a contoured foam head support with an opening for the endotracheal tube and cutouts for the eyes is effective. If the tube is secured with tape that encircles the neck, make sure that it does not become so tight that cerebral venous drainage is obstructed. The eyes, ears, and nose are individually inspected and verified to be free of any externally applied pressure from the padding.

Cervical Spine

The cervical spine is maintained in a neutral to slightly flexed position during the procedure. Neutrality of the cervical spine is easily verified by observing symmetry of the skin

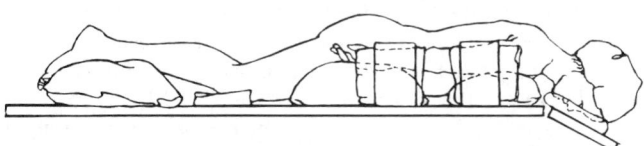

FIGURE 30–7. Prone position with arms at the side. (From Positioning the Surgical Patient. Anderton JM, Keen RI, Neave R (eds). London, Butterworths, 1988, p 50.)

folds between the neck and shoulder on each side and by ensuring that several inches of space are present between the mandible and the suprasternal notch.

Arms

Arm position in the prone position should also be assessed. All efforts should be made not to abduct the arms beyond a 90° angle to the sagittal plane of the body so as to avoid brachial plexus stretch injury. Be sure that no skin crease is visible over the posterior shoulder. If it is, the arm probably is in an overly abducted position. We prefer to see both arms somewhat abducted so that they are slightly in front of the plane of the body. This position is made possible by use of a chest support at sufficient height.

Chest/Abdomen

Chest rolls or a Wilson-type laminectomy frame help to position a patient for prone surgery. However, complications can result from the use of either. The most prevalent complication is the occurrence of pressure ulcers on that portion of the chest wall that is in contact with the chest roll or frame. This problem is related to the duration of surgery and is sometimes unavoidable if the patient cannot be repositioned in a scheduled fashion during the operation. These skin injuries likely represent a combination of traction and pressure. Despite attempts to eliminate traction on the skin and to pad the weight-bearing areas (see Table 30–1), pressure ulcers are still common, especially in procedures that last longer than 4 hours.

The chest rolls or laminectomy frame should be placed so that the iliac crests and lateral hemithoraces bear the weight. The clavicles should not be involved; otherwise, the brachial plexus becomes compressed between them and the underlying ribs. Either support system allows the abdomen to hang freely. Care should also be taken to verify that breast tissue and genitalia are not trapped; once the patient is draped, reassessment and repositioning are extremely difficult.

Bone Prominences

Ample padding of bone prominences is efficacious, especially in the ulnar nerve region on the medial aspects of the arms. The iliac crests, knees, ankles, and tibial portions of the lower legs should also be padded.

The Patient with Cervical Instability

On occasion, surgery is performed on the posterior cervical spine of a patient with radiculopathy or myelopathy. In such a case, the endotracheal tube should be placed using either a nasal or oral approach while the patient is supine and awake. The patient is then helped to roll facedown onto the padded frame or rolls. Positioning is performed while the patient indicates that no aggravation of symptoms or pain is occurring in any extremity. Only after this is done is anesthesia induced.

While the patient is still awake, move both arms and legs into the surgical position that will be used throughout the procedure and ask for feedback from the patient concerning these adjustments. Usually, the patient is the best judge of what position can be tolerated; once an acceptable position is found, every effort should be made not to change it.

What Problems Are Associated with the Lateral Decubitus Position?

The lateral decubitus position is most often used for chest, renal, or hip procedures. It is designated as left or right to identify the side of the patient in contact with the operating room table. Ventilation/perfusion ($\dot{V}/\dot{Q}$) mismatches are significant. The dependent lung receives the majority of pulmonary blood flow and is compressed by mediastinal contents and a cephalad shift of the diaphragm. The nondependent lung receives the majority of ventilation (during positive-pressure ventilation). This $\dot{V}/\dot{Q}$ mismatch can lead to hypoxemia and a larger than usual arterial versus end-tidal carbon dioxide gradient.

Precautions

Dependent Arm and Axilla

The dependent arm should be well padded and a chest roll placed just *below* the axilla to support the upper part of the rib cage, to ensure decompression of the axillary neurovascular bundle, and to remove pressure from the head of the humerus (see Fig. 30–5). If the chest roll is placed too cephalad, brachial plexus compression can occur, and a postoperative neuropathy can result. If an open space is present between the axilla and the chest roll and if the pulse in that arm is palpable, the arm and axilla are likely in appropriate position. The usual considerations apply for protecting the ulnar nerve. The nondependent arm is positioned over the dependent one, and one or two pillows are placed between the two.

Head and Neck

The patient's head must be kept in a neutral C-spine position, and the ear must be checked for excessive cartilaginous pressure. Our experience is that a pad thicker than one would expect is required to support the head in a normal position. Neutrality is easily checked by comparing the skin creases for symmetry on each side of the neck posteriorly. The dependent eye and ear should be checked to ascertain that no pressure is exerted upon them.

Hip and Leg

Considerable pressure is exerted on the dependent iliac crest, greater trochanter, and knee. We place a foam eggcrate pad or gel-filled pad on top of the mattress to protect these points. The dependent leg is also flexed, and the safety strap is placed so that it is across the waist or the thigh rather than the hip or knee. The peroneal nerve at the knee is especially vulnerable; padding is placed so that no pressure is exerted over the course of the nerve around the fibular head.

Moving Supine to Decubitus

When the patient is placed in the lateral decubitus position, there must be an adequate number of persons to assist in lifting, and each person must be assigned a task. The patient is anesthetized on the operating room table rather than on a gurney; from that point onward, the anesthesiologist is responsible for control of the head and endotracheal tube. The head, shoulders, and body are turned as a unit under the anesthesiologist's direction, and the patient is in effect log-rolled into position. This maneuver requires at least three and preferably four persons. If an ether screen is used, the patient's arms should not rest against it.

After the chest roll is in place, an easy (although imperfect) test for vascular compromise to the dependent arm and hand is to place the pulse oximeter on one of its fingers. Pulse oximeter technology is sufficiently sensitive that unless perfusion is <10% normal, an adequate signal is recorded. Although a palpable pulse and normal oxygen saturation alone are not adequate to verify acceptable positioning, when used in conjunction with visual inspection and palpation of pressure points, they complete the assessment routine.

What Problems Are Associated with the Head-Up Position?

The head-up position is used in order to facilitate exposure and enhance venous drainage for posterior fossa craniotomies and some operations of the cervical spine, face, neck, and shoulders. The position also predisposes to venous air embolism. Initially, the patient is supine for anesthetic induction and then is moved into the lawnchair position. The neck is flexed, and the head is placed in a pinning head holder by the neurosurgeon, with the anesthesiologist having control of the airway at all times. The back of the table is raised to create the sitting position while the table is tilted downward (see Fig. 30–6).

Neck flexion is limited to allow at least two fingerbreadths between the sternum and the chin and to preserve some slack in the cervical musculature. Gluteal padding should be maximized with foam, and the knees should be flexed with the feet in the slightly dorsiflexed position. The patient's arms are either secured to padded armboards at the sides, or they are placed across the chest. In both instances, the courses of the ulnar nerves should be inspected.

Air Embolism

The risk of air embolism from the surgical field is always present. Since the surgical field is higher than the right atrium, holes made in the skull with pin-type head holders, the craniotomy, and retractors or bone canals potentially allow air to be entrained into an open vein, causing venous air embolism. Therefore, patients in the sitting position are routinely monitored for early detection of air embolism.

Monitors

Continuous monitors include a precordial Doppler ultrasound probe, which is secured over the heart in a position that is known to detect air; capnography, which identifies any sudden decrease in expired carbon dioxide; and placement of a central venous catheter at the superior vena cava right atrial junction, which aids in confirmation of the diagnosis and, possibly, in removal of entrained air.

Other indicators of air embolism include dysrhythmias, hypotension, and the very late, relatively uncommon, pathognomonic "mill-wheel" murmurs. If the patient has a patent foramen ovale, air embolism is extremely hazardous. Air can pass from the right side of the heart to the left side (paradoxically) and enter the coronary or cerebral circulation, causing ischemia and permanent injury.

A patient with physical findings or history suggestive of an intracardiac defect or patent foramen ovale preferably should be operated on in a non–head elevated position (e.g., in the prone or three-quarter prone position) to minimize (but not eliminate) the likelihood of venous and paradoxic air embolism. If this approach is not feasible, a transesophageal echocardiography probe is the most sensitive indicator of venous air embolism and should be considered for use in conjunction with the other monitors.

An additional consideration in head elevated cases is transducer positioning. Blood pressure transducers are referenced to the external auditory meatus and central venous pressure transducers to the heart. If blood pressure is referenced to the heart, as it is in the supine position, the hydrostatic pressure difference between the heart and the brain may be such that the brain is hypoperfused, even though cardiac perfusion is adequate.

What Problems Are Associated with the Lithotomy Position?

The lithotomy position is most commonly used for gynecologic and urologic surgery. The first consideration for lithotomy positioning is to make sure that the equipment fits the patient. A leg support system is preferable (Fig. 30–8); however, an ankle strap system can also be used. When using either system, attention should be given to the patient's height, age, and weight and to estimates of the knee-to-ankle and thigh lengths.

If the patient is properly positioned supine, the gluteal folds are at the hinge between the thigh and torso sections of the operating room table before anesthesia is induced. This preparation avoids the need to move the patient toward the foot of the bed after induction of anesthesia, but it does require that the headpiece of the table be attached to the foot of the bed so that the patient's feet do not hang over the edge. The patient's arms are then secured to the armrests in a comfortable position that allows surgical and equipment access. During laparo-

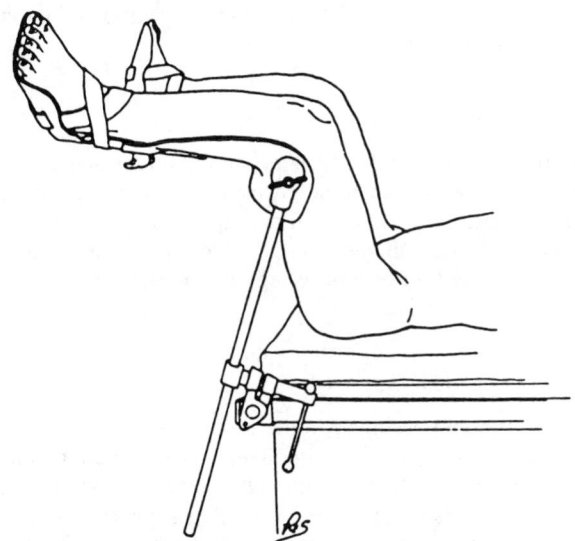

FIGURE 30–8. Proper lithotomy position. There is minimal external rotation of the legs, the thighs are minimally flexed toward the abdomen, and the legs symmetrically positioned. Protective padding is not shown. (From Martin JT: Positioning in Anesthesia and Surgery. 2nd ed. Philadelphia, WB Saunders, 1987, p 45.)

scopic procedures, one arm is often tucked and padded at the patient's side to allow equipment positioning while the other is abducted.

Once anesthesia commences, the legs are simultaneously elevated, flexed at the hips and knees, and then positioned in either the stirrups or leg supports. Care should be taken to cushion both ankles and knees with eggcrate padding or gel-filled foam padding to prevent pressure injury to the peroneal nerve where it crosses the head of the fibula (see Fig. 30–3).

Precautions

The lithotomy position is associated with positioning-related complications that should be carefully considered. They include nerve injuries and compartment syndromes in the lower extremities.[9]

Obturator Nerves

Injury to the obturator nerve results in weakness or paralysis of the adductors of the thigh. Usually, sensory loss does not occur. Injury to the obturator nerve is best prevented by avoiding acute flexion (>90°) of the thigh onto the groin, especially in obese patients; otherwise, this position risks stretching and compression of the obturator nerve at the inguinal ligament.

Saphenous Nerves

The saphenous nerve is sensory to the medial portion of the leg, and its compression at the medial portion of the thigh can lead to loss of sensation along its distribution.

Femoral Nerves

More common than obturator or saphenous nerve injury is trauma to the femoral nerve as it is trapped under the inguinal ligament following acute flexion and angulation of the thigh.[10] Injury to this nerve is manifested by abnormal gait, loss of quadriceps sensation, numbness, and hyperesthesia over the quadriceps. This complication can be prevented by avoiding excess abduction of the thigh and external rotation of the hip by lateral thigh supports.

Sciatic Nerves

Sciatic nerve injury can occur when the thighs and legs are externally rotated or when the knees are extended. Clinically, all muscles below the knee, and perhaps even the hamstrings, are paralyzed, and numbness of the lateral half of the calf and almost all of the foot occurs, except at the inner border of the arch.

Common Peroneal Nerves

The most common injury to the lower extremity associated with the lithotomy position involves the common peroneal nerve (see Fig. 30–3). It is vulnerable to compression along the lateral aspects of the knee by the leg support rods or by the supports themselves. Common peroneal nerve injury is manifested by weakness to the intrinsic muscles of the foot, sensory deficit to the sole of the foot, and foot drop.

A rare but serious complication is compartment syndrome of the lower extremities, which is caused by direct pressure on calf muscle tissue. This complication is best prevented by devoting close attention to padding adequacy and uniform weight distribution over weight-bearing areas. Remember that the perfusion pressure in the legs, especially in the calves and feet, is reduced in proportion to the height to which they are elevated above the heart (0.7 mm Hg for every 1 cm of elevation).

What Problems Are Associated with the Trendelenburg Position?

The Trendelenburg position, or head-down position, is used most commonly to improve exposure of pelvic organs during gynecologic or urologic surgery. Classically, this position was characterized by a steep 30° to 40° tilt and necessitated shoulder braces to prevent the patient from sliding off the table. These braces were often implicated in brachial plexus injury.

In modern practice, the tilt is usually limited to 10° to 15°, and thus it does not require any additional patient restraints. With the Trendelenburg position, arterial pressure in the legs is decreased while relative engorgement occurs in the vessels of the mediastinum and head. Preload to the heart is increased, and in the patient with intracranial pathology, intracranial pressure increases because of the interference with cerebral venous drainage; cerebral perfusion pressure also may be decreased.

Resuscitation

Use of the head-down position to treat hypotension and shock has not been shown to provide any consistent beneficial effect.[11] In fact, data from animal studies suggest that all forms of shock are made worse by the Trendelenburg position. When hypovolemia is present, this position does not improve blood pressure but may improve cardiac output slightly. Simple elevation of the patient's legs to increase preload is a more prudent measure.

Cardiovascular

In addition to increasing intracranial pressure, placing a patient with congestive heart failure in the head-down position for cannulation of a central vein may also result in increased pulmonary artery occlusion pressure, which exacerbates acute congestive heart failure or produces myocardial ischemia, or both.[12]

Respiratory

The head-down position also decreases functional residual capacity, decreases pulmonary compliance, and increases the work of breathing. Atelectasis is aggravated, and hypoxemia may follow, especially when the patient is obese or elderly. Because of the cephalad shift of the mediastinum, endotracheal tube position should be reconfirmed when an intubated patient is placed in the head-down position. This shift can displace the lungs and the carina cephalad, causing the tip of the endotracheal tube to migrate distally into the right mainstem bronchus.

TABLE 30–2. Prevention of Brachial Plexus Injuries

Avoid abduction of the arm >90°.
If the arms are above the head (prone position or supine position for cardiac surgery), keep abduction and anterior flexion of the arm <90°.
Minimize combination of the abduction, external rotation, and dorsal extension of the arm.
Minimize combination of dorsal extension of the arm and opposite lateral flexion of the head.
Avoid downward pressure on the head of the humerus.
Avoid placing the humerus behind the plane of the body, such as with a sagging armboard.
With the lateral or three-quarter prone position, minimize compression between the lateral thorax and the head of humerus with a roll placed under the lateral thorax (*not* in the axilla).

(From Mahla ME: Nervous system. *In* Manual of Complications During Anesthesia. Gravenstein N (ed). Philadelphia, JB Lippincott, 1991, p 386.)

PERIPHERAL NERVE INJURY

The principal cause of peripheral nerve injury in anesthetized patients is ischemia of the intraneural vasonervorum (a topic that has been discussed previously). This problem results from nerve stretching or compression, or both. Stretching and compression are more likely to occur in anesthetized rather than awake patients because muscle tone is reduced and the patients are unable to complain of pain secondary to inappropriate posture.

In the conscious patient, abduction of the arm by >90° may quickly become painful and intolerable. After a few minutes, the radial pulse disappears in 83% of volunteers.[13] Because as little as 20 minutes of inappropriate posture or compression in an unfavorable position can produce a nerve palsy, virtually every anesthetized patient is at some risk.

Factors that contribute to the likelihood of peripheral nerve injury include hypotension, diabetes mellitus, peripheral vascular disease, vasoconstriction, and hematoma. Tables 30–2, 30–3, and 30–4 describe considerations that are useful in the prevention of specific peripheral nerve injuries.

How Is a Postoperative Peripheral Nerve Complaint Evaluated?

Assessment of Injury Mechanism

The differential diagnosis for peripheral nerve injury should consider trauma sustained prior to hospitalization (i.e., prior to

TABLE 30–3. Prevention of Median, Ulnar, and Radial Nerve Injuries

Median: Avoid antecubital fossa as intravenous infusion site, if possible. If unavoidable, observe site frequently for infiltration. This nerve is also vulnerable at the wrist. If possible, avoid severe wrist dorsiflexion or insertion of intravenous tubes in the volar veins.
Radial: Avoid pressure against the posterior and lateral aspects of the humerus.
Ulnar: Avoid stretching nerve by acute elbow flexion, and keep medial epicondyle and surrounding tissues free of pressure and well padded. This nerve is also vulnerable at the wrist; use the radial artery (separate from the nerve) rather than the ulnar artery (adjacent to the nerve) when feasible.

(From Mahla ME: Nervous system. *In* Manual of Complications During Anesthesia. Gravenstein N (ed). Philadelphia, JB Lippincott, 1991, p 387.)

TABLE 30–4. Prevention of Lower Extremity Nerve Injuries

Sciatic nerve: Knees should be flexed whenever the hips are flexed. Minimize external rotation of hips.
Common peroneal nerve: Avoid compression against the head of the fibula (especially in lateral position and in the lithotomy position [pressure from stirrups]).
Superficial and deep peroneal nerves: Maintain the foot in dorsiflexion.
Tibial nerve: Avoid compression of the popliteal fossa.
Saphenous nerve: Avoid pressure against the medial aspect of the upper one-third of the tibia.
Lateral femoral cutaneous nerve: Avoid pressure on the anterior superior iliac spine (pad this area in prone patients).

anesthesia); compression by a hematoma from a pre-existing disease; and misplaced needles inserted by personnel other than anesthesiologists (e.g., sciatic nerve injury from a misplaced gluteal injection). A nerve palsy also may result from direct needle probing of a nerve or from chemical irritation caused by an injected drug. Intraoperative positioning or surgically mediated injury is also included in the differential diagnosis.

Neurologic Consultation

When a nerve injury is suspected postoperatively, a neurologist should be consulted. Electrophysiologic testing can be performed to obtain information concerning the injury site and to give some indication of the duration of the injury (e.g., whether it was present before the procedure). A patient's electromyogram does not change until at least 1 week after the injury.[6]

In many instances, nerve conduction studies allow the location of the nerve injury to be delineated. They also give some indication of its severity (e.g., conduction delay versus absence). Thus, a patient with a perioperative nerve injury initially has normal results on electromyographic study but several weeks later would manifest an abnormal electromyographic response that consists of reduced amplitude of the evoked motor and sensory responses.

Spinal Anesthesia

Spinal anesthesia can result in a dural cerebrospinal fluid leak, which leads to low cerebrospinal fluid pressure and cranial nerve palsies. Paralysis of all but the vagus nerve has been reported; however, in 90% of cranial nerve palsies, the abducens nerve is affected. Symptoms associated with low cerebrospinal fluid pressure and abducens palsy are diplopia (since the lateral rectus muscle of the eye is affected); severe postural occipital headache; stiff neck, nausea, and dizziness; and photophobia. This palsy may occur up to 21 days postoperatively, and recovery may not be complete for up to 2 years.

Epidural Anesthesia

Administration of local anesthetics in the epidural space is another cause of postoperative lower extremity nerve dysfunction. This problem occurs several days into a course of epidural analgesia and can be caused by dilute local anesthetics (even though 0.0625% bupivacaine is not sufficient to cause a motor or sensory block). Over time, however, bupivacaine's lipid solubility enables it to become concentrated in the nerves that run through the epidural space. Treatment consists of removing the local anesthetic solution from the epidural infusion. These cases usually resolve in 6 to 8 hours after the local anesthetic has been cleared from the nerve tissue.

Surgical Manipulation

The femoral nerve is prone to damage by pressure, lateral deflection, and direct trauma during lower abdominal procedures that employ self-retaining retractors. On examination, loss of hip flexion, knee extension, and musculus quadriceps femoris palsy are noteworthy.

Postpartum

In the early 1900s, femoral neuropathy following childbirth reportedly was as high as 4.7%.[14] Although the condition is less common now, it still occurs as a result of prolonged lithotomy positioning and the exertion of undue pressure on the patient's legs by surgeons performing pelvic and perineal surgery.[14]

Why Is the Brachial Plexus Commonly Injured?

Anatomic Relationship

The brachial plexus apparently is the nerve group that is most susceptible to damage from malpositioning during anesthesia. This is for two reasons: first, the plexus has a relatively long and mobile superficial course in the axilla between two firm points of fixation, the vertebrae and prevertebral fascia above and the axillary fascia below; second, the plexus lies in proximity to a number of freely movable bone structures (see Fig. 30–1).

Mechanism of Injury

The chief cause of injury is thought to be stretching from dorsal extension and lateral flexion of the humeral head. This problem can best be avoided by maintaining the arm on an armboard that is level with the plane of the body and by never abducting the arm to an angle >90° from the sagittal plane.

Clinical Presentation

Brachial plexus injury is characterized by shoulder pain and tenderness in the supraclavicular area from 1 to several days postoperatively. If the entire plexus is involved, the arm hangs flaccidly, and the skin of the whole limb is numb. If only the upper roots (C5-7) are injured, Erb's paralysis (internal rotation of the arm, extension of the forearm, and pronation of the hand) results. Rarely, the lower roots (C-8 and T-1) are affected, and Klumpke's paralysis (loss of finger flexion, paralysis of the hand muscles, and perhaps Horner's syndrome) results.

Why Is the Radial Nerve Vulnerable?

The radial nerve may be traumatized if it is compressed as it passes around the lateral border of the middle of the humerus. Radial nerve palsy is characterized by wrist drop, ina-

bility to extend the metacarpal joints, and inability to abduct the thumb. Sensation may be lost over the lateral three and one-half fingers and the hand.

How Is the Median Nerve Traumatized?

The median nerve, which lies adjacent to the medial cubital and basilic veins in the antecubital fossa, may be traumatized by direct needle penetration or by drug extravasation. The patient is unable to oppose the thumb and little finger, has decreased ability to abduct the thumb, and loses flexion of the distal phalanx of the second finger. Sensation and sweating are diminished over the palmar surface of the lateral three and one-half digits and the adjacent palm.

How Does Ulnar Nerve Damage Occur?

The ulnar nerve may be damaged by compression against the operating room table or an armboard or by a tightly applied draw sheet. However, cases of postoperative ulnar nerve palsy occur in which, based on all available information, appropriate padding was used.[1] Therefore, as was discussed previously, the specific etiology of most ulnar neuropathies is yet to be determined.[8]

The result of ulnar nerve injury is decreased ability to grip with the hand and inability to abduct or oppose the little finger to the thumb. Decreased sensation occurs over both surfaces of the medial one and one-half fingers in the adjacent hand. In severe cases, the intrinsic hand muscles atrophy and contractures develop, resulting in the characteristic "claw hand."

The ulnar nerve may also be injured at the wrist during ulnar artery puncture or catheterization. Unlike the radial nerve, which becomes separate from the radial artery proximal to the wrist, the ulnar artery and nerve lie in close proximity at this location. Distal placement of a noninvasive blood pressure cuff on the arm where the cuff impinges on the antecubital fossa can result in ulnar nerve injury, especially if a 1-minute or shorter cycle time is used.[15]

THE PATIENT WITH A NECK INJURY

Patients who come to the operating room with a radiculopathy or myelopathy are, whenever possible, positioned while they are awake. Once the appropriate position is assumed, all efforts should be made to maintain it throughout the operation. Documentation should be detailed so as to avoid possible legal ramifications postoperatively.

If a patient is in a cervical collar or splint upon arrival in the operating room, the device is left in place during the operation and documented to be so. If headpins are to be placed, the neurosurgeon involved in the case should direct the positioning in order to minimize further trauma.

RHEUMATOID DISORDERS

The rheumatoid patient should be assessed for cervical pathology prior to intubation and positioning. If neurologic compromise is present (or thought possibly to exist), the patient is intubated and positioned while he or she is awake. Patients with a rheumatoid disorder undergoing monitored anesthesia care should be positioned as comfortably as possible with the knowledge that they may have difficulty because of multiple joint involvement.

References

1. Kroll DA, Caplan RA, Posner K, et al: Nerve injury associated with anesthesia. Anesthesiology 1990; 73:202.
2. Brown EM, Elman DS: Postoperative backache. Anesth Analg 1961; 40:683.
3. Courington FW, Little DM: The role of posture in anesthesia. Clin Anesth 1968; 3:24.
4. Denny-Brown D, Doherty MM: Effects of transient stretching of peripheral nerve. Arch Neurol Psychiatr 1945; 54:116.
5. Britt BA, Gordon RA: Peripheral nerve injuries associated with anaesthesia. Can Anaesth Soc J 1964; 11:514.
6. Dawson DM, Krarup C: Perioperative nerve lesions. Arch Neurol 1989; 46:1355.
7. Vander Salm TJ, Cereda J-M, Cutler BS: Brachial plexus injury following median sternotomy. J Thorac Cardiovasc Surg 1980; 80:447.
8. Stoelting RK: Postoperative ulnar nerve palsy: is it a preventable complication? Anesth Analg 1993; 76:7.
9. Martin JT: Compartment syndromes: concepts and perspectives of the anesthesiologist. Anesth Analg 1992; 75:275.
10. Tondare AS, Nadkarni AV, Sathe CH, et al: Femoral neuropathy: a complication of lithotomy position under spinal anaesthesia. Can Anaesth Soc J 1983; 30:84.
11. Sibbald WJ, Patterson NAM, Holliday RL, et al: The Trendelenburg position: hemodynamic effects in hypotensive and normotensive patients. Crit Care Med 1979; 7:218.
12. Kubal K, Komatsu T, Sonchala V, et al: Trendelenburg position used during venous cannulation increases myocardial oxygen demand (Abstract). Anesth Analg 1984; 63:239.
13. Wright S: The neurovascular syndrome produced by hypertension of the arms. Am Heart J 1945; 29:1.
14. Vargo MM, Robinson LR, Nicholas JJ, et al: Postpartum femoral neuropathy: relic of an earlier era. Arch Phys Med Rehab 1990; 71:591.
15. Sy W: Ulnar nerve palsy possibly related to use of automatically cycled blood pressure cuff. Anesth Analg 1981; 60:687.

CHAPTER 31

Regional Anesthesia

DAVID L. BROWN, M.D.

Anesthetic prescription is often made with more thought about institutional tradition than individualization of technique for a specific patient. General anesthetic proponents often suggest that in the large majority of patients, no measurable outcome differences can be demonstrated between general and regional anesthesia. If the focus of anesthetic prescription and clinical outcome simply includes the intraoperative period, perhaps they are correct. Nevertheless, when anesthesiologists are questioned about their preference for anesthetic prescription, they overwhelmingly choose regional anesthesia for themselves.[1, 2] Perhaps they recognize there is more to anesthetic prescription than just a consideration of the intraoperative period. Experimental and clinical evidence is increasingly accumulating that preventing painful intraoperative neural impulses from reaching the central nervous system (CNS) minimizes pain transmission in the immediate as well as distant postoperative period.[3–5]

PHILOSOPHY OF REGIONAL ANESTHESIA

When Is It Indicated?

If anesthetic prescriptions take into consideration the prevention of dorsal horn wind-up and central sensitization of pain pathways, almost every surgical patient is a candidate for some form of regional anesthesia. If an anesthetic is selected on the basis of other factors, such as the applicability of regional anesthesia to the surgical procedure in question, the group of patients may be slightly different.

Kopacz and Nickel suggest that almost 60% of patients older than 65 years are candidates for regional anesthesia.[6] They developed this estimate by calculating the number of Medicare patients undergoing specific operations in the United States (Fig. 31–1). Because those over 65 years of age undergo the majority of surgical procedures in many practices, the possibility for widespread use of regional anesthesia seems evident.

When Is It Contraindicated?

Patient Refusal/Inability to Cooperate

Are there situations in which regional anesthesia is contraindicated? One obvious and absolute contraindication to regional anesthesia is patients' refusal. Often, however, such refusal results because the technique is presented to them in an unfavorable light by anesthesiologists uncomfortable with their own abilities.[7]

Many patients are concerned because they are led to believe they will be "awake" during the surgical procedure. In my experience, it is a rare adult who is unwilling to receive a regional block if it is presented as an option with confidence, if it is administered humanely and comprehensively, and if anxiolytics and opioids are titrated according to the patient, surgical procedure, and anesthetic technique chosen.

Another absolute contraindication to regional anesthesia is a patient's inability to cooperate. Risks are unnecessarily increased by attempting a regional block in a patient who is either unable or unwilling to hold still while the regional anesthetic is induced.

Aortic Stenosis

Patients in whom regional anesthetics should be cautiously prescribed are those with significant aortic stenosis. This is not an absolute contraindication to a centroneuraxis block. However, the pathophysiology of aortic stenosis (thickened left ventricle requiring higher perfusion pressures) needs to be seriously considered before a centroneuraxis block is considered.[8]

Coagulopathy

Another group of patients who often are excluded from regional anesthetic prescription are those with any signs of coagulopathy. Automatic exclusion of anyone receiving drugs that may affect the coagulation system may be convenient; however, appropriate risk-benefit partitioning needs to be considered if regional anesthesia is to be appropriately prescribed. For example, most orthopedic surgical patients undergoing total joint replacement have received platelet-active drugs, and regional anesthetics are often safely used. Some patients receiving oral preoperative anticoagulants, such as Coumadin, have prothrombin times not yet returned to a normal range. They still may be candidates for expertly performed regional anesthetics.

My preference is to consider small-gauge, midline, single-

SURGICAL SITES IN PATIENTS >65 YEARS

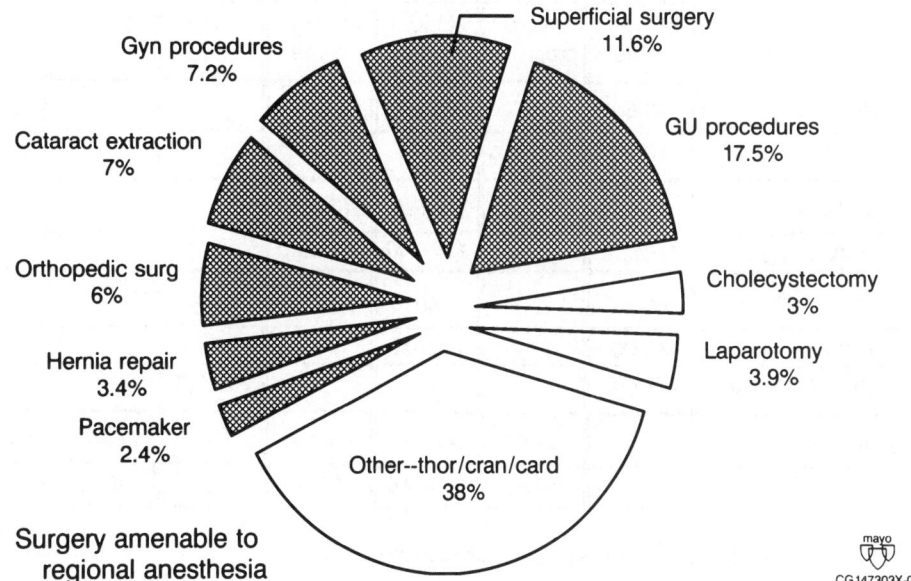

FIGURE 31–1. Proportion of surgical procedures performed in patients over age 65 years. Gyn = gynecologic; GU = genitourinary; thor = thoracic; cran = cranial; card = cardiac. (Modified from Sourcebook of Aging, Chicago, Marquis Academica Media, 1979, p 422.)

shot spinal anesthetics when prothrombin times are up to 1.5 times normal (approximately 16–17 s), and the anesthetic provides clear advantages. Such patients include individuals with significant reactive airway disease or those with a pertinent history of deep venous thrombosis following prior surgical procedures. Each anesthesiologist must develop a risk-benefit equation to suit his or her practice and patient subgroups.

Sepsis

Patients who are considered septic are often excluded from consideration for spinal or epidural blockade because the needle may allow infected blood to enter either the epidural or subarachnoid space,[12] resulting in either epidural abscess or meningitis. If a patient has received antibiotic therapy and shows a positive response and the risk-benefit of spinal or epidural versus general anesthetic favors a regional technique, it is acceptable.[9]

Neuropathy

Patients with neuropathy often are similarly excluded. This judgment does not seem entirely logical, because little or no evidence shows that carefully administered regional anesthetics carry a higher risk of neuropathy for a particular patient and procedure than well-administered general anesthetics. To develop this concept even further, patients with painful neuropathies often visit a comprehensive pain clinic where local anesthetic injections are made near the neuropathic neural structures. Many of the patient subgroups with a high incidence of coexisting neuropathies, such as diabetic and alcoholic individuals, are excellent candidates for regional anesthetic prescription.

MAKING IT WORK

Why Should an Induction Area Be Available?

Performance of regional anesthesia demands an integrated approach to its induction if one is successfully to incorporate

varied techniques into a daily practice. An essential component of comprehensive regional anesthesia is an area of the operating suite that can be used for induction. Many regional blocks can be administered while the operating room is still being readied.

If dedicated areas for regional anesthesia induction are not available in your operating suite, an area of the postanesthesia care unit or a partitioned area in the preoperative holding area can be used. Any area that is chosen must be equipped with the full array of resuscitative aids.

If one's practice involves teaching regional anesthesia, an induction area is even more essential than for an individual in private practice. My clinical impression is that trainees are able to remember and incorporate more aspects of regional anesthesia in a nonstressful induction area than in a hectic operating theater with an audience of impatient surgeons in attendance.

What Factors Govern Local Anesthetic Choice?

Selecting the appropriate local anesthetic for a given regional anesthetic requires consideration of a number of factors, including the duration of surgery, postoperative analgesia requirements, the operative site (including the degree of motor block required), and a patient's status (outpatient versus inpatient).

Local anesthetics range from short, to medium, to long acting, and the degree of motor blockade increases with increasing local anesthetic concentration; thus, individualization of local anesthetic choice is possible. Figure 31–2 outlines one method of "walking across the local anesthetic time line."

Another factor that affects the duration of local anesthetics is the addition of vasoconstrictors or α-adrenergic agonists (at least for centroneuraxis blocks). Epinephrine or phenylephrine may prolong useful local anesthetic action from 30% to 50%.[10]

A patient's weight, the volume of anesthetic needed to achieve the block, and avoidance of toxic doses are additional factors (Table 31–1).

LOCAL ANESTHETIC TIME LINE (in minutes)

	Pro-caine	Chloro-procaine	Lido-caine	Mepiva-caine	Tetra-caine	Etido-caine	Bupiva-caine
Infiltration	45-60		75-90				180-360
+ epi	60-90		90-180				200-400
Peripheral			90-120	100-150			480-780
+ epi			120-180	120-220			600-900
SAB*	60-75		60		70-90		90-110
+ epi	75-90		75-100		100-150		100-150
phenylephrine†	90-120				200-300		
Epidural		45-60	80-120	90-140		120-200	165-225
+ epi		60-90	120-180	140-200		150-225	180-240

*Subarachnoid block, †For lower extremity surgery

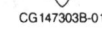

CG147303B-01

FIGURE 31–2. Local anesthetic time line. Understanding the length of time that specific local anesthetics can be expected to provide surgical anesthesia can be extremely helpful in matching local anesthetic choice to patient, procedure, surgeon, and so on.

What Constitutes a Successful Block?

Perhaps the most important concept in successful use of regional anesthesia is an understanding of what constitutes a successful block. For too many individuals, a regional anesthetic is considered successful only if no additional sedative drugs are administered. This concept needs rethinking. Supplementation of a regional anesthetic with intravenous or inhaled agents should not be considered a marker of a failed block but rather an appropriate use of balanced anesthesia. Anxiolysis is an extremely important part of any perioperative anesthetic experience, and patients undergoing regional anesthesia are no different from patients undergoing general anesthetic techniques.

One analogy that may help to focus this issue follows: An anesthesiologist would not be expected to select an arbitrary concentration of isoflurane before administering a general anesthetic and, on discovering that the concentration needed to be altered during the anesthetic, consider the technique a failure. Regional anesthesia is no different; after its initial induction, supplementation should be administered to provide opti-

mal operating conditions for the patient, surgeon, and anesthesiologist. The intravenous agents that are available for appropriate regional anesthesia sedation include benzodiazepines, opioids, propofol, and barbiturates.

CENTRONEURAXIS BLOCKADE: SPINAL ANESTHESIA

How Is a Spinal Anesthetic Performed?

Spinal anesthesia is unrivaled in the way a small amount of drug, almost devoid of systemic pharmacologic effect, produces profound, reproducible surgical anesthesia. Further, by altering the drug choice, different levels of spinal anesthesia can be produced. Low spinal anesthesia, a block below T-10, carries with it a different physiologic impact than does a block performed to produce higher spinal anesthesia (above T-5).

The block is unsurpassed for lower abdominal or lower extremity surgical procedures. However, for operations in the mid to upper abdomen, "light" general anesthesia may be needed to supplement the spinal block. Stimulation of the

TABLE 31–1. Comparative Pharmacology of Local Anesthetics

Classification	Potency	Maximum Single Dose			Toxic Plasma Concentration (μg · mL⁻¹)
		Plain (mg)	(mg · kg⁻¹)	With Epinephrine (mg · kg⁻¹)	
Esters					
Procaine	1	500	7–8	10–12	
Chloroprocaine	4	600	8–9	10–12	
Tetracaine	16	100		2	
Amides					
Lidocaine	1	300	4–5	7–8	>5
Mepivacaine	1	300	4–5	7–8	>5
Prilocaine	1	400	5–6	8–9	>5
Bupivacaine	4	175	2–3	3–4	~1.5
Etidocaine	4	300	4–5	5–6	~2

(Data abstracted from Covino BG, Vassalo HL: Local Anesthetics: Mechanisms of Action and Clinical Use. New York, Grune & Stratton, 1976, p 151.)

diaphragm during upper abdominal procedures often causes patients discomfort. The area is difficult to block completely through high spinal anesthesia (to do so requires blockade of the phrenic nerve, not a very desirable goal).

Patient Selection

Patient selection for spinal anesthesia often places too much focus on a side effect—namely, spinal headache—than on the applicability of the technique.[11] The incidence of spinal headache increases with decreasing age and female gender; however, with proper technique and needle selection, it should not preclude spinal anesthesia in young, healthy patients if the block has advantages over epidural anesthesia. Almost any patient who is to have a lower extremity operation is a potential candidate for spinal anesthesia, as are most patients scheduled for lower abdominal surgery (gynecologic, urologic, and obstetric procedures and inguinal herniorrhaphy).

Drug Choice

In North America, three local anesthetics are commonly used to produce spinal anesthesia: lidocaine, tetracaine, and bupivacaine. Lidocaine produces a short- to intermediate-acting spinal anesthetic; tetracaine and bupivacaine provide intermediate to long duration block.

Lidocaine

Lidocaine, without epinephrine, is often chosen for procedures that can be completed in 1 hour or less. The mixture most commonly used is a 5% solution in 7.5% dextrose. When epinephrine (0.2 mg) is added, the useful length of clinical anesthesia in the lower abdomen and lower extremities is approximately 90 minutes.[12]

Tetracaine

Tetracaine is packaged as both niphanoid crystals (20 mg) and as a 1% solution (2-mL ampule). When dextrose is added to make the solution hyperbaric, tetracaine generally produces effective clinical anesthesia for procedures lasting up to 1.5 to 2 hours in the plain form, for up to 2 to 3 hours when epinephrine (0.2 mg) is added, and up to 5 hours for lower extremity procedures when phenylephrine (5 mg) is added as a vasoconstrictor.[9]

Bupivacaine

Bupivacaine spinal anesthesia is commonly carried out with 0.5% or 0.75% solution, either plain or in 8.25% dextrose. My impression is that the clinical difference between 0.5% tetracaine and 0.75% bupivacaine as hyperbaric solutions is minimal.[13] Bupivacaine is useful for procedures lasting from 2 to 2.5 hours.

Hypobaric Techniques

Local anesthetics can be mixed to produce hypobaric spinal anesthesia. The most common method of formulating a hypobaric solution is to mix tetracaine in a 0.1% to 0.33% solution with sterile, preservative-free water. Lidocaine also can be mixed to provide useful hypobaric spinal anesthesia.[14] This drug is diluted from a 2% solution with sterile, preservative-free water to make a 0.5% solution, and a total of 30 to 40 mg is used.

Anatomic Considerations

The spinous processes of the lumbar vertebrae have an almost perpendicular relationship to the long axis of their respective vertebral bodies. When a needle is inserted between lumbar vertebral spines, it should be placed almost perpendicular to the long axis of the back. To facilitate spinal anesthesia, an anesthesiologist must constantly keep in mind the relationship of the midline of the patient (centroneuraxis) and the needle.[15] As illustrated in Figure 31–3, the needle must puncture skin, subcutaneous tissue, supraspinous ligament, interspinous ligament, ligamentum flavum, epidural space, and finally the dura and arachnoid mater to reach the cerebrospinal fluid (CSF).

What Induction Positions Are Common?

Induction of spinal anesthesia is carried out in three positions: lateral decubitus, sitting, and the prone jackknife. In both the lateral decubitus and sitting positions, a well-trained assistant is essential if the block is to be easily and safely administered in a time-efficient manner.

Lateral Decubitus Position

The assistant should help the patient to assume the position with the legs flexed on the abdomen and chin flexed on the chest. This goal is most effectively accomplished by pulling the head toward the chest, placing an arm behind the patient's knees, and pushing the head and knees together. The position is facilitated by an appropriate amount of sedation that permits a patient to be relaxed yet cooperative.

Sitting

The sitting position can make location of the midline easier in obese patients or those with scoliosis. The patient should assume a comfortable sitting position with legs placed over the edge of the operating table and feet supported by a stool. A pillow should be placed in the lap, and the arms allowed to drape over the pillow, resting on the flexed lower extremities. An assistant should be positioned immediately in front of the patient, supporting the shoulders and allowing the patient to minimize lumbar lordosis, all the while ensuring that the vertebral midline remains in a vertical position.

Prone Jackknife

It is sometimes more time efficient to place a patient in a prone jackknife position before administering the spinal anesthetic. An assistant is not as essential for this technique as for the lateral decubitus and sitting positions. However, to improve efficiency, an assistant can position the patient while the anesthesiologist readies the equipment and drugs.

What Factors Govern Needle Choice?

One of the first choices with spinal anesthesia is to decide what kind of needle to use. Although many eponyms are

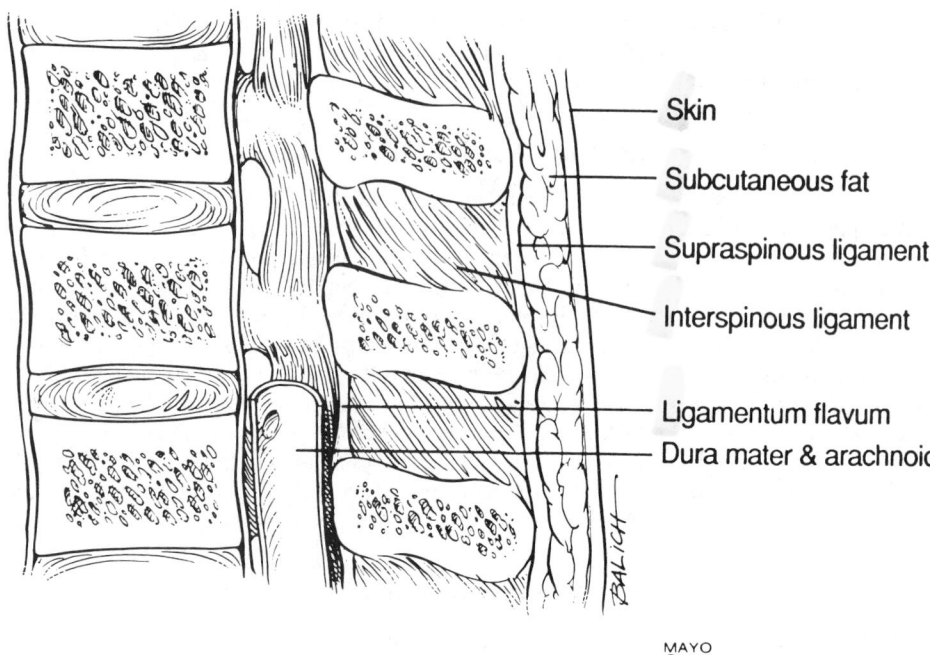

FIGURE 31–3. Spinal block; sagittal lumbar anatomy. From the surface inward, a spinal needle must puncture skin, subcutaneous fat, supraspinous ligament, interspinous ligament, ligamentum flavum, epidural space, dura mater, and arachnoid.

applied to spinal needles, they are divided into two main types: those that cut the dura and those that spread dural fibers. The former category includes the traditional, disposable, Quincke-Babcock needle; the latter category contains the Whitacre, Greene, and Sprotte needles (Fig. 31–4). If a continuous spinal technique is chosen, a Tuohy or other thin-walled needle facilitates passage of the catheter.

To make a logical choice of spinal needle, one must understand the risks and benefits of each. Small needles reduce the incidence of postdural puncture headache. Larger needles im-

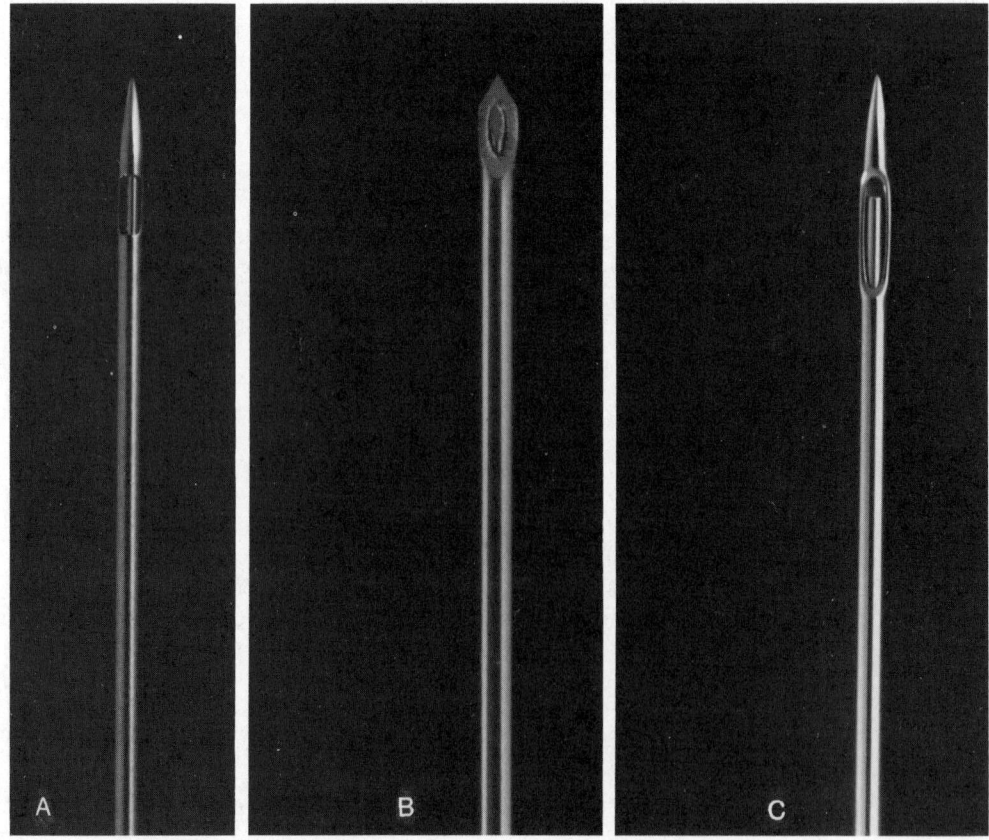

FIGURE 31–4. Collage of spinal needles in oblique and anteroposterior views. A, No. 25 Whitacre needle designed to spread dural fibers. B, No. 25 Quincke needle designed to cut dural fibers. C, No. 24 Sprotte needle designed to spread dural fibers.

prove the tactile ''sense'' of needle placement, thus increasing operator confidence. However, these risk-benefit ratios are relative. For example, a small, 26-gauge needle does not decrease headache incidence in younger patients if a number of passes through the dura are required until CSF flow is recognized. Likewise, a larger needle, such as a 22-gauge Whitacre, may result in a lower post–dural puncture headache incidence if subarachnoid needle localization occurs on the first pass.

Different needle tip designs likely are a factor in post–dural puncture headache incidence, even when needle sizes are comparable. The most recent data suggest that the pencil point, dural, fiber spreading–type needles are associated with the lowest incidence of post–dural puncture headache.

To avoid multiple passes through the dura with the smaller-gauge needles, it is probably advantageous to perform the block with the patient sitting up to increase hydrostatic pressure and thereby assist CSF flow into the needle. If flow is not spontaneous, intermittently aspirate the needle with a small syringe to overcome surface tension and tissue plug effects that inhibit CSF flow.

How Is The Needle Placed?

Midline Approach

With a patient positioned properly, the palpating hand identifies the intervertebral space and midline. As illustrated in Figure 31–5, this important maneuver is carried out by moving the fingers in an alternating cephalocaudal direction, as well as rolling them side to side. The latter maneuver confirms the middle of the midline. Once the appropriate intervertebral space has been clearly identified, a skin wheal is raised over it.

Next, an introducer needle is inserted into the substance of the interspinous ligament, taking care to seat it firmly in the midline. The introducer is grasped and steadied with the palpating fingers, while the other hand holds the spinal needle,

somewhat like a dart (see Fig. 31–5). With the fifth finger of the needle hand used as a tripod against the patient's back, the needle, with the bevel (if present) parallel to the longitudinal dural fibers, is advanced slowly to heighten the sensation of tissue planes traversed, as well as to avoid skewering nerve roots. A characteristic change in resistance is noted as the needle passes through the ligamentum flavum and again as it passes through the dura.

The stylet is then removed, and CSF should appear at the needle hub. If it does not, rotate the needle in 90° increments until CSF appears. If CSF does not appear in any quadrant, the needle should be advanced a few millimeters and rechecked in all four quadrants. If CSF still has not appeared and the needle is at an apparently appropriate depth, it should be gently aspirated. If this is unsuccessful, the needle and introducer should be withdrawn and insertion steps repeated. The most common reason for lack of CSF return is needle insertion off the midline. Another common error is needle insertion at too great a cephalic angle.

Once CSF flows freely, the dorsum of the anesthesiologist's nondominant hand steadies the spinal needle against the patient's back while the syringe containing the therapeutic dose is attached. CSF is again freely aspirated into the syringe, and the dose injected.

Paramedian Approach

The midline approach to subarachnoid block is the technique of first choice because it requires anatomic projection in only two planes and is relatively avascular. When difficulties with needle insertion are encountered, however, the paramedian route, which does not require the same level of patient cooperation or reversal of lumbar lordosis, may be used.

As illustrated in Figure 31–6, the paramedian approach exploits the larger subarachnoid target that exists if a needle is

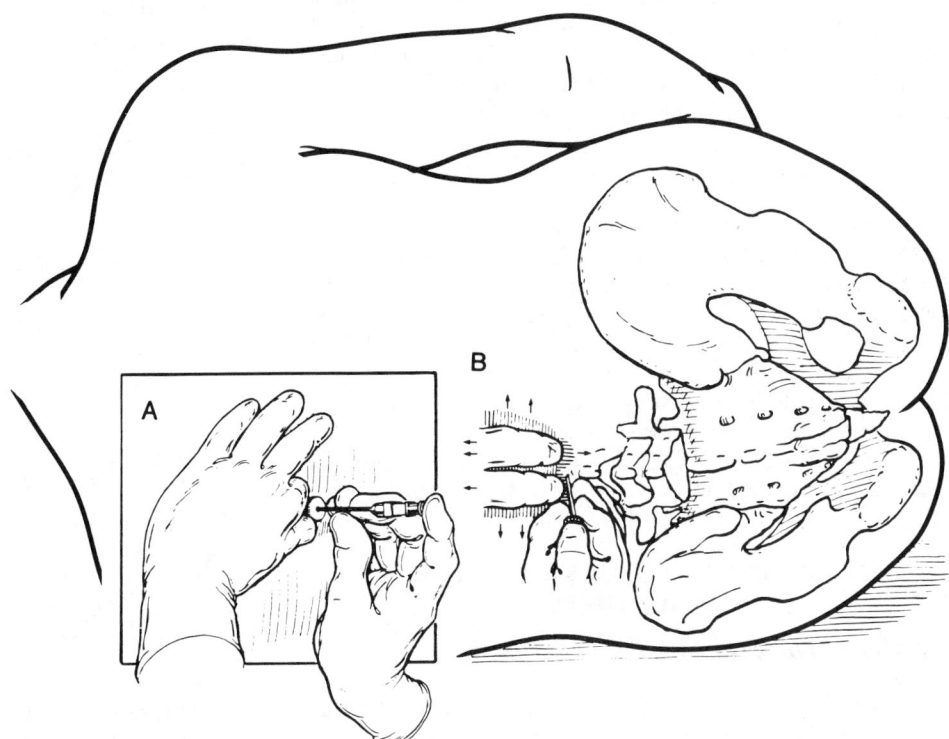

FIGURE 31–5. Spinal needle insertion. *A*, During needle insertion, the needle should be stabilized in a tripod fashion while held in the hand (as if it were a dart to be thrown). *B*, The palpating fingers are ''rolled'' in both a side-to-side and cephalic-to-caudal direction to identify interspinous space.

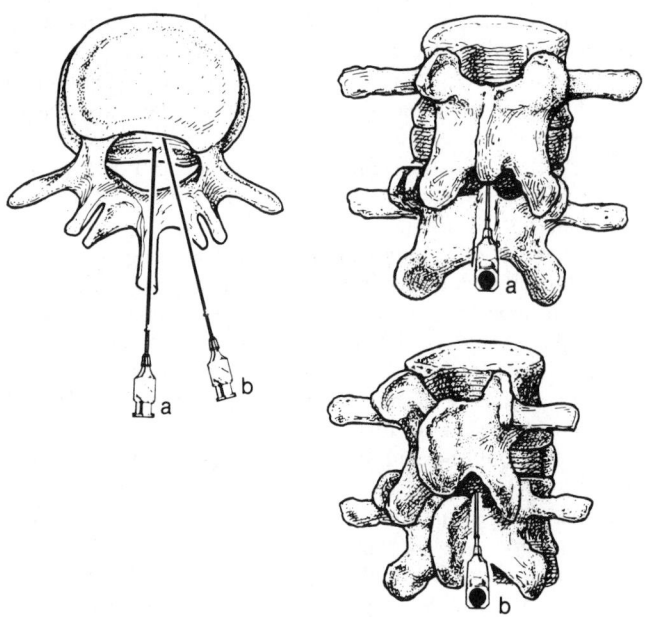

FIGURE 31–6. The advantage of a larger paramedian target (b) with the centroneuraxis technique compared with the midline approach (a).

inserted slightly lateral to the midline. The palpating fingers should identify the caudal edge of the cephalic spinous process of the intervertebral space chosen; a skin wheal is raised 1 cm lateral and 1 cm caudad to this point. A 4-cm 22-gauge short-beveled needle is then used to infiltrate deeper tissues in a cephalomedial plane. The spinal introducer and needle are then inserted 10° to 15° off the sagittal plane in a cephalomedial plane. The most common error with this technique is also to angle the needle either too cephalic or too medial on the initial insertion. In the latter case, it encounters either the contralateral vertebral lamina or paraspinous muscles.

Once the needle contacts bone, it is redirected in a slightly cephalic or medial direction. If bone is again contacted but at a deeper level, incremental redirection is continued, because it is likely that the needle is being "walked" up the lamina toward the intervertebral space. When CSF is obtained, the block is similar to that described for the midline approach.

Lumbosacral Approach

A modification of the paramedian approach is the lumbosacral approach of Taylor.[16] The technique is carried out at the L5–S1 interspace, the largest interlaminal interspace of the vertebral column. As illustrated in Figure 31–7, the skin insertion site is 1 cm medial and 1 cm caudal to the ipsilateral posterior superior iliac spine. Through this point, a 12- to 15-cm spinal needle is inserted in a cephalomedial direction toward the midline. If bone is encountered on the first insertion, the needle is walked off the sacrum into the subarachnoid space, similar to the method for a lumbar paramedian approach.

CENTRONEURAXIS BLOCKADE: EPIDURAL ANESTHESIA

How Is an Epidural Anesthetic Performed?

Epidural anesthesia is the second major type of centroneuraxis block. In contrast to spinal anesthesia, epidural block

requires pharmacologic doses of local anesthetics, making local anesthetic systemic toxicity a concern. In skilled hands, the incidence of postdural puncture headache should be lower with epidural anesthesia than with spinal anesthesia. Most commonly, spinal anesthesia is a single-shot technique, whereas frequent intermittent injection often is performed through an epidural catheter, allowing prolongation of the block. Another difference is that epidural block permits segmental anesthesia but a spinal block does not. Thus, if a thoracic injection is made with an appropriate amount of local anesthetic, a band of anesthesia can be produced that does not block the lower extremities.

Patient Selection

Epidural block is appropriate for virtually the same patients as is spinal anesthesia, with the exception that it can be used in the cervical and thoracic areas—levels at which spinal anesthesia is not often performed. As with spinal anesthesia, if epidural block is to be used for intra-abdominal procedures involving the upper abdomen, it is advisable to combine the technique with a light general anesthetic; diaphragmatic irritation can make the patient, surgeon, and anesthesiologist uncomfortable.

Other patients for whom epidural anesthesia is useful are those receiving a continuous technique, which is maintained with local anesthetic or opioid analgesia postoperatively after major surgical procedures. This application alone probably explains the increased interest in epidural block.[17]

Drug Choice

Effective use of epidural local anesthesia also requires an understanding of local anesthetic potency and duration and a realistic estimate of the operation's length and the postoperative analgesia requirements. Drugs for epidural use can be categorized into short-, intermediate-, and long-acting agents; with the addition of epinephrine, surgical anesthesia ranging from 45 to 240 minutes is possible (see Fig. 31–2).

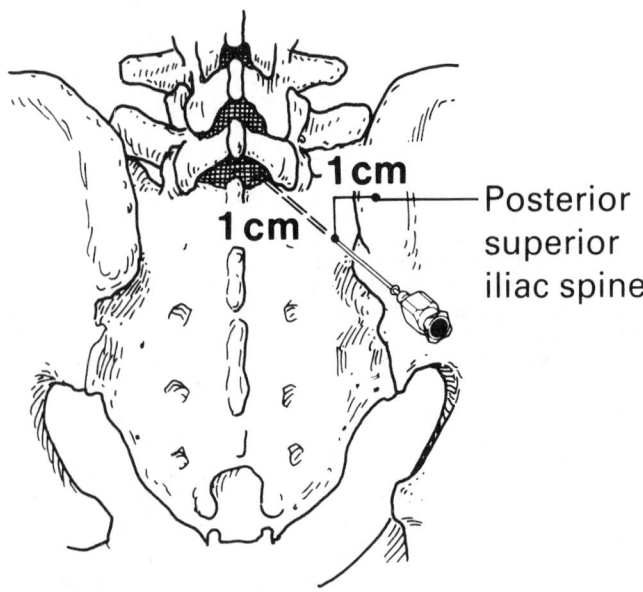

FIGURE 31–7. Anatomy of the Taylor approach, which is really a paramedian approach at the L5-S1 level.

2-Chloroprocaine

2-Chloroprocaine, an amino ester local anesthetic, is a short-acting agent that allows efficient matching of surgical procedure length and duration of epidural analgesia, even in outpatients. It is available in 2% and 3% concentrations, with the latter preferable for surgical anesthesia and the former for techniques not requiring muscle relaxation.

Lidocaine and Mepivacaine

Lidocaine is the prototypical amide local anesthetic and is used in 1.5% and 2% concentrations. Mepivacaine concentrations are similar to lidocaine but last from 15 to 30 minutes longer at equivalent dosages. Epinephrine significantly prolongs the duration of surgical anesthesia with 2-chloroprocaine, lidocaine and mepivacaine (i.e., approximately 50%).

Bupivacaine

Bupivacaine, an amide in 0.5% and 0.75% concentrations, is the most widely used long-acting drug for epidural anesthesia. Analgesic techniques can be performed with concentrations from 0.125% to 0.25%. Its duration of action is not as consistently prolonged by the addition of epinephrine, although up to 240 minutes of surgical anesthesia can be obtained when epinephrine is added.

Anatomic Considerations

The key to carrying out successful epidural anesthesia is an understanding of midline centroneuraxis anatomy. The anesthesiologist should create a cross-sectional image of the centroneuraxis midline structures underlying the palpating fingers (Fig. 31–8). When a lumbar approach is used, the depth from the skin to the ligamentum flavum commonly is 4 cm; 80% of patients have their epidural space cannulated between 3.5 and 6 cm from the skin. In the lumbar region, the ligamentum flavum is 5 to 6 mm thick in the midline; in the thoracic region, it is somewhat thinner, 3 to 5 mm thick. If needles are kept in the midline, the ligamentum flavum is perceived as thicker than if it is inserted off the midline.

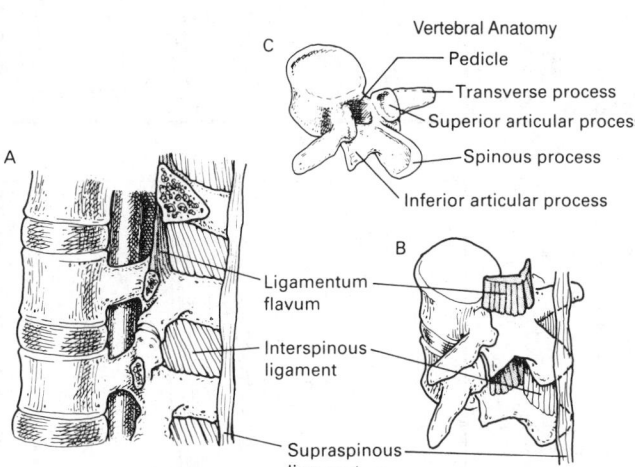

FIGURE 31–8. Vertebral anatomy. *A*, Sagittal view. *B*, Oblique view of lumbar vertebra showing ligamentum flavum thickening in the caudad extent of intervertebral space and in the midline. *C*, Oblique view of a single lumbar vertebra.

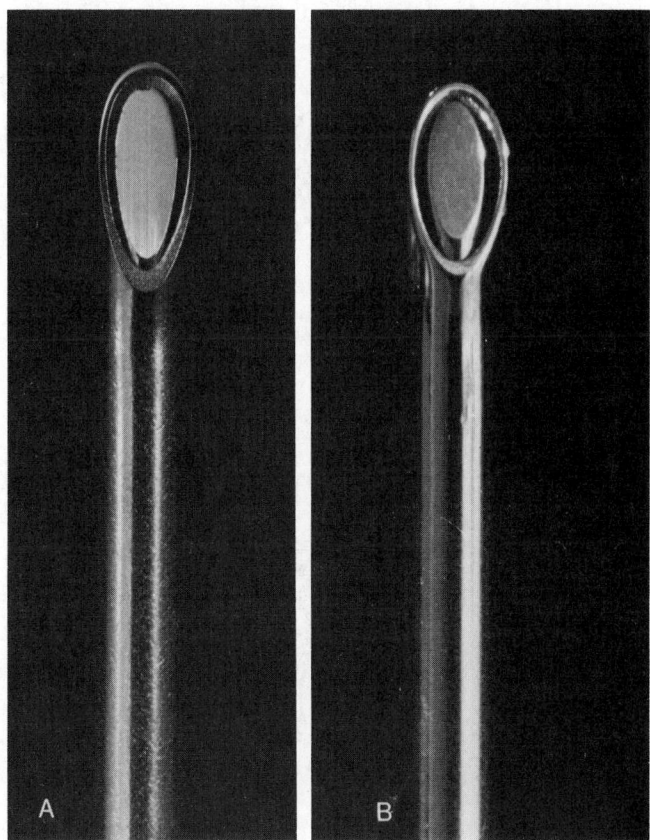

FIGURE 31–9. Collage of epidural needles in oblique and anteroposterior views. *A*, No. 17 Tuohy needle designed with a laterally facing opening. *B*, No. 18 Hustead needle designed with a laterally facing opening.

Positioning

Positioning for epidural anesthesia is similar to that for spinal anesthesia, with lateral decubitus, sitting, and prone jackknife approaches all applicable. The lateral decubitus position is applicable to both lumbar and thoracic techniques, whereas the sitting position allows lumbar and thoracic as well as cervical epidural anesthesia to be administered. The prone jackknife position permits access to the caudal epidural space.

Needle Placement

A palpation technique similar to that used for spinal anesthesia should be used to identify midline structures. If a single-shot technique is chosen, a Crawford needle is appropriate; if a continuous catheter technique is indicated, a Tuohy or other needle with lateral face opening is appropriate (Fig. 31–9).

Loss of Resistance

For lumbar epidural anesthesia, the midline approach is easiest. The needle is inserted into the midline in the same way as for spinal anesthesia. It is slowly advanced until a change in tissue resistance is noted as the needle abuts the ligamentum flavum. At this point, a 3- to 5-mL low-resistance glass or plastic syringe is filled with 2 mL of saline and a small (0.25 mL) air bubble. The syringe is attached to the needle. If the needle tip is in the substance of the ligamentum flavum, the air bubble is compressible. If it is not in the

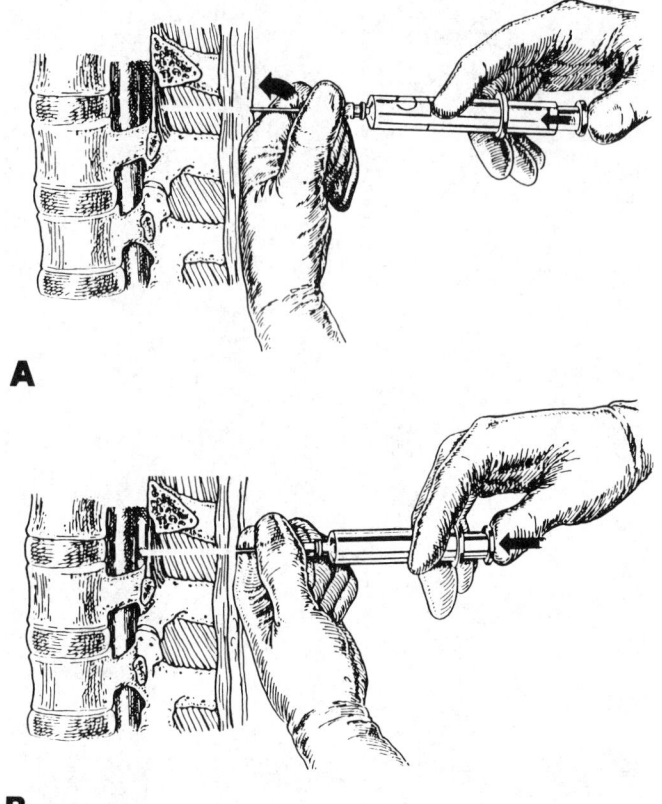

A

B

FIGURE 31–10. Loss of resistance technique. *A*, Needle is "seated" in interspinous ligament and ligamentum flavum while constant, steady pressure is applied to the syringe plunger. *B*, Entry of the needle into epidural space is confirmed by the loss of resistance to syringe plunger pressure and by the easy entry of the solution into the space.

ligamentum flavum, pressure on the syringe plunger does not compress the air bubble.

Once compression of the air bubble is achieved, the needle is grasped with the nondominant hand and pulled slowly toward the epidural space while the dominant hand (thumb) applies constant steady pressure on the syringe plunger. On entry into the epidural space, pressure applied to the syringe plunger allows the solution to flow without resistance (Fig. 31–10).

Hanging Drop

Another technique (although I believe with a less precise end point) is the hanging drop identification of entry into the epidural space. When the needle is inserted into the ligamentum flavum, a drop of solution is placed within the hub. As the needle is slowly advanced into the epidural space, the solution should be "sucked in" as the dura is tented away from the ligament, creating negative pressure in the epidural space (Fig. 31–11).

Catheter Insertion

When the epidural space is cannulated, the frequency of successful catheter insertion may be increased by advancing the needle an additional 1 to 2 mm. Additionally, the incidence of unintentional intravenous cannulation with an epidural catheter may be lessened by distending the epidural space by

injecting 5 to 10 mL of solution before threading the catheter.[18-20]

The catheter should be inserted only 2 to 3 cm into the epidural space to decrease the likelihood of catheter malposition. If analgesia is the primary indication for an epidural catheter and the surgical procedure is primarily upper abdominal or thoracic, thoracic catheter placement may be necessary. If this is the case because of the longer, overlapping urethral spinous processes, a paramedian approach at T6–7 often allows a more time-effective placement than a midline approach. My preference is to use a loss-of-resistance technique for thoracic catheter placements as well, although others recommend the hanging drop technique.

What Are Potential Problems?

Intravascular Injection

One of the most feared complications of epidural anesthesia is systemic toxicity resulting from intravenous injection of the intended epidural anesthetic dose. One way to identify intravenous injection is to administer a test dose of 3 mL of local anesthetic solution containing 1:200,000 epinephrine (i.e., 15 µg of epinephrine). If a tachycardiac response occurs, consider either the needle or catheter tip to be in an epidural vein and reposition. Subsequently, inject incrementally, be vigilant for unintentional intravascular injection, and have all necessary equipment and drugs available to treat local anesthetic-induced systemic toxicity.

Inadvertent Spinal

Another problem is unintentional administration of an epidural dose into the CSF via either needle or catheter. Aspirating before injecting any anesthetic usually identifies CSF. As

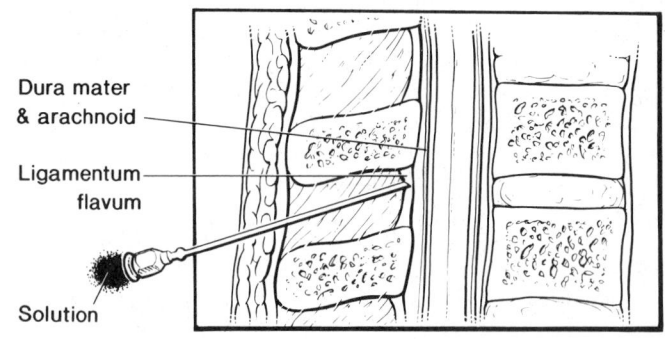

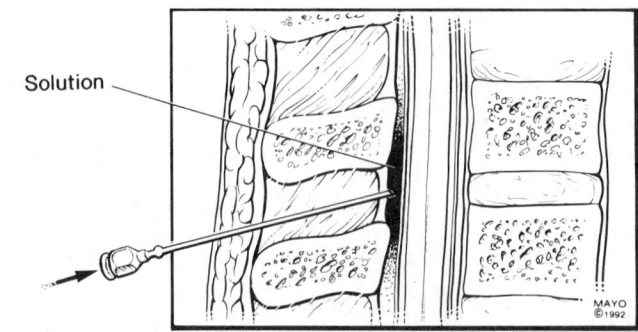

FIGURE 31–11. Hanging drop technique of epidural block needle insertion. Once the epidural needle tip enters the epidural space, the solution placed in the hub will be "sucked" into the needle.

with any centroneuraxis block that reaches high sensory levels, blood pressure and heart rate should be supported pharmacologically and ventilation assisted as required. Atropine and ephedrine usually suffice or at least provide the time to administer more potent catecholamines. If the entire dose (20–25 mL) of local anesthetic is administered into the CSF, tracheal intubation and mechanical ventilation are indicated. Approximately 1 to 2 hours will pass before a patient can consistently maintain adequate spontaneous ventilation after such an event.

When epidural anesthesia is performed and a higher than expected block develops only after a delay of 15 to 30 minutes, subdural placement of the local anesthetic must be considered. Treatment is symptomatic, and the most difficult aspect is recognizing that a subdural injection may have occurred.

CENTRONEURAXIS BLOCKADE: CAUDAL ANESTHESIA

How Is a Caudal Anesthetic Performed?

Caudal anesthesia can be effectively used for anorectal, perineal, and some lower extremity operations.

Patient Selection

Patient selection should be determined by the anatomy of the sacral hiatus. In approximately 5% of patients, the sacral hiatus is nearly impossible to cannulate with a needle or catheter; thus, in 1 of 20 patients the technique is impractical.[21] In some patients, the tissue mass overlying the sacrum makes the technique difficult; if another technique is applicable, caudal block should be deferred. Probably more so than for any other block, experience and confidence with the technique are necessary in order to carry it out effectively.

Drug Choice

When local anesthetics are prescribed for caudal anesthesia, the same considerations as those for epidural anesthesia apply. Volumes of local anesthetic of 25 to 35 mL are necessary to provide a sensory level of T-12 to T-10.

Anatomic Considerations

The sacral hiatus can be localized by finding the posterior superior iliac spines bilaterally, drawing a line to join them, and then completing a caudally directed equilateral triangle, the tip of which overlies the hiatus (Fig. 31–12). Overlying the sacral hiatus is a fibrous elastic membrane, which is the functional equivalent of the ligamentum flavum.

Positioning

Caudal block is carried out in a lateral decubitus position or prone position. In adults, the prone position, with a pillow placed beneath the lower abdomen, seems most effective. Localization of the sacral hiatus in a prone patient is aided by having the legs abducted to a 20° angle and the toes rotated inward. This maneuver helps to relax the gluteal muscles and allows easier identification of the sacral hiatus (Fig. 31–13). Patients can be sufficiently sedated to make the block comfort-

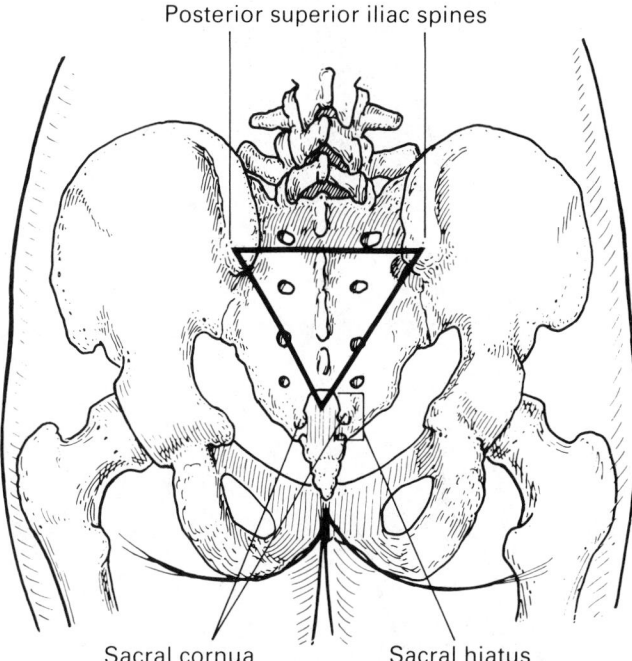

FIGURE 31–12. Sacral surface anatomy. An equilateral triangle can be drawn to connect the posterior superior iliac spines and the sacral hiatus. This can be useful in confirming palpation of the sacral hiatus.

able, and midline identification is easier than in the lateral position.

In contrast, pediatric caudal anesthesia is commonly carried out with a child in the lateral decubitus position. Because most pediatric caudal blocks are performed after induction with general anesthesia, the lateral position is almost mandatory. Identification of the midline and performance of the block are less complicated in pediatric patients.

Needle Placement

If a single-shot caudal anesthetic is to be performed, almost any needle of sufficient length to reach the caudal canal is appropriate. In adults, a needle at least 22 gauge or larger is recommended, because it is large enough to allow sufficiently rapid injection of solution to help detect a misplacement. If a through-the-needle catheter is to be used, a needle of sufficient size to allow catheter passage is required; otherwise, a 1.5-inch 20-gauge intravenous catheter is adequate.

After the sacral hiatus is identified, the index and middle fingers of the palpating hand are placed on the sacral cornu, and the caudal needle is inserted at an angle of approximately 45° to the sacrum. While the needle is advanced, a decrease in resistance should be appreciated as it enters the caudal canal. It is then further advanced until the dorsal aspect of the ventral plate of the sacrum is contacted.

Next, the needle is withdrawn slightly and redirected so that the angle of insertion relative to the skin surface is decreased. In male patients, this angle ends up almost parallel to the skin; in females, a slightly steeper angle is necessary (Fig. 31–14). During redirection after loss of resistance, the needle should be advanced approximately 1 to 1.5 cm into the caudal canal. Further advancement is not suggested, because dural puncture and unintentional intravascular cannulation become more likely.

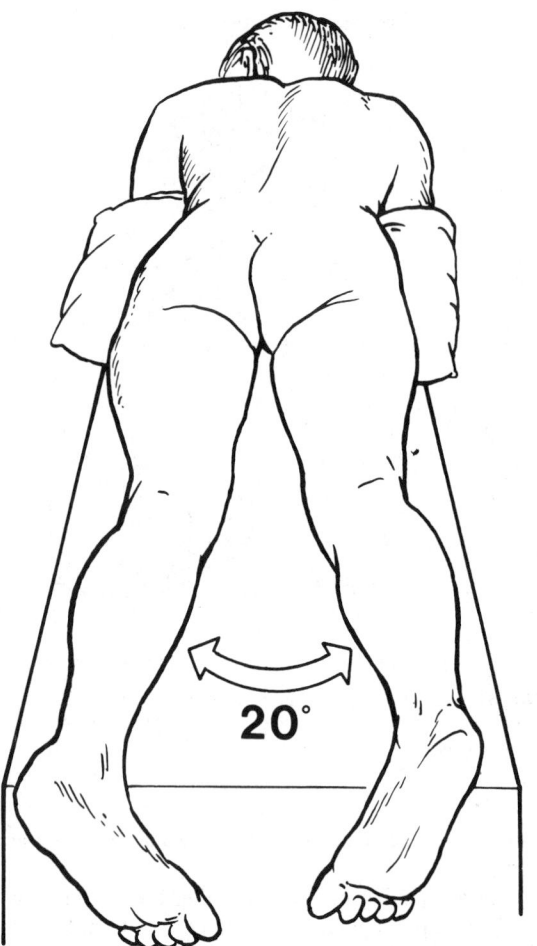

FIGURE 31–13. Prone position for performing the caudal technique. A pillow is used under the anterior iliac crests to rotate the pelvis, the legs are spread 20° to ease identification of the sacral hiatus, and the heels are rotated laterally to relax the gluteal musculature.

Testing Needle Location

Before administration of the therapeutic dose of local anesthetic, aspiration and a test dose injection should be performed. A helpful technique that confirms needle location during caudal anesthesia is a test injection of preservative-free saline. Once the needle has been placed into what is thought to be the caudal canal, apply a palpating hand across the dorsal sacral region and inject 5 mL of saline rapidly through the caudal needle. Subcutaneous needle positioning overlying the sacrum is immediately apparent, because a bulge during injection develops over the midline during injection. If the needle is correctly positioned within the caudal canal, no midline bulge should be palpable.

In thin individuals, accurate needle placement in the caudal canal followed by rapid injection of solution may cause small pressure waves more laterally overlying the sacral foramina. Do not confuse these smaller pressure waves with those associated with a misplaced subcutaneous needle.

What Are Potential Problems?

Caudal anesthesia embodies most of the same complications that can accompany lumbar epidural anesthesia. One distinct difference, however, is that the incidence of subarachnoid puncture is exceedingly low with caudal techniques. The dural

sac ends at approximately the S-2 level; thus, unless a needle is inserted deeply within the caudal canal, subarachnoid puncture is unlikely. In children, the dural sac extends more distally in the caudal canal; this fact should be considered when carrying out pediatric caudal anesthesia.

UPPER EXTREMITY BLOCKS

What Is the Relevant Anatomy?

The brachial plexus is formed by the ventral rami of the fifth to eighth cervical nerves and the greater part of the ramus of the first thoracic nerve (Fig. 31–15). Additionally, small contributions may be made by the fourth cervical and the second thoracic nerves.

Trunks

After the cervical nerve roots pass the lateral margin of the scalene muscles, they reorganize into brachial plexus trunks—superior, middle, and inferior.

Divisions

The trunks continue toward the first rib, at the lateral edge of which they undergo a primary separation into ventral and dorsal divisions. This is also the point at which an understanding of brachial plexus anatomy frequently gives way to frustration and unnecessary descriptive complexity. Nevertheless, this anatomic division is functionally significant, because nerves destined to supply the originally ventral part of the upper extremity separate from those that supply the dorsal part.

Cords

As these divisions enter the axilla, they give way to cords. The posterior divisions of all three trunks unite to form the posterior cord; the anterior divisions of the superior and middle trunks form the lateral cord; and the medial cord is the ununited, anterior division of the inferior trunk. These cords are named according to their relationship to the second part of the axillary artery.

Peripheral Nerves

At the lateral border of the pectoralis minor muscle, the three cords reorganize to give rise to the peripheral nerves of the upper extremity. The branches of the lateral and medial cords are all ''ventral'' nerves to the upper extremity. The posterior cord, in contrast, provides all ''dorsal'' innervation to the upper extremity. Thus, the radial nerve supplies all the dorsal musculature in the upper extremity below the shoulder. The musculocutaneous nerve supplies muscular innervation in the arm and cutaneous innervation to the forearm.

In contrast, the median and ulnar nerves are nerves of passage in the arm, but in the forearm and hand they provide the ventral muscles with motor innervation. These nerves can be further categorized: The median nerve innervates more heavily in the forearm, whereas the ulnar nerve innervates more heavily in the hand.

Fascial Investments

Some investigators have focused attention on the fascial investment of the brachial plexus. As the brachial plexus nerve

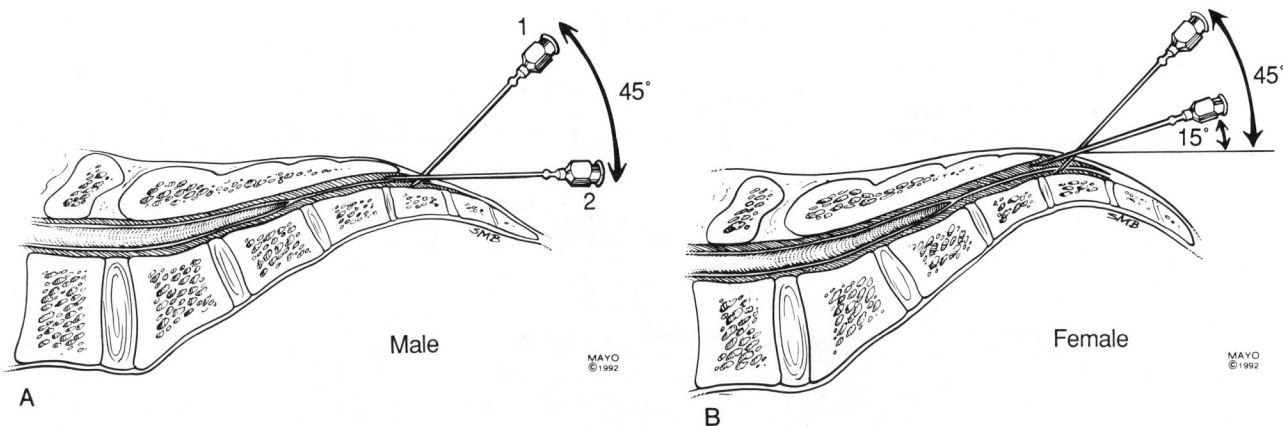

FIGURE 31–14. Caudal block anatomy and technique. The initial needle insertion angle for both males and females is 45° from the horizontal plane with the patients in a prone position. *A*, In males, the final needle position within the caudal canal will often end in the horizontal plane. *B*, In females, the final needle position within the caudal canal will often end approximately 15° off the horizontal plane.

roots leave the transverse processes, they do so between prevertebral fascia that divides to invest both the anterior and middle scalene muscles. This prevertebral fascia surrounding the brachial plexus is said to be tubular in form throughout its course, thus allowing needle placement within the "sheath" to produce brachial plexus blockade easily.

The brachial plexus certainly is invested with prevertebral fascia; however, it appears that the fascial covering is discontinuous, with septa subdividing portions of the sheath into compartments that may prevent adequate spread of local anesthetics. My clinical impression is that the discontinuity of the sheath increases from the transverse process to the axilla.

Vertebral Arteries

As the cervical nerve roots exit via the transverse processes on their way to form the brachial plexus, they pass through the gutter in the transverse process immediately posterior to the vertebral artery. The vertebral arteries leave the brachiocephalic and subclavian arteries on the right and left, respectively, and travel cephalad to enter a bony canal in the transverse process at the level of C-6 and above. Thus, one must be constantly aware of needle tip location in relationship to the vertebral artery during interscalene brachial plexus blocks. For emphasis, the vertebral artery lies anterior to the roots of the brachial plexus as they leave the cervical vertebrae.

Phrenic Nerves

Another structure of interest to brachial plexus anatomy is the phrenic nerve. It is formed from branches of the third, fourth, and fifth cervical nerves and passes through the neck on its way to the thorax on the ventral surface of the anterior scalene muscle. It is almost always blocked during interscalene anesthesia and less frequently with supraclavicular techniques. Avoidance of phrenic blockade is important in only a small percentage of patients, although its functional location should be kept in mind for those with significantly decreased pulmonary function—that is, those whose day-to-day activities are limited by their pulmonary impairment.

How Is an Interscalene Block Performed?

Interscalene block is indicated for surgery of the shoulder or upper arm, because the upper roots of the brachial plexus

are most easily blocked with this technique.[22, 23] The ulnar nerve is often spared, unless one makes a special effort to inject local anesthetic caudad to the site of the initial paresthesia.

The block is ideal for reduction of a dislocated shoulder and often can be achieved with as little as 10 to 15 mL of local anesthetic. It can also be performed with a patient's arm in almost any position and thus can be useful when brachial plexus block needs to be repeated during a prolonged upper extremity procedure.

Patient Selection

Interscalene blockade is appropriate in almost all patients, because even obese individuals usually have identifiable scalene and vertebral body anatomy. However, it should be avoided in patients with significantly impaired pulmonary function. This point is likely moot if one is planning to use a combined regional and general anesthetic technique, which allows control of ventilation intraoperatively. Even when a long-acting local anesthetic is chosen for the interscalene technique, phrenic nerve and pulmonary function usually have returned to a level that patients can tolerate by the time the surgical procedure is completed.

Drug Choice

Lidocaine and mepivacaine produce 2 to 3 hours of surgical anesthesia without epinephrine and 3 to 5 hours when epinephrine is added. These drugs are useful for less involved or outpatient surgical procedures. For extensive surgical procedures requiring hospital admission, a longer-acting agent such as bupivacaine is appropriate.

More complex surgical procedures on the shoulder often require muscle relaxation; thus, bupivacaine concentrations of at least 0.5% are needed. Plain bupivacaine produces surgical anesthesia lasting from 4 to 6 hours; the addition of epinephrine may prolong this duration to 8 to 12 hours.

Anatomic Considerations

Surface anatomy of importance involves the larynx, sternocleidomastoid muscle, and external jugular vein. Interscalene blockade is most often performed at the level of the C-6 vertebral body and cricoid cartilage.[23] By projecting a line laterally from the cricoid cartilage, the level at which one

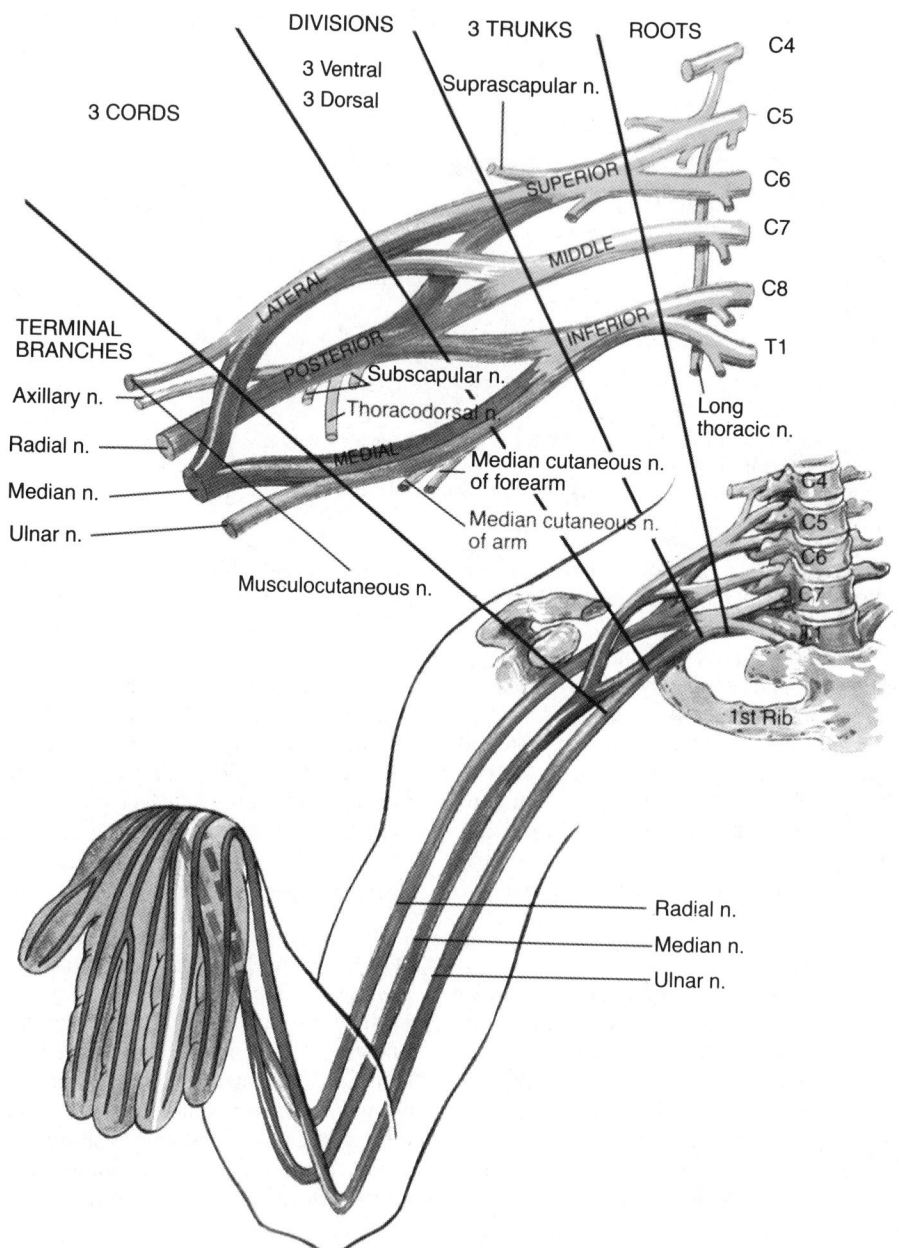

FIGURE 31–15. The brachial plexus anatomy. (From Brown DL: Atlas of Regional Anesthesia. Philadelphia, WB Saunders, 1992, p 15.)

should roll the fingers off the sternocleidomastoid muscle onto the belly of the anterior scalene and then into the interscalene groove can be identified. With firm pressure, it is possible to feel the transverse process of C-6 in most individuals, and in some, it is possible to elicit a paresthesia by deep palpation. The external jugular vein often overlies the interscalene groove at the level of C-6, although this relationship should not be relied on.

Always create a mental image of what lies under the palpating fingers. The key to success is identifying the interscalene groove. The closeness of the lateral border of the anterior scalene muscle and the posterior border of the sternocleidomastoid should be constantly kept in mind.

Positioning

The patient lies supine, with the neck in the neutral position and the head turned slightly opposite the site to be blocked,

and is asked to lift the head off the table. This movement tenses the sternocleidomastoid and allows identification of its lateral border. Roll the fingers onto the belly of the anterior scalene and subsequently into the interscalene groove in the horizontal plane through the cricoid cartilage.

Needle Placement

When the fingers are firmly pressing into the interscalene groove, the needle is inserted in a slightly caudal and posterior direction. If a paresthesia is not elicited on insertion, the needle is walked (maintaining the same angulation) in a plane joining the cricoid cartilage to the C-6 transverse process. Because the brachial plexus is traversing the neck at virtually a right angle to this plane, a paresthesia is almost certain if small enough steps of needle reinsertion are carried out (Fig. 31–16).

In anesthetic procedures for shoulder surgery, this probably

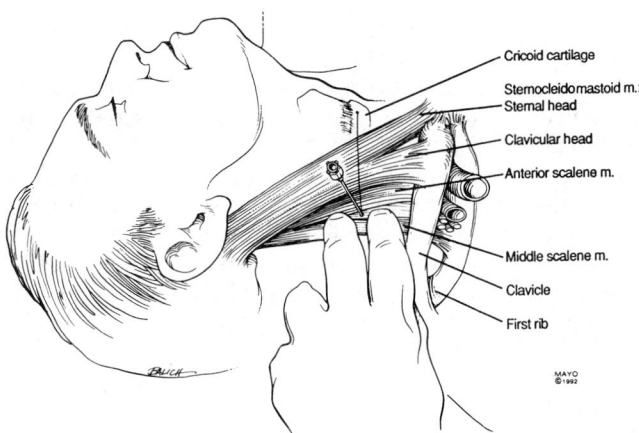

FIGURE 31–16. Interscalene block technique. The anesthesiologist's fingers are inserted overlying the interscalene groove at the level of the cricoid cartilage (C-6), and the needle is inserted in a slightly posterior and caudal direction. The needle orientation is maintained in the same plane as it is withdrawn and reinserted and is "walked" in an anteroposterior direction if a paresthesia is not obtained on the first pass.

is the one brachial plexus block in which a large volume of local anesthetic, coupled with a single needle position, allows effective anesthesia. Thirty to 40 mL of lidocaine, mepivacaine, or bupivacaine can be used.

Potential Problems

Problems that can arise from interscalene blockade are related to subarachnoid injection, epidural blockade, intravascular injection (especially in the vertebral artery), pneumothorax, and phrenic block.

If the operation requires ulnar nerve blockade, this is not my choice of brachial plexus block. The ulnar nerve is difficult to anesthetize with the interscalene approach because it is derived from the eighth cervical nerve, which is seldom blocked by injection at a more cephalic site. Also, be cautious in a patient with significant pulmonary impairment, because phrenic blockade is almost guaranteed to occur. If an epidural block occurs, consider also that it is likely to result in a bilateral phrenic nerve block and be prepared to ventilate the patient.

How Is a Supraclavicular Block Performed?

Supraclavicular block provides anesthesia of the entire upper extremity in the most consistent, time-efficient manner of any brachial plexus technique.[22] It is the most effective block for all portions of the upper extremity and is carried out at the "division" level of the brachial plexus, explaining why limited sparing of peripheral nerves may occur even if an acceptable paresthesia is obtained. If this block is to be used for shoulder surgery, it should be supplemented with a superficial cervical plexus technique to block the cutaneous innervation of the shoulder.[24]

Patient Selection

Almost all patients are potential candidates for this block, with the exception of those who are uncooperative. In addition, in less experienced hands, it may be inappropriate for outpa-

tients. Although pneumothorax is an infrequent complication of the block, it often becomes apparent only after a delay of several hours, when an outpatient might already be at home.

Drug Choice

As with other brachial plexus blocks, the prime consideration of drug selection should be the length of the procedure and the degree of motor blockade desired. Mepivacaine (1–1.5%), lidocaine (1–1.5%), and bupivacaine (0.5%) all are applicable. Lidocaine and mepivacaine produce from 2 to 3 hours of surgical anesthesia without epinephrine and 3 to 5 hours when epinephrine is added. These drugs can be useful for less involved or outpatient surgical procedures.

For more involved surgical procedures requiring hospital admission, a longer-acting agent like bupivacaine can be chosen. Plain bupivacaine produces surgical anesthesia lasting from 4 to 6 hours, and adding epinephrine may prolong this period to 8 to 12 hours.

Anatomic Considerations

The relevant anatomy involves the relationship between the brachial plexus and the first rib, subclavian artery, and cupula of the lung. My experience suggests that this block is more difficult to teach than many of the other regional blocks, and for that reason two approaches to the supraclavicular block are illustrated: the classic Kulenkampff approach and the plumb-bob approach. The plumb-bob approach has been developed in an attempt to overcome the difficulty and prolonged learning curve that seems attendant to the classic supraclavicular block approach. Despite that caution, either of the techniques is clinically useful, once mastered.

The subclavian artery and brachial plexus pass over the first rib between insertion of the anterior and middle scalene muscles onto the first rib. The nerves lie in a cephaloposterior relationship to the artery; thus, paresthesia may be elicited before the needle contacts the rib. At the point where the artery and plexus cross the first rib, it is broad and flat, sloping in a caudad direction as it moves from posterior to anterior. Although the rib is a curved structure, a needle can be walked in an anterior-posterior direction for a distance of 1 to 2 cm. Remember, immediately medial to this first rib is the cupula of the lung; when the needle is angled too medially, pneumothorax may result.

Classic Approach

Positioning

The patient is supine without a pillow, with the head turned opposite to the side to be blocked. The arms are at the sides, and the anesthesiologist can stand either at the head of the table or at the patient's side near the arm to be blocked.

Needle Puncture

The needle insertion site is approximately 1 cm superior to the clavicle at the clavicular midpoint (Fig. 31–17). This entry site is closer to the middle of the clavicle than to the junction of the middle and medial third, as is often described. Additionally, if the artery is palpable in the supraclavicular fossa, it can be used as a landmark.

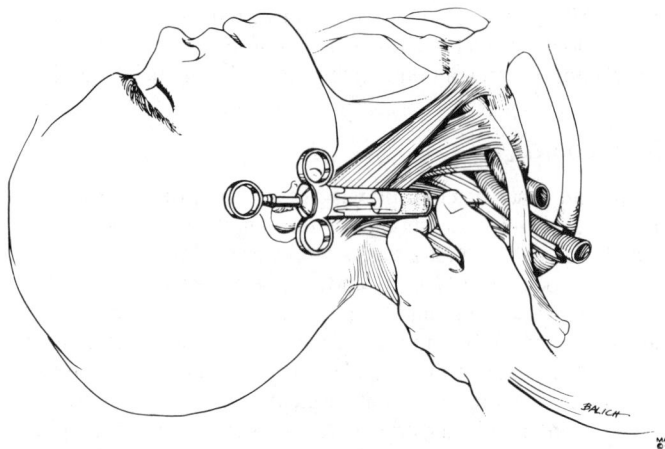

FIGURE 31–17. Classic supraclavicular block technique. A point 1 cm superior to the clavicular midpoint is marked, and the needle and syringe assembly are inserted in a cephalocaudal plane approximately parallel to the patient's neck. It is emphasized that care must be taken to ensure that the needle-syringe assembly is not angled medially toward the cupula of the lung.

The needle and syringe are inserted in a plane approximately parallel to the patient's neck and head, with care taken that the axis of syringe and needle does not aim medially toward the cupula of the lung.[22] The needle should be a 22-gauge 5-cm length that typically contacts the rib at a depth of 3 to 4 cm, although it sometimes requires a depth of 6 cm in a very large patient.

Initial needle insertion should not be carried out past 3 to 4 cm until a careful search in an anteroposterior plane does not identify the first rib. During insertion, the assembly should be controlled with the hand, as illustrated in Figure 31–17. The hand rests lightly against a patient's supraclavicular fossa to prevent unintentional deeper insertion, because with elicitation of a paresthesia, patients often move their shoulder.

Plumb-Bob Supraclavicular Block

Positioning

The plumb-bob approach resulted from efforts to simplify the anatomic projections necessary for the block.[25] A patient is positioned similarly to that for the classic approach, lying supine without a pillow, with the head turned slightly away from the side to be blocked. The anesthesiologist should stand lateral to the patient at the level of the upper arm. This block involves inserting the needle and syringe assembly at approximately a 90° angle to the classic approach.

Needle Puncture

Patients should raise their head slightly off the table so that the lateral border of the sternocleidomastoid muscle can be marked as it inserts onto the clavicle. From that point, a "mental" plane is imagined running parasagittally. Through a skin mark, the needle-syringe assembly is then inserted in the parasagittal plane at a 90° angle to the table top.

If paresthesia is not elicited on the first pass, the needle and syringe are redirected cephalad in small steps through an arc of approximately 30°. If a paresthesia still has not been obtained, they are reinserted at the starting position and then moved in small steps through an arc of approximately 30° in a caudal direction (Fig. 31–18).

Because the brachial plexus lies cephaloposterior to the artery as it crosses the first rib, a paresthesia often can be elicited before contacting either the artery or the first rib. If that occurs, approximately 30 mL of local anesthetic is inserted at this single site.

If a paresthesia is not elicited with the maneuvers described but the first rib is contacted, the block is carried out just like the classic approach—walking along the first rib until paresthesia is elicited. As in the classic approach, care should be taken not to aim the syringe and needle assembly medially toward the cupula of the lung.

Potential Problems

Pneumothorax

The most feared complication of these blocks is pneumothorax. The principal cause of this problem is needle-syringe angles that drift medially toward the cupula of the lung. Special attention should be directed toward walking the needle in a strict anteroposterior direction.

Pneumothorax often takes a number of hours to develop; thus, it is likely related to impingement of the needle on the lung rather than air entering the pleural space as the needle is inserted.

If a pneumothorax does occur after supraclavicular block, it can most often be observed while the patient is reassured. If the pneumothorax is large enough to cause dyspnea or discomfort, aspiration through a small-gauge catheter is often all that is necessary. The patient should be admitted for observation; however, it is the exceptional patient who needs formal chest tube placement for re-expansion of the lung.

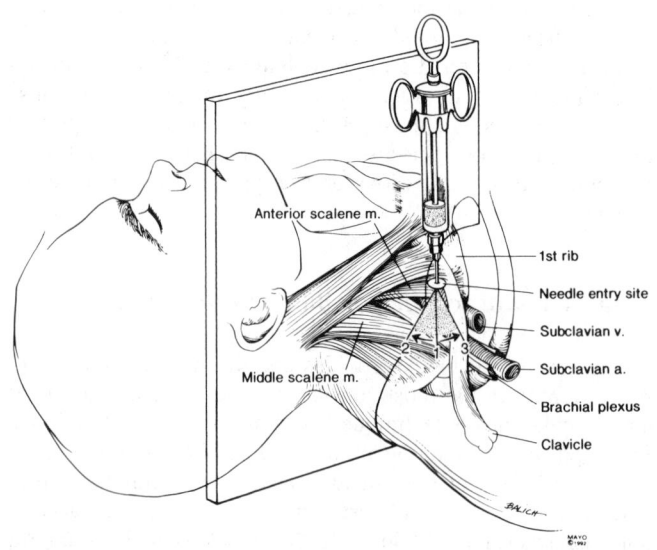

FIGURE 31–18. Plumb-bob (vertical) supraclavicular block technique: A point is marked at the junction of the lateral border of the sternocleidomastoid muscle as it attaches onto the clavicle. Patients should be instructed to turn their heads slightly opposite of the side to be blocked. The needle-syringe assembly is then inserted in the parasagittal plane of the skin entry site and at 90° to the table top (position 1). If paresthesia is not obtained on the initial needle insertion, the needle-syringe assembly is withdrawn and reinserted in small steps through an arc of 30° cephalad (position 2). If a paresthesia is still not obtained, this process is repeated in a caudad direction through another 30° arc (position 3). Again, it is important to avoid angling the needle-syringe assembly medially toward the cupula of the lung.

Phrenic Nerve Blockade

Phrenic nerve blockade does occur, probably in 30% to 50% of cases, and the block's use in patients with significantly impaired pulmonary function must be weighed individually.

Subclavian Artery Puncture

The development of hematoma after supraclavicular block, as a result of puncture of the subclavian artery, usually requires only observation.

Applicability

The predictability and rapid onset of this block allow its use even in a busy practice. As previously outlined, a longer learning curve is associated with it than with most other regional blocks. For that reason, anesthesiologists should develop a system for its use. Unfocused probing at the root of the neck is not the way to approach this block. Choose either the classic or plumb-bob approach early, and give each a fair trial before abandoning it.

How Is an Axillary Block Performed?

Axillary brachial plexus block is most useful for surgical procedures distal to the elbow.[22] In selected patients, procedures on the elbow or distal humerus can be carried out with an axillary block, but strong consideration should be given to supraclavicular block for more proximal operations. To carry out a successful axillary block only to find the surgical procedure extends outside the area of block is discouraging.

The block is most appropriate for hand and forearm surgery; thus, it is often the technique of choice for outpatients in a hand surgery practice. Because this block is performed remote from both the centroneuraxis and the lung, complications attendant to those areas are avoided.

Patient Selection

To receive an axillary block, patients must not have an infection in the axilla and must be able to abduct their arm at the shoulder. As operator experience increases, the necessity for this requirement diminishes, but the block cannot be carried out with a patient's arm at the side. Because the block is most appropriate for forearm and hand surgery, it is a rare patient with a surgical condition at those sites who cannot abduct the arm.

Drug Choice

Hand and wrist operations often require less motor block than do those on the shoulder. As a result, the local anesthetic concentration can usually be slightly decreased, in contrast to supraclavicular or interscalene block. Appropriate drugs are lidocaine (1–1.5%), mepivacaine (1–1.5%), and bupivacaine (0.5%).

Lidocaine and mepivacaine produce from 2 to 3 hours of surgical anesthesia without epinephrine and 3 to 5 hours when epinephrine is added. These drugs are useful for less involved or outpatient surgical procedures. For more extensive procedures requiring hospital admission, a longer-acting agent such as bupivacaine can be chosen. Plain bupivacaine produces surgical anesthesia lasting from 4 to 6 hours; the addition of epinephrine may prolong this duration to 8 to 12 hours.

Anatomic Considerations

In the distal axilla or upper arm, where axillary block is performed, the axillary artery can be imagined as indicating the center of a four-quadrant neurovascular bundle. It seems useful to conceptualize these nerves in a quadrant (or clock face) manner, because multiple injections during axillary blockade may result in more predictable and rapid clinical anesthesia than does injection at a single site (Fig. 31–19).

The musculocutaneous nerve is in the 9 to 12 quadrant in the substance of the coracobrachial muscle. The median nerve is most often in the 12 to 3 quadrant; the ulnar nerve is inferior to the median nerve in the 3 to 6 quadrant; and the radial nerve is in the 6 to 9 quadrant. From radiographic and anatomic study of the brachial plexus and the axilla, it is clear that separate and distinct sheaths are functionally associated with the plexus at this point.

Positioning

A patient is placed supine with the upper arm forming a 90° angle with the trunk and the forearm forming a 90° angle with the upper arm. This position allows the anesthesiologist to stand at the level of the patient's upper arm and easily palpate the axillary artery or neurovascular cord. A line should be drawn tracing the course of the artery from the midaxilla to the lower axilla. The anesthesiologist's fingers overlying this line identify the artery and displace the subcutaneous tissue surrounding the neurovascular bundle. In this manner, one can develop a sense of the longitudinal course of the artery, which is essential for axillary blockade.

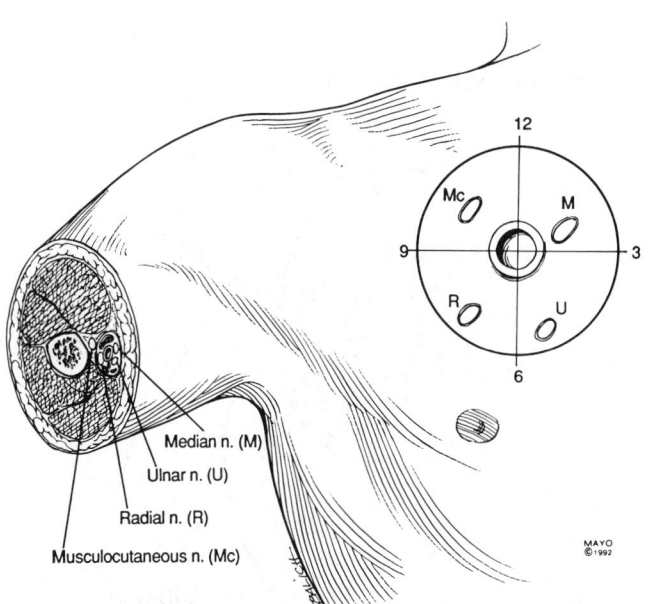

Median n. (M)
Ulnar n. (U)
Radial n. (R)
Musculocutaneous n. (Mc)

FIGURE 31–19. Axillary block anatomy; functional quadrant anatomy. It is useful to imagine the perivascular axillary anatomy in a cross-sectional plane of the upper arm as if it were the face of a clock. In a patient's right arm, the median, ulnar, radial, and musculocutaneous nerves are found approximately in the 12-to-3-o'clock, 3-to-6-o'clock, 6-to-9-o'clock, and 9-to-12-o'clock quadrants, respectively.

Needle Puncture

Undue expenditure of time and patient discomfort should not occur during attempts to elicit a paresthesia. As illustrated in Figure 31–20, this technique of axillary block is produced by using the axillary artery as an anatomic landmark and infiltrating in a fanlike manner around it. Anesthesia of the musculocutaneous nerve is best achieved by identifying the coracobrachial muscle and injecting into its substance or by inserting a longer needle until it contacts the humerus and injecting in a fanlike manner.

For axillary blockade to be as effective as possible, an understanding of the organization of the peripheral nerves at the level of the lower axilla is necessary. The axillary sheath at this level is discontinuous. A single injection may produce useful surgical anesthesia; however, I believe the most consistently effective axillary blockade results from depositing smaller amounts of local anesthetic in multiple sites.

How Is Intravenous Regional Anesthesia Performed?

This technique, also called Bier's block, can be used for various upper extremity operations, including both soft tissue and orthopedic procedures, primarily in the hand and forearm. It also has been used for foot procedures with a calf tourniquet.

Patient Selection

Intravenous regional anesthesia is best suited for patients with no disruption in the involved upper extremity, because the technique relies on an intact venous system. It can be used for distal orthopedic fractures and soft tissue operations. It may not be appropriate for patients in whom movement of the upper extremity causes significant pain, because such movement is required to exsanguinate the venous system adequately.

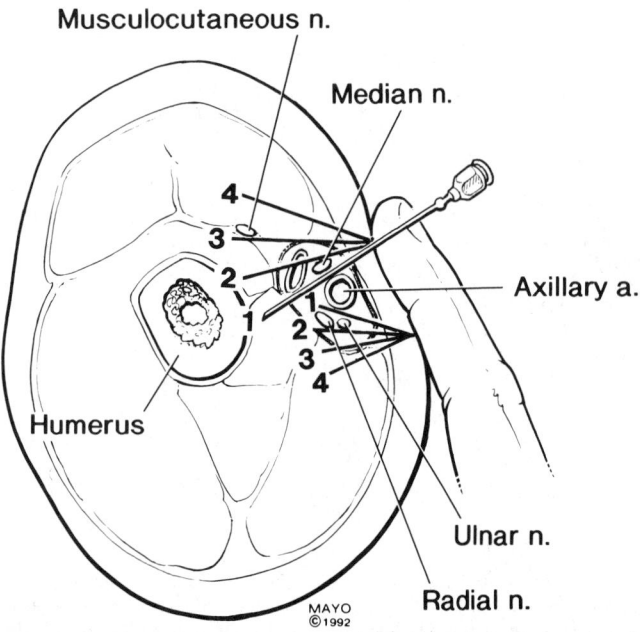

FIGURE 31–20. Needle placement for performance of axillary block. Numbers refer to the fanlike infiltration pattern to block the several nerves listed, using the axillary artery as the point of reference.

Pharmacologic Choice

The agent most commonly used for an upper extremity block is a dilute (0.5%) concentration of lidocaine, approximately 50 mL. Because of the risk of toxic reaction, bupivacaine is not an appropriate drug for this technique.

Anatomic Considerations

The only requirement is access to a peripheral vein in the involved extremity.

Positioning

A patient should be resting supine on the operating table with an intravenous infusion established in the nonoperative arm. The involved arm should be extended on an arm board.

Needle Puncture, Exsanguination, and Tourniquet Inflation

A double or single tourniquet should be placed around the operative upper arm. An intravenous cannula is inserted in the operative extremity, as distally as possible. Two methods are acceptable for exsanguination of venous blood from the operative extremity: The traditional technique requires the wrapping of an Esmarch bandage from distal to proximal. When an Esmarch bandage is not available or a patient has too much pain to allow its placement, another method is to raise the arm for 3 to 4 minutes, allowing gravity to produce venous exsanguination.

After exsanguination, the tourniquet is inflated. If a single tourniquet is used, it is inflated. If a double tourniquet is used, the upper tourniquet is inflated at this point. Recommendations for tourniquet inflation vary and include 50 mm Hg above systolic blood pressure with a wide cuff; a cuff pressure double the systolic blood pressure; or 300 mm Hg pressure regardless of blood pressure. A calibrated tourniquet manometer should be used, and regardless of technique, pressures >300 mm Hg should not be used.

If an Esmarch bandage has been wrapped and the tourniquet is inflated, the elastic bandage is then unwrapped, and 50 mL of 0.5% lidocaine without a vasoconstrictor is slowly injected in an average adult. Onset of the block is usually within 5 minutes. When a double tourniquet is used, the lower (distal) one is now inflated, after which the upper one is deflated. This usually affords an additional 20 minutes of relief before tourniquet pain again is an issue. It is my clinical impression that use of propofol to provide conscious sedation during intravenous regional anesthesia postpones the onset of tourniquet pain. The intravenous cannula is removed before preparation for operation. The block persists as long as the cuff is inflated and disappears shortly after deflation.

Potential Problems

The principal potential problem of intravenous regional anesthesia is that associated with premature accidental tourniquet release, causing local anesthetic-induced systemic toxicity. The tourniquet should not be deflated for at least 20 minutes after an anesthetic injection, even if the operation is completed before that; otherwise, the risk of toxicity is excessive. After that, the tourniquet can be cycled with several deflation-reinflation cycles to allow redistribution of the anesthetic. During upper extremity intravenous regional anesthesia, many patients complain about tourniquet pressure even when a double tourniquet is used; this often is the clinically limiting feature of this technique. Important for patients' acceptance is appropriate use of intravenous sedatives.

LOWER EXTREMITY BLOCKS

How Is a Sciatic Nerve Block Performed?

The sciatic nerve is one of the largest nerves in the body, yet few surgical procedures can be performed with sciatic block alone. It is most often combined with femoral, lateral femoral cutaneous, or obturator nerve blocks to produce analgesia or surgical anesthesia of the lower leg.

Patient Selection

This block may be indicated for patients requiring analgesia before transport for definitive repair of lower leg or ankle fractures. In selected patients, it may be desirable to avoid the sympathectomy accompanying spinal or epidural block. Sciatic block combined with femoral nerve block often allows ankle and foot procedures to be carried out. It is also useful in patients undergoing distal amputations of the lower extremity if their vascular compromise is based on diabetes or peripheral vascular disease.

Drug Choice

Sciatic nerve block requires 20 to 25 mL of local anesthetic solution. When this volume is added to that required for other lower extremity peripheral nerve blocks, the total may reach the upper end of the acceptable local anesthetic dose range (see Table 31–1). If motor block is needed, either 1.5% mepivacaine or lidocaine is necessary; also, ≥0.5% bupivacaine is effective.

Anatomic Considerations

The sciatic nerve is derived from the L-4 through S-3 spinal nerve roots (sacral plexus) on the anterior surface of the lateral sacrum. The "medial" sciatic nerve functionally is the tibial nerve, which forms from the ventral branches of the anterior rami of L-4 to L-5 and S-1 to S-3. The posterior branches of the ventral rami of these same nerves form the "lateral" sciatic nerve, which functionally is the peroneal nerve.

As the sciatic nerve exits from the pelvis, it is anterior to the piriform muscle and is joined by the posterior cutaneous nerve of the thigh. At the inferior border of the piriform muscle, the nerve is approximately equidistant from the ischial tuberosity and the greater trochanter. It continues on a downward course through the thigh to lie along the posterior medial aspect of the femur.

At the cephalic portion of the popliteal fossa, it usually divides to form the tibial and common peroneal nerves. This division occasionally occurs much higher, and the tibial and peroneal nerves sometimes are separate through their entire course.

In the popliteal fossa, the tibial nerve continues its downward course into the lower leg, and the common peroneal nerve travels laterally along the medial aspect of the short head of the biceps femoris muscle.

Positioning

A patient is typically placed in Sims' position with the side to be blocked uppermost. The flexed, nondependent leg supports the patient with its heel opposed to the knee of the dependent leg (Fig. 31–21).[26]

Needle Puncture

A line is drawn from the posterior superior iliac spine to the midpoint of the greater trochanter. Perpendicular to the midpoint of this line, another line is extended caudomedially for 5 cm. The needle is inserted through this point. As a cross-check for proper placement, an additional line may be drawn from the sacral hiatus to the previously marked point on the greater trochanter. The intersection of this line with the 5-cm perpendicular should coincide with the needle insertion site (see Fig. 31–21).

A 22-gauge 10- to 12-cm needle is inserted and directed toward an imaginary point where the femoral vessels cross the inguinal ligament. The needle is inserted until a paresthesia is

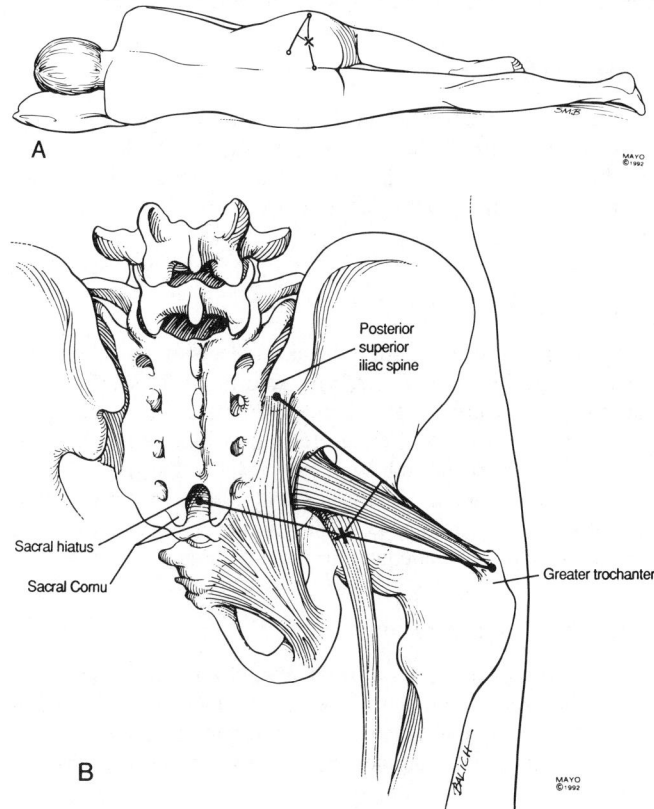

FIGURE 31–21. Sciatic nerve block technique. *A,* The patient is positioned in Sims' position, rotated slightly away from the anesthesiologist and the side to be blocked. The patient's nondependent heel should oppose his or her dependent knee. *B,* Surface markings for sciatic block are made by joining the posterior-superior iliac spine and the greater trochanter with a line. At the midpoint of this line, a second line is drawn caudomedially, and a point 5 cm off the original line is marked. The needle is then inserted through this point toward an imaginary point where the femoral vessels cross under the inguinal ligament. As a cross-check for the needle insertion site, a line is drawn from the sacral hiatus to the greater trochanter. It should cross the caudomedially directed line at the previously marked needle site.

elicited or until bone is contacted. If bone is encountered before eliciting a paresthesia, the needle is redirected along the line joining the sacral hiatus and the greater trochanter until paresthesia is elicited.

During this needle redirection, the needle should not be inserted more than 2 cm past the depth at which bone was originally contacted, or it will be anterior to the sciatic nerve. Once a paresthesia to the lower leg is elicited, 20 to 25 mL of local anesthetic is injected.

Potential Problems

When the block is used after injury to the lower extremity, Sims' position is sometimes difficult to achieve. This block can be long lived, and patients should be warned of this possibility preoperatively to prevent undue concern postoperatively about slow return of function.

How Is a Femoral Block Performed?

Superficial and deep surgical procedures may be carried out on the anterior thigh with this block. It is most frequently combined with other lower extremity peripheral blocks to provide anesthesia for operations on the lower leg and foot. It is useful as an analgesic technique for femoral fractures.

Patient Selection

Because a patient is in the supine position when this block is performed, virtually anyone undergoing a surgical procedure of the lower extremity is a candidate. Paresthesias are not necessary for this block; therefore, even anesthetized patients are candidates.

Drug Choice

As with all lower extremity blocks, a decision must be made about the desired extent of sensory and motor block. If motor blockade is essential, higher concentrations of local anesthetic are necessary. The requirement for motor block must be considered in light of the total volume of local anesthetic necessary if femoral, sciatic, lateral femoral cutaneous, and obturator blocks are combined. Approximately 20 mL of local anesthetic should be adequate to produce femoral block.

Anatomic Considerations

The femoral nerve traverses the pelvis in the groove between the psoas and iliac muscles. It becomes more superficial beneath the inguinal ligament, posterolateral to the femoral vessels. It frequently divides into its branches at or above the level of the inguinal ligament.

Needle Puncture

The patient is in a supine position, and the anesthesiologist should stand at the side to palpate the femoral artery. A line is drawn connecting the anterosuperior iliac spine and the pubic tubercle. The femoral artery is palpated on this line, and a 22-gauge 4-cm needle is inserted (Fig. 31–22). The initial insertion should abut the femoral artery in a perpendicular fashion and then produce a "wall" of local anesthetic in a fanlike

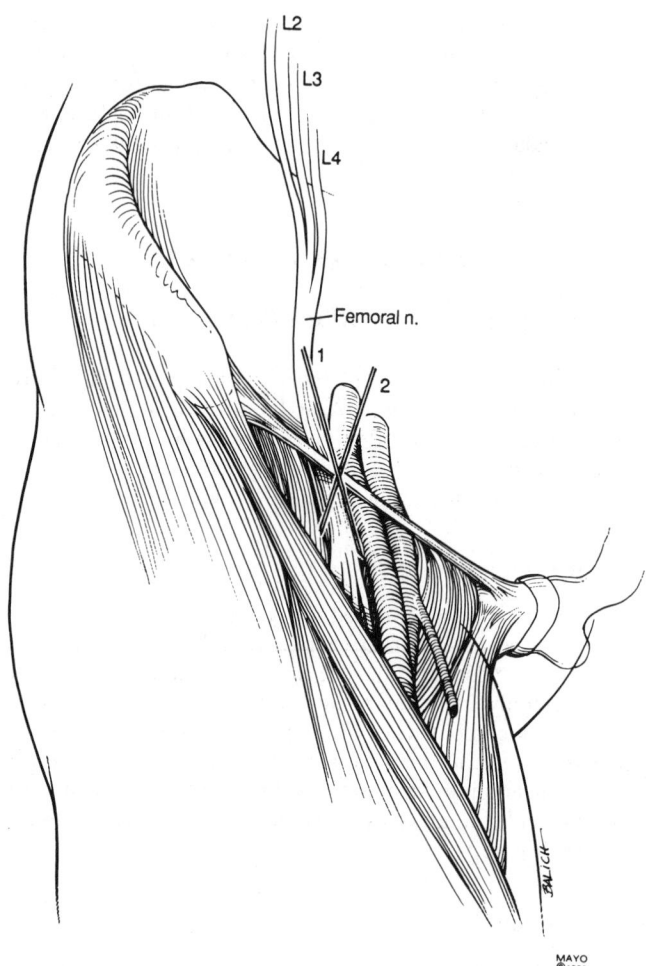

FIGURE 31–22. Femoral nerve block technique. The femoral artery should be located and the needle-syringe assembly inserted to abut the femoral artery in the sagittal plane *(position 1)*. During local anesthetic injection, the needle is withdrawn and reinserted in small steps to build a "wall of anesthesia" through an arc ending at *position 2*.

manner, by redirecting the needle in progressive steps. Because the injection is made adjacent to two large vessels, one must aspirate repeatedly to allow immediate identification of intravascular needle placement. Approximately 20 mL of local anesthetic is injected incrementally in this fashion. The needle entry can also be directed laterally 1 cm and aimed immediately posterior to the femoral artery; an additional 2 to 5 mL of drug is then injected to block those nerve fibers that may be more posterior to the femoral artery.

Potential Problems

Unilateral lower extremity blocks are often indicated for patients with peripheral vascular disease. If a patient has recently undergone placement of a prosthetic femoral artery graft, efforts should be made to avoid the prosthesis.

How Is a Lateral Femoral Cutaneous Block Performed?

If this block is used together with other lower extremity blocks, procedures can be carried out with fewer complaints of tourniquet pain. It also allows superficial procedures on the lateral thigh, including skin graft harvesting. The diagnosis of meralgia paresthetica, a neuralgia involving the lateral femoral cutaneous nerve, can be made if the pain resolves when the nerve is blocked.

Patient Selection

This block also is carried out with the patient in the supine position. Thus, almost all patients are candidates.

Drug Choice

The same concerns about total local anesthetic dose outlined in the sciatic and femoral sections apply to the lateral femoral cutaneous blockade. If multiple nerves to the lower extremity are to be anesthetized, be aware of the total mass of drug administered. Because this nerve does not have motor components, a lower concentration of 10 to 15 mL is effective.

Anatomic Considerations

The lateral femoral cutaneous nerve emerges along the lateral border of the psoas muscle immediately caudad to the ilioinguinal nerve. It courses deep to the iliac fascia and anterior to the iliac muscle to emerge from the fascia immediately inferior and medial to the anterior superior iliac spine. After passing beneath the inguinal ligament, it crosses or passes through the origin of the sartorius muscle and travels beneath the fascia lata, dividing into anterior and posterior branches at variable distances below the inguinal ligament. The anterior branch supplies skin over the anterolateral thigh, and the posterior branch supplies the skin laterally from the greater trochanter to midthigh.

Positioning

Positioning is the same as for femoral nerve block.

Needle Puncture

The anterior superior iliac spine is marked, and a 22-gauge 4-cm needle is inserted at a site 2 cm medial and 2 cm caudal to the mark. The needle is advanced until a pop is felt as it passes through the fascia lata. Local anesthetic is then injected in a fanlike manner above and below the fascia lata, from medial to lateral (Fig. 31–23).

How Is an Ankle Block Performed?

An ankle block is useful for surgical procedures carried out on the foot, especially when high tourniquet pressure is not required.

Patient Selection

An ankle block is principally an infiltration block, not demanding elicitation of paresthesia. A patient's cooperation is not mandatory for success.

Drug Choice

Because motor block is not often needed for procedures carried out during ankle block, lower concentrations of local

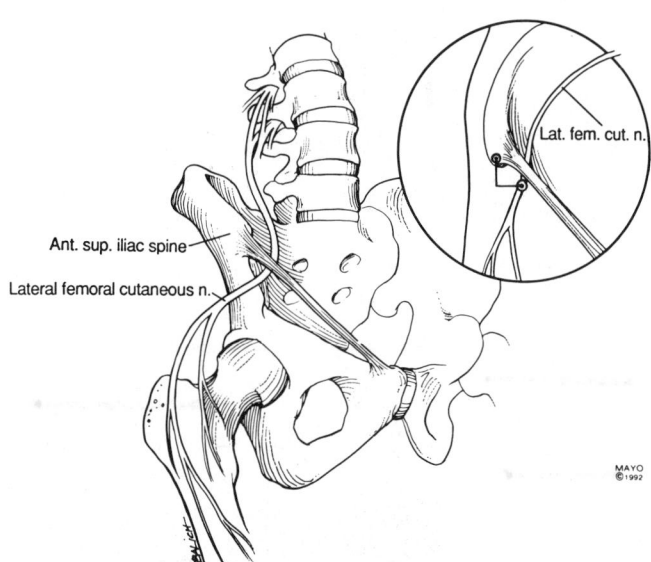

FIGURE 31–23. Lateral femoral cutaneous nerve block technique. The lateral femoral cutaneous nerve emerges from beneath the inguinal ligament immediately inferior and medial to the anterior superior iliac spine. A point is marked 2 cm inferior and 2 cm medial to the anterior superior iliac spine, and the needle is inserted through this site to develop a wall of anesthetic above and below the fascia lata.

anesthetics may be used. Practical choices are 1% lidocaine, 1% mepivacaine, and 0.25% to 0.5% bupivacaine. Epinephrine should not be used, especially if injection is circumferential.

The peripheral nerves requiring block during ankle block all are derived from the sciatic nerve, except for the saphenous nerve (the only branch of the femoral nerve below the knee). It courses superficially anterior to the medial malleolus, providing cutaneous innervation to an area of the medial ankle and foot. The remaining nerves requiring block are the common peroneal and tibial. The tibial nerve divides into posterior tibial and sural nerves, and the common peroneal nerve divides into its terminal branches, the superficial and deep peroneal nerves, in the proximal portion of the lower leg.

Needle Puncture

The block can be performed with a patient in the supine position if the foot is placed on a padded support (Fig. 31–24).

Deep Peroneal, Superficial Peroneal, and Saphenous Nerves

The anterior tibial artery pulsation is located at the superior level of the malleoli. A 22-gauge 4-cm needle is advanced posteriorly and immediately lateral to this point. Alternatively, insert the needle between the tendons of the anterior tibial and extensor hallucis longus muscles. Approximately 3 to 5 mL of local anesthetic is injected in this area. From this midline skin wheal, using the same or a longer 22-gauge 8-cm needle, the infiltration is advanced subcutaneously laterally and medially to the malleoli, injecting 2 to 3 mL of local anesthetic as the needle is advanced in each direction. These lateral and medial approaches block the superficial peroneal and saphenous nerves, respectively.

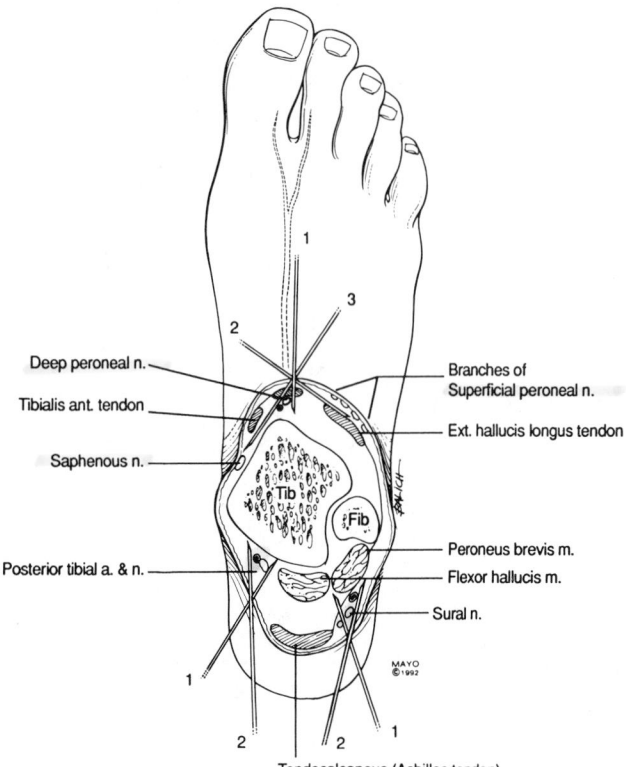

FIGURE 31–24. Ankle block technique. This block can be performed with the patient in the supine position if the ankle is supported, or it can be performed in two stages with the patient in both the supine and prone positions. In either case, three injections are made. First, the deep and superficial peroneal and saphenous nerves are blocked by inserting a needle between the anterior tibial and extensor hallucis longus tendons *(position 1)* and by developing a wall of local anesthetic from tibia to skin. The needle is then inserted subcutaneously both medial and lateral from the original skin insertion site to anesthetize the subcutaneous branches of superficial peroneal *(position 2)* and saphenous nerves *(position 3)*. Second, the tibial nerve is anesthetized by inserting a needle immediately medial to the Achilles tendon *(position 1)* at the level of the medial malleolus and by developing a wall of anesthesia through an arc *(position 2)*. Third, the sural nerve is anesthetized by inserting a needle immediately lateral to the Achilles tendon *(position 1)* at the level of the lateral malleolus and by developing a wall of anesthesia through an arc *(position 2)*.

Posterior Tibial Nerve

After the ankle is rotated laterally, a 22-gauge 4-cm needle is directed anteriorly at the cephalic border of the medial malleolus, just medial to the Achilles tendon. The needle is inserted near the posterior tibial artery; if a paresthesia is obtained, 3 to 5 mL of local anesthetic is injected. If no paresthesia is obtained, the needle is allowed to contact the medial malleolus, and 5 to 7 mL of local anesthetic is deposited in a fanlike pattern near the posterior tibial artery.

Sural Nerve

Rotate the ankle medially and insert a 22-gauge 4-cm needle anterolaterally immediately lateral to the Achilles tendon at the cephalad border of the lateral malleolus. If no paresthesia is obtained, the needle is allowed to contact the lateral malleolus, and 5 to 7 mL of local anesthetic is injected in a fanlike manner.

Potential Problems

The ankle block can be painful if a patient is not adequately sedated. This problem should be infrequent, because an alert patient is not essential for the block.

TRUNCAL BLOCKS

How Is Intercostal Nerve Block Performed?

Intercostal nerve block provides excellent body wall analgesia. Thus, the technique is appropriate for relieving pain after unilateral upper abdominal and thoracic surgery or for rib fracture analgesia. Minor surgical procedures can be performed on the chest or abdominal wall using only intercostal blocks, but in general, some supplementation is most often appropriate. This block can also be used when chest tubes or feeding gastrostomy tubes are inserted.

Patient Selection

All patients are candidates for this block, although it is more difficult in obese patients.

Drug Choice

If intercostal nerve block is combined with light general anesthesia for intra-abdominal surgery and the intercostal block is expected to provide abdominal muscle relaxation, a higher concentration of local anesthetic is needed. In this setting, 0.5% bupivacaine, 1.5% lidocaine, or 1.5% mepivacaine is an appropriate choice. Conversely, if sensory analgesia is all that is required, 0.25% bupivacaine, 1% lidocaine, or 1% mepivacaine is appropriate.

Anatomic Considerations

Intercostal nerves are formed from the ventral rami of T-1 through T-11. The 12th thoracic nerve is technically a subcostal nerve.

Positioning

The intercostal nerves are most easily blocked if the patient is placed in the prone position. A pillow should be inserted under the midabdomen to reduce the lumbar lordosis and to accentuate the intercostal spaces posteriorly. The arms should be allowed to hang dependently from the edge of the block table (or gurney) to allow the scapula to rotate as far laterally as possible. If the block is for postoperative analgesia, the same positions used for performing a lumbar puncture provide adequate access.

Needle Puncture

Before needle puncture, appropriate intravenous sedation should be administered to produce amnesia and analgesia during the multiple injections needed for the block. Barbiturates, benzodiazepines, ketamine, or short-acting opioids can be combined.

Use a marking pen to outline the pertinent anatomy. The midline should be marked from T-1 to L-5. Two paramedian lines should be drawn at the posterior angle of the ribs. These lines should angle medially in the upper thoracic region, paralleling the medial edge of the scapula. By successfully palpating and marking the inferior edge of each rib along these two paramedian lines, a diagram like that in Figure 31–25 is created.

Skin wheals are raised with a 30-gauge needle at each of the previously marked sites of injection. As illustrated in Figure 31–25, a 22-gauge short-beveled 3- to 4-cm needle is attached to a 10-mL control syringe. Be sure to use the hand and finger positions illustrated.

Beginning at the most caudal rib to be blocked, the index and third fingers of the left hand are used to retract the skin up and over the rib. The needle should be introduced through the skin between the tips of the retracting fingers and advanced until it contacts the rib. Do not allow the needle to enter to a depth greater than what the palpating fingers define as rib.

Once the needle contacts the rib, the right hand firmly maintains this contact while the left hand is shifted to hold the needle's hub and shaft between the thumb, index, and middle fingers. The left hand's hypothenar eminence should be firmly

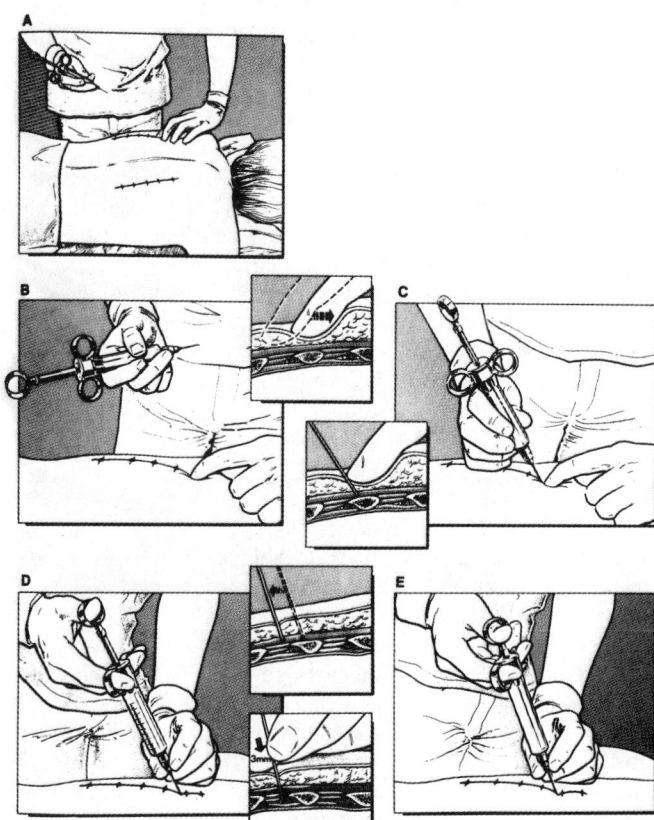

FIGURE 31–25. Technique for intercostal block and corresponding deep anatomy (see text). *A,* Skin markings at lateral edge of sacrospinalis muscle (6–8 cm from midline). Note the medial curve of the line superiorly to avoid the scapulae. Ribs and interspaces are palpated. The lowest (most inferior) intercostal nerve is blocked first because the lower ribs are easy to palpate. (Diagrams *A–E* show the second last intercostal nerves to be blocked in this patient.) *B,* Skin at the lower edge of the rib is retracted superiorly onto the rib. *C,* The needle is inserted onto rib (see also inset). Note that the finger palpating the rib is still in place and that the hand holding the syringe is firmly braced against the back. *D,* The position of the hands now changes. Note that the left hand now rests against the back and holds the needle as it is walked off the inferior edge of the rib and advanced 3 mm. The right hand is free to aspirate and inject. *E,* Injection is completed with the left hand still firmly braced against the patient's back while the needle is controlled.

placed against the patient's back. This hand placement allows maximum control of the needle depth as the left hand walks the needle off the inferior margin of the rib and into the intercostal groove, a distance of 2 to 3 mm past the edge of the rib.

With the needle in position, 3 to 5 mL of local anesthetic solution is injected. The process is then repeated for each of the nerves to be blocked. In certain patients with cachexia or severe barrel chest deformity, the intercostal injection can be most effectively carried out with an even shorter 23- or 25-gauge needle.

Potential Problems

The principal concern with intercostal nerve block is pneumothorax. Many physicians avoid this block because of the imagined high frequency and seriousness of this complication. Data suggest that the incidence of pneumothorax is <0.5%, and even when it occurs, careful clinical observation is usually all that is necessary.[27]

The incidence of symptomatic pneumothorax following intercostal block is even lower, approximately 1:1000. If treatment is deemed necessary, needle aspiration can often be carried out with successful lung re-expansion. Chest tube drainage should be performed only after failure of lung re-expansion after observation or percutaneous aspiration.

As a result of the vascularity of the intercostal space, local anesthetic blood levels are higher for multiple-level intercostal block than for any other regional anesthetic technique. Because these peak blood levels may be delayed for 15 to 20 minutes, patients should be closely monitored after the completion of a block for at least that interval.

How Is Interpleural Block Performed?

Interpleural anesthesia is a technique to provide body wall and visceral analgesia after upper abdominal or thoracic surgery. Accurate stratification of the risks and benefits of interpleural anesthesia currently remains elusive, perhaps in large part because of the success and popularity of epidural opioid analgesia.

Patient Selection

Patients undergoing upper abdominal or flank surgery or those recovering from fractured ribs have been selected most frequently for interpleural block. Appropriate selection remains ill defined.

Drug Choice

Most commonly, 20 to 30 mL of 0.25% to 0.5% bupivacaine solution is injected via the interpleural needle or catheter.

Anatomic Considerations

The pleural space extends from the apex of the lung to the inferior reflection of the pleura at approximately L-1. It also invests the posterior and anterior mediastinal structures (Fig. 31–26).

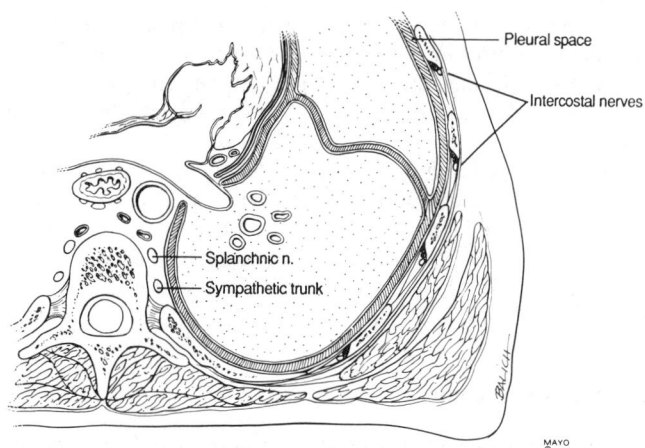

FIGURE 31–26. Interpleural block cross-sectional anatomy. The block likely results in both intercostal nerve block and block of deep splanchnic nerves.

Positioning

A patient is most often turned to an oblique position, with the side to be blocked uppermost.

Needle Puncture

Once a patient is positioned and supported by a pillow, a skin wheal is raised immediately superior to the eighth rib in the seventh intercostal space, approximately 10 cm lateral to the midline. If a continuous technique is selected, a needle allowing passage of a catheter (often epidural) is selected. If a single-injection technique is to be used, a short, beveled needle of sufficient length to reach the pleural space can be used. Before inserting the needle, a syringe-needle assembly containing approximately 2 mL of saline is inserted immediately superior to the eighth rib, using a loss of resistance technique much like that used during epidural anesthesia. When the needle tip is in the pleural space, the local anesthetic solution is very easy to inject.

Once the needle is in position, the local anesthetic is injected, if it is to be a single-shot technique, or a catheter is threaded through the needle approximately 10 cm into the pleural space, taking care to minimize the volume of air entrained through the needle. The catheter is then taped in a position that does not interfere with the surgical procedure, and the local anesthetic, typically 20 to 30 mL, is injected. Finally, the patient is rolled into the supine position to allow distribution of the local anesthetic.

Potential Problems

Although pneumothorax would seem to be associated with any technique that violates the pleural space, it is reported to be an infrequent problem with interpleural anesthesia.[28] A second potential problem is the unpredictable nature of analgesia accompanying what otherwise seems to be an acceptable technique.

At this time, the mechanism behind interpleural anesthesia remains uncertain. One theory proposes that the local anesthetic diffuses from the pleural space through the intercostal membrane to reach the intercostal nerves along the chest wall. A second proposal is that the local anesthetic is distributed through the pleura and into the region of the posterior medias-

tinum, at which point it provides visceral analgesia by anesthetizing the splanchnic nerves.

COMPLICATIONS

Why Does Neurologic Injury Occur?

Neurologic injury is a complication of regional anesthesia that frequently is not evaluated in a comprehensive manner. If an appropriate risk-benefit analysis is undertaken, the incidence of neuropathy accompanying general anesthesia, which is not zero, also must be considered. Similarly, many perioperative nerve injuries are unrelated to anesthetic care. Some of these include surgical positioning problems, surgical trauma, tourniquet sequelae, pressure from extremity casts, pre-existing neurologic conditions, and postoperative nerve injury.[28]

Do Paresthesias Have a Role?

Some have suggested during the past 15 years that paresthesia-seeking techniques are more likely to cause nerve injury. This impression needs perspective. The original report by Selander and colleagues concluding that paresthesia should be avoided during regional block was a nonrandomized, unblinded study in which no statistical difference between paresthesia-seeking and nonparesthesia-seeking patient groups was found.[29]

One would suppose that if regional anesthesia can be successfully conducted without elicitation of a paresthesia, the occasional needle-induced nerve injury can be avoided. Nevertheless, even in situations in which paresthesias were not being sought, a paresthesia was obtained unintentionally in almost half of the patients.[29] Persistent neuropathy after peripheral nerve block is usually temporary and resolves with time. A number of large series demonstrate the relative neurologic safety of these techniques.[30, 31]

Are Centroneuraxis Blocks Problematic?

Large series of centroneuraxis blocks also highlight the relative neurologic safety of these techniques.[32, 33] Reports have focused attention on neurologic injury following continuous spinal anesthesia.[34]

Centroneuraxis neurologic complications have a long and colorful history. Many Medicare-age patients remember the publicity in the lay press associated with the well-publicized Wooley and Roe case in England in the late 1940s.[35] What most are unaware of is the report by Marinacci from Los Angeles shortly after that era in which 99% of the neurologic lesions believed due to postspinal anesthetic changes were found on neurologic and electromyographic (EMG) examination to be related to other factors.[36]

Neurologic injury can occur with centroneuraxis blocks, but a rational risk-benefit analysis requires that those neurologic injuries associated with general anesthesia be included in the equation.

Continuous Spinal Catheters

Continuous spinal anesthesia with small-bore catheters resulted in a sufficient number of cases of cauda equina syndrome to prompt the Food and Drug Administration (FDA) to issue a safety alert on May 29, 1992, ''advising against the use of *any* small-bore catheter for continuous spinal administration of *any* local anesthetic agent.''[37] The mechanism by which this occurs is uncertain but may relate to the slow rate at which one injects through these catheters, resulting in poor mixing (dilution) of the anesthetic in the CSF and thereby creating pockets of toxic concentrations of local anesthetic.[38, 39]

One additional concern I have about potential centroneuraxis nerve injury involves the use of continuous spinal catheters for postoperative analgesia. Many substances are used in the subarachnoid space to improve postoperative analgesia. Nevertheless, I believe this is a risk-filled endeavor.

We have found that if a continuous epidural catheter is in place out of the immediate operating theater, various unintentional drug injections occur.[40] The epidural space is likely more forgiving of misapplied drugs than is the subarachnoid space. For these reasons, anesthesiologists should be extremely cautious about continuing subarachnoid catheters in a setting where drug swaps and unintentional drug injection may be more likely to occur.

When Should Neurologic Consultation Be Obtained?

If neurologic injury occurs after regional anesthesia, an important decision that needs to be made involves the request for a neurologic consultation. Anesthesiologists who use regional anesthesia should have a close working relationship with at least a few neurologists in their practice setting.

A frequent dilemma is caused by a neurologist who provides a well-focused consultation but then suggests that an EMG would not be useful immediately postoperatively, because ''all physicians know, the neurologic changes may take from 14 to 21 days to develop after injury.'' That is exactly the point! As noted previously, Marinacci found that 99% of the neurologic lesions believed related to spinal anesthesia that were found (often with EMG help) actually represented pre-existing neurologic deficits.

If a neurologic deficit develops after operation, a baseline EMG may help to outline that neurologic abnormalities were present before operation, rather than being solely attributable to the anesthetic technique. Neurologic injury related to anesthesia has been well outlined in a report formatted from the American Society of Anesthesiologists Closed Claims database; the concluding statement in that report suggests that for the majority of perioperative nerve injuries, the cause is not apparent.[28]

What Are the Cardiovascular Effects of Regional Anesthesia?

The most frequent cause of cardiovascular side effects is autonomic blockade. Reduced blood pressure and heart rate during centroneuraxis blocks are primarily attributable to the vasodilation (especially venous) produced by sympathetic blockade. The second major mechanism for cardiovascular side effects is direct actions of the local anesthetic (or its additives) on the cardiovascular system.

One of the advantages of peripheral regional blocks is that they have minimal cardiovascular side effects because they are most often administered at sites remote from autonomic neural pathways. Therefore, the cardiovascular side effects attributed to peripheral blocks are almost exclusively a result of local anesthetic or vasoconstrictor side effects.

Should Epinephrine Be Used?

When one plans a peripheral block, a decision that needs to be made is whether to add epinephrine to the local anesthetic mixture. An epinephrine dilution of 1:200,000 (5 µg of epinephrine per milliliter of local anesthetic solution) provides adequate prolongation of the local anesthetic block without undue side effects.[41]

In situations when more than 45 mL of local anesthetic solution is administered during a peripheral regional block, the total dose of epinephrine should be limited to 0.25 mg (250 µg) to minimize epinephrine-related side effects.[24]

How Is Hypotension Defined?

Although centroneuraxis blocks almost always routinely lower blood pressure, what level of lowered blood pressure should be defined as hypotension? Arterial blood pressure decreases should approximate 15% of preblock levels, if euvolemia is maintained.[42]

Complicating clinical decisions about the augmentation of blood pressure during centroneuraxis block is the recognition that for many of the patients we are most concerned about, those with ischemic heart disease, reduction of blood pressure normally is a desirable long-term goal to minimize myocardial oxygen demands. In one sense, a centroneuraxis block is similar to β-blockade—that is, blood pressure is lowered as is heart rate, albeit acutely.

At present, clinical judgment and tradition, as well as some experimental evidence, suggest that mean arterial blood pressure should not be allowed to decline more than 30% after a centroneuraxis block. Most anesthesiologists aim to keep mean arterial blood pressure at or above 65 mm Hg even in nonhypertensive patients. If patients have pre-existing hypertension, this minimum level is necessarily shifted upward.

What Is Profound Bradycardia?

Considerable attention has been focused on what has been described as an unrecognized entity: profound bradycardia following centroneuraxis blockade.[43] When viewed over time, this problem is neither new nor unrecognized by most anesthesiologists performing regional anesthesia.[32, 44, 45] Symptomatic bradycardia and even asystole are possible after autonomic interruption by centroneuraxis block.

Appropriate therapy usually includes an anticholinergic drug, such as atropine, and verification that the bradycardia is not secondary to hypoxemia. If atropine is not successful in raising the heart rate to an acceptable level, epinephrine, 25 to 100 µg, is indicated. If these treatment options, together with adequate volume replacement, are used, profound bradycardia is manageable.[46]

What Is Local Anesthetic Toxicity?

Local anesthetic systemic toxicity usually results from unintentional intravascular injection or use of an excessive dose during regional block. Manifestations are primarily reflected in the CNS and cardiovascular system. Approximately four to

TABLE 31–2. Comparative Central Nervous System and Cardiovascular Toxicity of Local Anesthetics in Dogs

Drug	Cumulative Convulsive Dose (mean ± SEM)	Cumulative Lethal Dose (mean ± SEM)	CV/CNS
Lidocaine	22.0 ± 6.7	76.2 ± 15.1	3.5
Etidocaine	8.0 ± 2.2	40.4 ± 6.0	5.1
Tetracaine	4.0 ± 2.2	26.9 ± 4.6	6.7
Bupivacaine	5.0 ± 0	20.4 ± 2.4	4.1

Abbreviations: CV = cardiovascular; CNS = central nervous system; SEM = standard error of the mean.

seven times as much local anesthetic is required to produce cardiovascular collapse as to initiate convulsions (Table 31–2).[47] Systemic effects occur on a continuum (Fig. 31–27).

Central Nervous System Effects

The CNS toxic effects range from sedation to seizure. They are plasma concentration dependent. In general, the CNS toxic-to-therapeutic ratio of local anesthetics is quite similar after intravenous administration. Convulsions result from inhibitory fiber depression in the subcortical brain structures, probably the amygdala, with subsequent amplification to grand mal seizures.[48] Modification of CNS toxicity can be achieved by the use of barbiturates, benzodiazepines, and even inhalational anesthetics.[49–53]

The decision to administer benzodiazepines prophylactically before regional block affects the risk-benefit relationship of systemic toxicity in two ways. CNS toxicity is less likely in an individual who has received benzodiazepines. Conversely, the early signs of CNS toxicity may be observed in a patient who has not been so "prophylaxed," allowing earlier intervention before the cardiovascular effects become apparent.

Cardiotoxic Effects

The sodium-blocking action of local anesthetics produces dose-related decreases of myocardial contractility and cardiac conduction. At low concentrations, a small increase in mean arterial pressure often occurs, whereas at high concentrations, vasodilation or vasoconstriction can be noted.[54–58]

For many years, the potential for cardiac toxicity related to local anesthetics was believed to parallel their anesthetic potency.[59] It has now become apparent, however, that the long-acting local anesthetics, bupivacaine and etidocaine, are proportionally more cardiotoxic than their relative anesthetic potencies suggest.[60, 61] This increase in cardiac toxicity appears to result from proportionally more and longer-lasting sodium channel blockade.

Sodium channel block typically develops during systole and resolves during diastole. However, the long-acting agents such as bupivacaine do not leave the sodium channels as rapidly during diastole, and the sodium channel block accumulates.[62] CNS activity also may influence cardiac toxicity.[63, 64]

Treatment

Local anesthetic-induced systemic toxicity ranges from minor alterations in sensorium to significant tonic-clonic seizures that result in profound hypoxemia, hypercarbia, and acidosis. These metabolic and acid-base changes can develop quite rapidly (seconds to minutes) and can significantly increase toxicity.[65–67] If you suspect that toxicity is developing, the first drug to administer is oxygen. Oxygen alone occasionally is sufficient treatment,[68] but positive-pressure breathing with a bag and mask may be necessary.

A CNS depressant (barbiturate or benzodiazepine) is all that is usually necessary to treat local anesthetic-induced seizures. If a CNS depressant and rapid-acting neuromuscular relaxant, such as succinylcholine, are deemed necessary, the latter should be administered first to prevent seizure-induced muscle activity and the accompanying acidosis. Furthermore, after administration of succinylcholine, the airway is more easily managed and oxygen more effectively delivered.

Most anesthesiologists encounter local anesthetic-induced toxicity rarely during their entire career. Hence, they should practice a local anesthetic-induced seizure management drill, much like the recommendations for failed intubation drills.

As outlined earlier, local anesthetic systemic toxicity progresses to cardiovascular toxicity. The ABCs of resuscitation should be followed in this setting, recognizing that larger than usual doses of epinephrine may be needed. Ventricular dysrhythmias (especially those related to the long-acting local anesthetics, bupivacaine and etidocaine) are likely more effectively treated with bretylium than lidocaine.[69–71]

A fundamental modification of local anesthetic use that may reduce the number of systemic toxic reactions is to use a test dose whenever possible or techniques to inject local anesthetics incrementally. If an intravascular injection occurs, only a small mass of drug is injected at any one time.

Why Do Spinal Headaches Occur?

One of the principal reasons anesthesiologists recommend epidural over spinal anesthesia in patients for whom either technique is an option is concern that spinal anesthesia will lead to a significant incidence of position-related headaches. The loss of CSF through the dural puncture site is the principal cause of postdural puncture headache.[72] Why certain patient subgroups are more or less likely to develop headaches after spinal anesthesia remains speculative. The factors listed in Table 31–3 seem to be associated with an increased incidence.

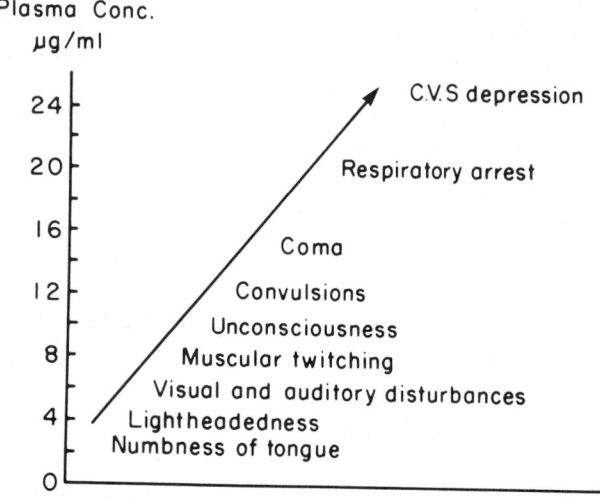

FIGURE 31–27. Local anesthetic systemic toxicity continuum. Symptoms begin with changes in sensorium and with perioral numbness. They progress along the continuum to seizures and eventually cardiovascular depression. C.V.S. = cardiovascular.

TABLE 31–3. Factors in Spinal Headaches

Factors increasing incidence of headache	Age
	Gender
	Needle size
	Needle bevel
	Younger > older
	Females > males
	Larger > smaller
	Cutting bevel > "spreading" bevel greater when dural
	Fibers cut transversely
	Pregnancy
	Number of dural passes
	Greater when pregnant
	Greater with multiple punctures
Factors unrelated to incidence of headache	Continuous epidural
	Timing of ambulation

Characteristics

The onset of headaches typically ranges from immediate to approximately 1 week after the spinal anesthetic. The peak incidence appears to be on postoperative day 2 or 3, often just when a surgeon would like to discharge an inpatient from the hospital.[73] Postdural puncture headaches developing more than 1 week after spinal anesthesia are unusual, and additional reasons for the headaches should be sought. The diagnosis is supported if the headache is most pronounced in an upright or sitting position; it should lessen or be significantly relieved in the supine position. As with all medical conditions, spinal headache symptoms exist on a continuum that must be kept in mind when a diagnosis is made or ruled out.

Before the development of epidural blood patch therapy, the typical headache lasted from 2 to 3 days to approximately a week. On rare occasions, they persisted for weeks to months.[74–76]

Prevention

The most important means to minimize the incidence of postdural puncture headache is appropriate matching of patients, equipment, and techniques. Postdural puncture headaches are more frequent in women (especially parturients) and are two times more common in females than males in the under-50 age group.[77] Younger individuals have headaches more frequently than older patients.

A critical factor is an operator's skill. If one is able to identify the subarachnoid space easily with one pass of the spinal needle, a lower headache incidence likely results than when a novice is unable to recognize subarachnoid placement and perforates the dura a number of times before achieving obvious subarachnoid placement.

One clinical dictum that seems unrelated to the incidence of postdural puncture headache is the prescription for bed rest following spinal anesthesia. This approach may delay the onset of the headache, but it does not appear to reduce the incidence.[74, 78]

Increasing evidence suggests that splitting dural fibers by using pencil-point side hole needles rather than cutting them with conventional needle points reduces the incidence. Additionally, for similar-tipped needles, the incidence of headache decreases as needle size decreases.[79] It may also be decreased by using a paramedian rather than a midline approach.[80]

Postdural puncture headache following continuous spinal anesthesia may be lower than one would anticipate from the needle size used to perform the dural puncture.[81–83] For this reason, I am concerned about the push to develop increasingly smaller spinal catheters. Their appropriate use (and indications) need much further clarification as well as resolution of the issues leading to the FDA Safety Alert[37] before we introduce them widely into our practices, especially for postoperative analgesia.

Treatment

Finally, if spinal anesthesia is to be used successfully and postdural puncture headaches are not allowed to limit your choice, epidural blood patch therapy must be provided in a time-efficient manner. Although bed rest is often an appropriate short-term treatment, it should not be unnecessarily prolonged before undertaking an epidural blood patch.

The prescription for hydrating (possibly overhydrating) patients intravenously needs rethinking. Little evidence supports the concept that hydration actually treats postdural puncture headaches.

Caffeine (7 mg · kg^{-1}) relieves some headaches, often needs to be repeated, and thus seems to be a temporizing treatment.[84] Any question about the efficacy of caffeine also should not delay definitive epidural blood patch therapy.

Is There a Role for Nerve Stimulator–Assisted Regional Anesthesia?

Clearly, regional anesthesia is routinely and successfully implemented based on knowledge of the local anatomy and occasionally also elicitation of paresthesias. In some circumstances, however, a patient is unable to respond adequately to interrogation about either onset of block or occurrence of paresthesia. There are also patients whose anatomic landmarks are indistinct and occasions when one is asked to place an infrequently performed block. In such instances, a nerve stimulator is quite helpful to verify that the tip of the block needle is located precisely adjacent to the desired nerve. This localization is manifested as an evoked motor response—that is, a twitch for a motor nerve or a burning sensation if it is a sensory nerve referable to the intended nerve. If the nerve is a mixed sensory and motor nerve, then the motor response predominates as large myelinated fibers (motor) are stimulated by lower currents than their smaller unmyelinated sensory nerve counterparts.

Needle Placement

In order to obtain maximum utility out of nerve stimulator-assisted peripheral nerve identification, one should first use an insulated or shielded needle. The insulation serves to localize the densest current at the needle tip, compared with an insulated needle, which emits some current along its entire shaft. A conducting portion of this needle is then connected to the negative terminal of the nerve stimulator, usually via an alligator clamp. The positive terminal is connected to an electrocardiograph pad placed on the lateral ipsilateral shoulder for upper extremity block or buttock for lower extremity block.

The nerve stimulator should have a discreetly adjustable current output with a display of the output. The stimulator is then set to deliver one pulse per second of 10 to 20 mA. Placement of the needle is based on the needle path predicted by the anatomic landmarks. Because this current is relatively large, a desired motor response only suggests that the needle is within several centimeters of the intended nerve. The current is then progressively reduced, and the needle position adjusted in trial-and-error fashion until <1 mA of current still elicits the desired response. Abolition of the twitch response on injection of 1 mL of local anesthetic solution confirms appropriate placement.

References

1. Katz JA: A survey of anesthetic choice among anesthesiologists. Anesth Analg 1973; 52:373.
2. Broadman LM, Mesrobian R, Ruttimann U, et al: Do anesthesiologists prefer a regional or general anesthetic for themselves? Reg Anaesth 1986; 11:A57.
3. Bach S, Noreng MF, Tjellden NU: Phantom limb pain in amputees during first 12 months following limb amputation, after preoperative lumbar epidural blockade. Pain 1988; 33:297.
4. Dickenson AH, Sullivan AF: Subcutaneous formalin-induced activity of dorsal horn neurones in the rat: differential response to an intrathecal opiate administered pre or post formalin. Pain 1987; 30:349.
5. Tverskoy M, Cozacov C, Ayache M, et al: Postoperative pain after inguinal herniorrhaphy with different types of anesthesia. Anesth Analg 1990; 70:29.
6. Kopacz DJ, Nickel P: Regional anesthesia in the elderly patient. Probl Anesth 1989; 3:602.
7. Bridenbaugh LD: Are anesthesia resident programs failing regional anesthesia? Reg Anaesth 1982; 7:26.
8. O'Keefe JH, Shub C, Rettke SR: Risk of noncardiac surgical procedures in patients with aortic stenosis. Mayo Clin Proc 1989; 64:400.
9. Chestnut DH: Spinal anesthesia in the febrile patient. Anesthesiology 1992; 76:667.
10. Caldwell C, Nielsen C, Baltz T, et al: Comparison of high-dose epinephrine and phenylephrine in spinal anesthesia with tetracaine. Anesthesiology 1985; 62:804.
11. Gielen M: Post dural puncture headache (PDPH): a review. Reg Anaesth 1989; 14:101.
12. Moore DC, Chadwick HS, Ready LB: Epinephrine prolongs lidocaine spinal: pain in the operative site the most accurate method of determining local anesthetic duration. Anesthesiology 1987; 67:416.
13. Moore DC: Spinal anesthesia: bupivacaine compared with tetracaine. Anesth Analg 1980; 59:743.
14. Greene NM: Hypobaric, isobaric, and hyperbaric spinal anesthesia. Curr Rev Clin Anesth 1985; 5:99.
15. Brown DL: An Atlas of Regional Anesthesia. Philadelphia, WB Saunders, 1992.
16. Taylor JA: Lumbosacral subarachnoid tap. J Urol 1940; 43:561.
17. Brown DL, Carpenter RL: Perioperative analgesia: a review of risks and benefits. J Cardiothorac Anesth 1990; 4:368.
18. Philip BK: Effect of epidural air injection on catheter complications: experience in obstetric patients. Reg Anaesth 1985; 10:21.
19. Verniquet AJW: Vessel puncture with epidural catheters. Anaesthesia 1980; 35:660.
20. Mannion D, Walker R, Clayton K: Extradural vein puncture—an avoidable complication. Anaesthesia 1991; 46:585.
21. Trotter M: Variations of the sacral canal: their significance in the administration of caudal anesthesia. Anesth Analg 1947; 26:192.
22. Lanz E, Theiss D, Jankovic D: The extent of blockade following various techniques of brachial plexus block. Anesth Analg 1983; 62:55.
23. Winnie AP: Interscalene brachial plexus block. Anesth Analg 1970; 49:455.
24. Moore DC: Regional Block: A Handbook for Use in the Clinical Practice of Medicine and Surgery. 4th ed. Springfield, IL, Charles C Thomas, 1965.
25. Brown DL, Cahill DR, Bridenbaugh LD: Supraclavicular nerve block: anatomic analysis of a method to prevent pneumothorax. Anesth Analg 1993; 76:530.
26. Labat G: Regional Anaesthesia: Its Technique and Clinical Application. Philadelphia, WB Saunders, 1923.
27. Moore DC, Bridenbaugh LD: Pneumothorax: its incidence following intercostal nerve block. JAMA 1960; 174:842.
28. Kroll DA, Caplan RA, Posner K, et al: Nerve injury associated with anesthesia. Anesthesiology 1990; 73:202.
29. Selander D, Edshage S, Wolff T: Paresthesia or no paresthesia. Acta Anaesthesiol Scand 1979; 23:27.
30. Winchell SW, Wolfe R: The incidence of neuropathy following upper extremity nerve blocks. Reg Anaesth 1985; 10:12.
31. Thompson AM, Newman RJ, Semple JC: Brachial plexus anaesthesia for upper limb surgery: a review of 8 years experience. J Hand Surg 1988; 13B:195.
32. Moore DC, Bridenbaugh LD: Spinal (subarachnoid) block: a review of 11,574 cases. JAMA 1966; 195:907.
33. Vandam LD, Dripps RD: Long-term follow-up of 10,098 spinal anesthetics: incidence and analysis of minor sensory neurological defects. Surgery 1955; 38:463.
34. Rigler M, Drasner K, Yelich S, et al: Cauda equina syndrome after continuous spinal anesthesia. Anesth Analg 1991; 72:275.
35. Cope RW: The Wooley and Roe case: Wooley and Roe versus the Ministry of Health and others. Anesthesia 1954; 9:247.
36. Marinacci AA: Neurologic aspects of complications of spinal anesthesia. Los Angeles Neurological Society Bulletin 1960; 25:170.
37. FDA Safety Alert: Cauda equina syndrome associated with use of small-bore catheters in continuous spinal anesthesia. Rockville, MD, Food and Drug Administration, 1992.
38. Ross BK, Coda B, Heath CH: Local anesthetic distribution in a spinal model: a possible mechanism of neurologic injury after continuous spinal anesthesia. Reg Anaesth 1992; 17:69.
39. Rigler ML, Drasner K: Distribution of catheter-injected local anesthetic in a model of the subarachnoid space. Anesthesiology 1991; 75:684.
40. Bickler P, Spears R, McKay W: Intralipid solution mistakenly infused into epidural space (Letter to the editor). Anesthesiology 1990; 71:712.
41. Tucker GT, Moore DC, Bridenbaugh PO, et al: Systemic absorption of mepivacaine in commonly used regional block procedures. Anesthesiology 1972; 37:277.
42. Greene NM: Physiology of Spinal Anesthesia. 3rd ed. Baltimore, William & Wilkins, 1981.
43. Caplan RA, Ward RJ, Posner K, et al: Unexpected cardiac arrest during spinal anesthesia: a closed claims analysis of predisposing factors. Anesthesiology 1988; 68:5.
44. Wetstone DL, Wong KC: Sinus bradycardia and asystole during spinal anesthesia. Anesthesiology 1974; 41:87.
45. Thompson KW: Fatalities from spinal anesthesia. Anesth Analg 1934; 13:75.
46. Mackey DC, Carpenter RL, Thompson GE, et al: Bradycardia and asystole during spinal anesthesia: a report of three cases without morbidity. Anesthesiology 1989; 70:866.
47. Liu PL, Feldman HS, Giasi R, et al: Comparative CNS toxicity of lidocaine, etidocaine, bupivacaine, and tetracaine in awake dogs following rapid IV administration. Anesth Analg 1983; 62:375.
48. Wagman IH, de Jong RH, Prince DA: Effects of lidocaine on the central nervous system. Anesthesiology 1967; 28:155.
49. de Jong RH, Wagman IH, Prince DA: Effect of carbon dioxide on the cortical seizure threshold to lidocaine. Exp Neurol 1967; 17:221.
50. Ausinsch B, Malagodi MN, Munson ES: Diazepam in the prophylaxis of lignocaine seizures. Br J Anaesth 1976; 48:309.
51. de Jong RH, Heavner JE: Local anesthetic seizure prevention: diazepam vs. pentobarbital. Anesthesiology 1972; 36:449.
52. Feinstein MB, Lenard W, Mathias J: The antagonism of local anesthetic induced convulsions by the benzodiazepine derivative diazepam. Arch Int Pharmacodyn Ther 1970; 187:144.
53. de Jong RH, Heavner JE, de Oliveira LF: Effects of nitrous oxide on the lidocaine seizure threshold and diazepam protection. Anesthesiology 1972; 37:299.
54. Gibbs CP, Noel SC: Response of arterial segments from gravid human uterus to multiple concentrations of lignocaine. Br J Anaesth 1977; 49:409.
55. Johns RA, DiFazio CA, Longnecker DE: Lidocaine constricts or dilates rate arterioles in a dose-dependent manner. Anesthesiology 1985; 62:141.
56. Johns RA, Seyde WC, DeFazio CA, et al: Dose-dependent effects of bupivacaine on rat muscle arterioles. Anesthesiology 1986; 65:186.
57. Fleisch JH, Titus E: Effect of local anesthetics on pharmacologic receptor systems of smooth muscle. J Pharmacol Exp Ther 1973; 186:44.
58. Klein SW, Sutherland RI, Morch JE: Hemodynamic effects of intravenous lidocaine in man. Can Med Assoc J 1968; 99:472.
59. Block A, Covino B: Effect of local agents on cardiac conduction and contractility. Reg Anaesth 1981; 6:55.
60. de Jong RH, Ronfeld RA, DeRosa R: Cardiovascular effects of convulsant

and supraconvulsant doses of amide local anesthetics. Anesth Analg 1982; 61:3.

61. Kotelko DM, Shnider SM, Dailey PA, et al: Bupivacaine-induced cardiac arrhythmias in sheep. Anesthesiology 1984; 60:10.

62. Clarkson CW, Hondeghem LM: Mechanism for bupivacaine depression of cardiac conduction: fast block of sodium channels during the action potential with slow recovery from block during diastole. Anesthesiology 1985; 62:396.

63. Thomas RD, Behbehani MM, Coyle DE, et al: Cardiovascular toxicity of local anesthetics: an alternative hypothesis. Anesth Analg 1986; 65:444.

64. Heavner JE: Cardiac dysrhythmias induced by infusion of local anesthetics into the lateral cerebral ventricle of cats. Anesth Analg 1986; 65:133.

65. Munson ES, Tucker WK, Ausinsch B, et al: Etidocaine, bupivacaine, and lidocaine seizure thresholds in monkeys. Anesthesiology 1975; 42:471.

66. Moore DC, Crawford RD, Scurlock JE: Severe hypoxia and acidosis following local anesthetic-induced convulsions. Anesthesiology 1980; 53:259.

67. Morishima HO, Covino BG: Toxicity and distribution of lidocaine in nonasphyxiated and asphyxiated baboon fetuses. Anesthesiology 1981; 54:182.

68. Moore DC, Bridenbaugh LD: Oxygen: the antidote for systemic toxic reactions from local anesthetic drugs. JAMA 1960; 174:842.

69. Kendig JJ: Clinical implications of the modulated receptor hypothesis: local anesthetics and the heart. Anesthesiology 1985; 62:382.

70. Kasten GW, Martin ST: Bupivacaine cardiovascular toxicity: comparison of treatment with bretylium and lidocaine. Anesth Analg 1985; 64:911.

71. Kasten GW, Martin ST: Comparison of resuscitation of sheep and dogs after bupivacaine-induced cardiovascular collapse. Anesth Analg 1986; 65:1029.

72. Kunkle EC, Ray BS, Wolf HG: Experimental studies on headaches: analysis of the headache associated with changes in intracranial pressure. Neurol Psychiatr 1943; 49:323.

73. Vandam LD, Dripps RD: A long-term follow-up of patients who received 10,098 spinal anesthetics. II: incidence and analyses of minor sensory neurologic defects. Surgery 1955; 38:463.

74. Jones RJ: The role of recumbency in the prevention and treatment of postspinal headache. Anesth Analg 1974; 53:788.

75. Driessen A, Mauer W, Fricke M, et al: Prospective studies of the postspinal headache. Reg Anaesth 1980; 3:38.

76. Kortum K, Nolte H, Kenkmann HJ: Beschwerden nach Spinalanaesthesie. Sex difference related complication rates after spinal anesthesia. Reg Anaesth 1982; 5:1.

77. Gielen M: Postdural puncture headaches: a review. Reg Anaesth 1989; 14:101.

78. Thornberry EA, Thomas TA: Posture and post-spinal headache: a controlled trial in 80 obstetric patients. Br J Anaesth 1988; 60:195.

79. Mulroy MF: Spinal headaches: management and avoidance. Probl Anesth 1987; 1:602.

80. Ready LB, Culpin S, Haschke RH, et al: Spinal needle determinants of rate of transdural fluid leak. Anesth Analg 1989; 69:457.

81. Denny N, Masters R, Pearson D, et al: Postdural puncture headache after continuous spinal anesthesia. Anesth Analg 1987; 66:791.

82. Peterson DO, Borup JL, Chestnut JS: Continuous spinal anesthesia. Case review and discussion. Reg Anaesth 1983; 8:109.

83. Kallos T, Smith TC: Continuous spinal anesthesia with hypobaric tetracaine for hip surgery in lateral decubitus. Anesth Analg 1972; 51:766.

84. Sechzer PH, Abel L: Post spinal anesthesia headache treated with caffeine. Curr Ther Res 1978; 24:307.

32

Vascular Access

CHRISTINE A. CZEPIZAK, M.S., P.A.-C.

JAMES M. O'CALLAGHAN, P.A.-C., B.M.Sc.

BAHMAN VENUS, M.D., F.C.C.M., F.C.C.P.

NIKOLAUS GRAVENSTEIN, M.D.

In 1952, Aubaniac described modern percutaneous central venous cannulation.[1] Since then, many new insertion techniques have been developed, and major technologic advances have been made in the equipment used for cannulation.[2–8] Despite these advances, controversies regarding vascular catheterization remain in most areas. Current standard practices for peripheral and central venous cannulation are reviewed in this chapter. Included are recommendations and modifications of some procedures under certain clinical situations.

EQUIPMENT

What Is Necessary?

Peripheral Catheterization

For peripheral catheterization, the smallest-gauge catheter that is appropriate for the clinical situation should be used. Choices include stainless steel/butterfly needles and plastic over-the-needle catheters. They are typically 2 inches or less in length. The Centers for Disease Control (CDC) recommend that stainless steel cannulas be used for peripheral access to reduce the incidence of phlebitis.[9] If plastic catheters are used for cannulation, the CDC recommends replacement every 48 to 72 hours. The National Intravenous Therapy Association (NITA) recommends steel catheters for single or short-term use and plastic catheters for long-term access.[10] Recommendations suggest replacement every 48 to 72 hours to reduce the incidence of infection. Steel catheters have not gained acceptance for routine use during anesthesia out of concern for mechanical vessel trauma and associated loss of venous access, as well as the potential for infiltration/extravasation.

Refer to Table 32–1 for additional necessary equipment. Most is contained in commercial kits manufactured by many different companies. Wearing gloves has become standard for all invasive procedures as part of universal precautions, even for insertion of a peripheral intravenous catheter.[9] In addition,

a 3-mL syringe attached to a Luer-Lok T-connector filled with bacteriostatic normal saline solution is recommended to assist with withdrawal of blood, flushing, and intravenous tube changes in children.[11]

For arterial catheter flush solutions, heparin and bacteriostatic normal saline should be available. No standardization for the type of flush solution or volume necessary to maintain access has yet been determined. Multicenter studies are currently under way to establish such recommendations.[12]

Central Venous Catheterization

Equipment for central venous cannulation is usually available in sterile prepackaged kits. Time and cost reduction for setup are two advantages of these kits. They vary depending on the type of central access required. Most include an 18-gauge thin-walled needle or a 16-gauge catheter over a 20-gauge needle, a 0.89-mm (0.036-inch) diameter J-wire, and a single- or multilumen central venous catheter. Table 32–2 lists the recommended equipment. Masks, caps, and sterile gowns should be donned. Although their effectiveness in reducing infection has not been proved, they decrease the chance of

TABLE 32–1. Peripheral Intravenous Equipment Set

Povidone-iodine, 70% isopropyl alcohol swabs, or chlorhexidine
Two intravenous cannulas
Tourniquet
Sterile or nonsterile gloves
Tape
Sterile 2×2-cm or 4×4-cm gauze
Flush or intravenous set
0.5 to 1 mL of 1% or 2% lidocaine without epinephrine as local anesthetic, or appropriate alternative syringe with 23-gauge or smaller needle

Optional equipment
Infusion cap
Antimicrobial ointment

TABLE 32–2. Central Venous Catheterization Equipment

Central venous catheter
Povidone-iodine or chlorhexidine and applicator
Mask with sterile gown and sterile gloves
Sterile drapes and several 4 × 4 gauze pads
5-mL syringe with 1.5-inch 21- or 23-gauge locator needle (for use with IJV cannulation)
Guidewire 10 cm longer than the cannula to be inserted
Scalpel
Vessel dilator
Heparinized saline for catheter flush
2-0 or 3-0 silk suture on cutting needle
Needle holder (sterile) if curved needle is used
Sterile dressing

Optional equipment
Sterile pencil probe Doppler and gel
Sterile tubing for manometry

---

accidental contamination of the equipment during the procedure.

Arterial Cannulation

Arterial catheterization can be performed with much the same equipment used for peripheral venous access. These and additional items are listed in Table 32–3. For distal extremities, 1.25- to 1.5-inch 20-gauge Teflon catheters over 18-gauge or smaller needles are usually used. Some are available with a built-in guidewire or simply an intracatheter. If an intracatheter is used, addition of a 15-cm length of extension tubing filled with heparinized saline, a three-way stopcock, and a 10-mL syringe containing heparinized saline are recommended.[13] Attachment of this setup to the intracatheter before catheterization probably reduces the risk of contamination from blood for the operator and other personnel.

For femoral artery catheterization, a 0.35-mm guidewire fed through an 18-gauge cannulating needle may be used. The catheter should be 3.75 to 4.5 inches long, depending on the patient's body size. Larger cannulas are used for procedures such as cardiac catheterization but are not recommended for routine monitoring. In children, particularly infants, the use of a Doppler pulse monitor on the dorsalis pedis artery may assist with cannula passage and guide arterial compression for hemostasis.[14]

Pulmonary Artery Catheterization

Equipment for pulmonary artery catheterization is similar to that used for central venous catheter placement, in addition to an introducer sheath and pulmonary artery catheter. Special introducers made from polyurethane or polyethylene have been developed for easier passage of the Swan-Ganz catheter and are available with a side port that can be used as an additional infusion site. Pulmonary artery catheters are made from polyvinylchloride, which softens somewhat at body temperature. They are available in sizes ranging from 5 to 8 French and are approximately 110 cm long. A sterile plastic sleeve to protect the external portion of the catheter is available in the introducer kits. An additional pressure transducer and monitoring system are also needed.[15, 16]

PREPARATION

What Steps Are Necessary?

Informed Consent

In a nonurgent situation, written consent should be obtained from the patient or from the legal guardian or next of kin if a patient is unable to consent. The discussion must include the potential benefits, risks, and alternatives. If access is urgent, consent is unnecessary and only serves to delay treatment. Informed consent is not required for peripheral venous cannulation.

After consent is obtained, gather the essential equipment before beginning the procedure to avoid delay. Answer any questions the patient may have, and determine if the patient has had adverse reactions to any medication or skin preparation that you plan to use. Place the patient in a supine position. If the patient is nervous or uncomfortable, a sedative or narcotic may be administered.

Positioning

Once a venous site is selected, positioning a patient is the key to success. For clavicular or jugular approaches, modified Trendelenburg's position is recommended unless contraindicated by elevated intracranial pressure or cardiorespiratory insufficiency. Ventilation and oxygenation must be monitored at all times during the procedure. Historically, a patient's head has been turned to the contralateral side for the internal jugular vein (IJV) approach, and the shoulders retracted by placing a towel roll vertically between the scapula when the subclavian vein (SCV) approach is attempted.

These recommendations should be reconsidered in view of data that show that rotation of the head moves the IJV on top of the carotid artery, predisposing it to incidental puncture and the attendant complications during IJV cannulation[17] (Table 32–4). Thus, the current recommendation is to leave the head in as neutral a position as possible. Leaving a patient's head

---

TABLE 32–3. Arterial Catheterization Equipment

Antiseptic preparation solution: povidone-iodine, 70% isopropyl alcohol, or chlorhexidine
Sterile or nonsterile gloves
1% or 2% xylocaine without epinephrine or alternative for local anesthesia
20-gauge catheter over 22-gauge needle or smaller (with or without guidewire) for peripheral artery
18-gauge thin-walled needle for femoral artery
3.125- or 4.75-inch 20-gauge catheter for femoral artery
0.021-mm guidewire
5-mL syringe
Heparin-flushed tubing, transducer, flushing system, and pressure monitor
2-0 or 3-0 silk suture on cutting needle if femoral artery is cannulated
Needle holder (sterile) if curved needle is used
Sterile dressing

Recommended
Sterile drapes and several 4 × 4 gauze pads
Arm board
Towel roll
Tape
15-cm flushed extension tubing with three-way stopcock and 10-mL syringe containing heparinized saline
Pencil probe Doppler monitor for dorsalis pedis artery in children

TABLE 32–4. Per Cent Overlap of the Carotid Artery by the Internal Jugular Vein As Shown by Ultrasound with Different Degrees of Head Rotation

Side of Neck	0°	40°	80°
Right	1.5 ± 0.8	6.5 ± 2.8	27.5 ± 7.4*
	0 to 17.4	0 to 48	0 to 100
Left	5.2 ± 2.9	11.5 ± 4.9	44.7 ± 7.2*
	0 to 54	0 to 76.5	0 to 100

(Modified from Sulek CA, Weiss L, Gravenstein N, et al: Influence of head position on relationship between internal jugular vein and carotid artery. Crit Care Med 1993; 21:A218.)
*$P < .05$ compared with 0% and 40% on the same side of the neck.

in a neutral position is also ideal for subclavian catheterization when turning a patient's head away from the side of catheterization reduces the acute angle between the internal jugular and subclavian veins, thereby predisposing the catheter to going into the neck as opposed to the superior vena cava.

As a corollary, turning the head also makes it easier for an internal jugular catheter to end up in the subclavian vein.[18] In point of fact, turning a patient's head toward the side of catheterization during subclavian catheterization makes passage of the catheter into the neck least likely. Use of a shoulder roll is similarly counterproductive in that it actually decreases the dimension of the SCV by compressing it between the clavicle and the first rib.[18]

Operator preparation is also essential. Adequate lighting should be available, and all possible obstructions removed. For supraclavicular approaches, we suggest that the operator be positioned at the head of the bed on the side of the procedure. For infraclavicular approaches, the operator should be positioned lateral to the patient's shoulder on the side of the cannulation site. A qualified assistant with training and experience should be in attendance.

Skin Preparation

If excessive hair is present over the insertion site, its removal should be considered. The hair should be clipped with sterile scissors or removed chemically. Shaving with a razor blade is easiest but not recommended because it increases the risk of skin irritation and infection.[19] The insertion site must be scrubbed with appropriate antimicrobial solution. Choices include povidone-iodine, chlorohexidine 0.5% in 70% isopropyl alcohol, 70% alcohol, and tincture of iodine. Chlorohexidine or 70% isopropyl alcohol is an acceptable alternative for those patients allergic to iodine.

Whichever solution is used, standard surgical protocol must be followed. Operators must wash their hands with an antimicrobial soap before sterilizing the skin. From the intended site of insertion, scrub in a continuous circular motion outward to cover a margin approximately 5 cm peripheral to the area of fenestration in the drapes used. This approach allows coverage over the external jugular vein (EJV), IJV, and SCV sites. Scrub the area twice and wait for the solution to dry for bactericidal action to be complete. Final preparation may be completed at this time.

Local Anesthetics

For central cannulation, infiltration of the skin and catheter path with a local anesthetic is advisable for conscious patients. One percent or 2% lidocaine without epinephrine is most commonly used. With a 25-gauge needle, make a 1-cm skin wheal at the site of insertion. Change to a 1.5-inch 22-gauge needle and inject subsequent 0.2-mL boluses after advancing the needle in 2-mm increments. Aspirate the plunger before injecting to exclude free-flowing blood, and inject slowly to minimize burning and pain from tissue distention in sensitive patients. Between 2 and 4 mL is usually adequate for analgesia. When infiltrating for IJV cannulation, it is possible to anesthetize the ipsilateral phrenic nerve if large volumes and deep infiltration are used.

Mepivacaine and bupivacaine are other local anesthetic options but are longer acting and probably unnecessary. For those rare individuals who are allegedly allergic to the amide local anesthetics just listed, alternatives are the aminobenzoate esters, procaine and tetracaine. Diphenhydramine (Benadryl) can also be used for patients with previous adverse reactions to local anesthetics. A local anesthetic may not be required for small-gauge peripheral cannulation unless multiple attempts are anticipated. Regardless of one's personal philosophy, patients appreciate being given the option to choose whether or not a local anesthetic is used.

Sedation

Uncooperative, delirious, or anxious patients may require sedation for their protection. Sedatives and narcotics are used to reduce complications; however, they all have potentially lethal adverse effects. These agents must not be used without experience and careful monitoring.

For delirium and psychotic agitation, droperidol, $0.1 \text{ mg} \cdot \text{kg}^{-1}$ can be administered intravenously and repeated in 5 to 10 minutes until the desired effect is achieved. Haloperidol is another available neuroleptic agent, but its onset of action is slower and titration is more difficult. In hypotensive patients with severe agitation, ketamine, 1 to $3 \text{ mg} \cdot \text{kg}^{-1}$ can be substituted. Midazolam, a short-acting benzodiazepine, is favored for patients with substantial anxiety. Doses of 0.5 to 2.5 mg intravenously over a 2-minute period are recommended; they can be repeated every 2 minutes up to 5 mg total. Narcotics like morphine (2-mg boluses) or fentanyl (50–100 µg boluses) can also be effective.

Patients must be continuously monitored for potentially adverse reactions. Ventilation and oxygenation should also be closely observed. Reduced doses are highly recommended for unstable patients and the elderly. To reverse oversedation from benzodiazapines, flumazenil, a competitive benzodiazepine antagonist, is given in an initial dose of 0.2 mg intravenously and is repeated every minute until sedation is reversed. Naloxone in 40-µg increments can be titrated to effectively antagonize oversedation from narcotics. In general, if the procedure is supplemented with sedatives, it is preferable to sedate patients with either benzodiazepines or narcotics because specific pharmacologic antagonists are available.

VENOUS CATHETERIZATION

What Factors Should Be Considered When Choosing a Site?

Peripheral Placement

A peripheral vein is usually the first choice for intravenous infusion. In emergency situations, any vein available may be used for resuscitation. During cardiorespiratory arrest, central placement is preferable, because resuscitative drugs are more effective when administered directly into the central circulation.[20] In nonemergent cases, central venous access may be necessary for diagnostic or therapeutic purposes or if peripheral sites are inadequate. Table 32–5 summarizes the indications for central catheter placement.[21]

Factors of concern in peripheral placement include the condition of available veins and skin sites and the types and duration of intravenous therapy. Alert patients can often recommend the best site based on their prior experience. Catheterization of arm veins is safer than head, neck, or leg veins and should be attempted first. If possible, the nondominant arm should be used. The veins of the antecubital fossa should ideally be reserved for venipuncture and used for intravenous access only in emergencies or when other sites cannot be identified or cannulated.

Central Placement

Table 32–6 summarizes the advantages and disadvantages of various central insertion sites.[21] The clinical situation often determines the site to be used. Supraclavicular sites interfere less with cardiopulmonary resuscitation (CPR) than infraclavicular or jugular sites. A long (30-cm) femoral line inserted so that its tip lies above the diaphragm is an acceptable alternative.

Patients with short or edematous necks or with tracheotomy appliances in place may not be suitable candidates for IJV catheters because the landmarks are obscured and tracheal secretions increase contamination and risk of infection. Subclavian or femoral sites are generally preferred in these patients.

Patients who have a chest tube in place and who need a central venous catheter should have a site chosen on the same side as the chest tube if possible in order to reduce the risk of iatrogenic pneumothorax. Those with severe unilateral lung disease should be catheterized on the ipsilateral side. A pneumothorax on the nonaffected side severely compromises the already marginal pulmonary status.

Subclavian sites are best avoided in patients with chronic obstructive lung disease or in those receiving high-level positive end-expiratory pressure. These patients are at high risk for pneumothorax, because the cupulae of the pleural cavities are often higher than normal. An external jugular vein, if prominent, would be the first choice in this group. It is also the first site choice in patients with a bleeding diathesis. However, a series of 1000 patients who had documented coagulopathy and underwent IJV catheterization showed that this is also a safe approach in this setting. The only significant complication

TABLE 32–5. Common Indications for Central Venous Cannulation

---

Hemodynamic evaluation and management (e.g., central venous pressure monitoring or pulmonary artery Swan-Ganz catheterization)
The need for multiple concomitant intravenous lines
Infusion of thrombogenic material (e.g., potassium, calcium chloride, hyperalimentation solutions)
Inability to cannulate peripheral veins
Immediate or potentially massive fluid resuscitation
Diagnostic techniques (e.g., cardiac catheterization, endomyocardial biopsy)
Emergency transvenous pacing
Treatment of air embolism (e.g., sitting craniotomy)
Temporary venous access (e.g., hemodialysis, plasmapheresis)

(From Novak RA, Venus B: Clavicular approaches for central vein cannulation. Prob Crit Care 1988; 2:248.)

encountered in this series was a large thyroid venous hematoma in a patient with a large goiter despite a 7% incidence of accidental carotid artery puncture in the series.[22] The subclavian sites are avoided in this circumstance because compression is impossible if the subclavian artery is inadvertently punctured. Table 32–7 lists central venous insertion sites in a proposed order of preference for common clinical situations.[21]

ARTERIAL CATHETER PLACEMENT

What Are the Indications?

Indications and contraindications for arterial catheterization are summarized in Table 32–8. Direct monitoring of arterial pressure is often necessary in critically ill or hemodynamically unstable patients or in patients with severe hypertension. Patients requiring frequent arterial blood gas analysis or frequent blood analysis benefit from an arterial catheter as well. In patients undergoing a procedure with cardiopulmonary bypass, an arterial catheter is the only way available to monitor blood pressure because automated noninvasive methods all require pulsatile flow.

Advantages and disadvantages of common arterial catheter sites are listed in Table 32–9.[23] Radial and femoral sites are most commonly chosen because of their relatively easy access and generally good collateral flow. Allen's test is commonly used to assess collateral arterial flow. To perform the test, compress the radial and ulnar arteries as a patient opens and closes his or her hand. Once the hand is blanched, the ulnar artery is released, and the time it takes for the blush to reappear is measured. Normally, the blush should reappear in <7 seconds. Seven to 15 seconds is considered borderline, and >15 seconds is considered to reflect an absence of adequate collateral flow via the ulnar artery.

The reliability of this test as a predictor of good collateral flow is questionable, because neither the presence nor the absence of a normal Allen's test response reliably predicts absence or occurrence, respectively, of thrombotic complications.[24] Nevertheless, it remains common practice to perform the test; if significant interarm discrepancy is noted, cannulate preferentially the wrist with the more normal Allen's test response.

PULMONARY ARTERY CATHETERIZATION

What Are the Indications?

Indications for pulmonary artery cannulation are outlined in Table 32–10. The catheter is designed to give information useful in assessing cardiac function. In addition, some catheters allow continuous mixed venous oxygen saturation monitoring, atrial or ventricular pacing, calculation of right ventricular volumes and ejection fractions, or continuous cardiac output determination. Pulmonary artery catheterization and monitoring is recommended whenever a patient's status cannot be determined adequately by clinical means and by central venous pressure monitoring or when deterioration occurs despite treatment and intervention.

TABLE 32–6. Advantages and Disadvantages of Various Central Vein Approaches

Approach	Advantages	Disadvantages
External jugular vein	Part of surface anatomy Clotting abnormalities not prohibitive Pneumothorax avoided Head-of-table access Prominent in elderly	High failure rate Not ideal for prolonged central venous access Dressing and maintenance are difficult Poor landmarks in obese patients Unsuccessful in young patients Difficult approach for threading central catheters
Internal jugular vein	Pneumothorax rare High success rate Head-of-table access (general anesthesia) Control of bleeding is easier Right internal jugular straight path to superior vena cava (easier to pass catheters, less malposition) Continued chest compression during CPR is possible Less failure with inexperienced operator	Not ideal for prolonged central venous access (e.g., total parenteral nutrition) Uncomfortable Dressing and catheter difficult to maintain Left internal jugular increases risk of thoracic duct injury Poor landmarks in obese or edematous patients Difficult access with tracheostomies Contraindicated with intracranial hypertension Vein more prone to collapse with volume depletion or shock Not ideal for temporary hemodialysis Difficult access during emergencies when airway control is being established Carotid artery puncture incidence is relatively frequent (4%)
Supraclavicular	Low incidence of pneumothorax High success rate Easier to pass catheters Head-of-table access Good landmarks No interference with CPR Anatomic landmarks constant Short path from skin to vein	Control of bleeding is difficult Pneumothorax possible Not ideal for prolonged venous access More uncomfortable Dressing and catheter maintenance difficult Thoracic duct puncture possible Not ideal for temporary hemodialysis
Infraclavicular	Easier to maintain dressing and more comfortable for patients Better landmarks in obesity Large vein does not collapse during volume depletion or shock Better access when airway control is being established simultaneously Multiple catheter insertions easier when massive volume resuscitation needed Femoral pulse just lateral is constant landmark	Higher risk of pneumothorax Compression of bleeding site difficult Decreased success rate with inexperience Long distance from skin to vein Catheter malposition common Relatively inaccessible from head of table Interference with chest compressions during CPR
Femoral	Fast, easy access; high success rate Does not interfere with chest compressions Does not interfere with airway management No risk of pneumothorax Supine or head-down position not necessary during insertion	Delayed circulation of drugs during CPR Higher risk of complications in patients with abdominal pathology Prevents patient mobilization Arteriovenous fistula possible Difficult to keep the site sterile Greater difficulty with Swan-Ganz catheter flotation

(Modified from Novak RA, Venus B: Clavicular approaches for central vein cannulation. Probl Crit Care 1988; 2:249–250.)
Abbreviation: CPR = cardiopulmonary resuscitation.

TECHNIQUES OF PERIPHERAL VENOUS CATHETERIZATION

How Is Venous Distention Obtained?

The most commonly used method for venous distention is application of a tourniquet or blood pressure cuff proximal to the intended cannulation site. Other useful distention methods include placing the limb in the dependent position, milking the vein from proximal to distal, lightly tapping the vein, and applying moist heat or a thin film of nitroglycerin ointment.

When distention by these methods is inadequate, a very small-bore catheter may be placed and used to infuse fluid to effect venous distention or a larger catheter may be inserted via a guidewire exchange technique.

How Is the Catheter Inserted?

After the necessary equipment has been assembled, gloves are donned, the limb is positioned, the intended vein is dis-tended by one of the previously mentioned methods, and the site cleansed. Local anesthetic is infiltrated, and the vein is stabilized by applying distal traction.

The needle is inserted at a 30° to 45° angle to the skin with the bevel up. Of note is that it is probably counterproductive first to loosen the catheter from the needle stylet. This is because the manufacturer goes to considerable effort to build a smooth transition between catheter and stylet. Loosening the catheter defeats this and makes threading more difficult. Entry may be from the side or directly over the vein. Once blood return is noted, the needle is advanced slightly so the bevel is completely within the vessel. Thus, large-bore needles need to be advanced farther into the vein than smaller ones. The needle is then brought down parallel to the skin, and the catheter is rotated and advanced off the needle. After satisfactory placement, the tourniquet (if used) is released. The catheter is flushed, or an intravenous infusion tubing is attached, and the site is dressed. If swelling occurs around the intravenous site, the catheter must be removed and a new site chosen.

TABLE 32–7. Preferred Techniques for Specific Clinical Situations

Clinical Situation	Choices (Order of Preference)				
	1st	*2nd*	*3rd*	*4th*	*5th*
Bleeding diathesis	EJ	Femoral* Peripheral large-vein cannulation	IJ†	High clavicular notch‡	SC
Obesity or edema	SC	IC	IJ	Femoral	EJ
Decreased pulmonary reserve; hyperinflation or positive end-expiratory pressure	EJ	IJ†	Femoral	SC	IC
Parenteral nutrition	IC	SC	IJ	EJ	Short-term femoral
Hypovolemia; shock	IC or SC	Femoral	IJ	Peripheral large-vein cannulation	EJ
Cardiopulmonary resuscitation	IJ	SC	EJ	IC	Femoral
Emergency airway management§	Femoral	IC	SC	IJ	EJ
Temporary hemodialysis	IC	Femoral	IJ	SC	EJ
Multiple catheter insertion	IC	SC	IC or SC	IC or IJ	SC or IJ
Swan-Ganz catheter insertion	IC or RIJ	SC or IJ	IJ	EJ	Femoral
Temporary pacemaker‖	RIJ	RSC	LIC	EJ	Femoral
Tracheotomy or sternal wounds	EJ	IJ	Femoral	SC	IC
Short diagnostic techniques	IJ/femoral	SC	IC	—	—
Inability to lower head	Femoral	EJ	SC	IC	—

(Modified from Novak RA, Venus B: Clavicular approaches for central vein cannulation. Probl Crit Care 1988; 2:249–250.)

*Femoral approach is most useful for emergency large-vein access for volume resuscitation and rarely used for hemodynamic monitoring or temporary pacing.

†Higher (i.e., nearer the cricoid than the clavicle) IJ approaches recommended.

‡High clavicular notch refers to skin puncture 1–2 cm above clavicle, thereby allowing easier tamponade for arterial bleeding. The skin puncture site is close to that in the central IJ technique.

§Situations where airway is unstable and control is highest priority. Simultaneous large-vein access is next to highest priority; however, interference with airway control is contraindicated.

‖Order of vein preference would be the same as for Swan-Ganz catheterization if balloon-tipped Swan or Paceport Swan is used. The semi-rigid pacing catheter using fluoroscopy increases the preferability of the femoral approach. If SC or IJ is used, the preferred site is the right side.

Abbreviations: EJ = external jugular; IJ = internal jugular; SC = supraclavicular; IC = infraclavicular; R = right; L = left when one is preferred.

INTRAOSSEOUS ACCESS

For intraosseous access, a sturdy needle is required for successful penetration. In infants and children, the needle is placed into the medial tibia just below the tibial tubercle below the epiphysis, whereas in adults either the tibial site or the medial malleolus is used. In neonates and young infants, a standard 16- to 19-gauge short-bevel spinal or hypodermic needle may be used.[23] In older children and adults, a 13-gauge bone marrow needle with a stylet is required. Using sterile technique, the operator inserts the needle perpendicular to the bone and advances it using firm rotary pressure until loss of resistance is noted. At this point, the stylet is removed and a syringe attached to aspirate blood and marrow. An intravenous tubing is then attached, and the site dressed. A preassembled intraosseous infusion set (Sur-Fast, Cook Critical Care, Bloomington, IN) has been introduced.[25] It overcomes some of the difficulties of hypodermic needle aspiration (Fig. 32–1).

ARTERIAL CATHETERIZATION TECHNIQUES

How Is the Radial Artery Approached?

To cannulate the radial artery selected, the wrist is gently hyperextended 30° to 60° and the hand supinated. Rolled gauze

TABLE 32–8. Indications and Contraindications for Arterial Catheterization

Indications	Contraindications
Direct arterial pressure measurement	Local infection or injury
Access for repeated blood sampling	Presence of an arterial graft
Hemodynamic instability	Inadequate collateral flow
Cardiopulmonary bypass	

or a washcloth can be placed beneath the wrist, and the arm immobilized by taping the hand and forearm to an arm board. After gloves have been donned, the radial area is then cleansed and anesthetized using a small-gauge needle. Lidocaine serves two purposes by decreasing patients' discomfort and reducing arterial vasospasm.[26] If the pulse is lost while the local anesthetic is injected, massaging the wheal should restore it. The catheter device may be flushed with heparinized saline before use to reduce clotting during placement.

It is helpful to palpate the artery with two fingers alongside and not over the pulse to fix it in place and to help the operator visualize the path of the vessel. The needle is introduced, bevel up, through the skin at a 15° to 30° angle and advanced toward the palpated pulse until blood return is noted. Once again, the needle is advanced sufficiently so that the entire bevel is within the vessel. If threading is unsuccessful, the technique may be changed to one of transfixation, in which the needle and catheter are passed through both walls of the artery, after which the needle is completely withdrawn. The catheter is then slowly withdrawn until pulsatile blood flow is observed. Then the needle is gently reinserted three quarters of its length to act as a stylet. The catheter can then usually be easily advanced. The catheter is advanced with a rotating (spinning) motion as the needle is held still. Inconsistent blood return may be resolved by rotating the bevel of the needle 90° or more to exclude partial occlusion by an intimal flap.

Liquid Stylet

Alternatively, the radial artery can be cannulated using a liquid stylet. The catheter over the needle is advanced through the far side of the artery. A syringe filled with heparinized saline is attached, and the needle and catheter withdrawn until blood return is noted. The needle is removed, and the catheter

TABLE 32–9. Peripheral Arterial Cannulation Sites: Advantages and Disadvantages

Site	Advantages	Disadvantages
Radial	Highly accessible Easily visible No adjacent nerve	Relatively high complication rate High degree of disability if complication occurs
Femoral	Relatively low complication rate Longer catheter function More accurate readings High cannulation success rate	Decreased mobilization of patient Possibly higher contamination rate Occult bleeding
Axillary	Low complication rate Longer catheter function More accurate readings	Low accessibility and visibility High degree of disability if complication occurs Adjacent nerves Occult bleeding
Dorsalis pedis	Easily visible Highly accessible	Congenital absence in >12% of population High rate of cannulation failure Decreased mobilization of patient
Temporal	Low thrombotic complication rate A preductal site	Difficult cannulation Short catheter function Risk of cerebral embolization
Brachial	Highly accessible	Inadequate collateral circulation High degree of disability if complication occurs Adjacent median nerve Not recommended by most authors

(Modified from Venus B, Mallory DL: Vascular cannulation. *In* Critical Care. Civetta JM, Taylor RW, Kirby RR (eds). Philadelphia, JB Lippincott, 1988, p 165.)

advanced while the heparinized saline solution is gently flushed.[27]

Guidewire Technique

Some catheters have a guidewire that is advanced through the needle into the artery, after which the catheter is threaded. This is an especially useful approach when other techniques have failed.

Pressure Monitoring

Another technique for cannulating difficult radial arteries uses the pressure-monitoring system while the catheter is placed. The system is connected directly to the catheter-over-needle. As the needle enters the arterial lumen, an arterial pressure curve is displayed on the screen. The catheter is advanced while observing the screen. Once it is in place, the needle is removed and the tubing to the monitor is reconnected to the catheter, which is then secured, and the site dressed.[28]

TABLE 32–10. Indications for Pulmonary Artery Cannulation

Cardiovascular	Complicated cardiac surgery Dissecting abdominal aneurysm Thoracic aorta aneurysmectomy Emergency or extensive surgery Cardiogenic shock
Respiratory	Pneumonectomy Acute pulmonary edema Acute lung injury Complicated mechanical ventilation
Miscellaneous	Severe burns Multiple trauma Septic shock Research Preoperative optimization (e.g., pheochromocytoma)

(Modified from Venus B, Mallory DL: Vascular cannulation. *In* Critical Care. Civetta JM, Taylor RW, Kirby RR (eds). Philadelphia, JB Lippincott, 1988, p 164.)

How Is the Femoral Artery Approached?

To cannulate the femoral artery, the leg is extended and slightly abducted. Folded towels are placed under the ipsilateral hip of obese individuals to help elevate the inguinal area. Large abdominal folds may be taped out of the working field, or a helper may hold them away from the inguinal area. Once the leg is positioned, the inguinal region is cleansed. Clipping the hair is optional. Local anesthesia is infiltrated using a small-gauge skin needle. In obese individuals, a longer 1.5-inch 22-gauge needle may be necessary.

The artery is palpated 0.3 to 1.5 cm below the inguinal fold, and the needle advanced toward the pulse at a nearly perpendicular 75° angle. Once pulsatile flow is obtained, the needle and syringe are lowered against the skin while maintaining blood flow. The syringe is removed, and a flexible guidewire is inserted through the needle into the vessel. If difficulty advancing the wire is encountered, the needle may be advanced 1 mm or rotated to free the bevel if it is covered by an intimal flap. The needle is withdrawn, and if necessary, the skin at the site of wire entry may be nicked to create a larger opening. A 5-cm or longer catheter is then advanced over the wire by rotating it in to its full length. The wire is removed, and the catheter connected to the monitoring equipment. In distinction to other arterial catheter sites, the femoral catheter is sutured in place and the site cleansed and dressed.

How Is the Dorsalis Pedis Artery Approached?

If the dorsalis pedis artery is chosen, the foot is positioned in plantar flexion. The pulse is located, and after the site is prepared, the artery is cannulated using the same technique as that used for radial artery catheterization, except that it is more common to use a 22-gauge catheter. After placement and confirmation of flow, the catheter is secured and the site dressed.

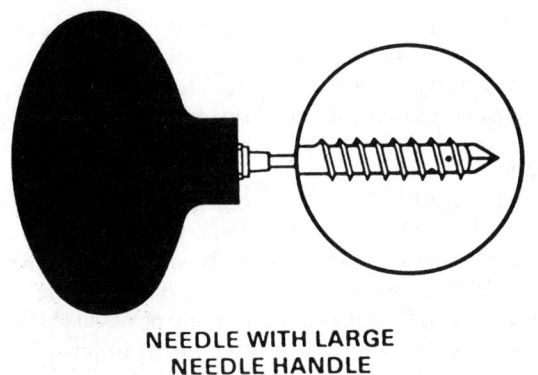

NEEDLE WITH LARGE
NEEDLE HANDLE

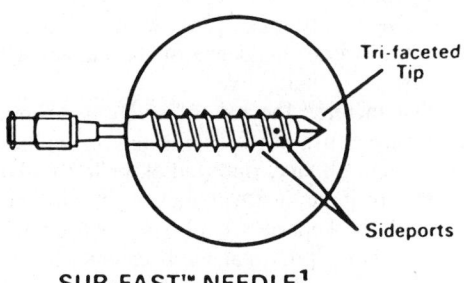

SUR-FAST™ NEEDLE[1]
Stainless Steel
12 gage 2.3 cm long

FIGURE 32–1. Sur-Fast intraosseous components. Removable handle permits controlled intraosseous placement and intravenous tubing attachment to a Luer connector. The threaded screw permits relatively atraumatic advancement through the cortex and provides stabilization. Sideports minimize the risk of obstruction and permit free flow of infused fluids. (Courtesy of Cook Catheter, Bloomington, IN.)

How Is the Axillary Artery Approached?

The left axillary artery is preferred over the right because the risk of inadvertent cerebral embolization is higher with right axillary artery catheterization. Any retrograde emboli that enter the adjacent central aortic circulation by way of the right axillary and subclavian artery traverse the aortic arch and the origins of the vertebral and carotid arteries, but those that enter via the left axillary and subclavian arteries do not.

The arm is extended and externally rotated. The elbow may be flexed, with the patient's head resting in his or her hand. The artery is located at its highest palpable point and entered at a 30° to 45° angle. Once adequate flow is confirmed, the catheter is connected to the monitoring system, secured, and dressed. Because it is difficult to immobilize this site, it is also advantageous to wire a longer (e.g., 5-cm) catheter and to suture it in place. Only small volumes of solution at very slow flush rates should be used, to lower the risk of cerebral embolization.

How Is the Brachial Artery Approached?

Brachial artery catheterization is generally avoided because of concern for inadequate collateral flow and an assumed increased risk of complications. If one chooses to use the brachial artery, the arm is positioned fully extended. The artery is palpated above the antecubital fossa medial to the bicipital tendon. In an adult, a 2-inch 20-gauge catheter-over-needle is inserted using the same technique as for the radial artery; a modified Seldinger's technique may also be used. Once the artery is cannulated, the arm must be splinted in the extended position.

What Factors Predispose to Complications?

Complications of arterial cannulation are summarized in Table 32–11. Factors predisposing to complications are summarized in Table 32–12. This section addresses the more common or serious complications.

Bleeding, Thrombosis, and Embolization

Risk of bleeding is increased in anticoagulated patients or after multiple puncture attempts. The risk of thrombosis is increased with large-gauge catheters and with a duration of catheterization >48 hours.[29] More catheterization attempts also increase the risk of thrombosis.[30]

Vessel size appears to affect the incidence of thrombosis.

TABLE 32–11. Complications of Peripheral Arterial Cannulation

Local ischemia, inflammation, or infection
Arterial spasm
Hematoma formation and infection
Bleeding from cannula disconnection
Thrombosis
Proximal or distal embolization
Limb ischemia and necrosis
Sepsis
Pseudoaneurysm
Arteriovenous fistula
Peripheral neuropathy

(Modified from Venus B, Mallory DL: Vascular cannulation. *In* Critical Care. Civetta JM, Taylor RW, Kirby RR (eds). Philadelphia, JB Lippincott, 1988, p 167.)

TABLE 32–12. Factors Increasing the Chance of Complications After Peripheral Arterial Cannulation

Low perfusion state
Use of vasopressors
Intrinsic vascular disease
Female gender
Cannula/vessel diameter ratio near unity
Tapered catheters
Catheter material (non-Teflon)
Long duration of cannulation
Repeated cannulation attempts
?Abnormal Allen's test results
Insertion by cutdown
Presence of bacteremia
Bleeding diathesis or hypercoaguable states
Use of dextrose solutions for flush systems
Flush system close to insertion site

(Modified from Venus B, Mallory DL: Vascular cannulation. *In* Critical Care. Civetta JM, Taylor RW, Kirby RR (eds). Philadelphia, JB Lippincott, 1988, p 167.)

Because the femoral and axillary arteries have a larger radius, thrombosis is relatively rare.[28] Continuous heparin flush systems reduce the overall incidence of thrombosis, whereas intermittent flushing is ineffective.[30]

Factors that increase the risk of cerebral embolization include small stature; use of (in decreasing order) the temporal, right axillary, left axillary, right radial, or left radial site; and rapid flush rate or large flush volumes.[26] The flush or irrigation flow rate should be kept at <1 mL $\cdot$ s^{-1} especially in infants or children or when a proximal site is cannulated.

Infection and Sepsis

Arterial catheter infection occurs infrequently as a complication of catheterization if the site is used <96 hours.[31] Guidewire exchange is a safe alternative if new sites are not available. Sepsis secondary to nosocomial bacteremia is an important but uncommon complication of arterial cannulation. It does not occur in the absence of catheter-related infection. Conversely, pre-existing bacteremia may not resolve until a colonized arterial catheter is removed.[32] Local inflammation as a predictive sign of catheter infection is not consistent.[33–35] Local inflammation may be the result of irritation by the dressing, topical antibiotics, or reaction to the catheter.

Skin flora are usually the source of catheter-related infections, although contaminated infusate and monitoring equipment are also significant sources.[26] Organisms isolated from arterial catheter infections are usually gram negative and include *Pseudomonas, Serratia, Enterobacter,* and *Flavobacterium. Candida* is occasionally isolated. Catheter-related infection causing delayed radial artery rupture has been described.[36] Such complications are infrequent but can lead to hemorrhage or pseudoaneurysm formation.[37]

TECHNIQUES OF CENTRAL VENOUS CATHETERIZATION

What Considerations Are Generally Applicable?

Strict aseptic technique must be used. The site is prepared as previously described. Hat, mask, sterile gloves, and gown are donned after hand washing. Patients, unless they have elevated intracranial pressure, are placed in a 15° to 30° Trendelenburg's position with the operator at the head of the bed for jugular, supraclavicular, or SCV approaches, or by a patient's side for infraclavicular SCV insertion. If the femoral site is chosen, a patient may be left flat or even in reverse Trendelenburg's position, with the operator to the patient's side. After the area is prepared and if the patient is awake, the site is anesthetized using a small-gauge needle.

For the IJV, we recommend a pencil probe Doppler or finder needle to locate the vessel and to avoid arterial puncture or minimize complications should inadvertent arterial puncture occur. If a Doppler probe is used, the strongest signal occurs when the probe is held in the plane of the intended needle path. The probe is then moved from side to side so that both artery and vein are identified, and the center of the vein is located. The needle is then advanced in a path designed to intersect the Doppler beam 2 cm below the skin. If a finder needle is used, blood return is confirmed with the finder needle, the angle and depth of the finder needle are carefully noted, and the needle is removed. A catheter-over-needle is then inserted using the same angle and depth at the exact site. Alternatively, the needle may be left in place with the syringe attached to prevent air embolism, and the catheter-over-needle advanced directly behind it at the same angle to the same depth.

Once free-flowing venous blood is obtained, the catheter-over-needle is advanced 2 to 3 mm with the needle in a plane parallel to the vein. The catheter is advanced into the vein, the needle/syringe apparatus is removed, and blood return is confirmed. The hub of the catheter should be occluded at all times, if the patient is breathing spontaneously, to prevent air embolism.

A J-tipped guidewire is then advanced (with the J-tip leading) to a maximal distance of 20 cm. The short catheter is removed, and a small skin cut is made at the lateral side of the guidewire entry site. The dilator should then be passed smoothly through the skin and the subcutaneous tissues. It should not be advanced farther than necessary to dilate the path to the vessel itself (i.e., 1–2 cm beyond the depth of the previous needle insertion). With skin traction held over the incision, the catheter is advanced over the guidewire, which is extracted until it may be grasped from the distal port. The catheter is then advanced to the desired length while the guidewire is held firmly.

After removal of the guidewire, blood return is confirmed from each port before flushing with heparinized saline. The ports should be flushed within 1 to 2 minutes of insertion to prevent catheter thrombosis. The catheter is held in place until it is securely sutured at a depth chosen to ensure superior vena cava and not intra-atrial placement, after which a dressing is applied. The catheter site is dressed according to protocol after suturing the catheter.

How Is the External Jugular Vein Catheterized?

The patient's head is positioned facing 30° to 45° away from the EJV selected. The right EJV is generally preferred because of easier catheter passage. The vein may be better visualized if the patient performs Valsalva's maneuver or is placed in a 20° Trendelenburg position. If it cannot be visualized or palpated, another site should be selected.

The large-bore needle or catheter-over-needle is inserted at a 15° to 20° angle above the skin along the vein course. Slight negative pressure is kept on the syringe while the vein is sought. As the vein is entered, blood return is noted. The needle is then advanced 1 to 2 mm. If a catheter-over-needle is used, the catheter is advanced into the vein. If a longer catheter is to be inserted, a guidewire is passed through the catheter or a large-bore needle used. It has been reported that the guidewire is easiest to pass if the J-tip is advanced and the wire is rotated during passage to allow the J to find its way. Several attempts may be necessary to advance the guidewire beyond the EJV-SCV junction.

How Is the Internal Jugular Vein Catheterized?

The patient's head is positioned facing no more than 20° away from the selected site. The following landmarks are identified and palpated: the sternal notch, carotid artery, cricoid cartilage, and the two heads of the sternocleidomastoid (SCM) muscle.

The course of the IJV is from the apex of the triangle outlined by the clavicle inferiorly, the sternal head of the SCM medially, and the clavicular head of the SCM laterally through the middle or medial portion of this triangle just lateral to the carotid artery and 1 to 3 cm deep to the skin.

Three basic approaches are used for IJV cannulation. A high or low site may be selected for each approach. Higher sites have low risk of pneumothorax or hemothorax but have slightly lower success rates because the vein is smaller at the entry site.

Anterior Approach

Using an anterior approach, the finder needle (22-gauge 1.5-inch) is placed medial to the sternal head of the SCM between the apex of the triangle and the cricoid cartilage and lateral to the carotid artery. The needle is advanced at a 10° to 20° angle to the skin toward the ipsilateral shoulder. Negative pressure is applied to the syringe until blood return is noted. If the first pass is unsuccessful after insertion to 3 cm depth, the needle is slowly withdrawn while aspirating. If blood is still not encountered, it is redirected medially 10° to 15° and advanced again. The procedure is repeated until blood appears in the syringe. The needle path should not cross the sagittal plane nor enter the area where the carotid artery is palpated. The carotid should not be palpated during actual venipuncture, because this action decreases the IJV diameter. If multiple passes with the finder needle are unsuccessful, venipuncture with a larger needle should not be attempted. Instead, a new site approximately halfway down the SCM should be selected.

Median Approach

For the median approach, the finder needle is placed at the apex of the triangle formed by the two bellies of the SCM. The apex is easiest to locate by palpation. The needle is advanced at a 30° angle to the skin toward the ipsilateral nipple. The vein is usually <2.5 cm deep but the needle may occasionally have to be advanced up to 4 cm. If the first pass is unsuccessful after insertion to 3 cm, the needle is slowly withdrawn while continuing to aspirate with the syringe. If blood is not encountered, the needle is redirected 10° to 15° closer to the midline. This approach may be repeated up to five times before choosing a lower site. As with the anterior approach, to avoid complications the needle should not be directed across the sagittal plane to lessen the chance of carotid artery puncture.

Posterior Approach

The posterior approach theoretically poses an increased risk of carotid artery, tracheal, and sympathetic chain puncture; however, these complications have not been reported frequently.[38] The finder needle is positioned 15° to 20° above the skin, 4 cm above the clavicle, and lateral to the clavicular head of the SCM. The needle is advanced beneath the SCM toward the contralateral nipple. Venous return is usually noted before a maximum depth of 4 to 5 cm is reached. Deeper insertion angles may be necessary to pass the needle beneath the SCM. If unsuccessful, the process may be repeated at a point along the lateral border of the SCM closer to the clavicle.

Carotid Artery Puncture

The incidence of unintentional carotid artery puncture is at least 4%, even in experienced hands. It is, therefore, important to verify that the vessel entered is not the artery. We have found that when using a pencil probe Doppler, the artery is reliably avoided. If landmarks and palpation are used, it is wise to attach a piece of intravenous tubing to the needle, aspirate blood into the tubing, elevate the tubing, remove the syringe, and verify that blood flows back into the vessel. We routinely perform this manometry because the absence of pulsatile blood does not preclude arterial puncture because the needle bevel may be against the artery wall, blood color is unreliable, and the consequences of dilation and catheterization of the carotid artery can be devastating.[39]

How Is the Subclavian Vein Catheterized?

Supraclavicular Approach

Patients are positioned either with the head turned slightly to the contralateral side or straight up. The right side is preferred to avoid the thoracic duct and because catheter placement is easier. Three supraclavicular approaches are determined by landmarks and skin puncture sites. The anatomic relationships and proper and improper needle insertions for supraclavicular and inferior clavicular approaches are shown in Figures 32–2 to 32–6.

Junctional

The finder needle is placed at a 45° angle between the lateral border of the clavicular head of the SCM and the clavicle and is advanced beneath the clavicle toward the sternal notch (see Figs. 32–3 to 32–5). The depth of puncture is usually between 0.5 and 5 cm. If the first pass is unsuccessful, the needle may be repositioned three ways: (1) 2 to 3 cm superior to the clavicle, close to the lateral border of the SCM, (2) 1 to 1.4 cm above the junction of the clavicle and the lateral border of the SCM, or (3) 1 cm above the clavicle and 1 cm lateral to the lateral border of the SCM.

In a variation of the technique, after venipuncture, the large-bore needle or catheter-over-needle apparatus and syringe are "swung" laterally 35° from the sagittal plane and depressed slightly before passage of the guidewire or cannula.[8]

Anterior Scalene/First Rib

For the anterior scalene/first rib approach, a patient's head is turned 45° to the opposite side and the neck flexed approximately 15° (see Fig. 32–3). The ipsilateral arm may be crossed over the abdomen. These maneuvers enlarge the costoclavicular space. The landmarks are identified by placing the nondominant index finger on the scalene tubercle located behind the insertion point of the clavicular head of the SCM.

The finder needle is inserted lateral to the scalene tubercle over the first rib and advanced until blood appears in the syringe. The process is repeated using the catheter-over-

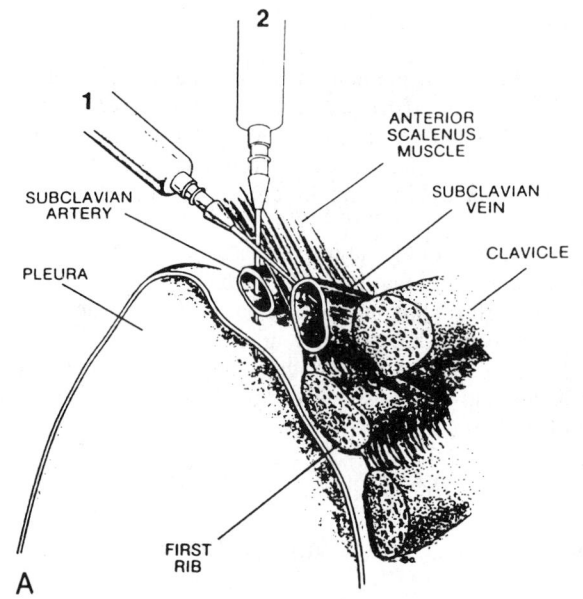

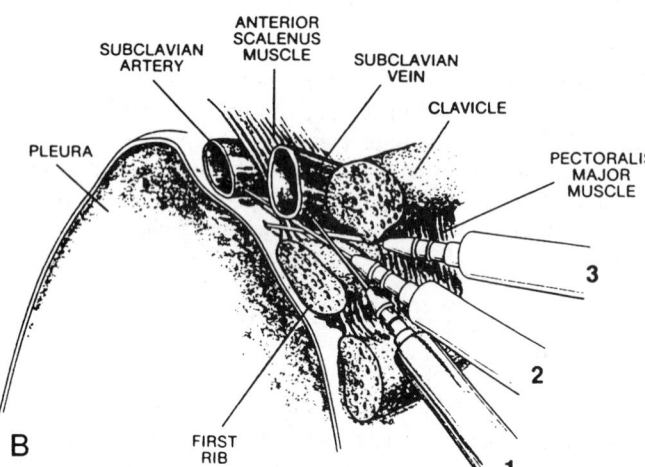

FIGURE 32–2. Sagittal view of subclavian vein and pertinent superficial and deep perivascular anatomy. Safe and unsafe insertions are demonstrated for supraclavicular and infraclavicular approaches. *A*, Supraclavicular approaches. 1 = Safe angle and depth of insertion, anterior to the anterior scalenus muscle; 2 = unsafe angle and depth of insertion prone to arterial and pleural puncture after traversing the anterior scalenus muscle. *B*, Infraclavicular approaches. 1 = Safe angle and depth of insertion; 2 = unsafe depth and angle predispose to arterial puncture; 3 = insertion prone to pleural puncture. (From Novak RA, Venus B: Clavicular approaches for central vein cannulation. Probl Crit Care 1988; 2:245.)

needle. When venipuncture is accomplished, the catheter-over-needle is lowered toward the shoulder to align the needle with the course of the vein, and the catheter or guidewire is advanced into the vein.

A modification of this technique is described by Parsa and Tabora.[40] The needle is directed perpendicular to the scalene tubercle and advanced until venipuncture is achieved. The needle/syringe is aligned with the course of the vein before catheter or guidewire passage.

Clavicular Notch

For the clavicular notch approach, a patient is positioned with a towel roll placed under the shoulders to extend the neck slightly. The head is turned away from the site. The clavicular notch is located by palpating the sternal notch then sliding a

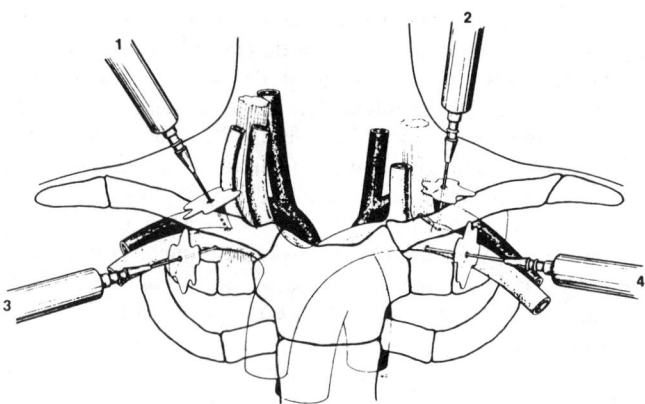

FIGURE 32–3. 1 = Supraclavicular, junctional approach (Yoffa); 2 = supraclavicular, anterior scalene–first rib approach; 3 = midclavicular approach, sternal notch orientation; 4 = infraclavicular, medial approach–sternal notch orientation. (From Novak RA, Venus B: Clavicular approaches for central vein cannulation. Probl Crit Care 1988; 2:254.)

finger along the anterior superior edge of the clavicle. It may also be palpated just lateral to the carotid artery along the anteriosuperior edge of the clavicle.

The finder needle is advanced at a 30° to 45° angle to the skin parallel to the sagittal plane (see Fig. 32–6). The vein is usually located between 2 and 4 cm below the skin. Venipuncture is noted by a click and venous blood return. If the first attempt is unsuccessful, the needle is redirected and advanced in a slightly more lateral plane.

Alternatively, the insertion point may be extended 1 to 2 cm above the notch. Using the same angle and direction of insertion, the needle is "marched" down the clavicle and advanced as it slips beneath the clavicle until blood return is noted.

Infraclavicular Approach

The patient is positioned supine. A towel between the scapulae may actually decrease the size of the subclavian vein by compressing it between the clavicle and first rib.[18] The head is left in a neutral position or turned toward the side being cath-

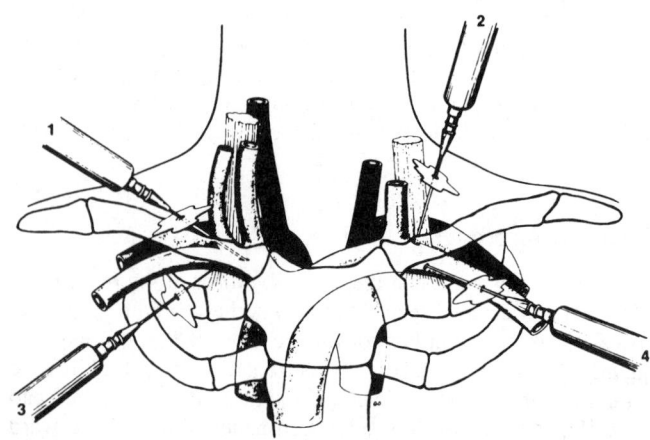

FIGURE 32–4. 1 = Supraclavicular, modified junctional approach (Brahos); 2 = supraclavicular, modified junctional approach (Haapaenimi and Slatis); 3 = infraclavicular, midclavicular approach—clavicular sternocleidomastoid (CSCM) triangle orientation; 4 = infraclavicular, medial approach—CSCM triangle orientation. (From Novak RA, Venus B: Clavicular approaches for central vein cannulation. Probl Crit Care 1988; 2:255.)

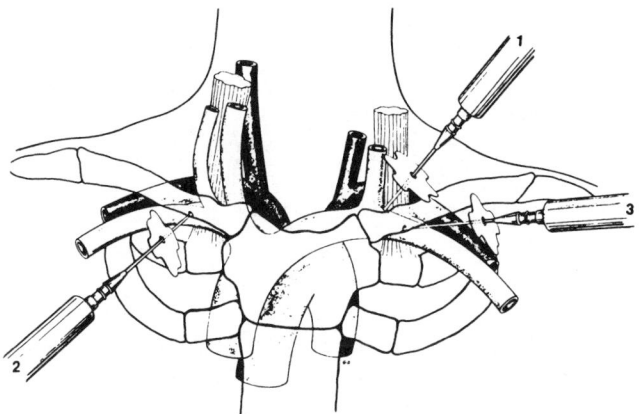

FIGURE 32–5. 1 = Supraclavicular, modified junctional approach (Helmkamp); 2 = infraclavicular, midclavicular approach—scalene tubercle orientation; 3 = infraclavicular, lateral approach. (From Novak RA, Venus B: Clavicular approaches for central vein cannulation. Probl Crit Care 1988; 2:256.)

eterized in order to decrease the angle between the subclavian and ipsilateral jugular vein to make it more difficult for the guidewire to find its way into the IJV. The following landmarks are identified: the inferior border of the clavicle, the sternal notch, and the SCM-clavicular triangle. Infraclavicular approaches may be divided into three basic insertion points.

Lateral

The lateral insertion point is lateral to the midclavicular line at the junction of the lateral and middle thirds of the clavicle (see Fig. 32–5). A large-bore needle is directed beneath the clavicle by marching it down the clavicle or by inserting it 1 to 2 cm inferior to the clavicle and slipping beneath it. The needle/syringe assembly is kept parallel to the skin surface as it is gently advanced toward the sternal notch. The index finger of the nondominant hand is kept on the sternal notch as a guide during venipuncture, and the thumb is held over the needle to help guide it under the clavicle. It is often helpful to bend (curve) the needle gently to facilitate passing it under the

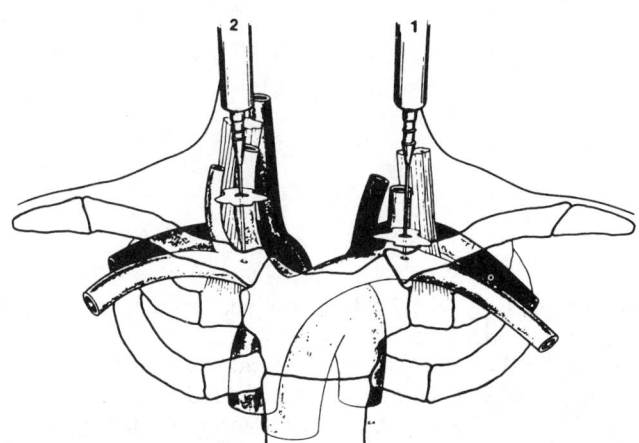

FIGURE 32–6. 1 = Supraclavicular, clavicular notch approach; 2 = supraclavicular, modified clavicular notch approach. (From Novak RA, Venus B: Clavicular approaches for central vein cannulation. Probl Crit Care 1988; 2:257.)

clavicle. Once venous return is noted, the bevel of the needle should be oriented caudally to minimize guidewire malposition.

Midclavicular and Medial

The procedure is the same for the second subclavian insertion point (midclavicular) (see Figs. 32–3 to 32–5) and for the third point (medial) (see Figs. 32–3 to 32–4), which is at the junction of the middle and medial thirds of the clavicle. If venipuncture is unsuccessful on the first pass at any point, the needle path may be redirected 5° to 10° above the sternal notch and advanced, keeping the needle/syringe assembly parallel to the skin surface. No more than five passes at each insertion point should be attempted.

After successful venipuncture, the basic procedure outlined earlier is used to insert the introducer and then the catheter.

How Is the Femoral Vein Catheterized?

The patient is positioned supine, with the leg rotated externally slightly. In an obese individual, an assistant may be needed to retract abdominal folds away from the inguinal field. Placing a folded towel under the hip may help elevate the inguinal field into better view.

The finder needle is positioned at a 45° angle above the skin medial to the femoral artery (Fig. 32–7). The skin site should be distal enough so that the tip of the needle does not traverse the inguinal ligament (i.e., enter the abdominal cavity) as it is advanced cephalad. The needle may be directed slightly toward the palpable artery as it is advanced. Gentle negative pressure is applied on the syringe while advancing. If venipuncture is unsuccessful on the first pass, the needle is redirected a few degrees closer to the femoral artery as it is advanced. As many as five passes may be necessary.

Once the vein is located, a large-bore needle is introduced at the same site and inserted to the same depth. After confirmation of adequate venous flow, a guidewire is introduced and the needle removed. The skin is nicked at the site of guidewire entry, and the vein dilated. The catheter is inserted to its full length and secured.

How Far Should a Central Venous Catheter Be Advanced?

Catheter tip position is of utmost importance after central venous catheter placement. Cardiac tamponade and vessel perforation are well-known, potentially lethal complications of catheter tip malposition.[41–43] Both are preventable by ensuring proper positioning. Erosion and perforation occur either when the catheter tip is perpendicular to the vessel wall or when the tip enters the right atrium or ventricle.[38, 42–45] This problem is particularly likely with left-sided approaches.[43] The critical angle of incidence between catheter tip and superior vena cava is probably 40°; thus, any catheter with a contact angle ≥40° should be repositioned.

The catheter tip should lie within the superior vena cava but outside the right atrium. The distance between the puncture site and the superior vena cava–atrial junction can vary considerably, depending on the site selected and a patient's height and body habitus. Central venous catheters should be inserted

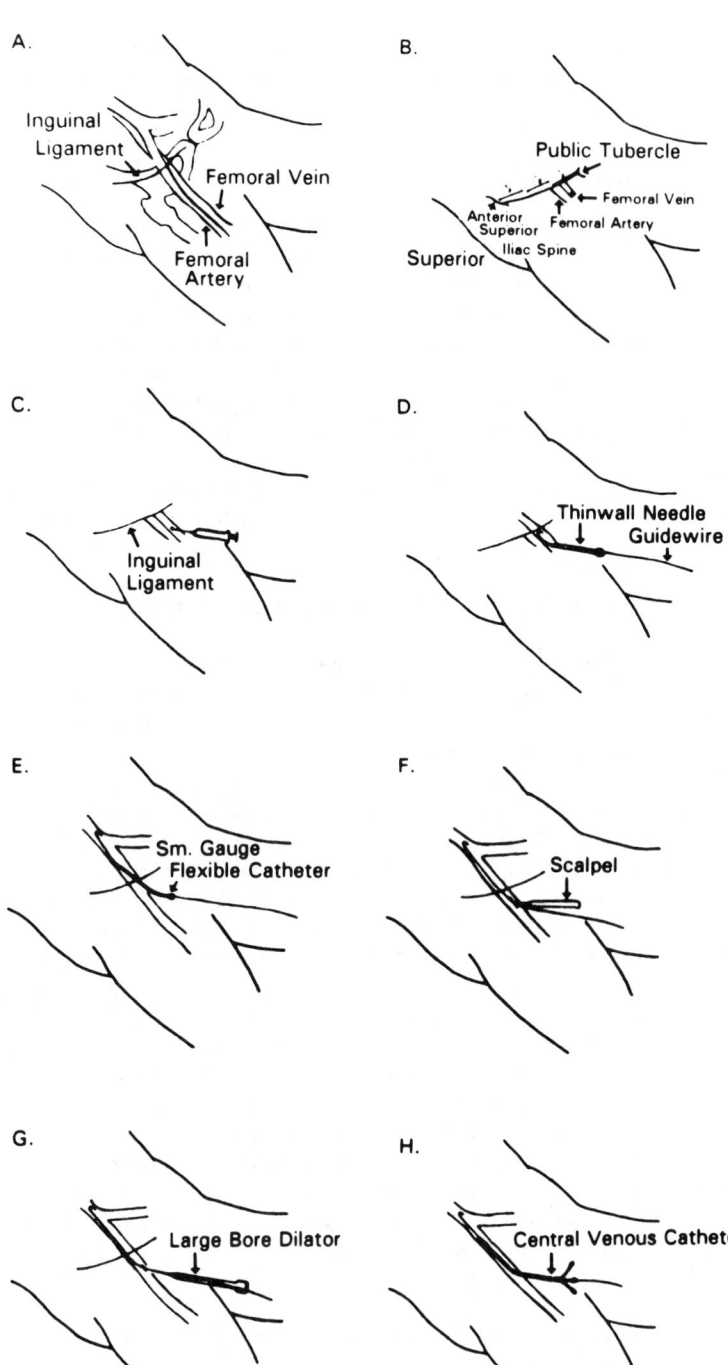

FIGURE 32–7. *A*, Femoral vein location. At the level of the inguinal ligament, the femoral vein is located medial to the femoral artery. *B*, Femoral vein anatomy. At a level 2 to 3 cm below the inguinal ligament, the femoral artery can be found 1 to 2 cm medial to the artery. *C*, Anesthetic administration and femoral vein localization. Lidocaine is infiltrated over the insertion site, and the femoral vein is located. Always withdraw on the syringe plunger prior to injection of lidocaine to avoid inadvertent intravascular injection. The syringe should be directed at 45° cranially, staying below the inguinal ligament. *D*, Femoral guidewire insertion. The femoral vein is cannulated with a needle capable of accommodating a flexible guidewire. The guidewire is gently inserted through the needle. There should be no resistance to passage of the guidewire. The needle is then removed, leaving the guidewire in place. *E*, Confirmation of intravenous location prior to dilation. Intravenous location of the guidewire is confirmed prior to dilation of the cannulation site by passing a small flexible catheter over the guidewire. The guidewire is then removed, and blood is withdrawn through the catheter. The guidewire is again placed through the catheter, and the catheter is removed (leaving the guidewire in place again in the vein). *F*, Skin incision. A small (0.25-cm) skin incision is made adjacent to the site of entry of the guidewire. *G*, Insertion of venous dilator. A large-bore dilator is passed over the guidewire. The dilator is then removed, leaving the guidewire in place in the vein. *H*, Insertion of venous catheter. The central venous catheter is placed over the guidewire. The guidewire is removed, and the catheter is sutured securely in place. (From Tribett D, Brenner M: Peripheral and femoral vein cannulation. Probl Crit Care 1988; 2:279.)

13 to 16 cm for right SCV and jugular vein approaches and 15 to 20 cm for left-sided approaches. Thus, it makes little sense to use a 20-cm or longer catheter from the right side. One may approximate the insertion distance by placing the catheter over the chest, traveling over the envisioned path from the insertion site to a point 2 to 3 cm below the sternoclavicular joint. Several formulas based on a patient's height and the insertion site have been proposed to provide a potentially more accurate method for determining insertion distance. A chest film is necessary to reliably assess and predict catheter tip position and orientation.[46]

Right atrial electrocardiography is an alternative method to determine catheter position.[47, 48] An electrode is placed on the end of a saline-filled catheter during insertion, and lead II is monitored. An increase in P wave size occurs as the catheter enters the right atrium. Withdrawing the catheter 1 cm beyond the point where the P wave size becomes normal ensures correct placement outside the heart, unless a patient's neck is subsequently flexed or the shoulder is adducted with jugular and subclavian catheters, respectively.

Catheter Orientation

The risk of vessel perforation is minimized by positioning the catheter tip so that it lies parallel to the superior vena cava. This is most easily accomplished with right-sided placements. Left-sided catheterizations are more prone to result in acute impingement of the catheter tip against the vena cava (Fig. 32–8).[48] A review of reported cases and in vitro data suggests that any catheter tip that is at a >40° impingement angle to the superior vena cava should be repositioned.[49, 50]

Is a Chest Radiograph Necessary After Central Catheter Placement?

Controversy surrounds use of a chest radiograph because it exposes patients to radiation, is relatively expensive, and is potentially not cost effective, considering the low complication rate with jugular vein approaches. However, chest radiographs are used not only to rule out immediate complications such as pneumothorax but also to confirm that the catheter is not lying in the heart or at an unacceptable angle to the wall of the superior vena cava.[51] We recommend immediate chest radiography after subclavian catheterization out of concern for pneumothorax. Chest radiographs following uncomplicated IJV catheterization can be delayed until the end of the operative procedure, because their primary utility is to allow catheter position to be assessed.

If a Catheter Is Malpositioned, Can It Be Repositioned Without Contamination?

Malpositioning is a well-known complication of central venous catheterization. Catheters are malpositioned in the ipsilat-

eral IJV or contralateral SCV 11% to 19% of the time.[51] Placement in the brachiocephalic, azygos, and pericardiophrenic veins, among others, also has been reported. Perhaps the easiest way to reposition the catheter is to remove it and recatheterize. Extenuating circumstances such as hypovolemia, poor landmarks, and coagulopathy, as well as exposing patients to further risk, make such attempts less desirable. To reduce these risks during the initial attempt, electrocardiographic and ultrasound real-time guidance, fluoroscopic placement, and flow-directed techniques can be used.[52–54] However, additional equipment is required and may not be immediately available.

Catheter Rewiring and Replacement

A simple method for repositioning a wayward catheter requires minimal additional equipment or personnel and is useful, rapid, and relatively safe.[55] Obtain another central venous catheter preparation kit and drape the in situ catheter and patient in the usual sterile fashion. Ensure that all exposed areas in the field are sterile. Remove the suture and withdraw the catheter 2 to 3 cm. A portable chest radiograph obtained earlier helps to determine the distance for withdrawal.

Using a scalpel, cut the catheter into two pieces, 1 cm above the insertion site. The catheter that remains in the central vein must at all times be visible and tightly held to prevent vascular embolization. A J-wire is then advanced through the distal port to approximately 15 cm.

Remove the malpositioned catheter tip entirely, withdraw the J-wire, and readvance it with the patient's head turned toward the side of the catheter. This reduces the likelihood of its going into the subclavian from the jugular, or vice versa. A new catheter is then inserted over the J-wire. If this does not result in appropriate positioning, then manipulation during fluoroscopy is recommended. A portable chest radiograph should be taken to confirm proper positioning.

What Should I Do If I Have Difficulty with Cannulation?

Difficulties are occasionally encountered despite proper patient positioning, careful selection of approach, and meticulous attention to detail. Hypovolemia, altered anatomy, vein thrombosis, patient's movement, and operator inexperience are among the many reasons for difficulties.

Internal and External Jugular Veins

For IJV and EJV approaches, difficulty in locating the vein may be secondary to head position. Maintain the patient's head rotation to the contralateral side to <45°. The SCM begins to obstruct the IJV, and the EJV becomes compressed at angles greater than this.[54] Again, the use of a sterile pencil probe Doppler is encouraged. This identifies the thrombosed vein (no Doppler signal) or location of an aberrant vein. Use of a 22-gauge 1.5-inch finder needle is a less precise option for determining the location of the vein, barring congenital anomalies.

Another approach is to use a "pull" maneuver, especially in patients with multiple skin folds. Pull the skin in the opposite direction of the needle to help prevent vein collapse in response to an advancing needle. Under certain circumstances,

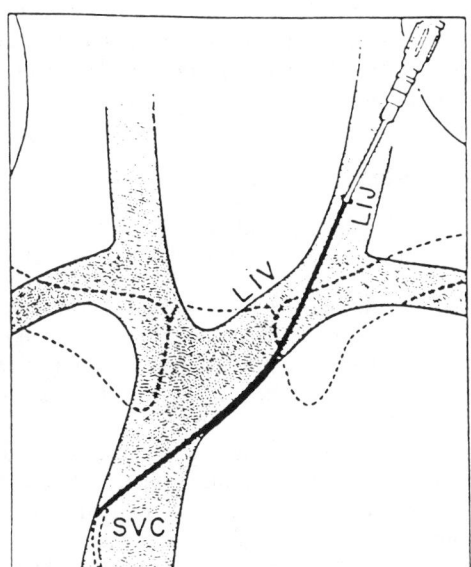

FIGURE 32–8. Schematic drawing of central venous catheter. Course is along the left internal jugular vein (LIJ), left innominate vein (LIV), and superior vena cava (SVC). The sharp angle of the catheter tip against the SVC may lead to perforation of the vessel. *Dotted lines* at bottom demonstrate proper position of catheter tip, which lies parallel to the vessel wall. (From Iberti TJ, Katz B, Reiner MA: Hydrothorax as a late complication of central venous indwelling catheters. Surgery 1983; 94:845.)

Valsalva's maneuver, volume challenge, or expiratory hold for those patients who are mechanically ventilated may be of assistance. If the vein has been traversed, apply slight negative pressure intermittently on the syringe during slow withdrawal. Two-dimensional Doppler ultrasonography used for guiding IJV and SCV cannulations has been suggested as well.[52, 54] If these trials fail, another site should be selected for cannulation.

Subclavian Veins

Several maneuvers to expedite difficult SCV catheter insertion are available. For patients with poor landmarks, a towel roll placed longitudinally between the shoulder blades has been recommended, but this should be done with the understanding that it is likely to bring the clavicle and first rib closer together and may thereby actually make it more difficult.

The operator may have an assistant pull the ipsilateral arm caudally without abduction. This maneuver prevents shoulder retraction in Trendelenburg's position, places a patient in a neutral posture, and allows optimal needle entry parallel to the frontal plane. Applying slight intermittent pressure on the syringe should be tried. A more medial or lateral approach from the initial attempt and re-evaluation of direction, angle of insertion, and depth may be helpful as well.

Femoral Vein

In femoral vein catheterization, success may be facilitated by placing the ipsilateral leg in slight abduction and external rotation. Once again, if the femoral pulse landmark is difficult to palpate or the vein is possibly thrombosed, a sterile Doppler probe is invaluable. Have an assistant lift an obese patient's abdominal folds. A towel roll placed posteriorly between the anterosuperior and posterosuperior iliac spines may improve the landmarks.

What Should I Do If I Have Difficulty Threading the J-Wire?

A guidewire should never be forcibly inserted when resistance is encountered. Once the vein is entered, advance the needle 1 to 2 mm farther to be sure the entire needle bevel is within the vessel. Rotate the needle so that the proximal portion of the bevel is positioned caudally in SCV attempts. Thread the J-wire with the J configuration also facing caudally. If difficulty is still encountered, maintain the needle close to the frontal plane. If it is flexible, we also try the straight end of the J-wire because it passes more readily through a small vein. However, if *any* resistance is met, this method is abandoned, the wire is removed, and the needle is repositioned. Several unsuccessful attempts suggest that the needle is in a very small neck vein, and a new puncture is performed at an adjacent or different site. Guidewires are available separately and in various diameters. When possible, a smaller, flexible angiographic wire can also be used to advantage.

Subclavian guidewire placement from the EJV can also be difficult. Maneuvers such as medial and lateral flexion of the neck, abduction and adduction, plus external and internal rotation of the ipsilateral arm provide some help. Withdrawal of the J-wire approximately 1 cm followed by concomitant rotation of the wire medially by 90° during readvancement is occasionally useful. If resistance is met when the J-wire is retracted, be sure that the needle/cannula and wire are removed simultaneously to prevent shearing.

When Should a Central Venous Catheter Be Replaced?

Considerable controversy surrounds this important issue. Catheter-related sepsis is a serious complication with significant morbidity and mortality. Infection has been reported in approximately 10% to 14% of all catheter sites[56]: 0.2% to 0.5% for peripheral catheters, up to 7% for central parenteral nutrition catheters, and subsequent bacteremia and septicemia in 4% to 12% of central venous catheters.[56–59]

The type of catheter, number of lumina, type of fluid infused, site and duration of catheterization, and catheter maintenance techniques all have been studied in detail to determine those factors that lead to infection. New central venous catheters have been developed with a silver-impregnated cuff (VitaCuff) or silver sulfadiazine with chlorohexidine (Arrowgard) bonded to the catheter in an attempt to reduce these risks. Studies are currently under way to determine their efficacy in reducing catheter-related infection. Recommendations are difficult considering the variables, conflicting data, and the diverse patient population between different hospital centers. Certainly when purulent drainage is noted at the insertion site, the catheter should be removed.

Duration of Catheterization

Studies of when a catheter should be changed have been either inconclusive or conflicting. Maki and colleagues showed that the potential for infection increases after 72 hours in catheters not used for hyperalimentation in critically ill patients.[57] A study by Gil and associates revealed that colonization and bacteremia increase significantly after 6 days.[60] Others maintain a catheter to a later date or until a complication develops. Individuals and institutions should evaluate their patient populations, type and number of catheters placed, and incidence of infection to determine policies for replacement.

Recommendation

Based on our experience and that of others, we recommend the following protocol:

1. In critically ill patients with adequate access available, a catheter change using a different site after 72 hours appears reasonable for infection control. Low infection rates using single- or multilumen catheters have been reported with this approach.[36, 58, 60–62]

2. If access is limited (e.g., obesity, extreme burns, scar tissue), an option is to leave the catheter for an extended period with close daily observation or to change the catheter after 72 hours over a J-wire and to culture the tip. If the culture result is positive, a new site and catheter should be chosen. If the catheter is to be left for an extended period, replace it before signs of infection are evident. A maximum of 6 days is suggested unless otherwise indicated.

3. Central venous catheters placed via the antecubital fossa should be removed after 72 hours. Studies report a higher frequency of complications, 12.5% to 23%, via this site.[63]

4. Replace both pulmonary artery catheters *and* their introducers after 72 hours. The risk of infection is reported to increase for those catheters left >3 days.[63, 64]

5. Discontinue central catheters as soon as they are no longer required.

What Are the Complications of Central Venous Catheterization?

Complications are many, varied, and potentially lethal. They, together with those associated with pulmonary artery catheterization, are listed in Table 32–13. Most can be avoided by meticulous attention to detail, careful preparation, and a sound knowledge of the involved anatomy.

PULMONARY ARTERY CATHETERIZATION TECHNIQUES

Various dilator-sheath assemblies are available. After venipuncture, we use modified Seldinger's technique to place a 9 French sheath with a one-way valve at the outer end and a side arm for blood sampling and infusion of fluids or drugs. The introducer and sheath are advanced gently to avoid venous perforation. After placement, the introducer is removed and the sheath is sutured to the skin.

Before insertion and after the sterility sheath is placed over it, the catheter should be tested for bends or kinks and balloon integrity. The catheter is then connected by means of a three-way stopcock and pressure tubing to an appropriately balanced and calibrated pressure transducer. All lumina are flushed and filled with sterile heparinized saline solution. The balloon should remain deflated until the catheter tip is beyond the end of the sheath. Once the tip is advanced 20 cm, the balloon is inflated with 1.5 mL of air. The catheter is then slowly and monotonously advanced with continuous electrocardiographic

TABLE 32–13. Complications of Central Venous and Pulmonary Artery Catheterization

Immediate	Multiple puncture
	Pneumo/hemo/hydro/chylothorax-mediastinum
	Arterial puncture—hematoma or bleeding
	Air embolism
	Cardiac dysrhythmias
	Catheter malposition
	Catheter knotting
	Subcutaneous and mediastinal emphysema
	Tracheal puncture or laceration
Late	Pulmonary artery rupture
	Pulmonary infarction
	Catheter-related sepsis
	Balloon rupture
	Endocardial or valvular damage
	Venous thrombosis
	Infections (cellulitis, osteomyelitis, endocarditis, thrombophlebitis)
	Nerve injury
	Cerebrovascular compromise
	Cardiac or vena cave perforation and pleural effusion or cardiac tamponade
	Arteriovenous fistula
	Thrombocytopenia

(Modified from Venus B, Mallory DL: Vascular cannulation. *In* Critical Care. Civetta JM, Taylor RW, Kirby RR (eds). Philadelphia, JB Lippincott, 1988, p 157.)

TABLE 32–14. Factors Predisposing to Pulmonary Artery Rupture

Age >60 years
Female gender
Cardiopulmonary bypass
Hypothermia
Anticoagulation
Pulmonary hypertension
Peripheral catheter tip location (i.e., >5 cm lateral to mediastinum)
Multiple wedge pressure determinations
Atypical pulmonary artery pressure waveform (mitral valve disease)

(From Gravenstein N (ed): Manual of Complications During Anesthesia. Philadelphia, JB Lippincott, 1991, p 290.)

and pressure waveform monitoring across the tricuspid valve and into the pulmonary artery via the right ventricle. The right ventricular tracing should appear about 45 to 55 cm from the antecubital fossa, 40 to 55 cm from the femoral vein, 35 to 40 cm from the IJV, and 30 to 40 cm from the SCV (lower numbers represent right-sided approaches). Characteristic pressure changes should accompany passage from the right ventricle to the pulmonary artery and into the occlusion position. The occlusion position should be obtained when the balloon is inflated with 1.5 mL of air. If occlusion is obtained with <1 mL inflation, the catheter is too far in the pulmonary artery and needs to be retracted to a distance where 1.5 mL is required to wedge the tip.

Once the catheter is in position, secure it in place. Obtain a chest radiograph to document the tip location and to check for pneumothorax either immediately if a subclavian approach was used or immediately postoperatively if an internal jugular vein approach was used. Placement may be difficult in the presence of right atrial or ventricular dilatation, low cardiac output, pulmonary hypertension, or tricuspid regurgitation. Passage during deep spontaneous inspiration in the sitting position may facilitate entrance to the right ventricle.[65] Catheter passage is also facilitated by placing the patient in a 5° head-up position with a right lateral tilt.[66] Stiffening the catheter in a cold solution before passage or use of a guidewire (length 120 cm, outer diameter 0.021 inches) under fluroscopy can help as well. Distal migration of the catheter tip should be anticipated as the catheter warms and softens. If it migrates to a wedge position, it should again be withdrawn. Because of the anticipated distal migration, it is critical to inflate the balloon very gradually any time a wedge pressure determination is made during continuous pulmonary artery pressure waveform monitoring.

What Are the Complications?

Table 32–13 lists early and late complications of central venous and pulmonary artery catheterization.[67–72] Sustained ventricular dysrhythmias are usually due to catheter slack and should be treated by withdrawing the catheter to relieve any slack. A knotted catheter usually can be removed in a cardiac catheterization laboratory without much difficulty. The incidence of pulmonary artery rupture is very low but has a high mortality. It should be suspected whenever hemoptysis occurs, especially if it is temporally related to balloon inflation. Factors predisposing to pulmonary artery rupture are listed in Table 32–14. Mechanical damage to the cardiac valves and endocardium may occur as a result of prolonged catheterization. Valvular ruptures have been reported when the catheter is entrapped in the trabeculae. The balloon must always be deflated before withdrawing the catheter.

Pulmonary artery catheters predispose to bacterial colonization and systemic infection. The degree of catheter manipulation and the length of time it is in place are important factors. In critically ill patients, entrapment of platelets by the catheter may also cause clinically significant thrombocytopenia, which responds to removal of the catheter.

References

1. Aubaniac R: Einjection intraveneuse souseclavculare advantage et technique. Presse Med 1952; 60:1456.
2. Seldinger SL: Catheter replacement of the needle in percutaneous arteriography: a new approach. Acta Radiol 1953; 39:368.
3. Yoffa D, Melb MB: Supraclavicular subclavian venipuncture and catheterization. Lancet 1965; 2:614.
4. Moncrief J: Femoral catheters. Ann Surg 1958; 147:166.
5. English CW, Frew RM, Pigott JF, et al: Percutaneous catheterization of the internal jugular vein. Thorax 1969; 24:521.
6. Rao TL, Wong AY, Salem MR: A new approach to percutaneous catheterization of the internal jugular vein. Anesthesiology 1977; 46:362.
7. Hermasura B, Vanagas L, Dichey MW: Measurement of pressure during intravenous therapy. JAMA 1966; 195:321.
8. Haapaniemi L, Slatis P: Supraclavicular catheterization of the superior vena cava. Acta Anaesthesiol Scand 1974; 18:12.
9. Forber B: Infection control in intensive care. In Centers for Disease Control Guidelines for the Prevention of Intravascular Infections. New York, Churchill Livingstone, 1987, pp 50–56.
10. National Intravenous Therapy Association: Intravenous Nursing Standards of Practice. Vol. 4. Cambridge, MA; National Intravenous Therapy Association, 1981, p 9.
11. O'Brian R: Starting intravenous lines in children. J Emerg Nurs 1991; 17:4.
12. Garrelts J, LaRocca J, Ast D, et al: Comparison of heparin and 0.9% sodium chloride injection in the maintenance of indwelling intermittent i.v. devices. Clin Pharm 1989; 8:34.
13. Lyon MT, Armstrong A: Correspondence. Anaesth Intensive Care 1990; 18:579.
14. Becher C, Toulin RB: Doppler flow monitoring of the dorsal artery of the foot facilitates puncture of the femoral artery in children. AJR 1990; 155:131.
15. Chatterjie K, Swan J, Ganz W, et al: Use of a balloon-tipped flotation electrode catheter for cardiac monitoring. Am J Cardiol 1975; 36:56.
16. Baele P, McMechan J, Marsh H, et al: Continuous monitoring of mixed venous oxygen saturation in critically ill patients. Anaesth Analg 1982; 61:513.
17. Sulek CA, Weiss L, Gravenstein N, et al: Influence of head position on relationship between internal jugular vein and carotid artery. Crit Care Med 1993; 21:A218.
18. Jesseph JM, Conces DJ, Agustyn GT: Patient positioning for subclavian vein catheterization. Arch Surg 1987; 122:1207.
19. Murphy LM, Lipman TO: Central venous catheter care in parenteral nutrition. A review. JPEN J Parenter Enteral Nutr 1987; 11:190.
20. Emerman CL, Bellon EM, Lukens TW, et al: A prospective study of femoral versus subclavian vein catheterization during cardiac arrest. Ann Emerg Med 1990; 19:26.
21. Novak RA, Venus B: Clavicular approaches for central vein cannulation. In Problems in Critical Care. Venus B, Mallory DL (eds). Philadelphia, JB Lippincott, 1988, pp 242–265.
22. Goldfarb G, Lebreq D: Percutaneous cannulation of the internal jugular vein in patients with coagulopathies: an experienced based on 1,000 attempts. Anesthesiology 1982; 56:321.
23. Venus B, Mallory DL: Vascular cannulation. In Critical Care. Civetta JM, Taylor RW, Kirby RR (eds). Philadelphia, JB Lippincott, 1992, pp 149–169.
24. Slogoff A, Keats AS, Arlund BS: On the safety of radial artery cannulation. Anesthesiology 1983; 59:42.
25. Melker RJ: Complications of intraosseous infusion. Ann Emerg Med 1990; 19:731.
26. Seneff M: Arterial line placement and care. In Intensive Care Medicine. Rippe JM, Irwin RS, Alpert JS, Fink MP (eds). Boston, Little, Brown & Co, 1991, pp 37–47.
27. Stirt JA: "Liquid stylet" for percutaneous radial artery cannulation. Can Anaesth Soc J 1982; 29:492.
28. Kondo K: Percutaneous radial artery cannulation using a pressure-curve-directed technique. Anesthesiology 1984; 61:639.
29. Mallory DL, Sapienza R, McGee WT, et al: "State-of-the-art" vascular cannulation in the ICU. Res Medica 1988; 4:5.
30. Sladen A: Complications of invasive hemodynamic monitoring in the intensive care unit. In Current Problems in Surgery. Ravitch MM (ed). Chicago, Year Book Medical Publishers, 1988, pp 69–145.
31. Norwood SH, Cormier B, McMahon NG, et al: Prospective study of catheter-related infection during prolonged arterial catheterization. Crit Care Med 1988; 16:836.
32. Clark CA, Harman EM: Hemodynamic monitoring: arterial catheters. In Critical Care. Civetta JM, Taylor RW, Kirby RR (eds). Philadelphia, JB Lippincott, 1988, pp 289–292.
33. Moyer MA, Edwards LD, Farley L: Comparative culture methods on 101 intravenous catheters. Arch Intern Med 1983; 143:66.
34. Thomas F, Burke JP, Parker J, et al: The risk of infection related to radial vs femoral sites for arterial catheterization. Crit Care Med 1983; 11:807.
35. Ducharme FM, Gauthier M, Lacroix J, et al: Incidence of infection related to arterial catheterization in children: a prospective study. Crit Care Med 1988; 16:272.
36. Arnow PM, Costas CO: Delayed rupture of the radial artery caused by catheter-related sepsis. Rev Infect Dis 1988; 10:1035.
37. Russell RC, Steichen JB, Sook EG: Radial artery pseudoaneurysms: their diagnosis, treatment and prevention. Orthop Rev 1979; 8:49.
38. McGee WT, Mallory DL: Cannulation of the internal and external jugular veins. In Problems in Critical Care. Venus B, Mallory DL (eds). Philadelphia, JB Lippincott, 1988, pp 217–241.
39. Schwartz AJ, Jobes DR, Greenhow DE, et al: Carotid artery puncture with internal jugular cannulation using the Seldinger technique: Incidence, recognition, treatment, and prevention. Anesthesiology 1979; 51:S160.
40. Parsa MH, Tabora F: Central venous access in critically ill patients in the emergency department. Emerg Med Clin North Am 1986; 4:709.
41. Ellis L, Vogel S, Copeland E: Central venous catheter vascular erosions. Diagnosis and clinical course. Ann Surg 1989; 209:475.
42. Long R, Kassum D, Donen N, et al: Cardiac tamponade associated with a multi-lumen central venous catheter. Crit Care Med 1987; 2:39.
43. Sheep R, Guiney W: Fatal cardiac tamponade. Occurrence with other complications after left internal jugular vein catheterization. JAMA 1982; 248:1632.
44. Dane TE, Kreig EG: Fatal cardiac tamponade and other mechanical complications of central venous catheters. Br J Surg 1975; 62:6.
45. Purdue GF, Hunt JL: Placement and complications of monitoring catheters. Surg Clin North Am 1991; 71:4.
46. Peres PW: Positioning central venous catheters—a prospective survey. Anaesth Intens Care 1990; 18:4.
47. McGee WT, Mallory DL, Johans TG, et al: Safe placement of central venous catheters is facilitated using right atrial electrocardiography. Crit Care Med 1988; 16:4.
48. Iberti TJ, Katz R, Reiner MA: Hydrothorax as a late complication of central venous indwelling catheters. Surgery 1983; 94:842.
49. Blackshear RH, Gravenstein N: Critical angle of incidence for delayed vessel perforation by central venous catheter: A study of in vivo data (Abstracted). Ann Emerg Med 1992; 21:659.
50. Gravenstein N, Blackshear RH: In vitro evaluation of relative perforating potential of central venous catheters: comparison of materials, selected models, number of lumens, and angle of incidence to simulated membrane. J Clin Monit 1991; 7:1.
51. Deital M, McIntyre J: Radiographic confirmation of site of central venous pressure catheters. Can J Surg 1971; 14:42.
52. Nolsoe C, Nielsen L, Korstrup S, et al: Ultrasonically guided subclavian vein catheterization. Acta Radiol 1989; 30:108.
53. Babikian G, Byron R, Hassett J Jr: Redirection of central venous catheters using a flow-directed technique. Surg Gynecol Obstet 1986; 163:482.
54. Tryba M, Kleine P, Zeng M: Sonographic studies for optimizing cannulation of the internal jugular vein. Anaesthetist 1982; 31:626.
55. Kayal TJ, Sallaum LJ, Snyker AB, et al: A simple method for repositioning the wayward central venous catheter. JPEN J Parenter Enteral Nutr 1989; 13:438.
56. Snyder RH, Archer FJ, Endy T, et al: Catheter infection: a comparison of two catheter maintenance techniques. Ann Surg 1988; 208:651.
57. Maki DG, Goldman DA, Rhome RS: Infection control in intravenous therapy. Ann Intern Med 1973; 79:867.
58. Kelly CS, Ligas JR, Smith CA, et al: Sepsis due to triple lumen central venous catheters. Surg Gynecol Obstet 1986; 14:163.
59. Prayer RL, Silva J: Colonization of central venous catheters. South Med J 1984; 77:458.
60. Gil RT, Krause JA, Thill-Baharozian MC, et al: Triple versus single lumen central venous catheters. Arch Intern Med 1989; 149:1139.

61. Hilton E, Haslett T, Borenstein M, et al: Central catheter infections: single versus triple lumen catheters. Am J Med 1988; 84:667.
62. Elliott TS: Intravascular-device infections. J Med Microbiol 1988; 27:161.
63. Myers M, Austin T, Sibbold W: Pulmonary artery catheter infections: a prospective study. Ann Surg 1985; 201:237.
64. Miller J, Venus B, Mathru M: Comparison of the sterility of long term central venous catheterization using single lumen, triple lumen, and pulmonary artery catheters. Crit Care Med 1984; 12:634.
65. Venus B, Mathru M: A maneuver for bedside pulmonary artery catheterization in patients with right heart failure. Chest 1982; 82:803.
66. Keusch DJ, Winters S, Thys DM: The patient's position influences the incidence of dysrhythmias during pulmonary artery catheterization. Anesthesiology 1989; 70:582.
67. Childs D, Wilkes RG: Puncture of the ascending aorta: a complication of subclavian venous cannulation. Anesthesia 1986; 41:331.
68. Herbst CA: Indications, management, and complications of percutaneous subclavian catheters. Arch Surg 1978; 113:1421.
69. Brown CQ: Inadvertent prolonged cannulation of the carotid artery. Anesth Analg 1982; 61:150.
70. Bernard RW, Stahl WM: Subclavian vein catheterization: A prospective study. I. Non-infectious complications. Ann Surg 1971; 173:184.
71. Jay AWL, Aldridge HE: Perforation of the heart or vena cava by central venous catheters inserted for monitoring or infusion therapy. Can Med Assoc J 1986; 135:1143.
72. Aldridge HE, Jay AWL: Central venous catheters and heart perforation. Can Med Assoc J 1986; 135D:1145.

Pharmacologic Considerations and Anesthetic Administration

CHAPTER **33**

Basic Pharmacologic Applications in Anesthesia

W. JERRY MERRELL, M.D.

Pharmacology is a basic and clinical science that can be broadly defined as the study of the interactions between drug substances and living systems. In this chapter, we assume that the response to a medication is related to the concentration of active drug in plasma. The terms *drug level* or *drug concentration* refer to a concentration of a medication in blood, serum, or plasma. This chapter focuses on the following three major fields of pharmacology as they relate to the practice of anesthesia:

- *Pharmacokinetics,* derived from the Greek words for *drug* and *motion,* refers to the movement of drugs throughout the body and to what the body does to the drug.
- *Pharmacodynamics,* from the Greek words for *drug* and *action,* refers to the effects of drugs on the body. These effects involve the relationship between drug concentration and pharmacologic responses. Pharmacodynamic effects frequently are mediated by interactions between drugs and receptors.
- *Pharmacogenetics* is the study of genetic factors that affect drug disposition.

DRUG DISPOSITION: PHARMACOKINETICS

What Happens After a Patient Receives a Medication?

When administered orally or parenterally, medications usually are first absorbed into the systemic circulation. They are distributed throughout the body, reach a site of action, and produce a pharmacologic response. Finally, they are cleared (or removed) from the body by biotransformation or elimination (Fig. 33–1).

Not all medications are administered systemically, however. For example, local anesthetics may be administered "selectively" to the following sites: epidural space; skin, muscle, or wounds (by infiltration); intra-arterial; interpleural space; peripheral nerves; subarachnoid space; and cornea, skin, or mucosa (by topical application).

Even though a medication may be administered near the site of action, it may still be absorbed systemically and may produce adverse effects. Eye drops containing phenylephrine or timolol may produce clinically significant hemodynamic effects,[1] and those containing echothiophate may impair succinylcholine biotransformation.

How Does the Route of Administration Affect Drug Disposition?

The route of drug administration affects

1. The amount of drug entering the systemic circulation
2. The time of onset and duration of drug effect
3. The peak drug concentration and hence the intensity of the drug effect.

The effect of route of administration on drug concentration is demonstrated for local anesthetics in Figure 33–2.[2]

Drugs administered orally or topically may be incompletely

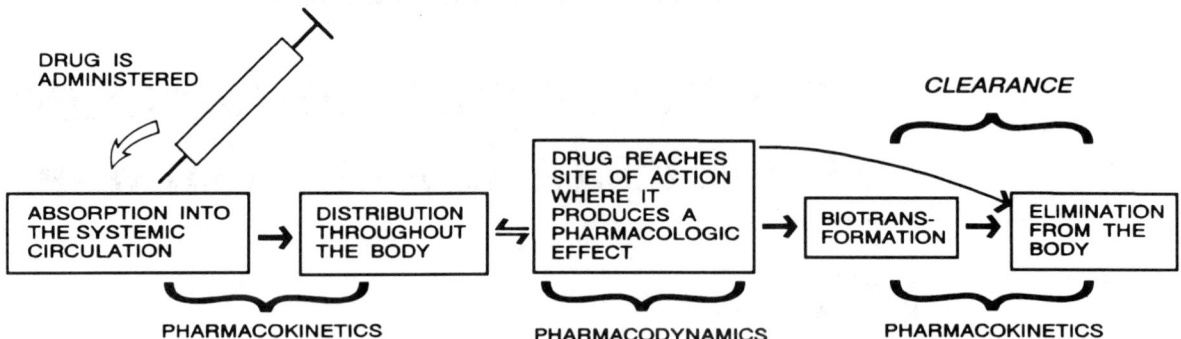

FIGURE 33–1. Pathway of drug distribution and elimination.

absorbed or else metabolized before entering the systemic circulation. Consequently, only a fraction of a given dose of medication may reach the systemic circulation. We define *bioavailability* (F) as follows:

$$F = \frac{\text{amount of medication reaching the systemic circulation}}{\text{amount of medication administered}}$$

Equation 1

The *extraction ratio* (ER) is the fraction of a dose that is cleared from the body before reaching the systemic circulation. The following equation illustrates the relationship between extraction ratio and bioavailability:

$$ER = 1 - F$$

Equation 2

How Is Bioavailability Measured?

A medication is usually administered on separate days by two routes (e.g., orally and parenterally). Multiple drug levels are then measured and plotted against time after administration. The areas under the plasma concentration versus time curves (AUCs) are then determined and corrected for any differences in dose. Bioavailability is determined by comparing the ratio of these two areas (Fig. 33–3). For instance, if

the AUC after oral administration is 25% of that following parenteral administration, the bioavailability is 25%. The bioavailability of parenterally administered drugs is always considered to be 100%.

Why Are Extraction Ratio and Bioavailability Clinically Important?

Consider the following hypothetical problem:

Problem 1. A patient taking the antihypertensive medication labetalol (Trandate or Normodyne) must fast for several days before and after surgery. During this period, you wish to maintain a parenteral dose of labetalol that is comparable to her usual oral dose of 300 mg · day^{-1}. You refer to a pharmacology reference and note that the extraction ratio is 0.75 (i.e., three fourths of a dose of orally administered labetalol is extracted by the liver before reaching the systemic circulation).[2] You then calculate that bioavailability (F) = 1 − 0.75 = 0.25 (Equation 2). In other words, only 25% of a dose of orally administered labetalol reaches the systemic circulation (because of a high first-pass effect by the liver). Therefore, if this patient responds like an average patient, of the 300 mg of labetalol administered orally, about 225 mg (75%) is cleared during the first pass through the liver and 75 mg (25%) reaches the systemic circulation. A reasonable intravenous dose for this patient would therefore be 75 mg · day^{-1} given in divided doses.

Interindividual Variability

Considerable interindividual variability is usually noted in pharmacokinetic parameters such as bioavailability. Interindividual pharmacokinetic differences may be exaggerated by factors such as smoking, age, disease processes, race, hormones, other medications, and even surgery and anesthesia. We can anticipate, therefore, that for a given individual, the appropriate drug dose may change over time, depending on the effects of these other factors; drug responses in patients may be quite different from those in young, healthy, unanesthetized volunteers who are often the subjects of drug studies.

Pharmacologic Responses

A second effect of interindividual variability is that for many drugs, the pharmacologic response is related to the logarithm of the dose (Fig. 33–4). That is to say, clinically significant changes in drug response are often related to orders-of-

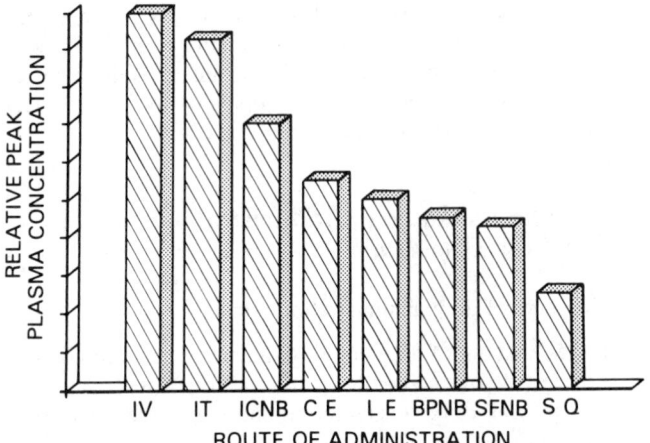

FIGURE 33–2. Effect of route of administration of local anesthetics on peak plasma concentration. IV = intravenous; IT = intratracheal; ICNB = intercostal nerve block; CE = caudal epidural; LE = lumbar epidural; BPNB = brachial plexus nerve block; SFNB = superficial nerve block; SQ = subcutaneous.

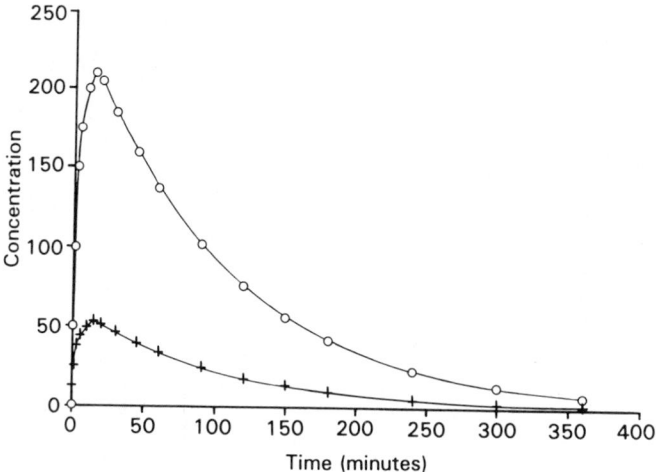

FIGURE 33–3. Plasma concentrations following parenteral (○) and oral (+) drug administration. Bioavailability is determined by the ratio of the areas under the curves.

magnitude changes in dose. Consequently, doses do not always have to be titrated as precisely as we might presume.

Whenever possible, drug dosage should be titrated to response: For example, the response to a peripheral nerve stimulator may be used to guide the dosing of muscle relaxants. Sometimes, however, it is not practical to base drug dosages on pharmacologic response. In these cases, an alternative may be to base dosing on measured drug levels.

> **Problem 2.** What doses of orally administered morphine might be comparable to an intravenously administered dose of 24 mg · d⁻¹? From a pharmacology reference source, you discover that the bioavailability of morphine varies between 10% and 40%.[3] Consequently, in order for 24 mg of a daily oral dose to reach the systemic circulation, an administered oral dose ranging between 60 and 240 mg · d⁻¹ could be required (i.e., 24 mg divided by 0.40 or 0.10, respectively; refer to Equation 1).

Why Should We Be Concerned About Drug Distribution?

Once absorbed into the systemic circulation, a medication distributes throughout the body. Drug distribution is affected by factors such as body composition, regional organ blood flow, protein binding, tissue diffusion, and physicochemical characteristics of a medication. Clinicians are interested in the process of distribution because drug distribution influences two critical determinants of drug response: peak drug concentration and duration of pharmacologic response. Peak drug concentration, in turn, affects the intensity of drug response and of adverse drug effects.

Apparent Volume of Distribution

Although not an actual compartment or volume, the *apparent volume of distribution* (V_D) is a convenient value that can be used to understand drug distribution. Drug dose, *initial drug concentration* (C_0), F, and V_D are related by the following equation:

$$C_0 = \frac{Dose \cdot F}{V_D}$$

Equation 3

Although mathematic relationships such as this one may be intimidating, the implication of Equation 3 simply states that C_0 is increased when a larger dose is administered (more of the administered dose is absorbed into the systemic circulation), and the V_D is decreased (Fig. 33–5).

Half-Life

As indicated, drug distribution also affects the duration of pharmacologic response, often expressed as a *half-life* ($t\frac{1}{2}$). Half-life may be defined simply as the amount of time required for drug concentration to be reduced by 50% (Fig. 33–6). Many drugs have a rapid distribution $t\frac{1}{2}$ and a longer terminal elimination $t\frac{1}{2}$: when the type of $t\frac{1}{2}$ is unspecified, it is usually assumed to be a terminal elimination $t\frac{1}{2}$.

The relationship between $t\frac{1}{2}$ and V_D is shown by the following equation:

$$t\frac{1}{2} = \frac{V_D \cdot 0.693}{Cl}$$

Equation 4

where Cl is drug clearance from the body by all routes and 0.693 represents the natural logarithm of 2. In this equation,

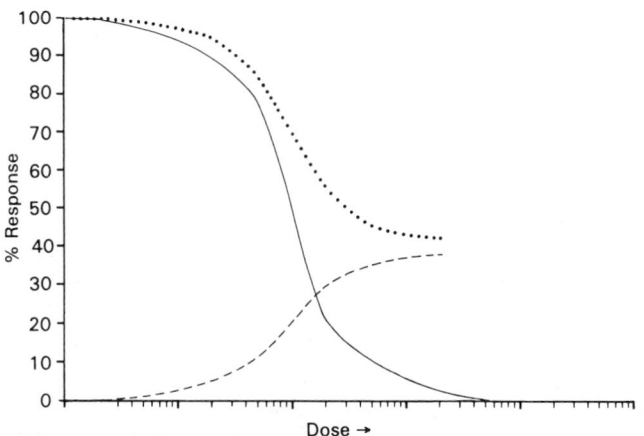

FIGURE 33–4. Pharmacologic responses to some drugs may vary greatly with logarithmic changes in dose.

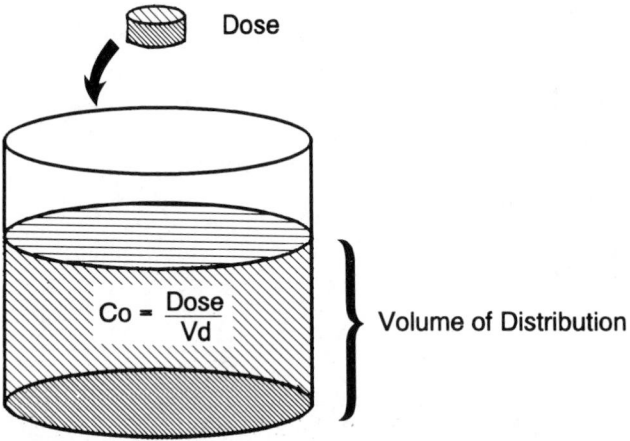

FIGURE 33–5. Relationship among drug dose, initial drug concentration (Co), and volume of distribution (Vd). A larger dose and smaller Vd increase the Co.

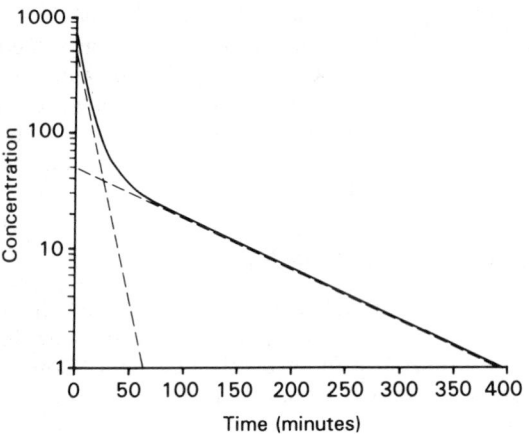

FIGURE 33–6. The half-life of a drug can be represented by a log plot of plasma concentration against time and is defined as the amount of time for the drug concentration to be reduced by 50%.

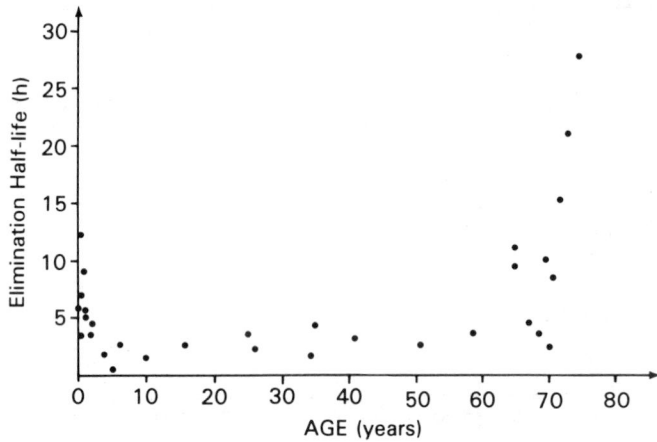

FIGURE 33–8. Increase in elimination half-life in infants (increased V_D) and in the elderly (decreased Cl).

$t\frac{1}{2}$ is a dependent variable, and the V_D and clearance are independent variables.

From this very important relationship, we infer that the only ways to alter the $t\frac{1}{2}$ of a medication are to change the V_D or the clearance. The following examples illustrate the clinical importance of this relationship:

Example 1. Alfentanil (Alfenta) and fentanyl (Sublimaze) are structurally similar narcotic analgesics that have markedly different pharmacokinetic profiles. Specifically, the $t\frac{1}{2}$'s of alfentanil and fentanyl are approximately 90 min and 220 min, respectively.[4, 5] We deduce that for $t\frac{1}{2}$ to be reduced, clearance must be increased or V_D must be decreased. In this case, the large difference in $t\frac{1}{2}$ is due to alfentanil's much smaller V_D.

Example 2. The $t\frac{1}{2}$ of midazolam (Versed) is prolonged in obese patients compared with nonobese individuals. This increase in $t\frac{1}{2}$ is due to an increased V_D (Fig. 33–7).[6] The V_D in turn, is increased because midazolam is a lipophilic drug that has a larger volume in which to distribute in obese patients.

Example 3. The $t\frac{1}{2}$ of atropine is longer in infants or the elderly than in young adults (Fig. 33–8).[7] The increased $t\frac{1}{2}$ in infants is due to a larger V_D of this drug in infants; in contrast, $t\frac{1}{2}$ is prolonged in the elderly because atropine's clearance is decreased in senescence.

Why Do Drugs with Long Half-Lives Often Produce Short-Lived Biologic Effects?

The key to this question is distribution. After administration, drugs distribute throughout the body. As a rule, lipophilic medications rapidly distribute into fat, and only a small portion of the dose remains as unbound (i.e., active or free) drug in plasma. The effect of distribution is most pronounced for the first dose of a medication and for relatively small doses of a medication.

Example. Thiopental is a lipophilic drug with an elimination $t\frac{1}{2}$ of about 5 to 12 hours. The minimum blood concentration that produces a hypnotic effect is higher than the concentration reached after rapid distribution for a small but not a large dose (Fig. 33–9).[8, 9] Therefore, a small dose of thiopental produces a short-lived effect, whereas a large dose or repetitive small doses produce long-lasting effects.

Multiple small doses of thiopental achieve steady-state conditions after three to five $t\frac{1}{2}$ (i.e., 18–60 h). After steady state is reached, as much drug enters as leaves the plasma. In other words, distribution is complete. Therefore, when discontinuing a long-term infusion of thiopental, drug levels decrease at a rate equal to the terminal elimination $t\frac{1}{2}$.

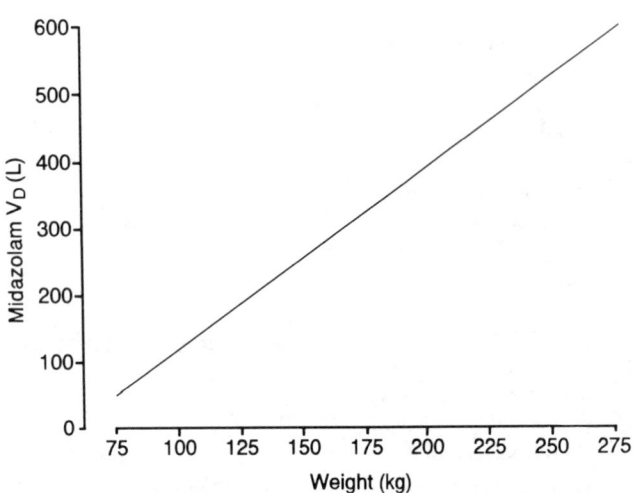

FIGURE 33–7. Prolonged half-life of midazolam with increasing weight owing to increased V_D.

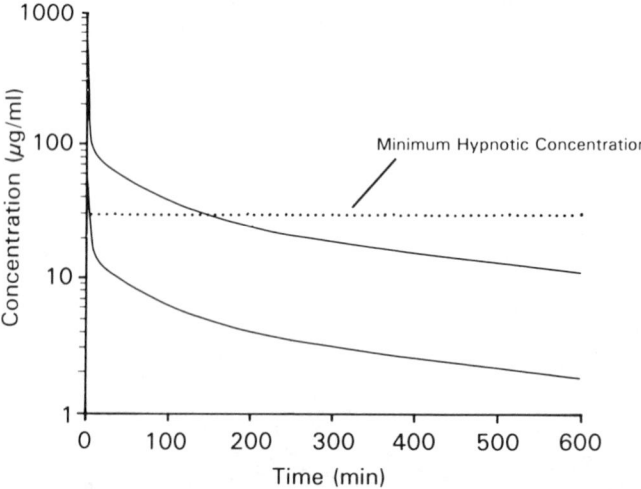

FIGURE 33–9. The effect of rapid redistribution of thiopental (a lipophilic drug) on small and large doses. A small dose quickly falls below the minimum hypnotic concentration, whereas a large dose maintains plasma level above this concentration for a longer period of time.

How Do Changes in Volume of Distribution Affect Water-Soluble Drugs?

When corrected for weight (i.e., when expressed as volume per kilogram), the V_D of water-soluble drugs *generally* is

- Larger in men than in women
- Larger in children than in adults
- Larger in younger adults than in older adults
- Larger in lean individuals than in obese individuals

The basis for these changes is the differences in body composition. In particular, changes in the ratio of body fat to body water may change the V_D of a hydrophilic medication. From the relationship illustrated in Equation 3, we deduce that as V_D increases, peak drug level decreases. The maximum intensity of pharmacologic response parallels changes in peak drug levels; hence, the maximum drug effect usually decreases as the V_D increases. In addition, the t½ increases as the V_D increases (see Equation 4).

> **Example.** Ethanol and succinylcholine are hydrophilic drugs that distribute primarily in body water. After a given dose of alcohol, blood levels generally are higher in older than in younger adults (Fig. 33–10)[10] and higher in women than in men. This fact explains why women or the elderly may appear to be more sensitive to alcohol than young adult men.
>
> Similarly, in the case of succinylcholine, a given dose (in mg · kg^{-1}) usually is associated with lower blood levels in young children than in adults.[11] Hence, the intubating dose of succinylcholine is higher in infants than in adults.

How Do Changes in the Volume of Distribution Affect Fat-Soluble Drugs?

In general, the t½ of lipophilic medications increases as body fat composition increases (because of an increased V_D; see Equation 4). Peak drug levels and hence the intensity of drug effect decrease as body fat composition increases (see Equation 3).

> **Example.** The t½ of the lipophilic benzodiazepine diazepam increases with age owing to age-related changes in body fat com-

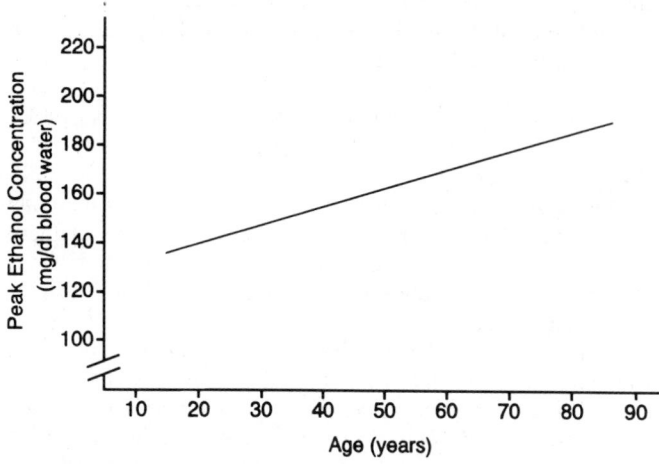

FIGURE 33–10. A given dose of a water-soluble drug such as ethanol will produce a higher blood level in older adults because their ratio of body water to body fat is reduced. Thus, the V_D for water-soluble drugs is reduced.

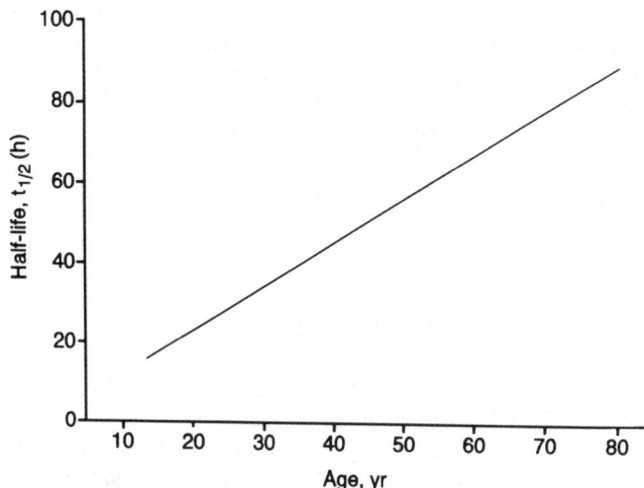

FIGURE 33–11. Increased half-life of diazepam (a lipophilic drug) because of increased fat stores associated with aging. Similar findings apply in obese individuals.

position (Fig. 33–11).[12] For similar reasons, the t½ of midazolam has been found to be prolonged in obese individuals.

How Does Protein Binding Affect the Volume of Distribution?

A drug in blood may be present as free, unbound drug in plasma; taken up into red blood cells and other cellular blood elements; or bound to plasma proteins, especially albumin or α_1-acid glycoprotein (AAG). The latter is an acute phase reactant protein that binds many *basic* drugs, such as propranolol, and many of the local anesthetics. Its concentration may be increased after trauma, infection, myocardial infarction, or inflammation. Albumin, on the other hand, binds many *acidic* drugs such as benzodiazepines, warfarin, and thiopental.

As the degree of binding to plasma proteins increases, less drug leaves the intravascular space; therefore, the V_D decreases.[13] In addition, a smaller fraction of drug exists in plasma in the free, unbound form. We would expect, therefore, that drug concentrations in other organs, such as the central nervous system (CNS), will be decreased as protein binding increases. Conversely, as protein binding decreases, the V_D increases and the free fraction increases.[14]

The net effect of these changes is that the response to a medication decreases as the amount of protein binding increases.

> **Example.** Thiopental is highly bound to albumin. If albumin levels are decreased, we can expect a larger fraction of this drug to be in the free, unbound form in the circulation.[15] More thiopental thus is able to leave the circulation and enter the CNS. We can predict, therefore, that hypoalbuminemic patients will appear to be extremely sensitive to the sedative-hypnotic effects of thiopental.

MEMBRANE TRANSPORT

How Do Acid-Base Changes Affect Transport?

Most drugs enter cells by diffusion of the un-ionized moiety through a lipid membrane. Because medications often are either weak acids or weak bases, the degree of ionization is dependent on the dissociation constant (pKa) of the medication and the pH of the medium. The *Henderson-Hasselbalch* equation demonstrates the relationship between pKa, pH, and the ratio of charged to uncharged forms of a molecule:

$$pKa = pH + \log \frac{[acid]}{[base]}$$

Equation 5

How Does Transport Occur?

Drugs may penetrate cellular membranes by passive diffusion, facilitated diffusion, active transport, or endocytosis. Endocytosis refers to intracellular drug transportation via a vacuolar apparatus. An example of this relatively minor process of drug transport is the intracellular transport of insulin.

In active transport and facilitated diffusion mechanisms, drug transport is mediated by a macromolecule that is saturable and specific for certain molecules. The principal differences between active transport and facilitated diffusion are that facilitated diffusion does not require energy and cannot move a drug from an area of low concentration to an area of high concentration. The source of energy for active drug transport is frequently a sodium-potassium adenosine triphosphatase enzyme.

Fick's Law of Diffusion

Fick's law of diffusion relates the rate of drug diffusion (D) to the temperature-dependent permeability coefficient (P), the area across which diffusion occurs (A), and the concentration gradient of unbound drug across the membrane (ΔC):

$$D = P \cdot A \cdot \Delta C$$

Equation 6

The permeability coefficient is inversely proportional to the thickness of the membrane and the size of the drug molecule; it is directly proportional to the degree of lipophilicity of the medication.

The degree of protein binding also affects drug transport across a membrane. Because only the free or unbound form of a drug is available to cross a membrane, the rate of drug diffusion decreases as protein binding increases. In order for highly ionized or highly protein-bound drugs to cross a membrane, a very large concentration gradient must be achieved.

What Factors Control Placental Drug Transfer?

These principles can be applied to drug transport across the placenta. During a cesarean section, large amounts of thiopental rapidly cross the placenta because this agent is extremely lipophilic.[16] In contrast, relatively little succinylcholine crosses the placenta because this muscle relaxant is highly ionized in plasma. In the case of local anesthetics, the degree of protein binding is an important determinant of whether a particular drug is or is not acceptable for use during epidural analgesia. Bupivacaine, for instance, is acceptable for analgesia during

labor because it is highly protein bound in the maternal circulation.[17]

Fetal Protection

Several important mechanisms help to protect a fetus from drugs present in the maternal circulation. First, the human placenta contains a number of enzymes that are involved in drug biotransformation reactions. In addition, drugs that cross the placenta pass through the umbilical vein and through the fetal liver before entering the fetal circulation. As a result of these two mechanisms, many drugs present in the maternal circulation are biotransformed before entering the fetal circulation.

DRUG REMOVAL

How Are Drugs Removed?

Drug levels in blood or plasma may decrease because of

1. Distribution into other body compartments
2. Biotransformation
3. Elimination from the body

The processes of biotransformation and elimination remove drugs from the body and are referred to as *clearance* (see Fig. 33–1). Elimination denotes the removal of an *unchanged* substance from the body. In contrast, the term *biotransformation* is usually associated with the transformation of a lipophilic compound into a more hydrophilic compound: The hydrophilic metabolite is then more easily eliminated.

Which Organs Are Responsible for Drug Clearance?

The major organs responsible for drug clearance are the liver, kidneys, and lungs; however, other organs may have a role in clearing drugs from the body, including the gastrointestinal tract, sweat glands, and breasts (milk secretion). For drugs that are metabolized, the amount of blood that may be cleared of a drug by an organ is limited by the blood flow to the organ and the intrinsic capacity of the enzymes in the organ to biotransform the medication. By applying *Fick's principle* to drug clearance, we can state

$$Clearance = blood\ flow \cdot ER$$

Equation 7

(See also Equation 2.)

During surgery, drugs may also be removed from the body by nonphysiologic clearance mechanisms. Examples of these mechanisms include blood loss, loss through washing via a cell saver, and absorption or adsorption to the cardiopulmonary bypass circuit.[18]

Clearance values have units of volume divided by time. Clearance signifies the volume of blood or plasma that is cleared of drug per unit time. *The total body clearance is the sum of all the individual clearances.* If, for example, a drug is removed from the blood by the kidneys and liver at rates of 100 mL · min^{-1} and 500 mL · min^{-1}, respectively, then total clearance is 600 mL · min^{-1}.

DOSING REGIMENS

How Are Appropriate Intravenous Regimens Devised?

Three steps are involved in developing a dosing regimen for an intravenously administered medication. Values of the three pharmacokinetic parameters required for this process (target concentration, clearance, and V_D) may be obtained from a pharmacology reference text or the package insert.

STEP 1: *Select a target drug concentration.*

The tacit assumption here is that beneficial and adverse drug effects are related to plasma drug concentrations. Therefore, consider the minimum drug concentration that will produce a therapeutic response and the minimum concentration that will likely produce an unacceptable toxic response. This range of acceptable plasma drug concentrations defines a *therapeutic window* (Fig. 33–12) and presupposes a knowledge of the dose-response effects of a given drug. From the therapeutic window, we can determine the acceptable amount of fluctuations in plasma drug levels.

STEP 2: *Determine the loading dose.*

The loading dose (L_D) may be calculated from Equation 3. For drugs administered intravenously, bioavailability is equal to 1. Therefore, loading dose equals target plasma concentration multiplied by the V_D.

STEP 3: *Calculate the maintenance dose.*

Under steady-state conditions, the amount of drug entering the body is equivalent to the amount being removed from the body and can be written as follows:

$$X_0 = Cl \cdot C_{SS}$$

Equation 8

X_0 is the amount of drug given per unit time, and C_{SS} is the mean steady-state drug concentration. Equation 8 is used to calculate the maintenance dose of a medication. Note that rearrangement of this equation gives the more familiar relationship:

$$C_{SS} = \frac{X_0}{Cl}$$

Equation 9

Example. Consider the case of lidocaine. Values for therapeutic concentration (3 mg $\cdot$ L^{-1}), clearance (0.95 L $\cdot$ min^{-1}) and V_D (90 L) determine the loading and the maintenance doses. Specifically, the loading dose is 3 mg $\cdot$ L^{-1} times 90 L = 270 mg; the maintenance infusion rate is 3 mg $\cdot$ L^{-1} times 0.95 L $\cdot$ min^{-1} = 2.9 mg $\cdot$ min^{-1} ($\approx$ 3 mg $\cdot$ min^{-1}). This loading dose should be given over 15 to 30 minutes, and the infusion commenced when initiating therapy. While a patient is maintained with a constant infusion of lidocaine, the steady-state concentration may be measured after three to five t½s (i.e., after 4.5–7.5 h), and appropriate dosage adjustments may then be made.

The concepts described earlier are not peculiar to pharmacology. In fact, the concept of clearance is found throughout medicine. Note that Equation 7 relates the determinants of clearance, and Equations 8 and 9 illustrate the effect of clearance on the steady-state concentration of a substance.

In What Other Areas Are These Principles Used?

Other examples of these principles include the following:

1. *Oxygen uptake (i.e., Cl)* by the body is the familiar application of Equation 7 (i.e., oxygen uptake is the product of cardiac output and oxygen extraction ratio).

2. The *removal (i.e., Cl) of carbon dioxide (CO_2)* by the lungs is analogous to Equation 9 (i.e., the fraction of CO_2 in blood can be obtained by dividing CO_2 production by minute alveolar ventilation).

3. *Glomerular filtration rate (GFR)* can be determined from creatinine clearance by application of Equation 8. For example, if steady-state serum creatinine concentration is 1 mg $\cdot$ 100 mL^{-1} and the amount of creatinine collected is 1 mg $\cdot$ min^{-1} (or 1440 mg $\cdot$ d^{-1}), from Equation 8, the GFR must be 100 mL $\cdot$ min^{-1}. However, if the GFR is then reduced by 50% but no change in creatinine production occurs, after steady-state conditions are achieved, the serum creatinine concentration must double.

PERIOPERATIVE CONCERNS

What Factors Decrease Clearance?

Clearance is decreased by reducing organ blood flow or inhibiting enzymes that are involved in drug biotransformation (see Equation 7). The following factors may reduce drug clearance in surgical patients:

1. Use of inhalational anesthetics that reduce either cardiac output, liver blood flow, or renal blood flow (e.g., most currently available inhalational anesthetics)[19]

2. Use of inhalational anesthetics that inhibit the activity of microsomal enzymes involved in drug biotransformation (e.g., the effects of halothane on oxidative enzymes located in the liver)[20, 21]

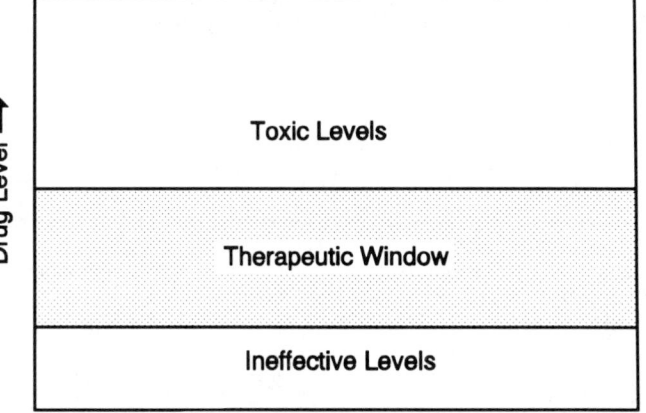

Therapeutic Window

Drug Level →

Toxic Levels

Therapeutic Window

Ineffective Levels

FIGURE 33–12. Schematic representation of the therapeutic window above which an unacceptable toxic response or responses will occur and below which the drug will likely be ineffective.

3. Surgical manipulations that decrease cardiac output or organ blood flow (e.g., cross-clamping the aorta, retracting the liver)

4. Positive-pressure ventilation and positive end-expiratory pressure (PEEP) (reduce cardiac output and renal and hepatic blood flow)[22]

5. Hyperventilation (autoregulatory reduction of liver blood flow)

6. H_2 blockers by either reduction of liver blood flow (e.g., cimetidine) or competitive inhibition of certain enzymes (e.g., cimetidine, which inhibits certain hepatic microsomal P_{450} enzymes; ranitidine, which inhibits the activity of the enzyme alcohol dehydrogenase)[23]

7. Congestive heart failure (reduces liver blood flow)

8. Advanced age (alterations in hepatic and renal function)

9. Malnutrition (reduces levels of certain enzymes that are involved in drug biotransformation) (e.g., pseudocholinesterase)

What Factors Increase Clearance?

In contrast, drug clearance occasionally may be increased when enzymes involved in biotransformation are induced. For example, theophylline clearance is increased by cigarette smoking,[24, 25] and enflurane biotransformation is increased in patients receiving the antituberculous agent isoniazid (INH).[26] Muscle relaxant transformation is increased in patients receiving the anticonvulsant phenytoin. The clinical ramifications of these changes are that maintenance theophylline dose requirements are increased in smokers, and in patients receiving INH, enflurane administration may result in potentially nephrotoxic concentrations of free fluoride ions in plasma (fluoride ion is a byproduct of enflurane metabolism).

How Are Half-Lives, Time Constants, and Rate Constants Related?

Consider the case of an ideal one-compartment system that behaves according to a first-order differential equation. In this system, drug concentration at any given time (C_t) will be related to C_0 according to the following equation (Fig. 33–13):

$$C_t = C_0 e^{-kt} \qquad \text{Equation 10}$$

The rate constant, $-k$, is equal to the slope of the $\log_e$ AUC. Because these data usually are plotted as $\log_{10}$ and not $\log_e$, $-k$ is equal to slope/2.303. This rate constant has units of time^{-1} and indicates the fraction of drug removed per unit time. For instance, $k = 0.01 \cdot \text{min}^{-1}$ means that 1% of the drug is removed from the body every minute.

By definition, if $t = t\frac{1}{2}$, then $C_t/C_0 = 0.5$. Therefore, $0.5 = e^{-kt\frac{1}{2}}$, and $t\frac{1}{2} = \ln2/k$, or:

$$t\frac{1}{2} = 0.693/k \qquad \text{Equation 11}$$

Thus, $t\frac{1}{2}$ is inversely related to the rate constant.

Example. Consider the case of thiopental. If the elimination $t\frac{1}{2}$ of this agent is 12 hours, how much thiopental is removed from the body each hour? Solve this problem by substituting 12 hours for $t\frac{1}{2}$ into equation 11, and $k = 0.06 \text{ h}^{-1}$. Therefore, 6% of the amount of thiopental in the body is cleared each hour.

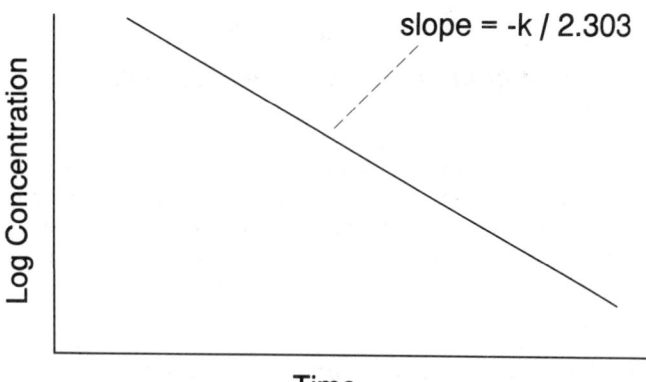

FIGURE 33–13. Logarithmic decline in concentration of administered drug plotted against time from administration according to the relationship $C_t = C_0 e^{-kt}$.

In this model, the time constant, K, is the amount of time equal to $1/k$. (Pay attention to the upper and lower cases: Rate constant = k, time constant = K.) From Equation 10, at time = K, $C_K = C_0 e^{-1} = C_0 \cdot 0.37$. (Recall that e is a number roughly equal to 2.7.) From this relationship, we see that approximately 63% of a drug is removed from this system after a period of time equal to one time constant.

To summarize (Table 33–1):

1. This one-compartment system may be used to model the pharmacokinetics of some but not all drugs.

2. The rate constant indicates the fraction of drug removed per unit time.

3. The rate constant is mathematically related to both $t\frac{1}{2}$ and K.

4. After each $t\frac{1}{2}$, drug concentration is reduced by 50%.

5. After each K, drug concentration is reduced by 63%.

6. The K for a given medication will always be greater than the corresponding $t\frac{1}{2}$.

DRUG ACCUMULATION

After repetitive dosing, all drugs accumulate in the body until steady-state conditions are obtained. The amount of accumulation is determined principally by the dose, the *dosing interval* (DI), the apparent V_D, and clearance. Fortunately, if only the dosing interval and elimination $t\frac{1}{2}$ are combined, the degree of accumulation after multiple dosing can be predicted (Table 33–2).[27]

TABLE 33–1. Comparison of Drug Concentration Versus Half-Life or Time Constant for an Ideal One-Compartment System

Time (Multiple of Half-Life)	Drug Concentration (%)	Time (Multiple of Time Constant)	Drug Concentration (%)
$0 \cdot t\frac{1}{2}$	100	$0 \cdot K$	100
$1 \cdot t\frac{1}{2}$	50	$1 \cdot K$	36.7
$2 \cdot t\frac{1}{2}$	25	$2 \cdot K$	13.5
$3 \cdot t\frac{1}{2}$	12.5	$3 \cdot K$	5.0
$4 \cdot t\frac{1}{2}$	6.25	$4 \cdot K$	1.8
$5 \cdot t\frac{1}{2}$	3.125	$5 \cdot K$	0.7

TABLE 33–2. Degree of Accumulation After Multiple Dosing Based on the Ration of the Dosing Interval to the Elimination Half-Life (DI/t½)

DI/t½	Degree of Accumulation
0.5	3.41
1.0	2.00
2.0	1.33
5.0	1.03

(From Thompson GA: Dosage regimen design: a pharmacokinetic approach. J Clin Pharmacol 1992; 32:210.)

What Are the Primary Determinants?

The following generalizations are useful in understanding drug accumulation:

1. The time to reach steady state is independent of the dosing interval and solely determined by the elimination t½.[27]
2. For practical purposes, steady state will be reached after a period of time equal to three to five elimination t½s.
3. As the ratio of the dosing interval to elimination t½ increases, the degree of accumulation decreases (see Table 33–2).

Example. Consider a patient who receives 10 mg of morphine intravenously every 3 hours. Assume that the t½ of morphine is 3 hours. Three hours after the initial dose, 5 mg of morphine remains (half has been cleared from the body). Immediately after the second dose, 15 mg of morphine is present. Similarly, just before and after the third dose, 7.5 mg and 17.5 mg of morphine are present, respectively; and before and after the fourth dose, 10 mg and 20 mg of morphine are present, respectively. After steady state has been achieved, 10 mg of morphine will be present before and 20 mg of morphine will be present after each dose is given.

Note that the degree of accumulation in this case is 2.0 (see Table 33–2). Accordingly, if a 10-mg dose is administered every 90 minutes (i.e., DI/t½ = 0.5), about 34 mg of morphine will accumulate when steady state has been obtained.

THE RESPONSE TO ANESTHESIA

Drug response may be affected by aging, smoking, disease processes, other medications, nutritional status, surgery, anesthesia, and even mechanical ventilation. Besides these factors, genetically determined differences in drug response are also important in affecting the manner in which a given individual responds to anesthesia.

How Do Genetic Differences Affect Drug Regimens?

Most genetic differences affecting drug response can be accounted for by deficiencies in certain enzymes or proteins. For example, 5% to 10% of all patients do not have the cytochrome P_{450} microsomal enzyme that biotransforms *codeine* to its active metabolites. Consequently, about 1 of every 10 to 20 patients does not have a therapeutic response to this particular narcotic analgesic.[28] Other examples of pharmaco-

genetic conditions that may alter response to anesthesia include the following:

1. *Pseudocholinesterase* is a circulating enzyme that is responsible for the hydrolysis of acetylcholine. Approximately 1 in 3000 individuals has an atypical form of this enzyme and is not able to metabolize substances such as succinylcholine or ester-type local anesthetics.
2. *Acetylation.* Individuals may be classified as either slow or fast acetylators. The manner in which individuals acetylate certain compounds explains the relatively selective toxicity of medications such as procainamide, INH, and hydralazine.[29]
3. *Cytochrome P_{450} enzymes* are a family of hepatic microsomal enzymes that are involved in specific oxidative reactions. These reactions normally transform lipophilic compounds into more hydrophilic substances that may be eliminated by the kidneys. As noted previously, the presence or absence of these enzymes may have an important role in controlling the way individuals metabolize medications. Besides codeine, other drugs that may be affected by genetically impaired cytochrome P_{450} activity include dextromethorphan, caffeine, propranolol, debrisoquin, and mephenytoin.[30]
4. *Ethnic differences.* Many examples of altered drug response due to ethnic differences exist. For instance, Chinese individuals are known to have enhanced sensitivity to β-adrenergic agonists and antagonists.[31, 32] Also, black men are more prone to have essential hypertension.[33, 34] In addition, the low incidence of alcoholism among Japanese may be due in part to reduced activity of enzymes that are involved in alcohol metabolism.[35]
5. *Malignant hyperthermia* (see Chapter 49).
6. *Glucose-6-phosphate dehydrogenase deficiency.* This is one of the most common disorders in the world, with a prevalence of up to 10% among black males and individuals from the Mediterranean littoral.[36] In patients with this disorder, red blood cells are susceptible to drug-induced hemolysis.
7. *Intermittent porphyria.* This condition is inherited in an autosomal dominant pattern and is associated with the absence of porphobilinogen deaminase. Barbiturates may trigger abdominal pain, polyneuropathies, and acute psychiatric disturbances.

CHARACTERISTICS OF DRUG RESPONSE

Most drugs produce their pharmacologic effects by binding reversibly to saturable, stereospecific, membrane-bound receptors.

What Is Affinity?

The degree to which a compound binds to a receptor is termed *affinity*. The importance of the affinity may be demonstrated by the antihypertensive agent labetalol.[37] Labetalol is a compound that has two chiral centers; consequently, racemic labetalol consists of four stereoisomers. Two of these isomers are pharmacologically inactive. One stereoisomer has affinity for β-adrenergic receptors and another for α-adrenergic receptors. The β-receptor effect is greater than the α-receptor response, primarily because the agent that binds to the β-receptor has greater affinity for that receptor than does the one that binds to the α-receptor.

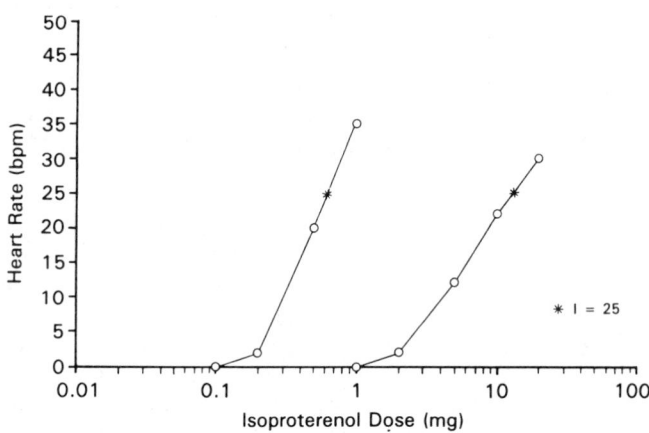

FIGURE 33–14. Efficacy of β-blockade based on response to increasing doses of isoproterenol. *Left,* Responses before blockage. *Right,* Responses after blockade. In these examples, the dose to produce a 25-beat · min⁻¹ (bpm) increase in heart rate is the end point.

What Is Efficacy?

Not all drugs that bind to receptors produce the same type of response. Some drugs produce a maximum response; these drugs are said to have a high degree of *efficacy*. Other drugs produce only a partial response, and some drugs produce no response.

Drugs are classified as either *agonists, partial agonists,* or *antagonists,* depending on whether they produce a maximum, partial, or negligible response, respectively. The degree of response produced by various doses of medication can be depicted by dose-response curves, in which the intensity of drug effect is plotted against the logarithm of the dose (see Fig. 33–14).

> **Example.** Suppose you wished to know whether a patient was adequately β-blocked. You could administer progressively larger doses of isoproterenol and note the dose that produces a 25-beats-per-minute increase in heart rate (I-25).[38] Figure 33–14 compares log isoproterenol dose versus heart rate dose-response curves in a patient before and after β-blocker administration. The degree of β-blockade is related to how far the dose-response curve is shifted to the right. The antagonism of a pharmacologic effect by an antagonist or partial agonist is illustrated in Figure 33–15.

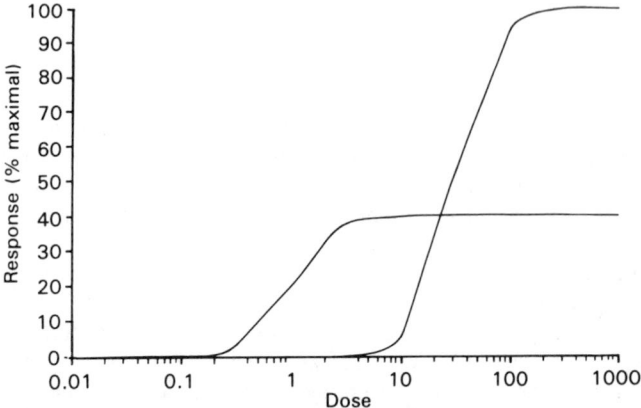

FIGURE 33–15. Antagonism of pharmacologic effect by an antagonist *(left)* or a partial agonist *(right).*

ANESTHETIC AGENTS

What Characteristics Are Important?

Lipid Solubility

The potency of anesthetic agents is related to lipid solubility. The minimum alveolar concentration (MAC) decreases as lipid solubility increases (Meyer-Overton principle). Lipid solubility can be expressed as either a *blood:brain partition coefficient* or as a *blood:oil solubility coefficient.* From the blood:brain partition coefficient, the K for anesthetic uptake by and removal from the brain is determined by dividing the V_D of the anesthetic for the brain by the brain blood flow. Alternatively, K, as was noted previously, may be defined as the amount of time required to produce a 63.2% change in brain anesthetic concentration.[39]

Blood:Gas Partition Coefficient

The blood:gas partition coefficient defines the amount of anesthetic that enters the circulation from the lungs and the amount of anesthetic that moves from the circulation into a closed space. A small blood:gas partition coefficient indicates that very little anesthetic moves from the lungs or an air-filled space into the systemic circulation. Consider what happens when nitrous oxide is administered to a patient with a pneumothorax. Because nitrous oxide is 34 times more soluble in blood than nitrogen, nitrous oxide enters the pneumothorax faster than the nitrogen can leave and enter blood. The result is that the pneumothorax becomes substantially larger.

Boiling Point

The boiling point of the anesthetic determines whether an anesthetic agent is available as a compressed gas or as a volatile liquid.

Vapor Pressure

For volatile liquids, the vapor pressure (which is dependent on temperature) affects the amount of anesthetic that enters the gas phase.

Flammability

The flammability of agents like diethyl ether (ether) or cyclopropane eliminates their use in modern operating rooms.

Minimum Alveolar Concentration

Anesthetic requirements are reduced in the elderly[40, 41] and by CNS depressants such as barbiturates, benzodiazepines, ethanol, and narcotic analgesics.[42] In animal models, anesthetic sensitivity has been found to correlate with CNS catecholamine levels: High CNS catecholamine levels are associated with higher MAC values.[43]

In keeping with this observation, MAC is decreased by medications that deplete CNS catecholamines such as clonidine, α-methyldopa (Aldomet),[44] reserpine,[45] and chronic amphetamine administration.[43] In addition, the anesthetic sparing actions of adenosine may also be due to the antiadrenergic actions of this nucleoside.[46]

In contrast, agents that deplete peripheral but not CNS catecholamine levels (e.g., guanethidine) do not alter MAC.[45] As expected, MAC is increased by acute administration of sympathomimetic agents like amphetamines.

Miscellaneous Properties

Other important characteristics of anesthetics include chemical stability, the need for preservatives to reduce decomposition, and the ability of specific agents to react with metal or soda lime.

ANESTHETIC INDUCTION

How Is the Speed of Induction Changed?

During the induction of anesthesia, a gradient of anesthetic partial pressure develops such that the partial pressure in the lungs exceeds partial pressure in the blood, which exceeds partial pressure in the brain. Increasing the alveolar fraction of an anesthetic produces a greater driving pressure of anesthetic into the brain. Consequently, anesthetic induction is speeded as more anesthetic is delivered to the lungs or less anesthetic is removed from the lungs.

Increased anesthetic delivery to the lungs is caused by

1. Increased minute ventilation[47]
2. Rapid uptake of nitrous oxide, producing a second gas or concentrating effect[48, 49]
3. High concentrations of anesthetic agents (i.e., overpressure)
4. High gas flows or nonrebreathing anesthetic systems
5. Decreased functional residual capacity (FRC) (e.g., in infants or pregnant women)

The rate at which anesthetics are removed from the lungs is decreased as the blood:gas solubility of the anesthetic is decreased or cardiac output is decreased.

ANESTHETIC DRUG SELECTION

Because the practice of medicine is not yet an exact science, this section must be prefaced by saying that the information presented is highly subjective and based as much on experience and philosophy as on scientific reasoning. The goal is to describe (and justify) why certain medications are selected in the course of a routine anesthetic. My basic premise is that the best anesthetic techniques are simple, adaptable, and controllable. Whenever practical, a relatively inexpensive agent is used instead of a more costly agent. Finally, medications are administered by the oral route when possible.

Most anesthetics include a benzodiazepine, an opioid, thiopental, succinylcholine, nitrous oxide, and isoflurane. Propofol is substituted for thiopental and isoflurane for cases that are expected to last <1 hour or for patients with a history of severe nausea and vomiting after anesthesia.

When Is Nitrous Oxide Not Used?

I omit nitrous oxide if intraoperative neurodiagnostic monitoring is used; if patients have severe cardiac disease or an impaired immune system or are donating bone marrow; if a high fraction of inspired oxygen (FIO_2) is indicated; or if induced arterial hypotension will be used. I also avoid nitrous oxide during the first trimester of pregnancy and when diffusion into a closed space could be problematic (e.g., patients with a pneumothorax, pneumocephalus, or bowel obstruction).

Thiopental

Even though the cardiac depressant effects of thiopental are highly questionable, I tend to avoid this agent in patients with impaired left ventricular function or severe coronary artery disease or if they are suffering from multiple trauma. I often substitute etomidate for thiopental for patients with hemodynamic instability and occasionally substitute ketamine for thiopental when inducing general anesthesia in a severely asthmatic patient.

What Factors Guide the Choice of Inhalational Anesthetics?

Enflurane

I never use enflurane (nor, in the future, will others, since it is no longer manufactured). This agent may produce seizures, is less potent than isoflurane or halothane, is a relatively potent cardiac depressant, and may produce nephrotoxic and hepatotoxic adverse effects.[26]

Halothane

I tend to use halothane as an induction agent in children or for certain cardiac patients (e.g., patients with idiopathic hypertrophic subaortic stenosis). Halothane is not used routinely because it is hepatotoxic (admittedly rarely) and sensitizes the heart to the dysrhythmogenic effects of catecholamines.

Isoflurane

My inhalational agent of choice is isoflurane. Unfortunately, it is quite expensive and therefore is used with low gas flows ($<1.5 \text{ L} \cdot \text{min}^{-1}$) as often as possible to reduce the amount administered. Except when washing oxygen into or out of the anesthesia circuit, the total gas flow never is $>3 \text{ L} \cdot \text{min}^{-1}$. This approach is possible because the intravenous induction agents selected gradually wear off during the early maintenance phase of anesthesia; consequently, rapid initial uptake of the inhalational agent after induction is unnecessary.

Why Are Benzodiazepines Used?

Four benzodiazepine-like medications are used in my practice: midazolam, lorazepam (Ativan), diazepam, and triazolam (Halcion). The most useful effects of these drugs are anxiolysis, sedation, amnesia, muscle relaxation, vasodilation, anticonvulsant effects,[50] and prevention and treatment of delirium tremens. They have a better safety profile than do other CNS depressants.

Midazolam

Midazolam is one of the most frequently administered medications. It is often used as a premedicant for pediatric patients (initial dose, 0.5 mg · kg^{-1} orally[51] or 0.2 mg · kg^{-1} intranasally[52]). This agent is not administered by the intramuscular route but is particularly useful for intravenous sedation during regional anesthetic techniques. The muscle relaxant effects seem to help patients tolerate lying still on the operating room table for long periods.

Like other benzodiazepines, midazolam may also offer some protection against the CNS side effects of large doses of local anesthetics (after an intravenous regional anesthetic or after inadvertent intravascular administration of a local anesthetic).

Midazolam is often administered in conjuction with fentanyl to patients with coronary artery disease. The vasodilation produced by benzodiazepines is useful. In these circumstances, a large dose of fentanyl is administered first (e.g., 20 μg · kg^{-1}), followed by 1-mg aliquots of midazolam every 30 to 90 seconds until the systolic blood pressure is between 100 and 110 mm Hg. If this end point is not reached after 10 mg of midazolam, a small dose of thiopental and possibly esmolol is given, followed by tracheal intubation. On the other hand, if this blood pressure is "overshot," phenylephrine (Neo-Synephrine) or "laryngosynephrin" (i.e., laryngoscopy and intubation) is administered for the treatment of hypotension.

Lorazepam

Lorazepam is chosen as an oral anxiolytic for young and elderly adults, when a medication with a long duration of effect is desirable; as a sleep medication; for patients with liver disease; and for treatment or prevention of delirium tremens.

Because lorazepam does not have active metabolites and undergoes glucuronidative (as opposed to oxidative) metabolism, the pharmacokinetic profile is preserved in elderly patients or patients with liver disease.[53] In addition, fewer drug-drug interactions occur with lorazepam than with most other benzodiazepines.

The onset of action is much longer than that of many other benzodiazepines. When used orally, lorazepam should be administered 60 to 90 minutes before the desired effect. After intravenous administration, at least 15 minutes should elapse for maximum effect. This agent is not given intramuscularly because of the pain and erratic absorption associated with this route. Note that lorazepam tablets may be administered sublingually (with considerable cost savings) to many patients.

Diazepam

Diazepam is usually not administered to elderly patients or to patients with liver disease,[54] nor is it given intramuscularly or intravenously because it is too painful. It is absorbed erratically after intramuscular injection. It is occasionally useful orally as an anxiolytic for children and adults.

Triazolam

A one-time dose of triazolam is occasionally given as a sleep medication the evening before surgery. Because of its short duration of action, this agent is less likely than most other benzodiazepines to produce a hangover effect or to interact with medications administered during the intraoperative period.

Why Is Succinylcholine Used?

I administer succinylcholine to facilitate tracheal intubation because of the rapid onset and offset of action; however, several side effects of this agent limit its use.

Absolute Contraindications. Succinylcholine is not chosen for patients with burns <6 months duration, hyperkalemia (potassium >5.5 mEq · L^{-1}), and various neuromuscular disorders (e.g., muscular dystrophies, malignant hyperthermia, and muscle deafferentation disorders such as cerebrovascular accidents).

Relative Contraindications. Succinylcholine is avoided in patients with open eye injuries or intracranial hypertension except in rare cases of difficult airways or emergency procedures in patients with a full stomach.

Minor Contraindications. Succinylcholine is avoided in young muscular individuals or adults who will be ambulatory shortly after surgery. This is the only certain way to avoid postoperative myalgias associated with the drug.

Why Are Defasciculating Doses of Nondepolarizing Relaxants Not Used?

A defasciculating dose of a nondepolarizing muscle relaxant is not given before administering succinylcholine because this therapy does not always prevent postoperative myalgias. In addition, a small dose of nondepolarizing muscle relaxant significantly prolongs the onset and offset of action of succinylcholine. Clinically, patients who receive a benzodiazepine before induction of anesthesia (i.e., most of my patients), as well as pregnant patients, appear to have fewer problems with muscle fasciculations after succinylcholine administration than other patients.

Which Narcotic Analgesics Are Chosen?

Alfentanil

Alfentanil is occasionally used for patients who have severe cardiac disorders and are undergoing short surgical procedures (e.g., a patient having severe coronary artery disease and undergoing direct laryngoscopy).

Morphine

Morphine is the narcotic analgesic of choice for obese patients without sleep apnea syndrome, patients with pulmonary edema, patients with liver disease, and some elderly patients. The pharmacokinetics of morphine are changed less by obesity, liver disease, and aging as compared with other opioids.[55] This stable pharmacokinetic profile is due to the relative hydrophilicity of this compound, as well as the manner in which it is metabolized (primarily by hepatic glucuronidation).[56] Morphine is also the agent of choice for patient-controlled intravenous analgesia.

Fentanyl

In almost all other circumstances, fentanyl is the narcotic analgesic of choice. I administer fentanyl (usually 50–150 μg doses) before anesthetic induction because it blunts airway reflexes and reduces the hypertension and tachycardia associated with laryngoscopy and intubation. Opioids also help to smooth maintenance and emergence from general anesthesia.

For intravenous sedation, a small dose of fentanyl provides analgesia for pain, followed by up to 5 mg of midazolam for sedation. Large doses of narcotic analgesics are not used to produce sedation; the respiratory depressant effects of these medications make this technique dangerous.

Whenever practical, narcotic analgesics are avoided in patients with sleep apnea syndrome, CO_2 retention, or a history of severe nausea and vomiting after narcotics or anesthetics, as well as in patients undergoing middle ear or ophthalmologic procedures.

> **Example.** A healthy 70-kg adult requiring *elective* hand surgery has an axillary block that is "setting up" very slowly. How would you manage this situation?

Because a very large dose of local anesthetic solution has been administered, the block is not repeated. Instead, fentanyl (50 or 100 μg) would be given for any pain that may be experienced, and midazolam would be titrated (1–5 mg) for anxiolysis and amnesia. This person should not leave the operating room thinking that he or she was operated on without anesthesia! If 5 mg of midazolam does not suffice, larger doses probably will not work either. With a partial block, these medications might be all that is necessary. Otherwise, nitrous oxide is added by face mask.

If a patient complains of pain, a small dose of thiopental (usually 1–2 mg · kg^{-1}) is given, followed by isoflurane by mask in doses of 0.4% to 0.6%, end tidal. Ideally, the patient should breathe spontaneously throughout this process, without manual assistance. For long procedures or for patients with difficult airways, I would administer succinylcholine and intubate the trachea before administering nitrous oxide and isoflurane.

Which Muscle Relaxants Are Chosen?

Any patient for whom surgical relaxation is unnecessary is not paralyzed unless a nitrous oxide/narcotic anesthetic technique is being administered or if the patient is unable to tolerate the hemodynamic side effects of the anesthetics. An inadequate anesthetic should not be "covered up" with a muscle relaxant.

Pancuronium

Pancuronium bromide is the nondepolarizing muscle relaxant of choice for most cases lasting more than 90 to 120 minutes; the antimuscarinic effects of this agent, manifested by an increased heart rate, are almost never problematic.

Atracurium

For shorter procedures or for patients with renal insufficiency, atracurium is chosen because of its predictable pharmacokinetic profile.

Vecuronium

Vecuronium is occasionally administered but is not used routinely because it becomes long acting in elderly patients,

patients with liver disease, patients with decreased cardiac output, and patients with reduced liver blood flow (e.g., during upper abdominal surgical procedures).[57]

Other Nondepolarizing Muscle Relaxants

Doxacurium (Nuromax) and pipecuronium (Arduan) are rarely used. In my practice, the clinical advantages generally do not justify these very expensive agents.

When Are Nondepolarizing Muscle Relaxant Reversal Agents Used?

Most of these anesthetics are reversed with neostigmine (2.5–5 mg · 70 kg^{-1}) and atropine (1–2 mg · 70 kg^{-1}). In obese patients, these doses are based on lean body weight. They are not mixed in one syringe because the atropine is drawn up as a resuscitative drug before induction of anesthesia (two syringes of this agent are unnecessary). In addition, poor technique leads to contaminated multidose vials of either atropine or neostigmine.

When Is Glycopyrrolate Indicated?

Glycopyrrolate (Robinul) is not substituted for atropine because the pharmacodynamic or pharmacokinetic differences between these drugs do not appear to be clinically significant. In particular, reliable evidence fails to document that the CNS effects of atropine are a problem in any patient population after general anesthesia. (Editors' note: Clinical experience sometimes suggests otherwise.)

Glycopyrrolate is a useful antisialagogue, particularly in patients placed in the prone position or in those who undergo awake or fiberoptic intubations. It is available in 1- and 2-mg tablets and may be administered orally in (adult) doses of 4 to 8 mg (depending on the desired effect); the dose should be administered 60 to 90 minutes before surgery.

What Is the Indication for Naloxone?

Narcotic analgesics are reversed with naloxone if the respiratory rate is less than eight breaths per minute or the end-tidal CO_2 is >55 mm Hg. In older or debilitated patients, the thresholds for respiratory rate and CO_2 are 10 breaths per minute and 50 mm Hg, respectively.

Should Antacids or Antihistamines Be Adminstered?

Clear, nonparticulate antacids (e.g., sodium bicitrate) are given for pregnant patients or patients with a full stomach who require anesthesia. Antihistamines are not routinely administered. Patients receiving antihistamines are continued on their medication until 1 hour before surgery. H_1 and H_2 blockers are given to patients who might have anaphylactic or anaphylactoid reactions during the perioperative period. The H_1 blocker of choice is diphenhydramine (Benadryl). H_2 blockers are indicated for patients who are at risk of acid aspiration or who have peptic ulcer disease (e.g., burned patients, patients receiving steroid therapy, and patients with severe esophageal reflux).

Is Metoclopramide Useful?

Metoclopramide (Reglan), 20 mg, is occasionally used before surgery when increased gastrointestinal motility is desirable. In usual doses, the antiemetic and gastrointestinal motility effects of metoclopramide are mediated by peripheral cholinergic receptors. Giving metoclopramide after administration of an anticholinergic agent (e.g., atropine or glycopyrrolate) is therefore illogical. Whether metoclopramide therapy can overcome the antimotility effects of narcotic analgesics or inhalational anesthetics is unclear.

Should Flumazenil Be Used to Reverse Benzodiazepines?

Benzodiazepines rarely require reversal because such therapy is not benign; acute abstinence reactions and seizures may occur after flumazenil (Romazicon) administration.[58] Furthermore, the risk of resedation after premature discharge from the recovery area is a potential problem.

Flumazenil is approved for reversal of the sedating but *not* the respiratory depressant effects of benzodiazepines. Physostigmine (Antilirium) and aminophylline have also been used to reverse the effects of benzodiazepines.[59]

Is Doxapram Useful?

There is no reason why doxapram would be indicated during emergence from general anesthesia. However, this agent is useful during fiberoptic intubation of spontaneously breathing patients. In patients who have received a narcotic analgesic, doxapram favorably alters the pattern of respiration—that is, the respiratory rate increases and the tidal volume decreases. The net effect is that patients maintain adequate ventilation while movement of the larynx is minimized.

Other possible uses of this medication include medical treatment of selected patients with chronic obstructive lung disorders. Small doses of doxapram ($0.25 \text{ mg} \cdot \text{kg}^{-1}$) may also be useful for the treatment of severe shivering.

References

1. Mishra P, Calvey TN, Williams NE, et al: Intraoperative bradycardia and hypotension associated with timolol and pilocarpine eye drops. Br J Anaesth 1983; 55:897.
2. Covino BG, Vasallo HL: Local Anesthetics: Mechanisms of Action and Clinical Use. New York, Grune & Stratton, 1976.
3. Gilman AG, Rall TW, Nies AS, et al (eds): Goodman and Gilman's The Pharmacological Basis of Therapeutics. 8th ed. New York, Pergamon Press, 1991.
4. Manufacturer's package insert: Alfenta. Piscataway, NJ, Janssen Pharmaceuticals, 1987.
5. Shafer SL, Varvel JR: Pharmacokinetics, pharmacodynamics, and rational opioid selection. Anesthesiology 1991; 74:53.
6. Greenblatt DJ, Allen MD, Harmatz JS, et al: Diazepam disposition determinants. Clin Pharmacol Ther 1980; 27:301.
7. Virtanen R, Kanto J, Usalo E, et al: Pharmacokinetic studies on atropine with special reference to age. Acta Anaesthesiol Scand 1982; 26:297.
8. Becker KE Jr: Plasma levels of thiopental necessary for anesthesia. Anesthesiology 1978; 49:192.
9. Christensen JH, Andersen F, Jansen JA: Pharmacokinetics and pharmacodynamics of thiopentone: a comparison between young and elderly patients. Anaesthesia 1982; 37:398.
10. Vestal RE, McGuire EA, Tobin JD, et al: Aging and ethanol metabolism. Clin Pharmacol Ther 1977; 21:343.
11. Cook DR, Fischer CG: Neuromuscular blocking effects of succinylcholine in infants and children. Anesthesiology 1975; 42:662.
12. Greenblatt DJ, Abernethy DR, Locniskar A, et al: Effect of age, gender, and obesity on midazolam kinetics. Anesthesiology 1984; 61:27.
13. Wood M: Plasma binding and limitation of drug access to site of action. Anesthesiology 1991; 75:721.
14. Marathe PH, Shen DD, Artru AA, et al: Effect of serum protein binding on the entry of lidocaine into brain and cerebrospinal fluid in dogs. Anesthesiology 1991; 75:804.
15. Burch PG, Stanski DR: The role of metabolism and protein binding in thiopental anesthesia. Anesthesiology 1983; 58:146.
16. Kosaka Y, Takahashi T, Mark LC: Intravenous thiobarbiturate anesthesia for cesarean section. Anesthesiology 1969; 31:489.
17. Thomas J, Long G, Moore G, et al: Plasma protein binding and placental transfer of bupivacaine. Clin Pharmacol Ther 1976; 19:426.
18. Holley FO, Ponganis KV, Stanski DR: Effects of cardiac surgery with cardiopulmonary bypass on lidocaine disposition. Clin Pharmacol Ther 1984; 35:617.
19. Reilly CS, Merrell J, Wood AJJ, et al: Comparison of the effects of isoflurane or fentanyl-nitrous oxide anaesthesia on propranolol disposition in dogs. Br J Anaesth 1988; 60:791.
20. Pessayre D, Allemand H, Benoist C, et al: Effect of surgery under general anaesthesia on antipyrine clearance. Br J Clin Pharmacol 1978; 6:505.
21. Reilly CS, Wood AJJ, Koshakji RP, et al: The effect of halothane on drug disposition: contribution of changes in intrinsic drug metabolizing capacity and hepatic blood flow. Anesthesiology 1985; 63:70.
22. Perkins MW, Dasta JF, DeHaven B, et al: A model to decrease hepatic blood flow and cardiac output with pressure breathing. Clin Pharmacol Ther 1989; 45:548.
23. DiPadova C, Roine R, Frezza M, et al: Effects of ranitidine on blood alcohol levels after ethanol ingestion. JAMA 1992; 267:83.
24. Vestal RE, Wood AJJ: Influence of age and smoking on drug kinetics in man. Clin Pharmacokinet 1980; 5:309.
25. Bukowskyj M, Nakatsu K, Munt PW: Theophylline reassessed. Ann Intern Med 1984; 101:63.
26. Mazze RI, Woodruff RE, Heerdt ME: Isoniazid-induced enflurane defluorination in humans. Anesthesiology 1982; 57:5.
27. Thompson GA: Dosage regimen design: a pharmacokinetic approach. J Clin Pharmacol 1992; 32:210.
28. Chen ZR, Somogyi AA, Reynolds G, et al: Disposition and metabolism of codeine after single and chronic doses in one poor and seven extensive metabolisers. Br J Clin Pharmacol 1991; 31:381.
29. Uetrecht JD, Woosley RL: Acetylator phenotype and lupus erythematosus. Clin Pharmacokinet 1981; 6:118.
30. Gonzalez FJ, Meyer UA: Molecular genetics of the debrisoquin-sparteine polymorphism. Clin Pharmacol Ther 1991; 50:233.
31. Zhou HH, Koshakji RP, Silberstein DJ, et al: Racial differences in drug response. Altered sensitivity to and clearance of propranolol in men of Chinese descent as compared with American whites. N Engl J Med 1989; 320:565.
32. Wood AJJ, Zhou HH: Ethnic differences in drug disposition and responsiveness. Clin Pharmacokinet 1991; 20:350.
33. Talmers FN, Cushman WC, Schnaper H, et al: Comparison of propranolol and hydrochlorothiazide for the initial treatment of hyertension. JAMA 1982; 248:1996.
34. Falkner B: Differences in blacks and whites with essential hypertension: biochemistry and endocrine. Hypertension 1990; 15:681.
35. Guttendorf RJ, Wedlund PJ: Genetic aspects of drug disposition and therapeutics. J Clin Pharmacol 1992; 32:107.
36. Schrier SL: Anemia: hemolysis. In Scientific American Medicine. Rubenstein E, Federman DD (eds). New York, Scientific American, 1988, pp 5, IV, 10–12.
37. Louis WJ, McNeil JJ, Drummer OH: Pharmacology of combined α-β-blockade I. Drugs 1984; 28S:16.
38. Coltart DJ, Shand DG: Plasma propranolol levels in the quantitative assessment of β-adrenergic blockade in man. Br Med J 1970; 26:731.
39. Lowe HJ, Ernst EA: The Quantitative Practice of Anesthesia. Baltimore, Williams & Wilkins, 1981.
40. Gregory GA, Eger EI II, Munson ES: The relationship between agent and halothane requirement in man. Anesthesiology 1969; 30:488.
41. Stevens WC, Dolan WM, Gibbons RT, et al: Minimum alveolar concentrations (MAC) of isoflurane with and without nitrous oxide in patients of various ages. Anesthesiology 1975; 42:197.
42. Orkin LR, Chen CH: Addiction, alcoholism, and anesthesia. South Med J 1977; 70:1172.
43. Mueller RA, Smith RD, Spruill WA, et al: Central monaminergic neuronal effects on minimum alveolar concentrations (MAC) of halothane and cyclopropane in rats. Anesthesiology 1975; 42:143.

44. Bloor BC, Flacke WE: Reduction in halothane anesthetic requirement by clonidine, an alpha-adrenergic agonist. Anesth Analg 1982; 61:741.

45. Miller RD, Way WL, Eger EI II: The effects of alpha-methyldopa, reserpine, guanethidine, and iproniazid on minimum alveolar anesthetic requriement (MAC). Anesthesiology 1968; 29:1153.

46. Seitz PA, ter Riet M, Rush W, Merrell WJ: Adenosine decreases the minimum alveolar concentration of halothane in dogs. Anesthesiology 1990; 73:990.

47. Stoelting RK, Eger EI II: The effects of ventilation and anesthetic solubility on recovery from anesthesia: an in vivo and analog analysis before and after equilibrium. Anesthesiology 1969; 30:290.

48. Eger EI II: Effect of inspired anesthetic concentration on the rate of rise of alveolar concentration. Anesthesiology 1963; 24:153.

49. Epstein RM, Rackow H, Salanitre E: Influence of the concentration effect on the uptake of anesthetic mixtures: the second gas effect. Anesthesiology 1964; 25:364.

50. Wood M: Intravenous anesthetic agents. *In* Drugs and Anesthesia, Pharmacology for Anesthesiologists. 2nd ed. Wood M, Wood AJJ (eds). Baltimore, Williams & Wilkins, 1990, pp 179–224.

51. Feld LH, Negus JB, White PF: Oral midazolam preanesthetic medication in pediatric outpatients. Anesthesiology 1990; 73:831.

52. Karl HW, Keifer AT, Rosenberger JL, et al: Comparison of the safety and efficacy of intranasal midazolam or sufentanil for preinduction of anesthesia in pediatric patients. Anesthesiology 1992; 76:209.

53. Kraus JW, Desmond PV, Marshall JP, et al: Effects of aging and liver disease on disposition of lorazepam. Clin Pharmacol Ther 1978; 24:411.

54. Klotz U, Avant GR, Hoyumpa A, et al: The effects of age and liver disease on the disposition and elimination of diazepam in adult man. J Clin Invest 1975; 55:347.

55. Patwardhan RV, Johnson RF, Hoyumpa A, et al: Normal metabolism of morphine in cirrhosis. Gastroenterology 1981; 81:1006.

56. Merrell WJ, Gordon L, Wood AJJ, et al: Relative contributions of the liver and kidney to morphine metabolism in the dog. Anesthesiology 1990; 72:308.

57. Lebrault C, Berger JL, D'Hollander AA, et al: Pharmacokinetics and pharmacodynamics of vecuronium (ORG NC 45) in patients with cirrhosis. Anesthesiology 1985; 62:601.

58. Klotz U, Kanto J: Pharmacokinetics and clinical use of flumazenil (Ro 15-1788). Clin Pharmacokinet 1988; 14:1.

59. Gallen JS: Aminophylline reversal of midazolam sedation (Letter to the editor). Anesth Analg 1989; 69:268.

CHAPTER 34

The Preoperative Visit and Premedication

SNO E. WHITE, M.D.

The preoperative visit provides the anesthesiologist with an opportunity to prepare the patient for surgery mentally as well as physically. Numerous studies suggest that patients benefit from a preoperative interview.[1-3] Personal interviews, even those conducted by nonanesthetists, are more effective than only giving patients printed instructional booklets.[2] Does this observation prove that the human factor is important? Or is it more important that counselors adjust their comments to meet individual needs?

PSYCHOLOGIC PREPARATION

The degree and etiology of patient anxiety must be assessed. Most patients face surgery with some trepidation. Certain procedures are especially anxiety-provoking. In a group of 218 patients, 85.7% of those undergoing cancer operations and 79% of those anticipating major genitourologic surgery were anxious as compared with 57.2% of patients undergoing other types of procedures.[1] When 260 other patients ranked their concerns, the number one fear was loss of sight. Diagnosis of cancer and loss of an organ ranked second and third, respectively. The absence of diagnosis and anxiety about pain followed close behind.[4]

How Should Pain Expectations Be Handled?

Allaying anxiety about metastatic disease or functional outcome is not a feasible goal of a preoperative anesthesia visit. Should postoperative pain be discussed, or does mentioning it create undue anxiety and negative expectations? Patients are reassured by the anesthesiologist's interest in their comfort when pain management is a stated priority. Postoperative narcotic requirements are reduced by preoperative counseling and follow-up.[5]

Figure 34–1 shows the amounts by which morphine utilization was decreased when ''special care counseling'' was used. ''Special care'' patients were told that they could control much of their pain by using relaxation techniques such as deep breathing. Reassurance was given that although not all the pain would be relieved by relaxation, the patients could request medication that would help them become comfortable. These

patients were taught that pain was not only normal but controllable and that they could take an active role in controlling it. Failure to appropriately describe expected postoperative discomforts can engender patient dissatisfaction and hostility.

What Is an Appropriate Level of Fear?

An extensive psychologic evaluation and follow-up of patients undergoing elective surgery has related the level of preoperative anxiety (fear) to patient satisfaction.[6] Figure 34–2 shows a significantly higher incidence of dissatisfaction in patients who preoperatively demonstrated a low level of fear. Patients with low levels of fear may have unrealistic expectations as a result of either lack of information or denial.

Although anesthesiologists may not be able to prevent denial, they can correct information deficits. Making the patient with low levels of anxiety aware of postoperative discomfort has several benefits. If subsequent events confirm predictions, confidence is boosted. When predicted postoperative pain is actually encountered, the prepared patient views the pain as a normal phase of recovery rather than a sign of impending disaster or complication resulting from negligence or malpractice. Further, only when the negative aspects of planned surgery are acknowledged can a patient make an informed decision whether to undergo the surgery.

Advance descriptions of perioperative events give patients time to develop coping strategies. Table 34–1 demonstrates the association of different levels of preoperative fear with different coping mechanisms. Extremely anxious patients may not tolerate further anxiety-provoking explanations. These patients do better when the protective resources available, such as the many modalities that provide pain relief, as well as the benefits of the upcoming procedure are emphasized.

Informational discussion alone may not be optimal for any patient, regardless of his or her underlying state of anxiety. In one investigation, simple cognitive coping skills were presented in addition to information and reassurance. This combination improved postoperative coping. Not only was postoperative anxiety diminished, but sedative and pain relief requirements were reduced as well.[7] In this study, patients were told that although most people are somewhat anxious before an operation, they can learn to control their thoughts

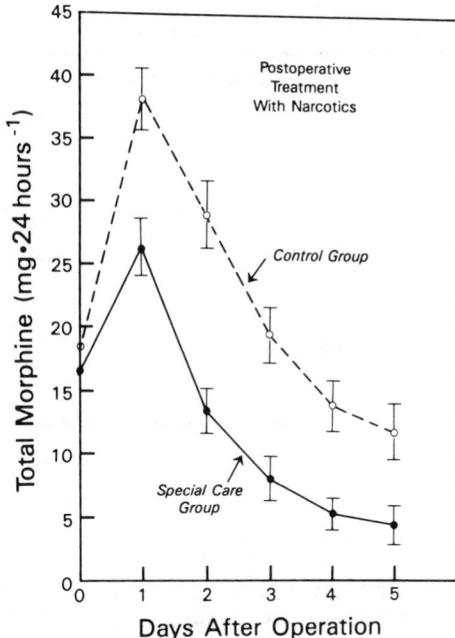

FIGURE 34–1. Ninety-seven patients who were to undergo abdominal surgery were divided into two groups. Each patient in the control group had a preoperative visit during which the anesthesiologist discussed his or her medical condition but did not explain postoperative events. Patients in the special care group were given a careful preoperative explanation about postoperative pain that addressed its character, intensity, and management; it was also stressed that pain was a normal occurrence. The special care group required significantly less morphine for pain relief than did the control group. This finding emphasizes the importance of the preoperative visit in postoperative care. (Reprinted from Egbert LD, Battit GE, Welch CE, et al: Reduction of postoperative pain by encouragement and instruction of patients: a study of doctor-patient rapport. N Engl J Med 1964; 270:825, by permission of the New England Journal of Medicine.)

What Coping Mechanisms Are Useful?

Active participation, demonstration of control over thoughts and physiologic functions, relaxation, and distraction can all be employed.

Active Participation

Patients function better if they consider themselves active participants in their health care team rather than helpless victims of disease. The first step in empowering patients is to ensure that their decision to have surgery means that they consider the benefits worth the expected discomfort as well as the possible risks. In answer to the question, ''Why are you having this procedure done?'' a patient may respond, ''I don't have any choice.'' One can remodel the patient's outlook by suggesting, ''You would like to know more about that growth so that you can make some decisions.'' One may be more succinct by asking, ''What do you hope to gain from this procedure?''

Exercise of Control

Exercise of control is an effective tool in stress tolerance. Perceived control over the delivery of aversive stimuli renders the stimuli more tolerable.[8, 9] Control over even minute details may be helpful for patients in the hospital, since so many variables are beyond the control of the medical team. The functions that patients can control should be emphasized. No matter what the circumstances, patients have control over what they choose to think about and how they view events that occur.

Patients can control the rate and depth of their breathing. Once the technique is demonstrated, control of breathing supports the assertion that other physiologic processes can be controlled as well. Psychologists recommend encouragement such as: ''You can relax now. You are in control. Take a deep breath.''[10] The deep breath that the patient takes reinforces the credibility of the suggestion that the patient is in control and can relax.

Precise wording is important. The simple command ''Relax'' may trigger a mental response of ''I can't.'' The temporal

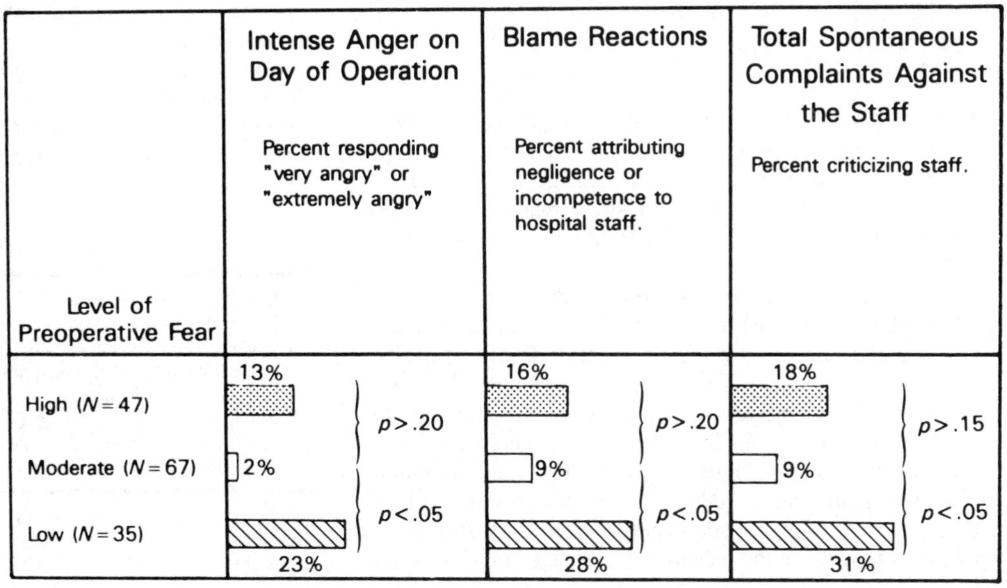

and focus their attention on things they would like to think about. To demonstrate distraction, patients were asked to imagine participating in an exciting sporting event and were asked if they thought they would notice receiving a minor cut. Patients were then asked what they hoped to accomplish by undertaking the proposed surgical procedures. Other benefits were suggested, such as ''the rare opportunity to relax, to have a vacation from outside pressures.''[7]

FIGURE 34–2. Relationship between the level of preoperative fear and subsequent aggressive reactions. (From Janis IL: Psychological Stress: Psychoanalytic and Behavioral Studies of Surgical Patients. New York, John Wiley & Sons, 1958.)

Level of Preoperative Fear	Intense Anger on Day of Operation Percent responding "very angry" or "extremely angry"		Blame Reactions Percent attributing negligence or incompetence to hospital staff.		Total Spontaneous Complaints Against the Staff Percent criticizing staff.	
High (N = 47)	13%	} p > .20	16%	} p > .20	18%	} p > .15
Moderate (N = 67)	2%	} p < .05	9%	} p < .05	9%	} p < .05
Low (N = 35)	23%		28%		31%	

TABLE 34–1. Association of Different Levels of Preoperative Fear With Different Coping Mechanisms*

Coping Mechanism	Level of Preoperative Fear		
	Low (N = 15)	Moderate (N = 21)	High (N = 27)
1. Adopted a joking or facetious attitude	40%	10%	0%
2. Thought that operation would be of a very minor or trivial nature	27%	10%	15%
3. Felt confident in surgeon or gained reassurance from talking with him or her	27%	48%	26%
4. Made effort to learn about the operative procedure or its effects	13%	29%	11%
5. Thought that pains and discomforts would be of short duration or that he or she would be free from medical complications	7%	19%	4%
6. Concentrated on anticipated gains from the operation	7%	19%	4%
7. Plunged into distracting games or fantasies	7%	5%	22%
8. Adopted an attitude of resignation, fatalism, or trust in God	0%	5%	15%
9. Miscellaneous contents	7%	10%	7%

(From Janis IL: Psychological Stress: Psychoanalytic and Behavioral Studies of Surgical Patients. New York, John Wiley & Sons, 1958.)
*The data are based on a content analysis of written answers obtained in a questionnaire survey of 63 major surgery cases.
Note: The percentages add up to more than 100% because some subjects mentioned more than one type of anesthesia.

cue ''now'' suggests that in addition to being able to relax, the patient can choose when to do so. The implications of specific word choice have long been recognized by anesthesiologists who carefully avoid the phrase ''put to sleep,'' which invokes memories of the demise of a beloved pet. Control, in addition to immediacy, is probably an important factor in the success of patient-controlled analgesia infusion devices.

Control is important for children and perhaps even more so for adolescents. Whenever possible, children should be given choices such as on which finger the pulse oximeter probe is placed. Combine challenges such as ''How high can you make those green (end-tidal carbon dioxide) mountains?'' with encouragement such as ''How big can you blow up the balloon? I'll help by adding some extra air.''

Relaxation Exercises

Relaxation exercises suggest that relaxation is a skill that can be developed. One simple relaxation technique is to have the patient tense or flex as tightly as possible the muscles in a very small area, such as in the toes or ankle, maintain the tension for a few seconds, and then release the tension and feel the difference. Doing this exercise, the patient can, on his or her own, start with the toes and progress through the body up to the facial muscles.

Mental Distraction

Subjects given a means of mental distraction have a higher level of tolerance for adverse conditions.[11] Distraction can take the form of selective attention, guided imagery, music, or the progressive relaxation described. A stress management adage is, ''Don't think about fear, just think about what you have to do.''[10]

Therapeutic benefit is derived from review with a patient of just what he or she does have to do. For example, on emergence, a patient needs to wake up, breathe deeply, and communicate his or her needs to receptive personnel. To speed recovery, patients must exert themselves with incentive spirometry and ambulation. By selectively attending to these tasks, they will be less bothered by anxiety and discomfort. Anesthesiologists can introduce these concepts as well as guided imagery. On induction and at other stressful times, what environment can the patient imagine that would be soothing and reassuring? Anesthesiologists can rehearse their role as facilitators when patients envision as many details as possible of their selected escape. Patients may want to bring a tape of some favorite music or programmed relaxation (Table 34–2).

PHARMACOLOGIC EVALUATION

When Are Pharmacologic Anxiolytics Indicated?

Patients who have much to gain from their operations can realistically learn to envision a positive outcome and concentrate on that goal to help tolerate stressful and painful procedures. However, patients facing disfiguring operations for palliation of incurable diseases may have less optimistic outcomes to consider. The prospect of an ostomy, limb loss, or mastectomy does not provide a favorable focus. A benzodiazepine may allow temporary distraction, although it interferes with the concentration necessary for guided imagery.

Patients with extremely high levels of anxiety may benefit greatly from anxiolytics. Small children given benzodiazepines are more likely to find a facemask acceptable. Anxiolytics can ease invasive catheter placement prior to induction and prevent anxiety-induced myocardial ischemia. On the other hand, pharmacologic depression of mental status is disadvantageous for the patient undergoing carotid endarterectomy or intracranial surgery, in which immediate postoperative neurologic status influences further management (Table 34–3).

TABLE 34–2. Psychologic Approach

1. Determine expectations
2. Assess anxiety, its level, and its cause
3. Correct information deficits
4. Describe pain relief modalities
5. Solicit active participation
   • Induction: Select ''escape,'' music
   • Emergence: Spirometry, ambulation
6. Demonstrate areas of control (breathing, thoughts, muscle tension)

(From Meichenbaum D, Cameron R: Stress inoculation training toward a general paradigm for training coping skills. In Stress Reduction & Prevention. Meichenbaum D, Jaremko ME (eds). New York, Plenum Press, 1983.)

TABLE 34–3. When Is Premedication Dangerous?

Extremes of age (less than 1 y or over 80 y)
Decreased level of consciousness
Increased intracranial pressure
Caution: (In the presence of) hypoxia, impaired ventilatory
    drive, chronic obstructive pulmonary disease, cardiac valvular
    disease, or cardiac failure

Lack of premedication may contribute to last minute refusal of surgery. Conversely, premedication, particularly with droperidol, has also been blamed for patient refusal.[12] Profound dysphoria can be induced by droperidol. Patient appearance has been found to be misleading following a variety of premedications.[13] Benzodiazepines are most likely to provide not only the appearance of tranquility but also the subjective sense of it.

What Routes of Administration Are Available?

Intramuscular injection has been the most common mode of premedicant delivery in adults. Complications of this approach include sciatic nerve damage and failure of medication absorption. Ninety-five per cent of injections in women and 85% in men deposit medication into adipose tissue rather than into muscle.[14] Newer oral and intravenous premedications virtually eliminate the need for intramuscular injections. Children particularly hate needles of any kind, usually citing them as the most noxious aspect of hospitalization.

In the days when children were accustomed to having their temperature measured rectally, rectal administration of premedication seemed rational. At present, many children have their temperature measured with heat-sensitive strips or infrared devices. These children may find rectal administration disturbing.

The intranasal approach in children is effective, does not require patient cooperation, has a more rapid onset than does oral medication with drugs such as midazolam, and may be especially useful when administration by the oral route fails.

The hazard to avoid with incremental intravenous sedation is the failure to allow enough time for the drug to take effect before a subsequent dose of it is given. Oral premedications may not have achieved peak effect prior to induction and may be associated with a prolonged emergence phase after short procedures. This phenomenon can be minimized by suctioning the stomach of residual premedication after induction is completed.

BENZODIAZEPINES

The main adverse effects of benzodiazepines are depression of ventilation and interference with normal cognitive as well as fine motor function. For inpatients whose neurologic functions need not immediately return to normal at the end of the surgical procedure and for whom memory of the postoperative period can be ablated, oral lorazepam can be given the morning of surgery in addition to or instead of its dosing the night before. For outpatients, diazepam (orally) and especially midazolam (intravenously) are more appropriate.

How Do Midazolam and Diazepam Differ?

The elimination half-life of midazolam is short (1–4 hours) compared with that of diazepam (20–100 hours). Although aging can increase the half-life of midazolam by as much as 8 hours, advanced age can prolong the half-life of diazepam by several days. Midazolam, like diazepam, is almost completely metabolized by microsomal oxidative enzymes in the liver.

Midazolam and diazepam both have active by-products, but those of midazolam are relatively weak. Both metabolites of diazepam—oxazepam and desmethyldiazepam—clinically prolong sedation. Desmethyldiazepam is only slightly less potent than its parent compound and accounts for the exacerbation of drowsiness that occurs 6 to 8 hours after diazepam administration.

Such facts suggest that midazolam might be a better sedative for the outpatient who needs to be free of residual sedation as soon as possible. In one study, 50 patients undergoing at least 2 outpatient dental procedures served as their own controls, receiving intravenous midazolam sedation for one procedure and intravenous diazepam for the other. Significantly greater amnesia and quicker recovery were associated with midazolam use[15] (Table 34–4; Figs. 34–3 and 34–4).

TABLE 34–4. Dosing and Characteristics of Midazolam, Diazepam, and Lorazepam*

	Midazolam	Diazepam	Lorazepam
Peroral Dose	3–5 mg · kg⁻¹	0.15–0.2 mg · kg⁻¹	0.015–0.03 mg · kg⁻¹
Peak effect	0.5–1 h	1–1.5 h	2–4 h
Duration	1–2 h	2–2.5 h	4–6 h
Elimination half-life	1–4 h	20–100 h	8–24 h
Apparent volume of distribution	1.1–1.7 L · kg⁻¹	0.7–1.7 L · kg⁻¹	0.8–1.3 L · kg⁻¹
Protein binding	94–97%	97–99%	—
Active metabolites	Weak	Strong	None
Metabolism	Hydroxylation Conjugation	Methylation Conjugation	Conjugation Less effect (age/hepatic)
Clearance	6–11 mL · kg⁻¹ · min⁻¹ (50% of hepatic blood flow)	0.2–0.5 mL · kg⁻¹ · min⁻¹	0.7–1.0 mL · kg⁻¹ · min⁻¹
Lipid solubility	High	High	Moderate
Elderly	1 dose 15% per decade	Hours half-life = years of age	Little change

*Intravenous midlatency is 2–3 minutes; frequency of amnesia is 70–80%, with duration of 20–30 minutes.

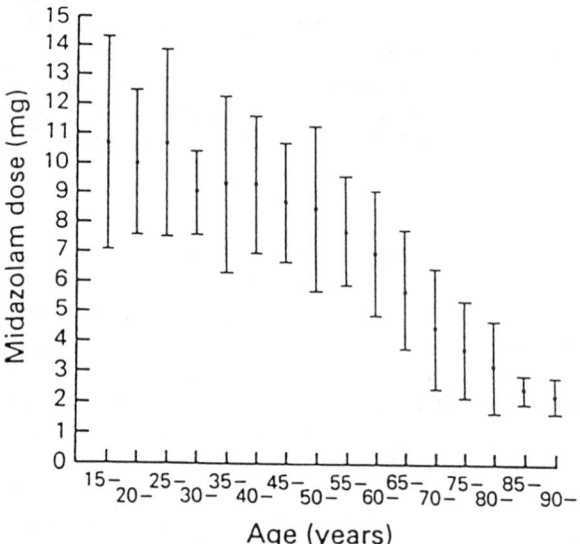

FIGURE 34–3. Relationship between age of patient and the mean dose (±1 SD) of intravenous midazolam required to produce adequate sedation prior to upper gastrointestinal endoscopy. (From Bell GD, Spickett GP, Reeve PA, et al: Intravenous midazolam for upper gastrointestinal endoscopy: a study of 800 consecutive cases relating dose to age and sex of patient. Br J Clin Pharmacol 1987; 23:242.)

Why Have So Many Deaths Been Associated with Midazolam?

Since 83 of 86 deaths reported to the U.S. Department of Health and Human Services occurred outside of the operating room, inattention to ventilation and oxygenation has been cited. Furthermore, in 38% of the patients who died, opioids had been given in addition to midazolam.[16] These facts emphasize the importance of monitoring oxygenation and ventilation after the administration of midazolam[16] and suggest that caution be exercised with the addition of opioids. If opioids are used, the best may be one that combines agonist as well as antagonist properties. Nalbuphine (0.2 mg · kg^{-1}) and midazolam (0.09 mg · kg^{-1}) have been used successfully without respiratory complications in patients undergoing minor oral surgery.[17]

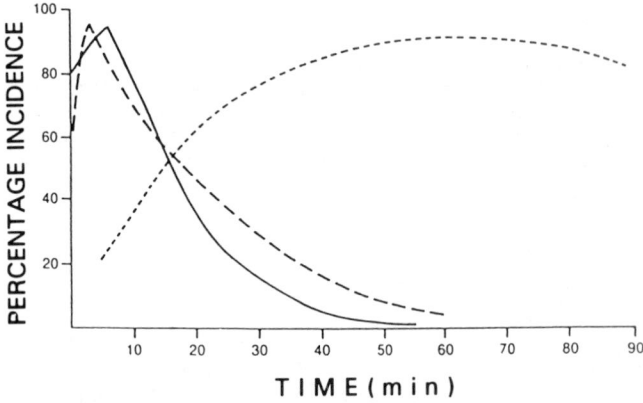

FIGURE 34–4. The extent and duration of amnesia following equipotent intravenous doses of 5 mg of midazolam (*solid line*), 10 mg of diazepam (*large dash line*), and 4 mg of lorazepam (*small dash line*). (From Dundee JW, Halliday NJ, Harper KW, et al: Midazolam: a review of its pharmacological properties and therapeutic use. Drugs 1984; 28:520.)

How Is Midazolam Used in Children?

Oral

Midazolam has revolutionized pediatric induction. No longer present is the worry that the cheerful cooperative child seen preoperatively will develop acute facemask phobia. In the past, intramuscular ketamine offered an alternative solution; now, oral midazolam, 0.5 mg · kg^{-1}, usually prevents the problem. In 80% of cases, 30 minutes after the oral administration of midazolam (0.5 mg · kg^{-1}), the pediatric patient easily separates from the parents and accepts monitors and mask. When the dose of midazolam is increased to 0.75 mg · kg^{-1}, 91% of patients undergo induction without crying or combativeness. The effects of oral midazolam start to dissipate in an hour, and neither of the doses appears to prolong recovery.[18] Palatability, particularly when midazolam is mixed with atropine (0.02 mg · kg^{-1}), is improved when the drugs are mixed with cherry syrup or melted popsicle.

Oral midazolam can be a blessing for children whose parents are extremely anxious and for those younger than 5 years of age who are likely to fear parental separation. It is also helpful for children who can not be psychologically prepared ahead of time, for example, when surgery is urgent or when the child did not attend the preoperative operating room tour.

Oral midazolam is quite useful in situations in which crying and stress may worsen the underlying condition, such as congenital heart disease associated with "tet spells." Many children with congenital heart disease show improvement in oxyhemoglobin saturation following midazolam use. Some, however, may undergo oxyhemoglobin desaturation (3 of 17 children with cyanotic heart disease had a decrease of more than 10% in saturation);[19] pulse oximetry monitoring is critical.

Although crying may worsen airway obstruction, as with epiglottitis or laryngeal papillomatosis, midazolam premedication for the patient with a compromised airway is inadvisable. Resultant apnea could be associated with inability to mask ventilate.

Nasal

Intranasal midazolam, 0.2 mg · kg^{-1}, requires less patient cooperation and has a quicker onset than does oral midazolam. In one study, only 3% of children younger than 5 years of age were crying or combative during induction of anesthesia 15 minutes after intranasal instillation of midazolam.[20] Intranasal administration may be helpful after an oral dose fails. Rarely, midazolam can cause a hyperexcitability reaction. Because of this possibility, some practitioners do not use it for cooperative and prepared children who can separate from their parents and concentrate on guided imagery.

What Can Be Expected from Lorazepam?

Lorazepam is the ortho chlorophenyl derivative of oxazepam, the main metabolite of diazepam. Unlike diazepam, lorazepam has no active metabolic products and has a relatively short half-life (about 15 hours) that is unaffected by patient age. The half-life of diazepam, in contrast, is roughly approximated (in hours) by the patient's age in years. Thus, the half-life of diazepam in a 72-year-old patient is about 3 days.

Why Is Lorazepam Longer Lasting Than Diazepam?

Lorazepam is less lipophilic than is diazepam; thus, it traverses the blood-brain barrier more slowly. However, with oral administration, the onset of action of both diazepam and lorazepam is between 30 and 60 minutes.[21] Lorazepam has less tissue affinity than does diazepam; thus, its effects are not dissipated as rapidly by tissue redistribution as are the effects of diazepam. Psychomotor impairment persists 12 hours after a single dose of lorazepam.[23] Lorazepam undergoes glucuronidation and is then renally excreted. Glucuronide conjugation is faster than oxidation (the elimination pathway of diazepam) and is more resistant to the effects of both aging and hepatocellular disease.

Lorazepam, 2 mg orally (about equal in potency to 10 mg diazepam), produces sedation that lasts 4 to 6 hours. Increasing the dose to 5 mg reliably adds antegrade amnesia that lasts up to 8 hours.[22] Most references suggest limiting the dose to 4 mg, since 40% of patients who received 5 mg were disoriented for as long as 17 hours.[23] Lorazepam is superior to diazepam in preventing recall.

Ten milligrams of oral diazepam provides almost no amnesia. Twenty milligrams of diazepam prevents recall in 30% of patients, whereas 4 mg of oral lorazepam prevents recall in 72%.[21] With intravenous administration, 3 mg of lorazepam impairs recall significantly, whereas 10 mg intravenous diazepam does not.[23]

Lorazepam use may not be advisable for outpatients, but it can be quite beneficial for patients undergoing major procedures followed by intensive care unit monitoring. An advantage for the critically ill patient is that lorazepam causes no myocardial depression or relaxation of vascular smooth muscle even at dosages as high as 9 mg.[22] When a traditional premedication for adult patients with heart disease—intramuscular morphine ($0.1 \text{ mg} \cdot \text{kg}^{-1}$) and scopolamine—was compared with lorazepam, $0.06 \text{ mg} \cdot \text{kg}^{-1}$, given orally 90 minutes prior to surgery, no difference in the levels of anxiolysis and sedation was detected.[24]

MODIFICATION OF GASTRIC CONTENTS

Physiologic preparation for surgery includes pharmacologic emptying and modification of gastric contents. The association of aspiration of gastric contents with maternal mortality represented an anesthetic breakthrough. Intubation of the trachea to protect the lungs from gastric acid has improved the outcome of obstetric anesthesia.

What Drugs Are Useful?

Animal experiments have shown that both volume and pH of gastric secretions are important variables. Hence, the goals of reducing gastric volume below $0.3 \text{ mL} \cdot \text{kg}^{-1}$ and elevating gastric pH above 2.5 have been proposed[25] (Fig. 34–5).

Detrimental pulmonary effects of particulate antacids were demonstrated, and the use of nonparticulate antacids such as sodium citrate was recommended. The ability to decrease gastric acidity without increasing volume became possible with histamine receptor blockade. The gastrokinetic agent metoclopramide was found not only to empty the stomach but also to increase lower esophageal sphincter tone simultaneously.

Who Needs Such Preparation?

With this multifaceted approach for preventing aspiration pneumonitis, the question of who needs it became pertinent. To answer this question, gastric pH and volume were measured in many groups of patients. Alarming results were reported. Gastric volumes $>0.4 \text{ mL} \cdot \text{kg}^{-1}$ with pH <2.5 were identified in 75% of pediatric patients[26] and in 50% of adult outpatients.[27, 28] Various regimens were investigated as was the recommendation that all outpatients receive some pharmacologic prophylaxis. However, despite the magnitude of the "at risk" population, numerous practitioners noted that the actual incidence of aspiration was low. One review of 40,240 anesthetic procedures in children revealed only 4 episodes of aspiration, 2 of which occurred intraoperatively and 2 of which occurred postoperatively.[29]

In a computerized review of 185,358 anesthetic procedures, only 83 cases of aspiration were noted, an incidence of 1 per 2000 cases. Furthermore, in 68 of these 83 cases, conditions associated with delayed gastric emptying (increased intracranial pressure, obesity, history of gastritis or ulcer, pregnancy, extreme pain or stress, emergency surgery, or upper abdominal surgery) were present.[30] Of the 15 cases in which no risk

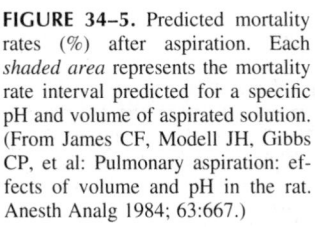

FIGURE 34–5. Predicted mortality rates (%) after aspiration. Each *shaded area* represents the mortality rate interval predicted for a specific pH and volume of aspirated solution. (From James CF, Modell JH, Gibbs CP, et al: Pulmonary aspiration: effects of volume and pH in the rat. Anesth Analg 1984; 63:667.)

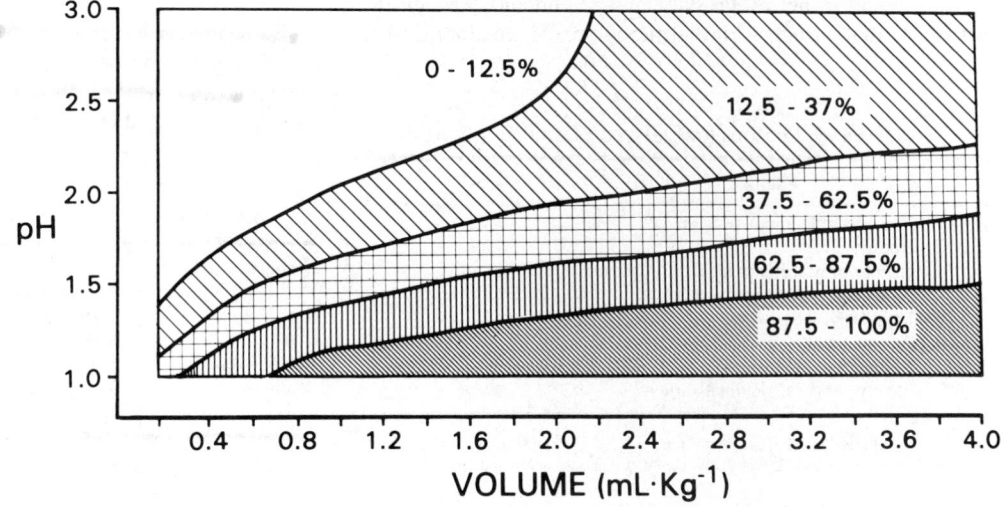

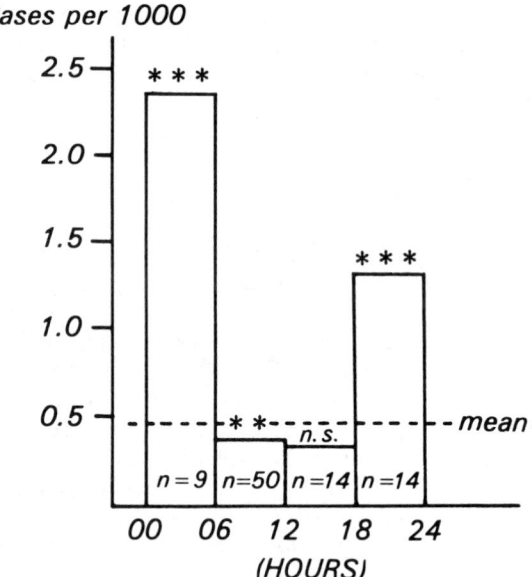

Cases per 1000

FIGURE 34–6. Incidence of aspiration during anesthesia according to the hour of day. n.s. = Difference between this group and the other groups not significant; * = $p < .05$; ** = $p < .01$; *** = $p < .001$. (From Olsson GL, Hallen B, Hambraeus-Jonzon K: Aspiration during anaesthesia: a computer-aided study of 185,358 anaesthetics. Acta Anaesthesiol Scand 1986; 30:86.)

factors existed, 10 involved difficulties with the airway. Timing of surgery was important as well. Operations performed at night carried 6 times the risk of those performed during daylight hours (see Fig. 34–6).

Because of the relatively low risk of aspiration in healthy patients without risk factors who are undergoing elective procedures, routine pharmacologic aspiration prophylaxis is not recommended. However, each patient should be scrutinized preoperatively for risk factors (Tables 34–5 to 34–7).

What Is the Role of Metoclopramide?

Metoclopramide is remarkable in its beneficial effects on the gastrointestinal tract. Prior to its availability, the main drugs used to increase gastrointestinal motility were parasympathomimetic agents such as bethanecol, which is given for postvagotomy gastric atony. Parasympathomimetics cause a diffuse and disorganized increase in intestinal activity that does not result in net progress of gastric contents through the gastrointestinal tract. Furthermore, parasympathomimetic

TABLE 34–5. Reasons for Delayed Gastric Emptying

Factor	Cases
Elevated intracranial pressure	15
Obesity	15
History of gastritis or ulcers	13
Emergency abdominal surgery	8
Pregnancy	7
Pain or stress	6
Nothing but emergency	5
Elective upper abdominal surgery	2

(From Olsson GL, Hallen B, Hambraeus-Jonzon K: Aspiration during anaesthesia: a computer-aided study of 185, 358 anaesthetics. Acta Anaesthesiol Scand 1986; 30:84.)

TABLE 34–6. Which Patients Need Aspiration Prophylaxis?

Anticipated difficult airway
Emergency surgery
Trauma
Depressed level of consciousness (e.g., drug ingestion, head trauma)
  Intestinal obstruction
  Increased intracranial pressure (edema or mass lesion)
  Impaired laryngeal reflexes (bulbar palsy, cerebrovascular accident, multiple sclerosis, Shy-Drager syndrome, amyotrophic lateral sclerosis, vocal cord paralysis)
Obesity (or history of gastric stapling)
History of ulcer disease, partial gastrectomy, or vagotomy (gastric paresis)
Hiatal hernia and reflux
Pregnancy
Upper abdominal surgery
Abdominal tumor or ascites
Other causes of gastric paresis (diabetes, dialysis)

agents increase both the acidity and volume of gastric secretions. Vomiting is a common side effect of bethanecol therapy.

Action

Metoclopramide, a dopamine antagonist, stimulates gastrointestinal motility in an organized fashion. It lowers the pressure threshold required for initiation of the peristaltic reflex, relaxes the pyloric sphincter as it increases antral contractions, and enhances duodenal and jejunal peristalsis. Metoclopramide does not increase gastric secretions.

In addition to emptying the stomach, metoclopramide increases lower esophageal sphincter tone and decreases reflux into the hypopharynx. All its actions decrease the risk of aspiration. Many commonly used anesthetic drugs decrease lower esophageal sphincter tone, as do the antiemetics droperidol and compazine.

Oral metoclopramide should be given 90 to 120 minutes preoperatively in a dose of 0.3 mg · kg^{-1}. Intravenous delivery decreases the onset of action to 3 minutes. Even without intravenous access, the onset of action occurs within 20 minutes of oral administration. In emergency situations, oral metoclopramide is clinically effective in decreasing gastric contents within 15 minutes. Metoclopramide is more effective in emptying the stomachs of children who have sustained trauma than is simply waiting 6 or 8 hours[30] (see Table 34–6).

Complications

Extrapyramidal side effects, including tremor, torticollis, opisthotonos, and oculogyric crisis, occur in about 1% of patients. They are more common in children and when higher dosages of metoclopramide are administered to prevent the

TABLE 34–7. Which Agent for Aspiration Prophylaxis?

Trauma victim	Sodium citrate, 30 mL (alkalinizes stagnant acid)
	Metoclopramide, 20 mg intravenously (empties stomach)
	Ranitidine, 50 mg intravenously
Elective difficult airway	Ranitidine, 150 mg perorally, at 7:00 PM and AM
	Metoclopramide, 20 mg perorally in AM
	Glycopyrrolate, 0.2 mg intravenously*

*To clear secretions for fiberoptic bronchoscopy.

vomiting associated with chemotherapy. Diphenhydramine can ablate these side effects.

Contraindications

Patients taking other dopamine antagonists, monoamine oxidase inhibitors, tricyclic antidepressants, or sympathomimetics should not receive metoclopramide. Metoclopramide has caused hypertensive crises in patients with undiagnosed pheochromocytomas.

MISCELLANEOUS DRUGS

What Are the Indications?

Anticholinergics

Anticholinergics are useful for drying secretions in preparation for awake intubation, procedures for which the upper airway must be topically anesthetized, and bronchoscopies. For children, atropine or glycopyrrolate, orally or intravenously, is indicated to prevent the bradycardia that results from laryngeal stimulation, laryngospasm, and hypoxia. In infants, oral atropine maintains hemodynamics during halothane induction.[31]

Critically ill adult patients such as those with dead bowel or ruptured aortic aneurysm, who can not tolerate an anesthetic of any sort may benefit from intravenous scopolamine, 0.4 mg. A patient who is already maximally catecholamine stimulated and tachycardic usually tolerates scopolamine without a clinically significant further increment in heart rate. If anticholinergic administration (atropine or scopolamine) results in postoperative delirium (since, unlike glycopyrrolate, both compounds cross the blood brain barrier), it is readily treated with physostigmine (antilirium) titrated in 0.6-mg increments.

Narcotics

Narcotics are necessary for patients who are in pain. The rapidity of action of intravenous narcotics is useful for patients for whom the move from stretcher to operating room table will likely be painful (patients with burns, fractures, and ischemic bowels or extremities). The preoperative intramuscular administration of narcotics, a prevalent practice in the past, is becoming uncommon; in many practices, it has been completely replaced by benzodiazepine use.

Clonidine

The centrally acting α-agonist clonidine has been promoted as a premedication for hypertensive patients. Clonidine effectively reduces sympathetic nervous system activity and diminishes cardiovascular responses to intubation and other noxious stimuli.[32, 33] Clonidine may be very useful for the patient with uncontrolled hypertension who requires urgent surgery. However, irreversibly impaired sympathetic responses can interfere both with the identification of hidden volume loss and compensation for it.

Beta-Blockers

Beta-blockers are the drugs most effective for preventing myocardial ischemia. The importance of continuing β-block-

ade in the perioperative period was realized decades ago. More recently, a single-vial dose of a β-blocker has been used as a premedication to decrease the incidence of intraoperative ischemia in hypertensive patients.[34]

SUMMARY

Historically, a premedication was an intramuscular injection of narcotic and sedative administered to facilitate induction. With less noxious modern anesthetics, other goals have emerged. Optimization of the psychologic and physiologic state of the patient requires careful assessment, active patient participation, pain management planning, and selective medication use.

References

1. Egbert LD, Battit GE, Turndorf H, et al: The value of the preoperative visit by an anesthetist. JAMA 1963; 185:553.
2. Leigh JM, Walker J, Janaganathan P: Effect of preoperative anaesthetic visit on anxiety. Br Med J 1977; 2:987.
3. Arellano R, Cruise C, Chung F: Timing of the anesthetist's preoperative outpatient interview. Anesth Analg 1989; 68:645.
4. Volicer BJ, Bohannon MW: A hospital stress rating scale. Nurs Res 1975; 24:352.
5. Egbert LD, Battit GE, Welch CE, et al: Reduction of postoperative pain by encouragement and instruction of patients. N Engl J Med 1964; 270:825.
6. Janis IL: Psychological Stress. Psychoanalytic and Behavioral Studies of Surgical Patients. New York, John Wiley & Sons, 1958.
7. Langer EJ, Janis IL, Wolfer JA: Reduction of psychological stress in surgical patients. J Exp Soc Psychol 1975; 11:155.
8. Corah NL, Boffa J: Perceived control, self-observation and response to aversive behavior. J Pers Soc Psychol 1970; 16:1.
9. Kanfer FH, Seidner ML: Self-control: factors enhancing tolerance of noxious stimulation. J Pers Soc Psychol 1973; 25:381.
10. Meichenbaum D, Cameron R: Stress inoculation training. Stress Reduction & Prevention. In Meichenbaum D, Jaremko ME (eds). New York, Plenum Press, 1983, pp 115–154.
11. Kanfer FH, Goldfoot DA: Self-control and tolerance of noxious stimulation. Psychol Rep 1966; 18:79.
12. Lee CM, Yeakel AE: Patient refusal of surgery following innovar premedication. Anesth Analg 1975; 54:224.
13. Forrest WH, Brown CR, Brown BW: Subjective responses to six common preoperative medications. Anesthesiology 1977; 47:241.
14. Cockshott WP, Thompson GT, Howlett LJ: Intramuscular or intralipomatous injection? N Engl J Med 1982; 307:356.
15. Barker I, Butchart DGM, Gibson J, et al: IV sedation for conservative dentistry: a comparison of midazolam and diazepam. Br J Anaesth 1986; 58:371.
16. Bailey PL, Pace NL, Ashburn MA, et al: Frequent hypoxemia and apnea after sedation with midazolam and fentanyl. Anesthesiology 1990; 73:826.
17. Hook PCG, Lavery KM: New intravenous sedative combinations in oral surgery: a comparative study of nalbuphine or pentazocine with midazolam. Br J Oral Maxillofac Surg 1988; 26:95.
18. Feld LH, Negus JB, White PF: Oral midazolam preanesthetic medication in pediatric outpatients. Anesthesiology 1990; 73:831.
19. DeBock TL, Davis PJ, Tome J, et al: Effect of premedication on arterial oxygen saturation in children with congenital heart disease. J Cardiothorac Anesth 1990; 4:425.
20. Wilton NCT, Leigh J, Rosen DR, et al: Preanesthetic sedation of preschool children using intranasal midazolam. Anesthesiology 1988; 69:972.
21. Kothary SP, Brown ACD, Pandit UA, et al: Time course of antirecall effect of diazepam and lorazepam following oral administration. Anesthesiology 1981; 55:641.
22. Ameer B, Greenblatt DJ: Lorazepam: a review of its clinical pharmacological properties and therapeutic uses. Drugs 1981; 21:161.
23. Heisterkamp DV, Cohen PJ: The effect of intravenous premedication with lorazepam (ativan), pentobarbitone or diazepam on recall. Br J Anaesth 1975; 47:79.

24. Thomson IR, Bergstrom RG, Rosenbloom M, et al: Premedication and high-dose fentanyl anesthesia for myocardial revascularization: a comparison of lorazepam versus morphine-scopolamine. Anesthesiology 1988; 68:194.

25. Olsson GL, Hallen B, Hambraeus-Jonzon K: Aspiration during anaesthesia: a computer-aided study of 185,358 anaesthetics. Acta Anaesthesiol Scand 1986; 30:84.

26. Coté CJ, Gouldsouzian NG, Liu LMP, et al: Assessment of risk factors related to the acid aspiration syndrome in pediatric patients: gastric pH and residual volume. Anesthesiology 1982; 56:70.

27. Manchikanti L, Colliver JA, Marrero TC, et al: Ranitidine and metoclopramide for prophylaxis of aspiration pneumonitis in elective surgery. Anesth Analg 1984; 63:903.

28. Ong BY, Palahniuk RJ, Cumming M: Gastric volume and pH in outpatients. Can Anaesth Soc J 1978; 25:36.

29. Tiret L, Nivoche Y, Hatton F, et al: Complications related to anaesthesia in infants and children: a prospective survey of 40,240 anaesthetics. Br J Anaesth 1988; 61:263.

30. Olsson GL, Hallén B: Pharmacological evacuation of the stomach with metoclopramide. Acta Anesth Scand 1982; 26:417.

31. Miller Br, Friesen RH: Oral atropine premedication in infants attenuates cardiovascular depression during halothane anesthesia. Anesth Analg 1988; 67:180.

32. Ghignone M, Calvillo O, Quintin L: Anesthesia and hypertension: the effect of clonidine on perioperative hemodynamics and isoflurane requirements. Anesthesiology 1987; 67:3.

33. Pouttu J, Scheinin B, Rosenberg PH, et al: Oral premedication with clonidine: effects on stress responses during general anaesthesia. Acta Anaesthesiol Scand 1987; 31:730.

34. Stone G, Foëx P: Myocardial ischemia in untreated hypertensive patients: effect of a single small oral dose of a beta-adrenergic blocking agent. Anesthesiology 1988; 68:495.

CHAPTER 35

General Anesthesia: Induction, Maintenance, and Emergence

J. S. GRAVENSTEIN, M.D.

ROBERT R. KIRBY, M.D.

In a study conducted in 1992, we examined how a preoperative evaluation can influence anesthetic choice and management.[1] In 27% of 2800 patients, features were found that were judged to be important for the anesthetist to know about before he or she started a routine general anesthetic procedure with sodium thiopental, succinylcholine, tracheal intubation, nitrous oxide and oxygen, and isoflurane for maintenance. The most common relevant historical findings are listed in Table 35–1. Other rarer findings that can influence the choice of technique and drugs include conditions such as allergies, diabetes, and hypertension, all of which may require special consideration in the anesthetic management. A review of the data contained in the preoperative evaluation also includes an assessment of the drugs a patient has been given or should have received before he or she is to be anesthetized (see Chapter 1).

PRELIMINARY CONCERNS

What Is Needed Before Inducing General Anesthesia?

A Few Preliminaries

A patient should be asked how long he or she has been fasting (but a patient should not be asked, "When did you have your last meal?"). Examine his or her face and check to see whether intubation is likely to present difficulties. Many patients are now seen preoperatively by someone who likely will not be providing the anesthetic. During the preanesthetic examination, a patient may have been sitting and facing the examiner; in the operating room, he or she is lying down, and such positioning may alter the appearance of the airway and the estimation of how easy or difficult intubation will be. In children and mentally retarded patients, make sure that nothing is in the mouth before inducing anesthesia. Chewing gum or the rubber cap from the plunger of a plastic syringe has been found at the last-minute check.

Dentures

Many patients come to the operating room holding a blanket in front of their mouths because they are embarrassed to be seen without their dental prostheses. In modern anesthesia, it is rather unlikely that the patient will "swallow" or aspirate a prosthesis. Often, we find it acceptable to leave the false teeth in place (to the considerable comfort of the patient) if we believe that not removing the teeth will not hinder anesthetic management. During intubation, dental prostheses often become dislodged and must be taken out; this is acceptable at this point, as the patient is asleep. However, special precautions must be taken to ensure that the teeth are not lost and that they are safely stored postoperatively. Admittedly, it is more convenient for the clinical team if the patient comes without removable teeth. However, before the removal of false teeth becomes a routine preanesthetic requirement, thought should be given to a patient's comfort and dignity.

TABLE 35–1. Common Findings During Preanesthetic Evaluation That Can Affect Anesthetic Technique

Findings	Precautions to Be Taken
Hiatal hernia	Use rapid-sequence induction to prevent aspiration
Asthma	Intubate under deep anesthesia to prevent bronchospasm
Difficult airway	Prepare for alternative to routine orotracheal intubation under direct visualization
Rheumatoid arthritis	Rule out ligamentous instability at Cl-2 with flexion-extension radiograph of cervical spine before submitting patient to routine orotracheal intubation
	Anticipate in 26% of patients the possibility of involvement of the cricoarytenoid joint[2], which may hinder intubation[3]
Stroke	Prevent changes in cerebral perfusion and intracranial pressure

Personal Interaction

Always address a patient by his or her name. If a patient prefers, and relatively few adults object, you can use the first name. Whether you are a man or a woman, do not call a female patient ''honey'' or other similar casual informality. Remember, patients are likely to be afraid; anything you can do to make them feel that they are in competent, professional hands helps to allay their fears.

Just before induction is not the time to present a patient with options. Patients expect you to know what you will do. Explain to him or her what you will do; do not ask for his or her opinion (even if the patient is a professor of anesthesiology!). Anesthesia, even though you administer it daily, is something very special for the individual patient. Options should have been discussed during the preoperative visit, not before the induction of anesthesia.

Tell patients that you will obtain blood pressure and heart rate measurements and other information before you collect it. Comment that the blood pressure is fine (if it is) or that the oxygen saturation is excellent (assuming that it is). Talk with patients so that they do not feel as if they are lying in a factory awaiting their turn in some impersonal and awful process.

When you are about to apply the mask or to inject the first drug, do not ask the patient if he or she is ready. This is a well-meaning phrase on your part, but it leaves some individuals with the unsettling feeling that you expect an intellectual contribution to an undertaking that should be entirely in your expert hands.

Requesting a patient to swallow everything in his or her mouth before starting anesthesia should be omitted if the patient has come dry-mouthed to the operating room. Let those patients with a productive cough clear their throats to remove phlegm poised to drop into the glottis and trigger laryngospasm on induction of anesthesia. Let them clear their throats to spit out what is lodged in the pharynx while they are sitting up, or at least let them turn a little to the side; expectoration is difficult for one who is lying in the supine position.

Equipment Check

Although this subject is discussed elsewhere, it cannot be overstressed that a last look at the anesthesia equipment is essential before it is used. Think about every step you are about to take and about the equipment you will use, from drug injection to intubation; from blood pressure recording to reversal of muscle relaxant; and from tongue blade insertion to emergency drug use. Check the light on the laryngoscope and the cuff on the endotracheal tube. You should have a flashlight ready should the main and emergency power fail (this can and does happen occasionally). Also, you should have emergency equipment handy to insufflate oxygen into the trachea, should this be necessary. If you do not have such equipment ready but find you need it, you will not have time to send someone to get it; it must be within easy reach at all times. Check Chapter 55 for details about what you should have on the anesthesia cart *before* you start a general anesthetic procedure.

Monitoring Before Induction

The anesthesiologist requires baseline data before beginning induction. The patient may have a pulse oximeter–monitored oxygen saturation of only 90%, electrocardiographic evidence of a silent myocardial infarction, or some other unexpected problem that has not yet been detected. The anesthesiologist also needs reference data for comparison should something go wrong during anesthesia, and again for comparison when the patient is discharged from the postanesthesia care unit.

PREOXYGENATION

Why Preoxygenate?

The rationale for preoxygenation or denitrogenation is simple: filling the lungs with oxygen (O_2) gains time should a patient's airway become obstructed during induction of anesthesia.[4] A simple calculation shows that a functional residual capacity (FRC) of 2500 mL filled with air contains roughly 250 mL of water vapor and carbon dioxide (CO_2); 2250 mL of air contains about 470 mL of O_2. Assuming that adult patients at complete rest consume 300 mL of O_2 per minute (and much more, should they struggle), it is not long before they become quite hypoxemic and stop breathing. At this point you cannot ventilate their lungs. Eliminating the nitrogen increases the reservoir of O_2 fivefold and thus generates a grace period of several minutes before a patient becomes hypoxic.

Techniques

Do not start preoxygenation until you are ready to devote your full attention to the task. Some anesthesiologists like to strap the mask to a patient's face and then complete other chores, leaving the patient on his or her own during the preoxygenation. If the mask fits tightly and comfortably, this approach may be acceptable. However, it is even better if you can talk during the preoxygenation period, holding the mask yourself rather than strapping it on the patient. Patients welcome the human contact during this time of high anxiety. More likely than not, a mask held in a hand cradling the patient's face is more comfortable than one secured with the help of a head strap. Finally, when you hold the mask properly, your fourth finger supports the mandible, and the fifth finger rests gently to detect motion of the floor of the mouth during patient talking, swallowing, or retching (Fig. 35–1).

Fresh Gas Flows

Preoxygenation will proceed most quickly if you can provide the O_2 without having the patient rebreathe any expired gas. This means using the highest flow rate of O_2 that the anesthesia machine can deliver (at least when you are dealing with an adult). Figure 35–2 shows computer-generated depictions of body compartments. Observe how long it takes to wash out the alveolar nitrogen to <10% of its original value if a fresh gas flow of 6 L · min^{-1} is administered with a semiclosed system and if the patient is breathing normally. Compare this value with that obtained with an open system (no rebreathing at all) and with hyperventilation. (Figure 35–2 assumes an average adult without lung disease.)

The lesson is simple: deliver enough O_2 to satisfy your patient's peak inspiratory flow rate. Many anesthesia machines will not deliver enough oxygen via the flow meter (it might take 16 L · min^{-1} for an adult) to accomplish this goal, and you must accept some rebreathing; hence, the recommendation

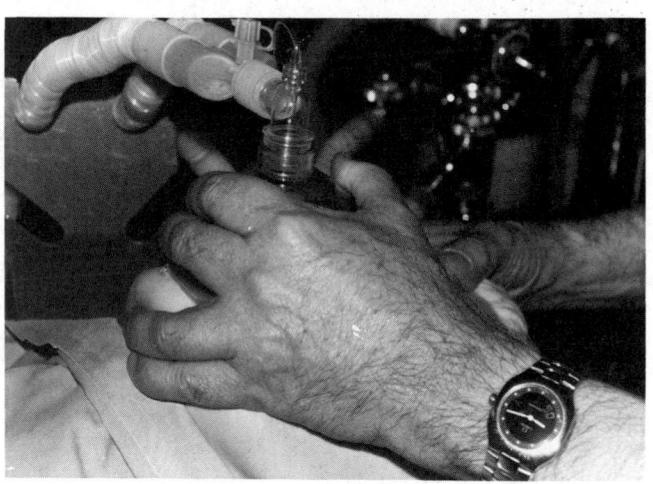

FIGURE 35–1. This photograph shows the position of the hand of the anesthesiologist as it holds a facemask. Observe that the fourth finger supports the chin, whereas the fifth rests gently to feel motion of the floor of the mouth; thus, the fifth finger can detect swallowing, which is often the forerunner to retching and vomiting. Thumb, index, and middle fingers adjust pressure to provide a comfortable but tight fit of the mask to the patient's face.

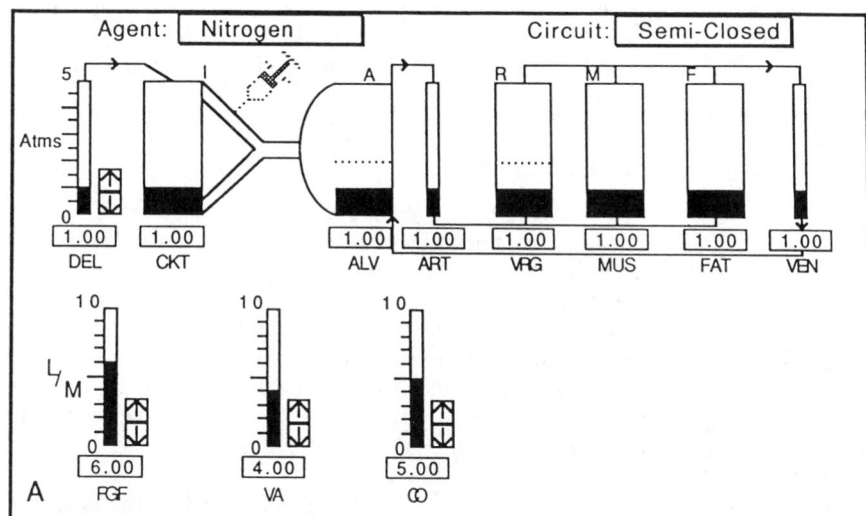

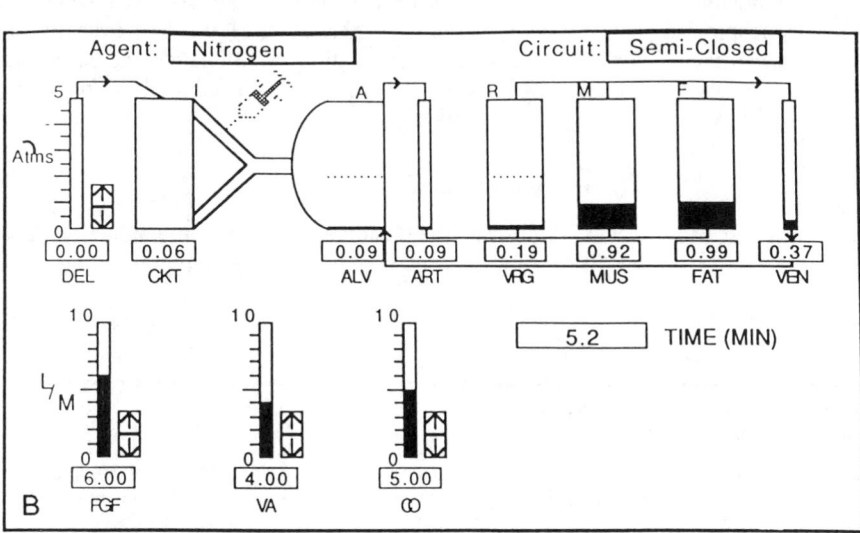

FIGURE 35–2. *A* and *B*, All panels are based on GasMan, a computer simulation of the uptake and distribution of gases in an average adult. The interconnected boxes at the top represent different compartments of the anesthesia machine and body; the numbers under the boxes represent the concentrations of the gases in the compartments. Boxes are blackened according to the concentration of gas in each. From left to right: DEL = the concentration of gases delivered into the anesthesia machine; CKT = the breathing circuit, the volume of which is assumed to be about 7 L; ALV = the FRC, 2.5 L, showing the alveolar concentration of the gas; ART = the arterial concentration of the gas; VRG = the concentration of the gas in the vessel-rich group (about 6 L) which receives 76% of the cardiac output; MUS = the concentration of gas in the muscle group (about 33 L), which receives only 18% of the cardiac output; and FAT = a fat compartment (14.5 L), which receives only about 0.06% of the cardiac output. The lower row of icons: FGF = fresh gas flow chosen by the anesthesiologist; $\dot{V}_A$ = the effective alveolar ventilation; CO = the cardiac output. The box on the right shows the time from the start of the simulation.

A, Before the simulation is started, nitrogen is in equilibrium in all compartments in the body. *B*, The FGF is 6 L · min^{-1}. The patient is assumed to breathe normally with an effective $\dot{V}_A$ of about 4 L · min^{-1}. After 5.2 minutes, preoxygenation is stopped because the concentration of nitrogen in the ALV is <10% of the starting value. Observe that muscle and fat, in particular, still show significant partial pressures of nitrogen. An open system (not shown) prevents rebreathing of any expired gas. The patient hyperventilates to bring the effective $\dot{V}_A$ to 10 L · min^{-1}. Washout of gas from the lungs is much faster. Less than 10% nitrogen remains in the alveoli after only about 0.5 minute. A little more nitrogen remains in the body compartments than in *B*.

is to run the highest O_2 flow rate that the machine can deliver. Ask the patients to breathe as if they are exercising at vital capacity effort (inhale maximally and exhale maximally).

Make sure that there is no leak around the mask. If the breathing bag does not fill completely and if the pop-off valve does not relieve pressure with every exhalation, a leak is present around the mask (of course, you had prechecked the breathing circuit and the mask and you know that they were tight!). When a leak is present, the patient inhales some air (with a large amount of nitrogen) in addition to the O_2 from the breathing circuit.

Has Preoxygenation Reached the Desired Goal?

Do not be satisfied if the pulse oximeter shows 100% O_2 saturation. Check the *exhaled* O_2 concentration. Once it is >90%, you know that most of the nitrogen has been washed out from the lungs. If you cannot monitor exhaled O_2, have patients produce at least three vital capacity breaths (if their lungs are healthy), or allow at least 3 minutes for patients with obstructive lung disease.[5]

INDUCTION OF ANESTHESIA

Table 35–2 gives a general overview of different patterns of inducing general anesthesia. All of these patterns may be modified by borrowing from one another or by substituting other drugs.

When Is Mask Anesthesia Acceptable?

Mask anesthesia is a rational option for relatively brief anesthesia administered to a patient with a freely patent airway who is breathing spontaneously, who is not at risk of aspirating stomach content, and who is positioned so that tracheal intubation can be accomplished with the slightest provocation. In other words, never rely on mask anesthesia when a muscle relaxant (even in a dose that enables the patient to breathe spontaneously) has been given; when the patient has respiratory insufficiency and requires assisted ventilation; when the upper airway is obstructed; and when the patient is in a position other than flat on his or her back with the face in easy reach of the anesthesiologist.

Long anesthetic procedures can be conducted using mask anesthesia, but maintenance of the airway becomes a chore. With fatigue, the clinician may slacken his or her support of the airway, and optimal ventilation is thus jeopardized.

Are Inhalation Induction Techniques Still Useful?

Induction of anesthesia by inhalation through a facemask is the oldest technique and is still used often in children, who abhor needle sticks. This method is discussed in greater detail in Chapter 61. Here is a tip concerning inhalation induction in adults, which is occasionally necessary if the patient has no accessible veins and if a surgical cut-down seems the greater of two evils: if you induce by mask and inhalation, *do not* ask the patient to hyperventilate during preoxygenation, as subsequent minute ventilation will be reduced and uptake of the inhalation anesthetic will be delayed.

Slow Induction

After completing preoxygenation (but before taking the mask off), select a high flow of nitrous oxide and O_2 (for example, 6 L $\cdot$ min^{-1} of nitrous oxide and 2 L $\cdot$ min^{-2} of O_2. Do not administer the nitrous oxide too long, as the patient might become excited. After just a few breaths, begin to add a halogenated inhalation agent. Halothane is the least irritating of these agents, but induction can be accomplished with any agent. Starting nitrous oxide and the halogenated agent together exploits the second gas effect (see Chapter 37). Warn the patient that the gas will smell a little strong. Talk but do not ask questions; it is not easy for the patient to answer with a mask over his or her face.

Three Breath Rule

With every third breath, increase the concentration of the inhalation anesthetic by about 0.125%. The *three breath rule* can help: the first breath gives the gas a chance to reach the patient; the second gives him or her an opportunity to react to it; and the third shows you whether he or she is going to breath-hold, cough, or retch in response to the irritating vapor. If the patient does tolerate the concentration, increase it. If the patient breath-holds, do not take the mask off; instead, wait until he or she once again is breathing normally, and then increase the concentration.

Do not encourage the taking of deep breaths. The patient is able to do so while he or she is responsive (i.e., when the concentration of the anesthetic is still low). However, by the time the anesthetic concentration is sufficiently increased, the patient will have hyperventilation-induced shallow breathing that slows gas uptake.

Manual Ventilation

Do not push on the breathing bag during the induction. You are likely to trigger a cough or laryngospasm. Once you think

TABLE 35–2. Common Patterns of Inducing General Anesthesia

Mask	Intravenous and Endotracheal Inhalation	Intravenous and Relaxant: Endotracheal Inhalation	Narcotic/Relaxant	Rapid-Sequence Induction
Start inhalation anesthetic	Small dose of thiopental, methohexital, or propofol Start inhalation anesthetic Intubation under deep anesthesia	Large dose of thiopental, methohexital, or propofol Inflate lungs Relaxant lubrication	Large dose of narcotic/ tranquilizer Inflate lungs Relaxant lubrication	Large dose of thiopental, methohexital, or propofol, relaxant, and intubation

that the patient is anesthetized (i.e., he or she has regular and perhaps depressed ventilation; no eye movement; and pupils that are moderately dilated [unless you have given a narcotic] and unresponsive to light), manually inflate the lungs with gas containing the high anesthetic concentration. If the patient tolerates this process without breath-holding, he or she is likely to be ready for intubation and certainly for the insertion of an intravenous catheter.

Tracheal Intubation

If you now intubate, remember that the patient is very early in the process of distributing the anesthetic into the different body compartments. Depth of anesthesia, therefore, rapidly decreases as the anesthetic in the vessel-rich group is redistributed to the other compartments that have not yet reached high anesthetic partial pressures. When you remove the mask (remember to turn off the agent delivery so as not to fill the operating room), the depth of anesthesia quickly decreases.

Be swift with intubation. As a rule, if you cannot intubate after one quick exposure of the larynx, do not persist; otherwise, the patient may experience laryngospasm. Take the laryngoscope out while the patient is still breathing spontaneously, reapply the mask, and reinstitute the delivery of high gas concentrations, once again deepening anesthesia. Then repeat laryngoscopy and intubation.

Rapid Induction

Alternatively, you can induce inhalation anesthesia directly with a very high concentration of a vapor, such as 5% isoflurane in O_2. For this technique, you need two systems, one for preoxygenation (e.g., a Mapleson D system with a high flow of O_2) and the other to provide anesthesia (i.e., the anesthesia machine, which stands ready with its system already filled with the desired high concentration of the anesthetic in O_2).

After preoxygenation, ask the patient to take a single vital capacity breath and blow it out down to the residual volume. At this point, switch systems so that the next vital capacity breath that the patient takes fills his or her lungs with the high concentration of the anesthetic. In order to lessen the likelihood of coughing, it may be useful (but not essential) to premedicate the patient with a narcotic.[6]

What Are the Characteristics of Intravenous Induction?

All other induction techniques employ intravenous agents. Intravenous agents have three advantages:

1. They spare the patient the discomfort of having to breathe a smelly vapor;
2. They can provide general anesthesia—alone or in conjunction with other drugs; and
3. They can quickly render the patient ready for tracheal intubation.

They have two disadvantages:

1. They require venous access, although this route is usually available; and
2. They are not as readily controlled as inhalation agents, which can be accurately measured in inhaled and exhaled gas and, if necessary, can be removed actively via the lungs.

When Is a Combination Intravenous/Mask Induction Useful?

This technique slightly modifies slow mask induction. Patients with significant reactive airway disease benefit if intubation is delayed until the bronchial smooth muscles are relaxed and bronchoconstrictive airway reflexes are obtunded. However, the use of an intravenous agent to ease the transition from the inhalation of oxygen to that of halogenated anesthetic is acceptable.

You need give only small amounts of sodium thiopental or other short-acting intravenous agent, such as propofol. A large, intubating dose of the agent (or narcotics) would depress ventilation and slow the inhalation induction. A typical dose for the average patient might be thiopental, 1 to 2 mg · kg^{-1}, or propofol, 200 to 400 µg · kg^{-1}. These doses can be repeated and must be adjusted to each patient's tolerance.

Once a patient is in the surgical stage of anesthesia and still breathing spontaneously, you can intubate. If necessary, you can now employ muscle paralysis to facilitate intubation; however, instead of giving a "usual" intubating dose, such as 1 mg · kg^{-1} succinylcholine, you now need only one-half to one-third of this dose. Remember that halogenated inhalation anesthetics reduce the need for large doses of relaxants.

What Is a Standard Intravenous Induction?

This is by far the most common technique currently in use. A relatively (i.e., adjusted for the patient's physical condition) large dose of thiopental, 4 to 5 mg · kg^{-1}, propofol, 2 mg · kg^{-1}, or methohexital, 2 mg · kg^{-1}, is injected rapidly. Within one circulation period (about 20 seconds), the patient feels the drug's effect and perhaps yawns. About a minute after injection, the lid reflex (gently touch the eye lashes to check it) is absent, ventilation is depressed, and arterial blood pressure is reduced. At this time, test the patency of the airway by inflating the patient's lungs with a few deep breaths (either of O_2 or of O_2 and a potent inhalation agent).

Airway Obstruction

Management of airway obstruction depends on whether the obstruction is due to laryngospasm or to soft tissue obstruction. The two cannot always be easily distinguished. Laryngospasm often comes on suddenly, secondary to irritation of the vocal cords. When the patient can get a little air through the vocal cords, a typical stridorous noise often occurs. High airway pressures often lead to stomach inflation. Soft tissue obstruction of the hypopharynx, if complete, prevents gas entry into the lungs or the stomach. Obstruction of the larynx or trachea due to tumor, trauma, a foreign body, or swelling may be impossible to distinguish from laryngospasm.

Soft Tissue

If the airway obstruction is caused by soft tissue, try simple maneuvers first. Sometimes, insertion of an oral airway is all that is required. However, caution should be exercised: if you insert the airway before adequate anesthesia is established, you may trigger a laryngospasm. A nasal airway may serve equally well, but do not force the nasal tube into the nose; this may cause troublesome nose bleeding.

If neither of these benign attempts helps, and if you cannot visualize the larynx and you cannot intubate, stop all efforts and let the patient awaken from the single dose of the induction agent. Even if momentarily rendered apneic by the drug, the patient is likely to recover muscle tone and, at about the same time, spontaneous ventilation before suffering harm. Here, a well-conducted preoxygenation period demonstrates its benefit by delaying hypoxemia for several minutes.

Laryngospasm

If the obstruction is due to laryngospasm, administer succinylcholine to relax the striated muscle of the mouth and pharynx and to enable tracheal intubation. Do not expect a relaxant to re-establish the ease of manual ventilation if:

1. Bronchospasm exists. Neuromuscular blocking drugs do not relax the airway smooth muscle or any other smooth muscle. Indeed, some relaxants may contribute to bronchospasm by releasing histamine. Start treating the bronchospasm. If it is so severe that you need very high airway pressures to deliver gas into the patient's lungs, let him or her wake up. Then optimize broncholytic therapy and start again when better conditions are present.

2. The obstruction is attributed to anatomic abnormalities or to edema or a tumor that blocks the upper airway. The prudent decision is to let the patient wake up and then to reassess the anesthetic approach. Ordinarily, such problems are discovered during a careful preanesthetic evaluation, and an awake intubation is chosen.

How Is Anesthesia Induced Without a Halogenated Inhalation Drug?

A technique that is gaining favor relies on O_2 and intravenous drugs, including muscle relaxants, and avoids inhalation agents altogether or uses them only as adjuvants. It calls for titration of the intravenous drug until the patient is induced, usually with concomitant depression of ventilation, and requires continuous encouragement of the patient to take deep breaths.

Doses of one of the major tranquilizers (e.g., midazolam) are used in preparation and are followed by sufentanil, ≤ 1 $\mu g \cdot kg^{-1}$; fentanyl, ≤ 10 $\mu g \cdot kg^{-1}$; or alfentanyl, ≤ 100 $\mu g \cdot kg^{-1}$. Some patients develop muscle rigidity after the administration of narcotics. Neuromuscular blocking drugs (e.g., succinylcholine) can be given to overcome this "tight chest" syndrome. Although small doses would suffice to relax the rigid chest, this is usually the time to intubate. Administration of a small dose of thiopental, 2 mg $\cdot kg^{-1}$, or an alternative intravenous induction agent to ensure amnesia may be necessary for intubation.

Instead of induction with narcotics, propofol can be used alone with O_2 or can be supported by narcotics and muscle relaxants as needed. Alternatively, propofol can be given with nitrous oxide, other inhalation agents, and muscle relaxants as required. A typical amount for induction is around 2 to 2.5 mg $\cdot kg^{-1}$, given in divided doses. In elderly or debilitated patients, lower doses are used.

When Is a Rapid-Sequence Induction Indicated?

A rapid-sequence induction (sometimes inelegantly called a "crash induction") is indicated in certain situations (Table 35–3).

Patients at Risk of Aspiration

Patients with Full Stomach

The patient who aspirates stomach contents may suffocate on the spot, or a piece of food may occlude the trachea or a bronchus, with the likelihood of causing first atelectasis and later an abscess. Signs and symptoms are listed in Table 35–4. All patients who, because of an emergency, have not fasted and are coming to the operating room must be suspected of having a full stomach.

Patients with Gastric Juice of Low pH

Patients who give a history of regurgitation, "heart burn," or hiatal hernia fall into this category. All have an incompetent gastroesophageal sphincter and are at risk of bringing the gastric juice (often silently—i.e., without retching or vomiting) into the hypopharynx, from where it can trickle into the larynx or can be aspirated. If enough material reaches the lungs and if it is sufficiently acidic (pH <2.5), lung tissue will suffer a chemical burn, and the so-called Mendelson syndrome will develop[7] (see Table 35–4).

Technique

For a rapid-sequence induction, the Sellick maneuver is used. We do not give a defasciculating dose of a nondepolarizing neuromuscular blocking drug. Such a dose might reduce the patient's ability to deal with reflux while still awake and will delay the onset of the effect of succinylcholine. To counteract that possibility and the antagonistic effects of succinylcholine and the nondepolarizing agent, one would have to give a large dose of succinylcholine, thereby increasing the duration of relaxation.

After preoxygenation, inject an intubating dose of thiopen-

TABLE 35–3. Risk Factors for Pulmonary Aspiration of Gastric Contents

Perioperative	Pregnancy
	Obesity
	Gastrointestinal dysfunction
	Intestinal obstruction
	Emergency surgery
Depressed Level of Consciousness	Head injury
	Drug overdose
	Coma
	Central nervous system infections
	Seizures
Laryngeal Incompetence	Bulbar dysfunction
	Multiple sclerosis
	Stroke
	Muscular dystrophy
	Myasthenia gravis
	Amyotrophic lateral sclerosis
	Vocal cord trauma

TABLE 35–4. Characteristics of Various Types of Aspiration

Particulate Obstruction	Total ("cafe coronary")
	  Inability to speak or breathe
	  Cyanosis
	  Rapidly fatal
	Partial
	  Stridor
	  Tachypnea
	  Wheezing

Particulate Nonobstructive	Tachypnea Wheezing Cyanosis Cough Cardiovascular collapse
Acidic (Liquid pH <2.5)	Tachypnea Dyspnea Wheezing Hypotension, often profound Pulmonary edema

tal, 5 mg · kg^{-1}, or ketamine, 1 mg · kg^{-1}, and immediately follow it with an intubating dose of succinylcholine, 1 mg · kg^{-1} (other relaxant drugs can be used, but none works as fast as succinylcholine).

As soon as the drugs are injected and before the patient loses consciousness, pressure is applied over the cricoid cartilage (the patient should be warned) and maintained until the cuff of the endotracheal tube is inflated and the correct position of the tube is confirmed by capnography (preferably) or by auscultation and other less reliable methods.

The Sellick Maneuver

The method of pressing on the cricoid cartilage to obstruct (not really occlude) the esophagus is not new.[8] It was originally used to prevent the inflation of the stomach with air during mechanical ventilation of the lungs by mask. It is therefore acceptable to ventilate the lungs during the seconds of apnea and before intubation.

Many anesthesiologists do not ventilate during the period of apnea with a rapid-sequence induction because of their fear of pushing gas into the stomach. We believe that gentle manual ventilation is not only acceptable but also preferable, as long as unusual pressures are not required to inflate the lungs (and, thus, presumably the stomach).

Patients Who Are Easy to Intubate

The technique of injecting the intubating doses of thiopental and succinylcholine in rapid succession can be employed in most routine anesthetic procedures. Indeed, an argument can be advanced in favor of the rapid sequence (with or without Sellick's maneuver): if thiopental and succinylcholine are injected together (do not mix them in the same syringe—the thiopental will precipitate!), their duration of action is likely to be about as long as the duration of either one given alone, provided that the patient has normal pseudocholinesterase activity. Hemodynamically, patients seem to fare best if the intubation is accomplished while the peak effects of thiopental and succinylcholine coincide.

Should a Defasciculating Drug Be Given Before Succinylcholine Is Injected?

No! Yet, some anesthesiologists are strong advocates of giving the average adult 3 mg of d-tubocurarine or an equivalent dose of another nondepolarizing agent about 3 minutes before injecting the intubating dose of succinylcholine. They point to studies showing that patients suffer less muscle pain if a defasciculating dose is used. However, almost as many studies report that pretreatment with a defasciculating dose failed to prevent so-called succinylcholine myalgia. Other reasons why we do not favor pretreatment with a nondepolarizing agent are summarized in Table 35–5.

What Should You Do When You Cannot Intubate and Ventilate?

If you have tried all the "tricks of the trade" (see Chapter 55) and absolutely cannot intubate the trachea orally, nasally, blindly, or fiberoptically and cannot ventilate the lungs, even with an oral or nasal airway in place, then:

1. Ask for help. Two persons may be required to ventilate using bag and mask: one to hold the mask with two hands while lifting the patient's chin, and the other to squeeze the bag. Positioning of the jaw is important. Sometimes it helps to lift and push the mandible forcefully forward, thus allowing the lower incisor teeth to be anterior to the upper incisors.

2. If the O$_2$ saturation begins to drift downward into unacceptable ranges below 80%, depending on the patient's physical condition, take steps at once to insufflate O$_2$ percutaneously into the trachea. The necessary techniques are described in detail in Chapter 55.

MAINTENANCE OF ANESTHESIA

A wise Creator has surrounded our vital organs with sensitive coverings. Thus, cutting through skin, dura, and peritoneum or scraping periosteum hurts more than does surgery on muscle, brain, gut, or bone. Consequently, a patient requires more analgesia (anesthesia) during incision and closure than he or she does during the middle of a procedure.

How Should Agents Be Administered?

Because we never fully equilibrate the anesthetic agents across all body compartments, anesthesia should be main-

TABLE 35–5. Defasciculating Pretreatment

Pro	Cons
• In many patients, it reduces postsuccinylcholine myalgia	• In many patients, it fails to reduce postsuccinylcholine myalgia • Nondepolarizing relaxants are antagonistic to depolarizing agents; therefore, succinylcholine dose has to be increased • Onset of succinylcholine action is slowed • Duration of succinylcholine is prolonged • Unpleasant effects of defasciculating dose include diplopia, inability to swallow, and sometimes dyspnea

tained as lightly as possible during the phases in which only moderate analgesic requirements must be met. The less time the patient spends in deep anesthesia (with high blood levels of anesthetic agents), the faster he or she recovers from the drugs, be they inhalation or intravenous agents.

Figure 35–3 presents a comparison of two 2-hour computer-simulated anesthetic procedures with isoflurane. All variables (fresh gas flow, ventilation, cardiac output, and induction concentrations) were kept the same for both cases, but in one case, isoflurane concentration was decreased to 1.5% during the maintenance phase. In the other case, it was kept at 2% (Table 35–6).

For the painful closure, anesthesia was deepened—in the first case to 4% for 5 minutes, and in the second case to only 3% (because the patient was already more deeply anesthetized). Once the isoflurane administration was discontinued and the ''patients'' had breathed room air for 5 minutes, the one who had been under light anesthesia during the maintenance phase had about one-fifth less anesthetic (1.4 L versus 1.7 L of isoflurane vapor dissolved in the tissues) than did the other who had been kept in a deeper stage during the maintenance phase.

For intra-abdominal procedures, the requirement for muscle relaxation is also greatest during exposure and closure. Again, recovery from relaxation is faster when less of the total drug amount has been given.

How Are Fluids Regulated?

Although drug requirements may be fairly small during the maintenance phase of anesthesia, fluid requirements are likely to be greatest at this time. While the wound is open to room air (fluid loss by evaporation); while the surgeon works on the tissue, which causes edema to form and fluids to be sequestered in traumatized tissue (third space losses); and while outright bleeding occurs, losses must be replaced (see Chapters 40 and 42).

When and Why Should Patients Be Allowed to Breathe Spontaneously?

Allowing spontaneous ventilation once was common during the maintenance phase of anesthesia, even for thoracic, upper abdominal, and intracranial operative procedures. However, the introduction of tracheal intubation, semi-closed systems, mechanical ventilators, and a wide variety of neuromuscular relaxants has changed this approach. Maintenance of spontaneous breathing, except during induction of and emergence from anesthesia, became a lost art.

Monitoring of Anesthetic Depth

In some respects, this approach is unfortunate. Many operative procedures do not require relaxants prior to incision of

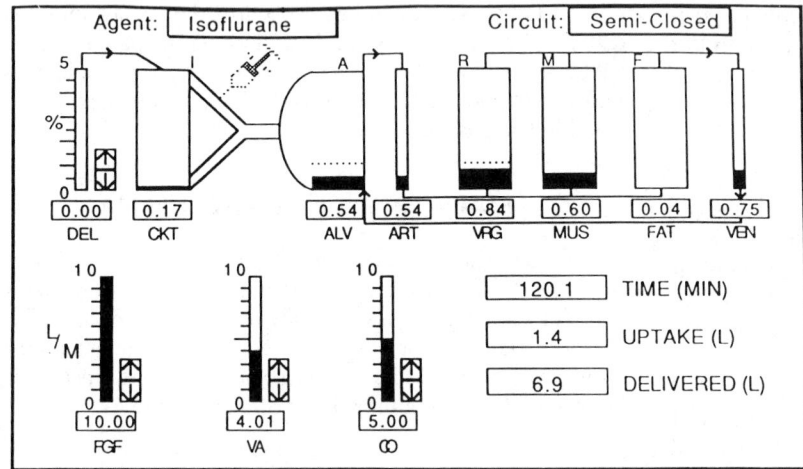

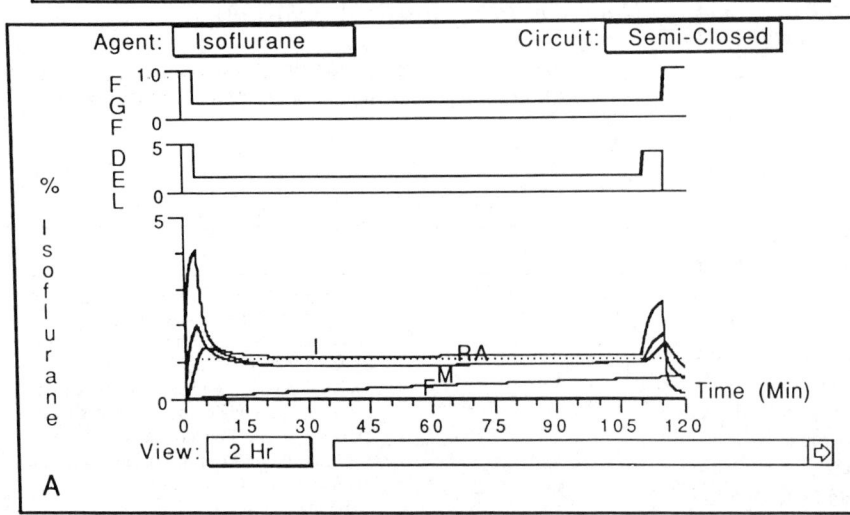

FIGURE 35–3. All panels are based on GasMan, a computer simulation of the uptake and distribution of gases in an average adult. *A and B, upper frames,* The boxes on the lower right show the elapsed time since the start of the simulation, the total volume of isoflurane vapor dissolved in the body (UPTAKE [L]), and the volume of isoflurane (in liters) delivered since the beginning of the simulation. *A and B, lower frames,* Graphic representations of the course of anesthesia with FGF on top (10 L · min⁻¹ for induction and emergence, 3 L · min⁻¹ for maintenance) and the setting of the vaporizer. V̇A and CO are constant. The curves show the concentration of isoflurane (in volume %) in the different compartments. I = inspired; A and R = artery and vessel rich group; M = muscle group; F = fat group. Two anesthetic procedures are simulated: *A,* Keeping the patient fairly deeply anesthetized. *B,* Keeping the patient fairly lightly anesthetized. The FGF and isoflurane concentration settings for induction, maintenance, and emergence were as shown in Table 35–6.

Observe that at the end of operation there are (in *A*) 1.7 L of dissolved isoflurane vapor in the tissues and (in *B*) 1.4 L of dissolved isoflurane vapor in the tissues (about one-fifth less). For a rapid recovery, it is worth adjusting the anesthetic administration to the minimal patient requirements.

TABLE 35–6. Fresh Gas Flow and Isoflurane Concentrations in Two Simulated Anesthetic Procedures During Induction, Maintenance, and Emergence

	Light Plane of Anesthesia During Maintenance					Deep Plane of Anesthesia During Maintenance			
Time (min)	0–3	90	110	115	120	0–3	110	115	120
Isoflurane (%)	5	2	1.5	3	0	5	2.0	4	0
Fresh gas flow (L · min⁻¹)	10	3	3	3	10	10	3	3	10

the fascia and following its closure. Many more require no relaxants whatsoever following tracheal intubation. Spontaneous ventilation provides an elegant means to assess the clinical depth of anesthesia; in many ways, the rate and volume of tidal breathing obtained during patient spontaneous ventilation are superior to conventional measurements of pulse and blood pressure. If a paralyzed patient is tachycardic during an isoflurane anesthetic procedure, is it because the anesthesia is "too light" or because this is simply a normal, autonomic response to the agent? However, if the spontaneous respiratory rate doubles and the tidal volume increases by 50% following incision (or if the patient moves), valuable information has been obtained.

Maintenance of Arterial Carbon Dioxide Partial Pressure and pH

Many anesthesiologists (mostly those recently trained) assume that spontaneous ventilation cannot be maintained adequately because of anesthetic-induced respiratory depression. Certainly, this may be true if large doses of narcotics are administered. However, an endotracheal tube reduces physiologic dead space by 50% or more. Thus, a smaller than normal tidal volume and a slower respiratory rate still maintain satisfactory arterial partial pressure of carbon dioxide ($Paco_2$), pH, and oxygenation, which can be verified and continuously monitored by measurement of end-tidal carbon dioxide partial pressure ($PETco_2$) and O_2 saturation.

Ventilation/Perfusion Relationships

Spontaneous breathing during general anesthesia maintains more normal ventilation/perfusion relationships.[10] In contrast, manual or mechanical ventilation increases dead space in nondependent lung areas and increases shunting in dependent ones. If you do not agree with this statement, ask yourself how

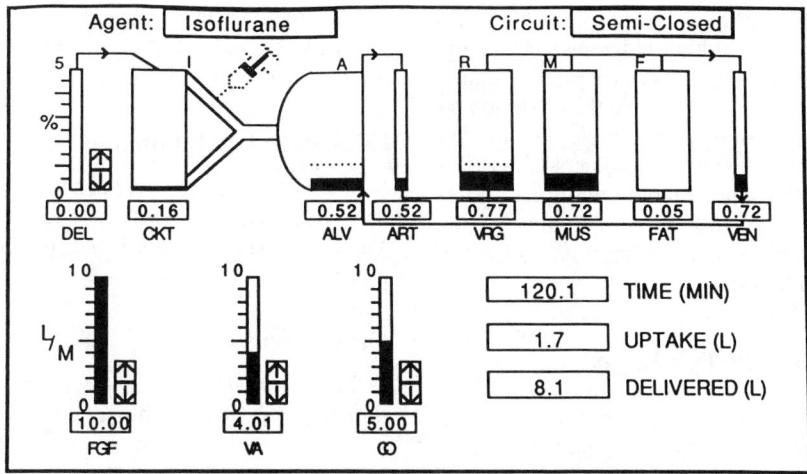

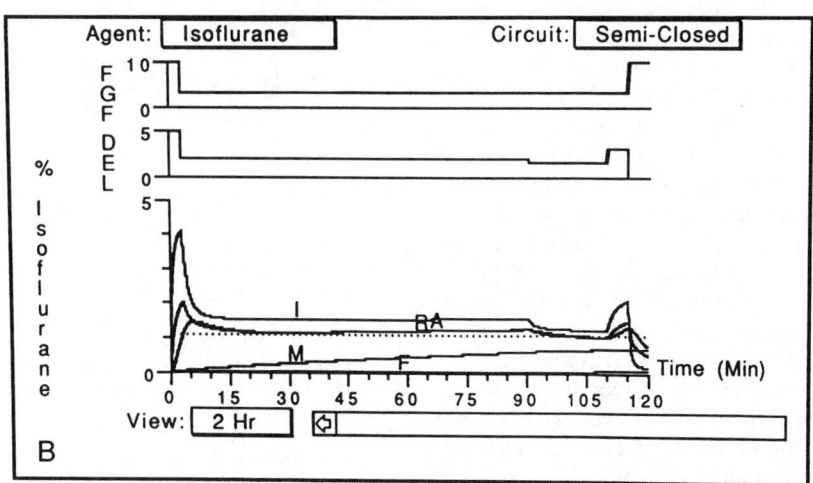

FIGURE 35–3. *Continued*

many patients have a normal, predicted arterial partial pressure of oxygen (PO_2) for any given inspired O_2 concentration? Then, consider why tidal volumes of 10 to 15 mL · kg^{-1} are necessary to maintain normal PCO_2 and pH during mechanical ventilation when volumes of 6 to 8 mL · kg^{-1} suffice in awake, spontaneously breathing individuals.

Finally, consider that positive-pressure manual or mechanical ventilation decreases venous return and cardiac output and thus exacerbates the myocardial depressant effects of many anesthetics. Spontaneous breathing, however, enhances venous return and helps to maintain cardiovascular function and to preserve normal ventilation/perfusion matching.

Thus, spontaneous breathing has much to offer in terms of maintaining cardiopulmonary integrity. It also provides satisfaction to the anesthesiologist who titrates anesthetic depth based on a patient's needs rather than using a ''cookbook'' approach or by reading the exhaled anesthetic concentration on a mass spectrometer. When the operative procedure allows, spontaneous breathing should be attempted.

EMERGENCE AND EXTUBATION

When Should Analgesics Be Administered?

Should you administer an analgesic before the end of the operation to cover the early postoperative period? The answer to this question depends largely on the operation and on what type of anesthesia the patient had received. If the primary anesthetic was an inhalation agent or propofol with nitrous oxide, you may want to give an intramuscular analgesic about 45 minutes before admission to the recovery room. Medication that has a longer plasma concentration plateau than that obtainable with a single intravenous dose is preferable. For the average adult, 10 mg morphine or 60 mg ketorolac is a reasonable choice. If the anesthesia included large intermittent doses or a continuous infusion of narcotics, do not administer more at the end of the case. Even the so-called ''short-acting narcotics'' have long elimination times.

When Should The Patient Be Extubated?

In the days when diethyl ether was the primary agent, all patients were slow to awaken. Extubation of patients still in surgical levels of anesthesia was common. This is no longer necessary, as we now use inhalation and intravenous agents that are more rapidly eliminated. In general, the trachea can be extubated if the patient is capable of protecting the airway and maintaining adequate ventilation. The latter can be tested by asking him or her to take a deep breath (about 15 mL · kg^{-1}). Muscle power needs to be checked by verifying that the patient can raise his or her head off the pillow for 5 seconds.

A patient who can execute these tasks can be safely extubated. However, a patient who received large doses of narcotics and relaxants may be able to lift his or her head, take a deep breath on command, and even answer questions after extubation but 10 to 30 minutes later may suffer respiratory arrest in the postanesthesia care unit. We assume that this happens when the respiratory depressant effect of the narcotic lingers while the respiratory stimulating effects of pain begin to subside in the postanesthesia care unit. Beware of the insidious tail effect of some intravenous anesthetics.

Be careful not to remove the bite block or oral airway before extubation. Once the patient begins to respond, he or she may bite down on the endotracheal tube and occlude his airway. If the bite block or oral airway has fallen out, and if the patient bites on the tube, try to pry the teeth apart using tongue blades. Insert one and then a second between the teeth. Even in patients with clenched teeth, this maneuver is usually possible. Then, wedge additional tongue blades between the first two, and in this way separate the incisors far enough that the endotracheal tube is protected.

How Do You Extubate If the Patient Should Not Cough or Struggle?

After regaining their reflexes, many patients strain and cough during extubation. This activity is occasionally very undesirable, for example, in a patient with an eye injury (straining → increased venous pressure → increased intraocular pressure → loss of vitreous). Three techniques can be used to abolish straining during extubation. All require preoxygenation (because once again the patient's airway may be jeopardized right after the tube is removed) and preparation for reintubation (should the patient lose his or her airway).

Deep Anesthesia

Keep the patient well anesthetized, and extubate under deep anesthesia. Then, put the patient on his or her side (Fig. 35–4) so that the tongue falls forward, preventing obstruction. Should the patient regurgitate or vomit, the gastric material will follow gravity and drain from the mouth instead of pooling in the hypopharynx.

Extubation-like Intubation

Repeat the induction sequence and extubate after the patient has been paralyzed with a small dose of succinylcholine. Ventilate manually until the patient has regained muscle power.

Cough Suppression

Deepen anesthesia briefly with intravenous agents that have short effects, such as thiopental, 1 to 2 mg · kg^{-1}; lidocaine,

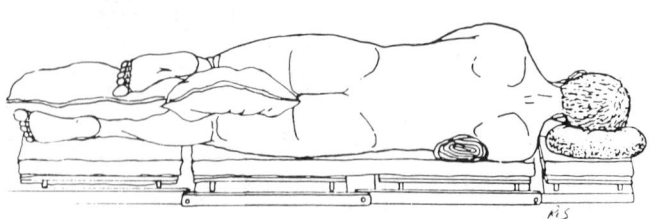

FIGURE 35–4. The optimal position of an unconscious patient during transport from the operating room to the postanesthesia care unit. The patient is placed on his or her side. If the patient was in a lateral position during the operation, the side with the incision is placed down. The lower leg is straightened, and the upper leg is flexed 90° at the hip and knee. This adjustment provides stability to the hip. Both arms and hands are brought forward to stabilize the shoulder girdle. The head is supported by the placement of a pillow or folded blanket under the occiput so that the face is turned slightly downward; this causes the jaw and tongue to fall forward, preventing obstruction while letting saliva, gastric juice, or vomitus to drain from the mouth rather than to pool in the hypopharynx.

1 mg · kg^{-1}; or propofol, 0.5 to 1.0 mg · kg^{-1}. Pull out the tube 1 minute after the bolus of one of these drugs reaches the vein. Ventilate manually as necessary.

When Is the Patient Ready to Be Taken to the Postanesthesia Care Unit?

We are sometimes too casual when taking a patient to the postanesthesia care unit. During general anesthesia, the patient breathed a gas mixture enriched with O_2. Now the patient is breathing room air and he or she may be exhaling nitrous oxide by the liter, presenting the very real risk of diffusion hypoxia. Intraoperatively, the patient stayed in one position; now, he or she is being moved and turned. Compensatory vascular reflexes may still be depressed by anesthetic after effects; with sudden turning, the patient may become hypotensive. Make sure that ventilation and circulation are adequate before leaving the operating room. If necessary, encourage deep breaths during transport. If patient breathing is deemed to be inadequate, give O_2.

When Should Oxygen Be Given During Transport?

Oxygen should be given if any of the following circumstances are applicable:

1. The patient's trachea is still intubated. This should be the case if ventilation is depressed by muscle relaxants and lingering anesthetic or narcotic effects.

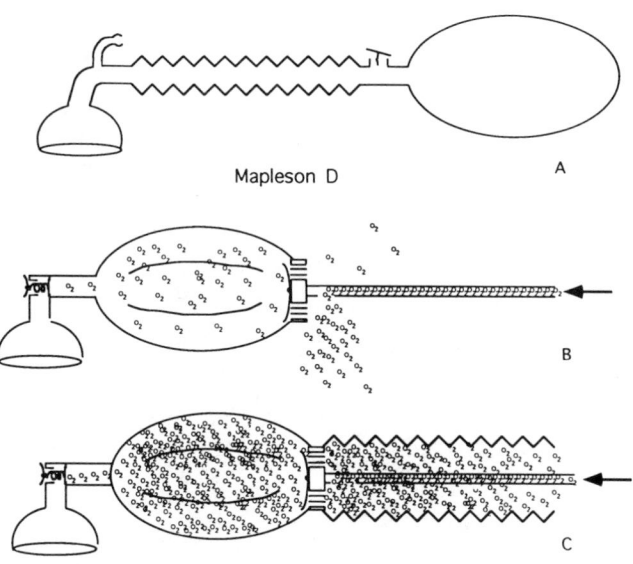

FIGURE 35–5. Bags and mask used for manual ventilation during transport, shown at end of exhalation. *A,* The Mapleson D system requires relatively high flow rates of oxygen to prevent rebreathing. Without a source of compressed gas, this system cannot be used. *B* and *C,* The self-inflating devices can be used to ventilate a patient's lungs with ambient air. If the patient's inspired gas is to be enriched with oxygen, it is necessary to have the extension bellows *(C)* attached because the oxygen delivered by the oxygen tube does not blow directly into the bag; instead, it deposits in front of the intake valve where it accumulates during expiration. Without the extension bellows, very little extra oxygen is made available to the patient *(B)*.

TABLE 35–7. Approximate Values of Inspired Oxygen for Different Devices

	100% Oxygen (L · min^{-1})	Oxygen in Inspired Gas (%)
Nasal cannula or catheter	1	24
	2	28
	3	32
	4	36
	5	40
	6	44
Oxygen mask	5–6	40
	6–7	50
	7–8	60
Mask with reservoir	6	60
	7	70
	8	80
	9	90
	10	99

2. The patient is extubated, awake, and breathing normally, but the pulse oximeter shows values that are reduced by more than 3% (more or less, depending on the patient's condition and control values) below the preanesthetic values. Lung pathology (shunting) should be expected.

3. The patient continues to exhale nitrous oxide. Remember that during an average case of nitrous oxide anesthesia, many liters of nitrous oxide are absorbed. When large volumes of nitrous oxide are exhaled, mostly during the first few minutes after the nitrous oxide flow meter is turned off, they replace O_2 and nitrogen in the lung; diffusion hypoxia is the consequence. Therefore, give O_2 during transport if nitrous oxide was given up until a few minutes before transport to the postanesthesia care unit. A gas analyzer shows how much nitrous oxide is left in the expired gas. If it is less than about 10%, diffusion hypoxia is not a concern.

4. Prolonged hyperventilation was used. A patient who had been hyperventilated for several hours will have depleted his tissue stores of dissolved CO_2. Instead of having to exhale CO_2 to maintain normal $PaCO_2$ values, much of the generated CO_2 is absorbed by the tissue.[10] Consequently, relatively low minute ventilation suffices to maintain the $PaCO_2$ within a normal range. Although this adjustment maintains normal $PaCO_2$, it may lead to inadequate oxygenation.

5. If you are aware of lung pathology, surgery (e.g., thoracotomy), tight bandages, or splinting secondary to pain and of their effects on ventilation. Give O_2 if you have any reason for concern.

Several devices are available. Most commonly used are nasal prongs, O_2 masks (not assuming a tight fit), and masks with reservoir bags. Table 35–7 shows approximate values of inspired O_2 with these devices for different flow rates of 100% O_2.

How Should Ventilation Be Supported?

A patient who is apneic or hypoventilating should not simply be supplied with O_2 but should have ventilation actively controlled or assisted. For this purpose, several devices are available. Commonly used is the so-called Mapleson D system, which requires a source of compressed O_2 (Fig. 35–5).

Gas flow rates should be twice the patient's normal minute ventilation. In adults, this value is often not obtained: the patient's alveoli contain enough O_2, but some rebreathing of expired gas occurs, and the Pa_{CO_2} rises.

Alternatively, one can use a self-inflating resuscitation bag. This bag can be used without O_2 because it fills itself with air. However, patients with pulmonary pathology may require an O_2-enriched atmosphere. To obtain significant concentrations of O_2 with such devices, the self-inflating bag must have a reservoir in which O_2 accumulates. Figure 35–5 shows this principle.

References

1. Gibby GL, Gravenstein JS, Layon AJ, et al: How often does the preoperative interview change anesthetic management (Abstract)? Anesthesiology 1992; 77:1174.
2. Lofgren RH, Montgomery WW: Incidence of laryngeal involvement in rheumatoid arthritics. N Engl J Med 1962; 267:193.
3. Gardner DL, Homes F: Anaesthetic and postoperative hazards in rheumatoid arthritis. Br J Anaesth 1961; 33:259.
4. Editorial: Preoxygenation: physiology and practice. Lancet 1992; 339:31.
5. Valentine SJ, Marjot R, Monk CR: Preoxygenation in the elderly: a comparison of the four-maximal breath and three minute techniques. Anesth Analg 1990; 71:516–519.
6. Loper K, Reitan J, Bennet H, et al: Comparison of halothane and isoflurane for rapid anesthetic induction. Anesth Analg 1987; 66:766.
7. Mendelson CL: The aspiration of stomach contents into the lungs during obstetric anesthesia. Am J Gynecol 1946; 52:191.
8. Sellick BA: Cricoid pressure to control regurgitation of stomach contents during induction of anaesthesia. Lancet 1961; 2:404.
9. Engbeak J, Viby-Mogensen: Precurarization: a hazard to the patient? Acta Anaesth Scand 1984; 28:61.
10. Froese AB, Bryan AC: Effects of anesthesia and paralysis on diaphragmatic mechanics in man. Anesthesiology 1974; 41:242.
11. Salvatore AJ, Sullivan SF, Papper EM: Postoperative hypoventilation and hypoxemia in man after hyperventilation. N Engl J Med 1968; 280:467.

CHAPTER 36

Intravenous Agents

JAY KOSKA, M.D., Ph.D.

Intravenous agents are at least part of virtually every anesthetic. Their administration represents the simplest pharmacokinetic form because no absorption phase exists, only distribution and elimination.

PHARMACOKINETIC PROPERTIES OF INTRAVENOUS AGENTS

What Factors Determine the Volume of Distribution?

The volume of distribution (Vd) is a hypothetical, apparent volume in which if a specific amount of drug were mixed, sampling of a portion of that volume (e.g., blood) would yield a specific concentration. This assumption is predicated on equal drug distribution to all parts of the body.

Actual distribution within the body depends on other chemical and biologic features of the drug administered. Table 36–1 lists the principal factors that affect distribution. Some are inherent in the drug, and others in patients who receive it.

Drugs with greater lipophilia distribute more to lipids and other fatty tissues than to hydrophilic tissues like blood. At equilibrium, the concentration of a lipophilic drug in the blood is, therefore much lower than would be expected if it were distributed only to the blood volume. Thus, the apparent Vd is many times larger than the predicted blood volume. Just as there is a spectrum of drug solubilities, ranging from highly lipophilic (e.g., fentanyl) to highly hydrophilic (e.g., ketorolac), there is a parallel range of Vds.

What Factors Affect Distribution?

Protein Binding

Distribution of highly lipophilic drugs is a dynamic process. After their initial administration into the blood, they are variably bound to the blood proteins. Some remain unbound and are distributed primarily to fatty tissues. If a substance is highly protein bound, this relationship in effect partially offsets its fat solubility; it has a smaller Vd because part remains in the blood, bound usually to albumin or α_1-glycoproteins. An aliquot of blood measured for drug concentration includes both the protein-bound and unbound components.

Redistribution and Equilibrium

Redistribution, the movement of drug from bound sites to unbound sites, occurs away from the blood proteins. An equilibrium is eventually reached between bound and unbound drug (in both the tissues and blood). Movement from blood to tissues takes time, during which, if blood samples are ana-

TABLE 36–1. Factors That Affect Drug Distribution

Property	Effect on Volume of Distribution (Vd)	Relative Effect
Lipophilia	Increases Vd.	+ + + +
Protein binding to blood or plasma	Decreases Vd, with increased protein binding in circulation.	+ + +
Tissue protein binding	Increases Vd with increased tissue protein binding.	+ +
Ionization	Decreases Vd for lipophilic compounds. May increase Vd for hydrophilic compounds.	+ +
Hypovolemia	Little effect on lipophilic unbound drugs. May decrease Vd in hydrophilic compounds.	+
Other drugs	May increase Vd if displacing from protein binding. May decrease if reduced circulating volume in hydrophilic compounds.	+
Temperature	Decreased Vd of hydrophilic compounds as circulating volume decreases.	+
Hemodilution	Increases Vd on highly protein-bound drugs. Little effect on true Vd of hydrophilic drugs.	+
Molecular size	Distribution varies with solubility. May not cross tissue barrier.	+

lyzed, a higher concentration of the drug is found than would be predicted based simply on its Vd and the dose administered. This movement is referred to as the *distribution* or *equilibrium phase.*

Figure 36–1 reflects two drugs given intravenously. Drug A is highly distributed, as evidenced by the long, sloping, initial part of the curve. Because we measure drug concentration in the blood compartment, we would expect that as the drug moves from the blood into fatty and other tissues, its concentration in the blood would decrease rapidly at first and then more slowly as tissue equilibrium is approached.

Elimination

Once blood and tissue equilibrium occurs, drug elimination by either metabolism or excretion accounts for the remainder of the curve. The elimination phase is the linear part of the log concentration versus time curve in Figure 36–1. The common log or natural log value usually is plotted versus time. Because the decay is so rapid, the decrease in concentration is an exponential function (see Chapter 33, Equation 10). By plotting the common log or natural log values of these concentrations, we convert a curve to nearly a straight line. The slope of the latter part of this line then represents the elimination constant for the drug, which is inversely proportional to the half-life ($t\frac{1}{2}$).

Drug B (see Fig. 36–1) has little or no distribution, as might occur with a water-soluble agent. Table 36–2 lists several commonly used intravenous anesthetic agents, their usual dose ranges for single-bolus administration, their relative lipophilia, and the $t\frac{1}{2}$ of their terminal elimination phase.

Clinical Implications

If a drug requires time to distribute from the blood to other organs, it is eliminated slowly. If an organ on which a drug

TABLE 36–2. Dose Range, Lipophilia, and Half-Lives of Several Intravenous Anesthetic Agents

	Dose Range (mg · kg^{-1})	Lipophilia	$t\frac{1}{2}$
Sodium pentothal	3–5	High	6.4–7.6
Methohexital	1.0–1.5	High	1.8–6.0
Propofol	1.0–2.0	High	7.7–8.3
Etomidate	0.3–0.5	High	1.8–4.0
Ketamine	0.5–1.5	High	3.1
Midazolam	0.1–0.4	Medium	1.9–3.5
Diazepam	0.3–0.6	Medium	32.4–60.8
Morphine	0.1–0.5	Medium	1.0–2.2
Fentanyl	0.001–0.075	High	3.1–4.4
Alfentanil	0.0005–0.10	Low	0.5–1.0
Sufentanil	0.0001–0.005	High	2.7
Meperidine	1.0–5.0	High	3.2–4.4

exerts its action (the target organ) is in the circulation and hence requires no distribution from blood to deep target tissues, the blood concentration rapidly reflects the target tissue concentration and the effective concentration.

Barriers to distribution, such as the epithelium of the vessels in the brain, abscess walls, and poorly perfused organ areas, increase the time it takes for a drug to reach the target tissue. Glycopyrrolate, a large polar molecule with limited lipophilia, has difficulty crossing the blood-brain barrier; therefore, its central nervous system (CNS) effects are limited. Conversely, atropine, a lipophilic molecule, rapidly crosses into the brain, has a rapid rate of onset of action, and produces CNS effects.

What Are the Effects of Continuous Drug Infusion?

Because intravenously administered drugs do not require absorption across a barrier to gain access to the bloodstream and demonstrate only distribution and elimination phases, they often require frequently repeated dosing to maintain some minimum drug concentration and effect. This requirement is particularly evident if they have a high clearance, due either to a large Vd or a rapid elimination phase.

To eliminate the "peak and valley" effect of frequent intermittent administration, a continuous-infusion technique is often preferable. Figure 36–2 shows the relationship of multiple injections versus a continuous infusion of a drug with rapid clearance. Note how continuous infusion dampens the oscillations in serum drug levels that may cause toxicity at the peak or inadequate effect at the valley (trough).

When Should Continuous Infusion Be Used?

The decision about whether an intermittent bolus or continuous-infusion technique is appropriate should be based on several key elements (Table 36–3).

Therapeutic Index

First, what is the therapeutic index of the drug—that is, the ratio of the toxic dose to the effective dose. If the therapeutic index is very high, there is less concern about overshooting the target concentration, and giving large, intermittent doses is

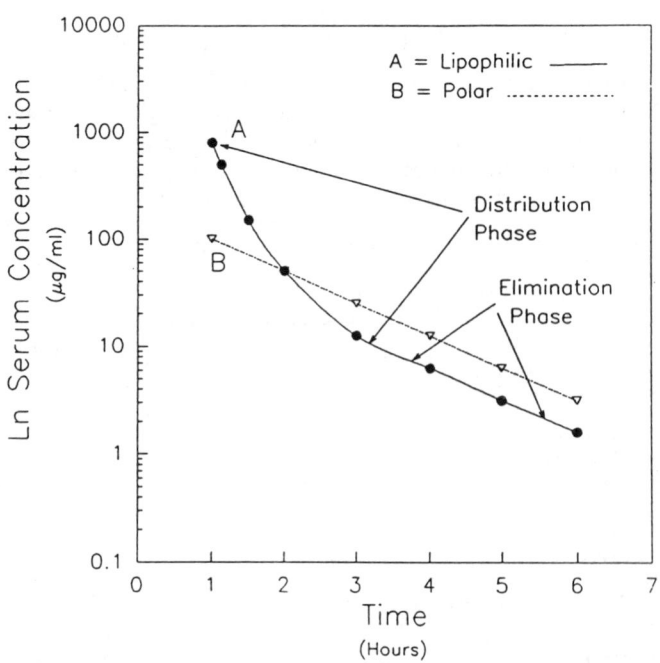

FIGURE 36–1. Lipophilic versus polar drug level profiles. A = Hypothetical lipophilic drug profile, with distribution phase and elimination phase; B = polar drug profile with only elimination phase.

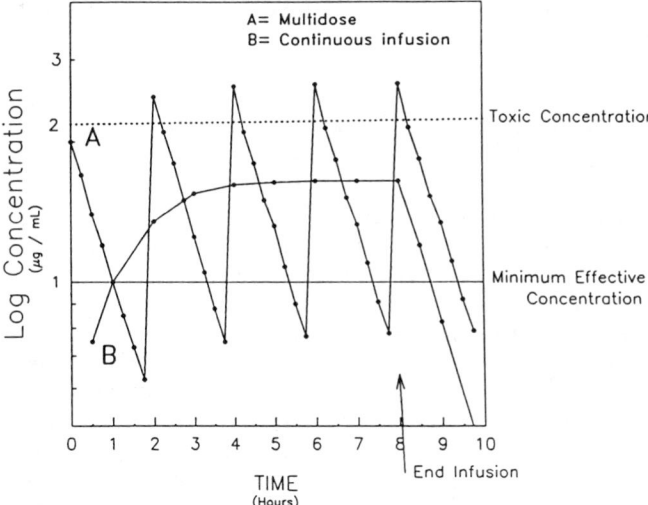

FIGURE 36–2. Multidose versus continuous infusions. A = Drug levels from multiple doses of a hypothetical drug; B = continuous infusion of same hypothetical drug. Note repetitive decay below minimum effective concentration with intermittent dosing.

acceptable. If, however, the therapeutic index is low, continuous infusions minimize overshooting the effective concentration and the resulting toxicity.

Saturable Effects

Second, if the desired effect is saturable or maximal and giving more drug does not produce further pharmacologic activity, intermittent dosing is acceptable. This is the case with H_2 blockers; once a maximum effective concentration is reached, no further blockade of acid production occurs, regardless of additional drug administration. However, if the process is not saturable, provision of the minimum concentration that gives the desired pharmacologic benefit is desirable and achievable with a continuous infusion.

Offset of Action

Next, if speed of offset—the time from discontinuing the drug until no further pharmacologic effect is noted—is critical, infusions may be preferable. If the drug concentration is maintained just above the minimum effective concentration, discontinuing the infusion quickly allows the concentration to fall a small amount to below the minimum effective concentration (see Figure 36–2). If an intermittent bolus technique were used, a prolonged distribution and elimination time would be required for a recently administered bolus.

Propofol administration demonstrates this point well. Maintenance of the level just high enough to provide anesthesia

TABLE 36–3. Factors Suggesting Efficacy of Continuous Infusions

High therapeutic index
No ceiling effect
Maintaining minimum effective concentration for rapid offset of action
Ability to maintain minimum effective concentration with rapidly cleared drugs
Cost, tendency to use less drug to achieve similar effect
Less labor intensive

allows rapid emergence as soon as the infusion is discontinued. In contrast, a more delayed arousal follows administration of a large bolus (see Fig. 36–2).

Clearance and Half-Life

Continuous infusions are best suited to drugs with rapid clearance and short t½. These compounds leave the blood rapidly and would require numerous intermittent boluses. Alfentanil is a prime example. With a 0.5 to 1.0 hour t½ and a small Vd, 0.5 to 1.0 L · kg⁻¹, it is cleared rapidly. Maintenance of effect by continuous infusion is superior to intermittent injections.

Conversely, morphine, which has a relatively long half-life of 1.7 to 2.2 hours and a large Vd of 3.2 to 3.4 L · kg⁻¹, is cleared relatively slowly and does not need repeated dosing to maintain adequate tissue levels.

No specific values of Vd, clearance, and t½ can be used to determine absolutely whether an intermittent bolus or continuous-infusion technique is preferable. However, if infusion pumps are available, most drugs that do not demonstrate cumulative toxicity or that do not benefit from peak and valley effects, such as the aminoglycoside antibiotics, can achieve better results when given by continuous infusion.

Continuous infusions are also more cost efficient. Because just enough drug is given to provide the desired effect, less total drug is given in the long run. The cost of administration is thereby reduced, a substantial benefit in the case of expensive drugs.

Continuous-infusion techniques also tend to be less labor intensive; once an infusion is started, fewer adjustments are required to maintain appropriate pharmacodynamic end points.

How Is the Correct Infusion Rate Determined?

To reach and maintain a particular level, drug going into the body must equal drug going out of the body; in other words, a steady state must be reached. We know from Chapter 33 that the concentration at steady state (C_{ss}) is determined by the following relationship:

$$C_{ss} = X_o/Cl$$

where X_o is the amount of drug given per unit time. Thus for fentanyl, with a clearance of 12.7 mL · kg⁻¹ · min⁻¹, administering 2 µg · kg⁻¹ · h⁻¹, or 0.033 µg · kg⁻¹ · min⁻¹ yields a steady state of 0.0026 µg · mL⁻¹ (2.6 ng · mL⁻¹). This value is within the minimum effective concentration range, 1 to 5 ng · mL⁻¹ for analgesia and minimal respiratory depression.[1] Knowledge of the clearance of a drug and the approximate minimum effective concentration in the blood allows prediction of the infusion rate necessary to achieve that level (Table 36–4).

What Factors Alter Clearance?

Ionization

Clearance is dependent on the Vd elimination constant. As mentioned earlier, the Vd of a drug is dependent on its relative

TABLE 36–4. Pharmacokinetic and Pharmacodynamic Parameters of Several Intravenous Anesthetics

Agent	Clearance Rate (mL · kg⁻¹ · min)	Volume of Distribution (L · kg⁻¹)	Minimum Effective Concentration (µg · mL⁻¹)
Sodium pentothal	3.0–3.8	1.92–5.0	12.9–25.5
Methohexital	7.0–13.0	3.68	10.0
Propofol	33.8–36.6	1.8–3.04	0.96–1.14
Etomidate	12.3–24.5	2.0–6.72	0.231–0.383
Ketamine	16.6–21.6	4.4–5.8	0.43–0.85
Midazolam	5.1–9.9	1.29–1.91	0.78–0.236
Diazepam	0.4	1.53	Not available
Morphine	15–23	3.2–3.4	0.02–0.2
Fentanyl	11–21	3.2–5.9	0.001–0.005
Alfentanil	5.0–7.9	0.5–1.0	0.05–1.5
Sufentanil	9.0–14	2.86	0.0005–0.001
Meperidine	8.0–18	2.8–4.2	0.1–0.5

lipophilia, the degree of protein binding, and its ionization. Ionization has an important role. Drugs are generally more soluble in the ionized state; however, they usually are not cleared from the body as well, because they have difficulty crossing cell membranes. They also tend to be more protein bound and are thus less available to their target tissues.

Weak acids like sodium thiopental (STP) are more ionized and more protein bound in a basic medium. Less is free to cross cell membranes, producing a smaller but prolonged effect because of reduced clearance. Patients maintained in an alkalotic state during hyperventilation therapy for closed head injury have less effect from similar levels of sodium thiopental than do nonalkalotic subjects. Increased ionization results in less drug available to cross into the brain. Conversely, on termination of hyperventilation therapy, as the blood becomes less alkalotic, more drug is available for both the therapeutic effect and for clearance. Table 36–5 gives the pKa, protein-binding, and acid-base characteristics of several commonly used intravenous agents.

Drug-Drug Interactions

Several other factors should be considered when assessing or predicting drug clearance. Drug-drug interactions also affect drug clearance (see Chapter 39). For example, general anesthesia with inhalational agents is known to reduce liver blood flow and to prolong the clearance of drugs such as lidocaine, which are metabolized primarily by the liver and may have a prolonged duration of action in hepatic failure. Drugs such as pancuronium, which are cleared primarily by the kidneys, may have prolonged effects in patients with renal failure.

Metabolism

Drug metabolism may be increased by enzyme induction. Certain enzymes are modulated and can increase their function, thus increasing clearance of some agents. An example of this type is the accelerated clearance of muscle relaxants when a patient takes anticonvulsants such as phenobarbital and phenytoin. These agents increase the metabolic rate of the cytochrome P_{450} enzymes in the liver responsible for metabolizing vecuronium and thus shorten its duration of action for any given dose. Enzyme induction generally takes days to

weeks to occur, so it is not usually a concern after the acute administration of barbiturates.

What Other Factors Affect the Amount of Drug Needed?

The serum level of a required intravenous agent varies with the degree of surgical stimulus.[1] Pharmacokinetic estimations in the drug package inserts must be modified by knowledge that in the operating room, drugs seldom are given to a patient without surgical stimulus and without other simultaneously administered drugs. The minimum required levels obtained from pharmacokinetic estimations in the package inserts are useful only as guidelines.

Titration of the analgesic according to vital sign changes after surgical stimulus is necessary to fine-tune the requisite dose. This process involves the science of pharmacodynamics. Sedation also is titrated to a clinical end point. Changes in electroencephalographic (EEG) tracings, esophageal motility, and skin impedance have been proposed to estimate the depth of sedation and anesthesia. To date, no simple method absolutely predicts the pharmacodynamic end point.

Titration of dose to desired effect provides the best method of reaching steady-state levels that are appropriate for the stimuli provided. Pharmacokinetic parameters alone may lead to insufficient levels but do serve as a starting point from which one can increase the dose to provide the desired effect.

What Happens If One's Estimates Are Off and Too Much Agent Is Given?

Numerous factors may contribute to an undesirable excess drug effect (Table 36–6). Too much agent or an agent with a long half-life that is given over a prolonged time causes accumulation; reversal of the drug, when possible, may be required. Often, this situation results from simple human error (wrong concentration, calculation error). Discontinuation of surgical stimuli may lead to a relative excess of drug postoperatively.

Ideally, one should titrate the dose to offset the maximal surgical stimuli, then, as the stimuli decrease, reduce the rate of administration. However, some surgical stimuli are extremely painful acutely, then stop altogether (e.g., bronchos-

TABLE 36–5. Chemical Properties of Several Intravenous Anesthetic Agents

Agent	pKa (pH)	Type (Acid-Base)	% Bound
Sodium pentothal	7.6	Acid	82.0–84.8
Methohexital		Acid	73
Etomidate	4.5	Base	75.9–77.9
Propofol	11.0	Base	96–98
Ketamine	7.5	Base	12.0
Diazepam	3.4	Base	96.8–98.8
Midazolam	6.15	Base	92.1–95.9
Morphine	7.93	Base	26–36
Fentanyl	8.43	Base	79–87
Alfentanil	6.5	Base	89–92
Sufentanil	8.01	Base	92.5
Meperidine	7.93	Base	64–82

TABLE 36–6. Causes of Excess Drug Effect

Administration error (too much drug given)
Loss of offsetting surgical stimuli
Early termination of surgical procedure
Unusual or idiosyncratic patient reaction
Drug-drug interaction

copy and biopsy). An extreme example is represented by a surgical procedure that is aborted just after premedications, anesthetic induction, and administration of a large dose of morphine. These situations can be avoided by using short-acting narcotics or inhalational agents (or both) that are eliminated rapidly.

Some patients have altered dose-response relationships in which small doses of narcotic or sedative produce excessive effects. This situation may be associated with limited patient exposure and, therefore, lack of tolerance to the agents or to unique pharmacokinetic variations. Titration with a small initially administered dose, increasing to the anticipated needs instead of administering a single large dose, minimizes the impact. Finally, certain drugs may interact with the narcotic or sedative, either blunting or magnifying their effects. This interaction can be avoided by practitioners who know the pharmacology of the agents they administer.

The best way to avoid excessive medication is by frequent monitoring of the pharmacodynamic end point: If giving an analgesic, watch the heart rate, blood pressure, respiratory rate, and tidal volume while titrating the drug. If a sudden increase in heart rate and blood pressure occurs with the surgical stimulus, in the absence of other factors (massive blood loss, exogenous catecholamine administration, baroreflex changes, pheochromocytoma, aortic cross-clamping, hyperthermia), insufficient analgesia probably is the cause, and more drug is required.

What Pharmacologic Reversal Agents Are Available?

Naloxone and Flumazenil

For narcotic reversal, naloxone is the drug of choice. This drug has a high affinity for the narcotic receptor. In the doses studied, it usually but not always reverses their effect. For the benzodiazepines, flumazenil, a specific receptor antagonist, is available. Unlike naloxone, it has a weaker affinity for its receptor. In the doses studied, it usually but not always reverses the effect of the offending benzodiazepine.[2]

Both naloxone and flumazenil have relatively short half-lives and may be metabolized before the primary drug, the agonist, loses its pharmacologic effect. Thus, renarcotization or sedation may occur. Intramuscular administration of naloxone provides a depot for a prolonged absorption phase and reversal effect. This relationship is not true of flumazenil, however, which requires frequent administration or a continuous infusion to provide a prolonged duration of effect.

Doxapram

Doxapram, a direct respiratory stimulant, counteracts the respiratory depression side effects seen with both narcotics and sedatives. It does not reverse the primary agent's action at the receptor but instead stimulates and overdrives the respiratory center.

INTRAVENOUS ANESTHETIC AGENTS

How Are Barbiturates Best Used?

Sodium Thiopental

Distribution

STP is the most commonly used intravenous anesthetic agent. It is rapidly distributed because of its lipophilic nature, accounting for the short duration of effect. Seltzer and colleagues[3] demonstrated the clinical usefulness of this distribution effect. A smaller dose given rapidly minimizes the distribution duration and yields a higher peak concentration. The same induction effect results as that from a 50% larger amount given in small incremental doses. Only small differences in hemodynamic side effects occur.

Duration of Effect

The short duration of action attributed to distribution is evident until large doses are given. At that point, after distribution has occurred, plasma concentrations still remain above the minimum effective concentration of 12.9 to 25.5 $\mu g \cdot mL^{-1}$. This level results when 30 to 40 $mg \cdot kg^{-1}$ is administered. Subsequently, the duration of action is dependent on elimination only. Because elimination is extremely slow, with a half-life of 6.4 to 17.6 hours, prolonged use or high-dose administration, as for barbiturate-induced coma, has a long-term effect even after the drug is discontinued. Elimination can be increased by alkalization of the urine with sodium bicarbonate. However, this approach speeds up recovery by only approximately 10%.

Beneficial Effects

Beneficial effects of STP include rapid distribution and efficacy and limited toxicity. STP is metabolized virtually 100% by the liver, with a low hepatic extraction. Approximately 10% to 24% of a single dose is metabolized per hour; therefore, it is subject to less variation by changes in liver blood flow.

Seizure Control

Like all barbiturates, STP reduces seizures by limiting the spread of epileptic brain activity. Thus, it is a useful and readily available agent for quick resolution of seizures.

Side Effects

Untoward effects of STP include reduction in myocardial contractility and blood pressure, which are transient in normovolemic patients but can be profound with hypovolemia. The reduction in myocardial contractility may also be significant in patients with limited function before induction.

Because STP is cleared exclusively by the liver, patients with hepatic coma manifest prolonged duration of action with repetitive dosing. It can be administered by continuous infusion at a rate of 1 to 2 mg · kg^{-1} · min^{-1} to maintain anesthesia while the EEG tracing is used as a pharmacodynamic monitor.

STP has relatively high protein binding, averaging 83.4%. Thus, other agents that compete for similar binding sites may be displaced, causing potentially increased toxicity of those drugs; conversely, they may prevent binding of thiopental, thereby increasing its effectiveness and rate of metabolism. Thiopental causes hyperalgesia, most often in low doses, yielding increased pain responses. Thus it must be administered with an analgesic agent if total intravenous anesthesia is desired. Last, it is a known triggering agent for porphyria.

Methohexital

Distribution and Duration

Because of its lipid solubility (slightly larger Vd) and rapid extraction in the liver, methohexital has a clearance that is three times that of STP. It has a lower minimum effective concentration, primarily because of its limited ionization at a pH of 7.4 (only 24% versus 39% for STP). This property allows smaller doses to produce similar pharmacodynamic end points. It has a rapid distribution phase, which produces a short duration of effect and a larger elimination constant, which accounts for its rapid recovery when it is administered as a continuous infusion. These properties combine to provide a drug that still has a short duration of action after repetitive dosing.

Side Effects

Untoward effects may include excessively rapid elimination of drug from the brain, leading to withdrawal syndrome, lower seizure threshold, and increasing excitatory activity such as hiccups and involuntary skeletal movement during induction.[4] The lowered seizure threshold may be a useful property during procedures to map seizure foci.

Summary

All barbiturates have important common properties. They cause and are affected by various degrees of liver enzyme induction. Histamine release is associated with large and rapidly administered doses. They lower cerebral oxygen consumption to some degree. STP is the usual drug of choice for this action, because it is readily available in the operating room and offers the most cerebral protection compared with myocardial depression (i.e., it has the highest therapeutic index). Finally, tolerance occurs with prolonged administration, probably because of liver enzyme induction and true tolerance at the cellular level.

How Are Other Agents Used?

Propofol

Propofol, a diisopropyl phenol compound, is a highly lipophilic drug with limited water solubility. This property necessitates its dissolution in Intralipid, a soybean-free lecithin diluent. The high osmolality of this solution makes rapid injection in peripheral veins painful unless patients are pretreated with a local anesthetic or narcotic or both. Like the

barbiturates, it can cause hypotension in approximately 17% of patients, primarily as a result of peripheral vascular dilatation.[5] Propofol is highly protein bound (97 ± 1%). It may displace or be displaced by small amounts of other highly bound compounds.

In extremely hypoalbuminemic patients (with fewer protein-binding sites), it has an enhanced effect. More rapid clearance and thus more rapid offset occur than with STP or methohexital, which depend less on protein binding. Also, because of its high elimination constant, significant accumulation is unlikely. Figure 36-3 compares the log concentration versus time curves of thiopental, methohexital, and propofol given as a single bolus. From this curve, we can see that propofol is eliminated faster and thus is associated with more rapid awakening than the other two agents at usual inductive doses.

Etomidate

Because of its highly lipophilic nature, etomidate is dissolved in propylene glycol. The latter vehicle makes it painful on injection, and it may be hepatotoxic in high doses. Also, etomidate may cause myoclonic movements and postoperative myalgias. These can be blocked with small doses of nondepolarizing neuromuscular-blocking agents.

In high doses or with prolonged, continuous administration, etomidate suppresses adrenocorticotropic hormone and, therefore, cortisol. This effect has been encountered even in single-dose administration.[6] One unique property of etomidate is its ability to preserve cardiovascular function without significant

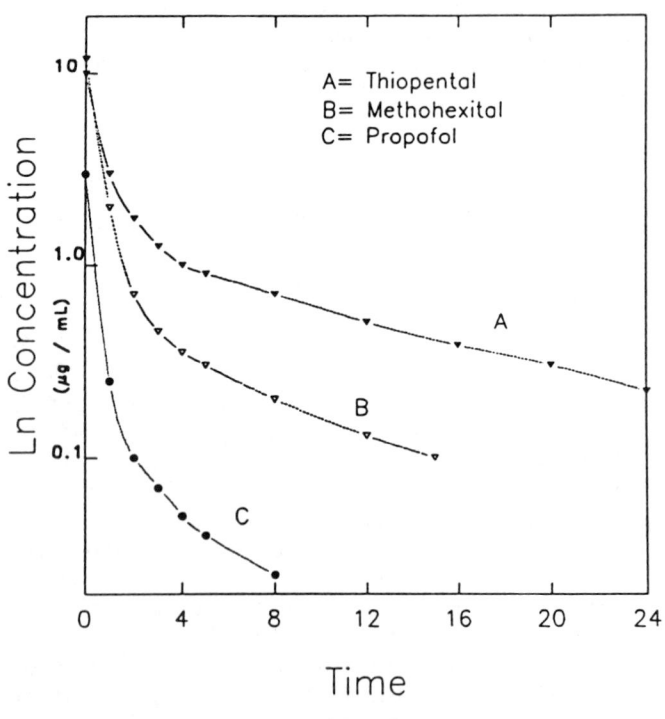

FIGURE 36-3. Thiopental, methohexital, and propofol level profiles. A = Thiopental level profile for a single dose, 6.1 mg · kg^{-1}, intravenous; B = methohexital level profile for a single dose, 2.9 mg · kg^{-1}, intravenous; C = propofol level profile for a single dose, 2.5 mg · kg^{-1}, intravenous. (Adapted from Cockshott ID: Propofol pharmacokinetics and metabolism: an overview. Postgrad Med J 1985; 61:45–50, and Hudson RJ, Stanski DR, Burch PG: Pharmacokinetics of methohexital and thiopental in surgical patients. Anesthesiology 1983; 59:215–219.)

TABLE 36–7. Bioavailability, Time to Onset, and Dosage Guidelines for Midazolam

Route	Bioavailability (%)	Time to Onset (min)	Dose (mg · kg^{-1})
Intravenous	100	0.5	0.05 to 0.5, given in divided doses, adjusting down (decreasing?) for elderly, neonates, and hepatic disease. Tolerance may occur, requiring increased doses.
Intramuscular	91	12–36	Same as intravenous dose; may burn slightly on injection. Onset dependent on vascularity of injection site.
Oral	40–50	15–45	0.5–1.0; bitter taste; best mixed in minimal volume of sweet diluent.
Intranasal	51	10–15	0.2–0.4; bitter taste; minimal volume suggested.
Rectal	Variable: 5–50	15–45	0.3; variable bioavailability; volume dependent.

hemodynamic changes. Myocardial oxygen consumption is not increased significantly. Etomidate may lower seizure thresholds; therefore, it must be used with caution in patients with seizure disorders.

Ketamine

Ketamine provides excellent analgesia, with profound amnesia and cardiovascular stability. However, it has a direct myocardial depressant effect that may cause hypotension in hypovolemic patients who already have maximal sympathetic stimulation. Because of its chemical similarity to phencyclidine, a hallucinogen, bizarre emergent reactions have been reported. These effects are easily blocked with coadministration of most benzodiazepines, but to be effective, their effects must outlast those of ketamine.

Ketamine also causes tachycardia by CNS stimulation. Blood pressure increases owing to an increase in systemic vascular resistance (SVR) and mild increase in cardiac output. It produces a larger increase in pulmonary vascular resistance than in SVR; thus, it may not be an ideal agent for induction in patients with resistance-dependent shunts (i.e., tetralogy of Fallot).

Ketamine also increases cerebral blood flow and thus may raise intracranial pressure (ICP). This effect can be blunted by coadministration of lidocaine, STP, or benzodiazepines. However, the drug should be used with caution in patients in whom ICP is of concern.

Midazolam

Benzodiazepines facilitate the central inhibitory action of γ-aminobutyric acid. They vary with respect to duration and onset of action. Midazolam is a short-acting water-soluble benzodiazepine. It possesses excellent qualities as an inductive or sedative-anxiolytic agent. It causes some venodilatation as well as alteration of the hypoxic and, to a lesser degree, hypercarbic ventilatory drive mechanisms.

Side effects associated with all benzodiazepines are more profound in the elderly and extremely young but can be encountered in all age groups. Extreme caution should be used when these agents are combined with other known respiratory depressants. The effects, in combination with narcotics, may be synergistic.

Midazolam has a rapid onset of action and can be given as a premedication via numerous routes. The relative rate of onset, from fastest to slowest, is intravenous > intramuscular > nasal > oral > rectal. Bioavailability differs, depending on the route chosen; the dose must be adjusted accordingly (Table 36–7).

Midazolam offers some advantages over other benzodiazepines. Its greater water solubility means it can be given intramuscularly and intravenously with less pain on injection and less venous irritation than can diazepam and lorazepam. It has a short t½ and rapid clearance, properties that make it ideal for quick procedures in which a clouded postoperative sensorium is undesirable. Its actions can be reversed with flumazenil. Little danger of resedation is present because the two agents have a similar duration of effect when equally potent doses are given.

Narcotics

Agonists

Narcotic analgesics activate specific receptors in the peripheral and central nervous system. Four general receptor types have been identified: mu, kappa, sigma, and delta (Table 36–8). Each has a pure receptor agonist, although the delta agonist is not available clinically. Each agent interacts with its specific

TABLE 36–8. Receptor Types and Properties

Receptor	Pharmacologic Property	Agonist	Antagonist
Mu	Supraspinal analgesia; depression of ventilation, euphoria, physical dependence	Morphine, fentanyl, meperidine	Naloxone, nalbuphine, naltrexone
Kappa	Spinal anesthesia, depression of ventilation, sedation, miosis	Morphine, pentazocine, nalbuphine, butorphanol	Naloxone, nalbuphine, naltrexone
Sigma	Vasomotor stimulation, stimulation of ventilation, hallucinations, dysphoria	Ketamine*, pentazocine*, morphine*	Naloxone, nalbuphine*, naltrexone
Delta	Modulation of mu receptor activity	Endorphins	Met-enkephalin

*Activity only partially explained by drug listed; no pure agent available.

receptor and produces specific effects. However, all available narcotics can variably activate all receptors. Some compounds, like fentanyl, are more pure receptor agonists—that is, they activate primarily one receptor and produce a positive response without activating multiple receptors or blocking other drug effects.

Antagonists

Conversely, drugs like naloxone are antagonists and can reverse the effect previously produced by an agonist. They have little inherent pharmacologic activity. Drugs like nalbuphine, pentazocine, butorphanol, and dezocine have both agonist and antagonist activity. They may produce a pharmacologic response like analgesia but can reverse the effect of previous narcotics. Buprenorphine, a partial agonist, only partially activates the receptor but in higher doses reaches a maximal pharmacologic (ceiling) effect that does not increase with additional drug.

Receptor Activation and Drug Effect

Each agent has a slightly different spectrum of receptor activation. For example, morphine has mostly mu but also some kappa and sigma activity in higher doses. Thus, it provides peripheral and central analgesia at both the spinal and brain levels. Sigma receptor activation accounts for the dysphoria experienced by some patients after morphine administration. The delta receptor modulates the effect on the mu receptor, thus causing some intersubject variation in effect. This modulation might account in part for some of the pharmacologic tolerance in patients administered narcotics for a long period.

Knowledge of receptor activation has a role in understanding the way a narcotic works but has little direct clinical application. With an understanding of each compound's activity, however, one can conceptualize how a new agent might work and how various other drugs may interact with it. For example, if epidural morphine is given, which primarily activates the kappa receptors in the spinal cord, intravenous nalbuphine can be administered to prevent undesirable pruritus or nausea. These effects are activated by peripheral receptors that can be blocked. The centrally mediated analgesia is unimpaired.

Other Properties

Morphine also causes release of histamine. In higher doses, this effect may cause hypotension, a quality inherent in most opioid derivatives but not the semi-synthetic narcotics, like fentanyl, sufentanil, and alfentanil. This hypotension can only partially be blocked by H_1 blockers like diphenhydramine and hydroxyzine but can be minimized by slow administration.

All narcotics can be used to blunt the hormonal response to surgical stimuli. The magnitude of blunting varies from agent to agent and is also dose dependent. Morphine in doses of 1 to 3 mg · kg^{-1} blocks cortisol and growth hormone responses to surgical stimuli.[3] In large doses, 5 to 10 mg · kg^{-1}, it blunts but does not block the release of antidiuretic hormone (ADH).[7, 8] Fentanyl, 50 to 75 µg · kg^{-1}, blunts the cortisol and epinephrine hormonal effects of surgical stimuli but does not affect the release of ADH.[9]

Induction of Anesthesia

Narcotic regimens have been used for induction of anesthesia in conjunction with neuromuscular-blocking agents. This approach requires extremely high doses of narcotics. Typical doses are 25 to 100 µg · kg^{-1}, for sufentanil, 10 to 20 µg · kg^{-1} for fentanyl, and 50 to 250 µg · kg^{-1} for alfentanil. These doses generally blunt hormonal effects and provide hemodynamic stability. They are quite broad because of the large intersubject variation in response and pharmacokinetics.

Although excellent analgesia is provided, high-dose narcotic techniques are not without problems. Muscle rigidity is common, and the exact cause is unknown. This property, in descending order, is inherent in sufentanil > alfentanil > fentanyl > morphine. Neuromuscular-blocking agents are often necessary to inhibit this effect and to allow ventilation.

Recall can be a substantial problem with pure narcotic techniques. Addition of a benzodiazepine, such as midazolam, 0.1 mg · kg^{-1}, or low-dose inhalational agents, 0.1 maximum allowable concentration, virtually eliminates this problem.

What Are the Alternatives to Narcotic Analgesics?

Nonsteroidal Anti-Inflammatory Drugs

Nonsteroidal analgesics are not narcotics. By and large, they are given orally, but indomethacin and ketorolac can be given intravenously. These agents block prostaglandin synthesis and therefore inhibit the swelling and pain associated with prostaglandin production. They are best administered before insult and are effective adjuncts to the narcotics for pain control.

Nonsteroidal analgesics possess no respiratory depressant qualities; thus they increase analgesia without compromising respiration. They do inhibit prostaglandin-mediated renal blood flow and must be used with caution in patients with limited intrinsic renal disease. They also inhibit prostaglandin-mediated platelet aggregation. This property appears to be reversible when the drug concentration diminishes; aspirin, however, irreversibly poisons the platelets.

Can Pure Intravenous Anesthesia Be Performed?

Continuous propofol infusion with low-dose narcotic background analgesia probably represents the best current total intravenous regimen. This combination allows rapid awakening and provides favorable intraoperative conditions. Amnesia is present with complete anesthesia, and recall seldom is an issue. The major drawback is cost, which is exorbitant for long cases but is acceptable for short procedures of 1 hour or less. The techniques are especially dependent on adequate intravenous access, which if lost causes undesired arousal.

Combinations of high-dose narcotics, neuromuscular-blocking agents, and amnestic agents provide excellent intravenous anesthesia. However, they may result in prolonged respiratory depression, especially if the surgical procedure is short. Continuous infusions of short-acting narcotics minimize this problem. Newer, even shorter-acting narcotics that are under development may resolve it completely.

Continuous infusion of STP, ketamine, or etomidate, in

combination with neuromuscular-blocking agents, also provides adequate anesthetic conditions. However, these drugs often require analgesic supplementation to blunt the cardiovascular response to noxious stimuli. In long cases, they can accumulate, causing prolonged anesthesia after the infusion is discontinued.

References

1. Hug CC Jr: Pharmacokinetics and dynamics of narcotic analgesics. *In* Pharmacokinetics of Anaesthesia. Prys-Roberts C, Hug CC Jr (eds). London, Blackwell Scientific, 1984, pp 187–234.
2. Brogden R, Goa K: Flumazenil: a reappraisal of its pharmacologic properties and therapeutic efficacy as a benzodiazepine antagonist. Drugs 1991; 42:1061.
3. Seltzer JL, Gerson JI, Allen FB: Comparison of the cardiovascular effects of bolus vs incremental administration of thiopentone. Br J Anaesth 1980; 52:527.
4. Barron DW: Effect of rate of injection on incidence of side effects with thiopental and methohexital. Anesth Analg 1968; 47:171.
5. Hug CC, McLeskey CH, Nahrwald ML, et al: Hemodynamic effects of propofol: data from over 25,000 patients. Anesth Analg 1993; 77(Suppl):521.
6. Wagner RL, White PF: Etomidate inhibits adrenocortical function in surgical patients. Anesthesiology 1984; 61:647.
7. George JM: Morphine anesthesia blocks cortisol and growth hormone response to surgical stress in humans. J Clin Endocrinol Metab 1974; 38:736.
8. Philbin DM, Coggins CH: Plasma antidiuretic hormone level in cardiac surgical patients during morphine and halothane anesthesia. Anesthesiology 1987; 49:95.
9. Stanley TH, Philbin DM, Coggins CH: Fentanyl-oxygen anaesthesia for coronary artery surgery. Cardiovascular and antidiuretic hormone responses. Can Anaesth Soc J 1979; 26:168.

CHAPTER 37

Inhalation Agents

WENDELL C. STEVENS, M.D.

Inhalation agents were the foundation of general anesthesia and were used without adjuvants for many decades. This practice changed in the 1920s, when Lundy[1] introduced the concept of *balanced anesthesia*, an approach to anesthesia care that involves the use of several techniques or agents simultaneously. Since that time, and increasingly since about 1970, general anesthesia has been performed with combined inhalation and intravenous anesthetics. The utility of regional anesthesia in decreasing the hormonal response to stress and controlling postoperative pain has renewed and extended the interest in combined regional and general anesthesia. Use of inhaled agents is one option for the general anesthesia component of the latter combination.

Thus, a drift away from pure inhalation techniques has occurred. Inhalation agents have become one alternative among many to provide narcosis, prevent recall, control reflex responses to noxious stimuli, and induce muscle relaxation. These drugs provide parts of these components of anesthesia but ordinarily not all of them. The context of this chapter assumes that one wants to provide as much of the anesthetic state as possible with inhalation agents, while recognizing that this may not be the way in which most anesthetics are given. Data are not available to demonstrate superior outcomes for a pure inhalation approach in comparison with the various balanced techniques, or vice versa.

Nevertheless, roles for pure inhalation techniques do exist. One is to allow gradual, breath-by-breath change in anesthetic level as the anesthesiologist assesses airway adequacy and circulatory changes that accompany anesthetic induction. Another is to improve the simplicity of anesthesia management, to allow one to ascribe more clearly a cause-and-effect relationship to intra-anesthetic events than might occur if multiple drugs were used. The use of inhalation agents provides a logical way to learn and to maintain airway management skills. These skills are the hallmark of capable anesthesiologists who must maintain a high level of proficiency if they are to manage all patients' airways successfully. Finally, if venous access cannot be obtained, a patient usually can be anesthetized with inhalation agents.

THE HISTORY OF INHALED ANESTHETICS

Why Were They Developed and Introduced?

Early experiments with drugs that became anesthetics were directed more toward scholarly explication of their chemical or physical properties, their application as medical therapies, or their use for pleasurable purposes than toward relief of the agony of surgery.[2] Sedation, sleep, and analgesia that occurred during medicinal or exhilarating uses of the drugs triggered trials of their use as anesthetics by physicians who had been looking for some ways to make surgery pain-free.[3]

Diethyl ether, nitrous oxide (N_2O), and chloroform —drugs introduced into clinical practice almost simultaneously in the 1840s—were the only anesthetics used regularly for nearly half a century. Around 1930, efforts were directed toward *biochemomorphology*,[4] which is the design of drugs based on structure-activity relationships. The first widely used anesthetic developed by this process was divinyl ether (Vinethene). Analysis of structure-activity relationships guided the explorations of fluorinated hydrocarbons by Robbins,[5] Van Poznak and Artusio,[6] and Krantz,[7] and the analysis of hundreds of fluorinated ethyl-methyl ethers by Terrell and coworkers.[8] Table 37–1 lists 20 inhalation anesthetics that have been given to humans. Some are of only historical interest, and some are in the developmental process.

Why Does the Search for New Agents Continue?

Probable reasons include the attractiveness of providing the entire anesthetic state with one agent and the ability to control anesthetic dose precisely. Improvements in efficacy and safety are paramount considerations in the ongoing search for new drugs and account for loss of interest in older ones. Testing must be exhaustive and, therefore, is expensive, since govern-

TABLE 37–1. A Chronology of Use of Inhaled Anesthetics

Drug	Date Use Reported in Humans	Status or Reason If Not Current
Diethyl ether	1842	Current (developing countries)
Nitrous oxide	1844	Current
Chloroform	1847	Hepatotoxicity
Ethyl chloride	1894	Flammability; cardiac dysrhythmias
Ethylene	1923	Flammability
Divinyl ether	1923	Flammability
Cyclopropane	1933	Flammability
Trichlorethylene (Trilene)	1935	Reacts with soda lime
Metopryl	1946	Flammability
Ethyl vinyl ether (Vinamar)	1947	Flammability
Trifluoroethyl vinyl ether (Fluroxene)	1953	Flammability; toxic metabolites
Halothane	1956	Current
Methoxyflurane	1960	Nephrotoxicity; high tissue solubility
Teflurane	1961	Cardiac arrhythmias
Halopropane	1962	Cardiac arrhythmias
Enflurane	1966	Current, but disappearing; seizures
Isoflurane	1971	Current
Aliflurane	1979	In development
Sevoflurane	1981	Current
Desflurane	1990	Current

ment approval of a drug must be obtained before widespread clinical use is permitted. Commercial goals definitely have a role in the search for new anesthetics.

PHARMACOKINETICS AND PHARMACODYNAMICS: CLINICAL IMPLICATIONS

What Makes Inhalation Agents Useful?

A significant feature of inhalation agents is the ease and predictability with which changes in anesthetic depth can be achieved with their use. Since these anesthetics are entirely administered and chiefly eliminated via the lungs, the alveolar concentration of these drugs governs concentrations in all tissues. Anesthesiologists can increase or decrease the alveolar concentration at will by changing the inspired concentration and ensuring adequate alveolar ventilation.

A key factor determining the depth of anesthesia is the rate at which the tissue anesthetic concentrations approach the alveolar concentration. This equilibration is rapid for tissues whose blood flow is high in relation to their capacity for the anesthetic. For these tissues, the alveolar concentration accurately reflects tissue concentration, and the equilibrium of concentrations occurs rapidly. For example, the anesthetic concentration in the brain is about 5% of the alveolar concentration within approximately 5 minutes, presuming that stable alveolar concentration, normal cardiac output, and distribution of output exist. Thus, in a short time, the anesthetic concentration in the brain can be estimated from the end-expired concentration.

Is the Rapidity of Equilibration Always an Advantage?

The answer to this question is "Yes" in that knowledge and control of the anesthetic dose at the site of action of the anesthetic are helpful. However, substantial risk of overdose occurs if delivery of anesthetic into the lungs is unopposed. When a patient breathes spontaneously during inhalation induction, alveolar ventilation decreases because the anesthetic depresses breathing. As a result, anesthetic delivery to the lungs decreases.[9] If ventilation is controlled and the inspired anesthetic concentration is high, this safety net is removed; the alveolar concentration can then increase rapidly to circulatory depressant levels. A positive feedback occurs as cardiac output (CO) and anesthetic uptake decrease, thus accelerating the rate of rise of alveolar concentration[10] (Fig. 37–1). At times of rapid increase in delivered anesthetic concentration, one probably should preserve spontaneous breathing or avoid a high inspired anesthetic concentration and make an effort not to hyperventilate the patient.

Is Anesthetic Elimination As Controllable As Uptake?

Overpressurization (the use of higher inspired concentrations during induction than are required to maintain anesthesia) provides excellent compensation for anesthetic uptake and allows inductions to occur rapidly and in a controllable manner. No similar assist can occur during emergence, since the inspired anesthetic concentration cannot be less than zero.

Cardiac output and its distribution are not controlled by the anesthesiologist. When the CO is low during emergence such that smaller than usual amounts of anesthetic are delivered to the lungs, continued ventilation rapidly lowers the alveolar anesthetic concentrations. The tissue-to-alveolar partial-pressure gradients may be large, and the low alveolar concentration may lead one to think arousal should occur quickly. However, the patient may still be anesthetized despite a subanesthetic alveolar concentration of anesthetic.

A clinical application of the problem of persistent tissue anesthetic levels is the continuation of drug-induced respiratory depression at a time when spontaneous ventilation is desired. The apneic threshold for carbon dioxide (CO_2) may be high despite low alveolar anesthetic concentrations, so that the

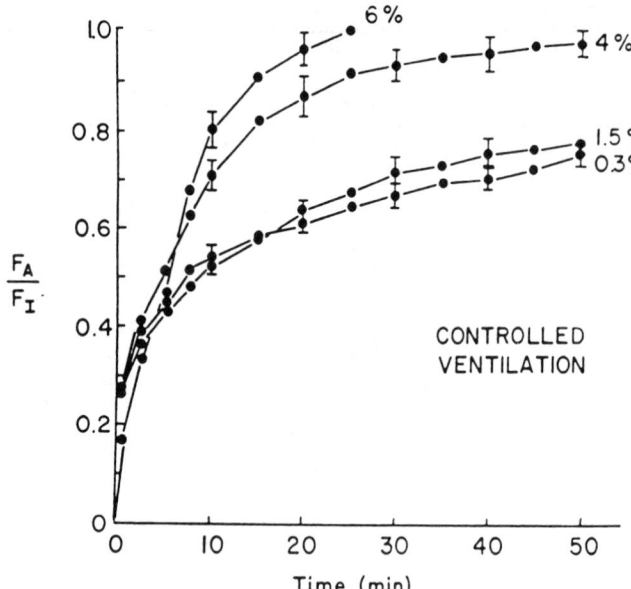

FIGURE 37–1. The rates of rise of FA/FI (ratio of alveolar fraction of halothane to inspired fraction of halothane) over time at various inspired halothane concentrations. After the first 5 minutes, the rates were more rapid at the higher inspired halothane concentrations in dogs receiving constant controlled ventilation. This is due to depression of cardiac output and to decreased anesthetic uptake. (From Gibbons RT, Steffey EP, Eger EI II: The effect of spontaneous versus controlled ventilation on the rate of rise of alveolar halothane concentrations in dogs. Anesth Analg 1977; 56:32–34. © International Anesthesia Research Society.)

patient fails to breathe as expected. This situation leads to a dilemma in the management of emergence: hypoventilation required to increase the arterial CO_2 partial pressure ($PaCO_2$) delays the removal of anesthetic from blood and tissues. A way to avoid this problem is to maintain end-tidal CO_2 at or only slightly below the CO_2 apneic threshold throughout the anesthetic procedure.

How Much Anesthetic Is Required for Surgery?

Assessment of Depth

Anesthetic depth can be considered in terms of the body's response to various alveolar or tissue levels of anesthetic drugs. The Guedel stages and planes of anesthesia, and the correlation of electroencephalogram (EEG) patterns with blood anesthetic levels are examples of this approach. Another approach is analysis of the anesthetic concentration required to block responses to stimuli.[11] The stimuli can be non-noxious, such as verbal commands, or noxious, such as skin incision or traction on abdominal viscera. The anesthetic doses required to block responses to various stimuli have been quantified[12–15] (Table 37–2). The data provide guidelines by which the anesthesiologist predicts the amount of anesthetic to administer or when awakening is to be expected.

External Factors

Maintaining the appropriate depth of anesthesia is not straightforward, however, because the stimulation from surgery and anesthesia procedures changes. A dynamic relation-

TABLE 37–2. Alveolar Halothane Concentrations (FA) Required to Prevent Responses to Various Stimuli in 50% of Subjects

Stimulus	Response	FA (%)
Verbal	Open eyes	0.41[12]
Skin incision	Gross muscle response	0.77[13]
Laryngoscopy	Extremity movement; relaxation of vocal cords	1.12[14]
Endotracheal intubation	Coughing	1.46[14]
Skin incision	Norepinephrine level	1.12*[15]

*Plus 60% nitrous oxide.

ship is present among the stimuli, the anesthetic, and the patient. Patient factors such as age, ongoing drug regimens, and temperature alter anesthetic requirement. Large differences in anesthetic requirement probably occur during different stages of the operation and for operations in different sites. This phenomenon has been shown clearly with intravenous agents,[16] but data are not as well developed for inhaled ones. Also, the anesthetic concentration in the body is constantly changing unless the inspired anesthetic concentration is decreased as uptake continues.

Inadequate or Excessive Anesthetic Depth

Achieving the appropriate depth of anesthesia in the face of so many variables can indeed be challenging. Inadequate anesthesia can lead to recall, some of which is not necessarily painful or disturbing to the patient.[17, 18] Excessive anesthesia can cause death.[19] If these extremes of the spectrum of anesthetic depth occur, the delivered concentration of anesthesia did not necessarily deviate from the usual or expected amounts. Rather, such outcomes reflect our inability to determine with certainty the appropriate depth of anesthesia for all patients at all times. Often, attention is focused on the maintenance of circulatory variables within chosen ranges because a better approach is lacking. It is generally accepted that tissue perfusion should be maintained above all else. Satisfactory management involves constant review of clinical signs and monitored data.

CONSIDERATIONS IN PATIENTS WITH CENTRAL NERVOUS SYSTEM DISEASES

The effects of inhalation anesthetics on the central nervous system (CNS) include alteration of the cerebral metabolic rate for oxygen ($CMRO_2$), direct effects on blood vessels, vascular effects by interaction with CO_2, effects on cerebrospinal fluid (CSF) dynamics, and alteration of neuronal function and electrical activity. Should these effects lead to the selection of one drug over another? If so, when?

Does Planned Interruption of Blood Supply Affect Anesthetic Choice?

All potent inhaled agents decrease $CMRO_2$[20] primarily by decreasing brain functional activity as reflected by EEG changes.[21] The effect of N_2O on $CMRO_2$ is not predictable and probably depends on the level of CNS depression produced by diseases or other drugs.[22] Decrease in electrical activity characterized as burst suppression occurs with all inhaled anesthetics. Of special significance is the finding that isoflurane and the new anesthetic desflurane begin to produce burst suppression at moderate levels of anesthesia, between 0.5 and 1.0 times the minimum alveolar concentration (MAC) (Fig. 37–2). When doses of these agents equivalent to 1.5 MAC are given, the EEG demonstrates burst suppression over 90% of the time.[23]

The electrical suppression produced by isoflurane is probably of clinical significance. Greater decreases in cerebral blood flow (CBF) are tolerated with isoflurane before cerebral ischemia occurs than with halothane or enflurane. This observation may reflect isoflurane's electrical effects (Fig. 37–3). The relationship between blood flow and EEG changes defines the critical regional CBF at which cerebral ischemia is detected.[24, 25]

Although reliance on cerebral protection from inhaled agents is not warranted,[21] isoflurane, and perhaps desflurane, offer the advantage of maximum depression of $CMRo_2$ at moderate commonly used levels of anesthesia. Other evidence of the favorable effect of isoflurane is better preservation of cerebral welfare during deliberate hypotension compared with halothane.[26]

How Are Cerebral Blood Volume and Intracranial Pressure Affected?

Anesthetic-Induced Cerebrovasodilation

The potent agents produce cerebrovasodilation: halothane > enflurane > isoflurane = desflurane.[27, 28] The smaller effect of isoflurane may be due to its prominent effect of decreasing $CMRo_2$.[29] N_2O produces vasodilation to a degree similar to that with an equivalent MAC multiple of potent agent.[30]

Hypocapnia-Induced Cerebrovasoconstriction

Cerebrovasodilation is modified by changes in $Paco_2$. With all inhaled anesthetics, cerebrovascular resistance increases as

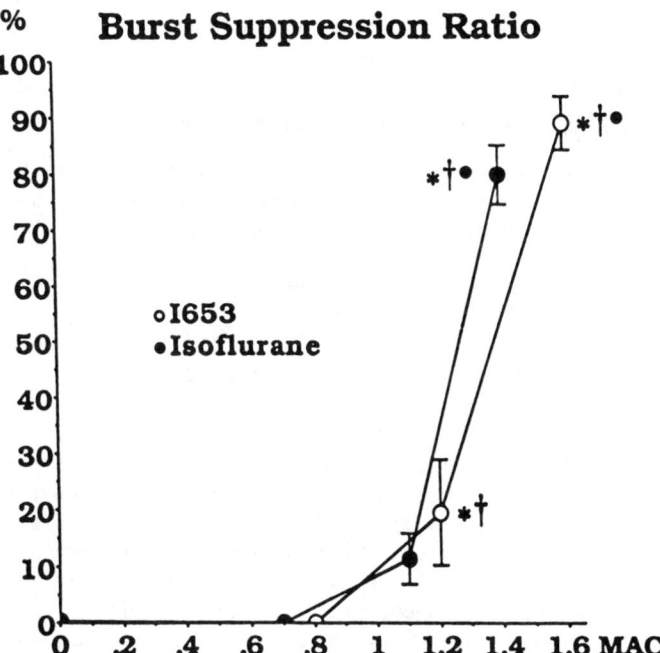

FIGURE 37–2. Burst suppression ratios for I653 (desflurane) and isoflurane at various multiples of MAC. Burst suppression ratio is the percentage of time in 4-second epochs during which the EEG voltage did not exceed 5.0 μV. (From Rampil IJ, Weiskopf RB, Brown JG, et al: I653 and isoflurane produce similar dose-related changes in the electroencephalogram of pigs. Anesthesiology 1988; 69:298.)

$Paco_2$ decreases to hypocapnic levels, resulting in decreased CBF. Control of intracranial pressure (ICP) by this mechanism is better with isoflurane than with halothane[31] or desflurane.[32] Hyperventilation must precede halothane administration if increases in ICP are to be attenuated in patients with intracranial tumors.[31] Hypocapnia effectively decreases CBF and ICP over a broad range of anesthetic depths.[33] Decreases in CBF from hypocapnia may decrease ICP less than expected because the

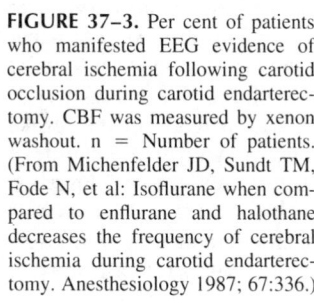

FIGURE 37–3. Per cent of patients who manifested EEG evidence of cerebral ischemia following carotid occlusion during carotid endarterectomy. CBF was measured by xenon washout. n = Number of patients. (From Michenfelder JD, Sundt TM, Fode N, et al: Isoflurane when compared to enflurane and halothane decreases the frequency of cerebral ischemia during carotid endarterectomy. Anesthesiology 1987; 67:336.)

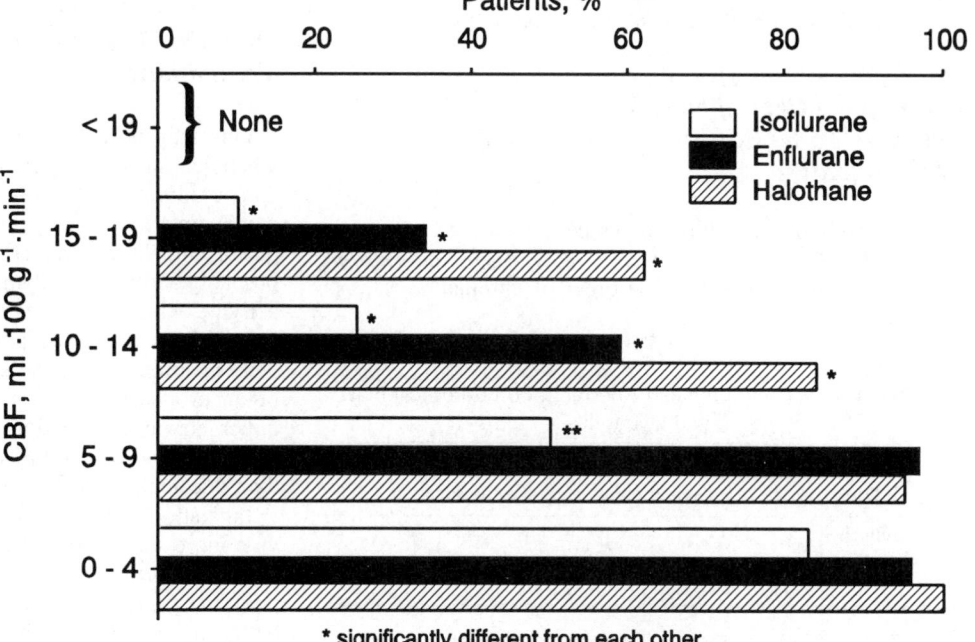

anesthetics may cause cerebrovenodilation that is not responsive to change in $Paco_2$.

Cerebrospinal Fluid Production/Reabsorption

The finding of increased ICP despite adequate depth of anesthesia and hypocapnia led to consideration of CSF dynamics as a factor governing ICP. The potent agents affect CSF production or reabsorption, or both (Table 37–3).[34–37] Enflurane is unfavorable in both respects.

Why Are the Electroencephalographic Effects of Interest?

Electroencephalographic patterns have long been recognized as an indicator of anesthetic depth.[38] A pattern of progressive cortical depression occurs as depth increases; that is, wave frequency decreases while amplitude increases.[39] The amount of time that the EEG is electrically silent progressively increases with the anesthetic dose.[40] Despite the predictability of these changes, the EEG is not yet used routinely to monitor depth of anesthesia, perhaps because burst suppression is a nonstationary event. A patient may have a highly variable degree of EEG suppression at given times.[40] Many agents cause EEG epileptiform activity.[41] At higher concentrations and with hypocapnia, enflurane causes EEG and muscular epileptiform activity.[42] However, enflurane is not contraindicated in patients who exhibit seizure foci preoperatively.[43]

Can Inhaled Agents Be Used with Evoked Potential Monitoring?

Inhalation anesthetics have a greater effect on cortical responses than on subcortical recordings.[44] They cause dose-related decreases in amplitude and increases in latency of cortical somatosensory evoked potentials.[45] The order of depression is enflurane > isoflurane > halothane. Of paramount importance is maintenance of stable alveolar concentration of all anesthetics throughout the period of recording.

Is Complete Central Nervous System Recovery To Be Expected After Elimination of the Agent?

Yes. Cerebral elimination of inhaled agents resembles the pattern of their elimination from alveoli. As predicted from blood and tissue solubilities, the order of elimination rates is

TABLE 37–3. Effect of Inhaled Anesthetics on Cerebrospinal Fluid Dynamics

Drug	Cerebrospinal Fluid Production	Resistance to Resorption
Enflurane[34]		
Halothane[35, 36]	↓	↑
Isoflurane[37]	→	→

Key: ↑ = increased; ↓ = decreased; → = unchanged.

TABLE 37–4. Influence of Inhalation Anesthetics on Respiration

Decrease whole body or individual organ metabolism
Obtund upper airway reflexes affecting airway patency
Depress peripheral chemoreceptors
Depress the central respiratory control center
Alter mechanical properties of the chest wall and diaphragm
Decrease bronchomotor tone
Alter volume and distribution of pulmonary blood flow

desflurane > isoflurane > halothane.[46] This ranking parallels the ranking of speed of recovery of animals from anesthesia.[47] Although CNS recovery is complete following elimination of inhaled anesthetics, several days may be required for all behavioral or mental effects to disappear. Neurologic signs, including transient hyperreflexia or a Babinski reflex, commonly exist in the first several minutes of recovery.[48] Their presence early in recovery is not necessarily or even usually a sign of CNS damage.

MANAGEMENT OF BREATHING

Inhalation agents affect breathing in multiple ways (Table 37–4).[49] In some instances, variables are changed toward more satisfactory gas exchange. Decreased CO_2 production and total body O_2 demand[50] reduce the ventilatory requirement. Another favorable effect is decreased bronchomotor tone, which reduces airway resistance.[51] Airway maintenance is a problem, however, because inhaled anesthetics relax upper airway muscles and disrupt reflexes intended to maintain patency.[52] Functional residual capacity (FRC) nearly always decreases with induction of anesthesia; increased intrapulmonary shunting of blood and increased airway resistance may result.[53] Intrapulmonary shunting may increase if the anesthetic attenuates hypoxic pulmonary vasoconstriction[54] or if lowered pulmonary artery pressure favors distribution of blood to less well ventilated parts of the lung.[57]

How Do These Factors Influence Ventilation?

One may need to preserve the patient's respiratory efforts when dealing with upper airway obstruction from supraglottitis and tumors or with more distal obstruction from cervical or mediastinal masses. A number of problems are likely to occur during inhalation induction in such instances. Anesthetics probably abolish reflexly maintained phasic pharyngeal muscle activity, which preserves upper airway patency in the awake state.[55] Loss of airway patency may require manipulation of head position, use of increased airway pressure, and insertion of an oropharyngeal or nasopharyngeal airway to overcome upper airway obstruction. If inhalation induction is chosen, isoflurane and desflurane induce more airway reflex responses than does halothane.[56]

Inhalation induction with spontaneous breathing may provide more satisfactory gas exchange than controlled breathing in patients with obstruction of the intrathoracic trachea; transpulmonary pressure and nonturbulent gas flow probably are better maintained with this approach.[57]

Is Spontaneous Breathing Useful During Maintenance?

Anesthetic dose–dependent depression of the ventilatory CO_2 response and increase in the apneic threshold are common to the potent agents.[58, 59] Consequently, $Paco_2$ will be elevated during spontaneous breathing. Substitution of some of the potent agents with N_2O lessens the respiratory depression and leads to a lower $Paco_2$.[60] The depression is antagonized by surgical stimulation such that $Paco_2$ returns toward (but ordinarily not to) normal levels when surgery begins[61] (Fig. 37–4).

Changes in ventilatory variables provide reliable guides to anesthetic depth.[62] Tidal volume decreases and frequency of breathing commonly increases as alveolar anesthetic concentration increases.[58] When the patient and anesthesiologist must be separated by some distance, monitors of breathing provide a useful indicator of anesthetic depth. Also, if a mechanical problem such as an airway disconnection occurs, the patient will continue to breathe.

The FRC decreases with onset of general anesthesia regardless of the anesthetic drugs that are selected or the mode of ventilation used.[53, 63] A major cause of the decrease is thought to be compression atelectasis. Similar amounts of atelectasis occur with spontaneous or controlled breathing.[63]

Will Increased Airway Resistance Affect Spontaneous Ventilation?

Anesthetics depress the normal immediate response to imposed resistance that is characterized by prolonged inspiration

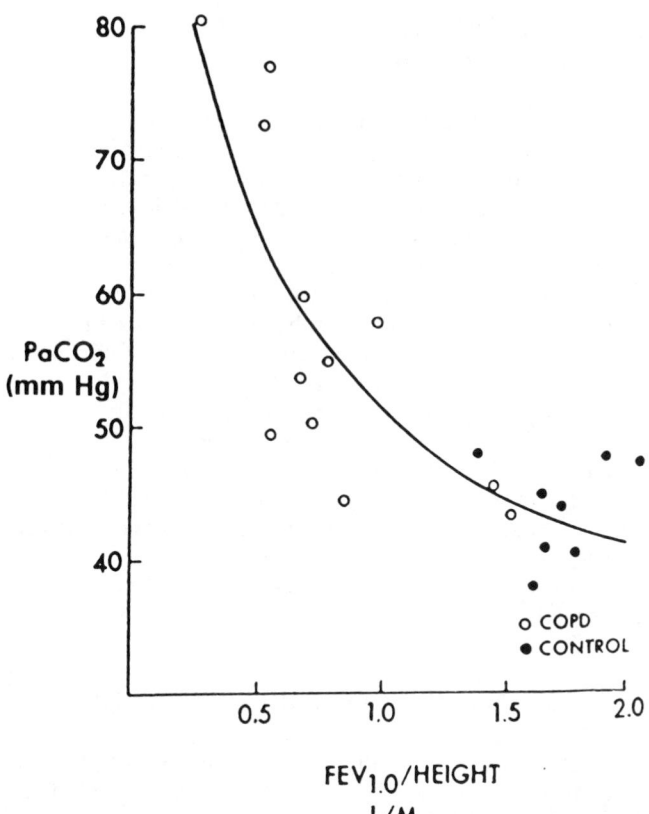

FIGURE 37–5. Relationship between $Paco_2$ levels during anesthesia with spontaneous ventilation and preoperative $FEV_{1.0}$ expressed in terms of body height. (From Pietak S, Weenig CS, Hickey RF, et al: Anesthetic effects on ventilation in patients with chronic obstructive pulmonary disease. Anesthesiology 1975; 42:160.)

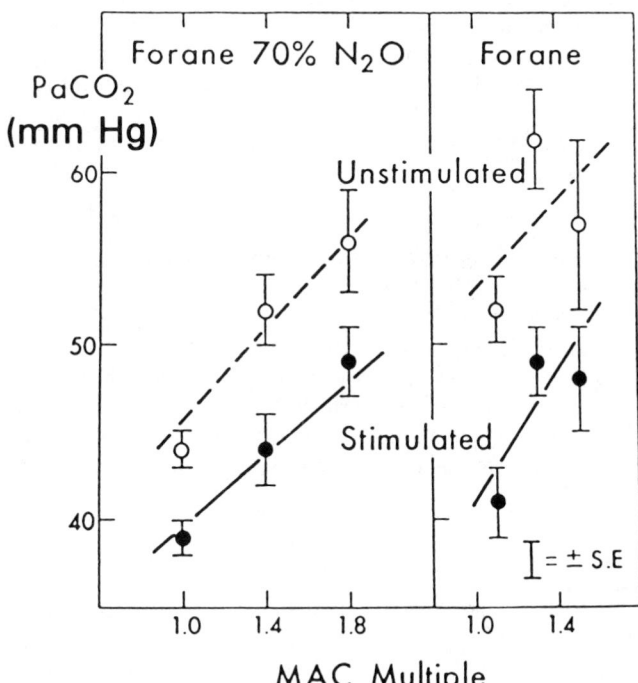

FIGURE 37–4. $Paco_2$ prior to and during operations (unstimulated and stimulated, respectively). Results are shown for several MAC multiples of nitrous oxide–Forane and Forane alone. (From Eger EI II, Dolan WM, Stevens WC, et al: Surgical stimulation antagonizes the respiratory depression produced by Forane. Anesthesiology 1972; 36:544.)

and maintained tidal volume and respiratory frequency.[64] During halothane anesthesia, less inspiratory compensation occurs than during anesthesia with other agents, and that which develops is delayed until the central hypercapnic drive is augmented. The anesthetized patient compensates poorly for weight placed on the chest.[65]

An inverse relationship exists between preoperative forced expiratory volume in 1 second (FEV_1) and intraoperative $Paco_2$. Although few data document this effect, those that do exist are convincing.[66, 67] Whether this effect is due only to impairment of mechanics of breathing or results in part from altered chemical control of respiration is unknown. In any event, allowing spontaneous ventilation in patients with chronic obstructive pulmonary disease and low FEV_1 almost certainly will result in elevated $Paco_2$, sometimes to inordinate levels (Fig. 37–5).

Is Halothane the Preferred Agent in Reactive Airway Disease?

The answer to this question is predicated on the accepted concept that tracheal intubation should not be attempted until deep anesthesia has been obtained.[68] Inhalation induction appears to be most easily accomplished with halothane. Once induction is completed, however, halothane, enflurane, and isoflurane are equally effective in preventing or reversing bronchoconstriction.[69, 70]

Should Inhalation Agents Be Avoided During One-Lung Ventilation?

The potent inhalation agents depress hypoxic pulmonary vasoconstriction and increase the alveolar-to-arterial oxygen partial-pressure difference.[54, 63] In the clinical setting, when relatively low doses of inhaled agents are used, intrapulmonary shunting is not increased by these drugs over the amount that occurs during primarily intravenous anesthesia.[71]

The ventilatory hypoxic drive mediated via peripheral chemoreceptors is attenuated at subanesthetic doses of potent agents and obliterated when the drugs are given at anesthetizing concentrations[72] (Fig. 37–6). The clinical significance of this effect is that a small increase or no increase in breathing might occur if hypoxia develops during anesthesia. Ventilation may even be depressed further. A recent study[73] disputed the lack of hypoxic ventilatory response shown in the earlier study.[72] I am unaware of data describing the ventilatory impact of persistent subanesthetic doses during recovery. Whether patients who become hypoxic during recovery from anesthesia are at risk for further depression of breathing is unknown.

MANAGEMENT OF THE CIRCULATION

For an inhaled agent to be used as the sole anesthetic, especially in adults, is rare in clinical practice. Consequently, the impact of inhaled agents on the circulation is modified by interaction with other drugs. In some circumstances, inhaled agents may be a favorable choice. The effects of inhaled agents alone on circulatory variables are listed in Table 37–5. Note that arterial pressure decreases with all agents except N_2O.

These effects can be expected to occur when inhaled agents are given concomitantly with other drugs. The specific properties of the agents can be used to advantage if an inhalation anesthetic is a component of a multiple-drug balanced technique. For example, isoflurane decreases peripheral resistance when added to a narcotic-based regimen.[74] If myocardial depression is desired, halothane reliably produces it and maintains heart rate to near control levels.[75]

Why Has the Use of Inhaled Agents As Sole Anesthetic Drugs Decreased?

The dose of anesthetic required to attenuate circulatory responses to stimulation from surgery or anesthetic procedures may be large, leading to an undesired decrease in systemic arterial pressure. For example, the dose of halothane required

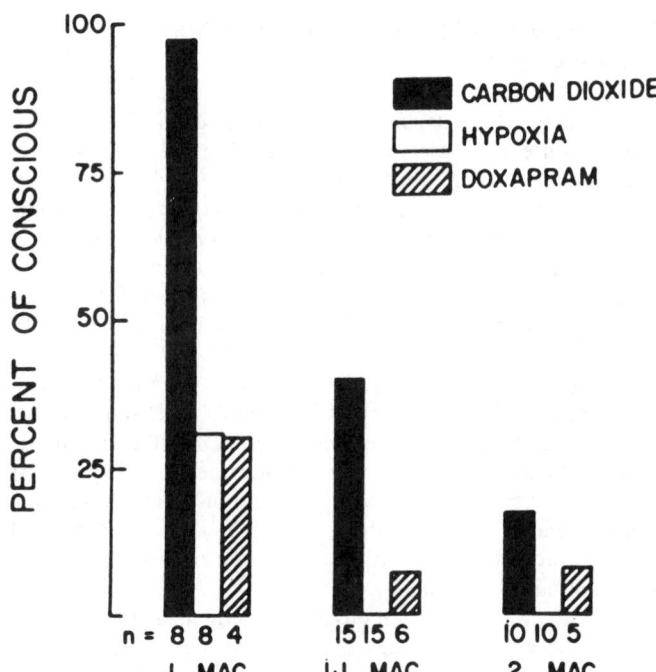

FIGURE 37–6. Relative activity of respiratory chemoreflexes in humans during various levels of halothane anesthesia. Responses are shown as a per cent of the ventilatory responses that occurred in subjects during the control state. (From Knill RL, Gelb AW: Ventilatory responses to hypoxia and hypercapnia during halothane sedation and anesthesia in man. Anesthesiology 1978; 49:244.)

to prevent movement during tracheal intubation is 1.33 MAC,[76] and the dose required to block the adrenergic response to skin incision is 1.45 MAC.[16] On average, these doses lead to at least a 25% to 30% decrease in arterial pressure, even in healthy patients,[77] and probably to greater decreases in patients with vascular or cardiac diseases. The adrenergic or laryngeal responses can be blocked in part by narcotics[78] or local anesthetics.[79] Use of adjuvants to allow lower doses of the inhaled agents during these procedures is preferred by many anesthesiologists.

Are Inhaled Agents Useful in Patients with Coronary Artery Disease?

If so, is one agent better than another? Much research has attempted to answer these questions. The major benefit of the research has been the increase in knowledge about coronary and myocardial physiology and the effects of anesthetic drugs on the heart. Much more is now known about the relative

TABLE 37–5. Changes From Awake Values of Circulatory Variables Produced by Inhalation Anesthetics*

	Desflurane[93, 94]	Enflurane[95]	Halothane[77]	Isoflurane[96]	Nitrous Oxide[85]	Sevoflurane[93]
Arterial pressure	↓	↓	↓	↓	→ or ↑	↓
Cardiac output	↓	↓	↓	→	→ or ↑	→
Heart rate	↑	↑	→	↓	→ or ↑	→
Systemic vascular resistance	↓	↓	→	↓	→ or ↑	↓
Central venous pressure	↑	↑	↑	→ or ↑	?	?

*The effects of nitrous oxide are those occurring when it is added to anesthesia with a volatile agent.
Key: ↓ = decreased; ↑ = increased; → = unchanged.

importance of factors affecting cardiac O_2 supply and demand relationships.

Although agreement is not universal, the anesthetic drug by itself probably is of minor importance as a determinant of outcome from surgery and anesthesia in patients with coronary artery disease.[80–82] Despite concern that anesthesia-induced coronary vasodilation (the steal phenomenon) from isoflurane may lead to myocardial ischemia, this phenomenon simply has not been a clinically significant problem. Anesthesia-induced negative inotropism actually may prevent the steal phenomenon.[83]

Are Inhaled Anesthetics Appropriate in Patients with Valvular Disease?

Potent Agents

For mitral regurgitation, the relatively rapid heart rate and decrease in systemic vascular resistance seen with isoflurane correspond well to the requirements for maintained myocardial performance. These same factors make isoflurane and, to some extent, enflurane weak choices for management of the patient with aortic stenosis or idiopathic hypertrophic subaortic stenosis. Such statements apply fully only if anesthesia is managed with inhalation agents alone. In practice, balanced anesthesia is commonly used. The inhalation agents provide an attractive component when myocardial depression (halothane) or vasodilation (isoflurane, enflurane) are needed in addition to somewhat deeper anesthesia.

Nitrous Oxide

The appropriate role for N_2O in patients with coronary artery or valvular disease is uncertain. The inspired O_2 concentration must necessarily be decreased when N_2O is used. Infants with high pulmonary vascular resistance may have further increases caused by N_2O.[84] Its direct myocardial effects are negligible, but systemic vascular resistance may increase.[85] The major advantage of N_2O is the prompt onset and emergence from the anesthesia that it provides.

Can Volatile Agents Be Used Safely During Catecholamine Administration?

The answer is a qualified "Yes." Qualifiers include the anesthetic, the catecholamine, and other drugs that are given for or during anesthesia. Although dysrhythmias associated with catecholamine administration are not rare, the frequency with which the rhythm deteriorates to ventricular fibrillation probably is very low, even if no treatment is given. Decrease of the dysrhythmic threshold of epinephrine produced with halothane is greater than that with enflurane, isoflurane, desflurane or sevoflurane.[86–88]

The interaction of anesthetics and epinephrine has been studied more extensively than the interaction of anesthetics with other vasoactive drugs. Although a risk of dysrhythmias exists with the use of many drugs,[89] the frequent use of epinephrine makes it the focus of greatest concern.

Other drugs administered during anesthesia can induce dysrhythmia because their infusion must continue for a long period of time; also, anesthesiologists may be less familiar with the properties of the drugs. An example of this circumstance is the administration of theophylline to decrease airway reactivity.[90] Finally, the induction agents may increase epinephrine sensitivity (thiopental)[91] or produce no change in sensitivity (midazolam).[92]

NEUROHUMORAL RESPONSE TO SURGERY

Do Inhaled Agents Alone Effectively Attenuate the Stress Response?

Anesthesia alone results in significant increases in plasma cortisol, growth hormone, and norepinephrine levels.[97] Sufficient levels of inhaled agents block the adrenergic response to surgical incision. The results of Roizen and coworkers[16] suggest that a reliable relationship exists between anesthetic dose and blockade of the response. However, other work with halothane[98] and isoflurane[99] indicates that the hormonal responses to 0.5 to 1.2 MAC as well as to doses approximately twice as large were similar. Thus, inhaled anesthetics can decrease the hormonal response to surgery,[100] but the dose required to do so reliably may be very large.

In current practice, adjuvants—including adrenergic antagonists and narcotics—often are used to decrease the sympathetic nervous system's response to surgery.[101] Although the response can be prevented by the use of inhaled agents alone, much experience supports the current practice of using such combinations.[101] Lower doses of inhaled agents can then be used, and the suppression of stress response may extend into the postoperative period.[102]

RENAL FUNCTION

Are Enflurane and Sevoflurane Contraindicated in Renal Disease?

This question arises because increases of inorganic fluoride to nephrotoxic levels can occur with the use of both of these drugs as a consequence of their metabolism.[103, 104] With both, the duration of the peak levels appears to be so brief that kidney injury does not occur. Prudence suggests their use should be avoided in patients with renal insufficiency, since alternatives to their use are available.[105] Also, the significance of the sometimes high levels of inorganic fluoride with sevoflurane anesthesia is not yet known in view of the limited experience with the agent.

Renal Perfusion

Disturbance of renal function in the perioperative period is related far less to toxicity of anesthetic metabolites than to changes in renal perfusion. The direct effects of anesthetic drugs on the kidney are small compared with the indirect effects of combined anesthesia and surgery acting through the renin-angiotensin system.[106, 107] In dog studies, when halothane was delivered at concentrations of 1% to 1.5%[108] and enflurane at doses as high as 1.75 MAC,[109] renal blood flow was preserved by autoregulation. However, if the anesthetic dose is high enough, decreases in CO may exceed the ability of the kidney to compensate, and renal blood flow decreases.

Anesthetics may attenuate the response to activation of the renin-angiotensin system caused by surgery or tracheal intubation, but they do not obliterate it. This response leads to intraoperative oliguria.[106] Oliguria may be an appropriate response to anesthesia and surgery and does not necessarily mean kidney injury is occurring.[110, 111] On the other hand, anuria that is not due to a simple problem such as an occluded urinary catheter is an ominous sign.

THE LIVER AND INHALED AGENTS

Is Halothane Contraindicated in Patients with Hepatic Insufficiency?

Although rare, severe hepatic injury can result from halothane use.[112] Since alternatives are available, halothane use logically should be avoided in patients with damaged livers, otherwise, it would be difficult to ascribe another cause if additional damage occurs. Even this rationale is difficult—even impossible—to support with data. Zinn and associates[113] did not detect a difference in hepatic effects of several anesthetic regimens in patients with alcoholic hepatitis.

Why Do Alterations in Hepatic Function Occur?

Alterations in hepatic function occur following most anesthetic procedures and appear to be related to the effects of anesthesia and surgery, and not to those of anesthesia alone. This general statement, however, obscures the differences among agents.[114] For example, hepatic artery flow is preserved during isoflurane but not halothane anesthesia.[115, 116] Hepatic artery perfusion in the presence of hemorrhage is better preserved during isoflurane than during halothane anesthesia.[117] If the surgical procedure interferes with hepatic blood flow, liver function may be decreased. Thus, alterations in liver function are greatest with upper abdominal operations.

Hepatic Perfusion and Metabolism

The effects just noted are related more to impairment of hepatic perfusion than to a cellular toxic effect of the anesthetics. Cellular toxicity is believed to be connected to anesthetic metabolism.[118, 119] Significant differences among agents are unknown. The fraction of an administered dose that is metabolized is in the order halothane > enflurane > isoflurane > desflurane. Sevoflurane is metabolized, but the implication of this process in hepatic damage is unknown.

The oxidative pathway of halothane metabolism can yield products that bind to proteins and lipids, leading to cellular damage.[118] The anesthetic metabolite–protein complex stimulates antibody formation so that future contact with halothane may produce hepatic injury. Christ and colleagues[120] recently showed that enflurane and possibly isoflurane metabolism can produce covalently bound adducts that are recognized by antibodies from patients who had halothane hepatitis. This mechanism of toxicity has provoked great interest in desflurane, which is minimally metabolized, is largely insoluble in body tissues, and is rapidly removed from the body. Whether this agent is truly less hepatotoxic than the more widely used anesthetics is unknown at this time.

ENDOCRINE EFFECTS

Will Inhalation Anesthetics Affect Diabetes or Vice Versa?

No evidence shows that the diabetic state is controlled best by any one inhaled agent. Few experimental data explore the impact of diabetes on anesthesia, a surprising fact in view of the frequency with which diabetic patients are anesthetized. One of the few research reports addressing this topic showed that diabetic patients with autonomic neuropathy have significantly wider swings in circulatory variable measurements than do diabetics without neuropathy.[121] The patients did not receive purely inhalation agents, however. Blood sugar increases during anesthesia, both from decreased insulin secretion and decreased tissue response to insulin.[122] The response is similar regardless of the inhalation agent being given.

Are Other Effects Significant?

Increase of adrenal cortical secretion during anesthesia was alluded to earlier.[97] Antidiuretic hormone output does not change significantly in response to the use of inhalation anesthetics alone, but these drugs may modify the output of antidiuretic hormone in response to surgery.[123] The direct effect of inhaled anesthetics on thyroid function is small or insignificant.[124]

OBESITY

Should the Administration of Inhaled Agents Be Altered?

Potential Disadvantages

Any anesthetic drug with significant lipid solubility—whether intravenous or inhaled—will accumulate in body fat. Evidence is lacking to show advantage of one technique over another in obese patients. Some factors are known, however. Adipose tissue is a reservoir for many anesthetic drugs and empties slowly when anesthesia is terminated. This effect does not significantly delay awakening, but it does impede total removal of anesthetic from the body. As a result, low concentrations in the blood persist for long periods and lead to continued metabolism of the anesthetic. Levels of metabolites are higher for longer periods of time in obese patients.[125, 126] This fact may be the explanation in part for the greater evidence of hepatic injury from halothane in obese patients. Obese patients may also be more liable to hypoxic episodes, which lead to the combined effects of larger amounts of reductive metabolites in obese than in nonobese patients.

Potential Advantages

Unproven advantages can be proposed for the use of inhaled agents over that of fixed anesthetics. First, smaller amounts of muscle relaxants should be required, since the inhaled agents potentiate the effects of neuromuscular blocking drugs.[127] Return of full skeletal muscle function should be more easily accomplished. Second, removal of anesthetic can be accomplished actively by ventilating the patient, perhaps simplifying the assessment of respiratory and mental function.

MUSCLE RELAXATION

Are Inhalation Agents Contraindicated in Patients with Neuromuscular Disease?

The answer to this question is "No."[128] Selection of an inhalation agent is logical in the management of a patient with neuromuscular disease because the anesthetic dose can be increased or decreased at will (providing relaxation as needed) and reversed simply by ventilating the drug away. In patients with muscle weakness, the additional relaxation needed for surgery may be small and provided easily by the use of inhalation agents. In contrast to intravenous anesthetics, inhaled drugs depress skeletal muscle function.[129, 130] Greater relaxation is produced by isoflurane, enflurane, and desflurane than by halothane, and the effect is related to the anesthetic dose.[131]

Potentiation of Effects

Volatile agent-induced muscle relaxation can be used to advantage when profound relaxation is needed. Volatile drugs potentiate the effects of depolarizing and nondepolarizing neuromuscular blocking drugs. As a result, smaller doses of blocking drugs are needed to provide equivalent conditions during anesthesia with inhalation agents than with intravenous anesthetics (Figure 37–7).[132]

The implications of this are twofold: (1) removal of the anesthetic reverses the neuromuscular blockade in part; and (2) less anticholinesterase reversal should be required to reverse the relaxant effect. If neuromuscular blockade was provided during a bowel resection, for example, administration of a smaller dose of an anticholinesterase may lessen the jeopardy to the intestinal anastomosis.

BONE MARROW TRANSPLANTATION

Are Effects on Hematopoiesis of Concern?

Concern exists for N_2O use, since detectable decrease in liver methionine synthetase level occurs when this drug is administered to humans at a concentration of 60% for 1.2 hours.[133] However, N_2O has not been shown to be detrimental to marrow survival. If N_2O at a concentration of 40% or greater is inspired for 3 to 5 days, predictable leukopenia occurs.[134] This event precludes the use of N_2O for prolonged anesthesia or analgesia in the intensive care setting. Despite these findings, no evidence shows that inhaled agents affect the survival or function of transplanted bone marrow.

TRAUMA

How Do Inhaled Agents Affect the Circulation?

A major issue in anesthesia for trauma is circulatory management. How do different volatile agents affect the reflex circulatory response to hypovolemia? Once a victim's airway is secure, if no underlying pulmonary trauma or other disease of greater priority is present, attention usually is directed to the maintenance of circulatory adequacy. From the anesthetic point of view, management of hypovolemia becomes a major consideration.

Hypovolemia

Circulatory baroreflex responses are blunted by volatile agents; thus, heart rate may not increase with hypovolemia.[135] Small amounts of blood loss can be tolerated during halothane, isoflurane, or enflurane anesthesia with an insignificant effect on systemic arterial pressure.[136] In animal studies, once blood loss exceeds 10% of estimated blood volume, blood pressure decreases in relation to the amount of blood lost.[136] With each of the anesthetics, loss of blood short of exsanguination in animals is tolerated quite well for short periods of time without development of metabolic acidosis.

Is Nitrous Oxide Appropriate?

Entry Into Closed Gas Spaces

N_2O necessarily lowers the inspired O_2 concentration. The consequences of this effect will be apparent by monitoring PaO_2 or hemoglobin saturation. Entrance of N_2O into closed gas spaces (such as pneumothorax or areas where gases are entrapped in veins) increases the trapped volumes in proportion to the alveolar N_2O concentration.[137, 138] The increase in volume occurs quickly in spaces surrounded by highly perfused tissues such as lung or brain tissue.[137] N_2O should be avoided in patients with pneumothorax or pneumocranium.

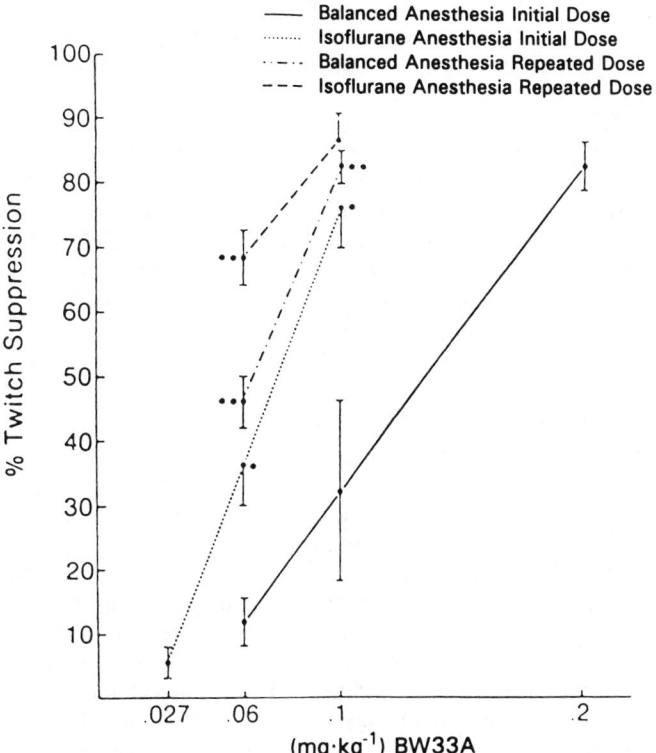

FIGURE 37–7. Twitch depression as a function of dose of atracurium (BW33A) during balanced and isoflurane anesthesia. Repeated doses were given after twitch tension had returned to 95% of the control level. Significantly greater blockade occurred with isoflurane than with balanced anesthesia (*) and with repeated doses of atracurium (**). (From Sokoll MO, Gergis SD, Mehta M, et al: Safety and efficacy of atracurium (BW33A) in surgical patients receiving balanced or isoflurane anesthesia. Anesthesiology 1983; 58:450.)

When Is Recall a Problem?

Awareness is more likely in trauma patients than in any group of patients that we care for routinely. Anesthesia may be withheld from the patient with inadequate circulation until function is restored. The incidence of recall, which was sometimes painful, was 43% in one group of patients who had 20-minute or longer periods of no anesthetic delivery.[17]

Can this problem be avoided by using volatile anesthetics alone? Probably not. In the markedly hypovolemic patient, a dose of inhalation anesthetic that is slightly greater than the awakening MAC may cause further hypotension, especially when combined with controlled ventilation and the attendant increase of intrathoracic pressure. The reader should note, however, that recall is not always a painful experience, but one that does need to be discussed openly with patients postoperatively.[139] All personnel in the operating theater should use gentle and encouraging language, especially in the setting just described.

PROLONGED ANESTHESIA

The requirements for procedures necessitating prolonged anesthesia, such as extremity reimplantation, include maintenance of arterial pressure at near-awake values, preservation of body temperature, and immobility of the operative site. Among the possible regimens to accomplish these goals is the use of inhalation agents without adjuvants. An immobile patient can be provided with inhalation anesthesia alone. Ordinarily, the dose of anesthesia can be sufficiently low to preserve circulatory variables at near-awake levels. Despite some anesthesia-induced decrease in metabolism and in vasodilation of skin vessels, body temperature can be maintained by heating the respired gases and keeping the room temperature near the thermoneutral point.

Will Recovery Be Prolonged If an Inhaled Agent Is Used?

The major determinants are the solubility of the anesthetic and the depth and duration of anesthesia. The greater the total dose of anesthetic—that is, the concentration delivered multiplied by the duration of delivery—and the greater the blood solubility of the drug, the longer the recovery time will be.[140]

If anesthesia is to be provided by the inhalation route alone, the alveolar anesthetic concentration must be approximately 1.25 times the MAC or greater to ensure nonmovement. Prolonged anesthesia at this level requires 30 to 40 minutes for awakening if halothane is used, and 15 to 20 minutes if isoflurane is used. With newer agents such as desflurane, whose solubilities are similar to the solubility of N_2O, duration of anesthesia has little effect on recovery time.[47, 141] Recovery time is nearly the same for both brief and prolonged anesthesia.

PREGNANCY AND THE PUERPERIUM

Inevitably, inhalation agents will be given to some patients during pregnancy or the puerperium despite the popularity of regional anesthesia for obstetric care. Choosing the best parameters for anesthesia care of the mother may be at odds with optimum care of the fetus. The potent inhalation agents have at least one advantage over other general anesthetic agents in this setting: they provide unconsciousness and uterine relaxation simultaneously. Hence, they offer a method to relax the uterus reversibly when manipulations such as cervical cerclage, delivery of an after-coming head, and manual removal of the placenta are required.

Should Inhalation Agents Be Used for Cervical Cerclage?

Although concern about teratogenicity or fetal loss may be a reason to avoid these agents during the earliest stages of pregnancy,[142, 143] this concern no longer exists by the time cerclage ordinarily is performed. Uterine relaxation provided by inhalation agents may be an advantage. A quiet, comfortable, nonstraining patient is probably more important than the technique used to provide these conditions.

What Are the Fetal Effects of Inhalation Agents?

Transfer of agent to the fetus is rapid.[144, 145] The umbilical vein–to–maternal artery anesthetic concentration ratio increases throughout the anesthetic procedure. When the anesthetic procedure is completed, the anesthetic drugs are removed quickly as well. Laboratory studies show that N_2O is fetotoxic to rats and may lead to increased reproductive loss when given at a specific time in the gestation.[146] The potent agents have not shown the same effects.[142]

On the other hand, in one study the presence of N_2O did not affect in vitro fertilization success rates.[147] It does not appear that inhalation anesthetic drugs by themselves influence fetal welfare when surgery must be done during pregnancy.[148] Once the gestation has progressed sufficiently for the mother to be certain that she is pregnant, probably only intervening complications such as hypotension and hypoxia have a detrimental effect on the fetus, uterus, or placenta.[149]

Is Any Potent Agent Preferable for Operative Deliveries?

The drugs are so similar in their ability to relax the uterus that no drug is preferable to the others.[150] In doses equivalent to 1.0 MAC, all of the agents significantly relax the uterus. When doses of 0.5 MAC or less were compared with respect to their effects on blood loss at cesarean section, no differences were found.[150, 151] In most studies, no greater loss occurred with inhalation agents compared with regional techniques.[152]

The maximum discrepancy in anesthetic goals for the mother and fetus exists during emergency cesarean section, when fetal welfare may already be compromised and anesthesia still must be provided. One study demonstrated that the stressed fetus may have an exacerbation of metabolic and respiratory acidosis when exposed to anesthetizing concentrations of isoflurane.[153] Anesthetizing the mother with an inhalation agent may be necessary, but the cost may include worsening the condition of the already depressed baby.

AMBULATORY SURGERY

Care in the ambulatory surgery setting requires prompt induction of and emergence from anesthesia. As the indications for operations in this setting are extended, rapid recovery of cognitive and psychomotor skills is increasingly relevant.[154] Some of the features of inhalation agents promote their use in outpatients. Induction of anesthesia can be conducted in a predictable and controlled manner. It can be accomplished rapidly, even with agents of moderately high solubility in blood by overpressurization technique. Emergence also is predictable. Inhaled anesthetics are removed largely via ventilation. Thus, one can ensure awakening by actively removing the drug.

Will Desflurane or Sevoflurane Significantly Enhance Emergence?

Considering only the pharmacokinetic properties of the inhaled agents, the rate of elimination of desflurane and sevoflurane is similar to that of N_2O and is more rapid than that of enflurane, isoflurane, or halothane.[141, 155] Hence, return of consciousness following anesthesia with desflurane and sevoflurane is more rapid than with the more soluble drugs. Caveats include a prolongation of recovery with any of the inhaled agents when premedication or intravenous induction drugs are used.[156, 157] For anesthetics of short duration given at low doses, anesthetic solubility is not of great significance in determining speed of recovery.[47] Although initial awakening may be more rapid with drugs of low solubility, discharge from the postanesthesia care unit and hospital may be influenced more by administration of analgesics or sedatives than by the inhaled agents.[158]

How Long Do Changes in Mental Function Persist After Anesthesia?

The greatest fractional recovery occurs in the first few minutes following anesthesia. Recovery is slower after prolonged anesthesia than after brief exposures.[141, 154] Nitrous oxide is not likely to have an important influence on psychomotor skills 1 hour after anesthesia. Recommended time periods that patients do not drive after anesthesia have varied from 24 to 48 hours.[154] Sedatives, hypnotics, and analgesic drugs given concomitantly with inhaled agents delay full recovery of cognitive and psychomotor skills.[154, 156]

Since persistence of emetic symptoms prolongs hospitalization and prevents resumption of activity, can these symptoms be avoided or prevented by selection of the appropriate anesthetic? Premedicant, intraoperative, or postoperative administration of narcotics increases the incidence of nausea.[159, 160] Of all the currently used inhaled agents, N_2O has been singled out as a cause of postoperative nausea. However, any enhancement caused by N_2O must be small, if it exists at all.[154, 157, 161]

CONCLUSION

We are fortunate to have access to many anesthetic drugs and to be able to apply a variety of techniques. When possible, confining an anesthetic to the area requiring operation seems wise. Thus, surgeries on a toe or a finger lend themselves to highly localized anesthesia. Exposure to drugs is thus minimal, and the physiologic effects of anesthesia are limited.

With operations of a more central nature, the ease of providing localized anesthesia diminishes. Furthermore, many patients simply do not tolerate being awake during surgery. Inhaled or intravenous anesthetics, alone or in combination, must be used. Advantages of pure inhalation techniques were noted at the beginning of the chapter. Clearly, general anesthesia can be provided safely with any one of several techniques.[162]

Will the New Potent Inhaled Agents Alter Our Practice?

Their impact may manifest itself in two ways. First, we will learn how to alter anesthesia depth quickly, since alterations in anesthetic dose should be easy to accomplish. Second, the rate of awakening from anesthesia will be influenced little by the duration of anesthesia. Anesthetic delivery can be continued to the end of surgery at full agent doses without delaying recovery greatly. Of course, recovery from brief anesthetic procedures will be prompt. Data as to whether postanesthesia recovery times will be shortened or hospital discharge of ambulatory surgery patients hastened are not conclusive.

References

1. Lundy JS: Balanced anesthesia. Minn Med 1926; 9:399.
2. Keys TE: The early pneumatic chemists and physicians: their influence on the development of surgical anesthesia. Anesthesiology 1969; 30:447.
3. Keys TE: The development of anesthesia. Anesthesiology 1941; 2:552.
4. Leake CD: The role of pharmacology in the development of ideal anesthesia. JAMA 1934; 102:1.
5. Robbins BH: Preliminary study of the anesthetic activity of fluorinated hydrocarbons. J Pharmacol Exp Ther 1946; 86:197.
6. Van Poznak A, Artusio JF Jr: Anesthetic properties of a series of fluorinated compounds. I. Fluorinated hydrocarbons. Toxicol Appl Pharmacol 1960; 2:363.
7. Krantz JC Jr: The rationale of the use of fluorinated hydrocarbons and ethers as volatile anesthetic agents. Anesth Analg 1965; 44:260.
8. Terrell RC, Speers L, Szur AJ, et al: General anesthetics. 1. Halogenated methylethyl ethers as anesthetic agents. J Med Chem 1971; 14:517.
9. Munson ES, Eger EI II, Bowers DL: Effects of anesthetic-depressed ventilation and cardiac output on anesthetic uptake. Anesthesiology 1973; 38:251.
10. Gibbons RT, Steffey EP, Eger EI II: The effect of spontaneous versus controlled ventilation on the rate of rise of alveolar halothane concentration in dogs. Anesth Analg 1977; 56:32.
11. Prys-Roberts C: Anaesthesia: a practical or impractical construct? Br J Anaesth 1987; 59:1341.
12. Stoelting RK, Longnecker DE, Eger EI II: Minimum alveolar concentration in man on awakening from methoxyflurane, halothane, ether and fluroxene anesthesia: MAC awake. Anesthesiology 1970; 33:5.
13. Saidman LJ, Eger EI II, Munson ES, et al: Minimum alveolar concentrations of methoxyflurane, halothane, ether and cyclopropane in man: correlation with theories of anesthesia. Anesthesiology 1967; 28:994.
14. Yakaitis RW, Blitt CD, Angiulo JP: End-tidal halothane concentration for endotracheal intubation. Anesthesiology 1977; 47:386.
15. Roizen MF, Horrigan RW, Frazer BM: Anesthetic doses blocking adrenergic (stress) and cardiovascular responses to incision—MAC BAR. Anesthesiology 1981; 54:390.
16. Ausems ME, Hug CC Jr, Stanski DR, et al: Plasma concentrations of alfentanil required to supplement nitrous oxide anesthesia for general surgery. Anesthesiology 1986; 65:362.
17. Bogetz MS, Katz JA: Recall of surgery for major trauma. Anesthesiology 1984; 61:6.
18. Breckenridge JL, Aitkenhead AR: Awareness during anaesthesia: a review. Ann Coll Surg Engl 1983; 65:93.
19. Keenan RL, Boyan CP: Cardiac arrests due to anesthesia. a study of incidence and causes. JAMA 1985; 253:2372.

20. Stullken EH Jr, Milde JH, Michenfelder JD, et al: The non-linear responses of cerebral metabolism to low concentrations of halothane, enflurane, isoflurane, and thiopental. Anesthesiology 1977; 46:28.
21. Warner DS: Volatile anesthetics and the ischemic brain. J Neurosurg Anesth 1989; 1:290.
22. Warner DS, Zhou J, Ramani R, et al: Nitrous oxide does not alter infarct volume in rats undergoing reversible middle cerebral artery occlusion. Anesthesiology 1990; 73:686.
23. Rampil IJ, Weiskopf RB, Brown IG, et al: I653 and isoflurane produce similar dose-related changes in the electroencephalogram of pigs. Anesthesiology 1988; 69:298.
24. Michenfelder JD, Sundt TM, Fode N, et al: Isoflurane when compared to enflurane and halothane decreases the frequency of cerebral ischemia during carotid endarterectomy. Anesthesiology 1987; 67:336.
25. Messick JM, Casement B, Sharbrough FW, et al: Correlation of regional cerebral blood flow (CBF) with EEG changes during isoflurane anesthesia for carotid endarterectomy. Anesthesiology 1987; 66:344.
26. Newberg LA, Milde JH, Michenfelder JD: Systemic and cerebral effects of isoflurane-induced hypotension in dogs. Anesthesiology 1984; 60:541.
27. Smith AL, Wollman H: Cerebral blood flow and metabolism: effects of anesthetic drugs and techniques. Anesthesiology 1972; 36:378.
28. Lutz LJ, Milde JH, Milde LN: The cerebral functional, metabolic, and hemodynamic effects of desflurane in dogs. Anesthesiology 1990; 73:125.
29. Drummond JC, Todd MM, Scheller MS, et al: A comparison of the direct cerebral vasodilating potencies of halothane and isoflurane in the New Zealand white rabbit. Anesthesiology 1986; 65:462.
30. Hansen TD, Warner DS, Todd MM, et al: Effects of nitrous oxide and volatile anaesthetics on cerebral blood flow. Br J Anaesth 1989; 63:290.
31. Adams RW, Gronert GA, Sundt TM, et al: Halothane, hypocapnia, and cerebrospinal fluid pressure in neurosurgery. Anesthesiology 1972; 37:510.
32. Muzzi DA, Losasso TJ, Dietz NM, et al: The effect of desflurane and isoflurane on cerebrospinal fluid pressure in humans with supratentorial mass lesions. Anesthesiology 1992; 76:720.
33. McPherson RW, Brian JE Jr, Traystman RJ: Cerebrovascular responsiveness to carbon dioxide in dogs with 1.4% and 2.8% isoflurane. Anesthesiology 1989; 70:843.
34. Artru AA, Nugent M, Michenfelder JD: Enflurane causes a prolonged and reversible increase in the rate of CSF production in the dog. Anesthesiology 1982; 57:255.
35. Artru AA: Effect of halothane and fentanyl on the rate of CSF production in dogs. Anesth Analg 1983; 62:581.
36. Maktabi MA, Elboki FF, Faraci FM, et al: Halothane decreases the rate of production of cerebrospinal fluid: possible role of vasopressin V_1 receptors. Anesthesiology 1993; 78:72.
37. Artru AA: Isoflurane does not increase the rate of CSF production in the dog. Anesthesiology 1984; 60:194.
38. Courtin EF, Bickford RG, Faulconer A Jr: The classification and significance of electroencephalographic patterns produced by nitrous oxide–ether anesthesia during surgical operation. Proc Staff Meet Mayo Clin 1950; 25:197.
39. Eger EI II, Stevens WC, Cromwell TH: The electroencephalogram of man anesthetized with Forane. Anesthesiology 1981; 35:504.
40. Rampil IJ, Lockart SH, Eger EI II, et al: The electroencephalographic effects of desflurane in humans. Anesthesiology 1991; 74:434.
41. Joas TA, Stevens WC, Eger EI II: Electroencephalographic seizure activity in dogs during anesthesia. Br J Anaesth 1973; 43:739.
42. Neigh JL, Garman JK, Harp JR: The electroencephalographic pattern during anesthesia with Ethrane: effects of depth of anesthesia, $Paco_2$ and nitrous oxide. Anesthesiology 1971; 35:482.
43. Opitz A, Brechts B, Stenzel E: Enflurane anesthesia for epileptic patients. Anaesthetist 1977; 26:329.
44. Peterson DO, Drummond JC, Todd MM: Effects of halothane, enflurane, isoflurane and nitrous oxide on somatosensory evoked potentials in humans. Anesthesiology 1986; 65:35.
45. Grundy BL: Intraoperative monitoring of sensory evoked potentials. Anesthesiology 1983; 58:72.
46. Lockhart SH, Cohen Y, Yasuda N, et al: Cerebral uptake and elimination of desflurane, isoflurane and halothane from rabbit brain: an in vivo NMR study. Anesthesiology 1991; 74:575.
47. Eger EI II, Johnson BH: Rates of awakening from anesthesia with I-653, halothane, isoflurane and sevoflurane: a test of effect of anesthetic concentration and duration in rats. Anesth Analg 1987; 66:977.
48. Rosenberg H, Clofine R, Bialik O: Neurologic changes during awakening from anesthesia. Anesthesiology 1981; 54:125.
49. Keats AS: The effect of drugs on respiration in man. Ann Rev Pharmacol Toxicol 1985; 25:41.
50. Theye RA, Tuohy GF: Oxygen uptake during light halothane anesthesia in man. Anesthesiology 1964; 25:627.
51. Heneghan CPH, Bergman NA, Jordan C, et al: Effect of isoflurane on bronchomotor tone in man. Br J Anaesth 1986; 58:24.
52. Jones JG: Mechanisms of some pulmonary effects of general anaesthesia. Br J Hosp Med 1987; 38:472.
53. Bergman NA: Distribution of inspired gas during anesthesia and artificial ventilation. J Appl Physiol 1963; 18:1085.
54. Domino KB, Borowec L, Alexander CM, et al: Influence of isoflurane on hypoxic pulmonary vasoconstriction in dogs. Anesthesiology 1986; 64:423.
55. Rodenstein DO, Stanescu DC: The soft palate and breathing. Am Rev Respir Dis 1986; 134:311.
56. Taylor RH, Lerman J: Induction, maintenance and recovery characteristics of desflurane in infants and children. Can J Anaesth 1992; 39:6.
57. Sibert KS, Biondi JW, Hirsch NP: Spontaneous respiration during thoracotomy in a patient with mediastinal mass. Anesth Analg 1987; 66:904.
58. Fourcade HE, Stevens WC, Larson CP Jr, et al: The ventilatory effects of Forane, a new inhaled anesthetic. Anesthesiology 1971; 35:26.
59. Hickey RF, Fourcade HE, Eger EI II, et al: The effects of ether, halothane and Forane on apneic thresholds in man. Anesthesiology 1971; 35:32.
60. Wahba WM: Analysis of ventilatory depression by enflurane during clinical anesthesia. Anesth Analg 1980; 59:103.
61. Eger EI II, Dolan WM, Stevens WC, et al: Surgical stimulation antagonizes the respiratory depression produced by Forane. Anesthesiology 1972; 36:544.
62. Cullen DJ, Eger EI II, Stevens WC, et al: Clinical signs of anesthesia. Anesthesiology 1972; 36:21.
63. Hedenstierna G: Causes of gas exchange impairment during general anaesthesia. Eur J Anaesthesiol 1988; 5:221.
64. Lindahl SGE, Charlton AJ, Hatch DJ, et al: Ventilatory responses to inspiratory mechanical loads in spontaneously breathing children during halothane anaesthesia. Acta Anaesthesiol Scand 1986; 30:122.
65. Nunn JF, Ezi-Ashi TI: The respiratory effects of resistance to breathing in anesthetized man. Anesthesiology 1961; 22:174.
66. Pietak S, Weenig CS, Hickey RF, et al: Anesthetic effects of ventilation in patients with chronic obstructive pulmonary disease. Anesthesiology 1975; 42:160.
67. Wahba WM: Influence of airway resistance and ventilatory pattern in $Paco_2$ during enflurane anaesthesia. Br J Anaesth 1979; 51:123.
68. Kingston HGG, Hirshman CA: Perioperative management of the patient with asthma. Anesth Analg 1984; 63:844.
69. Hirshman CA, Bergman NA: Halothane and enflurane protect against bronchospasm in an asthma dog model. Anesth Analg 1978; 57:629.
70. Hirshman CA, Edelstein G, Peetz S, et al: Mechanism of action of inhalational anesthesia on airways. Anesthesiology 1982; 56:107.
71. Benumof JL: One-lung ventilation and hypoxic pulmonary vasoconstriction: implications for anesthetic management. Anesth Analg 1985; 64:821.
72. Knill RL, Kieraszewicz HT, Dodgson BG, et al: Chemical regulation of ventilation during isoflurane sedation and anaesthesia in humans. Can J Anaesth 1983; 30:607.
73. Sjögren D, Ebberyd A, Sollevi A, et al: Ventilatory responses to hypoxia in awake and anesthetized humans. Anesthesiology 1991; 75:A1102.
74. Hess W, Arnold B, Schulte-Sasse U, et al: Comparison of isoflurane and halothane when used to control intraoperative hypertension in patients undergoing coronary artery bypass surgery. Anesth Analg 1983; 62:15.
75. Hamilton WK: Do let the blood pressure drop and do use myocardial depressants! Anesthesiology 1976; 45:273.
76. Yakaitis RW, Blitt CD, Angiulo JP: End-tidal halothane concentration for endotracheal intubation. Anesthesiology 1977; 47:386.
77. Eger EI II, Smith NT, Stoelting R, et al: Cardiovascular effects of halothane in man. Anesthesiology 1970; 32:396.
78. Crawford DC, Fell D, Achola KJ, et al: Effects of alfentanil on the pressor and catecholamine responses to tracheal intubation. Br J Anaesth 1987; 59:707.
79. Henderson PS, Cohen JI, Jarnberg PO, et al: A canine model for studying laryngospasm and its prevention. Laryngoscope 1992; 102:1237.
80. Tuman KJ, McCarthy RJ, Spiess BD, et al: Does choice of anesthetic agent significantly affect outcome after coronary artery surgery. Anesthesiology 1989; 70:189.
81. Slogoff S, Keats AS: Randomized trial of primary agents on outcome of coronary artery bypass operations. Anesthesiology 1989; 70:179.

82. Thomson IR, Bowering JB, Hudson RJ, et al: A comparison of desflurane and isoflurane in patients undergoing coronary artery surgery. Anesthesiology 1991; 75:776.

83. Lillehaug SL, Tinker JH: Why do "pure" vasodilators cause coronary steal when anesthetics don't (or seldom do)? Anesth Analg 1991; 73:681.

84. Hickey PR, Hansen DD, Strafford M, et al: Pulmonary and systemic hemodynamic effects of nitrous oxide in infants with normal and elevated pulmonary vascular resistance. Anesthesiology 1986; 65:374.

85. Eger EI II: Cardiovascular effects of nitrous oxide. In Nitrous Oxide. Eger EI II (ed). New York, Elsevier, 1985, pp 125–156.

86. Johnston R, Eger EI II, Wilson C: A comparative interaction of epinephrine with enflurane, isoflurane, and halothane in man. Anesth Analg 1976; 55:709.

87. Weiskopf RB, Eger EI II, Holmes MA, et al: Epinephrine-induced premature ventricular contractions and changes in arterial blood pressure and heart rate during I-653, isoflurane, and halothane anesthesia in swine. Anesthesiology 1989; 70:293.

88. Imamura S, Ikeda K: Comparison of the epinephrine-induced arrhythmogenic effect of sevoflurane with isoflurane and halothane. J Anesth 1987; 1:62.

89. Tucker W, Rackstein A, Munson E: Comparison of arrhythmic doses of adrenaline, metaraminol, ephedrine and phenylephrine during isoflurane and halothane anesthesia in dogs. Br J Anaesth 1974; 46:392.

90. Roizen MF, Stevens WC: Multiform ventricular tachycardia due to interaction of aminophylline and halothane. Anesth Analg 1978; 57:738.

91. Atlee JL, Malkinson CE: Potentiation by thiopental of halothane—epinephrine-induced arrhythmias in dogs. Anesthesiology 1982; 57:285.

92. Court MH, Dodman NH, Greenblatt DJ, et al: Effect of midazolam infusion and flumazenil administration on epinephrine arrhythmogenicity in dogs anesthetized with halothane. Anesthesiology 1993; 78:155.

93. James R: Desflurane and sevoflurane: inhalation anesthetics for this decade? Br J Anaesth 1990; 65:527.

94. Warltier DC, Pagel PS: Cardiovascular and respiratory action of desflurane: is desflurane different from isoflurane. Anesth Analg 1992; 75:S17.

95. Calverley RK, Smith NT, Prys-Roberts C, et al: Cardiovascular effects of enflurane anesthesia during controlled ventilation in man. Anesth Analg 1978; 57:619.

96. Stevens WC, Cromwell TH, Halsey MJ, et al: The cardiovascular effects of a new inhalational anesthetic, Forane, in human volunteers at constant arterial carbon dioxide tension. Anesthesiology 1971; 35:8.

97. Werder KV, Stevens WC, Cromwell TH, et al: Adrenal function during long-term anesthesia in man. Proc Soc Exp Biol Med 1970; 135:854.

98. Lacoumenta S, Paterson J, Burrin J, et al: Effects of two different halothane concentrations on the metabolic and endocrine responses to surgery. Br J Anaesth 1986; 58:844.

99. Gelman S, Rivas J, Erdemir H, et al: Hormonal and haemodynamic responses to upper abdominal surgery during isoflurane and balanced anaesthesia. Can J Anaesth 1984; 31:509.

100. Hamberger B, Jarnberg PO: Plasma catecholamines during surgical stress: difference between neurolept and enflurane anaesthesia. Acta Anaesthesiol Scand 1983; 27:307.

101. Bovill JG, Sebel PS, Stanley TH: Opioid analgesics in anesthesia: with special reference to their use in cardiovascular anesthesia. Anesthesiology 1984; 61:731.

102. Campbell B, Parikh R, Naismith A: Comparison of fentanyl and halothane supplementation to general anesthesia on the stress response to upper abdominal surgery. Br J Anaesth 1984; 56:257.

103. Frink EJ Jr, Ghantous H, Malan TP, et al: Plasma inorganic fluoride with sevoflurane anesthesia: correlation with indices of hepatic and renal function. Anesth Analg 1992; 74:231.

104. Mazze RI, Woodruff RE, Heerdt ME: Isoniazid-induced enflurane defluorination in humans. Anesthesiology 1982; 57:5.

105. Mazze RI: Fluorinated anaesthetic nephrotoxicity: an update. Can J Anaesth 1984; 31:S16.

106. Mirenda JV, Grissom TE: Anesthetic implications of the renin angiotensin system and angiotensin-converting enzyme inhibitors. Anesth Analg 1991; 72:667.

107. Miller ED Jr, Longnecker DE, Peach MJ: The regulatory function of the renin-angiotensin system during general anesthesia. Anesthesiology 1978; 48:399.

108. Priano LL: Effect of halothane on renal hemodynamics during normovolemia and acute hemorrhagic hypovolemia. Anesthesiology 1985; 63:357.

109. Bernard JM, Doursout MF, Wouters P, et al: Effect of enflurane and isoflurane on hepatic and renal circulations in chronically instrumented dogs. Anesthesiology 1991; 74:298.

110. Priano LL, Smith JD, Cohen JI, et al: IV fluid administration and urine output during radical neck surgery. Head Neck 1993 (in press).

111. Sweny P: Is postoperative oliguria avoidable? Br J Anaesth 1991; 67:137.

112. Subcommittee on the National Halothane Study: Summary of the National Halothane Study. JAMA 1966; 197:775.

113. Zinn SE, Fairley HB, Glenn JD: Liver function in patients with mild alcoholic hepatitis, after enflurane, nitrous oxide–narcotic, and spinal anesthesia. Anesth Analg 1985; 64:487.

114. Eger EI II, Johnson BH, Strum DP, et al: Studies of the toxicity of I-653, halothane, and isoflurane in enzyme-induced, hypoxic rats. Anesth Analg 1987; 66:1227.

115. Gelman S, Dillard E, Bradley E: Hepatic circulation during surgical stress and anesthesia with halothane, isoflurane and fentanyl. Anesth Analg 1987; 66:936.

116. Gelman S, Fowler KC, Smith LR: Liver circulation and function during isoflurane and halothane anesthesia. Anesthesiology 1984; 61:726.

117. Seyde WC, Longnecker DE: Anesthetic influences on regional hemodynamics in normal and hemorrhaged rats. Anesthesiology 1984; 61:686.

118. Brown BR: Hepatotoxicity and inhalation anesthetics: views in the era of isoflurane. J Clin Anesth 1989; 1:368.

119. Koblin DD: Characteristics and implications of desflurane metabolism and toxicity. Anesth Analg 1992; 75:S10.

120. Christ DD, Kenna JG, Kammerer W, et al: Enflurane metabolism produces covalently bound liver adducts recognized by antibodies from patients with halothane hepatitis. Anesthesiology 1988; 69:833.

121. Burgos LG, Ebert TJ, Asiddao C, et al: Increased intraoperative cardiovascular morbidity in diabetics with autonomic neuropathy. Anesthesiology 1989; 70:591.

122. Hirsch I, McGill J, Cryer P, et al: Perioperative management of surgical patients with diabetes mellitus. Anesthesiology 1991; 74:346.

123. Philbin D, Coggins C: Plasma antidiuretic hormone levels in cardiac surgical patients during morphine and halothane anesthesia. Anesthesiology 1978; 49:95.

124. Oyama T, Matsuki A, Kudo T: Effect of halothane, methoxyflurane anaesthesia and surgery on plasma thyroid-stimulating hormone (TSH) levels in man. Anaesthesia 1972; 27:2.

125. Young SR, Stoelting RK, Peterson C, et al: Anesthetic biotransformation and renal function in obese patients during and after methoxyflurane or halothane anesthesia. Anesthesiology 1975; 42:451.

126. Bentley JB, Vaughan RW, Gandolfi AJ, et al: Halothane biotransformation in obese and non-obese patients. Anesthesiology 1982; 57:94.

127. Miller RD, Eger EI II, Way W, et al: Comparative neuromuscular effects of Forane and halothane alone and in combination with d-tubocurarine in man. Anesthesiology 1971; 35:38.

128. Stoelting RK, Dierdorf SF, McCammon RL: Skin and musculoskeletal diseases. In Anesthesia and Co-Existing Disease. 2nd ed. Stoelting RK, Dierdorf SF, McCammon RL (eds). New York, Churchill Livingstone, 1988, pp 611–646.

129. Ali HA, Savarese JJ: Monitoring of neuromuscular function. Anesthesiology 1976; 45:216.

130. Waud BE, Waud DR: Effects of volatile anesthetics on directly and indirectly stimulated skeletal muscle. Anesthesiology 1979; 50:103.

131. Caldwell JE, Laster MJ, Magorian T, et al: The neuromuscular effects of desflurane, alone and combined with pancuronium or succinylcholine in humans. Anesthesiology 1991; 74:414.

132. Sokoll MD, Gergis SD, Mehta M, et al: Safety and efficacy of atracurium (BW33A) in surgical patients receiving balanced or isoflurane anesthesia. Anesthesiology 1983; 58:450.

133. Koblin DD, Waskell L, Watson JE, et al: Nitrous oxide inactivates methionine synthetase in human liver. Anesth Analg 1982; 61:75.

134. Lassen HCA, Henriksen E, Neukirch F, et al: Treatment of tetanus: severe bone-marrow depression after prolonged nitrous-oxide anaesthesia. Lancet 1956; i:527.

135. Kotrly K, Ebert T, Vucins E, et al: Baroreceptor reflex control of heart rate during isoflurane anesthesia in humans. Anesthesiology 1984; 60:173.

136. Weiskopf RB, Townsley MI, Riordan KK, et al: Comparison of cardiopulmonary responses to graded hemorrhage during enflurane, halothane, isoflurane and ketamine anesthesia. Anesth Analg 1981; 60:481.

137. Eger EI II, Saidman LJ: Hazards of nitrous oxide anesthesia in bowel obstruction and pneumothorax. Anesthesiology 1965; 26:61.

138. Munson ES, Merrick HC: Effect of nitrous oxide on venous air embolism. Anesthesiology 1966; 27:783.

139. Blacher RS: Awareness during surgery (Editorial). Anesthesiology 1984; 61:1.

140. Eger EI II: Recovery from anesthesia. *In* Anesthetic Uptake and Action. Eger EI II (ed). Baltimore, Williams & Wilkins, 1974, pp 228–248.

141. Smiley RM, Ornstein E, Matteo RS, et al: Desflurane and isoflurane in surgical patients: comparison of emergence time. Anesthesiology 1991; 74:425.

142. Lane GA, Nahrwold M, Tait A, et al: Anesthetics on teratogens: nitrous oxide is fetotoxic, xenon is not. Science 1980; 210:899.

143. Mazze RI, Fujinaga M, Rice SA, et al: Reproductive and teratogenic effects of nitrous oxide, halothane, isoflurane and enflurane in Sprague-Dawley rats. Anesthesiology 1986; 64:339.

144. Marx GF, Joshi CW, Orkin LR: Placental transmission of nitrous oxide. Anesthesiology 1970; 32:429.

145. Gregory GA, Wade JG, Beihl DR, et al: Fetal anesthetic requirement (MAC) for halothane. Anesth Analg 1983; 62:9.

146. Fink BR, Shepherd TH, Blandau RJ: Teratogenic activity of nitrous oxide. Nature 1967; 214:146.

147. Rosen MA, Roizen MF, Eger EI II, et al: The effect of nitrous oxide on in-vitro fertilization success rates. Anesthesiology 1987; 67:42.

148. Aldridge LM, Tunstall ME: Nitrous oxide and the fetus. Br J Anaesth 1986; 58:1348.

149. Duncan PE, Pope WDB, Cohen MM, et al: Fetal risk of anesthesia and surgery during pregnancy. Anesthesiology 1986; 64:790.

150. Warren TM, Datta S, Ostheimer GW, et al: Comparison of the maternal and neonatal effects of halothane, enflurane, and isoflurane for cesarean delivery. Anesth Analg 1983; 62:516.

151. Moir DD: Anaesthesia for cesarean section. Br J Anaesth 1970; 42:136.

152. Gilstrap LC III, Hauth JC, Hawkins GDV, et al: Effect of type of anesthesia on blood loss at cesarean section. Obstet Gynecol 1987; 69:328.

153. Baker BW, Hughes SC, Shnider SM, et al: Maternal anesthesia and the stressed fetus: effects of isoflurane on the asphyxiated fetal lamb. Anesthesiology 1990; 72:65.

154. Korttila K: Postanesthetic cognitive and psychomotor impairment. Int Anesth Clin 1986; 24:59.

155. Van Hemelrijck J, Smith I, White PF: Use of desflurane for outpatient anesthesia. Anesthesiology 1991; 75:197.

156. Fletcher JE, Sebel PS, Murphy MR, et al: Psychomotor performance after desflurane anesthesia: a comparison with isoflurane. Anesth Analg 1991; 73:260.

157. Wrigley SR, Fairfield JE, Jones RM, et al: Induction and recovery characteristics of desflurane in day case patients: a comparison with propofol. Anaesthesia 1991; 46:615.

158. Ghouri AF, Bodner M, White PF: Recovery profile after desflurane–nitrous oxide in outpatients. Anesthesiology 1991; 74:419.

159. Rising S, Dogson MS, Steen PA: Isoflurane versus fentanyl for outpatient laparoscopy. Acta Anaesthesiol Scand 1985; 29:251.

160. Hackett GH, Harris MNE, Plantevin OM, et al: Anaesthesia for outpatient termination of pregnancy: a comparison of two anaesthetic techniques. Br J Anaesth 1982; 54:865.

161. Hovorka J, Korttila K, Erkola O: Nitrous oxide does not increase nausea and vomiting following gynaecological laparoscopy. Can J Anaesth 1989; 36:145.

162. Forrest JB, Cahalan MK, Rehder K, et al: Multicenter study of general anesthesia. II. Results. Anesthesiology 1990; 72:262.

CHAPTER **38**

Local Anesthetics*

JAY S. ELLIS, M.D., Lt. Col., U.S.A.F., M.C.

Local anesthetics provide anesthetists with the ability to render patients insensible to pain without having to render them unconscious. This characteristic permits many procedures to be performed with minimal physiologic challenge. Such drugs significantly expand the number of anesthetic choices and contribute a great deal to the art of our specialty. Like all therapeutic agents, local anesthetics have their risks. This chapter discusses the rational use of these drugs, and particular attention is paid to their toxicity and therapeutic uses. Although local anesthetics are also useful in the treatment of cardiac dysrhythmias, this chapter deals exclusively with their anesthetic properties.

The chemical structure of local anesthetics in clinical use consists of three parts: an aromatic group, an intermediate chain, and an amine group (Fig. 38–1). The intermediate chain is either an ester or amide linkage. Local anesthetics are classified into major groups depending on the presence of the amide or ester linkage. The amide local anesthetics include lidocaine, mepivacaine, prilocaine, bupivacaine, and etidocaine (remember the amide local anesthetics as those drugs having an *i* in the drug name before the *caine*). The ester local anesthetics are cocaine, procaine, chloroprocaine, and tetracaine. Important differences characterize the esters and amide local anesthetics and are discussed later.

MECHANISMS OF ACTION

How Do Local Anesthetics Work?

Physiology of Nerve Conduction

Before the mechanism of action of local anesthetics can be discussed, the physiology of nerve conduction must be reviewed. The resting nerve fiber maintains a transmembrane potential between -70 and -80 mV. This transmembrane potential results from the high concentration of potassium ions inside the nerve relative to the surrounding extracellular fluid. A concentration gradient also exists for sodium ions, the extracellular concentration of which is much higher than the intracellular concentration.

When a nerve is stimulated, sodium ion channels in the nerve cell membrane undergo a voltage-dependent conforma-

tional change that opens the channel, allowing rapid influx of sodium ions into the cell. This movement changes the transmembrane potential. When a certain level (the threshold potential) is exceeded, an action potential is generated and an impulse is conducted down the fiber. The change in potential opens adjacent sodium channels, allowing propagation of the action potential and generation of the impulse.

The nerve reacquires its resting membrane potential through the efflux of potassium ions. The relative concentrations of sodium and potassium ions are then restored by the energy-dependent sodium-potassium adenosine triphosphate (ATP) pump.[1] Figure 38–2 summarizes these events.

Effect on the Action Potential

Local anesthetics bind to the sodium channels in the nerve cell membranes and inhibit the influx of sodium ions.[2] The limited influx of ions reduces the rate of rise of the action potential; if enough sodium channels are blocked, the action

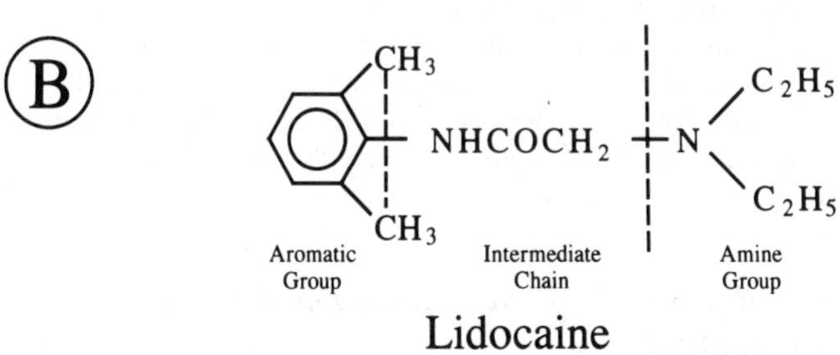

FIGURE 38–1. Chemical structure of *(A)* ester local anesthetic procaine and *(B)* amide local anesthetic lidocaine. Local anesthetics in clinical use all consist of an aromatic element, an intermediate element, and an amine element. Modification of the chemical structure of the three parts affects the clinical properties of the local anesthetic agent.

---

*All material in this chapter is in the public domain, with the exception of any borrowed figures or tables.

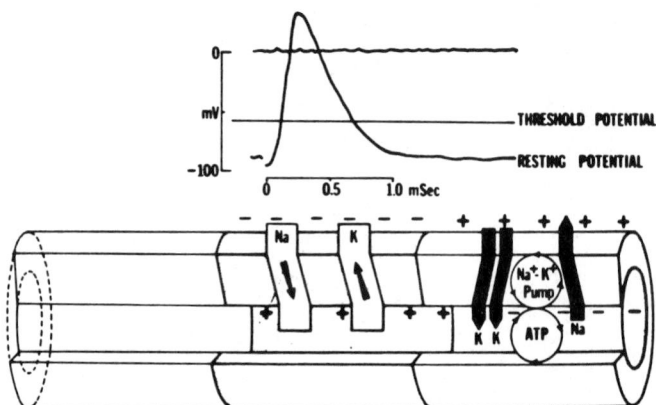

FIGURE 38–2. Summary of the ion and membrane potential changes during nerve conduction. (From Covino BG, Vassallo HG: General pharmacological and toxicological aspects of local anesthetic agents. *In* Local Anesthetics: Mechanisms of Action and Clinical Use. New York, Grune & Stratton, 1976, p 20.)

potential; if enough sodium channels are blocked, the action potential fails to reach the threshold level and no impulses are conducted. Local anesthetics, therefore, do not affect the resting membrane potential, but they do affect the rate of rise and the maximum level of the action potential.

The exact mechanism by which local anesthetics affect the sodium channels remains to be determined. Several theories have been proposed.[3] The most popular propose that local anesthetics bind to the protein subunits of the sodium channel and inhibit the voltage-dependent conformational changes that allow sodium influx into the cell (Fig. 38–3).

Use-Dependent Block

Any theory that describes local anesthetic action must account for the phenomenon of use-dependent block, in which the local anesthetic effect is much more pronounced after repeated action potentials than it is in resting nerves.

One explanation for this phenomenon is the modulated receptor hypothesis, which states that local anesthetics bind more tightly to the sodium channel during the open or inactive states than they do during resting states. An alternative proposal is the guarded receptor hypothesis. According to this hypothesis, the affinity of the local anesthetic for the sodium channel does not change. However, the channel itself limits the access of local anesthetic to its binding site during the resting state and allows more access to the binding site after an action potential (Fig. 38–4).

The differences between these theories are small; however, both indicate that the interaction between the drug and the sodium channel is a dynamic one in which local anesthetic molecules are moving in and out of the sodium channels, not simply acting as a simple plug that physically obstructs the sodium ion as it enters.

Are All Nerves Equally Susceptible to Local Anesthetics?

For many years, the conventional teaching was that large, myelinated nerves such as the A-α and A-β fibers required greater amounts of local anesthetic to effect a block than did the smaller A, B, or C fibers. This "requirement" was thought to be due to the greater diameter of the large fibers. Gissen and colleagues[4-6] demonstrated that the margin of safety for nerve transmission in vitro was greater for small fibers such as the pain-carrying A-δ and C fibers but that the larger fibers had more barriers to diffusion than did the smaller fibers. These barriers account for the clinical finding that small fibers are blocked more readily than large fibers. Fiber diameter is not a factor.

Differential Blockade

Although this information refuted conventional wisdom, it did not explain the phenomenon of differential block encountered with epidural and spinal anesthesia. With spinal anesthesia, the loss of temperature discrimination extends about two dermatomes higher than the loss of sharp/dull sensation, which is in turn about two dermatomes higher than the loss of sensation to light touch. With epidural anesthesia, similar effects are noted during the initial phases of the block, and dilute solutions of local anesthetic can block pain while preserving motor and some sensory function.

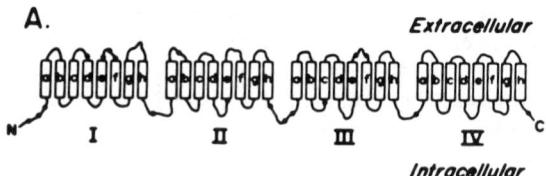

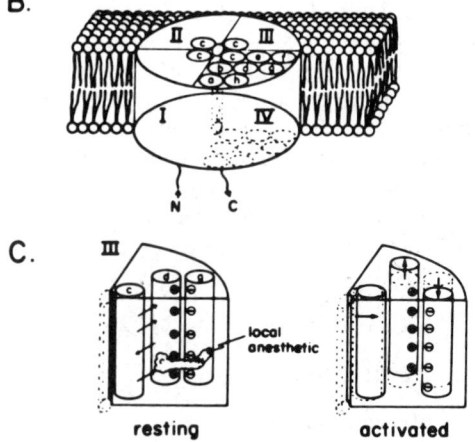

FIGURE 38–3. Speculative model for the molecular mechanism of local anesthetic action. *A*, The large protein subunit of the Na⁺ channel has four regions of six to eight repeating amino acids. *B*, The four regions align themselves with the polar edges, forming the lining of the ion pod. *C*, The amino acids form a strip of positive or negative charge owing to their arrangement in α-helical structures. When the membrane depolarizes, it causes movement in one helix that then causes movements in adjoining helices, resulting in the opening of the ion channel. Butterworth and Strichartz speculate that the local anesthetic molecule prevents the movement of these helices, impeding Na⁺ channel opening. (From Butterworth JF IV, Strichartz GR: Molecular mechanisms of local anesthesia: a review. Anesthesiology 1990; 72:729. Section B adapted from Greenblatt RE, Blatt Y, Montal M: The structure of the voltage sensitive sodium channel: inferences derived from computer aided analysis of the *electrophorus electricus* channel primary structure. FEBS Lett 1985; 193:125.)

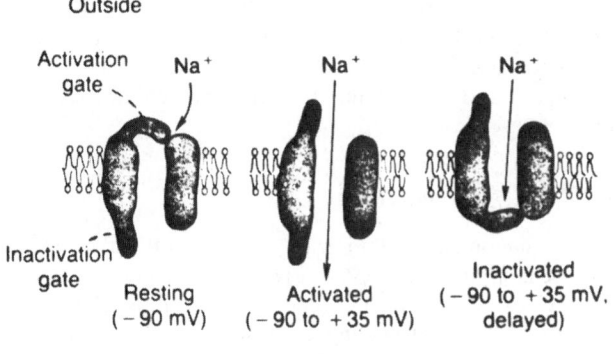

Outside

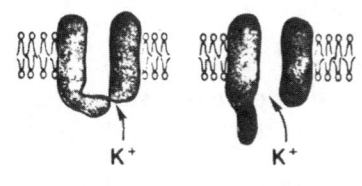

Inside

FIGURE 38–4. Representation of the voltage-dependent conformational changes of Na^+ and K^+ channel protein subunits. Note that during the resting phase, access of molecules to the interior of the Na^+ channel is limited by the activation gate. This is not true during the activated and inactivated states. This is one theoretical explanation for use-dependent block, with which local anesthetics are more effective after repeated stimulations of the nerve. Repeated stimulation leaves fewer Na^+ channels in the resting state. (From Guyton AC: Human Physiology and Mechanisms of Disease. 5th ed. Philadelphia, WB Saunders, 1992.)

Nodes of Ranvier

Fink attributes differential block to differences in the number of nodes of Ranvier bathed by the local anesthetic solution.[7] If a 2-mm segment of nerve is bathed by local anesthetic, the small nerve fibers, which have more nodes of Ranvier per millimeter, have more nodes bathed than do larger nerve fibers. Conducted impulses can skip two blocked nodes of Ranvier but not three. Therefore, the large nerves have fewer nodes exposed to the local anesthetic and are better able to conduct impulses than are the small fibers. Characteristics of nerve fibers are shown in Table 38–1.

Partial Blockade of Multiple Nodes

This explanation works well for epidural anesthesia, when a few millimeters of nerve segment are bathed by local anes-

thetic, but not for spinal anesthesia, when larger segments are involved. Fink explains differential block for spinal anesthesia with the theory that multiple partially blocked nodes decrementally reduce conduction sufficiently so that the impulse ultimately fails to conduct. The number of nodes to be blocked varies inversely with the concentration of the local anesthetic solution. High-concentration solutions need to bathe fewer nodes to block conduction.

At the extremes of local anesthetic diffusion in spinal anesthesia, large nerve fiber nodes would be blocked to the same degree as small fiber nodes, but because more of the nodes are present per millimeter in the small fibers, the small fibers are more likely to reach the critical combination of number of nodes blocked plus intensity of block to effect decremental conduction. Experimental evidence seems to support the theory of decremental conduction.[8]

What Are the Important Chemical Properties of Local Anesthetics?

The four key chemical properties of local anesthetics are lipid solubility, protein binding, capacity to produce vasodilation, and degree of ionization (Table 38–2).

Lipid Solubility

Local anesthetics that are more lipophilic than hydrophilic tend to be more potent. For example, tetracaine and bupivacaine differ from their congeners, procaine and mepivacaine, by having an additional butyl group on the molecule. This extra butyl group increases the lipid solubility of tetracaine 80-fold and the lipid solubility of bupivacaine 28-fold over the less potent drugs procaine and mepivacaine, respectively. Tetracaine is roughly eight times more potent than procaine, and bupivacaine is four times more potent than mepivacaine.

Protein Binding

Drugs that are highly protein bound have a longer duration of action than do drugs of low protein binding. The shortest-acting local anesthetic, procaine, has only 6% plasma protein binding. The long-acting local anesthetics, tetracaine, bupivacaine, and etidocaine, have protein binding of 76%, 96%, and 94%, respectively. Although high levels of plasma protein binding mean that less drug is available to diffuse across nerve membranes, the highly protein-bound drugs appear to bind to cell membrane proteins with much higher affinity once they reach the binding sites and therefore produce a much longer duration of block.

TABLE 38–1. Physical Characteristics of Nerve Fibers

Fiber	Diameter (μm)	Conduction Velocity (m · s⁻¹)	Internodal Distance (mm)	Function
C	0.5–1.3	0.5–2.0	Unmyelinated	Pain, temperature
B	1–3	3–14	0.1	Preganglionic, sympathetic
A-δ	2–5	12–30	0.2	Pain, touch, temperature
A-γ	3–6	30–70	0.5	Motor to muscle spindle
A-β	5–12	30–70	0.8	Touch, pressure
A-α	12–20	70–120	1.2	Proprioception, somatic motor

TABLE 38–2. Physical Properties of Local Anesthetics and Their Local Effects

Physical Property	Clinical Effect
Lipid solubility	Potency
Protein binding	Duration of action
Vasodilator activity	Duration of action
pKa	Onset time

Changes in protein binding due to the presence of other drugs or in hypoproteinemic states may substantially affect the amount of free drug available to exert its effect. Such alterations change not only the potency of the drug and its local anesthetic effect but also may result in toxic reactions at lower than expected doses.[9, 10]

Finally, protein binding may have some relation to toxicity per se. The two drugs that are most highly protein bound are bupivacaine and etidocaine. These drugs are associated with higher degrees of cardiovascular toxicity than the agents with lower levels of protein binding.[11] Whether this difference is related to the drug's high degree of protein binding or some other chemical characteristic is unclear.

Vasodilation

Vasodilation is another factor that affects duration of action. All local anesthetics except cocaine are vasodilators, but the relative ability to produce vasodilation differs among specific agents. For example, lidocaine shows protein-binding properties that are similar to mepivacaine and prilocaine. In isolated nerve preparations, these three drugs have a similar duration of action. In vivo, lidocaine has a shorter duration of action than prilocaine or mepivacaine because of the greater vasodilation produced by lidocaine. When a vasoconstrictor such as epinephrine is added, the durations of action are similar.[12]

Ionization

The degree of ionization determines the time to onset of action for a local anesthetic. It is determined by the drug's pKa, the pH at which the concentration of the uncharged base form of the local anesthetic equals the concentration of the positively charged cationic form.

Those drugs with pKa close to physiologic pH have the greater number of molecules in the uncharged, base form. For example, at pH 7.4, 35% of lidocaine, with a pKa of 7.9, is present in the uncharged base form, whereas only 5% of tetracaine, with a pKa of 8.5, is uncharged.[12] Because local anesthetics must cross several diffusion barriers before reaching their sites of action, drugs with a lower pKa and more uncharged molecules develop a local anesthetic effect faster. Charged molecules do not diffuse as readily across the epineurium, perineurium, endoneurium, and nerve membrane to reach the sodium channels.

This property does not mean that the charged, cationic form of the molecule is unimportant. It has been shown to bind with the sodium channel and to exert a local anesthetic effect.[13] A binding site also is present for uncharged molecules. They penetrate the sodium channel through the nerve membrane, not the cytoplasm, making both forms important for successful channel blockade.[13] Uncharged ions cross the numerous bar-

riers to diffusion to reach the cytoplasm. Once they are in the cytoplasm, the intracellular pH establishes a new equilibrium of ionized and non-ionized molecules. The ionized molecules then move into the sodium channel to prevent channel opening.

Acidic Environments

The phenomenon of ionization due to pKa also explains why local anesthetics work poorly in acidic environments such as those associated with abscesses or cellulitis. Because the local tissue pH surrounding an abscess is <7.4, more drug exists in the cationic form. Fewer local anesthetic molecules are available for diffusion across the nerve structures, resulting in a block that is slow to set up and of less intensity than would otherwise be expected.

How Are Local Anesthetics Metabolized?

Esters

Ester local anesthetics undergo ester hydrolysis in the plasma, red blood cells, and liver. The products of hydrolysis do not exert any significant pharmacologic effect, with the exception of *para*-aminobenzoic acid, which may be a source of allergic reactions associated with ester local anesthetic use.[14]

Procaine, chloroprocaine, and tetracaine undergo very rapid hydrolysis in blood; the half-lives of chloroprocaine and procaine in plasma are <1 minute.[15] Chloroprocaine in particular appears to be a very safe drug.

Case reports of even massive overdoses failed to show any serious effect despite high serum levels detected 10 minutes after injection.[16]

Atypical Cholinesterase

Some patients possess an atypical cholinesterase enzyme that is less efficient in drug hydrolysis. In theory, delayed metabolism of ester local anesthetics should result, depending on the severity of the atypical cholinesterase disorder. However, red blood cell esterases and liver metabolism may compensate for atypical cholinesterase deficiencies, and thus even patients with an atypical cholinesterase may not manifest a prolonged effect.

Liver Disease

Liver disease may also affect the metabolism of ester local anesthetics, because the plasma cholinesterase enzyme is produced in the liver. However, red blood cell esterase activity remains normal, and overall plasma hydrolysis is probably affected only at the extremes of liver disease, making ester-type local anesthetics possibly even safer than the amide drugs for these patients.

Neostigmine, Echothiophate, and Acetazolamide

Drugs that inhibit plasma pseudocholinesterase, such as neostigmine and echothiophate, a drug used in treatment of glaucoma, can decrease the clearance of the ester local anesthetics. Acetazolamide can also decrease ester local anesthetic

TABLE 38–3. Drugs Reducing Local Anesthetic Clearance

Drug	Local Anesthetic
Anticholinesterase agents	Ester agents
Echothiophate	Ester agents
Acetazolamide	Ester agents
Propranolol	Lidocaine*
Cimetidine	Lidocaine*

*Other amides may also be affected.

clearance because of inhibition of hydrolysis by red blood cell esterase enzymes[17] (Table 38–3). A prudent anesthetist exercises caution in using ester local anesthetics in these patients.

Amides

The amide local anesthetics undergo biotransformation within the liver by aromatic hydroxylation, *N*-dealkylation, and amide hydrolysis. The importance of each route of transformation varies greatly among the different drugs.

Lidocaine

Lidocaine primarily undergoes *N*-dealkylation to monoethylglycinexylidide (MEGX). MEGX is important because it has local anesthetic effects comparable to lidocaine.[18] In long-term infusions of lidocaine, MEGX may add to the potential toxicity of the parent drug.

Prilocaine

Prilocaine is metabolized to *o*-toluidine. If the total dose of prilocaine exceeds 600 mg in adults, methemoglobinemia can develop. In normal adults with normal oxygen-carrying capacity, prilocaine in doses <600 mg may be the safest amide local anesthetic because of its rapid hydrolysis and low level of central nervous system (CNS) toxicity.[12] It also may be the ideal drug for intravenous regional anesthesia because of these unique properties. Other amide local anesthetics have metabolic products with some of the pharmacologic activity of the parent drug.[14]

Liver Disease

Because of the dependence of amide local anesthetics on metabolism in the liver, any process that affects liver function or liver blood flow can dramatically alter the metabolism of local anesthetics. Disease states that are known to result in increased drug levels include congestive heart failure, severe hepatic cirrhosis, and the acute phase of viral hepatitis. Renal disease does not appear to affect the metabolism of local anesthetics.[19] However, metabolites of local anesthetics that depend on renal excretion, such as glycinexylidide, another metabolite of lidocaine, may accumulate in the blood. Evidence that such accumulation contributes significantly to drug toxicity is lacking.[20]

Drug Interactions

Like all therapeutic agents, local anesthetics are subject to interaction with other drugs. Beta-blockers, propranolol in par-

ticular, decrease the clearance of lidocaine owing to inhibition of the mixed-function oxidase enzymes and by decreasing liver blood flow.[21] Beta-blockers with intrinsic sympathomimetic activity (pindolol) and low lipid solubility (atenolol) tend to affect lidocaine metabolism less than propranolol.[22]

Cimetidine can reduce the clearance of lidocaine by 30%.[23, 24] This effect also appears to be due primarily to inhibition of the mixed-function oxidase enzyme system of the liver, although some reports suggest that cimetidine also reduces hepatic blood flow. Ranitidine, another H_2 antagonist, does not affect lidocaine clearance.[25]

CLINICAL APPLICATIONS

How Should a Local Anesthetic Be Chosen?

Type of Block

The choice of a local anesthetic agent depends on several factors. First is the type of block to be performed. Some local anesthetics, such as bupivacaine, are used in almost all local anesthetic procedures, including peripheral, spinal, and epidural anesthesia. Other agents, because of their slow onset of action and limited potential to diffuse across anatomic barriers surrounding peripheral nerves, are used only for spinal anesthesia. Tetracaine and dibucaine have limited usefulness in peripheral nerve blocks but are excellent spinal anesthetic agents.

Duration of Procedure

The second important factor is the duration of the procedure, which needs to be well matched to the duration of action of the local anesthetic. Local anesthetics can be categorized into three broad classes based on duration of action (Table 38–4). The duration of action of the drug varies with the technique and use of adjunctive agents (discussed later).

A good rule of thumb is to choose an agent with a duration of action at least 50% greater than the expected duration of the procedure. If the expected duration of the procedure is unknown or unpredictable, two choices are available. First, use the longest-acting agents such as bupivacaine or etidocaine. A bupivacaine brachial plexus block can last 12 hours or more. However, to keep a patient anesthetized for many hours after the completion of a procedure may be undesirable. The second choice is to use a catheter technique, which allows either continuous infusion or repetitive dosing of local anesthetics.

TABLE 38–4. Agents

Short-acting agents	Procaine
	Chloroprocaine
Intermediate-acting agents	Lidocaine
	Mepivacaine
	Prilocaine
Long-acting high-potency agents	Tetracaine
	Bupivacaine
	Etidocaine
	Ropivacaine

Motor Blockade

The third factor to be considered is the need for motor block. For some procedures (orthopedic joint surgery, intra-abdominal surgery, gynecologic surgery), motor blockade is desirable or necessary. In other situations, such as epidural analgesia for vaginal delivery, motor blockade is undesirable.

Of the long-acting local anesthetics, bupivacaine and ropivacaine appear to have less propensity for motor blockade than etidocaine.[12] Why bupivacaine permits selective sensory nerve block with less motor block is unclear but may be related to a unique relationship between its pKa and lipid solubility.[6] Etidocaine, on the other hand, causes dense motor blockade. As a result, it is much better suited for intra-abdominal and orthopedic procedures, whereas bupivacaine and ropivacaine are more useful to provide analgesia without interrupting motor function.

Toxicity

The last factor to consider is the potential for toxicity with a particular technique. Specific discussion of local anesthetic toxicity follows later, but a few words about toxicity and general selection are appropriate.

For special techniques such as intravenous regional anesthesia, certain drugs have specific advantages. Prilocaine has a low potential for toxicity, and the amount of prilocaine needed for intravenous regional anesthesia is usually 200 to 400 mg, well below the 600 mg usually associated with methemoglobinemia.

Chloroprocaine, which is probably the safest of the ester local anesthetics, might seem to be another ideal choice for intravenous regional anesthesia, based on its extremely short serum half-life. However, chloroprocaine can cause phlebitis on intravenous injection.[26]

Bupivacaine, which has a potential for serious cardiovascular toxicity, is not approved for intravenous regional anesthesia. The 0.75% concentration is not approved for obstetric anesthesia because of potentially severe cardiovascular toxicity, which has resulted in several maternal deaths.[12]

How Can Local Anesthetics Be Made To Work Better?

The ideal local anesthetic would have a rapid onset of action, predictable duration of action, reliable depth of anesthesia, and low toxicity. As with all things in life, the ideal does not exist, and local anesthesia is no exception. Fortunately, a wide selection of local anesthetics can be tailored to meet virtually all requirements for anesthesia and analgesia. In order to make the best use of these agents, the important principles that determine time of onset, quality of anesthesia, duration of action, and toxicity must be considered (Table 38–5).

Dosage

The single most important factor in determining time of onset, duration of action, and intensity of nerve blockade is the total dose of local anesthetic used. This fact was demonstrated in a study comparing the anesthetic effects of epidural prilocaine administered as 30 mL of a 2% solution and 20 mL of a 3% solution for a total dose of 600 mg with both techniques.[27] Time of onset, duration of anesthesia, and intensity of motor blockade were the same with both solutions.

The extent of anesthesia varies with increasing volumes; 30 mL of local anesthetic solution provides anesthesia over a greater area than does 20 mL of solution.[28] This characteristic can be used to advantage to provide intense anesthesia over a limited number of dermatomes. A highly concentrated solution in low volumes is useful, for example, in thoracic epidural techniques. Intense anesthesia is needed over the thoracic dermatomes with concomitant sparing of motor function in the lower extremities.

Other studies with epidural bupivacaine showed that increasing the dose of local anesthetic produced more rapid onset of anesthesia, increased motor blockade, and lengthened duration of action.[29] Clearly, increasing the mass (milligrams) of drug used magnifies the overall anesthetic effects.

Vasoconstrictors

Vasoconstrictors, epinephrine in particular, are added to local anesthetic solutions to increase the duration of action, serve as markers for intravascular injection, and reduce peak serum levels. The optimal dose of epinephrine appears to be a 1:200,000 solution or 5 μg $\cdot$ mL^{-1}.[30] Vasoconstrictors are thought to produce local vasoconstriction and reduce the vascular uptake of anesthetic solution.[12] This action leaves more local anesthetic molecules available to exert their effect locally and reduces the peak plasma levels (potential toxicity). In the spinal canal, epinephrine also may have actions of its own, directly modulating pain transmission in the spinal cord.[31]

Other vasoconstrictor drugs such as norepinephrine and phenylephrine are also used, but they are not more effective than epinephrine when used in equivalent doses.[32] Phenylephrine may produce less tachycardia than epinephrine, and some practitioners use phenylephrine in those patients thought to be especially sensitive to the β-adrenergic effects of epinephrine.

Epidural and Peripheral Blocks

Vasoconstrictors do not work for all local anesthetics in all situations (Table 38–6). Epinephrine prolongs the duration of action of all agents used for peripheral nerve blocks except ropivacaine.[33] It also prolongs the duration of action of chloroprocaine, lidocaine, and mepivacaine in epidural blockade but does not significantly prolong the effects of prilocaine, etidocaine, or bupivacaine.[34, 35]

The reasons for these differences are unclear. The uptake of prilocaine, which is less a vasodilator than lidocaine, is not significantly prolonged by epinephrine. Etidocaine and bupivacaine, which are highly lipid soluble, are thought to be taken up by epidural fat, which then acts as a depot for prolonged slow release of these local anesthetics. Because they are quickly absorbed into the local tissues and then slowly released, their duration of action may be so long that it is not extended by a vasoconstrictor.

Blood levels of epidural etidocaine and bupivacaine are not significantly altered by adding epinephrine; neither are the blood levels of ropivacaine when it is used in brachial plexus block.[36] Epinephrine appears to improve the incidence of satisfactory analgesia with low concentrations of epidural bupivacaine (0.125% and 0.25%) in labor analgesia; it does not alter

TABLE 38–5. Clinical Properties of Local Anesthetics

	Agent	Concentration (%)	Clinical Use	Onset	Usual Duration	Recommended Maximum Single Dose (mg)	Comments	pH of Plain Solutions*
Amides	Lidocaine	0.5–1.0	Infiltration	Fast	1.0–2.0 h	300	Most versatile agent	6.5
		0.25–0.5	IV regional			500 + epinephrine		
		1.0–1.5	Peripheral nerve block	Fast	1.0–3.0 h	500 + epinephrine		
		1.5–2.0	Epidural	Fast	1.0–2.0 h	500 + epinephrine		
		4	Topical	Moderate	0.5–1.0 h	500 + epinephrine		
		5	Spinal	Fast	0.5–1.5 h	100		
	Prilocaine	0.5–1.0	Infiltration	Fast	1.0–2.0 h	600	Least toxic amide agent	4.5
		0.25–0.5	IV regional			600		
		1.5–2.0	Peripheral nerve block	Fast	1.5–3.0 h	600	Methemoglobinemia usually occurs	
		2.0–3.0	Epidural	Fast	1.0–3.0 h			
	Mepivacaine	0.5–1.0	Infiltration	Fast	1.5–3.0 h	400	Duration of plain solutions longer than lidocaine without epinephrine. Useful when epinephrine is contraindicated	4.5
						500 + epinephrine		
		1.0–1.5	Peripheral nerve block	Fast	2–3 h			
		1.5–2.0	Epidural	Fast	1.5–3 h			
		4.0	Spinal	Fast	1.5	100		
	Bupivacaine	0.25	Infiltration	Fast	2–4 h	175	Lower concentrations provide differential sensory/motor block. Ventricular arrhythmias and sudden cardiovascular collapse reported after rapid IV injection	4.5–6
						225 + epinephrine		
		0.25–0.5	Peripheral nerve block	Slow	4–12 h	225 + epinephrine		
		0.25–0.5	Obstetric epidural	Moderate	2–4 h	225 + epinephrine		
		0.5–0.75	Surgical epidural	Moderate	2–5 h	225 + epinephrine		
		0.5–0.75	Spinal	Fast	2–4 h	20		
	Etidocaine	0.5	Infiltration	Fast	2–4 h	300	Profound motor block useful for surgical anesthesia but not for obstetric analgesia	4.5
						400 + epinephrine		
		0.5–1.0	Peripheral	Fast	3–12 h	400 + epinephrine		
		1.0–1.5	Surgical epidural	Fast	2–4 h	400 + epinephrine		
	Ropivacaine	0.5–1.0	Brachial plexus block	Slow	9–11 h	No recommended maximum dose	Less cardiovascular toxicity and less motor block than bupivacaine	
	Dibucaine	0.25–0.5 hyperbaric	Spinal	Fast	2–4 h	10	Recommended only for spinal and topical use	
		0.00067 hyperbaric	Spinal	Fast	2–4 h	10		
			Topical	Slow	0.5–1.0 h	50		

Table continued on following page

TABLE 38–5. Clinical Properties of Local Anesthetics *Continued*

Agent		Concentration (%)	Clinical Use	Onset	Usual Duration	Recommended Maximum Single Dose (mg)	Comments	pH of Plain Solutions*
Esters	Procaine	1.0	Infiltration	Fast	0.5–1.0 h	1000	Used mainly for infiltration and differential spinal blocks, allergic potential after repeated use	5–6.5
		1.0–2.0	Peripheral nerve block	Slow	0.5–1.0 h	1000		
		2.0	Epidural	Slow	0.5–1.0 h	1000		
		10.0	Spinal	Moderate	0.5–1.0 h	200		
	Chloroprocaine	1.0	Infiltration	Fast	0.5–1.0 h	800	Lowest systemic toxicity of all local anesthetics	2.7–4
		2.0	Peripheral nerve block	Fast	0.5–1.0 h	1000 + epinephrine	Intrathecal injection may be associated with sensory/motor deficits. Occasional back pain with epidural use	2.7–4
		2.0–3.0	Epidural	Fast	0.5–1.0 h	1000 + epinephrine		
	Tetracaine	0.5	Spinal	Fast	2–4 h	20	Use is primarily limited to spinal and topical anesthesia	4.5–6.5
		2.0	Topical	Slow	0.5–1.0 h	20	Use is primarily limited to spinal and topical anesthesia	4.5–6.5
	Cocaine	4.0–10.0	Topical	Slow	0.5–1.0 h	150	Topical use only, addictive, causes vasoconstriction, CNS toxicity, initially features marked excitation ("fight and flight") response. May cause cardiac arrhythmias	
	Benzocaine	Up to 200	Topical	Slow	0.5–1.0 h	200	Useful only for topical anesthesia	

*No maximum recommended dose is currently available. Doses of 3.1 mg · kg^{-1} for brachial plexus block and 200 mg for epidural use are reported without any signs of toxicity.
Abbreviations: CNS = central nervous system; IV = intravenous.

the effect of solutions of higher concentration.[37] Epinephrine also enhances etidocaine and bupivacaine motor blockade in epidural anesthesia.[38]

Subarachnoid Block

The effect of epinephrine when used as an adjunct for subarachnoid anesthesia is a bit confusing. If the duration of anesthesia is defined as the time for the sensory level to regress by two dermatomes from its maximum level of anesthesia, epinephrine does not prolong the effects of subarachnoid lidocaine or bupivacaine but does significantly extend the duration of action of tetracaine.[39–41]

This observation would be of most importance if spinal anesthesia were used for prolonged intra-abdominal procedures, in which the level of anesthesia could regress to such a point that a patient might become uncomfortable. However, anesthesia at the site of injection, specifically in the sacral areas and lower lumbar segments, is prolonged for all three local anesthetic agents.

The explanation for this phenomenon may be a difference between the three agents and their effects on spinal cord blood

TABLE 38–6. Effects of Epinephrine on Duration of Action of Different Local Anesthetics

Local Anesthetic	Spinal	Epidural	Peripheral Nerve Block
Tetracaine	+	0	+
Chloroprocaine	0	+	+
Lidocaine	–	+	+
Mepivacaine	0	+	+
Prilocaine	0	–	+
Bupivacaine	–	–	+
Etidocaine	0	–	+
Ropivacaine	0	0	–

+ = prolongation; – = no effect; 0 = not used.

flow. Subarachnoid tetracaine increases spinal cord blood flow in dogs.[42] Hence, a vasoconstrictor such as epinephrine may block the increase, reduce tetracaine uptake, and increase the duration of anesthesia.

The key point of this discussion is that epinephrine prolongs a tetracaine spinal anesthetic used for an intra-abdominal procedure but does not affect lidocaine or bupivacaine used in the same fashion. However, epinephrine prolongs the effects of all three agents when they are administered in the subarachnoid space for procedures on the lower extremities.

Physiologic Consequences

Addition of a vasoconstrictor not only changes the quality of nerve block but also may alter its physiologic effects. Epinephrine significantly affects the hemodynamic characteristics of a nerve block compared with the same block performed without epinephrine. Epidural anesthesia performed with epinephrine-containing solutions results in greater decreases in mean arterial pressure than do plain solutions.[43] This response is due to the predominantly β-adrenergic effects of epinephrine in the low doses (1:200,000) used with epidural solutions. When used in local anesthetic solutions for brachial plexus block, epinephrine also causes dose-related changes in pulse and mean arterial pressure, whereas brachial plexus block without vasoconstrictors produces no significant change.[30]

Precautions

When using epinephrine, many find it desirable to add it to the solution just before use. Commercial preparations of local anesthetics contain antioxidants that reduce the solution pH. This change results in a solution with slower time to onset. Epinephrine added just before use does not significantly change pH, but it does create the potential for a drug dosage error.

Can Local Anesthetic Solutions Be Modified to Improve Performance?

The answer is "Yes." Another method to improve local anesthetic performance is to modify the standard preparations with selected additives. Commercial preparations are packaged as hydrochloride salts with pH values from 3.6 to 5.6. This range increases the charged, cationic molecular form.

Alkalization

Sodium bicarbonate ($NaHCO_3$) is added immediately before injection, thus increasing the pH and the uncharged base form. Theoretically, this approach should improve the onset of action and possibly the quality of anesthesia.

Bupivacaine

Alkalization of bupivacaine for epidural analgesia during labor appears to reduce the onset time of sensory anesthesia and the duration of nerve block as well.[44] However, other studies of alkalized bupivacaine failed to demonstrate any benefit over the plain solution.[45, 46]

The addition of $NaHCO_3$ to solutions of bupivacaine for brachial plexus block improved onset time in one study[47] but not in another.[48] The study showing no improvement used 0.1 mL of 8.4% $NaHCO_3$ solution per 20 mL of local anesthetic, and the other study used 0.1 mL per 10 mL of solution. However, the final pH in both was at least 6.4 to 7.15.

Lidocaine and Mepivacaine

Alkalized lidocaine and mepivacaine for epidural anesthesia showed improved onset time and better quality of anesthesia.[49-51] The dose of $NaHCO_3$ was 1.0 mL of 8.4% per 10 mL of anesthetic solution.

In summary, alkalization of local anesthetics decreases the onset time and improves the quality of lidocaine and mepivacaine epidural anesthesia. However, the onset times of nonalkalized lidocaine and mepivacaine are fairly rapid; hence, the benefit of alkalization of these solutions seems small. Available information suggests that alkalization of bupivacaine is of dubious value.

Carbonation

When carbonated local anesthetics are injected near a nerve, carbon dioxide is believed to diffuse rapidly out of the solution, through the nerve into the cytoplasm, to lower the intracellular pH and raise the pH of the local anesthetic solution. When local anesthetic molecules subsequently diffuse into the cytoplasm, the lowered intracellular pH results in a higher proportion of ionized molecules. Because they diffuse poorly across the nerve membrane, these molecules are trapped inside the cell, providing a larger number to bind to their sites of action in the sodium channels.

Lidocaine

Studies evaluating the efficacy of carbonated solutions of lidocaine have produced conflicting results. Lidocaine carbonate appears to have a more rapid onset when used for brachial plexus anesthesia.[52] Studies comparing the onset of carbonated lidocaine anesthesia in epidural blockade yield conflicting data.[53, 54]

Bupivacaine

Carbonated bupivacaine appears to improve the profoundness of sensory and motor blockade during epidural anesthesia and may improve quality and spread of anesthesia in brachial plexus block.[55, 56]

Dextran

In a randomized study of intercostal nerve blockade, the mean duration of the intercostal nerve block was not significantly altered by the use of dextran.[57] Conflicting data on dextran result from the fact that it may alter the local anesthetic pH. One study compared bupivacaine and dextran at pH 8.0 with bupivacaine and dextran at a pH of 4.5 to 5.5 during coccygeal nerve block in rats.[58] The pH 8.0 solution significantly prolonged the duration of nerve block, but the more acidic solution did not, suggesting that the change of pH, not the dextran molecule, imparts the therapeutic benefit.

Hyaluronidase

Hyaluronidase breaks down extracellular hyaluronic acid, a component of connective tissue, to improve the diffusion of local anesthetic between tissue planes. It is commonly used for retrobulbar block[59] but also has been described for leg and upper extremity nerve blocks and epidural blockade. Hyaluronidase does not improve epidural anesthesia, and its advantages in peripheral nerve block are questionable.[60]

Local Anesthetic Mixtures

Some investigators combine two local anesthetics in an attempt to develop a solution with the rapid-onset characteristic of the short-acting component drug and the long-duration characteristic of the more potent but slower-onset component drug.

Chloroprocaine and Bupivacaine

One study combined 10 mL of 3% chloroprocaine with 20 mL of 0.5% bupivacaine for brachial plexus block. This mixture had quicker time to complete anesthesia, a similar duration of action, and a more intense block than 30 mL of 0.5% bupivacaine.[61] Two studies using mixtures of chloroprocaine and bupivacaine for epidural anesthesia reported no advantage of the mixture over either drug alone and further found that chloroprocaine may reduce the effectiveness of bupivacaine during labor.[62, 63]

Two studies suggest why chloroprocaine may inhibit the effectiveness of bupivacaine. In one, a mixture of the drugs was applied to isolated nerves and the pH varied.[64] At a pH of 3.6, the block had the characteristics of chloroprocaine alone. At a pH of 5.5, the block resembled bupivacaine alone. In another study of isolated nerves, a metabolite of chloroprocaine, 4-amino-2-chlorobenzoic acid, completely blocked the effects of bupivacaine.[65] In general, a mixture of chloroprocaine and bupivacaine has no advantage over either solution alone.

Lidocaine and Bupivacaine

In a randomized study of lidocaine and bupivacaine in various proportions for epidural anesthesia, no significant difference between bupivacaine alone and any of the other solutions of bupivacaine and lidocaine was observed.[66]

To summarize, no benefit accrues to mixtures of local anesthetics for epidural anesthesia. In brachial plexus block, a slight advantage in terms of time of onset may result from a mixture of chloroprocaine and bupivacaine compared with bupivacaine alone. However, large studies in support of this conclusion are lacking. Remember that the toxicity of local anesthetics is additive and that mixing of agents does not allow an increase of the total dose.

What Are the Differences Between Agents?

The most useful clinical division of local anesthetic agents is by duration of action and ability to produce a dense anesthetic block with adequate muscle relaxation. They can be divided into three categories: short-acting agents of low potency, agents with intermediate duration and potency, and agents with long duration and high potency (see Table 38–4).

Short-Acting Agents

Procaine

Before the discovery of lidocaine, procaine was the most commonly used local anesthetic. It now has limited clinical use. Procaine is available as a 1% or 2% solution for skin infiltration and peripheral nerve block. Blocks with procaine have a relatively slow onset and short duration of 30 to 60 minutes. Procaine is also available in a 10% solution for spinal anesthesia. It is still occasionally used as a spinal anesthetic for the diagnosis of chronic pain disorders and occasionally for vaginal delivery.

Chloroprocaine

Chloroprocaine is the least toxic local anesthetic agent.[12] It is used in concentrated solutions ranging from 1% to 3%. Chloroprocaine has a fast onset and duration of 30 to 60 minutes. It is used extensively in cesarean section; its low toxicity, rapid onset, and short duration make it ideal for epidural anesthesia.

Neurotoxicity. Prolonged and sometimes permanent neurologic deficits have been reported after inadvertent massive subarachnoid injections during attempted epidural anesthesia.[67, 68] These deficits were thought to result from the combination of low pH and the preservative sodium bisulfite.[69] Chloroprocaine is not neurotoxic.

Back Pain. Currently available solutions of chloroprocaine avoid the combination of sodium bisulfite and low pH. However, the new solutions, marketed under the trade name Nesacaine-MPF, have been associated with severe back pain after epidural anesthesia.[70–72] The back pain is described as a dull, deep lumbar ache, occasionally associated with spasm of the erector spinae muscles. It is hypothesized to be caused by ethylenediaminetetraacetic acid (EDTA) in Nesacaine-MPF solution.

EDTA is a chelator of calcium and may affect localized skeletal muscle calcium activity. One patient received calcium chloride in graduated doses to a total of 300 mg to relieve what was thought to be chloroprocaine-induced back pain after an epidural anesthetic.[73] In another report, 10 volunteers who received epidural chloroprocaine as part of a clinical investigation developed back pain as the anesthetic resolved. Epidural fentanyl, 100 to 200 µg, effectively treated the back pain.[72]

Factors thought to contribute to chloroprocaine-induced back pain are the large volumes of chloroprocaine and its use to infiltrate the intraspinous ligaments before insertion of the epidural needle.

Cocaine

Cocaine, which was the first clinically used local anesthetic, is now used almost exclusively for mucous membrane topical anesthesia. Unlike the other local anesthetics, cocaine blocks norepinephrine reuptake and has significant vasoconstrictor properties. The 4% solution is used as a topical anesthetic and vasoconstrictor for ear, nose, and throat surgery. However, the potential for abuse and serious toxic reactions, including hypertension and cardiac dysrhythmias, limit its clinical usefulness.

Intermediate-Acting Agents

Lidocaine

Lidocaine is the most versatile and widely used of all local anesthetics. Solutions of 0.5% are useful for skin infiltration, with a rapid onset and a duration of 1 to 2 hours. In 1% to 2% solutions, it provides excellent anesthesia for peripheral nerve blocks. The duration of action is 1 to 1½ hours for plain solutions and 2 to 2½ hours for solutions with epinephrine. Lidocaine is also used for epidural anesthesia (2% solution), as a topical anesthetic (4% solution), and for spinal anesthesia (5% solution).

Prilocaine

Prilocaine can be used for any technique except spinal anesthesia. It may be advantageous for intravenous regional anesthesia because of its lower systemic toxicity. Prilocaine without epinephrine also has a longer duration of action than lidocaine without epinephrine, making it a useful agent when epinephrine is contraindicated. Because prilocaine in doses of 600 mg can cause methemoglobinemia, its use has been discouraged in obstetric anesthesia. Otherwise, its spectrum of activity is equivalent to lidocaine.

Mepivacaine

Mepivacaine also has the same spectrum of action as lidocaine, although it is not effective as a topical anesthetic. Like prilocaine, solutions without a vasoconstrictor have a longer duration of action than solutions of lidocaine without a vasoconstrictor. Mepivacaine with epinephrine has the same duration of action as lidocaine with epinephrine. Mepivacaine is useful when epinephrine is contraindicated, as in patients with unstable angina or other cardiac conditions. It is not used for obstetric anesthesia because a fetus cannot metabolize it as well as the other local anesthetics.[12]

Long-Acting High-Potency Anesthetics

Tetracaine

Tetracaine is the most potent ester local anesthetic. Because of its slow onset of action, its use is virtually confined to spinal anesthesia as a 1% solution or as lyophilized crystals. The crystals allow tetracaine to be made into hypobaric, isobaric, or hyperbaric solutions, making it a versatile agent. As a 2% solution, tetracaine is an effective topical anesthetic agent. However, because of its high potency, the maximum recommended single dose is 20 mg. Case reports of deaths associated with the use of tetracaine as a topical anesthetic agent have been published. Thus, careful attention to dose and symptoms of toxicity is essential.[12]

Bupivacaine

Bupivacaine is a useful and versatile local anesthetic. It is available in 0.25%, 0.5%, and 0.75% solutions. The solutions of low concentration can be used to provide a differential block for analgesia during labor. Solutions of 0.125% combined with narcotic provide satisfactory labor analgesia with almost no motor block.[74] High concentrations of bupivacaine for peripheral nerve blocks provide anesthesia lasting 12 to 24 hours when used with a vasoconstrictor.

A 0.75% solution of epidural bupivacaine provides rapid onset of surgical anesthesia, and a commercially available hyperbaric spinal solution of 0.75% bupivacaine is an extremely effective anesthetic with a duration of action of 2 to 4 hours.

Bupivacaine's only drawback is its tendency to cause severe cardiovascular toxicity when administered inadvertently as a large intravenous dose (see *Toxicity*, later). Because of the risk of cardiovascular toxicity, bupivacaine is not recommended for intravenous regional anesthesia in any concentration, and the 0.75% solution is not recommended for use in obstetrics.

Etidocaine

Etidocaine is a long-acting local anesthetic characterized by profound motor block. This feature makes the agent extremely useful for surgical anesthesia but much less so as an analgesic in obstetrics. It is approximately half as potent as bupivacaine. Surgical anesthesia is achieved with a 1.5% solution. Etidocaine's duration of action is similar to that of bupivacaine. Cases of profound motor block without sensory anesthesia have been reported, a fact that has dampened some of the initial enthusiasm for this otherwise very useful agent.

Ropivacaine

Ropivacaine is a new amide local anesthetic with a chemical structure similar to that of bupivacaine and mepivacaine. It appears to be as potent as bupivacaine for sensory block but provides less motor block. It is prepared as the S isomer, which enhances the clinical properties of the drug compared with the racemic mixture.[75]

Cardiovascular Toxicity. Ropivacaine appears to have less cardiovascular toxicity than bupivacaine but more toxicity than lidocaine.[76] The dose producing CNS toxicity is the same for ropivacaine and bupivacaine, but ropivacaine causes fewer dysrhythmias and less myocardial depression.[77–79]

Clinical Properties. The drugs have equivalent potency and time to onset.[80] Compared with bupivacaine, ropivacaine has a slightly shorter duration of action (333 min versus 394 min) and less motor block when used as an epidural anesthetic.[81, 82] Ropivacaine does not appear to have increased toxicity in pregnant animal models, another advantage over bupivacaine.[83]

Comparative Features. Ropivacaine appears to be an equally effective yet less toxic drug than bupivacaine. However, cardiovascular toxicity from bupivacaine is still a rare event that usually occurs only when a large amount of bupivacaine is injected intravenously.

Bupivacaine has been used widely for many years. Many anesthetists are reluctant to trade a tried-and-true drug for a relative newcomer, although the equipotent dose of ropivacaine makes transition from bupivacaine that much easier. The determining factor regarding use may be the cost of ropivacaine relative to bupivacaine.

TOXICITY

Toxicity due to local anesthetics is rare but can be life threatening. It may take the form of systemic and local reactions. Systemic toxicity results from allergic reactions, drug overdose, and drug metabolites (i.e., prilocaine-induced methemoglobinemia). Tissue toxicity occurs at the site of injection because of drug irritation.

What Are the Central Nervous System Effects of Local Anesthetic Overdose?

Signs and symptoms of CNS toxicity appear before those of cardiovascular toxicity[84] (Fig. 38–5). The ability of any local anesthetic to produce CNS toxicity is related directly to the potency of the drug. For example, tetracaine, which is eight times more potent than procaine, requires only one eighth the amount of drug to produce an equivalent amount of CNS toxicity. This relationship is not always true for cardiovascular toxicity.

CNS toxicity is remarkably similar for all drugs. Test subjects who received intravenous infusions of local anesthetics reported initial circumoral numbness, numbness of the extremities and trunk, a lightheaded sensation, and tinnitus.[15, 84] Other visual and auditory disturbances were also reported. As the dose of infused local anesthetic becomes larger, more pronounced effects result. They include muscle twitching and, if doses are high enough, unconsciousness, seizures, and respiratory arrest.[84]

How Is Cardiovascular Toxicity Manifested?

The cardiovascular toxicity of local anesthetics manifests in three possible ways: direct action on cardiac muscle, affecting myocardial contractility; disturbance of the conduction system of the heart; and direct effects on peripheral vascular smooth muscle.[85]

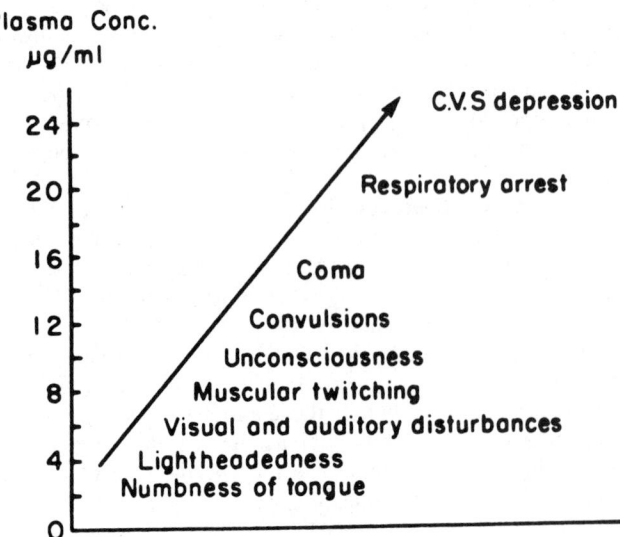

FIGURE 38–5. Relationship of signs and symptoms of local anesthetic toxicity to plasma concentrations of lidocaine. C.V.S. = Cardiovascular system. (From Covino BG: Clinical pharmacology of local anesthetic agents. *In* Neural Blockade in Clinical Anesthesia and Management of Pain. 2nd ed. Cousins MG, Bridenbaugh PO (eds). Philadelphia, JB Lippincott, 1988, p 122.)

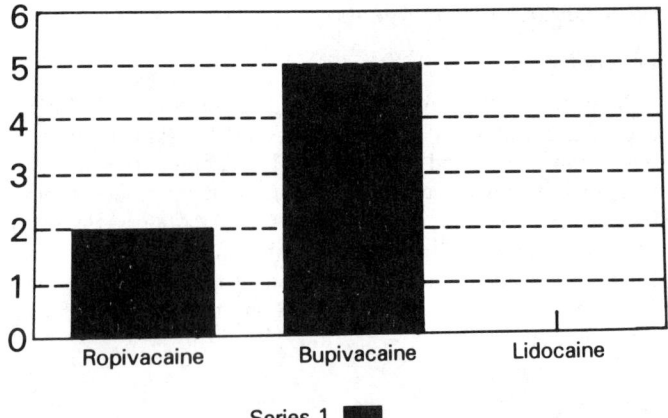

FIGURE 38–6. Six sheep in each of these groups received toxic doses of three different local anesthetic agents (ropivacaine, bupivacaine, or lidocaine). Almost all of the sheep in the bupivacaine-treated group developed ventricular dysrhythmias, whereas none of the lidocaine-treated sheep did. (From Nancarrow C, Rutten AJ, Runciman WB, et al: Myocardial and cerebral drug concentrations and the mechanisms of death after fatal intravenous doses of lidocaine, bupivacaine, and ropivacaine in the sheep. Anesth Analg 1989; 69:276.)

Contractility

Local anesthetics exert a negative inotropic effect on cardiac muscle that is dose and potency related.[86] As with CNS toxicity, the negative inotropic effect of tetracaine is about eight times that of procaine, reflecting the relative potency of the two drugs. Drug levels associated with the usual clinical doses of local anesthetics do not significantly affect myocardial contractility. However, the blood levels achieved with a rapid intravenous injection or from an absolute overdose of local anesthetics can result in decreased cardiac output.

Conductivity

The conduction system of the myocardium also has ion channels that are susceptible to the effects of local anesthetics. The antidysrhythmic effects of lidocaine are well known. Lidocaine decreases the action potential duration and, to a lesser degree, the effective refractory period. It increases the ratio of effective refractory period to action potential duration in ventricular muscle Purkinje's fibers.[87]

Not all local anesthetics are equal in their effects on the cardiac conduction system. In animal studies of massive intravenous overdoses of lidocaine, the sequence of events is a prolongation of conduction time in the heart followed by decrease in spontaneous pacemaker activity, profound bradycardia, and eventual cardiac standstill.[88]

Case reports of cardiac arrest following inadvertent intravenous administration of bupivacaine during epidural anesthesia led to a number of studies investigating its potential cardiac toxicity.[84, 85, 87] Bupivacaine and to a lesser degree etidocaine and ropivacaine produce cardiovascular effects that are quantitatively and qualitatively different from those of the local anesthetics of low and intermediate potency. Bupivacaine at toxic doses results in ventricular tachycardia and ventricular fibrillation in a significant percentage of animals.[89, 90] Similar effects to a lesser extent occur with etidocaine and ropivacaine but not with intermediate-potency local anesthetics such as lidocaine[79, 91] (Fig. 38–6). Resuscitation of animals with ventricular dysrhythmias is difficult, as it is in humans who receive inadvertent overdoses of bupivacaine.[11, 92]

Mechanisms

The reason why bupivacaine is more prone to cause ventricular dysrhythmias is unclear. Protein binding alone is not a factor, because etidocaine, which is more protein bound than bupivacaine, has a lower incidence of ventricular dysrhythmias. The piperidine ring is not responsible, because mepivacaine and ropivacaine also possess one. Mepivacaine does not cause ventricular dysrhythmias in animal models.[91] The incidence of ventricular dysrhythmias with ropivacaine is much less than with bupivacaine, despite the fact that the drugs are almost equipotent.[79]

Electrophysiologic Changes. Electrophysiologic studies in cardiac muscle show that bupivacaine binds to ion channels for much longer periods than do other local anesthetics.[93] Even at relatively slow heart rates, ion channels may not fully recover from bupivacaine-induced blockade, resulting in conditions that favor re-entrant–type cardiac dysrhythmias.

Serum Levels. An important feature of bupivacaine myocardial toxicity is the relatively low serum levels necessary. Morishima and colleagues[94, 95] studied the infusion rates of lidocaine, bupivacaine, and etidocaine needed to cause cardiovascular collapse (CC) and convulsions (CNS) in sheep. For lidocaine, the CC/CNS ratio was 7.1:1 (i.e., seven times more lidocaine was required to cause cardiovascular collapse than convulsions). The ratios for bupivacaine and etidocaine were 3.7:1 and 4.4:1, respectively. The CC/CNS ratio of blood levels of bupivacaine and etidocaine was also half the CC/CNS ratio of lidocaine.

In a separate study evaluating the ratio of fatal doses to convulsive doses for the three drugs, the values were lidocaine 4.5:1, bupivacaine 2.2:1, and ropivacaine 2.1:1[80] (Fig. 38–7).

These studies demonstrate that the margin for error is less with the potent, long-acting agents than with the agents of intermediate potency. Inadvertent intravenous injections of the long-acting potent agents can result in rapid progression from

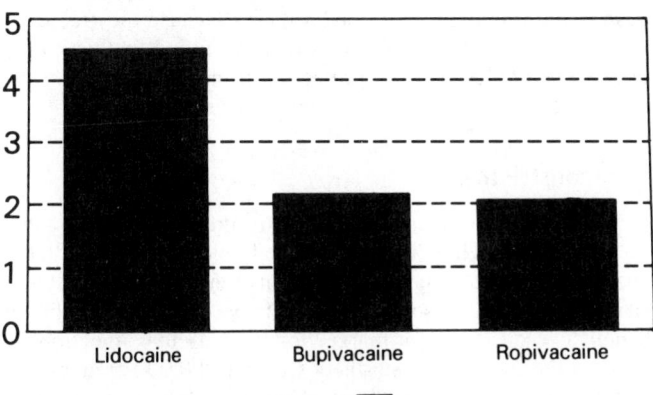

FIGURE 38–7. Bupivacaine and ropivacaine both demonstrate a lower ratio of fatal to convulsive doses of local anesthetics when compared with lower potency agents such as lidocaine. This indicates a lower margin of safety for toxic reactions from the onset of central nervous system symptoms to development of serious cardiovascular toxicity. (Extrapolated from Nancarrow C, Rutlen AJ, Runciman WB, et al: Myocardial and cerebral drug concentrations and the mechanisms of death after fatal intravenous doses of lidocaine, bupivacaine, and ropivacaine in the sheep. Anesth Analg 1989; 69:276. © International Anesthesia Research Society.)

TABLE 38–7. Factors in Local Anesthetic Toxicity

Total drug dose
Site of administration
Drug interactions
Patient disease
Alterations in protein binding
Inadvertent intravenous injection

CNS toxicity to cardiovascular collapse. If a patient is sedated or the dose injected is relatively large, no premonitory CNS symptoms may be noted before cardiac arrest occurs.

Although bupivacaine toxicity is a real and potentially dangerous problem, the drug remains one of the most widely used local anesthetics. If steps are taken to avoid inadvertent large intravenous doses, the chances of serious toxicity remain extremely small.

How Is Local Anesthetic Toxicity Avoided?

The key to avoiding local anesthetic toxicity is to identify those factors that contribute to high levels in the blood (Table 38–7) and then take steps to minimize them (Table 38–8).

Total Dose

Scott pointed out many of the problems associated with currently accepted "maximum recommended doses" of local anesthetics.[96] They include (1) failure to account for different sites of injection with their differing blood levels; (2) failure to account for the use of vasoconstrictors or, if vasoconstrictors are considered, allowing doses not supported by scientific study; and (3) recommendations not based on the relative potency of drugs, such as a maximum dose of bupivacaine that is half the dose of lidocaine despite the fact that bupivacaine is four times more potent than lidocaine. He suggested that (1) recommended maximum doses are unsatisfactory and poorly reflect the realities of clinical practice; (2) anesthetists should use recommended doses only as broad guidelines in the total perspective of patient health and anesthetic technique; and (3) the greatest threat to patients is a rapid, direct intravenous injection of local anesthetics, which can cause serious reactions even at recommended "safe" doses.

Site of Administration

Blood levels of local anesthetics vary greatly with site of administration.[97] Intercostal nerve blocks are associated with

TABLE 38–8. Prevention of Local Anesthetic Toxicity

Prepare emergency equipment
  Airway equipment
  Intravenous line
  Resuscitative drugs
Adjust drug dose for patient's disease
Monitor pulse, blood pressure, and oxygenation
Aspirate needle before injecting
Consider using a vasoconstrictor
  Reduces blood levels
  Marker for intravenous injection
Fractionate dose

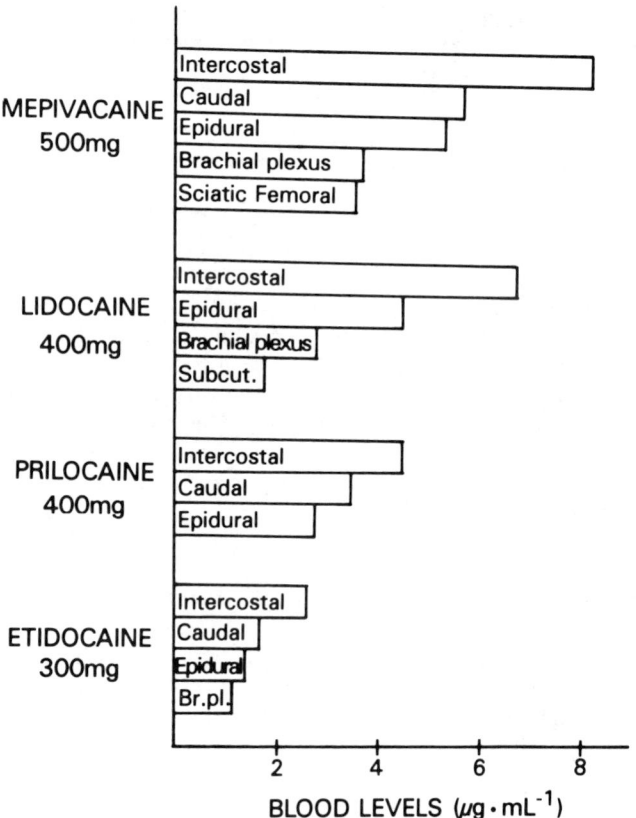

FIGURE 38–8. Comparative peak levels of various local anesthetic agents following administration for different local anesthetic techniques. Subcut. = Subcutaneous; Br. pl. = brachial plexus. (From Covino BG, Vassallo HG: General pharmacological and toxicological aspects of local anesthetic agents. *In* Local Anesthetics: Mechanisms of Action and Clinical Use. New York, Grune & Stratton, 1976, p 97.)

the highest levels of local anesthetic, followed by caudal, epidural, brachial plexus, and sciatic-femoral nerve blocks (Fig. 38–8). Spinal anesthesia produces very low levels in the blood. Anesthetic techniques with the highest blood levels usually require the highest drug doses to achieve effective anesthesia and are associated with high vascularity at the site of injection. An acceptable dose of local anesthetic for brachial plexus anesthesia could prove toxic if administered for intercostal nerve blocks. When feasible, lower concentrations of local anesthetics with vasoconstrictors should be used in highly vascular areas.

Drug Interactions

Interactions with other medications a patient may be using can be important. Propranolol and cimetidine decrease local anesthetic metabolism; both drugs increase blood levels of lidocaine. Patients with severe liver disease and congestive heart failure are also more prone to develop amide local anesthetic toxicity because of impaired metabolism. Individuals with atypical plasma cholinesterase enzymes may have some impairment of ester local anesthetic metabolism.

Pregnancy

Pregnancy affects the body's susceptibility to local anesthetic toxicity. Pregnant patients require a lower dose of local anesthetics for effective nerve blocks and reduced doses of local anesthetics for epidural and spinal anesthesia.[98, 99] The recommended dose of local anesthetics for spinal and epidural anesthesia during pregnancy is approximately 25% to 30% lower than in nonpregnant patients.[100] The altered response to local anesthetics in pregnancy may be related to increased levels of progesterone.[101]

Pregnant animals also are more susceptible to cardiovascular toxicity with bupivacaine but not lidocaine and ropivacaine.[83, 102] This susceptibility does not appear to be related to increased myocardial uptake of bupivacaine. It may result from the increase in circulating progesterone levels. Progesterone-treated animals show more depression of the maximum rate of Purkinje's fiber depolarization than do nontreated animals.[103] Progesterone has no effect on the electrophysiologic changes occurring with lidocaine.

Protein Binding

Protein binding of local anesthetics can affect the blood levels required to produce toxicity. The free local anesthetic drug, not the protein-bound form, crosses the blood-brain barrier to cause CNS toxicity.[104] Therefore, anything that alters protein binding also alters the amount of free drug.

Alpha₁-Acid Glycoprotein

Unfortunately, predicting which patients will have alterations in protein binding is not simple. The primary binding protein for local anesthetics is α_1-acid glycoprotein.[104] This substance is an acute phase reactant that is increased during sepsis, other acute illnesses, and cancer. Because α_1-acid glycoprotein is an acute phase reactant, it is elevated in almost all clinical situations in which local anesthetics are used, including surgery, trauma, and chronic pain states. This rise is theorized to protect most patients from local toxicity.

Support for this theory was provided by patients who received long-term infusions of epidural local anesthetics for postoperative pain relief.[105, 106] In one group of nine patients, four had bupivacaine levels exceeding 4.0 μg · mL^{-1}. Despite these high serum levels, no patient experienced symptoms of toxicity. Given the slow rate of rise of the drug levels, increased protein binding conceivably kept free drug levels low despite the relatively high total values. Because the free drug is responsible for toxic symptoms, postsurgical patients may have some degree of CNS protection from toxicity due to the increased levels of α_1-acid glycoprotein.

Vasoconstrictors

Vasoconstrictor agents are useful in preventing local anesthetic toxicity. They reduce the peak blood levels of local anesthetics by causing local vasoconstriction at the injection site and reducing vascular uptake of the drug. An additional benefit is their role as a marker for intravascular injection. A 3-mL solution of local anesthetics with 1:200,000 epinephrine contains 15 μg of epinephrine. This solution, when administered intravenously, augments the pulse by 20 to 30 beats per minute within 20 seconds of administration.[107] This change can be reliably detected and should prevent the subsequent administration of larger amounts of local anesthetic intravenously. Other β-agonist drugs, such as isoproterenol and ephedrine, have also been used as markers for intravascular injection, although none is convincingly superior to epinephrine.[108]

Pros and Cons of Use

Certain patients do not respond reliably to standard test doses of epinephrine, including those taking β-adrenergic antagonist agents,[109] children under halothane general anesthesia,[110] and pregnant patients in labor. In the latter group, Leighton and colleagues could not reliably identify heart rate changes in women given 15 μg of epinephrine intravenously.[111] The wide changes in pulse and blood pressure associated with labor make detection of transient changes in heart rate difficult.

Some practitioners believe that epinephrine test doses may cause dangerous reductions in uterine blood flow in all pregnant patients and severe hypertension in pre-eclamptic patients. Because a test dose is unreliable, they conclude it is dangerous and is of little use.[108]

The alternative opinion is that 15 μg of intravenous epinephrine has never been shown to cause adverse human fetal or maternal outcomes despite animal studies showing reductions in uterine blood flow. Even if epinephrine does not detect all intravenous injections, it detects some of them and does prevent more serious problems associated with subsequent inadvertent intravenous injections of local anesthetics. This latter view probably reflects the majority opinion.

How Can Inadvertent Intravenous Injection Be Avoided?

To avoid intravenous injection, (1) aspirate before injecting to ensure there is no blood return and (2) give the local anesthetic in fractional incremental doses over a period of time. Negative results on aspiration tests do not ensure the prevention of intravenous injections. Therefore, fractionation of the dose is important, usually in 3- to 5-ml increments every 30 seconds or more. This procedure allows detection of the early symptoms of toxicity before they progress to seizures and cardiovascular collapse.

What Is the Treatment?

The key to treatment of local anesthetic toxicity is early recognition. Any alteration in a patient's mental status should be viewed as local anesthetic toxicity until proved otherwise. The classic symptoms such as a metallic or strange taste in the mouth, circumoral numbness, tinnitus, and numbness of the trunk or extremities are almost diagnostic. Treatment follows that of virtually all anesthetic emergencies: (1) maintain a patent airway, (2) ventilate the patient, and (3) support the circulation (Table 38–9).

Hypoxia and Acidosis

Hypoxia and acidosis aggravate toxicity.[112] Administer 100% oxygen and ventilate the patient if breathing ceases. The initial cardiovascular effect is hypotension due to the vasodilating properties and negative inotropic effects of the offending agent. The legs should be elevated, volume expanders infused, and inotropic agents administered when appropriate. For mild hypotension, ephedrine in 5- to 25-mg doses is appropriate. More profound hypotension should be treated aggressively with epinephrine.

TABLE 38–9. Treatment of Local Anesthetic Toxicity

Establish an airway
Ventilate with 100% oxygen
Support circulation
   Elevate legs
   Volume expanders
   Ephedrine, 5–25 mg
Treat seizures
   Diazepam, 5–10 mg
   Midazolam, 2–5 mg
   Thiopental, 50–200 mg
Treat cardiovascular collapse
   Epinephrine
   Atropine
   Bretylium for ventricular dysrhythmias

Seizures

Sodium thiopental (50–200 mg), diazepam (2–10 mg), or midazolam (1–5 mg) should be effective treatment for most seizures. Seizures due to intravascular injection should be short lived, unless the dose is an especially large one, and may subside without treatment. If they persist, the accompanying acidosis and hypoxia aggravate the toxic effects. Hence, administration of a barbiturate or benzodiazepine is appropriate.

Tonic-clonic muscle activity accompanying seizures often makes ventilation difficult. A fast-acting muscle relaxant such as succinylcholine terminates the motor activity, making ventilation easier. Muscle paralysis does not terminate electrical seizure activity in the brain.

Cardiovascular Collapse

Profound cardiovascular collapse requires aggressive treatment with epinephrine and atropine. If malignant ventricular dysrhythmias result, immediate defibrillation is essential. Bupivacaine-induced ventricular dysrhythmias are especially difficult to convert. Animal models suggest that large doses of epinephrine, atropine, and bretylium increase the chance of successful resuscitation.[113] Lidocaine should not be administered as an antidysrhythmic for ventricular dysrhythmias associated with local anesthetic toxicity. Bupivacaine-induced cardiovascular collapse may require prolonged resuscitation for several hours. In some instances, heroic steps such as the use of cardiopulmonary bypass to maintain circulation may be considered.

Do Local Anesthetics Cause Allergic Reactions?

They can. Another variant of systemic toxicity is an allergic reaction. Allergic reactions are more common with the ester class of drugs.

Incidence

Esters are derivatives of *para*-aminobenzoic acid, a substance to which a percentage of the population has demonstrated allergic reactions. The number of patients who relate a history of local anesthetic allergy and actually demonstrate allergic phenomena during skin testing or subcutaneous challenge is extremely low. deShazo and Nelson reviewed their experience with 90 patients reported to be allergic to local anesthetics.[114] Of these 90 patients, only 14 had histories consistent with immediate hypersensitivity reactions. Of these 14, 12 patients had negative skin test responses and negative subcutaneous challenge to lidocaine. The investigators concluded that "the vast majority of patients labelled allergic to local anesthetics are, in fact, not."

Evaluation

When one evaluates patients with an alleged allergy to "caine" drugs, taking a history is the first step in determining the presence of true immediate hypersensitivity reactions (Table 38–10). Symptoms consistent with this diagnosis are wheezing, hives, angioedema, rhinorrhea, shock, and tachycardia.[115] Manifestations of vasoconstrictor effect may also be misinterpreted as allergy. Most commonly, these are described as palpitations and a sense of nervousness or anxiety. Bradycardia is not a symptom of anaphylaxis and can aid in differentiating immediate hypersensitivity from other toxic reactions such as intravenous injections of local anesthetics and local anesthetic overdose. Patient-generated symptoms such as vasovagal reactions and anxiety/hyperventilation syndrome can also masquerade as allergic reactions.

If the history is suggestive of allergy to local anesthetics, two approaches are open (Fig. 38–9). First, if the local anesthetic causing the reaction is known, an agent from the other class can be used. If the agent is unknown or if it is not possible to use an agent from the other class, skin testing should be performed, followed by subcutaneous challenge with the agent to be used.[114–116] Skin testing should be carried out by a consultant knowledgeable about local anesthetic allergy. False-negative skin test results are rare, but false-positive rates may be as high as 10%.[116]

Patients must be challenged with the local anesthetic solution proposed for use in the procedure. If the solution contains preservatives such as parabens and bisulfites, challenge with the drug including preservatives should be performed because preservatives are also responsible for allergic reactions.

If the skin test results are negative and graded subcutaneous challenges, including 1 mL of undiluted drug, produce no response, the risk of allergic reaction to that drug is no greater than the risk in the general population.[116] With this approach, a safe local anesthetic agent can be identified for every patient.[114–116]

TABLE 38–10. Differential Diagnosis of Local Anesthetic Reactions

Diagnosis	Signs and Symptoms
Local anesthetic toxicity	Central nervous system
Intravenous injection	toxicity, convulsions,
Drug overdose	bradycardia or
	tachycardia, rapid onset
Vasoconstrictor reaction	Tachycardia, hypertension,
	palpitations, nervousness
Patient's disease	Bradycardia
Vasovagal	Chest pain
Myocardial infarction	
Bronchospasm	
Allergic reactions	Tachycardia, urticaria,
	bronchospasm

Approach to the Patient with Suspected Local Anesthetic Allergy

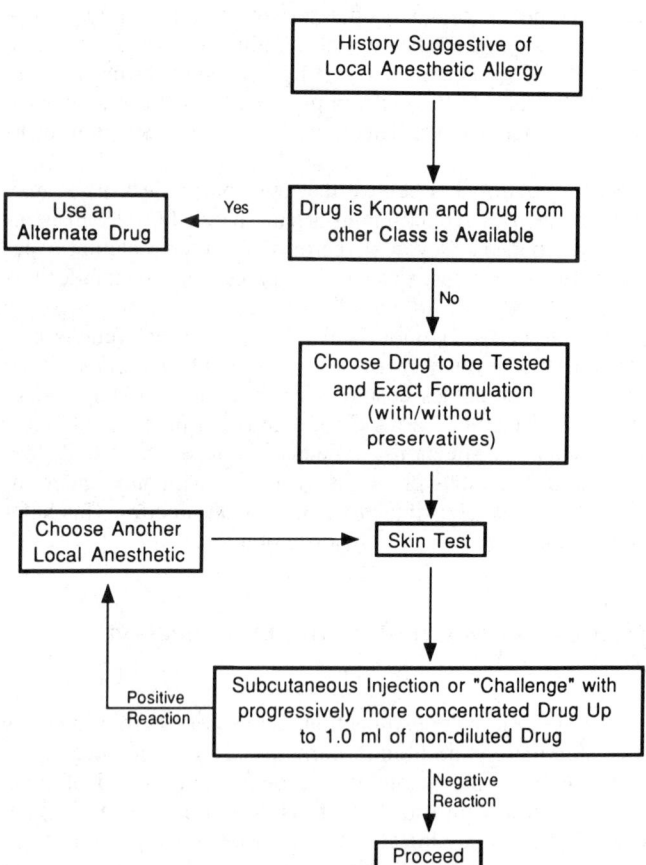

FIGURE 38–9. Algorithm for management of the patient with a history suggestive of local anesthetic allergy. If the patient has a history of reaction to a specific drug, then a drug from the other class (ester or amide) can be used safely. If the drug is unknown or if there is no acceptable alternative, then skin testing followed by subcutaneous injection of progressively more concentrated solutions of drug can help identify a local anesthetic for safe use. Skin tests are best done by a consultant experienced in allergy testing.

Do Local Anesthetics Cause Tissue Toxicity?

Standard solutions of local anesthetics rarely, if ever, cause nerve injury. Prolonged neurologic deficits after local anesthetic techniques are much more likely to be due to direct trauma to the nerves as a result of the anesthetic infiltration or the accompanying surgery.

Chloroprocaine Neurotoxicity

As mentioned previously, chloroprocaine solutions were associated with permanent neurologic deficits after inadvertent administration of large amounts of drug into the subarachnoid space during attempted epidural anesthesia. The manufacturer subsequently altered the solution to avoid the combination of the low pH and bisulfite solution that was the etiologic factor in chloroprocaine toxicity.

Spinal Microcatheters and High-Concentration Lidocaine Neurotoxicity

Another reported cause of prolonged neurologic deficits involves the use of microcatheters and large doses of 5% lidocaine in 7.5% dextrose for continuous spinal anesthesia. Several reports of cauda equina syndrome revealed the following elements common to these cases: (1) 5% lidocaine in 7.5% dextrose, with initial or total doses exceeding 100 mg, (2) unusually low or inadequate levels of anesthesia for a given amount of drug, and (3) use of a small-bore subarachnoid catheter.[117] In response to these reports, the Food and Drug Administration removed small-bore catheters for subarachnoid use from the U.S. market, pending further evaluation of their safety.[118] Significant controversy has followed this action.[119]

Skeletal Muscle Damage

Local anesthetics may cause damage to skeletal muscle. With bupivacaine in particular, intramuscular injections cause local skeletal muscle fiber reaction.[12] This damage is almost never associated with clinical symptoms, and muscle regeneration is complete within several weeks after the injection.

References

1. Wildsmith JAW: Peripheral nerve and local anaesthetic drugs. Br J Anaesth 1986; 58:692.
2. Taylor RE: Effect of procaine on electrical properties of squid axon membrane. Am J Physiol 1959; 196:1071.
3. Butterworth JF IV, Strichartz GR: Molecular mechanisms of local anesthesia: a review. Anesthesiology 1990; 72:711.
4. Gissen AJ, Covino BG, Gregus J: Differential sensitivity of fast and slow fibers in mammalian nerve fibers to local anesthetic drugs. Anesthesiology 1980; 53:467.
5. Gissen AJ, Covino BG, Gregus J: Differential sensitivity of fast and slow fibers in mammalian nerve. II. Anesth Analg 1982; 61:561.
6. Gissen AJ, Covino BG, Gregus J: Differential sensitivity of fast and slow fibers in mammalian nerve. III. Effects of etidocaine and bupivacaine on fast and slow fibers. Anesth Analg 1982; 61:570.
7. Fink BR: Mechanisms of differential axial blockade in epidural and subarachnoid anesthesia. Anesthesiology 1989; 70:851.
8. Raymond SA, Steffenson SC, Gugino LD, Strichartz GR. The role of length of nerve exposed to local anesthetics in impulse blocking action. Anesth Analg 1989; 68:563.
9. Marathe PH, Shen DD, Artru AA, et al: Effect of serum protein binding on the entry of lidocaine into brain and cerebrospinal fluid in dogs. Anesthesiology 1991; 75:804.
10. Tucker GT: Pharmacokinetics of local anesthetics. Br J Anaesth 1986; 58:717.
11. Albright GA: Cardiac arrest following regional anesthesia with etidocaine and bupivacaine. Anesthesiology 1979; 51:285.
12. Covino BG: Clinical pharmacology of local anesthetic agents. *In* Neural Blockade in Clinical Anesthesia and Management of Pain. 2nd ed. Cousins MG, Bridenbaugh PO (eds). Philadelphia, JB Lippincott, 1988, pp 111–144.
13. Courtney KR: Local anesthetics. Int Anesthesiol Clin 1988; 26:239.
14. Tucker GT, Mather LE: Properties, absorption, and disposition of local anesthetics. *In* Neural Blockade in Clinical Anesthesia and Management of Pain. 2nd ed. Cousins MG, Bridenbaugh PO (eds). Philadelphia, JB Lippincott, 1988, pp 47–110.
15. Foldes FF, Davidson GN, Duncalf D, et al: The intravenous toxicity of local anesthetic agents in man. Clin Pharmacol Ther 1965; 6:328.
16. Gross TL, Kuhnert PM, Kuhnert BR: Plasma levels of 2-chloroprocaine and lack of sequelae following an apparent intravenous injection. Anesthesiology 1981; 54:173.
17. Calvo R, Carlos R, Erill S: Effects of disease and acetazolamide on procaine hydrolysis by red cell enzymes. Clin Pharmacol Ther 1980; 27:175.
18. Blumer J, Strong JM, Atkinson AJ: The convulsant potency of lidocaine and its *N*-dealkylated metabolites. J Pharmacol Exp Ther 1973; 186:31.
19. Thompson P, Melmon KL, Richardson JA, et al: Lidocaine pharmacokinetics in advanced heart failure, liver disease, and renal failure in humans. Ann Intern Med 1973; 78:499.
20. Collinsworth KA, Strong JM, Atkinson AJ, et al: Pharmacokinetics and metabolism of lidocaine in patients with renal failure. Clin Pharmacol Ther 1975; 18:59.
21. Bax NDS, Tucker GT, Lennard MS, et al: The impairment of lignocaine clearance by propranolol—major contribution from enzyme inhibition. Br J Clin Pharmacol 1985; 19:597.
22. Tucker GT, Bax NDS, Lennard MS, et al: Effects of beta-adrenoreceptor antagonists on the pharmacokinetics of lignocaine. Br J Clin Pharmacol 1984; 17:21S.
23. Feely J, Wilkinson GR, McCallister CB, et al: Increased toxicity and reduced clearance of lidocaine by cimetidine. Ann Intern Med 1982; 96:592.
24. Webb TD, Ward DS: Elimination of lidocaine following regional block is inhibited by cimetidine. Anesthesiology 1983; 59:A213.
25. Feely J, Guy E: Lack of effect of ranitidine on the disposition of lignocaine. Br J Clin Pharmacol 1983; 15:378.
26. Harris WH: Choice of anesthetic agents for intravenous regional anesthesia. Acta Anaesthesiol Scand 1969; 36(Suppl):47.
27. Crawford OB: Comparative evaluation in peridural anesthesia of lidocaine, mepivacaine and L-67, a new local anesthetic agent. Anesthesiology 1964; 25:321.
28. Erdemir HA, Soper LE, Sweet RB: Studies of factors affecting peridural anesthesia. Anesth Analg 1965; 44:400.
29. Scott DB, McClure JH, Giasi RM, et al: Effects of concentration of local anesthetic drugs in extradural block. Br J Anaesth 1980; 52:1033.
30. Kennedy WF Jr, Bonica JJ, Ward RJ, et al: Cardiorespiratory effects of epinephrine when used in regional anesthesia. Acta Anaesthesiol Scand 1966; 23(Suppl):320.
31. Yaksh TL: Pharmacology of spinal adrenergic systems which modulate spinal nociceptive processing. Pharmacol Biochem Behav 1985; 22:845.
32. Concepcion M, Maddi R, Francis D, et al: Vasoconstrictors in spinal anesthesia with tetracaine. A comparison of epinephrine and phenylephrine. Anesth Analg 1984; 63:134.
33. Hickey R, Candido KD, Ramamurthy S, et al: Brachial plexus block with a new local anesthetic: 0.5 percent ropivacaine. Can J Anaesth 1990; 37:732.
34. Buckley FP, Littlewood DG, Covino BG, et al: Effects of adrenaline and the concentration of solution on extradural block with etidocaine. Br J Anaesth 1978; 50:171.
35. Kier L: Continuous epidural analgesia in prostatectomy: comparison of bupivacaine with and without adrenaline. Acta Anaesthesiol Scand 1974; 18:1.
36. Hickey R, Blanchard J, Hoffman J, et al: Plasma concentrations of ropivacaine given with or without epinephrine for brachial plexus block. Can J Anaesth 1990; 37:878.
37. Littlewood DG, Buckley P, Covino BG, et al: Comparative study of various local anesthetic solutions in extradural block in labor. Br J Anaesth 1979; 51:47.
38. Sinclair CJ, Scott DB. Comparison of bupivacaine and etidocaine in extradural blockade. Br J Anaesth 1984; 56:147.
39. Chambers WA, Littlewood DG, Scott DB: Spinal anesthesia with hyperbaric bupivacaine: effect of added vasoconstrictors. Anesth Analg 1982; 61:49.
40. Chambers WA, Littlewood DG, Logan MR, et al: Effect of added epinephrine on spinal anesthesia with lidocaine. Anesth Analg 1981; 60:417.
41. Concepcion M, Maddi R, Francis D, et al: Vasoconstrictors in spinal anesthesia with tetracaine. A comparison of epinephrine and phenylephrine. Anesth Analg 1984; 63:134.
42. Kozody R, Palahniuk RJ, Cumming MO: Spinal cord blood flow following subarachnoid tetracaine. Can Anaesth Soc J 1985; 32:23.
43. Cousins MJ, Bromage PR: Epidural neural blockade. *In* Neural Blockade in Clinical Anesthesia and Management of Pain. 2nd ed. Cousins MG, Bridenbaugh PO (eds). Philadelphia, JB Lippincott, 1988, pp 253–360.
44. McMorland GH, Douglas MJ, Jeffery WK, et al: Effect of pH adjustment of bupivacaine on onset and duration of epidural analgesia in parturients. Can Anaesth Soc J 1986; 33:537.
45. Benhamou D, Labaille T, Bonhomme L, et al: Alkalinization of epidural 0.5% bupivacaine for cesarean section. Reg Anaesth 1989; 14:240.
46. Stevens RA, Chester WL, Gruetter JA, et al: The effect of pH adjustment of 0.5% bupivacaine on the latency of epidural anesthesia. Reg Anaesth 1989; 14:236.
47. Hilgier M: Alkalinization of bupivacaine for brachial plexus block. Reg Anaesth 1985; 10:59.

48. Bedder MD, Kozody R, Craig DB. Comparison of bupivacaine and alkalinized bupivacaine in brachial plexus anesthesia. Anesth Analg 1988; 67:48.

49. Sweeney N, Denson D, Juneja MM, et al: The effect of pH on the onset and duration of epidural lidocaine in the parturient. Reg Anaesth 1989; 14:21.

50. Difazio CA, Carron H, Grosslight KR, et al: Comparison of pH adjusted lidocaine solutions for epidural anesthesia. Anesth Analg 1986; 65:760.

51. Galindo A: pH adjusted local anesthetics: clinical experience. Reg Anaesth 1983; 8:35.

52. Bromage PR: An evaluation of two new local anesthetics for major conduction blockade. Can Anaesth Soc J 1970; 17:557.

53. Bromage PR: A comparison of the hydrochloride and carbon dioxide salts of lidocaine and prilocaine in epidural analgesia. Acta Anaesthesiol Scand 1965; 16(Suppl):55.

54. Morrison DH: A double blind comparison of carbonated lidocaine and lidocaine hydrochloride in epidural anaesthesia. Can Anaesth Soc J 1981; 28:387.

55. Brown DT, Morrison DH, Covino BG, et al: Comparison of carbonated bupivacaine and bupivacaine hydrochloride for extradural anaesthesia. Br J Anaesth 1980; 52:419.

56. McClure JH, Scott DB. Comparison of bupivacaine hydrochloride and carbonated bupivacaine in brachial plexus block by the interscalene technique. Br J Anaesth 1981; 53:523.

57. Bridenbaugh LD: Does the addition of low molecular weight dextran prolong the duration of action of bupivacaine? Reg Anaesth 1978; 3:6.

58. Rosenblatt RM, Fung DL: Mechanism of action of dextran prolonging regional anaesthesia. Reg Anaesth 1980; 5:3.

59. Feitl ME, Krupin T: Neural blockade for ophthalmologic surgery. In Neural Blockade in Clinical Anesthesia and Management of Pain. 2nd ed. Cousins MG, Bridenbaugh PO (eds). Philadelphia, JB Lippincott, 1988, pp 577–592.

60. Bromage PR, Burfoot MF: Quality of epidural blockade. II. Influence of physio-chemical factors. Hyaluronidase and potassium. Br J Anaesth 1966; 38:857.

61. Cunningham NL, Kaplan JA: A rapid onset, long-acting regional anesthetic technique. Anesthesiology 1974; 41:509.

62. Cohen SE, Thurlow A: Comparison of a chloroprocaine-bupivacaine mixture with chloroprocaine and bupivacaine used individually for obstetric epidural analgesia. Anesthesiology 1979; 51:288.

63. Hodgkinson R, Husain FJ, Bluhm C. Reduced effectiveness of bupivacaine 0.5% to relieve labor pain after prior injection of chloroprocaine 2%. Anesthesiology 1982; 57:3A201.

64. Galindo A, Wichter T: Mixtures of local anesthetics bupivacaine-chloroprocaine. Anesth Analg 1980; 59:683.

65. Corke BC, Carlson LG, Dettbarn WD: The influence of 2-chloroprocaine on the subsequent analgesic potency of bupivacaine. Anesthesiology 1984; 60:25.

66. Seow LT, Lipps FJ, Cousins MJ, et al: Lidocaine and bupivacaine mixtures for epidural blockade. Anesthesiology 1982; 56:177.

67. Ravindran RS, Bond VK, Tasch MD, et al: Prolonged neural blockade following regional anesthesia with 2-chloroprocaine. Anesth Analg 1980; 58:447.

68. Moore DC, Spierdijk J, VanKleef JD, et al: Chloroprocaine neurotoxicity: four additional cases. Anesth Analg 1982; 61:155.

69. Gissen AJ, Datta S, Lambert D: The chloroprocaine controversy II. Is chloroprocaine neurotoxic? Reg Anaesth 1984; 9:135.

70. Fibuch EF, Opper SE: Back pain following epidurally administered Nesacaine-MPF. Anesth Analg 1989; 69:113.

71. Levy L, Randall GI, Pandit SK. Does chloroprocaine (Nesacaine MPF) for epidural anesthesia increase the incidence of backache? Anesthesiology 1989; 71:476.

72. Stevens RA, Chester WL, Artuso JD, et al: Back pain after epidural anesthesia with chloroprocaine in volunteers: preliminary report. Reg Anaesth 1991; 16:199.

73. Dikes WE: Treatment of Nesacaine-MPF induced back pain with calcium chloride. Anesth Analg 1990; 70:461.

74. van Steenberge A, DeBroux HC, Noorduin H: Extradural bupivacaine with sufentanil for vaginal delivery. A double blind trial. Br J Anaesth 1987; 59:1518.

75. Brown DL, Carpenter RL, Thompson GE: Comparison of 0.5% ropivacaine and 0.5% bupivacaine for epidural anesthesia in patients undergoing lower extremity surgery. Anesthesiology 1990; 72:633.

76. Hickey R, Hoffman J, Ramamurthy S: Comparison of ropivacaine 0.5% and bupivacaine 0.5% for brachial plexus block. Anesthesiology 1991; 74:639.

77. Ackerman B, Hellberg IB, Trassvik C: Primary evaluation of the local anesthetic properties of the amino amide agent ropivacaine (LEA 103). Acta Anaesthesiol Scand 1988; 32:571.

78. Moller R, Covino BG: Cardiac electro-physiologic properties of bupivacaine and lidocaine compared with those of ropivacaine, a new amide local anesthetic. Anesthesiology 1990; 72:322.

79. Feldman HS, Arthur GR, Covino BG: Comparative systemic toxicity of convulsant and supraconvulsant doses of intravenous ropivacaine, bupivacaine, and lidocaine in the conscious dog. Anesth Analg 1989; 69:794.

80. Nancarrow C, Rutlen AJ, Runciman WB, et al: Myocardial and cerebral drug concentrations and the mechanisms of death after fatal intravenous doses of lidocaine, bupivacaine, and ropivacaine in the sheep. Anesth Analg 1989; 69:276.

81. Scott DB, Lee A, Fagan D, et al: Acute toxicity of ropivacaine compared with that of bupivacaine. Anesth Analg 1989; 69:563.

82. Concepcion M, Arthur GR, Steele SM, et al: A new local anesthetic ropivacaine. Its epidural effects in humans. Anesth Analg 1990; 70:80.

83. Pederson H, Santos A, Morishima HA: Systemic toxicity of ropivicaine in pregnant and non-pregnant ewes. Anesthesiology 1988; 69:A344.

84. Covino BG, Vassallo HG: General pharmacological and toxicological aspects of local anesthetic agents. In Local Anesthetics: Mechanisms of Action and Clinical Use. New York, Grune & Stratton, 1976, pp 123–148.

85. Covino BG: Toxicity of local anesthetic agents. Acta Anaesthesiol Belg 1988; 39:159.

86. Courtney KR: Potentially toxic actions of local anesthetics in cardiac tissue. In Molecular and Cellular Mechanisms of Anesthetics. Roth SH, Miller KW (eds). New York, Plenum Medical Books, 1986, pp 377–384.

87. Reiz S, Nath S: Cardiotoxicity of local anesthetic agents. Br J Anaesth 1986; 58:736.

88. Feldman HS, Arthur RG, Covino BG: Toxicity of intravenously administered local anesthetic agents in the dog: cardiovascular and central nervous system effects. In Molecular and Cellular Mechanisms of Anesthetics. Roth SH, Miller KW (eds). New York, Plenum Medical Books, 1986, pp 395–404.

89. Kotelko DM, Shnider SM, Daily PA, et al: Bupivacaine induced cardiac arrhythmias in sheep. Anesthesiology 1984; 60:10.

90. Sage D, Feldman H, Arthur GR, et al: Cardiovascular effects of lidocaine and bupivacaine in the awake dog. Anesthesiology 1983; 59:A210.

91. Feldman HS, Arthur GR, Norway SB, et al: Cardiovascular effects of mepivacaine and etidocaine in the awake dog. Anesthesiology 1984; 61:A229.

92. Thigpen JW, Kotelko DM, Shnider SM, et al: Bupivacaine cardiotoxicity in hypoxic-acidotic sheep. Anesthesiology 1983; 59:A204.

93. Hondeghem LM, Clarkson CW: Modulated receptor theory and cardiac toxicity of local anesthetics. In Molecular and Cellular Mechanisms of Anesthetics. Roth SH, Miller SW (eds). New York, Plenum Medical Books, 1986, pp 385–393.

94. Morishima HO, Pederson H, Finster M, et al: Is bupivacaine more cardiotoxic than lidocaine? Anesthesiology 1983; 59:A409.

95. Morishima HO, Pederson H, Finster M, et al: Etidocaine toxicity in the adult, newborn and fetal sheep. Anesthesiology 1983; 58:342.

96. Scott DB: "Maximum recommended doses" of local anaesthetic drugs. Br J Anaesth 1989; 63:373.

97. Tucker GT, Moore DC, Bridenbaugh LD, et al: Systemic absorption of mepivacaine in commonly used regional block procedures. Anesthesiology 1972; 37:277.

98. Datta S, Lambert DH, Gregus J, et al: Differential sensitivities of mammalian nerve fibers during pregnancy. Anesth Analg 1983; 62:1070.

99. Flanagan HL, Datta S, Lambert DH, et al: Effects of pregnancy on bupivacaine-induced conduction blockade in the isolated rabbit vagus nerve. Anesth Analg 1987; 66:123.

100. Shnider SM, Levonson G: Anesthesia for cesarean section. In Anesthesia for Obstetrics. 2nd ed. Shnider SM, Levonson G (eds). Baltimore, Williams & Wilkins, 1987, pp 159–178.

101. Flanagan HL, Datta S, Moller RA, et al: Effect of exogenously administered progesterone on susceptibility of rabbit vagus nerves to bupivacaine. Anesthesiology 1988; 69:A676.

102. Morishima HO, Pederson H, Finster M, et al: Bupivacaine toxicity in pregnant and nonpregnant ewes. Anesthesiology 1985; 63:134.

103. Moller RA, Datta S, Fox J, et al: Effects of progesterone on the cardiac electrophysiologic action of bupivacaine and lidocaine. Anesthesiology 1992; 76:604.

104. Marathe PH, Shen DD, Artru AA, et al: Effect of serum protein binding on the entry of lidocaine into brain and cerebrospinal fluid in dogs. Anesthesiology 1991; 75:804.

105. Ross RA, Clarke JE, Armitage EN: Postoperative pain prevention by continuous epidural infusion. Anaesthesia 1980; 35:663.

106. Richter O, Glein K, Abel J, et al: The kinetics of bupivacaine (Carbostesin) plasma concentrations during epidural anesthesia following intraoperative bolus injection and subsequent infusion. Int J Clin Pharmacol Ther Toxicol 1984; 22:611.

107. Moore DC, Batra M: The components of an effective test dose prior to epidural block. Anesthesiology 1981; 55:693.

108. Mulroy MF: Epidural test doses. Anesthesiol Clin North Am 1992; 10:45.

109. Guinard JP, Mulroy MF, Carpenter RL, et al: Optimal epinephrine content with and without acute beta-adrenergic blockade. Anesthesiology 1990; 73:386.

110. Desparmet J, Mateo J, Ecoffey C, et al: Efficacy of an epidural test dose in children anesthetized with halothane. Anesthesiology 1988; 69:A774.

111. Leighton BL, Norris MC, Sosis M, et al: Limitations of epinephrine as a marker of intravascular injection in laboring women. Anesthesiology 1987; 66:688.

112. Thigpen JW, Kotelko DM, Shnider MS, et al: Bupivacaine cardiotoxicity in hypoxic-acidotic sheep. Anesthesiology 1983; 59:A204.

113. Kasten GW, Martin ST: Successful resuscitation after massive intravenous bupivacaine overdose in the hypoxic dog. Anesthesiology 1984; 61:A206.

114. deShazo RD, Nelson HS: An approach to patient with a history of local anesthetic hypersensitivity: experience with 90 patients. J Allergy Clin Immunol 1979; 63;387.

115. Glinert RJ, Zachary ZB: Local anesthetic allergy: its recognition and avoidance. J Dermatol Surg Oncol 1991; 17:491.

116. Schatz M: Drug allergy. *In* Allergic Diseases Diagnosis and Management. 3rd ed. Patterson R (ed). Philadelphia, JB Lippincott, 1985, pp 622–627.

117. Hurley RJ, Lambert D: Cauda equina syndrome after continuous spinal anesthesia. Anesth Analg 1991; 72:817.

118. Benson JS: FDA Safety Alert: Cauda equina syndrome associated with the use of small bore catheters in continuous spinal anesthesia. Rockville, MD, U.S. Food and Drug Administration, 1992.

119. Special Edition: FDA Safety Alert. ASRA News; July, 1992, pp 1–8.

CHAPTER **39**

Drug Interactions

MARK VEERMAN, Pharm.D.
SALVATORE R. GOODWIN, M.D.

In 1984, Levy[1] published a multicenter study on isoflurane that listed preoperative medications and included the smoking history of patients. Figure 39–1 shows the percentage of these patients receiving any of five classes of medications, the percentage of smokers, and the percentage of those that did not smoke or take any medications. Significantly, 45% of the patients were either smokers or were taking the listed medications, as well as other unlisted medications, prior to surgery. Considering that five or more drugs are commonly used during a typical anesthetic procedure, the potential for possible drug interactions, both desired and undesired, is significant.

Drug interactions can be beneficial or harmful. Although not all interactions must be avoided, the possible effects of combining drugs should be known by the anesthesiologist prior to surgery. This chapter asks questions that guide the reader into discussions of important drug interactions in three categories: drug compatibility, pharmacokinetic interactions, and pharmacodynamic interactions. The terms "pharmacokinetics" and "pharmacodynamics" refer to the effects of the body on drugs and the effects of drugs on the body, respec-tively. Questions apply not only to drug interactions during anesthesia but also those occurring during the perioperative period. Included in this chapter are expanded tables that list many of the potential drug interactions important to anesthesiologists.

DRUG COMPATIBILITY

The physical compatibility or, conversely, incompatibility of drugs often is not considered a drug interaction; in fact, incompatibility is quite significant and can lead to diminished response or an increase in adverse effects. Drug interactions of this type primarily involve the physical properties of injectable medications.

What Types of Incompatibilities Occur?

Drug incompatibilities are of two types. *Physical incompatibilities* result when a drug is no longer soluble. Visible examples include precipitation, haze, color change, and evolution of a gas from a drug. However, microcrystalline formation, which cannot be seen, can also occur; thus, the interaction is not observable. *Chemical inactivation* is the second form of incompatibility. This process results in chemical degradation of the active drug, prevents any pharmacologic response, and cannot be detected visually.[2-4] An example is physicochemical inactivation of gentamicin by complex formation with ticarcillin or carbenicillin.[5]

What Is the Major Cause of Physical Incompatibilities?

The solubility of many drugs is pH-dependent. Changes in pH that result from the addition of other drugs or the dilution of the drug in question can affect the drug's solubility.[3, 4] When injectable phenytoin (pH 12) is diluted with normal saline (pH 5 to 6), the resultant lowering of pH below 10 causes microcrystalline precipitation of the drug.[6]

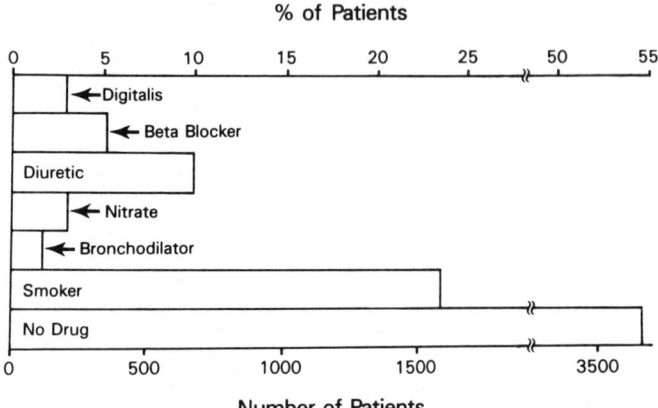

FIGURE 39–1. The incidence of preoperative medication with any of five classes of drugs, the percentage of smokers, and the percentage of those who did not smoke or take any medication. Almost half of the patients in this study were either smokers or took at least one of the listed medications. (From Levy WJ: Clinical anesthesia with isoflurane. Br J Anaesth 1984; 56:101s.)

Sodium thiopental has a pH of 10 to 11. The only intravenous solutions with which it should be mixed (according to manufacturer recommendations) are 5% dextrose in water (D_5W), normal saline, and sterile water for injection. When a 2.5% solution of sodium thiopental is added to lactated Ringer's solution, drug precipitation can result. This effect appears to be both concentration-dependent and time-dependent. When a sodium thiopental solution of greater concentration is mixed with lactated Ringer's solution, the rate of precipitation increases. The longer the sodium thiopental–lactated Ringer's solution is allowed to stand before use, the greater the probability that precipitation will occur.[7] Sodium thiopental also is incompatible with other medications, including morphine sulfate, fentanyl citrate, succinylcholine, atracurium, and vecuronium.

Most drugs are the salts of either a weak base and a strong acid or of a weak acid and a strong base. Examples of the former are morphine sulfate and midazolam hydrochloride, and those of the latter are sodium phenobarbital and sodium phenytoin. Midazolam hydrochloride has a solubility >22 mg · mL^{-1} of water at a pH of 2.8, whereas at a pH of 6.2, its solubility decreases to 0.24 mg · mL^{-1}. Thus, in a high-pH intravenous solution such as lactated Ringer's solution, it is both chemically and physically stable for only 4 hours at a concentration of 0.5 mg · mL^{-1}.[4, 8]

In contrast, injectable diazepam is even less soluble than midazolam, since diazepam is only available as a weak base rather than as a salt. Diazepam is soluble in propylene glycol but is only sparingly soluble in aqueous solutions. Thus, midazolam hydrochloride is the better of the two benzodiazepines to mix with intravenous solutions, since it is less likely to precipitate.

How Is the Anesthesiologist Alerted to Incompatibilities?

The package insert supplied by the manufacturer of a drug often contains information pertaining to intravenous solution compatibility. Most hospital pharmacies have several reference books that list drug compatibility information. We recommend the *Handbook of Injectable Drugs* by Lawrence Trissel[9] and *Guide to Parenteral Admixtures* by James C. King[10] as useful references for compatibility information. However, most of the information in these sources pertains to physical compatibility, not to chemical stability. The concentrations of drugs described in these references also may be different from those that are being used. Therefore, if one fails to observe the expected response, compatibility and stability problems are potential explanations.

When no compatibility information is available, comparing the salt types of the drugs to be combined may give some information on the compatibility. Drugs of the same salt type, such as morphine sulfate and midazolam hydrochloride (both of which are weak base and strong acid salts), are more likely to be compatible than are drugs of different salt types, such as morphine sulfate and sodium phenobarbital (which are strong base and weak acid salts). Infusion of drugs via the same catheter lumen or in solutions that may be incompatible should be avoided whenever possible. Figure 39–2 lists compatibility information for common medications used in the operating room, postanesthesia care unit, and intensive care unit.

How Can Incompatible Drugs Be Administered Concurrently?

Incompatible drugs can be given in the same intravenous infusion if, after the first drug is administered, the tubing is flushed with a compatible solution having a volume equal to twice the volume from the site of drug administration to the infusion site in the patient. Gauger and coworkers[11] determined that if a flush volume less than twice the tubing volume is used, residual amounts of the drug will remain in the tubing. Typical intravenous tubing extension sets with stopcocks have 3.5- to 4-mL volumes.

Can Intravenous Drug Incompatibilities Cause Harm to the Patient?

Intravenous mixtures that form a precipitate can cause venous irritation, embolism, and granuloma formation.[3] Notably, precipitation can also cause occlusion of the catheter or the infusion tubing, or both. This is especially likely with small-gauge catheters. Also, drugs that are chemically inactivated likely will not yield the desired pharmacologic response.[12] Thus, care should be taken not to infuse the precipitate into the patient. All anesthesiologists have observed the precipitate that forms when even a small amount of sodium thiopental comes into contact with either succinylcholine or atracurium. No observable untoward reactions have been reported as a consequence of these precipitates; however, it has been shown that thiopental-atracurium precipitates are prone to cause histamine release and may lead to serious systemic reactions as a result of aggregate anaphylaxis.[4]

PHARMACOKINETIC DRUG INTERACTIONS

Pharmacokinetic interactions are the effects of coadministered drugs on absorption, distribution, metabolism, and elimination. Figure 39–3 illustrates these interrelationships. Variations in these parameters may increase or decrease the pharmacologic response by changing the concentration of the active drug at the receptor site. Increased drug concentrations may also increase drug toxicities.[4, 13]

We emphasize that in most situations the potential for drug interactions does not preclude the use of the drug combinations. However, one should be aware of the possible interactions and be prepared to alter the dose and to respond appropriately should an undesirable response occur.

Table 39–1 highlights some of the clinically important pharmacokinetic drug interactions. Not all known drug interactions are listed, but many of those important to consider in the perioperative period are presented. Each interaction is coded to indicate its clinical significance, onset and severity of response, and documentation.

How Is Absorption Altered by Other Drugs?

Interactions that involve changes in the absorption characteristics of a drug are more of a potential problem for anesthe-

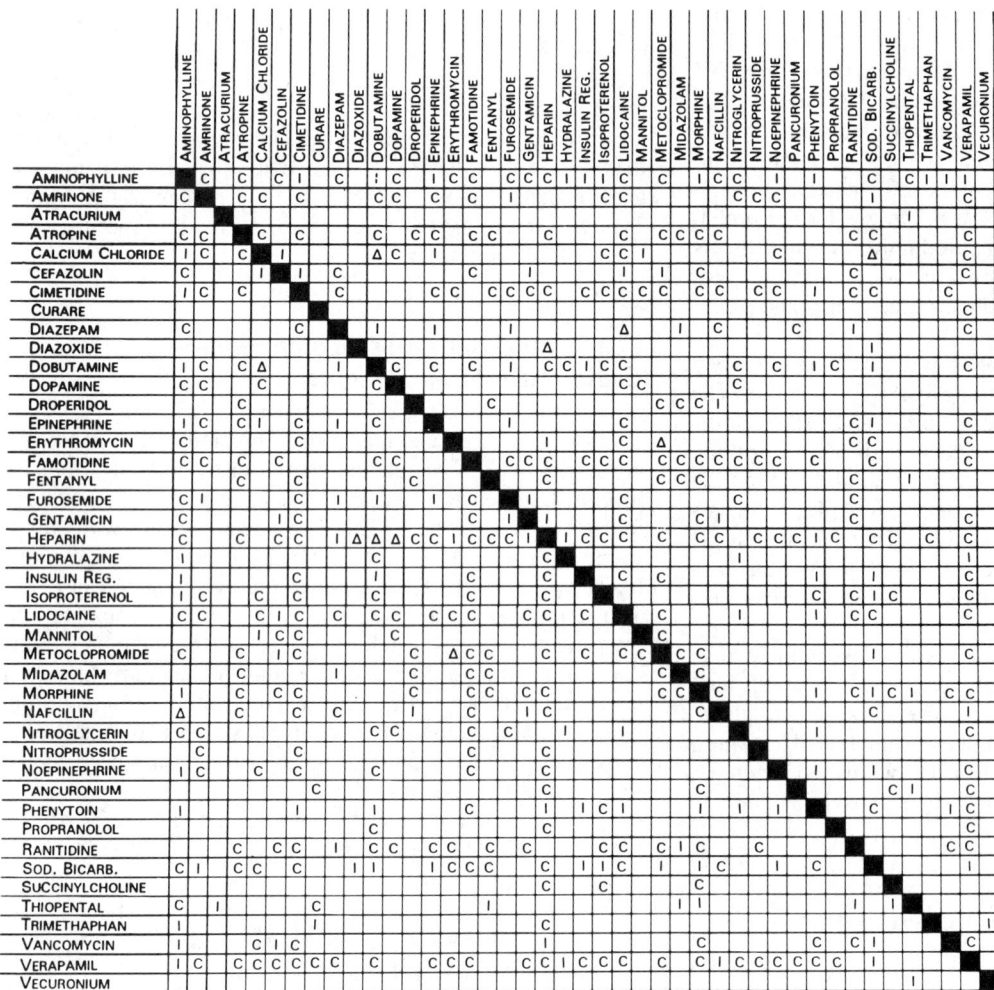

FIGURE 39–2. Drug compatibility chart.

DRUG INCOMPATIBILITY CHART
I = INCOMPATIBILITY
C = COMPATIBLE
Δ = CONCENTRATION DEPENDENT

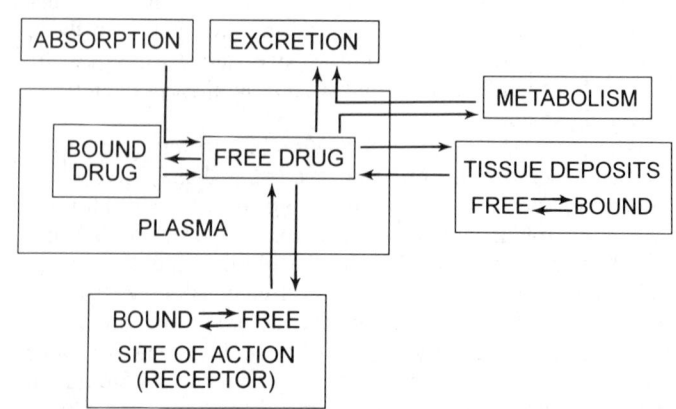

FIGURE 39–3. Schematic representation of drug disposition. (From Goodwin SR: Drugs and drug reactions. *In* Manual of Complications During Anesthesia. 1st ed. Gravenstein N (ed). Philadelphia, JB Lippincott, 1991, pp 479–508.)

siologists today than in the past, since more preoperative medications are given by the oral, intranasal, and rectal routes. The absorption of these drugs can be affected by the administration of other medications (sometimes this is done intentionally to achieve a desired response).

Enteral

Changes in absorption most commonly involve drugs administered via the gastrointestinal tract. An example is the combination of antacids with the oral antibiotics tetracycline or ciprofloxacin. Antacids significantly decrease absorption by forming complexes with these antibiotics.[13–15] Histamine$_2$ (H$_2$) blockers also may be more poorly absorbed when they are administered with antacids. However, their effectiveness does not appear to be affected significantly.

The absorption of orally administered cyclosporin can also be altered by several medications. Erythromycin increases the rate and extent of cyclosporin absorption in two ways: (1) it inhibits the cytochrome P$_{450}$-dependent metabolism of cyclosporin within the gastrointestinal mucosa; and (2) it decreases cyclosporin metabolism by the liver.[16]

Metoclopramide also can increase the rate of cyclosporin absorption in the small bowel, probably by accelerating the gastric emptying rate.[17] Conversely, phenytoin reduces the absorption of cyclosporin by ≤50%, possibly by increasing presystemic metabolism by the intestinal cytochrome P$_{450}$ enzymes.[18]

More common problems that concern the anesthesiologist involve the administration of topical, rectal, oral, and nasal medications prior to surgery. For example, when ranitidine or cimetidine is administered prior to giving a preoperative dose of oral midazolam, both the peak midazolam concentration and its bioavailability are increased, and the time to onset of action is decreased.[19]

Parenteral

Epinephrine

The addition of epinephrine to local anesthetics results in vasoconstriction, which delays drug absorption. Epinephrine, 1:200,000, decreases the plasma lidocaine concentration predictably (Fig. 39–4)[20] and thereby prolongs the block, de-

creases the peak lidocaine concentration, and allows higher doses of lidocaine to be used.

pH Adjustment of Local Anesthetics

The effect of pH adjustment of local anesthetics is complex. Local anesthetics cross biologic membranes more easily in their un-ionized form but are more active at the receptor in their ionized form. Since these anesthetics are weak bases, they are more likely to be ionized in an acidic milieu and un-ionized in a basic one. Thus, injection into an acid abscess limits transneural penetration and effectiveness. Carbonation also lowers pH and would seem to inhibit absorption. However, efficacy may be enhanced by other mechanisms. Carbon dioxide may have local anesthetic properties, its diffusion may reduce intracellular pH, and this gas may decrease pH and cause ion trapping intracellularly. Alkalinization of local anesthetics has also been shown to speed onset of action, although opinions regarding this practice and its efficacy have been mixed.

What Factors Alter Drug Distribution?

Distribution is a pharmacokinetic term that describes the process of drug movement from plasma to tissue spaces or binding sites. The distribution process is quantified by the volume of distribution (Vd) in liters per kilogram as expressed by the following formula:

$$Cp = Dose/Vd$$

.where Cp is the plasma concentration of the drug and Dose is the number of milligrams administered per kilogram. The greater the Vd, the lower the serum concentration for a given dose of a drug. The Vd may be greater or smaller than either the total body or plasma volume, depending on the drug's solubility and partition coefficient. Consider that sodium thiopental has a Vd of approximately 2.3 L · kg^{-1} (see Chapter 33).

Lipid and Water Solubility

Lipid-soluble drugs usually have a greater Vd than do water-soluble drugs. They also distribute more readily across the blood-brain barrier than do water-soluble drugs. Diazepam passes readily into the central nervous system (CNS), and this is followed by its rapid distribution out of the CNS into lipid tissues; it has an unbound Vd of about 1.33 L · kg^{-1}. This property leads to a rapid onset of action but also to a decreased duration of effect. The large Vd for diazepam compared with that of lorazepam is a result of its almost fourfold greater degree of lipophilicity.[20–25] Lorazepam, a more water-soluble benzodiazepine with an unbound Vd of only 12 L · kg^{-1}, penetrates less readily into the CNS but has a longer duration of effect.

Homer and Stanski[26] found that thiopental rapidly affects electroencephalographic recordings and has a mean pharmacodynamic half-life effect of 1.2 minutes. This observation indicates an almost immediate distribution of thiopental to

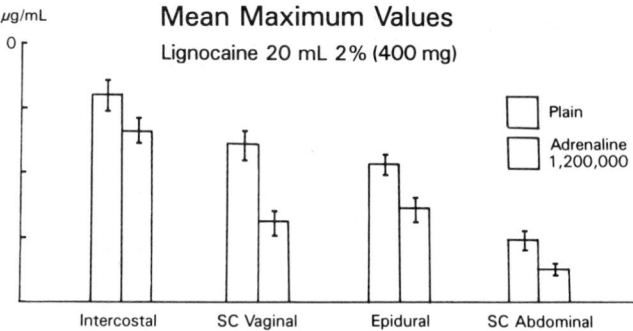

FIGURE 39–4. Plasma levels of lidocaine (= lignocaine) showing the effects of 1:200,000 epinephrine at four different injection sites: intercostal, subcutaneous vaginal, epidural, and subcutaneous abdominal. (From Scott DB, Jebson JR, Braid DP, et al: Factors affecting plasma levels of lignocaine and prilocaine. Br J Anaesth 1972; 44:1043.)

Text continued on page 648

TABLE 39–1. Pharmacokinetic Drug Interactions

Inhaled Anesthetics

Drug		Barbiturates	Rifampin	Isoniazid (INH)
Methoxyflurane	Significance:	Avoid		
	Onset:	<24 h		
	Effect:	Increase metabolism to nephrotoxic metabolites		
	Severity:	Moderate		
	Documentation:	Suspected		
Halothane	Significance:	Anticipate	Avoid	
	Onset:	>24 h	<24 h	
	Effect:	Increased metabolism to hepatotoxic metabolites in presence of hypoxia	Rifampin plus isoniazid with halothane anesthesia may lead to hepatotoxicity	
	Severity:	Major	Major	
	Documentation:	Possible	Possible	
Enflurane	Significance:			Avoid
	Onset:			<24 h
	Effect:			Hydrazine produced from the fast acetylation of INH facilitates the defluorination of enflurane, which may cause nephrotoxicity with prolonged exposure
	Severity:			Moderate
	Documentation:			Suspected
Isoflurane	Significance:			Be aware of
	Onset:			<24 h
	Effect:			Reported to increase fluoride concentration, but no adverse effects noted
	Documentation:			Suspected

Benzodiazepines (BZDs)

		Theophylline	Cimetidine	Oral Contraceptives	Ethanol	Omeprazole
Benzodiazepines (BZDs)	Significance:	Be aware of	Be aware of	Be aware of	Anticipate	Be aware of
	Onset:	<24 h	<24 h	>24 h	<24 h	>24 h
	Effect:	Sedative effect may be antagonized by theophylline, possibly through binding to intracerebral receptors	Inhibition of metabolism by cimetidine may increase BZD concentration, prolonging effect	Inhibition of BZD metabolism may prolong effect	Increased central nervous system effects from acute to chronic alcohol ingestion and decreased elimination secondary to impaired liver function	Decreased hepatic metabolism of BZD increases serum concentrations, prolonging effect
	Severity:	Minor	Minor	Minor	Minor	Minor
	Documentation:	Suspected	Probable	Suspected	Established	Suspected

Anticonvulsants

		Theophylline	Anticoagulants (Warfarin Dicumarol)	Barbiturates	Benzodiazepines (BZDs)	Carbamazepine (CBZ)	Cimetidine	Disulfiram	Fluconazole
Phenytoin	Significance:	Be aware of	Anticipate	Clinical changes unlikely	Clinical changes unlikely	Be aware of phenytoin effect on CBZ; clinical changes unlikely for CBZ effect on phenytoin	Anticipate	Anticipate	Be aware of
	Onset:	>24 h	>24 h	>24 h	>24 h	>24 h	>24 h	<24 h	>24 h
	Effect:	Increased metabolism of phenytoin by theophylline and vice versa, decreasing serum concentration of both	Increased phenytoin concentration and increased prothrombin times, with increased bleeding	Addition of barbiturates results in unpredictable phenytoin changes; seldom requiring changes, but phenytoin may increase phenobarbital concentration	Increase in phenytoin concentrations due to decreased metabolism	Decreased CBZ concentration from increased metabolism; variable changes of phenytoin concentration	Inhibits phenytoin metabolism, increasing phenytoin concentration	Inhibits phenytoin metabolism, increasing phenytoin concentration	May inhibit phenytoin metabolism, increasing phenytoin concentration
	Severity:	Moderate	Moderate	Minor	Minor	Moderate	Moderate	Moderate	Moderate
	Documentation:	Probable	Suspected	Possible	Possible	Suspected	Established	Established	Suspected

Nondepolarizing Muscle Relaxants (NDMRs)

Phenytoin

	Isoniazid (INH)	Omeprazole	Rifampin	Nondepolarizing Muscle Relaxants (NDMRs)
Significance:	Anticipate	Clinical changes unlikely	Anticipate	Anticipate
Onset:	>24 h	>24 h	>24 h	<24 h
Effect:	Inhibits hepatic metabolism of phenytoin; increases phenytoin concentrations	May inhibit phenytoin metabolism	Increases metabolism of phenytoin	Patients taking phenytoin increase NDMR metabolism, decreasing duration of muscle relaxant effects
Severity:	Moderate	Moderate	Moderate	Moderate
Documentation:	Established	Possible	Suspected	Suspected

Barbiturates (Pentobarbital Phenobarbital)

	Theophylline	β-Blockers (Propanol, Metoprolol only)	Carbamazepine (CBZ)	Valproic Acid	Cimetidine
Significance:	Be aware of	Anticipate	Be aware of	Anticipate	Clinical changes unlikely
Onset:	>24 h	<24 h	>24 h	>24 h	>24 h
Effect:	Barbiturates may increase theophylline metabolism, decreasing theophylline concentration	Barbiturates increase metabolism, possibly decreasing duration and effect	Barbiturates may enhance metabolism, decreasing CBZ concentrations	Inhibits barbiturate metabolism, increasing concentration	May inhibit metabolism of thiopental and phenobarbital, increasing serum concentrations of both
Severity:	Minor	Minor	Minor	Moderate	Minor
Documentation:	Suspected	Probable	Suspected	Established	Unlikely

Carbamazepine

	Cimetidine	Erythromycin	Barbiturates	Calcium Channel Blockers (Verapamil, Diltiazem)	Valproic Acid
Significance:	Anticipate	Anticipate	Be aware of	Anticipate	Anticipate
Onset:	>24 h	<24 h	>24 h	>24 h	>24 h
Effect:	Inhibits CBZ metabolism, increasing CBZ concentration	Inhibits CBZ metabolism, increasing CBZ concentration	May increase clearance of CBZ, decreasing CBZ concentration	May inhibit CBZ metabolism, increasing CBZ concentration	Both drugs may enhance metabolism of each other, decreasing serum concentrations of both
Severity:	Moderate	Moderate	Minor	Moderate	Moderate
Documentation:	Suspected	Established	Suspected	Suspected for verapamil; less likely for diltiazem	Suspected

Anticoagulants — Warfarin

	Amiodarone	Barbiturates	Cephalosporins (Cefoperazone, Cephamandole, Cefotetan, Moxalactam)	Cephalosporin (Cefazolin, Cefoxitin, Ceftriaxone)	Corticosteroids	Erythromycin	Cimetidine
Significance:	Avoid	Avoid	Avoid	Be aware of	Clinical changes unlikely	Anticipate	Avoid
Onset:	>24 h	>24 h	>24 h	>24 h	>24 h	>24 h	>24 h
Effect:	Inhibits metabolism, increasing anticoagulant effect	Increases the metabolism by induction, decreasing anticoagulant effect	Anticoagulant effects may increase due to warfarin-like activity of these cephalosporins	Increased anticoagulant effect by an unknown mechanism	Increase and decrease in coagulability have been reported	Increase anticoagulant effect of warfarin probably due to decreased warfarin metabolism	Increased anticoagulant effect due to inhibition of warfarin metabolism
Severity:	Major	Major	Major	Moderate	Minor	Major	Major
Documentation:	Established	Established	Suspected	Possible	Possible	Established	Established

Warfarin

	Furosemide	Metronidazole	Rifampin	Salicylates	Trimethoprim and Sulfamethoxazole (Bactrim, Septra)
Significance:	Clinical changes unlikely	Avoid	Anticipate	Avoid	Anticipate
Onset:	>24 h	>24 h	>24	>24 h	>24 h
Effect:	Possible displacement of protein-bound warfarin may occur	Increased anticoagulant effect due to decreased warfarin metabolism	Increases the metabolism of warfarin, decreasing its anticoagulant effect	Increases the anticoagulant effect of warfarin	Increased anticoagulant effect of warfarin due to decreased warfarin metabolism
Severity:	Moderate	Major	Moderate	Major	Major
Documentation:	Possible	Established	Established	Established	Established

Table continued on following page

TABLE 39–1. Pharmacokinetic Drug Interactions *Continued*

Drug	Interacting Drug	Significance	Onset	Effect	Severity	Documentation
Heparin	Cephalosporins (Parenteral)	Clinical changes unlikely	>24 h	Increased bleeding tendencies have been reported	Moderate	Possible
Heparin	Nitroglycerin (IV)	Clinical changes unlikely	<24 h	Decreased anticoagulation effects may occur	Moderate	Possible
Anti-infective Agents **Erythromycin**	Carbamazepine	(see under carbamazepine)				
Erythromycin	Warfarin	(see under warfarin)				
Erythromycin	Theophylline	Anticipate	<24 h	Decreases metabolism by inhibiting cytochrome P_{450} system	Major	Established
Erythromycin	Cyclosporin	Be aware of	>24 h	May inhibit the metabolism of cyclosporin	Moderate	Possible
Ciprofloxacin	Theophylline	Anticipate	>24 h	Inhibits the liver metabolism of theophylline by inhibition of cytochrome P_{450} system	Moderate	Probable
β-Blockers	Cimetidine	Anticipate	<24 h	Decreases first pass elimination of oral propranolol, increasing propranolol effects	Moderate	Probable
β-Blockers	Ranitidine	No interaction	>24 h	May have increased β-blocker effects	Minor	Unlikely
β-Blockers	Theophylline	Anticipate	<24 h	Propranolol may inhibit metabolism, increasing concentrations of theophylline	Moderate	Probable
β-Blockers **Metoprolol, Propranolol**	Hydralazine	Anticipate	>24 h	Serum concentration of propranolol is increased by decreasing first pass effect of orally administered propranolol	Moderate	Probable
Digoxin	Esmolol	Clinical changes unlikely	<24 h	Serum digoxin concentration may increase for unknown reasons	Moderate	Possible
Digoxin	Quinidine	Avoid	>24 h	Quinidine decreases both the volume of distribution and elimination, increasing digoxin concentrations	Major	Established
Digoxin	Verapamil	Avoid	<24 h	Decreases digoxin elimination, increasing concentrations	Major	Established
Digoxin	Acetylcholine Esterase Inhibitors (Captopril, Enalapril, Lisinopril)	Clinical changes unlikely	>24 h	Plasma concentrations of digoxin may be increased or decreased	Minor	Possible
Digoxin	Anticholinergics	Clinical changes unlikely	>24 h	Digoxin concentrations may increase owing to increased absorption of tablets	Moderate	Possible

Loop Diuretics (Furosemide, Bumetanide, Ethacrynic Acid)

Thiazide and Other Miscellaneous Diuretics (Chlorothiazide, Hydrochlorothiazide, Chlorothalidone, Metolazone, Acetazolamide)

Digoxin	Loop Diuretics	Thiazide and Other Miscellaneous Diuretics
Significance:	Anticipate	Anticipate
Onset:	>24 h	>24 h
Effect:	Increased potassium loss, potentially increasing the risk of digoxin toxicity	Increased potassium loss, potentially increasing the risk of digoxin toxicity
Severity:	Moderate	Moderate
Documentation:	Established	Established

Cyclosporine (CSA)	Barbiturates	Carbamazepine (CBZ)	Diltiazem	Erythromycin	Phenytoin	Ketoconazole	Ciprofloxacin (Quinolones)
Significance:	Clinical changes unlikely	Clinical changes unlikely	Anticipate	Anticipate	Anticipate	Anticipate	Clinical changes unlikely
Onset:	>24 h	>24 h	>24 h	>24 h	>24 h	>24 h	>24 h
Effect:	Induce hepatic enzymes, increasing clearance of CSA, decreasing CSA concentrations	Induces metabolism, decreasing CSA concentration	Inhibits metabolism, increasing CSA concentrations	Inhibits metabolism, increasing CSA concentration; erythromycin may also increase oral absorption of CSA	Decrease in CSA concentrations by either decreased elimination or metabolism, or both	Probably inhibits metabolism, increasing the CSA concentration	Some reports of increased concentrations caused by inhibition of cytochrome P_{450} system
Severity:	Moderate	Moderate	Moderate	Moderate	Major	Moderate	Minor
Documentation:	Possible	Possible	Established	Established	Probable	Probable	Possible

Succinylcholine	Echothiophate	Cyclophosphamide	Anticholinesterases (e.g., Edrophonium, Neostigmine)
Significance:	Anticipate	Anticipate	Anticipate
Onset:	<24 h	<24 h	<24 h
Effect:	Systemic absorption of echothiophate inhibits pseudocholinesterase, the enzyme responsible for metabolizing succinylcholine	Inhibits plasma pseudocholinesterase, the enzyme responsible for metabolizing succinylcholine	Inhibits pseudocholinesterase, increasing the duration of neuromuscular blockade
Severity:	Moderate	Moderate	Moderate
Documentation:	Established	Probable	Probable

Succinylcholine	Metoclopramide	Quinidine, Quinine
Significance:	Anticipate	Anticipate
Onset:	<24 h	<24 h
Effect:	Metoclopramide may inhibit plasma cholinesterase, prolonging neuromuscular blockade	Neuromuscular blockade may be prolonged secondary to decreases in plasma cholinesterase activity
Severity:	Anticipate	Avoid
Documentation:	Suspected	Suspected

brain tissue by rapid perfusion and partitioning from the blood. In fact, the distribution of thiopental to brain tissue is so rapid that it cannot be effectively measured pharmacokinetically; therefore, it can be considered to be instantaneous following administration. The redistribution of thiopental from brain tissue to muscle and fat is also rapid and is nearly complete after about 10 minutes.

Protein Binding

Plasma protein binding also represents a site of drug distribution. Changes in plasma protein binding can increase or decrease the unbound portion of the drug. The unbound or "free" drug is the active portion that is capable of diffusing across membranes and interacting with receptor sites.[3, 27, 28] Table 39–2 lists factors that influence drug plasma and tissue distribution.

Certain characteristics are necessary for an interaction to be of practical importance. The drug should be highly protein bound (>85%), have a narrow therapeutic range, and have a small Vd.[28] A good example is phenytoin, which is 90% bound to albumin, has a narrow therapeutic range (10–20 $\mu g \cdot L^{-1}$), and has a Vd of 0.7 $L \cdot kg^{-1}$.[29]

Albumin

Albumin constitutes 60% of the plasma proteins and is capable of binding drugs of different charges. Hypoalbuminemia is associated with burns, cancer, inflammatory diseases, liver disease, malnutrition, nephrotic syndrome, renal disease, premature and term infant birth, and extensive intra-abdominal surgery.[30]

Thiopental and phenytoin are usually at least 90% albumin-bound. The percentage of unbound or free phenytoin is higher than normal in patients with renal failure and hypoalbuminemia and in patients receiving drugs such as valproic acid, which displaces phenytoin from albumin. If the phenytoin concentration (unbound and protein-bound) remains constant, a higher unbound percentage results in an increase in effects just as if the total serum phenytoin concentration were elevated in a patient with normal protein binding or albumin stores.

Patients suspected of having a higher percentage of unbound phenytoin should have their serum unbound phenytoin levels monitored to determine whether they are in the therapeutic range of 1 to 2 $\mu g \cdot mL^{-1}$.[29] In the case of thiopental administration, it is wise to start with a reduced dose.

α_1-Acid Glycoprotein

The α_1-acid glycoprotein is an acute-phase reactant that increases in concentration in response to stresses such as trauma, inflammation, and acute myocardial infarction.[28, 30] Drugs that may have a decreased effect in response to an increase in α_1-acid glycoprotein include bupivacaine, lidocaine, meperidine, methadone, and propranolol. Phenytoin, quinidine, and meperidine displace bupivacaine in vitro; this increases its unbound fraction three- to fivefold. This effect may increase the toxicity of systemically absorbed bupivacaine from epidural administration, and possibly that of other local anesthetics, if the same interaction occurs in vivo.[31, 32]

TABLE 39–2. Physiologic Determinants of Drug Partition or Distribution Ratios Between Tissues and Plasma

Active transport
Donnon ion effect
pH difference
Plasma protein binding
Tissue binding
Lipid partitioning

(Reprinted by permission from Applied Pharmacokinetics: Principles of Therapeutic Drug Monitoring, third edition, edited by William E. Evans, Jerome J. Schentag, and William J. Jusko, published by Applied Therapeutics, Inc., Vancouver, Washington, © 1992.)

Can Other Medications Affect the Elimination of Anesthetic Agents?

Narcotic agents depress alveolar ventilation; this leads to delayed excretion of inhaled anesthetics and prolongs their effects in spontaneously breathing patients.[27] Probenecid can increase the duration of thiopental-induced anesthesia. Kaukinen and colleagues examined the effects of pretreatment with 0.5 to 1 g of probenecid on thiopental-induced anesthesia (4–7 mg $\cdot$ kg^{-1}).[33] The duration of the loss of the eyelid reflex increased by ≤109%.

The mechanism by which probenicid prolongs thiopental anesthesia may be related to increased penetration to the sites of action in the brain or to displacement of thiopental from plasma proteins. Thus, reduced doses of thiopental may be indicated for patients receiving this drug.[33, 34]

What Are the Effects of Drug Metabolism?

Metabolism is primarily a function of the liver, which biotransforms drugs to more readily excretable metabolites through a series of chemical reactions. Phase I reactions involve oxidation, reduction, or hydrolysis to a more polar compound. Further metabolism by conjugation, a phase II reaction, results in a more highly polar metabolite that can be excreted by the kidneys.

Metabolites generally have decreased or absent pharmacologic activity. However, some drugs, such as chloral hydrate, are transformed to an active metabolite. Also, although metabolized drug forms are generally less toxic than unmetabolized forms, in certain circumstances some drugs become more toxic, such as acetaminophen taken in overdose.[35]

Drug metabolism occurs within the hepatocyte. Cytochrome P$_{450}$ and NADPH (nicotinamide-adenine dinucleotide phosphate [reduced form]) cytochrome P$_{450}$ reductase are the responsible enzyme systems. Their induction or inhibition is affected by genetic factors, age, hormones, disease, nutrition, stress, and exogenous chemicals. Drugs initially metabolized by the body are more variably eliminated than are those excreted unchanged in the urine. Therefore, the effect of hepatic enzyme induction or inhibition on drug interactions varies considerably.[27, 35, 36] Table 39–1 lists drug interactions that result from changes in metabolism.

Volatile Anesthetics and Enzyme Induction
Halothane Hepatitis

Enzyme induction may play a role in halothane-induced hepatitis. Models in which animals were given hypoxic gas mixtures with halothane after phenobarbital pretreatment have caused liver injury. The proposed mechanism is a change from the normal oxidative pathway to a reductive pathway for halothane metabolism.[27, 37, 38] Although the exact mechanism is still a subject of controversy, the following factors seem to be required: drug-related enzyme induction; poor nutritional status; halothane anesthesia; reduced hepatic oxygenation associated with an anesthetic-related decrease in splanchnic blood flow; and a reduced concentration of oxygen during abdominal surgery.[27, 39]

Methoxyflurane Nephrotoxicity

Methoxyflurane metabolism yields a free fluoride ion that is nephrotoxic when present in sufficient concentrations. Patients taking phenobarbital may have enhanced metabolism of methoxyflurane, which increases the formation of fluoride ions to potentially toxic concentrations.[27, 40] Enflurane metabolism also releases fluoride ions but probably only results in increased nephrotoxicity after prolonged exposure in obese patients or in patients taking isoniazid who also acetylate rapidly. Enflurane metabolism and free fluoride ion release is not enhanced by other enzyme-inducing drugs such as phenobarbital.[41]

Drug Class Similarities and Differences

Often, the members of a given drug class alter metabolism similarly, but notable exceptions do occur.[42] The H_2 blockers cimetidine, famotidine, and ranitidine are available in the United States. Cimetidine is a consistent inhibitor of the cytochrome P_{450} system and can lead to increased concentrations of other drugs that are dependent on this system for metabolism.[43] These drugs include theophylline, cyclosporin, phenytoin, carbamazepine, and warfarin.

In a study comparing the inhibition of theophylline elimination, Powell and colleagues found that cimetidine, but not ranitidine, statistically decreased mean theophylline clearance.[43] Ranitidine inhibited theophylline metabolism in some subjects, but the magnitude of this effect was not as great as with cimetidine. Famotidine, the newest of the H_2 blockers, appears to be relatively free of effects on the cytochrome P_{450} system.[44] Since efficacy among the H_2 blockers is thought to be equivalent, famotidine may have some advantages in patients who are taking other medications subject to inhibition.[45, 46]

Time to Onset of Induction or Inhibition

The metabolic induction of drugs is most likely due to increased synthesis of cytochrome P_{450} system enzymes.[43, 47, 48] Studies of warfarin have demonstrated that phenobarbital and rifampin induction can be detected within 6 to 7 days and within 2 days, respectively. The maximum effect is seen at 14 to 21 days with phenobarbital and at 4 days with rifampin. Upon discontinuation of the inducing drug, the same time course is followed to the return of normal status.[49, 50]

Competitive and Noncompetitive Inhibition

Drug inhibition can be competitive or noncompetitive. In competitive inhibition, the inhibitor is an alternate substrate for the metabolizing enzyme, whereas in noncompetitive inhibition, the drug inactivates the enzyme. Most drugs that inhibit drug metabolism do so by inhibiting the cytochrome P_{450} system. Drug inhibitors that act directly on enzyme synthesis generally have a rapid onset of inhibition. Cimetidine reversibly binds to cytochrome P_{450} enzymes in a competitive or noncompetitive manner. It inhibits drug metabolism within 24 hours after administration of a single dose. As a general rule, inhibitory drugs exert their effect within a short period of time compared with those drugs that induce liver microsomal enzymes.[35]

Practical Considerations

An anesthesiologist must know when a drug treatment was begun (or discontinued) to know whether it will affect his or her ministrations. If a drug capable of changing liver metabolism is administered for several weeks before anesthesia, its effect can be seen during anesthesia. Dosage requirements of those drugs metabolized by the liver may change, depending on whether an inhibitor or inducer is used. Erythromycin inhibits cytochrome P_{450} microsomal enzymes and augments the action of drugs that undergo similar metabolism. Prolonged respiratory depression has been demonstrated with alfentanil in patients who have received erythromycin.[51]

Drug inducers given simultaneously with anesthetics such as sodium thiopental have no lasting effects unless they are continued for extended periods of time. In contrast, if cimetidine is given preoperatively, it can decrease the metabolism of drugs that were given several hours later, resulting in an exaggerated or prolonged response.

Echothiophate (phospholine iodide) is an organophosphate anticholinesterase that is used for the treatment of glaucoma. It is capable of depleting plasma pseudocholinesterase. Despite extraocular administration, sufficient amounts of echothiophate may be absorbed systemically, preventing succinylcholine metabolism by pseudocholinesterase. Glaucoma patients are thus at risk for prolonged neuromuscular blockade from succinylcholine. Discontinuation of echothiophate several weeks before surgery would be necessary to allow pseudocholinesterase activity to return to normal.[52, 53]

How Are Drugs Eliminated?

Drug elimination is primarily by renal excretion, but it can also proceed through the biliary and respiratory systems. Remarkably, few drugs interact to alter the elimination of other drugs. Diuretic administration can enhance the elimination of other renally excreted medications but can also impede elimination. Drugs that bind bile salts (cholestyramine) can enhance the elimination of those agents that undergo reabsorption via the enterohepatic circulation. Examples of such drugs include digoxin, thyroid compounds, and propranolol.

Diuretics and Lithium Excretion

Lithium elimination by renal excretion is decreased by diuretic therapy. The result is increased serum lithium concentrations. This interaction can occur perioperatively and requires careful monitoring of serum lithium concentrations.[54, 55]

PHARMACODYNAMIC INTERACTIONS

The changes in the effect of a drug brought on by concurrent use of another drug or drugs represents a pharmacodynamic interaction. Changes in drug responsiveness or an adverse effect may result. Pharmacodynamic interactions may be additive, synergistic, potentiating, or antagonistic. A purist might argue justifiably that additive drug interactions are not interactions; however, they are included for completeness (Table 39–3).

Pharmacodynamic drug interactions often prove important during anesthesia. Since many anesthetics have narrow therapeutic ranges, combining drugs produces an additive or synergistic response. The same desired pharmacologic effect results but with lesser risk to the patient. This goal is accomplished by decreasing the individual side effects of each agent. Obviously, certain combinations of agents can result in an increase in adverse effects.

Pharmacodynamic interactions can be grouped into drug categories or classes. Table 39–4 lists many of the classes that are important in the operating room and intensive care environments. The remainder of this chapter addresses some of the important aspects of these drug interactions.

How Are Inhalation Anesthetics Involved?

The combination of inhaled anesthetic agents with other medications is frequently used in balanced anesthesia techniques. Pharmacodynamic interactions between inhaled anesthetic agents and other CNS depressants usually decrease the minimum alveolar concentration (MAC) of the inhaled agents. Sometimes, however, they lead to antagonism of the inhaled anesthetic.[38]

Nitrous Oxide

The combination of nitrous oxide and a potent volatile agent results in an additive drug interaction. If nitrous oxide is delivered at 50% MAC, a 50% reduction in the MAC of the inhalation agent is to be expected. Furthermore, since the initial uptake of nitrous oxide is extremely rapid, the alveolar concentration of a coadministered volatile anesthetic is increased by the loss of alveolar gas volume. This phenomenon is known as the *second gas effect*[56, 57] and results in increased speed of induction. Discontinuation of nitrous oxide and its rapid elimination reverse this process, increasing minute ventilation and elimination of the inhaled volatile agent.

The addition of nitrous oxide decreases respiratory depression to a lesser degree than would be expected from higher concentrations of the volatile anesthetic alone. It also decreases cardiovascular depression. Bahlman studied the effects

TABLE 39–3. Mathematic Examples of Additive, Synergistic, Potentiating, and Antagonistic Interactions

Additive	$2 + 2 = 4$
Synergistic	$2 + 2 > 4$
Potentiation	$0 + 2 > 2$
Antagonism	$2 + 2 < 4$

of 1.2 and 2.4 MAC equivalents of halothane–oxygen compared with those of halothane–nitrous oxide.[58] Depression of cardiac output, mean arterial pressure, and ventricular work was greater with halothane alone than with halothane combined with nitrous oxide. The lesser degree of cardiovascular depression at the same MAC level when nitrous oxide is added makes this an appealing drug combination.

What Are the Effects of Antipsychotic Medications?

Antipsychotic medications include phenothiazines, thioxanthines, and butyrophenones. They are used for the treatment of a variety of problems, including schizophrenia and psychoses associated with organic brain syndromes. The antipsychotic mechanism of action of these drugs includes blocking of dopaminergic receptors within the CNS and other effects, some of which may be adverse. Table 39–5 lists the relative differences in sedative, cardiovascular, and extrapyramidal side effects of the various agents. Patients taking antipsychotics at the time of surgery may have exaggerated respiratory depression, sedation, and analgesia.[58, 59]

Alpha-adrenergic blockade caused by many antipsychotic agents is commonly associated with orthostatic hypotension.[60] This action theoretically can attenuate the pressor effects of norepinephrine and epinephrine or even lead to unopposed β-effects with subsequent hypotension, as demonstrated in dogs receiving epinephrine (0.005 mg · kg^{-1}) and chlorpromazine.[61] Additionally, dopaminergic blockade by phenothiazine and butyrophenones may decrease the vasopressor effect of dopamine infusions.[62]

Enflurane and isoflurane administration with chlorpromazine has resulted in hypotension that is disproportionate to that which might have been expected from the administration of each drug separately.[63] Should hypotension occur with any of the halogenated anesthetic and antipsychotic agents, treatment with sympathetic amines that possess α-adrenergic activity (norepinephrine, phenylephrine) or with fluids is recommended.[4]

What Problems May Be Associated with Antidepressants?

Tricyclic Agents

The tricyclic antidepressants are thought to work by increasing CNS concentrations of serotonin or norepinephrine, or both, through blockade of their reuptake in presynaptic nerve terminals.[64] Chronic use (i.e., >10–20 days) leads to significant receptor changes. Down-regulation of presynaptic α_2-adrenergic receptors occurs; this increases the release of norepinephrine from storage vesicles. Increased neuronal responsiveness of postsynaptic α_1-adrenergic receptors also occurs, as does increased sensitivity of the postsynaptic receptors to serotonin. The number of β-adrenergic binding sites and CNS responsiveness to β-adrenergic agonists are either reduced or down-regulated.[59] The overall result is that the β-receptors have increased sensitivity to drugs that stimulate postsynaptic α_1-receptors (e.g., ephedrine, epinephrine, and norepinephrine).

Tricyclic antidepressants also possess anticholinergic activity, which, along with the increase in adrenergic tone that they produce, can cause problems during anesthesia. Patients who are taking tricyclic antidepressants may be at greater risk for developing cardiac dysrhythmias. Edwards and associates found that dogs that received chronic imipramine therapy manifested a higher frequency of cardiac dysrhythmias during halothane anesthesia after they had received pancuronium.[65] They recommended the avoidance of pancuronium in patients who are treated with chronic tricyclic antidepressants and are anesthetized with halothane. Enflurane did not provoke cardiac dysrhythmias under the same conditions in this animal study.

Sympathomimetics (especially indirect acting agents) may result, at worst, in an exaggerated or, at best, unpredictable response from increased norepinephrine at the receptor site.[66, 67] Other potential problems in patients receiving tricyclic antidepressants include potentiation of opioid analgesics, decreased seizure threshold, and increased barbiturate sedative and depressant effects.[61, 68]

Newer Antidepressants

Newer antidepressant medications include amoxapine, maprotiline, fluoxetine (Prozac), and trazodone. The mechanisms of action of amoxapine and maprotiline are similar to those of the tricyclic antidepressants, with the exception that maprotiline does not block reuptake of serotonin.[7] Because of similar actions of amoxapine and maprotiline, anesthetic concerns for patients taking these drugs are the same as those for patients taking tricyclic agents. To date, however, no interactions have been reported. Amoxapine does not have as many cardiovascular side effects as does maprotiline. Maprotiline has significant adverse side effects in overdose situations. Maprotiline can also lower seizure threshold, which is a consideration in patients receiving enflurane or ketamine anesthetics.

Trazodone does not affect the reuptake of norepinephrine or dopamine and is thought to have a more benign effect than do the tricyclics.[69] No interactions with anesthetic agents have been reported. Fluoxetine primarily inhibits the reuptake of serotonin in the CNS and has little effect on other neurotransmitters. It does not have significant cardiotoxicity. The only major drug interaction that may affect the anesthetized patient is inhibition of diazepam metabolism. This possibility necessitates a reduction in diazepam dosage.[7]

Should Antidepressant Administration Be Discontinued Prior to Anesthesia?

No answer to this question is universally accepted. We feel that antidepressant use should be discontinued 72 hours before elective surgeries in nonsuicidal patients. In emergency situations or in suicidal patients, the anesthesiologist should be aware of the potential interactions and treat the patient accordingly (i.e., avoid halothane and pancuronium and, if a vasopressor is required, use titrated phenylephrine rather than ephedrine).

Does Lithium Administration Alter Neuromuscular Blockade?

Several case reports published in the 1970s suggested prolonged neuromuscular blockade followed the use of pancuro-

nium and succinylcholine in lithium-treated patients.[70, 71] A follow-up study conducted in lithium-treated dogs showed prolonged neuromuscular blockade with succinylcholine, decamethonium, and pancuronium but not with gallamine or d-tubocurarine. Therapeutic lithium concentrations in the guinea pig model showed no significant effect of pancuronium.[72] In a retrospective review of 17 lithium-treated patients who had received succinylcholine before electroconvulsive therapy, prolonged recovery from succinylcholine did not occur.[73]

Although the information is conflicting, therapeutic concentrations of lithium do not appear to prolong neuromuscular blockade significantly.

Should Monoamine Oxidase Inhibitors Be Discontinued Prior to Surgery?

Four monoamine oxidase inhibitors are available in the United States (Table 39–6). They are used as antidepressants because they inhibit oxidative deamination of the naturally occurring monoamines serotonin, dopamine, tyramine, norepinephrine, and epinephrine. The resultant catecholamine accumulation at the receptor site produces increased sympathetic stimulation.[3, 27] Sympathomimetics administered to patients taking monoamine oxidase inhibitors may cause the release and persistence of excessive amounts of neurotransmitters, resulting in cardiovascular instability, tachycardia, hypertensive crisis, severe headache, and hyperpyrexia.[74]

Meperidine is uniquely contraindicated in patients receiving monoamine oxidase inhibitors. Severe reactions, including hypertension, hypotension, sweating, coma, apnea, and even death, have occurred following its use. Other drugs that should be avoided in monoamine oxidase inhibitor–treated patients include phenothiazines, other antidepressants, and tyramine-containing food and cheese products.[27, 61]

Monoamine oxidase inhibitors fall into either the hydrazine or nonhydrazine class (see Table 39–6). This is of consequence, since the nonhydrazine compounds are considered to be reversible blockers devoid of pharmacologic effect 24 hours after discontinuation. The hydrazine compounds, however, bind to the enzyme irreversibly; thus, the recommendation is to discontinue therapy at least 2 weeks prior to elective surgery.[75] If this is not possible or if hemodynamic instability occurs despite drug discontinuation according to the recommended protocol, labetalol or sodium nitroprusside are recommended for hypertension, and fluid or titrated quantities of direct-acting vasopressor (phenylephrine), or both, are suggested for treatment of hypertension.

Should Antihypertensive Agents Be Discontinued Prior to Surgery?

The extensive number of antihypertensives on the market today present the anesthesiologist with many potential drug interactions. Understanding the interactions of these agents can affect the choice of anesthetic drugs.

Discontinuation of antihypertensive agents may lead to rebound hypertension from withdrawal. Unless specific circumstances dictate otherwise, antihypertensive therapy should not be discontinued before surgery.[71, 72]

Text continued on page 656

TABLE 39-4. Pharmacodynamic Interactions

Barbiturate Anesthetics (Thiopental, Methohexital, Thiamylal)	Benzodiazepines	Narcotic Analgesics (e.g., Alfentanil, Morphine, Pentazocine)	Phenothiazines (e.g., Chlorpromazine, Promethazine)
Significance:	Anticipate	Anticipate	Be aware of
Onset:	<24 h	<24 h	<24 h
Effect:	Synergistic central nervous system effects	Narcotic analgesics reduce the anesthetic dose of thiopental	Phenothiazines may increase frequency of neuromuscular excitation and hypotension with barbiturate analgesia
Severity:	Moderate	Moderate	Minor
Documentation:	Established	Suspected	Suspected

Ketamine	Theophylline	Halothane
Significance:	Be aware of	
Onset:	<24 h	
Effect:	Increased extensor-type seizures have occurred when patients taking theophylline received ketamine	Hypotension and decreased cardiac output can occur when ketamine and halothane are given together. Also reduces minimum alveolar concentration (MAC) of halothane.
Severity:	Moderate	Moderate
Documentation:	Possible	Established

Nondepolarizing Muscle Relaxants (NDMRs)	Trimethaphan	Verapamil	Lithium
Significance:	Anticipate	Anticipate	Clinical changes unlikely
Onset:	<24 h	<24 h	<24h
Effect:	Trimethaphan can prolong the neuromuscular blockade of NDMRs	Verapamil may prolong the neuromuscular blockade of NDMRs	Patients taking lithium may have prolonged effect from NDMRs
Severity:	Moderate	Moderate	Moderate
Documentation:	Suspected	Suspected	Possible

Nondepolarizing Muscle Relaxants (NDMRs)	Aminoglycosides	Benzodiazepines (BZDs)	β-Blockers	Carbamazepine (CBZ)	Clindamycin
Significance:	Anticipate	Clinical changes unlikely	Clinical changes unlikely	Anticipate	Be aware of
Onset:	<24 h	<24 h	<24 h	<24 h	<24 h
Effect:	Have synergistic effects on neuromuscular blockade	May have a variable effect on neuromuscular blockade	Variable effect by β-blockers on neuromuscular blockade	May cause shorter duration of action of neuromuscular blockade by nondepolarizing muscle relaxants	Potentiates neuromuscular blockade of NDMRs probably by inhibiting acetylcholine release
Severity:	Major	Moderate	Moderate	Moderate	Moderate
Documentation:	Established	Possible	Established	Suspected	Suspected

Nondepolarizing Muscle Relaxants (NDMRs)	Inhalation Anesthetics	Phenytoin	Ketamine	Magnesium Sulfate (Parenteral)	Polypeptide Antibiotics (Bacitracin, Polymyxin B, Vancomycin)
Significance:	Anticipate	Be aware of	Anticipate	Anticipate	Anticipate
Onset:	<24 h	<24 h	<24 h	<24 h	<24 h
Effect:	Potentiate the neuromuscular blockade of NDMRs	Neuromuscular blockade may be shortened in patients receiving phenytoin	Potentiates the neuromuscular blockade	Can potentiate the neuromuscular blockade	Enhance neuromuscular blockade by affecting presynaptic and postsynaptic blockade
Severity:	Major	Moderate	Moderate	Moderate	Moderate
Documentation:	Established	Suspected	Probable	Suspected	Probable

Nondepolarizing Muscle Relaxants (NDMRs)

	Quinidine, Quinine	Theophylline	Azathioprine
Significance:	Anticipate	Be aware of	Be aware of
Onset:	<24 h	<24 h	<24 h
Effect:	May enhance neuromuscular blockade of NDMRs	May antagonize the neuromuscular blockade	May inhibit phosphodiesterase at the nerve terminal and, increase cAMP, thereby antagonizing the neuromuscular blockade
Severity:	Moderate	Moderate	Moderate
Documentation:	Suspected	Suspected	Suspected

Succinylcholine

	Aminoglycosides	Cimetidine	Lithium	Ketamine	Lidocaine	Azathioprine
Significance:	Anticipate	Anticipate	Clinical changes unlikely	Be aware of	Anticipate	
Onset:	<24 h	<24 h	Established	Established	Established	
Effect:	Can be additive or synergistic neuromuscular block with succinylcholine	May potentiate the neuromuscular blocking effects of succinylcholine by inhibiting metabolism of succinylcholine	May potentiate neuromuscular blocking effects of succinylcholine	May prolong the neuromuscular block of succinylcholine	May prolong the neuromuscular block	
Severity:	Moderate	Moderate	Moderate	Moderate	Moderate	Moderate
Documentation:	Probable	Possible	Possible	Possible	Suspected	Suspected

Succinylcholine

	Propofol	Trimethophan
Significance:	Be aware of	Anticipate
Onset:	<24 h	<24 h
Effect:	Severe bradycardia has been reported during coadministration	Inhibits pseudocholinesterase by decreasing succinylcholine metabolism
Severity:	Moderate	Major
Documentation:	Possible	Probable

Benzodiazepines (BZDs)

	Barbiturates	Narcotics (e.g., Morphine, Fentanyl)	Halothane
Significance:	Anticipate	Anticipate	Anticipate
Onset:	<24 h	<24 h	<24 h
Effect:	Synergistic central nervous system effects occur when used concurrently	May cause hemodynamic depression; synergistic enhancement of BZD effect	Decreases the MAC of halothane
Severity:	Moderate	Moderate	Moderate
Documentation:	Established	Established	Suspected

Propofol

	Benzodiazepines	Theophylline
Significance:	Clinical changes unlikely	No interaction
Onset:	<24 h	<24 h
Effect:	Increase effects of propofol	May antagonize effects of propofol
Severity:	Moderate	Minor
Documentation:	Established	Possible

Halothane

	Labetalol	Theophylline
Significance:	Anticipate	Anticipate
Onset:	<24 h	>24 h
Effect:	Synergistic cardiodepressant effects, which also occur with enflurane and isoflurane	Catecholamine-induced arrhythmias in patients taking theophylline
Severity:	Moderate	Major
Documentation:	Probable	Probable

Table continued on following page

TABLE 39–4. Pharmacodynamic Interactions *Continued*

Drug	Interacting Agent	Significance	Onset	Effect	Severity	Documentation
Enflurane	Aminoglycosides	Clinical changes unlikely	>24 h	Nephrotoxicity of aminoglycosides may be increased	Moderate	
	Tetracyclines	?				Possible
Methoxyflurane	Aminoglycosides	Avoid	<24 h	May have synergistic nephrotoxicity when both agents are given together	Major	Possible
	Tetracyclines	Avoid	<24 h	Synergistic renal toxicity from both agents may occur	Major	Possible
Narcotic Analgesics (Morphine, Fentanyl, Sufentanil, Alfentanil)	Benzodiazepines (BZDs)	Anticipate	<24 h	Decreased mean arterial pressure and systemic vascular resistance synergistic of BZD effects	Moderate	Established
	Inhalation Anesthetics	Anticipate	>24 h	Decreases the MAC requirement for anesthesia	Moderate	Established
	Naloxone	Anticipate	<24 h	Reverses respiratory depression, analgesia, and other narcotic effects	Moderate	Established
β-Blockers	Nitrous Oxide	Anticipate	<24 h	Decreased cardiac output	Moderate	Probable
	Halothane (also Isoflurane, Enflurane)	Be aware of	<24 h	Hypotension can occur secondary to cardiac depression	Moderate	Suspected
	Ketamine	Avoid	<24 h	Hypotension may occur secondary to the heart's inability to respond to sympathetic stimulation	Major	Probable
	Epinephrine	Avoid	<24 h	Restrict epinephrine's effect to α-receptor stimulation	Major	Established
Digoxin	Loop Diuretics	Anticipate	>24 h	May induce electrode losses of K^+ and Mg^{2+}, which predispose to digoxin-related arrhythmias	Moderate	Established
	Succinylcholine	Be aware of	<24 h	Increased potential for cardiac arrhythmias when succinylcholine is given to digitalized patients	Moderate	Possible
Methyldopa	β-Blockers	Clinical changes unlikely	<24 h	Severe hypertension may occur due to unopposed vasoconstriction from α-methylnorepinephrine owing to β-blockade	Major	Possible
	Sympathomimetics	Anticipate	<24 h	Methyldopa may potentiate the pressor response of sympathomimetics	Major	Possible
	Inhaled Anesthetics	Be aware of	<24 h	MAC reduced	Moderate	Established

Drug	Interacting Agent	Significance	Onset	Effect	Severity	Documentation
Reserpine	Sympathomimetics	Anticipate	<24 h	Reserpine may potentiate the vasopressor response of direct-acting sympathomimetics	Moderate	Suspected
	Inhaled Anesthetics	Be aware of	<24 h	A decrease in MAC may occur in reserpine-treated patients	Moderate	Established
Clonidine	β-Blockers	Avoid	>24 h	Blockage of β-receptor–mediated vasodilation may result in unopposed vasoconstriction	Major	Suspected
	Inhaled Anesthetics	Anticipate	<24 h	Decreases the MAC requirement for inhaled anesthetics	Moderate	Established
	Narcotics	Be aware of	<24 h	Clonidine may potentiate the effects of narcotics	Moderate	Suspected
Prazosin	β-Blockers	Anticipate	<24 h	May have increased postural hypotension	Moderate	Probable
	Verapamil	Be aware of	<24 h	May have increased postural hypotension	Moderate	Suspected
Angiotensin-Converting Enzyme Inhibitors (Captopril, Enalapril, Lisinopril)	Propofol	Be aware of	<24 h	Prolonged hypotension has occurred with these agents	Minor	Possible
Monoamine Oxidase Inhibitors (Phenelzine, Nialamide, Isocarboxazid, Pargyline, Tranylcypromine)	Meperidine	Avoid	<24 h	Seizures, agitation, fever, coma, apnea, and death have occurred for unknown reasons	Major	Established
	Sympathomimetics (Epinephrine, Dopamine, Ephedrine, Pseudoephedrine, Metaraminol)	Avoid	<24 h	Inhibition of the enzyme monoamine oxidase decreases the breakdown of biogenic amines, increasing their activity	Major	Established

TABLE 39–5. Pharmacologic Profile of the Adverse Effects of Antipsychotic Agents

Class	Sedative	Cardiovascular*	Extrapyramidal†
Phenothiazine			
Aliphatic	3‡	3	2
Piperidine	2	2	1
Piperazine	1	1	3
Butyrophenone	1	1	3
Thioxanthine			
Aliphatic	3	3	2
Piperazine	1	1	3
Dihydroindolone	1	1	3
Dibenzoxazepine	2	2	3

(From Perry PJ, Alexander B, Liskow BI: Psychotropic Drug Handbook. Cincinnati, Harvey Whitney Books, 1988, p 17.)
*Orthostatic hypotension (2° to α-blockade) and electrocardiogram changes.
†Refers to dystonia, akathisia, and pseudoparkinsonism, but not to tardive dyskinesia.
‡Greatest relative incidence = 3.

Do Centrally Acting Antihypertensive Agents Decrease Minimum Alveolar Concentration?

Methyldopa, clonidine, and reserpine act centrally to treat hypertension. Abrupt discontinuation of methyldopa or clonidine use also can lead to rebound hypertension. Methyldopa and reserpine deplete central catecholamine stores, whereas clonidine is a central α-adrenergic agonist. Because of their central effects, each is capable of decreasing the MAC of anesthetic agents.[76, 77] A decrease in the MAC of halothane in dogs has been noted for both methyldopa and reserpine (Fig. 39–5).[78] The authors hypothesized that CNS norepinephrine depletion was responsible for the MAC decrease.

Clonidine decreases the MAC of inhalation agents and has been administered preoperatively to reduce the requirements for these agents and for narcotics.[79–81] Table 39–7 compares

TABLE 39–6. Monoamine Oxidase Inhibitors

Generic Name	Brand Name	Type
Isocarboxazid	Marplan	Hydrazine
Pargyline	Eutonyl	Nonhydrazine
Phenelzine	Nardil	Hydrazine
Tranylcypromine	Parnate	Nonhydrazine

the different requirements for isoflurane and fentanyl in patients not receiving clonidine (group 1) and in patients who received a 5 μg · kg⁻¹-dose preoperatively (group 2). The requirements for both isoflurane and fentanyl were markedly reduced in the clonidine-treated patients.[80] Clonidine, 0.6 mg, given preoperatively also reduces the dosage requirements of propofol during surgery.[82]

Discontinuation of antihypertensive agents may lead to rebound hypertension from withdrawal. Clonidine is an excellent example of this. The α-agonist stimulation results in decreased sympathetic outflow from the CNS. Abrupt withdrawal is often associated with profound rebound hypertension. Patients who must be of nil per os status should have an alternate antihypertensive regimen instituted and their blood pressure monitored frequently. Clonidine patches can be used under these circumstances, but their effects must be monitored closely. Transition from oral to patch delivery of clonidine must be titrated to effect as it is not completely predictable.

Do Special Considerations Apply to Patients Taking β-Blockers?

Currently, 12 β-adrenergic blockers are available in the United States as intravenous, oral, and ophthalmic preparations. These drugs have different indications, selectivity, pharmacokinetics, and other receptor site actions. Pharmacody-

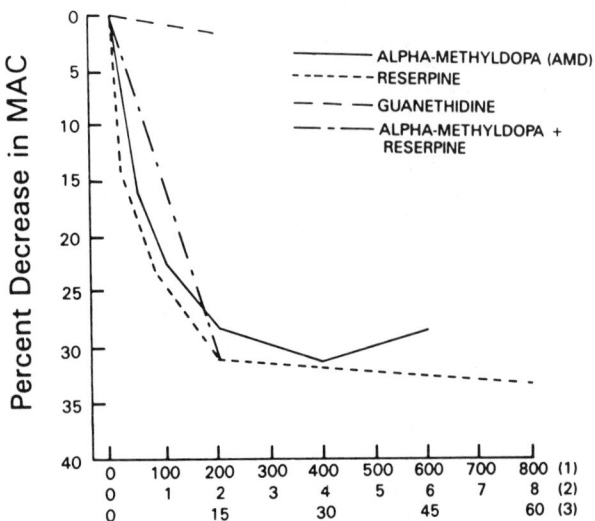

FIGURE 39–5. Per cent decreases in halothane MAC associated with prior administration of α-methyldopa, reserpine, guanethidine, and α-methyldopa in combination with reserpine. (From Miller RD, Way WL, Eger EI: The effects of α-methyldopa, reserpine, guanethidine, and iproniazid on minimum alveolar anesthetic requirement [MAC]. Anesthesiology 1968; 29:1156.)

DOSAGE:

(1) AMD, mg · kg⁻¹ · day⁻¹ × 3 DAYS

(2) RESERPINE, mg · kg⁻¹ (TOTAL DOSE)

(3) GUANETHIDINE, mg · kg⁻¹ · day⁻¹ × 3 DAYS

TABLE 39–7. Drug Requirements*

	Intraoperative				Postanesthesia Recovery Room (Morphine [mg])
	Isoflurane (End-Expiratory %)	*Fentanyl (μg)*	*Thiopental (mg)*	*Nitrous Oxide (%)*	
Group 1†	1.03 ± 16	250 ± 345	353 ± 93	51 ± 3.5	7.0 ± 7.7
Group 2‡	0.62 ± .2	61 ± 99	302 ± 112	49 ± 5	9 ± 5
P	*P* < 0.01	*P* < 0.005	Not significant	Not significant	Not significant

(From Ghignone M, Calvillo O, Quintin C: Anesthesia and hypertension: the effect of clonidine on perioperative hemodynamics and isoflurane requirements. Anesthesiology 1987; 67:7.)
*Mean ± SD.
†No clonidine.
‡Received clonidine (5 mg · kg⁻¹ preoperatively).

namic interactions of β-blockers with anesthetics result in changes in cardiac output and blood pressure.

Beta-blockers limit the heart's ability to respond to endogenous or exogenous catecholamines. If epinephrine is used in patients with β-blockade, unopposed α-constriction can result and potentially lead to hypertension and myocardial ischemia. Agents with β-agonist activity—such as dobutamine and isoproterenol or calcium, glucagon, and digoxin—can be used to counteract the effects of β-blockade.[4, 83, 84]

Some inhalation anesthetics can produce myocardial depression that may be intensified by β-blockers.[85–88] Animal studies have shown that methoxyflurane, cyclopropane, ether, and trichloroethylene produce significant myocardial depression when combined with β-blockers, a fact that obviously is of historical interest only in this country. Enflurane in high concentrations also produces increased circulatory depression in dogs administered β-blockers.[86] Although halothane and isoflurane are better tolerated in this situation, additive myocardial depression is still seen in patients receiving β-blockers. Use of these drugs should be continued up to the time of surgery, but the anesthesiologist should be prepared to adjust the dosage of volatile anesthetics to account for the aforementioned effects and to treat them if they occur.

Do Calcium Channel Blockers Affect Cardiovascular Function During Anesthesia?

Calcium channel blockers are useful in the treatment of hypertension, angina, dysrhythmias, and migraine headaches. They have significant interactions with a number of drugs used in general medical practice, and a knowledge of their potential interactions with other drugs is important. Hypotension, bradycardia, negative inotropic activity, and peripheral vasodilation may occur as a result of their use.

Inhalation and narcotic anesthetics can have additive adverse effects.[89, 90] In animal studies, verapamil, nifedipine, or diltiazem produces marked ventricular depression when given with isoflurane or halothane. More importantly, those animal studies that were conducted with open chest instrumentation showed left ventricular depression that was greater than that which occurred in other acutely anesthetized animals.[91–94] Patients with good ventricular function who are taking calcium channel blocking agents should be able to tolerate anesthetic agents well. However, those requiring open chest surgery could have a pronounced decrease in ventricular function with inhalation anesthetics.[95]

Calcium channel blocking agents can also affect neuromuscular blockade. Verapamil potentiates depolarizing and nondepolarizing blocking drugs. It may also inhibit the antagonism of neuromuscular blockade with neostigmine.[96, 97]

Do Other Antihypertensive Agents Have Potential Interactions?

Only one interaction of angiotensin-converting enzyme inhibitors, such as captopril or enalapril, has been reported (a case of prolonged hypotension with propofol,[98] which was thought to be due to decreased preload and systemic vascular resistance). Peripheral vasodilators such as hydralazine or minoxidil have no known interactions with anesthetic agents. Prazosin, an α-adrenergic blocker, may offer some protection against dysrhythmias produced as a result of halothane-epinephrine interaction. When prazosin is used for the first time, a low dose must be administered to minimize the first dose phenomenon that often results in exaggerated hypotension.[4]

What Medications Interact with Neuromuscular Blocking Agents?

Antidysrhythmic Agents

Many of the antidysrhythmic medications can potentiate neuromuscular blockade because they act at the prejunctional membrane.[99–101] This effect has occurred with quinidine in both nondepolarizing and depolarizing blockade, and with lidocaine and procainamide during nondepolarizing blockade.

Quinidine has significant anticholinergic and α-adrenergic blockade activity, and, thus, can potentially produce additive responses when combined with other similarly acting agents. Other concerns regarding the use of quinidine and procainamide are these drugs' ability to enhance conduction through the A-V node, which can potentially lead to ventricular tachycardia. If these agents are to be used to treat or suppress supraventricular tachydysrhythmias, pretreatment with digoxin should prevent ventricular tachycardia.[102]

Antibiotics

Aminoglycoside antibiotics (amikacin, gentamicin, tobramycin, neomycin, streptomycin, kanamycin) can produce synergistic neuromuscular blockade when used with nondepolar-

TABLE 39–8. Interaction of Antibiotics, Muscle Relaxants, Neostigmine, and Calcium

	Neuromuscular Block from Antibiotic Alone, Antagonized by		Increase in Neuromuscular Block of		Neuromuscular Block from Antibiotic and d-Tubocurarine, Antagonized by	
	Neostigmine	*Calcium*	*d-Tubocurarine*	*Succinylcholine*	*Neostigmine*	*Calcium*
Neomycin	Sometimes	Sometimes	Yes	Yes	Usually	Usually
Streptomycin	Sometimes	Sometimes	Yes	Yes	Usually	Usually
Gentamicin	Sometimes	Yes*	Yes	†	Sometimes	Yes*
Kanamycin	Sometimes	Sometimes	Yes	Yes	Sometimes	Sometimes
Paromomycin	Yes*	Yes*	Yes	†	Yes*	Yes*
Viomycin	Yes*	Yes*	Yes	†	Yes*	Yes*
Polymyxin A	No	No	Yes	†	No	No
Polymyxin B	No‡	No	Yes	Yes	No‡	No
Colistin	No	Sometimes	Yes	Yes	No	Sometimes
Tetracycline	No	†	Yes	No	Partially	Partially
Lincomycin	Partially	Partially	Yes	†	Partially	Partially
Clindamycin	Partially	Partially	Yes	†	Partially	Partially

(From Miller RD, Smith NT: Neuromuscular blocking agents. *In* Drug Interactions in Anesthesia. 2nd ed. Philadelphia, Lea & Febiger, 1986, p 366.)
*Despite this, difficulty with antagonizing the block from these antibiotics is still likely to occur.
†Not studied.
‡Block augmented by neostigmine.

izing agents.[103–104] This effect can occur if the aminoglycoside is given intraoperatively or preoperatively.[4, 104]

Other antibiotics (clindamycin, tetracycline, polymyxin B, vancomycin) may produce additive effects or potentiation of neuromuscular block. This enhanced neuromuscular blockade may not be antagonized by neostigmine and calcium. Table 39–8 lists the effects that neostigmine or calcium may have when used to antagonize the neuromuscular blockade caused by various anti-infective agents.[4, 105, 106]

Have Drug Interactions Occurred with Propofol?

Propofol is a short-acting anesthetic agent with an effective half-life of a few minutes. Only a few possible drug interactions have been reported. Hendley[107] noted convulsions following the use of topical cocaine and propofol. He stated that it was unclear whether the convulsions were caused by propofol alone. Halothane may prolong the elimination of propofol by decreasing hepatic blood flow, thereby decreasing the rate of metabolism of propofol.[108, 109] Fentanyl, 1.5 $\mu g \cdot kg^{-1}$, combined with propofol did *not* affect anesthetic duration, eye opening time, or the time to repeat correct birth date. It also did not affect propofol elimination.[110] The combination of pro-

pofol and benzodiazepines is synergistic (the combination of the two drugs has 1.44 times the potency of the use of the agents in isolation).[111] This observation can be used to advantage, that is, the propofol dose can be decreased during either conscious sedation or general anesthesia applications.

What Are Significant Benzodiazepine Interactions?

Benzodiazepines have been found to interact synergistically with barbiturates, narcotics, and propofol.[110, 112, 113] Table 39–9 illustrates the dramatic effect of the coadministration of midazolam and alfentanil. Analogous effects occur with any—and probably all—narcotic, benzodiazepine, propofol, and barbiturate combinations and should be considered, especially during concomitant administration in the induction of conscious sedation.

What Is the Role of Flumazenil?

Flumazenil was approved by the Food and Drug Administration in December 1991 to be used to bring about the com-

TABLE 39–9. Equieffective Doses (ED$_{50}$)

Groups	Alfentanil Component		Midazolam Component		Sum of Fractional Doses	Ratio*
	Fraction of ED$_{50}$	*Dose (mg/kg)*	*Fraction of ED$_{50}$*	*Dose (mg/kg)*		
Alfentanil	1.00	0.13 (0.11, 0.19)	0.00	0.00	1.00	—
Midazolam	0.00	0.00	1.00	0.22 (0.15, 0.50)	1.00	—
Alfentanil and midazolam	0.21	0.028 (0.018, 0.036)	0.33	0.07†	0.54 ($P < 0.0001$)‡	1.85

(From Vinik HR, Bradley EL Jr, Kissin I: Midazolam-alfentanil synergism for anesthetic induction in patients. Anesth Analg 1989; 69:216. © International Anesthesia Research Society.)
*Ratio of single drug fractional dose to combined fractional dose.
†Dose was kept constant.
‡P = Significance of deviation from additivity.

plete or partial reversal of benzodiazepine sedation. This drug acts by competitively binding to the benzodiazepine receptor.[112, 113] Flumazenil rapidly reverses sedation and antagonizes the effect of midazolam on tidal volume but does not correct the depressant effect of midazolam on the slope of the carbon dioxide response curve.[113]

In a manner similar to narcotic reversal with naloxone, the antagonistic effects of flumazenil may dissipate before the effects of the benzodiazepine are reversed, particularly when high doses of benzodiazepines have been taken. Flumazenil should also be used with caution in patients with a long-term history of benzodiazepine therapy or with a seizure disorder treated with a benzodiazepine, as they are more likely to develop withdrawal symptoms and seizure activity if given flumazenil.[114]

Flumazenil also has been shown to be an effective antidote in benzodiazepine poisoning or mixed drug overdosage. It may prevent other, more invasive interventions.[112] Flumazenil is effective in reversing sedation and some aspects of respiratory depression during or following conscious sedation, general anesthesia, and benzodiazepine poisoning. It does not have proven pharmacodynamic antagonistic properties for other medications.

SUMMARY

Drug interactions that the anesthesiologist can expect to see in practice include not only the frequently considered pharmacokinetic and pharmacodynamic drug interactions but also physical incompatibilities. Tables 39–1 and 39–4 list selected drug interactions of interest to anesthesiologists.

Whenever the administration of two or more drugs results in an unexpected effect, the anesthesiologist should consider a drug interaction as a potential explanation. Because of the myriad drug combinations that can occur during the perioperative period, all possible interactions cannot be known or predicted. Knowledge of drug classes, mechanisms of action, and potential adverse effects is helpful to predict possible drug interactions.

References

1. Levy WJ: Clinical anaesthesia with isoflurane. Br J Anaesth 1984; 56(Suppl):101.
2. Zeller FP, Anders RJ: Compatibility of intravenous drugs in a coronary intensive care unit. Drug Intell Clin Pharm 1986; 20:349.
3. Davie IT: Specific drug interactions in anaesthesia. Anaesthesia 1977; 32:1000.
4. Goodwin SR: Drugs and drug reactions. In Manual of Complications During Anesthesia. 1st ed. Gravenstein N (ed). Philadelphia, JB Lippincott, 1991, pp 479–508.
5. Schentag JJ, Simons GW, Schultz RW, et al: Complexation versus hemodialysis to reduce elevated aminoglycoside serum concentrations. Pharmacotherapy 1984; 4:374.
6. Bauman JL, Sieplen JK, Fitzloff J: Phenytoin crystallization in intravenous fluids. Drug Intell Clin Pharm 1977; 11:646.
7. Finch ME: Sodium thiopental in 5% dextrose in lactated Ringer's precipitate. Hosp Pharm 1979; 14:559.
8. McEvoy GK (ed): American Hospital Formulary Service Drug Information. 9th ed: Bethesda, American Society of Hospital Pharmacists, Inc, 1992, pp 1345–1351.
9. Trissel LA: Handbook of Injectable Drugs. 6th ed. Bethesda, American Society of Hospital Pharmacists, Inc, 1990.
10. King JC: Guide to Parenteral Admixtures. St Louis, Pacemarq, Inc, 1989.
11. Gauger LJ, Gibboney ER, Nordin BJ: Flow dynamics of a retrograde IV drug infusion system. Am J Hosp Pharm 1984; 41:492.
12. Horrow JC, Digregorio GJ, Barbieri EJ, et al: Intravenous infusions of nitroprusside, dobutamine, and nitroglycerin are compatible. Crit Care Med 1990; 18:858.
13. Evans WE: General principles of applied pharmacokinetics. In Applied Pharmacokinetics. 2nd ed. Evans WE, Schentag JJ, Jasko WJ (eds). Spokane, Applied Therapeutics, Inc, 1986, pp 1–8.
14. Höffken G, Borner K, Glatzel PD: Reduced enteral absorption of ciprofloxacin in presence of antacids. Eur J Clin Microbiol 1985; 4:345.
15. Garty M, Hurwitz A: Effect of cimetidine and antacids on gastrointestinal absorption of tetracycline. Clin Pharmacol Ther 1980; 28:203.
16. Yee GC, McGuire TR: Pharmacokinetic drug interactions with cyclosporin (Part 1). Clin Pharmacokinet 1990; 19:319–332.
17. Wadhwa NK, Schroeder TJ, O'Flaherty E, et al: The effect of oral metoclopramide on the absorption of cyclosporine. Transplant Proc 1987; 19:1730.
18. Freeman DJ, Laupacis A, Keown PA, et al: Evaluation of cyclosporin-phenytoin interaction with observations on cyclosporin metabolites. Br J Clin Pharmacol 1984; 18:887.
19. Fee JPH, Collier PS, Howard PJ, et al: Cimetidine and ranitidine increase midazolam bioavailability. Clin Pharmacol Ther 1987; 41:80.
20. Scott DB, Jebson PJR, Braid DO, et al: Factors affecting plasma levels of lignocaine and prilocaine. Br J Anaesth 1972; 44:1040.
21. DiFazio CH, Carron H, Grosslight KR: Comparison of pH-adjusted solutions for epidural anesthesia. Anesth Analg 1986; 65:760.
22. Greenblatt DJ, Allen MD, Harmatz JS, et al: Diazepam disposition determinants. Clin Pharmacol Ther 1980; 27:301.
23. Greenblatt DJ, Divoll M: Diazepam versus lorazepam: relationship of drug distribution to duration of clinical action. Adv Neurol 1983; 34:487–491.
24. Ameer B, Greenblatt DJ: Lorazepam: a review of its clinical pharmacological properties and therapeutic uses. Drugs 1981; 21:161.
25. Lacey DJ, Singer WD, Horwitz J, et al: Lorazepam therapy of status epilepticus in children and adolescents. J Pediatr 1986; 108:771.
26. Homer TD, Stanski DR: The effect of increasing age on thiopental disposition and anesthetic requirement. Anesthesiology 1985; 62:714.
27. Cullen BF, Miller MG: Drug interactions and anesthesia: a review. Anesth Analg 1979; 58:413.
28. Wood M: Plasma drug binding: implications for anesthesiologists. Anesth Analg 1986; 65:786.
29. Winter ME, Tozen TN: Phenytoin. In Applied Pharmacokinetics. 2nd ed. Evans WE, Schentag JJ, Jusko WJ (eds). Spokane, Applied Therapeutics, Inc, 1986, pp 493–539.
30. Svensson CK, Woodruff MN, Lalka D: Influence of protein binding and use of unbound drug concentrations. In Applied Pharmacokinetics. 2nd ed. Evans WE, Schentag JJ, Jusko WJ (eds). Spokane, Applied Therapeutics, Inc, 1986, pp 187–219.
31. Munson ES: Local anesthetics. In Drug Interactions in Anesthesia. 2nd ed. Smith NJ, Corbascio AN (eds). Philadelphia, Lea & Febiger, 1986, pp 391–406.
32. Ghoeneim MM, Pandya H: Plasma protein binding of bupivacaine and its interaction with other drugs in man. Br J Anaesth 1974; 46:435.
33. Kaukinen S, Eerola M, Ylitalo P: Prolongation of thiopentone anaesthesia by probenecid. Br J Anaesth 1980; 52:603.
34. McMurray JJ, Dundee JW, Henshaw JS: The influence of probenecid on the induction dose of thiopentone. Br J Clin Pharmacol 1984; 17:224.
35. Powell JR, Cate EW: Induction and inhibition of drug metabolism. In Applied Pharmacokinetics. 2nd ed. Evans WE, Schentag JJ, Jusko WJ (eds). Spokane, Applied Therapeutics, Inc, 1986, pp 139–186.
36. Rawling MD: General mechanisms of drug interactions. In Drug Interactions. Grahame-Smith DG, (ed). Baltimore, University Park Press, 1977, pp 35–44.
37. Brown BR, Sipes JC: Biotransformation and hepatotoxicity of halothane. Biochem Pharmacol 1977; 26:2091.
38. Halsey MJ. Drug interactions in anaesthesia. Br J Anaesth 1987; 59:112.
39. Neigh JL: Inhalation anesthetic agents. In Drug Interactions in Anesthesia. 2nd ed. Smith NT, Corbascio AN (eds). Philadelphia, Lea & Febiger, 1986, pp 340–362.
40. Mazze RI, Trudell JR, Cousins MJ: Methoxyflurane metabolism and renal dysfunction: clinical correlation in man. Anesthesiology 1971; 35:247.
41. Dooley JR, Mazze RI, Rice SA, et al: Is enflurane defluorination inducible in man? Anesthesiology 1979; 50:213.

42. Powell JR, Donn KH: Histamine H₂-antagonist drug interactions in perspective: mechanistic concepts and clinical implications. Am J Med 1984; 77(Suppl SB):57.

43. Powell JR, Rogers JF, Wargin WA, et al: Inhibition of theophylline clearance by cimetidine but not ranitidine. Arch Intern Med 1984; 144:484.

44. Feldman M, Barton ME: Histamine₂-receptor antagonists: standard therapy for acid-peptic diseases. N Engl J Med 1990; 323:1672.

45. Teem WR, Davis PM, Hyams JS: Suppression of gastric acid secretion by intravenous administration of famotidine in children. J Pediatr 1991; 118:812.

46. Feldman M, Barton ME: Histamine₂-receptor antagonists: standard therapy for acid-peptic diseases. N Engl J Med 1990; 323:1749.

47. Conney AH: Pharmacological implications of microsomal enzyme induction. Pharmacol Rev 1967; 19:317.

48. Gelehrter TD: Enzyme induction. N Engl J Med 1976; 294:522.

49. Breckenridge AM, Orme MLE: Clinical implications of enzyme induction. Ann N Y Acad Sci 1971; 179:421.

50. Dossing M, Pilsgaard H, Rasmassen B, et al: Time course of phenobarbital and cimetidine mediated changes in hepatic drug metabolism. Eur J Clin Pharmacol 1983; 25:215.

51. Bartkowski RR, McDonnell TE: Prolonged alfentanil effect following erythromycin administration. Anesthesiology 1990; 73:566.

52. Pantuck EJ: Ecothiophate iodide eye drops and prolonged response to suxamethonium. Br J Anaesth 1966; 38:406.

53. Eildenton TE, Farmati O, Zsigmond EK: Reduction in plasma cholinesterase levels after prolonged administration of echothiophate iodide eyedrops. Can Anaesth Soc J 1968; 15:291.

54. Himmelhoch JM, Poust RI, Mallinger AG, et al: Adjustment of lithium dose during lithium-chlorothiazide therapy. Clin Pharmacol Ther 1977; 22:225.

55. Hartig HI, Dyson WL: Lithium toxicity enhanced by diuresis (letter). N Engl J Med 1974; 290:748.

56. Stoelting RK, Eger EI: An additional explanation for the second gas effect. Anesthesiology 1969; 30:273.

57. Eyer EI: Surgical stimulation antagonizes the respiratory depression produced by Forane. Anesthesiology 1972; 36:544.

58. Bahlman SH: The cardiovascular effects of nitrous oxide: halothane anesthesia in man. Anesthesiology 1974; 35:274.

59. Perry PJ, Alexander B, Liskow BI: Psychotropic Drug Handbook, 1988. Cincinnati, Harvey Whitney Books, pp 3–43.

60. Lambertsen CJ, Wendel H, Longenhagen JB: The separate and combined respiratory effects of chlorpromazine and meperidine in normal men controlled at 46 mm Hg alveolar PCO₂. J Pharmacol Exp Ther 1961; 131:381.

61. Eggers GWN, Corssen G, Allen CR: Comparison of vasopressor responses in the presence of phenothiazine derivatives. Anesthesiology 1959; 20:261.

62. Stoelting RK: Drugs used in treatment of psychiatric disease. In Pharmacology and Physiology in Anesthetic Practice. Philadelphia, JB Lippincott, 1991, pp 365–383.

63. Gold MI: Profound hypotension associated with preoperative use of phenothiazines. Anesth Analg 1974; 53:844.

64. Baldessarin RJ: Drugs and the treatment of psychiatric disorders. In Goodman and Gilman's the Pharmacological Basis of Therapeutics. 8th ed. Gilman AG, Rall TW, Nies AS, et al (eds). New York, Pergammon Press, 1990, pp 383–435.

65. Edwards RP, Miller RD, Roizen MF, et al: Cardiac responses to impromine and pancuronium during anesthesia with halothane or enflurane. Anesthesiology 1979; 50:421.

66. Boakes AJ, Laurene DR, Teoh DC, et al: Interactions between sympathomimetic amines and antidepressant agents in man. Br Med J 1973; 1:311.

67. Wong KC, Puerto AX, Puerto BA, et al: Influence of imipramine and pargyline on the arrythmogenicity of epinephrine during halothane, enflurane, or methoxyflurane anesthesia in dogs. Anesthesiology 1980; 53(Suppl):25.

68. Dobkin AB: Potentiation of thiopental anaesthesia with tigan, panectyl, benadryl, gravol, marzine, histadyl, librium, and haloperidol. Can Anaesth Soc J 1961; 8:265.

69. Janowsky EC, Risch SC, Janowsky DS: Psychotropic agents. In Drug Interactions in Anesthesia. 2nd ed. Smith NT, Corbascio AN (eds). Philadelphia, Lea & Febiger, 1986, pp 261–281.

70. Borden H, Clarke M, Katz H: The use of pancuronium bromide in patients receiving lithium carbonate. Can Anaesth Soc J 1974; 21:79.

71. Hill GE, Wong KL, Hodges MR: Potentiation of succinylcholine neuromuscular blockade by lithium carbonate. Anesthesiology 1976; 44:439.

72. Waud BE, Farrell C, Waud DR: Lithium and neuromuscular transmission. Anesth Analg 1982; 61:399.

73. Martin BA, Kramer PM: Clinical significance of the interaction between lithium and neuromuscular blocker. Am J Psychiatry 1982; 139:1326.

74. Prys-Roberts C: Hypertension and anesthesia: fifty years on. Anesthesiology 1979; 50:281.

75. Hurt GR, Anderson RJ: Withdrawal syndromes and the cessation of antihypertensive therapy. Arch Intern Med 1981; 141:1125.

76. Stoelting RK: Antihypertensive drugs. In Pharmacology and Physiology in Anesthetic Practice. 2nd ed. Philadelphia, JB Lippincott, 1991, pp 311–323.

77. Stoelting RK: Antihypertensives and alpha-blockers. In Drug Interactions in Anesthesia. 2nd ed. Smith NT, Corbascio AN (eds). Philadelphia, Lea & Febiger, 1986, pp 147–175.

78. Miller RD, Woy WL, Eger EI: The effects of alpha-methyldopa, reserpine, guanethidine, and iproniazid on minimum alveolar anesthetic requirement (MAC). Anesthesiology 1968; 29:1153.

79. Engelman E, Lipszyc M, Gilbert ES, et al: Effects of clonidine on anesthetic drug requirements and hemodynamic response during aortic surgery. Anesthesiology 1989; 71:178.

80. Ghignone M, Calvillo O, Quintin L: Anesthesia and hypertension: the effect of clonidine on perioperative hemodynamics and isoflurane requirements. Anesthesiology 1987; 67:3.

81. Flacke JW, Bloor BL, Flacke WE, et al: Reduced narcotic requirements by clonidine with improved hemodynamic and adrenergic stability in patients undergoing coronary bypass surgery. Anesthesiology 1987; 67:11.

82. Richards MJ, Skaes MA, Jarcuis AP, et al: Total IV anaesthesia with propofol and alfentanil: dose requirements for propofol and the effect of premedication of clonidine. Br J Anaesth 1990; 65:157.

83. Stoelting RK: Alpha- and beta-adrenergic receptor antagonists. In Pharmacology and Physiology in Anesthetic Practice. 2nd ed. Philadelphia, JB Lippincott, 1991, pp 295–310.

84. Lowenstein E, Foey P: Beta-adrenergic blockers. In Drug Interactions in Anesthesia. 2nd ed. Smith NT, Corbascio AN (eds). Philadelphia, Lea & Febiger, 1986, pp 119–134.

85. Foey PL: Alpha- and beta-adrenoreceptor antagonists. Br J Anaesth 1984; 56:751.

86. Horan BJ, Prys-Roberts C, Hamilton WK, et al: Haemodynamic responses to enflurane anaesthesia and hypovolemia in the dog and their modification by propranolol. Br J Anaesth 1977; 49:1184.

87. Roberts JG, Foey P, Clarke TNS, et al: Haemodynamic interactions of high-dose propranolol pre-treatment and anaesthesia in the dog: III. The effects of haemorrhage during halothane and trichloroethylene anaesthesia. Br J Anaesth 1976; 48:411.

88. Saner CA, Foey P, Roberts JG, et al: Methoxyflurane and practolol: a dangerous combination. Br J Anaesth 1975; 47:1025.

89. Bosnjak ZJ, Kampine JP: Effects of halothane, enflurane, and isoflurane on the SA node. Anesthesiology 1983; 58:314.

90. Nussmeier NA, Curling PE, Murphy DA, et al: Nifedipine: cardiovascular effects after sublingual administration during fentanyl-pancuronium anesthesia in man. Anesthesiology 1983; 59:A34.

91. Tosone SR, Reves JG, Kissin I, et al: Hemodynamic response to nifedipine in dogs anesthetized with halothane. Anesth Analg 1983; 62:903.

92. Ramsay JG, Cutfield GR, Francis CM, et al: Halothane-verapamil causes regional myocardial dysfunction in the dog. Br J Anaesth 1986; 58:321.

93. Kapur PA, Bloor BC, Flacke WE, et al: Comparison of cardiovascular responses to verapamil during enflurane, isoflurane, or halothane anesthesia in the dog. Anesthesiology 1984; 61:156.

94. Priebe HJ, Skarvan K: Cardiovascular and electrophysiologic interactions between diltiazem and isoflurane in the dog. Anesthesiology 1987; 66:114.

95. Merin RG: Calcium channel blocking drugs and anesthetics: is the drug interaction beneficial or detrimental (editorial). Anesthesiology 1987; 66:111.

96. Jones RM, Cashman JN, Casson WR, et al: Verapamil potentiation of neuromuscular blockade: failure of reversal with neostigmine, but prompt reversal with edrophonium. Anesth Analg 1985; 64:1021.

97. Lawson NW, Kraynack BJ, Gintantas J: Neuromuscular and electrocardiographic responses to verapamil in dogs. Anesth Analg 1983; 62:50.

98. Littler C, McConachie I, Healy JEJ: Interaction between enalapril and propofol (letter). Anaesth Intens Care 1989; 17:514.

99. Harrah MD, Way WL, Katzung BG: The interaction of d-tubocurarine with antiarrhythmic drugs. Anesthesiology 1970; 33:406.

100. Miller RD, Way WC, Katzung BG: The potentiation of neuromuscular blocking agents by quinidine. Anesthesiology 1967; 28:1036.
101. Miller RD, Way WL, Katzung BG: The neuromuscular effects of quinidine. Proc Soc Exp Biol Med 1968; 129:215.
102. Atlee JL III: Antidysrhythmic agents. *In* Drug Interactions in Anesthesia. 2nd ed. Smith NT, Corbascio AN (eds). Philadelphia, Lea & Febiger, 1986, pp 225–244.
103. Waterman PM, Smith RB: Tobramycin-curare interaction. Anesth Analg 1988; 56:587.
104. Pittinger C, Adamson R: Antibiotic blockade of neuromuscular function. Ann Rev Pharmacol 1972; 12:169.
105. Burkett L, Bikhazi GB, Thomas KC, et al: Mutual potentiation of the neuromuscular effects of antibiotics and relaxants. Anesth Analg 1979; 58:107.
106. Fogdall RP, Miller RD: Prolongation of a pancuronium-induced neuromuscular blockade by clindamycin. Anesthesiology 1974; 41:407.
107. Hendley BJ: Convulsions after cocaine and propofol (letter). Anaesthesia 1990; 45:788.
108. Nies AS, Shand DG, Wilkinson GR: Altered hepatic blood flow and drug disposition. Clin Pharmacokinet 1976; 1:135.
109. Cockshott ID, Douglas EJ, Prys-Roberts C, et al: Pharmacokinetics of propofol during and after IV infusion in man. Br J Anaesth 1987; 59:941P.
110. Gill SS, Wright EM, Reilly CS. Pharmacokinetic interaction of propofol and fentanyl: single bolus injection study. Br J Anaesth 1990; 65:760.
111. Short TG, Chui PT: Propofol and midazolam act synergistically in combination. Br J Anaesth 1991; 67:539.
112. Brogden RN, Goa KL: Flumazenil: a reappraisal of its pharmacological properties and therapeutic efficacy as a benzodiazepine antagonist. Drugs 1991; 42:1061.
113. Amnein R, Leishman B, Bentzingen C, et al: Flumazenil in benzodiazepine antagonism, actions and clinical use in interactions and anesthesiology. Med Toxicol 1987; 2:411.
114. Gross JB, Weller RS, Conard P: Flumazenil reversal of midazolam. Anesthesiology 1991; 75:179.

Physiologic Aberrations and Their Control

CHAPTER 40

Shock

DAVID J. TORPEY, JR., M.D.

MICHAEL D. INGRAM, M.D.

A comprehensive understanding of the pathophysiology of shock is necessary if an anesthesiologist is to approach treatment in a rational manner. The clinical manifestations of shock are diverse because it may be caused by many diseases and modified by a patient's pre-existing physical status. It is understandable, therefore, that the literature contains a multitude of definitions of shock based on the etiology and pathologic changes involved. Classifying shock into the major categories of hypovolemic, cardiogenic, anaphylactic, spinal cord, and septic may aid in selecting proper therapy.

In this chapter, we review current theories of the pathophysiology of shock states and provide a practical orientation for anesthesiologists who may be involved in the management of patients in shock.

HYPOTENSION

What Role Does It Play?

Hardaway[1] aptly stated that shock is not synonymous with arterial hypotension, hypovolemia, low cardiac output, low peripheral vascular resistance, acidosis, anoxia, or lack of vascular tone. Indeed, these factors may or may not be present, and as a corollary, all patients who are hypotensive are not in shock. Factors such as marked obesity, improper (excessive) cuff size, severe atherosclerotic vascular disease, or peripheral vasoconstriction contribute to the inaccuracy of indirect cuff blood pressure measurement. Anesthesiologists are well aware of the adequacy of flow in patients in whom controlled hypotension has been induced. When combined with moderate hemodilution and a concomitant decrease in blood viscosity, flow to the tissues may be enhanced despite a low (but controlled) blood pressure.

How Is Tissue Perfusion Altered?

In shock, hypotension is associated with an inability of the terminal vascular bed to regulate the orderly distribution of blood flow.[2] Microcirculatory deterioration occurs secondary to adverse, myogenic, rheologic, or diffusion (cellular exchange) factors or a combination thereof. In the early stages of circulatory shock, a reduction in the mean arterial blood pressure (driving force in the vascular bed) stimulates reflex vasoconstriction (compensatory neuroendocrine feedback) of the arterioles and veins.

What Are the Intracellular Changes?

Tissues supplied by the constricted vessels eventually become ischemic and hypoxic, and metabolic by-products build up in localized areas. These metabolites eventually lead to relaxation of the precapillary sphincters; however, continued arteriolar constriction prevents increases in capillary blood flow. This loss of microcirculatory homeostasis changes the structural integrity of the terminal vascular beds.

If ischemia is prolonged, damage to the mitochondria, endoplasmic reticulum, and lysosomes occurs. Cell membrane ion pump regulation activity by Na^+-K^+ adenosine triphosphatase is inhibited, with resultant increases of extracellular potassium and intracellular sodium and water. Mitochondrial damage leads to uncoupling of oxidative phosphorylation and a resultant decrease in the ratio of high-energy phosphate bonds generated per mole of oxygen (O_2) consumed.[3]

Lysosomal disruption occurs in all types of circulatory shock. Disruption of lysosomal membranes causes the release of proteases, lipases, phosphorylases, and other acid hydrolases into the cytosol, eventuating in the loss of cellular structural integrity and metabolic function. The crucial factor and common denominator of all types of shock is cellular hypoperfusion with resultant impaired substrate transport from the extracellular fluid into the cell—a *cellular energy crisis.*

VASCULAR ENDOTHELIUM

How Is It Altered?

Normal vascular endothelial cells are permeable to water but variably restrictive to the transport of solute and plasma proteins. Ischemia or hypoxia damages the vascular endothelium, resulting in permeability edema. Plasma proteins may extravasate into the extracellular space. This pathologic permeability results from the accumulation of metabolic end products and fatty acids, arachidonic acid metabolites, and oxygen free radicals. Cellular swelling, which causes junctional openings between endothelial cells, also contributes. Cellular swelling further contributes to hypoperfusion because of capillary compression, even after the blood volume has been restored.

Why Does Platelet Adhesion Occur?

The derangement of endothelial cell function and its part in the pathophysiology of shock are subjects of intensive research. Under normal conditions, the endothelium not only acts as a barrier to solute, proteins, and cellular exchange but also maintains a nonthrombogenic surface because of its production of prostacyclin (PGI_2), an inhibitor of platelet aggregation.

Thrombus Formation

Removal of endothelial cells from the vessel wall produces platelet adhesion within minutes of the endothelial loss. Platelets that may have been activated by acidosis, ischemia, stagnated flow, or hypoxia during low-flow states are much more prone to adhere to the exposed receptor sites. The subendothelium (basement membrane of the endothelium) provokes platelet adhesion, as do the collagen and microfibrils around the subendothelial elastin. Endothelial cell injury suppresses PGI_2 production and stimulates the conversion of arachidonic acid to thromboxane A_2 within the vessel wall.[4]

Platelets primarily are involved in arterial hemostasis and thrombosis. Platelet aggregation is an important component of thrombus formation. In contrast, in venous thrombi, fibrin, generated from tissue factors and activation of factor VII, and red blood cells are most prominent in the formation of thrombi (red clot); however, fibrin also has an important role in the formation of arterial thrombi (white clot). If thrombi are of sufficient size, they may block circulation to the tissue or organ supplied by the involved vasculature.

In some instances, blood flow conditions at the area of vascular damage may actually limit thrombus formation or size. If a thrombus is not formed within approximately 24 hours of injury, the initial platelet monolayer disappears and the subendothelial surface originally exposed during injury to the vessel becomes unreactive with platelets.[5] The mechanism by which platelets become antithrombogenic is unknown.

Endothelial cells are also involved in clot lysis through the synthesis and release of plasminogen-activating factor and the production of plasmin, a fibrinolytic enzyme in the blood. Although normal endothelium regulates clot dissolution by the production of plasmin, damaged or deranged endothelium may be incapable of reversing the intravascular clotting process. The outcome may be occlusion in the microcirculatory beds.

Myocardial Infarction

Cardiologists are well aware of the role that the vascular endothelium and platelets have in the production of acute myocardial infarction and the acute or chronic reocclusion of the coronary vessel after thrombolytic therapy or percutaneous transluminal coronary angioplasty (PTCA).

Plaque disruption causes arterial injury and clot formation secondary to platelet adhesion and thrombus formation. The nature of the clot formed depends on the degree of injury. Minimal arterial damage results in formation of a platelet-rich clot, whereas deep arterial injury causes the formation of a mural thrombus. Pharmacologic therapy aimed at preventing clot thrombus formation (i.e., aspirin or heparin) needs to be based on this understanding.

Thrombolytic therapy using fibrin-selective agents such as tissue plasminogen activator or systemic agents such as urokinase, streptokinase, or acylated plasminogen streptokinase activator complex, instituted within 2 hours of the onset of angina and electrocardiographic (ECG) changes, has been successful in opening the thrombosed vessel in a large majority of patients so treated.

What Is Endothelium-Derived Relaxing Factor?

Lefer and colleagues[6] showed that in endotoxemia, macrophages and other cell types, when activated, are associated with the release of tumor necrosis factor (TNF). This substance may produce hypotension, hypoglycemia, hyperkalemia, and hemoconcentration. Both TNF and superoxide free radicals (released from neutrophils on reperfusion of ischemic tissues) alter surface receptors on endothelial cells and inhibit the release of endothelium-derived relaxing factor (EDRF). Superoxide radicals also inactivate EDRF once it has been released from the endothelial cells. This substance facilitates vascular smooth muscle dilatation in response to various vasoactive agents. Nitric oxide (NO) is thought to be a major component of EDRF.

TNF does not influence endothelium-independent dilators such as nitroglycerin or sodium nitroprusside; thus, these direct-acting smooth muscle vasodilators are often useful to improve microcirculatory blood flow.[7] However, in some patients, the doses needed to produce vasodilation may result in systemic hypotension, reduced perfusion pressure, and reflex tachycardia.

Myocardial Ischemia

Impairment of endothelium-derived relaxation has been demonstrated in myocardial ischemia during the reperfusion stage (reperfusion injury). TNF and other vasoactive substances such as leukotrienes and thromboxanes cause neutrophils to adhere to coronary vessel endothelium supplying the ischemic myocardium during the reperfusion period. These neutrophils release free radicals, which are in turn capable of inactivation of EDRF. Superoxide dismutase and endothelial protective agents such as transforming growth factor (β-TGF) protect the vascular endothelium of experimental animals from these harmful substances.

Johnson and colleagues[8] demonstrated that NO infusion provided significant myocardial protection after ischemia and reperfusion in cats. Nitric acid is incorporated into the circulating neutrophils and platelets, inhibiting their accumulation and adherence in the ischemic region of the myocardium.

The coronary arterial lumen at the site of an atheromatous plaque is not fixed in all cases. Seventy-four per cent of coronary artery lesions are eccentric, and 26% are circumferential; therefore, vasoreaction of the noninvolved wall segment is possible in 74% of the atherosclerotic vessels. Flow depends on the type and length of the lesion and the amount of diffuse disease along the vessel distal to the major obstruction. Longer lesions result in a greater reduction in flow. Thus, to estimate the reduction of flow in a coronary vessel, not only the per cent of stenosis must be known but also the per cent of the vessel lumen that is open.

Several vasoactive substances such as serotonin, platelet-generated thromboxane, and α-sympathetic agonists may cause constriction of that portion of the coronary artery capable of vasomotion. Loss of intrinsic EDRF by the noninvolved vessel wall segment at the area of plaque disruption results in a paradoxical response by that segment to vasoactive substances released endogenously or injected intravenously. Such vasoconstrictor responses have been demonstrated for substances normally associated with vasodilation (e.g., acetylcholine, histamine, and others).

Nitric Oxide Inhalation

Inhalation of NO relaxes pulmonary vessels without inducing concomitant systemic hypotension in experimental animals with pulmonary artery vasoconstriction.[9] This dilatory effect of NO on the pulmonary circulation is independent of cyclo-oxygenase substances such as PGI_2. The effectiveness of inhaled NO as a pulmonary vasodilator in neonates with pulmonary hypertension is well demonstrated. The heme structure of hemoglobin has such an affinity for NO that the inhaled gas is rapidly inactivated, thus confining the vasodilatory action to the lungs. Localized bronchodilatation occurs after NO inhalation as well.[10]

Inhaled NO has been used in patients with persistent pulmonary hypertension following mitral valve replacement.[11] Systolic, diastolic, and mean pulmonary artery pressures and pulmonary vascular resistance (PVR) were significantly reduced in six patients who breathed 40 ppm NO in 50% oxygen for 10 minutes. These hemodynamic changes were apparent immediately after beginning NO inhalation but had dissipated 30 minutes after inhalation was discontinued.

A study by Swedish investigators[12] in six healthy volunteers who breathed 12% oxygen to produce increases in pulmonary artery pressure demonstrated that the inhalation of 10 to 40 ppm of NO decreased hypoxic pulmonary vasoconstriction without affecting systemic hemodynamics.

Although anecdotal reports describe such findings, we are unaware of any large clinical trials in humans at this time. Methemoglobin production has not been shown to be a problem in the few studies to date. However, whether a critical duration of exposure and dose of NO produces potentially significant human blood cell abnormalities is unknown.

PHARMACOLOGIC TREATMENT

Because the underlying cause of most shock states is inadequate tissue or cellular perfusion, with the eventual loss of microcirculatory cellular integrity (leaky cell membranes), cell destruction, and death, it is reasonable to expect that potentially beneficial pharmacologic agents in shock therapy will have membrane-stabilizing properties. Glucocorticoids, when used early and in sufficiently large doses, have been thought to promote such effects, although most recent studies have reported little efficacy.

Calcium entry blockers, which regulate the transport of calcium ions across cell membranes, and agents that enhance or regulate endothelial function such as angiotensin-converting enzyme (ACE) inhibitors have been of limited value in humans. The calcium channel blocker nimodipine has been reported to improve neurologic outcome in patients with hypoxic or anoxic encephalopathy. In extensive clinical trials, however, its usefulness has not been convincingly proved.

Although ACE inhibitors such as captopril and enalapril are frequently used for the treatment of systemic hypertension and chronic congestive heart failure (CHF), fewer data on their effectiveness in patients with acute myocardial infarction are available. In animal models, ACE inhibitors reduce infarct size and enhance recovery of the stunned myocardium because they act as antioxidants or free radical scavengers.

Are Angiotensin-Converting Enzyme Inhibitors Useful in Acute Myocardial Infarction?

The Consensus-2 Trial

The Consensus-2 Trial,[13] in which enalaprilat was given intravenously followed by oral enalapril within the first 24 hours of an acute myocardial infarction, was stopped because of the lack of effect of the drug in the treatment group. The disappointing results of this trial emphasized the delicate situation prevailing in myocardial infarction. Although ACE inhibitors seem to decrease stress on the infarcted myocardium (scar) and to prevent or decrease ventricular remodeling (dilatation), the associated decrease in perfusion pressure may increase infarct size.

Critics of this trial state that the therapy may have been too aggressive and beneficial results might have been observed if enalaprilat and enalapril had been given in smaller doses (and with a more gradual increase in doses) to prevent hypotension and a concomitant increase in infarct size. Likewise, better patient selection might have improved outcome. Patients likely to benefit are those with the largest infarcts, who are most prone to ventricular dilatation. Therapy with ACE inhibitors should be followed by echocardiography to determine response and end point of therapy.

Other Benefits of Angiotensin-Converting Enzyme Inhibitor Therapy

ACE inhibitors are frequently used in patients with end-stage cardiomyopathies, especially those of ischemic origin, and in individuals awaiting cardiac transplantation. Captopril may actually improve the efficacy of vasodilators in the treatment of patients with cardiac failure, because it can block the vasodilator-induced increases in renin output.

In animals, ACE inhibitors have been shown to have a protective effect during hemorrhagic shock by reducing or inhibiting angiotensin II production by the vascular endothelium. The result is a reduction of systemic vascular resistance (SVR) and improved cardiac output. Such use in humans during acute hemorrhagic shock states has not proved to be efficacious.

Are Prostaglandins Useful?

Prostaglandins are capable of producing vasoconstriction or vasodilatation. The role of prostaglandins as mediators of effects on organ systems depends on the system under consideration.[14] PGI_2 has vasodilatory and membrane-stabilizing properties in animals. It is also a potent inhibitor of platelet aggregation. Thus, it may have a beneficial role in the treatment of shock as previously noted.

Prostaglandin E_1 and PGI_2 are currently used in patients with primary pulmonary hypertension to demonstrate vascular reactivity (vasoresponsiveness) and to predict the response to long-term vasodilatory therapy. PGI_2 is not inactivated in the lungs and is thus an effective vasodilator when administered intravenously. However, significant arterial hypotension may occur.

OXYGEN DELIVERY AND OXYGEN CONSUMPTION

The classic concept of the relationship between O_2 delivery ($\dot{D}O_2$), and O_2 consumption ($\dot{V}O_2$) assumes that under normal conditions, $\dot{V}O_2$ reflects metabolic demands. $\dot{V}O_2$ remains independent of $\dot{D}O_2$ over a wide range, until a critically low $\dot{D}O_2$ is reached. At that point, $\dot{V}O_2$ becomes supply dependent. Further reduction in $\dot{D}O_2$ below the critical level results in a fall in $\dot{V}O_2$, anaerobic metabolism, and lactic acidemia. Improved survival in low-flow states (i.e., cardiogenic and hemorrhagic shock) with elevation of $\dot{D}O_2$ to supernormal levels has been described.[15]

What Is Pathologic Oxygen Supply Dependency?

The theory underlying pathologic O_2 supply dependence is that at some critical $\dot{D}O_2$, compensatory mechanisms fail to maintain $\dot{V}O_2$.[16] Evidence validating the association of O_2-supply dependence—that is, $\dot{V}O_2$ varying directly with $\dot{D}O_2$ delivery—is indirect, because the invasive methods needed to prove the hypothesis are not clinically applicable. Lactate levels per se do not prove that tissue hypoxia exists.

Tissue hypoxia may be very "selective" in terms of the organ systems involved. Thus, when cardiogenic shock responds to treatment, large increases in $\dot{D}O_2$ may lead to only small increases in $\dot{V}O_2$ but marked increases in mixed venous oxygen saturation ($S\bar{v}O_2$), which reflects improved tissue O_2 availability.

Villar and colleagues[17] reported that spontaneous changes in $\dot{V}O_2$ and $\dot{D}O_2$ can occur in critically ill patients who have normal arterial lactate levels, even when no experimental intervention is performed. Such spontaneous changes complicate interpretation of studies demonstrating that delivery-limited $\dot{V}O_2$ occurs. A close overall correlation between $\dot{D}O_2$ and $\dot{V}O_2$ was found. Ten patients with a dependent relationship had normal blood lactate levels. A subset of patients within this group did not show this relationship.

The investigators cautioned that the therapeutic interventions involved in producing the increase in $\dot{D}O_2$ may also cause the increase in $\dot{V}O_2$. Blood transfusion, inotropic support, and some mechanical interventions are known to increase O_2 demands.

What Are Appropriate Oxygen Delivery and Consumption Goals in Hemorrhagic/Hypovolemic Shock?

The specific physiologic alterations that occur in hemorrhagic shock depend on the volume of blood loss, the rapidity with which it is lost, and the physical status and age of the patient before the hemorrhage occurred. Patients with significant acute blood loss have the greatest changes in hemodynamics and organ function and can be classified according to per cent of blood volume lost (Table 40–1).

Arterial vasoconstriction, which occurs secondary to the neuroendocrine response to hemorrhage, initially maintains the central aortic blood pressure at the expense of reduced flow to kidneys, liver, and skeletal muscle. During the early compensatory phase, despite the reduction in cardiac output, the heart and brain continue to receive a larger portion than other visceral organs because of selective redistribution of blood flow.

Therapy in the initial, compensated stage of hemorrhagic shock must be directed toward restoration of an adequate circulating blood volume in class III hemorrhagic shock and restoration of both fluid volume and red blood cell mass in class IV. The goal of resuscitation is to restore $\dot{V}O_2$ to whatever level is required to correct the shock-induced O_2 debt. If uncorrected, the latter results in multiorgan failure, eventual irreversible heart failure, and death.

PREHOSPITAL RESUSCITATION

What Are Military Antishock Trousers?

During field resuscitation after acute hemorrhage, inflatable military antishock trousers (MAST) have been recommended. Originally, they were thought to divert venous return from the subdiaphragmatic areas of the body to the heart and brain. Data now show that only about $4 \ mL \cdot kg^{-1}$ "autotransfusion" occurs in adults when MAST are inflated.[18] Therefore, blood volume displacement per se probably does not produce the hemodynamic changes associated with MAST inflation. The primary means by which central blood pressure is maintained is now thought to be reduction in the size of the perfused vascular bed and increase in SVR. Use of the MAST may reduce the time needed to control blood loss from the lower extremities and allow stabilization of pelvic and long bone fractures at the trauma site.[19, 20]

TABLE 40–1. Evaluation of Hemorrhage

Class	Amount (mL)	Blood Volume (%)	Pulse	Blood Pressure	Respiratory Rate	Skin	Urine (mL · h⁻¹)	Mental Status
I	≤750	15	↑ Possibly	No change	No change	No change	No change	Normal
II	1000–1250	20–25	100	↓ Pulse pressure	20–30	Capillary blanch	25–30	No change
III	1500–1800	30–35	120	↓ Systolic and ↓ pulse pressures	30–40	Prolonged blanch	5–15	Anxious, confused
IV	2000–2500	40–45	≥140	Systolic pressure <60 mm Hg	30–40	Pale and cool	0	Confused, lethargic

Are Military Antishock Trousers Dangerous?

Specific problems related to MAST use include interference with ventilation due to increased intra-abdominal pressure, an increase in intracranial pressure (ICP) secondary to impedance of venous return, possible pressure damage to tissues compressed beneath the MAST, and sudden severe hypotension, which may occur on MAST deflation. In head-injured patients, the potentially adverse effect of increased ICP may be outweighed by the benefits of maintaining cerebral perfusion pressure (CPP).[21]

MAST are contraindicated in cardiogenic shock and CHF with pulmonary edema, because the increase in SVR (afterload) and venous return (preload) produced by MAST inflation result in an increase in cardiac work and myocardial oxygen consumption ($M\dot{V}O_2$) and thereby aggravates the underlying problem.[21]

FLUID RESUSCITATION

The subject of fluid therapy is discussed extensively in Chapter 42 but is briefly reviewed here. Shoemaker and colleagues[22] believe that "fluid therapy controversies arise from a misconception: namely, the failure to differentiate clinically between excess and deficit of total body water, extracellular fluid (ECF), and plasma volume." Not uncommonly, a maldistribution of flow, with a contracted plasma volume and expanded interstitial water, occurs in trauma victims. Crystalloid should be used to replace ECF losses, and blood volume losses should be replaced with packed red blood cells and colloid plasma expanders.

Unfortunately, the values available for monitoring, such as arterial blood pressure, hemoglobin and hematocrit, central venous pressure (CVP), and pulmonary artery occlusion pressure (PAOP), often do not accurately reflect blood volume changes in hemorrhagic shock. Isotope dilution techniques, which are not available in clinical practice, are necessary to measure the distribution of water between the plasma, ECF, and intracellular fluid (ICF).

Our personal experience, research, and review of the current literature suggest that resuscitation in hemorrhagic shock is best accomplished with a combination of crystalloid and colloid solutions. Our colloid of choice is 5% albumin solution, although a 6% hetastarch has been used with comparable success. Our crystalloid of choice is lactated Ringer's solution. Electrolyte solutions alone probably are inadequate in profound shock.

What Are the Characteristics of Crystalloid Resuscitation?

When crystalloids are infused, the transient nature of intravascular volume expansion should be appreciated. Several factors must be considered.

Refill and Dispersal

Approximately one fourth of the infused crystalloid solution remains in the vascular bed, and three fourths is dispersed into the interstitial or intracellular space over time.

Sequestration

In hemorrhagic shock, sequestration of ECF occurs.[23] This fluid is not lost from the body but is "nonfunctional" in that it is no longer in dynamic equilibrium with the blood and ICF.

Volume Expansion Above Normal Levels

Sufficient volume must be infused to fill the expanded ECF and to provide adequate venous return to the heart. Weisel and colleagues[24] demonstrated that the large volume of crystalloid solution required to maintain satisfactory postoperative hemodynamics in 27 patients who had undergone coronary artery bypass grafting resulted in a delay in myocardial metabolic recovery. When compared with a similar group of patients who received colloid to maintain hemodynamic stability (i.e., mean arterial blood pressure, left atrial pressure, and cardiac index), the crystalloid-treated group required twice as much fluid to maintain normovolemia and developed more peripheral edema. Myocardial oxygen extraction and lactate production were delayed in their return to normal.

Dilutional Hypoproteinemia

Changes in colloid oncotic pressure (COP) may follow large-volume infusions of both crystalloids and colloids. How important this change is to individual organ function remains debatable.

Maintenance of Colloid Oncotic Pressure

Haupt and Rackow[25] examined the changes in plasma COP during resuscitation with 6% hetastarch solution, 5% albumin solution, or normal saline solution in 26 patients in hypovolemic circulatory shock. They reported that 1 L of hetastarch produced a 36% increase in COP; the same volume of 5% albumin solution resulted in an 11% increase. One liter of normal saline was associated with a 12% decrease in COP. The changes in COP persisted for 2 to 3 days after resuscitation. They concluded that a PAOP of 10 to 15 mm Hg as an end point for fluid resuscitation was more easily achieved, COP was increased more, and less volume was required when colloid solutions were used.

Nevertheless, the value of COP to guide the type and volume of fluid resuscitation needed is open to question. Davidson and colleagues[26] noted that COP is operationally determined under rather arbitrary and artificial in vitro laboratory conditions; therefore, it cannot be considered a direct indicator of in vivo effects, especially in shock associated with increased microvascular permeability.

What Are the Advantages of Hypertonic Saline?

Hypertonic 7.5% saline solution has been recommended as the initial fluid to be used for resuscitation in hemorrhagic shock. It produces similar results to lactated Ringer's solution, but the total volume of fluid required is much less. Sodium exerts its physiologic effect at the cell membrane and may restore toward normal the membrane potential, which has been altered during periods of hypotension. It may also prevent the cellular edema that occurs later in the shock phase secondary to the ICF shift.

Shimazaki and associates[27] measured respiratory function and body fluid changes in 46 burned patients for up to 6 days after burn. Patients were randomized into two groups. One group was resuscitated with hypertonic lactated saline solution and the other with lactated Ringer's. Extracellular distribution of the resuscitation fluid differed in the two groups. The ratio of plasma volume to interstitial fluid volume decreased with lactated Ringer's solution, and a deterioration in pulmonary function was noted compared with hypertonic saline.

What Are the Effects of Colloid Administration?

Pearl and colleagues[28] were unable to demonstrate any evidence that colloid solutions such as 5% albumin or 6% hydroxyethyl starch solutions differed from saline with respect to their effect on pulmonary function and extravascular lung water in dogs subjected to hemorrhagic shock. This similarity was thought to result from crystalloids and colloids having similar effects on plasma and interstitial COP. Hence, the net movement across the permeable pulmonary capillaries was equal with each fluid.

HEMOGLOBIN AND HEMATOCRIT

How Important Is Dilutional Anemia?

Oxygen is carried in the blood in two forms, dissolved and bound to hemoglobin. Dissolved oxygen amounts to 0.003 mL $\cdot$ dL^{-1} $\cdot$ mm Hg^{-1}. If one assumes a basal $\dot{V}O_2$ of 300 mL $\cdot$

min^{-1} and complete extraction of all dissolved O_2 (no hemoglobin present), cardiac output would need to approach 100 L $\cdot$ min^{-1} just to meet the basal need. Thus, hemoglobin is the important factor in O_2 transport, each gram combining with 1.39 mL of O_2. Tissue O_2 extraction is variable. Under basal conditions, 5 mL $\cdot$ dL^{-1} is consumed for every 20 mL $\cdot$ dL^{-1} delivered, leaving a "reserve" of 75%.

What Are the Determinants of Oxygen Transport?

The main determinants of O_2 transport are cardiac output, hemoglobin concentration, and the per cent saturation of oxyhemoglobin (HbO_2). Remember that although $\dot{D}O_2$ is a determinant of tissue oxygenation, it is not identical to the cellular O_2 supply. The latter may be inadequate despite a normal or elevated $\dot{D}O_2$ because of maldistribution of blood flow. Unfortunately, no clinically applicable methods by which cellular O_2 supply can be measured accurately are available. Nevertheless, the importance of maintaining adequate hemoglobin values (preventing excessive hemodilution) is apparent.

Hematocrit is a measure of the percentage of the red blood cells in a sample of arterial or venous blood. Initial and serial hematocrit values are frequently determined to assess the magnitude of initial blood loss and to monitor the course of fluid and blood volume replacement. Hematocrit is a static measurement of the amount of red blood cells in a sample, the absolute value of which may be influenced by sampling, techniques of measurement, fluid (crystalloid or colloid) infusion, red blood cell transfusion, and transcapillary refill or loss between the interstitial and intravascular spaces. Hence, it is not reliable during the acute, dynamic, and uncompensated phases of shock.

How Is Myocardial Oxygen Consumption Affected by Anemia?

During acute anemia, coronary blood flow increases out of proportion to the compensatory increase in cardiac output. This response is accomplished by coronary vasodilatation secondary to the imposed increase in myocardial oxygen consumption (M$\dot{V}O_2$) required to increase cardiac output. Coronary sinus partial pressure of oxygen (PO_2) is about 10 mm Hg when the hematocrit reaches 12.5%. Thus, almost complete extraction of coronary artery blood O_2 has occurred at this hematocrit level.

Ischemic coronary artery disease significantly affects the ability of this compensatory mechanism to provide adequate O_2. Myocardial ischemia with resultant decrease in cardiac output thwarts the heart in its quest to compensate for acute anemia. Patients who have reduced cardiac reserve secondary to cardiomyopathy (ischemic or nonischemic), valvular heart disease, or pharmacologic agents also may be unable to compensate for acute hemorrhage by increasing cardiac output.

What Is the Critical Oxygen Delivery?

Shibutani and colleagues[29] studied 58 anesthetized patients with known coronary artery disease during the prebypass period for coronary artery bypass surgery (Fig. 40–1). When the $\dot{D}O_2$ decreases to 330 mL $\cdot$ min^{-1} $\cdot$ m$^{2-1}$, a marked decrease in O_2 uptake occurs; therefore, mixed venous blood may remain saturated. At $\dot{D}O_2$ levels >330 mL $\cdot$ min^{-1} $\cdot$ m$^{2-1}$, a reduction of mixed venous O_2 partial pressure and saturation ($P\bar{v}O_2$ and $S\bar{v}O_2$) was found to be proportional to the decrease in $\dot{D}O_2$. They concluded that a reduction in $\dot{D}O_2$ below the critical level of 330 mL $\cdot$ min^{-1} $\cdot$ m$^{2-1}$ should be interpreted as evidence of tissue O_2 deprivation.

Wilkerson and associates[30] performed gradual total body hemodilution using 5% human serum albumin in baboons. Isovolemic hemodilution was well tolerated to a hematocrit of 10%. Below that level, a sharp drop in $\dot{V}O_2$ was associated with a similar decrease in $\dot{D}O_2$ (Fig. 40–2). Significant lactate production occurred (Fig. 40–3), and the whole body O_2 extraction ratio was 50%, compared with the normal 25%. The total body extraction ratio thus appears to be a valid indicator of myocardial metabolism in anemic states.

What Are Acceptable Hemoglobin/Hematocrit Values?

Hypovolemic and Normovolemic Anemia

Acute hypovolemic anemia (hemorrhage) differs considerably from normovolemic hemodilutional anemia.[31] In the latter case, an increase in cardiac output and stroke volume results from a decrease in blood viscosity and SVR. In acute hemorrhage, the neuroendocrine compensatory response produces an increase in SVR and the cardiac output usually decreases because of volume loss and reduced venous return to the heart.

Blood viscosity may not change initially, because both plasma and red blood cells are lost together. Over time, it may actually increase if significant traumatic ECF sequestration occurs. Thus, the work of the heart increases.

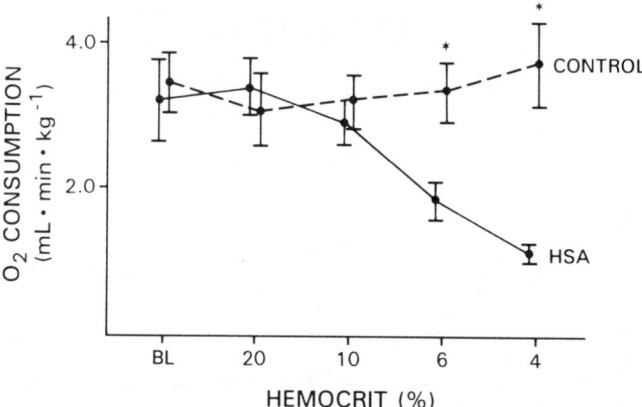

FIGURE 40–2. Total O_2 consumption versus hematocrit for the experimental human serum albumin (HSA) group. Control group data were obtained at equivalent volume-exchange points. Difference between groups is significant ($P < 0.05$) at hematocrits of 6 and 4%. BL = Baseline. (From Wilkerson DK, Rosen AL, Gould SA, et al: Oxygen extraction ratio: a valid indicator of myocardial metabolism in anemia. J Surg Res 1987; 42:629–634.)

Viscosity

Viscosity is a measure of the thickness or consistency of a liquid. Blood is a non-newtonian fluid, and its viscosity is shear/flow rate dependent[32] (Fig. 40–4). Changes in blood temperature also affect viscosity. At a hematocrit of 45%, a decrease in blood temperature from 37°C to 25°C results in a 50% increase in blood viscosity. The temperature change may counteract the viscosity benefit of reductions in hematocrit and is another reason to maintain body and blood temperature during resuscitation.

What Levels Can Normal Patients Tolerate?

Can arbitrary levels for minimum hemoglobin and hematocrit levels that are safe for all individuals be set? Obviously, the answer is no. Oxygen content (CaO_2) is an important deter-

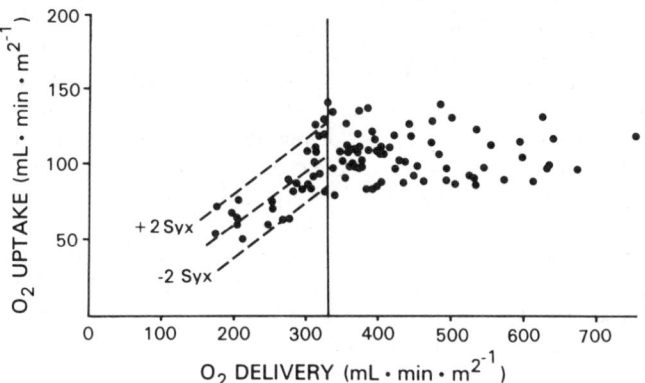

FIGURE 40–1. Relationship between $\dot{D}O_2$ and $\dot{D}O_2$ based on 99 sets of measurements in 58 patients. The *vertical line* is a linear regression calculated from the data points where $\dot{D}O_2$ was less than 330 mL/min $\cdot$ m^2. The *dashed lines* show 2 SE of estimate. (From Shibutani K, Komatsu T, Kubal K, et al: Critical level of oxygen delivery in anesthetized man. Crit Care Med 1983; 11:640–643, © Williams & Wilkins, 1983.)

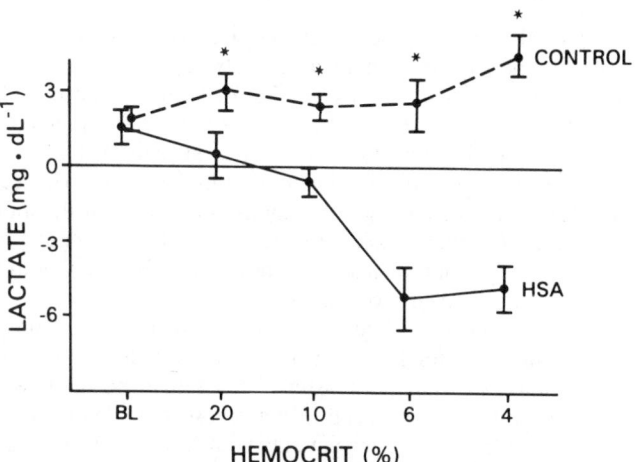

FIGURE 40–3. Net lactate concentration across the left ventricle versus hematocrit for the experimental human serum albumin (HSA) group. Control group data were obtained at equivalent volume-exchange points. Difference between groups is significant ($P < 0.05$) at hematocrits of 20, 10, 6, and 4%. (From Wilkerson DK, Rosen AL, Gould SA, et al: Oxygen extraction ratio: a valid indicator of myocardial metabolism in anemia. J Surg Res 1987; 42:629–634.)

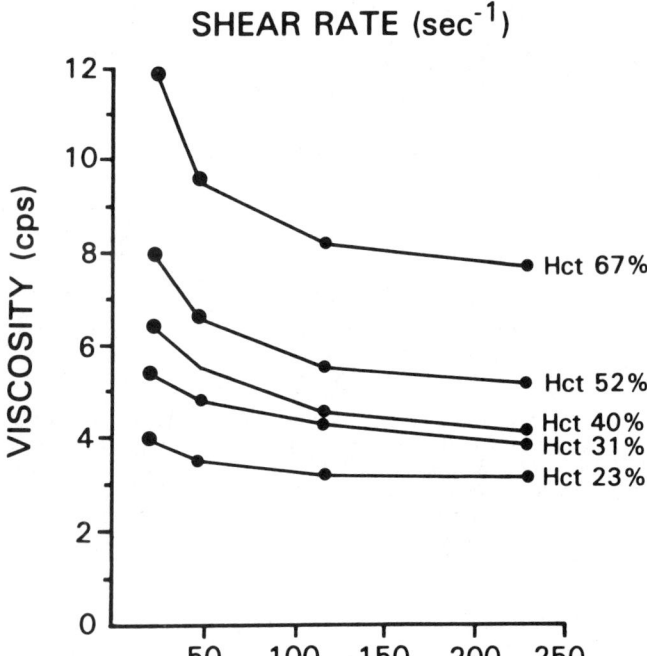

FIGURE 40–4. Relationship of apparent viscosity to shear rate for blood samples obtained from five subjects with different hematocrits. It is important to note that the higher the hematocrit, the greater the shear rate dependence of viscosity; that is, a decrease in shear rate from 46 to 23 s^{-1} results in a considerably greater increase in viscosity for blood with a hematocrit of 67% than for blood with a hematocrit of 23%. (From Burch GE, De Pasquale NP: Hematocrit, viscosity, and coronary blood flow. Dis Chest 1965; 48:225–232. © Williams & Wilkins, 1965.)

minant of tissue O_2 transport. Clinical and experimental evidence show that patients who have satisfactory cardiac reserve and are normovolemic may tolerate a hemoglobin of 6 g · dL^{-1} and hematocrit of 18%.[33]

What Levels Can Critically Ill Patients Tolerate?

Survival among critically ill surgical patients is highest when the hematocrit is maintained between 27% and 33%.[15] Several factors must be considered to determine an acceptable or optimal hematocrit (or what level a particular patient can tolerate). They include (1) age and physical status, (2) coexisting disease (especially pulmonary, cardiac, or cerebrovascular), (3) degree of anemia, (4) rapidity of onset and duration of anemia, (5) blood volume status, (6) extent of injury or trauma, and (7) additional surgical procedures that are required as part of the resuscitative process.

Indirect evidence of human tolerance may be drawn from a case-control study of 125 surgical patients who declined blood transfusions for religious reasons.[34] Operative mortality was found to be inversely related to the preoperative hemoglobin level, rising from 7.1% for patients with levels >10 g · dL^{-1} to 61.5% for those with levels <6 g · dL^{-1}. Mortality rates were also related to the amount of blood lost during surgery. No patient died who had a hemoglobin level >8 g · dL^{-1} and operative blood loss <500 mL.

Animal or human studies that define physiologic changes and limits during isovolemic hemodilution may not be transferable to hypovolemic, anemic shock states. Clinical and he-

modynamic response to acute bleeding and resuscitative efforts are more important than hemoglobin and hematocrit levels. CVP measurements may be helpful during early resuscitative efforts. However, many factors influence the CVP. The often poor relationship between CVP and blood volume suggests that caution be exercised in relying on this parameter to assess blood volume in critically ill patients (Fig. 40–5).

Are Blood Substitutes Helpful?

Recombinant Hemoglobin

Recombinant hemoglobin solutions used during hemodilution could have numerous advantages, most notably reduction of transfusion-related infection. In addition to sterility and availability, they also have a longer storage life compared with blood. However, these solutions probably will not be available for human use until the mid-1990s at the earliest.[35, 36]

Perfluorocarbon Emulsions

The perfluorocarbon chemical emulsion Fluosol-DA 20%, an acellular oxygen carrier, has had limited use in humans as a red blood cell substitute in acute anemia. Studies of Jehovah's Witnesses who refused blood on religious grounds indicate that the inadequate total oxygen content of the 20% Fluosol solution renders it ineffective as a red blood cell substitute.

What Are the Effects of Isovolemic Hemodilution on the Brain?

Nago and associates[37] carried out hemodilution in stepwise fashion in ten anesthetized normocarbic (35–40 mm Hg Paco$_2$) baboons by isovolemic exchange transfusions using 6% normal-molecular-weight dextran. Neural activity during hemodilution and after reinfusion was assessed by monitoring somatosensory evoked potentials (SSEP) and visual evoked potentials (VEP).

At hematocrit levels from 10% to 15%, the SSEP latencies were significantly increased, probably as a result of peripheral nerve and spinal cord hypoxia. Oxygen supply to the brain was maintained, however, owing to an increase in cerebral blood flow (CBF). This effect was attributed to vasodilation and decreases in blood viscosity caused by cerebral hypoxia. However, at hematocrit values <10%, a significant increase in all latencies and decreases in amplitude of both SSEP and VEP occurred. These were believed to result from the brain's neural function being adversely effected by such severe anemia.

Reinfusion of packed red blood cells did not immediately lead to recovery of neural function in these animals. Based on these primate data, the investigators recommend that hemodilution be limited to hematocrit values >15%.

Most shock states represent incomplete global brain ischemia. When CBF is reduced to <10% of normal, the elevated intracellular lactate and decrease in washout of tissue catabolites may result in greater cellular damage than would occur with global ischemia. Likewise, very low blood flow to the ischemic tissues may allow increased free radical production and a reperfusion-type membrane injury.

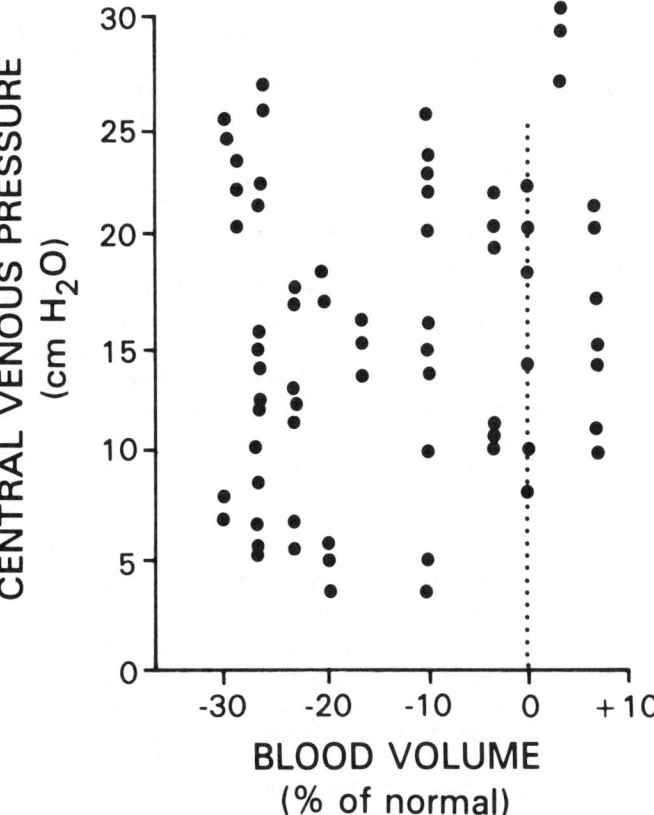

FIGURE 40–5. CVP values plotted against their corresponding measured blood volumes in a consecutive unselected series of intensive care unit patients. Note the lack of relationship of CVP to blood volume; many high CVP values are associated with low blood volumes, and many low CVP values are associated with normal blood volumes. (From Shoemaker WC, Thompson WL, Holbrook PR: Textbook of Critical Care. WB Saunders, 1984, p 111.)

What Is the Effect of Hypocapnia on Dilutional Anemia?

Mitchenfelder and Theye[38] studied the effects of profound hypocapnia and dilutional anemia on canine cerebral metabolism and blood flow. They found that although CBF was well maintained in dogs subjected to a $PaCO_2$ of 11 mm Hg and isovolemic anemia to a hemoglobin of 5 g $\cdot$ dL^{-1}, a reduction in the cerebral metabolic rate for consumption of oxygen ($CMRO_2$) occurred. The reduction in $CMRO_2$ was thought to result from a reduction in O_2 extracted from the blood secondary to the effect of alkalosis on HbO_2 dissociation. This decrease in $CMRO_2$ occurred despite the fact that the amounts of O_2 delivered to the brain, during both normocarbia and hypocarbia, were virtually unchanged. Neither the reduction in $PaCO_2$ nor hemodilution independently resulted in reduced $CMRO_2$.

Therefore, data suggest that the brain can safely tolerate normovolemic anemia to 6 g $\cdot$ dL^{-1}, but that hypocapnia with resultant respiratory alkalosis should be avoided because of its effect on HbO_2 dissociation. The applicability of these data to patients with occlusive cerebral vascular disease is uncertain.

What Effect Does Acute Normovolemic Anemia Have on the Myocardium?

The subendocardium of the left ventricle is perfused mainly during diastole. Oxygen delivery is determined by the CaO_2 and coronary blood flow. Brazier and colleagues[39] studied the effects of normovolemic anemia in anesthetized dogs with normal coronary arteries. When hemoglobin was reduced to 5

g $\cdot$ dL^{-1} or lower, total left ventricular coronary blood flow increased; however, the proportion of subendocardial flow fell by 35%, and the endocardial/epicardial flow ratio diminished below 1.0. When CaO_2 was normal, subendocardial O_2 delivery per unit of demand was significantly higher.

Subendocardial ST segments were elevated 5 mm above baseline, whereas those from the epicardial area remained isoelectric at the time when the endocardial/epicardial flow ratio was <1.0 (Fig. 40–6).

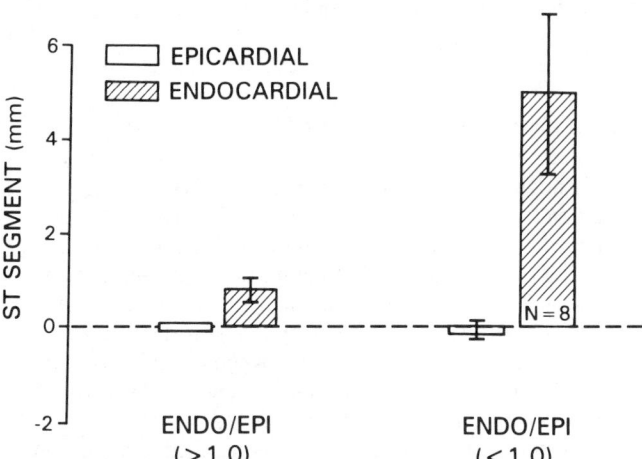

FIGURE 40–6. The change in ST segment (from isoelectric) during control (Hgb > 10 g $\cdot$ dL^{-1}) and with severe anemia (Hgb < 5 g $\cdot$ dL^{-1}). *Note*: Although the ST segment of the epicardial lead remains isoelectric during control (endocardial/epicardial flow ratio > 1.0), with severe anemia (endocardial/epicardial flow ratio < 1.0) the ST segment on the intracavitary lead becomes significantly elevated. (From Brazier J, Cooper N, Maloney JV, et al: The adequacy of myocardial oxygen delivery in acute normovolemic anemia. Surgery 1974; 75:508–516.)

One must once again be cautious in transferring these animal data to patients. The normal human coronary vasculature has the ability to "autoregulate" between mean arterial pressures of 60 and 140 mm Hg. Once maximal coronary vasodilatation has occurred, coronary blood flow is directly related to perfusion pressure.

Hypertension, valvular heart disease, elevated circulating catecholamines, and fever may cause an increase in O_2 demand. Concurrently, an inability to increase O_2 supply may result from coronary artery disease or β-blockers. Coronary vasodilatation may be maximal; therefore, no coronary vasodilatory reserve remains to compensate for the imposition of acute anemia.[40] Subendocardial ischemia (in these patient subsets) may therefore occur at much higher hemoglobin levels.

Reductions in systolic and diastolic perfusion pressure usually accompany acute blood loss. A significant reduction in coronary perfusion pressure decreases a patient's tolerance to acute anemia.

CARDIOGENIC SHOCK

To make the diagnosis of cardiogenic shock, specific criteria must be met. The definition proposed by the National Heart, Lung and Blood Institute includes patients who, despite optimal preload levels, maximum inotropic support, and intra-aortic balloon support, are unable to maintain a cardiac index >1.8 L $\cdot$ min^{-1} $\cdot$ m$^{2-1}$, SVR <2100 dynes $\cdot$ s^{-1} $\cdot$ cm^{-5-1}, systolic blood pressure >90 mm Hg, right and left atrial pressures <20 mm Hg, and urinary output >20 mL $\cdot$ h^{-1}.

The incidence of cardiogenic shock complicating acute myocardial infarction ranges from 5% to 15%. Cardiogenic shock is the most frequent complication leading to death in the coronary care unit after acute myocardial infarction. Despite dramatic improvements in coronary care, in-hospital mortality still remains in the 80% to 90% range when treatment consists of only pharmacologic intervention. Standard drug therapy with sympathomimetic amines has not significantly improved survival. Although the β-adrenergic agonists may increase both the force and velocity of myocardial contraction, their positive inotropic effect is achieved only at the expense of increased $M\dot{V}_{O_2}$.

What Are Its Characteristics?

Cardiogenic shock most frequently occurs in the following situations[41]: (1) when 40% or more of the myocardial mass is damaged; (2) in occlusion of the proximal left anterior descending coronary artery (left main trunk equivalent) with lack of adequate collateral circulation; (3) when more than one infarct is present; (4) in severe multivessel disease with both previous and recent infarct; and (5) when acute left or bilateral bundle branch block develops after an anterior Q wave infarction has occurred.

Beyersdorf and colleagues[42] demonstrated that in cardiogenic shock, the immediate and persistent failure of ischemic muscle to contract and contribute to systemic blood flow places the hemodynamic burden of supporting the circulation elsewhere. A significant amount of shortening of remote, nonischemic muscle is expended in stretching the ischemic zone during isovolumetric systole, thus reducing the available shortening during the ejection phase. Systolic shortening of the nonischemic muscle must increase to 150% or more of control values in order to maintain preischemic hemodynamic function.

Beyersdorf's group also demonstrated that anaerobic metabolism and signs of energy depletion may occur in the normally perfused remote cardiac muscle segments. Flow may have been insufficient to meet metabolic demands, perhaps because of autoregulatory failure. A depletion of substrate and energy stores in remote muscle occurs despite the maintenance of normal or increased blood flow. Thus, remote hypokinesis, which precedes hemodynamic deterioration, should be viewed as a warning sign of cardiogenic shock.

Noninvasive echocardiographic monitoring may be used to evaluate the myocardial contractile state and may also be helpful to monitor improvement, or lack thereof, in wall motion in the infarct-related arterial distribution after thrombolytic therapy or direct percutaneous transluminal coronary angioplasty (PTCA) has been performed.

What Is the Mortality Rate?

Goldberg and colleagues[43] found that neither the incidence nor the prognosis of cardiogenic shock resulting from acute myocardial infarction improved between 1975 and 1988. They reported cardiogenic shock in 7.5% of a study population with acute myocardial infarction and an in-hospital mortality of 81.7%. However, aggressive and timely use of thrombolytic agents or interventional techniques, such as primary angioplasty or emergency coronary artery bypass surgery, may improve outcome.

Are the New Therapeutic Modalities Effective?

More than 90% of the patients who develop cardiogenic shock may not show signs of left ventricular power failure until 1 hour or more after coronary occlusion has occurred. Vasodilators, β-blockers, and afterload reduction agents, which are considered a temporizing procedure, do not salvage ischemic muscle or permanently improve blood flow to remote muscle. The infarct-related vessel must be acutely opened, either by thrombolysis, direct primary PTCA, or coronary artery bypass grafting, in order to reduce infarct size, relieve ischemia in the myocardium supplied by the infarct-related artery as well as remote muscle, and prevent progressive ventricular dysfunction and cardiogenic shock. Early reperfusion is the sine qua non of enhanced early and late survival.

Time Constraints

Data from the ISIS-3[44] and EMIRAS[45] studies support a reduction in the time of the therapeutic window previously reported for the successful application of thrombolytic therapy or direct PTCA. Early studies indicating that treatment was effective if instituted within a 12- to 24-hour time frame were incorrect. Current data show that the infarct-related artery must be opened within 1 hour of the onset of symptoms for maximum benefit. However, even late use of thrombolytic therapy appears to limit myocardial remodeling and possibly to reduce ventricular aneurysm formation and dysrhythmias (late sequelae).

Effective thrombolytic therapy, adjunctive thrombin inhibitors and platelet antagonists, PTCA or surgical revascularization, and, where necessary, mechanical circulatory assistance and appropriate pharmacologic therapy reduce the incidence of developing cardiogenic shock and the mortality due to extensive myocardial infarction.

Note, however, that although thrombolytic agents may be helpful in prevention, once cardiogenic shock has developed, they have not been consistently shown to improve survival rates. Furthermore, although early surgical revascularization has been reported to improve survival,[46] the mortality rate is 30% to 60%, unless the cause is a surgically correctable mechanical complication of acute myocardial infarction such as ventricular septal defect, rupture of papillary muscle, or rupture of ventricular free wall.

Limiting Factors in Surgical Revascularization

The limiting factor in surgical revascularization may be that the myocardium supplied by the infarct-related artery has limited tolerance to further ischemia. During bypass surgery, despite myocardial preservation during aortic cross-clamping, the myocardium may suffer additional intraoperative damage. For this reason, some surgeons suggest that aortic cross-clamping be avoided in this high-risk subset of patients and that instead, ventricular fibrillation be induced during the distal anastomosis while maintaining core body temperature at ≤ 32 °C.

Thrombolysis and Angioplasty

Several studies report that thrombolysis or coronary angioplasty or both reduce the mortality of cardiogenic shock. Mortality in patients whose infarct-related artery was acutely opened and reperfused after thrombolytic therapy was reduced to 42% in one large series.[47] Likewise, the success rate for acute intervention with primary PTCA is reported to approximate 75% or higher. In those patients with an open artery after PTCA, mortality rate varied between 25% and 30%; when the infarcted artery could not be opened, mortality was 80% to 90%.

The GISSI trial,[48] reported in 1986, however, showed high mortality in patients who were treated with intravenous streptokinase alone. Indeed, thrombolytic therapy, either conventional or intracoronary, in many reported studies has been associated with low success rates of recanalization for patients in cardiogenic shock. Some trials have demonstrated that only 70% of the thrombolytic attempts are successful; 15% to 20% of those arteries reocclude silently and often very early after intervention. Even those attempts that were successful may leave significant residual stenosis in >85% of treated lesions.

Direct PTCA in acute myocardial infarction is used in many institutions throughout North America because of the higher success rate in opening the infarct-related artery and lower residual stenosis when compared with thrombolytic therapy (estimated 70% success rate). Lee and colleagues[49] reported successful reperfusion with direct coronary angioplasty in 80% to 90% of acute myocardial infarctions, especially in single-vessel cases. Others have used immediate coronary angioplasty with success rates approximating 78%; hospital mortalities were 35% in those patients for whom perfusion was possible, versus >72% when the infarct-related artery was unable to be perfused.

Reperfusion and Myocardial Salvage

Because myocardial infarction is an evolving process, starting in the endocardium and progressing to the epicardium, early reperfusion of the infarct-related injury should be expected to reduce myocardial necrosis and mortality. However, controversy about the relationship between myocardial salvage and mortality persists. Salvage depends on such variables as the presence or absence of collateral circulation to the infarct-related area and the $M\dot{V}O_2$. In patients who lack collaterals and have a high $M\dot{V}O_2$, reperfusion, to be successful, probably has to be accomplished within 40 to 60 minutes from the onset of symptoms.

If myocardial salvage is the end point of therapy, early opening of the infarct-related artery is of paramount importance, and the techniques by which this is accomplished are probably secondary. Similar success has been demonstrated for all interventions, although specific factors (e.g., the presence or absence of left ventricular dysfunction, available facilities, multivessel disease) may influence one's choice of therapy.

Reocclusion

The rate of success in restoring patency of an infarct-related artery may be higher with primary PTCA than with thrombolytic therapy, but the rate of reocclusion is higher after PTCA than after thrombolytic therapy. Reocclusion after either therapy is associated with a significant increase in mortality. Direct primary PTCA may also cause distal embolization into peripheral vessels, leading to microinfarctions; therefore, some clinicians use intracoronary thrombolytic agents during the primary PTCA to prevent or reduce embolization.

What Are the Major Problems/Complications of Therapy?

Acute Closure and Restenosis

Acute closure and restenosis remain the major limiting problems following angioplasty in nonemergent situations. Acute closure occurs in 4% to 8% of the patients undergoing balloon angioplasty, and restenosis in 30% to 40% of the patients who have had successful dilatation. Acute closure is usually manifested within the first 6 to 12 hours after PTCA and is most commonly due to spasm, mechanical dissection or disruption of the coronary arterial wall by the balloon, or plaque separation and development of a thrombus.[50] Moderate injury to the subendothelium of the coronary vessel during angioplasty stimulates platelet, thrombus, and fibrin deposition, whereas deep injury to the media of the vessel wall is an even more powerful stimulus to thrombosis from platelet aggregation and activation of the coagulation cascade.

Stent Placement

Numerous interventions to prevent or manage acute closure after angioplasty, including scaffolding of the interior vessel wall by stents or laser balloon angioplasty, have been applied with various degrees of success. The most experience with stents to treat acute closure has been at Emory University. Approximately 140 stents were placed between 1988 and 1991. Poststent complications were significant. Of the patients in whom stents were placed for the treatment of acute closure, 18.9% required coronary artery bypass. Bleeding that required transfusion occurred in 10% to 25% of these patients.

A significant number, on restudy, showed restenosis in the stented artery. Stents are thrombogenic and therefore require anticoagulation after their placement. Various methods to control or prevent the bleeding associated with anticoagulant therapy after stent placement are being studied. Specific antithrombin agents to reduce heparin dosage, as well as local antithrombolytic therapy at the site of stent implantation, may obviate systemic anticoagulation.

Laser Balloon Angioplasty

Grines[51] reported a technical success rate of 95% in 154 attempts with laser balloon angioplasty for the management of acute closure or restenosis after balloon angioplasty. Her end points were a 50% residual stenosis and adequate flow within the coronary blood vessel. However, in one series of 25 patients in whom Grines used laser balloon angioplasty, 16% required emergency coronary artery bypass, and an additional 16% had Q wave infarction; the overall death rate was 8%. Thus, significant morbidity and mortality are associated with acute coronary occlusion after balloon angioplasty, even with the rather heroic modalities for management that are currently available.

How Effective Is Heparin Therapy?

Residual thrombus may remain after thrombolytic therapy. Heparin does not prevent the formation or evolution of an arterial thrombus in all patients with deep arterial injury after trauma or PTCA. A residual thrombus can cause continued activation of clotting factors, most notably factor V, and platelet deposition. This sequence perpetuates continued thrombin generation and eventual restenosis of the vessel. Intravenous heparin, 30,000 USP units per 24 hours, is usually necessary to produce therapeutic plasma heparin levels. Partial thromboplastin time must be maintained above 1.5 times normal to reduce the incidence of thrombosis.

Specific inhibitors to thromboxane A_2 and serotonin also do not prevent acute arterial thrombosis. Hirudin, a potent thrombin inhibitor, however, does inhibit fibrin and platelet deposition to less than a single layer, thus preventing arterial thrombosis in injured arteries despite conditions of high or low flow.[52]

Remember that thrombosis occurs in seconds, but lysis of a thrombus requires hours. To reduce the incidence of restenosis from intravascular thrombus formation, a steady-state blood level of antithrombin agents must be provided. A bolus of heparin followed by continuous infusion is superior to intermittent bolus injections. Anesthesiologists should be aware of this fact and avoid discontinuation of the heparin infusion in the operating room before the establishment of invasive monitoring and the induction of anesthesia.

What Is the Scope of Thrombolytic Therapy?

In the United States, only 20% of patients with acute myocardial infarction meet the eligibility requirements for thrombolytic therapy; the main contraindication is a period >6 hours since the onset of symptoms. Among those few patients eligible for thrombolytic therapy, only a minority actually receive it. Mortality rates among patients who are ineligible for thrombolytic therapy are greater than for those who are eligible to receive it.

In the TIMI-2B study,[53] among a subset of 1471 patients with acute myocardial infarction, only 15.6% met the eligibility criteria. This group had a 3.9% in-hospital mortality, whereas that of patients with contraindications to thrombolysis was 18.7%. Patients with ST segment depression accompanying their anginal symptoms did not respond well to thrombolytic therapy. They had a higher mortality rate than those with ST segment elevations.

Probable reasons included a longer period of symptoms, a higher number of females in the subset, a history of multiple prior infarctions, and the presence of multivessel disease with collateral blood flow that prevented ST segment elevation. Also of note is that patients who were older than 75 years and who had no other contraindications to thrombolytic therapy and who therefore were treated had a significantly reduced mortality compared with those in the same age range who were not treated.

Beta-Blockers Following Thrombolytic Therapy

In the ISIS-2 Study,[54] early death (day 0 and 1) in those patients who received thrombolytic therapy with streptokinase was associated with an increase in the incidence of cardiac rupture and stroke. In a subset of these patients treated with β-adrenergic blockers, the incidence of early cardiac ruptures was reduced. Afterload reducers such as ACE inhibitors may also decrease the incidence of early cardiac rupture.

When β-blockers and ACE inhibitors are used after thrombolytic therapy, the hemodynamic effects must be monitored carefully. Although some reduction in systolic and diastolic blood pressure is beneficial, marked reduction may reduce coronary artery perfusion and worsen the infarction.

What Is the Success Rate of Percutaneous Transluminal Coronary Angioplasty in Multiple- Versus Single-Vessel Disease?

Results of direct angioplasty in patients with cardiogenic shock and multivessel disease have been disappointing when compared with patients with single-vessel disease. Therefore, many investigators recommend acute surgical revascularization for patients with multivessel disease and cardiogenic shock.

When primary angioplasty is unsuccessful or when acute closure or a dissection occurs and immediate rescue bypass grafting is scheduled, "bail-out" catheters may be of value. If they can be passed by the coronary artery obstruction, blood flows in the proximal holes and out the distal holes of these catheters, perfusing the infarct-related area until surgical revascularization can be accomplished.

What Is the Benefit of Surgical Revascularization?

In most centers, surgical revascularization in patients in cardiogenic shock is usually accomplished with reverse saphenous vein grafts for ease of operation and infusion of cardioplegia solution into the areas of ischemia. Some surgeons prefer not to arrest the heart and avoid cross-clamping of the aorta to avoid an ischemic period. Aortic anastomosis is accomplished first with partial cross-clamping, after which the saphenous vein is sutured to the infarct-related vessel during induced ventricular fibrillation. Surgery for cardiogenic shock also offers the benefit of revascularization of the stenotic, noninfarct-related arteries.

Guyton and colleagues[55] state that in patients who had cardiogenic shock and who had previously undergone coronary artery bypass graft, expeditious surgical revascularization is much more difficult. They recommend that an intra-aortic balloon pump be inserted at the time of coronary catheterization and that aggressive attempts be made to restore coronary flow by angioplasty techniques.

Patients who are considered for emergency surgical revascularization must be operable candidates, with angiographic visualization of at least one proximally stenosed coronary artery that supplies either viable or infarcting myocardium. Balooki[56] reported an operative mortality of 40% for infarctectomy and revascularization of patients in cardiogenic shock. He states that the goal of surgical therapy in cardiogenic shock is to revascularize all ischemic areas adjacent to the zone of acute myocardial infarction, as well as those disparate from it.

What Are the Endpoints for Resuscitation?

Shoemaker[57] states, "There is considerable concurrence with the concept that the essence of resuscitation from acute circulatory failure is not the return of so-called vital signs but the restoration of tissue perfusion, circulatory function and body metabolism." Forrester and colleagues[58] demonstrated that the direction and magnitude of the hemodynamic response to therapy in patients who had sustained acute myocardial infarction varied with the pretreatment level of cardiac index and PAOP.

Although the cardiac index and PAOP values show wide variability among patients with acute myocardial infarction, hemodynamically distinct subsets may be identified as having diagnostic, therapeutic, and prognostic relevance for management (Fig. 40–7). Mortality is highest in patients with pulmonary congestion and hypoperfusion. Patients with a cardiac index of $2.2 \ L \cdot min^{-1} \cdot m^{2-1}$ or greater have improved survival.

How high the cardiac index should be raised with inotropic and intra-aortic balloon counterpulsation (IABP) in patients in cardiogenic shock is more difficult to answer. Creamer and colleagues[59] studied hemodynamic and oxygen transport variables in patients in cardiogenic shock following acute myocardial infarction. They were able to improve cardiac index from $1.2 \ L \cdot min^{-1} \cdot m^{2-1}$ to $2.5 \ L \cdot min^{-1} \cdot m^{2-1}$ in some patients by maximizing inotropic support. This improvement in cardiac index, however, was associated with a minimal increase in Do_2 from $230 \ mL \cdot min^{-1} \cdot m^{2-1}$ to $397 \ mL \cdot min^{-1} \cdot m^{2-1}$. Oxygen use only increased from $103 \ mL \cdot min^{-1} \cdot m^{2-1}$ to $124 \ mL \cdot min^{-1} \cdot m^{2-1}$, and $S\bar{v}o_2$ from 56% to 69%. The O_2 extraction ratio decreased from 48% to 31%. Hence, the increase in Do_2 was considerably greater than the increase in Vo_2. The heart, therefore, may have been driven harder than was needed. Attempts to provide supranormal hemodynamic values, as has been recommended, are unnecessary for patients in cardiogenic shock and may be detrimental.

Cardiac index and O_2 delivery should be increased sufficiently to maintain a $S\bar{v}o_2$ of 60% or greater and to reverse hyperlactacidemia. A cardiac index of 2 to $2.2 \ L \cdot min^{-1} \cdot m^{2-1}$ with a hematocrit of 32% or greater usually suffices. Remember that isovolemic anemia with very low hematocrit values may cause a reversal in the epicardial/endocardial blood flow ratio and a reduction in pressure across significant coronary artery stenotic lesions (viscosity effect).

What Is the Role of Mechanical Assistance?

Intra-Aortic Balloon Counterpulsation

In patients with cardiogenic shock or low cardiac output syndromes, IABP may increase coronary artery perfusion, reduce $M\dot{V}o_2$, increase coronary collateral blood flow, and increase cerebral and coronary perfusion pressure in early diastole. The reduction in left ventricular end-diastolic pressure (LVEDP) and volume is accomplished by a reduction in aortic

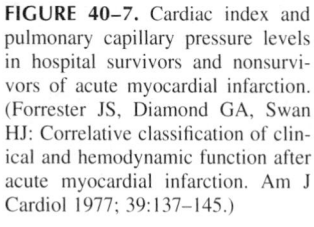

FIGURE 40–7. Cardiac index and pulmonary capillary pressure levels in hospital survivors and nonsurvivors of acute myocardial infarction. (Forrester JS, Diamond GA, Swan HJ: Correlative classification of clinical and hemodynamic function after acute myocardial infarction. Am J Cardiol 1977; 39:137–145.)

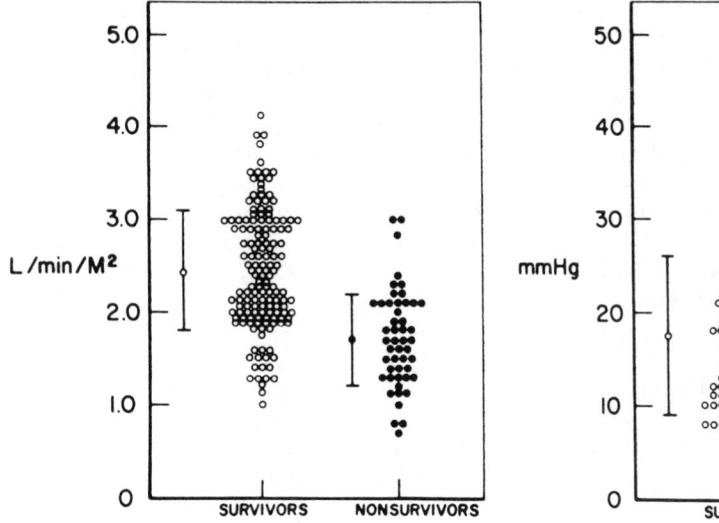

impedance at end-diastole. Thus IABP simultaneously enhances myocardial O_2 supply and diminishes myocardial O_2 demand, in contrast to catecholamine therapy, which generally increases myocardial blood supply at the expense of increased myocardial O_2 demand.

This therapy is most beneficial when used in patients with moderate and reversible left ventricular dysfunction. It is not capable of generating forward flow by itself; therefore, sufficient pump function of the native myocardium must exist. In cardiogenic shock or acute myocardial infarction, IABP may delay the onset of myocardial necrosis and reduce infarct size if prompt reperfusion of the ischemic myocardium can be accomplished.

Application

The intra-aortic balloon is filled with helium or carbon dioxide and is positioned in the descending aorta, just distal to the left subclavian artery. Care should be taken to avoid placing the balloon tip in the aortic arch, because aortic dissection may result from trauma to the arch on repeated inflations. Inflation of the balloon may be timed or triggered from the arterial pressure waveform or from the ECG. Proper timing of inflation and deflation is vitally important if maximum benefit is to be achieved.

Timing

The balloon should be inflated after the closure of the aortic valve (at the beginning of diastole), which occurs approximately 40 milliseconds before the dicrotic notch inscribed on the pressure pulse wave contour from a radial or femoral artery. Early balloon inflation may cause premature closure of the aortic valve secondary to an increase in pressure in the ascending aortic arch (increased left ventricular afterload) and result in a decreased stroke volume and an increase in end-systolic volume. Late balloon inflation decreases perfusion pressure and flow to the coronary and cerebral arteries.

Deflation of the balloon should occur just before mechanical systole. If the balloon is deflated too early, afterload reduction is impaired. If it is deflated too late, an increase in the workload of the left ventricle may result, because the balloon mechanically obstructs the descending aorta during the early systolic ejection phase. To properly time inflation and deflation, the difference between dicrotic notch inscription on the pressure pulse contour of the central aorta and a peripheral artery must be appreciated (Fig. 40–8).

The dicrotic notch on the central aortic trace is due to closure of the aortic valve. That of a peripheral artery results from the summation of incident and reflected waves and occurs later than the true, central aortic dicrotic notch (see Fig. 40–8). Thus, the balloon should be inflated before the dicrotic notch inscribed on a radial or femoral artery trace, which occurs several milliseconds after the closure of the aortic valve. If inflation of the balloon is timed to occur after the peripheral dicrotic notch, inflation is late and may not optimally increase coronary blood flow and pressure. When the ECG is used, inflation should be timed with the peak of the T wave and deflation with the PR interval.

Complications related to IABP range from 5% to 15%, with aortic dissection and ipsilateral limb ischemia being the most serious.

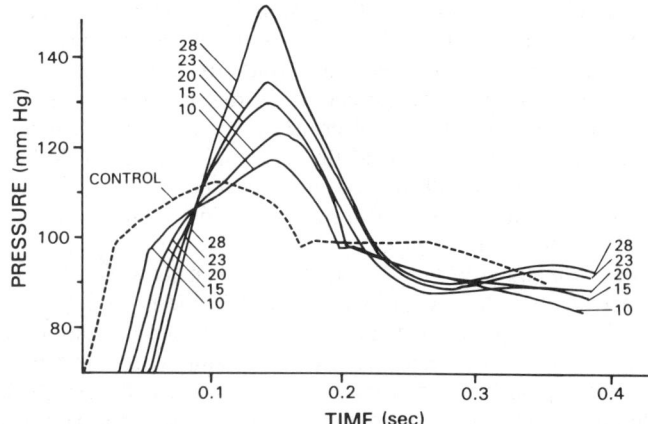

FIGURE 40–8. Increase in pressure pulse amplitude with increasing distance from aortic arch. Control *(dotted line)* is aortic arch tracing. Numbers on *solid lines* indicated distances (cm) down the aorta from the arch in dogs. "At its maximum in this experiment the pulse pressure exceeds that in the arch by more than 90 percent," but the mean pressures "are identical within the limits of error." Frequency response greater than 100 Hz is claimed for catheter and manometer system in this classic study. (From Hamilton WF, Dow P: Experimental study of standing waves in pulse propogated through the aorta. Am J Physiol 1939; 125:48–59.)

Ventricular Assist Devices

In those patients with profound, refractory ventricular failure despite maximal pharmacologic therapy and IABP, total circulatory support may be provided by a ventricular assist device. Ventricular assist devices provide substituted systemic and pulmonary circulation and allow time for cardiac recovery. When surgical revascularization is not possible or proves unsuccessful, these devices may be used to sustain life. They function to reduce the work of the noncontractile but viable or stunned myocardium, in the hope that contractility will return with time.

In our 10 years of experience with centrifugal ventricular assist devices, we have found a significant number of patients with postcardiotomy ventricular failure who have reversible cardiac injury.[60] Recoverability of the damaged myocardium lies in the use of available high-energy substrates for cellular repair instead of for pump function.

Capabilities

Most left ventricular assist devices have the capacity to support 80% to 100% of the workload required to maintain hemodynamic stability. When the left ventricle is completely decompressed and the entire left ventricular output is from the device, $M\dot{V}O_2$ may be reduced to 50% of control values. Left or right ventricular assist devices or both have also been used as a bridge to heart transplantation until a donor heart becomes available. Left ventricular assist devices are often capable of maintaining coronary and intramyocardial blood flow during cardiogenic failure and myocardial ischemia.

Efficacy

Various types of ventricular assist devices are currently being studied in selected centers throughout the United States. All have been reported to improve survival of patients in cardiogenic shock. The Hemopump can be applied by way of peripheral vascular access, can decompress the left ventricle, and can support up to 80% of the left ventricular workload. It is capable of providing 3.5 L · min⁻¹ without left ventricular contribution or synchronization.

During Hemopump assistance, the left ventricular work index reflects the combined work of the Hemopump and the left ventricle. It may be used, therefore, to assess the adequacy of Hemopump assistance and the level of left ventricular recovery. Wampler and colleagues[61] have shown that the hemodynamic response to Hemopump assistance and the prognosis for left ventricular recovery and survival may be correlated with the cardiac index and the PAOP. In Wampler and coworkers' series of 41 patients in cardiogenic shock, despite maximal pharmacologic therapy and IABP, survival rates were 32% after Hemopump insertion.

Clinical Experience

From January 1980 to April 1991, of the 15,500 patients in whom cardiopulmonary bypass was used during cardiac surgery at Allegheny General Hospital, 77 (0.5%) developed refractory cardiac failure that required extended support with a centrifugal ventricular assist device. Thirty-seven patients had left, 4 right, and 36 biventricular assist. Concomitant IABP and pharmacologic support were used in all patients.

Pump flow rates, which in this system are dependent on preload, were manipulated to maintain a cardiac index of 2.0 L · min⁻¹ · m²⁻¹ or greater. High flow rates were maintained to unload and therefore "rest" the ventricle, as well as to minimize or eliminate the need for heparin. Activated clotting times were maintained between 150 and 200 seconds. The average durations for left-sided, right-sided, and biventricular assistance were 45, 49, and 60 hours, respectively.

Twenty-seven patients (35%) survived for 30 days or longer and were discharged from the hospital. Long-term survival among the 27 patients who were "salvaged" was 67%. They were equally distributed between left-sided and biventricular assistance (34% and 37%, respectively). Duration of assistance was not significantly different between survivors and nonsurvivors.

Thirteen years of experience with assist devices in postcardiotomy patients who develop refractory ventricular failure has led Magovern and colleagues[60] to advocate a "continued focused effort toward the development of more effective ventricular assist devices for application in the post cardiac surgery patient who develops refractory ventricular failure."

Causes of Death

The main cause of death in patients treated with ventricular assist devices is irreversible left or right ventricular failure. In those who require support for long periods, death may result from multiple organ failure.

Right Heart Function During Left Ventricular Assistance

A left ventricular assist device used to manage left ventricular failure may improve or decrease right ventricular function owing to changes in right ventricular preload, afterload, or contractility.[62] Monitoring of the CVP and PAOP and, when possible, direct left atrial pressure is indicated.

Left ventricular assist devices may increase the volume presented to the right ventricle (right ventricular preload) by increasing the output from the failing left ventricle. If the right ventricle is unable to handle this increased preload, right ventricular failure occurs. More commonly, however, the right ventricle is helped by decompression of the left ventricle and left atrium. The concomitant reduction in pulmonary artery pressure, in turn, reduces right ventricular afterload work.

Decompression of the left ventricle also permits a leftward shift of the interventricular septum, resulting in improved compliance of the right ventricle (ventricular interdependence). Finally, as arterial blood pressure improves, an increase in coronary blood flow to the right ventricle may also result in improved right ventricular function.

In a small subset of individuals with fixed pulmonary hypertension and left ventricular failure, left ventricular assist devices may unmask right ventricular failure or actually cause deterioration in right ventricular function. This problem results from the increase in right ventricular preload without a concomitant decrease in pulmonary artery pressure (afterload). In such patients, biventricular assist devices are necessary. In those patients with fixed pulmonary hypertension in whom a right ventricular assist device is used, be aware that a probe-patent foramen ovale may promote right-to-left shunting of blood, with resultant hypoxemia.

MECHANICAL COMPLICATIONS OF ACUTE MYOCARDIAL INFARCTION

What Are the Types, Incidence, and Mortality?

Patients who sustain mechanical complications of acute myocardial infarction such as right ventricular infarction with rupture of the right ventricular free wall, rupture of the left ventricular free wall and papillary muscles, or ventricular septal defect have an infarct size that is substantially less than that which occurs with cardiogenic shock primarily due to pump function.

Left Ventricular Free Wall Rupture

Rupture of the left ventricular free wall is primarily a complication of the first myocardial infarction and is associated with considerably smaller amounts of coronary narrowing than fatal, acute myocardial infarction without rupture.[63] It has been reported to occur in 1% to 3% of all acute myocardial infarctions, with 32% of the ruptures being subacute—that is, occurring more than 24 hours after the onset of symptoms. In the acute myocardial infarction study, 67% of myocardial rupture occurred in the left ventricular free wall, 27% in the septum and 2% in papillary muscle rupture.[64]

Ventricular Septal Rupture

Cardiogenic shock occurring shortly after ventricular septal rupture was usually associated with acute inferior wall infarction and carried a 90% mortality. Complex rupture (i.e., combined right ventricular and ventricular septal involvement secondary to acute inferior wall infarction) was associated with a higher mortality rate than was septal rupture complicating an anterior infarction.

Diagnosis

Diagnosis is usually confirmed by clinical symptoms of acute left ventricular failure, a loud systolic murmur, and concomitant right heart failure. Transesophageal echocardiography is an invaluable aid to diagnosis. Angiography is usually reserved for surgical candidates. Increased oxygen saturation occurs in the right ventricle or the proximal pulmonary artery. An increase in O_2 saturation of >10% as a pulmonary catheter is passed from the right atrium to the right ventricle is diagnostic of ventricular septal rupture.

Surgical Intervention

Early surgical intervention, although associated with increased surgical mortality, produces the best overall survival and patient salvage.[65] If surgical repair is planned, it should be performed without delay to avoid further multisystem deterioration.[66] Some data support an inverse relationship between the timing of surgery and mortality.

The physical status of a patient at the time of the rupture is an important independent variable for survival. A marked increase in mortality in patients 75 years of age and older has been reported. Those patients who survive surgical closure and revascularization may have a survival rate as high as 45% at 8 years.

Urgent surgery is indicated in patients with severe CHF who are not in cardiogenic shock, after initial stabilization with vasodilators and IABP. In the small subset of patients with compensated heart failure, stabilization by medical therapy and elective surgical repair may be performed at 2 weeks.

Papillary Muscle Rupture

Papillary muscle rupture occurs in approximately 2% of all acute myocardial infarctions and is associated most commonly with an inferior myocardial infarction. Because the posterior papillary muscle has only a single blood supply from the posterior descending coronary artery, its rupture is usually associated with acute left ventricular failure and pulmonary edema. Because the left atrium is small and does not have time to dilate, an acute rise in left atrial pressure occurs and large V waves appear on the PAOP trace.

Deterioration after papillary muscle rupture is rapid and unpredictable and may result from a partial rupture becoming a complete rupture or further ischemia and the onset of acute respiratory distress syndrome.

Outcome

The mortality of patients with shock who receive only medical therapy approaches 100%. Therefore, insertion of an intraaortic balloon pump to maintain hemodynamic function during cardiac catheterization, followed by emergency cardiac surgery, is indicated. At the Mayo Clinic, urgent surgery for acute mitral regurgitation secondary to papillary muscle rupture, even in patients with moderate failure and pulmonary edema, has reduced the acute mortality to 15%.[65] Some patients who develop acute pulmonary edema may also develop the adult respiratory distress syndrome (ARDS) or other pulmonary complications and become balloon pump dependent.

RIGHT VENTRICULAR INFARCTION

How Does It Cause Shock?

Right ventricular infarction may cause cardiogenic shock and death. Hypotension and shock occur in three ways: (1) inadequate left ventricular filling from reduced right ventricular output, (2) interventricular septal dysfunction, and (3) deranged left ventricular pump function from associated left ventricular ischemia.

How Is It Treated?

Bradycardia or heart block may occur with right ventricular infarction; therefore, atrioventricular sequential pacing may be of great value in improving the cardiac index. IABP, which directly affects only left ventricular afterload, may provide transient stabilization of right ventricular infarction.

Inotropic Support

Inotropic agents sometimes improve right ventricular function (improve right ventricular ejection) in patients with right ventricular failure. Dopamine, dobutamine, norepinephrine, and amrinone, alone or in combination, have been used with various degrees of success. Amrinone, which has inotropic and pulmonary vasodilator effects, should be considered in those patients not sufficiently responding to other inotropic agents, especially in the presence of increased pulmonary artery pressure and PVR. Amrinone may improve diastolic relaxation in the right and left ventricles.

Right Ventricular Afterload Reduction

After right ventricular ischemia, the ventricle may dilate, causing an increase in myocardial O_2 demand, which is not matched by a concomitant increase in coronary blood flow to the right ventricle (supply/demand imbalance). Although optimization of right ventricular preload is an important aspect of the management of acute right heart failure, if it results in right ventricular overload, left ventricular function may be compromised. Decreases in left ventricular filling, stroke volume, cardiac output, and mean arterial pressure further aggravate right ventricular failure, setting up a vicious downhill cycle.

At a specific right ventricular end-diastolic volume, a "falloff" of right ventricular stroke volume occurs (Fig. 40–9). However, right ventricular myocardial O_2 demand, here represented as right ventricular stroke work index, continues to increase, because a decrease in right ventricular perfusion may occur coincidentally with the increase in right ventricular myocardial O_2 demand. Adequate aortic pressure must be maintained for perfusion of the right ventricle; thus, judicious use of vasoactive agents that raise mean arterial pressure is often necessary.

Right ventricular afterload reduction may be tried in patients with elevated PVR. Unfortunately, no ideal pulmonary vasodilator currently exists. Prostaglandin E_1 has been used and often causes a temporary increase in cardiac index, but outcome studies suggest that survival is worse than that of pla-

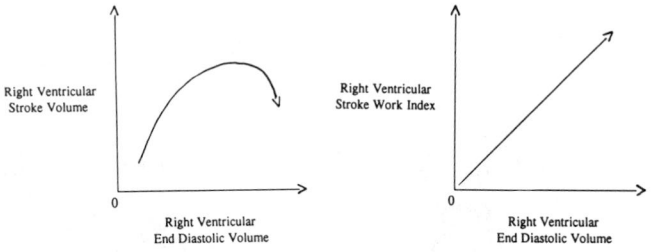

FIGURE 40–9. Relationship between right ventricular stroke volume or work and end-diastolic volumes.

cebo-treated control patients. Dobutamine or dopamine plus amrinone currently remains the most useful combination to improve right ventricular contractility. Right ventricular assist devices may be used when hope is held for eventual recovery of the stunned myocardium.

OTHER CAUSES OF ACUTE RIGHT VENTRICULAR DYSFUNCTION

Acute right ventricular dysfunction also may occur in multiple trauma and after an acute increase in impedance to right ventricular ejection (i.e., pulmonary embolism, severe acute respiratory failure, intermittent positive-pressure ventilation [IPPV] with positive end-expiratory pressure [PEEP], severe hypoxemia).

Eddy and colleagues[67] studied 17 patients who had sustained severe multiple trauma and found an early decrease (3 to 6 h after trauma) in right ventricular ejection fraction secondary to a concomitant increase in pulmonary artery pressure. In the five nonsurvivors, the decrease in right ventricular ejection fraction was significantly greater than that of the survivors and was not detected by the usual methods used for hemodynamic monitoring.

As the pulmonary artery pressure increased, the right ventricle progressively dilated, and right ventricular end-systolic volume, ventricular wall tension, and myocardial oxygen demand increased. If right ventricular perfusion pressure decreases in the setting of increased right ventricular wall tension and afterload, myocardial ischemia and decreased ventricular compliance ensue.

How Are the Relationships Between Pulmonary Artery Occlusion Pressure, Left Ventricular End-Diastolic Pressure, and Left Ventricular End-Diastolic Volume Affected?

The decrease in right ventricular compliance renders filling pressures suspect as a guide to fluid volume resuscitation and inotropic support. Pressure/volume relationships show poor correlation. The relationship between end-diastolic volume and end-diastolic pressure is curvilinear, not linear; therefore, changes in volume are not predictable by changes in pressure. A small change in volume may be reflected by a large change in pressure.

In such patients, evaluation of right ventricular performance by measurement of right ventricular ejection fraction and vol-

ume, two-dimensional echocardiography, or radionuclide angiocardiography provides the most accurate information.

MONITORING IN SHOCK

What Are the Limitations of Pulse Oximetry?

Pulse oximetry uses optical plethysmography and spectrophotometry to estimate O_2 saturation (SpO_2). Therefore, it may be affected by poor peripheral pulsations, low-flow states, or dark skin pigmentation. Hypothermia, low cardiac output, and vasoconstrictor drugs—all usually present in patients in shock—may combine to reduce the plethysmographic pulsation and the portion of the total signal that a pulse oximeter must detect to record saturation.

Pulse Amplitude and Flow

Current pulse oximeters have built-in automatic signal gain controls, thus making them relatively insensitive to changes in peripheral pulse amplitude and flow. Hence, the presence of a pulse recording does not ensure that adequate flow exists in the monitored tissues.[68] Pulse oximetry can estimate O_2 saturation over a wide range of peripheral blood flow and cardiac output if a pulse can be sensed by the monitor.

Lawson and colleagues[69] showed that peripheral blood flow could be reduced to 8.6% of normal before the SpO_2 was no longer measurable. Pälve and Vuori[70] showed that the accuracy of saturation readings during low cardiac index states (i.e., <2.2 L · min^{-1} · m^{-2}) may not be affected until significantly lower flows are reached.

Vasoconstriction

Vasoconstriction of the digit due to any cold vasoconstrictors or high sympathetic tone sometimes interferes with SpO_2 monitoring. In such instances, a digital nerve block may increase circulation to the finger and thus render pulse oximetry useable under these conditions.

Sensitivity

Hemoglobin O_2 saturation determined by pulse oximetry allows an estimation of oxygen content, if the hemoglobin concentration is known. Because of the shape of the HbO_2 dissociation curve, information on the directional change of PaO_2 is not obtained until it falls below 75 mm Hg. Thus, large changes in PaO_2 may occur above 75 mm Hg and are not detected by the pulse oximeter.

Accuracy in Traumatic and Hemorrhagic Shock

Calibration curves developed for most oximeters were established by measuring saturation in normal human volunteers. Therefore, their accuracy is ensured only above 85% saturation. Saturation values $<85\%$ were extrapolated from the calibration curve and are questionable. In healthy humans, SpO_2 is accurate within 2% of the true O_2 saturation determined by co-oximetry unless significant HbO_2 is present.

How Useful Is Capnography?

A sudden decrease in the partial pressure of end-tidal carbon dioxide ($PETCO_2$) may result from decreased blood flow to the lungs caused by hypovolemia, embolization, or myocardial dysfunction. The gradient between $PaCO_2$ and $PETCO_2$ increases because the poorly perfused areas of the lungs during situations of low flow or severe hypovolemia may have a $PaCO_2$ approximating zero. The dead space to tidal volume (VD/VT) ratio increase owing to the increase in dead space ventilation.

A favorable response to resuscitation (i.e., increase in cardiac output, increase in pulmonary blood flow, and correction of anemia and hypovolemia) is mirrored by increases in the $PETCO_2$ if ventilation remains constant and a trend toward normal for the VD/VT ratio.

What Is the Value of Electroencephalography?

Spackman and colleagues[71] compared an analysis of the processed Life Scan electroencephalogram (EEG) with a standard EEG and measurement of CBF to detect cerebral ischemia (Fig. 40–10). Their study verified the ability of processed EEG monitoring to detect cerebral ischemia. Other modalities of processed EEGs, such as the compressed spectral array and density-modulated spectral array, have likewise shown close correlation with cerebral function (see Chapter 22).

Ischemia Detection

$CMRO_2$ is high, 3.0 to 3.5 mL $\cdot$ 100 g tissue^{-1} $\cdot$ min^{-1}. Oxidative metabolism is mandatory because anaerobic glycolysis cannot satisfy the brain's energy demands. CBF of 20 mL $\cdot$ 100 g^{-1} $\cdot$ min^{-1} produces an alteration of the normal EEG. Absence of EEG activity occurs in normal persons when the CBF falls to <15 mL $\cdot$ 100 g^{-1} $\cdot$ min^{-1} or the CPP is <20 mm Hg. A flow threshold of 40% of normal may also be associated with the beginning of ischemic brain edema.

Brain edema begins when the cerebrovascular endothelium has been structurally damaged. Inhalation anesthetics such as isoflurane may extend the lower limit of CBF to 10 mL $\cdot$ 100 g^{-1} $\cdot$ min^{-1} before cerebral electrical activity ceases. Within 10 seconds of total brain ischemia, the available O_2 is consumed; high energy stores of adenosine triphosphate (ATP) are depleted by 4 minutes, and cellular disruption begins at 5 minutes.

Hypoxemia

In awake humans, the EEG pattern does not begin to change until the HbO_2 saturation falls below 60%. Hemoglobin saturations less than 60% to 65% and PaO_2 of <40 mm Hg cause decreases in brain high-energy ATP stores and loss of high-frequency EEG activity. A PaO_2 of 25 mm Hg results in flattening of the EEG pattern.

We have used processed EEG (Life Scan) to study the response and effect of acute cessation and return of circulation secondary to induced ventricular fibrillation and defibrillation during electrophysiologic testing of the automatic implantable defibrillator (AICD).

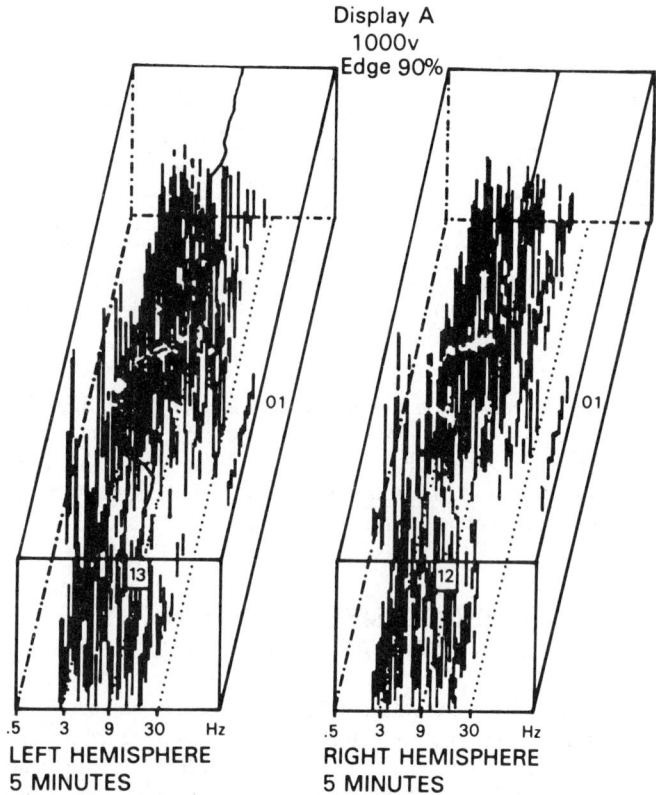

FIGURE 40–10. Processed EEG (Lifescan) tracings recorded during testing of implantable cardioverter defibrillator (AICD). Note bilateral absence of electrical activity and drop in spectral edge *(solid line)* during ventricular fibrillation (Event 01) with return to baseline upon defibrillation.

The electrical activity of the brain ceases immediately with the onset of ventricular fibrillation. The absence of cardiac output during ventricular fibrillation and return after defibrillation were documented by systemic and pulmonary artery pressure monitoring and transesophageal echocardiography. After various periods of induced ventricular fibrillation (20 to 90 s), defibrillation resulted in immediate recovery of EEG activity (see Fig. 40–10).

Similar changes and response to total circulatory arrest during normothermic or hypothermic cardiopulmonary bypass have been recorded by processed EEG monitoring. It is of value to determine the presence, absence, and degree of depression of cerebral electrical activity in one or both hemispheres during shock and resuscitation.

ANAPHYLACTIC SHOCK

What Is an Anaphylactic Reaction?

Anaphylaxis represents an immediate and frequently catastrophic manifestation of immune hypersensitivity. Although most organ systems are involved, the common manifestations are cutaneous, pulmonary, cardiovascular, central nervous system (CNS), and gastrointestinal disturbances. The exact prevalence or frequency of the syndrome is unknown because of underreporting; however, rates of occurrence have been placed as high as 1 in 3000 in hospitalized patients. Deaths directly attributable to anaphylaxis may be on the order of 500 patients annually.[72–74]

The term *anaphylaxis* is derived from the two Greek words, *ana*, meaning ''backward,'' and *phylaxis*, meaning ''protection.'' It is somewhat of a misnomer and a historical holdover from original research in immunization, when during attempts to provide immunity (or improved tolerance) to sea anemone toxin in dogs, repeat challenges with the toxin at greatly reduced doses frequently led to the fulminant response of anaphylaxis and death within minutes. Instead of the planned protective effects, an undesired increased sensitivity was generated—hence the coining of the term *anaphylaxis*.

Subsequently developed was the concept that anaphylactic sensitivity was an acquired disease. It required previous exposure to the sensitizing agent, with a mandatory delay of several weeks between original exposure and re-exposure in order to elicit the fulminant response. This is what is now commonly recognized as ''true'' or ''classic'' anaphylaxis. Only later was the role of immunoglobin E (IgE) in this response elucidated.

What Is an Anaphylactoid Reaction?

Since this original description, ''anaphylactoid'' reactions have been described as well. These responses have all the hallmarks of anaphylaxis, being indistinguishable clinically, but they do not involve the presence of IgE, nor do they require prior exposure. For convenience of discussion, most authors group all these responses under the umbrella term *anaphylaxis* while keeping in mind the divergent etiologies. Additional discussion of anaphylaxis with specific reference to anesthesia is covered in detail in Chapter 44.

What Are the Mechanisms?

Immunoglobulin E Antibody Production

Bochner and Lichtenstein[74] described three well-documented mechanisms through which anaphylaxis may occur. In the first, foreign proteins are presented to the immune system, either directly or as haptens covalently bound to carrier proteins. This exposure stimulates B lymphocytes to proliferate and differentiate into monoclonal plasma cells, producing a specific IgE antibody. The IgE antibody subsequently binds with high-affinity sites on basophils and mast cells. During re-exposure, antigen-generated cross-linking leads to cell degranulation with release of both stored and rapidly synthesized anaphylaxis mediators. This mechanism represents the classic anaphylaxis response.

Complement Activation

In a second mechanism, the response is initiated through direct antigen stimulation by the antigen of the complement cascade. The latter proteins may produce direct cell lysis and, as a by-product, peptide fragments C3a and C5a. These fragments are designated *anaphylatoxins* because of their action in stimulating further release of mediators from basophils and mast cells. As a variation of this response, specific drugs may directly induce the release of C3a, with subsequent degranulation of mast cells and basophils.

Direct Triggering of Mast Cells and Basophils

A third mechanism involves direct triggering of mast cells and basophils with release of mediators by a mechanism that appears to be independent of either IgE or the complement system. A typical inciting agent might be radiocontrast medium or a hyperosmolar solution.

Other Causes

A poorly defined fourth clinical picture has also been identified. In this response, many of the stigmata of anaphylaxis, including bronchospasm, cutaneous manifestations, and angioedema, are present, but no clearly identified immune mediators have been elucidated. These reactions typically occur after the use of aspirin or nonsteroidal anti-inflammatory drugs and may be induced with exercise as well. Table 40–2 lists those common agents in the operating room that have been implicated in anaphylaxis.

What Is the Pathophysiologic End Point?

Calcium Dependence

Regardless of its inciting agent or mechanism of action, clinical presentation of anaphylaxis seems to depend on the pharmacologic and physiologic effects of the mediators released from tissue mast cells and circulating basophils. The mediators seem to be either stored or immediately derived by methylation of membrane phospholipids. The process of release appears to be calcium dependent and requires an influx of calcium ions through channels in the cell wall.

The calcium-dependent release sequence appears to be inhibited by the action of cyclic adenosine monophosphate (cAMP), which is created by the action of the enzyme adenylate cyclase on the substrate ATP. Adenylate cyclase activity may be increased through the stimulation of cell surface prostaglandin, β-adrenergic, and histamine type 2 receptor sites. This fact explains in part the rationale for treatment that is outlined later.

Mediators

To date, the list of released and formed mediators includes the following: histamine, prostaglandin, leukotrienes, tryptase, chymase, heparin, chondroitin sulfate, and platelet-activating factor. The released mediators are extremely potent in their systemic action. Table 40–3 shows some typical mediators and their concentrations in basophils or mast cells.[75–79]

TABLE 40–2. Agents More Likely to Be Implicated in Perioperative Anaphylaxis

Antibiotics	Narcotics
Blood and blood products	Opiates
Plasma volume expanders	Aminoester local anesthetics
Iodinated radiocontrast material	Chymopapain
Induction agents	Methylmethacrylate cement
Muscle relaxants	Protamine
Insulin	Cyclosporine
Streptokinase	Nonsteroidal anti-inflammatory drugs

(Modified from Sage D: Anaphylactoid reactions during anesthesia. *In* Wellcome Trends In Anesthesiology. Burroughs-Wellcome Co., Research Triangle Park, NC, 1991.)

TABLE 40–3. Mast Cell-Derived and Basophil-Derived Mediators of Potential Importance in Anaphylaxis in Humans

Mediators Generated	Basophils	Mast Cells	
		Lung	Skin
Histamine (pg/cell)	1	3–4	3–4
Prostaglandin D$_2$ (pg/cell)	<1	60	60
Leukotriene C$_4$ (pg/cell)	60	60	2–3
Platelet-activating factor (pg/cell)	ND*	1	ND*
Tryptase (pg/cell)	<0.1	10	35
Chymase (pg/cell)	0	0	4.5
Heparin (pg/cell)	<1	4	ND
Chondroitin sulfate (pg/cell)	10	2	ND

(Data obtained from references 74–79.)
*The production of platelet-activating factor has been detected but has not been quantitated.[74]
Abbreviations: ND = not determined.

What Are the Signs and Symptoms?

Cardiovascular Dysfunction

The clinical picture of anaphylaxis reflects the systemic release of potent vasoactive mediators. The response usually is immediate (within minutes after exposure), dramatic, and consistent with the effects of the released mediators on the various organ systems. After exposure to the inciting agent, pronounced hypotension, tachycardia, and cardiovascular collapse occur. These changes are secondary to decreased vascular tone and increased capillary permeability leading to loss of intravascular volume. Decreased myocardial contractility may also be an element of the cardiovascular response.

Respiratory Compromise

Respiratory compromise, although less common, is responsible for the majority of immediate deaths due to anaphylaxis and may include intense bronchospasm, wheezing, shortness of breath, and associated life-threatening upper airway obstruction due to laryngeal edema. Pulmonary edema may occur but is relatively uncommon.

Other Manifestations

Cutaneous manifestations include urticaria, pruritus, rash, and edema. Awake patients may have abdominal pain, cramps, nausea, vomiting, diarrhea, hematemesis, and an impending sense of doom. Other manifestations include a ''histamine'' headache and coagulopathy.

What Is the Treatment?

Immediate Steps

Management of anaphylaxis involves removal of the inciting agent, ventilation and oxygenation if required, restoration of cardiovascular function, and treatment of the systemic effects of the released mediators. As soon as anaphylaxis is suspected, all medications being injected should be stopped. Anesthetic agents should be discontinued if profound cardiovascular changes are present. Patients should be ventilated with 100% O$_2$. Tracheal intubation may be required for airway control and ventilation if a patient is awake or undergoing a mask anesthetic.

Rapid infusion of crystalloid or colloid solutions to restore circulating volume should be instituted, along with the titrated administration of epinephrine, 0.1 to 0.5 mg intravenously for moderate hypotension or 1 mg intravenously for cardiovascular collapse. If blood pressure or pulse is not detectable, cardiopulmonary resuscitation should be instituted immediately. The cornerstone of treatment is graded doses of epinephrine.[75, 81] Epinephrine stops mast cell degranulation and acts as a bronchodilator and positive inotrope, with vasoconstriction occurring at higher doses.

Secondary Therapy

Secondary measures include intravenous bronchodilators such as aminophylline, 5 to 7 mg · kg^{-1}, intravenous H$_1$ and H$_2$ blockers such as diphenhydramine, 0.5 to 1 mg · kg^{-1}, and cimetidine, 4 mg · kg^{-1}. Hydrocortisone in doses as high as 1 g intravenously is also advocated as part of the secondary therapy. Steroids and antihistamines have little immediate effect but may improve the recovery phase.

In patients with refractory hypotension, titrated doses of norepinephrine, starting at 1 to 2 μg · min^{-1} may prove useful. Glucagon, at 5 to 15 μg · min^{-1} has also been used to good effect in patients with refractory hypotension.[80, 81] Arterial blood gas measurements should be obtained to monitor the adequacy of ventilation and to guide the treatment of metabolic abnormalities.

Coagulopathy has been reported and should be investigated if an abnormality is suspected. Those patients with major reactions require intensive care observation and management. Bochner and Lichtenstein[74] proposed a pharmacologic rationale for the treatment of anaphylaxis (Table 40–4). One must have more than a passing familiarity with the dosages and uses of the primary and adjuvant agents if calamity is to be avoided in the emergent treatment of anaphylactic shock.

SPINAL CORD SHOCK

What Is the Epidemiology?

More than 10,000 new cases of spinal cord injury occur in the United States every year.[82, 83] Mechanisms of injury can be roughly grouped as vehicular (automobile and motorcycle), sports related (diving), and high-velocity missile (gunshot). The demographics of spinal cord injury reveal a predilection for males, with the majority of the injuries occurring between the ages of 11 and 30 years. The estimated cost of medical care of the acute injury may be as high as $50,000 to $100,000, with a lifetime cost of more than $750,000.[83] Although spinal cord injuries have devastating personal consequences, societal implications of this condition must be considered as well.

A statistical breakdown of the actual level of the injuries shows the cervical spine being the most common (C-4 to C-7; 48%), followed by high thoracic (T-3 to T-6; 13%) and low thoracic (T-10 to T-12; 18%). Knowledge of the level of the injury is important for optimum care of patients during the acute and chronic phases of their injury. Although definitive care is often rendered in a specialized tertiary care facility, as many as half of the patients require initial evaluation and stabilization at a community hospital before transfer is possible. Anesthesiologists must be familiar with the initial stabilization and management.

TABLE 40–4. Pharmacologic Treatment of Systemic Anaphylaxis in Adults*

		Agents	Indications	Dosages	Goals	Complications
Airway or cutaneous reactions	Initial therapy	Epinephrine	Bronchospasm, laryngeal edema, urticaria, angioedema	0.3–0.5 mL of 1:1000 dilution (0.3–0.5 mg) subcutaneously every 10–20 min	Maintain airway patency, reduce fluid extravasation and pruritus	Dysrhythmias, hypertension, nervousness, tremor
		Oxygen	Hypoxemia	40–100%	Maintain $Po_2 \geq 60$ mm Hg	None
		Metaproterenol	Bronchospasm	0.3 mL (5% solution) in 2.5 mL of saline, inhaled through nebulizer	Maintain airway patency	Same as for epinephrine
	Secondary therapy	Aminophylline	Bronchospasm	Loading dose if necessary (6 mg · kg^{-1}) intravenously as maintenance dose§	Maintain airway patency	Dysrhythmias, nausea, vomiting
		Corticosteroids	Bronchospasm	250 mg of hydrocortisone or 50 mg of methyl-prednisolone intravenously every 6 h for 2–4 doses	Block or reduce prolonged or late-phase reactions	Hyperglycemia, fluid retention
		Antihistamines	Urticaria	25–50 mg of hydroxyzine or diphenhydramine intramuscularly or orally every 6–8 h as needed	Reduce pruritus, antagonize H_1 effects of histamine	Drowsiness, dry mouth, urinary retention
				300 mg of cimetidine intravenously or orally every 6 h	Antagonize H_2 effects of histamine	
Cardiovascular reactions	Initial therapy	Intravenous fluids (saline, colloid)	Hypotension	1 L every 20–30 min as needed	Maintain systolic blood pressure ≥ 80–100 mm Hg	Congestive heart failure, pulmonary edema
		Ephedrine	Hypotension	1 mL of 1:1000 dilution in 500 mL of D_5W intravenously at a rate of 0.5–5 μg (0.25–2.5 mL · min^{-1})	Same as for intravenous fluids	Dysrhythmias, hypertension, nervousness, tremor
	Secondary therapy	Norepinephrine	Hypotension	4 mg in 1 L of D_5W intravenously at a rate of 2–12 μg (0.5–3 mL · min^{-1})	Same as for intravenous fluids	Same as for epinephrine
		Antihistamines	Hypotension	25–50 mg of hydroxyzine or diphenhydramine intramuscularly or orally every 6–8 h as needed	Antagonize H_1 and H_2 effects of histamine on myocardium and peripheral vasculature	Drowsiness, dry mouth, urinary retention
				300 mg of cimetidine intravenously or orally every 6 h		
		Glucagon‖	Refractory hypotension	1 mg in 1 L of D_5W intravenously at a rate of 5–15 μg (5–15 mL · min^{-1})	Increase heart rate and cardiac output	Nausea

(From Bochner BS, Lichtenstein LM: Anaphylaxis, current concepts. N Engl J Med 1991; 324:1788, reprinted by permission of the New England Journal of Medicine.)
*Dosages, choice of specific agents, efficacy, and safety must be individualized.
†Albuterol (0.5 mL of the 0.5% solution in 2.5 mL of saline) or isoetharine (0.5 mL of the 1% solution in 2 mL of saline) can also be used.
‡These agents have little or no efficacy during the acute anaphylactic reaction; they may reduce or prevent recurrent or prolonged reactions.
§Lower rates are suggested for older patients, those taking medications that reduce metabolism, those with hepatic dysfunction, and those with congestive heart failure; higher rates should be used in younger persons or cigarette smokers.
‖May be particularly useful in patients taking β-adrenergic blockers, because its ability to stimulate both inotropic and chronotropic cardiac function may be unaltered by β-adrenergic blockade.
Abbreviations: Po_2 = partial pressure of oxygen; D_5W = 5% aqueous dextrose solution.

What Is the Pathophysiology?

Physical Forces

The pathophysiology of acute spinal cord injury most frequently involves axial or translational forces applied to the spinal column, with subluxation or fracture of the bony processes, disruption of the ligamentous elements, and secondary damage to the spinal cord itself.

In the acute injury, direct mechanical trauma to the spinal cord is common; however, complete transection is uncommon.[84] Although the spinal cord is relatively strong anatomically, it is very vulnerable physiologically. Despite the fact that it often remains intact, an almost immediate autodestructive process results in acute, widespread necrosis of its substance, with eventual replacement by fibrosis and scar tissue. This cascade of events produces anatomic, physiologic, and biochemical changes.

Anatomic Changes

Anatomically, the spinal cord may be deformed by direct injury, with subsequent axonal swelling, central hemorrhage, edema, and white matter necrosis. Physiologically, immediate loss of autoregulation, with ischemia, hypoxia, and infarction result. Evoked potentials cannot be elicited across the lesion.

Biochemical Changes

Biochemically, a release of biogenic amines and leukotactic factors from the injured cells is noted. Serum endorphin levels are dramatically elevated. Lipid peroxidation occurs after disruption of myelin lipid bilayers and may enhance the generation of free radicals, as well as PGI_2 and thromboxanes.[84]

Studies have addressed the idea that endoperoxidases may, in fact, be the final common pathway for the injury process, with all of the other inciting agents being branches of this final pathway. The effect of high-dose steroids likely relies on inhibition of endoperoxidase activity.[83, 84] Table 40–5 shows the time frame and expected injury mechanisms in the evolution of acute spinal cord injury.

TABLE 40–5. Pathophysiologic Response to Spinal Cord Injury

Time	Anatomic	Physiologic	Biochemical
Immediate	Cord deformation		
1 min		Loss of evoked potentials	Lipid perioxidation, free radical formation
5 min	Axonal swelling	Vasoconstriction	
15 min		Decreased gray and white matter blood flow	Increased thromboxane levels, increased tissue norepinephrine levels
30 min	Central hemorrhages	Ischemia	Profound tissue hypoxia
1 h			
4 h	Blood vessel necrosis, white matter edema		
8 h	Central hematoma formation		
24 h	White matter necrosis		

(From Wilberger JE: Spinal Cord Injuries in Children. Mt. Kisco, NY, Futura Publishing Company, 1986, p 113.)

Secondary Injury

Research efforts and clinical trials in acute injury are centered on prevention of the secondary injury process by early administration of specific inhibitors.[85] Despite these efforts, improvements in neurologic salvage after spinal cord injury have evolved slowly, with only modest gains in the past 20 years. Improved long-term outcome probably is more a function of better chronic care management than a pharmacologic impact on the acute injury phase.[86]

What Is the Clinical Presentation?

The presentation of acute spinal shock may be biphasic. Immediately after the injury a brief period of arterial hypertension and accompanying bradycardia follows. This response is evanescent, lasting 10 to 30 minutes.[82, 87]

Subsequently, the more familiar clinical presentation occurs and is presumably due to impaired sympathetic outflow below the level of the injury. The loss of sympathetic tone leads to arterial and venodilatation, with decreased arterial pressure and increased venous capacitance. At high levels of cord injury, disruption of the cardiac sympathetic fibers occurs as well, leading to impaired cardiac accelerator activity and occasionally profound bradycardia.

Loss of sympathetic tone in the presence of hypovolemia due to associated injuries is particularly threatening to patients with spinal cord shock. At the same time, these patients are highly sensitive to fluid administration, the effects of anesthetic drugs, and perioperative stress. Aggressive fluid management often produces pulmonary edema.

What Is the State of Pharmacotherapy?

Steroids and Naloxone

Only in the past decade have large multicenter investigations such as the National Acute Spinal Cord Injury Study 1 and 2 (NASCIS)[83, 88, 89] and individual investigators attempted to document treatment modalities that may enhance recovery. Encouraged by data from animal models, Faden and others studied the effects of endorphin inhibitors in humans during the postinjury phase of spinal cord trauma.[88] Unfortunately, although the animal model was promising, no quantifiable improvement was demonstrated in the NASCIS 2 human trial.

NASCIS 2 examined the role of both high-dose naloxone and methylprednisolone. The latter drug was begun within 8 hours after injury and was given as a bolus of 30 mg $\cdot$ kg^{-1} in the first hour, followed by 5 to 6 mg $\cdot$ kg^{-1} continuous infusion over the subsequent 23 hours. In this study, naloxone showed no advantage, but quantifiable improvements were seen at 6-month follow-up in the steroid treated patients.[83] The improvements, although real, were far from the total recovery of preinjury function.

Endoperoxidase Inhibitors

These investigators have initiated a new multicenter study, the end point of which is improvement in neurologic outcome after endoperoxidase inhibitors administered in the acute phase of spinal cord trauma. Although some early, encouraging effects have been noted in patients sustaining closed head injuries, the results in spinal cord–injured patients are not yet available.[90]

Ganglioside GM₁

A study by Geisler and colleagues[91] demonstrated that ganglioside GM₁ (a CNS glycolipid thought to enhance neuritic growth) may improve neurologic recovery after spinal cord injury. The investigators caution that further study is needed before widespread use can be recommended.

At present, the therapeutic modalities that can be offered with confidence to spinal cord trauma victims are few. As anesthesiologists, we must recognize injured patients, take all precautions to prevent the progression of the injury while managing other attendant injuries, and be aware of the physiologic consequences of spinal cord injury in both its acute and chronic phases.

How Is a Patient Managed?

Neurologic Compromise

The acute care of spinal cord trauma is begun in the field at the site of the injury. Paramedical personnel generally have first patient contact. All personnel must have a high degree of suspicion for occult spinal cord injury and presumptively treat all patients with the appropriate precautions.[82, 85] Nothing is more tragic than a patient who suffers spinal cord injury during treatment or transport because of an unrecognized vertebral column injury. The goal should be early recognition and prevention of progression of an incomplete spinal cord injury.

In-Line Stabilization

For this reason, all patients suspected of having spinal cord injury should be afforded the use of immediate in-line stabilization or traction. They should be moved as a single unit, using backboards and cervical collars when appropriate. As soon as feasible, they should be transported to a medical center capable of the diagnostic and therapeutic modalities that such patients demand.

Initial management on arrival at the hospital includes standard assessment of the extent of trauma with additional attention to signs and level of neurologic compromise. Patients often need additional diagnostic and therapeutic interventions. Therefore, the adequacy of spinal immobilization should be confirmed in the emergency room and maintained during transport and testing in these often remote areas of the hospital (see Chapter 59).

Cardiorespiratory Compromise

A second component of the management of these patients includes the possibility of cardiac and respiratory embarrassment.[87, 92–94] Although such abnormalities may be present in any traumatized patient, they require extra consideration in this patient group. Patients sustaining a high thoracic or cervical injury should be considered to have cardiorespiratory compromise until proven otherwise. Tracheal intubation and mechanical ventilation should be instituted if observable deterioration occurs.

Injuries at the level of the sixth cervical vertebra result in loss of intercostal muscle activity and a pattern of paradoxical breathing, with recruitment of the accessory muscles (because their innervation is from higher in the cervical cord) to assist respiration.

Diaphragmatic innervation via the phrenic nerves is maintained at levels of injury below the fourth cervical vertebra. Although patients with a C-4 injury may be able to maintain satisfactory ventilation initially, those elements of innervation required for generation of an effective cough and to prevent fatigue of the diaphragm are missing. As a result, such patients may be unable to clear secretions. These deficiencies lead to poor airway maintenance and early susceptibility to pneumonic processes.

How Should the Airway Be Secured?

Nasal Intubation

The literature is divided on the best way to secure the airway in patients with cervical cord injury.[87, 92, 93] The advocated choices include topical anesthetic and blind or fiberoptic nasal intubation. Proponents claim this approach is less likely to cause motion of the neck and head and has obvious benefits for patients.

Oral Intubation

The second commonly advocated method is awake topical oral intubation. Proponents of this technique point out the possible existence of basilar skull fracture. This approach avoids the subsequent development of maxillary sinusitis, which may act as a nidus for infection and is relatively common with indwelling nasotracheal tubes.

Rapid-Sequence Induction and Intubation

A third group advocates the use of anesthetized and paralyzed intubation in these patients (rapid-sequence induction), with in-line cervical traction held during laryngoscopy and intubation.

The means for emergent cricothyrotomy or tracheotomy must always be available with any of the techniques discussed. Treatment of such patients at our institution has evolved from an awake nasal technique to oral intubation with in-line traction, anesthesia, and paralysis. Obviously, each patient presents a unique situation and may require variation from any protocol. Such situations mandate a discussion between all members of the trauma team, with anesthesiologists bringing their expertise in airway management to bear on the issue.

What Are the Systemic Effects Following Spinal Cord Injury?

Traumatic spinal cord injury disrupts the normal afferent and efferent nerve impulses at the level of the injury. Immediately after spinal cord trauma, evanescent arterial hypertension may be present, as was noted previously. However, by the time most patients are seen in the emergency department, marked hypotension or spinal shock usually is present.[87, 94]

Cardiovascular changes are due to the loss of descending sympathetic control and a preponderance of parasympathetic tone below the level of the injury. These physiologic imbalances result in increased venous capacitance, arterial hypotension, profound bradycardia, and ventricular dysfunction. This clinical presentation, along with poikilothermia and flaccid paralysis, represents spinal shock.

Cardiovascular Alterations

This clinical presentation may mask other injuries. The typical response of tachycardia in the presence of hypovolemia is blunted, and patients are unable to compensate for loss of intravascular volume by the usual mechanisms of increased sympathetic tone. The loss of normal sympathetic tone also produces dramatic hypotensive responses following postural changes.[82, 87, 92–94] Subjective and reflexive signs of abdominal and thoracic injury may be absent in quadriplegic patients. The mechanisms and patterns of injury should prompt early investigation and treatment. Volume administration typically improves hypotension; however, aggressive resuscitation frequently produces pulmonary edema and ventricular failure.

Invasive monitoring (arterial and pulmonary artery catheters) is an invaluable management tool, particularly in seriously injured patients. In the presence of depressed ventricular function and hypotension, the combination of inotropic support with judicious volume administration may be required to re-establish normal hemodynamic function. Remember that direct-acting vasoactive and inotropic agents are required to produce optimum effects in patients devoid of sympathetic innervation.

Gastrointestinal Dysfunction

Gastrointestinal changes due to spinal cord injury include gastric atony, dilation, and ileus and a hypersecretory state. Gastric dilatation may produce respiratory embarrassment in already compromised patients. The ileus, atony, and hypersecretory state place patients at high risk for aspiration in the perioperative period.[93, 94] Early decompression and suctioning of the gastric contents are advisable in patients slated for emergency operative intervention.

Temperature Control

With the loss of sympathetic control, patients suffering from spinal cord injuries lose the ability to control vasodilatation and vasoconstriction necessary for temperature control. They become functionally poikilothermic. These changes make it imperative that measures be taken to control and preserve body temperature in the operating room as well as the intensive care unit. Significant hypothermia is one of the most frequently observed complications in patients with spinal cord injury.

How Should Anesthesia Proceed?

Anesthetic management entails consideration of the foregoing changes, as well as the anesthetic agents that are to be used for the procedure. Recall that patients have a limited capacity to respond to the potent effects of most anesthetic agents as well as the usual physiologic stress of the perioperative experience. No clear choice of one best anesthetic agent or technique has been promulgated despite considerable debate. Most investigators prefer gentle induction, typically

using judicious doses of narcotics, benzodiazepines, and attenuated doses of sedative-hypnotics.[92]

Induction

Ketamine, with its direct myocardial depressant effects in the absence of an intact sympathetic nervous system, would be a poor choice for induction or maintenance. Barbiturates and volatile agents in hypotensive or relatively hypovolemic patients must be considered carefully. In the acute phase of injury, depolarizing muscle relaxants appear to be safe, although many prefer to avoid the issue altogether by using nondepolarizing agents for intubation and maintenance.

Induction and maintenance of anesthesia mandate constant reassessment of the information provided by the arterial and pulmonary artery catheters. Frequent examination of serum chemistry values and careful accounting of blood loss, urine output, and volume administration are required as well.

Tracheal Extubation

Postoperative extubation criteria should be well established. A cavalier approach to early (premature) extubation must be avoided. Our usual preference has been postoperative, volume-controlled, or assisted mechanical ventilation. Weaning is gradual in those patients with high cord injuries or those who have undergone extensive spinal instrumentation for stabilization. This approach ensures airway maintenance, provides a mechanism for pulmonary toilet, and prevents patient fatigue and the need for emergent reintubation.

SEPTIC SHOCK

Septic shock is not as commonly encountered by anesthesiologists as hypovolemic or cardiogenic shock. Nonetheless, an adequate understanding of the inciting agents and management is critical for practicing anesthesiologists.

Trauma is the leading cause of death in persons younger than 45 years in the general population.[95] Patients can be further stratified by the time of their death into one of the following categories:

1. Immediate death (e.g., aortic disruption, massive CNS trauma). Most of these patients are pronounced dead at the scene or immediately on arrival in the emergency department.
2. Early death (e.g., hypovolemic shock, tamponade). These patients survive to arrive in the hospital and succumb in the emergency department or operating room after initial resuscitative attempts.
3. Late death (e.g., sepsis with subsequent multiorgan failure).[17, 95]

In the late death group, sepsis is the major contributing factor. The cost of caring for patients with septicemia is estimated to be between 5 and 10 billion dollars each year in the United States.[96]

What Are the Inciting Agents?

Despite advances in acute trauma management and improvements in critical care, the mortality in septic shock is

40% to 60%.[17, 95, 97–99] A multitude of infective agents elicit the characteristic syndrome. Distinguishing between fungal, viral, or bacterial agents is often next to impossible. A striking uniformity in the clinical presentation supports the idea that numerous chemical mediators lead to a common final pathway defined as the septic shock state.

Two important features are currently thought to be responsible for the clinical syndrome. The first involves direct tissue damage produced by the infective agent. Second and more important is the resultant ischemia and inflammation that release potent chemical mediators.[97] To date, the list of mediators is extensive (more than a dozen) and includes endotoxins, kinins, endorphins, anaphylatoxins, eicosanoids, interleukin, and TNF.[97–100] The net effect of the various mediators includes systemic arterial vasodilatation, increased capillary permeability, consumptive coagulopathy, pulmonary vasoconstriction, decreased myocardial contractility, and cellular destruction.

What Are the Hemodynamic Derangements?

The hemodynamic manifestations of septic shock involve a two-phase process. The first is a hyperdynamic state, with elevated cardiac output and associated peripheral vasodilatation (so-called warm shock).[97] Responsible mediators are thought to include endorphins, kinins, and PGI_2.[99, 100] The second phase involves a hypodynamic state, with low cardiac output and marked peripheral vasoconstriction (so-called cold shock).[97] Typical associated mediators include the thromboxanes and leukotrienes.

The hypodynamic state is frequently regarded as an ominous preterminal sign by clinicians, although either state may be present at death. Early, hyperdynamic septic shock usually involves macrocirculatory and microcirculatory failure, with inadequate tissue perfusion and resultant lactic acidosis. Oxygen use is thought to be supply limited. The picture in late, hypodynamic shock is less clear. Some investigators suggest the existence of a supply-independent depression of O_2 use at the tissue level.[16, 57, 99, 101] Proposed mechanisms include reduced delivery because of arteriovenous shunting, capillary plugging by thrombotic microaggregates, and loss of the normal vascular autoregulatory functions.[16, 97]

What Happens at the Cellular Level?

Aggressive volume re-expansion, adequate oxygenation, and support of pump function are the keys to successful management.[57, 101] However, correction of the hemodynamic dysfunction does not ensure patients' survival,[16, 17, 57, 102] suggesting that a primary metabolic derangement at the cellular level is an important component of the septic shock state.[16, 102, 103] Accumulation of toxic metabolites and depletion of ATP lead to eventual cell death. This deranged cellular metabolism, coupled with ongoing sepsis, leads to multiorgan system failure and death despite correction of the major hemodynamic derangement.

Specific sites where depression of cellular O_2 use may be affected are shown in Figure 40–11.

Newer therapy uses monoclonal antibodies directed specifically against toxic mediators by the formation of inactive antibody-antigen complexes.[96, 104] Although clinical trials allegedly show improved outcome in patients with demonstrated gram-negative shock, definitive proof of efficacy awaits further study.

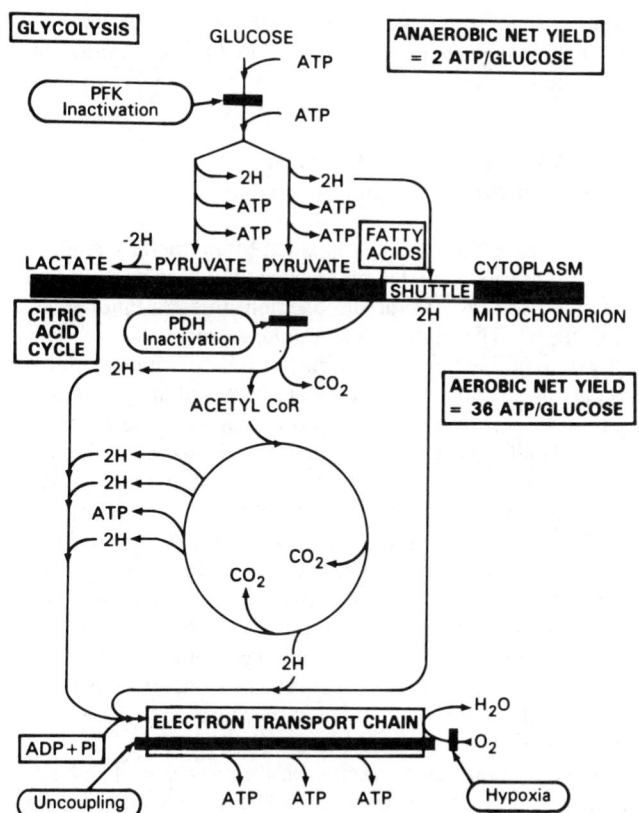

FIGURE 40–11. Schematic drawing showing four key areas where blocks in metabolism might occur. PFK = Phosphofructokinase; PDH = pyruvate dehydrogenase; ADP = adenosine diphosphate; PI = inorganic phosphate; Uncoupling = dissociation of oxidation from phosphorylation; Hypoxia = where oxygen becomes limiting to energy production. (From Cain SM, Curtis SE: Crit Care Med 1991; 19:608, © Williams & Wilkins, 1991.)

Repletion of high-energy substrates using magnesium-adenosine phosphate infusions has improved cellular and organ function in experimental sepsis, ischemia, and shock. This concept may add a new dimension to the treatment of sepsis in the future. However, no "magic bullet" is yet available, and clinicians must rely on supportive therapies as the mainstay of acute management.

What Are the Management Goals?

Acute management demands a multifaceted approach that addresses (1) restoration of hemodynamic stability through intravascular volume expansion and pharmacologic support of myocardial pump function[95, 97, 101]; (2) improved tissue oxygenation (mechanical ventilation, PEEP/continuous positive airway pressure, bronchodilators, correction of anemia); (3) correction of coagulopathy (appropriate component therapy, follow-up laboratory determinations); and (4) surgical intervention to remove the source of infection if a definite site can be identified.

With regard to volume expansion, the debate about crystalloid and colloid use rages on[105–107] (see Chapters 42 and 59). If a patient is anemic, infusion of packed red blood cells to produce a final hematocrit of 40% has been advocated.[18]

Fresh-frozen plasma and platelets may be appropriate therapy for documented coagulopathy but should not be used indiscriminately.

How Are Oxygen Delivery and Consumption Optimized?

Appropriate fluid therapy is aided by pulmonary artery and systemic arterial catheter monitoring. Ventricular dysfunction is manifested by decreased ejection fraction and elevated LVEDP.[95, 97] The high cardiac output in sepsis frequently is a reflection of increased heart rate. Clinical acumen alone to manage these patients is often inaccurate and inconsistent with optimum clinical practice.[108] Information from pulmonary artery catheter measurements permits optimization of preload and cardiac output by construction of modified ventricular function curves. A simplified algorithm suggests that patients with low filling pressures and cardiac index benefit from a volume infusion. With intermediate filling pressures and a depressed cardiac index, an initial volume challenge can be administered, followed by inotropic support if the cardiac index does not respond to the volume therapy.[98, 109–111] High filling pressures not productive of incremental increases in the cardiac index should be avoided, because they contribute to interstitial pulmonary edema formation.

Concern about renal function in the presence of intense α-adrenergic stimulation has prompted concomitant infusion of "renal dose" dopamine to ameliorate these changes. Animal studies suggest that this combination provides arterial pressure support while preserving renal blood flow and function in subjects with normal cardiac output.[112]

INTRAOPERATIVE MANAGEMENT OF SHOCK

Is There a Best Anesthetic?

Two questions are pertinent with regard to the anesthetic management of shock: (1) Is a specific anesthetic agent or technique indicated? (2) Is morbidity or mortality altered based on anesthetic technique? The first question engenders several theoretic issues with regard to anesthetic pharmacology and physiology; the second would necessitate a large multicenter study (which has not been performed) to provide a definitive answer.

"Shock Anesthesia": A Study in Reverse Engineering

The anesthetic management of a patient in shock can be considered situational "reverse engineering." We are presented with a decompensated and inherently unstable patient and have the goal of stabilizing the physiologic aberrations and reversing the decompensation.[113] This problem is the opposite of that encountered in most anesthetics and operations, in which we begin with a stable patient and then induce a controlled, "globally toxic state" while our surgical colleagues work their (potential) physiologic chaos. The question of which anesthetic is most suitable in a shock state becomes an analysis of how to provide the least noxious trespass while the other physiologic derangements are addressed and incurred.

Theoretic Considerations

In the best of all possible worlds, an anesthetic for patients in shock would be neutral with respect to its effects on the peripheral circulation and myocardium, while providing analgesia, amnesia, and protection from unwanted sympathetic responses. This preference would be based on the assumption that a patient in shock has decompensated pump function, profound hypovolemia, or dramatic alterations in SVR and venous capacitance.[114, 115]

With these assumptions in mind, major regional anesthesia (spinal or epidural) is not within the stated goal of neutral effects on the circulation. The attendant sympathectomy predisposes to further decompensation with potentially dramatic adverse physiologic consequences. Similarly, anesthetic technique based *solely* on the use of volatile anesthetic agents would be unacceptable. Myocardial depression and the potential for changes in afterload or preload encountered with usual anesthetizing concentrations make them an unsuitable choice.

Van der Linden and colleagues[116] studied four anesthetic agents (halothane, isoflurane, alfentanil, and ketamine) in an animal model of early septic shock. Their data showed that cardiovascular function and tissue oxygenation were best preserved by ketamine. Halothane was associated with dramatic reduction in hemodynamic function and led to increased lactate production. Ketamine as the sole anesthetic in a patient with cardiogenic shock would be a debatable choice. This agent supports cardiovascular function by virtue of an indirect sympathomimetic action. When the sympathomimetic effects are blocked or are already maximal, ketamine's effect is one of direct myocardial depression.[117]

Induction Agents

Etomidate

Ultrashort-acting sedative-hypnotic induction agents may cause significant hypotension. Etomidate is associated with minimal cardiovascular depression in doses of 0.3 mg $\cdot$ kg^{-1} for patients with good ventricular function. When added to fentanyl, the combined induction regimen produced decreases in SVR and cardiac output and an average decrease of 20% in arterial blood pressure.[120]

Propofol

The use of propofol in shock is of no proven superiority and may be counterproductive because it produces significant decreases in SVR with typical induction doses, even in patients with preserved ventricular function.[121, 122]

Benzodiazepines

Benzodiazepines as sole agents for induction are remarkably free of significant hemodynamic consequences[123, 124] but do not provide analgesia and sympathetic blunting. When they are added to a narcotic-based anesthetic, the synergistic effects can produce myocardial depression and decreases in cardiac index and SVR.[125]

Do Epidemiologic Data Support a "Best" Anesthetic?

In summary, no ideal anesthetic can be prescribed for shock. Each technique, agent, or combination of agents has potentially undesired effects on the myocardium, the peripheral vasculature, and the autonomic nervous system. For most patients, titrated doses of potent synthetic narcotics, with added benzodiazepines or trace quantities of volatile anesthetic agents to provide amnesia, seem prudent.

The overall mortality of patients in shock is high regardless of any medical intervention. Anesthetic-related mortality in itself is very low in incidence. Thus, defining the anesthetic contributions to shock mortality would require multivariate analysis of an immense, perhaps unobtainable population. Furthermore, ethical considerations might prevent such a study. Who would feel comfortable randomly assigning patients in shock and undergoing exploratory laparotomy to a spinal anesthetic group?

A number of studies have examined morbidity and mortality in patients undergoing elective or emergency coronary artery bypass grafting. Various anesthetic agents (narcotics, volatile agents, ketamine, barbiturates, benzodiazepines) were used individually or in combination for patients at high risk of cardiac failure or impending cardiogenic shock.[126-128] An analysis of these studies by Mangano[129] revealed no distinct pattern of anesthetic-related morbidity or mortality. Thus, in the anesthetic management of shock, it may indeed be true that the important factor is not what anesthetics are given but who gives what anesthetic.

INTRAOPERATIVE HEMODYNAMIC STABILIZATION

Hemodynamic abnormalities fall into the general categories of cardiogenic, hypovolemic, and hyperdynamic shock (Fig. 40–12). Cardiogenic shock is most frequently related to myocardial ischemia or infarction. Hypovolemic shock occurs primarily in trauma. Hyperdynamic shock is encountered with sepsis or, less commonly, anaphylaxis.

These categories are not mutually exclusive, and any patient may be included in more than one. For example, a septic patient with known coronary artery disease may start with a hyperdynamic state but subsequently develop evidence of frank cardiac dysfunction because of increased $M\dot{V}O_2$ and circulating myocardial depressant toxins. Management is complex and cannot be handled by a predetermined algorithm.

The goals of hemodynamic management involve an assessment of intrinsic cardiac function and its interaction with the peripheral circulation. With this information, manipulation of ventricular preload, afterload, contractility, rhythmicity, and systemic oxygenation produces the desired end point. Interventions include volume infusion, cardiotonic and vasoactive agents, changes in $\dot{D}O_2$, and, in applicable circumstances, surgical correction of the causative factor (emergent cardiac surgery or excision/drainage of a septic focus).

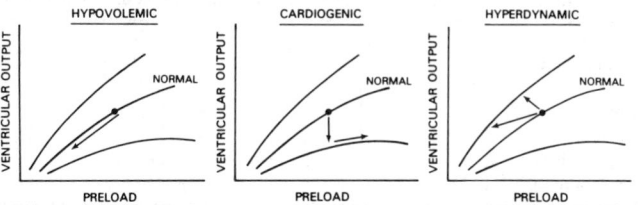

FIGURE 40–12. Hemodynamic patterns (Starling curves) in hypovolemic, cardiogenic, and hyperdynamic shock. (Modified from Rosenthal MH: Shock: diagnosis and treatment. ASA 1991 Annual Refresher Course Lectures. San Francisco, CA, October 26–30, 1991.)

Which Patients Benefit from Preload Optimization?

The majority of shock episodes result from trauma and hypovolemia. As noted previously, trauma is the leading cause of death in patients younger than 35 years.[115, 130] Typical causes are vehicular accidents, penetrating (gunshot and stabbing) wounds, falls from a height, and industrial accidents. These features have promoted the establishment of the shock trauma centers in most urban centers.

Intraoperative volume resuscitation is used to optimize preload in hypovolemic patients. In most cases, the working presumption is that ventricular function is preserved and that volume restitution will restore normal circulation. Although this generalization is not true for all patients, recall that in all categories of shock, some role for optimization of cardiac preload is definable[114, 115, 131] (see Fig. 40–12).

Preserved Ventricular Function

In hypovolemic patients with preserved ventricular function, a nearly linear response in arterial pressure and cardiac output follow volume infusion. The heart is "operating" on the steep part of the ventricular function curve. Hence, volume restoration improves preload and moves the patient "up the curve" (perhaps even to a higher curve). Patients with hyperdynamic shock also may demonstrate increases in arterial pressure and improvement in tissue oxygenation with volume infusion, if relative hypovolemia from vasodilatation or fluid translocation is coupled with decreased afterload.[114]

Compromised Ventricular Function

In contrast, a component of intrinsic ventricular dysfunction is manifested in some patients with advanced sepsis.[97] The response to volume augmentation may produce initial improvement in arterial pressure; however, the cardiac output remains depressed and the PAOP rises. Here, a patient functions on a relatively flat portion of the ventricular function curve; large changes in preload produce small or no changes in cardiac index. These patients require other modalities to effect restoration of hemodynamic stability.

Cardiogenic Shock

Patients with cardiogenic shock also may demonstrate initial improvement in cardiac output with preload augmentation. However, persistence in volume infusion effects no further changes in ventricular performance and may be detrimental. The rising LVEDP impedes coronary perfusion pressure (diastolic blood pressure minus LVEDP), adding to left ventricular ischemia and work. These patients require additional therapeutic modalities to effect change in ventricular performance and cardiac index.

How Should Vasoactive Agents Be Selected?

For patients with a low cardiac index in the presence of adequate volume repletion, the use of cardiotonic agents must be considered.[114, 121, 132] Early and prudent use of epinephrine is life saving in anaphylaxis. However, the situation is less clear in cardiogenic shock or the hyperdynamic phase of septic shock.

Classification

Agents to support the failing cardiovascular system fall into three categories: (1) true catecholamines (e.g., epinephrine or norepinephrine), (2) sympathomimetic agents (e.g., dobutamine or isoproterenol), and (3) noncatecholamine (e.g., amrinone or milrinone). Sites of action of cathecholamines and sympathomimetic agent are usually cell surface adrenoreceptors (α, β, and dopaminergic, with subdivision into types 1 and 2 in each group).

Adrenoreceptors

The adrenoreceptors in vivo respond to specific ligands, most notably norepinephrine (α_1), epinephrine (β_1 and β_2), and dopamine (dopaminergic sites). Sympathomimetic agents presumably bind in a stereospecific fashion at the same adrenoreceptor sites. The effect of this binding is a cascade of intracellular events, including activation of adenylate cyclase and increased production of intracellular cAMP (Fig. 40–13). Subsequent changes in transmembrane calcium flux occur as well.

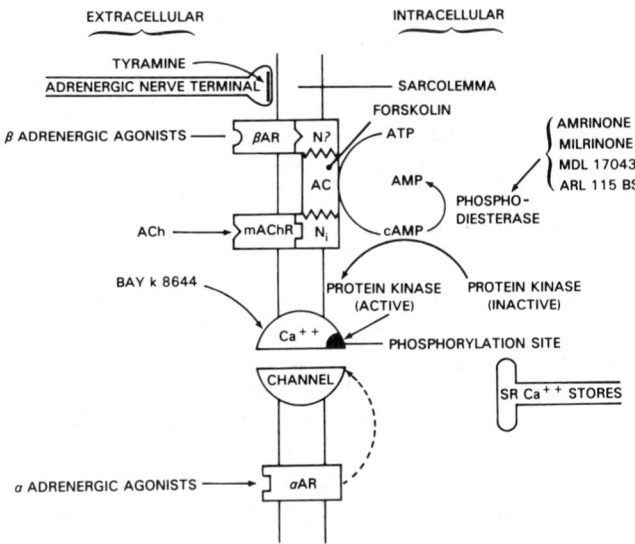

FIGURE 40–13. Diagram illustrating the sites of action of several positive inotropic agents. Circulating catecholamines, catecholamines released from adrenergic nerve terminals, and exogenous sympathomimetic drugs act on β-adrenergic and α-adrenergic receptors (β-AR and α-AR, respectively). Stimulation of β-adrenergic receptors causes activation of adenylate cyclase (AC), resulting in increased cyclic AMP (cAMP) production, which in turn causes an increase in calcium influx through slow calcium channels, presumably owing to the activation of protein kinases that phosphorylate the slow calcium channel. The mechanism by which stimulation of α-adrenergic receptors causes an increase in myocardial contractility is not fully understood, but it may also involve an action on the slow calcium channel. Tyramine acts on adrenergic nerve terminals to release catecholamines, which then act on adrenergic receptors. Calcium-channel agonists (e.g., the drug Bay k 8644) act directly on the calcium channel to increase calcium influx. Intracellular cAMP is degraded by phosphodiesterases and, therefore, phosphodiesterase inhibition results in an increase in intracellular cAMP levels. Several of the newer positive inotropic agents appear to act largely by this mechanism. cAMP can also be increased independently of β-adrenergic receptors by direct stimulation of adenylate cyclase with forskolin. N? = Guanine nucleotide stimulatory subunit; ACh = acetylcholine; mAChR = muscarinic ACh receptor; N_i = guanine nucleotide inhibitory subunit; SR = sarcoplasmic reticulum. (Reprinted from Calacci W, Wright R, Braunwald E: New positive inotropic agents in the treatment of congestive heart failure: mechanisms of action and recent clinical developments (first of two parts). N Engl J Med 1986; 314:290–292, by permission of the New England Journal of Medicine.)

TABLE 40–6. Comparison of Hemodynamic Effects of Sympathomimetic Agents

Agonists	HR	SV	CO	MAP	SVR	PCWP
Dopamine	→↑↑*	↑↑	↑↑↑	→↑↑↑*	↓→↑*	→↑
Dobutamine	↑	↑↑↑	↑↑↑↑	→↑*	↓	→↓
Isoproterenol	↑↑↑↑	↑↑↑↑	↑↑↑↑	→↓↓↓	↓↓↓	↓
Epinephrine	↑↑↑	↑↑	↑↑↑	↑↑*	↓↑*	→↑
Levarterenol	→↓	↑	→↑	↑↑↑↑	↑↑↑↑	→↑

(From Barrett J, Nyhus LM: Treatment of Shock: Principles and Practice. 2nd ed. Philadelphia, Lea & Febiger, 1986, p 198.)
*Dose = dependent effects.
Abbreviations: HR = heart rate; SV = stroke volume; CO = cardiac output; MAP = mean arterial pressure; SVR = systemic vascular resistance; PCWP = pulmonary capillary wedge pressure; ↑ = increase; → = no change; ↓ = decrease.

Conversely, the action of noncatecholamine agents involves inhibition of phosphodiesterase, resulting in decreased degradation of cAMP[133] (see Fig. 40–12).

Receptor Down-Regulation

Cell surfaces are not static but instead undergo a continuous process of rapid remodeling. The α- and β-receptors can be down-regulated—that is, the density of receptor sites is decreased over the cell surface with a resultant decreased activity in response to unchanged stimuli. Down-regulation has been observed in septicemia and in patients with chronically elevated catecholamine levels (as in chronic congestive failure).[97] In septicemia down-regulation probably involves endotoxin binding at the receptor site with subsequent disruption of function.

In cardiac failure, the decrease in sites presumably results from long-term elevation of the native ligand. It may explain the insensitivity that such patients appear to have in response to catecholamine or sympathomimetic agent administration.

Which Agents Are Effective?

Once pertinent information is obtained about a patient's cardiac status, a cardiotonic agent can be chosen on the basis of the physiologic alterations and the desired response at the organ and tissue levels. Management for patients with cardiac failure involves assessment of the myocardial contractile state, correction of the imbalance of $M\dot{V}O_2$ and $\dot{D}O_2$, and augmentation of systolic and diastolic function. A further goal (although it is difficult to assess clinically) is the adequacy of peripheral blood flow and oxygenation.[99, 101] Tables 40–6 and 40–7 reflect the hemodynamic effects and the expected changes in organ

TABLE 40–7. Comparison of Sympathomimetic Effects on Regional Blood Flow

Agonists	Renal	Cerebral	Splanchnic	Skeletal	Cutaneous
Dopamine	↑↑↑↓*	↑	↑	↑	↓
Dobutamine	→	↑	↑↓*	↑↓*	→↓*
Isoproterenol	→↓	↑	↑	↑	↑
Epinephrine	↓	↑	↑↓*	↑↓*	↓
Levarterenol	↓	↑	↓	↓	↓
Phenylephrine	↓	↑	↓	↓	↓
Metaraminol	↓	↑	↓	↓	↓

(From Barrett J, Nyhus LM: Treatment of Shock: Principles and Practice. 2nd ed. Philadelphia, Lea & Febiger, 1986, p 197.)
*Dose = dependent effects.
Abbreviations: ↑ = increase; → = no change; ↓ = decrease.

blood flow for several catecholamines and sympathomimetic agents used in the treatment of shock states.[134]

Dopamine

Dopamine has a long history of use in septic patients. The pharmacologic profile shows mixed α- and β-activity depending on the dose administered. Dopaminergic activity is usually associated with dosages of 0.5 to 3.0 $\mu g \cdot kg^{-1} \cdot min^{-1}$. Experimental work has documented aberrations in tissue oxygenation that lead to microcirculatory shunting of blood from ischemic tissues and ultimately to organ dysfunction. Additional vasopressor therapy may add to these abnormalities to the detriment of a patient.[57, 68, 98, 101]

Dobutamine

Because of undesired vasoconstriction at high doses of dopamine, increasing interest has been focused on dobutamine. In the dosage range of 5 to 15 $\mu g \cdot kg^{-1} \cdot min^{-1}$, the drug exhibits mixed β_1- and β_2-activity. Some investigators have postulated a weak α-activity in doses exceeding 15 $\mu g \cdot kg^{-1} \cdot min^{-1}$.[135] Nevertheless, the β-effects are by far more important and include improved peripheral circulation, myocardial contractility, and, if ventricular wall tension is decreased, a lowering of $M\dot{V}O_2$. Less tachycardia occurs than with dopamine or epinephrine. In early shock, improvements in $\dot{D}O_2$ are usually accompanied by improved $\dot{V}O_2$. In conjunction with intravascular volume augmentation, dobutamine may be the mainstay in the management of septic shock. Its value in the treatment of cardiogenic shock is well established.

Epinephrine

Epinephrine enjoys a venerable history in the management of shock. In the myocardium, the β_1- and β_2-effects produce increased contractility and a positive chronotropic effect. Increases in heart rate are associated with increased $M\dot{V}O_2$ and may be poorly tolerated in patients with fixed coronary obstruction. Alpha-activity is marked in the renal vasculature and

has been a source of concern in shock. We prefer to initiate biomechanical assist devices in cardiogenic shock rather than to persist with high doses of epinephrine.

Norepinephrine

Norepinephrine is predominantly an α-agonist. Dramatic improvement in arterial blood pressure is achieved at the expense of peripheral vasoconstriction and reduced vital organ perfusion.[134] Stimulation of β-receptors produces improved contractility, but the absolute increase is less than that achievable by many other sympathomimetic agents. Prolonged infusion of high-dose norepinephrine is associated with decrements in renal function and manifestations of mismatched $\dot{V}O_2$ and $\dot{D}O_2$.

In summary, the ultimate goal of therapy in septic or cardiogenic shock is not slavish maintenance of arterial blood pressure but rather improved matching of myocardial performance to peripheral circulatory needs.[16, 17, 57, 68, 136] Knowledge of the measured and derived parameters of cardiac performance and oxygen use and the effect of the prescribed therapy is essential to the rational use of pharmacologic support (Tables 40–8 and 40–9).[136]

How Should Ongoing Volume Losses Be Replaced?

Early restitution of intravascular volume can be life saving in major trauma. The choice of fluids and the rationale for their use were discussed earlier. Independent investigators have been unable to demonstrate differences in mortality according to the types of fluid used.[138–143] However, disadvantages of specific solutions are recognized.

Our preference is to commence resuscitation with a combination of colloid (5% albumin and 6% hetastarch) and crystalloid (lactated Ringer's) solutions. This philosophy is in keeping with the earlier work by Shoemaker and others, which showed a decrease in the time required for the restitution of intravascular volume and blood pressure[138, 143] when colloid

TABLE 40–8. Derived Hemodynamic Parameters*

Term	Formula	Units	Normal Range
Cardiac index	$CI = \dfrac{CO}{BSA}$	$L \cdot min \cdot m^{2^{-1}}$	2.8–4.2
Stroke volume	$SV = \dfrac{CO}{HR}$	$mL \cdot beat^{-1}$	(Varies with size)
Stroke index	$SI = \dfrac{SV}{BSA}$	$mL \cdot beat \cdot m^{2^{-1}}$	30–65
Mean arterial pressure	$MAP = DP + \dfrac{(SP - DP)}{3}$	mm Hg	70–105
Systemic vascular resistance	$SVR = \dfrac{MAP - CVP^3}{CO} \times 80$	$dyne \cdot s \cdot cm^{-5}$	900–1400
Pulmonary vascular resistance	$PVR = \dfrac{MPAP - PAOP}{CO} \times 80$	$dyne \cdot s \cdot cm^{-5}$	150–250
Left ventricular resistance	$OVSWI = SI (MAP - PAOP) \times 0.0136$	$g \cdot m \cdot m^{2^{-1}}$	43–61
Right ventricular stroke work index	$RVSWI = SI (MPAP - CVP) \times 0.0136$	$g \cdot m \cdot m^{2^{-1}}$	7–12
Coronary perfusion pressure	$CPP = DP - PAOP$	mm Hg	60–90

(From Barrett J, Nyhus LM: Treatment of Shock: Principles and Practice. 2nd ed. Philadelphia, Lea & Febiger, 1986, p 44.)
*Hemodynamic parameters derived from intravascular pressure and flow measurements are used to select the optimal management for patients with inadequate cardiac output.
Abbreviations: CO = cardiac output; BSA = body surface area; HR = heart rate; DP = diastolic pressure; SP = systolic pressure; CVP = central venous pressure; MPAP = mean pulmonary artery pressure; PAOP = pulmonary artery occlusion pressure.

TABLE 40–9. Cardiorespiratory Formulas Derived from Analysis of Gases

Term	Formula	Units	Normal Range
Arterial O_2 content	Cao_2 (Hb × 1.39 × Sao_2) + (0.0031 × Pao_2)	mL $O_2 \cdot dL^{-1}$	16–22
Mixed venous O_2 content	$C\bar{v}o_2$ = (Hb × 1.39 × $S\bar{v}o_2$) + (0.0031 × $P\bar{v}o_2$)	mL $O_2 \cdot dL^{-1}$	12–17
Pulmonary capillary O_2 content	$C\acute{c}o_2$ = (Hb × 1.39) + (0.0031 × Pao_2)	mL$O_2 \cdot dL^{-1}$	(Varies with Fio_2)
Alveolar O_2 tension	Pao_2 = (PB − PH_2O) Fio_2 − $\dfrac{Paco_2}{RQ}$	mm Hg	(Varies with Fio_2)
Arterial-venous O_2 content difference	$C(a - \bar{v})o_2$ = Cao_2 − Cvo_2	mL $O_2 \cdot dL^{-1}$	3–5
Respiratory quotient	$RQ = \dfrac{\dot{V}co_2}{\dot{V}o_2}$	Fraction	0.7–1.0
CO_2 production	$\dot{V}co_2$ = VE × $Feco_2$	mL $\cdot$ min^{-1}	140–250
O_2 consumption (Fick)	$\dot{V}o_2$ = $C(a - v) Do_2$ × CO × 10	mL $\cdot$ min^{-1}	180–280
O_2 consumption (measured)	$\dot{V}o_2$ = VE $\dfrac{(Fio_2 - Feo_2 - [Fio_2 × Feco_2])}{1 - Fio_2}$	mL $\cdot$ min^{-1}	180–280
Physiologic right-to-left shunt (venous admixture)	$\dot{Q}sp/\dot{Q}t = \dfrac{C\acute{c}o_2 - Cao_2}{C\acute{c}o_2 - C\bar{v}o_2}$	Fraction	0.03–0.05

(From Barrett J, Nyhus LM: Treatment of Shock: Principles and Practice. 2nd ed. Philadelphia, Lea & Febiger, 1986, p 36.)
*Cardiorespiratory measurements derived from the analysis of blood and expired gases form the basis for understanding oxygen transport balance.
Abbreviations: HB = hemoglobin concentration; Sao_2 = arterial O_2 saturation; Pao_2 = arterial O_2 tension; $S\bar{v}o_2$ = mixed venous O_2 saturation; $P\bar{v}o_2$ = mixed venous O_2 tension; PB = barometric pressure; PH_2O = partial pressure of water vapor (47 mm Hg at 37 °C); VE = expired minute ventilation; $Feco_2$ = mixed expired CO_2 fraction; CO = cardiac output; Fio_2 = inspired O_2 fraction; Feo_2 = expired O_2 fraction.

solutions were used. Hypertonic solutions may also be useful.[144–147] They typically include saline (7.5%) or a combination of hypertonic saline and hetastarch or albumin. These fluids supply more sustained improvements in intravascular volume and colloid oncotic pressure, with lower total amounts required.

What Is the Goal of Red Blood Cell Transfusion?

Augmentation of red blood cell mass must be part of the acute and ongoing resuscitation of trauma.[148] Our goal is to restore the hematocrit to a level between 27% and 32% within the framework of a normal intravascular volume. These recommendations are flexible but are based on our view that lower levels are disadvantageous for patients with intrinsic coronary or cerebrovascular disease. In such individuals, compensatory increases in $\dot{V}o_2$ are limited by already high levels of extraction in the brain and myocardium. When such compensation is exhausted, increased demands without increased supply lead to tissue ischemia and injury or death. Higher hematocrit values may be "wasted" in the presence of ongoing blood losses.

What Is the Value of Serum Electrolyte Measurement?

Specific electrolytes of interest include sodium, potassium, ionized calcium, and magnesium. Acute dilutional hyponatremia is associated with seizures and cerebral edema. Hypernatremia often results from repeated administration of sodium bicarbonate and, less commonly, from infusion of hypertonic saline solutions.

Significant hypokalemia may occur with prolonged resusci-

tation and the use of solutions containing little or no potassium. The likelihood of cardiac dysfunction and dysrhythmias increases in hypokalemic patients. Serum potassium levels may decrease significantly after prolonged epinephrine infusion[149] and other β_2 inotropic support. Hyperkalemia is associated with cardiac dysrhythmias and ventricular fibrillation at serum concentrations >7.0 mEq $\cdot$ L^{-1}. In acutely traumatized patients, however, it is uncommon.

Interest in calcium centers on the decreases in ionized levels that may occur in response to the rapid infusion of citrated blood products.[150] Hypocalcemia is associated with cardiac depression and coagulopathy.

Magnesium is important for its role in maintaining the transmembrane electrical stability of the myocardium. Low serum levels are dysrhythmogenic, especially when coupled with hypokalemia. Correction of the latter often necessitates concomitant administration of magnesium.

PULMONARY DYSFUNCTION

Pulmonary dysfunction may occur as an early or late sequela of shock. Early dysfunction is primary, related to direct parenchymal injury, or secondary, as a manifestation of other injury. Primary dysfunction includes blunt thoracic trauma and pulmonary contusion, as well as aspiration of gastric contents. Secondary dysfunction includes neurogenic pulmonary edema following acute head injury, acute pulmonary edema following cardiogenic shock, and bronchospasm accompanying anaphylaxis. Elimination of the inciting cause should take first priority (CHF, cerebral edema, anaphylaxis). Subsequently (or often concurrently), abnormalities of gas exchange should be addressed, using conventional therapeutic regimens. Typical problems include interstitial pulmonary edema, alveolar collapse, decreased compliance, increased dead space, $\dot{V}/\dot{Q}$ mismatch, and decreased functional residual capacity (FRC).

When Is Positive End-Expiratory Pressure Effective?

Recommended therapy includes graded application of PEEP and an enriched fraction of inspired oxygen (Fio_2).[151, 152] The rationale for PEEP is based primarily on improvement of pulmonary compliance and recruitment and stabilization of atelectatic alveoli, problems that are not corrected by IPPV alone (Fig. 40–14) (see Chapter 47). PEEP increases the FRC and promotes arterial oxygenation at a lower Fio_2.

Prophylactic Positive End-Expiratory Pressure

Because PEEP is useful for the treatment of acute respiratory failure, one must ask whether its prophylactic use is indicated to prevent ARDS. This question was addressed in a randomized study that reaffirmed the value of PEEP in the treatment of ARDS but showed no benefit of early application to patients at high risk for its development.[153]

HYPOTHERMIA

Unintentional hypothermia, the undesired and nontherapeutic decrease in core body temperature to <34.5 °C, remains a critical operating room problem in shock and trauma.

Temperature homeostasis involves a complex system of receptors and feedback loops that are integrated at the hypothalamic level to produce normal body temperature. In its most rudimentary form, body temperature reflects the balance between heat loss and heat gain. In shock, the intrinsic metabolic processes become deranged, thermoregulatory set-points are altered, and the efficient control of heat loss by behavior or physiologic mechanisms is disrupted. These alterations, compounded by the cold environment of the operating room, predispose to hypothermia (see Chapter 49).

Hypothermia exacerbates acidosis, induces platelet dysfunctional coagulopathy, predisposes to dysrhythmias, and potentiates neuromuscular blockade. In awake or unparalyzed patients, shivering dramatically increases $\dot{V}o_2$, placing unwanted demands on the myocardium and leading to potential ischemia and infarction when coronary arterial blood supply is marginal.

How Does Heat Loss Occur?

Evaporation

Evaporative losses are a reflection of the latent heat of vaporization. For every gram of water evaporated from the body surface, 0.58 Kcal of heat is lost. Such losses occur with skin preparation solutions, exposed viscera (lung and bowel in particular), and humidification of cold, dry inspired respiratory gases as they pass through the airways. Decreases of evaporative losses are achieved with barrier draping for exposed bowel, warming and humidifying the inspired anesthetic gases, and maintaining the operating room at a higher relative humidity and temperature.

Conduction

Conductive losses reflect heat transferred to objects in direct contact with a patient. An extension of this concept involves

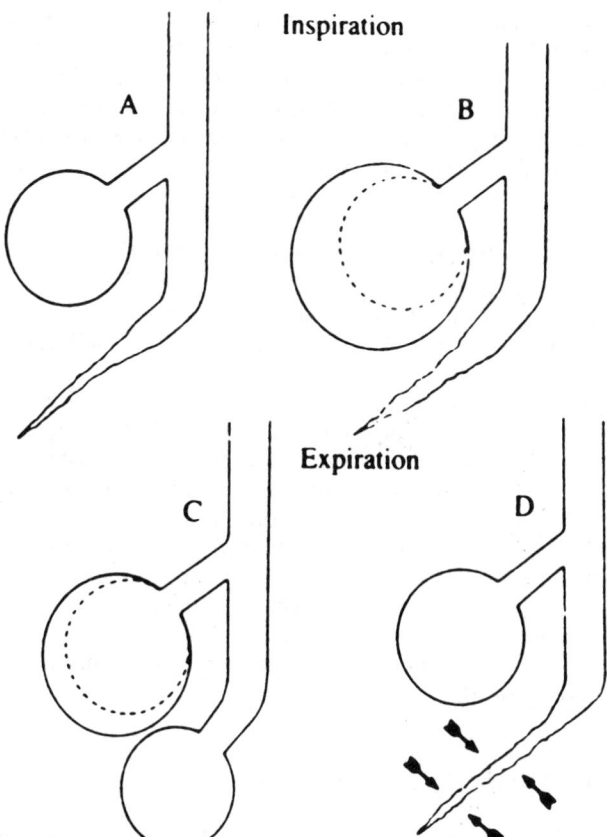

FIGURE 40–14. Limitation of intermittent positive-pressure ventilation (IPPV). Suggested events occurring in two adjacent lung segments (or alveoli), one of which (A) is normally inflated and the other of which is collapsed or fluid-filled. Initial inflation (B) tends to increase volume in the normal area preferentially. Later in the cycle (C), continued gas delivery may partially inflate the abnormal area. During exhalation (D), whatever forces were predisposing to airway closure are again unopposed, and a return to the baseline abnormal condition results. (From Kirby RR: Mechanical ventilation in the newborn: pitfalls and practice. Perinatol Neonatol 1981; 5:47.)

heat loss related to the infusion of cold intravenous solutions and blood products. Prevention involves the use of insulating blankets, appropriate draping, increased room temperature, and the warming of all administered intravenous solutions and blood products. The use of high-volume countercurrent fluid warmers for the treatment of shock and trauma is standard in our institution.

Convection

Convective losses occur with air movement over exposed skin. Because most operating rooms have high levels of air exchange or laminar flow conditions, the conditions of air movement cannot be modified. Thus, patients must be well covered with blankets and draping materials. Additional drafts should be prevented by closing corridor and hall doors to the operating room.

Radiation

Radiant heat loss is based on the principle that any body above the temperature of 0 °K emits electromagnetic energy. Energy loss is a function of the temperature differential between the patient and the surrounding environment (windows, walls, and ceiling). Loss of radiant heat is prevented by using insulating barriers and increasing the temperature of the surrounding environment. In small infants and children, radiant heaters are useful. Perforated blankets that bathe a patient with warmed air are also effective but not widely used.

ORGAN RESPONSES TO SHOCK

Throughout this chapter, it has been reiterated that shock is a disease with multiple progenitors, mediators, and effects. The common element is decreased perfusion, causing tissue hypoxia and deprivation of metabolic substrates. As ischemia persists, the cascade of events leading to cell death is set in action. These include loss of high-energy intermediates, formation of free radicals, massive cellular calcium influx, autolysis, and the loss of intracellular organelles.

Well-established evidence documents that cells that were only compromised during the initial insult may be fatally injured during the reperfusion stage.[134, 154] Blunting of the reperfusion injury through the use of free radical scavengers, membrane stabilizers, and prostaglandin inhibitors is a major focus of shock research.

How Are the Kidneys Affected?

The kidneys display a great deal of heterogeneity in both the tubular and cortical response to shock.[155, 156] As arterial pressure drops, sympathetic nervous system outflow reduces and redistributes renal blood flow. Redistribution occurs primarily from the outer to the inner cortex. Tubular flow also is altered, but no specific pattern of change is noted.

Damage Sites

Glomerular capillary cells and those of the pars recta of the proximal tubule are most susceptible to injury. The tubules vary in their susceptibility to ischemia. This variability, coupled with the redistribution of flow, probably accounts for the diverse patterns of renal injury after shock. The time frame of ischemia and injury suggests that 25 minutes of normothermic ischemia produces mild, reversible injury, whereas 40 to 60 minutes produces severe dysfunction, with some elements of recovery requiring several weeks.[157] These are rough guidelines, however, and not all patients sustain the same magnitude of injury for similar ischemic insults. Indeed, as little as 10 minutes of significant hypotension has been associated with acute renal failure.

Postischemic Injuries

Typical renal tubular postischemic injuries include (1) damaged tubules promoting interstitial edema and tubular collapse, (2) tubular necrosis, and (3) tubular blockage with debris or cellular casts.[134, 157] Alterations in the glomerular filtration rate (GFR) occur as well.[158] The majority of such cases evolve to a short bout of nonoliguric renal failure, and no other renal support is required.

A subset of patients, however, fail to achieve normal GFR after resuscitation and may develop tubular dysfunction with oliguric renal failure. This syndrome, referred to as *acute tubular necrosis* (ATN), requires dialysis therapy. The combined insult of trauma and postresuscitation ATN carries a mortality of 70% compared with a mortality of 25% to 30% for nonoliguric renal failure.[159]

How Is the Gut Affected?

The bowel is particularly susceptible to the effects of ischemia. As with the kidneys, a significant component of the overall injury is related to reperfusion. As ischemia evolves, the bowel loses motility, and massive volumes of fluid may be sequestered both intraluminally and in the bowel wall (third space losses). With necrosis, toxins and ischemia-related metabolites are absorbed, adding to the shock state and having direct effects on the function of other organ systems as well.[160]

When Does Liver Injury Occur?

Hepatic damage also occurs early as a result of hypotension or hypoxia and subsequently during the reperfusion phase. The earliest manifestation may be changes in the intracellular energy substrates and metabolic decompensation of the cellular organelles.[161] As intracellular high-energy substrates are depleted, free radical formation, calcium influx, and lipid peroxidation lead to mitochondrial damage and cell injury or death[136] (Fig. 40–15).

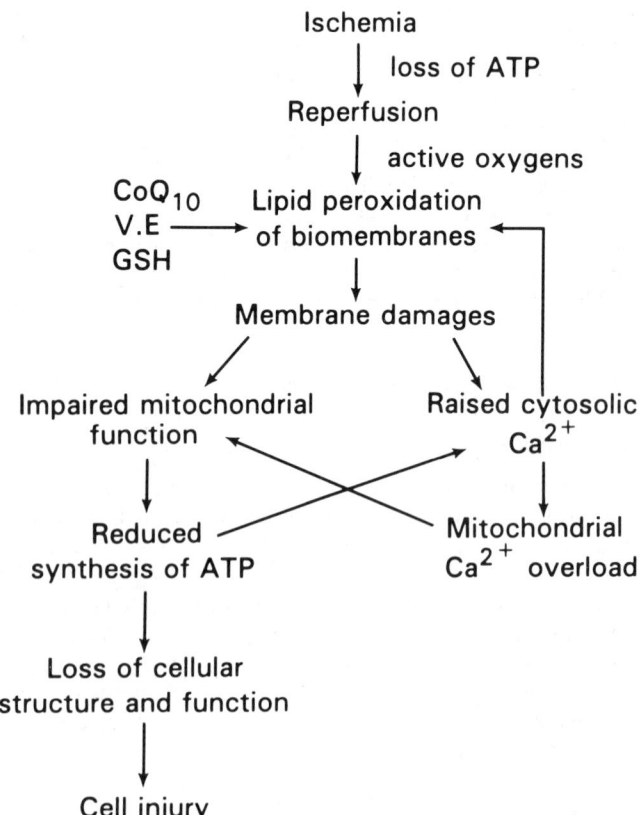

FIGURE 40–15. Schematic representation of the sequence of events leading to ischemic liver cell injury. (From Barrett J, Nyhus LM: Treatment of Shock: Principles and Practice. 2nd ed. Philadelphia, Lea & Febiger, 1986, p 159.)

As the liver fails, its metabolic function decreases and predisposes other organ systems to failure as well. Parenchymal injury affects the reticuloendothelial system (RES), with a resultant decrease of phagocytic activity[134, 162–164] and production of fibronectin, a tissue opsonic protein.

Normally, the RES acts as a filter for blood-borne particulate matter, including bacteria, leukocyte and platelet aggregates, and tissue debris. The combination of decreased opsonic activity and the loss of the RES filtering capacity allow particulate matter to circulate for longer periods, adding to the propensity for complications in other organ systems (pulmonary insufficiency, renal failure, septicemia, and coagulopathy).

What Are the Causes of Acute Pulmonary Failure?

Acute pulmonary failure or ARDS following shock is multifactorial in origin[165–168] (Table 40–10). It is a major contributor to morbidity in shock and has an associated mortality of >50% in most reported series. Although the mediators of ARDS are not fully elucidated, isolated hypotension and resuscitation are not causative. Rather, soft tissue trauma or frank sepsis, combined with hypotension, is a necessary progenitor. Once initiated, the cascade of events includes the expected features of complement and platelet activation, leukotactic response (migration of polymorphonuclear neutrophils to the pulmonary microvascular bed), and the release of cytotoxic products (prostaglandins, thromboxanes, free radicals, and proteolytic enzymes) (Fig. 40–16).

Pathologic Features

The key pathologic abnormality in ARDS appears to be leakage of protein-rich fluid at the capillary endothelial basement membrane and the resultant generation of interstitial edema in the perivascular and peribronchial tissue.[167, 168] Interstitial accumulation of this proteinaceous fluid leads to changes in lung compliance and subsequent alveolar flooding, loss of surfactant, and atelectasis. The associated loss of lung volume and progression of $\dot{V}/\dot{Q}$ mismatching produces hypoxemia. Associated damage to the alveolar epithelium, together with the accumulated protein and fibrin, predisposes to the formation of hyaline membranes and, in the final stages of resolution, to interstitial fibrosis.

TABLE 40–10. Causes of Adult Respiratory Distress Syndrome

Thoracic and nonthoracic trauma
Gram-negative sepsis
Fat embolism—fractures
Aspiration
Pancreatitis
Intestinal infarction
Burns
Cardiopulmonary bypass
Viral and bacterial pneumonia
Oxygen toxicity
Neurogenic factors
Massive blood transfusion

(From Barrett J, Nyhus LM: Treatment of Shock: Principles and Practice. 2nd ed. Philadelphia, Lea & Febiger, 1986, p 60.)

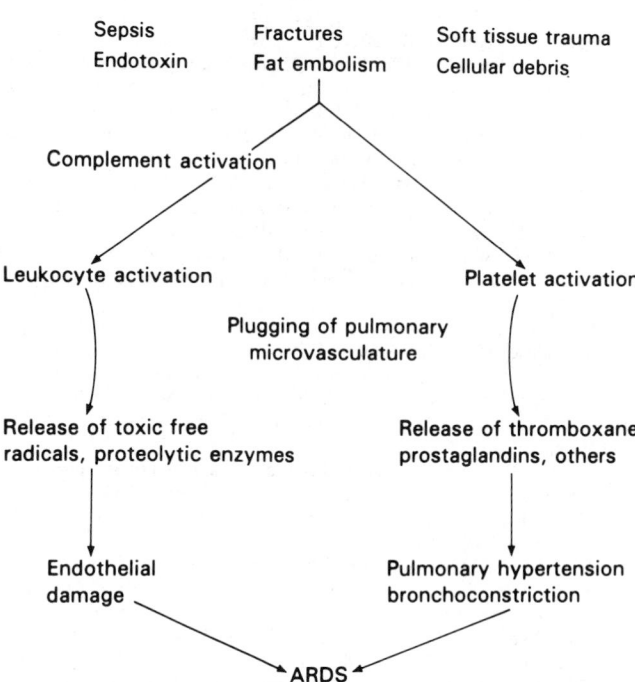

INITIATING EVENT

FIGURE 40–16. Pathogenesis of ARDS. (From Barrett J, Nyhus LM: Treatment of Shock: Principles and Practice. 2nd ed. Philadelphia, Lea & Febiger, 1986, p 68.)

Treatment

Treatment is entirely supportive and, as discussed previously, is focused on restoration of the FRC and correction of the associated $\dot{V}/\dot{Q}$ abnormalities (see Chapters 47 and 48).

References

1. Hardaway RM: Treatment of shock from a clinical viewpoint. *In* Circulatory Shock: Basic and Clinical Implications. Janssen HF, Barnes CD (eds). San Diego, Academic Press, 1985, pp 197–235.
2. Lefer AM, Williams SK. Microcirculation in shock. *In* Treatment of Shock. 2nd ed. Barrett J, Nyhus LM (eds). Philadelphia, Lea & Febiger, 1986, pp 3–21.
3. White RR, Mela L, Bacalzo LV, et al: Hepatic ultrastructure in endotoxemia, hemorrhage and hypoxia: emphasis on mitochondria changes. Surgery 1973; 73:525.
4. White JG: Platelet structural physiology: the ultrastructure of adhesion, secretion, and aggregation in arterial thrombus. *In* Thrombosis and Platelets in Myocardial Ischemia. Mehta JL (ed). Philadelphia, FA Davis, 1987, pp 13–33.
5. Packham MA, Mustard JF. Platelet adhesion. *In* Progressive Hemostasis and Thrombosis. Vol. 17. Spaet TH (ed). Orlando, Grune & Stratton, 1984, p 211.
6. Lefer AM, Tsao PS, Ma XL. Shock and ischemia-induced mechanisms of impairment of endothelium-mediated vasodilation. Chest 1991; 100(Suppl):161S.
7. Palmer RMJ, Ferrige AG, Moncada S: Nitric oxide release accounts for the biological activity of endothelium-derived relaxing factor. Nature 1988; 327:524.
8. Johnson G, Tsao PS, Mulloy D, et al: Cardioprotective effects of acidified sodium nitrite (NaNO$_2$) in myocardial ischemia with reperfusion. J Pharmacol Exp Ther 1989; 252:35.
9. Frostell C, Fratazzi M, Wain J, et al: Inhaled nitric oxide: a selective pulmonary vasodilator reversing hypoxic pulmonary vasoconstriction. Circulation 1991; 83:2038.
10. Vanhoutte PM: Epithelium-derived relaxing factors and bronchial reactivity. Am Rev Respir Dis 1988; 138:524.

11. Girard C: Inhaled nitric oxide, potent and selective pulmonary vasodilator (Abstract 984). ASA 1991 Annual Meeting. San Francisco, CA, October 26, 27, 1991.

12. Forestell C: Nitric oxide: effect on hypoxic pulmonary vasoconstriction (Abstract 989). ASA 1991 Annual Meeting. San Francisco, CA, October 26, 27, 1991.

13. Consensus Trial Study Group: Effects of enalapril on mortality in severe congestive heart failure. Results of cooperative north Scandinavian enalapril survival study. N Engl J Med 1987; 316:23.

14. Lefer AM, Ogletree ML, Smith JB, et al: Prostacyclin: profile of a potentially valuable agent for preserving jeopardized myocardial tissue in acute myocardial ischemia. Science 1978; 200:52.

15. Shoemaker WC, Kram HB, Appel PL: Therapy of shock based on pathophysiology, monitoring, and outcome prediction. Crit Care Med 1990; 18:19.

16. Cain SM, Curtis SE: Experimental models of pathologic oxygen supply dependency (Mini Symposium). Crit Care Med 1991; 19:5.

17. Villar J, Slutsky AS, Hew E, et al: Oxygen transport and oxygen consumption in critically ill patients. Chest 1990; 98:687.

18. Stene JK, Grande CM (eds): Trauma Anesthesia. Baltimore, Williams & Wilkins, 1991.

19. Holcroft JW, Link OP, Lantz BM, et al: Venous return and pneumatic anti-shock garment—hypovolemic baboons. J Trauma 1984; 24:928.

20. McSwain NE: Pneumatic trousers and the management of shock. J Trauma 1977; 17:719.

21. Mackersie RC: The pneumatic anti-shock garment. *In* Clinical Procedures in Anesthesia and Intensive Care. Benumof J (ed). Philadelphia, JB Lippincott, 1992, p 549.

22. Shoemaker WC, Thompson WL, Holbrook PR: Textbook of Critical Care. Philadelphia, WB Saunders, 1984.

23. Shires GT, Carrico CT, Cohn D: The role of extracellular fluid in shock. Int Anesthesiol Clinic 1964; 2:435.

24. Weisel RD, Charlesworth DC, Mickleborough LL, et al: Limitations of blood conservation. J Thorac Cardiovasc Surg 1984; 88:26.

25. Haupt MT, Rackow EC: Colloid osmotic pressure and fluid resuscitation with hetastarch, albumin and saline solution. Crit Care Med 1982; 10:159.

26. Dawidson I, Gelin L, Haglind E: Plasma volume, intravascular protein content, hemodynamic and oxygen transport changes during intestinal shock in dogs. Crit Care Med 1980; 8:73.

27. Shimazaki S, Yukioka T, Matuda H: Fluid distribution and pulmonary function following burn shock. J Trauma 1991; 31:623.

28. Pearl RG, Halperin BD, Mihm FG, et al: Pulmonary effects of crystalloid and colloid resuscitation from hemorrhagic shock in presence of oleic acid-induced pulmonary capillary injury in dog. Anesthesiology 1968; 68:12.

29. Shibutani K, Komatsu T, Kubal K, et al: Critical level of oxygen delivery in anesthetized man. Crit Care Med 1983; 11:640.

30. Wilkerson DK, Rosen AL, Gould SA, et al: Oxygen extraction ratio: a valid indication of myocardial metabolism in anemia. J Surg Res 1987; 42:629.

31. Laks H, Pilon RN, Klovekorn P, et al: Acute hemodilution: its effect on hemodynamics and oxygen transport in anesthetized man. Ann Surg 1984; 3:103.

32. Burch GE, DePasquale NP. Hematocrit, viscosity and coronary blood flow. Dis Chest 1965; 48:225.

33. Robertie PG, Gravlee G: The limits of isovolemic hemodilution and recommendations for erythrocyte transfusion. Int Anesthesiol Clin 1990; 28:197.

34. Carson JL, Spence RK, Poses RM, et al: Severity of anemia and operative mortality and morbidity. Lancet 1988; i:727.

35. Gould SA, Rosen AL, Sehgal LR, et al: Fluosol-DA as a red cell substitute in acute anemia. N Engl J Med 1986; 314:1653.

36. Sehgal LR, Rosen AL, Gould SA, et al: Artificial blood: current status of fluorocarbon and hemoglobin solution. Anesth Rev 1990; 17(Suppl 3):38.

37. Nago S, Roccaforte P, Moody R: The effects of isovolemic hemodilution and reinfusion of packed erythrocytes on somatosensory and visual evoked potentials. J Surg Res 1978; 25:530.

38. Michenfelder JD, Theye RA: The effects of profound hypocapnia and dilutional anemia on canine cerebral metabolism and blood flow. Anesthesiology 1969; 31:449.

39. Brazier J, Corper N, Maloney J, et al: The adequacy of myocardial oxygen delivery in acute normovolemic anemia. Surgery 1974; 75:508.

40. Crystal GJ, Salem RM: Myocardial oxygen consumption and sequential shortening during selective coronary hemodilution in dogs. Anesth Analg 1988; 67:500.

41. Willerson JT, Frazier OH: Reducing mortality in patients with extensive myocardial infarction. N Engl J Med 1991; 325:1666.

42. Beyersdorf F, Buckberg GD, Acar C, et al: Cardiogenic shock after acute coronary occlusion. Thorac Cardiovasc Surg 1989; 37:28.

43. Goldberg RJ, Gore JM, Alpert JS, et al: Cardiogenic shock after acute myocardial infarction: incidence and mortality from a community-wide perspective 1975–1988. N Engl J Med 1991; 325:1117.

44. ISIS-3: A randomized comparison of streptokinase vs tissue plasminogen activator vs anistreplase and of aspirin plus heparin vs aspirin alone among 41,299 cases of suspected acute myocardial infarction. Third International Study of Infarct Survival, Collaborative Group. Lancet 1992; 339:753.

45. Arnold AE, Brower RW, Collen D, et al: Increased serum levels of fibrinogen degradation products due to treatment with recombinant tissue-type plasminogen activator for acute myocardial infarction are related to bleeding complications, but not to coronary patency. European Co-operative Study Groups for rt-PA. J Am Coll Cardiol 1989; 14:581.

46. Athanasuleas CL, Geer DA, Arciniegas JG: A reappraisal of surgical intervention for acute myocardial infarction. J Thorac Cardiovasc Surg 1987; 93:405.

47. Mueller HS: Reperfusion therapy in acute myocardial infarction. Present status and controversy. Clin Cardiol 1990; 13:239.

48. Gruppo Italiano Per Lo Studio Della Streptochinasi Nell' Infarcto Miocardio (GISSI). Effectiveness of intravenous thrombolytic treatment in acute myocardial infarction. Lancet 1986; 1:397.

49. Lee L, Bates ER, Pitt B, et al: Percutaneous transluminal coronary angioplasty improves survival in acute myocardial infarction complicated by cardiogenic shock. Circulation 1986; 78:1345.

50. King SB: American College of Cardiology—Cardiovascular Conference at Snowmass. Aspen, CO, January 1992.

51. Grines CL: Current thrombolytic options for myocardial infarction. Prim Cardiol 1991; 17:62.

52. Chesebro JH: American College of Cardiology—Cardiovascular Conference at Snowmass. Aspen, CO, January 1992.

53. Roberts R, Rogers WJ, Mueller HS, et al: Results of thrombolysis on myocardial infarction (TIMI) II-B study. Immediate verses deferred β-blockade following thrombolytic therapy in patients with acute myocardial infarction. Circulation 1991; 83:422.

54. ISIS-2 Collaborative Group: Randomized trial of intravenous streptokinase, oral aspirin, both or neither, among 17,187 cases of suspected acute myocardial infarction. Lancet 1988; 2:349.

55. Guyton RA, Arcidi JM, Langford DA, et al: Emergency coronary bypass for cardiogenic shock. Circulation 1987; 76(Suppl V):V22.

56. Balooki H: Surgical treatment of complications of acute myocardial infarction. JAMA 1990; 263:1237.

57. Shoemaker WC: Tissue perfusion and oxygenation: a primary problem in acute circulatory failure and shock states. Crit Care Med 1991; 9:595.

58. Forrester JS, Diamond GA, Swan HJC: Correlative classification of clinical and hemodynamic function after acute myocardial infarction. Am J Cardiol 1977; 39:137.

59. Creamer J, Edwards JD, Nightingale P: Hemodynamic and oxygen transport variables in cardiogenic shock following acute myocardial infarction and their response to treatment. Am J Cardiol 1990; 65:1297.

60. Magovern GJ, Magovern JA, Sakert T, et al: Long-term follow up of 27 centrifugal circulatory support survivors (Abstract). Society of Thoracic Surgeons 1991. Annual Meeting.

61. Wampler RK, Frazier OH, Lansing AM, et al: Treatment of cardiogenic shock with the hemopump left ventricular device. Ann Thorac Surg 1991; 52:506.

62. Kronenfeld MA: Mechanical circulatory assist devices. Prog Anesthesiol 1989; Jan III(2).

63. Mann JM, Roberts WC: Rupture of the left ventricular free wall during acute myocardial infarction. Am J Cardiol 1988; 62:847.

64. AIMS Trial Study Group: Long-term effects of intravenous anistreplase in acute myocardial infarction: final report of the AIMS study. Lancet 1990; 335:427.

65. Gersh B: American College of Cardiology—Cardiovascular Conference. Snowbird, UT, 1990.

66. Moore CA, Nygaard TW, Kaiser DL, et al: Post infarction ventricular septal rupture: the importance of location of infarction and right ventricular function in determining survival. Circulation 1986; 74:45.

67. Eddy AC, Rice CL, Anardi DM: Right ventricular dysfunction in multiple trauma victims. Am J Surg 1988; 155:712.

68. Edwards JD: Oxygen transport in cardiogenic and septic shock. Crit Care Med 1991; 19:658.

69. Lawson D, Norley I, Korbon, et al: Blood flow limits and pulse oximeter signal detection. Anesthesiology 1987; 67:599.

70. Pälve H, Vuori A: Accuracy of three pulse oximeters at low cardiac index and peripheral temperature. Crit Care Med 1991; 19:560.

71. Spackman TN, Faust RJ, Cucchiara RF, et al: A comparison of the life scan EEG monitor with EEG and cerebral blood flow for detection of cerebral ischemia. Anesthesiology 1985; 63:A187.

72. Boston Collaborative Drug Surveillance Program. Drug-induced anaphylaxis. JAMA 1973; 224:613.

73. Wasserman SI, Marquardt DL: Anaphylaxis. In Allergy: Principles and Practice. Vol. 2. Middleton E Jr, Reed CE, Ellis EF, et al (eds). St Louis, CV Mosby, 1988, pp 1365–1376.

74. Bochner BS, Lichtenstein LM: Anaphylaxis, current concepts. N Engl J Med 1991; 324:1785.

75. Castells MC, Irani AM, Schwartz LB: Evaluation of human peripheral blood leukocytes for mast cell tryptase. J Immunol 1981; 138:2184.

76. Metcalfe DD, Bland CE, Wasserman SI: Chemical and functional characterization of proteoglycans isolated from basophils of patients with chronic myelogenous leukemia. J Immunol 1984; 132:1943.

77. Schwartz LB, Irani AM, Roller K, et al: Quantitation of histamine, tryptase, and chymase in dispersed human T and TC mast cells. J Immunol 1987; 138:2611.

78. Stevens RL, Fox CC, Lichtenstein LM, et al: Identification of chondroitin sulfate E proteoglycans and heparin proteoglycans in the secretory granules of human lung mast cells. Proc Natl Acad Sci USA 1988; 85:2284.

79. Triggiani M, Hubbard WC, Chilton FH: Synthesis of 1-acyl-2-acetyl-sn-glycero-3-phosphocholine by an enriched preparation of the human lung mast cell. J Immunol 1990; 144:4773.

80. Zaloga GP, DeLaney W, Holmboe E, et al: Glucagon reversal of hypotension in a case of anaphylactoid shock. Ann Intern Med 1986; 105:65.

81. Hirshman CA: Anaphylaxis and anesthesia. ASA 1985 Refresher Course Lectures. San Francisco, CA, October 1985.

82. Smith D: Perioperative management of the patient with acute spinal cord injury. ASA 1988 Refresher Course Lectures. San Francisco, CA, October 1988.

83. Bracken MB, Shepard MG, Collins WF, et al: A randomized, controlled trial of methylprednisolone or naloxone in the treatment of acute spinal-cord injury. N Engl J Med 1990; 222:1411.

84. Vertosik F, Willberger JE: Pharmacotherapy of spinal cord injury. In Spinal Cord Injuries in Children. Wilberger JE Jr (ed). New York, Futura, 1986, pp 111–130.

85. Young W, Ransohoff J: Injuries to the cervical cord. In The Cervical Spine, The Cervical Spine Research Society Editorial Committee. Philadelphia, JB Lippincott, 1989, pp 464–495.

86. Collins WF, Peipmeier J, Ogle E: The acute spinal cord injury problem—a review. Central Nervous System Trauma 1986; 3:317.

87. Albin MS: Acute spinal cord trauma. In: Textbook of Critical Care. Shoemaker WC, Thompson WL, Holbrook PR (eds). Philadelphia, WB Saunders, 1984, pp 928–936.

88. Faden AI: Opiate antagonists and thyrotropin-releasing hormone. II. Potential role in the treatment of central nervous system injury. JAMA 1984; 252:1452.

89. Bracken MB, Collins WF, Freeman DF, et al: Efficacy of methylprednisolone in acute spinal cord injury. JAMA 1984; 254:45.

90. Willberger J: Personal communication.

91. Geisler FH, Dorsey FC, Coleman WP: Recovery of motor function after spinal-cord injury—a randomized, placebo-controlled trial with GM-1 ganglioside. N Engl J Med 1991; 324:1829.

92. Frost EM: Anesthesia for neurosurgical emergencies. Anesthesiol Rev 1991; 27:21.

93. Ruben BH, Greenberg J: Neurologic injury: prevention and initial care. In Critical Care. Civetta J, Taylor RW, Kirby RR (eds). Philadelphia, JB Lippincott, 1992, pp 725–746.

94. Luce JM: Medical management of spinal cord injuries. Crit Care Med 1985; 13:126.

95. McGuire GP, Pearl RG: Sepsis and the trauma patient. Crit Care Clin 1990; 6:121.

96. Bone RC: A critical evaluation of new agents for the treatment of sepsis. JAMA 1991; 266:1686.

97. Boyd JL, Stanford GC, Chernow B: The pharmacotherapy of septic shock. Crit Care Clin 1989; 5:133.

98. Rosenthal MH: Shock: Diagnosis and treatment. ASA 1991 Refresher Course Lectures. San Francisco, CA, October 26, 27, 1991.

99. Tuchschmidt J, Oblitas D, Fried J: Oxygen consumption in sepsis and septic shock. Crit Care Med 1991; 19:664.

100. Slotman GJ, Quinn JV, Burchard DS: Thromboxane, prostacyclin and the hemodynamic effects of graded bacteremic shock. Circ Shock 1985; 16:395.

101. Shoemaker WC, Appel PL, Kram HB: Oxygen transport measurements to evaluate tissue perfusion and titrate therapy: dobutamine and dopamine effects. Crit Care Med 1991; 19:672.

102. Gutierrez G: Cellular energy metabolism during hypoxia. Crit Care Med 1991; 19:619.

103. Harkema JM, Chaudry IH: Magnesium-adenosine triphosphate in the treatment of shock, ischemia, and sepsis. Crit Care Med 1992; 20:263.

104. Ziegler EJ, Fisher CJ, Spring CL, et al: Treatment of gram-negative bacteremia and septic shock with HA-1A human monoclonal antibody against endotoxin. N Engl J Med 1991; 324:429.

105. Armstead CW, Vincent JL, Preiser JC, et al: Hypertonic saline solution—hetastarch for fluid resuscitation in experimental septic shock. Anesth Analg 1989; 69:714.

106. Prough DS, Johnston WE: Fluid resuscitation in septic shock: no solution yet. Anesth Analg 1989; 69:699.

107. Kimchi A, Ellrodt AG, Berman D, et al: Right ventricular performance in septic shock: a combined radionuclide and hemodynamic study. J Am Coll Cardiol 1984; 4:945.

108. Redl G, Zadrobilek E, Schindler I: Judgment of central hemodynamics with and without Swan Ganz catheter in septic shock states. First Vienna Shock Forum. New York, Alan R Liss, 1987, pp 123–128.

109. Dhainaut JF, Edwards JD, Grootendorst AF, et al: Practical aspects of oxygen transport: conclusions and recommendations of the round table conference. Intensive Care Med 1990; 16(Suppl 2):S179.

110. Martin C, Saux P, Eon B, et al: Septic shock: a goal directed therapy using volume loading, dobutamine and/or norepinephrine. Acta Anesthesiol Scand 1990; 34:413.

111. Vincent JL, Van Der Linden P, Domb M: Dopamine compared with dobutamine in experimental septic shock: relevance to fluid administration. Anesth Analg 1987; 66:565.

112. Schaler GL, Fink MP, Parrillo JE: Norepinephrine alone versus norepinephrine plus low dose dopamine: enhanced renal blood flow with combination pressor therapy. Crit Care Med 1985; 13:492.

113. Shoemaker W, Appel P, Kran H: Tissue oxygen debt as a determinant of lethal and nonlethal postoperative organ failure. Crit Care Med 1988; 16:1117.

114. Rosenthal M: Shock: diagnosis and treatment. ASA 1991 Refresher Course Lectures. San Francisco, CA, October 26, 27, 1991.

115. RA Cowley, CM Dunham (eds): Shock Trauma/Critical Care Manual: Initial Assessment and Management. Baltimore, University Park Press, 1987.

116. Van der Linden P, Gilbart E, Engelman E, et al: Comparison of halothane, isoflurane, alfentanil, and ketamine in experimental septic shock. Anesth Analg 1990; 70:608.

117. Pagel P, Schmeling W, Kampine J, et al: Alteration of canine left ventricular diastolic function by intravenous anesthetics in vivo. Ketamine and propofol. Anesthesiology 1992; 76:419.

118. Blackburn JP, Conway CM, Leigh M, et al: The effects of anesthetic induction agents upon myocardial contractility. Anesthesia 1982; 26:93.

119. Gooding J, Corssen G: Effect of etomidate on the cardiovascular system. Anesth Analg 1977; 56:717.

120. Lindeburg T, Spotoff H, Sorensen MB, Skovsted P: Cardiovascular effects of etomidate used for induction and in combination with fentanyl and pancuronium for maintenance of anesthesia in patients with valvular heart disease. Acta Anesthesial Scand 1982; 26:205.

121. Goodchild CS: Cardiovascular effects of propofol and relevance to use in patients with compromised cardiovascular function. Semin Anesth 1992; 11:37–38.

122. Williams JP, McArthur JD, Walker WE, et al: The cardiovascular effects of propofol in patients with impaired cardiac function. Anesth Analg 1986; 65:S166.

123. Schulte-Sasse U, Hess W, Tarnow J: Hemodynamic responses to induction of anesthesia using midazolam in cardiac surgical patients. Br J Anaesth 1982; 54:1053.

124. Reves JG, Samuelson PN, Lewis S: Midazolam maleate induction in patients with ischemic heart disease. Hemodynamic observations. Can Anesth Soc J 1979; 26:402.

125. Tomicheck FC, Rosow CE, Philbin DM, et al: Diazepam-fentanyl interaction: hemodynamic and hormonal effects in coronary artery surgery. Anesth Analg 1983; 62:881.

126. Sloggoff S, Keats A: Randomized trial of primary anesthetic agents on outcome of coronary artery bypass operations. Anesthesiology 1989; 70:179.

127. Tuman K, McCarthy R, Spiess B, et al: Does choice of anesthetic agent significantly affect outcome after coronary artery surgery? Anesthesiology 1989; 70:189.

128. Mangano D: Anesthetics, coronary artery disease, and outcome: unresolved controversies. Anesthesiology 1989; 70:175.

129. Mangano D: Perioperative cardiac morbidity. Anesthesiology 1990; 72:153.

130. Trunkey D: Trauma. Sci Am 1983; 249:28.

131. Billhardt R, Rosenbush S: Cardiogenic and hypovolemic shock. Med Clin North Am 1986; 70:853.

132. Stene J, Girard C, Giesecke A: Shock resuscitation. *In* Trauma Anesthesia. Stene GK, Grande CM (eds). Baltimore, Williams & Wilkins, 1981, pp 100–132.

133. Colacci W, Wright R, Braunwald E: New positive inotropic agents in the treatment of congestive heart failure: mechanisms of action and recent clinical developments (second of two parts). N Engl J Med 1986; 314:349.

134. Barret J, Nyhaus L (eds): Treatment of Shock: Principles and Practice. 2nd ed. Melvern, PA, Lea & Febiger, 1986.

135. Hoff JV, Beatty PA, Wade JL: Dermal necrosis from dobutamine. JAMA 1980; 243:1145.

136. Schaer G, Fink M, Parrillo J: Norepinephrine alone versus norepinephrine plus low dose dopamine: enhanced renal blood flow with combined pressor therapy. Crit Care Med 1985; 13:492.

137. Guillermo G: Cellular energy metabolism during hypoxia. Crit Care Med 1991; 19:619.

138. Shoemaker W, Schlucter M, Hopkins J, et al: Comparison of the relative effectiveness of colloids and crystalloids in emergency resuscitation. Am J Surg 1981; 142:73.

139. Pearl R, Halperin B, Mihm F, et al: Pulmonary effects of crystalloid and colloid resuscitation from hemorrhagic shock in the presence of oleic acid-induced pulmonary capillary injury in the dog. Anesthesiology 1988; 68:12.

140. Lowery B, Cloutior C, Carey L: Electrolyte solutions in resuscitation in human hemorrhagic shock. Surg Gynecol Obstet 1971; 133:273.

141. Nees J, Hauser C, Shippy C, et al: Comparison of cardiorespiratory effects of crystalline hemoglobin, whole blood, albumin, and Ringer's lactate in the resuscitation of hemorrhagic shock in dogs. Surgery 1978; 83:639.

142. Hankelin K, Radel C, Beez M, et al: Comparison of hydroxyethyl starch and lactated Ringer's solution on hemodynamics and oxygen transport of critically ill patients in prospective crossover studies. Crit Care Med 1989; 17:133.

143. Tait A, Larson L: Resuscitation fluids for the treatment of hemorrhagic shock in dogs. Effect on myocardial blood flow and oxygen transport. Crit Care Med 1991; 19:1561.

144. Armistead C, Vincent JL, Preiser JC, et al: Hypertonic saline solution-hetastarch for fluid resuscitation in experimental shock. Anesth Analg 1989; 69:714.

145. Oswaldo L, Velasco T, Guertzenstein P, et al: Hypertonic sodium chloride restores mean circulatory filling pressures in severely hypovolemic dogs. Hypertension 1986; 8(Suppl 1):I–195.

146. Velasco I, Silva M, Oliveira M, et al: Hypertonic and hyperoncotic resuscitation from severe hemorrhagic shock in dogs: a comparative study. Crit Care Med 1989; 17:261.

147. Stanford G, Patterson R, Payne L, et al: Hypertonic saline resuscitation in a porcine model of severe hemorrhagic shock. Arch Surg 1989; 124:733.

148. Schwab C, Civil I, Shayre J, et al: Saline-expanded group O uncross-matched packed red blood cells as an initial resuscitation fluid in severe shock. Ann Emerg Med 1986; 15:1282.

149. Brown M, Brown D, Murphy M: Hypokalemia form beta$_2$-receptor stimulation by circulating epinephrine. N Engl J Med 1983; 309:1414.

150. Coté C: Ionized hypocalcemia after fresh frozen plasma administration to thermally injured children: effect of infusion rate, duration and treatment with calcium chloride. Anesth Analg 1988; 67:152.

151. Suter PM, Fairley HB, Isenberg MD: Effect of tidal volume and positive and expiratory pressure on compliance during mechanical ventilation. N Engl J Med 1975; 292:284.

152. Rinaldo JE, Rogers RM: Adult respiratory distress syndrome: changing concepts in lung injury and repair. N Engl J Med 1982; 306:900.

153. Pepe P, Hudson L, Carrico J: Early application of positive and expiratory pressure in patients at high risk for the adult respiratory distress syndrome. N Engl J Med 1984; 311:281.

154. Hearse D: Reperfusion of the ischemic myocardium. J Mol Cell Cardiol 1977; 9:605.

155. Passmore JC: Role of the kidney in shock: current views. *In* Handbook of Shock and Trauma. Vol. 1. Basic Science. Altura BM (ed). New York, Raven Press, 1983.

156. Brezis M, Rosen S, Silva P, et al: Renal ischemia: a new perspective. Kidney Int 1984; 26:375.

157. Venkatachalam MA, Rennke HG, Sandstrom DJ: The vascular basis for acute renal failure in the rat. Circ Res 1967; 38:267.

158. Levinsky NG: The pathophysiology of acute renal failure. N Engl J Med 1979; 296:1453.

159. Stene JK: Renal failure in the trauma patient. Crit Care Med 1990; 6:111.

160. Sobel BE: Cardiac and non-cardiac forms of acute circulatory failure (shock). *In* Heart Disease: A Textbook of Cardiovascular Medicine. Braunwald E (ed). Philadelphia, WB Saunders, 1984, pp 578–604.

161. Pass LJ, Schloerb PR, Chow FT, et al: Liver adenosine triphosphate (ATP) in hemorrhagic shock in rats. J Trauma 1982; 22:730.

162. Nakatani T: The pathophysiology of septic shock: studies of the reticuloendothelial system and liver high-energy metabolism in rats following sublethal and lethal escherichia coli injection. Adv Shock Res 1982; 7:147.

163. Kaplan JE: Reticulo-endothelial phagocytic response to bacterial challenge after traumatic shock. Circ Shock 1977; 4:1.

164. MacLean LD: Shock: a century of progress. Ann Surg 1985; 201:407.

165. Billhardt RA, Rosenbush SW: Cardiogenic and hypovolemic shock. Med Clin North Am 1986; 70:853.

166. Balk R, Bone RC: The adult respiratory distress syndrome. Med Clin North Am 1983; 67:685.

167. Rinaldo JE, Rogers RM: Adult respiratory distress syndrome: changing concepts in lung injury and repair. N Engl J Med 1982; 306:900.

168. Pontoppidon H, Geffin B, Lowenstein E: Acute respiratory failure in the adult (first of three parts). N Engl J Med 1982; 287:690.

CHAPTER 41

Thermal Injuries: Pathophysiology and Anesthetic Considerations

MAXIMILIAN W.B. HARTMANNSGRUBER, M.D.

A. JOSEPH LAYON, M.D.

Major burns pose a challenge to patients and to members of the burn team. Anesthesiologists are often involved early in the resuscitation phase, repeatedly during the chronic phases, and increasingly in the challenging field of continuous acute pain care.

Citizens of the United States have a 1 in 70 chance of being hospitalized for a burn during their lifetime. In 1982, more than 2 million patients with burns required medical attention. There were 4710 accidental deaths due to fires and burns in 1987.[1] Many centers now report that patients with burns as large as 70% to 80% total body surface area (TBSA) survive.[2] A 27% reduction in accidental deaths due to fires and burns occurred from 1979 to 1989, and a 6% reduction from 1988 to 1989. This reduction in mortality is believed to be primarily a result of research advances and the promulgation of preventive information since 1970.[3] Children younger than 5 years and adults older than 65 years have the highest fire and burn death rates. About three fourths of fire deaths occur in the home.[1]

PATHOLOGY

What Is a Burn?

Excessive thermal exposure causes characteristic changes in the damaged tissues.[4] Three distinct zones of tissue injury have been described.[5]

Zone of Coagulation

The zone of coagulation is the area closest to the site of heat. Blood flow has ceased, and the tissue is nonviable.

Zone of Stasis

The zone of stasis comprises tissue that is seriously damaged but at least initially still viable and represents an area that shows signs of increasing vascular occlusion. This zone is interesting because of the possibility of intervening therapeutically, thereby preventing further cell death and enlargement of the zone.[6] This partially injured tissue zone is thought to be capable of recovery up to 48 hours after a burn.

The zone of stasis can be further subdivided into two zones. A zone of early stasis (the upper one third of the zone of stasis) results from formation of early edema within the first 4 hours. A zone of delayed stasis (the deeper two thirds of the zone of stasis) results from delayed edema formation. It develops 4 to 24 hours after a burn as a result of vascular occlusion.

Zone of Hyperemia

The zone of hyperemia is reactive, responding to damage in the first two zones; thus it is not directly injured.

Only in relatively small burns is the zone of hyperemia restricted to the immediate site of injury. Larger burn injuries are more appropriately viewed as a whole body inflammatory response to injury.[3] Acute therapy is initially concerned with resuscitation from hypovolemic shock and treatment of concurrent injuries. Subsequently, the treatment of integumentary defects, multiple organ systems deterioration, and iatrogenic or psychiatric damage must be addressed. Many of these problems are potentially lethal and are discussed in detail.

What Are the Effects of Electrical Injury?

Electrical burns constitute nearly 5% of all admissions to burn centers in the United States. For current to flow, a closed pathway (circuit) and a difference in potential (voltage) must exist between two points. Bone and skin offer relatively high resistance to current flow, but skin resistance can be decreased by moisture. Blood, muscle, and nerve, on the other hand, are good conductors.

Cardiovascular

The pathway of current through the body is unpredictable. If the heart is involved, dysrhythmias are possible. Low-voltage death may result from relatively small amounts of current that produce ventricular fibrillation. High-intensity current can result in cardiac asystole and respiratory arrest, probably due to injury of medullary centers in the brain. An echocardiographic study of survivors of electrical injury demonstrated wall motion abnormalities.[7] In selected patients with a history of electrical injuries, determination of the ejection fraction may be indicated before elective operative procedures.

Soft Tissues

Extensive carbonification of the skin and underlying tissues may obscure damage to striated muscle and blood vessels. The current may also travel via blood vessels and muscles; thus, thromboses may result at sites distant from the body surface. In general, one should always be suspicious that the electrical injury is more extensive than appreciated on first inspection.

Neuromuscular

Fractures of bone may result from convulsive muscle contractions or falls after an electric shock. Nervous system injuries are frequent and include partial or complete transection of the spinal cord due to vertebral fractures. The latter injuries result from tetanic muscular contractions produced by alternating current or are sustained in falls (i.e., from utility poles, transmitter towers, and so forth). A careful neurologic evaluation must be performed before manipulation or tracheal intubation of these patients. If this is not possible, as in comatose patients, patients should be treated as though a spinal column/cord injury is present.

Renal

Renal tubular damage from myoglobin and hemoglobin pigments liberated during massive muscle necrosis and hemolysis may lead to acute renal failure. The mechanism by which myoglobinuria causes renal damage is not entirely clear. It probably involves more than mechanical obstruction of the tubules by precipitated myoglobin. However, intravenous administration of sodium bicarbonate (e.g., 100 mEq in a liter of D_5W run at maintenance fluid) to alkalize the urine protects the kidneys by preventing the formation of myoglobin casts.

If myoglobinuria is present, hydration and the use of mannitol, initially 25 g intravenously (about $0.5 \ g \cdot kg^{-1}$) followed by $12.5 \ g \cdot h^{-1}$ (about $0.25 \ g \cdot kg^{-1} \cdot h^{-1}$) are indicated. Alkalization of the urine with sodium bicarbonate to a pH ≥ 9 is recommended.[8] A urine output of 50 to 100 mL $\cdot h^{-1}$ (≥ 1.5 mL $\cdot kg^{-1} \cdot h^{-1}$) should be maintained.[8-10] If mannitol alone is insufficient to establish diuresis, furosemide is added. Hammond and Ward reported an 8% incidence of renal complications when this aggressive therapy was used in patients who suffered high-voltage electrical injury.[10]

What Are the Effects of Chemical Injury?

Chemical burns pose additional problems to the previously mentioned injuries because of the possibility of systemic absorption of the caustic agent through the injured skin. In particular, after alkali burn, processes may continue for a relatively long time, until all of the agent is combined with tissue. Phosphorus burns require immediate debridement and washing

under regional or general anesthesia to avoid further particle spread. Calcium and phosphorus levels may be seriously deranged after chemical burns with phosphorus because the increased phosphate level induces a decrease in the calcium level.[11]

CLASSIFICATION

What is the Depth of Injury?

First Degree

First-degree burns are superficial injuries involving the outer epidermis and causing mild pain. Healing occurs within 5 to 10 days. Pain may be extensive in superficial injuries. It is thought to be caused by local prostaglandin production.

Second Degree

Second-degree burns involve the epidermis and variable portions of the dermis. Superficial second-degree burns are also known as *superficial partial-thickness* burns. These burns include the epidermal and upper one third of the dermal layers of the skin. They heal in 7 to 10 days, and scarring is absent or minimal. Deep second-degree burns are also referred to as *deep partial-thickness* burns and extend farther into the dermis. However, skin appendages (e.g., ears) are spared; therefore, skin regenerates over 3 to 5 weeks, but significant scarring results.

Third Degree

In third-degree or *full-thickness* burns, skin is destroyed down to the subcutaneous tissue. Re-epithelialization does not occur, and grafting must be carried out to cover the defect.[12]

In deeper burns, destruction of the nerve endings usually results in absence of pain. An exception is a chemical burn in which the burning process continues for minutes to hours. Pain with this type of injury may be severe.

Increasing evidence suggests that early excision and coverage of third-degree burns with skin autograft are desirable. However, the estimation of burn wound depth is difficult and is often possible only in retrospect. Burn wound depth has been determined by histologic examination of biopsy specimens. This examination is most accurate 3 days after a burn. Admission laser Doppler flowmetry noninvasively measures the rate and volume of blood cells moving through tissues. It accurately predicts later deep second- or third-degree burns that require excision in 98.4% of injuries.[13]

What Is the Body Surface Area Involved?

The *rule of nines* approximates the size of burn wounds in adults. The relative percentages of the total body surface area (TBSA) differ between adults and infants (Table 41–1). In infants, the *rule of elevens* is a better approximation. The surface of a patient's hand approximates 1% of the patient's TBSA. The TBSA burn is simply the arithmetic sum of the burned areas. It is convenient to use a diagram to depict the involved area and make the calculation (Fig. 41–1).

TABLE 41–1. Calculation of Percentage of Body Surface Area Burned

Adult burned patient: body surface area (rule of nines)	Head and neck	9%
	Left arm	9%
	Right arm	9%
	Anterior chest	9%
	Posterior chest	9%
	Anterior abdomen	9%
	Posterior lower back	9%
	Anterior left leg	9%
	Posterior left leg	9%
	Anterior right leg	9%
	Posterior right leg	9%
	Perineum	1%
Infant burned patient: body surface area (rule of elevens)	Anterior head and neck	11%
	Posterior head and neck	11%
	Left arm	11%
	Right arm	11%
	Anterior torso	11%
	Posterior torso	11%
	Left leg	11%
	Right leg	11%
	Buttocks	11%
	Perineum	1%

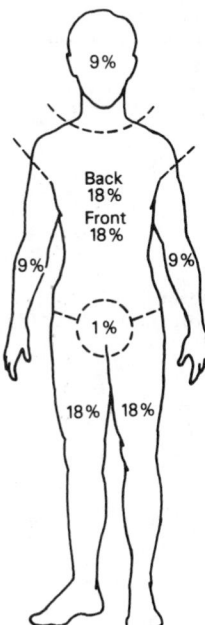

FIGURE 41–1. Burn TBSA picture from burn unit. (From Demling RH: Fluid resuscitation. *In* The Art and Science of Burn Care. Boswick JA Jr (ed). Rockville, MD, Aspen Publishers, 1987.)

How Is Severity Assessed?

Major burns are categorized in Table 41–2. Prediction of burn mortality is closely approximated by the abbreviated burn severity index developed by Tobiasen and colleagues (Table 41–3).[14] Sex, age, inhalation injury, depth of burn, and TBSA are correlated with survival.

PATHOPHYSIOLOGY

How Are Hypermetabolic States Manifested?

Endocrine Response

Immediately after a burn, cellular nutrient and oxygen (O_2) delivery to the injured area are decreased. The adrenal medulla and the autonomic nervous system release large amounts of catecholamines, leading to increased systemic vascular resistance. Glucagon and corticosteroid release, coupled with decreased responsiveness of peripheral tissues to insulin, lead to hyperglycemia.[15] Renin and aldosterone production are increased owing to burn-induced hypovolemia, leading to decreased free water clearance and increased urine concentration. Hypothermia, due to heat loss through the injured skin, and pain and anxiety potentiate the stress response.

Metabolic Rate

The metabolic rate, which is initially suppressed, begins to increase after resuscitation and may peak between days 7 and 12 after injury. It increases linearly in patients with thermal injuries <40% of TBSA. For those with injuries <50% TBSA, basal metabolic rate and O_2 consumption may reach values twice normal.[16]

Nutritional Changes

The hypermetabolic state results in catabolic protein loss, impaired immune function, and delayed wound healing. To offset this metabolic demand, wound closure and enteral feeding are critical. Enteral feeding via a nasogastric tube is safe and can be instituted within 1 hour of admission.[17] This approach not only provides nutrients but also helps to maintain intestinal barrier function, thus preventing bacterial and fungal translocation, a common cause of sepsis in these patients. Early feeding of burned patients is also believed to enhance a patient's ability to control a septic insult.[18]

High-protein diets, including fatty acids of the ω-3 series and arginine, are beneficial.[19–21] They improve immunologic function and thus may decrease infectious complications. The data of Herndon and colleagues suggest that enterally fed burned patients have a survival rate approximately twice that of patients supplemented with parenteral nutrition.[22] This decreased mortality in burned patients is likely due to an increase in secretory immunoglobulin production, with a resultant decrease in bacterial translocation across the gut wall.

Decisions for early feeding must be weighed against the increased risk of aspiration in case of emergent intubation or surgery. In the future, anesthesiologists likely will see more burned patients with a "full stomach."

TABLE 41–2. Categorization of Major Burns

Total body surface area	Adults: ≥25%
	Children: ≥20%
	Children <2 years: ≥10%
Full thickness	Adults: ≥15%
	Children 2–15 years: >10%
	Children <2 years: >2%
Miscellaneous	Burns on the face, hands, feet, perineum
	Electrical burns
	Burns with inhalation injuries
	Burns with associated injuries
	Burns of patients with major chronic illnesses

TABLE 41–3. Burn Severity Index and Calculated Threat to Life

Gender	Score
Female	1
Male	0
<20	1
21–40	2
41–60	3
61–80	4
>80	5
Inhalation injury	1
Full-thickness burn	1
Total body surface area involved (%)	
≤10	1
11–20	2
21–30	3
31–40	4
41–50	5
51–60	6
61–70	7
71–80	8
81–90	9
>90	10

Total Burn Score	Threat to Life	Probability of Survival
2–3	Very low	99%
4–5	Moderate	98%
6–7	Moderate–severe	80–90%
8–9	Serious	50–70%
10–11	Severe	20–40%
12–13	Maximal	<10%

(Modified from Tobiasen J, Hiebert JH, Edlich RF: Prediction of burn mortality. Surg Gynecol Obstet 1982; 154:711. By permission of Surgery, Gynecology, & Obstetrics.)

What Are the Effects of Burn Toxins?

Immune Function

Once dermal integrity is compromised owing to the acquired derangement in the normal host immune system, the body may become substrate to many infectious processes. In most patients with burns >40% TBSA, virtually all specific (cell-mediated and humoral) and nonspecific (polymorphonuclear leukocyte [PMNL], macrophage) immune functions are deranged. Every effort must be made to treat these patients as immunocompromised.

Histamine Release and Complement Activation

At the local site of thermal injury, histamine release and complement activation lead to increased vascular permeability. Interaction of histamine with xanthine oxidase leads to formation of toxic OH^- radicals and hydrogen peroxide.[23] It has been speculated that increased vascular permeability may be attenuated by xanthine oxidase inhibitors (allopurinol) or cromolyn sodium, an inhibitor of histamine release.

The complement cascade and xanthine oxidase cause activation of PMNLs, mast cells, and endothelial cells, further increasing histamine and xanthine oxidase activity. Release of cytokines such as tumor necrosis factor (TNF)/cachectin, a polypeptide product of activated macrophages, also occurs. TNF is implicated in the hyperdynamic hypermetabolic state following burns.[24] Interleukin-1 (IL-1), another important cytokine and a polypeptide product of activated macrophages,

acts as a primary mediator of the acute phase organ response to infection and injury.[24]

Sepsis and Multiple System Organ Failure

The effects of IL-1 and TNF are additive. These cytokines have properties that mimic the clinical presentation of sepsis and multiple system organ failure (MSOF). Sepsis and MSOF have many characteristics in common with thermal injuries; indeed sepsis, MSOF, and the adult respiratory distress syndrome (ARDS) remain major causes of death after burn injury.[25] Secretion of the these cytokines results in various responses[26-28] (Table 41–4).

Later Changes

During the second to fourth postburn week, the activation, proliferation, and differentiation processes of B lymphocytes are impaired in severely injured patients. This impairment may contribute to enhanced susceptibility to infection and sepsis.[29] Burn mortality is highly correlated with failure of T cell function and with the presence of a serum toxic lipoprotein that affects IL-2 dependence after the first postburn week. The production and action of IL-2 are inhibited by postburn serum. Finally, subeschar-tissue fluid is even more immunosuppressive than is the serum of a burned patient. Because of slow reabsorption, this fluid may be at least partially responsible for maintaining the immunocompromised state of patients with open burn wounds.[30] These observations argue in favor of aggressive repetitive debridement/dressing changes, many of which require the involvement of members of the department of anesthesiology.

Decreased particulate filtering by hepatic macrophages (Kupffer's cells) and splenocytes occurs, but accumulation of particulate material by lung macrophages is increased.[31] This alteration may explain the increased incidence of ARDS in burned patients, even in the absence of an inhalation injury. Although increased numbers of PMNLs are noted, they are functionally impaired.[32]

Blood Transfusion

Blood transfusion–induced immunosuppression seems to be an additional nonspecific component of the immune dysfunction encountered with thermal injuries.[33, 34] The observed impairment of immune function is indomethacin sensitive and is possibly induced by series E prostaglandins. Increased risk may result when large volumes of donor blood are used over a short period of time.[35] However, successful coverage of the integumentary defect (debridement and grafting) requires the

TABLE 41–4. Effects of Release of Interleukin-1 and Tumor Necrosis Factor

Fever
Production of hepatic acute phase reactants
T and B lymphocyte activation
Fibroblast proliferation
Cyclooxygenase gene expression
Shock
Induction of interleukin-6 and interleukin-8
Complement system activation
Coagulation and fibrinolytic activation
Further release of interleukin-1 and tumor necrosis factor

liberal use of blood and blood products. Tourniquets should be used whenever possible during debridement and grafting of extremities to help decrease a patient's exposure to donor blood products.

Neurologic and Immunologic Coupling

Increasing evidence suggests a coupling of neurologic and immunologic functions. Endogenous opioids have a role in the altered immune response after injury, and morphine sulfate has been linked to altered cell-mediated immune response. In vitro morphine sulfate–induced impairment of lymphocyte function, as measured by delayed-type hypersensitivity assay, was prevented by concurrent treatment with the opioid antagonist naloxone.[36] The relevance of this in vitro study to the clinical setting in the burn intensive care unit is unclear but clearly merits further study.

Eicosanoids

Eicosanoids, especially series E prostaglandins, prostacyclin, thromboxane, and the leukotrienes, are likely involved in many of the physiologic alterations observed in shock and trauma. Infusion of bacteria or endotoxin increases plasma prostaglandin levels in animals. Clinical trials to evaluate the potential utility of nonsteroidal anti-inflammatory drugs (NSAIDs) to favorably modify the stress response in severe illness are currently under way. The immunomodulator thymopentin, although useful in a murine model of thermal injury, has been unsuccessful in improving survival in burned patients.[37]

Conclusions

Given the immunocompromised state of burned patients, it is no surprise that sepsis remains a major cause of death despite major improvements in burn survival rates and antibiotic therapy. Of those who die after a burn, infection is the cause of death in almost 100% of children and >75% of adults.[38] In addition to focused, specific intravenous and topical antibiotic coverage and aseptic technique, the immune response may be improved by early enteral nutrition and early excision of burn wounds.[39, 40]

How Is Cardiovascular Function Affected?

Immediately after a burn, regardless of the cause of the burn, cardiac output falls to approximately 50% to 60% of the normal resting value. This decrease is likely due to a combination of reduced preload, impaired contractility, and increased arterial resistance.[41] Although some controversy exists, impaired contractility has been attributed to a low-molecular-weight myocardial depressant factor.[42] Increased arterial resistance is due to increased plasma catecholamines.

In an untreated animal, cardiac output falls to approximately 20% of normal resting values. This observation underscores the need for aggressive fluid resuscitation, despite which cardiac output still remains below normal until the beginning of the hyperdynamic phase, which begins about 24 hours after the initial injury. It may then climb to values as high as 200% of normal.

Why Do Fluid Shifts Occur?

The marked tissue swelling observed in the burned area is due to leaky capillaries and is essentially complete within 12 hours. Diffuse edema (anasarca) is also frequently encountered after fluid resuscitation of patients with >30% TBSA burns. The processes that lead to edema formation are not entirely understood and cannot be blamed entirely on fluid resuscitation, which is necessary to restore intravascular volume. The prudent practice is to err on the side of too much rather than too little fluid because the sequelae of inadequate fluid resuscitation (e.g., acute tubular necrosis) are more serious.

Microvascular Injury

Edema occurring within the first few minutes of a thermal injury is thought to be secondary to direct injury of the microvasculature. Endothelial gaps form and lead to transvascular loss of fluid, electrolytes, and proteins; this fluid shift results in increased volume of both the interstitial and intracellular compartments.

Cell Membrane Dysfunction

Vasoactive agents such as prostaglandins, leukotrienes, histamine, and kinins promote continued fluid loss from the intravascular to the interstitial and intracellular compartments. Cellular swelling probably results from a generalized impairment in cell membrane function with subsequent sodium and water movement into the cells. This initial defect is reversed within about 12 hours. Further fluid shifts and edema are a result of burn- and resuscitation-induced hypoproteinemia.[43] After the 12-hour period has elapsed, the use of a colloid-containing fluid can be considered.

What Are the Effects of Fluid Translocation?

Extracellular fluid shifts from the circulating plasma volume result in decreased venous return and preload. If the resulting hypovolemia and hypotension are not reversed, conversion of a viable but ischemic (zone of stasis) deep partial-thickness burn to one that is full thickness and nonviable may occur. Unfortunately, even carefully managed fluid resuscitation may be followed by massive edema formation, resulting in increased tissue pressure and decreased tissue O$_2$ partial pressure. Increased work of breathing may also occur from edema of the thorax imposing a *restrictive* load, whereas upper respiratory tract edema imposes a *resistive* load. The latter may be quite serious. Edema formation at sites other than those that were burned may be due to overhydration, decreased oncotic pressure, or a vascular leak linked to circulating vasoactive mediators, adherence of leukocytes to vascular endothelium, and activation of the alternate complement pathway.[44]

Can Edema Formation Be Controlled?

Cyclooxygenase inhibitors, such as 5% ibuprofen or 5% flurbiprofen creams, applied topically, have been shown to reduce local lymph flow about 3.5-fold in a sheep model of treated scald burns.[45] Flurbiprofen, a much longer-acting agent than ibuprofen, additionally inhibits leukocyte migration. Interestingly, although topical flurbiprofen decreases burn hypermetabolism, much like early excision and closure of burn wounds, it does not attenuate local burn wound vascular permeability.[46] Burn-induced thromboxane release enhances permeability edema and can be decreased, at least in an experimental model, by thromboxane synthetase inhibition.[47]

Despite these data, pharmacologic manipulation of the previously mentioned vasoactive mediators has not resulted in reproducible modification of edema.[48] Presumably, additional factors other than those responsible for vasoactive changes are involved in postburn edema formation as well.

PULMONARY INJURY

Inhalation injury is a significant contributor to mortality.[49] Airway mucosal sloughing and pulmonary edema, with atelectasis caused by increased microvascular permeability, result in progressive pulmonary deterioration.[50] The extent of injury due to smoke inhalation is less than that due to steam. Smoke is usually hot enough to injure only the larynx and upper trachea. Steam, on the other hand, has a heat content that is sufficiently high to injure alveoli directly.

Nonsteam smoke injury in small airways is usually due to chemical irritation. Early decreased arterial O_2 partial pressure (PaO_2) results from direct injury of the alveoli by the products of combustion. The chemical components of smoke may lead to airway irritation and severe bronchospasm. This problem may be treated by albuterol or other bronchodilator by nebulizer or metered dose inhaler. Prophylactic steroids in inhalational injury are controversial and in general have not proved to be beneficial.[51]

Early increases in extravascular lung water occur only with very severe inhalation injury or as a result of toxic inhaled gases. Major increases in extravascular lung water are more frequently noted 4 to 24 days after injury and are usually due to wound or pulmonary sepsis.[52] The impact of smoke inhalation on later complications may be significant. Wroblewski and Bower found that 85% of patients with facial burns developed pneumonia, compared with only 12% of those without such injury.[53]

What Are the Effects of Carbon Monoxide Intoxication?

Most deaths (80%) resulting from smoke inhalation are due to asphyxia or carbon monoxide intoxication.[54] Cellular respiration is often impaired by the carbon monoxide or cyanide inhalation associated with smoke inhalation. Carbon monoxide, with 200 times greater affinity for hemoglobin than O_2, displaces the latter and produces a leftward shift in the oxyhemoglobin (HbO_2) dissociation curve. Further, it likely causes direct cellular damage as well by interference with the cytochrome oxidase system.

Treatment

The half-life of carbon monoxide during room air breathing is approximately 250 minutes; this time can be shortened to 40 to 60 minutes by breathing 100% O_2, and to 20 minutes in a hyperbaric chamber. Carbon monoxide poisoning should always be suspected in thermal injury, especially if a patient

demonstrates even subtle neurologic changes. A blood sample subjected to co-oximeter analysis for carboxyhemoglobin is diagnostic if the level is $\geq 10\%$ and should be part of the routine laboratory screen for any smoke-associated burn injury.

In suspected intoxication, 100% O_2 (or treatment in a hyperbaric chamber if availability and patient stability allow) should be used until the carboxyhemoglobin level is less than about 3%.

How Is Cyanide Intoxication Managed?

After other differential diagnostic possibilities are ruled out, unless prolonged exposure to carbon monoxide has occurred, cyanide intoxication should be suspected when a patient remains comatose with carboxyhemoglobin levels <30% to 40%. Empiric therapy should begin with inhalation from amyl nitrite ampules held under the patient's nose and mouth for 15 to 30 seconds every 1 to 3 minutes until sodium nitrite and sodium thiosulfate are available. Ten milliliters of 3% sodium nitrite and 50 mL of 25% sodium thiosulfate should then be infused slowly. If symptoms persist, one half of the original dose may be repeated 30 minutes later. Pediatric doses are 3% sodium nitrite, 6 to 8 mL $\cdot$ m$^{2-1}$ or 0.2 mL $\cdot$ kg^{-1}; and 25% sodium thiosulfate, 7 g $\cdot$ m$^{2-1}$ to a dose of no more than 12.5 g.

INITIAL THERAPY

When Is Hospitalization Required?

Not all burned patients require hospitalization.[55] Minor burns, defined as a partial thickness (<15% TBSA) or full thickness (<2% TBSA), unless the face, genitalia, hands, or feet are involved, may be treated in an outpatient facility. In small children, a short period of observation may be appropriate even in cases of minor injury.

Moderate burns, defined as partial-thickness injury of from 15% to 25% TBSA or full thickness <10% TBSA, require hospitalization. However, a community hospital is adequate for the care of these injuries as long as experienced and interested nursing and medical personnel are available.

A major burn is one with a burn severity index (BSI), which depends on a patient's age, underlying medical problems, and the proportion that is full thickness (see Table 41–2) and requires care in a designated burn unit, either immediately or after initial stabilization.

Patients with TBSA involvement that would allow classification into moderate or minor categories but with serious underlying medical problems such as diabetes mellitus, ischemic heart disease, and obstructive or restrictive lung disease should be treated as if they had more severe burns. These individuals do not easily withstand the stresses imposed by thermal injury.

What Should Be Done in the Emergency Department?

History and Physical Examination

For a severely burned individual, as for any acute trauma victim, the initial care provided involves special attention to the airway to ensure that oxygenation and ventilation are not compromised. A patient's cervical spine must be considered at risk until proven otherwise, especially if a fall or trauma was involved.

As soon as a patient is moved into the emergency department treatment room, while the initial evaluation is ongoing, a focused history must be obtained. Necessary information includes details of the burn (where it occurred, how it started, whether the area was open or closed, what the patient did to extinguish the fire) underlying medical problems, allergies, and medicinal or recreational drug use. If the patient is unable to provide the necessary information, one of the health team members must obtain the history from a family member, the police, firefighters, or emergency medical technicians.

A history of fire in a closed space has important implications when considering the possibility of major airway or inhalation injury. Symptoms and signs include burnt facial hair or eyebrows, face and neck burns, hoarseness, stridor, wheezing, bronchorrhea, carbonaceous sputum, and mental changes; dyspnea and cyanosis are late findings.

Fiberoptic Bronchoscopy and Direct Laryngoscopy

If a patient is not in respiratory distress on admission yet has one or more of the previously mentioned findings suggestive of an airway or inhalation injury, we perform fiberoptic bronchoscopy. Positive findings include erythema and edema in superficial burns; blister formation, hemorrhage, and ischemia in partial-thickness injury; and ulceration and necrosis of the mucous membrane in full-thickness burns.[55-57] Although these findings do not correlate with later mortality, severity of respiratory failure, and subsequent requirement for mechanical ventilatory support, they allow identification of patients who have upper airway injury and will require intubation out of concern for edema.[58]

Fluid resuscitation of patients with large burns can cause sufficient tracheal edema to jeopardize a later intubation, even if the neck and face appear not to be involved. Thus, even when we determine that fiberoptic bronchoscopy is not required, direct laryngoscopy is performed to evaluate erythema and edema; only rarely is this procedure contraindicated.

Tracheal Intubation

The decision about whether to intubate a burned patient on arrival in the emergency department or simply to observe may be difficult. We are often impressed with the extent of airway and lung changes within 24 hours of admission. When in doubt, our policy is to opt for intubation. In any patient with upper airway erythema or blisters, *not* intubating imposes substantial risk, because upper airway injury may not become apparent until almost complete occlusion takes place.

The use of muscle relaxants to facilitate intubation of a patient with upper airway edema is fraught with risks and may be fatal because bag-mask ventilation and intubation may be extremely difficult after neuromuscular paralysis. Awake intubation or intubation over a bronchoscope is the safest approach if there is any question about the ease of airway exposure. After intubation, be sure to document the endotracheal tube cuff volume necessary to barely occlude the endotracheal tube cuff or to obtain a slightly audible leak around it. This value/volume serves as an indicator of progressive or residual airway edema. We do not hesitate to "prophylactically" intubate an individual for 2 to 4 days if upper airway erythema or edema is evident.

Cricothyrotomy Versus Tracheotomy

A cricothyrotomy, using the Melker cricothyrotomy kit (Cook Catheter Co.), or an emergent bedside tracheotomy may be performed if needed. *However, our experience is that the former rather than the latter procedure is more likely to save a patient's life if the airway is lost acutely. Even in the hands of a very experienced surgeon, an emergent tracheotomy in an edematous burned patient will require 5 to 15 minutes because of the distorted anatomy* (see Chapter 50).

Fluid Resuscitation

As soon as the airway has been secured, attention is turned to the circulation. Several large-bore peripheral intravenous catheters should be placed, and infusions of lactated Ringer's or other solutions begun. Appropriate fluid resuscitation must be ensured. An indwelling urethral catheter should be placed as well. Resuscitation is adequate, all other things being equal, when the urine output is no less than $0.5 \text{ mL} \cdot \text{kg}^{-1} \cdot \text{h}^{-1}$ and the patient is oriented and lucid. Invasive monitoring may be required if cardiopulmonary disease is present. We usually place an arterial and central venous catheter in all patients with moderate to severe burns to guide the fluid and hemodynamic resuscitation. Because these patients are often quite intravascularly volume depleted, the subclavian or femoral approach is more easily executed than the internal jugular vein because the latter tends to be collapsed in this setting.

Miscellaneous Considerations

With the airway secured and volume infusion begun, attention may be turned to a more detailed physical examination, tetanus prophylaxis, sedation/analgesia, and cleansing of the burn wound. A nasogastric tube should be placed in order to decrease gastric volume and in anticipation of the ileus that commonly accompanies significant burns. Preliminary baseline laboratory studies should be ordered (hematocrit, electrolytes, blood urea nitrogen, creatinine, arterial blood gases, and pH, as well as co-oximetry to determine the carboxyhemoglobin level if smoke was involved, plus urinalysis and a chest radiograph).

DEFINITIVE THERAPY

How Should Resuscitation Be Managed?

Prevention of hypovolemic shock and renal failure poses a major challenge in the first 24 hours after a burn is sustained. Fluid requirements tend to decrease after this time. Early work by Kilgore and colleagues suggested that the origin of edema fluid in thermal injuries <24 hours old was the extracellular rather than the intracellular compartment.[59] This determination was made using ^{51}Cr-labeled red blood cells, ^{131}I-labeled serum, ^{35}S-labeled sodium sulfate (Na_2SO_4), and the Na^+:K^+ ratio in rhesus monkeys with 35% to 40% TBSA burns caused by flame (kerosene gauze for 25 s) or scald (70 °C for 15 s). These investigators found decreases in the red blood cell mass

(10.5%), plasma volume (25%), and functional extracellular volume (44%) 18 hours after injury. Loss of red blood cell mass is likely due to lysis. Electrolytic concentration of the edema fluid suggested that its origin was from the extracellular fluid compartment.

Replacement Formulas

Numerous fluid formula recommendations have been suggested for initial replacement guidance; these are shown, primarily for historical interest, in Table 41–5. The crucial issue with each of these formulations is that they are approximations. The actual volume administered may be increased or decreased depending on a patient's mental status and urine output.

The Evans and Brooke formulas called for increasing fluid as needed to keep the urinary output between 30 and 50 mL · h^{-1}. The Parkland formula requires administration of fluid to a urine output of 50 to 100 mL · h^{-1}. Each of these regimens assumes that urine output is a reliable indicator of volume status. Although this maxim generally holds true, in some clinical situations (e.g., patients with uncontrolled blood sugar and a resultant diuresis, or after mannitol therapy) it does not. In these circumstances or when urine output is inadequate despite apparently adequate fluid administration, central venous pressure measurement can be used to monitor and guide fluid resuscitation.

The Parkland formula (see Table 41–5) maintains a leading position in the resuscitation of thermal injuries. This regimen met the requirements of 70% of adult patients and 98% of pediatric burn victims when half of the calculated volume was replaced during the first 8 postburn hours and the other half during the next 16 hours.[60]

Hypertonic Solutions

Many investigators have demonstrated a significant reduction in fluid requirement and maintenance of adequate urine output after the administration of concentrated sodium solutions.[61–64] Although approximately the same amount of sodium was administered (0.5–0.6 mEq · kg^{-1} · %TBSA^{-1}) the decreased water load was thought to decrease edema, a significant advantage because excessive edema, as noted previously, has been implicated in increasing burn depth.

We often use hypertonic lactated Ringer's as well as the standard solution. This solution is obtained by placing 100 mEq of sodium lactate into each 1000-mL bag of lactated Ringer's; the result is 230 mEq of sodium, 3 mEq of calcium, 4 mEq of potassium, 128 mEq of lactate, and 109 mEq of chloride. We calculate sodium requirement at 0.6 mEq · kg^{-1} · %TBSA^{-1}. This amount is then administered over 24 hours.

We continue to use this solution until metabolic alkalosis supervenes, then change to 3% saline solution (513 mEq each of sodium and chloride). If alkalosis occurs, it is usually after the first 8 to 12 hours; the 3% saline solution usually corrects it within another 8 to 12 hours. In general, hypertonic solutions are used so long as the serum sodium level does not exceed 155 to 160 mEq · L^{-1}. A paucity of reported complications occurs at these levels.[65] We then change to lactated Ringer's solution.

Invasive Monitoring

Data suggest that urine output and vital sign changes may be inadequate for optimal resuscitation. Dries and Waxman studied 14 patients with average 61% TBSA burns.[66] Flow-directed balloon-tipped pulmonary artery (PA) catheters were placed in all patients. Measured wedge pressure, cardiac output, and calculated systemic vascular resistance, O$_2$ delivery ($\dot{D}O_2$), and O$_2$ consumption ($\dot{V}O_2$) parameters were obtained during resuscitation. They found that within the first 48 hours, urine output and vital signs, as assessed by heart rate and mean arterial pressure, did not correlate with the invasively determined physiologic parameters. In some patients, fluid boluses increased $\dot{V}O_2$, further suggesting that despite other clinical parameters being normal, O$_2$ delivery was not optimized. These individuals could not be predicted based on clinical criteria. The investigators suggested that PA catheters may be helpful in the resuscitation of patients with ≥28% TBSA burns.

A shortcoming of this study was that no control group was reported so that readers could not determine if the discrepancy in vital signs and urine output, and therefore fluid management, affects outcome. We do not, as a matter of course, place PA catheters in our thermally injured patients.

How Are Compartment Syndromes Assessed?

Full-thickness injury is associated with almost complete loss of skin elasticity, leading to encasement of tissue compart-

TABLE 41–5. Resuscitation Formulas*

Fluid Type	Evans Formula	Brooke Formula	Parkland Formula
	First 24 Hours		
Colloid	1 mL · kg^{-1} · %TBSA^{-1} (2800)	0.5 mL · kg^{-1} · %TBSA^{-1} (1400)	None
Electrolyte solution (solution: lactated Ringer's or normal saline)	1 ml · kg^{-1} · %TBSA^{-1}	1.5 mL · kg^{-1} · %TBSA^{-1} (4200)	4 mL · kg^{-1} · %TBSA^{-1} (11,200)
Glucose (H$_2$O) (D$_5$W)	(2000)	(2000)	None
	Second 24 Hours		
Colloid	0.5 mL · kg^{-1} · %TBSA^{-1} (1400)	0.25 mL · kg^{-1} · %TBSA^{-1} (700)	As needed for urine output (70–100 mL · h^{-1})
Electrolyte solution	0.5 mL · kg^{-1} · %TBSA^{-1} (1400)	0.75 mL · kg^{-1} · %TBSA^{-1} (2100)	None
Glucose/H$_2$O	(2000)	(2000)	Urine output tested as needed

*Assumes a 70-kg male with a 40% TBSA thermal injury. Number in parentheses ( ) is volume for that particular fluid; total volume for each 24-h period may be calculated by summation of numbers in parentheses in each column.

ments. This change can impede venous outflow, arterial inflow, or both. Physical assessment of peripheral pulses and skin temperature is unreliable in severely vasoconstricted patients with edema due to burn wounds and resuscitation fluids; hence, distal extremity blood flow, arterial and venous, should be assessed hourly with an ultrasonic Doppler probe.

Indications For Decompression

Even if distal Doppler pulses are present, nutrient flow into the muscle compartments may be inadequate. Indications for surgical decompression, aside from the loss of distal pulses, include delayed capillary refilling; paresthesias or motor weakness; cyanosis of distal, uninjured skin; and tense edema with rigid muscle compartments.[67] Intracompartmental pressure is easily measured by sterile placement of a fluid-filled hollow needle attached to a pressure transducer zeroed to the tip of the needle into the compartment. Interstitial pressure—that is, subescharotic or compartmental pressure—consistently >25 mm Hg warrants escharotomy; pressures >40 mm Hg require immediate decompression by escharotomy or fasciotomy. One option is to reassess compartment pressure after escharotomy. If it is <25 mm Hg, then escharotomy was therapeutic; if it remains >25 mm Hg, consider proceeding to fasciotomy.[68] Elevation of the extremities may reduce edema formation, but an escharotomy is indicated when vascular impairment is apparent.

Escharotomy

An escharotomy is simply an incision over the arteries and veins through the full depth of the burn eschar. These incisions are usually performed on the lateral and medial aspects of the extremity and should be continued across the joints. Once performed, return of peripheral perfusion is to be expected. Continued absence of peripheral blood flow requires reassessment of intravascular fluid status and the extent and depth of the escharotomies. Rarely, fasciotomy is necessary after swelling in the muscle compartment. Electrical burns are more prone to compartment edema, requiring fasciotomy, than are thermal burns.

What Is the Burn Wound Sepsis?

Surface microflora of the skin changes after burn injury, with eventual predominance of more pathogenic organisms. Immediately after thermal injury, the burn wound may be sterile, but within 48 hours it becomes colonized. Subsequent growth into the burn wound (supraeschar, intrafollicular, and intraeschar colonization) may lead to invasion of viable non-burned tissue, termed *burn wound sepsis*.[69] This condition is diagnosed pathologically from biopsy samples of skin (including eschar and subcutaneous fat). Microscopic invasion into viable tissue is seen, and culture of the specimen demonstrates $\geq 10^5$ bacterial colonies per gram of tissue.

Offending Organisms

Many organisms cause burn wound colonization and infection, including *Pseudomonas* species, β-hemolytic *Streptococcus*, *Staphylococcus aureus*, *Klebsiella* species, *Proteus* species, *Escherichia* species, *Providencia* species, and *Enterobacter cloacae*. Yeast, fungal, and viral pathogens may also be present. Because primary wound closure often cannot be achieved, topical antimicrobial therapy is an important component of wound care before and after debridement of nonviable tissue.

Therapeutic Agents

Silver Sulfadiazine

Silver sulfadiazine is a bacteriostatic material synthesized from silver nitrate and sodium sulfadiazine. It is available as a 1% cream and has a broad antimicrobial spectrum of activity. Treatment failures occur, especially in burns >50% TBSA. Eschar penetration is intermediate between the relatively poor penetration of silver nitrate and the deep penetration of mafenide. This agent is painless on application and is generally used in the initial hours after injury. When treatment failure occurs, another agent, such as mafenide, is used.

Transient leukopenia 2 to 3 days after initiation of therapy is often noted. This change, however, may well be an intrinsic response to the burn injury itself rather than an untoward effect of drug therapy. A maculopapular rash may also be seen. It usually does not require cessation of the agent.

Mafenide

Mafenide is a broad-spectrum bacteriostatic topical agent with superior eschar-penetrating properties. It is helpful for early treatment of a burn wound; a significant drawback is the pain it causes on application. Mafenide is available as an 11% cream in a water-soluble base. Side effects include inhibition of carbonic anhydrase, which may result in hyperchloremic metabolic acidosis.

The drug is highly absorbed from the base within about 3 hours of application. Metabolism of the parent drug results in the presentation of a large osmotic load to the kidneys, with resultant osmotic diuresis; the diuresis is enhanced by the drug's carbonic anhydrase effect. The metabolic acidosis and diuretic effects generally become clinically important in thermal injuries of $\geq 40\%$ TBSA and serve to further confound fluid management. This is another instance when central venous pressure monitoring can be used to guide therapy.

Cerium Nitrate–Silver Sulfadiazine

This agent primarily enhances control of enteric flora in a burn wound. It apparently is not as useful in control of staphylococci. In addition to superior control of enteric bacteria compared with silver sulfadiazine, it may enhance cell-mediated immunity.[70] The untoward effects occurring with silver sulfadiazine may be complicated further by methemoglobinemia. It should be suspected if the skin or blood appears cyanotic or gray and the pulse oximeter identifies a desaturation in the presence of a normal PaO_2.

Honey

We have no experience with using honey to treat burns. Nevertheless, honey was recently compared with silver sulfadiazine in patients with 21% to 40% TBSA burns. In 52 patients treated with honey, 91% of wounds were rendered sterile within 7 days. In the 52 patients treated with silver sulfadiazine, 7% showed control of infection within 7 days. Healthy granulation tissue in the honey-treated group was observed in 7.4 days, versus 13.4 days in the silver sulfadiazine–treated patients. Finally, 87% of the honey-treated group healed within 15 days, compared with only 10% in the group treated with silver sulfadiazine. Relief of pain and a lower incidence of hypertrophic scar and postburn contracture were observed with honey.[71] These are intriguing findings but do not have any particular anesthetic implications.

Silver Nitrate

Although effective against most strains of *S. aureus, Staphylococcus epidermidis,* and *Pseudomonas aeruginosa,* silver nitrate is infrequently used today because of poor eschar penetration and the association of electrolyte disturbances secondary to its hypotonicity. Rarely, methemoglobinemia occurs through bacterial reduction of nitrate to nitrite, which is subsequently absorbed.[72]

What Are the Effects of Burn Debridement and Skin Grafting?

Open burn wounds initiate and perpetuate tissue oxidant changes and hypermetabolism. Immediate removal and closure of a wound minimize these effects. Early excision and grafting of burn wounds, rather than separation over 2 to 6 weeks after a burn, was popularized in the early 1970s and was shown to decrease the duration of hospitalization, pain, and the need for future reconstructive procedures.[73]

How Is Operative Blood Loss Managed?

Major burn debridement is a very bloody procedure that may require replacement of an entire blood volume in the first 30 minutes after incision. Loss of between 200 and 600 mL of blood for every 1% of the TBSA excised by tangential excision technique has been estimated.[74, 75] Adequate amounts of crossmatched blood must be in the operating room before incision.

Because blood and blood products are potentially infectious and these patients are immunocompromised, they should be used judiciously. Arterial tourniquets should be applied whenever possible during extremity debridement. Hypertension should be meticulously avoided during debridement (which is usually not a problem), as well as postoperatively in order to decrease oozing. Aggressive intraoperative monitoring of the coagulation status (i.e., prothrombin time, partial thromboplastin time, platelets, fibrin degradation products, fibrinogen) and appropriate treatment of coagulopathies help to decrease blood product requirements.

Topical Vasoconstrictors

A significant reduction in blood loss is obtained by application of topical vasoconstrictors immediately after debridement and before skin grafting. Epinephrine-soaked sponges, 1:200,000 concentration, are superior to thrombin when applied to the donor site.[76] If ventricular dysrhythmogenicity is a concern, epinephrine can be replaced by phenylephrine solutions (1 mL of 1% phenylephrine in 1000 mL normal saline).

Miscellaneous Regimens

Major burns have been successfully managed without blood or blood products using a high-calorie high-protein diet, iron supplementation, and pediatric blood sampling techniques and allowing spontaneous eschar separation rather than performing early debridement.[77] We have used this approach successfully, together with the administration of recombinant erythropoietin, when treating Jehovah's Witnesses.

ANESTHETIC MANAGEMENT

What Are the Vascular Access Requirements?

We do not anesthetize patients for wound debridement without adequate vascular access. Because temperature regulation is difficult after significant thermal injuries, we prefer to have all catheters placed at the bedside, before moving a patient to the operating room (OR).

The decision about what constitutes "adequate" venous access is subjective. In our experience, whenever any patient with a major thermal injury ($\geq$20% to 25%) is taken to the OR for anything more than the final "touch-up" work (i.e., debridement and grafting of small areas of eschar after all of the major debridement has been performed), significant blood loss is highly probable. We use, at a minimum, two large-bore catheters, at least one of which is a 9 French bore placed in a central vein. An arterial catheter is necessary as well for blood pressure monitoring and for drawing blood.

A central venous catheter is useful for several reasons. Vasoactive drugs must frequently be used, and we want these to be infused into the central circulation. Calcium chloride is also often used to counteract myocardial depression attendant to rapid transfusion of citrate-containing blood.[78] It can cause serious soft tissue damage even without extravasation when administered peripherally and is therefore always given centrally. Because "line sepsis" is a common problem in these patients who have recurrent bacteremias, we either remove catheters placed for operative resuscitation as soon as they are no longer considered necessary, usually 12 to 24 hours postoperatively, or exchange them via guidewire exchange every 3 days.

What Should Be Monitored During Anesthesia?

Monitoring of patients about to undergo debridement and split-thickness skin grafting requires consideration of several factors.

Electrocardiography

Monitoring for rhythm and ischemia is made difficult in severely burned patients because unburnt skin may be unavailable for placement of electrocardiographic (ECG) electrode pads. Commercially available needle electrodes should be used in these patients. Serious dysrhythmias are uncommon, perhaps because we use, as a matter of course, rapid infusion and warming devices for the administration of all blood products and fluids.

Continuous ECG recording allows rapid diagnosis of hypocalcemia, which causes prolongation of the QT interval. Myocardial depression due to rapid transfusion of citrate-containing blood can be rapidly corrected by intravenous administration of calcium chloride. Our practice is to administer as an intravenous bolus 500 mg to 1 g of calcium chloride when blood products are administered at a rate ≥ 1 unit every 5 minutes.

Myocardial ischemia should be monitored as well because of the predisposition of these patients to a baseline myocardial dysfunction aggravated by tachycardia and frequent changes in blood pressure.

Pulse Oximetry

Pulse oximetry is essential; the probe may be applied to fingers, toes, ears, the nose, or even the cheek or tongue when suitable extremity sites are unavailable.

Temperature

Esophageal stethoscope/temperature monitoring is also essential. Because patients with significant thermal injuries have difficulty with temperature regulation and because hypothermia can cause severe dysrhythmias, we monitor temperature in all patients. We stop the operative procedure if a patient's temperature decreases to $<35\ °C$ or falls by more than $1.5\ °C$ below baseline. The operating room temperature is monitored as well and always kept $>29\ °C$.

Exhaled Gases

Monitoring of the respired gases is vital. In our burn unit OR, we have identified low cardiac output syndromes, partial endotracheal tube obstruction, and inadequate minute ventilation by virtue of continuous capnography for all patients.

Urine Output

A Foley catheter provides an indication of adequate renal perfusion, provided the urine output is $>0.5\ mL \cdot kg \cdot h^{-1}$ and an osmotic diuresis does not contribute to urine flow.

Neuromuscular Blockade

Monitoring of neuromuscular blockade provides useful information. The ulnar nerve may be used for this purpose. However, if both wrists are burned, we use the facial or posterior tibial nerves. After induction and intubation, we do not completely relax our patients because neuromuscular blockade is not necessary for debridement and split-thickness skin grafting. Deep anesthesia often is difficult to achieve because of the tenuous hemodynamic status of these patients. The normal signs of light anesthesia—tachycardia, hypertension, and diaphoresis—frequently are obscured in thermally injured patients. Thus, a patient's movement can be an excellent monitor of inadequate anesthesia.

Transesophageal Echocardiography

We have inserted transesophageal echocardiographic probes in patients about to undergo major debridement. Our intention is to determine if this device is more sensitive than clinical judgment or a PA catheter, which we have found to be unwieldy in the burn OR, in determining fluid requirements. This device, if available, is helpful in the differential diagnosis of hypovolemia versus myocardial dysfunction and in the rapid diagnosis of air embolization.

Which Resuscitation Drugs Are Essential?

A thermally injured patient undergoing debridement is potentially as hemodynamically unstable as any acute trauma victim. Accordingly, we have ready for use the drugs listed in Table 41-6.

When Is Air Embolization Problematic?

Rapid-infusion warming devices, such as the Level 1 Fluid Warmer (Level 1 Technologies), help to maintain hemodynamic and temperature stability through immediate replacement of large amounts of warmed blood, blood products, and fluids. Our experience is that the air eliminator of this device is rapidly overwhelmed by residual air in fluid bags or by entrained air during fluid bag exchange.[79] At infusion flow rates of 1000 mL $\cdot$ min^{-1}, $>50\%$ of even small 5-mL air boluses pass beyond the air eliminator. If the bolus is large (e.g., 60 mL), up to 50 mL passes through the eliminator. Sixty milliliters is approximately the amount of air found in every bag of crystalloid before it is spiked, if no effort has been made to vent this gas during spiking.

If the air eliminator has been exposed to protein-containing fluid or blood products, its ability to eliminate air is further compromised. Low flows make the passage of air through the eliminator and into the patient less likely, but debridement of a severely burned patient frequently necessitates the use of high flow rates. When this device is used, one must adhere to a rigorous protocol to eliminate air from fluid bags and to monitor the infusion path for bubbles distal to the air eliminator. The Level 1 air eliminator, once overwhelmed, does not recover its air elimination capabilities and must be replaced.

How Is Body Temperature Maintained Intraoperatively?

Because maintenance of body temperature is a problem in thermally injured patients and because multiple potential problems may occur in cold patients (ineffective coagulation, dysrhythmias, increased myocardial O_2, consumption secondary

TABLE 41–6. Resuscitation Drug Use During Debridement and Skin Grafting

Drug	Concentration	Volume
Atropine	400 μg $\cdot$ mL^{-1}	30 mL
Ephedrine	5 mg $\cdot$ mL^{-1}	10 mL
Epinephrine	10 μg $\cdot$ mL^{-1}	10 mL
	100 μg $\cdot$ mL^{-1}	10 mL
Calcium chloride	100 mg $\cdot$ mL^{-1}	10 mL
Phenylephrine	40 μg $\cdot$ mL^{-1}	1-mL ampule of 10% concentration taped to 250-mL bag of lactated Ringer's

to shivering), we keep the thermostat in the OR at 29°C during debridement. We always use an actively warmed airway humidifier (although its efficacy has been questioned[80]), maintain a low fresh gas flow rate, cover all body parts not involved in the surgical procedure, and warm all fluids going into the patient. Overhead warming lights and a warming blanket are used during operative procedures in children.

How Is Ventilation Supported?

Edema of the chest and abdominal walls and ARDS may result in a very noncompliant lung-thorax unit, requiring high inspiratory pressures to maintain adequate gas exchange. Preoperative evaluation of mechanically ventilated burned patients must include a measurement of the peak inspiratory pressures and minute ventilation. Many OR ventilators cannot predictably generate peak pressures >50 cm H_2O or minute ventilations >15 L $\cdot$ min^{-1}.[81] If the patient requires higher pressure or minute ventilation, the intensive care unit ventilator should be brought to the OR.

What Factors Govern the Choice of Anesthetic?

When anesthetic agents have to be administered within the first 24 postburn hours, circulatory instability should be anticipated owing to the previously described marked vasoconstriction and depressed cardiac output. Acute fluid resuscitation must be continued in the operating room in addition to the appropriate replacement of intraoperative fluid and blood losses. Establishment of large-bore intravenous catheters, especially in children or obese patients, may be difficult. Intravenous access without penetrating burn eschar is optimal but cannot always be avoided.

General Considerations

Intravenous drug and inhaled anesthetic agent administration need careful titration. An increase in the anesthetic dose requirement is very frequently noted after resuscitation during the acute stage of a thermal injury. Sodium thiopental, narcotic, and ketamine requirements may be increased for months after burn injury.[82, 83] We routinely use a nondepolarizing muscle relaxant.

Ketamine, at a dose of 0.25 to 1 mg $\cdot$ kg^{-1} intravenously, is used frequently for bedside dressing changes. We often coadminister an anticholinergic drug (glycopyrrolate, 0.2–0.4 mg intravenously) to minimize salivation and midazolam ($\leq$0.25 mg $\cdot$ kg^{-1} intravenously) to minimize the potential for emergence hallucinations. We avoid the use of nitrous oxide because of its potentially adverse effect on hematopoiesis and wound healing by inhibition of methionine synthase activity in these patients who usually undergo multiple procedures.[84]

Why Do We Prefer Intravenous Techniques?

Inhaled volatile anesthetic agents allow rapid adjustments in the depth of anesthesia and have been used successfully in many burned patients. However, we prefer intravenous anesthetic techniques for debridement of burns $\geq$20% TBSA. We

interpret the admittedly controversial data on the immunosuppressive effects of the inhaled agents as sufficient reason to avoid them whenever possible.[85] Instead, we use one of two major intravenous techniques (Table 41–7). We have found hemodynamic function with these techniques to be very stable, provided blood loss is rapidly corrected. An additional advantage is that continued sedation or analgesia in the postoperative period may be provided by either technique by simply titrating the infusion rate downward.

When Is Continuation of Anesthesia and Surgery Contraindicated?

Of crucial importance in providing anesthesia for burn debridement is good rapport with the surgical team. They need to be informed when blood loss due to debridement is approaching or exceeding either replacement availability or capability. Their interruption of further debridement to focus attention on control of bleeding for a few minutes often is all that is required in order to catch up with blood and fluid replacement.

Surgical duration probably has a significant impact on outcome in large burns. Thus, we usually limit our surgical colleagues to approximately 2 hours of operative time. We recommend discontinuation of surgery even before this time period has expired if more than two blood volumes have been lost or, as noted previously, the body temperature falls to 35 °C or by >1.5 °C from baseline. Even with adherence to these limits, massive postoperative resuscitation and correction of continued bleeding problems may require the continued involvement of the anesthesiologist long after the patient has left the operating room.

How Should Neuromuscular Blockers Be Used?

Succinylcholine

Succinylcholine in burned patients can cause massive potassium efflux from the muscle cells and result in acute lethal hyperkalemia. It is speculated that after burn injury, a denervation phenomenon occurs, with spreading of acetylcholine receptors throughout the muscle membranes. This hyperkalemic response is related to the dose of succinylcholine, time elapsed since injury, and severity of the burn injury.[86] The hyperkalemia and subsequent cardiac arrest usually occur within minutes of the administration of a paralyzing dose of succinylcholine.[87] We simply do not use this agent in thermally injured patients.

Nondepolarizing Agents

In thermal injury, resistance to nondepolarizing neuromuscular blockers, proportional to the TBSA involved (from 25% TBSA upward), has been demonstrated. Resistance is not observed in the first postburn week; maximum resistance occurs between 15 and 40 days after the initial thermal injury.[88] To achieve a given level of paralysis, a longer onset time is required; both the dose administered and serum concentrations required are increased two- to threefold.

Early *local* resistance to atracurium in muscles under ther-

TABLE 41–7. Intravenous Anesthetic Regimens Used at the University of Florida/Shands Hospital Burn Operating Room

Period	Ketamine-Based Regimen	Narcotic-Based Regimen
Preoperative medication (8 AM case)	Lorazepam 1–3 mg IV (6 AM) Metoclopramide 10 mg IV (OCOR) Famotidine* 20 mg IV (6 AM)	Lorazepam 1–3 mg IV (6 AM) Metoclopramide 10 mg IV (OCOR) Famotidine* 20 mg IV (6 AM)
Induction	Midazolam 0.1–0.2 mg · kg^{-1} Ketamine 2.0 mg · kg^{-1} Vecuronium 0.2 mg · kg^{-1}	Midazolam 0.1–0.2 mg · kg^{-1} Fentanyl 5.0–10.0 μg · kg^{-1} Vecuronium 0.2 mg · kg^{-1}
Maintenance	Midazolam 0.1–0.2 mg · kg^{-1} · h^{-1} infusion Ketamine 1.0–2.0 mg · kg^{-1} · h^{-1} infusion	Midazolam 0.1–0.2 mg · kg^{-1} · h^{-1} infusion Fentanyl 1.0–5.0 μg · kg^{-1} · h^{-1} infusion
Midazolam infusion	20 mg in 100 ml 0.9% saline = 0.2 mg/mL	
Ketamine infusion	200 mg in 100 ml 0.9% saline = 2 mg/mL	
Fentanyl infusion	500 μg in 250 mL 0.9% saline = 2 μg/mL	
Sufentanil (may be used in place of fentanyl, if desired)	0.5–1 μg · kg^{-1} load, followed by 0.1–0.5 μg · kg^{-1} · h^{-1}	

Abbreviations: OCOR = on call to the operating room.
*Ranitidine and cimetidine are equally effective; famotidine is cheaper in our institution.

mally injured skin in rats (2% TBSA burn only!) was shown by Pavlin and colleagues.[89] Ligand binding with bungarotoxin showed that at 2 weeks, acetylcholine receptors in the gastrocnemius muscle under the burned skin were four times denser than in the gastrocnemius in the contralateral uninjured leg. This group suggested that facial burns might be associated with unexpected resistance to nondepolarizing neuromuscular blockers due to the nature of the muscles in the area. Using facial nerve rather than ulnar nerve stimulation to assess adequacy of relaxation for intubation may be of value in the setting of a facial burn.

Tracheal Intubation

For intubation, we commonly use vecuronium, 0.3 mg · kg^{-1}; pancuronium, 0.3 mg · kg^{-1}; or atracurium, 1.0 mg · kg^{-1}. With these doses, relaxation sufficient for intubation is achieved within about 60 seconds.

Although hypotension is a concern with an atracurium dose >0.5 mg, it was not noted when 0.8 mg · kg^{-1} was used in burned patients.[90] Frequent monitoring with a nerve stimulator is necessary if continued muscle relaxation is desired. Debridement and grafting, however, usually do not require profound muscle relaxation.

THE CHRONIC PHASE

How Are Repetitive Anesthetics Managed?

Pain Control

Pain control, in particular, is of critical importance during the acute and chronic phases of burn injury. Enlisting the help of an acute pain service to assist members of the burn care team must be considered. As mentioned earlier, use of keta-

mine during dressing changes and whirlpool procedures is critical.

Psychologic support during the period of acute, chronic, and rehabilitative care must be considered as important as volume resuscitation and debridement. There is no magic to this phase of burn care; we must treat our patients as we would want our family members treated.

A critical stage in the treatment of patients with burns is control of the hypertrophic scarring that is responsible for deformities and contractures. With burns that involve the face, hypertrophic scarring can be disfiguring and painful. This problem can be ameliorated by the use of a contoured pressure mask. Fabrication of this mask in children often requires sedation or general anesthesia.

Intravenous anesthesia with ketamine, in which tracheal intubation is not performed, has been used frequently. However, apnea may occasionally occur, engendering significant risk if the alginate mold material completely covers the face.[91] Because rapid-sequence induction with succinylcholine is contraindicated in these patients secondary to potential problems with hyperkalemia, we recommend inhalation anesthesia and nasotracheal intubation, with or without nondepolarizing muscle relaxants.[92]

References

1. Accident Facts. Chicago, National Safety Council, 1990.
2. Demling R: Burns. N Engl J Med 1985; 313:1389.
3. Burke JF: From desperation to skin regeneration: progress in burn treatment. J Trauma 1990; 30:S36.
4. Zimmermann TJ, Krizek TJ: Thermally induced dermal injury—a review of pathophysiologic events and therapeutic intervention. J Burn Care Rehabil 1984; 5:193.
5. Jackson DM: The diagnosis of depth of burning. Br J Surg 1953; 40:588.
6. Zawacki BE: Reversal of capillary stasis and prevention of necrosis in burns. Ann Surg 1974; 180:98.
7. Homma S, Gillam L, Weyman A: Echocardiographic observations in survivors of acute electrical injury. Chest 1990; 97:103.

8. Dixon GF: The evaluation and management of electrical injuries. Crit Care Med 1983; 11:384.

9. Bingham H: Electrical burns. Clin Plast Surg 1986; 13:75.

10. Hammond JS, Ward CG: High-voltage electrical injuries—management and outcome of 60 cases. South Med J 1988; 81:1351.

11. Kaufman T, Yehuda U, Yaron H-S: Phosphorus burns—a practical approach to local treatment. J Burn Care Rehabil 1988; 9:474.

12. Demling RH, Lalonde C: Burn Trauma. New York, Thieme Medical Publishers, 1989, pp 43–45.

13. O'Reilly TJ, Spence RJ, Taylor RM, et al: Laser Doppler flowmetry evaluation of burn wound depth. J Burn Care Rehabil 1989; 10:1.

14. Tobiasen J, Hiebert JH, Edlich RF: Prediction of burn mortality. Surg Gynecol Obstet 1982; 154:711.

15. Parker CR Jr, Baxter CR: Divergence in adrenal secretory pattern after thermal injury in adult patients. J Trauma 1985; 25:508.

16. Wilmore DW: Metabolic changes after thermal injury. In The Art and Science of Burn Care. Boswick JA Jr (ed). Rockville, Aspen Publishers, 1987, pp 137–144.

17. McDonald WS, Sharp CW, Deitch EA: Immediate enteral feeding in burn patients is safe and effective. Ann Surg 1991; 213:177.

18. Saito H, Trocki O, Alexander JW: The effect of route of nutrient administration on the nutritional state, catabolic hormone secretion, and gut mucosal integrity after burn injury. JPEN J Parenteral Enteral Nutr 1986; 11:1.

19. Alexander JW, MacMillan BG, Stinnett JD, et al: Beneficial effects of aggressive protein feeding in severely burned children. Ann Surg 1980; 192:505.

20. Alexander JW, Peck MD: Future prospects for adjunctive therapy—pharmacological and nutritional approaches to immune system modulations. Crit Care Med 1990; 18:S159.

21. Madden HP, Breslin RJ, Wasserkrug HL, et al: Stimulation of T-cell immunity by arginine enhances survival in peritonitis. J Surg Res 1988; 44:658.

22. Herndon DN, Barrow RE, Stein M, et al: Increasing mortality with intravenous supplemental feeding in severely burned patients. J Burn Care Rehabil 1989; 10:309.

23. Ward PA, Till GO: Pathophysiologic events related to thermal injury of skin. J Trauma 1990; 30:S75.

24. DeCamp MM, Demling RH: Posttraumatic multisystem organ failure. JAMA 1988; 260:530.

25. Pitman JM III, Thurman GW, Anderson BO, et al: WEB2170, a specific platelet-activating factor antagonist, attenuates neutrophil priming by human serum after clinical burn injury. J Burn Care Rehabil 1991; 12:411.

26. Dinarello CA: The proinflammatory cytokines interleukin-1 and tumor necrosis factor and treatment of the septic shock syndrome. J Infect Dis 1991; 163:1177.

27. Barton R, Cerra FB: The hypermetabolism multiple organ failure syndrome. Chest 1989; 96:1153.

28. Cerra FB: The systemic septic response—concepts of pathogenesis. J Trauma 1990; 30:S169.

29. Schlüter B, König W, Köller M, et al: Studies on B-lymphocyte dysfunctions in severely burned patients. Trauma 1990; 30:1380.

30. Ferrara JJ, Dyess DL, Luterman A, et al: The suppressive effect of subeschar tissue fluid upon in vitro cell-mediated immunologic function. J Burn Care Rehabil 1988; 9:584.

31. Trop M, Schiffrin EJ, Jung WK, et al: Effect of acute burn trauma on phagocytic activity of the reticuloendothelial system in rats. J Burn Care Rehabil 1989; 10:388.

32. Gruber DF, D'Alesandro MM: Alteration of rat polymorphonuclear leukocyte function after thermal injury. J Burn Care Rehabil 1989; 10:394.

33. Schriemer PA, Longnecker DE, Mintz PD: The possible immunosuppressive effects of perioperative blood transfusion in cancer patients. Anesthesiology 1988; 68:422.

34. Waymack JP, Miskell P, Gonce S: Alterations in host defense associated with inhalation anesthesia and blood transfusion. Anesth Analg 1989; 69:163.

35. Shelby J: Transfusion-induced immunosuppression. J Burn Care Rehabil 1987; 8:546.

36. Hendrickson M, Shelby J, Sullivan JJ, et al: Naloxone inhibits the in vivo immunosuppressive effects of morphine and thermal injury in mice. J Burn Care Rehabil 1989; 10:494.

37. Waymack JP, Jenkins M, Warden GD, et al: A prospective study of thymopentin in severely burned patients. Surg Gynecol Obstet 1987; 164:423.

38. Alexander JW: The body's response to infection. In Burns—A Team Approach. Artz CP, Moncrief JA, Pruitt BA Jr (eds). Philadelphia, WB Saunders, 1979, pp 107–119.

39. Deitch EA, Berg R: Bacterial translocation from the gut—a mechanism of infection. J Burn Care Rehabil 1987; 8:475.

40. Dobke MK, Simoni J, Ninnemann JL, et al: Endotoxemia after burn injury—effect of early excision on circulating endotoxin levels. J Burn Care Rehabil 1989; 10:107.

41. Suzuki K, Nishina M, Ogino R, et al: Left ventricular contractility and diastolic properties in anesthetized dogs after severe burns. Am J Physiol 1991; 260:H1433.

42. Moncrief JA: Burns. N Engl J Med 1973; 288:444.

43. Demling RH, Kramer GC, Gunther R, et al: Effect of non-protein colloid on post-burn edema formation in soft tissues and lung. Surgery 1984; 95:593.

44. Zimmerman TJ, Krizek TJ: Thermally induced dermal injury—a review of pathophysiologic events and therapeutic intervention. J Burn Care Rehabil 1984; 5:193.

45. Demling RH, Lalonde C: Topical ibuprofen decreases early postburn edema. Surgery 1987; 102:857.

46. Lalonde C, Knox J, Daryani R, et al: Topical flurbiprofen decreases burn wound-induced hypermetabolism and systemic lipid peroxidation. Surgery 1991; 109:645.

47. Alexander F, Mathieson M, Teoh KHT, et al: Arachidonic acid metabolites mediate early burn edema. J Trauma 1984; 24:709.

48. Deitch EA: The management of burns. N Engl J Med 1990; 323:1249.

49. Haponik EF, Crapo RO, Herndon DN, et al: Smoke inhalation. Am Rev Respir Dis 1988; 138:1060.

50. Herndon DN, Traber DL, Linares H, et al: Etiology of the pulmonary pathophysiology associated with inhalation injury. Resuscitation 1986; 14:43.

51. Moylan JA, Chan CK: Inhalation injury—an increasing problem. Ann Surg 1978; 188:34.

52. Tranbaugh RF, Elings VB, Christensens JM, et al: Effect of inhalation injury on lung water accumulation. J Trauma 1983; 23:597.

53. Wroblewski DA, Bower GC: The significance of facial burns in acute smoke inhalation. Crit Care Med 1979; 7:335.

54. Zikria BA, Budd DC, Floch F, et al: What is clinical smoke poisoning? Ann Surg 1975; 181:151.

55. Moylan JA: Diagnostic techniques and steroids. J Trauma 1979; 19:11s.

56. Vossmann H: Das inhalationstrauma beim Brandverletzten Handchirurgie, Mikrochirurgie. Plastische Chirurgie 1988; 20:229.

57. Zellner PR: The 1990 Everett Idris Evans Memorial Lecture—the inhalation injury. J Burn Care Rehabil 1990; 11:487.

58. Bingham HG, Gallagher TJ, Powell MD: Early bronchoscopy as a predictor of ventilatory support for burned patients. J Trauma 1987; 27:1286.

59. Kilgore E, Baxter CR, Shires GT: Changes in body fluid compartments in full thickness burns. Surg Forum 1965; 16:29.

60. Curreri PW, Luterman A, Braun DW, et al: Analysis of survival and hospitalization time for 937 patients. Ann Surg 1980; 192:472.

61. Monafo WW, Halverson JD, Schechtman K: The role of concentrated solutions in the resuscitation of patients with severe burns. Surgery 1984; 95:129.

62. Monafo WW, Chuntrasakul C, Ayvazian VH: Hypertonic sodium solutions in the treatment of burn shock. Am J Surg 1973; 126:778.

63. Moylan JA, Reckler JM, Mason AD: Resuscitation with hypertonic lactate saline in thermal injury. Am J Surg 1973; 125:580.

64. Caldwell FT, Bowser BH: Critical evaluation of hypertonic and hypotonic solutions to resuscitate severely burned children—a prospective study. Ann Surg 1979; 189:546.

65. McGough EK: Resuscitation in shock, trauma, and burns—hypertonic saline solutions. In Innovative Fluid and Electrolyte, Nutritional, and Transfusion Therapy. Kirby RR (ed). Problems in Critical Care 1991; 5:346.

66. Dries DJ, Waxman K: Adequate resuscitation of burn patients may not be measured by urine output and vital signs. Crit Care Med 1991; 19:327.

67. DiVincenti FC, Moncrief JA, Pruitt BA: Electrical injuries—a review of 65 cases. J Trauma 1969; 9:497.

68. Monafo WW, Freedman BM: Electrical and lightning injury. In The Art and Science of Burn Care. Boswick JA (ed). Rockville, Aspen Publishers, 1987, pp 247–248.

69. Teplitz C: The pathology of burns and the fundamentals of burn wound sepsis. In Burns—A Team Approach. Artz CP, Moncrief JA, Pruitt BA Jr (eds). Philadelphia, WB Saunders, 1979, pp 45–94.

70. Peterson VM, Hansbrough JF, Wang XW, et al: Topical cerium nitrate cream prevents postburn immunosuppression. J Trauma 1985; 25:1039.

71. Subrahmanyam M: Topical application of honey in treatment of burns. Br J Surg 1991; 78:497.

72. Monafo WW, West MA: Current treatment recommendations for topical burn therapy. Drugs 1990; 40:364.

73. Janzekovic Z: A new concept in the early excision and immediate grafting of burns. J Trauma 1970; 10:1103.

74. Moran KT, O'Reilly TJ, Furman W, et al: A new algorithm for calculation of blood loss in excisional burn surgery. Am Surg 1988; 54:207.

75. Goodwin CW, Maguire MS, McManus WF, et al: Prospective study of burn wound excision of the hands. J Trauma 1983; 23:510.

76. Brezel BS, McGeever KE, Stein JM: Epinephrine vs thrombin for split-thickness donor site hemostasis. J Burn Care Rehabil 1987; 8:132.

77. Schlagintweit S, Snelling CFT, Germann E, et al: Major burns managed without blood or blood products. J Burn Care Rehabil 1990; 11:214.

78. Coté CJ, Drop LJ, Hoaglin DC, et al: Ionized hypocalcemia after fresh frozen plasma administration to thermally injured children—effects of infusion rate, duration, and treatment with calcium chloride. Anesth Analg 1988; 67:152.

79. Hartmannsgruber MWB, Gravenstein N: Performance of Level 1 air eliminator at high and low flow rates (Abstract). Anesthesiology 1992; 77:A1051.

80. Hynson JM, Sessler DI: Comparison of intraoperative warming devices (Abstract). Anesth Analg 1991; 72:S118.

81. Marks JA, Schapera A, Kraemer RW, et al: Pressure and flow limitations of anesthesia ventilators. Anesthesiology 1989; 71:403.

82. Coté CJ, Petkau AJ: Thiopental requirements may be increased in children reanesthetized at less than one year after recovery from extensive thermal injury. Anesth Analg 1985; 64:1156.

83. Martyn J: Clinical pharmacology and drug therapy in the burned patient. Anesthesiology 1986; 65:67.

84. Royston BD, Nunn JF, Weinbren HK, et al: Rate of inactivation of human and rodent hepatic methionine synthase by nitrous oxide. Anesthesiology 1988; 68:213.

85. Layon AJ, Peck AB: Anesthetic effects on immune function—Where do we stand? *In* Advances in Anesthesia. Stoelting RK, Barash PG, Gallagher TJ (eds). St Louis, Mosby-Year Book (in press).

86. Schaner PJ, Brown RL, Kirksey TD, et al: Succinylcholine hyperkalemia in burned patients. Anesth Analg 1969; 48:764.

87. Tolmie JD: Succinylcholine danger in the burned patient. Anesthesiology 1967; 28:467.

88. Dwersteg JF, Pavlin EG, Heimbach DM: Patients with burns are resistant to atracurium. Anesthesiology 1986; 65:516.

89. Pavlin EG, Howard ML, Slattery JT: Resistance to atracurium in muscles under thermally injured skin in the rat (Abstract). Anesthesiology 1991; 75:A779.

90. Dwersteg JF, Pavlin EG, Haschke R: High dose atracurium does not produce hypotension in the burned patient (Abstract). Anesthesiology 1986; 65:A293.

91. White PF, Way WL, Trevor AJ: Ketamine—its pharmacology and therapeutic uses. Anesthesiology 1982; 56:119.

92. Layon AJ, Vetter TR, Hanna PG, et al: An anesthetic technique to fabricate a pressure mask for controlling scar formation from facial burns. J Burn Care Rehabil 1991; 12:349.

CHAPTER 42

Fluids and Electrolytes

EDWARD K. MCGOUGH, M.D.
ROBERT R. KIRBY, M.D.

The human body is 60% to 70% water. In obese patients, the percentage of water decreases, whereas in very thin patients it increases. It is also affected greatly by disease states such as renal failure, hepatic failure, congestive heart failure, and sepsis, as well as by age. Body water is divided into various compartments (Fig. 42–1). A means to remember this division is the "rule of thirds." Approximately two thirds of total body weight (in a lean patient) is water; of this quantity, two thirds is intracellular, and one third is extracellular. Of the extracellular water, approximately two thirds to three quarters is extravascular, and the remaining one third to one quarter is intravascular. Although this rule is only an approximation, it presents an easy way to remember body water composition.

FLUID COMPARTMENTS

The intracellular and extracellular compartments are separated by cell membranes. These membranes are permeable to water but are relatively impermeable to ionized particles (elec-

trolytes). Therefore, water crosses membranes freely. The equilibrium between the intracellular and extracellular body compartments is determined by osmotic gradients. These osmotic differences determine the size of each compartment.

Intravascular and extravascular spaces are separated by capillary endothelium that is freely permeable not only to water but also to electrolytes and other small molecules. However, it is normally less permeable to large molecules such as albumin. Permeability to ions and proteins varies from organ to organ, being least in the brain (blood-brain barrier) and highest in the liver.

How Do Extracellular and Intracellular Compartments Differ?

Each of the fluid compartments has a different composition (Table 42–1). The intravascular compartment contains water and electrolytes, a high concentration of proteins, and the formed blood elements (red blood cells, white blood cells, and platelets). This fluid space is accessible to the anesthesiologist for drug administration and for the measurement of various body components, and it is essential for oxygen transport. The principal difference between the intravascular and extravascular fluid compartments is the absence of much of the protein and most of the formed blood elements in the latter.

Since fluids and electrolytes pass freely between these compartments, the electrolyte composition is approximately the same. However, because of the previously described, relatively impermeable cellular membranes and the membrane-bound sodium-potassium pump, the concentration of electrolytes in the

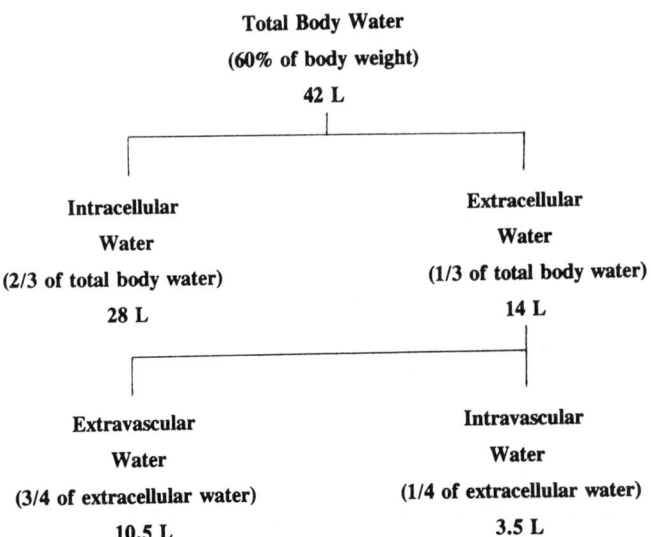

FIGURE 42–1. Distribution of body water in an "ideal" 70-kg man.

TABLE 42–1. Approximate Electrolyte Concentrations

	Extracellular Fluid* (mEq · L^{-1})	Intracellular Fluid (mEq · L^{-1})
Sodium	140	10
Potassium	4.5	150
Calcium	5	1
Magnesium	2	40

*Plasma and interstitial.

intracellular compartment is very different from that in the extracellular compartment (see Table 42–1). The importance of some of these differences is discussed in the section on electrolyte disturbances.

Regulation of Body Fluid Composition

Normally, the body's fluid composition is carefully regulated. Figure 42–2 represents the major factors of importance. Water balance is intimately associated with solute balance. The human kidneys can produce urine with a solute concentration of between 50 mOsm $\cdot$ L^{-1} and 1400 mOsm $\cdot$ L^{-1}.[1] These changes in concentration are caused by changes in the level of antidiuretic hormone (ADH; also known as arginine-vasopressin).

The production of ADH is controlled by extracellular fluid volume, osmoreceptors, and perfusion to various organ systems, including the central nervous system and the kidneys. In awake patients, thirst and drinking control the intake of both solutes and water. However, during anesthesia, thirst is eliminated. Furthermore, during major operative procedures, the fluid shifts and blood loss that occur are often much greater than could be corrected by the usual drinking response and oral intake.

The observation of urine output provides a rough but often imprecise indication of fluid balance; this topic is discussed later in this chapter in the section on monitoring of adequacy of replacement. For a more complete description of the regulation of body water, the reader is referred to other sources.[2]

ORIGINS OF THERAPEUTIC MISCONCEPTIONS

Does "Salt Intolerance" Exist?

Throughout the 1940s and 1950s, patients in the immediate postoperative period received salt-free solutions such as 5% dextrose in water (D$_5$W). This practice was derived from the hypothesis that these patients were salt intolerant, that is, that they were unable to excrete an administered sodium load. Most of these assumptions were based on small numbers of case reports in which patients were felt to have received sufficient amounts of intravenous saline but had major complications, including abdominal distention, somnolence, lethargy, coma, shock, and sometimes, death.[3] Salt intolerance was blamed. However, on later review it was realized that the complications reported were those of hyponatremia and hyposmolarity associated with the administration of excess D$_5$W. Nevertheless, for years thereafter surgical patients underwent forced sodium restriction in the immediate postoperative period, and as a result severe hyponatremia and water intoxication continued to occur.

Hormonal Fluxes

The identification and characterization of ADH, the 17-OH corticosteroids, and aldosterone as well as more precise delineation of intraoperative fluid shifts and renal function resulted in significant changes in the concepts underlying fluid and electrolyte therapy. Nonstressed patients can form as much as 10 mL of urine for each milliosmole of solute excreted by the kidneys. However, stressed surgical patients can only excrete 1.2 to 1.6 mL $\cdot$ mOsm^{-1} of solute.[4] Thus, when such individuals are given a fluid such as D$_5$W with minimal solute, they are unable to excrete a large water load and retain large amounts of free water; consequently, they develop a dilutional hyponatremia, hyposmolarity, and water intoxication.

Additionally, in the operative and postoperative periods, significant fluid losses occur. These include continued bleeding and so-called "third space" losses. The latter represents the loss of isotonic fluid, that is, fluid with the same electrolyte composition as that in plasma. Current recommendations are to replace these losses with fluid of a composition that is similar to that of the fluid being lost, (i.e., balanced electrolyte solutions, colloid solutions, or both).

Our better understanding of the hormonal control of fluid balance, improved invasive and noninvasive monitoring, and rapid measurements of serum and urine electrolytes and hematocrit allow more precise titration of fluid therapy than was ever possible when urine output was the primary determinant of fluid status and renal function.[5]

FLUID BALANCE DURING SURGERY

What Changes Occur with Regional Anesthesia?

If patients had no physiologic changes during anesthesia and surgery, there would be little need for fluid therapy other than to replace blood loss. However, physiologic alterations do occur. When spinal, epidural, or caudal anesthesia is induced, a variable degree of sympathetic blockade results. The stress response to general anesthesia and mechanical ventilation, which is associated with increased ADH production, is blocked. Peripheral vasodilatation results in venous pooling and effectively removes circulating blood from the central intravascular compartment. Sufficient fluid must be administered to maintain venous return, blood pressure, and cardiac output.

Most young patients tolerate this sympathectomy well if

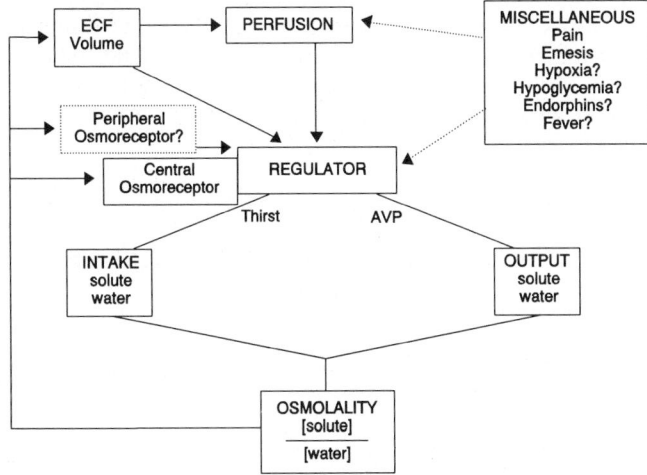

FIGURE 42–2. Factors affecting water balance. *Question marks* and *dashed lines* indicate factors that are not clearly understood. ECF = Extracellular fluid; AVP = arginine-vasopressin. (From Tonneson AS: Water balance and control of osmolality. *In* Fluid and Electrolyte Management in Critical Care. Askanazi J, Starker PM, Weissman C (eds). Boston, Butterworths, 1986, p 99.)

they have been sufficiently hydrated prior to the induction of anesthesia. However, elderly patients with underlying heart disease or patients taking diuretics or antihypertensive drugs may not be able to mount the responses necessary to overcome the sympatholytic effects of regional anesthesia. Careful fluid administration and judicious use of anticholinergic drugs (atropine, glycopyrrolate) or vasopressors (dopamine, phenylephrine hydrochloride, ephedrine, epinephrine) are sometimes essential to the successful use of such techniques.

Regional anesthesia involving small areas of the body, such as brachial plexus blocks, requires much less fluid replacement. When spinal anesthesia is chosen, up to 1 L of fluid is usually administered prior to the start of the anesthesia because the onset of sympathetic blockade is rapid. With epidural techniques, especially when a catheter and incremental doses are used, the fluid administration can occur concomitantly with the slower onset of anesthesia.

What Changes Occur with General Anesthesia?

General anesthesia has two components of importance to fluid management. First are the anesthetic effects, and second are the effects of positive-pressure ventilation.

Anesthetic Effects

No commonly used anesthetics cause increased fluid losses. Nevertheless, all anesthetics may blunt the normal response to absolute or relative hypovolemia, especially during induction. A moderately hypovolemic patient with a normal blood pressure may suddenly become hypotensive after anesthesia has been induced. These effects are exaggerated when myocardial depressants, such as barbiturates or propofol, or agents with potent vasodilatory properties, such as isoflurane, are used. However, even a usually sympathomimetic agent such as ketamine can produce similar effects if the sympathetic response prior to induction is already maximal, thereby uncovering its myocardial depressant effect.

Mechanical Ventilation

Mechanical ventilation also affects fluid balance by decreasing the release of atrial natriuretic hormone and, particularly when administered with positive end-expiratory pressure, by increasing the release of ADH (as noted previously). Thus, patients retain slightly more sodium and fluid. Of more importance are the reduction of venous return and blood pressure, which, when added to the anesthetic-induced decreases, may be profound. In general, these changes are rapidly reversed upon discontinuation of the anesthetic and resumption of spontaneous breathing. They rarely lead to prolonged postoperative fluid shifts and decrease in urine output.

What Surgical Factors Are Important?

The major fluid and electrolyte shifts result from the "trauma" of surgery. In addition to blood replacement, third space losses (edema, intracellular translocation, ascites, and so forth) must be replenished. Such losses are not easily quantified and do not exist in nor move to specific anatomic areas.

The involved fluid, although still physically present in the body, is no longer functional in terms of its contribution to intravascular volume, oxygen and nutrient delivery, and waste removal.

Trauma-Induced Fluid Loss

A convenient way to think about this problem is to consider the fluid that is lost from the area of surgical trauma. An increase of capillary permeability and localized swelling (edema) occurs much the same as is seen when one's thumb is struck with a hammer. The leaked fluid is still present but is in a new location and is obviously no longer functional in fluid homeostasis. If the area of involvement is sufficiently large, as it is with bowel resection, retroperitoneal exploration, radical prostatectomy or hysterectomy, or major trauma, several liters of fluid are lost and must be replaced so that functional activity is maintained. Successful management results in an obligatory increase in total body water in order to restore the functional component to normal.

Bleeding and Third Space Fluid Loss

Third space fluid loss also occurs with major bleeding. In a classic resuscitation experiment, Shires and coworkers[6] showed that replacement of all lost blood in a dog model of hemorrhagic shock produced only 30% survival. When a quantity of lactated Ringer's solution equal to 5% of the body weight was given with the shed blood, survival increased to 70% (Fig. 42–3). Simple restoration of shed blood volume alone is insufficient to restore function and ensure survival when major blood loss and large fluid shifts have occurred.

Patients undergoing major surgery, therefore, need fluid replacement in addition to that required for the lost blood. This additional fluid must eventually be excreted, usually between the second and the fifth postoperative days in uncomplicated cases. The third space losses are "mobilized" at this time into the intravascular compartment, and a brisk spontaneous diuresis ensues. Patients with tenuous cardiac or renal function may not tolerate this mobilization, and congestive heart failure sometimes results. Such a complication, although undesirable, is often a necessary consequence of appropriate fluid administration in the operative and immediate postoperative periods. Careful fluid restriction and diuretic use in this phase is indicated in such cases.

INTRAOPERATIVE AND POSTOPERATIVE FLUID THERAPY

In addition to blood, commonly used fluids for intraoperative use are divided into three categories:

1. Conventional crystalloids
2. Colloids
3. Hypertonic solutions

Some less commonly used fluids include blood substitutes. In this section, the choice of initial fluids and the question of glucose utilization are addressed.

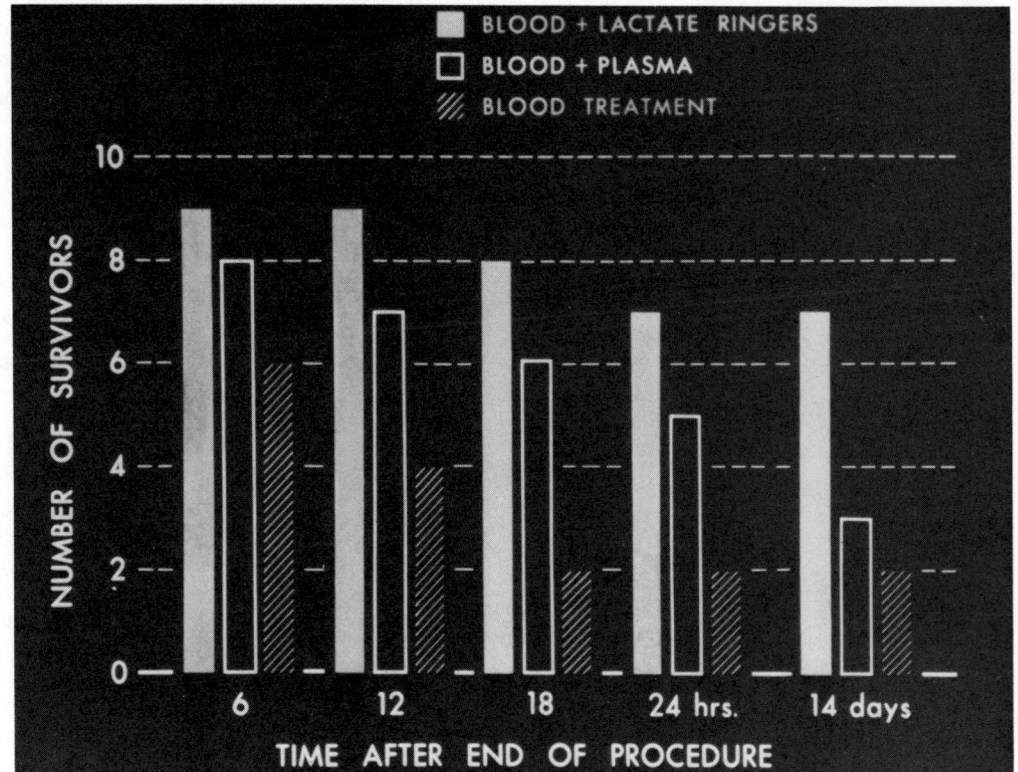

FIGURE 42–3. Survival from hemorrhagic shock following resuscitation with blood alone; with blood and plasma; and with blood and lactated Ringer's solution. (Redrawn from Shires T, Cohn D, Carrico J, et al: Fluid therapy in hemorrhagic shock. Arch Surg 1964; 88:688. Copyright 1964, American Medical Association.)

What Are Conventional Crystalloids?

Conventional crystalloids are fluids that contain a combination of water and electrolytes. They are divided into "balanced" salt solutions and hypotonic salt solutions. Balanced salt solutions include lactated Ringer's solution, Plasma-Lyte, and Normosol (Table 42–2). Either their electrolyte composition approximates that of plasma, or they have a total calculated osmolality that is similar to that of plasma.

Normal saline (0.9%) is frequently considered to be balanced but is actually hypertonic with respect to sodium and especially to chloride, if the osmolality is calculated. However, when normal saline is subjected to a freezing point depression test in an osmometer, its osmolality is approximately 285 mOsm · L^{-1}. The *calculated* value is derived by simple addition of its ionic constituents, whereas the *measured* value is affected by ionic association/dissociation. Thus, sodium chloride has a relative osmolality of 1 compared with that of Na$^+$ and Cl$^-$, the value of which is 2. Other balanced electrolyte solutions are slightly hypotonic in vitro (~265 mOsm · L^{-1}) in comparison with their calculated values and normal plasma. Solutions that contain less than the concentration of electro-

TABLE 42–2. Composition of Selected Intravenous Fluids

	Na$^+$ (mEq · L^{-1})	Cl$^-$ (mEq · L^{-1})	K$^+$ (mEq · L^{-1})	Mg^{2+} (mEq · L^{-1})	Ca^{2+} (mEq · L^{-1})	Lactate (mEq · L^{-1})	Other	Approximate pH	mOsm · L^{-1} (calculated)
D$_5$W							Dextrose, 5 g · L^{-1}	5.0	253
0.9 Sodium chloride	154	154						4.2	308
Lactated Ringer's solution	130	109	4.0		3.0	28		6.5	273
Plasma-Lyte	140	98	5.0	3.0			Acetate, 27 mEq · L^{-1} Gluconate, 23 mEq · L^{-1}	7.4	294
Hespan	154	154					Hydroxyethyl starch, 6.0 g · dL^{-1}	5.5	310
Dextran 70	154	154						5.5	308
5% Albumin	145	145					Albumin, 5.0 g · dL^{-1}		308
3% Sodium chloride	513	513						5.0	1027
5% Sodium chloride	855	855						5.6	1710

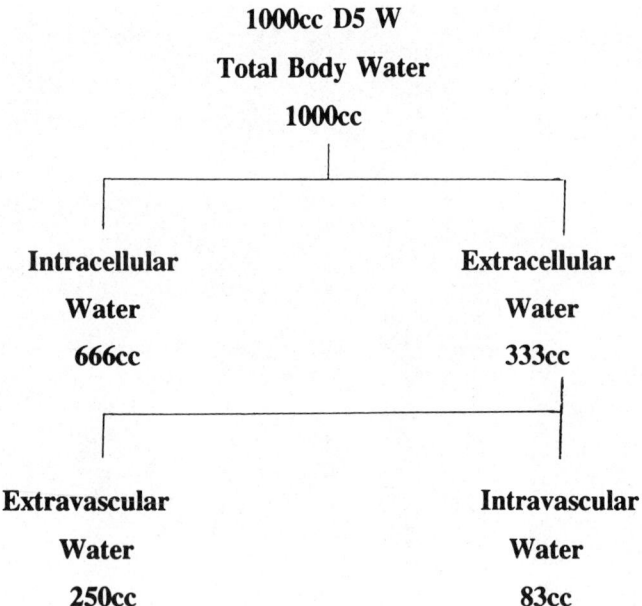

FIGURE 42–4. Distribution of 1 L of an administered solution of D₅W in an "ideal" 70-kg man (in cc).

lytes found in lactated Ringer's solution are not used as often intraoperatively.

How Are Crystalloids Distributed?

The distribution of water after the administration of D₅W, lactated Ringer's solution, hypertonic saline, and albumin is shown in Figures 42–4 to 42–7. Note that when an electrolyte-free solution such as D₅W is administered, less than 10% stays intravascular. A large amount of fluid, approximately two thirds, is distributed to the intracellular space. Thus, "intravascular resuscitation" is minimal, and cellular swelling occurs. The administered free water causes a decrease in the serum and interstitial electrolyte concentrations (dilutional effect) and may lead to symptomatic hyponatremia.

When solutions such as 0.2% or 0.45% saline are adminis-

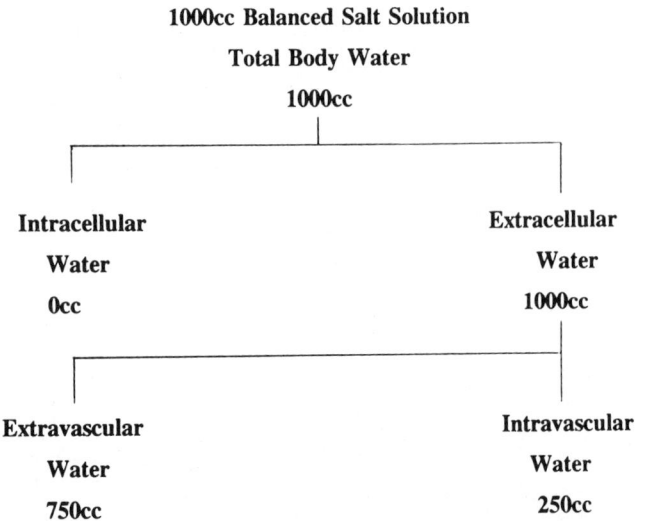

FIGURE 42–5. Distribution of 1 L of an administered balanced salt solution, such as lactated Ringer's solution or normal saline.

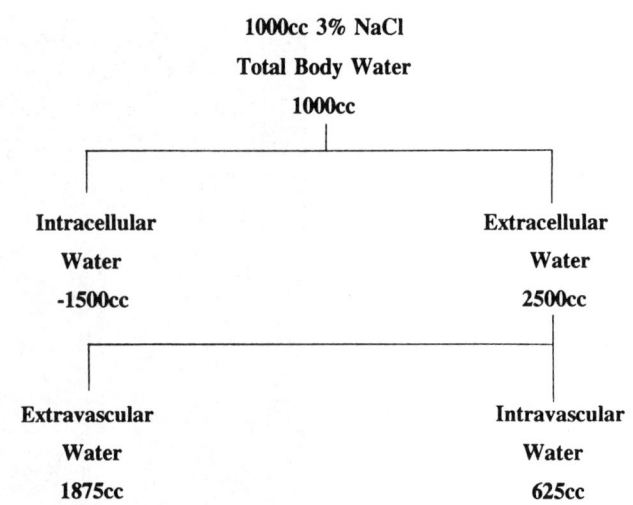

FIGURE 42–6. Distribution of 1 L of an administered solution of hypertonic saline (3% sodium chloride) in an "ideal" 70-kg man.

tered, similar although slightly less pronounced redistribution occurs. Therefore, a balanced salt solution with a sodium concentration of ≥130 mEq · L⁻¹ is normally chosen when major operative procedures are performed and when excessive blood loss is anticipated. Hypotonic solutions and D₅W should be restricted (if they are used at all) to very minor procedures and for pediatric surgery (see Chapters 60 and 61).

What Are Colloids?

Colloids commonly used in the United States include albumin, hydroxyethyl starch (HES; also known as *hetastarch* [Hespan]) and dextran. In Europe, gelatin derivatives are available as well. Colloid molecules are sufficiently large that they normally do not cross capillary membranes in significant numbers. Therefore, under normal conditions, most of an adminis-

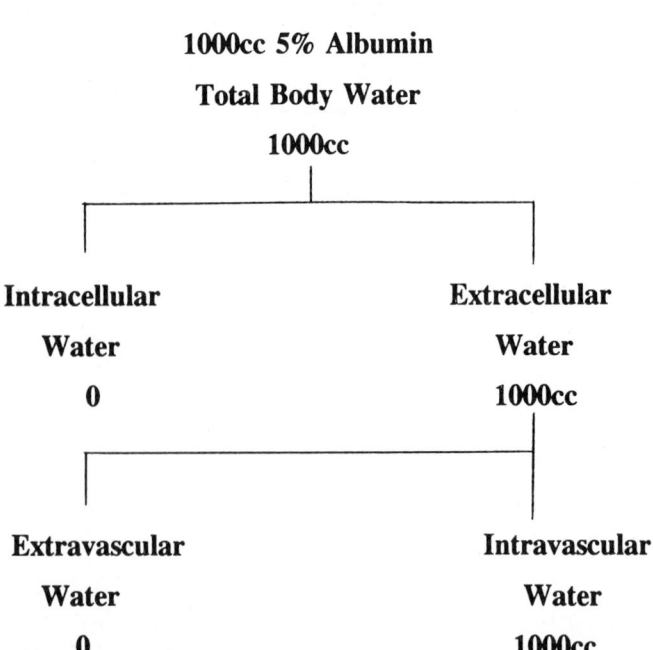

FIGURE 42–7. Distribution of 1 L of an administered 5% albumin solution in an "ideal" 70-kg man.

tered colloid remains intravascular (see Fig. 42–4). Distribution of fluid throughout the body is dependent on the forces represented in the Starling equation,

$$J_V = K[(P_{MV} - P_T) - \delta(COP_{MV} - COP_T)],$$

in which J_V represents the rate of filtration of fluid across the capillaries; K is the ultrafiltration coefficient (a measure of permeability); P_{MV} is the hydrostatic pressure within the microvasculature (i.e., the capillaries); P_T is the hydrostatic pressure in the interstitial space (the tissues); δ is the reflection coefficient and is a relative value expressing the ability of the semipermeable membrane to prevent movement of a given solute (in this case, the colloids of interest); COP_{MV} is the colloid oncotic pressure in the microvasculature; and COP_T is the colloid oncotic pressure in the tissue.

How Are Colloids Distributed?

For colloids "to work," δ must be very large (approaching 1.0), that is, the colloids must not cross the capillary membranes into the extravascular space. The value of δ varies greatly among tissues; for example, the lungs are moderately permeable ($\delta = 0.6$); muscle is moderately impermeable ($\delta = 0.9$); and the brain and glomeruli are essentially impermeable to protein entry ($\delta = 0.99$ and 1.0, respectively). The δ value for other tissues, such as liver, is very low ($\delta \approx 0$).[7]

Changes in Capillary Permeability

During trauma or sepsis, these δ values may change significantly. A classic example is the increase in capillary permeability to albumin in the lungs during the adult respiratory distress syndrome. In such a case, administered colloid may freely move across what ordinarily would be moderately permeable membranes in much the same fashion as does a balanced electrolyte solution. Increased capillary permeability (a "capillary leak") also occurs at the site of surgical trauma, and administered colloid moves out of the capillaries into the involved interstitium. In this setting, colloids are less effective than would otherwise be expected for intravascular expansion and may actually increase interstitial edema.

Oncotic Pressure Gradients

Once colloid molecules have leaked into the interstitial space, they must be removed or they will exert a reverse oncotic pressure gradient, resulting in further swelling of the involved tissue. Rarely, if ever, does a concentration gradient exist for colloid movement from the interstitial space back into the capillaries. Instead, it must be removed by the lymphatic system. Although many tissues, especially lung tissue, have a large capacity for lymphatic drainage, others, including skeletal muscle tissues, do not. Removal of colloid is much slower than that of crystalloids, and persistent edema, even to the point of blood flow interruption, sometimes results. This situation is particularly problematic in major trauma and burns.

Are Colloids or Crystalloids Preferable?

Few topics in anesthesia and surgery have generated as much controversy as the relative merits of colloids and crys-

talloids for intraoperative fluid replacement and resuscitation. Numerous animal and human studies have been undertaken to attempt to prove that one or the other is superior.[8–13] In many cases, the choice is based more on personal opinion and dogma rather than on scientific merit.

One noteworthy attempt to sort out this controversy was undertaken by Valanovich.[8] He performed a meta-analysis of mortality for eight previously published human trials in patients receiving either crystalloid or colloid for resuscitation. (A meta-analysis is a statistical technique that involves the combining of data from multiple studies in an attempt to increase the overall statistical power of the data.) These pooled data showed an overall 5.7% decrease in mortality in patients who were resuscitated with crystalloid rather than colloid solutions. When the data were divided into subgroups of trauma/sepsis and elective surgery, a 12.3% decrease in mortality in the former group was demonstrated. Conversely, a 7.8% increase in mortality was found in the crystalloid group undergoing elective surgical procedures (Fig. 42–8).

Valanovich believed that patients with trauma and sepsis have an increase in capillary permeability that allows the administered colloid to leak out of the vasculature, to be less effective as an intravascular volume expander, and to slow resolution of edema from the affected tissues (mentioned earlier). In patients undergoing elective procedures, the amount of capillary leak, in contradistinction to that in major trauma, is more discretely limited to the surgical site; thus, the use of colloids may be more efficacious in increasing intravascular volume. This study does not settle the controversy, but it does provide some insight into specific situations when one or the other may be preferable.

How Are Comparisons Made?

Most advocates of colloid use do not recommend colloid substances as the sole resuscitative fluid. The usual protocol involves the initial administration of crystalloids, followed by the administration of colloid solutions when large volumes are

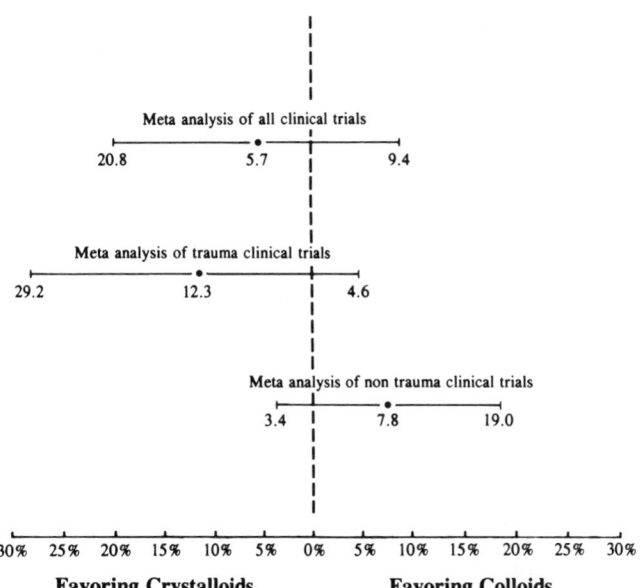

FIGURE 42–8. Meta-analysis of mortality rates for colloid versus crystalloid fluid resuscitation. (From Valanovich V: Crystalloid vs. colloid fluid resuscitation: a meta-analysis of mortality. Surg 1989; 105:70.)

necessary to reduce the amount of crystalloid. In general, crystalloid needs to be administered in volumes that are approximately 2 to 3 times that of colloid to obtain the same hemodynamic effect when iso-oncotic colloid solutions such as 5% albumin or HES are used. When more concentrated colloid solutions, such as 25% albumin, are used, this ratio is no longer valid.

Is the Role of Colloid Therapy Delineated?

The most comprehensive evaluation of colloid therapy was presented in a recent workshop on the assessment of plasma volume expander.[14] All of the pertinent clinical trials involving albumin, dextran, and HES were carefully evaluated in terms of efficacy, cost, indications for use, and complications. Very little evidence was found for either a short-term or long-term benefit from the use of supplemental colloidal agents in the clinical situations listed (blood loss, burns, cardiopulmonary bypass, pulmonary edema, trauma, and nutrition). No evidence suggested that serum albumin levels as low as 3.0 g · dL^{-1} were deleterious, and even values as low as 2.0 g · dL^{-1} have not been clearly shown to be problematic.

Pulmonary Edema

Of particular interest was the discussion relating pulmonary edema and the fact that administration of albumin in hypoalbuminemic patients, by abruptly increasing pulmonary artery perfusion pressure, may produce the very complication it is designed to prevent—interstitial and alveolar flooding.[14]

Renal Function

The workshop also emphasized the fact that raising the colloid oncotic pressure a remarkably small amount above normal significantly impairs renal salt and water excretion. No congenital hyperalbuminemic states are known, and the body reacts to transient elevations of albumin by immediately stopping production and accelerating catabolism. The adverse renal effects may be associated with the absence of naturally occurring states of excess albumin, whereas those in which albumin level is low are common. However, with one exception,[15] in which albumin supplementation of 900 g occurred over several days, no "toxic" effect of albumin therapy has been shown. The effects of colloidal products on bleeding and clotting have been mentioned and are discussed in detail later.

Costs

Cost is another consideration when considering the use of crystalloid and colloid solutions. Table 42–3 gives the approx-

TABLE 42–3. Approximate Hospital Cost of One Liter of Various Fluids*

Plasma-Lyte	$ 1.66
Lactated Ringer's solution	$ 0.80
Normal saline	$ 0.65
5% Albumin	$236.00
Hespan	$ 83.06
Dextran 70	$ 17.50
3% Sodium chloride	$ 1.40

*Prices as of January 1992 in Denver, CO.

imate *hospital* cost of the various crystalloid and colloid solutions. Note that balanced electrolyte solutions are inexpensive (a 1-L bag costs approximately $1.00). The cost of colloid solutions is as much as 200 times that for an equal volume of crystalloid solution or 50 to 100 times that for an "equipotent" volume of crystalloid solution. The cost to patients, of course, is much higher.

HYPERTONIC SOLUTIONS

What Are Hypertonic Saline Solutions?

Hypertonic saline solutions (sodium concentration greater than that found in normal saline) include 1.8%, 3%, 5%, 7.5%, and 10% sodium chloride solutions. Other anions such as lactate and acetate may be incorporated. They are sometimes mixed with colloids such as dextran.

How Are These Fluids Distributed?

Figure 42–6 shows what happens when 1 L of 3% sodium chloride solution is administered to a normal 70-kg adult. Because the osmolality of the administered solution exceeds that of intracellular water and because sodium and chloride ions cannot freely cross cell membranes, the extracellular fluid becomes slightly hyperosmolar. A gradient for water to pass from the cells into the extravascular compartment is established, and the extracellular volume is expanded by approximately 2.5 L.

Because electrolytes freely cross capillary membranes, the fluid is divided between the intravascular and extravascular compartments according to their relative volumes. Although hypertonic saline solutions increase the intravascular volume more than would the same volume of a balanced salt solution, they do so at the expense of a decreased intracellular volume. If large volumes of previously administered balanced electrolyte solutions have already increased intracellular volume (remember that most are, in effect, slightly hypotonic), hypertonic saline is therapeutic. If not, cellular dehydration can result.

What Are Potential Complications?

Hypertonic saline solution use is not widespread. However, there has been a resurgence of interest in these solutions for both intraoperative administration and trauma resuscitation.[16–19] A major concern is the potential development of hypernatremia. However, complications associated with hypernatremia have not been reported in the clinical trials. Hypernatremia, when it occurs, is usually transient, especially when these solutions are used with balanced electrolyte or colloid solutions.[16] A comprehensive review of many of the aspects of hypertonic saline solution has been published.[20]

What Other Hypertonic Solutions Are Useful?

Hyperosmotic solutions, such as 20% mannitol or urea, are used as osmotic diuretics and to reduce cerebral edema, most commonly during neurosurgical procedures. In the latter case, an osmotic gradient must be established between the intravascular and extravascular compartments. This goal is easily accomplished in the brain, where the normally functioning blood-brain barrier with its tight intercellular junctions excludes passive ion transport. However, in tissues such as muscle and lung that are more permeable, an effective gradient cannot be established or is only transient, and little or no edema fluid is removed.

BLOOD SUBSTITUTES

Discovery of the human immunodeficiency virus and recognition of transfusion complications have prompted the search for alternatives to blood administration. Oxygen-carrying solutions that can be stored without refrigeration for long periods of time and stocked in large amounts have been investigated. Such substances could be carried in ambulances and used for mass trauma resuscitation in times of war or civil disasters.

What Types Are Available?

Perfluorochemical Emulsions

Perfluorochemical emulsions have a linear oxygen-carrying capability as opposed to the sigmoid affinity of naturally occurring red blood cells.[21] Their oxygen-carrying capacity alone is insufficient to support cellular respiration at concentrations that can be tolerated in humans,[22-24] and they do not appear to be clinically useful at this time.

Stroma-Free Hemoglobin

The second class of red blood cell substitutes includes stroma-free hemoglobin solutions that are produced by processing human or animal red blood cells. Following polymerization of the hemoglobin molecules and addition of pyridoxal phosphate, a solution with a reasonable colloid oncotic pressure and an oxygen-carrying capacity that approximates that of normal hemoglobin is obtained. Initial clinical studies of stroma-free hemoglobin substances suggested a detrimental effect on renal function after their administration.[24, 25] Currently available stroma-free hemoglobin solutions are not approved for clinical use in the United States.

Synthetic Hemoglobin

Synthetic hemoglobin, manufactured using recombinant deoxyribonucleic acid (DNA) technology, is in beginning phase 1 of Food and Drug Administration trials. For an excellent review of red blood cell substitutes, the reader is referred to Gould and associates.[26]

INDICATIONS FOR GLUCOSE IN WATER

Routine fluid administration in the operating room frequently includes D_5W combined with a balanced electrolyte solution. The logic behind this approach is that patients usually are in nil per os (NPO) status for variable lengths of time prior

to arrival in the operating room and are thus prone to intraoperative hypoglycemia. However, many nondiabetic patients on entry to the operating room are actually hyperglycemic.[27] Addition of glucose to the intravenous (IV) infusions results in further hyperglycemia that may exceed the kidney's ability to reabsorb glucose, leading to a forced osmotic diuresis. Routine use of dextrose in IV solutions for nondiabetic adults is, therefore, discouraged.

How Should Diabetic Adults Be Managed?

Diabetic adults present special problems. The continuation of oral antihyperglycemic agents or insulin may cause significant hypoglycemia if glucose is not administered. Several approaches are commonly used in caring for these patients.

Non–Insulin-Dependent Diabetics

Oral hypoglycemic agents are discontinued at midnight the night before surgery. A nonglucose IV infusion is started, and blood sugar measurements are obtained on arrival to the hospital for outpatients or in the operating room for inpatients. Insulin (glucose >300 mg $\cdot$ dL^{-1}), IV glucose (glucose <100 mg $\cdot$ dL^{-1}), or both, are added based on the patient's serum glucose concentration.

For most patients maintained on an oral antihyperglycemic agent, this approach is simple and safe. However, some of the oral hyperglycemic agents have very long half-lives; therefore, patients who are scheduled for surgery late in the afternoon require periodic glucose monitoring throughout the day and need to be cautioned about the possibility of hypoglycemia.

Insulin-Dependent Diabetics

Management of insulin-dependent diabetics is more complicated. One standardized approach is to administer one half of their usual morning dose of regular insulin and to start an IV infusion of a glucose solution at either midnight the night before surgery or early in the day upon arrival in the hospital. Sequential monitoring of serum glucose follows, and the appropriate quantity of dextrose or insulin is added as needed. The limits of serum glucose fluctuation are broad; most recommendations suggest no treatment for serum glucose levels <200 to 300 mg $\cdot$ dL^{-1}.

Although this approach is simple, it does not provide tight glucose control. Outpatients scheduled for surgery late in the day may remain in NPO status for a prolonged period of time after taking insulin in the morning. This situation is especially problematic for particularly diabetic patients. Scheduling surgery early in the day for such patients is prudent.

Another approach is more complicated but provides for tighter blood glucose control. Patients are maintained in NPO status from midnight and do not take insulin in the morning. Two infusions, one containing dextrose and one containing insulin, are started, and frequent serum glucose determinations are made. The insulin infusion is adjusted to maintain euglycemia. This approach is preferred by some clinicians because of its ability to maintain very tight glucose control. However, because of the difficulty and labor intensiveness of the continuous glucose and insulin infusions, this technique is not very popular. Furthermore, tight glucose control has not been shown to be of benefit in the short-term operative management of most diabetics.[28]

Should Glucose Solutions Be Used in Children?

The management of glucose infusions in pediatric patients differs from that in adults in several ways. Very young children have limited glycogen stores and do not tolerate long periods with no oral intake. In these situations, the use of intravenous glucose, combined with a balanced salt solution, may be indicated.

D_5W often induces hyperglycemia.[27] Therefore, formula can be given by mouth until midnight, and clear glucose-containing solutions can be given orally until approximately 3 to 6 hours prior to surgery. In very young patients, a 2.5% glucose *maintenance* infusion should be provided. Glucose should *not* be included in the *replacement* balanced electrolyte solution, because large glucose loads may result from glucose-containing fluid boluses.[27]

ESTIMATION OF FLUID REQUIREMENTS

When considering patients undergoing surgery, it is helpful to divide fluid needs into several categories and, at least in theory, to deal with each category separately. Four areas of major concern are:

1. Preoperative fluid deficit
2. Intraoperative blood loss
3. "Third space" needs
4. Other (unusual) needs

In practice, a unified approach is necessary despite the need for individual considerations.

What Is the Preoperative Fluid Deficit?

Most patients scheduled for elective surgical procedures have a simple preoperative fluid deficit equal to the amount of fluid that would have been required during the NPO period. A simple approach is summarized in Figure 42–9. The hourly fluid requirement is calculated by taking the first 10 kg of the patient's weight and multiplying it by 4 mL · h⁻¹ times the number of hours; the second 10 kg of the patient's weight is

4 mL·kg⁻¹·h⁻¹ for the 1st 10 kg of weight
2 mL·kg⁻¹·h⁻¹ for the next 10 kg of weight
1 mL·kg⁻¹·h⁻¹ for all weight over 20 kg

Examples:

7-kg child   7 kg x 4 mL·kg⁻¹·h⁻¹ = 28 mL·h⁻¹

60-kg adult   10 kg x 4 mL·kg⁻¹·h⁻¹ = 40 mL·h⁻¹
                 10 kg x 2 mL·kg⁻¹·h⁻¹ = 20 mL·h⁻¹
                 (60 kg – 20 kg =) 40 kg x 1 mL·kg⁻¹·h⁻¹ = 40 mL·h⁻¹
                                                      100 mL·h⁻¹

FIGURE 42–9. A simple formula for calculating maintenance fluid requirements.

multiplied by 2 mL · h⁻¹ times the number of hours; and the remaining number of kilograms is multiplied by 1 mL · h⁻¹ times the number of hours.

Thus, a 7-kg child who was in NPO status for 6 hours would have a preoperative fluid deficit of 7 kg × 4 mL · h⁻¹ × 6 hours, or 168 mL. A 60-kg adult in NPO status for 8 hours would have a fluid requirement of 10 kg × 4 mL · h⁻¹ × 8 hours, plus 10 kg × 2 mL · h⁻¹ × 8 hours, plus 40 kg × 1 mL · h⁻¹ × 8 hours, or a total 800 mL deficit. Normally, one half of this preoperative fluid deficit is replaced during the first hour of surgery and the remainder over the next 2 hours.

Other preoperative deficits may result from chronic diuretic use, nasogastric suction, vomiting, diarrhea, bleeding, a bowel preparation, intravenous contrast agents, fever, or losses from gastrointestinal fistulas.

Clinical Evaluation

Because the deficit in each of these situations is different, no prediction can quantitate it precisely.

Urine Output

A workable estimate may be made using urine output as a guide. A urine volume <0.5 mL · kg⁻¹ · h⁻¹ suggests a significant deficit. An adult who has not voided in the preceding 6 to 8 hours often has a 1- to 3-L overall deficit. A urine specific gravity <1.020 indicates a normally hydrated patient, whereas specific gravities >1.030 to 1.040 suggest a 1- to 3-L deficit. Urine-specific gravity >1.040 indicates a severe dehydration fluid deficit in excess of 3 L.

Vital Signs

Pulse and blood pressure measurements with the patient lying supine provide useful information. If a >20% change in either parameter occurs when the patient stands, significant dehydration is indicated. However, the reliability of orthostatic changes is interfered with by many commonly used antihypertensive drugs (β-blockers or direct-acting vasodilators).

One useful piece of information obtained from continuous, direct blood pressure monitoring is the amount of change in the patient's blood pressure during the respiratory cycle. This phenomenon is often referred to as "cycling" or systolic pressure variation (Fig. 42–10).[29, 30] In patients who are hypovolemic, the decrease in venous return may be significant. A greater than 10-mm Hg reduction in systolic pressure associated with each mechanical breath is presumptive but indirect evidence of relative hypovolemia.

Physical Assessment

Other signs and symptoms are helpful. Dry mucous membranes and significant thirst indicate dehydration and may still be helpful in patients whose urine output or orthostatic changes are questionable. Patients with jugular venous distention probably are not significantly dehydrated, whereas those with flat jugular veins, especially when they are supine or in a slightly head down tilt, may be.

Invasive Monitoring

When all else fails, placement of a central venous or pulmonary artery catheter may be indicated to assess fluid status

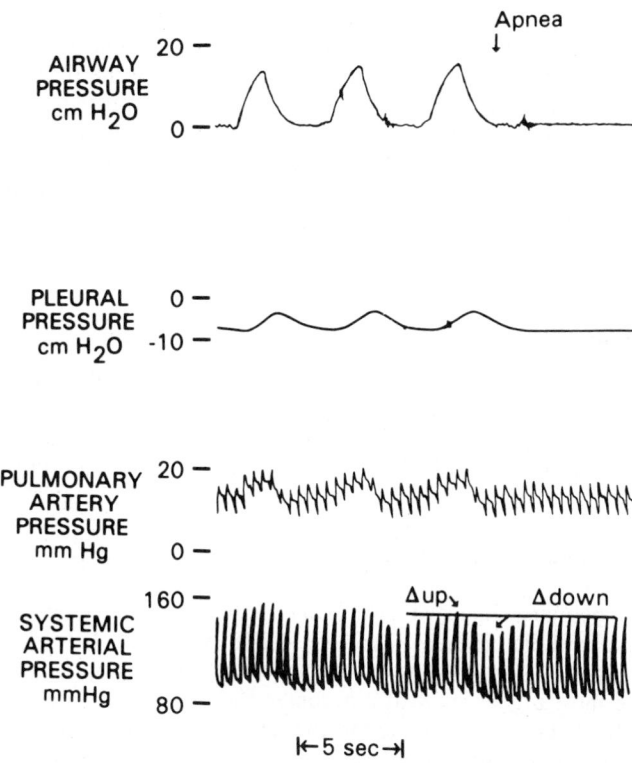

FIGURE 42–10. Variations in airway, pleural, pulmonary artery, and systemic pressures with positive-pressure ventilation following a 10% hemorrhage. (Reproduced with permission from Perel A, Pizov R, Cotev S: Systolic blood pressure variation is a sensitive indicator of hypovolemia in ventilated dogs subjected to graded hemorrhage. Anesthesiology 1987; 67:498.)

perioperatively. However, significantly fewer of such invasive devices should be used than are in reality, at least for this purpose.

Anesthetic Effects

Marked dehydration is associated with hypotension and hemodynamic instability. Young, healthy patients often compensate for hypovolemia while they are awake. However, most induction agents blunt these compensatory reflexes, predisposing patients to significant hypotension. The administration of 1 to 2 L of a balanced electrolyte solution often alleviates this problem.

How Should Intraoperative Blood Loss Be Replaced?

If significant amounts of blood are lost, the anesthesiologist has two choices. The first is to administer fresh or stored autologous or homologous blood in the form of reconstituted packed red blood cells. The second is to eschew the use of blood and to give instead crystalloid solutions, colloid solutions, or both.

With colloid solutions, an equal volume of an iso-oncotic solution, such as 5% albumin or HES, is indicated. If a balanced electrolyte solution is utilized, a volume at least equal to three times that of the lost blood is necessary to maintain a euvolemic state. In general, blood loss should be replaced by such solutions as it occurs.

When Are Third Space Fluid Losses Replaced?

During major surgical procedures, a large third space fluid loss occurs that, as was noted, is not anatomic in the usual sense. Replacement of this loss necessitates administration of a fluid with an electrolyte profile similar to that of plasma and interstitial fluid. The protein concentration in third space fluid is variable and usually unknown but is probably less than that of plasma. The volume of fluid required to replace such losses varies considerably.[31]

Calculations

Most clinicians recommend various replacement formulas based on the perceived degree of trauma of the surgery. For surgical procedures associated with minimal trauma (e.g., herniorrhaphies or superficial procedures), administration of 1 to 3 $mL \cdot kg^{-1} \cdot h^{-1}$, in addition to the amount given to satisfy the maintenance requirement and the accumulated fluid deficit, should be sufficient.

For those operations involving moderate trauma (e.g., open cholecystectomy), administration of approximately 4 to 6 $mL \cdot kg^{-1} \cdot h^{-1}$ is appropriate. For extensive and traumatic procedures (e.g., radical intraperitoneal resections, or in the presence of severe peritonitis), infusion rates of 7 to 9 $mL \cdot kg^{-1} \cdot h^{-1}$ or greater are necessary.

These recommendations represent an initial estimate of third space losses. Patients must be carefully monitored, and the rate of replacement must be adjusted up or down based on their clinical response (see later).

What Other Fluid Losses Occur?

During surgery, exposure of peritoneal or pleural surfaces to the operating room environment predisposes the patient to major evaporative loss. Anesthetic gases are anhydrous, and respiratory water loss will occur unless adequate humidification is provided.

Patients treated with diuretics, acutely or chronically, may have continued urinary losses that must be replaced with appropriate fluids. Intravenous contrast agents, mannitol, and large glucose loads often induce an osmotic diuresis, even in the presence of relative hypovolemia, thus further increasing the fluid requirements.

PERIOPERATIVE ELECTROLYTE AND GLUCOSE MANAGEMENT

What Are Common Sodium Disorders?

Sodium is the predominant extracellular cation (see Table 42–1). Total body sodium content is approximately 5000 mEq. The average daily requirement for sodium is 1 to 2 $mEq \cdot kg^{-1}$. However, the kidneys can compensate for a very wide range of intake, from approximately 0.25 $mEq \cdot kg^{-1} \cdot d^{-1}$ to more than 6 $mEq \cdot kg^{-1} \cdot d^{-1}$.

Sodium is also one of the major cations involved in intravascular volume regulation. Disorders in sodium concentration often reflect disorders of intravascular volume status more than actual changes in total body sodium. Normally, the intake of

TABLE 42–4. Causes of Hypernatremia

Excess Free Water Loss
  Sweating
  Respiratory losses (nonhumidified gases)
  Fever
  Diarrhea
  Vomiting
  Gastrointestinal fistula losses
  Renal losses
    Diabetes insipidus (nephrogenic or decreased vasopressin production)

Inadequate Water Intake
  Inability to drink (mental status or NPO status changes)
  Environmental (no access to water)

Excess Sodium (Rare)
  Increased salt intake
  Iatrogenic (hypertonic saline or bicarbonate)

Decreased Renal Excretion
  Renal failure

sodium via the diet is adequate to meet the body's needs. Therefore, the kidneys regulate sodium concentration in relation to water balance.

Sodium and its accompanying cations account for about 93% of serum osmolality, which may be approximated by the following formula:

$$\text{Osmolality (mOsm} \cdot \text{kg}^{-1} \text{ H}_2\text{O}) = 2 \times [\text{Na}^+] + [\text{glucose}]/18 + [\text{BUN}]/28,$$

in which BUN is blood urea nitrogen.

Hypernatremia

Patients with hypernatremia present a wide range of signs and symptoms, including mental status changes, increased thirst, peripheral edema, myoclonus, and possibly cardiovascular decompensation. Most commonly, hypernatremia is caused by excess renal excretion of free water or extrarenal free water losses such as sweating, diarrhea, fever, and increased respiratory evaporation (Table 42–4).

Treatment

In the patient with hypernatremia, hypotonic fluids (e.g., 0.45–0.20% saline), administered at a rate sufficient to reduce serum Na$^+$ concentration by approximately 2 mEq · h^{-1}, will restore volume and electrolyte status to normal. In case of excess total body sodium, as might be seen following the administration of large amounts of sodium bicarbonate or hypertonic saline solutions, administration of a loop diuretic such as furosemide and fluid replacement with hypotonic solutions will restore equilibrium.

Hyponatremia

Hyponatremia is more often caused by a water excess than a sodium deficit. Common causes include renal failure, congestive heart failure, and replacement of fluid losses (vomiting or diarrhea) with sodium-deficient solutions (Table 42–5). Patients with the syndrome of inappropriate antidiuretic hormone have inappropriate water retention, a decrease in serum osmolality, and an increase in urine osmolality.

When evaluating patients with hyponatremia, one must be certain to exclude possible laboratory error. Laboratories calculate the sodium concentration based on the total volume of plasma rather than on the volume of water in the plasma. In patients with extreme hyperlipidemia, hyperproteinemia, or hyperosmolarity (hyperglycemia or mannitol intoxication), a significant portion of the plasma is occupied by these interfering substances so that the *measured* sodium concentration is much lower than the *effective* sodium concentration.[32]

Treatment

In patients with mild hyponatremia (an absolute serum sodium level greater than approximately 125 mEq · L^{-1}, and normal mental status), treatment is usually conservative. Evaluation of the patient's volume status and restriction of fluid intake suffice. If patients are significantly hypervolemic, diuretic use may be indicated. Sodium intake can be increased by administering isotonic or slightly hypertonic fluids.

The management of severe, *acute,* symptomatic hyponatremia is much different. Absolute sodium values <110 to 120 mEq · L^{-1} may represent a true medical emergency. All but the most urgent surgical procedures should be cancelled, the patient should be admitted to the intensive care unit, and the hyponatremia should be corrected in a very careful and controlled manner.

Debate regarding the speed of correction is widespread.[33-39] An increase in sodium level to 120 to 125 mEq · L^{-1} can proceed relatively rapidly (1–2 mEq · L^{-1} · h^{-1}) in cases of acute hyponatremia, followed by a slower increase into the low normal range. Normal or hypertonic saline is used while intravascular volume status is carefully monitored. Diuretics are useful to increase the excretion of free water.

Rapid correction of severe hyponatremia is believed by some to predispose the patient to central pontine myelinolysis, a myelin degenerative disease that is associated with paraparesis or quadriparesis. A cause-effect relationship, however, is not well established. Nevertheless, a 1992 paper by Sterns[39] suggests that rapid correction of even severe *chronic* hyponatremia (serum sodium as low as 98 mEq · L^{-1}) is seldom, if ever, indicated and may lead to an osmotic demyelination syndrome. In such cases, he recommends correction by no more than 0.5 mEq · L^{-1} · h^{-1}.

TABLE 42–5. Causes of Hyponatremia

Free Water Excess
  Congestive heart failure
  Hepatic failure
  Renal failure
  Excessive ADH (vasopressin)
    Pain, blood loss, dehydration, hypotension
  Syndrome of inappropriate antidiuretic hormone (SIADH)
  Replacement of fluid losses (e.g., sweating, vomiting, diarrhea) with hypotonic fluid (e.g., beer, soda, tea, plain water)
  Inappropriate IV fluids
  Psychogenic water drinkers
  Syndrome of transurethral resection of the prostate (TURP syndrome)

Sodium Deficit
  Renal losses (e.g., with use of diuretics)
  Excessive losses (e.g., sweating, vomiting, diarrhea)
  Inadequate intake
  Inappropriate IV fluids

What Are Common Potassium Disorders?

Total body potassium averages 3500 mEq, most of which is intracellular (see Table 42–1). Therefore, measurements of serum potassium concentration represent a very small fraction of total body potassium. However, potassium equilibrium is important in the maintenance of cell membrane potentials, particularly in excitable cells such as those of the myocardium.

Normal regulation of potassium concentration occurs in the kidneys, which can alter urinary potassium from less than 5 to more than 100 mEq $\cdot$ L^{-1} under the influence of aldosterone. As is to be expected, most abnormalities of potassium concentration occur when the kidneys' ability to regulate potassium is compromised by renal failure or by the administration of diuretics. Other nonrenal losses include excessive sweating and diarrhea.

Hyperkalemia

Hyperkalemia can be life threatening. Common causes are listed in Table 42–6. Hemolysis of red blood cells in a laboratory specimen may cause an artifactually high reported serum potassium concentration (see Table 42–6). Thus, a patient's clinical status must be correlated with the laboratory value. In patients with chronic renal failure, a potassium concentration of 5.0 to 6.0 mEq $\cdot$ L^{-1} may have few physiologic effects. The same level of potassium in patients who are not chronically exposed to such high levels may cause dysrhythmias.

The most sensitive indicator of hyperkalemia is the electrocardiogram (ECG). Peaked T waves are often followed by a prolonged PR interval and absent P waves. In severe hyperkalemia, a widened QRS complex precedes a sine wave pattern, ventricular tachycardia, and ventricular fibrillation.

Treatment

Initial treatment includes alkalization with sodium bicarbonate and hyperventilation, which induces an extracellular-to-intracellular potassium shift. Calcium chloride should be administered under ECG guidance to counteract the cellular membrane effects of hyperkalemia. Glucose (25 g) and regular insulin (10 USP units) also promote an intracellular potassium shift.

TABLE 42–6. Common Causes of Hyperkalemia

"False" Cases
   Hemolysis of blood sample

Inadequate Excretion
   Renal failure
   Potassium-sparing diuretics
   Angiotensin-converting enzyme (ACE) inhibitors

Excessive Intake
   Salt substitutes
   IV administration
   Rapid, massive blood transfusion

Extracellular Redistribution
   Acidosis
   Hemolysis
   Cellular destruction (electrical burns, rhabdomyolysis)
   Succinylcholine
   β-Blockers

TABLE 42–7. Common Causes of Hypokalemia

Increased Losses
   Diuretics
   Vomiting
   Sweating
   Diarrhea, bowel preparation, enemas
   Magnesium deficiency
   Alcoholism
   Amphotericin B therapy

Redistribution
   Alkalosis (metabolic or hyperventilation)
   Insulin activity
   Glycogen

Inadequate Intake
   Iatrogenic (chronic IV fluids with no K^{+})
   Inadequate postoperative intake (rare)

None of these measures decrease total body potassium content. A potassium-binding resin, diuretics, or dialysis must be utilized for this purpose. However, these approaches are much slower than the acute interventions that are necessary in an emergent situation. Succinylcholine should be avoided in patients with pre-existing, significant hyperkalemia (>5.5 mEq $\cdot$ L^{-1}).

Hypokalemia

Hypokalemia frequently is a iatrogenic problem (Table 42–7) most commonly caused by the chronic use of diuretics with inadequate potassium replacement. Patients with chronic hypokalemia often have significant total body potassium depletion. The initial volume of distribution of intravenously administered potassium, however, is the extracellular volume. Therefore, correction of large potassium deficits must take place over several days to avoid acute hyperkalemia.

Delay of Elective Surgery

A few years ago, patients with potassium levels of 3.0 to 3.5 mEq $\cdot$ L^{-1} would have their operations cancelled and their potassium levels corrected to the normal range because of the perceived risk of increased intraoperative dysrhythmias. However, studies from the mid- and late 1980s[40, 41] indicate that chronic hypokalemia as low as 2.5 to 3.0 mEq $\cdot$ L^{-1}, if without side effects, is not associated with increased risk. Current recommendations suggest that patients receiving diuretic therapy have their potassium levels checked on the day before surgery.

Intraoperatively, hypokalemia may be exacerbated by hyperventilation-induced respiratory alkalosis. This situation represents an intracellular shift of potassium and should not be corrected with potassium administration. Instead, ventilation should be adjusted to a normal value, using arterial pH as the primary guideline.

Treatment

In patients with severe hypokalemia, an associated magnesium deficiency can be inferred. These patients may receive very large amounts of supplemental potassium with limited increase of the serum level. Administration of supplemental magnesium sulfate usually corrects the deficit.

The link between potassium and magnesium movements is

unclear, but cellular levels tend to rise and fall together during periods of a deficiency in either. It may be that magnesium deficiency prevents cells from establishing a normal transcellular gradient for potassium. Magnesium deficiency perhaps selectively affects membrane-bound magnesium, which, in turn, regulates permeability to potassium. In hypokalemia, replacement of magnesium, even in the absence of potassium replacement, often corrects the deficiency.

Because potassium is irritating to peripheral vessels, it normally should be administered through a central vein unless it is diluted. In adults, up to 40 mEq of potassium chloride diluted in a volume of 100 mL or greater is given over approximately 1 hour when rapid correction is deemed necessary. A very dilute solution (e.g., $40 \text{ mEq} \cdot \text{L}^{-1}$) can be administered peripherally. The rate of potassium administration to pediatric patients should not exceed $0.5 \text{ mEq} \cdot \text{kg}^{-1} \cdot \text{h}^{-1}$ and should be followed by continuous ECG monitoring.

What Are Common Chloride Disorders?

Chloride is the major extracellular anion. Its chief importance is in acid-base regulation. Primary disorders of chloride without associated acid-base disorders are unusual. Hyperchloremia is commonly associated with metabolic (nonrespiratory) acidosis, and hypochloremia is associated with metabolic alkalosis.

Hyperchloremia

Hyperchloremic metabolic acidosis often is seen in conjunction with renal tubular acidosis or as a result of the administration of excessive amounts of chloride. Therapy for renal tubular acidosis consists of evaluation of the underlying acid-base disorder and of the avoidance of solutions containing excessive chloride.

Treatment

Substitution of phosphate, bicarbonate, or acetate for chloride as the major anions usually should be made in hyperalimentation fluids or other chronically administered solutions. In the operating room, the major concern is the potential hyperchloremic acidosis and whether it should be corrected with sodium bicarbonate.

Hypochloremia

Hypochloremia and its associated alkalosis result from excessive loss of chloride following diuretic administration and nasogastric suction. It is seen frequently in patients with pyloric stenosis and small bowel or gastric outlet obstruction. It may also follow the administration of large-volume blood transfusions. The associated metabolic alkalosis can present significant problems when one attempts to wean patients from mechanical ventilation. Such individuals often hypoventilate as a compensatory response to the metabolic alkalosis.

Treatment

Administration of an appropriate volume of saline and potassium or ammonium chloride usually corrects hypochloremia. At one time, dilute hydrochloric acid (0.1 N) was infused

slowly through a central vein but is seldom used now. Acetazolamide (Diamox), a carbonic anhydrase inhibitor, can be given in a dose of 250 to 500 mg that is repeated once or twice at 4-hour intervals. This treatment corrects the alkalosis but not the hypochloremia.

As long as the patient's acid-base status is acceptable, surgery need not be postponed because of moderate degrees of hyperchloremia or hypochloremia. However, a work-up for the basis of the disorder should be undertaken.

What Are Common Calcium Disorders?

Ninety-nine per cent of the body's calcium is contained in bone and is not immediately available to the circulation. Calcium's major function is the maintenance of cell membrane integrity, membrane excitability, and excitation-contraction coupling. It is also involved in the coagulation cascade. Calcium is highly protein bound; therefore, ionized calcium, which can be measured with ion-specific electrodes, is a more reliable indicator of activity than is the total serum calcium level.

Calcium binding is decreased by acidosis and increased by alkalosis. Normal calcium metabolism is under the control of parathyroid hormone and vitamin D. Fluid resuscitation in patients in shock tends to lower total and ionized calcium concentrations. Infused albumin, with its calcium-binding sites, and transfusion of large amounts of citrate-containing banked blood also decrease the level of ionized calcium.

Hypercalcemia

Hypercalcemia is associated with a variety of conditions (Table 42–8). The primary signs are mental status changes, weakness, and renal failure.

Treatment

Treatment must be directed at the underlying condition; otherwise, it is relatively ineffective. Diuresis and administration of large volumes of normal saline are the mainstays of supportive therapy. Patients with symptomatic hypercalcemia should have elective surgery postponed until the underlying condition can be evaluated and treated. Those with mild hy-

TABLE 42–8. Causes of Hypercalcemia

Redistribution
  Osteolysis
    Malignancy
    Sarcoidosis
    Tuberculosis
    Vitamin D excess
    Parathyroid hormone excess (often seen with renal failure)
  Immobilization
  Adrenal insufficiency
  Hypophosphatemia

Excess Intake
  Vitamin D intoxication
  Milk-alkali syndrome
  Iatrogenic

Decreased Excretion
  Parathyroid hormone excess
  Renal failure

percalcemia and no symptoms may undergo surgical procedures, but ionized calcium level should be sequentially determined.

Hypocalcemia

Hypocalcemia (Table 42–9) is much more common in the operating room than is hypercalcemia. The major signs and symptoms relate to the irritability of electrically active cells and include mental status changes, tetany, Chvostek's and Trousseau's signs, and dysrhythmias. Abnormal excitation-contraction coupling, manifested by a prolonged QT interval on the ECG, depressed myocardial contractility, and associated hypotension may result.

In the operating room, rapid infusion of citrated blood (usually in excess of 1.5 mL $\cdot$ kg^{-1} $\cdot$ min^{-1}) or albumin, coupled with acute hyperventilation are the most common acute causes of symptomatic hypocalcemia.

Treatment

Treatment with intravenous calcium chloride (15 mg $\cdot$ kg^{-1}), through a central venous catheter, or with calcium gluconate (45 mg $\cdot$ kg^{-1}), via a peripheral or central venous catheter, should be accompanied by careful and continuous ECG monitoring. Note that except in cases of documented hypocalcemia, recommendations for calcium salts during resuscitation from cardiac arrest have been virtually eliminated.[42]

What Are Magnesium Disorders?

Magnesium is a predominantly intracellular cation that is involved in membrane excitability as well as in the regulation of potassium concentration. Magnesium supplementation in the acute setting is indicated for dysrhythmias associated with hypomagnesemia or hypokalemia, with uncorrectable hypokalemia, or with pre-eclampsia or eclampsia.

Rapid administration of magnesium may cause symptomatic hypotension. High magnesium levels are associated with muscle weakness and potentiate neuromuscular blocking agents. Patients receiving chronic diuretic therapy are sometimes severely magnesium-depleted. Hypermagnesemia is usually iatrogenically induced and is associated with the treatment of pre-eclampsia or eclampsia.

TABLE 42–9. Common Causes of Hypocalcemia

Redistribution
Alkalosis
Citrate (banked blood) infusion
Rapid albumin infusion
Phosphate infusion
Sepsis
Hemodialysis
Pancreatitis
Hypomagnesemia

Inadequate Intake or Inability to Mobilize from Bone
Vitamin D deficiency
Parathyroid hormone deficiency
Inadequate diet (rare)

What Are Phosphate Disorders?

Eighty-five per cent of the body's phosphate is contained in bone. The remaining 15% is involved in energy flux (adenosine triphosphate) and in the production of nucleic acids and proteins. Hyperphosphatemia may induce hypocalcemia through calcium binding.

Significant phosphate abnormalities are uncommon in the operating room. When seen, they are usually associated with chronic malnutrition or iatrogenic complications of hyperalimentation. Intravenous phosphate is infused slowly to avoid vascular tissue calcification or acute hypocalcemia.

What Are Common Glucose Disorders?

Although glucose is not an electrolyte, disorders of glucose concentration can severely affect the perioperative fluid status. The most common cause for alterations in glucose status is diabetes mellitus. However, acute alterations in serum glucose level can result from fluid and electrolyte therapy as well.

Hyperglycemia

Hyperglycemia is more common in the operating room than is hypoglycemia and usually follows the administration of large amounts of glucose in intravenous fluids. The stress response to surgery also increases serum glucose concentration. Transient, moderate hyperglycemia is less dangerous than hypoglycemia. However, glucose in excess of approximately 300 mg $\cdot$ dL^{-1} places patients at increased risk of osmotic diuresis and of a worsened neurologic outcome after an anoxic or ischemic event (see Chapter 73).

Treatment

Because of unpredictable skin perfusion, the administration of subcutaneous insulin to control hyperglycemia is not recommended in the operating room. Small intermittent doses of intravenous regular insulin or a continuous insulin infusion should be used instead.

Hypoglycemia

Hypoglycemia in normal adults, even after prolonged periods with no oral glucose intake, is uncommon. Exceptions include patients with severe liver disease, those undergoing major hepatic resections, and neonates, all of whom frequently are depleted of glycogen stores and therefore prone to hypoglycemia.

Diabetics who have received long-acting (neutral protamine Hagedorn [NPH]) insulin or oral antihyperglycemic agents are also at risk for significant intraoperative hypoglycemia. General anesthesia masks the usual clinical signs and symptoms of hypoglycemia but does not protect the central nervous system and other organ systems from its effects. Patients at increased risk for hypoglycemia should have frequent monitoring of their blood glucose levels.

FLUID THERAPY AND COAGULATION

How Do Colloids Affect Hemostasis?

Patients who undergo surgery with significant blood loss often have problems with coagulation. However, not all coagulation deficits seen in surgical patients can be related to the use of blood. Colloid solutions have been reported to be responsible in many settings. These deficits are in addition to those expected purely from the dilution associated with large-volume resuscitation.

Albumin

Johnson and coworkers[46] treated severely injured patients with a standardized resuscitation protocol. Approximately one half of the patients received $150 \ g \cdot d^{-1}$ of additional albumin for 3 to 5 days. The patients given supplemental albumin required greater volumes of whole blood and fresh frozen plasma to obtain normal clotting studies than did those who were resuscitated with crystalloid solutions. Albumin-treated patients had a significant decrease in fibrinogen concentration and prolongation of the prothrombin time that could not be explained by dilution. In contrast, the prolonged thromboplastin time and decreased platelet counts that also occurred in the albumin-treated group were ascribed to dilution.

The amount of albumin administered in this study was much greater than that usually given in clinical settings. Other investigators, using smaller doses of albumin, reported clotting abnormalities that could be explained solely on the basis of dilution.[45] In addition, in vitro studies found that albumin did not adversely influence clotting nor did it affect the structure of fibrin clots.[47]

Overall, albumin may exert some mild effects on hemostasis; however, these effects seem to be primarily dilutional as a result of volume expansion. When large amounts of albumin are infused, the degree of volume expansion exceeds that obtained with a comparable amount of crystalloid solutions. Therefore, a more pronounced coagulation defect is likely.

Dextran

Dextran is used not only for volume expansion but as a form of antiaggregant in patients undergoing vascular and microvascular surgical procedures. Clotting deficits associated with dextran probably are related to defects in platelet interaction and to an antithrombotic effect. The platelet-vascular interaction is believed to be primarily associated with an effect on factor VIII.[48–50] Dextran also seems to be incorporated into the polymerizing fibrin clot so that it alters clot structure and enhances fibrinogenolysis.[51–54]

Types

Dextran is commonly supplied in two forms, dextran 70 and dextran 40. The numbers 70 and 40 refer to the average molecular weights (70,000 and 40,000, respectively) of the molecules in solution. Dextran 40 appears to have greater inhibitory effects on coagulation than does Dextran 70. It is used in vascular surgery to prevent thrombosis but is rarely employed as a primary volume expander. Dextran 70, on the other hand, is used as a primary volume expander, alone or in combination with hypertonic saline.

Hydroxyethyl Starch

HES is derived from carbohydrate (usually corn). It is available in the United States as a 6% solution in 0.9% sodium chloride (Hespan).

Clotting Factors

The effects of HES have been studied in two major groups of patients. The first group consists of healthy patients undergoing leukopheresis for donation of white blood cells. These patients usually receive small amounts (approximately 500 mL) of HES. In one study, 10 donors who received HES during leukopheresis had slight but significant prolongation of their prothrombin time and prolonged thromboplastin time (mean increases of 0.6 and 2.5 seconds, respectively).[43] Levels of fibrinogen, factor VIII:C, and factor V were similarly reduced but remained within the normal range. In another report, no defects in platelet function were noted.[44]

The second group of patients includes those who receive larger doses of HES for trauma and surgery. In these patients, a prolonged partial thromboplastin time and up to a 50% decrease in factor VIII:C occurs with an infusion of 1 L HES.[45]

Clot Formation

In addition to its effect on levels of factor VIII, HES appears to cause changes in fibrin clot formation and fibrinogenolysis. This characteristic may be related to incorporation of the HES molecules into the clot with subsequent prevention of solid clot formation.

Pentastarch

Pentastarch is a new lower molecular weight version of HES that has fewer hydroxyethyl groups per molecule. It is unavailable for volume expansion in the United States but is undergoing clinical trials. It is available in Europe. The anticoagulant effects of pentastarch seem to be similar in type and magnitude to those observed with HES.

Summary

All of the synthetic colloids have some adverse effects on clotting, especially when administered in large quantities. Albumin seems to have a purely dilutional effect that is less than that of any of the synthetic agents. If the latter are to be used for volume expansion, one of the HESs is recommended in a maximum volume between 1 and $1.5 \ L \cdot ^{-1}$. If additional colloid is desired, a switch to albumin is probably indicated.

The synthetic colloids are relatively contraindicated in patients in whom small amounts of bleeding would be potentially devastating (e.g., neurosurgical patients). Dextran 40 is not commonly used for volume expansion but may be used for its anticoagulant effects in vascular surgery patients and other patients prone to thrombosis.

COMPLICATIONS OF FLUID THERAPY

Why Do Electrolyte Changes Occur?

When balanced electrolyte solutions are administered, minimal electrolyte changes should occur because the composition of the fluids approximates that of normal plasma (see Tables 42–1 and 42–2). However, when solutions that contain non-balanced electrolytes are used (0.25%, 0.5%, or 0.9% saline, hypertonic saline, or colloid), significant changes can occur. All products that are suspended in 0.9% saline (albumin and synthetic colloids) have a chloride composition higher than that of normal plasma (see Table 42–2). Patients who are given large volumes of these solutions often develop a transient hyperchloremic acidosis that, although usually mild, may worsen other acidotic conditions (see Chapter 43).

Should Hypotonic Solutions Be Used?

If hypotonic solutions such as 0.45% or 0.2% saline or D_5W are used, patients can develop significant hyponatremia and hyposmolar states. Although isosmotic when administered, D_5W provides a large free water excess as the glucose is metabolized. These complications are much more common and severe than is the transient hyperchloremia associated with normal saline. As noted previously, hypotonic solutions are not recommended for major surgical procedures. They are acceptable for minor surgery with minimal fluid shifts.

Should Glucose Solutions Be Used?

Glucose-containing solutions can produce hyperglycemia with resultant electrolyte abnormalities. Hyperglycemia, if untreated, may lead to a hyperosmolar state in susceptible patients. In addition, it promotes an osmotic diuresis. Because of these problems, routine use of glucose-containing solutions during major surgery in adults, as has been noted repeatedly throughout this chapter, is not recommended.

Why Does Renal Failure Occur?

Physiologic responses "attempt" to correct hypovolemia. The kidney is one of the major organs that is affected. If patients are inadequately volume-resuscitated in the operating room, urine output will fall. Significant hypotension for as little as 10 minutes has resulted in acute renal failure.[55]

Mortality associated with acute postoperative renal failure, even with dialysis, is high. The cornerstone of prevention is to provide adequate fluid replacement in patients undergoing surgical procedures. There are many therapeutic interventions for fluid overload and congestive heart failure but relatively few for renal insufficiency. When in doubt, one should err on the side of too much fluid rather than too little. Both the type and volume of fluid are important. As long as patients produce at least 0.5 to 1 $mL \cdot kg^{-1} \cdot h^{-1}$ of urine, renal function, although not optimal, is generally preserved.

When Is Congestive Heart Failure Likely?

Healthy patients can receive large volumes of fluid with no change in cardiac function. However, elderly patients and patients with underlying cardiac disease may suffer significant cardiac complications from even moderate amounts of fluid. Because these patients have limited cardiac reserve, increasing their intravascular volume may overdistend the heart, or the heart may not be able to compensate for the increased volume, leading to congestive heart failure. In addition, these patients have difficulty in the postoperative mobilization phase of edema and other third space fluids.

Advocates of colloid therapy suggest that because the total volume of fluid administered is lower than that with crystalloid resuscitation, less stress is placed on a compromised heart. However, no good experimental studies back up this claim, and the problems encountered with such therapy have been discussed.

Which Factors Lead to Pulmonary Dysfunction?

Pulmonary dysfunction after large volume resuscitation is multifactorial. Fluid overload and an increase in pulmonary capillary permeability (sepsis, anaphylaxis, or other inflammatory reactions) place patients at much greater risk for this phenomenon. Those with limited myocardial reserve or impaired renal function also are at increased risk.[14, 15]

Is Peripheral Edema a Problem?

Massive peripheral edema sometimes accompanies large-volume fluid resuscitation, particularly following trauma and burns. It represents a classic example of third space loss. A frequently posed question is whether this edema is detrimental. It is certainly cosmetically unappealing, but the medical implications are unclear. A major consideration involves wound healing and burn conversion. If edema is significant, the distance between capillaries and cells increases, and cellular hypoxia is a distinct possibility.

Another potential but fortunately uncommon complication is the development of a compartment syndrome. When edema in a closed space such as an extremity increases sufficiently, interstitial pressure rises; this pressure eventually exceeds the venous pressure, at which time ischemia will follow. This problem occurs in circumferential burns and extremity trauma.

How Is Hypothermia Produced?

Fluids stored at "room temperature" are actually cool compared with body temperature. One liter of room-temperature fluid decreases a 70-kg patient's body temperature by about 0.2%. Even if warmed prior to infusion, these fluids may undergo significant cooling while passing through the IV tubing.

Cold fluids such as stored blood can induce hypothermia when infused rapidly. Therefore, large volume infusions should be passed through fluid warming devices. However, it should be remembered that although important, warming of fluids is a relatively inefficient means to prevent, and especially to treat, hypothermia (see Chapter 49).

TRANSURETHRAL RESECTION OF THE PROSTATE

What Problems Arise?

Transurethral resection of the prostate (TURP) entails the infusion of large volumes of electrolyte-free irrigation fluid through the surgical resectoscope to provide a clear field of view for the surgeon. Multiple prostatic sinuses are opened, and significant volumes of this irrigation fluid, up to 20 to 30 mL · min^{-1}, are absorbed into the circulation. Patients can develop severe hyponatremia, hypotonicity, and hypervolemia.[56] In addition, if glycine is used in the irrigating solution, glycine intoxication, which presents as transient blindness, may result (see Chapter 70).

Presentation

Major aberrations in the so-called "TURP syndrome" involve mental status changes, which result from hyponatremia, and congestive heart failure, which results from fluid overload. This syndrome usually occurs only after large or prolonged (>30–45 minutes) prostatic resections. Spinal anesthetics for TURP are recommended, in part so that mental status can be assessed. Sequential measurement of serum sodium is indicated in longer procedures.

SEPSIS

How Is Fluid Therapy Altered?

Patients with sepsis develop widespread increases in capillary permeability. They often translocate so much fluid into the third space that they are severely hypovolemic, even when their total body water is increased. Fluid therapy is a challenge, particularly when urgent or emergent surgery is performed to drain abscesses or look for a source of infection. This in combination with the myocardial depressant factors that are present underscores the complexity of the situation.[57] These problems are mentioned again to emphasize their importance and ubiquity.

LIVER FAILURE

What Are the Effects on Fluid Requirements?

Complications of end-stage liver disease include ascites, severe hypoproteinemia, and the hepatorenal syndrome. When patients with massive ascites undergo intra-abdominal surgery, several liters of protein-rich fluid are drained. During surgery, ascitic fluid continues to form and is lost. This combination of events means higher fluid requirements than in a patient with no liver disease undergoing the same type of surgical procedure. Because of the severe associated hypoproteinemia, these patients are prone to a hypo-oncotic state and, therefore, are subject to increased peripheral edema. However, as was discussed previously, colloid administration does not seem to ameliorate this situation.

When Is Hypervolemia a Problem?

Some patients with uncontrollable ascites may undergo insertion of a peritoneovenous shunt, allowing fluid to be siphoned from the abdomen and returned to the vasculature. Initially, this procedure results in a hypervolemic state. After a period of several days to weeks, the kidneys will excrete the additional fluid load, and a new equilibrium will be established. Intraoperatively and perioperatively, therefore, these patients should receive minimal amounts of fluid and may be candidates for the use of diuretics in the immediate postoperative period.

NEUROSURGERY

Is Glucose Contraindicated?

Human and animal studies suggest that recovery from a central nervous system ischemic event is worse when hyperglycemia is present prior to the development of the ischemia.[58] Because of the possibility of localized (and occasionally generalized) ischemia related to surgical retraction and the operative procedure, glucose solutions are believed by many to be contraindicated in neurosurgical patients. Glucose monitoring and aggressive control of stress-induced hyperglycemia are indicated in these patients. This approach is very different from that used two to three decades ago, when electrolyte solutions were believed to be contraindicated in such cases and when D_5W or $D_{10}W$ was advocated as the fluid of choice.

How Should Cerebral Edema Be Minimized?

Normally, the blood-brain barrier excludes translocation of fluid and prevents the formation of cerebral edema. However, during neurosurgical procedures or in the presence of trauma and tumors, this barrier function often is abnormal. Mannitol or other osmotic agents are often administered in an attempt to induce some degree of cerebral dehydration and to prevent edema formation. Intraoperative fluid management should be tailored to produce mild hypovolemia to minimize additional cerebral swelling. Because of the osmotic diuretics, urine output may not be an accurate indicator of overall fluid status.

How Is Diabetes Insipidus Controlled?

Patients undergoing pituitary surgery often develop diabetes insipidus because of a lack of ADH. Large volumes of dilute urine may result in a postoperative hyperosmolar state. Measurement of serum sodium and urine and serum osmolality is indicated. The administration of adequate volumes of 0.25% saline or, when possible, allowing the patient to drink large volumes of liquids, maintains a euvolemic state and electrolyte balance.

PEDIATRIC PATIENTS

Chapters 60 and 61 deal with neonatal and pediatric surgical patients. The newborn's kidneys have limited capability for concentrating or diluting urine; as a result, electrolyte balance may be more difficult to achieve during and following surgery. Invasive monitoring in these patients often is more problematic than in adults. Clinical examination is essential to determine the adequacy of perioperative hydration, but orthostatic changes in vital signs are unreliable, and an age-related baseline tachycardia is present. Changes in moisture of the mucous membranes and skin turgor are important signs.

BURN PATIENTS

Patients who sustain thermal or electrical burns present special problems with respect to fluid therapy; these are discussed in Chapter 41. Few situations present greater problems in management than burns, including their potential for producing severe and often life-threatening complications.

References

1. Pitts RF: Physiology of the Kidney and Body Fluids. 3rd ed. Chicago, Year Book Medical Publishers, 1974.
2. Askanazi J, Starker PM, Weissman C: Fluid and electrolyte management in critical care. Boston, Butterworths, 1986.
3. Coller FA, Campbell KN, Vaughan HH, et al: Postoperative salt intolerance. Ann Surg 1944; 119:533.
4. Hayes MA, Goldenberg IS: Renal effects of anesthesia and operation mediated by endocrines. Anesthesiology 1963; 24:487.
5. Bernards WC, Kirby RR: A brief history of fluid and electrolyte therapy in the surgical patient. Probl Crit Care, 1991; 5:331.
6. Shires T, Cohn D, Carrico J, et al: Fluid therapy in hemorrhagic shock. Arch Surg 1964; 88:688.
7. Gabel JC, Drake RE: Plasma proteins and protein osmotic pressure. In Staub NC, Taylor AE (eds). Edema. New York, Raven Press, 1984, p 371.
8. Valanovich V: Crystalloid versus colloid fluid resuscitation: a meta-analysis of mortality. Surgery 1989; 105:65.
9. Gammage GW: Crystalloid versus colloid: is colloid worth the cost? Int Anesthesiol Clin 1987; 25:32.
10. Vincent JL: Fluids for resuscitation. Br J Anaesth 1991; 67:185.
11. Nearman HS, Herman ML: Toxic effects of colloids in the intensive care unit. Crit Care Clin 1991; 7:713.
12. Falk JL, Rackow EC, Astiz M, et al: Fluid resuscitation in shock. J Cardiothorac Anesth 1988; 2(Suppl):33.
13. London MJ: Plasma volume expansion in cardiovascular surgery: practical realities, theoretical concerns. J Cardiothorac Anes 1988; 2(Suppl):39.
14. Workshop on Assessment of Plasma Volume Expanders. Center for Biologics, Food and Drug Administration and National Heart, Lung, Blood Institute, Division of Blood Diseases and Resources. Bethesda, MD, March 25 and 26, 1991.
15. Lucas CE, Ledgerwood AM, Higgins RF: Impaired pulmonary function after albumin resuscitation from shock. J Trauma 1980; 20:446.
16. Holcroft JW, Vassar MJ, Turner JE, et al: 3% NaCl and 7.5% NaCl/Dextran 70 in the resuscitation of severely injured patients. Ann Surg 1987; 206:279.
17. Maningas PA, Mattox KL, Pepe PE, et al: Hypertonic saline–Dextran solutions for the prehospital management of traumatic hypotension. Am J Surg 1989; 157:528.
18. Jelenko C, Williams JB, Wheeler ML, et al: Studies in shock and resuscitation, I: use of a hypertonic, albumin-containing, fluid demand regimen (HALFD) in resuscitation. Crit Care Med 1979; 7:157.
19. Cross JS, Gruber DP, Gann DS, et al: Hypertonic saline attenuates the hormonal response to injury. Ann Surg 1989; 209:684.
20. McGough EK: Resuscitation in shock, trauma, and burns. Probl Crit Care 1991; 5:346.
21. Gould SA, Rosen AL, Sehgal LR, et al: Red cell substitutes: hemoglobin solution or fluorocarbon? J Trauma 1982; 22:736.
22. Spence RK, McCoy S, Costabile J, et al: Fluosol DA-20 in the treatment of severe anemia: randomized, controlled study of 46 patients. Crit Care Med 1990; 18:1227.
23. Gould SA, Rosen AL, Sehgal LR, et al: Fluosol-DA as a red-cell substitute in acute anemia. N Engl J Med 1986; 314:1653.
24. Savitsky JP, Doczi J, Black J, et al: A clinical safety trial of stroma-free hemoglobin. Clin Pharmacol Ther 1978; 23:73.
25. Moss GS, Gould SA, Sehgal LR: Hemoglobin solution—from tetramer to polymer. Surgery 1984; 95:249.
26. Gould SA, Moss GS, Rosen AL, et al: Red cell substitutes. In Critical Care. Civetta JM, Taylor RW, Kirby RR (eds). Philadelphia, JB Lippincott, 1992, pp 1719–1726.
27. Welborn LG, McGill WA, Hannallah RS, et al: Perioperative blood glucose concentrations in pediatric outpatients. Anesthesiology 1986; 54:543.
28. Roizen MF: Anesthetic implications of concurrent disease. In Anesthesia. 3rd ed. Miller RD (ed). New York, Churchill Livingstone, 1990, p 795.
29. Perel A, Pizov R, Cotev S: Systolic blood pressure variation is a sensitive indicator of hypovolemia in ventilated dogs subjected to graded hemorrhage. Anesthesiology 1987; 67:498.
30. Perel A, Segal E, Pizov R: Assessment of cardiovascular function by pressure waveform analysis. In Update in Intensive Care and Emergency Medicine. Vincent JL (ed). Berlin, Springer Verlag, 1989, pp 541–550.
31. Shires T, Williams J, Brown F: Acute change in extracellular fluids associated with major surgical procedures. Ann Surg 1961; 154:803.
32. Alpern RJ, Saxton CR, Seldin DW: Clinical interpretation of laboratory values. In Fluids and Electrolytes. 2nd ed. Kokko JP, Tannen RL (eds). Philadelphia, WB Saunders, 1990, pp 3–69.
33. Arieff AI: Hyponatremia, convulsions, respiratory arrest, and permanent brain damage after elective surgery in healthy women. N Engl J Med 1986; 314:1529.
34. Sterns RH, Riggs JE, Schochet SS: Osmotic demyelination syndrome following correction of hyponatremia. N Engl J Med 1986; 314:1535.
35. Narins RG: Therapy of hyponatremia: does haste make waste? (Editorial). N Engl J Med 1986; 314:1573.
36. Ayus JC, Krothapalli RK, Arieff AI: Treatment of symptomatic hyponatremia and its relation to brain damage. N Engl J Med 1987; 317:1190.
37. Chung HM, Kluge R, Schrier RW, et al: Postoperative hyponatremia: a prospective study. Arch Intern Med 1986; 146:333.
38. Sterns RH: Severe symptomatic hyponatremia: treatment and outcome. A study of 64 cases. Ann Intern Med 1987; 107:656.
39. Sterns RH: Severe hyponatremia: the case for conservative management. Crit Care Med 1992; 20:534.
40. Vitez TS, Soper LE, Wong KC, et al: Chronic hypokalemia and intraoperative dysrhythmias. Anesthesiology 1985; 63:130.
41. Hirsch IA, Tomlinson DL, Slogoff S, et al: The overstated risk of preoperative hypokalemia. Anesth Analg 1988; 67:131.
42. American Heart Association: Guidelines for cardiopulmonary resuscitation and emergency cardiac care. JAMA 1992; 268:2209.
43. Kisker CT, Strauss RG, Kaepke JA, et al: The effects of combined platelet and leukopheresis on the blood coagulation system. Transfusion 1978; 19:173.
44. Maguire LC, Henriksen RA, Strauss RG, et al: Platelet function in donors undergoing intermittent-flow centrifugation plateletpheresis or leukapheresis. Transfusion 1980; 20:549.
45. Strauss RG: Volume replacement and coagulation: a comparative review. J Cardiothorac Anesth 1988; 2(Suppl 1):24.
46. Johnson SD, Lucas CE, Gerrick SJ, et al: Altered coagulation after albumin supplements for treatment of oligemic shock. Arch Surg 1979; 114:279.
47. Carr ME: Turbidimetric evaluation of the impact of albumin on the structure of thrombin-mediated fibrin gelation. Haemostasis 1987; 17:189.
48. Aberg M, Hedner U, Bergentz S: Effects of dextran on factor VIII (antihemophilic factor) and platelet function. Ann Surg 1979; 189:243.
49. Aberg M, Hedner U, Bergentz S: The antithrombotic effect of dextran. Scand J Haematol 1979; 34:61.
50. Batlle J, del Rio F, Lopez-Fernandez F, et al: Effect of dextran on factor VIII/von Willebrand factor structure and function. Thromb Haemost 1985; 54:697.
51. Carr ME, Gabriel DA: The effect of dextran 70 on the structure of plasma derived fibrin gels. J Lab Clin Med 1980; 96:985.
52. Katsuda K, Maeno H: Mechanism for the inhibitory effect of dextran on α_2 plasmin inhibitor activity. Thromb Res 1980; 19:655.
53. Carlin G, Saldeen T: On the interaction between dextran and the primary fibrinolysis inhibitor α-antiplasmin. Thromb Res 1980; 19:103.
54. Carlin G, Bang NU: Enhancement of plasminogen activation and hydrolysis of purified fibrinogen and fibrin by dextran 70. Thromb Res 1980; 19:535.
55. Beck C: Disordered renal function. In Critical Care. Civetta JM, Taylor RW, Kirby RR (eds). Philadelphia, JB Lippincott, 1988, pp 1315–1322.
56. Berger JJ: Transurethral resection of the prostate. Probl Crit Care 1991; 5:376.
57. Schuster DP, Lefrak SS: Shock. In Critical Care. Civetta JM, Taylor RW, Kirby RR (eds). Philadelphia, JB Lippincott, 1992, pp 407–426.
58. Sieber FE, Traystman RJ: Special issues: glucose and the brain. Crit Care Med 1992; 20:104.

CHAPTER 43

Acid-Base

DAVID R. BEVAN, M.B., M.R.C.P., F.F.A.R.C.S.

Interpretation of laboratory acid-base values is perceived as difficult. In part this view reflects a confusing nomenclature that developed from the problems of measurement. It is not possible to measure hydrogen ion concentration ($[H^+]$) or its activity in biologic systems directly. Instead, measurements are made of the differences in electrical potential generated between unknown and standard buffered solutions to which pH numbers have been assigned at fixed temperatures.[1] These numbers are considered to be equivalent to assessments of H^+ activity and concentration.

The relationship between $[H^+]$ and the partial pressure of carbon dioxide (Pco_2) has been expressed with a multiplicity of simplified diagrams and equations in an attempt to make interpretation easy. The diagrams gave rise to an associated jargon (buffer base, base excess, base deficit, standard bicarbonate, and so forth) with the intention of simplifying therapeutic actions.

Unfortunately, some of these diagrams were based on erroneous interpretation of the complicated physicochemical concepts underlying acid-base data. For example, it was believed that the relationship between $[H^+]$ and Pco_2 was similar in blood (in vitro), to that in the whole body (in vivo). In the past 15 years, there has been considerable re-evaluation of the roles of the kidneys and the liver in the maintenance of acid-base homeostasis in health and disease. Also, interpretation of acid-base variables has shifted from a graphic to a mathematic format, giving a false appearance of accuracy to the evaluation.

Opinions differ about the optimal sampling site for acid-base evaluation (venous, central venous, arterial) in certain conditions and whether the values should be "corrected" according to a patient's temperature.

The purpose of this chapter is to provide a current review of the pathophysiology of acid-base balance, to produce a framework for the recognition of acid-base disorders, and to suggest a rational approach to their management.

PHYSIOLOGY

What Is an Acid?

An acid ionizes in solution to produce H^+ and anions (A^-). The more H^+ produced, the stronger the acid. Acids are proton donors, and bases are proton acceptors.

What Are Buffers?

When acids or bases are added to solutions, they tend to cause a change in H^+ of the solution. Buffers are substances that limit the change in H^+. When an acid is presented to the body, the change in H^+ is titrated by intracellular (proteins and polypeptides) and extracellular (hemoglobin, plasma proteins, and bicarbonate $[HCO_3^-]$) buffers. The arterial blood pH (pHa) is normally maintained within fairly close limits, 7.35 to 7.45. For venous blood, the range is 7.32 to 7.42. When the pHa is <7.35, *acidemia* is present; when it is >7.45, *alkalemia* is present.

The Henderson-Hasselbalch Equation

The key to the understanding of acid-base terminology lies in the relationship between changes in H^+, Pco_2, and HCO_3^- as expressed in the Henderson-Hasselbalch equation.[2, 3]

$$pH = pK + \log\frac{[HCO_3^-]}{H_2CO_3}$$

where H_2CO_3 is carbonic acid and pK equals the pH (6.1) at which the HCO_3^- and H_2CO_3 are present in equal amounts.

How Does Buffering Occur?

Buffering of H^+ in the extracellular fluid is achieved by HCO_3^-, which is also responsible for 50% of the buffering in the blood; hemoglobin (35%), plasma protein (6%), and phosphates are also important. The activity of a buffer is greatest when the pH is at the pK of the particular system, which for HCO_3^-/H_2CO_3, as noted previously, is 6.1. The buffer reaction is as follows:

$$H^+ + HCO_3^- \leftrightarrow H_2CO_3 \leftrightarrow H_2O + CO_2$$

At physiologic pH (7.4), this system is relatively weak. Its importance lies in the ability of the lungs to excrete CO_2 so that the addition of H^+ or elimination of CO_2 drives the foregoing equation to the right. H_2CO_3 can be formed by the addition or failure of elimination of either CO_2 (respiratory load) or nonvolatile acids (nonrespiratory, metabolic load).

What Are Metabolic and Respiratory Compensation?

In situations in which the tendency to develop acidemia by either a respiratory or metabolic component is matched, at least in part, by metabolic or respiratory compensation, the disorders are known, respectively, as *respiratory acidosis* with metabolic compensation or *metabolic acidosis* with respiratory compensation. Such compensations make acidemia and alkalemia uncommon.

The Henderson-Hasselbalch equation may be rearranged to relate the H^+ (but not pH) to P_{CO_2} and HCO_3^-:[4]

$$H^+ (nmol \cdot L^{-1}) = 24 \times \frac{P_{CO_2}}{HCO_3^-}$$

This rearrangement facilitates mathematic manipulation of acid-base data and demonstrates that changes in H^+ are determined by the ratio of P_{CO_2} to HCO_3^-, not by either alone.

How Is Acidity Measured?

$[H^+]$ in body fluids ranges from 10^{-1} to 10^{-15} mol $\cdot L^{-1}$. For convenience, these values are expressed by exponential arithmetic so that pH is the negative logarithm of the $[H^+]$ (Table 43–1).

The Relationship Between pH and [H⁺]

Within the pH range of 7.10 to 7.50, an almost linear relationship exists between pH and $[H^+]$. For each 0.01-unit change in pH from 7.4, the $[H^+]$ alters by 1 nmol $\cdot L^{-1}$. For example, a decrease in pH from 7.4 to 7.2 increases $[H^+]$ by 20 nmol $\cdot L^{-1}$. Alternatively, a more precise estimate is obtained by multiplying the $[H^+]$ at a pH of 7.4 (40 nmol $\cdot L^{-1}$) by 1.25 for each 0.1 decrease in pH. Thus, the $[H^+]$ at pH 7.2 is $40 \times 1.25 \times 1.25 = 63$ nmol $\cdot L^{-1}$. For each 0.1 increase in pH, the $[H^+]$ is multiplied by 0.8, so that at pH 7.6, the $[H^+]$ is $40 \times 0.8 \times 0.8 = 26$ nmol $\cdot L^{-1}$.

Temperature Correction

The P_{CO_2} and pH of a blood sample are temperature dependent. As the sample is warmed, the pH decreases and the P_{CO_2} increases as it comes out of solution, but the total CO_2 content of the sample does not change. Most laboratories maintain the measurement electrodes at 37 °C; they may correct the values according to a patient's temperature in certain situations such as hypothermic cardiopulmonary bypass.

It has been suggested that the uncorrected values should be used in the ventilatory management of hypothermic patients.[5]

TABLE 43–1. Conversion of Hydrogen Ion Concentration ($[H^+]$) to pH Units

$[H^+]$ nmol $\cdot L^{-1}$	$[H^+]$ mol $\cdot L^{-1}$	pH
1,000,000	$0.001 = 10^{-3}$	3
10,000	$0.000\ 01 = 10^{-5}$	5
100	$0.000\ 000\ 1 = 10^{-7}$	7
1	$0.000\ 000\ 001 = 10^{-9}$	9

TABLE 43–2. Differences in Arteriovenous Values During Anesthesia With Three Inhalation Anesthetics*

	Isoflurane (N = 15)	Enflurane (N = 16)	Halothane (N = 17)
P_{CO_2}	-1.2 ± 1.6	-1.5 ± 2.1	-1.6 ± 1.6
pH	0.01 ± 0.01	0.01 ± 0.01	0.02 ± 0.02
BE (mEq $\cdot$ L)	0.09 ± 0.56†	0.03 ± 0.75†	0.20 ± 0.33
P_{O_2}	49.5 ± 36.9	39.4 ± 29.1	56.9 ± 52.1
O_2 (% vol)	0.65 ± 0.98	0.57 ± 0.44	0.69 ± 0.45

(From Williamson DG, Munson ES: Correlation of peripheral venous and arterial blood gas values during general anesthesia. Anesth Analg 1982; 61:951.)
*Values are mean $\pm$ SD.
†With these exceptions, all arteriovenous values were significantly different at the 0.05 level.
Abbreviation: BE = base excess.

This practice has some physiologic merit, because in nonhomeothermic animals the pHa varies inversely with temperature.[6]

Cerebral Perfusion and Cerebral Metabolic Rate of Oxygen with Temperature Correction

In practice, it is difficult to demonstrate much advantage with respect to cerebral or myocardial function with either approach. However, during hypothermic cardiopulmonary bypass, if the values are corrected for temperature (pH stat) by then administering CO_2, induces hypercapnia and produces cerebral vasodilation despite a decrease in cerebral metabolic rate of oxygen uptake (CMR_{O_2}). In contrast, the decrease in CMR_{O_2} is matched by a decrease in cerebral perfusion so that coupling of blood flow and metabolism is preserved when the values are not corrected (α-stat). On balance, it appears to be unnecessary to correct measured acid-base values for temperature.[7, 8]

Should Arterial or Venous Sample Be Used?

Usually, arterial blood is sampled for acid-base analysis, in part because this practice enables the simultaneous measurement of partial pressure of arterial oxygen (Pa_{O_2}). However, arterial blood may also be viewed as easily obtained "arterialized" mixed venous blood. Blood from warm, vasodilated peripheral veins (arterialized capillary blood) has been used as a close estimate of arterial blood, at least for the measurement of pH and P_{CO_2} during inhalation anesthetics (Table 43–2).

Advantages to Using Venous Blood

The acid-base status of most body tissue is best reflected in the blood draining that tissue. (The brain is an exception because lactate, from anaerobic metabolism, is confined to the brain cells and cerebrospinal fluid by the blood-brain barrier). Arterial and mixed venous acid-base variables may differ considerably in states of impaired tissue perfusion or cardiac arrest.[9, 10] In this situation, mixed venous (pulmonary artery) or central venous sampling may be more representative than arterial for acid-base evaluation.[11]

What Is Intracellular pH?

The measurement of intracellular pH (pHi), although desirable, is not possible in clinical practice. The methods available (insertion of microelectrodes, calculations from the distribution of weak acids, examination of pH-dependent reactions) are neither robust nor repeatable. Normally, pHi is less than extracellular pH, but the magnitude of the difference may change considerably in acid-base disorders. CO_2 but not highly ionized acids or alkalis is permeable across cell membranes.

What Is the Anion Gap?

The anion gap (AG) is estimated as the difference between serum sodium and the sum of chloride and HCO_3^- concentrations[12]:

$$AG = Na^+ - (Cl^- + HCO_3^-)$$

The normal range is 12 ± 2 mmol $\cdot$ L^{-1} and is a reflection of anions other than chloride that balance the positive charge of sodium. HCO_3^- may be replaced with endogenous (lactate, keto acids) or exogenous (salicylate, paraldehyde, formate, glycolate) organic and inorganic acids and toxins. An AG that is >30 mmol $\cdot$ L^{-1} is usually indicative of significant organic acid acidosis.

What Is Lactic Acidosis?

Lactic acidosis is defined as the combination of pH <7.25 and blood lactate concentration >5 mmol $\cdot$ L^{-1} and may result from either increased production or decreased metabolism of lactic acid. High levels of lactic acid (>9 mmol $\cdot$ L^{-1}) are associated with a very high mortality. Lactic acidosis is discussed later.

VENTILATION AND ACID-BASE STATUS

What Happens When the Body Carbon Dioxide Changes?

The Henderson-Hasselbalch equation enables the change in pH following an acute alteration in P_{CO_2} to be predicted. An in vivo CO_2 titration curve can be constructed when a steady state has been reached after a step increase or decrease in P_{CO_2} (Fig. 43–1).[13]

Mathematically, $\Delta[H^+]$ (nmol $\cdot$ L^{-1}) is approximately $0.8 \times \Delta P_{CO_2}$ (mm Hg). In addition, $\Delta[HCO_3^-]$ can be predicted: The $[HCO_3^-]$ increases by 1 mEq $\cdot$ L^{-1} for every 10 mm Hg increase in P_{CO_2} above 40 mm Hg and decreases by 2 mEq $\cdot$ L^{-1} for each 10 mm Hg decrease in P_{CO_2} below 40 mm Hg. When the change in $[H^+]$ or $[HCO_3^-]$ differs from that predicted, an additional metabolic (nonrespiratory) disorder is implied.

How Can These Changes Be Displayed?

When such P_{CO_2} titrations are performed in acidotic subjects or in animals made acid by the infusion of hydrochloric acid (HCl), a family of in vivo CO_2 titration curves is produced parallel and to the left of the normal curve. Similarly, in alkalotic situations, the curves are shifted to the right. The more acid or alkaline the subject, the more the lines are shifted from normal (Fig. 43–2).[14]

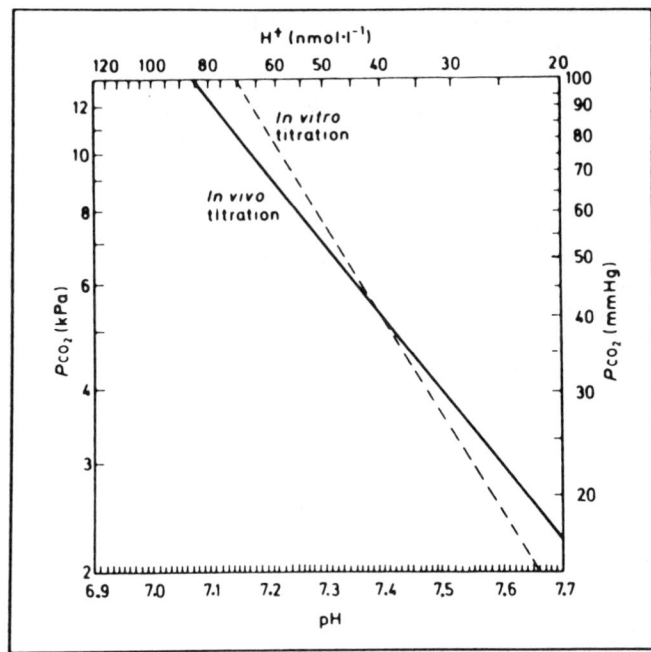

FIGURE 43–1. In vivo and in vitro CO_2 titration curves.

What Happens When the Blood P_{CO_2} Changes?

A similar CO_2 titration may be performed by changing the P_{CO_2} of a blood sample rather than P_{CO_2} of the whole body. Such an in vitro CO_2 titration curve formed the basis of the early assessment of acid-base status using a pH electrode before the availability of the CO_2 electrode. Blood was equilibrated in a tonometer with two known concentrations of CO_2 (high gas, 10% CO_2; low gas, 0.5% CO_2), the pH was measured after each equilibration, and a CO_2 titration line was

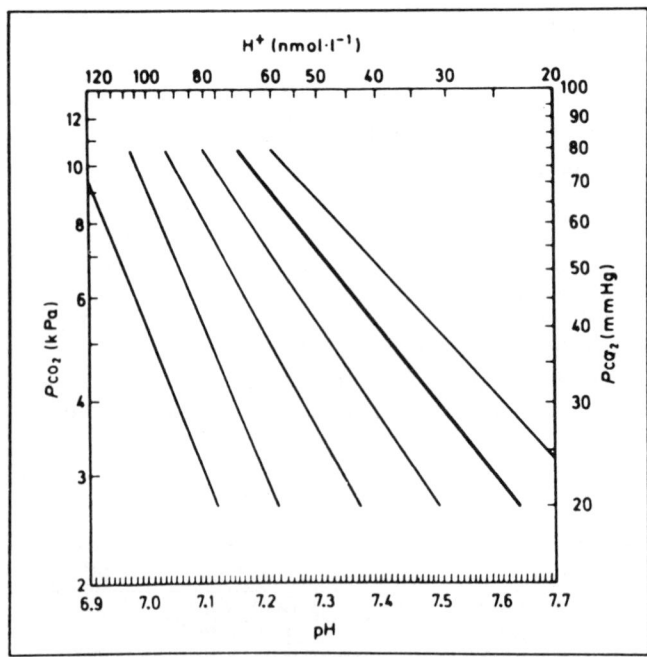

FIGURE 43–2. Family of in vivo CO_2 titration curves after addition of acid or alkali.

plotted. The P_{CO_2} of the original sample was then determined by interpolation, if its pH was measured before equilibration (Fig. 43–3).

The CO_2 titration lines lie to the left of the normal in acidotic and to the right of the normal in alkalotic conditions. Also, it was realized that the slope of the line was modified by a change in hemoglobin concentration. A number of indices were introduced to account for these variations in an attempt to produce a numeric indication of the metabolic disturbance.

Base Excess

The most common of these indices, which is still in use, is the *base excess*.[15] A series of CO_2 titration lines at several hemoglobin concentrations was constructed before and after adding known quantities of strong acid or alkali (Fig. 43–4). When the intersections of each family of curves were joined, a base excess curve was produced related to the amount of acid or alkali that had been added. Thus, when a CO_2 titration was performed in the determination of pH, the position of the line allowed the base excess or base deficit (negative base excess) to be determined from the position at which the line crossed the base excess curve.

Buffer Base and Standard Bicarbonate

Earlier indices of acid-base status included the calculation of the sum of all the buffer anions (HCO_3^-, plasma proteins, and hemoglobin). They are the *buffer base*.[16] The influence of hemoglobin was also estimated by *standard bicarbonate*, which was the $[HCO_3^-]$ in plasma equilibrated to a P_{CO_2} of 40 mm Hg.[17]

How Should Acid-Base Changes Be Assessed?

Base excess, *standard bicarbonate*, and *buffer base* are outdated, and these terms should no longer be used. The terminology is confusing and seldom understood. More important, the indices are based on the in vitro titration of blood and do

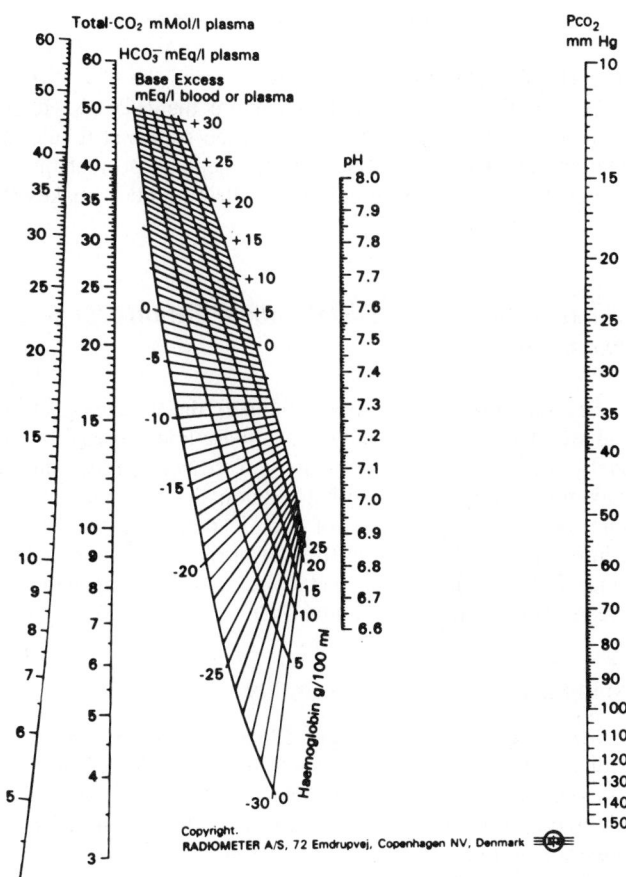

FIGURE 43–4. Base excess curve (Astrup P, Jorgensen K, Siggaard-Andersen O, et al: The acid-base metabolism: a new approach. Lancet 1960; 1:1035. Copyright RADIOMETER A/S, Emdrupvej, Copenhagen NV, Denmark.)

not reflect the changes in pH that might be expected when the whole body P_{CO_2} is changed: In vitro CO_2 titration curves have a steeper slope than in vivo curves (see Fig. 43–1) and thus may introduce considerable errors into the measurement. It is recommended that acid-base assessment be based on predictions from the Henderson-Hasselbalch equation using either a graphic (see Fig. 43–4) or mathematic representation for the calculation of actual bicarbonate.

RENAL RESPONSES TO ACID-BASE DISTURBANCE

Classically, renal control of acid-base homeostasis has been explained in terms of reabsorption of bicarbonate (5000 mmol · d^{-1}), which reduces systemic acidity, and the excretion of nonvolatile acid (50–100 mmol · d^{-1}) by trapping H$^+$ with phosphate buffers and ammonium salts. However, there are several confusing observations that do not fit with these simple explanations.

What Is Bicarbonate Reabsorption?

H$^+$ is produced in the renal tubular cells in the presence of carbonic anhydrase (CA):

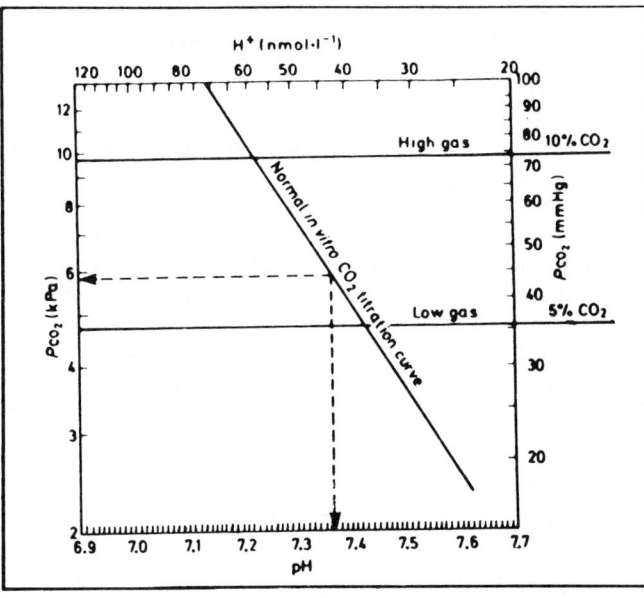

FIGURE 43–3. Assessment of P_{CO_2} by interpolation technique.

$$CO_2 + H_2O \leftrightarrow H_2CO_3 \leftrightarrow H^+ + HCO_3^-$$

The H^+ neutralizes the filtered HCO_3^-, and the CO_2 diffuses back into the tubular cell to recapture the HCO_3^-. HCO_3^- reabsorption takes place primarily in the proximal tubule, although acidification occurs along the nephron so that the H^+ secreted into the distal tubule and collecting ducts makes the urine as acid as pH 4.5.

What Is the Role of Distal Tubule Cation Exchange?

Several observations do not support the concept that the kidneys act primarily to defend acid-base homeostasis. In animals, urine pH decreases acutely if sodium in the diet is accompanied by nonreabsorbable anions—phosphate and sulfate. Also, in the presence of sodium depletion, the chronic administration of H^+ in the form of nitric (H_2NO_3) or sulfuric acid (H_2SO_4) causes less metabolic acidosis and, therefore, greater acid excretion than after HCl.

Maintenance of Electroneutrality

Schwartz and Cohen[18] suggest that the primary role of the kidneys is to preserve electroneutrality, not pH. Reabsorption of sodium must be accompanied either by reabsorption of accompanying anions or secretion of cations. Thus, in the presence of nonreabsorbable anions (nitrate, phosphate, or sulfate), sodium reabsorption is associated with secretion of H^+ or K^+, and renal acid excretion becomes dependent on Na^+-H^+ exchange[18] (Fig. 43–5).

In humans, continuous gastric drainage is associated with loss of acid and dehydration, producing metabolic alkalosis and, paradoxically, aciduria. Saline administration corrects the decreased extracellular fluid volume, as well as the metabolic acidosis, by decreasing urine acid excretion. Again, Na^+-H^+ exchange is invoked as the cause of the aciduria and its correction with volume replacement.

This hypothesis is not supported by micropuncture techniques of individual nephron segments (or other tissues resembling the distal tubular cell), which have shown that the tubule is capable of responding to acid-base disturbance indepen-

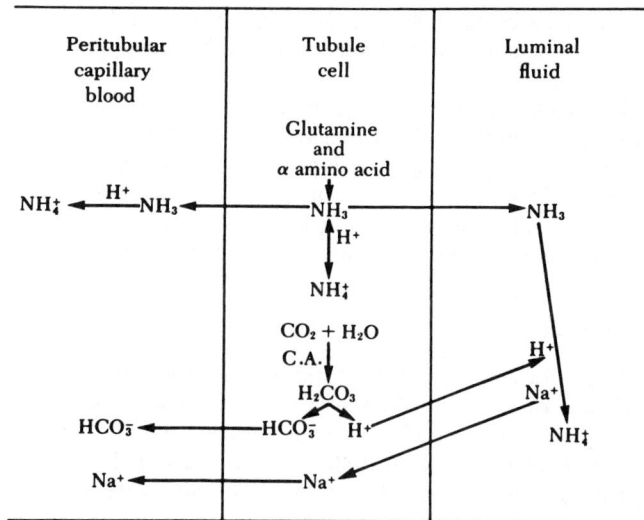

FIGURE 43–6. Suggested mechanism for the secretion of NH_3 by tubular cells and the excretion of NH_4^+ in urine (From Masoro EJ, Seigel PD: Acid-Base Regulation: Its Physiology, Pathophysiology, and the Interpretation of Blood-Gas Analysis. Philadelphia, WB Saunders, 1977, p 76.)

dently of sodium reabsorption.[19] Thus, although the cation exchange mechanism may account for some chronic acid-base disturbances, renal acid excretion is not solely a byproduct of electrolyte homeostasis.

Are Phosphate Buffers Important?

Approximately 30 to 40 mmol $\cdot$ d^{-1} of H^+ is excreted as "titratable acid" bound to monohydrogen phosphate (see Fig. 43–5):

$$HPO_4^{-2} + H^+ \leftrightarrow H_2PO_4^-$$

At pH 6.8, the phosphate buffer is only 50% titrated, but it is nearly fully titrated at pH 5, a more acid condition.

How Are Ammonium Salts Used?

Similarly, H^+ is buffered by ammonia (NH_3) (Fig. 43–6):

$$NH_3 + H^+ \leftrightarrow NH_4^+$$

The rate of excretion of ammonium (NH_4^+) may be increased 5 to 10 times in diabetic ketoacidosis.[20]

It has been suggested that this equation represents a fundamental error. Urinary NH_4^+ is formed from glutamine, but at the pH in the tubule, glutamine already is ionized to NH_4^+ and cannot further buffer H^+.[21] Thus, the increased excretion of NH_4^+ in acidosis should not be regarded as a means to excrete additional H^+ but rather as a means of depriving the liver of a source of NH_3 for urea synthesis and the consequent increase in H^+ production.[22] The importance of this observation requires further evaluation.[23]

THE LIVER AND ACID-BASE REGULATION

Each day, approximately 20 mmol $\cdot$ kg^{-1} of lactate and its accompanying cation are produced. The H^+ is titrated with

---

Peritubular capillary blood	Renal tubule cell	Luminal fluid
	$CO_2 + H_2O$ C.A.$\downarrow$	
	H_2CO_3	$H_2PO_4^-$
$HCO_3^- \leftarrow$	$HCO_3^- \quad H^+ \longrightarrow$	H^+
$Na^+ \leftarrow$	Na^+	Na^+
		HPO_4^-

FIGURE 43–5. Distal tubule cation exchange; acidification of the phosphate buffer system in the renal tubule. (From Masoro EJ, Seigel PD: Acid-Base Regulation: Its Physiology, Pathophysiology, and the Interpretation of Blood-Gas Analysis. Philadelphia, WB Saunders, 1977, p 75.)

HCO_3^-, as described earlier, and the lactate is metabolized mainly in the liver (70%) but also in the kidneys by gluconeogenesis or oxidation. Either pathway consumes 1 mol H^+ for each mole of lactate that is metabolized. In effect, this process leads to the generation of 1 mol HCO_3^-.

Why Is Urea Synthesis Important?

Urea is synthesized in the liver:

$$CO_2 + 2NH_4^+ \leftrightarrow CO(NH_2)_2 + H_2O + H^+$$
$$(urea)$$

Each mole of urea produces 2 mol of H^+, which are used to neutralize HCO_3^- generated from the metabolism of amino acids. A decrease in the availability of NH_4^+ resulting from the increased renal NH_4^+ excretion associated with diabetic ketoacidosis reduces H^+.[23] In addition, acidosis decreases urea synthesis directly.

Alterations in Liver Disease

Liver disease is often associated with decreased urea synthesis and metabolic alkalosis. The acidosis of uremia is not necessarily a consequence of decreased NH_4^+ excretion but also of increased urea synthesis. Compensation for acute respiratory acidosis may result from depression of urea synthesis and a failure to titrate the HCO_3^- from amino acid metabolism.[24] The disposal of lactate is impaired by acidosis, high lactate concentrations ($>3-5$ mmol $\cdot$ L^{-1}), and decreased hepatic perfusion. However, metabolism is increased through stimulation of gluconeogenesis by the stress hormones (catecholamines, angiotensin, vasopressin, glucagon).[25]

ACID-BASE DISTURBANCES

If Ventilation Changes, What Happens?

Respiratory Acidosis

When the elimination of CO_2 is less than its production, the PCO_2 increases. Apnea results in an increase of PCO_2 of 3 mm Hg $\cdot$ min^{-1} at normal metabolic rate. In surgical patients, the most common causes are respiratory center depression by anesthetic agents or narcotics, as well as persistent neuromuscular blockade; these changes may be augmented by pulmonary disease or instability of the rib cage.

Compensation

The change in pH in response to an increase in PCO_2 can be predicted according to the in vivo CO_2 titration curve (see Figs. 43–1 and 43–2). Renal and hepatic compensation is slow and is not complete for 48 hours. In chronic respiratory acidosis, the increase in H^+ averages only 0.3 times the increase in PCO_2, compared with 0.8 times the increase in PCO_2 during acute disturbances (Fig. 43–7). An increase in extracellular H^+ is associated with H^+-K^+ exchange across the cell membrane so that hypercapnia is commonly associated with hyperkalemia.

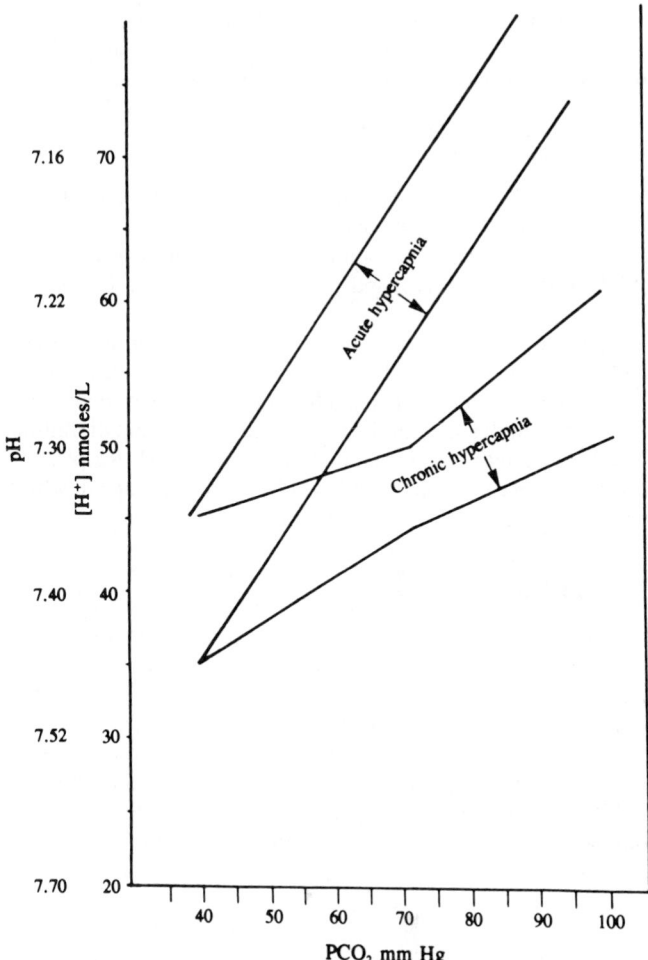

FIGURE 43–7. Changes in H^+ and pH during acute and chronic hypercapnia (95% confidence limits). The ameliorating effects of renal and hepatic compensation in the chronic state are shown clearly. (From Masoro EJ, Seigel PD: Acid-Base Regulation: Its Physiology, Pathophysiology, and the Interpretation of Blood-Gas Analysis. Philadelphia, WB Saunders, 1977, p 116.)

Appropriate Treatment

Correction of respiratory acidosis, as for all acid-base disturbances, should be achieved slowly and, primarily, by correcting the underlying cause, particularly when the persistent effects of respiratory depressant or neuromuscular blocking drugs are responsible.

Chronic CO_2 retention is associated with decreased central drive to ventilation, which then becomes dependent on peripheral chemoreceptors. If the PCO_2 is reduced rapidly in these patients, the sudden increase in cerebrospinal fluid pH may produce convulsions and unconsciousness.[26] Thus, PCO_2 should be reduced slowly (e.g., over 48 h).

Respiratory Alkalosis

Hypocapnia occurs when the effective pulmonary ventilation is increased. The most common cause seen by anesthesiologists is mechanical hyperventilation. However, the condition occurs frequently when the respiratory center is stimulated by pain, anxiety, fear, pregnancy, or salicylate intoxication. Peripheral hypoxic chemoreceptor stimulation occurs at high altitude and probably also accounts for the hypocapnia of sepsis, anemia, and heart failure. Although CO_2 depletion is common in hepatic failure, decreased lactate and urea metabolism causes more important metabolic than respiratory disturbances of acid-base status, as noted previously.

Compensation

The initial change in H^+ and HCO_3^- can be predicted from the in vivo CO_2 titration curves (see Figs. 43–1 and 43–2). In acute disturbances, each 1 mm Hg decrease in P_{CO_2} decreases $[H^+]$ by 0.8 nmol $\cdot$ L^{-1} and decreases HCO_3^- by 0.2 nmol $\cdot$ L^{-1}.

In chronic disturbances, H^+ decreases by 0.4 nmol $\cdot$ L^{-1} and HCO_3^- by 0.4 mmol $\cdot$ L^{-1} for each 1 mm Hg decrease in P_{CO_2}.[27] Within hours, renal and hepatic mechanisms counteract the change in pH so completely that the hypocapnia of altitude is accompanied by a normal or nearly normal pH. Respiratory alkalosis appears to be the only acid-base disturbance in which compensation restores pH to normal.[12]

Appropriate Treatment

Respiratory alkalosis is better prevented than treated by avoiding increased central or peripheral ventilatory drive. In particular, mechanical ventilation should be guided by end-tidal or arterial P_{CO_2} monitoring.

It may be difficult to maintain Pa_{O_2} when ventilation is reduced to correct profound hypocapnia, because the depletion in CO_2 stores causes an apparent reduction in the respiratory quotient (R). Consequently, as predicted from the alveolar air equation,

$$P_{AO_2} = F_{IO_2}(P_B - P_{H_2O}) - Pa_{CO_2}\left[F_{IO_2} + \frac{1 - F_{IO_2}}{R} \right]$$

P_{AO_2} and hence Pa_{O_2} decrease, providing further justification for additional oxygen when patients are weaned from mechanical ventilation.[28]

Respiratory alkalosis results in hypokalemia from both H^+-K^+ exchange across the cell membrane and an increase in renal potassium excretion.

If Metabolic Changes Occur, What Happens?

Metabolic Acidosis

Metabolic acidosis is commonly classified according to the AG (Table 43–3). Those conditions associated with an in-

TABLE 43–3. Causes of Metabolic Acidosis

Increased Anion Gap	Normal Anion Gap
Lactic acidosis*	Renal tubular acidosis
Circulatory arrest*	Diarrhea
Pulmonary edema*	Biliary/pancreatic fistulas
Gram-negative sepsis*	Saline excess
Ketoacidosis	
Toxins	
Nitroprusside	
Fructose	
Acid-citrate-dextrose blood	

*Associated with hypoxia.

TABLE 43–4. Causes of Type B Lactic Acidosis

Systemic Disease B1	Drugs and Toxins B2	Inherited B3
Diabetes mellitus	Biguanides	Glycogen storage
Renal failure	Salicylates	Fructose-1, 6-diphosphate deficiency
Hepatic failure	Parenteral nutrition	Methylmalonic acidemia
Leukemia		Pyruvate dehydrogenase deficiency

creased AG may be further divided, depending on the presence or absence of hypoxia, and this subdivision may have important therapeutic implications. The toxic causes listed are the result of the addition of organic acids or substances that produce acid by their metabolism (paraldehyde, ethylene glycol, methanol).

Alternatively, some conditions may result from an increased loss of base (diarrhea, biliary/pancreatic fistulas). Administration of large volumes of stored blood, particularly when acid-citrate-dextrose was used as an anticoagulant, produced an acute metabolic acidosis that was converted into a metabolic alkalosis during the next 2 to 3 days as the citrate was metabolized to HCO_3^-. Infusion of several liters of saline during resuscitation may result in a mild metabolic acidosis from dilution of extracellular HCO_3^-. Although the pH of saline is decreased compared with the normal blood value, the titratable acidity (actual acid load) is minuscule. The pH is low because there are no buffers in saline; thus a very small amount of acid causes a significant reduction of pH.

Lactic Acidosis

Type A lactic acidosis is the result of tissue hypoxia and anaerobic metabolism and is more common than type B, which results from other causes[29] (Table 43–4). In shock, if the blood lactate concentration is > 5 mmol $\cdot$ L^{-1}, the mortality is >75%; it is only 18% when the concentration is 1.3 to 4.4 mmol $\cdot$ L^{-1}.[30]

Type A Lactic Acidosis. Lactic acidosis is commonly associated with hypoxia because the available oxygen is inadequate for a patient's needs. In shock, hypovolemia, and sepsis, overall oxygen consumption may not be altered because the decrease in cardiac output is offset by an increase of oxygen extraction. However, the distribution of oxygen uptake is modified: Extraction by the liver, muscle, kidneys, and gut decreases while that of the heart and brain increases.[11] Decreased oxygen availability in the affected tissues leads to anaerobic glycolysis and the accumulation of lactate. In addition, as previously noted, decreased lactate uptake by the liver leads to decreased clearance.

After cardiac arrest, the increase in myocardial H^+ is the result of CO_2 accumulation and failure of sufficient adenosine triphosphate generation to drive the Na^+-H^+ exchange.[31, 32] If sodium bicarbonate ($NaHCO_3$) is given to correct the acidosis, the result is liberation of CO_2, which causes further increase in intracellular H^+ and acidosis.[33]

Type B Lactic Acidosis. The lactic acid in type B lactic acidosis originates from metabolic causes and is not associated with hypoxia (see Table 43–4). Severe renal and hepatic disease is associated with lactate accumulation. Acidosis may cause very rapid lactic acidosis in uremia; hepatic gluconeogenesis is decreased, but renal gluconeogenesis, which increases lactic acid production, is increased.

Biguanides (oral hypoglycemic agents) act by reducing alimentary absorption of glucose and amino acids; they increase glycolysis and decrease hepatic gluconeogenesis. Normally, lactate concentrations are <2 mmol $\cdot$ L^{-1}, but they may increase considerably in the presence of renal or hepatic disease.

Fructose, sorbitol, and xylitol all have been used in parenteral nutrition as a source of carbohydrate because they are metabolized in the absence of insulin and produce less venous irritation. However, all lead to an increase in lactate production; consider that 30% to 40% of a fructose load is converted to lactate.

Finally, several congenital diseases of the liver, such as pyruvate dehydrogenase deficiency, are associated with impaired hepatic lactate metabolism.

Compensation

Metabolic acidosis stimulates ventilation, producing hypocapnia, which limits the decrease in pH. The P_{CO_2} decreases slowly to reach its nadir at 12 to 24 hours. Although the change in P_{CO_2} is variable, it is related to the ΔHCO_3^- [anticipated P_{CO_2} (mm Hg) = 1.5 (ΔHCO_3^- mEq $\cdot$ L^{-1}) + 8] and to the pH. A useful rule of thumb is that the anticipated P_{CO_2} is approximately equal to the last two numbers of the pH (e.g., at pH 7.20, the anticipated P_{CO_2} is 20 mm Hg).

Appropriate Treatment

Sodium Bicarbonate. Traditionally, metabolic acidosis has been treated by $NaHCO_3$ titration. The quantity required can be estimated from the numeric expression of the Henderson-Hasselbalch equation, assuming that the HCO_3^- is distributed through the extracellular fluid volume (20% body weight). Half the estimated deficit was given slowly over 10 minutes, and subsequent therapy was dictated by frequent acid-base assessment.

For example, a 70-kg patient has a 14-kg extracellular fluid volume. If normal HCO_3^- is 24 mEq $\cdot$ L^{-1} and the patient's HCO_3^- is 14 mEq $\cdot$ L^{-1}, each kilogram (liter) of extracellular fluid has a deficit of 10 mEq $\cdot$ L^{-1}, or a total deficit of 140 mEq. One half of this value (70 mEq) would be infused slowly over 10 minutes, followed by assessment.

Although such therapy may be appropriate for some causes of metabolic acidosis (uremia, diarrhea and fistulas, renal tubular acidosis), administration of $NaHCO_3$ in the presence of hypoxia neither corrects the acidosis nor improves the cardiovascular status. In experimental metabolic acidosis, $NaHCO_3$ leads to an increase in intracellular H$^+$ in the heart, liver, muscle, and red blood cells.[11] In addition, $NaHCO_3$ promotes cerebrospinal fluid acidosis, hypoxia, circulatory depression, hyperosmolality, and hypernatremia.

$NaHCO_3$ has no place in the treatment of diabetic ketoacidosis. It does not decrease ketone body concentration, increase pH, or improve patients' survival. Management is with fluid and insulin to restore glucose metabolism, which has the additional advantage of improving hepatic metabolism of accumulated lactate, itself a store of HCO_3^-.

Several promising alternatives to $NaHCO_3$ have been tried experimentally, although none is currently approved for clinical use.

Sodium Dichloroacetate. Sodium dichloroacetate (DCA) has been shown to decrease lactate concentration and to improve cardiovascular function in several hypoxic states without an increase in P_{CO_2} and thus, presumably, without an increase in intracellular H$^+$. It acts by stimulating pyruvate dehydrogenase, which encourages the conversion of lactate to pyruvate for eventual removal via the Krebs cycle in the liver.

Carbicarb. An equimolar mixture of $NaHCO_3$ and sodium carbonate buffers acid in a similar manner to $NaHCO_3$ but without an increase in P_{CO_2}. It produces little hemodynamic effect but improves acid-base status and decreases intracellular H$^+$ and lactate production.

Tris(hydroxymethyl)aminomethane Buffer. This substance (also called *THAM*) is unusual in that it crosses cell membranes and buffers intracellular as well as extracellular H$^+$, again without an increase in P_{CO_2}.

Sodium DCA, carbicarb, and THAM do not possess the problems associated with $NaHCO_3$, particularly with regard to intracellular H$^+$ increase, and are currently undergoing clinical evaluation. At present, it appears that the safest treatment of metabolic acidosis in hypoxia is removal of the cause and aggressive cardiorespiratory support. Survival depends on the ability of the individual to increase cardiac output and oxygen delivery in the presence of tissue hypoxia and anaerobic metabolism.

Metabolic Alkalosis

Severe metabolic alkalosis has a mortality as high as 65% when the pH is >7.65.[34] The causes of metabolic alkalosis include loss of gastrointestinal fluid, adrenal hyperplasia, and administration of loop diuretics, cortisone, or alkali (Table 43–5).

Compensation

The in vivo CO_2 titration curve (see Fig. 43–2) is shifted to the right in metabolic alkalosis. Respiratory compensation does occur but often is variable. The resulting P_{CO_2} is seldom >50 mm Hg but can be predicted:

$$P_{CO_2} \text{ in mm Hg} = 0.9 \times HCO_3^- + 9 \text{ mmol} \cdot L^{-1}$$

Appropriate Treatment

The management of metabolic alkalosis is removal of the cause. Many patients respond to rehydration with saline, suggesting that the principal abnormality was related to loss of Cl$^-$ and not H$^+$. Ammonium chloride, one-sixth molar, may act as a source of acid by the production of urea and H$^+$, but normal hepatic function is required. Ammonium chloride should be avoided in hypokalemic patients, because further potassium loss may be induced. Infusion of HCl has been attempted, but it is not part of conventional therapy.

TABLE 43–5. Causes of Metabolic Alkalosis

Saline Responsive	Saline Unresponsive
Gastrointestinal losses	Aldosterone
Diuretics	Cortisone
	Alkali

Mixed Disturbances

The acid-base disturbances previously discussed placed considerable emphasis on the ability to predict the compensatory changes that are induced by a primary alteration in P_{CO_2}, H^+, or HCO_3^-. Such predictions may be made using mathematic or graphic representations of the in vivo CO_2 titration curves. An acid-base map plots the 95% confidence limits of the relationship between pH and P_{CO_2} in various acute and chronic respiratory and metabolic disorders (Fig. 43–8).[35] In some situations, this approach may make it easier to determine the cause of the disturbance.

For example, using such a map, the finding of a pH of 7.25 and a P_{CO_2} of 25 mm Hg suggests metabolic acidosis. However, a pH of 7.2 and P_{CO_2} of 80 mm Hg could represent either acute *respiratory acidosis* and slight *metabolic alkalosis* or chronic *respiratory acidosis* and slight *metabolic acidosis*. Clearly, a clinical history is essential in making a correct diagnosis; acid-base values cannot be evaluated in isolation.

Metabolic and Respiratory Acidosis

The most common disturbance is metabolic and respiratory acidosis. It is frequently encountered when the presence of chronic lung disease prevents the appropriate ventilatory compensation for a metabolic acidosis (e.g., cardiac arrest, pulmonary edema, chronic lung disease with hypoxia). Some substances (sodium nitroprusside, carbon monoxide, ethylene glycol) depress ventilation and induce metabolic acidosis. The importance of the combination is that administration of $NaHCO_3$ leads to further increase in P_{CO_2}, which cannot be removed because of impaired ventilation. Such patients require mechanical ventilatory support.

Metabolic Alkalosis and Respiratory Acidosis

Administration of diuretics to patients with chronic lung disease induces potassium loss and metabolic alkalosis that results in a compensatory respiratory acidosis. Treatment with ammonium chloride corrects the alkalosis and reduces P_{CO_2}.

Respiratory Alkalosis and Metabolic Acidosis

The combination of respiratory alkalosis and metabolic acidosis may be induced by salicylate poisoning. It also occurs in critically ill patients when the ventilatory response to lactic acidosis is excessive. This condition is difficult to recognize, although a normal pH with an increased AG may be suggestive. Again, the clinical history is important in making the diagnosis.

EFFECTS OF ACID-BASE DISTURBANCES

Is the Circulation Impaired?

The effects of acid-base disturbance on the circulation depend on the origin. For respiratory disturbances, the direct depressant actions of P_{CO_2} may be offset by the associated sympathetic stimulation. CO_2 acts as a peripheral vasodilator and a pulmonary vasoconstrictor. However, in the presence of an intact autonomic system, its secondary sympathetic stimulation leads to vasoconstriction of those organs such as the kidneys with a rich sympathetic innervation. Thus, hypoventilation induces renal vasoconstriction and cerebral vasodilation. Also, sympathetic activation leads to increases in stroke volume, heart rate, and cardiac output.

When the P_{CO_2} is maintained constant, the cardiovascular effect of pH depends on the source and distribution of H^+. In general, a decrease in pH leads to myocardial depression with decreased stroke volume and cardiac output. However, in the presence of myocardial ischemia, intracellular H^+ decreases from hydrolysis of adenosine triphosphate and the local production of CO_2.[11] In this situation, the heart is particularly vulnerable to attempts at correcting the acidosis with $NaHCO_3$.

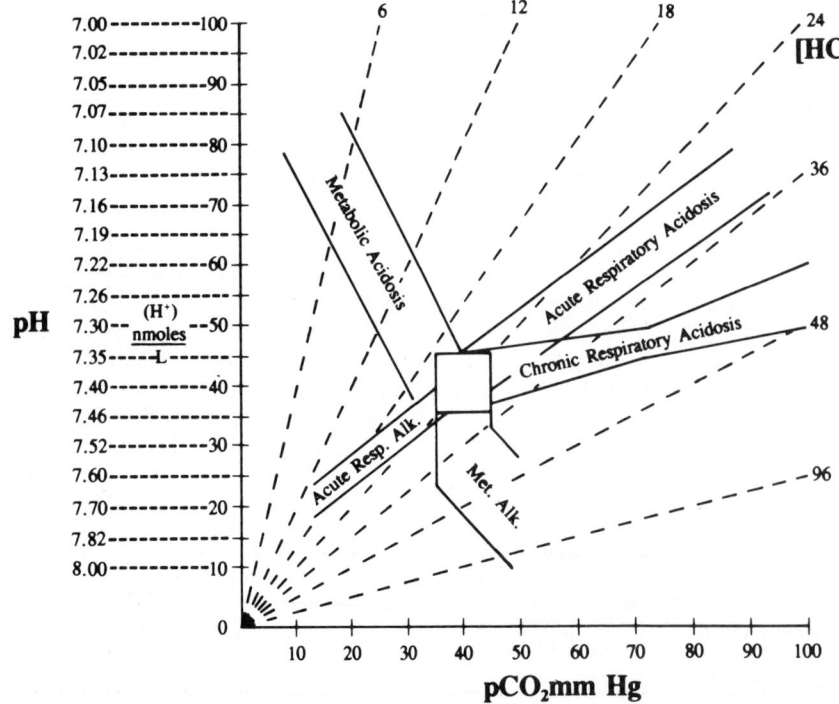

FIGURE 43–8. An acid-base "map" used to define mixed metabolic and respiratory disturbances. (Reproduced with permission from Masoro EJ, Seigel PD: Acid-Base Regulation: Its Physiology, Pathophysiology, and the Interpretation of Blood-Gas Analysis. Philadelphia, WB Saunders, 1977, p 142.)

The resulting increase in P_{CO_2} leads to further increase in intracellular H^+, myocardial depression, and impaired tissue oxygenation.

How Is Ventilation Affected?

Hypercapnia stimulates central and peripheral chemoreceptors maximally at a P_{CO_2} of about 80 mm Hg. Above that level, ventilation is depressed. Elevated P_{CO_2} induces a rapid increase in ventilation from stimulation of the aortic and carotid bodies. The accompanying decrease in pH produces a slower but additional central stimulus to ventilation. CO_2 and H^+ produce separate and additive rightward shifts of the oxyhemoglobin dissociation curve. The P_{50} (normal 26 mm Hg) is increased by about 2 mm Hg per 0.1 pH unit reduction.

Tissue oxygen delivery is the product of cardiac output and arterial oxygen content. To some extent, the shift in the oxygen dissociation curve induced by hypercapnia and acidosis compensates for the hemodynamic depression. Consequently, it is preferable, in the correction of metabolic acidosis, to produce a slight undercorrection rather than overcorrection, because metabolic alkalosis has a detrimental effect on both cardiac output and the oxygen dissociation curve.

What Neurologic Changes Occur?

CO_2 and H^+ have no direct effect on cerebral metabolism except as a consequence of altered cerebral perfusion. Hypocapnia has been shown to have some effect on increasing pain threshold. Tetany, in alkalotic states, is secondary to a decrease in the ionized calcium concentration.

Are Pharmacologic Actions Altered Significantly?

Drug activity is modified by pH as a result of the degree of ionization. This fact has some therapeutic application: Absorption of drugs is increased in the un-ionized state. At the pH of the stomach, salicylates (weak acids) are mainly un-ionized and, consequently, well absorbed. Conversely, absorption of quinidine (weak base) is enhanced by alkalization of the gastric pH. Similarly, alkalization of the urine increases the ionization of weak acids (salicylates, phenobarbitone), decreases their tubular reabsorption, and increases renal excretion.

The extent of ionization also modifies protein binding and the amount of active free drug. The duration of action of *d*-tubocurarine but not other muscle relaxants is prolonged by acidosis. Curare normally has a single quaternary NH^+_4 grouping, but in acidotic situations it becomes a bis-quarternary compound, which increases its potency.[36]

Although metabolism of atracurium by Hoffman's elimination is pH dependent, hypercapnia induces only a small increase in its duration of action, and recovery is only marginally more rapid in alkalotic conditions.[37] Thus, the effect of acid-base disturbances on pharmacologic activity is multifactorial and difficult to predict.

CONCLUSION

Acid-base disturbances are common in clinical practice. Interpretation of laboratory values may be difficult. However, when the compensatory responses to primary disturbances can be predicted, either graphically or mathematically, it is usually possible to determine the initiating mechanisms.

The effects of the disturbances are wide ranging and include major organ dysfunction and abnormal responses to several drugs. Correction should be directed primarily at reversing the underlying defect. Respiratory disturbances are usually managed by appropriate mechanical ventilation. Metabolic disturbances are more difficult. Although $NaHCO_3$ has been used for more than 50 years to correct metabolic acidosis, it appears that its use has been excessive. In particular, it is ineffective in hypoxia-induced acidosis and may actually worsen the disturbance. The most important goal of therapy is to improve tissue oxygen delivery.

References

1. Bates RG: Determination of pH. Theory and Practice. New York, John Wiley & Sons, 1964.
2. Henderson LJ: The theory of neutrality regulation in the animal organism. Am J Physiol 1908; 21:427.
3. Hasselbalch KA: Die Berechnung der Wasserstoffzahl des Blutes aus der freien und gebundenen Kohlensäure desselben und die Sauerstoffbindung des Blutes als Funktion der Wasserstoffzahl. Biochemie 1917; 78:112.
4. Kassirer JP, Bleich HL: Rapid estimation of plasma carbon dioxide tension from pH and total carbon dioxide content. N Engl J Med 1965; 272:1067.
5. Ream AK, Reitz BA, Silverberg G: Temperature correction of P_{CO_2} and pH in estimating acid-base status. Anesthesiology 1982; 56:41.
6. Rahn H, Reeves RB, Howell BJ: Hydrogen ion regulation, temperature, and evolution. Am Rev Respir Dis 1975; 112:165.
7. Bassein G, Townes BD, Nessly ML, et al: A randomized study of carbon dioxide management during hypothermic cardiopulmonary bypass. Anesthesiology 1990; 72:7.
8. Murkin JM, Farrar JK, Tweed WA, et al: Cerebral autoregulation and flow/metabolism coupling during cardiopulmonary bypass: the influence of Pa_{CO_2} management. Anesth Analg 1987; 66:825.
9. Androgue HJ, Rashad MN, Gorin AB, et al: Assessing acid-base status in circulatory failure. N Engl J Med 1989; 320:1312.
10. Weil MH, Rackow EC, Trevino R, et al: Difference in acid-base state between venous and arterial blood during cardiopulmonary resuscitation. N Engl J Med 1986; 315:153.
11. Arieff AI: Indications for use of bicarbonate in patients with metabolic acidosis. Br J Anaesth 1991; 67:165.
12. Narins RG, Emmett M: Simple and mixed acid-base disorders: a practical approach. Medicine 1987; 56:161.
13. Prys-Roberts C, Kelman GR, Nunn JF: Determination of the in vivo carbon dioxide titration curve of anaesthetized man. Br J Anaesth 1966; 38:500.
14. Kappagoda CT, Linden RJ, Snow HM: An approach to the problems of acid-base balance. Clin Sci 1970; 39:169.
15. Astrup P, Jorgensen K, Siggaard-Andersen O, et al: The acid-base metabolism. A new approach. Lancet 1960; 1:1035.
16. Singer RB, Hastings AB: An improved method for the estimation of disturbances of the acid-base balance of human blood. Medicine 1948; 27:223.
17. Jorgensen K, Astrup P: Standard bicarbonate: its clinical significance, and a new method for its determination. Scand J Clin Lab Invest 1957; 9:122.
18. Schwartz WB, Cohen JJ: The nature of the renal response to chronic disorders of acid-base equilibrium. Am J Med 1978; 64:417.
19. Levine DZ, Jacobson HR: The regulation of renal acid secretion: new observations from studies of distal nephron segments. Kidney Int 1986; 29:1099.
20. Pitts RF: Physiology of the Kidney and Body Fluids. 3rd ed. Boston, Year Book Medical Publishers, 1974.
21. Oliver J, Bourke E: Adaptations in urea and ammonium excretion in metabolic acidosis in the rat. Clin Sci Mol Med 1975; 48:515.
22. Atkinson DE, Bourke E: Metabolic aspects of the regulation of systemic pH. Am J Physiol 1987; 252:F947.
23. Cohen RD: Roles of the liver and kidney in acid-base regulation and its disorders. Br J Anaesth 1991; 67:154.
24. Oliver J, Koelz AM, Costello J, et al: Acid-base alterations in glutamine

metabolism and ureagenesis in perfused muscle and liver of the rat. Eur J Clin Invest 1977; 7:445.

25. Pilkis SJ, El-Maghrabi MR, Claus TH: Fructose-2, 6-diphosphate in control of hepatic gluconeogenesis. Diabetes Care 1990; 13:582.
26. Cotev S, Severinghaus JW: Role of cerebrospinal fluid pH in management of respiratory problems. Anesth Analg 1969; 48:42.
27. Krapf R, Beeler I, Hertner D, et al: Chronic respiratory alkalosis: the effect of sustained hyperventilation on renal regulation of acid-base equilibrium. N Engl J Med 1991; 324:1394.
28. Sykes MK, McNicol MW, Campbell EJM: Respiratory Failure, 2nd ed. Oxford, London, Edinburgh, Melbourne, Blackwell Scientific, 1976.
29. Cohen RD, Woods HF: Clinical and Biochemical Aspects of Lactic Acidosis. Oxford, Blackwell Scientific, 1976.
30. Peretz DL, Scott HM, Duff J: The significance of lactic acidemia in the shock syndrome. Ann NY Acad Sci 1965; 119:1133.
31. Johnson DG, Alberti KGMM: Acid-base balance in metabolic acidosis. Clin Endocrinol Metabol 1983; 12:267.
32. Zilva JF: The origin of acidosis in hyperlactaemia. Ann Clin Biochem 1978; 15:40.
33. Graf H, Leach W, Arieff AI: Evidence for detrimental effect of bicarbonate therapy in hypoxic lactic acidosis. Science 1985; 227:754.
34. Wilson RF, Gibson D, Percinel AK, et al: Severe alkalosis in critically ill surgical patients. Arch Surg 1972; 105:197.
35. Goldberg M, Green SB, Moss ML, et al: Computer-based instruction and diagnosis of acid-base disorders. JAMA 1973; 223:269.
36. Hughes R: The influence of changes in acid-base balance on neuromuscular blockade in cats. Br J Anaesth 1970; 42:658.
37. Hughes R, Chapple DJ: The pharmacology of atracurium: a competing neuromuscular blocking agent. Br J Anaesth 1981; 53:31.

General Reading

Masoro EJ, Seigel PD: Acid-Base Regulation: Its Physiology, Pathophysiology, and the Interpretation of Blood-Gas Analysis. Philadelphia, WB Saunders, 1977.

CHAPTER 44

Allergy and Immunology

JERROLD H. LEVY, M.D.

An allergic reaction is one form of an adverse drug reaction that can occur in humans. Often, however, patients complain of being ''allergic'' to a drug when what they actually have experienced is a form of predictable adverse drug reaction.[1] For example, patients often state they are allergic to an opioid, because it causes nausea. Opioids, however, are known to produce nausea as one of their side effects, by stimulating receptors in the chemotrigger zones. True allergy to a drug is an untoward response that is mediated by an immune mechanism[1] (Table 44–1).

An immune reaction involves activation of either cellular or humoral processes that can interact with many different types of foreign molecular structures called *antigens* to provide host defense. Immunologic mechanisms involve interaction of antigens with either antibodies or specific effector cells or both. If a patient has antibodies against a specific drug or protein, exposure to that agent activates the patient's immune system.[1]

The immune system normally functions to protect the body against external microorganisms and toxins and internal threats from neoplastic cells.[2] However, the immune system can also respond inappropriately and cause allergic reactions. Clinically observed life-threatening allergic reactions to drugs and other foreign substances may represent different types of immune responses.[1, 3] This chapter reviews the life-threatening allergic reactions an anesthesiologist may encounter.

ANTIGENS AND ANTIBODIES

What Are Antigens?

Molecules capable of stimulating an immune response when injected are called *antigens*. Only a few drugs administered by anesthesiologists, such as large polypeptides (chymopapain, latex) and other large macromolecules (dextrans), are complete antigens (Table 44–2).

Neuromuscular blocking agents are one of the few small-molecular-weight compounds or drugs that are complete antigens. The presence of biquarternary ammonium structures allows for bridging of two IgE antibodies to trigger mast cell activation.[1]

Haptens

Most commonly used drugs are simple organic compounds of low molecular weight, usually less than 1000. For such a small molecule to become a complete antigen capable of sensitizing a patient, it must bind to circulating host proteins such as albumin or cellular membranes. Such anesthetic drugs or drug metabolites are called *haptens* and, by themselves, are not antigenic.[4] Some reactive drug metabolites (e.g., the penicilloyl derivative of penicillin) are thought to bind with macromolecules to become antigens, but for most drugs this relationship has not been proved.

What Are Antibodies?

Antibodies are proteins with a molecular weight of approximately 150,000. They are also called *immunoglobulins* and can recognize and bind with specific antigens.[1] The basic structure of the antibody molecule is illustrated in Figure 44–1. Each antibody has at least two heavy chains and two light chains that are bound together by disulfide bonds. The Fab fragment has the ability to bind antigen. The Fc fragment is responsible for the unique biologic properties of the different classes of immunoglobulins (cell binding and activation of the complement system).[5, 6] Once antibodies bind with antigens, they undergo conformational changes to activate either mast cells or the complement cascade.

TABLE 44–1. Characteristics of an Allergic Reaction

Adverse response of host
Produced after injection of a foreign drug/blood product
Mediated by antibodies or sensitized cells
Can be reproduced if foreign substance reinjected

TABLE 44–2. Drugs and Macromolecules That Can Be Foreign Antigens

Chymopapain
Latex
Muscle relaxants
Protamine
Dextrans

743

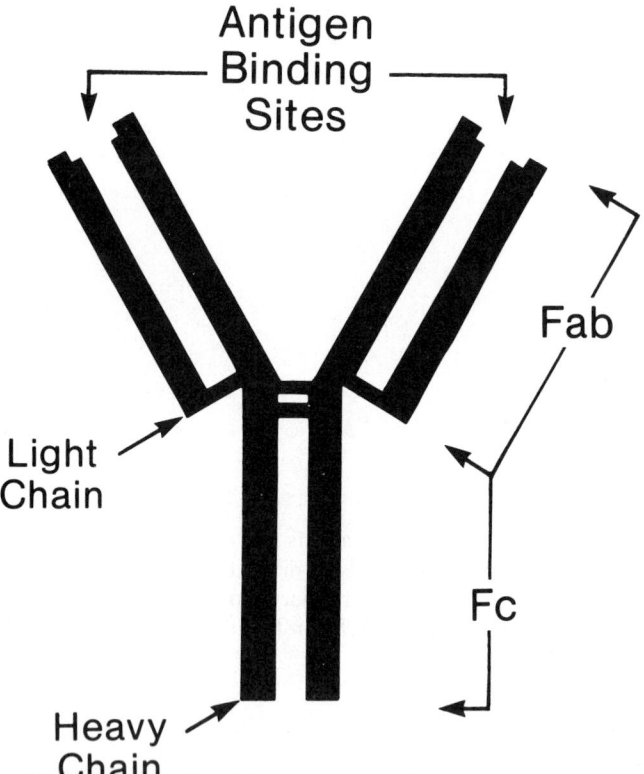

Antigen Binding Sites

Fab

Light Chain

Fc

Heavy Chain

FIGURE 44–1. Simplified basic structural configuration of an antibody molecule representing human immunoglobulin G. Immunoglobulins are composed of two heavy chains and two light chains bound by disulfide linkages (represented by *cross bars*). Papain cleaves the molecule into two Fab fragments and one Fc fragment. Antigen binding occurs on the Fab segments; the Fc segment is responsible for membrane or complement activation. (From Levy JH: Anaphylactic Reactions in Anesthesia and Intensive Care. 2nd ed. Boston, Butterworth-Heinemann, 1992, with permission.)

Antibodies have been developed in the laboratory and used clinically to treat nonimmunologic disorders. Monoclonal antibodies with binding sites directed against endotoxin are clinically available for use in combatting septic shock. Fab antibody fragments are also clinically available for treating digoxin overdose. Because digoxin cannot be dialyzed, the only current therapy in overdoses is to administer Fab fragments that selectively bind to digoxin to inactivate its biologic activity.

ANAPHYLAXIS

What Is the Pathophysiology?

Acute cardiovascular and pulmonary collapse occurs in anaphylaxis, the most severe form of allergic reaction.[1] Studies suggest approximately one in every 2700 hospitalized patients experiences drug-induced anaphylaxis.[7] In 1902, Portier and Richet first used the word *anaphylaxis* (*ana*, ''against,'' and *prophylaxis*, ''protection'') to describe the profound shock and subsequent death that sometimes occurred in dogs immediately after a second parenteral challenge with a foreign antigen.[8]

Life-threatening allergic reactions mediated by antibodies are described as anaphylactic. When antibodies are not responsible for the reaction, when other antibody-independent mechanisms of mast cell or complement activation occur, or when

we are unable to prove antibody involvement, the reaction is called *anaphylactoid*.[1] One cannot distinguish between anaphylactic and anaphylactoid reactions on the basis of clinical observation.

Immunoglobulin–Mediated Reactions

Antigen binding with IgE antibodies initiates anaphylaxis (Fig. 44–2).[6, 9, 10] Prior exposure to the antigen or to a substance of similar structure is required to produce sensitization, although an allergic history may be unknown to the patient. When the foreign substance is reintroduced in the patient, the antigen binds with and bridges two IgE antibodies located on the surfaces of mast cells and basophils. Antigen-antibody binding on these cell surfaces releases stored mediators.[1, 5, 10]

Other chemical mediators, including the lipid-derived compounds—arachidonic acid metabolites (leukotrienes and prostaglandins), platelet activating factor—and the peptide-derived mediators, kinins, subsequently are synthesized and released in response to cellular activation.[11–18] The liberated mediators produce a unique symptom complex of bronchospasm and upper airway edema in the respiratory system; vasodilation and increased capillary permeability in the cardiovascular system; and urticaria in the cutaneous system. Various mediators are released from mast cells and basophils after activation.

What Are the Cardiopulmonary Effects of the Chemical Mediators?

Histamine

Histamine is the most commonly studied mediator of anaphylaxis (Fig. 44–3). Stored in mast cell granules before release, it stimulates H_1 and H_2 receptors. H_1 receptor binding activates vascular endothelium to release endothelium-derived relaxing factor and prostacyclin, potent short-acting mediators that produce vasodilation.[1] H_1 receptor stimulation also causes increased capillary permeability, bronchoconstriction, and smooth muscle contraction.[11, 12]

H_2 receptor activation causes gastric secretion and inhibits mast cell activation.[19] Vasodilation results from the interaction of both H_1 and H_2 receptors. When injected into skin, histamine produces the classic wheal (increased capillary permeability producing tissue edema) and flare (cutaneous vasodilation) response in humans.[20]

Histamine has a very short half-life and undergoes rapid metabolism in humans, catalyzed by the enzymes histamine *N*-methyltransferase and diamine oxidase located in endothelial cells.[1]

Chemotactic Factors of Anaphylaxis

Peptide and lipid products are released from mast cells and basophils, causing granulocyte migration (chemotaxis) and collection at the site of the inflammatory stimulus. Eosinophilic and neutrophilic chemotactic factors of anaphylaxis are small-molecular-weight peptides that produce chemotaxis and activation of polymorphonuclear leukocytes. Eosinophils release enzymes that can inactivate histamine. Granulocyte activation may be responsible for recurrent manifestations of anaphylaxis. Other lipid mediators, including leukotrienes and prostaglandins, may cause activation and directed migration of polymorphonuclear leukocytes.[15, 21]

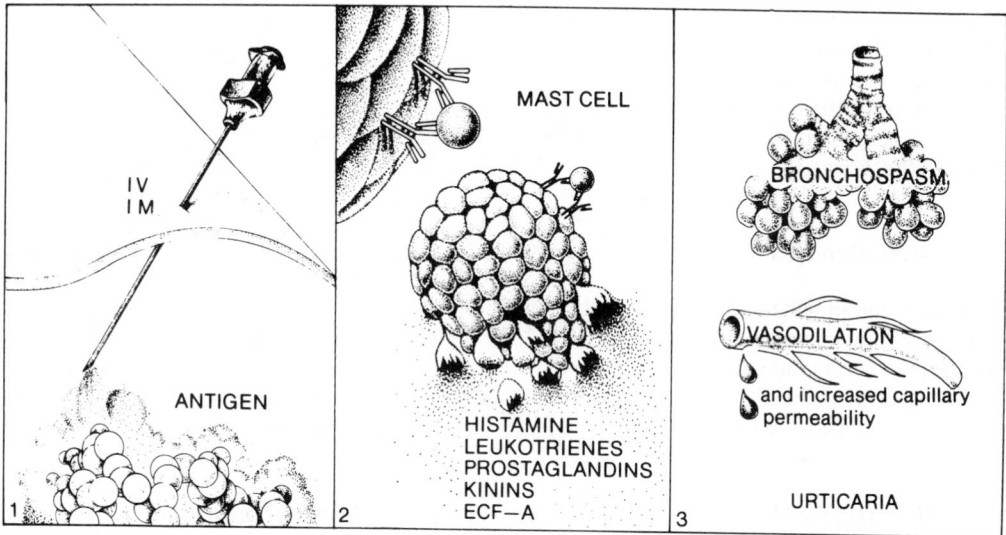

FIGURE 44–2. IgE anaphylaxis (type I immediate hypersensitivity reaction). When an antigen enters a patient parenterally—either intravenously or intramuscularly—it bridges two IgE antibodies on the surface of the mast cells and basophils. In a calcium- and energy-dependent process, cells release various substances (histamine, eosinophilic and other chemotactic factors, lipid mediators [including prostaglandins and leukotrienes], and bradykinin), producing the characteristic pulmonary, cardiovascular, and cutaneous effects. The most severe and life-threatening effects of these vasoactive mediators occur in the respiratory and cardiovascular systems. (Reprinted from Levy JH: Identification and treatment of anaphylaxis. *In* Chemonucleolysis Anaphylaxis: Mechanisms of Action and Strategies for Treatment under General Anesthesia. Chicago, Smith Laboratories, 1982, with permission.)

Leukotrienes

Various leukotrienes are synthesized from arachidonic acid metabolism of phospholipid cell membranes via the lipoxygenase pathway following mast cell activation.[1] The slow-reacting substance of anaphylaxis is a combination of leukotrienes C_4, D_4, and E_4.[13] Leukotrienes produce bronchoconstriction, increased capillary permeability, vasodilatation, coronary vasoconstriction, and myocardial depression.[21]

Prostaglandins

Prostaglandins are the products of arachidonic acid metabolism synthesized by the cyclooxygenase pathway.[23] They are potent mast cell mediators that produce vasodilation, bronchospasm, pulmonary hypertension, and increased capillary permeability.[15, 21] Prostaglandin D_2, the major metabolite of mast cells, produces bronchospasm and vasodilation.[21] Elevated plasma levels of thromboxane B_2 (the metabolite of thromboxane A_2), also a prostaglandin synthesized by mast

cells as well as polymorphonuclear leukocytes, have been demonstrated after protamine reactions associated with pulmonary hypertension.[1, 16]

Kinins

Small peptides called *kinins* are synthesized in mast cells to produce vasodilation, increased capillary permeability, and bronchoconstriction. The exact part that kinins play in anaphylaxis is not well understood. Bradykinin, a potent activator of vascular endothelium, stimulates the release of endothelium-derived relaxing factor and prostacyclin in a manner analogous to H_1 receptor stimulation.[1]

Platelet-Activating Factor

Platelet-activating factor (PAF), an unstored lipid synthesized in activated human mast cells, is an extremely potent biologic material, producing physiologic effects at concentrations as low as 10^{-10} molar.[15] PAF aggregates and activates human platelets, and perhaps leukocytes, to release inflammatory products. PAF causes a profound wheal and flare response, smooth muscle contraction, and increased capillary permeability.[21]

How Is Anaphylaxis Recognized?

When mast cells and basophils are activated and release mediators, their specific end-organ effects produce the clinical syndrome. Antigenic challenge in a sensitized individual usually produces immediate clinical manifestations of anaphylaxis, but the onset may be delayed 2 to 20 minutes.[1, 22, 23] The reaction may include symptoms and signs primarily in the cardiovascular and pulmonary systems.

The manifestations and course of anaphylaxis vary greatly from one affected individual to another.[1] A spectrum of reactions exist, ranging from minor clinical changes through acute

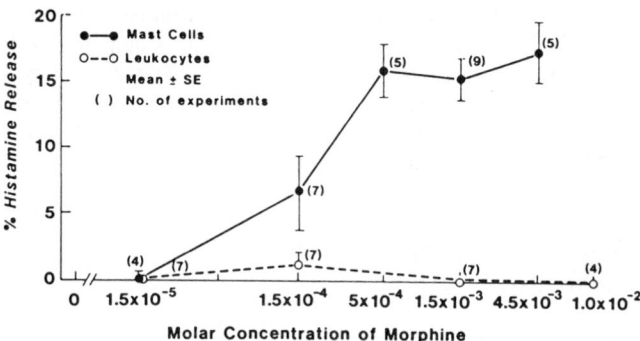

FIGURE 44–3. Per cent histamine release from plasma leukocytes and human skin at increasing concentrations of morphine sulfate. Morphine sulfate induces dose-related histamine release from skin mast cell preparations but not from leukocyte preparations. (From Hermens JM, Eberty JM, Hanifan JM, et al: Comparison of histamine release in human skin mast cells by morphine, fentanyl, and oxymorphone. Anesthesiology 1985; 62:124.)

cardiovascular or pulmonary dysfunction to cardiopulmonary arrest and death.[1] The problems clinicians face when anaphylactic reactions develop in the perioperative period are (1) the unpredictability of an attack, (2) the severity of the attack, and (3) the improbability that the patient will be aware of a prior allergy to an implicated drug.

What Are Non–IgE-Mediated Reactions?

Other immunologic and nonimmunologic mechanisms liberate many of the mediators previously discussed, independent of IgE, creating a clinical syndrome identical to anaphylaxis. Specific pathways important in producing the same spectrum of clinical manifestations are considered later.

What Is Complement Activation?

Triggering Mechanisms

Complement activation can be triggered by either immunologic (antibody mediated, i.e., classic pathway) or nonimmunologic (alternative) pathways. The complement system is a series of multimolecular, self-assembling proteins that resemble the coagulation cascade. Activation of either pathway can liberate biologically active complement fragments of C3 and C5.[24]

Effects

C3a and C5a are called *anaphylatoxins* because they release histamine from mast cells and basophils, contract smooth muscle, and increase capillary permeability.

Granulocytes

In addition, C5a interacts with specific receptors on polymorphonuclear leukocytes and platelets, initiating granulocyte chemotaxis, aggregation, and activation.[25] Aggregated polymorphonuclear leukocytes can form microemboli that sequester in various organs, producing microvascular obstruction. When granulocytes aggregate, they also liberate inflammatory products such as arachidonic acid metabolites, oxygen-free radicals, and lysosomal enzymes.

Antibodies of the IgG class directed against antigenic determinants or granulocyte surfaces can also produce leukocyte aggregation.[1] These antibodies are called *leukoagglutinins* (white blood cell aggregation) and are implicated in the acute lung injury and respiratory distress that often follow transfusions.[1]

Investigators have also implicated complement activation and polymorphonuclear leukocyte aggregation in producing the clinical manifestations of acute pulmonary hypertension and right ventricular dysfunction following protamine reactions,[16] transfusion reactions,[26] adult respiratory distress syndrome,[27] and septic shock.[27]

NONIMMUNOLOGIC RELEASE OF HISTAMINE

Various drugs administered during the perioperative period release histamine in a dose-dependent, nonimmunologic fash-

TABLE 44–3. Drugs That Release Histamine from Human Cutaneous Mast Cells

Antibiotics	Vancomycin
Hyperosmotic agents	Mannitol, ionic radiocontrast media
Induction agents	Sodium thiopental, thiamylal
Muscle relaxants	Atracurium, *d*-tubocurarine, mivacurium, doxacurium
Opioids	Morphine, meperidine, codeine
Polybasic compounds	Protamine

ion (Table 44–3).[28–33] Intravenous administration of morphine, thiopental, atracurium, or vancomycin can release histamine, producing vasodilation, systemic hypotension, and urticaria along the vein of administration.[28, 30, 33]

What Are the Mechanisms?

The mechanisms involved in nonimmunologic histamine release are not well understood but appear to represent noncytotoxic degranulation of mast cells (but not basophils).

Opioids and Neuromuscular Blocking Agents

The opioids, morphine, meperidine, and codeine release histamine in human skin equipotently.[20, 32] However, sufentanil, fentanyl, and alfentanil, all μ-receptor agonists, do not appear to release histamine when administered intravenously.[20]

Different molecular structures release histamine in humans, suggesting that both opioid and nonopioid receptors are involved.[20, 33] The benzylisoquinoline structure of neuromuscular blocking agents appears to be the structure responsible for histamine release in humans.[33]

Our studies evaluating both opioids and neuromuscular blocking agents indicate they all possess, on an equimolar basis, the ability to release histamine.[20, 33] Differences in histamine release reported represent different doses administered and not different abilities to release histamine (Fig. 44–3).

Precautions During Administration

Because mast cells reside in the perivascular spaces of the skin and other tissues, any drug known to release histamine should be given slowly and in a diluted solution (e.g., vancomycin). Prior administration of antihistamines before injecting drugs that are known to release histamine in humans does not directly inhibit histamine release but rather competes with histamine at the receptor and may attenuate decreases in systemic vascular resistance.[34] However, the effect of any drug on systemic vascular resistance may be dependent on other factors in addition to histamine release.[35, 36]

What Is the Appropriate Treatment for Anaphylaxis?

A plan for the treatment of anaphylactic or anaphylactoid reactions is outlined in Table 44–4. These life-saving interventions are essential to treat the hypotension and hypoxia that result from vasodilation, increased capillary permeability, and bronchospasm.[1] The treatment plan is the same for life-threatening anaphylactic or anaphylactoid reactions.

TABLE 44–4. Initial Therapy of Anaphylactic/Anaphylactoid Reactions

Stop administration of antigen if known or suspected
    Blood products
    Muscle relaxants
    Narcotics
    Antibiotics
Secure airway; administer 100% oxygen
Discontinue *all* anesthetic drugs
Infuse volume rapidly
Administer *epinephrine*

Drugs must be *titrated* with careful monitoring. Severe reactions require aggressive therapy and may be associated with refractory shock, pulmonary vasoconstriction and right heart failure, lower respiratory obstruction, or laryngeal obstruction that persist 5 to 32 hours despite appropriate and aggressive therapy.[37] All patients who have had an anaphylactic reaction should be admitted to a postanesthesia care unit (PACU) or intensive care unit for 24 hours of monitoring, because they can develop a recurrence of manifestations after successful treatment.[1, 37]

Initial Therapy

Stop Antigens

Blood products, antibiotics, protamine, or any other infusion should be stopped immediately at the first sign of anaphylactic reaction. Limiting antigen administration may prevent further recruitment of activated mast cells and basophils.

Oxygenation, Ventilation

Profound hypoxemia, airway obstruction, and air trapping can occur during anaphylaxis, as well as ventilation/perfusion abnormalities producing hypoxemia.[1, 38] Always administer 100% oxygen along with airway and ventilatory support as needed. Pulse oximetry, end-tidal carbon dioxide, and arterial blood gases should be monitored during the reaction resuscitation and into the intensive care unit or PACU.[1]

Discontinue All Anesthetic Drugs

Inhalation anesthetic drugs are not the drugs of choice in treating allergy-mediated bronchospasm following anaphylaxis, especially when hypotension is present. These drugs interfere with the body's compensatory response to cardiovascular collapse. Furthermore, halothane sensitizes the myocardium to catecholamines, which must be administered in severe reactions.

Volume Expansion

Hypovolemia rapidly ensues during anaphylactic shock. Fisher has reported a loss of up to 40% of intravascular fluid into the interstitial space during reactions, as demonstrated by hemoconcentration.[39] Therefore, volume expansion is extremely important, in conjunction with epinephrine, in correcting the acute hypotension.

Hypotension. Initially, 2 to 4 L of lactated Ringer's solution, normal saline, or colloid solutions should be administered, keeping in mind that an additional 25 to 50 mL $\cdot$ kg^{-1}

may be necessary with persistent hypotension. Refractory hypotension following volume and epinephrine administration requires additional hemodynamic monitoring, including pulmonary and radial arterial catheterization for accurate assessment of intravascular volume and to guide rational therapeutic interventions.

Pulmonary Edema. Fulminant noncardiogenic pulmonary edema due to acute increases in pulmonary capillary permeability volume can occur after anaphylaxis.[1, 38] This condition is due to loss of intravascular volume into pulmonary interstitial spaces in tissue and requires PEEP or CPAP as well as intravascular volume repletion with careful hemodynamic monitoring until the capillary defect improves.

Epinephrine

Epinephrine is the drug of choice in the initial resuscitation of patients during anaphylactic shock. Epinephrine stimulates α-, β_1-, and β_2-adrenergic receptors. Alpha-adrenergic effects constrict both venous capacitance and arterial resistance vessels to reverse hypotension; β_2-receptor stimulation bronchodilates and inhibits mediator release by increasing cyclic adenosine monophosphate (cAMP) in mast cells and basophils; and β_1-receptor stimulation increases myocardial contractility.

Epinephrine dosage and method of administration depend on a patient's condition. Rapid and timely intervention with common sense is crucial when treating anaphylaxis. During regional or general anesthesia, patients may have altered sympathoadrenergic responses to acute anaphylactic shock. Spinal or epidural anesthesia may partially sympathectomize patients, necessitating earlier intervention with larger doses of catecholamines.[40]

Dosage. In hypotensive patients, 5- to 10-μg intravenous boluses of epinephrine should be titrated to restore blood pressure. Additional volume and incrementally increased doses of epinephrine should be administered until hypotension is corrected.[1] Although an epinephrine infusion is the ideal method to administer the drug, it is usually impossible to infuse the drug through peripheral intravenous routes during acute volume resuscitation.

With cardiovascular collapse, full intravenous cardiopulmonary resuscitative doses of epinephrine, 0.5 to 1.0 mg, should be administered and repeated until hemodynamic stability occurs. In patients without intravenous access, epinephrine can be administered into the endotracheal tube. Epinephrine should not be administered intravenously to patients with normal blood pressure.[1, 41]

Secondary Treatment

After initial treatment, additional therapy may be useful (Table 44–5).

TABLE 44–5. Secondary Therapy for Anaphylactic/Anaphylactoid Reactions

Antihistamines
Catecholamine infusions
Phosphodiesterase inhibitors
Corticosteroids
Sodium bicarbonate
Airway evaluation

Antihistamines

Because H$_1$ receptors mediate many of the adverse effects of histamine, intravenous administration of 0.5 to 1 mg · kg^{-1} of an H$_1$ antagonist, such as diphenhydramine, may be useful in treating acute anaphylaxis. The H$_1$ antagonists currently available for parenteral administration may have antidopaminergic effects and should be given slowly to prevent precipitous hypotension in potentially hypovolemic patients.[1] The indication for administering an H$_2$ antagonist once anaphylaxis has occurred remains unclear.

Catecholamine Infusions

Catecholamines are important first- and second-line therapeutic agents in the treatment of anaphylaxis. Specific direct-acting catecholamines—epinephrine, norepinephrine, and isoproterenol—should be administered as needed for their α-, β$_1$-, and β$_2$-adrenergic effects. Indirect-acting catecholamines, such as dopamine, should not be first-line therapeutic agents.

Epinephrine. Epinephrine infusions may be useful in patients with persistent hypotension or bronchospasm after initial resuscitation.[1] Epinephrine infusions should be started at 4 to 8 μg · min^{-1} and titrated to correct hypotension.

Norepinephrine. Norepinephrine infusions of 4 to 8 μg · min^{-1} may be required in patients with refractory hypotension due to decreased systemic vascular resistance. They should be adjusted to correct hypotension.[1]

Isoproterenol. Isoproterenol infusions can be used in patients with refractory bronchospasm, pulmonary hypertension, or right ventricular dysfunction. The usual starting dose is 0.5 to 1 μg · min^{-1}. Isoproterenol has profound β$_2$-adrenergic effects that can produce systemic vasodilation; therefore, it must be used cautiously in hypotensive or hypovolemic patients.[1]

Phosphodiesterase Inhibitors

Phosphodiesterase inhibitors prevent the catabolism of cyclic nucleotides in cells. The net effect is to increase intracellular levels of cAMP and cyclic guanosine monophosphate.[42] These drugs also act additively with catecholamines to augment the production of intracellular nucleotides.

Aminophylline. Aminophylline is the most commonly used phosphodiesterase inhibitor. Its therapeutic effectiveness in patients with asthma and chronic obstructive pulmonary disease may be due to improvements in diaphragmatic contractility, augmentation of right and left ventricular ejection fraction, and reduction in pulmonary vascular resistance.

Amrinone, Milrinone, Enoximone. The newer cAMP-specific phosphodiesterase inhibitors—drugs such as amrinone, milrinone, and enoximone—also increase biventricular contractility and decrease pulmonary and systemic vascular resistance.

In patients with persistent pulmonary hypertension and right ventricular dysfunction following anaphylactic reactions, these drugs are important therapeutic considerations and should be administered in addition to the catecholamines.

Corticosteroids

Mechanisms of Action. Although corticosteroids are not first-line therapeutic agents, they help to correct anaphylaxis by mechanisms that include decreasing arachidonic acid metabolites, inhibiting phospholipid membrane breakdown, and preventing or attenuating the activation and migration of polymorphonuclear leukocytes.[43, 44]

Corticosteroids may require from 12 to 24 hours to work, and despite their unproven usefulness in treating acute reactions, they often are administered as adjuncts to therapy when refractory bronchospasm or shock occurs after anaphylaxis.

Dosage. The appropriate corticosteroid dose and preparation are not established to treat anaphylaxis; however, 0.25 to 1 g of hydrocortisone appears to be an appropriate dose for IgE-mediated reactions. Alternatively, 1 to 2 g of methylprednisolone (30–35 mg · kg^{-1}) may be useful in treating reactions that are thought to be complement mediated, such as acute pulmonary hypertension following protamine administration, or transfusion reactions.[44] Administering corticosteroids after an anaphylactic reaction may also be important in attenuating the late-phase reactions reported to occur 12 to 24 hours after anaphylaxis.[37]

Sodium Bicarbonate

During anaphylactic shock, acidosis develops rapidly, diminishing the beneficial effects of epinephrine on the heart and systemic vasculature. With refractory hypotension or acidemia, sodium bicarbonate, 0.5 to 1 mEq · kg^{-1}, should be given and repeated every 5 minutes or as indicated by arterial blood gas and pH analysis. (For a detailed analysis of new guidelines for bicarbonate therapy, see Chapter 50.)

Airway Evaluation

Laryngeal edema and airway obstruction can occur after anaphylactoid reactions; therefore, the airway should be evaluated before extubation of the trachea.[1, 37] In patients with persistent facial edema, underlying airway edema can also occur; they should remain intubated until the edema subsides. The development of a significant air leak after endotracheal tube cuff deflation is useful in assessing airway patency before extubation of the trachea. If there is any question of airway edema, direct laryngoscopy should be performed before extubation.

PERIOPERATIVE ANAPHYLAXIS

What Drugs Are Implicated?

Many of the potentially offending agents have already been discussed. Almost every drug, at some time, has been implicated in producing an anaphylactic reaction.[1, 45–61] The incidence of perioperative anaphylaxis varies, depending on the country reporting, but appears to be approximately 1 in 5000 to 25,000 anesthetized patients.

Agents most often implicated are listed in Table 44–6. Latex (rubber) is an environmental antigen that is ubiquitous in anesthetic, intravenous, and operative equipment. Patients who have spina bifida and who have undergone multiple surgical procedures, as well as health workers, are potentially at increased risk for anaphylaxis to latex. These individuals appear to be sensitized from repeated exposure to this large, foreign plant antigen.

Drugs that are nonimmunologic histamine releasers may cause a higher incidence of adverse drug reactions and produce

TABLE 44–6. Agents Most Often Implicated in Perioperative Anaphylaxis

Antibiotics
Blood products
Chymopapain
Induction agents
Latex
Neuromuscular blocking agents
Protamine

acute cardiovascular dysfunction with rapid intravenous administration. Vancomycin, which produces its adverse effects by histamine release, is an important example. Slow administration of a diluted solution is important to prevent severe reactions.

How Is an Allergic Reaction Recognized?

Only a small percentage of adverse drug reactions are allergic in nature (Table 44–7).

Signs and Symptoms

Observed clinical signs and symptoms of the allergic reaction do not resemble known pharmacologic actions of the drug. The temporal relationship between exposure to the drug and clinical manifestations of the adverse drug reaction is the most important information to determine which administered drugs were the cause of a suspected allergic reaction.[62]

Although the reaction may produce a life-threatening response in the cardiopulmonary system (anaphylaxis), other clinical presentations of drug allergy include cutaneous eruptions, fever, and pulmonary reactions.[62] The reaction can usually be reproduced by giving very small doses of the suspected drug or other agents possessing similar or cross-reacting chemical structures.

On occasion, drug-specific antibodies or lymphocytes that react with the suspected drug have been identified, although this test is seldom diagnostically useful in practice. As with adverse drug reactions in general, the reaction usually subsides within several days after discontinuation of the drug.[62]

Historical Factors

Life-threatening allergic reactions are more likely to occur in patients with a history of allergy, atopy, or asthma.[46] Nevertheless, because the incidence is low, the presence of such a history is not a reliable predictor that an allergic reaction will occur and does not mandate that these patients should be investigated or pretreated or that specific drugs be selected or avoided. Drugs and foreign substances implicated in producing adverse drug reactions may have both immunologic and non-immunologic mechanisms.

TABLE 44–7. Characteristics of an Allergic Reaction

Occur in a small percentage of patients
Unrelated to known pharmacologic drug actions
Temporally related to the suspected drug administration
Produced by the presence of an immunospecific antibody

How Should Patients Be Evaluated?

Identification of the drug responsible for a suspected allergic reaction still depends on a high degree of clinical suspicion implicating the temporal sequence of drug administration. Conventional in vivo and in vitro methods to diagnose allergic reactions to most anesthetic drugs are either unavailable or not applicable to supporting the diagnosis of an allergic reaction.

The most important factor in diagnosis is a physician's awareness that an untoward event may be related to a drug that a patient received.[1, 62] Always be aware that any drug may produce a life-threatening anaphylactic reaction.

A clinical history is extremely important when evaluating whether an adverse drug reaction is allergic and whether the drug can be readministered. Although a prior allergic reaction to the drug in question is important, it is rarely ascertained. Although an anesthesiologist commonly administers small "test" doses of anesthetic drugs, these doses represent large numbers of molecules and have nothing to do with immunologic doses.[1]

Specific Tests

The demonstration of drug-specific IgE antibodies is generally accepted as evidence that a patient may be at risk for anaphylaxis if the drug is administered.[62] Different clinically available tests to confirm or diagnose drug allergy have been reported and are individually considered in Table 44–8.

For a patient who has had a suspected anaphylactic reaction, the causative agent should be identified to prevent readministration. When one particular drug has been administered and a clear correlation between time of administration and occurrence of reaction can be demonstrated, then testing may be unnecessary and the drug should not be readministered. However, when patients simultaneously receive multiple drugs (e.g., induction agent, opioid, muscle relaxant, and antibiotic), determining which particular drug caused the reaction is more difficult.

When patients want to know which drug was the culprit or when patients are scheduled for several other procedures, some degree of allergy evaluation should be undertaken to determine the implicated drug. Unfortunately, few in vitro tests exist for anesthetic drugs. Currently available allergy tests are discussed.

Radioallergosorbent Test

The radioallergosorbent test detects specific IgE antibodies directed toward particular antigens.[63] In this test, antigens are linked to an insoluble matrix such as sepharose, cellulose, or paper to make an immunoabsorbent and are then incubated with the serum from the patient to be evaluated so that immunospecific antibodies directed toward the antigen can bind. After washing, the antigen-antibody complex on the immunoabsorbent is incubated with radioactive iodine–labeled anti-

TABLE 44–8. Tests Used to Evaluate Patients After Anaphylaxis

Radioallergosorbent testing
Enzyme-linked immunosorbent assay testing
Intradermal testing (skin testing)

bodies directed against human IgE, and the complex is counted in a scintillation counter to evaluate the concentration of specific IgE.

The radioallergosorbent test is more quantitative than skin tests and avoids the risk of re-exposure of an antigen to a patient who had a life-threatening anaphylactic reaction. However, it is more expensive, and the antigens available for anesthetic drug testing are limited. Radioallergosorbent testing has been used to detect the presence of IgE antibodies to meperidine, protamine, muscle relaxants, propofol, and thiopental.[1, 64, 65] Two major limitations of this test are the commercial inavailability of a drug prepared as an antigen and potential false-positive test results.

Enzyme-Linked Immunosorbent Assay

The enzyme-linked immunosorbent assay also measures antigen-specific antibodies. The basis of this test is similar to the radioallergosorbent test. IgE antibodies directed against the antigen in question are determined by the addition of an anti-IgE coupled to peroxidase, an enzyme that acts as a chromogen. A colorless substrate is converted by peroxidase to produce a colored by-product.

The enzyme-linked immunosorbent assay has been used to demonstrate IgE antibodies to chymopapain and protamine and has been developed to screen patients for other antibodies to infectious agents such as the human immunodeficiency virus, but no tests for anesthetic drugs are clinically available.[1]

Intradermal Testing (Skin Testing)

Skin testing is the method most widely used to confirm specific sensitivity in patients who have had anaphylactic reactions to anesthetic drugs.[66–69] After intradermal antigen injection, histamine released from cutaneous mast cells causes flare and wheal.

Fisher has used this technique extensively, and multiple reports from his group and others suggest that it is a safe and useful method for establishing a diagnosis in most cases of suspected anaphylactic reactions.[66, 67] Intradermal testing can determine cross-sensitivity among drugs of similar structures, an especially important factor when evaluating patients after reactions to the neuromuscular blocking agents.

Skin testing for local anesthetics is considered a direct challenge or provocative dose testing.[69] Local anesthetic drugs are injected in increasing quantities under controlled circumstances. This test determines if an individual can safely receive amide derivatives (e.g., lidocaine), and it can also be used to determine sensitivity to the *para*-aminobenzoic ester agents (e.g., tetracaine or procaine).

SUMMARY

Allergic reactions are adverse drug reactions that are produced by pathologic activation of the immune system. The most life-threatening form of allergic reaction is anaphylaxis, which can manifest as acute cardiovascular and pulmonary dysfunction produced by physiologic responses to the mediators released from mast cells and basophils. Other immune and nonimmune pathways may also be activated to produce a similar clinical syndrome of cardiopulmonary dysfunction.

Recognition and appropriate therapy are important clinical considerations. Because any drug can potentially produce ana-

phylaxis, anticipation that a drug may be implicated in perioperative cardiovascular collapse is important. Certain drugs and environmental antigens are more likely to be implicated.

Although different tests have been studied to evaluate patients after anaphylaxis, skin testing is the most often reported and readily available method.

References

1. Levy JH: Anaphylactic Reactions in Anesthesia and Intensive Care. 2nd ed. Boston, Butterworth-Heinemann, 1992.
2. Stevenson GW, Hall SC, Rudnick S, et al: The effect of anesthetic agents on the human immune response. Anesthesiology 1990; 72:542.
3. Walton B: Anaesthesia, surgery, and immunology. Anaesthesia 1978; 33:322.
4. Roitt I, Brostoff J, Male D (eds). Immunology. St Louis, CV Mosby, 1989.
5. Metcalf DD: Effector cell heterogeneity in immediate hypersensitivity reactions. Clin Rev Allergy 1982; 1:311.
6. Ishizaka T: Analysis of triggering events in mast cells for immunoglobulin E-mediated histamine release. J Allergy Clin Immunol 1981; 67:90.
7. Porter J, Jick H: Drug-induced anaphylaxis, convulsions, deafness, and extrapyramidal symptoms. Lancet 1977; 1:587.
8. Portier MM, Richet C: De l'action anaphylactique de certains venins. C R Soc Biol 1902; 54:170.
9. Gomez E, Corrado OJ, Baldwin DL, et al: Direct in vivo evidence for mast cell degranulation during allergen-induced reactions in man. J Allergy Clin Immunol 1986; 78:637.
10. Kazimierczak W, Diamant B: Mechanisms of histamine release in anaphylactic and anaphylactoid reactions. Prog Allergy 1978; 4:295.
11. Ginsburg R, Bristow MR, Stinson EB, et al: Histamine receptors in the human heart. Life Sci 1980; 26:2245.
12. Majno G, Palade GE: Studies on inflammation. I. The effect of histamine and serotonin on vascular permeability: an electron microscopic study. J Biosphys Biochem Cytol 1961; 11:571.
13. Parker CW: Leukotrienes: Their metabolism, structure, and role in allergic responses. In Leukotrienes and Other Lipoxygenase Products. Samuelsson B, Paoletti R (eds). New York, Raven Press, 1982, pp 115–126.
15. Schulman ES, Newball HH, Demers LM, et al: Anaphylactic release of thromboxane A$_2$, prostaglandin D$_2$, and prostacyclin from human lung parenchyma. Am Rev Respir Dis 1981; 124:402.
16. Morel DR, Zapol WM, Thomas SJ, et al: C5a and thromboxane generation associated with pulmonary vaso- and bronchoconstriction during protamine reversal of heparin. Anesthesiology 1987; 66:597.
17. Meier HL, Kaplan AP, Lichtenstein LM, et al: Anaphylactic release of a prekallikrein activator from human lung in vitro. Clin Invest 1983; 72:574.
18. Weiss ME, Adkinson NF, McFadden R Jr, et al: Airway constriction in normal humans produced by inhalation of leukotriene D. JAMA 1983; 249:2814.
19. Reinhardt D, Borchard V: H$_1$ receptor antagonists: comparative pharmacology and clinical use. Klin Wochenschr 1982; 60:983.
20. Levy JH, Brister NW, Shearin WA, et al: Wheal and flare responses to opioids in humans. Anesthesiology 1989; 70:756.
21. Pavek K, Wegmann A, Nordström L, et al: Cardiovascular and respiratory mechanisms in anaphylactic and anaphylactoid shock reactions. Klin Wochenschr 1982; 60:941.
22. Delage C, Irey NS: Anaphylactic deaths: a clinicopathologic study of 43 cases. J Forensic Sci 1972; 17:525.
23. Goldberg M: The allergic response and its treatment. Curr Rev Clin Anesth 1985; 5:153.
24. Frank MM. Complement: a brief review. J Allergy Clin Immunol 1988; 84:411.
25. Dubois M, Lotze MT, Diamond WI, et al: Pulmonary shunting during leukoagglutinin-induced noncardiogenic pulmonary edema. JAMA 1989; 244:2186.
26. Teissner B, Brandslund I, Grunnet N, et al: Acute complement activation during an anaphylactoid reaction to blood transfusion and the disappearance rate of C3c and C3d from the circulation. J Clin Lab Immunol 1983; 12:63.
27. Hammerschmidt DE, Weaver LJ, Hudson LD, et al: Association of complement activation and elevated plasma-C5a with adult respiratory distress syndrome. Lancet 1980; 1:947.
28. Rosow CE, Moss J, Philbin DM, et al: Histamine release during morphine and fentanyl anesthesia. Anesthesiology 1982; 56:93.

29. Hirshman CA, Edelstein RA, Eastman CL: Histamine release by barbiturates in human mast cells. Anesthesiology 1985; 63:353.

30. Levy JH, Kettlekamp N, Goertz P, et al: Histamine release by vancomycin: a mechanism for hypotension in man. Anesthesiology 1987; 67:122.

31. Hermens JM, Ebertz JM, Hanifin JM, et al: Comparison of histamine release in human skin mast cells by morphine, fentanyl, and oxymorphone. Anesthesiology 1983; 62:124.

32. Casale TB, Bowman S, Kaliner M: Induction of human cutaneous mast cell degranulation by opiates and endogenous opioid peptides: evidence for opiate and nonopiate receptor participation. J Allergy Clin Immunol 1984; 73:775.

33. Levy JH, Adelson DM, Walker BF: Wheal and flare responses to muscle relaxants in humans. Agents Actions 1991; 34:302.

34. Philbin DM, Moss J, Akins CW, et al: The use of H_1 and H_2 histamine antagonists with morphine anesthesia: a double-blind study. Anesthesiology 1981; 55:292.

35. Hirshman CA, Downes H, Butler J: Relevance of plasma histamine levels to hypotension. Anesthesiology 1982; 57:424.

36. Levy JH, Hug CC: Cardiopulmonary bypass as a model to study the effects of drugs on myocardial function. Br J Anaesth 1988; 60:35S.

37. Stark BJ, Sullivan TJ: Biphasic and protracted anaphylaxis. J Allergy Clin Immunol 1986; 78:76.

38. Levy JH, Rockoff MR: Anaphylaxis to meperidine. Anesth Analg 1982; 61:301.

39. Fisher MM: Blood volume replacement in acute anaphylactic cardiovascular collapse related to anaesthesia. Br J Anaesth 1977; 49:1023.

40. Barnett A, Hirshman CA: Anaphylactic reaction to cephapirin during spinal anesthesia. Anesth Analg 1979; 58:337.

41. Levy JH: Cardiovascular changes during anaphylactic/anaphylactoid reactions in man. J Clin Anesth 1989; 1:426.

42. Levy JH, Ramsay JM, Bailey JM: Pharmacokinetics and pharmacodynamics of phosphodiesterase III inhibitors. J Cardiothorac Anesth 1990; 4(S):7.

43. Hammerschmidt DE, White JG, Craddock PR, et al: Corticosteroids inhibit complement-induced granulocyte aggregation. A possible mechanism for their efficacy in shock states. J Clin Invest 1979; 63:798.

44. Sheagren JN: Septic shock and corticosteroids (Editorial). N Engl J Med 1981; 305:456.

45. Laxenaire MC, Moneret-Vautrin DA, Vervloet D, et al: Accidents anaphylactoides graves peranesthetiques. Ann Fr Anesth Reanim 1985; 4:30.

46. Fisher M McD, Outhred A, Bowey CJ: Can clinical anaphylaxis to anaesthetic drugs be predicted from allergic history? Br J Anaesth 1987; 59:690.

47. Fisher M McD, Munro I: Life-threatening anaphylactoid reactions to muscle relaxants. Anesth Analg 1983; 62:559.

48. Laxenaire MC, Moneret-Vautrin DA, Watkins J: Diagnosis of the causes of anaphylactoid anaesthetic reactions. Anaesthesia 1983; 38:147.

49. Vervloet D, Nizankowska E, Arnaud A, et al: Adverse reactions to suxamethonium and other muscle relaxants under general anesthesia. J Allergy Clin Immunol 1983; 71:552.

50. Assem ESK, Frost PG, Levis RD: Anaphylactoid-like reaction to suxamethonium. Anaesthesia 1981; 36:405.

51. Bennet MJ, Anderson LK, McMillan JC, et al: Anaphylactic reaction during anesthesia associated with positive intradermal skin test to fentanyl. Can Anaesth Soc J 1986; 33:75.

52. Hilgard P: Immunological reactions to blood and blood products. Br J Anesth 1979; 51:45.

53. Sheffer AL, Pennoyer DS: Management of adverse drug reactions. J Allergy Clin Immunol 1984; 74:580.

54. Levy JH, Zaidan JR, Faraj B: Prospective evaluation of risk of protamine reactions in NPH insulin-dependent diabetics. Anesth Analg 1986; 65:739.

55. Doolan L, McKenzie I, Krafchek J, et al: Protamine sulphate hypersensitivity. Anesth Intensive Care 1981; 9:147.

56. Goldberg M: Systemic reactions to intravascular contrast media. A guide for the anesthesiologist. Anesthesiology 1984; 60:46.

57. Isbister JP, Fisher M McD: Adverse effects of plasma volume expanders. Anesth Intensive Care 1980; 8:145.

58. Colman WR: Paradoxical hypotension after volume expansion with plasma protein fraction. N Engl J Med 1978; 299:97.

59. Ring K, Messmer K: Incidence and severity of anaphylactoid to colloid volume substitutes. Lancet 1977; 1:466.

60. Gold M, Swartz JS, Braude BM, et al: Intraoperative anaphylaxis: an association with latex sensitivity. J Allergy Clin Immunol 1991; 87:662.

61. Nguyen DH, Burns MW, Shapiro GG, et al: Intraoperative cardiovascular collapse secondary to latex allergy. J Urol 1991; 146(2):571.

62. De Swarte RD: Drug allergy—problems and strategies. J Allergy Clin Immunol 1984; 74:209.

63. Johansson SGO: In vitro diagnosis of reagin-mediated allergic diseases. Allergy 1978; 33:292.

64. Baldo BA, Fisher MM: Detection of serum IgE antibodies that react with alcuronium and tubocurarine after life-threatening reactions to muscle relaxants. Anaesth Intensive Care 1983; 11:194.

65. Harle DG, Baldo BA, Smal MA, et al: Detection of thiopentone-reactive IgE antibodies following anaphylactoid reactions during anesthesia. Clin Allergy 1986; 16:493.

66. Fisher MM: Intradermal testing after anaphylactoid reaction to anaesthetic drugs: practical aspects of performance and interpretation. Anaesth Intensive Care 1984; 12:115.

67. Fisher MM, Munro I: Life threatening, anaphylactoid reactions to muscle relaxants. Anesth Analg 1983; 62:559.

68. Sage D: Intradermal drug testing following anaphylactoid reactions during anesthesia. Anaesth Intensive Care 1981; 9:381.

69. Shatz M: Skin testing and incremental challenge in the evaluation of adverse reactions to local anesthetics. J Allergy Clin Immunol 1984; 74:606.

CHAPTER 45

Myocardial Ischemia and Dysfunction

MARTIN J. LONDON, M.D.

MARK RYAN, M.D.

Perioperative myocardial ischemia presents a complex and often frustrating series of diagnostic and therapeutic problems for an anesthesia practitioner. An increasing number of clinical studies suggest that vigorous detection and therapy of perioperative ischemia significantly improve patients' outcome. Although patients with manifest or occult coronary artery disease (CAD) are the largest group at risk for developing ischemia and postoperative infarction, clinical situations occur in which ischemia may develop *in the absence* of CAD. ST segment changes suggestive of ischemia have been reported in neonates undergoing cardiac surgery for congenital lesions and in otherwise healthy parturients undergoing cesarean section. However, the implications of ischemia in patients with CAD are the primary emphasis here. They are discussed in detail in the following pages.

PERIOPERATIVE MYOCARDIAL ISCHEMIA

What Are the Hemodynamic Causes?

In the simplest pathophysiologic terms (i.e., assuming normal coronary arteries and myocardium), ischemia results from a significant imbalance of myocardial oxygen (O_2) supply and demand (Fig. 45–1). Although the basic determinants appear to be straightforward, the relations between them are not. Recall that they are components of a remarkably complex homeostatic system; they exert either negative or positive "gains" within the system; and they act in varying combinations. Thus, a clinician must strive to "dissect" the system to its simplest level first. This process is usually straightforward, although in sicker patients, complex interactions are more likely to occur.

Heart Rate

Although indices derived from various parameters, either noninvasive (e.g., rate pressure product, the product of heart rate and systolic blood pressure) or invasive (e.g., tension-time index, the product of mean systolic pressure and systolic duration), have been used to estimate myocardial O_2 consumption ($M\dot{V}O_2$), the bulk of evidence suggests that tachycardia is the most important clinical variable.[1] A distinct trend in clini-

cal practice is to emphasize control of heart rate as a major goal of perioperative hemodynamic management. Heart rate is not only a key determinant of myocardial O_2 demand; it is also a critical determinant of myocardial O_2 supply, moderating the time during which coronary blood flow occurs (diastolic perfusion time). In the left ventricle, blood flow is restricted almost exclusively to diastole because systolic compression of intramural coronary arteries "throttles" forward blood flow. The relationship between heart rate and diastolic time is nonlinear, with small changes in rate producing large increases in diastolic time, especially at lower heart rates[2] (Fig. 45–2).

Blood Pressure

That control of heart rate is more important than blood pressure was emphasized by Loeb and colleagues, who paced awake patients with CAD to heart rates of approximately 140 beats per minute, followed by elevation of blood pressure with methoxamine to systolic values of approximately 200 mm Hg.[3] Chest pain occurred in 85% of patients with pacing, versus only 30% with hypertension. Similarly, ST segment depression occurred in 70% with pacing but only 15% with hypertension. The critical lesson here is that hypertension (with maintenance of a normal preload) increases rather than decreases coronary perfusion pressure.

Buffington, using a highly controlled canine model, demonstrated that the ratio of mean arterial blood pressure (MAP) to heart rate, rather than their product, is more closely correlated with regional ischemia.[4] Between MAPs of 60 and 120 mm Hg, ischemia occurred only when heart rate exceeded the MAP (MAP/heart rate ratio <1.0). This observation is a useful rule of thumb to consider when one treats ischemia believed to be related to hemodynamic insufficiency, rather than that mediated by local factors, vasomotor tone, or platelet plug. Despite these laboratory findings, clinical studies have been conflicting, most likely because of the complexity of measuring ischemia.

What Is the Ischemic Cascade?

The *ischemic cascade* is a progressive sequence of pathophysiologic events triggered by ischemia.[5] It is commonly

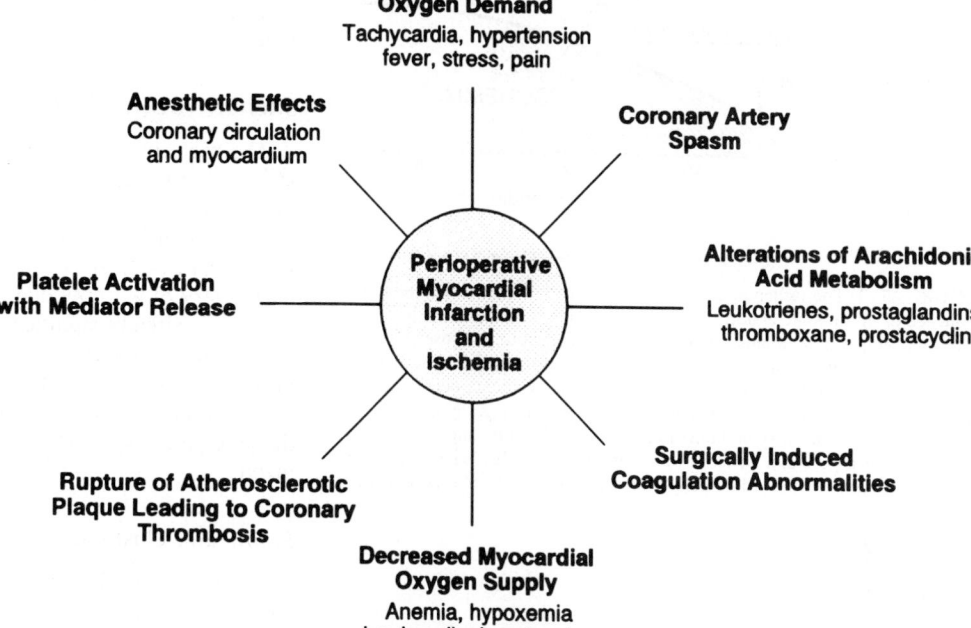

FIGURE 45–1. Many factors, both morphologic and physiologic, influence myocardial oxygen balance. The anesthesiologist can effectively manipulate most of the physiologic and hemodynamic factors. However, our ability to influence the many factors involved in the pathogenesis of ischemia directly related to coronary artery disease is very limited. (From London MJ: Silent ischemia and postoperative infarction. J Cardiothorac Vasc Anesth 1990; 4(Suppl 1):60.)

displayed as a temporal sequence starting at the onset of ischemia (Fig. 45–3), although it can also be depicted by plotting myocardial O_2 supply versus demand. It illustrates the most sensitive signs of ischemia, as well as the temporal relations between them.

The earliest steps of the cascade include alterations of diastolic compliance with an increase in left ventricular end-diastolic pressure (LVEDP). After this change, systolic function is altered and regional wall motion abnormalities occur. The latter may be observed with echocardiography. Subsequently, surface electrocardiographic (ECG) changes occur,

and later still, anginal chest pain (in awake patients). A global reduction in ventricular function occurs only if the compensatory response of adjacent nonischemic myocardium is inadequate or if the ischemia is global (i.e., subendocardial ischemia due to severe hypotension).

Although the cascade is best considered a continuum, in certain instances, various signs may not occur (e.g., no angina with silent myocardial ischemia [SMI]). Also, the signs of ischemia may not reverse in the same temporal order in which they occurred (e.g., consider the persistence of wall motion abnormalities despite resolution of ECG changes with stunned myocardium).

What Is the Most Useful Clinical Tool to Detect Ischemia?

Three major clinical tools are used to detect myocardial ischemia: ECG, two-dimensional transesophageal echocardiography (TEE), and pulmonary artery (PA) catheterization.[5] The characteristics and limitations of these monitors are considered in Table 45–1. TEE is the most sensitive monitor. However, ECG is the most useful clinical tool because it can be used continuously during the perioperative period; it is truly noninvasive; it is easily automated, quantitated, and trended; and a wealth of literature documents its sensitivity and specificity.

What Types of Ischemia Occur Perioperatively?

Subendocardial

Subendocardial ischemia, manifested as ST segment depression (horizontal or downsloping of >1 mm at 60–80 msec after the J point, or slowly upsloping depression of >1.5–2.0 mm), is the most common type of perioperative ischemia.[6]

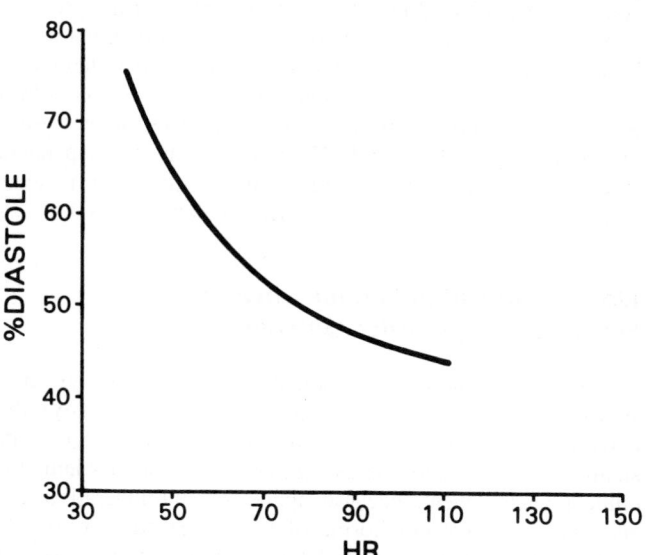

FIGURE 45–2. The relation between heart rate and the per cent of the cardiac cycle spent in diastole is shown. Note the nonlinear relationship in which small changes in heart rate produce large increases in diastolic time especially at low heart rates (e.g., 15% increase from 70 to 50 bpm). HR = Heart rate (in bpm). (From Boudoulas H, Rittgers SE, Lewis RP, et al: Changes in diastolic time with various pharmacologic agents. Circulation 1979; 60:165.)

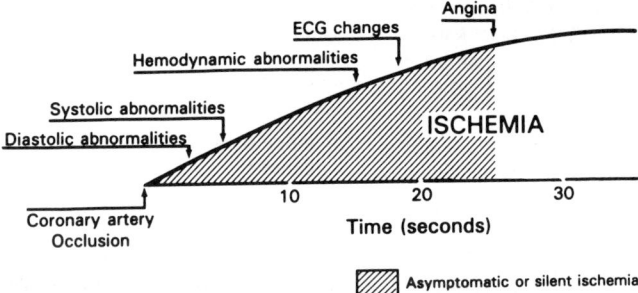

FIGURE 45–3. The ischemic cascade depicted as the approximate temporal sequence of physiologic abnormalities following onset of ischemia. Note that the exact sequence is variable, particularly with regard to the onset of ECG, hemodynamic changes, and angina. In the majority of instances, ECG changes occur earlier than depicted here. Hemodynamic changes (e.g., decreased cardiac output) only occur after compensatory mechanisms (e.g., hyperkinesis of adjacent nonischemic myocardium) fail. In many patients, angina does not occur ("silent myocardial ischemia"). (From Kennedy HL, Wiens RD: Ambulatory (Holter) electrocardiography and myocardial ischemia. Am Heart J 1989; 117:165.)

Transmural

With more profound imbalance of the supply/demand ratio, transmural ischemia, manifested as ST segment elevation of similar magnitude, may occur (in leads without a pre-existing Q wave). In patients undergoing cardiac surgery, particularly coronary artery bypass grafting, transmural ischemia is common and may result from various processes including coronary vasospasm or coronary embolism (air or particulate debris) (Fig. 45–4).

What Characteristics of Ischemia Are Unique to Patient's with Coronary Artery Disease?

In patients with CAD, a unique set of factors may complicate the straightforward O_2 supply/demand schema. CAD is a complex morphologic process. Thus, an understanding of how its pathophysiology can result in various clinical presentations (i.e., chest pain, unstable angina, subendocardial or transmural

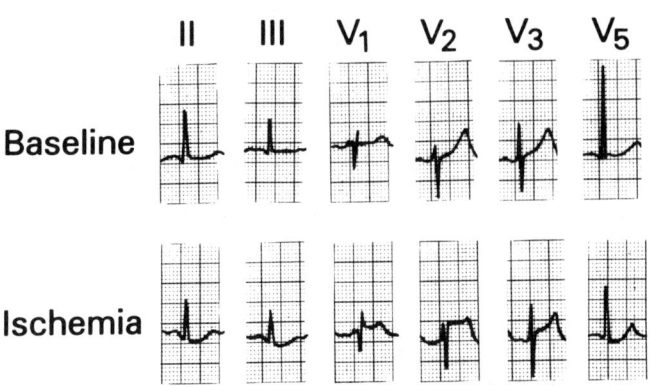

FIGURE 45–4. Ischemic episode diagnostic of transmural ischemia in the distribution of the left anterior descending artery with ST segment elevation in $V_1–V_3$ (verified by anterior wall akinesis on transesophageal echocardiography). Changes in the routine monitoring leads (II and V_5) are reciprocal and of much lower magnitude and do not engender the same degree of clinical concern. (From London MJ, Hollenberg M, Wong MG, et al: Intraoperative myocardial ischemia: localization by continuous 12 lead electrocardiography. Anesthesiology 1988; 69:233.)

infarction) is essential (Fig. 45–5).[7, 8] Further complicating simple analysis are the concepts of SMI and stunned/hibernating myocardium.

Silent Myocardial Ischemia

The majority of patients with CAD have most of their episodes of ST segment depression, suggestive of myocardial ischemia, in the absence of chest pain, with only minor or no alterations in heart rate and blood pressure.[9] The underlying mechanism of SMI is a transient reduction in regional coronary artery blood flow due to increased vasomotor tone at the site of an already significant coronary lesion (i.e., >70% reduction in cross-sectional area). Increased α-adrenergic tone is probably responsible, although other hormonal mediators may be important. In the past, SMI was believed to be unique to diabetic patients, in whom painless infarction was well recognized.

Stable and Unstable Angina

A number of clinical studies using differing diagnostic modalities including exercise treadmill testing, ambulatory ST segment monitoring, invasive catheterization (i.e., coronary sinus sampling), and radionuclear perfusion scanning have conclusively proved the existence of SMI in patients with CAD.[10, 11] It is prognostic for adverse outcomes in certain subgroups of patients with CAD, particularly those with unstable angina and in those recovering from a recent myocardial infarction (MI). However, controversy surrounds its significance in patients with stable angina pectoris; the extent to which various cardiac medications are effective in suppressing it; and how aggressive to be in its treatment.

Silent Perioperative Myocardial Ischemia

Recent perioperative studies using various ECG techniques for perioperative monitoring (e.g., ambulatory ST segment monitors, "routine" operating room [OR] ECG monitors, computerized 12-lead monitors), have confirmed the presence of SMI in the surgical population,[12–16] documenting that it is at least as common as hemodynamically mediated ischemia. In this setting, SMI may not be entirely benign. Patients with it are at significantly increased risk for postoperative cardiac morbidity or mortality (Table 45–2). Its role as an independent risk factor is underscored by its similar frequency in patients with and without preoperative clinical markers of CAD.

Does Treatment of Perioperative ST Segment Changes Alter Outcome?

Despite the finding that patients with ischemia are at a statistically increased risk for morbidity (high sensitivity), the percentage of those who actually suffer an infarct is very small. This observation poses significant logistic problems for clinical management, because aggressive intraoperative and early postoperative monitoring of very large numbers of patients would be necessary to detect a single patient who will have an infarct (low positive predictive value).

Probably the most important information from these studies is that patients without perioperative ischemia are at exceedingly low (or no) risk for morbidity (very high negative predictive value). This finding has particular significance in guid-

TABLE 45-1. Clinical Assessment of Perioperative Myocardial Ischemia

	ECG	TEE	PAOP
Ischemia detection	Electrical: QRST abnormalities	Wall motion, compliance changes (Doppler)	Compliance changes
Other uses	Rhythm, conduction	Volume, contractility, CO, valve function	CO, pressures, resistances
Invasiveness	Low	Medium	High
Limitations	Bundle branch and other conduction blocks, Q wave leads, open chest	Esophageal disease, technical factors (spatial relations of heart to esophagus)	Valvular pathology, severe pulmonary hypertension
Sensitivity for ischemia	Medium	High	Low
Specificity for ischemia	High	Medium	Low
Analysis	Easy, automated	Difficult, not automated	Medium
Expense	$5000-10,000/unit	$100,000-200,000/unit	$50-250/catheter
Utility	Perioperative	Intraoperative	Perioperative

Abbreviations: TEE = transesophageal echocardiography; PAOP = pulmonary artery occlusion pressure; CO = cardiac output.

ing the length of intensive care unit (ICU) stay necessary for postoperative cardiac monitoring of high-risk patients. Remember, however, that these studies have not yet answered the most important question: Does treatment of perioperative ST segment changes alter adverse outcome, or is it simply a marker of a pathophysiologic process over which we may have little control?

When Is a Patient with Coronary Artery Disease Ready for Surgery?

Deciding whether a patient with CAD is ready for surgery is a continually evolving science (see also Chapter 9). In the past, it was left up to an internist or cardiologist to "clear" a patient for surgery. This approach usually was based on several simple rules commonly accepted among cardiologists: First, no patient should undergo elective surgery within 6 months of an MI; second, no patient should go to the OR with any degree of heart failure; and third, no patient should go to the OR while taking β-blockers because of their myocardial depressant effects.

The first rule has been challenged (see *What Is the Incidence?*). The second has been modified, because we are able to treat patients with heart failure safely as long as it is "compensated." The third rule has been totally debunked.

As our specialty becomes more sophisticated and technical, we are being consulted about patients' readiness for surgery with increasing frequency. In fact, in many situations, anesthesiologists institute consultation and further work-up because we are more acquainted with the cardiovascular system than most surgeons.

Ischemic Burden

A newly evolving issue that relates closely to the third question mentioned earlier deals with a patient's "ischemic burden"—that is, how much and how easily a patient develops reversible ischemia, either as angina pectoris or as silent ischemia. It is being closely examined as a risk factor.

Beta-Blockers

Clinical evidence suggests that patients who are β-blocked before surgery develop less ischemia than those who are not

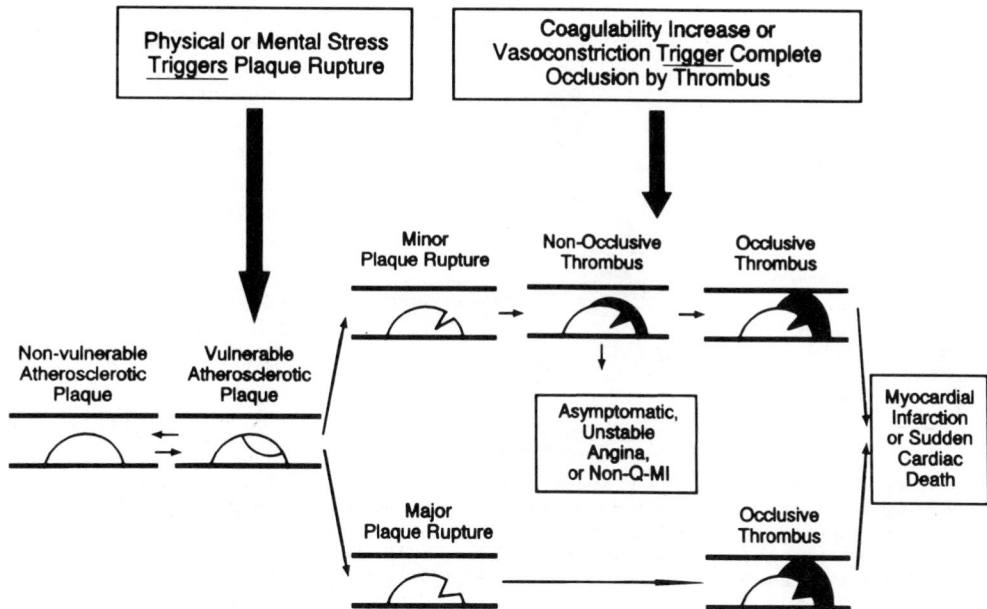

FIGURE 45-5. Sequence of events leading to clinical syndromes of coronary artery disease. Recent clinical studies on silent myocardial ischemia have more clearly delineated the major role of mental stress in triggering plaque rupture that would place the patient at risk for a major thrombotic event. (From Muller JE, Tofler GH: Introduction: a symposium: triggering and circadian variation of onset of acute cardiovascular disease. Am J Cardiol 1990; 66(Suppl):4G.)

TABLE 45–2. Cardiac Morbidity and Mortality in Patients with Silent Myocardial Ischemia

Study	N	Monitor Leads/Duration	Ischemia (% Patients)	Events— Ischemic Group	Events— Nonischemic Group	Predictors of Outcome
McCann and Clements[14]	50 Vasc	Q-Med 1 lead/pre to late POD3	38%, > post	4/19 (21%)	None	None
Ouyang et al[12]	24 Vasc	Holter 2 leads/17 h pre, 29 h intra/post	63%, all had postoperative ischemia	8/15 (53%)	1/9 (11%)	None
Pasternack et al[13]	200 Vasc	Q-Med 1 lead/18 h pre, 37 h intra/post	64%, > post	10/127 (8%)	None	Preoperative ischemia, rest angina
Raby et al[15]	176 Vasc	Holter 2 leads/pre only	18%, pre only	12/32 (38%)	1/144 (<1%)	Preoperative ischemia: RR 24.4
Mangano et al[16]	172 Vasc	Holter 2 leads/48 h pre, 48 h intra/post	20% pre, 25% intra, 41% post	Post: 12/167 (7%)	0–2 (<1%)	Postoperative ischemia: RR 9.2
	474 Total					

Abbreviations: Vasc = vascular surgery; Q-Med = real-time digital Holter monitor; Holter = standard analog recorder; RR = relative risk.

or who are receiving calcium entry blockers only. This difference appears to be related to lower heart rates or, more precisely, less tachycardia in β-blocked patients, a supposition that is supported by the results of several major studies of postinfarction β-blockade in medical patients.

Calcium Entry Blockers

In similar epidemiologic studies, calcium entry blockers have resulted in worse outcome, perhaps related to their negative inotropic effects. Newer, nondepressant agents may yield better results. However, calcium entry blockers may have beneficial effects by preventing stunned myocardium (discussed later).

Nitrates

Curiously, no firm data on the value of preoperative nitrate therapy are available, and results of studies of its prophylactic intraoperative use are conflicting.[10, 11] The value of these agents prophylactically in patients with known CAD but no angina (i.e., remote MI or SMI only) is currently under investigation by a number of research groups in both anesthesiology and cardiology.

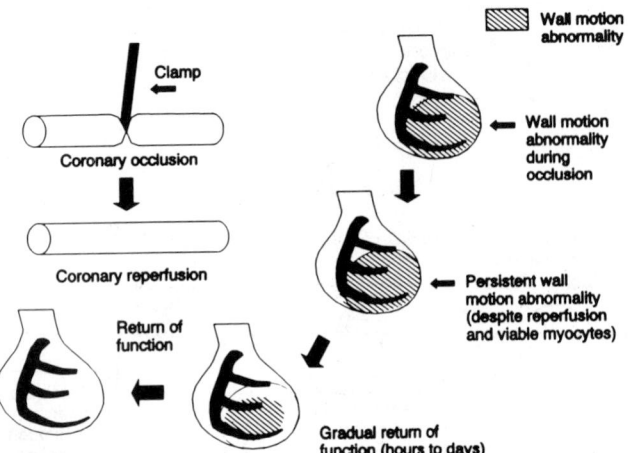

FIGURE 45–6. Schematic representation of stunned myocardium following coronary reperfusion. This syndrome is now well recognized as a common clinical event. It may have significant prognostic implications for postoperative myocardial dysfunction. (From Kloner RA, Przyklenk K, Patel B: Altered myocardial states: the stunned and hibernating myocardium. Am J Med 1989; 86(Suppl 1A):15.)

What Is Stunned Myocardium?

In certain patients, after return of normal coronary blood flow to a previously ischemic region, ST segment changes, regional wall motion abnormalities, or impaired ventricular function may persist for extended periods, lasting up to several days (Fig. 45–6). This interesting phenomenon is termed *stunned myocardium* and is most common after brief, repetitive episodes of ischemia.[17] It may occur during a "stormy" surgical procedure, such as thoracic aortic aneurysm repair or repetitive high aortic cross-clamping. The latter procedure markedly increases afterload and wall stress, decreases coronary perfusion pressure, and increases myocardial O_2 demand. Hypovolemia due to hemorrhage or vasodilation distal to the clamp decreases preload, markedly reducing cardiac output and systemic pressure and further compromising coronary perfusion.

That myocardial stunning occurs clinically is suggested by a study in which we observed that the majority of patients who were found to have new akinetic segments persisting at the conclusion of surgery did not suffer an infarct (i.e., no new Q waves or increases in creatine kinase [CK] isoenzymes).[18] However, such a process is not likely entirely benign either, because it may result in significant postoperative ventricular dysfunction.

What Is Hibernating Myocardium?

Hibernating myocardium is chronic regional dysfunction (i.e., severe hypokinesis or akinesis) distal to a significant coronary stenosis.[19] This process, occurring in the absence of infarction, is considered an adaptive response to chronic ischemia. Wall motion frequently normalizes after myocardial revascularization or with reduction in myocardial O_2 demand during anesthesia. Thus, wall motion assessed by intraoperative TEE may appear substantially better than that observed by preoperative precordial echo, multigated angiogram (MUGA) scan, or contrast ventriculogram.

ANESTHESIA AND INTRAOPERATIVE ISCHEMIA

Is There a "Best" Technique?

In few areas of anesthesiology does clinical art diverge so far from academic science. The literature is replete with carefully controlled, invasive animal studies and clinical trials rigorously evaluating the effects of different anesthetic agents on hemodynamic function and signs of ischemia. In these highly controlled studies, a significant number of agents have been shown to precipitate ischemia, either via direct myocardial effects (coronary steal with isoflurane) or peripheral effects (vagolytic effects of pancuronium causing tachycardia).

Despite these studies, little conclusive evidence shows that any anesthetic agent is more likely to precipitate ischemia than any other when it is used by experienced clinicians. More importantly, no evidence shows that one technique is associated with better outcome. The basic adage "It's not what you use, but how you use it" remains the most important rule for anesthetic management. This generalization does not imply that any agent can be used with impunity; rather, it suggests that a clinician must properly dose agents to achieve desired physiologic end points despite varying effects on the myocardium and autonomic nervous system.

Control of Heart Rate

Despite the multiplicity of factors involved in the development of ischemia, particularly in patients with CAD, the heart rate should be maintained at the lowest level consistent with adequate cardiac output meeting peripheral and myocardial O_2 demand. This is most often a heart rate of 70 beats per minute or less.

Control of Blood Pressure

Recommendations for maintenance of blood pressure are more controversial, including which pressure is most important: systolic, diastolic, or mean. Some authorities vigorously recommend maintaining blood pressures within 20% of the preoperative "mean."

This approach suffers from several problems. First is a lack of validation about what constitutes a representative mean value for hospitalized patients. Second, during a well-conducted anesthetic, O_2 demands of all organs are significantly reduced. Thus, autoregulatory responses should allow adequate perfusion at a lower pressure.

Although autoregulatory responses distal to a significant coronary lesion may be markedly impaired or even abolished, because maximal vasodilation is already present, other moderating factors influence ischemia.[20] Obviously, elevated heart rate at a low pressure places a patient at greater risk than lower heart rate at an equivalent pressure. Also, the effects of blood pressure on afterload and wall stress (direct relation) must be considered. A factor of particular importance in today's climate, with the ever present risk of transfusion-associated infections, is that higher blood pressures result in greater blood loss, increasing the probability of transfusion.

Magnitude and Duration of Hypotension

Although Goldman and colleagues suggested that profound hypotension of more than a 50% decrease below control was a major risk factor, the duration also was important. Reductions of pressure >33% for periods >10 minutes were statistically related to adverse postoperative cardiac outcome.[21] However, in healthy patients, even cardiac arrest on induction, if treated promptly, is rarely associated with adverse sequelae.

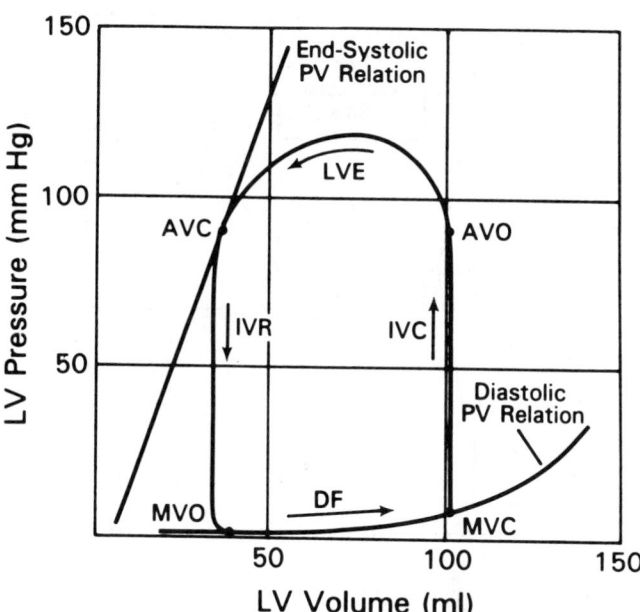

FIGURE 45–7. Pressure-volume loop illustrating the change in left ventricular pressure and volume during a single cardiac cycle in a normal ventricle. A point of significant importance in assessing myocardial contractility is the pressure-volume relation at end-systole. PV = Pressure-volume; LV = left ventricular; AVO = aortic valve opening; AVC = aortic valve closure; MVO = mitral valve opening; MVC = mitral valve closure; LVE = left ventricular ejection; IVC = isovolumic contraction; IVR = isovolumic relaxation; DF = diastolic filling. (From Hutter AM: Congestive heart failure. *In* Scientific American Medicine. Rubenstein E (ed). New York, Scientific American, 1988, p 4. Scientific American Medicine, Section I, Subsection II. © 1988 Scientific American, Inc. All rights reserved.)

MYOCARDIAL DYSFUNCTION

Myocardial dysfunction is commonly equated with an abnormally low cardiac output, resulting in impaired systemic O_2 delivery. However, cardiac output is modulated by both myocardial and peripheral vascular factors. To diagnose and treat low cardiac output, clinicians must have a firm grasp of normal cardiac physiology.[22] The temporal relation between ventricular pressure and volume throughout the cardiac cycle can be effectively displayed as a pressure-volume loop (Fig. 45–7). From this plot, both stroke volume (the volume ejected during systole) and stroke work (the energy expended to eject it) can be visualized by examining the difference between the end-systolic and end-diastolic volumes (for stroke volume) and the area enclosed by the loop (for stroke work).

What Are the Determinants of Stroke Volume?

The major determinants of stroke volume are preload, afterload, and contractility.[1] Alterations of one or more of these factors alter cardiac output (Fig. 45–8). *Preload*, the stretch on the myofibrils at end-diastole, and *afterload*, the force resisting systolic shortening of the myofibrils, under most clinical conditions are modulated primarily by the peripheral vasculature: venous return and aortic impedance, respectively. *Contractility* (inotropy), the intrinsic property of the cardiac muscle cells to generate force, is modulated by hormonal catecholamine and drug (e.g., digoxin) effects. Heart rate (*chronotropy*) is also modulated by hormonal and chemical effects, as well as direct

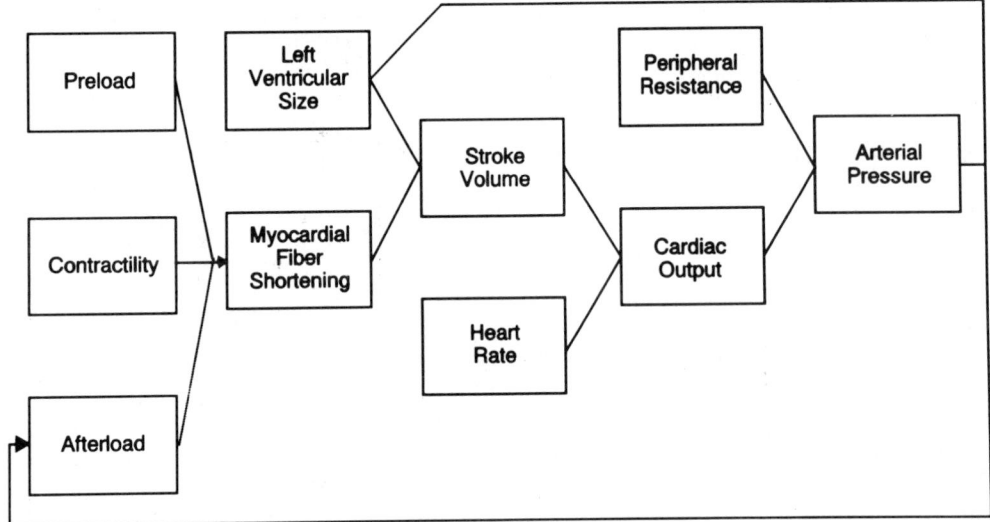

FIGURE 45–8. Relation between major factors modulating cardiac function. The *solid line* indicates positive effect, and the *dashed line* indicates negative effect. Left ventricular size influences both stroke volume and preload. (From Braunwald E: Regulation of the circulation. N Engl J Med 1974; 290:1129, reprinted by permission of the New England Journal of Medicine.)

and indirect autonomic innervation (i.e., sinoatrial node automaticity and peripheral baroreceptors).

Stroke volume and preload are directly related. The Frank-Starling relation (or ventricular function curve) illustrates this point. In humans, throughout a physiologic range of pressures, little evidence of a distinct plateau portion of the curve is seen. The relationship between stroke volume and afterload is inverse. A ventricle with significant depression of contractile function may generate normal cardiac output if preload is optimized and afterload reduced (Fig. 45–9).

How Is Myocardial Dysfunction Assessed?

When approaching a patient with abnormal hemodynamics, a clinician must first attempt to localize the problem to the appropriate component of the cardiovascular system (i.e., the peripheral vasculature or the cardiac pump). If the cardiac pump appears to be primarily affected, the focus of this discussion, the abnormality should be characterized as either systolic or diastolic. Systolic dysfunction is by far the more common clinical problem and is characterized by abnormalities of one or more of the determinants of stroke volume.

Diastolic Dysfunction

Recognition of diastolic dysfunction as a clinical entity has increased in recent years, especially with the use of calcium entry blockers. Certain patients develop pulmonary edema or congestion despite normal systolic function. In these patients, abnormalities of ventricular relaxation (lusitropy) or filling are present. A number of diseases have been associated with diastolic dysfunction (Table 45–3). The pathophysiologic hallmark of this disorder, impaired ventricular filling, is significantly worsened by tachycardia because it so dramatically decreases diastolic filling time (see Fig. 45–2).[22]

As complex forms of cardiovascular monitoring, such as PA catheterization (invasive) and TEE (noninvasive), become almost routine in clinical practice, emphasis on the interrelations between hemodynamic variables increases. End-diastolic wall stress (EDWS), an estimate of the force stretching the myocardial fibers at end-diastole, can be assessed. It is derived from

wall thickness (h), ventricular radius (R), and end-diastolic pressure or preload (P):

$$EDWS = \frac{PR}{2h}$$

Equation 1

The EDWS is a critical variable modulating systolic ejection; end-systolic wall stress (ESWS) is a critical determinant of afterload effects.

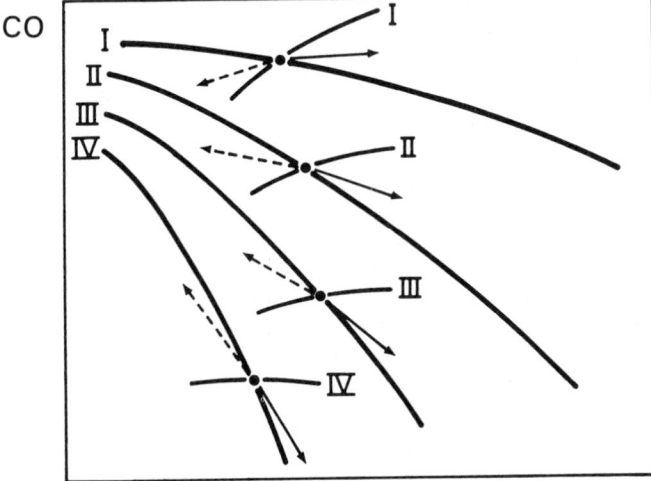

FIGURE 45–9. Relation between preload (*short segments*) and afterload effects (*longer segments*) on ventricular function is shown. The classical Frank-Starling curve for either parameter is the relation of the parameter (either left ventricular filling pressure/volume for preload or outflow resistance/impedance for afterload) to a measure of ventricular output (e.g., cardiac output, stroke volume, or stroke work). A balanced arteriolar and venous vasodilator such as nitroprusside will reduce both preload and afterload. In patients with normal ventricular function (*curves I and II*), the effects of preload reduction predominate over those of afterload reduction and cardiac output may fall (*hatched arrows*). With impaired function (*curves III and IV*), afterload reduction predominates and cardiac output increases. CO = Cardiac output; LVFP = left ventricular filling pressure. (From Cohn JN, Franciosa JA: Vasodilator therapy of cardiac failure (part II). N Engl J Med 1977; 297:28, reprinted by permission of the New England Journal of Medicine.)

TABLE 45–3. Diseases Associated with Diastolic Dysfunction

> Myocardial ischemia
> Hypertrophic cardiomyopathies
> Systemic hypertension with left ventricular hypertrophy
> Infiltrative systemic disorders
> Diabetes mellitus
> Hypothyroidism

What Are the Effects of Inhalational Anesthetics?

The volatile agents differ in their circulatory and myocardial effects, with halothane and isoflurane generally representing opposite ends of the spectrum.[23] Enflurane is intermediate between the two in many of its effects and is not considered further.

Halothane

Halothane has significant negative inotropic effects that are either desirable or dangerous, depending on a clinician's perspective. These effects reduce myocardial and peripheral O_2 demand, decreasing the risk of ischemia unless the decrement in cardiac output is severe. If end-diastolic volume and pressure increase, however, an increase in wall tension and O_2 demand may result, together with decreased coronary perfusion pressure.

The heart rate is usually unchanged or may decline. However, a greater potential for atrioventricular dissociation and junctional rhythm exists owing to slowing throughout the conduction system. Cardiac output is decreased from the negative inotropic and chronotropic effects, as well as from loss of the atrial kick if a nodal rhythm ensues. The coronary vasculature is unaffected, although coronary blood flow falls in proportion to the lower myocardial O_2 demand.

Isoflurane

Isoflurane's negative inotropic effects are much less than halothane's, although in the elderly the differences are not as marked (i.e., both exert significant effects). It is a potent peripheral and coronary vasodilator. The heart rate is unchanged or may increase, and in rare instances, frank tachycardia may occur. Sinus rhythm is usually maintained, given a lack of effect on the cardiac conduction system.

Coronary Steal

The clinical significance of isoflurane's coronary vasodilating properties has been hotly debated during the past decade. A few well-publicized clinical and animal studies suggested a "coronary steal" syndrome[24, 25]; other studies have not.[26, 27] More importantly, epidemiologic studies and widespread clinical use have confirmed its safety. This property should properly be considered "luxury perfusion," because in most instances, global $M\dot{V}o_2$ is significantly reduced.

Myocardial Depression

The lesser myocardial depressant properties of isoflurane compared with halothane are occasionally a liability. Control

of hemodynamic function is often difficult during acute hyperadrenergic states. Thus, myocardial ischemia may occur as a result of elevated demand. In this situation, a brief period of halothane administration or treatment with esmolol or propranolol can provide rapid control and resolution of ischemia.

What Are the Effects of Narcotics?

The narcotics are commonly cited as the "best" agents for at-risk patients because of their lack of intrinsic myocardial depression. Their vagotonic effects cause bradycardia, improving diastolic perfusion time. Blood pressure falls only to a minor degree consistent with a reduction in sympathetic tone.

Recall and Amnesia

As sole anesthetic agents, narcotics must be administered in very high doses to ensure unconsciousness. However, even at these doses, recall can occur. Administration of other agents to ensure amnesia, most commonly benzodiazepines, can cause significant hypotension owing to peripheral vasodilation.

Adrenergic Responses

The dose-response relationship between plasma level of opioid and suppression of adrenergic responses is extremely variable. Thus, "breakthrough" hypertension and tachycardia can occur, placing patients at risk for myocardial dysfunction and ischemia. This effect is less likely with the more potent agent sufentanil.

Narcotics used in a balanced technique with a benzodiazepine (particularly midazolam) or a low-dose potent inhaled anesthetic, a nondepolarizing muscle relaxant (particularly those lacking vagolytic effects), and nitrous oxide represent an appealing technique because a very low O_2 demand state can be achieved. This technique is also associated with improved early postoperative analgesia.

Is Regional Anesthesia "Safer" than General Anesthesia for At-Risk Patients?

The merits of regional compared with general anesthesia have been vigorously debated within the specialty for many years. Recent clinical studies and the explosive growth of postoperative epidural analgesia have rekindled the controversy.[28]

Unfortunately, regional anesthetic techniques frequently are championed by well-intentioned but decidedly ignorant preoperative consultants. The rationale is based not on the safety of regional anesthesia but on the perceived hazards of general anesthesia (with its attendant hypoxemia and hypotension). The arguments are at times carried to ludicrous extremes when a stressful local anesthetic technique is performed for major surgery. Luckily, a distinct trend has developed away from preoperative consultants who pontificate on anesthetic selection.

Advantages

The potential advantages of regional anesthesia alone, in the case of amenable peripheral surgery, or in combination with general anesthesia, for major intra-abdominal or thoracic surgery, are many. Relatively small doses of drug, particularly with spinal anesthesia, provide predictable and long-lasting surgical anesthesia and muscle relaxation.

The stress response during a well-performed regional anesthetic is reliably attenuated or completely blocked. Vasodilation during vascular surgery can facilitate surgical anastomoses and graft flow. The propensity for deep venous thrombosis is attenuated, although few surgeons rely on this approach. Evidence for enhanced patient outcome (i.e., decreased incidence of MI, stroke, death, and so forth) has been advanced but remains strongly contested.

Disadvantages

As was noted, a poorly performed regional (or local) anesthetic, in which placement of the block causes considerable discomfort, as well as one in which spontaneous ventilation is allowed during lengthy surgery in a compromised patient, can induce much greater stress than a well-performed general anesthetic. Hypotension and bradycardia from a high sympathectomy may be a significant hazard if excessive doses of intrathecal or epidural anesthetic are used or if appropriate supportive therapy is not rapidly provided.

The evidence for improved outcome and patient comfort with postoperative epidural analgesia (narcotic or narcotic/local anesthetic combinations) is rapidly accumulating. In the author's opinion, this fact provides ample reason for preoperative placement of epidural catheters for major surgery whenever feasible. Their use intraoperatively (i.e., epidural anesthesia), in combination with a "light" general anesthetic, may maximize the benefits of both techniques.

INTRAOPERATIVE ISCHEMIA

How Should It Be Treated?

Beta-Blockers

Effective treatment of intraoperative ischemia entails a rapid assessment of the clinical situation and a decision about which determinant(s) of myocardial O_2 balance have been compromised. In the majority of instances, tachycardia, elicited through excessive adrenergic activity from a host of factors (e.g., light anesthesia, hypercarbia, hypovolemia, or acute anemia), is the offending factor.

Although treatment is most effective when directed at the underlying cause, management of tachycardia can be enhanced by the judicious use of β-blockers (Table 45–4), initially with the ultrashort-acting agent esmolol. Inappropriate use of β-

blockers can be disastrous, especially in the setting of unrecognized hypovolemia (thus the rationale for starting with esmolol). However, they are invaluable when myocardial O_2 demand and adrenergic tone are clearly increased.

Although additional anesthesia or analgesia is indicated in many instances, most commonly with opioids, poor correlation of plasma opioid levels with adrenergic suppression demonstrated by Philbin and colleagues supports the use of both analgesia and β-blockade.[29]

Nitroglycerin

Assessment of preload is also crucial. Coronary perfusion pressure decreases with increased preload, especially if severe ischemia impairs global ventricular function, cardiac output, and MAP, a major variable influencing coronary perfusion pressure. Adverse effects of ischemia on diastolic function include decreased ventricular compliance due to impaired relaxation, and thus increased LVEDP. Beta-blockers also can decrease contractility enough to increase LVEDP, especially if the dose is excessive (i.e., bradycardia and hypotension occur).

The most effective agent to lower preload is nitroglycerin. Its potent venodilating effects lower end-diastolic volume and pressure. If a PA catheter is in place, the PA occlusion pressure (PAOP) should be reduced to a level just adequate to maintain cardiac output. Reduction below this level predisposes to a significant increase in heart rate in a normal ventricle. Hypotension results from an excessive dose in a normal ventricle or at low doses in an impaired one.

Because hypovolemia, relative or absolute, is common in the perioperative period, cautious intravascular volume expansion is almost always indicated during nitroglycerin administration. When ischemia has resulted in significant impairment of ventricular function, with acute ventricular dilation causing altered geometry of the mitral valve apparatus and a significant reduction in atrial compliance, acute mitral regurgitation is common (Fig. 45–10). Nitroglycerin, via its salutary effect on end-diastolic volume, is very effective in reducing the degree of regurgitation. In this particular situation, intravascular volume expansion may be contraindicated.

Although technically complex, TEE can provide similar information. Assessment of ventricular cross-sectional area is achieved with short-axis views of the left ventricle, and mitral function is analyzed with color flow Doppler imaging and spectral Doppler tracings of diastolic inflow velocities (E-to-A ratio).

Sodium Nitroprusside

A primary reduction in afterload may also be indicated, especially during severe uncontrolled hypertension. Several

TABLE 45–4. Cardiovascular Effects of Nitrates, β-Blockers, and Calcium Entry Blockers

Agent	Coronary Vasodilation	Peripheral Vasodilation	Myocardial Contractility	Heart Rate	Atrioventricular Conduction
Nitrates	↑	↑	0/↑	0/↑	0
Beta-blockers	0	↓	↓↓	↓↓	↓
Calcium entry blockers					
Verapamil	↑	↑	0/↓	0/↓	↓
Diltiazem	↑	↑	↓	0/↓	0/↓
Nifedipine	↑	↑↑	↓	↑	0
Nicardipine	↑↑	↑↑	0	↑	0

NTG Effects on Abnormal PCWP "V" Waves

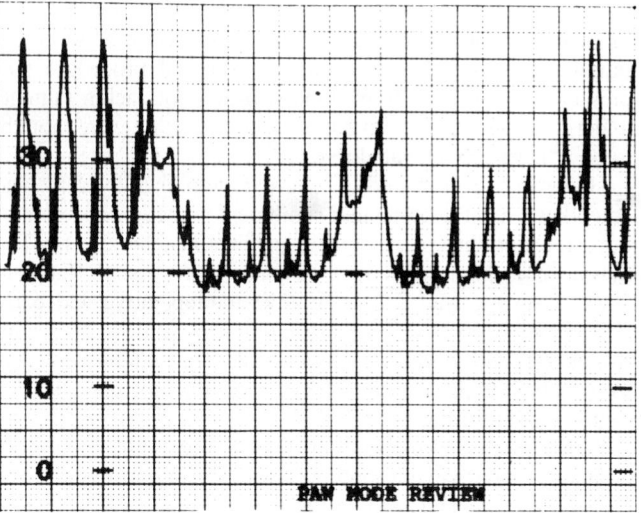

Pre-NTG

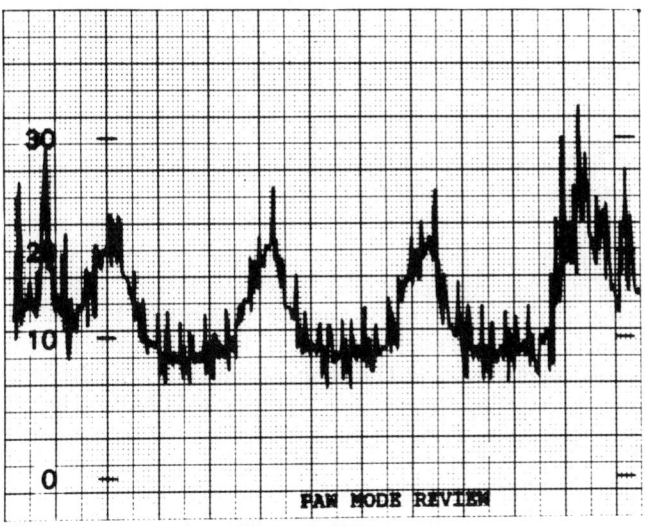

Post-NTG

FIGURE 45–10. Compressed pulmonary capillary wedge pressure (PCWP) tracings from a patient with severe inoperable coronary artery disease undergoing aortofemoral bypass grafting. Elevated PCWP with 10-mm Hg V waves are indicative of impaired ventricular function most likely resulting from chronic ischemia, mitral regurgitation, and decreased left atrial compliance. Following intravenous institution of low-dose nitroglycerin (NTG), PCWP fell dramatically, V waves resolved, and cardiac output increased. (From London MJ: Monitoring for myocardial ischemia. *In* Vascular Anesthesia. Kaplan JA (ed). New York, Churchill Livingstone, 1991, p 281.)

arteriolar vasodilators are available. Sodium nitroprusside (SNP) is most commonly used but has a relatively low therapeutic index, especially at high doses (i.e., cyanide toxicity or cardiovascular collapse). An uncommon effect of sodium nitroprusside is acute coronary steal, either between two coronary perfusion zones or from the subendocardium to the epicardium.

Calcium Entry Blockers

The so-called second-generation dihydropyridine calcium entry blockers, nicardipine and isradipine, lack negative ino-

tropic effects, in marked contrast to the first-generation agent, nifedipine. They are very potent systemic and coronary vasodilators. However, they have much longer half-lives than SNP and thus are more difficult to titrate clinically.

How Is Cardiogenic Shock Managed?

An uncommon situation but one in which failure to act appropriately and aggressively may be disastrous occurs when ischemia depresses global ventricular function and cardiac output to such a degree that severe hypotension results from cardiogenic shock. Nitroglycerin is still helpful, although it may be contraindicated with severe hypotension.

Inotropic Support

In this case, inotropic support with epinephrine, dopamine, dobutamine, or amrinone is indicated. The dose should be carefully titrated to a point where blood pressure and cardiac output are sufficiently elevated that nitroglycerin can be started. Epinephrine infusion can be begun at 0.02 $\mu g \cdot kg^{-1} \cdot min^{-1}$. This can be accomplished on short notice by putting 1 mg of epinephrine in 250 mL of diluent and beginning the infusion with a pump set to deliver the number of milliliters per hour equal to the patient's weight in kilograms, divided by three. The dose should be continuously monitored to avoid worsening the ubiquitous tachycardia accompanying low cardiac output states.

Intra-Aortic Balloon Counterpulsation

If inotropic therapy alone fails to increase cardiac output or if the doses used produce adverse effects, such as oliguria or severe tachycardia, intra-aortic balloon counterpulsation therapy should be instituted.

Balloon counterpulsation acts in several different, mutually beneficial ways to improve coronary perfusion and decrease myocardial O_2 demand.[30] Its most important function is to augment diastolic coronary perfusion. This goal is accomplished by inflating the balloon in the thoracic aorta during diastole, pushing blood in the aortic root from the preceding systolic ejection into the coronary vessels.

With rapid deflation of the balloon during early systole (isovolumic contraction), afterload is significantly reduced, allowing more efficient systolic ejection (i.e., end-systolic volume is diminished) (Fig. 45–11). This effect, in turn, reduces end-diastolic volume (i.e., preload). Despite these beneficial effects, the use of this device must be tempered by its high cost and its propensity for major vascular complications.

POSTOPERATIVE MYOCARDIAL INFARCTION

What Are the Clinical Presentation and Timing?

As noted previously, the morphologic correlates of myocardial ischemia span the spectrum from stable angina pectoris through unstable angina, to acute subendocardial or transmural MI. Based on epidemiologic studies, perioperative infarction is most common by the third postoperative day.[11, 31] In fact, actual *intraoperative* infarction is much less common than early postoperative infarction, emphasizing the significant degree of stress that patients undergo postoperatively compared with the well-controlled and relatively stress-free intraoperative period.

The incidence of Q wave and non–Q wave infarction is similar, as is their associated mortality of roughly 50%. With more aggressive therapy and intervention, this mortality should be substantially reduced. Chest pain is relatively uncommon, occurring in <50% of patients. Most, however, manifest a significant change in their clinical picture, particularly new or worsened heart failure, hypotension, or significant ventricular dysrhythmias. In the landmark study by Goldman and colleagues, only 1 of 1001 patients had a completely silent infarction, manifested only by asymptomatic ECG changes.[21]

What Is the Incidence?

Infarction following noncardiac surgery in the general surgical population is a rare event, with an incidence of 0 to 0.7%. In patients with documented CAD, the incidence of infarction is most closely related to the type of surgery; patients undergoing major vascular surgery are at greatest risk. The recent flood of articles evaluating the role of dipyridamole thallium scanning as a predictive tool provides important data on the substantial cardiac risk these patients face today.[31] Compiled data from nine studies of 776 patients revealed an incidence of nonfatal MI and cardiac death of 5% and 4%, respectively.

Prior Myocardial Infarction

Patients with prior MI are at significantly increased risk over those with stable angina alone. The time interval between the initial (or latest) infarction and the surgical procedure was previously considered to be a major prognostic factor. Patients undergoing surgery within 6 months of infarction were thought to be at markedly elevated risk.

However, several studies, starting with that by Rao and coworkers, have documented significant reduction in reinfarction and mortality rates in these patients (Table 45–5).[32] The reasons for these reductions remain controversial. Rao and associates suggested that aggressive intraoperative and early postoperative invasive pressure monitoring and therapy with β-blockers and nitrates were critical. This study was performed before the advent of TEE and did not consider ST segment monitoring.

Because most clinicians are able to accomplish this goal without as aggressive a routine as Rao's group proposed, better preoperative management, as well as lighter, less-depressant anesthetic regimens, may be more important. Significant improvement in postoperative pain management, especially routine patient-controlled analgesia or epidural opioids, is also likely to be of significance, based on measured reductions in postoperative hormonal stress responses.

When and How Should a Patient Be Ruled Out for Myocardial Infarction?

Ruling out a MI because of intraoperative findings suggestive of ischemia or infarction is a common clinical "exercise," especially in the geriatric surgical population. In most instances, the anesthesiologist triggers this drill, based on suspicious intraoperative ECG findings or abnormal hemodynamics (e.g., unexplained hypotension with elevated PAOP). This observation leads to the patient's being admitted directly to an ICU for monitoring of vital signs and cardiac rhythm and performance of serial 12-lead ECGs and CK isoenzyme determinations. In patients already scheduled for postoperative intensive care, the additional expense of several 12-lead ECGs and CK enzyme assays is relatively minor. However, if a patient was undergoing *minor* surgery, this exercise is costly and psychologically stressful.

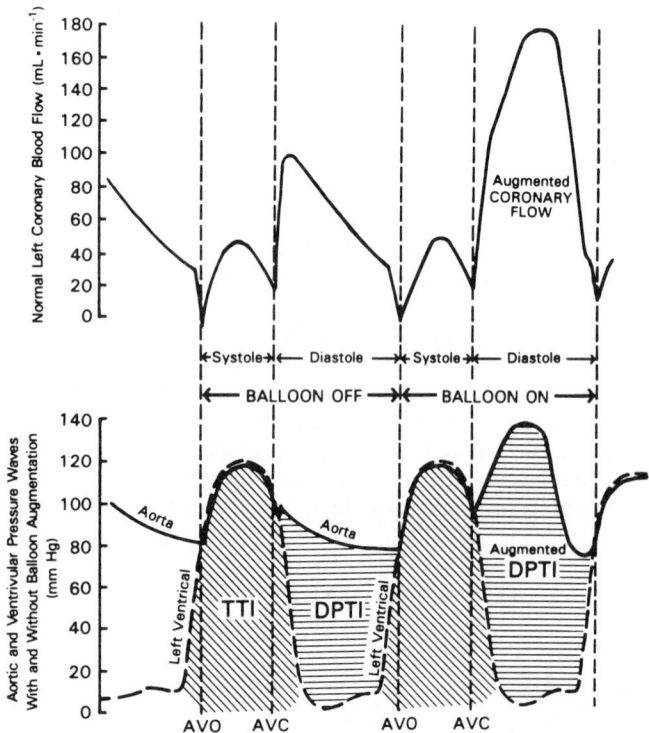

FIGURE 45–11. Effects of intra-aortic balloon counterpulsation on coronary blood flow and intracardiac pressures. *Top panel,* Coronary flow tracings during diastolic augmentation. *Bottom panel,* Augmentation of diastolic pressure time index (DPTI; a measure of myocardial oxygen supply) versus systolic tension-time index (TTI; a measure of myocardial oxygen demand). (From Maccioli GA, Lucas WJ, Norfleet EA: The intra-aortic balloon pump: a review. J Cardiothorac Vasc Anesth 1988; 2:369.)

TABLE 45–5. Reinfarction Following Anesthesia in Patients with Myocardial Infarction

Interval Between Infarction and Anesthesia (Months)	% of Patients with Postoperative Reinfarction	
	Group I*	*Group II**
0–3	36	5.8†
4–6	26	2.3‡
7–12	5	1
13–24	5	1.6
25	5	1.7
Total	7.7	1.9‡

(From Rao T, Jacobs K, El-Etr A: Reinfarction following anesthesia in patients with myocardial infarction. Anesthesiology 1983; 59:499.)
*Group I = historical control group (1973–1976); group II = prospective study group (1977–1982).
† = P < 0.05.
‡ = P < 0.005.

Indications

Most of these decisions are based on a clinician's bias and experience. Different clinicians may have various levels of concern about the intraoperative findings, how long they were present, and to what magnitude. The most common indications for ruling out MI are intraoperative ECG changes, particularly ST segment depression, T wave inversions, and frequent premature ventricular contractions. ST segment elevation is rarely encountered in patients undergoing noncardiac surgery. It should be considered diagnostic of infarction until proven otherwise.[5, 6]

Diagnostic Measures

For accurate diagnosis, the change should be observed in the diagnostic mode (0.05 Hz low-frequency response) rather than the monitoring mode (0.5 Hz response) of the ECG monitor. The monitoring mode quite strikingly exaggerates ST segment responses (Fig. 45–12). If the particular monitor does not have a diagnostic mode, a common deficiency of small 3-lead monitors used in many ORs, the change must be carefully compared with a 12-lead ECG done in the immediate postoperative period.

Careful consideration to lead placement is essential. Although standard torso mounting of the limb leads provides a lead II very similar to the 12-lead ECG, many clinicians fail to take the time to locate the precordial leads properly, particularly V_5. Placement of the precordial V_5 is often several interspaces above or below and far to the right or left of the true position. Correct placement is the fifth intercostal space in the anterior axillary line. The sensitivity and specificity of a response in an aberrantly placed precordial lead, particularly in cases involving changes in the axis of the heart (i.e., thoracotomy or upper abdominal surgery), are dubious.

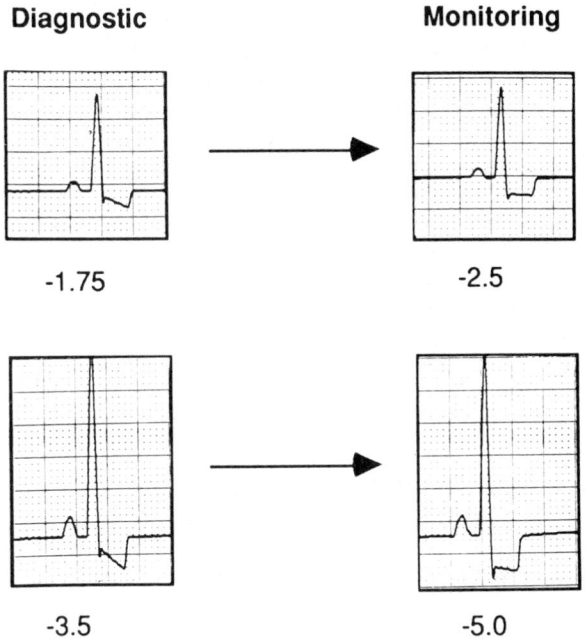

FIGURE 45–12. Effects of monitoring versus diagnostic mode on ST segment morphology (PC2 monitor, SpaceLabs, Inc., Redmond, WA). Note change in slope and augmentation of ST segment depression. This occurs with any monitor when the low-frequency response is altered. Fortunately, all segment trending devices default to the diagnostic mode during analysis. (From Cardiothoracic and Vascular Anesthesia Update, Vol. 3, p 5.)

Sensitivity and Specificity of Electrocardiographic Changes

In many instances, transient intraoperative ECG changes, particularly minor ST depression, are likely to be false-positive responses or transient episodes of subendocardial ischemia and need not be ruled out. T wave changes are less specific for ischemia, given their marked sensitivity to various autonomic stimuli. However, when symmetrically inverted, particularly in the anterior precordial leads, they are likely to represent ischemia.

Frequent ventricular ectopy accompanying ECG changes is particularly worrisome and probably represents ischemia. Significant intraoperative ischemia is likely to manifest on the postoperative 12-lead ECG, although intraoperative therapy may have attenuated or aborted it. Thus, at times, a clinician may have to recommend a rule-out protocol despite a normal postoperative 12-lead ECG.

How Is Myocardial Dysfunction Assessed and Quantitated?

Preload

Precise quantitation of the determinants of stroke volume is difficult, and clinical estimations are to various degrees imprecise. Preload is the easiest to estimate using central venous pressure or PAOP measurements. However, these pressures provide only indirect assessment of left or right ventricular end-diastolic volume, the relation being defined by ventricular compliance ($\Delta V/\Delta P$). Although this approximation is useful in most instances, marked abnormalities of compliance occur commonly (e.g., left ventricular hypertrophy, after cardiopulmonary bypass, and so forth). In these instances, compliance is usually reduced. Thus, to obtain a similar ventricular volume, a significantly higher intraventricular pressure is necessary and may reduce coronary perfusion pressure and lead to subendocardial ischemia.

Afterload

Afterload is often equated with systemic vascular resistance. This approximation is a gross oversimplification of a very complex phenomenon. In fact, a precise definition of afterload has yet to be universally accepted by physiologists. Some equate afterload with ESWS, whereas others relate it to instantaneous aortic impedance during ventricular ejection. A more recent approach involves estimating arterial elastance, defined as end-systolic pressure divided by stroke volume.

Contractility

Contractility, the variable of most interest to clinicians, is also the most difficult to quantitate. It must be assessed at known loading conditions (i.e., constant preload and afterload). A number of indices unique to each phase of systole (isovolumetric contraction and systolic ejection) have been proposed to quantitate contractility.

dP/dt

The maximum rate of rise of systolic pressure during isovolumic contraction ($\delta P/\delta t$) has been widely used by cardiologists because it can be easily measured during cardiac catheterization. However, its use is limited by its dependence on preload (increasing from 5–10% with an acute increase in preload). The rate of rise of systolic wall stress is more robust because it takes into account left ventricular geometry and mass, factors that vary greatly between individuals.

Ejection Fraction

The most commonly used ejection phase index is the ejection fraction, the percentage of change in ventricular volume from end-diastole to end-systole. This noninvasive measurement is easily made using radionuclide or echocardiographic techniques and is widely used clinically.[22] It also is dependent on loading conditions and may remain normal despite deteriorating contractility, especially if preload is augmented or afterload is reduced. Conversely, it may be low, despite normal contractile function, with increased afterload (so-called afterload mismatch).[33] However, in an intact organism, preload and afterload do not vary independently. An increase in preload simultaneously increases afterload, counterbalancing the theoretic increase in ejection fraction.

End-Systolic Pressure-Volume Relation

During the past decade, the end-systolic pressure-volume relation (ESPVR), a series of pressure-volume measurements at end-systole from a series of cardiac cycles obtained by rapidly reducing preload, has received considerable acceptance as a useful model to characterize contractility, independent of loading conditions (Fig. 45–13). These points lie on a straight line, the slope of which is end-systolic elastance (E_{es}). E_{es} is the reciprocal of compliance and is proportional to contractility. It is unaffected by changes in preload or afterload. In a

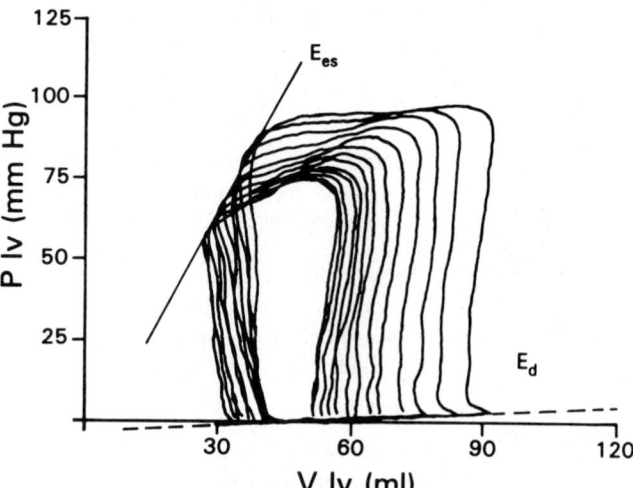

FIGURE 45–13. Pressure-volume loops from a patient undergoing cardiac surgery as measured by an intraventricular catheter capable of determining pressure (micromanometer tip) and volume (electrical impedance). The slope of the line joining a series of end-systolic pressure-volume points (obtained by a rapid decrease in preload during inferior vena cava occlusion) termed *end-systolic elastance* (E_{es}) is a measure of contractility unaffected by alteration in loading conditions. End-diastolic elastance (E_d) is determined from the same series of points at end-diastole and will change with alterations of ventricular stiffness. P lv = LV pressure; V lv = LV volume. (From Schreuder JJ, Biervliet JD, van der Velde ET, et al: Systolic and diastolic pressure-volume relationships during cardiac surgery. J Cardiothorac Vasc Anesth 1991; 5:543.)

similar fashion, end-diastolic elastance (E_d) is determined from the same series of points at end-diastole and changes with alterations of ventricular stiffness. Although complex and invasive, this assessment has been used during cardiac surgery via a specialized ventricular catheter capable of measuring both pressure (micromanometer tip) and volume (electric conductance).[34]

Which Patients Are at Greatest Risk?

Clinical signs of congestive heart failure (CHF) or a significant reduction in ejection fraction following acute MI are important predictors of short- and long-term survival.[31] In patients with heart failure secondary to nonischemic causes such as hypertension and infiltrative diseases, the degree of functional impairment assessed by the New York Heart Association (NYHA) classification is also predictive.

Outcome Analysis

Goldman and colleagues prospectively evaluated patient outcome after noncardiac surgery, finding preoperative S_3 gallop and jugular venous distention to be the most important multivariate predictors.[21, 35] Not unexpectedly, the preoperative NYHA classification was also predictive. Patients with significant valvular disease were at increased risk as well.

Interestingly, preoperative cardiomegaly in the absence of clinical signs was not significant. More than half of the patients with postoperative pulmonary edema had no preoperative signs of failure, although almost all were older than 60 years, underwent either major vascular or abdominal surgery, and had abnormal ECGs. These patients fared very poorly, with 40% dying of cardiac causes. In contrast, no cardiac deaths occurred in patients with new postoperative heart failure but no pulmonary edema.

Other clinical studies using various techniques to quantitate ventricular function have confirmed many of these findings. However, with the trend in anesthesiology toward less depressant anesthetic techniques, frequent intraoperative monitoring of PA pressures or ventricular function (via TEE), and more effective postoperative pain management, these patients can be anesthetized with low morbidity and mortality. At the time of Goldman and colleagues' 1975 study,[21] halothane was the primary anesthetic agent for most cases, PA catheterization with thermodilution cardiac output measurements was a specialized procedure, TEE did not exist, intravenous nitroglycerin was not widely available, and epidural narcotics were not used. Clearly, these advances have made a substantial impact on patients' safety and outcome.

TREATMENT OF PERIOPERATIVE MYOCARDIAL DYSFUNCTION

What Are the Pharmacologic Options?

The treatment of intraoperative myocardial dysfunction involves proper diagnosis of the underlying problem and correction of reversible etiologic or exacerbating physiologic abnormalities (i.e., acid-base disorders, particularly acidosis, impaired oxygenation or ventilation, severe anemia, sepsis, acute dysrhythmias, and so on). If these interventions are insufficient, pharmacologic or mechanical support of the circulation is indicated.[36–38]

Therapy is tailored to a patient's pathophysiologic state. In the majority of clinical situations encountered perioperatively, it requires augmentation of contractility; reduction of preload to decrease ventricular dimensions, wall stress, and myocardial O_2 demand; and optimization of diastolic filling, primarily by maintaining or establishing sinus rhythm and controlling heart rate. In certain instances, afterload reduction is indicated (i.e., regurgitant valves and severe cardiomyopathy), whereas in others (i.e., aortic stenosis) it is hazardous.

Inotropes

Inotropic agents include the catecholamines, either endogenous (epinephrine, norepinephrine, and dopamine) or synthetic (isoproterenol, dobutamine), that act on adrenergic receptors. A noncatecholamine inotrope such as ephedrine acts on adrenergic receptors as well but lacks the catecholamine structure (catechol nucleus and amine side chain) or works via nonadrenergic mechanisms (i.e., amrinone via phosphodiesterase inhibition; digoxin via inhibition of sodium-calcium countertransport; or calcium chloride via direct augmentation of excitation-contraction coupling).

Mechanisms of Action

Catecholamines and other adrenergic agonists act to stimulate the enzyme adenyl cyclase adenosine triphosphate, which converts to cyclic adenosine monophosphate (cAMP), thereby increasing intracellular calcium concentration. Phosphodiesterase inhibitors achieve a similar effect via a different mechanism, inhibiting phosphodiesterase, the enzyme responsible for inactivation of cAMP.

Adrenergic Receptors

Three major classes of adrenergic receptors, α, β, and dopaminergic (Table 45–6), modulate the diverse physiologic functions of the autonomic nervous system.[38] Receptor concentration is dynamic in number and responds to various physiologic factors, particularly plasma catecholamine concentrations and neural innervation of an organ. This upregulation or downregulation markedly affects the response of a particular organ to exogenous catecholamines. Almost all of the cate-

cholamines, endogenous or synthetic, activate both α- and β-receptors, although affinity varies with the particular agent and its concentration. Phenylephrine and isoproterenol are notable exceptions with exclusive α and β affinity, respectively.

Calcium Chloride

Calcium chloride has long been used for acute management of myocardial dysfunction in the OR (particularly during cardiac surgery) and during cardiopulmonary resuscitation. Severe depression of extracellular *ionized* calcium levels causes myocardial depression and peripheral vasodilation.

Ionized calcium may be reduced after massive transfusion with citrated blood products. It is also reduced during cardiopulmonary bypass because of hemodilution from the pump prime and calcium binding by citrate, albumin, and heparin. However, considerable controversy exists about the level at which hemodynamic effects occur and, curiously, what hemodynamic effects are associated with its acute administration.

Studies performed after cardiopulmonary bypass have shown that small doses ($5 \text{ mg} \cdot \text{kg}^{-1}$) increase MAP but not cardiac output.[39] Also, administration before β-adrenergic inotropes (particularly epinephrine) significantly attenuates their hemodynamic effects.[40] Calcium chloride also has been implicated in development of acute coronary spasm.

Advanced Cardiac Life Support. Routine administration of calcium chloride has been eliminated from the advanced cardiac life support protocols of the American Heart Association. As the cellular role of calcium has become more clearly defined during the past decade, theoretic arguments against its use have been advanced. A major consideration is the adverse role of increased intracellular calcium levels during ischemic reperfusion on subsequent cellular viability and function. Diastolic relaxation, an energy-requiring process involving transport of calcium out of the cell, may be adversely affected by exogenous calcium. Increased intracellular levels of calcium are believed to be the primary mechanism for stunned myocardium, which in animal models can be prevented by pretreatment with calcium entry blockers.

Indications. Despite these theoretic concerns, indications for the use of calcium do exist, particularly after massive transfusion (especially in pediatric patients) and for the treatment of the acute effects of hyperkalemia on cardiac conduction. Although its value during cardiac surgery has been challenged, studies have not been directed at patients with impaired ventricular function, in whom it is most likely to be of benefit. Thus, cautious administration of calcium chloride should not be universally condemned at this time.

Choice of Agent

When choosing an inotrope, one must consider the net effect of a particular agent in regard to its direct inotropic actions, its effects on arteriolar and venous resistance, its effects on heart rate (chronotropy) and conduction velocity (dromotropy), and its effects on renal dopaminergic receptors (Table 45–7). The actual high and low dose ranges in the table are arbitrary owing to relatively wide variability between patients.

Note that potent physiologic modifiers of "expected" responses exist based on receptor affinity alone. In anesthetized patients, baroreceptor-mediated vagal bradycardia, due to marked increase in MAP (α_1 stimulation), may not occur (although it often does, particularly during narcotic or isoflurane anesthesia).

TABLE 45–6. Adrenergic Receptors

Receptor Type	Location	Actions
α_1	Postsynaptic—vascular smooth muscle	Vasoconstriction
α_2	Presynaptic	Inhibition of norepinephrine release, decreased central sympathetic outflow
β_1	Postsynaptic—myocardium	Increased inotropy, chronotropy, dromotropy
β_2	Postsynaptic—vascular bronchial, uterine smooth muscle	Vasodilation, bronchodilation, uterine relaxation
DA_1	Postsynaptic—renal mesenteric smooth muscle	Renal, mesenteric vasodilation
DA_2	Presynaptic	Inhibition of norepinephrine release

TABLE 45–7. Inotropes

Inotrope		Dose Range	α_1	β_1	β_2	DA	Dose (Titrate to Effect)	Clinical Effects
Catecholamines	Epinephrine	Low	0/+	+ + +	+ +	0	0.025–0.15 $\mu g \cdot kg^{-1} \cdot min^{-1}$	Natural hormone; increased CO, SVR, HR; may increase PVR (rare)
		High	+ + + +	+ + + +	+ + +	0		
	Norepinephrine	Low	+ + + +	+	0	0	0.025–0.15 $\mu g \cdot kg^{-1} \cdot min^{-1}$	Natural neurotransmitter; preserves cerebral and coronary flow; may be effective in combination with "inodilators"
		High	+ + + +	+ +	0	0		
	Dopamine	Low	0/+	+	+	+ + + +	1–3 $\mu g \cdot kg^{-1} \cdot min^{-1}$	Enhanced renal flow
		High	+ + +	+ + + +	+ +	+ + + +	4–20 $\mu g \cdot kg^{-1} \cdot min^{-1}$	Effects of DA stimulation unclear at high doses
	Isoproterenol	Low	0	+ + + +	+ + + +	0	0.025–0.05 $\mu g \cdot kg^{-1} \cdot min^{-1}$	Use restricted to refractory bradydysrhythmias and elevated PVR; expect ventricular dysrhythmias
		High	0	+ + + +	+ + + +	0		
	Dobutamine	Low	0	+ +	+	0	1–10 $\mu g \cdot kg^{-1} \cdot min^{-1}$	So-called inodilator may be helpful in right and left ventricular failure due to afterload reduction
		High	+	+ + + +	+ + +	0	10–20 $\mu g \cdot kg^{-1} \cdot min^{-1}$	
Noncatecholamines	Ephedrine		+ + +	+ +	+	0	5–10 mg bolus	Mixed α- and β-agonist; bronchodilator, preserves uterine blood flow
	Phenylephrine		+ + + +	0	0	0	50–100 μg bolus or as infusion	Pure α-agonist, potent baroreceptor effects on heart rate
	Amrinone		0	0	0	0	0.75–1.5 mg $\cdot kg^{-1}$ bolus load; 2–20 $\mu g \cdot kg^{-1} \cdot min^{-1}$ infusion	Inodilator; phosphodiesterase inhibitor; peripheral vasodilation more potent than inotropic action

Abbreviations: DA = dopamine; SVR = systemic vascular resistance; HR = heart rate; PVR = pulmonary vascular resistance; CO = cardiac output.

Dopaminergic Effects. Dopaminergic stimulation, in the absence of strong α-stimulation, causes increased renal blood flow (usually preserving urine output). At high doses or with other α agents, effects on renal blood flow are controversial. At least one animal study suggests that when administered concomitantly with norepinephrine, dopamine maintains renal blood flow (i.e., prevents norepinephrine-mediated vasoconstriction). However, in clinical use, few data support these findings, and oliguria is common during high-dose α-adrenergic therapy even used together with low-dose dopamine.

Alpha-Receptor Stimulation. An additional factor to be considered is the difference between arterial and venous α-receptor activation. Venoconstriction has direct effects on preload (increasing it), whereas arteriolar constriction has effects on afterload. In general, most α agents cause venoconstriction at lower doses than are necessary for arteriolar effects.

Clinical Application. During the past 20 years, a shift away from rigorous maintenance of a "normal" MAP, as was done previously with primary vasoconstrictors such as norepinephrine, and toward optimization of cardiac output has occurred. MAP is then titrated to the minimum level consistent with major organ perfusion. Dopamine and dobutamine are the most widely used agents, although many clinicians rely on epinephrine because it is the "natural agent." However, this property is also a limitation because of its other, noncardiac physiologic effects (hyperglycemia and hypokalemia).

The phosphodiesterase inhibitor amrinone has received substantial attention and promotion. Its inotropic actions appear to be less than those of dobutamine, whereas its vasodilating effects are greater. Use with dobutamine has been suggested. However, the resulting, potentially excessive vasodilation may substantially reduce MAP. Some clinicians, therefore, recommend concurrent administration of primary vasoconstrictors such as phenylephrine. Indeed, addition of norepinephrine, which also has potent inotropic effects, may provide an optimal combination.

How Should Actual or Potential Perioperative Dysfunction Be Monitored?

An intra-arterial catheter should be placed in patients with myocardial dysfunction for beat-to-beat monitoring of arterial pressure. Indirect assessment of contractility is also possible by observation of the systolic upstroke and pulsus alternans, when it occurs.

Pulmonary Artery Catheterization

In patients who have marginally impaired function and are undergoing minor surgery, a central venous catheter is usually adequate, especially if the dysfunction is predominantly right sided (i.e., cor pulmonale). However, in patients with significant left ventricular dysfunction and in any at-risk patient undergoing major surgery involving significant blood loss or high aortic cross-clamping, a PA catheter is mandatory. Such monitoring also allows measurement of cardiac output by thermodilution.

Although the clinical signs of low cardiac output may be obvious in awake patients, they are difficult to assess during anesthesia. For example, anesthetic-induced alterations of renal autoregulation may reduce urine output unrelated to cardiac output. Further, the increased work of breathing associated with increased pulmonary extravascular fluid is not obvious during controlled ventilation. Thus, direct measurement of cardiac output and calculation of cardiac index for diagnosis and precise titration of therapeutic agents are essential. Noninvasive technologies for measuring cardiac output are available (i.e., esophageal or tracheal Doppler probes, bioelectric impedance), although none is as reliable as thermodilution measurement.

Continuous mixed venous O_2 saturation measurement provides additional assessment of cardiovascular function (i.e., O_2-carrying capacity and consumption) but is primarily used as a warning system for changes in cardiac output.

Transesophageal Echocardiography

TEE can be helpful. Indeed, some have proposed that it can replace the PA catheter or allow use of a central venous pressure catheter alone. However, substantial clinical limitations are inherent in TEE. Determinations of cardiac output via spectral Doppler analysis during transmitral or PA imaging is difficult, time-consuming, and highly operator dependent. PA pressures can be estimated, but this technique is also complex and discontinuous.

Assessment of intracavitary area by observing the left ventricular short-axis view allows qualitative estimation of ventricular volumes. Measurement of ejection fraction is possible but requires careful tracing of endocardial borders in two orthogonal views. Continuous on-line assessment of ventricular area to estimate volume is possible using automated edge detection software. Overall, however, the clinical utility of this approach awaits further literature confirmation.

PREOPERATIVE "OPTIMIZATION" OF PATIENTS WITH MYOCARDIAL DYSFUNCTION

How Should It Be Done?

Because of the significant risk of postoperative infarction in patients with preoperative dysfunction, optimization of ventricular function before surgery is crucial. In recent years, medical management of chronic CHF has focused on pharmacologic afterload reduction rather than digoxin and diuretics alone. More efficacious oral inotropic agents, such as the phosphodiesterase inhibitors amrinone and milrinone, will replace digoxin, which has a comparatively low therapeutic index.

Hydralazine has been used with good results. However, angiotensin-converting enzyme (ACE) inhibitors are now used almost exclusively. Although it is believed that all preoperative surgical candidates with CHF should be treated with ACE inhibitors, prospective study of the issue is clearly indicated. To what degree ACE inhibitors impair compensatory vasoconstrictive reflexes, particularly during weaning from cardiopulmonary bypass, with its attendant vasodilation during rewarming, is unclear.

Preoperative Admission to the Intensive Care Unit

For elective surgical patients with CHF, outpatient evaluation with serial ejection fractions (echo or MUGA) and medical management with ACE inhibitors for a period of weeks are all that is usually required to optimize a patient's condition before surgery. In urgent or emergent cases or in patients with significant decompensation due to intercurrent surgical illness, admission to an ICU for PA catheterization is frequently recommended to assess filling pressures, cardiac output, and the response to a fluid challenge.

Therapeutic Interventions

If the PAOP is elevated, nitroglycerin should be used to lower it while the corresponding cardiac index is assessed. Generally, PAOP should be maintained in the range of 10 to 15 mm Hg. Lower pressures may result in a precipitous decline in cardiac index if intravascular volume falls during surgery. Higher pressures are likely to result in a significant decline in coronary perfusion pressure and pulmonary vascular congestion. However, selected patients may tolerate lower or higher wedge pressures based on their particular pathophysiology.

In patients with profound degrees of dysfunction, inotropic augmentation, diuretics, and afterload reduction should be used to increase cardiac index above the range of 2.0 to 2.2 L · m^{-2}. A common approach is to use low-dose dopamine ($3\mu g \cdot kg^{-1} \cdot min^{-1}$) to improve renal perfusion and facilitate diuresis. An inotropic agent with predominant β effects and a low dose of an arteriolar vasodilator such as SNP are frequently added. Increased emphasis also has been placed on "inodilator" agents such as dobutamine and amrinone. However, their superiority over a primary inotrope such as epinephrine or dopamine, plus a primary vasodilator such as nitroglycerin or SNP, has not been demonstrated conclusively.

Hazards

A word of caution about preoperative placement of catheters and optimization of hemodynamics is necessary. These techniques and assessments are often performed by surgeons or cardiologists. Many permutations of this approach are recognized, ranging from very helpful to nearly destructive. Patients frequently are stressed and are given little if any sedation or analgesia during invasive catheterization. Curiously, little attention is paid to the hemodynamic changes or significant tachycardia that may be induced by this stress.

Surgeons generally prefer the subclavian approach to PA catheterization, with its attendant hazards. Many cardiologists prefer femoral cannulation, which is not accessible to the anesthesiologist during surgery, thereby placing the patient at risk of PA perforation if the catheter cannot be manipulated during hypovolemic states or cardiopulmonary bypass. In some instances, adapters, tubing, fittings, and so on differ from those used in the OR, presenting additional problems to the anesthesiologist, who must then make on-the-spot adjustments or changes.

References

1. Buckberg GD, Robertson JM, McConnell DH, et al: Determinants of myocardial performance and the adequacy of subendocardial blood flow. *In* Perioperative Cardiac Dysfunction. Utley JR (ed). Baltimore, Williams & Wilkins, 1985, p 139.
2. Boudoulas H, Rittgers SE, Lewis RP, et al: Changes in diastolic time with various pharmacologic agents. Circulation 1979; 60:164.
3. Loeb HS, Saudye A, Croke RP, et al: Effects of pharmacologically induced hypertension on myocardial ischemia and coronary hemodynamics in patients with fixed coronary obstruction. Circulation 1978; 57:41.
4. Buffington CW: Hemodynamic determinants of ischemic myocardial dysfunction in the presence of coronary stenosis in dogs. Anesthesiology 1985; 63:651.
5. London MJ: Monitoring for myocardial ischemia. *In* Vascular Anesthesia. Kaplan JA (ed). New York, Churchill Livingstone, 1991, p 249.
6. London MJ, Kaplan JA: Advances in electrocardiographic monitoring. *In* Cardiac Anesthesia. 3rd ed. Kaplan JA (ed). Philadelphia, WB Saunders, 1993.
7. Fuster V, Badimon L, Badimon JJ, et al: The pathogenesis of coronary artery disease and the acute coronary syndromes (1). N Engl J Med 1992; 326:242.
8. Fuster V, Badimon L, Badimon JJ, et al: The pathogenesis of coronary artery disease and the acute coronary syndromes (2). N Engl J Med 1992; 326:310.
9. Epstein SE, Quyyumi AA, Bonow RO: Myocardial ischemia—silent or symptomatic. N Engl J Med 1988; 318:1038.
10. London MJ: Preoperative Assessment: the role of ambulatory electrocardiography, imaging techniques, and cardiac catheterization. J Cardiothorac Vasc Anesth 1990; 4(Suppl 1):2.
11. London MJ: Silent ischemia and postoperative infarction. J Cardiothorac Vasc Anesth 1990; 4(Suppl 1): 58.
12. Ouyang P, Gerstenblith G, Furman WR, et al: Frequency and significance of early postoperative silent myocardial ischemia in patients having peripheral vascular surgery. Am J Cardiol 1989; 64:1113.
13. Pasternack PF, Grossi EA, Baumann FG, et al: The value of silent ischemia monitoring in the prediction of perioperative myocardial infarction in patients undergoing peripheral vascular surgery. J Vasc Surg 1989; 10:617.
14. McCann RL, Clements FC: Silent myocardial ischemia in patients undergoing peripheral vascular surgery: incidence and association with perioperative cardiac morbidity and mortality. J Vasc Surg 1989; 9:583.
15. Raby KE, Goldman L, Creager MA, et al: Correlation between preoperative ischemia and major cardiac events after peripheral vascular surgery. N Engl J Med 1989; 321:1296.
16. Mangano DT, Browner WS, Hollenberg M, et al: Association of perioperative myocardial ischemia with cardiac morbidity and mortality in men undergoing noncardiac surgery. N Engl J Med 1990; 323:1781.
17. Kloner RA, Przyklenk K, Patel B: Altered myocardial states. The stunned and hibernating myocardium. Am J Med 1989; 86(Suppl 1A):14.
18. London MJ, Tubau JF, Wong MG, et al: The "natural history" of segmental wall motion abnormalities in patients undergoing noncardiac surgery. Anesthesiology 1990; 73:644.
19. Rahimtoola SH: The hibernating myocardium. Am Heart J 1989; 117:211.
20. Bradley JA, Alpert JS: Coronary flow reserve. Am Heart J 1991; 122:1116.
21. Goldman L, Caldera D, Nussbaum S, et al: Multifactorial index of cardiac risk in noncardiac surgical procedures. N Engl J Med 1977; 297:845.
22. Grossman W: Evaluation of systolic and diastolic function of the myocardium. *In* Cardiac Catheterization and Angiography. Grossman W (ed). Philadelphia, Lea & Febiger, 1986, p 301.
23. Hickey RF, Sybert PE, Verrier ED, et al: Effects of halothane, enflurane, and isoflurane on coronary blood flow autoregulation and coronary vascular reserve in the canine heart. Anesthesiology 1988; 68:21.
24. Reiz S, Balfors E, Sorenson MB, et al: Isoflurane—a powerful coronary vasodilator in patients with coronary artery disease. Anesthesiology 1983; 59:91.
25. Buffington CW, Romson JL, Levine A, et al: Isoflurane induces coronary steal in a canine model of chronic coronary occlusion. Anesthesiology 1987; 66:280.
26. Cason BA, Verrier ED, London MJ, et al: Effects of isoflurane and halothane on coronary vascular resistance and collateral myocardial blood flow: their capacity to induce coronary steal. Anesthesiology 1987; 67:665.
27. Priebe HJ: Isoflurane and coronary hemodynamics. Anesthesiology 1989; 71:960.
28. Breslow MJ, Jordan DA, Christopherson R, et al: Epidural morphine decreases postoperative hypertension by attenuating sympathetic nervous system hyperactivity. JAMA 1989; 261:3577.
29. Philbin DM, Rosow CE, Schneider RC, et al: Fentanyl and sufentanil anesthesia revisited: how much is enough? Anesthesiology 1990; 73:5.
30. Maccioli GA, Lucas WJ, Norfleet EA: The intra-aortic balloon pump: a review. J Cardiothorac Vasc Anesth 1988; 2:365.
31. London MJ, Mangano DT: Assessment of perioperative risk. *In* Advances in Anesthesia. Stoelting RK (ed). Chicago, Year Book Medical Publishers, 1988, p 53.
32. Rao T, Jacobs K, El-Etr A: Reinfarction following anesthesia in patients with myocardial infarction. Anesthesiology 1983; 59:499.
33. Ross JJ: Afterload mismatch in the perioperative period. *In* Perioperative Cardiac Dysfunction. Utley JR (ed). Baltimore, Williams & Wilkins, 1985, p 139.
34. Schreuder JJ, Biervliet JD, van der Velde ET, et al: Systolic and diastolic pressure-volume relationships during cardiac surgery. J Cardiothorac Vasc Anesth 1991; 5:539.
35. Goldman L: Multifactorial index of cardiac risk in noncardiac surgery: ten year status report. J Cardiothorac Vasc Anesth 1987; 1:237.
36. Lawson NW: The use of inotropes and vasopressors. *In* ASA Refresher Courses in Anesthesiology. Barash PG (ed). Philadelphia, JB Lippincott, 1990, p 195.
37. Royster RL: Intraoperative administration of inotropes in cardiac surgery patients. J Cardiothorac Vasc Anesth 1990; 4(Suppl 5):17.
38. Breslow MJ, Ligier B: Hyperadrenergic states. Crit Care Med 1991; 19:1566.
39. Royster RL, Butterworth J, Prielipp RC, et al: A randomized, blinded, placebo-controlled evaluation of calcium chloride and epinephrine for inotropic support after emergence from cardiopulmonary bypass. Anesth Analg 1992; 74:3.
40. Zaloga GP, Strickland RA, Butterworth J, et al: Calcium attenuates epinephrine's beta-adrenergic effects in postoperative heart surgery patients. Circulation 1990; 81:196.

CHAPTER **46**

Abnormal Intracranial Pressure

SUSAN BLACK, M.D.

ROY CUCCHIARA, M.D.

Intracranial pressure (ICP) results from the combination of tissue, fluid, and blood pressures within the cranial vault. Investigators and clinicians have long used the term as if no gradients exist within the vault and as if one value for pressure represents "ICP." This is often the case because of the fluid nature of the brain and its surrounding cerebrospinal fluid (CSF). Pressure changes are transmitted throughout the fluid and result in an overall higher baseline pressure.

Although this concept is useful, one must recognize that clinical situations arise in which local tissue pressure is higher in one part of the brain than the generic overall ICP value might indicate. For example, an area of edema around and including a tumor may have a higher pressure than the surrounding tissue, perhaps because it is contained by that tissue. Not infrequently, we see patients whose ICP is normal yet in whom the area around the tumor is clearly tense. The other compartments of the system compensate for an increase of pressure in one compartment by decreasing their own volumes.

Thus, when we think of abnormal ICP, we should remember that local increases in pressure can cause a somewhat different set of responses and problems than do general increases in ICP. These responses are the material from which we make clinical decisions during the administration of anesthesia.

DETERMINANTS OF INTRACRANIAL PRESSURE

The normal central nervous system (CNS) membranes provide a watertight containment of the CSF which, in addition to fulfilling other functions, surrounds the brain and serves as a fluid cushion for the hydraulic forces that act upon it. These forces result from changes in blood pressure and blood volume; rotation and shear; and acceleration and deceleration. Simplistically, the CSF can be thought of as "floating" the brain so as to reduce traction forces on the meninges and vascular structures.

What Are the Cranial Vault Contents?

The contents of the cranial vault are the CSF, brain blood volume, brain tissue content, and interstitial brain water (Fig.

46–1). Some ability to alter CNS volume without noticeable change in ICP is possible—that is, the underlying nature of the "vault" is not a totally accurate physiologic and pathologic concept. For practical purposes, the capacity of the organism to adjust to an increase in volume of one of the components within the vault is primarily limited by the amount of reduction possible in other components. Most discussions of ICP are based on the premise that the cranial vault is intact, a situation that exists only at the beginning of the surgical procedure for elective craniotomy patients and one that may not exist at all for a trauma patient with skull damage or for an infant with open fontanelles.

Normal and Abnormal Values for Intracranial Pressure

ICP is usually measured in millimeters of mercury (mm Hg). Values between 5 and 15 mm Hg are considered normal, whereas those from 15 to 20 mm Hg are considered to be elevated and may be characterized as intracranial hypertension. Resting values from 20 to 40 mm Hg are clearly abnormal. Sustained elevations greater than 40 mm Hg are prognostic of a poor outcome.

In addition to abnormal ICPs, abnormal pressure waveforms

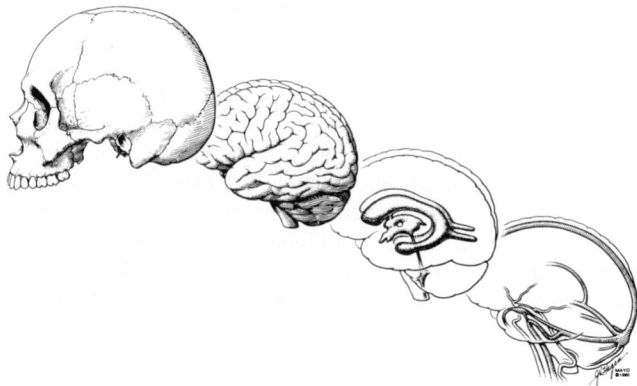

FIGURE 46–1. The cranial vault with its contents of brain tissue, CSF, and major cerebral vascular structures. These are the primary components that contribute to ICP.

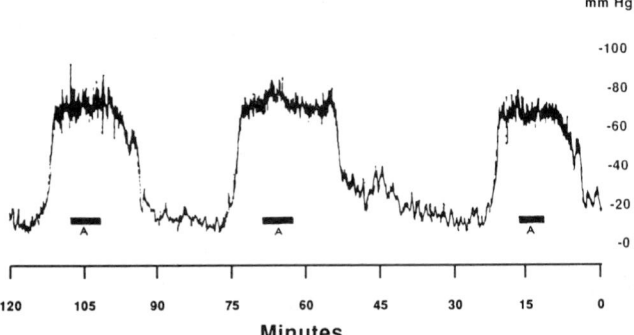

FIGURE 46–2. Spontaneous plateau waves in a patient with an intracranial tumor and elevated ICP. (From Lundberg N, Cronquist S, Kjallquist A: Clinical investigation on interrelations between intracranial pressure and intracranial hemodynamics. Prog Brain Res 1968; 30:70.)

are sometimes observed. They are called *plateau waves* and occur in patients with intracranial hypertension. The characteristic plateau wave consists of a rapid and significant increase in ICP that persists for a matter of minutes but then rapidly returns to a baseline level (Fig. 46–2). Plateau waves are often associated with the onset or worsening of neurologic symptoms. They typically occur at irregular intervals, with a duration of minutes to hours between waves. Increasing frequency of plateau waves may be associated with deteriorating neurologic status.[1, 2]

How Are Intracranial Pressure and Cerebral Perfusion Pressure Related?

The ICP can be thought of as the pressure against which the blood pressure must act to perfuse the brain. The general formula for determining the cerebral perfusion pressure (CPP) is:

$$CPP = MAP - ICP$$

in which MAP is the mean arterial pressure.

Decreases in Cerebral Perfusion Pressure

If we examine one extreme of this relationship, which unfortunately occurs in the patient with a severely injured brain, the ICP may actually equal or be greater than the MAP. As an example, a patient with a severe head injury and shock may have an ICP of 38 mm Hg and an MAP of 38 mm Hg. The resultant CPP is zero. Inadequate cerebral perfusion will result unless and until the pressures are brought back into a physiologic rather than pathologic relationship. (The CPP does not become negative, even though mathematical analysis indicates a negative value if the ICP is higher than the MAP.) Unless the ICP was measured, an anesthesiologist would be unaware of this circumstance and of the possibility that the CPP might be too low to perfuse the brain.

Increases in Cerebral Perfusion Pressure

Conversely, a very low ICP might be present following substantial catheter drainage of CSF, and the MAP might rise quite high during surgical stimulation. The CPP might then exceed the limits of autoregulation (50–150 mm Hg MAP). ''Breakthrough'' with very high cerebral blood flow (CBF), edema formation, hemorrhage, and seizure activity might ensue.

Therapeutic Dilemmas

A third and more difficult situation exists when an intracerebral hematoma raises the ICP, and the MAP increases in response to this insult (Cushing's reflex). The clinical decision to lower the MAP in an effort to reduce further bleeding risks cerebral ischemia because of the high ICP and impaired CPP. The decision is more difficult because one seldom (almost never) has knowledge of all the variables of the equation. Furthermore, the equation does not consider the cause of the elevation in ICP, a factor that clinical decision-making must incorporate.

How Is Intracranial Pressure Measured?

ICP measurements have two general features: the type of measurement device used and its location. Two basic monitor types are available: the fluid-coupled (or fluid-filled) system, in which the transducer is external to the skull; and the electronic implantable transducer, in which the transducer is placed at the intracranial site where the pressure is to be measured. Fluid-coupled systems must be calibrated frequently. Implanted transducers are electronically calibrated; recalibration is necessary less often than with fluid-coupled systems (Fig. 46–3).

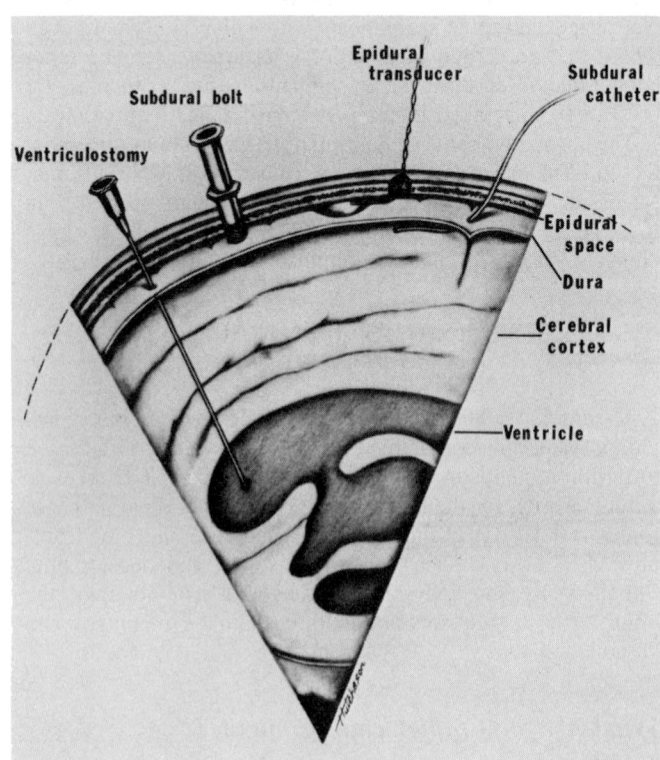

FIGURE 46–3. Clinical methodology for measurement of ICP. (From Cucchiara RF, Black S, Steinkeler JA: Anesthesia for intracranial procedures. *In* Clinical Anesthesia. Barash PG, Cullen BF, Stoelting RK (eds): JB Lippincott, Philadelphia, 1989, p 853.)

Measurement Sites

The location of the site of measurement may be the cerebral ventricles, the subdural or epidural space, or the lumbar subarachnoid space. The cerebral ventriculostomy has long been considered the gold standard of ICP measurement. Lumbar subarachnoid space measurements are a reflection of this pressure, but only if the spaces are continuous. More recently, subdural bolt and the epidural transducer have become popular for longer-term measurement techniques.

Potential Problems

Problems with all of these systems include the need for recalibration, interference of the signal by occlusion of the catheter, damage to the brain on insertion, infection, and dislodgement with faulty readings (Table 46–1). When proper calibration has been performed and appropriate waveforms are present on the tracings, the clinical ICP monitor can be used to select therapeutic modalities.

Why Is Intracranial Hypertension Dangerous?

Although intracranial hypertension is a clinical diagnosis, the pathophysiology of brain injury is of a more direct and specific nature. The major processes by which intracranial hypertension causes brain injury are cerebral ischemia and herniation of brain tissue.

Cerebral Ischemia

The likelihood of permanent tissue damage depends on both the severity and duration of ischemia. The relationship between CPP and ICP (see the previous section) reminds us that if the ICP either locally or globally reaches levels that prevent the inflow of blood at the existing MAP, cerebral ischemia will develop. When the ICP is high enough to collapse the brain's venous system, blood inflow is very slow, since blood cannot escape by the usual high-volume low-resistance routes. Total obstruction of flow is unnecessary; significant reductions

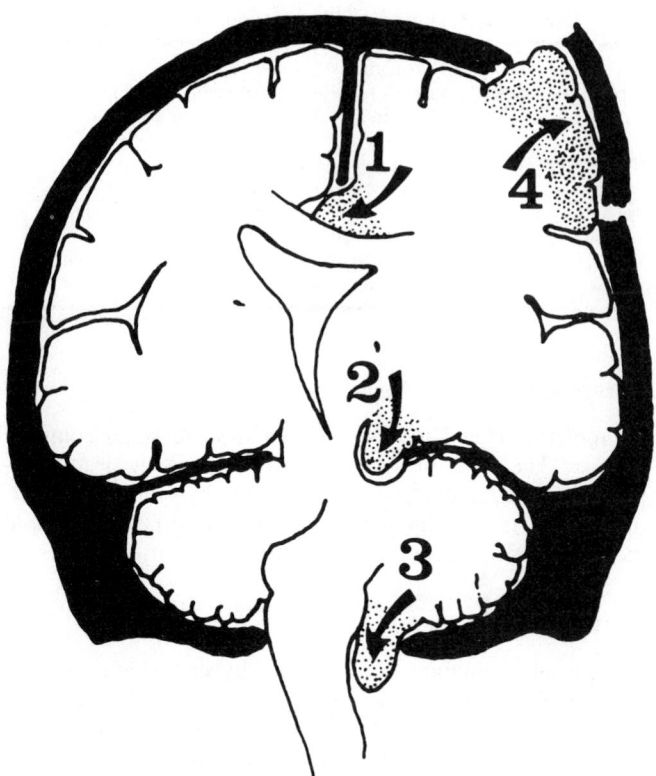

FIGURE 46–4. Schematic representation of different types of brain herniation. 1 = Cingulate gyrus; 2 = temporal lobe (uncal); 3 = cerebellar; 4 = transcalvarial (postoperative or traumatic). (From Fishman RA: Brain edema. N Engl J Med 1975; 293:706. Reprinted by permission of the New England Journal of Medicine.)

can also cause cerebral ischemia but over a slightly longer time period.

Herniation of the Brain

Brain herniation can occur through or around any fixed structure in the skull (Fig. 46–4). In major cranial trauma, injured brain frequently herniates through the fractured skull. This situation is extremely serious, and decompression usually requires resection of some brain tissue.

The falx is a rigid, midline intracranial structure under which the cingulate gyrus can herniate. Temporal lobe (uncal) herniation through the tentorium results in ipsilateral impingement and contralateral compression of the brainstem against the tentorium, producing a mixed neurologic picture.

Classic herniation of the cerebellum through the foramen magnum, which compresses the medulla, is termed *coning* and produces cardiorespiratory signs that precede death. Because each type of herniation produces a pressure gradient within the calvarium, brain tissue in some areas is at greater risk of ischemic damage than that in other areas.

What Factors Cause Abnormal Intracranial Pressure?

Grouping of patients with numerical or clinical signs of intracranial hypertension according to etiology is helpful. The management, intraoperative problems, and outcome are, to some degree, predictable within groups (Table 46–2).

TABLE 46–1. Monitoring of Intracranial Pressure

Location	Advantages	Disadvantages
Intraventricular	"Gold standard"	Increased risk of infection
	Reliability	Potential for brain injury
	CSF drainage	Placement
	Waveform	Fluid-filled system
		Transducer repositioning
Intraparenchymal	Ease of placement	Potential for brain injury
	Non–fluid-filled	Increased risk of infection
		No CSF drainage
		Catheter breakage
Subarachnoid	Ease of placement	Questionable accuracy
	No brain penetration	No CSF drainage
	Less risk of infection	Fluid-filled system
		Brain tissue obstruction
Epidural	Dura remains intact	Questionable accuracy
	Non–fluid-filled	No CSF drainage
	Ease of insertion	"Wedge" effect

(Used by permission from Lyons MK, Meyer FB: Cerebrospinal fluid physiology and the management of increased intracranial pressure. Mayo Clin Proc 1990; 65:684–707.)

TABLE 46–2. Etiologies of Intracranial Hypertension

CSF regulation	Hydrocephalus
	Posterior fossa lesion obstructing CSF flow
Tumors	Neoplasm
	Hematoma
Head trauma	Edemal hematoma
Mixed	Bleeding cerebral aneurysm
	Hemorrhage within an area of tumor of cerebral arteriovenous malformation (AVM)
	Medical conditions (e.g., hepatic encephalopathy, malignant hypertension)

Cerebrospinal Fluid Regulation

Problems related to CSF regulation share some common features. The onset of symptoms with neurologic decompensation is quite rapid; relief of the pressure by venting or shunting of CSF is, in principle, a straightforward task; and rapid recovery usually occurs when the pressure is lowered.

Tumors

Signs and symptoms of intracranial hypertension associated with neoplastic lesions are of slower onset; when they present, nearly complete exhaustion of compensatory mechanism has occurred. Surgical procedures are more complex and are complicated by the tendency of the brain to extrude through the craniotomy site. Because simple lowering of the ICP is seldom the only surgical goal, recovery is slower despite the return to a numerically normal ICP postoperatively. Subdural and epidural hematomas have their own varied clinical patterns within the basic larger tumor pattern.

Head Trauma

Intracranial hypertension associated with head trauma has a rapid onset. Cranial surgical procedures sometimes are minimally efficacious and may be limited to the insertion of nontherapeutic monitoring devices. The patient frequently undergoes other surgery that is not directed at the intracranial problem. We assume that the patient emerges from such surgery with the same ICP that was present when he or she was anesthetized, but we frequently have no monitors from which to draw information about the ICP. Immediate postoperative recovery is difficult to relate to the anesthetic technique, since the patient may remain comatose.

Anesthetic Management

Clinical impressions (but insufficient data) suggest the relative impact of anesthetic management on most of these patient groups. Those patients with CSF regulation problems seem to tolerate decidedly inferior neuroanesthesia induction techniques and generally emerge fairly well. Perhaps their compensatory mechanisms are not really exhausted, or perhaps the effect of our technique in these patients is not the same as in other neurosurgical patient populations. In addition, the surgery is short compared with other brain surgeries, with complete correction of the ICP problem.

Patients in the neoplastic group have changes in ICP during induction that may be reflected intraoperatively by a so-called "tight brain." They seem to have reached the very edge of their compensatory mechanisms such that our techniques can produce visible clinical improvement or degradation in the operating conditions. The time period between induction and surgical correction of the intracranial hypertension is long enough that damage to the brain can reasonably be expected to occur.

We know little about the impact of anesthesia on the head trauma victim's neurologic outcome. We still have much to learn in this important area.

Why Are Acute and Chronic Processes Different?

Signs and symptoms of increased ICP depend on the disease process responsible for the abnormal intracranial dynamics. Slowly progressive processes such as intracranial tumor growth may present without any signs or symptoms until quite late in the course, whereas more rapidly progressive pathologic states (e.g., an intracerebral hematoma) may present with signs of increased ICP at the onset.

Compensatory Changes

In order for clinicians to understand the progression of symptoms and the clinical importance of any change in symptomatology, the intracranial pressure-volume curve must be analyzed (Fig. 46–5).[3] Initial increases in intracranial volume are not associated with an increase in ICP because of compensatory changes (i.e., a decrease in CSF and cerebral blood volume). However, once these changes are exhausted, further increases in intracranial volume result in exponential increases in ICP.

Slowly progressive lesions allow greater time for compensation to occur. Acute processes are represented by a shift of the curve to the left, whereas chronic processes would be represented by a shift to the right. Thus, large, slowly growing lesions may be present without signs or symptoms of increased ICP. Patients with normal ICP and a mass lesion may be at the "knee" of the curve (Point 2) with respect to their ability to compensate for further increases in volume. Any interven-

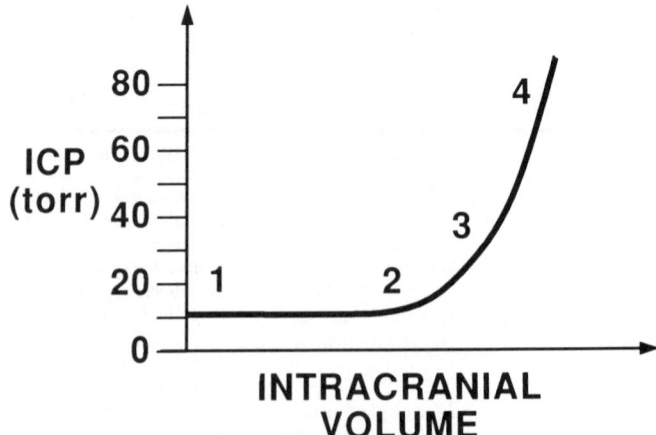

FIGURE 46–5. Intracranial pressure-volume curve. At *point 1*, ICP and intracranial volume are normal. With initial increases in volume, ICP does not change owing to compensatory mechanisms until intracranial elastance is decreased *(point 2)*. Further increases in volume will result in elevated ICP *(point 3)*. Once ICP is elevated, further increases in volume will lead to exponential increases in pressure *(point 4)*. (From Shapiro HM: Intracranial hypertension: therapeutic and anesthetic consideration. Anesthesiology 1975; 43:445.)

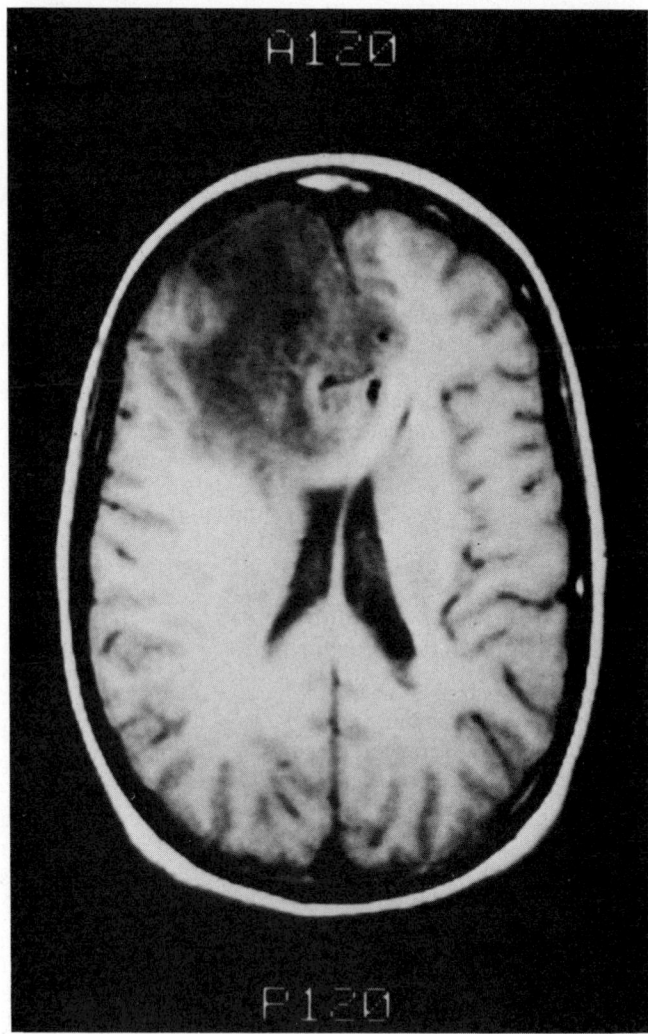

FIGURE 46–6. Magnetic resonance image of a large intracranial tumor with peritumor edema, midline shift, and compression of the ventricles.

tion that causes even small increases in intracranial volume can lead to devastating increases in ICP (Fig. 46–6).

Signs and Symptoms of Increased Intracranial Pressure

Signs and symptoms of increased ICP may be the initial presenting features for patients with intracranial pathology, or they may be present in combination with other findings specific to the pathologic process itself. Symptoms include headache (which is often worse on rising in the morning), nausea, vomiting, and drowsiness. Signs include papilledema and personality changes, especially lethargy (Table 46–3). In the unconscious patient, hypertension and bradycardia suggest elevated ICP (Cushing's triad).[4]

How Is the Level of Brainstem Involvement Assessed?

To access the progression of neurologic deterioration in an unconscious patient, brainstem function must be evaluated. Pupil size and reactivity, oculovestibular reflex, respiratory pattern, and response to painful stimuli should be assessed (Fig. 46–7).

Midbrain

Midbrain compression is characterized by abnormal pupillary responses, changes in the oculomotor reflex, decerebrate motor response to painful stimuli, and central hyperventilation. Early midbrain compression results in loss of the pupillary response to light. With further midbrain involvement, complete oculomotor palsy occurs—either unilaterally or bilaterally as the oculomotor nerve or nerves are compressed by uncal herniation. Hyperthermia often develops, signifying involvement of the hypothalamus.

Pons

Involvement of the pons is indicated by a change to irregular, apneustic ventilation; with low pontine compression, flaccidity, and complete loss of the oculomotor reflex occur.

Medulla

Medullary compression results in ataxic respiration and cardiovascular instability, which progress to apnea and cardiovascular collapse.[3]

What Diagnostic Studies Are Useful?

Most patients with suspected intracranial pathology will undergo computed tomography (CT) or magnetic resonance imaging (MRI). Findings suggestive of increased ICP include peritumor edema (the degree of surrounding edema can be measured); shift of midline structures; ventricular compression and loss of the basilar cisterns with mass lesions; and dilation of the cerebral ventricles in hydrocephalus (Table 46–4). Following head trauma, CT findings that can be useful in predicting ICP include the size of the hematoma, ventricular and basilar cistern compression, and the degree of midline shift (see Table 46–4).[5, 6]

How Is Intracranial Elastance Assessed?

Some investigators suggest that an evaluation of intracranial elastance (change in ICP with a given change in intracranial volume) is useful. This information provides an indication of where a particular patient "lies" on the ICP volume curve and may identify those individuals with mass lesions, normal ICP, and exhausted compensation (i.e., at the knee of the curve; see Fig. 46–5).

To obtain this information, one must inject or withdraw a known volume of fluid from the intracranial vault while measuring the ICP response to that change in volume. This procedure can be accomplished with an intraventricular catheter. Usually, 1 mL of normal saline is injected. If the ICP does not change, residual elastance is available. If the ICP increases by >5 mm Hg, elastance is markedly diminished, as represented by Points 3 and 4 in Figure 46–5.

Recent work suggests that continuous monitoring and computerized frequency analysis of the ICP waveform provide an estimation of intracranial elastance.[7] Review of the history

TABLE 46–3. Findings Suggestive of Increased Intracranial Pressure in Nontrauma Patients

Clinical		Radiologic	
Symptoms	*Signs*	*Skull Films*	*CT/MRI*
Headache	Papilledema	Calvarium suture spread	Shift of mildine structures
Nausea, vomiting	Personality change	Increased convolutional marking ("beaten silver" skull); thinning of sella turcica	Edema around lesion; hydrocephalus; ventricular compression

may be helpful to identify an individual with a normal ICP at the knee of the pressure-volume curve. A patient who presents with signs or symptoms of elevated ICP but who has been treated with diuretics or steroids may have no signs of elevated ICP at the time of surgery. However, he or she is likely to have limited or no ability to compensate for any further increase in intracranial volume.

INTRACRANIAL PRESSURE AND ANESTHESIA

Why Is a Knowledge of Intracranial Pressure Important to the Anesthesiologist?

To anesthetize a patient with intracranial pathology safely, the anesthesiologist should know the actual (or probable) ICP. This knowledge is as important as (or perhaps more important than) a knowledge of a hypertensive patient's usual blood pressure or of the cardiac function in a patient with heart disease. Without accurate knowledge of a patient's baseline state, one cannot provide optimal perioperative care.

Elevations in ICP can lead to decreases in CPP and the potential for both focal and global cerebral ischemia. Unchecked severe intracranial hypertension can result in herniation of the intracranial contents. Without knowledge of the initial ICP, the relative risk of such complications is unknown as are the particular steps necessary to lower that risk.

How Is a Quick Clinical Intracranial Pressure Status Check Performed?

Preoperative measurement of ICP is not always practical or possible. Clinical examination and review of diagnostic evaluations can provide an indication of likely ICP levels. If the patient tolerates having the bed placed in the Trendelenburg position prior to induction, evidence for residual compensatory mechanisms may be obtained. Should the patient become more symptomatic, compensatory mechanisms are close to exhaus-

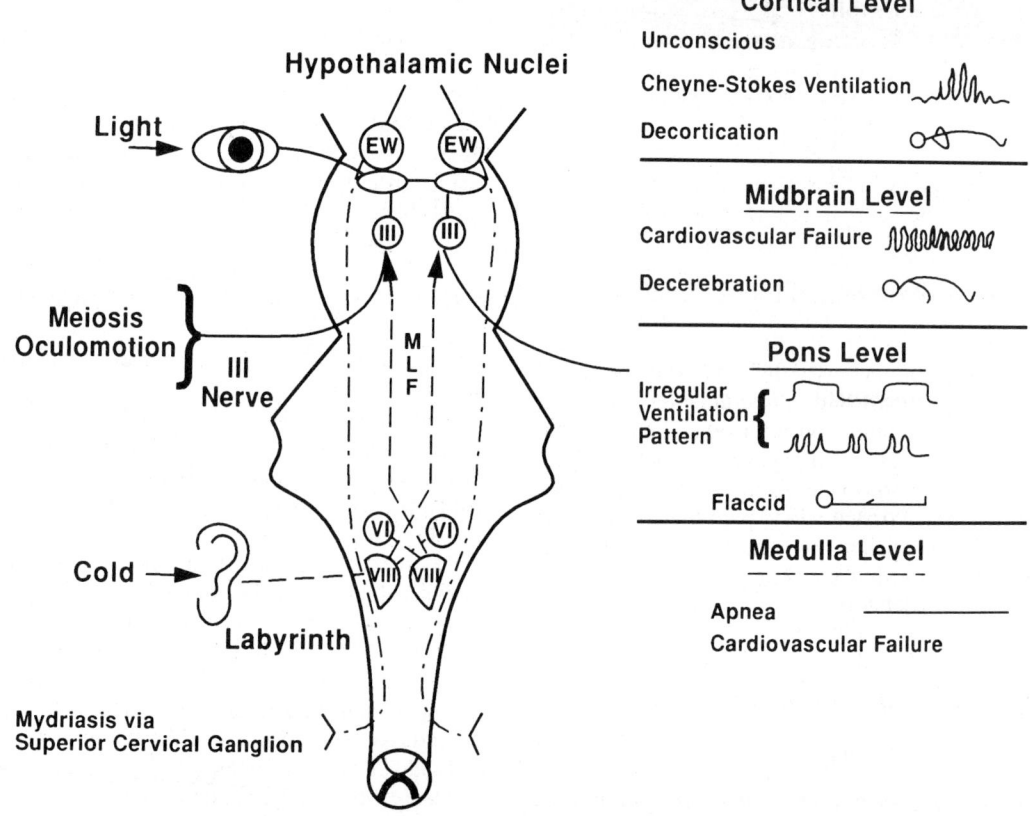

FIGURE 46–7. Brainstem reflexes and abnormal responses. *Abbreviations:* EW = Edinger-Westphal nucleus; MLF = medial longitudinal fasciculus. (From Shapiro HM: Intracranial hypertension: therapeutic and anesthetic considerations. Anesthesiology 1975; 43:445.)

TABLE 46–4. Computed Tomography Findings Aiding Assessment of Intracranial Pressure Following Closed Head Injury

Presence of intraventricular clot
Ventricular compression
Disappearance of cisterns
Size of a subdural hematoma
Degree of subarachnoid hemorrhage
Severity of cerebral contusion

tion, and additional maneuvers or interventions associated with an increase in ICP may not be tolerated.

What Are the Implications for Anesthetic Management?

For the patient with normal ICP, a lowering of ICP perioperatively may not be necessary unless the surgical procedure can be facilitated by a decrease in the volume of the intracranial contents. For a patient with normal ICP but reduced ability to compensate for increases in intracranial volume, anesthetic management must be planned meticulously to avoid an increase of intracranial volume.

Any degree of cerebral vasodilation induced by hypoventilation or by the use of volatile anesthetic agents or nitrous oxide without hyperventilation can have a significant adverse impact. If intracranial hypertension is present preoperatively, the anesthetic plan must include means for reducing ICP and for avoiding any potential for increases of intracranial volume in the perioperative period. Without attention to these factors, significant morbidity can result.

What Are the Prognostic Implications?

The ICP and time course for development of any increase in ICP may be of prognostic value. A neoplasm presenting with a rapid onset of intracranial hypertension that is not associated with obstructive hydrocephalus is likely rapidly growing and may be associated with a poor prognosis. Following head trauma, the ICP and CT scan findings can be used to indicate the need for surgical intervention.[8] The duration and severity of intracranial hypertension following head trauma are predictive of long-term neurologic function as well as of mortality.[9–11]

How Is Abnormal Intracranial Pressure Managed?

Management of patients with elevated ICP depends on the cause of the intracranial hypertension, the time course of its development, the severity of the increase, and the signs and symptoms associated with it. Common to all management strategies of patients with abnormal ICP is the avoidance of any increase of intracranial volume and ICP. The type of lesion will determine the likelihood of success with different interventions.

Aggressive (Emergent) Intervention

Rapid development or worsening of intracranial hypertension and altered level of consciousness demands prompt intervention (Table 46–5).

Bleeding

An epidural hematoma following head trauma or spontaneous intracerebral bleeding necessitates immediate operative intervention in most cases. Patients with slowly progressing mass lesions may develop sudden and severe increases in ICP, such as when bleeding into a tumor occurs. Prompt surgical evacuation is necessary to minimize neurologic morbidity.

In the postoperative period, dramatic increases in ICP and neurologic deterioration can occur with bleeding at the operative site or into areas with impaired cerebral autoregulation. The blood vessels distal to the carotid artery after endarterectomy or regions of the brain that had been subject to a steal phenomenon as with a large arteriovenous malformation do not have normal autoregulation.

Hydrocephalus

Hydrocephalus usually causes a more gradual increase in ICP; however, children with chronic hydrocephalus who have undergone multiple shunt revisions have small scarred ventricles with reduced periventricular compliance. If shunt malfunction occurs, these children tolerate increases in CSF volume poorly; neurologic deterioration may occur rapidly, requiring emergent placement of a ventricular shunt or drain.[3]

Diffuse Cerebral Contusion

Causes of severe and sudden increases in ICP not associated with a discrete mass lesion, such as diffuse cerebral contusion following trauma, require intensive medical management.

Perioperative and Postoperative Care

Patients requiring emergency surgery for severe intracranial hypertension require intensive management in the perioperative period to decrease or control ICP. Multiple modalities are utilized including hyperventilation; osmotic and loop diuretics; and the use of drugs such as barbiturates to decrease cerebral metabolic rate, blood flow, and volume. Similar measures are implemented in the intensive care unit in the postoperative period and for those patients with involvement that is not amenable to surgical intervention.

Elective Intervention

For patients with more slowly developing increases in ICP, surgical intervention can occur electively. The principles of management and the therapeutic modalities utilized to control ICP are the same as those utilized in more emergent situations. However, fewer interventions may be necessary. In some situations, operative treatment of intracranial hypertension may be separate from the definitive surgery.

TABLE 46–5. Processes Requiring Emergent Treatment of Intracranial Hypertension

Traumatic epidural or subdural hematoma
Large spontaneous intracerebral bleeding with severe elevation in ICP
Hemorrhage into a tumor or AVM with severe increase in ICP
Aneurysmal subarachnoid hemorrhage with large clot and severe increase in ICP
Ventriculoperitoneal (VP) shunt malfunction with neurologic deterioration
Postoperative bleeding with neurologic deterioration
Intracerebral bleed following carotid endarterectomy

Infratentorial Mass Lesions

In patients with infratentorial mass lesions, obstruction of CSF flow may lead to hydrocephalus. These patients often benefit from placement of a ventricular shunt or drain to normalize ICP prior to the procedure to resect the tumor.

Subarachnoid Hemorrhage

Subarachnoid hemorrhage from rupture of an intracranial aneurysm can lead to increased ICP due to cerebral edema or the presence of a large clot. Severe increases in ICP may require surgical removal of the clot, placement of a ventricular drain, or intensive medical management to reduce ICP.

It should be remembered that ICP is a component of the transmural pressure gradient of an aneurysm (MAP minus ICP). Although marked elevations of ICP are dangerous, sudden and dramatic decreases in ICP that increase the transmural pressure may lead to an increased risk of rebleeding from the aneurysm. This concern is probably more theoretic than actual, since the MAP changes are usually many times larger than the ICP changes associated with the hyperventilation and barbiturate use that accompany induction. Preoperative and intraoperative therapy to control or lower ICP must balance these risks.

Preinduction Control of Intracranial Pressure in Acute Lesions

Conventional therapy of the patient with severe head injury and elevated ICP includes the administration of osmotic diuretics such as mannitol and glycerol, fluid restriction, elevation of the head of the bed, maintenance of the head in a neutral position, muscle paralysis, ventricular CSF drainage, mechanical hyperventilation to maintain a $PaCO_2$ of 25 to 30 mm Hg, and barbiturate therapy if other modalities have not been effective in lowering ICP.[12] Steroids have no proven benefit in the treatment of severe closed head injury.[13]

Hyperventilation

Decreases in $PaCO_2$ increase brain extracellular pH and result in linear decreases in CBF between a $PaCO_2$ of 25 and 80 mm Hg. Hyperventilation is an effective means of lowering ICP. However, with time (hours to days), extracellular pH returns toward baseline and hyperventilation may become less effective. Abrupt discontinuation of hyperventilation after several days may cause significant increases in CBF, cerebral blood volume, and ICP.

Muscle Relaxants

Muscle relaxants do not directly affect ICP. However, by eliminating straining against the endotracheal tube or mechanical ventilation, muscle paralysis can decrease the intra-abdominal and intrathoracic pressure, the venous pressure, and ultimately the ICP of an intubated, mechanically ventilated patient.

Diuretics

Mannitol and glycerol both are effective in lowering elevated ICP when administered in a dose of 0.5 to 1.0 g · kg⁻¹. The dose and rapidity of infusion influence the degree of ICP reduction and rebound increases following therapy.[14] Furosemide also effectively decreases ICP in a dose of 1 mg · kg⁻¹. This dose of furosemide caused fewer electrolyte abnormalities and no transient increase in ICP before the onset of diuresis compared with mannitol.[15]

Head Elevation

A 20° to 30° elevation of the patient's head is effective in decreasing ICP, but the anesthesiologist should be sure that an untoward decrease in CPP with resultant cerebral ischemia does not occur. To prevent this complication, always reference the arterial pressure transducer to the level of the head at the external auditory meatus.[16, 17]

Barbiturates

Barbiturates decrease the cerebral metabolic rate for oxygen ($CMRo_2$) and lead to a coupled decrease in CBF and ICP. They may be effective in lowering ICP when other modalities fail. The $CMRo_2$ is reduced by about 50% when the electroencephalogram is isoelectric. Beyond this point, further reduction in $CMRo_2$ is not possible without hypothermia. A further reduction in $CMRo_2$ of approximately 7% occurs with each 1 °C drop in temperature. The best way to use barbiturates is to titrate them to an electroencephalogram isoelectric endpoint. This method helps to avoid the use of higher dosages that lead to myocardial depression and hypotension and the resultant decrease in CBF not matched by a decrease in $CMRo_2$.

Fluid Therapy

Crystalloids and Colloids. In the head trauma patient, other associated injuries frequently result in hemorrhagic shock. Aggressive fluid resuscitation is often necessary to restore and to maintain hemodynamic stability. Limitation of crystalloid infusions has been a common practice in neurosurgical patients; when resuscitation is necessary, colloids have been recommended. This practice was based on the idea that lowering of oncotic pressure with large volumes of crystalloid solutions could increase brain swelling.

Infusions of hypotonic solutions do cause an increase in ICP in this setting. However, no difference in the ICP effects of resuscitation are seen with the use of isotonic crystalloids compared with that of colloids following head injury. Maintenance of a normal *osmotic* (not *oncotic*) pressure appears to be the important concern. Infusions of hypertonic saline are also effective in resuscitating multiple trauma patients and result in a lowering of ICP.[18, 19]

Although conventional therapy of the head trauma patient includes fluid restriction, a recent study in which normovolemia and relatively high levels of CPP were maintained reported good results.[20] ICP was monitored, and patients were resuscitated with adequate fluid to maintain a normal CPP. Infusions of inotropes were utilized if necessary. The investigators suggested that fluid restriction can result in hemodynamic instability, which leads to inadequate CPP, especially in the presence of increased ICP. They proposed that a vasodilatory cascade occurs in the presence of low CPP and cerebral ischemia, resulting in further increases in ICP (Fig. 46–8). Conversely, a vasoconstriction cascade occurs with higher CPP and further lowers ICP (Fig. 46–9). Table 46–6 contains

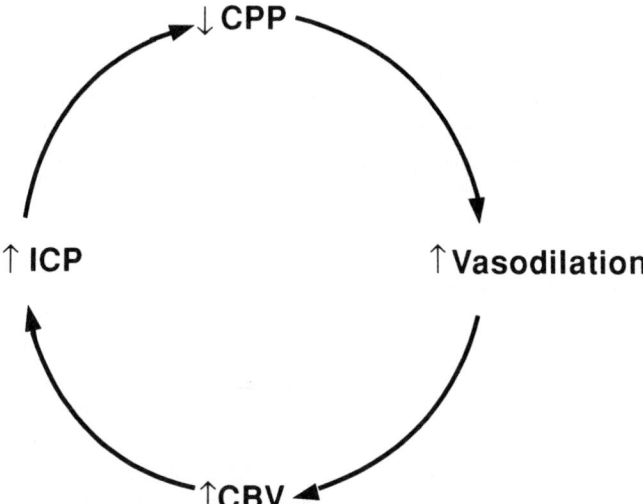

FIGURE 46–8. Vasodilatory cascade. With inadequate CPP, cerebral vasodilation occurs, causing an increase in cerebral blood volume (CBV). This leads to further increases in ICP; this, in turn, causes additional decreases in CPP. Once activated, this cycle may be self-perpetuating until maximum vasodilation occurs. (From Rosner MJ, Daughton S: Cerebral perfusion pressure management in head injury. J Trauma 1990; 30:993. © Williams & Wilkins, 1990.)

a summary of preoperative interventions to control ICP in the head trauma patient.

Preinduction Control of Intracranial Pressure in Chronic Lesions

Modalities commonly used to lower preoperative ICP in patients with more chronic lesions such as tumors differ from those used in acute head trauma patients (Table 46–7).

Diuretics

Preoperative therapy with diuretics begins to reduce ICP with the onset of diuresis.

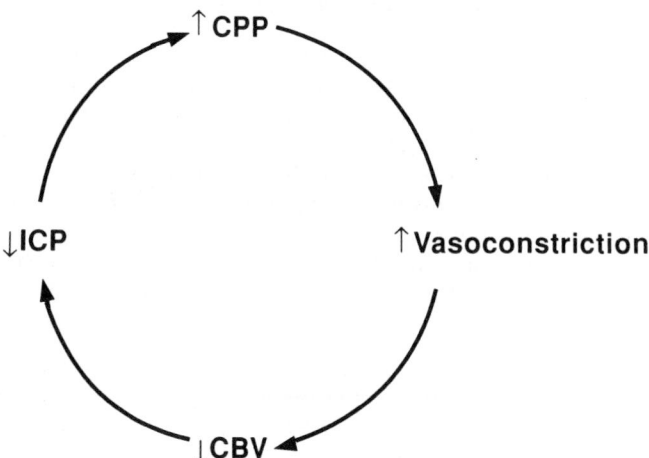

FIGURE 46–9. Vasoconstriction cascade. Restoration of adequate CPP leads to cerebral vasoconstriction, which results in a decrease in CBV. With this further decrease in volume, ICP decreases; this causes further elevation of CPP. This cycle is self-sustaining until maximum vasoconstriction occurs. (From Rosner MJ, Daughton S: Cerebral perfusion pressure management in head injury. J Trauma 1990; 30:993. © Williams & Wilkins, 1990.)

TABLE 46–6. Preoperative Control of ICP Following Head Trauma

Head-elevated and in neutral position
Hyperventilation ($Paco_2$ 25–30 mm Hg)
Furosemide (0.5–1 mg/kg)
Mannitol (0.5–1.0 g/kg over 15–30 min)
Sodium pentothal (titrated to EEG, if available)
Hypertonic saline for resuscitation
Maintain adequate cerebral perfusion pressure
100% oxygen

Steroids

Steroids given preoperatively result in a decrease in peritumor edema, reduction in shift of midline structures, reopening of compressed ventricles, and improvement of the ICP volume relationship.[21] The onset of effect occurs after several days rather than after minutes or hours as might be seen with diuretics.

Anesthesiologists must be aware that patients coming for tumor resection are likely to have been on high-dose steroid therapy for some time before surgery and are at risk for a suppressed perioperative adrenocortical stress response if the steroids are not continued. Remember also that the resolution of symptoms of increased ICP in preoperatively treated tumor patients does not imply that the ICP-volume relationship is normal. In all likelihood, the patient still has reduced cerebral elastance.

Preoperative Sedation

Sedation may result in a decreased level of consciousness and hypoventilation. Any degree of hypercarbia and resultant increase in CBF can initiate a dangerous cycle of increased ICP and a further depressed level of consciousness.

Avoidance of preoperative sedation in patients at risk for elevated ICP is a prudent course. If for any reason sedation is considered necessary, the patient should be closely monitored, and narcotics should not be utilized. Once the patient arrives in the operating suite, judicious use of sedation with continuous monitoring by anesthesia personnel can be safely undertaken.

How Is Intracranial Pressure Controlled During Anesthetic Induction?

Many events occur sequentially during anesthetic induction (Table 46–8). Approaches that seem generally similar may produce very different patient responses because of the timing and duration of pharmacologic interventions designed to offset stimulation.

TABLE 46–7. Preoperative Therapy for Improvement of Intracranial Pressure for Patients with Chronic Lesions

Mannitol
Furosemide
Steroids
Avoid preoperative sedative medications

TABLE 46–8. Control of Intracranial Pressure

Sodium thiopental, etomidate
Narcotic
Nondepolarizing muscle relaxant
Hyperventilation, assure high SpO_2
Blunt stress of intubation
   Deepen anesthetic
      Narcotic, sodium thiopental
Lidocaine
      β-Blockade (short-acting), labetalol
Prompt intubation

Preinduction Hyperventilation

Preinduction voluntary hyperventilation is popular. Although hyperventilation decreases ICP, application of a facemask to some awake brain tumor patients has been shown to elevate ICP transiently, perhaps owing to the patients' anxiety. Since we cannot predict which response will occur in a given patient, we ask him or her to hyperventilate before we apply the facemask.

Such an approach may not be critical because sodium thiopental dramatically reduces ICP when administered in doses commonly used for induction. This effect on ICP makes sodium thiopental a valuable induction agent in tumor patients. In addition, it rapidly produces unconsciousness, is well tolerated by most patients, and is a drug familiar to everyone in anesthesia. A potential shortcoming of its use is its short duration of action.

Timing

One of the most common mismatches in timing relative to ICP control is the use of sodium thiopental and nondepolarizing muscle relaxants. Techniques that use this approach are valuable and are to be recommended. However, total loss of train-of-four response is desirable to avoid an elevation of ICP during tracheal intubation. Depending on the dose of relaxant employed, this response may take ≥3 minutes. In this time, the CNS effects of sodium thiopental are decreasing; the anesthetic level is lightening; CBF is returning toward control; the reduction in ICP has peaked; and ICP is returning to its baseline level. Intubation at this point likely results in elevation of blood pressure and a probable increase in ICP. Thus, the proper selection of drugs may not give the anticipated results. Administration of additional sodium thiopental just before intubation blunts these responses.

Adjuvant Drugs

The induction drugs may be supplemented with fentanyl or a β-blocker. Fentanyl is a cerebral vasoconstrictor and reduces ICP; β-blockade prevents hypertension and the high CPP that allows breakthrough in autoregulation.

Oxygen

A very high PaO_2 is associated with an approximate 10% decrease in CBF and, thus, is a useful adjunct in the patient with increased ICP.

Nitrous Oxide

Some clinicians express concern about the use of nitrous oxide because it decreases the FIO_2 that can be used and be-cause some studies suggest that nitrous oxide causes an increase in $CMRO_2$, CBF, and ICP. These effects have been demonstrated but are not very worrisome because they are easily offset by the concomitant use of sodium thiopental or of hyperventilation during induction, or both. When nitrous oxide is used as part of an inhalation induction in a child, an intravenous infusion should be started as soon as possible to allow the administration of sodium thiopental.

Muscle Relaxants

Succinylcholine can cause an elevation in ICP by inducing contraction of the abdominal muscle or by virtue of a complex afferent mechanism that affects muscle spindles. Again, these effects can be clinically eliminated by induction doses of sodium thiopental and do not contraindicate the use of succinylcholine if other factors (e.g., full stomach) suggest its usefulness. Nondepolarizing muscle relaxants are generally preferred because they do not directly or indirectly increase ICP.

Blood Pressure

Blood pressure control during induction may be important both in normal brain and in areas where a loss of autoregulation results from the pathologic problem. Flow is pressure-dependent in areas without autoregulation, and ICP is related to CBF. Since we do not know which, if any, areas have lost autoregulation, clinical prudence suggests that blood pressure be maintained at levels that the patient sustained while awake.

Blunting the hemodynamic response to intubation can be achieved with additional anesthetic agents such as sodium thiopental, fentanyl, and lidocaine, or with vasoactive agents such as esmolol or labetalol. Trimethaphan, which also does not dilate cerebral blood vessels, is another option; however, this drug is rarely used. Sodium nitroprusside and nitroglycerin should be assiduously avoided because they are potent cerebral vasodilators and reliably increase ICP while reducing MAP, a potentially catastrophic combination, but these concerns become moot once the dura is opened.

How Is Intracranial Pressure Controlled During Anesthetic Maintenance?

Observation of the surgical site burr hole or craniotomy allows local ICP to be assessed. If the brain falls away from the dura, it is, by definition, slack. If the brain is at the edge of the craniotomy, it is difficult to "make a call." In this case, the anesthesiologist should ask the surgeon to palpate it and offer his or her assessment. When the brain or dura, or both, protrude beyond the wound's edges, pressure is high; the surgeon should be informed by the anesthesiologist that he or she is aware of the problem and is addressing it (Table 46–9).

TABLE 46–9. Therapeutic Maneuvers to Improve "Tight Brain"

Position patient to enhance cerebral venous drainage
  ↓ PCO_2, ↑ PaO_2
  ↓ Anesthetic agent, nitrous oxide
  ↑ Sodium thiopental
  ↑ Muscle relaxants
  ↑ Diuretics
  ↑ Spinal fluid drainage
  ↓ Pneumocephalus

Signs

Intracranial hypertension can result in the extrusion of brain tissue when craniotomy is performed or when difficulty is encountered in exposing a deep lesion. The first sign of difficulty is usually noted by the neurosurgeon as the craniotomy flap is removed and the dura is bulging and tense. The term "tight brain" gives no clue as to etiology nor does is suggest a probable course of treatment.

Some observations can help to assess the severity and intractability of the situation: (1) the dura is tense and bulging only at the lower portion of the craniectomy; (2) palpation may reveal that the brain tissue is easily displaced upward; and (3) the superior dura is tense only because it is being pushed out at the lower level. Surgical exposure may be slightly compromised, and certain maneuvers may improve the situation (see Table 46–9).

If the dura is tense at all edges of the craniectomy and if palpation reveals fairly immobile brain tissue beneath, surgical exposure may be severely compromised. Therapeutic interventions may help the situation but are unlikely to bring the brain profile back to the bone edge. A large dural incision will result in brain extrusion with trapping at the edges and little room to achieve exposure.

Although such extreme tenseness of the dura usually is not amenable to anesthetic manipulation, correctable problems should, nevertheless, be ruled out. The usual cause is intracranial hypertension related to the tumor mass. As resection is performed, the dural opening can be enlarged and the offending mass removed, eventually leaving a cavity where a bulging brain previously was present. An ominous cause of such swelling is occult, acute bleeding into the tumor. Hypertension without apparent cause that is unusually resistant to increasing anesthetic depth may develop. Heart rate may initially rise but then slows (Cushing's response). This response is somewhat masked by the complexity of pharmacologic and surgical interventions superimposed during anesthesia.

Timing is also important. If the brain begins to bulge vigorously where it had previously been slack, intracerebral hemorrhage must be strongly suspected. The surgeon should be informed of the subtle vital sign changes that suggest this etiology and will need to proceed more rapidly and boldly with decompression. Because of the relationship of CPP to ICP and to blood pressure, blood pressure should not be reduced before decompression, despite the probability of bleeding.

Head Position

While using the operating microscope, the surgeon may adjust the position of the table for best exposure without realizing that the patient is slowly being placed horizontal or head-down. Readjustment of the operating table to allow the head to be slightly elevated can dramatically improve the situation. Venous drainage may be compromised by extreme head positions and remain unnoticed until the dura is exposed. Repositioning the alignment of head and chin more neutrally with respect to the rest of the body may be necessary.

Control of Paco₂ and Pao₂

Because it is a powerful cerebral vasodilator, an increase in Paco₂ usually causes a dramatic increase in ICP. Hypoxic cerebral vasodilation may produce the same effect. Reassur-

ance that hypocarbia is present is only possible with blood gas analysis; capnography suggests the value, but in this situation, in which the precise Paco₂ is so important, confirmatory blood gas analysis is mandated.

Volatile Anesthetics

Despite the overall evidence supporting the safety of volatile anesthetics, these drugs probably should be discontinued and an opiate utilized in the presence of tight brain. No causal connection may exist between the use of volatile drugs and brain size, but change to an opioid-based anesthetic eliminates any such possibility.

In theory, sequential changes in anesthetics can help identify the agent responsible, although rarely is this helpful clinically. It is usually more practical to make several changes at once to effect a reduction in intracranial mass as quickly as possible.

Nitrous Oxide

Nitrous oxide may increase CBF, but its effect is likely to be less pronounced and is easily altered by sodium thiopental or opioids. Nonetheless, discontinuance of nitrous oxide completely eliminates any concern of its being causative to the problem.

Sodium Thiopental

Acute administration of a sleep dose of sodium thiopental can be expected to reduce ICP. Lack of any visible response of the brain to sodium thiopental suggests a serious problem.

Muscle Relaxants

Patients receiving antiseizure medications often have an accelerated clearance of these drugs and a shortened response to nondepolarizing muscle relaxants. Return of abdominal and thoracic muscle tone during light anesthesia can raise central venous and cerebral venous pressures (the presumed origin of the saying that "curare relaxes the brain"). Evaluation of the level of neuromuscular blockade is a subtle but important step in seeking a cause for tight brain.

Diuretics

Osmotic diuretics have long been shown to be effective in reducing normal brain tissue size by drawing water from the interstitial tissue. In a patient with intact autoregulation, mannitol results in no change in CBF and a decrease of ICP by 27% at 25 minutes. However, in patients with impaired autoregulation, the CBF increases by 5% and a lesser decrease in ICP (18%) occurs at 25 minutes.[22] Furosemide, 1 mg · kg⁻¹, intravenously reduces ICP and has a more rapid onset of effect than mannitol. Its mechanism of action is not entirely clear.[23]

Cerebrospinal Fluid Drainage

Drainage of CSF is a rapid and effective method to reduce intracranial bulk. Generally effective methods include subarachnoid needle and catheter techniques. Pneumocephalus may occur during the procedure, especially when the patient is in the sitting position, or it may be present from some previous diagnostic test. It can increase with the use of nitrous oxide.

How Is Intracranial Pressure Controlled During Anesthetic Emergence?

Neurologic Examination

The emergence strategy following neurosurgical procedures often includes a neurologic examination promptly upon completion of the operative procedure. This approach promotes early detection of any deterioration in neurologic function. Rapid diagnosis and definitive therapy to correct the etiology of unexpected postoperative neurologic changes is essential to decrease operative morbidity and mortality.

Tracheal Extubation

Frequently, the first examination occurs prior to removal of the endotracheal tube. A number of events that have the potential for causing increases in ICP may result (Table 46–10). As a patient emerges from anesthesia, the presence of the endotracheal tube may result in coughing and straining, which cause hypertension and an increase in ICP. This sequence is especially likely if the head dressing is applied during emergence while the endotracheal tube is still in place.

Emergence should be planned so that the patient is either extubated prior to placement of the head dressing or remains adequately anesthetized during the dressing application so that he or she does not respond. The latter approach can be accomplished with intravenous lidocaine or sodium thiopental, since each slows subsequent arousal.

Hypertension

Hypertension on emergence from anesthesia occurs in up to 90% of patients following neurosurgical procedures. If increases in blood pressure exceed the autoregulatory range, or if impaired autoregulation exists, increases in cerebral blood flow and ICP occur. Many agents have been shown to be effective in controlling or preventing hypertension during emergence from anesthesia, including labetalol and esmolol.[24, 25] Sympathetic blocking agents have an advantage over direct vasodilators such as nitroprusside and hydralazine in that they are less likely to cause cerebral vasodilation and increases in cerebral blood volume.

Hypoventilation

Hypoventilation also results in increases of ICP. It can result from excessive sedation or from airway obstruction. Patients undergoing posterior fossa operative procedures are at increased risk for airway obstruction and aspiration of gastric

TABLE 46–10. Management of Intracranial Pressure on Emergence

Problems	Management
Coughing	Extubate prior to dressing placement, or maintain adequate anesthesia during placement of dressing
Hypertension	Labetalol, esmolol
Hypoventilation	Assess airway reflexes prior to extubation Avoid excessive sedation
Intracerebral hemorrhage	Frequent neurologic examination, prompt diagnosis and return to operating room

contents. Impairment of cranial nerve function may occur postoperatively; patient's ability to protect the airway should be carefully verified prior to extubation. Lack of response to the endotracheal tube after arousal suggests that airway protection is at least transiently disturbed and extubation should be delayed.

Rarely following surgery involving the brainstem, the centers controlling respiratory function will have been damaged intraoperatively. Patients with such impaired function have inadequate respiratory drive and require intubation and assisted ventilation until this function improves.

How Should the Patient with Increased Intracranial Pressure Be Managed During Transport?

During transport of critically ill patients within the hospital, untoward events often occur. These events frequently are in part due to inadequate monitoring or to discontinuation of necessary therapy during the transport.[26] For the patient with elevated ICP, problems of particular concern include hypoventilation, inability to monitor the adequacy of ventilation and oxygenation, interruption of monitoring of ICP, and undetected decreases or increases in CPP.

The ideal transport should provide continued therapy (drug infusions, effective hyperventilation, and sedation if indicated) and monitoring (of ICP, oxygenation, and ventilation). With such a transport, decreases in morbidity and mortality associated with transport are demonstrated.[26] A transport ventilator, set up in the intensive care unit or operating room and titrated to a capnometer, is desirable.

Diagnostic Studies

Often, neurosurgical patients require diagnostic studies prior to or following the operative procedure. Patients with mass lesions for stereotactic neurosurgery often have the stereotactic head frame placed under local anesthesia (or in the case of pediatric patients, general anesthesia) and then travel from the operating room to the radiologic suites for multiple diagnostic procedures. These patients present a special challenge, since several hours may be required to complete all diagnostic studies. During this period, patients may be sedated or anesthetized, and are in locations remote from the main operating rooms; also, airway access may be compromised by the head frame.

Adequate monitoring should be available for transport. The diagnostic procedures are carried out in areas that are often not sufficiently well equipped to care for the anesthetized or critically ill patient. A time of particular concern is just after the patient is moved to the examining table. The patient is supine, whereas previously he or she was in a head-elevated position. An increase in ICP results. Maintenance of appropriate hyperventilation in this setting is even more important than in the operating room; access to equipment that meets the same standards as those applied to the operating room is also crucial.

Magnetic Resonance Imaging

MRI scanners are used commonly for patients with neurosurgical disorders. Because of the magnetic field, adequate monitoring may be difficult. All ferromagnetic materials must be avoided. A brass precordial stethoscope can be utilized. Automated blood pressure monitors may malfunction, but oscillatory blood pressure can be measured if the dial of the sphygmomanometer is kept away from the magnet. The electrocardiogram can be monitored utilizing telemetry (some scanners have an incorporated electrocardiograph). Special pulse oximeters can function within the scanner. However, standard pulse oximeters interfere with the scanner.

Capnography can be utilized to monitor the adequacy of ventilation by using a longer sampling line. Fluidic ventilators are useful if mechanical ventilation is indicated. Infusion pumps and pressure transducers used in the operating room are not reliable. Nonferromagnetic anesthesia machines are commercially available. To properly equip an MRI suite, anesthesiologists should be involved in the planning stages. Equipment must be evaluated in the suite on an individual basis.[27]

SUMMARY

Optimal management of the patient with increased ICP requires understanding of the pathophysiology of the process. Anesthesiologists caring for patients with neuropathology should have a thorough understanding of the intracranial pressure-volume relationship, the effect of ICP on CPP, and the impact of drugs and other interventions on these parameters. They should be knowledgeable of each patient's pathology, neurologic status, probability for developing increased ICP, and potential perioperative problems. Attention to these principles and careful monitoring of the patient in the perioperative period rather than choice of a specific technique or agent are the keys to success.

References

1. Lundberg N: Continuous monitoring and control of ventricular fluid pressure in neurosurgical practice. Acta Psychiatr Neurol Scand Suppl 1960; 36:1.
2. Lundberg N, Cronqvist S, Kjaliquist: Clinical investigations on interrelations between intracranial pressure and intracranial hemodynamics. Prog Brain Res 1968; 30:69.
3. Shapiro HM: Intracranial hypertension: therapeutic and anesthetic considerations. Anesthesiology 1975; 43:445.
4. Cushing H: Concerning a definite regulatory mechanism of the vasomotor center which controls blood pressure during cranial compression. Bull Johns Hopkins Hosp 1901; 12:290.
5. Mizutani T, Manaka S, Tsutsumi H: Estimation of intracranial pressure using computed tomography scan findings in patients with severe head injury. Surg Neurol 1990; 33:178.
6. Tadaddor K, Danziger A, Wisoff HS: Estimation of intracranial pressure by CT scan in closed head trauma. Surg Neurol 1982; 18:212.
7. Robertson CS, Narayan RK, Constant CF, et al: Clinical experience with a continuous monitor of intracranial compliance. J Neurosurg 1989; 71:673.
8. Bullock R, Golek J, Blake G: Traumatic intracerebral hematoma—which patients should undergo surgical evacuation? CT scan features and ICP monitoring as a basis for decision making. Surg Neurol 1989; 32:181.
9. Miller JD, Becker DP, Ward JD, et al: Significance of intracranial hypertension in severe head injury. J Neurosurg 1977; 47:503.
10. Uzzell BP, Orbist WD, Dolinskas CA, et al: Relationship of acute CBF and ICP findings to neuropsychological outcome in severe head injury. J Neurosurg 1986; 65:630.
11. Levin HS, Eisenberg HM, Gary HE: Intracranial hypertension in relation to memory functioning during the first year after head injury. Neurosurgery 1991; 28:196.
12. Stone JL: Nonsurgical management of increased intracranial pressure. Semin Neurol 1989; 3:218.
13. Braakman R, Schouten HJA, Dishoeck MB et al: Megadose steroids in severe head injury: results of a prospective double-blind clinical trial. J Neurosurg 1983; 58:326.
14. Node Y, Nakazawa S: Clinical study of mannitol and glycerol on raised intracranial pressure and on their rebound phenomenon. Adv Neurol 1990; 52:359.
15. Cottrell JE, Robustelli A, Post K, et al: Furosemide and mannitol induced changes in intracranial pressure and serum osmolality and electrolytes. Anesthesiology 1977; 47:28.
16. Kenning JA, Toutant SM, Saunders RL: Upright patient positioning in the management of intracranial hypertension. Surg Neurol 1981; 15:148.
17. Ernst PS, Albin MS, Bunegin L: Intracranial and spinal cord hemodynamics in the sitting position in dogs in the presence and absence of increased intracranial pressure. Anesth Analg 1990; 70:147.
18. Prough DS, Whitley JM, Taylor CL, et al: Regional cerebral blood flow following resuscitation from hemorrhagic shock with hypertonic saline: influence of a subdural mass. Anesthesiology 1991; 75:319.
19. Ducey JP, Mozingo DW, Lamiell JM, et al: A comparison of the cerebral and cardiovascular effects of complete resuscitation with isotonic and hypertonic saline, hetastarch, and whole blood following hemorrhage. J Trauma 1989; 29:1510.
20. Rosner MJ, Daughton S: Cerebral perfusion pressure management in head injury. J Trauma 1990; 30:933.
21. Miller JD, Leech P: Effects of mannitol and steroid therapy on intracranial volume-pressure relationships in patients. J Neurosurg 1975; 42:274.
22. Muizelaar JP, Lutz HA, Becker DP: Effect of mannitol on ICP and CBF and correlation with pressure autoregulation in severely head-injured patients. J Neurosurg 1984; 61:700.
23. Samson D, Beyer CW: Furosemide in the intraoperative reduction of intracranial pressure in the patient with subarachnoid hemorrhage. Neurosurgery 1982; 10:167.
24. Muzzi DA, Black S, Losasso TJ, et al: Labetalol and esmolol in the control of hypertension after intracranial surgery. Anesth Analg 1990; 70:68.
25. Gibson BE, Black S, Maass L, et al: Esmolol for the control of hypertension after neurologic surgery. Clin Pharmacol Ther 1988; 44:650.
26. Link J, Krause H, Wagner W, et al: Intrahospital transport of critically ill patients. Crit Car Med 1990; 18:1427.
27. Trankina MF, Houser WO, Cucchiara RF: Neurodiagnostic procedures. *In* Clinical Neuroanesthesia. Cucchiara RF, Michenfelder JD (eds). New York, Churchill Livingstone, 1990, pp 421–435.

CHAPTER 47

Hypoxemia

ROY D. CANE, M.B., B.Ch., F.F.A. (S.A.)

JUKKA RÄSÄNEN, M.D.

Hypoxemia is traditionally defined as a relative deficiency of oxygen (O_2) in the arterial blood. In clinical practice, arterial O_2 is quantified by measurement of the partial pressure exerted by the O_2 dissolved in plasma (PaO_2) or by the relative O_2 saturation of hemoglobin present in the blood as measured by pulse oximetry (SpO_2). In terms of these measurements, the classic definition of hypoxemia is a PaO_2 of <80 mm Hg or a SpO_2 of <95% when a patient breathes room air. Because the content of O_2 is minimally changed by increases in oxyhemoglobin (HbO_2) saturation above 90%, many clinicians consider hypoxemia as a PaO_2 of <60 mm Hg or a SpO_2 of <90%.

HYPOXEMIA, ARTERIAL OXYHEMOGLOBIN SATURATION, AND OXYGEN CONTENT

Most blood O_2 is in combination with hemoglobin. The affinity of hemoglobin for O_2 varies with the degree of oxygenation of the hemoglobin molecule. Thus, the relationship between the partial pressure of O_2 (PO_2) and HbO_2 saturation (SaO_2) is not linear. Figure 47–1 illustrates the relationship between PO_2 and SaO_2.

The affinity of hemoglobin for O_2 is increased (leftward shift of the HbO_2 dissociation curve) by reduced: temperature, partial pressure of carbon dioxide (PCO_2), hydrogen ion concentration (alkalemia), and red blood cell concentration of 2,3-diphosphoglycerate (2,3-DPG); increases in these factors decrease the HbO_2 affinity (rightward shift of the HbO_2 dissociation curve) (Fig. 47–2.) These alterations in hemoglobin-O_2 affinity have the potential to impair tissue O_2 availability significantly under conditions of acute severe acidemia or hypercarbia.

How Do PaO₂ and SpO₂ Correlate?

Pulse oximetry measures the SpO_2 in vivo and is an indirect reflection of the PaO_2. Note that the magnitude of change in SpO_2 secondary to changes in PaO_2 is greater at PaO_2 <60 mm Hg (SpO_2 <90%) and decreases with increasing PaO_2 above 60 mm Hg. Thus, pulse oximetry is a sensitive monitor of arterial oxygenation in the critical range of PaO_2 <60 mm Hg but a relatively insensitive monitor at higher and supranormal PaO_2.

How Do PaO₂ and Arterial Blood Oxygen Content Correlate?

The actual volume of O_2 in the arterial blood (CaO_2) is the sum of the amount of O_2 in combination with hemoglobin and the amount dissolved in the plasma. The O_2 content of an arterial blood sample ($mL \cdot dL^{-1}$) can be calculated as follows:

$$CaO_2 = Hb \times 1.34 \times SaO_2 + PaO_2 \times 0.003$$

Equation 1

Assuming a PaO_2 of 100 mm Hg and a hemoglobin concentration of 15 $g \cdot 100 mL^{-1}$, the CaO_2 is approximately 20.3 $mL \cdot dL^{-1}$, 20 mL of which is in combination with hemoglobin and 0.3 mL of which is in solution in the plasma. Because of the nonlinear relationship between PaO_2 and SaO_2, increasing PaO_2 above 60 mm Hg (SpO_2 >90%) results in small increases in CaO_2. Figure 47–3 shows the relative amounts of dissolved O_2 and HbO_2 relative to PaO_2 and SaO_2.

Dyshemoglobinemias

Pathologic forms of hemoglobin (e.g., carboxyhemoglobin, methemoglobin) that are unable to combine reversibly with O_2 reduce the CaO_2 even if the PaO_2 is normal. Calculation of CaO_2 should be based on direct measurement of the SaO_2 by co-oximetry rather than obtained from values derived from nomograms if any form of abnormal hemoglobin is suspected.

What Are the Causes of Hypoxemia?

O_2 moves from the alveolar gas to the plasma by diffusion down a partial pressure gradient. When O_2 dissolves in the plasma, it is almost immediately taken up by combination with hemoglobin. O_2 continues to move from alveolar gas to pulmonary capillary blood until the partial pressure gradient no

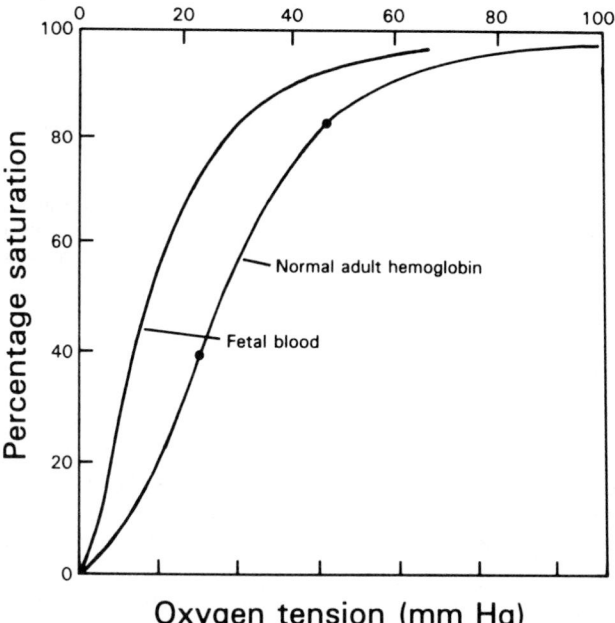

FIGURE 47–1. Graphic depiction of the relationship between Pa_{O_2} and oxyhemoglobin saturation for adult and fetal hemoglobin.

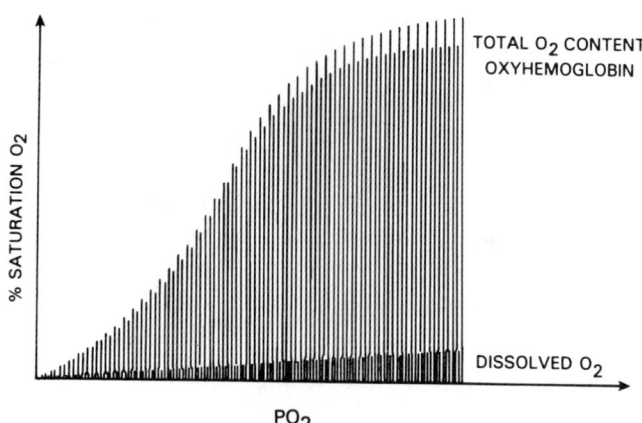

FIGURE 47–3. Graphic depiction of the contributions of the dissolved O_2 and the oxyhemoglobin content to the total O_2 content of blood at different oxyhemoglobin saturations and P_{O_2}. (Reproduced from Shapiro BA, Harrison RA, Cane RD, et al: Arterial oxygenation. *In* Clinical Application of Blood Gases. 4th ed. Chicago, Year Book Medical Publishers, 1989; p 66.)

longer exists. At this equilibrium point, the hemoglobin is maximally saturated for that P_{O_2}.

Development of adequate P_{O_2} in the pulmonary capillary blood is dependent on maintenance of an adequate alveolar O_2 partial pressure (PA_{O_2}); given that the P_{O_2} at the end of a pulmonary capillary should be equal to the PA_{O_2}, inadequate oxygenation of the pulmonary capillary blood occurs if the PA_{O_2} is <80 mm Hg.

Appropriate matching of alveolar ventilation ($\dot{V}A$) and perfusion ($\dot{Q}$) is also essential for adequate gas exchange. Hypox-emia commonly develops because of pulmonary abnormalities that impair $\dot{V}A$ and/or $\dot{Q}$.

Pulmonary Mechanisms

Alveolar gas is a mixture of O_2, nitrogen (N_2), water vapor, carbon dioxide (CO_2), and various trace inert gases. The partial pressure of the individual gases in a mixture of gases contained in a closed space is equal to the total pressure within that space. The total pressure of gas in an alveolus is equal to barometric pressure (PB).

Ventilation

The PA_{O_2} is determined by $\dot{V}A$, the fraction of inspired O_2 (FI_{O_2}), and alveolar O_2 uptake. Ideal alveolar gas cannot be sampled; however, the ideal PA_{O_2} may be calculated:

$$PA_{O_2} = PB \times (FI_{O_2} - [O_2 \text{ uptake}/\dot{V}A])$$

Equation 2

The alveolar CO_2 tension (PA_{CO_2}) is determined by the level of $\dot{V}A$ (see Chapter 48). Assuming that the PA_{CO_2} is equal to the Pa_{CO_2} and that the O_2 in the inspired gas is exchanged for the CO_2 in exhaled gas, the PA_{O_2} can be approximated by the following equation:

$$PA_{O_2} = \text{inspired } P_{O_2} - Pa_{CO_2}$$

Equation 3

Application of correction factors to compensate for the fact that CO_2 production is less than O_2 consumption (reflected by the respiratory quotient [RQ]) produces the following clinically practical relationship:

$$PA_{O_2} = \text{inspired } P_{O_2} - (Pa_{CO_2}/RQ)$$

Equation 4

Note that although this equation does not account for the difference between inspired and expired gas volumes, it allows bedside calculations of the ideal PA_{O_2}. The inspired P_{O_2} is equal to the PB minus the partial pressure of N_2 and water

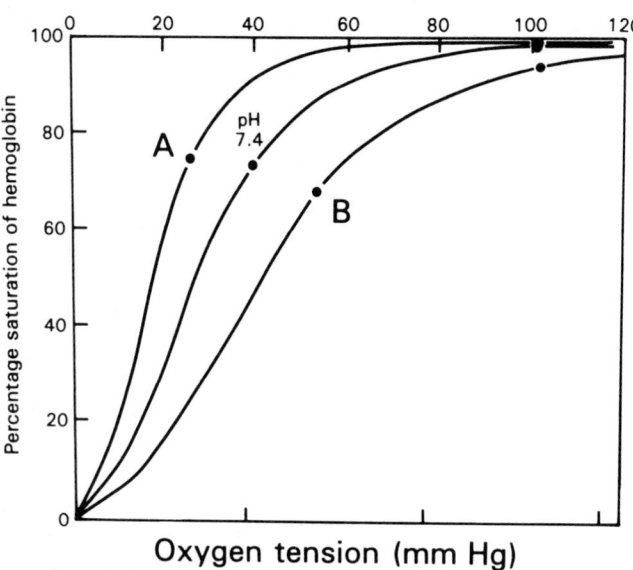

FIGURE 47–2. Graphic representation of the shift in the HbO_2 curve associated with changes in pH, P_{CO_2}, temperature, and 2,3-DPG. The *center curve* is the normal curve under standard conditions; the other two curves show the leftward displacement *(Curve A)* caused by a decrease and the rightward shift *(Curve B)* caused by an increase in hydrogen ion concentration, temperature, P_{CO_2}, and 2,3-DPG concentration.

vapor (47 mm Hg)—that is, $P_{IO_2} = (P_B - P_{H_2O}) \times F_{IO_2}$; a clinically useful form of the equation follows:

$$P_{AO_2} = [(P_B - 47) \times F_{IO_2}] - [P_{aCO_2}/0.8]$$

Equation 5

Thus lower P_B (high altitude) or F_{IO_2} and higher P_{aCO_2} (hypoventilation) result in reduced P_{AO_2}. Figure 47–4 graphically represents the relationship between P_{AO_2}, F_{IO_2}, and alveolar ventilation ($\dot{V}_A$).

Ventilation/Perfusion Mismatching

For any given level of $\dot{V}_A$, the distribution of ventilation relative to the distribution of pulmonary perfusion determines the effective gas exchange hence has a role in determining the P_{aO_2}.

A normal pulmonary gas exchange unit consists of an alveolus and an associated pulmonary capillary. Normal gas exchange between blood and alveolar gas depends on matching of relatively equal $\dot{V}_A$ and $\dot{Q}$ (i.e., a $\dot{V}_A/\dot{Q}$ ratio of approximately one). Figure 47–5 depicts the spectrum of alveolar ventilation and pulmonary perfusion relationships.

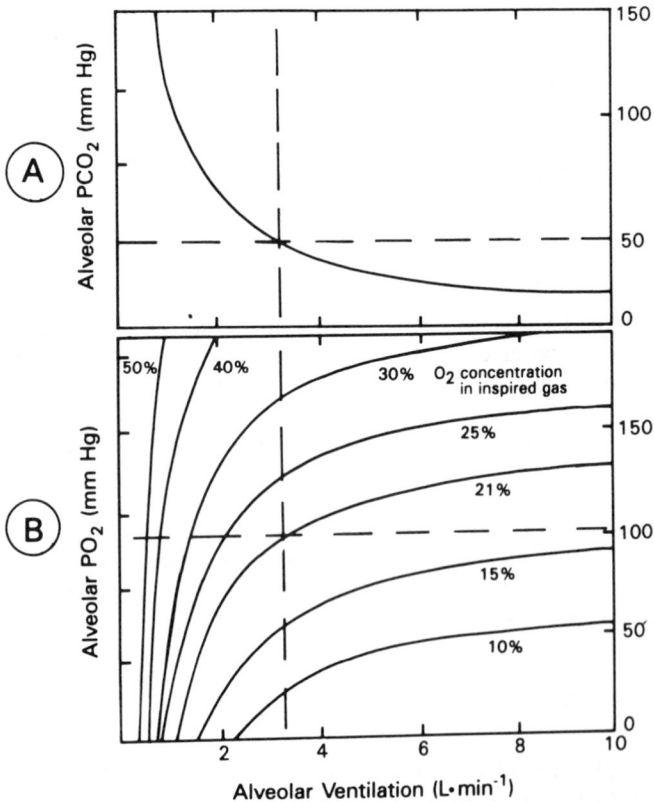

FIGURE 47–4. Alveolar gas tensions produced by different levels of alveolar ventilation. *A*, The hyperbolic relationship between alveolar P_{aCO_2} and $\dot{V}_A$. *B*, The relationship between P_{AO_2} and $\dot{V}_A$ for different levels of oxygen concentration in the inspired gas. The *broken vertical line* indicates a $\dot{V}_A$ of 3.2 L · min⁻¹. Dry barometric pressure = 713 mm Hg; CO_2 output = 180 mL · min⁻¹ (BTPS); oxygen uptake = 225 mL · min⁻¹ (BTPS). No allowance has been made for the difference between inspired and expired volumes. (Reproduced from Nunn JF: Pulmonary ventilation. *In* Applied Respiratory Physiology. 3rd ed. Nunn JF (ed). London, Butterworth-Heinemann Ltd, 1987; p 111.)

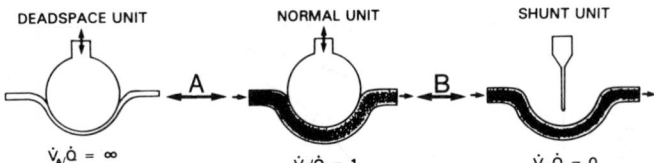

FIGURE 47–5. Ventilation to perfusion relationships. *A*, The spectrum of ventilation in excess of perfusion. *B*, The spectrum of perfusion in excess of ventilation. The true deadspace unit is represented by $\dot{V}_A/\dot{Q} = \infty$; the normal unit is represented by $\dot{V}_A/\dot{Q} = 1$; the shunt unit is represented by $\dot{V}_A/\dot{Q} = 0$.

Dead Space Ventilation. Ventilation in excess of $\dot{Q}$ results in increased dead space ventilation ($\dot{V}_D$) and primarily impairs CO_2 excretion (see Chapter 48).

Shunt Effect. Diminished $\dot{V}_A$ relative to $\dot{Q}$ results in a reduced P_{AO_2} and, hence, a reduced P_{O_2} in the pulmonary capillaries. Figure 47–6 demonstrates the incomplete oxygenation of pulmonary capillary blood in regions of lung with $\dot{V}_A/\dot{Q}$ of <1 but >0, and $\dot{V}_A/\dot{Q} = 0$.

When the partial pressure of pulmonary capillary blood O_2 ($P\acute{c}O_2$) is reduced, a lower O_2 content ($C\acute{c}O_2$) results. This change, in turn, reduces the C_{aO_2} in left heart blood and results in hypoxemia. The magnitude of hypoxemia is a function of the amount and degree of lung with reduced $\dot{V}_A/\dot{Q}$ matching; the lower the $\dot{V}_A/\dot{Q}$, the lower the P_{AO_2}. Gas exchange units with a $\dot{V}_A/\dot{Q}$ of <1 but >0 are termed *shunt effect units*.

Shunt. A gas exchange unit with no ventilation that is still perfused ($\dot{V}_A/\dot{Q} = 0$) results in mixed venous blood returning to the left heart and is termed a *shunt unit*. The magnitude of hypoxemia secondary to shunt units is a function of their number and the O_2 content of the shunted mixed venous blood.

Cardiopulmonary Pathology

Cardiopulmonary pathology results in various degrees of $\dot{V}_A/\dot{Q}$ mismatching. The magnitude of hypoxemia depends on the relative ratio of shunt to shunt effect units and the amount of lung tissue with abnormal $\dot{V}_A/\dot{Q}$ relationships. Factors that affect the distribution of pulmonary blood flow and ventilation are summarized in Table 47–1. Maldistribution of ventilation secondary to regional differences in airway resistance and lung

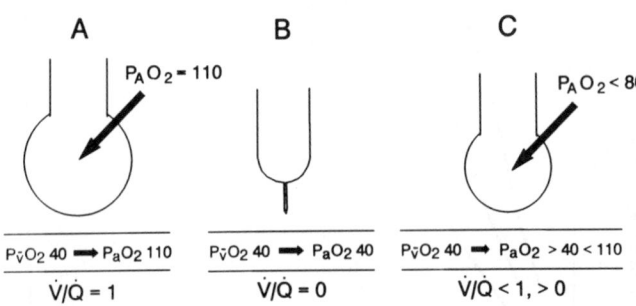

FIGURE 47–6. Diagrammatic representation of ventilation/perfusion relationships. *A*, A normal $\dot{V}_A/\dot{Q}$ relationship with a ratio of 1. This $\dot{V}_A/\dot{Q}$ relationship is associated with complete saturation of hemoglobin in the blood passing through this alveolocapillary unit. *B*, A shunt unit ($\dot{V}_A/\dot{Q} = 0$). The HbO_2 saturation of blood passing through this unit is unchanged. *C*, A shunt effect unit with a $\dot{V}_A/\dot{Q}$ of <1, but >0. Hemoglobin in the blood passing through this unit is only partially saturated. (From Cane RD: Oxygen challenge. *In* Handbook of Critical Care Procedures and Therapy. Cane RD, Davison R, Albrink MH (eds). St Louis, Mosby–Year Book, 1992.)

TABLE 47–1. Factors That Affect Pulmonary Blood Flow and Ventilation

Body position
Cardiac output
Hypoxic pulmonary vasoconstrictor reflexes
Pulmonary vascular resistance
Alveolar ventilation
Regional variations in airway resistance
Regional variations in lung compliance
Inspired oxygen concentrations

TABLE 47–2. Factors That Determine the Rate of Oxygen Diffusion

The tension gradient between alveolar gas and pulmonary capillary plasma ($P_{AO_2}-P\acute{c}o_2$)
The surface area across which gas exchange occurs
The length of the diffusion pathway (i.e., thickness of the alveolar-capillary membrane)
The solubility of oxygen in the plasma
The rate at which hemoglobin takes up oxygen from the plasma
The transit time of blood in the capillary bed

compliance associated with pulmonary disease is the most common cause of $\dot{V}_A/\dot{Q}$ mismatching.

Diffusion Block

O_2 moves from alveolar gas to capillary blood by a process of diffusion. The rate of diffusion is determined by the factors listed in Table 47–2. Whether a diffusion block is a cause of hypoxemia is controversial. However, a $\dot{V}_A/\dot{Q}$ mismatch can result in reduction of P_{AO_2} and in the surface area across which gas diffusion occurs. Thus, impairment of diffusion may be a factor in the hypoxemia associated with $\dot{V}_A/\dot{Q}$ mismatching.

Electron microscopic studies of the alveolar-capillary membrane in pulmonary edema and fibrosis have not revealed appreciable thickening of the area of membrane across which gas exchange occurs, suggesting that lengthening of the diffusion pathway is not a clinical reality.

Mean Transit Time. The mean transit time of blood in the pulmonary capillary is about 0.8 seconds, although the range around the mean is great. An average transit time of 0.3 seconds is thought to be necessary to develop a maximal $P\acute{c}o_2$. Blood from capillaries with very short transit times (<0.2 s) will be desaturated and may contribute to hypoxemia. Capillary transit times vary throughout the lungs, and a wide spread of transit times increases the gradient between the P_{AO_2} and Pa_{O_2}.[1, 2]

Hemoglobin-Oxygen Uptake. The rate at which hemoglobin takes up O_2 from the pulmonary capillary plasma is sufficiently slow so that at normal pulmonary capillary transit times, HbO_2 uptake is the rate-limiting factor for diffusion of O_2.

Nonpulmonary Mechanisms

Changes in Cardiac Output and Oxygen Consumption

The relationship between cardiac output, O_2 consumption ($\dot{V}_{O_2}$), and the O_2 content difference between arterial and mixed venous blood, $C(a-\bar{v})_{O_2}$ may be represented by Fick's equation:

$$\text{Cardiac output} = \dot{V}_{O_2}/C(a-\bar{v})_{O_2} \qquad \text{Equation 6}$$

If cardiac output remains unchanged and $\dot{V}_{O_2}$ increases or $\dot{V}_{O_2}$ remains constant but cardiac output decreases, the amount of O_2 extracted from the arterial blood increases. A decrease in the $C\bar{v}_{O_2}$ and an increase in $C(a-\bar{v})_{O_2}$ result. Table 47–3 shows the relationship of cardiac output to O_2 extraction.

Intrapulmonary shunting of mixed venous blood results in hypoxemia, the magnitude of which varies directly with the amount of shunt and inversely with the $C\bar{v}_{O_2}$. For any given intrapulmonary shunt ($\dot{Q}sp/\dot{Q}t$), a lower $C\bar{v}_{O_2}$ increases the degree of hypoxemia.

Cardiac output normally is adjusted to meet the tissue O_2 demand. However, in patients with limited myocardial function, this physiologic mechanism fails, and hypoxemia results in response to an increase in tissue O_2 demand. Primary myocardial failure (cardiogenic shock) causes hypoxemia because of the low $C\bar{v}_{O_2}$. Table 47–4 shows the relationship between cardiac output and Pa_{O_2}.

Anemia

Anemia reduces Ca_{O_2}. Tissue O_2 delivery ($\dot{D}_{O_2}$) is the product of cardiac output and Ca_{O_2}. Normally, a decrease in Ca_{O_2} is compensated for by an increase in cardiac output, thus maintaining $\dot{D}_{O_2}$. If cardiac output cannot be increased and $\dot{V}_{O_2}$ remains constant, the net result is a reduction in $C\bar{v}_{O_2}$ with the potential for hypoxemia described earlier.

Anemia is likely to be a factor in hypoxemia if limited myocardial function or an increase in $\dot{V}_{O_2}$ exceeds a patient's ability to increase cardiac output. In patients with good myocardial function, hemoglobin concentrations as low as $7 \text{ g} \cdot 100 \text{ mL}^{-1}$ are well tolerated. When myocardial failure is present, consideration should be given to maintaining $\dot{D}_{O_2}$ by increasing the O_2-carrying capacity and Ca_{O_2}; hemoglobin concentrations of 10 to $11 \text{ g} \cdot 100 \text{ mL}^{-1}$ may be necessary.

Right-to-Left Intracardiac Shunting

Right-to-left intracardiac shunts result in mixed venous blood entering the left heart and a reduction in the Ca_{O_2}. The magnitude of hypoxemia that results depends on the size of the shunt and the $C\bar{v}_{O_2}$.

TABLE 47–3. Relationship of Cardiac Output to Oxygen Extraction

	Oxygen Consumption ($\text{mL} \cdot \text{min}^{-1}$)	Cardiac Output ($\dot{Q}t$) ($\text{L} \cdot \text{min}^{-1}$)	Oxygen Extraction $C(a-\bar{v})_{O_2}$ [$\text{mL} \cdot \text{dL}^{-1}$ ($\text{mL} \cdot \text{L}^{-1}$)]
Normal cardiac output	250	5	5 (50)
Increased cardiac output	250	10	2.5 (25)
Decreased cardiac output	250	2.5	10 (100)

TABLE 47–4. Comparison Effect of Cardiac Output on Arterial Oxygen Tension

$\dot{Q}sp/\dot{Q}t$ (%)	$\dot{V}O_2$ (mL · min^{-1})	$\dot{Q}t$ (L · min^{-1})	$C(a–\bar{v})O_2$ (mL · dL^{-1})	PaO_2 (mm Hg)
25	250	10	2.5	127
25	250	5	5.0	84
25	250	2.5	10.0	55
PAO_2 = 335 mm Hg	FIO_2 = 50%	Hemoglobin = 15 g · 100 mL^{-1}	$C\acute{c}O_2$ = 2.17 vol%	

ASSESSMENT OF HYPOXEMIA

What Are Conventional Blood Gas Measurements?

Modern blood gas analyzers incorporate electrodes that measure pH, PCO_2, and PO_2.[3] Bicarbonate concentration and base deficit are derived from nomograms based on the Henderson-Hasselbalch equation.

pH

If two solutions of different pH are separated from each other by a pH-sensitive glass membrane, a potential difference develops across the glass membrane and can be measured as a voltage. If the pH of one solution is known, that of the second solution can be determined from the measured potential difference.

PCO_2

When a CO_2-containing solution is separated from an aqueous bicarbonate solution by a semi-permeable membrane, CO_2 diffuses across the membrane and undergoes the following chemical reaction:

$$CO_2 + H_2O \rightarrow H_2CO_3 \rightarrow H^+ + HCO_3^-$$

Equation 7

The hydrogen ion concentration ($[H^+]$) developed is proportional to the PCO_2 of the CO_2-containing solution. This principle is applied in the Severinghaus electrode.

PO_2

The polarographic PO_2 electrode (Clark's electrode) consists of a silver anode and a platinum cathode in a potassium chloride solution. Oxidation of the anode to form silver chloride results in a flow of electrons and a measurable current.

At the cathode, O_2 is reduced to hydroxyl ions, a reaction that consumes electrons and, in turn, accelerates the oxidation reaction at the anode. The electrode is separated from the blood sample by a polypropylene membrane that allows slow diffusion of O_2 into the electrode.

The change in the current flow from cathode to anode is related to the number of electrons consumed at the cathode, which in turn is proportional to the amount of O_2 reduced. Thus, the PO_2 in the blood is proportional to the change in current measured at the anode.

What Are the Alternatives to Conventional Analysis?

Conventional blood gas analysis has the disadvantage of being an interval monitor that requires collection of an arterial blood sample for analysis at a remote site with a significant time delay. Newer developments in blood gas monitoring allow continuous on-line monitoring at patients' bedsides.

Pulse oximetry and transcutaneous blood gas measurements are well defined and characterized. Optical fluorescence techniques have enabled development of bedside blood gas analyzers for intermittent, on-demand, ex vivo arterial blood gas (ABG) measurement with response times <2 minutes. Continuous intra-arterial monitors are technically feasible.[4] These optical fluorescence–based techniques have just become available for routine clinical application.

Transcutaneous Gas Measurement Limitations

Transcutaneous PO_2 ($PtcO_2$) electrodes (modified Clark's electrodes), measure the flux of O_2 across the skin.[5] Perfusion of the dermis involves capillary loops that extend up into the epidermal papillae.

Arterial Venous Mixing

As well-oxygenated arterial blood flows up the loop, O_2 diffuses out of the ascending limb of the capillary into the less well-oxygenated blood in the descending limb of the loop. Thus the blood at the skin surface has a PO_2 approximately 15% less than the PaO_2. Figure 47–7 illustrates this principle.

Skin Perfusion

The $PtcO_2$ is also dependent on skin perfusion and is a reliable reflector of PaO_2 only when the cardiac index is >2 L · min^{-1}/m$^{2-1}$. Available transcutaneous monitors all use heated electrodes that raise the skin temperature to 40 °C to 44 °C.

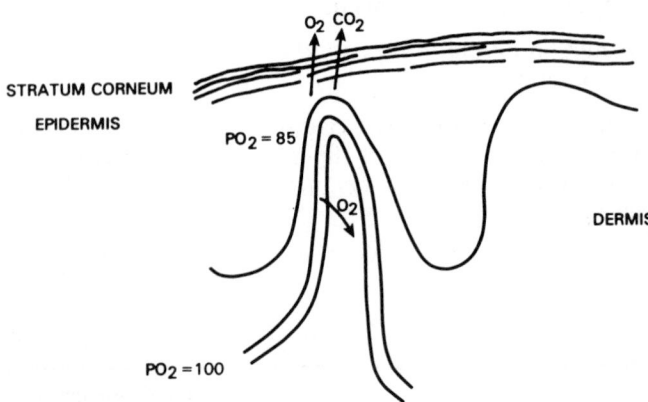

FIGURE 47–7. Diagrammatic representation of the countercurrent flow of O_2 in a capillary of a dermal papilla. The PO_2 at the base of the capillary loop is approximately 100 mm Hg; as blood ascends in the capillary loop, O_2 diffuses across to the descending limb of the capillary loop, resulting in a PO_2 at the tip of the loop of only approximately 85 mm Hg.

Blood flow rate and transcutaneous flow of O_2 are thereby enhanced.

Although transcutaneous monitoring of Po_2 provides reliable trend information in patients with adequate cardiovascular function, pulse oximetry is the more widely used technique for continuous monitoring of the arterial oxygenation status.

Oximetry

Oximetry describes various spectrophotometric techniques that determine the HbO_2 saturation. If blood is exposed to light of a particular wavelength and intensity, measurement of the light absorbed by the HbO_2 moiety is proportional to the relative amount of HbO_2 present. This relationship can be expressed mathematically as follows:

$$A = alc \qquad \text{Equation 8}$$

where A is the amount of light absorbed, a is the absorption of HbO_2 at a given wavelength, l is the length of the light path, and c is the concentration of HbO_2. Rearranging this equation gives the following mathematic relationship for absorption:

$$a = A/lc \qquad \text{Equation 9}$$

A calibration constant can be derived by comparison of absorption between two substances with identical absorption at a given wavelength:

$$A/lc \ (standard[st]) = A/lc \ (unknown[u])$$

$$\text{Equation 10}$$

If the light path length is held constant, the concentration of the unknown substance is determined by the following relationship:

$$c_u = A_u \times C_{st}/A_{st} \qquad \text{Equation 11}$$

Application of these principles to patient monitoring assumes that the measured change in absorption is a function of the different forms of hemoglobin present in the blood only. The presence of other substances with spectral activity in the light wavelengths used results in erroneous measurements. Two applications of these principles are routinely used in the clinical management of anesthetized and critically ill patients: pulse oximetry and mixed venous oximetry.

Pulse Oximetry

Principles of Operation. Pulse oximeters are dual-wavelength spectrophotometers that use light-emitting diodes as a light source and photodiodes for light detection. When the light source and detector are separated by a pulsating arterial vascular bed, the degree of change in the transmitted light (light emitted minus light absorbed) is proportional to the size of the arterial pulse, the wavelengths of light, and the HbO_2 concentration. If the pulse is considered to be entirely due to the passage of arterial blood and the appropriate light wavelengths (660 and 940 nm) are used, the SpO_2 can be continuously measured.

Accuracy. The clinical accuracy of pulse oximeters compared with laboratory co-oximeters is excellent for HbO_2 saturations >80%.[11-19] At saturations <80%, agreement between the pulse oximeter and co-oximeter is diminished; however, the pulse oximeter still reliably trends the changes in HbO_2 saturation.

Table 47–5 shows the range of bias and precision of four different commercially available pulse oximeters. Note that the precision is best at HbO_2 saturations >95% and deteriorates at lower levels.

Applicability. The noninvasive nature, almost universal applicability, and real-time measurements of pulse oximetry, coupled with the lack of any calibration routine and sensor site preparation, have resulted in widespread use of this monitor for continuous assessment of patients' arterial oxygenation status in the operating room and intensive care unit.

Reliability. Pulse oximetry may be unreliable under the following circumstances:

Spectrophotometric Limitations. Substances other than reduced hemoglobin and HbO_2 with spectral activity in the light wavelengths used for pulse oximetry give spurious results. Methylene blue, indocyanine green, and indigo carmine have been reported to interfere.[6] Intralipid has spectral activity in the wavelengths used for co-oximetry and may interfere with pulse oximetry.[7]

Significant amounts of other hemoglobin moieties (carboxy-hemoglobin; methemoglobin) may impair pulse oximetry. The algorithm used in most pulse oximeters contains a correction factor that compensates for fetal hemoglobin; thus, pulse oximetry can be reliably used to monitor neonates and infants.

Severe anemia (hemoglobin <5 g · 100 mL^{-1}) results in unreliable pulse oximeter readings. High levels of ambient infrared light from heating lamps used in pediatric care can interfere with pulse oximetry if the sensor is not properly shielded.[8]

Absence of Pulsatile Flow. Absence of arterial pulsation, as may occur with cardiopulmonary arrest, severe hypotension, cardiopulmonary bypass, and significant hypothermia, renders pulse oximetry unreliable.[9, 10] Similarly, significant venous pulsations can impair the validity of pulse oximetry readings. Clinical circumstances in which this aberration may occur include severe right ventricular failure, obstruction to venous drainage, tricuspid incompetence, markedly increased intrathoracic pressures, and placement of a pulse oximetry probe on a dependent limb.[10]

Interference Artifact. Motion of the digit to which the sensor is applied may be interpreted as pulsatile motion and lead

TABLE 47–5. Ranges of Bias and Precision of SpO_2 Measured with Four Different Pulse Oximeters

Range of Sao_2	<85	85–89%	90–95%	>95%
Bias	0.02–2.41	0.12–1.12	0.35–1.45	−0.16–1.09
Precision	± 2.7 to ± 4.5	± 1.97 to ± 3.68	± 1.55 to ± 2.1	± 0.98 to ± 1.95

(Unpublished data courtesy of David Thrush, M.D.)

to spurious readings. Electrocautery can interfere with the instrument, a problem readily overcome by having the electrocautery device on a separate alternating current circuit or running the pulse oximeter from an internal battery.[9]

Mixed Venous Oximetry. Incorporating fiberoptic techniques in flow-directed pulmonary artery catheters enables continuous measurement of the HbO_2 concentration of mixed venous blood in the pulmonary artery. Mixed venous oximetry is an application of reflectance spectrophotometry, in which light of appropriate wavelengths is flashed down a fiberoptic path; the resultant reflected light from the hemoglobin passes back up the fiberoptic path. The ratio of reflected light between the different wavelengths is proportional to the mixed venous HbO_2 saturation ($S\bar{v}O_2$).[20]

Calibration. The catheter must be calibrated. Stability of the calibration is unaffected by temperature variations and by hemoglobin concentration, provided the hematocrit is >40%.[21] Calibration curves are shifted by 1% for every 0.1 change in pH.[21] Thus, calibration, either against a standard sample of known HbO_2 saturation before insertion[22] or against a measured $S\bar{v}O_2$ obtained from a blood sample taken after catheter placement[20] is feasible and reliable. Technical limitations of mixed venous oximetry are listed in Table 47–6.[20, 23]

Mixed venous fiberoptic oximetry correlates well with co-oximetric measurement of $S\bar{v}O_2$.[23, 24] Clinically acceptable accuracy is unaffected by body temperature, hemoglobin concentration, cardiac index, and method of calibration.

Clinical Significance of $S\bar{v}O_2$

The $S\bar{v}O_2$ is proportional to the $C\bar{v}O_2$ and thus reflects the balance between $\dot{D}O_2$ and $\dot{V}O_2$. Because tissue oxygenation depends on cardiac output, CaO_2, tissue perfusion, and tissue $\dot{V}O_2$, any change in these factors may alter the $S\bar{v}O_2$.

Changes in Cardiac Output. Significant decreases in CaO_2 secondary to reductions in PaO_2 or hemoglobin concentration usually result in an increase in cardiac output and no change in $S\bar{v}O_2$. If a patient's cardiovascular function is limited, a reduction in PaO_2 or hemoglobin concentration may result in a fall in $S\bar{v}O_2$. If hemoglobin concentration and pulmonary gas exchange remain constant, changes in $S\bar{v}O_2$ readings reflect changes in cardiac output or $\dot{V}O_2$ or both.

Table 47–7 lists average values for measurements of the oxygenation of mixed venous blood under different conditions of cardiovascular function. These guidelines are rendered unreliable by anemia, hypoperfusion, acidemia, and sepsis.

Adequacy of Tissue Perfusion. Any change in $S\bar{v}O_2$ requires complete evaluation of the patient's cardiopulmonary function.[25] However, the ranges of $S\bar{v}O_2$ reflecting the adequacy of O_2 reserves if the $\dot{V}O_2$ demand increases are reliable (Table 47–8).

TABLE 47–6. Limitations of Mixed Venous Oximetry

Catheter breakage.
Vessel wall interference secondary to the catheter's tip lying against the vessel wall.[23] Repositioning of the catheter usually corrects this problem.
Thrombus formation over the catheter.tip; appropriate continuous flushing of the catheter minimizes this problem.
Presence of other substances with spectrophotometric activity in the light wavelengths used. In vivo calibration of the catheter against a co-oximeter measured $S\bar{v}O_2$ corrects this problem, provided the concentrations of carboxyhemoglobin and methemoglobin remain relatively constant.[20]
Hemodilution. Hematocrits between 40% and 30% result in $S\bar{v}O_2$ readings that vary by approximately 3%.

When Is Physiologic Shunt Calculation of Value?

The foregoing discussion has demonstrated the interrelated aspects of cardiopulmonary function and the multiple factors that affect PaO_2. Evaluation of the relative contribution of cardiac and pulmonary dysfunction to hypoxemia is frequently useful in guiding management of disorders of tissue oxygenation in critically ill patients. Assessment of how well the lungs are functioning as an oxygenator is best accomplished by calculation of the $\dot{Q}sp/\dot{Q}t$.

The concept behind this calculation is best stated as a question: How much of the cardiac output would have to pass directly from the right heart to the left heart to produce this degree of hypoxemia?

Methodology

Calculation of the $\dot{Q}sp/\dot{Q}t$ requires simultaneous arterial and mixed venous blood gas measurements. The formula for the calculation is as follows:

$$\dot{Q}sp/\dot{Q}t = (C\acute{c}O_2 - CaO_2)/(C\acute{c}O_2 - C\bar{v}O_2)$$

Equation 12

The $C\acute{c}O_2$ is calculated assuming that $P\acute{c}O_2$ equals PAO_2 and the O_2 saturation of pulmonary capillary blood equals 100% (generally true if the PAO_2 is at least 150 mm Hg). If the PAO_2 is <150 mm Hg, correction factors can be applied to enable calculation of $C\acute{c}O_2$.[26] Figure 47–8 illustrates the O_2 content relationships expressed in the $\dot{Q}sp/\dot{Q}t$ calculation.

The $\dot{Q}sp/\dot{Q}t$ incorporates both the true shunt ($\dot{V}A/\dot{Q} = 0$) and the shunt effect ($\dot{V}A/\dot{Q} >0$ but <1) contributions to hypoxemia.

Limitations

The $\dot{Q}sp/\dot{Q}t$ originally was calculated from blood gas measurements made with a patient breathing 100% O_2 in an attempt to separate the relative contribution of true shunt and shunt

TABLE 47–7. Reference Values Relating to Pulmonary Artery Oxygenation in the Critically Ill

Cardiovascular Status	$P\bar{v}O_2$	$S\bar{v}O_2$	$C(a-\bar{v})O_2$
Healthy resting human volunteer	40 (37–43)	75 (70–76)	5.0 (4.5–6.0)
Critically ill, adequate cardiovascular status	37 (35–40)	70 (68–75)	3.5 (2.5–4.5)
Critically ill, borderline cardiovascular status	32 (30–35)	60 (56–68)	5.0 (4.5–6.0)
Critically ill, inadequate cardiovascular status	<30	<56	>6.0

TABLE 47–8. Relationship Between Ranges of $S\bar{v}O_2$ and Reserve of Oxygen Available to the Tissues

$S\bar{v}O_2$	Oxygen Reserve
>65%	Adequate
51–65%	Limited
35–50%	Inadequate
<35%	Tissue hypoxia

effect. Unfortunately, breathing of O_2 in concentrations >50% is associated with iatrogenic increases in shunt (Fig. 47–9).[27, 28]

Practical Considerations

Calculation of $\dot{Q}sp/\dot{Q}t$ with a patient breathing a maintenance FIO_2 (other than 1.0) provides a reliable means of assessing the degree of lung dysfunction and of tracking progression of the disease and the effect of therapy. Intrapulmonary shunt fractions of <0.1 (10%) are normal; shunts >0.19 (19%) are associated with significant pulmonary dysfunction. Shunts of >0.30 (30%) are potentially life threatening and usually require aggressive cardiopulmonary supportive care.

Effect of the FIO_2

Calculation of the $\dot{Q}sp/\dot{Q}t$ theoretically considers the FIO_2 and cardiac output. However, the $\dot{Q}sp/\dot{Q}t$ does vary with the FIO_2. Figure 47–9 reveals that increasing FIO_2 up to 0.4 to 0.5 corrects for the component due to shunt effect by increasing PaO_2 and thereby reduces the calculated total $\dot{Q}sp/\dot{Q}t$. At a FIO_2 >0.5, this value increases, probably because of loss of hypoxic pulmonary vasoconstriction (HPV) or denitrogenation atelectasis.

The HPV reflexes reduce blood flow to those areas of the lungs with decreased or absent ventilation. These reflexes are initiated by a low PaO_2 (areas of lung with low but finite $\dot{V}A/\dot{Q}$) and low $P\bar{v}O_2$ (areas of lung with $\dot{V}/\dot{Q} = 0$).

$$\frac{\dot{Q}_{SP}}{\dot{Q}_T} = \frac{Cc'O_2 - CaO_2}{Cc'O_2 - C\bar{v}O_2} = \frac{\text{DIFF N}}{\text{DIFF D}}$$

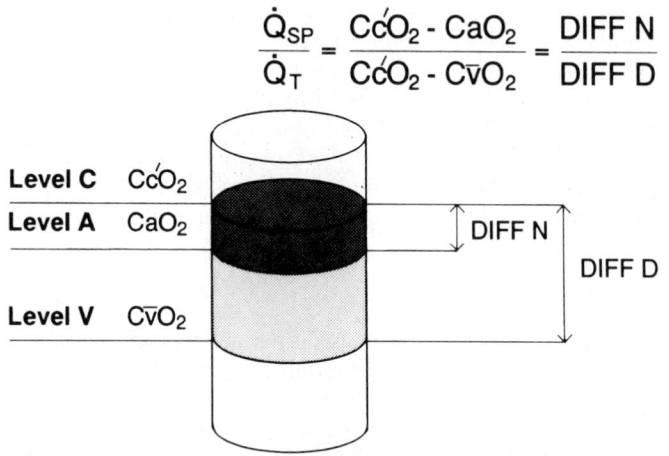

FIGURE 47–8. Diagrammatic representation of the oxygen content levels of end-pulmonary capillary ($Cc'O_2$), arterial (CaO_2) and mixed venous ($C\bar{v}O_2$) blood. The relationship of these contents to each other as expressed by the equation for calculation of the intrapulmonary shunt ($\dot{Q}sp/\dot{Q}t$) is shown. N = numerator; D = denominator. (From Shapiro BA, Harrison RA, Cane RD, et al: Applying the physiologic shunt. *In* Clinical Application of Blood Gases. 4th ed. Chicago, Year Book Medical Publishers, 1989; p 152.)

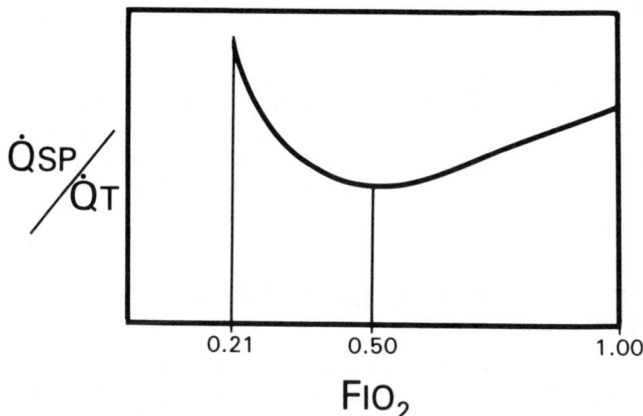

FIGURE 47–9. Graphic depiction of the relationship between intrapulmonary shunt fractions ($\dot{Q}sp/\dot{Q}t$) and inspired O_2 concentration (FIO_2). As the FIO_2 is increased from 0.21 (room air) toward 0.50, $\dot{Q}sp/\dot{Q}t$ decreases because the hypoxemic effect of shunt effect units ($\dot{V}A/\dot{Q} < 1$, but > 0) decreases as the PaO_2 increases. As the FIO_2 is increased from 0.50 toward 1.0, the shunt fraction increases. (From Shapiro BA, Harrison RA, Cane RD, et al: Hypoxemia and oxygen therapy. *In* Clinical Application of Blood Gases. 4th ed. Chicago, Year Book Medical Publishers, 1989; p 120.)

Cardiovascular Changes

Intrapulmonary shunting tends to change directly with cardiac output. It usually increases with the administration of vasoactive drugs (e.g., sodium nitroprusside, dopamine, dobutamine).

What Are Oxygen Partial Pressure–Based Indices?

The major drawback to $\dot{Q}sp/\dot{Q}t$ calculation is the need to obtain a mixed venous blood sample. Several alternative means of assessing the degree of lung dysfunction based on PaO_2 have been described.

Estimated Shunt

The shunt equation can be mathematically manipulated to enable substitution of an assumed value for $C(a-\bar{v})O_2$ as follows:

$$\dot{Q}sp/\dot{Q}t = (Cc'O_2 - CaO_2)/$$
$$[(Cc'O_2 - CaO_2) + C(a-\bar{v})O_2] \qquad \text{Equation 13}$$

Most critically ill patients with good cardiovascular function have a $C(a-\bar{v})O_2$ of 3.5 mL $\cdot$ dL^{-1}.[29] Thus, the estimated shunt is calculated as follows:

$$\dot{Q}sp/\dot{Q}t \text{ (Est)} = (Cc'O_2 - CaO_2)/$$
$$[(Cc'O_2 - CaO_2) + 3.5] \qquad \text{Equation 14}$$

Alveolar-to-Arterial Oxygen Partial Pressure Gradient

When the PaO_2 is >150 mm Hg, the $Pc'O_2$ must also be >150 mm Hg, and the arterial and pulmonary capillary HbO_2 is fully saturated with O_2. Under these circumstances, the difference between $Cc'O_2$ and CaO_2 reflect the amounts of dissolved O_2. Because the $Pc'O_2$ is assumed to be equal to the

PaO_2, to the extent that the PaO_2 is less, disruption of pulmonary O_2 transfer is indicated.[30]

The alveolar to arterial O_2 partial pressure gradient, $P(A-a)O_2$, is a useful index in patients who have stable cardiac function and are breathing room air. However, because this value varies directly with changes in the FIO_2, SaO_2, and $S\bar{v}O_2$ and because many critically ill patients have a PaO_2 <100 mm Hg, it is frequently unreliable.[31, 32]

Arterial-to-Alveolar Oxygen Partial Pressure Ratio

The arterial to alveolar O_2 partial pressure ratio (PaO_2/PAO_2) is less affected by FIO_2 changes than is the $P(A-a)O_2$[33] and is more reliable at a FIO_2 <0.55.[34] O_2 transfer abnormalities secondary to true shunts are better reflected by the PaO_2/PAO_2 than are those secondary to shunt effect.[35]

Arterial Oxygen Partial Pressure to FIO_2 Ratio

The PaO_2 to inspired FIO_2 ratio (PaO_2/FIO_2) varies with changes in $PaCO_2$.[36] It correlates poorly with $\dot{Q}sp/\dot{Q}t$ in patients with burns and respiratory tract disease and in critically ill pediatric patients.[37–39]

Respiratory Index

The respiratory index (RI) is a modification of the $P(A-a)O_2$ gradient. It is intended to improve accuracy in the presence of FIO_2 changes and is calculated by dividing the $P(A-a)O_2$ by the PaO_2.[40]

Table 47–9 shows the correlations between $\dot{Q}sp/\dot{Q}t$ and the previously described PO_2-based indices in a large heterogeneous group of critically ill patients.[41] Only the estimated shunt correlates acceptably with $\dot{Q}sp/\dot{Q}t$.

What Is Dual Oximetry?

Simultaneous pulse and mixed venous oximetric monitoring (dual oximetry) includes changes in PaO_2 as measured by pulse oximetry, thus allowing greater discrimination of the underlying reason for changes in $S\bar{v}O_2$. Furthermore, dual oximetry enables continuous real-time measurements of O_2 extraction and a $\dot{V}/\dot{Q}$ index.

Oxygen Extraction Index

O_2 extraction from arterial blood is reflected by the $C(a-\bar{v})O_2$. If the small amount of O_2 dissolved in the plasma ($PO_2 \times 0.003$) is ignored, the $C(a-\bar{v})O_2$ can be expressed as

$SaO_2 - S\bar{v}O_2$ or by substituting SpO_2 for SaO_2: $SpO_2 - S\bar{v}O_2$. Dividing this value by the SpO_2 gives the O_2 extraction index (O_2EI):

$$O_2EI = (SpO_2 - S\bar{v}O_2)/SpO_2 \qquad \text{Equation 15}$$

Because the SpO_2 is a reliable reflection of SaO_2 at values >90%, it is not surprising that the O_2EI correlates well with total body O_2 utilization.[42]

Ventilation/Perfusion Index

If the dissolved O_2 in the plasma is ignored and the hemoglobin concentration, common to all parts of the equation, is deleted, the calculation of $\dot{Q}sp/\dot{Q}t$ can be rendered in terms of SaO_2 and $S\bar{v}O_2$:

$$\dot{Q}sp/\dot{Q}t = (S\acute{c}O_2 - SaO_2)/(S\acute{c}O_2 - S\bar{v}O_2) \qquad \text{Equation 16}$$

Assuming complete saturation of pulmonary capillary blood (reasonable assumption at FIO_2 of 0.3 or greater) and substituting SpO_2 for SaO_2, the equation becomes

$$\dot{Q}sp/\dot{Q}t = (1 - SpO_2)/(1 - S\bar{v}O_2) \qquad \text{Equation 17}$$

This form of the equation has been termed the $\dot{V}/\dot{Q}$ index (VQI).[43]

Very close correlations between $\dot{Q}sp/\dot{Q}t$ and VQI have been reported in a large heterogeneous group of critically ill patients.[43, 44] The continuous real-time nature of the VQI enables more rapid, cost-effective titration of positive end-expiratory (PEEP) therapy than does serial calculation of $\dot{Q}sp/\dot{Q}t$.[45]

Why Is Hypoxemia a Problem?

Hypoxemia potentially affects normal physiologic processes by increasing cardiopulmonary work and impairing the maintenance of tissue oxygenation. Hypoxemia stimulates the peripheral chemoreceptors of the carotid bodies, resulting in increased ventilation. An increase in ventilation may increase the PAO_2, thereby correcting or improving the PaO_2. This compensatory mechanism is inefficient, however, because it only improves hypoxemia that is secondary to a reduced PAO_2 ($\dot{V}A/\dot{Q}$ <1, >0). Furthermore, the increase in $\dot{V}O_2$ by the increased ventilatory muscle work may exceed the additional O_2 uptake by the arterial blood. The cardiac response to hypoxemia and reduced CaO_2 is an increase in temperature.

Tissue Oxygenation

Tissue oxygenation depends on the delivery of an amount of O_2 sufficient to meet the tissue O_2 demands. Hypoxemia results in a reduced CaO_2, which can lead to reduced $\dot{D}O_2$. The usual physiologic response to a reduced CaO_2 is an increase in cardiac output and maintenance of $\dot{D}O_2$. If the patient is unable to increase cardiac output sufficiently to compensate for the reduced CaO_2, inadequate O_2 delivery leads to tissue hypoxia.

Figure 47–10 illustrates the changes in O_2 content of pulmonary capillary, arterial, and mixed venous blood consequent to changes of cardiac output and FIO_2.

TABLE 47–9. Comparison of Gas Exchange Indices

Parameter	(Mean ± SD)	Range (Min–Max)	R² Value
$\dot{Q}sp/\dot{Q}t$	22.3 (11.2)	3.0–53.0	
Estimated shunt	27.6 (11.3)	2.7–62.3	+0.88
Respiratory index	3.1 (2.6)	0.3–14.0	+0.55
PaO_2/PAO_2	0.3 (0.2)	0.06–0.77	−0.52
PaO_2/FIO_2	1.8 (0.9)	0.1–4.3	−0.50
$P(A-a)O_2$	222.8 (141.7)	32–611	+0.38

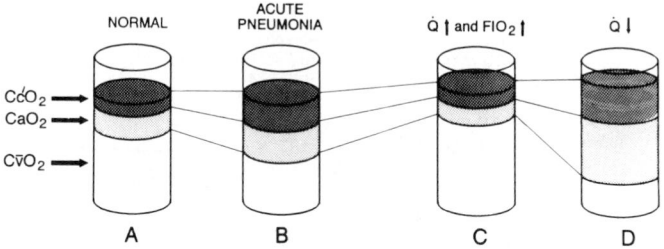

FIGURE 47–10. Diagrammatic representation of the relative changes in O_2 contents from normal *(A)* with the development of pneumonia *(B)*. *C*, The changes in O_2 content secondary to the physiologic response of an increase in CO and provision of O_2 therapy. *D*, What would happen if the CO were to fall. Note that although the $C\acute{c}O_2$ in *D* remains unchanged because of the O_2 therapy, the CaO_2 falls as the CO declines. (From Shapiro BA, Harrison RA, Cane RD, et al: Applying the physiologic shunt. *In* Clinical Application of Blood Gases. 4th ed. Chicago, Year Book Medical Publishers, 1989; p 154.)

How Is Hypoxemia Corrected?

Increasing the F_{IO_2}

Breathing of gas mixtures with an increased F_{IO_2} may correct hypoxemia and reduce the work of breathing required to maintain a given PaO_2. The myocardial work necessary to maintain a given PaO_2 may also be decreased.

Change in the Shunt Effect

Figure 47–11 illustrates the effect of breathing 100% O_2 on the hypoxemia associated with shunt effect. Alveolus A represents a shunt effect unit ($\dot{V}A/\dot{Q}$ <1 but >0), whereas alveolus B is normal ($\dot{V}A/\dot{Q}$ = 1). Denitrogenation associated with breathing 100% O_2 increases PaO_2 in the underventilated alveolus to a level sufficient to ensure complete HbO_2 saturation; thus, hypoxemia is corrected.

The F_{IO_2} needed to elevate PaO_2 enough to saturate the hemoglobin to >80 mm Hg depends on the magnitude of $\dot{V}A/\dot{Q}$ discrepancy; the lower the $\dot{V}A/\dot{Q}$, the higher the required F_{IO_2}. For practical purposes, hypoxemia secondary to shunt effect is responsive to O_2 therapy and is usually corrected with a F_{IO_2} up to 0.5.

Effect on True Shunt

Hypoxemia caused by true shunt ($\dot{V}A/\dot{Q}$ = 0) is barely responsive to an increased F_{IO_2}. Blood passing through shunt units is *not* exposed to alveolar gas; therefore, it is unaffected by an increase in F_{IO_2}. The PaO_2 in undiseased lung areas usually is >80 mm Hg, even with breathing room air; therefore, little additional O_2 can be added to the exposed blood by an increase in PaO_2. Overall, then, shunt-induced hypoxemia is refractory to O_2 therapy. The possibility that a refractory hypoxemia is present should be considered when the PaO_2 is <55 mm Hg and the F_{IO_2} is >0.35.

Oxygen Challenge

Most hypoxemia results from combinations of shunt and shunt effect mechanisms. Because a F_{IO_2} >0.5 is potentially harmful, identification of hypoxemic states that are relatively refractory to O_2 therapy is important. The O_2 challenge is a useful clinical technique that helps to differentiate between those patients with refractory hypoxemia (predominantly

caused by shunt) from those with hypoxemia that is responsive to O_2 therapy (predominantly caused by shunt effect).

To perform an O_2 challenge, obtain baseline ABG values, then increase the F_{IO_2} by 0.2; repeat the ABG measurements after approximately 30 minutes. If the PaO_2 has increased by >10 mm Hg from baseline, the patient has responsive hypoxemia; if the change in PaO_2 is <10 mm Hg, the hypoxemia is refractory.

Figure 47–12 illustrates the O_2 challenge. Patients with responsive hypoxemia can usually be managed with increases in F_{IO_2} up to 0.5, with or without low levels of positive airway pressure (+5 to +10 cm H_2O). Table 47–10 lists the common pathologic entities that are associated with refractory hypoxemia.

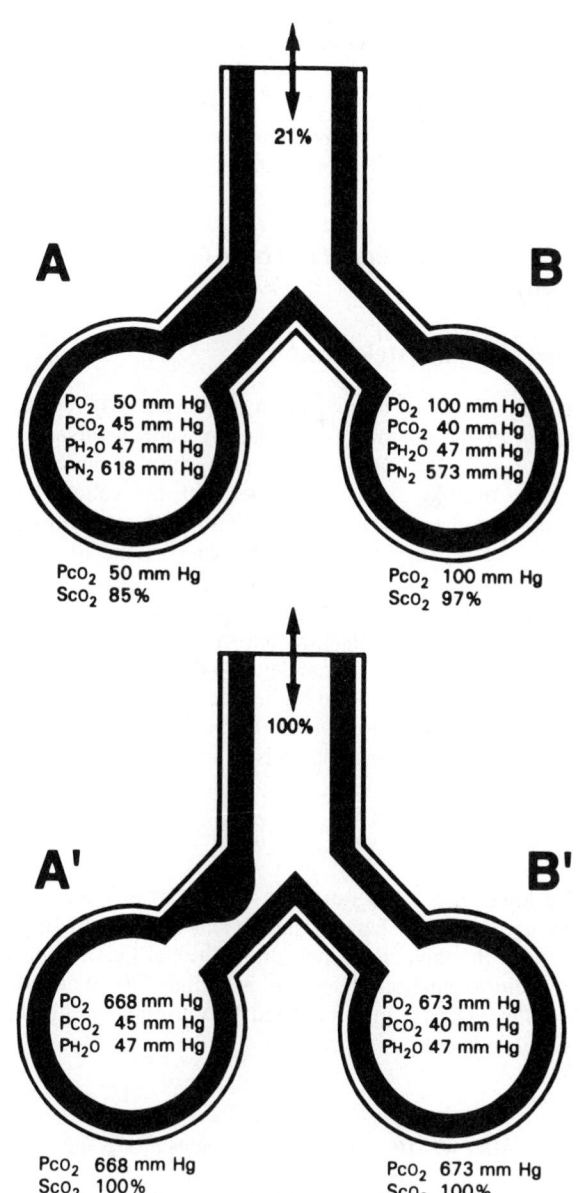

FIGURE 47–11. Alveoli A and A′ represent diminished ventilation with normal perfusion; alveoli B and B′ represent normal ventilation and perfusion. After 15 minutes of breathing 100% O_2, the lung is denitrogenated (A′ and B′). Note that any meaningful PaO_2 difference is ablated after denitrogenation. (From Shapiro BA, Harrison RA, Cane RD, et al: Hypoxemia and oxygen therapy. *In* Clinical Application of Blood Gases. 4th ed. Chicago, Year Book Medical Publishers, 1989; p 113.)

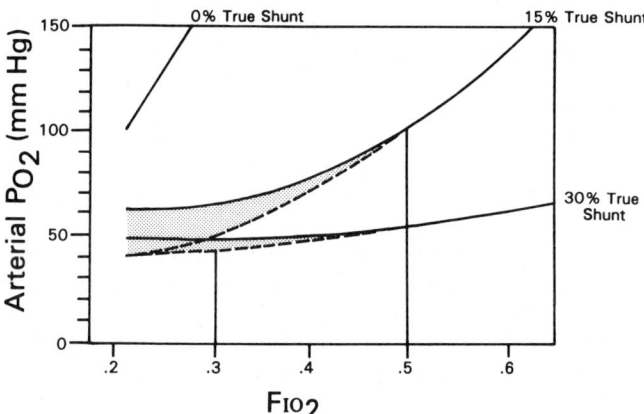

FIGURE 47–12. Representation of two patients with a Pao_2 of 40 mm Hg while breathing room air. Patient A's hypoxemia is due to a .30 shunt with a small additional component of shunt effect. Patient B's hypoxemia is due to a shunt of .15 with a large additional component of shunt effect. The *broken lines* represent the Pao_2–Fio_2 relationships from both the shunt and shunt effect, whereas the *solid lines* represent the Pao_2–Fio_2 relationships from the shunt alone. The O_2 challenge (increasing Fio_2 from 0.3 to 0.5) results in an increase in Pao_2 of <10 mm Hg for patient A (refractory hypoxemia) and of >10 mm Hg for patient B (responsive hypoxemia).

What Are the Adverse Effects of Oxygen Therapy?

Denitrogenation Atelectasis

Increases in Pao_2 secondary to increased Fio_2 result in a reduction of the alveolar N_2 partial pressure. In alveoli with reduced ventilation but good perfusion, the volume of O_2 removed by the blood may be greater than the volume of gas that enters with each tidal ventilation. In this circumstance, reduction of N_2 may allow the alveolar volume to decrease below a critical value, resulting in collapse.

Figure 47–13 illustrates the development of denitrogenation atelectasis. Patients with low but finite $\dot{V}A/\dot{Q}$ ratios who breathe a high Fio_2 (>0.5) can develop this problem in as little as 15 to 30 minutes.[46, 47] The higher the Fio_2, the greater is the degree of denitrogenation and the more likely is the development of denitrogenation atelectasis.

Effect of Low $\dot{V}A/\dot{Q}$

The lower the $\dot{V}A/\dot{Q}$ ratio, the lower the alveolar volume following significant denitrogenation and the more likely is the collapse of that alveolus. Thus, an additional factor contributing to denitrogenation atelectasis is a high Fio_2 that reduces HPV reflex activity. In turn, blood flow to underventilated or nonventilated regions is increased.

TABLE 47–10. Common Pathologies Producing Refractory Hypoxemia

Cardiovascular	Right-to-left intracardiac shunt
	Pulmonary arteriovenous fistula
Pulmonary	Consolidated pneumonitis
	Lobar atelectasis
	Large neoplasm
	Adult respiratory distress syndrome

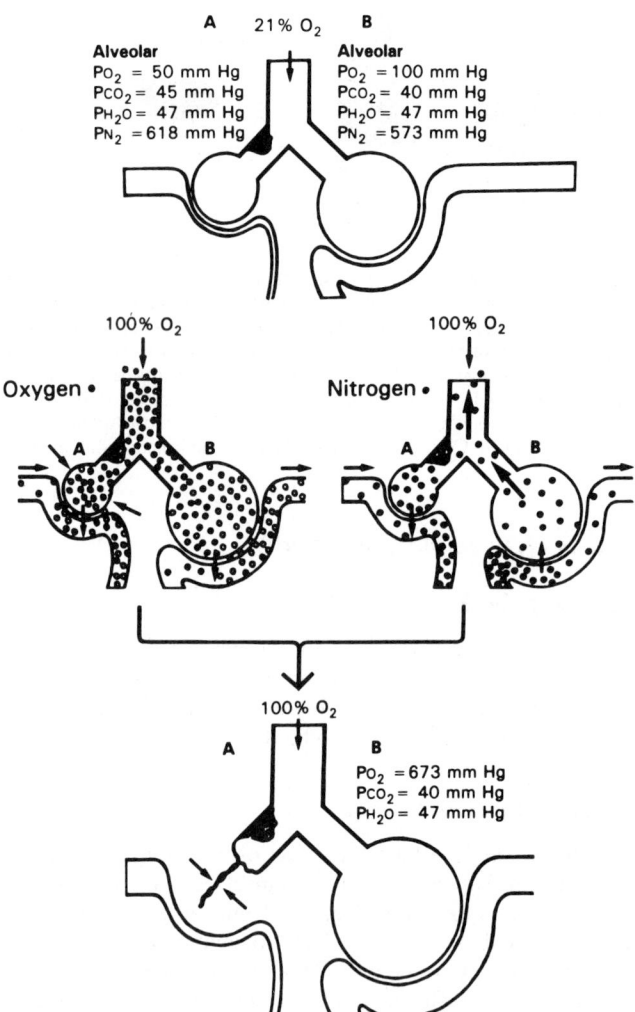

FIGURE 47–13. Diagrammatic representation of the mechanism of denitrogenation absorption atelectasis. Alveolus A has low $\dot{V}/\dot{Q}$ relationships (minimal ventilation); alveolus B has normal $\dot{V}/\dot{Q}$ relationships. The *top panel* shows the alveolar partial pressures on breathing room air. The *center panel* shows the effect of breathing 100% oxygen. The high Fio_2 results in a loss of hypoxic pulmonary vasoconstriction (HPV), and blood flow to alveolus A increases. The increased blood flow to this poorly ventilated alveolus results in significantly increased O_2 extraction, which in turn results in a diminished gas volume in alveolus A. *Black circles* represent nitrogen, which is rapidly depleted from all units because the inspired nitrogen concentration is now zero. Initially, more nitrogen leaves the blood and the body via unit B because it is better ventilated. As the blood Pn_2 level progressively decreases, however, nitrogen starts to leave alveolus A via the blood. This process results in further loss of gas volume from alveolus A because it remains poorly ventilated but well perfused. Thus, nitrogen is depleted from all units within 5 to 15 minutes. The *bottom panel* represents final steady state in which increased O_2 and nitrogen extraction has caused alveolus A to collapse. Thus, a poorly ventilated, poorly perfused unit, A, becomes a nonventilated, poorly perfused unit after administration of 100% inspired oxygen. (From Shapiro BA, Harrison RA, Cane RD, et al: Hypoxemia and oxygen therapy. *In* Clinical Application of Blood Gases. 4th ed. Chicago, Year Book Medical Publishers, 1989; pp 121, 123.)

Oxygen Toxicity

The inherent toxicity of O_2 to tissue was demonstrated almost a century ago.[48, 49] Intracellular O_2 metabolism involves serial reduction of O_2 to water, a process that involves the formation of highly reactive free radicals, the superoxide molecule (O_2^-) and hydroxyl ion (OH^-).

These toxic free radicals are capable of unregulated reactions with organic molecules that can result in damage to cell membranes and mitochondria and inactivation of cytoplasmic and nuclear enzymes.[50]

Protection Against Free Radicals

Mammalian tissue contains enzyme systems (e.g., superoxide dismutase) that catalyze the reduction of O_2 and prevent accumulation of these toxic O_2 radicals.[51] In small mammals, exposure to 100% O_2 for several days results in rapid depletion of these enzyme systems, accumulation of O_2-free radicals, and development of severe lung injury.[52]

Lung capillary endothelial cells are affected earlier and to a greater extent than are epithelial cells. The clinical syndrome of ''ventilator lung,'' reported in the 1950s when patients were first maintained on mechanical ventilation with 100% O_2 for prolonged periods, was probably a manifestation of pulmonary O_2 toxicity.[53]

Normal humans appear to have adequate enzyme reserves and do not manifest pulmonary parenchymal damage after prolonged exposure to a F_{IO_2} <0.6. However, pulmonary pathology may result in reduction of cellular enzyme reserves that could potentially lead to accumulation of toxic O_2 radicals and hyperoxic lung cell damage.

Many clinicians believe that the potential for hyperoxia-related lung damage is increased in diffuse lung injury (e.g., the adult respiratory distress syndrome [ARDS]) and attempt to maintain a patient's arterial oxygenation with a F_{IO_2} <0.5. Given that responsive hypoxemia, associated with shunt effect, is usually fully corrected by increases in F_{IO_2} to 0.4 to 0.5, this approach seems prudent.

Retinopathy of Prematurity

A special case of O_2 toxicity is the retinopathy that develops in premature neonates when the Pa_{O_2} is >100 mm Hg. O_2 therapy must be carefully titrated to prevent this disastrous consequence of hyperoxia.

What F_{IO_2} Should Be Used?

In emergent situations (during cardiopulmonary resuscitation), when a patient manifests acutely unstable cardiopulmonary function, or while transporting patients, administration of 100% O_2 is advisable. Remember that O_2 toxicity develops only after significant periods of exposure to a high F_{IO_2} (>72–96 h).

In all other circumstances, the therapeutic efficacy of O_2 generally is limited to F_{IO_2} from 0.21 to 0.5 because

1. O_2-responsive hypoxemia secondary to shunt effect is usually reversed with a F_{IO_2} of 0.5 or less
2. Denitrogenation atelectasis developing at a F_{IO_2} >0.5 increases true $\dot{Q}sp/\dot{Q}t$ and results in worsening hypoxemia that is refractory to O_2 therapy

Hypoxemia due to true shunting ($\dot{V}A/\dot{Q} = 0$) requires therapy to improve $\dot{V}A/\dot{Q}$ matching. Hypoxemia due to nonpulmonary causes (low cardiac output, with or without high $\dot{V}O_2$ or severe anemia) is improved by correction of the underlying pathology in conjunction with a F_{IO_2} <50%.

How Should Oxygen Be Administered?

O_2 may be delivered by rebreathing or nonrebreathing systems. Modern anesthesia machines commonly use a rebreathing circle circuit in which exhaled CO_2 is scrubbed by soda lime. For discussion of the gas delivery circuits, see Chapter 16.

The Postanesthesia Care Unit

O_2 for critically ill patients or patients in a postanesthesia care unit (PACU) is properly administered by nonrebreathing systems.

High-Flow Systems

High-flow O_2 systems supply the total inspired gas (patients breathe only gas supplied by the apparatus). They provide a warmed and humidified consistent F_{IO_2}, irrespective of a patient's ventilatory pattern. Adequate flows are achieved by inclusion of some form of inspiratory reservoir that supplies additional amounts of gas during the transient times when a patient's inspiratory flow demand exceeds the uniform flow delivered by the apparatus. Alternatively, an extremely high flow of gas may be provided, but this approach is wasteful and expensive. A total gas flow at least three times a patient's measured minute volume usually ensures that the peak inspiratory flow demand is met.

Many systems use air entrainment to provide a specific F_{IO_2} and gas flow. Air entrainment is achieved by constant-pressure jet mixing, in which a rapid velocity of gas passing through a restricted orifice creates viscous shearing forces that entrain air into the main gas stream. The air entrainment ratio (and hence F_{IO_2}) depends on orifice and entrainment port sizes. Variation in the O_2 flow rate through the orifice determines the total gas flow delivered by the device.

Table 47–11 lists approximate air entrainment ratios for different O_2 concentrations. A F_{IO_2} from 0.24 to 0.35 is most frequently provided by air entrainment devices. Higher values are best provided by systems that deliver adequately high flows of gas at known F_{IO_2}.

Commonly used high-flow O_2 delivery systems include T-piece circuits, face masks with wide-bore gas delivery circuits, and air entrainment masks (often referred to as *Venturi masks*) (Fig. 47–14).

Low-Flow Systems

Low-flow O_2 systems do not provide sufficient gas flow to supply the entire inspired atmosphere; thus, part of each breath is received from the room air. F_{IO_2} from 0.21 to 0.8 can be provided by a low-flow system. The F_{IO_2} is determined by the size of the available O_2 reservoir (usually the nose, nasopharynx, and oropharynx), the O_2 flow ($L \cdot min^{-1}$), and ventilatory pattern.

TABLE 47–11. Approximate Air Entrainment Ratios for Different Oxygen Concentrations

Oxygen Concentration (%)	Air/Oxygen ($L \cdot min^{-1}$)
24	25/1
28	10/1
34	5/1
40	3/1
60	1/1
70	0.6/1

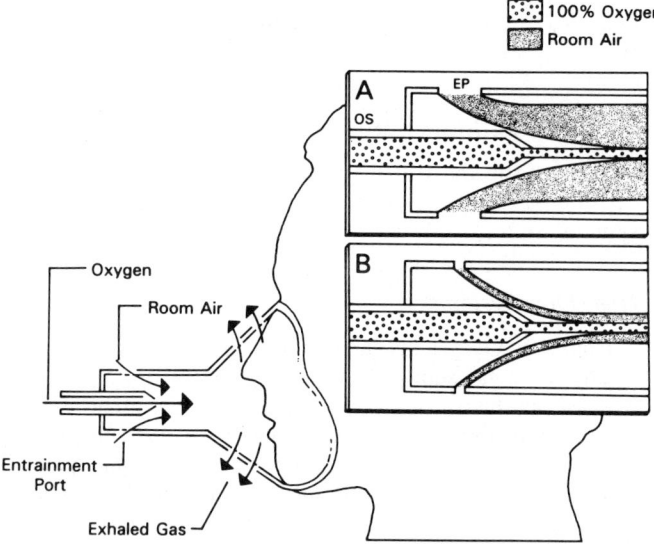

FIGURE 47–14. Operational principle of a Venturi mask. A high-pressure jet of O_2 is directed down the center of the mask. Entrained air is drawn into the mixing tube by viscous interaction with the jet flow. The percentage of O_2 is determined by the size of the entrainment ports controlling the flow of ambient air. In some masks, these are fixed; in others, they are variable.

Practical Applications

With a preset O_2 flow, the F_{IO_2} varies inversely with minute ventilation. Larger tidal volume (V_T) or faster respiratory rate decreases the F_{IO_2}; the smaller the V_T or the slower the respiratory rate, the higher the F_{IO_2}. Critically ill patients frequently manifest an unstable ventilatory pattern. If delivery of a consistent F_{IO_2} is deemed important, a high-flow system should be used.

Equipment

Commonly used systems for low-flow O_2 delivery include nasal cannulas, simple O_2 masks, and O_2 masks with a reservoir bag. Table 47–12 shows the approximate F_{IO_2} that will be achieved with commonly used low-flow (O_2 delivery systems (provided a patient has a relatively normal ventilatory pattern).

Anatomic Reservoir

Mouth breathing does not affect the F_{IO_2} delivered by nasal cannulas, provided the nasal passages are patent. Airflow in the oropharynx creates a jet mixing effect in the nasopharynx that draws air through the nose. The anatomic reservoir is usually completely filled with O_2 by flows of 6 L · min^{-1}; further increases in O_2 flow through nasal cannulas seldom result in a higher F_{IO_2}.

Increased F_{IO_2}

Masks. To provide a higher F_{IO_2} with a low-flow system, the O_2 reservoir has to be increased by placing a mask over the nose and mouth. A potential risk with a low-flow face mask is accumulation of exhaled gas in the mask, leading to rebreathing of CO_2. Provision of an O_2 flow >5 L · min^{-1} flushes most of the exhaled air from the mask. O_2 flows of 8 L · min^{-1} usually fill the mask reservoir and provide the highest F_{IO_2} possible with a low-flow face mask.

Reservoir Bags. To deliver a F_{IO_2} >0.6 with a low-flow system, the O_2 reservoir has to be further increased by attaching a reservoir bag to the mask. The first one third of the exhaled gas (dead space gas free of CO_2) enters the reservoir bag and is rebreathed; thus, a mask with a reservoir bag is a partial rebreathing system. For proper function, the mask should be close fitting and the flow of O_2 sufficient to prevent the reservoir bag from totally emptying during inspiration (>6 L · min^{-1}).

What Are the Clinical Guidelines for Oxygen Therapy?

Patients Without Chronic Lung Disease and Hypoventilation

Provision of a F_{IO_2} of 0.4 via a high-flow delivery system is a reliable starting point. The adequacy of therapy must be evaluated by patient assessment *and* measurement of arterial oxygenation status. The F_{IO_2} should be adjusted to maintain a Pa_{O_2} of 60 to 80 mm Hg or a Sp_{O_2} of 90% to 94%.

When a patient's arterial oxygenation and cardiopulmonary function have stabilized and an appropriate pattern of breathing with a F_{IO_2} of <0.4 is achieved, switch to a low-flow O_2 delivery system can be considered.

Performance of an O_2 challenge before initiation of therapy is strongly recommended to identify patients with predominant shunt and refractory hypoxemia.

TABLE 47–12. Approximate F_{IO_2} Delivered by Different Low-Flow Oxygen Delivery Systems*

Nasal Cannula		Oxygen Mask		Mask with Reservoir Bag	
O_2 Flow (L · min^{-1})	F_{IO_2}	O_2 Flow (L · min^{-1})	F_{IO_2}	O_2 Flow (L · min^{-1})	F_{IO_2}
1	0.24	5–6	0.4	6	0.6
2	0.28	6–7	0.5	7	0.7
3	0.32	7–8	0.6	8	0.8
4	0.36				
5	0.4				
6	0.44				

*Assumes a normal ventilatory pattern.

Patients with Chronic Lung Disease and Chronic Elevation of P_{ACO_2}

Patients with chronic CO_2 retention represent a particular challenge with respect to O_2 therapy. First, they may hypoventilate in response to arterial hyperoxia. The mechanism of hyperoxia-induced hypoventilation is not understood.

Second, worsening hypoxemia is difficult to assess, because these patients often have a markedly reduced Pa_{O_2} (usually <60 mm Hg) when they are ''well.'' Suspect acute hypoxemia if examination reveals acute respiratory distress in the early phase of an acute cardiopulmonary problem. ABG analysis often shows acute alveolar hyperventilation superimposed on chronic alveolar hypoventilation (Pa_{CO_2} elevated, with pH >7.40). Careful monitoring of respiratory rate, heart rate, and a patient's subjective feelings of ease or difficulty in breathing provide the best indicators of oxygenation.

Third, because the hypoxemia usually is due to shunt effect and is responsive to increases in the FIO_2, do not perform an O_2 challenge. Finally, recall that the FIO_2 of a low-flow system varies inversely with minute ventilation. Hence, transient and inadvertent hyperoxia resulting in hypoventilation leads to an increase in FIO_2 that potentially results in further hypoventilation.

Because these patients seldom require a high FIO_2 or high minute ventilation, air entrainment masks are reliable. Start with a FIO_2 of 0.24 and evaluate the patient's response. Titrate the FIO_2 in increments of 0.04 to 0.05. The desirable end point is best determined by normalization of the respiratory rate, heart rate, and pHa.

Patients usually state that their breathing feels easier when appropriate arterial oxygenation is restored. The actual value of Pa_{O_2} or Sp_{O_2} depends on the degree of underlying lung disease and, invariably, is <60 mm Hg or 90%, respectively. Prior knowledge of a patient's usual ABG values is of considerable benefit.

When Is Mechanical Ventilation Indicated?

Airway pressure therapy includes the application of positive pressure to the airway during the inspiratory phase only (mechanical ventilation) or during the entire ventilatory cycle (i.e., continuous positive airway pressure [CPAP]). Hypoxemia that is secondary to hypoventilation and acute ventilatory failure is readily corrected by mechanical ventilatory support. If the O_2 cost of breathing is extremely high, ventilatory support may also be beneficial. However, increased work of breathing is associated with various causes, and alternative therapeutic options can be used.[54]

When Is Continuous Positive Airway Pressure Indicated?

Hypoxemia in anesthetized and critically ill surgical patients is most frequently associated with an acute process. Restriction of lung function and volume, particularly the functional residual capacity (FRC), results. Maintenance of airway pressure above ambient pressure increases FRC. If a patient can maintain adequate spontaneous breathing, hypoxemia secondary to $\dot{V}_A/\dot{Q}$ mismatching is best treated with increase of the FIO_2 and CPAP, not with mechanical ventilation.

Mechanism of Action

CPAP increases the FRC by expansion of patent alveoli or re-expansion of collapsed alveoli, a process termed *alveolar recruitment*. Lower levels of CPAP (+5 to +15 cm H_2O) improve shunt effect. Higher levels (>15 cm H_2O) are required to recruit collapsed alveoli. Re-expansion of collapsed alveoli converts true shunt into shunt effect units, thereby changing hypoxemia from refractory to responsive.

Benefits

Judicious use of CPAP, when it is indicated, invariably enables reduction of the FIO_2, minimizing the risks associated with high FIO_2. It provides the additional benefit of improved lung compliance that was reduced by a loss of intrathoracic gas volume. Improvement of compliance reduces the inspiratory work of breathing.

Techniques of Administration

CPAP can be provided by face mask, nasal prongs, nasal mask, or an endotracheal tube. In patients with particularly severe restrictive lung pathology (e.g., ARDS), augmentation of ventilation may be required despite improved lung function secondary to CPAP therapy. Improvement in the FRC with intermittent positive-pressure ventilation (IPPV) is achieved by the addition of PEEP.

How Is Hypoxemia Prevented During Apnea?

In anesthetic practice, patients are frequently rendered apneic by the administration of neuromuscular blocking agents to facilitate tracheal intubation and surgery. Gas exchange across the alveolar-capillary membrane continues, resulting in a rise in P_{ACO_2} and a fall in the P_{AO_2}. If the pulmonary O_2 reserve is augmented by increasing the P_{AO_2}, arterial oxygenation can be maintained; hypercarbia and acidosis then become the limiting factors. An apneic patient with a patent airway connected to a high-flow 100% O_2 delivery circuit can maintain arterial oxygenation for at least 20 minutes.[55]

Preoxygenation

Preoxygenation increases the P_{AO_2} and minimizes apnea-induced hypoxemia. Complete denitrogenation of the lungs requires breathing of 100% O_2 for at least 15 minutes. However, to protect against hypoxemia during intubation, 3 to 5 minutes of O_2 breathing usually is sufficient. Alternatively, having a patient take four maximum breaths of pure O_2 provides similar protection to 3 minutes of preoxygenation with normal ventilation.[56]

Rate of Rise of Carbon Dioxide

Table 47–13 shows the approximate rate of rise of Pa_{CO_2} with apnea.[57] These data suggest that up to 5 minutes of apnea can occur before acidosis becomes significant.

TABLE 47–13. Predicted Pa_{CO_2}-pH Relationships with Apnea

Apnea Time (min)	Pa_{CO_2} (mm Hg)	pH (Units)
0	40	7.400
1	52	7.340
2	55.5	7.323
3	59	7.305
4	62.6	7.288
5	66	7.260
10	83.5	7.183
15	101	7.095

Why Does Hypoxemia Occur During Anesthesia?

Several factors may contribute to the development of hypoxemia during anesthesia.

Reduction of the Functional Residual Capacity

Supine Positioning

Induction of anesthesia in supine patients is associated with a reduction of approximately 15% to 20% in the FRC.[58] This reduction occurs within minutes of induction, irrespective of the anesthetic agents used, is not progressive, and appears to be unaffected by neuromuscular blocking drugs and a high F_{IO_2}.

The supine position clearly is a factor, because the FRC is unchanged by anesthesia administration to patients in the sitting position. Active expiration secondary to increased expiratory muscle tone in anesthetized patients may contribute in nonparalyzed patients. The reduction in FRC persists into the first 4 to 6 hours after emergence.

Diaphragmatic Tone

Loss of end-expiratory diaphragmatic tone during anesthesia results in a cephalad diaphragmatic shift.[59] The reduction in FRC correlates with the observed increase in the $P_{(A-a)O_2}$ gradient and as such probably has a role in the development of hypoxemia under anesthesia.

Shunt Increases

A reduction in FRC may reduce the end-expiratory lung volume below the closing capacity, particularly in older patients. Premature airway closure, absorptive collapse, and shunting can result. Whether significant increase of $\dot{Q}sp/\dot{Q}t$ occurs under anesthesia is controversial. If shunting does increase, it is probably related to changes in HPV and not simply to changes in the FRC-closing capacity relationships.

Tube Malpositioning

Esophageal and bronchial intubation lead to profound hypoxemia and a potentially lethal outcome if not detected early and corrected immediately.

Ablation of Hypoxic Pulmonary Vasoconstriction

Inhalation but not intravenous anesthetics[60, 61] depress HPV in an isolated lung and may contribute to increased $\dot{V}_A/\dot{Q}$

mismatching and hypoxemia. Because HPV is modulated by the partial pressure of O_2 in mixed venous blood ($P_{\bar{v}O_2}$) as well as Pa_{O_2}, concomitant decrements in cardiac output with reduction in $P_{\bar{v}O_2}$ may override the effect of inhalation agents on HPV in intact animals and humans.[62]

Intermittent Positive-Pressure Ventilation

IPPV is a common adjunct to anesthesia delivery. It is associated with increased volume of gas distribution to nondependent lung areas. Reduced dependent lung ventilation increases the number of lung regions with low $\dot{V}_A/\dot{Q}$ relationships. A high F_{IO_2} may exaggerate this effect by inhibiting HPV. Pre-existing $\dot{V}_A/\dot{Q}$ relationships are important; lower values before administration of a high F_{IO_2} make the development of increased shunting secondary to denitrogenation more likely.

Equipment Malfunction

Disconnection of a patient from the anesthesia circuit and O_2 supply probably is the most common technical mishap that results in hypoxemia. A wide variety of errors related to anesthesia machine, gas supply, and machine-patient interface have been described.[63, 64]

Oxygen Administration

For patients without pre-existing cardiopulmonary disease, a F_{IO_2} between 0.25 and 0.3 usually is sufficient. A higher F_{IO_2} is required for patients with pre-existing cardiopulmonary disease or for specific surgical procedures that impair ventilation (e.g., airway endoscopy or one-lung anesthesia). Patients maintained with CPAP or IPPV plus PEEP preoperatively should receive similar support intraoperatively and postoperatively.

Why Does Hypoxemia Occur Postoperatively?

In the immediate postanesthetic period, patients may develop hypoxemia. The previously discussed mechanisms productive of intraoperative hypoxemia often persist into the postanesthetic period. Additional factors that have a role include residual anesthesia, neuromuscular blockade, induced hypoventilation, and increased $\dot{V}_{O_2}$ secondary to shivering.

Diffusion Hypoxia

When nitrous oxide is discontinued, large amounts enter the alveoli and dilute the alveolar O_2 concentration. This so-called diffusion hypoxia is short-lived and easily corrected by maintaining a F_{IO_2} of 0.5 to 1.0 for 3 to 5 minutes. However, if this period of high O_2 delivery is prolonged (>15 min), lung denitrogenation may predispose to atelectasis. This problem is of particular significance if a patient hypoventilates. The risk is reduced by washing out the nitrous oxide with a F_{IO_2} of approximately 0.5 in nitrogen (i.e., 4 L O_2 in 6 L air).

What Is the Value of Pulse Oximetry in the Postanesthesia Care Unit?

Monitoring a patient's oxygenation status with pulse oximetry is a standard practice in modern anesthesia. The ease of application and the low cost, coupled with the continuous real-time nature of SpO$_2$ monitoring, make it an ideal monitor for the PACU.

As discussed previously, the sensitivity of pulse oximetry is greatest when the SaO$_2$ is between 90% and 93%. Thus, the almost routine practice of administering 30% to 40% O$_2$ to all postoperative patients in the PACU reduces the sensitivity by increasing the PaO$_2$ to >100 mm Hg. Pulse oximetry removes the need for routine O$_2$ therapy in the PACU.

One study showed that only 25% of patients who had general anesthesia with narcotics and inhalation agents transiently had a decrease in SpO$_2$ below 90% when managed without O$_2$ in the PACU. Only 2% of these patients required therapy other than verbal stimulation to maintain a SpO$_2$ >90%.[65]

We recommend that routine O$_2$ therapy not be used in the PACU, that all patients be monitored with pulse oximetry, and that significant hypoxemia (persistent SpO$_2$ >90%) be appropriately investigated. The indicated therapy must be based on the underlying cause.

References

1. Piiper J: Variations of ventilation and diffusing capacity to perfusion determining the alveolar-arterial O$_2$ difference: theory. J Appl Physiol 1961; 16:507.
2. Piiper J, Haab P, Rahn H: Unequal distribution of pulmonary diffusing capacity in the anesthetized dog. J Appl Physiol 1961; 16:499.
3. Shapiro BA, Harrison RA, Cane RD, et al (eds): Blood gas analyzers. In Clinical Application of Blood Gases. 4th ed. Chicago, Year Book Medical Publishers, 1989, pp 265–273.
4. Shapiro BA, Cane RD, Chomka CM, et al: Preliminary evaluation of an intra-arterial blood gas system in dogs and humans. Crit Care Med 1989; 17:455.
5. Tremper KK, Waxman KS, Bowman R: Continuous transcutaneous oxygen monitoring during respiratory failure, cardiac decompensation, cardiac arrest and CPR. Crit Care Med 1980; 8:377.
6. Scheller MS, Unger RJ, Kelner MJ: Effects of intravenously administered dyes on pulse oximetry readings. Anesthesiology 1986; 65:550.
7. Cane RD, Harrison RA, Shapiro BA, et al: The spectrophotometric absorbance of Intralipid. Anesthesiology 1980; 53:53.
8. Brooks TD, Paulus DA, Winkle WE: Infrared heat lamps interfere with pulse oximeters. Anesthesiology 1984; 61:630.
9. New W: Pulse oximetry. J Clin Monit 1985; 1:126.
10. Kim J-M, Arakawa, K, Benson KT, et al: Pulse oximetry and circulatory kinetics associated with pulse volume amplitude measured by photoelectric plethysmography. Anesth Analg 1986; 65:1333.
11. Hess D, Kochansky M, Hassett L, et al: An evaluation of the Nellcor N-10 portable pulse oximeter. Respir Care 1986; 31:796.
12. Yelderman M, New W: Evaluation of pulse oximetry. Anesthesiology 1983; 59:349.
13. Mihm FG, Halperin BD: Non-invasive detection of profound arterial desaturations using a pulse oximetry device. Anesthesiology 1985; 62:85.
14. Fait CD, Wetzel RC, Dean JM, et al: Pulse oximetry in critically ill children. J Clin Monit 1985; 1:232.
15. Taylor MB, Whitham JG: The current status of pulse oximetry. Anesthesiology 1986; 41:943.
16. Fanconi S, Doherty P, Edmonds JF, et al: Pulse oximetry in pediatric intensive care: comparison with measured saturations and transcutaneous oxygen tension. J Pediatr 1985; 107:362.
17. Ramanthan R, Durand M, Larrazabal C: Pulse oximetry in very low birth weight infants with acute and chronic lung disease. Pediatrics 1987; 79:612.
18. Jenni MS, Peabody JL: Pulse oximetry: an alternative method for the assessment of oxygenation in newborn infants. Pediatrics 1987; 79:524.
19. Durand M, Ramanathan R: Pulse oximetry for continuous oxygen monitoring in sick newborn infants. J Pediatr 1986; 109:1052.
20. Martin WE, Cheung PW, Johnson CC, et al: Continuous monitoring of mixed venous oxygen saturation in man. Anesth Analg 1973; 52:784.
21. Johnson CC, Palm D, Stewart DC, et al: A solid state fiberoptics oximeter. J Assoc Advan Med Instrumentation 1971; 5:77.
22. Taylor JB, Lown B, Polanyi M: In-vivo monitoring with a fiber optic catheter. JAMA 1972; 221:667.
23. Divertie MB, McMichan JC: Continuous monitoring of mixed venous oxygen saturation. Chest 1984; 85:423.
24. Baele PL, McMichan JC, Marsh HM, et al: Continuous monitoring of mixed venous oxygen saturation in critically ill patients. Anesth Analg 1982; 61:513.
25. Shapiro BA, Harrison RA, Cane RD, et al: Oximetric measurement. In Clinical Applications of Blood Gases. 4th ed. Chicago, Year Book Medical Publishers, 1989, pp 283–294.
26. Shapiro BA, Harrison RA, Cane RD, et al: Applying the physiologic shunt. In Clinical Application of Blood Gases. 4th ed. Chicago, Year Book Medical Publishers, 1989, p 157.
27. Douglas ME, Downs JB, Dannemiller FJ, et al: Changes in pulmonary venous admixture with varying inspired oxygen. Anesth Analg 1976; 55:688.
28. Shapiro BA, Cane RD, Harrison RA, et al: Changes in intrapulmonary shunting with the administration of 100% oxygen. Chest 1980; 77:138.
29. Harrison RA, Davison R, Shapiro BA, et al: Reassessment of the assumed A-V oxygen content difference in the shunt calculation. Anesth Analg 1975; 54:198.
30. Lilienthal JL, Riley RL, Proemmel DD, et al: An experimental analysis in man of the oxygen pressure gradient from alveolar air to arterial blood. Am J Physiol 1946; 147:199.
31. Peris LV, Boix JH, Salom JV, et al: Clinical use of the arterial/alveolar oxygen tension ratio. Crit Care Med 1983; 11:888.
32. Kanber GJ, King FW, Eshchar YR, et al: The alveolar-arterial oxygen gradient in young and elderly men during air and oxygen breathing. Am Rev Respir Dis 1968; 97:376.
33. Hess D, Maxwell C: Which is the best index for oxygenation: P(A–a)O$_2$, PaO$_2$/PAO$_2$ or PaO$_2$/FIO$_2$? Respir Care 1985; 30:961.
34. Gilbert R, Keighley JF: The arterial/alveolar oxygen tension ratio: an index of gas exchange applicable to varying inspired oxygen concentrations. Am Rev Respir Dis 1974; 109:142.
35. Gilbert R, Auchincloss JH, Juppinger M, et al: Stability of the arterial/alveolar oxygen partial pressure ratio: effects of low ventilation/perfusion regions. Crit Care Med 1979; 7:267.
36. Lawrence M: Abbreviating the alveolar gas equation: an argument for simplicity. Respir Care 1985; 30:964.
37. Cohen A, Taeusch HW Jr, Stanton C: Usefulness of the arterial/alveolar oxygen tension ratio in the care of infants with respiratory distress syndrome. Respir Care 1983; 28:169.
38. Martyn JAJ, Aikawa N, Wilson RS, et al: Extrapulmonary factors influencing the ratio of arterial oxygen tension to inspired oxygen concentration in burn patients. Crit Care Med 1979; 7:492.
39. Wallfisch HK, Tonnesen AS, Huber P: Respiratory indices compared to venous admixture. Crit Care Med 1981; 9:147.
40. Sjanga G, Seigal JH, Coleman W, et al: Physiologic meaning of the respiratory index in various types of critical illness. Circ Shock 1985; 17:179.
41. Cane RD, Shapiro BA, Templin R, et al: The unreliability of oxygen tension based indices in reflecting intrapulmonary shunting in the critically ill. Crit Care Med 1988; 16:1243.
42. Räsänen J, Downs JB, Seidman P, et al: Estimation of oxygen utilization by dual oximetry. Crit Care Med 1987; 15:404.
43. Räsänen J, Downs JB, Malec DJ, et al: Oxygen tensions and oxyhemoglobin saturations in the assessment of pulmonary gas exchange. Crit Care Med 1987; 15:1058.
44. Bandala LC, Cane RD, Shapiro BA: Validation of the VQI in critically ill patients. Crit Care Med 1989; 17:S21.
45. Räsänen J, Downs JB, Dehaven B: Titration of continuous positive airway pressure by real time dual oximetry. Crit Care Med 1987; 15:395.
46. Suter PM, Fairley HB, Schlobohm RM: Shunt, lung volume and perfusion during short periods of ventilation with oxygen. Anesthesiology 1975; 43:617.
47. Markello P, Winter P, Olszowka A: Assessment of ventilation-perfusion inequalities by arterial-venous nitrogen differences in intensive care patients. Anesthesiology 1972; 37:4.
48. Smith JL: The influence of pathological conditions on active absorption of oxygen by the lungs. J Physiol 1897; 22:307.
49. Smith JL: The pathological effects due to increase of oxygen tension in the air breathed. J Physiol 1899; 24:19.
50. Crapo J, Tierney D: Superoxide dismutase and pulmonary oxygen toxicity. Am J Physiol 1974; 226:1401.
51. Stevens JB, Autor AP: Oxygen induced synthesis of ethylene oxide. Anesthesiology 1969; 30:349.
52. Kistler GS, Caldwell PRB, Weibel ER: Development of fine structural damage to alveolar and capillary lining cells in oxygen-poisoned rat lungs. J Cell Biol 1967; 32:605.

53. Winter P: The toxicity of oxygen. Anesthesiology 1972; 37:210.
54. Cane RD: Detrimental work of breathing. *In* Case Studies in Critical Care Medicine. 2nd ed. Cane RD, Shapiro BA, Davison R (eds). Chicago, Year Book Medical Publishers, 1990, pp 30–51.
55. Frumin MJ, Epstein RM, Cohen G: Apneic oxygenation in man. Anesthesiology 1959; 20:789.
56. Gambee, AM, Hertzka RE, Fisher DM: Preoxygenation techniques: comparison of three minutes and four breaths. Anesth Analg 1987; 66:468.
57. Stock MC, Schisler JQ, McSweeney TD: The Pa_{CO_2} rate of rise in anesthetized patients with airway obstruction. J Clin Anesth 1989; 1:328.
58. Don H: The mechanical properties of the respiratory system during anesthesia. Int Anesth Clin 1977; 15:113.
59. Muller N, Volgyesi G, Becker L, et al: Diaphragmatic muscle tone. J Appl Physiol 1979; 47:279.
60. Sykes MK, Loh L, Seed RF, et al: The effect of inhalational anesthetics on hypoxic pulmonary vasoconstriction and pulmonary vascular resistance in the perfused lungs of the dog and cat. Br J Anesth 1972, 44:776.
61. Bjertnaes LJ: Hypoxia-induced vasoconstriction in isolated lungs exposed to injectable or inhalation anesthetics. Acta Anaesthesiol Scand 1977; 21:133.
62. Marshall BE, Marshall C: Anesthesia and pulmonary circulation. *In* Effects of Anesthesia. Covino BG, Fozzard HA, Rehder K, et al (eds). Bethesda, MD, American Physiological Society, 1985.
63. Eger EI, Epstein RM: Hazards of anesthetic equipment. Anesthesiology 1964; 25:490.
64. Ward CS: The prevention of accidents associated with anesthetic apparatus. Br J Anaesth 1968; 40:692.
65. Cane RD, Johnson MT: Is routine postoperative oxygen therapy necessary or desirable? Anesthesiology (in press).

CHAPTER 48

Abnormal Ventilation

JUKKA RÄSÄNEN, M.D.
ROY D. CANE, M.B., B.Ch., F.F.A. (S.A.)

Hypoventilation is present when a patient's alveolar ventilation ($\dot{V}_A$) is insufficient to maintain arterial blood carbon dioxide partial pressure (Pa_{CO_2}) at or below the upper limit of the normal range (45 mm Hg). Hyperventilation is defined as excessive $\dot{V}_A$ that lowers the Pa_{CO_2} below the lower limit of the normal range (35 mm Hg). By definition, hypoventilation is associated with hypercapnia and respiratory acidosis, and hyperventilation is linked to hypocapnia and respiratory alkalosis.

The terms *hypoventilation* and *hyperventilation* are sometimes used incorrectly to denote low minute ventilation and high minute ventilation, respectively. However, a patient with a slow ventilatory rate (bradypnea) or low tidal volume (hypopnea) does not necessarily have hypoventilation; likewise, hyperventilation may not be present even if a patient's ventilatory rate is fast (tachypnea) or his or her tidal volume (V_T) is high (hyperpnea). An unusually high or low minute ventilation may be appropriate for maintaining CO_2 homeostasis when the CO_2 output or the ratio of dead space to tidal volume (V_{DS}/V_T) is altered.

VENTILATORY WORK

What Is Ventilatory Work?

Ventilatory work is required to maintain minute ventilation. The physical definition of work as the product of force and distance or pressure and volume is only applicable to situations in which a change in distance or volume occurs. Therefore, an isovolemic change in intrathoracic pressure during inspiration against a closed airway or respiratory circuit does not constitute "work" in the physical sense, even though it may be associated with forceful muscle contraction and considerable energy expenditure.

Respiratory Effort

To account for isovolemic work, the total muscle activity of breathing is sometimes referred to as "respiratory effort." Inspiratory work is stored as potential energy in the respiratory system to be expended during the following exhalation or is used to overcome resistive forces during lung inflation.

Exhalation usually occurs passively using the energy stored in inspiratory deformation of the lungs and the chest wall. However, when increased resistance to exhalation or increased expiratory flow requirement calls for additional energy expenditure, the expiratory muscles are recruited and contribute to the respiratory work.

Assessment

If changes in lung volume and the pressure differential distending the lungs or the lung-thorax combination can be measured, ventilatory work can be calculated. During spontaneous breathing or full mechanical ventilatory support, work to inflate the lungs can be separated from work to displace the chest wall and the diaphragm.[1]

During partial ventilatory support, when the ventilatory muscles and the mechanical ventilator are simultaneously active, total ventilatory work can be calculated, but ventilator work and spontaneous work of breathing are difficult to separate accurately. Various techniques, such as calculation of time-tension relationships of airway and transdiaphragmatic pressure and measurement of total body oxygen (O_2) consumption ($\dot{V}_{O_2}$), have been used. The utility of these estimates is questionable at best.

A portable monitor that measures airway and esophageal pressures, gas flow, and V_T, and then provides automated pressure-volume loops has been introduced. Published work indicates that patient and ventilator work differentiation is easily determined with this device under most clinical circumstances.[2] At least some work of breathing is expended whenever spontaneous breathing is present, even with mechanical ventilatory support.[2] Whether the patient should be subjected to this work must be evaluated clinically.

Clinical Correlates

The presence or absence of ventilation is determined clinically by listening to breath sounds, observing chest wall movement, and feeling gas movement at the airway. When the patient is intubated and connected to an anesthesia circuit, observation of inspiratory deflation of the reservoir bag and expiratory fogging of the transparent tracheal tube wall provides additional proof of ventilation.

Alveolar hypoventilation and hyperventilation are assessed with arterial blood gas analysis. Their presence may be inferred from capnography data, but because of the virtually inevitable arterial versus end-tidal CO_2 differences that occur with this method, blood gas analysis is the gold standard.

Signs and Symptoms

Clinical signs and symptoms of these conditions vary widely, depending on their etiology and modifying factors. However, tachycardia, hypertension, wide pulse pressure, and dysrhythmias during acute hypercapnia as well as tachycardia, hypotension, carpopedal spasms, chest discomfort, and paresthesias in acute hypocapnia are seen with some consistency.

An acute increase in the patient's $Paco_2$ by more than 10 mm Hg from baseline that is accompanied by a fall in arterial blood pH by at least 0.1 unit below normal represents acute ventilatory failure. These values should lead to consideration of pharmacologic intervention (e.g., muscle relaxant antagonism) or of mechanical ventilatory support.

Capnography and Pulse Oximetry

Under most circumstances, the $Paco_2$ can be estimated from a capnogram or from the output of a transcutaneous CO_2 monitor, taking into account the limitations of these devices (see Chapter 20). Monitoring of oxygenation with a pulse oximeter can be used to indicate ventilatory adequacy only when the patient is breathing room air. An oxyhemoglobin (Hbo_2) saturation of 90% suggests hypoventilation and a $Paco_2$ and Pao_2 of approximately 60 mm Hg each (in the absence of other factors that produce hypoxemia).[3]

This approximation arises out of the prediction made by the alveolar gas equation and assumes a physiologic degree of shunting. The simplified form of this equation states that

$$Pao_2 = Pio_2 - \frac{Paco_2}{R} \qquad \text{Equation 1}$$

where Pio_2 is inspired O_2 partial pressure; $Paco_2$ is alveolar CO_2 partial pressure; and R is the respiratory exchange ratio (normally 0.8).

If the Pao_2 is 85 mm Hg, a 20–mm Hg increase in $Paco_2$ decreases the Pao_2 by 20/0.8, or about 25 mm Hg. However, even minimal O_2 supplementation compensates for such hypoventilation-induced hypoxemia and invalidates the pulse oximeter as a monitor of ventilation (Fig. 48–1).

Respiratory Mechanics

Ventilatory work is evaluated by studying the patient's respiratory mechanics (chest wall expansion, use of accessory ventilatory muscles, intercostal and suprasternal retractions, ventilatory rate, and the ratio of inspiratory time to expiratory time). Additional clues to increased ventilatory work are tachycardia, hypertension, anxiety, and the patient's refusal of an O_2 mask, which he or she feels is an added resistance to breathing (Table 48–1).

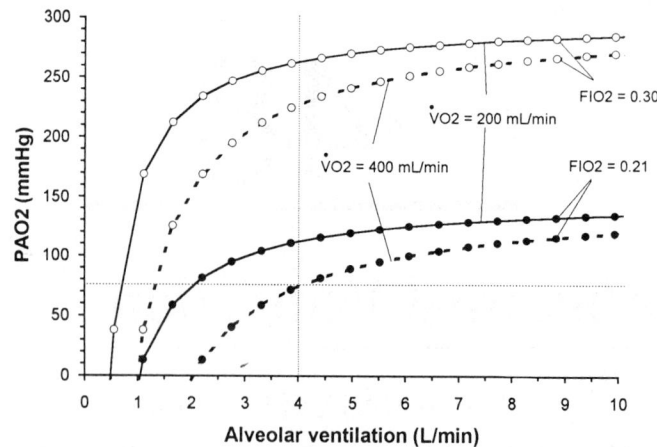

FIGURE 48–1. The effect of Fio_2 and $\dot{V}o_2$ on the relationship between alveolar ventilation and Pao_2. The *dotted vertical line* represents normal alveolar ventilation (4 L · min^{-1}) and a Pao_2 that produced an arterial blood oxyhemoglobin saturation of 90% in the absence of pulmonary pathology. Oxygen supplementation *(open circles)* corrects hypoventilation-induced hypoxemia unless ventilation is reduced to a very low level. Increased oxygen consumption may cause hypoxemia during room air breathing even when alveolar ventilation is only slightly depressed.

Patients often attempt to assume a sitting, forward-leaning position with their arms supported to minimize inspiratory effort. When increased ventilatory work is secondary to increased airway flow resistance, the ventilatory rate is decreased and the V_T increased in order to minimize turbulent air flow. In contrast, a reduction in respiratory system compliance usually leads to rapid, shallow breathing.[4]

Impending ventilatory failure from excessive work is characterized by an erratically variable rate and depth of breathing that rapidly progress to bradypnea and apnea if mechanical ventilatory support is not instituted.

ALVEOLAR HYPOVENTILATION

What Are the Consequences?

Hypoxemia develops during hypoventilation when O_2 transfer into the alveoli is insufficient to maintain the alveolar O_2 partial pressure (Pao_2) for a given O_2 uptake. The interdependence of Pao_2 and $Paco_2$ is expressed in the alveolar air equation, the long version of which is as follows:

$$Pao_2 = (P_B - P_{H_2O}) \times Fio_2 - Paco_2 \times 1 - Fio_2 \times (1 - R)/R \qquad \text{Equation 2}$$

TABLE 48–1. Clinical Signs of Increased Ventilatory Work

Tachypnea
Anxiety
Tachycardia
Hypertension
Sitting, forward-leaning position
Intercostal and suprasternal retractions during inspiration
Use of accessory respiratory muscles
Refusal of oxygen mask
Erratically variable V_T

where P_B is barometric pressure; P_{H_2O} is water vapor pressure; and F_{IO_2} is the fraction of inspired O_2. Given a stable metabolic rate and unchanged composition of inspired gas, the inverse and linear relationship between P_{AO_2} and P_{ACO_2} is evident. The P_{ACO_2} is dependent on CO_2 production ($\dot{V}_{CO_2}$) and on alveolar ventilation ($\dot{V}_A$):

$$P_{ACO_2} = (P_B - P_{H_2O}) \times \dot{V}_{CO_2}/\dot{V}_A \qquad \text{Equation 3}$$

$\dot{V}_{CO_2}$ can be derived from O_2 consumption ($\dot{V}_{O_2}$) and R:

$$\dot{V}_{CO_2} = \dot{V}_{O_2} \times R \qquad \text{Equation 4}$$

Thus, P_{AO_2} can be expressed as a function of $\dot{V}_A$ and $\dot{V}_{O_2}$:

$$P_{AO_2} = (P_B - P_{H_2O}) \times [F_{IO_2} - \frac{\dot{V}_{O_2}}{\dot{V}_A} \times [1 - F_{IO_2} \times (1 - R)]]$$

Equation 5

which defines a hyperbolic relationship between P_{AO_2} and $\dot{V}_A$ (see Fig. 48–1). This relationship is shifted by changes in the F_{IO_2} and $\dot{V}_{O_2}$. Consequently, hypoventilation-induced hypoxemia is easily masked by O_2 supplementation, and dangerous hypoxemia may be precipitated in a hypercapnic patient if the inspired O_2 concentration is suddenly lowered.

Alveolar hypoventilation leads inevitably to respiratory acidemia. However, the consequences of hypercapnia and acidosis vary, depending on the effects of compensatory mechanisms on intracellular and extracellular pH and on factors that modify the normal response of the various organ systems.

What Are the Central Nervous System Effects?

Hypercapnia has profound direct and indirect effects on the central nervous system (CNS).[5] In experimental animals, the anesthetic effect of CO_2 becomes apparent when the P_{ACO_2} reaches 90 to 100 mm Hg. With increasing hypercapnia, the minimum anesthetic concentration of inhalation anesthetics is reduced, and the ventilatory stimulant effect of CO_2 decreases.

Carbon dioxide narcosis likely is a consequence of intraneuronal acidosis, which interferes with normal cellular processes. Thirty per cent CO_2 alone produces general anesthesia with an isoelectric electroencephalogram. However, the use of CO_2 as an anesthetic in humans has been abandoned because it frequently produces seizures at anesthetic concentrations.

Cerebral Blood Flow

Increasing the P_{ACO_2} from its normal range up to 100 mm Hg is associated with a nearly linear increase in cerebral blood flow secondary to cerebral arteriolar vasodilation. This effect is accentuated by inhalation anesthetics that have a cerebral vasodilating effect of their own. Hypercapnia-induced augmentation of cerebral blood flow and volume cause an immediate rise in intracranial pressure, which may be detrimental to patients with space-occupying intracranial lesions or generalized cerebral edema.

Sympathetic Nervous System

The sympathetic nervous system is stimulated by hypercapnia both directly and by way of increased release of epineph-

rine and norepinephrine from the adrenal medulla. This sympathomimetic response almost completely reverses the direct effects of hypercapnia on circulatory function. Although CO_2 has negative myocardial inotropic and chronotropic effects, the net effect of moderate hypercapnia in humans with a functioning autonomic nervous system is an increase in heart rate, blood pressure, pulse pressure, and cardiac output as well as a slight decrease in systemic vascular resistance.

In the elderly, in patients with cardiovascular disease, and in individuals receiving β-adrenergic antagonists, respiratory acidosis may impair circulatory function both directly and by attenuating the circulatory response to circulating catecholamines.

What Are the Effects on Cardiac Rhythm?

Dysrhythmias—most commonly ventricular premature contractions—may occur in hypercapnic patients as a result of a direct effect of CO_2 and low pH on the heart, elevated catecholamine levels, or electrolyte abnormalities, particularly hyperkalemia. The likelihood of hypercapnia-induced dysrhythmias increases during halothane anesthesia.[6]

What Electrolyte Changes Occur?

Acute respiratory acidemia is accompanied by an increase in serum potassium concentration by an average of 0.1 mEq · L^{-1} for every 0.1 unit decreases in pH.[7] This change is variable but generally smaller than that seen in metabolic acidosis of similar magnitude. In chronic ventilatory failure, the serum potassium level is normal or slightly decreased.

What Is the Effect on Oxyhemoglobin Affinity?

The decrease in blood pH during alveolar hypoventilation decreases HbO_2 affinity. Therefore, unloading of O_2 into the peripheral tissues is facilitated because a lower HbO_2 saturation can be reached at tissue O_2 partial pressures. However, simultaneous impairment of O_2 loading in the lungs may decrease the O_2 content of arterial blood, resulting in a net reduction in tissue O_2 delivery. Compromise in tissue O_2 delivery is accentuated if hypoventilation leads to a concurrent decrease in P_{AO_2} (see Fig. 48–1 and Equation 2).

How Are Pulmonary Vascular Resistance and Bronchomotor Tone Affected?

In the lungs, respiratory acidemia effects an increase in the tone of both the pulmonary vasculature and small airways. After cardiopulmonary bypass, the increase in pulmonary vascular resistance with rising P_{ACO_2} is markedly accentuated and can be demonstrated even within the range of normal ventilation.[8] A combination of hypercapnia and hypoxemia may elevate pulmonary vascular resistance sufficiently to cause right ventricular failure in a compromised patient. A coexisting reduction in airway caliber further aggravates respiratory failure by increasing ventilatory work and ventilation/perfusion ($\dot{V}_A/\dot{Q}$) mismatching.

TABLE 48–2. Factors Contributing to Respiratory Acidosis

Equipment malfunction and misuse
Impaired transport of carbon dioxide to the alveoli
   Hypoperfusion of ventilated lung
   Right-to-left shunting of blood
   Diffusion block
Inadequate respiratory drive
   Metabolic alkalosis
   Respiratory depressant drugs
   Injury to the respiratory center
   Altered responsiveness of the respiratory center
Failure of neuromuscular transmission
   Injury to the neural pathway
   Disease of the neuromuscular junction
   Neuromuscular blockade
Respiratory muscle dysfunction
   Muscular dystrophy
   Poor muscle strength/fatigue
   Excessive ventilatory load
Structural abnormality of the respiratory system
   Inability to generate negative intrathoracic pressure
   Restriction of lung or chest wall expansion

Why Does Hypoventilation Occur?

The causes of hypoventilation may lie at one level or at more than one level in the chain of events that maintain and control spontaneous breathing (Table 48–2). In a patient rendered apneic during anesthesia, a host of potential iatrogenic causes of hypoventilation require attention.

When ventilatory problems are suspected in an intubated patient, a useful differential diagnostic procedure entails manual ventilation of the lungs with a FIO_2 equivalent to or higher than that previously used. If the patient is receiving positive end-expiratory pressure (PEEP), it too should be continued.

Equipment Malfunction or Misuse

Manual ventilation with simultaneous auscultation of breath sounds and observation of chest wall motion and the response of the pulse oximeter and capnograph usually allow one to distinguish between ventilatory problems associated with the ventilator and those caused by the artificial airway or a change in the patient's clinical condition. "Feeling" the mechanics of manual ventilation usually directs attention appropriately to tracheal tube misplacement, airway obstruction, or reduction in respiratory system compliance.

Tracheal Tube Malpositioning

Misplacement of the tracheal tube should always be suspected as a cause of a ventilatory problem until correct placement is confirmed.

Physical Findings. Manual ventilation and auscultation of breath sounds bilaterally below the clavicles frequently detect esophageal intubation. However, ventilation of the stomach may feel and sound deceptively similar to ventilation of the lungs. Therefore, confirmation of tracheal intubation should be sought whenever possible with capnography, by direct visualization of the larynx and of the tracheal tube passing between the vocal cords, or using fiberoptic bronchoscopy.

Capnography. A stable, normal capnogram during positive-pressure ventilation indicates that the tip of the tracheal tube is in the trachea or a bronchus. Carbon dioxide may be present in the stomach as a result of earlier mask ventilation or ingestion of CO_2-releasing material. However, the end-tidal concentration of CO_2 is low and decreases rapidly during continued ventilation of the stomach.[9, 10]

During spontaneous ventilation, exhaled CO_2 can be detected at the tracheal tube even when the tube is not in the trachea as long as its tip is at or above the laryngeal opening. In this situation, exhalation around the tracheal tube, low insertion depth of the tube, and unsuccessful manual ventilation usually indicate tube misplacement.

Bronchial intubation may not produce alveolar hypoventilation if the ventilated lung is normal, but it can do so in patients with pulmonary disease. Signs alerting to bronchial intubation include an increase in peak airway pressure and asymmetric motion of the chest during inspiration. Inadvertent advancement of the tracheal tube below the carina can usually be detected by bilateral auscultation of the lungs.

Circuit Problems

If manual ventilation is possible without difficulty, the cause of ventilatory problems should be sought in the breathing circuit or in the ventilator (Table 48–3). Anesthesiologists should be thoroughly familiar with how to troubleshoot the equipment they use and should know how to obtain technical assistance or acquire replacement parts so that a problem can be quickly located and corrected.

Leaks and Disconnections. The multiple connections between the different parts of an anesthesia machine allow leaks and disconnections to develop easily in the breathing circuit (see Chapter 16). Equipment-related mishaps tend to occur during times of cardiopulmonary instability, when the activity level is high and multiple tasks require simultaneous attention from the anesthesiologist. During these periods, it is particularly important to maintain vigilance and to ensure that a combination of alarm systems can signal failure of adequate ventilation, whatever its cause may be. A backup plan that allows continuation of anesthesia and cardiopulmonary support, regardless of failure of electrical or pneumatic equipment, should always be formulated prior to inducing anesthesia.

Mechanical Ventilation. The operating principle of the mechanical ventilator may contribute to the development of alveolar hypoventilation during changing clinical circumstances. The VT delivered by a pressure-cycled ventilator at a given peak airway pressure decreases if lung compliance is reduced or if airway resistance is increased.

The VT delivered by time-cycled and volume-cycled ventilators also is affected by changes in lung compliance and

TABLE 48–3. Causes of Equipment-Related Hypoventilation

Misplaced artificial airway
Power or gas supply failure
Inadequate ventilator settings
   Ventilator turned off
   Failure to adjust to changes in pulmonary
     mechanics
   Failure to adjust to changes in metabolic rate
Circuit leak
Rebreathing of exhaled gas
   Inadequate fresh gas flow in a rebreathing circuit
   Carbon dioxide absorber off or not functioning
   Circuit valve dysfunction
Misinterpretation/calibration of the capnogram

airway resistance but only to the extent that the increased peak airway pressure results in inspiratory circuit distention and gas compression within the breathing circuit.

Metabolic and Mechanical Interactions. Factors that produce an increase in CO_2 output may cause alveolar hypoventilation during anesthesia. Decreasing the depth of anesthesia or level of neuromuscular blockade and the development of hypermetabolic states such as septicemia and malignant hyperthermia cause profound respiratory acidosis unless the increased CO_2 output is promptly compensated for with an adjustment in minute ventilation.

Standard Circle Systems. Equipment-related causes of alveolar hypoventilation during anesthesia vary between different types of breathing circuits. A standard circle system that incorporates a functioning in-line CO_2 absorber prevents rebreathing of CO_2 as long as minute ventilation and gas volume in the circuit are adequate. However, incompetence of the one-way valves that are intended to ensure unidirectional flow of exhaled gas through the absorber quickly leads to hypercapnia secondary to rebreathing.

If the inspiratory unidirectional valve seats permanently in the closed position, ventilation is impossible, and the canister pressure rises while pressure in the patient's airway remains low. An obstructed expiratory valve or closed overflow (pop-off) valve increases pressure in the breathing circuit and in the patient's airway.

Partial Rebreathing Circuits. In circuits that allow rebreathing of exhaled gas, the fresh gas flow rate relative to the patient's CO_2 output is an essential factor in determining CO_2 removal. Insufficient fresh gas flow in these circuits results in increased Pa_{CO_2} owing to rebreathing. As with the circle system, a combination of hypercapnia and dangerous hyperinflation occurs if the fresh gas flow is allowed to accumulate in the system owing to excessive closure of the pop-off valve.

Interpretive Errors. An equipment-related cause of pseudoalveolar hypoventilation is related to misinterpretation of the capnogram. Although abnormally high exhaled CO_2 concentrations virtually always indicate alveolar hypoventilation, the end-tidal CO_2 tension may be low for several reasons, including low blood flow to the lungs, increased dead space ventilation, inadequate expiratory time, or sensor calibration/function. These conditions result in a change in the difference between end-tidal and arterial CO_2 concentrations. Responding to low end-tidal CO_2 by reducing minute ventilation without appropriate differential diagnostic attention may subject the patient to serious underventilation and respiratory acidemia.

What Is the Effect of Failed Carbon Dioxide Transport?

Excretion of CO_2 is possible only if sufficient blood flow through the ventilated lungs can be maintained. The efficiency of CO_2 transport and considerable ventilatory reserve suggest that only extreme impairment of pulmonary blood flow will result in increased Pa_{CO_2} if ventilation is not depressed.

Causes

Reduced Pulmonary Blood Flow

Severe reduction in pulmonary blood flow may result from right or left ventricular failure, blood volume loss, obstructed

venous return, or pulmonary artery obstruction. Hypoperfused but ventilated alveoli (zone 1 units) constitute alveolar dead space and require a compensatory increase in minute ventilation.

Zone I lung units can also be created from the alveolar side by excessive lung inflation (ventilation with high tidal volume, inappropriately high PEEP, or a rapid ventilatory rate that does not allow complete emptying of the alveoli during exhalation). Increased expiratory flow resistance secondary to bronchoconstriction or technical problems that cause increased flow resistance in the expiratory limb of the breathing circuit may lead to dynamic hyperinflation of the lungs, even with a normal ventilatory rate.

Increased Shunting

Right-to-left shunting of blood constitutes another potential mechanism for failure of CO_2 to reach the alveoli. Shunting may occur through nonventilated lung units in patients with pulmonary disease, or it may be extrapulmonary, making part of the cardiac output bypass the lungs completely.

The effect of shunting must be compensated for by functioning lung units to maintain normoventilation. Since CO_2 diffuses rapidly through the alveolocapillary membranes, areas of low but finite $\dot{V}A/\dot{Q}$ ratio have less effect on CO_2 excretion than they do on oxygenation.

What Are the Causes of Respiratory Center Depression?

Several acute and chronic disease processes result in ventilatory failure, particularly in patients receiving anesthetics or analgesics.

Chronic Lung Disease

Chronic ventilatory failure associated with many types of pulmonary disease causes respiratory depression by poorly understood mechanisms that resemble depression of the respiratory center. Hypoxemia, not hypercarbia, becomes the major driving force of ventilation. Correction of chronic hypoxemia with O_2 therapy in such patients may lead to severe acute hypoventilation and respiratory acidemia.

Morbid Obesity

Patients with morbid obesity or chronic upper airway obstruction also frequently have abnormalities of ventilatory drive and may be particularly prone to develop alveolar hypoventilation during recovery from anesthesia or upon receiving narcotic analgesics.

Respiratory Center Impairment

Any acute condition that results in the compression of the respiratory center or impairs its blood supply (e.g., hypotension) may lead to ventilatory failure of central origin. Although impairment of ventilatory control by neoplasms, vascular disease, or CNS trauma frequently is known when a patient presents for surgery, the possibility of CNS catastrophies developing during anesthesia must be considered in the differential diagnosis of postanesthetic ventilatory failure.

Metabolic Alkalosis

Metabolic alkalosis produces alveolar hypoventilation as a compensatory change to attenuate the increase in blood pH. The response is variable, ranging between 0.4 and 0.9 mm Hg increase in $PaCO_2$ for each 1 mEq $\cdot$ L^{-1} increase in plasma bicarbonate concentration. Respiratory compensation for metabolic alkalosis occurs slowly, reaching its maximum in 12 to 24 hours. Alveolar hypoventilation to a $PaCO_2$ greater than 50 mm Hg occurs rarely in conscious and alert individuals but may be encountered in patients with depressed consciousness.

Drug Effects

Respiratory depression is one of the most common and serious side effects of drugs used by anesthesiologists. Therefore, the severity and expected duration of the respiratory effects of each drug that one uses in practice must be known, and modifying factors in individual patients must be taken into account.

Monitoring of ventilatory function after anesthesia and during the administration of postoperative pain medication must be arranged to cover the period of respiratory depression with a sufficient margin of safety.

What Role Do Abnormalities of Impulse Conduction Play?

Conduction of the electrical impulse from the respiratory center to the ventilatory muscles can be interrupted by several conditions.

Spinal Cord Trauma

Spinal cord trauma below the C-5 level spares the phrenic nerves but results in a degree of paralysis of the intercostal muscles, which depends on the extent, type, and level of injury. Transection of the spinal cord above the C-3 level results in the permanent inability of a patient to maintain spontaneous ventilation.

Nontraumatic Problems

Several nontraumatic conditions, including infections, demyelinating CNS diseases, poliomyelitis, and the Guillain-Barré syndrome, may lead to ventilatory failure secondary to impaired neural impulse conduction at different levels of the efferent neural pathway.

Phrenic Nerve Damage

The phrenic nerves are subject to damage from neoplastic disease, regional anesthesia (interscalene block in particular), and surgery that involves the neck and thorax. Topical cooling and distention of mediastinal structures during cardiac surgery may render one or both phrenic nerves nonfunctional for several months and may result in the need for prolonged postoperative ventilatory support.[11]

Intercostal Muscle Function

Regional anesthesia extending to the thoracic nerve roots may compromise intercostal muscle function sufficiently to reduce ventilatory reserve and contribute to ventilatory failure when other abnormalities such as airway obstruction or parenchymal lung injury are present.

Neuromuscular Coupling

The neuromuscular junction is a common target of anesthetic management and, therefore, a frequent site of derangements that lead to ventilatory failure. Incomplete reversal of neuromuscular blockade is a common problem in the postanesthesia recovery period, especially in patients with preexisting disorders of neuromuscular function such as myasthenia gravis, the Eaton-Lambert syndrome, and muscular dystrophies.

Uncommon Problems

Rare acute disorders that disable the neuromuscular junction include botulism, organophosphate insecticide poisoning, and exposure to some nerve gases. Infection with *Clostridium tetani* may cause ventilatory failure by inducing spasm of ventilatory and laryngeal muscles.

Inability to Reverse Relaxants. Reversal of nondepolarizing neuromuscular blockade may be difficult in patients who are receiving large doses of some antibiotics (particularly the aminoglycosides) and in those with electrolyte and acid-base abnormalities (particularly hypokalemia, hypocalcemia, hypermagnesemia, and acidosis).[12]

Inadequate or Atypical Pseudocholinesterase. Succinylcholine and miracurium may effect prolonged muscle relaxation in patients with inadequate levels of pseudocholinesterase or a hereditary condition that results in production of an atypical form of this enzyme. A partially paralyzed patient exhibits a characteristic discoordinated breathing pattern in which diaphragmatic contraction pushes the flaccid abdominal muscles outward while the anterior chest wall moves paradoxically inward.

Tests of Neuromuscular Function

Several tests of neuromuscular function have been proposed to predict when a patient will be able to maintain spontaneous ventilation. A forced vital capacity of $\geq$15 mL $\cdot$ kg^{-1}, a negative inspiratory pressure of <25 cm H_2O, and the patient's ability to keep the head elevated for 5 seconds while he or she is lying supine are commonly considered as indications of the presence of adequate muscle strength for spontaneous breathing. However, these tests do not ensure normal muscle strength. Endurance and ventilatory muscle failure may still ensue if the work of breathing is increased.

When Is Ventilatory Muscle Dysfunction Problematic?

Ventilatory muscle weakness may be a primary cause of hypoventilation in patients with muscular dystrophies or hypothyroidism. More commonly, ventilatory muscle weakness contributes to the development of alveolar hypoventilation. Strength can be compromised by disuse atrophy after long periods of mechanical ventilation, by malnutrition, or by imbalances in nutritional homeostasis, particularly hypokalemia and hypophosphatemia.[13, 14]

Fatigue

Ventilatory muscle fatigue is defined as loss of ventilatory muscle contractile force during exercise. Since a V_T of 500 mL in a normal individual only requires a 4- to 6-cm H_2O decrease of intrathoracic pressure, fatigue is usually caused by abnormal muscle loading, deranged lung or chest wall mechanics, or high ventilatory demand.

Exposure to conditions requiring prolonged development of 40% or more of maximum transdiaphragmatic pressure from a normal functional residual capacity eventually leads to fatigue and ventilatory failure.[15] If muscle contraction is started from a volume higher than the normal functional residual capacity, as may be the case in patients with chronic obstructive lung disease, the initial overstretching of the ventilatory muscles at the start of the contraction puts them at a disadvantage for pressure development (Fig. 48–2). Fatigue in such patients develops at lower workloads than it does in patients with normal resting lung volume. Patients with conditions that impair neuromuscular function may not tolerate any increase in ventilatory load.

Energy Supply and Demand Imbalance

Muscles may fail to contract because of an imbalance between energy supply and demand. Fatigue occurs more readily when patients with diminished systemic blood flow or blood O_2 content are subjected to an increased respiratory workload. In fact, ventilatory muscle fatigue and ventilatory failure can be induced in experimental animals by reducing O_2 even when lung mechanics are normal.[16] When muscle cells revert to anaerobic metabolism, the accumulation of lactic acid further impairs contractile function and accelerates the development of fatigue.

Repetitive Neuronal Firing

Failure of neuromuscular transmission secondary to repeated firing of the neurons has been shown to occur in the phrenic nerves of experimental animals.[15, 17]

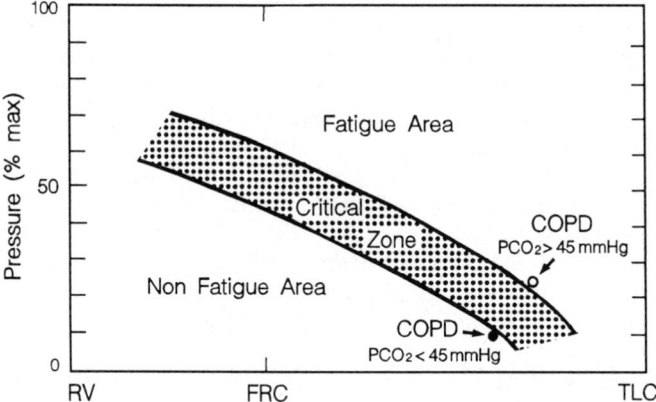

FIGURE 48–2. A schematic diagram of respiratory system pressure and volume demonstrating the dependence of critical intrathoracic or transdiaphragmatic pressure at which respiratory muscle fatigue occurs on expiratory lung volume. At normal functional residual capacity, the critical zone is 40 to 60% of maximum load. If the inspiratory phase is started at higher lung volume, fatigue occurs at much smaller load. Patients with COLD and chronic alveolar hypoventilation are placed in the fatigue area. FRC = Functional residual capacity; TLC = total lung capacity; COPD = chronic obstructive pulmonary disease. (Redrawn from Roussos C: Respiratory muscle fatigue and ventilatory failure. Chest 1990; 97:89S, with permission.)

Inhibition of Muscle Stimulation

Evidence suggests that afferent impulses from the ventilatory muscles, when transmitted to the respiratory center, inhibit the electrical stimulation of the muscles before actual muscle contractile failure sets in.[18] This CNS "fatigue" may be a mechanism by which the ventilatory muscles are protected from exhaustion. The exact role of transmission fatigue and respiratory center failure in humans is not known.

What Are the Effects of Structural Derangement?

Adequate ventilation requires that contraction of ventilatory muscles results in lung inflation. If intrathoracic pressure fails to decrease during spontaneous inspiration, movement of gas into the lungs will not occur despite adequate respiratory drive, neural and neuromuscular impulse transmission, and muscle strength.

Pneumothorax

Equilibration of intrathoracic and ambient pressure following an open pneumothorax and the loss of chest wall rigidity after multiple rib fractures may disrupt the structural integrity of the respiratory system sufficiently to impair spontaneous ventilation. Conditions such as pneumothorax or hemothorax restrict inspiratory lung expansion, making breathing difficult or impossible until the air or fluid is evacuated from the pleural space.

Pulmonary Contusion

A crushing injury to the chest wall that produces these conditions usually also decreases the distensibility of the lung parenchyma (pulmonary contusion), requiring large increases in transpulmonary pressure to provide a normal V_T.

Pendelluft

Unilateral disruption of chest wall integrity may lead to a "pendelluft" phenomenon in which the functioning lung receives a large part of its V_T by deflating the contralateral lung. During exhalation, gas returns into the traumatized lung from which it is rebreathed during the next inspiration. Rebreathing of exhaled gas results in inefficient removal of CO_2 and in respiratory acidemia.

Congenital Deformities and Abdominal Distention

Restriction of lung expansion leads to chronic alveolar hypoventilation in patients with congenital or acquired chest wall or thoracic spine deformities. In pulmonary interstitial fibrosis, minimal lung expansion is accomplished despite increased effort. Distention of the abdominal cavity during laparoscopy or in patients with large amounts of ascites may restrict diaphragmatic movement sufficiently to cause ventilatory failure.

Diffusion Block

Reduction in the gas exchanging area of the lung eventually leads to impaired excretion of CO_2. Since CO_2 moves through the alveolocapillary membrane much more readily than does O_2, conditions that affect transfer of CO_2 from capillary blood to alveolar gas usually present first with hypoxemia (see Chapter 47).

Because of the rapid diffusion of CO_2, intrapulmonary shunting of blood and an increase in dead space volume, rather than diffusion block, are the predominant mechanisms impairing removal of CO_2 during acute lung injury.

How Should Hypoventilation Be Corrected?

When acute ventilatory failure with respiratory acidemia is evident, mechanical ventilatory assistance should be instituted without further delay. In less severe cases, correction with measures directed at the cause of hypoventilation and without mechanical ventilatory support often suffice.

Postanesthetic Depression

Mild postanesthetic respiratory depression can frequently be corrected by verbal and tactile stimulation. Ventilation may be improved by having the patient assume a semi-sitting position that allows the diaphragm to move with less impedance from the abdominal organs. However, patients who have been extubated following deep inhalation anesthesia should be placed in a lateral recumbent position to maintain patency of the upper airway and to allow drainage of the pharynx should regurgitation of gastric contents occur.

Opiate-induced respiratory depression can be reversed with opiate antagonists or with doxapram. Neuromuscular blockade should be evaluated in any patient with alveolar hypoventilation during recovery from anesthesia involving muscle relaxants. In patients with chronic lung disease, O_2 therapy must be planned and conducted carefully to avoid loss of the hypoxic drive to breathe.

Pneumothorax and Hydrothorax

A pneumothorax or hydrothorax may require immediate needle or chest tube drainage before positive-pressure ventilation is instituted. Tracheal intubation and mechanical ventilation delay definitive treatment and, in the case of a pneumothorax, may result in further cardiopulmonary compromise.

Airway Management

Several measures can be taken to reduce increased work before mechanical ventilatory support is initiated if ventilatory fatigue is not imminent. Components of the circuit should be checked and changed to minimize equipment-related dead space and resistance. Airway obstruction to the midtrachea can frequently be alleviated with an artificial airway without mechanical ventilation.

Continuous Positive Airway Pressure

Decreased Compliance. When increased ventilatory work is caused by decreased lung compliance, an increase in end-expiratory lung volume by continuous positive airway pressure (CPAP) often improves lung mechanics and decreases the work of breathing sufficiently to obviate mechanical ventilatory support (Fig. 48–3). CPAP can be applied with a face-mask, even for prolonged periods of time.[19, 20] The beneficial

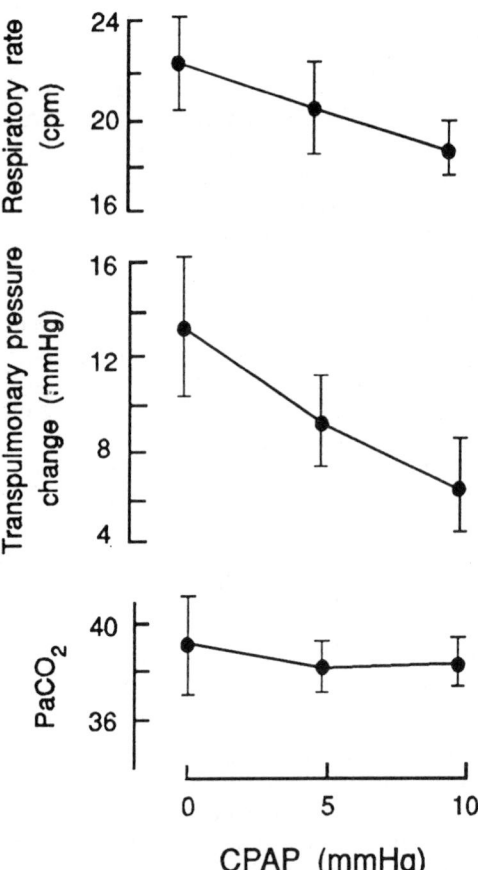

FIGURE 48–3. Changes in ventilatory rate, inspiratory fall in transpulmonary pressure, and $PaCO_2$ on application of up to 10 mm Hg CPAP in 14 patients with respiratory failure secondary to acute myocardial infarction. Improvement in pulmonary mechanics results in an almost linear decrease in ventilatory rate and transpulmonary pressure change and normalization of $PaCO_2$. (Redrawn from Räisänen J, Väisänen I, Heikkila J, et al: Acute myocardial infarction complicated by left ventricular dysfunction and respiratory failure: the effects of continuous positive airway pressure. Chest 1985; 87:158, with permission.)

effects probably result from recruitment of previously collapsed alveoli, increase in the distensibility of patent lung units, increase in the caliber of conducting airways, reduced intrapulmonary shunting of blood, and correction of hypoxemia.[21, 22]

The improvement in lung mechanics is instantaneous and can easily be recognized in the responding patient by a reduction in respiratory rate, less inspiratory intercostal retraction, absence of accessory ventilatory muscle contraction, and subjective relief of breathing effort (Fig. 48–4). Simplicity of the equipment and the rapid onset of a favorable effect make a trial of CPAP therapy applicable, even in patients with overt ventilatory failure, unless respiratory exhaustion is imminent.[23, 24]

Mask CPAP should not be used in patients with obtunded protective laryngeal reflexes because of the possibility of regurgitation and aspiration of gastric contents. In hypovolemic patients, CPAP may decrease stroke volume and require restoration of venous return with fluid therapy.

Cardiogenic Ventilatory Failure. In patients with cardiogenic ventilatory failure, decreased muscle work, alleviation of hypertension and tachycardia, and augmentation of left ventricular function secondary to decreased afterload are also important advantages of CPAP.[25, 26]

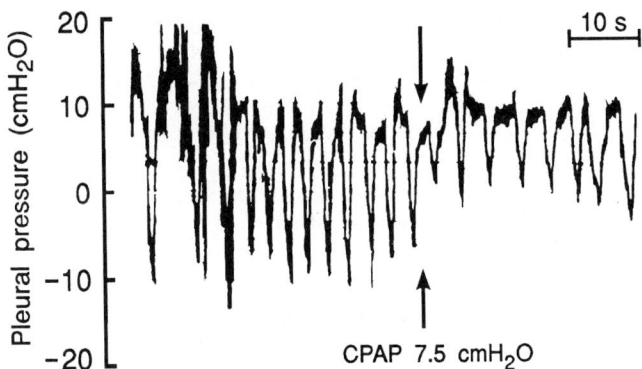

FIGURE 48–4. A tracing of directly measured intrathoracic pressure in a patient with cardiogenic pulmonary edema before and after application of 7.5 cm H_2O CPAP. Within one respiratory cycle from the institution of CPAP therapy, the ventilatory rate and the inspiratory fall in intrathoracic pressure decrease dramatically.

Relief of Airway Obstruction. Airway obstruction due to accumulation of secretions can be alleviated by thorough bronchial suctioning using a tracheal tube with a catheter or a flexible bronchoscope. Obstructive pulmonary disease may require the use of topical or systemic bronchodilators.

When bronchoconstriction occurs during anesthesia, the bronchodilating effects of inhalation anesthetics and ketamine may be useful. In fact, inadequate anesthesia is a frequent cause of operative bronchoconstriction and wheezing, particularly in children.

Mechanical Ventilation

Mechanical ventilation must be instituted if ventilatory failure is caused by a factor for which another immediate remedy is not available. It is also indicated if increased ventilatory work is likely to lead to ventilatory failure before its cause can be removed. Several techniques are available to provide total or partial ventilatory support. The reader is referred to specific texts for detailed description of their application.[27]

Extracorporeal Carbon Dioxide Removal

Severe reduction in the gas-exchange area following acute lung injury may not allow matching of $\dot{V}A$ and $\dot{V}CO_2$. Extracorporeal removal of CO_2, with or without simultaneous extracorporeal oxygenation, has been used in children and adults in this rare and extreme case.[28, 29]

ALVEOLAR HYPERVENTILATION

What Are the Consequences?

The sequelae of alveolar hyperventilation depend on whether the patient is hyperventilating spontaneously or is mechanically hyperventilated. In all patients, a reduction in $Paco_2$ will increase Pao_2 (see Equation 2).

Oxygenation

If the patient is mechanically ventilated, a potential improvement in the oxygenation of arterial blood is frequently offset by the detrimental effects of positive airway and intrathoracic pressure on the distribution of ventilation and perfusion in the lungs. Therefore, deliberate hyperventilation is not effective treatment for hypoxemia. The deleterious effects of hypocapnia frequently outweigh the advantages of slightly increased Pao_2 and Pao_2, even in spontaneously breathing patients.

Carbon Dioxide

An increase in alveolar ventilation beyond the needs of CO_2 production produces hypocapnia and respiratory alkalosis. When induced with artificial ventilation, hypocapnia usually results in apnea when the $Paco_2$ decreases below 32 mm Hg.

What Are the Central Nervous System Effects?

Respiratory alkalemia generally increases CNS excitability and lowers the threshold for seizures.

Tetany

Tetany in patients with severe respiratory alkalemia has been attributed to decreased ionized calcium ion (Ca^{2+}) concentrations in the plasma. However, tetany is seen at higher Ca^{2+} concentrations in patients with respiratory alkalemia than in those in other hypocalcemic states, suggesting that the Ca^{2+} level alone is not responsible for this problem.[30]

Cerebral Vasoconstriction

A decrease in $Paco_2$ produces cerebral vasoconstriction, reduces the cerebral blood flow and volume, and lowers intracranial pressure (ICP). The decrease in cerebral blood flow is nearly linear down to a $Paco_2$ of 20 mm Hg. Below this level, further vasoconstriction probably is limited by concurrent hypoxia effected by reduced O_2 delivery.

Induction of cerebral vasoconstriction with hypocapnia can be used to reduce ICP when it is elevated by intracranial disease and to counteract the vasodilatory properties of inhalation anesthetics in patients who cannot tolerate a perioperative rise in ICP.

How Is Cardiovascular Activity Affected?

Myocardial Function

Although mild hyperventilation has little effect on cardiovascular function, moderate to severe respiratory alkalemia may indirectly depress myocardial contractility by reducing the Ca^{2+} concentration in the blood and by causing coronary artery vasoconstriction.[31, 32]

Systemic Vascular Resistance

The systemic vascular resistance is increased by the peripheral effects and lowered by the central effects of hypocapnia. If hyperventilation is accomplished with positive-pressure ventilation, the increased intrathoracic pressure decreases right and left ventricular filling and causes a reduction in cardiac output.

Dysrhythmias

Respiratory alkalemia is associated with electrical irritability of the myocardium and with an increased incidence of cardiac dysrhythmias. The dysrhythmogenicity of increased blood pH is further accentuated by a fall in serum potassium concentration that is effected by intracellular translocation in exchange for hydrogen ions. The likelihood of serious hypokalemia-induced dysrhythmias is of particular concern in patients who receive digitalis glycosides.

What Is the Effect on Oxyhemoglobin Affinity?

An increase in blood pH during alveolar hyperventilation increases the HbO_2 affinity. Consequently, O_2 uptake by hemoglobin in the lungs is facilitated, whereas unloading of O_2 from blood to tissues is impeded. Concurrently, alkalosis increases $\dot{V}O_2$ by uncoupling oxidative phosphorylation. Diminished systemic blood flow, shifting of the HbO_2 dissociation curve to the left, and increased $\dot{V}O_2$ produce a potentially deleterious impairment in the matching of O_2 supply ($\dot{D}O_2$) and demand.

How Are Pulmonary Vascular Resistance and Bronchomotor Tone Affected?

Acute respiratory alkalosis increases bronchomotor tone and airway flow resistance and decreases pulmonary vascular resistance. The combination of regional reductions in ventilation and reversal of hypoxic pulmonary vasoconstriction further decreases the $\dot{V}A/\dot{Q}$ ratios of such poorly ventilated lung units and may contribute to hypoxemia.

Why Does Alveolar Hyperventilation Occur?

Common etiologic factors leading to alveolar hyperventilation are listed in Table 48–4. Iatrogenic hyperventilation fre-

TABLE 48–4. Factors Contributing to Alveolar Hyperventilation

Equipment malfunction and misuse
  Mechanical overventilation
  Excessive fresh gas flow
Increased central stimulation of the respiratory center
  Anxiety
  Injury to the respiratory center
  Pain
  Fever
  Liver failure
  Pharmacologic agents
  Gram-negative septicemia
  Hormonally mediated (catechols, thyroxine)
  Pregnancy (hyperprogesteronemia)
Hypoxia
Hypotension
Metabolic acidosis

quently follows from an attempt to avoid hypoventilation in a mechanically ventilated patient. Since both hypoventilation and hyperventilation have deleterious consequences, patients should be ventilated to a near normal $PaCO_2$ and pH, unless there are specific reasons to do otherwise.

Equipment Malfunction or Misuse

Mechanical Ventilation

Modern mechanical ventilators rarely deliver excess minute ventilation when properly used. However, in anesthesia breathing circuits, an increase in fresh gas flow during mechanical ventilation may lower the $PaCO_2$ to a hypocapnic level because the fresh gas flow augments the ventilator-delivered V_T. This is most commonly an issue immediately following induction and prior to emergence, when the highest fresh gas flows are used.

Volume-Cycled and Time-Cycled Ventilators. Conventional volume-cycled or time-cycled patient-triggered mechanical ventilatory support may produce hypocapnia and respiratory alkalemia as a side-effect because the V_T is controlled by the ventilator and not by the patient.[33] The ventilator delivers the set V_T and eventually lowers the CO_2 partial pressure below the apneic threshold. When, after a period of apnea, the patient again triggers the ventilator, the fixed V_T again lowers the $PaCO_2$. Thus, the $PaCO_2$ ultimately fluctuates slightly above and below the apneic threshold, and hypocapnia is predictable.

Pressure-Cycled Ventilators. Failure to adjust the settings of a pressure-cycled ventilator also may lead to inadvertent hyperventilation if the patient's respiratory system compliance increases or if airway resistance decreases during recovery.

Changes in Dead Space and Carbon Dioxide Production. Decrease in respiratory V_{DS} or CO_2 production during mechanical ventilation leads to alveolar hyperventilation if ventilator settings are maintained unchanged. Carbon dioxide production may decrease significantly with increasing depth of anesthesia, neuromuscular blockade, or decreasing body temperature.

Respiratory Center Stimulation

Respiratory center stimulation may be induced by higher level centers (i.e., cerebral cortex), by neural feedback mechanisms that affect it directly, or by blood-borne chemical or pharmacologic effectors. Many factors act simultaneously in some clinical situations; others are counteracted by respiratory center depressants. Therefore, the ventilatory status in a given clinical setting may vary.

Anxiety

Anxiety-related primary hyperventilation syndrome is a common cause of emergency room admission. Although this condition usually is characterized by the absence of any signs of illness other than those related to the anxiety and alveolar hyperventilation, the associated chest discomfort, dyspnea, and ST segment changes in the electrocardiogram sometimes produce differential diagnostic problems. Alveolar hyperventilation also is a common response to stimuli that cause physical pain and discomfort.

Central Nervous System Factors

CNS lesions such as tumors, infections, hemorrhage, or loss of blood supply in the brainstem region may produce alveolar hyperventilation by direct mechanical or chemical stimulation.

Central Hyperventilation

Central hyperventilation may take the form of a stable increase in ventilatory rate and V_T, or it may present as a periodic fluctuation in the rate and depth of ventilation (Cheyne-Stokes respiration). The former is more likely to result from localized disease, whereas the latter is usually caused by diffuse CNS lesions.

Periodic hyperventilation also may accompany conditions in which the circulation time is prolonged sufficiently to prevent efficient control of blood CO_2 tension.[34]

Hypoxemia

The most important respiratory center chemical stimulants are hypoxemia and acidosis. When the Pa_{O_2} falls below 55 to 60 mm Hg for any reason, minute ventilation begins to increase until a maximum stimulating effect is reached at a Pa_{O_2} of approximately 40 mm Hg.[35] The stimulating effect of hypoxemia overrides the normal controlling effects of pH and Pa_{CO_2} and results in respiratory alkalosis.

Plasma Bicarbonate

A $1\text{-mEq} \cdot L^{-1}$ fall in plasma bicarbonate concentration—that is, a metabolic acidosis—produces a compensatory 1- to 1.4-mm Hg decrease in Pa_{CO_2}. The last two digits of blood pH provide a rough estimate of the expected Pa_{CO_2}.[36] Ventilatory changes in response to acidosis occur relatively slowly (over 12–24 hours). The reversal of this compensation occurs equally slowly, which explains the respiratory alkalosis seen following rapid correction of metabolic acidosis.

Fever

Fever produces alveolar hyperventilation by directly stimulating the respiratory center neurons through neural connections from the hypothalamus or by causing the release of neurotransmitters. Fever-induced hyperventilation may lead to chronic respiratory alkalosis if the fever persists for a long period of time.

Mechanoreceptors

Feedback from pulmonary mechanoreceptors frequently causes alveolar hyperventilation in the early stages of acute pulmonary diseases such as asthma, acute lung injury, pulmonary embolus, pulmonary edema, and pneumonia. Anxiety, hypoxemia, acidosis, pain, and fever provide further stimuli for such patients. As pulmonary gas exchange deteriorates and ventilatory work increases, the initial alveolar hyperventilation is replaced by ventilatory failure and respiratory acidemia.

Stimulation of baroreceptors by hypotension and circulating mediators, the nature of which is poorly defined, has been implicated in alveolar hyperventilation by critically ill patients with systemic infections.

Drugs

Alveolar hyperventilation can be induced pharmacologically by doxapram hydrochloride through peripheral chemoreceptor stimulation. The increase in minute ventilation results mainly from an augmentation of V_T, although an increase in ventilatory rate also is seen.

Epinephrine, norepinephrine, and theophylline cause alveolar hyperventilation but only when they are used in very large doses. Administration of more than 12 g of salicylate within a 24-hour period will produce respiratory alkalemia in the average adult.[37] The mechanism is unclear but probably is related, at least in part, to the anion gap acidosis that results from salicylate intoxication.

How Is Hyperventilation Corrected?

Mechanical overventilation is corrected by decreasing ventilator rate or V_T, or both. Spontaneous hyperventilation usually resolves when the underlying cause of the abnormality is corrected. If respiratory alkalemia is detrimental to a critically ill patient with spontaneous hyperventilation, correction can be accomplished by inducing deep sedation or neuromuscular blockade in conjunction with a gradual return to normal ventilation with mechanical ventilatory support.

The time-honored treatment for psychogenic hyperventilation is rebreathing of exhaled gas to increase the Pa_{CO_2}. This treatment is effective and safe in patients with true anxiety-related hyperventilation, but it is not effective and may be hazardous in patients who hyperventilate in response to other stimuli such as hypoxemia.

VENTILATORY WORK

What Are the Consequences?

Increased ventilatory work may lead to ventilatory failure and respiratory acidemia when the ventilatory muscles are no longer able to maintain adequate $\dot{V}_A$. However, even in the absence of overt failure, increased ventilatory work has considerable deleterious effects, particularly on cardiovascular function (Table 48–5).[38]

Increased Ventilatory Muscle Work

The increased muscle effort during respiratory distress not only requires an increase in CO (cardiac output) but also diverts blood flow to the ventilatory muscles at the expense of other organ tissues, including the myocardium.[38] Consequently, myocardial O_2 demand is increased in the face of reduced supply. The tachycardia and hypertension associated with the anxiety of suffocation and acidosis secondary to anaerobic muscle metabolism further load the circulation.[39, 40]

Pleural Pressure Fluctuations

Increased respiratory effort is always associated with ''negative'' (subambient) fluctuations of intrathoracic pressure that have additional direct effects on cardiac function.[41] The negative pressure surrounding the left ventricle raises transmyocar-

TABLE 48–5. Factors Contributing to Development of Left Ventricular Dysfunction During Increased Ventilatory Work

Anxiety
　　Hypertension
　　Tachycardia
　　Myocardial ischemia
Negative intrathoracic pressure
　　Increased muscle work
　　Increased cardiac output requirement
　　Redistribution of blood flow
　　Left ventricular distention
　　Increased left ventricular afterload
　　Myocardial ischemia
Respiratory muscle fatigue
　　Lactic acidosis
　　Hyperkalemia
　　Arrhythmias
　　Myocardial ischemia
Ventilatory fatigue
　　Respiratory acidosis
　　Hypoxemia
　　Hyperkalemia
　　Arrhythmias
　　Myocardial ischemia

dial pressure, increases the ventricle's size, and effects a reduction in wall thickness (Fig. 48–5). These changes are related according to the law of Laplace:

$$Ptm = \frac{2h\ W}{r}$$

Equation 6

where Ptm is transmural chamber pressure, W is wall stress, r is chamber radius, and h is wall thickness. Rearrangement of these terms results in the following expression:

$$W = Ptm \times \frac{r}{2h}$$

A patient with normal left ventricular function can tolerate the increase in afterload because the function of a normal heart is primarily dependent on preload. However, myocardial ischemia, left ventricular failure, and cardiogenic pulmonary edema may be induced by negative intrathoracic pressure secondary to increased ventilatory work in a patient with pre-existing left ventricular dysfunction.[42, 43] Further impairment in lung mechanics and gas exchange from pulmonary vascular congestion may trigger a vicious cycle of cardiopulmonary failure and quickly lead to the patient's demise unless ventilatory work is reduced effectively and promptly.

TABLE 48–6. Sources of Increased Ventilatory Work

Breathing circuit–related work
　　Demand valve resistance
　　Circuit resistance
　　Tracheal tube size and length
　　Resistance of the exhalation valve and PEEP valve
　　Type of positive airway pressure therapy
　　Maximum inspiratory flow
Airway obstruction
Lung compliance
Chest wall compliance
Volume of functional dead space
Carbon dioxide production

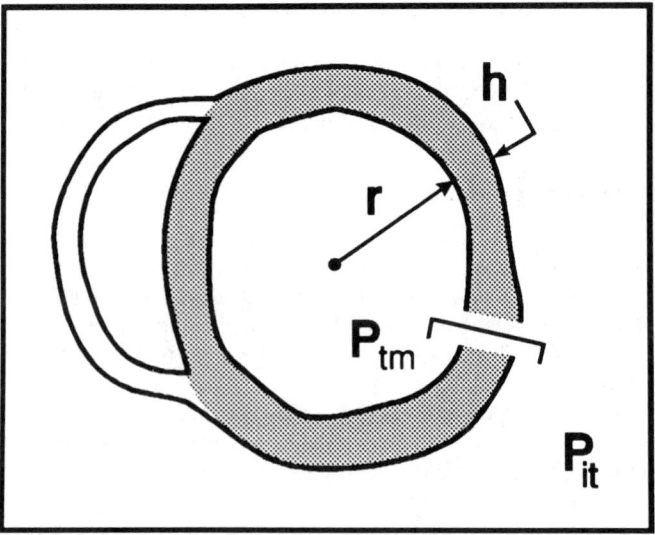

FIGURE 48–5. A schematic cross-section of the left ventricle *(shaded)*. A decrease in intrathoracic pressure (Pit) increases the transmural chamber pressure (Ptm) and the chamber radius and decreases wall thickness (h). These three factors change in a direction that will increase wall stress (W) according to the Laplace's law: W = Ptm·r/2h. An elevation in wall stress (afterload) will increase myocardial oxygen consumption and may produce ischemia and wall motion abnormalities in a susceptible patient.

Why Does Ventilatory Work Occur?

Common causes of increased ventilatory work are listed in Table 48–6. Work imposed by the breathing circuit is in addition to that required to effect pulmonary ventilation in the absence of the circuit. The most important characteristics in terms of added work of breathing are the mechanisms by which inspiratory gas flow is made available; the flow resistance of the circuit; the tracheal tube; and the exhalation valve. When PEEP is used during spontaneous breathing, two additional factors must be taken into account: the flow-resistance of the PEEP valve and the stability of airway pressure during the respiratory cycle (Fig. 48–6).

Generation of Inspiratory Flow

Inspiratory flow and volume can be made available from a continuous, free flow of gas or by the patient's triggering of the opening of a demand valve in the inspiratory limb.

Continuous Gas Flow

Continuous flow circuits usually incorporate a reservoir to collect gas during exhalation for the subsequent inspiratory phase. This arrangement allows the fresh gas flow to be reduced considerably and to be immediately available at all times.

Demand Valves

In a demand valve circuit, no gas is available to the patient unless inspiratory effort activates the flow. The signal to open the demand valve is usually the initial fall in airway pressure at the beginning of inspiration.

These circuits supply gas with minimal inspiratory effort as long as the fresh gas flow and the reservoir volume are sufficient to meet the patient's demand. However, if the VT and

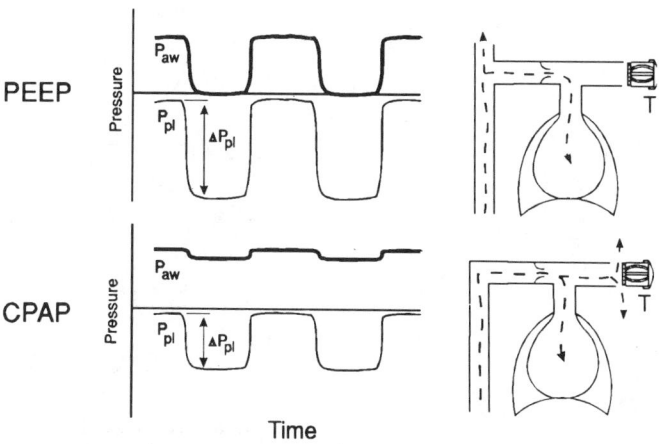

FIGURE 48–6. Changes in airway (Paw) and pleural (Ppl) pressure during spontaneous breathing with PEEP and CPAP circuits. Positive circuit pressure is created by the threshold resistor valve (T) only when gas flows through it. The necessity of bringing airway pressure to ambient status before start of lung inflation during breathing with PEEP as compared to CPAP increases the required change in intrathoracic pressure (DPpl) and ventilatory work.

inspiratory flow rate exceed the capacity of the breathing circuit, gas flow stops. The patient continues the inspiratory effort against what amounts to a closed airway.

Breathing with a demand valve circuit requires additional effort, the magnitude of which depends on the time required to initiate flow from the ventilator, the trigger sensitivity, and the valve design. The maximum inspiratory flow and volume available after the valve opens are also important determinants of inspiratory work. Considerable differences reflect the functional characteristics of commercially available circuits.[44] Some have been shown to impose a significantly larger inspiratory load on the spontaneously breathing patient than do continuous-flow circuits.[45, 46]

Circuit Flow Resistance

Components of the anesthesia circuit, tubing, elbow connectors, valves, and humidifiers may offer significant flow resistance. Such resistance must be overcome by the patient during spontaneous breathing and by the ventilator during mechanical ventilation.

When turbulent gas flow occurs, flow resistance is directly proportional to the flow rate. Therefore, a rapid ventilatory frequency and high flow rate increase the resistive effect of a given circuit configuration. Although the resistance of a single component may not appear significant, the additive effect of the different components arranged in series may contribute to ventilatory fatigue and failure.

The Tracheal Tube

The size and length of the tracheal tube have a significant effect on the resistance of the breathing circuit. Depending on gas flow, each 1-mm decrease in an adult-size tracheal tube diameter increases ventilatory work by 34% to 154%, depending on the ventilatory flow rate.[47]

Fiastro and coworkers[48] reported that the mechanically generated inspiratory pressure required to overcome resistance from the ventilator circuit and tracheal tube was 6 cm H_2O for a 9-mm diameter tube and 15 cm H_2O for a 7-mm diameter tube at a gas flow rate of 40 L · min^{-1}. Tube resistance also

increases with length, which is usually alterable and therefore should be minimized.

Christie and Leon[49] reported that spontaneous breathing through an endotracheal tube and standard circle system without positive airway pressure during inhalational anesthesia was associated with a twofold increase in the work of breathing. A demand-flow circuit was associated with a work of 690 mJ · L^{-1} which decreased to 170 mJ · L^{-1} following the application of 5 cm H_2O inspiratory pressure support.

This amount of work represents only 0.5% to 1% of the resting total body energy expenditure; therefore, the changes are not significant for a healthy individual. However, minimizing the extrinsic, equipment-related work may be of considerable importance in patients with pulmonary insufficiency, for whom intrinsic ventilatory work already represents significant energy expenditure.

The Exhalation Valve

The flow resistance of the exhalation valve can increase inspiratory and expiratory ventilatory work.[50, 51] Resistance to exhalation is overcome first by increasing VT so that more elastic energy is available for subsequent exhalation. As the load increases further, expiratory muscles are recruited to contract actively during exhalation.[52]

Spontaneous Breathing with Positive Pressure

When positive airway pressure is applied with a continuous flow system, the pressure/flow characteristics of the valve that generates the positive circuit pressure become important (see Fig. 48–6).[53] During exhalation, the valve must accommodate a patient's expiratory flow and the continuous flow; an increase in pressure above the baseline occurs when a flow-resistor valve is used.

If the valve has significant flow resistance, a reduction in flow through the valve as it is diverted into the patient's lungs leads to a fall in circuit pressure (Fig. 48–7). This drop in pressure must be generated by the patient and, therefore, requires increased respiratory effort.[54]

Conversely, a threshold resistor valve does not depend on flow to generate pressure. Therefore, airway pressure does not

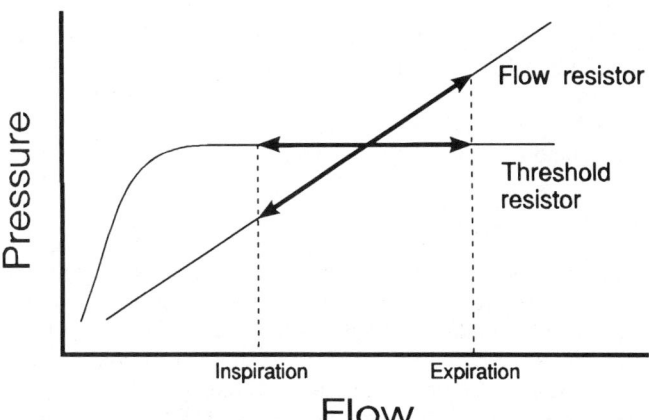

FIGURE 48–7. The mechanism by which inspiratory work is increased by the resistance of the positive-pressure valve during continuous-flow CPAP therapy. Fluctuation in flow through a flow resistor PEEP valve causes fluctuations in airway pressure that increase ventilatory effort. A threshold resistor PEEP valve does not increase effort because it can accommodate variation in flow without a change in circuit pressure.

fluctuate significantly during the respiratory cycle, and the valve-induced work of breathing is reduced.

Positive End-Expiratory Pressure. The technique used to apply PEEP also has implications for ventilatory work during spontaneous breathing.[55] PEEP can be applied to a spontaneously breathing patient by attaching a PEEP valve to the expiratory limb of a nonrebreathing circuit (i.e., a resuscitator bag equipped with a nonrebreathing valve). This valve pressurizes the airway and the expiratory limb as long as expiratory flow is present.

At the beginning of the next inspiration, the airway pressure must fall by an amount equivalent to the applied PEEP before gas flows into the lungs. A tidal breath requires an even greater reduction of intrathoracic pressure, the amount of which is dependent on the V_T, respiratory system compliance, and airway resistance.

The fall in intrathoracic pressure necessary to bring the airway pressure down from the PEEP level to ambient represents additional energy expenditure and increases the magnitude of negative intrathoracic pressure fluctuations (see Fig. 48–6). Both of these effects are detrimental, particularly to patients with compromised left ventricular function.

Continuous Positive Airway Pressure. If the entire circuit is pressurized to the prescribed level throughout the respiratory cycle, CPAP results. The early inspiratory drop in airway and intrathoracic pressure is avoided, and ventilatory work decreases (see Fig. 48–6). Therefore, when positive airway pressure is indicated for a spontaneously breathing patient and work of breathing is a concern, CPAP should be used. If only a PEEP circuit is available—for example, during transport of a patient supported with a PEEP-equipped resuscitator bag—controlled ventilation should be applied or the PEEP valve should be removed, whichever is less detrimental to the patient's overall cardiopulmonary function.

What Are the Effects of Airway Obstruction?

Airway obstruction increases ventilatory work in a variety of conditions characterized by pathologic airway reactivity, altered structure of the air passages, or reduced lung volume. Localized airway obstruction may occur at any level secondary to external compression by tumors and hematomas or to intraluminal narrowing from scarring, edema, secretions, and foreign bodies. Reduction in airway caliber imposes an abnormal load to ventilation during inspiration, expiration, or throughout the entire respiratory cycle, depending on the degree, localization, and dynamic characteristics of the obstruction.

Fixed Obstructions

A fixed resistance in the airway does not change in diameter or length regardless of changes in the distending pressure. Therefore, a similar resistance to flow occurs during inspiration and expiration, and its effects do not depend on whether the resistance is intrathoracic or extrathoracic. The pressure differential required to drive flow through the obstruction is directly and linearly related to the flow rate.

Tracheal or bronchial stenosis secondary to fibrosis or tumor infiltration and mediastinal masses represent typical fixed airway obstructions. Increased work of ventilation, auscultatory evidence of obstruction, and flow limitation proportional to the

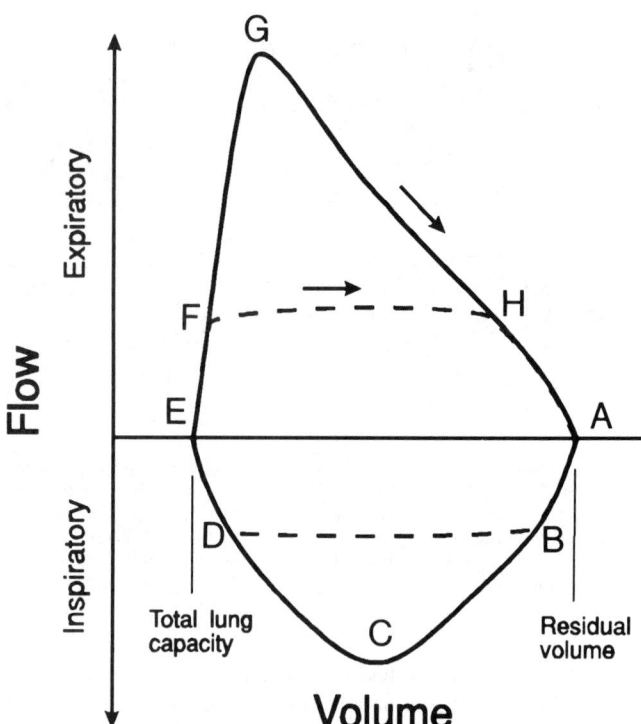

FIGURE 48–8. Maximum flow-volume curve under normal conditions (*continuous line*, ACEGA) and during fixed airway obstruction (*broken line*, ABDEFHA). With variable intrathoracic airway obstruction, the curve follows the *broken line* during expiration while inspiratory flow-volume characteristics may be nearly normal (ACEFHA). During variable extrathoracic airway obstruction, inspiratory flow is limited while expiratory flow may be unobstructed (ABDEGA).

degree of obstruction are noted during inspiration and expiration (Fig. 48–8).

Variable Obstructions

A variable airway obstruction allows the distending pressure of the airway to modify flow resistance.

Intrathoracic

Intrathoracic variable airway obstruction, which is seen for example in a patient with bronchial asthma or bronchomalacia, is alleviated during inspiration; the negative intrathoracic pressure increases the distending pressure and the diameter of the obstructed segment. This effect opposes the decrease in intraluminal pressure effected by gas flow through the narrow airway segment, which promotes airway collapse (the Bernoulli effect).

During exhalation, the flow-related decrease in intraluminal pressure is not opposed by intrathoracic pressure, and the obstruction worsens. In fact, forced positive intrathoracic pressure may contribute to increased obstruction, even though the intraluminal pressure distal (upstream) to the obstruction may be positive.

Extrathoracic

Extrathoracic variable airway obstruction, which is seen, for example, with laryngomalacia, is not affected by changes of intrathoracic pressure. Therefore, the inspiratory fall in intraluminal pressure worsens the obstruction. During expiration, positive intraluminal pressure distal (upstream) to the obstruction promotes gas flow, making expiration less obstructed than inspiration.

The differences in gas flow limitation between respiratory phases, depending on the location of the obstruction, are evident in flow/volume loop studies (see Fig. 48–8) and during clinical examination. Regardless of the type of airway obstruction, a functioning respiratory center "attempts" to make an adjustment toward a slow ventilatory rate with an increase in V_T to minimize the work of breathing. Since low flow allows gas to pass through the obstruction with a smaller pressure differential (less turbulence), the phase in which the obstruction is worse is prolonged.

What Are the Effects of Decreased Respiratory System Compliance?

The remarkably small effort required for normal breathing is largely a result of the high distensibility of the lung-thorax combination.

In a normal, upright adult, lung-compliance (C_L) is 200 mL $\cdot$ cm H_2O^{-1}, and chest wall compliance (C_{CW}) is 200 mL $\cdot$ cm H_2O^{-1}. Total respiratory system compliance (C_{RS}) is determined according to the following equation:

$$\frac{1}{C_{RS}} = \frac{1}{C_L} + \frac{1}{C_W} \qquad \text{Equation 9}$$

Solving for C_{RS},

$$\frac{1}{C_{RS}} = \frac{1}{200} + \frac{1}{200}$$

$$= \frac{1}{100}, \quad \text{and}$$

$$C_{RS} = 100 \text{ mL} \cdot \text{cm } H_2O^{-1}$$

However, in a normal, supine, anesthetized adult, the C_L is reduced to approximately 150 mL $\cdot$ cm H_2O^{-1} because of pressure from the abdominal viscera and cephalad displacement of the diaphragm. Chest wall compliance is unchanged. The result is a reduction of C_{RS} to 85 mL $\cdot$ cm H_2O^{-1}. A V_T of 500 mL can be achieved by applying 8 cm H_2O positive-pressure to the airway or by decreasing intrathoracic pressure by an additional 6 cm H_2O beyond the -2 cm H_2O baseline level (Fig. 48–9).[56]

Any process that reduces lung compliance necessitates a larger change in intrathoracic pressure during spontaneous breathing or a higher positive airway pressure during mechanical ventilation. Increased ventilatory work results. If chest wall compliance is reduced, the transpulmonary pressure change during tidal breathing is not increased, but more muscle work is required to generate a given change in intrathoracic pressure.

Causes of Reduced Lung Compliance

Lung compliance is reduced by factors that effect a decrease in the volume or distensibility of inflated lung tissue, or both.

Most acute parenchymal lung diseases are associated with decreased lung compliance and increased ventilatory work.

Regardless of whether the acute lung injury is caused by infection, by damage to the alveolocapillary membranes, or by hydrostatic vascular congestion and edema, a mixture of inflated, recruitable, and nonrecruitable lung parenchyma is present. The distensibility of the lungs and the impact of the injury on ventilatory work at different lung volumes depend on the relative magnitude of these components and on the mechanical characteristics of gas-containing areas of the lung.[57, 58]

Causes of Reduced Chest Wall Compliance

Chest wall compliance is reduced by the prone position, obesity, abdominal distention, chest deformities, and chronic disease states that alter the structure and configuration of the thoracic cage.

A. INTERMITTENT POSITIVE PRESSURE VENTILATION

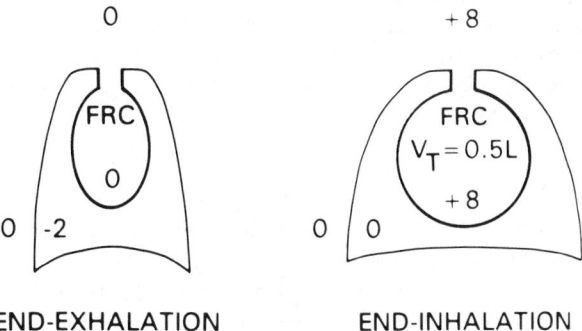

END-EXHALATION   END-INHALATION

B. SPONTANEOUS VENTILATION

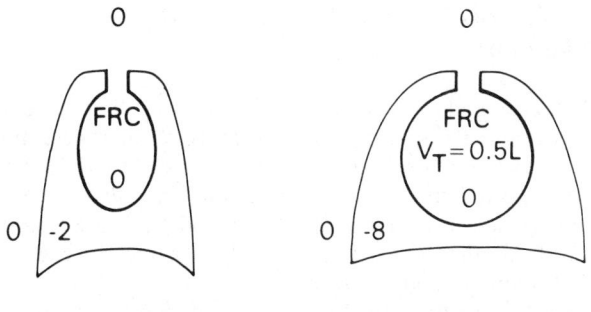

END-EXHALATION   END-INHALATION

FIGURE 48–9. Changes in airway and intrathoracic pressure in a supine, anesthetized adult whose C_{RS} is 85 mL $\cdot$ cm^{-1} H_2O. The initial end-exhalation transpulmonary pressure (airway pressure minus intrathoracic pressure) is $0-(-2 \text{ cm } H_2O) = 2 \text{ cm } H_2O$. With a positive-pressure inflation, airway pressure increases to 8 cm H_2O and intrathoracic pressure increases to 0. The transthoracic pressure is now 8 cm $H_2O-0 = 8$ cm H_2O at end-inhalation. The *change* in transpulmonary pressure (end-inhalation minus end-exhalation) is 8 cm H_2O-2 cm $H_2O = 6$ cm H_2O. Tidal volume is:
V_T = transpulmonary pressure $\times$ C_{RS}
    = 6 cm $H_2O \times 85$ mL $\cdot$ cm^{-1} H_2O
    = 510 mL
    = 0.5 L
With a spontaneous breath, the change in transpulmonary pressure is also $[0-(-8)]-[0-(-2)] = 6$ cm H_2O, the same value as that achieved with IPPV. An identical V_T of approximately 0.5 L results.

Morbid Obesity

Ventilatory function in morbidly obese patients is often markedly sensitive to position. Such patients may only be able to breathe spontaneously in the upright or semi-sitting position because abdominal pressure in the supine position limits diaphragmatic descent.

Hyperinflation. Hyperinflation of the lungs leads to reduced respiratory system compliance when the lung-thorax combination approaches the limits of its expansion. This factor is significant in patients with chronic lung disease and asthma.

What Are the Effects of Increased Dead Space?

Increase in physiologic dead space (i.e., the ventilated but not perfused parts of the respiratory system) requires augmentation of minute ventilation and increased ventilatory work for effective $\dot{V}_A$. An increase in minute ventilation to compensate for moderate increases in dead space can easily be accomplished if the respiratory mechanics and ventilatory muscle reserves are normal. However, in patients with compromised cardiopulmonary function, such compensation may not be possible, and ventilatory failure may ensue.

Causes

Common causes of increased physiologic dead space include reduced pulmonary perfusion due to a pulmonary embolus, hypovolemia or low cardiac output, hyperinflation of the lungs with mechanical ventilation or excessive PEEP, and disruption of the pulmonary architecture in emphysematous lungs. Breathing circuits may add considerable dead space and impose an unnecessary ventilatory burden during weaning from mechanical ventilatory support.

What Factors Increase Carbon Dioxide Production?

Carbon dioxide production is influenced by the metabolic rate and by the nature of metabolic processes that determine CO_2 production ($\dot{V}CO_2$) and $\dot{V}O_2$. Maintenance of CO_2 and pH homeostasis requires matching changes in $\dot{V}_A$ with $\dot{V}CO_2$. Factors associated with increased $\dot{V}CO_2$ include fever, decreasing depth of anesthesia, rapid administration of bicarbonate-containing solutions, and overfeeding.

Since ventilation normally requires little work, fluctuations in metabolic rate generally are well tolerated. However, in patients with borderline ventilatory function, a nutrition-related increase in $\dot{V}CO_2$ and rapid correction of metabolic acidosis with sodium bicarbonate may lead to acute ventilatory failure.

"ABNORMAL" VENTILATORY THERAPY

When Is It Indicated?

Control of Intracranial Pressure

The physiologic effects of alveolar hyperventilation can be used for therapeutic purposes in specific clinical circumstances. The most common example is to control ICP. Since hyperventilation is the most rapid method available to consistently reduce ICP, it can be used as first-line therapy without monitoring when life-threatening intracranial hypertension is suspected. However, such monitoring should be instituted as soon as possible to allow accurate titration of this and other forms of therapy.

Acceptable Limits

When continued control of ICP is attempted, the minimum level of hyperventilation that produces the desired effect should be used. This strategy allows further lowering of $PaCO_2$ to counteract tachyphylaxis and to control sudden further elevations in ICP with minimum side-effects.

The effect of respiratory alkalosis on ICP probably is mediated both by changes in pH and by a direct effect of hypocapnia. The primary mechanism is cerebral arterial vasoconstriction, which decreases cerebral blood flow. Such therapy may prevent herniation and other pressure-related detrimental sequelae inside the cranium, but it does not necessarily improve brain tissue oxygenation, even when it results in an increase in the calculated cerebral perfusion pressure.

To prevent cerebral ischemia, the $PaCO_2$ should not be reduced below 20 mm Hg. If ICP monitoring is not available, the $PaCO_2$ should be maintained between 25 and 30 mm Hg and verified by arterial blood gas analysis. Equilibration of pH between blood and cerebrospinal fluid causes an attenuation of hypocapnic cerebral vasoconstriction within 24 to 72 hours. Subsequent return to normal ventilation then has a vasodilating effect. Therefore, hyperventilation should be discontinued gradually to avoid a sudden rise in ICP.

Reduction of Pulmonary Vascular Resistance

The pulmonary vasculature also is sensitive to changes in blood pH and $PaCO_2$. Increases of blood pH up to 7.50 are frequently helpful in infants with pulmonary hypertension; resistance to pulmonary blood flow is decreased without systemic hypotension.[59]

Considerable sensitivity to alveolar hypoventilation has been demonstrated in the adult pulmonary circulation after open heart operations requiring cardiopulmonary bypass.[8] Even though these data suggest the importance of avoiding hypoventilation in such patients, deliberate hyperventilation with respiratory alkalemia has not been consistently successful in reducing the pulmonary vascular resistance.

Hyperventilatory Compensation for Metabolic Acidosis

The hazards of treating metabolic acidosis with sodium bicarbonate emphasize the importance of maintaining adequate oxygenation and slight to moderate hyperventilation.[60] Carbon dioxide diffuses readily in and out of cells; thus, changes in $PaCO_2$ rapidly translate into similar directional changes in intracellular CO_2 tension and pH. The hyperventilatory response to metabolic acidosis is, therefore, a key element in compensating for metabolic acidosis inside the cell.

Sodium Bicarbonate

If blood pH is corrected rapidly with sodium bicarbonate administration and if compensatory hyperventilation decreases simultaneously, the resultant increase of intracellular P_{CO_2} may lower intracellular pH significantly. Worsening intracellular acidosis has detrimental effects, particularly in the CNS and the myocardium. These considerations favor slow correction of metabolic acidosis, preferably by eliminating its cause; partial compensation for acidosis with hyperventilation; and avoidance of aggressive sodium bicarbonate therapy unless the acidosis is severe (pH <7.10) or other reasons (e.g., hyperkalemia) require rapid correction.

References

1. Annat G, Viale J.-P: Measuring the breathing workload in mechanically ventilated patients. Intensive Care Med 1990; 16:418.
2. Banner MJ, Kirby RR, Blanch PB, et al: Decreasing imposed work of the breathing apparatus to zero using pressure support ventilation. Crit Care Med 1993; 21:1333.
3. Räsänen J, Cane RD: Continuous oximetry: is it beneficial? Commentary. Perspect Crit Care 1991; 4:133.
4. McIlroy MB, Eldridge FL, Thomas JP, et al: The effect of added elastic and non-elastic resistances on the pattern of breathing in normal subjects. Clin Sci 1956; 15:337.
5. Nunn JF: The effects of changes in the carbon dioxide tension. In Applied Respiratory Physiology. 3rd ed. Nunn JF (ed). London, Butterworths, 1987, pp 460–470.
6. Black GW, Linde HW, Dripps RD, et al: Circulatory changes accompanying respiratory acidosis during halothane anesthesia in man. Br J Anaesth 1959; 31:238.
7. Molony DA, Jacobson HR: Respiratory acid-base disorders. In Fluids and Electrolytes. Kokko JP, Tannen RL (eds). Philadelphia, W.B. Saunders, 1986, pp 305–381.
8. Salmenperä M, Heinonen J: Pulmonary vascular responses to moderate changes in Pa_{CO_2} after cardiopulmonary bypass. Anesthesiology 1986; 64:311.
9. Linko K, Paloheimo M, Tammisto T: Capnography for detection of accidental oesophageal intubation. Acta Anesthesiol Scand 1983; 69:199.
10. Sum-Ping ST, Mehta MP, Anderton JM: A comparative study of methods of detection of esophageal intubation. Anesth Analg 1989; 27:627.
11. Curtis JJ, Nawarawong W, Walls JT, et al: Elevated hemidiaphragm after cardiac operations: incidence, prognosis, and relationship to the use of topical ice slush. Ann Thorac Surg 1989; 48:764.
12. Cronnelly R: Muscle relaxant antagonists. In Muscle relaxants: basic and clinical aspects. Katz RL (ed). Orlando, Grune & Stratton, 1985, pp 197–213.
13. Roussos C, Macklem PT: The respiratory muscles. N Engl J Med 1982; 307:786.
14. Aubier M, Murciano D, Lecocguic Y, et al: Effect of hypophosphatemia on diaphragmatic contractility in patients with acute respiratory failure. N Engl J Med 1985; 313:420.
15. Roussos C: Respiratory muscle fatigue and ventilatory failure. Chest 1990; 97:89S.
16. Aubier M, Trippenbach T, Roussos C: Respiratory muscle fatigue during cardiogenic shock. J Appl Physiol; Respir Environ Exerc Physiol 1981; 51:499.
17. Aubier M, Farkas G, De Troyer A, et al: Detection of diaphragmatic fatigue in man by phrenic nerve stimulation. J Appl Physiol 1981; 50:538.
18. Bellemare F, Bigland-Ritchie B: Central components of diaphragmatic fatigue assessed from bilateral phrenic nerve stimulation. J Appl Physiol 1987; 62:1307.
19. Räsänen J, Heikkilä J, Downs JB, et al: Continuous positive airway pressure by face mask in the treatment of cardiogenic pulmonary edema. Am J Cardiol 1985; 55:296.
20. Branson RD, Hurst JM, DeHaven CB: Mask-CPAP: state of the art. Respir Care 1985; 30,846.
21. Kirby RR, Downs JB, Civetta JM, et al: High level positive end-expiratory pressure (PEEP) in acute respiratory insufficiency. Chest 1975; 67:156.
22. Katz JA, Marks JD: Inspiratory work with and without continuous positive airway pressure in patients with acute respiratory failure. Anesthesiology 1985; 63:598.
23. Perel A, Williamson DC, Modell JH: Effectiveness of CPAP by mask for pulmonary edema associated with hypercarbia. Intensive Care Med 1983; 9:17.
24. Bersten AD, Holt AW, Vedig AE, et al: Treatment of severe pulmonary

25. Räsänen J, Väisänen I, Heikkilä J, et al: Acute myocardial infarction complicated by left ventricular dysfunction and respiratory failure: the effects of continuous positive airway pressure. Chest 1985; 87:158.
26. Väisänen I, Räsänen J: The cardiopulmonary effects of continuous positive airway pressure and supplemental oxygen in patients with acute cardiogenic pulmonary edema. Chest 1987; 92:481.
27. Kirby RR, Banner MJ, Downs JB (eds): Clinical Applications of Ventilatory Support. New York, Churchill Livingstone, 1990.
28. Gattinoni L, Pesenti A, Bombino M, et al: Extracorporeal carbon dioxide removal. In 91–113.
29. Dalton HJ, Thompson AE: Extracorporeal membrane oxygenation. In Mechanical Ventilation and Assisted Respiration. Contemporary Management in Critical Care, 1(1). Grenvik A, Downs JB, Räsänen J, et al (eds). New York, Churchill Livingstone, 1990, pp 115–137.
30. Edmondson JW, Brashear RE, Li TK: Tetany: quantitative interrelationships between calcium and alkalosis. Am J Physiol 1975; 228:1082.
31. Coetzee A, Holland D, Foëx P, et al: The effect of hypocapnia on coronary blood flow and myocardial function in the dog. Anesth Analg 1984; 63:991.
32. Rasmussen K, Bagger JP, Bottzauw J, et al: Prevalence of vasospastic ischaemia induced by the cold pressor test or hyperventilation in patients with severe angina. Eur Heart J 1984; 5: 354.
33. Downs JB, Douglas ME, Ruiz BC, et al: Comparison of assisted and controlled mechanical ventilation in anesthetized swine. Crit Care Med 1979; 7:5.
34. Brown HW, Plum F: The neurologic basis of Cheyne-Stokes respiration. Am J Med 1961; 30:849.
35. Hey EN, Loyd BB, Cunningham DJC, et al: Effects of various respiratory stimuli on the depth and frequency of breathing in man. Respir Physiol 1966; 1:193.
36. Narins RG, Emmett M: Simple and mixed acid-base disorders: a practical approach. Medicine 1980; 59:161.
37. Farber HR, Yiengst MJ, Shock NW: The effect of therapeutic doses of aspirin on the acid-base balance of the blood in normal adults. Am J Med Sci 1949; 217:256.
38. Lemaire F, Teboul J-L, Cinotti L, et al: Acute left ventricular dysfunction during unsuccessful weaning from mechanical ventilation. Anesthesiology 1988; 69:171.
39. Viires N, Sillye G, Rassidakis A, et al: Effect of mechanical ventilation on respiratory muscle blood flow during shock. Physiologist 1980; 23:1.
40. Mason DT, Spann JF Jr, Zelis R, et al: Alterations of hemodynamics and myocardial mechanics in patients with congestive heart failure: pathophysiologic mechanism and assessment of cardiac function and ventricular contractility. Prog Cardiovasc Dis 1970; 12:507.
41. Pinsky MR, Matuschak GM, Klain M: Determinants of cardiac augmentation by elevations in intrathoracic pressure. J Appl Physiol 1985; 58:1189.
42. Scharf SM, Bianco JA, Tow DE, Brown R: The effects of large negative intrathoracic pressure on left ventricular function in patients with coronary artery disease. Circulation 1981; 63:871–875.
43. Weber KT, Janicki JS, Hunter WC, et al: The contractile behavior of the heart and its functional coupling to the circulation. Prog Cardiovasc Dis 1982; 24:375.
44. Katz JA, Marks JD: Inspiratory work with and without continuous positive airway pressure in patients with acute respiratory failure. Anesthesiology 1985; 63:598.
45. Beydon L, Chasse M, Harf A, et al: Inspiratory work of breathing during spontaneous ventilation using demand valves and continuous flow systems. Am Rev Respir Dis 1988; 138:300.
46. Christopher KL, Neff TA, Bowman JL, et al: Demand and continuous flow intermittent mandatory ventilation systems. Chest 1985; 87:625.
47. Bolder PM, Hedy TEJ, Bolder AR, et al: The extra work of breathing through adult endotracheal tubes. Anesth Analg 1986; 65:853.
48. Fiastro JF, Habib MP, Quan SF: Pressure support compensation for inspiratory work due to endotracheal tubes and demand continuous positive airway pressure. Chest 1988; 93:499.
49. Christie JM, Smith RA: Pressure support ventilation decreases inspiratory work of breathing during general anesthesia and spontaneous ventilation. Anesth Analg 1992; 75:167.
50. Banner MJ, Downs JB, Kirby RR, et al: Effects of expiratory flow resistance on inspiratory work of breathing. Chest 1988; 93:795.
51. Marini JJ, Culver BH, Kirk W: Flow resistance of exhalation valves and positive end-expiratory pressure devices used in mechanical ventilation. Am Rev Respir Dis 1985; 131:850.

52. Abbrecht PH, Rajagopal KR, Kyle RR: Expiratory muscle recruitment during inspiratory flow-resistive loading and exercise. Am Rev Respir Dis 1991; 144:113.

53. Pinsky MR, Hrehocik D, Culpepper JA, et al: Flow resistance of expiratory positive-pressure systems. Chest 1988; 94:788.

54. Mecklenburgh JS, Latto IP, Al-Obaidi TAA, et al: Excessive work of breathing during intermittent mandatory ventilation. Br J Anaesth 1986; 58:1048.

55. Downs JB, Mitchell LA: Pulmonary effects of ventilatory pattern following cardiopulmonary bypass. Crit Care Med 1976; 4:295.

56. Nunn JF: Elastic forces and lung volumes. *In* Applied Respiratory Physiology. 3rd ed. Nunn JF (ed). London, Butterworths, 1987, pp 23–45.

57. Gattinoni L, Pesenti A, Torresin A, et al: Adult respiratory distress syndrome profiles by computed tomography. J Thorac Imaging 1986; 1:25.

58. Gattinoni L, Pesenti A, Bombino M, et al: Relationships between lung computed tomographic density, gas exchange, and PEEP in acute respiratory failure. Anesthesiology 1988; 69:824.

59. Drummond WH, Gregory GA, Heymann MA, et al: The independent effects of hyperventilation, tolazoline and dopamine on infants with persistent pulmonary hypertension. J Pediatr 1981; 93:603.

60. Grekin RJ: Ketoacidosis, hyperosmolar states and lactic acidosis. *In* Fluids and Electrolytes. Kokko JP, Tannen RL (eds). Philadelphia, W.B. Saunders, 1986, pp 688–711.

CHAPTER 49

Temperature Fluctuations

RICHARD B. LILLY, Jr., M.D.

Assuming the care of both healthy and critically ill patients requires basic knowledge and an understanding of human physiology. As such, routine temperature monitoring to detect hypothermia and hyperthermia during anesthesia administration can assist in formulating a more streamlined differential diagnosis of problems that may arise.

THERMOREGULATORY RESPONSES IN ANESTHETIZED PATIENTS

Classic teaching suggests that anesthetized patients become poikilothermic—that is, their body temperature passively approaches ambient temperature. Thus, in a cool operating room (OR) environment, hypothermia is to be expected. In the past few years, however Daniel Sessler and his associates have published a series of reports[1-8] that greatly improve our understanding of thermoregulation under anesthesia.

In awake humans, body temperature is maintained within a narrow range of 37 °C ± 0.4 °C. When temperature rises above that range, the body responds by vasodilation and sweating. When temperature falls, the normal response is vasoconstriction, shivering, and, in babies, nonshivering thermogenesis.

During anesthesia, initial cooling is not accompanied by any thermoregulatory response (Fig. 49–1). However, when the temperature reaches 34.5 °C, significant peripheral vasoconstriction occurs and the temperature decline decreases. This observation led to the description of an expanded "interthreshold" range under anesthesia. The 0.8 °C range in awake humans expands more than fivefold, from 34.5 °C to 39 °C (see Fig. 49–1). Within that range, an anesthetized patient is indeed poikilothermic. However, once the range is exceeded, normal thermoregulatory responses *do* occur in anesthetized patients.

In fully anesthetized adults, shivering is unlikely, especially when muscle relaxants are used; nonshivering thermogenesis is confined to neonates. Therefore, vasoconstriction is the only response to hypothermia. Once temperature falls below 34.5 °C, vasoconstriction decreases cutaneous heat loss by 25%.[9] Sweating and vasodilatation occur in response to hyperthermia just as in awake patients, but they do not occur until hypothalamic temperature approaches 39 °C.[10]

How Does Hypothermia Develop?

Three predictable phases occur in the development of hypothermia under anesthesia.[9] (Table 49–1).

Phase I

Phase I is a rapid linear temperature decrease of 1.5 °C during the first hour of anesthesia. The greatest heat loss occurs during this period. Heat production decreases because of decreased muscle tone and metabolism. Heat loss increases because of vasodilation. Most of a patient's clothing is removed in a cold, drafty room, and wet preparation solution is poured over the body surface.

Interestingly, measurements of the heat lost during the first hour show that heat loss alone is not enough to explain the decrease of core temperature. In fact, much of this temperature decline is caused by redistribution of core heat to the periphery.[11] Phase I temperature decline is hard to prevent because of this redistribution phenomenon. The best way to control temperature loss is to warm the periphery actively, thereby decreasing the core to periphery heat gradient.

Phase II

Phase II is a steady decline of 0.5 °C per hour for 3 to 4 hours until temperature approaches 34.5 °C. This is the period of poikilothermia, in which body temperature passively drifts toward ambient temperature.

Phase III

Phase III occurs when the lower limit of the interthreshold range (i.e., 34.5 °C) is reached and active thermoregulation (vasoconstriction) resumes. At this point, temperature decline diminishes, and temperature may even begin to increase.

How Is Temperature Regulated During Spinal or Epidural Anesthesia?

The thermoregulatory set-point is located in the hypothalamus and should not be affected by spinal or epidural anes-

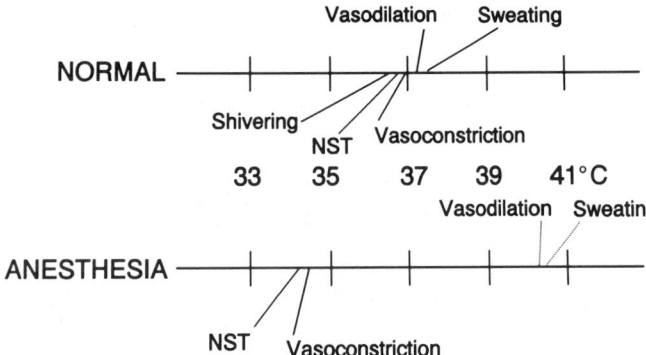

FIGURE 49–1. A schematic drawing illustrating thresholds and gains for common thermoregulatory responses in awake and anesthetized humans. The *angled lines* represent different effector responses, and the *thick horizontal lines* show mean body temperature. The intersection of each line with the temperature scale is the threshold, and the slope indicates the gain of that response. Thermoregulatory sensitivity is shown as the distance between the first cold response (vasoconstriction) and the first warm response (active vasodilation); temperatures within this range do not elicit thermoregulatory compensation. Actual thresholds in unanesthetized individuals are closer than illustrated (i.e., ~0.4 °C), and the gains are higher. The slope of the line that represents shivering is relatively small because there is a broad range of shivering intensity and intensity increases in proportion to hypothermia. Non-shivering thermogenesis (NST) is not triggered until vasoconstriction is nearly complete. The slope of the line that represents vasoconstriction is large because the response is an "all-or-nothing" phenomenon. Because each thermoregulatory effector has its own threshold and gain, there is an orderly progression of responses, with response intensities in proportion to need. During general anesthesia (bottom part of figure), shivering is not shown because it is inhibited by muscle relaxants and local effects of inhaled anesthetics. The thresholds for vasoconstriction and nonshivering thermogenesis are shifted down to ~ 34.5 °C (depending on anesthetic type and dose). The effects of anesthetics on active vasodilation and sweating are unknown, but the thresholds are probably several degrees above normal. (From Sessler DI: Temperature monitoring. *In* Anesthesia. 3rd ed. Miller RD (ed). New York, Churchill Livingstone, 1990, 1227–1242.)

thetics. However, spinal or epidural anesthesia can have several effects on thermoregulation. Vasodilatation below the level of the block causes heat loss; motor block reduces the muscle mass and activity available for heat production; and sensory block of thermal afferents occurs as well. Thus, patients who receive spinal or epidural anesthetics, not surprisingly are also at risk of developing hypothermia.

Vasodilatation increases cutaneous heat loss about 16%, but shivering generates more than enough heat to offset this loss.[12] Nevertheless, central hypothermia develops because of redistribution of core heat to the cooler periphery, analogous to phase I in general anesthesia.

Tremor occurring during epidural anesthesia meets all of the criteria for thermoregulatory shivering. No other tremor patterns or etiologies have been identified. Shivering during epidural anesthesia is less vigorous than after general anesthesia and therefore has fewer hemodynamic and metabolic consequences.

TABLE 49–1. Three Phases of Heat Loss During General Anesthesia

Phase I: redistribution	Rapid core temperature decline 1.5 °C during first hour of anesthesia owing to redistribution of core heat to the periphery.
Phase II: poikilothermia	Slower, linear decline over next several hours until temperature reaches 34.5 °C.
Phase III: thermoregulation	At 34.5 °C, peripheral vasoconstriction occurs, slowing heat loss dramatically. Temperature may begin to increase.

Patients' perception of cold does not correlate with central hypothermia. Hynson and colleagues' volunteers perceived a feeling of warmth despite maximal central hypothermia and shivering. They speculated that the conflicting signals of central hypothermia and subjective peripheral warmth may delay the onset of thermoregulatory shivering in some patients.[12]

Epidural Anesthesia and Shivering

Does the Temperature of the Epidural Drug Cause Shivering?

No clear answer can be given to this question. In Hynson's nonpregnant volunteers, injectate temperature had no influence on the incidence of shivering.[12] However, others studying parturients have believed that cool epidural injectate was more likely to cause shivering than drug injected at body temperature.[13, 14]

Epidural narcotics may reduce the shivering associated with epidural anesthesia. Epidural sufentanil in large doses of up to 100 μg is so effective in blocking shivering that it may cause patients to develop significant hypothermia.[15]

What Is the Clinical Significance of This Information?

Hypothermia and shivering are as much of a problem during spinal and epidural anesthesia as they are during general anesthesia. Patients having similar procedures under general or regional anesthesia arrive in the postanesthesia care unit (PACU) at the same temperature, but those who received regional anesthesia take twice as long to rewarm. Obviously, the mechanisms of heat loss persist in the regional anesthesia group until the block wears off, whereas the general anesthesia group begins to rewarm immediately on emergence. The skin should be kept warm in patients having regional anesthesia until the block wears off.

HEAT LOSS

What Are the Mechanisms?

Four mechanisms of heat loss occur in anesthetized patients (Table 49–2).

Radiation

Radiation is loss of heat in the form of electromagnetic radiation to cooler objects in the room. It is responsible for 70% of the body's heat loss but can be greatly reduced by any simple covering.

TABLE 49–2. Mechanisms of Heat Loss in Order of Importance

Radiation	70% of heat loss	Prevented by simple covering
Convection	Wind chill effect of cool, drafty operating room	Prevented by simple covering
Conduction	Small losses unless patient is wet. Wetness increases conduction loss 25-fold	Keep patient dry
Evaporation	Sweating, insensible loss, humidification of gases; normally a small factor	Use heat and moisture exchanger or humidifier

Convection

Convection reflects loss of heat to air currents flowing over the body—the so-called wind chill effect. In an OR with high air turnover rates and poorly designed air vents, a significant breeze may blow over a patient. Again, simply covering patients dramatically reduces convection losses.

Conduction

Conduction represents loss of heat to objects that the body is touching. This source of loss usually is much less because the OR table mattress is an effective insulator. However, wetness increases conduction losses 25-fold, and many patients are wet by the time surgical preparation is completed.

Evaporation

Evaporative heat loss results from sweating, insensible fluid losses, airway humidification of dry gases, and evaporation from large wound surfaces. Combined, they usually account for only a small portion of total heat loss. However, losses from extensive wounds can become significant.

Which Patients Are at Particular Risk of Hypothermia?

Sixty per cent to 80% of all patients arriving in PACUs are hypothermic. Because the greatest core heat loss (redistribution) is during the first hour of surgery, as previously mentioned, all patients but those undergoing the shortest procedures are at risk. Conahan and colleagues studied a group of patients undergoing laparoscopy in an ambulatory surgery setting.[16] They showed that heated humidification during the procedure allowed them to bring patients to the recovery room 0.5 °C warmer and more importantly to discharge them 1 hour sooner. In a busy facility, this practice can have significant economic benefit. Thus, even patients having short ambulatory procedures can benefit from heat conservation measures.

Infants

Infants are clearly at high risk of developing hypothermia because of large surface area (for heat loss) relative to their small body mass. Because nonshivering thermogenesis is a real factor in infants, it can cause significant increases in oxygen (O_2) consumption in hypothermic infants even when muscle relaxants prevent shivering.

The Elderly

Elderly or debilitated patients are at special risk because they have less insulating subcutaneous tissue and less muscle mass available for heat generation. On the other hand, they shiver less vigorously than younger patients and therefore may suffer fewer hypothermia-induced metabolic consequences.

Burn Victims

Burn victims lack insulating subcutaneous tissue in areas of full-thickness wounds; tremendous evaporative heat loss often results.

TABLE 49–3. Influence of Hypothermia on Oxygen Consumption

Temperature decrease of 0.3 °C	Increases O_2 consumption 7%
Temperature decrease of 0.3–1.2 °C	Increases O_2 consumption 92%
Violent shivering	Increases O_2 consumption 200–500%

Trauma Victims

Trauma victims often become hypothermic in the field before they are rescued. Large-volume room temperature fluid resuscitation further contributes to heat loss unless fluids are aggressively warmed. These individuals present some of the most severe cases of hypothermia. Patients subjected to large volumes of irrigating solution and those with large abdominal wounds lose heat rapidly.

PATHOPHYSIOLOGY OF HYPOTHERMIA

The effects of temperature changes on O_2 consumption in awake, nonparalyzed patients are summarized in Table 49–3.[17] Table 49–4 details the diverse physiologic consequences of hypothermia.

Why Is Hypothermia Clinically Significant?

A very nervous patient brought to a cold, drafty OR and uncovered for catheter and monitor placement may shiver violently from a combination of anxiety and thermoregulatory compromise. At best, this sequence is acutely uncomfortable for patients and may make peripheral venous access difficult. At worst, the hemodynamic and metabolic consequences of shivering can precipitate myocardial ischemia in a patient with minimal coronary reserve. Covering patients with a warmed blanket to keep the skin warm before induction helps prevent this scenario. The pathophysiologic effects of hypothermia are outlined in Table 49–5.

TABLE 49–4. Physiologic Effects of Hypothermia

Cardiovascular	↓ CO (↑ CO if shivering), ↑ SVR, central redistribution of blood → CHF, bradycardia → ventricular arrhythmias
Metabolic	↓ Metabolic rate (↑ if shivering), ↓ tissue perfusion → metabolic acidosis, lipolysis → ↑ FFA, ↓ glucose use → hyperglycemia
Pulmonary	↑ PVR, ↓ hypoxic pulmonary vasoconstriction, ↑ anatomic dead space, ↓ ventilation (apnea in newborns)
Hematologic	↑ blood viscosity, shift of O_2 dissociation curve to left (↑ availability)
Neurologic	↑ CVR, ↓ CBF, EEG slowing → coma, ↓ MAC
Drug disposition	↓ Hepatic blood flow, ↓ hepatic metabolism, ↓ renal blood flow, ↓ excretion, ↑ solubility of anesthetics, prolonged muscle relaxant effect
Shivering	↑ Oxygen consumption up to 500%. ↑ CO_2 production

Abbreviations: SVR = systemic vascular resistance; CHF = congestive heart failure; FFA = free fatty acids; PVR = pulmonary vascular resistance; CVR = cerebral vascular resistance; CBF = cerebral blood flow; EEG = electroencephalogram; MAC = minute alveolar concentration; CO = cardiac output. (From Kaplan RF: Hypothermia/hyperthermia. *In* Manual of Complications During Anesthesia. Gravenstein N (ed). Philadelphia, JB Lippincott, 1991, p 127.)

TABLE 49–5. Pathophysiology of Hypothermia

Organ/System	Major Effects
Heart	Bradycardia, myocardial depression, ventricular irritability leads to fibrillation at 28 °C.
Vascular system	Initial vasoconstriction and hypertension, hemoconcentration, late hypotension.
Coagulation	Decreased activity of humoral clotting factors, but more importantly reversible sequestration of platelets and decreased platelet function.
Kidney	Vasoconstriction may lead to antidiuretic hormone suppression and diuresis. Depressed tubular reabsorptive function with normal glomerular filtration rate also promotes diuresis of dilute urine.
Metabolism	Decreases 7% per 1 °C if not shivering.
Minute alveolar concentration	Decreases 7% per 1 °C if not shivering.
Neurologic	Short-term memory decline at 35 °C. Semi-consciousness at 33 °C. Shivering stops at 33 °C. Coma at 30 °C.

The Cardiovascular System

Hypothermia causes vasoconstriction, may increase blood pressure, and affects myocardial O_2 consumption. As a patient's temperature declines below 34 °C, bradycardia and myocardial depression follow, leading to hypotension. Fluid shifts out of the vascular space; with severe hypothermia (25 °C), hematocrit may increase 150%. The ensuing increase in blood viscosity and reduction in blood volume further contribute to decreased cardiac output.

The initial electrocardiogram (ECG) changes are sinus bradycardia with prolonged PR, QRS, and QT intervals. As body temperature approaches 30 °C, about 30% of patients develop a J wave after the QRS (Fig. 49–2). This event is a precursor to ventricular fibrillation between 28 °C and 25 °C. At temperatures <30 °C, mechanical stimulation of the heart also may provoke ventricular fibrillation.

Coagulation

Hypothermia may cause coagulopathy. Decreasing temperature reduces the activity of humoral clotting factors. More importantly, as temperature falls, the liver sequesters platelets, causing relative thrombocytopenia.[18] As a patient rewarms, these platelets are released back into the circulation and function normally within an hour. Valeri and colleagues[19] showed that wound cooling depresses platelet function and that wound rewarming restores platelet functions to normal. These findings support warming the OR and directing a radiant heat source at large operative wounds.

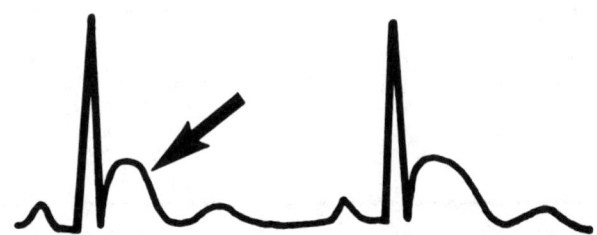

FIGURE 49–2. Osborne J wave (*arrow*) after the QRS complex (pathognomonic of hypothermia). (From Farmer JC: Temperature-related injuries. *In* Critical Care. 2nd ed. Civetta JM, Taylor RW, Kirby RR (eds). Philadelphia, JB Lippincott, 1988, p 695.)

The Kidneys

Cold-induced vasoconstriction can mimic volume overload, leading to antidiuretic hormone (ADH) suppression and diuresis. Hypothermia also depresses tubular reabsorbtive functions but not glomerular filtration, factors that also cause diuresis.

Metabolic Functions

All metabolic processes slow by 7% per 1 °C fall in temperature, and liver blood flow decreases. Therefore, all drugs dependent on the liver for metabolism have prolonged effects during hypothermia. Nondepolarizing muscle relaxant clearance is prolonged by hypothermia. The minimum alveolar concentration (MAC) of inhalation anesthetic agents also decreases 7% per 1 °C; thus, anesthetic concentration must be decreased as a patient cools to avoid excessive anesthetic depression on arrival in the PACU.

Neurologic Function

Short-term memory declines at 35 °C and is decreased 70% by 34 °C. At 33 °C, shivering ceases and patients can no longer actively warm themselves. Reduction in consciousness begins at 33 °C, and coma develops by 30 °C. As a result, postoperative hypothermia causes delayed emergence from anesthesia that becomes clinically significant when the temperature is <34 °C.

The Oxygen Dissociation Curve

Cold shifts the O_2 dissociation curve to the left, meaning that O_2 binds more tightly to hemoglobin and is not released as readily to tissues. The affinity of hemoglobin for O_2 increases 6% per 1 °C decrease. Cold-induced vasoconstriction makes pulse oximeter readings difficult to obtain. A temperature decrease of 2 °C to 3 °C increases the latency of somatosensory evoked potentials and complicates their interpretation.

SPECIAL POSTOPERATIVE PROBLEMS

The serious consequences of intraoperative hypothermia occur not in the OR but in the PACU or intensive care unit (ICU) during rewarming. Metabolic and cardiovascular changes caused by hypothermia, shivering, and rewarming are potentially detrimental to sick patients with limited cardiorespiratory reserve.

Is Postanesthesia Shivering Always Caused by Hypothermia?

All shivering patients are not hypothermic, and all hypothermic patients do not shiver. Sessler and colleagues studied the electromyography (EMG) patterns of muscular activity during emergence from anesthesia and described three distinct patterns: (1) tonic stiffening, (2) clonus, and (3) waxing and waning shivering.[20, 21] Tonic stiffening is believed to be a pure anesthetic effect not at all related to thermoregulation. Waxing and waning shivering is associated with an EMG pattern identical to thermoregulatory shivering in nonanesthetized individuals.

Clonic Shivering

Clonic shivering is more difficult to explain. Its EMG pattern resembles that of pathologic clonus in patients with spinal cord injury. It is most common at end-tidal isoflurane concentrations of 0.2% during emergence from general anesthesia. Initially, clonic shivering was postulated not to be thermoregulatory in origin. It was thought to represent a normally suppressed spinal cord reflex that became apparent at low end-tidal isoflurane concentration because "the spinal cord was waking up before the brain."[20] As the brain subsequently awakened, it again suppressed spinal cord clonus. Peripheral cold receptors were presumed to initiate these "pathologic" reflex tremors. Subsequently, the suggestion was advanced that clonic shivering is also purely thermoregulatory but is modified by low end-tidal anesthetic concentrations.

Thermoregulation During Emergence

At end-tidal isoflurane concentration >0.4% normal thermoregulation is inhibited unless core temperature is <34.5 °C (Table 49–6). Therefore, no shivering or vasoconstriction is expected until end-tidal isoflurane concentration drops below 0.4%. At <0.1% end-tidal values, normal thermoregulation recovers and all shivering is thermoregulatory. From 0.1% to 0.4% end-tidal isoflurane partially suppressed or abnormal clonus-like shivering is seen with normal shivering.[21] In summary, hypothermia is a contributory cause of all postanesthesia shivering. However, the presence and type of shivering are also influenced by residual anesthetic effects on thermoregulation.

What Are the Consequences of Postanesthesia Shivering?

Whatever the cause of postanesthesia shivering, the metabolic and cardiorespiratory consequences and treatment are the same (Table 49–7).[22] Shivering increases the metabolic O_2 requirement 200% to 500%, in turn increasing the demand for cardiac output and ventilation to provide increased O_2 to the shivering muscles. If a patient is unable to increase ventilation because of disease or residual anesthesia, respiratory acidemia supervenes. Likewise, failure to increase cardiac output appropriately predisposes to metabolic acidosis and venous desaturation. The latter, when combined with ventilatory depression, ultimately leads to arterial hypoxemia. Furthermore, the demand for increased cardiac output in a patient with minimal myocardial reserve can precipitate congestive heart failure or myocardial ischemia.

TABLE 49–6. Phases of Thermoregulation During Emergence from Anesthesia

End-Tidal Isoflurane	Thermoregulation
>0.4%	Inhibited completely unless temperature <34.5 °C.
0.1–0.4%	Normal thermoregulatory shivering begins to occur. "Abnormal" partially suppressed clonus-like shivering also present.
<0.1%	Normal thermoregulation; normal shivering.

(Adapted from Sessler DI, Rubenstein EH, Moayeri AM: Physiologic response to mild perianesthetic hypothermia in humans. Anesthesiology 1991; 75:594.)

TABLE 49–7. Problems Caused by Hypothermia in the Postanesthesia Care Unit

Severe shivering	May cause venous and arterial hypoxemia and acidosis.
Peripheral vasoconstriction	Can cause hypertension.
Rewarming vasodilation	Can cause hypovolemia and hypotension.
Ventilator adjustments	Shivering may interfere with ventilation. As patients rewarm and metabolism increases, minute ventilation needs to increase as well.

What Problems Occur with Rewarming?

Severely hypothermic patients have peripheral vasoconstriction and frequent postoperative hypertension. Fluid shifts combined with vasoconstriction reduce intravascular volume. As a patient rewarms and vasodilation occurs, relative hypovolemia and hypotension may necessitate aggressive fluid therapy to prevent hypotension.

Cardiac Surgery

After hypothermic cardiopulmonary bypass (CPB), patients tend to remain hypothermic. Their core temperature often is not fully restored even though the blood temperature may be 37 °C when they are weaned from bypass. Therefore, body temperature diminishes during wound closure and the early recovery period. If such patients are not fully paralyzed, they often shiver. Sladen and colleagues[23, 24] reported two ventilatory problems. With shivering, mechanical ventilator function was compromised, and patients tended to be underventilated. Conversely, paralyzed hypothermic patients tended to be hyperventilated while cold and subsequently hypoventilated as they rewarmed, unless careful adjustment of the ventilator accompanied rewarming. The rewarming period for patients recovering after open heart surgery was 12 hours, with an overshoot to above normal temperatures at the end of the period.

Increased O_2 consumption, energy expenditure, carbon dioxide (CO_2) production, and venous desaturation have been reported during postoperative rewarming of patients after cardiac surgery.[25, 26] Holtzclaw and Green[27] noticed that masseter muscle fasciculations precede these deleterious respiratory and metabolic phenomena. Patients undergoing cardiac surgery clearly are at increased risk of postoperative hypothermia and its attendant cardiorespiratory consequences. Prudence seems to dictate either warming these patients to a higher core temperature before separation from CPB or keeping them paralyzed until they are fully warm.

Radiant heat sources, forced hot-air warmers, intravenous meperidine, and prolonging bypass to allow full core rewarming are effective measures to decrease postoperative increases in energy expenditure due to rewarming. The same principles apply to any other cold, sick, intubated, mechanically ventilated postoperative patient.

What Are the Effects of Shivering in Febrile Patients?

Fever represents a resetting of the body thermostat to a new, higher level. Shivering maintains temperature at that higher level. However, violent fever-induced shivering has the same negative metabolic and cardiorespiratory consequences previously described. Active cooling of a febrile patient makes no sense if doing so serves only to increase shivering. Rather, one should administer antipyretics to restore the thermostat to normal before active cooling. Active cooling may be needed if the temperature reaches dangerous levels. However, its use should be monitored with an eye to the negative consequences of shivering.

PREVENTION AND TREATMENT OF HYPOTHERMIA

Minimization of heat loss should be a priority of the entire OR staff (Table 49–8). Nurses should learn that patients' skin must never be unnecessarily exposed. They must consider getting a patient a warm blanket a higher priority than tying the surgeon's gown. Surgeons must learn to tolerate the temporary discomfort of a warm OR in order to avoid the unfavorable consequences of postoperative hypothermia.

Remember that the initial temperature decrease does not reflect heat loss to the environment but redistribution from a warm body core to a cooler periphery. This translocation is difficult to prevent. However, active peripheral warming helps to minimize the initial reduction in temperature. Most heat loss involves radiation from uncovered parts of the body. Keeping patients covered, including the head and shoulders, is an important factor in avoiding hypothermia.

What Specific Modalities Should Be Used?

Warm the Operating Room

Most OR temperatures are around 19 °C. At least 21 °C and preferably 25 °C is needed to prevent heat loss. If surgeons cannot tolerate the warm room, it may be cooled again once a patient is draped.

Keep Patients Covered

Various covering materials including simple cotton blankets, plastic wrap, aluminum foil, space blankets of aluminum

and Mylar, and special reflective OR garments are available. Each reduces heat loss about 30%, with no great difference in efficacy. The cheapest and most convenient is probably the best.[28]

Use Heated Humidifiers or Heat and Moisture Exchangers

Only 10% of a patient's heat loss is via airway evaporation. A passive heat and moisture exchanger (HME) or active heated humidifier can prevent this loss. Increased humidity also maintains ciliary activity. Numerous studies show the dramatic effects of heated humidification in preventing heat loss and rewarming cold patients.[16, 29, 31] HMEs probably are as effective in preventing heat loss but do not actively transfer heat to patients to rewarm them. Sessler doubts the efficacy of heated humidification.[32] Nevertheless, such devices are only one of the forms of active heating readily available for use in the OR.

Use Radiant Heat Lamps

Radiant heat lamps have long been popular in pediatric ICUs and ORs to help keep neonates warm. If several are used, they may be helpful in adults as well. They serve as a useful adjunct to warming the OR during extensive preparation and draping periods or while invasive catheters are placed.

The disadvantage of infrared heat lamps is that surgical draping usually prevents enough skin surface exposure to the heat source. Furthermore, convection and conduction losses persist in cold, drafty ORs. Radiant heat lamps are not as effective as forced hot-air systems.[33] However, a radiant heat source on the skin can instantly stop postanesthesia shivering even without raising core temperature.[34, 35]

Use Forced Hot-Air Heating Systems

A plastic and paper disposable blanket with multiple openings placed on the patient allows warm air (up to 43 °C) to be blown through the blanket and over the patient. This system is ideally suited to the PACU. Its use in the OR is limited by the need to cover the patient. An OR version covers the shoulders, chest, and outstretched arms of patients positioned for abdominal or lower extremity surgery.

Forced hot-air systems eliminate radiation and convection heat loss by surrounding a patient with a warmed microclimate. They provide a cutaneous heat source that is at least as effective as radiant heat lamps, reduces shivering, and enables earlier PACU discharge.[36] Prophylactic use after cardiac surgery also decreases shivering episodes.[37] Sessler compared a forced hot-air system (the Bair Hugger) with radiant heat sources and with a water circulating blanket placed *over* a patient. The forced hot-air system was most effective in warming. On the ''high'' setting, it raised body temperature 1.5 °C per hour.[38]

Use Fluid Warmers

Administration of 1 L of room temperature fluid requires the patient to expend 15 Kcal to warm the fluid to 37 °C. This expenditure is 20% of a patient's hourly caloric production. Because anesthetized patients cannot increase caloric production, body temperature falls. A liter of blood at 4 °C administered over 15 minutes reduces body temperature 0.5 °C. Thus,

TABLE 49–8. Modalities to Prevent Heat Loss

Warm the operating room until patients are draped.	25 °C is ideal; 21 °C is better than the typical, which is 19 °C.
Keep patients covered.	*Any* covering material reduces heat loss 30%.
Use:	
Radiant heat lamps	Use during preparation and catheter placement when patients cannot be covered.
Forced hot-air heating blankets (Bair Hugger)	Limited by need for surgical exposure, but a chest and shoulder model is available for use in abdominal surgery.
Heat and moisture exchangers or heated humidifiers	The former slows heat loss; the latter were effective in some studies in rewarming cold patients.
Fluid warmers	1 L of 0.4 °C blood product over 15 min decreases body temperature 0.5 °C
Water-circulating warming blankets	Of little or *no* value when placed under adults. May be of value placed on top of patients.

fluid warmers are mandatory for blood administration and desirable for large fluid infusions if hypothermia is to be avoided. Use of a blood warmer should continue in the PACU if further transfusions are needed. The ideal fluid warmer must be easy to set up and to transport to the PACU. It should warm large volumes without reducing flow rate. The Level One device meets these criteria.

Use Water-Circulating Warming Blankets

Several studies show that water-circulating warming blankets are of no value when placed under adults on the OR table.[29, 30] Reasons include limited contact of the body with the blanket, limited circulation through areas in contact with the body, and limited total circulation of water through the blanket (12–15 gallons per hour). However, they are efficacious when placed on top of a patient in the PACU. In this application, they are more effective than radiant heat lamps but less effective than forced hot-air warmers.

How Is Shivering Treated in the Postanesthesia Care Unit?

Several measures can be used to minimize hypothermia and shivering (Table 49–9). The PACU should be comfortably warm, and patients should be kept covered. Supplemental O_2 must be provided to all hypothermic patients. Cutaneous warming stops shivering.[35] Rapid increase of cutaneous temperature, especially in the blush area of the face and chest, is most effective. Thermal comfort correlates with peripheral rather than central temperatures. Cutaneous warming stops shivering before it raises core temperature. If the cutaneous heat source is removed, the patient shivers again.

Meperidine

Intravenous meperidine, 12.5 to 50 mg, is very effective in rapidly terminating or decreasing the severity of shivering after general anesthesia.[39, 40] No other narcotic has this effect. The mechanism of action is unknown. This approach is the quickest, most efficacious, least costly, and most benign treatment for ordinary postanesthesia shivering. The efficacy of intravenous meperidine for shivering associated with epidural anesthesia is unclear.

HYPERTHERMIA

In ancient Greece, fever was viewed as a beneficial sign during infection, partly because of the humoral theory of disease. It was believed to promote purification and elimination of the evil body humors. In fact, considerable data support the hypothesis that temperature elevation can be beneficial in enhancing a host's defense mechanisms by promoting the mobility of leukocytes and their bactericidal and chemotactic properties and by enhancing lymphocyte transformation and interferon activity.[41] Fever may represent the body's response to viral, bacterial, or fungal infection; malignancy; drug toxicity; dehydration; connective tissue disease; hypersensitivity to foreign protein; endocrinopathy; and medication or substance withdrawal. However, regardless of its origin, fever is a very costly metabolic process.

What Is Hyperthermia?

Hyperthermia can be defined as a regulated elevation of central body temperature from a baseline temperature. In formulating this definition, consideration must be given to circadian rhythms, exercise, menstruation, and environmental factors. Although not constant, an oral temperature of 37 °C (98.6 °F) can be considered normal under most circumstances. An evening increase to 38 °C may be perfectly normal if multiple readings are scrutinized for a circadian trend.

The importance of temperature recording in anesthesia practice is to determine a baseline value and to investigate any acute trend that may develop (keeping in mind that body temperature typically decreases on commencement of anesthesia). The magnitude and rate of temperature elevation can lend helpful assistance in determining its source. For clarification, any acute rise of 2 °C per hour merits rapid evaluation.

Extreme pyrexia with temperatures in excess of 41 °C (106 °F) is rare from an infection; meningitis, pneumonia, acquired immunodeficiency syndrome (AIDS), and bacteremia may be the culprit. High fever is often caused by dysfunctional thermoregulation, represented by (1) increased heat production (thyrotoxicosis, pheochromocytoma, exercise, neuroleptic malignant syndrome [NMS], and malignant hyperthermia [MH]); (2) decreased heat dissipation (dehydration, heatstroke, autonomic dysfunction, excessive occlusive coverings, atropine); and (3) hypothalamic influences (stroke, tumor, trauma, infection, and antipsychotic medications).[42]

What Are the Physiologic Alterations Induced by Increased Temperature?

Metabolic

A 1 °C elevation of body temperature raises the basal metabolic rate by 10% to 12%, with a parallel increase in O_2 consumption, CO_2 production, and fluid and nutritional requirements. An alkalotic state due to respiratory compensation may be superseded by a cellular source of acid byproducts, leading to metabolic acidosis. This increased systemic demand can impose a great burden on a marginal cardiovascular system. Hence, the protective immune effects resulting from a temperature elevation may be overshadowed by diminished lymphocyte function and cell viability induced by a high fever.

Cardiovascular

The cardiovascular system responds to extreme pyrexia with myocardial hemorrhages, myofibril degeneration, and occa-

TABLE 49–9. Treating Hypothermia and Shivering in the Postanesthesia Care Unit

Supplemental oxygen until patients are fully warm.
Stop shivering:
  Intravenous meperidine
  Cutaneous heat source—forced hot-air system (Bair Hugger) warming blanket over the patient, or radiant heat lamps
  Paralysis and mechanical ventilation in severely hypothermic, sick patients.

TABLE 49–10. Differential Diagnosis of Hyperthermia

Metabolic imbalance
Excessive ambient, occlusive coverings
Drug reaction
Instrument malfunction/misuse
Central nervous system aberration
Malignant hyperthermia

sional necrosis, especially in the left ventricular myocardium. Elevated catecholamine levels are primarily responsible for the tachycardia, dysrhythmias, conduction changes, and demand-induced myocardial ischemia.[42]

Endocrine

The endocrine system may respond by increasing the release of ADH, aldosterone, growth hormone, corticosteroids, and thyroid hormone.

Central Nervous System

Central nervous system (CNS) deterioration may be evidenced by alterations in sensorium and cognitive skills and by seizure activity. Microscopically, neuronal degeneration, cellular edema, and parenchymal hemorrhages have been noted at necropsy following hyperpyrexia.

Hematologic

Hematologic changes may include decreases in platelets, prothrombin, fibrinogen, and coagulation factors (V, VI, VIII), as well as spontaneous fibrinolysis and a consumptive coagulopathy.[42]

What Is the Differential Diagnosis of Hyperthermia?

The vast array of causes can be limited to a manageable few by a quick review of a patient's past medical history, medications and allergies, personal and family anesthetic history, current illness necessitating surgical intervention, and the an-

esthetic care rendered (Table 49–10). Although MH could be categorized under drug reactions, its importance in anesthetic practice is indisputable. The differential diagnosis of hypermetabolic states is summarized in Tables 49–10 and 49–11.

What Metabolic Aberrations Lead to Hyperthermia?

Acute Thyroid Crisis (Thyroid Storm)

Thyroid storm is a life-threatening state of decompensated thyrotoxicosis that can appear abruptly on induction of anesthesia, during the course of surgery, or postoperatively (see Table 49–11).[43] The usual manifestations of hyperthyroidism are coupled with an extreme hypermetabolic and adrenergic-like state leading to marked increases in cardiac output, O_2 consumption, and CO_2 production. Thyroxine, in animal models, increases sodium-potassium-adenosine triphosphatase activity, enhances adenosine triphosphate–supported calcium transport, and maximizes calcium storage capacity in the sarcoplasmic reticulum.

Tachycardia, dysrhythmias, tachypnea, extreme pyrexia, diaphoresis, and mental status changes are hallmarks of this acute response to excess thyroid hormones. Fortunately, this presentation is rare as a consequence of adequate preoperative preparation. Acute thyroid crisis can promote muscle rigidity in its extreme form and mimic MH.[44] Dantrolene has been used successfully as an antipyretic, to relieve rigidity, and to decrease the hypermetabolic state when acute thyroid crisis could not be clinically differentiated from MH.

Pheochromocytoma

Pheochromocytoma and its extra-adrenal variants, similar to thyroid storm, stimulate an increase in metabolism with acute onset of diaphoresis, extreme tachycardia and hypertension, dysrhythmias, and pyrexia. Paroxysmal signs and symptoms due to episodic release of catecholamines can be precipitated by anesthesia, surgery, and labor. The elevated temperature may originate from the body's increased metabolic rate and the catecholamine-induced peripheral vasoconstriction that diminishes cutaneous heat loss, subsequently elevating the core temperature. As with thyroid storm, the constellation of clini-

TABLE 49–11. Hypermetabolic Syndromes—Differential Clinical Signs

	Malignant Hyperthermia	Neuroleptic Malignant Syndrome	Pheochromocytoma	Thyroid Crisis
Onset	Rapid, slow	Hours to days	Rapid	Rapid
Triggers	Succinylcholine, inhalation	Butyrophenones	Surgical stress	Surgical stress
Fever	Rapid, extreme	Slow, mild, moderate	Mild, moderate	Mild, moderate
Rigidity	75%, rapid	Yes, slow	Rare/none	Rare/none
Tachycardia	Yes	Yes	Yes	Yes
Arrhythmias	Yes	Yes	Yes	Yes
Labile blood pressure	Yes	Yes	Yes	Yes
Hypermetabolic	Extreme	Yes	Yes, moderate	Yes, moderate
Rhabdomyolysis	Yes	Often	Rare	Rare
Diaphoresis	Yes	Yes	Yes	Yes
Creatine kinase elevation	Yes, extreme	Often	Unlikely	Unlikely
Familial/genetic	Yes	Doubtful	Often	Possible
Altered central nervous system	Yes	Yes	Possible	Often
Therapy (plus supportive treatment)	Dantrolene	Dantrolene/bromocriptine	Alpha-, beta-blockers; surgical excision	Beta-blockers, iodide, propylthiouracil

cal changes associated with these two metabolic derangements can masquerade as MH (see Table 49–11).[45]

Pre-Existing Infection

Whether it is community acquired or nosocomial in origin, pre-existing infection is a common denominator in many patients who present for anesthetic care. Superficial skin infections requiring debridement, intrathoracic or intra-abdominal infectious processes, urinary tract contamination, pulmonary emboli and infection, pericarditis and infective endocarditis, and perforated viscus and biliary tract involvement are but a few of the many conditions that may necessitate surgical care or be present as a result of coexisting disease.

A patient in the ICU in septic shock may have markedly increased metabolic demands coupled with increased fluid requirements. Initial difficulties involve replenishment of the intravascular ''tank'' toward a euvolemic state. Subsequent problems involve maintenance of fluid balance to offset the profound insensible and third space losses associated with the ''capillary leak'' commonly seen in sepsis.

Recipients of Blood or Blood Components

Recipients of blood or blood components can experience a wide array of transfusion reactions leading to temperature elevation. Allergic reactions based on leukocyte-antibody interaction (donor versus recipient) and febrile reactions, most likely due to recipient antibodies and surface antigens of the donor platelet and leukocyte populations, occur in up to 3% of transfusions. Incompatible blood may lead to a hemolytic reaction resulting in a low- to moderate-grade fever, among other characteristic morbidities. Bacterial contamination of the blood product causing sepsis, although quite rare, is another possibility to be kept in mind.[46]

Bacterial Transfer

Bacteria infused from outdated or ''set up in advance'' intravenous fluid may be a source, as is contaminated intravenous fluid (by a needle, dirty administration set, uncapped and contaminated stopcock sites, and ports). Cross-contamination between patients can result from the ill-advised practice of reusing single-use vials and infusion sets (continuous infusion propofol, short-acting opioids and muscle relaxants) for multiple patients. Outdated medications and unused yet clean syringes saved from a previous case also increase the possibility of introducing contaminated material and causing an acute febrile episode. Propofol and its carrier medium have been noted to promote the growth of microorganisms and should be disposed of within a reasonable time after opening the vial (4–6 h).

Osteogenesis Imperfecta

Several publications mention the observation that the pyrexia associated with osteogenesis imperfecta may be related to an inherent hypermetabolic state leading to increased heart rate, respiratory rate, temperature, and metabolic rate. These changes perhaps are coincidental, but the suggestion that osteogenesis imperfecta is related to MH should be recognized and appreciated.[47]

What Drug Reactions Should Be Considered?

Neuroleptic Malignant Syndrome

NMS is caused by a neuroleptic-induced alteration of dopamine action in the basal ganglia and hypothalamus. It occurs in up to 1.5% of patients who are treated chronically with psychotropic drugs such as phenothiazines, butyrophenones, and monoamine oxidase (MAO) inhibitors. It has a less abrupt onset (days to weeks) and a longer duration (1–2 wk) than MH. The problem is characterized by a slow onset of akinesia, muscle rigidity, hyperpyrexia, and mental status fluctuations that may last from 5 to 10 days. Autonomic dysfunction leads to diaphoresis, labile hemodynamics, and tachycardia. The mortality of such an event (15%) may be precipitated by dysrhythmia, respiratory failure, myocardial ischemia/infarction, pulmonary embolism, rhabdomyolysis-induced renal failure, or a combination of these events (see Table 49–11). Despite a typical leukocytosis, elevated liver enzymes and increased creatine kinase (CK) levels, no diagnostic tests exist.

Therapy includes discontinuation of neuroleptics and initiation of supportive measures to control temperature, acid-base imbalance, muscle tone, and fluid requirements. No consensus has been reached about specific therapy, yet combination therapy with centrally acting bromocriptine and peripherally acting dantrolene may have clinical usefulness. Despite similarities between MH and NMS, the relatively small clinical sample of patients fails to demonstrate a clear relationship through muscle contracture testing.[48, 49]

Central Anticholinergic Syndrome

Central anticholinergic syndrome is an extreme complication of routine doses of anticholinergics. Presenting signs range from excitatory or agitated behavior to respiratory depression and coma. Mild pyrexia may exist in 25% of episodes, but one case report suggests extreme temperature elevation to 41.3 °C associated with scopolamine administration.[50] After routine administration of atropine, one must recognize the common response of temperature elevation because of diminished sweating and tachycardia, both of which may raise suspicion of MH.

Monoamine Oxidase Inhibitors

MAO inhibitors used in the therapy of various psychotic-depressive disorders, are a potential source of serious drug interactions when patients receiving them are anesthetized. Blockade of the MAO enzyme complex promotes the accumulation of catecholamines (norepinephrine, epinephrine, dopamine, 5-hydroxytryptamine). Excessive doses of MAO inhibitors can induce hyperpyrexia via two possible pathways: (1) excessive sympathetic α-stimulation with undue peripheral vasoconstriction, leading to limited cutaneous heat transfer; and (2) central effects with altered hypothalamic influence. Meperidine and morphine, which cause catecholamine and histamine release, respectively, can induce a hypertensive, hyperpyrexic, rigid state with marked CNS aberration. Meperidine is to be avoided and morphine avoided or severely restricted in patients receiving MAO inhibitor medications.

Tricyclic Antidepressants

Tricyclic antidepressants block neuronal norepinephrine uptake centrally and peripherally and promote anticholinergic activity. The potential to foster dysrhythmias, tachycardia, cardiac decompensation, and hyperpyrexia is evident.

Cocaine and Amphetamines

These agents alter the presynaptic reuptake of neurotransmitters, leading to myriad cardiovascular and CNS effects. Acute toxicity presents as agitation, paranoia, hallucinations, and combative behavior. It is coupled frequently with severe hypertension, dysrhythmias, stroke, and myocardial ischemia, even in patients with no history of previous cardiovascular disease. Hyperthermia can occur in response to increased basal metabolic rate and decreased peripheral heat loss due to cutaneous vasoconstriction. Further, cocaine can initiate the central anticholinergic syndrome and its inherent effect on thermoregulation.

Drug Withdrawal

Withdrawal from drugs, prescribed or illicit, can elevate core temperature. Ethanol and opioid abstinence during the perioperative period can elicit tachycardia, hypertension, and hyperpyrexia. Clonidine withdrawal, theoretically, can lead to catecholamine-induced temperature changes. Abrupt discontinuation of levodopa in the parkinsonian population can lead to either a simple elevation in temperature or, more seriously, to NMS.

When Are Mechanical Factors a Problem?

Conductive and convective heat gain through radiant warmers, warm-air convection systems, or a warmed mattress, when in excess of the actual heat loss, promotes heat gain and temperature elevation. Techniques that minimize heat loss when losses are smaller than anticipated (e.g., laparoscopic appendectomy) can induce further elevations in body temperature beyond the already present febrile state.

Warming blankets or heated humidifying systems with an excessively high set-point contribute to elevated temperatures. More importantly, the danger of cutaneous thermal burns at skin contact points and tracheal and bronchial mucosal drying may lead to damage with subsequent edema, inflammation, and hemorrhage.

Automated rapid-infusion (warm fluid) devices are a useful adjunct to resuscitation, but temperature elevation related to equipment use should be kept in mind. A >1 °C central temperature elevation may occur after significant fluid replacement incorporating a rapid-infusion device, for example, during a radical prostatectomy.

When Is the Central Nervous System a Source of Fever?

The anterior hypothalamus contains the body's thermoregulatory center, which receives input from cutaneous skin receptors, the spinal cord, and the sympathetic nervous system. These receptors may contribute to alterations in central temperature. Various clinical conditions in neurosurgical patients exemplify central influence on body temperature. Any disruption of the blood-brain barrier that allows blood and cerebrospinal fluid to contact each other can initiate a febrile reaction, such as after a stroke, an intracerebral hemorrhage, or surgical and traumatic manipulation of the brain. Also, direct trauma to the hypothalamus or surrounding tissue, edema, or vascular compromise can initiate "brain storming," with profound elevations in body temperature.

MALIGNANT HYPERTHERMIA

Ombrédanne noted the relationship of anesthesia and hyperthermia in 1929 (Ombrédanne's syndrome), yet it was not until 1960 that Denborough and Lovell published their classic description of a familial trend in anesthetic-induced death.[51] In 1966, Wilson coined the term *malignant hyperpyrexia*.[52] The term *malignant* was appropriate at the time owing to an incomplete understanding of the disease, the lack of a specific antidote, and the high mortality rate. Characteristic findings are listed in Table 49–11.

What Is the Incidence?

The estimated incidence of fulminant MH is 1 in 250,000 anesthetics (Table 49–12).[53] A combination of succinylcholine (SCH) and potent inhaled anesthetics increases the incidence to 1 in 60,000 exposures. A 15-fold increase (1 in 4200) is noted in cases of "suspected" MH with this combination (see Table 49–11).[54] The presenting signs and symptoms can be so variable, singly or in combination, that the suspicion of MH differs among individual patients according to the practitioner's interpretation. Although all age groups can experience MH, the incidence appears higher in children ages 3 to 12 years. However, a case of severe muscle rigidity has been

TABLE 49–12. Incidence of Different Forms of Malignant Hyperthermia (MH) in Relation to Type of Anesthesia

Type of Anesthesia	Fulminant MH	Abortive MH (All Subgroups Included)	Overall Incidence of Suspected Malignant Hypothermia
Total number of anesthetics	1:251,063	1:17,435	1:16,303
General anesthesia	1:221,811	1:15,404	1:14,403
Anesthesia with administration of succinylcholine	1:140,006	1:8,819	1:8,297
Anesthesia with potent inhalation agent	1:84,488	1:6,653	1:6,167
With succinylcholine	1:61,961	1:4,506	1:4,201
Without succinylcholine	1:174,597	1:20,541	1:18,379

(From Ording H: Incidence of malignant hyperthermia in Denmark. Anesth Analg 1985; 64:704. © International Anesthesia Research Society.)

described in a premature infant born via cesarean section after a triggering general anesthetic.

How Is the Diagnosis Made?

Clinical Assessment

One word is the key to diagnosis—*suspicion.* Survival from an MH episode requires early treatment; the crucial element in early treatment is heightened awareness of the possibility of MH and a keen suspicion based on clinical signs while other potential causes are ruled out. The onset may occur immediately after induction with potent inhalation agents or SCH or both, or it may be delayed by the use of nondepolarizing relaxants and barbiturates until later in the case or even as long as 18 to 24 hours postoperatively. The appearance of tachycardia, tachypnea (increased metabolism of onboard relaxants), muscle rigidity, rising partial pressure of end-tidal CO_2 (PETCO$_2$) in the presence of constant ventilation, and fever (frequently delayed onset) should stimulate the evaluation of arterial and venous blood samples for respiratory or metabolic acidosis (Table 49–13).

Capnography is a sensitive indicator of an evolving hypermetabolic state, but other causes should be ruled out. A single clinical sign does not usually implicate MH susceptibility (MHS) correctly, although generalized rigidity alone may be the only single sign that suggests susceptibility.[55] The maximum temperature attained during a MH episode has a direct correlation to the mortality rate (Table 49–14). Remember, however, that rapid temperature elevation may be delayed in onset and should not be the sole criterion to suggest or confirm a diagnosis of MH.

The North American MH Registry is currently attempting to clarify diagnostic criteria (clinical signs) and to formulate a grading system that assesses both the likelihood of a clinical case representing true MH and a patient's chances of being MH susceptible through contracture testing. The MH clinical grading system will use clinical information exclusively, without reference to the results of the MH muscle biopsy. This approach will allow researchers to compare patients continent-wide and to consolidate investigative efforts.

What Anesthetic Agents Are Triggers?

Triggers are volatile agents, including desflurane and SCH. MHS in swine can be triggered by nonanesthetic factors (e.g., stress, exercise, fright). Evidence is accumulating that families with MHS may have a higher incidence of sudden death and a predisposition to a nonspecific cardiomyopathy. Additionally,

TABLE 49–13. Frequency of Early Clinical Signs

Clinical Sign	Number of Patients	% with Sign
Tachycardia	409	91
Hyperventilation	209	83
Muscle rigidity	448	79
Altered blood pressure	254	78
Fever	201	72
Cyanosis	273	69

(Data from Britt BA, Lwong FHF, Endrenyi L: The clinical and laboratory features of malignant hyperthermia management: a review. *In* Malignant Hyperthermia Syndrome. Henschel EO (ed). New York, Appleton-Century-Crofts, 1977, pp 9–45.)

TABLE 49–14. Maximum Temperature Attained and Mortality Rates

Maximum Temperature (°F)	(°C)	Number of Patients	% Mortality
99–100.9	37.2–38.2	57	3.5
101–102.9	38.3–39.3	79	8.9
103–104.9	39.4–40.5	103	16.5
105–106.9	40.6–41.6	99	38.4
107–108.9	41.7–42.7	159	66.7
109–110.9	42.8–43.8	57	86.0
>110.9	>43.8	19	94.7

(Data from Britt BA, Lwong FHF, Endrenyi L: The clinical and laboratory features of malignant hyperthermia management: a review. *In* Malignant Hyperthermia Syndrome. Henschel EO (ed). New York, Appleton-Century-Crofts, 1977, pp 9–45.)

although MH is rare in conscious humans, associations linking MH to heatstroke, unusual stress states, and myalgias are surfacing.[52]

The list of potential triggering agents has been modified with continued clinical testing and experience. Because amide local anesthetics can raise intracellular calcium levels, they were once considered unsafe. Now, after extensively testing swine with MHS and common use of amide local anesthetic techniques in patients with MHS during biopsies for MH, they have been reclassified to the "safe" group (Table 49–15). However, it has been suggested they be avoided during an acute episode, if possible, because of their induction of calcium shifts.[56]

How Is an Acute Episode of Malignant Hyperthermia Treated?

Alterations in the sarcoplasmic calcium flux induced by triggering agents can lead to increases in metabolism, heat production, and acidic waste generation. If exposure to the triggers persists, the regulation of energy production and enzymatic control is lost. Cellular demand for O_2 and energy substrates outstrips supply, culminating in acidosis, cellular and interstitial edema, loss of perfusion, and further membra-

TABLE 49–15. Safe Anesthetic Agents in Patients with Malignant Hyperthermia and Malignant Hyperthermia Susceptibility

Barbiturates/intravenous anesthetics	Thiopental (Pentothal)
	Methohexital (Brevital)
	Thiamylal (Surital)
	Propofol (Diprivan)
	Etomidate (Amidate)
Narcotics (Opioids)	Morphine
	Meperidine (Demerol)
	Hydromorphone (Dilaudid)
	Fentanyl (Sublimaze)
	Sufentanil (Sufenta)
	Alfentanil (Alfenta)
Tranquilizers	Diazepam (Valium)
	Midazolam (Versed)
Amides	Lidocaine (Xylocaine)
	Mepivacaine (Carbocaine)
	Bupivacaine (Marcaine)
	Etidocaine (Duranest)
	Prilocaine (Citanest)
Esters	Procaine (Novocain)
	Chloroprocaine (Nesacaine)
	Tetracaine (Pontocaine)
	Propoxycaine and procaine

TABLE 49–16. Emergency Therapy for Malignant Hyperthermia (Revised 1993)

Acute Phase Treatment

1. Immediately discontinue all volatile inhalation anesthetics and succinylcholine. Hyperventilate with 100% oxygen at high gas flows; at least 10 L · min⁻¹. The circle system and CO_2 absorbent need not be changed.
2. Administer dantrolene sodium 2–3 mg · kg⁻¹ initial bolus rapidly with increments up to 10 mg · kg⁻¹ total. Continue to administer dantrolene until signs of MH (e.g., tachycardia, rigidity, increased end-tidal CO_2, and temperature elevation) are controlled. Occasionally, a total dose greater than 10 mg · kg⁻¹ may be needed. Each vial of dantrolene contains 20 mg of dantrolene and 3 g mannitol. Each vial should be mixed with 60 mL of sterile water for injection USP without a bacteriostatic agent.
3. Administer bicarbonate to correct metabolic acidosis as guided by blood gas analysis. In the absence of blood gas analysis, 1–2 mEq · kg⁻¹ should be administered.
4. Simultaneous with the above, actively cool the hyperthermic patient. Use IV iced saline (not lactated Ringer's solution), 15 ml · kg⁻¹ q 15 min × 3.
   a. Lavage stomach, bladder, rectum, and open cavities with iced saline as appropriate.
   b. Surface cool with ice and hypothermia blanket.
   c. Monitor closely, since overvigorous treatment may lead to hypothermia.
5. Dysrhythmias will usually respond to treatment of acidosis and hyperkalemia. If they persist or are life threatening, standard antiarrhythmic agents may be used, with the exception of calcium channel blockers (may cause hyperkalemia and cardiovascular collapse).
6. Determine and monitor end-tidal CO_2, arterial, central or femoral venous blood gases, serum potassium, calcium, clotting studies, and urine output.
7. Hyperkalemia is common and should be treated with hyperventilation, bicarbonate, intravenous glucose and insulin (10 units regular insulin in 50 mL 50% glucose titrated to potassium level). Life-threatening hyperkalemia may also be treated with calcium administration (e.g., 2–5 mg · kg⁻¹ of $CaCl_2$).
8. Ensure urine output of greater than 2 mL · kg⁻¹ · h⁻¹. Consider central venous or PA monitoring because of fluid shifts and hemodynamic instability that may occur.
9. Boys younger than 9 years of age who experience sudden cardiac arrest after succinylcholine administration in the absence of hypoxemia should be treated for acute hyperkalemia first. In this situation, calcium chloride should be administered along with other means to reduce serum potassium. They should be presumed to have subclinical muscular dystrophy.

Postacute Phase

1. Observe the patient in an intensive care unit setting for at least 24 h since recrudescence of MH may occur, particularly following a fulminant case resistant to treatment.
2. Administer dantrolene 1 mg · kg⁻¹ IV q 6 h for 24–48 h postepisode. After that, oral dantrolene 1 mg · kg⁻¹ q 6 h may be used for 24 h as necessary.
3. Follow arterial blood gases, creatine kinase, potassium, calcium, urine and serum myoglobin, clotting studies, and core body temperature until such time as they return to normal values (e.g., q 6 h). Central temperature (e.g., rectal, esophageal) should be continuously monitored until stable.
4. Counsel the patient and family regarding MH and further precautions. Refer the patient to MHAUS. Fill out an Adverse Metabolic Reaction to Anesthesia (AMRA) report available through the North American Malignant Hyperthermia Registry (717) 531-6936.

CAUTION: This protocol may not apply to every patient and must of necessity be altered according to specific patient needs.

(Used with permission from Malignant Hyperthermia Association of the United States.)

nous breakdown. Fulminant MH requires urgent therapy to ensure survival. The clinical signs can be noted within minutes, and despite appropriate and timely treatment, deterioration can be so rapid that death ensues. Conversely, the course may be less rapid, allowing resuscitative measures and dantrolene to prove their worth. A suggested clinical plan for therapy of an acute MH episode is presented in Table 49–16.

What Are the Serious Late Complications?

Rhabdomyolysis, with its associated muscle breakdown and pigment-induced acute tubular necrosis, is preventable or can at least be limited with adequate and timely dantrolene therapy and supportive measures to ensure adequate urine output (fluid, diuretics, mannitol, alkalization). A consumptive coagulopathy can be induced by the release of mediators, endothelial thromboplastins, hemolysis, inadequate capillary blood flow, and tissue destruction.

Appropriate therapy includes supportive and therapeutic care during the MH episode, which may control or eliminate the instigating mediator. Treatment with intravenous heparin, blood components, and ε-aminocaproic acid should be reserved for difficult cases unresponsive to standard MH resuscitative measures. Insufficient oxygenation and perfusion (hypermetabolic state) and loss of cell membrane integrity may lead to cerebral edema, cellular ischemia and destruction, increased intracranial pressure, coma, paralysis, and other serious neurologic sequelae.

How Does Dantrolene Work?

Dantrolene inhibits calcium release from the sarcoplasmic reticulum without altering the reuptake mechanism. Hence, it can foster a reversal of the calcium accumulation that occurs in the skeletal muscle sarcoplasm during a triggered MH episode. Originally investigated as an antibiotic, dantrolene found use in spastic muscle disorders by virtue of its muscle relaxation properties. It also is a very effective antipyretic.

Various hypercatabolic disorders presenting with clinical signs similar to MH can be treated with dantrolene with marked improvement. Its use in NMS, heatstroke, and MAO inhibitor overdose for reversal of the hyperpyrexia and hypermetabolic signs suggests a potentially wider array of clinical applications.[57] Likewise, clinical signs that are suggestive of MH and that appear during anesthetic administration and are treated successfully with dantrolene have proved, on occasion, not to represent MH but cases of acute thyroid crisis and pheochromocytoma.[44, 45]

Prophylactic Use in Patients with Malignant Hyperthermia

The Malignant Hyperthermia Association of the United States (MHAUS) suggests that prophylactic dantrolene administration should be considered on an individual basis. Questions to be addressed when making this decision should include the following: (1) Is the surgery emergent, and will the added stress involved initiate an MH episode? (2) What coexisting disease is present, and how well will the patient tolerate a potential multifocal increase in O_2 consumption, lactate production, tachycardia, fever, and hypercatabolic problems? (3) Does the patient have a pre-existing muscular disorder in which muscle weakness could be exacerbated by dantrolene administration (e.g., muscular dystrophy or myasthenia gravis)?

Susceptible parturients should receive dantrolene, if indicated, preferably after cord clamping to minimize fetal and newborn exposure. A well-informed patient and individual practitioners may be reluctant to leave the patient "unprotected," feeling more comfortable with pretreatment. However, no case of severe or fatal MH has been reported when the anesthesia team was informed of the patient's risk and a nontriggering technique was used either with or without dantrolene prophylaxis.[56]

If prophylactic therapy is instituted, 2.5 mg · kg^{-1} should be given intravenously 30 minutes before induction of anesthesia.[58] This recommendation is based on the data collected from a multicenter study in which a mean dose of 2.5 mg · kg^{-1} was shown to be sufficient to reverse MH reactions.[59] The current trend is away from dantrolene prophylaxis (except in the previously mentioned circumstances), depending instead on monitoring temperature, Petco$_2$, and muscle tone.[60] Additionally, standard recommendations for intraoperative care should be followed (Table 49–17).

Oral Dantrolene

Prophylactic coverage with dantrolene by the oral route is believed by some to be inadequate for patients with MHS. This opinion appears to be founded on case reports in which breakthrough MH episodes surfaced despite preoperative oral dose coverage. However, the dose given may have been inadequate, considering total dose and the time sequence of administration.[61] Based on studies of swine with MHS, Flewellen and Nelson suggested that a dose of dantrolene that produces at least 95% of the maximum muscle twitch depression (serum level of 2.8 μg · mL^{-1}) provides protection against MH.[62]

Attainment of an adequate serum level with oral dantrolene may require the Food and Drug Administration's recommended 5 mg · kg^{-1} · d^{-1}, with proper timing of the last preinduction dose. Allen and colleagues incorporated this amount in four divided doses, with the last given 4 hours preinduction. Appropriate plasma levels were reached at induction and maintained for 6 to 18 hours thereafter.[63]

TABLE 49–17. Treatment for Malignant Hyperthermia–Susceptible Patients—Known or Suspected

- Anesthesia machine: Remove or drain/disconnect vaporizers. High-flow O$_2$ (10 L · min^{-1}) for 20 min through circuit, 10 min if fresh gas line is replaced. Use a new or disposable breathing circuit.
- Preoperative creatine kinase determination and complete blood count.
- Cooling blanket on operating room table, nearly iced fluids, a posted MH plan in a conspicuous site, an MH cart or kit with necessary medications, i.e., dantrolene, at least 36 vials.
- Dantrolene prophylaxis (controversial) should be considered on an individual basis.
- Technique of choice: regional or local. Avoid triggering agents. Monitor routine American Society of Anesthesiologists guidelines, capnography, temperature. Invasive monitoring as appropriate for surgery.
- Uneventful anesthetic course: postoperative minimum 4 h electrocardiography, temperature monitoring. No further dantrolene is necessary.
- MH episode postoperative: Titrate dantrolene to normalize clinical signs, continue for 36 h after stabilization (suggested dose of 1 mg · kg^{-1} every 6 h). Monitor vitals, capnography, core temperature; check venous and arterial blood gases, baseline creatine kinase, electrolytes, calcium, lactate, blood urea nitrogen, creatinine, coagulation profile, platelets, urine for color, myoglobin.

(Modified from Malignant Hyperthermia Association of the United States (MHAUS). Darien, CT, MHAUS, 1991.)

Despite this study and the fact that oral dantrolene is less costly, requires no reconstitution, and avoids the large dose of mannitol required to make intravenous dantrolene solution isotonic, the intravenous preparation prevents any uncertainty about adequacy of serum levels. It may also decrease the incidence of preoperative muscle weakness, lethargy, and gastrointestinal distress and negate lengthy preoperative hospitalization. Although no anesthetic regimen can guarantee immunity to MH, provision of adequate preoperative sedation and preparation with oral or intravenous dantrolene does allow the use of a nontriggering anesthetic.[64]

Dosing Recommendations

The initial dose of intravenous dantrolene, as discussed, is 2.5 mg · kg^{-1}.[62] Subsequent dosing is based on clinical signs. After the initial dose, if objective clinical evidence does not support improvement (resolved dysrhythmias and hemodynamic stability, less rigidity, decreased Petco$_2$, lower temperature), repeating the dose is recommended, up to 20 mg · kg^{-1}. Although most cases respond to 4 mg · kg^{-1} or less, an occasional patient requires higher doses for control. Also, recrudescence is possible within a few hours to days after the episode. After reversal and stabilization, continued administration of intravenous dantrolene (1 mg · kg^{-1} every 4–6 h) is warranted for at least 36 and possibly 48 hours. Oral dosing may be used after successful treatment.[65]

Side Effects

The potential side effects or adverse reactions include lethargy, altered sensorium, and muscle weakness. Gastrointestinal distress with nausea and vomiting, skin rash, and phlebitis are other concerns. Concurrent dantrolene administration may potentiate the action of neuromuscular blocking agents. Likewise, significant hyperkalemia and cardiac depression can occur with concurrent calcium channel blocker therapy. Placental transfer with subsequent fetal and neonatal lethargy and weakness, and the association of dantrolene and uterine atony leading to postpartum hemorrhage, are concerns in obstetric cases.[59]

What Preoperative Conditions Suggest Risk?

General Considerations

Factors that suggest MH risk include a personal or family history of anesthetic problems (high fever, dark urine, or rigidity), unexplained anesthetic deaths, and masseter muscle spasm. Screening CK values are elevated in 70% of affected people but have proved less useful in predicting MHS than was previously thought. If a "resting" serum CK level is elevated in a close relative of a patient with MHS, that relative could be considered susceptible without a documenting contracture test. However, a normal CK level has less predictive value; therefore, a biopsy specimen should be secured for testing.

Associated Characteristics

Other characteristics noted to occur with higher frequency in individuals with MHS include squinting, backache, muscle weakness and cramps, ptosis, strabismus, kyphoscoliosis, inguinal hernia, pectus abnormalities, and others. Smith[67] suggested that a combination of 20 such variables was capable of predicting MHS with 61.5% reliability, compared with muscle biopsy results (considered 95% reliable in estimating susceptibility).[68] Closer scrutiny of these characteristics on a single basis, not as a group, does not reliably reflect a significant difference between patients with MHS and control groups.[69]

Related Disease Conditions

Many conditions and clinical signs have been suggested to have a higher incidence in those patients with MHS. Central core disease and King-Denborough syndrome are related to MH, and patients with Duchenne's muscular dystrophy and other myopathies may develop any or all of the signs across the MH spectrum (Table 49–18).

Fewer causal or coincidental relationships exist with osteogenesis imperfecta, NMS, glycogen storage diseases, lymphoma, and sudden infant death syndrome (SIDS).[70] Myotonic conditions that respond to SCH with rigidity and contracture could be confused with MH. However, they cause rigidity in the absence of serious metabolic derangements. Myotonic states may have positive results after MH contracture testing, further adding to the confusion and controversy.

Duchenne's Muscular Dystrophy

Patients with Duchenne's muscular dystrophy may respond to potent inhalation agents, with or without SCH, with sudden cardiac arrest or rhabdomyolysis. Although the incidence of MH in such patients is not confirmed, Sethna and Rockoff reported that six patients receiving a "safe" technique had no complications whereas 5 of 19 patients receiving volatile agents had problems (2 cardiac arrests, 3 unexplained fever or tachycardia responsive to withdrawal of the volatile agents).[66]

The Newington Children's Hospital, in a 10-year retrospective review of 84 anesthetics administered to 36 biopsy-diagnosed cases of Duchenne's muscular dystrophy, reported that only two patients had premature ventricular contractions (one patient had a potassium level of 2.9 mEq · L^{-1}). One had hyperthermia (skin temperature 102 °F, responsive to discontinuation of a warming blanket and surface cooling measures). The remainder of the procedure was uneventful, and the patient's temperature in the PACU was 98 °F. Of the 84 anesthetics, 83 were considered "triggering" (potent inhalation agents: 62% halothane, 26% isoflurane, 11% enflurane); SCH was used once without sequelae (Peluso A, Bianchini A: Personal communication, 1992). Nonetheless, cautious handling of these cases is warranted.

How Should Patients with Malignant Hyperthermia Be Anesthetized?

The key to success in anesthetizing a patient with MHS is preoperative preparation and perioperative heightened awareness for clinical clues suggestive of an MH episode in its early stages. To provide reassurance, one should discuss the perioperative management plan with the patient and family while emphasizing the anesthesia team's knowledge of MH recognition and its therapy.

TABLE 49–18. Disorders Associated with Malignant Hyperthermia

Duchenne's dystrophy
Central core disease
Neuroleptic malignant syndrome
Myotonia congenita
King-Denborough syndrome
Schwartz-Jampel syndrome
Osteogenesis imperfecta

Techniques

The anesthetic technique is chosen on the basis of the surgical site and the patient's condition, understanding that local and regional methods are safe and recommended. Berkowitz and Rosenberg reported their success with femoral nerve block for muscle biopsy in patients with MH, eliminating the need for dantrolene pretreatment, even in a high-risk patient.[70]

General anesthesia must consist of nontriggering agents. It is no longer necessary to use a new or uncontaminated anesthetic machine by flushing high-flow O_2 for an extended period. Removing the vaporizers (or draining and disconnecting them), replacing the fresh gas hose, and using a new disposable circuit make the machine safe to use after 5 to 20 minutes of high-flow O_2.[71–73] Dantrolene prophylaxis is considered on an individual basis. Central temperature monitoring is suggested.

A written treatment plan, as suggested by the MHAUS, can conserve time and be life saving. During surgery, any unexpected tachycardia, tachypnea, dysrhythmia, muscle rigidity, or P_{ETCO_2} elevation needs urgent evaluation. Postoperative care for an uneventful anesthetic course should consist of at least 4 hours of observation in the PACU, with continuous temperature and ECG monitoring.

What Is the Relevance of Masseter Muscle Rigidity?

Although the appropriate management and the clinical significance of masseter muscle rigidity (MMR) are controversial, further confusion has surfaced because of differing definitions of what masseter muscle "stiffness" truly represents. To determine the incidence, one must first adequately define the meaning of the term *MMR*. The degree of masseter stiffness can vary among individual patients under various clinical conditions, as can the practitioner's assessment of the rigidity.

Characteristic Responses

Kaplan has elegantly categorized the spectrum of masseter stiffness into three areas[56] (Fig. 49–3). This relationship is pertinent to our clinical practice of anesthesia because MMR has been associated with MH and may herald its onset. The first category is characterized by a degree of masseter muscle stiffness that can be physically overcome (with some difficulty). With a special mastication traction device, Van Der Spek and colleagues determined that SCH, when combined with halothane, consistently reduces mouth opening and increases masseter muscle tone, most often to a subclinical degree.[74] This response may be regarded as a normal phenome-

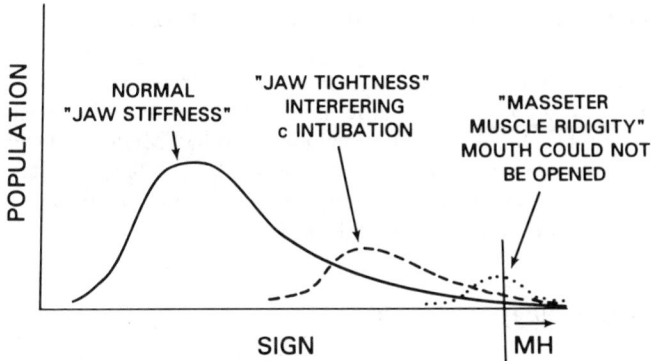

FIGURE 49–3. The spectrum of masseter muscle response to succinylcholine and the relationship to MH. (From Kaplan RF: Hypothermia/hyperthermia. *In* Manual of Complications During Anesthesia. Gravenstein N (ed). Philadelphia, JB Lippincott, 1991, p 138.)

non in children given both halothane and SCH and apparently does not portend a marked increase in risk for MH.[74]

The second category is a response to SCH in which jaw tightness interfering with intubation occurs. Retrospective review suggests that the incidence is as high as 1% among children receiving both SCH and halothane. The precise risk of MH in patients who manifest this response is undetermined, yet it is considered to be small.

The third response can be described as "the mouth cannot be opened." This reaction to SCH most likely represents true MMR and may correspond to a high risk (~50%) for MHS, based on halothane contracture testing.[75, 76] Other causes of limited jaw mobility should be ruled out. Nevertheless, with any degree of perceived MMR, MH could follow immediately or after a delay of 20 minutes or more. Any patient experiencing MMR should be observed in the PACU for at least 4 hours, with attention paid to temperature, muscle tone, and hemodynamic alterations, and then overnight, with periodic serum CK determinations (every 6–8 h for 24 h) and urine checked for color and the presence of myoglobin.

Cancellation of Operation

Three schools of thought have been published concerning this controversy. The most conservative approach suggests to stop the anesthetic and abort the surgery if it is an elective procedure. If surgery must continue, switch to nontriggering agents with precautionary measures and monitoring for MH (Table 49–19). The second, less conservative, plan is to switch to nontriggering agents (elective procedure) and continue with MH precautions and monitoring. The third approach is to continue the triggering agents while instituting appropriate MH monitoring.[77, 78]

In the absence of another myopathy, all patients who were not receiving dantrolene for MMR and who had CK levels >20,000 IU · L^{-1} after SCH use were MH-positive by muscle biopsy.[75] In one review, all patients with MMR who had anesthesia halted after induction fared well whether or not they received dantrolene.[56]

Until these arguments are better supported with adequate data and contracture testing, prudency suggests handling this enigma in the most conservative manner, with follow-up

serum CK determinations and urine evaluations. Providing patients with reassurance and education is essential.

Anesthetic Management

Ideally, such patients will have undergone muscle contracture testing to determine their risk of MH; most, however, will likely not have had this procedure performed. Thus, SCH should definitely be omitted from the anesthetic plan. Until proven otherwise, all patients who experience MMR and their close relatives should be treated as MHS. Intraoperative PETCO$_2$ and temperature monitoring, muscle tone evaluation, close clinical scrutiny, heightened MH awareness, and a nontriggering anesthetic should suffice. Controversy exists about whether muscle biopsy testing for MH should be performed on all those experiencing MMR and their families and if intravenous dantrolene should be administered after the occurrence of MMR in the absence of other signs of MH.

What Should Be Known About the Biochemistry of Malignant Hyperthermia?

MH is a disease affecting seemingly all skeletal muscle membranes once a triggering agent initiates the calcium (Ca^{2+})-related cascade. Excessive Ca^{2+} in the myoplasm may result when the overly sensitive sarcoplasmic reticulum is exposed to halothane. Potentiation of Ca^{2+} released by increased phospholipase A$_2$ activity and its effect on free unsaturated fatty acids from mitochondria have been linked with halothane exposure, thus leading to a further elevation of myoplasmic Ca^{2+}.

An abnormal Ca^{2+}-release channel protein in the sarcoplasmic reticulum, known as the *ryanodine receptor protein,* bridges the transverse tubules and the SR terminal cisternae membranes and may have a role in excitation-contraction coupling by promoting Ca^{2+} release. Nelson suggested that human MHS muscle may have a defect in the ryanodine-sensitive Ca^{2+} release channel.[79] Halothane causes inactive Ca^{2+} channels to open, leads to an increase in channel conductance, and effects the activation and inactivation process of the Ca^{2+} release from MHS muscle. Further investigations are evaluating the ryanodine receptor (via antibody-specific proteins) and its relationship to Ca^{2+} release in MHS muscle. If this work bears fruit, a serum test for MHS may be possible.

TABLE 49–19. Suggested Therapy for Masseter Muscle Rigidity

1. Stop triggering agents.
2. Abort the procedure if elective (most conservative approach).
3. Ventilate with high-flow 100% oxygen, switch to a clean machine or Mapleson system.
   Emergency case: Hyperventilate, use a clean machine, alert for assistance.
4. Monitor vital signs, capnography, core temperature; check venous and arterial blood gases; baseline creatine kinase, electrolytes, calcium, lactate, blood urea nitrogen, creatinine; urine for myoglobin, color.
5. If stable, hold dantrolene and observe in controlled setting (postanesthesia care unit, minimum of 4 h).
   Emergency case: Consider dantrolene to control a potential malignant hyperthermia crisis triggered by the emergency situation.
6. Give liberal fluids to force diuresis; creatine kinase determinations at 6, 12, 24 h. Additional laboratory studies as indicated.
7. Advise family counseling (noncontroversial), muscle biopsy (controversial).

What Genetic Factors Influence the Occurrence of Malignant Hyperthermia?

Initial genetic testing in swine with MHS showed an autosomal dominant pattern of inheritance. Subsequent studies have suggested other patterns as well. McPherson and Taylor believed that an autosomal dominant pattern was the most typical pattern present in 93 families with MH. An example of an MH-susceptible family tree is presented in Figure 49–4. It seems appropriate to assume that 50% of offspring of an individual with MHS are at risk. Relatives of individuals with MHS and elevated serum CK levels have a >70% chance of being at risk.[80] Remember that baseline CK levels may be of no predictive value, and likewise, offspring with normal levels may still be at risk for MH.

Ongoing research efforts are concentrating on the possibility that MH is caused by different genes in different families. Two possible gene candidates are the ryanodine receptor and the hormone-sensitive lipase. Determination of the genetic mechanisms of regulation will provide further knowledge about MH and its link to familial transmission and muscle development.

What Guidance and Counseling Are Available?

The MHAUS and its counterpart in Canada are dedicated to the control of MH via several services available to families and physician caregivers. Ongoing education for physicians and patients and their families is a prime objective, as are encouragement of MH research and emotional support and guidance for affected families. A hot line is available to physicians who desire expert advice concerning their urgent MH needs (tel.: [209] 634-4917, ask for Index Zero; mailing address: MHAUS, P.O. Box 3231, Darien, CT 06820). Physicians are encouraged to report MH cases, suspected or otherwise, to the North American MH Registry, Pennsylvania State University, Department of Anesthesia, Hershey, PA 17033-0850 (tel.: [717] 513-6936).

An MH susceptible family tree might look something like this:

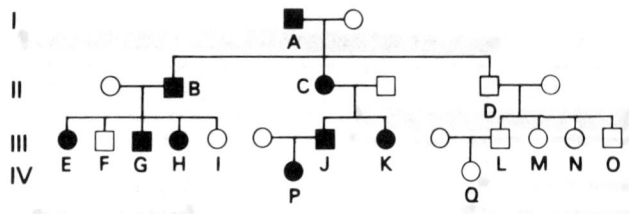

■ affected male
● affected female
□ unaffected male
○ unaffected female

FIGURE 49–4. The father (A) in generation I is MH-susceptible. He passes the MH gene to his oldest son (B), who then transmits MH to three of his five children (E, G, and H). The father (A) also transmitted the MH gene to his daughter (C), who bore two children (J and K), both of whom were MH-susceptible. The younger son (D) did not inherit the MH gene, so his children (L, M, N, and O) are unaffected as is his granddaughter (Q).

What Is the Basis of Contracture Testing?

The currently accepted standard for muscle contracture testing was suggested by Kalow and colleagues in 1970, when they noted that muscle from patients who had MHS and were exposed to caffeine responded abnormally.[81] Soon thereafter, other groups demonstrated similar striated muscle response abnormalities on exposure to halothane.

Methodology

One group of four to eight strips of muscle with intact fascicles of appropriate length and weight, according to protocol typically from the vastus lateralis group, is exposed to 3% halothane, and a second group is exposed to incremental caffeine concentration (hence the term *caffeine halothane contracture test* [CHCT]). A positive test for MHS occurs when at least one of the muscle strips undergoes contracture, thus generating a force greater than or equal to set protocol values (i.e., halothane, 0.7 g within a 5-min exposure).

Sensitivity and Specificity

Dantrolene can alter the muscle response to contracture testing and should not be given, if possible, when a biopsy specimen is obtained in a high-risk individual. The sensitivity of the threshold values currently accepted by the North American MH registry is >90% (frequency of true results in true positives), and the specificity (frequency of negative results in true negatives) is >70%.[82] False-positive results due to unusually cautious readings are difficult to follow up, discover, or disprove, because these patients most likely will never be exposed to triggering anesthetics.

Some myopathies express positive contracture test results with no direct relationship to MH.[83] A patient's true susceptibility is difficult to ascertain in such cases. To date, no patients with false-negative results have been reported to have experienced MH. Continued data collection could uncover a falsely negative group of patients; an improved specificity rating of the CHCT will become known as these patients undergo exposure to triggering agents. Additionally, continued data collection from high-risk subjects may allow further refinement in CHCT guidelines and testing thresholds to increase the sensitivity toward 100% and improve specificity.[82]

Are Other Tests Useful in Predicting Malignant Hyperthermia Susceptibility?

Many tests have been suggested, tested, and ultimately discredited for human use, including phosphorylase ratio, platelet adenosine triphosphate depletion, thin-strip muscle Ca^{2+} uptake, assay of glutathione peroxidase, hypotonic red blood cell lysis, and abnormal protein in MH muscle.[84] More recent testing protocols for MH include a monocyte-Ca^{2+} release test, intracellular inorganic phosphate-to-phosphocreatine ratio measured by magnetic resonance imaging, and measured intracellular Ca^{2+} concentrations.[85] These tests need further evaluation to confirm or disclaim their applicability. The ideal test should be easily reproducible, inexpensive, noninvasive, highly reliable, and available at most large hospitals.

When Should Muscle Biopsy Be Recommended?

Ideally, all patients who have had a MH or MH-like experience, those with an episode of MMR, and those siblings and offspring of MH-positive patients or patients with MMR should be tested. Considering that only 13 centers are accredited in the United States and that the logistics and expenses involved in travel and medical care are extreme, most patients will not undergo testing. Physicians should be cognizant and compassionate toward those many patients and their families who have emotional and financial difficulties when a family member is labeled MH positive.

The very least that should be offered to patients and their families is referral to MHAUS for educational purposes. Relatives must be informed of the implications and risks as well. They then should communicate this potential risk with a medical bracelet, a physician's letter carried on their person, or an explanatory notation in their medical record. Testing should be performed on any person who will be reassured by it, as well as on anyone who is denied insurance, employment, or other benefits on the basis of suspected but not biopsy-proven MH.

References

1. Sessler DI, Moayeri A: Skin-surface warming: heat flux and central temperature. Anesthesiology 1990; 73:218.
2. Sessler DI, Olofsson CI, Rubinstein EH, et al: The thermoregulatory threshold in humans during halothane anesthesia. Anesthesiology 1988; 68:836.
3. Sessler DI, Olofsson CI, Rubinstein EH: Active thermoregulation during isoflurane anesthesia (Abstract). Anesthesiology 1987; 67:A405.
4. Sessler DI, Olofsson CI, Rubinstein EH: The thermoregulatory threshold in humans during nitrous oxide-fentanyl anesthesia. Anesthesiology 1988; 69:357.
5. Sessler DI, Ponte J: Disparity between thermal comfort and physiological thermoregulatory responses during epidural anesthesia (Abstract). Anesthesiology 1989; 71:A682.
6. Sessler DI, Rubinstein EH, Eger EI II: Core temperature changes during N_2O fentanyl and halothane/O_2 anesthesia. Anesthesiology 1987; 67:137.
7. Sessler DI, Stoen R, Glosten B: Thermoregulatory vasoconstriction significantly decreases heat loss to the environment (Abstract). Anesth Analg 1990; 70:S362.
8. Sessler DI: Temperature monitoring. In Anesthesia, 3rd ed. Miller RD (ed). New York, Churchill Livingstone, 1990, p 1228.
9. Sessler DI, Moayeri A, Stoen R, et al: Thermoregulatory vasoconstriction decreases heat loss. Anesthesiology 1990; 75:656.
10. Bissonnette B: Body temperature and anesthesia. Anesth Clin North Am 1991; 19:849.
11. Sessler DI, McGuire F, Moayeri A, et al: Isoflurane-induced vasodilation minimally increases cutaneous heat loss. Anesthesiology 1991; 74:226.
12. Hynson JM, Sessler DI, Glosten BI, et al: Thermal balance and tremor patterns during epidural anesthesia. Anesthesiology 1991; 74:680.
13. Ponte J, Sessler DI: Extradurals and shivering. Br J Anaesth 1990; 64:731.
14. Walmsley AJ, Giesecke AH, Lipton JM: Centrilation of extradural temperature to shivering during extradural anaesthesia. Br J Anaesth 1986; 58:1130.
15. Sevarine F, Johnson M, Lima M, et al: Effect of epidural sufentanyl on shivering and body temperature in the parturient. Anesth Analg 1989; 68:530.
16. Conahan TJ, Williams CD, Apfelbaum JL: Airway heating reduces recovery room time (cost) in outpatients. Anesthesiology 1987; 67:128.
17. Rome CF, Goldberger MJ, Blair CS, et al: Influence of body temperature on early postoperative oxygen consumption. Surgery 1966; 60:85.
18. Thames: Platelet function during and after deep surface hypothermia. J Surg Res 1981; 31:314.
19. Valeri R, Casidy G, Shabri K, et al: Hypothermia-induced platelet dysfunction. Ann Surg 1987; 205:175.
20. Sessler DI, Israel D, Pozoo RS: Spontaneous post anesthesia tremor does not resemble thermoregulatory shivering. Anesthesiology 1988; 68:843.
21. Sessler DI, Rubenstein EH, Moayeri AM: Physiologic response to mild perianesthetic hypothermia in humans. Anesthesiology 1991; 75:594.
22. Lilly RB: Significance and recovery room management of post anesthesia hypothermia and shivering. Anesthesiol Clin North Am 1990; 18:373.
23. Sladen R: Temperature changes and ventilation after hypothermic cardiopulmonary bypass. Anesth Analg 1983; 62:283.
24. Sladen R, Renaghan RRT, Ashton JP, et al: Effect of shivering on mechanical ventilation. Anesthesiology 1985; 63:A140.
25. Guffin A, Girad D, Kaplan J: Shivering following cardiac surgery—hemodynamic changes and reversal. J Cardiothorac Anesth 1987; 1:24.
26. Joachinsson PO, Nystrom SO, Tyden H: Extended rewarming during cardiopulmonary bypass. Acta Anaesthesiol Scand 1987; 31:543.
27. Holtzclaw BJ, Green RT: Shivering after heart surgery: assessment of metabolic effects. Anesthesiology 1986; 65:A18.
28. Sessler DI, McGuire J, Sessler AM: Perioperative thermal insulation. Anesthesiology 1991; 74:875.
29. Tollofsrod SC, Andersen Y, Andersen N: Perioperative hypothermia. Acta Anaesthesiol Scand 1984; 28:511.
30. Stone DR, Downs JB, Paul WL, et al: Adult body temperature and heated humidification. Anesth Analg 1981; 60:736.
31. Pflug AE, Aasheim GM, Foster C, et al: Prevention of post anesthesia shivering. Can Anaesth Soc J 1978; 25:43.
32. Sessler DI: Temperature regulation and anesthesia. ASA 1991 Annual Refresher Course Lecture Series. Park Ridge, IL, 1991.
33. Sessler DI, Moayeri A: Skin surface warming, heat flux and control of temperature. Anesthesiology 1990; 73:218.
34. Murphy MT, Lipton JM, Longhron MB, et al: Post anesthesia shivering in primates: inhibition by peripheral heating. Anesthesiology 1985; 63:161.
35. Sharkey A, Lipton JM, Murphy MT: Inhibition of post anesthetic shivering with radiant heat. Anesthesiology 1987; 66:249.
36. Lennon RL, Hosking MP, Conover MA, et al: Evaluation of forced hot air systems for rewarming hypothermic post operative patients. Anesth Analg 1990; 70:424.
37. Mort TC, Rintel TD, Altman MD: Shivering in the cardiac patient: evaluation of the Bair Hugger. Anesthesiology 1990; 73:A239.
38. Sessler DI, Moayeri A: Skin surface warming, heat flux and control of temperature. Anesthesiology 1990; 73:218.
39. Oquna JM: A study of patient's temperature. AORN J 1978; 28:240.
40. Pauca AL, Savage RT, Simpson S, et al: Effect of pethedine, morphine and fentanyl on post operative shivering in man. Acta Anaesthesiol Scand 1984; 28:138.
41. Kluger MJ, Kauffman CA: Biologic mechanisms of fever. In FUO, Fever of Undetermined Origin. Murray H (ed). Mt Kisco, NY, Futura Publishing, 1983, pp 1–35.
42. Issac B, Kernbaum S, Burke M: Pathophysiology of fever. In Unexplained Fever. Boca Raton, FL, CRC Press, 1991, pp 23–45.
43. Bennett MH, Wainwright AP: Acute thyroid crisis on induction of anaesthesia. Anaesthesia 1989; 44:28.
44. Stevens JJ: A case of thyrotoxic crisis that mimicked malignant hyperthermia. Anesthesiology 1983; 59:263.
45. Allen GC, Rosenberg H: Pheochromocytoma presenting as acute malignant hyperthermia—a diagnostic challenge. Can J Anaesth 1990; 37:593.
46. Stoelting R, Dierdorf S, McCammon R: Transfusion therapy. In Anesthesia and Coexisting Disease. 2nd ed. Stoelting RK, Dierdorf SF, McCammon RL (eds). New York, Churchill Livingstone, 1988, pp 602–603.
47. Brownell AKW: Malignant hyperthermia: relationship to other diseases. Br J Anaesth 1988; 60:303.
48. Hermesh H, Aizenberg D, Lapidor M: The relationship between malignant hyperthermia and neuroleptic malignant syndrome. Anesthesiology 1989; 70:171.
49. Geiduschek J, Cohen S, Kahn A, et al: Repeat anesthesia for a patient with neuroleptic malignant syndrome. Anesthesiology 1988; 68:134.
50. Torline R: Extreme hyperpyrexia associate with central anticholinergic syndrome. Anesthesiology 1992; 76:470.
51. Denborough MA, Lovell RRH: Anesthetic deaths in a family. Lancet 1960; 2:45.
52. Gronert GA, Schulman SR, Mott J: Malignant hyperthermia. In Anesthesia. 3rd ed. Miller RD (ed). New York, Churchill Livingstone, 1990, pp 935–956.
53. Britt BA, Locher WG, Kalow W: Hereditary aspects of malignant hyperthermia. Can Anaesth Soc J 1969; 16:89.
54. Ording H: Incidence of malignant hyperthermia in Denmark. Anesth Analg 1985; 64:700.
55. Larach MG, Rosenberg H, Larach DR, et al: Prediction of malignant hyperthermia susceptibility by clinical signs. Anesthesiology 1987; 66:547.

56. Kaplan RF: Hypothermia/hyperthermia. *In* Manual of Complication during Anesthesia. Gravenstein N (ed). Philadelphia, JB Lippincott, 1991, pp 121–150.
57. Ward A, Chaffman MO, Sorkin EM: Dantrolene. Drugs 1986; 32:130.
58. Malignant Hyperthermia Association of the United States: Preventing Malignant Hyperthermia. Darien, CT, MHAUS, 1991.
59. Kolb ME, Horne ML, Martz R: Dantrolene in human malignant hyperthermia. Anesthesiology 1982; 56:254.
60. Brownell AKW: Malignant hyperthermia: relationship to other diseases. Br J Anaesth 1988; 60:303.
61. Wingard DW: Controversies regarding the prophylactic use of dantrolene for malignant hyperthermia. Anesthesiology 1983; 58:489.
62. Flewellen EH, Nelson TE, Jones WP, et al: Dantrolene dose response in awake man: implications for management of malignant hyperthermia. Anesthesiology 1983; 59:275.
63. Allen GC, Cattran CB, Peterson RG: Plasma levels of dantrolene following oral administration in malignant hyperthermia-susceptible patients. Anesthesiology 1988; 69:900.
64. Gronert GA: Puzzles in malignant hyperthermia. Anesthesiology 1981; 54:1.
65. Malignant Hyperthermia Association of the United States: The Specific Treatment for Malignant Hyperthermia. Darien, CT, MHAUS, 1991.
66. Sethna NF, Rockoff MA: Cardiac arrest following inhalation induction of anesthesia in a child with Duchenne's muscular dystrophy. Can Anaesth Soc J 1986; 33:799.
67. Smith RJ: Preoperative assessment of risk factors. Br J Anaesth 1988; 60:317.
68. Ording H: Diagnosis of susceptibility to malignant hyperthermia in man. Br J Anaesth 1988; 60:287.
69. Ranklev E, Henriksson KC, Fletcher R, et al: Clinical and Muscle Biopsy Findings in Relation to Malignant Hyperthermia Susceptibility; Investigation of Malignant Hyperthermia in Sweden. Lund, Sweden, Dept. of Anaesthesiology, University Hospital, 1986, p 109.
70. Berkowitz A, Rosenberg H: Femoral block with mepivacaine for muscle biopsy in malignant hyperthermia patients. Anesthesiology 1985; 62:651.
71. Beebe JJ, Sessler DI: Preparation of anesthesia machines for patients susceptible to malignant hyperthermia. Anesthesiology 1988; 69:395.
72. Ritchie PA, Cheshire MA, Pearch NH: Decontamination of halothane from anaesthetic machines achieved by continuous flushing with oxygen. Br J Anaesth 1988; 60:859.
73. McGraw TT, Keon TP: Malignant hyperthermia and the clean machine. Can J Anaesth 1988; 36:530.
74. Van Der Spek AFL, Fang WB, Ashton-Miller JA et al: The effects of succinylcholine on mouth opening. Anesthesiology 1987; 67:459.
75. Rosenberg H, Fletcher JE: Masseter muscle rigidity and malignant hyperthermia susceptibility. Anesth Analg 1986; 65:161.
76. Flewellen EH, Nelson TE: Masseter spasm induced by succinylcholine in children: contracture testing for malignant hyperthermia: report of six cases. Can J Anaesth 1982; 29:42.
77. Gronert GA: Management of patients in whom trismus occurs following succinylcholine (with reply by Rosenberg H). Anesthesiology 1988; 68:653.
78. Littleford JA, Patel LR, Bose D, et al: Masseter muscle spasm in children: implications of continuing the triggering anesthetic. Anesth Analg 1991; 72:151.
79. Nelson TE: Halothane effects on human malignant hyperthermia skeletal muscle single calcium-release channels in planar lipid bilayers. Anesthesiology 1992; 76:588.
80. McPherson EW, Taylor CA: The genetics of malignant hyperthermia; evidence for heterogenicity. Am J Med Genet 1982; 11:273.
81. Kalow W, Britt BA, Terreau ME, et al: Metabolic error of muscle metabolism after recovery from malignant hyperthermia. Lancet 1970; 2:895.
82. Malignant Hyperthermia Association of the United States: The Communicator. Vol. X, No. 2, March, 1992.
83. Heiman-Patterson TD, Rosenberg H, Fletcher JE, et al: Halothane-caffeine contracture testing in neuromuscular diseases. Muscle Nerve 1988; 1:453.
84. Ording H: Diagnosis of susceptibility to malignant hyperthermia. Br J Anaesth 1988; 60:287.
85. Rosenberg H, Seitman D: Pharmacogenetics. *In* Clinical Anesthesia. Barash PG, Cullen BF, Stoelting RK (eds). Philadelphia, JB Lippincott, 1989, pp 459–484.

CHAPTER 50

Cardiopulmonary Resuscitation

RICHARD J. MELKER, M.D., Ph.D.

ROBERT R. KIRBY, M.D.

J. R. MARSHALL, M.D.

Desperate measures have long been used in attempts to restore life to the dead and dying.[1] Early techniques included placing burning materials on the chest and abdomen to restore warmth to a cold body and flagellation with whips or stinging nettles to revive the victim. Carrying the person on the back of a trotting horse or rolling him or her over a barrel was thought to mimic a normal respiratory pattern. Not until the 19th century were true anatomic and physiologic principles incorporated into resuscitative techniques.

GOALS

Cardiopulmonary resuscitation (CPR) is intended to support or restore respiration and, in cardiac arrest, to provide some perfusion of the brain and heart. It consists of basic, intermediate, and advanced life support techniques.

What Is Basic Life Support?

Basic life support (BLS) includes creating a patent airway, using mouth-to-mouth ventilation, and, in the setting of cardiac arrest, performing closed chest cardiac massage. These techniques were introduced in the early 1960s. The ABC steps of CPR—A, *a*irway; B, *b*reathing; and C, *c*irculation—constitute the initial management of unconscious patients. Properly executing these skills in the prescribed sequence is essential.

What Is Intermediate Life Support?

Intermediate life support constitutes a situation in which some adjuncts of advanced life support (ALS) are available but not others. This is frequently the case in prehospital care, when emergency medical service personnel may be trained to ventilate with a bag-valve-mask but not perform tracheal intubation, or they may be trained to use an automatic external defibrillator but not to start intravenous infusions or give drugs.

What Is Advanced Life Support?

ALS, the techniques of which are in a state of constant revision, comprises additional methods of airway management and the prompt diagnosis and, when appropriate, treatment of life-threatening dysrhythmias. Definitive management of these dysrhythmias may require defibrillation, cardioversion, pacemaker insertion, and pharmacologic therapy.

AIRWAY

How Should Support Be Provided?

Patency

After establishing that a patient is unconscious, the rescuer must evaluate airway patency. If possible, the patient should be placed in the supine position, preferably on a firm surface, with the neck slightly flexed at the shoulders and extended at the atlantoaxial joint in the so-called sniffing position (Fig. 50–1). This position can be maintained by placing a towel or roll under the victim's occiput.

Observe the chest and abdomen for signs of spontaneous respiration or evidence of airway obstruction, such as paradoxical movement of the chest and abdomen, intercostal retraction, and absent or noisy upper airway respiratory sounds. The tongue, epiglottis, and soft tissues of the posterior pharynx may completely obstruct the upper airway of an unconscious patient unless the head is maintained in the sniffing position. This simple maneuver, which is often all that is necessary to establish a patent airway, must be executed carefully so that the cervical vertebrae, spinal cord, and nerves are not injured.

When unconscious patients are spontaneously breathing, rolling them on their side into the "recovery position" is now recommended in order to decrease the likelihood of obstruction and aspiration.

Cervical Fractures

If cervical fractures are suspected (i.e., in a trauma victim), the head should not be hyperextended because of an even

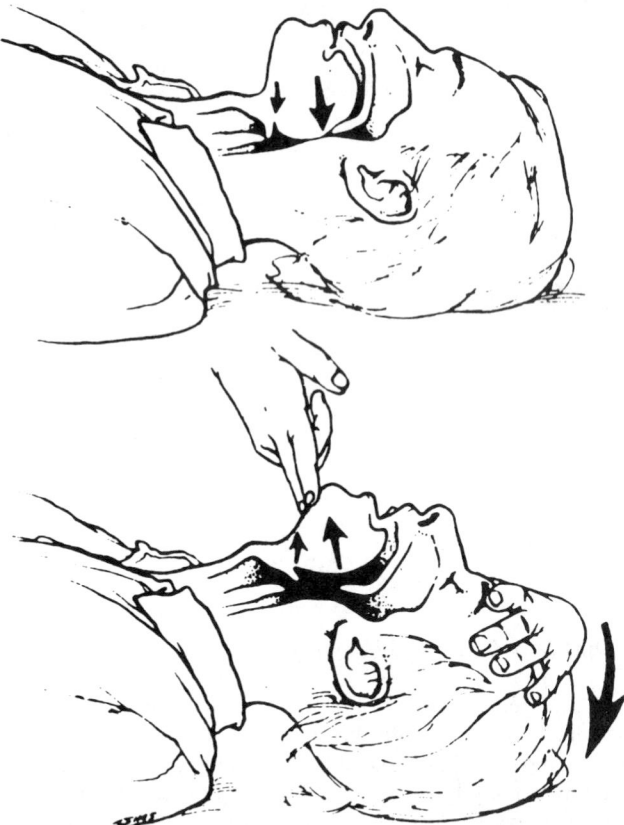

FIGURE 50–1. A patent airway is best created by extending the head and lifting the mandible anteriorly. (Reproduced with permission from Adjuncts for airway control, ventilation, and supplemental oxygen. *In* Textbook of Advanced Cardiac Life Support. 2nd ed., 1987, p 27. © American Heart Association.)

greater chance of damaging the spinal cord. Lifting or thrusting the jaw forward may move the tongue anteriorly and create a patent airway without hyperextension of the head (Fig. 50–2). When the patient's condition allows both maneuvers to be used, however, the combination of jaw lift and hyperextension usually is more successful.

Infants

The upper airway is most patent in infants when the head is maintained in the sniffing position. Hyperextension may collapse the soft trachea, which does not have well-formed rigid cartilaginous rings. Spontaneously breathing unconscious infants and children also can be placed in the recovery position.

What Is the Role for Nasal and Oropharyngeal Airways?

When airway adjuncts are available, additional procedures may be performed if the patient shows signs of airway obstruction despite proper positioning of the head or lifting the jaw. Any obvious foreign materials that obstruct the airway, such as food, vomitus, or a loose dental prosthesis, should be removed. A nasal or oropharyngeal airway may relieve the obstruction caused by soft tissue. Insertion of a nasal airway, however, may traumatize the nasal mucosa and cause bleeding, which exacerbates the existing obstruction.

Semi-conscious patients may tolerate a nasal airway better than an oral airway, which predisposes to gagging and vomiting. On the other hand, an oral airway is probably more effective in unconscious patients. When improperly inserted, however, it can push the tongue back into the pharynx and worsen the airway obstruction.

How Is a Foreign Body Removed?

Since 1976, subdiaphragmatic abdominal thrusts (the Heimlich maneuver) have been recommended to dislodge and expel a foreign body that is not readily visible. Slapping blows with the open palm on the midposterior thorax, which may increase airway pressure enough to dislodge the object, are recommended only in infants. Midsternal chest thrusts, in erect or supine patients, may generate enough expulsive air movement from the chest to expel the foreign body and can be used in pregnant or obese patients or in pediatric patients. Abdominal thrusts should not be used in these patients because they increase the risk of injury to the fetus or the abdominal organs.

After these maneuvers are completed, the mouth should be gently probed for any dislodged materials. A child's mouth should not be probed for foreign objects, because they can easily be forced more deeply into the airway. Instead, the pharynx can be examined if the rescuer places his or her thumb over the child's tongue and lifts the jaw forward. The foreign body, once visualized, should be removed.

BREATHING

In some situations, a patient's life may be saved by simply creating a patent airway. In many cases, however, it is necessary to assist or to control a patient's ventilation. This is the second step in the resuscitation plan.

Is the Victim Apneic?

If a victim is not breathing, give two slow lung inflations (i.e., the inflation takes at least 2 s) of approximately 800 mL

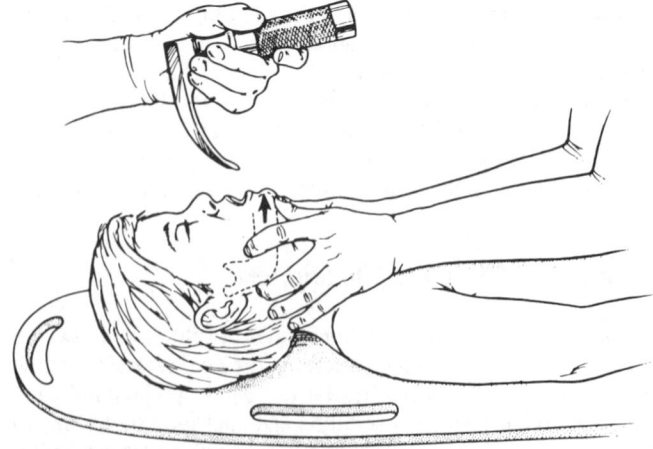

FIGURE 50–2. Cervical spine stabilization and intubation. One person holds the head and neck with both hands, lifting the jaw and immobilizing the neck. The other performs the intubation. (From Emergency Cardiac Care Committee and Subcommittee, American Heart Association: Guidelines for cardiopulmonary resuscitation and emergency cardiac care. VII: Neonatal resuscitation. JAMA 1992; 268:2271.)

with sufficient time for exhalation between breaths. Positive airway pressure increases the chance of gastric inflation in patients with an unprotected airway and greatly increases the incidence of regurgitation and aspiration. One should strive, therefore, to keep it as low as possible by using long inspiratory times. Gastric inflation may also cause restriction of diaphragmatic excursion, and thus ventilation, particularly in infants.

Ventilation should then continue with inflation of the lungs approximately every 5 to 6 seconds (10–12/min) in adults and every 3 seconds (20/min) in infants. Inspiratory time for ventilation in adults should be 1.5 to 2 seconds and in children should be 1 second. The tidal volume recommended for unintubated victims is significantly greater than that used in intubated patients because of the increased dead space produced by dilation of the soft tissues of the mouth and nasopharynx.

What Methods Are Available?

Mouth-to-Mouth

Mouth-to-mouth (or mouth-to-nose) ventilation delivers a fraction of inspired oxygen (FIO_2) of about 0.16; this amount usually is sufficient to maintain a life-sustaining arterial oxygen partial pressure. Nevertheless, supplemental oxygen must be given as soon as possible. The increased pulmonary shunting and ventilation/perfusion ($\dot{V}/\dot{Q}$) mismatching that are common in victims of cardiac arrest greatly reduce oxygenation. The mouth-to-mouth procedure can be used, however, until other ventilatory devices are available.

Mouth-to-Mask

Studies have demonstrated the superiority of mouth-to-mask ventilation over bag-valve-mask ventilation. Most masks are fitted with one-way valves to prevent rebreathing of exhaled gas by the rescuer. Mannequin studies show that all groups of rescuers (emergency medical technicians, paramedics, physicians) deliver higher tidal volume (V_T) with longer inspiratory time (T_I) with masks. A port to deliver supplemental oxygen is also recommended.

These devices are not to be confused with the ubiquitous "face shields," which have not been subjected to careful study and have not been shown to prevent contamination from a victim's secretions.

Bag-Valve-Mask

Many bag-mask devices that deliver a FIO_2 between 0.21 and 1.0 are available. The highest possible FIO_2 should be administered. A patient's head should be maintained in the hyperextended position whenever possible, and the chest observed for adequate lung inflation. If inflation of the stomach is noted, reassessment of airway patency is needed.

Close attention must be paid to positioning the mask properly on a patient's face. A loose-fitting mask may allow air to escape from beneath it, resulting in inadequate ventilation. Mask pressure on a patient's eyes may interrupt adequate blood flow to the eyes and cause retinal detachment.

Bag-mask devices have been evaluated in mannequins and unprotected airway models. They have repeatedly been shown to deliver the lowest tidal volumes and the shortest T_I of all

devices. Whenever possible, they should be used by two rescuers to ensure adequate mask seal, and two hands should squeeze the bag.[2] Additionally, cricoid pressure should be used during ventilation of unintubated patients.

Tracheal Intubation

Tracheal intubation is indicated for patients with an otherwise difficult to manage airway and for patients who remain unconscious. In every case, an attempt should be made to ventilate and oxygenate patients before intubation. After intubation, ventilation and chest compression can be performed independently.

Airway Adjuncts

The esophageal obturator airway (EOA) (Fig. 50–3) and other devices are adjuncts for airway management if tracheal intubation is impossible or the rescuer is not skilled in this technique. These include the esophageal gastric tube airway (EGTA) (Fig. 50–4), the pharyngotracheal lumen airway (PTL), and the esophageal-tracheal double-lumen airway (ETC—the "combitube"). These devices have been classified as IIb by National Institutes of Health (NIH) criteria and are therefore considered to be acceptable and possibly helpful; however, the full extent of complications is not yet known, nor have they been well studied. Tracheal intubation remains the technique of choice for airway control. As much training is needed to properly use alternative adjuncts as to accomplish tracheal intubation.

The Esophageal Obturator Airway

The EOA is a 15-cm flexible tube that resembles an endotracheal tube; its tip is occluded with an obturator (see Fig. 50–3). It is blindly inserted through a patient's mouth into the esophagus. To ensure that the tube is not inadvertently placed in the trachea, the adequacy of breath sounds must be confirmed before the cuff is inflated. The distal cuff is inflated

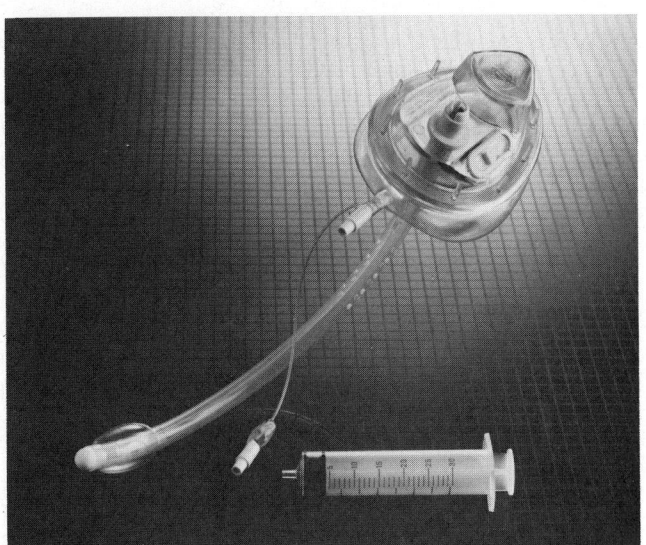

FIGURE 50–3. The esophageal obturator airway facilitates ventilation and prevents regurgitation.

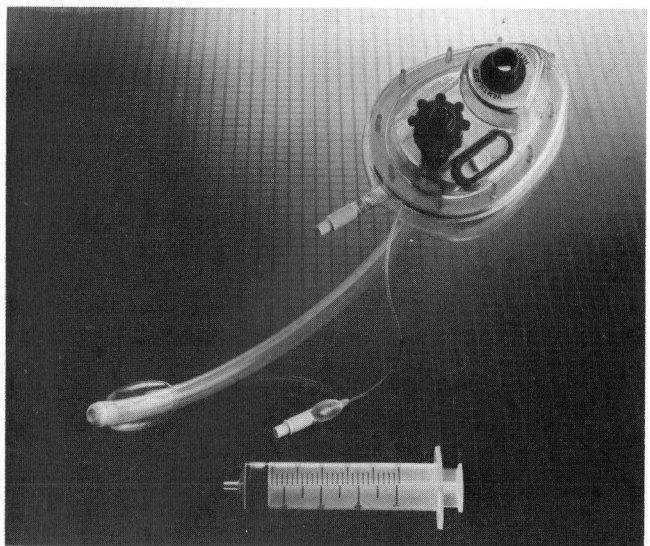

FIGURE 50–4. The esophageal gastric tube airway allows emptying of the stomach.

with approximately 35 mL of air, which both occludes the esophagus and minimizes the risk of regurgitation.[3]

The proximal tip of the tube extends through a face mask that is securely placed over the victim's mouth and nose. Because the tube is occluded at the tip, the inspiratory volume enters the tube at the mask and exits through multiple perforations in the tube wall, which is positioned in a patient's posterior pharynx. If a patient has a patent upper airway with an adequate mask fit and the tube was not inadvertently placed in the trachea, the lungs will be inflated. Careless insertion of the tube may cause esophageal perforation.[4]

This tube should not be used in children younger than 16 years or in patients with known esophageal disease. Inadvertent placement into the trachea is a potentially lethal complication.[5]

The Esophageal Gastric Tube Airway

The EGTA, which is a modification of the EOA, has two separate ports in the mask (see Fig. 50–4).[6] One is used for ventilation, and the other allows direct access to the esophageal tube. Because a separate port in the mask is used for ventilation, perforations in the pharyngeal segment of the tube are not necessary. The distal cuff is inflated. As with the EOA, breath sounds must be confirmed after cuff inflation to verify that the esophagus and not the trachea is obstructed by the tube.

This tube does not have a blind end, so a small nasogastric tube can be inserted through the mask and tube for removing air and liquid from the stomach. Electrodes can also be placed in the tube for transesophageal cardiac monitoring, pacing, and defibrillation.

If a patient requires ventilatory assistance for >2 hours, placement of an endotracheal tube should be attempted. Regurgitation and aspiration can easily occur when the EOA or EGTA is removed. Therefore, the endotracheal tube should be inserted and effective ventilation established before these tubes are removed.

When Are Emergency Surgical Techniques Indicated?

Cricothyroidotomy[7, 8] and transtracheal catheter ventilation[9] may be required in patients who cannot be ventilated with a mask or cannot be intubated, as may occur after face and neck trauma.

Cricothyroidotomy

Cricothyroidotomy is performed by puncturing the cricothyroid membrane with either a cricothyroidotomy blade and tube or a knife blade (Fig. 50–5). A cricothyroidotomy set for the placement of tubes by Seldinger's technique has recently been introduced (Fig. 50–6).[8] Once a tube has been placed through the cricothyroidotomy, a patient should be able to breathe spontaneously or with controlled ventilation through this opening.

Transtracheal Catheter Ventilation

For transtracheal catheter ventilation, a 14-gauge catheter-over-needle is inserted in a caudal direction through the cricothyroid membrane into the larynx.[9, 10] A high-pressure jet of oxygen introduced through this catheter into the trachea inflates the lungs (Fig. 50–7). A high-pressure gas source of at

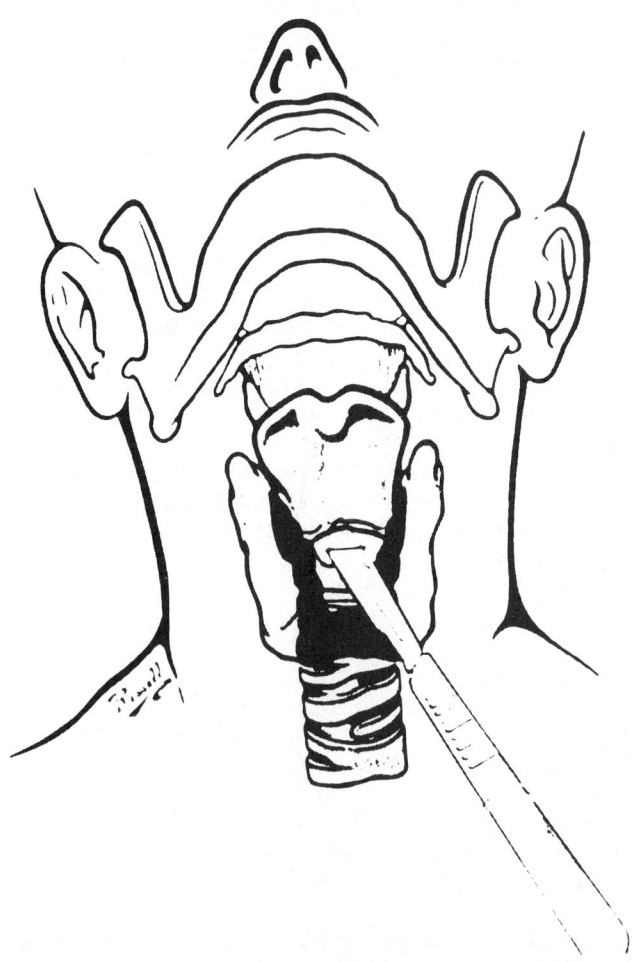

FIGURE 50–5. Cricothyroidotomy can be performed with a scalpel. (Reproduced with permission from Adjuncts for airway control, ventilation, and supplemental oxygen. *In* Textbook of Advanced Cardiac Life Support. 2nd ed., 1987. © American Heart Association.)

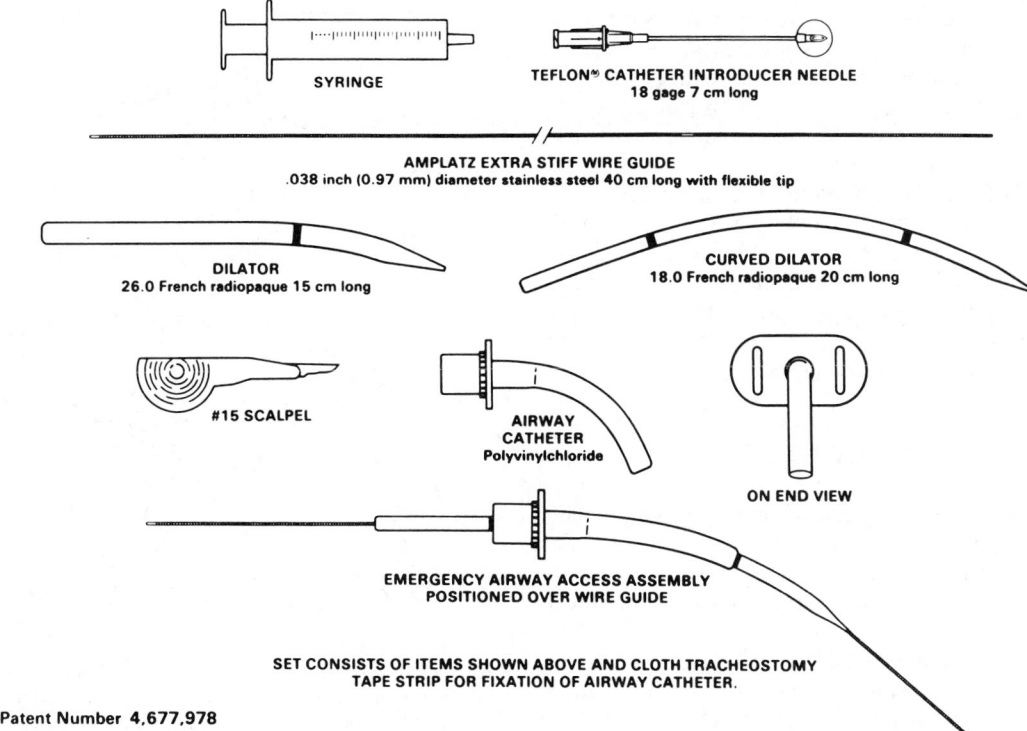

SYRINGE

TEFLON® CATHETER INTRODUCER NEEDLE
18 gage 7 cm long

AMPLATZ EXTRA STIFF WIRE GUIDE
.038 inch (0.97 mm) diameter stainless steel 40 cm long with flexible tip

DILATOR
26.0 French radiopaque 15 cm long

CURVED DILATOR
18.0 French radiopaque 20 cm long

#15 SCALPEL

**AIRWAY
CATHETER**
Polyvinylchloride

ON END VIEW

**EMERGENCY AIRWAY ACCESS ASSEMBLY
POSITIONED OVER WIRE GUIDE**

**SET CONSISTS OF ITEMS SHOWN ABOVE AND CLOTH TRACHEOSTOMY
TAPE STRIP FOR FIXATION OF AIRWAY CATHETER.**

Patent Number 4,677,978

FIGURE 50–6. Melker emergency cricothyrotomy catheter set (courtesy of Cook Critical Care, Bloomington, IN). Airway access is gained by percutaneous entry via the cricothyroid membrane. Subsequently, dilatation of the trachea and tracheal entrance site permits insertion of 6-mm-ID airway. Positive-pressure ventilation and spontaneous breathing are permitted.

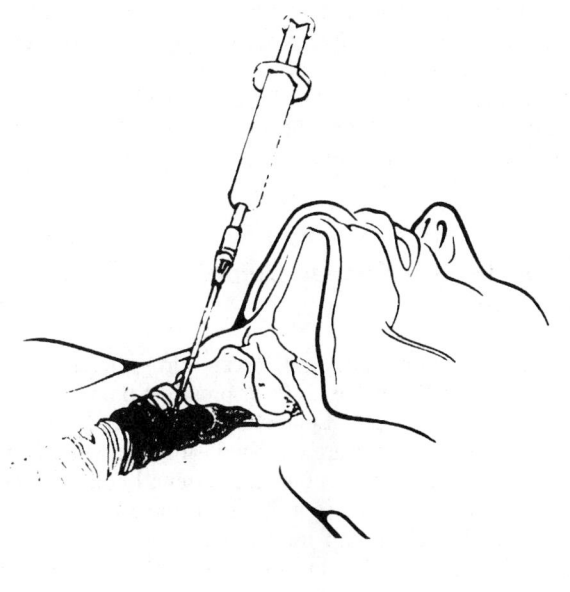

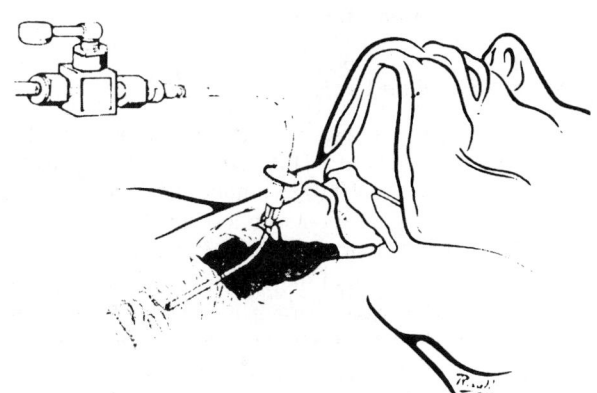

FIGURE 50–7. Ventilation with a transtracheal catheter attached to a high pressure gas source with a valve. (Reproduced with permission from Adjuncts for airway control, ventilation, and supplemental oxygen. Textbook of Advanced Cardiac Life Support. 2nd ed., 1987, p 34. © American Heart Association.)

least 20 pounds per square inch gauge is necessary for this technique to be successful. The pressure generated in the airway with this technique is dissipated (i.e., exhaled) through the glottis and mouth. If upper airway obstruction occludes this escape route, extremely high intrapulmonary pressures with resulting barotrauma can occur.

These procedures can be life saving, but they are not without hazards. They should be used only when other, less traumatic methods are not feasible and should be performed only by trained individuals. Potential complications include hemorrhage, creation of a false passage, subcutaneous or mediastinal emphysema, perforation of the esophagus, infection, pneumothorax, and subsequent tracheal stenosis.

CIRCULATION

If a patient has respiratory arrest only, creating a patent airway for life support or providing adequate ventilation may be all that is necessary. In many situations, though, respiratory arrest occurs in conjunction with cardiac arrest or life-threatening dysrhythmia.

After establishing a patent airway and giving an apneic patient the initial lung inflations, the rescuer should evaluate cardiac function by feeling for a carotid pulse. The carotid pulse can easily be palpated just lateral to the thyroid cartilage. Because of peripheral vasoconstriction associated with a shock state, the radial pulse may be difficult to palpate. The femoral pulse may also be difficult to locate in some patients because of body habitus.

In pediatric patients, the precordial, brachial, or temporal artery pulse may be more easily monitored. If the pulse is absent and the patient is unconscious, external cardiac compression should be initiated. In cases with significant hypovolemia (hemorrhagic shock, and so on), no benefit accrues to Trendelenburg's (head-down) position. Instead, the legs should be elevated to enhance venous return.

How Is Closed Chest Cardiac Massage Performed?

Adults

External cardiac compression is a relatively simple technique that can be performed after appropriate training. However, it may be totally ineffective or even hazardous if performed improperly. After positioning at the side of the patient, the rescuer should place the heel of one hand over the lower half of the sternum approximately 1 to 1.5 inches above the tip of the xiphoid. The heel of the second hand is then placed on top of the first. The arms must be extended with the rescuer's finger tips off the patient's chest. A vertical thrust that displaces an adult's sternum approximately 1.5 to 2 inches should be delivered. Closed cardiac massage must be performed in a regular, deliberate, uninterrupted manner; quick, jabbing thrusts are far less effective.[11]

Infants

In infants, the middle and index finger tips of one hand traditionally were recommended to compress the midsternum a distance of 0.5 to 0.75 inches. Some rescuers prefer to place

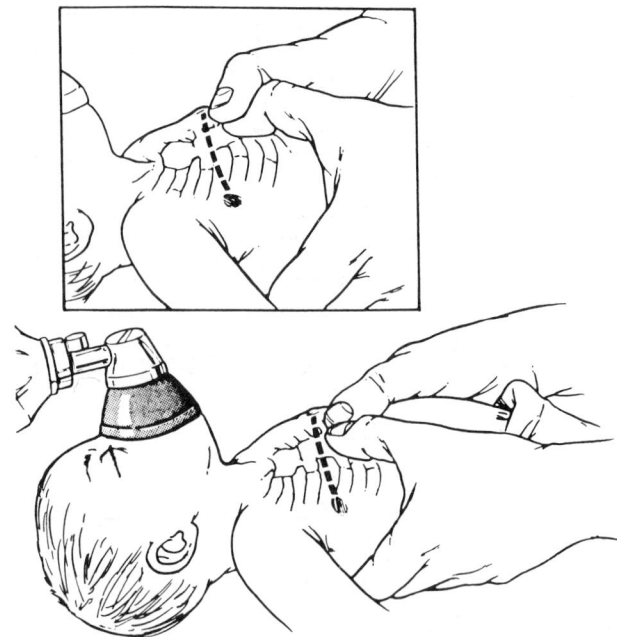

FIGURE 50–8. Method of external cardiac compression in neonates and small infants. (From Emergency Cardiac Care Committee and Subcommittee, American Heart Association. Guidelines for cardiopulmonary resuscitation and emergency cardiac care. VII: Neonatal resuscitation. JAMA 1992; 268:2279. Copyright 1992, American Medical Association.)

their hands around an infant's chest, positioning both thumbs on the midsternum and exerting a vertical thrust with the thumb tips (Fig. 50–8). Although studies suggest that the compression should take place over the distal sternum, as is the case in adult resuscitation,[12] the 1992 standards for infant resuscitation do not recommend this procedure because of potential damage to abdominal organs.[13] In small children, only the heel of one hand is used.

How Effectively Is Cardiac Output Maintained?

Under ideal circumstances of CPR and drug therapy, a cardiac output of approximately 30% of prearrest blood flow can be maintained with effective external compression; therefore, only minimal interruptions are tolerated. Both the compression of the heart between the sternum and vertebral column (chest pump model) and the increase in intrathoracic pressure during compression (thoracic pump model) may cause the forward flow of blood from the chest in some instances; in others, one mechanism or the other predominates.

Compression/Relaxation Cycle

The duration of the compression should be 50% of the compression/relaxation cycle. This ratio is most easily achieved at a rate of 80 to 100 per minute. Maintaining this ratio of compression to relaxation with a manual technique is physically exhausting. A commercially available oxygen-powered automatic compression unit may be more effective and is not subject to human fatigue. These portable units provide effective compressions interposed with appropriate ventilation.[14]

G-Suits

An additional adjunct is the application of a G-suit over the abdominal cavity. It is thought to improve cardiac output by retarding the retrograde movement of blood from the heart into the large venous plexus in the peritoneal cavity during compression.[15] This suit can be used in combination with the automatic compression unit for an even greater improvement in cardiac output, but clinical studies have not shown improved resuscitation success. Intermittent abdominal compression during the relaxation phase of chest compressions has been shown to improve survival compared with standard CPR on in-hospital patients.[16]

Compression Rate

Two Rescuers

If two rescuers are present, one can perform cardiac compressions while the second ventilates the patient. The rate of cardiac compression in this case is 80 to 100 per minute for adults, with a compression-to-ventilation ratio of 5:1. A 1.5- to 2-second pause should be provided for inspiration. Exhalation occurs during chest compression. Simultaneous compression and ventilation previously was evaluated as a means of further increasing cardiac output; it did not improve survival[17] and is not currently recommended.

Although close attention must be paid to both the rate of compression and the ratio of compression to relaxation, the latter probably has a greater influence on cardiac output. The second rescuer must periodically check the carotid pulse to evaluate the effectiveness of the cardiac compressions and to note the return of spontaneous cardiac activity. Bear in mind, however, that a palpable carotid pulse may reflect only external, not internal, carotid artery flow; thus, it does not guarantee effective cerebral circulation.

Single Rescuer

Fifteen chest compressions are performed at a rate of 80 to 100 per minute, followed by two breaths of 1.5 to 2 seconds each. This cycle is repeated four times, followed by reassessment. If CPR is continued, the rescuer should reassess for pulse and spontaneous breathing every few minutes. In infants, compressions are performed at approximately 100 to 120 per minute, with one breath interposed after every fifth compression.

BLS should be continued until the patient has recovered, the rescuers are exhausted, relief rescuers have arrived, or a medical decision to discontinue resuscitative efforts has been made.

Complications

Complications related to closed chest compression are listed in Table 50-1.

How Is the Efficacy of Cardiopulmonary Resuscitation Monitored?

No reliable prognostic indicator exists for the efficacy of ongoing CPR efforts. Experimental studies suggest that aortic diastolic and coronary perfusion pressures correlate with suc-

TABLE 50–1. Complications Associated with Closed Chest Compression

Fracture of the xiphoid and sternum
Costochondral separation
Pneumothorax
Hemothorax
Lung contusion
Laceration of the liver, stomach, heart, and lungs
Fat embolization
Cardiac contusion

cessful resuscitation.[18] These findings have been corroborated in a small number of humans. When arterial catheters are present, the diastolic pressure should be optimized, and in instances in which a pulmonary artery catheter is available, arterial minus right atrial diastolic pressure may be an indicator of CPR efficacy and survival.

Capnography is promising to evaluate blood flow during CPR[19, 20] and for confirming endotracheal tube placement (Fig. 50–9). Unfortunately, many drugs given during resuscitation and a variable minute ventilation, unless a patient is mechanically ventilated, interfere with the interpretation of end-tidal carbon dioxide (CO_2) measurements during CPR. Despite these caveats, a sudden increase in end-tidal CO_2 is generally the earliest sign of return of spontaneous ventilation, unless sodium bicarbonate (see Fig. 50–9) has just been given.[21] Further study is necessary to determine the utility of capnography during CPR.

What Is the Role of the Precordial Thump?

Indications

A precordial thump is most effective when it is performed as soon as possible after the onset of ventricular tachycardia or fibrillation and when the dysrhythmia is not secondary to hypoxia.[22] This technique is used only when the rescuer observes the onset of the dysrhythmia and a defibrillator is not immediately available, as may occur in monitored patients in the operating room, postanesthesia care unit, or intensive care unit or in unmonitored patients who suffer an arrest in the presence of someone who can initiate therapy immediately.

Technique

A precordial thump is performed by delivering a single blow to the midsternum with the fleshy portion of the clenched fist from a distance of 8 to 12 inches. Repeated precordial thumps are not indicated. An effective precordial thump interrupts ventricular tachycardia and ventricular fibrillation by causing ventricular depolarization. The cardiac activity may then return with a coordinated contraction, frequently of supraventricular origin. Performing the thump in a patient with ventricular tachycardia can, unfortunately, also cause conversion to ventricular fibrillation, asystole, or electromechanical dissociation (EMD).

How Is Ventricular Defibrillation Performed?

Defibrillation is most successful when it is performed immediately after the onset of ventricular fibrillation.[23] However,

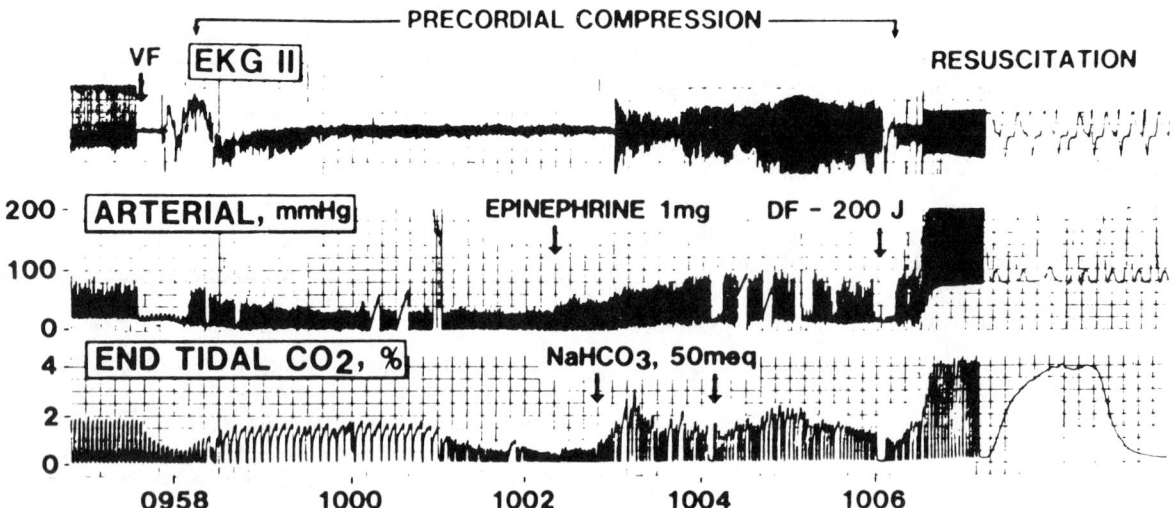

FIGURE 50–9. Serial changes in the end-tidal carbon dioxide concentration (E_{TCO_2}), arterial blood pressure, and ECG in a patient before and immediately after a cardiac arrest, during precordial compression, and after defibrillation (DF) and resuscitation. The transient increase in the E_{TCO_2} after the administration of sodium bicarbonate (NaHCO₃) is also demonstrated. The original tracing has been modified because of space limitations. (Modified from Falk JL, Rackow EC, Weil MH: End-tidal carbon dioxide concentration during cardiopulmonary resuscitation. N Engl J Med 1988; 318:607–611, with permission from The New England Journal of Medicine.)

regardless of the time lapse between the onset of ventricular fibrillation and the initiation of therapy, electrical defibrillation should be performed as soon as possible. If a defibrillator is not available for immediate use, BLS should be instituted until defibrillation can be accomplished. A coarse fibrillation pattern, which is usually of more recent onset, may be more easily corrected than a fine pattern. In many cases, a fine fibrillation pattern can be converted to a coarse pattern with an intravenous injection of epinephrine.

Precautions

Defibrillation is frequently unsuccessful in the anoxic myocardium and may be more effective after the initiation of CPR. This situation often prevails when a patient suffers cardiac arrest outside the hospital or when it is secondary to hypoxia, as may occur in drug overdose, asphyxiation, or near-drowning. Defibrillation also is less successful when it is performed in a patient who is acidotic. However, immediate defibrillation should be attempted in all situations if feasible, even before initiating BLS or administering drugs. Electrical defibrillation is not indicated in the treatment of asystole unless there is uncertainty about whether the rhythm is fine ventricular fibrillation or asystole.[24] More than one electrocardiogram (ECG) lead should be viewed to make this determination.

Technique

Before the paddles are placed on a patient's chest, conductive electrode paste or saline sponges should be applied. Skin impedance is thereby decreased, and the efficiency of current passage through the thorax is increased. The risk of skin burns is also reduced. The electrode paste or saline of one paddle must not come into contact with the conductive material of the other paddle. Otherwise, the amount of current delivered through the myocardium will be reduced and the effectiveness of the defibrillation minimized. The risk of skin burns will also be increased. Alcohol-soaked sponges should never be used as a conductor because the current may cause them to burst into flames.

Paddle Placement

Two 8- to 12-cm-diameter paddles should be placed on the patient's chest, with one paddle to the right of the upper sternum just below the clavicle and the other to the left of the left nipple in the midaxillary line.[25] If the design of the paddles permits, one may be placed anteriorly over the heart and the other posteriorly.[25, 26] This positioning is preferred by some rescuers, but it is not practical in most emergencies. The paddles should be firmly placed against the patient's skin, using an estimated 20 to 25 lb of pressure on each. Smaller paddles should be used in pediatric patients—4.5 cm diameter for infants and 8.0 cm for older children.

Energy Level

The initial defibrillation should be attempted with 200 J of delivered energy.[27] If unsuccessful, a second shock at 200 to 300 J should be attempted immediately. Because the transthoracic resistance is decreased by the first defibrillation attempt, a greater amount of energy is transmitted to the heart during the second attempt, even if the energy level is not increased.[28] If unsuccessful, a third attempt at 360 J is performed (Fig. 50–10).

If a third attempt also is unsuccessful, BLS should be initiated. After the administration of epinephrine, a fourth attempt at 360 J is indicated. If it, too, is unsuccessful, intravenous administration of lidocaine or bretylium or both may terminate the fibrillation or allow subsequent defibrillation attempts to be successful (see Fig. 50–10). For patients who weigh <50 kg, the initial attempt should be with 2 J · kg⁻¹ and should be doubled if the first attempt is unsuccessful.[28]

During open chest defibrillation in adults (such as during cardiac surgery), defibrillation should be attempted with 10 J of delivered energy through paddles specifically designed for internal use.[30] The energy may be increased stepwise, if necessary.

Complications

Damage to the myocardium is related to the following factors:

VENTRICULAR FIBRILLATION

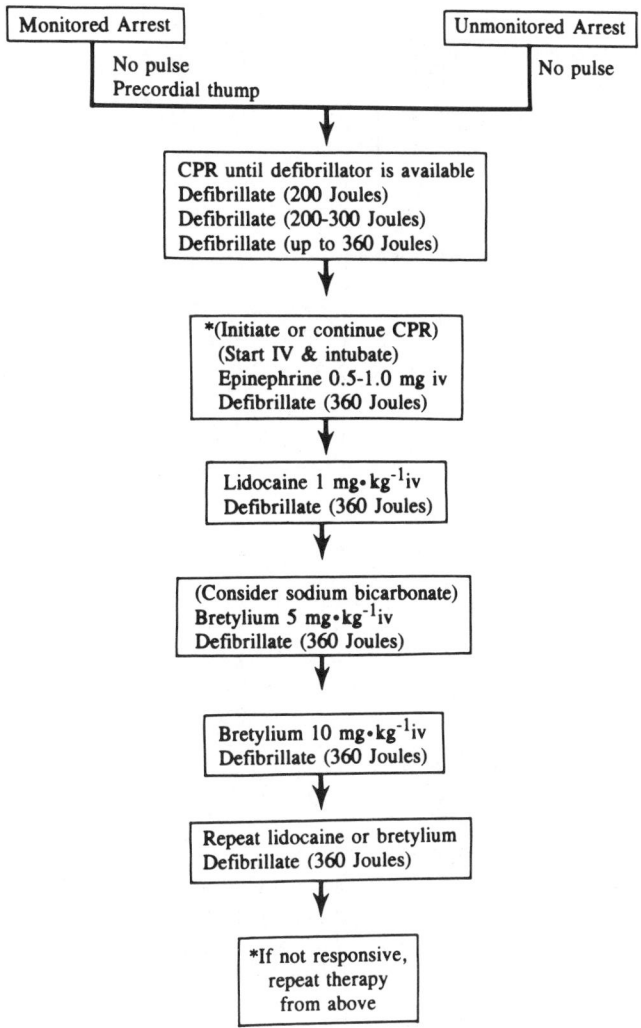

FIGURE 50–10. Algorithm for treatment of ventricular fibrillation or pulseless ventricular tachycardia.

1. *Energy level.* The higher the energy level, the greater the potential for myocardial damage. Delivered energy may not be the same as the energy level selected on the defibrillator dials, however. Because internal energy loss may occur in the machine, all defibrillators must be tested periodically for the amount of energy actually delivered through a 50-ohm resistance (the approximate resistance of the body).

2. *Frequency of shocks.* Multiple defibrillation attempts in quick succession may be associated with a higher incidence of myocardial damage.

3. *Electrode paddle size.* Large paddles are associated with less myocardial and skin damage than small paddles. Internal paddles, which have a small surface area, should never be used for external defibrillation.

When Is Electrical Cardioversion Performed?

Indications

Electrical cardioversion rather than pharmacologic therapy may be the treatment of choice for life-threatening dysrhyth-mias causing rapid cardiovascular deterioration. These include ventricular tachycardia (Fig. 50–11) and supraventricular tachycardias (i.e., paroxysmal atrial tachycardia [PAT], atrial flutter, or atrial fibrillation with a rapid ventricular response).

Technique

Unlike defibrillation, cardioversion must be synchronized with the patient's ECG. The ideal discharge point is during the upstroke of the R wave of the QRS. Delivery of the energy during the T wave of the QRS may result in ventricular fibrillation. Most commercially available defibrillators automatically coordinate the discharge to the patient's ECG if the machine is placed in the synchronized mode and if the QRS complex is of adequate size. If the defibrillator does not "sense" the QRS complex, the ECG gain should be increased so that the sensing algorithm functions. Cardioversion should never be attempted with "quick-look" paddles, because ECG artifact may make synchronization impossible. Unsynchronized cardioversion should only be used when the equipment at hand does not allow synchronization.

Energy Level

The amount of energy recommended for emergency cardioversion varies with the rhythm.[28, 31] An initial energy of 100 J is recommended for atrial fibrillation, and 50 J for atrial flutter.[32] Monomorphic ventricular tachycardia responds well to cardioversion, and 100 J should be attempted first. Polymorphic ventricular tachycardia behaves like ventricular fibrillation, and 200 J should be used initially (see Fig. 50–11). For cardioversion in conscious patients, sedation with intravenous diazepam or midazolam, or methohexital, is indicated, and the cardioversion accomplished with the lowest energy possible (50 and 200 J).

How Is Pulseless Electrical Activity Managed?

The treatment of pulseless electrical activity (including EMD) is outlined in Table 50–2.

How Is Bradycardia Managed?

Treatment of bradycardia is summarized in Table 50–3.

PHARMACOLOGIC THERAPY

What Is the New Role for Epinephrine?

Mechanism of Action

The pharmacologic actions of epinephrine are complex, because this drug has both α- and β-stimulating properties. The primary cardiovascular effect mediated through stimulation of the α_1-receptors is peripheral vasoconstriction, which increases systemic vascular resistance (SVR). Stimulation of β-receptors increases heart rate and myocardial contractile force.

A combination of increased contractile force, increased rate, and increased SVR increases blood pressure, cardiac output, and work of the heart. Most importantly, large doses of epinephrine promote cerebral perfusion more effectively than any

VENTRICULAR TACHYCARDIA

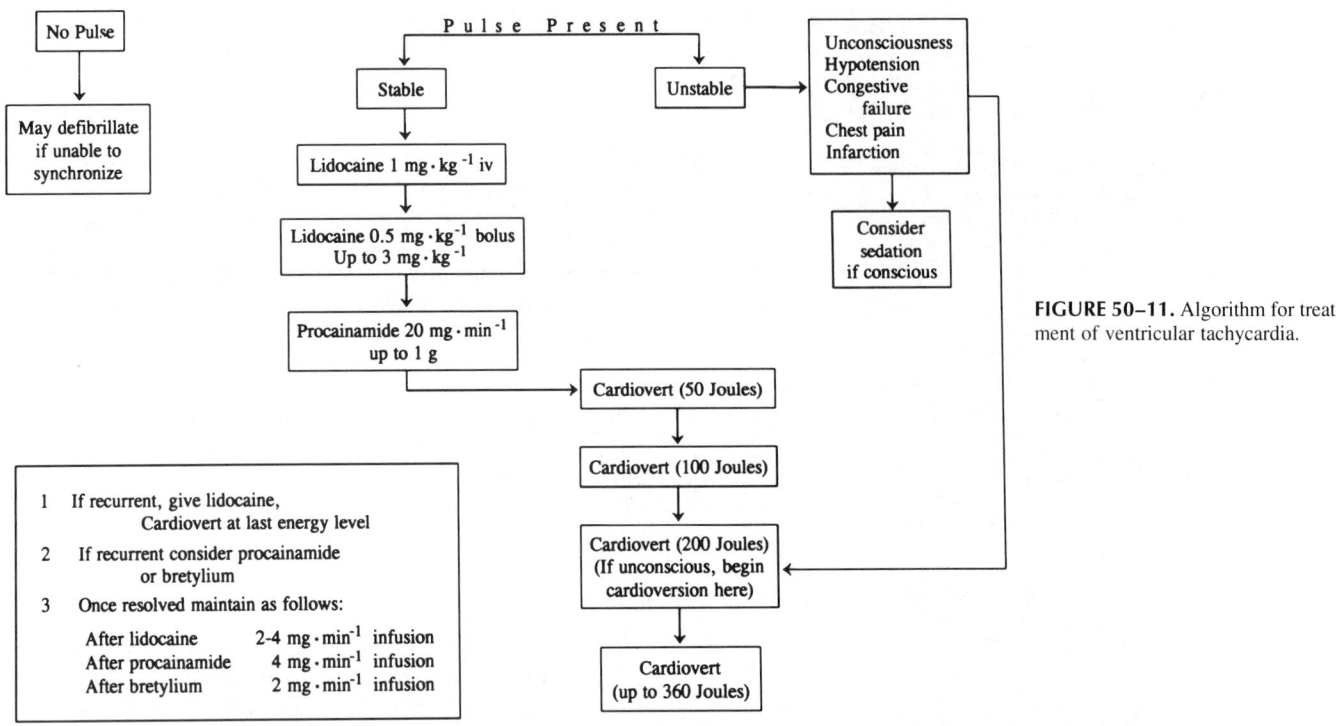

FIGURE 50–11. Algorithm for treatment of ventricular tachycardia.

other drug and are particularly useful to increase internal carotid artery blood flow.[33] Epinephrine increases myocardial irritability and automaticity and may initiate rhythms originating from various ectopic foci, especially the ventricles.

Indications

Pulseless Electrical Activity (Electromechanical Dissociation)

Epinephrine effectively improves cardiac output in a failing myocardium. Such is the case in patients with pulseless electrical activity due to poor cardiac output (see Table 50–2). In these patients, even though the ECG may appear normal, ventricular contractility is so impaired that a patient is without an effective pulse or blood pressure.

TABLE 50–2. Pulseless Electrical Activity

- Establish unresponsiveness, apnea, pulselessness.
- Initiate CPR: Intubate, deliver 100% oxygen, start IV, epinephrine 1 mg IV or 2.5 mg via endotracheal tube. (Consider bicarbonate and calcium chloride, but not via endotracheal tube.)
- Continue CPR (consider volume infusion).
- Consider cause secondary to hypovolemia, cardiac tamponade, tension pneumothorax, cardiac rupture, pulmonary embolism, hypoxemia, or acidosis.
- Repeat epinephrine, 1 mg ever 3–5 min.*
- If absolute bradycardia (<60 beats per minute), give atropine, 1.0 mg IV; repeat every 3–5 min up to 0.04 mg · kg⁻¹.

*If this approach fails, epinephrine in escalating doses (1–3–5 mg IV, 3 min apart); intermediate doses (2–5 mg IV every 3–5 min); or high doses (0.1 mg · kg⁻¹ IV every 3–5 min) may be used.
Abbreviations: CPR = cardiopulmonary resuscitation; IV = intravenous(ly).

Cardiac Standstill

Epinephrine's ability to increase automaticity is useful when one attempts to convert cardiac standstill to spontaneous contractions (Table 50–4). Even though the rhythm it produces may be another life-threatening dysrhythmia (which can be treated appropriately), the alternative (a dead heart) is less acceptable.

Fine Ventricular Fibrillation

Epinephrine, as noted previously, also may be useful in converting a fine ventricular fibrillation pattern to a coarse

TABLE 50–3. Treatment of Bradycardia: Absolute (<60 Beats Per Minute) or Relative

Serious Signs and Symptoms	
Chest pain	
Shortness of breath	
Decreased consciousness	
Shock	
Pulmonary congestion	

No	Yes
Type II second-degree block or third-degree block: Prepare for transvenous pacer; use transcutaneous pacer as bridge	1. Atropine, 0.5 to 1.0 mg every 3–5 min up to 0.04 mg · kg⁻¹* 2. Transcutaneous pacer if available 3. Dopamine, 5–20 µg · kg⁻¹ 4. Epinephrine, 2–10 µg · min⁻¹ 5. Isoproterenol (use with caution if at all; at high doses it is harmful)

*Atropine should be used with caution in type II second-degree atrioventricular block and new third-degree block with wide QRS complexes.

TABLE 50–4. Treatment of Cardiac Standstill

- Establish unresponsiveness, apnea, and pulselessness, initiate CPR.
- Contine CPR, intubate, deliver 100% oxygen. Start IV, epinephrine, 1 mg IV or 2.5 mg by endotracheal tube.
- Continue CPR, atropine 1 mg IV.
- Continue CPR, atropine 1 mg IV (consider sodium bicarbonate, 1 mEq · kg^{-1} IV)
- Continue CPR, consider transvenous pacer, consider that rhythm may be fine ventricular fibrillation, which may respond to defibrillation.
- Repeat epinephrine 1 mg IV every 3–5 min.

Abbreviations: CPR = cardiopulmonary resuscitation; IV = intravenous(ly).

pattern, which is more responsive to electrical defibrillation. This effect may be less significant than originally thought. The exact mechanism of this change in rhythm is not known.

Recommended Dosage

The recommended dose of epinephrine until 1992 was 0.5 to 1 mg (5–10 mL of a 1:10,000 solution) intravenously or 10 mL (1 mg) intratracheally. Because of the drug's short duration of action, this dose was administered as often as every 5 minutes, and a continuous infusion of 0.04 μg · kg^{-1} · min^{-1} used to sustain improved contractility in some patients.

The new guidelines recommend an epinephrine dose of 1.0 mg (10 mL of a 1:10,000 solution) every 3 to 5 minutes.[34] Each peripheral injection should be followed by a 20-mL flush of intravenous fluid to ensure that it is delivered to the central circulation. Studies suggest that an even higher dose of epinephrine is needed for tracheal administration. Although the optimal dose is unknown, it is at least 2.5 times greater than the intravenous dose. The dose should be drawn up from a 1:1000 solution, diluted to 10 mL with sterile water, and administered by a catheter to the tip of the endotracheal tube.

Preliminary results from unpublished studies using high-dose epinephrine (0.07–0.2 mg · kg^{-1}) on more than 2400 patients in cardiac arrest are disappointing. They show no statistically significant difference in survival compared with patients treated with standard doses of epinephrine. Thus, higher doses of epinephrine should be considered a class IIb recommendation (i.e., they are acceptable but are neither recommended or discouraged) and should be used at the discretion of the physician.[34]

Route of Administration

Epinephrine is best administered through a central venous catheter. It may be given into the tracheobronchial tree through an endotracheal tube if an intravenous route is not available, but this is not nearly as efficient and requires 2.5–10 times the intravenous dose. If the endotracheal route is used, peripheral bronchial administration via a catheter is much more efficient

TABLE 50–5. Hazards of Intracardiac Epinephrine Injection

Interruption of cardiac compression and ventilation
Pneumothorax
Coronary artery laceration
Cardiac tamponade
Intramyocardial injection and intractable ventricular fibrillation

than endotracheal.[35] An intracardiac injection of epinephrine may be indicated in a patient in asystole who is unresponsive to intravenous or endotracheal administration. However, the needle piercing the myocardium may be more of a cardiac stimulant than the epinephrine itself. Possible hazards of this route of administration are listed in Table 50–5.

Should Sodium Bicarbonate Be Used?

Both respiratory and metabolic acidosis usually develop during cardiac arrest. All patients maintained with external cardiac compression have decreased tissue perfusion and tissue hypoxia. Lactic acid is generated through anaerobic metabolism, producing metabolic acidosis. At the same time, inadequate ventilation, as well as the administration of sodium bicarbonate, which causes the release of >1 L of CO_2 per 50 mEq sodium bicarbonate, leads to hypercarbia and respiratory acidosis. Respiratory acidosis is best treated through improved ventilation by reducing CO_2; metabolic acidosis is best managed by a combination of bicarbonate administration, if the arterial pH is <7.10, and hyperventilation.

An elevated CO_2 probably is more detrimental to myocardial performance than is metabolic acidosis. Because CO_2 diffuses readily, it enters the myocardial cells rapidly; intracellular acidosis quickly develops, causing life-threatening derangements of myocardial function. Likewise, cerebrospinal fluid acidosis may occur secondary to the diffusion of CO_2 across the blood-brain barrier, producing postarrest cerebral acidosis. Therefore, administration of sodium bicarbonate without sufficient ventilation and circulation to remove the CO_2 that it produces is more detrimental than helpful.[36]

Mechanism of Action

Administration of sodium bicarbonate results in a simple acid-base reaction:

$$H^+ + HCO_3^- \rightleftarrows H_2CO_3 \rightleftarrows H_2O + CO_2$$

The carbonic acid dissociates into water and CO_2, which is eliminated through the lungs, thereby elevating the pH of the blood and surrounding tissues. However, if ventilation is marginal and widespread ventilation/perfusion ($\dot{V}/\dot{Q}$) abnormalities are present, as is usually the case during resuscitation efforts, the CO_2 cannot be eliminated and increases to as much as 300 to 400 mm Hg in the mixed venous blood and the myocardial cells. Profound intramyocardial acidosis then develops.

Indications

Untreated acidosis causes the suppression of spontaneous cardiac activity. It decreases the electrical threshold required for the onset of ventricular fibrillation, decreases ventricular contractile force, and may decrease cardiac responsiveness to catecholamines such as epinephrine. Under these circumstances, bicarbonate therapy may be useful but should only be used after confirmed interventions such as defibrillation, cardiac compression, intubation, ventilation, and more than one trial of epinephrine have been used.[37]

Recommended Dose

If arterial blood gas measurements are not available, the recommended initial dose of sodium bicarbonate is 1 mEq · kg^{-1} intravenously; half this dose may be repeated at 10-minute intervals. For pediatric patients, this 1 mEq · kg^{-1} dose should be diluted 1:1 with sterile water to reduce the osmolality.

During the initial stage of patient management, when sodium bicarbonate is given empirically, the rescuer must be careful to avoid an excessive dose. As soon as possible, arterial blood gas measurements should be obtained as a guide to further therapy.

Route of Administration

Sodium bicarbonate should be given as incremental bolus injections rather than as a continuous infusion. This method allows better minute-to-minute control of the quantity administered. It also reduces the possibility of inactivating other drugs such as calcium chloride and the catecholamines that cannot be mixed directly with bicarbonate.

Complications

Administration of excessive amounts of sodium bicarbonate results in the problems listed in Table 50–6. If sodium bicarbonate is administered in undiluted form via a peripheral vein, it is sufficiently hypertonic that vein and soft tissue injury occur.

When Is Atropine Useful?

Mechanism of Action

Atropine is a drug that long has been used for its vagolytic actions. A reduced vagal influence on the heart improves both the rate of firing of the sinoatrial node and impulse conduction through the atrioventricular (AV) conduction system, with a resulting increase in heart rate.

Indications

Atropine is most useful in treating sinus bradycardia when it occurs with hypotension or frequent premature ventricular contractions (PVCs) secondary to unsuppressed ectopic electrical activity arising in the area of injured tissue during the prolonged period after repolarization (see Table 50–3). Sinus bradycardia following a myocardial infarction (MI) may predispose the heart to the onset of ventricular fibrillation.[38]

When profound bradycardia is present, acceleration of the heart rate above 60 beats per minute (bpm) may improve cardiac output and reduce the incidence of ventricular fibrillation. Atropine may also be useful for treating a high-degree AV block with a slow ventricular rate.

TABLE 50–6. Effects of Excess Sodium Bicarbonate

Metabolic alkalosis; leftward shift of oxyhemoglobin dissociation curve; interference with tissue oxygenation
Hypernatremia
Hypokalemia
Worsening of respiratory, myocardial acidosis if adequate ventilation cannot be maintained

Asystole subsequent to increased parasympathetic tone that results in suppression of the electrical activity to the heart also frequently responds to atropine.[18] Because heart rate is a major determinant of myocardial oxygen consumption, however, any excessive increase in heart rate in an ischemic myocardium may result in frank infarction. Therefore, care should be taken in selecting the proper dose.

Recommended Dosage

The recommended dose for bradycardia is 0.5 to 1.0 mg intravenously repeated every 5 minutes until the desired pulse rate is obtained or a maximum of 0.04 mg · kg^{-1} has been given. A larger dose has little therapeutic value, and a smaller dose may actually slow the heart rate. Atropine may also be given intratracheally, in which case the dose is 2 to 2.5 mg. In the treatment of asystole, incremental doses of 1 mg are preferred.

Complications

Ventricular tachycardia and fibrillation following intravenous administration have been reported. In second-degree type II heart block, a paradoxical decrease in ventricular response may result.[36]

When Should Lidocaine Be Given?

Mechanism of Action

By raising the electrical stimulation threshold of the ventricle during diastole, lidocaine renders the myocardial tissue less prone to ectopic electrical activity. In ischemic myocardial tissue following infarction, it may also suppress re-entrant dysrhythmias such as ventricular tachycardia or fibrillation. This effect occurs by an induced delay of conduction through damaged myocardial tissue in the ischemic areas until the surrounding normal tissue is depolarized and refractory to the propagation of an abnormal impulse.

Indications

Lidocaine, an amide local anesthetic, is the drug of choice for the treatment and prevention of dysrhythmias of ventricular origin. Because of its reliability, relatively low incidence of side effects, and ease of administration, it is frequently used for the treatment of unifocal and multifocal PVCs, ventricular tachycardia, and ventricular fibrillation.

Recommended Dosage

The recommended loading dose is approximately 1 to 1.5 mg · kg^{-1} given as an intravenous bolus. To control the dysrhythmia and to prevent its recurrence, the bolus dose may have to be repeated, up to a total of 3 mg · kg^{-1}, followed by a continuous infusion of 20 to 40 μg · kg^{-1} · min^{-1} (2–4 mg · min^{-1} in a 70-kg patient).[39] Only bolus therapy should be used during cardiac arrest.

Complications

Used in the recommended doses, lidocaine has no significant effect on myocardial contractility, arterial blood pressure, or AV and intraventricular conduction. On the other hand, excessive doses may induce heart block or depression of sinus node discharge, especially in patients with pre-existing conduction disturbances.

Overdose

An overdose can occur either from administration of too large a dose or from high plasma levels because of reduced redistribution, metabolism, or excretion of the drug. A decreased lidocaine dose may be indicated in patients with hepatic dysfunction, such as occurs with cirrhosis, or in patients with compromised hepatic blood flow secondary to reduced cardiac output or congestive heart failure. These conditions result in decreased metabolism of lidocaine by the liver, producing a gradual accumulation of the circulating drug, if an infusion is instituted.

Toxicity

Likewise, toxicity may occur more easily in oliguric or anuric patients, because the degradation products of lidocaine, which also have pharmacologic effects and toxic potential, cannot be adequately eliminated from the plasma.

Early clinical signs of lidocaine toxicity are related to the drug's central nervous system (CNS) effects (Table 50–7). They may be followed by collapse of the cardiovascular system. If CNS irritability occurs, lidocaine therapy should be withdrawn. A barbiturate or a benzodiazepine may be administered if deemed necessary and if a patient's circulatory status is sufficiently stabilized.

When Is Procainamide Useful?

Mechanism of Action

The mechanism of action of procainamide is similar to that of lidocaine. It may decrease the rate of discharge of an ectopic irritable focus. It also blocks re-entrant dysrhythmias by slowing electrical conduction in the damaged myocardial tissue and by creating a bidirectional block.

Indications

A second-line agent, procainamide is used in the management of PVCs, ventricular tachycardia, and persistent ventricular fibrillation unresponsive to lidocaine or when lidocaine is contraindicated.

Recommended Dosage

Incremental bolus injections are slowly infused at 20 mg · min^{-1} until (1) the dysrhythmia is controlled, (2) hypotension

TABLE 50–7. Lidocaine Toxicity

Drowsiness
Slurred speech
Disorientation
Paresthesias
Muscle twitching
Focal or grand mal seizures

occurs, (3) the QRS complex is widened 50%, or (4) a total dose of 17 mg · kg^{-1} has been given.[39] After initial control of the dysrhythmia with the bolus injection, a continuous infusion of 1 to 4 mg · min^{-1} may be required to prevent recurrent dysrhythmias. Other effective administration schedules have been tested and approved, but all are designed to maintain a therapeutic plasma level of 4 to 8 μg · mL^{-1}.

Complications

Because of the profound myocardial depressant effects that may occur during administration of procainamide, continuous ECG and arterial blood pressure monitoring are mandatory. Patients may be especially prone to these side effects after an MI, and their treatment requires extreme caution. End points of therapy include hypotension and >50% widening of the QRS complex.

When Should Bretylium Tosylate Be Used?

Mechanism of Action

The pharmacologic effects of bretylium tosylate, a quaternary ammonium compound, are complex. It has both postganglionic adrenergic-blocking properties and a positive inotropic action. After the administration of an initial dose, catecholamine release may increase peripheral resistance and central inotropy. This response is followed by adrenergic blockade and a decrease in peripheral resistance, which frequently produces postural hypotension when the drug is administered to a conscious patient.

A large body of data documents the antifibrillatory effect of bretylium in animals, but this concept has been challenged. Clinically, bretylium has been found to be useful in the treatment of both ventricular tachycardia and fibrillation. In direct comparisons, it has been found to be no better than lidocaine; thus, it is considered to be a second-line drug.[40]

Indications

Bretylium is recommended only if

1. Lidocaine and defibrillation fail to convert ventricular fibrillation
2. Ventricular fibrillation recurs despite lidocaine therapy
3. Lidocaine and procainamide fail to control ventricular tachycardia associated with a pulse

Recommended Dosage

In refractory ventricular fibrillation, 5 mg · kg^{-1} are given intravenously as a bolus, followed by attempts at electrical defibrillation. If ventricular fibrillation persists, the dose may be increased to 10 mg · kg^{-1} and repeated every 5 minutes up to a maximum dose of 35 mg · kg^{-1}.

In persistently recurring ventricular tachycardia, 5 to 10 mg · kg^{-1} can be diluted to 50 mL with 5% dextrose in water and given intravenously over 8 to 10 minutes. After the loading dose, bretylium can be administered as a continuous infusion at a rate of 1 to 2 mg · min^{-1}.[40]

Is Calcium Chloride Useful?

Mechanism of Action

Calcium chloride has long been used for improving myocardial contractility, but the mechanisms of its effects on the myocardium are still poorly understood. Research into the part that calcium plays in malignant hyperthermia has shown that calcium ions enter the sarcoplasm of muscle from the extracellular space via an intracellular tubular network called the *sarcoplasmic reticulum.*

On spread of the excitation impulse in cardiac muscle, the calcium ions travel from the sarcoplasmic reticulum to the points of interaction between the actin and myosin filaments of the sarcomere. Calcium interacts there with troponin, a regulatory protein that inhibits the formation of cross-bridges between actin and myosin. When this inhibition is terminated by the action of calcium on troponin, cross-bridges form between the contractile elements of the muscle, and contraction ensues. It is probably through this mechanism that calcium has its positive inotropic effect.

Indications

Calcium chloride is most beneficial in reversing the cardiac effects of hyperkalemia, hypocalcemia, and toxicity due to the administration of calcium channel blockers.

Recommended Dosage

The use of calcium chloride is controversial because of the fear that it may produce a tetanic contraction of an irritable myocardium or depression of the sinus node, resulting in asystole. It has been hypothesized that the drug may pass through the cell membranes of cells with marginal viability, denaturing intracellular proteins and hastening cell death. This effect is particularly worrisome because the brain is so sensitive to hypoxia.

If it is to be used, the recommended dose is 2 mL of a 10% solution of calcium chloride (2–4 mg $\cdot$ kg^{-1}). A bolus may be repeated at 10-minute intervals, if necessary. Calcium salts cannot be mixed directly with bicarbonate solution because they precipitate as calcium carbonate.

Several calcium preparations are available for intravenous use; calcium chloride, calcium gluceptate, and calcium gluconate are the most popular. Calcium gluceptate can be given in a dose of 5 to 7 mL, and calcium gluconate in a dose of 6 to 8 mL.

Complications

Rapid administration of a large bolus of calcium chloride, especially through a central venous catheter, may produce severe sinus bradycardia or sinus arrest. Undiluted calcium chloride given via a peripheral vein causes sclerosis and tissue injury; therefore, if a central site is not available, it should either be markedly diluted or in a less irritating form (e.g., calcium gluconate). Calcium must also be used cautiously in digitalized patients, because it can produce or accentuate digitalis toxicity. Much controversy surrounds the issue about whether calcium is indicated at all in the management of cardiac arrest, unless documented hypocalcemia is present or

a calcium channel blocking drug is known to have been taken. Otherwise, it should not be used.[41]

When Should β-Adrenergic Blockers Be Used?

Mechanism of Action

Three β-blockers (atenolol, metoprolol, and propranolol) have been shown to significantly reduce the incidence of ventricular fibrillation in post-MI patients who did not receive thrombolytic agents. Studies suggest a potential benefit in patients receiving thrombolytics as well. Beta-blockers act to control rate and to limit infarct size. They also have a role in chronic therapy after MI to reduce mortality rates.

Indications

Beta-blockers are used in paroxysmal supraventricular tachycardia (PSVT) after the rate is initially controlled, as well as in uncomplicated MI.

Recommended Dosage

In patients who have had a MI and are not receiving thrombolytic agents, the recommended dose of atenolol is 5 to 10 mg intravenously over 5 minutes. Alternatively, metoprolol can be used. Doses of 5 to 10 mg are given as slow intravenous boluses at 5-minute intervals to a total of 15 mg; an oral regimen can then be initiated. Propranolol, in a dose of 0.1 mg $\cdot$ kg^{-1}, divided into three equal, slowly administered doses, can also be used, as can esmolol in a dose of 1 to 2 mg $\cdot$ kg^{-1}, followed by an infusion titrated to maintain the heart rate at the desired level. Oral therapy can then be initiated.

Complications

Side effects that should be monitored include bradycardia, AV conduction delays, and hypotension. Cardiovascular decompensation to cardiogenic shock is rarely observed. Contraindications include bradydysrhythmias, greater than first-degree heart block, conduction delays, hypotension, overt congestive heart failure, and lung disease caused by bronchospasm.

What Is the Role of Calcium Channel Blocking Agents?

Mechanism of Action

Verapamil and diltiazem are the calcium channel blocking agents of choice in emergency cardiac care. Both agents slow conduction and increase refractoriness in the AV node. These actions may terminate re-entrant dysrhythmias requiring the AV node for their continuation. Verapamil and diltiazem may also be used to control ventricular response rate in atrial fibrillation and flutter. Because these agents decrease myocardial contractility, they may exacerbate congestive heart failure in patients with severe left ventricular dysfunction, despite their vasodilatory effects.

Indications

Intravenous verapamil is effective in terminating narrow-complex PSVT and can be used to control the ventricular rate in atrial fibrillation. It may not be as effective in controlling atrial flutter. Less clinical experience has been accrued with diltiazem. It appears to be equally efficacious and may produce less myocardial depression than verapamil.

Recommended Dosage

The initial dose of verapamil is 2.5 to 5 mg intravenously over 2 minutes. In the absence of a response or a drug-induced adverse event, repeated doses of 5 to 10 mg may be administered every 15 to 30 minutes to a maximum of 20 mg. Diltiazem is given at a dose of $0.25 \text{ mg} \cdot \text{kg}^{-1}$, followed by a second dose of $0.35 \text{ mg} \cdot \text{kg}^{-1}$.

Complications

Verapamil may produce significant hypotension, which can be reversed with calcium chloride, 0.5 to 1 g, given slowly via a central catheter, or 1.5 to 3 g calcium gluconate, given slowly via a peripheral vein.[42]

When Is Adenosine Indicated?

Mechanism of Action

Adenosine, available in the United States only since 1990, is an endogenous purine nucleoside that depresses AV node and sinus node activity. It is effective in terminating common forms of PSVT because they involve a re-entry pathway including the AV node. It does not terminate dysrhythmias that are not due to re-entry involving the AV node (e.g., atrial flutter, atrial fibrillation, atrial or ventricular tachycardia) but may produce transient AV or ventriculoatrial block that clarifies the diagnosis.

Indications

Adenosine is indicated in PSVT and may also be used to differentiate PSVT from other tachydysrhythmias, including ventricular tachycardia.

Recommended Dosage

The recommended initial dose is 6 mg as a bolus over 3 to 5 seconds, followed by a 20-mL saline flush. If no response is observed in 1 to 2 minutes, a 12-mg dose should be given. Larger doses have not been well studied.

Complications

Side effects are common but transient. Flushing, dyspnea, and chest pain are frequently encountered. These side effects rarely last more than 1 to 2 minutes. Sinus bradycardia and ventricular ectopy are common transiently after termination of PSVT. Because the half-life of adenosine is <5 seconds, PSVT may recur and require additional adenosine or calcium channel blocker.

Adenosine produces few hemodynamic effects because of its short duration of action. However, its use should be reserved for situations in which suppression of AV nodal activity will be of therapeutic or diagnostic value.

Adenosine interacts with methylxanthines, which block the receptor responsible for adenosine's effects. Dipyridamole blocks adenosine uptake and potentiates its effects. Alternative therapy is warranted for patients receiving these drugs.

DRUGS TO IMPROVE CARDIAC OUTPUT AND BLOOD PRESSURE

When Should Nitroglycerin Be Used?

Mechanism of Action

Nitroglycerin relaxes vascular smooth muscle. It is the nitrate of choice for acute angina pectoris. In patients with congestive heart failure, intravenous nitroglycerin produces hemodynamic effects similar to those of sodium nitroprusside. Low doses ($30-40 \text{ }\mu\text{g} \cdot \text{min}^{-1}$) produce predominantly venodilation; high doses ($150-500 \text{ }\mu\text{g} \cdot \text{min}^{-1}$) lead to arteriolar dilation as well.

Indications

Indications for the use in nitroglycerin in emergency cardiac care include congestive heart failure and unstable angina associated with MI.

Recommended Dosage

For suspected angina pectoris, one nitroglycerin tablet is administered sublingually. It may be repeated at 3- to 5-minute intervals if discomfort is unrelieved. Safe administration of intravenous nitroglycerin usually requires hemodynamic monitoring. The initial intravenous dosage is 10 to 20 $\mu\text{g} \cdot \text{min}^{-1}$, and the dosage may be increased by 10 $\mu\text{g} \cdot \text{min}^{-1}$ until the desired response occurs.[40]

Complications

The principal toxic side effect of nitroglycerin is hypotension, which may exacerbate myocardial ischemia. Other potential complications include tachycardia, paradoxical bradycardia, hypoxemia due to increased pulmonary $\dot{V}/\dot{Q}$ mismatch, increased intracranial pressure, and headache.

What Are the Roles of Vasoconstrictor Drugs?

Norepinephrine is one of a number of α-stimulators that produce vasoconstriction by acting directly on peripheral vessels. (Isoproterenol, in contrast, is a purely β-stimulating drug that causes peripheral vasodilation and increased heart rate, electrical conduction, and contractility.)

Drugs such as ephedrine have both a direct α-stimulating effect and an indirect effect through the release of catecholamines, which in turn stimulate the α- and β-receptors. Dopamine, a precursor of norepinephrine, has direct α- and β-effects. It also stimulates dopamine receptors in low dosages ($3-5 \mu g \cdot kg^{-1} \cdot min^{-1}$) and improves renal blood flow.

Indications

Much debate centers on the indications for the use of vasoconstrictors in patients in shock, particularly those with coronary artery disease. Potent vasoconstrictors predispose to ischemic damage of vital organs. Although an elevation in systemic blood pressure may improve cerebral, coronary, and renal perfusion, this beneficial effect frequently is accompanied by increased cardiac work and oxygen consumption. These opposing effects must be considered in any decision to use vasoconstrictor therapy. It is probably better to have a low cardiac output with centralization from α-stimulation–induced peripheral vasoconstriction than a low cardiac output without preferable shunting of flow to the brain and heart. Alpha-stimulation is generally reserved until after an inotrope has been tried.

Isoproterenol administration is limited to the rare situation in which a bradydysrhythymia is refractory to atropine and a pacemaker is not immediately available.

LIFE-THREATENING DYSRHYTHMIAS

How Are Atrial Fibrillation and Paroxysmal Supraventricular Tachycardia Managed?

Atrial fibrillation or PSVT with a rapid ventricular response may be associated with such a fast ventricular rate that diastolic filling time is shortened and ventricular volume is markedly reduced. The result is decreased cardiac output and decreased coronary artery perfusion. If the patient does not develop life-threatening cardiovascular decompensation, pharmacologic therapy is recommended.

Calcium Channel Blockers and Digitalis

A calcium channel blocker (verapamil or diltiazem) or digitalis is usually the first therapeutic intervention for atrial fibrillation or atrial flutter. Sufficient drug is given so that an AV block is created, thereby reducing the ventricular response to atrial stimulation. These drugs do not convert the dysrhythmia. Verapamil and diltiazem may decrease myocardial contractility and precipitate congestive heart failure. Diltiazem is less of a myocardial depressant than is verapamil.

Beta-Blockers and Adenosine

Beta-blockers can be used to slow the ventricular rate if calcium channel blockers or digitalis is not effective. They also slow the atrial rate in PSVT. However, adenosine is the choice for narrow complex PSVT.

Cardioversion

Patients who are refractory to pharmacologic therapy or who are symptomatic may require elective cardioversion. In compromised patients with hypotension or pulmonary edema, sinus rhythm must be restored rapidly. In this situation, cardioversion is the indicated initial therapy.

How Are Ventricular Dysrhythmias Controlled?

Premature Ventricular Contractions

PVCs can be monomorphic and polymorphic, and they can occur in salvos. The proximity of a PVC to the preceding T wave is critical; if it falls on the T wave, it can initiate ventricular tachycardia or ventricular fibrillation.

When PVCs in a patient with suspected MI are frequent, occur in salvos, or are closely coupled to a previous T wave, intravenous lidocaine, 1 to 1.5 mg $\cdot$ kg^{-1}, is the recommended initial therapy. Procainamide, propranolol, or quinidine can also be used. If bradycardia is present, the heart rate should be maintained above 60 bpm, with intravenous atropine in 0.5-mg increments.

Ventricular Tachycardia

Ventricular tachycardia is defined as three or more consecutive beats of ventricular origin at a rate usually exceeding 100 bpm. Management is outlined in Figure 50–11. Drug therapy includes intravenous lidocaine, procainamide, and bretylium in order of priority. If no response occurs or if a patient's condition is critical, cardioversion or insertion of a transvenous pacemaker and overdrive pacing may be beneficial.

PSVT with aberrant conduction is often difficult to differentiate from ventricular tachycardia. Guidelines for differentiating these dysrhythmias are useless in acutely ill patients and divert attention from appropriate care. Critical points to remember include the following:

1. Do *not* administer verapamil, because it can accelerate heart rate and lower blood pressure, especially in Wolff-Parkinson-White syndrome.
2. Do *not* rely on clinical criteria to distinguish PSVT from ventricular tachycardia. Many patients with ventricular tachycardia may appear stable.
3. Treat hemodynamically significant, wide-complex tachycardias as ventricular tachycardia.
4. Adenosine may have a role in distinguishing PSVT from ventricular tachycardia in hemodynamically stable patients, but further study is necessary.

Ventricular Fibrillation

Ventricular fibrillation is the most common cause of cardiac arrest. It is classified as *coarse* or *fine,* terms that describe the amplitude and the frequency of the ECG waveform. Coarse fibrillation (high-amplitude, slow-frequency waveforms) is usually of recent onset and frequently is more responsive to therapy. Fine fibrillation (low amplitude, fast frequency) may be refractory to defibrillation. Epinephrine administration sometimes converts the fine pattern to coarse ventricular fibrillation, which is more responsive to defibrillation.

If the onset is observed, a defibrillator is not available, and hypoxia is not the precipitating event, a precordial thump may be effective. If not, defibrillation should be performed as quickly as possible. BLS must be administered until defibrillation can be accomplished or until an effective rhythm supervenes (see Figure 50–10).

Ventricular Asystole

Ventricular asystole, or cardiac standstill, is a total absence of ventricular electrical or mechanical activity and usually results from extensive myocardial ischemia, hypoxia, hyperkalemia, severe acidosis, extreme parasympathetic activity (e.g., drug overdose), or hypothermia.

CPR must be initiated immediately. Pharmacologic measures that should be considered include intravenous administration of epinephrine, sodium bicarbonate when the arterial pH is <7.10, and atropine. If response to these modalities does not occur, a transvenous or transcutaneous pacemaker is necessary. Because fine ventricular fibrillation may appear as asystole, an attempt at electrical defibrillation should be considered (see Table 50–4).

How Is Sinus Bradycardia Managed?

Sinus bradycardia is characterized by a heart rate <60 bpm. Unless hypotension or ventricular ectopic beats are present, therapy is unnecessary. However, intravenous atropine in 0.5-mg increments is used when patients are symptomatic or if ectopy appears. A dopamine infusion or a transvenous or transcutaneous pacemaker may be needed in the absence of a response to atropine (see Table 50–3).

How Is Second-Degree Atrioventricular Block Managed?

Mobitz type II second-degree AV block usually occurs in the conductive pathway below the AV node. Because it is frequently associated with myocardial damage rather than increased vagal tone, the prognosis is usually poor. Temporary pacer placement followed by a permanent pacemaker is often required for a patient with this form of second-degree AV block, because a complete heart block commonly ensues (see Table 50–3).

How Is Third-Degree Atrioventricular Block Managed?

Third-degree AV block is characterized by complete cessation of electrical conduction between the atria and ventricles. The conduction block may occur at or below the AV node. A block at the node is frequently associated with acute inferior MI, increased vagal tone, or toxic drug effect. In this instance, the prognosis is usually favorable, and the block may be corrected with intravenous atropine. If no response is seen, a temporary pacer is used.

When the block occurs below the AV node, it is often secondary to an extensive anterior MI. A pacemaker or intravenous atropine or epinephrine may be used (see Table 50–3).

How Is Pulseless Electrical Activity Managed?

Pulseless electrical activity is characterized by ineffective ejection of blood even though myocardial electrical activity is normal. The result is a pulseless patient with a normal ECG pattern. The prognosis for these patients is poor. If the etiology is myocardial failure, the patient may respond to CPR and the intravenous administration of epinephrine, or dobutamine in-fusion. In the absence of a response, hypovolemia should be considered and a fluid bolus given. Other causes include tension pneumothorax, cardiac tamponade, cardiac rupture, pulmonary embolism, hypoxemia, acidosis, massive MI, drug overdoses, and hypothermia.

References

1. Mörch ET: Mechanical ventilation. *In* Clinical Applications of Ventilatory Support. 2nd ed. Kirby RR, Banner MJ, Downs JB (eds). New York, Churchill Livingstone, 1990, pp 1–61.
2. Jesudian MCS, Harrison RR, Keenen RL, et al: Bag-valve-mask ventilation: two rescuers are better than one: preliminary report. Crit Care Med 1985; 13:122.
3. Smith JP, Bodai BI, Seifkin A, et al: The esophageal obturator airway. JAMA 1983; 250:1081.
4. Kassels SJ, Robinson WA, O'Bara KJ: Esophageal perforation associated with the esophageal obturator airway. Crit Care Med 1980; 8:366.
5. Michael TAD: The esophageal obturator airway—a critique. JAMA 1981; 246:1098.
6. Goldenberg IF, Campion BC, Siebold CM, et al: Esophageal gastric tube airway vs endotracheal tube in prehospital cardiac arrest. Chest 1986; 90:90.
7. Walls RM: Cricothyroidotomy. Emerg Clin North Am 1986; 6:725.
8. Melker RJ, Banner MJ: Work imposed by breathing through cricothyrotomy tube. Sixth World Congress on Emergency and Disaster Medicine, Hong Kong, September 1989.
9. Scuderi PE, McLeskey CH, Comer PB: Emergency percutaneous transtracheal ventilation during anesthesia using readily available equipment. Anesth Analg 1982; 61:867.
10. Gammage G: Airway management. *In* Critical Care. Civetta JM, Taylor RW, Kirby RR (eds). Philadelphia, JB Lippincott, 1988, pp 197–208.
11. Babbs CF, Voorhees WD, Fitzgerald KR, et al: Relationship of blood pressure and flow during CPR to chest compression amplitude: evidence for an effective compression threshold. Ann Emerg Med 1983; 12:527.
12. Orlowski JP: Optimum position for external cardiac compression in infants and young children. Ann Emerg Med 15:667, 1986.
13. Emergency Cardiac Care Committee and Subcommittee, American Heart Association: Guidelines for cardiopulmonary resuscitation and emergency cardiac care, VII: neonatal resuscitation. JAMA 1992; 268:2276.
14. McDonald JL: Systolic and mean arterial pressures during manual and mechanical CPR in humans. Ann Emerg Med 1982; 11:292.
15. Halperin HR, Tsitlik JE, Guerci AD, et al: Determinants of blood flow to vital organs during cardiopulmonary resuscitation in dogs. Circulation 1986; 73:539.
16. Sack JB, Kesselbrenner MB, Bregman D: Survival from in-hospital cardiac arrest with interposed abdominal counterpulsation during cardiopulmonary resuscitation. JAMA 1992; 266:379.
17. Krischer JP, Fine EG, Weisfeldt ML, et al: Comparison of prehospital conventional and simultaneous compression-ventilation cardiopulmonary resuscitation. Crit Care Med 1989; 17:1263.
18. Paradis NA, Martin GB, Rivers EP, et al: Coronary perfusion pressure and the return of spontaneous ventilation in human cardiopulmonary resuscitation. JAMA 1990; 263:1106.
19. Falk JL, Rackow EC, Weil MH: End-tidal carbon dioxide concentration during cardiopulmonary resuscitation. N Engl J Med 1988; 318:607.
20. Callaham M, Barton C: Prediction of outcome of cardiopulmonary resuscitation from end-tidal carbon dioxide concentration. Crit Care Med 1990; 18:358.
21. Martin GB, Gentile NT, Paradis NA, et al: Effect of epinephrine on end-tidal carbon dioxide monitoring during CPR. Ann Emerg Med 1990; 19:396.
22. Befeler B: Mechanical stimulation of the heart: its therapeutic value in tachyarrhythmias. Chest 1978; 73:832.
23. Kerber RE: Statement on early defibrillation. American Heart Association: Medical Scientific Statement from the Emergency Cardiac Care Committee. Circulation 1991; 83:2233.
24. Ewy GA, Dahl CF, Zimmerman M, et al: Ventricular fibrillation masquerading as ventricular standstill. Crit Care Med 1981; 9:841.
25. American Heart Association standards and guidelines for cardiopulmonary resuscitation (CPR) and emergency cardiac care (ECC). JAMA 1986; 255:2841.
26. Kerber KE, Grayzel J, Kennedy J, et al: Elective cardioversion; influence of paddle-electrode location and size on success rates and energy requirements. N Engl J Med 1981; 305:658.

27. Weaver WD, Cobb LA, Copass MK, et al: Ventricular defibrillation: a comparative trial using 176-J and 320-J shocks. N Engl J Med 1982; 307:1101.

28. Sirna SJ, Ferguson DW, Charbonnier F, et al: Electrical cardioversion in humans: factors affecting transthoracic impedance. Am J Cardiol 1988; 62:1048.

29. Gutgesall LHP, Zacker WP, Geddes LA, et al: Energy dose for ventricular defibrillation of children. Pediatrics 1976; 58:898.

30. Kerber RE, Carter J, Klein S, et al: Open-chest defibrillation during cardiac surgery: energy and current requirements. Am J Cardiol 1980; 46:393.

31. Kerber RE, Martins JB, Kienzle MG, et al: Energy, current, and success in defibrillation and cardioversion: Clinical studies using an automated impedance-based energy adjustment method. Circulation 1988; 77:1038.

32. Kerber RE, Kienzle MG, Olshansky B, et al: Ventricular tachycardia rate and morphology determine energy and current requirements for transthoracic cardioversion. Circulation 1992; 85:158.

33. Brown CG, Werman HA, Davis EA, et al: Comparative effects of graded doses of epinephrine or regional brain blood flow during CPR in a swine mode. Ann Emerg Med 1986; 15:1138.

34. Emergency Cardiac Care Committee and Subcommitte, American Heart Association: Guidelines for cardiopulmonary resuscitation and emergency cardiac care: III. Adult advanced cardiac life supprt. JAMA 1991; 268:2208.

35. Mazkereth R, Paret G, Ezra D, et al: Epinephrine blood concentrations after peripheral bronchial versus endotracheal administration of epinephrine in dogs. Crit Care Med 1992; 20:1582.

36. Kette F, Weil M, Gazmuri R, et al: Buffer solutions may compromise cardiac resuscitation by reducing coronary perfusion pressure. JAMA 1991; 266:2121.

37. Emergency Cardiac Care Committee and Subcommittee, American Heart Association: Guidelines for cardiopulmonary resuscitation and emergency cardiac care: III Adult advanced cardiac life support. JAMA 1992; 268:2210.

38. Gunnar RM, Passamani ER, Bourdillon PD, et al: American College of Cardiology/American Heart Association Guidelines for the early management of patients with acute myocardial infarction: report of the ACC/AHA Task Force on Assessment of Diagnostic and Therapeutic Cardiovascular Procedures. Circulation 1990; 82:664.

39. Haynes RE, Chinn TL, Copass MK, et al: Comparison of bretylium tosylate and lidocaine in management of out of hospital ventricular fibrillation: a randomized clinical trial. Am J Cardiol 1981; 48:353.

40. Emergency Cardiac Care Committee and Subcommittee, American Heart Association: Guidelines for cardiopulmonary resuscitation and emergency cardiac care: III. Adult advanced cardiac life support. JAMA 1992; 268:2206.

41. Emergency Cardiac Care Committee and Subcommittee, American Heart Association: Guildelines for cardiopulmonary resuscitation and emergency cardiac care: III. Adult advanced cardiac life support. JAMA 1992; 268:2209.

42. Weiss AT, Lewis BS, Halon DA, et al: The use of calcium with verapamil in the management of supraventricular tachyarrhythmias. Int J Cardiol 1983; 4:275.

SECTION IX

Hazardous Environments

CHAPTER **51**

Occupational Hazards in the Operating Room

SALVATORE LOPALO, C.R.N.A., M.S.Ed., M.A.

A. JOSEPH LAYON, M.D., F.A.C.P.

The operating environment is a hazardous place. Risks include infectious as well as chemical and psychologic threats. This chapter reviews the most important of these, identifying methods to minimize risk while at the same time providing optimal patient care.

HIV INFECTION

The central issue with regard to human immunodeficiency virus (HIV) infection and the anesthesiologist involves two specific points: (1) Should a different anesthetic technique be used for patients who are HIV infected, and (2) what are the risks of HIV transmission from patient to physician or from physician to patient?

What Is the Relevant Epidemiology?

As of March 1992, 218,301 cumulative cases of acquired immunodeficiency syndrome (AIDS) were reported in the United States,[1] and approximately 65% of the afflicted individuals have died. As of May 30, 20,284 new cases of AIDS were reported in 1992.[2] An approximate 5% to 10% increase in the cases of AIDS reported yearly has occurred; each week, between 200 and 600 new cases are reported to the Centers for Disease Control (CDC).[3, 4] Cases continue to be seen predominantly in the following groups: (1) homosexual/bisexual men, 55%; (2) intravenous drug abusers (heterosexual), 24%; and (3) heterosexuals, 7%. The remainder occur in children, are transfusion related, or are of indeterminate cause (Tables 51–1 and 51–2).

Use of the term *AIDS* is for convenience. HIV infection encompasses a spectrum of disease, of which AIDS is the end stage. Nonetheless, because of common usage, we use *HIV* infection and *AIDS* interchangeably. When it is important to differentiate early from end-stage infection, we so designate.

Pediatric AIDS

Cases of pediatric AIDS (defined as AIDS in children younger than 13 y) have been of concern and are on the rise. In 1988, 574 cases were reported; this number was 648 cases (+13%), 788 cases (+22%), and 683 cases (−13%) in 1989, 1990, and 1991, respectively.[5] The prevalence of HIV infection in newborns, based on surveys of blood specimens, is estimated at 0.5 per 1000 births.[6] Most perinatal AIDS is

TABLE 51–1. The March of HIV: Comparison of the First 100,000 and Second 100,000 Cases in the United States

Group	First 100,000 Cases (June 1981–August 1989)	Second 100,000 Cases (September 1989–November 1991)
Homosexual/bisexual men	61%	55%
Intravenous drug abusers	20%	24%
Heterosexuals	5%	7%
Transfusion	2.5%	1.9%
Children	11%	5.6%
Other/undetermined	0.5%	6.5%

(Modified from Centers for Disease Control: The Second 100,0000 cases of acquired immunodeficiency syndrome—United States, June 1981–December 1991. MMWR 1992; 41:28.)

TABLE 51–2. The March of HIV: Case Increases (1983–1991)

Group	1983	1987	1989	1991
Homosexual/bisexual men	1249	10,777	19,652	23,960
Intravenous drug abusers	330	2473	7970	11,155
Heterosexuals	22	426	1562	3387
Undetermined	56	599	1848	2925

(1991 figures from Centers for Disease Control. HIV/AIDS Surveillance Report, January 1992, p 9.)

thought to occur from mother to child via transplacental infection.[7]

What Treatment Is Available?

Extensive work has resulted in elucidation of the viral causative agent of AIDS. HIV is generally recognized as the causative agent for the immunodeficiency that results in the spectrum of complications we term AIDS, although some controversy exists.[8–11] The molecular biology of this agent has been extensively detailed, including the steps by which the viral particle binds to and is incorporated into the CD4+ cell.[12–20] Although much work has been done, research is ongoing to determine optimal types and use of anti-HIV agents, including the substituted nucleosides, zidovudine (AZT), dideoxyinosine (ddI), and dideoxycytidine (ddC), as well as nonnucleoside inhibitors of HIV.[21–33] Reduced sensitivity of HIV to AZT after prolonged therapy has been reported.[34]

Vaccine Development

Work continues in an effort to examine the feasibility of a vaccine against this viral agent.[35–37] Recombinant gp160 (a major envelope gene product) has been shown to induce antibody formation in both healthy and asymptomatic HIV-infected subjects; whether this effect will be protective is unclear.[36, 37] The potential availability of a vaccine is still sufficiently remote that it is premature to be anything more than cautiously optimistic.

What Is the Role of Prevention?

Despite these advances, HIV infection continues to take a significant toll, both in the United States and worldwide. HIV infection is now one of the top five leading causes of death in women 15 to 44 years of age and the second leading cause of death in men 25 to 44 years of age.[38] Further and perhaps of most concern, in 1989, AIDS became the sixth leading cause of death for adolescents and young adults (ages 15–24 y) of both sexes.[39–41]

The CDC estimates of HIV prevalence in projected AIDS cases are certainly disturbing.[42] Approximately one million HIV-infected individuals are thought to reside in the United States at this time. Remember, however, that the HIV-infected individuals who are identified today were likely infected 8 to 10 years ago. Thus, any prophylaxis that has a chance of success must prevent cases that we will only begin to diagnose in a decade. In the next 2 to 3 years, the cumulative incidence of AIDS will probably range between 390,000 and 480,000

cases. During 1994, between 150,000 and 225,000 patients with AIDS will require medical care, and the number of AIDS-related deaths will likely range between 53,000 and 76,000. Clearly, prevention of HIV disease is, in many regards, more important than its treatment.

Education

To date, attempts to deal with HIV disease have placed significant emphasis on treatment. Prevention, specifically with regard to education on and discussion of sexual behaviors, "safe sex," and needle exchange programs, has received inadequate attention.

This problem, recognized as a political rather than a medical one, is accorded by us and others to the shortsightedness of political leadership of our country. Indeed, Donald P. Francis, who recently retired from the CDC's AIDS Division of the National Center for Prevention Services, stated emphatically that the CDC was forced "to follow political dogma rather than sound public health principles."[43]

HIV is not an agent that respects sexual orientation. The virus is transmitted by exchange of body fluids; whether it be semen or blood, and whether transmission occurs between homosexual or heterosexual lovers, is unimportant.

Heterosexuals engaging in high-risk behaviors such as promiscuous or unprotected sex or intravenous drug abuse put themselves at risk for HIV infection. Thus, limiting educational measures to prevent this disease puts at risk broad segments of our population. HIV respects sexual preference no more than did syphilis in the 15th and 16th centuries. Syphilis was initially called the *Neapolitan disease,* then the *French pox,* because it was first described in Italians, then in the French.[44] This sexually transmitted disease eventually infected individuals of many ethnic groups, although contemporary accounts voiced the hope it would be restricted to "others." That such thinking now about HIV still exists at the dawn of the 21st century is both remarkable and sobering.

What Is the Virology of HIV?

HIV, a retrovirus, initiates its life cycle by recognizing and binding to the CD4 molecule on the T helper lymphocyte. These molecules are also found on macrophages and certain elements of the central nervous system (CNS).[45] Thus, these cells may also be HIV infected. After recognition and binding, the virus enters the host cell, is uncoated, and its genomic RNA is transcribed into DNA. Some of this is integrated into the host cell DNA, and other pieces remain in the cytoplasm.

Infection and Infectivity

Because the viral genome is integrated into that of the host, infection and infectivity persist throughout an infected individual's life. As many as 1 in 100 T4+ (helper) lymphocytes may be infected with HIV in patients with advanced disease.[46, 47] The helper lymphocyte is a central player in the immune system, intimately involved in the functioning of the monocyte/macrophage, the cytotoxic T cell, the natural killer cell, and B cells. Thus, a selective quantitative or qualitative depletion of the former cell line can lead to severe and recurrent infections. This process occurs in HIV infection of the T helper cell and results in cellular death. The infected monocyte/macrophage, however, is relatively resistant to cytolysis and appears to be the HIV reservoir.

Signs and Symptoms of Infection

Infection with and seroconversion to HIV is often associated with a virus-like syndrome. The most common symptoms include fever, sore throat, and lymphadenopathy. Less commonly, rash, myalgias, diarrhea, and symptoms of CNS involvement are encountered. Thrombocytopenia and leukopenia are occasionally noted as well. The incubation period of the virus, from exposure to the development of viral syndrome type of symptoms, is approximately 2 weeks. Most frequently, the antibody response occurs 4 weeks after the initial viral exposure; however, some data suggest that seroconversion may, on rare occasions, not occur until 18 to 36 months after infection.[48, 49]

How Is the Diagnosis Made?

Serology

Enzyme-Linked Immunosorbent Assay

For individuals who engage in high-risk behavior, a strongly reactive enzyme-linked immunosorbent assay (ELISA) has a positive predictive value of 93%.[50] However, for individuals who do not practice high-risk behavior and thus have a relatively low disease prevalence, the positive predictive value for a strongly reactive specimen may be only 67%.[51] The importance of a confirmatory study is thus obvious.

Western Blot

Although the ELISA tests for antibody to one of several viral antigens, the confirmatory test most commonly used is the Western blot. In this assay, viral antigen is electrophoretically dispersed, and a patient's serum specimen is then evaluated to determine if antibodies to the specific viral particles are present. In order to have a positive result, bands must be positive for any two of the following: p24 (core antigen), gp41 (envelope antigen), or gp120/gp160 (envelope antigen).[52] A negative result is the absence of all bands, and one that is indeterminate signifies the presence of bands on the Western blot that fail to meet the specific criteria for positivity. A patient with an indeterminate test result for at least 6 months may, in the absence of any known risk factors or clinical symptoms, be considered negative for HIV. Such an individual is almost certainly not infected with HIV, although no large-scale studies have confirmed this view.[50]

Polymerase Chain Reaction

The polymerase chain reaction (PCR), which identifies viral DNA integrated into the host genome, is a newer analytic technique that is quite sensitive in determining early HIV infection.[49] The methodology of PCR is reasonably difficult to master; thus, results must be interpreted with this fact in mind.

History

The predictive value of any of these studies is greater when coupled with a carefully taken history. Thus, when a test for HIV is to be performed, patients must be gently and nonjudgmentally queried about whether they engage in any high-risk behaviors such as intravenous drug use, sexual contact with an intravenous drug user, prostitution, or nonmonogamous homosexual or heterosexual contacts. Heterosexual promiscuity should be considered high-risk behavior.

What Are the Risks of HIV Transmission from Patients to Health Care Workers?

Several series suggest that the risk of HIV seroconversion after a single puncture wound with a blood/secretion-contaminated instrument is on the order of 0.5%.[53–56] However, given the frequency of blood contamination and needle sticks during a working lifetime, the cumulative risk of occupationally acquired HIV disease may range from <1% to as high as 10%.[57–59] The following example illustrates this point.

Assume an HIV seroprevalence of 1% (present range is 0.02–5.2%), a frequency of puncture wounds of 1% (conservative), and an overall risk of seroconversion of 1% (currently quoted at approximately 0.5%) after a needle-stick injury from a patient who is HIV positive. Thus,

$$0.01 \times 0.01 \times 0.01 = 0.000001 = 10^{-6}$$

Hence, the risk of HIV infection after one needle-stick injury is one in a million. However, an anesthesiologist cares for approximately four patients per day for 250 workdays per year. Thus,

$$4 \times 250 = 1000 = 10^{3}$$

$$10^{-6}/10^{3} = 10^{-3}$$

Thus, over 1 year, the risk increases to 1 in 1000. In a 40-year career, it increases by

$$40 \times 10^{-3} = 0.04$$

Thus, the risk of HIV disease over a lifetime is more like 1 in 25. In a program the size of ours at the University of Florida (90 residents), 3 or 4 will be projected to die eventually of HIV disease.

Despite this epidemiologic calculation, current data show that unlike the prevalence of hepatitis B virus (HBV),[60] no excess prevalence of HIV infection in health care workers now exists; whether this observation will remain so in the future is unclear at this time.[60]

Prevention

Many although not all exposures to HIV infection are preventable if reasonable precautions are taken. However, we are cognizant that no matter how careful one is, the nature of surgical procedures is such that accidental punctures, caused by bone fragments, scalpel blades, or unseen needles, will occur. The best we can do is strive to minimize these incidents.

This approach becomes critically important unfortunately, because of an apparently asymptomatic pool of HIV-positive individuals who, depending on geography and age, range from 16% to 18% of the population studied.[31, 48, 49, 61] Such information should make us ever more compulsive in our attention to

TABLE 51–3. Universal Precautions

Barriers	Gloves, masks, eyewear as appropriate.
Needles	Do not resheathe, bend, or break. Dispose of in a puncture-proof container.
Dermatologic conditions	Weeping or exudative lesions as well as cuts and abrasions imply a breach in the integumentary barrier. This may increase risk if the area involved is not protected with a barrier.
Decontamination	Wash hands.
Pregnant health care workers	Be especially careful because intrauterine transmission occurs.

TABLE 51–5. Laboratory Precautions in Addition to Universal Precautions

Material handling	• Use a biologic safety hood. • Use only mechanical pipettes. • Use needle/syringes only if there is no alternative. • Use well-constructed containers with well-fitting lids.
Cleanup	• Decontaminate work space after spills; household bleach works well. • Decontaminate/clean equipment before transport/ repair. • Discarded liquids/solids should be appropriately neutralized (i.e., via autoclave).

detail in order to prevent inadvertent inoculation with HIV-positive material, especially in the emergency room and operating room (OR). Thus, health workers are at highest risk of inoculation with HIV-positive material not from an individual who is known to have AIDS but, perhaps, from a young trauma victim or routine elective surgical patient for whom we are caring.

Precautions

All patients and all blood/body fluid specimens *must be considered to be infectious at all times.* The CDC has promulgated precautions that we should strive to follow while caring for all patients:

1. Universal precautions (Table 51–3): Those taken with all patients because HIV-infected individuals cannot reliably be identified by history and physical examination. Of particular significance are cases in emergency care settings, such as trauma resuscitation, when exposure to blood or body fluids is likely and the patient's infectious status is unknown.

2. Invasive precautions (Table 51–4): Those taken in addition to the universal precautions when such a procedure is to be performed. An invasive procedure is defined by the CDC as any surgical entry into tissues, cavities, or an organ or repair of any traumatically induced lesions. These include but are not limited to traumatic lesions, cardiac catheterization and other angiographic procedures, vaginal or cesarean delivery, intravenous catheter placement, and dental surgical procedures. We also consider nasogastric and airway intubation to be invasive because of the possibility of blood contamination.[62]

3. Laboratory precautions (Table 51–5): Those recommended for health workers involved in clinical laboratories. Blood and body fluids from all patients, regardless of known HIV status, must be considered infectious until proven otherwise. The precautions noted supplement universal precautions.

Let's Discuss Reality

If easy answers were available to the question of whether we are put at risk for HIV infection by our patients and by how much, a separate section of this chapter would not be

TABLE 51–4. Invasive Precautions

Universal precautions plus additional barriers	Liquid-repellent gown over a repellent apron, repellent leggings and shoe covers. Consider double gloving. Watch for glove tears.

needed. Although only limited data exist, some of the following material represents nothing more than obvious good sense; the rest is our educated opinion.

Any integumentary contamination with a patient's blood must be washed with germicidal soap as soon as practical and safe to do so. Gloves must be worn whenever patients are administered care. This practice, in our view, does not include the initial portion of the patient encounter, in which one greets and shakes the patient's hand in the preoperative area, or when further contact is made in the OR before anesthetic induction. In addition to gloves, plastic eyewear or prescription glasses are certainly appropriate in the prevention of mucous membrane contamination.

Types of Injuries

Different types of exposures may carry different risks. Cutaneous contamination, barring breaks in the skin, are usually without great risk; they are, nonetheless, handled as noted previously.

Needle Punctures. Exposure via hollow-tipped needles, such as those used to start intravenous infusions, are recognized to be responsible for approximately 61% of contamination events occurring in OR personnel; most of these occur in anesthesiologists.[63]

Sharp Injuries. Among surgical personnel, sharp injuries are more often inflicted by a solid instrument such as a scalpel or a sharp clamp. Wright and colleagues noted that three mechanisms accounted for almost 60% of sharp injuries: (1) those caused by instruments left on the surgical field but not in use (24%); (2) those caused to hands used in directly retracting tissue (17%); (3) those of a stationary hand holding an instrument that was injured by a second instrument (16%).[64] Only 6% of sharp injuries occurred during passage of instruments between the scrub nurse and surgeon.

We cannot overemphasize that needles should never be resheathed, because this practice may lead to puncture wounds. All sharp objects should be discarded in a puncture-proof container immediately after use. This puncture-proof container should be placed as close to the procedure site as possible. Instruments not in use must be removed from the surgical field; the use of hands as retractors must be minimized; and double gloving should be the norm.[65] Although we appreciate intellectually that these precautions should be followed, recent data suggest these preventive measures are too frequently ignored by health workers during patient care.[66, 67] Of even more significance, up to 84% of blood contacts are preventable by barriers such as face masks/shields and fluid-resistant gowns and gloves.[68]

Should Testing Be Performed After Possible Exposure?

The issue of testing after possible exposure to an individual with HIV infection is an even more difficult problem than prevention. Should health workers be tested after possible exposure? At least two answers can be provided.

The Ideal World

Let us first hypothesize an ideal world with no bias against individuals with HIV infection. A rational health care system would be in place to provide a residence for exposed health workers, and a disability system would exist so that health workers who become HIV positive would not become destitute as a result of the loss of their jobs. In this ideal world, testing should occur at least every 6 to 12 months.

After traumatic exposure to a potentially HIV-positive patient, an immediate sample of blood should be obtained and held, and another sample obtained approximately 4 to 6 weeks later. These should be tested, as should a blood specimen from the patient in question, in the same manner. Even if the patient were HIV positive, one would have some security in the knowledge that so far, only about 0.5% of traumatic exposures of health workers result in seroconversion.

Whether an HIV-exposed health worker should begin prophylactic therapy with AZT or another antiviral agent is unclear, because failure of AZT prophylaxis has been reported.[69] However, our opinion is that the consequences of HIV infection are so severe and the risk of AZT is so low that a short course of the antiviral agent is appropriate in the previously mentioned setting. Other therapies might be appropriate to use if they become available—for example, a short course of blocking antibody (anti-CD4).

The Real World

In the real world, the questions are not so easy to answer. At least two issues of concern arise with regard to the best course of action after exposure to an infected or possibly infected patient. If you test positive, will you lose your job? In the most enlightened institution, health workers would be protected by their chairperson and hospital director; however, this sequence does not always happen.

Furthermore, the issue of disability insurance for house officers and medical students is entirely unclear at this point. At Shands Hospital, the University of Florida, medical students are not covered by disability insurance, because they often have no income, and house officers have coverage that may not be adequate. Insurance companies frequently do not cover "pre-existing" conditions. Thus, we would not be surprised if an insurance company, in order to minimize financial risk, attempted to deny benefits to an individual based on a history of exposure, seroconversion, or a question of alleged promiscuous behavior, whether heterosexual or homosexual.

With these possibilities in mind, a health worker exposed to a patient potentially infected with HIV should obtain testing in the not-so-perfect world, but in a slightly different manner. Anonymous testing is available throughout the United States and should be used when questionable exposure has occurred. This approach may have implications regarding insurance coverage, if the clinician later seroconverts and has neither been tested at the work site nor filed an incident report of an occurrence. We believe, therefore, that an incident report should be filed in any event, even if HIV testing is carried out anonymously. The issue of AZT prophylaxis remains as mentioned earlier.

Our view is that testing and AZT prophylaxis are appropriate when a questionable exposure has occurred. However, the precise means by which the sequence should be carried out is somewhat vague, given the emotional, political, and financial implications of seroconversion. We recognize that the delicate treatment of the issue offered here is not entirely acceptable to many individuals. However, the "right answer," whatever it may be, is still to be found among the shadows.

Patient Testing

Patients should also be studied serologically. In Florida, this is done in one of two ways: (1) Informed consent is given, the test result entered in the patient's chart, and the patient given pre- and post-test counseling. (2) When consent is not possible, as is the case of a comatose patient without family, the serologic study may be performed on a "leftover" blood specimen originally obtained for another reason. In this case, the result is not entered in the patient's chart. Clearly, the first of the two options is the more appropriate one.

What Is the Risk to Patients of HIV-Positive Health Care Workers?

Cases studied by the CDC have suggested HIV transmission to patients from their dentist.[70, 71] The most well-known case is likely that of Kimberly Bergalis. This young woman from a small town in Florida appears to have been infected with HIV by her seropositive dentist before he died. Precisely how infection occurred remains unknown. The dentist's office records are unclear about the precise technique used for instrument sterilization. Inadequate cleaning of instruments may have resulted in the transmission of the viral agent. Purposeful infection based on behavioral changes induced by HIV CNS disease is a possibility. The result of this case, however, was a very emotional and powerful call by some, including Ms. Bergalis, that all health care workers be serologically tested for HIV and that patients be informed about the workers' HIV status.[72] This approach has found little support from those of us providing health services.

Physicians' Duties to Patients

A patient, under a strictly defined concept of autonomy, has the right to know the HIV status of the physician providing care. Furthermore, under the principle of nonmalfeasance, physicians ought not put their patients at risk by being HIV positive.[68] Nevertheless, we believe that mandating HIV testing would, in the long term, worsen rather than enhance both patients' rights and medical care.

One of the authors of this chapter has argued on several occasions that it is a health care worker's strict duty to look after any patient who requires care, regardless of the patient's HIV status and with the full realization of the possible, though unlikely, risk that the health worker might become HIV positive.[72-74] Our concept was, and remains so to this day, that this small risk was part of the responsibility taken on when the mantle of physician was assumed.

Protection of Physicians and Health Care Workers

Demanding that physicians care for all patients, including those who are HIV infected, is reasonable; further demanding that physicians put at risk livelihood and family is not. To do so would result, we fear, in physicians' turning away patients who appear in any way to be at risk. This view has been eloquently argued and termed the *switching dilemma*.[75] The appropriate steps, in our opinion, are as follow:

1. As a matter of safety and concern for the well-being of patients, health workers should undergo testing for HIV at 6- to 12-month intervals.

2. Any health worker who seroconverts from HIV negative to positive will remain on the job until his or her superior and a committee of colleagues (including a lay person), agreed on by both the infected health worker and the administration, determine that it is no longer in the institution's, health care worker's, or patients' best interest for the infected worker to do so.

3. At that time, the health worker would then be moved to a new job at the same salary. The job would be within the department or health center and would be considered appropriate by all concerned.

4. When the health care worker is no longer able to work, disability insurance would continue to pay the salary previously earned.

Any shortfall in departmental funds would be made up by disability insurance payment or federal/state funds from a special tax. It would seem inappropriate to spend any time attempting to determine whether the infection was obtained as a result of occupational exposure or in some other way, because this process could lead to abuse of an ill colleague.

These suggestions are neither radical nor unworkable.[76] They attempt to address the concerns of our frightened citizenry as well as those of health care workers who must provide the care to HIV-positive and HIV-negative patients. The keys to success with this proposal are consistency and fairness of the committees and the trust of our fellow citizens that we are watching out for their welfare as well as ours.

HIV-NEGATIVE CD4+ LYMPHOPENIA

The CDC has received reports of 14 persons with HIV-negative CD4+ lymphopenia; another 21 people suspected of having this condition have been described.[77] For the 14 CDC cases, the condition was reported between 1985 and 1992. Individuals range in age from 31 to 70 years (median 48 y). Males make up 57% of the cases. Risk factor information was available for 13 people and was positive in 4 (31%): Three had received blood transfusions, and one had a male homosexual contact.

AIDS-defining illnesses were diagnosed in eight (57%); six had other illnesses. Only one of these individuals has died of an AIDS-defining illness. As of August 7, 1992, the other 13 were alive. HIV antibody and supplemental studies were negative. The cause of HIV-negative CD4+ lymphopenia is unknown. Both the CDC and National Institutes of Health are studying this process. Whether the disease complex even exists has been questioned.

HEPATITIS

What Is the Relevant Epidemiology?

If we are appropriately concerned about the possibility of HIV infection in the health care setting, we must be even more vigilant with regard to the hepatitides. HIV infects only with great difficulty outside of actual body fluid or blood-borne transmission. Hepatitis B virus (HBV), on the other hand, is approximately 100 times more infectious than HIV when blood borne and is 10 times more prevalent among health workers than is HIV.[78]

According to the CDC, in 1988, approximately 57,000 cases of hepatitis occurred. Of these, 28,500 were hepatitis A; 23,200 were hepatitis B; 2600 were hepatitis non-A non-B (including hepatitis C); and 2500 were unspecified.[79] By the middle of 1992, 9605 cases of hepatitis A, 7772 cases of hepatitis B, 3735 cases of non-A non-B hepatitis, and 340 unspecified cases were reported.[80]

The hepatitides may be divided into two main groups—those that are considered primary and those that are secondary. The primary hepatitides account for approximately 95% of cases of hepatitis encountered in clinical practice. As the name suggests, these organisms have little effect other than on the liver. The secondary hepatitides account for only approximately 5% of hepatitis encountered in clinical practice and have clinical effects that are distant from the liver.

What Are the Primary Hepatitides?

Hepatitis A

Hepatitis A virus (HAV) is an RNA virus found in the stool of acutely infected individuals.[81, 82] In the United States, the seroprevalence increases with age, so that by age 50 years, approximately 50% of individuals are seropositive. Specific IgG is found in the plasma of previously infected individuals.

Clinical and Serologic Features

Symptoms of infection caused by HAV are seen 2 to 6 weeks after inoculation; for this reason, it has been termed *short incubation hepatitis*. During this symptomatic period, elevated serum levels of transaminases are noted. Jaundice may follow several days after the initiation of symptoms, but anicteric disease is common. Just before the onset of symptoms, viral particles are noted in the stool and serum. This shedding of the virion, as well as infectiousness, stops with the onset of jaundice. The clinical and serologic features of HAV infection are summarized in Figure 51–1.

Transmission

HAV is transmitted via the fecal-oral route, although parenteral transmission does occur uncommonly. This agent is not thought to be of any significance in post-transfusion hepatitis; it only rarely causes fulminant hepatitis; chronic carrier states and chronic hepatitis do not occur with HAV. The reservoir for this infectious process is thought to consist of the

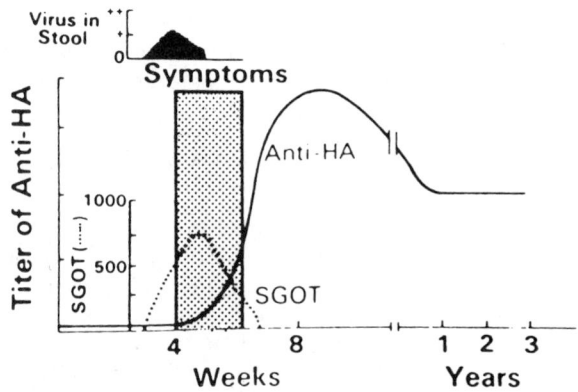

FIGURE 51–1. The sequence of events of HAV infection. Note that virus excretion in stool predates any symptom. The SGOT (aspartate transaminase) level is elevated prior to and anti-HAV is elevated after onset of symptomatology. (From LaMont JT: Viral hepatitis. *In* Internal Medicine. Stein JH (ed). Boston, Little, Brown & Co, 1983.)

large number of clinically inapparent cases from which the organism is transmitted to uninfected individuals.

An increase in hepatitis A among homosexual men has recently been noted.[82] This observation may indicate a return to unsafe sexual practices that result in fecal contamination, misperception in the gay community about the relative safety of certain sexual activities, or a susceptible population of homosexual men with an increased number of sexual partners.

Hepatitis B

HBV infection is a major cause of acute and chronic hepatitis, cirrhosis, and primary hepatocellular carcinoma in the United States, Western Europe, and Australia. The disease occurs primarily in adults; approximately 0.1% to 0.5% of the population are chronic viral carriers. This low incidence of viral carriage is in contrast to the approximately 10% incidence of individuals in the same populations who are positive for hepatitis B surface antibody (HBsAb). The implication is that most HBV infection is self-limited and followed by immunity; only occasionally does the chronic carrier state result. However, these chronic carriers appear to be the reservoir that perpetuates the virus.

Composition

HBV is a DNA virus consisting of a core region containing viral DNA, DNA polymerase, and core antigen; the outer coat consists of the surface antigen (HBsAg).[83] The complete and infectious virus is termed the *Dane particle*. Another antigen, termed *e* (HBeAg), is present only in serum containing the Dane particle. Although the biologic significance is not entirely clear, HBeAg correlates well with infectivity.

Risk of Infection

The risk of infection with HBV depends on one's activities (Table 51–6). Anesthesiologists, who as a group have frequent blood contact, are considered to be at intermediate risk for HBV, with 1% to 2% of that population being positive for HBsAg and approximately 10 times that many individuals in the same population positive for any serologic marker of HBV infection. Data suggest that individuals with multiple sexual partners increase their risk of HBV infection.[84, 85]

TABLE 51–6. Prevalence of Hepatitis B Serologic Markers in Various Population Groups

	Population Group	Prevalence of Serologic Markers of HBV Infection	
		HBsAg (%)	All Markers (%)
High risk	Immigrants or refugees from areas of high HBV endemicity	13	70–85
	Clients in institutions for the mentally retarded	10–20	35–80
	Users of illicit parenteral drugs	7	60–80
	Homosexually active men	6	35–80
	Household contacts of HBV carriers	3–6	30–60
	Patients on hemodialysis units	3–10	20–80
Intermediate risk	Health care workers with frequent blood contact	1–2	15–30
	Prisoners (male)	1–8	10–80
	Staff of institutions for the mentally retarded	1	10–25
Low risk	Health care workers with infrequent or no blood contact	0.3	3–10
	Healthy adults (first-time volunteer blood donors)	0.3	3–5

(Reproduced with permission from Centers for Disease Control: Recommendations for protection against viral hepatitis. Ann Intern Med 1985; 103:395.)

Abbreviations: HBV = hepatitis B virus; HBsAg = hepatitis B surface antigen.

Clinical and Serologic Features

The incubation period of HBV is variable, ranging between 6 and 24 weeks. The reason for this variable period of incubation relates to both the size of the inoculum and its portal of entry. For example, an infusion of 50 mL of infected blood may result in a patient's becoming HBsAg positive in only a few weeks; a 50-μL inoculation most frequently results in surface antigenemia only after 3 to 4 months.

Serologic features are important in the diagnosis of this viral infection.[86] The first marker noted is HBsAg (Fig. 51–2) before any other clinical or laboratory findings are observable.

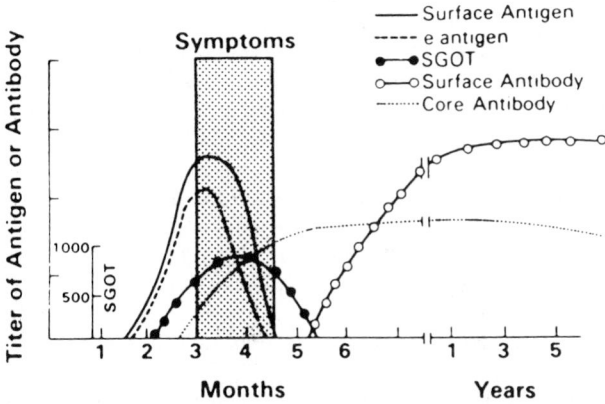

FIGURE 51–2. The sequence of events of infection with HBV. Both HB_sAg and HB_eAg (which correlate with infectivity) are in relatively high concentrations prior to onset of symptoms. Note the late appearance of HB_sAb, which usually implies a successful host response to HBV. (From LaMont JT: Viral hepatitis. *In* Internal Medicine. Stein JH (ed). Boston, Little, Brown & Co, 1983.)

The Dane particle markers, HBeAg and DNA-polymerase, parallel the rise of HBsAg. Approximately 2 weeks after the appearance of these markers, liver enzymes including aspartate transaminase begin to rise. Approximately 6 weeks after the onset of antigenemia, clinical symptoms may be noted.

Antibody Formation. As HBV-associated DNA-polymerase becomes detectable, HBsAg levels peak. The first antibody against HBV, noted within 2 to 4 weeks after initiation of antigenemia, is an IgM core antibody (HBcAb). The IgG isotype of HBcAb may persist for months to years after the antigenemia has cleared. Except in those patients who eventually develop chronic viral disease, HBsAb is noted several weeks after clearing of viral antigen. The presence of HBsAg indicates unequivocally either acute or chronic HBV infection. On the other hand, the presence of HBsAb generally implies a successful response to HBV and confirms lifelong protection against further infection.

A small group of individuals with HBV infection is negative for both surface antigen and antibody but positive for HBcAb. These individuals are capable of transmitting HBV until HBsAb is produced. Most infected individuals, however, clear the viral antigen, usually implying complete eventual recovery.

Chronic Carriers. Unfortunately, a small percentage of HBV-infected individuals become chronic carriers. Carriers are most frequently patients who have developed mild anicteric acute hepatitis followed by gradual return of normal results of liver function studies. Despite these normalizing biochemical parameters, patients are unable to clear the antigen. No HBsAb is detected. Of significance here is that chronic carriers are most frequently asymptomatic and are thus likely to infect others. Approximately 10% of HBV-infected patients have clinical manifestations for longer than 6 months. These individuals are classified as having chronic hepatitis.

Epidemiology

The fecal-oral or urine-oral route of HBV transmission is thought unlikely, because HBV particles are most frequently not found in stool and urine. However, viral particles have been found in saliva, semen, vaginal secretions, tears, and breast milk. Thus, the major routes of transmission are thought to be parenteral and mucosal (including sexual).

The parenteral route is most frequently identified in cases that are acquired in the hospital or by intravenous drug abusers. Only 10% of cases of post-transfusion hepatitis are caused by HBV. In these cases, the viral antigen is present in such low titer that the immunoassay used to screen blood cannot detect it or the blood donor may be a member of that small group with undetectable HBsAg and HBsAb but a positive titer for HBcAb.

Health care workers are put at risk for HBV infection via accidental needle sticks. That the infection rate is only 10% seems to be because of the small amount of inoculated blood present on these sharp objects. Transmission may occur when inapparent cuts or abrasions are inoculated with infectious material; conjunctival contamination followed by infection may also occur.

When health care workers are compared with the general population, the serologic evidence of previous infection with HBV ranges from 15% to 30% for the former group, compared with only 3% to 5% in the latter.[60, 81] Thus, distinctly unlike HIV infection, an excess prevalence of HBV infection occurs in health care workers. One study, in which serum of patients presenting to an inner-city emergency room were tested for HBV, HCV, and HIV-1, showed that the seroprevalence of HBsAg was 5%.[87] This incidence is more than 10 times the figure quoted for healthy adult first-time blood donors.[81]

Non-A Non-B Hepatitis

Non-A non-B hepatitis may be due to more than one viral agent.[88] It is the major cause of post-transfusion hepatitis, which occurs at a rate of approximately 5 to 10 cases per 1000 transfusions.[89, 90] This incidence seems to be decreasing because of our ability to test for anti-HCV. Until recently, no clinical serologic test for the detection of infected blood was available. Data suggesting that HBcAb and perhaps serum alanine transaminase could serve as markers for hepatitis C allowed them to be used as surrogates to screen blood.[89–91]

When these markers were used, for equal numbers of units transfused, recipients of HBcAb-positive blood had an approximately twofold higher incidence of post-transfusion hepatitis. Specifically, the incidence was from 4% to 6% in HBcAb-negative blood to 8% to 14% in blood that was positive. Elimination of blood positive for HBcAb from the donor pool removed about 5% of the donated units and resulted in a decrement of approximately 20% of cases of non-A non-B hepatitis.

Hepatitis C virus (HCV), which is one of what are likely several agents responsible for non-A non-B hepatitis, has recently been cloned and sequenced.[92] This agent appears to be a member of the togavirus family. A second-generation serologic assay detects anti-HCV in post-transfusion non-A non-B hepatitis approximately 60% of the time when used in conjunction with the first-generation assay.[76]

Clinical and Serologic Features

Although the viral agent may be rarely transmitted by the oral-fecal route, it is of an epidemiologic pattern more commonly resembling HBV than HAV. Specifically, HCV is most commonly transmitted through needle sticks and transfusions. The period between inoculation and onset of symptoms ranges from 2 to 20 weeks and averages 8 weeks. Although symptoms range from mild to fulminant, non-A non-B hepatitis is typically milder than HBV during the acute stage. Up to 50% of cases are anicteric, with only moderate biochemical abnormalities. Spontaneous resolution occurs approximately 12 weeks after infection in most patients. In a variable percentage of cases, ranging from 20% to 70%, one can find biochemical and pathologic abnormalities suggestive of chronic disease.

The diagnosis of non-A non-B hepatitis has been by exclusion, but with the development of the assay for HCV, this is no longer the case. One study noted that in an inner-city population, the prevalence of anti-HCV is 18%.[87] Interferon-α, 2 to 3 $\times$ 10^6 units three times weekly, has been shown to be effective in normalizing results of liver function studies and histology in patients with HCV infection; the drug may have to be continued for prolonged periods to prevent relapses.[93]

Delta Hepatitis

Delta hepatitis is an infection that occurs of necessity with HBV infection.[82, 94] The agent, hepatitis D virus (HDV), is an incomplete RNA virus requiring antecedent or concomitant infection with HBV in order to infect the host; it is sometimes considered a complication of HBV infection. Delta hepatitis is most frequently encountered in intravenous drug abusers or patients who are recipients of multiple transfusions. A chronic carrier state and chronic hepatitis are known to occur, as does massive hepatic necrosis. Anti-HDV antibody is similar to HBcAb in that it signifies that infection has occurred but is not protective. Prevention is most important with regard to HDV disease. Without HBV, HDV does not occur.

What Protective and Therapeutic Measures Should Be Undertaken?

Anesthesiologists are at intermediate risk for hepatitis infection as classified by the CDC.[81] Thus, a prevalence of approximately 1% to 2% of HBsAg is noted in anesthesiologists and other health care workers, with a 15% to 30% prevalence of all markers, such as HBsAb. Once again, we emphasize that the risk of patient to health care worker transmission of HIV is much less than the same transmission of HBV.

Immunization

Based on the foregoing data, anesthesiologists (and, in our opinion, all health care workers) should be immunized with hepatitis B vaccine. This is given as 20-μg intramuscular injections three times, with the second and third doses 1 and 6 months after the first. Once blood exposure has occurred, the series of events that should be followed depend on both the source of the exposure and the immunization status of the health care worker exposed.

Unknown Source

If the source of the needle stick were unknown, treatment of an exposed, nonimmunized health care worker would be to initiate the hepatitis B vaccine series immediately. If the worker had been vaccinated against hepatitis B, no specific treatment would be required.

Known, Low-Risk Source

If the exposure source was from an individual at low risk of being HBsAg positive, an unvaccinated health care worker would have the vaccine series initiated, and a vaccinated person, once again, would require no treatment.

Known, High-Risk Source

If the source of the exposure was an individual at high risk of being HBsAg positive, several things would be done. In an unvaccinated individual, the hepatitis B vaccine series would be initiated. Further, the source of the exposure would be tested for HBsAg status. If the source proved to be positive, a dose of hepatitis B immune globulin (HBIG) would immediately be given to the exposed individual. The dose for HBIG is $0.06 \text{ ml} \cdot \text{kg}^{-1}$, given intramuscularly.

If the exposed individual had been vaccinated in the past and was a vaccine nonresponder, the source would be tested for HBsAg status. If the source is indeed HBsAg positive, a dose of HBIG would be given immediately, as well as a booster dose of hepatitis B vaccine.

Known Serologic Positive Source

If the source was known to be HBsAg positive, as opposed to simply being at high risk, the unvaccinated individual would be given a dose of HBIG immediately and the series of HBV vaccine immunizations begun. If the exposed individual had been vaccinated, he or she would be tested for anti-HBV antibody. An inadequate antibody level (less than 10 sample ratio units by radioimmunoassay or by enzyme immunoassay) would necessitate a dose of HBIG immediately, plus a hepatitis B vaccine booster dose.

The risk of hepatitis B vaccine to the recipient is minimal. The doses for perinatal, sexual, percutaneous, and dialysis exposures and exposure of immunocompromised patients are listed in Table 51–7.

What Are the Secondary Hepatitides?

In the differential diagnosis of viral hepatitis, one must consider the possibility of an agent that affects the liver secondarily rather than primarily. Such agents include cytomegalovirus (CMV), disseminated herpes simplex virus (HSV), coxsackievirus A and B, Epstein-Barr virus, and yellow fever virus. These infectious agents account for approximately 5%

TABLE 51–7. Hepatitis B Virus Postexposure Recommendation

| Exposure | Hepatitis B Immunoglobulin | | Inactivated Vaccine | | |
| | Dose | Recommended Timing | Plasma-Derived Hepatavax-B Dose | Recombinant | |
				Dose	Recombivax Engerix-B Dose
Perinatal	0.5 mL IM	Within 12 h	10 μg IM*	5 μg IM*	10 μg IM*
Sexual	0.06 mL · kg⁻¹ IM	Single dose within 14 d of sexual contact	20 μg IM†	20 μg IM†	20 μg IM†
Percutaneous	N/A	N/A	20 μg IM	10 μg IM	20 μg IM
Dialysis and immunocompromised patients	N/A	N/A	40 μg IM (20 μg in each of two sites)	—	40 μg IM

*The first dose can be given at the same time as the dose of hepatitis B immune globulin (HBIG) but at a different site.
†Vaccine is recommended for homosexual men and for regular sexual contacts of hepatitis B virus carriers and is optional in initial treatment of heterosexual contacts of persons with acute hepatitis B.
(Data from Centers for Disease Control: Recommendations for protection against viral hepatitis. Ann Intern Med 1985; 103:399; *and* Facts and Comparisons. Philadelphia, JB Lippincott, 1990, pp 467–468.)
Abbreviations: IM = intramuscular; N/A = not applicable.

of clinical hepatitis and are termed *secondary hepatitides* because they only secondarily affect the liver.

HERPETIC WHITLOW

Herpetic whitlow is herpes simplex virus (HSV) infection of the finger. Infection by this viral agent does not necessarily result in the death of the host cell; rather, latency may be induced. In this state, the viral genome is maintained in a largely repressed state that is compatible with survival and normal activity of the host cell. Reactivation of the viral genome results in reappearance of the herpetic lesion.

Individuals who are positive for HSV antibody may not report symptoms during an acute infection. In fact, asymptomatic salivary excretion of HSV type 1 (HSV-1) is encountered in 2% to 9% of adults and 5% to 8% of children. Although herpetic whitlow has been reported as being more common in health care workers,[95] more recent data suggest that health care workers account for only about 8% of cases, whereas children/students (31%) and adults in non–health care occupations (45%) account for 76%.[96]

How Does It Occur?

Herpetic whitlow can occur as a complication of primary oral or genital herpes through a break in the skin when a digit contacts lesions on either the mouth or genitalia. Clinically, one may see abrupt onset of erythema, edema, and tenderness of the involved digit. Vesiculopustular lesions, which are indistinguishable from those of a pyogenic infection, may result. Fever, lymphadenitis, and lymphadenopathy of the epitrochlear and axillary chains are common. Herpes simplex pharyngitis may be encountered in up to 37% of infected individuals.

How Is It Treated?

Although studies are few, oral acyclovir has been shown to be effective in shortening the duration of symptoms both in immunocompetent and immunocompromised individuals with mucocutaneous HSV. The possibility of immunization is currently under investigation. For now, the most rational preventive measures are those suggested by universal precautions.[97]

CHICKENPOX/HERPES ZOSTER

Varicella-zoster virus (VZV), sometimes referred to as herpesvirus type III, is a member of the herpesvirus family. The primary clinical form of VZV is chickenpox, and the reactive form is seen as herpes zoster, or shingles. The virion contains a core of double-stranded DNA. Once within the human cell, the virus induces specific enzymes collectively termed *thymidine kinase*. These act to phosphorylate nucleosides, and indeed nucleoside analogues are preferentially phosphorylated by these enzymes. From this activity stems our ability to use acyclovir and ganciclovir against this agent.

What Is the Relevant Epidemiology?

VZV is highly communicable. It is epidemic in large urban centers and, interestingly, in temperate climates. Humans are the only known species naturally infected; all races and both sexes are equally affected, although the attack rate for children is the highest of any population group.

The viral agent is spread by close contact with an infected person in the early stages of disease. Attack rates in susceptible siblings at home range from 70% to 87% and are lower in the school environment. VZV does not survive in scabs or crusts; thus, once the vesicles are crusted over, usually 5 to 7 days after their appearance in normal children, transmission is unlikely. Aerosol spread is documented, particularly in the hospital environment, because the virus is shed in respiratory secretions.

Incidence

In the United States, approximately three million cases of this infection occur yearly, with the highest incidence of infection noted in children ages 5 to 9 years. Most people show evidence of infection by adulthood, and very sensitive antibody assays have shown that the seroprevalence of antibody to VZV ranges from 95% to 100%. Clinical varicella infection has been demonstrated by increases in antibody titer after exposure to VZV. Indeed, even though the subclinical attack rate is thought to be <5%, many who have protective titers of antibody have no history of clinical disease.[98]

For unclear reasons, in tropical regions, varicella has been noted to have a higher morbidity and mortality, perhaps because childhood infection is less frequent. Infection thus occurs in an older population than is noted in temperate climates. Pregnant women from nontemperate regions may not be immune to VZV; they have a higher risk of bearing children with congenital varicella.[99]

Patients who have recurrent VZV in the form of herpes zoster may transmit the viral agent to previously uninfected individuals, thus resulting in primary varicella. Previously unexposed adults who have a negative varicella titer and are exposed to either a child with chickenpox or an adult with herpes zoster may develop VZV infection. Therefore, recognition of the signs and symptoms of this infection is important.[100]

How Is Varicella (Chickenpox) Manifested?

As noted previously, a history of exposure is common either in school or in the family. In a normal child, varicella is a relatively benign process. The incubation period ranges from 10 to 21 days, averaging 15 days. The prodromal stage, consisting of fever and malaise, is noted about 24 hours before the onset of rash. This stage is often more severe in adolescents and adults. The fever is usually ≤39 °C, and affected children do not appear acutely ill. However, pruritus is common.

Skin Lesions

Initially, the lesions may be seen on the scalp, mucous membranes, face, and neck. They often are most numerous on the trunk. The classic lesion of chickenpox is a superficial vesicle surrounded by a halo of erythema. The lesions may change very rapidly, within hours, from maculopapules to vesicles. With this change, the pruritus becomes intense. In an immunologically normal child, new lesions continue to form for approximately 5 days after the initial eruption, with the lower extremities often the last to be involved. Gradual healing of lesions occurs over a period of approximately 3 weeks. Disfigurement is very uncommon with this process.

As a result of under-reporting, the number of children hospitalized for varicella infection is unclear. Probably 2000 to 5000 hospitalizations occur annually. Approximately 10% of the children hospitalized for this process die, primarily from secondary bacterial infections or VZV CNS involvement.

Bacterial Infections

Bacterial infections are most frequently caused by *Staphylococcus aureus* or *Streptococcus pyogenes*. In adults, approximately 1 in 400 patients with varicella require hospitalization owing to pneumonia.[87, 88] This pneumonic process is usually noticed while integumentary lesions are actively forming. Findings on a chest radiograph, which shows the diffuse nodular infiltrations as well as bilateral peribronchial processes, frequently appear worse than the physical findings themselves. Nonetheless, hypoxia as well as reactive airways disease may be seen.

Central Nervous System Involvement

In normal children, the CNS is involved in approximately 1 of 5000 cases. Involvement ranges from cerebellar ataxia, which is self-limited and benign, to Reye's syndrome. Rarely, one may see other CNS syndromes caused by VZV, including optic neuritis, transient spinal cord dysfunction, and Guillain-Barré syndrome. Other, much less common, complications include thrombocytopenic purpura, purpura fulminans, nephritis, myocarditis, and arthritis.[99]

Maternal Varicella

Maternal VZV is uncommon in the United States, being noted in fewer than 1 in 1000 pregnancies. Although it may cause some maternal morbidity and immunologic evidence of fetal infection is present in 17% to 24% of infants, most neonates born with evidence of intrauterine VZV infection are asymptomatic.

Congenital Varicella

The risk of congenital varicella syndrome following a case of maternal varicella is difficult to estimate but has been reported between zero and 2.6%. Infection in the first trimester is thought to be more frequently associated with congenital varicella, although even in these cases, <10% of infants are affected.

Neonatal

The onset of maternal varicella from 5 days before to 48 hours after delivery may result in neonatal infection. Infection that occurs within the first 10 days of life is considered to be congenitally acquired. The course of chickenpox in neonates ranges from mild varicella to very severe disease. Mortality ranges from 20% to 30%, and even after treatment with VZV immune globulin or acyclovir, deaths have been reported.

How Is Infection Diagnosed?

Although the diagnosis of VZV infection is most frequently based on the history and clinical findings, isolation of the viral agent is definitive. Cells are obtained from vesicular lesions or from biopsy samples; the latter should be examined microscopically. The presence of multinucleated giant cells with eosinophilic intranuclear inclusions is suggestive of either HSV or VZV infection; studies with monoclonal antibody differentiate the two.

Measurement of specific antibody against VZV may be used to determine the susceptibility to infection. The most sensitive methods are either ELISA or indirect immunofluorescence against membrane antigen (IFAMA).[99]

What Is the Prognosis?

In most immunologically normal children, varicella resolves without sequelae in 5 to 10 days. The complication rate in this group of patients is approximately 5%, with CNS involvement being the major cause of morbidity and mortality. Severity of infection and complications increase with age, including visceral dissemination of the virus resulting in, among other things, respiratory failure. This progression is fairly common in either older adults or pregnant women.

Adults have a more serious complication rate with this infection, including visceral dissemination in otherwise healthy individuals. Thus, treatment with acyclovir may be instituted when the diagnosis of VZV is considered. Because varicella during pregnancy carries with it significant risk of maternal morbidity and mortality, treatment with acyclovir may also be necessary in this situation. Although this agent is not teratogenic in animal models, its use to decrease the risk of congenital varicella may be neither safe nor effective.[98] Antiviral therapy is likely to be necessary in immunocompromised individuals. Further, if a patient is receiving steroids or other immunomodulating agents, the dose should be decreased or the agent discontinued, if possible.

How Is It Prevented?

An attenuated varicella vaccine is under evaluation and may be available in the near future. Until then, VZV immune globulin may be used in high-risk patients. Although it has a failure rate of nearly 20%, it does appear to modify the ensuing infection. In addition, VZV immune globulin may prolong the incubation period for as long as 42 days after exposure to the virus.

Immunization

Individuals at high risk should receive VZV immune globulin within 96 hours of exposure, at a dose of 125 units per 10 kg of body weight (minimum dose 125 units, maximum dose 625 units) via intramuscular injection. This agent is distributed by the Red Cross blood service. Before receiving VZV immune globulin, adults should be evaluated on an individual basis. This evaluation should take into consideration the possibility of exposure, the geographic background, the health status, and the likelihood of previous infection. Health care workers with a negative history of VZV infection and significant exposure to children may benefit from laboratory testing to determine whether or not they have an antibody to VZV. Seronegative health care workers should not care for patients with varicella or herpes zoster.

Isolation

Hospitalized patients with VZV infection should be isolated until their lesions have crusted. If possible, this isolation should be in a negative-pressure room to decrease or prevent the possibility of dissemination of viral particles to other patients.

If I Have a Negative Varicella Titer and Am Exposed to Chickenpox, What Should I Do?

Seropositivity to VZV is extremely common in the United States. It is likely, even in an adult who has no recollection of symptoms, that exposure has occurred. However, for those who are unsure, testing for the antibody via either ELISA or IFAMA may be used to determine antibody titer. In a high-risk individual who has no titer, VZV immune globulin may be used to modify the attack rate and severity of symptoms. If visceral dissemination of this virus occurs, such as varicella pneumonia, acyclovir should be initiated. Until an adequate vaccine is available, an individual with a negative titer should not care for an infectious patient.

CYTOMEGALOVIRUS INFECTION

What Is the Relevant Epidemiology?

CMV also is a member of the herpesvirus group. In an intact human, CMV growth occurs in epithelial or endothelial cells and in macrophages. Because a very high titer of virus is produced in the salivary glands and kidneys, protracted CMV shedding is noted in oral secretions and urine; the viral agent can, however, be found in essentially all organs and body fluids.[101] CMV infection occurs commonly throughout the world; most patients are without symptoms. The incidence of infection in children ranges from 15% in Seattle to 99% in Tanzania.[102] The exact means of transmission is not completely elucidated.

Young children asymptomatically shed the virus in urine and saliva. In daycare centers, for example, up to 69% of children may be so affected. Daycare workers and nurses caring for hospitalized children who shed CMV are infected at a rate that is similar to that of the general population. However, parents of children who are in daycare centers and are shedding acquire the infection at a very high rate. This observation may have implications for mothers of childbearing age, because serious congenital infection may occur in children born to infected mothers.

Pregnancy

In apparently healthy pregnant women infected with CMV, the rate of recovery of the virus from vaginal secretions is increased. Infants born to such mothers frequently are infected during passage through the vaginal canal. Most often, these infants develop antibody without obvious illness. Severe interstitial pneumonia occasionally occurs.

Congenital Infection

Pregnant women infected with CMV transmit the virus to their children approximately 50% of the time.[103] Most of these infections are silent, and the children are usually normal. However, approximately 10% have obvious CMV inclusion disease at birth. Of these 10%, approximately 20% develop moderate to severe deficiencies of intelligence, sensorineural hearing loss, seizure disorders, or psychomotor retardation. In addition to these CNS findings, one may encounter hepatosplenomegaly, jaundice, interstitial pneumonia, and thrombocytopenia with petechiae or purpura. Many of these infants die shortly after birth; others require lifelong institutional care.

Blood Transfusion

Transmission of the viral agent via blood transfusion occurs on occasion. The risk of infection from a single unit of blood may range from 3% to 6%. Although most of these infections are subclinical, in immune-suppressed patients or transplant recipients, infection with CMV may have catastrophic consequences. This can be avoided by using CMV-seronegative blood. Use of high-titer anti-CMV γ-globulin decreases the severity of an infection, although not the infection itself. The use of ganciclovir to treat infection or CMV vaccine to prevent it may be appropriate in the future.

How Is Cytomegalovirus Infection Diagnosed?

The presence of circulating antibodies to CMV suggests prior infection, whereas seroconversion indicates more recent acquisition of the viral agent. Testing in this manner may be helpful in counseling pregnant women (e.g., health care workers) who may have been exposed to CMV. This form of testing may not be helpful, however, to diagnose patients who are immune suppressed. Detection of CMV IgM antibody is possible in up to 70% of infants who are infected with the agent in utero.

What Is the Prognosis?

The prognosis for congenital CMV inclusion disease is relatively poor, because death or permanent institutionalization is frequently the end result. Therapy for active infection is unsatisfactory, because CMV is resistant to agents such as vidarabine and acyclovir; ganciclovir is useful in some cases. Relapses are common, however, and multiple courses of therapy or prolonged maintenance therapy must be considered.

Are Preventive Measures Effective?

Although prevention of the primary viral infection in seronegative women of childbearing age would be important to decrease morbidity and mortality, such measures are generally limited. From the epidemiologic data at hand, it appears that pregnant mothers are at greatest risk from their daycare-attending children, compared with the risk from infected health care workers. Nonetheless, although the data are unclear, seronegative pregnant women should use extreme caution in caring for patients infected with CMV. Because one does not always know who is infected with CMV, universal precautions are appropriate. As always, transfusion should be minimized in all patients, but in those who are seronegative, only CMV-negative blood should be used.[104]

TUBERCULOSIS

Since 1990, nosocomial (Florida and New York) and correctional system transmission of multidrug-resistant tuberculosis (MDR-TB) has been reported to the CDC.[105] All eight of the correctional facility patients identified in a retrospective epidemiologic study have died; seven were HIV positive, and one was a state correctional facility employee who had recently been treated for cancer with radiation. All of these individuals had profoundly subnormal $CD4^+$ lymphocyte counts, and all died before (mean 25 d, range 3–42 d) the hospital was notified that their isolates were MDR-TB (mean time from collection of sputum to notification of the referring hospital: 18 wk, range 13–23 wk). MDR-TB is reported to be resistant to isoniazid, rifampin, pyrazinamide, ethambutol, streptomycin, kanamycin, and ethionamide. The CDC identified no effective drug regimen to treat patients in this outbreak.

As a result of this outbreak, health care workers need to be aware of their tuberculin status. Annual tuberculin skin tests should be carried out on all staff who previously tested negative or do not know their tuberculin status. The HIV status of all patients with tuberculosis should be evaluated, because immunocompromised individuals with MDR-TB may die very rapidly. The role of anesthesia equipment in transmitting tuberculosis is unclear and deserves to be studied. Specifically, does the use of a disposable carbon dioxide absorber decrease the possibility of tuberculosis transmission between patients?

DRUG ABUSE

No occupational hazard in the practice of anesthesiology is more devastating than the abuse of drugs (Table 51–8).[106–125] Those who have been involved in anesthesiology for a few years can, almost without exception, relate at least one tragedy due to drug abuse. Abuse of chemical substances, both licit and illicit, can lead to addiction. Although addiction is considered to be a disease process in enlightened circles, sanctions, including criminal justice processes, potentially await abusers or addicts.[106] Loss of medical licensure and incarceration in state or federal penal institutions loom as possible legal measures levied by government bodies.

Why Are Drugs Used and Abused?

One must ask the question, "Why would anyone use or abuse drugs?" Historical reasons are summarized in Table 51–9.[107]

Occupational Factors

Many times, more than one reason enters into the use/abuse of drugs by an anesthesia practitioner. Some common factors are cited by practitioners who abuse drugs.[106, 109] First, drugs are easily available. Narcotics, a primary component in the armamentarium of most anesthesia practitioners, give any potential abuser the vehicle for drug acquisition. Second, many stresses are involved in providing anesthesia care. Anesthesiology is one of the few specialties of medicine or nursing in which an act of omission or commission can lead to immediate catastrophe. The need to act quickly in many situations only increases the level of stress. Third, a common feeling among

TABLE 51–8. Common Terms Defining Drug Use

Term	Definition
Appropriate	Medication taken as prescribed by physician or manufacturer for specific indication.
Misuse	Unintended or inappropriate drug use.
Habituation	Continued taking of a drug after the initial reason for taking it has resolved. Intervals between taking drugs are sufficiently long to prevent dependence, but discontinuance of the drug causes anxiety.
Abuse	Intentional use of a psychoactive chemical to the extent that it interferes with a person's health or economic or social function.
Dependence	An altered physiologic state produced by repeated exposure to a drug requiring continued administration in order to prevent the occurrence of withdrawal or abstinence syndrome characteristic of the particular drug.
Addiction	Abuse characterized by compulsion, loss of control, and continued use despite adverse consequences. An overwhelming preoccupation with its use and securing its supply denotes increased tolerance and withdrawal reactions on cessation of drug intake.
Tolerance	Progressively larger doses of a drug are required to produce the same effect.

some anesthesia practitioners is that they are not held in the same esteem as other specialists.[109] This outlook has been called the *Rodney Dangerfield syndrome* because of this entertainer's famous saying, "I don't get no respect."

What Are the Warning Signs and Symptoms?

A number of clues may give rise to suspicion that a practitioner is abusing chemical substances. The disease process has a predictable course, with progressive manifestations in certain settings.[102] Problems often arise first at home. Harmonious relations are replaced with those characterized by strife and a concomitant increase in fights and spouse or child abuse.

Behavior often becomes inappropriate and embarrassing. Vehicular accidents occur, as do arrests for driving while intoxicated. Withdrawal from friends, family, and social gatherings is common. Previously gregarious individuals isolate themselves from the closest of friends. An individual's physical status changes. Numerous health complaints occur, as do frequent needs for medical attention. Prescription drug use increases dramatically. Emotional control becomes extremely difficult.

Finally, signs and symptoms become evident in the professional setting. When such changes are noted in the workplace,

Table 51–9. Reasons For Drug Use (and Abuse)

To treat disease
To aid in religious practices
To explore the self
To alter moods
To promote and enhance social interactions
To stimulate artistic creativity and performance
To improve physical performance
To rebel
To go along with peer pressure
To establish an identity

the disease process is in a very advanced stage. Evidence of addictive behavior and drug abuse is summarized in Tables 51–10 and 51–11.

What Is Enabling Behavior?

A pattern that occurs at any or all levels in this progressive process has been termed *enabling behavior*.[109] Whether practiced by members of the family, by friends, or by professional colleagues, denial and rationalization of behavior enable an impaired professional to become more embroiled in a potentially fatal process. Having been involved personally with this process on a number of occasions, we can trace it as follows.

Behavior that is out of the ordinary in a colleague with whom one has worked and socialized for several years is often justified as ''just a bad day.'' As this behavior continues, it becomes clear that a problem exists, but it is often excused as the result of probable marital discord. As other symptoms surface, the rationale becomes, ''Maybe he or she is drinking a bit too much.'' Not until one is slapped in the face with irrefutable proof, such as walking into a room and seeing the individual with a needle in a vein, does everything coalesce.

The feelings that surface are devastating. Self-recrimination occurs as the observer asks, ''Why did I not recognize it before?'' The individual is frankly amazed that all of the signs, which should have been obvious much earlier, were only recognized when denial was no longer an option to deal with the problem.[111, 112]

How Is the Problem Recognized?

In order for this problem to be recognized, the potential for its occurrence must be appreciated; signs and symptoms must be noted when they occur. Recognition is possible through education of hospital personnel. They need to be familiar with the nature of addictive disease and the appropriate responses to impaired colleagues. They also need to be aware that resources are available for prevention, treatment, and rehabilitation.

Drugs are rarely abused as a single entity.[109, 110, 113] The drug that is the most commonly abused is alcohol. Fentanyl is also widely used, and its oral ingestion has been reported.[114] Even propofol, a noncontrolled substance, has been reported to

TABLE 51–11. Signs of Drug Abuse by Anesthesia Providers

Unusually heavy narcotic technique
Frequent breakage of ampules
Frequent illness and absence from work
Sloppy, illegible anesthesia records
Inappropriate temperature sensitivity
Need for a bathroom break (every two hours)
Desire and request to work alone
Refusal of lunch breaks
Heavy use of adjunctive drugs
Anesthetic mishaps (harm to patient at end stage of the disease)
Hostility

cause chemical dependency.[115] Combinations of alcohol and other substances are extremely common. When one confronts an impaired colleague, denial occurs, usually accompanied by belligerence and hostility. Do not use such confrontation alone. The ''platoon'' technique, in which a number of people elicit an admission of use or abuse, is necessary.[106]

How Is Treatment Provided?

Identification

Successful treatment is dependent on early recognition and identification of the impaired individual. According to the disease model of chemical dependency, there is no cure for addiction. However, successful treatment can lead to recovery, followed by social and occupational rehabilitation and an eventual return to a useful and productive career. Identification of addicted physicians is very important, because they rarely seek help on their own. Denial is a key behavioral factor in addiction. Moreover, peers are reluctant to confront suspected abusers because they do not want to be responsible for the abuser's loss of license or job. Early intervention, however, may prevent serious or irreversible consequences for an addicted individual.

Intervention

Drug dependence and alcoholism are treatable, if not curable. First, the individual must acknowledge his or her dependency and the need for treatment. A confrontational approach involving multidisciplinary chemical dependency specialists, psychiatrists, psychologists, and other health professionals is usually required in order to make impaired physicians realize the extent of their illness.[101] This intervention should be conducted in a caring, factual, nonjudgmental manner. Such confrontation is a very successful method for enrolling addicted physicians into recognized treatment programs.

Referral

All states now have impaired physicians' assistance committees. The Medical Association of Georgia's Disabled Doctor Program[109, 116] and the California Diversion Program[117] are examples of state medical society programs that have demonstrated great success in returning impaired physicians to productive careers. Recovery rates range from 60% to 80% in these types of programs. Recovery is a lifelong process, however, and relapses are common. Data from several programs demonstrate a relapse rate of approximately 40%; however,

TABLE 51–10. Signs of Addiction

Social	• Withdrawal from leisure activities, friends, family. Uncharacteristic or inappropriate behavior in social gatherings
	• Impulsive behavior (overspending, gambling)
	• Domestic turmoil (separation, spouse or child abuse, sexual dysfunction)
	• Change in behavior of spouse or children
	• Legal problems (arrests for driving while intoxicated)
Health	• Deterioration of personal hygiene
	• Accidents
	• Numerous health complaints, frequent need for medical attention for unrelated conditions
Professional	• Unreliability
	• Complaints by patients or staff; subject of hospital gossip
	• Unstable work history (frequent relocations)
	• Working at less than par performance

relapses do not necessarily predict a negative treatment outcome.

Methods of achieving long-term recovery are many and are shown in Table 51–12.

Pharmacologic Measures

Pharmacologic manipulation of behavior is useful but must be undertaken only in the context of a multidisciplinary approach to the problem of substance abuse. Out of this context, it is no panacea.

Disulfiram

Disulfiram blocks the metabolism of ethanol, resulting in formation of the intermediate metabolite acetaldehyde. It is relatively nontoxic when administered alone. However, when ethanol is ingested, blood acetaldehyde concentration rises 5 to 10 times higher than normal, resulting in the acetaldehyde syndrome. This reaction is very unpleasant, producing intense vasodilation, headache, respiratory distress, sweating, blurred vision, nausea, copious vomiting, hypotension, vertigo, and confusion. An individual treated with disulfiram usually does not ingest alcohol again after experiencing these adverse reactions.

Naltrexone

This oral opiate antagonist with no agonist properties can block the effects of narcotics for 48 to 72 hours. If a narcotic is self-administered during this period, no unpleasant side effects occur, but the desired effect from the narcotic is not obtained either. Therefore, this agent may be a valuable adjunct in deterring physicians prone to the compulsive use of narcotics. Anesthesiologists in particular may benefit from such therapy, because they can continue to prescribe and administer narcotics to patients without the temptation to self-administer.

What Is the Narcotic Withdrawal Syndrome?

Acute narcotic withdrawal can produce various signs and symptoms, some of which are very intense (Table 51–13). Addicted individuals often resort to extreme measures to avoid this withdrawal syndrome. Treatment of acute withdrawal reactions relies substantially on the use of pharmacologic therapies. Once again, however, the use of drugs to "withdraw" a drug abuser is only acceptable in the context of a multidisciplinary approach to the treatment of the problem.

TABLE 51–12. Achievement of Long-Term Recovery

- Group psychotherapy sessions with other chemically dependent persons.
- Individual and family therapy with a psychiatrist or psychologist.
- Participation in Alcoholics Anonymous (AA) or Narcotics Anonymous (NA).
- Routine urine screening for alcohol and other drugs. Screening should be performed randomly and at least weekly for the first 6 months, with a gradual reduction in frequency as therapy progresses.
- Use of specific blocking agents to prevent abuse.

TABLE 51–13. Signs and Symptoms of Narcotic Withdrawal

Early (first 10 h)	Anxiety
	Sweating
	Tachypnea
	Rhinorrhea
	Dilated, reactive pupils
Late (>10 h)*	Excessive lacrimation and rhinorrhea
	Tachycardia
	Hypertension
	Tremor
	Abdominal pain
	Nausea, vomiting, diarrhea
	Piloerection
	Muscle spasms
	Fever

(Adapted from Stimmel B: Pain, Analgesia, and Addiction. The Pharmacological Treatment of Pain. New York, Raven Press, 1983, p 120.)
*Symptoms can last 5 months.

Clonidine

An α_2-adrenergic agonist, clonidine is an effective agent in controlling the excessive sympathetic response associated with acute opiate withdrawal. A total of 0.4 to 1.2 mg is given orally in divided doses on day 1, followed by the application of two Catapres-TTS-2 patches. The release of clonidine from the patches is constant and is approximately equivalent to 0.4 mg orally per day for 7 days. The patches should be replaced once, for a total of 14 days of therapy.

Methadone

Methadone is another effective drug used for detoxification and maintenance. In essence, it replaces the narcotic and thereby prevents the abstinence syndrome. A daily dose of 20 mg may be sufficient in alleviating symptoms to facilitate long-term rehabilitation. The majority of patients can be withdrawn completely from opioids in <10 days.

What Measures Are Useful for Prevention?

Addiction and substance abuse have so many serious consequences that prevention is of prime importance. Several steps can be taken to help reduce the growing numbers of chemically dependent anesthesiologists and nurse anesthetists.

Increased Control and Accountability of Narcotics

Many large hospitals have established OR satellite pharmacies. One of the many important functions provided by an OR pharmacy is greatly increased control of narcotics. Dispensing narcotics on a per case basis and issuing individual anesthesia drug boxes to each anesthesiologist are examples of greater narcotic control.[119] Documentation of administered doses is recorded, and unused drugs in syringes are returned to the satellite pharmacy rather than "wasted." Routine use of a refractometer or random assays on syringe contents can readily detect abusers.[120] Audit of individual practices can identify other prescribing patterns. Unfortunately, as has been well documented, control and accountability are anything but precise, uniform, and effective.[125, 126]

Summary

Early identification of substances abusers is critical. Look for the warning signs and behavioral changes in coworkers. Not every resident who is a sloppy dresser nor every partner who is short-tempered is an addict, but dismissing warning signs among peers can lead to disability or even death of an addicted individual. Alerting the department chairperson or chief of staff of a potentially impaired colleague is the first step in intervention. Enrollment in a state-sponsored program for impaired physicians is a nonpunitive therapeutic alternative for ultimate rehabilitation without loss of license and career.[107, 108]

FATIGUE

How does one define fatigue?[127, 128] In a dictionary, it may be characterized as weariness and physical or mental exhaustion or as the cause of weariness, such as labor or toil. To fatigue is to tire out; to weary with labor or any bodily or mental exertion; to harass with toil; to exhaust the strength of and finally to weaken by continued use. Many factors add to fatigue, such as stress, both internal and external, and the ambiance within which one functions.[128–131]

How Is It Perceived?

The perception of fatigue in anesthesiology appears as a continuum that is, to some extent, dependent on professional status. Is the individual an actively practicing resident or a person close to retirement? In a residency setting, listen to the perceptions and attitudes about fatigue. "They're not making residents like they used to." "These kids have no stamina." "They're coddled and are given every break in the world." "When I was a resident (and dinosaurs walked the earth), things were different. We were cut from a different cloth. We walked to and from the hospital in the snow (uphill both ways). We were on call 24 hours and then worked a full shift before going home for a few hours and came back to repeat the cycle. We never complained. We never fatigued."

One's perception of one's own indefatigability is somewhat colored by the number of years that have passed since serving as a house officer. Often forgotten are the 3 AM catnaps that were taken while diethyl ether and nitrous oxide were administered. Such agents, with a wide margin of safety, were "forgiving" when a resident's mind wandered or his or her eyes closed for a minute or two. However, in today's anesthetic milieu, agents with a narrow margin between therapy and overdose necessitate a clear-thinking, vigilant individual if they are to be administered safely.

What Factors Influence Fatigue?

Any number of factors influence fatigue in an anesthesia care provider.[128] First is individual variance. Some people simply tire more rapidly than others, and signs of fatigue are manifested in a shorter period of time. Factors such as physical and emotional well-being also enter into the picture. A common cold or influenza virus can sharply reduce effectiveness. Transient slight depression often leads to disproportionate fatigue. Dealing with the day-to-day stresses of patient care

responsibility also has an impact. Concerns about one's physical state, multisystem problems, psychologic well-being, family matters, and morbidity and mortality wear heavily on the psyche.

The surgical suite is an environment in which external stimuli such as daylight or darkness are not apparent. No windows allow confirmation of circadian rhythm. Trace gases may be in the inspired air.[129–131] Sleeplessness and long working hours are major factors. Fatigue of the anesthesia provider can lead to abuse of alcohol and other substances.[109] The suicide rate among physicians is two to three times higher than among the general population.[123] Suicide is the penultimate response to stress and fatigue.

Workable Schedules

Collective bargaining units have negotiated workable schedules for house officers. What is fair, equitable, and safe has not been defined exactly, but a 12-hour workday with call every third night appears not to have any deleterious results that are measurable by present technology. Obviously, the central concern is patients' safety. Because 95% of the reported problems in anesthesiology are related to human error, vigilance should be as close to optimal as possible.[132] Fatigue factors can predispose to therapeutic misadventures with potentially disastrous results.

Parker[127] has made the following suggestions to attenuate fatigue factors:

1. Any anesthesiologist involved in a procedure lasting more than 3 hours should be relieved every 2 hours for short periods.
2. No anesthesiologist should work longer than 17 hours without a full 12-hour recovery period.
3. No anesthesiologist should be on call more often than every third night.
4. One must not hesitate to say "no" to unreasonable workloads.

TRACE GAS EXPOSURE

Chronic low-level exposure to anesthetic agents has for years been a concern among anesthesia care providers.[129–131, 135–148] Studies have suggested that carcinogenic and teratogenic hazards, spontaneous abortions, neurologic symptoms, miscarriages, hepatitis, renal disease, and decreased mental performance are due to chronic exposure to the potent inhaled anesthetic agents.[135–142] Because of these findings, the National Institute of Occupational Safety and Health (NIOSH) recommended standards for occupational exposure of trace anesthetic gas contamination in the operating room.[141]

A number of studies describing the hazards of chronic exposure to inhalation agents have often conflicted with one another. Many of the studies were epidemiologic surveys or animal series using extremely high concentrations of the potent inhaled anesthetic agents. Human studies have used health surveys of practicing anesthesiologists, nurse anesthetists, dentists, and operating room nurses.[136, 138–140]

What Are the Suspected Deleterious Effects?

Dose-related bone marrow depression developing from chronic exposure to nitrous oxide was described by Eastwood and colleagues in 1963.[142] Increased mortality among anesthesiologists due to malignancies of the lymphoid and reticuloendothelial system has been reported.[108] Knill-Jones and associates reported an 18.2% frequency of spontaneous abortions in married female nurse anesthetists, versus a 13.7% rate in married female physician controls unexposed to anesthetic agents.[143] A survey of anesthesiologists and OR nurses, using similar control groups, revealed an abortion rate of 38% for anesthesiologists, 30% for OR nurses, and 10% for the controls.[144] It also revealed an increased incidence of congenital malformations in the live births of anesthesiologists working (6.5%) versus those not working (2.5%) during pregnancy.

A survey jointly conducted by the American Society of Anesthesiologists (ASA) and NIOSH revealed a statistically greater incidence of spontaneous abortions, congenital anomalies, cancer, and hepatic disease than among controls.[145] The survey showed a 1.3 to 2 times greater risk of spontaneous abortion in women exposed to the operating room environment during the first trimester of pregnancy. An increase of 60% to 100% in the reported incidence of congenital anomalies in the offspring of exposed female anesthetists, as well as a 25% greater incidence of anomalies in the offspring of the wives of exposed male anesthetists, was noted.

The incidence of cancer was 1.3 to 2 times greater in exposed female respondents. Hepatic disease was also 1.3 to 2 times greater in exposed females than in nonexposed females. A 1.2- to 1.4-fold increase in renal disease was noted among nurse anesthetists. These findings, although impressive, must be interpreted cautiously because of the voluntary and noncontrolled nature of the survey.[145] None has been verified by prospective controlled and randomized studies.

Performance Studies

Performance studies in human volunteers after exposure to nitrous oxide were conducted by Bruce and Bach.[130] Nitrous oxide alone at 500 ppm and at 500 ppm plus halothane or enflurane, 15 ppm, were studied. Also studied were patients exposed to nitrous oxide at 50 ppm plus halothane, 1 ppm, and 25 ppm of nitrous oxide plus 0.5 ppm of halothane. Significant deterioration of memory, recognition, decision-making ability, and action were demonstrated for concentrations as low as 50 ppm of nitrous oxide and 1 ppm of halothane.

These data were challenged by Smith and Shirley, who were unable to reproduce the reported findings.[131] A study of ambient concentrations of anesthetic gases in the ORs of 20 hospitals revealed nitrous oxide levels ranging from <10 to 3000 ppm.[146] The mean was 388.5 ppm, and halothane concentrations were <0.1 to 60 ppm, with a mean value of 2.8 ppm. As a result of this study, NIOSH recommended that levels be maintained at <25 ppm for nitrous oxide and <0.5 ppm for halothane.[141]

What Are the Sources of Trace Gases?

The sources of trace gas exposure are well described. Leakage from high-pressure nitrous oxide tanks to the flowmeters on anesthesia machines can produce substantial ambient contamination. The most common leakage sites are the quick connects on the central inflow lines resulting from faulty pipe threads, spring seals, or crimped joints. Leaks from the low-pressure side of the system, beginning with the flowmeters, can be so great that an otherwise effective control system is

TABLE 51–14. Common Low-Pressure Leak Sites

Improperly connected or leaking tubing
Improperly sealed valve domes
Deformed gas delivery lines or machine connection joints
Leaking delivery lines
Leaking Y-connector joints

negated (Table 51–14). Even if no gas leaks result from mechanical malfunction, significant anesthetic agent pollution of the OR environment can occur as a result of improper technique by the anesthesiologist or nurse anesthetist. Suggested measures that can avoid or significantly reduce gas contamination are noted in Table 51–15.

How Are Anesthetic Agents Scavenged?

Control measures designed to capture gas overflow exist as a part of every modern anesthesia machine.[149–152] The central mechanism is the scavenging system. The system connects to the expiratory limb of the breathing circuit and consists of a gas-capturing assembly, an interface, and a disposal route (Figs. 51–3 and 51–4).[153] Excess gas from the breathing circuit, ventilator, sidestream gas analyzer, or extracorporeal oxygenator is collected via the gas-capturing assembly and conducted to the disposal system.

Variation in anesthetic gas flow and effluent volumes requires that the scavenging system and the anesthesia circuit be appropriately matched in terms of capacity and flow. The interface is a pressure-regulating device designed to prevent significant positive or negative pressures within the circuit (see Fig. 51–4). It has two components: a reservoir to collect transient overflow of gas that occurs when the outflow exceeds the disposal rate and a one-way valve designed to prevent the suction of gas from the breathing circuit.

Disposal

In ORs with a nonrecirculating ventilation system, disposal is uncomplicated because waste gas can simply be directed to the exhaust grill for elimination to the outside. ORs with a recirculating ventilation system, however, should have an alternate disposal route, such as an independent vacuum line vented outside the hospital. Central vacuum lines are not used

TABLE 51–15. Measures to Minimize Operating Room Pollution with Anesthetic Agents

- Ensure proper mask fit to patient.
- Avoid turning on the nitrous oxide or the vaporizer until a tight mask seal is obtained or the patient is intubated and connected to the circuit.
- Discontinue gas flows (while continuing oxygen) and empty the reservoir bag via the pop-off valve (not by emptying it into the room) before suctioning or intubation.
- Administer oxygen as long as possible before extubation or removal of the mask.
- Avoid spillage of volatile agents during vaporizer filling by using a vaporizer-specific filling device.
- Do not disconnect and empty the reservoir bag into the room during emergence.
- Return the sidestream gas analyzer's exhaust flow to the circuit or scavenger system.
- Scavenge oxygenator from cardiopulmonary bypass circuit if a vaporizer is in line.

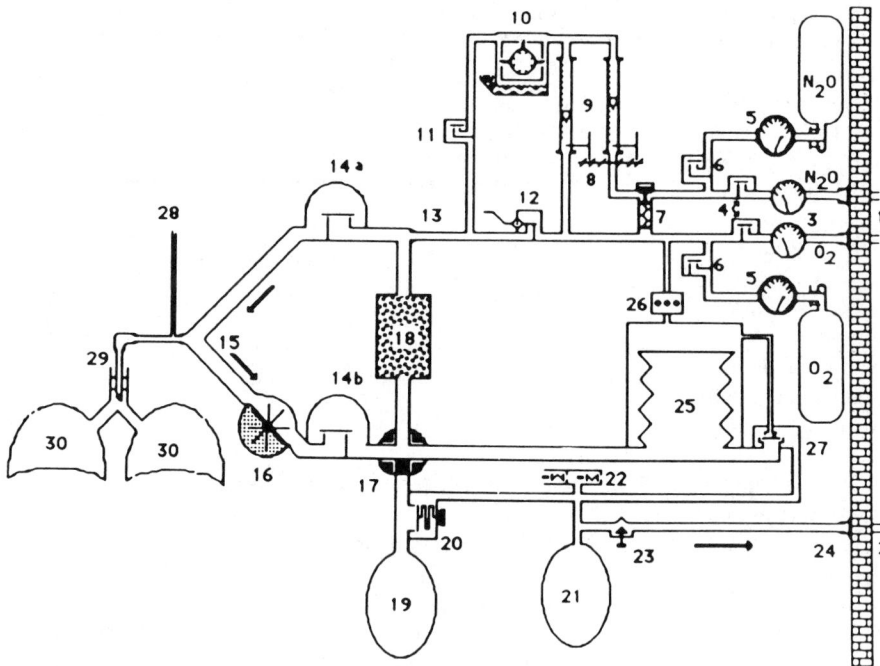

FIGURE 51–3. Schematic drawing of gas supply and anesthesia machine with a circle system. Anesthesia machine (1–13), breathing circuit (14–20), scavenging system (21–24), anesthesia ventilator (25–27), and patient interface (28–30). (From Gravenstein N, Lampotang S: Ventilation during anesthesia. *In* Clinical Applications of Ventilatory Support. Kirby RR, Banner MJ, Downs JB (eds). New York, Churchill Livingstone, 1990, p 282.)

because of fire code regulations. Charcoal absorbers are of limited usefulness because they are expensive, have a short life span, and do not remove nitrous oxide.

Maintenance

Periodic maintenance of anesthesia machines should be performed by factory-trained technicians every 4 to 6 months. Nevertheless, anesthesia personnel should be vigilant for faulty connections, torn gaskets, and other potential flaws that can become evident between routine service checks.[132] Efficient OR ventilation systems are important to ensure a high number of OR air turnovers; more than 15 turnovers per hour prevent areas of air stagnation.

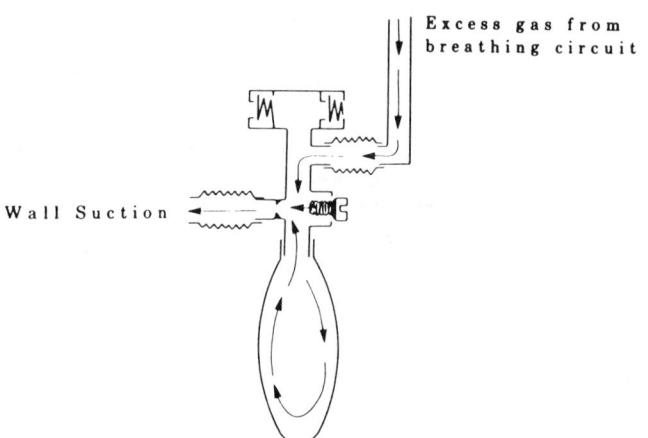

FIGURE 51–4. Anesthesia scavenger system. Note the incorporation of a positive-pressure (overpressure) governor (*right*) and a negative pressure valve (*left*) to prevent the transmission of either positive or negative pressure from the scavenger system to the ventilator or breathing circuit. (From Gravenstein N, Lampotang S: Ventilation during anesthesia. *In* Clinical Applications of Ventilatory Support. Kirby RR, Banner MJ, Downs JB (eds). New York, Churchill Livingstone, 1990, p 282.)

Testing

Routine environmental monitoring of trace gas concentrations should be conducted several times per year. Gas chromatographic or infrared analysis of ambient air samples provides quality assurance of the effectiveness of trace gas control measures in the institution. Monitoring should be carried out with specialized equipment, because nitrous oxide is both colorless and odorless. The olfactory threshold for halogenated agents is approximately 50 ppm, which is 100 times greater than the NIOSH standard dictates.

In our institution, the clinical engineering department performs quarterly sampling of nitrous oxide concentrations using a time-weighted average method. Levels >25 ppm are considered unacceptable by both our and NIOSH standards. All OR personnel should be educated about the potential hazards of trace anesthetic gases. Results of periodic monitoring under NIOSH conditions should be made available to all involved. Institutional guidelines for scavenging should be strictly followed by all personnel in order to minimize levels of exposure.

References

1. Case watch. AIDS Clinical Care 1992; 4:51.
2. Centers for Disease Control: Summary—Cases of specified notifiable diseases, United States, cumulative, week ending June 20, 1992. MMWR 1992; 41:446.
3. Centers for Disease Control: Summary—cases of specified notifiable diseases, United States, cumulative, week ending May 16, 1992. MMWR 1992; 41:356.
4. Centers for Disease Control: Summary—cases of specified notifiable diseases, United States, cumulative, week ending May 30, 1992. MMWR 1992; 41:392.
5. Centers for Disease Control: HIV/AIDS Surveillance Report, January 1992. Atlanta, Centers for Disease Control, 1992, pp 9, 17.
6. Centers for Disease Control: Estimates of HIV prevalence and projected AIDS cases—summary of a workshop, October 31–November 1, 1989. MMWR 1990; 39:110.
7. Oxtoby MJ: Perinatally acquired human immunodeficiency virus infection. Pediatr Infect Dis J 1990; 9:609.

8. Francis DP, Curran JW, Essex M: Epidemic acquired immune deficiency syndrome—Epidemiologic evidence for a transmissible agent (Editorial). J Natl Cancer Inst 1983; 71:1.

9. Barre-Sinoussi F, Chermann JC, Rey F, et al: Isolation of a T-lymphotropic retrovirus from a patient at risk for acquired immune deficiency syndrome (AIDS). Science 1983; 220:868.

10. Gallo RC, Sarin PS, Gelmann EP, et al: Isolation of human T-cell leukemia virus in acquired immune deficiency syndrome (AIDS). Science 1983; 220:865.

11. Duesberg PH: Human immunodeficiency virus and acquired immunodeficiency syndrome—correlation but not causation. Proc Natl Acad Sci USA 1989; 86:755.

12. Klatzmann D, Champagne E, Chamaret S, et al: T-lymphocyte T4 molecule behaves as the receptor for human retrovirus LAV. Nature 1984; 312:767.

13. Dalgleish AG, Beverly PCL, Clapham PR, et al: The CD4 (T4) antigen is an essential component of the receptor for the AIDS retrovirus. Nature 1984; 312:763.

14. McDougal JS, Kennedy MS, Sligh JM, et al: Binding of HTLV-III/LAV to T4⁺ T cells by a complex of the 110K viral protein and the T4 molecule. Science 1986; 231:382.

15. Ho DD, Pomerantz RJ, Kaplan JC: Pathogenesis of infection with human immunodeficiency virus. N Engl J Med 1987; 317:278.

16. Fauci AS: The human immunodeficiency virus—infectivity and mechanisms of pathogenesis. Science 1988; 239:617.

17. Levy JA: Human immunodeficiency viruses and the pathogenesis of AIDS. JAMA 1989; 261:2997.

18. El-Farrash MA, Masuda T, Harada S: Synergistic infectivity of highly and minimally infectious clones of human immunodeficiency virus in vitro. J Infect Dis 1990; 161:1010.

19. Greene WC: The molecular biology of human immunodeficiency virus type I infection. N Engl J Med 1991; 324:308.

20. Fauci AS, Schnittman SM, Poli G, et al: Immunopathogenic mechanisms in human immunodeficiency virus (HIV) infection. Ann Intern Med 1991; 114:678.

21. Yarchoan R, Mitsuya H, Myers CE, Broder S: Clinical pharmacology of 3'-azido-2',3'-dideoxythymidine (Zidovudine) and related dideoxynucleosides. N Engl J Med 1989; 321:726.

22. Hirsch MS: Chemotherapy of human immunodeficiency virus infections—current practice and future prospects. J Infect Dis 1990; 161:845.

23. Broder S, Mitsuya H, Yarchoan R, et al: Antiretroviral therapy in AIDS. Ann Intern Med 1990; 113:604.

24. Krasinski K: Retroviral therapy and clinical trials for HIV-infected children. J Pediatr 1991; 119:S63.

25. Volberding PA, Lagakos SW, Koch MA, et al: Zidovudine in asymptomatic human immunodeficiency virus infection—a controlled trial in persons with fewer than 500 CD4-positive cells per cubic millimeter. N Engl J Med 1990; 322:941.

26. Collier AC, Bozzette S, Coombs RW, et al: A pilot study of low-dose zidovudine in human immunodeficiency virus infection. N Engl J Med 1990; 323:1015.

27. Fischl MA, Parker CB, Pettinelli C, et al: A randomized controlled trial of a reduced daily dose of zidovudine in patients with the acquired immunodeficiency syndrome. N Engl J Med 1990; 323:1009.

28. Cooley TP, Kunches LM, Saunders CA, et al: Once-daily administration of 2',3'-dideoxyinosine (ddi) in patients with the acquired immunodeficiency syndrome or aids-related complex—results of a phase I trial. N Engl J Med 1990; 322:1340.

29. Lambert JS, Seidllin M, Reichman RC, et al: 2',3'-dideoxyinosine (ddi) in patients with the acquired immunodeficiency syndrome or AIDS-related complex—a phase I trial. N Engl J Med 1990; 322:1333.

30. Butler KM, Husson RN, Balis FM, et al: Dideoxyinosine in children with symptomatic human immunodeficiency virus infection. N Engl J Med 1991; 324:137.

31. Merigan TC, Skowron G, Bozzette SA, et al: Circulating p24 antigen levels and responses to dideoxycytidine in human immunodeficiency virus (HIV) infections—a phase I and II study. Ann Intern Med 1989; 110:189.

32. Merluzzi VJ, Hargrave KD, Labadia M, et al: Inhibition of HIV-1 replication by a non-nucleoside reverse transcriptase inhibitor. Science 1990; 250:1411.

33. Abrams DI, Kuno S, Wong R, et al: Oral dextran sulfate (ua001) in the treatment of the acquired immunodeficiency syndrome (AIDS) and AIDS-related complex. Ann Intern Med 1989; 110:183.

34. Larder BA, Darby G, Richman DD: HIV with reduced sensitivity to zidovudine (AZT) isolated during prolonged therapy. Science 1989; 243:1731.

35. Javaherian K, Langlois AJ, LaRosa GJ, et al: Broadly neutralizing antibodies elicited by the hypervariable neutralizing determinant of HIV-1. Science 1990; 250:1590.

36. Dolin R, Graham BS, Greenberg SB, et al: The safety and immunogenicity of a human immunodeficiency virus type 1 (HIV-1) recombinant gp160 candidate vaccine in humans. Ann Intern Med 1991; 114:119.

37. Redfield RR, Birx DL, Ketter N, et al: A phase I evaluation of the safety and immunogenicity of vaccination with recombinant gp160 in patients with early human immunodeficiency virus infection. N Engl J Med 1991; 324:1677.

38. Centers for Disease Control: Update: acquired immunodeficiency syndrome—United States, 1981–1990. MMWR 1991; 40:358.

39. Centers for Disease Control: The HIV/AIDS epidemic—the first 10 years. MMWR 1991; 40:357.

40. Chu SY, Buehler JW, Berkelman RL: Impact of the human immunodeficiency virus epidemic on mortality in women of reproductive age, United States. JAMA 1990; 264:225.

41. Centers for Disease Control: Selected behaviors that increase risk for HIV infection among high school students—United States, 1990. MMWR 1992; 41:231.

42. Centers for Disease Control: HIV prevalence estimates and AIDS case projections for the United States: report based upon a workshop. MMWR 1990; 39(#RR-16):1.

43. Francis DP: Toward a comprehensive HIV prevention program for the CDC and the nation. JAMA 1992; 268:1444.

44. Osler W, McCrae T: The Principles and Practice of Medicine. New York, Appleton, 1920, p 269.

45. Fauci AS: The human immunodeficiency virus—infectivity and mechanisms of pathogenesis. Science 1988; 239:617.

46. Ho DD, Moudgil T, Alam M: Quantitation of human immunodeficiency virus type 1 in the blood of infected persons. N Engl J Med 1989; 321:1621.

47. Coombs RW, Collier AC, Allain J-P, et al: Plasma viremia in human immunodeficiency virus infection. N Engl J Med 1989; 321:1626.

48. Wolinsky SM, Rinaldo CR, Kwok S, et al: Human immunodeficiency virus type 1 (HIV-1) infection median of 18 months before a diagnostic Western blot. Ann Intern Med 1989; 111:961.

49. Imagawa DT, Lee MH, Wolinsky SM, et al: Human immunodeficiency virus type 1 infection in homosexual men who remain seronegative for prolonged periods. N Engl J Med 1989; 320:1458.

50. Weiss R, Their SO: HIV testing is the answer—What's the question? (Editorial). N Engl J Med 1988; 319:1010.

51. Meyer KB, Pauker SG: Screening for HIV—Can we afford the false positive rate? N Engl J Med 1987; 317:238.

52. Centers for Disease Control: Interpretation and use of Western blot assay for serodiagnosis of human immunodeficiency virus type 1 infection. MMWR 1989; 38(S-7):1.

53. Lifson AR, Castro KG, McCray E: National surveillance of AIDS in health care workers. JAMA 1986; 256:3231.

54. McCray E: Occupational risk of the acquired immunodeficiency syndrome among health workers. N Engl J Med 1986; 314:1127.

55. Centers for Disease Control: Update: acquired immuno-deficiency syndrome and human immunodeficiency virus infection among health care workers. MMWR 1988; 37:229.

56. Henderson DK, Fahey BJ, Willy M, et al: Risk for occupational transmission of human immunodeficiency virus type 1 (HIV-1) associated with clinical exposures—a prospective evaluation. Ann Intern Med 1990; 113:740.

57. Jones ME: A thing about AIDS. Anaesth Intensive Care 1989; 17:253.

58. McKinney WP, Young MJ: The cumulative probability of occupationally acquired HIV infection—the risks of repeated exposures during a surgical career. Infect Control Hosp Epidemiol 1990; 11:243.

59. Lowenfels AB, Wormser GP, Jain R: Frequency of puncture injuries in surgeons and estimated risk of HIV infection. Arch Surg 1989; 124:1284.

60. Berry AJ, Isaacson IJ, Kane MA, et al: A multicenter study of the prevalence of hepatitis B viral serologic markers in anesthesia personnel. Anesth Analg 1984; 63:738.

61. Baker JL, Kelen GD, Silverton KT: Unsuspected human immunodeficiency virus in critically ill emergency patients. JAMA 1987; 257:2609.

62. Kristensen MS, Sloth E, Jensen TK: Relationship between anesthetic procedure and contact of anesthesia personnel with patient body fluids. Anesthesiology 1990; 73:619.

63. Harrison CA, Rogers DW, Rosen M: Blood contamination of anesthetic and related staff. Anaesthesia 1990; 45:831.

64. Wright JG, McGeer AJ, Chyatte D, et al: Mechanisms of glove tears and sharp injuries among surgical personnel. JAMA 1991; 266:1668.

65. Matta H, Thompson AM, Rainey JB: Does wearing two pairs of gloves protect operating theatre staff from skin contamination? Br Med J 1988; 297:597.
66. Hammond JS, Eckes JM, Gomez GA, et al: HIV, trauma, and infection control—universal precautions are universally ignored. J Trauma 1990; 30:555.
67. Gerberding JL, Schecter WP: Surgery and AIDS—reducing the risk (Editorial). JAMA 1991; 265:1572.
68. Panlilio AL, Foy DR, Edwards JR, et al: Blood contacts during surgical procedures. JAMA 1991; 265:1533.
69. Lange JMA, Boucher CAB, Hollak CEM, et al: Failure of zidovudine prophylaxis after accidental exposure to HIV-1. N Engl J Med 1990; 322:1375.
70. Centers for Disease Control: Update: transmission of HIV infection during an invasive dental procedure—Florida. MMWR 1991; 40:21.
71. Centers for Disease Control: Update: transmission of HIV infection during invasive dental procedures—Florida. MMWR 1991; 40:377.
72. Lo B, Steinbrook R: Health care workers infected with the human immunodeficiency virus—the next steps. JAMA 1992; 267:1100.
73. Layon AJ, D'Amico R: Intensive care for patients with acquired immunodeficiency syndrome—medicine versus ideology. Crit Care Med 1990; 18:1297.
74. D'Amico R, Layon AJ: AIDS and the politics of morbidity. Telos 1988 (Summer); 76:115.
75. Daniels N: HIV-infected professionals, patient rights, and the "switching dilemma." JAMA 1992; 267:1368.
76. Rogers DE, Osborn JE: Another approach to the AIDS epidemic. N Engl J Med 1991; 325:806.
77. Centers for Disease Control: Update: CD4$^+$ T-lymphocytopenia in persons without evident HIV infection—United States. MMWR 1992; 41:578.
78. Centers for Disease Control: Summary of notifiable diseases—United States 1988. MMWR 1988; 37:3.
79. Centers for Disease Control: Summary of selected notifiable diseases—United States week ending June 27, 1992 (26th week). MMWR 1992; 41:471.
80. Lemon SM: Type A viral hepatitis. N Engl J Med 1985; 313:1059.
81. Centers for Disease Control: Recommendations for protection against viral hepatitis. Ann Intern Med 1985; 103:391.
82. Centers for Disease Control: Hepatitis A among homosexual men—United States, Canada, and Australia. MMWR 1992; 41:15.
83. Ockner RK: Acute viral hepatitis. In Cecil Textbook of Medicine. 18th ed. Wyngaarden JB, Smith LH (eds). Philadelphia, WB Saunders, 1988, pp 818–826.
84. Alter MJ, Ahtone J, Weisfuse I, et al: Hepatitis virus B transmission between heterosexuals. JAMA 1986; 256:1307.
85. Rosenblum L, Darrow W, Witte J, et al: Sexual practices in the transmission of hepatitis B virus and prevalence of hepatitis delta virus infection in female prostitutes in the United States. JAMA 1992; 267:2477.
86. Czaja AJ: Serologic markers of hepatitis A and B in acute and chronic liver disease. Mayo Clin Proc 1979; 54:721.
87. Kelen GD, Green GB, Purcell RH, et al: Hepatitis B and Hepatitis C in emergency department patients. N Engl J Med 1992; 326:1399.
88. Aach RD, Stevens CE, Hollinger FB, et al: Hepatitis C virus infection in post-transfusion hepatitis—an analysis with first- and second-generation assays. N Engl J Med 1991; 325:1325.
89. Stevens CE, Aach RD, Hollinger FB, et al: Hepatitis B virus antibody in blood donors and the occurrence of non-A non-B hepatitis in transfusion recipients. Ann Intern Med 1984; 101:733.
90. Czaja AJ, Davis GL: Hepatitis non-A non-B. Mayo Clin Proc 1982; 57:639.
91. Koziol DE, Holland PV, Alling DW, et al: Antibody to hepatitis B core antigen as a paradoxical marker for non-A non-B hepatitis agent in donated blood. Ann Intern Med 1986; 104:488.
92. Choo QL, Kuo G, Weiner AJ, et al: Isolation of a cDNA clone derived from a blood-borne non-A, non-B viral hepatitis genome. Science 1989; 244:359.
93. Baron S, Tyring SK, Fleischmann WR Jr, et al: The interferons—mechanisms of action and clinical applications. JAMA 1991; 266:1375.
94. Lettau LA, McCarthy JG, Smith MH, et al: Outbreak of severe hepatitis due to delta and hepatitis B viruses in parenteral drug abusers and their contacts. N Engl J Med 1987; 317:1256.
95. Goldberg ME, Brajer J, Seltzer JL: Herpetic whitlow—hazard for the anesthesiologist and an unusual complication. Anesthesiol Rev 1985; 12:26.
96. Gill MJ, Arlette J, Buchan K: Herpes simplex virus infection of the hand—a profile of 79 cases. Am J Med 1988; 84:89.
97. Corey L, Spear PG: Infections with herpes simplex viruses. N Engl J Med 1986; 314:686.
98. England JA, Balfour HH Jr: Varicella and herpes zoster. In Infectious Diseases—A Modern Treatment of Infectious Processes. 4th ed. Hoeprich PD, Jordan MC (eds). Philadelphia, JB Lippincott, 1989, pp 942–953.
99. Brunell PA: Varicella. In Cecil Textbook of Medicine. 18th ed. Wyngaarden JB, Smith LH (eds). Philadelphia, WB Saunders, 1988, pp 1788–1790.
100. Weller TH: Varicella and herpes zoster. N Engl J Med 1983; 309:1362.
101. Lang DJ: Cytomegalovirus infection. In Cecil Textbook of Medicine, 18th ed. Wyngaarden JB, Smith LH (eds). Philadelphia, WB Saunders, 1988, pp 1784–1786.
102. Weller TH: The cytomegaloviruses—ubiquitous agents with protean clinical manifestations. N Engl J Med 1971; 285:267.
103. Jordan MC: Cytomegalovirus infections. In Infectious Diseases—A Modern Treatise of Infectious Processes. 4th ed. Hoeprich PD, Jordan MC (eds). Philadelphia, JB Lippincott Company, 1989, pp 805–811.
104. Tegtmeier GE: Transfusion transmitted cytomegalovirus infections—significance and control. Vox Sang 1986; 51(Suppl):22.
105. Centers for Disease Control: Transmission of multidrug-resistant tuberculosis among immunocompromised persons in a correctional system—New York, 1991. MMWR 1992; 41:507.
106. Spiegelman WG, Saunders L, Mazze RJ: Addiction and anesthesiology. Anesthesiology 1984; 60:335.
107. Weil A, Rosen W: Chocolate to morphine—understanding mind-active drugs. Boston, Houghton Mifflin, 1976.
108. Bruce DL, Eide KA, Linde HW, et al: Causes of death among anesthesiologists—a 20 year survey. Anesthesiology 1968; 29:565.
109. Talbott GD, Benson EB: The impaired physician. Postgrad Med 1980; 68:56.
110. Ward CF, Ward GC, Saidman LJ: Drug abuse in anesthesia training programs—a survey: 1970 through 1980. JAMA 1983; 250:922.
111. Herrington RE: The impaired physician—recognition, diagnosis and treatment. Wis Med J 1979; 78:21.
112. Lew EA: Mortality experience among anesthesiologists, 1954–1976. Anesthesiology 1979; 51:195.
113. Gravenstein JS, Kory WP, Marks RG: Drug abuse by anesthesia personnel. Anesth Analg 1983; 62:467.
114. Hays LR, Stillner V, Littrell R: Fentanyl dependence associated with oral ingestion. Anesthesiology 1992; 77:819.
115. Follette JW, Farley WJ: Anesthesiologists addicted to propofol. Anesthesiology 1992; 77:817.
116. Herrington RE, Benzer DG, Jacobson GR, et al: Treating substance-use disorders among physicians. JAMA 1982; 247:2253.
117. Gualtieri AC, Dosentino JP, Becker JS: The California experience with a diversion program for impaired physicians. JAMA 1983; 269:226.
118. Talbott GD, Richardson AC, Mashburn JS, et al: The medical association of Georgia's disabled doctor program—a 5 year review. J Med Assoc Ga 1981; 70:545.
119. Adler GA, Potts FE, Kirby RR, et al: Narcotics control in anesthesia training. JAMA 1985; 253:3133.
120. Moleski RJ, Easley S, Barash PG, et al: Control and accountability of controlled substance administration in the operating room. Anesth Analg 1985; 64:989.
121. Goodman and Gilman's the Pharmacologic Basis of Therapeutics. 7th ed. New York, MacMillan, 1985.
122. Johnson VE: The dynamics of intervention, I'll quit tomorrow. New York, Harper & Row, 1980, pp 43–55.
123. Blachly PH, Osterud HT, Josslin R: Suicide in professional groups. N Engl J Med 1963; 268:1278.
124. Garb S: Drug addiction in physicians. Anesth Analg 1969; 48:129.
125. Klein RL, Stevens WC, Kingston HGG: Controlled substance dispensing and accountability in United States anesthesiology residency programs. Anesthesiology 1992; 77:806.
126. Ward CF: Substance abuse: now and for some time to come (Editorial). Anesthesiology 1992; 77:619.
127. Parker JBR: The effects of fatigue on physician performance—an underestimated cause of physician impairment and patient risk. Can J Anaesth 1987; 34:489.
128. Hawkins MR, Vichick DA, Silsby HD, et al: Sleep and nutritional deprivation and performance of house officers. J Med Educ 1985; 60:530.
129. Bruce DL, Bach MJ, Arbit J: Trace anaesthetic gases on perceptual, cognitive, and motor skills. Anesthesiology 1974; 40:453.
130. Bruce DL, Bach MJ: Effects of trace anaesthetic gases on behavioral performance of volunteers. Br J Anaesth 1976; 48:871.

131. Smith G, Shirley AW: Failure to demonstrate effects of low concentrations of nitrous oxide and halothane on psychomotor performance (Abstract). Br J Anaesth 1976; 48:271.

132. Cooper JB, Newbower RS, Kitz RJ: An analysis of major errors and equipment failures in anesthesia management—considerations for prevention and detection. Anesthesiology 1984; 60:34.

133. McCue JD: The effects of stress on physicians and their medical practice. N Engl J Med 1982; 306:458.

134. Vaillant GE, Sobowale NC, McArthur C: Some psychologic vulnerabilities of physicians. N Engl J Med 1972; 287:372.

135. Lecky JH: Problems of trace anesthetic levels. *In* Complications in Anesthesia. Orkin FK, Cooperman LH (eds). Philadelphia, JB Lippincott, 1980, pp 715–732.

136. Axelsson G, Rylander R: Exposure to anesthetic gases and spontaneous abortion—response bias in a postal questionnaire study. Int J Epidemiol 1982; 11:250.

137. Lane GA, Nahrwold ML, Tait AR, et al: Nitrous oxide is teratogenic—xenon is not! Anesthesiology 1979; 51:S260.

138. Cohen EN, Brown BW, Wu ML, et al: Occupational disease in dentistry and chronic exposure to trace anesthetic gases. J Am Dent Assoc 1980; 101:21.

139. Vessey MP, Nunn JF: Occupational hazards of anesthesia. Br Med J 1980; 281:696.

140. Ferstandig LL: Trace concentrations of anesthetic gases—a critical review of their disease potential. Anesth Analg 1978; 57:328.

141. National Institute for Occupational Safety and Health, DHEWC (NIOSH): Criteria for a Recommended Standard. Occupational Exposure to Waste Anesthetic Gases and Vapors. Publication 77–140, 1977.

142. Eastwood DW, Green CD, Lamblin MA, et al: Effect of nitrous oxide on the white cell count in leukemia. N Engl J Med 1963; 268:297.

143. Knill-Jones RP, Moir DB, Rodrigues LV, et al: Anaesthetic practice and pregnancy—a controlled survey of women anaesthetists in the United Kingdom. Lancet 1972; 2:1326.

144. Cohen EN, Belville JW, Brown BW: Anesthesia, pregnancy, and miscarriage—a study of operating room nurses and anesthetists. Anesthesiology 1971; 35:343.

145. American Society of Anesthesiologists: Report of an ad hoc committee on the effect of trace anesthetics on the health of operating room personnel. Occupational disease among operating room personnel—a national study. Anesthesiology 1974; 41:321.

146. Davenport HT, Halsey MJ, Wardley-Smith B, et al: Occupational exposure to anaesthetics in 20 hospitals. Anaesthesia 1980; 35:354.

147. Linde HW, Bruce DL: Occupational exposure of anesthetists to halothane, nitrous oxide, and radiation. Anesthesiology 1969; 30:363.

148. Corbett TH: Retention of anesthetic agents following occupational exposure. Anesth Analg 1973; 52:614.

149. Gravenstein JS, Paulus DA: Monitoring practice in anesthesia. Philadelphia, JB Lippincott, 1982, pp 336–354.

150. Petty C: The anesthesia machine. New York, Churchill Livingstone, 1987, pp 108–113.

151. Dorsch JA, Dorsch SE: Understanding Anesthesia Equipment. 2nd ed. Baltimore, Williams & Wilkins, 1984, pp 254–266.

152. Bowie E, Huffman LM: The anesthesia machine: Essentials for understanding. Madison, WI, Ohmeda Corp, 1985, pp 137–139.

153. Gravenstein N, Lampotang S: Ventilation during anesthesia. *In* Clinical Applications of Ventilatory Support. Kirby RR, Banner MJ, Downs JB (eds). New York, Churchill Livingstone, 1990, pp 277–300.

CHAPTER 52

Battlefield Surgery and Anesthesia*

AZRIEL PEREL, M.D.

ERAN DOLEV, M.D.

JAY S. ELLIS, M.D., Lt. Col., U.S.A.F., M.C.

ROBERT R. KIRBY, M.D.

SALVATORE LOPALO, C.R.N.A., M.S.Ed., M.A.

Perhaps the only beneficial effect of trauma is that it contributes to medical knowledge; almost every specialty has realized major advances from the experience gained in the management of injuries. Wound treatment advanced surgical techniques; bandaging was an art by the 5th century BC,[1] and cautery-thermal debridement was developed during that period.[2] Alexandrian physicians around 300 BC used ligation to control bleeding.[3] Celsus in the first century AD described wounds, extraction of foreign bodies, and surgical instruments.[4] Galen (130–201) used sutures for wound closure.

WARTIME SURGERY

Wound surgery always has been war surgery, and war advanced the management of trauma. The old Ionian word for physician, *Iatros*, as mentioned by Homer, meant "an extractor of arrows." The hippocratic advice to those who would be surgeons was to follow the army.[2, 5]

In the Dark Ages, ligation and suturing were supplanted by cautery.[1] Gunpowder was introduced during the 14th century. Most military surgeons were convinced that gunshot wounds were poisoned. Giovanni de Vigo (1460–1520) probably introduced boiling oil as the treatment of choice for these wounds.[6]

What Were the Major Advances?

Wound Management

Ambroise Paré (1510–1590) was the greatest military surgeon during the Renaissance period. Through his experience, he came to the conclusion that treatment of wounds with

boiling oil was wrong.[6] Paré in France and Maggi in Italy recognized that tissue injured by bullets was not poisoned but simply crushed. Paré reintroduced the ligature, allowing the performance of amputations.[7] He realized the importance of reporting surgical results and other data in order to improve treatment.[8]

Early Treatment and Transport

Dominique Jean Larrey (1766–1842) recognized the importance of early battle wound treatment during the Napoleonic Wars. Previously, wounded soldiers were unattended on the field until the battle was concluded. Larrey began to treat casualties during fighting and introduced a system of battle casualty transportation ("flying ambulances") to medical stations and field hospitals. This rapid evacuation of casualties allowed surgery to be performed as soon as possible.[8, 9] Larrey also treated casualties according to medical priorities, ignoring rank and distinction.[10]

Jonathan Letterman (1824–1867) was the Medical Director of the Army of the Potomac during the American Civil War. He planned ambulance corps for evacuating casualties from the front line and organized mobile field hospitals manned by adequate surgical personnel. By further shortening the time between injury and treatment, he contributed significantly to the care of battle casualties. Letterman realized that echeloning is mandatory in any military medical organization, and he established the concept that evacuation of casualties did not just represent transportation but was itself a medical process.[11, 12]

During the Russo-Japanese War (1904–1905), Princess Vera Gedroitz, a Russian surgeon, also shortened the time between injury and surgery by operating on battle casualties at the field. For abdominal penetrating wounds, the importance of early operation was demonstrated, and urgency was accepted as a new concept in trauma surgery.

---

*The opinions expressed are those of the authors and do not necessarily reflect the views of the United States Air Force or the Department of Defense.

Anesthesiology

Trauma surgery also helped to advance anesthesiology. Although the first widespread use of ether previously was thought to have occurred during either the Crimean or German-Danish conflicts after 1848, recent information suggests that it was first used during the Mexican-American War in the spring of 1847.[13] During World War I, nitrous oxide (N_2O) use on the western front marked an important advance in acceptance of this anesthetic.[14]

Fluid Therapy and Transfusion

Intravenous fluid therapy was initiated during World War I by George Crile of Cleveland, who used seawater to resuscitate hypovolemic injured soldiers.[15] Now, over 70 years later, the effectiveness of hypertonic saline therapy in various traumatic injuries is again being evaluated. In the early years of the 20th century, the principles of crossmatching and preparation of whole blood were developed. During World War II, large amounts of whole blood were prepared and shipped under refrigeration to the battlefield. These techniques were refined to an even higher degree in the Vietnam conflict and ultimately led to the popularization of frozen red blood cell preparations.

Management of Shock

Recognition of the endocrine-metabolic response to trauma is also credited to Crile, who realized in World War I that the nervous system must be intact for the metabolic response to occur.[16] Trauma care improved significantly during World War II. By that time, the meaning of *shock* caused by blood loss was realized. Major innovations included the administration of whole blood and antibiotics. Special shock units were established in field hospitals, and the essential unity of resuscitation and operation was recognized. The understanding of hypovolemic shock, the pathophysiology of wounding, and the complications of injury, mainly infections, advanced to a new level.

Triage

Wilson was the first to propose military triage in 1846.[17] He held that immediate life-saving surgery often could be provided for severely injured casualties only if treatment for lesser injuries was deferred. Palliative measures were given to those whose injuries were likely to prove fatal. The military medical system adopted the concept of triage as a mode of operation during World War II, the goal being rescue of the maximum number of lives. This goal was achieved by prioritization of urgent care after identification of battle casualties according to the severity of their injuries and the estimation of their chances of survival. Discerning readers will note that this approach is in counterdistinction to that in civilian practice, in which most severely traumatized individuals are transported to trauma centers; those less severely injured often are managed at lower-level institutions.

Air Evacuation Versus Prompt Initial Care

Modern military and civilian experience confirms that any reduction in the time period between injury and surgery is one of the main factors contributing to higher survival rates. Helicopters, first used during the Korean War, had a major role in Vietnam. Critically injured patients were evacuated from the site of injury directly into the definitive surgical hospital, bypassing the battalion aid station and the divisional surgical hospital. The average time from injury to surgery in Vietnam was about 80 minutes,[18] compared with 2 to 4 hours during the Korean War and 6 to 12 hours during World War II.[19–21]

The high survival rate in Vietnam has been attributed by some solely to rapid helicopter evacuation. However, other factors contributed to that success: Units were available for resuscitation and definitive surgery, and mass casualty situations that jeopardized their ability to attend every patient rarely were encountered by surgical units.

Acting according to the "scoop and run" policy, in Vietnam battle casualties were evacuated to a hospital without being resuscitated, a practice that ignored the military principle of echeloning. Although this approach was justified in many instances in Vietnam, it also has been criticized. Could the Vietnam survival rate have been even better if first aid, resuscitation, and stabilization had been used before evacuation?[22, 23] Here are the sources of a future dispute: Is the contribution of rapid evacuation greater than that of prompt and proper initial care that potentially interferes with the speed and efficiency of the evacuation process?[2]

THE MISSION

Battlefield military medicine has a threefold mission: (1) to save lives, (2) to alleviate suffering, and, (3) to return soldiers to duty. A task of military medicine is the study of previous wars, which allows prediction of the number and types of future battle casualties. To achieve this end, military physicians should be familiar with the military scenario, the types of weapons used, and the meaning of tactical situations. They also should understand the pathophysiology of trauma and the epidemiologic and statistical methods used to analyze battlefield casualties.

How Are Mortality and Morbidity Analyzed?

The following terms are commonly used:

Killed in action (KIA). The number of soldiers who die before being seen by a medical officer.
Died of wounds (DOW). The number of soldiers who die after being attended by a medical officer.
Total rate of mortality. The number of soldiers who die (i.e., KIA + DOW)/total number of casualties.

Mode of Warfare

Many factors account for the differences in injuries reported in different wars. During June 1966, in Vietnam, 49.6% of the "hits" were caused by shell fragments and 42.7% by small arms. In June 1970, 80% of the hits were caused by shell fragments and only 10% by small arms.[24]

When data are compared from the Israeli experience during the 1973 October War and the 1982 Lebanon War, the most significant difference was the rate of multitrauma cases. Because warfare modes changed, multitrauma accounted for only

6.9% of battle casualties in 1973, compared with 19% in 1982. In 1973, open fighting involved armored units. Conversely, in 1982, the conflict was largely a closed-area battle in which the use of small arms, grenades, mines, and explosives was common.[25, 26]

Reorganization of Medical Care

Reorganization of the medical delivery system may also alter injury patterns. During the first phase of the 1969 Israeli War of Attrition, 25.4% of the casualties were KIA. To lower this KIA incidence, the front lines were reinforced by physicians. In the second phase of the war, the KIA rate was reduced to 18.1%. Conversely, the DOW rate, which was 3% during the first phase, increased to 3.7% during the second phase. This increase was attributed to the initial resuscitation of casualties so severely wounded that they could not survive. The mortality rate decreased from 28.6% in the initial phase to 21.8% in the second phase.[27]

Type of Injury

Most combat deaths occur on the battlefield before treatment by a medical officer. Exsanguination causes 50% of these deaths. The majority of the remaining early deaths are unavoidable because of severe central nervous system injury. Thus, the most important goal of combat casualty care is to reduce the death rate secondary to hemorrhage.[28] As the 1967 Israeli War showed, the proximity of medical care to the front line contributed to a reduction in mortality but also accounted for the paradoxical increase in DOW rates.

Source of Injury

The extent of missile injury is based on their velocity. Weapons with muzzle velocities >760 m · s^{-1} are high velocity, whereas those below that speed are low velocity.[29] The primary effect of low-velocity missiles is laceration and crushing of tissues. Tissue damage is a result of immediate contact with the bullet or fragment.

High-velocity missiles cause extensive tissue destruction in two ways. First is the formation of a temporary cavity as a result of rapid transfer of energy from the missile to the tissues. Second is the formation of a tissue shock wave that compresses the tissue in front of the missile. Solid tissues are particularly susceptible to this form of energy transfer. Tissues and organs also can be damaged at remote locations, in which case the injury is unrelated to the missile track per se.[30] Most weapons used on the modern battlefield are high velocity and have potentially devastating wounding power.

During the Vietnam conflict, artillery was responsible for 65% of the injuries but only 36% of the deaths. Small arms, primarily high velocity, were responsible for only 16% of the injuries yet caused 51% of the deaths.[24] In the 1982 Lebanon War, artillery was responsible for 53% of the injuries but <10% of the fatalities. Small arms, conversely, caused only 11.7% of the injuries yet produced 31.7% of the fatalities.[25, 31]

Mechanized battles are composed of large formations of tanks and other armored vehicles that move rapidly across any terrain. Tank guns fire large-caliber high-velocity rounds that can penetrate the opponent's armor, destroy other tanks, and injure or kill the tank crews. Tank bullets have high energy; their fragments may be large; and if they strike a soldier in the head, neck, or trunk, death is immediate. Injuries caused by antitank missiles are similar to those produced by tank bullets; however, they carry an additional threat. Severe facial burns may result, and smoke inhalation within the tank may cause pulmonary injury.[32]

Protective Measures

Today, infantry soldiers are highly skilled, operate sophisticated weapons, fight in small, efficient units, and may even wage battle against tanks. Versatile infantrymen in helmets and flak jackets are largely protected from fragment injuries but not usually from high-velocity missiles. Substitution of Kevlar vests and helmets probably will improve this situation. Because infantrymen may be involved in any kind of warfare, they exhibit no typical injuries as a group.

URBAN WARFARE

How Does It Differ?

Experience has demonstrated the consequence of military operations in urbanized terrain (MOUT).[33] As a result of extensive urbanization in areas where battles traditionally have been fought, this type of warfare is difficult to avoid. However, MOUT is not just another way of fighting; this violent combat involves several units simultaneously engaged in close-range conflict. During battle, soldiers are exposed to snipers, explosives, small arms fire, and grenades, resulting in a high rate of head, neck, and chest injuries.

Blast Injury

Blast injury results from changes in air pressure (shock wave) that originate from an explosion.[34] During the 1982 Lebanon War, 2.3% of the Israeli battle casualties sustained blast injuries.[25]

Crush Syndrome

The crush syndrome, or traumatic rhabdomyolysis, is commonly found in persons trapped under fallen masonry. Terrorist activities in Lebanon, including the bombing of a barracks that killed more than 200 United States Marines, caused the destruction of populated buildings, buried inhabitants under rubble, and created increased interest in the syndrome.

Most victims of a building collapse die immediately from the direct effects of falling walls, blast effect, or fire or through compression of their head, neck, and trunk. The survivors are those whose limbs have been trapped under rubble, with resulting symptoms of local and systemic injury.

Local injury includes tissue destruction and neurologic extremity deficits.[35] Systemic manifestations also result from compression of the muscles. Release of intracellular muscle constituents into the circulation bellows (e.g., myoglobin, phosphate, potassium, uric acid, lactic acid), producing a severe metabolic acidosis. The crushing of blood vessels may cause hypovolemia and coagulation defects.[35]

In the past, the common outcome of this injury was acute renal failure and a grave prognosis. In 1982, the Israelis treated traumatic rhabdomyolysis with early infusion of alkaline solutions and antibiotics. With such therapy, most victims did not require hemodialysis.[35, 36]

MULTITRAUMA

Since the Korean conflict, the pattern of injuries from military encounters has been similar (Table 52–1). The only significant difference is in the number of mixed-injury or multi-trauma cases. When data from the Korean and Vietnam Wars and from the 1973 and 1982 Israeli Wars are compared, the increase in multitrauma is significant. This increase is probably a result of the type of warfare encountered—that is, an increase in MOUT. Injuries primarily were caused by fragments. Two thirds of the casualties were lightly wounded, 20% moderately wounded, and 7% severely wounded. The remaining wounds were undefined.[24–26]

What Is Its Significance?

The change in incidence of chest injuries between specific conflicts also highlights the importance of multitrauma (Table 52–2). It was present in 85.5% of Vietnam battle casualties. In chest-injured Israeli soldiers, 41.6% also suffered from abdominal injury, 23.4% from head and neck injury, and 89.1% from extremity injury.[37] This large overlap means that most injured Israelis sustained multitrauma. Data from the Iran-Iraq Gulf War showed that 23% of patients with spinal injury also sustained chest injury.[38, 39] The KIA rate has remained approximately 20% to 25% since World War II (Table 52–3).

TERRORISM

Terrorism has reached such epidemic proportions that it has become a threat to society. When one terrorism success leads to another terrorist event, at a different location and time, no society can be immune from its destruction. This point was demonstrated pointedly in the United States by the 1993 World Trade Center bombing in New York City. Because of increasing terrorist activity, the line between civilian and military trauma medicine is increasingly difficult to define.

What Are the Results of Bomb Blast Injuries?

Bomb blast injuries in Northern Ireland from 1969 to 1977 resulted in 50% of the casualties sustaining injuries while inside buildings. Injuries occurred in vehicles 25% of the time. The major hazards of terrorism in Northern Ireland were

TABLE 52–2. Cause of Battlefield Chest Injuries in Recent Conflicts

Agent	Vietnam (%)	1982 Israel (%)	Iran–Iraq Gulf (%)
Fragments	81	64.1	83
Bullets	14	10.9	10
Blunt injury	5	9.4	7
Mixed	—	15.6	—

shown to be high-velocity fragments and falling debris. Among the fatalities, 66% had brain injuries, 51% had skull fractures, 47% had diffuse lung contusions, and 34% had liver lacerations.[34] Thirty-seven people were injured in 1975 as a result of the Tower of London bombing. Nineteen (51.3%) of the injured were hospitalized. Ten (52.6%) of those admitted had severe multiple injuries.[40]

Twenty-four terrorist explosions produced 511 victims in Jerusalem from May 1975 until November 1979. Two thirds of the victims were evacuated to hospitals; 26 (7.7%) died before arrival. Hospitalization was required for 112 patients (32.9%), and the average length of stay was 16.2 days. Children younger than 13 years represented 6.2% of the injured, and those older than 65 years accounted for 6.8%. Head and neck injuries were found in 19.3% of the patients.[41]

ANESTHESIA PRACTICE

Anesthesiologists and nurse anesthetists who are placed in a combat environment for the first time encounter problems that no amount of civilian peacetime or military experience can adequately simulate. If ever the term *on-the-job training* was applicable, it is in this situation. Yet forewarned is forearmed, and knowledge of the nature of events to be encountered will be useful and potentially life saving.

What Are the General Problems?

Casualties

Hollywood has presented a skewed version of combat through the art of movie production. Viewing of portrayed battle scenes leads one to believe that large numbers of combat casualties occur in every battle, most of which descend, en masse, on the medical facilities portrayed. In fact, disease and nonbattle injuries account for 60% to 75% of all casualties. In Operations Desert Shield and Desert Storm (1990–1991), this figure was even higher because of the extremely low number of United States and allied battle injuries. Much more common are endemic diseases ranging from sand fly bites to hepatitis,

TABLE 52–1. Types of Injuries In Military Conflicts

Injury	Korea (%)	Vietnam (%)	Israel 1982 (%)	Israel 1973 (%)	Falklands (%)
Head and neck	17	14	13.5	13.3	14
Thorax	7	7	5	4.4	7
Abdomen	7	5	4.9	7.3	11.5
Extremities	67	54	41.4	40.9	67.5
Burns	—	—	3.9	9.3	—
Mixed	2	20	19	6.9	—
Soft tissues	—	—	8.2	9.1	—
Psychiatric	—	—	4.1	8.8	—

TABLE 52–3. Killed in Action Rate

Conflict	KIA Rate (%)
World War II	22.7
Korean War	19.7
1973 Israeli War	26.2
1982 Israeli War	20.5
Falklands War	23.4

TABLE 52–4. United States Deaths in Operations Desert Shield and Desert Storm (1990–1991)

Service	Battle Deaths	Non-Battle Deaths	Total
Army	98	105	203
Navy	6	8	14
Marines	24	26	50
Air Force	20	6	26
Total	148	145	293

amebiasis, typhus, and malaria. Mortality figures show similar distributions (Table 52–4). Battle- and non–battle-related injuries in Operations Desert Shield and Desert Storm were almost equal.

Security

Battlefield casualties, whether friendly forces or enemy, are likely to be armed. One cannot count on a well-intentioned physician or nurse to be perceived as a benefactor. Language barriers, fear, pain, and physiologic instability make an armed patient a potentially dangerous adversary. Security personnel must search and disarm all casualties, preferably before they enter the compound. Listen to and obey the security people. They are trained and know what to do. Do not try to be a hero.

Communication and Supply

Be familiar with your equipment and equipment needs. The battlefield is no place to discover that some of your essential gear is missing or does not work. Although satellite communication systems can put one in touch with any part of the world, they will likely have higher priority use than to request a vaporizer or soda lime canister. Know your supply personnel. A good noncommissioned officer is worth his or her weight in gold. Such a person can find material where it seemingly does not exist.

What Specific Problems Are Related to Anesthesia Practice?

Anesthesia practice in the field environment is a challenge for any provider. The keys to success are a complete understanding of anesthesia principles, flexibility, and ingenuity. Remember that field triage involves two additional steps generally not present in civilian practice: decontamination and search for weapons.

High Volume of Cases

On occasion, a large influx of casualties can be overwhelming. In Vietnam, mass casualty situations, particularly during the Tet Offensive, sometimes required anesthetists to administer two anesthetics simultaneously by placing operating tables head to head. Dentists, medical technicians, and nurses who are not Certified Registered Nurse Anesthetists (CRNAs) can be used as anesthesia "expanders." During nonpeak periods, anesthesia providers can enter other roles (physicians covering sick call, CRNAs performing ward duties). In between periods of high casualties, periods of intense boredom often

are sandwiched. Effective leaders use this time to prepare, train, and equip their units for the next surge.

Lack of Full Range of Equipment and Drugs

The basic anesthesia machine (Ohmeda 885 Field Anesthesia Machine) appears archaic but is functional (Fig. 52–1). It provides N_2O and oxygen (O_2) from compressed tank sources and has a VerniTrol vaporizer suitable for isoflurane or halothane use.[42] Advantages and disadvantages of this device are listed in Table 52–5. This machine generally is unfamiliar to most anesthesia personnel trained from the early 1970s to the present. It is scheduled for upgrading and eventual replacement, perhaps by the year 1999 or 2000.

Monitoring is spartan but includes automated noninvasive blood pressure, an electrocardiogram (ECG), and pulse oximetry (be aware, however, that pulse oximeters are tricky to use in environments outside the standard operating room [OR] and intensive care unit [ICU]). End-tidal carbon dioxide (CO_2) monitoring is not available.

As with equipment, drug inventories are limited, as are laboratory and blood bank facilities (Table 52–6). Logistic considerations limit availability. Ask yourself if the items provided are satisfactory for the job at hand. The answer, almost uniformly, is yes. Be aware that OR and anesthesia supplies are stored together. An unfamiliar piece of anesthesia equipment may be lost during unpacking. Search all OR stores if something is missing.

The VerniTrol Vaporizer

The VerniTrol vaporizer has been declared obsolete and is no longer serviced in civilian practice. However, it is the mainstay of the Ohmeda 885 machine. It is a bubble-through type vaporizer that is not temperature or pressure compensated. To know how much of an agent is delivered, one must calculate the output:

$$\text{Anesthesia concentration (\%)} = \frac{(VF)(VA)}{P_B(VF + DF) - (VA)(DF)} \times 100$$

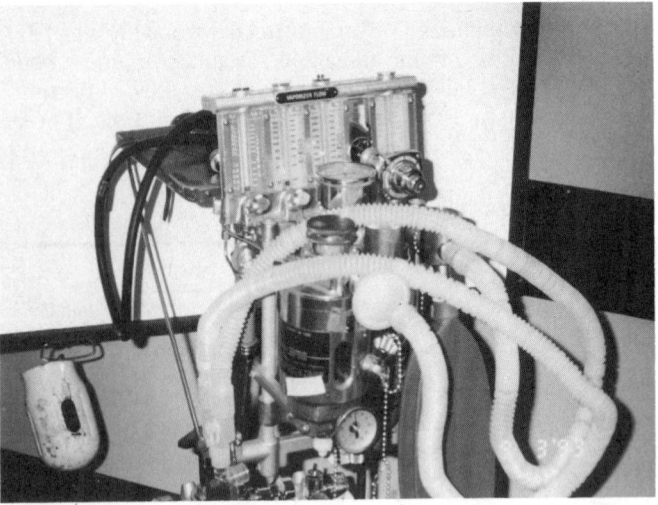

FIGURE 52–1. The Ohmeda 885 Field Anesthesia Machine. (Ohmeda, Madison, WI.)

TABLE 52–5. The Ohio 885 Field Anesthesia Machine

Advantages	Rugged, simple operation; multiple agent capacity; low-flow capable
Disadvantages	Lack of familiarity; requires compressed gas; heavy; no proportional flow; can deliver lethal concentrations of agent

where VF is vaporizer flow (mL · min^{-1}), DF is diluent flow (mL · min^{-1}), V_A is vapor pressure of the anesthetic (mm Hg), and P_B is barometric pressure (mm Hg).

Example. Calculate the vaporizer flow necessary to deliver 1% isoflurane at 22 °C with a total gas flow of 5000 mL · min^{-1}:

$$1\% = \frac{VF \times 238}{760 (5000) - 238 (5000)}$$

$$FV = \frac{(522) 5000}{23,800}$$

$$= 110 \text{ mL}$$

A flow calculator is provided by the manufacturer to simplify the process (Fig. 52–2). However, for someone who has never had to calculate vaporizer output (or has not done so for many years), the task, although simple, may seem daunting.

Drawover Vaporizer

The Universal PAC drawover vaporizer (Figs. 52–3 and 52–4) is also available.[43, 44] It incorporates a lightweight drawover vaporizer with a self-inflating bag that does not require a compressed O_2 source. However, hypoxia is a real danger if supplemental O_2 is not provided.

Battlefield Concerns: The Air Transportable Hospital

Remember that dust and humidity are the enemies of all electronic devices. Do your best to keep the immediate environment as contamination free as possible. The modern air transportable hospital (ATH) makes this task considerably easier than in past wars when tents were used. The ATH is a hard-walled modular building with enclosed connecting walkways. Depending on the availability of electrical generators, the environment it provides can be quite comfortable. Limited pressurization is possible (not enough to prevent chemical entry [e.g., nerve agents] but at least sufficient to exclude dust and dirt).

The echelon concept of operations is North Atlantic Treaty Organization (NATO) based and describes the level of care available at each location (Table 52–7). The ATH is second echelon, close to the site of casualties, has limited capacity

TABLE 52–6. Anesthesia Practice Problems

> High volume of cases
> Lack of full range of equipment and drugs
> Unfamiliarity with equipment
> Battlefield unique problems
> Personal motivation

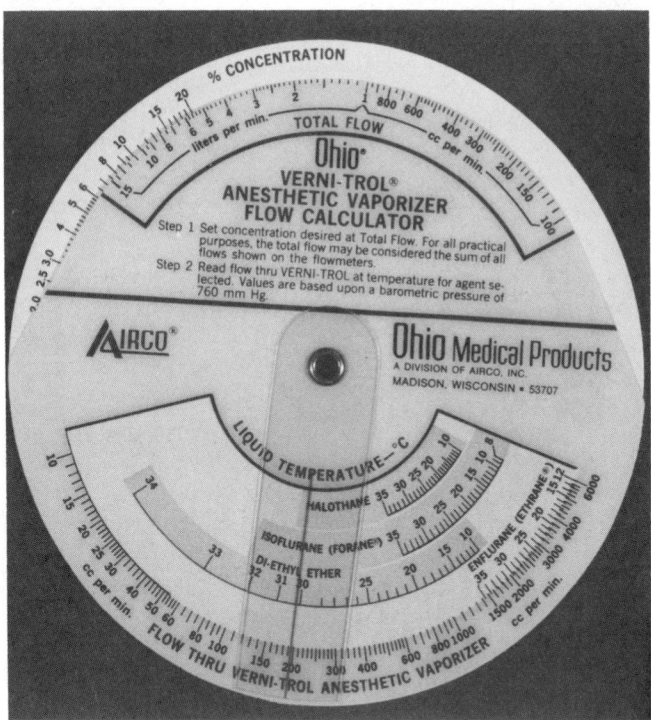

FIGURE 52–2. Flow calculator used to determine flow through the VerniTrol vaporizer. (Ohmeda, Madison, WI.)

(14–50 beds), and is designed only for life- or limb-saving surgical procedures. General surgeons, nurse anesthetists, or anesthesiologists are a part of the approximately 130 total personnel. Procedures include decontamination, emergency control of the airway, tube thoracostomy, and control of hemorrhage. Some idea of the size and complexity of the ATH may be obtained from the knowledge that 7 to 14 C-141 transports are necessary to ferry it to the destination.

What Are Common Management Problems?

During elective surgery, the scope of procedures performed has reflected the available anesthesia. Anesthesiologists on the battlefield, however, frequently have been confronted with severe shock and trauma beyond their accustomed state-of-the-art ministrations. Attempts to use standard peacetime drugs and techniques led to the appreciation that such drugs could

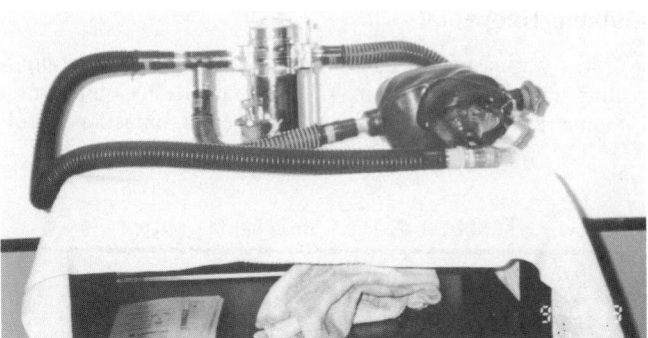

FIGURE 52–3. The Ohmeda Universal PAC drawover vaporizer and self-inflating bag. (Ohmeda, Madison, WI.)

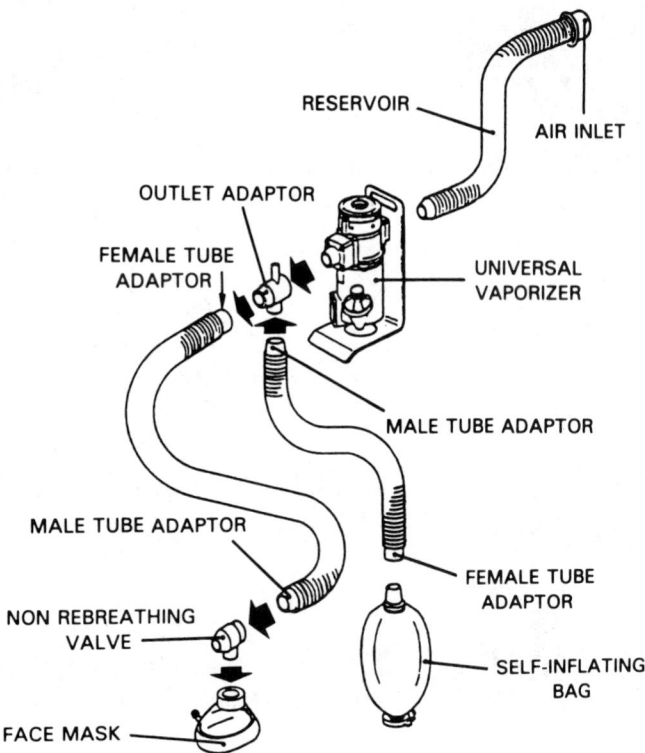

RESERVOIR
AIR INLET
OUTLET ADAPTOR
FEMALE TUBE ADAPTOR
UNIVERSAL VAPORIZER
MALE TUBE ADAPTOR
MALE TUBE ADAPTOR
FEMALE TUBE ADAPTOR
NON REBREATHING VALVE
SELF-INFLATING BAG
FACE MASK

FIGURE 52–4. Schematic "exploded" view of the PAC unit.

be fatal to hemodynamically unstable patients (chloroform, sodium thiopental, and spinal anesthetics).[45, 46]

Failure to recognize and treat hypovolemia is the most common management error.[47, 48] Overtransfusion is managed relatively easily with diuretics and positive end-expiratory pressure. Thus, fast and aggressive fluid administration should be carried out before emergency surgery. Once hemodynamic stabilization is evident, additional volume infusion should be performed before induction, because both anesthetic agents and positive-pressure ventilation can cause further hemodynamic deterioration.

Hemorrhaging patients should receive large fluid volumes before operation. These fluids should be administered warm, if possible, and should include blood, preferably fresh when available, lactated Ringer's solution, and plasma expanders.[49, 50]

How Should Induction Be Performed?

Sodium Thiopental

Most war casualties have "full stomachs," further complicating anesthetic induction. A rapid-sequence technique after volume resuscitation with sodium thiopental, immediately fol-

TABLE 52–7. The Four-Echelon Concept

First Echelon	Buddy care
Second Echelon	Medical personnel; limited surgical care
Third Echelon	Definitive surgical care
Fourth Echelon	Comprehensive medical care; subspecialists; rehabilitation

lowed by succinylcholine while cricoid pressure is maintained, usually is appropriate. However, severely injured battle casualties often cannot tolerate a large thiopental bolus, a point that was painfully demonstrated during World War II when this agent purportedly contributed to numerous fatalities.[46, 51] Thus, "when pentothal sodium is administered intravenously to patients who are in a state of shock . . . small doses (1 or 2 mL of 2.5% solution) administered slowly, with intervals . . . is the only rational scheme of dosage."[52]

Ketamine

Ketamine has become the most widely used induction agent for trauma victims in recent years. Because it causes sympathetic stimulation, ketamine may be less likely than other agents to cause hypotension during induction. Ketamine also acts quickly and can be used as a rapid-sequence induction agent.

Weiskopf and colleagues challenged the usefulness of ketamine for hypovolemic trauma victims.[53, 54] They contend that ketamine depresses the myocardium; produces sympathoadrenal stimulation leading to reduced peripheral perfusion, hence more lactic acidosis; and has no advantage over low doses of sodium thiopental. However, ketamine was compared with thiopental in hypovolemic swine, each drug administered in a dose of approximately $6 \text{ mg} \cdot \text{kg}^{-1}$. The investigators stated that "Other doses of ketamine or thiopental could have produced different effects during hypovolemia."

Thus, ketamine probably is still indicated for anesthetic induction in hemodynamically unstable, war trauma casualties. The large body of clinical experience with ketamine in battle casualties attests to its usefulness and safety in such conditions.[49, 55, 56]

How Is Anesthesia Maintained?

Nitrous Oxide

N_2O is of questionable value in battlefield conditions. It is supplied in heavy cylinders that are a logistic problem for forward medical units. It must be administered with O_2; thus, when O_2 is unavailable, N_2O is of no use.

Potent Inhalation Agents

The potent inhalation agents have a limited role during induction but are useful intraoperatively. Traditionally, halothane has been most commonly used, although it may not be ideal because of its tendency to induce cardiovascular depression. Isoflurane is an increasingly popular alternative and will supersede halothane in future conflicts. We believe that inhalation agents have a major role in battlefield anesthesia. When administered in low doses with narcotics, they produce easily controlled and reversible anesthesia.

Intravenous Anesthetic Agents

Narcotics always have been used on the battlefield; their prompt administration comforts patients and supports the morale of their unharmed colleagues. A narcotic-relaxant technique can be used as the only anesthesia for patients in shock. Narcotic amounts should be titrated, because total relief of "stress" may produce severe hypotension because of decreased sympathetic outflow and narcotic-induced vasodilation. When hypothermic battle casualties in shock receive intramuscular narcotics, delayed absorption may occur, causing postoperative respiratory depression. This reaction is also possible after postoperative administration, even when narcotics are not administered intraoperatively.[46, 55]

Muscle Relaxants

The ideal battlefield muscle relaxant should be thermostable and have a long shelf life. Because they do not require refrigeration, succinylcholine bromide and vecuronium bromide are superior to succinylcholine chloride and pancuronium or atracurium, respectively. In practice, a larger than usual dose of nondepolarizing muscle relaxant is needed for unstable trauma patients because they will receive little or no anesthesia. Nevertheless, deliberate pancuronium underdosing has proved adequate in combat casualties.[50]

Sedatives and Tranquilizers

Tranquilizers, such as diazepam and midazolam, can be useful in perioperative management, although they have little role in anesthetic maintenance. Their amnesic properties are advantageous, because patients may have operative recall after a ''light'' anesthetic is administered.[57] Other patients need sedation to prevent ketamine emergence reactions.

How Should Patients Be Ventilated?

Nearly all patients undergoing battlefield surgery should be manually or mechanically ventilated, although the ideal battlefield ventilator has yet to be designed. Such a ventilator should be small, lightweight, robust, and battery powered. Many wartime ventilators depend on an external power source, either compressed gas or electricity. The consumption of compressed gas by gas-powered ventilators familiar to us in civilian ORs makes them impractical for field mobility use.

Other anesthetic ventilators, prevalent in many parts of the world, remain manually driven. One such system, the previously described Tri-Service Anesthetic Apparatus,[43, 44] received wide acclaim after its use in the Falklands.[55] This system uses a draw-over vaporizer and self-inflating bag that is simple, practical, and useful in remote or battlefield environments (see Figs. 52–3 and 52–4).[58]

Such anesthetic systems might seem esoteric antiques to current anesthesia residents. Their attractiveness, though, is that they are independent of any power source, dependable, and easy to maintain. Under battlefield conditions, they may be more useful than manual or mechanical anesthetic systems that depend on a supply of compressed N_2O and O_2.

What Are the Major Postoperative Concerns?

Arousal/Awakening

Patients should be readied for rapid reversal of relaxants and extubation at the end of the operation. However, they may remain deeply anesthetized as a result of drug overdose, most commonly from narcotics. Reversal of sedation/narcosis and

respiratory depression with naloxone, doxapram,[50] and flumazenil, should it be available, perhaps minimizes recovery times and prepares the OR most rapidly for the next patient.

Pulmonary Edema

Pulmonary edema can develop perioperatively.[57] Such pulmonary edema, unlike the classic delayed nonspecific inflammatory process of the adult respiratory distress syndrome, probably is caused by sudden changes in microvascular permeability resulting from direct parenchymal or vascular pulmonary insults. It can appear after excessive sympathetic discharge, such as in neurogenic pulmonary edema, or after administration of naloxone. It may follow direct pulmonary injury, including contusion, penetration, or blast, and can occur after airway injury caused by the inhalation of toxic fumes. Any increase in microvascular permeability is greatly exaggerated during liberal fluid resuscitation, thus making the appearance of postoperative pulmonary edema a relatively frequent event.[59]

Analgesia

Another common postoperative problem is lack of analgesia. Analgesia can be achieved by further administration of narcotics, although the risk of respiratory depression cannot be overestimated. As a result, alternative techniques, such as ketamine infusions, have been tried in acute war injuries.[60]

Transport

An important component of postoperative care is preparation of patients for safe evacuation. This process includes ensuring adequate ventilatory support, providing fluid replacement, securing catheters or endotracheal tubes, and reporting relevant information to the transport personnel.

FUTURE CONSIDERATIONS

What Problems Must Be Addressed?

Quality Assurance

The question of quality assurance during battlefield medical operations may seem out of place. However, success in treating combat casualties improved dramatically from World War II through Korea and Vietnam. Table 52–8 shows the mortality

TABLE 52–8. Per Cent Mortality of Wounds

	World War II	Korea	Vietnam
Large bowel	37	15	6.5
Small bowel	30	13	5.6
Liver	27	16	8.5
Stomach	41	18	7.3
Kidneys	35	25	7.8
Spleen	25	15	4.5
Bladder	30	9	9.7
Pancreas	58	22	5.7
Ureters	41	50	10.5
All abdominal wounds	21	12	4.5
All wounds	3.3	2.4	1.8

(Data from Hardaway RM: Vietnam wound analysis. J Trauma 1978; 18:635.)

rates for various wound types in these periods. The mortality rate for abdominal wounds in World War II was 21%, declining to 12% during the Korean conflict and 4.5% in Vietnam. These figures reflected improvements in treatment of battlefield casualties. Soldiers injured in future conflicts should also benefit from advances in medical technology that have occurred in the years since the Vietnam conflict. Quality assurance reporting provides data to verify that this improvement is occurring and, if not, can provide the insight to allow changes to be instituted.

Evacuation and Triage

One of the essential elements in providing this care, rapid evacuation of casualties from the battlefield by helicopter, resulted in significant improvement in survival and has been discussed in some detail already. A second element, rapid evaluation and treatment of life-threatening airway, breathing, and circulation problems, is essential to maintaining high survival rates. Finally, when large numbers of casualties are present, personnel must work quickly to do the greatest good for the greatest number of injured patients. Careful triage, as expressed by Wilson,[17] must be performed to separate those patients with a high likelihood of survival from those with virtually no chance of survival in order to avoid wasting precious resources and time.

How Are These Goals Met?

What is the best way to implement this strategy in the modern battlefield? First, surgical services must be provided as far forward as possible. One of the lessons learned in Operation Desert Storm was that large, heavily equipped hospitals could not keep pace with the fast movement of modern armored and mechanized units.

Forward Surgical Teams

In response to these deficiencies, the United States armed services are developing concepts of forward surgical teams, small units consisting of 20 individuals (usually several surgeons, anesthesia personnel, nurses, and technicians) who can take surgical capability right to the edge of the battlefield. The goals of these units are to provide only immediate life-saving procedures such as emergency airways and hemorrhage control, along with intravascular volume resuscitation. In concept, they are similar to the units deployed by the Israelis in 1969.[27]

Organization

Units of this type have been in operation as part of contingency plans in all three services of the United States Department of Defense. An example is the Air Force Flying Ambulance Surgical Trauma (FAST) teams stationed at medical facilities in Europe (Table 52–9). Their total equipment weighs 5000 pounds, is carried on two air-transportable cargo pallets, and is stored in footlockers that can be taken off the pallets and easily packed in one or two trucks. These units are designed to operate independently without resupply for 48 hours and to provide up to 50 life-saving operations. For situations in which more than 50 casualties are anticipated, several teams may operate together, increasing their total capacity accordingly.

TABLE 52–9. Flying Ambulance Surgical Trauma Team Personnel

General surgeon	1
Orthopedic surgeon	1
Anesthesiologist	1
Flight medical officer	1
Operating room nurse	1
General duty nurse	5
Operating room technicians	3
Emergency medical technicians	7
Total	20

(Desert Storm. Defense 91. Sept–Oct 1991, p 56.)

Because the equipment and number of personnel are relatively small, they may fit in standard vehicles and aircraft and move quickly to any point in the battlefield. Medical operations are set up in a "shelter of opportunity," using an available fixed structure such as a house or school. When no fixed structures are available, favorable terrain features or tents may substitute.

Technology

Although these units have yet to be put to a full test of their capability, their advantage lies in their simplicity and selective use of technology. For example, the FAST teams provide their own electricity using small gasoline-powered electric generators. These generators are used to operate a combination ECG-defibrillator, a pulse oximeter, and a noninvasive automated blood pressure device. The anesthesia machine is the previously described Ohmeda 885 Field Unit. Surgical lighting is provided with battery-powered headlamps; batteries are recharged from the portable generators. The headlamps provide good lighting conditions yet save space and weight over more cumbersome standard OR lights.

Anesthetic Agents

The anesthetic formulary is limited but adequate, consisting of isoflurane as the sole inhalation anesthetic agent; succinylcholine, vecuronium, and pancuronium as the muscle relaxants; thiopental and ketamine for anesthetic induction; and fentanyl and morphine. A selection of various regional block needles, lidocaine, and bupivacaine are available for regional anesthesia as appropriate. With these units, future combat casualties may only be minutes away from a life-saving operation.

How Should Anesthesia Providers Prepare for the Battlefield?

Personal Motivation

Anesthesiologists and nurse anesthetists possess sufficient knowledge and skill to handle most situations that occur related to combat casualties. Although traumatic injuries often are impressive in appearance, their management is relatively straightforward, because most soldiers are healthy young individuals who are free of other systemic disease. The biggest challenge to anesthesia providers may be the ability to keep themselves healthy, physically conditioned, and psychologically prepared to meet the rigors of battlefield life.

Disease Prevention

Disease may pose the biggest threat to medical and nonmedical personnel alike. History is replete with examples of armies decimated by disease before they ever entered battle. Anesthesia personnel must pay close attention to endemic diseases and strategies designed to prevent illness. Simple commonsense advice is to avoid local cuisine, no matter how bad standard military fare might taste. Protection against biting insects, proper immunizations, chemoprophylaxis against disease, and maintenance of good personal hygiene will prevent >90% of communicable disease. Physical health can be further maintained by taking full advantage of all opportunities to engage in regular exercise and, whenever possible, trying to get a good night's sleep.

Activities

The biggest threat to well-being may not be the enemy or disease but inactivity. Battlefield operations are almost always characterized by brief periods of intense activity followed by prolonged periods of boredom. Anesthetists who prepare to leave for prolonged deployment benefit greatly from taking such items as books, playing cards, portable tape players, and stationery. Many individuals have kept themselves sane by maintaining a journal and a photographic record of their life during those difficult times. Without doubt, physicians and nurses who cannot take care of themselves are of little benefit to their patients.

SUMMARY

The entire scope of military medicine and anesthesiology cannot be presented in a single chapter. Additional succinct and informative references enlarge on the subject matter presented here and are recommended for interested readers.[61–64]

References

1. Forrest RD: Early history of wound treatment. J R Soc Med 1982; 75:198.
2. Wangensteen OH, Wangensteen SD: Military surgeons and surgery, old and new: an instructive chapter in management of contaminated wounds. Surgery 1967; 62:1102.
3. Drapanas T, Litwin MS: Trauma: management of the acutely injured patient. *In* Progress in Critical Care Medicine: Multiple Trauma. Dudley HAF (ed). Bristol, UK, John Wright & Sons, 1967, pp 47–57.
4. Garrison F: Short Notes on the History of Military Medicine. Washington, DC, Association of Military Surgeons, 1922, p 57.
5. Garrison F: Short Notes on the History of Military Medicine. Washington, DC, Association of Military Surgeons, 1922, p 41.
6. Forrest RD: Development of wound therapy from the Dark Ages to the present. J R Soc Med 1982; 75:268.
7. Garrison F: Short Notes on the History of Military Medicine. Washington, DC, Association of Military Surgeons, 1922, p 116.
8. Cales RH, Trunkey DD: Preventable trauma deaths. JAMA 1985; 254:1059.
9. Kennedy RH: Ambulances are more than vehicles. J Trauma 1965; 5:393.
10. Brewer LA III: Baron Dominique Jean Larrey (1766–1842). J Thorac Cardiovasc Surg 1986; 92:1096.
11. Joy RJT: Jonathan Letterman of Jefferson: Medical Director of the Army of the Potomac. Topic: A Journal of the Liberal Arts (Medical-Science Colloquium). 1983, pp 26–38.
12. Garrison F: Short Notes on the History of Military Medicine. Washington, DC, Association of Military Surgeons, 1922, p 174.
13. Aldrete JA, Marron GM, Wright AJ: The first administration of anesthesia in military surgery: on occasion of the Mexican-American War. Anesthesiology 1984; 61:585.
14. Courington FW, Calverley RK: Anesthesia on the western front: the Anglo-American experience of World War I. Anesthesiology 1986; 65:642.
15. Davis JH: History of trauma. *In* Trauma. Mattox KL, Moore EE, Feliciano DV (eds). Norwalk, CT, Appleton, 1988, p 3.
16. Crile GW: Phylogenetic association in relation to certain medical problems. Boston Med Surg J 1910; 103:893.
17. Watt J: Doctors in the wars. J R Soc Med 1984; 77:265.
18. Jacobs LM, Berrizbeitia LD: Prehospital trauma care. Emerg Med Clin North Am 1984; 2:717.
19. Trunkey DD: Trauma. Sci Am 1983; 249:28.
20. Trunkey DD: Overview of trauma. Surg Clin North Am 1982; 62:3.
21. Trunkey DD: Shock trauma. Can J Surg 1984; 27:429.
22. Dolev E, Llewellyn CH: The chain of medical responsibility in battlefield medicine. Milit Med 1985; 150:471.
23. Bzik KD, Bellamy RF: A note on combat casualty care statistics. Milit Med 1984; 149:229.
24. Neel S: Vietnam Studies: Medical Support of the US Army in Vietnam, 1965–1970. Washington, DC, Department of the Army, 1973, pp 51–54.
25. Danon YL, Nili E, Dolev E: Primary treatment of battle casualties in the Lebanon War, 1982. Isr J Med Sci 1984; 20:300.
26. Dolev E: The October 1973 War: Organization of medical services, types of casualties and their management. *In* The Management of War Casualties: A Symposium by Eight Israeli Medical Officers. Penn J (ed). Johannesburg, South Africa, Hugh Heartland, 1976, pp 1–8.
27. Naggan L: Medical planning for disaster in Israel. Injury 1976; 7:279.
28. Bellamy RF: The causes of death in conventional land warfare: implications for combat casualty care research. Milit Med 1984; 149:55.
29. Dimond FC Jr, Rich NM: M-16 rifle wounds in Vietnam. J Trauma 1967; 7:619.
30. Owen-Smith MS: High velocity missile wounds. London, Edward Arnold, 1981, pp 19–24.
31. Rogov M: Pathological evaluation of trauma in fatal casualties of the Lebanon War, 1982. Isr J Med Sci 1984; 20:369.
32. Ben-Hur N: The antitank missile burn syndrome. Harefuah 1974; 87:543.
33. Llewellyn CH, Dolev E: Health service support for military operations in urbanized terrain. Med Bull US Army Europe 1985; 42:3.
34. Hill JF: Blast injury with particular reference to recent terrorist bombing incidents. Ann R Coll Surg Engl 1979; 61:4.
35. Ron D, Taitelman U, Michaelson M, et al: Prevention of acute renal failure in traumatic rhabdomyolysis. Arch Intern Med 1984; 144:277.
36. Michaelson M, Taitelman U, Bursztein S: Management of crush syndrome. Resuscitation 1984; 12:141.
37. Rosenblatt M, Lerner J, Best LA, et al: Thoracic wounds in Israeli battle casualties during the 1982 evacuation of wounded from Lebanon. J Trauma 1985; 25:350.
38. Kurukchy T: High velocity missile injuries to the spine. Int Rev Army Navy Air Force Med Serv 1985; 53:159.
39. Suleman ND, Rasoul AH: War injuries of the chest. Injury 1985; 16:382.
40. Tucker K, Lettin A: The Tower of London bomb explosion. Br Med J 1975; 3:287.
41. Adler J, Golan E, Yitzhaki M, et al: Terrorist bombing experience during 1975–1979. Isr J Med Sci 1983; 1:189.
42. Model 885A Anesthesia Apparatus Instruction and Service Manual. Madison, WI, Ohmeda, 1990.
43. Ohmeda Universal PAC Operation and Maintenance Manual. Madison, WI, Ohmeda, 1991.
44. Houghton IT: The triservice anesthesia apparatus. Anaesthesia 1981; 36:1094.
45. Gray TC: Another side of Mars (the Mitchiner Memorial Lecture). J R Army Medical Corps 1984; 130:3.
46. Beecher HK: Resuscitation and Anesthesia for Wounded Men: The Management of Traumatic Shock. Springfield, IL, Charles C Thomas, 1949.
47. Dove DB, Stahl WM, DelGuercio LRM: A five-year review of deaths following urban trauma. J Trauma 1980; 20:760.
48. Foley RW, Harris LS, Pilcher DB: Abdominal injuries in automobile accidents: review of care of fatally injured patients. J Trauma 1977; 17:611.
49. Davidson JT, Cotev S: Anesthesia in the Yom Kippur War. Ann R Coll Surg Engl 1975; 56:304.
50. Jowitt MD, Knight RJ: Anaesthesia during the Falkland campaign. Anaesthesia 1983; 38:776.
51. Halford FJ: A critique of intravenous anesthesia in war surgery. Anesthesiology 1943; 4:67.
52. The question of intravenous anesthesia in war surgery (Editorial). Anesthesiology 1943; 4:74.
53. Weiskopf RB, Bogetz MS, Roizen MF: Cardiovascular and metabolic

sequelae of inducing anesthesia with ketamine or thiopental in hypovolemic swine. Anesthesiology 1984; 60:214.

54. Weiskopf RB, Townsley MI, Riordan KK, et al: Comparison of cardiopulmonary responses to graded hemorrhage during enflurane, halothane, isoflurane, and ketamine anesthesia. Anesth Analg 1981; 60:481.

55. Jowitt MD: Anaesthesia ashore in the Falklands. Ann R Coll Surg Engl 1984; 66:197.

56. Jago RH, Restall J, Thompson MC: Ketamine and military anesthesia: the effect of heavy premedication and althesin induction on the incidence of emergence phenomena. Anaesthesia 1984; 39:925.

57. Bogetz MS, Katz JA: Recall of surgery for major trauma. Anesthesiology 1984; 61:6.

58. Boulton TB: Editorial. Anaesthesia 1978; 33:769.

59. Perel A: Pulmonary edema in combat casualties. *In* Intensive Care and Critical Care Medicine 1981–1985–1989. Proceedings of the 4th World Congress on Intensive Care Medicine. Jerusalem, Israel, June 15, 1985.

60. Bion JF: Infusion analgesia for acute war injuries: a comparison of pentazocine and ketamine. Anaesthesia 1984; 39:560.

61. Dolev E: The management of trauma: historical perspective. *In* Trauma. Problems in Critical Care. Shackford S, Perel A (eds). Philadelphia, JB Lippincott, 1987, pp 527–537.

62. Perel A: Battlefield anesthesia. *In* Anesthesia for Trauma. International Anesthesiology Clinics. Kirby RR, Brown DL (eds). Boston, Little, Brown & Co, 1987, pp 175–189.

63. Dolev E: Wartime trauma: lessons and perspectives. Int Anesthesiol Clin 1987; 25:191–203.

64. Capan LM, Miller SM, Turndorf H: Trauma overview. Trauma Anesthesia and Intensive Care. Philadelphia, JB Lippincott, 1991, pp 3–28.

CHAPTER **53**

Electrical Safety

JAN C. HORROW, M.D.

HISTORICAL CONSIDERATIONS

An explosion or fire requires the presence of three components: a fuel, an oxidizing substance, and an ignition spark. Several decades ago, anesthetic gases were explosive. Ether, cyclopropane, or one of the other flammable anesthetics constituted the fuel. They were almost always combined with oxygen or nitrous oxide, both oxidizing substances. Because this mixture leaked into the operating room atmosphere, prevention of sparks assumed great importance. Static electricity was the enemy.[1]

Hydraulics powered the anesthesia machine. Monitoring rarely used more than a manually operated blood pressure cuff, chest stethoscope, and finger on the pulse. Electrosurgery had not achieved universal use. Thus, operating rooms did not need extensive electric power. The few electric outlets permitted in operating rooms were placed 5 feet above floor level to limit their exposure to dense explosive gases. These special electric outlets ensured contact within an explosion-proof encasement. Personnel wore conductive shoes to dissipate any static charges through a conductive floor and tore adhesive tape above their heads in case that act generated static charge. A special power supply, isolated from ground, prevented sparks from line-powered devices.

Today, the environment of flammable anesthetics exists no longer. Static electric discharge carries no explosion risk now, and conductive shoes are antiques. Nonflammable anesthetics permit free use of electrically powered devices, which have proliferated. What protective devices provide a safer electric environment? This chapter discusses electrical safety and the basis for protective devices.

ELECTROCUTION

Forget about the operating room for the moment, and consider electrical safety in your own home or office. To understand what makes an environment electrically safe, let us first consider what makes the home environment hazardous. This understanding follows from a relatively painless review of physics.

What Are the Laws of Current Flow?

An understanding of electrical safety does not require an in-depth review of the physical laws and equations governing electric energy. Only four principles pertain to this topic.

Energy

First, electricity is energy, and energy performs work. Misapplied, this energy can be destructive. Uncontrolled electric energy harms property by starting fires. People may suffer burns or electrocution. The latter occurs when electric energy confounds the biopotentials that permit proper cardiovascular function.

Circuit Components

Second, electric charges can flow only within an unbroken electric circuit. This circuit usually contains physically connected elements, such as wires, lamps, or speakers. Electrical hazards relate to unintentional flow of electric charge. The magnitude of this flow, measured in amperes, depends on the driving force for the electric charges (their voltage) and the resistance in their path, measured in ohms. Ohm's law defines this relationship:

$$\text{Potential difference (V)} = \text{current (I)} \times \text{resistance (R)}$$

This equation is familiar to us in its cardiovascular analogy: Pressure difference (mean arterial pressure minus central venous pressure) equals the product of cardiac output and systemic vascular resistance (Fig. 53–1). Note that just as the vascular bed with a smaller resistance receives greater blood flow, so does the limb of a circuit with less electric resistance receive greater current flow.

Capacitance

The third physical principle needed to appreciate electrical safety is the operation of a capacitor. Conductive surfaces in close physical proximity separated by an insulator form a

885

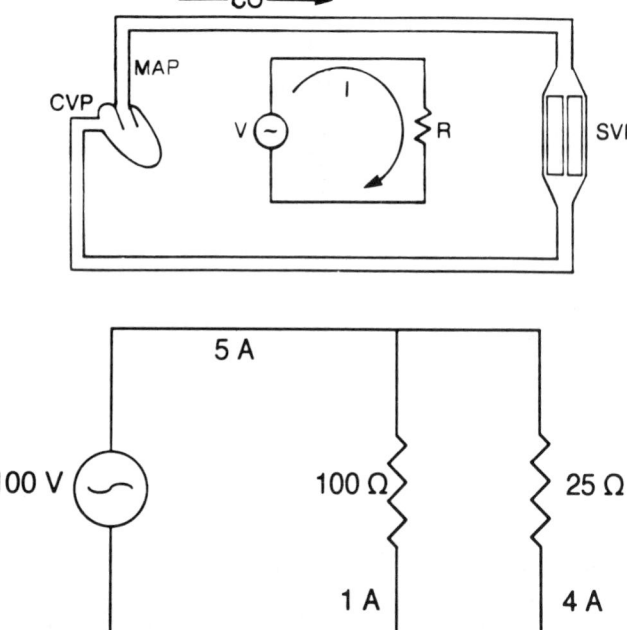

FIGURE 53–1. The *upper panel* displays the cardiovascular analogy of Ohm's Law. The force driving blood through the systemic vasculature is the mean arterial pressure (MAP) less the central venous pressure (CVP). It is analogous to the potential difference (V) at the voltage source in the *lower panel*. The systemic vascular resistance (SVR) corresponds to the device resistive load (measured in ohms). Flow in the cardiovascular circuit (measured in liters per minute of cardiac output [CO]) corresponds to the flow of charge (I) in the electrical circuit (measured in amperes). The *lower panel* demonstrates Ohm's Law. The 100-V potential difference produces a current of 1 A through the 100-Ω resistance, and 4 A through the 25-Ω resistance. Note that since a total of 5 A of current flows in the circuit, the equivalent resistance of the two parallel resistors is 20 Ω. (Reproduced from Horrow JC, Seitman DT: Electrical safety and device calibration. Anesthesiol Clin North Am 1988; 6:699.)

capacitor. Capacitance depends on the ability of the insulator between the conductive surfaces to block the flow of charge from one surface to the other despite a potential difference. Thus, the capacitor must tolerate a certain amount of electrical "stress."

Direct Current

What happens when a constant voltage (as from a battery) is applied across a capacitor? Positive charges leave one conductive surface and travel toward the negative pole of the battery, and negative charges leave the opposite surface, being attracted by the positive pole of the battery. This nearly instantaneous flow occurs such that the potential difference appearing across the capacitor's surfaces equals that applied by the battery (Fig. 53–2). This equal and opposite potential difference creates a net driving force of 0 V in the circuit, so that no current flows. Application of an unvarying voltage source such as a battery reveals that capacitors block direct current, just as if the circuit were open.

Alternating Current

The behavior of alternating current differs. When the voltage applied across the capacitor varies with time, charges are continuously flowing between the capacitor's conductive sur-

face and the voltage source. The voltage across the capacitor moves to oppose that of the changing voltage source. Although no current flows across the capacitor (between its conductive surfaces), current flows around it, in the circuit. In fact, the more quickly the voltage source changes (i.e., the higher its frequency), the more easily current flows. Should the circuit also contain resistive elements (which consume electric energy), this current produces work. Application of a varying voltage source reveals that capacitors permit the flow of alternating current.

Capacitive Coupling

The fourth electrical concept is that of capacitive coupling. Because any two conductors in proximity form a capacitor, the wires carrying electricity from a power outlet form a weak capacitor. It is weak because they are separated by a very poor conductor—in fact, an insulator. Air is also an effective insulator.

Such unintentional elements are termed *stray capacitors*, and the paths inadvertently formed are considered to be capacitively coupled. The extremely low capacitance and high resistance in these circuits determine extraordinarily small "leakage" currents. These leakage currents assume greater importance, however, when they pass through myocardium (discussed later).

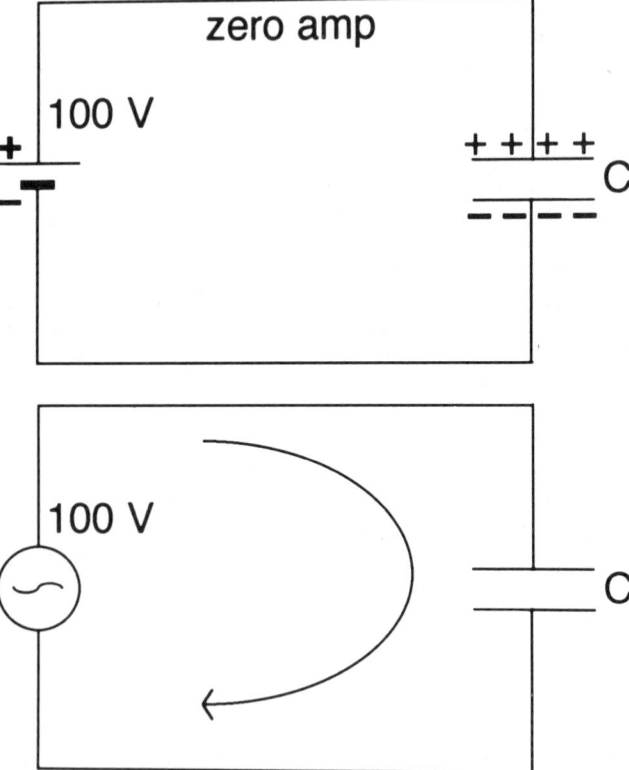

FIGURE 53–2. In the *upper panel*, a fixed voltage applied across the capacitor (C) yields zero current flow after a near-instantaneous equilibration. Charges move to the capacitor's plates to exactly oppose the applied voltage. However, a finite current flows with an alternating voltage source (depicted in the *lower panel*). The impedance to flow in this circuit (X) depends on the frequency of the applied voltage (f) and the capacitor's capacitance (C): X = $1/(2\pi fC)$.

What Is a Grounded Electrical System?

Generating stations distribute electric power as alternating current at high voltage. This method minimizes the amount lost as heat during transmission. Power is the product of current and voltage ($P = IV$), but heat loss varies with the square of the current. Thus, optimal power transmission uses low current and high voltage. At a nearby utility pole or ground enclosure, a transformer decreases this 2400- to 8000-V supply to 110 V.[2] At the entrance of electrical service to a building, one but not both of the two wires carrying this 110-V supply is permanently connected to a conductor that unmistakably contacts the earth (i.e., ground) (Fig. 53–3).[3]

Why Is a Ground Necessary?

The connection to ground prevents unwanted high voltages from residing in the end-user system. High voltages relative to ground are dangerous because they can overcome the insulating properties of air. The resulting spark may ignite a fire. High voltage in one conductor might occur from lightning or from insulation failure in the high-voltage transformer. Without this ground connection, high voltage, relative to ground, would usually occur in each of the two conductors. Even though the voltage between them remains 110 V, their source at the transformer is several thousand volts. Any conductive object connected to the earth in proximity to one of the conductors might then receive a voltage arc. The grounded system

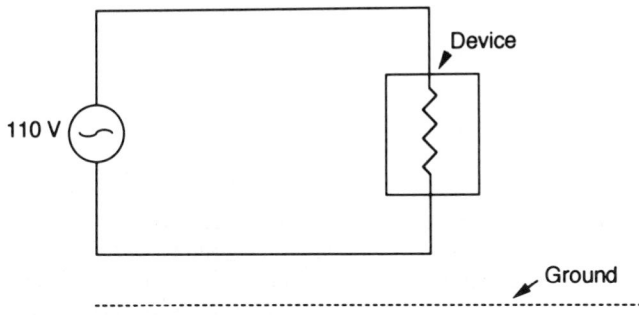

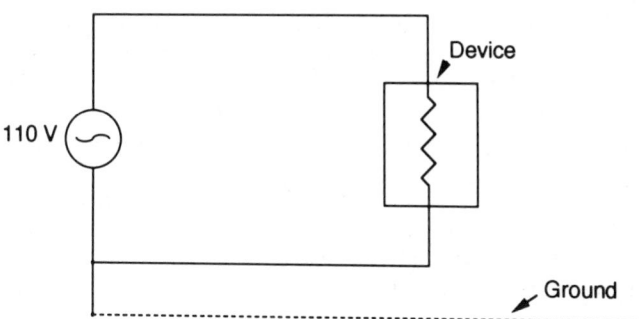

FIGURE 53–3. Ungrounded and grounded electrical systems. The upper panel depicts a typical electrical circuit in an ungrounded system. The lower panel shows the grounded system universally present in North America in which one of the power lines is connected to the ground. The ungrounded line is called "hot," and the grounded line is described as "neutral" or "grounded."

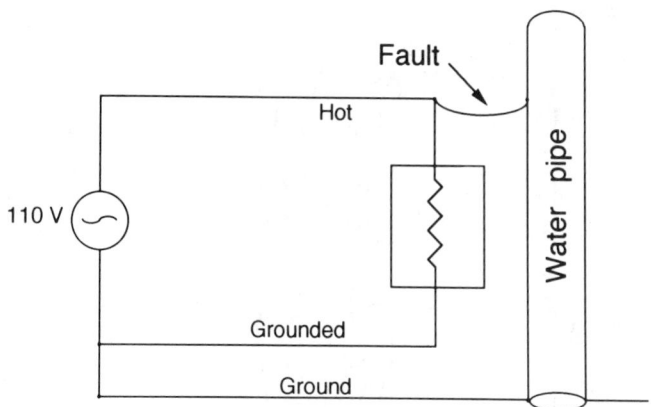

FIGURE 53–4. A fault situation in which the hot power line is connected to the ground via a conductor such as a metal water pipe. Current may flow uninterrupted from the voltage source via the connection between the ground and the other ("grounded") power line. A large current will flow, causing a fuse to blow or a circuit breaker to trip, interrupting power to all devices grouped on that line.

keeps these sources of high voltage away from the household conductors.

The grounded system also provides a low-resistance circuit when a live wire mistakenly contacts any conductor at ground potential, such as a water pipe (which is connected to ground) or the housing of any properly grounded device (Fig. 53–4). This low-resistance circuit is desirable because the resulting high current then triggers a fuse or circuit breaker, opening the circuit to protect the system from damage. Thus, the grounded system of electrical supply protects equipment and property, or in the case of the operating room, it protects people. Misapplied electric energy risks burns and electrocution.

What Are the Determinants of Electric Shock?

Frequency

High-frequency electric energy passes through the body harmlessly. Rapidly changing signals (>3 kHz) vary too quickly to confound the endogenous biopotentials that govern the orderly depolarization and repolarization of critical tissues (heart and nervous system). In contrast, direct current applied as a pulse to the chest wall can defibrillate the heart. In this situation, simultaneous depolarization of all myocardial tissue permits the dominant pacemaker to recover control.

Frequencies between 0 Hz (direct current) and roughly 1 kHz, however, easily induce ventricular fibrillation. The current needed to interfere with cardiac electrophysiology to yield ventricular fibrillation depends on the frequency of the energy, with more current needed for higher frequencies.[4] Figure 53–5 displays the relative biologic hazards of alternating currents of different frequency in an animal model. Note that the current needed to induce ventricular fibrillation is least when the frequency of the electric energy coincides with that of commercially supplied electric power (60 Hz), an unfortunate coincidence.

Macroshock and Microshock

The current that induces fibrillation also depends on the point of entry. It is current density (flow per unit cross-sec-

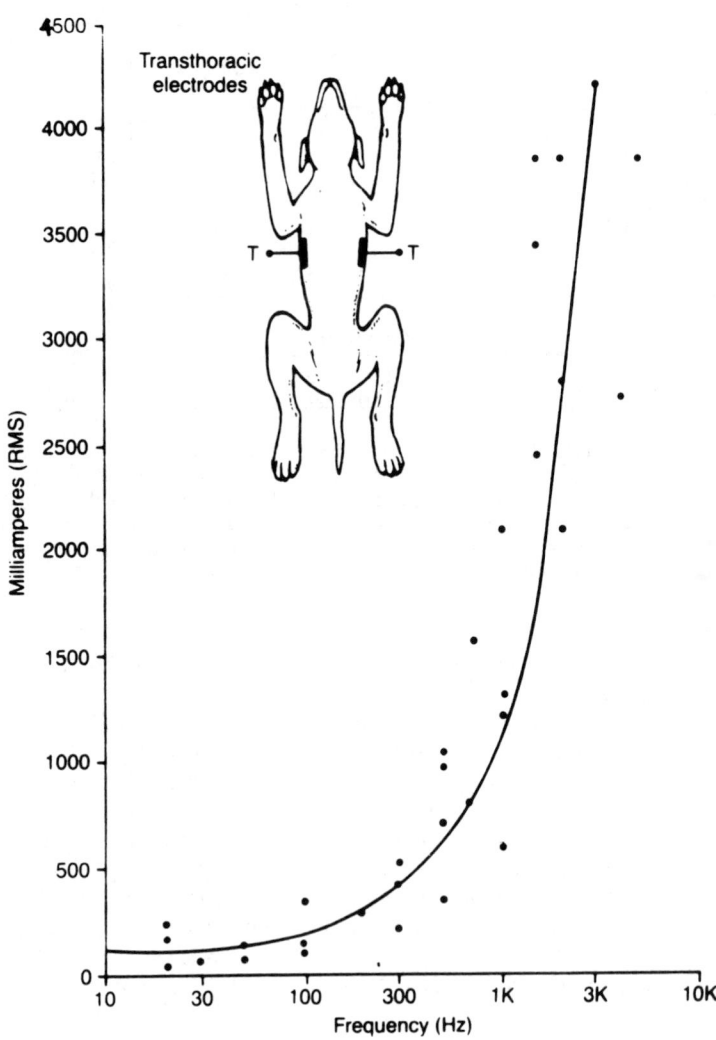

FIGURE 53–5. The hazard of alternating current applied across the thorax of a dog depends on the current's frequency, with lower frequency signals requiring smaller currents to induce ventricular fibrillation. (Reproduced from Geddes LA, Baker LE: Response to passage of electric current through the body. J Assoc Adv Med Instrument 1971; 5:13.)

tional area) and not current itself that causes harm. Thus, 100 to 2500 mA applied across the trunk when the skin is wet induces fibrillation, but only 100 μA suffices when conducted via a saline-filled catheter in contact with the myocardium.[5] The latter current enters through a much smaller area and has no opportunity to disperse across additional tissue before reaching the organ at jeopardy. *Macroshock* describes the former situation, in which larger currents travel across the body, and *microshock* applies to minute currents entering myocardium directly.

What Are the Circuit Requirements for Electric Shock?

Figure 53–6 displays several possibilities. In the first, the victim interposes his body between the "hot" and "neutral" conductors. Should the natural barrier of intact skin be defeated by wet hands, its resistance falls to about 1 KΩ, yielding a current of 110 mA on application of 110 V.

The second case displays a more subtle opportunity for electrocution. Here, direct physical contact with only the "hot" conductor occurs. The connection to the neutral side arises from contact with ground, because the neutral conductor is connected to ground at the entrance of power to the building. For this reason, shoes, which are electrical insulators,

provide protection from electric shock. Likewise, the rubber tires of a car isolate the vehicle from ground, decreasing the likelihood that lightning will seek a path through the vehicle.

In the third case, an overt fault within the electrical system has not occurred. Rather, the device contains a capacitive coupling that enables flow of sufficient current to cause microshock.

Safety Measures

Can safety be provided for these three situations? Yes, in some cases. Unfortunately, no system currently provides the ability to differentiate between an electrical appliance and the human body when the latter is interposed between the two current-carrying conductors. Fortunately, few people create this situation.

In contrast, modern electrical wiring can avert electrocution in the second situation, that of line-to-ground contact. In the third case, complete safety does not accrue even with radical alteration of electric energy supply.

How Are Grounding and Grounded Systems Used?

Grounding provides protection from shock. It results from the practice of providing a third wire, usually green, in the

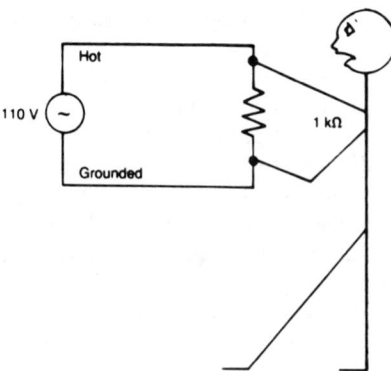

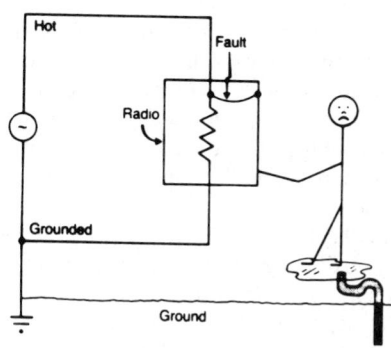

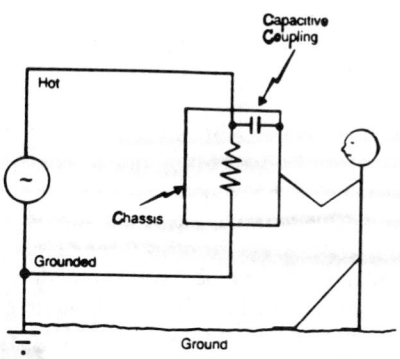

FIGURE 53–6. Three ways that electrocution can occur. In the *upper panel*, an ignorant victim simultaneously contacts both conductors, placing his or her body in parallel with the device supplied by the power cord. Regardless of the device's resistance, a current of 110 V ÷ 1 kΩ = 110 mA will flow across the trunk if the victim's hands are wet. The *middle panel* demonstrates how shock occurs in a grounded system when the victim contacts only one conductor. The insulation of the "hot" conductor of this radio has worn away so that the conductor contacts the radio's enclosure ("chassis"). Should the victim touch the chassis and be in electrical contact with ground, as easily happens in wet environments, he creates a parallel current path through his or her body to ground and back to the voltage source via the connection of the second power conductor to ground. The *lower panel* depicts a similar current path. In this case, the "hot" conductor insulation is intact. However, capacitive coupling permits a small current to flow via the device enclosure and through the victim as in the middle panel. The small current is of no consequence unless a direct path to the myocardium exists. (Reproduced from Horrow JC, Seitman DT: Electrical safety and device calibration. Anesthesiol Clin North Am 1988; 6:699.)

power cord of an appliance. This wire, connected to ground at the service entrance of a building in a fashion similar to that of the neutral conductor, attaches to those parts of each appliance that should not be part of a current path, such as the covering (chassis).

Should defective insulation in the hot conductor cause contact of that wire with the chassis, current completes a circuit from the power source via the hot wire to the chassis and then through the grounding wire back to the power source (Fig. 53–7). As a result, a circuit breaker or fuse then breaks the circuit.

This design supplies safety by breaking the circuit before a person can touch the chassis, inadvertently providing a path through his or her body via ground. Without the grounding wire, the device chassis sits at hot wire potential, awaiting the victim.

Why Aren't All Power Cords Three Pronged?

A reader may note with some bewilderment that not all marketed appliances carry a three-prong grounding power cord. Some devices constructed with plastic or insulating materials obviate a grounding wire; they may or may not feature a polarized plug, which ensures that the neutral, grounded side of the circuit never becomes the hot side by inverting the plug.

If a device carries a three-prong grounding plug, interposed "cheater plugs," which interrupt contact with the grounding receptacle (the rounded hole), pose a risk of electrocution should a fault occur from the hot wire within the device. Such interruptions degrade safety.

Are Fuses and Circuit Breakers Effective?

Do fuses and circuit breakers provide sufficient safety? Because electrocution may occur with 100 mA, the protection afforded by a fuse that breaks the circuit at 15 A appears woefully inadequate. Partial insulation faults, or current leaks within a device, could provide macroshock-range currents in

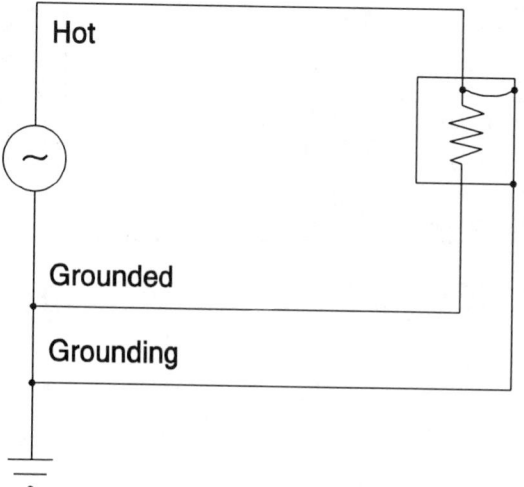

FIGURE 53–7. A grounded electrical system with ground depicted merely by its electrical symbol. Note the additional connection between the device enclosure and the grounded conductor. This additional wire, termed the *grounding conductor*, appears as a third prong, somewhat longer and rounded, on the plug of the power cord. A fault to the chassis now causes a large current to flow without a victim touching the chassis, providing additional protection from faults to the chassis. Unfortunately, this protection occurs at the expense of power interruption. (Reproduced from Horrow JC, Seitman DT: Electrical safety and device calibration. Anesthesiol Clin North Am 1988; 6:699.)

contact with personnel that go undetected by fuses or circuit breakers.

For situations requiring additional safety, such as bathrooms, kitchens, basements, and outdoor areas, all places where wet conditions may prevail, ground fault circuit interrupters (GFCI) furnish further protection. These devices monitor the currents flowing in the hot and grounded wires. Should those currents differ by at least 6 mA for at least 25 msec, a scenario in which the discrepant current may be traveling in a path via ground, the device breaks the circuit.[3] The isolated power supply, originally used to prevent sparks, furnishes a solution superior to that of a GFCI.

THE OPERATING ROOM

What Is an Isolated System?

This approach to preventing electric shock via ground pathway nullifies the grounded electrical systems—that is, provides an isolated system. Transformers isolate electric circuits easily by converting electric energy to magnetic energy. If the number of windings on each limb of a transformer is equal, the output and input voltages will be equal. Energy transfer through the transformer occurs in the absence of a contiguous path for current flow.

Figure 53–8 demonstrates the placement of an isolation transformer to isolate a power supply from ground. Current flows separately in each part of the transformer (left and right) but not between them.[6] Energy, but not current, is transferred. Notice the lack of an unbroken path from the voltage source,

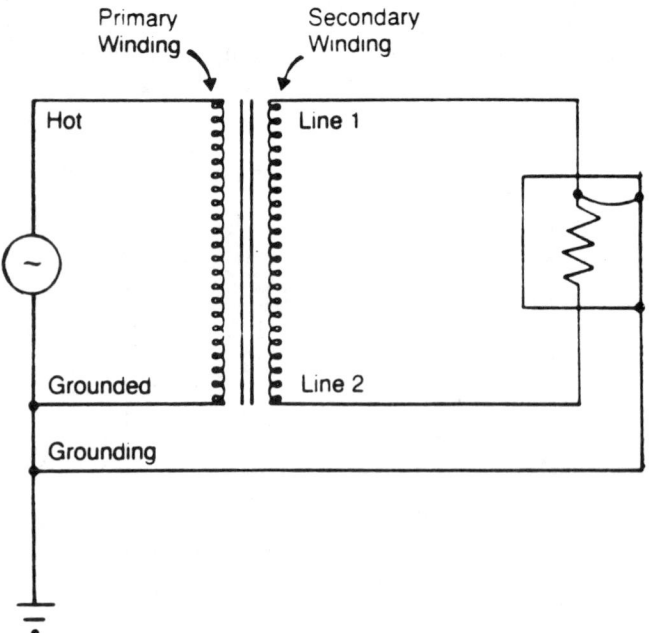

FIGURE 53–8. The isolated power supply. The isolation transformer permits electrical energy, but not electric current, to transfer from the primary to the secondary windings. The path beginning at the Line-1 end of the secondary winding, through the device fault, and via grounding wire cannot return to the Line-2 end of the secondary winding because the isolation transformer does not permit current to flow across it. Similarly, a victim touching the chassis and in contact to ground would not form part of an electrical circuit. The isolation transformer effectively ungrounds the grounded system. (Reproduced from Horrow JC, Seitman DT: Electrical safety and device calibration. Anesthesiol Clin North Am 1988; 6:699.)

via ground, back to the voltage source, despite the short circuit in a device, because current does not flow from the primary to the secondary limb of the transformer.

Why not instead simply omit the connection between the neutral power line and ground at the service entrance? This approach would risk supplying conductors with potentially high voltage with respect to ground. The step-down utility pole transformer secondary limb would then "float" at an average potential of 2400 to 8000 V relative to ground.[2] The isolation transformer primary and secondary limbs, however, contain 120 V relative to ground because they originate from a grounded system. The secondary limb conductors are termed *line 1* and *line 2*.

Isolation of the grounded system brings both the good and the bad. True, a solitary short circuit from hot to ground becomes harmless. The defect does not cause electrocution, nor is power interrupted, a valuable feature during critical operating room procedures. Unfortunately, the fault also remains undetected, because a complete circuit via ground no longer exists. Thus, faulty equipment remains in service until a fault occurs from the other conductor to ground. In this case, electrocution becomes possible, and the fuse or circuit breaker interrupts service.

Another drawback of the isolated system arises from capacitive coupling. All equipment contains stray capacitances between the conductors and surfaces connected via grounding wires, thereby degrading the isolation. To account for these deficiencies, the isolated system also contains a special monitor that detects when a fault to ground occurs.

What Is the Purpose of a Line Isolation Monitor and Alarm?

Should either limb of the isolated system contain a fault or leakage to ground, no current would flow because the isolation transformer negates the connection of ground to the power supply. The line isolation monitor (LIM) measures the current that would flow if the system were still grounded. This measurement is obtained by momentarily grounding line 1 and measuring the current in line 2, then grounding line 2 and measuring the current in line 1 (Fig. 53–9). An analog or digital ammeter displays this current, with an alarm sounding when it exceeds 2 mA.

To avoid nuisance alarms resulting from an accumulation of small leakage currents from the many electrically powered devices in the operating room, the National Fire Protection Association (NFPA) code increased the threshold from 2 mA to 5 mA in 1981. The most recent edition of the code also specifies that the monitor should not alarm for a fault current <3.7 mA, a condition not satisfied by systems with 2-mA thresholds.[7] Few clinicians, however, agree that the 2-mA level constitutes a nuisance. Thus, an LIM alarm may indicate that the last device plugged in has a serious electrical fault, or it may merely reflect "the straw that broke the camel's back"— namely, simultaneous use of many devices, each with a reasonable leakage current.

What Are the Disadvantages and Limitations of Isolated Systems?

The isolation transformer allows a single fault to ground to occur without interrupting power or creating the potential for

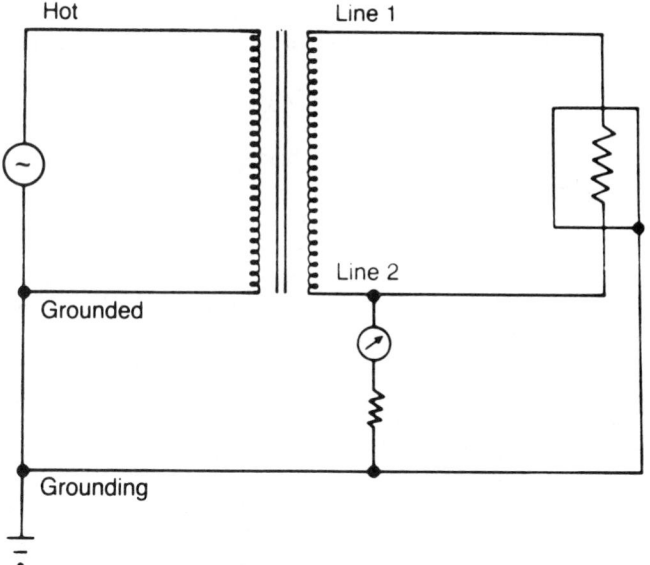

FIGURE 53–9. An isolated power system in which a line isolation monitor tests the current that would flow to ground from Line-1 should Line-2 be grounded. The ammeter displays the current that would flow back to the Line-2 side of the secondary winding from the grounding conductor, whereas the series resistor limits the actual current flow. The line isolation monitor alternately tests each line by connecting its partner to ground through the ammeter, and displays the average leakage current. The current displayed does not actually flow but would flow had the isolation transformer not ungrounded the system. (Reproduced from Horrow JC, Seitman DT: Electrical safety and device calibration. Anesthesiol Clin North Am 1988; 6:699.)

shock. The LIM warns of a situation that could cause electrocution or power interruption in a grounded system.

Does this isolated system with its monitor always provide protection? No system can protect from two-conductor contact (gripping line 1 in one hand and line 2 in the other). Furthermore, although the 2-mA threshold protects from macroshock (it is significantly below the 100 mA that induces ventricular fibrillation when applied across the trunk), but it is several orders of magnitude too large to protect from microshock (~100 μA).

Thwarted Line-to-Ground Fault Detection

Some device circuit designs thwart line-to-ground fault detection. For example, if a device itself contains a transformer, it breaks the path of a complete circuit via grounding wire when a short occurs from the power line to ground. The LIM cannot detect the fault under those conditions. Devices with two-prong plugs (no grounding wires) provide no return path for stray currents to be measured by the LIM. The NFPA code (American National Standards Institutes [ANSI]/NFPA 99) forbids the use of two-prong devices in all patient care areas.[7]

Expense

Expense constitutes another limitation of the isolated power supply. This factor, coupled with doubts about the need for an additional layer of electrical safety for patients and personnel, resulted in removal of the requirement for isolated power in the NFPA guidelines. Facilities constructed after 1984 may omit isolated power in all patient care areas, including operating rooms and intensive care units. Immediate access to circuit

breakers becomes imperative in the absence of an isolated system, because power interruption may occur without warning in the course of critical procedures. Anesthesiologists need to know the kind of power supplied to their patient care area.

Why Does the Isolated Power Debate Continue?

Because a grounded system cannot tolerate a single fault to ground, immediate access to replacement equipment becomes imperative. An isolated system clearly provides extra protection and should be preferred despite increasing the total cost of an operating room by approximately 1%.

Even when flammable agents became obsolete and special measures protecting from static electricity hazards such as conductive shoes and flooring disappeared, the isolated power system remained. Its final abolition in 1984 occurred with great debate. Some experts advocate continued use of isolated systems despite the NFPA code change.[8]

Can a GFCI substitute for the isolated power supply? Although superior to the grounded system, the GFCI furnishes less protection than the isolated system: It breaks the circuit only after the hazardous current has flowed for 25 msec. In contrast, the isolated system prevents that current from flowing, warns that it could flow, and maintains power all the while. For these reasons, a GFCI scheme ranks inferior to an isolated one in terms of safety.

ELECTROSURGERY

How Does It Work?

The industrial revolution of the late 19th century provided a substrate for many applications of alternating current that came of age in the early 20th century, including the transatlantic telegraph, transcontinental telephone service, and electrosurgery.

Initial successes in controlling surgical hemorrhage in Europe were rediscovered by the Philadelphia surgeon William L. Clark and published in 1910.[9] Independent of these events, Harvey Cushing, Surgeon-in-Chief at the Peter Bent Brigham Hospital in Boston, collaborated with the Harvard biologist and physicist William T. Bovie, in an effort to control bleeding during neurosurgery. After their first operative success in 1965, the electrosurgical instrument took many years to gain popularity.[10] Electrosurgery now enjoys nearly universal application and has become known as the *Bovie*.

What Is an Electrosurgical Unit?

Electrosurgery differs from electrocautery in that the latter uses electricity to heat a wire. Touching the hot wire to tissue transfers heat to the tissue. No current flows through the patient. With electrosurgery, however, the patient forms part of a circuit through which alternating current passes.

An electrosurgical unit (ESU) can cut or coagulate tissue. When tissue cutting is desired, voltage sufficiently high to generate a spark between electrode and tissue arcs into the cells. The high voltage instantly turns intracellular water to steam, exploding the cell and leaving a gap in the cellular

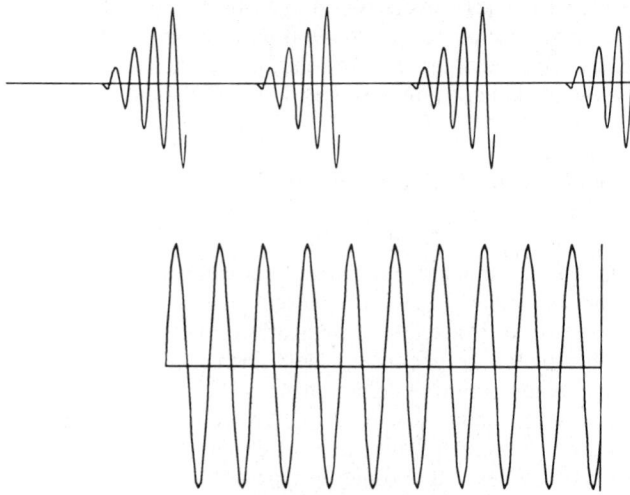

FIGURE 53–10. The current flowing from the electrosurgical unit during the cutting mode *(upper panel)* and during the coagulation mode *(lower panel).*

matrix. The electrode travels on a blanket of steam, destroying cells as it moves. A continuous sinusoidal wave of constant amplitude provides the high power needed to vaporize intracellular water.[11]

What Is Electrocautery?

In contrast, the coagulation mode provides electric output consisting of bursts of dampened sine waves (Fig. 53–10). These pulses are at higher voltage, although the total power is less than that of cutting current, because the pulsed nature of the output provides 0 V more than half the time.

Pulses of current desiccate the cells rather than exploding them. The resultant cellular debris clogs the vessels, providing hemostasis. Because desiccated cells provide higher resistance, the coagulation signal's peak voltage must be nearly twice as high as that of the continuous voltage supplied in the cutting signal.

Is the Patient Grounded?

Perhaps the most misunderstood principle of electrosurgery is patient "grounding." Current applied to a patient's tissues via the active electrode enters at a small surface area, producing enormous current density. Heat from this current density then desiccates or explodes the cells. The current then returns to the ESU via a large surface area at the "dispersive" electrode. This plate or pad provides the necessary return path for ESU energy. It does not ground the patient. In fact, neither the patient nor any part of the circuit through which the ESU current passes should be grounded.

In order to restrict tissue heating to its intended site only, the ESU current must exit via a large surface area, so that the current density, now many orders of magnitude diminished, produces little heat as it travels through tissue. If this condition does not exist, unintended tissue thermal damage ("burn") occurs.

As long as the current density remains low, high-frequency currents pass through the body without harm. In fact, D'Arsonval demonstrated nearly 100 years ago that radio frequency current at 500 kHz can enter via one hand and power an electric light bulb held in the other.[9] Remember, these rapidly changing signals do not confound endogenous biopotentials.

Why Not Ground the Electrosurgical Unit and the Patient?

Under these circumstances, the ESU current can find many opportunities to return from the patient to the ESU: Connections from patient to equipment and furniture and from equipment to ground are ubiquitous. Even though the current may be split into many paths, should a contact supply a small surface area, such as would occur with the head of the fibula touching a leg stirrup, or the back of the scalp on a conductive mattress, the resultant current density achieves sufficient intensity to burn the skin.

High-frequency signals easily form circuits via capacitive coupling; only moderate impedance exists at high frequency despite low capacitance (Fig. 53–11). High-frequency signals can reach ground by traveling from the operating room table to the steel rods of the reinforced concrete of the operating room floor! Rather than grounding the patient and device, prevention of contact between patients and equipment and establishment of a reliable, large surface area dispersive electrode maximize the current returning to the ESU via the desired dispersive electrode pathway.

How Is Proper Dispersive Electrode Placement Verified?

Most dispersive electrodes contain not one but two wires that are connected at the pad applied to the patient. The device sends a small current out one wire and expects it will return on the other. If not, the wire is broken or the electrode is not plugged into the device. For this reason, one always plugs the electrode into the ESU *after* applying it to the patient. Otherwise, the device would sense electrode integrity, even though the pad may be nowhere near the patient.

A refinement of this scheme uses two separate surfaces in the dispersive electrode. The device sends a small high-fre-

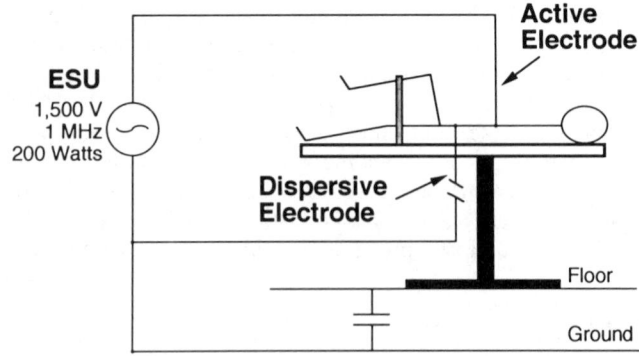

FIGURE 53–11. A patient undergoing surgery with the leg contacting a stirrup that is connected to ground via capacitive coupling to steel-reinforced concrete in the operating room floor. Should the dispersive electrode not supply a low resistance path for current to return to the electrosurgery unit (ESU), current may flow from the active electrode into the patient, then out of the patient at the head of the fibula, via the stirrup, table, and floor to ground, back to the ESU. A skin burn at the contact point of the fibula will result. For this reason, ESU devices with ungrounded circuits are safer.

quency current into one and expects it will return from the other, traversing the patient in between. A pad connected to the device but not to the patient does not return the signal.

In yet a third attempt to prevent inadvertent tissue injury, one device compares the currents leaving and returning to the patient. If they are sufficiently different, the device shuts off current. Note that this feature is identical to the operation of a GFCI. Devices provide the greatest safety by isolating the high-frequency ESU signal from ground.

What Is a Bipolar Electrosurgical Unit?

If both active and return electrodes are placed in close proximity, the applicator is termed a *bipolar electrode.* Here, current enters via one electrode and returns to the ESU via the other, heating the tissue held between. This arrangement does not obviate a dispersive electrode, however. The tissue quickly desiccates, thus increasing the resistance of the current path enormously.

The low-resistance return path provided by a dispersive electrode prevents current from taking some unsuspected alternate pathway. Furthermore, a surgeon may not always touch both prongs of the bipolar electrode to tissue before activating the device. Finally, a bipolar electrode's return wire may have an undetected fault.

Why Are Electrosurgical Unit–Electrocardiographic Monitor Interactions Problematic?

In the past, an electrocardiographic (ECG) monitor served as a common partner with an ESU in causing unintended burns. Connection of the right leg lead of the ECG to ground explains this association: Current entering a patient from the active electrode of the ESU could exit via the small surface area of the ECG electrode and return to the ESU via ground (Fig. 53–12). Early ECG designs featured circuitry to protect the ECG machine from large voltages such as defibrillating shocks. Unfortunately, these designs also provided a path for high-frequency signals via the ECG to ground.

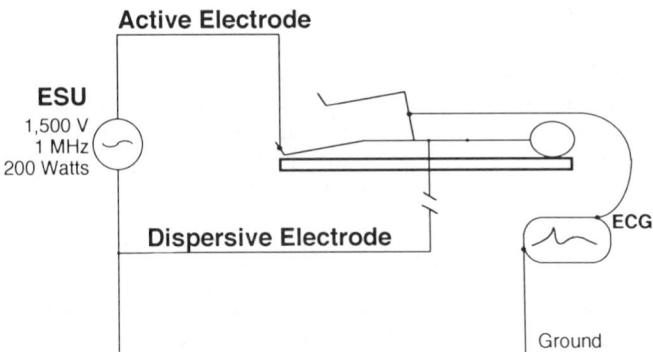

FIGURE 53–12. In this case, the right leg electrocardiogram (ECG) electrode provides a path to ground for ESU current that cannot return to the device because of a defective dispersive path. A skin burn at the electrode site will result. The high frequency ESU currents cannot be prevented by most ECG "isolated" circuits.

Do Electrocardiographic Devices with Isolated Circuits Prevent Electrosurgical Unit Burns?

Unfortunately, they do not. These isolated circuits filter out 60-Hz signals, not the radio frequencies used in electrosurgery. When the ESU is activated, the ECG signal disappears from the monitor. It is possible to obtain ECG equipment with radio frequency squelching circuitry. In this way, ECG monitoring continues despite ESU use.

Even battery operation of a device does not obliterate the possibility of ESU current traveling through a device to ground. Any conductive material leading from a patient may capacitively couple to ground via mounting brackets or proximity to power cords. The most notable offenders in this category are temperature probes.[12–14]

To prevent unintended burns, place the dispersive electrode over well-perfused nonbony tissue, preferably a muscle mass. Electrodes contain a conductive gel that facilitates current flow and improves physical contact with skin. Dispersive electrodes with dried out gel should be discarded. Never substitute ultrasound gel, which is not conductive, for the original gel.

ECG leads also require conductive gel. The same rules apply to placement of ECG electrodes as apply to placement of the ESU dispersive electrode. Failure of the latter may result in ESU current returning via the ECG electrodes. Isolated circuit ECG machines do not render the practice of placing ECG electrodes over bony prominences safe.

How Can an Electrosurgical Unit Cause Fires?

By providing a spark, an ESU contributes one of the three requirements for a fire or explosion. Of course, flammable anesthetics preclude the use of electrosurgery. Yet conditions may still exist by which the ESU starts a fire.

Consider laparoscopic tubal ligation, in which electrosurgery closes the fallopian tubes. The gas used to distend the abdomen should not be nitrous oxide, as originally used, because it supports combustion.[15] A misapplied active electrode that cuts the bowel can release intestinal gas containing the fuel methane. Spark, fuel, and oxidizing substance all coexist, resulting in an abdominal explosion. For this reason, laparoscopic surgery today uses carbon dioxide as the insufflating gas.

LIVING WITH PACEMAKERS

How Do They Work?

Pacemakers are battery-powered devices that supply depolarizing pulses directly to the myocardium to correct or treat cardiac dysrhythmias. An external pacemaker resides outside the body, with only the wire electrodes entering the heart, usually through the vasculature. Internal pacemakers are implanted under the skin: Both the device and the electrodes are physically inaccessible except when specifically approached during surgery.

Superlative engineering design has yielded reliable performance in even the most unfriendly electric environments. So-

TABLE 53–1. Pacemaker Nomenclature*

Position	Indicator	Choices
1st	Chamber paced	O = none; A = atrium; V = ventricle; D = dual (A and V)
2nd	Chamber sensed	O = none; A = atrium; V = ventricle; D = dual (A and V)
3rd	Response to sensing	O = none; T = triggered; I = inhibited; D = dual (T and I)
4th	Programmability	O = none; P = simple programmable†; M = multiprogrammable; C = communicating‡; R = rate modulation
5th	Antitachydysrhythmia functions	O = none; P = pacing; S = shock; D = dual (P and S)

	Examples	
VOO	Fixed-rate pacer. Used occasionally for temporary pacing.	
VVI	Demand pacer. Stimulates ventricle when ventricular spike is not detected within set interval.	
VAT	Atrial tracking pacer. Senses the atrium and stimulates the ventricle, thus supporting sinus rhythm with atrioventricular conduction block.	
DOO	Fixed-rate atrioventricular sequential pacing. Often used after cardiopulmonary bypass in the absence of any intrinsic rhythm.	
DDD	"Universal pacer." Can be set to perform most pacemaker functions, including atrial tracking.	
DDDR	Rate-responsive pacemaker, in which the rate varies with some other input sensor, such as respiration rate, temperature, or movement. Useful to mimic the physiologic response to exercise.	
DDDMS	An automatic implantable cardioverter/defibrillator (AICD).	

*North American Society of Pacing Electrophysiology/British Pacing and Electrophysiology Group.
†Can reprogram parameters such as pulse width or atrioventricular interval.
‡Can be interrogated for summary historical rhythm and pacing data.

phisticated digital circuitry provides not only rhythm sensing, interpretation, and therapeutic responses but also noise detection and elimination, as well as strategic responses to overwhelming interference and to battery depletion. Table 53–1 displays the code by which pacemakers are described and the common types likely to be encountered.

Power Transmission

Battery power to permanent pacers derives from lithium cells, which last approximately 5 years. Plutonium-powered devices, popular many years ago, are now rarely used. Nuclear-powered devices undergo stringent regulatory control, and appropriately so. For example, what happens to the plutonium if the patient is cremated on death?

The wires attached to the control unit are used both to sense the endogenous rhythm (i.e., provide incoming signal to the pacemaker) and pace the heart (i.e., transmit the electric pulses output from the unit). Unipolar pacemakers feature a single electrode to the target chamber (atrium or ventricle), using body tissues for return of current to the control unit.

With bipolar leads, two conductors terminate a few millimeters apart in the target chamber.[16] The latter arrangement eliminates much interference, because the proximity of the two electrodes minimizes any potential difference between them.

Sources of Interference

Oversensing and crosstalk are the major sources of interference in unipolar systems. Oversensing occurs when other sig-

nals such as pectoral muscle potentials (whether physiologic or succinylcholine induced) or myocardial repolarization (ECG T wave) become interpreted as the ECG R wave.

With crosstalk, an atrial stimulus sent out via an atrial electrode is sensed by the ventricular unipolar lead as an R wave, thus inappropriately inhibiting the ventricular stimulus. Intelligent programming of the control unit easily overcomes each of these confounding influences.

Circuit Protection

Modern pacemaker control units protect their integrated circuits from electrical harm, such as occurs when a patient receives countershock. Patients with pacemakers preferably receive countershock with the paddles applied in an anterior-posterior direction rather than across the chest, so that the applied electricity is perpendicular to the plane of the electrodes.

These units effectively handle the electromagnetic interference from high-intensity electric fields such as power lines and from airport security magnetometers, microwave ovens, and automobile ignition systems. Only the ESU, with its intense radio frequency output, can confound these clever devices. How and why this occurs is discussed after introducing the concept of the magnet.

What Does a Magnet Do?

Historically, pacemakers began as fixed-output devices that sent pulses out at regular intervals, regardless of the underlying rhythm. Once component miniaturization permitted, the control units inhibited an output pulse when an endogenous depolarization (R wave) occurred. This process conserved battery power and obviated fibrillation from the R-on-T phenomenon.[17]

External interference that stimulated cardiac depolarization, however, would fool the control unit into inappropriately inhibiting output, resulting in cardiac asystole. The control unit design thus incorporated a safety feature: Placing a magnet on the skin overlying the control unit caused the unit to revert to a fixed (VOO) mode (see Table 53–1), ensuring ventricular stimulation.

What Is the Impact of Electrosurgical Unit Interference?

When a patient with an implanted pacemaker becomes part of the high-voltage, high-frequency-current electrosurgical circuit, the pacemaker senses enormous interference.[18] Is it imperative to use a magnet in this circumstance to prevent asystole? No, for several reasons that follow.

Pacing During Anesthesia

Few patients with implanted pacemakers actually depend on them during anesthesia and surgery. It is the exception rather than the rule for the pacemaker, in fact, to be pacing the patient. First, monitor the patient to determine the underlying rhythm. A pulse oximeter or intra-arterial catheter (our modern equivalents of the traditional "finger on the pulse") proves invaluable to determine the persistence of effective cardiac contraction when the ESU wipes out the monitored ECG waveform. Only asystole requires intervention.

Modern Pacemaker Design

Modern pacemaker design far surpasses the older versions. Once they detect significant interference, they automatically revert to a fixed mode (VOO), after pausing for several seconds in hopes that the interference will abate. Because implantable defibrillators sense an ESU as a ventricular dysrhythmia, these devices *should* be disabled before using an ESU. Thus, the magnet is superfluous. Does this risk R-on-T induction of ventricular fibrillation? Theoretically, yes, but decades of pacer use have effectively disproved the risk of this occurrence clinically.

Pacemaker Reprogramming

Some modern pacemakers use a magnet to reprogram the unit.[19, 20] Placing a magnet over the pacemaker not only induces fixed-mode VOO pacing but may direct the control unit to receive a manufacturer's password. Most likely, nothing will come of this, but the intense, erratic ESU radio frequency environment could reprogram the pacemaker. Even in the absence of a magnet, reprogramming might occur. For this reason, many cardiologists recommend that patients with pacemakers undergo pacemaker evaluation after operative procedures.

These considerations do not argue against preparing for the unexpected by having a magnet available, but its use should usually be avoided, despite its presence.[21] ESU-pacemaker interaction can be minimized by the precautions listed in Table 53–2.

HOW TO THINK ELECTRICALLY

The Line Isolation Monitor Sounds— Now What?

Remember that the isolation transformer provides an added level of protection from electrical hazards. Although only one fault to ground can disable the grounded electrical system, two faults to ground are required in the isolated system. At worst, an LIM alarm indicates that the level of safety has reverted to that normally present with the grounded system.

What Not to Do

Most important is an understanding of what *not* to do.[22] Do not evacuate the operating room or discontinue the administra-

TABLE 53–2. How to Minimize Electrosurgical Unit–Induced Pacemaker Malfunction

- Use a bipolar pacemaker.
- Use a bipolar ESU.
- Maintain the lowest ESU power output needed.
- Keep the active electrode as remote from the pacer electrodes as possible.
- Place the ESU dispersive electrode between the ESU active electrode and the pacemaker electrodes.
- Limit the ESU duty cycle to bursts of several seconds of operation alternating with equal periods of inactivity.
- If the ESU causes asystole, place a magnet over the control unit.

tion of any anesthetic gases. Indeed, surgery should not pause. Do not, under any circumstance, ground the patient, the surgeon, the anesthetist, or any other person, because that increases the risk of electrocution under any condition. Instead, think of the possible causes of the alarm.

What to Do

The most likely reason for an LIM alarm is recent connection to the power supply of a device with significant leakage current to ground. To verify the cause, simply unplug the last device plugged in while watching the LIM ammeter. If it drops substantially, the device is defective and should be sent for repair at the next convenient opportunity. If the device is absolutely indispensable at the moment, as would be true for a cardiopulmonary bypass machine, it should be removed for service only when doing so does not place the patient at risk. Remember, the isolated power supply will protect the electric environment from this fault to ground.

A true fault to ground may not occur specifically within a device. In one case, intravenous fluid slowly leaking onto the face of a multiple-outlet extension cord triggered the LIM by shorting the power supply. Treatment involved drying the outlet and moving it away from the hazardous wet environment.

The second most likely reason for the LIM alarm is that a multitude of electrically powered devices have been plugged into a common receptacle. Although each devices carries an acceptable amount of leakage current, when combined they exceed the LIM threshold. In this case, redistribute the load among several outlets.

How Can You Survive When the Lights Go Out?

Sudden interruption of the power supply to the operating room can be a frightening experience for all personnel. Remember, however, that almost no anesthesia machine in current use depends on electric power for delivery of a gas mixture or for hydraulic operation of the mechanical ventilator (although the ventilator timing circuits may require battery backup).

A battery backup may permit at least partial operation of monitors such as inspired oxygen concentration and ventilatory parameters. Battery backup commonly exists for independent pulse oximeters but not for integrated operating room monitors. Thus, despite loss of electric power, patients' safety can be maintained. Even the anesthesia record can be continued: Keep a flashlight in the drawer of the anesthesia machine.

Why Does Sudden Power Loss Occur?

What causes sudden loss of power? Emergency power generators should enable recovery from global outages or an institution-wide loss of power. Because restoration of power occurs within a few minutes, avoid invoking drastic measures such as immediate closure of a surgical wound or postponement of surgery soon after induction of anesthesia.

Locally, a short between conductors within a device activates the circuit breaker for that outlet, resulting in discrete power loss to a group of devices. (The isolated system prevents power interruption from a single fault to ground but not from contact of both conductors. Review Figure 53–8 to understand why.) In this case, remove the errant device and reset the tripped circuit breaker to restore power.

What Should Be Done When a Device Stops Working?

Even in the absence of a global or regional power failure, a device occasionally fails to work. Immediate replacement of the presumed defective device usually constitutes the first response. Unfortunately, this extreme reaction is often unnecessary. Minimal probing of the device commonly yields information that leads to prompt repair.

First, verify that failure has in fact occurred. Has the brightness to the output screen merely been adjusted too low, or has a secondary enabling switch been overlooked?

Second, turn the device off, wait a few seconds, and then turn it on again. Complex microprocessor-controlled instruments may "crash" from software malfunction. Resetting internal indicators by reapplication of power usually restores function, although at the risk of losing previously acquired data.

Finally, check the fuse. Many devices have a fuse that limits power consumption. Mechanical trespass (in whose operating room does this not occur?) can sever the delicate wire in the fuse, interrupting power to the device. Simply replacing the fuse restores function.

SUMMARY

The household electric environment protects equipment but not people from live to ground faults. The operating room isolation transformer and LIM increase patient and personnel safety by warning of a potential fault to ground without interrupting power. The ESU cuts or coagulates tissue by purposefully making the patient part of a high-voltage, high-frequency electric circuit. Pacemakers enjoy sophisticated programming to filter out electric interference that confounds their ability to sense dysrhythmia and to restore effective cardiac function.

Knowledge of how these devices function enhances an anesthesiologist's ability to react and to direct the operating room team appropriately in an unexpected circumstance.

References

1. Dripps RD, Eckenhoff JE, Vandam LD: Introduction to Anesthesia. The Principles of Safe Practice. 3rd ed. Philadelphia, WB Saunders, 1967, pp 406–414.
2. Bruner JMR, Leonard PF: Electricity, Safety, and the Patient. Chicago, Year Book Medical Publishers, 1989, p 19.
3. Richter HP, Schwan WC: Wiring Simplified. 35th ed. St Paul, Park Publishing, 1986, pp 47–56.
4. Geddes LA, Baker LE: Response to passage of electric current through the body. J Assoc Advancement Med Instrument 1971; 5:13.
5. Bruner JMR: Hazards of electrical apparatus. Anesthesiology 1967; 28:396.
6. Leeming MN: Protection of the "electrically susceptible patient." Anesthesiology 1973; 38:370.
7. National Fire Protection Association: ANSI/NFPA 99. Health Care Facilities. Quincy, MA, National Fire Protection Association, 1990, pp 99–137.
8. Bruner JMR, Leonard PF: Electricity, Safety, and the Patient. Chicago, Year Book Medical Publishers, 1989, p 310.
9. Geddes LA: The beginnings of electromedicine. IEEE Engineering in Medicine and Biology Magazine 1984; 3:8.
10. Cushing H: Electrosurgery as an aid to the removal of intracranial tumors. With a preliminary note on a new surgical current generator by W.T. Bovie. Surg Gynecol Obstet 1928; 47:751.
11. Bruner JMR, Leonard PF: Electricity, Safety, and the Patient. Chicago, Year Book Medical Publishers, 1989, p 229.
12. Brock-Utne JG, Downing JW: Rectal burn after the use of an anal stainless steel electrode/transducer system for monitoring myoneural junction (Letter to the editor). Anesth Analg 1984; 63:1141.
13. Schneider AJL, Apple HP, Braun RT: Electrosurgical burns at skin temperature probes. Anesthesiology 1977; 47:72.
14. Wald AS, Mazzia VDB, Spencer FC: Accidental burns associated with electrocautery. JAMA 1971; 217:916.
15. Neufeld GR: Principles and hazards of electrosurgery including laparoscopy. Surg Gynecol Obstet 1978; 147:705.
16. Zaidan JR: Pacemakers. Anesthesiology 1984; 60:319.
17. Engle TR, Meister SG, Frankl WS: The "R-on-T" phenomenon. An update and critical review. Ann Intern Med 1978; 88:221.
18. Levine PA, Balady GJ, Lazard HL, et al: Electrocautery and pacemakers: Management of the paced patient subject to electrocautery. Ann Thorac Surg 1986; 41:313.
19. Domino KB, Smith TC: Electrocautery-induced reprogramming of a pacemaker using a precordial magnet. Anesth Analg 1983; 62:609.
20. Goldberg ME, McSherry RT, O'Connor ME: Electrocautery and pacemaker reprogramming (Letter to the editor). Anesth Analg 1984; 63:541.
21. Shapiro WA, Roizen MF, Singleton MA, et al: Intraoperative pacemaker complications. Anesthesiology 1985; 63:319.
22. Horrow JC, Seitman DT: Electrical safety and device calibration. Anesthesiol Clin North Am 1988; 6:699.

CHAPTER 54

Radiologic Procedures, Computed Tomography Scans, Magnetic Resonance Imaging, and Radiation Therapy

MARK E. ROMANOFF, M.D.*

Anesthesia performed out of the operating room (OR) entails many considerations. These issues include patients' characteristics, equipment, support personnel, transport, the environment where the procedures take place, and postanesthesia recovery (Table 54–1).

Many patients thought *too* sick for surgery may undergo diagnostic or therapeutic procedures out of the OR because these procedures are perceived to be less invasive. Unstable patients may need emergent diagnostic studies or therapeutic interventions. Their anesthetic management can rival complex cases in the OR. In patients undergoing transhepatic cholecystotomy, acute cholestasis and hepatic dysfunction may be present. Emergent computed tomography (CT) scans or magnetic resonance imaging (MRI) may be performed in patients with elevated intracranial pressure (ICP) or after blunt trauma.

The American Society of Anesthesiologists (ASA) guidelines for standard monitoring of oxygenation, ventilation, circulation, and temperature must be adhered to when one performs any anesthetic, regardless of procedure site. As in an OR case, additional appropriate patient-specific monitors are also important. Provision of such care can be difficult in settings where space is at a premium.

Early inspection of the procedure site before the procedure is crucial. The anesthesia equipment used for these procedures often is older, thought not to be adequate for the OR, and in need of repair. Upkeep of machines must be documented; the use of hazardous equipment, which may need to be transported to the location of the anesthetic, cannot be tolerated. The route taken must be investigated for obstructions (such as small doorways or stairs) that may impede movement.

"Crash cart" locations should be known. We assume their proximity in the OR. In the radiology suite or radiation therapy department, these carts may be stocked improperly or may not be present. Other emergency equipment, such as for malignant

hyperthermia therapy, or special airway equipment may be brought to the site.

Electrical safety concerns include the lack of isolation transformers, which are commonplace in the OR, thus increasing the risk of macroshock. Invasive catheters used by the radiologist or for monitoring present potential microshock hazards. Anesthesia machines and standard monitors require multiple electrical outlets and proper grounding. The number of outlets and the capacity of circuit breakers should be investigated before the anesthetic to avoid losing power during the procedure (see Chapter 53).

ENVIRONMENTAL HOSTILITY

What Are the Risk Factors?

Support Personnel

The usual support personnel are lacking. We define the role of anesthesia technicians in the OR; however, during radiologic procedures, it is unlikely that such individuals will be present. Other personnel are in the room but often are not helpful. Their role is to assist other providers, such as the radiologist. Even if available to help, they frequently do not understand our needs or equipment.

Radiologists (not unlike surgeons) are appropriately concerned with the technical aspects of their intervention and cannot always participate when an unstable situation arises. We often count on our colleagues to help or act as "educated hands" when difficulties arise in the OR. If procedures are performed in the MRI scanner, help may be in another building or so far away that it is essentially unattainable. Protocols should be in place to allow a swift response from other anesthesia providers.

Physical Constraints

The physical environment has been set up to provide an ideal, procedure-oriented working space. In the special proce-

*The opinions expressed are those of the author and do not necessarily reflect the views of the United States Air Force or the Department of Defense.

TABLE 54–1. Preanesthetic Site Evaluation

Physical plant	Interview room
	Induction area
	Lighting
	Monitor location
Patient positioning and access	
Equipment	Permanent: oxygen supply; suction; monitors; anesthesia machine
	Transportable: airway equipment, medications, monitors, reserve oxygen
Transport considerations	Monitors
	Portable oxygen
	Route
	Protection from elements
Emergency plans	Code cart
	Special airway equipment
	Training of on-site personnel
	Availability of additional support
Protection from site hazards	Equipment
	Temperature
	Noise
	Radiation
	Magnetic field

(Adapted from Greenberg DJ, Romanoff ME: Anesthesia in the radiology suite. Prob Anesth 1992; 6:413.)

dures room, fluoroscopy monitors are placed in locations convenient to the radiologist. These overlie the field, limiting access to a patient. Such constraints often require locating anesthesia equipment in positions that are not ideal or even convenient. The room lights are dimmed to allow viewing of x-ray screens. This process limits visibility of the patient, the monitors, and the anesthesia record. Appropriate directed lighting should be available to improve this situation.

Temperature

Ambient temperature in the rooms where these procedures take place is often cold, and thermostat changes may not be possible. Children (and even adults) are at risk for hypothermia unless precautions are observed. Heating blankets can be used but may interfere with the image quality. Radiant heating may be acceptable, as are other adjunctive measures (airway humidification, fluid warmers).

Radiation

The risks of radiation are of special concern. A wide range of electromagnetic radiation produces ion pairs that react with tissues and can transmit enough energy to alter chemical bonds. X-rays and gamma rays are the most common forms of radiation. The dose of radiation absorbed is measured in grays. One gray (Gy) equals 1 joule (J) $\cdot$ kg^{-1}. *Rad* is an acronym for "radiation absorbed dose." One rad is equivalent to 0.01 J $\cdot$ kg^{-1}, and 1 Gy equals 100 rads. Different particles have various biologic effects, so dose equivalents are measured in sieverts (Sv) and rems (rad equivalent mammal). Sieverts are equal to grays multiplied by a quality factor to account for the activity of the ionization produced. Rems have a similar relationship to rads. Ionizing radiation produced by clinical imaging has a quality factor of one. This relationship simplifies the equations:

$$Sv = Gy$$

$$Rem = rad[1]$$

Mechanisms of Damage

Ion pairs cause damage by two mechanisms. *Direct action* involves breaking the chemical bonds of an essential biologic compound. *Indirect action* occurs when these biomolecules are damaged by the high-energy chemical species produced by ion pairs. Ionization of water forms hydroxyl free radicals, which react with oxygen (O$_2$) to form peroxide. These free radicals have an unpaired electron and can damage chemical bonds. DNA is the only important molecule affected by free radicals. Types of destruction include single- or double-strand breakage, cross-linking of two strands, or the deletion of a base. Cells that are undergoing rapid mitotic activity are most likely to express damage. Nonlethal damage causes mutations; lethal damage causes cell death.[1]

Acute Effects

The clinical effects of radiation are classified as acute or late. Acute effects include death if a whole-body radiation dose of 5 Gy is absorbed. Other acute changes involve the hematologic system, central nervous system (CNS), bone marrow depletion, loss of intestinal crypt cells, and burns. They are manifested in hours to weeks after a "critical population" of cells is destroyed. Despite the fact that whole-body doses as low as 0.2 to 0.5 Gy can cause these changes, diagnostic imaging never has been implicated. Table 54–2 presents typical radiation exposures from common imaging studies.

Late Changes

Late changes are caused by damage to DNA; the latent period (time from radiation to expression) may be months or years. Cataracts and sterility are of concern, but carcinogenesis from DNA damage is the most relevant issue. Only "naturally occurring" cancers are induced by radiation. Organs and tissues at risk are listed in Table 54–3. The thyroid is extremely sensitive to radiation-induced malignancies. Use of a lead collar during exposure is often overlooked by anesthesia personnel but is important in protecting the thyroid. The latent period may be as long as 30 years for some tumors. Population-based studies suggest that 2300 additional cancer deaths result from medical imaging, compared with the 400,000 usual cancer deaths per year in this country.

Genetic Effects

The genetic effects of radiation result from chromosomal anomalies. Most common are reciprocal translocations caused by the exchange of broken chromosome pieces.[1] As in radiation-induced tumors, only naturally occurring mutations are observed after exposure to radiation. Males are twice as sensitive to these changes as are females. Fractionated doses appear to have less effect than sustained high doses. Mature spermatozoa are at highest risk; if one waits to conceive until at least a year after a significant radiation exposure, the risk decreases significantly.

Although animal data reveal radiation-induced genetic defects, no conclusive human evidence exists. Extrapolation of the animal data to humans suggests that a diagnostic study producing a gonadal dose of 10 mGy would increase the birth risk of a seriously genetically diseased child from 10.6% to 10.602%.[1] This risk can be applied to the general population

TABLE 54–2. Radiation Exposure from Imaging Studies

Examination	Skin Exposure (mR)	Thyroid	Active Marrow	Lungs	Breasts	Testes	Ovaries	Embryo
Chest	15–20	20	30	50	30		1	
Skull	105–210	220	30	2				
Extremities	10–100		10					
Abdomen	375–700		200	50		60	850	1050
Intravenous pyelography	475–850		220	65		90	1200	1500
Thoracic spine	300–500	160	100	800	1050		1	550
Lumbar/sacral spine	450–800		200	30		40	550	550
Mammography (film screen)	750–1100				400			
Xeromammography	800–1700				3700			
Fluoroscopy	500–5000/min		Depends on site and duration of exposure					
Head CT	2000–5000	2000	15000			70	70	70
Body CT	1000–3000		Depends on site, midline structures 25–75% of entrance exposure					

(Adapted from Edwards FM: Risks of medical imaging. *In* Textbook of Diagnostic Imaging. Putman CE, Ravin CE (eds). Philadelphia, WB Saunders, 1988, pp 91–110.)
mR = milliroentgen. All measurements except skin exposure are in micrograys (10 μGy = mrad).

using a formula developed by the United Nations Scientific Committee on the Effects of Atomic Radiation. Their conclusion was that diagnostic imaging would cause 10 serious genetic defects out of the 3.5 million births per year in the United States. A male patient's risk can be further reduced by shielding his gonads; however, a female's gonads are more difficult to protect because their location varies, and shielding usually obscures the image. The lead aprons worn by clinicians offer good protection.

TABLE 54–3. Sensitivity of Tissues to Carcinogenic Effects of Radiation

Site/Type of Cancer	Spontaneous Incidence	Relative Sensitivity to Radiation
Major Radiation-Induced Cancers		
Female breasts	Very high	High
Thyroid	Low	Very high (females)
Lungs (bronchi)	Very high	Moderate
Leukemia	Moderate	Very high (myeloid)
Alimentary tract	High	Moderate-Low
Minor Radiation-Induced Cancers		
Pharynx	Low	Moderate
Liver/biliary tract	Low	Moderate
Pancreas	Moderate	Moderate
Lymphomas	Moderate	Moderate
Kidney/bladder	Moderate	Low
Brain and central nervous system	Low	Low
Salivary glands	Very low	Low
Bone	Very low	Low
Skin	High	Low
Uncertain Radiation-Induced Risk		
Larynx	Moderate	Low
Nasal sinuses	Very low	Low
Parathyroid	Very low	Low
Ovaries	Moderate	Low
Connective tissue	Very low	Low
No Radiation-Induced Risk		
Prostate	Very high	Absent
Uterus/cervix	Very high	Absent
Testes	Low	Absent
Mesentery/mesothelium	Very low	Absent
Chronic lymphocytic leukemia	Low	Absent

(Adapted from Edwards FM: Risks of medical imaging. *In* Textbook of Diagnostic Imaging. Putman CE, Ravin CE (eds). Philadelphia, WB Saunders, 1988, pp 91–110.)

Fetal Risks

The risk of fetal radiation is high because a fetus is rapidly growing. However, teratogenic effects are dependent on the timing of the radiation exposure. During the first 2 weeks of life, an embryo is sensitive to the lethal but not the teratogenic effects of ionizing radiation. Fetal death causing a failure to conceive would be experienced. Organogenesis occurs from 15 to 50 days. During this time, a fetus can experience teratogenic effects and growth retardation. Mental retardation, eye malformations, and microcephaly can be documented after a fetal dose of 100 mGy.

Few human data implicate doses of <50 mGy as being harmful.[1] After the second month of development, a fetus is less sensitive to organ abnormalities. The risk at this time involves development of a childhood cancer. Diagnostic abdominal examinations rarely expose a fetus to doses >10 to 20 mGy owing to absorption by maternal tissues. The risk of developing a childhood cancer probably increases from a baseline of 1 in 1000 to 1 in 200 after an abdominal diagnostic examination. Radiation to other areas of the body presents almost no risk to a fetus.

Why Are Transport Issues Important?

Patients usually must travel long distances, often to another building, to reach the radiation therapy department or MRI suite. Remote areas are chosen to reduce the risks of exposure. Figure 54–1 reveals the *outside* distance a patient must travel from the main hospital to the portable MRI scanner at the author's institution. Protection of patients from the elements, including temperature changes, rain, snow, or accidents, must be ensured. Ambulances are often used for transport.

Getting patients to the drop-off and pick-up locations may be difficult because of elevator size, lack of personnel, or other obstacles. These problems are magnified when a patient is unstable or recovering from the effects of anesthesia. To minimize difficulties, the route of travel must be planned before the patient is moved. Emergency equipment should be available during this vulnerable time as well (see Chapter 24).

The location of the recovery area should be as close to the anesthetizing location as is safe. However, this arrangement is not always possible. Transportation may need to be arranged back to a suitable location. Appropriate monitoring and per-

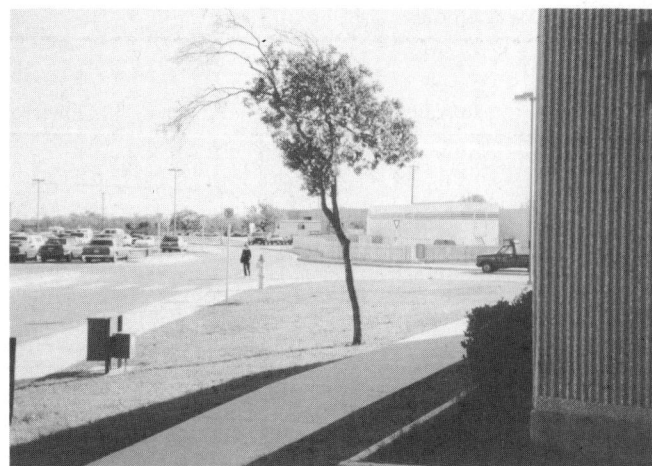

FIGURE 54–1. Patients must be transported from the main entrance of the hospital to the MRI trailer in the distance. (See text for details.)

sonnel should accompany a patient at all times. Ventilation requirements at the site of the examination as well as during transport must be well thought out.

ANESTHETIC CONCERNS

As with any anesthetic, monitoring, airway maintenance, analgesia, sedation or anesthesia, and prevention of movement during the intervention are the major concerns. Cardiovascular instability may be induced by the procedure (bleeding), from the use of contrast material (hypotension), from changes in positioning (sitting), or deterioration of the patient's underlying disease (elevated ICP).

Control of the airway can be difficult because access to the patient is limited or impossible (e.g., a small child in the MRI gantry) (Fig. 54–2). Pulmonary aspiration of gastric contents may occur after changes in mental status induced by sedation or progression of disease. Patients predisposed to aspiration need chemical prophylaxis to decrease their risk. An appropriate nil per os (NPO) period should be ensured for any patient undergoing sedation or anesthesia for a radiologic procedure.

Immobile conditions are necessary for optimal imaging or

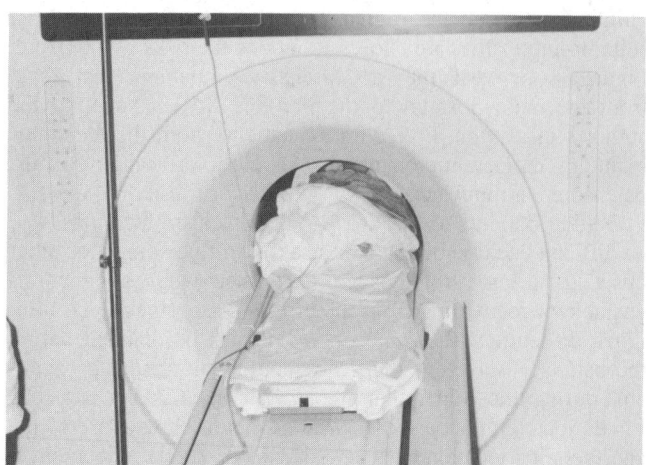

FIGURE 54–2. Access to this patient's airway is severely limited. Note the pulse oximeter probe on the left toe.

to perform the planned procedure adequately. Children almost always need sedation or general anesthesia to accomplish these goals. Most adults do not require anesthesia for diagnostic studies, but those who have CNS changes, who are uncooperative, or who have communication barriers may have requirements similar to children.

What Are the Goals of Sedation?

Conscious sedation, deep sedation, and general anesthesia are defined in Table 54–4. The most important priority is patients' welfare. Control of behavior to allow the procedure to be completed successfully is necessary. If possible, generation of a positive mental attitude toward treatment is also desirable, especially in patients receiving multiple treatments such as radiation therapy. Finally, patients should be returned to the pretreatment level of consciousness by the time of discharge.

Many medications have been used to achieve these goals, but the ideal sedative is yet to be discovered (Table 54–5). Each new medication introduced into anesthesia practice is thought of as the solution to this problem (e.g., midazolam, alfentanil, and propofol). However, these medications have side effects that may be exaggerated in patients with limited cardiovascular or respiratory reserve. They are generally safe owing to a large therapeutic index, but patients respond to medications in unique ways, thereby limiting the margin for error.[2]

How Is Sedation Provided?

An O_2 delivery device that can supply a fraction of inspired O_2 (FIO_2) of ≥ 0.9 for 60 minutes at 5 L $\cdot$ min^{-1} is necessary.

TABLE 54–4. Definitions of Levels of Consciousness

Conscious sedation	Conscious sedation is a minimally depressed level of consciousness that *retains* a patient's ability to maintain a patent airway independently and continuously and to respond appropriately to physical stimulation and/or verbal command (e.g., "Open your eyes"). For very young or handicapped individuals incapable of the usually expected verbal responses, a minimally depressed level of consciousness for that individual should be maintained. The caveat that the loss of consciousness should be unlikely is a particularly important part of the definition of conscious sedation, and the drugs and techniques used should carry a margin of safety wide enough to render unintended loss of consciousness unlikely.
Deep sedation	Deep sedation is a controlled state of depressed consciousness or unconsciousness from which a patient is not easily aroused, which *may* be accompanied by a partial or complete loss of protective reflexes, including the ability to maintain a patent airway independently and respond purposefully to physical stimulation or verbal command.
General anesthesia	General anesthesia is a controlled state of unconsciousness accompanied by a loss of protective reflexes, *including* the ability to maintain an airway independently and respond purposefully to physical stimulation or verbal command.

(From American Academy of Pediatrics Committee on Drugs, Section on Anesthesiology: Guidelines for the elective use of conscious sedation, deep sedation, and general anesthesia in pediatric patients. Pediatrics 1985; 76:317. Copyright 1985.)

TABLE 54–5. Characteristics of the Ideal Sedative

Safe
Easy to administer
Painless
Consistency of action
Complete immobilization
Rapid action
Controlled duration of action
Reversible
No residual central nervous system depression
No side effects

(Adapted form Thompson JR, Schneider S, Ashwal S, et al: The choice of sedation for computed tomography in children. A prospective evaluation. Radiology 1982; 143:475.)

A system to administer inhalation sedation must also be able to deliver an FIO_2 of 1.0 (never <0.2). A fail-safe system is mandatory.

Informed consent should be obtained from all patients who are to receive sedation. A responsible adult should accompany the patient to the procedure, remain during the procedure, and take the patient home. NPO policies should be established at each institution. Suggested guidelines include no milk or solids after midnight. Clear liquids are allowed up to 4 hours before the procedure in patients from birth to 3 years old. A 6-hour period from the time of last clear liquid intake in patients from 3 to 6 years old is acceptable. Patients older than 6 years should have an 8-hour fast.[3] In many procedures, large amounts of oral contrast material are given within the NPO period. This issue must be addressed and generally suggests that if sedation is provided, the airway should be protected.

Monitoring

Monitoring during conscious sedation should include continuous observation of heart and respiratory rates. A precordial stethoscope and observation of nail bed color are also recommended. Patients undergoing deep sedation should have an intravenous catheter in place. Additional monitors include those for pulse oximetry and noninvasive blood pressure measurement. Temperature monitoring capability should be available. The American Academy of Pediatrics suggests monitoring the electrocardiogram (ECG) and having a defibrillator available. Patients should never be left unattended.[3]

The need for pulse oximetry monitoring has been repeatedly emphasized for any patient receiving sedation.[2] Capnography should be considered in patients receiving deep sedation. The end-tidal carbon dioxide (CO_2) partial pressure (P_{ETCO_2}) can be used as a trend monitor for changes in arterial partial pressure of CO_2 (Pa_{CO_2}) as well as respiratory rate. Capnography is a standard of care for intubated patients; however, it is not yet a standard of care for patients undergoing conscious sedation. If in doubt, be reminded that both the Joint Commission on the Accreditation of Healthcare Organizations (JCAHO) and the ASA clearly state that patients are to receive the same level and quality of care during a procedure, regardless of where it occurs in an institution.

Remember that procedures can be noninvasive but the anesthetic is not. The largest patient risk is often from the medications used for sedation or anesthesia. Complications occur commonly but are markedly underreported in the literature.[3]

Is Sedation or a General Anesthetic Required?

The type of procedure and a patient's characteristics dictate different approaches to achieve one's anesthetic goals. In adults undergoing diagnostic procedures, sedation for anxiety or claustrophobia may be all that is necessary. If deep sedation is required, airway concerns assume greater importance. Patients at risk for aspiration or airway compromise should be intubated and anesthetized. The same considerations are important in children. A prospective study showed that 30% of CT scans fail in 6- to 9-year-old children who are not sedated.[4]

Therapeutic procedures in adults may be accomplished using local anesthesia administered at the site by the radiologist. However, supplemental sedation is often required.[5] Regional or general anesthesia may be necessary for particularly painful procedures, for uncooperative adults, and for children.

REACTIONS TO CONTRAST AGENTS

Many radiologic procedures require contrast agents to delineate structures or define anatomy. The composition of these agents and their unique risks are important.

What Is the Chemical Structure of Intravascular Contrast Dyes?

Many compounds have been used, but only iodine is a satisfactory intravascular radiocontrast agent. It has a molecular weight of 127. All ionic contrast agents are salts of a sodium or meglumine cation and a tri-iodinated substituted benzoate anion.[6] The chemistry of contrast agents is presented in Table 54–6. The substituted amines in these molecules do not add to the radiodensity (only iodine does) but are necessary to reduce toxicity and improve solubility.

The total amount of iodine in the body is 0.01 g. The dose of iodine needed for an angiogram may be as high as 80 g

TABLE 54–6. Contrast Material Characteristics

Product	Composition	Iodine (mg/mL)
Ionic		
Conray 280	Meglumine iothalamate 60%	280
Conray 325	Sodium iothalamate 54%	325
Conray 420	Sodium iothalamate 70%	420
Hypaque 45%	Sodium diatrizoate 45%	270
Hypaque 65%	Meglumine diatrizoate 50%	390
	Sodium diatrizoate 45%	
Urografin 325	Sodium diatrizoate 40%	325
	Meglumine diatrizoate 18%	
Urografin 370	Meglumine diatrizoate 66%	325
	Sodium diatrizoate 10%	
Nonionic		
Amipaque	Metrizamide	280
Omnipaque	Iohexol	280
Nipam	Iopamidol	300

(Adapted from Grainger RG: Intravascular contrast media. *In* Diagnostic Radiology, an Anglo-American Textbook of Imaging. Grainger RG, Allison DJ (eds). New York, Churchill Livingstone, 1986, pp 99–110.)

delivered in <1 hour. Because iodine accounts for only 50% of the content of contrast media, 160 g of contrast is necessary. Meglumine salts are less toxic than sodium salts, but meglumine is more viscous and is a strong diuretic, both properties that may be undesirable. Contrast agents can compete with other medications for protein-binding sites. One study demonstrated barbiturate potentiation when contrast agents were administered.[7] This interaction may increase the incidence of hypotension.

Contrast media readily pass through capillary walls into all organs except the brain if the blood-brain barrier is intact. Intravenous urography is performed with sodium salts (iodine content 280–440 mg · mL^{-1}). Cerebral and peripheral angiography are performed with meglumine because a low osmolar agent is preferred (iodine content 280–320 mg · mL^{-1}). Cardiac and aortic procedures ordinarily are performed with mixtures of sodium and meglumine salts (iodine content 370–440 mg · mL^{-1}). A compromise between a low-osmolar agent and a physiologic sodium content is thus maintained.

What Are the Differences Between Ionic and Non-Ionic Contrast Media?

The advantages of ionic agents are their long record of relative safety and low cost. Disadvantages include the high osmolality, up to 1500 mOsm · kg^{-1} (physiologic osmolality is approximately 285 mOsm · kg^{-1}). The osmotic load is responsible for many of the adverse reactions. Non-ionic agents have been available for approximately 20 years. Substitutions in the structure of the ionic salts result in non-ionic salts with a higher iodine-to-particle ratio (3:1 compared with 3:2). This chemical change substantially decreases the osmolality. These agents have less toxicity and a lower incidence of adverse reactions and are more stable in solution. Their significant disadvantage is higher cost (up to 40 times higher than that of ionic compounds).[6]

What Types of Reactions Are Seen with Contrast Material?

Most complications in the radiology suite are from the technical aspects of the procedure (bleeding, vessel damage, organ perforation), not from the contrast agent.

Allergic

Intra-arterial injections are associated with one third of all anaphylactic reactions. This problem may result from the delivery of a high concentration of antigen complexes to the lungs with less time for dilution, or from a greater liberation of vasoactive substances (histamine, serotonin, bradykinin).

Cardiovascular

Hypervolemia can result from the osmotic effects of contrast agents. Blood volume may actually increase 10%. Cardiac depression can occur from a loss of contractility, changes in calcium availability, and conduction abnormalities from direct effects of the contrast agent on the heart. This problem may compound the hypotension resulting from vasodilation.[8] Patients with pulmonary hypertension have developed significant right ventricular failure after ionic media examinations. In these patients, a low-osmolar agent is preferable.

TABLE 54–7. Occurrence of Nausea and Vomiting with Major Contrast Agent Reactions

Complication	Nausea (%)	Vomiting (%)
Laryngeal edema	7.7	4.2
Hypotension	17.5	9.2
Pulmonary edema	0	0
Angina	22	8.2
Ventricular fibrillation	3.7	7.4
Circulatory collapse	10	8.5
Cardiac arrest	6.5	4.3

(Adapted from Shehadi WH: Contrast media adverse reactions: occurrence, recurrence, and distribution patterns. Radiology 1982; 143:11.)

Contrast agents are among the safest intravenous medications. The risk of death is quoted at 1 in 14,000 to 1 in 75,000. However, in one large Japanese study, only 2 deaths occurred in 337,647 patients receiving contrast agents (1 in 168,000).[9] Most contrast media reactions occur within the first 5 minutes of injection; 47% occur during the injection. One in seven reactions occurs later, so vigilance must be kept high, and the contrast agent should be suspected when cardiovascular compromise occurs.[10] Nausea and vomiting may be minor complications, but they often are associated with the start of a more severe reaction (Table 54–7).

Chemotoxic

Chemotoxic reactions are rare with ionic and non-ionic contrast agents. Iodine is tightly bound, so it does not usually cause problems. Patients consuming a low-iodide diet can develop thyrotoxicosis from the small amount of *iodide* (not *iodine*) present.

Osmolar

Reactions occur as a result of the very high osmolality of ionic contrast media (five to eight times higher than normal). Non-ionic agents exert one third the osmolality of conventional ionic agents but contain the same amount of iodine. The use of non-ionic media reduces the incidence of osmolar reactions, all of which are dose dependent. Reactions include erythrocyte damage, endothelial disruption, vasodilation, hypervolemia, and cardiac depression. Loss of erythrocyte water can induce rigidity and the loss of deformability that is needed for capillary passage.

Signs and symptoms include bronchospasm, systemic vasodilation, changes in capillary permeability (peripheral and pulmonary edema), hypotension, tachycardia, cardiovascular collapse, cardiac arrest, and death. These reactions are not dose dependent. They may develop after as little as 1 mL of contrast. The percentage of patients exhibiting symptoms after exposure to intravenous contrast is depicted in Figure 54–3.

Central Nervous System

Endothelial damage can cause increases in permeability and the extravascular movement of toxic agents into tissues. The blood-brain barrier normally excludes contrast agents from the brain. However, tumors, cerebral infarcts, and other CNS insults affect this barrier and allow contrast to pass and predispose to toxic effects on neural tissue. Seizures can occur.

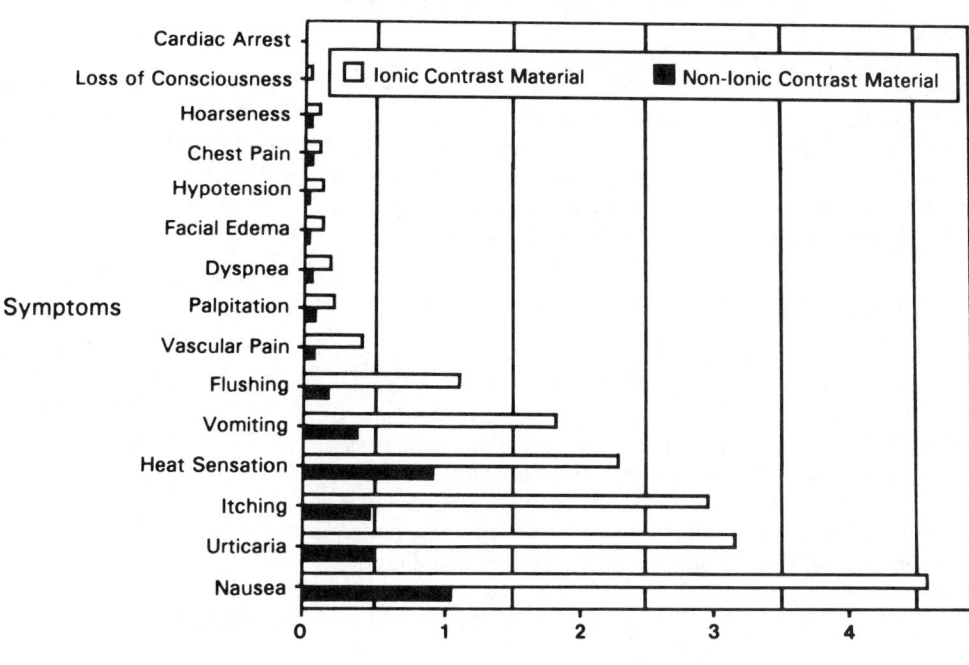

Contrast Media Adverse Reactions

□ Ionic Contrast Material   ■ Non-Ionic Contrast Material

FIGURE 54–3. Percentage of patients exhibiting symptoms following administration of intravenous contrast medium. (Adapted from Katayama H, Yamaguchi K, Kozuka T, et al: Adverse reactions to ionic and nonionic contrast media. Radiology 1990; 175:621.)

Meglumine iothalamate appears to have the lowest neurotoxicity of the ionic agents. Metrizamide has been used in the past but is associated with headaches in 30% of patients. Vasodilation of capillary beds and arterioles increases blood flow, so patients feel warmth, heat, or pain locally. Global vasodilation causes a loss of venous return and hypotension.

Renal

Renal impairment causing oliguria and uremia may be induced with contrast media. Patients at highest risk are those with pre-existing renal disease, diabetic nephropathy, or hypovolemia. The damage to the glomeruli and tubules is *not* related to the osmolality of these medications.[6, 11]

Which Mediators Are Involved?

As in other allergic reactions, histamine, complement, serotonin, bradykinin, and leukotrienes have major roles. Contrast agents have a relatively low molecular weight and act as haptens to induce antibody formation and cause the degranulation of mast cells and basophils.[12] True anaphylactic reactions are IgE mediated. Anaphylactoid reactions result from protein binding of the contrast material. Inhibition of plasma cholinesterase by contrast agents may also play a part. Higher levels of acetylcholine and increasing vagal tone conceivably result in bradycardia, bronchospasm, and cardiovascular collapse. Activation of other cascade systems is also implicated in these reactions. Complement (C3a, C5a, anaphylatoxins), kinins, consumption coaguloapthy, and the fibrinolytic systems may be involved. The association of these reactions with a patient's anxiety and fear, perhaps through hypothalamic activation, has been suggested but is not well worked out.[8]

How Often Do Reactions Occur?

The incidence and severity of contrast agent reactions are presented in Table 54–8. The likelihood of developing a reaction is dependent on the procedure being performed. Peripheral arteriography has a 2.5% incidence of reactions, intravenous pyelograms have a 5.7% incidence, and intravenous cholangiography has a 10.1% incidence.[5]

How Are Severe Reactions Treated?

Minor complications include symptoms of a short duration that are usually self-limited. The incidence of these reactions is as high as 13%.[6] No specific treatment is necessary. Pain, anxiety, skin flushing, and rash are examples. An antihistamine, anxiolytic, or analgesic may limit a patient's discomfort. Moderate reactions include bronchospasm, hypotension, or ur-

TABLE 54–8. Incidence and Severity of Reactions with Contrast Media

	Ionic (%)	Non-Ionic (%)
Incidence	4–13	0.7–3
Severity		
Mild	2.5	0.58
Moderate	1.2	0.11
Severe	0.2–0.4	0–0.004
Treatment required?		
Yes	1.3	0.2
No	2.7	0.5

(Adapted from Wolf GL, Arenson RL, Cross AP: A prospective trial of ionic vs. nonionic contrast agents in routine clinical practice: Comparison of adverse effects. AJR 1989; 152:939, *and* Katayama H, Yamaguchi K, Kozuka T, et al: Adverse reactions to ionic and nonionic contrast media. Radiology 1990; 175:621.)

ticaria, which are not life threatening. Treatment may involve corticosteroids in addition to the previously mentioned medications.[6]

Marked cardiovascular compromise including significant hypotension, dysrhythmias, pulmonary edema, or cardiac arrest may be encountered. Laryngeal edema and severe bronchospasm can lead to respiratory compromise. Treatment must be swift and aggressive. Effective medications include adrenergic agents, anticholinergic medications, corticosteroids, antihistamines, methylxanthine derivatives, and fluids.

Catecholamines

Early use of epinephrine and other pressors is often successful. Increasing contractility, systemic vascular resistance (SVR), and heart rate is necessary to treat cardiovascular collapse. Epinephrine also produces bronchodilation and may decrease subsequent histamine release from basophils and mast cells. Phenylephrine, an α-agonist, can be given to treat severe hypotension associated with a loss of SVR or venodilation. Pulmonary edema also improves with inotropes and diuretics. Beta$_2$-adrenergic agonists are effective in the treatment of bronchospasm. They can be given down the endotracheal tube. Because much of the medication adheres to the tube, substantially larger doses are necessary to achieve results. These agents have a high therapeutic index, and toxicity is rare.

Anticholinergic Agents, Corticosteroids, and Antihistamines

Anticholinergic agents decrease secretions, reverse bronchoconstriction, and offset bradycardia. Corticosteroids stabilize mast cells and decrease the further release of histamine. Their peak effect is in hours; hence, they are not useful for initial resuscitation. Antihistamines may be given but are probably of little use during a severe reaction because histamine already has been liberated.

Theophylline

Theophylline preparations have been used as first-line agents for bronchospasm, but their effectiveness has been questioned. They may be helpful as secondary agents, but their potentially high toxicity limits their usefulness.

Fluids

Supportive therapy with fluid to restore intravascular volume is usually required. Increased capillary permeability leading to generalized edema and vasodilation substantially increases volume requirements. Crystalloid or colloid resuscitation is appropriate, and several liters of fluid may be required to restore intravascular volume.

Mortality

The death rate, as noted previously, has been quoted as high as 1 in 14,000 patients and as low as 1 in 168,000.[9, 12] In recent years, it may have increased, perhaps because an increasing number of studies are performed on an older and more debilitated population.

What Are the Risk Factors?

Previous Reactions

Patients with previous adverse reactions are 4 to 10 times more likely to have a new reaction.[9, 12] Such reactions are often minor, and severe reactions tend not to be repeated.[11] In one study, approximately 44% of previous responders had second reactions with ionic media compared with 11% with non-ionic media. Severe reactions occurred in only 0.73% and 0.18% of previous responders with ionic and non-ionic agents, respectively.[9]

Patients with a history of allergies have a fourfold increase in the risk of developing contrast media reactions.[12] Previous laryngeal edema and bronchospasm appear to be important risk factors. Bronchospasm confers almost a fourfold increase in reactions. Fifteen per cent of patients with asthma exhibit signs of reactions, compared with 4% of patients without risk factors. Contrast agents containing meglumine (Conray 280, Hypaque 65%, Urografin 370) should be avoided in these patients.[11]

Cardiac Disease

Cardiac disease, especially congestive heart failure, is associated with a fivefold increase in the risk of adverse reactions. Slow injection of contrast and avoidance of a high sodium load is prudent. Patients with sickle cell disease may develop a sickle crisis from the induced osmotic changes.[13] Cerebral and coronary angiography have produced significant reactions, including cerebral or myocardial infarction from thrombosis. Non-ionic (low osmolar) agents in these patients are mandatory.

Miscellaneous

Other conditions that may predispose to adverse reactions include pheochromocytoma and a hypertensive crisis. Prophylactic treatment with α- and β-adrenergic blocking agents is suggested. Patients with multiple myeloma may develop renal failure from the precipitation of Bence Jones and Tam-Horsfall proteins. Those at the extremes of ages, with multiorgan system failure or diabetes, tend to have a higher incidence of reactions.[6] One study showed that the highest incidence of reactions was in the 20- to 29-year-old range, with severe reactions peaking in the 10- to 19-year age group.[9] The amount of contrast agent used does not affect the reaction rate. One fifth of all reactions occur with <20 mL of agent.

Can Reactions Be Prevented?

Many studies show that routine test dosing is ineffective in identifying patients at risk. Intradermal or subcutaneous testing does not predict those who will react to contrast media.[14] Although non-ionic agents significantly decrease the number of severe reactions, they are expensive and add approximately $70 to the cost of each study. If they are used in low-risk individuals, 1 severe reaction will be prevented in every 555 patients, a cost of $44,000 per reaction saved.[15] Non-ionic agents in high-risk patients prevent a severe reaction in 1 of 182 patients. This cost is $14,000 per severe reaction saved.[15]

Treatment for even one severe reaction approximates this cost. Most authors suggest that high-risk patients should receive non-ionic contrast media.

Prophylactic Medication

Prophylactic medication regimens have been studied, and they prevent high-risk patients from developing severe reactions. Commonly used drugs include corticosteroids and antihistamines. One double-blind randomized study evaluated prophylactic corticosteroids in preventing these reactions. More than 6500 patients were enrolled, and patients were divided into four groups. One group received methylprednisolone, 32 mg, 12 hours and 2 hours before the contrast injection. A second group received methylprednisolone only 2 hours before the study. The other two groups received placebo. Severe reactions were reduced by 62%, and reactions requiring treatment were decreased by 42% only in the group receiving two doses of corticosteroid. High-risk patients had the same results. In fact, corticosteroid prophylaxis reduced the risk of reactions from ionic media to a level similar to that of non-ionic media.[16]

Corticosteroids appear to reduce reactions by increasing C1 esterase inhibitor levels, thereby inhibiting the kallikrein and bradykinin systems.[17] Antihistamines (diphenhydramine and hydroxyzine) have obvious benefit when given before the histamine challenge, but the time course, dosage, and optimum dosing intervals have not been well worked out. In animals, other medications have been evaluated, including quinidine, lidocaine, and diazepam. These agents have decreased the median lethal dose in animals but have not been applied to humans.[17]

DIAGNOSTIC RADIOLOGIC PROCEDURES

What Are the Risks of Cerebral and Spinal Angiography?

Hyperosmolar contrast agents can pass through a damaged blood-brain barrier and cause cerebral or spinal cord edema as well as neural toxicity including seizures. Electroencephalographic (EEG) suppression has been documented after intravenous contrast.[18] The incidence of permanent neurologic defects is 0.65% after cerebral angiography in patients with symptomatic cerebrovascular disease.[19]

One of the more devastating complications is vasospasm in patients with cerebral aneurysms. Angiography-induced spasm can significantly worsen already altered cerebral function. Ischemic events occur in up to 2% of patients after the study.[20] Risk factors include advanced age, diabetes mellitus, the volume of contrast agent used, hypertension (systolic blood pressure >160 mm Hg), and a procedure duration longer than 1 hour.[20] During spinal angiography, acute lower extremity spasm can be induced. This problem usually resolves with an anterior spinal artery injection of diazepam. Arterial spasm can precipitate motor or sensory deficits during localization of the spinal vessels.[21]

Which Anesthetic Techniques Are Appropriate?

Most patients can tolerate these procedures with sedation plus local anesthesia at the site of arterial puncture. Conscious sedation is preferred so that communication can be maintained during the study. Anesthetic agents with a short half-life (propofol, alfentanil, midazolam) are recommended to facilitate neurologic evaluation after the procedure.

General anesthesia with tracheal intubation appears to be well tolerated. Hyperventilation decreases spinal cord and cerebral blood flow, effectively concentrating the contrast media and improving the recorded image.[22] However, in patients with vasospasm, hypocapnia is contraindicated. A nitrous oxide–narcotic technique avoids high-dose inhalation agents that can cause cerebral vasodilation and a poorer quality study from contrast media dilution. Monitoring of the EEG and somatosensory evoked potentials (SSEPs) can be helpful in assessing these patients while they are anesthetized.

How Were Pneumoencephalography and Ventriculography Performed?

Pneumoencephalography was first described in 1913 and was performed until 1975. At that time, CT scanning made this test rare; the introduction of MRI has made it obsolete. When it was performed, both negative and positive contrast agents were used. The negative contrast agents were air and O_2. The positive contrast agent was Pantopaque. Up to 120 mL of air was injected, but usually only 15 to 20 mL was necessary to complete the procedure. (The entire volume of cerebrospinal fluid [CSF] is 150 mL.)

CSF was removed through a needle placed in the lumbar subarachnoid space with the patient in the sitting position. Air was then injected into the needle. Less air was injected than CSF removed to allow expansion. The patient's position was then changed to allow the air to enter the appropriate area in the cranial vault. A cisternal puncture was used if the lumbar approach was untenable. This was a high-risk procedure because of the location of the needle. Furthermore, the neck posture could not be changed even when one wished to adjust the location of the contrast agent.

Ventriculography was performed when pneumoencephalography was contraindicated. The procedure was accomplished in the OR. Bur holes were made, and contrast was injected into the lateral ventricles. Moving the patient's head ensured proper position of the contrast.[22] The reported risks of these procedures included air embolism, nausea and vomiting, syncope, cardiovascular compromise, and brainstem herniation.[23] Nitrous oxide was obviously contraindicated during the test because of the risk of expansion of the air-containing cavity and also for at least a week after the study because of residual air.

THERAPEUTIC VASCULAR INTERVENTIONS

When Is Embolization Used?

The development of materials (Table 54–9) and catheter equipment has led to an increase in percutaneous embolization. Cerebral, spinal, splenic, esophagogastric, and hepatic vascular beds have been so treated. Intracranial aneurysms and arteriovenous malformations are embolized only if they are surgically inaccessible. If a patient is thought to be a poor risk for surgery and anesthesia, embolization is considered. Hyper-

TABLE 54–9. Embolic Material Used for Vascular Embolization

Natural agents (obsolete)	Autogenous blood clots (regular)
	Autogenous blood clots (modified)
	Tissue fragments (muscle, fat, other)
Synthetic	Solid (resorbable)
	Gelatin sponge (Gelfoam)
	Oxidized cellulose (Oxycel)
	Occlusion gel (Ethibloc)
	Collagen suspensions
	Microfibrillar bovine collagen (Avitene)
	Equine collagen (Tachotop)
Solid (permanent)	Polyvinyl alcohol (Ivalon)
	Silicone beads
	Plastic beads
	Metal beads
	Glass beads
Solid (mechanical)	Coils (stainless steel)
	Wool threads
	Silk threads
	Dacron threads
	Springs (stainless steel)
Solid (balloon systems)	Nondetachable balloon systems
	Detachable balloon systems
	Controlled leak balloon systems
Liquid	Isobutyl-2-cyanoacrylate (IBCA; bucrylate)
	Silicone elastomer
	Absolute ethanol
	Barium sulfate
	Hot contrast agents
Chemoembolization	Micromycin C microcapsules
Electrocoagulation	

(Data from Snopek AM: Vascular interventional procedures. *In* Fundamentals of Special Radiographic Procedures. 3rd ed. Snopek AM (ed). Philadelphia, WB Saunders, 1992, pp 330–350.)

splenism can be treated with partial splenic embolization. Surgery in such patients has a mortality rate approaching 10%; in those patients who develop postsplenectomy sepsis, it rises to 50%.[24] Patients with esophageal varices that continue to bleed despite sclerotherapy can undergo emergency shunting procedures, with mortality rates >50%. Embolization of gastric and gastroepiploic arteries is successful in up to 40% of cases. Hepatic artery embolization is used for surgically unresectable hepatic carcinoma or metastases.[25] This procedure is limited in use because of the severe epigastric pain that develops during and after the maneuver.

Complications

The risks of these interventions depend on the location of the artery. Complications common to all approaches include pain, fever, restlessness, tachycardia, and tachypnea. Embolization of nontarget organs can lead to myocardial infarction, pulmonary embolus, neurologic deficits, and death. Perforation of vessels with hemorrhage has been noted.[26] Technical difficulties can cause premature detachment of balloons and embolic material.

Direct occlusion of an intracranial aneurysm is associated with a stroke rate of 10% and mortality rate of 18%.[27] Embolization for control of bleeding esophageal varices is associated with a 63% rebleeding rate and a 20% mortality rate.[28] Uncontrollable bleeding from acute portal vein thrombosis occurred in 4% of patients. Complications following splenic artery embolization include pleural effusions, pneumonia, and severe abdominal pain requiring a narcotic infusion.[24]

Which Anesthetic Techniques Are Appropriate?

In patients undergoing intracranial procedures, neurologic evaluation during and after the intervention is important to assess and limit the extent of damage from emboli.[29] Conscious sedation and local infiltration should be sufficient for these studies. Injections of amytal or lidocaine or temporary balloon inflations can be performed to simulate permanent embolization and to document any neurologic deficits. If severe deficits occur, the vessel to be occluded is rejected.[27] If a parent vessel was the primary target, moving more distally can be attempted. If a patient requires general anesthesia, comprehensive neurologic monitoring should be performed.

Most other embolization techniques can be performed with minimal sedation and local anesthesia at the site of skin entry. Children and uncooperative adults may require general anesthesia. Hepatic embolization is an exception. The severe pain that occurs during this procedure demands regional or general anesthesia. Of note is that celiac plexus blocks have been used with favorable results.[25]

Many of these procedures carry a risk of significant hemorrhage. Adequate intravenous access plus additional monitoring (arterial, central venous, or pulmonary artery pressures) may be necessary. Blood products must be available. Remember that most of these techniques are carried out because the patients are at high risk for surgical mortality. The procedures are invasive, produce significant side effects, and remain a significant anesthetic challenge.

THERAPEUTIC NONVASCULAR INTERVENTIONS

Nonvascular therapeutic radiologic interventions are summarized in Table 54–10.

How Is a Percutaneous Nephrostomy Performed?

Patients with supravesicular obstructions often have the obstruction relieved with a percutaneous nephrostomy as initial therapy. However, patients who are extremely debilitated

TABLE 54–10. Nonvascular Interventional Procedures

Location of procedures	Urinary system
	Biliary system
	Abdominal cavity
Percutaneous drainage	Dilate stenotic channels (ureter)
	Occlude areas of leakage
	Close off fistulas
	Aspirate fluid collections (abscess, cyst, seroma)
	Remove dissolved calculi
Drug instillation	Antibiotics
	Chemotherapy
	Calculi dissolution
Special procedures	Basket extractions
	Biopsy brushings
	Visualization (nephroscope)
	Diagnostic studies

(Data from Snopek AM: Nonvascular interventional procedures. *In* Fundamentals of Special Radiographic Procedures. 3rd ed. Snopek AM (ed). Philadelphia, WB Saunders, 1992, pp 351–368.)

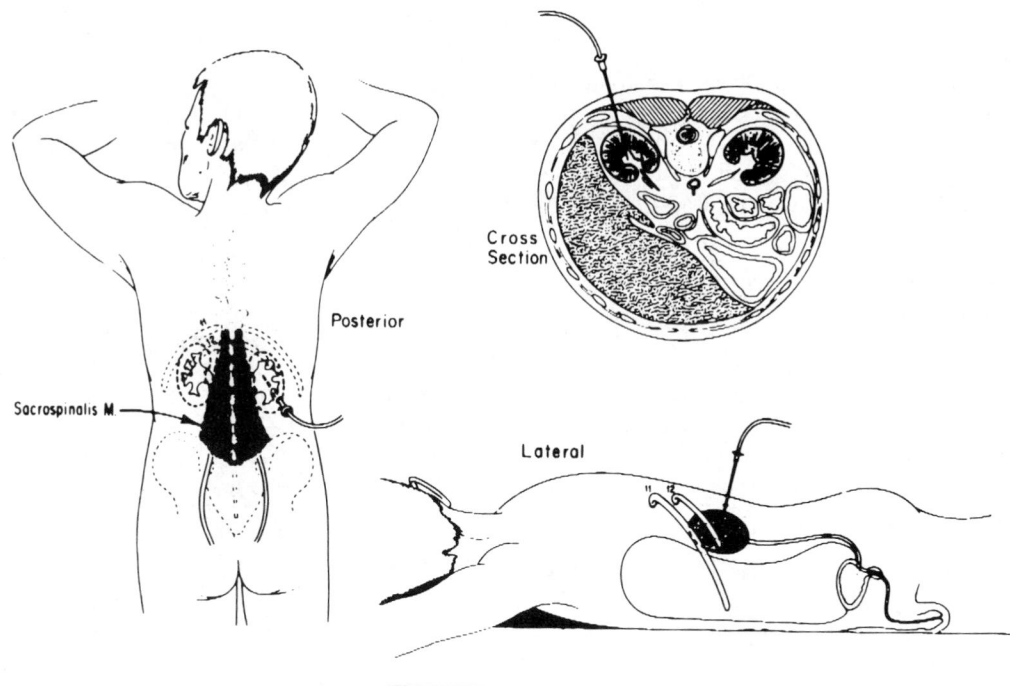

FIGURE 54–4. The technique of percutaneous nephrostomy. (From Newhouse JH, Pfister RC: Antegrade pyelography. *In* Interventional Radiology. Athanasoulis CA, Pfister RC, Greene RE, Roberson GH (eds). Philadelphia, WB Saunders, 1982, p. 438.)

sometimes undergo temporizing procedures because they may not survive a more invasive surgical procedure. Acute renal failure is often present. Patients with spinal cord disease and bladder dysfunction are predisposed to the development of renal calculi that can be removed percutaneously. Autonomic hyperreflexia has been reported to occur during this procedure.[30]

The procedure commonly is carried out in the prone position (Fig. 54–4). The kidney is localized with fluoroscopy, ultrasonography, or CT scan. The skin is anesthetized with local anesthetic, a 22-gauge spinal needle is inserted, and the kidney is punctured. An anterograde pyelogram is obtained with contrast.

Once this aspect is accomplished, a skin nick 2 cm deep is made just lateral to the insertion of the spinal needle. A trocar

is inserted and advanced into the kidney. An 8 to 12 French Silastic catheter is placed inside the trocar, and the trocar is removed. The final intervention may be nephroscopy; removal of renal calculi from the pelvis, calyx, or ureter; or progressive ureteral dilation.[31] Nephroscopy and irrigation of the urinary system can require the use of copious amounts of fluid. The catheter is left in place for drainage after the procedure. Ureteral dilation cannot be completed in a single session. These patients often have larger cannulas inserted at 1- to 2-week intervals (Fig. 54–5).

Risks

Pain at the insertion site and from expansion of the urinary system with irrigation is common. Blood loss, when it occurs,

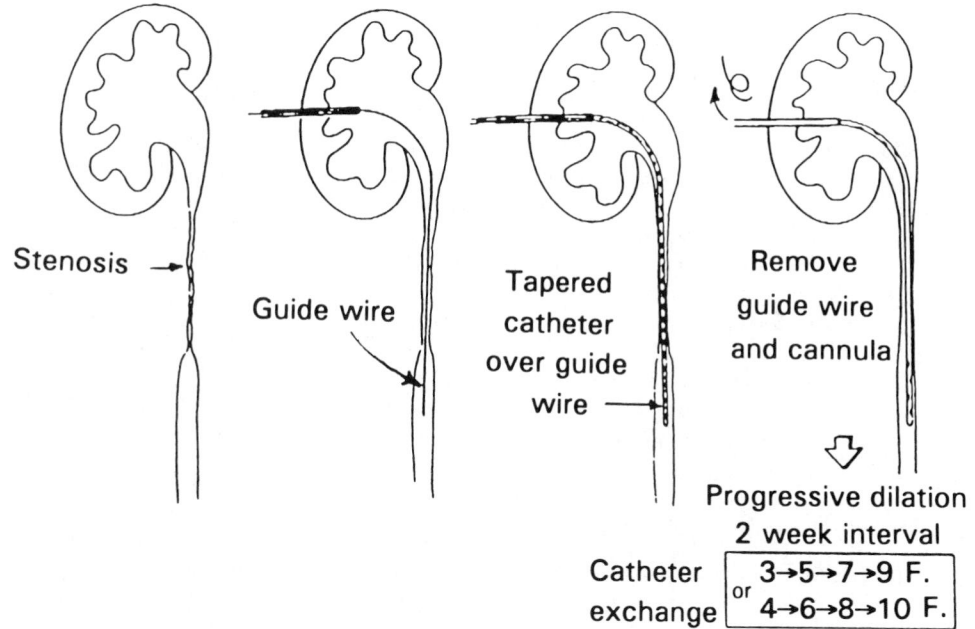

FIGURE 54–5. The technique of progressive ureteral dilation. (From Pfister RC, Newhouse JH: Percutaneous nephrostomy: Types of catheters for drainage, occlusion, dilatation and fiberoptics for endoscopy. *In* Interventional Radiology. Athanasoulis CA, Pfister RC, Greene RE, Roberson GH (eds). Philadelphia, WB Saunders, 1982, p 483.)

is often concealed and may be manifested only by hypotension and tachycardia. Pneumothorax has been documented. Large amounts of irrigation fluid can lead to fluid overload, hyponatremia, and hypothermia. Because of the large volumes of fluid used, it is worthwhile to use warmed fluids. The same signs and symptoms as for the transurethral resection of the prostate (TURP) syndrome can be witnessed and should be anticipated.

What Anesthetic Techniques Are Appropriate?

Patients must be immobile, especially during trocar insertion and manipulation. Intravascular dehydration should be avoided to minimize the renal toxic effects of the contrast medium. Intravenous sedation and local infiltration at the site of needle insertion are usually adequate. However, the pain from dilation of the tract may not be blunted by sedation. If deep sedation is contraindicated because of potential airway risk problems or other reasons, general anesthesia or a regional technique is required.

Regional

For a regional technique to be successful, the kidney's afferent nerve supply must be blocked. A T-10 sensory block should be sufficient. Bladder afferents arise from S-2 to S-4; if bladder manipulation is performed, these nerves should be blocked as well. Spinal and epidural anesthesia provide excellent conditions for this procedure. Hypobaric spinal anesthesia has been reported to be effective because patients are in the prone position.[32] Another method suggested when the epidural or subarachnoid approach is contraindicated is an L-1 paravertebral block combined with a lumbar sympathetic block.[33]

General

Any general anesthetic technique appropriate for patients with renal dysfunction can be used. Because of the possibility of hyponatremia with prolonged irrigation, sodium levels should be monitored if a hyponatremic irrigating solution is used. If signs of the TURP syndrome occur, the procedure should be terminated quickly and treatment effected immediately.

What Are Transhepatic Procedures?

These interventions can be nonsurgical or may require a minilaparotomy. The most common indication is for access to the gallbladder for stone removal, drainage, or decompression. They are often used in seriously ill patients. Common diagnoses include cholelithiasis, obstructive jaundice, sclerosing cholangitis, biliary cirrhosis, and a calculous cholecystitis. Operative mortality for open cholecystectomy is 0.5% to 1.8%. Patients older than 65 years account for 70% of all gallbladder mortality. Emergent cholecystectomy has a 13% mortality. Patients at high risk are those with empyema of the gallbladder, liver disease, and recent myocardial infarction, as well as the elderly.[34] Success rates vary from 40% to 90%.

Percutaneous Cholecystotomy

Under fluoroscopic or ultrasonographic guidance, the gallbladder is visualized. Transhepatic or transperitoneal ap-

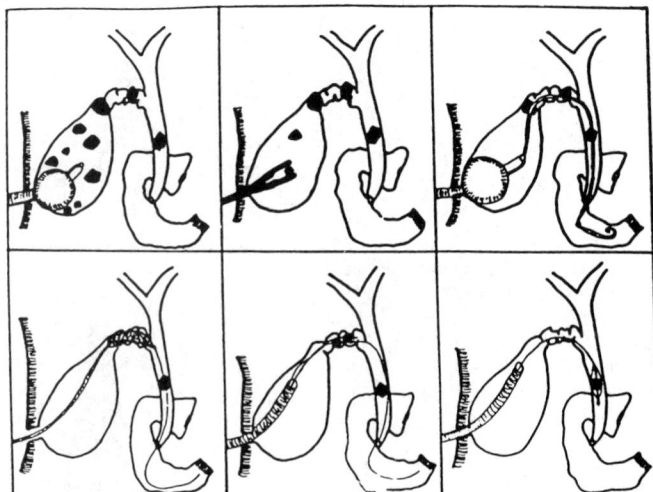

FIGURE 54–6. Basket extraction of gallbladder and common duct calculi through a transhepatic percutaneous cholecystotomy. (Adapted from Sacks BA, Vine HS: Postoperative instrumentation of the biliary tree. *In* Interventional Radiology. Athanasoulis CA, Pfister RC, Greene RE, Roberson GH (eds). Philadelphia, WB Saunders, 1982, p 526.)

proaches have been described. A 22-gauge spinal needle is inserted through the skin after local infiltration. The needle is advanced into the gallbladder, or a 6 French catheter is inserted into the biliary system. Dilation of the tract to a 14 French diameter can be done if necessary. Contrast is injected when the catheter is in the gallbladder. A basket extraction of gallbladder stones and common duct stones can be performed (Fig. 54–6). If calculus dissolution is required, it can be achieved with methyl-tert-butyl ether (MTBE). Monooctanoin, which acts on cholesterol, can also be infused but requires 10 days for successful therapy of cholesterol stones.[34]

Another technique involves the rigid nephroscope. The surgeon and radiologist work together using this approach. A needle is inserted into the gallbladder after ultrasonographic visualization. A wire is placed through the needle, and the needle removed. Catheters are advanced over the wire until it is dilated up to 28 French. A rigid nephroscope is introduced, and stones are removed with forceps. Success rates are quoted as 75%.

Complications

Complications include nausea and vomiting, vasovagal reactions, abdominal pain due to bile spillage into the peritoneal cavity, sepsis, endotoxemia, wound infection, and colon or duodenal puncture. Liver puncture may cause hemorrhage, arteriovenous fistula formation, or pleural contamination. Damage to arteries or veins may produce an aneurysm, tear, or significant bleeding. Hemorrhage in many cases is not visible. MTBE is flammable and has a strong smell. It can causes sedation if it is absorbed into the peritoneum or intestines and may potentiate the effects of sedatives or general anesthetics.[34]

Minicholecystectomy

This combined surgical and interventional technique is used when a strong, wide tract is necessary for calculus extraction. The surgeon makes a small incision over the gallbladder after ultrasonographic visualization. A 24 French Foley catheter is inserted into the gallbladder for drainage. Typically, the tract is allowed to become established for 5 to 7 days before stone manipulation. If a transperitoneal approach is used, the tract requires 5 weeks to mature before manipulation. The operative mortality approaches zero for these procedures.[34]

Anesthetic Techniques

Although stoic individuals may be able to tolerate this procedure with local infiltration and sedation, such an approach is not recommended. It is quite painful even if local anesthetic is placed in the biliary tree for analgesia. In most cases, pain limits the procedure to one or two attempts, after which it must be rescheduled. Regional anesthesia is effective if the liver and gallbladder afferents are blocked. This technique can require a somatic block up to T-6. In patients with pulmonary disease, the loss of accessory muscle use may preclude this approach. Patients who cannot tolerate a decline in SVR are better served by a general anesthetic. The anterior approach (i.e., transabdominal) to the celiac plexus, although not familiar to most anesthesiologists, provides excellent pain relief.[35] Any general anesthetic technique that takes into account a patient's hepatic dysfunction should prove acceptable.

COMPUTED TOMOGRAPHY SCANS

CT scans are now so prevalent that they warrant a separate discussion from other diagnostic radiologic interventions. The first working model was operational in 1971. Since then, new generations have improved detection systems that have decreased scan time from 5 minutes to 2 to 10 seconds per slice. CT scanners are ubiquitous because of the detailed images they produce of any part of the body, their precise demonstration of abnormalities, most patients' lack of discomfort, and the ease of performance.[36] Dynamic CT scanning is becoming more common. With scan times of as little as 50 microseconds, 17 scans per second can be done. This capability allows analysis of cardiac motion, airway studies, and aortic dissections and minimizes movement artifact.

How Does a CT Scanner Work?

Inside the gantry is an x-ray tube, collectors and equipment for movement control, and a hole for the patient. Movement of the patient table can be controlled manually or by the computer to make a "scout" film and imaging slices. The detectors use gas ionization or scintillation. Radiation not absorbed by the body (remnant radiation) hits the collector and is converted to an electric current (Fig. 54–7). The amount of radiation collected correlates with the current generated. The current is then amplified and sent to the computer for processing.[36]

Three methods are used for image reconstruction: back projection, iterative reconstruction, and analytic reconstruction. Analytic methods are preferred because they use two-dimensional Fourier reconstruction, which is very accurate and quicker than the other methods. "Reference" detectors are

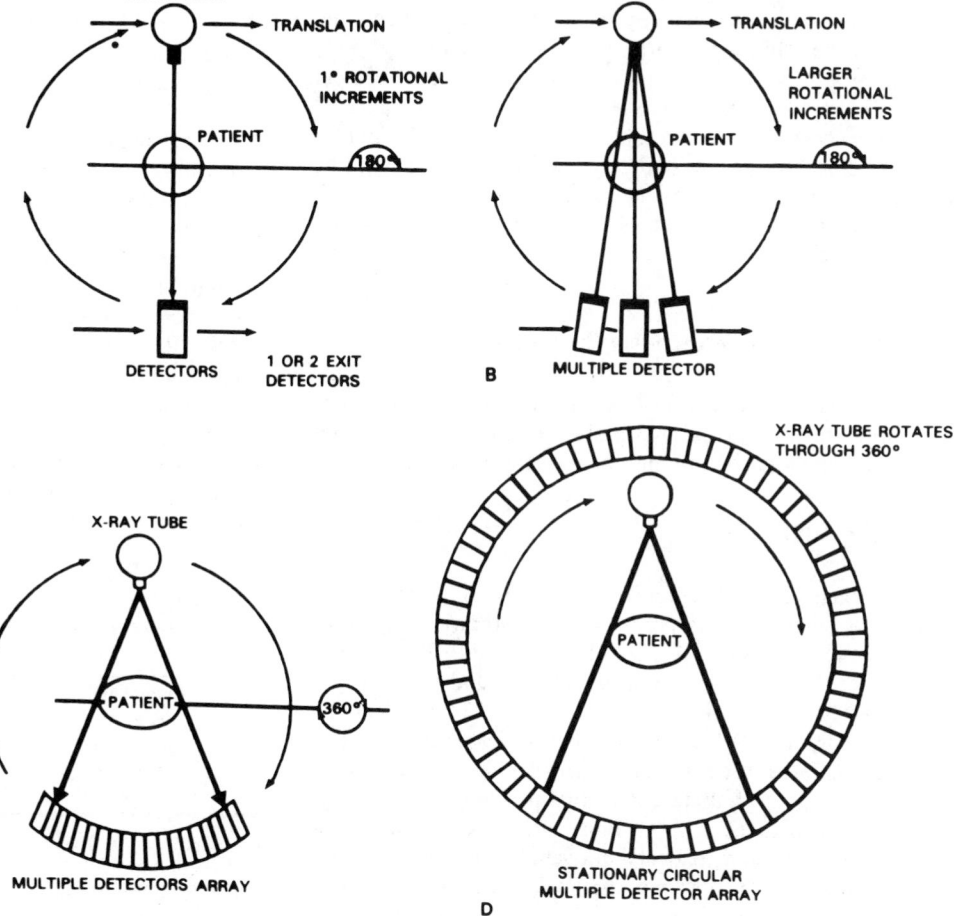

FIGURE 54–7. A, Rectilinear pencil-beam scanning typical of first-generation CT scanners. B, Rectilinear multiple pencil-beam scanning used in second-generation CT scanners. C, Continuously rotating pulsed fan-beam scanning typical of third-generation CT scanners. D, Fourth-generation CT scanning scheme. (From Seeram E: Computed Tomography Technology. Philadelphia, WB Saunders, 1982, pp 46–49.)

TABLE 54–11. Types of Sedation Used for CT Scanning*

Sedation	Young Infant	Older Infant	Toddler	Young Child	Older Child
None	60	31	20	38	75
Light	33	56	61	48	20
Deep	6	12	16	12	4
General anesthetic with	0	0	1	1	0
endotrocheal intubation	1	1	2	1	1

(Adapted from Keeter S, Bernator RM, Weinberg SM, et al: Sedation in pediatric CT: national survey of current practice. Radiology 1990; 175:745.)
*All numbers are percentages.

used to compare remnant radiation with the x-ray tube intensity so that relative values can be identified after digitalization. Tissue attenuation values are related to those of water and are arranged on a scale (EMI or Hounsfield). These numbers are actually indicators of brightness or a gray scale. The gray scale or contrast can be adjusted to show the relative differences between tissues. This procedure is called *windowing* or *setting a window.* This relative scale for tissue is as follows[36]:

Bone → congealed blood → gray matter →
white matter → blood → water → fat → air

How Are CT Scans Performed?

Head CT scans are one of the most requested procedures. They can be performed with and without intravenous contrast agents. Patients may have a wide range of actual or suspected CNS pathology. Considerations must be given to anticonvulsant medications, increases in ICP from placing the patient in a supine position, and changes in mental status. Patients are placed on the table with the head inside the gantry, severely restricting access to the airway. Scan time for each 1-cm cut or slice is approximately 60 to 90 seconds. Approximately 22 scans are necessary for a complete study. Up to 45 minutes may be needed to finish a study, especially if scans need to be repeated because of movement artifact. Because of the high level of radiation, the anesthesia provider does not usually remain in the room.

How Is Sedation/Anesthesia Provided?

The typical CT room size is 300 square feet, a size that does not allow much room for anesthesia equipment. The location of monitors and machinery must be thought out in advance.

Premedication

A national survey categorized the types of sedation and general anesthesia usually performed in children to help complete CT scans (Table 54–11).[37] In this study, 9% of light sedation cases progressed to deep sedation, and in some patients airway compromise was evident.[37] Oral premedications used for CT and MRI scans are listed in Table 54–12. The most common one used by radiologists is chloral hydrate in a dose of 80 mg · kg^{-1}, up to 2 g maximum. Onset time is long, averaging 55 minutes. A 15% failure rate includes many failures due to excessive patients' movement during the scan. Rectal thiopental, 25 to 45 mg · kg^{-1}, has been used to avoid

the pain associated with intramuscular (IM) injections. This technique is successful in 86% of children. Side effects included hyperactivity, vomiting, and fecal incontinence.

Intramuscular Regimens

In children unwilling to take oral medications, or if oral premedication is unsuccessful, IM regimens can be used (Table 54–13). Methohexital sedation, 10 mg · kg^{-1} IM, was evaluated in children up to 5 years old.[6] The injections were made with a 5% solution. Peak effect was noted in 3 minutes, and patients were alert enough to be discharged in 86 minutes. This technique was successful in 92% of children. No cardiovascular, respiratory, or CNS complications were noted. Disadvantages included the need for additional dosing in 6% of patients and pain during injection. In patients taking anticonvulsant medications, no difference in arousal times was noted. Previous studies revealed increased metabolism of barbiturates with a shorter duration of action. This observation was not confirmed.[40]

Another IM regimen is referred to as *DPT.* This "cocktail" includes Demerol (meperidine, 2 mg · kg^{-1}), Phenergan (promethazine, 1 mg · kg^{-1}), and Thorazine (chlorpromazine, 1 mg · kg^{-1}).[39] It is successful in 86% of patients but is associated with a 16% incidence of agitation, disorientation, and respiratory depression.[7] In another study, DPT produced sedation in 70% of patients for >7 hours.[8] A combination of atropine, meperidine, promethazine, and secobarbital (AMPS) is advocated by some investigators. It must be given in two syringes and takes 53 minutes to reach peak effect. Disadvantages include a 12% failure rate; 10% of patients required additional sedation to complete the study.[38]

If an intravenous catheter is necessary for contrast media injection or because of anesthetic concerns, intravenous medications can be used for sedation (Table 54–14). These regimens have a higher success rate and fewer complications. Bypassing the absorptive phase by direct intravenous administration allows much easier titration to the desired drug effect.

TABLE 54–12. Oral Premedication Regimens for CT/MRI

Medication	Dose
Chloral hydrate	75–100 mg · kg^{-1}
Diazepam	0.1–0.3 mg · kg^{-1}
Lorazepam	0.05 mg · kg^{-1}
Midazolam	0.25–0.8 mg · kg^{-1}
Pentobarbital	4 mg · kg^{-1}

(Data from Brann CA, Janik DJ: Anesthesia in the radiology suite. Probl Anesth 1992; 6:413, *and* Nahata MC: Sedation in pediatric patients undergoing diagnostic procedures. Drug Intell Clin Pharm 1988; 22:711.)

TABLE 54–13. Intramuscular Medications for CT/MRI

Medication*	Dose
Meperidine	$2 \text{ mg} \cdot \text{kg}^{-1}$
Promethazine	$1 \text{ mg} \cdot \text{kg}^{-1}$
Chlorpromazine	$1 \text{ mg} \cdot \text{kg}^{-1}$
Atropine	$0.016 \text{ mg} \cdot \text{kg}^{-1}$
Meperidine	$1 \text{ mg} \cdot \text{kg}^{-1}$
Promethazine	$1 \text{ mg} \cdot \text{kg}^{-1}$
Secobarbital	$4 \text{ mg} \cdot \text{kg}^{-1}$
Ketamine	$3–15 \text{ mg} \cdot \text{kg}^{-1}$
With or without atropine	$0.02 \text{ mg} \cdot \text{kg}^{-1}$
With or without glycopyrrolate	$0.01 \text{ mg} \cdot \text{kg}^{-1}$
Meperidine	$50 \text{ mg} \cdot \text{m}^{-2}$
Pentobarbital	$90 \text{ mg} \cdot \text{m}^{-2}$
Midazolam	$0.025–0.08 \text{ mg} \cdot \text{kg}^{-1}$
Methohexital	$5–10 \text{ mg} \cdot \text{kg}^{-1}$
Morphine sulfate	$0.1–0.3 \text{ mg} \cdot \text{kg}^{-1}$
Pentobarbital	$4–6 \text{ mg} \cdot \text{kg}^{-1}$

(Adapted from Brann CA, Janik DJ: Anesthesia in the radiology suite. Probl Anesth 1992; 6:413, *and* Nahata MC: Sedation in pediatric patients undergoing diagnostic procedures. Drug Intell Clin Pharm 1988; 22:711.)
*Medications grouped together are given together.

One very effective approach in children is to premedicate with $0.5 \text{ mg} \cdot \text{kg}^{-1}$ midazolam orally followed by intravenous catheter placement and then a propofol infusion titrated to effect.

What Are the Complications?

The complications reported with all sedation techniques include respiratory depression, respiratory arrest, bradycardia, activation of seizure disorder, excessive vomiting, urinary retention, and prolonged sedation. This list underscores the fact that no ideal sedative agent exists.[41, 42] Many patients have developed life-threatening difficulties with the "appropriate" dosage of medications, and others are not sedated enough to cooperate.[2] Each sedation regimen must be tailored to the patient and the type and length of study contemplated. Appropriate monitoring is mandatory and has been discussed previously.

MAGNETIC RESONANCE IMAGING

More than 2500 MRI scanners are present in the United States. Soft tissue MRI images reveal more detail than do CT scans. Some pediatric indications for MRI scanning are pre-

TABLE 54–14. Intravenous Sedation Techniques for CT/MRI

Medication		Dosage
Diazepam	Bolus	$0.07–0.09 \text{ mg} \cdot \text{kg}^{-1}$
Meperidine	Bolus	$1.5–2.0 \text{ mg} \cdot \text{kg}^{-1}$
Pentobarbital	Bolus	$1–6 \text{ mg} \cdot \text{kg}^{-1}$
Propofol	Bolus	$0.5–2.0 \text{ mg} \cdot \text{kg}^{-1}$
	Infusion	$1–9 \text{ mg} \cdot \text{kg}^{-1} \cdot \text{h}^{-1}$
Midazolam	Bolus	$0.05–0.35 \text{ mg} \cdot \text{kg}^{-1}$
	Infusion	$0.01–0.15 \text{ mg} \cdot \text{kg}^{-1} \cdot \text{h}^{-1}$
Ketamine	Bolus	$1–4 \text{ mg} \cdot \text{kg}^{-1}$
	Infusion	$2–4 \text{ mg} \cdot \text{kg}^{-1} \cdot \text{h}^{-1}$
Methohexital	Bolus	$0.5–2 \text{ mg} \cdot \text{kg}^{-1}$
	Infusion	$1–6 \text{ mg} \cdot \text{kg}^{-1} \cdot \text{h}^{-1}$
Thiopental	Bolus	$1–6 \text{ mg} \cdot \text{kg}^{-1}$
	Infusion	$2–9 \text{ mg} \cdot \text{kg}^{-1} \cdot \text{h}^{-1}$

(Adapted from Brann CA, Janik DJ: Anesthesia in the radiology suite. Probl Anesth 1992; 6:413, *and* Nahata MC: Sedation in pediatric patients undergoing diagnostic procedures. Drug Intell Clin Pharm 1988; 22:711.)

TABLE 54–15. Pediatric Indications for MRI

Brain	Aneurysm
	Arteriovenous malformation
	Blunt head trauma
	Cerebral atrophy
	Demyelinating lesion
	Tumor
Spinal cord	Meningocele
	Meningomyelocele
	Syringomyelia
	Tethered cord syndrome
	Intervertebral disk space infection
Congenital heart disease	Aortic aneurysm/dissection
	Coarctation
	Hypertrophic cardiomyopathy
	Pericardial disease
	Septal defects
	Systemic pulmonary shunts
	Vascular rings
	Ventricular function
Pulmonary disease	Bronchus
	Diaphragm
	Mediastinum
	Pleura
	Trachea
Orthopedic	Bone cysts
	Knee (post-traumatic, juvenile rheumatoid arthritis)
	Hip (Legg-Perthes disease, avascular necrosis)
	Neurofibromatosis
	Rhabdoid sarcoma
	Solitary neoplasms

(Data from Oh KS, Newman B, Bender TM, Bowen A: Pulmonary pseudofibrosis and pseudomass lesions. Radiol Clin North Am 1988; 26:365–375.)

sented in Table 54–15. The unique environment of the MRI scanner and the anesthetic implications are important to understand.

How Does an MRI Scanner Produce an Image?

MRI was initially designated *nuclear magnetic resonance,* but the *nuclear* was taken out after the Three Mile Island incident. Atomic nuclei contain a charge because of protons and possess mass because of protons and neutrons. The nuclei of some atoms spin. This spin creates a magnetic field because of proton and neutron gyrations. The nuclei act similarly to a bar magnet; when placed in a static magnetic field, they align along the longitudinal axis of the field.[43] Approximately half of the nuclei are parallel, and half are antiparallel. Some nuclei (1 or 2 out of 10^6) are not matched with a parallel or antiparallel partner. This minute fraction of nuclei accounts for all the magnetic resonance activity[43] (Fig. 54–8).

Nuclei spin on their own axes but also rotate around the strong magnetic axis of the scanner; this movement is called *precession* (Fig. 54–9). Precession creates a resonant frequency that can identify the specific type of nuclei spinning in that particular magnetic field. Addition of another strong magnetic field that oscillates at right angles to the first field produces a current. This current is also characteristic of specific nuclei. When the perpendicular second field is turned off, the current decays. The curve of this decay is known as the spin-spin relaxation time constant, or T_2. The spin-lattice relaxation time constant, or T_1, is produced by the rapidity of nuclei

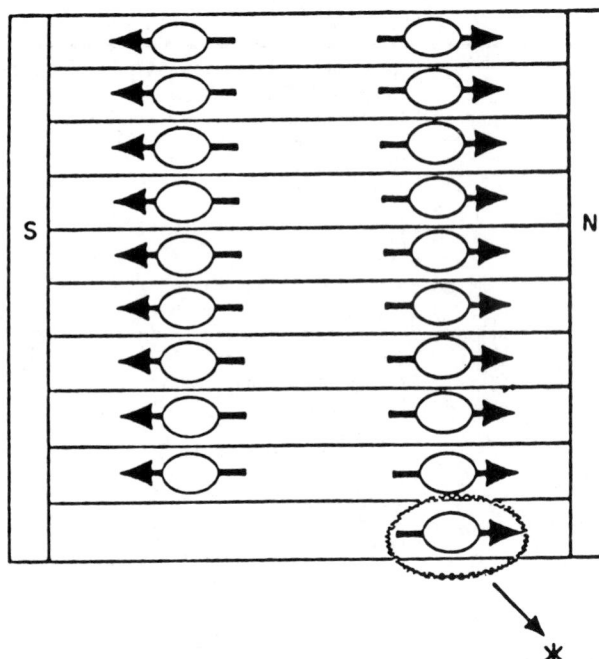

FIGURE 54–8. Diagrammatic representation of NMR-sensitive nuclei aligned in a magnetic field. Nuclei are either aligned parallel or antiparallel to the field. A small excess of nuclei are parallel to the field (*) and are responsible for the NMR phenomenon. (From Menon DK, Peden CJ, Hall AS, et al: Magnetic resonance for the anaesthetist: Part 1: physical principles, applications, safety aspects. Anaesthesia 1992; 47:240.)

response to a repetitive, right-angle, varying magnetic field. The unique properties of particular nuclei are used to produce the images seen with MRI.

Large amounts of carbon (C) are present in the body, but ^{12}C is not MR sensitive and ^{13}C is not abundant enough to produce an image. The most abundant and sensitive nuclei in the body are hydrogen (in water). They are used for the signals in MRI. Hence, the intensity and resolution of the MRI signal are dependent on the density of water in the region.

T_1- and T_2-weighted scans can be performed in any plane (sagittal, transverse, coronal, or oblique). The usual data collection time per scan is 1 to 3 minutes. Newer technology will permit collection in milliseconds, allowing dynamic scanning of the heart and lungs. The shorter times, as with CT scanning, will reduce artifact from voluntary movement, as well as breathing or peristalsis.

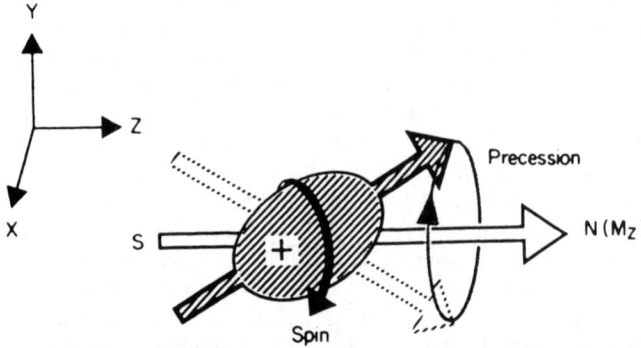

FIGURE 54–9. Movement of NMR-sensitive nucleus in a magnetic field. The nucleus spins on its own axis and precesses about the magnetic axis. (From Menon DK, Peden CJ, Hall AS, et al: Magnetic resonance for the anaesthetist: Part 1: physical principles, applications, safety aspects. Anaesthesia 1992; 47:240.)

Physical Characteristics

The field strengths of MRI magnets range from 0.05 to 2.0 tesla (T).[43] One tesla equals 10,000 gauss (G). The earth's magnetic field is measured at 0.5 to 1.0 G. The stronger the magnetic field, the higher the resolution of the MRI. Magnets of >0.5 T use superconducting coils cooled with liquid helium and nitrogen and present special risks. The patient opening is 2 m in length and, unlike CT scanners, is only 50 to 65 cm in diameter. For increased resolution, the head can be placed into a smaller coil, which further limits access to the airway, especially in children. Obese patients may not fit comfortably in the scanner.

Operational Problems

High-frequency electromagnetic radiation (FM radio waves) disrupts the low-intensity MR signals. A Faraday's cage (radio frequency [RF] shield) protects the information to be recorded.[43] Any wire or cable leaving the cage acts as an antenna and defeats the shield's purpose. Special copper-lined RF ports are available to allow nonconducting material such as anesthetic circuit tubing to exit without affecting the field.

Monitors that pass information out of the room must have electronically filtered wires or use optical or radio links with frequencies that do not disrupt the MRI.[43] Some equipment items deliver inaccurate information when electronic filters are placed on their cables. The power supply to anesthesia equipment also produces interference; an isolated transformer or battery-operated equipment should be acquired.

What Are the Risks of the Magnetic Field?

These risks include concerns about ferromagnetic items, heat production, hearing loss, psychologic changes, biologic effects, the use of contrast agents, and the properties of the superconducting magnets used to generate the fields (Table 54–16).[44]

Ferromagnetic Materials

The anesthesia team should not accept care for a patient unless they know that it is safe to place the patient in the magnetic field. Checklists have been established to identify high-risk patients (Table 54–17).

TABLE 54–16. MRI Risks

Effects on ferromagnetic material
External
Internal
Foreign bodies
Implanted material
Heat production
Effects on hearing
Psychologic effects
Biologic effects
Contrast agents
Quenching of superconducting magnets

(Adapted from Kanal E, Shellock FG, Talagala L: Safety considerations in the MR. Imaging Radiology 1990; 176:593.)

TABLE 54–17. Patient Questionnaire: Ferromagnetic Objects

Cerebral aneurysm or other hemostatic clip*
Cochlear implants*
Known metal fragments in head/eyes, postoperative/post-trauma
Has the patient ever been a machinist, welder, metal worker?
Colored contact lenses*
Ocular prosthesis (false eyes)*
Dentures or removable bridgework
Heart pacemaker
Prosthetic heart valves (Starr-Edwards pre 6000)*
Implantable automatic cardiac defibrillators
Shrapnel
Orthopedic implants (pins, plates, wires)*
Neurostimulators (chronic pain, spasticity)*
Implantable pumps*
Penile implants*
Contraceptive devices (diaphragm, intrauterine device)*
Interventional radiology devices (coils, filters, stents)*

(Adapted from Menon DK, Peden CJ, Hall AS, et al: Magnetic resonance for the anesthetist. Part I: physical principles, applications, safety aspects. Anaesthesia 1992; 47:240.)
*Indicates possible material that may be safe to allow in MRI scanning room.

Rotation (torque) or translation (attractive forces) is applied to ferromagnetic compounds around the MRI magnetic field. Torque occurs because ferromagnetic objects align their long axes parallel to the direction of the field.[43] Attraction to the magnet does not occur with shifting fields, only with static ones. The amount of attraction or translation of an object is associated with the field strength and gradient, the distance from the center of the magnet, and the shape of the object. To determine whether a material is ferromagnetic, attach a string to it and place it near a strong hand-held magnet to see if deflection occurs.

External

External ferromagnetic materials can exhibit a projectile or missile effect. Kinetic energy is produced from the attraction to the magnet, which can cause damage to personnel or equipment.[44] Table 54–18 lists objects that can become projectiles.

Internal

Internal ferromagnetic materials also are affected by the magnetic field, so torque and translation can occur. Even stainless steel may be ferromagnetic. Other implanted metals may not be ferromagnetic and should not undergo movement; this

TABLE 54–18. Possible Projectiles in the MRI Scanner

Pulse oximeter
Stethoscope
Pager
"Sandbag"
Calculator
Intravenous pole
Chest tube stand
Pen, paper clip
Infusion pump
Laryngoscope (including plastic with ferromagnetic batteries)
Clipboard
Keys
Watch

(Adapted from Kanal E, Shellock FG, Talagala L: Safety considerations in MR imaging. Radiology 1990; 176:593.)

fact needs to be documented before the scan. Ferromagnetic intraocular foreign bodies have caused blindness and retinal damage; MRI is contraindicated.[45] In patients who have been shot, the location of bullets should be known (if they are ferromagnetic), and a CT scan performed instead of MRI.

Implanted material such as intracranial aneurysm clips and other surgical clips should be documented. Ferromagnetic clips that have been in situ for years are considered safe if scar tissue has surrounded them and movement is not possible. However, a patient at my institution developed an intracerebral bleed from movement of what was thought to be a nonferromagnetic aneurysm clip. Any clip in a vulnerable or strategic location should be thought of as a contraindication to MRI until its composition can be determined.

Cardiac Devices and Pacemakers

Prosthetic cardiac valves are probably safe because even the attraction forces of the strong magnet on the small mass of the valve are less than the dynamic forces generated in the heart.[46] Pulmonary artery catheter thermistors and pacemakers are absolute contraindications to all MRI (even low field strength). These patients should not get within the 5 to 20 G line of a magnetic field. Pacemakers use a reed relay switch to sense cardiac activity and can be inactivated by a strong magnetic field.[47] This maneuver is performed all the time in the OR with a donut magnet to convert the pacemaker to VOO status. Loss of sensing capability can predispose a patient to an R-on-T phenomenon.

The lithium battery used to power a pacemaker is ferromagnetic; attraction of the generator toward the magnet can occur. One controversial aspect of pacemaker function is whether the leads can generate current in a changing magnetic field and produce ventricular fibrillation. Two reports filed with the Food and Drug Administration deal with sudden death during MRI in patients with pacemakers.[48] After coronary artery bypass surgery, patients often have epicardial leads left in place; these may be of theoretic risk. However, low-field MRI has been performed on such individuals without difficulty.[43]

How Is Heat Generated During MRI?

Energy can be absorbed from proton resonance, but it is not of clinical importance. The RF-induced currents produced by the MRI magnetic fields can induce tissue heat. Induced currents from RF and magnetic field gradient switching differ. RF currents but not switched gradients generate thermal energy. The basal metabolic rate of adults is 1 to 2 $W \cdot kg^{-1}$. The MRI scanner can produce 0.4 to 2 $W \cdot kg^{-1}$.

Tissue Damage

Skin surfaces experience the most dramatic heating; none occurs at the core. Adult structures are not at major risk for thermal injury except for the eyes and testes. A long scan duration may place children at risk for deep organ thermal injury, based on a study of anesthetized dogs.[49] Spermatogenesis may be impaired if testicular temperature is increased. In one study, scrotal temperature was elevated by 2 °C.[50] Cataracts have been induced in animals by RF fields. Corneal temperatures when measured are not more than 2 °C above normal.[51] Ocular thermal damage is unlikely to occur.

Burns

Focal heating effects have been documented. All types of thermal burns have been reported after MRI scans. Burns can be caused by loops of cables in which current is generated by the magnetic field and heat is produced within the wires. A case report documented a third-degree burn on an adult's finger from a pulse oximeter probe.[52] No damage was noted on the cable or probe. The patient required skin debridement and a full-thickness skin graft. Metallic implants may absorb heat and produce burns, as can an external apparatus (e.g., halo, external fixator).[44] Recommendations to avoid burns are listed in Table 54–19.

What Are the Effects on Hearing?

Loud banging sounds heard during MRI are from the rapid changes in the magnetic current produced in the coils. Motion is induced, and the vibration causes the noise. Loudness is associated with the kind of examination, pulse sequence, amount of current, and slice thickness.[53] The sound level of the noise produced near the magnet is 65 to 95 dB. Children and adults can be frightened by noise, and anxiety is common. Patients undergoing general anesthesia have relaxation of the muscles holding the stapes, thus are more sensitive to loud noises and are at higher risk for hearing damage. Tinnitus and temporary or permanent hearing loss have been reported. One prospective study showed a temporary (15-min duration) mild (10 dB) hearing loss in 43% of patients undergoing MRI.[53]

A number of strategies have been used to decrease noise for patients and personnel in the MRI scanning room. Earplugs and headphones are the cheapest and easiest remedies. Phase cancellation using Fourier's analysis of noise wavelengths to generate an opposite sound wave can be effective.

What Are the Psychologic Effects of MRI?

Claustrophobia and panic attacks have been documented in 5% to 10% of patients. The causes of discomfort include the restrictive dimensions of the magnetic bore, which is only a few inches above the face. Examinations can be twice as long as similar CT scans. The loud noise is disconcerting, as is the vaultlike door when it is closed and bolted. One patient described the experience as similar to being slid into an open-ended coffin.[48] Psychologic effects are usually temporary, but permanent damage has been noted.

Patients' anxiety can be reduced and less intravenous sedation can be used if simple steps are followed.[54] Discuss the MRI environment (noise, lack of space) before the scan. Allow a parent, spouse, or friend in the examination room. Talk with the patient during the examination. The prone position appears to be well tolerated. Mirrors that allow the patient to see more of the area may be helpful. Blindfolding may be effective in some individuals. Permit patients to take their pain medications. Psychologic desensitization or hypnosis is effective in resistant cases.[55]

What Are the Biologic Effects?

Changes in living organisms caused by MRI are controversial. Some animal and human studies have shown adverse effects. Increases in chick embryo malformations; altered rat behavior, including changes in growth and activity; increased sensitivity to implanted tumor cells in mice; and reduced fentanyl requirements have been reported.[57] In human cell culture experiments, lymphocyte chromosomal changes, pancreatic cell insulin release abnormalities, and changes in sickle cell red blood cells have been observed.[57] Other studies have shown no changes in behavior, memory, or nerve function in rats or guinea pigs. No studies have documented an increase in cancer risk with static magnetic fields. Although controversial, pregnancy is not an absolute contraindication to MRI, which may be safer than ionizing radiation. Although the question of safety is not totally answered, static magnetic fields probably do not have adverse biologic effects.

What Contrast Agent Is Used?

The only contrast agent used in MRI is gadopentetate dimeglumine (gadolinium). Gadolinium increases signal density on T1-weighted images. It does not cross a normal blood-brain barrier; when it does cross, it identifies where the breakdown is located. This agent has a high safety margin. The median lethal dose in dogs is 10 mmol $\cdot$ kg^{-1} (100 times the usual dose of 0.1 mmol $\cdot$ kg^{-1}). As with ionic contrast media, gadolinium is highly hyperosmotic. Adverse reactions have been reported in 2.4% of patients (Table 54–20). Extravasation of >10 mL has not caused tissue damage.

What Are the Potential Hazards of Superconducting Magnets?

Cryogenic

Cryogen hazards, the risks of quenching, and the effects of shielding should be understood by personnel working with MRI scanners. Superconducting magnets use liquid helium for cooling down to −268.93 °C (4.22 °K). If the temperature should increase, helium turns to a gas, producing 760 mL for each milliliter of liquid. A pop-off valve allows gas to vent to the atmosphere, but it could possibly escape into the room. Helium is odorless, cold, and lighter than air. Although it should rise to the top of the room, asphyxiation and frostbite can occur. In fact, opening the door to evacuate the room may be difficult because of the increased pressure within.

TABLE 54–19. MRI Monitor Safety Recommendations

Cables that touch a patient should not have loops (to prevent conduction and burns).

Monitoring devices not working well should be removed from the MRI scanner.

Equipment should be checked before each anesthetic to make sure insulation is intact.

Monitoring devices should be used only by trained individuals.

Potential conductors should not touch a patient twice to decrease loop formation.

Monitors should be as far as possible from magnet (pulse oximeter on foot instead of ear for head MRI).

All unnecessary equipment and cables should be brought out of the scan room before the scan.

(From Shellock FG, Slimp GL: Severe burn of the finger caused by using a pulse oximeter during MR imaging. Am J Radiol 1989; 153:1105, *and* Kanal E, Shellock FG: Burns associated with clinical MR examinations. Radiology 1990; 176:585.)

TABLE 54–20. Adverse Reactions to Gadolinium Contrast

Local	Burning or cool sensation
	Erythema
	Swelling
	Pain
	Phlebitis
Systemic	Headache
	Nausea
	Vomiting
	Urticaria
	Serum iron elevation (transient)
	Serum bilirubin elevation (secondary to hemolysis)
	Severe hypertension
	Anaphylactoid reaction (1:100,000 incidence)
	Death (six reported by 1990)

(Adapted from Kanal E, Shellock FG, Talabala L: Safety considerations in MR imaging. Radiology 1990; 176:593.)

Liquid nitrogen (77.3 °K) is used as a buffer around the helium. If nitrogen enters the room, it settles to the floor. Pure nitrogen causes unconsciousness in seconds. Oxygen monitors with an audible alarm must be in the MRI room at an appropriate height.[44]

Induction of Electric Currents

Quenching is a loss of cryogen, which causes a quick shift in the magnetic field. Induction of electric currents with this unexpected rapid field change is possible, but no deleterious effects have been noted.

Magnetic Effects

Shielding is used to limit the influence of the strong magnetic fields. It causes the field to be highly concentrated and decreases the possibility of the field's affecting ferromagnetic material far from the magnet. In shielded systems, the G lines around the magnet are smaller, but a larger gradient is present between lines. Hence, the magnetic field can change by hundreds of gauss in just a few centimeters. Shielding can lead to a sense of false security in personnel working near the magnet. However, as can be seen, one step closer to the magnet may mean the difference between no apparent magnetic field and one that is dangerous.[44]

What Equipment Can Be Used Near the MRI Scanner?

General Considerations

Once large metallic objects are brought into the room, they cannot be moved because to do so changes the magnetic field density and affects scan images. Within the strong magnetic field, all components of machinery must be nonferromagnetic. Anesthesia machines that meet this requirement are available from a number of sources. Gas tanks must be aluminum. Battery-powered equipment is usually used. The batteries are ferromagnetic; thus, monitors must be secured so that they do not become projectiles.[56] Members of the anesthesia team must determine the distance of the 50-G line from the magnet. Outside the 50-G line, ferromagnetic items can be used.

Circuits/Ventilators

A nonmodified anesthesia machine can usually be located several meters away from the patient. One provider cannot monitor both the patient and the anesthesia machine, so additional help is required. Long tubing from the fresh gas source to the patient is necessary. The tubing should be meticulously checked for leaks, and all connections must be plastic or rubber. RAE endotracheal tubes may be needed if clearance around the mouth is compromised, as when the head coil is used. A loss of tidal volume from the compressibility of the gas in the longer length of tubing should be anticipated.

Solenoid positive end-expiratory pressure (PEEP) valves may fail if placed too close to the magnet. Pressure-limited ventilators should not be used in the MRI suite. The long tubing may cause changes in compliance and drastically affect the tidal volume delivered.[56] Be sure to watch chest excursion to minimize the possibility of hypoventilation. Long Bain's circuits can be used in children but produce 1.7 cm $H_2O \cdot L^{-1} \cdot s^{-1}$ of expiratory resistance for each 10 m of tubing.

Electrocardiogram

ECG alterations are seen in a static magnetic field. Peaked T wave abnormalities are common, but any part of the ECG may be affected, depending on lead placement. This change is related to the interaction between blood in the aortic arch and the magnet. No clinical significance of blood attraction to the magnet is known at fields <2 T.[58] The best way to get acceptable ECG signals is to put the leads in the center of the field, where the least amount of shifting occurs; keep limb leads in the same plane, one to the others; braid or twist leads to prevent them from forming a loop; and monitor V_5 and V_6. These leads have the least artifact owing to their location away from the transverse aorta.[58] Long monitor leads are also necessary and must be shielded.

Infusion Pumps

Infusion pumps cannot be placed too close to the magnet because their motors will be damaged and the pump will malfunction. However, most pumps work properly if kept 2 m away from a 1.5-T MRI scanner.[59] Dial-a-Flow devices are an effective alternative for delivering sedative medications (Fig. 54–10).

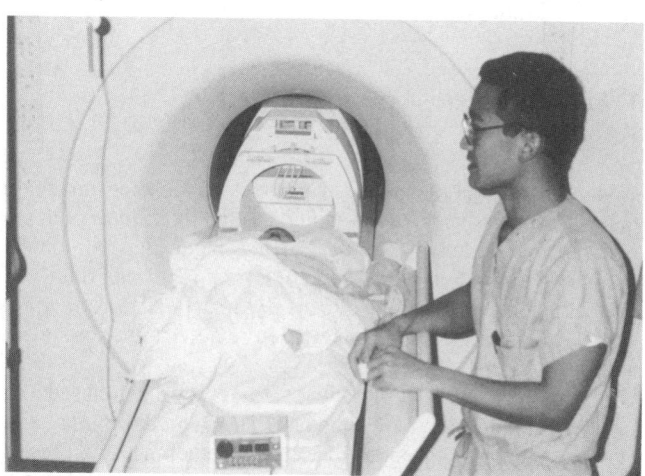

FIGURE 54–10. The anesthesiologist is monitoring the patient during an MRI scan. The pulse oximeter can be seen on the bed, and the Dial-a-Flow device can be seen delivering propofol for sedation. Supplemental oxygen is given by blow through the Styrofoam cup. (The cup was moved so that the patient's head could be visualized.)

Blood Pressure Monitors

Blood pressure can be measured with standard noninvasive methods. Automated cuffs can be used with long tubing but without metal connectors. Invasive pressure monitoring can also be used, but the pressure transducer cable must be passed through an RF filter. Tubing length should be as short as possible to reduce dampening. The MRI scanner produces RF in the kilohertz range and does not interfere with the transducer, which should have a natural frequency of <150 Hz.[60]

Pulse Oximeters/Capnometers

All manufacturers produce a pulse oximeter that can work in this environment (see Fig. 54–10). Capnography can be used if the machinery is kept far away from the magnet. Mainstream analysis cannot be used because of the ferromagnetic material in the analyzer. A sidestream device with a long sampling line placed 11 m from the patient works without difficulty but has a lag time of 10 seconds. Temperature monitoring has been carried out without difficulty.

Miscellaneous

Other equipment effects include erasure of magnetic tape media, including computer disks and credit cards. Color cathode ray tube screens are distorted by magnetic fields >1 to 2 G, but monochrome screens are resistant to fields <5 G. Liquid crystal displays appear not to undergo significant changes as a result of the magnetic field. Rechargeable batteries tend not to work well. These batteries often turn on and off with changes in magnetic field gradients.

For Whom Are MRI Scans Performed?

Some of the pediatric indications for MRI are presented in Table 54–15. Indications for adults are similar. One study has shown that MRI is more sensitive than CT in detecting cerebral parenchymal lesions in acute head injury.[61] MRI detected more cerebral abnormalities associated with traumatic loss of consciousness as well. More trauma victims may be presenting for MRI in the future.

What Anesthetic Techniques Are Appropriate?

Remember that plastic laryngoscopes contain ferromagnetic batteries (unless specially modified to contain lithium) and can become projectiles. The choice of anesthetic depends on the patient. Most adult patients do not require more than oral premedication if anxiety is effectively treated. Children require sedation. These techniques have been reviewed previously and summarized in Tables 54–12 to 54–14.

Seriously ill patients or patients not appropriate for sedation need general anesthesia. General anesthesia includes inhalation agents with the appropriate anesthesia machine and precautions. Total intravenous anesthesia has been used effectively in acutely ill patients.[62] Propofol, midazolam, and alfentanil have been recommended. An antisialagogue is often suggested to decrease secretions because of limited access to the airway. General anesthetics may influence MRI of the brain.[63]

RADIATION THERAPY

The most common pediatric tumors treated with radiation therapy are retinoblastoma, cerebrospinal malignancies, Wilms' tumor, and embryonic sarcomas. Many of these patients have cushingoid features due to corticosteroid use.

How Is Radiation Therapy Performed?

Anesthesia providers must remain outside of the room because of the high level of radiation emitted. Video monitoring of patients is necessary. The procedure usually lasts only 30 to 90 seconds, but patients must be completely immobile during this time. Patients often undergo daily treatment for 5 to 8 weeks. They may be supine, lateral, or prone. Treatment of retinoblastoma is performed with a lateral external beam (lens sparing), and the head is immobilized in a shell. The eye is kept immobilized by a contact lens attached to the linear accelerator. In this situation, access to the head is obviously quite restricted, and airway protection is required.[64]

What Are the Risks?

Multiple procedures are performed on these patients; they often fail to thrive during therapy because of sequential intubations, awakening after protracted anesthesia, a lack of appetite due to nausea and vomiting, or changes in sleeping and feeding cycles. Intravenous access is a concern during the weeks of therapy if one is to avoid multiple IM injection, and placement of a long-term catheter is advantageous. Maintaining an adequate airway without trauma is also crucial. The risks of radiation have been discussed.

What Anesthetic Techniques Are Applicable?

Inhalation

Inhalation agents offer an anesthetic that is rapid and well tolerated by both the patient and parents. The depth of anesthesia can be changed quickly, and recovery is usually fast and complete. Disadvantages include the difficulty of maintaining an adequate airway without an endotracheal tube.

One technique to overcome this problem is insufflation.[65] Anesthesia is induced with 70% nitrous oxide and 30% O_2 along with halothane or isoflurane. An oral airway is inserted, and a soft, single-orifice 8 to 10 French catheter is inserted into the posterior pharynx through a naris. The catheter is taped to the chest, and halothane 0.7% to 2.0% or isoflurane 0.5% to 1.5% is delivered using a fresh gas flow of 5 L · min^{-1}. After the procedure, patients are given 100% O_2 until awake. All patients reported were alert, discharged in 15 to 20 minutes after treatment, and continued to grow normally during therapy. However, one fourth of the patients had complications including hypoxemia, laryngospasm, and apnea during induction.

If the nasal catheter is misplaced, complications such as laryngospasm or coughing may occur. Esophageal placement may insufflate the stomach and precipitate pulmonary aspiration. This technique should not be used in patients with abnor-

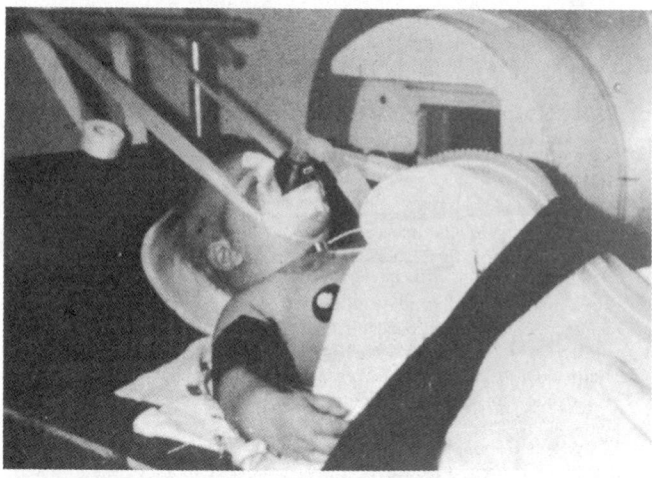

FIGURE 54–11. Airway maintained with the aid of a sling of tape suspended from the crossbar. (From Glauber DT, Audenaert SM: Anesthesia for children undergoing craniospinal radiotherapy. Anesthesiology 1987; 67:801.)

mal airways (Treacher Collins syndrome and others) or with a full stomach. Scavenging was not addressed in this study. Multiple exposures to halothane appear to be well tolerated by children.[66, 67] The small risk of posthalothane hepatitis leads many practitioners to recommend the use of isoflurane.

Airway Management

Airway frames have been used in the past to maintain the child in the correct position.[68, 69] The frame holds the chin forward and the head in the extended position during mask anesthesia or the use of a T-piece (Fig. 54–11).

The laryngeal mask airway has been used to prevent the complications of multiple intubations and positioning and is now available in this country. One report of 312 anesthetics in

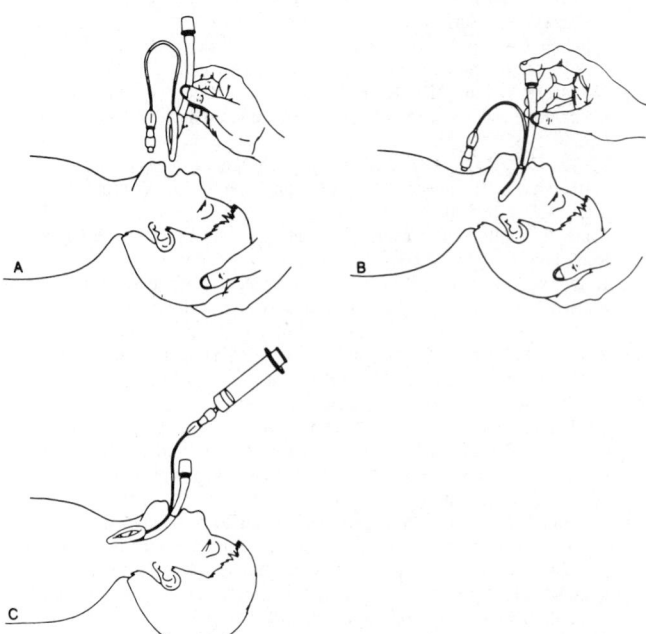

FIGURE 54–12. The technique of laryngeal mask insertion (steps A, B, and C). (From Grebenik CR, Ferguson C, White A: The laryngeal mask airway in pediatric radiotherapy. Anesthesiology 1990; 72:474.)

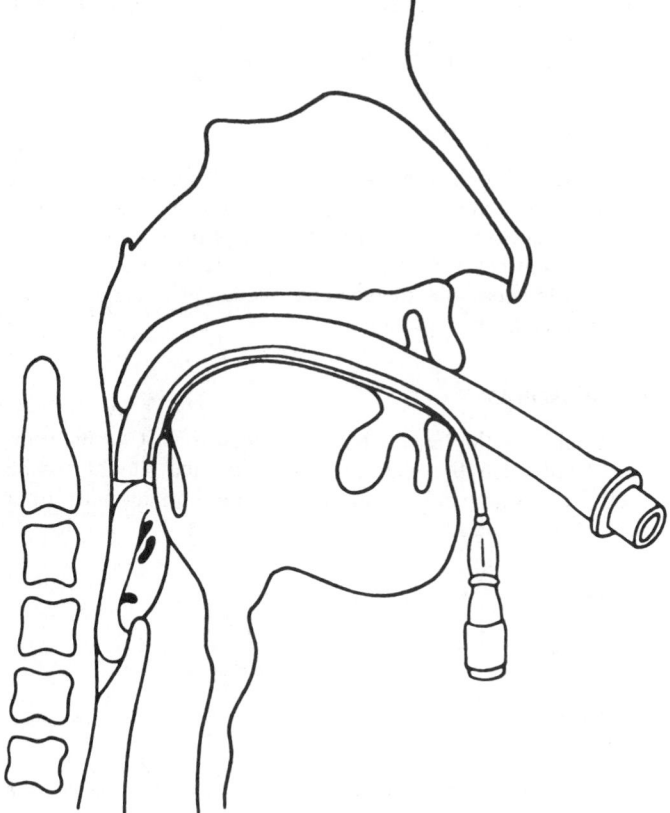

FIGURE 54–13. The correctly positioned laryngeal mask. (From Grebenik CR, Ferguson C, White A: The laryngeal mask airway in pediatric radiotherapy. Anesthesiology 1990; 72:474.)

25 children has been published.[70] Patients 3 weeks to 3 years old were included in the study, and most received more than 20 anesthetics. They were premedicated with atropine, 0.03 mg · kg^{-1} orally after a 4-hour fast. An inhalation induction was performed, and the laryngeal mask was inserted (Figs. 54–12 and 54–13). Monitoring consisted of a pulse oximeter and closed-circuit television. The patients recovered with supplemental O$_2$ and were then discharged home. The only complication noted was laryngospasm when the mask was inserted too soon in one patient. In only 7% of cases was more than one attempt needed to insert the mask. It was ineffective for ventilation of 8% of patients.

Intramuscular Ketamine

IM ketamine is quick and effective but may be associated with tachyphylaxis, nystagmus (which would be especially detrimental in the treatment of retinoblastoma), increased oral secretion, and dysphoria. A study of 28 children 6 months old to 3.5 years old used ketamine injection, 7 to 15 mg · kg^{-1}, with atropine.[71] The peak effect was evident in 1.5 to 4 minutes, and all patients had adequate sedation. Recovery time varied from 1 to 2.5 hours. One child exhibited tachyphylaxis when a maximum dose of 22.3 mg · kg^{-1} was required. Only 6% of patients required supplemental doses of medication. Seven per cent had purposeless movements that required stopping treatment for repositioning. Upper airway obstruction was noted in one patient. One child had a nightmare on one occasion. An equal number of patients gained weight, lost weight, or had no change in weight during therapy. No symptomatic tachycardia developed, and no patients had local irritation at injection sites. Ketamine use in patients with cerebral pathology and increased ICP is contraindicated.

Intravenous Agents

Intravenous inductions are smooth and simple but require a long-term central or peripherally inserted catheter. Thiopental has been used successfully for induction followed by an inhaled anesthetic. Complications include sepsis, air embolism, thromboembolic phenomena, dislodgment, catheter fracture, and catheter migration.

Rectal Agents

Rectal induction agents have also been used. Chronic thiopental administration can cause proctitis and should not be used. Midazolam and brevital may be appropriate, but further studies are required.

References

1. Edwards FM: Risks of medical imaging. *In* Textbook of Diagnostic Imaging. Putman CE, Ravin CE (eds). Philadelphia, WB Saunders, 1988, pp 91–110.
2. Fisher DM: Sedation of pediatric patients: an anesthesiologist's perspective. Radiology 1990; 175:613.
3. Committee on Drugs, Section on Anesthesiology: Guidelines for the elective use of conscious sedation, deep sedation and general anesthesia in pediatric patients. Pediatrics 1985; 76:317.
4. Cohen MD: Pediatric sedation. Radiology 1990; 175:611.
5. Thompson JR, Schneider S, Ashwal S, et al: The choice of sedation for computed tomography in children: a prospective evaluation. Radiology 1982; 143:475.
6. Grainger RG: Intravascular contrast media. *In* Diagnostic Radiology, an Anglo-American Textbook of Imaging. Grainger RG, Allison DJ (eds). New York, Churchill Livingstone, 1986, pp 99–110.
7. Lasser EC, Elizonda-Martel G, Granke RC: Potentiation of pentobarbital anesthesia by competitive protein binding. Anesthesiology 1965; 24:665.
8. Bettmann MA: Ionic versus nonionic contrast agents of intravenous use: are all the answers in? Radiology 1990; 175:616.
9. Katayama H, Yamaguchi K, Kozuka T, et al: Adverse reactions to ionic and nonionic contrast media. Radiology 1990; 175:621.
10. Goldberg M: Systemic reactions to intravascular contrast media. Anesthesiology 1984; 60:46.
11. Shehadi WH: Adverse reactions to intravascularly administered contrast media. A comprehensive study based on a prospective survey. AJR 1975; 124:145.
12. Ansell G, Tweedie MCK, West CR, et al: The current status of reactions to intravenous contrast media. Invest Radiol 1980; 15(Suppl):S32.
13. Rao VM, Rao AK, Steineer RM, et al: The effect of ionic and nonionic contrast media on the sickling phenomenon. Radiology 1982; 144:291.
14. Arroyave CM: An in vitro assay for radiographic contrast media idiosyncrasy. Invest Radiol 1980; 15(Suppl):S21.
15. Lasser EC, Berry CC: Nonionic vs ionic contrast media: what do the data tell us? Am J Radiol 1989; 152:945.
16. Lasser EC, Berry CC, Talner LB, et al: Pretreatment with corticosteroids to alleviate reactions to intravenous contrast material. N Engl J Med 1987; 317:845.
17. Harnish PP, Morris TW, Fischer HW, et al: Drugs providing protection from severe contrast media reactions. Invest Radiol 1980; 15:248.
18. Artu AA, Stout D, Katz RA, et al: EEG suppression and increased BBB permeability following intracarotid injection of iothalamate meglumine (Conray) in dogs. J Neurosurg Anesth 1990; 2:105.
19. Earnest F IV, Forbes G, Sandok BA, et al: Complications of cerebral angiography: prospective assessment of risk. AJR 1984; 142:247.
20. Dion JE, Gates PC, Fox AJ, et al: Clinical events following neuroangiography: a prospective study. Stroke 1987; 18:997.
21. Trankina MF, Houser WD, Cucchiara RF: Neurodiagnostic procedures. *In* Clinical Neuroanesthesia. Cucchiara RF, Michenfelder JD (eds). New York, Churchill Livingstone, 1990, p 442.
22. Snopek AM: Central nervous system radiography. *In* Fundamentals of

Special Radiographic Procedures. 3rd ed. Snopek AM (ed). Philadelphia, WB Saunders, 1992, pp 267–271.
23. Jacoby J, Jones JR, Ziegler J, et al: Pneumoencephalography and air embolism: simulated anesthetic death. Anaesthesia 1959; 20:336.
24. Shah R, Mahour GH, Ford EG, et al: Partial splenic embolization: an effect alternative to splenectomy for hypersplenism. Am Surg 1990; 56:774.
25. Coldwell DM, Loper KA: Regional anesthesia for hepatic arterial embolization. Radiology 1989; 172:1039.
26. Snopek AM: Vascular interventional procedures. *In* Fundamentals of Special Radiographic Procedures. 3rd ed. Snopek AM (ed). Philadelphia, WB Saunders, 1992, pp 330–350.
27. Higashida RT, Halbach VV, Dowd CF, et al: Intracranial aneurysms: interventional neurovascular treatment with detachable balloons—results in 215 cases. Radiology 1991; 178:663.
28. Berman HL, DelGuercio LRM, Katz SG, et al: Minimally invasive devascularization for variceal bleeding that could not be controlled with sclerotherapy. Surgery 1988; 104:500.
29. Tarr RW, Horton JA: Embolization of intracranial and extracranial tumors. *In* Current Practice of Interventional Radiology. Kadir S (ed). Philadelphia, BC Decker, 1991, p 141.
30. Chang C-P, Chen M-T, Chang LS: Autonomic hyperreflexia in spinal cord injury patient during percutaneous nephrolithotomy for renal stone: a case report. J Urol 1991; 146:1601.
31. Snopek AM: Non-vascular interventional procedures. *In* Fundamentals of Special Radiographic Procedures. 3rd ed. Snopek AM (ed). Philadelphia, WB Saunders, 1992, pp 331–376.
32. Rosenblatt M, Merai B, Robalino J, et al: Hypobaric spinal anesthesia in percutaneous nephrostomy (Abstract). Can J Anaesth 1989; 56:S56.
33. Morgan PD, Strong WE, Menk EJ: Anesthesia for percutaneous renal procedures. Reg Anesth 1991; 16:296.
34. Burhenne HJ: Interventional radiology of the biliary tract. Rad Clin North Am 1990; 28:1100.
35. Lieberman RP, Nance PN, Cuka DJ: Anterior approach to celiac plexus block during interventional biliary procedures. Radiology 1988; 167:562.
36. Snopek AM: Computed tomography. *In* Fundamentals of Special Radiographic Procedures. 3rd ed. Snopek AM (ed). Philadelphia, WB Saunders, 1992, pp 110–132.
37. Keeter S, Bernator RM, Weinberg SM, et al: Sedation in pediatric CT: national survey of current practice. Radiology 1990; 175:745.
38. Thompson JR, Schneider S, Ashwal S: The choice of sedation for computed tomography in children: a prospective evaluation. Radiology 1982; 143:475.
39. Burchart GJ, White TJ, Siegel RL, et al: Rectal thiopental versus an intramuscular cocktail for sedating children before computerized tomography. Am J Hosp Pharm 1980; 37:222.
40. Varner PD, Ebert JP, McKay RD, et al: Methohexital sedation of children undergoing CT scan. Anesth Analg 1985; 64:643.
41. Mitchell AA, Louik C, Lacouture P, et al: Risks to children from computed tomographic scan premedication. JAMA 1982; 247:2385.
42. Nahata MC, Coltz MA, Krogg EA: Adverse effects of meperidine, promethazine, and chlorpromazine for sedation in pediatric patients. Clin Pediatr 1985; 24:558.
43. Menon DK, Peden CJ, Hall AS, et al: Magnetic resonance for the anaesthetist. Part 1: physical principles, applications, safety aspects. Anaesthesia 1992; 47:240.
44. Kanal E, Shellock FG, Talagala L: Safety considerations in MR imaging. Radiology 1990; 176:593.
45. Kelly W, Paglen PG, Pearson JA, et al: Ferromagnetism of intraocular foreign body causes unilateral blindness after MR study. AJNR 1986; 7:243.
46. Shellock FG, Curtis JS: MR imaging and biomedical implants, materials and devices: an updated review. Radiology 1991; 180:541.
47. Pavlicek W, Geisinger M, Castle L, et al: The effects of nuclear magnetic resonance on patients with cardiac pacemakers. Radiology 1983; 147:149.
48. Center for Devices and Radiological Health MR Product Reporting Program and Medical Device Report Program. Washington, DC, US Food and Drug Administration, 1989.
49. Shuman WP, Haynor DR, Guy AW, et al: Superficial and deep tissue temperature increases in anesthetized dogs during exposure to high specific absorption rates in a 1.5 T MR imaging. Radiology 1988; 167:551.
50. Shellock FG, Rothman B, Sarti D: Heating of the scrotum by high field strength MR imaging. Am J Radiol 1990; 154:1229.
51. Shellock FG, Crues JV: Corneal temperature changes induced by high-field strength MR imaging with a head coil. Radiology 1987; 167:809.
52. Shellock FG, Slimp GL: Severe burn of the finger caused by using a pulse oximeter during MR imaging. Am J Radiol 1989; 153:1105.

53. Brummett RE, Talbot JM, Charuhas P: Potential hearing loss resulting from MR imaging. Radiology 1988; 169:539.

54. Flaherty JA, Hoskinson K: Emotional distress during magnetic resonance imaging. N Engl J Med 1989; 320:467.

55. Friday PJ, Kubal WS: Magnetic resonance imaging: improved patient tolerance utilizing medical hypnosis. Am J Clin Hypn 1990; 33:80.

56. Menon DK, Peden CJ, Hall AS, et al: Magnetic resonance for the anaesthetist. Part II: anaesthesia and monitoring in MR unit. Anaesthesia 1992; 47:508.

57. Buddinger TF: Nuclear magnetic resonance (NMR) in vivo studies: unknown thresholds for health effects. J Comput Assist Tomogr 1981; 5:800.

58. Dimick RN, Hedlund LW, Herfkens RJ, et al: Optimizing electrocardiograph electrode placement for cardiac-gated magnetic resonance imaging. Invest Radiol 1987; 22:17.

59. Karlaic SJ, Heatherley T, Pavan F, et al: Patient anesthesia and monitoring at a 1.5 T MRI installation. Magn Reson 1988; 7:210.

60. Barnett GH, Ropper AH, Johnson KA: Physiological support and monitoring of critically ill patients during magnetic resonance imaging. J Neurosurg 1988; 68:24.

61. Hadley DM, Teasdale GM, Jenkins A, et al: Magnetic resonance imaging in acute head injury. Clin Radiol 1988; 39:131.

62. Smith DS, Askey P, Young ML, et al: Anesthetic management of acutely ill patients during magnetic resonance imaging. Anesthesiology 1986; 65:710.

63. Whitfield A, Douglas RHB: Effect of general anesthesia on the magnetic resonance imaging signal from the brain. Br J Anaesth 1989; 62:694.

64. Harnett AN, Hingerford J, Lambert G, et al: Modern lateral external beam (lens sparing) radiotherapy for retinoblastoma. Ophthalmic Paediatr Genet 1987; 8:53.

65. Brett CM, Wara WM, Hamilton WK: Anesthesia for infants during radiotherapy: an insufflation technique. Anesthesiology 1986; 64:402.

66. Stock JGL, Strunin L: Unexplained hepatitis following halothane. Anesthesiology 1985; 63:424.

67. Wark HJ: Postoperative jaundice in children. The influence of halothane. Anaesthesia 1983; 38:237.

68. Browne CHW, Boulton TB, Crichton TC: Anaesthesia for radiotherapy: a frame for maintaining the airway. Anaesthesia 1969; 24:42.

69. Clauber DT, Audenaert SM: Anesthesia for children undergoing craniospinal radiotherapy. Anesthesiology 1987; 67:801.

70. Grebenik CR, Ferguson C, White A: The laryngeal mask airway in pediatric radiotherapy. Anesthesiology 1990; 72:474.

71. Cronin MM, Bousfield JD, Jewett EB, et al: Ketamine anesthesia for radiotherapy in small children. Anaesthesia 1972; 27:135.

Anesthetic Considerations, Special Problems, Approaches, and Problem-Solving

CHAPTER 55

Management of the Difficult Airway

ROGER S. MECCA, M.D.

This chapter focuses on recognition and management of the "difficult airway" during anesthesia. For ease of analysis, various stages of airway management are considered separately. These include ventilation and oxygenation by facemask, tracheal intubation, ventilation and oxygenation after intubation, and extubation. For each of these stages, clinical conditions or complicating factors that interfere with successful airway management are reviewed, along with various techniques for dealing with them. Finally, criteria for determining success of interventions are discussed.

GENERAL PRINCIPLES

What Does Airway Management Provide?

Oxygen Delivery

The most immediate goal of airway management is delivery of sufficient oxygen to replete uptake by pulmonary arterial blood from ventilated alveoli (Table 55–1). Airway patency and adequate fresh gas ventilation of perfused air spaces are required. If effective ventilation fails, both the alveolar partial pressure of oxygen (P_{AO_2}) and systemic arterial partial pressure of oxygen (Pa_{O_2}) rapidly fall. Because gas in the functional residual capacity (FRC) and hemoglobin molecules are the only reservoirs of available oxygen, progressive hypoxia in peripheral tissues must inevitably follow. Anaerobic generation of high-energy phosphate compounds ensues and generates a metabolic (i.e., lactic) acidemia by converting pyruvate to lactic acid. Acidemia is fulminant because poor minute ventilation precludes hyperventilation and compensatory respiratory alkalosis.

The initial sympathetic nervous system (SNS) response to hypoxemia and acidemia causes hypertension, tachycardia, and dysrhythmia, increasing morbidity in patients with cardiovascular disease. Severe acidemia interferes with interaction of catecholamine molecules with SNS receptors, leading to cardiovascular collapse and further reduction of oxygen delivery to tissues. Profound hypoxemia causes cerebral, myocardial, hepatic, and renal ischemia, leading to major disruption of function and irreversible tissue damage. Fatal dysrhythmias can occur in a matter of minutes.

Carbon Dioxide Removal

A second goal of airway management is sufficient effective alveolar ventilation to match carbon dioxide (CO_2) production. Again, both airway patency and adequate alveolar minute ventilation are important. Insufficient alveolar ventilation causes a progressive increase in the arterial partial pressure of CO_2 (Pa_{CO_2}). There is no effective immediate metabolic compensation for acute respiratory acidemia because the kidneys require hours to days to generate a compensatory alkalosis.

Hypercarbia in itself is relatively benign when compared with hypoxemia; however, very high Pa_{CO_2} can cause narcosis and volume displacement of oxygen from the alveoli. Consider the alveolar air equation:

$$P_{AO_2} = F_{IO_2} - \frac{Pa_{CO_2}}{R}$$

TABLE 55–1. Intraoperative Airway Management

End Point	Factors Required	Consequences of Failure
Adequate oxygenation (maintain PaO₂)	Airway patency O₂ delivery ≥ uptake	Reduced PaO₂; decreased PaO₂; metabolic acidemia; vital organ ischemia or infarction; fatal dysrhythmia
Adequate ventilation	Airway patency Effective minute ventilation CO₂ excretion ≥ production	Hypercarbia; respiratory acidemia; increased sympathetic nervous system activity with hypertension/tachycardia; severe cardiovascular depression; fatal acidemia/dysrhythmia
Airway protection	Prevent matter from accumulating in pharynx Prevent matter from entering trachea	Pulmonary aspiration; bronchospasm; mechanical airway obstruction; hypoxemia; chemical pneumonitis/adult respiratory distress syndrome; chronic pulmonary morbidity
Conduct of anesthesia	Ability to alter minute ventilation and adjust inspired gas composition	Delayed induction; inability to control responses; undesirable variation in anesthesia depth; difficult airway management

Abbreviations: PaO₂ = partial pressure of arterial oxygen; PAO₂ = partial pressure of alveolar oxygen.

Respiratory acidemia generates a profound SNS response but subsequently interferes with SNS function. Even in the absence of hypoxemia, ventricular fibrillation, secondary to progressive acidemia, can occur after 15 to 30 minutes of severe hypoventilation.

Protection of the Airway and Prevention of Aspiration

The third goal of airway management is to prevent aspiration of foreign material into the airways. Normally, solid or liquid matter near the glottic inlet elicits airway responses such as swallowing, coughing, gagging, or laryngospasm. The effectiveness of these protective reflexes is diminished by general anesthesia and eliminated by neuromuscular paralysis. If aspiration occurs, mechanical obstruction of small airways and diffuse bronchospasm causes ventilation/perfusion ($\dot{V}/\dot{Q}$) mismatching and increased airway resistance.

A profound reflex SNS response to foreign matter in the airway increases the risk of cardiovascular morbidity. The effectiveness of pulmonary surfactant is impaired after aspiration, leading to a marked reduction in pulmonary compliance. Chemical pneumonitis from aspirated acidic gastric contents often progresses to severe adult respiratory distress syndrome, and aspiration of particulate matter greatly enhances the risk of infection and chronic granulomatous changes.[1]

Delivery of Inhalation Anesthesia

The fourth goal of airway management during surgery is reliable delivery of a known anesthetic mixture, allowing con-

trol of anesthetic depth. Hypoventilation during anesthetic induction decreases the rate at which the alveolar partial pressure of an inhalation anesthetic rises. This effect is accentuated when a moderately to highly soluble agent is used if the SNS response to hypoxemia or hypercarbia increases cardiac output.

Inadequate anesthetic depth increases upper airway irritability, secretions, and bronchospastic responses to airway interventions. During emergence from anesthesia, hypoventilation slows alveolar washout of the agent. The risk of diffusion hypoxia, caused by rapid transfer of nitrous oxide from pulmonary arterial blood into the alveoli, is also increased.

FACEMASK VENTILATION

When Is Ventilation by Facemask Appropriate?

Ventilation by facemask is an important initial phase of airway management during induction of anesthesia, and it sometimes provides complete support of pulmonary function throughout a surgical procedure. Difficulty with initial facemask ventilation delays more definitive airway interventions and may ruin the timing and coordination of an induction. Depletion of oxygen reserves in the FRC and significant hypercarbia can occur, leaving less time for subsequent attempts to secure the airway. Gastric distention from insufflation of gas into the stomach increases the risk of regurgitation and aspiration. Even a seasoned practitioner can be unnerved when dealing with an unmanageable facemask airway.

Risks

An initial step in planning a patient's airway management is to decide whether facemask ventilation is appropriate after the loss of consciousness.

Regurgitation and Aspiration

The Full Stomach. Increased potential for regurgitation of gastric contents into the pharynx is a strong contraindication to prolonged facemask ventilation, especially when airway reflexes are compromised. The definition of a full stomach remains elusive, but ingestion of solid food within 6 to 8 hours of an anesthetic induction makes facemask ventilation with general anesthesia unsafe, especially if eating was proximate to trauma or onset of painful symptoms. Whether ingestion of clear liquids by elective surgical patients within a few hours of induction influences risk is unclear.

Patients at Particular Risk. Parturients, patients with bowel obstruction, and those with nausea and vomiting are at increased risk for regurgitation. An incremental risk in moderately obese fasted patients or those with asymptomatic hiatal hernia is questionable. To err on the safe side, consider that all patients who relate oral intake within 8 hours of induction and all emergency patients are likely to regurgitate.

Contraindications

Brisk post-tonsillectomy airway bleeding or severe epistaxis is a relative contraindication to facemask ventilation during induction. Evolving conditions that might compromise upper airway patency, such as airway burns, hereditary angioedema, or upper airway trauma, may also preclude this technique.

Feasibility

It is also important to decide if facemask ventilation is feasible. A fresh gas source must be available to provide sufficient volume to compensate for any leak around the facemask and to provide sufficient positive pressure to overcome resistance to gas flow. A seal between the facemask and the patient's face is required to sustain airway pressure during positive-pressure ventilation or to prevent dilution of the fresh gas mixture with ambient air during spontaneous ventilation. A low-resistance pathway must exist for fresh gas to reach distal air spaces so that spontaneous work of breathing or delivered positive pressure is minimized. Finally, the airway must be clear of secretions, blood, gastric contents, or other matter.

Facemask Seal

Inability to generate sufficient pressure under the mask during controlled ventilation is a common problem. Assuming that pressure integrity of the anesthesia circuit was assiduously checked before induction and the circuit pop-off valve is set to an appropriate outflow resistance, pressure dissipation invariably indicates a volume leak caused by a faulty seal between the facemask and the patient's face.

Improper Cushion Inflation

Most adult facemasks are fitted with an inflatable cushion to conform to facial contours. With proper inflation, it should be easy to dimple the cushion with a finger tip but difficult to palpate the rigid edge of the mask through the cushion. Both underinflation and overinflation make achieving a seal more difficult. With many masks, the cushion inflation volume is user adjustable via a valve, analogous to the pilot valve on a cuffed endotracheal tube. If the facemask is too large, leakage occurs near the orbits, chin, or cheeks; if too small, leakage often occurs along the nose.

Facial Features

Evaluation of facial features helps to predict difficulties with facemask seal. Facial hair under the mask edge can cause remarkable leakage, which prevents generation of sufficient positive pressure to support ventilation. In edentulous or cachectic patients and those with prominent noses or thin, "hatchet" facial features, lateral seal is problematic. A seal is also difficult in patients with severely recessed chins or mandibular fractures. If very high airway pressures are delivered to overcome airway obstruction, even the best seal will be broken and leakage will occur.

What Supportive Maneuvers Are Useful?

Various simple maneuvers can improve the seal. Properly sized and inflated masks usually seal with the weight of the operator's hand. A slight tip of the mask toward the leak often improves a faulty seal with no increase in downward force, as does a slight caudad shift of the cushion onto the chin. Using excessive pressure to force the mask cushion over facial contours risks corneal abrasion, pressure neuropathy of superficial facial nerves, and soft tissue damage. Pressure of the fingers under the mandible can lead to soft tissue trauma and neuropathy.

Mask Fit

Spreading the sides of the cushion before placement on the face pulls soft tissue slightly up into the mask once the sides rebound, thereby improving the seal. Circumferential mask straps can hold slack cheek tissues against the mask cushion, although straps should not be used to exert excessive downward pressure. In the author's opinion, however, the facemask should always be held by hand. Using straps to free the hands during anesthesia can jeopardize airway patency and allow the mask to migrate onto the patient's eyes.

Dentures and Padding

Leaving dentures in place or stuffing the cheeks with cotton or gauze serves to support flaccid tissues, but one should always be cautious about potentially loose foreign bodies in the mouth during facemask ventilation. An assistant's hands placed on the sides of the patient's face in order to pucker the cheeks upward against the mask is sometimes helpful. This maneuver is especially useful when trying to effect a seal through facial hair. Application of gauze soaked in petroleum jelly might help fill facial contours under the mask cushion.

Increased Gas Inflow

Despite all these maneuvers, facemask seal may be impossible. Fresh gas flow into the circuit can be increased to counteract the volume lost through the leak. Whenever possible, increase the metered flow of the selected mixture instead of using the oxygen flush valve repeatedly to refill the circuit. This technique avoids diluting the delivered anesthetic mixture and reduces the possibility that high flow from the flush will transiently generate excessive peak pressures.

What Factors Contribute to Airway Obstruction?

History and Physical Assessment

A preoperative history and physical examination often unearth conditions that predispose to difficulty in maintaining airway patency. Heavy snoring, sleep apnea, or airway surgery suggests anatomic obstruction. Records from previous anesthetics may reveal difficulty that occurred. In obese patients, facemask ventilation is often difficult because a bulky, muscular tongue interferes with airway patency and a thick, stiff neck interferes with head and jaw manipulation.

Acquired and Congenital Abnormalities

Patients with reactive airways secondary to asthma, chronic obstructive pulmonary disease, or smoking are more prone to protracted coughing, laryngospasm, or increased small airway resistance. Congenital conditions such as Pierre Robin syndrome or trisomy 21 predispose to obstruction, as do chronic conditions like sarcoidosis and myxedema. Acute problems characterized by upper airway edema or inflammation, such as smoke inhalation, croup, epiglottitis, or peritonsillar abscess, can cause severe life-threatening airway obstruction. Unexpected glottic or tracheal obstruction from hematoma, tumor, goiter, or radiation therapy can also severely impede ability to ventilate by facemask after induction.

Why Is Increased Airway Resistance Problematic?

Excessive airway resistance that obstructs gas flow from the mouth and nose to small airways is a dangerous problem (Table 55–2). High resistance in the upper airway necessitates high positive pressure in the mouth to achieve ventilation. High mouth pressure interferes with facemask seal and causes gastric distention if esophageal opening pressure is exceeded.[2] Conversely, if the pressure gradient is constant, high resistance decreases fresh gas delivery.

In the extreme, airway resistance may become so high that complete airway obstruction occurs. In addition to the risk of acute hypoxemia and hypercarbia, forceful spontaneous inspiratory efforts against an obstructed upper airway often lead to fulminant postobstructive pulmonary edema resulting from very low negative intrathoracic pressure.[3, 4]

How Is the Cross-Sectional Area of the Airway Reduced?

Increased resistance to gas flow usually indicates a decreased cross-sectional area at some level in the airway.[5] Upper airway caliber is frequently reduced by the tongue falling back against the soft palate or by soft tissues occluding the pharynx. Laryngospasm secondary to glottic or vocal cord stimulation during light anesthesia can also be responsible. Vomitus or a foreign body in the mouth can mechanically block airflow. Acute onset of severe bronchospasm secondary to mechanical stimulation or unrecognized aspiration can increase small airway resistance and mimic upper airway obstruction, as does poor pulmonary compliance secondary to coughing, straining, or chest wall rigidity.

How Is an Obstructed Airway Recognized?

Various clinical signs appear during airway obstruction (Table 55–3).

TABLE 55–2. Factors That Increase Resistance to Airflow

Equipment	Occluded inspiratory limb in circuit
	Closed pop-off valve with lung overinflation
Pharynx/larynx	Soft tissue obstruction
	Laryngospasm
	Foreign body obstruction
	Inflammatory disease
Airway/air spaces	Bronchospasm
	Gas trapping
	Abdominal pressure
	Foreign body blockage
Pulmonary mechanics	Pneumothorax
	Chest wall rigidity
	Coughing/gagging

TABLE 55–3. Signs of Upper Airway Obstruction

Auditory	Gurgling (esophageal ventilation)
	Crowing or stridor (laryngeal)[1]
	Stridor (laryngeal)[1]
	Snoring (pharyngeal)[1]
	Wheezing (small airway)
	Absent breath sounds[1]
Tactile	Decreased reservoir compliance[2]
	Decreased expiratory return
	Airway vibration
	Large facemask leak[2]
Visual	Chest wall/abdominal excursion
	Accessory muscle recruitment[3]
	Puffed cheeks/neck[2]
	Abdominal rocking[3]
	Abdominal distention[2]
	Cyanosis
	Nasal flaring
	Suprasternal retraction
Objective	Increased airway pressure[2]
	Absence of CO_2 waves on capnograph[1]
	Low measured expired volume
	Hypoxemia (pulse oximeter)

Abnormal Sounds

Turbulent gas flow past an airway obstruction often generates noise, so auscultation with a pretracheal or precordial stethoscope is invaluable to assess upper airway patency during facemask ventilation. Snoring or inspiratory stridor may indicate significant obstruction in the nasopharynx or larynx, respectively, although these sounds can occur when ventilation is adequate.

Gurgling secondary to esophageal ventilation may also be audible when excessive positive airway pressures are being delivered. High airway resistance in the larynx often generates a high-pitched crowing sound, whereas small airway obstruction causes audible prolonged expiratory wheezing. Diminished or absent breath sounds should mean that facemask ventilation is inadequate until proven otherwise.

Chest and Abdominal Motion

Absence of coordinated chest expansion often indicates that the airway is obstructed, as does a prolonged inspiratory or expiratory interval. However, the adequacy of ventilation, as gauged by chest or abdominal excursion, is unreliable in obese or draped patients.

During spontaneous ventilation, partial airway obstruction often elicits accessory muscle recruitment, intercostal or suprasternal retraction, nasal flaring, abdominal withdrawal during inspiration, and other signs of increased work of breathing. More severe obstruction generates a characteristic "rocking" motion as the chest wall and diaphragm compete to achieve chest cavity expansion.

In a patient receiving positive-pressure ventilation, bulging of the cheeks or lateral neck tissues is caused by high pressures proximal to the obstruction. Progressive abdominal distention is an ominous sign that airway obstruction is causing gastric insufflation.

Palpation

Tactile signs are also valuable for recognizing airway obstruction. Vibrations caused by flapping of the tongue or soft tissues during partial or intermittent obstruction can be felt when hand-holding the mask. Excessive, noisy leak under a tight facemask seal is another indicator.

Palpation of the reservoir bag is a valuable diagnostic index. The rate of volume reduction during inspiration qualitatively indicates flow adequacy through the upper airway, and palpation of a tight, distended bag indicates high inspiratory pressure and is a reasonable sign of increased airway resistance.

One should be cautious about using peak pressure alone to evaluate obstruction, for at high pressures, the circuit "pops off" past the mask into the scavenging system or into the stomach. Increased inspiratory pressure from changes in chest wall or abdominal compliance can be difficult to differentiate from airway obstruction.

Exhaled Carbon Dioxide Monitoring

Although clinical signs are useful, nothing substitutes for monitoring exhaled CO_2 when airway patency is evaluated. A capnograph is an essential anesthesia monitor that should be used during facemask ventilation as well as after intubation. Evaluation of the expired CO_2 waveform is more useful than recording only the end-expired partial pressure. During facemask ventilation, the absence of exhaled CO_2 waveforms usually indicates a high degree of airway obstruction, unless there is significant leak around the mask, such as when the pop-off valve is closed down. In this event, both exhaled gas and fresh gas inflow preferentially exit the circuit via the leak around the mask and thus bypass the CO_2 monitoring in the intubated patient when mask ventilation occurs during use of high fresh gas flows.

Pulse Oximetry

Pulse oximetry should not be relied on to monitor airway patency. Arterial desaturation indicates that obstruction has already been present long enough for the P_{AO_2} to fall. Similarly, if the diagnosis of airway obstruction is delayed until tachycardia, hypertension, or dysrhythmia is caused by the SNS response to hypoxemia or hypercarbia, valuable time will have already been lost. Recognition of airway obstruction should never be delayed until the observation of cyanosis or dark blood in the surgical field.

How Is Upper Airway Obstruction Avoided?

Certain precautions minimize the chances that problematic airway obstruction will occur during induction. Before every anesthetic induction, oral and nasal airways, facemasks, intubating equipment, strong suction, and appropriate medications should be assembled and readily available. Administration of a vagolytic antisialagogue such as atropine or glycopyrrolate reduces the chance that excessive secretions will cause obstruction or laryngospasm during induction.

Creating a relaxed environment for the patient is important, because preinduction anxiety probably increases the incidence of coughing and laryngospasm during induction. Judicious sedation in anxious patients can smooth induction, although caution must be exercised in patients who depend on arousal to maintain patency of a marginal airway.

What Does Preoxygenation Achieve?

Denitrogenation with 100% oxygen may not be necessary before every anesthetic induction, although it is seldom inappropriate to apply this safety measure.[6-9] Every patient at increased risk of airway obstruction should undergo rigorous denitrogenation, because the most immediate and serious complication of airway obstruction is acute hypoxemia. Replacing nitrogen in the FRC with the highest possible concentration of oxygen increases the time interval between the onset of airway obstruction and dangerous hypoxemia by a factor of four. These extra minutes often permit restoration of airway patency without the risk or complication associated with emergency airway interventions.

Which Induction Agents Are Preferable?

Inhalation Agents

Induction agents affect the incidence of airway obstruction, although comparisons often reflect variation in individual technique more than pharmacologic properties. Irritation from pungent inhalation agents can promote coughing, laryngospasm, and occasionally bronchospasm during inhalation induction. Of the commonly available agents, halothane is the least noxious, followed in order by enflurane and isoflurane.

Intravenous Anesthetics

Among intravenous induction agents, propofol appears to offer a high degree of "airway tolerance" for irritation from inhaled agents, positive-pressure ventilation, and airway insertion immediately after induction. Intravenous lidocaine may decrease airway reactivity in selected patients. (Part of propofol's airway-sparing characteristic might be attributable to intravenous lidocaine administered to counter irritation at the intravenous site.) Release of histamine after induction with sodium thiopental may increase airway resistance in patients with severe reactive airways diseases.

An anaphylactoid or anaphylactic reaction to an induction agent or neuromuscular relaxant can precipitate life-threatening refractory bronchospasm. Induction techniques using high doses of synthetic narcotics sometimes cause chest wall rigidity that mimics airway obstruction, although it is unclear whether this problem occurs with dosages used for routine inductions.

What Manipulations Are Detrimental?

Soft Tissue Stimulation

Stimulation of the palate, glottis, or vocal cords should be avoided during light levels of anesthesia. Head positioning immediately after induction can precipitate laryngospasm, as does impingement of rigid oral airways or suction devices against the pharynx or larynx.

Ventilatory Waveforms

Rapid generation of positive pressure and turbulent high gas flow rates caused by brisk, clenching compressions of the reservoir bag should be avoided. A gradual rate of pressure change that generates a low-flow, sighing inflation reduces vocal cord movement that leads to laryngospasm, brisk diaphragmatic descent that causes reflex contraction (hiccup), and high peak pressure that predisposes to gastric insufflation. To achieve a gentle positive-pressure inspiration, an inexperienced operator can match delivery of the patient's tidal volume against his or her own slow, deep inspiration.

High Ventilatory Rate

Inadvertent ventilation of a patient at high rates may not allow sufficient time for complete exhalation, especially if small airway resistance is increased. Thoracic expansion caused by trapped gas dramatically reduces chest wall compliance and necessitates high airway pressures for delivery of subsequent tidal volumes.

Increased physiologic dead space, coupled with decreased effective minute ventilation, leads to clinically significant hypercarbia. In some patients, neuromuscular paralysis allows the soft palate to obstruct the nasopharynx during exhalation, and tight closure of the mouth during expiration then causes gas trapping.[10] Gas trapping prevents adequate capnometry, because incomplete exhalation precludes sampling of undiluted alveolar gas.

How Should Upper Airway Obstruction Be Managed?

If airway patency decreases after unconsciousness is induced, first ensure that an open passage exists for gas to flow from the mask into the pharynx. Tight apposition of the lips in a patient with occluded nares precludes free gas entry. Next, ensure that obstruction is not secondary to vomitus or a foreign object in the pharynx. Direct visualization of the posterior pharynx through the mouth and auscultation with a pretracheal stethoscope are useful.

Vomiting and Aspiration

Discovery of vomitus in the airway generally necessitates cessation of facemask ventilation, suction of the airway, and immediate tracheal intubation. The only possible exception to this dictum is a patient with a life-threatening upper airway condition such as epiglottitis, in whom a failed intubation attempt could precipitate life-threatening airway obstruction, or a patient in whom previous unsuccessful attempts at intubation have precipitated severe hypoxemia. Under these circumstances, one might have to accept the risk of aspiration during continued facemask oxygenation until the airway can be safely secured.

Reduced Pulmonary Compliance

If the upper airway is clear, ensure that difficulty with ventilation is not caused by a sudden reduction in pulmonary compliance secondary to coughing, abdominal straining, or breath holding. Attempting to generate sufficient airway pressure to overcome such low compliance is fruitless and only causes gastric inflation. Generally, waiting a few moments or deepening the anesthetic with rapidly acting intravenous agents returns compliance to normal and facilitates facemask ventilation.

Soft Tissue Obstruction

The most common cause of increased upper airway resistance is obstruction by the tongue or epiglottis by loss of airway muscle tone or flexion of the head.[11, 12]

Therapeutic Measures

Extension, Elevation, and Head Turning

Anatomic obstruction can usually be overcome with simple mechanical airway maneuvers such as extending and elevating the head into a "sniffing" position to raise the hyoid bone, the tongue, and the epiglottis.[13] However, obstruction may not improve if cervical spine stiffness moves the pharynx and larynx along with the head. Head extension and elevation may worsen obstruction in young children. In some cases, turning a patient's head to the side relieves soft tissue obstruction by making these tissues tauter. The head should always be repositioned slowly and with minimal force to avoid inadvertent injury to the cervical vertebrae or spinal cord, especially in patients with osteoporosis, osteoarthritis, bony lesions in the neck, or potential cervical trauma.

Jaw Thrust

If soft tissue airway obstruction persists, elevating the ramus of the mandible can further elevate the hyoid bone and tongue. Mandibular elevation can sometimes be provided by hooking the fifth finger of the hand holding the mask underneath the ramus and levering up toward the ceiling. In obese or very large patients, the third through fifth fingers of both hands can be used to elevate the mandible while holding the mask between the thumbs and index fingers. This approach often improves seal as well but obviously requires an assistant to supply compression of the reservoir bag.

Minimum force should be used, and the flat pad of the fingers rather than the tips should contact the patient's mandible. Significant bruising or neuropathy can result from digging the finger tips or nails into the tissues of the neck.

Skillfully applied upper airway maneuvers eliminate soft tissue airway obstruction in the majority of normal unconscious patients. However, if obstruction persists or excessive force is required to maintain marginal airway patency, insertion of an oral or nasal airway is indicated. The choice between these adjuncts is affected by individual preference and circumstances specific to each patient.

Nasal Airways

Because a nasal airway causes less pharyngeal stimulation during light anesthesia, it is often useful to maintain a marginal airway in a sedated or emerging patient. Nasal airways can also be used when dental appliances or crowns make use of a rigid oral airway undesirable. However, nasal airways usually do not provide a useful portal for airway suctioning and are often ineffective at overcoming airway obstruction that has not responded to airway maneuvers. In addition, insertion of a foreign body through the nasal passages can precipitate epistaxis, which significantly complicates management and increases the risk of laryngospasm or blood aspiration. Although nasal airways are soft and pliable, insertion in patients with basilar skull fractures can lead to serious, potentially life-threatening central nervous system complications, and in this situation, an oral airway is preferred.[14]

Oral Airways

An oral airway, although more rigid and stimulating to the pharynx, generally provides better tongue displacement and a larger airway opening than does a nasal airway. Selecting the proper size of oral airway significantly improves its effectiveness. If the airway is too small, it does not reach far enough to hold the tongue off the posterior pharyngeal wall. A small airway can also be lost in the oral cavity and cause laryngospasm or obstruction. If the airway is too large, it either protrudes from the mouth and interferes with facemask seal or pokes into the posterior pharynx and causes unnecessary pharyngeal trauma and stimulation. An airway can be sized by placing it adjacent to the face and picking one that reaches from the incisors to just beyond the angle of the jaw.

Improper insertion of an oral airway worsens airway obstruction if the tip forces the tongue back against the posterior pharyngeal wall. This complication can be avoided by inserting a properly sized airway with a twisting motion or by using a tongue blade to ensure proper tongue positioning.

Insertion of an oral airway in an inadequately anesthetized patient may precipitate coughing, laryngospasm, or bronchospasm, all of which interfere with airway management. Potential gagging and vomiting increase the risk of aspiration. Incidental trauma to the lips, tongue, teeth, or oral mucosa is also greater. A laryngeal mask airway may help to maintain a difficult facemask airway if intubation is undesirable or difficult to complete.[15]

If airway obstruction is secondary to epiglottitis, croup, peritonsillar abscess, laryngeal edema, hereditary angioedema, encroaching tumor, or hematoma, great care must be exercised when artificial airways are used. These conditions often require gas to flow through circuitous channels around the obstruction. Any trauma that occurs during airway insertion or other manipulations might cause increased swelling and dramatically worsen the degree of obstruction.

What Are Other Important Causes of Airway Obstruction?

If the preceding measures fail to improve airway patency, it is likely that obstruction is caused by bronchospasm or laryngospasm assuming that an unrecognized anatomic abnormality such as epiglottitis or pharyngeal abscess is not present.

Bronchospasm

Generally, bronchospasm must be severe to interfere significantly with positive-pressure inspiration. Because acute small airway constriction during induction is almost always triggered by mechanical stimulation of the tracheal mucosa, bronchospasm is rarely a cause of inability to ventilate with a facemask. However, in patients with reactive airway diseases, significant bronchospasm can occur in response to an unexpected drug reaction, minor aspiration of secretions or gastric contents, irritation from inhaled agents (especially isoflurane), or laryngeal stimulation from an airway or suction catheter.

Signs of acute bronchospasm are similar to those of an obstructed upper airway, although auscultation of diffuse wheezing helps to differentiate. Also, obstruction secondary to bronchospasm does not improve after head maneuvers or artificial airway placement unless a component of soft tissue obstruction is superimposed.

Laryngospasm

Laryngospasm is a far more common cause of severe facemask airway obstruction than bronchospasm. It is a complex protective reflex that tenses constrictor muscles of the larynx, causing tight apposition of the vocal cords and closure of the tracheal inlet.[16] Laryngospasm prevents solid or liquid matter from entering the tracheal inlet, so the reflex is often triggered by stimulation of the laryngeal mucosa. During induction, light anesthesia interferes with central integration of airway reflexes and severe spasm can be triggered by minor stimulation from brisk positive-pressure ventilation, oral secretions, or airway realignment. Peripheral noxious stimuli can also precipitate laryngospasm.

Laryngospasm is usually a self-limited process that resolves spontaneously. Airway patency often can be quickly restored by removing the offending stimulus and deepening the anesthetic. Application of a sustained low level of positive pressure (10–15 cm H_2O) often helps to "break" the airway obstruction. High-pressure spikes in the airway should be avoided, both to decrease esophageal ventilation and to reduce further airway stimulation. Before application of positive pressure, it is important to ensure that laryngospasm was not *appropriately* triggered by vomitus or a foreign body in the airway.

Hypoxemia

The evolution of hypoxemia determines how long one can wait for laryngospasm to resolve. If the initial P_{AO_2} was sufficient to maintain arterial saturation, more invasive interventions to restore airway patency can be avoided. This fact alone is an excellent justification for elective denitrogenation.

The advisability of administering nitrous oxide during induction varies with individual circumstances and technique, as does the point at which nitrous oxide should be eliminated if airway obstruction occurs. Elimination of nitrous oxide administration might slow induction or lighten the anesthetic, making facemask management more difficult. However, it is always defensible to maximize the fraction of inspired oxygen (FIO_2) in the presence of a marginal airway. There is less obvious justification (i.e., it does not interfere with oxygen administration unless the goal is to allow the patient to wake up) for eliminating a potent inhalation agent, because the volume percentage of vapor is low.

Muscle Relaxants

If hypoxemia or hypercarbia occurs, neuromuscular relaxation can resolve the obstruction. Administration of relaxants to a patient who cannot be easily ventilated by facemask is fraught with the risk of aspiration, worsening the obstruction, or being unable to intubate if ventilation cannot be restored.

The smallest effective dose of the shortest-acting available agent should be given. This problem represents one of the few remaining uncontested indications for the administration of succinylcholine. If the cause is laryngospasm, it is usually relieved with marginal paralysis from a small dose (0.1 mg · kg^{-1}; 5–10 mg in an adult). Fasciculation or bradycardia seldom occurs after these doses, and the duration of paralysis is short. If the offending stimuli and depth of anesthesia have been appropriately adjusted, laryngospasm should not recur.

How Is Refractory Airway Obstruction Managed?

When a decision is made to administer succinylcholine to relax an obstructed airway, a prudent anesthesiologist should be planning what emergency steps to take to restore ventilation if relaxation fails to improve airway patency (i.e., if the diagnosis of laryngospasm is incorrect). Anticipation and preparation are important, for this complex decision might need to be made within seconds.[17]

The degree of airway obstruction is one key factor that affects this choice. If marginal oxygenation can be maintained, one might choose to persist with attempts to ventilate the patient by facemask while evaluating other possible causes of obstruction. However, previous failure of airway maneuvers, artificial airways, and neuromuscular relaxation make the chance of achieving adequate facemask ventilation small. If obstruction is complete or if hypoxemia is imminent, a more definitive approach to restoring airway patency should be taken.

Arousal

One alternative approach to a refractory airway obstruction is to "back out" of the anesthetic and restore a level of arousal that allows the patient to maintain airway patency and ventilation spontaneously. Unfortunately, at this point in an induction, the anesthesiologist has usually attempted to deepen the anesthetic with additional doses of induction agents and high concentrations of inhaled agents. With a partial obstruction, it might be possible to maintain oxygenation while the effects of these anesthetics wear off. However, complete obstruction produces severe hypoxemia long before a patient can emerge sufficiently to restore airway control.

Tracheal Intubation

Another alternative is to proceed with tracheal intubation. Again, the degree of obstruction and individual clinical circumstances affect the approach to intubation (see *Emergency Intubation,* later), but a few general principles apply. The most experienced operator available should perform the intubation, using the most expeditious route. In the majority of cases, oral intubation under direct vision is the fastest technique, yielding the highest chance of immediate success and the lowest incidence of further airway compromise. Caution must be exercised during laryngoscopy to avoid soft tissue trauma, which may convert a marginal airway into a completely obstructed one.

The advisability of using neuromuscular relaxants to facilitate intubation varies with clinical circumstances. If relaxation is deemed appropriate, again the smallest appropriate dose of a short-acting relaxant should be given. A practitioner should be exceptionally cautious about administering intubating doses of relaxants to a patient who cannot be easily ventilated by facemask, especially when the ability to intubate is also unproven.

DIFFICULT INTUBATION

What Are the Purposes of Tracheal Intubation?

Tracheal intubation involves insertion of a tubular airway into the trachea, thereby effectively extending the tracheal lumen outside the body. Intubation facilitates prolonged positive-pressure ventilation without gastric distention or major leakage of fresh gas. In addition, intubation simplifies airway management, for the relatively rigid tube should maintain patency. An inflated cuff, which isolates the pulmonary air spaces from the pharynx, significantly decreases but does not eliminate the risk of aspiration secondary to ablation of airway reflexes.[18, 19]

What Are the Consequences of Failure to Intubate?

Failure to successfully complete an intubation can cause various complications, some of which are catastrophic. The risk to the patient varies with the practitioner's ability to ventilate by facemask and with the patient's underlying condition. If no contraindications are present and a patient can be well ventilated and oxygenated using a facemask, inability to intubate may cause only minor airway trauma, a shift in anesthetic technique, or cancellation of the operative procedure if intubation is essential. However, if facemask ventilation is contraindicated or ineffective, failed intubation can lead to rapidly evolving hypoxemia and hypercarbia, with profound morbidity or mortality.

Why Does Failed Intubation Occur?

The process of intubation includes locating the tracheal inlet and inserting the tube. The most frequent cause of failed intubation is difficulty locating the tracheal inlet. Because the majority of intubations are performed under direct observation, this problem usually equates with inability to visualize the vocal cords or glottic opening.

In order to establish a line of sight from the mouth to the vocal cords, one must align the three axes of the airway (mouth to pharynx, pharynx to glottis, glottis to trachea) along one common direction (Fig. 55–1). Given that alignment is possible, one must then see past any anatomic obstructions to the vocal cords.

What Factors Interfere with Visualization of the Glottis?

Careful historical assessment can uncover potential difficulties with laryngoscopy and visualization. When reviewing a patient's records, search for documentation of previous difficult intubations, cancellation of surgery, or complications secondary to loss of airway patency.

The value of this information is an excellent reason for carefully recording on the anesthesia record not only the technique used during intubation (i.e., route, blade size, tube size) but also the degree of difficulty and any qualitative recommendations that might make the next practitioner's approach more successful. Feedback from consultants such as otolaryngologists or maxillofacial surgeons who are familiar with a patient's airway anatomy can be very useful, particularly if the intended procedure involves the jaw, mouth, or oropharynx.

Mouth Opening

When evaluating the many anatomic pathologic characteristics that interfere with aligning the airway axes or visualizing

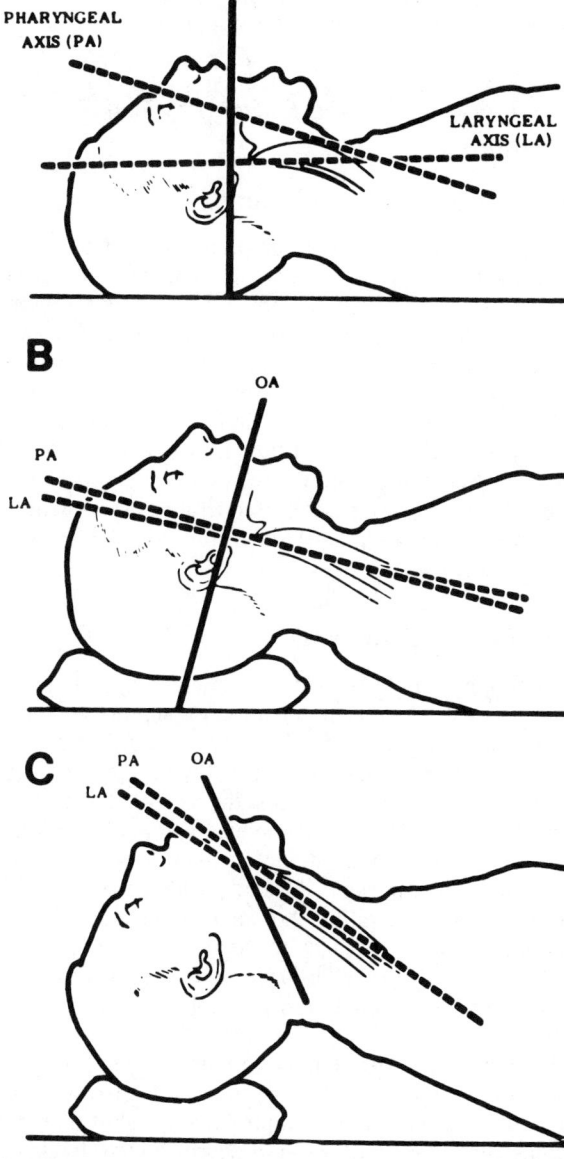

FIGURE 55–1. Head position for endotracheal intubation. *A,* Poor alignment of oral, pharyngeal, and laryngeal axes in supine position. *B,* Elevation of the head aligns the pharyngeal and laryngeal axes. *C,* Extension of the head at the atlanto-occipital joint rotates the oral axis and allows visualization of the glottis. (Adapted from Stoelting RK: Endotracheal intubation. *In Anesthesia.* Miller RD (ed). 3rd ed. New York, Churchill Livingstone, 1986, p 525.)

the tracheal opening, it is helpful to consider the basic maneuvers necessary to perform a successful laryngoscopy. Any characteristic that interferes with one of these steps can impede visualization (Table 55–4). For example, to view the vocal cords, one must open the mouth sufficiently to insert the laryngoscope blade and see around it. Patients with small oral openings or large protuberant teeth often present difficulties.

Jaw and Mouth Movement

Mandibular motion can be severely limited at the temporomandibular joint by arthritis, idiopathic joint dysfunction, or trismus secondary to infection or trauma.[20, 21] Another impor-

tant determinant of mouth opening is the degree of mandibular subluxation that is possible.[22]

Circumoral eschars, neck stabilization, or mandibular fixation devices also limit mouth opening. Contraction of the masseter muscles secondary to voluntary clenching or spasm during induction also interferes. Mandibular fractures or soft tissue injury impedes mandibular motion either directly or by causing pain.

It is important to differentiate between splinting of the mouth caused by pain and actual limitation, because the entire approach to intubation might hinge on how far the mouth can be opened after induction of anesthesia (and relief of pain). Large breasts or a massive anterior chest wall can also impede insertion of the laryngoscope blade and subsequent visualization.[23]

Head Movement

Bull Neck

Achieving head extension and elevation is another important maneuver necessary to achieve easy visualization.[24, 25] Obese or thick-necked patients often exhibit decreased mobility of the cervical spine caused by muscle mass or a cervical fat pad.

TABLE 55–4. Conditions That Interfere with Visualization of the Glottis

Anatomic variation	Small oral opening
	Limited temporomandibular joint motion
	Protuberant front teeth
	Recessed mandible
	Short, thick neck
	Limited neck extension
	High arched palate
	Large immobile tongue
Inherited syndromes	Trisomy 21
	Pierre Robin
	Goldenhar's
	Klippel-Feil
	Treacher Collins
	Turner's
	Angioedema
	Dwarfism
Chronic pathology	Rheumatoid arthritis
	Obesity
	Thyromegaly
	Acromegaly
	Scleroderma
	Sarcoidosis
	Ankylosing spondylitis
	Radiation fibrosis
	Cervical spine fusion
	Cervical traction
	Temporomandibular joint ankylosis
	Tonsillar hypertrophy
Acute pathology	Trismus
	Mandibular fracture
	Lingual trauma
	Epiglottitis
	Pharyngeal abscess
	Epistaxis
	Bleeding tonsil
	Airway tumor mass
	Airway inflammation
	Tetanus/seizures
	Cervical spine injury

A decrease in the occiput–C-1 distance to <5 mm as determined by a cervical spine film impedes extension and makes laryngoscopy difficult.[26]

Acquired and Congenital Cervical Disease

Patients with cervical arthritis, ankylosing spondylitis, or cervical fusions have decreased neck mobility, as do patients wearing external fixation devices such as cervical collars or halos.[27–29] Large space-occupying lesions in the neck or upper back such as head and neck tumors, severe subcutaneous emphysema, or edema can also impede motion. Many congenital or acquired skeletal abnormalities also decrease the cervical range of motion.[5, 30]

In some circumstances, neck movement to facilitate visualization is physically possible but relatively contraindicated because cervical fractures, subluxation of cervical vertebrae, or spinal column instability might pose a threat to spinal cord viability. However, instability of the spinal column does not preclude oral intubation when it is indicated.[31] Neck extension should also be restricted in patients suffering from vertebrobasilar artery syndrome or cervical radiculopathy.

Tongue Displacement

During laryngoscopy, lateral displacement of the tongue is important, so any factor that restricts tongue movement impedes visualization. Obese patients and those with congenital abnormalities often have unusually large tongues that can be difficult to manipulate during laryngoscopy. Head and neck surgery or radiation therapy frequently leaves a relatively immobile or ''wooden'' tongue. Significant lingual trauma or infections can also render the tongue difficult to manipulate, as can lingual tumors.

Mandibular Abnormalities

Mandibular abnormalities can interfere with visualization. An unusual degree of mandibular recession makes alignment of the airway axes difficult because the recessed mandible impedes elevation of the hyoid and tongue. Many patients exhibit some degree of mandibular recession as a normal variant.

Several congenital abnormalities (including Pierre Robin, Treacher Collins, and Goldenhar's syndromes) are notable for severe mandibular abnormalities.[5, 32, 33] Developmental abnormalities such as cleft lip or cleft palate may also be problematic.

Anatomic variations in otherwise unremarkable patients can sometimes cause completely unexpected problems with visualization of the vocal cords. A prominent thyroid cartilage or a larynx that is more cephalad than normal are anatomic variants that can impede visualization.

Other Factors

Pregnancy may increase difficulty with intubation secondary to laryngeal and tongue edema.[34] Pathology that enlarges or distorts pharyngeal or laryngeal structures can block visualization of the vocal cords. Conditions that impede visualization include epiglottitis, croup, peritonsillar abscess, laryngeal edema, airway burns, cervical trauma, hereditary angioedema, and tumors or hematomas impinging on the upper airway.[35, 36]

These conditions are particularly difficult to manage because the airway is essentially blocked with an anatomic obstacle that cannot be realigned to improve visualization.

What Should Be Assessed During Physical Examination?

Visualization of Mouth and Pharynx

A compulsive physical examination often predicts potential difficulties with intubation. Patients should always be asked to open the mouth to a point of minor discomfort in order to assess both orifice size and temporomandibular joint mobility. If the faucial pillars and uvula cannot be easily seen with the tongue fully extended, visualization of the glottis may be difficult.[30, 37] Patient posture, phonation, and variability among observers affect the accuracy of this determination.[38] This observation emphasizes the need always to assess the airway yourself, because someone else's preoperative assessment may differ from your own, perhaps suggesting a different airway management plan.

Neck Mobility and Anatomy

Neck mobility should be evaluated in anterior-posterior, lateral, and rotary motions, with attention to pain or paresthesias that limit neck motion. Check also for swelling or stiffness in soft tissues of the neck and for immobility or lateral deviation of the trachea. The distance from the notch of the thyroid cartilage to the tip of the mandible is a relatively valuable predictor of difficult visualization. A patient with a distance of 6.5 cm or less often presents difficulty with visualization.[39, 40] A bedside measurement along the ramus of the mandible from the anterior surface of the neck to the tip of the chin can also be predictive. Generally, a distance of less than three finger breadths (5 cm) in an adult warns of potential difficulty with visualization.

During a preinduction examination, one should also gently palpate the cricothyroid membrane to establish its location in the individual patient and to improve one's skill at rapidly identifying this vital portal to the tracheal lumen. Evaluation of the nares may reveal trauma or obstruction by inflammation or polyps.

When Is Adjunctive Radiologic Assessment Useful?

Radiologic assessment of the airway by lateral radiograph, computed tomography, or magnetic resonance imaging to ascertain potential problems with intubation is generally used in patients with unusual airway problems such as croup, epiglottitis, cervical spine abnormalities, or head and neck tumors.[41–43]

Should Endoscopic Examination Be Performed?

Judicious use of indirect laryngoscopy can reveal characteristics of the upper airway with minimal trauma or preparation. Preinduction endoscopic evaluation probably should be reserved for those instances when a decision must be made about whether to perform a tracheotomy before anesthetizing the patient.

In most other circumstances, if endoscopic evaluation is necessary, one should probably proceed directly with awake endoscopic intubation using appropriate sedation and topical anesthesia. Preinduction airway instrumentation should not be performed in patients with lesions such as epiglottitis or pharyngeal abscess. Even a small increase in edema secondary to trauma during evaluation can convert marginal patency into complete obstruction.

What Are the Technical Errors of Concern?

Flaws in technique can impede visualization regardless of the airway anatomy (Table 55–5). The impact of not opening the mouth sufficiently or failing to achieve proper head position is obvious, as is that of using a laryngoscope with weak batteries or a faulty light source. Selecting a blade of appropriate size is also essential to ensure that it can reach appropriate structures and yet not fill the oral opening with an unnecessarily large "footprint."

Blade Placement

Inappropriate placement of the laryngoscopic blade tip significantly impairs visualization. Placement of a straight blade tip between the epiglottis and tongue does not render sufficient stretch of the hyoepiglottic ligament to lift the epiglottis. Placing the tip of a curved blade under the epiglottis to force it against the tongue pulls the entire larynx into a more anterior position, again impeding visualization.

Inexperienced endoscopists often insert the laryngoscope blade too deeply into the pharynx, passing the epiglottis and perhaps even the laryngeal opening. Subsequent efforts to locate the epiglottis or to identify anatomic landmarks are fruitless. This problem is especially prevalent with straight blades, which can easily be inserted to the esophagus. When faced with completely unfamiliar anatomy, it is often advisable to withdraw the blade gradually. The larynx or epiglottis often falls down into view, and one can proceed without repeating laryngoscopy.

Alignment of the Blade Axis

Failure to align the blade axis with the midline is another common error. If the blade is oriented into the lateral pharynx,

TABLE 55–5. Technical Errors That Interfere with Intubation

Position and Approach	Laryngoscopy
Table is too low for easy visualization	Blade placed on center of tongue
Head is too far posterior	Blade not well oriented into the midline
Neck is not sufficiently extended	Blade too short to reach proper position
Mouth is not opened wide enough	Blade inserted far beyond epiglottis
Excess cricoid pressure distorts anatomy	Blade tip positioned wrong with epiglottis
Excess secretions obstruct view	Low batteries yield dim laryngoscope light
View of glottis is obstructed by tube	Light goes out during laryngoscopy
Tube not rigid enough	
Practitioner unfamiliar with anatomy	

visualization of the larynx is often impossible. Failure to insert the blade along the right margin of the tongue often allows a curtain of tongue to hang over the right side and obstruct a clear view. Pivoting the blade like a lever around its junction with the handle usually distorts the airway anatomy or pulls the larynx upward out of view. Visualization is much better served by pulling along the axis of the handle, as if the handle were sliding along a rigid wire fixed to a point about 2 feet above the patient's knees. Levering the laryngoscope blade also increases the risk of dental trauma.

Why Won't the Tube Pass Through the Vocal Cords?

Once the glottis has been located, inability to pass a tracheal tube into the trachea is a major impediment to securing the airway. Sometimes there is insufficient room to pass the tube past the laryngoscope blade, or the tube obstructs the view of the larynx when inserted into the mouth. This latter difficulty frequently occurs in patients with small oral openings or protuberant teeth. However, it is most often caused by failure to introduce the blade along the right margin of the tongue or to displace the blade and tongue sufficiently to the left. Correcting these errors in technique usually provides ample room to observe the tube passing through the vocal cords. Having an assistant retract the right corner of the mouth can also widen the portal available for tube introduction. A pliable tube may prevent adequate tip positioning or direction to be transmitted to the tip. These problems are solved through the use of a tube stylet. Laryngeal or tracheal pathology occasionally prevents passage of the anticipated size tube. Decreasing tube size by 1 French size increments until one fits is helpful.

Alignment of the Tube and Tracheal Axes

Inability to pass the tube through the vocal cords under direct visualization is frequently caused by misalignment of the tracheal lumen and the tube.

With appropriate head positioning and laryngoscopic technique, a view directly down the tracheal lumen sometimes allows a bright laryngoscope light to reflect off the carina. If the head is positioned too far posteriorly, the trachea may be visible but the lumen is oriented toward the floor, forcing the tip of the endotracheal tube to impinge on the posterior arytenoids or the tracheal wall. Keeping the head as mobile as possible (even suspended) during laryngoscopy allows minor adjustments in position to facilitate passage of the tube.

A solo operator may need to adjust head and neck orientation by using the laryngoscope as a pivot point. Having a skilled assistant to help manipulate the head can markedly improve the operator's ability to achieve proper orientation while decreasing laryngoscopic trauma. An assistant also can use his or her free hand to facilitate observation or to manipulate the orientation of the larynx.

Stylets

Curvature of the endotracheal tube itself can cause misalignment between the tracheal lumen and the tube tip. The tube tip often impinges on the anterior commissure when a sharp, hooklike stylet curvature is used or when the tube is introduced with its curvature in the sagittal plane. Straight stylets

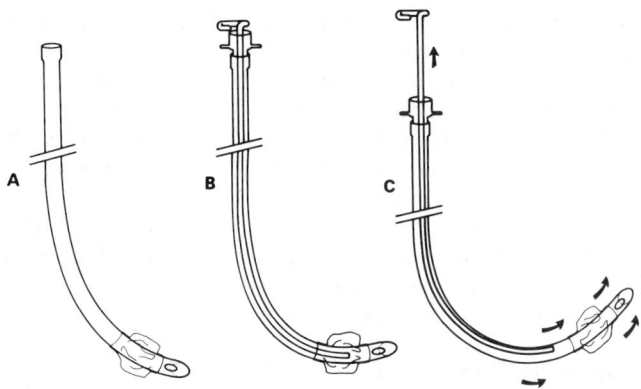

FIGURE 55–2. Effect of partial stylet withdrawal on the shape of an endotracheal tube. *A*, Tube without stylet. *B*, Tube with stylet inserted and tip angulated. *C*, Tip of tube displaced anteriorly as a result of partial stylet withdrawal.

cause posterior impingement. A gradual hockey stick configuration in the stylet and introduction of the tube with its curvature oriented more toward the coronal plane may help to orient the tip down the axis of the trachea. This coronal orientation also reduces visual obstruction from the tube and helps hold the right mouth border out of the way. If the stylet is the culprit, causing the tube to hang up at the laryngeal inlet, partial withdrawal in effect softens the tip of the tube and allows passage into the trachea. An additional benefit of partial stylet withdrawal is that if the stylet tip is bent into a J configuration, withdrawing it several centimeters brings the tip of the tube anterior (i.e., toward the difficult-to-visualize glottis) (Fig. 55–2).

Lubrication

Lack of lubrication is probably inconsequential when considering difficulty in passing a tube through the vocal cords. However, appropriate lubrication may reduce abrasion of the

vocal cord edges and the tracheal mucosa. The effect on post-intubation sore throat is unclear. Apposition of the vocal cords secondary to laryngospasm obstructs passage of a tracheal tube tip. The tube should not be forced past a laryngospasm, because it is possible to abrade, tear, or avulse the vocal cords. It is more appropriate to wait for the laryngeal muscles to relax or to use positive pressure or neuromuscular relaxation to resolve laryngospasm.

Tube Diameter

In a normal adult airway, tracheal diameter seldom limits passage of a tube, given minimal attention to choice of an appropriate tube size. However, tube diameter is often a problem in small pediatric patients, because the narrowest portion of the trachea is subglottic. Table 55–6 serves as a guide for selecting an endotracheal tube of appropriate diameter. An abnormal subglottic narrowing caused by unrecognized tracheal stenosis, tracheal webs, or tracheomalacia occasionally impedes passage of an appropriately sized tube in an adult, as does a vascular malformation or a tumor in the tracheal wall.

Tracheal Cross-Sectional Area

Reduction of tracheal cross-sectional area caused by mucosal edema from inhalation injuries, pregnancy, or prolonged bronchospasm usually does not interfere with passage of a tube of appropriate size, although choosing a slightly smaller tube than usual may decrease mucosal injury.

The trachea is relatively rigid, but an external mass can compromise the lumen, especially if pressure is on the posterior wall or the mass has gradually eroded the cartilaginous rings. More often, an external mass causes tracheal deviation, which interferes with tube passage by either realigning the tracheal axis laterally or actually bending the lumen. Tracheal fracture or crush injury secondary to blunt trauma also impedes or prevents intubation.

TABLE 55–6. Approximate Tracheal Tube Diameter and Length

| Age | Weight | Tracheal Tube Size Diameter | | | Anatomic Distance | | |
		Inside Diameter (mm)	*French*	*Lengths (cm)**	*Teeth to Cords (cm)*	*Teeth to Carina (cm)*	*Sagittal Diameter Trachea (mm)*
Premature	<5 lb	2.5	12	10	7	11	
Term infant to 3 mo	8	3	14	11	8	12	4
3–12 mo	10–20	3.5	16	12	8.5	13	7
2 y	20–25	4	18	14	9	14	8
3 y	30–35	4.5	20	15	9	14	
4 y	35–40	5.0	22	16	9		
6 y	40–45	5.5	24	16	9.5	15.5	9
8 y	55–60	6	26	18	9.5	16	9
10 y	65–70	6.5	28	18	10	17	4
12 y	80–90	6.5	28	20	10	17	
14 y	90–140	7	30	22	11	18	10
16 y	100–150	7.5	32	24	12	20	11–15
Adults	130–200	F 8	34	24	15		13–23
		M 8.5	36	24			
60 +		F 8.5	38	24		22	
		M 9	40	24			

(From Dripps RD, Eckenhoff JE, Vandam LD: Anesthesia: The Principles of Safe Practice. Philadelphia, WB Saunders, 1988, p 19.)
*Add 2–3 cm for nasotracheal tube.

NASAL INTUBATION

What Problems Are Unique?

Unexpected difficulty is often encountered when passing an appropriately sized nasotracheal tube through the nostril into the posterior pharynx. The tube must be inserted perpendicular to the plane of the face in order to avoid turbinate impingement. The bevel should face the septum to avoid catching on the inferior turbinate. Once the turbinates have been passed, turning the tube so that the bevel faces the occiput helps deflect it into the oropharynx.

Nostril Preference

If the left nostril is either more patent or equally patent, it is to be recommended for nasal intubation. This is a consequence of the orientation of the bevel at the tip of the tube. Thus, if one enters via the left side, contact anywhere within the glottic opening or up to one tube diameter left of it results in deflection of placement through the cords (Fig. 55–3). Placement via the right nostril requires that the tube tip (i.e., the right side of the tube) enter the airway opening, in effect decreasing the target size by the diameter of the tube. This approach presupposes that tubes placed via the nose enter the oropharynx via the midline or biased toward the side from which they are inserted.

Anatomic Abnormalities

Various anatomic abnormalities can interfere with passage, including a deviated nasal septum, mucosal edema, or tumor mass. Cystic fibrosis or aspirin allergy suggests the possibility of nasal polyps, and a history of drug abuse might warn of septal ischemia or necrosis. If the radius of curvature of the tube is markedly different from that of the nasopharynx, the tip may impinge against the posterior wall. Specialized tubes allow shortening of the tube curvature using a pull ring installed in the tube wall.

Excessive Force of Insertion

Gentle sustained pressure along the tube often overcomes a minor degree of tissue resistance without undue trauma. Use of excessive force increases the incidence of epistaxis, nasal trauma, submucosal dissection, or perforation of the cribriform plate. Force can be limited during insertion by holding the tube loosely between the thumb and index finger and inserting with a slow, smooth, rotary motion of the wrist. Be prepared to use the other nostril or a smaller tube or to switch techniques if unusual resistance is encountered, because assessment of nasal patency by history or observation of airflow is relatively unreliable.

Infectious Complications

Transient bacteremia usually occurs after nasal intubation.[44, 45] The risk of sinusitis or otitis is also increased by tubal obstruction of sinus openings or eustachian passages.[46, 47] Nasal intubation is relatively contraindicated in immunocompromised patients, and prophylactic antibiotics are indicated in those at risk for endocarditis.

Epistaxis

Epistaxis precipitated by passage of a relatively rigid nasotracheal tube through the highly vascular nasal passages can significantly interfere with subsequent visualization and upper airway management. Severe bleeding in a paralyzed or deeply anesthetized patient may lead to blood aspiration and hypoxemia in extreme cases.

Appropriate Tube Size

The risk of hemorrhage can be greatly reduced by choosing an appropriate nasotracheal tube size (6.0–6.5 mm inside diameter [ID] in adult women, 6.5–7.5 mm ID in adult men), by warming the tube before insertion in order to decrease its stiffness, and by generously lubricating both the nares and the tube. One should avoid introducing lubricant into the tube lumen, especially when using lidocaine jelly, which can dry and harden and decrease tube patency.

Topical Vasoconstrictors

Use of a topical vasoconstrictor in the nares is strongly recommended before insertion of a nasotracheal tube. Administering a few drops of 4% cocaine solution yields effective vasoconstriction with negligible systemic uptake, as well as desirable topical anesthetic in awake patients. Spray or droplet administration of phenylephrine or oxymetazoline mixed with a local anesthetic is also useful.[48, 49] Application of vasoconstrictor using cotton-tipped swabs, a vaporizer, or nasal spray distributes the drug on the nasal mucosa and affords an opportunity to gently probe and dilate the nasal passage (Table 55–7).

Submucosal Dissection

During passage of a nasotracheal tube, an operator occasionally feels the subtle "give" of the tube passing into the pharynx and yet is unable to locate the tube tip during subsequent laryngoscopy. The tube has sometimes not been advanced far enough for the tip to appear in the pharynx. However, disappearance of a nasotracheal tube can indicate dissection of the tube tip along a fascial plane at the sharp angulation of the posterior nasopharynx (Fig. 55–4). More careful scrutiny of

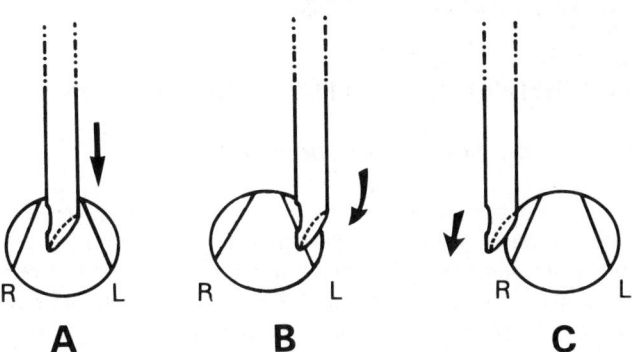

FIGURE 55–3. Effect of endotracheal tube bevel orientation on ease of nasal intubation. *A*, Tube tip in midline. *B*, Tube tip biased toward the right (note that it would deflect laterally away from the glottic opening). *C*, Tube tip biased to left (note that if bias is not greater than one tube diameter, the bevel deflects it medially).

TABLE 55–7. Common Topical Nasal Decongestants

- Prophylhexedrine (Benzedrex) inhaler (250 mg)
- Naphazoline HCl (Privine), 0.05% nasal spray or solution
- Tetrahydrozoline HCl (Tyzine), 0.05% and 0.1% nasal solution
- Oxymetazoline HCl (Afrin, others), 0.025% and 0.05% nasal solution (spray or drops)
- Xylometazoline HCl (Otrivin, others), 0.05% and 0.1% nasal solution (spray or drops)
- Epinephrine 1:50,000 to 1:2000 nasal solution (spray)
- Phenylephrine HCl, 0.125% to 1% nasal drops and 0.25% to 1% nasal spray

(Data from Weiner N: Norepinephrine, epinephrine, and the sympathomimetic agents. *In* Goodman's and Gilman's the Pharmacological Basis of Therapeutics. Gilman AG, Goodman LS, Dall TW, et al (eds). New York, Macmillan, 1985, p 145–180.)

the posterior pharynx may reveal the tube lying under a translucent layer of tissue. Because this fascial plane communicates with the mediastinum and chest cavity, it is important to observe the tube tip in the pharynx during laryngoscopy, or to hear breath sounds during "blind" intubation before advancing the tube toward the glottis.

A shallow dissection limited to the upper pharynx usually resolves with only observation and perhaps prophylactic antibiotic coverage. However, a deeper dissection may precipitate hematoma formation, mediastinitis, or pneumothorax. Attempted ventilation through a dissected nasotracheal tube can precipitate a life-threatening pneumomediastinum.

Cribriform Plate Perforation

Perforation of the cribriform plate is another, more serious, cause of a "lost" nasotracheal tube tip. Subsequent brainstem injury or central nervous system infection can lead to serious postintubation morbidity. Potential for perforation is the major

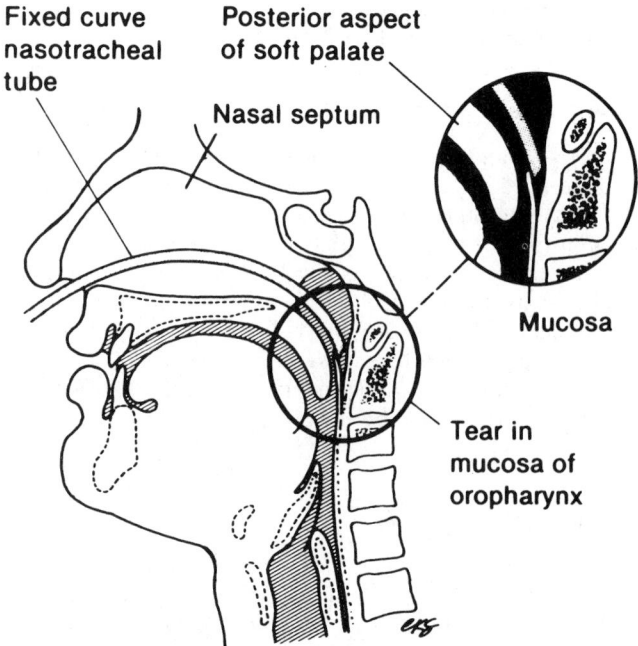

FIGURE 55–4. Laceration of the pharyngeal mucosa at the posterior edge of the soft palate allows a nasotracheal tube tip to dissect along a fascial plane outside the pharynx. (From Benumof JL: Special intubating techniques for adults (blind nasotracheal intubation). *In* Clinical Procedures in Anesthesia and Intensive Care. Philadelphia, JB Lippincott, 1992, p 153.)

reason why passage of a nasotracheal tube is inadvisable if a patient exhibits evidence of basilar or Le Fort's skull fractures, nasal fracture or contusion, cerebrospinal fluid rhinorrhea, or other head trauma.[50]

Orientation of the Tube Tip

Passage of a nasotracheal tube tip from the pharynx into the trachea can present significant difficulty. Orientation of the tube along the posterior pharynx may make it difficult to bring the tip sufficiently anterior to pass the posterior commissure and enter the trachea. Use of a McGill's forceps or some other instrument to grasp the tube tip so that its orientation can be changed is helpful. Having an assistant gradually advance the tube while the operator manipulates the head or directs the tip with forceps is effective.

When Is Blind Nasal Intubation Indicated?

In circumstances in which laryngoscopy proves impossible or the stress of laryngoscopy might be particularly detrimental, a blind nasal approach; that is, intubation of the trachea without aid of direct visualization may be indicated.[51] This technique involves a "hit-or-miss" effort using breath sounds heard through the tube or palpation of the neck to assess tube tip position.

Failure of Blind Nasal Intubation

Difficulty in intubating the trachea during blind nasal intubation is usually secondary to misalignment of the tube axis with respect to the tracheal inlet. Obstruction to passage usually indicates tip advancement into the vallecula, pyriform sinus, or supraglottic structures. Slight flexion or extension of the head usually assists with anteroposterior positioning, and rotation of the tube rectifies a problem with impingement on the lateral pharyngeal wall or in the pyriform sinus.

Be particularly gentle while probing the pharynx to locate the tracheal inlet, because major vocal cord or laryngeal trauma can occur secondary to repeated attempts at insertion. In a cooperative patient, attempts to guide the tube tip using forceps are sometimes useful, although success is less than with direct visualization. Threading a smaller catheter or a flexible stylet through the tube lumen and between the vocal cords and having a cooperative patient sit slightly forward may facilitate passage into the trachea.[52]

POTENTIALLY DIFFICULT INTUBATION

What Is the Best Anesthetic Plan?

Unfortunately, no reliable, easily measured index predicts difficult intubation.[22, 34, 38, 53–55] Many problems become evident only when intubation is actually attempted. The most worrisome airways often prove straightforward to manage, whereas relatively normal-appearing patients can present marked difficulties. In many instances, an ancillary medical condition such as a full stomach, a history of bronchospastic airway disease, decreased FRC, or cervical spine pathology limits options for dealing with the airway.

The anesthetic plan must be tailored to the skill and experience of the individual anesthesiologist, the severity of the patient's underlying medical conditions, and the type and urgency of the planned surgical procedure. There is no optimal clinical approach. Each time one is faced with a potentially difficult intubation, a clinical plan must be "customized" after weighing all of these factors. However, a practitioner should always have a well-conceived and practiced drill to use in case life-threatening airway emergencies arise.[56]

General Considerations

A few general principles are worth considering. Comprehensive preparation before induction of an anesthetic is essential when faced with a potentially difficult intubation.

Equipment

An assortment of endotracheal tubes, laryngoscope blades, and ancillary equipment (e.g., stylets, forceps), necessary to meet every conceivable problem with the intubation, should be at hand. Backups should also be available in case equipment fails or becomes contaminated during a difficult induction. Aids such as light wands or fiberoptic instruments and supplies required to secure an emergency transtracheal airway; for example, cricothyroidotomy or tracheotomy kits should be available on the anesthesia cart for immediate use.

Assistants

Whenever possible, one or more skilled assistants with experience in airway management should be mobilized. It may be appropriate to ensure availability of a skilled surgeon in emergency airway intervention, especially when dealing with anatomic abnormalities that might compromise airway patency. Before induction, the primary surgeon must be fully apprised of the anesthesiologist's concerns about intubation. Open communication solicits the primary surgeon's input and defuses potential interprofessional disagreements about operating room delays or subsequent complications.

Patient Preparation

Whatever approach one chooses, patients must be carefully prepared. Therapy for a patient's underlying medical conditions should be optimized because physiologic stresses elicited during a difficult intubation can be greater than usual. Exaggerated SNS-mediated reactions to repeated airway manipulation, transient hypoxemia and hypercarbia, or vacillating anesthetic depth can cause marked tachycardia or hypertension, increasing the risk of perioperative ischemia.[55, 58]

Medications. Risk also is increased if therapy with nitrates, β-adrenergic blockers, or calcium channel blockers was interrupted during preparation for surgery. Taking the appropriate time to supplement medication regimens and to use invasive monitoring before induction can decrease the comorbidity associated with management of a difficult airway.

Patients with bronchospastic airway conditions also demand compulsive preparation. Peri-induction treatment with inhaled β-mimetic drugs and topical anesthesia of the airway should reduce the possibility of bronchospasm in response to upper airway manipulations. Similarly, delay of surgery or administration of histamine$_2$ blockers, metoclopramide, or antacids is appropriate in patients considered at increased risk for gastric aspiration.

Nasogastric Tubes. A previously inserted nasogastric tube can be left in place.[59, 60] However, the relatively rigid tube crossing facial contours interferes with achieving a seal if facemask ventilation becomes necessary. Because the tube might also interfere with gastroesophageal sphincter integrity and increase the likelihood of regurgitation, it may be preferable to remove it before induction. The efficacy of inserting a gastric tube to decompress the stomach before induction is doubtful.

Which Anesthetic Techniques Are Preferable?

Selecting an anesthetic technique for a patient who might be difficult to intubate is a highly individualized matter.

Anesthetic Risks

A regional technique to avoid the need to deal with a problematic airway is sometimes selected. However, the potential always exists for an intravascular injection or an excessively high anesthetic level that necessitates emergency airway management and controlled ventilation.

If a regional technique is chosen, all equipment needed to immediately secure the airway must still be at hand. Whenever possible, lower-risk regional techniques should be used (e.g., monitored anesthesia care, digital or ankle blocks versus axillary or spinal, respectively) to minimize the chances of precipitating an airway disaster. Excessive sedation of a patient to achieve sufficient anesthesia with a "safe" minor regional technique can cause equally dangerous airway problems.[61]

General Anesthesia

If a general anesthetic is selected or required, the height of the table, the head position relative to the edge, and shoulder elevation all should be arranged according to the operator's preference before induction. A 2- to 3-inch head support usually yields sufficient extension without creating an exaggerated sniffing position.

In patients at risk for aspiration, the relative value of Trendelenburg's or reverse Trendelenburg's positions is unclear. Placing a patient in head-up position may reduce the risk of passive regurgitation, but it also establishes a gravitational gradient for vomitus from the mouth into the trachea. Conversely, placing a patient in the head-down position allows vomitus to gutter out the side of the mouth but may enhance passive regurgitation. The author prefers to keep the table in a level position while constantly assessing for foreign matter in the pharynx.

Should a Difficult Airway Be Secured Before Induction?

When inducing a general anesthetic for a patient with a difficult airway, a conservative approach is often the safest. Take as few irrevocable steps as possible. Initially, a decision must be made whether to secure the airway before inducing unconsciousness with "awake" intubation or to induce the anesthetic and then perform intubation.

Problems with Awake Intubation

Awake intubation can reduce the risks of aspiration, because airway reflexes are intact, and the risk of hypoxemia or hypercarbia, because spontaneous ventilatory drive and intrinsic airway patency are undisturbed. However, awake laryngoscopic intubation can be psychologically and physiologically more stressful than intubation after induction. Patients' struggling markedly reduces the chance of successful intubation, increases morbidity from cervical or cranial fractures, and accentuates the degree of oral, dental, or laryngeal trauma. Laryngoscopic stimulation also precipitates vomiting, breath holding, or laryngospasm, which further interferes with airway management.

Irritation of the larynx or tracheal mucosa during attempted intubation causes significant increases in airway resistance, especially in patients with reactive airways disease or those recovering from upper respiratory tract infections.[62–64] Hypertension, tachycardia, or dysrhythmia secondary to SNS responses may precipitate myocardial ischemia, as well as unacceptable increases in intraocular or intracranial pressure.[65–67]

Sedation and Analgesia

The impact of awake laryngoscopy and intubation can be minimized. Judicious administration of sedatives and analgesics can decrease the psychologic stress of the procedure and the autonomic response to direct airway stimulation. When administering sedatives, avoid suppressing upper airway reflexes, spontaneous ventilatory drive, or airway patency and choose from those for which a pharmacologic antagonist is available. Application of topical local anesthetics to the pharyngeal mucosa in gel or nebulized form can reduce the afferent stimulus from airway manipulation.[68–71]

Superior laryngeal or glossopharyngeal nerve blocks, intravenous lidocaine, or translaryngeal local anesthetic solution also reduces the sensitivity of the upper airway.[72–74] Again, be wary of interfering with a patient's ability to deal with regurgitation or vomiting during attempted intubation. Intravenous fentanyl or esmolol can also help control hypertension and tachycardia secondary to laryngoscopy and intubation.[36, 75]

How Should the Trachea Be Intubated?

In patients exhibiting morbid obesity or restricted neck mobility, gentle direct laryngoscopy can be performed with a patient awake to determine whether key landmarks are easily identified. Depending on the degree of difficulty visualizing the epiglottis or posterior arytenoids, one might choose to remove the laryngoscope and intubate after induction, to perform the awake oral intubation directly, or to retrench and use a different approach.

Awake Blind Nasal

In a conscious patient, stress and trauma from laryngoscopy can be decreased with an awake blind nasal technique. Nevertheless, this approach may still cause significant cardiovascular responses.[76] It is particularly useful when excess sedation or cardiovascular stress might be threatening (e.g., a patient with pulmonary edema due to acute ischemic cardiomyopathy).

Technique

After appropriate sedation and application of topical anesthetics and vasoconstrictors (see Table 55–7), a well-lubricated nasotracheal tube is gently introduced into the naris and passed into the posterior pharynx. The tube is then incrementally advanced during inspiration without direct laryngeal visualization. The position of the tube tip is assessed by palpation of the neck, by listening for breath sounds through the open tube end, or by capnometry.[77]

Phonation or palpable mouth ventilation after passage of the tube tip below the level of the glottis almost invariably indicates esophageal intubation. Inadvertent esophageal intubation is relatively inconsequential during blind nasal intubation, because a patient is still ventilating spontaneously through the vocal cords (assuming that the stomach is not distended with gas during subsequent attempts to corroborate tube placement).

Contraindications

Blind nasal intubation is relatively contraindicated in patients with facial trauma, potential skull fractures, coagulopathy, or nasal anatomic abnormalities. Absence of spontaneous ventilation significantly decreases the chances of successful blind nasal intubation, so caution should be used while administering medications that depress ventilatory drive. During blind nasal intubation, coughing, gagging, or transient laryngospasm can induce significant arterial desaturation. Every patient should undergo denitrogenation with 100% oxygen at high flows and inspire the highest possible oxygen concentration during intubation attempts. One approach is to attach the tube to the anesthesia breathing circuit with the pop-off valve in the open position to provide a high FIO_2 during awake nasal intubation.

Light Wands

Another approach involves use of a lighted stylet passed through the endotracheal tube and out the tip.[78–81] The stylet/tube combination is advanced through the mouth toward the anterior glottis, probing gently for the tracheal inlet. In a darkened room, it is obvious when the brightly lit stylet tip enters the tracheal lumen because transillumination of the tracheal wall is observed over the cricothyroid membrane. The tube is then advanced over the stationary stylet into the trachea. A flexible fiberoptic bronchoscope can be used in analogous fashion if blood and secretions obscure the view.

Transillumination can also be used to corroborate placement of a tube within the trachea, although false-positive findings can occur in thin individuals.[82] Illuminated rigid stylets can cause pharyngeal or laryngeal trauma while the tracheal opening is probed and are generally not applicable for use during nasal intubation. Flexible lighted tubes and stylets are available to facilitate blind nasal intubation.

Fiberoptic Techniques

Use of a fiberoptic instrument is probably the most definitive approach for viewing the larynx during a difficult intuba-

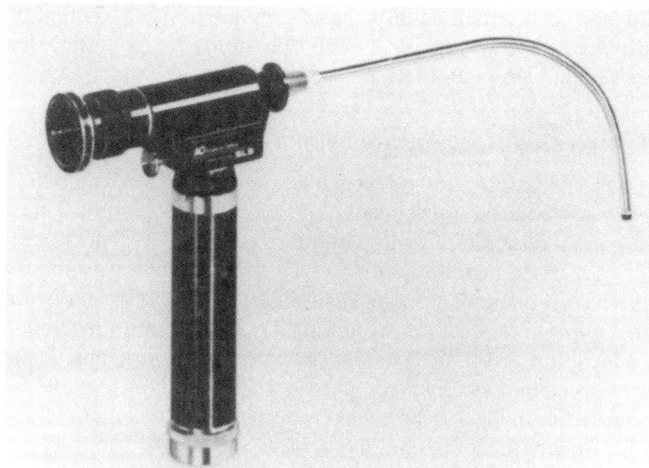

FIGURE 55–5. A flexible fiberoptic stylet for orotracheal intubation. (From Patil VU, Stehling L, Zauder HL: Instrumentation and auxiliary equipment. *In* Fiberoptic Endoscopy in Anesthesiology. Chicago, Year Book Medical Publishers, 1983, p 15.)

tion. Although fiberoptic intubation aids are available in various configurations, they generally fall into malleable and flexible categories.

Malleable Fiberoptic Laryngoscopy

A malleable fiberoptic intubating laryngoscope is basically a stylet containing fiberoptic bundles that both illuminate the stylet tip and transmit a magnified image from the tip to an eyepiece in the handle (Fig. 55–5).

Technique. An appropriately sized endotracheal tube is threaded over the stylet, and the tube/stylet combination is advanced through the mouth toward the glottis.[83] The stylet tip is maneuvered under direct visualization by manipulating the entire instrument. Once the operator observes the stylet tip pass through the vocal cords, the endotracheal tube is advanced into the tracheal lumen and the fiberoptic stylet is removed.

Limitations. Malleable fiberoptic stylets are easy to maintain and can be used with minimal preparation. They are particularly useful when visualization is impeded by unusual head and neck anatomy (thick neck, micrognathia, temporomandibular joint limitations, or a large, relatively immobile epiglottis). However, the relatively small fiberoptic tip is prone to obstruction with secretions or blood, and some models do not offer a suction port. Friable or inflamed airway tissues can be acutely traumatized by the stylet tip during attempted intubation. The stylet is too stiff for nasal introduction and cannot be easily manipulated unless introduced through the mouth.

Flexible Fiberoptic Laryngoscopy and Bronchoscopy

A flexible fiberoptic laryngoscope or bronchoscope is the most versatile and useful intubating aid available.[39, 84–86]

Technique. An appropriately sized endotracheal tube is threaded over the fiberoptic trunk of the scope, which is then gently advanced into the pharynx via either the oral or nasal route. Under direct visualization through the scope, the scope is guided toward the glottis and through the cords, using both handle rotation and built-in guide filaments to adjust orienta-

tion. Once the tip passes into the tracheal rings, the endotracheal tube is advanced into the trachea, and the scope is removed.

Indications. Flexible fiberoptic instruments are particularly useful to assist with intubation in the presence of anatomic distortion in the upper airway or when temporomandibular joint mobility is severely compromised by trismus or oral fixation. They offer a suction port to assist with clearance of secretions and, when properly used, cause minimum tissue trauma in airways compromised by tumors or inflammatory processes.

Transtracheal Approaches

For particularly difficult intubations, it may be necessary to electively use a transtracheal approach to secure the airway.

Retrograde Intubation

One technique involves identification of the tracheal lumen through the cricothyroid membrane and retrograde passage of a thin catheter or guidewire from the trachea past the vocal cords into the pharynx (Fig. 55–6). This guide is then extracted from the mouth and threaded through the lumen or Murphy's eye of the tracheal tube.[87–89] The tube is advanced over the guide through the vocal cords into the trachea, and the guide is then gently withdrawn through the cricothyroid membrane.

Antegrade Intubation

Alternatively, the initial thin guide can be used to pull a second, more rigid guide anterograde into the trachea to facilitate passage of the tracheal tube past the glottis.

Another approach involves passing a suture retrograde into the pharynx, fixing it through the end of the tube, and "pulling" the tube through the vocal cords. The suture can then be cut and the remaining small nub extracted with extubation. Numerous variations of this technique are possible.[90–93]

Elective Tracheotomy

An elective tracheotomy is probably the safest and most efficacious means of securing a difficult airway by a transtra-

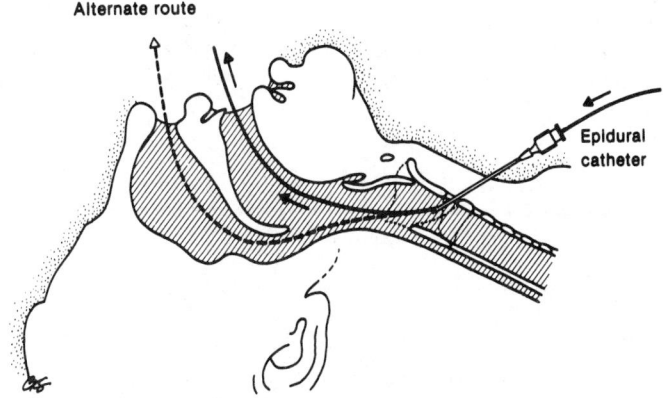

FIGURE 55–6. Retrograde intubation. A pliable wire or catheter is threaded retrograde across the cricothyroid membrane into the oropharynx or nasopharynx to guide a tracheal tube through the glottis. (From Benumof JL: Special intubating techniques for adults (retrograde intubation). *In* Clinical Procedures in Anesthesia and Intensive Care. Philadelphia, JB Lippincott, 1992, p 161.)

cheal route in an awake patient. However, the intrinsic risk of the procedure and the potentially undesirable long-term sequelae of tracheotomy must be weighed against the risks of other approaches. At this point in a patient's care, the need for the proposed surgical procedure should also be considered. It may on occasion be safer and more ethical for the surgeon and anesthesiologist first to confer and then convince the patient that a purely elective or discretionary procedure is not worth the inordinate risk of the required anesthetic.

INTUBATION AFTER ANESTHETIC INDUCTION

An alternative approach to a potentially difficult intubation is to attempt intubation *after* induction of general anesthesia. This course is often chosen when airway difficulties do not appear severe or when the potential stress of awake intubation poses an unusually high risk of morbidity.

Difficulties with visualization or intubation are often discovered after induction and an initial attempt at laryngoscopy, at which time there is no choice but to proceed. Whether one anticipates difficulty with intubation or not, it is always prudent to observe basic conservative approaches to airway management. Assiduous attention to setup, patient positioning, and denitrogenation is vital.

The choice of technique must be predicated on the unique spectrum of potential airway problems each individual patient presents. Before induction, an anesthesiologist must have a clear therapeutic plan that includes a series of alternatives should the primary intervention prove impossible to achieve. Indications for intubation are listed in Table 55–8.

Is General Anesthesia with a Mask Acceptable?

If none of the conditions or requirements enumerated in Table 55–8 is present, difficult intubation may be avoided by performing a general anesthetic using a facemask technique.

A decision to proceed with a facemask anesthetic as an alternative to securing a difficult airway should not be made lightly. Anatomic variations that interfere with visualization during laryngoscopy often render maintenance of a facemask airway difficult as well. When the anesthetic depth increases, a marginal facemask airway frequently deteriorates as pharyngeal tissues relax or fatigue decreases the operator's ability to maintain mechanical airway support. Attempts to overcome

TABLE 55–8. Indications for Intubation

- Requirement for prolonged positive-pressure ventilation (e.g., use of muscle relaxants)
- Surgical manipulation
- Patient positioning
- Table positioning
- Body habitus
- Respiratory depression due to general anesthetics
- Airway protection in the presence of a full stomach
- Symptomatic esophageal reflux
- Upper airway trauma
- Requirement to avoid surgical field during upper airway, head, or neck surgery

airway obstruction using positive-pressure assisted ventilation often cause air insufflation into the stomach, increasing the risk of sudden regurgitation.

Unexpected Need for Intubation

On occasion, an unexpected indication for intubation emerges as surgery proceeds. The anesthesiologist must then attempt a difficult intubation under relatively emergent circumstances when conditions for airway management are suboptimal. Such manipulations or resuscitative measures can disrupt the surgical procedure, promoting breaks in sterile technique or technical errors by relatively inexperienced surgeons. If the airway cannot be secured, the option of backing out of the anesthetic and using an awake approach or rescheduling the operative procedure is not available.

Given these risks, it is sometimes more prudent to secure the airway by electively performing a difficult intubation without a firm indication rather than to commence a facemask general anesthetic and risk disaster during the surgical procedure. This decision can be made only after weighing the quality of the patient's airway, the nature and duration of the surgical procedure, and the skill and confidence of the anesthesiologist.

What Steps Are Useful If Direct Laryngoscopy Fails?

Changes in Position

If initial attempts at laryngoscopy fail, several straightforward interventions may facilitate intubation in individual circumstances. A shift in a patient's position sometimes improves visualization, especially if the head is insufficiently elevated. Extreme posterior displacement of the head over the edge of the table, as during rigid bronchoscopy, occasionally facilitates visualization of the glottis, although passage of the tracheal tube is often difficult from this orientation.

Manipulation of the larynx may also help, either by clarifying the anatomy or by moving the glottis into view.[53, 94, 95] Gentle displacement of the thyroid cartilage posteriorly and in a caudad or cephalad direction sometimes yields good results. Having a colleague attempt intubation provides a fresh orientation or a slight variation in technique that can yield a successful intubation in a significant number of instances. Never let pride stand in the way of seeking such help.

Change in Laryngoscope Blade

A change in the laryngoscope blade configuration sometimes dramatically improves visualization. When the distance from the oral opening to the glottis is inordinately long, merely choosing a larger blade often improves one's ability to manipulate the epiglottis and achieve visualization. Controversy about the relative merits of different laryngoscope blades is often rooted in an individual practitioner's experience and level of confidence with one type. It is unclear whether cardiovascular response varies with the type of blade used during a well-executed laryngoscopy.[96]

Advantages of a Straight Blade

A slender, straight blade such as the Miller's 3 often optimizes tissue displacement and yields the clearest view, especially in a patient with a thick, immobile neck or a large, floppy epiglottis. A straight blade is easier to insert through a narrow oral opening or past protuberant teeth and has a lesser propensity to obstruct vision.

Successful use of straight blades generally requires more assiduous attention to placement. Absence of a large flange is an advantage (insertion into a small mouth) but allows a curtain of tongue to drape over the right edge of the blade unless it is correctly advanced along the right tongue margin. The blade may be advanced laterally or past the epiglottis into the esophagus.

Special Handles and Blades

Various custom blades and handle attachments are available to enhance visualization during difficult intubation.[97] Some practitioners increase mechanical advantage of the blade tip or change the angle of the blade to the handle, and others rely on indirect vision with prisms or mirrors. The efficacy of any one device is predicated on individual experience and opinion. If a practitioner believes such devices are useful, he or she should choose one or two and become intimately familiar with them by using them in many routine intubations. The worst time to learn how to use an innovative laryngoscope is during attempted intubation of a difficult airway.

A short laryngoscope handle may be more efficacious in difficult intubations.[98] It is easier to manipulate over the upper chest in patients with limited neck mobility or obesity, and it may improve grip and feel. However, a regular laryngoscope handle angled 45° to the right during blade insertion has a similar effect and facilitates passage.

Blind Approaches

If visualization is still problematic, completion of intubation may be achieved without a clear view of the tube passing through the vocal cords. Attempting a "blind shot" orotracheal intubation when visualization is poor often results in esophageal intubation, increasing the risk of aspiration and wasting valuable time. Blind nasal intubation in the absence of spontaneous ventilation also carries an inordinately high risk of esophageal intubation.

Esophageal Visualization

It is sometimes necessary to visualize the esophagus and then to gently probe with the tube tip above the area of visualization where the trachea must be located. Using the styletted tube to lift the epiglottis can yield a slightly better view of the arytenoids and facilitate placement.

Stylets and Light Wands

Another useful blind approach is to thread the stylet or the long plastic tip of a disposable laryngotracheal anesthesia (LTA) syringe through the Murphy's eye of the endotracheal tube (Fig. 55–7). The stylet or syringe tip is used to probe gently for the tracheal inlet.[95, 99, 100] Once it is introduced into the trachea, the endotracheal tube can be advanced over it through the vocal cords. A similar approach can be taken using a light wand. Great caution must be exercised with these techniques to avoid trauma to the vocal cords or perforation of the pharynx or trachea.

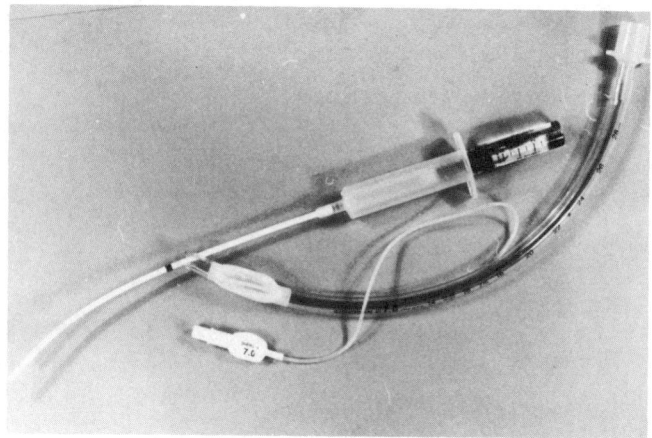

FIGURE 55–7. Laryngotracheal anesthesia (LTA) device threaded through the Murphy eye of an endotracheal tube as an aid to insertion through the vocal cords.

Fiberoptic Techniques

Intubation techniques can be switched after induction as long as the patient can be ventilated and oxygenated safely by facemask. Intubation may be avoided if a laryngeal mask airway provides adequate ventilation and airway protection.[15, 101] Fiberoptic techniques can be successfully used after induction, although lack of spontaneous ventilation imposes time constraints that may make such intubation more difficult to complete.

Direct Glottic Palpation

In special circumstances, directly palpating the glottis and guiding the tracheal tube tip with the finger tips can facilitate intubation. This tactile approach is most useful with severe forms of facial trauma or when the anesthesiologist is forced to attempt intubation from a disadvantageous position (e.g., replacement of a displaced tube in a prone patient). Great caution should be used to prevent the fingers from being trapped should the patient suddenly react to the stimulus with clenching of the masseter muscles.

When Are Transtracheal Approaches Indicated?

Ideally, transtracheal techniques for securing the airway should be used electively under controlled circumstances. Retrograde cannulation can be used after induction but probably is more effective in conscious patients. If tracheotomy or cricothyroidotomy is required to secure the airway after induction, the patient should first be awakened whenever possible. Tracheotomy can then be calmly performed under local anesthesia.

Emergency transtracheal intubation should be performed only when all other techniques to secure the airway have failed and severe hypoxemia is imminent. Anesthesiologists should be familiar with transtracheal intubation techniques and should always have a clear plan of action in case they are required under emergency circumstances.

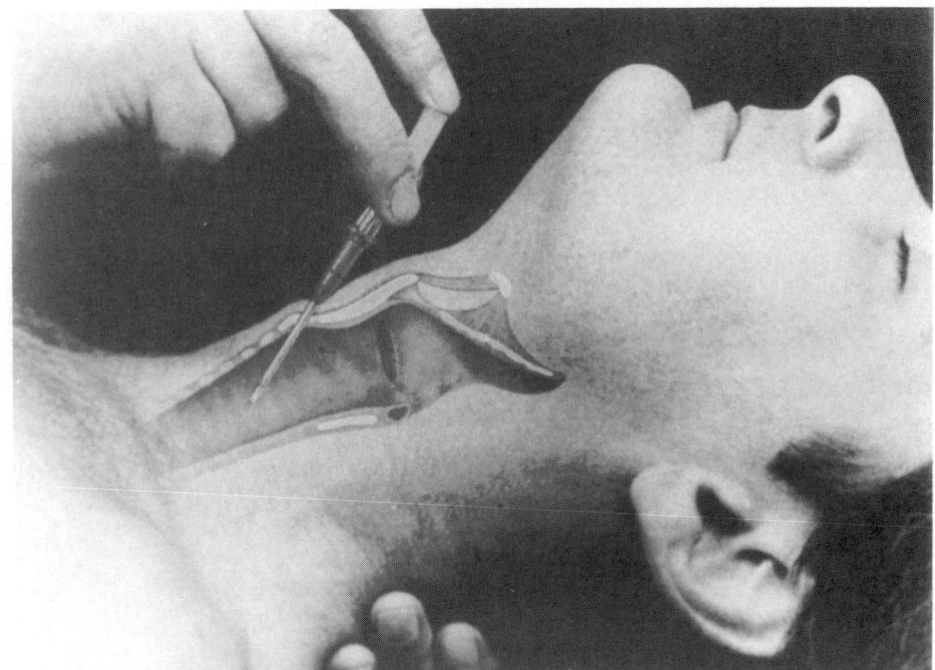

FIGURE 55–8. Cricothyroidotomy using a large-bore (12–14-gauge) intravenous catheter. (From Benumof JL: How to do transtracheal ventilation. *In* Clinical Procedures in Anesthesia and Intensive Care. Philadelphia, JB Lippincott, 1992, p 199.)

Techniques

Cricothyroid Catheter Insertion

If transtracheal intubation is essential, insertion of a large-caliber intravenous catheter (2–3 inch, 12–16 gauge) through the cricothyroid membrane into the tracheal lumen is the most reliable way to deliver 100% oxygen (Fig. 55–8). Although it is possible to maintain oxygenation through such a catheter, sustained CO_2 excretion is marginal.[102–106]

Even though aspiration of air through a fluid-filled syringe signals catheter entry into the tracheal lumen, the catheter can easily perforate the trachea and enter the esophagus or advance into a fascial plane in the neck. Corroboration of tracheal placement is difficult, because breath sounds are faint.

It is important to have a readily available means of attaching the catheter hub to a high-pressure oxygen source and of

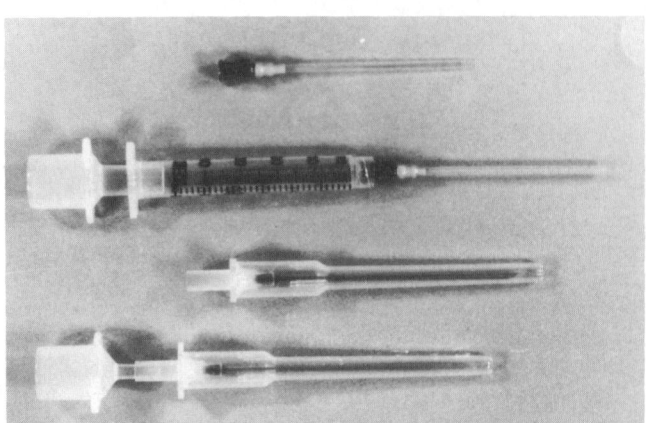

FIGURE 55–9. Devices for attaching a cricothyroidotomy catheter to a positive-pressure source for ventilation. An adapter from a 3.0 mm–ID pediatric tracheal tube fits directly into the Luer-Lok on the catheter (*lower*). An adapter from a 7.0 mm–ID endotracheal tube fits into the barrel of a 3-mL syringe, which in turn engages the Luer-Lok on the catheter (*upper*).

stabilizing the catheter so it is not dislodged or kinked (Fig. 55–9). A 3-mL syringe barrel fitted with an adapter from a 7.0-mm internal diameter tracheal tube provides an easily grasped connection to an anesthesia fresh gas hose (high-pressure source).[107] A 3-mm tracheal tube adapter also fits tightly into standard Luer-Lok catheters.[108]

High driving pressure is required to overcome flow resistance through the small-diameter catheter; use of the reservoir bag is ineffective. If a jet ventilator is not readily available, the oxygen flush apparatus on the anesthesia machine can deliver an adequate pressure-flow profile.[109]

Care should be taken to ensure that passive exhalation can occur through the normal airway. A complete airway obstruction that prevents escape of gas via the glottis greatly increases the risk of pneumothorax, subcutaneous emphysema, and other barotrauma during transtracheal jet ventilation.[110]

Cricothyroidotomy

Cricothyroidotomy and intubation with a small tracheal tube may be considered.[111–113] Custom kits with a trocar and tube are commercially available.

When successful, this approach allows sufficient ventilation to control hypercarbia and sustain oxygenation. However, under emergency circumstances, the success rate for an inexperienced operator is relatively low. Lack of appropriate instruments to spread and maintain the portal into the tracheal lumen often complicates tube insertion. Perforation of the esophagus or dissection into neck tissues is a common complication, as is hemorrhage, which interferes with subsequent attempts to secure the airway.

Tracheotomy

Emergency tracheotomy is a complicated, risky procedure that carries a high morbidity rate even when performed by skilled surgeons.[114] This alternative should be used only by anesthesia personnel with extensive experience and when less invasive approaches across the cricothyroid membrane are judged to be inappropriate.

Should Neuromuscular Relaxants Be Used in Difficult Intubation?

Visualization is improved through better anatomic displacement of neck structures after paralysis of striated muscles in the pharynx and neck. The necessary force to achieve visualization is reduced, decreasing trauma during laryngoscopy. Paralysis prevents development of laryngospasm in response to airway manipulation, facilitating better facemask ventilation and easier passage of a cannula into the trachea.

One negative aspect of neuromuscular relaxation is that it nullifies pharyngeal and laryngeal reflexes that protect against aspiration and reduces the contribution of striated muscle tone toward maintaining upper airway patency. Paralysis of the diaphragm, intercostal, and abdominal rectus muscles eliminates the ability to ventilate spontaneously or to clear the airway with forceful expiration.

General Considerations

Indications for neuromuscular relaxation and appropriate dosages and timing of administration vary widely with clinical circumstances and individual preference. A few general concepts warrant discussion when considering management of a difficult intubation.

Facemask Ventilation

Whenever feasible, be absolutely confident of your ability to adequately ventilate a patient by facemask before administering neuromuscular relaxants. The quality of a facemask airway should be assessed using capnography and precordial auscultation. Clinical impressions derived from evaluation of chest wall movement, vapor condensation in clear masks, or compliance of the reservoir bag are poor substitutes.

Demonstrating one's ability to ventilate by facemask before paralysis does not guarantee that ventilation after paralysis will be problem free, because relaxation may decrease airway patency. However, it is almost always possible to maintain arterial oxygen saturation until paralysis wears off and the patient resumes spontaneous ventilation.

Succinylcholine

Before a difficult intubation, a small dose of a very short-acting relaxant such as succinylcholine produces the shortest duration of paralysis consistent with achieving laryngoscopy and tracheal intubation. With this approach, a failed intubation does not require the anesthesiologist to ventilate through a facemask for a prolonged period. If additional laryngoscopy is necessary, one must proceed without paralysis or repeat the relaxant administration.

Nondepolarizing Agents

An alternative approach to relaxant use for a difficult intubation involves administration of an intermediate-duration nondepolarizing relaxant such as atracurium, vecuronium, or mivacurium. Although these medications necessitate pro-

longed facemask management of a paralyzed patient if the airway is not secured, they ensure reliable paralysis for subsequent intubation attempts. This approach should probably be used only when the ability to ventilate by facemask is absolutely certain and when the anesthesiologist is confident that repeated attempts at laryngoscopy will lead to successful intubation.

Long-acting nondepolarizing drugs like pancuronium or pipecuronium should not be used to facilitate intubation of a difficult airway. The duration of paralysis from intermediate-acting drugs can always be extended by readministration.

Does a Full Stomach Change the Approach to Difficult Intubation?

The risk of pulmonary aspiration following recent food or liquid ingestion or as a result of increased intra-abdominal pressure, hiatal hernia, pregnancy, or bowel obstruction presents unique challenges. A potentially difficult airway compounds the complexity and risk inherent in an anesthetic induction.

Awake Intubation

Anesthesiologists generally use one of two approaches to secure the airway in patients at risk for regurgitation and aspiration. The first involves awake intubation using one of the previously discussed blind or fiberoptic techniques in conjunction with appropriate sedation and airway anesthesia. Preservation of airway reflexes (i.e., limiting anesthesia to above the vocal cords) offers some protection against aspiration if regurgitation occurs during intubation attempts. Spontaneous ventilation is maintained, decreasing the risk of hypoventilation and hypoxemia if the intubation proves difficult.

Because sedation and airway anesthesia must be limited to maintain airway reflexes, awake intubation is unpleasant and is associated with significant hypertension and tachycardia. Optimal conditions for laryngoscopic intubation, which are achieved with induction of unconsciousness and neuromuscular paralysis, are precluded by this approach.

Rapid-Sequence Induction and Intubation

As an alternative, rapid-sequence induction, specifically conceived to reduce the risk of regurgitation, may be attempted. As the name implies, this technique is, by design, rapid in onset to allow quick laryngoscopy and short in duration to allow quick resolution of sedation and paralysis in case it is necessary to abort and allow the patient to regain consciousness. Important elements include compulsive denitrogenation, application of cricoid pressure to inhibit passive regurgitation, avoidance of mask ventilation before paralysis to minimize gastric insufflation, and aggressive laryngoscopy and intubation at the earliest possible moment.

Risks

Several risks are inherent in rapid-sequence induction.

Cardiovascular Stress. The short time between commencement and intubation precludes reliably establishing an anesthetic level sufficient to blunt physiologic responses to airway stimulation, so cardiovascular stress can be problematic.

Aspiration. Airway reflexes are completely obliterated, so the risk of aspiration is increased if regurgitation occurs. Although Sellick's maneuver is relatively effective in preventing passive regurgitation, increased gastric pressure secondary to distention and active vomiting before onset of paralysis can force gastric contents into the pharynx.[115]

Inability to Ventilate. Failure to intubate the trachea necessitates facemask ventilation. At best, this action prolongs the interval of risk for aspiration and promotes insufflation of air into a potentially distended stomach. In the worst-case scenario, ventilation may be impossible.

There is still no substitute for succinylcholine for rapid-sequence induction.[116] In this circumstance, one must choose immediately between another, often desperate attempt at intubation, cricothyroidotomy, or waiting for resolution of paralysis and airway obstruction. Unfortunately, these measures must often be performed in the presence of rapidly evolving hypoxemia or during cardiopulmonary resuscitation.

Alternative Approaches

When the risk of vomiting and aspiration is low, a few cautious low-pressure inflations can be given before laryngoscopy. Intravenous lidocaine in conjunction with short-acting β-adrenergic blocking agents minimizes cardiovascular responses. Topical anesthetics, superior laryngeal nerve blocks, or translaryngeal lidocaine administration before rapid-sequence induction may also attenuate these acute responses. Rapid-sequence induction should always be followed by oral intubation. If a nasal approach is required, intubation should be performed using an awake technique.

Does Reactive Airways Disease Affect the Approach to Difficult Intubation?

Unusual airway reactivity complicates difficult airway management. Patients with reactive airways disease manifest an inordinate reflex response to a stimulus in the airways, most likely triggered by rapidly adapting irritant receptors in the trachea.[68] Stimuli include blunt mechanical stimulation from laryngoscopy, suctioning, or intubation; release of histamine by drug reactions; "chemical" irritation of airway mucosa from inhalation anesthetics; or poor central integration of airway reflexes during light anesthesia. Potential responses to these stimuli include gagging, laryngospasm, and bronchospasm. The presence of any of the clinical conditions listed in Table 55–9 suggests a higher likelihood of increased airway reactivity.

Upper airway irritability with increased propensity to cough and laryngospasm often is evident in patients with predisposing factors (Table 55–9).

General Considerations

Whenever possible, a procedure should be delayed until an upper respiratory tract infection has cleared. Cessation of smoking for a period before surgery is frequently recommended, but its value is unclear with respect to airway reactivity. Appropriate preoperative control of anxiety and fear smooths postinduction airway management. Bronchodilator and steroid regimens should be optimized, and consultation for additional modalities should be secured whenever a patient's baseline condition warrants. Preinduction inhalation therapy

TABLE 55–9. Predisposition to Increased Airway Reactivity

Smokers
High level of preinduction anxiety
Upper respiratory tract infections, inflammatory conditions
Asthma
Bronchospastic chronic obstructive pulmonary disease

with nebulized β-mimetic medications or steroids decreases the baseline airway smooth muscle tone in patients with bronchospastic disease.

Induction Agents

Propofol seems to reduce upper airway reactivity immediately after induction, facilitating facemask ventilation in patients prone to coughing or laryngospasm. Intravenous lidocaine as part of the induction sequence decreases reactivity of both the upper and the small airways.[68, 117] Sodium thiopental may cause histamine release and bronchospasm, although this phenomenon is rarely significant. Gradual deepening of anesthesia with a potent inhalation agent delivered through a facemask, especially halothane, because it is least pungent, promotes bronchodilation and decreases airway receptor sensitivity. Small incremental increases in the inhaled concentration usually do not elicit cough, laryngospasm, or bronchospasm.

Techniques

Awake Intubation

Awake intubation involves greater difficulty and risk in patients with reactive airways because it is often impossible to fully attenuate airway sensitivity. Excessive coughing or gagging impedes laryngoscopy or passage of a tracheal tube while increasing the cardiovascular sequelae of the manipulation. Stimulation of the larynx or tracheal mucosa may also trigger bronchospasm, which can be so severe that spontaneous and controlled ventilation through the tracheal tube is impossible.

General Anesthesia

Intubation after induction of anesthesia is usually desirable. Progressive deepening of the anesthetic with an inhalation agent is difficult if problems are encountered with initial facemask ventilation. Accentuation of airway responses as the induction agent wears off further impedes airway management. However, a sufficiently deep level of anesthesia and bronchodilation usually can be achieved to allow laryngoscopy and intubation with minimal airway response.

If one chooses to induce anesthesia before intubation, a compromise must be struck between the risks of aspiration and severe bronchospasm. In general, the morbidity of aspirating gastric contents is far greater than that of intraoperative bronchospasm; therefore, most practitioners orient the induction toward securing the airway as quickly as possible.

Addition of a low concentration of potent inhalation anesthetics to the oxygen flow during denitrogenation attenuates bronchospasm without seriously affecting airway reflexes or the level of consciousness. In severely asthmatic patients, an inhalation induction can be initiated, followed by a switch immediately to a rapid-sequence intravenous technique just before airway protection or consciousness is lost.

TUBE PLACEMENT

How Is It Verified?

Various indices can be used to ensure intubation of the trachea.[25, 118] Which is most reliable or yields the smallest number of false-positive determinations is inconsequential. None is categorically foolproof; thus, each entails a variable risk of an error in diagnosis. Because the consequences of not recognizing a misplaced tracheal tube are catastrophic, a comprehensive, logical string of several different assessments is in order to minimize the chances of overlooking an esophageal intubation (Table 55–10).[119]

Direct Observation

The most effective means of ensuring tracheal placement is direct observation of the tube tip and cuff passing through the vocal cords. This sign obviously is not useful during blind nasal or tactile intubation and can be unreliable if distorted anatomy or difficult exposure precludes a clear view of the vocal cords.

A high degree of intellectual objectivity must be exercised when relying on this observation, for on occasion a practitioner honestly recalls what was desired rather than what actually was observed. If a clear, unobstructed view of the inserted tube resting between the spread vocal cords is not obtained, confidence in the observation is misguided.

Before removal of the laryngoscope, it is also valuable to visualize the esophageal opening to ensure that the tube has not been introduced into this orifice. These observations can be completed without lengthening the duration of laryngoscopy. After removal of the laryngoscope and attachment of a positive-pressure ventilation source to the tracheal tube, a second series of critical observations should be made.

Compliance and Volume Return

Pulmonary inflation usually can be accomplished at low pressures (<20 cm H_2O), with a slight decrease in perceived compliance toward the end of the expansion. During exhalation, the same volume should be returned to the reservoir.

Gastric ventilation usually feels different from pulmonary ventilation, but not in any predictable way. Initial inflation of a flaccid, empty stomach may mimic a lung inflation with respect to pressure and compliance, but gas return usually is dramatically decreased, because the stomach is a ''nonelastic'' organ without any retractile characteristics. Inflation of a distended stomach requires inordinately high pressures and yields a stiff and noncompliant feeling. However, gas still moves more freely than it does if high pressure is secondary to airway resistance or straining. Return from a distended stomach can feel halting and abrupt, lacking the sustained quality of a passive, retractile lung deflation.

Perceived compliance is affected by a patient's muscle tone, FRC, intra-abdominal pressure, and airway resistance. Increased airway resistance interferes with the evaluation of volume return, and loss of volume through the pop-off valve during inflation renders evaluation of compliance and expiratory return essentially useless. Assessment of compliance and volume return using any pressure source other than a quality anesthesia reservoir bag and a low-compliance circuit is unreliable.

This assessment is subjective and affected by experience and concentration. However, it requires no additional time or effort. More quantitative analysis of inflation pressures is time-consuming and difficult to interpret, given the variability among patients and clinical conditions.

Chest Wall Excursion

Lateral and anterior excursion of the chest wall should also be evaluated with the first compression. At the same time, observe that the stomach is not incrementally expanding. A clear view of the chest wall and epigastrium is essential, and the observations are unreliable if these areas are covered by clothing, piled blankets, or surgical drapes. Reliability also varies with body habitus and clinical condition.

Patients with severe chronic obstructive lung disease often exhibit marked epigastric excursion but relatively little chest wall movement during positive-pressure ventilation. Chest wall versus abdominal movement is difficult to assess in obese or pregnant patients and patients with abdominal distention. If a patient is straining or coughing, expansion is absent.

Because of its relative unreliability, this sign must always be used in conjunction with more definitive observations. However, assessment can be accomplished during the first attempt at ventilation, so it does not lengthen the time necessary to confirm tube placement.

Moisture Condensation

As the first breath is exhaled, glance at the endotracheal tube to observe condensation of vapor on the tube wall. A dense vapor haze that clouds the tube wall indicates that exhaled air is fully humidified and, therefore, most likely emanates from the airways rather than the stomach. However, gastric ventilation generates some vapor condensation, especially if exhaled gas from the lungs has been introduced into the stomach during difficult facemask ventilation.

Although observation of vapor is comforting and does not consume valuable time, it is sufficiently nonspecific to be an unimportant criterion for corroborating tube placement.

Auscultation of Breath Sounds

Auscultation of the lungs is an important index of tracheal tube position. Hearing clear airflow over the lung fields indicates tracheal placement, and comparison of breath sound intensity over each lung evaluates potential mainstem intubation. Accurate results can be obtained with various approaches.

TABLE 55–10. Suggested Sequence to Corroborate Tracheal Intubation

1. The tube tip is observed passing through the vocal cords.
2. The esophageal opening is observed and is not intubated.
3. Compliance of initial hand inflation seems appropriate.
4. Return of delivered tidal volume into the reservoir is rapid and smooth.
5. Chest inflation and deflation are noted with compression/release.
6. The stomach does not distend with inflation.
7. Vapor is observed condensing on the internal tube wall.
8. Clear inspiratory sounds are auscultated in the right axilla.
9. Inspiratory sounds are clearly absent or softer over the stomach.
10. Uniform, high-amplitude carbon dioxide waves appear on capnography.
11. Appropriate oxygen saturation persists on oximetry for 10 minutes.

If doubt persists, perform laryngoscopic confirmation or reintubation!

Auscultation between the mid and anterior axillary lines at approximately the level of the third rib, lateral to the pectoralis major muscle, is easily accessible and sufficiently removed from the contralateral lung to minimize transmitted breath sounds. In addition, the thoracic fat pad is notably thin under the arms, allowing auscultation close to the ribs.

To minimize the time necessary, auscultate the right side first. Because the vast majority of mainstem intubations occurs in the right bronchus, absence of breath sounds on the right immediately signals a high likelihood of esophageal intubation. In contrast, absence of left-sided breath sounds may be attributable to either an esophageal intubation or a right mainstem intubation.

Evaluation of breath sounds is not foolproof. The intensity of sounds varies with the thickness of insulating tissue, distance of conducting airways from the chest wall, inflation volume, airway caliber, flow rates, and a host of other factors. No matter how intensive the breath sounds are over the lung fields, it is essential to auscultate over the stomach as well. If more intense breath sounds are heard over the stomach than over the lung fields, assume that an esophageal intubation has occurred until proven otherwise.

Exhaled Carbon Dioxide

Analysis of exhaled CO_2 content using a capnograph is undoubtedly the most reliable index of tracheal intubation, but it can yield both false-negative and false-positive findings.[120] CO_2 evolution is preferable as the final confirmation rather than the initial evaluation of tube placement. A short delay between the first inflation and the appearance of the first few CO_2 tracings on the capnogram reflects the time necessary for the aspirated sample to arrive at the machine and to be processed. In these few seconds, the entire previously mentioned analysis (i.e., observation of chest excursion and vapor in the tube, evaluation of compliance and return, auscultation of breath sounds) can be completed.

If the stomach has been inflated with expiratory gas, several small-amplitude CO_2 curves can appear after an esophageal intubation. Initial assessment of more traditional indices such as breath sounds and compliance permits several CO_2 tracings to appear on the capnograph, and any progressive decrease in amplitude is then readily evident.

Other devices qualitatively indicate the presence of CO_2 in expired gas. Although these devices facilitate diagnosis of tracheal intubation when a capnograph is not available, they are inferior to capnographic analysis.

Miscellaneous Observations

Do not rely on pulse oximetry as an early way to corroborate tracheal intubation. Diagnosis and intervention for esophageal intubation should be completed before hypoxemia generates arterial desaturation. The role of esophageal detector devices, which use the ability to aspirate air freely from the tracheal tube as an indicator of tracheal placement, is unclear.[121, 122]

Other clinical observations indicate tracheal intubation but are relatively nonspecific, require additional time for assessment, and do not significantly improve the yield of the analysis. For example, before attaching the circuit, one can lightly press on the anterior chest wall while listening to the end of the tracheal tube. A soft whoosh of displaced air from the tube suggests tracheal placement.

Ease of achieving a cuff seal is another index of tube placement. Because the esophagus is a flaccid structure, a seal is difficult to obtain with usual degrees of cuff inflation. A persistent leak during positive-pressure inspiration may indicate esophageal intubation.

Observation of tracheal rings with a fiberoptic bronchoscope advanced through the tube is a reliable method of corroboration but is rather impractical for day-to-day use.

Direct Laryngoscopy

The final assessment involves immediate laryngoscopy and confirmation that the trachea has been intubated. If laryngoscopy does not absolutely confirm tracheal placement, consider immediate reintubation. Although this decision must be made in view of specific circumstances, it is often appropriate to secure the airway rather than to temporize. Resist momentary indecision, denial, or false hope that matters will improve by themselves. Understandable reluctance to again tackle a difficult airway only wastes valuable time, making the inevitable intervention far riskier and more difficult to complete.

Summary

When all signs indicate appropriate tracheal placement, one should still carefully watch for hypoxemia or disappearance of CO_2 curves for several minutes, because no combination of assessments is guaranteed correct in every instance. Even though this evaluation is comprehensive and involves multiple cross-checks, circumstances occasionally leave some doubt about the location of a tracheal tube. Always assume that difficulty with ventilation or oxygenation after intubation could be the result of an esophageal intubation.

ESOPHAGEAL INTUBATION

A well-conceived plan of action is essential in case the esophagus has been intubated. Ventilation and oxygen delivery to the lungs must be immediately restored with minimum risk of aspiration. A few different approaches to this problem are acceptable, depending on individual circumstances.

Is Immediate Extubation of the Esophagus Indicated?

The most common response is immediate extubation of the esophagus and reintubation of the trachea. Cricoid pressure and ventilation with 100% oxygen before laryngoscopy should be used. The risk of hypoxemia during subsequent laryngoscopy must be balanced against the risk of regurgitation under the facemask caused by possible gastric distention.

Candidates for facemask ventilation include elective surgical patients at lower risk for aspiration, patients who presented difficulty with visualization during the initial laryngoscopy, and those who exhibit signs of arterial hypoxemia or hypercarbia on extubation of the esophagus.

When Should the Esophageal Tube Be Left in Place?

An alternative approach to resolving esophageal intubation is to leave the esophageal tube in place with the cuff inflated while another tracheal tube is inserted into the trachea. The esophageal tube isolates the stomach from the airway relatively well, leaving only the correct orifice available for intubation during subsequent laryngoscopy. The esophageal tube can also vent the stomach or provide ready access for gastric decompression after reintubation. This approach is most appropriate in patients with significant gastric dilation who are at high risk for regurgitation and aspiration, although it can be used in any patient.

Problems

The esophageal tube can interfere with subsequent laryngoscopy and visualization, especially if the oral opening is small or temporomandibular joint motion is limited. The tube also interferes with achieving a mask seal if one chooses to attempt facemask ventilation before or between subsequent laryngoscopies. A marginal seal can sometimes be achieved by placing the esophageal tube across the soft portion of the cheek and pressing the facemask pillow over it. It should not be advanced into the mouth to fit under the facemask.

Leaving the esophageal tube in place may also increase the risk of incidental trauma during subsequent intubation of the trachea, because two rigid bodies with inflated cuffs will be occupying a relatively limited space and entrapping delicate tissue between them. After intubation, be sure to keep the two tubes clearly identified, in order to avoid inadvertently attaching the esophageal tube to the breathing circuit or accidentally removing the tracheal tube when the time comes to extubate the esophagus.

No matter which approach one chooses, caution must be exercised when the esophageal tube is finally removed. Extubation of the esophagus is sometimes immediately followed by regurgitation, which increases the risk of aspiration even if the trachea has already been secured with a second tube.

DIFFICULT VENTILATION AND OXYGENATION

Inability to ventilate a patient immediately after tracheal intubation is another harrowing airway difficulty occasionally encountered. Extraction of oxygen by pulmonary blood flow progressively reduces the PaO_2 during the intubation process.[123, 124] Interruption of ventilation during tube placement also fosters a gradual rise in $PaCO_2$, with a coincident fall in arterial pH. After a period of marginal facemask ventilation or a prolonged intubation sequence, the arterial oxygen saturation rapidly decreases and hypercarbia may be well advanced.

Once tracheal intubation is completed and the tube is attached to a positive-pressure gas source, a relatively large volume of fresh gas should flow into the lungs with a relatively small change in pressure at the tube inlet. If ventilation cannot be effected, only seconds are available to implement a solution.

How Is Ventilation Assessed?

Cyclic positive airway pressure (<30 cm H_2O) should create smooth, large-volume expansions of the chest with passive return of delivered volume after each cycle. Auscultation of precordial breath sounds should indicate low-velocity flow in

TABLE 55–11. Inability to Ventilate After Intubation

| Can Pressure Be Generated in the Circuit? | |
No	Yes
Likely Causes of Loss of Gas Volume from the Circuit	*Likely Causes of Obstruction of Gas Flow into the Lungs*
• Pop-off valve is open	• Inspiratory limb is occluded
• Feed from machine to circuit is disconnected	• Tracheal tube is kinked or bitten closed
• Reservoir bag is disconnected	• Tube is occluded by secretions or foreign body
• Connection of circle to tube is disconnected	• Tube tip is jammed against airway wall
• Capnograph or temperature probe port is open	• Foreign body has been forced into trachea
• Tracheal tube cuff is deflated	• Intubation has caused severe bronchospasm
• Tracheal tube is displaced into pharynx	• Patient is coughing or straining
• Tracheal tube is in esophagus	• Tension pneumothorax has developed
• Fresh gas flow is not turned on	• Rigid chest has developed
• Ventilator reservoir bag selector switch is in intermediate position	• Tube is in esophagus or closed tissue space

an uninterrupted to-and-fro pattern. Capnographic sampling reveals a series of CO_2 curves with uniform amplitude and steep upstroke.[125]

Is a Circuit Leak Present?

Determine whether it is possible to generate positive pressure in the circuit or ventilating device (Table 55–11). If gas volume is dissipated without the generation of positive pressure, a major leak exists between the gas source and the lungs.

Circuit Connections

The potential sources for leakage increase with the complexity of the ventilating device. In an anesthesia circuit, the most likely points are at removable circuit connections (circle fresh gas line from the machine, circuit tubes to valve inlets and outlets, reservoir bag, and the circuit Y-piece to the tracheal tube). If the integrity of the anesthesia machine circuit was carefully checked immediately before induction, it is unlikely that the reservoir bag has ruptured or that an internal machine leak has suddenly developed.

Open Ports

Small caps on circuit ports for capnography tubing or temperature probes can be displaced during circuit manipulations, causing large leaks. Other common sources include an open pop-off valve or a deflated endotracheal tube cuff. In some breathing circuits, if the anesthesia reservoir-ventilator detector switch is in an intermediate position, this acts as a low-pressure pop-off valve into the ventilator.

Cuff Leaks

A cuff that was checked before induction may lose its integrity during the intubation process. Cuffs can be lacerated on dental appliances or on sharp bony spicules during passage through the nasal cavity. Improvements in cuff design have made spontaneous cuff rupture on inflation an exceedingly rare event.

Herniation of a portion of the endotracheal cuff above the cords sometimes presents as a "recurring cuff leak," but loss of gas volume from the circuit generally is inconsequential. Cautious deflation, tube advancement, and reinflation rectify this problem.

A large leak may indicate that head movement or traction caused the endotracheal tube tip to slip back into the pharynx[13, 126] or that the tube was inserted into the esophagus. Corroboration of correct tube placement is obviously of the utmost importance.

What Alternative Sources of Ventilation Can Be Used?

If a cause of the lack of pressure in the circuit is not found, an alternate pressure source should be immediately secured to ventilate the patient rather than to waste more valuable time trying to find the leak. Every anesthetizing location should have either a self-inflating breathing bag or a transport oxygen tank with a ventilating device immediately available for emergency use, as well as a circulating nurse or assistant free to obtain it.

In the event that an alternative pressure source fails, the anesthesiologist can always inspire 100% oxygen from the circuit fresh gas flow (the anesthetic agents *must* be turned off) and perform mouth-to-tube ventilation.

Is Impedance to Gas Flow Present?

Compression of the reservoir bag may generate high pressure in the circuit but not cause sufficient airflow into a patient's lungs. Impedance to gas flow generally results from a dramatic increase in resistance along the flow pathway or from a significant decrease in the patient's pulmonary compliance.

Assessment of the potential causes helps to divide a large number of problems into smaller categories (Table 55–11). Excessive airway pressure increases the potential for pneumothorax or subcutaneous emphysema.[127] High airway pressure can also impede venous return, decreasing cardiac output and increasing intracranial or intraocular pressure.

Why Does Increased Resistance Occur?

High resistance to gas flow must occur in the circuit or between the tracheal tube inlet and the patient's exchanging air spaces. Because circuit patency and proper machine valve function are checked before induction, a significant increase in resistance appearing in the circuit immediately after intubation is unlikely. Nevertheless, the inspiratory limb must be checked to make sure it has not been pinched closed.

Endotracheal Tube Kinking

The cross-sectional area of the tracheal tube may be reduced by kinking, clamping between the patient's clenched teeth, or entrapment in a mouth gag. It is unlikely that a tube kink would occur immediately after intubation, because bending of tracheal tubes in the mouth and pharynx generally occurs with warming or unusual head positioning. At this point, the tube is still relatively cool and rigid and should lie along a large, smooth radius of curvature in the pharynx. However, kinking may occur if the tube is bent in half against the posterior pharyngeal wall rather than inserted into the trachea.

Luminal Obstruction

An alternative cause is occlusion of the tube lumen by secretions or by an unrecognized foreign body in the pharynx or trachea. Herniation of an inflated cuff over the end of the tube, although a historical problem, is nearly impossible with contemporary tubes. Doubt about endotracheal tube patency can be quickly dispelled by passing a suction catheter or stylet down the tube.

Outlet Obstruction

A final cause of endotracheal tube obstruction results from impingement of the tube tip against the carina, tracheal wall, or some other pliable tissue mass. Although rare, outlet occlusion can occur even in tubes with both end and side ports, especially if they are advanced too far.

Impingement is difficult to diagnose by passing a catheter down the lumen. Gently withdrawing an adult endotracheal tube 0.5 to 1.0 cm essentially eliminates the possibility that impingement is causing luminal obstruction. This small movement should not cause inadvertent extubation with an appropriately placed tube. However, withdrawal should be stopped if resistance is felt from the inflated cuff pulling against the vocal cords.

Bronchospasm

If the circuit and tracheal tube are patent, high resistance to gas flow must reside somewhere in the distal trachea or branching airways. Excepting rare possibilities such as critical tracheal stenosis, occluding tumors, or an unrecognized foreign body pushed down into the trachea during intubation, increased airway resistance almost always resides in small airways.

Characteristics

Bronchospasm is usually moderate in severity, so some fresh gas can be delivered to peripheral air spaces using increased airway pressure. However, in patients with severe airway disease, increased resistance to gas flow can be so marked that it becomes impossible to deliver appreciable ventilation. High-pitched sounds of turbulent gas flow through constricted airways can sometimes be auscultated, but absence of wheezing does not indicate absence of bronchospasm when gas flow is so attenuated that no sound is produced.

Management

When bronchospasm interferes with ventilation, oxygen should be administered using a very gradual inspiration with medium airway pressures, in order to optimize oxygen delivery with low inspiratory flow rates. This approach also maximizes laminar and minimizes turbulent gas flow. Long expiratory pauses should be provided to allow complete emptying of distal air spaces, even if ventilation is insufficient to maintain CO_2 excretion for the first few minutes. Hypercarbia from moderate hypoventilation is less significant than that caused by trapping of expired gas when a subsequent breath is delivered before exhalation is complete.

Moderate concentrations of a potent inhalation anesthetic are effective in reducing constriction of airway smooth muscle, both through a direct effect and by reducing the stimulus causing bronchospasm. Halothane, enflurane, and isoflurane are essentially equivalent with respect for efficacy for bronchodilation. It is usually possible to deliver some inhaled anesthetic through the constricted airways, so deepening anesthesia often resolves the bronchospastic episode. Addition of an aerosolized β-mimetic agent into the fresh gas mixture can also be effective. Commercially available metered dose inhalers can be introduced directly into the Y-piece of the circuit using special adapters or readily constructed fittings.

Severe bronchospasm also impedes the delivery of bronchodilating medications to the small airways. Although subcutaneous terbutaline or epinephrine might be efficacious, rapid bronchodilation can be achieved with intravenous epinephrine. Continuous infusion is preferable, both to avoid dysrhythmias and hypertension from inadvertent high serum levels and to allow easy discontinuation should complications arise. As little as 0.0025 to 0.005 $\mu g \cdot kg^{-1} \cdot min^{-1}$ causes sufficient smooth muscle relaxation to allow restoration of ventilation and delivery of other bronchodilating medications to the airways. Intratracheal administration also yields a rapid effect, but with less control of serum levels. Neuromuscular relaxants have no effect on bronchial smooth muscle and are not useful in the therapy of acute bronchospasm.

Why Is Compliance Reduced?

Acute reductions caused by postobstructive or hydrostatic pulmonary edema increase the work of breathing and peak airway pressure but seldom interfere with manual ventilation. However, acute tension pneumothorax or hemothorax impedes lung expansion as if lung compliance were reduced.

Reduction of compliance immediately after intubation generally is caused by straining, coughing, breath holding, or gagging.[128] When neuromuscular function is intact, these responses can prevent ventilation. However, they are generally self-limited and resolve spontaneously within moments, especially if the level of anesthesia is deepened quickly with intravenous agents.

Chest wall rigidity caused by a narcotic agent such as fentanyl may appear coincident with intubation. Because these phenomena involve striated muscle contraction, they do not reduce compliance if adequate neuromuscular relaxation was used in the intubation technique.

Gas Trapping

Any factor that impedes exhalation traps gas volume in the lungs and leads to hyperinflation. Subsequent ventilation occurs on a much flatter portion of the chest wall compliance curve and requires higher inflation pressure.

High-Pressure Ventilation

If the pop-off valve on the anesthesia circuit is closed or set to release at very high pressure, fresh gas flow pressurizes the circuit and distends the patient's lungs. Subsequent attempts to add a tidal volume to the already distended lungs require higher than normal pressures.

This circumstance sometimes occurs when intubation is preceded by a period of difficult facemask airway management,

during which the pop-off valve was closed to balance volume loss from mask leaks or to allow generation of relatively high mask airway pressures. It also results when the outlet valve or tubing that vents the circuit is obstructed.

High Ventilatory Rate

An insufficient expiratory pause also traps gas and causes a more gradual decrease in compliance. This problem occurs in patients with increased airway resistance or with ventilation at high rates with insufficient time for full exhalation. Gas trapping is occasionally caused by a tracheal tube tip that acts like a ball valve against the airway wall, allowing fresh gas to be forced into the lungs under positive pressure but obstructing return during exhalation.

Tube Placement

Incorrect placement of the endotracheal tube must always be considered when completing a differential analysis of difficult ventilation after intubation. Intubation of the esophagus seldom presents as high circuit pressure and no gas flow. Because the esophagus is a relatively flaccid structure, it is difficult to achieve a firm seal without gross overinflation of the cuff. Therefore, when positive pressure is applied, fresh gas usually distends the stomach and then leaks past the cuff with a gurgling or fluttering sound.

Compression of the reservoir bag often gives an impression of inflating relatively noncompliant lungs, with an exhaled volume that is much less than the inhaled volume. Peak pressure varies with the degree of gastric distention, intra-abdominal pressure, and integrity of the cuff seal in the esophagus.

The endotracheal tube may dissect down various fascial planes and inflate the mediastinum or a poorly defined closed tissue space. Such dissections appear most frequently after nasal intubations but can also occur during oral and transtracheal intubations, particularly when a rigid stylet inadvertently protrudes from the tube tip.

Why Does Oxygen Saturation Fall Despite Adequate Ventilation?

After tracheal intubation is completed and ventilation instituted, arterial oxygen saturation sometimes decreases without apparent cause (Table 55–12). When the low saturation reading is corroborated, nitrous oxide should be eliminated from

TABLE 55–12. Causes of Hypoxemia After Intubation

Profound, Relentless Fall in Hemoglobin Saturation	Plateau of Hemoglobin Saturation at Low Level
• Esophageal intubation	• Oximeter probe is poorly positioned
• Oximeter probe is disconnected from oximeter	• A mainstem bronchus has been intubated
• Tracheal tube is disconnected from the circuit	• Fresh gas flow is diverted to one lung
• Mechanical ventilation is not being provided	• A mucus plug has occluded a large airway
• Hypoxic fresh gas mixture is being delivered	• Anesthesia uncovered a ventilatory/perfusion abnormality
• Unrecognized cardiopulmonary collapse has occurred	

Tracheal tube has been placed in the esophagus!

the inspired mixture. Generally, the change caused by eliminating nitrous oxide for a short period is inconsequential. Next, assess the degree and rate of desaturation.

Esophageal Intubation

If saturation is rapidly decreasing despite brisk ventilation, the tracheal tube is most likely in the esophagus. Rapidly evolving hypoxemia secondary to mainstem intubation or hypoventilation through a tube properly placed in the trachea and attached to a source of 100% oxygen is unlikely.[129]

An immediate machine check can assess whether the tube is disconnected from the circuit, the ventilator is nonfunctional, or the patient is receiving a hypoxic mixture. If not, the next most important step is to verify tube placement, preferably with a combination of laryngoscopic visualization and capnographic analysis of expired gas. If tracheal placement cannot be immediately and absolutely confirmed, the most prudent intervention is to remove the tube and provide face-mask ventilation or reintubate.

Another, more common problem after intubation is a gradual fall in oxygen saturation to a worrisome but stable level, which usually appears after verification of tracheal intubation. Moderate, stable desaturation is consistent with venous admixture caused by a $\dot{V}/\dot{Q}$ mismatch. Hypoxic pulmonary vasoconstriction is ablated by every technique that supports tracheal intubation; hence, relatively small $\dot{V}/\dot{Q}$ abnormalities cause inordinately large decreases in arterial saturation.

Bronchial Mainstem Intubation

Another cause of moderate desaturation after intubation is hypoventilation of one lung secondary to tube advancement into a mainstem bronchus.[130, 131] Complete mainstem intubation isolates the contralateral lung from fresh gas delivery, creating a true transpulmonary shunt. Desaturation secondary to a true shunt should not improve with an increase in FIO_2.

Mainstem intubation occurring during the initial tube placement should be readily discovered on auscultation of breath sounds. However, it can occur insidiously after minor tube movement during taping or head positioning.[126, 132] Bilateral auscultation of breath sounds should be rechecked after the patient is in final position and repeatedly each time after subsequent movement with the tracheal tube in place.

Right Upper Lobe Bronchial Occlusion

Occlusion of the right upper lobe bronchus by the endotracheal tube tip or cuff aggravates venous admixture after right mainstem intubation. In a small percentage of otherwise normal patients, the right upper lobe bronchus arises from the distal trachea rather than the right mainstem bronchus, so occlusion of the bronchus can occur even if the tube tip is above the carina. It is also possible to ventilate one lung preferentially without actual mainstem intubation if the tube tip is directed into one mainstem bronchus but the cuff does not completely isolate the other (Fig. 55–10).

Preferential flow diversion to one lung is often difficult to diagnose with auscultation, because marginal retrograde ventilation is delivered to the contralateral lung as well. $\dot{V}/\dot{Q}$ mismatch can be caused both by relative hypoventilation of the contralateral lung and by unrecognized right upper lobe atelectasis. High flow velocities past the orifice of the right

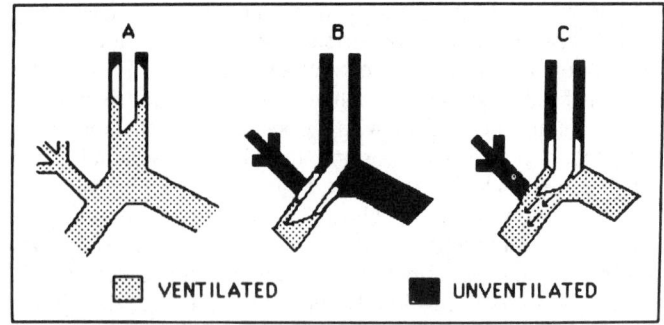

FIGURE 55–10. Right mainstem intubation. *A,* An appropriately positioned tracheal tube allows ventilation of both lungs. *B,* Advancement of a tracheal tube into the right mainstem bronchus prevents ventilation to the left lung and obstructs the right upper lobe bronchus as well. *C,* Preferential direction to flow down the right mainstem bronchus ventilates the right lung directly and the left lung by retrograde flow. High flow rates passing the orifice of the right upper lobe bronchus promote negative pressure in the right upper lobe (Venturi effect) and gradual atelectasis.

upper lobe bronchus may generate relatively negative pressures in the right upper lobe (Venturi's effect), promoting loss of lung volume and atelectasis. Unilateral ventilation can also occur if a mainstem bronchus is occluded by an aspirated foreign body or a tumor mass encroaching on the lumen.

Assessment

Care must be taken to differentiate actual ventilation from transmitted breath sounds originating in the other lung. Observation of unilateral chest expansion is a less reliable indicator of mainstem intubation, especially in patients with obesity or chronic obstructive lung disease. Because unilateral ventilation is almost always caused by advancement of the tube too far into the trachea, empirically withdrawing the tube 1 to 2 cm into better position usually improves hemoglobin saturation. Be cautious about inadvertent extubation, especially if resistance is felt as the cuff is pulled against the cords.

What Are Other Causes of Ventilation/Perfusion Mismatch?

Mucus Plugs

Another cause of moderate hypoxemia after intubation is mucus plugging of a relatively large airway. Brisk lung inflation or high inspiratory flow rates may lodge pulmonary secretions distally and obstruct flow to an area of lung tissue, creating a true shunt with hypoxemia that is resistant to increasing FIO_2. Mucus plugging is generally benign and often treatable with a few sustained inflations, followed by sterile suctioning of secretions if appropriate.

Infections

Moderate hypoxemia is sometimes encountered in children undergoing ear, nose, and throat surgery with a resolving upper respiratory tract infection.[133, 134] The effects of mild pneumonitis on $\dot{V}/\dot{Q}$ matching are unmasked if hypoxic pulmonary vasoconstriction is rendered ineffective by anesthetics. Similarly, patients with mild to moderate bronchospasm may present with transient regional $\dot{V}/\dot{Q}$ mismatch that can cause moderate decreases in saturation.

In contrast to hypoxemia caused by mainstem bronchial ventilation, desaturation due to these causes often responds to increased F_{IO_2} because low $\dot{V}/\dot{Q}$ units result where ventilation is present but is insufficient to match perfusion rather than true shunt. Little can be done to improve saturation other than to increase the F_{IO_2} and to ensure that another reversible problem is not contributing.

PROBLEMS AFTER EXTUBATION

Why Does Extubation Fail?

Extubation of the trachea is one of the final steps in withdrawal of therapeutic support for oxygenation, ventilation, and airway maintenance. Difficulty is seldom related to actual inability to remove the tube, although a grossly overinflated cuff, a sutured tube, a tethered pilot balloon, or various other mechanical problems can interfere with extraction.[135, 136] A "failed" extubation implies a need to reintubate the trachea to support a basic ventilatory function that the patient was unable to maintain.

To evaluate which patients might be at risk for failed extubation, first identify what indices can be used for assessment. Criteria for elective extubation reflect a judgment that the patient is capable of maintaining spontaneous ventilation, upper airway patency and protection, and oxygenation with low levels of supplemental oxygen.

What Problems Appear After Extubation?

Inability to sustain spontaneous ventilation after extubation is a common cause of failed extubation. Patients require intact ventilatory drives (i.e., sufficient central nervous system sensitivity to pH/Pa_{CO_2} to regulate minute ventilatory volume), appropriate work of breathing (i.e., acceptable pulmonary compliance and airway resistance), and adequate muscle strength. Assessment of these factors before extubation is often purely subjective, based on knowledge of the individual patient and the expected clinical course.

Extubation Criteria

Measured indices are seldom used to justify extubation of routine elective surgical patients before transfer to a postanesthesia care unit. However, doubt about a patient's capacity for spontaneous ventilation should trigger a more comprehensive evaluation before extubation.

Pulmonary Function

When using ventilatory criteria for extubation, one is attempting to predict whether a patient can sustain ventilation indefinitely by observation over a short period. For example, ability to achieve a peak negative inspiratory pressure of at least -25 cm H_2O (normal -80 to -100 cm H_2O) and a minimum forced vital capacity of 15 mL $\cdot$ kg^{-1} (normal 50–70 mL $\cdot$ kg^{-1}) indicates that a patient probably has sufficient muscle strength to sustain prolonged spontaneous ventilation.

Failure to achieve these thresholds does not reliably predict that a patient will fail to sustain ventilation, because many patients with chronic respiratory conditions cannot meet these standards at baseline.

Neuromuscular Function

Grosser tests of neuromuscular function such as head lift for 5 seconds or hand strength can be helpful to assess reversal of neuromuscular paralysis but do not reflect factors such as diaphragmatic fatigue and impairment of diaphragmatic excursion.

A trial period of spontaneous ventilation through the tracheal tube is frequently used to assess ventilatory drive and work of breathing. If a patient can maintain an appropriate arterial pH without evidence of fatigue or excess ventilatory effort, ventilatory drive and work of breathing are probably appropriate for extubation. The level of arousal may not correlate with ventilatory drive, especially after stimulus from a tracheal tube is withdrawn.[137]

Duration of the observation period varies, but most acute problems with ventilatory drive or pulmonary mechanics should manifest within 1 or 2 hours. The impact of subtler problems caused by baseline or evolving medical conditions must be predicted on a case-by-case basis. Objective evaluations should be monitored by the individual responsible for extubation. Observation of the forced vital capacity can yield valuable qualitative assessment of expiratory time and effort (indicative of airway resistance) as well as effort required to achieve full expansion (indicative of pulmonary compliance).

Why Don't Patients Breathe Adequately?

Failure to assess neuromuscular relaxant reversal or the impact of surgical manipulations on ventilatory mechanics leads to overestimation of a patient's ability to sustain ventilation.[138] Medications that depress ventilatory drive interfere with spontaneous ventilation, as can a cerebrovascular accident. Pulmonary edema, pneumonia, aspiration, and abdominal distention reduce pulmonary compliance and increase work of breathing, promoting respiratory muscle fatigue and ventilatory failure.

Increased airway resistance can also lead to fatigue. A significant increase in pulmonary dead space caused by the adult respiratory distress syndrome or pulmonary embolization reduces the effectiveness of minute ventilation, increasing the effort required to sustain CO_2 excretion. Similarly, an increase in CO_2 production due to sepsis, fever, or hyperalimentation can make marginally adequate ventilatory function insufficient to meet increased demands.

What Other Factors Should Be Considered?

Incision

Patients with large upper abdominal or thoracic incisions are prone to gradual decreases in compliance, especially if obesity or increased intra-abdominal pressure is a complicating factor. Diaphragmatic function also is impaired.

Intrinsic Lung Disease

Patients with chronic obstructive lung disease are often intolerant of an increment in work of breathing or ventilatory demand. Although asthma or other bronchospastic conditions increase the risk for ventilatory insufficiency, if proper management of airway tone is used, postextubation failure should be relatively low. Failure to oxygenate is a less frequent cause of failed extubation primarily.

Acute Respiratory Problems

Assuming adequate ventilation and airway patency, failure to sustain oxygenation after extubation is usually related to an unrecognized requirement for expiratory positive pressure (i.e., positive end-expiratory pressure or continuous positive airway pressure) to help maintain lung volume and $\dot{V}/\dot{Q}$ matching. Inability to clear secretions spontaneously after extubation also promotes $\dot{V}/\dot{Q}$ mismatch and hypoxemia.

Loss of lung volume or accumulation of secretions is often insidious, occurring over 24 to 48 hours. Patient groups at risk for impaired ventilation are also at risk for impaired oxygenation. Upper abdominal incisions reduce FRC, and chronic obstructive lung disease increases secretions. A new condition that interferes with $\dot{V}/\dot{Q}$ matching (pneumonia, pulmonary edema, pneumothorax) can precipitate marked hypoxemia unrelated to extubation.

What Treatment Is Indicated?

General Measures

Treatment of postextubation pulmonary dysfunction should first be oriented toward resolution of the underlying problems. With appropriate observation and anticipation, sufficient time should be available to improve pulmonary function with conservative measures. Treatment of increased airway resistance with bronchodilators or treatment of pulmonary edema with diuretics often improves work of breathing to a point that spontaneous ventilation can be maintained. Similarly, aggressive chest physiotherapy and incentive spirometry can increase lung volume and oxygenation.

Reintubation

Avoid reintubation whenever possible. Replacement of the tracheal tube and reinstitution of positive-pressure ventilation generally counteract sequelae of the condition that caused the failure but do less to rectify the problem itself. In addition, both the immediate complications of laryngoscopy and tube insertion (airway trauma, SNS responses, aspiration) and delayed morbidity from positive-pressure ventilation and prolonged intubation (pulmonary infection, ventilator dependence, barotrauma) can markedly affect long-term outcome. Nevertheless, the rate and degree of respiratory deterioration must be carefully assessed. If noninvasive measures do not generate a clear reversal of a negative trend or if respiratory acidemia or hypoxemia reaches serious proportions, reintubation should be performed electively under controlled conditions rather than delayed until circumstances reach emergency proportions.

How Should Postextubation Airway Obstruction Be Managed?

Postextubation airway obstruction is a serious problem. Most failures of ventilation or oxygenation evolve gradually, but airway obstruction is an emergency that must be rectified within moments, often in circumstances where equipment and personnel are not immediately available. An obstructed airway interferes with reintubation, making the severity of the emergency far greater.

Airway Patency

Edema

Inability to maintain upper airway patency usually manifests immediately after extubation, especially in the postoperative period. Obstruction can be minor, as occurs with moderate postintubation edema or underlying inflammatory conditions of the upper airway such as croup.[139] Topical vasoconstrictors such as racemic epinephrine often increase airway patency to a point that resistance to airflow disappears.

Laryngospasm

Obstruction can also be transient secondary to functional factors such as laryngospasm, swallowing, or gagging. These problems either resolve spontaneously after a few moments or can be quickly solved with basic airway management.

Residual Drug Effects

Obstruction might be the presenting sign of a more global problem such as inadequate reversal of neuromuscular relaxants or excessive sedation. Additional reversal or decreased sedation with temporary airway support should resolve the problem.

Intrinsic Conditions

Loss of airway patency can also be caused by intrinsic conditions that are not amenable to straightforward treatment. Fortunately, such circumstances are rare, especially if a conservative approach to extubation is used. Great care must be taken when extubating patients whose initial indication for intubation was upper airway obstruction due to epiglottitis, croup, airway burns, or obstructing lesions. Upper airway surgery or trauma increases the risk of postextubation obstruction.

When doubt exists about resolution of the original problem, extubation optimally should be performed in an operating room with a full setup for emergency airway control at hand and an otolaryngologist on standby. Severe glottic edema secondary to prolonged intubation decreases airway patency, especially in patients whose position or anatomy predisposes to airway obstruction. The presence of an unrecognized hematoma, blood clot, or foreign body can also cause airway obstruction, as can lingual swelling.

Therapy

Therapy must be timely and definitive. Reversible contributing conditions such as excess sedation, neuromuscular paralysis, and airway edema should be identified and treated. Avoid reintubation whenever possible, because even minor additional swelling due to laryngoscopy or attempted intubation can convert a marginally patent upper airway into a complete, refractory obstruction that necessitates cricothyroidotomy or tracheotomy. However, if obstruction precludes effective ventilation or oxygenation, the airway must be secured with intubation. Morbidity is high, so every effort should be made to keep the procedure controlled and effective, observing the previously espoused guidelines for difficult intubation.

Preventive Measures

Extubation of patients who presented significant airway problems during intubation is particularly worrisome. Emergency reintubation most likely will present an even greater degree of difficulty. The risk of death from sequelae of a failed extubation is significant. Every precaution should be taken to minimize the chance that extubation might fail, even if prolonged intubation causes increased anxiety and discomfort.

A conservative approach should be used in patients whose surgical procedures might interfere with reintubation. Patients with mandibular fixation, rigid cervical traction, mandatory prone positioning, or other limiting circumstances should be fully awake and cooperative before extubation. In selected instances, it is prudent to have patients demonstrate the ability to suction their own upper airway and to supply them with bedside suction apparatus in case secretions or vomitus accumulates in the upper airway after extubation.

Protection Against Aspiration

Inability to protect against aspiration is another upper airway problem that sometimes causes difficulty after extubation. Protective airway function is severely compromised by airway trauma or surgical procedures, laryngeal paresis secondary to instrumentation or prolonged intubation, and sedation, cerebral pathology, and insufficient neuromuscular function.[140, 141] Circumstances that interfere with clearing the airway, such as mandibular fixation or cervical traction, compound the risk.

Patients with refractory vomiting, massive gastric distention, or large amounts of oral secretions may have difficulty protecting the airway despite adequate reflexes. Although assessment of airway reflexes is less objective than that for ventilation or oxygenation, it is often easier to predict which patients are at risk.

Because aspiration carries a high morbidity and cannot be easily treated, it is always wise to delay extubation until the underlying cause of decreased airway protection improves. In circumstances in which deterioration of airway protection is irreversible, it may be necessary to perform an elective tracheostomy.

Future Clinical Course

When deciding whether to extubate, consider the patient's future clinical course. Delay in elective extubation of a patient in an intensive care unit is often reasonable if a surgical procedure is scheduled the next day. Transport of critically ill patients to other facilities is usually safer if the airway is secured.

Suspicion that a clinical problem may be evolving and could jeopardize pulmonary function may suggest delaying extubation, even though other criteria indicate that it is timely. However, when a patient performs an unplanned self-extubation, a trial of spontaneous ventilation usually is worthwhile. Reintubation often is unnecessary.[142]

Why Should Endotracheal Tubes Be Changed?

Electively changing an indwelling tracheal tube is one of the most hazardous airway interventions undertaken in a critically ill patient. Tube changes are often attempted at the bedside in a cramped intensive care cubicle or in a busy postanesthesia care unit, with less than optimal equipment and support. By definition, the patient is not a candidate for extu-

bation, and the risks of extubation (e.g., loss of patency, aspiration, inability to ventilate) are magnified. Added to these considerations is the additional risk inherent in attempting reintubation.

Tube Malfunction

If the indwelling tube is not functioning properly, it must be replaced. However, few elements of tracheal tube function actually fail.

Cuff Leak

Requests for consultation frequently are based on a perception that a leak has developed in the tube cuff and is preventing a reliable seal. When questioned, staff relate that addition of air to the pilot tubing generates a seal temporarily, but leakage recurs within minutes.

Cuff Location

Modern tracheal tube cuffs are remarkably durable and seldom spontaneously develop leaks. A compromise in cuff integrity usually results in complete failure rather than gradual deflation. Most cuff leaks are related to herniation of the cuff through the vocal cords. The problem can be eliminated by suctioning the mouth, deflating the cuff, and advancing the tube so the entire cuff is below the vocal cords. This procedure entails far less risk than extubation and reintubation. An inappropriately cut tracheal tube may not have sufficient length to permit advancement for a cuff seal, so care must be taken to leave sufficient (but not excessive) length to allow repositioning.

Pilot Tube Valve Dysfunction

On occasion, a defect develops in the valve of the pilot tubing and prevents closure. Subsequent leak from the valve allows gradual cuff deflation. This problem can be solved by occluding the pilot tube with a rubber-shod clamp, by leaving a stopcock or the inflating syringe attached to the valve, or by removing the valve and inserting a blunt needle attached to the stopcock into the lumen.[143] None of these solutions involves the risk in changing the tube, although none is entirely satisfactory.

Tube Size

Another common justification for tube change is that the indwelling tube is too small. Uncuffed tubes in children can be associated with significant leaks when their external diameter is significantly less than the tracheal diameter, but this problem is almost always identified and solved with a tube change at the time of intubation.

If an inappropriately small cuffed tube is inserted in a larger child or adult, high cuff pressures might be required to seal the cuff. In this instance, the risk of trauma to the tracheal wall must be balanced against the risk of tube change. Resistance to gas flow in adult tracheal tubes almost never causes intraoperative clinical problems. However, reduction in tube diameter due to secretions or kinking should be eliminated by cleaning or straightening the lumen. A tube change should be attempted only when all attempts to restore patency have failed.

Marginal occlusion of small pediatric tubes may be a valid indication for a tube change because small changes in cross-sectional area have proportionally greater impact on overall resistance, and suctioning is both difficult and risky for patients. Tube diameter can also be a limiting factor if fiberoptic bronchoscopy through the tracheal tube is planned, although most bronchoscopes easily fit through a 7.5-mm ID tube. One should consider these facts when the initial choice of endotracheal tube is made.

What Equipment Should Be Available?

Various aids that are available can be useful to reduce the risk of being unable to reintubate a patient.

Tube Changers

A long flexible tube changer stylet, an esophageal bougie, a clean nasogastric tube, or any semi-rigid tubing can be gently advanced through the existing tube down to the tip.[144–147] The first tracheal tube is then withdrawn over this guide, leaving it in place to guide the second tube back into the tracheal opening.

Although usually effective, this technique can fail if the stylet is inadvertently pulled out with the first tracheal tube or if one is unable to slide the second tube through the vocal cords. It probably should be reserved for instances when extubation and reintubation under direct visualization are impossible to achieve. Stylet modifications to hollow stylets allow marginal insufflation of oxygen during the tube change.[148, 149]

Flexible Fiberoptic Bronchoscopes

Tube changes can also be accomplished using a fiberoptic bronchoscope threaded through the new tube and passed alongside the existing tracheal tube. The glottis is visualized, and the first tube is removed.[150, 151] The fiberoptic scope is then advanced through the vocal cords, and the new tube introduced over it.

If it is essential to use the same route for placement of the new tube, the bronchoscope can be used as a tube changer and passed through the lumen of the original tube.[150] This approach requires that the original tube be sliced along its full length after withdrawal and removed from the bronchoscope to allow passage of the new tube. Indications for this technique are rare.

References

1. Wever JG, Warner MA, Warner ME: Perioperative pulmonary aspiration: incidence and risk factors. Anesthesiology 1990; 73:A1017.
2. Lawes EG, Campbell I, Mercer D: Inflation pressure, gastric insufflation, and rapid sequence induction. Br J Anaesth 1987; 59:315.
3. Jackson FN, Rowland V, Corssen G: Laryngospasm induced pulmonary edema. Chest 1980; 78:819.
4. Warner MA, Wever BA, Warner ME: Etiologies and incidence of acute pulmonary edema in the immediate perioperative period. Anesth Analg 1990; 70:S421.
5. Jones AEP, Pelton PA: An index of syndromes and their anesthetic implications. Can Anaesth Soc J 1976; 23:207.
6. Gambee AM, Hertzka RE, Fisher DM: Preoxygenation techniques: comparison of three minutes and four breaths. Anesth Analg 1987; 66:468.
7. Gold MI, Duarte I, Muravchick S: Arterial oxygenation in conscious patients after 5 minutes and after 30 seconds of oxygen breathing. Anesth Analg 1981; 60:313.
8. Carmichael FJ, Cruise CJE, Crago RR, et al: Preoxygenation: a study of denitrogenation. Anesth Analg 1989; 68:406.
9. Symreng T, Mehta MP, Sum-Ping JS, et al: Preoxygenation time—the influence of anthropometric and pulmonary variables? Anesth Analg 1991; 72:S288.
10. Safar P, Bircher NG: Cardiopulmonary Cerebral Resuscitation. Philadelphia, WB Saunders, 1988, pp 13–92.
11. Boidin MP: Airway patency in the unconscious patient. Br J Anaesth 1985; 57:306.
12. Morikawa S, Safar P, DeCarlo J: Influence of head position upon upper airway patency.
13. Liistro G, Stanescu D, Dooms G, et al: Head position modifies upper airway resistance in men. J Appl Physiol 1988; 64:1285.
14. Muzzi DA, Lossasso TJ, Cucchiara RF: Complication from a nasopharyngeal airway in a patient with a basilar skull fracture. Anesthesiology 1991; 73:366.
15. Brian AIJ: The laryngeal mask—a new technique in airway management. Br J Anaesth 1983; 55:801.
16. Suzuki M, Sasake CT: Laryngeal spasm: a neurophysiologic redefinition. Ann Otolaryngol 1977; 86:150.
17. Turnstall ME: Failed intubation drill. Anesthesia 1976; 31:850.
18. Bernard WN, Cottrell JE, Sivakumaran C, et al: Adjustment of intracuff pressure to prevent aspiration. Anesthesiology 1979; 50:363.
19. Petring OV, Adelhoj B, Jensen BN, et al: Prevention of silent aspiration due to leaks around cuffs of endotracheal tubes. Anesth Analg 1986; 65:777.
20. Redick LF: The temporomandibular joint and tracheal intubation. Anesth Analg 1987; 66:675.
21. Block C, Brechner VL: Unusual problems in airway management. II. The influence of the temporomandibular joint, the mandible, and associated structures on endotracheal intubation. Anesth Analg 1981; 50:114.
22. Wilson ME, Spiegenhalter D, Robertson JA, et al: Predicting difficult intubation. Br J Anaesth 1988; 61:211.
23. Kay NH: Mammomegaly and intubation. Anaesthesia 1982; 37:221.
24. Nichol HC, Zuck D: Difficult laryngoscopy. The ''anterior'' larynx and the atlanto-occipital gap. Br J Anaesth 1983; 55:141.
25. King TA, Adams AP: Failed tracheal intubation. Br J Anaesth 1990; 65:400.
26. White A, Kander PL: Anatomic factors in difficult direct laryngoscopy. Br J Anaesth 1975; 47:468.
27. Brechner VL: Unusual problems in the management of airways. Flexion-extension mobility of the cervical vertebrae. Anesth Analg 1986; 47:362.
28. Jenkins CL, McGraw RW: Anaesthetic management of the patient with rheumatoid arthritis. Can Anaesth Soc J 1969; 16:407.
29. Sinclair JR, Mason RA: Ankylosing spondylitis. The case for awake intubation. Anaesthesia 1984; 39:3.
30. Samson GLT, Young JRB: Difficult tracheal intubation, a retrospective study. Anaesthesia 1987; 42:487.
31. Rhee KJ, Green W, Holcroft JW, et al: Oral intubation in the multiply injured patient: the risk of exacerbating spinal cord damage. Ann Emerg Med 1990; 19:511.
32. Berkowitz ID, Raja SN, Bender KS, et al: Dwarfs: pathophysiology and anesthetic implications. Anesthesiology 1990; 73:739.
33. Herick IA, Rhane EJ: The mucopolysaccharidoses and anesthetics. A report of clinical experience. Can J Anaesth 1988; 35:67.
34. Cormack RS, Lehane J: Difficult tracheal intubation in obstetrics. Anaesthesia 1984; 39:1105.
35. O'Leary AM: Acute upper airway obstruction due to arterial puncture during percutaneous central venous cannulation of the subclavian vein. Anesthesiology 1990; 73:780.
36. Helfman SM, Gold MI, DeLisser EA, et al: Which drug prevents tachycardia and hypertension associated with tracheal intubation: lidocaine, fentanyl, or esmolol? Anesth Analg 1991; 72:482.
37. Mallampati RS, Gatt SP, Gugino LD, et al: A clinical sign to predict difficult tracheal intubation: a prospective study. Can Anaesth Soc J 1985; 32:429.
38. Tham EJ, Gildersleve CD, Sanders LD, et al: Effects of posture, phonation, and observer on Mallampati classification. Br J Anaesth 1992; 68:32.
39. Patil VU, Stehling L, Zauder HL: Fiberoptic endoscopy in anesthesiology. Chicago, Year Book Medical Publishers, 1983.
40. Mathew M, Hanna LS, Aldrete JA: Predictive indices to anticipate difficult tracheal intubation. Anesth Analg 1989; 68:518.
41. Hotchkiss RS, Hall JR, Braun IF, et al: An abnormal epiglottis as a cause of difficult intubation: airway assessment using magnetic resonance imaging. Anesthesiology 1988; 68:140.
42. Neuman GG, Wellington AE, Abramowitz RM: The anesthetic manage-

ment of the patient with an anterior mediastinal mass. Anesthesiology 1984; 60:144.

43. Bouget D, Boukobza M, Metzger M, et al: Difficult intubation for cervical spine surgery: airway assessment with magnetic resonance imaging. Anesthesiology 1988; 69:A725.

44. Berry FA, Blankenbaker WL, Ball CG: A comparison of bacteremia occurring with nasotracheal and orotracheal intubation. Anesth Analg 1973; 52:873.

45. Dinner M, Tjeaw M, Artusio JF: Bacteremia as a complication of nasotracheal intubation. Anesth Analg 1987; 66:460.

46. Arens JF, Lejeune FE, Webre DR: Maxillary sinusitis: a complication of nasotracheal intubation. Anesthesiology 1974; 40:415.

47. Deutschman CS, Wilton P, Sinow J, et al: Paranasal sinusitis associated with nasotracheal intubation: a frequently unrecognized and treatable source of sepsis. Crit Care Med 1986; 14:111.

48. Katz RI, Hovagim AR, Finklestein HA: A comparison of cocaine, lidocaine with epinephrine, and oxymetazoline for prevention of epistaxis during nasal intubation. Anesth Analg 1988; 67:S100.

49. Hertigon ML, Clearly JL, Gross JB, et al: Is nasal cocaine superior to a lidocaine-phenylephrine mixture for blind nasotracheal intubation? Anesth Analg 1984; 63:227.

50. Seebacher J, Nozik D, Mathieu A: Inadvertent intracranial introduction of a nasogastric tube, a complication of severe maxillofacial trauma. Anesthesiology 1975; 42:100.

51. Elder CK: Nasotracheal intubation: advantages and technic of "blind intubation." Anesthesiology 1944; 5:392.

52. Berry FA: The use of a stylet in blind nasotracheal intubation. Anesthesiology 1984; 61:469.

53. Williams KN, Carli F, Cormack RS: Unexpected difficult laryngoscopy: a prospective survey in routine general surgery. Br J Anaesth 1991; 66:38.

54. Cobley M, Vaughan RS: Recognition and management of difficult airway problems. Br J Anaesth 1992; 68:90.

55. Oates JDL, Oates PD, Pearsall RJ, et al: Comparison of two methods for predicting difficult intubation. Br J Anaesth 1991; 66:305.

56. Horton WA, Fahy L, Charters P: Disposition of cervical x-ray laryngoscopy. Br J Anaesth 1989; 63:435.

57. Davies MJ, Cronin KD, Cowie RW: The prevention of hypertension at intubation: a controlled study of intravenous hydralazine on patients undergoing intracranial surgery. Anaesthesia 1981; 36:147.

58. Derbyshire DR, Chielewski A, Fell D, et al: Plasma catecholamine responses to tracheal intubation. Br J Anaesth 1983; 55:855.

59. Tryba M, Zenz M, Milasowsky B, et al: Does a stomach tube enhance regurgitation during general anesthesia? Anaesthetist 1983; 32:407.

60. Salem MR, Joseph NJ, Heyman HJ, et al: Cricoid pressure is effective in obliterating the esophageal lumen in the presence of a nasogastric tube. Anesthesiology 1985; 63:443.

61. Bailey PL, Pace NL, Ashburn MA: Frequent hypoxemia and sedation with midazolam and fentanyl. Anesthesiology 1990; 73:826.

62. Gal TJ, Surrat PM: Resistance to breathing in healthy subjects following endotracheal intubation under topical anesthesia. Anesth Analg 1980; 59:270.

63. Cohen MM, Cameron CB: Should you cancel the operation when a child has an upper respiratory tract infection? Anesth Analg 1991; 72:282.

64. Jacoby DB, Hirschman CA: General anesthesia in patients with viral respiratory infections: an unsound sleep? Anesthesiology 1991; 74:969.

65. Shribman AJ, Smith G, Achola KJ: Cardiovascular and catecholamine responses to laryngoscopy with and without tracheal intubation. Br J Anaesth 1987; 59:295.

66. Bedford RF: Circulatory responses to tracheal intubation. Probl Anesth 1988; 2:201.

67. Burney RG, Winn R: Increased cerebrospinal fluid pressure during laryngoscopy and intubation for induction of anesthesia. Anesth Analg 1975; 54:687.

68. Camporesi EM, Mortola JP, SantAmbrogio F, et al: Topical anesthesia of tracheal receptors. J Appl Physiol 1979; 47:1123.

69. Bourke DL, Katz J, Tonneson A: Nebulized anesthesia for awake endotracheal intubation. Anesthesiology 1985; 63:690.

70. Kautto UM, Heinonen J: Attenuation of the circulatory response to laryngoscopy and tracheal intubation. A comparison of two methods of topical anesthesia. Acta Anaesthesiol Scand 1982; 26:559.

71. Stoelting RK: Circulatory changes during direct laryngoscopy and tracheal intubation: influence of viscous or intravenous lidocaine. Anesth Analg 1978; 57:197.

72. Woods AM, Lander CJ: Abolition of gagging and the hemodynamic response to awake laryngoscopy. Anesthesiology 1987; 647:A220.

73. Hamill JF, Bedford RF, Weaver DC, et al: Lidocaine before endotracheal intubation: intravenous or laryngotracheal? Anesthesiology 1981; 55:578.

74. Bidwai AV, Bidwai VA, Rogers CR, et al: Blood pressure and pulse rate responses to endotracheal extubation with and without prior injection of lidocaine. Anesthesiology 1979; 51:171.

75. Gold MI, Brown M, Coverman S, et al: Heart rate and blood pressure effects of esmolol after ketamine induction and intubation. Anesthesiology 1986; 64:718.

76. Finfer SR, MacKenzie SIP, Saddler JM, et al: Cardiovascular responses to tracheal intubation: a comparison of direct laryngoscopy and fiberoptic intubation. Anaesth Intensive Care 1989; 17:44.

77. Omoigui S, Glass P, Martel DLJ, et al: Blind nasal intubation with audio capnometry. Anesth Analg 1991; 72:392.

78. Ellis DG, Jakymec A, Kaplan RM, et al: Guided orotracheal intubation in the operating room using a lighted stylet. A comparison with direct laryngoscopic technique. Anesthesiology 1986; 64:823.

79. Rayburn RL: Light wand intubation. Anaesthesia 1979; 34:677.

80. Fox DJ, Castro T, Rastrelli AJ: Comparison of intubation techniques in the awake patient: the Flexi-lum surgical light (lightwand versus blind) nasal approach. Anesthesiology 1987; 66:69.

81. Williams RT: Lighted stylet and endotracheal intubation. Anesthesiology 1987; 66:851.

82. Stewart RD: Use of alighted stylet to confirm correct endotracheal tube placement. Chest 1987; 92:900.

83. Katz RL, Berci G: The optical stylet—a new intubation technique for adults and children with specific reference to teaching. Anesthesiology 1979; 51:251.

84. Rogers SN, Benumof JL: New and easy techniques for fiberoptic endoscopy-aided tracheal intubation. Anesthesiology 1983; 59:569.

85. Ovassapian A, Yelich SJ, Dykes MHM, et al: Fiberoptic nasotracheal intubation: incidence and causes of failure. Anesth Analg 1983; 62:692.

86. Vaughan RS: Teaching fiberoptic laryngoscopy. Br J Anaesth 1991; 66:538.

87. Ward CF, Salvatierra CA: Special intubation techniques for the adult patient. *In* Clinical Procedures in Anesthesia and Intensive Care. Benumof JL (ed). Philadelphia, JB Lippincott, 1992, pp 149–177.

88. Butler FS, Cirillo AA: Retrograde tracheal intubation. Anesth Analg 1960; 39:333.

89. Bourke D, Levesque PR: Modification of retrograde guide for endotracheal intubation. Anesth Analg 1974; 53:1013.

90. Dhara SS: Guided blind endotracheal intubation. Anaesthesia 1980; 35:80.

91. King HK: Translaryngeal guide intubation using a sheath stylet. Anesthesiology 1985; 63:576.

92. Freund PR, Rooke A, Schwide H: Retrograde intubation with a modified Eschman stylet. Anesth Analg 1988; 67:605.

93. Abou-Madi MN, Trop D: Pulling vs guiding: a modification of retrograde guided intubation. Can J Anaesth 1989; 36:336.

94. Salem MR, Heyman HJ, Liuschutz V, et al: Cephalad displacement of the larynx facilitates tracheal intubation. Anesthesiology 1987; 67:A453.

95. McIntyre JWR: The difficult tracheal intubation. Can J Anaesth 1987; 34:204.

96. Cozantis DA, Nuttila K, Merrett JD, et al: Influence of laryngoscope design on heart rate and rhythm changes during intubation. Can Anaesth Soc J 1984; 31:155.

97. Bellhouse CP: An angulated laryngoscope for routine and difficult tracheal intubation. Anesthesiology 1988; 69:126.

98. Thomas DV: Laryngoscopy technique in obese patients (Letter to the editor). Anesthesiology 1987; 66:583.

99. Cahen CR: An aid in cases of difficult tracheal intubation. Anesthesiology 1991; 74:197.

100. Rosenberg MB, Levesque PR, Bourke DL: Use of the LT kit as a guide for tracheal intubation. Anesth Analg 1977; 56:287.

101. Maltby JR, Loken RG, Watson NC: The laryngeal mask airway: clinical appraisal in 250 patients. Can J Anaesth 1990; 37:509.

102. Jocobs HB: Needle catheter brings oxygen to the trachea. JAMA 1972; 222:1231.

103. Spoerel WE, Narayanan PS, Singh NP: Transtracheal ventilation. Br J Anaesth 1971; 433:932.

104. Smith RB, Macmillan BB, Petruscak J, et al: Transtracheal ventilation for laryngoscopy. Ann Otol Rhinol Laryngol 1973; 82:347.

105. Wagner DJ, Coombs DW, Doyle SC: Percutaneous transtracheal ventilation for emergency dental appliance removal. Anesthesiology 1985; 66:664.

106. Benumof JL, Scheller MS: The importance of transtracheal jet ventilation in the management of the difficult airway. Anesthesiology 1989; 71:769.

107. Stinson TW: A simple connector for transtracheal ventilation. Anesthesiology 1977; 47:232.

108. Patel R: Systems for transtracheal ventilation. Anesthesiology 1983; 59:165.

109. Delisser EA, Muravchick S: Emergency transtracheal ventilation. Anesthesiology 1981; 55:606.

110. Spoeri WE, Greenway RE: Technique of ventilation during endolaryngeal surgery under general anesthesia. Can Anaesth Soc J 1973; 20:369.

111. Toye FJ, Weinstein JD: Clinical experience with percutaneous tracheostomy and cricothyroidotomy in 100 patients. J Trauma 1986; 26:1034.

112. Ciaglia P, Firsching R, Syniec C: Elective percutaneous dilational tracheostomy: a new simple bedside procedure. Chest 1985; 87:715.

113. DeLaurier GA, Hawkins ML, Treat RC, et al: Acute airway management: role of cricothyroidotomy. Ann Surg 1990; 56:12.

114. Heffner JE, Miller KS, Sahn SA: Tracheostomy in the intensive care unit. Part 2: Complications. Chest 1986; 90:430.

115. Sellick BA: Cricoid pressure to control regurgitation of stomach contents during induction of anesthesia. Lancet 1961; 2:404.

116. Boulanger A, Hardy JF, Lepage Y: Rapid induction sequence with vecuronium: should we intubate after 60 or 90 seconds? Can J Anaesth 1990; 37:296.

117. Tam S, Chung F, Campbell M: Intravenous lidocaine: optimal time of injection before tracheal intubation. Anesth Analg 1987; 66:1036.

118. Birmingham PK, Cheney FW, Ward RJ: Esophageal intubation: a review of detection techniques. Anesth Analg 1986; 65:886.

119. Utting JE, Gray TC, Shelley FC: Human misadventure in anesthesia. Can Anaesth Soc J 1979; 26:472.

120. Dunn SM, Mushlin PS, Lind LJ, et al: Tracheal intubation is not invariably confirmed by capnography. Anesthesiology 1990; 73:1285.

121. Wee MYK: The esophageal detector device. Anaesthesia 1988; 43:27.

122. Williams KN, Nunn JF: The oesophageal detector device. Anaesthesia 1989; 44:412.

123. Drummond GB, Park GR: Arterial oxygen saturation before intubation of the trachea. Br J Anesth 984; 56:987.

124. Gold MI: Arterial oxygenation during laryngoscopy and intubation. Anesth Analg 1981; 60:316.

125. Turner AKE, Sandler AN, Vosu HA, et al: Noninvasive monitoring of carbon dioxide in nonintubated patients: comparison of $Paco_2$ versus $ETco_2$ and $Paco_2$ versus $Tcco_2$. Anesthesiology 1990; 73:A53.

126. Conrady PA, Goodman LR, Lainge F, et al: Alteration for endotracheal tube position. Crit Care Med 1976; 4:8.

127. Haake R, Schlichtig R, Ulstad DR, et al: Barotrauma: pathophysiology, risk factors, and prevention. Chest 1987; 91:608.

128. Gal TJ: Effects of endotracheal intubation on normal cough performance. Anesthesiology 1980; 52:324.

129. Slutsky AS, Watson J, Leith DE, et al: Tracheal insufflation of oxygen (TRIO) at low flow rates sustains life for several hours. Anesthesiology 1985; 63:278.

130. Kerr JH, Crampton Smith AC, Prys-Roberts C: Observations during endobronchial anaesthesia. II: Oxygenation. Br J Anaesth 1974; 46:84.

131. Owen RL, Cheney FW: Endobronchial intubation: a preventable complication. Anesthesiology 1987; 67:255.

132. Toung TJK, Grayson R, Saklad J, et al: Movement of the distal end of the endotracheal tube during flexion and extension of the neck (Letter to the editor). Anesth Analg 1985; 64:1029.

133. Pandit UA, Levy L, Randel GI, et al: Perioperative respiratory complications in children with upper respiratory infection. Anesthesiology 1989; 71:A1011.

134. Desoto H, Patel RI, Soliman IE, et al: Changes in oxygen saturation following general anesthesia in children with upper respiratory infection signs and symptoms undergoing otolaryngological procedures. Anesthesiology 1988; 68:276.

135. Hilley MD, Henderson RB, Giesecke AH: Difficult extubation of the trachea. Anesthesiology 1983; 59:149.

136. Strung J, Conley S, Brown M: An unusual cause of difficult extubation. Anesthesiology 1991; 74:796.

137. Boerner TE, Torjman M, Bartkowski RR, et al: Does cognitive function predict respiratory depression? Anesthesiology 1989; 71:A1101.

138. Stanec A, Nuesa W, Akturk A, et al: Recovery of respiratory muscle function in surgical outpatients. Anesthesiology 1990; 73:A878.

139. Koka BV, Jeon IS, Andre JM, et al: Post intubation croup in children. Anesth Analg 1977; 56:501.

140. Pavlin EG, Holle RH, Schoene RB: Recovery of airway protection compared with ventilation in humans after paralysis with curare. Anesthesiology 1989; 70:381.

141. Arora NS, Gal TJ: Cough dynamics during progressive expiratory muscle weakness in healthy curarized subjects. J Appl Physiol 1981; 51:464.

142. Coppolo DP, May JJ: Self-extubations: a twelve month experience. Chest 1990; 98:165.

143. Alfrey DD: Changing an endotracheal tube. *In* Clinical Procedures in Anesthesia and Intensive Care. Benumof JL (ed). Philadelphia, JB Lippincott, 1992, pp 177–194.

144. Desai SP, Fencl V: A safe technique for changing endotracheal tubes. Anesthesiology 1980; 53:267.

145. Finucane BT, Kupshik HL: A flexible stylette for replacing damaged tracheal tubes. Can Anaesth Soc J 1978; 25:153.

146. McCarroll SM, Lamont BJ, Buckland MR, et al: The gum elastic bougie: old but still useful. Anesthesiology 1988; 68:643.

147. Montgomery G, Dueringer J, Johnson C: Nasal endotracheal tube change with an intubating stylette after fiberoptic intubation. Anesth Analg 1991; 72:713.

148. Badger RC, Chiang J: A jet stylet endotracheal catheter for difficult airway management. Anesthesiology 1987; 66:221.

149. Arndt GA, Ghani GA: A modification of an Eschmann endotracheal tube changer for insufflation. Anesthesiology 1988; 69:282.

150. Hudes ET, Fisher JA, Guslitz B: Difficult endotracheal reintubations: a simple technique. Anesthesiology 1986; 64:515.

151. Rosenbaum SH, Rosenbaum LM, Cole RP, et al: Use of the flexible fiberoptic bronchoscope to change endotracheal tubes in critically ill patients. Anesthesiology 1981; 54:169.

56

Anesthesia for Patients with Bronchial Asthma

S. S. MOORTHY, M.D.

STEPHEN F. DIERDORF, M.D.

Bronchial asthma is a chronic lung disease that episodically manifests as signs and symptoms of airway obstruction. Between the episodes, the patient is generally free of symptoms. The incidence of bronchial asthma in the general population is between 4% and 5%, and evidence suggests that this incidence is increasing. Fifty per cent of patients develop their disease during childhood, and 75% of patients are below the age of 40 years.[1, 2]

Although the morbidity produced by this disease is high, the mortality is, fortunately, low (0.3 deaths per 10,000 patients). However, here also evidence suggests that the mortality from asthma is increasing.[3] Bronchial asthma generally does not produce a progressive deterioration in pulmonary function as do chronic bronchitis and emphysema.

PATHOPHYSIOLOGY

Characteristic features of bronchial asthma include (1) reversible or partially reversible airway obstruction, (2) airway inflammation, and (3) hyperreactivity of airways to a variety of stimuli. Repeated exposure to inciting stimuli produces a bronchial tree that is responsive to many nonspecific stimuli as well. Inhalation of cold anesthetic gases, tracheal intubation, and suctioning of the tracheobronchial tree during light planes of anesthesia can precipitate bronchospasm in susceptible patients.

What Factors Cause Airway Hyperreactivity?

The mechanisms by which airways become sensitized and hyperreactive are not well known. However, once present, this hyperreactivity persists. Airway reactivity varies markedly during the day. Bronchospasm or overt asthmatic attacks usually occur at night and in the early morning hours. Consequently, it may be advantageous to defer elective surgery in asthmatic patients until late morning or midday, when bronchomotor tone is optimal. The origin of this diurnal variation is not known.

Known Stimuli

A number of stimuli can precipitate an acute episode of bronchial asthma in a sensitive individual; these include allergens, exercise, infection, emotional stress, and occupational, environmental, and pharmacologic agents. The patient who is prone to bronchial asthma generally has a genetic predisposition to the disease and responds to an antigenic challenge by developing bronchospasm. The inheritance of bronchial asthma is complex, and our knowledge of it is incomplete. Patients who develop allergic or atopic (extrinsic) asthma usually have a family history of atopy. Immunoglobulin E secreted by B cells attaches to receptors on mast cells and basophils. Activation of these receptors on mast cells results in the release of potent biologic mediators that trigger an asthmatic attack.[1]

What Are the Mediators?

The biologic mediators released from mast cells, macrophages, and respiratory epithelial cells of the bronchioles produce bronchoconstriction and increased capillary permeability, which results in airway edema. In addition, chemotactic factors recruit cells from which cyclooxygenases and leukotrienes are released. These mediators produce their effects by activating cell surface receptors. The end result is bronchoconstriction, inflammation, increased production of mucus, and destruction of ciliated epithelium.[4, 5] Various mediators are listed in Table 56–1.

What Types of Asthma Are Known?

Several types of bronchial asthma are identified (Table 56–2).

TABLE 56–1. Mediators of Bronchospasm in Asthma

Factors that produce bronchoconstriction	Prostanoids (PGD_2, PGF_{2K}) Thromboxane A_2 Leukotrienes (LTC_4, LTD_4) PAF Adenosine Bradykinin Substance P Calcitonin gene-related peptide
Factors that produce increased capillary permeability	Prostanoids (prostacyclin) PAF
Factors that produce increased secretion of mucus	Leukotrienes (LTC_4, LTD_4) PAF
Chemotactic agents that produce inflammatory response (Infiltration with neutrophils and eosinophils)	Leukotrienes (LTB_4) Adenosine Bradykinin Eosinophilic chemotactic factor Lymphocyte chemotactic factor High-molecular-weight neutrophil chemotactic factor of anaphylaxis

Abbreviation: PAF = platelet activating factor.

Atopic

Atopic or extrinsic asthma manifests in patients younger than 30 years of age. A family history of atopy, elevated blood levels of immunoglobulin E, and positive results on skin and bronchial challenge tests are diagnostic. This disease often remits in later years of life.

Intrinsic

Intrinsic asthma manifests in older individuals without a family history of atopy. The blood and sputum of these patients contain increased numbers of eosinophils. These patients may also have autoantibodies to smooth muscle as well as autoimmune diseases. Treatment is less effective than in other asthmas, and the disease is relentless in its effects.

Exercise-Induced

Exercise-induced asthma is precipitated by hyperpnea and by heat and water loss from respiratory mucosa. Increased osmolality of secretions is associated with hyperemia and congestion of bronchioles and alveoli.

Environmental/Infectious/Occupational

A number of environmental and infectious causes of bronchospasm are known. Viral respiratory tract infections damage the bronchial epithelium and release arachidonic acid metabolites that can precipitate asthma. In addition, organic dusts (e.g., from wood and vegetables), inorganic dusts (e.g., metal

TABLE 56–2. Types of Asthma

Atopic (extrinsic)
Intrinsic
Exercise-induced
Environmental/infectious
Occupational
Aspirin-induced
Psychogenic

salts and pharmaceutical dusts), and environmental pollutants can also precipitate bronchospasm in susceptible individuals.

CHARACTERISTICS

What Are the Clinical Features?

During an acute attack of bronchial asthma, patients present with dyspnea and cough. Physical examination reveals tachypnea, wheezing, and tachycardia. Some patients also exhibit diaphoresis and pulsus paradoxus. Excessive production of mucus causes plugging of bronchioles, which leads to air trapping. Consequently, the chest radiograph reveals hyperinflation of the lungs, subsegmental atelectasis, and an increase in the anteroposterior diameter of the chest. Mucus secretions and mucus plugs contain eosinophils, ciliated epithelium, Charcot-Leyden crystals (L150 phospholipase), and Curschmann's spirals (strands of mucus). As the attack resolves and symptoms abate, the patient develops a productive cough to clear the obstructed airways.

What Changes in Pulmonary Function Occur?

Spirometry

Pulmonary function testing during an asthmatic attack reveals increases in total lung capacity, functional residual capacity, and residual volume.[6, 7] Decreases in forced vital capacity (FVC), forced expiratory flow during the middle half of the FVC ($FEF_{25\%-75\%}$), maximum expiratory flow rates, and forced expiratory flow between 200 mL and 1200 mL of the FVC ($FEF_{200-1200}$) are also indicative of airway obstruction.[6, 8, 9]

The response to bronchodilator therapy can be measured as a guide to therapy (Fig. 56–1). FVCs are dependent not only

	PRE-DILATOR	POST-DILATOR	% CHANGE
FVC (L)	4.92	4.97	1
FEV₁ (L)	3.25	4.12	27
FEF₂₅₋₇₅	1.97	4.34	121

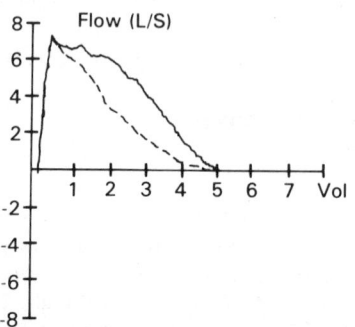

FIGURE 56–1. Spirometric tracings in a patient with asthma before (PRE) and after (POST) treatment with an inhaled bronchodilator. Significant improvement of FEV_1 and $FEF_{25\%-75\%}$ occurs following bronchodilator administration (*dashed line* = PRE; *solid line* = POST).

on airway obstruction but also on lung elastic properties, absolute volume of air in the lungs, and voluntary patient effort. Maximum expiratory flow rates and $FEF_{25\%-75\%}$ are effort-independent ($<75\%$ of FVC) and can be used for quantification of airway obstruction. Closing volume is elevated, and this leads to premature airway closure.

Relationship Between Airway Resistance and Work of Breathing

Airway resistance increases and specific conductance decreases during an asthmatic attack. As a result of these resistance changes, the work of breathing (both resistive and elastic) increases.[9, 10] In addition, abnormal ventilation-perfusion patterns develop; this leads to decreases in the arterial partial pressure of oxygen (PaO_2) and increases in the arterial partial pressure of carbon dioxide ($PaCO_2$). An increase in $PaCO_2$ is indicative of a severe episode. Abnormal ventilatory control may also be present.

What Cardiovascular Changes Occur?

The acute airway obstruction of asthma with air trapping can produce a deterioration in cardiovascular function. The electrocardiogram may demonstrate sinus tachycardia, premature ventricular contractions, P-pulmonale syndrome, right axis deviation, right bundle branch block, clockwise rotation of the heart, right ventricular strain pattern, and ST-T wave changes. The ST-T wave changes can be nonspecific or indicative of myocardial ischemia. Pulsus paradoxus and leftward shift of the interventricular septum with decreased left ventricular stroke volume are manifestations of severe airway obstruction.

What Conditions Aggravate Asthma?

Pregnancy, psychiatric disorders, sinusitis with nasal polyposis and aspirin allergy, obesity, cardiac disease, sleep apnea, and gastroesophageal reflux have an adverse effect on the asthmatic patient. Chronic obstructive pulmonary disease has an obviously negative impact. In some instances, treatment produces an unexpectedly adverse effect. For example, the use of β-adrenergic agonists can close small airways and leads to mucoid impaction of larger airways, resulting in deterioration in overall pulmonary function.

What Are Challenge Tests?

A number of challenges test the reactivity of bronchial airways. Nonantigenic agents such as histamine and methacholine can be used to elicit bronchoconstriction and to evaluate the adequacy of therapy. Inhalation of cold air and voluntary hyperpnea are used to provoke exercise-induced asthma. Inhalation of gases such as sulfur dioxide and ozone as well as exposure to occupational agents may provoke bronchospasm in susceptible individuals.

TREATMENT

What Are the Goals?

The primary goals of therapy are reversal of bronchospasm and control of the airway inflammatory reaction.[11-13] As noted, bronchospasm is due to airway hypersensitivity and hyperreactivity. Inflammation and release of inflammatory mediators not only produce edema and cellular infiltration of the airways but also contribute to bronchial hypersensitivity. Inflammation and loss of respiratory epithelium exposes autonomic and nonautonomic nerve endings. Stimulation of these nerve endings results in the release of neuropeptides (substance P), neurokinin A, calcitonin, and gene-related peptides that contribute to airway hyperreactivity. Pharmacologic therapy includes four major drug categories: (1) bronchodilators (β$_2$ agonists); (2) anti-inflammatory agents (adrenocorticosteroids); (3) inhibitors of mediator release (cromolyn sodium); and (4) anticholinergic agents.

Bronchodilators

The primary drugs for the treatment of bronchial asthma are bronchodilators. Airway smooth muscle contains large numbers of β$_2$-adrenergic receptors. Beta-adrenergic compounds increase intracellular cyclic adenosine monophosphate, activate protein kinase, inhibit myosin phosphorylation, and lower intracellular calcium levels, all of which lead to bronchial smooth muscle relaxation and bronchodilation. Beta-adrenergic agonists also stabilize cell membranes (mast cells, cholinergic nerve endings) and prevent release of mediators.

Several classes of β-adrenergic drugs exist (Table 56–3). Selected β$_2$-adrenergic agonists can be given in inhalation form. Inhaled drugs are effective and tend to be less toxic than parenteral preparations (Table 56–4).[14-16] Subcutaneous epi-

TABLE 56–3. Inhaled β-Adrenergic Agonist Bronchodilators

	Receptor Activity	Dose		Activity Duration (h)
		*Metered Dose Inhaler**	*Aerosol*	
Catecholamines				
Epinephrine	$\alpha_1, \beta_1, \beta_2$	160–250 µg	1% to 2.25% solution, 0.01 mL · kg^{-1} tid–qid	<1
Isoproterenol	β_1, β_2	120–130 µg (chloride) 80 µg (sulfate)	0.5% solution, 0.02 mL · kg^{-1} qid	<1
Isoetharine	β_2	340 µg	1% solution, 0.02 mL · kg^{-1} qid	1
Resorcinols				
Metaproterenol	β_2	650 µg	5% solution, 0.01–0.03 mL · kg^{-1} tid–qid	3
Albuterol	β_2	90 µg	0.5% solution, 0.01 mL · kg^{-1} tid–qid	4

*The usual patient dose with a metered dose inhaler is two puffs.
Abbreviations: tid = 3 times daily; qid = 4 times daily.

TABLE 56–4. Parenteral Bronchodilators

	Dose and Route of Administration
Methylxanthines	6 mg · mg^{-1} IV loading dose
Aminophylline	0.5–0.9 mg · kg^{-1} · h^{-1} maintenance
β-Adrenergic Agonists	0.1–0.5 mg SC
Epinephrine	1–4 µg · min^{-1} IV (10–50 ng · kg^{-1} · min^{-1})
Isoproterenol	0.5–5 µg · min^{-1} IV
Ephedrine	25–50 mg IM or SC
	5–25 mg IV
Terbutaline	Maximum of 0.5 mg in 4 h
Albuterol	10 µg · min^{-1} IV

Abbreviations: IV = intravenous; SC = subcutaneous; IM = intramuscular.

nephrine, in particular, is more toxic than inhaled epinephrine when administered to the hypoxic patient. Oral preparations (syrups and tablets) are also available for the resorcinols (terbutaline, metaproterenol) and albuterol.

Methylxanthines

The methylxanthines once were the most commonly used bronchodilators. They are synergistic with β-adrenergic agonists. Theophylline is most frequently used and can be administered orally or parenterally (Table 56–4).[17, 18] Their precise mechanism of action is not known; however, methylxanthines increase cyclic adenosine monophosphate by inhibition of phosphodiesterase.

The late response to allergens is also inhibited by an anti-inflammatory action. Theophylline, oxtriphylline, anhydrous theophylline (elixophyllin), and dyphylline are rapid-acting methylxanthines. Slow-release compounds that contain anhydrous theophylline are available.

Intravenous aminophylline is administered with a loading dose of 6 mg · kg^{-1} over 20 minutes, followed by an infusion of 0.9 mg · kg^{-1} · h^{-1} to maintain a serum level of 10 to 20 µg · mL^{-1}. Rapid improvement generally occurs within 15 minutes of administration of the loading dose. Side effects include nausea, vomiting, diarrhea, restlessness, insomnia, irritability, headache, seizures, tachycardia, dysrhythmias, hypotension, hypertension, diuresis, flushing, and fever.[19–21]

Several factors may affect the clearance of aminophylline from the bloodstream. Viral infections, cardiac failure, hepatic disease, and drugs (erythromycin, troleandomycin, cimetidine) decrease aminophylline clearance.[18] Increased clearance may result from cigarette smoking and hepatic enzyme induction (phenobarbital).

Adrenocorticosteroids

Corticosteroids are effective for the treatment of bronchial asthma because they suppress inflammation and prevent the release of mediators from mast cells.[22–24] Neither oral nor inhaled preparations are effective for acute attacks of bronchospasm. Inhaled steroids are useful in maintenance therapy to reduce the systemic effects of orally administered steroids.

Side effects of corticosteroids are protean and include sodium and chloride retention, gastric hyperacidity, hypertension, psychosis, hypokalemia, gluconeogenesis, increased intraocular pressure, growth retardation, muscle atrophy, poor wound healing, diabetes mellitus, osteoporosis, cataracts, and adrenal suppression. Several preparations are available (see Table 56–5).

Cromolyn Sodium

Cromolyn sodium is not a bronchodilator, but long-term use of this drug has been shown to reduce the number of acute episodes of asthma.[25] Cromolyn sodium stabilizes mast cell membranes and prevents the release of the mediators of immediate hypersensitivity.[26] It blocks or attenuates bronchoconstriction after the patient has been exposed to allergens or irritants. The protective effect lasts for 3 to 4 hours. It can be administered before exposure (for prevention of bronchoconstriction) by inhalation in the form of a powder or solution or with a metered dose inhaler. Side effects include throat irritation, cough, transient skin rashes, and, occasionally, bronchospasm.

Anticholinergic Agents

Anticholinergics block muscarinic airway receptors, inhibit vagal cholinergic tone, and produce bronchodilation.[27] These drugs are useful for the prevention of reflex cholinergic bronchospasm.

Ipratropium bromide (administered with a metered dose inhaler) and atropine methyl nitrate and glycopyrrolate methyl bromide (administered as aerosols) are three inhaled bronchodilators that are currently available. The quaternary anticholinergics have fewer side effects because of their low level of systemic absorption. Although the anticholinergics are not primary bronchodilators for the treatment of asthma, they are useful when given in conjunction with other bronchodilators, particularly β-adrenergic agonists.[28] They act on the larger airways and have a somewhat slower onset than do the β-adrenergic agents.

Unclassified Drugs

Anti-inflammatory drugs such as ketotifen, methotrexate, gold, and troleandomycin are currently under investigation. Experimental drugs such as leukotriene D4-receptor antagonist and 5-lipooxygenase inhibitors are also being studied.[29, 30] Nedocromil sodium is unrelated to cromolyn but has a similar action.

PERIOPERATIVE MANAGEMENT

Bronchial asthma is a relatively common disease, and the anesthesiologist must be prepared to manage asthmatic pa-

TABLE 56–5. Corticosteroid Preparations for Treatment of Asthma

	Potency Equivalents
Systemic Steroids	
Hydrocortisone	1
Prednisone	5
Prednisolone	4
Methylprednisone	4
Triamcinolone	5
Dexamethasone	30
Inhaled Steroids	
Beclomethasone (Beclovent), 250 µg per puff	800 µg · d^{-1}
Flunisolide (Aerobid), 250 µg per puff	1000 µg · d^{-1}
Triamcinolone acetonide (Azmacort), 100 µg per puff	1000–1600 µg · d^{-1}

tients. These individuals, including those who are asymptomatic, are more likely to develop postoperative pulmonary complications. Cardiac arrest is also more common in asthmatic patients than in normal individuals.

What Are the Elements of Preanesthetic Assessment?

Preanesthetic evaluation should include identification of precipitating factors and seasonal variation, frequency of attacks, time and duration of the last attack, and maintenance medications.[31] The physical examination should include observation of respiratory rate, use of accessory respiratory muscles, heart rate and blood pressure, auscultation of the chest for wheezing and rhonchi, elicitation of pulsus paradoxus, and awareness of the possible presence of physical signs of pulmonary hypertension.[32, 33]

Additional information may be obtained from examination of the sputum and from chest radiography, arterial blood gas partial pressure measurement (Pao_2 and $Paco_2$), and pulmonary function testing. Arterial blood gas measurement and measurement of pulmonary function are frequently beneficial, since a very poor correlation is often noted between the patient's subjective evaluation and the degree of pulmonary dysfunction.

Pulmonary function testing assesses the type and degree of airway obstruction, evaluates the response to bronchodilators, helps to determine perioperative risk, and provides guidelines for postoperative care. Measurement of the FVC, forced expiratory volume in 1 second (FEV_1), and $FEF_{25\%-75\%}$ indicates the severity of airway obstruction. A strong correlation exists among the FEV_1, the Pao_2, and the $Paco_2$: the lower the FEV_1, the higher the $Paco_2$.

What Are the Effects of Preanesthetic Preparation?

Preanesthetic preparation with respiratory therapy, cessation of smoking, treatment with bronchodilators, and physical training with deep breathing exercises reduce the incidence of postoperative complications in patients with obstructive lung disease. The asymptomatic patient who does not require maintenance medications can undergo anesthesia and surgery with little risk of postoperative complications. Avoidance of allergens, active or passive smoke, infection, alcohol, and nonsteroidal anti-inflammatory drugs is helpful in the management of asymptomatic patients.[33, 34]

Symptomatic patients without active disease should continue use of maintenance medications. Chest physiotherapy, postural drainage, and adequate hydration may be required to optimize preoperative preparation. The effect of therapy can be assessed by clinical, spirometric, and arterial blood gas evaluation. In particular, comparison of preoperative and postoperative data on pulmonary function tests allows the determination of whether a patient will respond to a change in the therapeutic regimen. Serum aminophylline levels should be measured and maintained between 10 and 20 $\mu g \cdot mL^{-1}$.[33]

Patients with active bronchospastic disease should be aggressively treated, and elective surgery for them should be postponed. If emergent surgery is required, bronchospasm can be treated with β-adrenergic agonists, aminophylline, and cor-

ticosteroids. The need for postoperative ventilatory support should be anticipated.

ANESTHETIC MANAGEMENT

What Factors Are Important?

General Considerations

In planning an anesthetic for the patient with asthma, the anesthesiologist must answer several questions (Table 56–6). Functional recovery from an acute episode of asthma may require several days to a week. Consequently, induction of anesthesia soon after an acute episode may provoke another attack.

Airway resistance in the asthmatic patient is greatest in the early morning hours. Although few data are available concerning the interaction of this diurnal pattern and anesthesia, delaying anesthesia and surgery until the late morning hours may be beneficial. Obviously, exposure to known irritants and allergens must be avoided during the perioperative period.

Interactions between anesthetics and bronchodilators such as β-adrenergic agonists and aminophylline may result in cardiac dysrhythmias. Changes in aminophylline levels and clearance may also occur during anesthesia.

Preanesthetic Medication

Preanesthetic medication should include the continuation of any agents that the patient is receiving for treatment of asthma, such as bronchodilators, corticosteroids, sedatives (barbiturates, benzodiazepines), and anticholinergics (atropine, glycopyrrolate). Patients receiving chronic corticosteroid therapy (oral or inhalation) may require supplemental corticosteroids during the perioperative period if they are considered to be at risk for steroid-induced adrenal suppression.

Administration of inhaled bronchodilators immediately before the induction of anesthesia may also be beneficial. Auscultation of the lungs immediately before induction should be performed to determine whether bronchoconstriction has developed since the preoperative examination. In patients with a history of atopy, antihistamines (histamine$_1$-receptor antagonists) may be beneficial. Histamine$_2$-receptor antagonists should be used with caution, since the histamine$_2$ receptors are necessary for inhibitory feedback for histamine$_1$ receptors.[33] Thus, sodium citrate may be preferable to cimetidine or other drugs of that class if an antacid is used.

When Is Regional Anesthesia Useful?

Regional anesthesia is preferred by many anesthesiologists for extremity, perineal, and lower abdominal surgery. It avoids

TABLE 56–6. Planning the Anesthetic Management of Patients with Asthma

- When was the last acute episode?
- What time of day is best for anesthesia and surgery?
- What allergens or irritants precipitate bronchospasm?
- What medications are used for treatment of asthma?
- What potential drug interactions can occur during anesthesia?

some potential bronchoconstrictive stimuli, such as tracheal intubation, and minimizes potential drug interactions. However, the occurrence of bronchospasm after spinal anesthesia suggests that unopposed vagal effects following sympathetic blockade as well as depression of adrenal function with decreased levels of endogenous steroids and catecholamines may be responsible.

What Are the Potential Problems with General Anesthesia?

Induction Agents

If general anesthesia is necessary, several considerations merit attention. Thiopental, methohexital, and propofol in usual clinical doses have no direct effects on bronchomotor tone and can be used in the asthmatic patient. Bronchospasm that occurs after the administration of these drugs is secondary to other stimuli (e.g., tracheal intubation). Ketamine is a bronchodilator and may be advantageous for the patient with bronchospasm. Nasotracheal intubation should be avoided in patients with an aspirin allergy and bronchial asthma owing to the great likelihood of the presence of nasal polyps.

Muscle Relaxants

Succinylcholine can be used for muscle relaxation in patients requiring tracheal intubation. Although d-tubocurarine, mivacurium, and atracurium can provoke histamine release, little clinical evidence suggests that these drugs are contraindicated. Vecuronium and pancuronium have also been used safely in asthmatic patients. Theoretically, the additive effects of pancuronium, β-adrenergic agonists, and aminophylline could result in tachydysrhythmias. Reversal of neuromuscular blocking drugs with neostigmine or pyridostigmine has not been shown to produce any adverse effects.

Inhalation Agents

Halogenated inhalation anesthetics (halothane, isoflurane, enflurane, desflurane) produce bronchodilation and are efficacious for the asthmatic patient.[35] In fact, these anesthetics have been used in the intensive care unit for the treatment of status asthmaticus.

Lidocaine

Lidocaine decreases bronchomotor tone. However, the direct instillation of lidocaine into the tracheobronchial tree may produce reflex bronchoconstriction. Consequently, use of intravenous lidocaine is preferable.

Drugs That Promote Bronchospasm

A number of drugs can release histamine, provoke bronchospasm, or produce anaphylactoid reactions (Table 56–7). They must be used with caution or avoided in patients with asthma.

What Monitoring Is Indicated?

Routine intraoperative monitoring of the asthmatic patient should include blood pressure and end-tidal CO_2 measurement,

TABLE 56–7. Drugs Associated with Histamine Release and/or Bronchoconstriction

Vancomycin
Histamine$_2$ antagonists
β-adrenergic blockers (propranolol, esmolol)
Anticholinesterases without concomitant anticholinergic agents
α- and β-adrenergic blockers (labetalol)
Radiopaque dyes
Prostaglandins with bronchoconstrictor effects
Protamine

pulse oximetry, and a chest or esophageal stethoscope evaluation. If wheezing is present, insertion of an arterial catheter and periodic measurement of arterial blood gas partial pressures are highly recommended.

When Should Tracheal Extubation Be Performed?

Extubation of the trachea during deep levels of anesthesia has the potential advantage of preventing reflex bronchospasm from tracheal irritation. However, many patients, such as those with gastroesophageal reflux or poor pulmonary function, are not good candidates for "deep extubation." These patients must be extubated when protective airway reflexes have returned.

INTRAOPERATIVE BRONCHOSPASM

How Should It Be Treated?

Intraoperative bronchospasm can present a significant challenge to the anesthesiologist. Bronchospasm results in air trapping; intrinsic positive end-expiratory pressure; decrease in cardiac output; hypotension; and increases in pulmonary arterial, right ventricular, and right atrial pressures.

Differential Diagnosis

The hallmark sign of bronchospasm is wheezing. However, a number of causes of intraoperative wheezing are not related to intrinsic bronchoconstriction (Table 56–8). These other causes must be considered and evaluated before treatment is begun. If they have been eliminated and asthmatic bronchoconstriction is suspected, treatment with bronchodilators should be initiated.

TABLE 56–8. Causes of Intraoperative Wheezing

Bronchial asthma
Chronic obstructive lung disease
Fluid overload
Acute left ventricular failure
Mechanical obstruction of the tracheal tube
Endobronchial intubation
Foreign body aspiration
Pulmonary aspiration of gastric acid
Persistent coughing against the tracheal tube
Pulmonary embolism

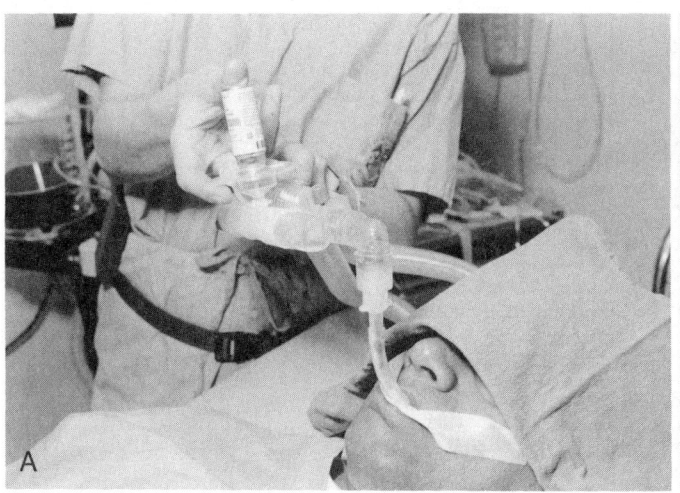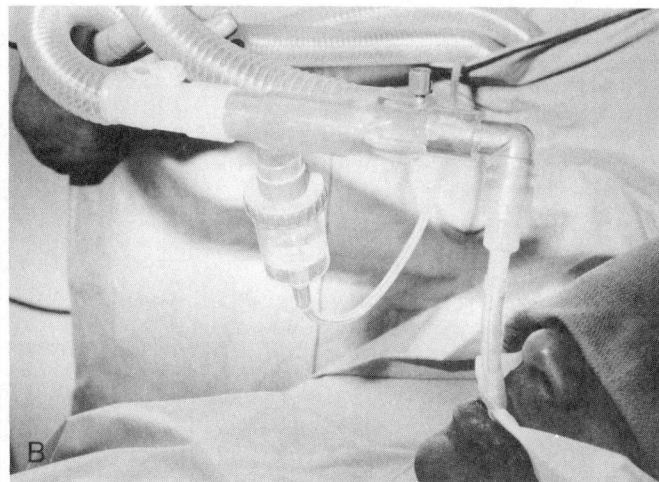

FIGURE 56–2. An efficient way of administering an inhaled bronchodilator through the inspiratory limb of the anesthesia circuit. A metered dose inhaler *(A)* or aerosol dispenser *(B)* can be attached without special adaptors. If an adaptor is available, the devices may be attached between the Y-connector and the tracheal tube.

Inhaled Bronchodilators

Inhaled bronchodilators can be administered with a metered dose inhaler attached to the tracheal tube or in aerosol form. The inhaled bronchodilator should be administered near the tracheal tube through the inspiratory limb of the breathing circuit or at the junction of the elbow connector and the tracheal tube (Fig. 56–2).

This treatment is best accomplished during manual ventilation, particularly if a metered dose inhaler is used, so that the respiratory effect can be optimized (i.e., by a deep inspiration with the drug delivery into the circuit at the midpoint, followed by an end-inspiratory pause). Metered dose or aerosol administration is equally effective.[36–40] How much bronchodilator is actually delivered to the airway when it is given through an endotracheal tube is unclear. Considerable deposition of the drug on the tube occurs. Thus, 5 to 10 metered doses may be required rather than the usual 1 to 2 puffs.

Beta$_2$-adrenergic agonists can produce tachycardia and must be used cautiously in patients with ischemic heart disease.[41, 42] Intravenous aminophylline is a very effective bronchodilator but requires more time to onset of action than do inhaled bronchodilators. Adjunctive therapy consists of promotion of a slow ventilatory rate and a low ratio of inspiratory to expiratory rate, application of expiratory retard, and adequate preload.[43–45]

POSTOPERATIVE CARE

The degree of postoperative ventilatory support is totally dependent on the preoperative status and intraoperative events. For example, the patient with active bronchospasm who requires emergent surgery may require postoperative mechanical ventilation. The asymptomatic patient with an uneventful intraoperative course requires no special postoperative care. Bronchodilator therapy should be continued in all asthmatic patients. Postoperative analgesia can be provided with neuraxial or parenteral narcotics.

References

1. McFadden ER Jr: Asthma: general features, pathogenesis, and pathophysiology. *In* Pulmonary Diseases and Disorders. 2nd ed. Vol. 2. Fishman AP (ed). New York, McGraw-Hill, 1988, pp 1295–1310.
2. Dawson A, Simon RA: Bronchospastic disorders: an overview. *In* The Practical Management of Asthma. Dawson A, Simon RA (eds). Orlando, Grune & Stratton, 1984, pp 3–18.
3. Weiss KB, Gergen PJ, Hodgson TA: An economic evaluation of asthma in the United States. N Engl J Med 1992; 326:862.
4. Barnes PJ: Inflammatory mediator receptors and asthma. Am Rev Respir Dis 1987; 135:526.
5. Kaliner MA, McFadden ER Jr: Bronchial asthma. *In* Immunological Disease. Vol. 2. Samter M, Talmage DW, Frank MM, et al (eds). Boston, Little, Brown & Co, 1988, pp 1067–1119.
6. McFadden ER Jr: Asthma: airway dynamics, cardiac function, and clinical correlates. *In* Allergy, Principles and Practice. 3rd ed. Vol. 2. Middleton E Jr, Reed CE, Ellis EF, et al (eds). St Louis, CV Mosby, 1988, pp 1018–1036.
7. Peres L, Sybrecht G, Maclem PT: The mechanism of increase in total lung capacity during acute asthma. Am J Med 1976; 61:165.
8. McFadden ER Jr, Kiser R, DeGroot WJ: Acute bronchial asthma: relations between clinical and physiologic mechanisms. N Engl J Med 1973; 288:221.
9. Bates DV: Respiratory Function in Disease. 2nd ed. Philadelphia, WB Saunders, 1989, pp 139–146.
10. Sheffer AL, Bailey WC, Bleecker UR, et al: Executive summary: guidelines for diagnosis and management of asthma. Bethesda, MD: National Institutes of Health; 1991. U.S. Department of Health and Human Services, pp 1–44.
11. McFadden ER Jr: Asthma: acute and chronic therapy. *In* Pulmonary Diseases and Disorders. 2nd ed. Vol. 2. Fishman AP (ed). New York, McGraw-Hill, 1988, pp 1311–1323.
12. Webb-Johnson DC, Andrew JL Jr: I. Bronchodilator therapy. N Engl J Med 1977; 297:476.
13. Webb-Johnson DC, Andrew JL Jr: II. Bronchodilator therapy. N Engl J Med 1977; 297:758.
14. Summer W, Elston R, Tharp L, et al: Aerosol bronchodilator delivery methods: relative impact on pulmonary function and cost of respiratory care. Arch Intern Med 1989; 149:618.
15. Newman SP, Clark SW: The proper use of metered dose inhalers. Chest 1984; 86:342.
16. Orgel HA, Kemp JP, Tinkelman DG, et al: Bitolterol and albuterol metered dose aerosols: comparison of two long acting beta-2 adrenergic bronchodilators for treatment of asthma. J Allergy Clin Immunol 1985; 75:55.
17. McFadden ER Jr: Methylxanthines in the treatment of asthma: the rise, the fall, and the possible rise again. Ann Intern Med 1991; 115:323.

18. Barnes PJ: A new approach to the treatment of asthma. N Engl J Med 1989; 321:1517.

19. Piafsky KM, Ogilvie RI: Dosage of theophylline in bronchial asthma. N Engl J Med 1975; 292:1218.

20. Hendeles L, Weinberger M: Theophylline: a "state of the art" review. Pharmacotherapy 1983; 3:2.

21. Bukowsky M, Nakatsu K, Munt PW: Theophylline reassessed. Ann Intern Med 1984; 101:63.

22. Morris HG: Mechanisms of action and therapeutic role of corticosteroids in asthma. J Allergy Clin Immunol 1985; 75:1.

23. Spector SL: The use of corticosteroids in treatment of asthma. Chest 1985; 87:73S.

24. Fanta CH, Rossing TH, McFadden ER Jr: Glucocorticoids in acute asthma: a critical controlled trial. Am Rev Respir Dis 1982; 125:94S.

25. Patalano F, Ruggieri F: Sodium cromoglycate: a review. Eur Respir J 1989; 2:556S.

26. Berman BA: Cromolyn: past, present, and future. Pediatr Clin North Am 1983; 30:915.

27. Gross NJ, Skorodin MS: Anticholinergic, antimuscarinic bronchodilators. Am Rev Respir Dis 1984; 129:856.

28. Chapman KR: Anticholinergic bronchodilators for adult obstructive airways disease. Am J Med 1991; 91:13S.

29. Manning PJ, Watson RM, Margolsku DJ, et al: Inhibition of exercise-induced bronchoconstriction by MK-571, a potent leukotriene D_4-receptor antagonist. N Engl J Med 1990; 323:1736.

30. Israel E, Dermarkarian R, Rosenberg M, et al: The effects of a 5-lipoxygenase inhibitor on asthma induced by cold, dry air. N Engl J Med 1990; 323:1740.

31. Geiger K, Hedley-White J: Preoperative and postoperative considerations. *In* Bronchial Asthma. 2nd ed. Ewiss EB, Segal MS, Stein M (eds). Boston, Little, Brown & Co, 1985, pp 892–907.

32. Hirshman CA: Perioperative management of the asthmatic patient. Can J Anaesth 1991; 38:R26.

33. Kingston HGG, Hirshman CA: Perioperative management of the patient with asthma. Anesth Analg 1984; 63:844.

34. Fung D, Smith NT: Anesthetic considerations in asthmatic patients. *In* Bronchial Asthma. Principles of Diagnosis and Treatment. Gershwin EE (ed). Orlando, Grune & Stratton, 1986, pp 525–540.

35. Behrakis PK, Higgs BD, Baydur A, et al: Respiratory mechanics during halothane anesthesia and anesthesia-paralysis in humans. J Appl Physiol 1983; 55:1085.

36. Bush G: Aerosol delivery devices for the anesthesia circuit (Letter). Anesthesiology 1986; 65:240.

37. Crogan SJ, Bishop MJ: Laboratory reports: delivery efficiency of metered dose aerosols given via endotracheal tubes. Anesthesiology 1989; 70:1008.

38. Tarala RA, Madsen BW, Patterson JW: Comparative efficacy of salbutamol by pressurized aerosol and wet nebulizer in acute asthma. Br J Clin Pharmacol 1980; 10:393.

39. Gay PC, Patel HG, Nelson SB, et al: Metered dose inhalers for bronchodilator delivery in intubated, mechanically ventilated patients. Chest 1991; 99:66.

40. Christensson P, Arborelius M Jr, Lilija B: Salbutamol inhalation in chronic asthma bronchiale: dose aerosol vs jet nebulizer. Chest 1981; 70:416.

41. Spitzer WO, Suissa S, Ernst P, et al: The use of beta-agonists and the risk of death and near death from asthma. N Engl J Med 1992; 326:501.

42. Neville E, Corris PA, Vivian J, et al: Nebulized salbutamol and angina. Br Med J 1982; 285:796.

43. Qvist J, Anderson JB, Pemberton M, et al: High level PEEP in severe asthma. N Engl J Med 1982; 307:1347.

44. MacDonnell KF, Moon HS, Sekar TS, et al: Extracorporeal membrane oxygenator support in case of severe status asthmaticus. Ann Thorac Surg 1981; 31:171.

45. Westerman DE, Benatar SR, Potgieter PD, et al: Identification of the high-risk asthmatic patient: experience with 39 patients undergoing ventilation for status asthmaticus. Am J Med 1979; 66:565.

CHAPTER **57**

Anesthesia for Patients with Chronic Obstructive Pulmonary Disease

S. S. MOORTHY, M.D.
STEPHEN F. DIERDORF, M.D.

Chronic obstructive pulmonary disease (COPD) includes several disease processes: chronic bronchitis, emphysema, asthmatic bronchitis, and bronchiolitis.[1, 2] The pathophysiologic hallmark of these disease processes is irreversible or partially reversible airway obstruction.

In addition to airway obstruction, each disease has other distinguishing features (Table 57–1). Chronic bronchitis is associated with cough, excessive expectoration of mucus, and a varying pattern of obstruction to airflow. Emphysema produces chronic enlargement of air spaces distal to terminal bronchioles, loss of lung elastic recoil, airflow obstruction, hyperinflation, and gas trapping. Asthmatic bronchitis is chronic persistent asthma with no symptom-free interval; airway inflammation; and hypertrophic, desquamative eosinophilic changes in bronchi. Bronchiolitis is usually a viral disease of childhood that is characterized by small airway narrowing secondary to inflammation. A number of viruses, including respiratory syncytial virus, influenza, rhinovirus, and mumps, can cause bronchiolitis.

COPD is much more common in men than in women (100:1) because of their greater genetic predisposition, occupational exposure to causative factors, and cigarette smoking (the last clearly being the most important factor). Deficiency of α_1-antitrypsin in homozygous individuals has an incidence of 1:2000 to 1:4000; in heterozygous individuals, this incidence is 1:100 to 4:100. This deficiency produces a specific type of emphysema. Inhalation of passive smoke and the smoking of marijuana or opium can also lead to emphysema. Air pollution (atmospheric and occupational), chronic lower respiratory infections, climatic factors, and heredity are associated with COPD. Also, persons with blood types A and O are at increased risk.

PATHOPHYSIOLOGY

What Are the Features of Chronic Bronchitis?

Chronic bronchitis is characterized by cough, sputum production, recurrent infection, and airway obstruction. Excessive smoking causes hyperplasia of mucous glands in the trachea and large bronchi; this results in production of copious quantities of mucoid secretions. Obstruction to airflow results from changes in small airways, associated emphysematous changes, an increased number of epithelial goblet cells, edema of mucous membranes, and muscular hypertrophy.[3]

TABLE 57–1. Characteristic Features of Bronchial Asthma, Chronic Bronchitis, and Emphysema

	Bronchial Asthma	**Chronic Bronchitis**	**Emphysema**
Age of onset	<30 y	>50 y	>60 y
History of smoking	No	Yes	Yes
Symptoms	Paroxysmal	Chronic	Chronic
Chest radiograph	Normal	Increased markings	Hyperinflation
FEV_1	Decreased during attack	Decreased	Decreased
TLC	Usually normal	Usually normal	Increased
RV	Usually normal	Usually normal	Increased
Pao_2	Normal	Decreased	Decreased
$Paco_2$	Normal	Elevated	Normal
D_{LCO}	Normal	Normal	Decreased

Abbreviations: FEV_1 = forced expiratory volume in 1 second; TLC = total lung capacity; RV = residual volume; Pao_2 = partial pressure of oxygen, arterial; $Paco_2$ = partial pressure of carbon dioxide, arterial; D_{LCO} = diffusing capacity of the lung for carbon monoxide.

In the early phases of an acute episode of bronchitis, the sputum is nonpurulent and airway obstruction is absent. Eventually, the sputum is colonized by bacteria and becomes purulent, although bacterial invasion of lung tissue does not occur. The degree of airway obstruction parallels infection of the sputum. Transudation of serum proteins and glycoproteins into the sputum occurs. Tracheal mucus velocity decreases secondary to reduced mucociliary activity. Normal ciliated epithelium is replaced by goblet cells and nonciliated squamous epithelial cells.

What Are the Features of Emphysema?

Emphysema produces abnormal and permanent enlargement of air spaces distal to the terminal bronchioles. The walls of these air spaces are destroyed, but no fibrosis occurs.[2, 3] Destruction of the elastic and collagen framework of the lung is caused by a proteolytic enzyme (elastase), which is secreted by neutrophils and other inflammatory cells. Normally, lung elastin is protected by a glycoprotein (α_1-antitrypsin) and a macroglobulin (α_2-antitrypsin).

Smoking produces a low-grade inflammatory reaction and increases the number of neutrophils in the blood and lung tissue; this produces elastolytic injury. Smoking can also alter the inhibitory effects of glycoproteins on elastase. Smokers with α_1-antitrypsin deficiency may develop emphysema by age 40 years (centrilobular emphysema). Nonsmokers with this deficiency may develop emphysema by age 60 years (panacinar emphysema).

What Are the Features of Asthmatic Bronchitis?

The diagnosis of asthmatic bronchitis is applied to patients with airway obstruction, chronic productive cough, and considerable difficulty with episodic bronchospasm. This syndrome may be a result of severe progressive classic asthma or a variant of chronic bronchitis. These patients have frequent and severe recurrences of bronchospasm.

SIGNS AND SYMPTOMS

Patients with a history of cigarette smoking and a family history of COPD are highly likely to have some component of COPD. Symptoms include progressive dyspnea, anorexia, nausea, chest pain, and, occasionally, hemoptysis.[4, 5] Signs include tachypnea, pursed-lip breathing, use of accessory muscles of respiration, tracheal tug, and pulsus paradoxus. Auscultation of the chest usually reveals distant breath sounds, rhonchi, crackles, and wheezing. Progressive chronic hypoxemia results in pulmonary hypertension and cor pulmonale. Cor pulmonale may be evidenced by hypoxemia, P-pulmonale syndrome on the electrocardiogram, and right ventricular hypertrophy.

What Does Pulmonary Function Testing Reveal?

Symptomatic patients with COPD invariably have abnormalities in pulmonary function (Table 57–2). As a general

TABLE 57–2. Features of Emphysematous Patients

Decreased	Increased
Lung recoil	RV
D_{LCO}	FRC
FEV_1	
MEFV	
$FEF_{25\%-75\%}$	
$\pm\ Pa_{O_2}$	

Abbreviations: MEFV = maximum expiratory flow volume; FRC = functional residual capacity.

guideline, pulmonary function testing reveals evidence of airway obstruction and parenchymal hyperinflation. A reduction in the forced expiratory volume in 1 second (FEV_1), forced expiratory flow, mid–expiratory phase ($FEF_{25\%-75\%}$), maximum flow at 75% of vital capacity, and mid–maximum expiratory flow, as well as prolonged expiration are indicative of obstructive airway disease.

Increases in residual volume, total lung capacity, and the ratio of residual volume to total lung capacity also occur.[5, 6] Specific airway compliance and dynamic compliance are reduced. An increased alveolar-to-arterial oxygen partial pressure gradient secondary to abnormal regional ventilation in the lower lobes results from poor compliance.

Emphysematous patients without hypersecretion of mucus exhibit the features listed in Table 57–2. In patients with pure chronic bronchitis, areas of low ventilation/perfusion matching dominate and produce hypoxemia and hypercarbia. Characteristically, the airway obstruction in patients with COPD does not improve significantly after the administration of bronchodilators as it does in patients with asthma (Fig. 57–1).

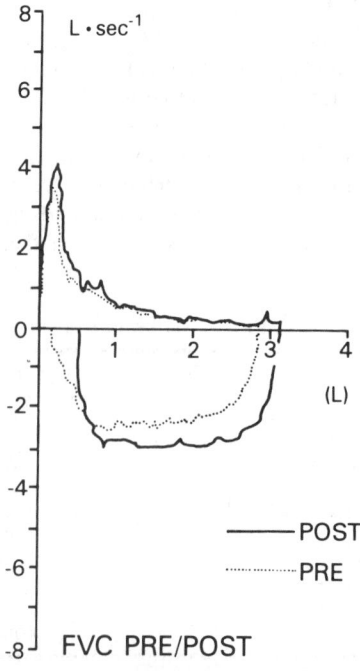

FIGURE 57–1. Flow-volume loops in a patient with COPD before (PRE) and after (POST) bronchodilator administration. No appreciable improvement in pulmonary function occurred after the bronchodilator was given. FVC = Forced vital capacity.

TREATMENT

Principles of treatment of patients with COPD include cessation of smoking, treatment of reversible bronchospasm, chest physiotherapy, and treatment of complications.[1] Complications include hypoxemia, hypercarbia, respiratory tract infection, and cor pulmonale.

What Drugs Are Useful?

Bronchodilators

Use of bronchodilators is the mainstay of treatment for managing reversible bronchospasm or bronchospasm that produces airflow limitation. Ipratropium bromide, β-adrenergic agonists, and aminophylline are commonly used.[7] Ipratropium has been found to be much more effective in patients with COPD than in patients with asthma.[8]

Corticosteroids

Corticosteroids, administered either as inhaled aerosols or systemically, are useful for reduction of inflammatory airway changes in patients with asthmatic bronchitis.[9] Preoperative administration of corticosteroids for 3 days prior to surgery has been associated with improved pulmonary function.

Do Ancillary Measures Help?

Observance of appropriate bronchial hygiene, cessation of smoking, avoidance of allergens and airway irritants, and antibiotic therapy for airway infection result in further improvement of pulmonary function.

Mobilization of Secretions

Mobilization of airway secretions is an important goal of adjunctive therapy for COPD. Adequate systemic hydration, effective cough training, and chest physiotherapy (chest percussion, vibration, postural drainage) aid in mobilization of airway secretions.

Iodinated glycerol is useful as an expectorant and mucolytic. Other oral mucolytic agents include thiopronine and 2-mercaptoethane. Acetylcysteine is an excellent mucolytic agent that can be administered as an aerosol or by direct instillation into the tracheobronchial tree. Considerable benefit, including improved exercise tolerance, can be derived from voluntary exercise and training of respiratory muscles (including upper abdominal muscles).

Oxygen

Hypoxemia should be treated promptly with administration of supplemental oxygen. Patients with pulmonary hypertension, cor pulmonale, polycythemia, exercise intolerance, impaired cognition, nocturnal restlessness, and morning headache benefit considerably.

PERIOPERATIVE MANAGEMENT

Patients with a history of smoking, COPD, and abnormal results on pulmonary function tests are at increased risk for developing pulmonary complications following surgery.[10, 11] Patients undergoing upper abdominal and thoracic surgery are at greatest risk.[11–13]

What Are the Important Historical Factors?

The preliminary evaluation of the patient with COPD should include the taking of a medical history that focuses on ascertaining the presence of dyspnea and its severity, smoking history, productive cough, wheezing, and the effects of previous anesthesia. The patient's ability to cough and clear secretions is also of considerable importance. Age over 60 years and obesity are also factors that increase perioperative risk.

What Should the Physical Examination Assess?

The physical examination should focus on the patient's breathing pattern (e.g., rate and depth, and accessory muscle use) and chest auscultation. A chest radiograph that demonstrates lung hyperinflation, cardiac enlargement, atelectasis, pneumonia, or pleural effusion is indicative of increased perioperative risk.

What Are the Guidelines for Pulmonary Function Testing?

Objective guidelines for performing pulmonary function testing are unclear, but clinical experience in concert with knowledge of the type of surgery generally is sufficient to suggest when to pursue arterial blood gas measurement and routine spirometry.

Spirometry

A patient with a clinical history of moderate COPD may not require spirometry prior to upper extremity surgery, but spirometry would certainly be necessary before laparotomy. Testing should include measurement of forced vital capacity (FVC), FEV_1, FEV_1/FVC, and $FEF_{25\%-75\%}$. The results can then be compared with normal predicted values. A typical flow-volume loop and spirometric measurements for a patient with COPD are shown in Figure 57–1.

Arterial Blood Gas Analysis

An arterial blood gas measurement during room air breathing is an excellent method to determine the patient's ability to exchange oxygen and carbon dioxide at rest. A partial pressure of arterial carbon dioxide ≥45 mm Hg is associated with greater postoperative risk.[11] Remember, however, that a surgical incision markedly affects respiratory function postoperatively. Consequently, isolated arterial blood gas measurement, which is not a good measure of pulmonary reserve, is an inadequate preoperative evaluation for the COPD patient undergoing upper abdominal or thoracic surgery.

More sophisticated measures of pulmonary function, such as split lung function testing, may be required for pulmonary resection.

What Is the Outcome After Upper Abdominal Surgery?

An upper abdominal incision is associated with reduced diaphragmatic excursion, and the effectiveness of cough is decreased by pain. These two factors lead to atelectasis, bronchitis, and pneumonia. After upper abdominal surgery, these complications occur in 25% of patients without COPD. Those with COPD and abnormal pulmonary function tests have a postoperative complication rate of 42%.

Proper preoperative preparation of patients with COPD can reduce the postoperative complication rate from 60% to 22%.[12] An increased likelihood of postoperative complications can be anticipated if the FVC is <75% predicted, the FEV_1 is <70% of the FVC, the $FEF_{25\%-75\%}$ is <50% of the FVC, and the maximum voluntary ventilation is <50% of predicted values (Table 57–3).

If preoperative preparation does not improve pulmonary function, a high incidence of complications should be anticipated. No pulmonary function values absolutely contraindicate surgery. Each patient with severe dysfunction must be considered on an individual basis, and the risk/benefit ratio of each patient for a given surgical procedure must be determined.

What Factors Increase the Risk of Thoracic Surgery?

Multiple factors contribute to the overall perioperative risk following thoracic surgery (see Table 57–3). Traditional pulmonary function testing has been used for many years in an attempt to correlate preoperative function with perioperative risk. Patients undergoing thoracic surgery for lobectomy or pneumonectomy have an increased postoperative risk with an FVC <2 L, an FEV_1 <1.2 L, an FEV_1/FVC <35%, an $FEF_{25\%-75\%}$ <1.6 L, a mid–expiratory flow rate <200 L · min^{-1}, and a maximum voluntary ventilation <50% of predicted (see Table 57–3).

Other pulmonary function values indicative of high risk include an increased residual volume, a diffusing capacity of the lung for carbon monoxide <50%, a partial pressure of arterial carbon dioxide >45 mm Hg, mean pulmonary artery pressure >22 mm Hg, and pulmonary vascular resistance >190 dynes · s^{-1} · cm^{-5}.[13, 14] Since the pulmonary tissue intended for resection may be noncontributory to ventilation, split pulmonary function testing that employs ^{133}Xe radiospi-

TABLE 57–3. Pulmonary Function Criteria Indicative of Increased Perioperative Risk

	Predicted Value (%)	
	Abdominal Surgery	*Thoracic Surgery*
FVC	<70%	<70%
FEV_1	<70%	<1.0 L
$FEF_{25\%-75\%}$	<50%	<50%
MVV	<50%	<50%
RV		>47%
$Paco_2$	>45 mm Hg	>45 mm Hg
Mean PAP		>22 mm Hg

(Modified from Gass GD, Olsen GN: Preoperative pulmonary function testing to predict postoperative morbidity and mortality. Chest 1986; 89:127.)
Abbreviations: MVV = maximum ventilatory volume; PAP = pulmonary artery pressure.

TABLE 57–4. Therapy to Reduce Pulmonary Risk

- Cessation of smoking
- Treatment of pulmonary infection
- Bronchodilator therapy
- Nutritional support
- Respiratory/chest physiotherapy
- Decreased anesthesia/surgical time (risk increased with operations >3 h)
- Effective postoperative analgesia (systemic and/or neuraxial narcotics)
- Maximum breathing exercises (incentive spirometry, nasal/mask continuous positive airway pressure)
- Early postoperative mobilization/ambulation
- Heparin prophylaxis in selected cases

rometry may be useful for predicting the effect of the actual loss of functional pulmonary tissue.

How Is the Patient Prepared for Surgery?

A number of therapeutic modalities can be employed preoperatively to improve perioperative outcome (Table 57–4).[15–19] Improved outcome is, however, predicated on the presence of a reversible component to the patient's COPD. Since most treatment requires more than overnight preparation, an adequate amount of time must be available for effective therapy.

Smoking

Cessation of smoking for 12 to 24 hours prior to surgery does not improve pulmonary function but does reduce the effects of nicotine. Reduced carboxyhemoglobin levels decrease the likelihood of erroneous pulse oximeter readings. To significantly reduce perioperative pulmonary morbidity related to smoking, cessation must occur at least 8 weeks before surgery. Pulmonary morbidity may actually increase if the duration of cessation is less than 8 weeks.[19]

ANESTHETIC MANAGEMENT

What Are the Advantages of Regional Anesthesia?

Regional anesthesia is advantageous for patients with COPD undergoing surgery on the limbs, lower abdomen, and perineum. The patient maintains relatively normal ventilation without alteration of ventilatory control mechanisms. Sedation, however, may negate many of these benefits. Spinal or epidural anesthesia at a level higher than T-10 may produce enough abdominal muscle dysfunction that the effectiveness of the patient's cough is reduced.

Continuous spinal or epidural techniques have the advantage of allowing the anesthesiologist to control the level of anesthesia. Brachial plexus anesthesia or more specific nerve block is associated with a very low perioperative pulmonary morbidity.

How Is General Anesthesia Utilized?

Induction Agents

If general anesthesia is required, no specific contraindications relate to commonly used induction agents such as thiopental, methohexital, propofol, etomidate, or ketamine.[20–22]

Maintenance Agents

Volatile Agents

Volatile halogenated agents (halothane, isoflurane, enflurane, desflurane) produce bronchodilation and are suitable for patients with COPD.[23-25]

Intravenous agents such as narcotics and benzodiazepines require more time for elimination than do inhaled anesthetics. Consequently, they may have a greater postoperative effect on respiratory control mechanisms than do inhaled agents. Despite these considerations, considerable individual patient variation and other factors (e.g., coexisting cardiac disease) have a significant influence on the selection of such drugs.

Nitrous Oxide

Since nitrous oxide has been shown to increase pulmonary vascular resistance and pulmonary artery pressures in patients with coexisting pulmonary hypertension, it should not be used in patients with cor pulmonale. It also may increase the volume and pressure of emphysematous blebs or bullae, or both, theoretically increasing the risk of barotrauma. In patients with blebs or bullae, nitrous oxide probably should not be administered.

Muscle Relaxants

Muscle relaxation can be produced with succinylcholine or nondepolarizing muscle relaxants. Muscle relaxants known to produce histamine release, such as d-tubocurarine and atracurium, have theoretic disadvantages, although no clear clinical evidence shows that these drugs are contraindicated. Pancuronium can produce tachydysrhythmias and should be used with caution. Vecuronium may be preferable because of its relative lack of cardiovascular effects and histamine release. Reversal of neuromuscular blockade with anticholinesterase agents does not have adverse effects.

What Problems Might Arise?

Cardiovascular

Intraoperative cardiovascular changes such as hypertension or supraventricular tachydysrhythmias should not be treated with β-adrenergic blockers because these drugs may provoke bronchospasm. Such bronchospasm is very unpredictable but can be severe. Atrial tachycardia can be treated with verapamil, 1 to 2 mg intravenously, to a total dose of 5 mg.

Respiratory

A slow respiratory rate with a prolonged expiratory time (a ratio of inspiratory to expiratory time of at least 1:3) is rec-

TABLE 57–5. Causes of Acute Increases in Airway Pressure with or Without Hemodynamic Changes During Anesthesia

- Bronchospasm from bronchial asthma or COPD
- Pulmonary edema with wheezing
- Pulmonary embolism with wheezing
- Partial obstruction of tracheal tube
- Inspissated secretions in the tracheobronchial tree
- Tension pneumothorax
- Endobronchial intubation

TABLE 57–6. Treatment of Intraoperative Wheezing and Increasing Airway Pressure

1. Stop nitrous oxide administration and ventilate lungs with 100% oxygen.
2. Discontinue mechanical ventilation and begin manual ventilation.
3. Increase expiratory time (ratio of inspiratory to expiratory rate >1:3).
4. Decrease respiratory rate.
5. Increase depth of anesthesia.
6. Administer intravenous lidocaine (1 mg · kg⁻¹).
7. Administer inhaled bronchodilator (use metered dose inhaler or aerosol).
8. Permit spontaneous ventilation, if feasible.
9. Perform tracheal extubation at a deep level of anesthesia at conclusion of procedure if not contraindicated.

ommended during controlled ventilation to prevent air trapping. Humidification of inspired anesthetic gases prevents inspissation of secretions. Administration of dry inhaled gases can lead to acute tracheal tube obstruction with impacted secretions, severe hypoxemia, and hypercarbia if not promptly recognized. Meticulous attention to ventilatory parameters is crucial during the perioperative period.

An increase in airway pressure and systemic hypotension should alert the anesthesiologist to the possibility of air trapping or tension pneumothorax. The conditions associated with intraoperative air trapping are listed in Table 57–5. Use of a pulse oximeter and capnograph are essential during general anesthesia, and insertion of an arterial catheter for periodic measurement of arterial blood gas partial pressures is highly recommended.

A number of causes of intraoperative wheezing must be eliminated before it can be assumed that intrinsic bronchospasm has developed. If bronchospasm is the cause, an inhaled bronchodilator (e.g., ipratropium, β-adrenergic agonist, or halogenated inhaled anesthetic) can be administered. Treatment of intraoperative bronchospasm is outlined in Table 57–6.

POSTOPERATIVE MANAGEMENT

How Is Weaning Accomplished?

The level of postoperative ventilatory care depends on the severity of the COPD and on the surgical site. Patients with severe COPD should be weaned from ventilatory support and managed with extubation as is any patient with respiratory failure. Measurement of arterial blood gases and bedside pulmonary function testing may provide very useful guidelines for extubation.

Careful consideration must be given to the effect of surgery on the respiratory "pump." Upper abdominal surgery, for example, produces significant disturbances in respiratory muscle coordination. The residual effects of anesthetics, narcotics, and muscle relaxants must also be considered.

Patients with mild to moderate COPD benefit from postoperative respiratory therapy such as chest physiotherapy or incentive spirometry, or both. Continuous positive airway pressure treatment and pressure support ventilation may reduce respiratory complications after upper abdominal and thoracic surgery.[26-30] Considerable individualization in postoperative care is necessary in patients with COPD.

How Is Pain Controlled?

Aggressive postoperative analgesia also appears to be of benefit in these patients as well, since it allows more aggressive pulmonary toilet. Epidural narcotic administration is of particular benefit after thoracotomy and upper abdominal procedures, particularly if the site of analgesic administration matches the dermatomes corresponding to the incision. As COPD patients are often particularly sensitive to the respiratory depressant effects of narcotics, consider an analgesic regimen that includes a narcotic and a nonsteroidal component (e.g., ketorolac).

References

1. Petty TL: Definitions in chronic obstructive pulmonary disease. Clin Chest Med 1990; 11:363.
2. Pierce JA, Niewoehner DE, Thurlbeck WM, et al: Standards for the Diagnosis and Care of Patients with Chronic Obstructive Pulmonary Disease (COPD) and Asthma. New York, American Thoracic Society, 1986, pp 225–244.
3. Thurlbeck WM: Pathophysiology of chronic obstructive pulmonary disease. Clin Chest Med 1990; 11:389.
4. Flenley DC: Chronic obstructive pulmonary disease. Dis Mon 1988; 34:543.
5. Georgopoulous D, Anthonisen NR: Symptoms and signs of COPD. *In* Chronic Obstructive Pulmonary Disease. Cherniack NS (ed). Philadelphia, WB Saunders, 1991, pp 357–362.
6. Hoppin FG Jr: Pulmonary function tests for diagnosis and evaluation of COPD. *In* Chronic Obstructive Pulmonary Disease. Cherniack NS (ed). Philadelphia, WB Saunders, 1991, pp 363–373.
7. Ziment I: Pharmacologic therapy of obstructive airway disease. Clin Chest Med 1990; 11:461.
8. Wesseling G, Mostert R, Wouters EF: A comparison of the effects of anticholinergic and beta 2-agonist and combination therapy on respiratory impedance in COPD. Chest 1992; 101:166.
9. Callaham CM, Dittus RS, Katz BP: Oral corticosteroid therapy for patients with stable chronic obstructive pulmonary disease. Ann Intern Med 1990; 114:216.
10. Gold MI, Schwam ST, Goldberg M: Chronic obstructive pulmonary disease and respiratory complications. Anesth Analg 1983; 62:975.
11. Harman E, Lillington G: Pulmonary risk factors in surgery. Med Clin North Am 1979; 63:1289.
12. Gass GD, Olsen GN: Preoperative pulmonary function testing to predict postoperative morbidity and mortality. Chest 1986; 89:127.
13. Zibrak JD, O'Donnell CR, Marton KL: Indications for pulmonary function testing. Ann Intern Med 1990; 112:763.
14. Frost EAM: Preanesthetic assessment of the patient with respiratory disease. Anesth Clin North Am 1990; 8:657.
15. Rehder K, Sessler AD, Marsh HM: General anesthesia and the lung. Am Rev Respir Dis 1975; 112:541.
16. Stein MA: Preoperative pulmonary function evaluation and therapy for surgical patients. JAMA 1970; 211:787.
17. Tisi GM: Preoperative evaluation of pulmonary function. Am Rev Respir Dis 1979; 119:293.
18. Van de Meter JM, Watring WG, Linton LA, et al: Prevention of postoperative pulmonary complications. Surg Gynecol Obstet 1972; 135:229.
19. Egan TD, Wong KC: Perioperative smoking cessation and anesthesia: a review. J Clin Anesth 1992; 4:63.
20. Nunn JF, Milledge JS, Chen D, et al: Respiratory criteria of fitness for surgery and anesthesia. Anesthesia 1988; 43:543.
21. Milledge JS, Nunn JF: Criteria of fitness for anesthesia in patients with chronic obstructive lung disease. Br Med J 1975; 3:670.
22. Tarhan S, Moffitt EA, Sessler AD, et al: Risk of anesthesia and surgery in patients with chronic bronchitis and chronic obstructive pulmonary disease. Surgery 1973; 74:720.
23. Hamilton WK, Sokoll MD: Choice of anesthetic techniques in patients with acute pulmonary disease. JAMA 1977; 197:789.
24. Pietak S, Weenig CS, Hickey RF, et al: Anesthetic effects of ventilation in patients with chronic obstructive pulmonary disease. Anesthesiology 1975; 42:160.
25. Rodrigues R, Gold MI: Enflurane as a primary anesthetic for patients with chronic obstructive airway disease. Anesth Analg 1976; 55:806.
26. Risser NL: Preoperative and postoperative care to prevent pulmonary complications. Heart Lung 1980; 9:57.
27. Bartlett RH, Gazzamga AB, Geraghty TR: Respiratory maneuvers to prevent postoperative pulmonary complications. JAMA 1973; 224:1017.
28. Banner MJ, Blanch PB, Kirby RR: Imposed work of breathing and methods of triggering a demand-flow continuous positive airway pressure system. Crit Care Med 1993; 21:183.
29. Stock MC, Downs JB, Gaver PK, et al: Prevention of postoperative pulmonary complications with CPAP, incentive spirometry, and conservative therapy. Chest 1985; 87:151.
30. Roukema JA, Carol EJ, Prins JG: The prevention of pulmonary complications after upper abdominal surgery in patients with non-compromised pulmonary status. Arch Surg 1988; 123:30.

CHAPTER 58

Pulmonary Edema

ERAN SEGAL, M.D.

AZRIEL PEREL, M.D.

Pulmonary edema is defined as the abnormal accumulation of fluid in the extravascular space of the lung. It is associated with disturbances of lung volumes, lung mechanics, and gas exchange; can be the result of diverse causes (Table 58–1); and always represents a potential threat to life.

In the perioperative period, pulmonary edema is a relatively rare event. Cooperman and Price described 40 cases of pulmonary edema and calculated that its overall incidence is 1:4500.[1] The true incidence is probably higher, since many patients have an increase in extravascular lung water (EVLW) without overt alveolar pulmonary edema. In their series of 1004 patients that formed the basis of the cardiac risk index, Goldman and coworkers found 36 patients who developed perioperative pulmonary edema, 58% of whom had no prior history of congestive heart failure (CHF).[2] The mortality in this subgroup was 57%, whereas those patients who developed heart failure without pulmonary edema had a lower overall mortality of 15%.

Since the impact of pulmonary edema on surgical outcome is significant, anesthesiologists must be familiar with its diagnosis and management. The majority of patients can be treated successfully if appropriate care is promptly initiated.

PATHOGENESIS

What Are the Important Anatomic Considerations?

Major structures involved in the pathogenesis of pulmonary edema are the microvascular endothelium, alveolar epithelium, interstitium, and pulmonary lymphatic system (Fig. 58–1).

Microvascular Endothelium

The endothelium is composed of a monolayer of cells situated on a basement membrane. Junctions between endothelial cells contain pores that allow the free passage of water and ions. They act as a sieve for protein molecules; of these molecules, only the smaller ones, such as albumin, normally can

pass with relative freedom, whereas larger ones, such as globulin and fibrinogen, cannot.

Alveolar Epithelium

Alveolar epithelial cells, which are situated on their own basement membrane, are composed of type 1 and type 2 pneumocytes. *Type 1 pneumocytes* are large, flat cells that line the alveoli as a continuous sheet and that have very tight gaps (pores) in their junctions. Thus, the alveolar wall is much less permeable than is the endothelial wall; this explains the many instances in which pulmonary edema remains in the interstitium without filling the alveoli. *Type 2 pneumocytes* are cuboidal stem cells that produce surfactant.

Pulmonary Interstitium

Between the endothelial and alveolar layers lies the thin part of the interstitium; its thicker component surrounds the larger blood vessels and airways. This space is a fibrin and collagen matrix that contains the pulmonary lymphatic vessels that drain the pulmonary microvascular filtrate.

PATHOPHYSIOLOGY

How Does Pulmonary Edema Present?

Pulmonary edema can be classified into three stages. The first involves EVLW accumulation in the interstitial space. Cuffs of fluid appear around bronchi and blood vessels, but oxygenation often is not severely impaired. During the second stage, fluid enters the alveoli, and hypoxemia appears owing to increased ventilation/perfusion ($\dot{V}/\dot{Q}$) mismatching. The third and most dramatic stage is that of airway flooding (Fig. 58–2).

What Is the Starling Equation?

The Starling equation incorporates the major forces that take part in transvascular (microvascular [mv] and interstitial [is])

TABLE 58–1. Some Conditions Associated with Perioperative Pulmonary Edema

CHF
Coronary ischemia
Fluid overload
Sepsis
Aspiration
Embolism
Neurogenic pulmonary edema
Re-expansion pulmonary edema
Negative-pressure postobstructive pulmonary edema
Aortic clamping
Lung resection
Cardiopulmonary bypass

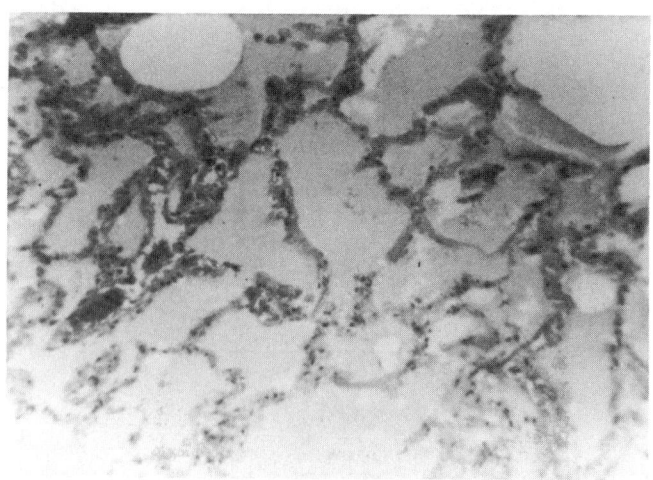

FIGURE 58–2. Histologic section of a lung from a patient with severe cardiogenic pulmonary edema. Note that the alveolar spaces were almost completely filled with pulmonary edema fluid (Photograph courtesy of J. Kopolovic, M.D., Chairman, Department of Pathology, Sheba Medical Center, Tel-Hashomer, Israel).

fluid exchange (Q̇f) (Fig. 58–3). These include the hydrostatic pressure gradient (Pmv minus Pis), which favors transudation of fluid from the microvessels; and the colloid oncotic pressure gradient (COPmv minus COPis), which normally draws water into the microvessels. The resulting balance, Q̇f, is the total amount of fluid that traverses the endothelial membrane. The equation is dominated by Kf, the fluid filtration coefficient that expresses the number and size of the endothelial membrane pores and the surface area available for fluid exchange.

Pulmonary edema usually is caused either by an increase in the pulmonary Pmv (cardiogenic) or by a change in the permeability characteristics of the microvascular membrane (noncardiogenic). The practical value of the Starling equation is conceptualization of pulmonary edema formation.

Microvascular Hydrostatic Pressure

The main determinant of filtration across the endothelium is the Pmv. When the left side of the heart fails, its end-diastolic volume increases owing to incomplete ejection. The resultant elevated pressure leads to increased left atrial, pulmonary venous, and pulmonary microvascular pressures.

Other downstream factors that can also affect Pmv include left atrial myxoma, mitral and aortic valve disease, decreased left ventricular compliance, and sudden increases in the peripheral vascular resistance. Clinically, Pmv is often estimated by the pulmonary artery occlusion pressure (PAOP), although it may be more accurately calculated as:

$$Pmv = LAP + 0.4 (PAP - LAP)$$

where PAP and LAP are the mean pulmonary artery and left atrial pressures, respectively. The constant, 0.4, denotes the estimated fraction of pulmonary vascular resistance that is downstream from the exchange vessels.

Pmv is influenced by gravity; in the upright position, it may be as much as 30 cm H_2O higher at the bases than at the apices of the lungs. Since fluid and protein probably cross pulmonary arterioles and venules as well as the capillaries, the operative Pmv within different segments of the pulmonary microvasculature can be quite different. Very high pulmonary perfusion pressures increase the passage of tracer substances into the interstitium from the intravascular space.

This observation forms the basis for the "stretched pores" theory, which suggests that high pressure and flow within the microvessels may cause physical shear damage to the endothe-

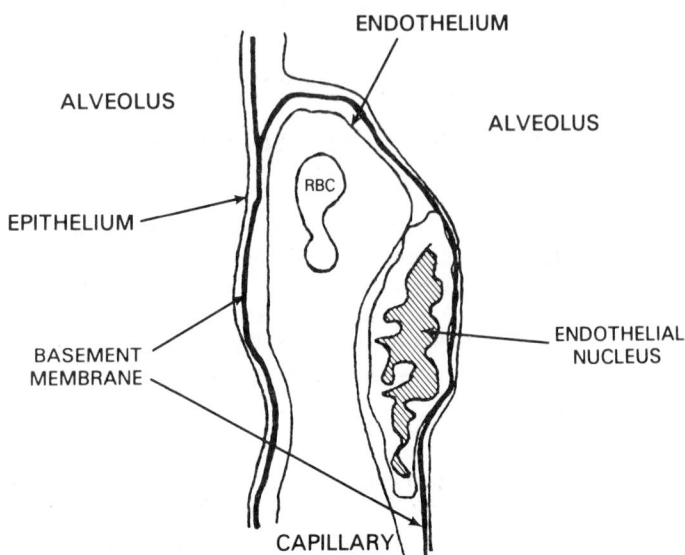

FIGURE 58–1. Schematic representation of the alveolocapillary membrane microanatomy. Note the basement membrane, which lies between the endothelial and the epithelial sides of the membrane.

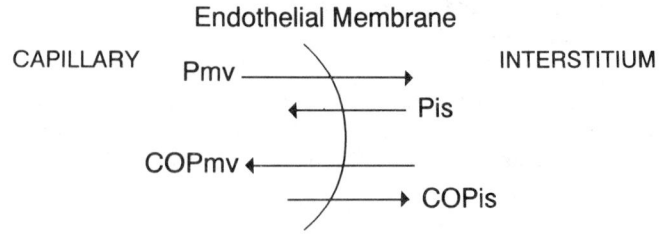

$$\dot{Q}f = Kf \left[(Pmv - Pis) - \sigma (COPmv - COPis) \right]$$

FIGURE 58–3. The Starling equation describes the forces involved in the transvascular fluid flux. The microvascular hydrostatic (Pmv) and the interstitial oncotic (COPis) pressures act in concert to drive fluid into the interstitium. The interstitial hydrostatic (Pis) and microvascular colloid oncotic (COPmv) pressures oppose this shift. σ = Reflection coefficient.

lium. Such a concept blurs the distinction between high pressure and increased permeability as precise causes of pulmonary edema. However, even when the entire cardiac output is diverted experimentally into a segment of the pulmonary vasculature, the ensuing edema appears to result primarily from high pressure with minimal evidence of physical damage to the endothelium.

Plasma Colloid Oncotic Pressure

The COPmv, which is generated by plasma proteins against the semi-permeable endothelial membrane, draws water into the microvessels from the interstitium. Because COPmv tends to negate Pmv, this gradient has been used in clinical studies of critically ill patients as an approximation of the net pulmonary fluid balance.[3] Hypoproteinemia does not affect steady-state filtration across the endothelial membrane. However, it makes the lungs more susceptible to pulmonary edema when Pmv is elevated.

Interstitial Hydrostatic Pressure

The Pis is believed to be more ''negative'' in the lung hilum than in the periphery.[4] This gradient within the interstitium probably is a major force in the mobilization of interstitial lymph from the periphery to its more central drainage sites. It acts in concert with the Pmv in the promotion of filtration from the microvessels into the interstitium and is important in negating the alveolar surface tension force and in keeping the alveoli dry.

Interstitial Colloid Oncotic Pressure

Data concerning COPis are derived mainly from analysis of lung lymph.[5] The pulmonary lymph, which is normally produced at a rate of $10 \ mL \cdot h^{-1}$, contains about 60% as much protein as the plasma. Distribution of proteins is determined by their capacity to cross the microvascular barrier. Thus, lymph albumin concentration is about 80% of the serum albumin concentration, but fibrinogen is almost absent in lymph.

The drainage capacity of the pulmonary lymphatic system may be overcome when large amounts of filtrate enter the interstitium from the intravascular space, leading to an increase in EVLW and interstitial edema, with or without overt alveolar edema.

CLINICAL IMPLICATIONS

How Are Pressure and Permeability Pulmonary Edema Differentiated?

Elevated left atrial pressure increases both lymph flow and EVLW content.[6] Pulmonary edema associated with an increase in hydrostatic pressure is relatively low in protein content because water primarily leaves the microvessels and passes into the interstitium. During increased permeability edema, the Kf is the primarily deranged variable, so that increased water and protein traverse the endothelial membrane. Since the membrane, in essence, loses its barrier function with respect to the passage of protein molecules, the normal oncotic pressure gradient between the plasma and interstitium may be abolished.

Etiology

Although the clinical picture of pulmonary edema is quite consistent, important etiologic differences must be distinguished if the response to therapy is to be enhanced. Thus, more than academic interest should spur clinicians to differentiate between high-pressure edema (as occurs in CHF) and permeability edema (as occurs in the adult respiratory distress syndrome [ARDS]) (Table 58–2). Such distinction is often difficult because patients may present with pulmonary edema owing to increases in both pressure and permeability.

Edema Fluid Analysis

When pulmonary edema results in flooding of the airways, its analysis may be helpful in differentiating the cause. With increased pressure, the fluid has a transudate-like quality and a low edema fluid/plasma protein ratio. When increased permeability is responsible, the edema fluid/plasma protein concentration ratio is usually >0.60.[7] Remember, however, that within 1 to 2 days, resorption of alveolar fluid will increase the ratio, even in high-pressure edema. Hence, the usefulness of this test is limited to the initial presentation.[8]

How Does Pulmonary Edema Affect Lung Volumes and Mechanics?

Accumulation of lung fluid has dramatic effects on volumes and mechanics. The functional residual capacity (FRC) in patients with pulmonary edema is greatly decreased; this leads to increased venous admixture and hypoxemia, even before alveolar flooding occurs. The reduction in FRC also activates stretch receptors that are responsible for the characteristic dyspnea. Finally, the reduced FRC causes markedly reduced lung compliance and a significant increase in the work of breathing.

Patients with pulmonary edema, therefore, revert to a pattern of rapid, shallow breathing and usually develop acute respiratory alkalosis. If the ratio of dead space to tidal volume is increased because of pre-existing chronic obstructive pulmonary disease (COPD) or other factors, carbon dioxide (CO_2) retention may eventually develop.[9] Increased airway resistance also may contribute to the increased work of breathing.

How Can Pulmonary Edema Be Recognized?

Awake Patients

The clinical presentation in awake patients can be quite variable. Initial signs and symptoms may include unexplained

TABLE 58–2. Differentiating High-Pressure and Increased-Permeability Pulmonary Edema

	High-Pressure Pulmonary Edema	Increased-Permeability/ Low-Pressure Edema
Filling pressures	High	Usually normal or low
Cardiac output	Often low	Often high
Edema fluid protein/ protein plasma	<0.5	>0.6
Heart size (on radiograph)	Large	Normal

agitation, increased blood pressure and heart rate because of generalized stress, and hypoxemia. Patients are dyspneic and tachypneic because of reduced lung compliance, activation of pulmonary interstitial stretch receptors, and shallow, rapid ventilation. Increased inspiratory effort is associated with intercostal retractions and accessory muscle activation.

When the respiratory rate exceeds 30 breaths per minute, the resistive work of breathing increases as well, leading to eventual fatigue and ventilatory failure. Inspiratory crackles reflect the sound of gas flowing through the fluid-filled distal airways. If pulmonary edema is mainly interstitial, the auscultatory findings are usually minimal.

Anesthetized Patients

Recognition of intraoperative pulmonary edema in the anesthetized patient is more difficult than in the awake patient, since few of the physical signs and none of the symptoms are present. Pulmonary edema should be suspected whenever an increase in airway pressure is associated with an apparent sudden decrease in compliance. Increased airway resistance also may cause sudden increases in airway pressure and is characterized by a large difference between the peak and plateau airway pressures pressure. This can be assessed by ventilating the patient with a respiratory pattern that includes an end-inspiratory hold.

The most common sign of pulmonary edema in the anesthetized patient is progressive hypoxemia that is relatively unresponsive to an increase in the fraction of inspired oxygen (FIO_2). Hypoxemia is not a specific sign of edema; it may be caused by bronchial intubation, atelectasis, or tube obstruction. Nevertheless, its appearance during anesthesia warrants careful investigation to rule out the possibility of pulmonary edema. Rarely, filling of the breathing circuit with edema fluid, which is often heard rather than seen, may be the initial presenting sign.

Oxygenation and Ventilation

Hypoxemia

The functional impairment associated with pulmonary edema usually is evaluated based on the degree of hypoxemia relative to the administered FIO_2 (PaO_2/FIO_2). In normal lungs, or in those in which $\dot{V}/\dot{Q}$ is low but finite (i.e., >0, implying that the airspaces are open), the partial pressure of arterial oxygen (PaO_2) rises when the FIO_2 is increased, so that PaO_2/FIO_2 remains relatively constant. With pulmonary edema, however, right-to-left shunting of blood through nonventilated lung regions often occurs. Therefore, the low PaO_2 may not respond appropriately to an increase in FIO_2, implying the presence of lung areas with a $\dot{V}/\dot{Q}$ ratio of 0.

Minimal pulmonary edema may be associated with only slight lowering of the PaO_2, which can remain unnoticed if the patient is breathing O_2-enriched gas; the decrease in the PaO_2 may be missed despite monitoring with a pulse oximeter, since arterial O_2 saturation decreases only when reductions in PO_2 <100 mm Hg occur. Thus, pulse oximetry does not replace periodic measurement of arterial blood gases to examine the response to therapy in the patient who develops intraoperative pulmonary edema.

Hypercapnia

A gradual increase in the partial pressure of arterial carbon dioxide ($PaCO_2$) may signify the worsening of edema, diminished alveolar minute ventilation, or both. This change can result from an increase in the anesthesia circuit's gas compression and compliance-related volume because of the higher airway pressures.

Lung Mechanics

Other parameters that reflect the functional impairment during pulmonary edema include alterations in lung mechanics—particularly lung compliance and work of breathing—that can be continuously monitored with advanced software (Fig. 58–4). Plateau airway pressure can be readily measured and used in the repeated calculation of static compliance. This parameter provides a good indication of the severity of the edema as well as a means to assess changes in the patient's clinical state.

Chest Radiography

High Pressure

In the absence of airway flooding, and because of the often nonspecific clinical picture, chest radiography is a major diagnostic tool.[10] In high-pressure edema, radiographic progression is predictable, with increased vascular markings appearing in the upper lung regions when the PAOP is about 15 mm Hg and signs of interstitial edema at a PAOP of 15 to 25 mm Hg. These signs include peribronchial cuffing or thickening of the peribronchial walls and Kerley B lines, which represent thickened interlobular septae.

When the PAOP is >25 mm Hg, alveolar flooding that appears as patchy air space opacification is usually seen. Such opacification may be most prominent near the mediastinum and take the form of a "butterfly," with the peripheral lung fields remaining relatively clear. The butterfly pattern is due to the greater degree of ventilation in the periphery of the lungs, which reduces the presence of fluid in the air spaces. A higher Pmv in the proximal pulmonary vessels may also contribute to this phenomenon. A large heart size is also typical of alveolar flooding of cardiogenic origin (Table 58–3).

Increased Permeability

The chest radiograph or a computed tomography (CT) scan during permeability edema often shows diffuse inhomogeneous infiltrates (Fig. 58–5). The picture may vary according to the underlying pathology.

Extravascular Lung Water Measurement

The direct measurement of EVLW can be done with a double dilution technique, using a cold solution with indocyanine green dye. The difference in the volume of distribution of both indicators (temperature and dye) is the volume of the EVLW. This technique requires the use of specially designed catheters and equipment and thus is impractical for routine clinical use.

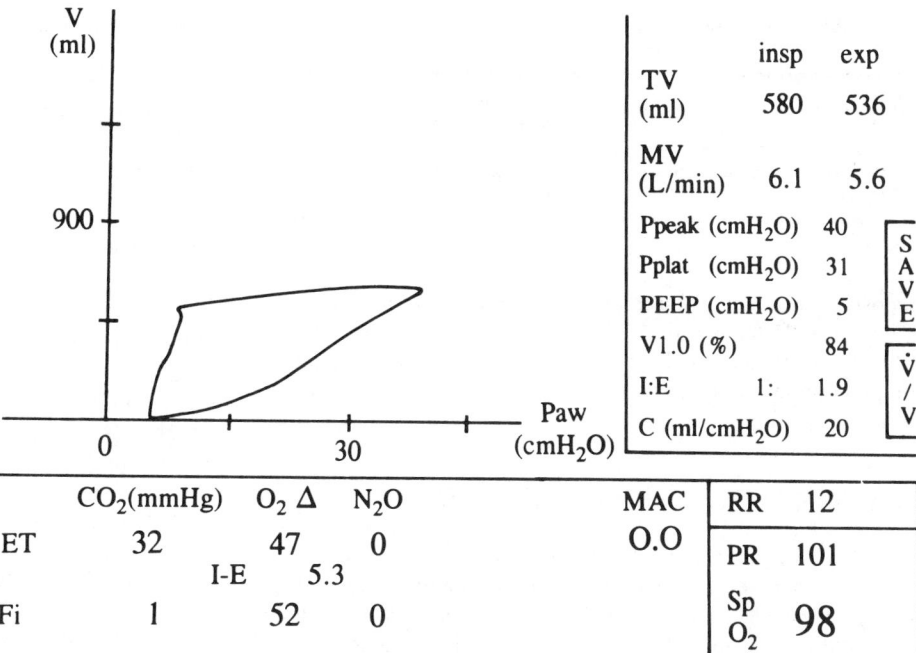

	insp	exp
TV (ml)	580	536
MV (L/min)	6.1	5.6
Ppeak (cmH$_2$O)	40	
Pplat (cmH$_2$O)	31	
PEEP (cmH$_2$O)	5	
V1.0 (%)	84	
I:E	1:	1.9
C (ml/cmH$_2$O)	20	

S A V E

$\dot{V}$ / V

	CO$_2$(mmHg)	O$_2$ Δ	N$_2$O	MAC O.O	RR	12
ET	32	47	0		PR	101
	I-E	5.3			Sp O$_2$	98
Fi	1	52	0			

TRACES FROZEN 08:31

FIGURE 58–4. Printout of a lung mechanics monitor. The compliance of the patient is 20 mL/cm H$_2$O. The resistive component of the patient's lung can also be appreciated by the large difference between the peak and plateau airway pressures.

PREOPERATIVE TREATMENT

The therapeutic approach to pulmonary edema includes three major elements: (1) normalization of oxygenation and ventilation, (2) reduction of excessive EVLW, and (3) identification and treatment of the underlying disease. Since the major pathophysiology of pulmonary edema is well understood, and since its response to certain therapeutic maneuvers is well established, treatment should begin immediately, even when the actual cause is still unclear.

Oxygen therapy, improvement of FRC and lung mechanics by continuous positive airway pressure (CPAP), and, if necessary, intubation and mechanical ventilation constitute the first therapeutic measures. The use of diuretics to rapidly achieve a negative water balance may be indicated if the patient's condition allows a decrease in preload in high-pressure edema. When possible, the cause should be determined. Identification of the causative mechanism may be of utmost importance in assessing the edema's natural course and prognosis and in directing more definitive therapy.

When pulmonary edema is suspected or diagnosed, several general supportive measures should be taken (Table 58–4).

What Is the Role of Positioning?

Patients with pulmonary edema should be placed in a head-up position whenever possible. In this position, the pulmonary Pmv is minimized and lung mechanics improve through gravitational augmentation of diaphragmatic descent. The head-up position, especially when combined with lowering of the legs, also reduces venous return, a factor of importance in patients with high-pressure edema. Immediate partial relief of dyspnea often follows.

These positional considerations are especially important in the surgical patient. Preoxygenation and induction should be performed with the patient sitting upright until loss of consciousness is achieved. The patient should then be rapidly

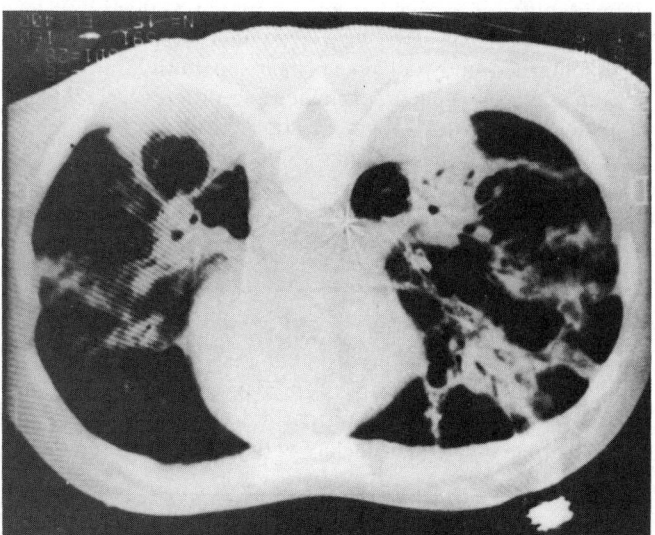

FIGURE 58–5. Computed tomography scan of a patient with severe ARDS, demonstrating the inhomogeneous type of injury in this disorder. (Photograph courtesy of Professor J.J. Rouby, Department of Anesthesiology, Hôpital Pitie-Salpetrier, Paris, France.)

TABLE 58–3. Commonly Found Radiologic Differences Between High-Pressure and Increased-Permeability Pulmonary Edema

	High-Pressure Pulmonary Edema	Increased-Permeability
Pleural effusion	Yes	No
Butterfly pattern	Yes	No
Peripheral distribution	No	Yes
Air bronchogram	No	Yes
Heart size	Large	Small

TABLE 58–4. Therapeutic Measures for the Patient with Pulmonary Edema

Positioning	Head-up position
Oxygen	High FIO_2
Negative fluid balance	When tolerated
Positive end-expiratory pressure	With mask or endotracheal tube
Drugs	Diuretics, vasodilators, inotropes

repositioned and tracheal intubation performed. If insertion of a central catheter is indicated, a modest Trendelenburg position is appropriate for the short duration of the venipuncture. Preparation and draping should be done with the patient in a head-up position.

How Should Oxygen Be Administered?

Although characteristically the hypoxemia that occurs during pulmonary edema does not respond significantly to O_2 therapy because of shunting, O_2 administration is still the first therapeutic measure. This is so because elevating the PaO_2 even slightly in very hypoxemic patients may significantly increase O_2 saturation and delivery. The highest FIO_2 possible should be delivered. During anesthesia, the patient must be ventilated with 100% O_2 until evidence of adequate oxygenation with a lower FIO_2 is demonstrated. The administration of 100% O_2 also has direct therapeutic value during the acute phase of pulmonary edema associated with air embolism because it promotes resorption of intravascular nitrogen.

Why Is Positive-Pressure Ventilation of Value?

Continuous Positive Airway Pressure

The ultimate supportive measure in pulmonary edema is facemask-administered CPAP in patients who have adequate spontaneous minute ventilation and an intact sensorium. Increasing the FRC by keeping the airway pressure positive at end-expiration often is sufficient to reduce the work of breathing and "flatten" the edema fluid on the walls of the tracheobronchial tree.

Use of the CPAP mask should be considered in the preoperative period, when the patient is prepared for surgery, or in the postoperative period, when pulmonary edema appears after extubation. In the latter instance, the anesthesiologist should be sure that the patient is fully conscious, has adequate pharyngeal reflexes, and shows adequate respiratory drive.

Mechanical Ventilation and Positive End-Expiratory Pressure

Intraoperative ventilation during pulmonary edema should include positive end-expiratory pressure (PEEP) delivered via a breathing circuit that is fitted with one of the various available "aftermarket" PEEP valves. The continuous administration of PEEP during transport to the postanesthesia care unit (PACU) is mandatory and should be performed with an appropriate transport ventilator, a PEEP valve attached to the self-inflating bag, or a Mapleson D circuit with an attached manometer so that PEEP can be continuously provided and monitored.

Although mechanical ventilation and PEEP can be dramatically effective, the attendant reduction of preload must be taken into consideration in hypovolemic patients. Once mechanical ventilation has been instituted, its gradual discontinuation (weaning) should be started when the patient is stabilized and the edema has resolved.

How Should Fluid Management Proceed?

Positive Balance

Fluid management in cases of pulmonary edema has been the subject of much controversy in critical care medicine. The most common approach is the aggressive reduction of filling pressures (i.e., keeping the patient "dry"). This approach, however, may cause hemodynamic instability and dangerously reduce perfusion to other organs, such as the kidneys.

Schuller and associates[11] retrospectively analyzed 89 patients with pulmonary edema in a medical intensive care unit (ICU). They found that survivors had no significant fluid gain or increases in EVLW. Patients with a low fluid gain (<1 L) had a better chance of survival, a shorter duration of mechanical ventilation requirement, and a shorter ICU stay compared with patients with a highly positive fluid balance.

The question to be answered is whether positive fluid balance is a marker or a cause of poor outcome. The investigators concluded that increased fluid administration is partially responsible for some patients' poor outcomes, and that if it is hemodynamically tolerated, a strategy of keeping patients dry is appropriate.

Intraoperatively, when active bleeding occurs in the presence of pulmonary edema, adequate fluid resuscitation should be carried out, even at the price of worsening edema. However, short bursts of rapidly administered fluids should be avoided, as they may locally increase pulmonary Pmv.

Colloid Therapy

Another approach is to attempt to increase the COPmv by infusing colloid solutions. This approach has been criticized because of the risk of infused colloid leaking into the interstitium, resulting in delayed edema resolution. Colloid infusions are also more expensive than crystalloid solutions, and no well-controlled study documents their superiority.

Shires and associates[12] examined the difference in EVLW in patients receiving colloid solutions compared with those who were given lactated Ringer's solution intraoperatively. No difference in EVLW occurred between the two groups. Although the patients receiving crystalloid solutions required twice as much fluid to achieve the same hemodynamic goals, this difference had no significance with respect to lung function.

Whatever fluid is chosen, attention should be given to maintaining adequate organ perfusion. Acute postoperative renal failure or critical illness carries grave prognostic implications, whereas worsening of $\dot{V}/\dot{Q}$ mismatch due to increased EVLW can usually be treated adequately with positive-pressure ventilation.

Which Drugs Are Potentially Beneficial?

The most useful drugs are diuretics, which can have a strikingly therapeutic effect in some patients. Besides reducing total body water, they may exert a beneficial effect owing to venodilation and increased COPmv.[13] When pulmonary edema is due to CHF, other measures for preload reduction, such as intravenous nitroglycerin administration or regional anesthesia to the lower half of the body, may be of value.

The reduction of pulmonary artery pressure with vasodilators may be of benefit as well and has been suggested to improve outcome in acute respiratory distress syndrome (ARDS) patients.[14] However, vasodilators can increase the production of lung lymph and may also increase shunt and hypoxemia by blunting hypoxic pulmonary vasoconstriction.

Other useful drugs are those directed at specific problems, such as sepsis, cardiac decompensation, or ischemia. Drugs that directly influence increased microvascular permeability are still considered experimental.

How Is the Patient with Cardiac Disease Managed?

Cardiac disorders, in particular ischemic heart disease, constitute a frequent cause of morbidity and mortality during anesthesia and surgery.[15] In adults undergoing cardiac or non-cardiac surgery, perioperative myocardial infarction, CHF, and pulmonary edema are among the most common causes of perioperative mortality.[16] Anesthesiologists, therefore, should carefully assess the patient with suspected heart disease preoperatively so that they may anticipate episodes of cardiac decompensation and optimize therapy.

History

The patient history is extremely important. Goldman and colleagues showed that a history and physical signs of CHF (an S3 gallop or the presence of jugular venous distention) are the strongest predictors of a cardiac complication in the perioperative period.[2] Information should be sought concerning daily activities and the patient's functional capacity. Since most patients are seen while they are at rest, those with mild to moderate CHF may be comfortable during the preoperative visit but may become dyspneic while walking into the examination room, undressing, or lying flat for a few minutes.

Physical Examination

Patients with chronic CHF are usually malnourished. They often show evidence of increased adrenergic activity that is reflected by peripheral vasoconstriction; pale, cold extremities; and a rapid but weak peripheral pulse. Examination of the lung fields may reveal fine inspiratory crackles at both lung bases. Ankle or sacral edema, an enlarged liver, and hepatojugular reflux due to right heart failure are often present.

Diagnostic Studies

The preoperative evaluation is also enhanced by objective measurements of left ventricular function (such as echocardiography) or radionuclide studies (to assess ejection fraction). Echocardiography is probably the better of the two methods because it also shows wall motion abnormalities and valvular function.

Preoperative Medication

A critical issue in the management of patients with ischemic heart disease concerns preoperative medication. Episodes of

ischemia often are unrecognized. The natural preoperative increase in stress can increase the frequency of ischemia. During such ischemic episodes, the associated acute reduction in left ventricular function may bring about an acute episode of pulmonary edema. Thus, patients should be adequately sedated when arriving for surgery. Some patients, however, may not tolerate heavy sedation that compromises respiratory drive and function. Hypoxemia in the preoperative admitting area should be prevented by administering O_2 to those patients who are suspected of having heart failure. The development of acute pulmonary edema in the immediate preoperative period is illustrated by the following case presentation.

CASE HISTORY NO. 1

A 67-year-old man arrived in the preoperative admitting area for a total hip replacement. The patient's previous medical history included ischemic heart disease and an acute myocardial infarction 3 years previously. He was seen the previous evening by an anesthesiologist who decided that he was not in optimal condition for surgery. Therefore, the anesthesiologist postponed the case. Owing to administrative error, the patient was brought to the operating room without having received his regular medications. Upon his arrival in the admitting area, he immediately started to complain of shortness of breath. A chest radiograph revealed pulmonary edema (Fig. 58–6).

Preparation of patients with CHF for surgery includes optimization of cardiac medications. Intravenous nitrates may improve coronary perfusion as well as preload and afterload conditions for the failing left ventricle. Intravenous dopamine or dobutamine may be started even before surgery to improve cardiac contractility.

Pulmonary Artery Catheterization

Elective surgery must be delayed until CHF is controlled. A pulmonary artery catheter may be inserted preoperatively, since gross aberrations of hemodynamic function are frequently unrecognized during clinical examination alone.[17] The pulmonary artery catheter should be used to establish the op-

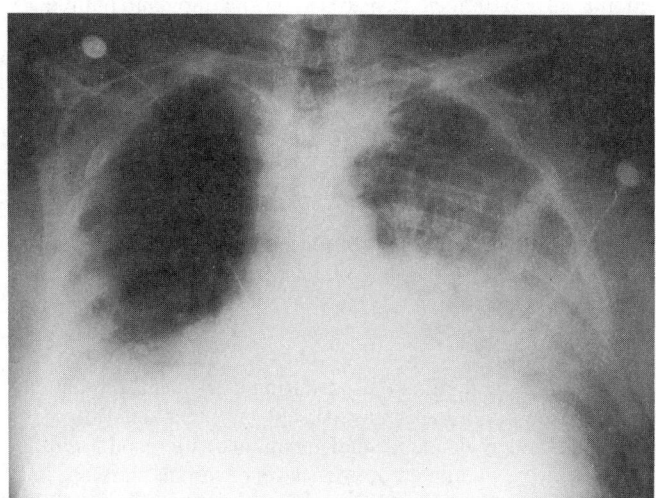

FIGURE 58–6. Chest radiograph of a patient who arrived in the operating room without being prepared for surgery. The patient developed chest pain and shortness of breath in the admitting area. The radiograph shows diffuse interstitial and intra-alveolar opacifications. Peribronchial cuffing may be seen in the right lung field.

timal filling pressures for the failing heart and to titrate drug therapy.

Patients in pulmonary edema should undergo surgery only in an emergency and when a conservative alternative is not available. The minimal possible procedure is the one that should be performed in these instances.

INTRAOPERATIVE PULMONARY EDEMA

How Is the Patient with Acute Respiratory Failure Managed?

The patient with pulmonary edema and ARDS who requires surgery usually comes from the ICU and may suffer from trauma, sepsis, aspiration, and other life-threatening conditions. Operative procedures may range from aggressive, stressful surgery for trauma or sepsis to "minor" procedures such as tracheotomy. Evaluation of the ICU patient with ARDS includes familiarization with the respiratory status and ventilatory parameters, since most patients need similar levels of support during transport and surgery.

Transport

Transport of the patient from the ICU to the operating room can be a serious challenge. The anesthesiologist should be involved in planning the transport and make sure that an adequate O_2 supply is available and that appropriate PEEP levels are provided throughout the transport. Use of a transport ventilator capable of providing CPAP and the required inspiratory pressures and minute ventilation is highly desirable (see Chapter 24).

Oxygenation

A major problem in many ARDS patients is the maintenance of adequate oxygenation during surgery. Biery and co-workers[18] reviewed 200 surgical procedures on patients who required mechanical ventilation for respiratory failure. The patients were divided into those with ARDS (n = 49), pneumonia (n = 20), atelectasis (n = 65), cardiogenic pulmonary edema (n = 11), and acute ventilatory failure that was due mostly to neurologic dysfunction (n = 55).

Most of the patients who developed intraoperative hypoxemia had ARDS and sepsis and were undergoing laparotomy. However, hypoxemia was usually short-lived and returned to preoperative values a few hours after surgery. The mortality within the first 3 postoperative days was quite low compared with overall in-hospital mortality. Thus, most of even the sickest patients survive the operative procedure.

Ventilation

The type of ventilator used during anesthesia for patients with pulmonary edema may present an unexpected problem. Schapera and associates[19] studied patients with respiratory failure who were ventilated during surgery with an Ohio anesthesia ventilator (Ohmeda, Madison, WI) or with a Siemens 900C critical care ventilator (Schaumberg, IL). Those ventilated with the Siemens 900C did better in terms of oxygenation and reduction of pulmonary shunt intraoperatively.

Choice of Ventilator

The same investigators conducted a bench study of different anesthesia ventilators and concluded that in situations of reduced compliance, increased resistance, and high minute ventilation, many anesthesia ventilators fail to provide the required ventilation parameters.[20] They recommended that for patients with a preoperative minute ventilation >15 L and a peak inspiratory pressure >50 cm H_2O, a critical care–type ventilator should be used intraoperatively.

Choice of Mode

Since patients frequently are given neuromuscular blocking agents during surgery, partial ventilatory support measures such as synchronized intermittent mandatory ventilation or pressure support ventilation must be replaced by controlled mechanical ventilation. Such change may lead to the development of excessive airway pressure as well as an increase in the compressible volume within the anesthetic circuit. A diminution of the patient-delivered tidal volume may result. Ideally, minute volume should be measured at the airway to obviate the effect of gas compression and circuit compliance. An arterial blood gas analysis after stabilization in the operating room is also useful because it is common for ARDS patients to have significant differences between arterial and end-tidal CO_2.

How Should Anesthesia Be Induced and Maintained?

The administration of anesthesia to the patient with pulmonary edema is a major feat. Anesthetic-induced stress reduction from a high adrenergic state, if not immediately accompanied by ventilatory and hemodynamic support, may cause hypotension and a vicious cycle that is difficult to control. Induction of anesthesia, therefore, requires agents that, at least in theory, maintain cardiac output (narcotics, ketamine, or etomidate). Care must be taken to prevent further myocardial ischemia in patients with coronary artery disease. In these patients and those with mitral stenosis, agents that may cause tachycardia are best avoided.

The maintenance of anesthesia may be complicated by hemodynamic instability and thus requires careful titration of anesthetic and vasoactive drugs. Consideration must be given to the effects of ventilation or different anesthetics on pulmonary vascular resistance and venous admixture, since hypercarbia increases pulmonary vascular resistance and because all inhalation agents depress hypoxic pulmonary vasoconstriction.

How Should the Patient with Pulmonary Edema Be Monitored?

All patients with or at risk of developing pulmonary edema intraoperatively should be monitored with pulse oximetry, capnography, and an arterial catheter. When cardiac ischemia is the cause of pulmonary edema, automated ST segment analysis and transesophageal echocardiography should be used when available.

Pulmonary Artery Catheterization

The insertion of a pulmonary artery catheter usually is indicated. Measurement of left ventricular filling pressures may be invaluable for both diagnosis and management, especially for patients with CHF undergoing major surgery associated with blood loss and large fluid shifts.

Differential Diagnosis of Pulmonary Edema

A major reason for performing pulmonary artery catheterization is to differentiate high-pressure from increased permeability pulmonary edema. Fein and colleagues[21] reported that in 70 consecutive patients, 40% of those suspected of having cardiogenic pulmonary edema had left ventricular filling pressures that were actually low. In contrast, patients with increased pulmonary microvascular permeability were, for the most part, diagnosed correctly on clinical grounds alone.

The overall value of pulmonary artery monitoring has been scrutinized in recent years. No objective evidence for improved outcome has been shown for this relatively expensive and invasive technology. However, some studies have shown a definite outcome difference when patients are managed with aggressive monitoring and goal-directed therapy outside of the operating room.[22]

Detection of Ischemia

Another potential benefit from pulmonary artery catheterization is its ability to detect ischemia. Although a rise in PAOP is a relatively late marker, most ischemic episodes are ''silent'' and are not accompanied by hemodynamic changes. Thus, the pulmonary artery catheter may help to diagnose subendocardial ischemia, even if it is not apparent in the electrocardiogram.

A major problem is that physicians who care for patients with pulmonary artery catheters on an irregular basis do not have adequate knowledge to make the most of this technique.[23] In addition, pulmonary artery catheter use is not without risks and complications. In the previously mentioned series described by Fein and colleagues, almost 25% of the patients had a major complication associated with pulmonary artery catheterization.[21]

What Is Neurogenic Pulmonary Edema?

Following severe injury to the central nervous system (trauma, subarachnoid hemorrhage, stroke, or seizures), an acute form of neurogenic pulmonary edema may occur. The classic explanation for neurogenic pulmonary edema is that the severe damage to the brain induces a ''sympathetic storm.'' The high levels of catecholamine cause a sudden increase in the pulmonary Pmv because of reduced left ventricular compliance and the shift of a large portion of the blood volume from the systemic circulation into the pulmonary circulation. The large increase in perfusion of the pulmonary microvessels is thought to cause pore stretching, which is, in turn, responsible for the high protein content in the edema fluid that is recovered. Thus, neurogenic pulmonary edema results from a combination of high pressure and increased permeability.

This syndrome frequently is short-lived and resolves rapidly with appropriate supportive therapy. However, it carries a grave neurologic prognosis.[24] Clinicians should be aware that the use of PEEP during neurogenic pulmonary edema may compromise cerebral perfusion by reducing cardiac output and impeding cerebral venous return.

How Does Embolization Produce Pulmonary Edema?

Air

Air embolism can be encountered during neurosurgical procedures that are carried out with the patient in the sitting position and also during spine, hip, and prostate gland surgery. It is occasionally seen following an inspiratory effort in the presence of a disconnected central venous catheter or after infusion of air via a pressurized fluid bag or as a result of the malfunction of an infusion system.

If a large amount of air suddenly enters the venous circulation, cardiac arrest may ensue owing to dysrhythmias, to airlock in the right ventricle, or to both. However, when air enters at a slower rate, the bubbles reach the pulmonary microvessels, and significant pulmonary edema may develop.

An early diagnosis should prompt an effort to remove as much air as possible through a central venous or right atrial catheter if one is present and if the source is from the upper half of the body.[25] The administration of 100% O_2 improves bubble reabsorption and oxygenation. PEEP should be immediately employed, as it prevents further entry of air into the venous circulation until the porta of entry is identified and sealed. However, in the presence of a probe-patent foramen ovale, paradoxic left-sided embolism may occur. Corticosteroids have been found to be effective in reducing the pulmonary damage only when they are administered prior to air embolism, and thus they have no role in the therapy of neurogenic pulmonary edema.[26]

Fat

The fat embolism syndrome usually appears 24 to 72 hours after long bone fracture and is characterized by mental confusion, thrombocytopenia, and petechiae in addition to respiratory failure. Increased pulmonary microvascular permeability is caused not only by the embolization of fat globules released from the bone marrow, since this is found after every bone fracture, but also by an as yet unidentified factor that causes activation of the complement or coagulation cascade. Moreover, intravenously administered fat globules do not produce the syndrome in experimental animals unless associated massive soft tissue trauma is also present. The release of free fatty acids by the action of lipase on neutral fat may also play a role in this process.

The incidence of severe fat embolism syndrome seems to be decreasing, most likely as a result of better and earlier fixation of fractures, careful administration of fluids, and earlier diagnosis. If a fracture has not been stabilized, it should be stabilized to stop this source of further embolization. Some investigators recommend the use of corticosteroids in the early management of fat embolism syndrome. Otherwise, the treatment is entirely supportive. Development of intraoperative pulmonary edema due to fat embolism during orthopedic surgery is extremely rare.

POSTOPERATIVE PULMONARY EDEMA

Why Does It Occur?

Acute pulmonary edema may develop in the immediate postoperative period. Of the 40 cases of perioperative edema studied by Cooperman and Price,[1] most occurred within the first 30 to 60 minutes postoperatively and were usually due to increased blood pressure in patients with previously known, poorly controlled hypertension. The following report illustrates such a case.

CASE HISTORY NO. 2

A 76-year-old man underwent endoscopic ureterectomy for stricture. His past medical history included ischemic heart disease with a myocardial infarction 4 years previously and coronary artery bypass graft 1 year later. He had been asymptomatic and was not receiving any cardiac medications. During the procedure, which was performed under general anesthesia, he was stable but had elevated blood pressure (180–190/115 mm Hg) even after fentanyl administration. Labetalol was administered in 5-mg increments until blood pressure and pulse rate were well controlled.

The patient was easily aroused at the end of the procedure and, therefore, was extubated and transported to the PACU. His O₂ saturation while he breathed room air was 87%. He complained of mild shortness of breath, and a chest radiograph revealed pulmonary edema (Fig. 58–7). The postoperative electrocardiogram was unchanged compared with a preoperative electrocardiogram, and creatine kinase (MB) levels were not elevated. He was treated with 100% O₂ and furosemide, and his status improved over a few hours.

The immediate postoperative period may be the first time that intraoperative pulmonary edema is diagnosed. It should be suspected when the patient exhibits signs and symptoms of respiratory failure following reversal of muscle paralysis and cessation of mechanical ventilation. When respiratory difficulty is encountered, the endotracheal tube should be kept in place while further doses of narcotics are administered. A chest radiograph should be obtained as soon as possible. If pulmonary edema is seen, adequate mechanical ventilatory support should be maintained while the cause is sought.

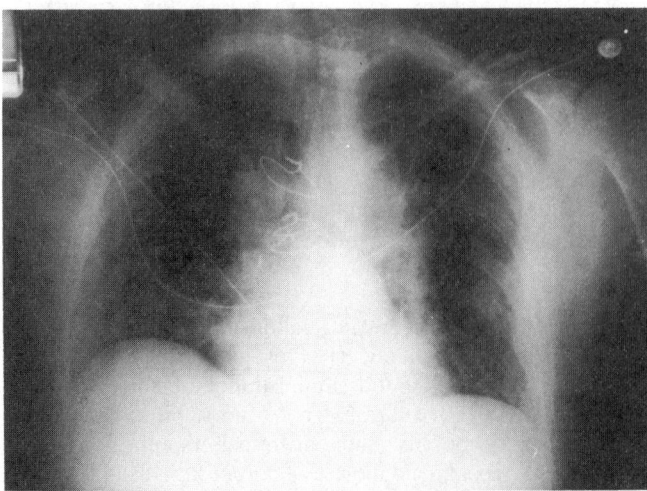

FIGURE 58–7. Chest radiograph of a patient with ischemic heart disease and a previous coronary artery bypass graft who developed hypertension and hypoxemia following a urologic procedure. The radiograph demonstrates enlargement of the vascular pedicles with cephalization of the pulmonary vascular markings consistent with cardiogenic pulmonary edema.

The cause is not always apparent; common problems in the differential diagnosis include overhydration, aspiration, and sympathetic overstimulation. Even when the reason cannot be defined, the prognosis is usually good if general principles of therapy are maintained (i.e., negative fluid balance, tailored respiratory support, and cautious weaning).

Hyperadrenergic State, and the Use of Naloxone

Emergence from anesthesia is characterized by significant sympathetic discharge, even in patients whose hemodynamic responses were well controlled during surgery. This sympathetic overstimulation can lead to hypertension and myocardial ischemia in those individuals with pre-existing heart disease. The excess catecholamine flux is further increased by pain, shivering, inadequate reversal of muscle paralysis, and anxiety. Adequate analgesia probably decreases the incidence and severity of these episodes.

Excessive catecholamine discharge also has been implicated as the reason for pulmonary edema following the administration of naloxone at the end of surgery. When naloxone is administered in doses that eliminate analgesia, the sudden, overwhelming sensation of pain results in a massive discharge of catecholamines, which may cause severe dysrhythmias as well as pulmonary edema. Postoperative respiratory depression, therefore, should be treated with small (20-μg) increments of naloxone, so as to achieve a relatively selective reversal of respiratory depression without elimination of analgesia.

This phenomenon serves as further evidence for the role of catecholamine-induced pulmonary edema, which is probably the result of a severe, nonhomogeneous constriction of segments of the pulmonary microvasculature. The administration of barbiturates and narcotics has been shown to prevent adrenaline-induced pulmonary edema in experimental models.

Relief of Airway Obstruction (Negative-Pressure Pulmonary Edema)

Pulmonary edema that appears following acute or prolonged airway obstruction is an intriguing problem.[27,28] It may appear in patients who develop airway obstruction during induction or emergence, particularly young adults who generate large "negative" intrapleural pressures during the period of obstruction. The relief of such obstruction by intubation or by resolution of laryngospasm can be followed by acute pulmonary edema.[29,30] Dyspnea, tachypnea, hypoxemia, and pink, frothy sputum are common within the first hour after arrival in the PACU. All patients with laryngospasm during induction or emergence should be watched for at least 2 hours. Pulmonary edema can appear as long as 4 hours after an episode of airway obstruction.[31]

Etiology

Pulmonary edema that develops following airway obstruction is due most probably to the large negative pericapillary inspiratory pressures that favor the transudation of fluid from the intravascular to the interstitial and airway spaces of the lung. Other factors also play a role. Among these are the increase in venous return and pulmonary blood volume secondary to the negative intrathoracic pressures as well as the

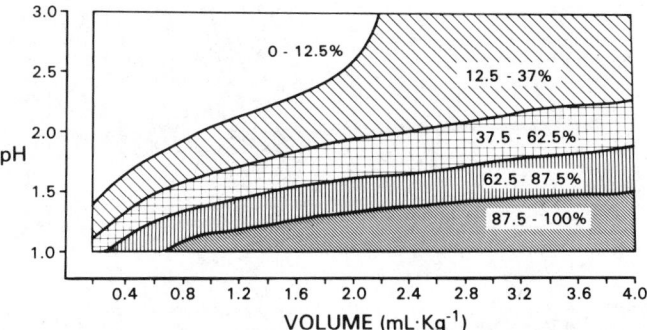

FIGURE 58–8. Predicted mortality rates (%) after aspiration. Each *shaded area* represents the mortality rate interval predicted for a specific pH and volume of solution aspirated. (From Janiec CF, Modell JH, Gibb CP, et al: Pulmonary aspiration: effects of volume and pH in the rat. Anesth Analg 1984; 63:667. © International Anesthesia Research Society.)

activation of hypoxic pulmonary vasoconstriction, which elevates pulmonary Pmv and promotes the efflux of fluid to the extravascular space.[28,31]

Increased sympathetic tone during episodes of airway obstruction causes further systemic vasoconstriction and additional increases in pulmonary blood volume. Intraoperative fluid overload also has been implicated, although documented PAOP values in patients with negative-pressure pulmonary edema have usually have been low.

Aspiration of Gastric Contents

Aspiration of gastric contents usually occurs during induction and emergence. At these times, patients are prone to aspirate because they are unconscious and do not mobilize their protective airway reflexes. Aspiration during induction usually manifests itself during surgery. Aspiration during emergence appears in the first minutes or hours postoperatively. Aspiration is not always accompanied by obvious signs of regurgitation.

The time from aspiration to its clinical presentation and the degree of pulmonary dysfunction depend on the pH and the quantity of the aspirate.[32] (Fig. 58–8). An aspirate with a pH of <2.5 and a quantity of >20 mL is thought to cause a clinically significant problem in an adult patient based on extrapolation of animal data. Particulate matter in the aspirate also causes serious damage as it can result in airway obstruction or granulomatous pneumonia. Risk factors for aspiration are listed in Table 58–5.

CASE HISTORY NO. 3

A 34-year-old man underwent emergency appendectomy. His previous medical history included familial Mediterranean fever with recurrent episodes of peritonitis. The patient had not received oral

TABLE 58–5. Some Conditions Associated with High Risk of Aspiration

Full stomach
Intestinal obstruction
Pregnancy
Trauma
Large intra-abdominal mass
Diabetes

intake for the previous 8 hours. Induction and surgery were uneventful, and the patient was extubated in the operating room while still somewhat somnolent. Upon arrival in the recovery room, he vomited a large amount of clear greenish fluid. He was turned on his side and his oropharynx immediately suctioned.

Ten minutes later, he experienced severe respiratory distress. He was intubated and ventilated with an FIO$_2$ of 1.0 and a PEEP of 10 cm H$_2$O. A chest radiograph revealed pulmonary edema with widespread opacification of both lung fields (see Fig. 58–9A). After 12 hours of therapy, a repeat chest radiograph taken during 5-cm H$_2$O PEEP showed marked improvement (see Fig. 58–9B).

Aspiration is the most important complication to prevent. Elective surgery patients at high risk should receive histamine$_2$ antagonists preoperatively to reduce gastric acidity. A single dose of metoclopramide (10 mg for a 70-kg patient) increases lower esophageal sphincter tone and improves gastric emptying. We routinely administer 200 mg of cimetidine or 50 mg of ranitidine intravenously, together with 10 mg of metoclopramide, 30 to 45 minutes before induction of high-risk patients. A nonparticulate antacid should be added to this regimen in emergency patients in order to neutralize what is already in the stomach. Placement of a nasogastric tube preinduction is advocated by some. This measure certainly decreases the gastric volume but does not predictably empty the stomach.

MISCELLANEOUS CAUSES

What Is Re-Expansion Pulmonary Edema?

Rapid evacuation of the pleural space in cases of pneumothorax or pleural effusion sometimes leads to pulmonary edema in the re-expanded lung. The exact mechanism that causes this entity is unclear but may involve the production of very negative interstitial pressures during the re-expansion that lead to a permeability defect.[33] It can occur in a single lung or even a single lobe after evacuation of air or fluid from the pleural space.[34] It is also occasionally seen as a bilateral phenomenon after evacuation of a single lung.

The disorder probably can be prevented by evacuating a longstanding pneumothorax or pleural effusion slowly. When a patient complains of chest pain following insertion of a chest tube (in the situation of longstanding lung collapse), the tube should be intermittently clamped and evacuation accomplished gradually over 10 to 15 minutes.[35]

Why Does Unilateral Pulmonary Edema Occur?

Mechanical Causes

A number of causes are possible for unilateral pulmonary edema. Most are mechanical factors and include the aforementioned cases of pulmonary edema following re-expansion and the relief of obstruction to a single lobe (as by laser surgery of an obstructing neoplasm).[36] Mechanical obstruction of the pulmonary veins following open heart surgery for congenital heart disease has been suggested as a cause.[37] Previous sympathectomy, which prevents edema in the denervated side, may result in contralateral manifestations.[38]

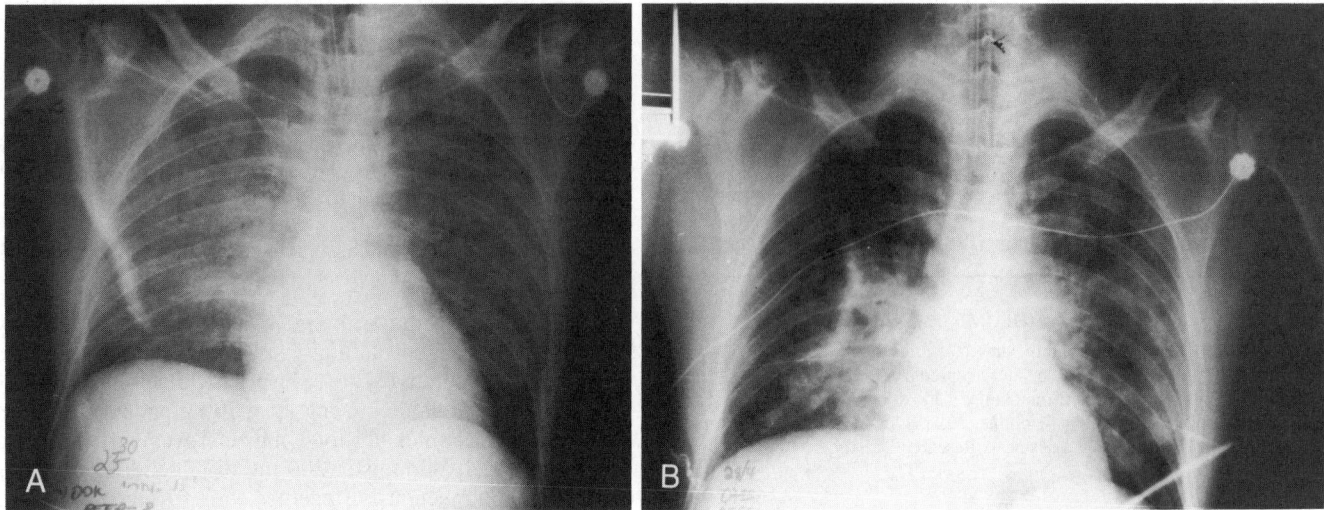

FIGURE 58–9. *A,* Chest radiograph of a patient who aspirated in the recovery room. The film was taken 15 minutes after the aspiration, and shows widespread interstitial and intra-alveolar opacification consistent with acid aspiration. *B,* Radiograph of the same patient taken 12 hours later. Substantial improvement is apparent.

Position

Patients in the lateral decubitus position tend to develop edema in the dependent lung because of increased hydrostatic pressure; this is described in the following case.

CASE HISTORY NO. 4

A 20-year-old man underwent surgery to remove a plate that had been placed for internal fixation of a fracture of the femur 6 months previously. The procedure was performed under general anesthesia with the patient in the right lateral decubitus position. The surgery lasted 2 hours, and the patient received 2 L of crystalloid solution during surgery. Upon arrival in the PACU, his O_2 saturation was low, and he required an O_2 mask with a FIO_2 of .40 to .50 to maintain saturation above 90%. His chest radiograph revealed predominately right-sided edema (Fig. 58–10).

Why Does Lung Resection Lead to Pulmonary Edema?

Pulmonary edema may appear in the first postoperative hours following lung resection. This entity has been described following both pneumonectomy and lobar resection. Manipulation of the lung, altered hemodynamics, intraoperative fluid overload, and reduced lymphatic capacity play a part in the formation of this disorder. Mathru and coworkers reported patients in whom the protein fraction in the edema fluid was >0.6 of that in plasma and suggested that this was caused by increased permeability.[39] The normal cardiac output that flows through a much smaller pulmonary vascular bed is associated with increased PAP and PAOP. Thus, the permeability defect can be caused by the increased shearing forces at microvascular junctions.

What Are the Effects of Aortic Cross-Clamping?

In patients who undergo aortic surgery, pulmonary edema may be caused by a number of factors. These patients often have intrinsic heart disease, and cardiac decompensation can

follow aortic cross-clamping. In addition, following aortic clamping, the problems of reperfusion may occur. In a number of studies, Hechtman's group showed that ischemia and reperfusion of a large body mass cause production of arachidonic acid metabolites. These metabolites, in particular, thromboxane, cause an elevation of PAP, margination of polymorphonuclear leukocytes in the lung, and an increase in EVLW.[40] Four to 8 hours following clamping, a decrease in oxygenation and an increase in airway pressures and EVLW (as assessed with chest radiography) were noted. The investigators described a protective effect of mannitol, which was ascribed to this drug's free radical scavenging properties.[41]

Why Does Pulmonary Edema Follow Open Heart Surgery?

Cardiopulmonary Bypass

Pulmonary edema may appear in the immediate postbypass period secondary to severe left ventricular dysfunction. The

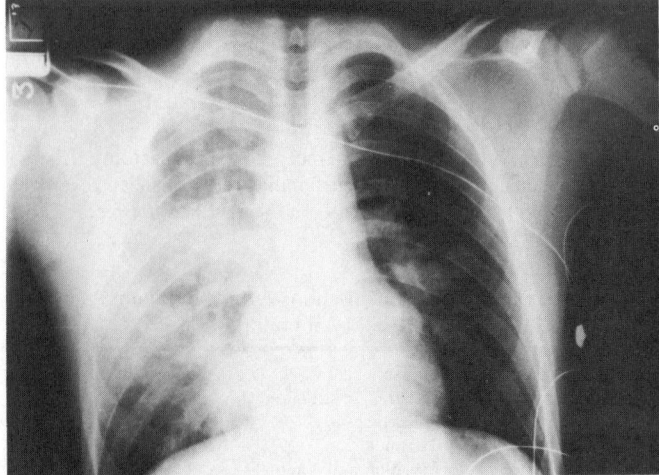

FIGURE 58–10. Chest radiograph of unilateral pulmonary edema in a patient who presented with moderate hypoxemia in the recovery room following a lengthy orthopedic procedure performed in the right lateral decubitus position.

heart-lung machine predisposes to hemodilution and a reduction of COP and also causes a permeability defect secondary to activation of complement and the sequestration of polymorphonuclear leukocytes and platelets.[42] The incidence and severity of pulmonary dysfunction increase with increasing bypass times. In procedures with mammary artery takedown, the commonly associated pleurotomy causes a pneumothorax and a lung that is atelectatic and immersed in ice solution for a prolonged time, thereby predisposing it to physiologic and mechanical insults.

Silent Ischemia

Another reason for post–open heart surgery pulmonary edema may be the ischemia that occurs in patients in the first few days following surgery. This ischemia, which is usually silent, has been correlated with adverse cardiac outcome, including pulmonary edema. The efficacy of intensive postoperative analgesia with a continuous infusion of sufentanil to reduce ischemia has been shown.[43] This approach may also reduce the risk of pulmonary edema due to such ischemic episodes.

References

1. Cooperman LH, Price HL: Pulmonary edema in the operative and postoperative period: a review of 40 cases. Ann Surg 1970; 172:883.
2. Goldman L, Caldera DL, Nussbaum SR, et al: Multifactorial index of cardiac risk in noncardiac surgical procedures. N Engl J Med 1977; 297:845.
3. Rackow EC, Fein IA, Siege J: The relationship of the colloid osmotic pulmonary artery wedge pressure gradient in pulmonary edema and mortality in critically ill patients. Chest 1982; 82:433.
4. Guyton AC, Parker JC, Taylor AE, et al: Forces governing water movement in the lung. In Pulmonary Edema. Fishman AP, Renkin EM (eds). Bethesda, MD, American Physiological Society, 1979, p 65.
5. Staub NC, Flick M, Perel A, et al: Lung lymph as a reflection of interstitial fluid. In Tissue Fluid Pressure and Composition. Hargens AR (ed). Baltimore, Williams & Wilkins, 1981, p 113.
6. Erdmann AJ III, Vaughn TR Jr, Brigham KL, et al: Effect of increased vascular pressure on lung fluid balance in unanesthetized sheep. Circ Res 1975; 37:271.
7. Sprung CL, Long WM, Marcial EH, et al: Distribution of proteins in pulmonary edema: the value of fractional concentrations. Am Rev Respir Dis 1987; 136:957.
8. Matthay MA, Wiener-Kronish JP: Intact epithelial barrier function is critical for the resolution of alveolar edema in humans. Am Rev Respir Dis 1990; 142:1250.
9. Perel A, Williamson DC, Modell JH: Effectiveness of CPAP by mask for pulmonary edema associated with hypercarbia. Intensive Care Med 1983; 9:17.
10. Morgan PW, Goodman LR: Pulmonary edema and adult respiratory distress syndrome. Radiol Clin North Am 1991; 29:943.
11. Schuller D, Mitchell JP, Calandrino FS, et al: Fluid balance during pulmonary edema: is fluid gain a marker or a cause of poor outcome? Chest 1991; 100:1068.
12. Shires GT III, Peitzman AB, Albert SA, et al: Response of extravascular lung water to intraoperative fluids. Ann Surg 1983; 197:515.
13. Wickerts CJ, Blomqvist H, Berg B, et al: Furosemide, when used in combination with positive end-expiratory pressure, facilitates the resorption of extravascular lung water in experimental hydrostatic pulmonary oedema. Acta Anesth Scand 1991; 35:776.
14. Humphrey H, Hall J, Sznajder I, et al: Improved survival in ARDS patients associated with a reduction in pulmonary capillary wedge pressure. Chest 1990; 97:1176.
15. Segal E: The preoperative evaluation of the patient with heart disease. Probl Anesth 1992; 6:22.
16. Browner WS, Li J, Mangano DT: Study of perioperative ischemia research group: in-hospital and long-term mortality in male veterans following non-cardiac surgery. JAMA 1992; 268:228.
17. Del-Guercio LRM, Cohn D: Monitoring operative risk in the elderly. JAMA 1980; 243:1350.
18. Biery DR, Marks JD, Schapera A, et al: Factors affecting perioperative pulmonary function in acute respiratory failure. Chest 1990; 98:1455.
19. Schapera A, Marks JD, Minagi H, et al: Perioperative pulmonary function in acute respiratory failure: effect of ventilator type and gas mixture. Anesthesiology 1989; 71:396.
20. Marks JD, Schapera A, Kraemer ARW: Pressure and flow limitations of anesthesia ventilators. Anesthesiology 1989; 71:403.
21. Fein AM, Goldberg SK, Walkenstein MD, et al: Is pulmonary artery catheterization necessary for the diagnosis of pulmonary edema? Am Rev Respir Dis 1984; 129:1006.
22. Shoemaker WC, Appel PL, Kram HB, et al: Prospective trial of supranormal values of survivors as therapeutic goals in high-risk surgical patients. Chest 1988; 94:1176.
23. Iberti TJ: Multicenter study of physician knowledge of the pulmonary artery catheter. JAMA 1990; 264:2928.
24. Wauchob TD, Brooks RJ, Harrison KM: Neurogenic pulmonary edema. Anaesthesia 1984; 39:529.
25. Artru A: Venous air embolism in prone dogs positioned with the abdomen hanging freely: percentage of gas retrieved and success rate of resuscitation. Anesth Analg 1992; 75:715.
26. Jerome EH, Bonsignore MR, Albertine KH, et al: Timing of corticosteroid treatment: effect on lung lymph dynamics in air embolism lung injury in awake sheep. Am Rev Respir Dis 1990; 142:872.
27. Kamal RS, Agha S: Acute pulmonary oedema: a complication of upper airway obstruction. Anaesthesia 1984; 39:464.
28. Sulek C: Negative pressure pulmonary edema. Curr Rev Clin Anesth 1992; 13:9.
29. Herrick IA, Mahendran B, Penny FJ: Postoperative pulmonary edema following anesthesia. J Clin Anesth 1990; 2:116.
30. Glasser SA, Siler JN: Delayed onset of laryngospasm-induced pulmonary edema in an adult outpatient. Anesthesiology 1985; 62:370.
31. Wilms D, Shure D: Pulmonary edema due to upper airway obstruction in adults. Chest 1988; 94:1090.
32. James CF, Modell JH, Gibbs CP, et al: Pulmonary aspiration: effects of volume and pH in the rat. Anesth Analg 1984; 63:665.
33. Timby J, Reed C, Zeilender S, et al: ''Mechanical'' causes of pulmonary edema. Chest 1990; 98:973.
34. Vuong TK, Dautheribes C, Robert J, et al: Reexpansion pulmonary edema localized to a lobe. Chest 1988; 93:1170.
35. Milano S, Tassi GF: Pneumothorax evacuation. Chest 1988; 93:443.
36. Miro AM, Shivaram U, Finch PJP: Noncardiogenic pulmonary edema following laser therapy of a tracheal neoplasm. Chest 1989; 96:1430.
37. Schiff GA, Simpson JI: Unilateral pulmonary edema after atrial septal defect repair. Anesthesiology 1991; 74:7851.
38. Flick MR, Kanzler GB, Block AJ: Unilateral pulmonary edema with contralateral thoracic sympathectomy in the adult respiratory distress syndrome. Chest 1975; 68:736.
39. Mathru M, Blakeman B, Dries DJ, et al: Permeability pulmonary edema following lung resection. Chest 1990; 98:1216.
40. Paterson IS, Klausner JM, Pugatch R, et al: Noncardiogenic pulmonary edema after abdominal aortic aneurysm surgery. Ann Surg 1989; 209:231.
41. Paterson IS, Klausner JM, Goldman G, et al: Pulmonary edema after aneurysm surgery is modified by mannitol. Ann Surg 1989; 210:796.
42. Klancke KA, Assey ME, Kratz JM, et al: Postoperative pulmonary edema in postcoronary artery bypass graft patients. Chest 1983; 84:529.
43. Mangano DT, Siliciano D, Hollenberg M, et al: Postoperative myocardial ischemia: therapeutic trials using intensive analgesia following surgery. Anesthesiology 1992; 76:342.

CHAPTER 59

Trauma

SCOTT H. NORWOOD, M.D.

MARY BETH MYERS, R.N., M.S.

Since the first recorded death from injury when Cain murdered his brother, Abel (Genesis 4:8, 4004 BC), trauma has remained the most common cause of premature death and disability. It is likely to remain the most common cause of death in young people until society mandates improvements in seat belt laws, automobile product design, preventive education, and gun control. Major improvements in emergency medical services throughout the United States have been instrumental in reducing immediate mortality due to trauma. Many injured patients who previously would have died of their injuries are now being rapidly transported to trauma centers for care.

It is unfortunate that the medical discipline of trauma care has evolved primarily as a result of peoples' inhumanity to each other. Many of the major advances in trauma care have evolved during global warfare. The first recorded use of anesthesia for military wounds was in 1847 under the direction of Edward H. Barton, when ether was administered to a soldier during a lower extremity amputation.[1]

Major advancements during the American Civil War included the first collection of records for a complete military medical history and development of a system for managing mass casualties with triage to aid stations, field hospitals, and general hospitals. This system set the pattern for the care of wounded soldiers in World War I, World War II, and the Korean War.[2] The importance of immediate definitive treatment of soft tissue wounds and fractures was also first recognized during the Civil War, when outcome from early extremity amputations was significantly improved if the amputations were performed within 24 hours after injury.[2]

Advances in homologous blood transfusion, recognition and treatment of renal failure, and management of the adult respiratory distress syndrome (ARDS) all are traced to the early experiences of military surgeons in World War II, Korea, and Vietnam.

Rapid air transport systems were first developed during the Korean War to evacuate soldiers from the front lines to field hospitals, and the extensive air evacuation system used during the Vietnam War was instrumental in improving survival from war wounds.

Although history has provided major improvements in pre-hospital care and emergency resuscitation, trauma continues to have an appalling toll in terms of morbidity and mortality in the Western World. Successful management of severely injured patients is dependent on rapid transport, early definitive resuscitation, operative intervention, comprehensive critical care, and early rehabilitation.

EPIDEMIOLOGY

How Is Trauma Categorized?

Classifying trauma by mechanism of injury is familiar to most physicians. The conventional categories are blunt (motor vehicle accidents, falls) and penetrating (gunshot wounds, stabbings). Another method focuses on the motive responsible for the injury—that is, intentional (deliberate) versus unintentional (accidental). This classification is often used by legal, statistical, and insurance systems. A third geographic category (urban versus rural) is useful in planning trauma care systems.

How Significant Is Trauma?

Injury is the primary cause of death in people ages 1 to 45 years and the fourth leading cause of death in all ages.[3] One study estimated the incidence to be 197 per 1000 population, with trauma accounting for as many as half of all emergency department visits.[4] Approximately 340,000 people per year are permanently disabled by injury.[3, 5] Because trauma afflicts primarily younger people, it is the primary cause of years of potential life lost as determined by the Centers for Disease Control and Prevention. Indeed, traumatic injury exceeds the years of potential life lost for cardiovascular disease and cancer *combined*.[3, 6, 7] The typical trauma patient in the United States is a young male involved in a motor vehicle accident.[5] The incidence of serious injury is three times greater in males than females.[8] Mortality rate for the "typical" age group (15–20 y) is 8.5%, based on data from 80,000 patients in the Major Trauma Outcome Study (MTOS).[5]

TABLE 59–1. Mortality Rate from Trauma by Age Group
(n = 80,529)

Age	Mortality Rate
>15	6.6
15–24	8.3
25–34	8.5
35–44	9.3
45–54	12.9
55+	31.3
Unknown	—

(Modified from Champion HR, Mabee MS: An American Crisis in Trauma Care Reimbursement. Washington, DC, The Washington Hospital Center, 1990.)

Mortality due to injury increases dramatically with age (Table 59–1), and despite the traditional correlation between trauma and youth, trauma in the elderly is increasing.[7, 8] Elderly patients are more likely to experience a complicated, prolonged hospital course owing to chronic underlying medical problems.[4, 5, 9, 10]

What Injury Patterns Occur in the Urban Setting?

Urban trauma is characterized by intentional, penetrating, and pedestrian injuries. Penetrating trauma outnumbers blunt trauma by two to one.[11] Forty per cent of trauma deaths in San Francisco were associated with violent crime.[11] In 1983, urban black males had a 5% chance of being murdered before the age of 30 years.[12] The risk is probably higher today. Homicides, assaults, burns, and pedestrian fatalities are highest among the poor,[3, 13] and large socioeconomic differences among urban populations increase the risk of intentional violent injury.

Urban trauma centers treat more patients than rural centers because of a large population base and tertiary care referral. Urban trauma centers also control helicopter transport programs, which further extend their normal catchment boundaries.

How Does Rural Trauma Differ?

Rural trauma is predominantly nonpenetrating. Two thirds of all traffic deaths occur in rural areas.[14] With the exception of homicide and suicide, death rates from other trauma are highest in rural areas.[3] Pennsylvania's trauma registry reflects a predominately rural trauma system and attributes only 11.9% of all statewide injuries to penetrating trauma.[15]

Maryland's trauma system population is also considered to be rural, because many acutely injured patients are transported from remote areas.[16] Their data reflect an incidence of 13.5% penetrating and 86.5% blunt trauma. Baker reported that 65% to 80% of rural hospital admissions secondary to injury were from blunt mechanisms.[11]

Rural trauma presents unique obstacles to care, including long transport distances, varied terrain, a smaller population base, predominance of basic and intermediate-level prehospital personnel, and limited access to professional and institutional resources.

What Is a Trauma System?

A trauma system is a network of informed professionals who work cooperatively to achieve a common goal: to get the right patient to the right hospital in the right time. The goal of a trauma system is to reduce mortality and morbidity by recognizing significant injury and integrating both prehospital emergency medical services and hospital resources to rapidly reverse the effects of injury. Thirty per cent to 40% of trauma deaths occur within a few hours after injury.[11, 12, 17] Hence, identification of patients at high risk for serious injury and development of standardized treatment strategies must be implemented throughout the spectrum of care.

Trauma systems are effective. Preventable deaths following trauma system development were reduced sevenfold in Orange County, California, during a 3-year period[17] and 12.1% in Dade County, Florida.[6] The trauma-related death rate declined 55% in San Diego over 1 year and 50% in Washington, DC, over 5 years of system operation.[17]

What Are the Costs?

Trauma care is phenomenally expensive to both individuals and society. The American Hospital Association reported the average charge for a trauma admission in 1988 to be nearly three times more expensive ($12,000 versus $4100) than a nontraumatic acute hospital admission.[15] McKenzie calculated that trauma in the United States cost 12.4 billion dollars in 1988.[18] This figure did not include the cost of rehabilitation and follow-up care.

Many Americans have no health insurance, and the uninsured sector is increasing three times faster than the population as a whole.[15] Medicare and Medicaid are unable to keep pace with rapidly inflating hospital costs. Penetrating trauma is frequently associated with violence and encompasses a much larger percentage of uncompensated care than blunt trauma.[19]

The lack of reimbursement for care has prompted many trauma centers to close, and inadequate, fragmented trauma care has resulted. During a 6-year period, the Los Angeles system lost 9 of the original 23 trauma centers.[20] Dade County, Florida, established a seven-hospital system in 1985. Within 2 years, only one institution, Jackson Memorial Hospital in Miami, continued to treat severely injured patients; their caseload rose to 6000 patients per year.[17] In 1986, the 66 hospitals throughout Florida that were treating trauma victims lost 39.5 million dollars in addition to operational costs.[6] San Diego County's six trauma centers estimated losses of 9 million dollars in 1987.[17] The Chicago trauma system estimated losses of 10 million dollars in 1989.[21]

Is Trauma Care Worth the Cost?

Given the costs and lack of reimbursement, one might question the benefits of providing trauma care. Champion and Mabee present a rational financial argument for developing trauma systems.[15]

"The most typical trauma patient, a 20 year old male, has an 80 percent chance of returning to full-time work post-injury, and will probably have a 40 year work history. Assuming an

average annual salary of $20,000 across his employment history, he will pay back in 7 years in federal, state, and local taxes the estimated $45,000 it cost (in 1988 dollars) for 1 year of acute and rehabilitative injury-related care. In addition, assuming a 6 percent discount, this rehabilitated trauma patient will contribute a total of $206,416 in taxes over his work history, and $554,918 in salary to the Gross National Product—12 times greater than the original $45,000 investment.''

Financial benefit to society can be defined. The benefit to individual trauma patients and their families defies calculation.

ASSESSMENT OF INJURY SEVERITY

Accurately identifying a severely injured trauma patient is essential for appropriately activating trauma system resources to achieve a reduced morbidity and mortality rate. Equally important is a standardized method for evaluating injury sever-

ity so that individual system performance may be compared with other systems and standard models of care.

What Defines a Severely Injured Trauma Victim?

Several scoring systems that assign a numeric value to physiologic indicators of injury are useful in identifying a severely injured patient. The Revised Trauma Score (Table 59–2), developed and statistically tested by Champion and Mabee, is widely used.[15] It uses systolic blood pressure, respiratory rate, and neurologic function (with the Glasgow Coma Scale) to determine the severity of injury.

Many Western states screen for severe injury using the CRAMS scale.[22] This scale requires assessment of circulation, respiration, abdominal signs, motor response, and sensory function. The Glasgow Coma Scale provides an objective measurement of global neurologic function through assess-

TABLE 59–2. The Revised Trauma Score

Systolic blood pressure (mm Hg)	Value	Score		
	>89	4		
	76–89	3		
	50–75	2	Points	
	1–49	1		
	0	0		

Respiratory rate (bpm)	Value	Score		
	10–29	4		
	>29	3		
	6–9	2	Points	
	1–5	1		
	0	0		

Glasgow Coma Scale (GCS)

Eye opening	Score	
Spontaneous	4	
To Voice	3	Points
To Pain	2	
None	1	

Verbal response	Score	
Oriented	5	
Confused	4	
Inappropriate words	3	Points
Incomprehensible words	2	
None	1	

Motor response	Score
Obeys commands	6
Localizes pain	5
Withdraw (pain)	4
Flexion (pain)	3
Extension (pain)	2
None	1

Total GCS Points [ ] = [ ]

Total GCS points = trauma points
13–15 = 4
9–12 = 3
6–8 = 2
4–5 = 1
3 = 0

A coded value less than 4 in any area should suggest transport to a trauma center.

(From Boyd CR, Tolson MA, Copes WS: Evaluating trauma care: the TRISS method. J Trauma 1987; 27:370. © Williams & Wilkins, 1987.)

ment of eye opening and verbal and motor responses. Tepas and colleagues developed a pediatric trauma score assessing size/weight, airway, the central nervous system (CNS), systolic blood pressure, wounds, and obvious skeletal injury.[23]

Scoring systems allow standardized injury severity classifications by both prehospital and trauma care providers. A threshold score can be determined (discussed in the triage section) to identify which patients activate the trauma system.

How Are Injuries and Outcomes Compared?

Several scoring systems that have been developed are based on studies that allow comparison among patient groups, institutions, and systems.[5, 24-26] The Injury Severity Score (ISS) numerically describes the overall severity of injury and may be applied to victims with multiple or isolated injuries.[24] It is calculated by rating each injury with the Abbreviated Injury Scale (AIS), then adding the squares of the highest AIS rating for each of the three most severely injured areas. The score ranges from 0 to 75 and correlates with expected mortality.

The TRISS score uses the ISS, age, Revised Trauma Score, and mechanism of injury (blunt or penetrating) to quantify the probability of survival.[25] This score is useful in quality assurance reviews: One should examine the deaths occurring in patients with predicted survival >50%. It provides a national standard that allows baseline comparisons among systems.

Which Patients Activate the System, and Who Goes to the Trauma Center?

Criteria for each system may vary slightly depending on unique characteristics, resources, and occasionally local politics. The major criteria include mechanism of injury; physiologic, anatomic, and comorbid factors (such as respiratory or cardiac disease); age; transport distances; and prehospital personnel expertise. The American College of Surgeons' Committee on Trauma developed and endorsed a general triage plan to determine which patients require trauma center care (Table 59-3).

EMERGENCY DEPARTMENT LOGISTICS AND OPERATING ROOM PREPARATION

Optimal trauma care requires team effort and a mechanism to ensure rapid team response to the resuscitation area when necessary. System criteria that direct patients to a trauma center are generally the same criteria used to activate the trauma resuscitation team. Prompt, optimum supportive care is crucial, and a system must be designed not to distract from this premise.

What Is the Trauma Alert?

The trauma alert is a notification system for activation of trauma team members. This may be an overhead page throughout the hospital or a series of individual pager activations. In our experience, simultaneous single pager activation quietly and effectively notifies the appropriate personnel without the heightened fanfare of an overhead page. Our current system

notifies both the primary responders and their backup personnel to increase each department's awareness and planning.

Team members are paged in their perceived order of importance (Table 59-4). Key areas (operating room [OR], blood bank) are also notified, even though no specific providers are dispatched to the resuscitation area. All responders have a predetermined time frame for response, generally 5 to 10 minutes based on institutional size and in-hospital personnel requirements. Any effective system must be carefully monitored and tested daily. Quality assurance monitoring and action on variances are imperative to prevent delays in providing care.

What Is the Trauma Team?

The composition and key roles of the resuscitation team are listed in Table 59-4. Trauma resuscitation requires a coordinated, organized team approach, and the resuscitation period is not the time for philosophic disagreements. Protocols of resuscitative care should be developed for common injury patterns, including delineation of specific team members' roles. This approach avoids confusion, assists in preparing for patients' arrival, and ensures a holistic approach.

The Team Leader

The team leader is usually a general surgeon, whose role varies based on the presence of a residency program. In teaching institutions, the team leader may be responsible for directing the resuscitation and providing minimum direct care, which is being performed by the third- and fourth-year residents. In nonresidency settings, the role is more comprehensive, providing overall direction and simultaneous direct care. The emergency department (ED) physician or anesthesiologist may also function as team leader under certain situations.

The Anesthesiologist's Role

In our institution, the anesthesiologist or certified registered nurse anesthetist (CRNA) is responsible for maintaining a patient's airway. Circumstances, pre-existing protocols, and experience of other team members dictate the actual techniques used.

The anesthesiologist's critical care experience provides a solid base for decision-making within the trauma resuscitation framework. Positioned at the head of the stretcher, anesthesia personnel have the best view of the progress in patient resuscitation. This role may continue during complicated diagnostic testing and, of course, into the operating suite.

Many anesthesiologists also contribute significantly to the critical care management of trauma patients in the surgical intensive care unit (SICU). For those reasons, a basic knowledge of traumatology, as presented in the Advanced Trauma Life Support (ATLS) course, is strongly recommended.[27, 28]

The Nurse's Role

Nurses provide continuous monitoring of patients throughout the spectrum of care from the emergency department to rehabilitation. Experienced nurses knowledgeable in trauma care are crucial to a patient's survival. Nurses may audit the ATLS course or participate in courses such as the Illinois Trauma Nurse Specialist Course[29] or Trauma Nurse Core Course.[30]

TABLE 59–3. Triage Decision Scheme

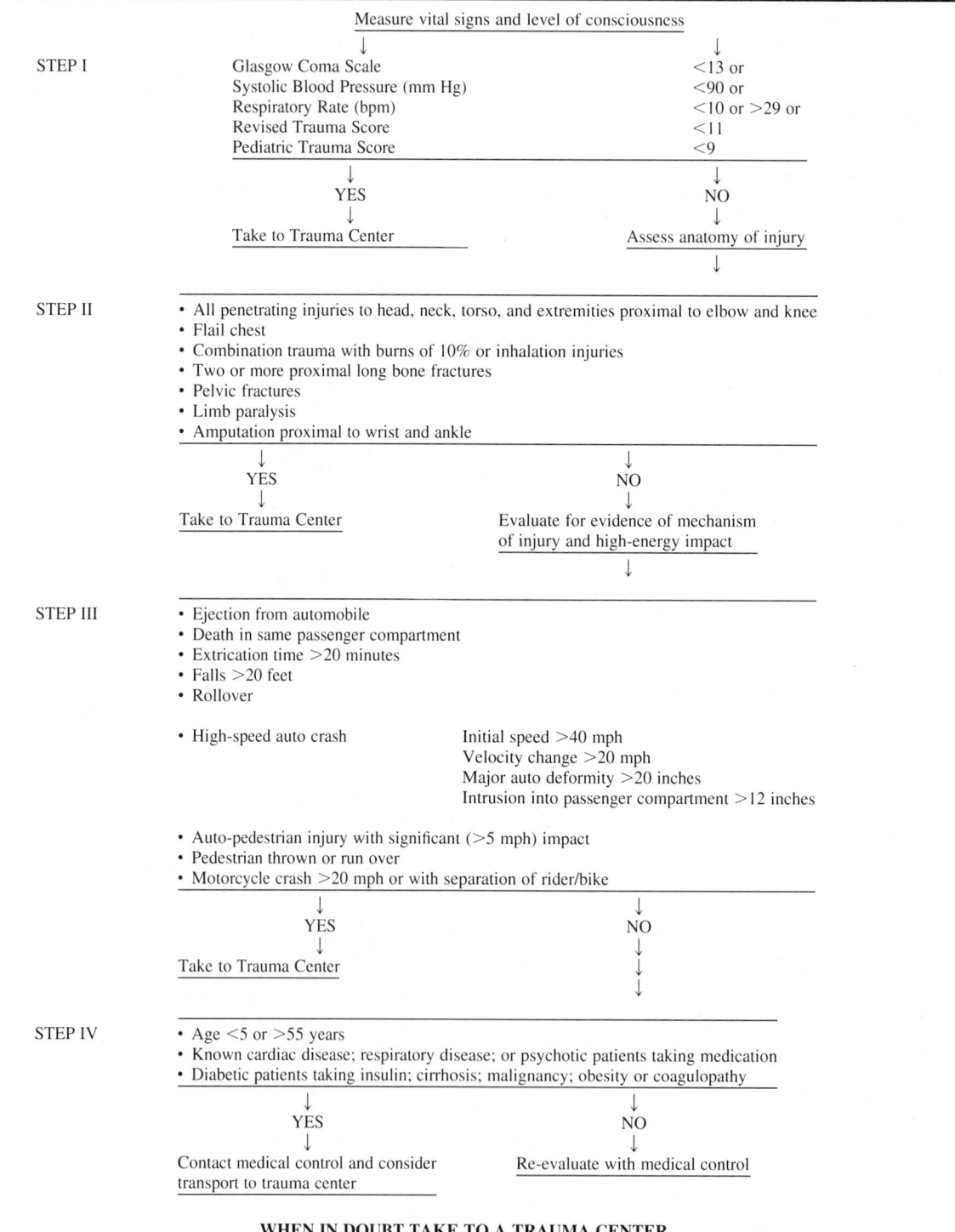

Measure vital signs and level of consciousness

STEP I

Glasgow Coma Scale	<13 or
Systolic Blood Pressure (mm Hg)	<90 or
Respiratory Rate (bpm)	<10 or >29 or
Revised Trauma Score	<11
Pediatric Trauma Score	<9

YES — Take to Trauma Center

NO — Assess anatomy of injury

STEP II

- All penetrating injuries to head, neck, torso, and extremities proximal to elbow and knee
- Flail chest
- Combination trauma with burns of 10% or inhalation injuries
- Two or more proximal long bone fractures
- Pelvic fractures
- Limb paralysis
- Amputation proximal to wrist and ankle

YES — Take to Trauma Center

NO — Evaluate for evidence of mechanism of injury and high-energy impact

STEP III

- Ejection from automobile
- Death in same passenger compartment
- Extrication time >20 minutes
- Falls >20 feet
- Rollover

- High-speed auto crash
  - Initial speed >40 mph
  - Velocity change >20 mph
  - Major auto deformity >20 inches
  - Intrusion into passenger compartment >12 inches

- Auto-pedestrian injury with significant (>5 mph) impact
- Pedestrian thrown or run over
- Motorcycle crash >20 mph or with separation of rider/bike

YES — Take to Trauma Center

NO

STEP IV

- Age <5 or >55 years
- Known cardiac disease; respiratory disease; or psychotic patients taking medication
- Diabetic patients taking insulin; cirrhosis; malignancy; obesity or coagulopathy

YES — Contact medical control and consider transport to trauma center

NO — Re-evaluate with medical control

WHEN IN DOUBT TAKE TO A TRAUMA CENTER

(From The Committee on Trauma, American College of Surgeons: Resources for optimal care of the injured patient. Chicago, American College of Surgeons, 1990, p 17.)

TABLE 59–4. Trauma Team Members and Their Roles

Personnel	Key Role
Trauma surgeon	Team leader; performs primary and secondary surveys and necessary procedures; directs resuscitation efforts and follow-through care
Emergency physician	Fulfills role of team leader if trauma surgeon not present; assists with procedures
Anesthesiologist/ anesthetist	Assess, establish and/or assist in maintaining airway while maintaining cervical spine integrity; assist with line access and hemodynamic monitoring if necessary
Primary nurse	Primary and secondary survey along with team leader; establish intravenous access on left; assist team leader with procedures; patient contact
Secondary nurse	Establish intravenous access on right; vital signs and cardiac monitoring; nasogastric tube/Foley catheter placement; wound care; splinting; family liaison
Respiratory care	Assist with airway management/securing; procedure arterial blood gases; set up ventilator; assist during transport
Laboratory	Procure, label, and transport blood specimens
X-ray/computed tomography	Procure radiographic studies; evacuate and prepare computed tomography scanner
Nursing supervisor	Documents all activities, interventions; initiates bed assignment
Operating room backup/ operating room team	Ensures preparation for potential surgery
Chaplaincy	Notification and support for family/significant others
Security	Secure valuables; crowd control
Trauma coordinator	Supervision/supportive assistance; direct care when necessary

Ancillary support staff are also crucial to a successful system. Each plays an important part, providing unique contributions. Teamwork is the key to optimal trauma care; mutual respect and cooperation are the foundation of that teamwork.

Must the Entire Team Always Respond?

Our system and others conserve resources by activating the entire team only when life-threatening injury is probable.[31, 32] Fewer resources are needed to manage patients with lesser injuries. Gomez and colleagues, using a two-tiered system, demonstrated an equally safe level of care, a 70% reduction in patient resuscitation charges, and incalculable savings in manpower.[31]

What Factors Are Considered in Preparing the Operating Room?

Ideally, there are always capable personnel to assist, a dedicated OR on standby, and advance warning; realistically, this scenario is the exception to the rule. Resources must be identified and dedicated to trauma care in advance. OR personnel familiar with trauma care should be available 24 hours a day.

Using the ED resuscitation area and personnel for surgery is reasonable to save time. However, this approach is only effective if there are sufficient numbers of patients to maintain the skills of the ED personnel. A dedicated OR provides the staff with a measure of familiarity and comfort that may be a crucial factor in critical situations.

What Should the Operating Room Do in Response to a Trauma Alert?

Advance notice of a patient's arrival is accomplished in most systems by including the OR in the trauma alert page system. Depending on the trauma case mix, the OR response may be two tiered. Initial activation must include ensuring an available OR suite (preferably one dedicated to trauma patients) and available staff preparing for a patient's arrival (case cart present, fluid warmer primed, and cell saver available). In many systems, a second call is then made to the OR confirming the need for surgery. At that time, the surgical technician and assistant rapidly prepare the room. In centers treating primarily blunt trauma victims, a two-tiered system is effective and economical.

Many experts support direct transport to the OR for resuscitation of patients with severe injuries.[33–38] In centers treating large volumes of penetrating trauma or when specific criteria are met (Table 59–5), all preparations commence with the first call; the patient should bypass the ED and be transported directly to the OR for evaluation and resuscitation. This approach may require dispatching an ED nurse to the OR or additional training of the OR staff because they now assume responsibility for screening and initial stabilizing interventions in addition to definitive surgery.

What Factors Modify the Ideal Situation?

Realistically, there are many variances from ideal situations, and the following suggestions may assist in resolving some problems.

Patient Volume

A small patient volume does not have to result in inadequate preparation. Commitment and a constant state of preparedness are the keys to avoiding problems. The trauma staff is accountable for checking the availability and working order of trauma room equipment and supplies at the beginning of each work shift. The degree of accountability correlates inversely with the amount of essential resources found to be missing during an emergency operation.

Supervisory Personnel

Trauma often occurs in the off-hours, when the on-call crew lack supervisory and support personnel. Continuous training and education are essential to maintain familiarity with patient preparation protocols and essential policies such as emergency

TABLE 59–5. Criteria for Direct Admission to Operating Room

Penetrating trauma with cardiac arrest
Witnessed arrest
Hypovolemic shock unresponsive to fluid resuscitation
Penetrating trauma to the torso
Major nonguillotine amputation or degloving injury
Evisceration of abdominal contents
Severe maxillofacial injuries
Interhospital transfer with known need for immediate surgery

blood procurement. Continuous in-service training and knowledge reassessment by both the system *and* the individual practitioner are essential in maintaining readiness.

What Can Be Done to Speed Up the System?

A good working knowledge of your system and resources combined with a little creativity can result in significant strides toward a more efficient system. The trauma alert system described earlier saves considerable time in notifying the appropriate personnel. A computer-generated group page occurs as fast as a verbal page and does not depend on the responder being within hearing range.

Patient Identification

A reliable patient identification system is crucial, because patients often arrive in groups and are occasionally unidentified. Our system uses computer-generated labels with three-digit numbers. A 4 × 6-inch sheet with approximately 15 labels is placed into a prepackaged laboratory test packet. The packets are heat sealed (to prevent scavenging) and contain the syringes, needles, and blood collection tubes necessary to process the standardized trauma panel laboratory studies.

One identification label is placed on a patient's blood bank bracelet, which is secured to an uninjured ankle. The lower extremity is used because upper extremity bracelets are frequently removed for venous and arterial access catheters. During the initial resuscitation, the ankle is usually more accessible. The patient is referred to by this emergency identification number throughout the resuscitation phase until he or she is positively identified and a hospital identification number is assigned.

Enhanced Communication

Few hospitals have the luxury of bedside computer terminals, but communications can be improved by using fax machines between the laboratory, radiology department, and ED or OR. Fax machines are also useful in rural systems with prolonged interhospital transport times.

Our system and others[21] advocate immediate patient transfer once the necessity is determined and stabilization occurs. Awaiting laboratory results should not delay transfer. Those patients requiring blood transfusions en route are usually clinically identifiable, and uncrossmatched O-negative blood may be sent with the patient. Laboratory data can be faxed to the receiving hospital ED when available.

Documentation

Information control and documentation are essential. Resuscitation procedures are concurrently recorded to document and assist with each phase of care. Accuracy is also paramount for litigation defense. The recorder may be a nurse or secretary; most important is that the person selected be a trained observer familiar with the terminology, personnel, and procedures involved in trauma resuscitation.

A flow sheet reduces the amount of narrative documentation and is useful to the recorder, primary nurse, and quality assurance auditor (Fig. 59–1). All data (e.g., resuscitation record, laboratory results, x-ray films) should remain *with the patient.* This procedure eliminates errors of mistaken identity and provides readily available data to consultants on their arrival.

Expedited Radiologic Procedures

Radiologic procedures have an important role in trauma diagnostics, especially in the blunt trauma population. Placing cassettes for chest and pelvic radiographs on the stretcher before a patient's arrival is a simple maneuver to save time in obtaining these often critical films. Developing a predetermined series and order for obtaining radiographs also minimizes diagnostic time.

Radiologic technicians can be trained to anticipate the common machine settings necessary (settings by weight are posted in the trauma room and on the portable machines for easy reference). A blunt trauma series is ordered for 90% of the severely injured patients at our facility (Table 59–6); adding extremity films or deleting one or more films from the series is a simple process.

Computed Tomography

Computed tomography (CT) scanning has become a standard of care for trauma victims. Maximum benefit is achieved if the scanner is rapid, readily available, and in close proximity to the resuscitation area. If the CT scanner is being used for an elective study, it should be evacuated as soon as possible when a trauma alert is paged and reserved until the scanner is either used or released by the trauma surgeon.

Many trauma surgeons are comfortable interpreting CT studies, but others are not. A radiologist's interpretation can be accelerated by using a modem that allows review of scans outside the hospital after hours, thus eliminating travel time.

Subspecialist Response

A subspecialist's response should not be a source of delay. A formal call list of subspecialists necessary for trauma care must be complete, accurate, and readily available. The American College of Surgeons' document advocates a prompt response by subspecialists in addition to the trauma surgeon and anesthesiologist.[14] Illinois' regulatory statute for trauma systems mandates a 30-minute response for level I centers and 60 minutes for level II centers. Variances from the expected response time must be documented and corrected if trends toward tardiness develop.

TABLE 59–6. Blunt Trauma Series of Radiographs*

Lateral cervical spine
Supine AP chest†
Lateral thoracic spine
Lateral lumbar spine
AP pelvis
AP cervical spine
AP skull
Lateral skull

*Any study may be deleted by the team leader based on a patient's presentation and stability.
†May be delayed until after spinal films are obtained if the patient is stable and an upright film is desired.
Abbreviation: AP = anteroposterior.

Carle
Carle Foundation Hospital

REVISED CHAMPION TRAUMA SCORE

Respiratory Rate	10-29/min	4
	29/min	3
	6-9/min	2
	1-5/min	1
	0	0
Systolic Blood Pressure	89 mm Hg	4
	76-89 mm Hg	3
	50-75 mm Hg	2
	1-49 mm Hg	1
	0	0

GLASGOW COMA SCALE

Eye Opening	Spontaneous	4	Total Glasgow Coma Scale Point
	To Voice	3	
	To Pain	2	
	None	1	
Verbal Response	Oriented	5	13-15 4
	Confused	4	9-12 3
	Inappropriate Words	3	6-8 2
	Incomprehensible Words	2	4-5 1
	None	1	3 0
Motor Response	Obeys Command	6	
	Localizes Pain	5	
	Withdraw (pain)	4	
	Flexion (pain)	3	
	Extension (pain)	2	
	None	1	

TOTAL REVISED TRAUMA

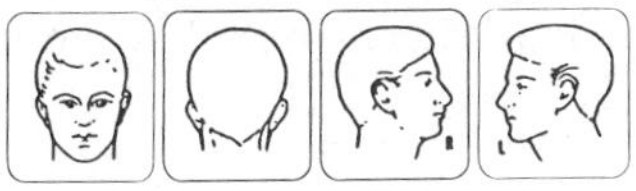

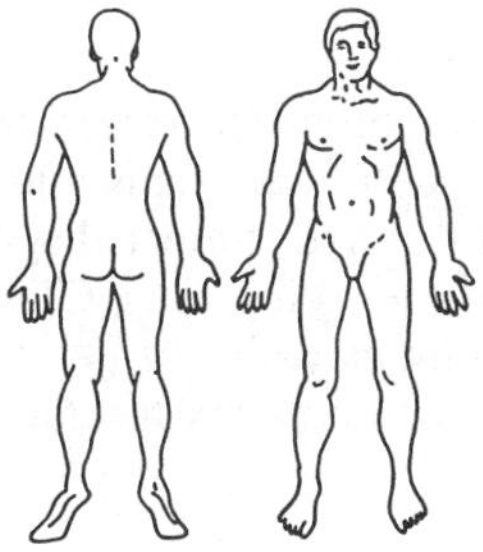

AB-Abrasion
Amp-Amputation
Av-Avulsion
B-Burn
Br-Bruise
F-Closed/Susp. Fx
H-Hematoma
L-Laceration
E-Edema

FIELD PERSONNEL REPORT
mechanism of injury

pertinent hx
meds
allergies
last meal   TOTAL FIELD INTAKE

PRESENTATION ON ARRIVAL

BACKBOARD   O ____ L ____ NC ____ MASK ____
C-COLLAR
SAND BAGS/KED/CID   AIRWAY ____ ORAL ____ NT ____ ET ____
BLEEDING CONTROL   SUPINE ____ PRONE ____
CPR
IVS   MAST LEGS/ABD
MEDS   INFLATED ____ DEFLATED ____
SPLINTS

DATE	TEAM ACTIVATED		TIME PATIENT ARRIVED
	Level	Time	
	O.R. Notified		Time Patient Arrived in OR

TRAUMA TEAM RESPONSE

	NAME	CALLED	ARRIVED
TRAUMA SURGEON			
E.D. PHYSICIAN			
PRIMARY R.N.			
SUPPORT R.N.			
SCRIBE			
ANESTHESIA			
X-RAY			
LAB			
R.T.			
HOUSE OFFICER			

TIME	MEDICATIONS	EFFECTS

SIGNATURES:
TRAUMA PRIMARY R.N. _____
SCRIBE _____

Copies: White - Chart   Yellow - ED   Pink - TNC

INITIAL ASSESSMENT

AIRWAY	___ CLEAR	___ NP AIRWAY	___ OP AIRWAY	___ ET TUBE (FIELD)
BREATHING	___ NORMAL	___ RAPID	___ SLOW	___ SHALLOW
	___ LABORED	___ DECREASED		

CIRCULATION   ___ NORMAL CAP REFILL   ___ PULSES PALP   Radial L R
              ___ DELAYED CAP REFILL   Femoral L R
              ___ RHYTHM   Pedal L R

SKIN SIGNS   ___ NORMAL   ___ WARM   ___ DRY   ___ PALE
              ___ CYANOTIC   ___ COOL   ___ DIAPHORETIC   ___ FLUSHED

LOC   ___ ALERT   ___ ORIENTED   ___ COOPERATIVE   ___ SOMNOLENT
              ___ COMATOSE   ___ CONFUSED   ___ COMBATIVE

RESPONDS TO   ___ VERBAL   ___ PAIN   ___ UNRESPONSIVE

PUPILS   ___ PERL   ___ UNEQUAL

HEAD   ___ CLEAR   ___ TM CLEAR   ___ ABNL
NECK   ___ CLEAR   ___ NON-TENDER   ___ TENDER   TRACHEA DEVIATED RT LT

CHEST   ___ CLEAR   ___ EXPANSION   ___ CREPITUS   ___ FLAIL R or L
              ___ PNEUMOTHORAX R or L   ___ HEMOTHORAX R or L

BREATH   ___ CLEAR   ___ DECREASED
SOUNDS   ___ RALES
              ___ RHONCHI   ___ WHEEZING

ABDOMEN   ___ SOFT   ___ FLAT   ___ NON-TENDER   BOWEL SNDS + -
              ___ RIGID   ___ DISTEN   ___ TENDER

PELVIS   ___ STABLE   ___ UNSTABLE   ___ RECTAL NEG   STOOL OB + -
GU   ___ MEATUS CLEAR   ___ BLOOD AT MEATUS

EXTREMITIES   ___ MAE   ___ DEFORMITY

BACK EXAM   ___ DONE   TETANUS STATUS   ___ CHECKED   ___ GIVEN   LAST TETANUS

COMMENTS

PROCEDURES

O L/MIN ____ BY ____
MASK ____ NASAL
CRICO
INTUBATION ET # ____

ART LINE SITE _____
CUTDOWN _____
CVP SITE _____
MAST DEFLATED AT _____
HOB Elevate 30-45
INSERTION ICP AT _____
Cervical Traction _____
EYE CARE _____

CHEST TUBE RT # _____
              LT # _____
DRAINAGE
PERICARDIOCENTESIS DONE AT _____
THORACOTOMY DONE AT _____
NG TUBE INSERTED _____
DIPSTICK BLOOD + -
PERITONEAL LAVAGE DONE AT _____
DRAINAGE

FOLEY INSERTED _____
DIPSTICK + -
DRAINAGE

WOUND CARE-SEE COMMENTS ☐
RESTRAINTS SOFT/LEATHER
LAST TETANUS

This is a sample of the 11"x24", 3-part form. It is shown smaller than actual size and divided because of space limitations.

Carle **TRAUMA CHART**

TIME			
VITAL SIGNS	CUFF B/P R		
	L		
	PULSE		
	RESP		
	TEMP		
	GCS		
MOTOR	RIGHT ARM		
	LEFT ARM		
	RIGHT LEG		
	LEFT LEG		
PUPILS	RIGHT		
	LEFT		

EM #
PUPIL SCALE mm
2●
3●
4●
5●
6●
7●
8●
9●

Name ___ Clinic # ___ Age ___ Date ___

STRENGTH OF MOVEMENT
0 No voluntary movement
1 Some voluntary movement cannot support weight of extremity
2 Supports weight of extremity has mild resistance
3 Slight weakness
4 Normal

PUPILLARY CODE
B Brisk
S Sluggish
N No Reaction

RESP KEY
V Ventilator
B Ambu Bag

CARLE FOUNDATION HOSPITAL

INTAKE — TRAUMA ROOM

Paren-teral	FLUIDS	Bag No.	Site	Time Start	Amount Start	Time Complete	Amount Complete
IV							
IV							
IV							
IV							
IV							
IV							
Blood							
Blood							
Blood							
Blood							
Blood							
Blood							
A-line or Other							
Other							

Total Crystalloids IV ____ cc   Total Blood/Blood Products ____ cc

DIAGNOSTIC TEST RESULTS

TIME DRAWN	TEST	TIME RETURNED TO TRAUMA ROOM
	Trauma Panel	
	T&C ____ units	
	CPK/MB	
	EKG	
	ABG's	

Blood Requested ____   Arrived ____

RADIOLOGY | REQUEST | TIME DONE | COMMENTS

C-Spine lateral		
Chest		
Skull		
Pelvis		
CT of ____		
KUB		
IVP		
Angiogram		
Arm R L		
Leg R L		
Spine T L		

OUTPUT — TRAUMA ROOM

TOTAL URINE	▶
NG/SALEM SUMP/EMESIS	▶
CHEST TUBE #1	▶
CHEST TUBE #2	▶
OTHER	▶
TOTAL OUTPUT	

DISPOSITION TO: _____   TIME: _____
VALUABLES: SEE BELONGINGS LIST
FAMILY NOTIFIED _____
ANCILLARY SERVICES _____
CORONER NOTIFIED _____

CONSULTS

NAME	TIME CALLED	TIME ARRIVED

2465-1291

FIGURE 59–1. Trauma Resuscitation Flow Sheet. (Courtesy of Carle Foundation Hospital, Urbana, IL.)

Environment and Leadership

The final components to expedite care are complementary: environment and leadership. The environment in the resuscitation room must be calm and controlled, allowing clear communication and coordination of team efforts. Raised voices, emotional outbursts, and lack of control only contribute to disorganization and poor care. A few short words of direction toward the resuscitation goal are far more productive than hysterical admonishment.

The person primarily responsible for providing direction and maintaining control is the team leader. The one-captain concept is vital for successful trauma resuscitation.[14, 27, 33, 35, 39] Fighting over a patient's parts is unacceptable and inefficient and detracts from the ultimate goal of resuscitation. The person with the most experience in treating the critically injured trauma patient—surgeon, anesthesiologist, emergency physician, or other—should assume the team leader role.

INITIAL PATIENT ASSESSMENT AND RESUSCITATION STRATEGY

What Is Advanced Trauma Life Support?

The Committee on Trauma of the American College of Surgeons, through the ATLS course, has developed guidelines for the initial assessment and resuscitation of critically injured patients.[40] Many of the recommendations and guidelines for therapy outlined in this chapter are derived from our experience using the techniques and recommendations so described.

Why Is Initial Assessment Critical?

The majority of injuries in patients presenting to an ED are usually not life threatening. The difficulty is differentiating the 10% to 15% of critically injured patients who, if not rapidly assessed and treated, can develop complications causing severe disability or death. Because the initial physiologic parameters may be misleading, especially in younger individuals with the capacity for hemodynamic compensation, the mechanism of injury must also be considered during triage and evaluation.

Assessment and resuscitation must occur simultaneously in unstable patients.[41] Effective initial management requires a basic knowledge of cardiopulmonary physiology and the kinematics of injury, together with the ability to perform certain manual tasks. A modicum of wisdom and understanding in dealing with patients and their families during very stressful situations is also helpful.[41]

Diagnostic and Therapeutic Priorities

During the initial phase of resuscitation, definitive diagnosis is usually low in priority; such an approach may significantly delay life-saving resuscitative measures. For example, it is important to quickly determine the presence of intra-abdominal bleeding but not the actual source of bleeding.[42] Similarly, determining that ventilation or oxygenation is inadequate is all that is required before starting appropriate therapy to correct the problem. Searching for the exact cause (other than simple mechanical factors) is unnecessary and may cause serious delays in treatment.

Because rapid assessment and resuscitation are crucial for survival, a systematic approach provides the best results. The ATLS guidelines provide an excellent framework for evaluation and treatment. This approach consists of a primary survey and resuscitation, secondary survey, and definitive management.

Primary Survey

The primary survey evaluates the ABC's of life support: A, *a*irway assessment (with cervical spine immobilization); B, *b*reathing assessment; C, establishment of *c*irculation and *c*ontrol of major hemorrhage; D, *d*isability assessment, with a brief neurologic examination; and E, *e*xposure of the patient by removing all clothing for complete evaluation.[40] Resuscitation for the correction of any physiologic abnormalities related to the ABC's should occur simultaneously as they are identified.

Secondary Survey

Once stabilization is achieved, a secondary survey is performed consisting of a complete head-to-toe examination and neurologic assessment. During this period, further diagnostic studies such as complete cervical spine radiographs, CT scans, and peritoneal lavage or angiography may also be performed. "A tube or finger in every orifice" describes the thorough nature of the secondary assessment.

Definitive Care

The definitive care phase usually occurs either in the OR or the intensive care unit (ICU) in severely injured patients. Continued reassessment during the first 24 hours of hospitalization is crucial; re-evaluation during the next several days may reveal other less serious injuries that were not apparent during the initial evaluation.

What Historical Information Should Be Sought?

A patient's history is obtained from any available source. Prehospital personnel are helpful in determining the mechanism of injury and describing important prognostic parameters including the patient's initial neurologic status, vital signs, and kinematics of injury (e.g., height of the fall, impact speed, and description of vehicular damage). Other events are also associated with a high probability of severe injury (Tables 59–3 and 59–7).

Witnesses

Individuals who witnessed the accident or were involved in it may also be helpful, along with family members who may be able to give the patient's medical history. A rapid AMPLE history is all that is required initially (Table 59–8). These data may be obtained by any member of the trauma team during the initial resuscitation (e.g., a social worker or chaplain) while the physicians and nursing staff are initially working with the patient.

TABLE 59–7. Injury Mechanisms Associated with a High Probability of Severe Injury

---

Ejection from vehicle
Pedestrian struck by vehicle
Death of another vehicle occupant
Separation of rider from motorcycle
Falls >12 feet
Gunshot wounds to the torso
Stab wounds to the torso

Patient

The approach to an awake, alert, cooperative patient is less complicated than the global evaluation necessary for a patient who has multiple injuries and arrives comatose, combative, or uncooperative. If a patient can answer appropriately, a series of questions can direct the physician to serious injuries that may be otherwise overlooked in a stable patient. Patients who can answer questions in a relaxed, calm fashion and can talk without difficulty probably do not have upper airway problems.

Questions should be directed toward identifying life-threatening or debilitating injuries. Alcohol- or drug-intoxicated patients cannot be relied on to give an appropriate response, and evaluation must be guided by other factors.

Combative or Uncooperative Trauma Victims

Combative, uncooperative behavior should never be assumed to be secondary to alcohol or drug intoxication if the mechanism of trauma is associated with a reasonable probability of head injury. Although drugs or alcohol may contribute to such behavior, closed head injury or hypoxemia may also be present. Our practice is to rapidly gain control of such patients with paralysis and orotracheal intubation to expedite the evaluation process. The incidence of significant intracranial pathology in our combative patient population is 42%; 64% were found to have either a major head injury or other life-threatening injuries.[43]

What Is the Primary Survey?

Trauma victims should be assessed and treatment priorities established based on the stability of their physiologic parameters and the mechanism of injury. The primary survey outlines a logical, sequential evaluation and treatment scheme based on a quick overall assessment of the patient. Vital signs (pulse, respirations, oxygen [O_2] saturation, and blood pressure) are quickly assessed, and treatment is initiated with the goal of rapidly normalizing physiologic parameters, alleviating hypoxia, and eliminating hypercarbia. The ABC's, as outlined earlier, are critical to success.

A: Airway and Cervical Spine Assessment

Establishment of a patent airway is the first priority of trauma resuscitation. If a trauma victim fails to respond appropriately to verbal questioning, one must immediately determine whether this finding indicates an airway problem or brain injury. Hypoxia may present as severe agitation, and extreme obtundation may be a manifestation of hypercarbia. Severely agitated patients who refuse to cooperate may have airway obstruction or hypoxia.

Unconscious or obtunded patients are intubated to protect the airway, deliver supplemental O_2, and support ventilation. Preventing hypercarbia and correcting hypoxemia are crucial in the initial management of trauma victims, especially if head injury is present. Proper oxygenation and hyperventilation to reduce arterial partial pressure of carbon dioxide ($PaCO_2$) reduces secondary brain injury. Indeed, in the prehospital setting, the only skill that has been consistently shown to improve outcome in trauma victims is the ability to provide a tracheal airway.[44]

Clinical Signs of Airway Obstruction

The examiner should listen for stridor from partial occlusion of the upper airway, gurgling or sonorous respirations, and the quality of breath sounds. Hoarseness or an inability to speak clearly is associated with laryngeal fractures. Immediate airway control should be obtained if any of these findings are identified or if the patient is extremely anxious or combative. If a laryngeal fracture is suspected, fiberoptic guided placement of an endotracheal tube is preferred if the equipment and expertise are available and time permits. This technique guards against possible false passage of the tube or aggravation of the injury.

Victims of falls, motor vehicle accidents, and isolated head injuries are assumed to have an associated cervical spine injury until appropriate studies can be performed. Therefore, whatever maneuver is used to obtain airway control, the cervical spine must remain immobilized.

Various noninvasive forms of airway control are presented in the ATLS manual. These techniques include chin lift, jaw thrust, and placement of oropharyngeal or nasopharyngeal airways. A "tonsil" suction tip should be available to clear the upper airway of all secretions and foreign bodies.

Most severely injured patients presenting with these symptoms require tracheal intubation. If time permits, a lateral cervical spine film can be obtained, but this procedure should not cause significant delays in establishing an airway.

Techniques of Intubation

Controversy exists about the safety of orotracheal intubation with in-line axial cervical traction for patients with potential cervical spine injury. Cadaver studies of patients immediately after traumatic cardiac arrest have yielded conflicting results about cervical spine stability with various methods of intubation.[45–47]

Orotracheal Intubation. A growing body of knowledge supports planned neuromuscular blockade in the emergency setting for orotracheal intubation.[48–51] Talucci and colleagues[50]

TABLE 59–8. AMPLE History

A	Allergies
M	Medications (current)
P	Past medical and surgical history
L	Last meal, last tetanus booster, last menses
E	Events and environment related to the injury

(Modified from The Committee on Trauma, American College of Surgeons: Advanced Trauma Life Support Course Manual. Chicago, American College of Surgeons, 1988, p 20.)

reported a series of 335 patients who required tracheal intubation. Rapid-sequence induction using sodium thiopental, 3 to 5 mg · kg^{-1}, followed by succinylcholine, 1 to 2 mg · kg^{-1}, was administered, with successful orotracheal intubation in 260 patients.

The authors departed from the traditional induction method for intubation in several ways. Cervical spine evaluation and nasogastric tube insertion usually were not performed before intubation. Their opinion was that stimulation of the oropharynx during passage of a nasogastric tube might induce vomiting and tracheal aspiration of gastric contents.[51]

We had similar success with orotracheal intubation. In our series of 229 trauma victims requiring emergency airway control, 223 were orotracheally intubated.[43] One hundred forty-one patients (61.5%) initially were paralyzed with high doses of vecuronium bromide (0.1–0.25 mg · kg^{-1}), and 33 patients (14.4%) initially were given succinylcholine. Only six patients (2.6%) required cricothyroidotomy. One patient (0.4%) aspirated a minimum amount of gastric contents during intubation. Cervical spine radiographs were not regularly obtained, and gastric decompression was not performed before orotracheal intubation. No neurologic complications occurred as a result of this technique.

The extensive experience of Stene and Grande, who use orotracheal intubation of trauma victims, has led to their general recommendation to avoid the nasotracheal route because orotracheal intubation in this setting is safe and usually successful.[52]

Nasotracheal Intubation. Nasotracheal intubation must be avoided in patients with obvious evidence of maxillofacial injury or if the mechanism of injury suggests that such an injury may be present. Any patient with suspected head injury may have an anterior fossa basilar skull fracture. Potential complications of nasotracheal intubation include inadvertent placement of the tube through the cribriform plate into the brain[53]; introduction of nasal bacteria through the skull fracture into the cranial vault, with subsequent bacteremia[54]; bacteremia due to nasal mucosal abrasion or transfer of nasal bacteria into the trachea[54]; and later complications of maxillary sinusitis[55] and otitis media.[56]

In addition to being technically more difficult, nasotracheal intubation is much more difficult to perform in intoxicated or combative patients. A smaller endotracheal tube is usually required, and it may cause increased work of breathing during spontaneous ventilation. Tube insertion may also increase intracranial pressure (ICP) if a patient is not adequately sedated. In combative trauma victims, adequate sedation is often not achieved without dangerously high doses of sedatives, which can severely depress spontaneous ventilation.

Our experience is that orotracheal intubation with planned neuromuscular blockade and in-line cervical traction before evaluation of the cervical spine or gastric tube placement is a safe and effective procedure in establishing airway control. It is our method of choice and has eliminated the need for nasotracheal intubation.

Emergency Cricothyroidotomy

Emergency cricothyroidotomy is reserved for patients with severe facial injuries that prohibit orotracheal intubation. It is performed by making either a vertical or horizontal skin incision over the area of the cricothyroid membrane. A scalpel blade (no. 11 or 15) is used to incise directly through the cricothyroid membrane, and either a curved hemostat or Trousseau's tracheal dilator is inserted to open the cricothyroid membrane for passage of an endotracheal or tracheostomy tube (7–8 mm). Percutaneous placement is also possible (see Chapter 50).

The neck must remain in neutral position during this procedure. Cricothyroidotomy is not recommended in children younger than 12 years because of potential damage to the cricoid cartilage, the only totally circumferential support for the upper trachea in children.

Cricothyroidotomy is recommended over formal tracheotomy because the technique is relatively simple, is easy to learn by individuals with a nonsurgical background, and, theoretically, is performed in a bloodless plane. Under emergency conditions, however, it can be a bloody procedure. Little and colleagues[57] studied the region anterior to the cricothyroid membrane in 34 adult cadavers. Seventy-nine per cent of the cadavers had vascular structures within the area of cricothyroidotomy. Other potential complications of cricothyroidotomy include permanent voice change, bleeding at the surgical site, wound infection, and the most serious complication, subglottic stenosis.

Emergency Tracheotomy

Controversy exists about the use of elective cricothyroidotomy versus tracheotomy for patients who require prolonged mechanical ventilatory support. Tracheotomy has no place in an emergency setting for airway control, except in patients with an obstructing laryngeal fracture, in which case cricothyroidotomy is usually unsuccessful in obtaining an adequate airway.

B: Breathing—Ventilation Assessment

Tension pneumothorax, flail chest, open pneumothorax, and massive hemothorax are conditions that significantly interfere with ventilation and blood return to the heart. They must be rapidly diagnosed and treated during the primary survey.

Tension Pneumothorax

Tension pneumothorax is usually a clinical rather than a radiologic diagnosis if a patient presents with severe respiratory distress and hypotension.

Pathophysiology. This abnormality occurs when a bronchial injury or, more commonly, a parenchymal lung injury allows air movement into the pleural space. As the amount of air in the pleural space increases, the lung collapses, causing inadequate ventilation. Increasing pressure on the mediastinum also causes decreased blood return to the heart and decreased cardiac output. The reported signs of tracheal deviation to the unaffected hemithorax, distended neck veins, unilateral absence of breath sounds, and cyanosis are not always present or detectable.

Diagnosis. The noisy ED environment often causes difficulty in assessing breath sounds unless the pneumothorax is massive. Distended neck veins are frequently absent if a patient is hypovolemic, and cyanosis is a very late manifestation. More commonly, patients present with grunting respirations, respiratory distress, and a decrease in pulse pressure.

Treatment. Tension pneumothorax requires immediate treatment; documentation of the abnormality with a chest radiograph is contraindicated if a patient is unstable. Rapid insertion of a 14- or 16-gauge intravenous catheter into the second intercostal space in the midclavicular line of the affected hemithorax is the initial emergency treatment. A sudden rush of air from the chest cavity confirms the clinical diagnosis.

A large-bore chest tube (36 to 40 French) should be inserted through the fifth intercostal space in the midaxillary line and directed posteriorly and superiorly for definitive care. This position adequately removes both air and blood. Smaller tubes generally are not recommended in adult trauma victims because clotted blood can render smaller tubes nonfunctional.

Open Pneumothorax

Large chest wall defects associated with pulmonary parenchymal injuries can result in an "open" pneumothorax (sucking chest wound).

Pathophysiology. If the opening in the chest wall is at least two thirds the diameter of the trachea, air passes preferentially through the chest defect with each respiratory effort, following the path of least resistance. This abnormal equilibration between intrathoracic and atmospheric pressure causes poor ventilation and hypoxia.

Treatment. Immediate management of open pneumothorax consists of covering the defect with air- and water-resistant bandages (such as petroleum jelly gauze) and tube thoracostomy to prevent tension pneumothorax.

Flail Chest

Pathophysiology. Flail chest occurs when a segment of the chest wall becomes completely disconnected from the remainder of the bony thorax. This problem usually results when two or more ribs are fractured in at least two places. Symbas[58] defines a flail chest as the fracture of three or more ribs in continuity and at more than one site, or a rib fracture at one site with costochondral separation or sternal fracture, which produces instability of the chest wall segment. This unstable chest wall segment moves paradoxically, independently, and in the opposite direction from the remaining thorax.

Management. Hypoxemia and hypercapnia can occur with flail chest. Immediate tracheal intubation and mechanical ventilation may be necessary. The ventilatory dysfunction results from a decrease in vital capacity, functional residual capacity, and total lung volume. The degree of underlying pulmonary contusion can lead to significant alterations in ventilation/perfusion matching and physiologic shunting.[58] The commonly held belief in pendelluft movement of air from one lung to the other without adequate external gas exchange has been disputed.[59]

Long-term therapy includes prolonged mechanical ventilation with continuous positive airway pressure (CPAP) until the underlying pulmonary abnormalities resolve. Splinting, traction, or operative stabilization is usually unnecessary.[58]

Massive Hemothorax

Pathophysiology. Massive hemothorax, defined as at least 1500 mL of blood loss into the chest cavity, presents signs and symptoms similar to tension pneumothorax, with the exception of distended neck veins. This abnormality is usually associated with penetrating chest trauma, but it may also result from blunt trauma.

Management. Initial management includes placement of one or more large-bore (36–40 French) chest tubes directed posteriorly through the fifth intercostal space, along with rapid volume resuscitation.

The need for thoracic exploration is based on the rate of continued blood loss rather than the initial volume removed. A continued blood loss of 200 mL $\cdot$ h^{-1} usually requires operative intervention.[40] Persistent bleeding at this rate is almost always from a lacerated intercostal or internal mammary artery, a branch of the pulmonary vein, or the aorta. Parenchymal lung bleeding usually subsides when the lung re-expands, because the pulmonary vascular system is relatively low pressure.

C: Circulation Assessment

Level of consciousness, skin color, rate and quality of peripheral pulses, mental status, and identification of bleeding sources are important assessment features. A quick overall assessment of the blood pressure, pulse, mental status, respiratory rate, and urine output allows classification of the level of circulatory dysfunction (Table 59–9). In younger patients and children, mental status and blood pressure may remain nearly normal until massive blood loss occurs and the patient suddenly "crashes." Children and younger adults have a tre-

TABLE 59–9. Classes of Hypovolemic Shock with Estimated Fluid and Blood Requirements (70-kg Male)

	Class I	Class II	Class III	Class IV
Blood loss (mL)	Up to 750	750–1500	1500–2000	2000 or more
Blood loss (% blood volume)	Up to 15%	15–30%	30–40%	40% or more
Pulse rate	<100	>100	>120	140 or higher
Blood pressure	Normal	Normal	Decreased	Decreased
Pulse Pressure (mm Hg)	Normal or increased	Decreased	Decreased	Decreased
Respiratory rate	14–20	20–30	30–40	>35
Urine output (mL $\cdot$ h^{-1})	30 or more	20–30	5–15	Negligible
CNS—mental status	Slightly anxious	Mildly anxious	Anxious and confused	Confused, lethargic
Fluid replacement (3:1 rule)	Crystalloid	Crystalloid	Crystalloid + blood	Crystalloid + blood

(Modified from Committee on Trauma, American College of Surgeons: Advanced Trauma Life Support Student Manual. Chicago, American College of Surgeons, 1993, p. 23.)

mendous capacity for prolonged vasoconstriction and hemo-dynamic reserve. Hypotension may not develop until as much as 30% to 40% of blood volume is lost.

Immediate Care Priorities

Immediate control of any external bleeding sites with direct pressure is initiated. Vascular clamps should not be used with open wounds, because such maneuvers may cause inadvertent nerve injury. Most wounds can be adequately controlled with sterile compressive dressings secured by either an air splint or elastic wrap until further definitive management is possible. Exceptions are major scalp and facial lacerations, which are difficult to control with direct pressure and are better managed with temporary large mattress sutures. Cosmetic closure can be performed later when the patient is stabilized and other life-threatening problems are resolved.

Restoration of Perfusion. The initial goal is to restore tissue perfusion to vital organs. Sophisticated monitoring systems are usually unavailable and initially superfluous. Persistent tachycardia ($\geq$120 beats per minute) following the infusion of 2 L of crystalloid usually indicates continued bleeding. Tachycardia may be blunted in elderly patients who are prescribed β-blockers or digoxin.

A narrowed pulse pressure is frequently the earliest sign of major bleeding but may also indicate cardiac tamponade. Muffled heart sounds, jugular venous distention, hypotension, and pulsus paradoxus all are indicative of the latter problem. These clinical findings are frequently absent if a patient is also hypovolemic, and a high index of suspicion is required, especially in those individuals with blunt chest injury.

Intravenous Catheter Sites. Patients whose mechanism of injury suggests the possibility of life-threatening injury should have at least two large-bore (12–16 gauge) peripheral intravenous catheters inserted immediately on arrival. The antecubital fossa is a reliable site for achieving rapid venous access. Central venous catheters are avoided during the initial resuscitation because of the potential complications.

If upper extremity access is unavailable owing to severe vasoconstriction, burns, or fractures, the femoral veins are useful and usually accessible in supine patients. An 8.5 or 9.0 French pulmonary artery catheter introducer can be easily and quickly inserted. These introducers are excellent for rapid volume resuscitation if the side port attachment is discarded and large-bore intravenous tubing is inserted directly into the introducer. Flow rates up to $1 \text{ L} \cdot \text{min}^{-1}$ are achieved if a pressure infusion device is used. The femoral route can be used successfully, even in the presence of intra-abdominal injuries.

As a last resort, the subclavian or internal jugular routes are cannulated. In a hypovolemic patient, the subclavian vein, because of its fascial attachments, is larger and easier to cannulate than the internal jugular vein. However, in the patients with multiple injuries, these areas are sometimes difficult to access, and pneumothorax can significantly complicate resuscitation efforts. (See Chapter 32.)

Blood Pressure. Systolic blood pressure can be estimated by palpating pulses at various levels (Table 59–10). Compensatory mechanisms generally maintain blood flow to the brain until systolic blood pressure is <60 mm Hg.[41]

Fluid/Transfusion Therapy. Initial fluid resuscitation is not only therapeutic but frequently prognostic. Two liters of lactated Ringer's solution or normal saline is administered over 5 to 10 minutes (thus the need for large-bore catheters).

TABLE 59–10. Estimation of Blood Pressure by the Presence of Pulses

Pulse	Blood Pressure
Radial	80 mm Hg
Femoral	70 mm Hg
Carotid	60 mm Hg
Heart tones	40 mm Hg

(Data from Standards and Guidelines for Cardiopulmonary Resuscitation and Emergency Cardiac Care. JAMA; 255:2905–2984.)

If the blood pressure increases together with an appropriate decrease in heart rate, hypovolemia as the cause of the shock state can be assumed. If the patient remains stable, ongoing hemorrhage is unlikely. If the heart rate later increases and the pulse pressure narrows or the systolic pressure again begins to decrease, major ongoing blood loss is probable.

During insertion of intravenous catheters, a blood sample is obtained for type and screen or crossmatch, along with electrolyte determinations and a complete blood count (CBC). If appropriate, a blood alcohol level and toxicology screen are also obtained. Generally, type-specific blood can be obtained in most busy EDs within 15 to 30 minutes.

If a patient is severely hypovolemic and is unresponsive to crystalloid resuscitation, uncrossmatched O-negative blood is given. Further assessment and treatment of inadequate hemoperfusion may necessitate emergent thoracotomy, exploratory laparotomy, or both.

Military Antishock Trousers. Prospective randomized studies by Mattox and colleagues have attenuated the initial enthusiasm for military antishock trousers (MAST) use when prehospital transport times are short.[60] Currently, the only strong indication for using the MAST is for splinting extremity and pelvic fractures (for control of bleeding).

At high pressures, increased systemic vascular resistance (SVR) may elevate systemic arterial pressure and, in some patients, decrease cardiac output by increasing afterload and stimulating bleeding at levels above the MAST application. Inflation of the abdominal portion may also compress the inferior vena cava and impair venous return.[60]

The MAST has been associated with compartment syndrome and limb loss in multiply injured patients with and without extremity injuries.[61] It still is useful in situations where prehospital transport time is prolonged (>20 min).

D: Disability—Neurologic Assessment

During the primary survey, neurologic assessment is limited to a patient's level of consciousness and pupillary reflexes. This assessment should take no more than a few seconds. The AVPU method[40] reliably describes a patient's level of consciousness (Table 59–11). Pupillary size and reaction are also recorded.

A more extensive neurologic assessment is performed during the secondary survey. If a patient requires neuromuscular blockade and tracheal intubation, a quick assessment of extremity motor strength should be performed. If a patient is uncooperative but moving all extremities appropriately, these facts are recorded and may be all that can be evaluated initially.

Movement of all extremities should be documented, in response to painful stimulation, if necessary, before administer-

TABLE 59–11. Brief Neurologic Assessment During the Primary Survey—AVPU

A	Alert
V	Responsive to verbal stimuli
P	Responsive to painful stimuli
U	Unresponsiveness

(From Committee on Trauma, American College of Surgeons: Advanced Trauma Life Support Student Manual. Chicago, American College of Surgeons, 1993, p. 86.)

ing neuromuscular blocking agents. Sluggish or absent movement of one or both lower extremities in response to painful stimulation may be the only initial sign of spinal cord injury. Remember, however, that a lower spinal reflex may be elicited, the presence of which does not completely rule out a higher level defect.

E: Exposure

Patients should be completely undressed and carefully log rolled to ensure that no penetrating injuries or other abnormalities of the posterior torso are present. Complete exposure is essential in order to assess for other injuries during the secondary survey.

What Is the Secondary Survey?

A secondary survey is performed after completing the primary survey and resuscitation, assuming the patient has responded appropriately and is stable. The secondary survey includes a complete but rapid head-to-toe physical examination to identify other non–life-threatening but potentially serious injuries.

Radiologic Studies

Further radiologic evaluation may be performed at this time. We have found that in patients involved in motor vehicle accidents or falls, a blunt trauma series of radiographs is helpful to identify certain injuries. The views routinely ordered in the blunt trauma series are listed in Table 59–6. Some of these studies may not be necessary if a patient is alert, oriented, and capable of giving a reliable history and an appropriate response to physical examination. Radiographs can then be directed to symptomatic areas identified on physical examination. Secondary evaluation of the extremities may identify other possible areas that need evaluation.

Cervical Spine

All patients with maxillofacial trauma and all combative, uncooperative, or unconscious patients must have an evaluation of their cervical spine. Initial assessment consists of anteroposterior (AP) and lateral cervical spine radiographs. If *any* question of cervical spine injury remains after these studies are obtained, the patient should remain in a cervical collar until further detailed evaluation can be performed.

The absence of neurologic deficit or severe pain does *not* always eliminate the possibility of cervical spine injury. Any patient wearing a sports or motorcycle helmet must have head

and neck immobilization in neutral position while the helmet is removed.[40]

Cardiac Tamponade and Tension Pneumothorax

Closer inspection, palpation, and auscultation of the chest may reveal subtle changes that were not initially apparent during the primary survey. Distant heart sounds and distended neck veins signify possible cardiac tamponade or tension pneumothorax. If a patient's physiologic condition warrants, pericardiocentesis may be necessary. This procedure may have already been performed during the primary survey if the patient arrived in a severely compromised state.

Pulmonary Contusion

Severe pulmonary contusion may present with hypoxia and unilateral or bilateral infiltrates seen on chest radiographs. Severe pulmonary contusions are usually associated with chest wall trauma. If multiple rib fractures or chest wall contusions are identified, an arterial blood gas analysis should be obtained.

The initial degree of hypoxemia may not be readily apparent, because most trauma victims are treated with 100% O_2. Patients may be tachypneic if hypoxemia is significant. Early management is supportive care with tracheal intubation and manual or mechanical ventilation. Treatment with positive end-expiratory pressure (PEEP) is beneficial in reducing the physiologic shunt fraction and restoring pulmonary function toward normal.

Myocardial Contusion

The diagnosis is often difficult because most patients present with multiple injuries. Myocardial contusion may be overlooked except in the unusual cases that present with multiple dysrhythmias or cardiogenic shock. The clinical manifestations are variable and dependent on the magnitude of myocardial injury. One should suspect myocardial contusion with any high-energy direct blow to the chest. Sternal fractures should increase the suspicion. The most common mechanism of injury is a direct blow to the anterior chest wall from a steering wheel.

Physical Findings

Conscious patients may complain of angina-like pain if the injury is severe. The clinical spectrum of symptoms found with myocardial infarction and occasionally cardiac failure may be present.[62] Cardiac failure associated with isolated myocardial contusion is rare, and its presence should suggest the possibility of ventricular septal or valve injury. Virtually any dysrhythmia can occur, but premature atrial or ventricular contractions are most common.

Laboratory Testing

Creatine kinase (CK)-MB elevation is also nonspecific and frequently nondiagnostic in multiply injured patients. Small amounts of the MB isoenzyme are found in skeletal muscle and other body tissues. The most reliable diagnostic test is two-dimensional echocardiography. Abnormal segmental heart wall motion, cardiac wall thinning, myocardial hematomas, chamber dilatation, intracavitary filling defects (from hematomas), valvular dysfunction, and increased pericardial fluid are some of the findings considered diagnostic of myocardial injury.[62]

No isolated laboratory or radiologic test absolutely confirms the diagnosis, and it is reasonable to obtain an electrocardiogram (ECG) and CK-MB isoenzyme test for any patient suspected of having a myocardial contusion. Two-dimensional echocardiography should be strongly considered after high-speed impact injury to the chest, regardless of the ECG or CK-MB results. The prognosis for most patients with myocardial contusion is excellent. Superficial or even limited full-thickness contusions usually heal without permanent deficit.

Aortic Disruption

Secondary assessment for injury to the thoracic great vessels is crucial, because 50% of patients with these injuries due to blunt trauma have no external signs of injury.[63] An ECG and portable supine AP 36-inch chest radiograph should be obtained in all patients with chest trauma. Stable patients who can tolerate the sitting position should have a 72-inch erect AP chest radiograph for better evaluation of the mediastinum.

Physical Findings

Several physical findings are usually absent but if present may confirm the diagnosis. These include decreased breath sounds in the left chest due to massive hemothorax, diminished or absent femoral pulses, and upper extremity hypertension. Patients may also complain of severe chest or back pain, along with shortness of breath.

Radiographic Findings

Various radiologic findings suggest aortic injury. The most reliable is loss of the aortic knob contour. A widened superior mediastinum of more than 8 cm at the level of the aortic isthmus, depression of the left mainstem bronchus >140°, a left apical hematoma (apical capping), and the presence of a massive hemothorax also suggest aortic injury (Fig. 59–2).

Although controversial, chest CT scanning is being used more frequently to diagnose aortic injury. It can be performed if a patient requires other CT scans and the diagnosis of aortic injury is questionable. A normal rapid-bolus contrast infusion chest CT scan has been helpful in our experience to rule out aortic injury. However, if the test is positive or nondiagnostic, an aortogram is required to further delineate the area of injury. The operative approach may be different, depending on the level of aortic injury.

Important Prognostic Factors

Autopsy series have shown that 50% of thoracic aortic tears occur at the aortic isthmus.[64] However, >90% of patients who survive to the ED have a tear at this site. Patients with injuries to the ascending aorta rarely survive, and repair requires total cardiopulmonary bypass.[65]

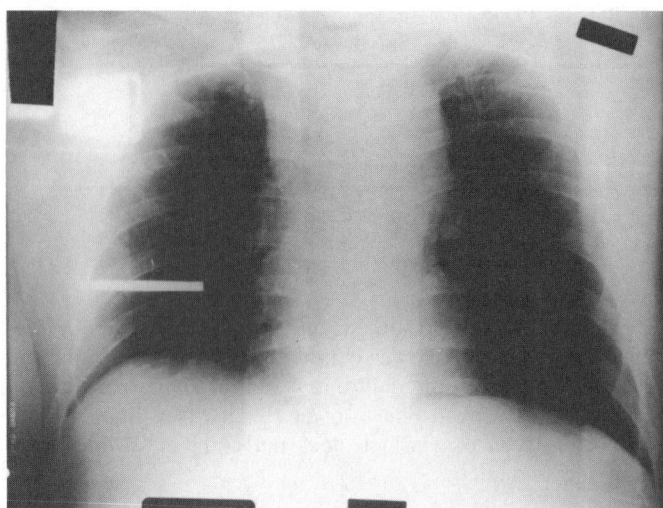

FIGURE 59–2. Chest radiograph depicting ruptured thoracic aorta. Note the widened upper mediastinum, tracheal deviation to the right, and loss of aortic knob contour.

Preoperative Treatment

Initial medical management of aortic injury may include sodium nitroprusside to lower the systolic blood pressure. Beta-blockers such as propranolol and esmolol may also be beneficial. These drugs are contraindicated if a patient is hypovolemic as a result of other injuries. Management is challenging and difficult, because multiple injuries are often present.

Diaphragmatic Injuries

Penetrating chest or abdominal wounds and blunt trauma causing a rapid rise in intra-abdominal pressure are mechanisms responsible for diaphragm injuries. Rapid deceleration against a poorly positioned lap belt restraint is a common cause. Crush injuries and falls are factors in diaphragmatic tears. Eighty-five per cent of injuries affect the left hemidiaphragm, because the right hemidiaphragm is relatively protected by the liver, which usually absorbs the force generated by compression of the right upper abdomen.

Physical Findings

Patients often present with severe tachypnea, hypoxemia, and hypercarbia. Decreased breath sounds may be found on the affected side, simulating a pneumothorax. The diagnosis is usually made by chest radiograph or CT scan. Findings on physical examination are rarely pathognomonic, because most patients have multiple injuries.

Radiographic Findings

A torn left hemidiaphragm can be diagnosed with chest radiographs if the stomach or a portion of bowel is seen within the left chest (Fig. 59–3). Injury to the right hemidiaphragm is less obvious, appearing as an elevated hemidiaphragm because of the herniation of the dome of the liver (Fig. 59–4). In this situation, the diagnosis is confirmed by either fluoroscopy or CT scan (Fig. 59–5).

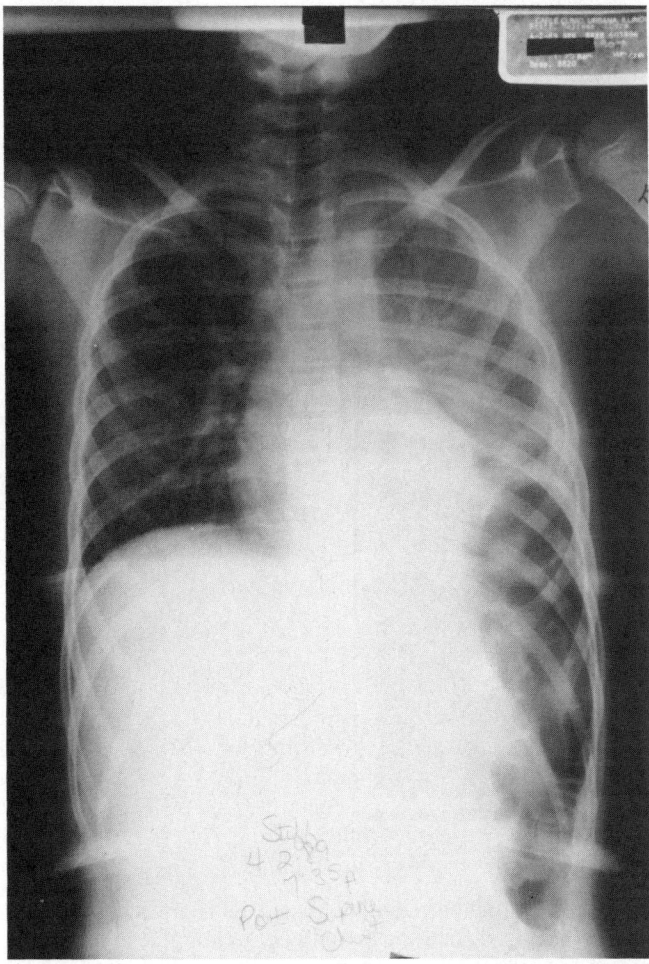

FIGURE 59–3. Chest radiograph demonstrating a ruptured left hemidiaphragm with herniation of small bowel into the left hemithorax.

Treatment

Diaphragm injuries require immediate surgery. Initial management includes nasogastric tube decompression of the stomach and endotracheal intubation for treatment of respiratory compromise.

Tracheobronchial Injuries

Direct trauma to the trachea can result in life-threatening upper airway obstruction. Stridorous respirations indicate partial airway obstruction; establishing a patent airway is crucial. Injury to the left or right mainstem bronchus or one of the major bronchioles is an unusual but frequently fatal injury.

These injuries are caused by blunt chest trauma, with the most life-threatening ones occurring within 1 inch of the carina. Patients generally present in severe respiratory failure, with subcutaneous emphysema, tension pneumothorax, hypotension, and frequently a massive mediastinal shift. Tube thoracostomy is usually diagnostic, because a massive air leak usually issues from the affected hemithorax. Immediate surgery to repair the defect is required.

Esophageal Injuries

Most injuries to the esophagus result from penetrating trauma and are usually diagnosed during thoracic exploration.

Blunt esophageal trauma is rare but frequently lethal if not rapidly diagnosed. The mechanism of injury with blunt trauma to the upper abdomen results from a forceful ejection of gastric contents, causing a linear tear in the lower esophagus. Mediastinal air or a left pneumothorax without pulmonary injury or rib fracture should suggest this injury. Diagnosis is confirmed by either an esophageal Gastrografin study or esophagoscopy.

Abdominal Injuries

Abdominal trauma is the third most common cause of death in patients with life-threatening injuries, ranking behind only those of the head and chest. All gunshot wounds to the abdomen resulting in peritoneal penetration require surgical exploration.

Stab wounds to the abdomen may require surgical exploration but can be treated initially by local wound exploration with or without diagnostic peritoneal lavage, before exploratory celiotomy. A significant number of stab wounds do not result in major intra-abdominal injury.[66]

Penetrating injuries to the chest in the area below the nipple line may also result in intra-abdominal injury. Further evaluation of the abdomen with either CT scanning or diagnostic peritoneal lavage (DPL) is indicated when these wounds are present. These tests often are complementary.

Diagnosis

Diagnostic Peritoneal Lavage. DPL has been criticized as being overly sensitive, occasionally detecting self-limited, solid visceral parenchymal injuries that may not require operative intervention.[67, 68] Henneman and colleagues,[69] in a retrospective review of 944 patients with blunt and penetrating abdominal trauma, reported an overall DPL accuracy of 93%, with a positive predictive value of 80% and a negative predictive value of 98% for intra-abdominal injury requiring surgical repair.

Positive criteria for blunt trauma were any of the following findings: aspiration of 10 mL or more of gross blood, red blood cell (RBC) count $\geq$100,000 · mL^{-1} white blood cell

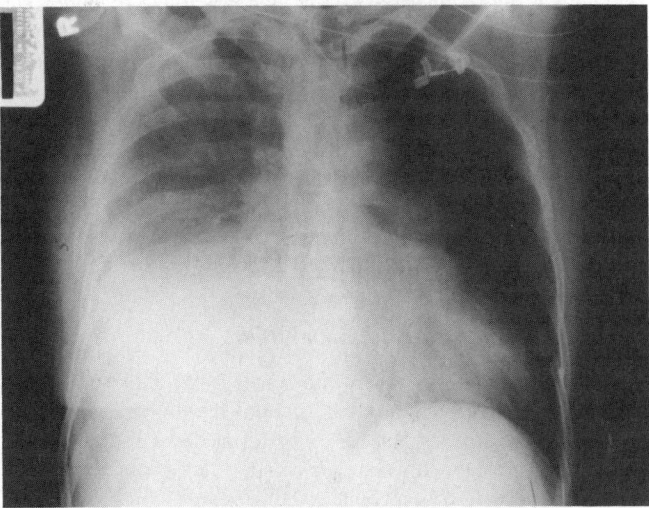

FIGURE 59–4. Chest radiograph demonstrating loss of right hemidiaphragm contour, consistent with right middle and lower lobe collapse of lung, hemothorax, or ruptured hemidiaphragm. Subsequent computed tomography scan (see Fig. 59–5) confirmed the latter diagnosis.

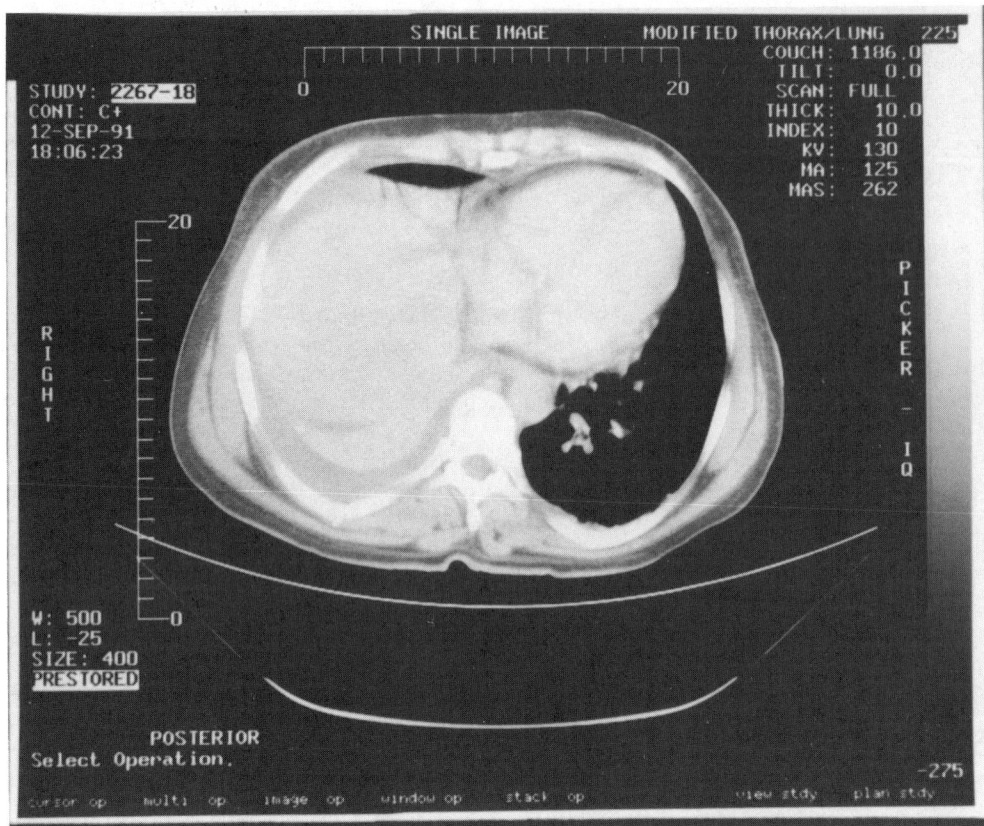

FIGURE 59-5. Computed tomography scan of chest demonstrating a ruptured right hemidiaphragm with herniation of the liver into the right hemithorax. This cut is at approximately the level of T7-T8. Note the right hemithorax filled with the contrast-enhanced liver and complete displacement of the right lung cephalad.

(WBC) count $\geq 500 \cdot mL^{-1}$, amylase level ≥ 200 U $\cdot L^{-1}$, or bacteria present on microscopic examination of the lavage fluid.

For stab wounds to the lower chest and abdomen and tangential gunshot wounds to the abdomen, the following values were considered positive: aspiration of ≥ 1 mL of gross blood, RBC count $\geq 5000 \cdot mm^{3-1}$, WBC count $\geq 500 \cdot mm^{3-1}$, amylase level ≥ 200 U $\cdot L^{-1}$, or the presence of bacteria in the lavage fluid.

CT Scanning. Matsubara and colleagues[70] reviewed their experience with CT scanning in the management of blunt abdominal trauma. A negative CT scan was found to be correct in 14 of 15 patients (93%), although one case of a perforated jejunum was overlooked. The overall accuracy rate for positive CT scans was found to be correct in 30 of 34 patients (88%).

CT scanning was found to be a valuable adjunct to clinical monitoring in hemodynamically stable patients after blunt abdominal trauma. The researchers warned, however, that if abdominal CT scanning did not include appropriate patient selection, standardized techniques, and accurate radiologic interpretation, a significant potential for serious error existed.[70]

Seat Belts And Intra-Abdominal Injury

An inappropriately applied lap belt is associated with intestinal injuries and associated fractures of the thoracic and lumbar spine (Chance's fractures).[71–73] Rapid deceleration during high-speed crashes can result in sudden flexion of the upper body around a fixed lap belt, causing severe compression of the abdominal viscera. Children who are restrained in the back seat of cars with only a lap belt are at especially high risk for such injuries.[73]

CT scanning may be unreliable for evaluating intestinal injury. Lateral spine radiographs and DPL are indicated if a patient has a mechanism or findings to suggest a seat belt–associated injury. The most serious injury, which may not be immediately identifiable, is avulsion of the bowel mesentery, causing avascular necrosis of a bowel loop. These injuries initially may not produce any abdominal tenderness or peritoneal irritation.

Prompt diagnosis is often difficult, requiring a very high index of suspicion as well as a determined approach that may include exploratory celiotomy.[71] Abdominal ecchymosis from the lap belt mandates further evaluation to rule out this potentially serious injury.

Summary

Our experience with CT scanning in blunt trauma victims has been very favorable. In hemodynamically stable patients, we prefer abdominal CT over DPL as an initial test unless a patient has a severe closed head injury requiring immediate treatment. Peritoneal lavage should be the test of choice in an unstable patient and can be a complementary test with CT scanning if the possibility of bowel injury exists.

Orthopedic Injuries

The first priority of care for patients with multiple injuries is restoration of hemodynamic function and life-saving support. Orthopedic injuries, unless very severe and obvious, are occasionally overlooked and temporarily neglected. If a patient is unable to demonstrate areas of pain, fractures can be missed, even after a well-performed secondary survey.

Certain orthopedic injuries require immediate care to prevent severe long-term disability, whereas others are of minimal initial importance. Those orthopedic injuries that, if not treated expeditiously, can result in severe morbidity and even limb loss must be identified. All open fractures require immediate attention and orthopedic consultation. Initial management consists of cleaning the wound with an antiseptic solution, followed by placement of dry sterile dressings and a pressure bandage if significant bleeding is present.

Physical Findings

The secondary survey should include a thorough examination of the extremities, the spine, and the pelvis. Inspection and palpation of the thoracic and lumbar spine and, if immobilization is not required, the cervical spine, can identify areas of deformity and tenderness. Inspection and palpation of the extremities may identify areas of edema, deformity, or crepitance, which indicate a possible fracture or joint dislocation. Any areas in question should undergo radiographic evaluation when the patient is stabilized. Temporary splinting should be performed during the secondary survey.

Radiographic Findings

If a patient has a possible unstable cervical spine injury, a rigid collar should remain in place until further definitive evaluation with a full cervical spine series (including flexion and extension views) can be obtained. A CT scan of the cervical spine may also be necessary to completely rule out cervical spine injury.

Thoracic and lumbar spine fractures also must be ruled out. If a patient is unable to report an adequate history or to respond appropriately to physical examination, screening lateral thoracic and lumbar spine radiographs should be obtained. Any evidence of severe thoracic or lumbar spine fracture requires orthopedic or neurosurgical evaluation.

If signs of associated spinal cord injury such as diminished motor or sensory function in the lower extremities are present, consultation should be obtained immediately after stabilization.

Critical Fracture Complications

Fractures and dislocations of the hip or knee, displaced fractures of the tibia and fibula, and severe fractures or dislocations of the ankle can cause compartmental syndrome problems and increased pressure on nerves, blood vessels, and skin. Permanent neurovascular injuries or skin sloughing may result.[74] Delays beyond 24 hours in reducing a dislocated hip are associated with virtually a 100% incidence of aseptic necrosis of the femoral head.

Failure to recognize an impacted or nondisplaced femoral neck fracture can result in displacement, which will require a much more extensive surgical procedure in the future.[74] Fractures and dislocations of the upper extremity, particularly at the elbow, can also be devastating, requiring immediate orthopedic consultation and reduction. Every attempt must be made to rule out associated vascular and neurologic injury as soon as possible in all extremity fractures and dislocations.

Open fractures are true emergencies and should undergo surgical treatment within 6 to 8 hours to minimize infection risks. Patients with open fractures should receive intravenous antibiotics immediately. We prefer cefuroxime, 1.5 g intravenously every 8 hours for 24 to 48 hours.

Acute Compartment Syndrome. Swelling and bleeding into the lower extremities associated with closed fractures, especially those below the knee, can result in acute compartmental syndrome. Severe pain in the extremity or pain distal to the fracture site (e.g., in the foot), often described as burning or a deep, throbbing, unrelenting pressure, are among the first signs of compartmental syndrome. The pain is often out of proportion to the apparent clinical situation and is unrelieved by rest or immobilization.

Sensory and motor changes may also be associated with compartment syndrome, but these are often difficult to evaluate and are usually late findings. Compartment pressure can be measured by various methods. A pressure transducer is attached to a fluid-filled extension tubing and needle that is inserted into the various compartments. A critical level of pressure that necessitates fasciotomy is not defined. The need for fasciotomy is usually based on clinical evaluation as well as compartment pressures.[75] (See Chapter 72.)

ALCOHOL AND DRUG INTOXICATION

Alcohol and drug intoxication have an important role in trauma-related injuries and death. Throughout recorded history, humans have constantly sought drugs and alcohol to make life more pleasurable and to avoid or decrease pain, discomfort, and frustration.[76] Assessment of a trauma victim who abuses drugs and alcohol is difficult, because these patients can present with a broad range of mental status changes ranging from depression, through emotional and violent behavior, to coma.

Although a ''watch and wait'' approach can be safe in patients who are not trauma victims, this approach leads to potentially disastrous consequences in patients with major injuries. Most abused drugs and alcohol are powerful respiratory depressants that can exacerbate the level of hypoxemia and respiratory acidosis. Alcohol and barbiturates are also cardiac depressants at higher doses, further enhancing the hemodynamic instability of hypovolemic shock.

Examination

Skin

The skin should be carefully examined during the secondary assessment for signs of needle tracks, abscess, ulcerations, or draining sinuses from deeper subcutaneous tissues. These signs may signify chronic, heavy drug abuse. Recent needle tracks suggest narcotic or cocaine abuse, although amphetamines and occasionally barbiturates may be used intravenously. The number of needle tracks allows estimation of the degree of drug use. Generally, if arm veins are not thrombosed, the patient is less likely to be physically addicted. Femoral and subclavian vein injection sites signify long-standing abuse. Other chronic abusers may resort to subcutaneous injections of drugs (skin popping).[76]

Nervous System

Neurologic assessment is especially difficult and unreliable in these patients, but a rapid evaluation of the neurologic status may help to determine what type of drug a patient used.

TABLE 59–12. Diagnostic Features of Commonly Abused Drugs

Drugs	Pupils	Respiratory	Central Nervous System	Seizures	Initial Evaluation	Withdrawal
Opioids	Pinpoint	Depressed	Lethargy, coma	+	Respiratory depression; drug-altered LOC	Withdrawal
Barbiturates	Small, reactive (not pinpoint)	Depressed	Lethargy, coma	+	Respiratory depression; hypotension; drug-altered LOC	Withdrawal (severe)
Anxiolytics	Normal, reactive	May be depressed	Lethargy, coma	–	Drug-altered LOC; respiratory depression (in elderly and when combined with ETOH)	Withdrawal
Amphetamines and cocaine	Dilated, reactive	Stimulated	Confusion, delusions, disorientation, paranoia	+	Seizures; ventricular arrhythmias; lack of cooperation	Withdrawal (mild); rhabdomyolysis (cocaine)
Marijuana	Dilated, reactive	No consistent changes	Euphoria, drowsiness, decreased attention span, paranoia	–	Dilated pupils; lack of cooperation	—
LSD	Dilated, reactive	No consistent changes	Euphoria, hallucinations, drowsiness	+	Lack of cooperation; altered mental status	—
PCP	Dilated, reactive	No consistent changes	Aggressive, violent behavior	+	Lack of cooperation; altered mental status; combativeness	Rhabdomyolysis
ETOH	Dilated, reactive	Depressed with high levels	Variable (initial aggressiveness, then somnolence)	–	Lack of cooperation, aggressiveness, or somnolence/lethargy	Withdrawal (mild to severe); seizures

(From Norwood SH, Dellinger RP: Managing substance abuse in the trauma patient. Probl Crit Care 1987; 1:117.)
Abbreviation: LOC = level of consciousness.

Clinical signs usually observed with the more frequently abused drugs are outlined in Table 59–12. These findings may not be helpful in patients with head injury. Despite a definite history of drug abuse, intracranial injury must always be ruled out before implicating substance abuse as the sole reason for a patient's comatose or altered mental state.

An emergency CT scan of the head should be obtained as soon as the patient has been stabilized. In our series of 229 patients who underwent emergency tracheal intubation, 76 were paralyzed and intubated because of combative or uncooperative behavior. In this group, 42% had significant intracranial injury detected by CT scan, and 22% had other life-threatening injuries requiring expedient therapy.[43]

Effects of Alcohol

Animal studies of alcohol intoxication associated with hypovolemic shock show a significant increase in mortality compared with hypovolemic shock without alcohol intoxication.[77] Others have shown depression of the respiratory response to shock in an intoxicated animal model and a definite decrease in the amount of blood loss necessary to cause severe hypovolemic shock.[78] This lack of normal physiologic response was associated with a higher mortality rate. Presumably, these same abnormalities occur in intoxicated patients after traumatic shock.

Cardiovascular

Alcohol causes peripheral vasodilation and a decrease in the SVR. This change, combined with the diuresis secondary to inhibition of antidiuretic hormone, can cause significant hypovolemia with even minimum blood loss. At high serum levels, alcohol also exerts a negative cardiac inotropic effect.

This depressant effect causes a reduction in the mean arterial blood pressure out of proportion to the actual volume of blood lost.[79]

Vasodilation can also lead to hypothermia. Patients may have a decreased perception of pain, thus making physical examination unreliable. Cirrhotic patients often exhibit a relatively low systolic blood pressure (90–110 mm Hg) associated with a high cardiac output and very low SVR. These findings must be taken into account when evaluating injured cirrhotic patients. Further studies may be indicated before rushing such patients to the OR for emergency laparotomy.[80]

Coagulation

Coagulation disorders may also complicate management of alcoholic patients. Although such abnormalities are well recognized in cirrhotic patients, less well known is the fact that acutely intoxicated patients demonstrate significant platelet coagulation abnormalities.[81]

Alcohol Withdrawal Syndrome

Recognition and management of alcohol withdrawal in hospitalized trauma victims are crucial. The syndrome usually begins after 12 to 36 hours of abstinence. Prophylactic regimens have been recommended to prevent alcohol withdrawal in its most severe form, delirium tremens, which even now has high morbidity and significant mortality.

THE FULL STOMACH

Aspiration

Trauma victims often arrive with an unsavory variety of gastric contents mixed with alcohol. In addition, anxiety, pain, and the metabolic response to trauma delay or completely arrest gastric emptying.[52] Patients with head injury and elevated ICP are also prone to vomiting. Trauma victims thus are at high risk for aspiration of gastric contents.

The most dangerous immediate complication of aspiration is obstruction of the upper airway by large food particles. Although various suggestions about management of a full stomach have been proposed, the most reliable method in obtunded trauma victims is to apply cricoid pressure, followed by rapid paralysis and intubation of the airway. The estimated risk of aspiration in patients with a full stomach during intubation for emergency surgery is approximately 5%, with an overall mortality rate of 0.2% per 10,000 anesthetics administered.[52, 82]

Are "Prophylactic" Measures Helpful?

The potential severity of the underlying traumatic injuries usually does not permit time for routine use of agents such as metoclopramide and H_2-blockers to decrease the risk of aspiration. Placement of a nasogastric tube may induce retching and for the most part is ineffective anyway. Such maneuvers markedly increase ICP and should be avoided at all costs in head-injured patients.

CERVICAL SPINE INJURY

Spinal cord injuries are uncommon compared with the incidence of head injuries. However, during the acute management and evaluation phase, the potential for serious iatrogenic injury is much higher with vigorous manipulation of an unstable cervical spine. Aggressive manipulation can cause a patient with an unstable fracture and no neurologic injury become completely quadriplegic. Thus, every precaution must be taken to ensure cervical spine stability until neck injury is definitely ruled out.

How Should the Trachea Be Intubated?

Patients can safely be orotracheally intubated with in-line cervical traction.[43, 52] Concern for a cervical spine injury should not, under any circumstances, prevent rapid establishment of a patent airway, but proper precautions must be taken. Neck flexion and extension must be avoided.

Is Methylprednisolone of Value?

Hypotension with bradycardia should immediately suggest the possibility of a cervical spine injury. It has been recommended that high-dose methylprednisolone be administered for the first 24 hours after spinal cord injury with motor deficits (30 mg $\cdot$ kg^{-1} in the first hour, followed by 5–6 mg $\cdot$ kg^{-1} $\cdot$ h^{-1} for 23 hours). Statistically significant improvement in neurologic outcome was noted.[83]

RETROPERITONEAL INJURIES

Bleeding into the retroperitoneal space can be severe and silent. As much as 4 L of blood can easily be sequestered.[84]

Irreversible shock secondary to massive retroperitoneal injury occurs in <1% of blunt trauma injuries, but its presence can be a major diagnostic and therapeutic dilemma.

What Are the Presenting Signs and Symptoms?

The most serious bleeding is usually associated with posterior disruption of the pelvis, creating venous plexus injuries.[84] This area is obscured from direct observation by the abdomen ventrally and by musculoskeletal structures dorsally. Hence, the diagnosis of retroperitoneal injuries is extremely difficult unless an obvious pelvic fracture is associated with the hemorrhage.

Conscious patients may complain of abdominal, back, or perineal pain, but often no specific symptoms are noted. Flank ecchymosis (Grey Turner's sign) and periumbilical ecchymosis (Cullen's sign) are usually absent during the initial resuscitative phase and may not appear until 48 hours after the time of injury. Pelvic instability noted on physical examination may be the first clue that significant retroperitoneal hemorrhage exists. Hematuria may also be an early sign.

Is CT Scanning Helpful?

Retroperitoneal hemorrhage can be confirmed either at laparotomy or by preoperative CT scanning. If a patient's condition permits, a CT scan is helpful in determining the nature of small or stable hematomas and their location. A CT scan using intravenous contrast is a more sensitive test for detecting retroperitoneal injuries and genitourinary injuries than is an intravenous pyelogram.

How Urgent Is Surgical Intervention?

The urgency of intervention depends primarily on the retroperitoneum's tamponading effect to limit progression of bleeding. Large retroperitoneal hematomas cause displacement of intraperitoneal organs, occasionally associated with secondary shearing of the attached vessels (i.e., the short gastric and gastroepiploic vessels). Secondary intra-abdominal hemorrhage may result. The need for operative intervention depends on which retroperitoneal organ is injured, the extent of bleeding, and the presence of hemodynamic instability.

HEAD INJURIES

What Are the Treatment Priorities?

Treatment should begin at the scene of the accident. Airway control and hyperventilation are started as soon as possible in order to attenuate further brain injury due to systemic insults. Hypotension, anemia, and hypercarbia are frequently present in patients with multiple injuries and significantly increase mortality and morbidity in head-injured patients.[85]

Patients who have a severe head injury and who arrive without an airway in place should be immediately intubated in a manner that avoids increased ICP.[45] The majority of patients brought to the ED with a suspected head injury have positive findings on CT scan; up to 15% of these patients require emergent neurosurgical intervention.[86]

What Should Be Done If Only a Loss of Consciousness Is Reported?

Many patients present with a history of questionable or brief loss of consciousness. Findings on neurologic examination and the Glasgow Coma Scale score are usually normal.[54] Ochsner and colleagues[87] reported a 5.7% incidence of serious intracranial pathology in patients with no history other than a brief loss of consciousness. Others[88, 89] have also reported a relatively high incidence of significant intracranial pathology after "minimum" head trauma. Because of these observations, a head CT scan is indicated in most patients who have had a brief loss of consciousness or whose mechanism of injury suggests a potentially serious head injury. The presence of intracerebral blood in patients who otherwise appear completely normal warrants admission to the hospital and careful observation.

What Therapy Is Indicated?

Patients who are comatose as a result of head injury need rapid resuscitation to improve oxygenation to the injured brain. Oxygen consumption in patients with isolated severe head injury is elevated and similar to that in patients with multiple injuries.[90]

Control of Intracranial Pressure

Rapid reduction of ICP and expedient transfer to a facility for surgical correction of intracranial lesions can be affected by prehospital and ED intervention. In one large series of patients with acute subdural hematomas, control of ICP and a patient's initial presenting neurologic status were the only variables predictive of improved morbidity and mortality[91] (see also Chapter 46).

Maintenance of Cerebral Perfusion Pressure

Rosner and Daughton[92] advocate intravascular volume expansion and inotropic support with various catecholamine infusions to maintain a target cerebral perfusion pressure of about 80 mm Hg. This approach is especially important if ICP cannot be reduced to <15 mm Hg. The results of this study, which showed morbidity and mortality to be equal or superior to the results from previous methods of therapy, bring into question many of the standard protocols of ICP management. Adequate intravascular volume resuscitation is crucial in the initial management of multiply injured patients and is usually not detrimental to head-injured patients.

Forced Diuresis

We recommend that patients receive 20% mannitol (0.5–1.0 g · kg^{-1} loading dose) if increased ICP is suspected. Patients with decorticate or decerebrate posturing and normal or elevated systolic blood pressure should be given mannitol even before an emergency CT scan is obtained. Further therapy is determined by the CT findings and serial physical examinations.

Penetrating Injuries

As with severe closed head injuries, penetrating injuries to the cranium should be treated aggressively using the same modalities as described previously. In addition to mannitol and hyperventilation, broad-spectrum antibiotic coverage should be started and immediate neurosurgical consultation obtained.

Blunt Cranial Injuries

Direct blows to the head associated with violence, motor vehicle accidents, and falls can result in linear skull fractures. Heavier impacts may also cause stellate fractures. Lacerations of the scalp over the fractured area convert the lesion to an open fracture.

These injuries should be treated with antibiotics and expeditious surgical repair. Depressed skull fractures are associated with a higher incidence of underlying brain and dural injuries. CT scanning to rule out underlying brain injury is indicated in all patients with skull fractures.

Bacterial Meningitis

Bacterial meningitis develops in about 1% of patients who suffer blunt head injury and who seek medical attention.[93] Patients at highest risk are those with fractures at the base of the skull. Dural disruption produces communication between the subarachnoid space and the nasal cavity, paranasal sinuses, or ear canal. This disruption allows bacteria to migrate from these areas to the meninges.

The frontal fossa at the level of the cribriform plate is the most common location for dural tears. Large fistulas are usually evident by cerebrospinal fluid (CSF) rhinorrhea or otorrhea. Several studies have demonstrated no benefit from prophylactic antibiotics in patients with basilar skull fractures.[93] Broad-spectrum antibiotics may generate resistance by the nasopharyngeal flora, resulting in a more serious form of meningitis.

The mortality rate from meningitis after blunt head injury is about 10%, which is considerably less than the 30% rate for patients with nontraumatic causes.[93] Most CSF leaks close spontaneously within about 2 weeks after the injury.

PREGNANT TRAUMA VICTIMS

The incidence of trauma occurring during pregnancy is reported to be about 7%, but the actual prevalence of pregnancy in trauma victims is unknown.[94] Pregnancy coincident with severe trauma is rare in our experience. The causes of traumatic injury are similar to those in the general population, with blunt mechanisms prevailing. However, penetrating injuries constitute a greater proportion of injuries at large urban hospitals.[94]

What Physiologic Changes Complicate Diagnosis and Resuscitation?

A number of hemodynamic alterations, along with changes in blood volume and composition, occur during pregnancy and can obscure the presence of injuries to the mother and fetus. Changes in other organ systems' function are also present (Table 59–13). Pregnancy per se may not adversely affect

TABLE 59–13. Physiologic Changes Associated with Pregnancy

Hemodynamic	Cardiac output	↑ 1.0–1.5 L · min⁻¹
	Heart rate	↑ 15–20 bpm
	Systolic/diastolic pressure*	↑ 5–15 mm Hg
Blood	Blood volume (34 weeks' gestation)	↑ 40–50%
	Hematocrit	↓ to 30–35%
	Leukocyte count	↑ to 20,000 · μL⁻¹
	Serum fibrinogen	↑
	Clotting factors	↑
	Serum albumin	↓ to 2.2–2.8 g · dL⁻¹
Respiratory	Tidal volume	↑ 40%
	PaCO_2	↓ to 30 mm Hg
Gastrointestinal	Delayed gastric emptying	
	Intestines displaced cephalad	

(Modified from Committee on Trauma, American College of Surgeons: Advanced Life Support Student Manual. Chicago, American College of Surgeons, 1993, p. 28.)
*Vena cava compression by the uterus when patient is in the supine position may cause severe hypotension and decreased cardiac output.

maternal outcome after a traumatic injury. However, its rare prevalence as an associated condition, trauma team members' unfamiliarity with the relevant physiologic changes, and the emotional overlay of the situation can lead to serious delays in diagnosis and treatment.[94]

Special Considerations

An aggressive approach to diagnosis and treatment is even more important in pregnant trauma victims. Maintenance of maternal systemic circulation after hypoxia or hemorrhage is accomplished in part at the expense of the uterine circulation.[95] Maternal intravascular volume progressively increases by 40% to 55% from the 6th to the 34th week of gestation.[95] This additional blood volume may improve maternal tolerance of hemorrhage and delay the signs and symptoms of shock. Hence, physiologic and laboratory parameters that are reliable indicators of shock in nonpregnant trauma victims may not accurately reflect the mother's status and are especially insensitive in determining fetal viability.

What Are the Causes of Fetal Death After Trauma?

Direct uteroplacental injury, direct fetal trauma, and the indirect effects of maternal trauma, including hypoxia and hypovolemia, are potential causes of fetal demise. Sympathetic nervous system stimulation and increased maternal serum levels of norepinephrine and epinephrine contribute to a decrease in uterine blood flow in both hypovolemic and normovolemic mothers. Isolated maternal head injury may also lead to indirect fetal injury by causing increased elaboration of thromboxane A_2 and prostaglandins. These powerful vasoconstrictors further decrease uterine blood flow.[95]

How Does Management Differ?

The initial evaluation and treatment of pregnant trauma victims are identical to those of nonpregnant patients. However, because of the increased blood volume, a normal blood pressure and pulse may be present even with severe injury. Preg-

nant patients whose histories suggest associated severe injury should be aggressively evaluated and resuscitated.

Supine Hypotension

The supine position can reduce venous return and aortic outflow because of vascular compression by the uterus. Unless a spinal injury is suspected, transportation and evaluation should occur with the patient positioned on her left side. If she must remain supine, the right hip should be elevated (unless injured) and the uterus manually displaced to the left side to relieve pressure on the inferior vena cava.[40]

Fetal Monitoring

In our institution, an obstetric nurse with experience in performing fetal heart rate monitoring and ultrasonography is dispatched to the ED as soon as a trauma victim is determined to be pregnant. Once the mother is stabilized, a quick assessment of the fetus is performed with both fetal heart monitoring and ultrasonography. An evaluation by an obstetrician is also performed at the earliest available time once the patient is stabilized. Various other tests can also be performed to help determine the presence of fetal injury (Table 59–14).

Fetal Risks from Diagnostic Studies

Teratogenic risk to the fetus from radiation exposure for diagnostic testing is an emotionally charged and occasionally irrationally discussed subject that must be dealt with in emergency situations. Diagnostic and therapeutic procedures cannot be withheld from the mother, regardless of her pregnancy status. DPL using a supraumbilical approach is a safe procedure.[94]

Although fetal heart rate and serum bicarbonate levels have been advocated as good indicators of fetal outcome, no one test has been found to be accurately predictive. Correction of hemodynamic abnormalities and hypoxemia in the mother offers the only chance for fetal survival. In a retrospective study, aggressive management of diagnosed maternal injuries has been shown to reduce the fetal mortality rate to approximately 10% to 30%.[94]

PEDIATRIC TRAUMA VICTIMS

Nothing is more emotionally distressing to medical personnel than treating a severely injured child. Although pediatric trauma centers have significantly improved the care of critically injured children in some areas of the country, the majority of injured children are still initially managed in hospital EDs without such expertise. Children should be approached in a systematic fashion so that proper and timely assessment and resuscitation occur.

TABLE 59–14. Laboratory Tests for Determining Fetal Injury in Pregnant Trauma Patients

- Fetal ECG monitoring
- Ultrasonography
- Kleihauer-Betke test (2nd and 3rd trimester)
- Diagnostic peritoneal lavage
- Pelvic CT scan

How Are Children Different?

Head injuries are common after blunt trauma. Because a child's head is large relative to the trunk, it is often the leading contact point in falls and high-speed motor vehicle accidents.[96] Children are also more likely to develop hypothermia because of their larger body surface area in relation to body mass.

Airway Considerations

The glottis lies in a more anterior and superior position in the pharynx, favoring orotracheal over nasotracheal intubation. Infants are obligate nasal breathers; nasal fractures, soft tissue injuries, and blood can occlude the upper airway. Nasogastric and nasotracheal tubes should not be placed in infants and younger children.

Endotracheal tube size can be gauged by the approximate diameter of the child's external nares or the size of the small finger.[97] The following formula is also useful:

$$\text{Internal diameter (mm) of tube} = [16 + \text{age (years)}] \div 4$$

In children, the airway is narrowest at the cricoid level. Therefore, uncuffed endotracheal tubes are used until approximately age 8 years.[96]

Normative Data

Because of age-related differences in size and physiologic parameters, prepublished normal ranges for pulse, blood pressure, and respiration should be available in the ED for each age group (Table 59–15).

The following relations are also useful in establishing dosage ranges and resuscitation measures. A child's weight in kilograms is approximately twice the age in years plus 8.[96] Blood volume is approximately $80 \text{ mL} \cdot \text{kg}^{-1}$.[96] Systolic blood pressure is estimated at approximately 70 mm Hg plus twice the age in years.[96]

TABLE 59–15. Parameters for Vital Signs in Pediatric Trauma Patients

Age	Average Weight (kg)	Normal Blood Pressure, Systolic/Diastolic	Heart Rate (bpm)
1 mo	4	60–90/40–60	120–160
3 mo	5	74–100/50–70	120–160
6 mo	7	74–100/50–70	120–160
9 mo	9	74–100/50–70	120–160
12 mo	10	80–112/50–80	90–140
15 mo	20–5	80–112/50–80	90–140
18 mo	11.5	80–112/50–80	90–140
21 mo	12	80–112/50–80	90–140
24 mo	12.5	80–112/50–80	90–140
30 mo	13.5	80–112/50–80	90–140
3 y	14.5	82–110/50–78	80–110
4 y	16.5	82–110/50–78	80–110
5 y	18	82–110/50–78	80–110
6 y	21	84–120/54–80	75–100
8 y	27	84–120/54–80	75–100
10 y	32	84–120/54–80	60–90
12 y	39	94–140/62–88	60–90
14 y	49	94–140/62–88	60–90
16 y	56	94–140/62–88	60–90

(Adapted from Donien J: Fear of floating to pediatrics. Nursing 1982; 12:56.)

TABLE 59–16. Pediatric Trauma Score*

Variable	+2	+1	−1
Weight (kg)	>20	10–20	<10
Airway patency	Normal	Maintained	Unmaintained
Systolic blood pressure	>90	50–90	<50
Neurologic status	Awake	Obtunded	Comatose
Open wound	None	Minor	Major
Skeletal trauma	None	Closed	Open or multiple

(From Tepas JJ III, Mollitt DL, Talbert JL, et al: The pediatric trauma score as a predictor of injury severity in the injured child. J Pediatr Surg 1987; 22:14.)
*A score of +2, +1, or −1 is given for each variable. Scores are added (range = −6 to +12). A score ≤8 indicates the potential for severe trauma.

What Factors Suggest Severe Injury?

Children whose triage assessment reveals a pediatric trauma score ≤8 (Table 59–16)[23] or a revised trauma score ≤11 should be extensively evaluated for serious injury or transferred to a facility that is able to perform such an evaluation.[96] Regardless of the trauma score, any child whose mechanism of injury involves high-energy impact, such as a fall from a height >10 feet and pedestrian or motor vehicle accidents, should also be carefully assessed for possible life-threatening injuries. Young adults and children have tremendous hemodynamic reserve, and normal vital signs do not rule out the possibility of severe injury. Liberal use of CT scanning and other diagnostic modalities is imperative. A "wait and see" approach is unacceptable.

How Is Venous Access Achieved?

Two percutaneous intravenous catheters should be placed in the upper extremities if possible. If this approach is unsuccessful, lower extremity intravenous catheters can also be used. If cutdowns are necessary, the vein with which the operating physician is most familiar should be used. Subclavian central venous catheters can be used, but they are often difficult to place under emergency situations and are generally reserved for children older than 2 years.[97]

When Is Intraosseous Infusion Useful?

Intraosseous infusion via cannulation of the medullary cavity of a long bone in an uninjured extremity is safe and effective for emergency vascular access.[98] The intraosseous route should be used early; when a child is in extremis, it should be considered after two unsuccessful attempts at peripheral venous cannulation.[98]

Technique

Intraosseous infusion is achieved by placing a rigid needle (preferably a 16-gauge disposable bone marrow aspiration needle) through the bony cortex into the medullary cavity of spongy bone. The proximal tibia and distal femur are the two most common sites used.[98] Fluid instilled into the marrow cavity is rapidly dispersed by the extensive network of venous sinusoids into the systemic circulation. Various fluids and medications can be successfully given by this route (Table 59–17).

TABLE 59–17. Fluids and Medications Given by Intraosseous Infusion

Fluids	Medications
5–10% Dextrose	Antibiotics
Packed red blood cells	Anticonvulsants
Plasma	Atropine
Lactated Ringer's solution	Catecholamines
Saline solution	Dextrose
Whole blood	Mannitol
	Sodium bicarbonate

(From Manley L, Haley K, Dick M: Intraosseous infusion: rapid vascular access for critically ill or injured infants and children. J Emerg Nurs 1988; 14:63.)

Contraindications

The only contraindications to this technique are bone disorders such as osteogenesis imperfecta and osteopetrosis, as well as infected burns, cellulitis, or recent fractures in the areas of insertion.[99]

AN APPROACH TO VICTIMS OF MULTIPLE TRAUMA

Isolated injuries are not the rule, especially in patients involved in motor vehicle accidents and falls. As much information as possible should be obtained in the shortest period of time after arrival in the ED. The trauma team leader can then assign priorities to life-threatening injuries and address each one definitively.[100]

Patients should undergo a rapid primary survey along with resuscitation as previously described in this chapter. Only those patients who become hemodynamically stable progress to the secondary survey, which focuses on a complete physical examination and further diagnostic studies.

Patients who remain unstable may require emergency surgery. The minimal diagnostic studies performed in unstable patients are a chest radiograph, lateral cervical spine film, and plain film of the pelvis.[100] Place the chest and pelvic portable film cassettes on the stretcher before a patient's arrival. These films can then be rapidly obtained after the primary survey.

What Are the Immediate Priorities?

Our approach in multiply injured patients is to obtain immediate airway control with neuromuscular blockade (if necessary) and orotracheal intubation. Two large-bore peripheral intravenous catheters are immediately placed on arrival in the ED by nursing personnel while the primary survey is performed by the trauma surgeon. Combative and uncooperative patients are controlled with neuromuscular blockade, because a high percentage of these patients have severe injuries.[43] If the patient stabilizes, progression to the secondary survey along with a full blunt trauma series is performed.

When a Patient Doesn't Stabilize, What Follows?

If a patient is not responding to initial resuscitative efforts with stabilization of blood pressure and decreasing pulse rate,

DPL is performed. We prefer using the percutaneous technique because it is quicker and has a complication rate similar to the open technique.

If a patient stabilizes, we prefer an abdominal CT scan initially over DPL. The majority of these patients also require a head CT scan. With a rapid CT scanner in close proximity to the ED, an abdominal CT scan with intravenous contrast does not require much time. Oral contrast medium is not routinely used for emergency abdominal scans. We have not found this omission to be detrimental in diagnosing bowel injuries.

When Is Aortography or Chest CT Scanning Appropriate?

If the initial chest radiograph shows a widened mediastinum or a large hemothorax, the decision to proceed with immediate aortography versus chest CT scan must be made. Unless aortic injury is obvious, we perform a chest CT scan with intravenous contrast *if* a patient requires other CT studies. In situations in which there is little question that aortic injury is present, aortography is mandatory. Aortography must also be performed if the CT scan does not definitely rule out aortic injury.

What Surgical Intervention Is Required?

Subdural and Epidural Hematomas

A large subdural or epidural hematoma requires immediate treatment in all cases. If a patient is in severe shock owing to an intra-abdominal injury, exploratory celiotomy and craniotomy may be done simultaneously. Patients with nonsurgical intracranial injuries should be treated with intraoperative hyperventilation if abdominal, thoracic, or orthopedic procedures are performed. Placement of a ventriculostomy catheter is helpful in monitoring ICP if time permits.

Combined Abdominal and Thoracic Injuries

Patients with combined abdominal and thoracic injuries, particularly those with traumatic rupture of the thoracic aorta, require a very well-coordinated resuscitative effort. The ABC's of resuscitation are more complicated because of the risk of free rupture of the aorta during routine resuscitation maneuvers.

Patients with intra-abdominal hemorrhage and traumatic rupture of the aorta should undergo immediate exploratory celiotomy. Townsend and colleagues[101] advocate a rapid-control laparotomy that consists of quick, simple maneuvers to control major blood loss and gross contamination. A towel clip closure of the abdomen is then performed, followed by placement of an adhesive drape. The aortic injury is then addressed, either with an angiogram, if not already performed, or with a thoracotomy. On completion of the aortic repair, the laparotomy incision is reopened and definitive repair of all injuries is completed.[101]

Other Procedures

Peripheral vascular injuries are assigned the next priority for surgery after head and torso injuries. Orthopedic injuries are fourth in priority. Because of the benefits of early mobilization, early fixation of most orthopedic injuries (within the first 24 h) should be undertaken.[100] Maxillofacial injuries generally receive the fifth priority of care.[101]

POSTOPERATIVE COMPLICATIONS

What Are the Goals of Management?

The fundamental goal of critical care in the postoperative or postresuscitative period is to maintain adequate O_2 delivery to vital tissues. The secondary survey may not be performed until the patient arrives in the SICU, if the patient required emergency surgery as part of the resuscitative effort. As in the ED, therapeutic interventions and diagnostic testing often proceed or are performed simultaneously to ensure adequate O_2 delivery.

Potential complications of surgically repaired injuries must be understood and evaluated postoperatively. The adverse physiologic effects of trauma on each organ system must also be understood. Sepsis and multiple system organ failure (MSOF) are the leading causes of death in the postoperative period. A logical mechanism for evaluating sepsis must be developed.

What Are the Homeostatic Responses to Injury?

Severe injury causes various complex homeostatic responses secondary to acute volume loss and inadequate hemoperfusion.

Hormonal Interplay

Acute volume reduction results in stimulation of pressor receptors located in the carotid artery and the aortic arch, as well as volume (stretch) receptors in the wall of the left atrium. In response to afferent input from these receptors, increased secretion of aldosterone from the zona glomerulosa of the adrenal gland and antidiuretic hormone (ADH) from the posterior pituitary gland occurs.[102]

Painful stimuli from the area of injury may also stimulate ADH output. Aldosterone and ADH, respectively, stimulate increased reabsorption of sodium and water by the kidneys. Afferent nerve stimulation also causes increased levels of adrenocorticotropic hormone (ACTH), which also stimulates aldosterone release.[102]

Continued Hypoperfusion

Decreased hemoperfusion results in elevated lactic acid production, which stimulates hyperventilation. Severe cellular damage and membrane dysfunction ensue if inadequate hemoperfusion persists. Membrane permeability defects are manifested by increased requirements for larger volumes of fluid to achieve adequate resuscitation. Reperfusion is associated with the generation of free O_2 radicals, further tissue injury, and cellular disruption.[102] (See Chapter 40.)

Why Are Metabolic Demands Increased?

Severely injured patients also show evidence of markedly increased metabolic demands, primarily owing to elevated levels of catabolic hormones and catecholamines (epinephrine and norepinephrine), which initially stimulate catabolism and accelerated loss of body fat and protein.

Protein and Fat Metabolism

The hypermetabolic response is characterized by increases in lipolysis, fat oxidation, and proteolysis. Dramatic loss of body cell mass from fat stores, skeletal muscle protein, and acute phase reactant proteins occurs if the metabolic response to injury persists. Activated polymorphonuclear leukocytes and macrophages release various mediator substances, including cytokines such as tumor necrosis factor (TNF) and the interleukins. Further activation of the cyclooxygenase pathway produces various prostaglandins that may cause adverse systemic effects.[102]

Thermoregulation

Hypothalamic alterations also occur, causing changes in thermoregulation. At any ambient temperature, core and skin temperature of injured or septic patients are greater than those in normal individuals.[102] Pharmacologic agents that affect the temperature set-point generally are not effective in reducing the hypermetabolism and hyperpyrexia that occur after injury.

Stress Hormone Increases

In all phases of injury, a marked rise in glucagon, cortisol, growth hormone, ACTH, and the catecholamines occurs. In contrast, plasma levels of insulin are low initially, but once a patient is stabilized, they return to normal or become elevated. Insulin release by the pancreas is inhibited, even in the presence of hyperglycemia, by α-adrenergic stimulation.[102] This inhibition accounts in part for the post-traumatic hyperglycemia that is commonly observed.

Why Does Sudden Unexplained Hypotension Occur?

Common causes of sudden hypotension in postoperative trauma victims are listed in Table 59–18. Immediate resuscitative efforts, rapid evaluation to rule out "mechanical" causes, and immediate notification of the surgical team are crucial for patients who develop sudden, unexplained postoperative hypotension. Hypotension associated with bradycardia indicates severe hypoxemia unless undiagnosed cervical spine injury is present. If hypotension and bradycardia occur as an acute event, loss of the airway, tension pneumothorax, or cardiac tamponade must be quickly ruled out.[103]

TABLE 59–18. Common Causes of Sudden Hypotension in Critically Ill Patients

Loss of airway
Tension pneumothorax
Cardiac tamponade
Hemothorax (massive)
Intra-abdominal hemorrhage
Acute myocardial infarction
Bacteremia and sepsis
Reaction to medication

Tension Pneumothorax

Decreased breath sounds, tracheal deviation, and a sharp rise in peak inspiratory pressure during mechanical ventilation are signs of tension pneumothorax. A chest radiograph should be obtained if time permits. However, if the systolic pressure falls below 70 mm Hg or a patient develops severe bradycardia, aspiration of the chest with a 14- or 16-gauge catheter should be performed. If air is withdrawn, surgical decompression should be performed immediately. A previously placed chest tube does not eliminate the possibility of ipsilateral tension pneumothorax. The tube may be clotted with blood, or the lung may be adherent to the tube openings. The clinical diagnosis of pneumothorax is often difficult to make in the SICU.

Hemothorax

Hemothorax can occur after the initial evaluation and resuscitation, or the rate of intrathoracic bleeding may be so slow that a significant deficit in blood volume does not occur until the patient arrives in the ICU. This problem may be diagnosed and treated in a manner similar to that for pneumothorax. Persistent bleeding may require further surgery.

Cardiac Tamponade

Muffled heart sounds, jugular venous distention, hypotension, increased systolic pressure variation with mechanical ventilation, and equalization of left and right atrial chamber pressures indicate cardiac tamponade. These signs can also occur with tension pneumothorax; if bilateral chest decompression does not result in clinical improvement, pericardiocentesis or pericardiotomy should be performed.

Intra-Abdominal Bleeding

If all extra-abdominal sources have been ruled out, intra-abdominal or retroperitoneal bleeding should be strongly considered in patients with blunt trauma or previous abdominal exploration. The abdomen should be rapidly assessed for any obvious signs such as distention or increased bloody discharge through the incision or from an abdominal drain.

Other catastrophic abdominal problems include ischemic bowel due to embolization or volvulus, missed or subsequent perforation of the alimentary tract, hemorrhagic pancreatitis, and streptococcal or clostridial wound infections. These complications require immediate surgical intervention.[103] Intravascular volume resuscitation is the most important therapy before abdominal re-exploration.

What Is Iatrogenic Post-Traumatic Hypothermia?

Iatrogenic post-traumatic hypothermia is a frequent complication after massive volume resuscitation. Anatomic and metabolic abnormalities inhibit temperature homeostasis. These abnormalities disrupt the skin–CNS–core negative feedback loops for temperature control. Patients becomes passive responders to ambient temperature and to the physics of heat loss.[104] Cellular enzymatic systems begin to fail as core temperature falls. Children and patients with head or spinal cord

TABLE 59–19. Organ System Dysfunction Associated with Hypothermia

Skin	Vasoconstriction (>32.2 °C), vasodilatation (≤32.2 °C)
Kidneys	$\downarrow$ Reabsorption Na$^+$ and H$_2$O (cold diuresis)
Mental status	Confusion, $\downarrow$ reflexes (<31.7 °C), coma (<26.7 °C)
Respirations	Progressive depression of respiratory center
Gastrointestinal	$\downarrow$ Gastrointestinal motility; stress ulcers, pancreatitis (<26.7 °C)
Lungs	Pulmonary edema (<26.7 °C)
Cardiac	Progressive bradycardia
O$_2$ consumption	Progressive decrease (4%/0.5 °C)
Blood pressure	$\uparrow$ Initially, then progressively $\downarrow$
Cardiac output	$\uparrow$ Initially, then progressively $\downarrow$
Serum electrolytes	Hyponatremia, hyperkalemia, hyperglycemia
Acid-base status	Progressive metabolic acidosis
Coagulation	Impaired coagulation; occasional disseminated intravascular coagulation

(Modified from Fischer RP, Souba WP, Ford EG: Temperature-associated injuries and syndromes. *In* Trauma. 2nd ed. Moore EE, Mattox KL, Feliciano DV (eds). Norwalk, CT, Appleton & Lange, 1991, pp 770–771.)

injury are particularly susceptible to hypothermia, even without associated hypovolemia and massive fluid resuscitation.

Iatrogenic post-traumatic hypothermia can be categorized into three groups: mild (35–32.3 °C; 95–90 °F), moderate (32.2–26.7 °C; 90–80 °F), and severe (<26.7 °C; <80 °F). A summary of the organ system dysfunctions associated with hypothermia is presented in Table 59–19. (See Chapter 49.)

Treatment

Standard Measures

The best treatment is prevention. For patients who are only mildly hypothermic, passive rewarming can be accomplished with warming blankets. Aluminum space blankets trap and reflect body heat back to a patient. Resuscitation areas in the ED and ORs should be kept warm. Patients should receive warm fluid and blood during the initial resuscitation, intraoperatively, and postoperatively.

Crystalloids and blood should be warmed to 37.7 °C to 40 °C (100–104 °F) with fluid- and blood-warming devices. Each liter of room temperature fluid (70 °C) decreases body temperature by approximately 0.2 °C in a 70-kg individual. In the OR, a heating blanket under the patient is helpful, and a heated humidifier should be used.

Core Warming

If moderate to severe hypothermia develops despite these preventive measures, active core warming should be performed. Warm lavage of the thoracic and peritoneal cavities is effective but gives very slow results.[104] Extracorporeal bypass is occasionally needed in situations of severe hypothermia. The most effective, easily managed, and readily available technique of active core warming is by inhalation.[104] Intubation and ventilation with warmed, humidified O$_2$ effectively and rapidly warms the heart and brain. The maximal inspired temperature should be in the 43.3 °C to 50 °C (110–122 °F) range to prevent thermal injury to the respiratory system. In an awake patient, the inspiratory temperature must be reduced to approximately 40 °C (104 °F).[105]

What Are the Origins of Coagulation Disorders?

Transfusion

Transfusion therapy is frequently required in trauma victims. Coagulopathy develops if >100% of a patient's blood volume is replaced with homologous blood.[106] Banked blood develops certain defects during storage. These defects assume greater clinical significance in massive transfusion situations. The major defect in massively transfused patients is dilutional thrombocytopenia. Factors V and VIII also decline rapidly during storage, but nonmechanical bleeding is usually due to thrombocytopenia during the early phase of resuscitation.[106] If more than 10 units of banked blood are required and the patient has active nonsurgical bleeding, a coagulation defect attributable to thrombocytopenia is likely.[106]

Injuries

Head injuries, gunshot wounds, severe blunt trauma, and stab wounds are all associated with coagulopathies.[107] Severe head injury lowers α_2-plasminogen activator inhibitor (α_2-PI) and elevates fibrinopeptides A (FPA) and B-β (FPB-β). Fibrinogen and antithrombin III are also decreased after traumatic injury.[106] Disseminated intravascular coagulation can be caused by primary brain injury as a result of extremely high levels of FPA and FPB-β levels and abnormally low α_2-PI and platelets.[106]

As many as 50% of patients with severe injuries may have signs of abnormal bleeding evidenced by diffuse oozing both at surgery and postoperatively. The most frequently abnormal test is the prothrombin time. Post-traumatic iatrogenic hypothermia further aggravates coagulation abnormalities, because the enzymatic reactions in the clotting cascade all are temperature sensitive.

Treatment involves careful monitoring and replacement with platelets and fresh-frozen plasma. A more detailed discussion of transfusion therapy and hemostasis is given in Chapters 40 and 42.

What Are the Causes of Acute Respiratory Failure?

The spectrum of pathophysiologic abnormalities associated with acute respiratory failure ranges from atelectasis to severe noncardiogenic pulmonary edema. Hypoxemia refractory to increasing levels of O_2 therapy and decreasing pulmonary compliance are common. The latter abnormality, often called ARDS, results from multiple causes that produce direct or indirect damage to the alveolar capillary interface.[103]

Risk Factors

Potential risk factors for developing ARDS specific to trauma victims include sepsis, aspiration of gastric contents, direct injury to the lungs due to pulmonary contusion, fat embolism, acute post-traumatic pancreatitis, and multiple blood transfusions.[103]

Initial Treatment

PEEP is still the most effective therapy for acute respiratory failure and ARDS. The functional residual capacity is increased, and hypoxemia is improved so that nontoxic levels of inspired O_2 may be used.

The goals of ventilatory support are adequate oxygenation at a safe fraction of inspired O_2 (<0.5) and adequate O_2 delivery to the peripheral tissues. Close monitoring in the early post-traumatic period, with interventions to restore pulmonary function, may improve outcome.[103]

What Are the Infectious Complications of Importance?

Fever in a critically injured patient often creates a sense of urgency to find the cause. Critically injured surgical patients who survive their initial injury often die of the complications of sepsis. Virtually 100% of severely injured patients develop fever after severe trauma because of elevated levels of interleukin-1 (previously known as *endogenous pyrogen*). Fever in trauma victims, however, does not equate with infection in all situations. Rational antibiotic therapy is often difficult to administer because of the diagnostic dilemmas involved in managing critically ill patients.

Diagnosis and Treatment

A high fever ($\geq$38.5 °C) in the immediate postsurgical or post-traumatic period mandates careful inspection of all surgical or traumatic wounds. Surgical dressings must be completely removed, and the wound carefully inspected and palpated for signs of infection. Life-threatening infections that cause gas gangrene or necrotizing fasciitis must be identified and rapidly treated.

Severe pain in the incision, erythema rapidly spreading from the edges of the wound, and serosanguineous drainage all are signs of possible early wound infection with group A streptococci or various clostridial organisms. These infections require immediate surgical intervention and antibiotic therapy to prevent death.

Septic Complications

Pneumonia

Pneumonia is one of the most common hospital-acquired infections, occurring in at least 12% to 15% of all patients in an ICU.[108] The presence of a new or significantly different infiltrate on a chest radiograph suggests the possibility of bacterial or fungal pneumonia. Confirmation of this diagnosis is often difficult in the presence of blunt chest trauma or ARDS.

If the sputum Gram's stain reveals a large number of WBCs or a predominant type of organism, appropriate specimens for culture should be obtained. Quantitative cultures using a bronchoscopically introduced, protected specimen brush probably give the most reliable information, along with bronchial washings from the affected areas. At least 10^3 colony-forming units per milliliter are generally considered diagnostic of pneumonia.

Urinary Tract Infections

The urinary tract is a possible source for infection. If a urinalysis reveals a large number of organisms or WBCs, urine cultures should be obtained and appropriate antibiotic therapy administered.

Catheter-Related Infections

Critically ill patients are at higher risk for developing venous and arterial catheter-related infections. If a catheter-related infection is suspected, the catheter should be removed and the intracutaneous 5-cm segment of catheter located just below the skin surface should be sent for semi-quantitative culture. A catheter source is considered positive if at least 15 colonies are present on semi-quantitative culture. The diagnosis is confirmed by the presence of the same organism recovered from peripheral blood cultures.

Meningitis

Meningitis must be considered in any patient who develops an altered mental status associated with high fever. Lumbar puncture with culture of the CSF should be obtained if this diagnosis is considered. Meningitis associated with head or spinal cord injury is an uncommon problem. Patients with basilar skull fractures and CSF leakage are at risk for developing meningitis.

Intra-Abdominal Infection

Intra-abdominal infection must always be considered in patients with previous exploratory laparotomy. A small bowel injury may be overlooked during the initial evaluation and resuscitation. Diagnostic peritoneal lavage can be performed in the SICU in patients who have not had recent abdominal exploration.

Abdominal CT scanning to rule out abscess is also an important adjunct to evaluation but should not be performed within the first week postoperatively. It should only be done if the information obtained will be used to direct therapy.

If the clinical examination and laboratory studies suggest the diagnosis, bedside ultrasonography is safe to diagnose acute acalculous cholecystitis.[103]

Why Does Acute Renal Failure Occur?

The most common cause of acute renal failure after trauma is acute tubular necrosis due to diminished renal blood flow. This complication may develop from systemic hypotension, sepsis, or a combination of both. Predisposing factors include renal hypoperfusion secondary to hypovolemia, sepsis, or inadequate intravascular volume resuscitation after the traumatic event. Other sources include nephrotoxic drugs, myoglobinuria, hemoglobinuria, and pre-existing renal or cardiac disease.[103]

Decreased urine output in the post-traumatic or postoperative period demands immediate evaluation because acute renal failure is a devastating complication with a high associated mortality. An approach to evaluating and treating postoperative oliguria in trauma victims is summarized in Table 59–20.

Incidence

A recent multicenter retrospective study evaluated the incidence of acute renal failure in the trauma population.[109] A total of 72,757 trauma admissions treated at nine regional trauma centers during a 5-year period were reviewed. Only 78 patients (0.098%) developed acute renal failure that required hemodi-

TABLE 59–20. Evaluating and Treating Oliguria in the Trauma Patient

Urine output <0.5 mL · kg^{-1} · h^{-1} for 2 consecutive hours
↓
Irrigate/replace Foley catheter
↓
Consider undiagnosed urologic injury
↓
Give 500-mL rapid bolus of crystalloid
↓
Consider repeating 500-mL fluid bolus
↓
Place pulmonary artery catheter if hypovolemia is no longer likely
↓
Continue fluid administration until PAOP = 15–18 mm Hg
↓
Send 5 mL urine and blood for diagnostic tests
(Do not wait for tests to return)
↓
Infuse dopamine 3 to 5 µg · kg^{-1} · min^{-1}
↓
Mannitol 25 g IV bolus
↓
Furosemide 40 mg IV bolus
↓
Furosemide 200 mg IV bolus
↓
Assume acute renal failure
↓
Consider hemodialysis as indicated

(From Norwood SH, Civetta JM: ICU Management of the trauma patient. *In* Trauma Management. Kreis DJ, Gomez GA (eds). Boston, Little, Brown & Co, 1989, p 444.)

alysis. Twenty-four of these 78 patients (31%) developed acute renal failure <6 days after injury. The remainder developed late renal failure, with a mean time to first dialysis of 23 days. The predominant cause of death in these patients was MSOF (82%).

The investigators concluded that post-traumatic renal failure requiring hemodialysis is rare, but the mortality rate remains very high (57% overall).[108] Two thirds of the cases develop late and are secondary to MSOF. One third of the cases of post-traumatic renal failure develop early and are probably secondary to inadequate volume resuscitation.[109]

What Is the Impact of Multiple System Organ Failure?

Dramatic improvements in the initial resuscitation and management of critically injured patients, together with therapeutic advances in the management of cardiovascular and respiratory problems, have resulted in improved survival from single organ system failure. However, patients with various acute insults and injuries are at risk for developing a syndrome characterized by progressive deterioration in the function of multiple organs.[110] MSOF is now the leading cause of death in the SICU.[111]

Acute respiratory failure is almost always present initially. The onset of other organ systems dysfunction is inconstant, and the magnitude of physiologic derangement is variable. The most common clinical manifestations of MSOF include azotemia, hyperbilirubinemia, ileus, thrombocytopenia, and altered mental status.[111]

Gastrointestinal tract failure, manifested by gastrointestinal hemorrhage, is now less common, although increasing evidence supports the concept that derangements in gut mucosal function contribute to the pathophysiology of MSOF. After severe injury and during prolonged critical illness, the gut mucosal barrier can atrophy or become damaged. Strong evidence suggests that gut perfusion decreases dramatically[112] and mesenteric ischemia is a likely occurrence in most forms of shock. Mucosal atrophy and migration of gram-negative bacteria into the mesenteric lymphatics and the portal system may follow.[110]

The outcome of patients with MSOF is determined by both the number of failed organ systems and the duration of organ system failure.[113] The death rate is approximately 80% when three or more organ systems are dysfunctional for 24 hours and increases to 100% if the organ dysfunction occurs for 4 days or more.[113]

Pathophysiologic Mechanisms

Polymorphonuclear Leukocytes

The presence of untreated infection is the most common cause of MSOF, although a documented infection is not a prerequisite for diagnosing the syndrome. Polymorphonuclear leukocytes and endogenous macrophages are responsible for introducing various molecular substances into the systemic circulation that can cause direct organ injury.

Data from numerous clinical studies implicate polymorphonuclear leukocytes as the primary etiologic factor in acute lung injury. Activated neutrophils release various O_2 metabolites including hydrogen peroxide, hypochloric acid, hydroxyl radicals, and superoxide ions. All of these factors are capable of injuring tissues by damaging DNA and cross-linking cellular proteins, and causing peroxidation of membrane lipids. Increased membrane permeability follows, with disastrous effects on cellular integrity and function.[110]

Cytokines

Cytokines are small proteins secreted by immune cells; they result in a wide variety of biologic actions. The most intensely investigated cytokines are TNF-α, interleukin-1, and interleukin-6. The cytokines have both unique and overlapping biologic activities and appear to represent an inflammatory mediator system, enhancing the injurious effects of neutrophils in addition to their own individual cellular effects. (See Chapter 41.)

Treatment

Reversal of Shock

The most common preceding event of MSOF in trauma victims is prolonged circulatory shock. The best treatment is prevention; rapid resuscitation to achieve normal O_2 delivery to the tissues is of paramount importance.

Infection Control

Sepsis is a common correlate of MSOF. Early identification and treatment of infectious complications are crucial to improve survival. Devitalized tissue appears to be a major risk factor. Careful debridement of necrotic wound tissue is an important preventive measure.

Fracture Stabilization

Early stabilization of major lower extremity fractures is thought to decrease the risk of respiratory failure and ARDS secondary to fat emboli. This practice should be considered standard care in the management of trauma victims.[110]

Miscellaneous Therapy

Thus far, corticosteroids, various prostaglandin inhibitors, immunotherapy, fibronectin, and several other agents have not proved useful in the prevention of or recovery from MSOF.[110]

References

1. Aldrete JA, Marrow GM, Wright AJ: The first administration of anesthesia in military surgery: on occasion of the Mexican-American War. Anesthesiology 1984; 61:585.
2. Blaisdell FW: Medical advances during the Civil War. Arch Surg 1988; 123:1045.
3. National Research Council and Institute of Medicine: Injury in America. Washington, DC, National Academy Press, 1985.
4. Barancik JI, Chatterjee BF, Greene YC, et al: Northeastern Ohio trauma study: I. Magnitude of the problem. Am J Public Health 1983; 73:746.
5. Champion HR, Copes WS, Sacco WJ, et al: The major trauma outcome study: establishing national norms for trauma care. J Trauma 1990; 30:1356.
6. Hammond J, Gomez G, Eckes J: Trauma systems: economic and political considerations. J Fla Med Assoc 1990; 77:603
7. Center for Disease Control: Leads from the MMWR: years of potential life lost before age 65—United States, 1987. JAMA 1989; 261:823.
8. Fischer DP, Miles DL: The demographics of trauma in 1995. J Trauma 1987; 27:1233.
9. Broos PLO, Stappaerts KH, Rommens PM, et al: Polytrauma in patients 65 and over: injury patterns and outcome. Int Surg 1988; 73:119.
10. Finelli FC, Jonsson J, Champion HR, et al: A case control study for major trauma in geriatric patients. J Trauma 1989; 29:541.
11. Baker CC: Epidemiology of trauma: the civilian perspective. Ann Emerg Med 1986; 15:1389.
12. Trunkey DD: Trauma. Sci Am 1983; 249:28.
13. Centers for Disease Control: Leads from the MMWR: differences in death rates among black and whites, 1984. JAMA 1989; 261:214.
14. Committee on Trauma, American College of Surgeons: Resources for Optimal Care of the Injured Patient. Chicago, American College of Surgeons, 1990.
15. Champion HR, Mabee MS: An American Crisis in Trauma Care Reimbursement. The Washington Hospital Center, Washington, DC, 1990.
16. Maryland Institute for Emergency Medical Services Systems: Annual Report. Baltimore, MD, 1988.
17. Uzych L: Trauma care systems. Am J Emerg Med 1990; 8:71.
18. McKenzie EJ: Acute Hospital Costs of Trauma in the United States: Implications for Regionalized Systems of Care. Presented at the American Association for the Surgery of Trauma Annual Meeting. Chicago, IL, October 1989.
19. Shapiro MJ, Keegan M, Copeland J: The misconception of trauma reimbursement. Arch Surg 1989; 124:1237.
20. Lee G: Trauma center "de-designation": a Los Angeles County update. J Emerg Nurs 1989; 15:20A.
21. Kim H: Trauma networks look for rescue. Mod Healthcare 1990; 20:33.
22. Gormican SP: CRAMS scale: field triage of trauma patients. Ann Emerg Med 1982; 11:29.
23. Tepas JJ, Mollitt DL, Talbert JL: The pediatric trauma score as a predictor of injury severity in the injured child. J Pediatr Surg 1987; 22:14.
24. Baker SP, O'Neill B, Haddon W, et al: The injury severity score: a method for describing patients with multiple injuries and evaluation of emergency care. J Trauma 1974; 14:187.
25. Boyd CR, Tolson MA, Copes WS: Evaluating trauma care: the TRISS method. J Trauma 1987; 27:370.
26. Copes WS, Champion HR, Sacco WJ, et al: Progress in characterizing anatomic injury. J Trauma 1990; 30:1200.
27. Grande CM, Stene JK, Bernhard WN, et al: Trauma anesthesia and critical care: the concept and rationale for a new subspecialty. Crit Care Clin 1990; 6:1.

28. DeMello W, Griffiths C: Anesthetists and trauma. Anesthesia 1991; 46:151.

29. Illinois Department of Public Health: Illinois Trauma Nurse Specialist Program Curricula, 1971–Present.

30. Rea R: Trauma Nursing Core Course Provider Manual. Chicago, Award Printing, 1986.

31. Gomez, MJ, Ferraro CA, Charlson DA, et al: The cost effectiveness of a two-tier trauma response (Abstract). J Trauma 1991; 31:1716.

32. Songne, EA: Trauma triage by mechanism of injury: a 30 month study. Presented at the California Trauma Conference, San Diego, CA, February 13, 1991.

33. Alexander RH: Treatment of the trauma patient: an overview. *In* Trauma Management. Kreis DJ, Gomez, GA (eds). Boston, Little, Brown & Co, 1989, pp 67–99.

34. Fischer RP, Perry JF Jr: Direct transfer to the operating room improves care of trauma patients: a simple economically feasible plan for large hospitals. JAMA 1978; 240:1731.

35. Maier RV: Evaluation and resuscitation. *In* Early Care of the Injured Patient. 4th ed. Moore E, Decker TB, Edlich RF, et al (eds). Philadelphia, BC Decker, 1990, pp 56–73.

36. Rhodes M, Gillett AR: Operating room resuscitation of the severely injured patient: direct transport to the operating room. *In* Advances in Trauma. Vol. 2. Maull K, Cleveland HC, Strauch GO, et al (eds). Chicago, Year Book Medical Publishers, 1987, pp 87–104.

37. Law DK, Lee JK, Brennan R, et al: Trauma operating room in conjunction with an air ambulance system: indications, interventions and outcomes. J Trauma 1982; 22:759.

38. Kim DH: Establishment of a voluntary trauma network: lessons learned. Emerg Care Q 1990; 6:1.

39. Harris BH, Latchaw LA, Murphy RE, et al: A protocol for pediatric receiving units. J Pediatr Surg 1989; 24:419.

40. Committee on Trauma, American College of Surgeons: Advanced Trauma Life Support Course Manual. Chicago, American College of Surgeons, 1989.

41. Collicott PE: Initial assessment of the trauma patient. *In* Trauma. 2nd ed. Moore EE, Mattox KL, Feliciano DV (eds). Norwalk, CT, Appleton & Lange, 1991, pp 109–125.

42. Stewart RD: Prehospital care of trauma. *In* Management of Blunt Trauma. McMurty RY, McLellan BA (eds). Baltimore, Williams & Wilkins, 1990, p 28.

43. Norwood SH, Myers MB, Butler J: The safety of emergency neuromuscular blockade and orotracheal intubation in the acutely injured trauma patient.

44. Rhodes M, Brader AH: Organization of a trauma resuscitation system. *In* Advances in Trauma. Vol. 4. Maull KI, Cleveland HC, Strauch GO, Wolferth CC (eds). Chicago, Year Book Medical Publishers, 1989, p 20.

45. Aprahamian C, Thompson BM, Finger WA, et al: Experimental cervical spine injury model: evaluation of airway management and splinting techniques. Ann Emerg Med 1984; 13:584.

46. Hauswald M, Sklar DP, Tandberg D, et al: Cervical spine movement during airway management: cinefluoroscopic appraisal in human cadavers. Am J Emerg Med 1991; 9:535.

47. Bivens HG, Ford S, Bezmalinovic Z, et al: The effect of axial traction during orotracheal intubation of the trauma victim with an unstable cervical spine. Ann Emerg Med 1988; 17:25.

48. Syverud SA, Borron SW, Storer DL, et al: Prehospital use of neuromuscular blocking agents in a helicopter ambulance program. Ann Emerg Med 1988; 236:99.

49. Roberts DJ, Clinton JE, Ruiz E: Neuromuscular blockade for critical patients in the emergency department. Ann Emerg Med 1986; 152:81.

50. Talucci RC, Shaikl KA, Schwab CW: Rapid sequence induction with oral endotracheal intubation in the multiply injured patient. Am Surg 1988; 54:185.

51. Ligier B, Buchman TG, Breslow MJ: The role of anesthetic induction agents and neuromuscular blockade in the endotracheal intubation of trauma victims. Surg Gynecol Obstet 1991; 173:477.

52. Stene JK, Grande CM, Barton CR: Airway management for the trauma patient. *In* Trauma Anesthesia. Stene JK, Grande CM (eds). Baltimore, Williams & Wilkins, 1991, pp 64–99.

53. Seebacher J, Nozik D, Mathieu A: Inadvertent intracranial introduction of a nasogastric tube, a complication of severe maxillofacial trauma. Anesthesiology 1975; 42:100.

54. Dinner M, Tjeuw M, Artusio JF: Bacteremia as a complication of nasotracheal intubation. Anesth Analg 1987; 66:460.

55. Bos AP, Tibboel D, Hazebroek FWJ, et al: Sinusitis: hidden source of sepsis in postoperative pediatric intensive care patients. Crit Care Med 1989; 17:886.

56. Dauphinee K: Nasotracheal intubation. Emerg Med Clin North Am 1988; 6:715.

57. Little CM, Parker MG, Tarnopolsky R: The incidence of vasculature at risk during cricothyroidostomy. Ann Emerg Med 1986; 15:805.

58. Symbas PN: Cardiothoracic Trauma. Philadelphia, WB Saunders, 1989, p 373.

59. Duff JH, Goldstein M, McLean APH, et al: Flail chest: a clinical review and physiological study. J Trauma 1968; 8:63.

60. Mattox KL, Bickell W, Pepe PE, et al: Prospective MAST study in 911 patients. J Trauma 1989; 29:1104.

61. Aprahamian C, Gessert G, Bandy KD, et al: MAST-associated compartment syndrome (MACS): a review. J Trauma 1989; 29:549.

62. Symbas PN: Cardiothoracic Trauma. Philadelphia, WB Saunders, 1989, p 63.

63. Mattox KL, Feliciano DV: Role of external cardiac compression in truncal trauma. J Trauma 1982; 22:934.

64. Mattox KL: Injury to the thoracic great vessels. *In* Trauma. 2nd ed. Moore EE, Mattox KL, Feliciano DV (eds). Norwalk, CT, Appleton & Lange, 1991, pp 393–408.

65. Reyes LH, Rubio PA, Korampai FL, et al: Successful treatment of transection of aortic arch and innominate artery. Ann Thorac Surg 1975; 19:468.

66. Thal ER: Evaluation of peritoneal lavage and local wound exploration in lower chest and abdominal stab wounds. J Trauma 1977; 17:642.

67. Federle MP, Crass RA, Jeffrey RB, et al: Computed tomography in blunt abdominal trauma. Arch Surg 1982; 117:645.

68. Goldstein AS, Sclafani SJA, Kupferstein NH, et al: The diagnostic superiority of computerized tomography. J Trauma 1985; 25:938.

69. Henneman PL, Marx JA, Moore EE, et al: Diagnostic peritoneal lavage: accuracy in predicting necessary laparotomy following blunt and penetrating trauma. J Trauma 1990; 30:1345.

70. Matsubara TK, Fong HMT, Burns CM: Computed tomography of abdomen (CTA) in management of blunt abdominal trauma. J Trauma 1990; 30:410.

71. Asbun HJ, Irani H, Roe EJ, et al: Intra-abdominal seat belt injury. J Trauma 1990; 30:189.

72. Anderson PA, Rivara FP, Maier RV, et al: The epidemiology of seat belt-associated injuries. J Trauma 1991; 31:60.

73. Newman KD, Bowman LM, Eichelberger MR, et al: The lap belt complex: intestinal and lumbar spine injuries in children. J Trauma 1990; 30:1133.

74. Rosenthal RE: lower extremity fractures and dislocations. *In* Trauma. 2nd ed. Moore EE, Mattox KL, Feliciano DV (eds). Norwalk, CT, Appleton & Lange, 1991, pp 623–638.

75. Tomkins GS, Hiatt JR: Compartment syndrome and fasciotomy. *In* Vascular Injuries in Surgical Practice. Bongard FS, Wilson SE, Perry MO (eds). Norwalk, CT, Appleton & Lange 1991, p 236.

76. Norwood SH, Dellinger RP: Managing substance abuse in the trauma patient. Probl Crit Care 1987; 1:115.

77. Gettler DT, Allbritten FF: Effect of alcohol intoxication on the respiratory exchange and mortality rate associated with acute hemorrhage in anesthetized dogs. Ann Surg 1963; 158:151.

78. Malt SH, Baue AE: The effects of ethanol as related to trauma in the awake dog. J Trauma 1971; 11:76.

79. Swan KG, Vidaver RM, Lavigne JE, et al: Acute alcoholism, minor trauma, and ''shock.'' J Trauma 1977; 17:215.

80. Lucas CE, Joseph AL, Ledgerwood AM: Alcohol and drugs. *In* Trauma. 2nd ed. Moore EE, Mattox KL, Feliciano DV (eds). Norwalk, CT, Appleton & Lange, 1991, pp 677–687.

81. Straus DJ: Hematologic aspects of alcoholism. Semin Hematol 1973; 10:183.

82. Majernick TG, Bieniek R, Houston JB, et al: Cervical spine movement during orotracheal intubation. Ann Emerg Med 1986; 15:417.

83. Bracken MB, Shepard MJ, Collins WF, et al: A randomized, controlled trial of methylprednisolone or naloxone in the treatment of acute spinal cord injury. N Engl J Med 1990; 322:1405.

84. Harrison AW, Whelan P: Retroperitoneal injuries. *In* Management of Blunt Trauma. McMurty RY, McLellan BA (eds). Baltimore, Williams & Wilkins, 1990, pp 272–275.

85. Miller JD, Sweet RC, Narayan R, et al: Early insults to the injured brain. Arch Surg 1978; 240:439.

86. Redan JH, Livingston DH, Tortella BJ, et al: The value of intubating and paralyzing patients with suspected head injury in the emergency department. J Trauma 1991; 31:371.

87. Ochsner MG, Cole F, Rozycki G, et al: The incidence of serious intracranial pathology in patients with low suspicion for significant head injury. Presented at the Fourth Scientific Symposium, Eastern Association for the Surgery of Trauma, January 16, 1991.

88. Livingston DH, Loder PA, Hunt CD. Minimal head injury: is admission necessary? Am Surg 1991; 57:14.

89. Mikhail MG, Levitt A, Christopher TA, et al: Intracranial injury following minor head trauma. Am J Emerg Med 1992; 10:24.

90. Feustal PJ, Fortune JB, Stratton H, et al: Oxygen delivery and consumption in head injured and multiple trauma patients. J Trauma 1990; 30:1259.

91. Wilberger JE, Harris M, Diamond DL: Acute subdural hematoma: morbidity and mortality related to timing of operative intervention. J Trauma 1990; 30:733.

92. Rosner MJ, Daughton S: Cerebral perfusion pressure management in head injury. J Trauma 1990; 30:933.

93. Hirschman JV. Meningitis following neurosurgery and blunt head trauma. Infections in Surgery 1990; 9:13.

94. Esposito TJ, Gens DR, Smith LG, et al: Trauma in pregnancy: a review of 79 cases. Arch Surg 1991; 126:1073.

95. Kissinger DP, Rozycki GS, Morris JA, et al: Trauma in pregnancy: predicting pregnancy outcome. Arch Surg 1991; 126:1079.

96. Jaffe D, Wesson D: Emergency management of blunt trauma in children. N Engl J Med 1991; 324:1477.

97. Pokorny WJ, Haller JA: Pediatric trauma. *In* Trauma. 2nd ed. Moore EE, Mattox KL, Feliciano DV (eds). Norwalk, CT, Appleton & Lange, 1991, pp 689–702.

98. Manley L, Haley K, Dick M: Intraosseous infusion: rapid vascular access for critically ill or injured infants and children. J Emerg Nurs 1988; 14:63.

99. Hodge D: Intraosseous infusions: a review. Pediatr Emerg Care 1985; 1:215.

100. Trunkey D: Initial treatment of patients with extensive trauma. N Engl J Med 1991; 324:1259.

101. Townsend RN, Colella JJ, Diamond DL: Traumatic rupture of the aorta: critical decisions for trauma surgeons. J Trauma 1990; 30:1169.

102. Wilmore DW: Homeostasis: bodily changes in trauma and surgery. *In* Textbook of Surgery. 14th ed. Sabiston DC (ed). Philadelphia, WB Saunders, 1991, pp 19–33.

103. Norwood SH, Civetta JM: ICU management of the trauma patient. *In* Trauma Management. Kreis DJ, Gomez GA (eds). Boston, Little, Brown & Co, 1989, pp 431–451.

104. Fischer RP, Souba WW, Ford EG: Temperature-associated injuries and syndromes. *In* Trauma. 2nd ed. Moore EE, Mattox KL, Feliciano DV (eds). Norwalk, CT, Appleton & Lange, 1991, pp 765–776.

105. Best R, Syverud S, Nowak RM: Trauma and hypothermia. Am J Emerg Med 1985; 3:48.

106. Rutledge R, Sheldon GF: Bleeding and coagulation problems in trauma. *In* Trauma. 2nd ed. Moore EE, Mattox KL, Feliciano DV (eds). Norwalk, CT, Appleton & Lange, 1991, pp 891–908.

107. Ordog GJ: Coagulation abnormalities in traumatic shock. Ann Emerg Med 1985; 14:650.

108. Tobin MJ, Grenvik A: Nosocomial lung infection and its diagnosis. Crit Care Med 1984; 12:191.

109. Morris JA, Mucha P, Ross SE, et al: Acute post-traumatic renal failure: a multicenter perspective. J Trauma 1991; 31:1584.

110. Heard SO, Fink MP: The multiple organ failure syndrome. *In* Intensive Care Medicine. 2nd ed. Rippe JM, Irwin RS, Alpert JS, Fink MP (eds). Boston, Little, Brown & Company 1991, pp 1515–1532.

111. Barton R, Cerra FB: The hypermetabolism multiple organ failure syndrome. Chest 1989; 96:1153.

112. Fink MP, Cohn SM, Lee PC, et al: Effect of lipopolysaccharide on intestinal intramucosal hydrogen ion concentration in pigs: evidence of gut ischemia in a normodynamic model of septic shock. Crit Care Med 1989; 17:641.

113. Knaus WA, Draper EA, Wagner DP, et al: Prognosis in acute organ system failure. Ann Surg 1985; 202:685.

CHAPTER 60

The Neonate

TIMOTHY W. MARTIN, M.D.*

The special considerations and unique features of pediatric anesthesia, discussed in Chapter 61, are most evident and affect anesthetic care most significantly in neonates; for this reason, a separate chapter is dedicated to neonatal anesthesia. The differences between anesthesia for neonates and adults may be viewed from several perspectives, as outlined in Table 60–1. The principal areas of contrast identified here serve as the basis for discussion of the clinical questions in neonatal anesthesia contained in this chapter.

PAIN AND ITS PERCEPTION

Do Neonates Require Anesthesia?

Only within the past decade has a significant volume of research addressed the issue of neonatal anesthetic requirements and the consequences of withholding appropriate anesthesia from surgical patients. Within the same period, we have come to terms with the realization that a great number of neonates born in the era of ''modern'' anesthesia have been and continue to be undermedicated; a double standard has existed in our approach to providing anesthesia and analgesia for newborns and adults.

To illustrate this point, in a 1970 discussion of anesthesia for premature neonates, the statement was made that ''Most of these babies do not need halothane. All they need is a little ventilatory support. They do not need much agent at all. A little bit of adhesive tape holds them down.''[1] A study in the United Kingdom demonstrated that even among anesthesiologists who spend more than half their time anesthetizing pediatric patients, only 80% believed that newborns younger than 1 week are able to perceive pain.[2] Eighty per cent of the respondents never or rarely prescribed opioid analgesia to neonates after major surgery, and nearly 70% never or rarely provided regional or local anesthesia for these patients.

How Is Pain Perceived by Neonates?

Because pain is generally defined as a subjective phenomenon, strongly influenced by previous emotional and painful

experiences, it is difficult to evaluate in neonates. For this reason, the suggestion has been made that nociceptive activity, or the perception of tissue damage, is more appropriately studied in neonates than is the phenomenon of pain.[3] Historically, reasons why neonates and sick infants have been provided little or no anesthesia have included poorly understood neonatal requirements for anesthesia, inadequate monitoring equipment, and fear of inducing cardiovascular instability with what previously had been a limited selection of anesthetic agents.[4]

Neural Development

Investigations in recent years have demonstrated that neonates possess the anatomic, functional, and neurochemical systems necessary for pain perception.[3] The neural pathways that transmit impulses from painful stimuli can be traced from sensory receptors in the skin to the cerebral cortex of newborn infants. A lack of complete myelination of the nervous system at birth has frequently served as an argument that neonates are not capable of pain perception, although even in adults nociceptive impulses are often transmitted by unmyelinated nerve fibers. The electroencephalographic (EEG) patterns of premature and term newborns allow distinction between wakefulness and sleep and demonstrate changes in response to tactile stimuli, indicating functional integrity of a neonate's nervous system. Additionally, neurochemical systems including the tachykinins and endogenous opioids (enkephalins and endorphins) are demonstrable in fetuses and neonates. The gestational timetable for maturation of pain pathways in a human fetus and neonate is illustrated in Figure 60–1.

What Are the Responses to Pain?

Physiologic and metabolic responses to pain and surgical stress similar to those observed in children and adults have been documented in neonates.[5] Parameters including heart rate, blood pressure, and respiratory rate and metabolic indicators such as serum glucose and lactic acid levels increase in the presence of pain or inadequate analgesia. Also apparently invalid is the argument that even if a neonate is able to perceive pain, he or she is unable to remember it and thus the anesthesia provided for adults is unnecessary for neonates. The anatomic

*The opinions expressed are those of the author and do not necessarily reflect the views of the United States Air Force or the Department of Defense.

TABLE 60–1. Contrasting Areas of Neonatal and Adult Anesthesia

Anesthetic requirements	
Anatomic and physiologic features	Airway and respiratory system
	Cardiovascular system
	Kidney and body fluid distribution
	Thermoregulation
Pre-existing or chronic medical problems	Infant respiratory distress syndrome
	Persistent pulmonary hypertension
	Intraventricular hemorrhage
	Anemia
	Retinopathy of prematurity
Preanesthetic preparation	Fasting requirements
	Premedication
	Equipment and operating room setup
Intraoperative management	Airway and ventilation
	Vascular access
	Fluid management
	Monitoring
Surgical disorders and procedures	Pyloric stenosis
	Tracheoesophageal fistula
	Gastroschisis and omphalocele
	Necrotizing enterocolitis
	Diaphragmatic hernia
	Patent ductus arteriosus
Postoperative problems	Apnea/bradycardia
	Pain
Neonatal resuscitation	

and functional requirements for long-term memory (principally the limbic system and diencephalon) are present in neonates; although painful experiences may not be subject to conscious recall, such events probably affect later development and behavior.[3]

THE RESPIRATORY SYSTEM

A number of a neonate's airway and respiratory system features have clinical implications. For purposes of discussion, these can be divided into the conductive airway, from

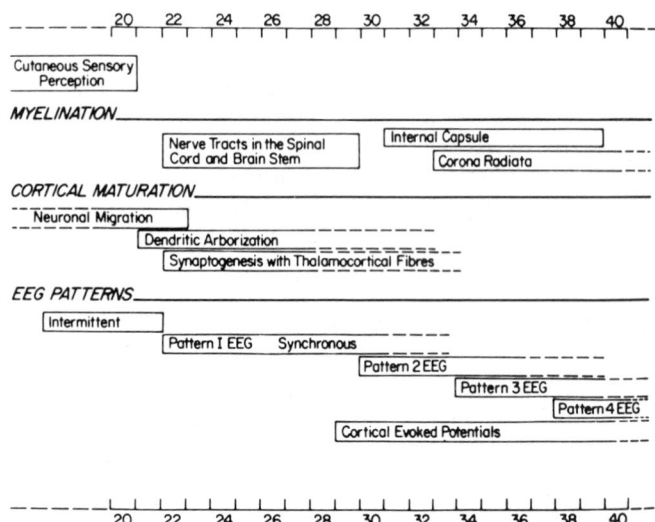

FIGURE 60–1. Schematic diagram of the development of structures and functions necessary for pain perception from weeks 20 to 40 of gestation. (Reprinted from Anand KJS, Hickey PR: Pain and its effects in the human neonate and fetus. N Engl J Med 1987; 317:1322, by permission of the New England Journal of Medicine.)

Significant Airway and Respiratory Differences of the Neonate

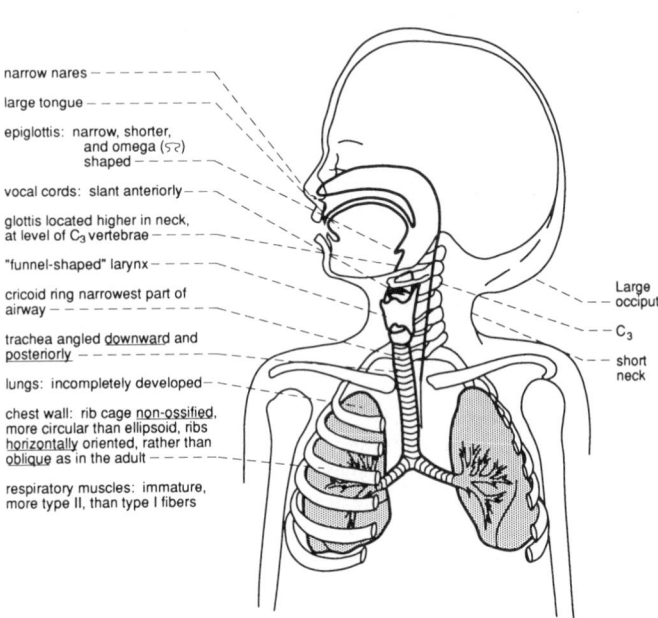

FIGURE 60–2. Diagram depicting the significant features of the neonatal airway and respiratory system that differ from those in adults.

the nares to the trachea, and the lower respiratory tract, including not only the lungs but also the chest wall and diaphragm (Fig. 60–2).

What Should Be Known About the Airway?

Nasopharynx

The nares are relatively narrow and, together with the nasal passages, account for nearly two thirds of the total airway resistance.[6] When not crying, neonates are obligate nose breathers. The relationship of the epiglottis to the soft palate allows infants to isolate the breathing and feeding channels effectively and to perform both processes simultaneously. Any anatomic abnormality, disease process, or artificial medical appliance (e.g., nasogastric tube) may significantly increase airway resistance and the work of breathing in spontaneously ventilating newborns.

Tongue and Epiglottis

The tongue is relatively large compared with the oral cavity and may predispose to airway obstruction and increase the difficulty of laryngoscopy during intubation. Because the epiglottis is integral to simultaneous breathing and swallowing, it is narrower, shorter, and somewhat omega shaped, and it has a tendency to protrude more into the hypopharynx.

Larynx

The larynx is located higher in the neck, as demonstrated by the position of the glottis at the level of the third cervical vertebra.[7] In adults, the glottis is at the level of C-5. The more cephalad location of the neonatal glottis creates the *impression* that the larynx is anterior during laryngoscopy, thus occasionally making laryngeal exposure and intubation more difficult. The neonatal cricoid ring is underdeveloped, imparting a funnel shape to the larynx and making this the narrowest segment of the upper airway.

This feature assumes significance in the selection of endotracheal tubes and the development of laryngeal and tracheal edema due to any of various causes. The fit of an endotracheal tube at the cricoid cartilage must not be so tight that it induces mucosal ischemia; otherwise, the short-term problem of increased resistance to airflow and the long-term problem of tracheal stenosis may result. In practice, intubating with an uncuffed endotracheal tube of a size that allows a small air leak at an inflation pressure of 20 to 30 cm H_2O appears to prevent this complication.

Trachea

A neonate's trachea is angled downward and posteriorly, unlike the straight downward projection in an adult.

Neck and Occiput

Although not parts of the airway, the occiput and neck of a newborn have features that affect airway management. The large occiput causes the head to be flexed anteriorly, sometimes making effective bag-valve-mask ventilation and laryngoscopy difficult; this problem is compounded if the head is elevated on folded towels or a headrest, as is frequently done before elective intubation in adults. Optimum positioning of the head, neck, and shoulders is achieved by placing a small rolled towel in a transverse position at the level of the shoulders.

What Should Be Known About the Lungs?

The lungs are incompletely developed at birth and do not attain their full complement of alveoli until approximately age 8 years.[8] The alveoli are composed of two types of pneumocytes: predominant type I cells, which provide the structure of the alveolus, and type II cells, which produce surfactant as early as the 24th week of gestation. Surfactant is a mixture of phospholipids and proteins; it reduces surface tension within the alveoli, preventing alveolar collapse as lung volumes are reduced during expiration.

On a weight basis, tidal volume, dead space, the ratio of dead space to tidal volume, and functional residual capacity (FRC) are nearly the same as in adults. Because of a neonate's elevated metabolic rate and an oxygen (O_2) consumption, which is two to three times an adult's rate of 3 mL · kg^{-1} · min^{-1}, alveolar ventilation also is two to three times an adult's volume.

The ratio of alveolar ventilation to FRC approaches 5:1 in neonates, compared with a ratio of approximately 1.4:1 in adults.[9] This significant difference explains the rapidity of oxyhemoglobin desaturation and hypoxemia after apnea and the increased rate of inhalation anesthetic uptake. Atelectasis and gas trapping can occur because closing volume, the lung volume at which terminal airway closure begins, is higher in infants. Even within the excursion of normal tidal volumes, some airway closure occurs, primarily as a result of underdevelopment of tissues that contribute to the elastic recoil of the lungs.[10]

What Should Be Known About the Chest Wall and Respiratory Muscles?

The chest wall and muscles of respiration must also mature. The nonossified rib cage is more circular than ellipsoid and is very compliant. The individual ribs are more horizontally oriented than oblique as in adults; hence, the accessory muscles of respiration have a shorter course and generate a less forceful contraction.[11] These features make a newborn essentially a diaphragmatic breather. The respiratory muscles are also different. In neonates, they are composed of a lower percentage of slow-twitch, high-oxidative muscle fibers (type I), which are capable of sustained activity; newborn infants are therefore predisposed to respiratory muscle fatigue.[12]

THE CARDIOVASCULAR SYSTEM

What Should Be Known About the Fetal Circulation?

A discussion of the neonatal cardiovascular system begins with an assessment of the fetal circulation (Fig. 60–3). The circulatory system must complete several adaptations to convert from the *parallel* pulmonary and systemic circuits of a fetus to the *series* components of an infant and adult.

The Ductus Venosus

In utero, unsaturated blood in the descending aorta is carried to the placenta via two umbilical arteries to pick up O_2. It then returns to the body via the umbilical vein. There, most blood enters the ductus venosus, then the inferior vena cava (IVC), effectively bypassing the liver.

The Foramen Ovale

Poorly oxygenated blood from the body and oxygenated blood from the placenta and IVC are *partially* mixed within the right atrium. It then may pass into the right ventricle or through the foramen ovale into the left atrium, bypassing the pulmonary circulation. Most of the oxygenated blood from the placenta and IVC is shunted through the foramen ovale, to the left atrium and ventricle, then into the ascending aorta, where it is primarily directed to the major arteries of the head and upper extremities.[13] Poorly oxygenated blood from the superior vena cava primarily enters the right ventricle and pulmonary artery.

The Ductus Arteriosus

Another anatomic shunt, the ductus arteriosus, serves to allow most of the blood in the pulmonary artery to bypass the lungs (and the high-resistance pulmonary vascular circuit) to enter the aorta. The flow dynamics are such that most of this blood courses into the descending aorta to the arteries of the abdomen and lower extremities or the umbilical arteries and placenta.

What Changes Occur at Birth?

At birth, the lungs are inflated with the onset of ventilation and intra-alveolar fluid is expelled, resulting in an elevation in

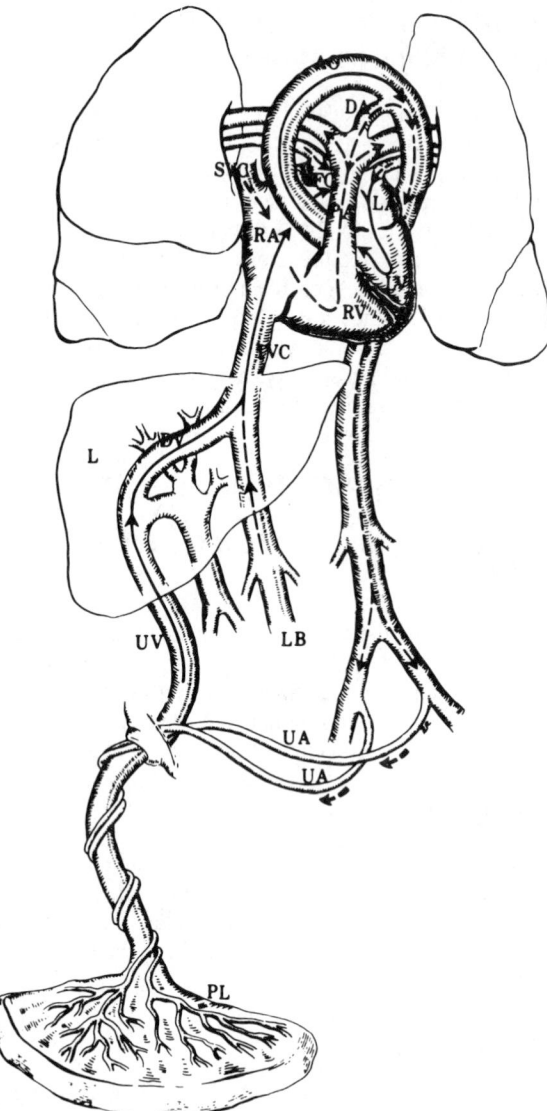

FIGURE 60–3. The fetal circulation. The *solid line with arrows* indicates the pathway that oxygenated blood follows from the placenta to the fetal heart. PL = Placenta; UV = umbilical vein; DV = ductus venosus; LB = lower body; IVC = inferior vena cava; SVC = superior vena cava; RA = right atrium; FO = foramen ovale; RV = right ventricle; PA = pulmonary artery; DA = ductus arteriosus; LA = left atrium; LV = left ventricle; AO = aorta; UA = umbilical artery; L = liver. (From Rimar S, Urban MK: Newborn physiology and development. *In* The Pediatric Anesthesia Handbook. Bell C, Hughes CW, Oh TH (eds). St Louis, CV Mosby, 1991, pp 1–17.)

How Does the Neonatal Heart Differ?

Several features of the neonatal heart and its innervation are unlike those of older children and adults.

Structure

The fetal and neonatal myocardium has a lower percentage of contractile mass than mature myocardium. Neonatal myocytes have a greater density of nuclei, mitochondria, and endosplasmic reticulum, which support cell growth but do not contribute to mechanical work. These noncontractile elements are gradually replaced with increasingly organized myofibrils in the first several months of extrauterine life as the left ventricle grows to meet the demands of the systemic circulation and becomes the dominant ventricular chamber.

Innervation

The parasympathetic innervation of the heart is well established at birth, but the sympathetic nervous supply is incomplete. The clinical implications of these observations are that a neonate's heart is less compliant and possesses a very limited ability to alter myocardial contractility; hence, stroke volume is relatively fixed.[15] For this reason, maintenance of cardiac output primarily depends on sustaining a normal heart rate, which, coupled with the cited predominance of parasympathetic vagal activity in neonates, explains the abrupt onset of hypotension and poor systemic perfusion observed in response to hypoxemia or noxious stimulation.

Heart Rate and Rhythm

The heart rate and cardiac index are considerably higher than in adults to compensate for the elevated O_2 consumption, metabolic rate, and limited myocardial contractility of the newborn. Despite the elevated neonatal heart rate and cardiac index, blood pressures of neonates are significantly lower than those of older patients, reflecting reduced SVR.[16] Table 60–2 indicates normally expected vital signs in neonates.

THE KIDNEYS

How Do They Differ?

The neonatal kidneys, like the heart and lungs, are functionally immature at birth and must continue to develop through-

arterial partial pressure of O_2 (PaO_2) and reduction in pulmonary vascular resistance (PVR). Simultaneously, the umbilical cord is clamped and the placenta is separated from the neonatal body and circulation. Systemic vascular resistance (SVR) immediately increases. The effect of these profound hemodynamic changes and oxygenation is to promote *functional* closure of the fetal shunts; permanent anatomic closure of the ductus arteriosus and foramen ovale may take several weeks, and in a small number of individuals it never occurs. Probe patency of the foramen ovale in older children and adults has been estimated to be as high as 34%.[14]

TABLE 60–2. Normal Neonatal Vital Signs*

Measurement	Premature	Term
Heart rate	150 ± 20	133 ± 18
Mean systolic blood pressure	50 ± 3	73 ± 8
Mean diastolic blood pressure	30 ± 3	50 ± 8
Respiratory rate	45	35

(Data derived from Goudsouzian NG: Anatomy and physiology in relation to pediatric anesthesia. *In* Anesthesia and Uncommon Pediatric Diseases. Katz J, Steward DJ (eds). Philadelphia, WB Saunders, 1987, pp 1–11, *and* Goldsmith JP, Karotkin EH (eds): Appendices 7 and 9. *In* Assisted Ventilation of the Neonate. 2nd ed. Philadelphia, WB Saunders, 1988, pp 435–436.)
*Significant variations may exist among and within individual neonates in the first hours and days of life.

out the first year of life to obtain adult levels of efficiency. Significant differences are noted in neonatal renal blood flow, glomerular filtration rate (GFR), and tubular function, as reflected in urine concentrating ability. During gestation, the fetal kidneys receive 3% to 7% of the cardiac output. This amount provides growth and developmental needs and the formation of a small amount of urine, which in turn becomes an important constituent of the amniotic fluid.

In contrast, mature kidneys receive approximately 20% of the cardiac output, a level not achieved until age 2 years. Renal blood flow increases rapidly in the first weeks of life as a result of mechanisms analogous to those in the pulmonary circulation at birth: increased cardiac output and mean arterial pressure and reduced renal vascular resistance.[17]

Glomerular Development

The adult number of nephrons, and hence glomeruli, is achieved by the 34th week of gestation. For this reason, a neonate's observed GFR of 30% of the healthy adult value is due to reduced glomerular surface area, ultrafiltration pressure, and glomerular capillary permeability.[18] Adult rates of GFR are reached at approximately 1 year of age.

Renal Tubular Development

The renal tubules, consisting of the proximal and distal convoluted tubules, loops of Henle, and collecting ducts, likewise demonstrates immature function at birth; premature infants at 30 weeks' gestational age can concentrate urine to an osmolarity only slightly greater than that of plasma. By 1 month of age, urine with a maximal osmolarity of 550 to 700 mOsm $\cdot$ L^{-1} may be produced. The clinical significance of this limitation is that neonates are more susceptible to dehydration when nonrenal water losses are increased.

Although a neonate's kidneys are widely reported to be obligate sodium losers, this "defect" seems to be present only in prematures; healthy term infants not subjected to stresses such as hypoxia, hyperbilirubinemia, or intrinsic renal disease are capable of maintaining a positive sodium balance. They may, however, experience difficulty excreting an excessive sodium load.[17] The normally expected levels of serum electrolytes, blood urea nitrogen, and creatinine are listed in Table 60–3.

HEAT LOSS

Why Does It Occur?

The problems of maintaining normal body temperature and avoiding hypothermia are pervasive in the care of all neonates, particularly in the operating room and during transport. Although neonates possess central regulatory mechanisms that respond to body and environmental temperature fluctuations, a number of factors predispose to hypothermia. These include an increased ratio of body surface area to mass, increased minute ventilation, poor body insulation, and a limited ability to shiver and generate heat.

Heat loss occurs through four mechanisms: radiation, evaporation of water within the respiratory tract or from the skin surface, conduction, and convection. Failure to maintain reasonably normal body temperature often results in depression of organ system function, hypoperfusion acidosis, apnea, and interference with normal metabolic processes. Recommendations for preventing hypothermia are listed in Table 60–4.

What Is Nonshivering Thermogenesis?

The phenomenon of nonshivering thermogenesis is a neonate's primary means of counteracting body heat loss.[19] This mechanism begins with the liberation of catecholamines (norepinephrine) as skin and mucosal temperatures decline. Norepinephrine induces the metabolism of fatty acids within a newborn's brown fat tissues, with resultant heat production.

PRE-EXISTING MEDICAL PROBLEMS

Critically ill neonates often have pre-existing medical problems that may be related to the indication for surgery. To the extent that these processes may affect intraoperative management or, conversely, that anesthetic maneuvers may influence the course of disease, the anesthesiologist must have an understanding of neonatal problems, including persistent pulmonary hypertension, infant respiratory distress syndrome (IRDS), intraventricular hemorrhage, and anemia.

TABLE 60–3. Normal Neonatal Laboratory Values*

	Determination	Premature	Term
Arterial blood gases	pH	7.35–7.46	7.35–7.45
	Po$_2$ (mm Hg)	45–75	50–80
	Pco$_2$ (mm Hg)	27–45	30–40
Blood chemistry	Sodium (mEq $\cdot$ L^{-1})	135–145	140–150
	Potassium (mEq $\cdot$ L^{-1})	4.5–6.5	4.5–6.5
	Chloride (mEq $\cdot$ L^{-1})	100–110	96–108
	Glucose (mg $\cdot$ dL^{-1})	7–10	7–11
	Blood urea nitrogen (mg $\cdot$ dL^{-1})	30–80	40–100
	Creatinine (mg $\cdot$ dL^{-1})	5–20	5–20
		0.5–1.5	0.3–1.2
Hematology	Hemoglobin (g $\cdot$ dL^{-1})	15–18	16–20
	Hematocrit (%)	45–55	48–60
	Platelets (1000s/mm^3)	100–300	150–350

(Data from multiple sources.)
*Values reflect range of "normal" measurements at approximately 24 hours of life; significant variations may exist, depending on birth weight, source of blood sampled, and age at time of sample.

TABLE 60–4. Recommendations for the Prevention of Hypothermia in Neonates During Anesthesia and Surgery

Warmed operating room*
Radiant heat lamp
Warming blanket or mattress
Humidified and warmed inspired gases
Warming of intravenous fluids and blood products
Warming of irrigating solutions
Covering exposed body parts with transparent plastic wrap

*Ideally, the operating room temperature is set as close as possible to the neonate's thermoneutral zone (32–37 °C), the environmental temperature range in which oxygen consumption is minimized.

What Is Persistent Pulmonary Hypertension of the Newborn?

Persistent pulmonary hypertension of the newborn (PPHN) is a condition that usually becomes apparent within the first day of extrauterine life in term or post-term newborns. It is characterized by the development or persistence of increased PVR, which is equal to or greater than SVR. Systemic hypoxemia often results because of right-to-left prepulmonary shunting through the ductus arteriosus or foramen ovale. For this reason, PPHN also has been referred to as *persistent fetal circulation*, although this term is a misnomer because the fetal circulation includes the umbilical vessels and placenta, which are no longer present.

Perioperative Contributory Factors

Several factors that are at least partially under the control of the anesthesiologist in the perioperative period may trigger or sustain the elevation in PVR and the ensuing worsening cycle of increased hypoxemia, right-to-left shunting, and congestive heart failure. They include acidemia, hypoxemia, hypercarbia, hypothermia, polycythemia, hypoglycemia, hypomagnesemia, and hypocalcemia.[20, 21]

Associated Clinical Disorders

A large number of clinical disorders or perinatal insults may be associated with PPHN. For purposes of classification, these can be organized according to their cause: (1) normal pulmonary vascular development, in which PVR is elevated in a reactive fashion (pulmonary vasoconstriction); (2) increased pulmonary vascular smooth muscle, as with chronic in utero hypoxemia; and (3) decreased vessel number or reduced pulmonary artery cross-sectional area, as in congenital diaphragmatic hernia.

Physical Findings

Physical findings in newborns with PPHN include increased respiratory effort; central cyanosis, prominent right ventricular impulse and loud pulmonary component (P_2) of the second heart sound, normal or decreased peripheral pulses, and normal systemic blood pressure until the late stages of congestive heart failure.[22] Diagnosis is made on the basis of the clinical setting; physical examination; demonstration of ductal right-to-left shunting with at least a 10 mm Hg stepdown in Pao_2 from the right arm (usually preductal) to the descending aorta or lower extremities (postductal)[23]; echocardiography; and, in a few cases, cardiac catheterization. Electrocardiography and chest radiography may help to confirm the diagnosis and to eliminate other possible causes of a neonate's clinical condition.

Treatment

The treatment of PPHN is directed at preventing or minimizing the triggering factors identified previously, reversing the increase in PVR, and addressing any associated conditions such as sepsis or pneumonia.

Oxygenation

Oxygenation must be optimized through delivery of a sufficient fraction of inspired oxygen (Fio_2) (100% O_2 initially and

as necessary) to induce a Pao_2 of at least 100 to 120 mm Hg,[24] maintenance of appropriate O_2-carrying capacity (hematocrit 40–45%), and support of cardiac performance.

Conventional Mechanical Ventilation

Mechanical ventilation may be required, frequently with sedation and muscle relaxation, to induce hypocarbia and respiratory alkalosis, promote pulmonary vasodilation, and support oxygenation. As long as adequate ventilation is ensured, metabolic alkalosis may be induced with a continuous infusion of sodium bicarbonate.[25]

Drugs

Pharmacologic pulmonary vasodilation is sometimes attempted with agents such as tolazoline or sodium nitroprusside; these drugs also induce systemic vasodilation and frequently require concomitant intravascular volume augmentation and administration of an agent such as dopamine, which supports myocardial contractility and increases SVR. Nitric oxide inhalation is used increasingly to reduce PVR.

Advanced Therapy

Advanced therapies that may be attempted in cases refractory to conventional management include extracorporeal membrane oxygenation (ECMO) and high-frequency ventilation. Surgical ligation of a patent ductus arteriosus in PPHN with right-to-left shunting is not indicated and may precipitate acute right ventricular failure.[26]

What Is Infant Respiratory Distress Syndrome?

IRDS, often referred to as *hyaline membrane disease*, is principally a disorder of premature infants.

Pathogenesis

It is caused by a deficiency of pulmonary surfactant, a mixture of phospholipids and proteins, produced by type II pneumocytes. Surfactant reduces surface tension at the air-water interface within the alveoli. A deficiency leads to alveolar and small airways collapse at end-expiration, preventing maintenance of the FRC necessary for gas exchange. With atelectasis and airway collapse, pulmonary compliance is reduced and the work of breathing is increased; the highly compliant neonatal chest wall, described earlier, makes efforts to expand the lungs and maintain FRC even more difficult.

Clinical Presentation

This syndrome is noted in premature infants within the first hours of life, particularly after perinatal asphyxia, maternal diabetes mellitus, or cesarean delivery. Physical signs include tachypnea, nasal flaring, grunting, and chest wall retractions. Breath sounds are often reduced.[27] Arterial blood gas analysis reveals hypoxemia and acidemia, which commonly is both respiratory (hypercarbia) and metabolic in origin. Chest radiography demonstrates the classic ground glass appearance, with scattered air bronchograms throughout both lungs.

Operating Room Problems

Neonates who have IRDS and who require a surgical procedure typically present with hypoxemia, increased O_2 requirement, hypercarbia, and reduced pulmonary compliance. Oxygenation and ventilation represent an added challenge to the usual problems of caring for premature infants, particularly if the ventilator or breathing circuit used is different from that in the neonatal intensive care unit (NICU). For unstable patients or neonates with advanced ventilatory requirements, consider using the NICU ventilator in the operating room for the surgical procedure or accomplishing the procedure within the NICU if possible.

Exogenous Surfactant

Research has focused on administering exogenous surfactant materials to premature infants, either at birth or with the onset of respiratory distress.[28] Surfactant replacement therapy, which improves oxygenation and pulmonary compliance within minutes, can significantly alter the course of IRDS and may result in a reduction of complications, including barotrauma, bronchopulmonary dysplasia (BPD), and pulmonary interstitial emphysema.

What Is Intraventricular Hemorrhage?

Intraventricular hemorrhage (IVH) actually refers to bleeding that begins around the capillaries of the subependymal germinal matrix and may then extend to the ventricles and brain parenchyma.[29] It occurs most commonly in premature infants but may also develop in severely asphyxiated term infants. Before the advent of computed tomographic (CT) scanning and intracranial sonography, the diagnosis of IVH was based on clinical findings of abrupt-onset hypotension, acute anemia, metabolic acidosis, full fontanel, apnea and bradycardia, altered sensorium, and seizures. Noninvasive CT and ultrasound scanning have demonstrated that many cases are asymptomatic and that as many as 90% of very low-birth-weight infants develop IVH at some point in the first hours or days of life.[30]

Predisposing Factors

A number of factors have been associated with IVH; most important among these are prematurity and IRDS. Premature infants typically have a germinal matrix that is poorly supported by connective tissue, a "pressure-passive" cerebral circulation, and altered blood coagulation status. Infants with respiratory distress syndrome may have variations in intrathoracic pressure and therefore venous drainage of the head; wide fluctuations in oxygenation and blood pH status; and frequent exposure to hypertonic solutions such as sodium bicarbonate, vasopressors, and intravascular volume expanders, which can result in sudden fluid and tissue shifts.

Procedures including tracheal suctioning, awake intubation, and poorly synchronized mechanical ventilation during spontaneous breathing have been associated with significant intracranial hypertension in premature neonates and may therefore predispose to the development of IVH.[31–32]

Anesthetic Contribution

Anesthesiologists who encounter a neonate with documented IVH or one who is at risk for developing IVH should attempt to use an anesthetic regimen, ventilator therapy, and a fluid management plan that minimizes the potential for abrupt changes in cerebral blood flow and intracranial pressure (ICP). Although an open anterior fontanel may help to protect against ICP elevations, wide fluctuations in arterial blood pressure during light anesthesia or stimulation are apt to be transmitted to the relatively fragile vasculature of the neonatal germinal matrix, with the potential for resulting hemorrhage. Correction of acid-base abnormalities, coagulation defects, and hypothermia is also important.[30]

Why Does Anemia Occur?

Healthy term neonates are born with a mean umbilical cord hemoglobin of 16.8 g · dL^{-1}, whereas preterm infants younger than 34 weeks' gestational age have somewhat lower mean values in the range of 15 to 16 g · dL^{-1}.[33] An occasional healthy neonate is born with a hemoglobin as high as 20 g · dL^{-1}. With birth and exposure to the O_2-rich environment of extrauterine life, erythropoiesis within the neonatal marrow comes to a virtual standstill.

Hemoglobin in term newborns typically reaches a nadir of 9.0 to 11.0 g · dL^{-1} in the third month of life, whereas premature infants may experience even lower hemoglobin concentrations within a shorter period. In addition to this "physiologic" anemia, critically ill neonates may develop anemia and consequent reductions in O_2-carrying capacity as a result of sepsis, hemolytic processes, nutritional deficiencies, and repeated blood sampling for laboratory studies.

Fetal and Adult Hemoglobin

Normally, the onset of physiologic anemia of early infancy is not accompanied by clinical evidence of tissue O_2 deficits because fetal hemoglobin, which has a relatively high O_2 affinity (P_{50} = 19 mm Hg), is being replaced by adult hemoglobin. Adult hemoglobin has a lower O_2 affinity, as reflected in its P_{50} value of approximately 27 mm Hg, implying that it more readily releases O_2 to the tissues. When one or more of the anemia-inducing processes mentioned earlier compound normal, physiologic anemia, a neonate may develop the clinical signs and problems of tachypnea, tachycardia, poor weight gain, apnea, bradycardia, pallor, and lethargy.[34]

The Minimally Acceptable Hemoglobin

Until recent years, common practice, particularly in NICUs, was to maintain hemoglobin values of at least 12 to 13 g · dL^{-1}. Although some investigations have supported the notion that transfusions improve the symptoms of anemia, particularly the incidence of apnea/bradycardia spells, others have failed to demonstrate any consistent benefit of red blood cell transfusions.[34, 35]

Concerns about the transmission of blood-borne infectious diseases have cast doubt on the wisdom of routinely transfusing neonates to achieve some arbitrary hemoglobin or hematocrit value. However, Welborn and colleagues showed that former preterm infants with hematocrit values of 25% to 30%

were much more likely to experience postoperative apnea than those with hematocrit >30%.[36]

Nevertheless, rigid and arbitrary requirements for preoperative hemoglobin values in neonates seem inappropriate; rather, each case should be approached on an individual basis, considering factors such as an infant's gestational and postconceptual ages, anticipated blood loss, history of apnea/bradycardia spells, and provisions for postoperative monitoring.

Transfusion Guidelines

In general, severely anemic neonates or former premature infants should be transfused if their preoperative hematocrit is <25%. Above this level, proceed with minimal blood loss procedures but make sure everyone knows that the patient may be more likely to experience postoperative apnea; therefore, appropriate monitoring with pulse oximetry, capnography, and an electrocardiogram (ECG) must be provided. To the extent that surgery in neonates or former premature infants in the first months of life is seldom purely elective, the possibility of postponing surgery is not often a practical option.

RETINOPATHY OF PREMATURITY

What Is It?

Retinopathy of prematurity (ROP) was formerly known as *retrolental fibroplasia*, a descriptive term that applies only to a subset of patients with advanced ROP. It is a disorder characterized by abnormal proliferation of small retinal vessels. As its name implies, ROP is almost exclusively a disease of premature infants (<37 wk gestational age), although a number of other factors have been associated with it, including low birth weight, O_2 therapy, shock, sepsis, poor nutritional status, and ambient light exposure.[37]

Pathogenesis

Although the exact cause and role of these factors in the pathogenesis of ROP is unclear, the fundamental problem appears to be that at the time of a premature birth, vascularization of the retina is incomplete; a variable area of the peripheral retina is avascular. At some point in early postnatal life, the delicately growing vessels at the margin of vascular development sustain an injury related to the previously mentioned factors. Vascularization of the remaining retina must then be accomplished through a repair response rather than normal angiogenesis. Abnormal vessel proliferation, retinal hemorrhage, scarring, and detachment may result. Possible sequelae of ROP include myopia, strabismus, glaucoma, amblyopia, and blindness.[38]

The Role of Oxygen

An understanding of ROP is essential for anesthesiologists because of the likely influence of O_2 therapy (specifically, hyperoxygenation) on the pathogenesis of the disease and because affected infants may require monitoring and sedation or a general anesthetic for retinal cryoablation or laser photocoagulation.

O_2 therapy is only one of many contributing factors in ROP, although it is one of the most widely recognized and one of the few that can be controlled. O_2 involvement in ROP is confused by the observation that many premature infants who receive it never develop the problems but others, including some term infants never exposed to O_2 supplementation, contract the disease.[39] After O_2 was first implicated in the early 1950s, therapy was widely restricted and exposure for premature infants was limited to 40% O_2 or less.[40] By the 1960s, although the incidence of ROP had fallen sharply, the problem of brain damage and death among premature infants had become more significant. In fact, for every case of ROP blindness prevented, 16 infants were estimated to have died in the United States.[41]

Administration Guidelines

The effect of O_2 on the incompletely vascularized retina is illustrated in Figure 60–4. Attempts to define a "safe" level or duration of supplemental O_2 exposure have been unsuccessful. O_2 and ventilatory therapy should maintain the preductal (right arm) Pao_2 between 50 and 80 mm Hg and the pulse oximetric O_2 saturation (Spo_2) between 85% and 92% until 44 weeks of conceptual age, when the retinal vasculature is mature.[42] Because of rapid changes in the degree of arterial oxygenation during surgical procedures, it is reasonable to allow some safety margin with Spo_2 values as high as 95%. During periods of airway manipulation (bronchoscopy, intubation) or profound hemodynamic instability, 100% O_2 should be provided even if it induces short periods of hyperoxygenation.[32]

Anesthetic Implications

Because 4 to 6 weeks normally must pass for ROP to become evident on ophthalmoscopic examination, older (or former) premature infants may require trans-scleral cryotherapy or photocoagulation to arrest the retinopathy.[43] These procedures may be performed with subconjunctival local anesthesia, sedation, or general anesthesia.[44] By this point, most infants are beyond the acute problems of prematurity such as IRDS and PPHN; they may, nonetheless, experience significant complications including bradycardia, cyanosis, seizures, and respiratory and cardiac arrest.[45]

For these reasons, despite the mode of analgesia or anesthe-

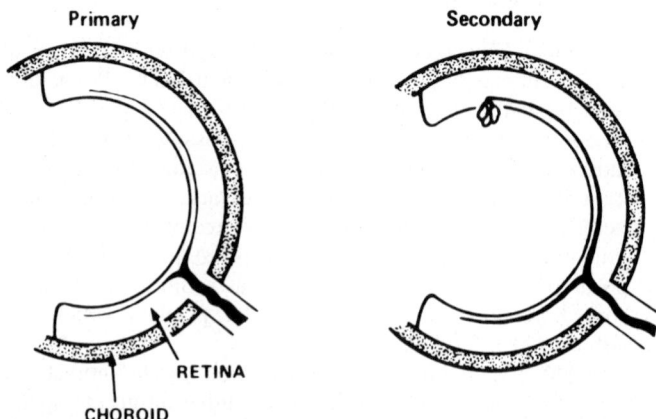

FIGURE 60–4. The mechanism of oxygen in retinopathy of prematurity. The primary response of vasoconstriction of the anterior retinal vessels and the later proliferation of remaining vascular components are demonstrated. (From Patz A: Retinopathy of prematurity. *In* Duane's Clinical Ophthalmology. Vol. 3. Rasman WS, Jaeger EA (eds). Philadelphia, JB Lippincott, 1990.)

sia selected, infants should be appropriately monitored with at least a pulse oximeter, ECG, and a noninvasive blood pressure device; *an individual other than the ophthalmologist should be primarily responsible for monitoring.* Resuscitation medications, including atropine and epinephrine, should be readily available in addition to equipment for airway support and positive-pressure ventilation.

ANESTHETIC PROBLEMS OF FORMER PREMATURE INFANTS

The dramatically increased survival of premature neonates in the past two decades has resulted in greater numbers of former premature infants presenting for surgical procedures. These patients have been demonstrated to be at higher risk of perioperative complications than term infants, and several scoring systems have been proposed to quantitate this risk.[46–48] Table 60–5 outlines the major anesthetic considerations that may apply to former premature infants. Most perioperative complications in this group are related to the airway and respiratory systems and include apnea, atelectasis, and aspiration.

What Is Bronchopulmonary Dysplasia?

BPD is a product of IRDS and its therapy, with resulting O_2 toxicity and pulmonary barotrauma. Former premature infants with BPD may demonstrate hypoxemia, hypercarbia, reactive airway disease, and increased PVR. Treatment includes fluid restriction, diuretics, digoxin, and bronchodilators.[49] These patients are particularly sensitive to fluid overload, and difficulty

TABLE 60–5. Anesthetic Considerations in Former Premature Infants

Effects of chronic organ system dysfunction	Pulmonary	Chronic lung disease; bronchopulmonary dysplasia
		Recurrent pneumonias
		Chronic aspiration (secondary to gastroesophageal reflux)
	Cardiac	Persistent patent ductus arteriosus
		Cardiomyopathy
	Central nervous system	Delayed development
		Impaired respiratory and cardiovascular reflexes
		Apnea
		Seizures
		Hydrocephalus
		Retinopathy of prematurity
Airway management problems		Subglottic stenosis
		Tracheobronchomalacia
		Impaired airway reflexes
Metabolic/fluid management problems		Poor nutritional status
		Tendency toward hypoglycemia
		Fragile bones, joints, and tissues
		Relative hypovolemia secondary to chronic fluid restriction and diuretics
		Difficult venous and/or arterial access
		Increased disposition to hypothermia (reduced amounts of brown fat and subcutaneous tissue)

may be experienced in providing effective controlled ventilation and restoration of normal oxygenation after oxyhemoglobin desaturation has occurred.

What Is the Significance of Perioperative Apnea?

Perioperative apnea is primarily a problem of premature and former premature infants and generally is inversely related to gestational age and weight. Isolated reports of postoperative apnea in otherwise healthy term infants have been published.[50] Even in the absence of anesthesia and surgery, a baseline incidence of apneic episodes >15 seconds' duration occurs in approximately 60% of premature infants.[51] This problem is thought to be due to immaturity of central respiratory control mechanisms and may be compounded by airway obstruction resulting from positioning and faulty control of soft tissues within the upper airway. Residual medications including potent inhalation agents, muscle relaxants, and opioids, as well as hypothermia, and electrolyte changes may contribute.

Postoperative Apnea Monitoring

The postconceptual age range of premature infants believed to be at increased risk of apnea has steadily increased during the past decade from 44 weeks to as late as 60 weeks.[52] Apnea will most likely appear within the first 12 hours after anesthesia, although it has been reported as late as 48 hours postoperatively. As with nil per os (NPO) guidelines, policies regarding postoperative apnea monitoring vary significantly among institutions. In the following infants, conservative practice requires monitoring for at least 12 (preferably 24) hours after anesthesia: former premature infants up to 60 weeks postconceptual age; patients with a history of episodic apnea; and survivors of sudden infant death syndrome and their siblings. At a minimum, monitoring should include an apnea/bradycardia monitor and pulse oximeter.

Prevention

Intravenous caffeine, $10 \, mg \cdot kg^{-1}$ intraoperatively, appears to stimulate central respiratory control centers and to minimize or eliminate the incidence of apnea in patients at risk.[53] Regional anesthetic techniques have been touted as a preferred alternative to general anesthesia, although infants have experienced apnea after regional anesthesia as well, particularly if intravenous sedation is provided to supplement the block.[54]

PREOPERATIVE FASTING GUIDELINES

Many surgical procedures in neonates are performed on an urgent or emergent basis. This fact, in combination with the knowledge that neonatal disease and surgical disorders often interfere with gastric emptying and normal gastrointestinal function, mandate that most neonates be considered to have a "full stomach," irrespective of the period of time since the last oral intake.

What Is the Appropriate NPO Interval?

For cases in which surgery is scheduled semi-electively or electively, formula administered by mouth or gavage should be withheld for 4 hours and clear fluids such as dextrose in water solutions for 2 hours before the anticipated time of induction of anesthesia.[32, 55] In determining the fasting interval, one must consider the risk of dehydration and hypoglycemia on the one hand and the possibility of increasing the volume of gastric contents and thereby increasing the potential for regurgitation and aspiration on the other. Because human breast milk passes through the stomach more rapidly than does formula, some practitioners allow human milk up to 2 to 3 hours before surgery.[56]

Modifying Factors

Neonates with disorders known to delay gastric emptying should be fasted for longer periods if the surgical condition allows. An intravenous infusion of 5% dextrose in quarter normal saline at a rate of $4 \text{ mL} \cdot \text{kg}^{-1} \cdot \text{hr}^{-1}$ should be instituted to prevent hypoglycemia and the development of an excessive fluid deficit. A similar practice is recommended for any neonatal surgical patient who is not otherwise at increased risk of aspiration and in whom the time of anesthetic induction is not known or delayed.

PREMEDICATION

Premedication, for practical purposes, is limited to anticholinergic agents. The goals of premedication in older children and adults, including anxiolysis, sedation, and preoperative amnesia, appear to have no application in neonates because separation anxiety does not become an issue until approximately age 6 to 9 months. The stress of separation and invasive procedures may influence later behavior such as feeding patterns and sleep cycles, but no evidence shows that preoperative sedation alters such effects.[57]

What Are the Desired Effects?

The anticholinergics atropine, glycopyrrolate, and scopolamine blunt the vagal cardiovascular responses to laryngoscopy, nasogastric suctioning, the potent inhalation anesthetics, and succinylcholine. Other effects of these drugs include drying of oral secretions, reduced gastric fluid volume and acidity, and sedation (atropine and scopolamine).[58]

Considerable variation exists with respect to the dosage, route of administration, and timing of premedication with these drugs. Although oral administration of atropine has achieved some popularity in older infants and toddlers, in the neonatal period, the anticholinergics are given intramuscularly (IM), subcutaneously (SC), or intravenously (IV).[59] The dose of atropine is 10 to 20 $\mu g \cdot kg^{-1}$ IV and 20 $\mu g \cdot kg^{-1}$ IM or SC (minimum total dose of 100 μg, or 0.1 mg). The dose of glycopyrrolate is 5 to 10 $\mu g \cdot kg^{-1}$ IV and 10 to 15 $\mu g \cdot kg^{-1}$ IM.

What Side Effects May Occur?

A number of potential drawbacks should be considered. These include the drying of lower respiratory tract secretions and the possibility that an endotracheal tube or lower natural airway may become plugged; persistent tachycardia; and ele-

vation of body temperature due to the inhibition of sweating. Historically, the routine preoperative use of anticholinergics was often questioned because their administration could mask the hypoxemia with its attendant bradycardia. The widespread use of pulse oximetry today largely has eliminated this concern.

AIRWAY MANAGEMENT

The techniques of airway management are based on the anatomic and physiologic features discussed previously. In addition to the specifics concerning tracheal intubation, controversial issues include the practice of awake versus anesthetized intubation and whether all neonates require intubation for general anesthesia.

What Are the Considerations for Awake Intubation?

Conventional neonatal anesthetic practice dictates that many newborns undergo intubation awake. This practice has been justified on the basis of immaturity of airway protective reflexes; the rapidity with which neonates develop oxyhemoglobin desaturation and hemodynamic instability once the airway is lost; and the fear that neonates may tolerate inhalation or intravenous induction poorly before securing the airway.

On the other hand, concern exists for arterial hypertension and the potential for intracranial hemorrhage, especially in premature infants, when awake intubation is accomplished.[60] Many practitioners also believe that newborns should be afforded the same benefit of anesthesia during this painful and stressful procedure as would older children or adults. To be sure, instances in which awake intubation is clearly preferred are delineated, such as during resuscitation, in situations involving profound hemodynamic instability, or when the airway is already compromised and mask ventilation is expected to be difficult or impossible.

Should Neonates Be Intubated Routinely?

Numerous justifications are offered for routine intubation of neonates who require general anesthesia. These include assurance of airway patency, reduction of dead space compared with mask ventilation, decreased likelihood of gastric distention and aspiration, and facilitated control of ventilation.

Is mask general anesthesia acceptable for neonates? Nearly every anesthesiologist has been faced with a vigorous, healthy term neonate who requires an anesthetic for a very brief procedure. In such cases, depending on the skill of the individual practitioner, mask anesthesia is a suitable alternative. In the vast majority of cases, however, tracheal intubation carries very low morbidity, and its advantages greatly exceed its disadvantages.[61]

What Techniques and Equipment Are Applicable?

Intubation requires an appropriately sized endotracheal tube and laryngoscope; the means to deliver positive-pressure ventilation with O_2; suction apparatus; appropriate monitoring devices; medications including atropine, succinylcholine, and an intravenous anesthetic; and, whenever possible, a skilled assistant.

Preoxygenation should be provided with 100% O_2 and a secure mask fit before intubation. Straight laryngoscope blades (usually Miller's 0 to 1) are preferred by most practitioners because they provide better glottic visibility and occupy less space in the mouth.

Endotracheal Tubes

Endotracheal tubes are commonly made of clear polyvinylchloride and should be nontapered and uncuffed. A selection above and below the anticipated required size should be available. Small premature infants <1000 g frequently require a tube of 2.5 mm inside diameter (ID), but most larger premature and term neonates accommodate 3.0-mm-ID tubes. An occasional large term infant may require a 3.5-mm-ID tube.

The range of clinically appropriate endotracheal tube lengths in neonates is from 7 cm (gum to midtrachea distance) in 1000-g premature infants to 10 cm in term newborns.[62] Endotracheal tubes typically are considerably longer; shortening them to 2 to 3 cm beyond the anticipated depth at the gum or alveolar ridge reduces the dead space and resistance to gas flow and the tendency for narrow tubes to kink. Making the cut at an oblique angle facilitates reattaching the endotracheal tube–breathing circuit adapter.

An audible leak should be detectable at <30 cm H_2O peak airway pressure; otherwise, tracheal mucosal ischemia may develop, with the potential for subglottic edema and delayed subglottic stenosis.[63] If the leak is too great (occurring at <10 cm H_2O pressure), effective positive-pressure ventilation may be difficult.

INTRAOPERATIVE VENTILATION

Should Manual or Mechanical Techniques Be Used?

How neonatal surgical patients should be ventilated entails the issues of manual versus mechanical support, the various available breathing circuits, and appropriate ventilator settings. In practice, a combination of manual and mechanical ventilation is frequently used in older children and adults. However, manual ventilation has been most strongly advocated as the principal means of ventilatory support.

Manual

The primary justification for this practice is that ventilation by hand allows rapid detection of the acute changes in compliance and resistance encountered during neonatal surgery and compensation for these changes. That manual ventilation or the use of an "educated hand" measures up to this claim and is superior to mechanical ventilation has been questioned.[64, 65]

Mechanical

Mechanical techniques are capable of predictable and constant ventilation over time (although this advantage is never guaranteed) and free the anesthesia practitioner's hands to perform other duties. Of course, if a change in ventilation is detected by the continuous assessment of breath sounds and chest movement or readings of monitoring devices, manual ventilation can be immediately restored.[66]

The important points to recall are that a means of providing manual ventilation must always be available and the limitations of the specific breathing circuit and ventilator in use must be understood. Regardless of whether a neonate is ventilated by manual or mechanical means, changes in lung-thorax compliance can significantly alter the actual tidal volume because of the compliance and compression volume of the breathing circuit as well as the leak around the uncuffed tube.

How Should Mechanical Ventilation Be Administered?

Neonatal Intensive Care Unit Ventilators

Several alternatives are available to provide mechanical ventilation in the operating room. One is to use any of the time-cycled, pressure-limited ventilators typically used in neonatal intensive care, in which case anesthesia must be provided by intravenous agents. A useful exception to this generalization is the Siemens 900C ventilator, which is available in modified form for use with inhalation agents as an anesthesia machine.

Anesthesia Ventilators

Volume-limited (or preset) ventilators found on most anesthesia machines can be used. Many are supplied with a smaller bellows for infant and pediatric use. In this case, the excursion volume of the ventilator bellows is reduced to its minimum setting, then gradually increased as the fresh gas flow and inspiratory-to-expiratory time (I:E) ratio are adjusted to provide adequate tidal volume.

Settings

The adequacy of tidal volume is assessed by observation of chest wall movement, breath sounds, and the capnograph and pulse oximeter readings. Although the ventilator settings are determined by the presence and stage of any cardiopulmonary disease processes, typical initial values include a peak inspiratory pressure (PIP) of 15 to 18 cm H_2O, positive end-expiratory pressure (PEEP) of 0 to 3 cm H_2O, ventilatory rate of 24 breaths per minute, and an I:E ratio of 1:2. The FIO_2 is adjusted to maintain SPO_2 between 88% and 95%. Requirements for fresh gas flow rate vary depending on the breathing circuit in use and the presence or absence of a carbon dioxide (CO_2) absorber. Fresh gas flow rates for common neonatal ventilators are typically 5 to 10 L $\cdot$ min^{-1}.[67]

What Circuits Are Available?

Nonrebreathing

Historically and in many institutions today, neonates have been ventilated during anesthesia with any of several "semi-open" nonrebreathing circuits, such as the Bain modification of the Mapleson D system (illustrated in Chapter 61) and the Jackson-Rees modification of the Ayres T-piece.[68] These systems lack unidirectional valves and a CO_2 absorber; hence, they eliminate much of the work of spontaneous ventilation and facilitate manual detection of subtle changes in lower airway resistance. CO_2 elimination and adequacy of ventilation are determined by fresh gas flow (which must be at least 2.5 L · min^{-1} and twice minute ventilation during spontaneous ventilation to prevent rebreathing), tidal volume, and respiratory rate.[69, 70]

Circle

Lightweight plastic pediatric circle systems with small-diameter tubing have become increasingly popular for use in infants and neonates and function identically to well-known adult circle systems. By necessity, pediatric circles include one-way valves that must be opened with each breath. Experts generally recommend that neonates not be allowed (or required) to breathe spontaneously without assistance for more than a few minutes.[71]

VASCULAR ACCESS

What Are the Indications?

Intravenous access is indicated in all anesthetized neonates for the purposes of administering anesthetic drugs, resuscitative medications, fluids, and blood products. When a patient is critically ill or has a significant thoracoabdominal disease process, intravenous access should be established before the induction of anesthesia.

The size and number of intravenous catheters are determined by the nature of the surgical procedure and the potential for major blood and third space fluid loss. For infants receiving infusions of parenteral hyperalimentation fluid or vasoactive medications, an additional venous access site or lumen of a central venous catheter is recommended for administration of anesthetic agents and bolus fluids.

What Sites Should Be Used?

Peripheral veins generally are easily seen and may be cannulated with 22- or 24-gauge intravenous catheters. Sequentially larger guidewires (0.18–0.25 mm) and catheters (18–20 gauge) may be placed. Alternatively, access to large central veins can be obtained at the femoral, axillary, and internal and external jugular veins.[72, 73] Common sites of peripheral access are the dorsum of the hand, antecubital fossae, greater saphenous vein on the medial surface of the ankle just anterior to the medial malleolus, and dorsal and lateral surfaces of the foot. Scalp vein needles may be used for administering medications and maintenance fluids but in my experience are not reliable for large-volume fluid infusions and boluses; they should only be used after depletion of sites on the extremities.

How Is Insertion Performed?

General Considerations

Thorough preparation and planning are essential to secure reliable venous access. A varied selection of appropriate-sized

catheters should be available and within reach of the individual attempting placement. The extremity should be immobilized by an assistant or padded support. Strict attention to asepsis should be ensured by the use of gloves and topically applied iodine solution or alcohol.

Helpful maneuvers include (1) nicking the skin at the site of anticipated entry of the catheter-over-the-needle device to prevent catheter drag at the skin surface; (2) removing the plastic cap from the hub of the intravenous needle assembly before venipuncture; and (3) after placement of the catheter, initially verifying correct intravenous location by hooking up an intravenous fluid-filled syringe attached to a T-connector extension set and injecting a small amount of fluid. If little or no resistance to injection is noted and the site does not become indurated or infiltrated, the intravenous tubing providing fluid administration is attached to the venous catheter.

Because all neonates can be assumed to have anatomic connections or shunts between the left and right sides of the heart, meticulous attention should be given to clearing the intravenous tubing of all bubbles. Microdrip (60 drops per milliliter) fluid administration sets with calibrated, limited-volume (100–150 mL) fluid chambers are typically used for neonates and infants. An electronic infusion pump may be used to provide more precise control of fluid administration rates.

Umbilical Catheterization

The umbilical vessels, including one vein and two arteries, provide an alternative source of vascular access in neonates and are typically used by the staff in the NICU before surgery. Umbilical venous catheters may be used to monitor central venous pressure and to administer fluids and medications. Catheters in the umbilical artery are used to monitor arterial pressure and to administer drugs and fluids in emergency situations.

The location of umbilical catheter tips must be verified before surgery and to minimize the potential for inward or outward migration of a catheter intraoperatively; disastrous complications including visceral artery thrombosis and liver necrosis or cirrhosis may result from many fluids and medications administered through an incorrectly located umbilical catheter.[74] The tip of an umbilical venous catheter may be either ''low'' just above the bifurcation of the femoral arteries (L-3–L-4) or ''high'' above the diaphragm (T-6–T-9). That of an umbilical venous catheter should rest in the IVC near the junction with the right atrium, beyond the ductus venosus.

Alternate Arterial Sites

Other sites for arterial cannulation include the radial, dorsalis pedis, posterior tibial, and femoral arteries. Arterial cannulation is indicated for continuous blood pressure monitoring and analysis of blood gases and pH. If possible, the right radial artery should be cannulated because it is representative of preductal blood flow for arterial blood gas measurements.

FLUID ADMINISTRATION

What Are the Basic Requirements?

Fluid management in neonatal surgical patients includes normal maintenance requirements, replacement of any pre-existing deficit, and both third space fluid and acute blood losses. A typical term neonate has a water content of 75% to 80% and a blood volume of 80 to 90 mL $\cdot$ $^{-1}$.[75] Premature infants may have a blood volume as great as 105 mL $\cdot$ kg^{-1}.

Maintenance

The average fluid requirement in a healthy neonate is approximately 100 mL $\cdot$ kg^{-1} $\cdot$ d^{-1}, or 4 mL $\cdot$ kg^{-1} $\cdot$ h^{-1}.[76] Various processes such as congenital heart disease, BPD, and the use of radiant warmers and phototherapy may increase or decrease this basic fluid requirement. Electrolyte replacement must be accounted for in maintenance fluids; appropriate amounts of sodium and chloride are usually provided by quarter normal saline. Potassium may be added (in the presence of adequate renal function) with 1 to 2 mEq per 100 mL of maintenance fluid.

Pre-Existing and Intraoperative Losses

Most critically ill neonates receive nothing by mouth and have received intravenous maintenance fluids for some time before surgery or have never taken oral fluids. Fluid deficits may result from incomplete or inadequate volume replacement before surgery. Third space fluid losses are particularly significant in patients with gastroschisis, omphalocele, necrotizing enterocolitis, and ruptured meningomyelocele.

What Fluids Are Indicated?

Balanced Electrolyte Solutions

During major operative procedures involving manipulation and exposure of large visceral surfaces, replacement with 2 to 15 mL $\cdot$ kg^{-1} $\cdot$ h^{-1} of balanced salt solution (normal saline or lactated Ringer's solution) is necessary to replenish intravascular fluid volume.[77] Pre-existing and intraoperative deficits associated with hypotension, metabolic acidosis, and oliguria require bolus fluid therapy; 10 to 20 mL $\cdot$ kg^{-1} of balanced salt solution or a colloid volume expander is repeatedly administered over 5 to 10 minutes as blood pressure, heart rate, and urine output are monitored. Large volumes of 100 to 200 mL $\cdot$ kg^{-1} or greater may be required to restore and maintain normal intravascular volume and hemodynamics.

Colloids

Colloid preparations, such as 5% albumin, plasma protein fraction, and fresh-frozen plasma (FFP) commonly are used in the fluid resuscitation of neonates, perhaps to a greater extent than in adults. The justification for this practice is not well defined but has been based on concerns that neonates are less tolerant of large fluid and salt loads, are perhaps more susceptible to the detrimental effects of interstitial edema, and are frequently experiencing at least a low-grade coagulopathy when critically ill. Colloids do remain in the intravascular compartment longer than crystalloids but are more expensive.[76]

Glucose and Hyperalimentation Solutions

Limited neonatal glycogen stores, the frequent absence of normal enteral nutrition, and the stress of the disease state and surgery necessitate that glucose be provided in a 5% to 12.5% concentration in the maintenance fluids to meet caloric requirements and prevent hypoglycemia. Critically ill neonates often receive all or a significant portion of their maintenance fluids from parenteral hyperalimentation solutions. Approaches to the management of hyperalimentation fluids vary, with some advocating administration of 10% dextrose in place of the hyperalimentation fluid during surgery to prevent rebound hypoglycemia. In most instances, the hyperalimentation fluid can be continued during surgery. In any case, blood glucose levels should be monitored at least hourly.

How Is Blood Loss Replaced?

Until recent years, hematocrit values were maintained in the minimum range of 35% to 40% because of a neonate's greater O_2 consumption and a limited ability to increase O_2 delivery by increases in cardiac output. The heightened concern of blood-borne infectious disease transmission has caused "target" hematocrit values in neonates to drift downward, as in older patients.

As blood is lost, intravascular volume replacement initially is provided in the form of isotonic crystalloid or colloid. Crystalloids are normally replaced in a 3:1 ratio to blood loss to compensate for the extravascular shift of fluid. Colloids and blood products are provided in a 1:1 ratio with blood loss after the allowable blood loss has been exceeded. Ten to 20 mL $\cdot$ kg^{-1} of packed red blood cells is commonly administered by a manual syringe or calibrated infusion pump, after which the clinical situation is reassessed.

Packed erythrocytes have a hematocrit of 65% to 75%; overzealous transfusion may induce a dangerously high hematocrit and hyperviscosity. One solution to this problem is to dilute the packed red blood cells with warm isotonic saline to a hematocrit of 45% to 50% before transfusion. All blood products and bolus crystalloids should be warmed before administration.

INTRAOPERATIVE MONITORING

What Are the Basics?

Monitoring during anesthesia and surgery includes two distinct but related functions: assessment of homeostasis of the patient's physiologic status and evaluation of equipment performance (breathing systems, ventilator, and intravenous infusion pumps). At a minimum, monitoring should comply with the American Society of Anesthesiologists' Standards for Basic Intra-Operative Monitoring; practically, this approach includes a precordial or esophageal stethoscope, continuous ECG, noninvasive blood pressure measurement, a temperature probe, and a pulse oximeter.[78] Monitoring of exhaled CO_2 has achieved widespread application in neonates. Additional measurements that may be required in selected patients include nerve stimulation, continuous invasive blood pressure, and urine output.

What Is the Value of Pulse Oximetry?

The most significant monitoring advances in the past decade are pulse oximetry and capnometry. Neonates and infants younger than 6 months are at greatest risk of experiencing at least one major episode such as accidental extubation, esophageal intubation, circuit disconnect, or kinking of the endotracheal tube.[79]

Pulse oximetry is relatively simple to use, particularly when compared with transcutaneous O_2 monitoring.[80] It provides early evidence of impending oxyhemoglobin desaturation before hypoxemia-induced changes in vital signs or clinically apparent cyanosis develops.[81] It may also be used to guide the F_{IO_2} selection and thereby lessen the risk of hyperoxia in premature neonates. This is the one situation in which the high Sp_{O_2} alarm setting can be used to advantage. Inferences concerning intravascular volume status, cardiac output, and peripheral vasoconstriction may be made when a well-placed oximeter cannot consistently detect arterial pulsations.[82]

From a practical standpoint, oximeter probes are often placed or wrapped (depending on the design of the probe) around the palm of the hand or the foot in neonates. In determining probe placement, consideration should be given to accessibility, potential for motion, compression, and light interference, as well as the vascular supply of the location (proximal or distal) to the ductus arteriosus.

What Is the Value of Capnometry/Capnography?

Indications

Capnometry, the measurement of CO_2 partial pressure in a gas mixture, and capnography, the representation of CO_2 partial pressure as a waveform over time, provide a large amount of information about a patient and the function of the artificial airway, breathing system, and ventilator. CO_2 analysis facilitates the detection of critical incidents, breathing system leaks, and rebreathing and assists the assessment of ventilation.

Limitations

Expired gas can be analyzed with a mainstream- or sidestream-type monitor; each has its limitations. Accurate measurements of true end-expired CO_2 partial pressure can be difficult with a sidestream analyzer in which the gas to be measured is aspirated from the airway or breathing circuit. This problem is particularly evident in nonrebreathing systems with relatively high fresh gas flows and in the presence of significant cardiopulmonary disease.[83] Accuracy is also decreased with low sampling flow rates (<100 mL $\cdot$ min^{-1}).[84] An endotracheal tube with a built-in distal sampling port or a mainstream analyzer improves the validity of CO_2 readings. A mainstream analyzer "reads" gas within the airway or circuit but is bulky and may lead to kinking or dislodgment of the endotracheal tube.

PYLORIC STENOSIS

Infantile hypertrophic pyloric stenosis is a relatively common gastrointestinal disorder, with an incidence that may approach 1 in 300 live births in some geographic locations.[85] It typically presents as nonbilious projectile vomiting between the second and sixth weeks of life. Boys are approximately four times more likely than girls to be affected.

The cause of pyloric stenosis is unknown, although a number of factors including genetic inheritance, infection, and pyloric irritation with subsequent edema and obstruction may play a part.[86] Infants with this disorder have been diagnosed increasingly early in the course of the disease in recent years. As a result, the profound metabolic derangement consisting of a hypochloremic, hypokalemic, hyponatremic metabolic alkalosis and hypovolemia is infrequently encountered. Diagnosis is made on the basis of history and physical examination and is confirmed by a barium contrast study of the stomach (Fig. 60–5) or ultrasonography of the upper abdomen.[87]

What Are the Primary Concerns?

Pyloric stenosis is a medical emergency first and surgical emergency second. As such, the initial point of management following diagnosis is to correct disturbances in acid-base, fluid, and electrolyte status.

Fluid Therapy

The exact nature and quantity of intravenous fluid required depend on the severity of these derangements. For mild to moderate hypovolemia (5–15% loss of body weight) 50 to 100 mL $\cdot$ kg^{-1} fluid replacement may be provided with normal saline. Half the deficit should be replaced during the first 8 hours, and the remaining half in the next 16 hours.

Acid-Base Status

For severe hypovolemia and alkalosis ($HCO_3 >42$ mEq $\cdot$ L^{-1}), several boluses of normal saline (20 mL $\cdot$ kg^{-1}) are

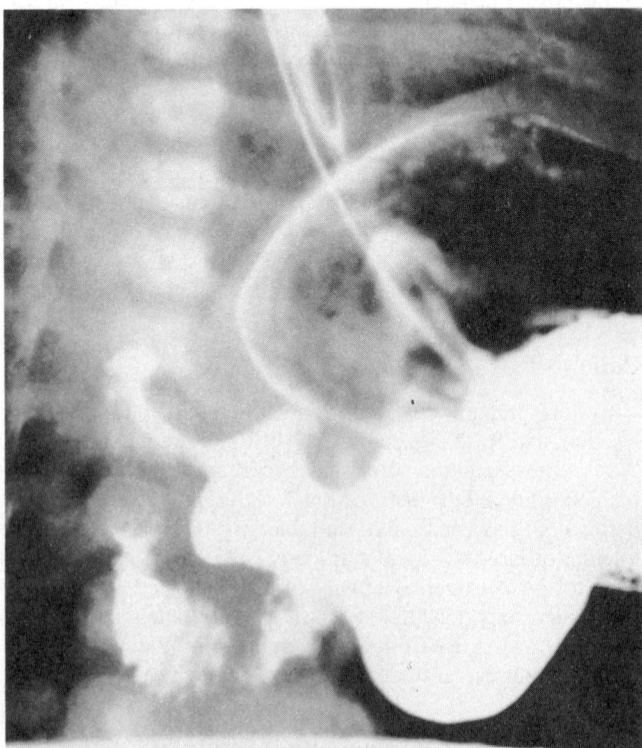

FIGURE 60–5. Barium contrast study of the stomach in a patient with pyloric stenosis. The fundus is at the upper right, and the area of the pylorus is seen on the left overlying the vertebra.

required, followed by replacement of the remaining deficit as outlined earlier. Potassium may be added to the intravenous fluid when urine output is adequate (>0.5–1 mL · kg⁻¹ · h⁻¹). A urinary chloride concentration >20 mEq · L⁻¹ following fluid resuscitation is proposed as a useful indicator of satisfactory volume replacement.[86]

How Is Anesthesia Managed?

A number of anesthetic considerations are implicit in the care of infants with pyloric stenosis in addition to the standard tenets of neonatal anesthesia. After fluid resuscitation and the correction of acid-base and electrolyte abnormalities, patients must be regarded as having a full stomach owing to impaired gastric emptying. Before either awake intubation or rapid-sequence induction and intubation, a *new* orogastric or nasogastric tube should be passed into the stomach and put to suction.

Muscle relaxants allow a reduction in the dose of inhalation anesthetics, improve surgical exposure, and minimize the risk of perforation of the duodenal mucosa. Some infants are prone to postanesthetic apnea, which may reflect uncorrected alkalosis within the blood or cerebrospinal fluid; for this reason, narcotics should be used sparingly (if at all).[88] Postoperative analgesia may be provided by rectal acetaminophen or infiltration of the surgical wound with a local anesthetic.

CONGENITAL ABDOMINAL WALL DEFECTS

What Are They?

Omphalocele and gastroschisis are congenital abdominal wall defects requiring emergent surgical repair. Considerable confusion exists about the terminology for these lesions and the distinction between them, with resultant difficulty in comparing treatments and outcomes in different patient series.

Omphalocele

Omphalocele (Fig. 60–6) is a herniation of the abdominal viscera that occurs into the base of the umbilical cord through

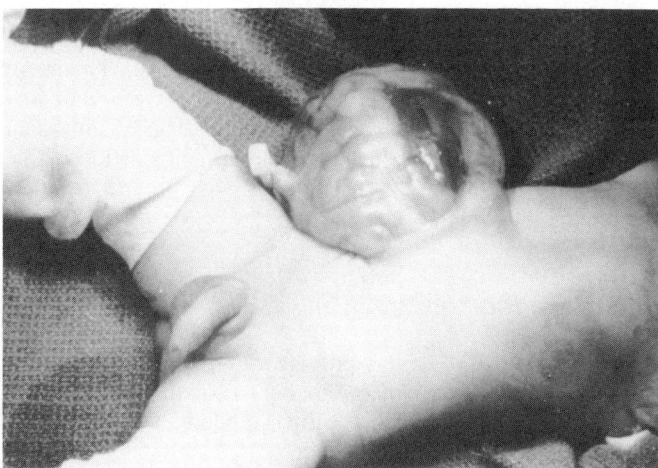

FIGURE 60–6. Omphalocele, with herniated abdominal organs covered by a translucent membranous sac.

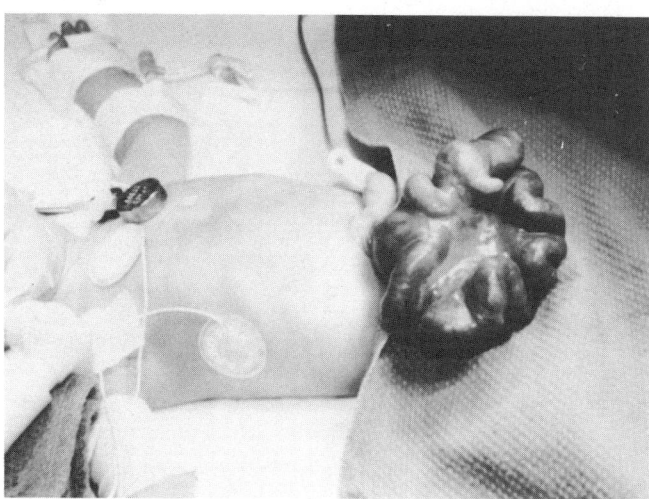

FIGURE 60–7. Gastroschisis. Note the lack of a membranous covering and the confluent appearance of the intestine. The herniation has actually occurred to the right of the umbilicus.

a central wall defect. Herniated organs are covered by a membranous sac and may include the intestine, stomach, liver, and spleen. Omphalocele has an incidence of 1 in 5000 to 10,000 live births and is frequently associated with other congenital anomalies (76%).[89] Potential coexisting defects include congenital heart disease, chromosomal trisomy, and the Beckwith-Wiedemann syndrome of hypoglycemia, macroglossia, and visceromegaly. Approximately 33% of patients with an omphalocele are premature.

Gastroschisis

Gastroschisis (Fig. 60–7) is an evisceration of bowel through a full-thickness defect in the abdominal wall, typically to the right of the umbilical cord. No membrane or sac covers the eviscerated organs, which characteristically are thickened and matted together. Fifty per cent of patients with this defect are premature, but it is less likely to be associated with other congenital defects.

What Are Potential Complications?

Patients with gastroschisis are most likely to die of processes related to prematurity or intestinal and wound complications, whereas mortality in patients with omphalocele is often related to their low birth weight and coexisting anomalies. With both disorders, the abdominal cavity may be small and underdeveloped, causing difficulty at the time of surgical repair. An artificial silo is occasionally required to enclose the viscera until all abdominal contents can later be returned to the abdomen (Fig. 60–8).[90]

What Are the Major Management Problems?

Problems encountered preoperatively persist into the operative period and include difficulty with maintenance of body temperature, significant fluid loss through the exposed viscera, and infection. Placing the exposed viscera into a plastic or gauze wrap preoperatively reduces heat and fluid loss. Addi-

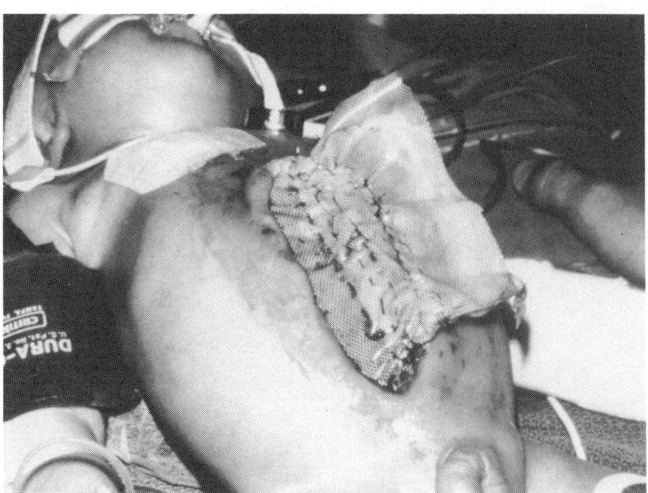

FIGURE 60–8. Artificial silo in place to contain abdominal viscera following omphalocele repair. This patient has undergone sequential reduction of the silo contents and is photographed prior to removal of the silo and closure of the abdominal wall.

tional measures such as warming the ambient environment, ventilator gases, and fluids to be infused are crucial.

Fluid Requirements

Fluid requirements vary depending on the size of the wall defect and the amount of exposed viscera. Parameters that can be monitored to guide fluid resuscitation include systolic blood pressure, heart rate, urine output, base deficit, and hematocrit. Hemoconcentration, as evidenced by increasing hematocrit, may denote hypovolemia. As in other instances of neonatal fluid resuscitation, colloid preparations are used frequently in 10 to 20 mL · kg^{-1} increments.[91] As much as 300 to 400 mL · kg^{-1} of crystalloid may be needed immediately preoperatively and during surgical repair. Significant amounts of blood loss usually are not encountered.

Airway

If they are not already intubated in the NICU, patients presenting for surgical repair of an abdominal wall defect may be intubated either awake or after rapid intravenous induction of anesthesia. Nasogastric or orogastric tube decompression of the stomach should precede induction.

How Is Anesthesia Managed?

Anesthesia is provided by a combination of a narcotic and a nondepolarizing muscle relaxant. A potent inhalation anesthetic may be used to supplement the intravenous agents if it is tolerated by the patient. Nitrous oxide should be avoided in these patients because of the possibility that it may contribute to intestinal distention and interfere with successful closure of the abdomen.

Adequacy of Ventilation

As the eviscerated or herniated organs are returned to the abdominal cavity, the PIP, adequacy of ventilation, and he-

modynamic stability must be closely monitored. Return of all herniated organs and primary closure of abdominal wall defects may be associated with severe limitation of diaphragmatic excursion and reduction of venous return of blood from the lower extremities and abdomen, with a subsequent reduction in cardiac output and impaired systemic perfusion.

Failure of primary operative repair of omphalocele and gastroschisis was associated with intragastric pressures exceeding 20 mm Hg, reductions of cardiac index of at least 0.78 L · min^{-1} · m$^{2-1}$, and increases in central venous pressure of at least 4 mm Hg in one report.[92] In the presence of such indices or a PIP significantly >30 cm H_2O, an artificial silo may be necessary to cover the eviscerated organs. The hernia may then be gradually reduced over a period of up to 10 days.

Extubation

The decision to extubate is influenced by the size of the defect, the extent of fluid loss and resuscitation, the residual effects of anesthetic agents, and the presence of other problems such as IRDS and congenital heart disease.

Monitoring

Monitoring includes all standard parameters. Invasive blood pressure monitoring is optional (but often required) and largely depends on pulmonary status, the size of the lesion, and the extent of existing or anticipated acid-base derangements.

NECROTIZING ENTEROCOLITIS

What Is It?

Neonatal necrotizing enterocolitis (NEC) is not a congenital anomaly. It is acquired and is primarily a disease of premature low-birth-weight infants, although 10% of patients are term.[93] The incidence and mortality of NEC vary among institutions, with clusters of "outbreaks" developing at different times.

Causes

A large number of conditions in addition to prematurity are associated with NEC, including perinatal asphyxia and hypoxemia, umbilical vessel catheterization, episodes of hypotension or shock, patent ductus arteriosus, exchange transfusions, polycythemia, and hyperosmolar feedings. The disease appears to involve hypoperfusion of the intestinal mucosa. The result is mucosal inflammation, ischemia, necrosis, bowel wall perforation, and sepsis. Other factors that appear to be important in the etiology of NEC include bacterial colonization of the gut and the presence of a substrate, usually formula feedings, within the gut lumen.[94]

What Are the Presenting Signs?

Neonates with NEC may present with a number of nonspecific signs, including lethargy, pallor, irritability, temperature instability, apnea, and bradycardia. Abdominal findings include distention (Fig. 60–9), tenderness, gastric retention, gastrointestinal hemorrhage, and erythema of the abdominal wall. Later in the disease, signs of sepsis and disseminated intravas-

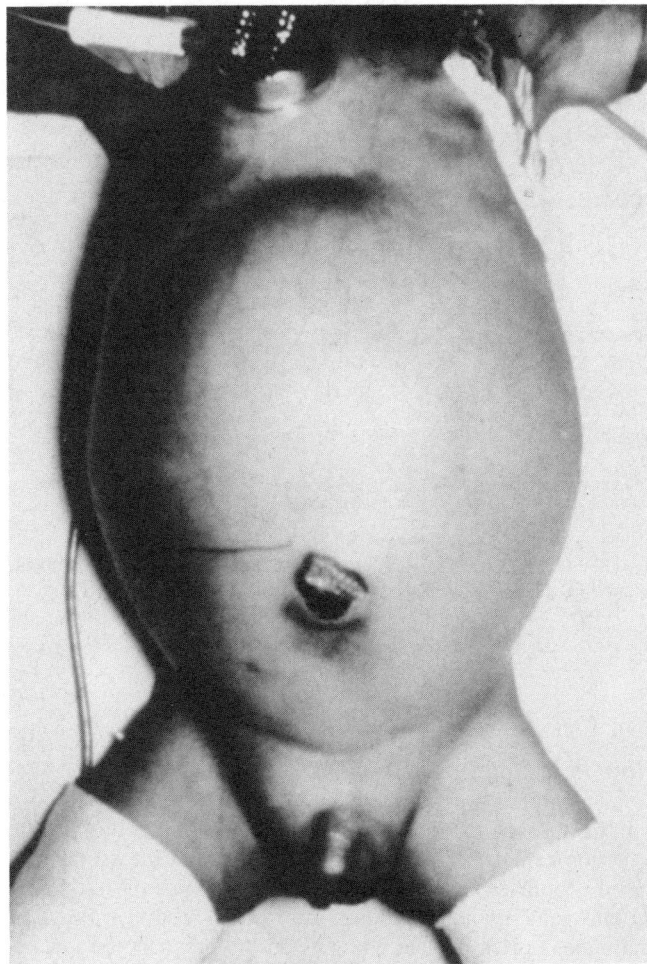

FIGURE 60–9. Photograph of chest and distended abdomen of a neonate with necrotizing enterocolitis prior to exploratory laparotomy.

cular coagulation may appear. Pneumatosis intestinalis (gas in the intestinal wall) is considered pathognomonic of NEC and may be associated with the presence of portal venous gas.

What Does Medical Management Entail?

Medical management of NEC includes discontinuation of enteral feeding, orogastric or nasogastric decompression of the stomach, intravenous antibiotics, and institution of parenteral hyperalimentation. Specific blood products, such as platelets and FFP, may be required to correct thrombocytopenia (platelets $<100,000 \cdot mm^{3-1}$) and any coagulopathy.

Indications for surgical intervention vary.[95] The only universally accepted criterion is perforation of the bowel wall with pneumoperitoneum. Other possible indications include positive findings on paracentesis, erythema of the abdominal wall, or a fixed abdominal mass. The appearance of the intestine at the time of laparotomy is shown in Figure 60–10.

How Is Anesthesia Managed?

Anesthetic management includes the same airway concerns and options previously discussed for the abdominal wall defects and pyloric stenosis. Most of these patients are prema-

ture; therefore, the usual problems and risks associated with hyperoxia and hypothermia apply. If the disease has evolved to sepsis and peritonitis, third space fluid losses may be large, necessitating vigorous fluid resuscitation. Invasive arterial pressure monitoring is usually necessary. Nitrous oxide is not used because it might contribute to intestinal distention and an increase in the volume of intraluminal gas pockets.

PATENT DUCTUS ARTERIOSUS

What Are the Characteristics?

The term *patent ductus arteriosus* (PDA) signifies only that a remnant of the normal fetal circulation remains open for an abnormally long period after birth. It provides no information about the direction of blood flow across the shunt or the underlying pathologic processes that may be responsible for continued patency of the ductus. Normally, the elevated Pao_2 after birth promotes functional (and later, anatomic) closure of the ductus within the first days of life.

Infants with a symptomatic PDA typically are premature and have left-to-right shunting of blood across the ductus and various degrees of respiratory distress syndrome and congestive heart failure. Infants with certain forms of congenital heart disease (e.g., tricuspid or pulmonary atresia) may depend on patency of the ductus to provide pulmonary blood flow. Those with PPHN have increased PVR causing a right-to-left shunt across the ductus. Ligation of a patent ductus in such patients generally is not indicated and may induce abrupt right ventricular failure.[96] A small number of otherwise healthy term infants also may have a PDA, but these cases are thought to be related to a defect in the quantity of smooth muscle in the ductal wall.[97]

What Are the Clinical Signs?

Clinical features of PDA with predominant left-to-right shunting include a typical continuous or systolic cardiac murmur, hyperactive precordium, widened pulse pressure (>35 mm Hg), bounding peripheral pulses, and findings of respira-

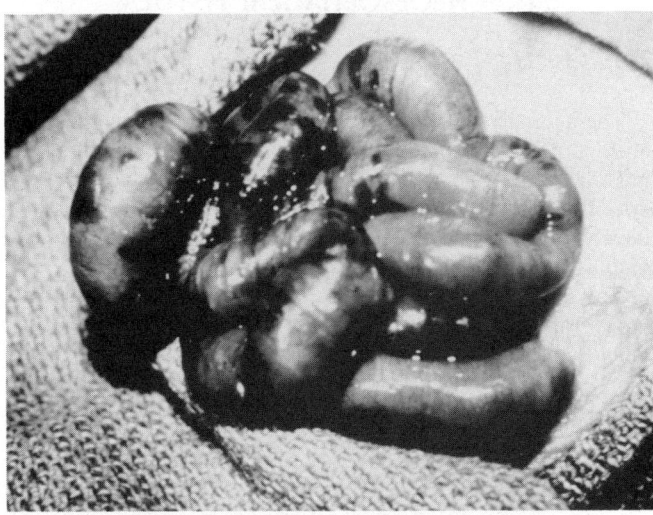

FIGURE 60–10. Intestine of a patient with necrotizing enterocolitis during exploratory laparotomy. Note dark patches of intestinal wall necrosis.

tory distress. The heart is enlarged (as seen on a chest radiograph), with evidence of volume overload of the pulmonary vasculature. Diagnosis is confirmed by echocardiography. Initial management includes fluid restriction, diuresis, mechanical ventilation, and treatment with a prostaglandin synthetase inhibitor, such as indomethacin, in appropriate candidates.[98]

How Is Anesthesia Managed?

Surgical ligation of the patent ductus is undertaken in patients who have refractory respiratory or cardiac failure and who have failed medical therapy. These neonates are usually critically ill. They frequently are already intubated and receiving conventional support or high-frequency ventilation and continuous infusions of inotropic agents.

Patients are placed in the right lateral decubitus position just before the procedure. Monitoring should include a right precordial stethoscope and an arterial line in most instances.

Fluids

Preoperative fluid restriction and diuretic therapy often induce a hypovolemic state. Many patients benefit from a bolus (10 mL · kg^{-1}) of crystalloid or colloid before the induction of anesthesia.[99]

Induction and Maintenance

Induction is typically accomplished with a combination of narcotic (fentanyl, 10–50 µg · kg^{-1}) and a nondepolarizing relaxant. It is usually necessary to increase the FIo$_2$ and mean airway pressure when the thoracic cavity is opened and the left lung is compressed. Occlusion of the PDA normally is associated with elevation of the systemic blood pressure and narrowing of the pulse pressure.

My practice is to monitor Spo$_2$ and peripheral pulses with a pulse oximeter both pre- and postductally in the event that the subclavian artery or aortic arch is occluded or ligated erroneously. The procedure of surgical ligation of the ductus arteriosus usually requires approximately 30 minutes.

TRACHEOESOPHAGEAL FISTULA

What Is It?

The anomaly of tracheoesophageal fistula (TEF) and esophageal atresia (EA) includes various anatomic defects; representative lesions are shown in Figure 60–11. In approximately 80% of cases, the defect consists of EA with a distal fistula between the lower trachea and the segment of esophagus extending upward from the stomach.

The disorder has an incidence of 1 in 3500 live births and an overall survival of 90%.[100] It is associated with other congenital anomalies in 30% to 50% of patients, the most common of these being cardiovascular and other gastrointestinal defects (imperforate anus). A complex of congenital anomalies known as the *VATER association* is found in approximately 10% of patients with TEF. In addition to TEF/EA, this "syndrome" consists of vertebral, anal, renal, and radial bony abnormalities.[101] Approximately one third of newborns with TEF/EA and esophageal atresia are premature.

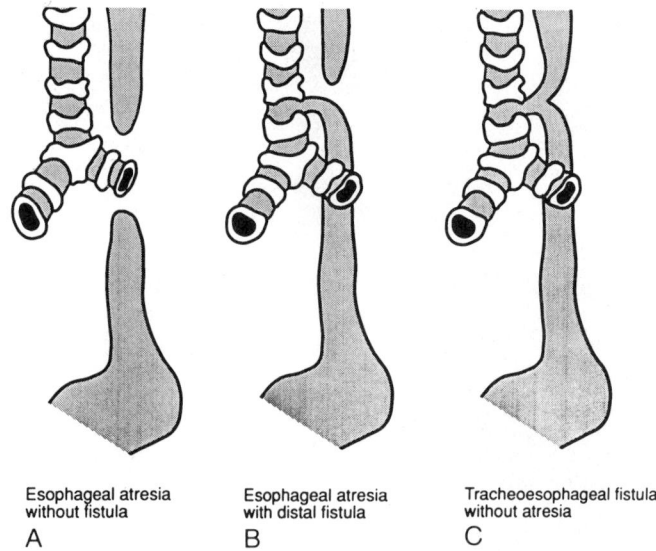

Esophageal atresia without fistula
A

Esophageal atresia with distal fistula
B

Tracheoesophageal fistula without atresia
C

FIGURE 60–11. Three configurations of the TEF/EA complex. *A*, EA without fistula. *B*, Depiction of the most common variant of TEF/EA. *C*, Depiction of an "H-type" fistula.

How Is It Diagnosed?

In most cases, the diagnosis is made shortly after birth when a suction catheter cannot be advanced through the esophagus into the stomach or when respiratory symptoms of coughing, choking, and cyanosis develop after initial feedings. Polyhydramnios is often present with EA during pregnancy. In cases without fistula, no gas is demonstrable within the abdomen.

Preoperative evaluation should include instillation of a small amount of contrast material (barium or metrizamide) into the blind esophageal pouch (Fig. 60–12) to help define the extent of atresia and any proximal fistula (rare). Additionally, ultrasonographic evaluation of the renal and cardiac systems is warranted to identify the existence of significant associated lesions.

What Should Be Done Preoperatively?

Before surgery, the goal of management in patients with TEF/EA is to minimize pulmonary complications through strict observance of NPO status. The patient's head is elevated, and continuous suction of the proximal esophageal pouch is carried out, along with provision of supplemental O$_2$ as required. Bronchoscopy is frequently performed to define the existence and location of the TEF (if present) and the presence of any other defects, such as a laryngeal cleft or tracheomalacia.

Spontaneous ventilation should be maintained during bronchoscopy before ligation of the fistula to minimize the passage of gas under positive pressure through the fistula and into the gastrointestinal tract. In the event of a large TEF with significant gastric distention, a small-caliber suction catheter may be passed through the fistula to decompress the stomach, after which a Fogarty's balloon catheter is advanced to occlude the fistula until the surgical ligation is performed. After bronchoscopy, the infant is intubated.

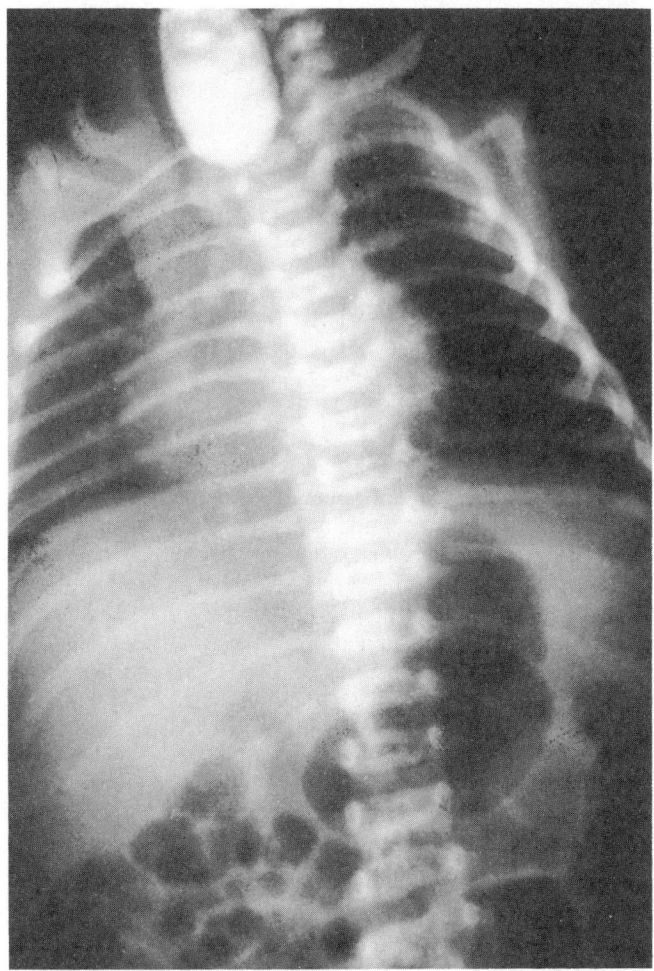

FIGURE 60–12. Chest radiograph of a patient with EA. The collection of barium in a dilated, blind upper esophageal pouch is demonstrated.

How Is Anesthesia Managed?

Intubation

When bronchoscopy is not required before the surgical procedure, the anesthesiologist is faced with the question of whether to perform awake intubation or a rapid-sequence induction with an intravenous agent and muscle relaxant. In light of improved monitoring techniques and recognition of neonatal anesthetic requirements, I intubate after administering intravenous anesthetics unless airway anomalies make intubation difficult or the patient is moribund. Succinylcholine is typically used to allow rapid return of spontaneous ventilation.

Endotracheal Tube Position

After intubation, the tip of the tracheal tube should be positioned distal to the fistula but above the carina. It is sometimes helpful to rotate the tube 90° from its usual insertion orientation so that the bevel is angled anteriorly, allowing the distal part of the tube to cover the fistula opening in the posterior tracheal wall.

Another approach is to place the tracheal tube intentionally into either mainstem bronchus and then withdraw it slowly to the point at which bilateral breath sounds are auscultated. This maneuver places the tip of the tube below the level of the fistula in all but the lowest of abnormalities.

Patient's Position

Patients are typically placed in the left lateral decubitus position and the procedure of fistula ligation and esophageal anastomosis is effected through a lateral thoracotomy incision, usually with a retropleural approach.

Maintenance

Anesthesia is maintained with inhaled anesthetics or intravenous narcotics or both, depending on a patient's condition and whether extubation of the trachea after surgery is anticipated. Nitrous oxide should be avoided because it may contribute to abdominal distention and often is tolerated poorly during thoracotomy when one lung is compressed and deflated.

Extubation

The decision to extubate is based on the knowledge of a patient's preoperative pulmonary status, the type of anesthetic administered, and any coexisting medical conditions. The passage of suction catheters into the trachea beyond the level of the fistula or the esophagus should be avoided out of concern that they may disrupt the fistula ligation or esophageal repair.

CONGENITAL DIAPHRAGMATIC HERNIA

What Is It?

Congenital diaphragmatic hernia (CDH) has an incidence of 1 in 2000 to 5000 live births. It most commonly involves the herniation of abdominal contents (stomach, spleen, liver, and intestine) through the left posterolateral diaphragm at the site of Bochdalek's foramen. It is thought to occur at approximately the eighth week of gestation as a result of the premature return of the midgut to the abdominal cavity from the umbilical stalk. Separation of the pleural and peritoneal cavities by closure of the diaphragm does not occur until the 9th to 12th week of gestation. In a small percentage of cases, herniation of abdominal organs also can occur through the substernal sinus (Morgagni's foramen) or the esophageal hiatus.

What Are the Effects?

The presence of midgut structures within the thoracic cavity impedes normal lung development, resulting in pulmonary hypoplasia, which is often bilateral but more severe on the ipsilateral side of the hernia. Pulmonary hypoplasia is marked by reduced lung weight, smaller numbers of terminal bronchioles and alveoli, and a significant reduction in the total cross-sectional area of the pulmonary vascular bed.[102] This abnormality and propensity to develop pulmonary hypertension, despite operative reduction of the hernia, are responsible for the persistent overall mortality of approximately 50%.

How Is It Diagnosed?

The diagnosis of CDH is based on the demonstration of gas-filled loops of bowel in the chest (Fig. 60–13), often with a shift of mediastinal structures to the opposite side. Clinical signs include a scaphoid abdomen, barrel chest, reduced or absent breath sounds on the side of the hernia, and, in a small number of patients, bowel sounds in the chest. Various degrees of respiratory distress may be observed, depending on the amount of herniated viscera and the degree of pulmonary hypoplasia. Other congenital anomalies frequently associated with CDH include malrotation of the intestine (50%), congenital heart disease (23%), and central nervous system and genitourinary disorders (15–20%).

How Is It Treated?

CDH historically was one of the true neonatal surgical emergencies requiring operative intervention within the first several hours of extrauterine life. In some cases and institutions, when a patient has severe respiratory distress shortly after birth, this approach is still followed. However, in many centers, the timing of surgery is varied depending on coexisting congenital problems, the degree of respiratory compro-

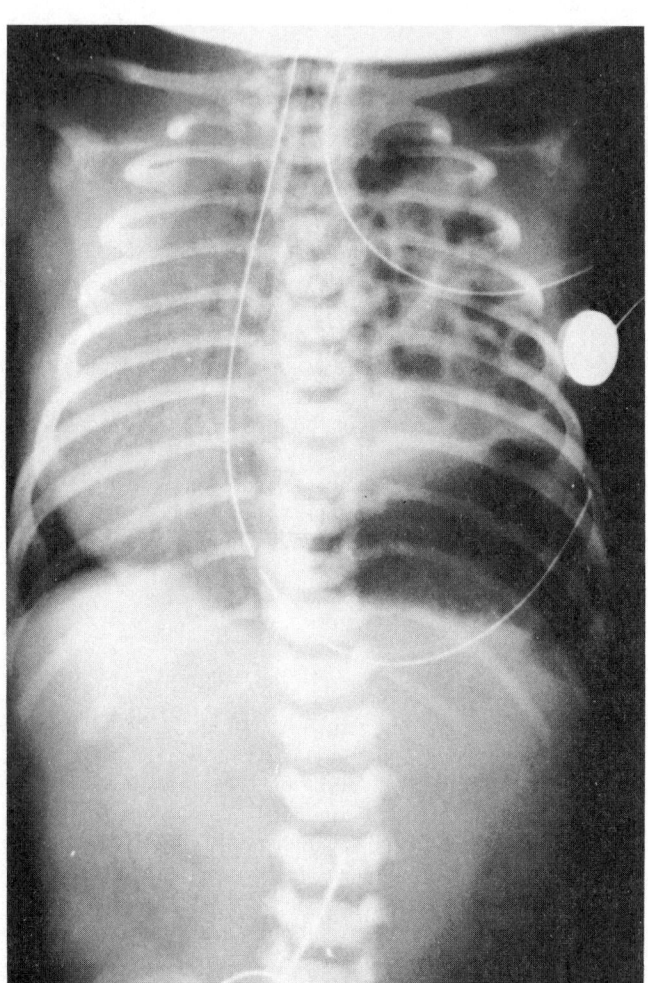

FIGURE 60–13. Left-sided congenital diaphragmatic hernia, with loops of intestine in left hemithorax.

mise, and the equipment and technology available to manage this group of critically ill neonates.

Preoperative Stabilization

Infants with respiratory distress cannot be expected to improve significantly without surgical repair of the hernia, but surgery alone usually does not "cure" these patients. Increased reactivity of the pulmonary circulation and pulmonary hypertension may persist or worsen postoperatively. For this reason, many neonates with CDH today undergo a period of stabilization and medical evaluation before surgery. If the equipment and appropriate personnel are available, patients may be supported by ECMO before, during, and after surgery.[103] Because of the high mortality rate among these babies, a range of management plans exists; no single standard or time for operative intervention is generally accepted.

Preoperative treatment includes orogastric or nasogastric tube decompression of the stomach, positioning in a semi-upright manner to minimize compression of lung tissue by abdominal contents, and conservative intravenous fluid therapy to avoid volume overload and exacerbation of pulmonary hypertension. Conditions that induce or contribute to pulmonary vasoconstriction, such as hypothermia, acidosis, hypoxemia, and hypercarbia, must be treated.[104] Infants with early respiratory distress generally require intubation and mechanical ventilation before surgery.

How Is Anesthesia Managed?

Induction

Mask ventilation should be avoided. This technique often forces gas into the gastrointestinal tract and exacerbates pulmonary compression.[89] Intubation may be accomplished either awake or, in stable patients, after rapid-sequence intravenous induction. After intubation, restriction of the PIP to 20 to 25 cm H_2O minimizes the chance of creating a pneumothorax. The temptation to inflate the atelectatic hypoplastic lung(s) aggressively must be resisted.

Rapid respiratory rates of 60 to 80 breaths per minute help to compensate for smaller than normal tidal volumes and restricted PIPs. This approach may also help to induce a mild state of hypocarbia and respiratory alkalosis, alleviating pulmonary vasoconstriction.

Nonventilatory strategies to reduce PVR include administration of direct vasodilating or α-blocking medications, such as sodium nitroprusside, nitroglycerin, prostaglandin E_1, tolazoline, or chlorpromazine. These vasodilators often are begun in the presence of poor systemic oxygenation and pulmonary hypertension refractory to nonpharmacologic manipulation. They predispose to systemic hypotension and frequently require simultaneous administration of increased fluid and a combined inotrope/vasopressor such as dopamine.

Maintenance

Anesthesia for CDH repair is usually provided with a combination of narcotics and nondepolarizing muscle relaxants. In some cases, anesthesia with a narcotic (fentanyl) or isoflurane may lower PVR and has been maintained postoperatively.[105] Most surgeons reduce the hernia and repair the diaphragm through an upper abdominal incision. The abdominal cavity may be underdeveloped, as in omphalocele and gastroschisis.

Tight abdominal closure sometimes contributes to postoperative respiratory compromise and vena caval compression, with concomitant reduction of venous return and cardiac output. Intraoperatively, close attention must be paid to body temperature maintenance, the possibility of pneumothorax with sudden cardiopulmonary compromise (particularly in the hemithorax opposite the hernia), intravascular fluid volume, and acid-base balance.

Postoperative Care

Completion of the operative procedure is not the end of the challenge in caring for these patients. The classic ''honeymoon period'' of improved ventilation and oxygenation observed immediately postoperatively is often abruptly terminated by recurrent bouts of pulmonary hypertension, hypercapnia, and hypoxemia. Intensive medical maneuvers to influence PVR are required.

NEONATAL RESUSCITATION

The subject of neonatal resuscitation encompasses the provision of life support and interventions within the delivery room, NICU, and operating room. Although the underlying disease or impaired physiologic processes leading to cardiorespiratory arrest or profound hemodynamic instability may vary in these settings, the fundamental principles of resuscitation outlined in the final section of this chapter are generally the same.

Six per cent of the approximately 3.8 million babies born each year in the United States require life support in the delivery room or nursery; in babies with a birth weight <1500 g, the requirement for resuscitation rises to 80%.[106] In most cases, the need for neonatal resuscitation can be anticipated on the basis of maternal history, antenatal diagnostic techniques, and fetal monitoring. Adequate resuscitation involves the skills of at least two to three people. For these reasons, anesthesiologists must have a sound understanding of neonatal resuscitation techniques.

When Is It Necessary?

Conditions that place a neonate at increased risk of asphyxia and requiring resuscitation are listed in Table 60–6; these may be divided into maternal, delivery-related, and fetal/neonatal factors.

Apgar Scoring

The Apgar scoring system remains in nearly universal use to assess a neonate's general condition and degree of compromise after delivery.[107] It is based on five objective measurements: (1) heart rate, (2) respiratory effort, (3) muscle tone, (4) reflex irritability, and (5) color. A score from 0 to 2 is assigned for each clinical sign, with a maximum possible score of 10, at 1- and 5-minute intervals after birth.

A number of caveats must be remembered in using Apgar scores. First, resuscitation must not be withheld until an Apgar

TABLE 60–6. Conditions That Place Neonates at Increased Risk for Requiring Resuscitation

Maternal	Delivery	Fetal/Neonatal
Age >35 years	Cesarean section	Meconium staining of amniotic fluid
Diabetes mellitus	Abnormal fetal presentations	Prematurity
Toxemia of pregnancy	Prolapsed umbilical cord	Multiple gestations
Hypertension	Cord compression	Intrauterine fetal growth retardation
Anemia	Maternal hypotension	Polyhydramnios
Blood type isoimmunization	Use of forceps (other than low elective)	Oligohydramnios
Antepartum hemorrhage (placenta previa or abruptio placentae)	Prolonged rupture of membranes	Immature lecithin-to-sphingomyelin ratio
Drug therapy (narcotics, lithium, recreational drugs, magnesium, alcohol)	Difficulty with delivery	Fetal malformation (diaphragmatic hernia, congenital heart disease)
Previous fetal or neonatal death	Prolonged labor	Gestation >42 weeks
Poor or no prenatal care		Indices of fetal distress during labor (low fetal scalp pH, abnormal fetal monitoring tracing)
Maternal infections		
Low estriol levels		

score is obtained; assessment of a patient begins immediately at birth, and appropriate interventions are applied as indicated. Second, the scoring system was not designed for premature infants, in whom several of the measurements can be difficult to apply meaningfully.[108] Third, scores should not be used in an attempt to predict long-term neurologic outcome.[109]

What Is the Basic Approach?

Successful neonatal resuscitation depends on appropriate anticipation of neonates at increased risk of asphyxia, proper preparation of equipment, the environment, personnel who will be caring for the patient, and prompt initiation of resuscitation maneuvers. Figure 60–14 provides an algorithm for resuscitation in the delivery room; with modification for specific patient problems and therapies, the outlined principles can be applied in the NICU or operating room.

Initial Maneuvers

The interventions that compose the neonatal resuscitation procedure begin with simple, noninvasive, and commonly required maneuvers and progress to the increasingly sophisticated steps required by smaller numbers of patients.[106] Simple initial steps include placing a patient in the supine or lateral position under a radiant warmer with the head in a neutral position as drying and suctioning are provided. Most newborns begin spontaneous ventilations with these maneuvers, but if necessary, additional stimulation can be achieved by slapping or flicking the soles of the feet and rubbing an infant's back. Assessment of heart rate, respiratory activity, and color is undertaken at this time.

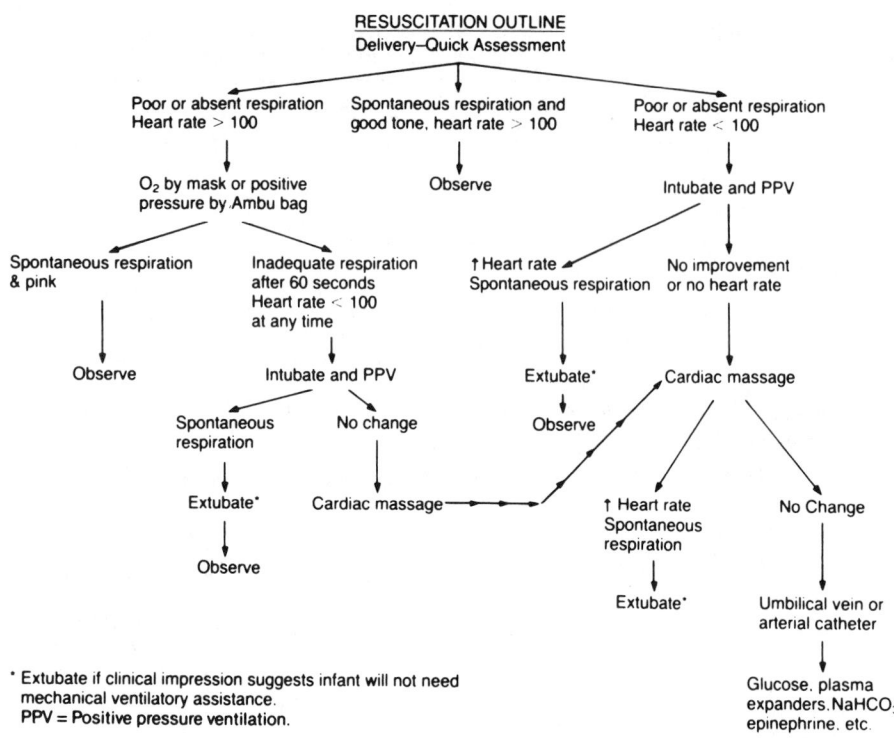

FIGURE 60–14. Algorithm for neonatal resuscitation. (From Patz A: Retinopathy of prematurity. *In* Duane's Clinical Ophthalmology. Vol. 3. Rasman WS, Jaeger EA (eds). Philadelphia, JB Lippincott, 1990.)

Ventilation

Bag-Mask

If a neonate remains apneic or has a heart rate <100 beats per minute, bag-valve-mask ventilation should be instituted. In newborns known or strongly suspected of having a diaphragmatic hernia, positive-pressure ventilation should be commenced through an endotracheal tube. Ventilations should be provided at a rate of 40 breaths per minute; initial lung inflation may require a peak pressure of 30 to 40 cm H_2O or higher, and subsequent breaths should require 15 to 20 cm H_2O pressure. Important is not so much what the airway pressure manometer shows but that gas exchange is accomplished at the lowest feasible inflation pressure.

Tracheal Intubation

If mask ventilation is difficult, causes including poor mask fit, obstruction of the airway by the tongue, or congenital airway abnormalities must be sought and the airway and head positions reassessed. In some cases, laryngoscopic examination of the upper airway and tracheal intubation are required.

After 15 to 30 seconds of adequate ventilation, the heart rate should be reassessed. Controlled ventilation may be stopped if the heart rate is >100 beats per minute and adequate spontaneous respirations are present. If the pulse is absent or the heart rate is <60 beats per minute, chest compressions should be started. If the heart rate is 60 to 100 beats per minute and rising, assisted ventilation should be continued but chest compressions may be withheld or stopped. In the event that a heart rate is <80 beats per minute and is not rising, both assisted ventilation and chest compressions should be provided.

Chest Compressions

Chest compressions in neonates should be provided at a rate of at least 120 beats per minute, with the goal of depressing the sternum ½ to ¼ inch with each stroke. Correct finger placement for compressions can be accomplished in two ways.[110] In one, the thumbs are placed side by side over the middle one third of the infant's sternum while the fingers on each side encircle the trunk and support the back. In the other, the resuscitator's middle and ring fingers are used to provide two-finger compressions one finger's breadth below the nipple line. The spontaneous heart rate (if any) should be checked periodically by auscultation or by lightly grasping the base of the umbilical cord. If it exceeds 80 beats per minute, compressions may be stopped.

What Is the Role of Drug Therapy?

Indicated Agents

Despite positive-pressure ventilation with O_2 and chest compressions, a small number of neonates may require drug and fluid therapy. Drugs that have a role in the acute phase of neonatal resuscitation include epinephrine, naloxone, glucose, sodium bicarbonate, and plasma volume expanders (Table 60–7). Calcium chloride or calcium gluconate should not be used without a specific diagnosis involving hypocalcemia or hyperkalemia. The vagolytic agent atropine, although useful in the initial resuscitation of older infants and children, is not a first-line drug in neonatal resuscitation.[111] It may have a role in the NICU after definitive therapies have begun.

Routes of Administration

Umbilical Vein

The preferred route of medication administration in neonatal resuscitation when no vascular access is in place is the umbilical vein.[112] This vessel can be located easily and cannulated with a 3.5 or 5 French umbilical catheter passed just below the skin level until free flow of blood is observed. Care must

TABLE 60–7. Primary Medications Useful in Neonatal Resuscitation

Medication	Indications	Dose	Concentration	Route
Epinephrine	Asystole, persistent heart rate <80 beats per minute	0.01–0.03 mg · kg^{-1} (perhaps as much as 0.2 mg · kg^{-1})	1:10,000 (0.1 mg · mL^{-1})	Intravenous, intratracheal
Naloxone	Documented or strongly suspected narcotic-induced ventilatory depression	0.1 mg · kg^{-1}	0.4–1.0 mg · mL^{-1}	Intravenous, intratracheal, intramuscular
Glucose	Confirmed or suspected hypoglycemia	200 mg · kg^{-1} to 1 g · kg^{-1}	200 mg · mL^{-1}	Intravenous
Sodium bicarbonate	Documented or strongly suspected metabolic acidosis	2 mEq · kg^{-1}	0.5 mEq · mL^{-1}	Intravenous
Volume expander	Hypovolemia or shock (weak pulses or hypotension)	10–20 mL · kg^{-1} (may require several doses)	Fresh whole blood (heparinized from placenta) Packed red blood cells (diluted with normal saline to 40% hematocrit) Fresh-frozen plasma 5% albumin Plasma protein fraction Lactated Ringer's solution Normal saline	Intravenous

be taken to locate the tip of the catheter either just below skin level or well beyond the liver into the high IVC so that hypertonic solutions are not infused into the liver.

Peripheral Veins

Peripheral veins in the scalp and extremities are difficult to cannulate during resuscitation, and medications administered into them may take a prolonged time to reach the central circulation.

Trachea

The intratracheal route can be used to administer epinephrine, naloxone, epinephrine, and lidocaine. Recommendations for intratracheal doses range from one- to fivefold the standard intravenous dose for the drug. The effectiveness of an intratracheal drug can be increased by diluting it with 2 to 3 mL of normal saline and injecting through a suction catheter or feeding tube passed to the tip of the endotracheal tube of the intubated patient.

References

1. Webb E (Quoted in audience participation discussion of Ward RJ, Crawford EW, Stevenson JK: Anesthetic experience for infants under 2500 grams weight. Anesth Analg 1970; 49:767.)
2. Purcell-Jones G, Dorman F, Sumner E: Paediatric anaesthetists' perceptions of neonatal and infant pain. Pain 1988; 33:181.
3. Anand KJS, Hickey PR: Pain and its effects in the human neonate and fetus. N Engl J Med 1987; 317:1321.
4. Berry FA, Gregory GA: Do premature infants require anesthesia for surgery? (Editorial). Anesthesiology 1987; 67:291.
5. Anand KJS, Aynsley-Green A: Measuring the severity of surgical stress in newborn infants. J Pediatr Surg 1988; 23:297.
6. Ferris BG, Mead J, Opie LH: Partitioning of respiratory flow resistance in man. J Appl Physiol 1964; 19:653.
7. Eckenoff JE: Some anatomic considerations of the infant larynx influencing endotracheal anesthesia. Anesthesiology 1951; 12:401.
8. Reid L: The lung: its growth and remodeling in health and diseases. Am J Roentgenol 1977; 129:777.
9. Cook DR, March JH: Pediatric anesthetic pharmacology. *In* Cook DR, Marcy JH (eds). Neonatal Anesthesia. Pasadena, CA, Appleton-Davies, 1988, pp 87–125.
10. Mansell A, Bryan AC, Levison H: Airway closure in children. J Appl Physiol 1972; 33:711.
11. Harris TR: Physiological principles. *In* Assisted Ventilation of the Neonate. Goldsmith JP, Karotkin EH (eds). Philadelphia, WB Saunders, 1988, pp 22–69.
12. Keens TG, Bryan AC, Levison H, et al: Developmental pattern of muscle fiber types in human ventilatory muscles. J Appl Physiol 1978; 44:909.
13. Friesen RH: Neonatal physiologic adaptations and their anesthetic implications. *In* Perinatal Anesthesia and Critical Care. Diaz JH (ed). Philadelphia, WB Saunders, 1991, pp 263–280.
14. Hagen PT, Scholz DG, Edwards WD: Incidence and size of patent foramen ovale during the first ten decades: a necropsy study of 965 normal hearts. Mayo Clin Proc 1984; 59:17.
15. Friedman WF: The intrinsic physiologic properties of the developing heart. Prog Cardiovasc Dis 1972; 15:87.
16. Goudsouzian NG: Anatomy and physiology in relation to pediatric anesthesia. *In* Anesthesia and Uncommon Pediatric Diseases. Katz J, Steward DJ (eds). Philadelphia, WB Saunders, 1987, pp 1–11.
17. Shaffr SE, Norman ME: Renal function and renal failure in the newborn. Clin Perinatol 1989; 16:199.
18. Larson L, Aperia A, Elinder G: Structural and functional development of the nephron. Acta Paediatr Scand (Suppl) 1983; 305:56.
19. Downes JJ, Heiser MS: Temperature regulation in the pediatric patient. Semin Anesth 1984; 3:37.
20. Borland LM: Persistent pulmonary hypertension of the newborn. *In* Neonatal Anesthesia. Cook DR, Marcy LH (eds). Pasadena, CA, Appleton-Davies, 1988, pp 49–61.
21. Rudolph A: High pulmonary vascular resistance after birth. Clin Pediatr 1980; 19:585.
22. Hagedorn MI, Gardner SL, Abman SH: Respiratory diseases. *In* Handbook of Neonatal Intensive Care. Merenstein GB, Gardner SL (eds). St Louis, CV Mosby, 1989, pp 365–426.
23. Levin DL, Heymann MA, Kitterman JA, et al: Persistent pulmonary hypertension of the newborn infant. J Pediatr 1976; 89:626.
24. Fox WW, Duara S: Persistent pulmonary hypertension in the neonate: diagnosis and treatment. J Pediatr 1983; 103:505.
25. Ward RM: Persistent pulmonary hypertension. *In* Current Therapy in Neonatal-Perinatal Medicine. 2nd ed. Nelson NM (ed). Toronto, BC Decker, 1990, pp 331–338.
26. Daberkow E, Washington RL: Cardiovascular diseases and surgical interventions. *In* Handbook of Neonatal Intensive Care. Merenstein GB, Gardner SL (eds). St Louis, CV Mosby, 1989, pp 427–465.
27. Thompson AE, Cook DR: Respiratory care. *In* Neonatal Anesthesia. Cook DR, Marcy JH (eds). Pasadena, CA, Appleton-Davies, 1988, pp 203–232.
28. Merritt TA, Hallman M, Bloom BT, et al: Prophylactic treatment of very premature infants with surfactant. N Engl J Med 1986; 315:785.
29. Minarcik CJ, Beachy P: Neurologic disorders. *In* Handbook of Neonatal

Intensive Care. 2nd ed. Merenstein GB, Gardner SL (eds). St Louis, CV Mosby, 1989, pp 501–530.

30. Hegyi T: Intraventricular hemorrhage. *In* Current Therapy in Neonatal-Perinatal Medicine. 2nd ed. Nelson NM (ed). Toronto, BC Decker, 1990, pp 289–292.

31. Friesen RH, Honda AT, Thieme RE: Changes in anterior fontanel pressure in preterm infants during tracheal intubation. Anesth Analg 1987; 66:874.

32. Diaz JH: Anesthetic management of premature neonates, term neonates, and infants. *In* Perinatal Anesthesia and Critical Care. Diaz JH (ed). Philadelphia, WB Saunders, 1991, pp 281–321.

33. Mosijczuk AD, Ellis-Vaiani C: Hematologic diseases. *In* Handbook of Neonatal Intensive Care. 2nd ed. Merenstein GB, Gardner SL (eds). St Louis, CV Mosby, 1989, pp 287–317.

34. Keyes WG, Donohue PK, Spivak JL, et al: Assessing the need for transfusion of premature infants and role of hematocrit, clinical signs, and erythropoietin levels. Pediatrics 1989; 84:412.

35. Joshi A, Gerhardt T, Shandloff P: Blood transfusion effect on the respiratory pattern of preterm infants. Pediatrics 1987; 80:79.

36. Welborn LG, Hannallah RS, Luban NLC, et al: Anemia and postoperative apnea in former preterm infants. Anesthesiology 1991; 74:1003.

37. Phelps DL: Retinopathy of prematurity. *In* Current Therapy in Neonatal-Perinatal Medicine. 2nd ed. Nelson NM (ed). Toronto, BC Decker, 1990, pp 350–353.

38. Porat R: Care of the infant with retinopathy of prematurity. Clin Perinatol 1984; 11:123.

39. Stafani FH, Ehalt H: Non-oxygen-induced retinitis proliferans and retinal detachment in full-term infants. Br J Ophthalmol 1974; 58:490.

40. Flynn JT: Retinopathy of prematurity. Pediatr Clin North Am 1987; 34:1487.

41. Cross KW: Cost of preventing retrolental fibroplasia. Lancet 1973; 2:954.

42. Martyn LJ: Pediatric ophthalmology. *In* Nelson Textbook of Pediatrics. 12th ed. Behrman RE, Vaughan VC III (eds). Philadelphia, WB Saunders, 1983, pp 1761–1762.

43. Kalina RE: Update on retinopathy of prematurity. West J Med 1990; 153:188.

44. Sternberg P, Lopez PF, Lambert HM, et al: Controversies in the management of retinopathy of prematurity. Am J Ophthalmology 1992; 113:198.

45. Brown GC, Tasman WS, Naidoff M, et al: Systemic complications associated with retinal cryoablation for retinopathy of prematurity. Ophthalmology 1990; 97:855.

46. Steward DJ: Preterm infants are more prone to complications following minor surgery than are term infants. Anesthesiology 1982; 56:304.

47. Welborn LG, Ramirez N, Oh TH, et al: Evaluation of anesthetic risks in premature infants. Anesthesiology 1984; 61:A417.

48. Mayhew JF, Bourke DL, Guinee WS: Evaluation of the premature infant at risk for postoperative complications. Can J Anaesth 1987; 34:627.

49. Kao LC, Durand DJ, Phillips BL, et al: Oral theophylline and diuretics improve pulmonary mechanics in infants with bronchopulmonary dysplasia. J Pediatr 1987; 111:439.

50. Noseworthy J, Duran C, Khine HH: Postoperative apnea in a full-term infant. Anesthesiology 1989; 70:879.

51. Daily WJR, Klaws M, Meyer HBB: Apnea in premature infants: monitoring, incidence, heart rate changes, and an effect of environment temperature. Pediatrics 1969; 43:510.

52. Kurth CD, Spitzer AR, Broennle AM, et al: Postoperative apnea in preterm infants. Anesthesiology 1987; 66:483.

53. Welborn LG, Hannallah RS, Fink R: High-dose caffeine suppresses postoperative apnea in former preterm infants. Anesthesiology 1989; 71:347.

54. Watcha MF, Thach BT, Gunter JB: Postoperative apnea after caudal anesthesia in an ex-premature infant. Anesthesiology 1989; 71:613.

55. Blumenthal I, Ebel A, Pildes RS: Effect of posture on the pattern of stomach emptying in the newborn. Pediatrics 1979; 63:532.

56. Tomomasa T, Hyman PE, Itoh K, et al: Gastroduodenal motility in neonates: response to human milk compared with cow's milk formula. Pediatrics 1987; 80:4343.

57. Richards MPM, Bernal JF, Brackbill Y: Early behavioral differences: gender or circumcision? Dev Psychobiol 1976; 9:89.

58. Salem MR, Wong AY, Mani M, et al: Premedicant drugs and gastric juice pH and volume in pediatric patients. Anesthesiology 1976; 44:216.

59. Noseworthy J, Duran C, Khine HH: Postoperative apnea in a full-term infant. Anesthesiology 1989; 70:879.

60. Marshall TA, Deeder R, Pai S, et al: Physiologic changes associated with endotracheal intubation in preterm infants. Crit Care Med 1984; 12:501.

61. Marcy TH, Cook DR: Basic neonatal anesthesia and monitoring. *In* Neonatal Anesthesia. Cook DR, Marcy JH (eds). Pasadena, CA, Appleton-Davies, 1988, pp 143–158.

62. Tochen ML: Orotracheal intubation in the newborn infant: a method for determining depth of tube insertion. J Pediatr 1979; 95:1050.

63. Finholt DA, Henry DB, Raphaely RC: Factors affecting leak around endotracheal tubes in children. Can Anaesth Soc J 1985; 32:326.

64. Gregory GA: Anesthesia for premature infants. *In* Pediatric Anesthesia. 2nd ed. Gregory GA (ed). New York, Churchill Livingstone, 1989, pp 803–832.

65. Spears RS, Yeh A, Fisher DM, et al: The ''educated hand''—can anesthesiologists assess changes in neonatal pulmonary compliance manually? Anesthesiology 1991; 75:693.

66. Steward DJ: Mechanical versus manual ventilation of the lungs of infants in the operating room (Response to letter to the editor). Anesthesiology 1992; 76:479.

67. Fox WW, Spitzer AR, Shutack JG: Positive-pressure ventilation: pressure- and time-cycled ventilators. *In* Assisted Ventilation of the Neonate. 2nd ed. Goldsmith JP, Karotkin EH (eds). Philadelphia, WB Saunders, 1988, pp 146–170.

68. Bain JA, Spoerel WE: A streamlined anesthetic system. Can Anaesth Soc J 1972; 19:426.

69. Miller DM: Breathing systems for use in anesthesia: evaluation using a physical lung model and classification. Br J Anaesth 1988; 60:555.

70. Badgwell JM, Wolf AR, McEvedy BA, et al: Fresh gas formulae do not accurately predict end-tidal P_{CO_2} in paediatric patients. Can J Anaesth 1988; 35:581.

71. Coté CJ: Pediatric equipment. *In* A Practice of Anesthesia for Infants and Children. 2nd ed. Coté CJ, Ryan JF, Todres ID, et al (eds). Philadelphia, WB Saunders Co, 1993, pp 483–504.

72. Metz RI, Lucking SE, Chaten FC, et al: Percutaneous catheterization of the axillary vein in infants and children. Pediatrics 1990; 85:531.

73. Coté CJ, Jobes DR, Schwartz AJ, et al: Two approaches to cannulation of a child's internal jugular vein. Anesthesiology 1979; 50:371.

74. Roberts JD, Todres ID, Coté CJ: Neonatal emergencies. *In* A Practice of Anesthesia for Infants and Children. 2nd ed. Coté CJ, Ryan JF, Todres ID, et al (eds). Philadelphia, WB Saunders, 1993, pp 225–246.

75. Furman EB, Roman GD, Lemmer LAS, et al: Specific therapy in water, electrolyte, and blood-volume replacement during pediatric surgery. Anesthesiology 1975; 42:187.

76. Liu LMP: Fluid management. *In* Coté CJ, Ryan JF, Todres ID, et al (eds). A Practice of Anesthesia for Infants and Children. 2nd ed. Philadelphia, WB Saunders, 1993, pp 171–182.

77. Shires T, Williams J, Brown F: Acute changes in extracellular fluids associated with major surgical procedures. Ann Surg 1961; 154:803.

78. American Society of Anesthesiologists: Standards for basic intraoperative monitoring. *In* Directory of Members, 1992. Park Ridge, IL, American society of Anesthesiologists, 1992.

79. Coté CJ, Rolf N, Liu LMP, et al: A single-blind study of combined pulse oximetry and capnography in children. Anesthesiology 1991; 74:980.

80. Rooth G, Huch A, Huch R: Transcutaneous oxygen monitors are reliable indicators of arterial oxygen tension (if used correctly). Pediatrics 1987; 79:283.

81. Coté CJ, Goldstein EA, Coté MA, et al: A single-blind study of pulse oximetry in children. Anesthesiology 1988; 68:184.

82. Partridge BL: Use of pulse oximetry as a non-invasive indicator of intravascular volume status. J Clin Monit 1987; 3:263.

83. Badgwell JM, McLeod ME, Lerman J, et al: End-tidal P_{CO_2} measurements sampled at the distal and proximal ends of the endotracheal tube in infants and children. Anesth Analg 1987; 66:959.

84. Gravenstein N: Capnometry in infants should not be done at lower sampling flow rates (Letter to the editor). J Clin Monit 1989; 5:63.

85. Katz S, Basel D, Branski D: Prenatal gastric dilatation and infantile hypertrophic pyloric stenosis. J Pediatr Surg 1988; 23:1021.

86. Bissonnette B, Sullivan PJ: Pyloric stenosis. Can J Anaesth 1991; 38:668.

87. Spicer RD: Infantile pyloric stenosis: a review. Br J Surg 1982; 69:128.

88. MacDonald NJ, Fitzpatrick GJ, Moore KD, et al: Anaesthesia for congenital hypertrophic pyloric stenosis: a review of 350 patients. Br J Anaesth 1987; 59:672.

89. Dierdorf SF, Krishna G: Anesthetic management of neonatal surgical emergencies. Anesth Analg 1981; 60:204.

90. Schwartz MZ, Tyson KRT, Milliorn K, et al: Staged reduction using a

Silastic sac is the treatment of choice for large congenital abdominal wall defects. J Pediatr Surg 1983; 18:713.

91. Philippart AI, Canty TG, Filler RM: Acute fluid volume requirements in infants with anterior abdominal wall defects. J Pediatr Surg 1972; 7:553.

92. Yaster M, Buck JR, Dudgeon DL, et al: Hemodynamic effects of primary closure of omphalocele/gastroschisis in human newborns. Anesthesiology 1988; 69:84.

93. Marcy JH, Cook DR: Common surgical conditions of the newborn. *In* Neonatal Anesthesia. Cook DR, Marcy JH (eds). Pasadena, CA, Appleton-Davies, 1988, pp 159–188.

94. Kosloske AM, Musemeche CA: Necrotizing enterocolitis of the neonate. Clin Perinatol 1989; 16:97.

95. Kliegman RM, Fanaroff AA: Necrotizing enterocolitis. N Engl J Med 1984; 310:1093.

96. Gersony WM: Patent ductus arteriosus in the neonate. Pediatr Clin North Am 1986; 33:545.

97. Gittenberger-de-Groot AC: Persistent ductus arteriosus: most probably a primary congenital malformation. Br Heart J 1977; 6:610.

98. Gersony WM, Peckham GJ, Ellison RC, et al: Effects of indomethacin in premature infants with patent ductus arteriosus: results of a national collaborative study. J Pediatr 1983; 102:895.

99. Robonson S, Gregory G: Fentanyl-air-oxygen anesthesia for ligation of patent ductus arteriosus in preterm infants. Anesth Analg 1981; 60:331.

100. Reyes HM, Meller JL, Loef D: Management of esophageal atresia and tracheoesophageal fistula. Clin Perinatol 1989; 16:79.

101. Barry JE, Auldist AW: The Vater association: one end of a spectrum of anomalies. Am J Dis Child 1974; 128:769.

102. Kitagawa M, Hislop A, Boyden EA, et al: Lung hypoplasia in congenital diaphragmatic hernia: a quantitative study of airway, artery, and alveolar development. Br J Surg 1971; 58:342.

103. Truog RD, Schena JA, Hershenson MB, et al: Repair of congenital diaphragmatic hernia during extracorporeal membrane oxygenation. Anesthesiology 1990; 72:720.

104. Tiefenbrunn LJ, Riemenschneider TA: Persistent pulmonary hypertension in the newborn. Am Heart J 1986; 111:564.

105. Vacanti JP, Crone RK: The pulmonary hemodynamic response to perioperative anesthesia in the treatment of high-risk infants with congenital diaphragmatic hernia. J Pediatr Surg 1984; 19:672.

106. American Heart Association: Neonatal resuscitation. JAMA 1992; 268:2276.

107. Apgar V: Proposal for method of evaluation of newborn infant. Anesth Analg 1953; 32:260.

108. Catlin EA, Carpenter MW, Brann BS IV, et al: The Apgar score revisited: influence of gestational age. J Pediatr 1986; 109:865.

109. Nelson KB, Ellenberg JH: Neonatal signs as predictors of cerebral palsy. Pediatrics 1979; 64:225.

110. Todres ID, Rogers MC: Methods of external cardiac massage in the newborn infant. J Pediatr 1975; 86:781.

111. Guidelines for cardiopulmonary resuscitation and emergency cardiac care. Part VII: Neonatal resuscitation. JAMA 1992; 268:2276.

112. Bloom RS, Cropley C: Textbook of Neonatal Resuscitation. Dallas, American Heart Association, 1987.

CHAPTER 61

The Pediatric Patient

TIMOTHY W. MARTIN, M.D.*

VINCENT G. JOHNSON, D.O.*

Physicians whose practices encompass both children and adults often must be reminded that pediatric patients are not simply "little adults." Within the realm of anesthetic practice, children pose a number of different problems and have requirements that separate them from adults, who are generally the foundation on which instruction and training in anesthesia are based.

Perhaps the most obvious differences between the juvenile and adult patient concern the physical size of the body and its constituent structures. Often related to variations in gross size are differences in physiologic processes and pharmacologic responses that have significant implications for the pediatric anesthesia practice. These differences are of greatest magnitude in the premature and term neonate and gradually diminish at varying rates over the first 10 to 15 years of life as anatomic, physiologic, and metabolic growth and maturation take place. By midadolescence, the teenage child may be considered physically (if not socially and psychologically) an adult for anesthetic purposes.

Because anatomic and physiologic differences are most profound in the neonatal and infant periods, they are considered in Chapter 60 ("The Neonate"). This chapter emphasizes the preoperative evaluation and preparation of the pediatric patient and common features of the induction, maintenance, and monitoring of anesthesia in children. Concluding sections discuss the postoperative problems encountered in the treatment of children as well as anesthetic approaches to pediatric laryngoscopy and bronchoscopy, tonsillectomy and pressure-equalizing tube insertion, and sedation for magnetic resonance imaging (MRI) procedures.

PREANESTHETIC ASSESSMENT: GENERAL CONSIDERATIONS

What Are Normal Vital Signs and Weights in Children?

Every clinician involved in providing anesthesia care for children should be aware of the actual and age-specific refer-

ence body weight and vital signs for each patient. Knowledge of this information provides the basis for a number of different anesthetic assessments and interventions in the preoperative, intraoperative, and postoperative periods. For example, the child's usual or baseline weight, heart rate, and blood pressure are useful in the evaluation of chronic disease states and fluid volume status during the preanesthetic assessment. Intraoperatively, the same parameters must be considered in determining drug dosages, intravenous fluid requirements, and appropriate hemodynamic responses to anesthesia and surgical stimulation. For these purposes, the data in Table 61–1 are provided as a reference.

What Information Must Be Exchanged Preoperatively?

The preanesthetic interview provides an opportunity for the anesthesiologist to obtain a great deal of information about the child's medical and surgical history, recent state of health, and general temperament, particularly as it relates to anticipated reactions to separation from the parents and to anesthetic induction. In addition, and as important, the interview serves to allow parents and older children an improved understanding of the anesthetic experience, perioperative period, and potential complications of anesthesia. Nothing substitutes for a frank, unhurried, and appropriately detailed discussion of what the patient and parents can expect on the day of surgery, both in and out of the operating room. To expect that the preoperative encounter should obviate the need for pharmacologic maneuvers to sedate the child prior to surgery is unrealistic. However, it should significantly allay parental anxieties and fears, which not uncommonly exceed those of the juvenile patient.

From the Parents and Child

Important information to be gathered includes current medications; any history of drug intolerances or allergies; previous surgical procedures or anesthetics, and the problems experienced with them; and general information that focuses on the

---

*The opinions expressed are those of the authors and do not necessarily reflect the views of the United States Air Force or the Department of Defense.

TABLE 61–1. Weights and Vital Signs for Children

Age	Resting Heart Rate (per minute)	Resting Blood Pressure (All Values ± 10 mm Hg)		Resting Respiratory Rate (per min)	Weight (kg), 50th Percentile	
		Males	Females		Males	Females
Newborn	120 (±25)	70/50	70/50	45 (±15)	3.4	3.2
6 mo	140 (±30)	95/50	90/50	40 (±10)	8	7
1 y	120 (±20)	95/55	95/50	35 (±10)	10	9.6
2 y	110 (±30)	95/60	95/60	35 (±5)	12.6	12
4 y	100 (±35)	90/55	90/55	25 (±8)	17	16
6 y	95 (±25)	95/60	95/60	22 (±7)	21	20
8 y	90 (±25)	100/60	100/60	22 (±7)	25	25
10 y	80 (±20)	100/65	100/65	22 (±7)	32	33
12 y	75 (±20)	105/65	110/70	20 (±5)	40	42
14 y	70 (±20)	110/65	110/70	20 (±5)	50	50

(Data from Hamill PW, Drizd TA, Johnson CL, et al: NCHS Growth Charts, 1976, Monthly Vital Statistics Report. US Department of Health, Education and Welfare, Washington, DC. Report of the Second Task Force on Blood Pressure Control in Children—1987. Pediatrics 1987; 79:1, *and* Baldwin GA: Vital signs for age. *In* Handbook of Pediatric Emergencies. Baldwin GA (ed). Boston, Little, Brown, & Co, 1989, p 46.)

cardiovascular and respiratory systems. For infants and toddlers, be sure to inquire about the gestational and neonatal periods and about any illnesses or difficulties that may have been encountered. If a chronic disease state or surgical condition with systemic manifestations is present, further specific questioning should be pursued to define the anticipated effect of the disorder on anesthesia and recovery. Postpubertal females should be specifically questioned for symptoms of anemia and the possibility of pregnancy.

To the Parents and Child

As indicated previously, information is exchanged bidirectionally during the preoperative interview. Specific points to be explained to the responsible adult or adults caring for the infant or school-age child include fasting guidelines, plans for premedication, the anticipated induction technique, vascular access and airway adjuncts (particularly if the latter are to remain in place postoperatively), plans for the use of blood products (if applicable), and any regional anesthetic techniques to be applied for anesthetic maintenance or postoperative analgesia. A description of what can be expected in the postanesthesia care unit (PACU) or intensive care unit (ICU) following surgery is also prudent.

What Pertinent Information Can Be Obtained from the Medical Record?

Previous Anesthetics

Although in the majority of cases sufficient information can be obtained in the course of the preanesthetic interview and the physical examination, in some instances, the medical record may provide invaluable data. This observation is perhaps most true with children who previously have experienced anesthesia; in this case, information regarding responses to premedication, ease of parental separation and induction, airway management, tolerance of anesthesia, and complications may be obtained.

Disease Processes

The records of children with disease processes likely to influence the response to anesthesia, such as cardiac and pul-

monary disorders, may contain details unavailable to or unknown by the parents. An example is cardiac catheterization or echocardiographic data in the child with congenital heart disease; such data may define anatomic abnormalities, the presence, direction, and degree of shunting, the existence of pulmonary hypertension, and an estimate of ventricular function. In children with symptoms of an upper respiratory tract infection (URI), an idea of the frequency and typical course of such infections can be obtained to assist in making the decision whether to proceed with or to reschedule surgery. The medical record also frequently indicates recent weights and vital signs and may list drug intolerances or allergies as well as any medications that are currently being taken.

Caretakers

The medical record of the child also typically contains information about the responsible caretaker, such as which adult or adults or agencies are legally responsible for the child, how the parent or consent-granting authority can be reached if that individual is not with the child, and how far the caretaker and pediatric outpatient must travel to reach a hospital should complications develop postoperatively.

What Does the Routine Preanesthetic Physical Examination Encompass?

Upper Airway

As is generally the case in adults, the emphasis of the preoperative examination of the child is on the cardiovascular and respiratory systems. The upper airway should be evaluated for two distinct reasons: first, to identify any evidence of upper respiratory infection that may place the child at increased risk of airway or pulmonary complications perioperatively; and second, to recognize any features that may make airway management and intubation difficult. In the absence of any of the several congenital abnormalities known to be associated with unusual or difficult facial and airway anatomy, such as the Pierre Robin, Treacher Collins, or Goldenhar syndromes, pediatric patients rarely are unable to be ventilated by mask and intubated.

In contrast to adults, no systematic classification scheme to assess the likelihood of difficulty with intubation has been developed for children. However, key elements of the airway examination include evaluation of the size of the mandible and potential displacement space for the tissues of the floor of the mouth, the size of the oral aperture, and the size of the tongue. The last of these is particularly important in children with any of several metabolic disorders that include macroglossia as a typical feature.

Chest

The chest should be physically inspected to detect use of any accessory muscles of respiration or asymmetry of chest wall excursion. It should be auscultated to detect any evidence of lower respiratory infection or reactive airways disease such as wheezing, rhonchi, crackles, or areas of diminished breath sounds. The heart should be auscultated during several inhalation/exhalation cycles to detect any murmurs.

Skin and Nailbeds

The skin and nailbeds merit examination to detect or evaluate a variety of conditions, including cyanosis, anemia, ecchymoses, hypovolemia, diffuse skin rashes (which may indicate the presence of any of several systemic diseases, such as measles or chicken pox), and the suitability of different sites for venous cannulation.

What Laboratory Studies Should Be Performed?

Most healthy children who are to undergo elective surgery require no routine laboratory testing, chest radiography, and electrocardiogram (ECG) in the absence of specific symptoms, signs, or known disease processes. Preoperative studies in children should largely be determined by the nature of any preexisting disease states and by the type and extent of the anticipated surgery.

Hemoglobin and Hematocrit

Although requirements vary among anesthesiologists and institutions, a strong case can be made for measuring hemoglobin or hematocrit in infants younger than 6 months of age and in postmenarchal females before all but the most minor of procedures. Infants typically experience the nadir of hemoglobin and hematocrit values at approximately 3 months of age (physiologic anemia of infancy), whereas adolescent females are prone to iron deficiency anemia if nutritional habits and iron intake are suboptimal.

What Are Appropriate Fasting Guidelines?

Historical Approach

The question of what constitutes an adequate preoperative fasting period in the child has been the subject of significant research and debate. The principal justification for prohibiting oral intake prior to surgery for nearly the past 50 years (since the work of Mendelson[1] and Teabeault[2]) has been to minimize the risk of pulmonary aspiration should the patient experience gastroesophageal reflux or vomiting in the perioperative period. Throughout most of this period, the "adult" fasting standard of "nil per os (NPO) after midnight" (or 6–8 hours) has been applied to children.

Gastric Fluid Characteristics

The characteristics of a gastric aspirate that are most closely associated with an increased risk of developing the pulmonary aspiration syndrome are a pH < 2.5, a volume > 0.4 mL $\cdot$ kg^{-1}, and a high level of particulate matter in the aspirate.[3] Since 1976, several investigators have demonstrated that despite "standard" preoperative fasts of at least 4 hours (and usually 8–12 hours), a high percentage of children continue to have gastric fluid characteristics that place them at increased risk of developing pulmonary aspiration syndrome, as shown in Table 61–2.[4–8]

Solid Foods Versus Clear Liquids

Keeping the information from Table 61–2 in mind, the question that one might ask is, Does allowing clear liquids preoperatively during the traditional fasting period adversely affect the risk of aspiration? Few would disagree that solid foods (including dairy products and pulp-containing juices) should continue to be withheld for at least 6 to 8 hours, even in children, since these foods require significantly longer gastric emptying times. However, several recent studies in children[9–11] demonstrated that clear liquids (e.g., water, apple juice, and Kool-Aid) administered in a variety of protocols up to 2 hours before induction do not significantly alter gastric residual volumes or pH. In fact, because clear liquids facilitate gastric emptying, gastric fluid volumes may actually be lower and pH values higher in patients allowed to consume clear liquids preoperatively.

The benefits of allowing clear liquids during the fasting period in children include providing a more humane experience for the patient and family, a reduced chance of anesthetic induction in a hypovolemic child, and a possibly reduced risk of intraoperative or postoperative hypoglycemia. The downside of a liberalized clear liquid policy includes the potential for delays in the surgical schedule should the patient be called to the operating room sooner than expected. Also, the possibility exists that allowing this exception to the traditional absolute NPO mandate may increase the likelihood that other food substances will be ingested in addition to clear liquids, increasing uncertainty as to the true nature of gastric contents in the individual patient.

TABLE 61–2. Pediatric Patients at Elevated Risk for Aspiration Following Standard Fast (>4 Hours)

Investigator	pH < 2.5 (%)	Mean Gastric Volume	Combined % at Risk*
Salem et al.[4]	90	0.6 mL $\cdot$ kg^{-1}	Not applicable
Goudsouzian et al.[5]	100	0.53 mL $\cdot$ kg^{-1}	64
Coté et al.[6]	96	0.78 mL $\cdot$ kg^{-1}	76
Manchikanti et al.[7]	92	0.49 mL $\cdot$ kg^{-1}	60
Meakin et al.[8]	100	0.25 mL $\cdot$ kg^{-1}	22

*Percentage of patients with both a gastric pH < 2.5 and a gastric volume > 0.4 mL $\cdot$ kg^{-1}.

Current Recommendations

At this time, anesthesiologists should continue to withhold solid foods at least 6 to 8 hours prior to elective surgery but allow clear fluids to be consumed up to 2 hours before induction. Children known to be at increased risk of having a full stomach or gastroesophageal reflux should continue to have even clear liquids withheld for the traditional period of at least 6 to 8 hours.

UPPER RESPIRATORY TRACT INFECTION

How Should It Be Assessed?

One of the most commonly encountered problems in the preoperative evaluation of children is the presence of symptoms or signs of a URI. Clinical findings, including a sore or scratchy throat, sneezing, malaise, fever, rhinorrhea, nonproductive cough, and nasal or sinus congestion may be nonspecific and overlap with manifestations of noninfectious disorders such as allergies and vasomotor rhinitis.

Acuity of Symptoms

The parent or other caretaker should be questioned regarding the presence of not only current URI symptoms but also those that have occurred within the preceding month. A recent, resolving URI is suggested to be associated with the same or an even greater risk of perioperative complications than is an existing infection.[12] When evidence of chronic allergy or URI symptoms is present, parents are frequently able to indicate whether the child's current clinical status is typical for the individual patient or unusual, as in the presence of a higher-than-normal fever, reduced activity level, or change in behavior.

As stated previously, some indications warrant routine preoperative laboratory or radiologic studies. Decisions concerning the management of children with URI symptoms must be based primarily on the clinical impression of whether the patient's condition is likely secondary to an infectious process. The white blood cell count may be depressed, normal, or elevated in the child with a viral URI. Therefore knowledge of it is of little help in the decision-making process. Chest radiographs are indicated only when symptoms such as a productive cough or findings on physical examination, including crackles, wheezing, or areas of decreased breath sounds, are present. In these cases, a lower respiratory tract process (pneumonia, asthma) more likely than not is present in addition to the URI.

Cancellation of Surgery

Because of airway reactivity and secretions, children with URIs are generally felt to be at risk of developing the complications described in the next section. The issue, once the diagnosis of a URI has been made, is whether to proceed with an elective surgical procedure or to postpone surgery for 4 to 6 weeks to allow resolution.

Con

One prospective investigation of 489 pediatric patients undergoing myringotomy under mask general inhalation anesthesia found no significant difference in perioperative compli-

cations between children without symptoms of URI, symptomatic children who met predetermined URI criteria, and symptomatic children who failed to meet URI criteria.[12] This study further suggested that the duration of certain URI symptoms, including sore throat, sneezing, and fever, was shorter in patients who underwent anesthesia and surgery than in a control group of patients with symptoms who did not undergo surgery but were evaluated over the course of a 3-week follow-up period. This finding was likely the result of the beneficial effect of myringotomy on upper respiratory tract physiology, although the possibility exists that the anesthetic itself may have exerted a beneficial influence on the course of the viral syndrome.

Pro

Conversely, another large retrospective review of prospectively gathered information demonstrated that children with a URI were 2 to 7 times more likely than healthy children to experience a respiratory complication in the perioperative period, depending on the specific respiratory event examined.[13] This investigation also demonstrated that tracheal intubation in children with URIs is associated with approximately twice the number of adverse respiratory events as is endotracheal intubation in the absence of URI.

Recommendations

The decision to proceed with elective surgery in the presence of a current or recent URI should be made only after the parents and surgeon understand the potential risks of perioperative respiratory complications. As with most medical judgments, it should be based on a risk-benefit analysis that includes such factors as the age of the patient, nature of the proposed surgery, frequency of URIs, history of previous respiratory complications, and any coexisting medical problems that may further complicate management. If the determination is made to postpone surgery, it should not be rescheduled until 4 to 6 weeks following the resolution of signs and symptoms.

What Perioperative Problems May Occur?

The child who has experienced a viral URI within the previous month or who currently exhibits evidence of a URI may be at increased risk of developing a number of perioperative problems and complications, although the data on this subject are frequently conflicting. Perhaps the first association between pre-existent respiratory infections and perioperative morbidity was made in 1936, when it was stated that the ''presence of any respiratory tract infection, even mild pharyngitis or oral sepsis, substantially increases the incidence of postoperative respiratory infections.''[14]

Airway

Potential problems that may be encountered include laryngospasm, airway obstruction, coughing, breath holding, hemoglobin desaturation, atelectasis, and bronchospasm. A 1984 study of laryngospasm during anesthesia indicated that children with URIs experienced nearly a 10-fold increase in incidence.[15] Inflammatory changes resulting from infection increase secretions, which may obstruct endotracheal tubes or predispose to the development of airway closure with atelectasis and pneumonia. Atelectasis and pulmonary dysfunction induced by URI may be manifested by hemoglobin desaturation in the operating room or PACU. One small study showed that 20% of children with a history or current signs and symptoms of URI had hemoglobin saturations below 95% while they breathed room air in the PACU.[16]

Pulmonary Function

Pulmonary function may be compromised during or after URI, despite the absence of overt evidence of lower respiratory tract involvement. Some changes may be subclinical as demonstrated by a longitudinal study of spirometric changes experienced by "healthy" children during periods both with and without a URI. Adjusted mean values of forced vital capacity, 1-second forced expiratory volume, peak expiratory flow, and several other variables all decreased during uncomplicated upper respiratory infections.[17]

Proposed mechanisms that account for observed spirometric changes and clinical wheezing or airway hyperreactivity are complex and likely interact to create the clinical picture of bronchospasm. They include viral stimulation of immunoglobulin E antibody production with resultant hypersensitivity, enhanced mediator release from basophils and mast cells, diminished β-adrenergic function in bronchial smooth muscle, and epithelial injury with sensitization of airway receptors, which may trigger cholinergic reflex bronchospasm.[18]

ASTHMA

How Is Reactive Airways Disease Assessed and Managed?

Asthma is a chronic disease of the tracheobronchial tree in which episodic increases in resistance to airflow result from heightened responsiveness to endogenous or exogenous stimuli, or both. It is one of the most common conditions encountered in children, with estimates of incidence of up to 12%, depending on diagnostic criteria, patient age, and geographic location.[19] As a clinical entity, asthma may occur in any of a variety of scenarios, from the older child or young adult with only a remote history of asthma or wheezing as a toddler, to the asymptomatic child who is well-controlled with bronchodilators, and, finally, to the patient with an exacerbation of asthma and respiratory distress who presents for emergency surgery or requires tracheal intubation in the course of treatment of status asthmaticus. The clinical approach depends primarily on the activity and time-course of the disease in the individual patient.

Classification

Several classification schemes have been proposed that are based on the causes or stimuli that induce bronchospasm. So-called "extrinsic" asthma is most common in children, in whom an allergy to some external substance and elevated levels of serum immunoglobulin E (IgE) can often be demonstrated. "Intrinsic" asthma, by contrast, has no apparent allergic cause but is rather a respiratory tract infection or some form of chronic lung disease, such as cystic fibrosis or bronchopulmonary dysplasia. It occurs more commonly in adolescents and adults. Other varieties of asthma include exercise- and aspirin-induced forms, which may overlap or coexist with extrinsic or intrinsic asthma.

Pathophysiology

The principal pathophysiologic features of asthma include a reduction in the diameter of the airways, thickening of the bronchial mucosa due to inflammation and edema, and the collection of thick secretions within the tracheobronchial tree. Several potential defects induce these changes, although the relative importance or applicability of a specific abnormality may vary from patient to patient. They include an "imbalance" of the autonomic nervous system's control of bronchomotor tone; alterations in the properties of the smooth muscle cells within the bronchial walls[20]; or abnormal immune function with increased IgE formation and mast cell degranulation, particularly in the case of extrinsic asthma in children.

The result of these underlying changes are gas trapping, ventilation/perfusion mismatching, atelectasis, and increased dead space ventilation. Pulmonary function studies reveal increased residual volume, functional residual capacity, and total lung volume and reduced expiratory flow rates, vital capacity, expiratory reserve volume, and inspiratory capacity.[21]

Therapeutic Implications

It is at the level of these defects that our somewhat incomplete understanding of the mechanism of action of the drugs used to treat asthma is found. Because parasympathetic-cholinergic or α-adrenergic stimulation promotes bronchoconstriction either by direct innervation or humoral passage of mediators, substances such as atropine or ipratropium may reverse or block bronchospasm induced by these mechanisms. Likewise, because β₂-adrenergic stimulation promotes bronchodilation, β-agonists such as epinephrine and albuterol may be used therapeutically as bronchodilators.

Theophylline, an agent commonly used as a bronchodilator, may have several different actions. The classical effect of intracellular phosphodiesterase inhibition with resultant elevation of cyclic adenosine monophosphate levels and consequent bronchodilation appears to be of minor importance at clinically useful theophylline concentrations of 10 to 20 $\mu g \cdot mL^{-1}$.[22] Other possible benefits of theophylline include inhibition of adenosine-induced bronchoconstriction and interference with the synthesis or effects of prostaglandins.[23]

Corticosteroids are thought to have a number of actions, including inhibition of the release of mediators of bronchoconstriction and inflammation, reduction of bronchial mucosal edema, and potentiation of β-adrenergic receptors.[19]

History and Physical Findings

Preoperative evaluation of the child with asthma is centered on determining the current activity of the disease and what is required (if anything) to improve the patient's condition. The history of the disease, which includes the child's age at onset, triggering stimuli, the number of clinic and hospital visits, the number of severe episodes requiring mechanical ventilation, and current medications, should be reviewed. Physical examination should include not only assessment of the chest and a search for wheezing, diminished breath sounds, and delayed expiration but also assessment of vital signs, the use of accessory muscles of respiration, hydration status, cyanosis, and any evidence of upper respiratory infection or pneumonia.

Laboratory Tests

As with the general preoperative evaluation of all patients, routine laboratory testing has no place; studies must be guided by the patient's condition. The asymptomatic patient with normal results on physical examination requires nothing; the child with a fever, focal chest findings, and some degree of respiratory distress may require a chest radiograph, complete blood count with white cell differential, and an arterial blood gas analysis. Older children may be able to undergo spirometry. If bronchospasm or symptomatic asthma is found, elective surgery should be postponed while the bronchodilator regimen is adjusted and any infectious process is treated or resolved.

Anesthetic Implications

Anesthetic management of the asthmatic child also depends on the patient's condition. Use of preoperative bronchodilators (oral or inhaled) should be continued until the time of surgery. If the patient is currently taking or has received systemic steroids within the 6-month period prior to surgery, "stress" steroid coverage for all but minor surgical procedures should be provided. An acceptable dosage is the equivalent of 2 to 3 mg · kg⁻¹ · d⁻¹ of methylprednisolone perioperatively.[24] Premedication with sedatives as outlined later in this chapter may be beneficial to the extent that anxiety and fear may contribute to the development of bronchospasm.

Regional Techniques

Asthmatic patients may be provided with either general or regional anesthesia. Regional techniques make it possible to avoid airway instrumentation and intubation, but in the case of moderately high levels of spinal or epidural anesthesia they may interfere with the patient's ability to cough or use some of the accessory muscles of respiration. The concern that thoracic pharmacologic sympathectomy secondary to spinal or epidural anesthesia may induce a predominance of parasympathetic tone to the tracheobronchial tree and thereby promote bronchospasm appears to be more theoretic than practical.

General Techniques

Induction Agents. In considering intravenous induction agents for general anesthesia, sodium thiopental, etomidate, ketamine, and propofol have been successfully used in asthmatic patients, despite the fact that thiopental has been demonstrated to induce histamine release in vitro.[25]

Inhalation Agents. The potent inhalation anesthetics—isoflurane, enflurane, and halothane—possess equivalent bronchodilating properties[26] and may be used for both mask induction and maintenance of general anesthesia. Halothane has the advantage of having the most tolerable odor and is therefore the most agreeable to children. However, because of its propensity to sensitize the myocardium to the effects of catecholamines,[27] it may induce problems with dysrhythmias in the asthmatic patient who has received β-agonists and theophylline preparations.

Narcotics and Muscle Relaxants. Some narcotics (mor-

phine, meperidine) and muscle relaxants (succinylcholine and the benzylisoquinolines [curare, atracurium, mivacurium, metocurine, doxacurium]) have the potential to cause histamine release, depending on dosage and speed of administration. As with thiopental, these agents have been safely used in patients with asthma, but in view of the wide variety of narcotics and muscle relaxants available today, the use of agents that are not associated with histamine release or exacerbation of bronchospasm is perhaps most prudent. Such drugs include fentanyl and related compounds and steroid muscle relaxants (pancuronium, vecuronium, pipecuronium). Nevertheless, circumstances may occur in which a drug like succinylcholine is indicated despite the presence of asthma, as when rapid muscle relaxation for tracheal intubation is essential.

Miscellaneous Considerations

Other maneuvers that are helpful in asthmatic patients include humidification of inspired gases, administration of intravenous lidocaine prior to intubation or tracheal suctioning,[28] and provision of mask anesthesia without intubation or deep extubation of the trachea at the conclusion of surgery in appropriate patients.

CONGENITAL HEART DISEASE

What Are the Implications for Noncardiac Surgery?

No other group of children, with the possible exception of those with an abnormal or difficult airway, elicit as much anxiety among anesthesiologists as pediatric patients with unrepaired or palliated congenital heart disease. For the most part, definitive surgical management of congenital cardiac lesions is reserved for pediatric centers; the anesthetic considerations in pediatric cardiac surgery are discussed in Chapter 66. However, a fundamental understanding of the nature of congenital cardiac lesions and of implications for anesthetic management of noncardiac surgery is essential.

Pathophysiologic Flow Characteristics

Various congenital cardiac lesions can be thought of in terms of their pathophysiologic flow characteristics (Table 61–3). In the first two of the categories, blood is shunted through abnormal circulatory connections or pathways as a function of pressure channels and of the relative pulmonary and systemic vascular resistances. In the third category, no shunting of blood occurs in the absence of coexisting lesions, although various cardiac chambers and vascular beds may be affected by the obstruction to forward blood flow.

Preanesthetic Management

The child with congenital heart disease scheduled for noncardiac surgery should have the same preoperative evaluation as previously discussed in addition to several further investigations. Specifically, the history and physical examination should seek any evidence of cyanosis or congestive heart failure. Cyanosis is typically found in lesions with reduced pulmonary blood flow, pulmonary hypertension, or both, and predominant right-to-left shunting of blood. Congestive heart

TABLE 61–3. Pathophysiologic Classification of Congenital Cardiac Lesions

Increased Pulmonary Blood Flow	Atrial septal defect
	Ventricular septal defect
	Patent ductus arteriosus
	Atrioventricular canal
	Anomalous coronary arteries
	Transposition of the great vessels*
	Anomalous pulmonary venous drainage
	Truncus arteriosus*
	Single ventricle*
Decreased Pulmonary Blood Flow	Tetralogy of Fallot
	Pulmonary atresia
	Tricuspid atresia
	Ebstein's anomaly
	Truncus arteriosus*
	Transposition of the great vessels*
	Single ventricle*
Obstruction to Blood Flow	Aortic stenosis
	Pulmonary stenosis
	Coarctation of the aorta
	Asymmetric septal hypertrophy

(From Schwartz AJ, Campbell FW: Pathophysiological approach to congenital heart disease in pediatric anesthesia. *In* Pediatric Cardiac Anesthesia. Lake CL (ed). Norwalk CT, Appleton & Lange, 1988, p 9.)
*Classification as an increased or decreased pulmonary blood flow lesion depends on absence or presence (respectively) of obstruction to pulmonary blood flow and relative pulmonary and systemic vascular resistance.

failure, conversely, usually results from increased pulmonary blood flow, increased pulmonary venous return, and left ventricular overload.

The nature and extent of previous palliative or corrective surgical procedures should be elucidated together with the child's current functional state as indicated by activity, symptoms, and objective measurements, including echocardiography and cardiac catheterization data. Chronic use of cardiac medications (digoxin, diuretics, antidysrhythmics) should be noted, continued until the time of surgery, and resumed postoperatively in either oral or parenteral form, as required. Patients demonstrating cyanosis are likely to have polycythemia secondary to chronic hypoxemia. An unusually high hematocrit places a child at risk of thrombotic complications. Platelet counts, although frequently elevated, may conceal platelet function abnormalities and potential defects in hemostasis.

Premedication

No lesion-specific approach to anesthesia and intraoperative management exists for children with congenital heart disease. Rather, the approach is dictated by the current degree of cardiopulmonary compensation, the anticipated surgical procedure, and the associated stresses. Preanesthetic sedation is nearly always indicated for the general reasons described later in this chapter and for the specific benefit of alleviating anxiety and sympathetic activation, which may impair cardiovascular function prior to and during induction.

What Are the Anesthetic Effects on Cardiopulmonary Function?

A number of anesthetic factors influence cardiovascular and pulmonary function perioperatively, any of which may be beneficial or deleterious, depending on the pathophysiology involved.[29]

Cardiac Output

Forward blood flow (cardiac output) may be enhanced by judiciously increased intravascular volume expansion and increasing heart rate, inotropic agents, and vasodilators (in normovolemia). Inhalation anesthetics and β-adrenergic blockers, which normally are myocardial depressants, may actually improve cardiac output in patients with hypertrophic cardiomyopathy and ventricular outflow obstruction. Cardiac output is reduced by hypervolemia, dysrhythmias, ischemia, and, in the presence of hypovolemia, vasodilators and increased mean airway pressures.

Systemic and Pulmonary Vascular Resistance

The resistances in the pulmonary and systemic circulations are influenced in numerous ways. Sympathetic stimulation (as in light anesthesia) and α-adrenergic agonists may increase both systemic and pulmonary vascular resistance. Pulmonary vascular resistance is also increased by hypoxemia, acidosis, hypercarbia, hypervolemia, and increased mean airway pressure. Both systemic vascular resistance and pulmonary vascular resistance are decreased by inhalation anesthetic agents, vasodilators, and α-adrenergic antagonists. Pulmonary vascular resistance additionally is reduced by oxygen, alkalosis, hypocarbia, prostaglandin E_1, prostacyclin, and nitric oxide.

What Other Factors Are Critical to Management?

Endocarditis Prophylaxis

Two further points in the care of children with congenital heart disease merit specific attention. Children undergoing surgery in which a transient bacteremia is possible (dental, ear, nose, and throat, gastrointestinal, and genitourinary procedures) require prophylaxis against bacterial endocarditis (Table 61–4). The only patients not requiring such prophylaxis are those who are more than 6 months postrepair of a secundum-type atrial septal defect (without patch) or postligation of a patent ductus arteriosus. Importantly, tracheal intubation alone is not an indication for bacterial endocarditis prophylaxis.

Air Embolization

With all forms of intravenous access, meticulous care should be provided to ensure that air does not enter the tubing or venous system. Once air gains access to the venous circulation, it may pass through a probe-patent foramen ovale or any other abnormal channel between the pulmonary and systemic circulations. A paradoxic air embolus, with resultant central nervous system or myocardial ischemia or infarction, can result.

MALIGNANT HYPERTHERMIA

An anxiety-provoking and potentially confusing clinical situation arises during the provision of anesthesia for the patient who is susceptible to malignant hyperthermia (MH).[30] Confusion is greatest when a personal or family history of MH is questionable or poorly documented. Management is relatively straightforward for patients with a history of a fulminant MH

TABLE 61–4. Bacterial Endocarditis Prophylaxis in Children

Dental, Oral, Upper Respiratory Tract Procedures

Standard oral regimen	Amoxicillin 50 mg · kg^{-1} 1 h before procedure, followed by 25 mg · kg^{-1} 6 h later
In patients unable to take oral medications	Ampicillin 50 mg · kg^{-1} IV or IM 30 min before procedure, followed by ampicillin 25 mg · kg^{-1} IV or IM or amoxicillin 25 mg · kg^{-1} PO 6 h later *or* Ampicillin 50 mg · kg^{-1} and gentamicin 2 mg · kg^{-1} IV or IM initially followed by amoxicillin 5 mg · kg^{-1} PO 6 h after initial antibiotic administration or a second dose of the IV/IM ampicillin and gentamicin combination 8 h later (for high-risk patients not considered candidates for the oral regimen)
In patients allergic to penicillin	Erythromycin 20 mg · kg^{-1} PO 2 h before the procedure, followed by erythromycin 10 mg · kg^{-1} PO 6 h later *or* If unable to take oral medications and penicillin-allergic, vancomycin 20 mg · kg^{-1} administered IV over 1 h before the procedure, followed by vancomycin 10 mg · kg^{-1} 8 h later *or* Clindamycin 10 mg · kg^{-1} IV 30 min before the procedure, followed by clindamycin 5 mg · kg^{-1} IV 6 h later

Genitourinary or Gastrointestinal Procedures

Standard regimen	Ampicillin 50 mg · kg^{-1} and gentamicin 2 mg · kg^{-1} IV or IM 30 min before the procedure, followed by ampicillin 25 mg · kg^{-1} and gentamicin 1 mg · kg^{-1} IV or IM 8 h later, or amoxicillin 25 mg · kg^{-1} PO 6 h after the intitial antibiotics
In patients allergic to penicillin	Vancomycin 20 mg · kg^{-1} administered over 1 h and gentamicin 2 mg · kg^{-1} IV 1 h before the procedure, followed by a second dose of vancomycin 10 mg · kg^{-1} IV and gentamicin 1 mg · kg^{-1} IV 8 h later
For low-risk patients undergoing minor procedures	Amoxicillin 50 mg · kg^{-1} PO 1 h before the procedure and amoxicillin 25 mg · kg^{-1} PO 6 h later

Abbreviations: IV = intravenously; IM = intramuscularly; PO = periorally.

crisis or a positive halothane-caffeine contracture test following muscle biopsy. Some controversy concerns the role of prophylactic administration of dantrolene and the use of drugs such as ketamine and the amide-type local anesthetics.

Who Is at Risk?

Patients considered at risk of developing a reaction include those who have survived an MH episode or who have positive muscle biopsy results; first-degree relatives of such patients; first-degree relatives with known muscle or skeletal abnormalities or chronically elevated creatine kinase levels; and patients who have experienced masseter spasm following the administration of halothane and succinylcholine. A number of other conditions have varying degrees of association with MH, including King-Denborough syndrome (the only disorder with a 100% MH association), Duchenne type muscular dystrophy, central core disease, and myotonia congenita.[31]

Why Does It Occur?

Malignant hyperthermia is a pharmacogenetic disease of skeletal muscle in which a hypermetabolic state that results in increased oxygen (O_2) consumption, carbon dioxide (CO_2) production, metabolic acidosis, and heat production is triggered by specific anesthetic agents. The only well-documented triggering agents are succinylcholine and the potent inhalation anesthetics. Although some controversy exists, the prevailing opinion is that all other anesthetic medications are safe (Table 61–5).

The inciting cellular event is a large increase in the level of intracellular ionized calcium secondary to a drug-induced disturbance or perturbation of membrane function. The elevated intracellular calcium then induces skeletal muscle contracture and acceleration of aerobic and anaerobic metabolism. Clinically, the MH episode is marked by hypercarbia, metabolic and respiratory acidosis, tachycardia, dysrhythmias, hemodynamic instability, muscle rigidity, masseter spasm, hyperthermia, and cyanosis. Late manifestations include central nervous system changes of cerebral edema and coma, renal failure, and disseminated intravascular coagulation. Not all of these clinical finding or complications may be evident in each individual patient. (See Chapter 49.)

How Is Preanesthetic Assessment Carried Out?

History and Physical Examination

The first priority is to obtain a detailed history, perform a physical examination, and review any available medical and anesthetic records. Parents should be counseled regarding the nature, diagnosis, and treatment of MH and how the impending anesthetic will be tailored to avoid triggering an episode. An increasing number of parents of MH-susceptible children are very knowledgeable of the disorder and its implications because of improved patient education and the activities of the Malignant Hyperthermia Association of the United States (MHAUS).

Laboratory Studies

Noninvasive or minimally invasive studies to evaluate potentially MH-susceptible patients do not exist, although molec-

TABLE 61–5. Anesthetic Drugs and Malignant Hyperthermia

Triggering Agents	Nontriggering Agents
Succinylcholine	Narcotics
Decamethonium	Benzodiazepines
Halothane	Barbiturates
Enflurane	Propofol
Isoflurane	Nitrous oxide
Sevoflurane	Etomidate
Desflurane	Nondepolarizing muscle relaxants
	Anticholinesterases
	Ketamine*
	Ester-type local anesthetics
	Amide-type local anesthetics*
	Anticholinergics (atropine)

*Agents considered to be safe in malignant hyperthermia–susceptible patients, but this belief is controversial.

ular genetic analysis[32] and MRI spectroscopy[33] may gain clinical utility in the future. Knowledge of serum levels is useful in that if they are elevated in a close relative of an individual known to be MH-susceptible, that relative may likewise be considered susceptible.

Postponement of elective surgery and insistence that a patient who may be MH-susceptible undergo a muscle biopsy and halothane-caffeine contracture testing is impractical. To do so would require the patient to travel to one of the few centers where standardized testing is performed and to undergo a surgical procedure. Such testing can and should be arranged for a later date, if indicated; in the meantime, such a patient may be safely anesthetized with nontriggering agents without the need to apply the label or diagnosis of MH.

What Are the Anesthetic Considerations?

Following evaluation and counseling, anesthesia may proceed with a variety of nontriggering anesthetic techniques. A common approach is to administer a rectal, oral, or intravenous barbiturate or benzodiazepine and to complete the induction with inhalation of nitrous oxide and O_2 administered by mask. Anesthesia is then maintained with a "balanced technique" that consists of the administration of nitrous oxide, O_2, narcotics, propofol,[34] and nondepolarizing muscle relaxants.

Routine monitors include pulse oximetry and capnography. A "clean" anesthesia machine with a fresh CO_2 absorber, disposable circuit, and no vaporizers that has been flushed with high-flow O_2 for 5 to 10 minutes may be used to ventilate the patient.[35] If a nontriggering anesthetic technique and appropriately prepared anesthesia machine or breathing circuit are used, dantrolene prophylaxis probably is unnecessary. If dantrolene is to be administered, it should be given intravenously in a dose of $2 \text{ mg} \cdot \text{kg}^{-1}$ within 30 minutes of anesthesia induction.[36] When applicable, regional anesthetic techniques may be employed as an alternative to general anesthesia. Management of an acute MH episode is outlined in Table 61–6.

PREMEDICATION

What Are the Goals?

Preinduction of Anesthesia

There has been an explosion of novel premedication techniques that utilize newly released agents and alternative routes of administration (or "orifices"). Approaches to pediatric premedication in the 1990s are altogether different than the techniques used 10 years earlier. Although the drugs and routes of administration have changed, the primary goals of premedication—or perhaps more appropriately, "preinduction of anesthesia"[37]—remain the same: to provide smooth and atraumatic separation of the child from the parents and to facilitate the induction of anesthesia. An additional benefit, although seldom a primary indication, is reduction of intraoperative anesthetic requirements.

Reduction of Stress

Beyond these objectives, several additional justifications can be suggested for preinduction pharmacologic preparation.

TABLE 61–6. Management of an Acute Malignant Hyperthermia Episode

1. Discontinue all anesthetic agents and request help from additional anesthesia and surgery personnel
2. Hyperventilate patient with 100% oxygen, preferably from a "clean" anesthesia machine with a fresh CO_2 absorber or from a nonrebreathing circuit with maximum oxygen flow
3. Terminate surgical procedure (if necessary) as soon as feasible
4. Mix each 20-mg bottle of dantrolene with 60 mL of sterile-water; administer intitial intravenous dose of $2.5 \text{ mg} \cdot \text{kg}^{-1}$
5. Obtain additional intravenous access and an arterial line for continuous measurement of blood pressure and arterial blood gas analysis
6. Begin surface cooling and lavage of body cavities with iced saline as necessary to reduce body temperature
7. Administer additional dantrolene in $2 \text{ mg} \cdot \text{kg}^{-1}$ increments up to a total of $10 \text{ mg} \cdot \text{kg}^{-1}$ every 10–15 min as needed based on resolution of tachycardia, hyperthermia, and muscle rigidity
8. Treat metabolic acidosis with sodium bicarbonate and persistent dysrhythmias with procainamide, after confirming adequate treatment with intravenous dantrolene
9. Monitor serum electrolytes, urinary output, and blood coagulation status; treat hyperkalemia with intravenous glucose and insulin, and treat oliguria with intravenous fluids (dantrolene preparation contains 3 g of mannitol per vial) and furosemide
10. Transfer to intensive care unit and monitor for 1–3 d for late effects of malignant hyperthermia episode. Continue intravenous dantrolene $1–2.5 \text{ mg} \cdot \text{kg}^{-1}$ for first 24 h after episode and for reappearance of features of malignant hyperthermia
11. Counsel family and discuss referral of relatives for muscle biopsy to MHAUS:

   MHAUS
   (Malignant Hyperthermia Association of the United States)
   P.O. Box 3231
   Darien, CT 06820
   (203) 655-3007

These include provision of amnesia for the period of separation and induction of anesthesia; vagolysis and reduction of secretions, as discussed in the section on anticholinergic agents; reduction of physiologic stress, as in patients with congenital heart disease; and provision of analgesia for preinduction placement of invasive catheters and monitors of postoperative pain.

Reduction of Anesthetic Requirements and Risk of Aspiration

Finally, specific agents such as clear, particulate-free antacids and histamine$_2$-receptor antagonists may be given to increase gastric pH and reduce gastric fluid volume, thereby minimizing the likelihood of aspiration of acidic stomach contents.

Which Patients Are or Are Not Candidates?

In determining which children should receive pharmacologic preparation prior to anesthesia and surgery, it is perhaps easier to identify those patients who are *not* candidates for preoperative sedation. Infants younger than 1 year of age traditionally have been premedicated with an anticholinergic agent alone, although many vigorous and healthy 9- and 10-month-old infants may benefit from a sedative.

Children with abnormal airways, respiratory distress, increased intracranial pressure, and hemodynamic compromise should receive premedication (if at all) only in the continuous presence of a practitioner skilled in airway management and in the presence of appropriate monitoring devices and resuscitative equipment.

Almost all other patients, from late infancy through adolescence, benefit from some form of preinduction medication. With the wide variety of agents and techniques available, little justification can be advanced for crying, kicking, and screaming children hauled off to the operating room where they are laid upon and restrained by two or three assistants while a mask is clamped onto their faces.

Should Anticholinergic Agents Be Administered?

A longstanding practice in pediatric anesthesia has been to administer an anticholinergic drug—usually atropine, but occasionally glycopyrrolate—prior to or at the time of induction. The primary justification for this practice is to block parasympathetically mediated reductions in heart rate or even asystole that may occur following the administration of intravenous succinylcholine and increasing concentrations of the potent inhalation anesthetics or after airway manipulation.

The cardiac output of newborns, infants, and small children is highly dependent on maintenance of an adequate heart rate because of a very limited ability to compensate with increases in stroke volume and myocardial contractility. Therefore, atropine commonly has been administered either orally, intravenously, intramuscularly, or rectally to promote hemodynamic stability.

Other benefits of preinduction anticholinergics include drying of oral secretions and a mild degree of sedation, which is observed only following the administration of atropine. Glycopyrrolate, a quaternary ammonium compound, is unable to pass the blood-brain barrier, and thus exerts no central nervous system effects.

Risks and Side Effects

The anticholinergic agents, although generally regarded as safe, are not without potential risks and side effects. In some patients, particularly those with congenital cardiac lesions such as aortic stenosis, the relative or absolute tachycardia induced by atropine and glycopyrrolate may reduce effective cardiac output. Atropine diminishes sweat gland activity and may interfere with thermoregulation, resulting in an elevation in body temperature. Newborns and patients with pulmonary disease such as cystic fibrosis may experience drying and impaired clearance of pulmonary secretions, which may promote atelectasis and pneumonia.

Although anticholinergic drugs reduce gastric fluid secretion,[38] they decrease lower esophageal sphincter tone, thereby producing opposing effects on the potential for gastric fluid reflux and pulmonary aspiration. Finally, although the effect is essentially cosmetic, atropine commonly causes flushing of the cheeks, neck, and trunk.

Indications

The administration of preoperative anticholinergic drugs must frequently be in accord with institutional guidelines and policies regarding the route and timing of dosing and the patients for which they are indicated. To state that any drug, including an anticholinergic, is always required for all infants or all children is too simplistic and is contrary to the concept of individually tailoring an anesthetic for each patient.

A reasonable approach is to provide a preinduction anticholinergic agent to infants and children with increased oral secretions; to newborns and small infants undergoing mask inhalation induction of anesthesia; and to any child undergoing mask induction in whom intravenous access is expected to be difficult. In an effort to avoid awake intramuscular injections, patients who are to receive intravenous succinylcholine or to undergo procedures likely to elicit vagal reflexes (e.g., laryngoscopy or bronchoscopy and strabismus surgery) may receive intravenous atropine immediately after intravenous access is obtained.

Doses

Several points concerning the dosing of anticholinergic agents require mention. Whether atropine or glycopyrrolate is administered prior to induction, predrawn syringes containing intravenous atropine and those containing intramuscular atropine should be readily available. A low threshold should prevail for administering a dose of atropine once the heart rate begins to decline below the lower acceptable limit. Such therapy may well offset the significantly reduced cardiac output and prolonged circulation time that accompany the onset of bradycardia.[39]

The minimum dose of atropine for an infant or child of any size is 0.1 mg. Smaller doses may induce a paradoxic slowing of the heart rate that is thought to be due to a weak peripheral muscarinic, cholinergic agonist effect.[40] The intravenous dose is 10 to 20 $\mu g \cdot kg^{-1}$, and the intramuscular dose is 20 $\mu g \cdot kg^{-1}$. Atropine also effectively dries secretions and attenuates the bradycardic responses to halothane in infants when it is given orally in a dose of 20 to 40 $\mu g \cdot kg^{-1}$,[41] although many practitioners find the oral route less efficacious than others. Glycopyrrolate is provided in a dose of 5 $\mu g \cdot kg^{-1}$ intravenously or 10 $\mu g \cdot kg^{-1}$ intramuscularly.

What Are the Alternatives for Preoperative Sedation?

Table 61-7 lists commonly used premedicant agents and their approximate doses, routes of administration, and onset times. As with most anesthetic drugs, intravenous administration (when appropriate) should be titrated to clinical effect. Because of significant patient variability, particularly among children who are chronically exposed to sedatives and anesthetics, individual requirements may fall below or well above the indicated ranges.

The expected clinical effects and uses of these agents depend on the dosage and route of administration. For example, ketamine in a low intramuscular dose of 2 $mg \cdot kg^{-1}$[42] and midazolam in an intravenous dose of 0.05 $mg \cdot kg^{-1}$ may be regarded as sedatives. In higher doses, ketamine (5 $mg \cdot kg^{-1}$ intramuscularly) and midazolam (0.3 $mg \cdot kg^{-1}$ intravenously) may be considered induction agents. The same principle applies for the rectal administration of the short-acting barbiturates methohexital and thiopental, which typically induce sleep and loss of consciousness rather than the anxiolysis, sedation, and euphoria usually observed with the indicated doses of midazolam.

Because of the availability of a variety of administration

TABLE 61–7. Current Preinduction Medications

Agent	Dose	Route	Onset
Benzodiazepines			
Midazolam	0.5–1.0 mg · kg⁻¹	PO	15–30 min
	0.02–0.1 mg · kg⁻¹	IV	1–3 min
	0.08–0.25 mg · kg⁻¹	IM	5–10 min
	0.2 mg · kg⁻¹	IN	10 min
	0.3–1 mg · kg⁻¹	PR	10–20 min
Diazepam	0.1–0.5 mg · kg⁻¹	PO, IM, PR	60 min
Narcotics			
Fentanyl	15–20 µg · kg⁻¹	OT	5–30 min
	0.5–1 µg · kg⁻¹	IV	1–3 min
	1–3 µg · kg⁻¹	IM	5–15 min
Sufentanil	1.5–4.5 µg · kg⁻¹	IN	7–10 min
Morphine	0.05–0.1 mg · kg⁻¹	IV	3–10 min
	0.1–0.2 mg · kg⁻¹	IM	30–45 min
Barbiturates			
Methohexital	6–10 mg · kg⁻¹	IM	3–5 min
	20–35 mg · kg⁻¹	PR	5–10 min
Thiopental	25–35 mg · kg⁻¹	PR	5–10 min
Pentobarbital	2–4 mg · kg⁻¹	PO, IM, PR	45–90 min
Dissociative Anesthetics			
Ketamine	6–10 mg · kg⁻¹	PO	10–20 min
	2–6 mg · kg⁻¹	IM	30 s to 2 min
	3 mg · kg⁻¹	IN	20 min
	10 mg · kg⁻¹	PR	10 min
Hypnotics			
Chloral hydrate	50–75 mg · kg⁻¹	PO	30–60 min

Abbreviations: OT = oral transmucosal; IN = intranasally; PR = per rectum.

techniques for agents with relatively rapid onsets of action and short durations of effect, such as midazolam, fentanyl, sufentanil, and ketamine, classical pediatric premedicants, including pentobarbital, secobarbital, and chloral hydrate, are infrequently used in modern anesthetic practice.

Midazolam

Midazolam administered by the oral, nasal, and rectal routes is very popular as a pediatric premedication. It may be given incrementally intravenously with great predictability and control. It may also be given intramuscularly,[43] although the needle stick is undesirable. In the interest of avoiding fear-inducing and painful intramuscular injections, less invasive and more tolerable routes of administration have been popularized.

Oral

Oral midazolam safely induces a state of tranquility and euphoria in children, but seldom sleep.[44, 45] It has a somewhat narrow "window" of optimum sedation that lasts from 15 to 45 minutes following administration; after this period, children appear to return to their baseline mental state quite rapidly. No oral midazolam preparation is commercially available in the United States; the intravenous formulation must be added to a small volume of clear juice or syrup and artificial sweetener. Despite this preparation, many children still complain that midazolam administered orally in this way is bitter.

Nasal

Midazolam may also be administered intranasally in drops or an aerosol. Intranasal administration has the advantages of

greater bioavailability (55%, in contrast to the 18% to 19% for the rectal and oral routes)[46] and, as a consequence, reduced dosage, lower cost, and a somewhat more rapid onset of action. The drawback of intranasal midazolam is that it burns and causes as many as 84% of patients to cry.[47]

Rectal

Rectal midazolam diluted with normal saline to a volume of 5 mL is perhaps most appropriate for infants and toddlers and for patients in whom an oral preparation is contraindicated.[48]

Fentanyl and Sufentanil

Fentanyl in the form of "lollipops" (which allow oral transmucosal absorption[49]) and intranasally administered sufentanil[37] also have attracted a great deal of interest as pediatric premedicants. These narcotic agents have the advantage of providing analgesia for preinduction vascular catheter insertion and postoperative analgesia following short procedures. The downside of the use of these agents as preinduction drugs includes an increased incidence of nausea and vomiting. Patients may also experience reduced ventilatory compliance ("stiff chest"), pruritis, and mild degrees of oxyhemoglobin desaturation (Spo₂ < 95%). Personnel skilled in airway management and appropriate resuscitative equipment must be immediately available following administration of these agents.

Ketamine

Ketamine, a dissociative anesthetic with sedative and analgesic properties, may be given via a number of alternative orifices in addition to the "standard" intravenous and intramuscular routes. Although it acts relatively rapidly, in our experience it has not been as predictable or reliable as similarly administered midazolam. We generally reserve its use for uncooperative and difficult-to-manage patients in whom it is given intramuscularly.

Should Pharmacologic Prophylaxis Against Aspiration Be Provided?

Incidence, Morbidity, and Mortality

The pulmonary aspiration of gastric contents remains one of the most feared of anesthetic complications. Historically, 26% of anesthesia-related mortality in children was related to the aspiration of blood or vomitus in the perioperative period.[50] A recent, large retrospective review of aspiration during anesthesia confirmed that children are more likely to experience aspiration than adults (8.6 aspirations per 10,000 children aged 1–9 years in contrast to 2.90 aspirations per 10,000 adults). However, despite the increased incidence and an overall mortality following aspiration of 5%, no deaths in pediatric patients were attributable specifically to aspiration.[51]

A large prospective study of anesthetic complications in infants and children revealed a lower aspiration incidence of approximately 1.2 per 10,000 anesthetics and no mortality attributable to aspiration.[52] Whether owing to increased awareness of the problem of pulmonary aspiration or to improved anesthetic practices and skill on the part of anesthesia practitioners, these data suggest that the incidence of aspiration and the associated mortality has decreased compared with those of previous years.

Antacids

The practice of routine prophylaxis against aspiration in pediatric patients has never been widespread. Sodium citrate, a clear, nonparticulate antacid, effectively increases the gastric content pH in children when administered in a dose of 0.4 mL · kg⁻¹.[53] Concern about antacids has been the increase of gastric fluid volume that follows their use; as a result, patients commonly present with significant gastric residual volumes following standard fasts. In addition, impaired gastric emptying may result.[54]

Histamine₂ Blockers and Metoclopramide

The histamine₂-receptor antagonists cimetidine and ranitidine reduce the volume and elevate the pH of gastric mucosal secretions and have demonstrated efficacy in children (Fig. 61–1).[55, 56] The dose of cimetidine is 5 to 7.5 mg · kg⁻¹ by either the intravenous, intramuscular, or oral routes; that of ranitidine is 0.5 to 1.0 mg · kg⁻¹ intravenously or intramuscularly and 2 mg · kg⁻¹ orally. Intramuscular and intravenous injections must be given at least 1 hour before the anticipated induction of anesthesia (1.5–3 hours for oral doses).

Metoclopramide, which increases the tension of the lower esophageal sphincter and facilitates gastric emptying, likewise may be given in a dose of 0.1 mg · kg⁻¹ intravenously or orally. This drug also exhibits an antiemetic effect and must be given at least 1 hour before induction when the oral preparation is used.

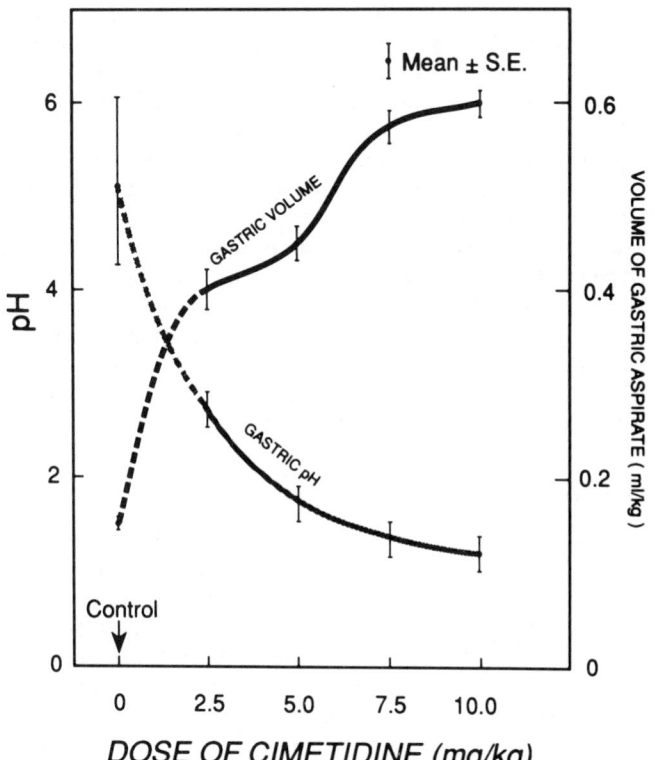

FIGURE 61–1. The effects of cimetidine on the volume and pH of gastric fluid in children. (Modified from Goudsouzian N: Aspiration in children: practical implications. Anesthesiology Rev 1984; 11:6.

The major drawback of the histamine₂-receptor antagonists and metoclopramide is the prolonged time they must be administered before surgery, which is particularly a problem with outpatients. If they are given earlier than 2 hours before induction, they must be administered by intramuscular injection or "awake" venous catheterization. Such injections may be beneficial and justified in a patient at increased risk of gastroesophageal reflux or with a full stomach but cannot be recommended for routine use in all pediatric surgical patients. Instead, one should focus attention on skillful airway management at the time of anesthetic induction and emergence, nasogastric and orogastric suctioning, and consideration of an alternate anesthetic technique (e.g., regional anesthesia) in the child at increased risk of aspiration.

A Practical Approach

A large percentage of healthy, fasted children have significant gastric residual volumes and pH values below 2.5; therefore, this condition may be considered "normal." A number of specific disease entities and conditions create the clinical setting of a "full stomach" and place the child at increased risk of aspiration. These include gastroesophageal reflux, recent ingestion of a meal with subsequent trauma or acute illness, hyperchlorhydria, peptic ulcer disease, extreme anxiety or fear, large abdominal tumors or ascites, and gastrointestinal obstruction (pyloric stenosis, volvulus, or obstructing intraperitoneal adhesions).

If time allows, children with full stomachs should undergo a 6- to 8-hour fast in the interest of maximizing any possible gastric emptying. Infants and small children should receive intravenous fluids during this period. If not contraindicated (e.g., metoclopramide in the presence of intestinal obstruction), pharmacologic agents, including sodium citrate, histamine₂-receptor antagonists, and metoclopramide, may be administered to increase gastric pH, reduce gastric volume, and facilitate gastric emptying.

Depending on the specific surgical condition, the patient's mental status, and coexisting medical problems, regional anesthetic techniques may be considered. Nasogastric or orogastric suctioning of gastric contents prior to induction and extubation may be attempted if general anesthesia is provided. However, multiorificed gastric tubes are not capable of removing large food particles, and one should never assume that because the stomach has been suctioned it is also empty.

ANESTHETIC INDUCTION

How Should the Airway Be Managed?

Awake Intubation

A variety of techniques may be used to secure the airway. Patients with hemodynamic instability or abnormal airways in whom tracheal intubation is expected to be difficult should be intubated while awake. Intubation may be accomplished blindly by the nasal route, orally or nasally with direct laryngoscopy, or, if time allows, with a pediatric fiberoptic laryngoscope. Appropriate monitors include a pulse oximeter and an electrocardiograph. Suction equipment and an assistant skilled in applying cricoid pressure (Fig. 61–2) should be available,[57, 58] and preoxygenation should be provided.

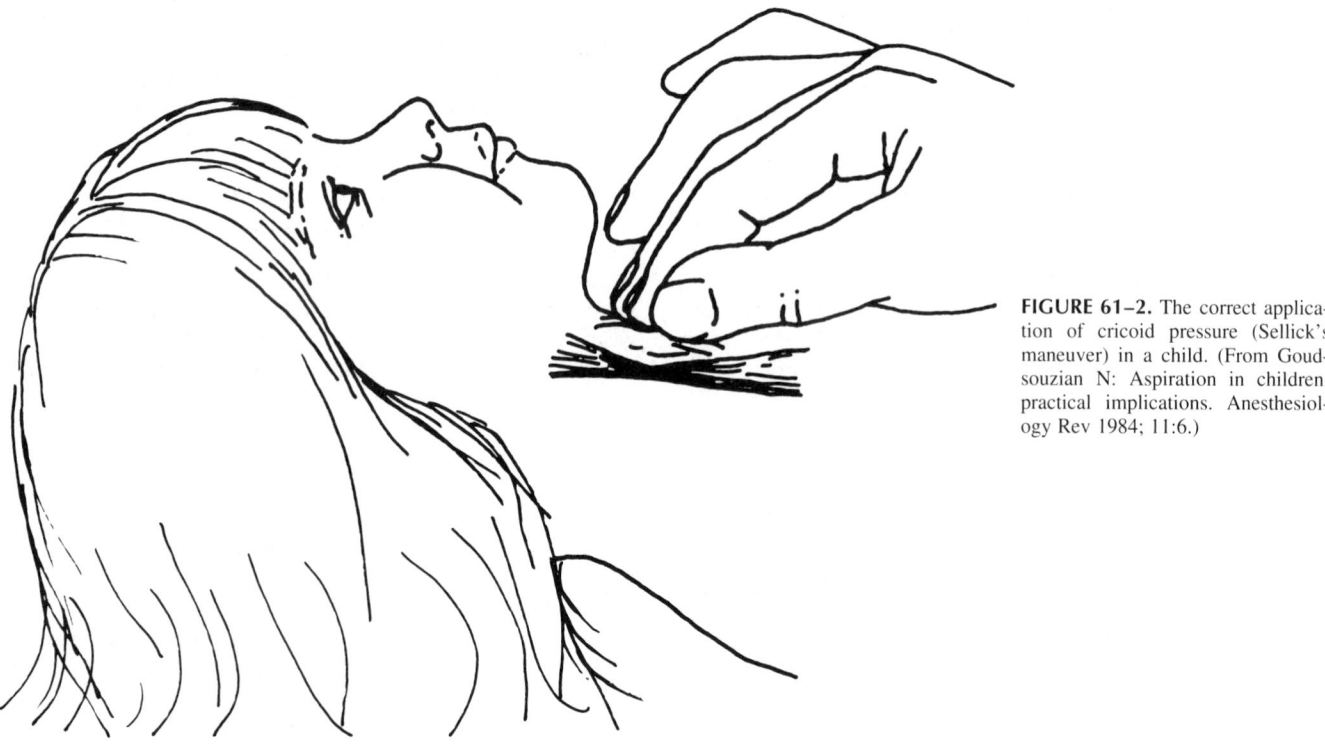

FIGURE 61–2. The correct application of cricoid pressure (Sellick's maneuver) in a child. (From Goudsouzian N: Aspiration in children: practical implications. Anesthesiology Rev 1984; 11:6.)

Rapid Sequence Induction

If the patient is hemodynamically stable and no difficulty is anticipated, intubation may be performed following induction of anesthesia. Preferably, and most commonly, a "rapid sequence" technique is used with a simultaneously administered intravenous induction agent (thiopental, ketamine, etomidate, or propofol) and a muscle relaxant, usually succinylcholine. Cricoid pressure is applied, and no positive-pressure mask ventilation is attempted; when the patient is induced and fully relaxed, ideally in less than 1 minute, direct laryngoscopy is performed, and the trachea is intubated with a styletted endotracheal tube. Following confirmation of appropriate tube placement by auscultation and detection of end-tidal CO_2, cricoid pressure is released, and the stomach is suctioned.

Inhalation Induction

Although a "rapid sequence" intravenous induction is the preferred method of inducing general anesthesia in a child with a normal airway and a full stomach, an occasional patient may be encountered in whom attempts at awake peripheral intravenous catheter placement have failed. The options in this case are to insert a percutaneous central line, perform a peripheral venous cutdown, or proceed with an inhalation induction and establish venous access after the child is anesthetized.

Each of these alternative approaches has its own merits and risks that must be considered in light of the specific clinical situation at hand. If a mask inhalation induction is chosen, one of the premedication techniques discussed previously should be utilized to smooth the induction. Spontaneous ventilation should be maintained as long as possible after beginning administration of the volatile agent, and an assistant should apply cricoid pressure until the trachea is intubated.

Should the Parents Be Present for Anesthetic Induction?

The practice of allowing one or both parents of a pediatric surgical patient to be present at the time of anesthetic induction has become increasingly popular in recent years, particularly at pediatric centers. Psychologists and pediatricians have been aware of the benefit of minimizing the period of parent-child separation for many years.[59] The provision of anesthetic and surgical care on an outpatient basis has focused attention on methods to get the child into the operating room, to induce anesthesia for the procedure, and to prepare the child for discharge with a minimum of premedication and recovery time. Several of the premedication schemes described earlier have resulted from this interest as has the preference of parental presence for anesthetic induction, which may minimize or alleviate the requirement for premedication and its potential for delayed recovery.[60, 61] Children of all ages but particularly those between the ages of 1 and 6 years (for whom separation anxiety is most likely to be a problem) benefit from having a parent in attendance at the time of induction.

Options

Allowing a parent to be present for anesthetic induction poses several potential logistic and management problems. Perhaps the most obvious is how to get the parent to the site of anesthetic induction, which is usually within or adjacent to the sterile environment of the operating room. Some operating suites are constructed with adjoining induction rooms into which parents may go dressed in street clothes; following induction, the parents leave, the airway is secured, and intravenous access is obtained (if necessary) either in the induction room or following transfer to the operating room.

An alternative but cumbersome approach is to have parents change into regular operating room scrub wear or put on a coverall "bunny suit" for access to the operating room. If bringing the parent to the induction site creates too many problems, the final option is to bring the induction site to the parent in the preoperative clinic or holding area. In this case, nearly any of the premedication techniques discussed previously may be employed with the goal of inducing anxiolysis and a state beyond sedation.

Precautions

Several caveats to allowing parental presence for induction of the child merit discussion. Wherever it is to occur, whether in an induction room or a holding area, airway equipment and resuscitative drugs must be readily available. The anesthetist caring for the patient should have an understanding of and be comfortable with parental presence. Provider concerns include fear of the parent watching or being critical during induction, having to divide one's attention between the child and parent, and fear that parental anxiety may make the child more upset.[61] With experience, these concerns are seldom an issue.

Finally, parents should be well informed prior to induction of their child as to what they may expect to see and experience and should be aware that they may be asked to leave the room immediately if a complication or emergency arises. A recent study demonstrated that a significant number of parents experience anxiety or become upset while observing their child's induction, particularly as the child loses consciousness and becomes limp.[62] However, the great majority felt their presence was beneficial to the child's emotional well-being (88%) and assisted the anesthesiologist (65%).

How Is an Inhalation Induction Performed?

Numerous methods are available for induction of general anesthesia; several are extensions of premedication techniques, and each has its own benefits and unique applications. The choice of technique is influenced by the patient's medical condition, ability to cooperate, the nature and duration of the surgical procedure, and the skill and training of the practitioner. Although mask inhalation of potent vapor agents is the most common means of inducing anesthesia in children below the age of approximately 10 years,[63] other techniques include intravenous, intramuscular, and rectal approaches.

The Classic Approach

A variety of inhalation induction techniques are available, many of which are facilitated by nasal, oral, intramuscular, or rectal premedication. The classical mask induction begins with the administration of a high-flow mixture of nitrous oxide and O_2 (60–70% nitrous oxide) through a cupped hand or loosely applied face mask. As the child becomes "stunned" or more sedated, the mask can be held snugly to the face and a potent agent, usually halothane, can be added in a low concentration of from 0.25% to 0.5%. The concentration of the volatile agent is increased in 0.25% to 0.5% increments with every fourth breath that the child takes.

If the potent agent is advanced too slowly or if the fresh gas flow is too low, the patient may experience a period of prolonged excitement (body movement, breathholding, agitation) during induction. If the anesthetic concentration is increased too rapidly, the child may likewise withdraw from the mask or develop breathholding or laryngospasm. The maximum indicated vaporizer "dial" concentration of volatile anesthetic administered is dependent on the medical condition and speed of induction of the patient. A healthy toddler or child readily tolerates a 3% to 4% concentration of halothane *with spontaneous ventilation* during induction, whereas an aggressively fluid-restricted infant does not.

Monitoring

Monitors applied prior to beginning a mask induction should include at a minimum a precordial stethoscope and a pulse oximeter; a noninvasive blood pressure cuff and ECG electrodes may be applied after the child loses consciousness. All healthy children need not be fully monitored prior to beginning a mask induction; the time and act of applying sticky pads and blood pressure cuffs may be the difference between the child who remains calm and cooperative and one who decompensates and becomes difficult to manage.

Full preinduction monitoring is reasonable in small infants and any older child with a significant cardiac or pulmonary abnormality that may affect the induction. Only after the child has reached a light plane of surgical anesthesia should an intravenous catheter be placed. Following placement, the anesthetic may be maintained by mask or the patient may be intubated with or without the use of a muscle relaxant.

Variations in Technique

As indicated previously, variations of the mask inhalation induction exist. These include the omission of nitrous oxide, the use of a potent agent other than halothane, and the "single-breath" technique.[64] In addition to some form of premedication, distraction with a story or game (e.g., a "blow-up the balloon" contest) or placement of a fruity scent inside of the mask is often helpful.

Many anesthesiologists omit nitrous oxide from their anesthetic regimens because of the wide variety of supplemental short-acting intravenous anesthetics, narcotics, and regional techniques now available; the reduction of inspired O_2 and the possibility that this low-potency agent may contribute to postoperative nausea and vomiting are two reasons for its omission.[65]

Isoflurane or enflurane may be administered in place of halothane. However, these agents are more pungent and less well tolerated by awake children and are more potent respiratory depressants than halothane.

The "single-breath" technique, somewhat of a misnomer, requires a cooperative and capable child to take a deep, vital capacity breath from a presaturated anesthesia circuit containing 5% halothane and 60% to 70% nitrous oxide. The patient must then take several regular breaths before eye closure and loss of the eyelid reflex are attained.

How Is an Intravenous Induction Performed?

General anesthesia may also be induced via the intravenous route.[66–69] Although it is the standard technique in some pediatric centers, intravenous induction generally is reserved for

TABLE 61–8. Intravenous Induction Agents in Children

Agent	Concentration	Dose	Comments
Thiopental	2.5%	4–6 mg · kg^{-1}	Rapid, smooth induction with blood pressure reduction similar to propofol Reduce dose in hypovolemic or compromised patients
Methohexital	1.0%	1–2 mg · kg^{-1}	May cause seizure activity; shorter elimination half-life than thiopental Frequent excitatory phenomena with induction
Ketamine	1.0%	1–2 mg · kg^{-1}	Useful in hypovolemic patients; increases oral secretions May induce dreaming, nystagmus, extremity movement
Propofol	2%	2–3 mg · kg^{-1}	Often burns on intravenous administration, less frequently with larger, more proximal veins Probably less nausea and vomiting than with other agents

small neonates and premature infants; for older children who may prefer awake placement of an intravenous catheter rather than a mask induction; for children who are considered at elevated risk of pulmonary aspiration or are hemodynamically unstable; and for patients who already have an intravenous catheter in place for treatment of a medical or surgical condition. Intravenous induction agents provide the most rapid loss of consciousness and can be titrated based on patient response and hemodynamic status. Commonly used agents and doses are indicated in Table 61–8.

How Are Intramuscular and Rectal Induction Performed?

The intramuscular and rectal routes are extensions of premedication techniques in which lower dosages of medications are used. The distinction between preanesthetic sedation and anesthetic induction with these approaches lies in a gray zone, however. Although they allow induction outside of the operating room in the parents' presence, they have the potential to induce airway obstruction and respiratory depression.

Intramuscular induction agents include methohexital (administration of 8–10 mg · kg^{-1} of a 5% solution, which is followed by loss of consciousness in 3–5 minutes)[70] and ketamine (administration of 3–10 mg · kg^{-1}, with loss of consciousness in 1–2 minutes). Rectal induction is usually accomplished with 25 to 35 mg · kg^{-1} of methohexital or thiopental administered with a well-lubricated, shortened suction catheter affixed to a syringe; loss of consciousness usually occurs within 10 minutes.

Our experience with intramuscular and rectal midazolam is that it provides effective sedation but seldom results in actual loss of consciousness with dosages of 0.3 to 0.5 mg · kg^{-1}.

How Is the Trachea Intubated?

Once the child has reached a satisfactory level of anesthesia, direct laryngoscopy is attempted; if the vocal cords and glottis

are visualized, the trachea is intubated with an appropriately sized endotracheal tube. If the glottis is not visualized, simple maneuvers, including a change in head and neck position, use of a different laryngoscope blade, and application of cricoid pressure, should be considered. If these adjustments fail to allow visualization of the glottis, alternative techniques of intubation, the need for which were anticipated prior to beginning the induction, are attempted.

At no time should the child receive a muscle relaxant until effective, controlled mask ventilation has been demonstrated. Unless contraindicated, succinylcholine is the preferred agent for use prior to securing the difficult airway, although mivacurium may serve as a suitable alternative.[71]

Failed Attempts

If at any time the patient is unable to be ventilated by mask or develops hemodynamic instability or oxyhemoglobin desaturation, consideration should be given to discontinuing anesthesia and attempting intubation while the patient is awake or on another day, or to proceeding to emergency percutaneous needle or surgical cricothyrotomy. Specific clinical circumstances and the experience of the anesthesiologist determine which of these alternatives is most appropriate. In some cases, awake intubation may be indicated from the start, as in the neonate with an obstructing airway mass or in the unstable trauma victim.

Alternative Techniques

Alternative techniques of intubation that may be applied in either the awake (with or without airway topicalization) or anesthetized child include (1) blind nasal intubation, which requires spontaneous ventilation; (2) use of several variations of small-caliber fiberoptic laryngoscopes[72] (Fig. 61–3); (3) use of devices such as a lighted stylet (''lightwand'')[73] or a Bullard laryngoscope[74]; and (4) ''retrograde'' intubation, in which the endotracheal tube is advanced through the nose or mouth and into the trachea over a guidewire that has been passed through an introducer in the cricothyroid membrane and into the upper airway[75] (see Fig. 61–3).

What Are the Essential Equipment Requirements?

In the course of preparing the operating room, a prepared checklist or predetermined routine should be followed so as not to omit any essential element of care. Valuable time and patient safety are jeopardized when appropriate checks and equipment preparation are not performed prior to the patient's arrival in the operating room.

Although a variety of different preanesthesia checklists have been developed in recent years, one published by the Food and Drug Administration in 1986 has achieved widespread use.[76] Additionally, it is suggested that the individual practitioner be thoroughly familiar with the manufacturers' recommendations and procedures for the start-up and use of all items. The mnemonic ''MS MAIDS'' (Table 61–9) serves as a useful guide to follow in ensuring that all areas of supply and equipment preparation have been considered.

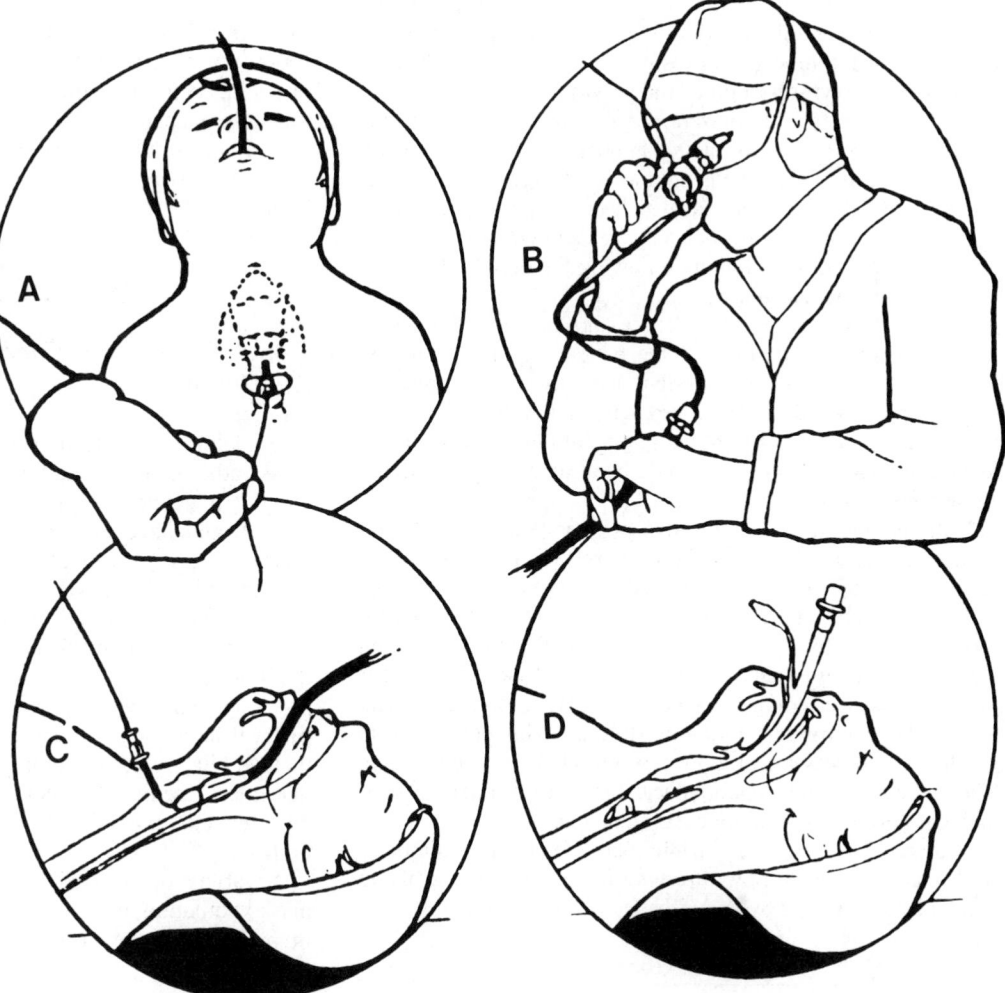

FIGURE 61–3. Technique of retrograde intubation in a child, using a fiberoptic laryngoscope. *A,* A flexible guidewire is introduced through a needle or intravenous catheter that has been inserted into the cricothyroid membrane, into the larynx, and up through the vocal cords and mouth. *B,* The guidewire is inserted into the suction channel of a fiberoptic laryngoscope over which an appropriately sized endotracheal tube has been placed. *C,* The fiberoptic laryngoscope is advanced over the guidewire into the larynx and upper trachea. *D,* The endotracheal tube is advanced over the fiberscope into the trachea, with fiberoptic visualization of the endotracheal tube tip within the trachea prior to removal of the guidewire and fiberscope. (Modified from Lechman MJ, Donahoo JS, Macvaugh H: Endotracheal intubation using percutaneous retrograde guidewire insertion followed by antegrade fiberoptic bronchoscopy. Crit Care Med 1986; 14:589. © Williams & Wilkins, 1986.)

Suction

Reliable central wall or portable suction must be continuously available in all anesthetizing locations. An appropriate selection of soft suction catheters in sizes 6, 8, and 10 French should be available for use with pediatric-sized endotracheal tubes in addition to rigid Yankauer suction instruments for large volumes of oral secretions. Soft, flexible catheters can be used to suction and decompress the stomach of infants and toddlers, whereas multiorificed tubes specifically designed for nasogastric or orogastric use may be required in older children and adolescents.

Airway

Airway supplies that must be available in a range of appropriate sizes include masks, oral and nasopharyngeal airways,

functional laryngoscope handles with blades, and endotracheal tubes with tube stylets. Suggested sizes of different items used in pediatric airway management are summarized in Table 61–10. Clear, see-through masks with an air-filled plastic cushion around the rim are in widespread use; allow visualization of lip color, oral secretions, and emesis; and provide a snug fit for most children.

Endotracheal Tubes

Uncuffed endotracheal tubes are commonly used in children up to approximately 8 years of age; before this age, the nar-

TABLE 61–9. Equipment Needs in the Operating Room

M	Machine, anesthesia
S	Suction
M	Monitors
A	Airway
I	Intravenous
D	Drugs
S	Special equipment

TABLE 61–10. Suggested Sizes of Pediatric Airway Equipment

Age	Oral Airways	Laryngoscope Blades	Endotracheal Tubes (mm ID)
Preterm neonate	40–50	Miller 0	2.5–3.0
Term neonate	50	Miller 0	3.0–3.5
3–6 mo	60	Miller 1	3.5
6–12 mo	60	Miller 1	4.0
2 y	70	Phillips 1, Miller 1	4.5
4 y	70	Phillips 1, Miller 2	5.0
6 y	70–80	Phillips 1, Miller 2, MacIntosh 2	5.5
8 y	80	Miller 2, MacIntosh 2	6.0
10 y	80	Miller 2, MacIntosh 2	6.5–7.0

rowest portion of the pediatric airway is in the subglottic region at the level of the cricoid cartilage, and proper placement of a cuffed tube would result in the inflated cuff resting above the narrowest portion of the airway.

Whether a "leak" is present around the endotracheal tube should be ascertained following intubation. Its presence implies that the fit of the tube is not too snug. Significant tracheal mucosal edema and ischemia, which may lead to postintubation croup in the recovery period[77] or acquired subglottic stenosis several weeks or months following the period of intubation, will thus be less likely.

The technique of checking the leak around an endotracheal tube should be standardized[78]; the patient should be supine, with the head in a neutral, straight and forward position, and deeply anesthetized or paralyzed with a muscle relaxant to minimize the effects of regional laryngeal muscle tone on the leak. The endotracheal tube should be at an appropriate depth for the age and size of the patient.

With the pop-off valve closed, airway pressure in the circuit is slowly increased as fresh gas enters the circuit or as the anesthesia bag is gently compressed. The anesthetist notes the leak pressure by auscultating over the larynx with a stethoscope or by listening near the patient's mouth while observing the airway pressure manometer. An audible leak should occur within the pressure range of 10 to 30 cm H_2O; too great a leak may make controlled ventilation difficult with normal fresh gas flows, whereas a leak above 30 cm H_2O or no detectable leak indicates a tight endotracheal tube-larynx interface and the potential for tracheal mucosal ischemia.

Endotracheal tube size (in millimeters of internal diameter [ID]) can be estimated by observing the circumference of the child's little finger or by using the following formula:

$$\text{mm ID} = \frac{16 + \text{age in years}}{4} \qquad \text{Equation 1}$$

The appropriate depth of insertion of an endotracheal tube in centimeters from the lips is calculated as the internal diameter of the tube multiplied by 3, or 10 plus the patient's age in years.

Intravenous Supplies

Necessary intravenous supplies include venous catheters in an assortment of sizes from 18 to 24 gauge, alcohol or iodine preparation pads, tourniquets, adhesive tape or clear plastic patches to secure and protect the catheter insertion site, and an infusion set with an appropriate intravenous fluid. For patients who weigh less than approximately 25 kg, a mini-drip set with a burette or small-volume fluid chamber that delivers 1 mL of fluid for every 60 drops affords more precise control of the fluid administration rate and reduces the maximum flow rate and potential for accidental administration of excessive intravenous fluid. Optional equipment that may be indicated for use with specific patients includes electronic infusion pumps and fluid warmers.

Temperature Control

Depending on the age and size of the patient and the nature and duration of the surgical procedure, consideration should be given to the use of some combination of techniques or devices to maintain or elevate core body temperature. These include increasing the ambient temperature of the operating room, use of a radiant heat lamp and heating blanket on the operating table, insertion of a humidifier or passive heat and moisture exchanger ("artificial nose") into the breathing circuit, administration of blood and fluids through warming devices, and covering the patient with plastic wraps or warmed blankets or towels.

ANESTHETIC MAINTENANCE

Which Patients Are Candidates for Mask Anesthesia?

Guidelines for selecting general anesthesia delivered by a mask rather than an endotracheal tube are similar to those for adults. In general, patients who are scheduled for elective surgery and have had an appropriate NPO interval, do not appear to have a difficult airway (e.g., micrognathia, macroglossia, or tracheal deviation) and are having surgery that does not compromise the airway nor affect pulmonary compliance are candidates for mask inhalation anesthesia. Although the duration of surgery is not an absolute determinant, cases that last longer than 1 hour tend to be more easily managed with tracheal intubation. Classic pediatric mask airway procedures include bilateral myringotomy with pressure equalization tube placement, inguinal hernia repair, circumcision, and short, distal orthopedic procedures (e.g., cast changes or wound irrigation).

A variety of congenital or acquired disorders may make mask ventilation or tracheal intubation difficult (Table 61–11). In most cases, the history and physical examination reveal

TABLE 61–11. Conditions Associated with Difficult Pediatric Airway Management

Congenital	Acquired
Choanal atresia	Infections
Subglottic stenosis (may be	Epiglottitis
acquired)	Laryngotracheitis
Cystic hygroma	Peritonsillar abscess
Tumors	Burns
Angiofibroma	Trauma (facial or cervical)
Hemangioma	Foreign body aspiration
Craniofacial syndromes	Tumors (oral cavity, neck, or mediastinum)
Crouzon's syndrome	Papillomatosis
Apert's syndrome	Juvenile rheumatoid arthritis
Goldenhar's syndrome	
Treacher Collins	
Pierre Robin	
Freeman-Sheldon	
Hallermann-Streiff	
Inborn errors of metabolism	
Hurler syndrome	
Pompe's disease	
Chromosomal abnormalities	
Trisomy-21 (Down's syndrome)	
Trisomy-13	
Trisomy-18	
Cri du chat (5p−) syndrome	
Turner's syndrome	
Beckwith-Wiedemann syndrome	
Mediastinal vascular rings	

conditions known to be associated with difficult pediatric airway management, and in many cases, it is the airway abnormality for which the patient is undergoing a surgical procedure. Unlike the case with adults, in our experience unanticipated difficult airways in children are very unusual. Physical features associated with difficult intubation include micrognathia, macroglossia, microstomia, maxillary hypoplasia, and a short neck with limitation of cervical spine mobility.

What Breathing Circuit Should Be Used?

Pediatric breathing circuits may be divided into circle systems and variations of the Mapleson classification of semi-open, nonrebreathing circuits. The work of breathing necessary to overcome the resistance of the one-way valves in an adult circle system by a spontaneously breathing neonate or infant may predispose to fatigue, hypoventilation, and atelectasis. The Bain circuit, a coaxial modification of the Mapleson D circuit (Fig. 61–4), contains no such valves and is therefore associated with less work of breathing. Other advantages include a degree of warming of inspired gases as they flow through tubing within the expiratory limb of the circuit and the rapidity with which change in the concentration of gases delivered to the patient can be achieved.

For the majority of pediatric cases, particularly infants and neonates, ventilation is assisted or controlled. Hence, a circle system can be used safely in most children. Adequate fresh gas flow is a critical factor to prevent rebreathing of CO_2 in any circuit without a CO_2 absorber. A minimum fresh gas flow of 2.5 to 3.0 L · min^{-1} with an additional 100 mL · kg^{-1} · min^{-1} is recommended for the Bain circuit.[79] Even higher fresh gas flow rates of 2 to 3 times the minute volume of ventilation also have been recommended, particularly during spontaneous breathing.[80]

How Do the Inhalation Agents Compare?

Anesthetic drugs and adjunctive agents such as muscle relaxants used to maintain the state of general anesthesia following one of the induction techniques discussed previously are essentially the same as those employed in adults. However, the dose-responses and clinical use of these medications frequently differ in children. Examples of such differences with the commonly used inhalation agent halothane are the higher minimum alveolar concentration values in infants and small children[81] and the widespread use of halothane for mask induction of general anesthesia.

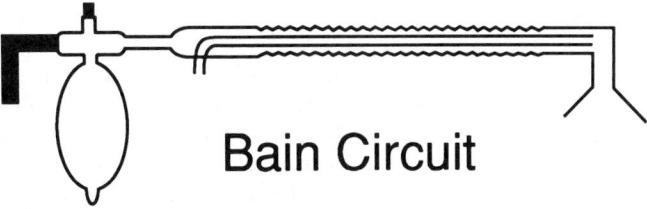

FIGURE 61–4. Schematic diagram of the Bain circuit demonstrating its coaxial design, with inner inspiratory flow tubing, outer (corrugated) flow channel, and anesthesia bag.

General Features

Halothane, enflurane, and isoflurane remain the only drugs that are individually capable of providing amnesia, analgesia, control of autonomic nervous system reflexes, and muscle relaxation. Halothane and isoflurane are used to the almost total exclusion of enflurane, primarily because enflurane offers no particular advantages and possesses a number of undesirable features. These include a somewhat pungent, disagreeable odor, low potency (higher minimum alveolar concentration) when compared with halothane and isoflurane, profound respiratory depression during spontaneous ventilation, and a small but significant degree of metabolism that results in liberation of potentially nephrotoxic free fluoride ions during prolonged administration.

Halothane has the most agreeable odor and is, therefore, associated with less breathholding, coughing, and laryngospasm than is isoflurane. Halothane and isoflurane minimum alveolar concentration values (at age 6 months, when minimum alveolar concentration peaks) are approximately 30% to 50% greater than adult values. A potent inhaled agent may be used alone or in combination with adjuvants such as nitrous oxide and narcotics for the maintenance of anesthesia.

Hemodynamic Effects

Halothane and isoflurane differ significantly in their hemodynamic effects, a fact that has implications for the anesthetic management of infants, who have limited myocardial contractile reserve, and of children with congenital heart disease. Halothane is a myocardial depressant and tends to reduce heart rate, whereas isoflurane tends to maintain or increase heart rate and to reduce peripheral vascular resistance, thus minimizing reductions in cardiac index. Greater cardiovascular reserve and ability to tolerate intravenous fluid challenges are said to occur with the use of isoflurane.[82]

Speed of Induction

Despite isoflurane's lower blood:gas solubility coefficient (1.4), which would be expected to provide more rapid anesthetic induction and recovery than halothane (the blood:gas solubility coefficient of halothane is 2.4), most clinical studies fail to demonstrate any significant difference between the agents. One report suggested shorter induction and elimination times for isoflurane.[83] This observation, in combination with many practitioners' clinical impressions that children anesthetized with isoflurane appear to wake up and recover more rapidly following cessation of administration, support the widespread practice of switching from halothane to isoflurane after induction. In general, however, halothane and isoflurane can be used interchangeably with similar results.

Of What Value Are Narcotics?

Narcotics are used both as supplements to inhalation anesthesia and, in higher dosages, as primary anesthetic agents. As adjuvants, doses include morphine, 0.05 to 0.1 mg · kg^{-1}; meperidine, 0.5 to 1.0 mg · kg^{-1}; fentanyl, 1 to 3 μg · kg^{-1}; sufentanil, 0.1 to 0.3 μg · kg^{-1}; and alfentanil, 10 to 50 μg · kg^{-1}. Narcotics blunt the cardiovascular responses to surgical stimulation, reduce the requirement for inhalation agents, and contribute to postoperative analgesia.

Fentanyl, 10 to 50 $\mu g \cdot kg^{-1}$, and sufentanil, 3 to 15 $\mu g \cdot kg^{-1}$, are frequently used as primary anesthetics in children with significant cardiovascular instability or in those who are undergoing cardiac surgery.[84] In these settings, these drugs must be used with muscle relaxants. Because the narcotics may not provide adequate amnesia, even with high dosages, they are supplemented with benzodiazepines or low concentrations of the potent inhalation agents.

Among the side effects are respiratory depression, chest wall rigidity, and bradycardia, particularly with rapid intravenous administration of higher dosages. Morphine and meperidine additionally induce histamine release, whereas meperidine induces tachycardia.

When Are Muscle Relaxants Indicated?

Muscle relaxants are used to facilitate tracheal intubation following anesthetic induction and to provide neuromuscular blockade throughout some procedures. They may be necessary for improved surgical exposure or to prevent patient movement should the level of anesthesia become unexpectedly "light." Differences in the pharmacokinetic and pharmacodynamic responses to muscle relaxants in pediatric and adult patients have received a great deal of attention in the anesthesia literature.[85] Most significant are the altered volumes of distribution of these water-soluble drugs and immaturity of the neuromuscular junction,[86] particularly in the neonatal and early infancy periods.

Nondepolarizing Agents

The nondepolarizing muscle relaxants are indicated in Table 61–12 along with their effective (ED_{95}) and intubating doses. Choice for a specific case is based on the anticipated duration of the procedure and the expected side effects of the agents. Because of significant variability in the individual response to muscle relaxants, monitors of neuromuscular function should be used to guide dosing.

Whether routine reversal of nondepolarizing relaxants (particularly atracurium and vecuronium) should be employed is controversial. Up to 70% of acetylcholine receptors at the neuromuscular junction may be blocked in the presence of an intact twitch response.[87] Infants and small children with increased O_2 consumption and ventilatory requirements may be predisposed to subclinical muscle weakness and respiratory failure. These facts suggest the advisability of reversal. Yet, if

an adequate interval has elapsed since the agent was last administered, and if adequate recovery of neuromuscular function can be demonstrated clinically[88] and with neuromuscular transmission (train-of-four) monitoring, the withholding of reversal agents such as edrophonium or neostigmine and close observation are probably satisfactory.[85]

Succinylcholine

Succinylcholine is the only depolarizing muscle relaxant in clinical use in the United States and is also the shortest acting of all relaxants. It is also the only agent that may be safely given intramuscularly when muscle relaxation is required but an intravenous route is lacking.[89]

Succinylcholine is associated with a number of potential side effects or complications that make its use less attractive. These include cardiac dysrhythmias such as bradycardia or sinus arrest, masseter spasm, rhabdomyolysis, and MH. In view of these potential problems, many anesthesiologists now reserve succinylcholine for use in specific circumstances, including rapid sequence inductions, when laryngospasm occurs, and in instances in which the longer duration of muscle relaxation provided by the nondepolarizing agents is undesirable. Mivacurium, a recently released short-acting nondepolarizing drug, may prove to be a suitable alternative to succinylcholine.[71]

How Should Ketamine and Propofol Be Used?

These intravenous drugs, which are typically used as induction agents, may also be used in incremental boluses or by continuous infusion for the maintenance of general anesthesia. Ketamine is particularly useful in hypovolemic patients and may also be given intramuscularly but is associated with several undesirable side effects, including dreaming, vomiting, increased intracranial pressure, and increased production of secretions.

Propofol is noted for the rapidity of recovery from its desired effects and for the low incidence of side effects, such as vomiting, headache, and confusion. It is particularly useful in short-duration procedures on outpatients and in situations when inhalation anesthetics are difficult or impossible to administer, such as when sedation must be provided for MRI procedures and jet ventilation for bronchoscopy or airway surgery.[90, 91]

FLUID THERAPY AND BLOOD TRANSFUSION

Which Children Require Intravenous Access?

If the question of intravenous access for a particular patient arises, it probably should be used. It should always be provided for any infant younger than 6 months of age; in children with any metabolic derangement (e.g., diabetes mellitus, dehydration, hyponatremia); for cases in which there exists the possibility of significant blood loss; for any procedure that is scheduled to last for more than 30 minutes; and for any patient in whom postoperative nausea or vomiting, or both, are antic-

TABLE 61–12. Effective (ED_{95}) and Intubating Doses of Nondepolarizing Muscle Relaxants in Children

Drug	Effective Dose (ED_{95}) ($\mu g \cdot kg^{-1}$)	Intubating Dose ($\mu g \cdot kg^{-1}$)
Atracurium	110–193	500–600
Doxacurium	27–32	500
Metocurine	180–340	300
Mivacurium	89–103	200
Pancuronium	81	100
Pipecuronium	56–70	100
Tubocurarine	320–600	600
Vecuronium	56–80	100

(Modified from Goudsouzian NG: Neuromuscular blocking agents in chilldren. Paediatr Anaesth 1991; 1:75.)

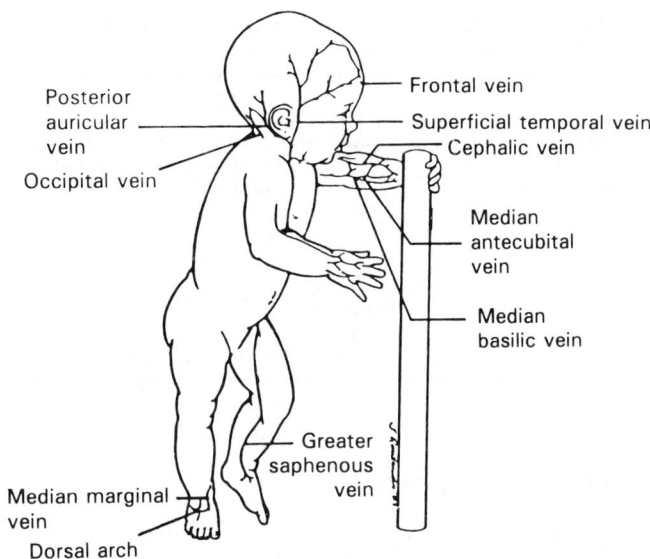

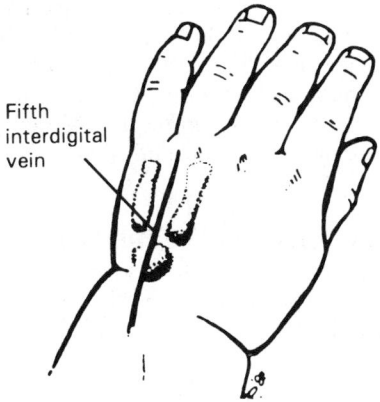

FIGURE 61–5. Peripheral intravenous access sites in the child. (From Baldwin GA: Handbook of Pediatric Emergencies. Boston, Little, Brown & Co, 1989, p 18.)

ipated. The only cases that do not routinely require intravenous access prior to the procedure are short, minimally invasive procedures in relatively healthy patients, such as pressure-equalizing tube placement and cast changes. Common sites of catheter placement are shown in Figure 61–5.

What Are the Available Alternatives to Vascular Access?

Central Venous Access

Pediatric vascular access frequently poses a daunting challenge. Along with the usual peripheral access sites, central venous access may be obtained through the external or internal jugular, subclavian, or femoral veins.

Intraosseous Access

Should these sites prove inaccessible, fluid resuscitation and the administration of medications may be accomplished via an intraosseous cannula in emergencies. Catecholamines, whole blood, calcium, antibiotics, digitalis, heparin, lidocaine, atro-

pine, and sodium bicarbonate have been infused via this route.[92]

A large (16- to 18-gauge) hypodermic needle, spinal needle with stylet, or bone marrow needle may be placed into the marrow cavity of any long bone. Typically, the tibia is chosen as the easiest and least complicated site. The technique is accomplished by placing the needle on the anterior surface of the tibia, 1 to 3 cm inferior to the tibial tuberosity. The needle is positioned perpendicular to the plane of the tibial surface and directed slightly caudad to avoid the epiphyseal plate (Fig. 61–6).[93] When the needle tip is in the bone marrow cavity, bone marrow aspirate should be obtainable, and a free flow of infusate should ensue. (See Chapters 32 and 50).

Endotracheal Access

Some medications may also be administered via the endotracheal tube. These include lidocaine, atropine, naloxone, and epinephrine.

What Are Maintenance Fluids?

Comprehensive fluid management includes consideration of maintenance fluid requirements, pre-existing water and electrolyte deficits, and intraoperative losses of fluid and blood. Maintenance fluids are those that would normally be consumed orally by the child to provide for the needs of caloric expenditure and metabolism, insensible water loss through the skin and respiratory tract, and measurable water loss through urinary and fecal excretion.

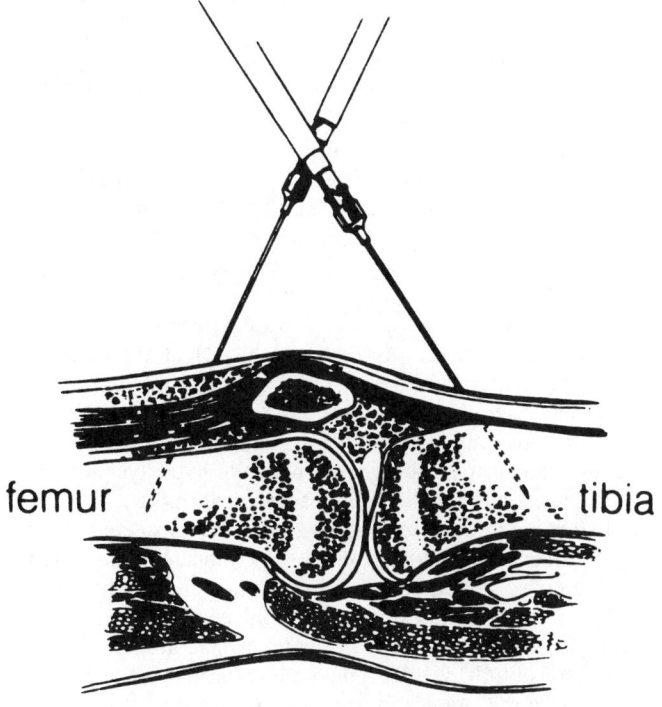

FIGURE 61–6. Placement of an intraosseous needle in the distal femur or proximal tibia. Note orientation away from the epiphyseal plate. (From Rosetti VA, Thompson BM, Miller J, et al: Intraosseous infusion: an alternative route of pediatric intravascular access. Ann Emerg Med 1985; 14:585.)

Infusion Rate

Administration rates may be calculated on the basis of weight, body surface area, or elaborate measures of metabolic rate.[94] For the initial 10 kg of body weight, 100 mL · kg^{-1} of water are needed for each 24-hour period. For the second 10-kg increment of weight, 50 mL · kg^{-1} are required per 24-hour period, and for every 1 kg above 20 kg, 25 mL · kg^{-1} per 24-hour period are needed.

If the 24-hour day is rounded up to 25 hours, the "4-2-1" rule may be applied to determine the hourly basal fluid requirement in any patient. For example, a 30-kg normothermic child in a normal indoor environment would require 70 mL · h^{-1} of maintenance fluid: 40 mL · h^{-1} for the initial 10 kg; 20 mL · h^{-1} for the next 10 kg; and 10 mL · h^{-1} for the final 10 kg.

Of course, water alone is not infused, since there are additional needs for electrolytes and glucose; the requirement for sodium is 3 mEq, that for potassium is 2 mEq, and that for chloride is 2 mEq per 100 mL of water. Quarter normal (0.22%) saline with 20 mEq · L^{-1} added potassium most closely approximates these requirements. Glucose is commonly added as well to meet part of the energy substrate need and to increase the tonicity of the intravenous fluid solution.

Glucose Requirements

The issue of how much (if any) glucose to provide in the intravenous fluids for a surgical procedure on a child remains controversial, and a wide variation of practice exists among pediatric anesthesiologists. On the one hand, routine administration of a 5% glucose-containing intravenous solution as the sole fluid during surgery frequently results in hyperglycemia.[95] Subsequent osmotic diuresis and the possibility of worsened neurologic outcome should a cerebral ischemic event occur intraoperatively are concerns. On the other hand, administration of glucose-free solutions presents the risk of having the patient become hypoglycemic while anesthetized, with consequent impairment of function or damage of the nervous[96, 97] or other organ systems.

The optimum glucose infusion concentration appears to range between 1.0% and 2.5%.[98, 99] That glucose requirements are lower during anesthesia and surgery than during the awake state is a result of the sympathoadrenal stress response to surgery, decreased glucose utilization, and increased gluconeogenesis.[100]

To insist that every pediatric patient receive intravenous glucose during surgery is unreasonable. Healthy, well-nourished children undergoing short procedures (shorter than 1 hour) may receive a glucose-free infusion as long as all caregivers involved understand that a small but real chance exists that the patient may be asymptomatically hypoglycemic prior to or during surgery. For this reason, performing a finger- or heel-stick blood glucose analysis should be considered following anesthesia induction; if the results indicate a low glucose level, glucose should be added to the intravenous infusion.

Patients at risk of developing hypoglycemia, as indicated in Table 61–13, should receive supplemental glucose in their intravenous fluids. Ideally, glucose is infused at a constant rate during surgery, preferably by "piggy-backing" the glucose-containing solution into the main intravenous infusion. Alternatively, a dedicated second intravenous catheter can be utilized.

TABLE 61–13. Children at Increased Risk of Developing Hypoglycemia During Anesthesia

Infants	Children
Preterm infants	Patients receiving total parenteral nutrition
Infants of diabetic mothers	Malnourished or chronically-diseased patients
Infants with erythroblastosis fetalis	Patients receiving insulin therapy
Infants small for gestational age	Patient who have been nil per os for prolonged periods
	Patients with certain glycogen storage diseases
	Patients undergoing prolonged surgical procedures
	Patients with insulin-secreting tumors

What Are Fasting Fluid Deficits?

The subject of preoperative fasting periods and resultant fluid deficits was discussed earlier in this chapter. The fasting fluid deficit is calculated by multiplying the hourly maintenance fluid rate by the number of hours since the patient last ingested oral fluids. One-half of this deficit is administered in addition to the maintenance fluid during the first hour of anesthesia; the remaining half is infused during the next 2 hours.[101] The fluid used to make up the fasting deficit is the same as that used for the maintenance infusion.

What Constitutes Intraoperative Fluid Loss?

Intraoperative fluid losses include so-called "third space" loss and actual blood loss.

Third Space Loss

Third space loss is the result of the transfer of isotonic fluid primarily from the extracellular compartment to a nonfunctional interstitial compartment. A number of conditions in addition to surgical tissue trauma may result in significant third space loss, including burns, gastrointestinal tract obstruction, infections, and blunt trauma. These fluid losses are difficult to quantify and must be estimated based on such factors as the size of the incision, the exposure of visceral surfaces, and the degree of inflammation present. Third space loss is replenished with non–glucose-containing isotonic fluid at rates that range from 1 mL · kg^{-1} · h^{-1} for minor procedures with minimal tissue injury to as much as 20 mL · kg^{-1} · h^{-1} for large abdominal incisions with extensive inflammation or tissue injury.

Blood Loss

Any intraoperative blood loss exceeding the minimum amount of 1% of estimated blood volume should be replaced in some fashion. The first step in replacement is to determine the allowable blood loss, that is, the volume of lost blood below which replacement will be provided by crystalloid or colloid preparations and above which a blood component such as packed red blood cells will be given. Calculation of the allowable blood loss requires an estimate of the patient's total blood volume, preoperative hematocrit, and the lowest acceptable hematocrit without a blood product transfusion. The total blood volume is approximately 90 mL · kg⁻¹ in the full-term infant; this value declines to 70 mL · kg⁻¹ by the age of 1 year.

Lowest Acceptable Hematocrit

The lowest acceptable hematocrit, or so-called "transfusion trigger," for all patients has steadily drifted downward because of the heightened concern of exposing patients to blood-borne infectious agents such as the human immunodeficiency and hepatitis viruses.[102] The hematocrit of an otherwise healthy child who is expected to make an uncomplicated recovery from surgery may be allowed to decrease to between 18% and 20% without transfusion. Some patients with chronic disease states may require higher minimum hematocrit values. With these considerations in mind, the allowable blood loss (ABL) is determined by the following relationship, in which the preoperative hematocrit (pre-Hct) and lowest acceptable hematocrit (la-Hct) are entered as decimals:

$$ABL = \frac{EBV \times (pre\text{-}Hct) - (la\text{-}Hct)}{(pre\text{-}Hct)} \qquad \text{Equation 2}$$

An expansion of this calculation, which also yields ABL, involves determining the difference of the red cell masses between the preoperative and lowest acceptable hematocrits (assuming that normovolemia is maintained) and multiplying this value by 3.

Replacement

Blood loss below the approximate ABL is replaced in the ratio of 2 to 3 mL of isotonic, non–glucose-containing crystalloid per 1 mL of blood loss or in a 1:1 ratio with a colloidal preparation such as 5% albumin or 5% plasma protein fraction. For patients with a pre-existing coagulopathy or a dilutional coagulopathy secondary to massive blood loss and transfusion, fresh frozen plasma may be used as an alternative colloid preparation, although dilutional coagulopathy is most commonly secondary to thrombocytopenia. Once the ABL has been exceeded, packed red blood cells should be administered.

Older children and adolescents may receive an entire unit of blood, not unlike adults. Infants and small children should receive packed red blood cells in 5- to 10-mL · kg⁻¹ increments by syringe or from subdivided units of blood. Serial hematocrit determinations, ongoing blood loss, and the hemodynamic response to the red blood cell infusion determine the speed and amount of transfusion. To the extent possible, a transfusion from a single-donor source should be continued once the child has been "exposed" to the blood. This approach optimizes the hematocrit and minimizes the chance of the patient requiring a second transfusion from another donor hours or days later. The justification for administration of all blood products should be clearly documented on the anesthetic record.

MONITORING

What Is Routine?

Routine monitoring in pediatric anesthesia includes, at a minimum, measures that satisfy the standards for basic intra-operative monitoring adopted by the American Society of Anesthesiologists.[103] These include (1) the presence of an anesthetist at all times; (2) monitoring of adequate oxygenation, as provided by an O_2 analyzer with audible alarm and pulse oximeter; (3) monitoring of adequate ventilation, as provided by a precordial or esophageal stethoscope, capnograph, and a functioning "disconnect" alarm if the patient is being mechanically ventilated; (4) a continuous ECG and arterial blood pressure measured at least every 5 minutes; and (5) a means to measure body temperature. To this list may be added monitoring of neuromuscular transmission in children receiving muscle relaxants in the course of anesthesia.

Pulse Oximetry and Capnography

Pulse oximetry has been shown to reduce the incidence of critical desaturation events in children undergoing general anesthesia.[104] Capnography provides the earliest diagnosis of esophageal intubation, accidental disconnections within the breathing circuit, inadvertent extubation, and endotracheal tube obstruction.[105] It also may reflect the onset of problems, including MH, venous air or particulate embolism, and acute changes in cardiac output.

What Common Intraoperative Problems May Be Detected?

Airway Obstruction

Airway obstruction in the narrow sense implies loss of upper airway patency from causes such as posterior displacement of the tongue into the oropharynx. Premature placement of an oral airway, the presence of blood and secretions in proximity to the larynx, and surgical manipulation during light anesthesia may trigger laryngospasm.

Management of upper airway obstruction includes placement of an artificial oral or nasal airway, administration of 100% O_2 with low-level continuous positive airway pressure (3–5 cm H_2O), and performing simple maneuvers such as a chin-lift or jaw-thrust. If laryngospasm fails to respond to these measures, a small dose of intravenous succinylcholine (0.2–0.5 mg · kg⁻¹) induces relaxation of the laryngeal muscles and facilitates assisted or controlled ventilation. Consideration should then be given to intubating the trachea.

In a broader sense, airway obstruction includes endotracheal tube occlusion by secretions or tissue; lower airway compromise due to bronchospasm or foreign bodies; and extrinsic compression of the intrathoracic airway by tumors or surgical manipulation.

Oxyhemoglobin Desaturation

Oxyhemoglobin desaturation indicated by a decreased SpO_2 results from any process that interferes with O_2 uptake or transport. Problems may involve the supply of O_2 to the breathing circuit, airway obstruction, cardiac dysfunction, and impaired perfusion of specific limbs or tissue beds. When desaturation develops abruptly during anesthesia, apnea, airway obstruction, endotracheal tube displacement, or malfunction of the ventilator and breathing circuit is commonly responsible.

The immediate response should be to administer 100% O_2

manually via mask or endotracheal tube, to assess airway patency, and to begin a sequential check of all elements from the O_2 source to the peripheral circulation. Remember that surgical maneuvers may be causative (positioning, packing, and clamping). Only after other possibilities are ruled out should the possibility of monitor inaccuracy or artifact be considered. Inaccuracies may result from excessive ambient light, impaired perfusion to the site of the oximeter probe, patient movement, partial probe displacement, and electrical interference.

Temperature Fluctuations

Pediatric patients may experience significant reductions or increases in body temperature during surgery. Because of their greater ratios of body surface area to weight, they are at higher risk of significant heat loss and hypothermia in the operating room. Because this risk is now generally well recognized by anesthesiologists and operating room nursing personnel, hyperthermia due to overzealous measures to maintain body temperature, in our experience, is as common a problem as significant hypothermia.

MH is distinguished from more common causes of intraoperative temperature elevation on the basis of findings that generally appear earlier, such as hypercarbia and nonrespiratory acidosis.

Blood Pressure Fluctuations

Intraoperative hypotension is commonly due to bradycardia, hypoxemia, hypovolemia, and relative anesthetic overdose. Myocardial dysfunction, in the absence of a known history of congenital cardiac disease, is an unusual cause. Other causes include inappropriately sized blood pressure cuffs, anaphylaxis, sepsis, and tension pneumothorax.

Hypertension may be secondary to pain or light anesthesia, excessive intravenous fluid administration, hypercarbia, or the use of inappropriately small blood pressure cuffs. A small number of pediatric patients have an organic source that is usually identified preoperatively, such as coarctation of the aorta, chronic renal disease, or a catecholamine-secreting tumor.

Cardiac Dysrhythmias

Bradycardia

Primary cardiac dysrhythmias are uncommon in the absence of structural heart disease. Sinus or junctional bradycardia or sinus tachycardia may occur in response to a host of acute clinical derangements. Prior to the popularization of pulse oximetry, the dictum that bradycardia reflects hypoxemia until proved otherwise prevailed. Although hypoxemia remains an important and common cause of bradycardia, it is now easier to exclude, allowing earlier consideration of other possibilities. These include light or inadequate anesthesia with consequent vagal stimulation; any of several neural responses such as the oculocardiac reflex; and drug effects (with the use of potent inhalation anesthetics, narcotics, or cholinesterase inhibitors).

Sinus Tachycardia

Sinus tachycardia, the diagnosis of which should include consideration of the patient's age and usual heart rate, may

occur secondary to hypovolemia, light anesthesia, hypoxemia (early), hypercarbia, temperature elevation, or drug effect.

Premature Ventricular Contractions

Premature ventricular contractions may appear in the setting of light anesthesia or impaired ventilation and usually resolve spontaneously with correction of these conditions. Halothane-induced sensitization of the heart to dysrhythmias should be considered, especially with concomitant use of epinephrine infiltration at the surgical site; however, children appear to be more resistant to dysrhythmias than adults in this situation.[106]

REGIONAL ANESTHESIA

What Is Its Role?

Regional anesthesia has proved to be useful as a primary technique and as an adjunct to general anesthesia. Physiologic considerations in patients 6 months of age or younger include a minimal hemodynamic response to extensive conduction blockade. Hypotension following sympathectomy is very rare, since cardiac output, blood pressure, and carotid blood flow are well maintained.[107] Myelinization of the central nervous system is not complete until approximately 18 months of age; hence, effective neural blockade may be achieved with lower concentrations of local anesthetics. Maximum recommended doses for local anesthetics are shown in Table 61–14.

Caudal

Caudal anesthesia appears to be the most commonly administered regional technique in children. Correct placement of a caudal epidural needle is illustrated in Figure 61–7. Because the distal end of the dura can be as low as the S-3 level in neonates, care should be taken when advancing the needle into the caudal space to avoid inadvertent dural puncture. Urinary retention is a possibility following this block, although most children void within 6 to 8 hours. Postoperative voiding, therefore, need not be a criterion for discharge from the PACU in the otherwise comfortable child.

For surgery below the diaphragm, 0.25% bupivacaine or

TABLE 61–14. Maximum Recommended Doses of Local Anesthetics in Children

| Drug | Maximum Dose of Local Anesthetic (mg · kg⁻¹) | | | |
	Caudal/Lumbar Epidural	Spinal	Peripheral Nerve	Intravenous Regional
Tetracaine (0.1–0.2%)	2	0.2–0.6	2	NR
Lidocaine (0.5–2.0%)	7–10†	1–2.5	7–10†	3–5
Bupivacaine (0.25–0.50%)	3–5†	0.3–0.4	3–5†	NR

*The higher dose is recommended only with the concomitant use of epinephrine (1:200,000).
†These are suggested safe upper limits for local anesthetic administration. Accidental intravenous or intra-arterial injection of even a fraction of these amounts may result in toxicity.
(From Yastr M, Maxwell LG: Pediatric regional anesthesia. Anesthesiology 1989; 70:324.)

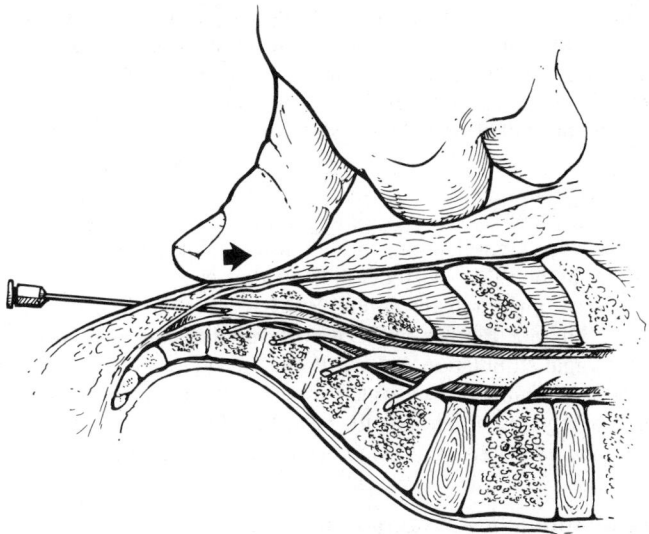

FIGURE 61–7. Sagittal view demonstrating placement of a needle within the caudal epidural space.

1.0% lidocaine (both with epinephrine, 1:200,000) in a dosage of 1 mL · kg⁻¹ (maximum 40 mL) provides good anesthetic conditions for surgery.[108] Postoperative analgesia with minimal motor blockade may be obtained with similar dosing of 0.25% bupivacaine. Analgesia of longer duration (8–24 hours) may be obtained with caudally administered preservative-free morphine in a dose of 0.05 to 0.1 mg · kg⁻¹ diluted in 5 mL of preservative-free normal saline. Ventilatory responses to CO_2 is attenuated with epidural doses of morphine as low as 0.05 mg · kg⁻¹; therefore, patients should be monitored for approximately 24 hours.[109]

Epidural

Lumbar and thoracic epidural anesthesia are becoming more popular in the pediatric age group. Technical difficulties with these approaches and the ability to obtain almost the same results by utilizing different local anesthetic and narcotic agents and volumes in the caudal space make these approaches less useful for the general anesthesiologist who may practice pediatric anesthesia infrequently.

Advantages include a decrease in the endocrine stress response to surgery[110] and the possibility of using more lipophilic narcotics (fentanyl, sufentanil) with their inherent advantages of less migration within the cerebrospinal fluid. For lumbar epidural administration, 0.75 mL · kg⁻¹ of 0.25% bupivacaine with 1:200,000 epinephrine provides good surgical analgesia; incremental dosing with 0.125% bupivacaine, with or without fentanyl, 1 to 2 μg · kg⁻¹, provides satisfactory postoperative analgesia.

Spinal

Intrathecal anesthesia for high-risk premature infants undergoing inguinal hernia repair has been suggested to avoid the risk of postoperative apnea if no incidental sedation is given. Nevertheless, studies maintain that apnea monitoring is required for all high-risk infants postoperatively.[111] Tetracaine in a dose of 0.5 to 0.6 mg · kg⁻¹ for infants less than 10 kg in weight provides adequate surgical anesthesia for approximately 75% of patients. When inadequate, the intrathecal block may be supplemented with intravenous or rectal sedation, local anesthesia, or general anesthesia.

Peripheral Nerve Blocks

Specific nerve blocks may be useful in pediatric anesthetic practice. Block of the dorsal nerve of the penis is easily performed with 0.8 mL of 1.0% plain lidocaine in the newborn and with 1 to 3 mL of 0.25% bupivacaine in older children. This nerve's major anterior and minor posterior divisions supply all but the base of the penis. The latter portion is innervated by branches from the genitofemoral and ilioinguinal nerves. Dorsal nerve block provides good anesthesia for circumcision and postoperative analgesia for hypospadias repair. The ilioinguinal and iliohypogastric nerves are also easily blocked and can provide excellent analgesia for inguinal hernia repair and orchiopexy.

Intravenous Regional

Intravenous regional anesthesia (Bier's block) is useful to provide extremity anesthesia for procedures of limited duration. Following limb exsanguination, tourniquet inflation should be twice the systolic blood pressure. Lidocaine in a dosage range of 2.5 to 5.0 mg · kg⁻¹ and in concentrations of 0.25% and 0.5% is the agent of choice.[108]

POSTANESTHETIC PROBLEMS

What Is Emergence Delirium?

Pediatric patients in the PACU experience complications unique to their age group as well as those seen in adults. Disorientation or emergence delirium is more common in children. Preoperative and intraoperative use of anticholinergics, ketamine, and the sole use of the potent inhalation anesthetics are associated with this phenomenon. Emergence delirium must be differentiated from abnormal behavior due to hypoxemia or pain; children normally pass through any period of disorientation in a short period of time.

How Is Pain Managed?

Pain is the most common problem seen in any patient population following surgery, although pediatric patients, particularly infants, tend to receive fewer analgesics intraoperatively and postoperatively. Pain can be attenuated prophylactically with adjunctive regional techniques (caudal, epidural, or intrathecal use of local anesthetics or narcotics, or both) or the parenteral administration of analgesic medications. Intravenous morphine (0.05–0.1 mg · kg⁻¹) or fentanyl (1–2 μg · kg⁻¹) is useful in ameliorating acute pain. Ketorolac, a nonsteroidal anti-inflammatory drug, is effective in alleviating postsurgical pain by the intramuscular (1 mg · kg⁻¹) and intravenous (0.9 mg · kg⁻¹) administration of a loading dose.[112]

Why Do Nausea and Vomiting Occur?

Nausea and vomiting occur commonly in postoperative pediatric surgical patients. Certain procedures, such as repair of strabismus, are associated with a high incidence (approaching 80% of patients) if no antiemetic therapy is provided. Administering droperidol, 25 to 75 $\mu g \cdot kg^{-1}$,[113] and metoclopramide, 0.1 $mg \cdot kg^{-1}$, as well as the pre-emergence suctioning of stomach contents decrease the incidence. Data are conflicting as to whether specific anesthetic agents such as nitrous oxide are associated with a greater incidence of nausea and vomiting. Anesthetics that include propofol as a primary agent appear to have a lower incidence of postoperative nausea and vomiting.

What Is the Treatment of Airway Obstruction?

Airway obstruction may also occur following anesthesia. Causes include displacement of the tongue into the oropharynx, laryngospasm, and postextubation subglottic edema. Obstruction of the airway by the tongue can be managed with head and jaw repositioning and support; oral airway insertion, although occasionally indicated, may precipitate laryngospasm in a lightly anesthetized or sedated child.

Laryngospasm

Laryngospasm is recognized by the presence of a paradoxic rocking motion of the abdominal and chest walls with ventilatory effort, sternal, and intercostal retractions. High-pitched, squeaky (partial obstruction) or absent (complete obstruction) breath sounds can result, leading to oxyhemoglobin desaturation and hypoxemia. Treatment consists of administering 100% O_2 and continuous positive airway pressure via a tight-fitting mask. If the laryngospasm does not abate, succinylcholine, 0.1 to 0.2 $mg \cdot kg^{-1}$ intravenously, often relieves the laryngospasm without necessitating reintubation.

Postintubation Croup

Postintubation croup is caused by mucosal edema, usually at the level of the cricoid cartilage. Patients with this disorder exhibit hoarseness, stridor, and suprasternal retractions. Although laryngospasm is typically seen during emergence, postintubation croup may be seen at anytime within the first 24 hours following extubation, with maximum airway edema occurring at about 4 hours.

Treatment consists of administering humidified O_2 and nebulized racemic epinephrine (0.5 mL of a 2.25% solution in 2–3 mL of normal saline). Severe cases may require reintubation with a smaller endotracheal tube (verifying a leak at < 30 cm H_2O pressure) and intravenous steroids (dexamethasone, 0.25–0.5 $mg \cdot kg^{-1}$).

COMMON ANESTHETIC PROCEDURES

What Are the Anesthetic Considerations for Laryngoscopy and Bronchoscopy?

Laryngoscopy and bronchoscopy may be performed with rigid or flexible instruments, or both. In most cases, rigid bronchoscopy requires general anesthesia, whereas flexible fiberoptic endoscopy can be accomplished with patient sedation and airway local anesthesia. Anesthetic goals for airway endoscopy include (1) provision of adequate oxygenation and ventilation; (2) control and inhibition of airway reflexes to prevent coughing, laryngospasm, and bronchospasm; (3) protection of the airway from gastric content aspiration; (4) rapid return of airway reflexes following the procedure; and (5) maintenance of hemodynamic stability.

Complications

Common complications in pediatric patients include bradycardia, hemoptysis, postoperative stridor, and dyspnea. Pneumothorax, pneumomediastinum, cardiac arrest, and death may occur but are rare.[114] Intraoperative bradycardia may result from vagal stimulation and should be considered secondary to hypoxemia until proved otherwise. Prophylactic use of atropine or glycopyrrolate has the dual benefit of attenuating vagally mediated bradycardia and of reducing airway secretions.

Ventilation and Oxygenation

Attention must be given to the adequacy of both ventilation and oxygenation during airway endoscopy. Considering the narrow diameter of pediatric airway instruments, the inherent high resistance to gas flow in ventilating bronchoscopes is much more readily overcome by compression of the anesthesia reservoir bag than by the passive elastic recoil of the chest wall. This combination may lead to "stacking of breaths" and resultant gas trapping with hypercarbia. Return of blood to the heart may be impaired, and hypotension may occur as a consequence.

Hypercarbia is further accentuated in infants by the increased minute production of CO_2 compared with that of adults.[115] If 100% O_2 is insufflated during periods of apnea, as when a telescope is inserted through the bronchoscope in an anesthetized and paralyzed patient, significant hypercarbia may occur before any hemoglobin desaturation is noted. For this reason, reliance on a decrease in SpO_2 as an end point for instrumentation of the airway in the apneic patient is not advisable and may significantly stress critically ill children.

A reasonable method of ventilating anesthetized and paralyzed patients during tracheoscopy and bronchoscopy is to limit the time that the telescope is inserted in the bronchoscope to 3 to 5 minutes in healthy patients, then to hyperventilate the patient with the telescope removed and the bronchoscope positioned above the tracheal carina. In neonates, significantly shorter periods of apneic oxygenation may be tolerated (from 20 seconds to 1 minute).

Anesthetic Agents

When the endoscopist requests that the patient breathe spontaneously so that he or she can evaluate the dynamic function of the airways, anesthesia may be maintained by insufflating O_2 and a potent inhalation agent through the side port of the laryngoscope or bronchoscope (Fig. 61–8). One drawback of this technique is that adequate scavenging of waste anesthetic gases is often not possible.

Although neither currently approved by the Food and Drug Administration nor specifically contraindicated for pediatric use in the United States, propofol infusion with insufflation of O_2 alone or with O_2 and air provides excellent operating conditions for most patients and has been utilized for procedures of short duration in children.[101]

Topical application of lidocaine to the vocal cords by the

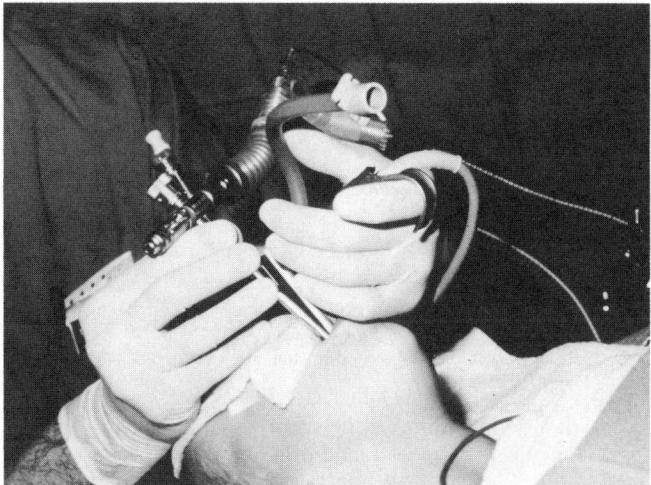

FIGURE 61–8. Pediatric patient in whom a suspension laryngoscope with insufflation side port (operator's left hand) is being exchanged for a ventilating bronchoscope (operator's right hand).

endoscopist may help to attenuate airway reflexes and to supplement the inhalation or intravenous anesthetic. Remember that the uptake of local anesthetic from the tracheal and pharyngeal mucosa is very rapid; lidocaine in a dose of 3 mg · kg^{-1} via this route produces a plasma level of 3 μg · mL^{-1}.[116]

Sedation

Flexible fiberoptic airway endoscopy can generally be accomplished with sedation and topical anesthesia. Sedation may be accomplished with oral, rectal, or intravenous agents. Midazolam given orally, 0.5 to 1.0 mg · kg^{-1}; rectally, 0.3 mg · kg^{-1}; or intravenously, 0.05 to 0.1 mg · kg^{-1}, titrated to effect may be used alone or with adjunctive agents such as ketamine, morphine, or fentanyl.

Supplemental O$_2$ should be given via facemask, nasal prongs, or the suction port of the fiberscope. When insufflating O$_2$, be sure to verify that egress can occur so that gas trapping, hypercarbia, and hemodynamic compromise are avoided. Should the fiberoptic endoscope occlude a significant portion of the trachea or endotracheal tube, endoscopic examination periods should be limited to allow intermittent, unrestricted spontaneous ventilation.

What Are the Anesthetic Considerations for MRI?

Anesthesiologists increasingly are asked to provide anesthesia care outside of the traditional confines of the operating room in such areas as the ICU, cardiac catheterization laboratory, and emergency department. Perhaps no location is more challenging than the MRI suite to provide safe sedation or general anesthesia while adhering to basic monitoring standards. MRI is a modality in which high-strength magnetic fields and pulses of radiofrequency energy are used to create digitalized tomographic imaging of the body. When compared with computed tomography, MRI provides superior images for neurologic and soft tissue examination[117] and does not expose patients or personnel to ionizing radiation.

Potential Problems

The technique requires placing a nonmoving patient within the bore of a large superconducting magnet that creates up to a 2.0-Tesla magnetic field. The magnetic field and impaired patient access introduce the challenges of providing anesthesia care in this situation. Ferromagnetic objects such as pacemakers and surgical clips that are implanted in the bodies of patients and personnel can malfunction or be displaced. Loose objects such as pens, paging devices, and laryngoscopes may be propelled to the center of the magnetic field, injuring people or damaging equipment in the path of the unintended projectile (see Chapter 54).

Although ferromagnetic monitors and other equipment may be bolted or otherwise secured in place, these same items have the capacity to act as radiofrequency antennae and to interfere with the image.[118] In return, the strong magnetic field can interfere with the function of monitors and equipment, including electrocardiographs, ventilators, and anesthesia machines that have moving ferromagnetic parts. Direct patient monitoring is limited by the distance of the patient from the observer and by the significant amount of noise produced when radiofrequency pulses are generated.

The anesthesiologist is consulted to (1) provide sedation or anesthesia for the purpose of limiting patient movement and to (2) monitor the patient, who may have any of a number of medical problems that may or may not be related to the indication for obtaining the MRI. The same standards that apply to elective anesthesia in the operating room regarding the use of monitoring modalities and availability of resuscitation equipment and medications must be satisfied when performing MRI. These include monitoring of oxygenation (pulse oximetry), ventilation (stethoscope or capnography), circulation (invasive or noninvasive blood pressure and ECG), and temperature. The reader is referred to an excellent review of anesthetic management for MRI that includes a detailed discussion and listing of MRI-compatible anesthesia equipment.[119]

Sedative and Anesthetic Agents

A variety of sedative and general anesthetic techniques are possible, depending on patient condition, requirements, and equipment availability. Most MRI facilities include a holding area where, with appropriate monitoring, initial sedation or anesthetic induction can occur; this site should be equipped to provide suction, emergency medications, and a means of administering positive-pressure ventilation with O$_2$ via mask or endotracheal tube. Sedation techniques include giving oral chloral hydrate, 50 to 80 mg · kg^{-1} 30 minutes prior to the study,[120] intramuscular ketamine, and combinations of several agents.

Two techniques are commonly used at our institution, both following initial sedation with an intramuscularly administered mixture of ketamine (2 mg · kg^{-1}), midazolam (0.1 mg · kg^{-1}), and atropine (0.01 mg · kg^{-1}). An intravenous catheter is placed, and further sedation with the goal of preventing spontaneous patient movement achieved either with incremental doses of pentobarbital, 1 mg · kg^{-1}, or a continuous infusion of low-dose propofol (20–50 μg · kg^{-1} · min^{-1}).[121]

When a patent airway, spontaneous ventilation, and adequate sedation are confirmed, the child is transferred to the MRI scanner and monitored. If at anytime during the imaging process airway obstruction, apnea, or hemodynamic instability occur, he or she should be rapidly removed from the bore of the magnet to the foot of the table or to the induction area where appropriate resuscitative interventions may be applied.

General anesthesia mandates tracheal intubation and can be provided with higher doses of the medications discussed above, with or without muscle relaxation. MRI-compatible vaporizers and anesthesia machines allow administration of inhalation anesthetics.[122]

What Are the Anesthetic Considerations in Tonsillectomy?

Anesthetic considerations for tonsillectomy include the need for a secured airway (oral RAE tubes are often utilized); close monitoring of breath sounds and inspiratory pressures while the surgeon places a mouth gag and elevates the mandible and tongue; annotation of placement of any packing in the posterior pharynx (confirmation of removal with surgeon prior to extubation); the need for an immobile patient for a relatively short surgical procedure; possible significant blood loss; and the need for postoperative analgesia. (See Chapter 72.)

Anesthetic Agents

Combinations of moderate doses of inhalation agents, short- or intermediate acting muscle relaxants (mivacurium, vecuronium, or atracurium), and small doses of intravenous narcotic ($2 \ \mu g \cdot kg^{-1}$ of fentanyl) or ketorolac ($1 \ mg \cdot kg^{-1}$) provide optimal surgical conditions and rapid return of airway reflexes. Extubation should proceed after stomach contents have been evacuated through an orogastric tube (which is often placed under direct vision by the surgeon), the tonsil beds are dry, and the patient is awake and protecting his or her own airway.

Bleeding

Emergent surgery for bleeding from the operative site after tonsillectomy adds to the concerns of hypovolemia, a difficult airway, and a full stomach. Securing a protected airway remains the primary concern for patients with a decreased level of consciousness while fluid resuscitation is ongoing. Hemodynamic stability and evacuation of the stomach are other management goals.

Fiberoptic intubation is usually difficult in the presence of active bleeding. Awake blind nasal or oral intubation with direct laryngoscopy and minimal topicalization are relatively safe means to secure the airway in obtunded or severely hypovolemic patients. Rapid sequence induction and intubation with cricoid pressure also have been advocated. The choice of technique must consider the individual patient and the anesthetist's expertise.

What Are the Anesthetic Considerations for Myringotomy and Pressure-Equalizing Tube Placement?

Surgical and anesthetic techniques for bilateral myringotomy and pressure-equalizing tube placement have changed little in the past several years. Children often have baseline symptoms of an upper respiratory infection. Rhinorrhea and coryza are not reasons to postpone pressure-equalizing tube placement in the absence of chest congestion, wheezing, or fever. The procedure is short and typically does not require placement of an intravenous catheter or an endotracheal tube in the otherwise healthy patient. Proper depth of anesthesia should be assured prior to myringotomy to prevent laryngospasm and patient movement. Postoperative analgesia may be provided with orally administered acetaminophen.

References

1. Mendelson CL: The aspiration of stomach contents into the lungs during obstetrical anesthesia. Am J Obstet Gynecol 1946; 52:191.
2. Teabeault JR: Aspiration of gastric contents: an experimental study. Am J Pathol 1952; 28:51.
3. Roberts RB, Shirley MA: Reducing the risk of acid aspiration during Cesarean section. Anesth Analg 1974; 53:859.
4. Salem MR, Wong AY, Mani M, et al: Premedicant drugs and gastric juice pH and volume in pediatric patients. Anesthesiology 1976; 44:216.
5. Goudsouzian N, Coté CJ, Liu LMP, et al: The dose-response effects of cimetidine on gastric pH and volume in children. Anesthesiology 1981; 55:553.
6. Coté CJ, Goudsouzian NG, Liu LMP, et al: Assessment of risk factors related to the acid-aspiration syndrome: gastric pH and residual volume. Anesthesiology 1982; 56:70.
7. Manchikanti L, Colliver JA, Marrero TC, et al: Assessment of age-related acid aspiration risk factors in pediatric, adult, and geriatric patients. Anesth Analg 1985; 64:11.
8. Meakin G, Dingwall AE, Addison GM: Effects of fasting and oral premedication on the pH and volume of gastric aspirate in children. Br J Anaesth 1987; 59:678.
9. Schreiner MS, Triebwasser A, Keon TP: Ingestion of liquids compared with preoperative fasting in pediatric outpatients. Anesthesiology 1990; 72:593.
10. Crawford M, Lerman J, Christensen S, et al: Effects of duration of fasting on gastric fluid pH and volume in healthy children. Anesth Analg 1990; 71:400.
11. Splinter WM, Stewart JA, Muir JG: Large volumes of apple juice preoperatively do not affect gastric pH and volume in children. Can J Anaesth 1990; 37:36.
12. Tait AR, Knight PR: The effects of general anesthesia on upper respiratory tract infections in children. Anesthesiology 1987; 67:930.
13. Cohen MM, Cameron CB: Should you cancel the operation when a child has an upper respiratory tract infection? Anesth Analg 1991; 72:282.
14. Rovenstine EA, Taylor IB: Postoperative respiratory complications: occurrence following 7874 anesthesias. Am J Med Sci 1936; 191:807.
15. Olsson GL, Hallen B: Laryngospasm during anesthesia: a computer-aided incidence study in 136,929 patients. Acta Anaesthesiol Scand 1984; 28:567.
16. DeSoto H, Patel RI, Soliman IE, et al: Changes in oxygen saturation following general anesthesia in children with upper respiratory infection signs and symptoms undergoing otolaryngological procedures. Anesthesiology 1988; 68:276.
17. Collier AM, Pimmel RL, Hasselblad V, et al: Spirometric changes in normal children with upper respiratory infections. Am Rev Respir Dis 1978; 117:47.
18. Busse WW: Respiratory infections: their role in airway responsiveness and the pathogenesis of asthma. J Allergy Clin Immunol 1990; 85:671.
19. Burrows FA, Lerman J: Immune and allergic disorders. In Anesthesia and Uncommon Pediatric Diseases. Katz J, Steward D (eds). Philadelphia, WB Saunders, 1987, pp 429–488.
20. Takiyawa T, Thurlbeck WM: Muscle and mucous gland size in the major bronchi of patients with chronic bronchitis, asthma, and asthmatic bronchitis. Am Rev Respir Dis 1971; 104:331.
21. Woolcock AJ, Read J: Lung volumes in exacerbations of asthma. Am J Med 1966; 41:259.
22. Goldberg P, Leffert F, Gonzalez M, et al: Intravenous aminophylline therapy for asthma: a comparison of two methods of administration in children. Am J Dis Child 1980; 134:596.
23. Horobin DF, Manku MS, Franks DJ, et al: Methylxanthine phosphodiesterase inhibitors behave as prostaglandin antagonists in a perfused rat mesenteric artery preparation. Prostaglandins 1977; 13:33.
24. Wilson DF: Asthma: In Anesthetic Management of Difficult and Routine Pediatric Patients. 2nd ed. Berry FA (ed). New York, Churchill Livingstone, 1990, pp 285–322.

25. Hirshman CA, Edelstein RA, Ebertz JM, et al: Thiobarbiturate-induced histamine release in human skin mast cells. Anesthesiology 1985; 63:353.

26. Hirshman CA, Edelstein G, Peetz S, et al: Mechanism of action of inhalational anesthesia on airways. Anesthesiology 1982; 56:107.

27. Munson ES, Tucker WK: Doses of epinephrine causing arrhythmias during enflurane, methoxyflurane, and halothane anesthesia in dogs. Can Anaesth Soc J 1975; 22:495.

28. Downes H, Gerber N, Hirshman CA: IV Lignocaine in reflex and allergic bronchoconstriction. Br J Anaesth 1980; 52:873.

29. Schwartz AJ, Campbell FW: Pathophysiological approach to congenital heart disease. *In* Pediatric Cardiac Anesthesia. Lake CL (ed). Norwalk, CT, Appleton & Lange, 1988, p 9.

30. Britt BA, Kwong IHF, Endrenyi L, et al (eds). Malignant Hyperthermia—Current Concepts. New York, Appleton-Century-Crofts, 1979, pp 63–77.

31. Brownell AKW: Malignant hyperthermia: relationship to other diseases. Br J Anaesth 1988; 60:303.

32. Levitt RC: Prospects for the diagnosis of malignant hyperthermia susceptibility using molecular genetic approaches. Anesthesiology 1992; 76:1039.

33. Olgin J, Argor Z, Rosenberg H, et al: Noninvasive evaluation of malignant hyperthermia susceptibility with phosphorus nuclear magnetic resonance spectroscopy. Anesthesiology 1988; 68:507.

34. Verburg MP, DeGrood PM: Safety of propofol in malignant hyperthermia (preliminary results). Anesthesia 1988; 43(Suppl):121.

35. Beebe JJ, Sessler DI: Preparation of anesthesia machines for patients susceptible to malignant hyperthermia. Anesthesiology 1988; 69:395.

36. Flewellen EH, Nelson TE, Jones WP, et al: Dantrolene dose-response in awake man: implications for management of malignant hyperthermia. Anesthesiology 1983; 59:275.

37. Henderson JM, Brodsky DA, Fisher DM, et al: Preinduction of anesthesia in pediatric patients with nasally administered sufentanil. Anesthesiology 1988; 68:671.

38. Salem MR, Wong AY, Mani M, et al: Premedicant drugs and gastric juice pH and volume in pediatric patients. Anesthesiology 1976; 44:216.

39. Zimmerman G, Steward DJ: Bradycardia delays the onset of action of intravenous atropine in infants. Anesthesiology 1986; 65:320.

40. Stoelting RK: Anticholinergic drugs. *In* Pharmacology and Physiology in Anesthetic Practice. 1st ed. Stoelting RK (ed). Philadelphia, JB Lippincott, 1987, pp 232–239.

41. Miller BR, Friesen RH: Oral atropine premedication in infants attenuates cardiovascular depression during halothane anesthesia. Anesth Analg 1988; 67:180.

42. Hannallah RS, Patel RI: Low-dose intramuscular ketamine for anesthesia preinduction in young children undergoing brief outpatient procedures. Anesthesiology 1989; 70:598.

43. Rita L, Seleny FL, Mazurek A, et al: Intramuscular midazolam for pediatric preanesthetic sedation: a double-blind controlled study with morphine. Anesthesiology 1985; 63:528.

44. Spahr-Schopfer IA, McMillan C, Sikich N, et al: Safety of oral midazolam premedication for use in children (abstract). Anesthesiology 1991; 75:A921.

45. Feld LH, Negus JB, White PF: Oral midazolam preanesthetic medication in pediatric outpatients. Anesthesiology 1990; 73:831.

46. Delaunay L, Murat I, Rey E, et al: Pharmacokinetics of intranasal and intravenous midazolam in young children (abstract). Anesthesiology 1991; 75:A923.

47. Karl HW, Keifer AT, Rosenberger JL, et al: Comparison of the safety and efficacy of intranasal midazolam or sufentanil for preinduction of anesthesia in pediatric patients. Anesthesiology 1992; 76:209.

48. Spear RM, Yaster M, Berkowitz ID, et al: Preinduction of anesthesia in children with rectally administered midazolam. Anesthesiology 1991; 74:670.

49. Conard PL, Rosenblum M, Weisman SJ, et al: Safety and efficacy of oral transmucosal fentanyl citrate (OTFC) for procedures in children (abstract). Anesthesiology 1991; 75:A954.

50. Graff TD, Phillips OC, Benson DW, et al: Baltimore anesthesia study committee: factors in pediatric anesthesia mortality. Anesth Analg (Cleveland) 1964; 43:407.

51. Olsson GL, Hallen B, Hambraeus-Jonzon K: Aspiration during anesthesia: a computer-aided study of 185,358 anaesthetics. Acta Anaesthesiol Scand 1986; 30:84.

52. Tiret L, Nivoche Y, Hatton F, et al: Complications related to anaesthesia in infants and children. Br J Anaesth 1988; 61:263.

53. Henderson IM, Spence DG, Clarke WN, et al: Sodium citrate in paediatric outpatients. Can J Anaesth 1987; 34:560.

54. Salem MR, Wong AY, Collins VJ: The pediatric patient with a full stomach. Anesthesiology 1973; 39:435.

55. Goudsouzian N, Coté CJ, Liu LMP, et al: The dose-response effects of oral cimetidine on gastric pH and volume in children. Anesthesiology 1981; 55:533.

56. Sandhar BK, Goresky GV, Maltby JR, et al: Effect of oral liquids and ranitidine on gastric fluid volume and pH in children undergoing outpatient surgery. Anesthesiology 1989; 71:327.

57. Sellick BA: Cricoid pressure to control regurgitation of stomach contents during induction of anesthesia. Lancet 1961; 2:404.

58. Salem MR, Wong AY, Fizzolti GF: Efficacy of cricoid pressure in preventing aspiration of gastric contents in pediatric patients. Br J Anaesth 1972; 44:401.

59. Vernon D, Schulman J, Foley JM: Changes in children's behavior after hospitalization. Am J Dis Child 1966; 111:581.

60. Schulman J, Foley JM, Vernon D, et al: A study of the effect of the mother's presence during anesthesia induction. Pediatrics 1967; 39:111.

61. Hannallah RS, Rosales JK: Experience with parents' presence during anesthesia induction in children. Can Anaesth Soc J 1983; 30:286.

62. Honig J, Maguire E, Hannallah RS: Parents' response to observing anesthesia induction in their children (abstract). Anesthesiology 1991; 75:A1051.

63. Gregory GA: Induction of anesthesia. *In* Pediatric Anesthesia. 2nd ed. Gregory GA (ed). New York, Churchill Livingstone, 1989, pp 539–560.

64. Liu LMP, Ryan JF: Modified single breath induction of anesthesia in children with and without nitrous oxide (abstract). Anesthesiology 1989; 71:A1008.

65. Alexander GD, Skupski JN, Brown EM: The role of nitrous oxide in postoperative nausea and vomiting. Anesth Analg 1984; 63:175.

66. Brett CM, Fisher DM: Thiopental dose-response relations in unpremedicated infants, children, and adults. Anesth Analg 1987; 66:1024.

67. Liu LM, Coté CJ, Goudsouzian NG, et al: Response to intravenous induction doses of methohexital in children (abstract). Anesthesiology 1981; 55:A330.

68. Hannallah RS, Baker SB, Casey W, et al: Propofol: effective dose and induction characteristics in unpremedicated children. Anesthesiology 1991; 74:217.

69. Sevel PS, Lowdon JS: Propofol: a new intravenous anesthetic. Anesthesiology 1989; 71:260.

70. Varner PD, Ebert JP, McKay RD, et al: Methohexital sedation of children undergoing CT scan. Anesth Analg 1985; 64:643.

71. Goudsouzian NG, Alifimoff JK, Eberly C, et al: Neuromuscular and cardiovascular effects of mivacurium in children. Anesthesiology 1989; 70:237.

72. Berthelsen P, Prytz S, Jacobsen E: Two-stage fiberoptic nasotracheal intubation in infants: a new approach to difficult pediatric intubation. Anesthesiology 1985; 63:457.

73. Holzman RS, Nargozian CD, Florence FB: Lightwand intubation in children with abnormal upper airways. Anesthesiology 1988; 69:784.

74. Borland LM, Casselbrant M: The Bullard laryngoscope: a new indirect oral laryngoscope (pediatric version). Anesth Analg 1990; 70:105.

75. Audenaert SM, Montgomery CL, Stone B, et al: Retrograde-assisted fiberoptic tracheal intubation in children with difficult airways. Anesth Analg 1991; 73:660.

76. Food and Drug Administration (FDA): Anesthesia apparatus checkout recommendations. Federal Register, Rockville, MD, Food and Drug Administration, February, 1987.

77. Koka BV, Jeon IS, Andre JM, et al: Postintubation croup in children. Anesth Analg 1975; 54:622.

78. Finholt DA, Henry DB, Raphaely RC: Factors affecting leak around tracheal tubes in children. Can Anaesth Soc J 1985; 32:326.

79. Bain JA, Spoerel WE: A streamlined anaesthetic system. Can Anaesth Soc J 1972; 19:426.

80. Miller DM: Breathing systems for use in anesthesia. Br J Anaesth 1988; 60:555.

81. Lerman J, Robinson S, Willis MM, et al: Anesthetic requirements for halothane in young children 0–1 month and and 1–6 months of age. Anesthesiology 1983; 59:421.

82. Murray D, Vandewalker G, Matherne GP, et al: Pulsed Doppler and two-dimensional echocardiography: comparison of halothane and isoflurane on cardiac function in infants and small children. Anesthesiology 1987; 67:211.

83. Wren WS, McShane AJ, McCarthy JG, et al: Isoflurane in paediatric anaesthesia: induction and recovery from anaesthesia. Anaesthesia 1985; 40:315.

84. Davis PJ, Cook DR, Stiller RL, et al: Pharmacodynamics and pharmacokinetics of high-dose sufentanil in infants and children undergoing cardiac surgery. Anesth Analg 1987; 66:203.

85. Goudsouzian NG: Neuromuscular blocking agents in children. Paediatr Anaesth 1991; 1:75.

86. Goudsouzian NG: The infant and the myoneural junction. Anesth Analg 1986; 65:1208.

87. Waud BE, Waud DR: The relation between the response to "train-of-four" stimulation and receptor occlusion during competitive neuromuscular block. Anesthesiology 1972; 37:413.

88. Mason LJ, Betts EK: Leg lift and maximum inspiratory force: clinical signs of neuromuscular blockade reversal in neonates and infants. Anesthesiology 1980; 52:441.

89. Liu LMP, DeCook TH, Goudsouzian NG, et al: Dose response to intramuscular succinylcholine in children. Anesthesiology 1981; 55:599.

90. Morton NS, Johnston G, White M, et al: Propofol in paediatric anaesthesia. Paediatr Anaesth 1992; 2:89.

91. Borgeat A, Popovic V, Meier D, et al: Comparison of propofol and thiopental/halothane for short-duration ENT surgical procedures in children. Anesth Analg 1990; 71:511.

92. Glaeseer PW, Losek JD: Emergency intraosseous infusions in children. Am J Emerg Med 1986; 4:36.

93. Rosetti VA, Thompson BM, Miller J, et al: An alternative route of pediatric intravascular access. Ann Emerg Med 1985; 14:885.

94. Lindahl SGE: Energy expenditure and fluid and electrolyte requirements in anesthetized infants and children. Anesthesiology 1988; 69:377.

95. Hongnat JM, Murat I, St Maurice C: Evaluation of current paediatric guidelines for fluid therapy using two different dextrose hydrating solutions. Paediatr Anaesth 1991; 1:95.

96. Sieber FE, Smith DS, Traystman RJ, et al: Glucose: a reevaluation of its intraoperative use. Anesthesiology 1987; 67:72.

97. Lanier WL, Stangland KJ, Scheithauer BW, et al: The effects of dextrose infusion and head position on neurologic outcome after complete cerebral ischemia in primates: examination of a model. Anesthesiology 1987; 66:39.

98. Welborn LG, Hannallah RS, McGill WA, et al: Glucose concentrations for routine intravenous infusion in pediatric outpatient surgery. Anesthesiology 1987; 67:427.

99. DuBois MC, Gouyet L, Murat I, et al: Lactated Ringer's with 1% dextrose: an appropriate solution for perioperative fluid therapy in children. Paediatr Anaesth 1992; 2:99.

100. Welborn LG, McGill WA, Hannallah RS, et al: Perioperative blood glucose concentrations in pediatric outpatients. Anesthesiology 1986; 65:543.

101. Furman EB, Roman DG, Lemmer LAS, et al: Specific therapy in water, electrolyte, and blood-volume replacement during pediatric surgery. Anesthesiology 1975; 42:187.

102. Ward JW, Holmberg SD, Allen JR, et al: Transmission of human immunodeficiency virus (HIV) by blood transfusion screened as negative for HIV antibody. N Engl J Med 1988; 318:473.

103. American Society of Anesthesiologists: Standards for Intraoperative Monitoring. Park Ridge, IL, American Society of Anesthesiologists, 1994.

104. Coté CJ, Goldstein EA, Coté MA, et al: A single-blind study of pulse oximetry in children. Anesthesiology 1988; 68:184.

105. Coté CJ, Rolf N, Liu LMP, et al: A single-blind study of combined pulse oximetry and capnography in children. Anesthesiology 1991; 74:980.

106. Karl HW, Swedlow DB, Lee KW, et al: Epinephrine-halothane interactions in children. Anesthesiology 1983; 58:142.

107. Payen D, Ecoffey C, Carli C, et al: Pulsed Doppler ascending aortic, carotid, brachial, and femoral artery blood flows during caudal anesthesia in infants. Anesthesiology 1987; 67:681.

108. Yaster M, Maxwell LG: Pediatric regional anesthesia. Anesthesiology 1989; 70:324.

109. Attis J, Ecoffey C, Sandouk P, et al: Epidural morphine in children: pharmacokinetics and CO_2 sensitivity. Anesthesiology 1986; 65:590.

110. Murat I, Walker J, Esteve C, et al: Effect of lumbar epidural anaesthesia on plasma cortisol levels in children. Can J Anaesth 1988; 35:20.

111. Welborn LG, Broadman LM, Rice LJ, et al: Postoperative apnea in former preterm infants: prospective comparison of spinal and general anesthesia. Anesthesiology 1990; 72:838.

112. Watcha MF, Jones MB, Lauguerela RG, et al: Comparison of ketorolac and morphine as adjuvants during pediatric surgery. Anesthesiology 1992; 76:368.

113. Eustis S, Lerman J, Smith DR: Effect of droperidol pretreatment on post-anesthetic vomiting in children undergoing strabismus surgery: the minimum effective dose. J Pediatr Ophthalmol Strabismus 1987; 24:165.

114. Puhakka H, Kero P, Valli P, et al: Pediatric bronchoscopy: a report of methodology and results. Clin Pediatr (Phila) 1989; 28:253.

115. Woods A: Pediatric bronchoscopy, bronchography, and laryngoscopy. In Anesthetic Management of Difficult and Routine Pediatric Patients. Berry F (ed). New York, Churchill Livingstone, 1986, pp 189–248.

116. Pelton DA, Daly M, Cooper PD, et al: Plasma lidocaine concentration following aerosol application to the trachea and bronchi. Can Anaesth Soc J 1970; 17:250.

117. Rejger VS, Cohn BF, Vielroye GJ, et al: A simple anesthetic and monitoring system for magnetic resonance imaging. Eur J Anaesthesiol 1989; 6:373.

118. Roth JL, Nugent M, Gray JE, et al: Patient monitoring during magnetic resonance imaging. Anesthesiology 1985; 62:80.

119. Patteson SK, Chesney JT: Anesthetic management for magnetic resonance imaging: problems and solutions. Anesth Analg 1992; 74:121.

120. Rumm PD, Takao RT, Fox DJ, et al: Efficacy of sedation of children with chloral hydrate. South Med J 1990; 83:1040.

121. Norreslet J, Wahlgren C: Propofol infusion for sedation of children. Crit Care Med 1990; 18:890.

122. Rao CC, Brandl R, Mashak JN: Modification of Ohmeda (R) Excel 210 anesthesia machine for use during magnetic resonance imaging. Anesthesiology 1988; 68:640.

CHAPTER 62

The Geriatric Patient

KENNETH M. JANIS, M.D.

Over the past several years, increased attention has been focused on the specific anesthetic problems associated with the elderly patient. Pediatric subspecialists have helped us to understand that the infant is not merely a small adult. By the same educational process, we have begun to conclude that the elderly patient is not just someone on Medicare who has multisystem illnesses and requires surgery.

In this chapter, the elderly patient is presented as an individual in whom age alone produces a specific set of changes that influence the response to anesthesia and surgery. I distinguish between the physiologic and pharmacologic changes associated with the aging process and the influence of systemic illness on the responses to anesthesia and surgery.

A clear distinction can be made between physiologic and chronologic age. It is possible to grow older with a minimum amount of deterioration in baseline physiologic function. The evidence presented in this chapter shows that chronologic age alone should never be considered a contraindication to surgery.

DEMOGRAPHICS

What Problems Do the Elderly Present As a Group?

With the increasing emphasis placed on the cost of health care and, in particular, on the cost of care for elderly Medicare patients, increasing attention focuses on the "graying of America." More health care is required by greater numbers of people who live past the age of 65 years. Large amounts of money are consumed in the management of elderly patients who have multisystem illnesses that are complicated by the need for surgical procedures.[1]

Currently, 11.3% of the American population is over the age of 65 years, and by the year 2030, 22% of the American population will be in this category. Older Americans as a group live longer, healthier, and financially more secure lives than did their parents or grandparents. Five thousand of them celebrate their 65th birthday every day! One-half of these individuals will require surgery.

Currently, this group of patients accounts for one-third of all health care costs. Their hospital surgical costs are rising at a rate that is fourfold that of the general population, with a large proportion of the cost generated during the last year of life. Elderly patients accounted for 38% of hospital bed days and 21% of inpatient surgical procedures. Women tend to outnumber men; in the population that is above the age of 85 years, the ratio is 100 women for every 39 men.

LIFE SPAN AND LONGEVITY

Fries focused our attention on the concept of "compression of morbidity" in discussing the rectangularization of mortality.[2] Life span is a species-specific, genetically determined, average limit to the life of the members of a species. Longevity, or life expectancy, is the ability of any individual member of a species to approach or to exceed the life span for that species. Improvements in medical care probably do not increase the life span of the human species but do allow an increasing proportion of a larger population pool to survive closer to the predetermined life span. Laboratory research has produced increased life spans in lower animals by genetic manipulation. The significance of this work for human beings is at best speculative.

Current data indicate that the average longevity at birth in the United States is 70.7 years for males and 78.3 years for females. Using this information and projecting maximum improvement in the rates of death from all causes, it remains improbable that life span for the human species from birth will ever exceed the currently projected value of 85 years, although many individuals do live longer.[3]

The fastest growing segment of our population at the present time is that including those who are between 80 and 85 years of age. Therefore, instead of larger numbers of sick elderly persons with severe chronic illnesses, we will likely see larger numbers of physiologically stable, elderly individuals who will demand operations that will enhance their lifestyle and make their later years more comfortable and productive.

What Are the Effects of Aging?

Medical progress has produced better control of chronic illness so that elderly patients come to surgery with improved baseline physiologic conditions. Nonetheless, aging alone results in a predictable and progressive decline in physiologic function accompanied by a decreased ability to overcome complications that require an augmented stress response. Age itself may be considered a legitimate cause of death; however, the ultimate, dominant factors in the survival of the elderly surgical patient are preoperative systemic illnesses and postoperative complications.

Normal physiologic functional decline is satisfactory to carry out the decreasing baseline functional demands of the aging person. It does not, however, allow enough compensatory response to overcome an increasing severity of systemic illness or surgical complications to the same degree that is possible in a younger patient. With advances in the care of chronic illness and improvement in surgical outcome for the elderly patient, larger numbers of elderly will approach the theoretic human life span while maintaining an enhanced physiologic reserve.

PERIOPERATIVE MORTALITY

What Are the Determinants?

Elective Procedures

The literature on perioperative risk for the elderly is extensive and confusing. Standardization of groups and knowledge of what is being compared by the experiences of different investigators is difficult to attain. Early data indicated that the perioperative mortality rate in patients over the age of 70 years averaged between 15% and 20%. Current experience indicates a mortality rate of 2% to 10% in patients over the age of 65 years undergoing elective operative procedures (Table 62–1). Overall operative mortality for all ages lies somewhere between 0.2% and 1.8%.

Emergency Procedures

Mortality rates for emergency procedures may be as high as 10% to almost 30% (see Table 62–1). In addition, the complication rate in the elderly is increased. These are the precise circumstances under which unstable systemic illness has the most dramatic role. Attention needs to focus on maximum stabilization of medical conditions without undue delay. The

TABLE 62–1. Mortality (%) by Age in Elective and Emergent Surgery

Condition	Age (y)		
	≤44	45–64	≥65
Healthy			
Elective	0.1	1.5	2.0
Emergent	1.0	3.0	9.4
Respiratory Infection			
Elective	1.5	2.5	5.0
Emergent	3.0	11.0	20.0
Ischemic Heart Disease			
Elective	2.0	3.5	6.0
Emergent	8.0	15.0	20.0
Renal Dysfunction			
Elective	2.5	8.0	10.0
Emergent	15.0	22.0	27.0

(Data from Fowkes FGR, Lunn JR, Farrow SC, et al: Epidemiology in anaesthesia. III: Mortality risk in patients with coexisting physical disease. Br J Anaesth 1982; 54:819.)

TABLE 62–2. Most Frequent Preoperative Medical Illnesses Associated with Aging

Hypertension
Renal disease
Atherosclerosis
Prior myocardial infarction
Chronic lung disease
Cardiomegaly
Diabetes mellitus

highest death rates follow intra-abdominal, intrathoracic, vascular, and cardiac procedures in patients over the age of 80 years who have unstable complicating medical illness and undergo emergency operations. Otherwise, the severity of complicating systemic illness is the dominant factor in risk analysis.

Patient Factors

In a large Canadian study, advanced age, male gender, extent of surgical procedure, physiologic condition, the need for emergency operations, and intraoperative complications were major determinants of mortality.[4] A trend toward increased mortality was observed with the use of narcotic anesthetics, although this relationship is likely secondary to the current trend toward selective use of "cardiac anesthesia–style" narcotic techniques in very compromised patients. The authors concluded that "patient and surgical risk factors were much more important in predicting 7-day mortality than the anesthesia factors we studied."[4] The intuitively expected bias in favor of regional anesthesia was not confirmed statistically. In this series, mortality increased by a factor of 10 from age 50 to 60 years. Other multicenter risk studies have produced similar results.[5]

What Is the Role of Systemic Disease?

The specific systemic conditions analyzed vary in numerous studies that attempt to pinpoint the most common individual preoperative medical findings. The most frequent preoperative medical illnesses are listed in Table 62–2. Cardiac failure, renal dysfunction, angina, diabetes, ischemic heart disease, and dementia are the conditions most commonly associated with an increased postoperative complication rate and death rate.

Prediction of Outcome

The degree of increased risk is determined not only by the severity of the complicating medical condition but also by the number of systems involved. Careful attention to the details of improving pre-existing impairment of function that is caused by systemic illness is the most important contribution to improvement in outcome in the elderly patient.

Physical Status Classification

The American Society of Anesthesiologists (ASA) physical status system repeatedly appears to predict both risk and outcome, even though determination of these parameters was not the purpose for which the system was designed. As an individual risk factor, age alone is not very useful. It reflects one facet of the "physiologic age," which is determined by the degree of systemic medical illness that accompanies or is associated with the surgical condition.[6]

Lifestyle

Preoperative independent lifestyle and the ability to carry out the activities of daily living without dependence on physical assistance are often predictive of outcome. Accordingly, physiologic age, and not chronologic age, should be used in determining the true risk of surgery in the elderly; no procedure should ever be denied to an elderly patient on the basis of chronologic age alone.

Risk Profiles

The data of Del Guercio and Cohn showed that it is possible to develop categories of risk for the elderly that are determined not only by the extent of physiologic impairment but also by the degree to which this impairment could be improved with aggressive monitoring and interventional therapy. The predictive ability of their risk profiles closely paralleled that of the ASA physical status evaluation system.[7] The conclusion must, therefore, be obvious: the greatest risk is not age alone, but the degree of physiologic impairment and the amount by which this functional impairment can be improved preoperatively and managed postoperatively.

Treatment Implications

Herein lies the answer to the question that is so often asked: What can be done to modify the risk of anesthesia and surgery in the elderly patient? This problem is particularly difficult in the emergency situation, in which time is limited because of the urgent nature of the surgical condition itself. We need, therefore, to obtain as much physiologic functional improvement as possible preoperatively, maintain this improvement in the intraoperative period, and extend it postoperatively in order to prevent complications that are tolerated less well by the elderly patient than by the younger patient. One complication often leads to another with a domino-like cascade, eventually resulting in an unnecessary, unfavorable outcome.

Is the Anesthetic Technique Important?

Attempts to distinguish between specific anesthetic-related mortality and overall surgical mortality have been cumbersome and inconclusive. Anesthesia itself contributes little to mortality compared with preoperative physical status and surgical factors. No consistent data link outcome to any specific choices of anesthetic technique or agent.

The debate regarding the benefits of general or regional anesthesia has produced volumes of opinion relative to very specific circumstances but not much in the way of comprehensive, conclusive data that shed light on the long-term survival of large groups of patients who undergo different operations. However, a clinical bias toward regional anesthesia for peripheral orthopedic procedures is clearly evident.

Experience and careful attention to detail of performance are more important than is the use of a particular technique or drug. If an anesthesiologist is not experienced with deep cervical plexus block, the patient with a recent myocardial infarc-

TABLE 62–3. Most Common Surgical Procedures

Total knee replacement
Open reduction and internal fixation of hip
Transurethral resection of prostate
Pacemaker
Vitrectomy
Bowel resection
Cholecystectomy
Coronary artery bypass graft
Total hip replacement
Carotid endarterectomy
Hernia

tion who needs a carotid endarterectomy is not the one upon whom to test a hypothesis regarding the advantages of local anesthesia for this operation.

COMMON SURGICAL PROCEDURES IN THE ELDERLY

Examination of the operating room logs at one hospital that serves as the main health resource for a large number of elderly patients (Saddleback Memorial Hospital, Laguna Hills, CA) indicates a common pattern (Table 62–3). The data in the logs are similar to those of previously published reports (Table 62–4). Elective total joint replacement to relieve pain and maintain independent ambulation is extremely popular, whereas repair of a fractured hip is the most common accident that requires surgical repair.

Transurethral resection of the prostate and, despite governmental reimbursement, pacemaker insertion and coronary artery bypass grafting are frequently performed. Several programs have published the results of cardiac procedures in the elderly; their statistics reflect highly successful outcomes and reasonable mortality rates. Successful coronary revascularization appears to improve the risk status for subsequent surgery.

The impact of laparoscopic intra-abdominal procedures has only begun to become apparent; when a sufficient number of these procedures have been performed, the data probably will show reduced risk of abdominal surgery in the elderly. Carotid endarterectomy seems to have survived recent adverse publicity. Results indicate that it remains a common procedure in patients at risk for ischemic stroke.

Cataract extraction would have appeared first on this list except that this procedure is increasingly performed in ambulatory surgical centers and private offices under local anesthe-

TABLE 62–4. Surgery in Patients Over 65 Years of Age

Operation	%
Genitourinary	17.5
Superficial	11.6
Gynecologic	7.2
Cataract extraction	7.0
Orthopedic	6.0
Laparotomy	3.9
Herniorrhaphy	3.4
Cholecystectomy	3.0
Pacemaker insertion	2.4
Thoracic or cardiac surgery, or craniotomy	38.0

(Data from Sourcebook of Aging. Chicago, Marquis Academica Media, 1979, p 422.)

sia. The same is true for herniorrhaphy, dilatation and curettage, and simple cystoscopy. Previously, mastectomy and hysterectomy were more frequent than they are today.

CHANGES THAT AFFECT ANESTHETIC MANAGEMENT

Which Anatomic Factors Are of Particular Concern?

Skin

Connective tissue losses in the elderly make their skin far more susceptible to trauma and injuries from tape than the skin of younger patients. Monitoring electrodes and dressings are a potential problem, and care must be taken in handling the skin of the elderly patient. Automated blood pressure cuffs can produce damage during long surgical cases. A thin layer of Webril underneath the cuff limits the extent of superficial skin trauma. Extra care must be taken when padding pneumatic tourniquets used in peripheral orthopedic surgery.

Joints and Pressure Points

Positioning for all surgical procedures must be done with extra attention to pressure points, particularly in long surgical cases in which patients are in the prone or lateral position. Heating blankets are potentially dangerous, particularly in patients with peripheral vascular disease. Care must also be taken in positioning patients, particularly when the lithotomy position is used in those with recently inserted or unstable total hip joints. External rotation of the hip can easily dislocate a prosthetic hip. These patients, as well as those with severe arthritis should be positioned while they are awake to verify that they are able to tolerate the necessary position during the procedure; it is also advisable to establish the comfortable limits of joint motion before inducing anesthesia (see Chapter 30).

Upper Airway

The combination of reduced periodontal support, dental deterioration, temporomandibular joint dysfunction, cervical spine stiffness, and alveolar bone mass reduction often makes mask fit and tracheal intubation more difficult in elderly than in younger patients. Many elderly patients have hiatal hernias with reflux. This problem, combined with a potential decrease in airway protective reflexes, makes aspiration a constant concern. Accordingly, facemask maintenance of anesthesia is decreasingly popular. If a patient normally sleeps with his or her dentures in, leaving them in place for induction of anesthesia often simplifies airway management. Autonomic responses to the stimulus of tracheal intubation may require aggressive management to prevent or treat hypertension and tachycardia. Small doses of esmolol ($0.5–1.0$ mg · kg^{-1}) or nitroglycerin ($0.5–1.0$ µg · kg^{-1}), or both, are helpful.

Body Composition

Other important anatomic changes include decreased total body water, decreased blood volume (20–30%), decreased skeletal muscle mass (10%), a tendency toward cellular dehydration, and increased body fat. These general changes in body composition contribute to the observation that the elderly patient is more sensitive to the depressant effects of anesthetic drugs when dosage is based on standard tables according to weight. Furthermore, the increase in body fat content produces greater storage capacity for lipophilic anesthetic drugs, which further increases the likelihood of the appearance of drug sensitivity secondary to the elimination time.

Body Temperature

Basal metabolic rate decreases at the approximate rate of 1% per year after the age of 30 years. These changes, along with a decrease in thermoregulatory compensation, make intraoperative and postoperative hypothermia more common in the elderly patient. Protection against hypothermia becomes a vital part of the care of the elderly patient in the operating room and the postanesthesia care unit (PACU). The elderly patient is particularly susceptible to the increase in oxygen consumption produced by shivering and to the demands this response places on the circulatory and ventilatory systems. Poorly controlled hypothermia may also impede elimination of anesthetic agents and prolong the awakening process (see Chapter 49).

New systems of forced heated air circulation through vented plastic blankets supplement the use of heated humidified gases, foil head and body coverings, careful use of circulating water heating blankets, use of warm intravenous fluids, and careful control of ambient operating room temperature in preventing heat loss.

How Is Central Nervous System Function Altered?

A common prevailing feeling is that elderly patients have decreased mental capacity. Alzheimer's disease has become a virtual diagnostic wastebasket into which are tossed all the varieties of age-related mental deterioration. This label is the most commonly applied diagnosis when mental changes lead to management problems. The patient's ability to control the activities of daily living without support is a major factor in recovery from major surgery.

Care must be taken in assigning this diagnosis because many of the causes of mental deterioration in elderly patients are actually clinically manageable problems (Table 62–5). Mental confusion is common postoperatively. However, a previously confused patient, in whom mental changes were not obvious preoperatively, may suddenly appear to be confused only because he or she is in a hospital setting and, hence, is more closely observed by trained observers. Anesthetic management of a regional technique may be difficult because of the patient's limited ability to comprehend and cooperate.

TABLE 62–5. Reversible Causes of Mental Deterioration with Aging

Drug interaction or side effect
Depression
Cerebral vascular insufficiency
Mass lesions
Head trauma
Metabolic imbalance

Medications

Sedative and depressant premedication should be limited. The sensitivity of the central nervous system to anticholinergic medications varies among patients. If an anticholinergic is used, glycopyrrolate is preferred over atropine or scopolamine because it does not cross the blood-brain barrier. Postoperative agitation is common, and management may be simplified by the careful use of small doses of haloperidol. The role of physostigmine is controversial, and the drug is of extremely limited use in the confused elderly patient unless atropine, scopolamine, or a belladonna preparation has been administered.

Brain Mass

Despite frequent confusion, many older individuals have excellent memories and are quite facile in the thought processes necessary for memory and constructive cognitive function. However, brain mass decreases with age, and this loss correlates with the loss in the number of neurons, particularly those involved in neurotransmitter production. These changes may well be in part responsible for the observations of the increased susceptibility of the elderly brain to the depressant effects of anesthetic agents as well as a potential explanation for postoperative mental confusion.

Embolization and Cerebral Blood Flow

Postoperative neurologic dysfunction following surgery that involves cardiopulmonary bypass is more likely to occur secondary to embolic phenomena rather than to ischemia related to cerebral flow. The elderly are two to three times more susceptible to these postoperative neurologic changes than are younger patients, and the outlook for their recovery is not as encouraging.[8] However, autoregulation of the cerebral circulation remains effective and allows a normal response of cerebral blood flow to changes in ventilation.

How Is the Circulation Affected By Aging?

Cardiac Output

Cardiac output has been thought to decrease by 1% every year after the age of 30 years. Newer information indicates that cardiac output in healthy elderly people often is well maintained. The apparent reduction may be related to the effects of chronic illness and sedentary lifestyles, since most of the original studies were performed on elderly hospitalized patients with systemic illnesses.

Older patients without significant cardiovascular disease do not always show a reduction of cardiac output in response to exercise testing and may demonstrate a positive training effect through the ninth decade of life. Elderly patients without evidence of overt coronary artery disease do not show extensive decremental changes in left ventricular force-length relationships.

The mechanism by which cardiac output increases in response to stress depends on increases in ventricular wall thickness (decreased compliance) and stroke volume; hence, older patients are more susceptible to heart failure following fluid administration. This response differs from that of younger individuals who rely more on heart rate increases, which are limited in the elderly.

Conduction Abnormalities

Degenerative changes in the conduction system and blunting of autonomic responses secondary to reduced β-receptor function sometimes impair heart rate response to catecholamines. These changes, as well as the gradual development of parasympathetic dominance, are responsible for the decreased tachycardic response associated with isoflurane administration, anticholinergic drugs, and pancuronium.

Arteriosclerotic changes in the conduction system are also responsible for reduced resting heart rates, prolonged PR interval characteristics of the sick sinus syndrome, and the need for a pacemaker. Tachycardic responses to hypoxia and hypercarbia are also blunted.

Ambulatory rhythm monitoring indicates that the elderly are more likely to have dysrhythmias at rest or with exercise. The types of rhythm disturbances vary; up to one-third of these patients have periods of supraventricular dysrhythmia. The significance of single-focus, premature ventricular contractions remains unclear.

Silent Myocardial Ischemia

The importance of silent myocardial ischemia in terms of anesthetic risk is unknown. A great deal of attention has focused on this abnormality. Until diagnostic techniques are more highly refined and predictive of ischemic coronary artery disease, we should suspect that silent myocardial ischemia may be present in elderly patients who do not have the classical signs of ischemia but who have risk factors such as a family history of the disease, obesity, cigarette smoking, hypertension, and diabetes.

Under many operative circumstances, background infusions of low doses of nitroglycerin are often helpful to protect the at-risk myocardium when silent myocardial ischemia or overt ischemia secondary to coronary artery disease is present.[9] Similar reasoning may suggest the use of calcium channel or β-blocking drugs in situations where increased myocardial oxygen demand occurs.

Miscellaneous Factors

Other cardiovascular changes that can influence the response to anesthetic drugs include arterial noncompliance, increased peripheral vascular resistance, and hypertension with exaggerated responses to normal adult doses of anesthetic drugs and volume infusions.

What Are the Effects of Aging on Ventilation?

Ventilatory changes are both anatomic (they affect the movement of gas in the airway) and physiologic (they influence gas exchange at the alveolar capillary membrane) (Table 62–6). The anatomic changes lead to increased work of breathing, reduced total lung and vital capacities, and decreased maximum voluntary ventilation. Gas exchange is less efficient. The parenchymal and mechanical changes markedly exacerbate functional ventilatory depression and make respiratory failure in the postoperative period more common.

TABLE 62–6. Age-Related Ventilatory Changes

Anatomic	Decreased chest wall compliance
	Decreased lung elastance
	Decreased ventilatory muscle strength
	Rib calcification
	Kyphosis
Physiologic	Increased work of breathing
	Decreased total lung capacity and vital capacity
	Decreased maximum breathing capacity
	Decreased maximum voluntary minute ventilation
	Decreased efficiency of gas exchange

Head-up positioning in the PACU, supplemental oxygen, and postoperative mechanical ventilation may help to prevent ventilatory failure and pneumonia. However, studies in this area are inconclusive, and routine oxygen use postoperatively has been challenged in other patient groups (see Chapters 7 and 47). Preliminary results suggest that epidural narcotics may reduce the incidence of postoperative ventilatory complications and the associated costs of hospital care.

Bronchoconstriction

Irritable airways with bronchoconstriction require aggressive bronchodilator therapy preoperatively, intraoperatively, and postoperatively. In patients over the age of 45 years, the functional residual capacity is reduced below closing volume when they are in the supine position; this increases small airway closure at normal tidal volumes (V_T). Having the patients assume the sitting position reverses this effect.[10] Therefore, whenever possible, elderly patients should be placed in the head-up position in the PACU in order to limit small airway closure. These patients should be transported to the PACU, monitored with pulse oximeters, and provided with supplemental oxygen in the presence of low hemoglobin oxygen saturation.

Ventilation/Perfusion Mismatching

The changes in gas exchange that occur with advancing age are marked by a progressive decline in arterial oxygen partial pressure (PaO_2). This deterioration is the result of increased alveolar air trapping and an increase in ventilation/perfusion ($\dot{V}/\dot{Q}$) mismatching. Other parenchymal changes include reductions in alveolar capillary blood flow, altered alveolar capillary membrane permeability, increased small airway closure, and decreased surface area for gas exchange.

The alveolar-to-arterial partial pressure gradient for oxygen ($P[A-a]O_2$) increases from 8 mm Hg at age 20 years to approximately 20 mm Hg at age 70 years. The relationship,

$$PaO_2 \ (mm\ Hg) = 100\ mm\ Hg - (0.4 \times age)$$

describes the reduction seen in PaO_2 of approximately 0.5 mm Hg per year after the age of 20 years.

Because of increased physiologic dead space, end-tidal carbon dioxide partial pressure ($PETCO_2$) monitoring can be misleading unless confirmation of the gradient between $PETCO_2$ and the arterial carbon dioxide partial pressure ($PaCO_2$) is obtained using blood gas measurement.

Elderly patients have decreased ventilatory responses to hypoxia and hypercarbia as well as an increased incidence of sleep apnea. In general, the alterations in ventilatory function

associated with aging mimic those of emphysema and are made more severe by heavy cigarette smoking. To improve cigarette smoking–related alteration in lung function significantly, smoking must be discontinued for 6 to 8 weeks. With general anesthesia, $\dot{V}/\dot{Q}$ abnormalities increase with advancing age, but atelectasis and intrapulmonary shunting are not age-dependent.[11]

Episodes of significant preoperative hypoxemia in patients with hip fractures are probably fat embolic in origin and often persist into the postoperative period. These patients should receive supplemental oxygen therapy prophylactically and be closely monitored until they are fully ambulatory.[12]

How Is Renal Function Impaired?

Renal function generally is sufficient for baseline needs. However, the kidneys' ability to respond to increased fluid loads or to compensate for dehydration is limited by the progressive decrease in creatinine clearance that occurs with advancing age. Renal blood flow and glomerular filtration rate decrease by between 1% and 2% per year after the age of 25 years.

Elderly patients with a serum creatinine level >1.0 mg · dL^{-1} may have significant impairment of renal function and increased susceptibility to postoperative renal failure and toxicity from the administration of nonsteroidal anti-inflammatory drugs (e.g., ketorolac). Therefore, the dosing interval should be increased or the dose decreased when using these agents in patients over the age of 60 years or when there is a documented decrease in renal function. Renal failure is a prominent cause of mortality in the postoperative elderly patient, particularly following vascular surgery.

Decreased renal blood flow may be related to a reduction in cardiac output and is the single most important factor in the reduction of renal function associated with aging. Patients at particular risk of renal failure often benefit from early use of low-dose dopamine infusion to support intraoperative and postoperative renal function. Urine output should be maintained between 0.5 and 1 mL · kg^{-1} · h^{-1}.

Decreased renal function delays the renal excretion of many anesthetic-related drugs and their metabolites and prolongs their effects. This problem can be significant in elderly patients with severe renal dysfunction who receive large doses of pancuronium and vecuronium. Reduced renal blood flow in the elderly also increases the renal threshold for glucose. Glycosuria, when it occurs in the elderly, reflects a serum glucose level that is higher than that occurring in younger patients.

What Changes In Liver Function Occur?

Despite the apparent lack of significant changes in baseline test results, progressive decrease in liver function seems to be associated with aging. A reduction in hepatic blood flow may be responsible for reduced hepatic clearance of anesthetic drugs and their metabolites. Conflicting evidence leaves in doubt conclusions about the efficiency of microsomal enzyme systems in the hepatic metabolism of anesthetic drugs.

Glucose Abnormalities

The ability to excrete glucose loads is impaired; therefore, elevated blood sugar is more likely to follow glucose inges-

TABLE 62–7. Monitoring

- Electrocardiogram (dual lead [precordial], ST segment analysis)
- Precordial stethoscope
- Blood pressure (automated, noninvasive, or intra-arterial line)
- Temperature
- Pulse oximetry
- $P_{ET}CO_2$
- Neuromuscular stimulator
- Urinary catheter
- Central catheter (venous or pulmonary artery)
- Transesophageal echocardiography
- Selected laboratory studies

tion, and the response to insulin is less predictable. Hyperglycemia in nondiabetic patients undergoing cardiopulmonary bypass is common and may require treatment with insulin placed into the pump circuit. In all major surgeries performed on elderly patients, close monitoring of blood glucose is helpful.

Decreased magnesium levels and the resultant cardiac rhythm disturbances may be associated with this tendency toward hyperglycemia and require aggressive intravenous replacement with magnesium sulfate (see Chapter 42). Unexpected hyperglycemia may also occur during extensive surgical procedures in nondiabetic elderly patients. Intravenous insulin therapy may be required under these circumstances. In addition, hypokalemia and hypocalcemia may occur, requiring replacement with intravenous infusions. Diabetic patients have been observed frequently to have generalized limitation of joint mobility that may be associated with difficult tracheal intubation.[13]

MONITORING

What Techniques Should Be Employed?

A variety of monitoring techniques provide useful information (Table 62–7).

Electrocardiography

Electrocardiographic monitoring has become increasingly sophisticated. Five-lead systems provide better visualization of ST segment morphology and are used simultaneously with the traditional limb lead II. Newer monitor systems allow automated ST segment analysis and trending. Aggressive therapy (e.g., nitroglycerin infusion) can thus be started at the first sign of ischemia and can be titrated to effect much better than was previously possible.

As has been noted, we are increasingly aware that many ischemic episodes are clinically silent in nature and probably unrelated to changes in patient care as it is currently monitored. Ambulatory (Holter) monitoring has identified up to one-third of elderly patients as having preoperative ischemic changes. Perioperative ischemia continues to be a significant predictor of outcome.

Blood Pressure

Automated noninvasive blood pressure recording is a standard of practice in most communities. Care must be taken, however, to avoid trauma and potential ischemic damage that is caused by frequent cuff compression during long surgical cases. Because blood pressure discrepancies may exist between arms, preoperative blood pressure measurements in both are helpful. Such discrepancies occur most commonly in patients with peripheral vascular disease.

When arterial catheters are used, waveform overshoot, commonly seen in elderly patients with peripheral vascular disease, can be prevented by attachment of a damping device (e.g., a Resonance OverShoot Eliminator [ROSE adaptor]). This simple device provides a more physiologically reliable direct blood pressure measurement. If a damper is unavailable, the mean blood pressure is much less affected by overshoot than is systolic or diastolic pressure.

Temperature

Temperature monitoring is crucial. Age impairs central temperature regulation. A large portion of heat loss occurs during induction of anesthesia and skin preparation before the patient is covered with drapes.[14] Keeping the operating room warm until the patient is draped and covering as much of the patient's body surface area as possible with reflective foil hats and blankets help to control heat loss. Warming blankets are potentially dangerous and have limited effectiveness. If they are used, insulated foam pads should be placed between the blanket and patient (see Chapter 49).

Pulse Oximetry

Pulse oximetry is a standard of care in the operating room and PACU and is unparalleled with regard to clinical usefulness in assessing oxygenation (Table 62–8). Severe peripheral vasoconstriction secondary to peripheral vascular disease or hypothermia may obliterate the signal. Digital block or topical application of nitroglycerin ointment under these circumstances often eliminates the regional vasoconstriction.[15]

Owing to the shape of the oxygen hemoglobin dissociation curve, small changes in oxygen saturation may mask significant changes in Pa_{O_2} above 60 mm Hg. Procedures such as cataract extraction are often felt to require less intensive monitoring of oxygenation, but hypoxemia is common, particularly immediately following the retrobulbar block.[16]

End-Tidal Carbon Dioxide

End-tidal carbon dioxide partial pressure measurement is a standard for the monitoring of intubated patients. It is also valuable for nonintubated individuals. An intravenous cannula or T-connector attached to the carbon dioxide sampling line is

TABLE 62–8. Assessment of Operation

Method	Sensitivity	Specificity	Speed	Usefulness
Cyanosis	1	2	3	2
Transcutaneous P_{O_2}	2	2	3	2
Pulse Oximetry	3	3	4	4
Capnometry	1	1	3	3
Arterial Blood Gas	4	4	1	3
Pa_{O_2} Probe	4	4	3	4

(Data from Scuderi PE, Prough DS: Indications for monitoring in the elderly. Probl Anesth 1989; 3:628–648.)
Key: 1 = poor; 2 = moderately poor; 3 = moderately good; 4 = good.

inserted into one prong of the nasal oxygen cannula. Although this method does not always provide a true PETCO$_2$, it does allow trend analysis for the early detection of apnea or ventilatory depression. It also gives information about the ambient environment. In eye procedures in which a plastic drape is used, a significant amount of carbon dioxide may accumulate under the drape. The carbon dioxide rebreathing that results can be identified with the carbon dioxide monitor (it manifests as inspired carbon dioxide >1 mm Hg), and the response to therapy can be verified. Taping either a suction hose to the patient's chest under the drape to entrain fresh air or providing a high flow of fresh gas to the patient via the anesthesia machine virtually eliminates carbon dioxide rebreathing in this setting.[17]

Nerve Stimulators

When muscle relaxants are used, monitoring with a neuromuscular stimulator is advisable because of the prolonged elimination half-life of some nondepolarizing muscle relaxants in elderly patients with reduced renal function.

Urine Output

Insertion of an indwelling urinary catheter is important for effective fluid management and to prevent bladder distention. Maintenance of urine output between 0.5 and 1.0 mL · h^{-1} *may* help to prevent acute renal failure. The role of small doses of furosemide or mannitol, or both, in maintaining adequate urine output is a topic of controversy.

Pulmonary Artery Pressure

Disparate ventricular function may exist; thus, a pulmonary artery catheter may be indicated. However, numerous potential complications, including dysrhythmias, pulmonary hemorrhage, infection, and catheter knotting, suggest that pulmonary artery catheterization should not be approached in a cavalier fashion. Age is a definite risk factor. If the internal jugular route is used, carotid entry is particularly dangerous in the presence of carotid ischemic disease.

Echocardiography

Two-dimensional transesophageal echocardiography can detect segmental wall motion abnormalities and left ventricular end-diastolic volume as indicators of myocardial ischemia and preload, respectively. Routine application of this technique is not justified and has yet to be fully evaluated in terms of its costs and benefits.

Laboratory Data

Selective intraoperative laboratory determinations are an important part of the monitoring process. Devices are available that perform simultaneous determination of blood gases, hematocrit, potassium, sodium, and ionized calcium. Serum glucose and magnesium determinations are also helpful.

During prolonged procedures, a clotting screen (determination of platelet count, fibrinogen, prothrombin time, partial thromboplastin time, and fibrin split products) helps to guide component therapy. Routine preoperative measurement of prothrombin time and partial thromboplastin time is of no value in the absence of a positive clinical bleeding history. When systemic heparinization is used for vascular procedures, serial hourly measurement of activated clotting time helps to monitor anticoagulation and guides reversal with protamine.

GENERAL ANESTHETIC DRUGS

Do Elderly Patients React Differently?

An increased volume of distribution associated with decreased clearance by the kidneys and the liver prolongs the elimination half-life of many intravenously administered anesthetic agents in elderly patients. These pharmacokinetic alterations are in part responsible for the increased sensitivity to commonly used medications. Not only must the initial dose be reduced but also an allowance should be made for prolonged response to average drug doses. Cumulative effects from repeated administration of many drugs, particularly barbiturates, opioids, benzodiazepines, and local anesthetics, are sometimes striking. Interindividual variability in dose-response relationships is more apparent in the elderly (see Chapter 33).

These effects are consequences of altered pharmacokinetics, which affect the initial distribution and subsequent transfer of drugs from central into peripheral compartments, and altered end-organ sensitivity to drug effects. Changes in medication receptor affinity may also occur. Finally, decreased protein binding, which increases the amount of free drug in the circulation, may be seen. These effects are enhanced by the increased proportion of body fat content and decrease in blood volume that occur with advanced age.

How Are the Actions of Specific Intravenous Anesthetic Drugs Influenced?

Sodium Thiopental

A reduction of approximately 30% of the dose necessary for induction of anesthesia is common, and a prolongation of effect resulting from a "sleep dose" frequently occurs. These changes are most likely pharmacokinetic and are related to a reduced initial volume of distribution and to reduced clearance. Brain end-organ sensitivity probably is unchanged.[18] Increased sensitivity to the cardiovascular depressant effects, combined with prolonged recovery, make thiopental a potentially "tricky" drug to use in the elderly patient, especially if hypovolemia or reduced circulatory function exists at the time of injection.

Opioids

The apparently increased sensitivity of elderly patients to opioids has a pharmacodynamic explanation. The elimination half-lives of fentanyl, sufentanil, and alfentanil are increased significantly, and clearance is reduced. Some of these changes may be associated with changes in protein binding. Clinically effective plasma alfentanil levels decrease with increasing age. Unlike thiopental, electroencephalographic evidence suggests increased brain sensitivity to these medications. Because of delayed elimination, decreased volume of distribution, and in-

TABLE 62–9. Pharmacokinetic Differences for Midazolam in Young and Old Individuals of Different Sex

Average Age (y)	Half-Life (h)	Clearance $(mL \cdot kg^{-1} \cdot m^{-1})$	Volume of Central Compartment $(L \cdot kg^{-1})$	Total Volume of Distribution $(L \cdot kg^{-1})$
28 y (male)	2.1	7.75	0.51	1.34
28 y (female)	2.6	9.93	0.70	2.00
68 y (male)	5.6	4.41	0.38	1.64
68 y (female)	4.0	7.50	0.65	2.11

creased brain sensitivity, a 50% reduction in the administered dose is appropriate.[19]

Elderly patients receiving β-blocking drugs may show a profound bradycardic response to intravenous opioids, particularly if these drugs are combined for induction with vecuronium or pipecuronium. This response is enhanced more with sufentanil than with fentanyl and may be further magnified if benzodiazepines or barbiturates are added to the induction mixture.

Benzodiazepines

Alterations in response to this group of drugs are more profound than in younger patients and are extremely variable. Doses that produce only sedation in young patients may result in significant ventilatory, cognitive, and vascular effects in older patients. The apparent increased end-organ sensitivity, combined with a marked increase in elimination half-life, indicates that pharmacokinetic and pharmacodynamic mechanisms are responsible (Table 62–9).[20]

After the initial release of midazolam to the general market, its manufacturer found it necessary to modify the package insert to reflect a reduction in the recommended dose for elderly patients. Up to a fivefold decrease in the dose of midazolam required to obtain sedation that is adequate for endoscopy has been observed in elderly patients (Fig. 62–1). When used for intravenous sedation to supplement local anesthetics (e.g., in cataract surgery) or regional blocks, maximum incremental doses of 0.5 mg should be used.

The combination of midazolam with fentanyl for intravenous sedation is popular; however, significant synergistic interaction among drugs is capable of producing exaggerated central nervous system effects. Diazepam and midazolam have a marked increase in elimination half-life in such combination, making them potentially long-acting in older individuals. Recent availability of flumazenil as a specific benzodiazepine antagonist may facilitate the management of situations in which excessive response or prolonged effects create a clinical problem.

Etomidate

Etomidate is an attractive drug because of its allegedly neutral hemodynamic effects following intravenous administration. Accordingly, it is suitable for rapid sequence inductions in elderly patients with compromised cardiovascular function.

No significant pharmacodynamic changes occur with advancing age; however, an increase in elimination half-life does occur. As with thiopental, the dose of etomidate necessary to reach the same electroencephalographic level of depression achieved in younger patients is reduced. Concern has been expressed about the effects of etomidate on immunologic function and about its interference with the adrenal response to stress. No evidence shows that this phenomenon is clinically important when the drug is administered as a single dose for the induction of anesthesia.

Propofol

Propofol has the clinical advantage over benzodiazepines of a more rapid patient awakening time, but the dose requirement is significantly reduced when it is used in the elderly. The drug has become quite popular to extend the benefits of outpatient management. Potential cardiovascular depression is a prominent feature, and successful use in the elderly requires slow intravenous administration of approximately one-half the dose recommended for younger patients.

How Are the Actions of Inhalation Agents Influenced?

A progressive reduction in the minimum alveolar concentration of inhalation agents occurs with advancing age (Fig. 62–2). This change seems to be associated with a progressive reduction in cerebral metabolic requirements and is equal to

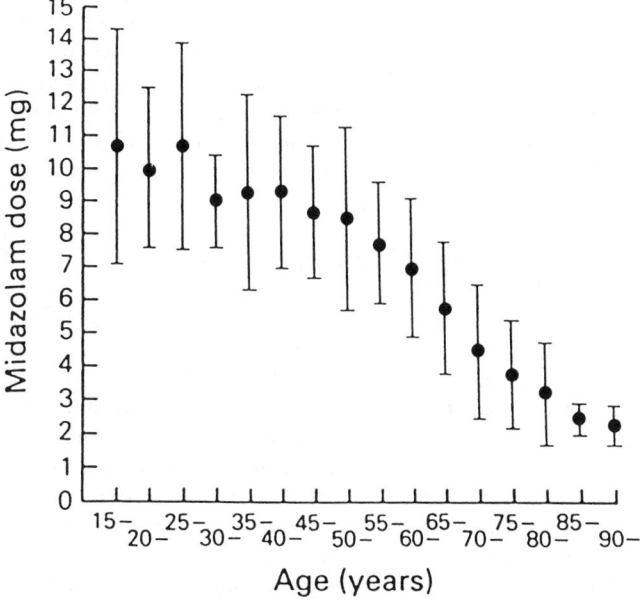

FIGURE 62–1. The relationship between age and the mean dose of midazolam required to obtain adequate sedation prior to upper gastrointestinal endoscopy. (Reprinted from Bell GD, Spickett GP, Reeve PA, et al: Intravenous midazolam for upper gastrointestinal endoscopy: a study of 800 consecutive cases relating dose to age and sex of patient. Br J Clin Pharmacol 1987; 23:241.)

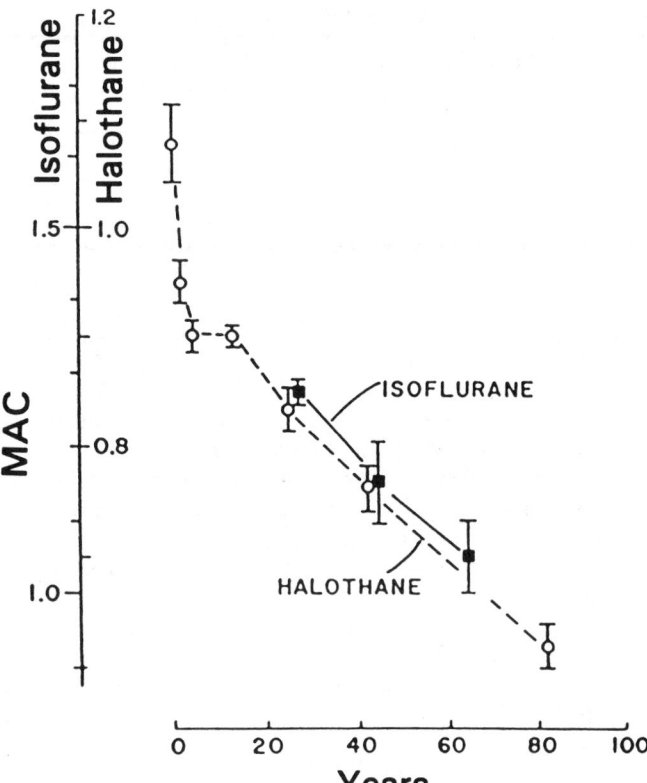

FIGURE 62–2. In humans, both isoflurane (Stevens and coworkers, 1975) and halothane (Gregory and associates, 1969) MAC decrease with increasing age. For adults, the decrease is parallel for the two agents. Data for isoflurane MAC in infants and children are not yet available. (Data from Gregory GA, Eger EI II, Munson ES: The relationship between age and halothane requirement in man. Anesthesiology 1969; 30:488–491, *and* Stevens WC, Dolan WM, Gibbons RT, et al: Minimum alveolar concentrations (MAC) of isoflurane with and without nitrous oxide in patients of various ages. Anesthesiology 1975; 42:197.)

approximately 4% for each decade after the age of 40 years. It is responsible for the extreme sensitivity of the elderly to increases in the partial pressure of the halogenated, volatile anesthetic agents.[21]

A trend toward increased cardiovascular depression is associated with volatile agents (i.e., reductions in cardiac output and perfusion pressure). The magnitude of this response is less with isoflurane than with halothane or enflurane.

Reductions in cardiac output produce a more rapid vascular uptake of volatile agents. Evidence suggests that the blood solubility of volatile agents increases with age.[22] However, the overall clinical effects of altered inhalation agent pharmacokinetics in elderly patients are not very important clinically. Of special note is the reduced tachycardic response of elderly patients to isoflurane, which limits their ability to maintain cardiac output in the face of reductions in contractility and stroke volume. Nevertheless, vasodilation of the systemic and coronary circulations limits this disadvantage of isoflurane compared with other halogenated volatile agents.

MUSCLE RELAXANTS AND REVERSAL AGENTS

No significant differences in the response of the elderly to succinylcholine occur despite their generally lower levels of pseudocholinesterase compared with those of younger patients. Most nondepolarizing relaxants show some prolongation of effect that is related primarily to the increased elimination half-life of this group of drugs.[23] Atracurium, however, is not eliminated differently in the elderly than in younger individuals. Initial response of the elderly patient to paralyzing doses of pancuronium and vecuronium is not substantially different from that of the younger patient.

Although mivacurium is structurally related to atracurium, it is associated with a 15% to 20% increase in the duration of neuromuscular block in elderly patients. Recent studies indicate a similar increase in the duration of effect of the chemically related long-acting drug doxacurium.[24] The intensity of the blockade, however, is not altered. No difference in the pharmacokinetic or pharmacodynamic effects of pipecuronium have been identified.[25]

Edrophonium, neostigmine, and pyridostigmine have a prolonged action with decreased clearance, which results in a prolonged elimination half-life in elderly patients.[26] The prolonged action of the nondepolarizing relaxants makes it most appropriate to use neostigmine or pyridostigmine.[27] Both agents show a markedly prolonged duration of maximum response in the elderly patient (>30 minutes) as compared with younger patients (<15 min).[27]

REGIONAL ANESTHETIC DRUGS

What Are the Effects of Local Anesthetics?

Several factors make older patients more sensitive to the effects of local anesthetics. Age-related reductions in the axon population of peripheral nerves and nerve conduction velocity occur. Evidence also exists for a reduction in the sensitivity of pain receptors to noxious stimulation. Myelin sheaths deteriorate with age, producing increased permeability to local anesthetics.

Several studies indicate a reduced requirement for local anesthetics injected into the epidural space; this is perhaps related to reduced clearance and increased terminal half-life of the agents, narrowing of the intervertebral disks, and reduction in volume of the epidural space. An increased end-organ sensitivity to the effects and side effects of the local anesthetics makes a decrease in the dose appropriate.

How Are Spinal and Epidural Blockade Affected?

Elderly patients are often more sensitive than are younger patients to the physiologic effects of sympathectomy following spinal anesthesia. Care with prehydration is necessary if acute circulatory overload is to be avoided. Once the spinal block with its related vasodilation has worn off, centralization of the excess fluid may precipitate myocardial dysfunction and pulmonary edema in patients with pre-existing heart disease.

Hypotension is related to the level of the block achieved and usually requires small doses of vasopressor drugs for correction. Advanced age appears to be associated with a faster onset and higher level of spinal anesthesia (Table 62–10). In elderly patients, the incidence of hypotension may not be influenced by preblock fluid administration.

Tetracaine, 10 mg; bupivacaine, 12 mg of a 7.5% dextrose

TABLE 62–10. Effect of Age on Spinal Anesthesia
(Bupivacaine, 15 mg)

Baricity	Concentration (%)	Onset Time	Dermatomal Spread	Duration
Hyperbaric	0.5	↑	↑	↑
Hyperbaric	0.375	↓	↑	↑
Isobaric*	0.5	↓	—	↑
Isobaric*	0.5	↓	↑	↑

(From Kopacz DJ, Nickel P: Regional anesthesia in the elderly patient. Probl Anesth 1989; 3:602–619.)
Key: ↑ = increased; — = no change; ↓ = decreased; * = different studies.

hyperbaric solution; and lidocaine, 70 mg of a 5% dextrose hyperbaric solution provide adequate analgesia for hip and genitourinary procedures. During orthopedic procedures on the lower extremities, less tourniquet discomfort seems to occur when hyperbaric bupivacaine is used for spinal anesthesia.

Spinal Microcatheters

Renewed interest has been voiced for continuous spinal anesthesia to provide slow, incremental elevations of spinal block that limit the amount of hypotension. However, spinal microcatheters that are 27 gauge and smaller have been ordered off the market by the Food and Drug Administration until full evaluation of a series of reports of cauda equina syndrome that is possibly related to their use is carried out.

Lumbar Puncture

Narrowing of the intervertebral spaces, the presence of osteophytes, reduced flexibility of the spine, and calcification of the interspinous ligaments make lumbar spinal and epidural puncture more difficult to perform in the elderly patient. The paramedian approach facilitates either procedure.

Spinal Headache

Spinal headache is less common in older patients, and the incidence is less dependent on the size of needle used for the lumbar puncture.[28, 29] Nonetheless, care should be taken to use a pencil-point needle or to insert the needle with the bevel parallel to the long axis of the body to facilitate splitting rather than cutting of the longitudinal fibers of the ligamentum flavum, thereby limiting prolonged cerebrospinal fluid loss and the associated headache.

Hip Fracture

Positioning of the patient with a hip fracture can be facilitated by placing the affected side down and flexing the upper thigh onto the trunk, thus splinting the fracture. This serves to keep the patient more comfortable and allows dependent positioning of the operative side during placement of the block if a hyperbaric solution is chosen. Oxygen should be provided during the block, and pulse oximeter and electrocardiographic monitoring should be performed. Small doses of midazolam or ketamine may help with patient cooperation. Sedation needs to be monitored carefully.

Epidural Catheters and Coagulation

Current wisdom holds that administration of an epidural anesthetic is safe when systemic anticoagulation is begun after placement of the needle or catheter, or both.[30] Care must be

taken, however, when manipulating or removing the catheter before laboratory confirmation of complete reversal of the systemic heparin effect is available.

Is Regional Anesthesia Advantageous?

A lot has been written about the advantages of regional over general anesthesia for various procedures. Hard data to support these views are sparse and limited for any procedure other than total hip replacement. Modig and coworkers established that unsupplemented epidural anesthesia for total hip replacement reduces the incidence of venous thrombosis and pulmonary embolism, which are the principal causes of death in hip replacement patients (Table 62–11). These dramatic data must be viewed with caution, since the epidural group received a local anesthetic and experienced its attendant sympathectomy for 24 hours postoperatively.[31] Numerous other studies show only a nonsignificant trend of more favorable outcome in the first 30 days for hip fractures repaired during regional anesthesia.

During the immediate postoperative period, a slower return of resting PaO$_2$ to normal is seen in patients who have received general anesthesia. By 6 months, the outcome after total hip replacement is equal for regional and general anesthesia. At the end of 2 years, survival is related more to the state of general health at the time of the fracture, as reflected by the ASA physical status profile, and to the degree to which patients were able to care for themselves than to the choice of general or regional anesthesia.

Yeager and colleagues attempted to show that reductions in mortality, complication rate, and cost for major surgical procedures occur when the procedures are performed with epidural anesthesia.[32] Tuman and coworkers support the long-held clinical impression that epidural anesthesia and maintenance of postoperative pain relief with epidural narcotics reduce the incidence of complications and mortality after major vascular surgery.[33] A mechanism for this reduction in complications appears to involve a decrease in postoperative hypercoagulability with an accompanying lower incidence of thrombosis. Some current speculation suggests that epidural anesthesia is associated with a lower reoperation rate for patients undergoing peripheral arterial revascularization. Clear-cut acceptance of the superiority of regional anesthesia awaits further documentation and study.

POSTOPERATIVE PAIN RELIEF

What Is the Role of Epidural Narcotics?

An important current subject in the general postoperative management of the elderly patient is the provision of postop-

TABLE 62–11. Incidence of Venous Thrombosis and Pulmonary Embolism After Total Hip Replacement

	Epidural Anesthesia (%)	General Anesthesia (%)
Popliteal veins	13	67
Calf and thigh veins	40	70
Pulmonary embolism	10	33

(From Modig J: The role of lumbar epidural anaesthesia as antithrombotic prophylaxis in total hip replacement. Acta Chir Scand 1985; 151:589–594.)

erative epidural narcotics following major operations. Relief of pain to an equivalent degree can be obtained with the administration of small doses of morphine (0.2–0.5 mg) into the subarachnoid space; such pain relief lasts for 18 to 24 hours. Small intrathecal doses of fentanyl or sufentanil (25 and 5 μg, respectively) also give an effective but shorter duration of pain relief.

Epidural morphine, fentanyl, and sufentanil infusions, with or without dilute solutions of local anesthetic, are successful as well and are now commonly used (in the absence of documented contraindications) for procedures such as radical prostatectomy, extensive colon resection, major vascular operations, and thoracotomy.

Elderly patients are more sensitive than younger patients to the potential respiratory depressant effects of epidural narcotics. Care must also be taken to watch for catheter migration into the subarachnoid space. Close clinical monitoring of ventilatory function for at least the first 24 hours is important, and continuous pulse oximetry is desirable.

How Effective Is Patient-Controlled Analgesia?

Patient-controlled analgesia systems are also quite effective in elderly patients who are not confused. Some patients actually claim more effective pain relief and greater satisfaction from patient-controlled analgesia than from epidural narcotics. Infusion pumps can be used to provide patient-controlled analgesia injections through an epidural catheter.

DRUG INTERACTIONS

How Do They Affect Anesthetic Management?

Prescription and Nonprescription Drugs

Drug interactions are of particular concern in this group of patients because so many of them receive numerous drugs for multisystemic illness. Compounding the problem is that many elderly patients are not aware of what drugs they take, nor are they always compliant with the instructions for administration. The question "What medications are you taking?" may be greeted by a shrug and the presentation of a paper sac full of half-empty medication vials. Heavy reliance on over-the-counter medications is also common.

Medication Reactions

Elderly patients often have a fixed bias about the effects of medications in general; this can lead to the self-administration of drugs in a manner different than that envisioned by the care team. Medication reactions are a frequent cause for hospital admission. The most common categories of drugs are listed in Table 62–12, and the 10 drugs most frequently prescribed to elderly patients are listed in Table 62–13.

Long-term use of thiazide diuretics leads to chronic contraction of the circulating blood volume, resulting in potentially extreme hypotension upon exposure to anesthetic agents that produce significant vasodilation. These drugs are also responsible for sometimes profound preoperative hypokalemia. Sim-

TABLE 62–12. Ten Most Common Categories of Drugs Prescribed to the Elderly

Analgesics
Antiarthritics
Antibiotics
Antispasmodics
Cardiovascular
Diabetic medications
Diuretics
Hormones
Sedatives and hypnotics
Tranquilizers

(Data from Stewart RB: Drug use in the elderly. *In* Therapeutics in the Elderly. Delafuente JC, Stewart RB (eds). Baltimore, Williams & Wilkins, 1988, p 55.)

ilar hypotension can result following long-term use of phenothiazine medications.

Maintenance of Drug Therapy

In general, the common management principle has shifted away from discontinuation of drugs that can potentially interact with anesthetics and toward the maintenance of such indicated drugs through the perioperative period. Potential interactions are anticipated and specifically treated, and this allows patients to continue to receive the benefits of the originally administered medication. This shift in emphasis recently has been extended to the use of tricyclic antidepressants and even monoamine oxidase inhibitors.

Anesthetic Implications

Many elderly patients drink large amounts of alcohol, which may have a strong additive interaction with the central nervous system depressant effects of many anesthetics. Beta-blocking drugs should be continued until the time of surgery to avoid sudden worsening of angina (or even myocardial infarction). Often, patients who consume large amounts of alcohol have low pulse rates. Significant bradycardia and hypotension can result from the use of fentanyl and related narcotics. These effects may occur particularly when intubation is performed after narcotic induction and after the administration of vecuronium or pipecuronium, which do not have the vagolytic effects of pancuronium. Similar problems have been anticipated with the use of calcium entry blockers; however, significant hemodynamic interactions with anesthetic agents have not been as common or severe as with the β-blocking drugs.

TABLE 62–13. Ten Most Frequently Prescribed Drugs for the Elderly

Hydrochlorothiazide
Digoxin
Furosemide
Triamterene
Aspirin
Propranolol
Methyldopa
Potassium
Vitamin B_{12}
Nitroglycerin

ALZHEIMER'S DISEASE

What Is Alzheimer's Disease?

Large amounts of media time have been devoted to Alzheimer's disease. Unfortunately, more heat than light has been created by this media attention. Less functional cerebral impairment is associated with aging than was previously thought. The presence of severe memory and cognitive impairment that is sufficient to interfere with the normal activities of daily living is necessary for a true diagnosis of Alzheimer's. Many cases of cognitive dysfunction in the elderly represent treatable mental depression.

How Is It Affected By Anesthesia?

Anesthetic management of patients with Alzheimer's disease is challenging because these patients' disorientation often makes them quite uncooperative and even combative. It is a mistake to think that pharmacologic sedation makes them docile; rather, sedation often leads to further problems with cooperation. Regional blocks, even with adequate pain relief, can result in a frustrating struggle to keep the patient from dangerous movement. However, anesthetic agents generally do not increase the amount of disorientation or agitation.

POSTOPERATIVE CEREBRAL DYSFUNCTION

Is It Anesthesia Related?

Numerous studies have attempted unsuccessfully to relate elderly patients' cerebral dysfunction in the postoperative period to specific anesthetic factors. Between 10% and 35% of elderly patients develop significant postoperative confusion. Postoperative mental outcome is more likely related to the initial preoperative functional state of the brain than to anesthesia. This conclusion obviously depends on the absence of events such as hypoxia, which are known to cause cerebral dysfunction. The problem of neurologic dysfunction is of particular concern in the elderly following cardiopulmonary bypass. It is far more likely to be caused by embolic rather than ischemic events; however, age alone also is related to the development of postoperative confusion after procedures during which cardiopulmonary bypass is instituted.

General and Regional Techniques

Repeated studies have failed to show any statistically reliable difference in postoperative mental function following general and regional anesthesia (Fig. 62–3). Individual studies hint at mental confusion being more common after general anesthesia than after regional blocks, but no reliable trend has been established. Some relationship is apparent, however, between the use of antidepressant, neuroleptic, or anticholinergic drugs and postoperative cerebral dysfunction, regardless of the type of anesthetic employed.[34]

Postoperative return of oxygenation toward normal appears to be more rapid following regional block. Whether this tendency toward better oxygenation in the postoperative period

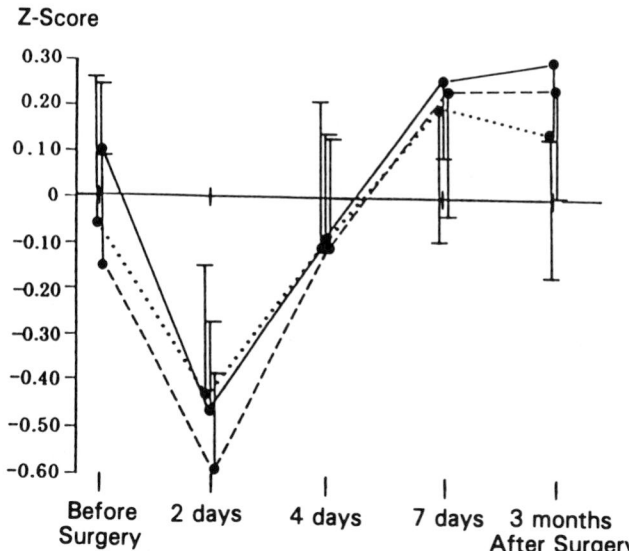

FIGURE 62–3. Comparison of attention test scores before and after hip replacement arthroplasty performed while utilizing general anesthesia (*solid line*, n = 9), epidural analgesia (*dotted line*, n = 10), and general anesthesia plus epidural analgesia (*dashed line*, n = 9) (mean ± SEM). (From Riis J, Lomholt B, Haxholdt D, et al: Immediate long term mental recovery from general vs epidural anesthesia in elderly patients. Acta Anaesthesiol Scand 1983; 27:44.)

minimizes hypoxemia that might produce changes in mental function remains speculative.

Care must be taken to avoid extreme passive hyperventilation during anesthesia, which may reduce $PaCO_2$ to levels that can impair cerebral perfusion. No operation should be denied to an elderly patient because of fear that anesthesia might in some way produce a harmful effect on postoperative mental function.

OUTPATIENT ANESTHESIA

How Safe Is It for the Elderly?

With careful selection of patients and operative procedures, no reason can be proposed to deny the benefits of outpatient surgery to elderly patients. Because they are more rapidly returned to their usual surroundings, the depersonalizing elements of the experience, which can be frightening, are minimized. Age alone influences neither the recovery from anesthesia nor the incidence of complications.[35] Certain items are of increased importance for the elderly patient in an outpatient setting. Timing of medications; assurance of nil per os status; stability of systemic illness (e.g., diabetes, angina, and asthma); and guaranteed availability of a ride home and a companion for the first night become crucial factors.

For Which Procedures Is It Suitable?

Cataract surgery has almost disappeared from the hospital setting. Minimal sedation is required to supplement a good retrobulbar block. In many areas, it is performed in physicians' offices with monitored anesthetic care.

Almost all inguinal hernia repairs are performed on an outpatient basis under field block local anesthesia and with small amounts of supplementary intravenous sedation. Transurethral resection of small bladder tumors is frequently performed on outpatients. Arthroscopy of the knee is increasingly common in elderly patients and lends itself well to outpatient management, particularly with the new interest in the use of local anesthesia for this operation. As techniques for laparoscopic intra-abdominal procedures become better defined and perfected, these procedures probably will be feasible in elderly outpatients. Increased sophistication in the use of propofol without significant hypotension expands the feasibility of outpatient programs oriented toward the elderly.

Finally, an outpatient center also can be the focal point for chronic pain management. Again, we see an example of medical progress that can be refined to serve the elderly and that should not be withheld on the basis of age alone.

PREOPERATIVE DO-NOT-RESUSCITATE ORDERS

How Should They Be Handled?

The more that is written about this delicate subject, the more questions arise and the fewer answers that follow. Many elderly patients approach surgery with a fear of becoming incapacitated and thus a burden to their families. More elderly patients are assertively insisting on the preparation of living wills and express their desires that life not be prolonged by extraordinary means. A recent study indicated that many institutions are not adequately prepared to deal with this growing problem. Although an overwhelming majority of surveyed departments of anesthesia suspended do-not-resuscitate orders prior to surgery, only half of them had a standing policy regarding the matter, and many of those that did not had no plans to develop one.[36]

The Anesthesiologist's Role

Confusion can be reduced if prior to the procedure the anesthesiologist develops a clear understanding with the surgeon, family physician, patient, and family members as to the extent of resuscitative maneuvers. Unfortunately, many procedures occur as emergencies, at times when family members are difficult to locate, or during situations in which the patient is unable to fully comprehend and agree to the proposed care. Better publicity of these issues has led to the execution of living wills by a greater number of elderly patients prior to admission to the hospital. Many hospitals have established distinct descriptions of resuscitative efforts (e.g., cardiopulmonary resuscitation, intubation with mechanical ventilation, treat dysrhythmias only, and no resuscitation).

The medicolegal implications and moral responsibilities of refusing to resuscitate a patient who has a cardiac arrest during anesthesia induction or during a surgical procedure are profound. One sensible approach is to discontinue do-not-resuscitate status upon the patient's arrival in the operating room and to fully treat situations that develop while he or she is there, and then to restore the do-not-resuscitate status when the patient is returned to the PACU or intensive care unit.

If a clear understanding cannot be reached or if the anesthesiologist finds himself or herself unable emotionally or intellectually to comply with the patient's and family's wishes, another anesthesiologist should be allowed to assume the responsibility for care. A clinical crisis in a desperately ill patient is not the time to try to resolve disagreement or confusion about resuscitative efforts.

Documentation

When possible, the accepted conditions of care should be carefully described in the chart and witnessed by the surgeon and the family. The signature of a third party should be obtained in order to avoid any ambiguity or postevent confusion about the extent of resuscitative care that is appropriate. Ambiguities can lead to longlasting and bitter disputes that often surface in a plaintiff attorney's office. In the event that a patient and family are unable to deal with this issue and state, "Do what you think best," the burden is placed directly upon the anesthesiologist and the surgeon.[37]

Future Direction

Legislative direction and judicial interpretation in the United States promote an analysis of responsibilities that favors the wishes of the patient rather than the moral sensibilities of the anesthesiologist. This is a burden that society wishes the medical profession to carry. Until the expected outcome is attained or until the point at which resuscitative efforts are to be discontinued is reached, care must be at the same level as that provided when full and prompt recovery is expected.

SUMMARY AND CONCLUSIONS

It is clear that elderly patients cannot be treated simply as individuals with organ dysfunction and a date of birth that is beyond the anesthesiologist's memory. Basic organ function in the elderly is generally sufficient for the daily activities of living, but the ability to increase organ function in response to stress is limited. The elderly do not read our literature nor do they know how they are supposed to react to our medications and interventions. Physiologic lability is the rule, not the exception, and response to medication can be profound and unpredictable.

Anesthesia is a clinical titration that is based on the principle that more of a drug can be given, but once it is given, it cannot be taken back. The elderly patient tolerates complications poorly, and extreme effort must be exercised to limit the incidence of complications that can, in a domino-like cascade, lead to death or permanent disability. Preoperative correction of physiologic defects is an important principle. No operation should ever be denied to an elderly patient based on his or her age alone. When care and compassion are provided, rewarding results after complex surgery are common.

References

1. Gardner B, Palasti S: A comparison of hospital costs and morbidity between octogenarians and other patients undergoing general surgical operations. Surg Gynecol Obstet 1990; 171:299.
2. Fries JF: Aging, natural death and the compression of morbidity. N Engl J Med 1980; 303:103.
3. Olshansky SJ, Carnes BA, Cassel C: In search of Methuselah: estimating the upper limits to human longevity. Science 1990; 250:634.
4. Cohen MM, Duncan PG, Tate RB: Does anesthesia contribute to operative mortality? JAMA 1988; 260:2859.

5. Forrest JB, Rehder K, Cahalan MK, Goldsmith CH: Multicenter study of general anesthesia: III. Predictors of severe perioperative adverse outcomes. Anesthesiology 1992; 76:3.

6. Jones RL: Anesthesia risk in the geriatric patient in perioperative geriatrics. Prob Anesth 1989; 3:527.

7. Del Guercio L, Cohn JD: Monitoring operative risk in the elderly. JAMA 1980; 243:1350.

8. Stump DA, Newman SP, Coker LH: The effect of age on neurologic outcome after cardiac surgery. Anesth Analg 1992; 74S:309.

9. Zaidan J: Hemodynamics of nitroglycerin during aortic clamping. Arch Surg 1982; 117:1285.

10. Don H: Measurement of gas trapped in the lungs at FRC and the effects of posture. Anesthesiology 1971; 35:582.

11. Gunnarsson L, Tokics L, Gustavsson H, Hedenstierna G: Influence of age on atelectasis formation and gas exchange impairment during general anesthesia. Br J Anaesth 1991; 66:423.

12. Dyson A, Henderson AM, Chamley D: An assessment of postoperative oxygen therapy in patients with fractured neck of femur. Anaesth Intensive Care 1988; 16:405.

13. Reissell E, Orko R, Maunuksela EL, Lindgren L: Predictability of laryngoscopy in patients with long-term diabetes mellitus. Anaesthesia 1990; 45:1024.

14. Sessler DI, Hudson S: Evaporative heat loss during surgical skin preparation. Anesth Analg 1992; 74S:276.

15. Bourke D, Grayson R: Digital nerve blocks can restore pulse oximeter signal detection. Anesth Analg 1991; 73:815.

16. Pälve H, Ali-Melkkilä T: Oxygenation during local anesthesia for cataract surgery. Acta Anaesthesiol Scand 1991; 35:181.

17. Zeitlin GL, Hobin K, Platt J: Accumulation of carbon dioxide during eye surgery. J Clin Anesth 1989; 1:262.

18. Homer TD, Stanski DR: The effect of increasing age on thiopental disposition and anesthetic requirement. Anesthesiology 1985; 62:714.

19. Scott JC, Stanski DR: Decreased fentanyl and alfentanil dose requirement with age. J Pharmacol Exp Ther 1987; 240:159.

20. Klotz U, Avant GR, Hoyumpa A: The effects of age and liver disease on the disposition and elimination of diazepam in the adult. J Clin Invest 1975; 55:347.

21. Hilgenberg JC: Inhalation and intravenous drugs in the elderly patient. Semin Anesth 1986; 5:44.

22. Lerman J, Gregory GA, Willis MM: Age and solubility of volatile anesthetics in blood. Anesthesiology 1984; 61:139.

23. Lien CA, Matteo RS, Ornstein E: Distribution, elimination, and action of vecuronium in the elderly. Anesth Analg 1991; 73:39.

24. Koscielniak-Nielsen ZJ, Law-Min JC, Donati F: Dose-response relations of doxacurium and its reversal with neostigmine in young adults and healthy elderly patients. Anesth Analg 1992; 74:845.

25. Ornstein E, Matteo RS, Schwartz AE: Pharmacokinetics and pharmacodynamics of pipecuronium in elderly surgery patients. Anesth Analg 1992; 74:841.

26. Matteo RS, Young WL, Ornstein E: Pharmacokinetics and pharmacodynamics of edrophonium in elderly surgical patients. Anesth Analg 1990; 71:334.

27. Young WL, Matteo RS, Ornstein E: Duration of action of neostigmine and pyridostigmine in the elderly. Anesth Analg 1988; 67:775.

28. Rasmussen BS, Blom L, Mikkelsen SS: Postspinal headache in young and elderly patients. Anaesthesia 1984; 44:571.

29. Stone DJ, DiFazio CA: Postspinal headache in older patients. Anesth Analg 1990; 70:222.

30. Rao TLK, El-Etr AA: Anticoagulation following placement of epidural and subarachnoid catheters. Anesthesiology 1981; 55:618.

31. Modig J, Maripuu E, Sahldtedt A: Thromboembolism after total hip replacement. Reg Anesth 1986; 11:72.

32. Yeager MP, Glass DD, Neff RK, Brinck-Johnsen T: Epidural anesthesia and analgesia in high-risk surgical patients. Anesthesiology 1987; 66:729.

33. Tuman KJ, McCarthy RJ, March RJ: Effects of epidural anesthesia and analgesia on coagulation and outcome after major vascular surgery. Anesth Analg 1991; 73:696.

34. Berggren D, Gustafson Y, Eriksson B: Postoperative confusion after anesthesia in elderly patients with femoral neck fractures. Anesth Analg 1987; 66:497.

35. Meridy H: Criteria for selection of ambulatory surgical patients and guidelines for anesthesia management. Anesth Analg 1982; 61:921.

36. Franklin CM, Rothenberg DM: Do-not-resuscitate orders in presurgical patients. J Clin Anesth 1992; 4:181.

37. Keffer MJ, Keffer HL: Do-not-resuscitate in the operating room: moral obligations of anesthesiologists. Anesth Analg 1992; 74:901.

CHAPTER 63

The Obstetric Patient

DONALD CATON, M.D.

Several factors make obstetric anesthesia different from other subspecialty areas. First, the patients are unique; pregnancy causes changes in body function that alter the character and magnitude of the response to many of our drugs and techniques.

Second, anesthesia affects *two* individuals, not just one. As a matter of fact, we tend to judge the quality of anesthesia by the response of the newborn rather than that of the mother. Of course, before delivery, the infant is far more difficult to evaluate than the mother.

Third, unlike situations in the operating room, during labor and delivery, obstetric anesthesiologists deal with a process that usually is normal and natural, one that will be carried to completion with a good outcome independent of our involvement. This fact puts on us the onus of showing that our efforts to relieve a woman of pain leave her and her child no worse off than if we had done nothing at all.

Fourth, our usual goal in obstetrics is to control pain, not necessarily to abolish it. Last—and this point may be the most important to women—the delivery of a child, including the pain associated with it, has very different social and personal implications from the pain associated with a surgical procedure such as an appendectomy or reduction of a fractured femur. For a brief period, the anesthesiologist enters a very intimate and emotional time in the life of the patient and her family. We must be very sensitive to the psychologic and physical needs and be ready to work with them.

The principles and standards of good anesthesia care apply to every patient, regardless of the location within the institution or the clinical situation. We must adapt these general rules to the circumstances of obstetric patients, to their physiology or pathophysiology, and to the surgical requirements. Such considerations help us to develop a special set of guidelines for this subspecialty (Table 63–1). These guidelines do not nullify general principles of good care but merely modify them.

We must occasionally ignore elements of the guidelines specific for obstetric anesthesia and revert to principles of general operating room care. This situation usually occurs when a patient has a concurrent medical or surgical problem—severe cardiac or pulmonary disease, for example—that overshadows the obstetric considerations. It sometimes results from an obscure medical problem for which there is no specific information to guide us in her anesthetic management, as with Marfan's syndrome or a rare metabolic disorder. In such circumstances, we may draw on the large body of information gained from our work in the operating room. This point will become clearer during discussion of specific problems.

NORMAL CHANGES IN PREGNANCY

Pregnancy involves significant change in virtually every maternal tissue and function. These changes form the basis for many aspects of our care of obstetric patients (Table 63–2).

Why Is the Maternal Metabolic Rate Increased?

Most important to understand is the increased maternal metabolic rate, which has two components: increased maternal oxygen (O_2) consumption to support the work of carrying so much extra tissue; and fetal, placental, and uterine tissue O_2 consumption, which directly supports growth and development.[1] The latter value is two to three times that of the mother per unit weight of tissue. Thus, a woman who weighs 50 kg when not pregnant uses about 150 to 200 mL of O_2 per minute ($3-4$ mL $\cdot$ kg^{-1} $\cdot$ min^{-1}) to maintain her own tissues. If her term infant weighs 3 kg and if the placenta and her uterus are of average weight for a child of that size, their combined O_2

TABLE 63–1. Guidelines for Obstetric Anesthesia

Goals of obstetric anesthesia	• Alleviate the pain of labor.
	• Provide optimum conditions for operative obstetrics.
	Cesarean section
	Vaginal deliveries
	Application of forceps
	Repair of lacerations and episiotomy
	Relaxation of the uterus
Constraints governing obstetric anesthesia	• Interfere as little as possible with progress of labor and delivery.
	• Minimize the effects of drugs on the infant.
	• Maintain fetal homeostasis, including reflexes involved in the adaptation to extrauterine life.

TABLE 63–2. Some Physiologic Changes of Pregnancy

Metabolic	Increased metabolic rate: O_2 consumption, CO_2 and heat production	Increased cardiac output, increased minute ventilation
	Altered liver metabolism	Changes in drug excretion and conjugation
	Increased glycolysis	Diabetogenic state
	Sodium and H_2 retention	Edema, expanded plasma volume
Smooth muscle	Tendency to hypertrophy	Most pronounced in uterus
	Decreased tone and irritability of most smooth muscle until term	
	Increased tone and irritability peripartum	
	Gastrointestinal (Delayed gastric emptying, relaxation of gastroesophageal sphincter)	Reflux
	Prolonged gastrointestinal transit time	Constipation
	Biliary stasis	Stone formation, acute cholecystitis
	Urogenital (Dilatation of ureters)	Stasis and infection
	Uterine enlargement	
	Cardiovascular (Myocardial hypertrophy and alterations, irritability)	
	Small blood vessel growth	Hypertrophy and hyperplasia
	Dilatation of arteries	Nasal stuffiness, thenar hyperemia, spider angiomas
	Venous enlargement	Hemorrhoids, varicose veins
	Pulmonary (Increased bronchiolar reactivity peripartum)	Bronchospasm
	Possible increase of pulmonary vascular resistance peripartum	
Glandular	Breast enlargement and onset of lactation	
	Increased salivation	Difficulty visualizing airway
	Increased activity of gastric glands	Heartburn, reflex
Central nervous system	Change in set-point of regulatory centers	Temperature, vomiting, appetite, respiration, and blood pressure
	Change in activity of cortex and reticular activating systems	Altered wake-sleep cycles, increased sensitivity to drugs

consumption may exceed 55 mL · min^{-1} (10–12 mL · kg^{-1} · min^{-1}). In other words, with only a 10% increase in total body weight, maternal metabolism may increase almost 30% above the basal nonpregnant rate (Fig. 63–1).

What Are the Effects of Increased Metabolic Rate?

Estimates of the increased metabolic rate serve as a useful approximation of the stress placed on various maternal organs. To support the increased O_2 demand, a commensurate increase in minute ventilation, cardiac output, heat dissipation, and excretion of metabolic waste products by the kidneys must occur.[2–8] Because the metabolism of a fetus is proportional to its weight, estimates of the latter also may be used to evaluate the ability of a woman to handle physiologic stress (Fig. 63–2).

Fetal Oxygen Consumption

To use concepts of metabolism, however, one must understand that fetal O_2 consumption has two functions. One part sustains the integrity of existing tissue; the other supports growth. The O_2 requirements of a fetus that is not growing are rather small, 3 to 4 mL · kg^{-1} · min^{-1}, almost identical to the rate of consumption of maternal tissue. On the other hand, O_2 consumption of a fast-growing fetus may be 12 mL · kg^{-1} · min^{-1}. The difference represents the metabolic cost of growth.

When growth stops, the fetal metabolic rate falls to the basal level needed to sustain tissue integrity. This decrease, in turn, lessens the load placed on the mother. Her respiratory, cardio-

vascular, and excretory systems no longer must work at the higher level needed to sustain rapid growth. Thus, women whose physiologic reserves are limited by disease tend to have low-birth-weight babies. The fetus may not have grown normally, but it has survived with the resources available to it.

"Small-for-Date" Infants

The previously mentioned facts help in evaluating patients whose reserves may be limited by disease. If estimates of an infant's weight are normal, the mother probably has sufficient cardiopulmonary function to sustain growth of a full-sized infant. In all likelihood, she will also be able to handle the increased stress associated with the work of labor (increased O_2 consumption, heat production, and cardiac output). On the other hand, if the present infant or previous infants were small for dates, one must suspect that maternal reserves are limited to the point of disrupting fetal growth.

The relationships between fetal growth, metabolic demands, and maternal reserves do not imply that all problems of fetal growth retardation are the result of altered maternal cardiopulmonary problems. However, they provide a convenient reference point to estimate physiologic stress and to evaluate maternal reserves in the event of pre-existing cardiopulmonary disease.

Why Do Ventilatory Changes Occur?

The uterus also grows in proportion to the growth of the fetus. Associated with this growth are changes in the mechanics of breathing.[9, 10] The anterior rib segments move up and

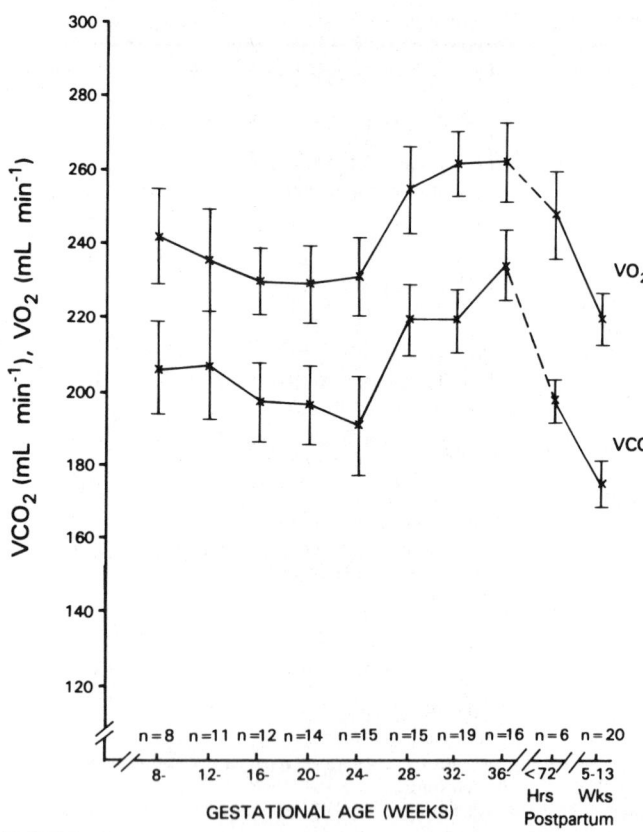

FIGURE 63–1. Oxygen consumption and carbon dioxide production of normal patients during pregnancy. Most of the increase during the third trimester reflects the high metabolic activity of the fetal, placental, and uterine tissues. (From Rees GB, Broughton Pipkin F, Symonds EM: A longitudinal study of respiratory changes in normal human pregnancy with cross-sectional data on subjects with pregnancy-induced hypertension. Am J Obstet Gynecol 1990; 162:826–830.)

out, the diaphragm elevates, and the functional residual capacity (FRC) decreases. These changes, in conjunction with the increase in O_2 consumption, create special problems for an anesthesiologist. Intubation of the trachea may be more diffi-

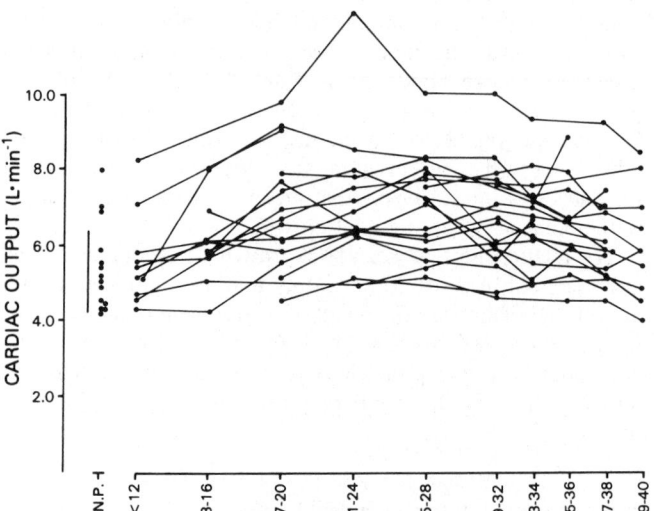

FIGURE 63–2. Cardiac output during pregnancy. *Lines* connect repeated measurements on individual patients. N.P. = Values for the same patient when she is "nonpregnant," 8 or more weeks after childbirth. (From Caton D, Banner TE: Doppler estimates of cardiac output during pregnancy. Bull N Y Acad Med 1987; 63:727–731.)

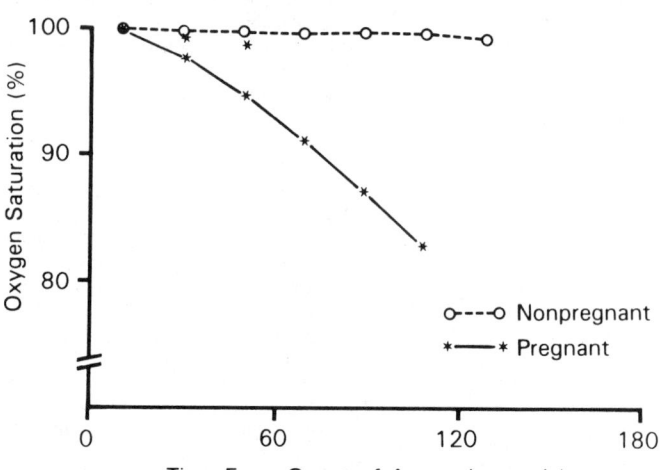

FIGURE 63–3. Oxygen saturation measured by pulse oximetry of a pregnant and nonpregnant patient. The pregnant patient was also obese. The rapid decline in saturation was caused by the decreased functional residual capacity and the increased metabolic rate.

cult simply because a woman's rib cage and enlarged breasts interfere with placement of the laryngoscope handle. Meanwhile, the combination of high metabolic rate and decreased FRC (and the physiologic anemia of pregnancy) combine to cause oxyhemoglobin desaturation to 70% or 80% during periods of apnea as short as a minute, despite preoxygenation (Fig. 63–3).

How Are Smooth Muscle Functions Altered?

Note in Table 63–2 how many alterations during pregnancy involve smooth muscle function.

Myometrium

Changes in the myometrium are most significant. This organ undergoes not only hyperplasia and hypertrophy but also systematic changes in function. Thus, several mechanisms combine to keep the myofibrils both inactive during pregnancy but then increasingly responsive as a patient approaches term.[11, 12]

Gastrointestinal Tract

Smooth muscles of other organs undergo similar changes of structure and function and are responsible for many of the clinical problems we encounter during pregnancy. For example, relaxation of the gastroesophageal sphincter and decreased gastric emptying (in association with increased gastric gland activity) increase the risk of regurgitation and aspiration of acidic gastric contents.[13] Decreased tone of the biliary tract[14-16] and ureters[17] increases the risks of cholecystitis and pyelonephritis.

Respiratory Tract

During the peripartum period, most smooth muscle becomes highly reactive. Bronchospasm among asthmatics and heavy smokers may become a significant problem when tracheal intubation is required.[18, 19]

How Are Set-Point Regulatory Functions Modified?

Pregnancy involves a systematic change in the set-point of many regulatory functions in the central nervous system (CNS). This phenomenon causes the sustained drop in the partial pressure of arterial carbon dioxide ($Paco_2$), the second trimester fall in mean arterial pressure and basal body temperature, the increased sensitivity of the vomiting center during the first trimester, and alterations in satiety throughout pregnancy.[9, 20]

How Are Central and Peripheral Nervous System Sensitivity Altered?

Changes in the central and peripheral nervous systems are great and cause increased sensitivity to many drugs used for anesthesia, including local anesthetics, inhalation anesthetics, narcotics, barbiturates, tranquilizers, and even muscle relaxants.[20–25] With all drugs, one should assume that the usual dose should be reduced by 25% to 30%.

How Is the Musculoskeletal System Affected?

Pregnant women experience significant changes even in the musculoskeletal system. Because the normal lordosis of the back tends to disappear, needles must be oriented more perpendicular to the plane of the back when a spinal or epidural block is performed. Ligaments soften, often to a remarkable extent, and make it difficult to use them as landmarks for regional block. Visible fasciculations after succinylcholine tend to disappear in a majority of patients.[24]

LABOR ANALGESIA: GENERAL CONSIDERATIONS

What Are the Major Anesthetic Constraints?

The primary goal of anesthesia for laboring patients is the control of labor pain. We also may try to create conditions that facilitate spontaneous labor or an operative vaginal delivery (see Table 63–1).

Several consideration are unique to obstetric anesthesia.

Fetal Drug Effects

We try to have as little effect as possible on the infant. Infants, like their mothers, tend to be very susceptible to the drug effects. Drugs and doses that have the least possible impact on the infant should be chosen, particularly during an infant's adaptation to extrauterine life.

Transplacental Drug Movement

Factors that affect the rate of transplacental movement of drugs are similar to those that affect drug movement across the blood-brain barrier and include molecular size, lipid and water solubility, and ionization. Several physical factors also

TABLE 63–3. Factors Affecting Maternal-Fetal Drug Equilibration

Maternal factors	Blood concentration
	Uterine blood flow
	Rate of delivery to placenta
Placental	Surface area of placenta
	Mean distance between maternal and fetal blood
Fetal	Blood concentration
	Umbilical blood flow
	pH (ion trapping)
	Rate of metabolism by fetus
Drug factors	Dosage
	Duration of exposure (time for equilibration)
	Binding
	pK
	Ionization
	Molecular size
	Lipid solubility

affect the process, including concentration gradients and protein binding (Table 63–3).[26] The relationships of these factors are shown in the following equation:

$$\text{Amount of drug diffusion per unit time} = \frac{K \, [C_1 - C_2] \, SA}{d}$$

where K is a constant influenced by the solubility of the drug in the intervening tissue and its molecular weight, $C_1 - C_2$ is the concentration gradient of the drug on either side of the placenta, SA is the surface area of the placenta, and d is the mean distance between maternal and fetal blood.

Although these factors are important, in practice we can do little to control them. We make our selection of a particular drug and dosage on the basis of other clinically important criteria such as duration of action, toxicity, rapidity of action, cost, and availability.

Effects of Greatest Concern

Drug effects on a newborn of most concern are those that depress or abolish the onset of ventilation. Investigators have suggested that drugs transmitted across the placenta also may disturb an infant's psychologic bonding with the mother, its eating patterns, and weight gain during the neonatal period.[27–37] Because an infant's liver does not metabolize drugs quickly, their effects may last longer than they would in an adult. Some investigators dispute the clinical significance of these data, and others doubt the existence of these phenomena altogether. Nevertheless, one guiding principle of obstetric anesthesia is to use only those drugs that are absolutely essential and to give no more than is absolutely necessary.

How Do Anesthesia/Analgesia Affect Labor?

We should interfere as little as possible with labor. Unfortunately, this problem is difficult to manage because we understand so little about the normal mechanisms that initiate and maintain labor. The hallmark of the onset of labor is uterine smooth muscle activation. This deceptively simple event involves several mechanisms, including changes in the synthesis and reflex release of oxytocin; catecholamines; steroid hormones, including estrogens, progesterone, and glucocorticoids; and prostaglandins.[38-41] Labor also involves skeletal muscle, many involuntary reflexes, and a certain amount of coordinated and semi-voluntary pushing.

Timing of Administered Analgesics

Some effects of analgesia on labor are obvious. For example, virtually any sedative, narcotic, tranquilizer, or regional anesthetic given too early can stop labor. For this reason, before giving any drug, anesthesiologists wait for the obstetrician to decide when labor is in the phase of rapid cervical dilatation. Unfortunately, the criteria for identifying this phase are, by necessity, somewhat vague. Generally, labor is considered well established for primiparas at 6 cm cervical dilatation and for multiparous women at 4 cm. An obstetrician may modify this estimate, however, based on the quality of the contractions or from some experience in managing a patient's previous labor pattern. If a patient is to receive a pitocin infusion, timing the anesthetic with the phase of labor is less important.

Depression

Anesthesia may interfere with labor in other ways. A woman given large doses of narcotics, sedatives, tranquilizers, or inhalation agents may be incapable of pushing during the second stage of labor. Complete anesthesia of the sacral fibers that innervate the perineum, as with spinal or epidural blockade, may inhibit the reflex release of oxytocin that normally occurs during the second stage of labor with passive dilatation of the cervix (Ferguson's reflex). Some regional anesthetics interfere with the "bearing down reflex," either because the woman cannot sense the infant's pressure on the perineum (the stimulus that normally initiates the reflex) or because she has lost strength of her abdominal muscles from a block that was too extensive.

Enhancement

Anesthesia may facilitate labor by reducing pain and thus inhibiting the reflex release of epinephrine, a hormone that has an adverse effect on myometrial function. Similarly, it may facilitate second-stage pushing by decreasing perineal pain.

Which anesthesic effects predominate and their clinical significance depend on factors beyond our control, such as the size and internal configuration of a women's bony pelvis, the size and presentation of an infant, the obstetrician's experience and expertise with forceps, and a woman's ability and will to push. The potential effects of anesthesia on the first and second stages of labor have been the subject of extensive debate between anesthesiologists and obstetricians. Many early studies are marred by inadequate descriptions of anesthetic and obstetric management.

Studies that take technique into account suggest that epidural anesthesia does not prolong the first stage of labor but may lengthen the second stage by 20 to 30 minutes.[42] These figures, however, represent averages compiled from large numbers of patients. What holds true for the group does not always apply to an individual. Physicians must be very cautious about the effects—or lack thereof—of any given anesthetic technique.

How Is Fetal Homeostasis Preserved?

At all times, we should interfere as little as possible with fetal homeostasis. In obstetrics, we have assumed that a diminished supply of O_2 is the mechanism most likely to damage an infant. Although this assumption oversimplifies the problem, we do place great emphasis on the preservation of maternal ventilation, maintenance of high maternal arterial O_2 content, and good perfusion of the placenta. Accordingly, we avoid unnecessary depression of maternal ventilation, give supplemental O_2, and make sure that maternal hemoglobin levels do not decrease. In addition, we work to maintain arterial pressure within normal limits, because perfusion of the placenta tends to vary directly with changes in mean arterial pressure (Fig. 63-4).[43-47]

The last point is particularly important because blockade of the sympathetic nervous system is a frequent cause of maternal hypotension. When maternal hypotension occurs, we treat it with the intent of increasing both maternal blood pressure and placental perfusion. Therefore, nonpharmacologic maneuvers such as left uterine displacement to relieve vena caval and aortic compression, as well as fluid resuscitation, generally precede pharmacologic intervention. Ephedrine is the drug of choice should a vasopressor be used.

What Methods Are Available for the Management of Labor Pain?

Psychologic methods of pain control remain important. In fact, all other techniques should be considered an adjunct to their use.[48] Studies in the obstetric literature demonstrate that

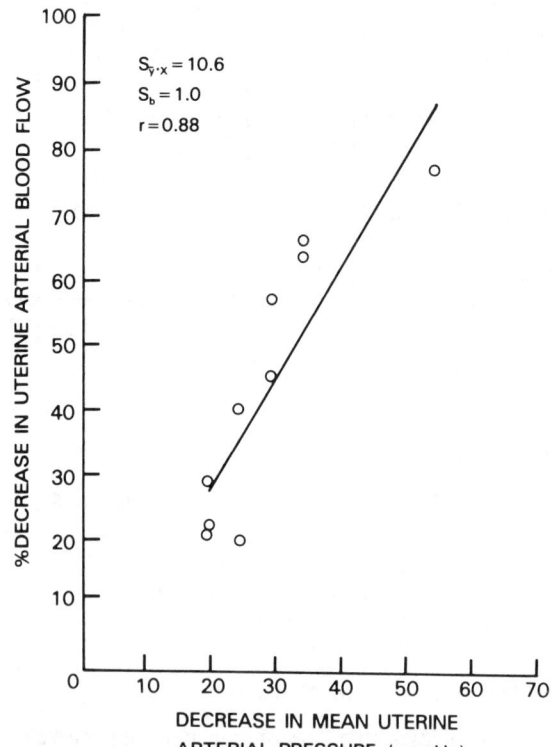

FIGURE 63-4. Pressure flow relationships in the uterine artery of the pregnant sheep. (From Berman W, Goodlin RC, Heymann MA, et al: Relationships between pressure and flow in the umbilical and uterine circulations of the sheep. Circ Res 1976; 38:262.)

good emotional support during labor lowers the incidence of problems such as forceps delivery, prolonged labor, and even cesarean section.

Analgesia may also be needed to control the pain of labor. The most logical way to classify analgesia is by route of administration.[49] Of the parenteral agents, narcotics are historically the oldest and still the most efficacious. Depending on a patient's needs, narcotics may be supplemented with sedatives, amnestic agents, or tranquilizers. Of the inhalation agents, nitrous oxide and methoxyflurane are all that remain; trichloroethylene, diethyl ether, chloroform, cyclopropane, and ethylene oxide have been eliminated for various reasons.

Regional techniques currently used are spinal and epidural anesthesia and their respective variants, saddle block and caudal; pudendal nerve block; and local infiltration of the perineum.

Factors Governing the Proper Choice

Coexisting Medical Problems

Perhaps the first question should be, Does the patient have a medical condition that eliminates any specific agent or technique? A bleeding disorder precludes a spinal or epidural anesthetic because it increases the risk of epidural hematoma. Similarly, pre-existing pulmonary problems such as asthma, pneumonia, or cor pulmonale could modify the use of narcotics and other agents that suppress respiration. Pre-existing medical problems should be explored during the routine preanesthetic history and physical examination. The same criteria and contraindications should be considered when dealing with obstetric patients as with any other group of patients.[49]

The Obstetrician's Experience

Options for obstetric anesthesia could be limited by the obstetrician's experience. Some obstetricians have not managed patients with an epidural anesthetic. Some may be concerned that the narcotics transmitted from mother to fetus might mask an important change in fetal heart rate beat-to-beat variability. Consultation with the obstetrician, therefore, is an important second step.

The Patient's Wishes

A third consideration is the patient's desires. Some women want natural childbirth, desire few if any medications, and consider anything else a personal failure. Others may have a morbid fear of needles or an irrational dread of pain. These factors should influence anesthetic choice. Many modern obstetric units have worked to include the father and other family members in the delivery process; their wishes and expectations should be considered also. Do not make assumptions about the desires of a given patient; too often you will be surprised.

The Anesthesiologist's Capabilities

Fourth, ask what you can do. This question really has two parts. First, what are you medically qualified to do? Second, what can you safely do with the existing circumstances? For example, you may be well qualified to perform an epidural block but decide it is unwise to do so because you do not have adequate nursing personnel to watch the patient. You may already have several laboring patients and cannot safely add another, or you may expect to be called away momentarily for some other emergency.

Who Is Responsible for Pain Management?

Until recently, obstetricians were responsible for pain management, often without any help from anesthesiologists. However, with the numbers of practicing anesthesiologists increasing, the pattern is shifting. In most institutions, obstetricians still order all parenteral medications and perform pudendal nerve blocks and local infiltration for delivery. Some even perform their own epidural blocks for labor and saddle blocks for delivery. In larger institutions with good coverage, however, anesthesiologists or nurse anesthetists take primary responsibility for epidural blocks for laboring patients and may give inhalation analgesia for delivery.

Nurses also share responsibility for pain management. We rely on them to prepare and assist laboring patients with most of the psychologic methods currently used. The nurse usually is the only professional at the bedside throughout all of labor. Often, the extent to which patients need the services of anesthesia personnel varies inversely with the nurses' skills.

EPIDURAL ANALGESIA

What Is the Relevant Anatomy and Physiology of Labor Pain?

The First Stage

Understanding the anatomy and physiology of labor pain helps with management. Keep in mind that labor pain has two components. The first stage of labor, from the onset of regular contractions to full dilatation of the cervix, consists of crampy, diffuse lower abdominal pain, sometimes referred to the back, legs, or a hip, and coincides with uterine contractions. This component is mediated by afferent sympathetic fibers that arise in the fundus of the uterus, converge on either side of the cervix (Frankenhauser's plexus), move cephalad in the retroperitoneal space, and finally join the spinal cord at the level of T-10 to T-12 (Table 63–4).

TABLE 63–4. Characteristics of First and Second Stage Labor Pain

First stage	Crampy, coincident with the contraction but starts slightly afterward and ends before
	Lower abdomen, occasionally accompanied by diffuse back or leg pain
	Dermatomes T-9–T-12; usually associated with drowsiness. Patients often go into rapid-eye-movement sleep between contractions.
	Patients usually hyperventilate; occasionally they push prematurely.
Second stage	Continuous but worse with contractions; sharp
	Perineal; well localized; dermatomes L-4–sacral
	Patients more alert. At full dilatation, diaphoresis (forehead and upper lip) associated with a brief bout of nausea and vomiting
	Bearing down reflex prominent, although pain may inhibit this in some women

The Second Stage

Pain during the second stage of labor, from full dilatation to delivery, is mediated by somatic afferent (and possibly parasympathetic) fibers that originate in the cervix and vagina and join the spinal cord in the sacral region. This pain is localized in the perineum, is sharper in nature, and is more likely to persist between contractions. This pain is often accompanied by nausea, vomiting, and diaphoresis on the forehead and upper lip.

What Factors Guide the Anesthetic Technique?

Anatomic and functional distinctions among the fibers mediating pain during the first and second stages of labor guide the anesthetic technique. For example, an ideal block for the first stage of labor would affect only sympathetic fibers that enter the cord at T-10 to T-12. Although it is not always possible to achieve this degree of precision, several variables can be manipulated to increase the probability.

Epidural Puncture Site

If a patient is in a very early stage of labor, choose an interspace as close as possible to T-12. A block this early in the labor will be used for a considerable time, so get as close as possible to the nerve roots involved. If the attempt is successful, a local anesthetic volume as low as 2 to 4 mL may suffice. Conversely, if the patient is fully dilated or crowning, consider a caudal approach or at least a lower lumbar interspace.

Drug Administration

Other factors that influence the dose of epidural blocks are the location of the tip of the catheter (you *cannot* control this variable with the needle), the volume of injectate, speed of injection (more rapid injection gives greater dispersal), and concentration of the local anesthetic (for a given volume, higher concentrations give a more extensive block than lower concentrations). Uterine contractions have no apparent effect on dispersal of the anesthetic agent; in this regard, epidural blocks differ from spinal blocks. With the latter technique,

injection of the drug during a contraction may cause total spinal blockade, even with doses of tetracaine as small as 4 mg.

Patient Positioning

The smaller the volume of injectate, the more gravity will influence the distribution of the block, even with epidural anesthesia. Thus, a patient lying on her right side during dosing may continue to have left-sided pain. If so, simply have her roll from one side to another to achieve more even distribution of the drug. Similarly, clinical observation suggests that sitting the patient upright during redosing may help to distribute the block to the perineum.

Progression of Labor

The goal of a regional anesthetic for labor and delivery is to *control* labor pain, not to eliminate all sensation or muscle control. As labor progresses, the character, distribution, and intensity of pain change, and the dose of local anesthetic must be adjusted accordingly. Premature dosing and overdosing are responsible for most of the problems that concern obstetricians: slowing or stopping labor, malrotation of the presenting part, and maternal inability to push during the second stage. The primary goal of anesthesia is to use the smallest dose to achieve the desired result at any given stage of labor.

What Drugs and Doses Are Appropriate?

Typical concentrations and volumes for different agents are given in Table 63–5. These figures should be used as guidelines, not rules. Requirements vary tremendously among patients and even within a patient, depending on the stage of labor. Perhaps the one consistent rule is to decide what effect you want, then dose to that end point but no further.

Aberrant Pain Patterns

Epidural Narcotics

Anesthesiologists have found it useful to add small doses of epidural narcotics to the local anesthetic to potentiate their effect (see Table 63–5). This approach seems particularly use-

TABLE 63–5. Dosing Epidural Anesthetics for Labor

Procedure	Drug	Concentration	Volume/Dose
Initiation of block	Lidocaine with epinephrine	1%, 1.5%, 2%	2–12 mL*
Maintenance of block			
Intermittent dose	Lidocaine with epinephrine	1%, 1.5%, 2%	2–12 mL*
	Carbocaine	1%, 1.5%, 2%	2–12 mL*
	Bupivacaine	0.25%, 0.5%	2–12 mL*
	2-Chloroprocaine	2%, 3%	2–12 mL‡
	Fentanyl	50–75 μg	1–1.5 mL†
Continuous infusion	Bupivacaine	0.062 to 0.125%	6–18 mL · h⁻¹*
	Fentanyl		0.5–1 μg · kg⁻¹ · h⁻¹†

*Volume and concentration must be adjusted for each patient depending on site of injection, severity of pain, stage of labor, need for a rapid onset, need for a motor as well as a sensory block.
†Epidural narcotics are not useful by themselves but may be added to a local anesthetic. They can help with difficult pain problems (see text) or help overcome problems of tachyphylaxis.
‡Some reports suggest 2-chloroprocaine may counteract the effects of epidural narcotics.

ful for management of some aberrant pain patterns (Table 63–6) and for patients who develop tachyphylaxis from local anesthetics. Current information suggests that narcotics given in the epidural space have very little effect on an infant.

Origin

Aberrant pain patterns are diverse (see Table 63–6). An occiput posterior presentation may cause severe continuous back pain even during the first stage of labor; back pain may also indicate abruption of a posteriorly implanted placenta. Diffuse abdominal pain may indicate a ruptured uterus or a distended liver due to eclamptic changes. Continuous suprapubic pain in a patient with an otherwise adequate block suggests bladder distention. Patients occasionally have severe, sharp pain in a leg or hip for a portion of labor as a result of direct pressure of the infant's presenting part on a sacral nerve root.

What Monitoring Is Appropriate?

Normal patients should have their blood pressure taken frequently as the block is taking effect. After that, 15-minute intervals are suitable if no other problems develop. Because an anesthesiologist may not be in attendance throughout labor, nurses must be trained to take blood pressure and to identify problems relating to the anesthetic, such as an excessive block, change in sensorium, an unexplained change in fetal heart rate pattern, or maternal hypotension. Nurses should be trained to initiate emergency treatment and to call for help.

Is the Approach Different for Delivery?

If a patient has an established epidural block, it may be extended to include the sacral nerves by having her sit up for redosing and by increasing the concentration or volume of infusate (keep in mind that somatic afferent fibers that mediate the pain of the second stage are larger and require a larger dose of local anesthetic).

The second stage of labor is not too late to initiate an epidural block. A caudal or low lumbar epidural block works well. Saddle blocks traditionally have been used for delivery, as have pudendal nerve blocks, local infiltration, and inhalation analgesia. Small doses of intravenous ketamine (0.25 mg · kg⁻¹) or inhalation analgesia with nitrous oxide or methoxyflurane may work by themselves or may be used to potentiate local infiltration or a pudendal nerve block.

The best choice often depends on the circumstances. If the patient has an existing block, use it. If not, is sufficient time available to establish a block? If so, will the obstetrician need a dense sensory and motor block of the perineal musculature for a difficult forceps delivery or extensive repair? Does the medical condition of the patient preclude a particular technique?

INHALATION ANALGESIA

Properly administered inhalation analgesia may be as effective as a dose of narcotic but without the risk of infantile respiratory depression. Placental transfer of gaseous agents tends to be slow, and a newborn quickly clears inhalation agents, particularly nitrous oxide, from its lungs.

In the past, inhalation analgesia was used extensively for the first stage of labor. Generally, this practice has been discontinued because it was inconvenient and exposed an infant to more drugs than necessary. Today, physicians tend to use inhalation agents primarily for delivery. The onset of action tends to be surprisingly fast, partly because of a pregnant woman's increased CNS sensitivity and partly because pulmonary uptake of the drugs is enhanced by the decreased FRC and by labor pain–associated hyperventilation. This method may work well even for a forceps delivery or for manual extraction of the placenta, particularly if combined with pudendal nerve block.

How Much Is Too Much?

An anesthesiologist must be very careful when using inhalation agents for analgesia, because concentrations that would be ineffective in nonpregnant patients can quickly put pregnant patients into stage two anesthesia. This effect constitutes a special danger, because pregnant women, as was described previously, often have gastroesophageal reflux, delayed gastric emptying, and increased gastric acidity.

Concentrations of nitrous oxide suitable for analgesia vary from 30% to 70%. Carefully adjust the dose for each patient. One end point is preservation of protective airway reflexes; another is the point at which the woman will no longer bear down on command. In either case, decrease the inhaled concentration until a safe depth of anesthesia is established. Despite adequate analgesia, some women react adversely to the pain of contractions; do not be distracted by this response and give them concentrations that might make them quiet but increase their risk for aspiration.

CESAREAN SECTION: GENERAL CONSIDERATIONS

For cesarean section, analgesia and relaxation of the abdominal wall are necessary as for any other intraperitoneal surgery. How these goals are achieved, however, is influenced by the general considerations governing obstetric anesthesia. We strive to maintain normal maternal and newborn physiology and to minimize an infant's drug exposure.

What Are the Anesthetic Options?

The choice of regional or general anesthesia depends on the circumstances. Do medical contraindications to one form or

TABLE 63–6. Aberrant Pain Sensation During Labor

Cause	Location
Distended bladder	Back pain
Occiput posterior	Back pain
Epidural hematoma	Back or leg pain
Abruption	Varies with placental implantation site
Uterine tetany	Abdominal pain
Uterine rupture	Abdominal pain
Direct nerve pressure by presenting part	Unilateral leg or thigh pain
Coccydynia	Coccygeal pain

the other exist? What are the desires of the patient and surgeon? How much time is available for preparation? (Regional block, even in the best of hands, takes longer.) Does the patient want a family member in the operating room for the delivery? (Many institutions allow this option only if the patient receives a regional anesthetic.) Does the surgeon anticipate problems with the newborn? What is the anesthesiologist's preference, given the medical circumstances?

Is One Form Advantageous?

This subject has been the topic of considerable debate. I believe that no current data show a clear medical advantage of either regional or general anesthesia among healthy patients. This was not always the case. Originally, all cesarean sections were performed using general anesthesia. With the drugs and techniques available at that time—sodium thiopental, muscle relaxants, and the primary agents diethyl ether, chloroform, or cyclopropane (tracheal intubation was not used)—regional anesthesia was shown to have less deleterious effect on the newborn. With modern drugs and techniques, however, this finding no longer holds, at least with respect to differences in Apgar scores or "time to sustained respiration," two standard methods used to evaluate outcome.[50]

What Factors Have a Role?

Even though no clear medical advantage accrues to either method, they are not entirely comparable. Problems for the patient, surgeon, and anesthesiologist tend to differ. Regional anesthesia allows a patient to experience the birth of her child (an extremely important consideration, particularly for those patients who have invested much time and emotional energy preparing for natural childbirth).

Drug Effects

Regional anesthesia probably exposes an infant to fewer effects from drugs (at least for spinal anesthesia, although some would contest this point for epidural anesthesia).

Postoperative Pain Relief

Postoperative spinal or epidural narcotics for pain control can be used, a technique that has become very popular. Patient-controlled analgesia is also popular among some groups.

Recovery

Women often recover from the effects of regional anesthesia more quickly than from those of general anesthesia.

Pain and Anxiety

With regional blocks, patients must endure placement of a catheter with little or no sedation, may experience unpleasant sensations during the surgery, and probably will have a sore spot in their back afterward. Some patients will not be able to handle the anxiety, and others may panic when they realize they have lost control of their limbs. In general surgery, the risk of these problems is reduced with premedication. In ob-

stetrics, however, premedication is avoided in order to minimize drug effects on the infant. If a patient must be heavily sedated in order to use a regional block, the advantages of reduced drug effects are lost.

Operative Anxiety

Some surgeons find it disconcerting to operate on an awake patient, or their technique with tissues may be too rough, even with a successful block, to make a patient comfortable. For anesthesiologists, regional blocks may take more time, the risk of hypotension with the onset of the sympathectomy may be as high as 30%, and they must continually reassure the patient.

General anesthesia is fast and allows the surgeon and anesthesiologist to concentrate on their work rather than on giving emotional support to the patient and family. On the other hand, it deprives a patient of the birth experience and subjects her to the risks of a rapid-sequence induction, tracheal intubation, and hypertension. In all likelihood, the patient will have a sore throat afterward. Patients often take longer to regain bowel function.

When Does One Form of Anesthesia Offer a Medical Advantage?

Anesthesia can provide three basic conditions for obstetricians: timing, relaxation of the perineal muscles, and relaxation of uterine musculature.

Timing

For the obstetrician, timing of an anesthetic may be crucial, such as when dealing with a prolapsed cord, placenta previa or abruption, ruptured uterus, or some other emergency. Moving quickly and surely can be life saving to both mother and fetus. Other, less obvious situations exist when an obstetrician may need an awake patient, cooperative and capable of pushing on command one moment and then being surgically anesthetized the next. Such cases include severe shoulder dystocia, application of Piper's forceps for an aftercoming head, version-extraction, or delivery of a second twin. In some instances, appropriate conditions are provided at a crucial time by additional dosing of an existing epidural block. If a block is not established, a general anesthetic might be necessary.

Perineal Relaxation

Obstetricians also may ask for profound perineal anesthesia and uterine relaxation. Relaxation of the striated muscles of the perineum may be important for a difficult forceps application, for added control during a breech delivery, or for repair of an extensive perineal tear. These situations have been less frequent in recent years as obstetricians resort more often to cesarean sections for difficult deliveries.

Relaxation of the perineum may be achieved with a saddle block or an epidural anesthetic. If the latter is used, high concentrations of local anesthetic (2% lidocaine or an equivalent dose of some other agent) are appropriate both for more rapid onset and greater ability to block the larger neural fibers that serve the striated muscles. Relaxation of the perineum can also be achieved with any of the neuromuscular blocking agents, although this approach virtually mandates a general anesthetic with tracheal intubation.

Uterine Relaxation

An obstetrician may need relaxation of the smooth muscle of the uterus in several situations (Table 63–7). Historically, uterine relaxation was achieved with a high concentration of an inhalation agent such as ether, halothane, or fluroxene. This approach, of course, necessitates general anesthesia with tracheal intubation because of the risk of aspiration. Clinicians also use inhalation of amyl nitrite from a capsule broken under the patient's nose or in the rebreathing bag, intravenous nitroglycerin (50-µg bolus), or subcutaneous terbutaline (250 µg) to achieve uterine relaxation without having to resort to general anesthesia and tracheal intubation.

GENERAL ANESTHESIA

The general approach conforms to the guidelines discussed for labor analgesia. The technique used should expose an infant to minimum amounts of drugs and cause the least possible derangement of maternal physiology. Techniques are also influenced by problems created by altered maternal physiology, particularly those that predispose pregnant women to vomiting and aspiration. Airway problems remain one of the most frequent causes of maternal death due to anesthesia.[51–53]

Should Maternal Deaths Due to Airway Problems Mitigate Against General Anesthesia?

The answer is unclear. We have relatively little information about anesthetic causes of maternal death. More parturients die during general than regional anesthesia; however, this fact must be interpreted cautiously because we do not know the *rate of deaths* in each group (i.e., the number who die relative to the number who received each type of anesthesia).

When case reports are examined, a large percentage of deaths are noted to occur during emergency procedures, often in patients who are obese or who have some other significant medical problem (Table 63–8). In such circumstances, the anesthesiologist must evaluate each patient and situation individually to decide on the safest course of action.

Equally competent and cautious physicians may make very different decisions. This fact can be illustrated by an obstetric patient who is difficult to intubate. Some may argue that awake intubation provides the safest management. Others may prefer an epidural anesthetic. We have no data that show the relative safety of each approach for a comparable set of circumstances. In this regard, the considerations for a high-risk obstetric pa-

TABLE 63–7. Situations That Require Uterine Relaxation

Internal version
Cesarean section
Relief of uterine tetany
Stopping of contractions before cesarean section
Difficult abdominal delivery (i.e., transverse lie)
Manual uterine exploration for retained placenta

TABLE 63–8. Problems Associated with Anesthesia Mortality Among Obstetric Patients (N = 15)

Emergency cesarean section	12/15
Obesity	12/15
Pregnancy-induced hypertension	6/15
Chronic hypertension	2/15
Diabetes	1/15
Heart failure	1/15

(Data from Endler GC, Mariona FG, Sokol RJ, et al: Anesthesia-related maternal mortality in Michigan, 1972 to 1984. Am J Obstet Gynecol 1988; 159:187.)

tient do not differ from those of any other patient with a similar set of problems.[54]

Which Preanesthetic Considerations Are Important?

Patient preparation should include all routine monitors and baseline measurements of oxygenation, pulse, and blood pressure.[55–60] In addition, place the patient in a 15° left lateral tilt to minimize supine hypotension and decreased placental perfusion due to compression of the abdominal aorta proximal to the origin of the uterine arteries. The weight of the uterus at term may be sufficient to occlude the arterial circulation.

How Is Anesthesia Provided?

Induction

Patients should be preoxygenated and then given sodium thiopental (4 mg · kg⁻¹) or a comparable agent, followed immediately by succinylcholine (1 mg · kg⁻¹). An assistant maintains cricoid pressure until the endotracheal tube is placed *and* its position confirmed.

Anesthesia is maintained with 50% oxygen, 50% nitrous oxide, and 0.5% or less of isoflurane or halothane. These doses may seem small, but remember that women have increased sensitivity to drugs during pregnancy. Also remember that an infant's drug exposure should be minimized and that concentrations of agents that cause unwanted uterine relaxation after delivery should be avoided.

After the cord is clamped and the infant is protected from drug exposure, the anesthetic may be deepened with higher concentrations of nitrous oxide, with narcotics, or with some combination thereof. The obstetrician usually asks to have oxytocin (40 U · L⁻¹) added to the intravenous solution to promote uterine contractions immediately after delivery of the placenta. Rarely, rapid administration of large doses of oxytocin may cause hypotension.

Muscle Relaxation

Neuromuscular relaxation can be maintained either with succinylcholine or with a short-acting nondepolarizing neuromuscular relaxant. Neither class of drugs crosses the placenta in sufficient quantity to affect a fetus clinically. Most cesarean sections rarely last longer than an hour. Moreover, the abdomen tends to be relaxed simply from chronic distention by the uterus. Therefore, do not err by giving too much muscle relaxant, and be particularly careful if a patient has received magnesium sulfate, because this drug potentiates the effect of all muscle relaxants.

Pregnant women tend to salivate excessively, sometimes to the point of making it difficult to visualize the vocal cords. Accordingly, patients may be pretreated with an antisialagogue, particularly if difficult intubation is anticipated.

Mental Awareness

Mental awareness has been a problem with general anesthesia for cesarean section. Originally, this observation prompted the use of low concentrations of isoflurane or halothane with nitrous oxide (high concentrations inhibit uterine contractions and increase blood loss after delivery). If high fresh gas flows and minute ventilation are not used at the beginning of the case, the induction dose of pentothal may dissipate before the onset of amnesia from the inhaled agents.[61, 62]

Potential Problems

With this technique, patients are lightly anesthetized, satisfying our stipulation to minimize fetal exposure to drugs. However, it entails some additional risks to the mother. As already discussed, the depth of anesthesia may be insufficient to provide amnesia. Hypertension and cardiac dysrhythmias associated with intubation and surgical incision may occur. In healthy patients, these risks are acceptable because the probability of medically significant problems is low. In high-risk patients, however, this technique may pose unacceptable problems. If so, the usual guidelines for obstetric patients have to be modified to suit the individual patient's medical problems. This topic is discussed in more detail in the section on coexisting medical or surgical problems.

REGIONAL ANESTHESIA

What Is the Risk of Hypotension?

The risk of hypotension exists in all patients but is exaggerated during pregnancy, not only because of reduced preload from the heavy uterus pressing on the inferior vena cava but also because of changes in autonomic reactivity, which are a normal part of pregnancy. Use regional anesthesia only in patients with normal blood volume. Patients with inadequate volume may be normotensive but only because they have compensated with increased sympathetic tone. A regional block removes the compensatory response and quickly results in profound hypotension.

Control of Blood Volume

Pretreat patients with large fluid volumes (1–2 L of balanced salt solution) before initiating the block. Do not use solutions containing glucose, because they cause the fetus to become hyperglycemic along with the mother. The fetus responds with a release of insulin that may precipitate severe hypoglycemia after the cord is clamped and the glucose source is lost.

Place the patient in at least a 15° left lateral tilt position to keep the uterus from interfering with flow in the inferior vena cava and aorta. Keep in mind that the origin of the uterine arteries is below the point at which the uterus may occlude blood flow in the descending aorta. Therefore, normal blood pressure in the arm may not reflect the uteroplacental perfusion pressure. In some circumstances, blood pressure should be monitored in the leg as well as the arm. Consider using a block technique that "sets up" more slowly, thereby allowing a patient more time to adapt to the loss of sympathetic tone.

Reduction of Drug Dosage

When performing a spinal or epidural block, remember that pregnant women need one-third to one-half the normal dose. Remember, too, that the block will distribute faster than in nonpregnant patients, presumably because of increased susceptibility of individual nerves to the local anesthetic. *Watch carefully for hypotension.*

Take a patient's blood pressure as often as possible during the first 10 to 15 minutes after administering the agent and remember that the uteroplacental circulation does not autoregulate (i.e., flow decreases with pressure; see Fig. 63–3). Depending on the technique and agent, as many as 30% of patients experience some hypotension despite all the normal precautions. Very often, the first sign of impending hypotension is nausea, even before a detectable drop in blood pressure.

Vasopressors

Be prepared to give a small dose of an appropriate vasoconstrictor. Ephedrine currently is the agent of choice because it appears to work as much by cardiac stimulation as by constriction of the peripheral vasculature with relative sparing of the uterine vessels.[44] Alpha-adrenergic agents maintain blood pressure but at the expense of uteroplacental vascular constriction.

What Toxic Effects May Occur?

In the first 15 minutes after administration of an epidural block, watch carefully for a maternal toxic CNS response to the local anesthetic (Fig. 63–5). During this time, maternal blood concentrations peak. To minimize drug effects on the fetus, do not sedate patients before the block. With this approach, the protective effect of sedatives against the local anesthetic-induced toxic CNS effects is lost. A few women experience a grand mal seizure, and many manifest early signs of toxicity, including an altered state of consciousness, tinnitus, or perioral paresthesia. Most anesthesiologists recommend an epidural test dose with a solution containing epinephrine. A sudden rise in maternal heart rate is used to indicate an inadvertent intravascular injection.

Is Spinal or Epidural Anesthesia Medically Advantageous?

An advantage has not been demonstrated for one form of regional anesthesia over another. Many clinicians prefer the rapid onset and well-defined level of spinal anesthesia and are willing to accept the increased risk of hypotension and postoperative headache. Others prefer the more controlled onset of an epidural block, particularly in the presence of certain maternal problems. More is said about this debate later in the section on medical or surgical problems.

Amount of Drug

Theoretically, a fetus is exposed to less drug with spinal than with epidural block; some investigators have described

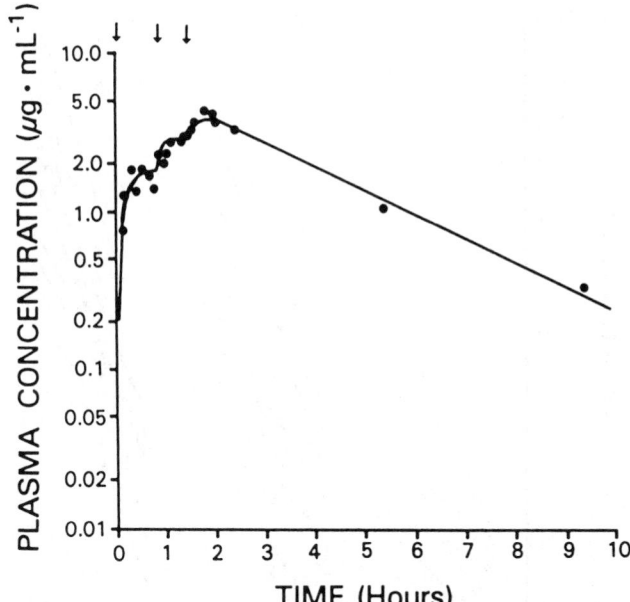

FIGURE 63–5. Plasma concentrations of lidocaine after three injections in the epidural space *(arrows)*. Highest concentrations occur during the first 15 minutes after injection. (From Inoue R, Suganuma T, Echizen H, et al: Plasma concentrations of lidocaine and its principal metabolites during intermittent epidural anesthesia. Anesthesiology 1985; 63:304–310.)

neurologic changes in infants whose mothers have received the latter anesthesia. To date, however, these effects have not been shown to persist beyond the neonatal period nor to be of sufficient importance to affect clinical practice.

Pharmacologic Differences

Rapid maternal metabolism of 2-chloroprocaine and increased protein binding of bupivacaine lower the effective concentration gradient of these drugs across the placenta, compared with lidocaine. In practice, however, most clinicians still favor lidocaine for epidural blocks because of its predictability and relative freedom from maternal side effects.

Among drugs currently used for spinal anesthesia, bupivacaine and lidocaine probably are most popular. However, neither adheres to tissue as quickly or avidly as does tetracaine. Accordingly, the level of the block may move dangerously high if the obstetrician asks for Trendelenburg's position during surgery.

MATERNAL COMPLICATIONS OF CESAREAN SECTION

Why Is Failure to Establish an Airway So Dangerous?

The greatest concern of most anesthesiologists is inability to establish an airway.[53] The anatomic and physiologic changes of pregnancy make this procedure technically more difficult. Reports suggest it is a major cause of maternal mortality. The considerations that hold for management of obstetric patients with a difficult airway are no different from those that apply in the operating room. In pregnancy, however, the possibility always exists that a situation requiring an emergency anesthetic will arise.

Proper preparation may help to avoid a problem. Advise the obstetrician early in labor of the need for an awake intubation. Surgery then can be planned before an obstetric problem becomes so serious that time becomes a crucial factor. In some instances, despite precaution, the need for surgery arises suddenly, without an opportunity for preparation. In these cases, the obstetrician and anesthesiologist must weigh the relative risks to the mother and fetus of proceeding quickly. No standard answers can be offered; each problem must be resolved on its own merits.

How Are Vomiting and Aspiration Minimized?

Vomiting and aspiration rank high as a serious problem but probably are less consequential as clinicians increase the routine administration of preanesthetic antacids,[55, 60] avoid mask ventilation, and use techniques of rapid-sequence induction and cricoid pressure during intubation. Tracheal intubation for general anesthesia is the usual standard of care. In rare instances, however, a general anesthetic administered by mask may be necessary and appropriate. In such instances, an assistant must hold cricoid pressure until the patient can once again protect her airway. These precautions decrease the risk of passive regurgitation and aspiration but do not abolish vomiting.

What Are the Manifestations of Amniotic Fluid Embolism?

Amniotic fluid embolism, although rare, can be fatal.[63–67] The manifestations usually are some combination of mechanical interference with pulmonary circulation (probably the lesser component) and a severe allergic response, which may progress to disseminated intravascular coagulation. Presenting signs are dyspnea, hypoxemia, and hypotension. Treatment is symptomatic. Air embolism may also occur through large, open uterine vessels, but this condition rarely constitutes a serious clinical problem. In the event of air embolism, be sure the uterus is below the level of the heart, flood the operative field with saline, and consider other standard methods for treatment of this problem.

How Is Hemorrhage Compensated?

As with any other abdominal operation, hemorrhage is always possible. Fortunately, pregnant women tend to tolerate a large volume loss because of their increased blood volume and their natural tendency to venoconstriction immediately after delivery. The expected blood loss with a normal vaginal delivery is approximately 500 mL and with a cesarean section about 800 mL; a 30% greater loss occurs during twin deliveries.

COEXISTING MEDICAL OR SURGICAL PROBLEMS

A special anesthetic approach for each disease or disorder that might occur in an obstetric patient is impossible.[68] We have specific information about anesthetic management for very few diseases. Most complications are so infrequent that no single investigator has the opportunity to carry out a controlled study to compare results with different types of management. Thus, a clinician faced with a new problem often must improvise and work out a course of therapy on the spot.

Several guidelines help clinicians to develop a plan of management for obstetric patients with a concurrent medical or surgical problem. Identify the type of dysfunction (e.g., hypertension, labile blood pressure, cardiac dysrhythmia, pulmonary insufficiency, or bleeding disorder) and make some estimate of its severity. Short-term management of a disease for the short duration of surgery usually is more important than is its immediate cure. Moreover, the nature of the underlying medical problem often dictates one or more major features of anesthetic management.

How Are the Rules of Obstetric Anesthesia Modified?

The normal "rules" of obstetric anesthesia really are guidelines. They are based on the assumption that a woman is healthy and able to tolerate the stress of minimum anesthesia; the techniques used are based on what is believed to be optimum for a fetus. In the presence of significant maternal disease, this approach must be abandoned, and reversion to basic principles of good operating room care must follow. That is, we must first ask, How would I deal with this problem in the operating room? Having answered that question, we then must decide how the pregnancy will alter the patient's response or influence what we do.

A patient who has severe cardiac dysfunction and who requires a cesarean section may best be served with a general anesthetic using very high doses of narcotic. This approach breaks the rule that a technique be used that has the least possible drug effect on the fetus; however, in the presence of cardiac disease, the mother's life may be at risk. Moreover, any significant narcotic depression of a neonate's respiration can be managed with attentive mechanical ventilatory support until the drug effects wear off, or a narcotic antagonist can be administered.

Rheumatic Heart Disease

Consider a pregnant patient at term with mitral stenosis and minimal mitral regurgitation. Several points of information about the normal course of pregnancy help with management. Pregnancy puts an extra burden on cardiac function. In normal patients, cardiac output may rise by as much as 30% by term (see Fig. 63–2) and increase even further during labor, partly in response to pain but also from the work associated with uterine contractions (Fig. 63–6). Output increases even more during the immediate postpartum period, with either abdominal or vaginal delivery, because of other physiologic changes that cause a redistribution of blood volume (Fig. 63–7).[69, 70]

This information suggests that the most significant danger to a pregnant woman with mitral valvular disease is development of congestive failure in the peripartum period. Anesthesia can be handled safely either with a regional block, because it might reduce preload, or with a general anesthetic, to control heart rate and maintain cardiac output. However, the specific method applicable to general anesthesia for cesarean section in normal patients is inappropriate, because the catecholamine response during intubation would cause severe tachycardia and

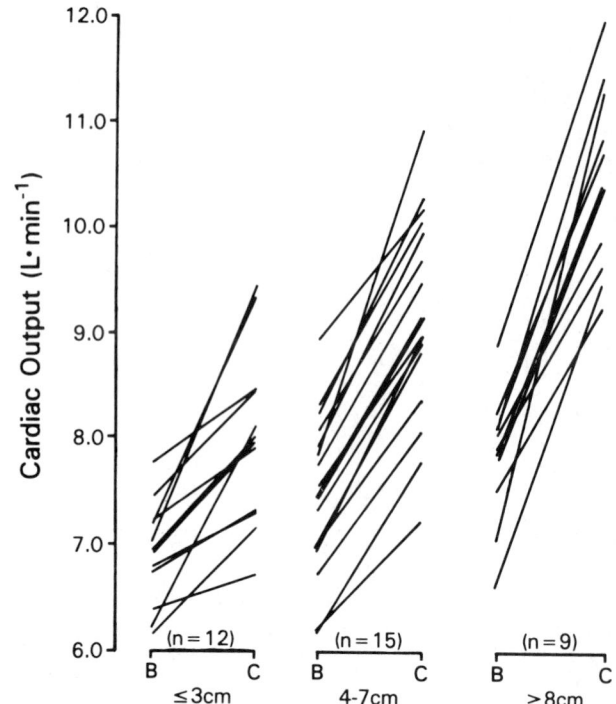

FIGURE 63–6. Cardiac output during different times of labor. The graph shows the tendency for output to increase (B). It also shows the rise in output that occurs with contractions (C). (From Robson SC, Dunlop W, Boys RJ, et al: Cardiac output during labour. Br Med J 1987; 295:1170.)

increased heart work. The plan should be modified to include a β-adrenergic blocking agent or pretreatment with intravenous narcotics to blunt the cardiovascular response. With the latter approach, respiratory depression of the newborn may result, but this is a small price to pay.

Congenital Heart Disease

In contrast, consider a patient with a congenital intracardiac defect, a left-to-right shunt, and some early changes of pulmonary hypertension. The greatest risk in such a patient is a reversal of the shunt, sudden severe O_2 desaturation, and death. Use of any anesthetic technique that decreases systemic arterial pressure could induce such conditions. Accordingly, regional anesthesia, whatever its benefits for labor or cesarean section, might be contraindicated.

Asthma

Consider also an asthmatic obstetric patient who has severe wheezing during general anesthesia. Normally, we avoid high concentrations of isoflurane or halothane because both agents relax uterine smooth muscle and predispose patients to increased uterine bleeding. In this case, however, the patient's pulmonary problem is of immediate concern. If her bronchospasm does not improve after a reasonable trial with a bronchodilator, consider using increased concentrations of inhalation agents. You can deal with uterine relaxation after you have managed her bronchospasm.

What Are the Special Problems of Pre-Eclampsia?

With pre-eclampsia, the primary physiologic derangements are as follow: diminished blood volume (not an entirely accu-

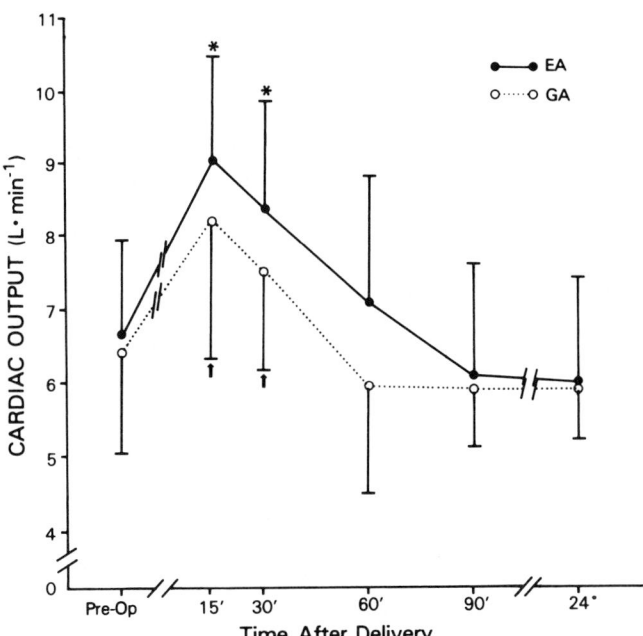

FIGURE 63-7. Cardiac output with cesarean section. The data illustrate the rise that occurs immediately following, several minutes after, and 1 day after delivery. The type of anesthesia used had no significant effect on the magnitude or pattern of response. (From James CF, Banner T, Caton D: Cardiac output in women undergoing cesarean section with epidural or general anesthesia. Am J Obstet Gynecol 1989; 160:1178–1184.)

rate term, because blood volume in pre-eclamptic patients is increased during pregnancy—not to the extent it should be, however, and patients often respond as if their blood volume were decreased); a vasculature that is hypersensitive to both endogenous and exogenous vasoconstrictors; and alterations of clotting mechanisms (sometimes) and of liver metabolism and electrolytes (less often). An element of renal insufficiency, either a result of primary renal artery constriction or secondary to diminished blood volume, may also be present.[71-74] The syndrome has other manifestations, but those mentioned are of greatest significance for anesthetic management.

These derangements, irrespective of the fact that they occur in a pregnant woman, dictate many aspects of anesthetic management. For example, a significant blood clotting deficiency eliminates the option of a regional anesthetic, as does insufficient blood volume, unless it can be corrected. Blood volume may be expanded with large volumes of fluids, but not if an element of primary renal insufficiency exists. To sort out this problem, the anesthesiologist may have to evaluate the need for central vascular access.

Should general anesthesia be necessary for a cesarean section, blood pressure must be controlled before induction. Because of blood pressure lability in such patients, the minimum dose of anesthesia customary for normal women is completely inappropriate. Untreated, the rise in blood pressure with intubation could be lethal.

Why Can't Specific Guidelines Be Established?

Inexperienced practitioners often want a precise list of guidelines for each medical problem they encounter. No such

lists exist for obstetric anesthesia problems. The literature often cites methods that a particular group found useful in managing a particular problem. However, few if any studies have systematically compared maternal and fetal outcome from one mode of therapy with another.

Thus, for cesarean section of severely pre-eclamptic patients, different experts may advocate regional or general anesthesia with equal verve. Some argue that central vascular catheters are not essential for good management. Still others debate the merits of one antihypertensive against another. In some respects, this lack of conformity is intimidating. On the other hand, it allows clinicians to focus on the goals of management and the best methods by which they can be achieved.

FETAL MONITORING

What Is the Anesthesiologist's Responsibility?

Fetal monitoring (electronic measurements of fetal heart rate in relation to uterine contractions and measurement of fetal scalp pH) are primarily tools used by obstetricians to identify fetal distress. Complete descriptions of the methods and their interpretation may be found in any standard obstetric textbook. The fact that they are primarily obstetric tools does not free others from the need to know something about them.

Significant changes occasionally take place in labor during placement of an epidural anesthetic. Anesthesiologists should be familiar with the interpretation of major patterns so that they can alert their colleagues about a potential problem and initiate appropriate therapy should it be necessary.

Which Fetal Heart Rate Patterns Are Significant?

Obstetricians look for several basic deviations from normal (Fig. 63–8).

Early Deceleration

In the second stage of labor, compression of the fetal head may initiate a sharp drop in fetal heart rate that coincides with the duration of the contraction. This pattern is believed to be a vagal response related to fetal head compression and is not thought to indicate fetal distress.

Late Deceleration

A reduction in fetal heart rate that begins late in the contraction and persists between contractions is thought to be indicative of uteroplacental insufficiency and fetal hypoxemia. It is commonly attributed to placental abnormalities like abruption or decreased uterine perfusion.

Variable Deceleration

Variable decelerations, literally a pattern that varies in severity and configuration, is attributed to umbilical cord compression, as with a nuchal or prolapsed cord.

Note that these are descriptive terms. No widely accepted criteria are available to differentiate significant from spurious

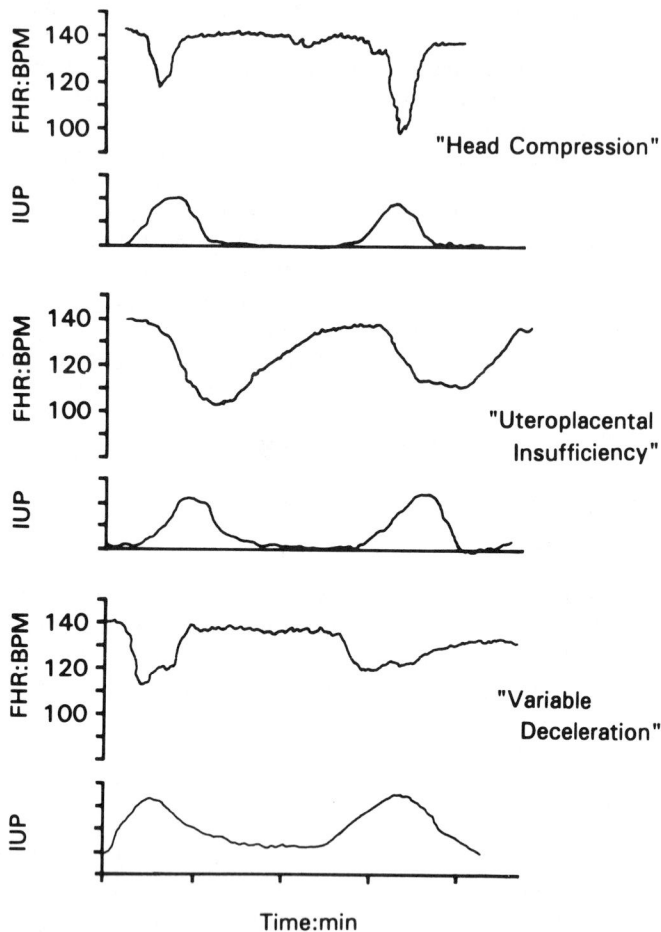

FIGURE 63–8. Three patterns of abnormal response of fetal heart rate tracings in relation to uterine contractions.

changes. In general, however, the more frequent, severe, and prolonged the decelerations, the more ominous the implication and thus the more likely that emergency cesarean section will be necessary.

Beat-to-Beat Variability

Obstetricians also look at the beat-to-beat variability associated with the previously mentioned interpretations. Variation is normal. Absence of variation is commonly attributed to hypoxia, congenital problems, or drugs. At present, variability is assessed simply by inspection. No widely accepted standards are available to measure or evaluate the changes (Fig. 63–9).

How Are "Fetal Distress" and Cesarean Section Related?

Anesthesiologists should recognize that the diagnosis of fetal distress is one of the major reasons for the high rate of cesarean sections now common in obstetric practice. Because patients are brought to us for anesthesia, often in unfavorable circumstances, we must understand the accuracy and reliability of these tests as predictors of permanent fetal damage. How fast must we move? Is the danger to the infant of sufficient magnitude to take risks with the mother's anesthetic management?

Significance of Alterations in Fetal Heart Rate

Until recently, patterns of variable and late fetal heart rate decelerations were believed to be reliable indicators of fetal hypoxemia and incipient brain damage. Studies in the obstetric and pediatric literature now question this concept. These data suggest that the most frequent causes of mental retardation and cerebral palsy are genetic in origin or occur early in pregnancy, before the onset of labor. Events during labor and delivery appear to have less influence on the incidence of cerebral palsy and mental retardation than originally was thought.

Parallel studies of the significance of fetal pH suggest that the original cutoff of 7.20 also may have been too stringent. Several investigators now suggest that the probability of fetal damage is not significant until values fall below 7.0.[75–83]

How Does This Information Affect Anesthesia Practice?

In the majority of patients, it does not. Anesthesiologists still must be prepared to anesthetize obstetric patients as rapidly as possible whenever our obstetric colleagues diagnose fetal distress. In the majority of normal patients, this approach presents no major problem for us and no significant danger to a patient.

On the other hand, some patients have medical or physical problems that constitute a significant risk for anesthesia. Such problems usually can be managed safely, given adequate time to prepare. In obstetrics, however, the emphasis on fetal well-being often makes us feel that we do not have that time. We feel rushed and, sometimes, forced to cut corners in the belief that such action may prevent irreparable fetal damage.

The data discussed earlier suggest that the sensitivity and specificity of current methods of fetal monitoring are not suf-

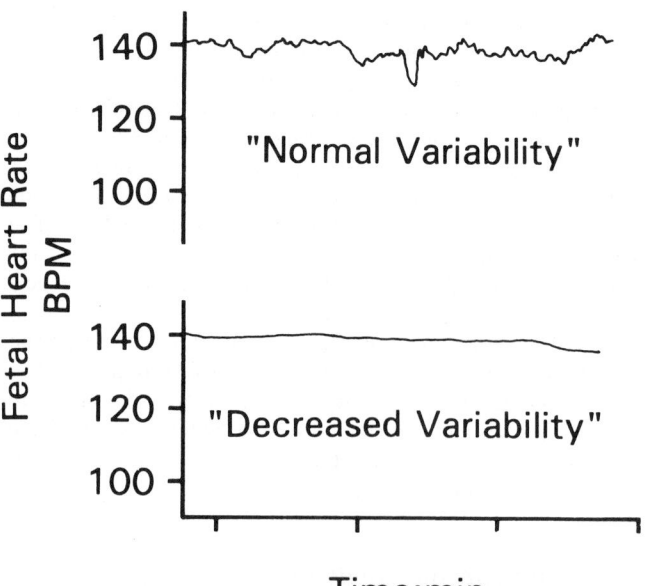

FIGURE 63–9. Illustration of normal and abnormal beat-to-beat variability. Loss of variability has been attributed to fetal brain injury, hypoxia, and drugs. At present, no accepted methods exist to measure variability or to establish limits of normal or abnormal change.

ficient to justify that approach. In other words, we may safely take more time, when needed, to prepare high-risk women. Anesthesiologists must recognize this fact, identify women for whom extra time to prepare a safe anesthetic is needed, inform the obstetrician of the problem, and together work out a plan of management that balances risks to the fetus with those to the mother. These problems are never easy, because neither anesthesiologists nor obstetricians have firm guidelines to help weigh risks. Each situation must be dealt with on its own merits.

NEONATAL RESUSCITATION

What Is the Anesthesiologist's Responsibility?

Our primary responsibility is to the patient we have anesthetized, the mother. In some circumstances, however, help with resuscitation of a depressed newborn may be possible. This help is usually limited to the establishment of an airway and maintenance of ventilation until infants starts breathing well on their own or until they can be mechanically ventilated. Keep in mind that a neonate's lungs are not only collapsed but also are fragile. Initial inflation pressure usually should be limited to 30 cm H_2O, if this level is adequate, to avoid pneumothorax. Remember that during initial lung expansion, a neonate generates negative intrathoracic pressures of about -80 cm H_2O. If in doubt, listen with a stethoscope and use whatever inflation pressure is needed to effect audible air movement in the chest.

Why Is the Newborn Distressed?

Remember also that a neonate may be in distress for various reasons, not simply from CNS depression. Definitive diagnosis and treatment include replacement of blood volume, management of respiratory distress syndrome, and diagnosis of intracranial hemorrhage or birth trauma, sepsis, jaundice, or problems with electrolyte and glucose metabolism. Unless the anesthesiologist is also skilled in the diagnosis and management of these problems in the newborn, he or she should see that the child is quickly turned over to someone who is.

References

1. Caton D, Henderson J, Wilcox CJ: Oxygen consumption of the uterus and its contents and weight at birth of lambs. *In* Fetal and Newborn Cardiovascular Physiology. Longo LD, Reneau DD (eds). New York, Garland STPM Press, 1978, pp 123–134.
2. Ueland K, Novy MJ, Peterson EN, et al: Maternal cardiovascular dynamics: IV. The influence of gestational age of the maternal cardiovascular response to posture and exercise. Am J Obstet Gynecol 1969; 104:856.
3. Ueland K, Novy MJ, Metcalfe J: Cardiorespiratory responses to pregnancy and exercise in normal women and patients with heart disease. Am J Obstet Gynecol 1973; 115:4.
4. Caton D, Banner TE: Doppler estimates of cardiac output during pregnancy. Bull NY Acad Med 1987; 63:727.
5. Easterling TR, Watts DH, Schmucker BC, et al: Measurement of cardiac output during pregnancy: validation of Doppler technique and clinical observations in preeclampsia. Obstet Gynecol 1987; 69:845.
6. Pirani BBK, Campbell DM, MacGillivray I: Plasma volume in normal first pregnancy. J Obstet Gynaecol Br Commonw 1973; 80:884.
7. Hytten FE, Paitin DB: Increase in plasma volume during normal pregnancy. Br J Obstet Gynaecol 1963; 70:402.
8. Duffus Gilliam M, MacGillivray I, Dennis KJ: The relationship between baby weight and changes in maternal weight, total body water, plasma volume, electrolytes and proteins, and urinary oestriol excretion. J Obstet Gynaecol Br Commonw 1971; 78:97.
9. Weinberger SE, Weiss ST, Cohen WR, et al: Pregnancy and the lung. Am Rev Respir Dis 1980; 121:559.
10. Hägerdal M, Morgan CW, Sumner AE, et al: Minute ventilation and oxygen consumption during labor with epidural analgesia. Anesthesiology 1983; 59:425.
11. Wynn RM (ed): Biology of the Uterus. New York, Plenum Press, 1977.
12. Carsten ME, Miller JD (eds): Uterine Function: Molecular and Cellular Aspects. New York, Plenum Press, 1990.
13. Fisher RS, Roberts GS, Crabowski CJ, et al: Inhibition of lower esophageal sphincter circular muscle by female sex hormones. Am J Physiol 1978; 234:E243.
14. Braverman DZ, Johnson ML, Kern F: Effects of pregnancy and contraceptive steroids on gallbladder function. N Engl J Med 1980; 302:362.
15. Reyes H, Kern F: Effect of pregnancy on bile flow and biliary lipids in the hamster. Gastroenterology 1979; 76:144.
16. Levyn L, Beck EC, Aaron AH: Further cholecystographic studies in the late months of pregnancy. Am J Roentgenol Radium Ther Nucl Med 1933; 30:774.
17. Hundley JM, Diehl WK, Diggs ES: Hormonal influences upon the ureter. Am J Obstet Gynecol 1942; 44:858.
18. Kochenour NK, Lavery JP: Managing asthma in the pregnant patient. Contemp Obstet Gynecol 1976; 7:27.
19. Turner ES, Greenberg PA, Patterson R: Management of the pregnant asthmatic patient. Ann Intern Med 1980; 93:905.
20. Kalra SP, Simpkins JW, Kalra PS: Progesterone-induced changes in hypothalamic luteinizing hormone–releasing hormone and catecholamines: differential effects of pentobarbital. Endocrinology 1981; 108:1299.
21. Falck B, Owman C, Rosengren E, et al: Reduction by progesterone of the estrogen-induced increase in transmitter level of the short adrenergic neurons innervating the uterus. Endocrinology 1969; 84:958.
22. Kuhnert BR, Kuhnert PM, Prochaska AL, et al: Meperidine disposition in mother, neonate, and nonpregnant females. Clin Pharmacol Ther 1980; 27:486.
23. Butterworth JF, Walker FO, Lysak SZ: Pregnancy increases median nerve susceptibility to lidocaine. Anesthesiology 1990; 72:962.
24. Cook WP, Schultetus RR, Caton D: A comparison of *d*-tubocurarine pretreatment and no pretreatment in obstetric patients. Anesth Analg 1987; 66:756.
25. Dalession DJ: Seizure disorders and pregnancy. N Engl J Med 1985; 312:559.
26. Faber JJ, Thornburg KL: Placental Physiology. Structure and Function of Fetomaternal Exchange. New York, Raven Press, 1983.
27. Poore M, Foster JC: Epidural and no epidural anesthesia: differences between mothers and their experience of birth. Birth 1985; 12:205.
28. Craft JB, Coaldrake LA, Bolan JC, et al: Placental passage and uterine effects of fentanyl. Anesth Analg 1983; 62:894.
29. Fisher JT, Mortalo JP, Smith B, et al: Neonatal pattern of breathing following cesarean section: epidural versus general anesthesia. Anesthesiology 1983; 59:385.
30. Lester BM, Als H, Brazelton TB: Regional obstetric anesthesia and newborn behavior: a reanalysis toward synergistic effects. Child Dev 1982; 53:687.
31. Kuhnert BR, Kennard MJ, Linn PL: Neonatal neurobehavior after epidural anesthesia for cesarean section: a comparison of bupivacaine and chloroprocaine. Anesth Analg 1988; 67:64.
32. Brazelton TB: Effect of prenatal drugs on the behavior of the neonate. Am J Psychiatry 1970; 126:1261.
33. Rosenblatt DB, Belsey EM, Lieberman BA, et al: The influence of maternal analgesia on neonatal behaviour: II. Epidural bupivacaine. Br J Obstet Gynaecol 1981; 88:407.
34. Abboud TK, Afrasiabi A, Sarkis F, et al: Continuous infusion epidural analgesia in parturients receiving bupivacaine, chloroprocaine, or lidocaine—Maternal, fetal, and neonatal effects. Anesth Analg 1984; 63:421.
35. Ralston DH, Shnider SM: The fetal and neonatal effects of regional anesthesia in obstetrics. Anesthesiology 1978; 48:34.
36. Amiel-Tinson C, Barrier G, Shnider SM, et al: A new neurologic and adaptive capacity scoring system for evaluating obstetric medication in full-term newborns. Anesthesiology 1982; 56:340.
37. Scanlon JW, Brown WU, Weiss JB, et al: Neurobehavioral responses of newborn infants after maternal epidural anesthesia. Anesthesiology 1974; 40:121.
38. Assali NS (ed). Biology of Gestation. New York, Academic Press, 1968.
39. Chard T: Fetal and maternal oxytocin in human parturition. Am J Perinatol 1989; 6:145.

40. Goodfellow CF, Hull MGR, Swaab DF, et al: Oxytocin deficiency at delivery with epidural anaesthesia. Br J Obstet Gynaecol 1983; 90:214.

41. Piper JM, Bolling DR, Newton ER: The second stage of labor: factors influencing duration. Am J Obstet Gynecol 1991; 165:976.

42. Chestnut DH, Vandewalker GE, Owen CL, et al: The influence of continuous epidural bupivacaine analgesia on the second stage of labor and method of delivery in nulliparous women. Anesthesiology 1987; 66:774.

43. Assali NS: Dynamics of the uteroplacental circulation in health and disease. Am J Perinatol 1989; 6:105.

44. Ralston DH, Shnider SM, deLorimier AA: Effects of equipotent ephedrine, metaraminol, mephenteramine, and methoxamine on uterine blood flow in the pregnant ewe. Anesthesiology 1974; 40:354.

45. Greiss FC, Anderson SG, Still JG: Uterine pressure-flow relationships during early gestation. Am J Obstet Gynecol 1976; 126:799.

46 Ladner C, Brinkman CR, Weston P, et al: Dynamics of uterine circulation in pregnant and nonpregnant sheep. Am J Physiol 1970; 218:257.

47. Clapp JF: Effect of epinephrine infusion on maternal and uterine oxygen uptake in the pregnant ewe. Am J Obstet Gynecol 1979; 133:208.

48. Sosa R, Kennell J, Klaus M, et al: The effect of a supportive companion on perinatal problems, length of labor, and mother-infant interaction. N Engl J Med 1980; 303:597.

49. Apgar V, Holaday DA, James LS, et al: Comparison of regional and general anesthesia in obstetrics. JAMA 1957; 165:2155.

50. Ong BY, Cohen MM, Palamnink RJ: Anesthesia for caesarian section. Anesth Analg 1989; 68:270.

51. Mabie WC, Sibai BM: Treatment in an obstetric intensive care unit. Am J Obstet Gynecol 1990; 162:1.

52. Morgan BM, Aulakh JM, Barker JP: Morbidity after cesarean section under epidural or general anesthesia. Intelligence Reports in Anesthesia 1984; 2:8.

53. Endler GC, Mariona FG, Sokol RJ, et al: Anesthesia-related maternal mortality in Michigan, 1972 to 1984. Am J Obstet Gynecol 1988; 159:187.

54. Benumof JL: Management of a difficult adult airway. Anesthesiology 1991; 75:1087.

55. Gibbs CP, Banner TC: Effectiveness of Bicitra as a preoperative antacid. Anesthesiology 1984; 61:97.

56. James CF, Gibbs CP, Banner T: Postpartum perioperative risk of aspiration pneumonia. Anesthesiology 1984; 61:756.

57. Gillett GB, Watson JD, Langford RM: Ranitidine and single-dose antacid therapy as prophylaxis against acid aspiration syndrome in obstetric practice. Anaesthesia 1984; 39:638.

58. Roberts RB, Shirley MA: Reducing the risk of acid aspiration during cesarean section. Anesth Analg 1974; 53:859.

59. Hodgkinson R, Glassenberg R, Joyce TH: Comparison of cimetidine (Tagamet) with antacid for safety and effectiveness in reducing gastric acidity before elective cesarean section. Anesthesiology 1983; 59:86.

60. Johnston JR, Moore J, McCaughey W, et al: Use of cimetidine as an oral antacid in obstetric anesthesia. Anesth Analg 1983; 62:720.

61. Tunstall ME: The reduction of amnesic wakefulness during caesarean section. Anaesthesia 1979; 34:316.

62. Bogetz MS, Katz JA: Recall of surgery for major trauma. Anesthesiology 1984; 61:6.

63. Clark SL, Pavlova Z, Horenstein J, et al: Fetal squamous cells in the maternal pulmonary artery circulation. Annual Meeting of the Society of Perinatal Obstetricians, Las Vegas, NV, February 1985.

64. Mulder JI: Amniotic fluid embolism: an overview and case report. Am J Obstet Gynecol 1985; 152:430.

65. Quance D: Amniotic fluid embolism: detection by pulse oximetry. Anesthesiology 1988; 68:951.

66. Girard P, Mal H, Laine JF, et al: Left heart failure in amniotic fluid embolism. Anesthesiology 1986; 64:262.

67. Peterson EP, Taylor HB: Amniotic fluid embolism. Obstet Gynecol 1970; 35:787.

68. James FM, Wheeler AS: Obstetric Anesthesia: The Complicated Patient. Philadelphia, FA Davis, 1982.

69. Niswonger JWH, Langmade CF: Cardiovascular changes in vaginal deliveries and cesarean sections. Am J Obstet Gynecol 1970; 107:337.

70. Robson SC, Dunlop W, Boys RJ, et al: Cardiac output during labour. Br Med J 1987; 295:1169.

71. Clark SL, Cotton DB: Clinical indications for pulmonary artery catheterization in the patient with severe preeclampsia. Am J Obstet Gynecol 1988; 158:453.

72. Cotton DB, Lee W, Huhta JC, et al: Hemodynamic profile of severe pregnancy-induced hypertension. Am J Obstet Gynecol 1988; 158:523.

73. Pritchard JA, Pritchard SA: Standardized treatment of 154 consecutive cases of eclampsia. Am J Obstet Gynecol 1975; 132:543.

74. Wright JP: Anesthetic considerations in preeclampsia-eclampsia. Anesth Analg 1983; 63:590.

75. Leveno KJ, Cunningham FG, Nelson S, et al: A prospective comparison of selective and universal electronic fetal monitoring in 34,995 pregnancies. N Engl J Med 1986; 315:615.

76. Dawes GS, Rosevear SK, Pello LC, et al: Computerized analysis of episodic changes in fetal heart rate varia.ion in early labor. Am J Obstet Gynecol 1991; 165:618.

77. Banta HD, Thacker SB: Assessing the costs and benefits of electronic fetal monitoring. Obstet Gynecol Surv 1979; 34:627.

78. Painter MJ, Scott M, Hirsch RP, et al: Fetal heart rate patterns during labor: neurologic and cognitive development at six to nine years of age. Am J Obstet Gynecol 1988; 159:854.

79. Shy KK, Luthy DA, Bennett FC, et al: Effects of electronic fetal heart rate monitoring, as compared with periodic auscultation, on the neurologic development of premature infants. N Engl J Med 1990; 322:588.

80. Low JA, Muir DW, Pater EA, et al: The association of intrapartum asphyxia in the mature fetus with newborn behavior. Am J Obstet Gynecol 1990; 163:1131.

81. Nelson K, Ellenberg JH: Antecedents of cerebral palsy. N Engl J Med 1986; 315:81.

82. Ellison PH, Foster M, Sheridan-Pereira M, et al: Electronic fetal monitoring, auscultation, and neonatal outcome. Am J Obstet Gynecol 1991; 164:1281.

83. Sykes GS, Molloy PM, Johnson P, et al: Do Apgar scores indicate asphyxia? Lancet 1982; i:494.

CHAPTER 64

Nonobstetric Surgery in the Pregnant Patient

CHRISTOPHER F. JAMES, M.D.
THOMAS W. LEBERT, II, M.D.

Not uncommonly, pregnant patients have to undergo surgery for nonobstetric reasons. In the United States, approximately 50,000 to 70,000 women per year, roughly 2% of those who are pregnant, require an anesthetic for a surgical procedure not related to parturition.[1, 2] Some of the more common reasons for surgical intervention are listed in Table 64–1. Intracranial procedures requiring induced hypotension and cardiac procedures requiring extracorporeal circulation have been reported with increasing frequency.[3] The prevalence of trauma during pregnancy is also increasing. In some areas of the United States, especially our inner cities, trauma is the leading cause of maternal mortality.

ANESTHETIC CONSIDERATIONS

Are They the Same As for Labor and Delivery?

Anesthetic management of the pregnant surgical patient, as with labor analgesia and cesarean section anesthesia, must ensure maternal safety and fetal well-being. Anesthesiologists taking care of obstetric and pregnant surgical patients must be concerned about the physiologic changes of pregnancy and their implications for the administration of a safe anesthetic (Table 64–2). However, several important differences between surgical and obstetric anesthesia are notable. In a laboring patient, one major goal is to avoid any disturbance of enhanced uterine contractility, whereas in the pregnant surgical patient, prevention of spontaneous contractions is a vital element.

For most instances of obstetric anesthesia, the anesthesiologist attempts to avoid any agent that might lead to neonatal depression after birth, whereas fetal central nervous system depression during or subsequent to surgical anesthesia is not as serious a problem.[4]

Finally, the avoidance of any agent that potentially could lead to fetal anomalies is self-evident.

What Are the Major Concerns?

The hormonal effects brought about by the placenta and ovaries represent the changes of greatest concern during the first trimester, whereas the mechanical effects of the gravid uterus, which begin in the second trimester, predominate during the third trimester.[5]

Aortocaval Compression

Aortocaval compression syndrome, which results from the impingement of the weight of the uterus on the aorta and vena cava, can occur as early as the 18th week of gestation. Usually, however, it is not significant until after the 24th week. Nevertheless, after the 18th week of gestation, pregnant patients should be placed in the left lateral tilt position rather than in the supine position.

Aortic compression may lead to decreased uterine perfusion with normal maternal upper extremity blood pressure measure-

TABLE 64–1. Reasons for Surgical Intervention During Pregnancy

Abdominal
Appendectomy
Ovarian surgery (cysto, torsion)
Cholecystectomy (laparoscopic)
Nonabdominal
Breast surgery
Thyroidectomy
Parathyroidectomy
Cardiac surgery
Neurosurgery
Trauma
Blunt (motor vehicle accident)
Penetrating (gunshot wound, stabbing)
Pregnancy-Related
Cervical cerclage
Fetal surgery
In vitro fertilization

TABLE 64–2. Physiologic Changes of Pregnancy That Affect Anesthetic Administration

	Increased	Decreased
Cardiac	Cardiac output Risk of aortocaval compression	Peripheral vascular resistance
Hematologic	Blood volume Plasma volume Risk of thromboembolism	"Physiologic" anemia
Respiratory	Minute ventilation Oxygen consumption	Functional residual capacity
Gastrointestinal	Acidity Gastric volume	Gastric motility Lower esophageal sphincter tone
Hepatic	Liver enzymes	Cholinesterase activity
Central nervous system	Sensitivity to inhalation, intravenous, and local anesthetic agents	Minimum alveolar concentration Regional anesthetic requirements

ments; thus, blood pressure measurement in the lower extremities may be prudent in the third trimester, especially if the procedure must be performed in the supine position.

Venous Thrombosis

During gestation, an approximate 1.8-fold increase occurs in Factors I, VII, VIII, X, and XII; this leads to a slightly hypercoagulable state and an increased risk for thromboembolism.[6] This hypercoagulable state is more prevalent in the immediate postpartum period. Therefore, pneumatic antiembolism stockings should be applied before anesthesia if the legs are to be immobile for several hours.

Airway Management

Progressive capillary engorgement and edema of the entire respiratory system are associated with pregnancy. Thus, smaller endotracheal tubes are often required. In addition, any airway manipulation or relatively minor trauma to the airway may lead to profuse bleeding, especially of the nasal passages. These factors, in addition to obesity, increased abdominal girth, increased anteroposterior chest dimension secondary to breast enlargement, and the urgency of many procedures, render tracheal intubation in the pregnant patient (especially at term) more difficult. Anesthesia-related mortality in obstetric patients is most commonly due to the inability to intubate the trachea, the aspiration of gastric contents, or to both.[7]

Pulmonary Function

Lung volumes undergo progressive changes beginning in the fifth month of gestation, eventually leading to a 20% reduction in functional residual capacity by term.[8] The reduction in functional residual capacity, coupled with an increase in oxygen (O_2) consumption ($\leq$20% in term patients) results in a quicker onset of hypoxemia associated with short periods of apnea during anesthetic induction. Thus, adequate preoxygenation (denitrogenation) is critical prior to a rapid sequence induction. Awake orotracheal intubation should be considered in pregnant patients who have a "difficult airway."

Minute ventilation increases early in pregnancy as a result of increases in tidal volume and respiratory rate.[9] The increase in alveolar ventilation coupled with a decrease in functional residual capacity increases the speed of induction with inhalation agents. Although inhalation induction usually is contrain-

dicated in pregnancy, the speed of induction combined with the decreased minimal alveolar concentration requirements associated with their use can lead to a state of "general anesthesia" when only supplemental mask analgesia was anticipated or intended.

Full Stomach

Increased gastric acidity, delayed gastric emptying, and a decrease in lower esophageal sphincter tone resulting from pregnancy-associated hormonal changes occur as early as the 8th to 10th week of gestation.[10] Administration of histamine₂ blockers and a nonparticulate antacid preoperatively, in addition to protection of the airway at the time of induction, is indicated to reduce the risk of aspiration or aspiration pneumonitis.[11, 12] The incidence of pulmonary aspiration in the obstetric patient is 15 per 10,000 cases (3 times that of the general surgical population).[13]

Do Pregnant Patients Have Reduced Anesthetic Requirements?

Gestation is associated with a decrease in drug requirement for both general and regional anesthesia. The reduction in minimum alveolar concentration for both halothane and isoflurane may be as great as 25% to 40%.[14] This change has been attributed to the sedative effects of high progesterone levels and, more recently, to increased levels of endogenous endorphins.[15]

Progesterone and other biochemical factors may also be responsible for an enhancement in membrane sensitivity to local anesthetics, thereby reducing requirements for these drugs as early as the first trimester.[16] Decreases in the total dose requirement for spinal or epidural anesthesia occur with increasing duration of gestation. These decreases probably are related to the decreased volume of the epidural space and cerebrospinal fluid that is brought about by epidural venous engorgement and the previously mentioned hormonal effects.[17]

The increase in vascularity increases the incidence of unintended epidural intravascular injection of local anesthetics to as much as 10%. Along with the increased sensitivity of local anesthetics in pregnancy is their increased systemic toxicity, which may in part be due to the increased free fraction of highly protein-bound drugs such as bupivacaine.[18, 19]

What Are the Primary Fetal Physiologic Concerns?

Whenever a pregnant patient undergoes surgery, two patients are placed at risk. Fetal hazards can be minimized by an understanding of the fetal effects of maternal drug administration and of the operation. The most important acute fetal risk related to maternal surgery and anesthesia is intrauterine asphyxia. Therefore, the anesthesiologist's primary concerns are the perioperative maintenance of maternal O_2-carrying capacity, O_2 affinity, arterial O_2 partial pressure (PaO_2), and uteroplacental blood flow. Maintenance of normal maternal PaO_2, arterial carbon dioxide partial pressure ($PaCO_2$), maternal blood pressure, and uterine vascular resistance is of paramount importance.[20]

Uteroplacental Perfusion

Uterine blood flow is described by the following equation that is based on Ohm's law:

$$\text{Uterine Blood Flow} = \frac{\text{Uterine Artery Pressure} - \text{Uterine Venous Pressure}}{\text{Uterine Artery Resistance}}$$

Equation 1

Normally, 10% of a pregnant patient's cardiac output goes to the uterus; this value is 1% in the nonpregnant patient. The placenta accounts for about 80% of this blood flow; the balance supplies the uterine smooth muscle. Autoregulation of uterine vessels does not occur; thus, flow is directly proportional to maternal mean arterial pressure. Interventions that increase uterine venous pressure or uterine artery resistance decrease uterine blood flow and may lead to placental hypoperfusion and fetal asphyxia (Table 64–3).

Uterine Vasoconstriction

The uterine vasculature normally functions in a state of near maximum vasodilation, and a significant reserve for vasoconstriction is present should maternal needs require it. Maternal hyperventilation leads to vasoconstriction and reduces placental perfusion. The rise in maternal pH associated with hyperventilation increases the affinity of maternal hemoglobin for O_2, thereby further reducing O_2 delivery to the fetoplacental unit.

Administration of direct acting vasoconstrictors such as phenylephrine reduces uterine perfusion by direct vasoconstriction; therefore, indirectly acting agents such as ephedrine,

which has fewer α-adrenergic receptor effects, are the drugs of choice.[21, 22] Hypoventilation and maternal hypercapnia lead to fetal respiratory acidosis, and maternal hypoxemia leads to fetal hypoxemia. Maternal hyperoxia, however, presents no fetal risk of retinopathy of prematurity or premature closure of the ductus arteriosus, since even in the presence of a maternal PaO_2 of 600 mm Hg, the fetal PaO_2 does not exceed 50 to 60 mm Hg.[23]

Maternal hypotension should be avoided when possible, and if it occurs the patient must be treated aggressively with intravenous fluids, lateral positioning, decreased levels of anesthesia, and aggressive use of ephedrine. Despite preblock hydration and positioning, the incidence of hypotension in the term pregnant patient under regional anesthesia is as high as 30%.[24]

FETAL RISKS

Fetal risks may be presented by an acute, single anesthetic exposure for a surgical procedure or by subacute or chronic low-dose occupational anesthetic exposure of a parent who works in an operating room. Numerous studies have been published, but conclusions are limited by these studies' retrospective nature, by inherent variables such as maternal health and multiple drug exposures, by the lack of needed control groups, and by the limited sample sizes.

What Is the Risk of Chronic Low-Dose Anesthetic Exposure?

Spontaneous Abortion

Although multiple reports have been published regarding an increased risk of both spontaneous abortion and congenital anomalies among operating room personnel, a causal relationship has never been demonstrated. The American Society of Anesthesiologists conducted an extensive nationwide survey in 1974 that appeared to demonstrate an increased rate of spontaneous abortion among female operating room personnel compared with their non–operating room hospital personnel counterparts.[25] Among female dentists who used inhalation agents in their practice, a reportedly higher incidence of spontaneous abortion existed than among those who limited their practice to the use of local anesthetics[26] (see Chapter 51).

Congenital Anomalies

Although multiple studies have alluded to a correlation between the occupational exposure of women to subanesthetic concentrations of inhalation anesthetics and an increased occurrence of spontaneous abortion, a correlation of such exposure with increased risk of congenital abnormalities has not been documented. Many factors such as maternal health, work-related stress differences, and the level and frequency of exposure to trace anesthetics could not be controlled. Furthermore, the efficient scavenging systems used today in all likelihood alter the relevance of this data in the current work environment.

TABLE 64–3. Factors That Decrease Uteroplacental Perfusion

Decreased Uterine Arterial Pressure
  Hypotension
  Hypovolemia

Increased Uterine Venous Pressure
  Inferior vena cava compression
  Increased uterine tone (hypercarbia, oxytocin, ergots, ketamine)

Increased Uterine Artery Resistance
  α-Adrenergic vasopressors
  Endogenous catecholamines
  Ketamine (>1 mg $\cdot$ kg^{-1} first trimester)

What Is the Risk of Acute Anesthetic Exposure?

Premature Labor and Abortion

Important questions regarding the anesthetic management of pregnant surgical patients must be addressed. Several studies have demonstrated an increased incidence of spontaneous abortion, most notably in procedures performed during the first trimester of pregnancy and especially in those involving the pelvic cavity. In one review of over 9000 patients, premature labor and subsequent delivery occurred 4 times more frequently in the 144 patients who underwent surgery than in their counterparts who did not.

In another retrospective review, 2500 pregnant patients who underwent surgery were matched against pregnant controls who did not.[27] The incidence of spontaneous abortion again was increased in the surgical cohort; patients undergoing intrapelvic procedures were at highest risk. Unfortunately, the majority of these patients were exposed to a general anesthetic, so no comparison of regional versus general anesthetic risk can be drawn.

Congenital Abnormalities

In a more recent review of a Swedish registry of 5405 cases, no increase in congenital malformations or stillbirths was noted in the offspring of patients having surgery, and no specific type of anesthesia or surgery was associated with adverse outcome. However, the incidence of low birthweight infants and neonatal deaths within the first 7 days of life was increased.[28] In these and other studies, an increased risk of congenital anomalies could not be demonstrated.[29]

Teratogenicity

Several premedicants and anesthetic drugs have been demonstrated to be teratogenic in some animal models under particular conditions.[30] Furthermore, certain physiologic risks associated with the administration of an anesthetic, such as hypoxia, hypotension, and hypercapnia, may be teratogenic in some animals. Multiple factors are involved in determining whether a particular drug or agent will be teratogenic in humans (Table 64–4). Drugs that have been shown to cause particular defects in animal models may have no such effect in humans. In addition, duration and dose of exposure play a significant role.

Although teratogenesis may occur after exposure to very high doses or prolonged chronic exposure to low doses, one cannot conclude that a single short exposure during the course of an anesthetic case will cause the same defect. The fetal gestational age is also a critical element. Susceptibility or enhanced sensitivity from exposure to a particular agent during one stage of fetal or embryonic development occurs rarely or not at all at a different stage.[30]

TABLE 64–4. Some Factors That Affect the Teratogenicity of Drugs

Dose of drug or agent
Duration of patient exposure
Embryonic/fetal stage at time of exposure
Genetic susceptibility to individual drug effects

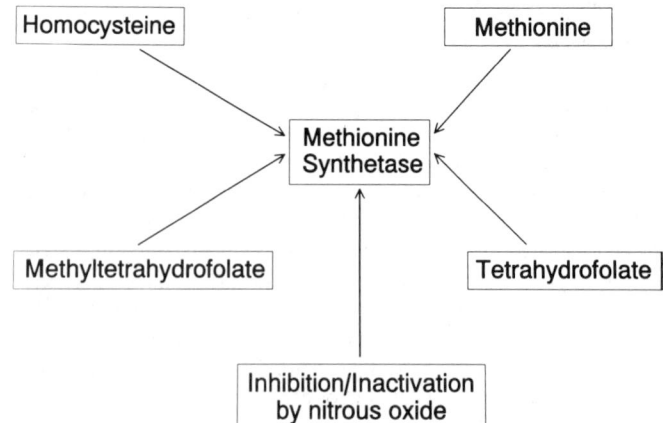

FIGURE 64–1. Abbreviated pathway demonstrating the inhibition of methionine synthase by nitrous oxide.

Organogenesis

In general, the most critical stage of development is thought to be during the period of organogenesis, which in humans occurs roughly from postconception days 15 to 56. Since the genitourinary system and the central nervous system continue to develop throughout the course of gestation, even into the neonatal period, extended periods of sensitivity are present throughout the course of pregnancy. Nevertheless, organogenesis represents the most critical period.[31]

What Are the Risks of Specific Agents and Other Factors?

Nitrous Oxide

Among the commonly used anesthetic agents, nitrous oxide use during pregnancy has been the subject of the greatest controversy. Concern stems from the potentially toxic effect nitrous oxide may pose relative to its ability to inactivate the enzyme methionine synthetase.[32] This enzyme is responsible for the production of methionine and tetrahydrofolate, which are important elements in the process of myelination. Hence, the potential for central nervous system aberration subsequent to the exposure to nitrous oxide is an important consideration (Fig. 64–1).

The inactivation of methionine synthetase by nitrous oxide appears to last for several days. However, its effect has not been demonstrated to be clinically significant in any human studies. Some investigators have advocated the administration of methionine, folinic acid, and vitamin B_{12} to patients undergoing anesthesia with nitrous oxide during pregnancy as a "rescue" technique because of the theoretic toxicity. Although this problem has not been proved to be clinically significant, most anesthesiologists in obstetrics advocate the avoidance of nitrous oxide for pregnant patients whenever possible but especially during the first trimester.

Potent Inhalation Agents

No major structural abnormalities could be found among rats exposed to 0.75 of the minimum alveolar concentration of halothane, enflurane, or isoflurane.[33] Single exposure for brief periods appears highly unlikely to produce fetal abnormalities.

A second, somewhat serendipitous advantage to the use of these agents during pregnancy is the fact that all three are known to reduce uterine contractility and, therefore, may provide some benefit to reduce the risk of intraoperative premature contractility.

Sodium Thiopental and Other Sedative Drugs

An increase in the incidence of congenital abnormalities following sodium thiopental use has been shown in some animal species. However, the administration of sodium thiopental to 152 women in their first trimester and undergoing cervical cerclage was not associated with any increase in the occurrence of fetal anomalies.[34]

Such has not been the case with the use of benzodiazepines. These drugs are among the most frequently administered medications in the United States. Although investigations of fetal outcome following in utero exposure have led to discrepant results, two separate retrospective studies have shown an association between high-dose maternal diazepam use and fetal cleft lip or cleft palate.[35, 36] No such linkage has been established in prospective studies with other benzodiazepines or sedative agents.[37]

Narcotics

The effects of in vitro and in vivo narcotics have been evaluated extensively. Chronic administration of morphine to pregnant rats did not lead to increased incidences of congenital anomalies, but it was found to be associated with decreased fetal and maternal weight gain, decreased litter counts, and an increased number of term stillbirths.[38] Parallel results have also been observed in human narcotics addicts and in those on methadone weaning.[39]

Animal studies involving the chronic administration of newer synthetic agents such as fentanyl have failed to demonstrate any impairment in reproductive capability or in the occurrence of fetal anomalies.[40] Little if any evidence shows that the short, single exposure of pregnant humans to narcotic agents in routine doses is associated with any adverse fetal outcome.

Muscle Relaxants

Despite the presence of skeletal abnormalities in chick embryos exposed to d-tubocurarine, no evidence suggests any adverse fetal effects in pregnant humans exposed to the usual range of clinically used muscle relaxants. Developmental abnormalities did not occur in cultured rat embryos until much greater than usual (30 times) clinical doses of d-tubocurarine, pancuronium, atracurium, and vecuronium were administered.[41]

Local Anesthetics

Although local anesthetics, even in very low concentrations, has been demonstrated in vitro to reversibly reduce cell division, studies have failed to demonstrate an increased rate of fetal malformation with amides or esters.[34] However, cardiac and neural sensitivity to local anesthetics is increased in pregnancy. Moreover, the myocardial depressant effects are enhanced with bupivacaine as opposed to with lidocaine.[18, 42]

Hypoxia and Hyperoxia

Hypoxia is teratogenic in several animal species.[43] Complications that might lead to maternal and fetal hypoxemia must be prevented with deliberate and careful anesthetic management. The fears of uterine and placental vasoconstriction in the face of maternal hyperoxia are unfounded.

No studies demonstrate fetal hypoxia in the face of maternal hyperoxia. Furthermore, as was noted earlier, increasing maternal Pao_2 to as high as 600 mm Hg cannot produce a fetal $Pao_2 > 60$ mm Hg because of the high metabolic activity of the placenta and the lack of autoregulation between the maternal and placental circulations.[44] Hyperbaric oxygen, however, does increase the incidence of fetal anomalies, although these effects appear to be more related to the high-pressure state than to maternal hyperoxia.[45]

Hypocarbia and Hypercarbia

Hypocarbia interferes not only with maternal and fetal acid-base balance but also with fetal development. Exposure of rats to elevated inhaled tensions of CO_2 for periods of 24 hours results in a high incidence of fetal cardiac anomalies.[46] Whether these effects are mediated in relation to direct exposure to higher levels of CO_2 or, more likely, as a result of the physiologic aberration that occurs in the face of hypercarbia (acidosis, vasoconstriction of uterine vessels, change in hemoglobin affinity for oxygen, and direct fetal myocardial depression) has not been determined.

Summary

Although surgery during pregnancy is associated with an increased incidence of spontaneous abortion and fetal demise, these outcomes cannot be attributed to the anesthetic. Rather, the increased risk appears to be related to the procedure itself, the site of maternal surgery, and the mother's underlying medical condition that may have precipitated the need for surgical intervention.

Obviously, hypoxia, hypercarbia, and hypotension have multiple deleterious effects, and careful anesthetic management of these factors is critical. No clinical evidence shows that any particular anesthetic type or technique is associated with improved fetal outcome.

What Is the Risk from Maternal Diagnostic Irradiation?

As with other potential teratogenic agents, the amount of radiation and the developmental stage of the fetus are the main factors of concern. Moreover, the type and location of the irradiation are also contributory. For example, fluoroscopic image intensifiers emit higher radiation doses than does routine chest radiography. Radiographic procedures of the abdomen, which expose the fetus' entire body to radiation, may be more detrimental than procedures that irradiate remote areas such as the extremities, head, or neck.

Large doses of radiation have led to congenital malformations, intrauterine growth retardation, childhood neoplasms, and death. The most common malformation in humans is microcephaly and eye abnormalities with associated mental retardation.[47] These anomalies manifest with doses > 100 rad. No apparent increase in congenital abnormalities or intrauterine growth retardation occurs with doses < 5 to 10 rad.

Fortunately, most diagnostic procedures emit significantly lower levels of radiation (20 mrad for a chest radiograph; 150 mrad for skull and neck films; and 1–2 rad for an abdominal computed tomography scan). Other radiographic procedures, such as contrast and radioisotope studies for venous thromboembolic disease, result in < 0.6 rad for contrast venography; < 0.375 rad for pulmonary angiography; and < 0.05 rad for lung scans.[47]

A possible increase in the relative risk of subsequent childhood cancers follows in utero exposure to low-dose irradiation (≤5 rad). However, all the applicable studies were retrospective with no control for confounding variables; thus, the question of whether irradiation was a causative or associated factor cannot be answered.

In summary, irradiation during pregnancy should be avoided whenever possible; however, diagnostic irradiation during pregnancy for medically indicated procedures should not be withheld if it is deemed necessary. Moreover, exposure of low-dose radiation (< 5 rad) to the fetus should not form the basis for termination of pregnancy.[48] Fortunately, ultrasonography often can replace radiographic procedures.

What Is the Risk of Preterm Labor?

As noted in the preceding discussion, several studies have suggested an increased incidence of preterm labor and spontaneous abortion in pregnant patients who must undergo surgery. In these reports, intra-abdominal procedures, especially those in which uterine manipulation or retraction is needed, yielded the highest risk of preterm labor. One study reported nearly a 10% incidence of spontaneous labor in patients who are pregnant and require surgery.[27] Furthermore, in those patients undergoing cervical cerclage, studies have demonstrated a 30% to 40% incidence of postoperative preterm labor.[49] Therefore, uterine activity should be monitored intraoperatively and postoperatively, and treatment should be initiated promptly if uterine contractions are noted.

Prophylactic Tocolysis During Anesthesia

Many obstetricians recommend prophylactic tocolysis in patients with a clinical history of preterm labor and in those undergoing cervical cerclage and intrapelvic procedures. Patients who are treated with tocolytic agents should continue to receive them for at least 24 to 48 hours postoperatively or until all signs of labor have resolved. All patients should be monitored for postoperative uterine activity, and tocolysis should be utilized if any change in cervical closure occurs. Other treatable causes of premature labor such as chorioamnionitis, urinary tract infection, or placental abruption must be ruled out.

Although no ideal tocolytic agent exists, the most commonly utilized drugs include the β-adrenergic agonists and magnesium sulfate. Each has the potential for adverse maternal and fetal side effects.

β-Adrenergic Agonists

The most commonly utilized β-agonists are ritodrine and terbutaline, whose side effects include hypokalemia, hypogly-

cemia, pulmonary edema, tachycardia, premature ventricular contractions, chest tightness, myocardial ischemia, ST and T wave electrocardiographic changes, atrial fibrillation, and, rarely, maternal death.[50]

Tachycardia associated with tocolysis makes it more difficult to assess the depth of anesthesia and hydration. Sympathomimetic or vagolytic agents such as halothane, ephedrine, ketamine, and pancuronium must be used with caution because of the increased risk for dysrhythmias. Further acceleration of the maternal heart rate makes the antisialagogues unattractive agents. Hyperventilation exacerbates the intracellular movement of potassium and thus compounds the relative hypokalemic state that is associated with these drugs.

Patients receiving terbutaline must have their fluid status evaluated closely because of the increased risk of pulmonary edema, especially when corticosteroids are used concomitantly to promote fetal lung maturity. This admonition is especially relevant during prehydration for regional anesthesia.

Magnesium Sulfate

Magnesium sulfate causes fewer maternal and fetal side effects than do the β-adrenergic agonists. Fetal side effects include hypotonia, hypocalcemia, and drowsiness. Mild maternal side effects include flushing, nausea, headache, and dizziness. More serious side effects associated with higher doses include arreflexia, pulmonary edema, and cardiorespiratory arrest.

Although the mechanism of action is unclear, magnesium sulfate is a smooth muscle relaxant and depresses neuromuscular conduction. It probably interferes with the cellular influx of calcium, which is normally necessary for excitation-contraction coupling. Magnesium also decreases the release of and sensitivity to acetylcholine at the motor endplate and depresses the excitability of the muscle membrane, thereby enhancing sensitivity to all muscle relaxants.

Since magnesium is excreted primarily by the kidneys, care must be taken to prevent toxicity in patients with renal failure. Toxic levels of magnesium lead to significant depression of cardiorespiratory function, although magnesium's effects can be antagonized by calcium salts.

Anesthetic Agents

No study has demonstrated that a specific anesthetic agent or technique is associated with a higher or lower rate of preterm delivery. Some vasopressors and doses of ketamine greater than 1 mg · kg^{-1} increase uterine tone and probably should be avoided.[51] Since anticholinesterase agents may also increase uterine tone, infusion of these drugs should be gradual and always after adequate pretreatment with atropine or glycopyrrolate.

PREPARING THE PREGNANT PATIENT FOR SURGERY

What Are the Major Concerns?

Five major concerns must be addressed before anesthesia is administered to a pregnant surgical patient (Table 64–5). Elective surgery should be postponed until after parturition. When surgery is deemed necessary, it should be avoided during the

TABLE 64–5. Key Anesthetic Concerns for the Administration of Anesthesia During Pregnancy

Maternal safety
Fetal well-being
Avoidance/prevention of preterm labor
Fetal and uterine monitoring
Maintenance of uteroplacental perfusion

first trimester, if at all possible, as long as the mother's health is not in jeopardy. Early second-trimester surgery also may be more appropriate if the peaks in blood volume, cardiac output, and aortocaval compression that occur in the third trimester are to be avoided. As was noted previously, procedures within the pelvic cavity pose the greatest risk of preterm labor.

Preoperative Management

A thorough preoperative evaluation is extremely important. In addition to the obviously important gathering of information, it allows the anesthesiologist to explain the relative risks involved and to reassure the patient that a safe and efficient anesthetic can be provided for the mother and fetus.

Anxiety and pain should be allayed with narcotics alone or in combination with a major tranquilizer. Diazepam and possibly other benzodiazepines should be avoided during organogenesis.

The preoperative administration of histamine$_2$ antagonists or metoclopramide, or both, may be well advised to decrease the risk of pneumonitis should aspiration occur. A clear, nonparticulate antacid such as sodium citrate is useful to neutralize pre-existing gastric secretions.[11] Uterine displacement is advisable from the second trimester onward during transport, anesthesia, surgery, and recovery in order to avoid aortocaval compression.

Monitoring

In addition to routine monitoring, as set forth in the guidelines of the American Society of Anesthesiologists for the administration of anesthetics, more serious conditions may dictate the need for invasive maternal monitors. The fetal heart rate should also be recorded continuously whenever possible. If the surgical field makes this an impossible task, presence of the fetal heart rate should be documented preoperatively and after induction of anesthesia with the surgeon or obstetrician present; subsequent continuous monitoring should be initiated at the end of surgery. During intra-abdominal cases, periodic fetal heart rate monitoring with a sterile ultrasonic transducer may be prudent.

The fetal heart rate can be detected as early as the 16th week of gestation with ultrasound. It is obviously a good indicator of uteroplacental function. Variability after the 25th week of gestation is a good indicator of fetal well-being. However, this variability is commonly lost following the administration of parenteral narcotics, barbiturates, sedative-hypnotics, and potent inhalation agents; regional anesthetic techniques do not usually affect variability.[52]

Whenever possible intraoperatively, and in all patients postoperatively, monitoring of uterine contractility with a tocodynamometer is advised for up to 24 hours. This technique is also most useful in assessing the need for tocolytic therapy.

Aggressive treatment of preterm labor is advised as was mentioned previously.

ANESTHETIC ADMINISTRATION

What Techniques Are Useful?

The choice of anesthesia should be based on the mother's condition and the extent of the planned surgery.

Subarachnoid Block

A subarachnoid block is our preferred method for those procedures that lend themselves to this technique. Spinal anesthesia is preferred, since maternal and fetal drug exposure is limited to a very small dose of local anesthetic. The risk of hypotension is, of course, a major consideration and makes prehydration and aggressive treatment essential.

Epidural and Caudal Block

Lumbar epidural or caudal anesthesia provides the same advantages as spinal anesthesia. However, more local agent (5–7 times the spinal dose) is necessary, increasing the risk of systemic local anesthetic toxicity. The incidence and degree of hypotension may be less owing to a slower onset of action. Other regional blocks should be utilized when possible, such as in upper extremity surgery.

General

General anesthesia is necessary when the operative procedure involves the head, neck, or thorax or when medical circumstances dictate its use. A combined epidural/general anesthetic offers several advantages. It provides loss of consciousness with a lower concentration of volatile anesthetic, thereby reducing fetal exposure. It further affords the opportunity to administer less systemic medication and to avoid the use of nitrous oxide. Finally, it provides an ideal approach to the control of postoperative pain through the use of neuraxial narcotics.

Table 64–6 lists recommended guidelines for the administration of these anesthetics to a pregnant patient.

TABLE 64–6. Guidelines for Administration of Anesthetics to Pregnant Patients

Spinal Epidural	General
Avoid premedicants if possible	Avoid premedicants if possible
30 mL 0.3-M sodium citrate preoperatively	30 mL 0.3-M sodium citrate preoperatively
Prehydrate with 1500–2000 mL of crystalloid solution	Left uterine displacement
Left uterine displacement	Fetal/uterine monitoring (with obstetrician present)
Fetal/uterine monitoring (with obstetrician present)	Preoxygenation
Supplemental O$_2$	Rapid sequence with cricoid pressure
Treat hypotension aggressively	Potent inhaled agent
Labor prophylaxis?	Narcotics
	Labor prophylaxis?

Can Hypotensive Anesthesia Be Provided Safely?

Inhalation Agents

Hypotensive anesthesia reportedly has been performed successfully, although some cases of its use have resulted in fetal distress and even death.[53, 54] Among the drugs commonly used for this purpose, the halogenated agents probably are contraindicated because of the myocardial depression and reduced cardiac output that result from the need for the administration of high concentrations.

Sodium Nitroprusside and Nitroglycerin

Although sodium nitroprusside is an effective and titrable agent, it rapidly crosses the placenta and is converted to cyanide ion that is potentially toxic to the fetus.[55] Nitroglycerin is probably the most frequently chosen agent during pregnancy. However, its onset is slower and may not be effective for severe hypertensive crisis. The drug is essentially nontoxic and has been demonstrated effective in clinical trials.[56]

Trimethophan

Trimethophan, with its large molecular weight, minimally crosses the blood-brain barrier and placenta. Thus, it has minor effects on maternal intracranial pressure (except in severe cases) and limited fetal involvement. However, control of hypertension may not be adequate owing to tachyphylaxis. Its side effects include pupillary dilatation and pseudocholinesterase inhibition.

Monitoring

When induced hypotension is needed, the reduction in maternal blood pressure should be limited in extent and duration. Maternal direct arterial pressure monitoring is advocated, and frequent assessment of maternal acid-base regulation is essential if fetal acidosis is to be avoided. The fetal heart rate must be monitored throughout the case.

Are Osmotic Diuretics Safe to Use During Pregnancy?

Osmotic diuretics such as mannitol are frequently used in neurosurgical procedures to optimize surgical exposure and reduce cerebral edema. Unfortunately, the use of these drugs leads to a net loss of water from the fetus to the mother through renal excretion and can result in severe fetal dehydration.[57] Hence, they should be used only when absolutely necessary.

Is Hypothermia Safe?

Hypothermia is utilized during certain cardiac and neurosurgical procedures in an attempt to reduce the metabolic O_2 requirements. Reports have indicated successful use of moderate hypothermia (30 °C) during pregnancy.[58] Although pla-

cental blood flow decreases secondary to increased uterine vascular resistance, O_2 transport remains unaffected. The fetus also becomes hypothermic and its metabolic requirements drop. Provided that maternal blood gases and acid-base status are optimized, the fetus appears to tolerate moderate hypothermia. Some evidence suggests that hypothermia during pregnancy may induce a fetal adrenocortical response. This effect has been suggested to be an inciting factor for the onset of labor in a normal term pregnancy.[59] Therefore, the possibility of preterm labor may also be greater in these individuals.

How Should Hyperventilation Be Provided?

As described previously, extreme hyperventilation causes decreases in uterine blood flow and placental O_2 delivery, which can potentially lead to fetal hypoxemia and acidosis. Mild hyperventilation (decreases in maternal $Paco_2$ of 5–7 mm Hg) may be well tolerated. This technique should be undertaken only with a fetal heart rate monitor in place and with the surgeon's understanding that ventilation will be returned to normal as soon as possible or if any sign of fetal distress is observed. Hyperventilation should be reserved for cases in which it is considered essential (i.e., in the presence of maternal cerebral edema and increased intracranial pressure).

How Is Cardiopulmonary Bypass Performed?

The incidence of cardiac disease during pregnancy is less than 2%. However, the problems of this disease are significant in pregnancy, since the cardiovascular demands are markedly increased. Although successful procedures with good outcomes have been performed on pregnant patients who require cardiopulmonary bypass, fetal mortality can be high. Whenever possible, these operations should be performed early in the second trimester, after organogenesis, and prior to the period of risk for premature labor and hemodynamic alterations, which peak in the third trimester.

High pump flows, upper limit pressures, and normothermic perfusion are recommended. Recall that the cardiac output of

TABLE 64–7. Basic Concerns During Anesthesia for Pregnant Patients

- The physiologic changes of pregnancy must be understood, and the anesthetic implications must be taken into account.
- Maternal blood pressure and uteroplacental perfusion must be maintained. Hypotension and aortocaval compression must be avoided, and, should they occur, aggressive treatment must be initiated promptly.
- Anesthetic techniques that limit the exposure of both mother and fetus should be chosen. Choose agents with a proven record of safety. Utilize regional anesthesia whenever possible.
- Discuss the implications of surgery and anesthesia during pregnancy, including our current knowledge regarding the lack of known teratogenicity among the commonly used anesthetic agents.
- Finally, monitor fetal heart rate and uterine activity intraoperatively and postoperatively, depending on the gestation. If changes are noted, appropriate action should be taken; this may include tocolysis for premature labor; alteration of anesthetic or surgical techniques, hemodynamics, or oxygenation for fetal distress; and cesarean delivery if fetal demise occurs.

a pregnant patient increases with increasing gestational age. Although moderate hypothermia (32 °C) is probably safe, more profound hypothermia may lead to fetal dysrhythmias and death. Moreover, despite adequate mean arterial pressure during cardiopulmonary bypass, increased uterine tone may decrease placental perfusion.

Fetal bradycardia often occurs with the onset of cardiopulmonary bypass and may continue throughout the pump run despite high flow rates, adequate pressures, and homeostatic control of acid-base balance. Frequently, a compensatory fetal tachycardia occurs after cardiopulmonary bypass. Uterine and fetal monitoring should be continued into the postbypass and postoperative periods.

SUMMARY

A number of concerns must be addressed when providing anesthetic care for the pregnant surgical patient. Basic considerations common to all such cases are summarized in Table 64–7. With these considerations in mind, safe, efficient, and uneventful anesthesia can be provided.

References

1. Shnider SM, Webster GM: Maternal and fetal hazards of surgery during pregnancy. Am J Obstet Gynecol 1965; 92:891.
2. Brodsky JM, Cohen EM, Brown BW, et al: Surgery during pregnancy and fetal outcome. Am J Obstet Gynecol 1980; 138:1165.
3. Conroy JM, Bailey MK, Hollon MF, et al: Anesthesia for open heart surgery in the pregnant patient. South Med J 1989; 82:492.
4. Steinberg ES, Santos AC: Surgical anesthesia during pregnancy. Int Anesthesiol Clin 1990; 28:58.
5. Bienarz J, Crottogini JJ, Curachet E: Aortocaval compression by the uterus in late pregnancy. Am J Obstet Gynecol 1968; 100:203.
6. Bell WR: Hematologic abnormalities in pregnancy. Med Clin North Am 1977; 61:165.
7. Morgan M: Anaesthetic contribution to maternal mortality. Br J Anaesth 1987; 59:842.
8. Prowse CM, Gaensler EA: Respiratory and acid/base changes during pregnancy. Anesthesiology 1965; 26:381–392.
9. Cugell DW, Frank NR, Gaensler EA, Badger TL: Pulmonary function in pregnancy: I. Serial observations in normal women. Am Rev Tubercul 1953; 67:568–597.
10. Simpson UH, Stakes AF, Miller M: Pregnancy delays paracetamol absorption and gastric emptying in patients undergoing surgery. Br J Anaesth 1988; 60:24.
11. Gibbs CP, Spohr L, Schmidt D: The effectiveness of sodium citrate as an antacid. Anesthesiology 1982; 57:44.
12. Colman RD, Frank M, Loughnan BA, et al: Use of IM ranitidine for the prophylaxis of aspiration pneumonitis in obstetrics. Br J Anaesth 1988; 61:720–729.
13. Olsson GL, Hallen B, Hambraeus-Jonzon K: Aspiration during anaesthesia: a computer-aided study of 185,358 anaesthetics. Acta Anaesthesiol Scand 1986; 30:84.
14. Palahniuk RJ, Shnider SM, Eger EI II: Pregnancy decreases the requirements for inhaled anesthetic agents. Anesthesiology 1974; 41:81–83.
15. Csontos K, Rust M, Holt V, et al: Elevated plasma beta-endorphin levels in pregnant women and their neonates. Life Sci 1979; 25:835–844.
16. Fagraeus L, Urban BJ, Bromage PR: Spread of epidural analgesia in early pregnancy. Anesthesiology 1983; 58:184.
17. Marx GF, Oka Y, Orkin LR: Cerebrospinal fluid pressures during labor. Am J Obstet Gynecol 1967; 84:213.
18. Morishima HO, Pedersen H, Finster M, et al: Bupivacaine toxicity in pregnant and nonpregnant ewes. Anesthesiology 1985; 63:134.
19. Santos AC, Pedersen H, Harmon TW, et al: Does pregnancy alter the systemic toxicity of local anesthetics? Anesthesiology 1989; 70:991.
20. Konieczko KM, Chapple JC, Nunn JF: Fetotoxic potential of general anesthesia in relation to pregnancy. Br J Anaesth 1987; 59:449.
21. Adamsons K, Mueller-Heubach E, Myers RE: Production of fetal asphyxia in rhesus monkeys by administration of catecholamines to the mother. Am J Obstet Gynecol 1971; 109:248.
22. James FM III, Griess FC Jr, Kemp RA: An evaluation of vasopressor therapy for maternal hypotension during spinal anesthesia. Anesthesiology 1970; 33:25.
23. Khazin AF, Hon EH, Hahre FW: Effects of maternal hyperoxia on the fetus: I. Oxygen tension. Am J Obstet Gynecol 1971; 109:628.
24. Brizgys RV, Dailey PA, Shnider SM, et al: The incidence and neonatal effects of maternal hypotension during epidural anesthesia for cesarean section. Anesthesiology 1987; 67:782.
25. American Society of Anesthesiologists Ad Hoc Committee on the Effect of Trace Anesthetics on the Health of Operating Room Personnel: Occupational disease among operating room personnel. Anesthesiology 1974; 41:321–340.
26. Cohen EN, Brown BW, Wu ML, et al: Occupational disease in dentistry and chronic exposure to trace anesthetic gases. J Am Dent Assoc 1980; 101:21.
27. Duncan PG, Pope WDB, Cohen MM, et al: Fetal risks of anesthesia and surgery during pregnancy. Anesthesiology 1986; 64:790.
28. Mazze RI, Kallen B: Reproductive outcome after anesthesia and operation during pregnancy: a registry study of 5,405 cases. Am J Obstet Gynecol 1989; 161:1178.
29. Brodsky JB, Cohen EN, Brown BW, et al: Surgery during pregnancy and fetal outcome. Am J Obstet Gynecol 1980; 138:1165.
30. Wilson JG: Experimental studies on congenital malformations. J Chron Dis 1959; 10:111.
31. Tuchmann-Duplessis H: The effects of drugs on the embryo. In Scientific Foundations of Obstetrics and Gynecology. Phillip E, Barnes J, Newton M (eds). Philadelphia, FA Davis, 1970.
32. Nunn JF, Chanarin I: Nitrous oxide inactivates methionine synthetase. In Nitrous Oxide/N$_2$O. Eger EI II (ed). New York, Elsevier, 1985.
33. Mazze RI, Funinaga M, Rice SA, et al: Reproduction and teratogenic effects of nitrous oxide, halothane, isoflurane, and enflurane in Sprague-Dawley rats. Anesthesiology 1986; 64:334.
34. Heinnen OP, Slone D, Shapiro S: Birth Defects and Drugs in Pregnancy. Littleton, MA, Publishing Sciences Group, 1977, p 337.
35. Safra M, Oakley GP: Association between cleft lip with or without cleft palate and prenatal exposure to diazepam. Lancet 1975; 2:478.
36. Saxen I, Saxen L: Association between maternal intake of diazepam and oral clefts. Lancet 1975; 2:498.
37. Hartz SC, Heinonen OP, Shapiro S, et al: Antenatal exposure to meprobamate and chlordiazepoxide in relation to malformation, mental development and childhood mortality. N Engl J Med 1975; 292:726.
38. Zagon IS, McLaughlin PJ: Effects of chronic morphine administration on pregnant rats and their offspring. Pharmacology 1977; 15:302–310.
39. Naeye RL, Blanc W, LeBlanc W, et al: Fetal complications of maternal heroin addiction: abnormal growth, infection and episodes of stress. J Pediatr 1973; 83:1055.
40. Fujinaga M, Mazze RI, Jackson EC, Baden JM: Reproductive and teratogenic effects of sufentanil and alfentanil in Sprague-Dawley rats. Anesth Analg 1988; 67:166.
41. Fujinaga M, Badden JM, Mazze RI: Developmental toxicity of nondepolarizing muscle relaxants in cultured rat embryos. Anesthesiology 1992; 76:999.
42. Moller RA, Datta S, Fox J, et al: Effect of progesterone on the cardiac electrophysiologic action of bupivacaine and lidocaine. Anesthesiology 1992; 76:604.
43. Grabowski CT: The teratogenic effects of graded doses of hypoxia on the chicken embryo. Am J Anat 1958; 103:313.
44. Khazin AF, Hon EH, Hahre FW: Effects of maternal hyperoxia on the fetus: I. Oxygen tension. Am J Obstet Gynecol 1971; 109:628.
45. Fern BH: Teratogenic effects of hyperbaric oxygen. Proc Soc Exp Biol Med 1964; 116:975.
46. Haring OM: Cardiac malformations in rats induced by exposure of the mother to carbon dioxide during pregnancy. Circ Res 1960; 8:1218.
47. Ginsberg JS, Hirsh J, Rainbow AJ, et al: Risks to the fetus of radiologic procedures used in the diagnosis of maternal venous thromboembolic disease. Thromb Haemost 1989; 61:189.
48. Brent RL: The effects of embryonic and fetal exposure to x-ray, microwaves, and ultrasound. Clin Obstet Gynecol 1983; 26:484.
49. Smith BE: Fetal prognosis after anesthesia during gestation. Anesth Analg 1963; 42:521.
50. Barden TP, Peter JB, Merkatz IR: Ritodrine hydrochloride: a betamimetic agent for use in pre-term labor: I. Pharmacology, clinical history, administration, side effects, and safety. Obstet Gynecol 1980; 56:1.

51. Oats JN, Vasey DP, Waldron BA: Effects of ketamine on the pregnant uterus. Br J Anaesth 1979; 51:1163.

52. Liu P, Warren TM, Ostheimer GW, et al: Foetal monitoring in parturients undergoing surgery unrelated to pregnancy. Can Anaesth Soc J 1985; 32:525.

53. Minielly R, Yupze AA, Drake CG: Subarachnoid hemorrhage secondary to ruptured cerebral aneurysm in pregnancy. Obstet Gynecol 1979; 53:64.

54. Robinson JL, Chir B, Hall CJ, et al: Subarachnoid hemorrhage in pregnancy. J Neurosurg 1972; 37:27.

55. Donchin Y, Amirav B: Sodium nitroprusside for aneurysm surgery in pregnancy. Br J Anaesth 1978; 50:849.

56. Wheeler AS, James FM III, Meis PJ, et al: Effects of nitroglycerin and nitroprusside on the uterine vasculature of gravid ewes. Anesthesiology 1980; 52:390.

57. Bruns PD, Linder RO, Brose VE, et al: The placental transfer of water from fetus to mother following intravenous administration of hypertonic mannitol to the maternal rabbit. Am J Obstet Gynecol 1963; 86:160.

58. Stange K, Halldin M: Hypothermia in pregnancy. Anesthesiology 1983; 58:460.

59. Levy DL, Warriner RA, Burges GE: Fetal response to cardiopulmonary bypass. Obstet Gynecol 1980; 56:112.

CHAPTER # 65

Abdominal Surgery

SERGIO GREGORETTI, M.D.

THE ABDOMINAL WALL

Why Does It Get Tight?

Muscle relaxation is essential in abdominal surgery to allow exposure of abdominal contents and minimize motion in the surgical field. The "tight" abdomen about which surgeons often complain is the result of a spinal polysynaptic reflex. It is evoked by painful stimuli applied to the abdominal wall and peritoneum and by traction of the intra-abdominal viscera.[1] Afferent pathways include the intercostal and splanchnic nerves, whereas efferent impulses travel through the intercostal and, if the stimulus is strong enough, the phrenic nerves, causing contraction of the abdominal wall muscles and diaphragm.[2]

This reflex is particularly noticeable during skin incision, peritoneal opening, placement of retractors, and intra-abdominal exploration. It tends to fatigue, becoming less effective with time despite continuous stimulation. This fact may explain why during surgery, once exposure is achieved, the need for additional relaxation is decreased.

Contraction of the abdominal wall can still be elicited late during an operation either by a strong sudden stimulus such as traction on the mesentery or when the viscera are repositioned in the abdomen and the peritoneum closed. Because a tight abdomen results from a spinal reflex, it can still be observed in patients with a spinal cord injury at T-5 and higher despite complete loss of abdominal wall sensitivity. It also can occur in brain-dead subjects during organ procurement for transplantation.

How Is It Relaxed?

Abdominal relaxation can be obtained by interrupting the spinal reflex at different sites. Regional techniques (intercostal nerve blocks combined with celiac plexus block, as well as spinal or epidural anesthesia) provide relaxation mainly by preventing afferent stimuli from reaching the spinal cord.[3] All inhalation and intravenous anesthetics, with the exception of the opioids and ketamine, provide some degree of relaxation by depressing the reflex pathways at the spinal cord level.[4]

Muscle relaxants act on the efferent side of the reflex, blocking motor impulses to the muscles. The intense degree of relaxation required during abdominal surgery can only be obtained by muscle relaxants or regional anesthesia techniques. The degree of relaxation that modern general anesthetics provide generally is inadequate for operations in the abdomen but enhances the relaxation provided by other drugs.

GENERAL ANESTHESIA

General anesthesia is most common for abdominal operations. Induction is usually achieved with an intravenous agent, followed by tracheal intubation facilitated by a muscle relaxant. Tracheal intubation is mandatory because of the high incidence of regurgitation of gastrointestinal (GI) contents during manipulation of the stomach, biliary tract, and other abdominal contents.

Is Hyperventilation Helpful?

Hyperventilation has been widely used during abdominal surgery because of empirical evidence that it enhances muscle relaxation and improves operating conditions. The mechanisms by which it affects muscle relaxation are largely unknown.[5] Hypocapnia, however, decreases cardiac output and blood flow to several organs, including the liver and intestine.[6, 7] Because intra-abdominal surgical manipulations and the anesthetic agents significantly decrease splanchnic blood flow,[8] it is perhaps preferable to maintain carbon dioxide (CO_2) tension within normal limits. Normocarbia also allows more rapid restoration of spontaneous breathing at the end of the procedure, particularly when opioids have been used.[9, 10]

What Are the Options?

Anesthesia can be maintained by intermittent doses or continuous infusions of intravenous agents such as thiopental,

1109

propofol, and opioids, usually combined with nitrous oxide. However, the halogenated anesthetics (halothane, enflurane, isoflurane) probably are the most commonly used drugs. They reliably control hemodynamic reflex responses elicited by the intense stimuli encountered during abdominal surgery, and their concentrations can be easily decreased when the stimuli are less intense or absent. In addition, they exhibit predictable pharmacokinetic activity, and even after very long procedures patients can be awakened within minutes after these agents have been discontinued.

Halogenated anesthetics also potentiate the effects of muscle relaxants.[4] Therefore, when a halogenated agent is used, less relaxant is required for adequate surgical conditions, and reversal of the residual block at the end of the procedure is easier. Furthermore, in the presence of a halogenated agent, recovery from neuromuscular blockade tends to be more gradual, more time is available to recognize the need for additional relaxant, and abrupt motion of the surgical field is avoided.

Which Halogenated Agent Is Best?

Any of the available halogenated agents can be satisfactory for abdominal surgery. Few would argue that the pharmacologic differences among anesthetics are much less important for a good outcome than the skill, clinical acumen, and vigilance of the anesthesia provider. However, isoflurane and enflurane maintain liver and intestinal blood flow better than halothane during abdominal procedures.[11–14] Thus, a case can be made in favor of the former agents when a decrease in visceral blood might be particularly detrimental. These circumstances include patients with severe liver disease, in whom further deterioration of liver function may result in overt failure, and patients undergoing major liver resections, in whom damage to the residual liver may jeopardize survival.

What Is the Role of Nitrous Oxide?

Although halogenated agents combined with a muscle relaxant can provide excellent anesthetic conditions during abdominal operations, they are often used in combination with nitrous oxide and opioids. Features that make nitrous oxide attractive are fast uptake and elimination, minimal cardiovascular effects, and its additive anesthetic effects to those of the halogenated agents.

Nitrous oxide can be used at the beginning of the procedure to ensure maintenance of the anesthetic state while the effects of the intravenous induction agents are dissipating. The halogenated agent may then be gradually introduced and titrated according to blood pressure changes. Nitrous oxide reduces the required concentration of the halogenated agent by approximately 50%. Therefore, hypotension is less likely, particularly during periods of minimum or absent surgical stimulation. Toward the end of the procedure, the potent agent can be discontinued well ahead of completion. Anesthesia is maintained with nitrous oxide, thus allowing more rapid awakening.

What Are the Roles of Opioids?

Opioids are used because of their "sparing" effect on the requirements for halogenated agents and their minimum car-

diovascular effects. These drugs are particularly useful at the beginning of the procedure when the most intense surgical stimulation occurs. Toward the end of the operation, one should rely more on the inhaled agents than the narcotic to control hemodynamic function, thus avoiding excessive narcotic-induced depression of the respiratory center. Opioids can be used to provide analgesia and to facilitate smoother emergence on completion of anesthesia.

MUSCLE RELAXANTS

Muscle relaxation during abdominal surgery is commonly obtained with nondepolarizing agents. If succinylcholine is used to facilitate tracheal intubation, the nondepolarizing agent preferably should be administered only after a patient shows some signs of recovery. This approach rules out the possibility of a generally abnormal pseudocholinesterase and provides useful information about anesthetic depth.

How Is the Muscle Relaxant Chosen?

The factors pertinent to abdominal surgery that influence the choice of a muscle relaxant are the duration of the procedure and pre-existing diseases that affect relaxant pharmacokinetics. Short procedures such as an appendectomy, which may be completed in 30 minutes, or an exploratory laparotomy that may be rapidly aborted call for a short- or intermediate-acting agent such as mivacurium or vecuronium and atracurium, respectively. For potentially short procedures, an infusion of succinylcholine is also appropriate.

Should the procedure become more complex and extended, a switch to a nondepolarizing agent is easily accomplished. Long-acting agents (e.g., metocurine, pancuronium, doxacurium) are appropriate for procedures lasting 2 hours or more. However, even when they are used in procedures of several hours' duration, the long-acting agents are associated with a significantly higher postoperative incidence of residual neuromuscular blockade than are the intermediate-acting agents.[15, 16] A case can be made, therefore, for the use of intermediate-acting agents in lengthy procedures.

What Factors Affect the Duration of Muscle Relaxation?

Obstructive Jaundice

Common situations that affect relaxant pharmacokinetics during abdominal surgery are obstructive jaundice (cholestasis) and cirrhosis of the liver. Obstructive jaundice prolongs the elimination half-life but does not affect the volume of distribution of pancuronium[17] and vecuronium.[18] Although this issue has not been specifically addressed, obstructive jaundice probably begins to affect the pharmacokinetics of these relaxants only when the bilirubin level is >5 mg · dL^{-1}.[18] In practice, the initial dose of pancuronium and vecuronium in patients with severe jaundice does not need to be adjusted, but the duration of the block is about 50% longer than normal.[17, 18]

To avoid an excessive dose, the maintenance doses need to be smaller than usual and administered only when signs of recovery from the block are noted. Apart from gallamine, whose kinetics are not altered in obstructive jaundice,[19] the pharmacokinetics of no other relaxant have been studied in patients with cholestasis. Clinical experience indicates that atracurium administered to these patients does not have a prolonged effect.

Cirrhosis

Cirrhosis and other severe liver diseases may prolong the duration of succinylcholine block because of the associated decrease in plasma pseudocholinesterase activity. In practice, succinylcholine use in the presence of liver disease does not pose any problem, because the increase in duration of the block amounts to a few minutes at most.[20]

A common clinical impression is that the initial dose of nondepolarizing relaxants needs to be larger than usual in patients with cirrhosis to achieve a given degree of block. The need for additional doses is decreased for pancuronium,[21] whereas for vecuronium this phenomenon becomes evident only after prolonged administration (i.e., after the third or fourth "top-up" dose).[22-24] The maintenance doses for atracurium are unchanged in cirrhosis.[25]

In patients with cholestasis and severe liver disease, although any relaxant can be safely used if it is titrated to effect, atracurium is "forgiving" because of its peculiar pharmacokinetics; therefore, it is an excellent choice.

How Should They Be Given?

The relaxants should be given in doses adequate to provide favorable surgical conditions, at the same time avoiding an overdose (i.e., excessive duration) and consequently a block difficult to reverse at the end of the procedure. The first dose of the nondepolarizing relaxant is given according to the known pharmacology of the drug. Subsequent doses, usually one third to one fifth of the initial one, are administered when evidence of block dissipation is noted. Neuromuscular blockade is best assessed by a peripheral nerve stimulator. Clinical criteria are also useful.

How Should the Nerve Stimulator Be Used?

The use of a peripheral nerve stimulator may be associated with several pitfalls that lead one to judge a block to be adequate, whereas in reality it is not. To avoid these pitfalls, the following factors are important.

First of all, a strong control twitch must be obtained before any relaxant is given. Use this response as a "control" against which to compare the twitches elicited during the onset, maintenance, and recovery of the block.

Second, although the motor responses evoked by peripheral nerve stimulation can be recorded on paper and examined very precisely, in clinical practice the evaluation is visual or tactile and, by nature, very imprecise. If the ulnar nerve is stimulated, as is most commonly done, tactile evaluation of the contraction of the adductor pollicis is preferred.

The best results are obtained if slight tension is applied to the thumb before the stimulus. Contractions of the fourth and fifth fingers are sometimes present while the thumb is completely paralyzed. These contractions probably occur because the hypothenar muscles are slightly more resistant to the relax-

ant than the adductor pollicis and should be disregarded when a train-of-four count assessment of the block is made.[26] If the facial nerve is stimulated, the contractions of the orbicularis oculi muscle are evaluated visually.

Third, when the neuromuscular block is monitored at the adductor pollicis, care should be taken to prevent cooling of the arm and hand examined. Cooling of the limb out of proportion to the rest of the body may cause a persistent block of the thumb at a time when the muscles in other parts of the body have recovered from the block.

Different muscles respond differently to muscle relaxants; therefore, the results obtained for one muscle cannot automatically be extrapolated to other muscles. The muscle usually monitored is the adductor pollicis, whereas in abdominal surgery the diaphragm and the abdominal muscles are of most concern. After a bolus dose of relaxant, the block of the diaphragmatic and abdominal muscles is probably as intense as that of the adductor pollicis.[27-29] However, both diaphragm and abdominal muscles recover from the block much faster than does the adductor pollicis (Fig. 65–1). This fact explains the frequent clinical situation in which contractions of the abdomen occur despite minimum or absent motor response of the thumb to ulnar nerve stimulation. The orbicularis oculi muscle shows the same response to relaxants as the diaphragm (see Fig. 65–1). Monitoring of this muscle may therefore be preferable to the adductor pollicis when intense diaphragmatic paralysis is important.

How Are Clinical Criteria Used?

Slight limb movements, small contractions of the abdominal wall or diaphragm, hiccups, and the surgeon's comments on the quality of the relaxation form the basis for clinical evaluation. Experience shows that other useful signs that the block is dissipating and will soon be inadequate are a sudden increase in heart rate and blood pressure during what otherwise appears to be a perfectly adequate anesthetic. That these hemodynamic changes are related to inadequate relaxation is confirmed by the fact that an additional dose of relaxant rapidly returns these parameters to the prior status quo. Validation of this clinical observation is left to the reader. Bucking on the endotracheal tube and elevated peak airway pressures are signs of inadequate relaxation.

Movements of the facial muscles (grimacing, winking, or wrinkling of the forehead), in view of the great resistance of these muscles to relaxants, are more likely signs of inadequate anesthesia than inadequate relaxation and are best treated by a small dose of thiopental or opioid or by increasing the concentration of the inhaled agent.

Finally, even when you use the peripheral nerve stimulator, look at the patient and surgical field and integrate the clinical observations with the information provided by the nerve stimulator. Should an apparent disparity arise, defer to the clinical observations.

When Is the Need for Relaxation Greatest?

The requirement for muscle relaxation encompasses the entire length of the operation. It is greatest at the beginning, when the peritoneum is opened and the surgical area exposed, and at the end, when the peritoneum is closed. Adequate relax-

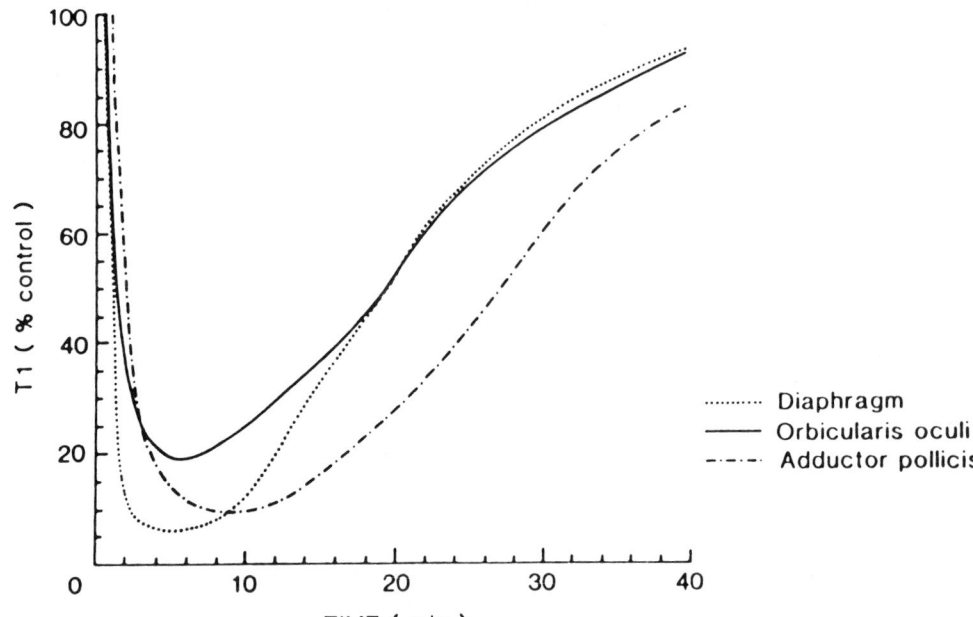

FIGURE 65–1. Intensity and time course of neuromuscular block at the diaphragm, orbicularis oculi, and adductor pollicis after administration of vecuronium, 0.07 mg/kg. The block is expressed as amplitude of the first twitch to train-of-four stimulation (T1) relative to control. The diaphragm recovers from the block much more quickly than does the adductor pollicis. The block at the orbicularis oculi is nearly identical to that at the diaphragm. The clinical implications of these observations are explained in the text. (From Donati F, Meistelman C, Plaud B: Vecuronium neuromuscular blockade at the diaphragm, the orbicularis oculi, and adductor pollicis muscles. Anesthesiology 1990; 73:870.)

ation for the beginning of surgery is present when no movement or only the first thumb or orbicularis oculi contraction can be barely detected in response to a train-of-four stimulation mode.[26] Later in the case, one or two twitches in response to train-of-four stimulation indicate adequate relaxation.

Remember, however, as was noted previously, even when no response of the thumb to ulnar nerve stimulation is present, diaphragmatic contractions can occur in response to intense surgical stimuli. If ulnar nerve stimulation is used to ensure diaphragmatic inactivity when the train-of-four count at the thumb is zero, the post-tetanic count method may be used.[30] If only two or three twitches are detected after the tetanic stimulus, even the strongest surgical stimulation does not evoke diaphragmatic activity.[31] Alternatively, the orbicularis oculi muscle, which responds to relaxants similarly to the diaphragm, can be monitored and sufficient relaxant given to suppress any response to facial nerve stimulation.[28]

Hiccups: a Minor Nuisance?

Hiccups are an intermittent spasm of the diaphragm of reflex origin.[32] The afferent limb of the reflex is composed of the vagus and phrenic nerves, with the "hiccup center" located in the spinal cord between the third and fifth cervical segments. The efferent limb is the phrenic nerve. Hiccups usually occur during procedures in the upper abdomen and are caused by visceral stimulation or irritation of the diaphragm.

Treatment

Hiccups signal that the diaphragm is not fully paralyzed and require treatment only if they are interfering with the surgeon's work. Although several pharmacologic treatments for hiccups have been suggested[33] (Table 65–1), the best treatment is to block the reflex pathway concerned by giving a further dose of muscle relaxant or by deepening the level of anesthesia with a small dose of thiopental or a higher concentration of inhaled agent. Hiccups may also be stopped by stimulation of the nasopharynx with a suction catheter.[34] A gentle to-and-fro

motion is used with the catheter inserted through one nostril to a depth of 3 to 4 inches.

How Should Inadequate Relaxation During Peritoneal Closure Be Handled?

Inadequate relaxation is occasionally present during peritoneal closure, when only 15 to 20 more minutes of anesthesia is needed. Several avenues can be followed to solve the dilemma of satisfying operative demands while at the same time avoiding an overdose of anesthetic or relaxant that makes awakening unduly prolonged or reversal of the block difficult.

A small intravenous dose of thiopental or lidocaine and an increase in the concentration of the inhaled agents sometimes are enough to solve the problem. Manual hyperventilation is also helpful. If the abdominal contractions are powerful, however, only a further dose of relaxant will bring the situation under control. When short-acting agents such as vecuronium and atracurium have been used throughout the procedure, a small dose of the same relaxant is appropriate.

Succinylcholine

When a long-acting relaxant has been used, however, an additional dose of the same drug probably would produce a

TABLE 65–1. Pharmacologic Treatments for Hiccups

Pharmacologic	Ketamine
	Ephedrine
	Chlorpromazine
	Doxapram
	Edrophonium
	Methylphenidate
	Smelling salts
	Muscle relaxants
Nonpharmacologic	Nasopharyngeal stimulation (catheter)
	Nasal iced saline instillation
	Nasogastric tube placement

block duration too long for the remaining procedure and cause difficulty with efficient reversal. In this situation, succinylcholine is a tempting but controversial choice. Some authorities object to the use of succinylcholine when the effect of a nondepolarizing block is dissipating because the block induced is somewhat variable and accompanied by a transient reversal of the residual nondepolarizing block.[35, 36] In addition, when neostigmine or a similar drug is administered to reverse the residual nondepolarizing block, it may potentiate the effect of the previous dose of succinylcholine. Furthermore, the admittedly remote possibility is that succinylcholine administration may be followed by a long-lasting block, should the patient have atypical plasma pseudocholinesterase.

Others argue that the brief antagonism of the nondepolarizing block is of little relevance, and provided a large enough dose of succinylcholine is administered (i.e., 1 mg $\cdot$ kg^{-1}), adequate relaxation can be consistently obtained for the few minutes needed.[36] Any succinylcholine/neostigmine interaction can be easily avoided if neostigmine is not administered until at least 10 minutes has elapsed after the administration of succinylcholine.[36] If a peripheral nerve stimulator is used, the residual nondepolarizing block is reversed only when the twitch has recovered to the level present before the administration of succinylcholine.

Vecuronium, Atracurium, Mivacurium

To avoid the succinylcholine controversy, the use of a shorter-acting nondepolarizing agent may seem to be a better choice. Unfortunately, vecuronium in a dose of 1 mg given during the recovery phase of a pre-existing metocurine or pancuronium block causes a profound block that lasts 30 to 60 minutes.[37, 38] Whether a similar potentiation of vecuronium occurs after the new long-acting agents pipecuronium and doxacurium is not known.

To the contrary, atracurium in a dose of 5 to 10 mg can be used after a long-acting agent with no untoward prolongation of the block.[39] The pharmacology of mivacurium suggests that it also may be used in a dose of 2 to 4 mg to provide brief relaxation. However, mivacurium is metabolized by plasma cholinesterase, and again, there is the remote possibility of a prolonged block even after such a low dose should the patient have atypical plasma pseudocholinesterase.[40]

Does Neostigmine Affect Bowel Anastomosis?

Neostigmine is an anticholinesterase agent commonly used to reverse the effects of nondepolarizing muscle relaxants. In addition to its action on the skeletal muscle, it also causes forceful contractions of the bowel that persist for several minutes.[41] These contractions are unaffected by the concomitantly administered anticholinergic drug[42, 43] but are completely prevented by inhalation agents.[43] The effects of edrophonium and pyridostigmine, the other common reversal agents, have not been investigated, but they are probably similar to those of neostigmine.

In patients undergoing bowel resection and anastomosis, the hyperperistalsis induced by neostigmine has been postulated to disrupt the newly constructed anastomosis by putting excessive traction on the suture line.[44] The suggestion that inhaled agents completely inhibit neostigmine-induced contractions

was discounted on the ground that these agents are usually discontinued before neostigmine administration and therefore cannot be relied on to prevent the hyperperistalsis caused by neostigmine. Several subsequent studies have failed to link the use of neostigmine to an increased incidence of anastomotic breakdown,[45–47] leading to current thinking that neostigmine is an unlikely cause of anastomotic complications.

Can Muscle Relaxation Be Re-Established Shortly After Reversal?

Shortly after a neuromuscular block has been reversed with an anticholinesterase agent, unexpected circumstances such as an incorrect sponge count may require a short period of intense muscle relaxation and re-exploration of the abdomen. In this situation, the anesthesiologist may be reluctant to use succinylcholine because of a fear that inhibition of plasma pseudocholinesterase by the anticholinesterase agent will result in an excessively prolonged block. This fear, however, is unfounded. The block caused by succinylcholine administered as 1 mg $\cdot$ kg^{-1} immediately after anticholinesterase administration (i.e., when pseudocholinesterase activity is maximally inhibited) lasts approximately 30 minutes.[48] If a shorter block is desired, a smaller dose (e.g., 0.5 mg $\cdot$ kg^{-1} provides about 15 minutes of relaxation.

Should the block recover before surgery is completed, additional doses of succinylcholine can be safely administered. The inhibitory effect of anticholinesterase agents on plasma pseudocholinesterase lasts only about 60 minutes.[49] Therefore, no prolongation of succinylcholine block is expected when an hour or more has elapsed since a previous dose of anticholinesterase.

SPINAL AND EPIDURAL ANESTHESIA

What Level of Sensory Block Is Needed for Upper Abdominal Procedures?

Upper abdominal procedures require an intense sensory block up to a T-4 level. In actuality, however, a sensory level at T-1 to T-2 is needed, because analgesia at the upper level of the block tends to be tenuous; only a sensory block to T-1 to T-2 ensures a "surgical" block at the lower level T-4. This high a level of anesthesia can be safely obtained only by a continuous epidural technique. Because an excessive dose of local anesthetic may be required if the injection is given at the lumbar level, the epidural puncture should be performed at T-6 to T-7, a technique that requires considerable skill.

Is Regional Anesthesia Alone Adequate for Upper Abdominal Surgery?

Despite an adequate sensory level, upper abdominal surgery under regional anesthesia is often marred by pain, nausea, and vomiting when the surgeon manipulates the viscera and by difficulty with respiration when retractors and packs are in place. In addition, relaxation of the abdominal muscles is not always satisfactory. For these reasons, regional anesthesia for an upper abdominal procedure is virtually always combined with inhalation anesthesia that eliminates patients' discomfort, ensures adequate ventilation, and allows the use of relaxants if the surgical field is unsatisfactory.

What Level of Sensory Block Is Needed for Lower Abdominal Procedures?

Surgery below the umbilicus requires a sensory block at T-4 to T-5 for both the patient's and surgeon's satisfaction. This sensory level can be obtained equally well by spinal or epidural anesthesia. If the operation time is estimated to be <2 hours, a spinal or a "single-shot" epidural anesthetic can be used. However, because the duration of operations cannot always be predicted reliably, a case can be made for routine placement of an epidural catheter that allows prolongation of the block if needed. Obviously, a continuous epidural technique is chosen if postoperative analgesia is to be provided by the epidural route. Continuous spinal anesthesia has several appealing features, but its use via spinal microcatheters has been linked to serious neurologic complications.[50]

Is Regional Anesthesia Alone Adequate for Lower Abdominal Procedures?

Although regional anesthesia can provide satisfactory conditions for lower abdominal surgery, it also is often combined with general anesthesia to improve patients' comfort. The combination prevents pain and nausea or the discomfort caused by a head-down position or by lying on the operating table for several hours. General anesthesia also allows administration of muscle relaxants should the abdominal relaxation provided by the regional block be inadequate.

Technique for Combined Regional with General Anesthesia

A spinal or a single-shot epidural block should be performed before the induction of general anesthesia in order to detect paresthesias or radicular pain during lumbar puncture and injection of the local anesthetic. If a continuous epidural technique is used, once the epidural catheter has been placed and the test dose administered, induction of general anesthesia first is expedient to allow placement of the Foley catheter and sterile preparation of the field without waiting for the block to be fully developed.

General anesthesia is induced with the intravenous agent of choice followed by tracheal intubation. Topical anesthesia of the larynx and trachea with 4% lidocaine enhances tolerance of the endotracheal tube. Light anesthesia is maintained with nitrous oxide supplemented as needed by minimal concentrations of a halogenated agent or small doses of intravenous agents.

Ventilation can be spontaneous[51] or controlled. Controlled ventilation is mandatory when muscle relaxants are used but can also be easily established without muscle relaxants after a small dose of fentanyl and moderate hyperventilation (end-tidal CO_2 of approximately 30 mm Hg). During such "light" anesthesia, insertion of a nasogastric tube invariably is associated with a patient's straining and bucking. This sequence can be avoided by inserting the nasogastric tube immediately after the endotracheal tube when the intubating level of muscle relaxant is still present.

How Is Hypotension Treated?

The combination of general and regional anesthesia is associated with a much greater decrease in blood pressure than when either technique is used alone. This hypotension responds poorly to fluid administration, and the preferred treatment is ephedrine.[52–54]

Is Regional Anesthesia Better Than General?

Numerous studies have addressed the question about whether regional anesthesia offers any significant advantage over general anesthesia in abdominal surgery. The techniques have been compared in relation to several intraoperative and postoperative factors, including blood loss and the need for transfusion,[55, 56] postoperative lung function and respiratory complications,[55, 57] wound dehiscence,[55] anastomotic breakdown after bowel resection,[56] incidence of deep venous thrombosis,[55, 58, 59] postoperative weight loss and nitrogen balance,[60] duration of postoperative ileus, and postoperative mental functioning.[61] No clinically important differences in these areas have been demonstrated. Although more studies perhaps are needed, at present, no convincing evidence favors one technique over the other for abdominal procedures. In skillful hands, either is acceptable; once again, a successful outcome is related more to careful monitoring and control of physiologic variables than to the method of anesthesia.

HYPOTENSION RELATED TO SURGICAL MANEUVERS

Why Does It Occur?

Surgical maneuvers, particularly during procedures in the upper abdomen, may cause hypotension that can be explained by mechanical, reflex, or humoral mechanisms.

Mechanical Causes

Placement of packs, retractors, or other instruments in the right upper abdominal quadrant or displacement of the liver can cause a drop in blood pressure by compression of the inferior vena cava and impedance to venous blood return. If invasive monitoring is used, the decrease in venous return is indicated by a rapid fall in filling pressures. Mechanical obstruction of the inferior vena cava should be promptly identified and relieved; treatment with fluids and vasopressors is seldom needed.

Reflex Mechanisms

Hypotension may follow traction and manipulation of the biliary tract, colon, uterus and ovaries, and parietal peritoneum.[62] If a patient is conscious during regional anesthesia, such maneuvers can also cause discomfort, nausea, and vomiting. The decrease in blood pressure caused by manipulation of intra-abdominal structures is associated with bradycardia in about 50% of patients.[62] Bradycardia is sometimes severe and appears to be the primary event that causes the reduction in blood pressure.[63]

These hemodynamic changes are usually ascribed to a reflex

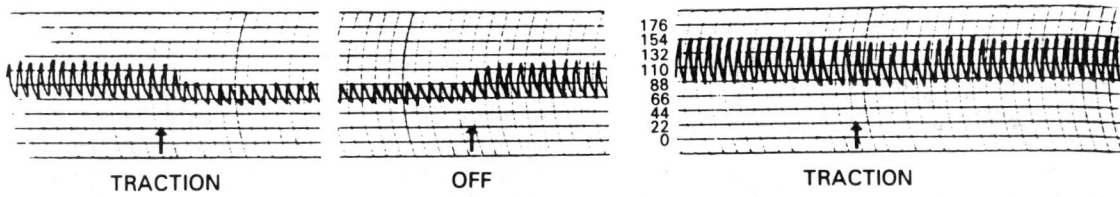

FIGURE 65–2. Continuous arterial pressure recordings during traction on the transverse colon (measured in mm Hg). Traction produced an immediate fall in blood pressure from 122/66 to 87/57, but the heart rate remained unchanged *(left tracing).* Note the prompt return to the control blood pressure upon release of traction *(middle tracing).* The *third tracing* illustrates the effect of similar traction after separation of the colon from its mesentery. The rapid changes in blood pressure when the stimulus was applied and released and the unchanged blood pressure after the mesentery was severed strongly suggest a reflex mechanism. (From Eather KF, Peterson LH, Dripps RD: Studies of circulation of anesthetized patients by new method for recording arterial pressure and pressure pulser contours. Anesthesiology 1949; 10:125.)

mechanism (Fig. 65–2). Impulses conducted by visceral and somatic pathways are postulated to increase parasympathetic tone or inhibit sympathetic activity. The ensuing hypotension is secondary to a decrease in heart rate or vasodilation in the splanchnic area, with blood pooling and decreased venous return.

Severe reflex bradycardia during intra-abdominal procedures seems to occur more commonly than in the past, particularly in younger patients who have greater vagal tone.[64] This observation probably is explained by the fact that in modern anesthesia practice, drugs with vagolytic activity (atropine, gallamine, pancuronium) are less frequently used, whereas opioids with vagotonic effects are commonly administered. As a consequence, the effects on the heart of vagal reflexes elicited during surgery are not only unopposed but also facilitated.

Humoral Mechanisms

Hypotension caused by systemic vasodilation and associated with a compensatory increase in heart rate and cardiac output characteristically follows traction on the small bowel mesentery.[65] These changes are commonly observed in patients undergoing aortic surgery when the small bowel is exteriorized and retractors are placed to expose the abdominal aorta (Table 65–2). In addition to the hemodynamic changes, about two-thirds of patients develop marked flushing of the skin in the head and neck areas. The greatest changes in blood pressure and heart rate occur 5 to 10 minutes after mesenteric traction and persist 30 minutes or longer. Pretreatment with aspirin and ibuprofen is effective in preventing these hemodynamic changes, supporting the hypothesis that they are mediated by intestinal release of prostacyclin.[66, 67]

TABLE 65–2. Hemodynamic Measurements and Derived Data (Means ± SD) Before and After Mesenteric Traction in 20 Patients Undergoing Aortic Surgery*

Hemodynamic Parameters	Premesenteric Traction	Postmesenteric Traction
Heart rate (beats per minute)	66.6 ± 13.7	77.3 ± 16.8
Mean arterial pressure (mm Hg)	105 ± 20	81 ± 19
Cardiac output (L · min⁻¹)	5.81 ± 1.93	7.66 ± 2.29
Stroke volume (mL)	88 ± 25	100 ± 22
Central venous pressure (mm Hg)	11 ± 4.7	9.7 ± 5.1
Pulmonary artery occlusion pressure (mm Hg)	17.9 ± 6.2	15.7 ± 5.8
Systemic vascular resistance (dynes · s · cm⁻⁵)	1423 ± 504	839 ± 405

(Modified from Seltzer JL, Ritter DE, Starsnic MA, et al: The hemodynamic response to traction on the abdominal mesentery. Anesthesiology 1985; 63:96.)
*All changes were statistically significant.

How Is It Treated?

When serious hemodynamic changes of reflex origin occur, any surgical maneuver should stop promptly. Treatment of severe bradycardia with intravenous atropine is preferable to glycopyrrolate because of its more rapid rate of onset.[68] If the heart rate is normal, ephedrine effectively restores blood pressure. Hypotension and tachycardia due to mesenteric traction may require fluid and phenylephrine administration.

NITROUS OXIDE AND BOWEL DISTENTION

Why Does It Occur?

The bowel contains variable proportions of nitrogen, hydrogen, and methane.[69] These gases are much less soluble in the blood than is nitrous oxide. When nitrous oxide is respired, it can enter the intestinal lumen far more readily than nitrogen and the other gases can be removed from it. As a result, the bowel, having highly compliant walls, increases its volume.

Concentration and Duration of Administration

The change in bowel volume depends on the nitrous oxide concentration and duration of administration. When 70% nitrous oxide is administered, a twofold increase in intestinal gas volume occurs in 2 hours, and up to a threefold increase occurs by 4 hours (Fig. 65–3). Bowel volume progressively increases until equilibrium is reached between the concentration of nitrous oxide in the blood and bowel lumen, a process that takes 5 to 6 hours. Should the administration of 70% nitrous oxide continue until equilibrium is reached, the bowel volume would at most increase fourfold.[70]

When nitrous oxide concentration is limited to 50%, the increase in volume is less; should nitrous oxide administration continue until equilibrium, the volume of intestinal gas doubles at most. Discontinuation of nitrous oxide reverses the gas expansion, but bowel deflation takes place slowly[71] (Fig. 65–4).

Is It a Problem in Normal Patients?

The potential for intestinal distention with nitrous oxide in normal persons is very limited. The intestine usually contains <200 mL of gas, mainly in the stomach and colon.[69] Even tripling this volume, which takes several hours, causes only a moderate expansion of the intestine; how this modest increase

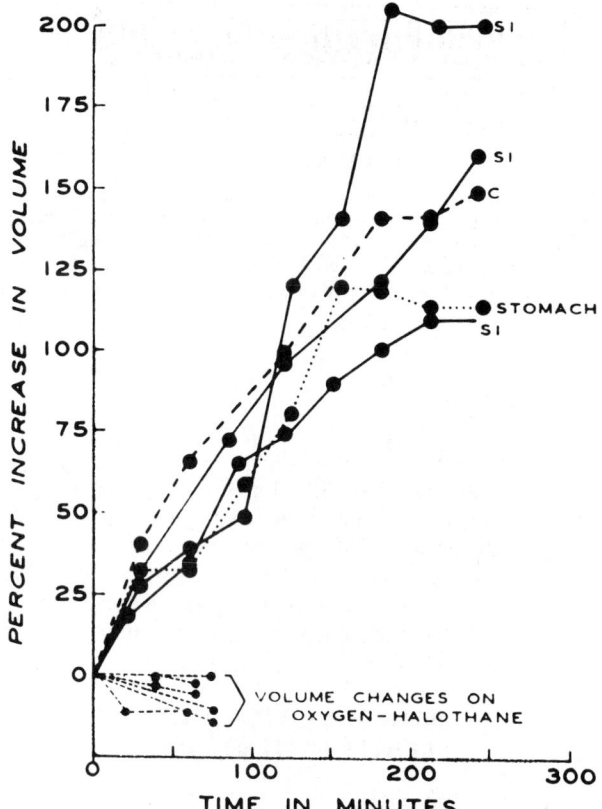

FIGURE 65–3. Changes in intestinal gas volume as a per cent of original volume with administration of 70% nitrous oxide *(large dots)* compared with the administration of halothane and oxygen *(small dots)*. The experiments were performed in isolated segments of animal stomach, small bowel (SI), and colon (C) into which a measured volume of air was injected. The animals were then given nitrous oxide to breathe. The volume changes in the bowel were then measured at intervals. (From Eger EI, Saidman LJ: Hazards of nitrous oxide anesthesia in bowel obstruction and pneumothorax. Anesthesiology 1965; 26:61.)

would interfere with exposure, closure, or ventilation is difficult to envisage.

A distended stomach, sometimes encountered at the beginning of a celiotomy, should be decompressed by inserting a nasogastric tube and does not pose a contraindication to the use of nitrous oxide. A distended bowel is occasionally noted when the abdomen is opened. In such patients, nitrous oxide concentration should be limited to 50% or the agent discontinued.

Can Nitrous Oxide Be Used with Intestinal Obstruction?

Nitrous oxide administration to patients with intestinal obstruction is more problematic. Further dilation of an already distended intestine carries several risks and should be avoided. Nitrous oxide, however, expands the bowel slowly, and the dilation observed during the first hour of administration is probably of little clinical relevance (see Fig. 65–4). According to Eger and Saidman, "It would seem prudent to consider bowel obstruction as a relative contraindication to nitrous oxide at inspired concentration exceeding 50%, particularly if it is anticipated that anesthesia will be prolonged."[70]

Nitrous oxide, therefore, is still acceptable in a patient with

bowel obstruction, provided it is administered for a short time (i.e., until the abdomen is open), the cause of the intestinal obstruction has been determined, and a plan has been made to relieve it. In most cases of severe abdominal obstruction, the surgeon effects some kind of decompression of the intestine (long intestinal tube or enterotomy) before proceeding to the rest of the operation. If the planned procedure is of long duration, nitrous oxide may be avoided, used in a concentration not exceeding 50%, or used only as an aid during induction and emergence.

NARCOTIC ADMINISTRATION AND BILIARY SPASM

Opioid analgesics such as morphine, meperidine, and fentanyl are known to cause contraction of the choledochoduodenal sphincter (sphincter of Oddi) and an increase in intrabiliary pressure. This effect, also present during anesthesia with potent inhaled agents, is promptly reversed by naloxone.[72] The agonist-antagonist agents butorphanol and nalbuphine have only negligible effects on the sphincter of Oddi.[72–74]

Is It a Problem?

Most surgeons operating on the biliary tract routinely perform intraoperative cholangiography to detect stones in the common bile duct and verify its patency. Narcotics are considered by many individuals to be contraindicated during biliary tract surgery because they may cause an intense contraction of the sphincter of Oddi. The resulting interference with the pas-

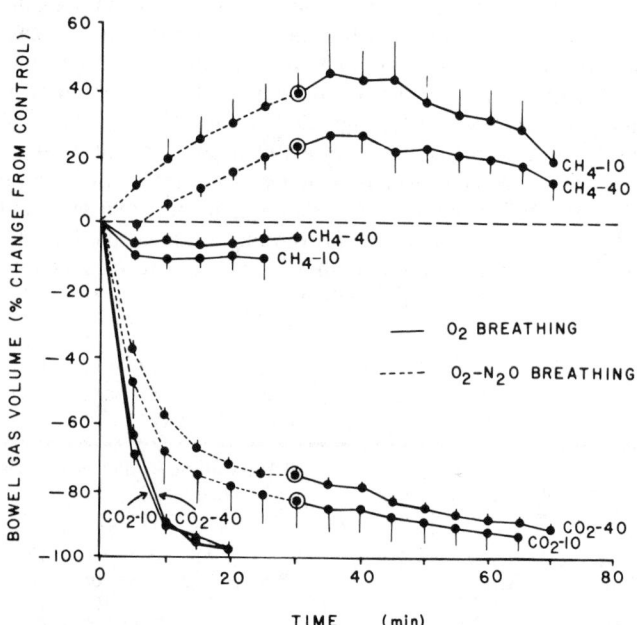

FIGURE 65–4. Effect of 100% O_2 or 21% O_2-balanced N_2O (O_2-N_2O) administration on bowel gas volume. Four bowel segments are represented, each of which was initially injected with 10 mL (ambient temperature and pressure, dry) or 40 mL of methane (CH_4-10, CH_4-40) or carbon dioxide (CO_2-10, CO_2-40). The changeover from O_2-N_2O to O_2 breathing at 30 minutes is indicated by a *circle*. The X ± SEM of the results from four dogs are given. (From Steffey EP, Johnson BH, Eger EI II, et al: Nitrous oxide: effect on accumulation rate and uptake of bowel gases. Anesth Analg 1979; 58:407.)

sage of contrast from the common bile duct into the duodenum can thereby simulate a mechanical obstruction, potentially leading to an unnecessary exploration of the biliary tract.

This concern seems largely unfounded. Surgeons are well aware that the contrast material may fail to enter the duodenum because of a spasm of the sphincter. This event is characterized radiologically by a smoothly tapered distal sphincter and a bile duct of normal diameter.[75] Failure of the dye to enter the duodenum as an isolated finding does not represent an indication for surgical exploration of the biliary tract. It must be associated with stones or other signs of long-standing mechanical obstruction such as a dilated common bile duct. Narcotics obviously do not have anything to do with these latter pathologic findings.

Are Other Factors Responsible?

The incidence of spasm of the sphincter of Oddi during operative cholangiography is low. Even when a fentanyl-based anesthetic was used, a spasm was detected in only about 3% of the patients.[76] The cause of this spasm is not clear. In addition to narcotics, surgical manipulation and the irritant effect of the contrast dye have been cited. When spasm of the sphincter of Oddi is suspected, administration of glucagon or cholecystokinin is invariable, followed by relaxation and flow of contrast medium into the duodenum.[75] Naloxone and nalbuphine[77] may be used if spasm is thought to be related to a previously administered opioid; they do not resolve spasm induced by other factors.

NASOGASTRIC TUBES

What Types Are Available?

Single Lumen

Nasogastric tubes are used to decompress the stomach by removing fluid and gas. A Levin tube is a single-lumen tube, the major drawback of which is that suction can be applied only intermittently. If continuous suction is applied, once the stomach is empty, the gastric mucosa is sucked into the distal orifice and occludes it. As a consequence, fluid or air that reaccumulates in the stomach cannot be removed.

Double Lumen

More popular but not necessarily more effective are nasogastric tubes designed to be used with continuous suction.[78] These tubes have a double lumen, one for suction and one, the ''sump,'' that is left open to ambient air. When continuous suction is applied and the stomach is empty, the sump lumen allows air to enter the stomach, preventing the gastric mucosa from obstructing the tube. A sucking sound around the proximal port of the sump lumen signals that the tube is properly functioning. Should fluid reaccumulate, air entrainment stops until the fluid has been suctioned out.

In elective abdominal surgery, the nasogastric tube is usually placed after induction of anesthesia for a patient's comfort, whereas in emergency procedures, a patient arrives in the operating room with a nasogastric tube already in place. Only the placement of gastric tubes in tracheally intubated and anesthetized patients is discussed here.

When Is the Tube Inserted Through the Mouth?

A gastric tube is usually placed through the nose, but if it is to be removed at the end of surgery, the oral route is preferred to avoid epistaxis. The oral route is also indicated in the presence of basal skull fractures to prevent accidental intracranial introduction[79] or when nasal deformities or facial fractures make transit through the nose impossible.

Are They Contraindicated in Patients with Esophageal Varices?

Placement of a gastric tube in patients with portal hypertension and esophageal varices is often considered to be contraindicated because of fear of variceal bleeding. Recent data indicate that this fear is largely unfounded, however, and patients with esophageal varices should not be denied the benefits of a nasogastric tube.[80] Obviously, utmost care is recommended.

How Are They Inserted?

Before insertion, a deep level of anesthesia or, preferably, intense neuromuscular block should be present to prevent straining and backing. When succinylcholine is used during induction of anesthesia, the nasogastric tube should be inserted either immediately after the endotracheal tube has been secured or delayed until neuromuscular block from the maintenance nondepolarizing agent is well established. If the gastric tube is placed later, deep neuromuscular block (i.e., no more than one twitch using a train-of-four count) keeps the patient from moving in response to this stimulus.

Technique

A nasogastric tube, properly lubricated, is inserted through the largest naris and advanced perpendicularly to the floor of the nasal cavity in an anteroposterior direction. Resistance is sometimes met in the posterior pharynx because the tube does not negotiate the sharp angle between the nasopharynx and oropharynx. If the resistance is not overcome by gentle manipulation, the tip of the tube can be retrieved in proximity to the soft palate and directed into the oropharynx by the operator's index finger.

Most of the time, the tube advances easily into the stomach. Proper position is confirmed by return of gastric juice with aspiration or by gastric palpation when the abdomen is open. The tube is then secured by a mesentery or umbilical bridge, thereby avoiding any pressure on the nostrils (Fig. 65–5).

Why Does the Ventilator Sometimes Alarm?

During attempts to negotiate a gastric tube in the esophagus of a mechanically ventilated patient, gas volume may sometimes be lost from the breathing circuit, the low-pressure alarm of the ventilator may sound, or the bellows may actually collapse, especially when the tube is attached to suction. These problems occur when the gastric tube accidentally enters the trachea, causing the air leak both around the endotracheal tube cuff and through the tube itself. Removal and repositioning solve the problem.

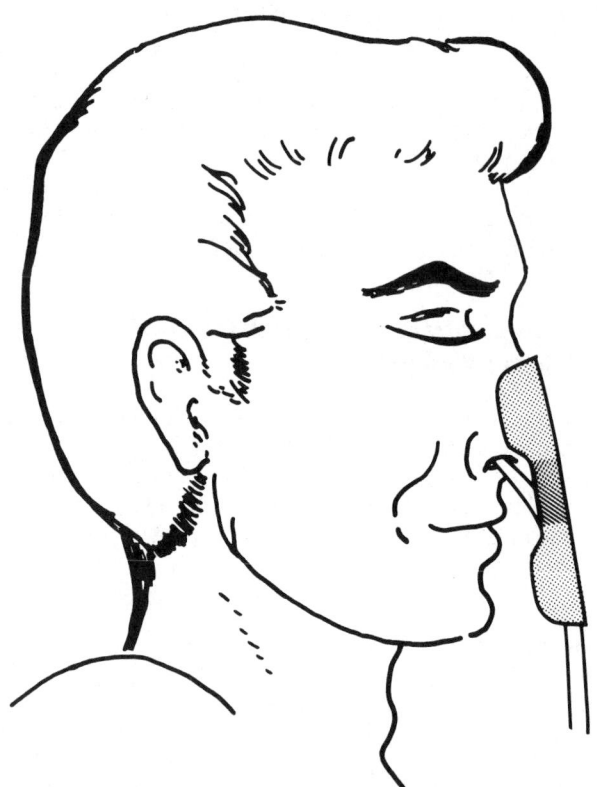

FIGURE 65–5. Umbilical bridge. Pinching the midsection of a strip of 1-inch tape so that it sticks to itself creates an umbilical bridge that allows the practitioner to secure a nasogastric tube to the nose without applying pressure to the tip of the nose. (From Guyton DC: Oral, nasopharyngeal, and gastrointestinal systems. *In* Manual of Complications during Anesthesia. Gravenstein N (ed). Philadelphia, JB Lippincott, 1991, p 632.)

What Can the Anesthesiologist Do To Pass a Tube That Won't?

Should the tube fail to enter the esophagus, several maneuvers may be attempted. If an esophageal stethoscope or other probe is already in place, it should be removed, then replaced after the nasogastric tube has been inserted. These tubes are sufficiently flexible that if their plastic surface contacts that of another, they stick and coil rather than advance.

A patient's head can also be turned to the side, or the thyroid cartilage can be grasped between the thumb and index finger and lifted anteriorly while the gastric tube is advanced. These maneuvers open an esophagus that is normally collapsed by gravity.[81] Should they fail, a laryngoscope is inserted into the oropharynx, the esophageal opening is visualized, and the tube is pushed in, possibly with the help of Magill's forceps.

Another technique uses a nasoesophageally placed endotracheal tube.[82] A 7.5-mm-internal diameter endotracheal tube with the connector removed is cut lengthwise along one side and inserted through the nose into the esophagus. A lubricated 18 French nasogastric tube is then passed through the lumen of the endotracheal tube into the stomach. The endotracheal tube is removed from the nose and, having been previously split, peeled away from the nasogastric tube.

How Is a Long Tube Passed?

A surgeon may sometimes wish to decompress a greatly distended bowel at the beginning of the procedure. Decompression can be accomplished by advancing a long tube from the stomach along the entire length of the small bowel to the ileocecal valve while suction is continuously applied.[83] The tube, approximately 120 inches long, is introduced into the stomach through the nose or mouth, depending on whether it is to be left in position. One or sometimes two balloons are present at the distal end and are inflated with air or water once the tube is in the stomach. This process enables the surgeon to grasp the tube and advance it past the pylorus into the small bowel. Once the tube is in place, the balloon(s) must be deflated.

RAPID-SEQUENCE INDUCTION IN EMERGENCY ABDOMINAL SURGERY

Patients requiring emergency abdominal surgery have a ''full stomach'' and therefore are at risk for pulmonary aspiration should regurgitation or vomiting occur during induction of anesthesia. These patients seldom have food in the stomach because vomiting is common. Gastric contents usually represent GI secretions, fecaloid fluid when bowel obstruction is present, or blood.

In these patients, a rapid-sequence induction technique[84] combined with cricoid pressure is indicated.[85] However, before initiating a rapid sequence, the anesthesiologist needs to assess a patient's anatomy to verify that tracheal intubation using conventional laryngoscopy is feasible. If uncertainty exists, awake intubation with local anesthesia may be the safest method to secure the airway.

Should the Patient Be Ventilated?

During rapid-sequence induction, mask ventilation before tracheal intubation is believed to be contraindicated by many anesthesiologists because positive-pressure ventilation may cause gastric insufflation and increases the chance of regurgitation. In addition, it is feared that should regurgitation occur mask ventilation can ''push'' the regurgitated material into the airways. However, properly applied cricoid pressure completely occludes the esophagus, preventing passive fluid regurgitation, and keeps air from being pushed into the stomach.[85–87] In this circumstance, *gentle* mask ventilation does not seem contraindicated.[85, 87]

Some patients, despite protracted preoxygenation, very rapidly develop hypoxemia when apneic during a conventional rapid-sequence induction.[88] Obesity, lung disease, and abdominal distention due to bowel obstruction or ascites greatly decrease the functional residual capacity (FRC) and hence the amount of oxygen (O_2) available when ventilation stops. To avoid hypoxemia, these patients may require a ''modified'' rapid-sequence induction, in which mask ventilation with O_2 is performed before intubation while cricoid pressure is continuously applied.

What Is Done If a Nasogastric Tube Is In Place?

Most of the time, patients have a nasogastric tube in place that should be suctioned before induction. It is then left open to ambient or connected to a continuous suction, if it is a sump type. However, this procedure does not guarantee that the stomach is empty.

Whether a nasogastric tube should be removed before induction is controversial. A gastric tube does not interfere with an adequate esophageal seal when cricoid pressure is applied.[86] In addition, it can act as a blow-off valve should intragastric pressure suddenly increase while cricoid pressure is applied (Fig. 65–6).[89]

A nasogastric tube, however, makes an airtight mask fit difficult and therefore may interfere with adequate preinduction oxygenation and mask ventilation. Hence, removal may be preferable when mask ventilation is likely because of low O_2 reserve (decreased FRC), high O_2 consumption (sepsis), or potentially difficult intubation.

Should Cricoid Pressure Be Released If the Patient Vomits?

Cricoid pressure should immediately be released if a patient actively vomits, lest esophageal rupture occur.[85, 90] Vomiting, which requires powerful abdominal contractions, should rarely if ever occur during rapid-sequence induction if succinylcholine is administered through a freely running intravenous catheter immediately after the intravenous induction agent.[85]

INTRAOPERATIVE FLUID MANAGEMENT

What Is the Preoperative Deficit and Basal Fluid Requirement?

The amount of fluid administered intraoperatively consists of the basal requirements, replacement of deficits incurred before anesthesia, and replacement of intraoperative losses. In adults, basal fluid requirements amount to 75 to 100 mL $\cdot$ h^{-1}

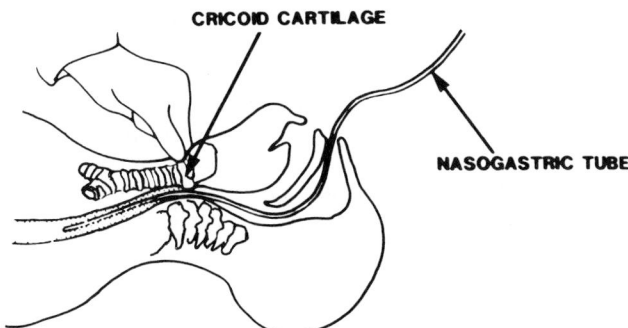

FIGURE 65–6. Firmly applied cricoid pressure is effective in sealing the esophagus around an esophageal tube against an intraesophageal pressure of up to 100 cm H_2O. (Modified from Salem MR, Joseph NJ, Heyman HJ, et al: Cricoid compression is effective in obliterating the esophageal lumen in the presence of a nasogastric tube. Anesthesiology 1985; 63:444.)

and represent the water needed for urine production and to replace that evaporated through the skin and lungs.[91] Pre-existing fluid deficits in patients undergoing elective surgery are caused by the 8 to 10 hours of preoperative fasting and total 500 to 750 mL.[92] Preoperative fluid deficits encountered in patients with acute intra-abdominal pathology are often significantly larger and should be replaced as much as possible before surgery (see Chapter 42).

What Is the Intraoperative Fluid Deficit?

Intraoperative water losses result from evaporation through the exposed surface of the bowel and humidification of dry respiratory gases. These losses usually are negligible. Additional loss that can be easily measured is represented by the fluid drained through the nasogastric tube.

What Are Third Space Losses?

More important is the extracellular fluid (ECF) that is lost internally in the so-called third space, the anatomic identity of which is unclear but includes the interstitial space in the wound and other areas traumatized during surgery. The amount of fluid accumulated in the third space is variable and depends in part on the severity of surgical dissection or trauma.[93] Most studies suggest that 1500 to 2000 mL of crystalloids is adequate to compensate for the fluid lost in the third space.[94–97]

How Are Fluids Replaced?

The total amount of fluids required for most abdominal procedures, in the absence of significant blood loss, is 2000 to 3000 mL, usually supplied as lactated Ringer's solution. Deficits due to fasting are quickly replaced just before or during anesthesia induction, and the rest is infused at a rate of 8 to 10 mL $\cdot$ kg^{-1} $\cdot$ h^{-1} of surgery. In addition, 2 or 3 mL of lactated Ringer's is infused for each milliliter of blood lost, until the blood loss has reached 800 to 1000 mL (15–20% of the circulatory volume). Should blood loss continue, packed red blood cells or additional crystalloids or colloids need to be administered. These guidelines are general; the amount and type of fluid administered may vary considerably according to specific clinical situations. The goal of fluid administration is to maintain stable hemodynamic function with adequate organ perfusion.

Limiting the volume of intraoperative fluids to what really is needed is based on two considerations. First, excess fluid is retained and accumulates as edema in the skin and other organs such as the intestine and skeletal muscle.[98] A growing consensus suggests that such edema may not be completely benign, as was previously thought.[99, 100] Second, retained fluids are mobilized on the second to third postoperative day and returned to the vascular compartment. Although mobilized fluids are well handled by patients with a normal heart and kidneys, pulmonary edema may occur should the cardiovascular system be unable to tolerate the increase in intravascular volume or the kidneys be unable to increase urine output.

USEFUL RULES OF THUMB

To maintain hemodynamic function and organ perfusion without excessive expansion of the ECF compartment, the following considerations may be useful:

1. If the procedure lasts several hours, not because of its inherent complexity but because the surgeon is particularly slow or the report on a specimen sent for tissue diagnosis is greatly delayed, for example, the hourly fluid rate should be decreased.

2. Low blood pressure during periods of minimal surgical stimulation probably is better treated by lightening the anesthetic or administering a vasopressor than by administering a fluid bolus.

3. If large amounts of crystalloids (i.e., >4000 mL) have been given in the absence of significant blood loss and the circulation is still unstable, colloids should be considered to minimize tissue edema.[101]

4. Colloids are useful to replace blood loss in elderly patients and in patients with cardiac diseases to decrease the fluid load and thus the risk of postoperative edema.

5. An hourly urinary output of >1 mL $\cdot$ kg^{-1} suggests that the fluid rate can be decreased.

6. Intraoperative oliguria (i.e., urinary output <0.5 mL $\cdot$ kg^{-1} $\cdot$ h^{-1}) does not always mean that the fluid rate needs to be increased. The first step is to rule out compression or kinking of the urine collecting system. A sudden drop in urine output can often be observed when a patient is placed in a steep head-down position. As a result, the bladder neck is moved uppermost, and urine pools at the bottom of the bladder rather than flowing through the Foley catheter into the collecting system. This situation does not require treatment; brisk flow of urine is observed when a patient's position is returned to horizontal.

In evaluating fluid replacement, observe the hemodynamic changes that occur over time (i.e., the trend rather than the absolute values) and resist the temptation to treat ''the numbers'' instead of the patient. For instance, a central venous pressure (CVP) of 3 mm Hg that has not changed in a patient with normal blood pressure, pulse rate, and adequate urinary output does not require treatment. Conversely, a drop in CVP from 9 to 6 mm Hg associated with sudden blood loss requires prompt intervention even if the blood pressure and heart rate have not changed significantly.

What Is Normovolemic Oliguria?

Intraoperative oliguria is often caused by hypovolemia but sometimes occurs in patients with normal kidneys, hemodynamics, and blood volume.[102] This ''normovolemic'' oliguria is a benign phenomenon that does not indicate poor kidney perfusion, nor is it associated with postoperative renal failure.[103, 104]

Low urinary output in the presence of normal kidney perfusion and adequate hydration probably is a consequence of the combined effects of the anesthetic agents and the neurohumoral changes set in motion by surgical trauma.[105] Normal urinary output resumes soon after completion of anesthesia.

If the volume status is uncertain, a bolus of 500 mL of crystalloid is administered over 5 to 10 minutes. Should urine output increase, the diagnosis of hypovolemia is confirmed

and additional fluid may be required.[102] If the urine output remains scanty after the fluid bolus and all else seems stable, normovolemic oliguria is likely. One may then do nothing, or a small dose (5 mg) of furosemide can be administered intravenously. Urine production generally increases within 15 to 20 minutes.

What Is the Effect of Preoperative Bowel Preparation?

In patients undergoing colon and rectal surgery, preoperatively cleansing the bowel of fecal material is important to decrease septic complications. The bowel can be effectively cleansed by oral administration of balanced electrolyte solutions to which osmotically active substances such as mannitol or polyethylene glycol are added. These solutions promptly cause watery diarrhea and are usually administered over several hours in large volumes until the rectal effluent is clear.

Fluid Deficits and Excesses

Depending on the composition of the solution, a positive or a negative fluid balance may result owing to water and electrolytes translocation through the intestinal mucosa.[106] Neither event is desirable; fluid absorption may result in hypervolemia and pulmonary edema, whereas fluid loss may cause hypovolemia and hypotension.

Currently, an electrolyte solution containing polyethylene glycol (marketed under the appropriate but inaccurate name of GoLytely) has gained widespread popularity because it leaves the fluid balance virtually unaffected. Water and electrolytes are neither absorbed nor secreted from the bowel.[107]

Patients treated with this solution usually do not manifest hypovolemia or hemodynamic instability during induction of anesthesia. This solution offers the additional advantage of not containing mannitol, which has been associated with explosions during surgery of the colon as a result of fermentation to hydrogen by intestinal bacteria.[108]

How Is Management Changed by Acute Intra-Abdominal Pathology?

Patients with acute intra-abdominal pathology often present with significant ECF deficits and electrolyte imbalance. External losses are secondary to vomiting, prolonged nasogastric suction, diarrhea, and intestinal fistulas. If the fluid lost is predominantly gastric juice, hypochloremic, hypokalemic metabolic alkalosis results. Potassium is present in the gastric juice, but the main reason for hypokalemia in vomiting is renal excretion as H$^+$ ions are conserved. The loss of intestinal and pancreatic juice, containing bicarbonate, tends to produce metabolic acidosis.

Where Does the Fluid Go?

Internal fluid losses occur in bowel obstruction, peritonitis, and acute pancreatitis. Bowel obstruction fluid, which is similar to plasma in protein and electrolyte content, accumulates in the intestinal lumen above the obstruction and in the walls of the involved bowel.

Peritonitis is associated with the loss of plasma-like fluid as edema of the parietal and visceral peritoneum and as exudate into the peritoneal cavity. Additional fluid loss occurs into the atonic bowel that invariably accompanies peritonitis. When the vascular supply to the bowel is compromised owing to strangulation or thromboembolism of the intestinal vessels, a significant amount of blood can extravasate into the wall and lumen of the necrotic bowel, further decreasing the circulating volume.

In acute pancreatitis, large amounts of fluid are sequestered in the retroperitoneal space and in the inflamed peritoneal cavity. In the hemorrhagic form of pancreatitis, a large amount of blood is also lost internally.

Fluid loss via the GI tract causes ECF contraction, the magnitude of which depends on the underlying disease process and its duration. Volume depletion is particularly severe in extensive peritonitis and pancreatitis, because of the large areas involved in the inflammatory process, and in bowel obstruction, because of both external and internal losses. Small bowel obstruction in this respect is more serious than large bowel obstruction because fluid losses are larger and progress more rapidly. The ECF volume reduction may eventually lead to shock with hypotension, tachycardia, and oliguria. Obvious signs of hypovolemia indicate an ECF deficit in excess of 20% to 25%.

Replacement

Fluid deficits secondary to GI pathology are replaced with lactated Ringer's solution or, if gastric juice loss is prominent, normal saline, because of its high chloride content. Potassium chloride is added when adequate urinary output is established.

Estimation of Deficit

The ECF deficit and, therefore, the volume of fluid replacement is difficult to estimate. A decrease in body weight represents external fluid losses but obviously does not provide information about the amount of internal fluid sequestration. Also, the body weight before dehydration took place frequently is unknown. In the absence of hemorrhage, the hematocrit increases in proportion to the ECF deficit. If the hematocrit before and after the fluid loss is known, calculation of the deficit is possible.[109]

Plasma electrolyte determinations give an idea of alterations in composition but not of the ECF volume deficit. In practice, according to the severity of the illness, several liters of crystalloids are rapidly infused after placement of a central catheter for pressure monitoring.

Adequacy of Replacement

Fluids are administered until the blood pressure, heart rate, heart filling pressures, and hourly urinary output have reached satisfactory values. Re-establishment of adequate perfusion is also indicated by warm dry skin, brisk capillary refill, improvement of metabolic acidosis, and an increase in cardiac output and mixed venous O_2 saturation. Blood pressure, heart rate, and heart filling pressures can be normal despite a considerable volume depletion.[110] Fluids are administered until the CVP and pulmonary artery occlusion pressures (PAOP) are 10 to 12 mm Hg and 15 to 18 mm Hg, respectively, and further

250-mL fluid boluses cause an excessive increase in filling pressures.

Another method to assess the adequacy of the circulatory volume is to measure blood pressure and heart rate changes in response to postural stress.[111] When a patient arises from a supine to a sitting position with both legs horizontal and the chest at an angle of 45°, an increase in heart rate of 10 beats per minute associated with a fall in blood pressure ≥15 mm Hg indicates a persistent volume deficit. Additional fluids are administered until the hemodynamic changes with alterations in posture are minimal.

Colloid Administration

Patients with peritonitis, ischemic bowel, or protracted bowel obstruction suffer large losses of protein-rich fluids. If they remain unstable despite large volumes of crystalloids, colloids such as 6% hetastarch or 5% albumin may be beneficial.

A combination of crystalloids and colloids should also be considered for elderly patients, in whom more rapid replenishment of the circulatory volume and re-establishment of adequate organ perfusion may be desirable. This combination also may be useful for patients with pre-existing cardiac disease to limit the volume of fluid required. With correction of the fluid deficit and plasma volume, the hematocrit may drop significantly, revealing pre-existent anemia or blood sequestration; blood transfusion may then be indicated.

Timing of Replacement

Patients who have incurred large fluid and plasma losses must be resuscitated as adequately as possible before induction of anesthesia. Otherwise, a dramatic fall in blood pressure will be associated with the loss of sympathetic tone and vasodilatation. The induction of anesthesia for emergency surgery should be delayed while crystalloids or colloids or both are rapidly infused. This preinduction volume resuscitation can usually be accomplished in <15 minutes. Although surgery is urgent, the extra time invested in stabilizing a patient before anesthesia may avert a disaster.

ACUTE GASTROINTESTINAL BLEEDING

Patients with GI bleeding require emergency surgery when they manifest persistent or recurrent bleeding despite conservative treatment, including endoscopic electrocoagulation or laser coagulation, selective intra-arterial vasopressin infusion, and transcatheter arterial embolization. These patients are almost invariably hypovolemic, often hypotensive or in frank shock, and require intravascular volume resuscitation before anesthesia can be safely induced.

What Should Be Done Before Induction?

The first step in management of hemorrhagic patients is to establish adequate venous access, preferably by placing two large-bore cannulas. The second step is to estimate the severity of blood loss and resuscitation needs based on blood pressure, heart rate, mental status, capillary refill, urinary output, and so on. Hemoglobin concentration is of no use in assessing blood volume status in patients who are acutely bleeding or in those who have been bleeding intermittently for 24 to 48 hours and have received multiple transfusions.

Patients with hypotension, tachycardia, apprehension, or mental cloudiness have lost at least 30% of their blood volume and require prompt resuscitation with crystalloids or colloids and blood.[112] Usually, 2 L of crystalloid is rapidly infused, followed by 2 units of blood. The situation is then re-evaluated, and additional fluids or blood is administered until a satisfactory blood pressure and heart rate are obtained. Colloids are also recommended because they allow a more rapid and sustained restoration of blood volume, cardiac output, and organ perfusion.[113]

Patients with less hemodynamic compromise are initially resuscitated with crystalloids or colloids; blood administration is less urgent. While volume resuscitation takes place, arterial and central venous catheters are placed for pressure monitoring and acid-base evaluation. After the blood volume has been restored, hemoglobin or hematocrit is measured to assess the need for additional blood transfusion.

How Should Anesthesia Be Induced?

Once adequate hemodynamics have been obtained, anesthesia is carefully induced with the agent of choice (e.g., etomidate, ketamine, or thiopental). The latter drug is used in a reduced dose, while the blood pressure is closely watched and additional fluids are promptly administered should it decrease. A rapid-sequence induction is mandatory.

Patients with acute GI bleeding sometimes arrive in the operating room with normal blood pressure and heart rate. By no means should this observation be considered proof of normovolemia. Younger patients in particular can compensate surprisingly well for a loss of up to 20% of their blood volume.[114] Induction of anesthesia in patients with compensated contraction of blood volume may be followed by a dramatic decline in blood pressure.

A prudent approach is to expand the circulatory volume rapidly just before induction of anesthesia by infusing 1 or 2 L of crystalloids to compensate for any hidden volume deficit. Anesthesia is then induced following the same precautions previously outlined.

What Should Be Done Intraoperatively?

Fluid resuscitation continues intraoperatively according to blood pressure, heart filling pressures, urinary output, and other clinical signs. These patients commonly have concurrent medical problems such as cirrhosis, sepsis, and renal failure that may compound the coagulopathy associated with massive blood loss. A coagulation profile should therefore be obtained at the earliest opportunity, and fresh-frozen plasma (FFP) and platelets administered as needed.

SPLENECTOMY

The majority of elective splenectomies are performed for hematologic diseases.[115] Conditions in which splenectomy may be beneficial include hemolytic anemias, idiopathic thrombocytopenic purpura, hypersplenism, and leukemias. In Hodg-

kin's disease, a staging laparotomy is performed, including splenectomy, liver biopsy, and abdominal lymph nodes sampling.

Patients scheduled for splenectomy, depending on the underlying pathology, may suffer from anemia, thrombocytopenia, and other coagulation disorders. Close cooperation with the surgeon and the hematologist is essential to make them ready for surgery. These patients also may have received recent chemotherapy, the implications of which should be recognized.

Removal of a spleen of normal size is usually an uncomplicated procedure. If the spleen is large, particularly in the presence of portal hypertension, intraoperative bleeding may be significant; venous access adequate for rapid volume replacement and transfusion is required.

When Should Platelet Transfusion Occur?

Patients presenting for splenectomy may be extremely thrombocytopenic. Thus, a preoperative platelet transfusion would seem advantageous. However, because the spleen is normally the cause of thrombocytopenia, platelet administration before ligation of the splenic artery is futile. If the platelet count is $<20,000 \cdot mm^{3-1}$ or bleeding is thought related to a platelet deficiency, infusion of platelets is reasonable after splenic artery ligation. The infused platelets will have a clinical effect within minutes of administration, and because the spleen has been removed, will have a normal life span of about 10 days.

OBSTRUCTIVE JAUNDICE

Patients with obstructive jaundice (cholestasis) present three problems.

1. Vitamin K malabsorption leads to coagulopathy with an increased prothrombin time (PT) secondary to a deficit of vitamin K–dependent clotting factors. Patients with obstructive jaundice are routinely treated for 2 to 3 days preoperatively with intramuscular vitamin K to normalize the PT. FFP should be used only in those patients who do not respond to vitamin K treatment.

2. Cholestasis modifies the pharmacokinetics of pancuronium and vecuronium.

3. Patients with obstructive jaundice are at increased risk of postoperative renal failure. Acute renal failure occurs in 5% to 10% of patients undergoing surgery for relief of obstructive jaundice. It is associated with a 75% mortality in this setting.[116] The risk of renal failure seems related to the severity of jaundice, particularly when bilirubin levels are $>12 \, mg \cdot dL^{-1}$.[116, 117]

Why Does Renal Failure Occur?

A number of studies have examined the effects of jaundice on renal function.[116, 118, 119] Overall, renal function and renal blood flow do not seem significantly altered by obstructive jaundice, per se. The mechanisms leading to kidney failure after surgery for obstructive jaundice remain uncertain.[116] A decrease in the ECF volume,[120] increased sensitivity of the kidneys to an ischemic insult,[121] and endotoxemia[116] have been suggested. Even if the merit of each of these mechanisms is uncertain, the message is clear.

How Is Renal Failure Treated/Prevented?

Anesthetic management of patients with jaundice requires liberal preoperative and intraoperative fluid administration,[122, 123] guided preferably by assessment of urinary output and heart filling pressures. Placement of a central venous catheter is recommended. In patients with severe jaundice (bilirubin >12 mg · dL^{-1}) or with pre-existing compromise in kidney function (increased levels of blood urea nitrogen and creatinine), a pulmonary artery catheter should be considered on the assumption that optimizing filling pressures and cardiac output may be beneficial in preventing kidney failure.

Hypotension should be avoided to prevent kidney hypoperfusion. Jaundiced patients seem to be unusually sensitive to a blood volume deficit. A moderate blood loss, usually well tolerated by normal subjects, may be followed in these patients by an exaggerated fall in blood pressure.[116] Accordingly, any blood loss needs to be carefully replaced, and early use of colloids and blood is recommended.

Mannitol

Mannitol administration has long been recommended to prevent renal failure in jaundiced patients.[124] One study, however, did not show any effect of this agent with respect to an increase in creatinine clearance or decrease in the incidence of postoperative renal failure.[125] Mannitol perhaps should be reserved for those patients in whom urine output is inadequate despite normal blood pressure and normal or slightly increased heart filling pressures. Should mannitol fail to improve urine output, dopamine in small doses is a reasonable choice, although no data are available to prove that such therapy is of any benefit in jaundiced patients.

Bile Salts and Lactulose

New research has focused on the importance of endotoxemia and sepsis as causes of renal dysfunction associated with obstructive jaundice. As a result, the bile salt sodium deoxycholate and lactulose, which are effective in decreasing endotoxemia in patients with cholestasis, have been administered preoperatively to these patients, with some success in preventing renal failure.[123]

HEPATIC RESECTION

Indications for hepatic resection include primary or metastatic tumors of the liver, cysts, granuloma, and vascular malformations.

What Factors Determine Surgical Risk?

Preoperative liver function has a fundamental role in determining the risk of this type of surgery, the outcome of which largely depends on the ability of the residual liver to undergo compensatory regeneration.

Patients with concomitant liver disease have a less favorable prognosis than those with normal preoperative liver function.

Severe liver dysfunction with ascites, low serum albumin levels, increased PT, and so on represents a serious contraindication to hepatic resection because of prohibitive operative mortality.

Isoflurane and fentanyl are sometimes the recommended anesthetic agents because they preserve intraoperative liver blood flow. However, extension of the hepatic resection and damage to the residual liver during surgical manipulations are far more important than any anesthetic agent in determining optimum operative recovery of hepatic function.

Intraoperative Problems

The main problems encountered intraoperatively are blood loss[126] and, infrequently, the need for the surgeon to clamp the inferior vena cava. Large-bore venous catheters placed in the upper body and arterial and central venous catheters for pressure monitoring are therefore recommended.

Hepatic resection is usually performed through a subcostal incision; rarely the incision needs to be extended into the right chest. The procedure consists in dissecting the porta hepatis to ligate the branches of the hepatic artery and portal veins supplying the area to be resected. Transection of the liver parenchyma then follows. The major hepatic veins are, for technical reasons, usually not ligated until transection across the hepatic parenchyma is completed.

How Is Blood Loss Minimized?

Blood loss is most common during dissection of the hepatic parenchyma and is mainly from the hepatic venous system. To decrease blood loss in this phase, a low pressure in the hepatic venous system may be beneficial. This approach translates in practice to maintaining the CVP at a low-normal level, carefully replacing the blood lost on a milliliter-per-milliliter basis.

What Is the Role of Vascular Exclusion?

Total vascular exclusion of the liver is sometimes used. This procedure allows dissection to be achieved in a virtually bloodless field. Vascular exclusion is obtained by placing clamps in turn on the hepatic pedicle to occlude the hepatic artery and portal vein, the inferior vena cava below the liver, and finally the inferior vena cava above the liver. Occlusion of the inferior vena cava sharply decreases venous return to the heart. It may be followed by hypotension that requires administration of large amounts of fluids.

Alternatively, the hemodynamic compromise due to vena caval occlusion can be prevented by the use of venovenous bypass similar to that used in orthotopic liver transplantation. At the end of the dissection, when proper hemostasis has been secured, the clamps are removed in the reverse order in which they were placed. A warm ischemia time of up to 60 minutes seems to be well tolerated by the liver.[127]

What Problems Occur After Liver Resection?

Clotting

During a major liver resection, three additional sets of problems encountered are related to the acute reduction of liver parenchyma. After surgery, until compensatory liver regeneration takes place, production of clotting factors and albumin by the residual liver is greatly diminished. Impaired protein synthesis usually lasts 2 or 3 weeks but may be more prolonged in patients with underlying liver disease or in those who underwent extensive resections such as trisegmentectomies. Accordingly, 5% albumin and FFP may be preferred for volume replacement in these patients, considering that clotting factors and albumin lost intraoperatively are not replaced by the liver as promptly as usual.

Citrate Metabolism

Citrate metabolism may be impaired, and citrate toxicity and hypocalcemia may follow rapid administration of blood and FFP. Treatment with calcium chloride, preferably guided by measurements of serum ionized calcium, may be indicated.

Glucose Metabolism

Hypoglycemia may also develop because of curtailed liver glycogen stores; blood glucose should be monitored intraoperatively and postoperatively.

PATIENTS WITH ASCITES

Patients with ascites who requires intra-abdominal surgery pose several problems. When the ascites is large, a conspicuous embarrassment of ventilation often is present, and tracheal intubation followed by mechanical ventilation is mandatory. Ventilatory encroachment is sometimes so great that patients do not tolerate the supine position even for a short time, making induction of anesthesia quite problematic. The problem can be prevented by performing paracentesis before surgery to remove enough fluid to allow patients to assume the supine position.

Another way to overcome the problem is to position patients on the operating table in a semi-sitting position as tolerated, preoxygenate, administer the intravenous induction agent, and then rapidly change the operating table position to allow mask ventilation and intubation. A rapid-sequence induction is advisable because of the increased intragastric pressure. Because of the distended abdomen, a rapid fall in O_2 saturation can occur during induction using a conventional rapid-sequence technique. A modified technique in which mask ventilation is used before intubation may therefore be considered.

What Happens Acutely When Ascitic Fluid Is Drained?

When the procedure requires a laparotomy, ascites is removed at the beginning of surgery through a small skin incision. Studies have investigated the immediate and delayed hemodynamic effects of removal of large volumes of ascitic fluid.[128] Most of the data have been obtained in patients with cirrhosis, but they apply equally to patients with malignancy-induced ascites.[129]

Ascitic fluid drainage is followed by an increase in cardiac output, mainly because of an increase in stroke volume, but the arterial blood pressure does not change because the systemic vascular resistance (SVR) decreases[130] (Fig. 65–7). The CVP and PAOP are unchanged or slightly decreased.[128–130] Renal function and urinary output remain unchanged or may improve[128, 130, 131] (Fig. 65–8). The circulatory blood volume is unchanged immediately after paracentesis.[132]

Mechanisms

These hemodynamic effects do not depend on the volume of ascitic fluid or the rate at which it is removed,[129] because they have been observed after the drainage of volumes in excess of 10 L and at a rate of up to 500 mL · min^{-1}. The results indicate that a large peritoneal effusion and the concomitant increase in intraperitoneal pressure are detrimental because they compress the inferior vena cava and possibly the portal vein, thereby decreasing venous return to the heart. The

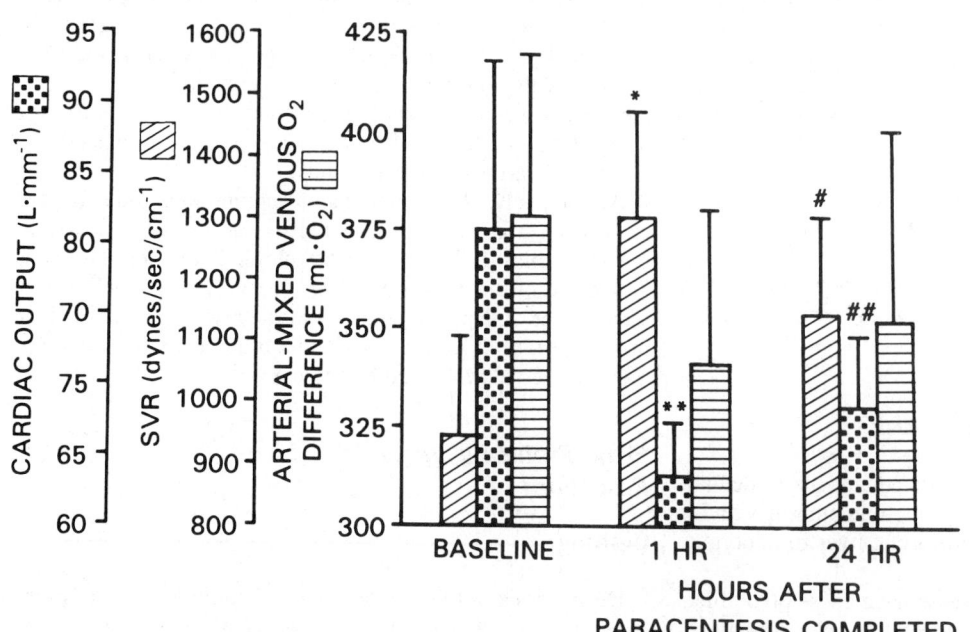

FIGURE 65–7. Changes in cardiac output, SVR, and the difference in arterial-mixed venous oxygen content observed 1 hour and 24 hours after large-volume paracentesis (range 4–15 L) in patients (n = 10) with cirrhotic ascites. (From Simon DM, McCain JR, Bonkovsky HL, et al: Effects of therapeutic paracentesis on systemic and hepatic hemodynamics and on renal and hormonal function. Hepatology 1987; 7:423.)

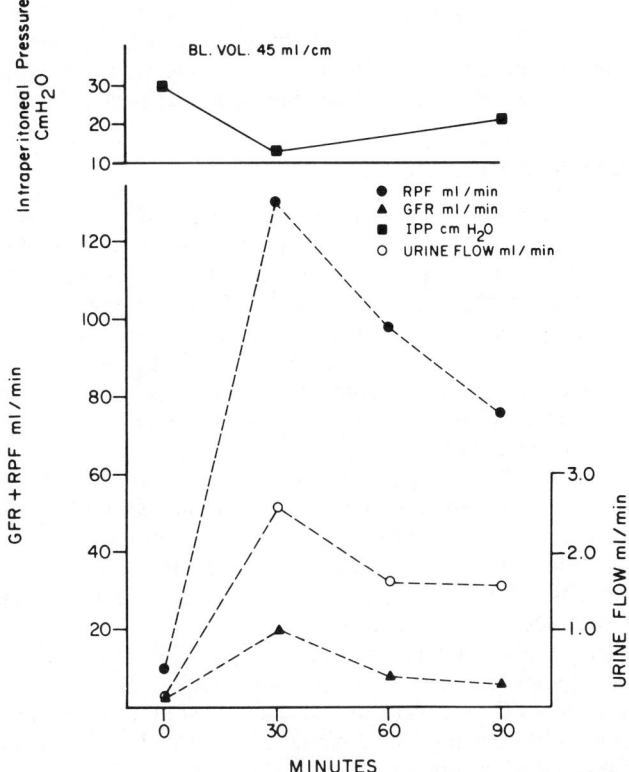

FIGURE 65–8. Change in intraperitoneal pressure, renal plasma flow (RPF), glomerular filtration rate (GFR), and urine flow in a representative patient with cirrhosis following a 2000-mL paracentesis. The deterioration in RPF and urine flow at 90 mm Hg is probably secondary to the reduction in circulatory volume caused by the continuous formation of ascitic fluid. (From Cade R, Wagemaker H, Vogel S, et al: Hepatorenal syndrome: studies of the effect of vascular volume and intraperitoneal pressure on renal and hepatic function. Am J Med 1987; 82:427.)

decrease in cardiac output elicits a compensatory SVR increase to maintain normal blood pressure.

The data also do not lend support to a commonly held belief that the removal of ascitic fluid is hazardous because of sudden hypotension or cardiovascular collapse. The sporadic reports of these untoward hemodynamic events date to more than 30 years ago, when paracentesis was performed with patients in a sitting position. The very infrequent episodes of collapse observed during paracentesis quite likely were syncopal (vasovagal) episodes.[128]

How Can the Delayed Intravascular Volume Contraction Be Avoided?

Despite the absence of immediate hemodynamic compromise after paracentesis, some evidence suggests that patients with advanced liver disease may develop hypovolemia a few hours later, causing deterioration in kidney function, oliguria, and avid sodium retention. This progressive decrease in circulatory volume is due to continuous formation of new ascitic fluid.[131] The delayed volume contraction and renal dysfunction that follow paracentesis in cirrhotic patients can be adequately prevented by administration of 50 g of albumin, preferably as a 25% solution, at the end of the ascites removal.[131]

When Is Ascitic Fluid Replaced Intraoperatively?

If surgery continues for several hours after ascites has been drained, such as during portacaval shunting, the amount of plasma lost in the peritoneum as newly formed ascites must be taken into account in order to maintain the blood volume normal. As a rule of thumb, colloids such as 5% albumin or FFP are administered at a rate of 500 mL per hour of surgery to compensate for the ascitic fluid that continuously forms.[131]

PERITONEOVENOUS SHUNTING

Peritoneovenous (PV) shunting is mainly used to treat refractory ascites secondary to cirrhosis or malignancy. A controversial but sometimes dramatically successful use of PV shunting is to reverse the functional renal failure (hepatorenal syndrome) that complicates end-stage liver disease.[133]

How Is It Performed?

The most common PV shunt in use today was developed by LeVeen and associates.[134] This shunt consists of one limb that is inserted through a small abdominal incision to lie free in the peritoneal cavity. The peritoneal limb is connected to a one-way valve placed extraperitoneally but underneath the abdominal wall muscles. A long tunneling instrument is used to pass the venous limb subcutaneously from the abdominal wound to the neck, where it is inserted into the internal jugular vein and positioned at the junction of superior vena cava and right atrium (Fig. 65–9). The one-way valve opens when a pressure gradient >3 cm H_2O is established between the peritoneal cavity and the venous system; ascitic fluid then flows into the systemic circulation. Effective decompression of the peritoneal cavity is obtained without the ensuing vascular volume depletion that often complicates paracentesis.

How Should Anesthesia Be Administered?

Patients undergoing PV shunt placement, besides having large ascites, are often in poor physical condition because of the underlying neoplastic or liver disease and are sometimes in kidney failure. The procedure can be performed under local anesthesia with sedation[134] or under general anesthesia. If the latter technique is chosen, rapid-sequence induction and tracheal intubation are mandatory, followed by mechanical ventilation. Anesthesia is maintained with nitrous oxide or isoflurane or both. Atracurium is an excellent choice for muscle relaxation. The ascitic fluid is drained at the beginning of the procedure so that patients can breathe more easily after surgery.

What Complications Follow Portovenous Shunting?

The placement of a PV shunt is followed by a wide array of complications.[133] Serious, albeit rare, complications occurring

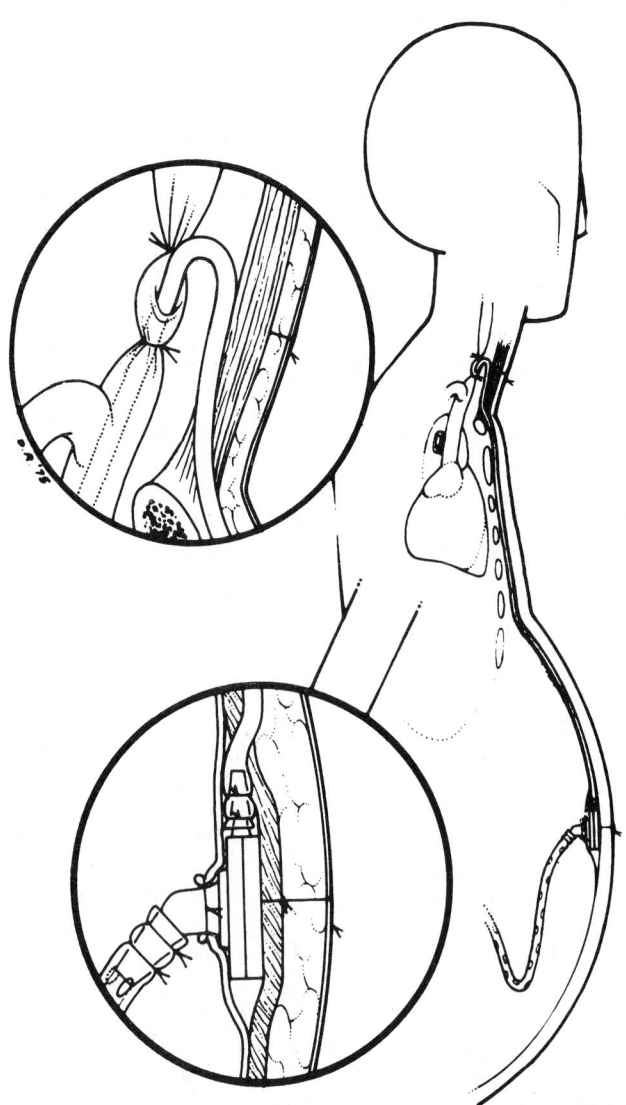

FIGURE 65–9. Schematic drawing of the LeVeen shunt following placement. Ascites is drained into the internal jugular vein via the intraperitoneal tubing. The one-way valve lies extraperitoneally and deep to the abdominal muscles *(lower enlarged view)*. The venous collecting tube traverses the subcutaneous tissue of the chest wall into the neck where it enters the internal jugular vein *(upper enlarged view).* (From LeVeen HH, Wapnick S, Grosberg S, et al: Further experience with peritoneo-venous shunt for ascites. Ann Surg 1976; 184:574.)

perioperatively include pneumothorax due to damage of the pleura when the tunneling instrument is pushed subcutaneously up the chest wall, trauma to the recurrent laryngeal nerve, air embolism, pulmonary edema, and coagulopathy.

Coagulopathy

The most worrisome complication is a coagulopathy manifested clinically by profuse bleeding from the surgical wounds and intravenous catheter sites. This coagulopathy occurs in up to one third of patients after shunt placement and has the laboratory features of disseminated intravascular coagulation.[133] It is ascribed to substances present in the ascitic fluid that interfere with coagulation when they are infused into the systemic circulation. However, the precise triggering mechanisms are unknown.[135]

A widely accepted practice to prevent postshunt coagulopathy consists in completely removing the ascites during surgery. Replacement of discarded ascitic fluid with normal saline infused into the peritoneal cavity before opening the shunt has been advocated to further decrease the incidence and severity of coagulopathy[136] (Fig. 65–10).

To prevent bleeding, the PT should be <6 seconds above normal and the platelet count >50,000 · mm$^{3-1}$ by the administration of FFP and platelets.[137] Treatment of the coagulopathy includes FFP, platelets, and possibly antifibrinolytic agents as aminocaproic or tranexamic acid.[135]

PORTOSYSTEMIC SHUNTS

Portosystemic shunts are usually performed to decompress the portal system in cirrhotic patients with bleeding esophageal varices caused by portal hypertension. The number of these procedures has decreased significantly because of the success in treating variceal bleeding by transesophageal sclerotherapy, a much less invasive and costly technique.[138] Emergency portacaval shunt, complicated by very high mortality, has in many institutions become virtually obsolete.

What Shunts Are Performed?

Several variants of portosystemic shunts have been described (Figs. 65–11 to 65–13). The most common are the

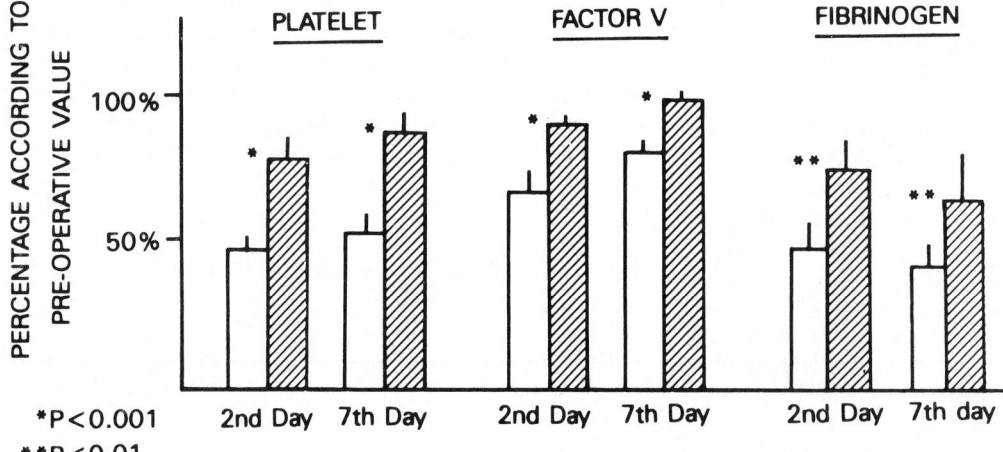

*P<0.001

**P<0.01

FIGURE 65–10. Mean percentage and standard error of the mean of the decrease of platelets, factor V, and fibrinogen in patients of group 1 (without replacement of ascitic fluids) and of group 2 (with replacement of ascitic fluids with normal saline solution) on the 2nd and 7th postoperative day. □ = group 1; ■ = group 2.

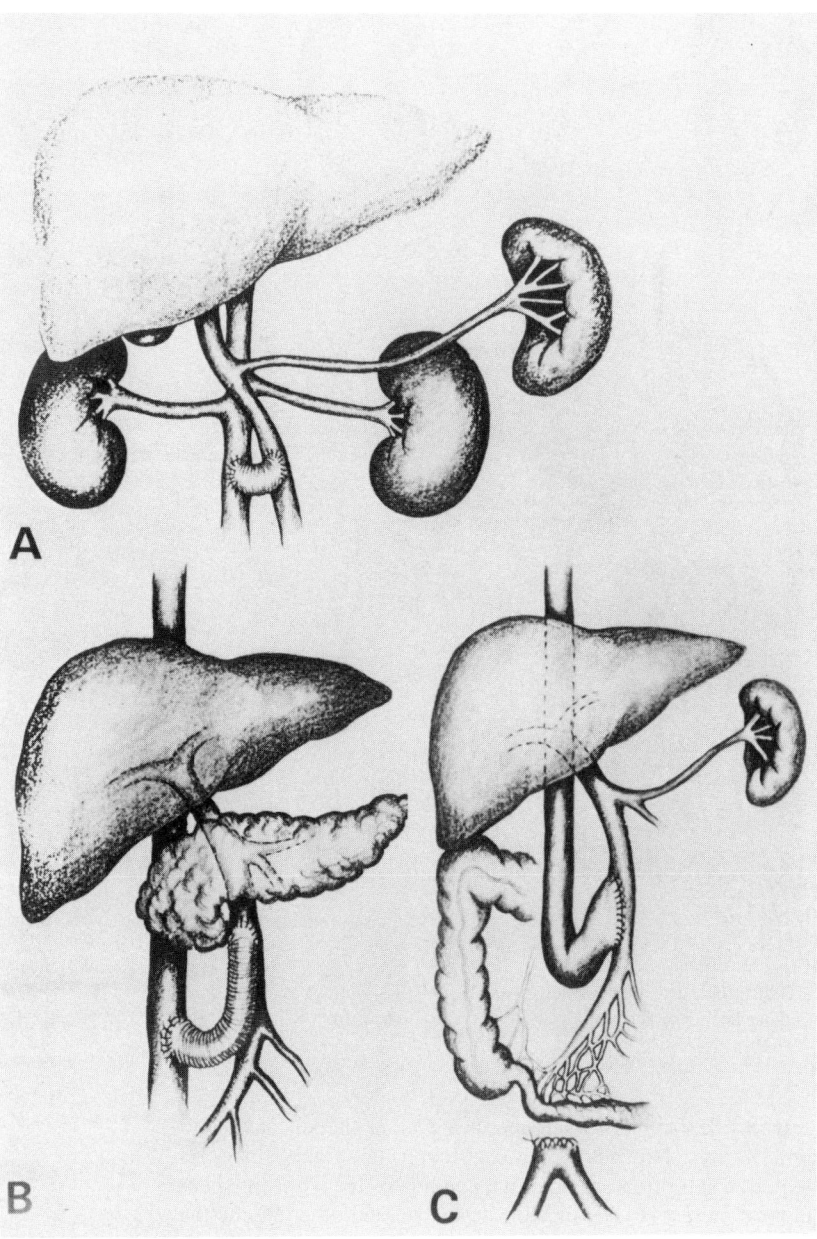

FIGURE 65–11. *A–C*, Portacaval shunts. *A*, End-to-side shunt. *B*, Side-to-side shunt. *C*, H-graft. (From Terblanche J: The surgeon's role in the management of portal hypertension. Ann Surg 1989; 209:381.)

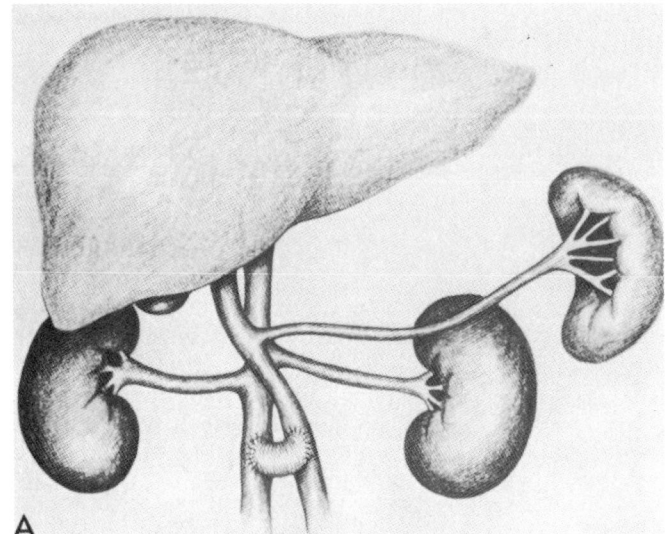

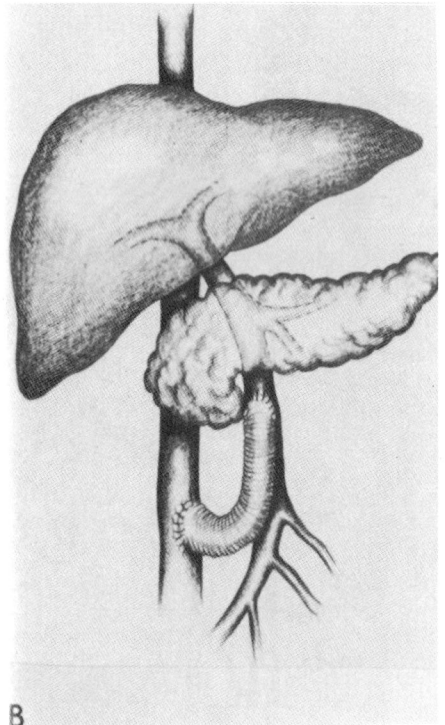

FIGURE 65–12. *A and B*, Mesocaval shunts. *A*, H-graft. *B*, C-graft. (From Terblanche J: The surgeon's role in the management of portal hypertension. Ann Surg 1989; 209:381.)

end-to-side or side-to-side portacaval and the distal spleno-renal shunts. Nowadays, patients requiring surgery for portal hypertension often are potential candidates for liver transplantation. Interest is growing for mesocaval and other shunts that interfere the least anatomically with a subsequent liver transplant.[139]

The hemodynamic effects of portosystemic shunts have been studied extensively, particularly in reference to liver blood flow.[140, 141] Of practical importance is that usually minimum systemic hemodynamic changes are observed intraoperatively when a newly fashioned portacaval shunt is opened. In general, the type of shunt chosen by the surgeon is irrelevant to the anesthetic management.

What Factors Predict Postoperative Outcome?

Surgical outcome is largely dependent on preoperative liver function. The risk assessment for cirrhotic patients undergoing portosystemic shunts is usually based on a slightly revised version of Child's classification[142, 143] (Table 65–3). Patients in group A, with good liver function, usually fare well, whereas patients in groups B and C, with poor liver function, have a much grimmer outcome.

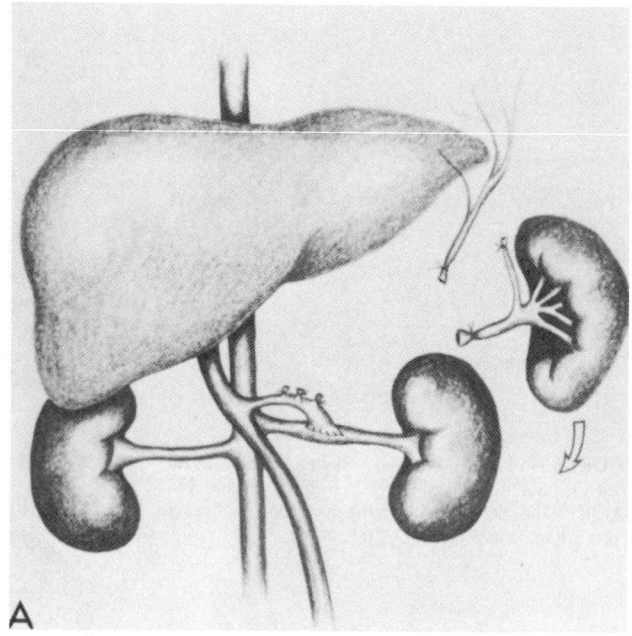

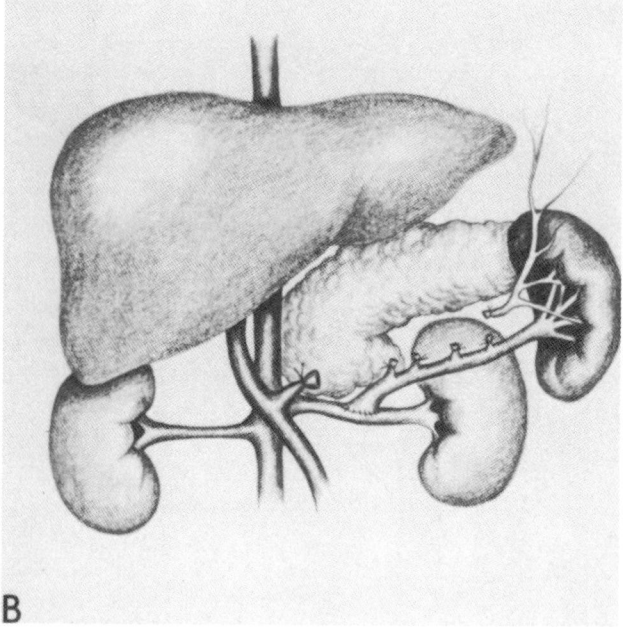

FIGURE 65–13. *A and B*, Splenorenal shunts. *A*, Central splenorenal shunt. *B*, Selective distal splenorenal shunt. (From Terblanche J: The surgeon's role in the management of portal hypertension. Ann Surg 1989; 209:381.)

TABLE 65–3. Risk Classification of Cirrhotic Patients Requiring Portosystemic Shunting

	Group A	Group B	Group C
Bilirubin (mg · dL^{-1})	<2.0	2.0–3.0	>3
Albumin (g · dL^{-1})	>3.5	3.0–3.5	<3
Ascites	None	Controlled	Poorly controlled
Encephalopathy	None	Minimum	Advanced
Nutrition	Excellent	Good	Poor
Prothrombin (seconds above control)	<4	4–6	>6
Surgical risk	Good (<5%)	Moderate (10%)	Poor (50%)

(Data from Child CG: Major problems in clinical surgery. *In* The Liver and Portal Hypertension. Child CG, Coon WW (eds). Philadelphia, WB Saunders, 1964, p 50, *and* Pugh RNH, Murray-Lyon IM, Dawson JL, et al: Transection of the esophagus for bleeding varices. Br J Surg 1973; 60:646.)

Can the Usual Drugs Be Used?

Liver cirrhosis significantly affects the pharmacodynamics and pharmacokinetics of a large number of drugs. In practice, however, any commonly used anesthetic drug can safely be used in these patients, provided they are titrated to the desired effect. The use of relaxants in patient with liver disease was discussed previously.

How Is Maintenance of Liver Function Optimized?

A specific goal during anesthesia in cirrhotic patients is to maintain an adequate O_2 supply to preserve whatever liver function remains. In addition to ensuring proper arterial oxygenation, hypovolemia and hypotension must be avoided because the liver blood supply will be severely curtailed. Maintenance of a normal circulatory volume is of paramount importance, because hypotension results after a moderate blood loss that normally would not cause blood pressure changes.

This poor tolerance to hypovolemia probably is due to impaired vasoconstriction in response to sympathetic stimulation,[144] as well as an inability to mobilize blood from the splanchnic pool into the systemic circulation.[145] Arterial partial pressure of CO_2 should be maintained within normal limits, because liver blood flow probably is best maintained with normocarbia.[7]

Anesthetic Choice

The anesthetic agents of choice are perhaps isoflurane and fentanyl because they better maintain the hepatic O_2 supply-demand relationship and possibly offer some liver protection during ischemia.[11, 14] Nitrous oxide, which has minimum cardiovascular depressant effects, is a useful addition because patients with cirrhosis are prone to hypotension and often do not tolerate isoflurane except at very low concentrations that may be inadequate to provide unconsciousness.

Monitoring

The main intraoperative problem is hemorrhage, due to venous congestion of the splanchnic area. The risk of profuse bleeding, combined with the need for maintaining the blood pressure and blood volume as close to normal as possible, mandates adequate venous access and placement of an arterial catheter for continuous pressure monitoring.

Whether a central venous or pulmonary artery catheter should be placed is controversial. My preference is to use a pulmonary artery catheter in patients in Child's groups B and C based on the assumption that aggressive hemodynamic management may better help to preserve liver and kidney function and improve outcome.

If a pulmonary artery catheter is used and cardiac output is measured, remember that cirrhotic patients often have a hyperdynamic circulation characterized by high cardiac output, low-normal systemic blood pressure, low SVR, and a narrow arteriovenous O_2 content difference because of a high mixed venous O_2 saturation. This hemodynamic pattern is characteristic of cirrhosis and does not require intervention. It does, however, establish a higher baseline and therefore sets the intraoperative hemodynamic maintenance goals differently than in a patient without cirrhosis.

What Are the Requirements for Fluid Management?

Intraoperative fluid management of cirrhotic patients is also somewhat controversial. Solutions of 5% dextrose in water (D_5W) are sometimes recommended instead of sodium-containing solutions based on the premise that these patients retain sodium and that the sodium retention is responsible for formation of ascites, generalized edema, and occasionally hypernatremia. Several arguments militate against this point of view.

1. First, the advocates of the intraoperative use of D_5W often equate crystalloid solutions to 0.9% normal saline that has a supranormal sodium concentration of 156 mEq · L^{-1}. Balanced electrolyte solutions currently used have a much lower sodium content. Lactated Ringer's has a sodium concentration of 130 mEq · L^{-1}, and its use is not associated with hypernatremia.

2. Those investigators who argue against the use of sodium-containing solutions recommend the use of colloids such as albumin and plasma to maintain adequate intraoperative hemodynamics. This recommendation does not seem very logical, because these colloids contain as much if not more sodium than balanced electrolyte solutions. For instance, 5% albumin is suspended in normal saline.

3. Therapeutic considerations that are valid in long-term treatment of cirrhotic patients may not apply to intraoperative management, when the priority is to maintain stable hemodynamics. The intraoperative use of lactated Ringer's or similar solutions may indeed be beneficial by preventing hypovolemia and liver hypoperfusion.

4. Cirrhotic patients are particularly prone to hyponatremia owing to their inability to excrete water normally.[146] Intraoperative administration of D_5W solutions to these patients may therefore be followed by severe hyponatremia. A serum sodium level <130 mEq · L^{-1} is considered an important cause of encephalopathy in cirrhotic patients.[147]

In my opinion, a safe and simple solution to this controversy is to use lactated Ringer's as the intraoperative maintenance fluid. The solution causes neither hypernatremia nor hyponatremia and may partially correct a pre-existing low serum sodium level.

Is Hypoglycemia a Problem?

Administration of D_5W also has been recommended to prevent intraoperative hypoglycemia. This phenomenon probably is rare and can be avoided by monitoring the blood glucose level and administering small volumes of 25% glucose solutions as needed. However, if you are not convinced by the position presented and choose to infuse D_5W, be sure to monitor the serum sodium concentration closely. Should the sodium level decrease to 130 mEq $\cdot$ dL^{-1}, discontinue the D_5W and replace it with lactated Ringer's solution.

How Is Oliguria Managed?

Urinary output should be monitored and maintained at >0.5 mL $\cdot$ kg^{-1} $\cdot$ h^{-1}. Oliguria is best prevented by careful replacement of intraoperative losses. In patients with ascites, an important and often overlooked cause of hypovolemia is represented by the loss of significant amounts of plasma-like fluid in the abdomen due to continuous formation of ascitic fluid. Poor urinary output is primarily due to inadequate volume replacement and needs to be treated as such.

Oliguria occasionally persists despite normal cardiac output and filling pressures. The approach to this condition consists in further expanding the circulatory volume, preferably with FFP,[131] until a CVP or PAOP of 18 to 20 mm Hg is reached. Oliguria refractory to volume expansion is very difficult to reverse. Low-dose dopamine as well as diuretics such as furosemide and mannitol may be tried, but the results are often disappointing.

Why Does Coagulopathy Occur?

Surgical bleeding may be compounded by coagulopathy associated with the underlying liver disease and the dilutional coagulopathy that follows resuscitation for large blood losses. During surgery, repeated assessments of the PT and platelet count may be needed to guide replacement therapy.

Postoperatively, these patients should be admitted to an intensive care unit because of significant continued fluid translocation and complications of bleeding, liver failure, encephalopathy, and kidney failure.

EFFECTS OF ABDOMINAL SURGERY ON PULMONARY FUNCTION

Pulmonary dysfunction is invariably present after laparotomy. The primary changes occur in lung mechanics, which in turn are responsible for impaired gas exchange.

What Abnormalities Occur?

Pulmonary abnormalities are characterized by a restrictive pattern, with a decrease in forced vital capacity (FVC) and FRC.[148, 149] The forced expired volume in 1 second (FEV$_1$) is

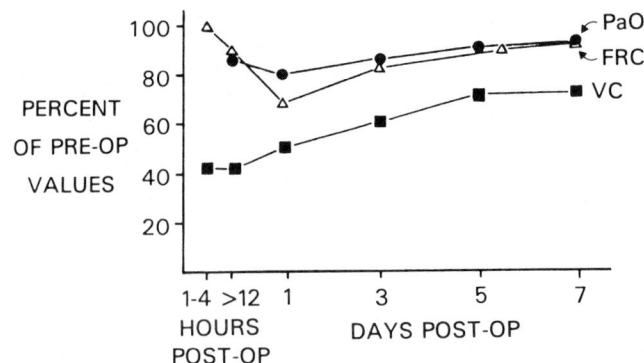

FIGURE 65–14. Postoperative vital capacity (VC), functional residual capacity (FRC), and Pao$_2$ (Fio$_2$ 0.21) as percent of preoperative values following upper abdominal surgery. (From Craig DB: Postoperative recovery of pulmonary function. Anesth Analg 1981; 60:46.)

also decreased, but the ratio of FEV$_1$ to FVC remains at preoperative values.[150]

The magnitude and duration of the postoperative lung abnormality depend on the site and, to a more limited extent, the type of surgical incision. After upper abdominal surgery, the FVC may decrease by 50% or more and the FRC by 20% to 25% (Fig. 65–14). The largest lung volume changes occur on the first postoperative day. Thereafter, they begin to recover, with a gradual return to normal by the seventh postoperative day.

The changes in FVC and FRC observed after lower abdominal surgery are much less and resolve more rapidly (Fig. 65–15). Lung function is slightly better preserved after laparotomies performed with a transverse rather than vertical incision.[151, 152]

What Causes the Restrictive Defect?

The restrictive deficit after abdominal surgery is believed to be primarily the result of dysfunction of the diaphragm combined with abnormal activity of the expiratory muscles (abdominal and low intercostal).[153–157] The impairment of diaphragmatic activity is best evidenced by the marked decrease in diaphragm excursion during maximum inspiration[153, 155] (Fig. 65–16). Diaphragmatic dysfunction probably is secondary to a reflex inhibition of phrenic nerve output mediated by stimuli originating in the abdominal cavity.

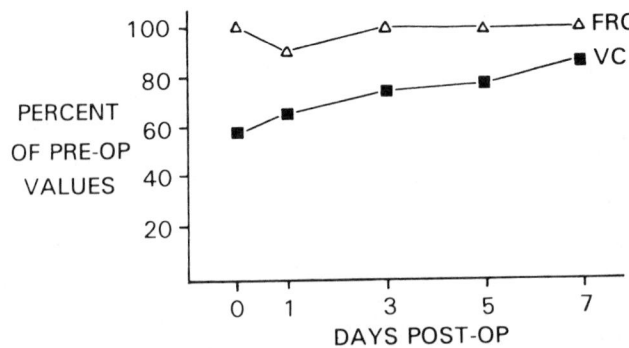

FIGURE 65–15. Postoperative VC and FRC as a per cent of preoperative values following lower abdominal surgery. (From Craig DB: Postoperative recovery of pulmonary function. Anesth Analg 1981; 60:46.)

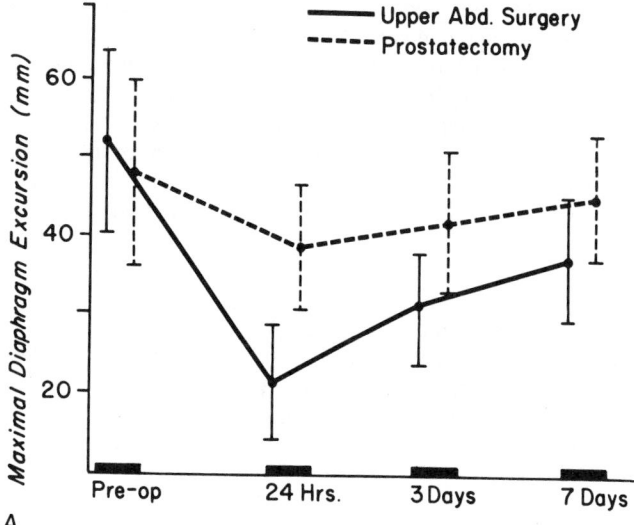

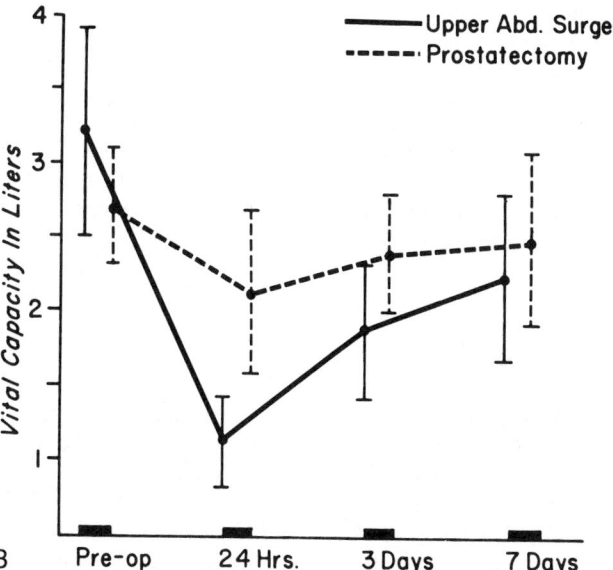

FIGURE 65–16. *A and B*, Mean changes in maximum diaphragmatic excursion *(A)* and vital capacity *(B)* after upper or lower (prostatectomy) abdominal surgery. The diaphragm excursion measured by fluoroscopy during maximum respiratory efforts was greatly decreased after upper abdominal surgery and correlated well with the decrease in vital capacity. The changes in diaphragmatic excursion and vital capacity were much less important after lower abdominal surgery. (From Tahir AH, George RB, Weil H, et al: Effects of abdominal surgery upon diaphragmatic function and regional ventilation. Int Surg 1973; 58:337.)

General anesthesia consistently decreases the FRC.[149] However, this effect is transitory, and the FRC rapidly returns to preoperative values shortly after a patient has regained consciousness.[149] Therefore, anesthesia is unlikely to have a role in causing the low FRC that persists for many days after abdominal surgery.

Does Postoperative Pain Influence Lung Function?

Postoperative pain has only a small contributory role in causing lung dysfunction, because with complete pain relief

FVC is only partially restored and FRC is virtually unchanged[149, 158, 159] (Table 65–4). Several studies have compared the effects of patient-controlled intravenous opioids,[160] epidural opioids,[161] epidural or interpleural local anesthetics,[162–164] and intercostal block[165] on postoperative lung volumes. The results indicate that no technique is superior in terms of improvement of respiratory function. The differences among techniques are modest and probably of little practical relevance.

Although postoperative pain relief does not seem to influence the recovery of lung function,[149] it is usually considered beneficial in decreasing the incidence of postoperative pulmonary complications because it enhances coughing, facilitates early ambulation, and improves patients' compliance with physiotherapy.

What Is the Effect of Abdominal Surgery on Oxygenation?

After abdominal surgery, arterial partial pressure of O_2 (Pao_2) is consistently lower than before operation. The average decrease in Pao_2 is accentuated more after upper than lower abdominal operations in patients breathing room air (15 mm Hg and 6 mm Hg, respectively).[166, 167] The decrease in Pao_2 is slightly greater in elderly patients.[166] It is lowest the first 24 to 48 hours after surgery, then recovers in parallel with the recovery of lung mechanics (see Fig. 65–14). The decrease in Pao_2 is not improved by postoperative pain relief (see Table 65–4). The defect in arterial oxygenation after abdominal operations is a consequence of the reduced FRC and is due to ventilation ($\dot{V}$) and perfusion ($\dot{Q}$) mismatch, with an increase in lung zones with zero (true shunt) or low $\dot{V}/\dot{Q}$ ratio.[149]

True right-to-left shunt probably is due to the development of small atelectases in the dependent lung regions.[168] Regions with low $\dot{V}/\dot{Q}$ develop when the closing capacity (i.e., the lung volume at which airway closure starts to occur) exceeds the FRC, resulting in small airway closure during normal tidal breathing.[148–149] The relative contributions of shunting and low $\dot{V}/\dot{Q}$ to postoperative hypoxemia vary from patient to patient in an unpredictable fashion.

This fact may explain the seemingly paradoxical observation that changing a patient's position from supine to sitting in the early postoperative period improves the FRC[169, 170] but does not consistently improve the Pao_2 (which in some patients may

TABLE 65–4. Lung Dysfunction and Postoperative Pain

| | | Postoperatively* | |
	Preoperatively (Control)*	Before Epidural Injection	1 h After Epidural Injection
FVC (mL)	3300 ± 208	1308‡ ± 115	1930‡ ± 144§
FRC (mL)	2500 ± 104	2208‡ ± 127	2220‡ ± 130
Pao₂ (mm Hg)	74 ± 3	64† ± 0.1	7.42 ± 0.1
Paco₂ (mm Hg)	39 ± 1	39 ± 1	38 ± 2

(Modified from Mankikian B, et al: Improvement of diaphragmatic function by a thoracic extradural block after upper abdominal surgery. Anesthesiology 1988; 68:379.)
*Values are expressed as mean ± standard error of the mean.
†*P* < 0.05.
‡*P* < 0.01 versus control.
§*P* < 0.01 versus before epidural injection.
Abbreviations: FVC = forced vital capacity; Pao₂ = partial pressure of arterial oxygen; Paco₂ = partial pressure of arterial carbon dioxide.

actually deteriorate).[171–173] It has been postulated that when the main cause of impaired oxygenation is an unfavorable FRC to closing capacity relation, change in position is followed by an increase in Pa_{O_2} because the FRC becomes larger and the $\dot{V}/\dot{Q}$ mismatch due to airway closure is reduced.[174] Conversely, when the main cause of hypoxemia is a true shunt, the sitting position is associated with a decrease in Pa_{O_2} because of a 10% decrease in cardiac output, which magnifies the effects of shunt on Pa_{O_2}.[173]

Who Needs Supplemental Oxygen Postoperatively?

The deficit in oxygenation that follows abdominal surgery usually is modest and well tolerated by the majority of the patients, who have no need for supplemental O_2 apart perhaps from the brief period while they recover from the anesthetic. Patients with low preoperative Pa_{O_2}, such as the elderly or those with significant lung disease, may show unacceptably low postoperative Pa_{O_2} values with O_2 saturation <90%. They require O_2 therapy for a few days, usually at moderate concentrations of 30% to 35%, until gas exchange improves. Pulse oximetry during the recovery period in the postanesthesia care unit identifies patients who still require O_2 after "recovery" from the anesthetic.

PULMONARY COMPLICATIONS

Pulmonary complications after abdominal surgery can be divided into two categories: acute ventilatory failure and atelectasis/pneumonia. Anesthesiologists commonly are more directly involved with the former; the latter complications are often in the domain of other physicians and are briefly discussed here.

Why Does Acute Ventilatory Failure Occur?

Acute ventilatory failure occurs immediately or shortly after surgery in patients who have severe underlying pulmonary disease and cannot tolerate the further impairment in lung function brought about by the surgical procedure.[175] The respiratory muscles, already chronically stressed, rapidly fatigue in the presence of the increased workload imposed by the acute reduction in lung volume that follows surgery.[175] Ventilatory failure then ensues, with hypercapnia and hypoxemia.

A surprising scarcity of data exists about the incidence of acute respiratory insufficiency requiring mechanical ventilation in patients who have compromised lung function and who undergo abdominal surgery. Similarly lacking are data about the outcome of these patients. However, patients with grossly abnormal spirometry (i.e., FEV_1 as low as 15% of predicted normal, FEV/FVC as low as 26%, and Pa_{O_2} <60 mm Hg) can undergo abdominal surgery without necessarily needing postoperative mechanical ventilation.

FVC and FEV_1 are often expressed in absolute values in the literature dealing with postoperative pulmonary complications. Because the same absolute value has a totally different meaning if applied to a small elderly woman or to a stocky younger man, it is more appropriate to express the spirometric indices

as a percentage of predicted normal values that take into account gender, age, and size of the patient.[176]

Timely identification of acute ventilatory failure requires continuous pulse oximetry and frequent clinical assessment in the acute postoperative period. If acute ventilatory failure requires ventilatory support, the effects of surgery on the lungs are temporary and reversible, and in the absence of other complications, patients usually can be extubated within a few days.

The outcome of patients with severe lung impairment undergoing abdominal procedures is, by and large, surprisingly good.[176] "Prohibitive" lung function that contraindicates abdominal surgery because of excessive mortality due to respiratory causes apparently does not exist. Patients should not be denied the benefits of an operation on the grounds of poor respiratory function.

Who Is at Risk for Ventilatory Failure?

Patients with an FVC or FEV_1 <50% of predicted normal or FEV_1/FVC <50% are at risk for ventilatory failure after upper abdominal procedures.[177] Although this risk has never been clearly quantified and overall seems to be relatively small,[176] these spirometric values should alert the anesthesiologist that acute failure is a distinct possibility. Preoperatively, these patients require vigorous care to optimize their residual lung function. Physiotherapy, antibiotics, and bronchodilators are indicated to clear purulent sputum and relieve airway obstruction.

What Anesthetic Technique Is Best?

The anesthetic technique (general or spinal/epidural) has no impact on postoperative lung function.[57] However, the anesthetic should be planned in order to have a patient awake and able to breathe spontaneously as soon as possible after surgery is completed. High-dose opioid techniques should be limited to cases in which ventilatory support is planned electively for the first 24 hours postoperatively.

When Is Extubation Performed?

Postoperatively, patients who do not immediately meet criteria for extubation are ventilated in the postanesthesia care unit until the compounding effects of residual anesthesia are dissipated, hypothermia and hemodynamic instability are corrected, and adequate pain relief has been obtained. Their ability to sustain adequate spontaneous ventilation is then reassessed.

Patients who require ventilatory support immediately after surgery commonly improve their respiratory function within a few hours, allowing rapid weaning and extubation. After extubation, they are maintained in a high-surveillance area for 24 hours to detect any deterioration.

If extubation cannot be accomplished, the patient is transferred to an intensive care unit and ventilated until lung function recovers. Patients with poor lung function are sometimes ventilated "prophylactically" for 18 to 24 hours. However, no evidence shows that prophylactic ventilation offers any advantage over a policy of extubating patients as soon as feasible.

Who Should Practice Breathing Exercises?

The acute restrictive deficit that follows abdominal surgery is associated with a decreased ability to breathe deeply and to cough efficiently. Plugging of the bronchi by retained sputum is followed by atelectasis and pneumonia. The incidence of these complications is higher after upper abdominal surgery and in patients with pre-existing lung disease, a history of smoking, and advanced age. However, they are so common that every patient, regardless of preoperative lung status, should practice some form of breathing exercises after an abdominal operation.[178]

Respiratory maneuvers used to decrease postoperative lung complications aim to re-expand lung volumes restricted by the abdominal procedure and to enhance the ability to clear secretions. The simplest method positions patients in a semi-sitting position, increasing the expiratory reserve volume and greatly improving the ability to cough.[169, 170]

Other techniques include intermittent positive-pressure breathing (IPPB), continuous positive airway pressure (CPAP) delivered at intervals by mask, incentive spirometry (sustained maximum inspiration), or simply deep-breathing exercises.

These techniques are equally effective in decreasing the incidence of pulmonary complications, but none enhances the restoration of normal lung volumes or Pao_2.[179, 180] Accordingly, techniques such as IPPB or CPAP requiring expensive apparatus or highly skilled personnel can hardly be justified. Surgical patients probably do not require more than the frequent use of an incentive spirometer or frequent deep-breathing exercises encourages by a nurse or respiratory therapist.[181]

POSTOPERATIVE INTESTINAL MOTILITY

Operations within the abdominal cavity are followed by a period of decreased GI motility, referred to as postoperative ileus and characterized by ineffective peristalsis and atony. The stomach and small bowel motor activity return within 24 hours after surgery. The colon shows a more profound inhibition that persists at least 48 hours. Decreased motility of the colon probably contributes most significantly to the duration of postoperative ileus.

What Causes Ileus?

Postoperative bowel dysfunction has been attributed to spinal reflexes originating from the abdomen and involving sympathetic efferent nerves to the gut. It also has been linked to reduced plasma concentrations of the intestinal hormone motilin.[182] The duration of ileus does not correlate with operative handling of the bowel, nor with the extent or duration of surgery.[183]

Anesthetic Effects

Inhalation anesthetic agents greatly depress bowel motility, but this effect is promptly reversed when they are withdrawn. Therefore, they do not seem to have any role in causing long-lasting postoperative ileus.[184] Whether intraoperative use of nitrous oxide delays the recovery of bowel function after abdominal surgery is controversial. Nitrous oxide has been found to have no effect on the return of bowel motility[185] or, con-

versely, to delay it by about 1 day.[186] How nitrous oxide that, per se, does not affect bowel motility[184] and is completely reabsorbed from the intestinal lumen long before peristalsis is resumed would influence the duration of postoperative ileus is difficult to envision.

Opioids

Opioids have a well-known depressant effect on bowel motility.[117] Because they are widely used to provide analgesia after abdominal surgery, separation of their effects on bowel function from those of the surgical procedure is difficult.

Although comparisons are lacking, no clinically significant difference is thought to exist between the various opioids in terms of duration of postoperative ileus. The route of administration also seems unimportant because the duration of ileus is the same after epidural or parenteral opioids.[188, 189] The agonist-antagonist opioids (pentazocine, nalbuphine, and others) apparently exert a depressant effect on bowel motility similar to the pure agonists; therefore, their use does not seem to offer any advantage.[190]

Epidural Analgesia

Whether continuous epidural analgesia with bupivacaine, by providing a visceral sympathectomy, leads to a shorter duration of postoperative ileus in comparison with conventional treatment with parenteral opioids is controversial. Some investigators found that postoperative epidural analgesia decreased the duration of ileus,[188, 189] but others were unable to confirm this finding.[190, 191]

Is Ileus Treatable?

Pharmacologic treatment of postoperative ileus has been attempted, with variable results.[192, 193] Metoclopramide is of no benefit and may be detrimental, probably because the contractions generated are uncoordinated and nonpropulsive.[194]

At present, whether faster recovery of bowel function after surgery is advantageous or whether postoperative ileus is a useful biologic response that "puts the bowel to rest" and enhances the healing process is unclear. Until this controversy is resolved, the value of pharmacologic interventions directed to shorten the duration of postoperative ileus remains speculative.

SURGERY OF THE ABDOMINAL WALL AND ABDOMINAL WALL HERNIAS

Which Anesthetics Are Appropriate?

Ventral Hernias

Ventral hernias (umbilical, epigastric, and postincisional) can be repaired under general or, if the incision is at or below the umbilicus, regional anesthesia. If regional anesthesia is chosen, a sensory block to T-5 is recommended in order to prevent pain when the peritoneum is opened. The repair of a giant ventral hernia may cause postoperative ventilatory problems that necessitate mechanical ventilation.

Inguinal and Femoral Hernias

Inguinal and femoral hernias can be operated on under local,[195] general, spinal, or epidural anesthesia. The degree of muscle relaxation required is usually moderate, and muscle relaxants can be used sparingly or avoided altogether. If regional anesthesia is used, a sensory block to T-5 is preferred to prevent pain when traction is applied to the spermatic cord or the peritoneum.

Hernia repairs performed under general or spinal anesthesia are followed by the same incidence of postoperative urinary retention, back ache, and respiratory complications.[196] The main difference is that the incidence of nausea, vomiting, and sore throat (if tracheal intubation has been performed) is greater after general anesthesia. Postspinal headache and other minor neurologic problems (temporary paresthesias or radicular pain) complicate spinal anesthesia.

Choice of Local Anesthetic

If hernia repair is performed under regional anesthesia, prompt recovery of motor and bladder function is desirable; therefore, short-acting local anesthetics are preferred. Hyperbaric 5% lidocaine and 0.75% bupivacaine are satisfactory agents for spinal anesthesia. Lidocaine, 2%, and chloroprocaine, 3%, both with 1:200,000 epinephrine, probably are the agents of choice for epidural anesthesia.[197] Very good and long-lasting postoperative analgesia can be obtained if, at the end of the herniorrhaphy, the surgical area is infiltrated with 30 to 40 mL of 0.25% bupivacaine.[198] This method of pain relief is particularly attractive for outpatients.[199]

Strangulated Hernias

Spinal anesthesia may be particularly advantageous for patients with strangulated hernias,[200] provided the circulatory volume is normal and no other specific contraindications are present. This technique negates the significant risk of pulmonary aspiration during the induction of general anesthesia in these patients.

During induction of anesthesia for repair of an incarcerated hernia, the bowel may retreat into the peritoneal cavity before the surgeon can confirm its viability. Under such circumstances, abdominal exploration may be indicated in order to examine the incarcerated segment.

Whether the untimely reduction of an incarcerated hernia is more likely during general or spinal anesthesia apparently never has been investigated. No data validate maneuvers sometimes used to prevent this event from occurring, such as inducing anesthesia with a patient in the head-up position or having the surgeon or an assistant hold the hernia during induction until the incision can be made.

References

1. Downman CBB: Skeletal muscle reflexes of splanchnic and intercostal nerve origin in acute spinal and decerebrate cats. J Neurophysiol 1955; 18:217.
2. Kugelberg E, Hagbarth KE: Spinal mechanism of the abdominal and erector spine skin reflexes. Brain 1958; 81:290.
3. Albano JP, Garnier L: Bulbo-spinal respiratory effects originating from the splanchnic afferents. Respir Physiol 1983; 51:229.
4. Ngai SH: Action of general anesthetics in producing muscle relaxation: interaction of anesthetics with relaxants. In Muscle Relaxants. Katz RL (ed). Amsterdam, North-Holland, 1975, pp 279–297.
5. Downes H: Hyperventilation and abdominal reflex inhibition. Anesthesiology 1963; 24:617.
6. Foex P: Effects of carbon dioxide on the systemic circulation. In The Circulation in Anaesthesia. Prys-Roberts C (ed). London, Blackwell Scientific Publications, 1980, pp 295–309.
7. Gelman S: Carbon dioxide and hepatic circulation. Anesth Analg 1989; 69:149.
8. Gelman S: Disturbances in hepatic blood flow during anesthesia and surgery. Arch Surg 1976; 111:881.
9. Cartwright P, Prys-Roberts C, Gill K, et al: Ventilatory depression related to plasma fentanyl concentrations during and after anesthesia in humans. Anesth Analg 1983; 62:966.
10. Schwartz AE, Matteo RS, Ornstein E, et al: Pharmacokinetics of sufentanil in neurosurgical patients undergoing hyperventilation. Br J Anaesth 1989; 63:385.
11. Nagano K, Gelman S, Parks DA, et al: Hepatic oxygen supply-uptake relationship and metabolism during anesthesia in miniature pigs. Anesthesiology 1990; 72:902.
12. Nagano K, Gelman S, Parks D, et al: Hepatic circulation and oxygen supply-uptake relationships after hepatic ischemic insult during anesthesia with volatile anesthetics and fentanyl in miniature pigs. Anesth Analg 1990; 70:53.
13. Goldfarb G, Debaene B, Ang ET, et al: Hepatic blood flow in humans during isoflurane-N_2O and halothane-N_2O anesthesia. Anesth Analg 1990; 71:349.
14. Bernard J-M, Doursout M-F, Wouters P, et al: Effects of enflurane and isoflurane on hepatic and renal circulations in chronically instrumented dogs. Anesthesiology 1991; 74:298.
15. Andersen BN, Madsen JV, Schurizek BA, et al: Residual curarization: a comparative study of atracurium and pancuronium. Acta Anaesthesiol Scand 1988; 32:79.
16. Bevan DR, Smith CE, Donati F: Postoperative neuromuscular blockade: a comparison between atracurium, vecuronium, and pancuronium. Anesthesiology 1988; 69:272.
17. Somogyi AA, Shanks CA, Triggs EJ: Disposition kinetics of pancuronium bromide in patients with total biliary obstruction. Br J Anaesth 1977; 49:1103.
18. Lebrault C, Duvaldestin P, Henzel D, et al: Pharmacokinetics and pharmacodynamics of vecuronium in patients with cholestasis. Br J Anaesth 1986; 58:983.
19. Westra P, Houwertjes MC, DeLange AR, et al: Effect of experimental cholestasis on neuromuscular blocking drugs in cats. Br J Anaesth 1980; 52:747.
20. Foldes FF, Rendell-Baker L, Birch JH: Cause and prevention of prolonged apnea with succinylcholine. Anesth Analg 1956; 35:609.
21. Duvaldestin P, Agoston S, Henzel D, et al: Pancuronium pharmacokinetics in patients with liver cirrhosis. Br J Anaesth 1978; 50:1131.
22. Lebrault C, Berger JL, D'Hollander AA, et al: Pharmacokinetics and pharmacodynamics of vecuronium (ORG NC 45) in patients with cirrhosis. Anesthesiology 1985; 62:601.
23. Hunter JM, Parker CJR, Bell CF, et al: The use of different doses of vecuronium in patients with liver dysfunction. Br J Anaesth 1985; 57:758.
24. Arden JR, Lynam DP, Castagnoli KP: Vecuronium in alcoholic liver disease: pharmacokinetic and pharmacodynamic analysis. Anesthesiology 1988; 68:771.
25. Parker CJR, Hunter JM: Pharmacokinetics of atracurium and laudanosine in patients with hepatic cirrhosis. Br J Anaesth 1989; 62:177.
26. Lee C: Train-of-4 quantitation of competitive neuromuscular block. Anesth Analg 1975; 54:649.
27. Derrington MC, Hindocha N: Comparison of neuromuscular block in the diaphragm and hand after administration of tubocurarine, pancuronium, and alcuronium. Br J Anaesth 1990; 64:294.
28. Donati F, Meistelman C, Plaud B: Vecuronium neuromuscular blockade at the diaphragm, the orbicularis oculi, and adductor pollicis muscles. Anesthesiology 1990; 73:870.
29. Saddler JM, Marks LF, Norman J: Comparison of atracurium-induced neuromuscular block in rectus abdominis and hand muscles of man. Br J Anaesth 1992; 69:26.
30. Viby-Mogensen J, Howardy-Hansen P, Chraemmer-Jorgensen B, et al: Posttetanic count (PTC): a new method of evaluating an intense nondepolarizing neuromuscular block. Anesthesiology 1981; 59:1089.
31. Fernando PUE, Viby-Mogensen J, Bonsu AK, et al: Relationship between posttetanic count and response to carinal stimulation during vecuronium-induced neuromuscular blockade. Acta Anaesthesiol Scand 1987; 31:593.
32. Lewis JH: Hiccups: causes and cures. J Clin Gastroenterol 1985; 7:539.

33. Bannon MG: Termination of hiccups occurring under anesthesia. Anesthesiology 1991; 74:385.

34. Salem M: An effective method for the treatment of hiccups during anesthesia. Anesthesiology 1967; 28:463.

35. Rouse JM, Bevan DR: Mixed neuromuscular block. Anesthesia 1979; 34:608.

36. Feldman SA: Rational use of muscle relaxants and anticholinesterase in clinical practice. *In* Muscle Relaxants. 2nd ed. Hamilton WK (ed). Philadelphia, WB Saunders, 1979, pp 221–222.

37. Rashkovsky OM, Agoston S, Ket JM: Interaction between pancuronium bromide and vecuronium bromide. Br J Anaesth 1985; 57:1063.

38. Ornstein E, Matteo RS, Weinstein JA, et al: The effect of maintenance dose vecuronium on preestablished metocurine- or vecuronium-induced neuromuscular blockade. Anesthesiology 1988; 69:954.

39. Aps C, Inglis MS: Peritoneal closure and atracurium. Anesthesia 1984; 39:187.

40. Ostergaard D, Jensen E, Jensen FS, et al: The duration of action of mivacurium-induced neuromuscular block in patients homozygous for the atypical plasma cholinesterase gene. Anesthesiology 1991; 75:A774.

41. Yellin AE, Newman J, Donovan AJ: Neostigmine-induced hyperperistalsis. Arch Surg 1973; 106:779.

42. Child CS: Prevention of neostigmine-induced colonic activity. Anesthesia 1984; 39:1083.

43. Wilkins JL, Hardcastle JD, Mann CV, et al: Effects of neostigmine and atropine on motor activity of ileum, colon, and rectum of anaesthetized subject. Br Med J 1970; 1:793.

44. Bell CMA, Lewis CB: Effect of neostigmine on integrity of ileorectal anastomoses. Br Med J 1968; 3:587.

45. Whitaker BL: Observations in the blood flow in the inferior mesenteric arterial system and the healing of colonic anastomoses. Ann R Coll Surg Engl 1968; 43:89.

46. Brown EN, Daughety MJ, Petty WC: Integrity of intestinal anastomoses following muscle relaxant reversal with neostigmine. Anesth Analg 1973; 52:118.

47. Morisot P, Loygue J, Guilmet EC: Effets de la décurarisation postopératoire par la néostigmine sur les anastomoses digestives. Can Anaesth Soc J 1975; 22:144.

48. Sunew KY, Hicks RG: Effects of neostigmine and pyridostigmine on duration of succinylcholine action and pseudocholinesterase activity. Anesthesiology 1978; 49:188.

49. Baraka A, Wakid N, Mansour R, et al: Effect of neostigmine and pyridostigmine on the plasma cholinesterase activity. Br J Anaesth 1981; 53:849.

50. Rigler ML, Drasner K, Krejcie TC: Cauda equina syndrome after continuous spinal anesthesia. Anesth Analg 1991; 72:75.

51. Morgan M, Norman G: The effect of extradural analgesia combined with light general anaesthesia and spontaneous ventilation on arterial blood gases and physiological dead space. Br J Anaesth 1975; 47:955.

52. Stephen GW, Lees MM, Scott DB: Cardiovascular effects of epidural block combined with general anesthesia. Br J Anaesth 1969; 41:933.

53. Germann PAS, Roberts JG, Prys-Roberts C: The combination of general anaesthesia and epidural block I: The effects of sequence of induction on haemodynamic variables and blood gas measurements in healthy patients. Anaesth Intensive Care 1979; 7:229.

54. Wright PMC, Fee JPH: Cardiovascular support during combined extradural and general anaesthesia. Br J Anaesth 1992; 68:585.

55. Hjortso NC, Neumann P, Frosig F, et al: A controlled study on the effect of epidural analgesia with local anaesthetics and morphine on morbidity after abdominal surgery. Acta Anaesthesiol Scand 1985; 29:790.

56. Worsley MH, Wishart HY, Brown P, et al: High spinal nerve block for large bowel anastomosis. A prospective study. Br J Anaesth 1988; 60:836.

57. Ravin MB: Comparison of spinal and general anesthesia for lower abdominal surgery in patients with chronic obstructive pulmonary disease. Anesthesiology 1971; 35:319.

58. Hendolin H, Tuppurainen T, Lahtinen J: Thoracic epidural analgesia and deep vein thrombosis in cholecystectomized patients. Acta Chir Scand 1982; 148:405.

59. Mellbring G, Dahlgren S, Reiz S, et al: Thromboembolic complications after major abdominal surgery: effects of thoracic epidural analgesia. Acta Chir Scand 1983; 149:263.

60. Kehlet H: Effect of pain-relieving techniques on postoperative protein economy. Br J Clin Pract 1988; 63:121.

61. Jones MJT: The influence of anesthetic methods on mental functioning. Acta Chir Scand 1988; 555(Suppl):169.

62. Rocco AG, Vandam LD: Changes in circulation consequent to manipulation during abdominal surgery. JAMA 1957; 16:14.

63. Doyle DJ, Mark PWS: Reflex bradycardia during surgery. Can J Anaesth 1990; 37:219.

64. Coventry DM, McMenemin I, Lawrie S: Bradycardia during inraabdominal surgery. Anaesthesia 1987; 42:835.

65. Seltzer JL, Ritter DE, Starsnic MA, et al: The hemodynamic response to traction on the abdominal mesentery. Anesthesiology 1985; 63:96.

66. Gottlieb A, Skrinska VA, O'Hara P, et al: The role of prostacyclin in the mesenteric traction syndrome during anesthesia for abdominal aortic reconstructive surgery. Ann Surg 1989; 209:363.

67. Hudson JC, Wurm WH, O'Donnell TF Jr, et al: Ibuprofen pretreatment inhibits prostacyclin release during abdominal exploration in aortic surgery. Anesthesiology 1990; 72:443.

68. Mirakhur RK, Jones CJ, Dundee JW: Effects of intravenous administration of glycopyrrolate and atropine in anaesthetized patients. Anaesthesia 1981; 36:277.

69. Levitt MD, Bond JH: Intestinal gas. *In* Gastrointestinal Disease. 4th ed. Sleisenger MH, Fordtran JS (eds). Philadelphia, WB Saunders, 1989, pp 257–603.

70. Eger EI II, Saidman LJ: Hazards of nitrous oxide anesthesia in bowel obstruction and pneumothorax. Anesthesiology 1965; 26:61.

71. Steffey EP, Johnson BH, Eger EI II, et al: Nitrous oxide: effect on accumulation rate and uptake of bowel gases. Anesth Analg 1979; 58:405.

72. Radnay PA, Duncalf D, Novakovic M, et al: Common bile duct pressure changes after fentanyl, morphine, meperidine, butorphanol, and naloxone. Anesth Analg 1984; 63:441.

73. McCammon RL, Stoelting RK, Madura JA: Effects of butorphanol, nalbuphine and fentanyl on intrabiliary tract dynamics. Anesth Analg 1984; 63:139.

74. Vatashsky E, Haskel Y: Effect of nalbuphine on intrabiliary pressure in the early postoperative period. Can Anaesth Soc J 1986; 33:433.

75. Carey LC, Ellison CE: Cholecystostomy, cholecystectomy, and intraoperative evaluation of the biliary tree. *In* Mastery of Surgery. 2nd ed. Vol. 1. Nyhus LM, Baker RJ (eds). Boston, Little, Brown & Co, 1992, pp 873–880.

76. Jones RM, Fiddian-Green R, Knight PR: Narcotic-induced choledochoduodenal sphincter spasm reversed by glucagon. Anesth Analg 1980; 59:946.

77. Humphreys HK, Fleming NW: Opioid-induced spasm of the sphincter of Oddi apparently reversed by nalbuphine. Anesth Analg 1992; 74:308.

78. Ikard RW, Federspiel CF: A comparison of Levin and sump nasogastric tubes for postoperative gastrointestinal decompression. Am Surg 1987; 53:50.

79. Galloway DC, Grundis J: Inadvertent intracranial placement of nasogastric tube through a basilar skull fracture. South Med J 1979; 72:240.

80. Ritter DM, Rettke ST, Hughes RW, et al: Placement of nasogastric tubes and esophageal stethoscopes in patients with documented esophageal varices. Anesth Analg 1988; 67:283.

81. Mundy DA: Another technique for insertion of nasogastric tubes. Anesthesiology 1979; 50:374.

82. Siegel IB, Kahn RC: Insertion of difficult nasogastric tubes through a nasoesophageally placed endotracheal tube. Crit Care Med 1987; 15:876.

83. Nelson RL, Nyhus LM: A new long intestinal tube. Surg Gynecol Obstet 1979; 149:581.

84. Stept WJ, Safar P: Rapid induction/intubation for prevention of gastric content aspiration. Anesth Analg 1979; 49:633.

85. Sellick BA: Cricoid pressure to control regurgitation of stomach contents during induction of anaesthesia. Lancet 1961; 2:404.

86. Salem MR, Joseph NJ, Heyman JH, et al: Cricoid compression is effective in obliterating the esophageal lumen in the presence of a nasogastric tube. Anesthesiology 1985; 64:443.

87. Salem MR, Wong AY, Mani M, et al: Efficacy of cricoid pressure in preventing gastric inflation during bag-mask ventilation in pediatric patients. Anesthesiology 1974; 40:96.

88. Lawes EG, Campbell I, Mercer D: Inflation pressure, gastric insufflation, and rapid sequence induction. Br J Anaesth 1987; 59:315.

89. Jense HG, Dubin SA, Silverstein P, et al: Effect of obesity on safe duration of apnea in anesthetized humans. Anesth Analg 1991; 72:89.

90. Ralph SJ, Wareham CA: Rupture of the esophagus during cricoid pressure. Anaesthesia 1991; 46:40.

91. Hayes MA, Goldenberg MD: Renal effects of anesthesia and operation mediated by endocrines. Anesthesiology 1963; 24:487.

92. Albert SN, Shibuya J, Economooulous B, et al: Simultaneous measurement of erythrocyte, plasma, and extracellular fluid volumes with radioactive tracers. Anesthesiology 1968; 29:908.

93. Shires T, Williams J, Brown F: Acute change in extracellular fluids associated with major surgical procedures. Ann Surg 1961; 154:803.

94. Shires T, Jackson DE: Postoperative salt tolerance. Arch Surg 1962; 84:703.

95. Roberts JP, Roberts JD, Skinner C, et al: Extracellular fluid deficit following operation and its correction with Ringer's lactate. Ann Surg 1984; 202:1.

96. Irvin TT, Hayter CJ, Modgill VK, et al: Plasma-volume deficits and salt and water excretion after surgery. Lancet 1972; 2:1159.

97. Shizgal HM, Solomon S, Gutelius JR: Body water distribution after operation. Surg Gynecol Obstet 1977; 144:35.

98. Pappova E, Bachmeier W, Crevoisier J-L, et al: Acute hypoproteinemic fluid overload: its determinants, distribution, and treatment with concentrated albumin and diuretics. Vox Sang 1977; 33:307.

99. Chan STF, Kapadia DR, Johnson AW, et al: Extracellular fluid volume expansion and third space sequestration at the site of small bowel anastomoses. Br J Surg 1983; 70:35.

100. Lowell JA, Schifferoecker C, Driscoll CF, et al: Postoperative fluid overload: not a benign problem. Crit Care Med 1990; 18:728.

101. Nielsen OM, Engell HC: The importance of plasma colloid osmotic pressure for interstitial fluid volume and fluid balance after elective abdominal vascular surgery. Ann Surg 1986; 203:25.

102. Zaloga GP, Hughes SS: Oliguria in patients with normal renal function. Anesthesiology 1990; 72:598.

103. Zaloga GP, Hughes SS: Oliguria in patients with normal renal function. Anesthesiology 1990; 72:598.

104. Mackenzie AI, Donald JR: Urine output and fluid therapy during anaesthesia and surgery. Br Med J 1969; 3:619.

105. Sladen RN: Effect of anesthesia and surgery on renal function. Crit Care Clin 1987; 3:373.

106. Ambrose NS, Keighley MRB: Physiological consequences of orthograde lavage bowel preparation for elective colorectal surgery: a review. J R Soc Med 1983; 76:767.

107. Davis GR, Santa Ana CA, Morawski SG, et al: Development of a lavage solution associated with minimal water and electrolyte absorption or secretion. Gastroenterology 1980; 78:991.

108. Zanoni CE, Bergamini C, Bertoncini M, et al: Whole-gut lavage for surgery. A case of intraoperative colonic explosion after administration of mannitol. Dis Colon Rectum 1982; 25:580.

109. Skillmann JJ, Critchlow JF: Postoperative hemorrhage and volume depletion. In Mastery of Surgery. 2nd ed. Nyhus LM, Baker RJ (eds). Boston, Little, Brown & Co, 1992, pp 48–54.

110. Shippy CR, Appel PL, Shoemaker WC: Reliability of clinical monitoring to assess blood volume in critically ill patients. Crit Care Med 1984; 12:107.

111. Amoroso P, Greenwood RN: Posture and central venous pressure measurements in circulatory volume depletion. Lancet 1989; 2:258.

112. Stene JK, Grande CM, Giesecke A: Shock resuscitation. In Trauma Anesthesia. Stene JK, Grande CM (eds). Baltimore, Williams & Wilkins, 1991, pp 100–131.

113. Dawson RB: Crystalloids versus colloids. In Trauma Care. Cowley RA, Conn A, Dunahri CM (eds). Philadelphia, JB Lippincott, 1987, pp 78–87.

114. Shenkin HA, Cheney RH, Govons SR, et al: On the diagnosis of hemorrhage in man. A study of volunteers bled large amounts. Am J Med Sci 1944; 208:421.

115. Vevon PA, Ellison EC, Carey LC: Splenectomy for hematological disease. Adv Surg 1989; 22:105.

116. Wait RB, Kahng KU: Renal failure complicating obstructive jaundice. Am J Surg 1989; 157:256.

117. Greig JD, Kurkowski ZH, Matheson NA: Surgical morbidity and mortality in one hundred and twenty-nine patients with obstructive jaundice. Br J Surg 1988; 75:216.

118. Green J, Beyar R, Bomzon L, et al: Jaundice, the circulation, and the kidney. Nephron 1984; 37:145.

119. Sitprija V, Kashemsant U, Sriratanaban A, et al: Renal function in obstructive jaundice in man: cholangiocarcinoma model. Kidney Int 1990; 38:945.

120. Martinez-Rodenas F, Oms L, Carulla X, et al: Measurements of body water compartments after ligation of the common bile duct in the rabbit. Br J Surg 1989; 76:461.

121. Dawson JL: Jaundice and anoxic renal damage: protective effect of mannitol. Br Med J 1964; 1:810.

122. McPherson GA, Benjamin IS, Blumgart LH: Improving renal function in obstructive jaundice without preoperative drainage (Letter). Lancet 1984; 1:511.

123. Pain JA, Cahill CJ, Gilbert JM, et al: Prevention of postoperative renal dysfunction in patients with obstructive jaundice: a multicentre study of bile salts and lactulose. Br J Surg 1991; 78:467.

124. Dawson JL: Postoperative function in obstructive jaundice. Effect of mannitol diuresis. Br Med J 1965; 1:32.

125. Gubern JM, Sancho JJ, Simo J, et al: A randomized trial on the effect of mannitol on postoperative renal function in patients with obstructive jaundice. Surgery 1988; 103:39.

126. Ekberg H, Tranberg K-G, Andersson R, et al: Major liver resection: perioperative course and management. Surgery 1986; 100:1.

127. Bismuth H, Garden OJ: Regular and extended right and left hepatectomy for cancer. In Mastery of Surgery. 2nd ed. Nyhus LM, Baker RJ (eds). Boston, Little, Brown & Co, 1992, pp 866–872.

128. Arroyo V, Gines P, Planas R, et al: Paracentesis in the management of cirrhotics with ascites. In The Kidney in Liver Disease. 3rd ed. Epstein M (ed). Baltimore, Williams & Wilkins, 1989, pp 578–590.

129. Cruikshank DP, Buchsbaum HJ: Effects of rapid paracentesis: cardiovascular dynamics and body fluid composition. JAMA 1973; 225:1361.

130. Simon DM, McCain JR, Bonkovsky HL, et al: Effects of therapeutic paracentesis on systemic and hepatic hemodynamics and on renal and hormonal function. Hepatology 1987; 7:423.

131. Cade R, Wagemaker H, Vogel S, et al: Hepatorenal syndrome: studies of the effect of vascular volume and intraperitoneal pressure on renal and hepatic function. Am J Med 1987; 82:427.

132. Kao HW, Rakov NE, Savage E, et al: The effect of large volume paracentesis on plasma volume—a cause of hypovolemia? Hepatology 1985; 5:403.

133. Epstein M: Role of the peritoneovenous shunt in the management of ascites and the hepatorenal syndrome. In The Kidney in Liver Disease. 3rd ed. Epstein M (ed). Baltimore, Williams & Wilkins, 1988, pp 593–612.

134. LeVeen HH, Christoudias G, Moon JP, et al: Peritoneo-venous shunting for ascites. Ann Surg 1974; 180:580.

135. LeVeen HH, Ip M, Ahmed N, et al: Coagulopathy post peritoneovenous shunt. Ann Surg 1987; 205:305.

136. Biagini JR, Belghiti J, Fekete F: Prevention of coagulopathy after placement of peritoneovenous shunt with replacement of ascitic fluid by normal saline solution. Surg Gynecol Obstet 1986; 163:315.

137. Fulenwider JT, Smith RB III, Reed SC, et al: Peritoneovenous shunts. Lessons learned from an eight-year experience with 70 patients. Arch Surg 1984; 119:1133.

138. Cello JP, Grendell JH, Crass RA, et al: Endoscopic sclerotherapy versus portocaval shunt in patients with severe cirrhosis and acute variceal hemorrhage. N Engl J Med 1987; 316:11.

139. Terblanche J: The surgeon's role in the management of portal hypertension. Ann Surg 1989; 209:381.

140. Reichel FA, Owen OE: Hemodynamic parameters in human hepatic cirrhosis. Ann Surg 1979; 190:523.

141. Steegmuller KW, Markin HM, Hollis HW Jr: Intraoperative hemodynamic investigations during portacaval shunt. Arch Surg 1984; 119:269.

142. Child CG: Major problems in clinical surgery. In The Liver and Portal Hypertension. Child CG, Coon WW (eds). Philadelphia, WB Saunders, 1964, p 50.

143. Pugh RNH, Murray-Lyon IM, Dawson JL, et al: Transection of the esophagus for bleeding varices. Br J Surg 1973; 60:646.

144. Lunzer MR, Newman S, Bernard AG, et al: Impaired cardiovascular responsiveness in liver disease. Lancet 1975; 2:382.

145. Greenway CV: Role of splanchnic venous system in overall cardiovascular homeostasis. Fed Proc 1983; 42:1678.

146. Vaamonde CA: Renal water handling in liver disease. In The Kidney in Liver Disease. 3rd ed. Epstein M (ed). Baltimore, Williams & Wilkins, 1989, pp 31–72.

147. Arieff A: Hyponatremia and hypernatremia in liver disease. In The Kidney in Liver Disease. 3rd ed. Epstein M (ed). Baltimore, Williams & Wilkins, 1989, pp 73–88.

148. Craig DB: Postoperative recovery of pulmonary function. Anesth Analg 1981; 60:46.

149. Wahba RWM: Perioperative functional residual capacity. Can J Anaesth 1991; 38:384.

150. Latimer RG, Dickman M, Day WC, et al: Ventilatory patterns and pulmonary complications after upper abdominal surgery determined by preoperative and postoperative computerized spirometry and blood gas analysis. Am J Surg 1971; 122:622.

151. Ali J, Khan TA: The comparative effects of muscle transection and median upper abdominal incisions on postoperative pulmonary function. Surg Gynecol Obstet 1979; 148:863.

152. Garcia-Valdecasas JC, Almenara R, Cabrer C, et al: Subcostal incision

versus midline laparotomy in gallstone surgery: a prospective and randomized trial. Br J Surg 1988; 75:473.

153. Tahir AH, George RB, Weil H, et al: Effects of abdominal surgery upon diaphragmatic function and regional ventilation. Int Surg 1973; 58:337.

154. Ford GT, Whitelaw WA, Rosenal TW, et al: Diaphragm function after upper abdominal surgery in humans. Am Rev Respir Dis 1983; 127:431.

155. Simmonneau G, Vivien A, Sartene R, et al: Diaphragm dysfunction induced by upper abdominal surgery. Am Rev Respir Dis 1983; 128:899.

156. Dureuil B, Cantineau JP, Desmonts JM: Effects of upper or lower abdominal surgery on diaphragmatic function. Br J Anaesth 1987; 59:1230.

157. Duggan JE, Drummond GB: Abdominal muscle activity and intraabdominal pressure after upper abdominal surgery. Anesth Analg 1989; 69:598.

158. Mankikian B, Cantineau JP, Bertrand M, et al: Improvement of diaphragmatic function by a thoracic extradural block after upper abdominal surgery. Anesthesiology 1988; 68:379.

159. Scott NB, Mogensen T, Bigler D, et al: Continuous thoracic extradural 0.5% bupivacaine with or without morphine: effect on quality of blockade, lung function, and the surgical stress response. Br J Anaesth 1989; 62:253.

160. Welchew EA: On-demand analgesia: a double-blind comparison of on-demand intravenous fentanyl with regular intramuscular morphine. Anaesthesia 1983; 35:19.

161. Bonnet F, Blery CH, Zatan M, et al: Effect of epidural morphine on postoperative pulmonary dysfunction. Acta Anaesthesiol Scand 1984; 28:147.

162. Pflug AE, Murphy TM, Butler SH, et al: The effects of postoperative peridural analgesia on pulmonary therapy and pulmonary complications. Anesthesiology 1974; 41:8.

163. Hendolin H, Lahtinen J, Länsimes E, et al: The effect of thoracic epidural analgesia on respiratory function after cholecystectomy. Acta Anaesthesiol Scand 1987; 31:645.

164. Frenette L, Boudreault D, Guay J: Interpleural analgesia improves pulmonary function after cholecystectomy. Can J Anaesth 1991; 38:71.

165. Ross WB, Tweedie JH, Leon YP, et al: Intercostal blockage and pulmonary function after cholecystectomy. Surgery 1989; 105:166.

166. Kitamura H, Sawa T, Ikezono E: Postoperative hypoxemia: the contribution of age to the maldistribution of ventilation. Anesthesiology 1972; 36:244.

167. Diament ML, Palmer KNV: Postoperative changes in gas tensions of arterial blood and in ventilatory function. Lancet 1966; 2:180.

168. Strandberg A, Tokics L, Brismar B, et al: Atelectasis during anaesthesia and in the postoperative period. Acta Anaesthesiol Scand 1986; 30:154.

169. Hsu HO, Hickey RF: Effect of posture on functional residual capacity postoperatively. Anesthesiology 1976; 44:520.

170. Moreno F, Lyons HA: Effect of body posture on lung volumes. J Appl Physiol 1961; 16:27.

171. Vaughan RW, Wise L: Postoperative arterial blood gas measurement in obese patients: effect of position on gas exchange. Ann Surg 1975; 182:705.

172. Russell WJ: Position of patient and respiratory function in immediate postoperative period. Br Med J 1981; 283:1079.

173. Bonnet F, Bourgain JL, Mtamis D, et al: The influence of position on ventilation-perfusion distribution after abdominal surgery. Acta Anaesthesiol Scand 1988; 32:585.

174. Craig DB, Wahba WM, Don HF, et al: "Closing volume" and its relationship to gas exchange in seated and supine position. J Appl Physiol 1971; 31:171.

175. Shapiro BA, Kacmarek RM, Cane RD, et al: The postoperative patient. *In* Clinical Application of Respiratory Care. 4th ed. St Louis, Mosby-Year Book, 1991, pp 256–264, 426–432.

176. Nunn JF, Milledge JS, Chen D, et al: Respiratory criteria of fitness for surgery and anaesthesia. Anaesthesia 1988; 43:543.

177. Gaa GD, Olsen GN: Preoperative pulmonary function testing to predict postoperative morbidity and mortality. Chest 1986; 89:127.

178. Roukema JA, Carol EJ, Prins JG: The prevention of pulmonary complications after upper abdominal surgery in patients with noncompromised pulmonary status. Arch Surg 1988; 123:30.

179. Celli BR, Rodriguez KS, Snider GL: A controlled trial of intermittent positive pressure breathing, incentive spirometry, and deep breathing exercises in preventing pulmonary complications after abdominal surgery. Am Rev Respir Dis 1984; 130:12.

180. Stock MC, Downs JB, Cooper RB: Comparison of continuous positive airway pressure, incentive spirometry, and conservative therapy after cardiac operations. Crit Care Med 1984; 12:969.

181. Hall JC, Tarala R, Harris J, et al: Incentive spirometry versus routine chest physiotherapy for prevention of pulmonary complications after abdominal surgery. Lancet 1991; 337:953.

182. Rennie JA, Christofides ND, Mitchenere P, et al: Neural and humoral factors in postoperative ileus. Br J Surg 1980; 67:694.

183. Graber JN, Schulte WJ, Condon RE, et al: Relationship of duration of postoperative ileus to extent and site of operative dissection. Surgery 1982; 92:87.

184. Condon RE, Cowles V, Ekbom GA, et al: Effects of halothane, enflurane, and nitrous oxide on colon motility. Surgery 1987; 101:81.

185. Giuffre M, Gross JB: The effects of nitrous oxide on postoperative bowel motility. Anesthesiology 1986; 65:699.

186. Scheinin B, Lindgren L, Scheinin TM: Preoperative nitrous oxide delays bowel function after colonic surgery. Br J Anaesth 1990; 64:154.

187. Wilson JP: Postoperative motility of the large intestine in man. Gut 1975; 16:689.

188. Scheinin B, Asantila R, Orko R: The effect of bupivacaine and morphine on pain and bowel function after colonic surgery. Acta Anaesthesiol Scand 1987; 31:161.

189. Ahn H, Bronge A, Johansson K, et al: Effect of continuous postoperative epidural analgesia on intestinal motility. Br J Surg 1988; 75:1176.

190. Wallin G, Cassuto J, Högström S, et al: Failure of epidural anesthesia to prevent postoperative paralytic ileus. Anesthesiology 1986; 65:292.

191. Bredtmann RD, Herden HN, Teichmann W, et al: Epidural analgesia in colonic surgery: results of a random prospective study. Br J Surg 1990; 77:638.

192. Verlinden M, Michiels G, Boghaert A, et al: Treatment of postoperative gastrointestinal atony. Br J Surg 1987; 74:614.

193. Hallerbäck B, Ander S, Glise H: Effect of combined blockage of β-adrenoceptors and acetylcholinesterase in the treatment of postoperative ileus after cholecystectomy. Scand J Gastroenterol 1987; 22:420.

194. Jepsen S, Klaerke A, Nielsen PH, et al: Negative effect of metoclopramide in postoperative adynamic ileus. A prospective, randomized, double blind study. Br J Surg 1986; 73:290.

195. Eriksson E (ed): Illustrated Handbook in Local Anaesthesia. 2nd ed. Philadelphia, WB Saunders, 1980, p 52.

196. Urbach KF, Lee WR, Sheely LL, et al: Spinal or general anesthesia for inguinal hernia repair? JAMA 1964; 190:137.

197. Kopacz DJ, Mulroy MF: Chloroprocaine and lidocaine decrease hospital stay and admission rate after outpatient epidural anesthesia. Reg Anaesth 1990; 15:19.

198. Tverskoy M, Cozacov C, Ayache M, et al: Postoperative pain after inguinal herniorrhaphy with different types of anesthesia. Anesth Analg 1990; 70:29.

199. Ryan JA Jr, Adye BA, Jolly PC, et al: Outpatient inguinal herniorrhaphy with both regional and local anesthesia. Am J Surg 1984; 148:313.

200. Lund PC: Principle and Practice of Spinal Anesthesia. Springfield, IL, Charles C Thomas, 1971, pp 462–463.

CHAPTER 66

Anesthesia for Pediatric Cardiovascular Surgery

LAURIE K. DAVIES, M.D.

Pediatric cardiovascular surgery is a challenging, continuously evolving field. In the 1960s, only a small fraction of patients with congenital heart disease (CHD) were offered surgical repair or palliation, and those that were experienced significant mortality and morbidity. Since the early 1970s, however, improvements in diagnostic capability, cardiopulmonary bypass techniques, and monitoring and perioperative care have permitted more complicated procedures to be performed on smaller, sicker children with remarkable success. Even today, operative procedures and technology are being constantly modified in an effort to further improve the safety and outcome of these very special children.

Each child presents a unique set of circumstances and pathophysiologic concerns. Thus, in today's environment of continual change, anesthesiologists caring for these patients must be flexible and innovative. Rigid protocols rarely are appropriate; instead, an individualized plan for each patient is mandatory. Another area of medicine in which team effort and good communication are as essential to the success of each case is difficult to conceive. Being a part of a successful team effort and caring for these patients are among the most exciting and rewarding experiences in medicine today.

MAJOR CONGENITAL HEART LESIONS

What Are Their Characteristics?

Incidence

CHD is relatively uncommon. It is estimated to occur in somewhat fewer than 1% of all live births (Table 66–1).[1] The true incidence is probably quite a bit higher. Much fetal wastage is thought to occur because of the presence of congenital heart defects that are incompatible with life. Also, some heart lesions (bicuspid aortic valve is an example) may be relatively asymptomatic early in life. Thus, the true incidence of CHD is unknown.

Available studies have tried to estimate CHD prevalence in selected populations.[2, 3] Certain lesions are more likely to become manifest early in life than are others. Thus, the prevalence of these symptomatic lesions is falsely elevated. With these caveats in mind, the lesions most likely to be encountered in the first year of life are ventricular septal defect (VSD), transposition of the great vessels, tetralogy of Fallot, coarctation of the aorta, and hypoplastic left-sided heart syndrome.[2]

Different reference populations may demonstrate different patterns of CHD. For instance, infants who are premature and small for their gestational ages have an increased prevalence of CHD (especially VSD and patent ductus arteriosus [PDA]) compared with full-term newborns.[4] Congenital heart defects are more common among infants of diabetic mothers than among those of normal mothers.[5] Infants with abnormal chromosomes have an increased frequency of congenital heart defects. The most common defects in children with Down's syndrome appear to be VSD, atrial septal defect (ASD), PDA, and atrioventricular septal defects.[6]

Severity

Patients with CHD present a broad spectrum of severity of illness. Some patients may be asymptomatic and found only incidentally to have an ASD defect or PDA. Others may be moribund with congestive heart failure (CHF) and cyanosis, or with a combination of the two. Keith studied 10,535 cases of cardiac defects at the Hospital for Sick Children in Toronto from 1950 to 1970.[7] Twenty-seven per cent of the patients died during the period of observation, and 34% died during the first month of life.

Prognosis

The outlook for these children in the 1990s has improved considerably over that of previous years. A better understanding of the pathophysiology of individual lesions allows a rational treatment care plan to be developed. Earlier complete repairs are being performed successfully, often resulting in the avoidance of the long-term sequelae of unrepaired CHD. Cardiac transplantation also has become a viable option for some children whose lesions cannot be surgically repaired. For any of these options to be successful, the patient's care must be

TABLE 66–1. Reported Estimate of Prevalence per 1000 Live Births for Specific Congenital Heart Defects

Defect	Prevalence
Ventricular septal defect	0.38
Transposition	0.21
Tetralogy of Fallot	0.21
Coarctation of aorta	0.18
Hypoplastic left-sided heart syndrome	0.16
Patent ductus arteriosus	0.14
Atrioventricular septal defect	0.12
Pulmonary stenosis	0.19
Pulmonary atresia	0.07
Secundum atrial septal defect	0.07
Total anomalous pulmonary venous drainage	0.06
Tricuspid atresia	0.06
Aortic stenosis	0.04
Double-outlet right ventricle	0.03
Truncus arteriosus	0.03
Other	0.18

(Modified from Daniels SR: Epidemiology. *In* Fetal and Neonatal Cardiology. Long WA (ed). Philadelphia, WB Saunders, 1990, p 430.)

thoughtfully individualized with vigilance, anticipation, and meticulous attention to detail.

PHYSIOLOGIC CONSIDERATIONS

What Is the Difference Between Fetal and Adult Circulation?

In order to develop an understanding of the clinical and anesthetic implications of CHD, one must be familiar with the fetal and the adult circulations. Three important channels characteristic of the circulation in utero allow preferential shunting of blood: the ductus venosus, foramen ovale, and ductus arteriosus (Fig. 66–1).

Ductus Venosus

Well-oxygenated blood from the placenta, with a partial pressure of oxygen [PO_2] of about 33 mm Hg, travels through the umbilical vein to enter the liver.[8] The ductus venosus allows about one-half of this blood to be shunted from the liver directly into the inferior vena cava.

Foramen Ovale

About one-third of the blood entering the right atrium from the inferior vena cava is preferentially shunted across the foramen ovale into the left atrium. On the other hand, superior vena cava blood (which is poorly oxygenated) primarily enters the right ventricle, with 2% to 3% crossing the foramen ovale.

Ductus Arteriosus

Right ventricular blood is largely shunted across the ductus arteriosus into the descending aorta (rather than perfusing the high-resistance pulmonary circulation).

Implications

The structure of the fetal circulation allows the well-oxygenated blood (which has a high glucose content) from the inferior vena cava to preferentially perfuse the brain, coronary circulation, and upper extremities. The lower portion of the body receives blood with a low oxygen content from the ductus arteriosus.[9] Hence, the systemic and pulmonary circulations in the fetus function in parallel, with each ventricle receiving only a portion of the systemic cardiac output.[10] The adult situation, in contrast, requires the two circulations to work in series, each processing the entire cardiac output.

What Is the Transitional Circulation?

At birth, remarkable changes occur rapidly in the circulation that allow the infant to adapt to the stresses of extrauterine life.[11] A period of transition in the neonatal circulation occurs before permanent adaptation to the normal adult pattern takes place. This transitional stage is unstable and may exist for a few hours or for many weeks, depending on the stresses imposed. Factors contributing to the instability of the transitional circulation are the state of the ductus arteriosus, foramen ovale, and pulmonary vascular bed as well as the immaturity of the neonatal heart. Conditions that may prolong the transitional circulation include hypoxia, hypothermia, acidosis, hypercarbia, sepsis, and CHD.[12]

Closure of the Ductus Arteriosus

Functional closure of the ductus arteriosus usually occurs within a few hours of birth, but anatomic closure may not occur for several weeks.[13] During this period, the resistance to

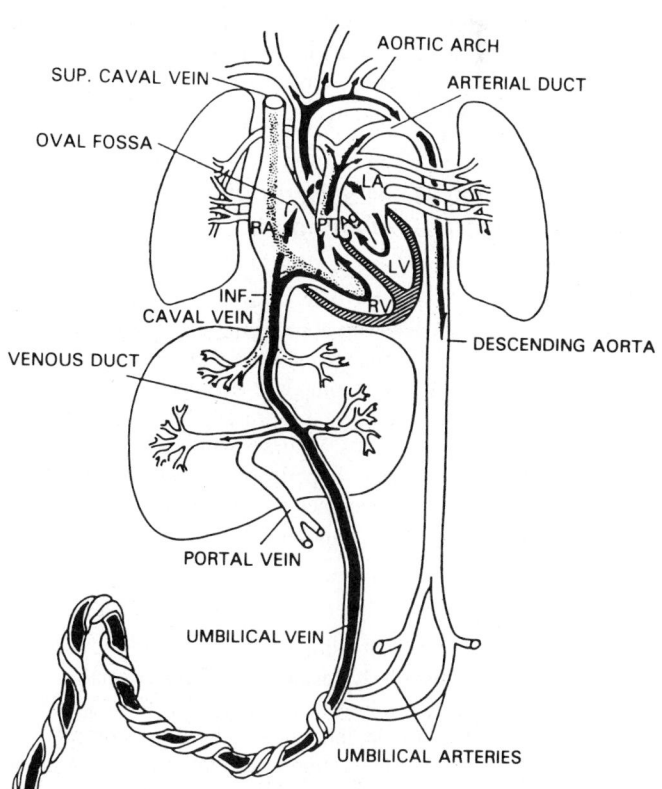

FIGURE 66–1. Diagram of the course of the fetal circulation. (From Ho SY, Angelini A, Moscoso G: Developmental cardiac anatomy. *In* Fetal and Neonatal Cardiology. 1st ed. Long WA (ed). Philadelphia, WB Saunders, 1990, p 4.)

ductus arteriosus blood flow is responsive to changes in arterial P_{O_2} (P_{aO_2}); that is, increased P_{aO_2} increases resistance, and decreased P_{aO_2} decreases resistance. Prostaglandin E_1 infusion relaxes the ductal musculature and increases ductal flow, which may be left-to-right, right-to-left, or bidirectional.[14] Maintenance of ductal patency may be important for the infant with cyanotic heart disease until repair or palliative surgery can be performed.

Closure of the Foramen Ovale and Ductus Venosus

The foramen ovale functionally closes when left atrial pressure exceeds right atrial pressure; this usually occurs within a few hours after birth. Anatomic closure does not occur for many months, and about 30% of adults demonstrate probe patency of the foramen ovale.[15] Right-to-left intracardiac shunting may occur across this area with coughing or the Valsalva maneuver or if pulmonary hypertension develops. Umbilical arteries and veins close shortly after birth, as does the ductus venosus. The latter forms the ligamentum venosum.

Pulmonary Vascular Resistance

Pulmonary vascular resistance is high in utero, but it declines rapidly after birth. Usually, it is lower than systemic levels within 24 hours of birth. Thereafter, it falls at a moderate rate for 5 to 6 weeks and then more gradually for the next 2 to 3 years.[16, 17] During this period, a child's pulmonary vascular bed is more reactive than an adult's, and a rise in pulmonary artery pressure can easily be produced by hypoxemia, hypercarbia, acidosis, or bronchospasm. If this reaction occurs shortly after birth, it may result in shunting across the ductus arteriosus or foramen ovale or in other cardiac defects. Later in life, only a patent foramen ovale or cardiac defect remains as a possible shunt site.

How Is a Child's Heart Structurally Different Than That of an Adult?

Size

At birth, both ventricles are approximately equal in size and wall thickness. With the change over from the fetal circulation, the left ventricle must accommodate a greater pressure and volume workload; conversely, the pressure load of the right ventricle is reduced, and its volume work is only slightly increased. The left ventricle hypertrophies in response to the increased workload and becomes roughly twice as heavy as the right ventricle by about 6 months of age.[18]

Ultrastructure

The neonate's heart is ultrastructurally immature. Myofibrils are arranged in a disorderly fashion and have a smaller percentage of contractile proteins than do those in the adult (30% versus 60%).[19] Autonomic innervation is also incomplete at birth. The sympathetic innervation to the heart is decreased as are cardiac catecholamine stores.[20] In contrast, the parasympathetic innervation of the neonatal heart is comparable with that of the adult heart.[21] These observations are often cited to explain the frequent vagal predominance that occurs in infants compared with adults. Sympathetic innervation also is imma-

ture in the peripheral vasculature. Therefore, control of vascular tone and myocardial contractility in infants depends largely on adrenal function and circulating catecholamines.

Compliance

The immature heart has a functionally decreased compliance when compared with the adult heart. This difference, in part, reflects the ultrastructure of the heart and the increased volume load that each ventricle must handle with the transition from a parallel fetal to an adult series circulation.[12] The right and left ventricles are more intimately interrelated as a result of this decreased compliance and similarity in size. Dysfunction of one ventricle very quickly leads to biventricular failure. Reduced compliance also means that the immature heart is more sensitive to volume overload. A neonate's ventricular function curve is shifted to the right compared with that of an adult. Over the physiologic range of ventricular filling pressures, stroke volume changes are, in fact, small.

This relatively fixed stroke volume makes a neonate highly dependent on heart rate and sinus rhythm for optimal cardiac output. In comparison, the adult heart is much more responsive to changes in preload to effect a change in stroke volume and thereby change cardiac output. Increases in pressure work are poorly tolerated by both the right and left sides of the immature heart. The neonate, therefore, responds poorly to either volume or pressure loading, because resting cardiac function is on or near the plateau of the cardiac function curve (Fig. 66–2).

How Are Congenital Cardiac Lesions Meaningfully Characterized?

Flow Pattern

Patients with congenital heart defects are a diverse group. Rather than memorize an approach to each lesion, one should group the many anatomic varieties into a few understandable categories (Table 66–2). Most defects can be assigned to one of three groups: (1) those resulting in increased pulmonary

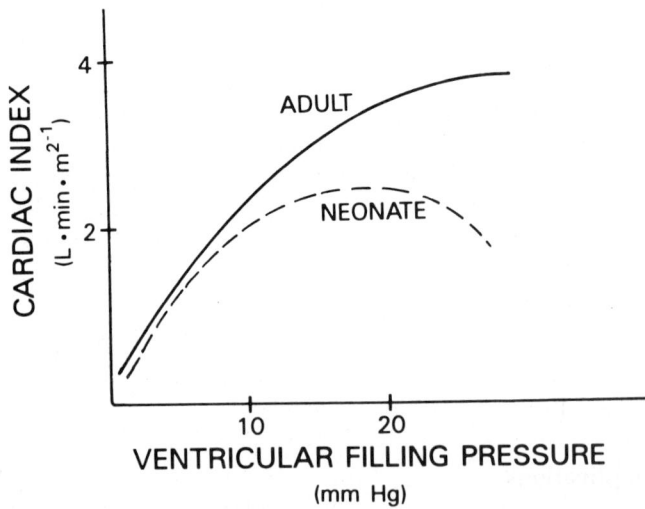

FIGURE 66–2. Schematic representation of the difference in ventricular function between neonates and adults.

TABLE 66–2. Flow Characteristics of Various Congenital Cardiac Lesions

Increased pulmonary blood flow lesions	ASD
	VSD
	PDA
	Endocardial cushion defect (atrioventricular canal abnormality)
	Anomalous origin of coronary arteries
	Transposition of the great arteries*
	Anomalous pulmonary venous drainage*
	Truncus arteriosus*
	Single ventricle*
Decreased pulmonary blood flow lesions	Tetralogy of Fallot
	Pulmonary atresia
	Tricuspid atresia
	Ebstein's anomaly
	Truncus arteriosus*
	Transposition of the great arteries*
	Single ventricle*
Obstructive lesions	Aortic stenosis
	Pulmonary stenosis
	Coarctation of the aorta
	Asymmetric septal hypertrophy

(Modified from Schwartz AJ, Campbell FW: Pathophysiological approach to congenital heart disease. *In* Pediatric Cardiac Anesthesia. Lake CL (ed). Norwalk, CT, Appleton & Lange, 1988, p 9.)
*Systemic hypoxemia occurs as a result of the mixing of systemic and pulmonary venous returns. Classification as an increased or decreased pulmonary blood flow lesion depends on the absence or presence within the anatomic variation of obstruction to pulmonary blood flow.

blood flow; (2) those resulting in decreased pulmonary blood flow; and (3) and those resulting in obstruction to blood flow. The first two groups feature an abnormal shunt pathway, whereas the third group has no shunting of blood. A fourth group could include lesions in which no pulmonary-systemic exchange of blood occurs (e.g., transposition of the great vessel [TGV]). However, infants with TGV have either naturally occurring or artificially induced mixing of systemic and pulmonary venous returns and often can be classified into one of the first two groups, depending on whether obstruction to pulmonary blood flow is present.

Cyanosis Versus Heart Failure

Cyanosis and CHF are the major manifestations of CHD. Thus, the pathophysiologic classification must be related to the clinical status. Cyanosis occurs most commonly with lesions in which pulmonary blood flow is anatomically decreased or functionally decreased as mixing of systemic and pulmonary venous blood occurs.

CHF occurs most commonly in shunt lesions with excessively increased pulmonary blood flow or obstructive lesions that stress the ventricle beyond its capacity to pump effectively.[22] Note that a child can be cyanotic, but the classification can still be that of a lesion with increased pulmonary blood flow and even CHF. An example of such a situation is an infant with TGV and a large VSD. Even the most complex lesions usually fall into one of the three categories, even if they are characterized by mixed features (see Table 66–2).[22]

When and Why do Patients Become Symptomatic?

Many types of CHD may not be detected immediately after birth. The age at which heart defects become manifest ob-

viously depends on the type of lesion, its severity, and the state of the infant's transitional circulation. Increased pulmonary blood flow lesions typically become symptomatic as pulmonary vascular resistance decreases and shunt flow to the lungs increases. These changes may take days to weeks to occur. Also, if the defect is small, it may remain asymptomatic.

Decreased pulmonary blood flow lesions often are detected earlier, usually because they result in significant cyanosis. If obstruction to pulmonary blood flow is severe, patients with such lesions may be dependent on left-to-right flow across their PDA. As the PDA closes in the first few days of life, hypoxemia becomes even more pronounced and may be incompatible with survival.

Infants with TGV and an inadequate intracardiac communication become extremely cyanotic as their PDA closes. On the other hand, if a large VSD or PDA is present, these patients develop excessive pulmonary blood flow as the pulmonary vascular resistance decreases during the first few weeks of extrauterine life. Left untreated, hypertrophic vascular changes and pulmonary hypertension will occur.

Left-sided obstructive lesions cause pulmonary congestion without pulmonary volume overload. They impede flow from the pulmonary venous system to the systemic arterial system and can precipitate CHF. The symptomatology and age at presentation depend on the severity of the lesion. If the ductus arteriosus is patent, it allows right-to-left shunting of blood around the lesion, improving systemic perfusion but causing cyanosis.

PREOPERATIVE ASSESSMENT

What Should the Anesthesiologist Look for?

In developing an anesthetic plan for these children, be sure to understand the pathophysiology of the individual lesion and to appreciate the degree of clinical symptomatology. As in any other assessment, taking of a careful history and the physical examination are probably the most important parts of the preoperative evaluation. Remember that the infant cannot tell you the symptoms experienced, and the parents often fail to understand the significance of some of their observations.

Age at Presentation

The age at presentation often provides a clue to the severity of the lesion. Infants with decreased pulmonary blood flow or inadequate mixing may be persistently cyanotic or may have intermittent episodes that are often associated with agitation, crying, or exercise. If a child is older, cyanotic episodes may be associated with "squatting" (which increases systemic vascular resistance). Particularly severe episodes can result in loss of consciousness or seizures.

Frequency of Episodes

The frequency of these episodes also suggests severity of the lesion. Knowledge that cyanotic episodes are intermittent confirms the dynamic nature of the shunt and should alert one to the fact that the same scenario is probable during anesthesia and surgical manipulations. Alterations in systemic and pulmonary vascular resistance may result in profound changes in the magnitude of the right-to-left shunt.

Cyanosis

During the physical examination, an important consideration is that clinical cyanosis depends on the absolute concentration of deoxygenated hemoglobin in the blood rather than on the oxygen saturation. More than $3 \text{ g} \cdot \text{dL}^{-1}$ of deoxygenated arterial blood hemoglobin should make central cyanosis recognizable.[23] The oxyhemoglobin saturation at which central cyanosis becomes clinically apparent varies from about 62% when hemoglobin level is $8 \text{ g} \cdot \text{dL}^{-1}$ to about 88% in the polycythemic infant whose hemoglobin level is $24 \text{ g} \cdot \text{dL}^{-1}$. Thus, cyanosis is more easily detected when the infant's hematocrit is elevated. However, recognition of cyanosis is more difficult if a newborn has a significant proportion of fetal hemoglobin because it is more highly saturated at a given Po_2 (Fig. 66–3).[23] Therefore, the newborn with a high proportion of fetal hemoglobin may have a very large reduction in Po_2 before central cyanosis is clinically apparent.[23]

Respiration

Infants with cyanotic heart disease often have an increased tidal volume. Clubbing of the fingers may also occur but may not be evident early in life. Children with decreased pulmonary blood flow usually have exercise intolerance. Progressive polycythemia and failure to thrive are also characteristic features of significant lesions. Infants with a preductal coarctation of the aorta may demonstrate cyanosis that is restricted to the lower half of the body, since the right ventricle supplies the descending aorta with deoxygenated blood via the PDA.

Congestive Heart Failure

Infants with too much pulmonary blood flow present with CHF early in infancy when the pulmonary vascular resistance

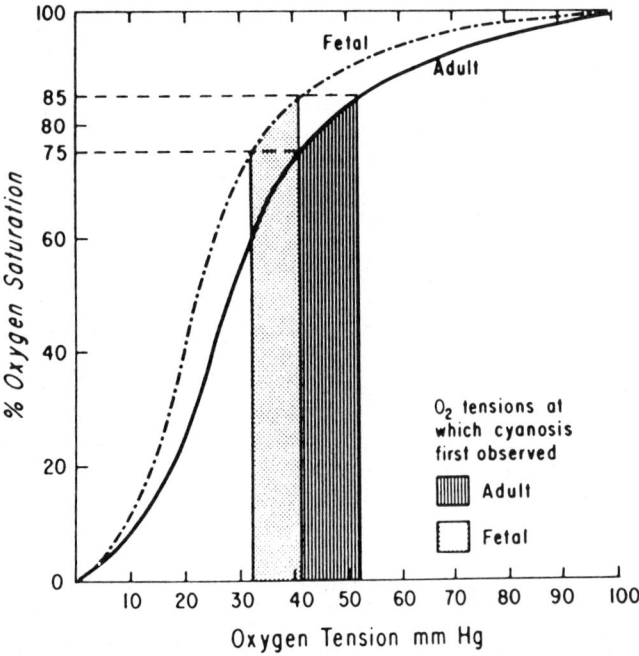

FIGURE 66–3. Hemoglobin-oxygen dissociation curves for fetal and adult hemoglobin. Note that an infant with a high proportion of fetal hemoglobin will have a very low Pao$_2$ (33–42 mm Hg) before cyanosis is observed. (From Lees MH, King DH: Heart disease in the newborn. *In* Heart Disease in Infants, Children and Adolescents. Adams FH, Emmanouilides GC, Riemenschneider TA (eds). Baltimore, Williams & Wilkins, 1989, p 844. © Williams & Wilkins, 1989.)

decreases. A history of feeding difficulties and failure to thrive are characteristic of CHF in infancy. Other features include tachypnea, tachycardia, inappropriate sweating (often with feeding), nasal flaring, sternal and intercostal retractions, cardiomegaly, and hepatomegaly. A history of wheezing, frequent respiratory infections, and pneumonia is common. The distinction between left-sided and right-sided heart failure in the newborn is less obvious than in the adult. Peripheral edema and rales are rarely present in the young infant. Systemic perfusion may be compromised as evidenced by decreased pulses, pallor, and poor capillary refill. A severely compromised infant may be apathetic and have a weak cry and little spontaneous movement.

Left-sided obstructive lesions may also cause CHF with clinical manifestations that are similar to those of pulmonary volume overload. Note, however, that the symptoms are a result of pulmonary venous congestion without abnormal shunting. If the lesion is located so that left ventricular *outflow* is obstructed, left ventricular hypertrophy will develop; if the site of obstruction involves the *inflow* to the left ventricle, left ventricular hypertrophy does not occur, and left ventricular end-diastolic pressure is normal.

Associated Anomalies

Look carefully for associated congenital anomalies, since they are common in newborns with cardiac disease. Other problems peculiar to the newborn or premature infant include difficulty with temperature regulation, impaired nutrition, susceptibility to dehydration and hypoglycemia, respiratory difficulties, coagulation abnormalities, and central nervous system disorders.

What Preoperative Laboratory Studies Are Helpful?

Laboratory studies of particular interest include hematocrit, white blood cell count, coagulation profile, and electrolyte and serum glucose determinations. Sickle cell screening and measurement of digoxin level should be included when applicable.

Hematocrit

The hematocrit progressively rises as hypoxemia becomes more profound. A high hematocrit can result in increased blood viscosity, which can lead to spontaneous thrombosis and resultant cerebral, renal, or pulmonary infarctions. This process may be aggravated by the relative dehydration produced by a long period without oral intake. If the polycythemia is sufficiently severe (i.e., hematocrit is >60–65%), phlebotomy may be required. Patients with cyanotic CHD are prone to develop coagulopathies because of platelet dysfunction and hypofibrinogenemia.[24, 25] These patients also have a blunted ventilatory response to hypoxia.[26]

White Blood Cell Count

Elevations in white blood cell count and a white blood cell shift in the differential should raise the suspicion of a systemic infection. Fever and upper respiratory infection must be ruled out. Children with elevated white blood cell counts should not be electively anesthetized, since immunologic function is compromised by cardiopulmonary bypass. Also, prosthetic material is frequently used in the surgical repair; if this material is inadvertently seeded by a bacteremia, its presence may have disastrous consequences.

Coagulation Studies

Results of coagulation studies must be normal before cardiopulmonary bypass can be performed. A family history of bleeding tendencies should be sought. Unsuspected factor deficiencies have manifested and caused uncontrollable bleeding following surgery, when it may be difficult to identify the source of the problem.

Electrolytes

Electrolyte problems may be present in the newborn, especially if the child is receiving medication or total parenteral nutrition. Hypokalemia, hypomagnesemia, hypocalcemia, and hypoglycemia should be ruled out. Hypocalcemia is common in children with DiGeorge's syndrome (a congenital disorder of the third and fourth branchial arches that is associated with thymic hypoplasia and congenital heart defects, especially aortic arch abnormalities).

Glucose

Hypoglycemia is especially common in infants with hypoplastic left-sided heart syndrome. The newborn's myocardium has an increased glucose dependence compared with the adult myocardium; thus, hypoglycemia may aggravate myocardial failure.[27]

Digoxin

Many children scheduled for heart surgery are receiving digoxin. Following cardiopulmonary bypass, both a rebound increase in digoxin level and an increased sensitivity to the drug have been reported.[28] Perioperative dysrhythmias are common and may be related to digoxin toxicity; other factors may play a role in this enhanced toxicity, including hypokalemia, calcium fluxes, hypomagnesemia, and decreased creatinine clearance. Therefore, verify that the digoxin level is within the normal range and withhold digoxin preoperatively.

Sickling Test

A sickling test should be performed in appropriate children. Hypothermia, acidosis, and anemia, as induced by cardiopulmonary bypass, as well as decreased perfusion enhance sickling if hemoglobin S is present. If the sickling test result is positive, hemoglobin electrophoresis should be performed to delineate the type of hemoglobinopathy. Depending on the type of defect, exchange transfusion may be indicated prior to cardiopulmonary bypass.

Electrocardiography

The electrocardiogram shows great variability, especially during the first 24 hours of life. In some instances, the electrocardiogram is diagnostically very helpful. For example, extreme left or right axis deviation with counterclockwise frontal vector and right ventricular hypertrophy suggests a form of endocardial cushion defect.

Echocardiography and Cardiac Catheterization

Two-dimensional echocardiography with quantitative Doppler and color flow mapping has revolutionized the diagnosis of CHD. In many institutions, the technology has become so refined that most surgical procedures are performed on the basis of this study alone. Cardiac catheterization is used to confirm the diagnosis and to provide information concerning vascular resistance, the magnitude of shunts, and coronary anatomy.

Chest Radiography

Chest radiography serves to evaluate the type and severity of the heart disease. It is also used to identify simulators of heart disease (e.g., meconium aspiration, mediastinal masses, pneumothorax, hyaline membrane disease, and diaphragmatic hernia) and to rule out significant pulmonary pathology.

What Should the Anesthesiologist Tell the Family About Risk?

Neurologic Sequelae

Morbidity and mortality vary with the lesion being repaired or palliated and with the institution involved. Neurologic sequelae occur in about 4.5% and seizures in approximately 20% of neonates following cardiopulmonary bypass.[29, 30] The seizures are generally self-limited, and some series have reported no long-term adverse sequelae.[31, 32] Apparently, the frequency of seizures and neuropsychologic abnormalities is unaffected by whether total circulatory arrest is used.

Anesthetic Risk

A comprehensive evaluation of anesthetic complications and outcome in 500 consecutive patients undergoing CHD operations has been performed.[33] Several anesthetic agents were used, including thiopental, ketamine, narcotics, and inhalation agents. No apparent differences in outcome were detected with these different agents. During hospitalization, a perioperative mortality of 6.3% occurred; no death was directly attributable to anesthesia. Anesthetic complications (major and minor) occurred in 2% of cases.

A 1991 abstract examined risk in patients with CHD undergoing noncardiac surgery.[34] A total of 135 anesthetic procedures in 110 patients were analyzed. Almost one-half of the patients (47%) experienced an adverse event, which was broadly defined as any unexpected event that was not part of a routine, uncomplicated anesthetic case (Table 66–3). Not all adverse events resulted in perioperative complications. Uncompensated CHF, cyanosis, and uncorrected heart disease were associated with a higher risk of adverse events. Patients with tetralogy of Fallot had the highest incidence of adverse events (9 of 13 patients); the most common complication involved airway difficulties. Thus, patients with CHD represent a challenge in both cardiac and noncardiac surgery.

TABLE 66–3. Perioperative Complications in Patients with or Undergoing 135 Operations for Congenital Heart Disease

Adverse Event	No. of Patients
Airway emergency	22
Bronchospasm	4
Dysrhythmias	17
Circulatory instability	16
Acidosis	2
Hypoglycemia	1
Delayed emergence	4
Nausea/emesis	5

(From Strafford MA, Henderson KH: Anesthetic morbidity in congenital heart disease patients undergoing noncardiac surgery [abstract]. Anesthesiology 1991; 75:A1056.)

When Should Oral Intake Stop?

Nil per os guidelines used for other infants and children can generally be used in patients with CHD. Recent evidence suggests that clear liquids can be continued until 2 to 4 hours before surgery.[35] In children with cyanotic heart disease, meticulous attention must be paid to the patient's state of hydration. Specifically, orders must be written to awaken the child 2 hours before surgery to offer clear liquids. If uncertainty exists concerning the precise time of surgery, place an intravenous catheter and begin an infusion to prevent dehydration in patients with cyanotic heart disease.

What Sedation Is Appropriate?

The need for sedation must be individualized, but certain guidelines can be offered. A thorough explanation to the patient and family may be in order, since the parents' anxiety is often transmitted to the child. Neonates and infants under the age of 6 months rarely require any sedation, since separation anxiety is not an issue. In older children, if intravenous access is already established and the child's parents are allowed to accompany him or her to the preoperative holding area, additional sedation may be unnecessary, since incremental intravenous agents can be titrated prior to transfer to the operating room.

Children between the ages of 1 and 5 years benefit most from judicious sedation. A variety of agents and routes can be used. I prefer to avoid intramuscular injections and use either intravenous or oral midazolam. If given intravenously, I titrate in 0.1- to 0.25-mg increments, whereas if given orally, I give 0.5 mg · kg^{-1}. Patient acceptance is improved if the drug is offered in sweetened apple juice. An oral dose of 0.5 mg · kg^{-1} typically results in easy separation from the parents at 15 to 30 minutes. If given intranasally, 0.2 mg · kg^{-1} will be effective at about 10 to 15 minutes. These patients must be monitored when sedation is given. Pulse oximetry and careful observation are mandatory, since the hemodynamic status may be adversely and unpredictably affected if hypercarbia or hypoxemia occur.

Some physicians routinely administer anticholinergics preoperatively. Others give atropine in the operating room only if clinically necessary. Keep in mind that slow heart rates are often not tolerated in infants whose stroke volume is relatively fixed.

When Does the Patient Need Intravenous Infusions?

Children requiring vasoactive infusions preoperatively come to the operating room with such access already available. For others, the timing of intravenous access is strictly up to the anesthesiologist involved. For many cases, a gentle inhalation induction with subsequent expeditious venous catheter placement prior to intubation is appropriate. Again, if the timing of surgery is uncertain, preoperative intravenous catheter placement is desirable to avoid dehydration, especially in children with cyanotic heart disease.

When Is Prostaglandin E₁ Indicated?

Prostaglandin E$_1$ is indicated whenever it is thought that maintaining, reopening, or enlarging an existing ductus arteriosus will benefit the neonate. Common situations in which it is used include the presence of (1) lesions with decreased pulmonary blood flow; (2) TGV; and (3) left-sided heart outflow obstruction.

With TGV, the response to prostaglandin E$_1$ is variable, but in some infants, mixing of systemic and pulmonary circulation improves sufficiently to reduce hypoxemia slightly and to relieve acidosis. With left-sided heart outflow obstruction (e.g., hypoplastic left-sided heart syndrome, coarctation) prostaglandin E$_1$ will open the ductus and allow right-to-left flow across it, improving systemic perfusion and perhaps even coronary blood flow. It also may dilate the pulmonary vascular bed.

Stabilization of the infant before surgical intervention and improved outcome often result from prostaglandin E$_1$ infusion. Side effects include apneic spells, seizures, systemic hypotension, inhibition of platelet aggregation, peripheral edema, and unexplained fever. Cortical proliferation in long bones can occur with chronic cases. Since prostaglandin E$_1$ is very rapidly metabolized, it must be continuously infused, usually at a dose of 0.05 to 0.1 µg · kg · min^{-1}. As much as 80% of circulating prostaglandin E$_1$ is metabolized in one pass through the lungs; thus, the ductal response diminishes within minutes after its discontinuation.

EQUIPMENT AND INFUSIONS

What Is Required?

Care for an infant undergoing heart surgery demands meticulous attention to detail and extreme vigilance. A well-thought-out plan should be developed prior to induction so that all equipment needed is available and in working order (Table 66–4).

Anesthetic and Surgical Considerations

The anesthesia machine and circuit should be checked as for all procedures. Multiple sizes of endotracheal tubes, masks, and laryngoscope blades must be available. Appropriate equipment to keep the infant warm may be needed, including a heating/cooling blanket, radiant warming lights, a fluid warmer, and a heated humidifier. A working operating room

TABLE 66–4. Equipment Used During Pediatric Cardiac Surgery

Heating blanket
Radiant warming lights
Fluid warmer
Heated humidifier
Defibrillator (external, internal)
Pacemaker generator
Cardiac output computer
Coagulation analyzer
Fibrillator
Infusion pumps

table that allows optimal positioning to facilitate surgical exposure is required. A defibrillator with both nonsterile (external) and sterile (internal) paddles, a dual-chamber pacemaker generator, a cardiac output computer, and a coagulation analyzer must be operational. A fibrillator is frequently needed intraoperatively to induce ventricular fibrillation during open chamber procedures.

Monitoring

Equipment needed to monitor the patient includes a pulse oximeter, a hemodynamic monitor, appropriate catheters for arterial and venous cannulation, transducers (zeroed and calibrated to mercury), a blood pressure cuff, a stethoscope, thermistors, and a mixed venous oxygen saturation monitor.

Intravenous Fluids

Two intravenous fluid sets should be prepared, and all air bubbles should be removed from the tubing. This task is made easier if one begins with warm fluid; microbubble formation seems to occur less frequently than if cold fluid is allowed to warm when the room temperature is raised. All intravenous and monitoring tubing must be bubble-free whenever a potential shunt is present, since intracardiac shunts can be bidirectional and may become right-to-left during surgery. Air filters can be used, but the same amount of effort must be expended to remove air from intravenous tubing, since air filters cannot be relied on to trap all air. Another drawback to air filters is that they slow down intravenous infusions significantly and may make it difficult to keep up with volume replacement.

A method to carefully control and limit intravenous fluid intake is important, since many patients have barely compensated excess pulmonary blood flow and volume. Infusion using a limited amount in a buret chamber and a minidripper, use of infusion pumps with set volumes, or administration of fluid via syringe in bolus increments are methods that can be used to limit intake. At least three infusion pumps that allow accurate titration of vasoactive drugs should be available.

Preparation of Infusions

Appropriate intravenous solutions for mixing infusions (e.g., normal saline and 5 per cent dextrose in water) and cassettes for the pumps should be on hand. Common infusions to be available on short notice include sodium nitroprusside, epinephrine, isoproterenol, dopamine, and amrinone.

Some thought should be given to the appropriate concentrations for the patient's body size so that fluid overload can be minimized. In general, I find it useful to mix the infusions

such that a starting dose infuses at about 2 to 3 mL · h⁻¹. In the following example for sodium nitroprusside, I solve for "concentration" so that my infusion pump rate is approximately 2 to 3 mL · h⁻¹.

$$\text{Rate } (2\text{–}3 \text{ mL} \cdot \text{h}^{-1}) = \frac{\mu g \cdot kg^{-1} \cdot min^{-1} \times \text{Weight (kg)} \times 60 \text{ min} \cdot h^{-1}}{\text{Concentration } (\mu g \cdot mL^{-1})}$$

If the patient weighs 10 kg and a starting dose of 1 μg · kg⁻¹ · min⁻¹ is desired, the formula is

$$3 \text{ mL} \cdot h^{-1} = \frac{1 \ \mu g \cdot kg^{-1} \cdot min^{-1} \times 10 \text{ kg} \times 60 \text{ min} \cdot h^{-1}}{200 \ \mu g \cdot mL^{-1}}$$

Therefore, I would mix 50 mg of sodium nitroprusside in 250 mL of diluent for a final concentration of 200 μg · mL⁻¹ and begin my infusion at 3 mL · h⁻¹. See Table 66–5 for commonly used drugs and bolus doses or initial infusion rates.

In general, infusions are not prepared unless they are needed. Instead, commonly needed drugs are mixed in syringes so that a small bolus can be given if required. If needed repetitively, an infusion is mixed. Table 66–6 shows drugs that should be available in syringes at the beginning of each pediatric cardiac surgical case. A narcotic, a benzodiazepine, and a muscle relaxant are also on hand for ready use.

Blood and Blood Products

Blood products appropriate to the particular procedure and patient size should also be readied in advance. Preparation may range from typing and screening for simple procedures to typing and cross-matching of multiple units of blood or platelets (or both) and fresh frozen plasma for complex pump cases. At the University of Florida, infants younger than 4 months of age undergo typing and screening and then preferentially receive type O blood without a cross-match, since the risk of transfusion reaction is very low.

Transfusion-acquired cytomegalovirus infection is generally a benign entity in immunocompetent patients who receive blood. However, immunologically immature patients (especially low-birth-weight infants) can become symptomatic if infected. Therefore, our routine is to use cytomegalovirus-negative blood products in children younger than 4 months of age. For infants with aortic arch abnormalities, blood products should be irradiated, since these cardiac lesions may be associated with DiGeorge's syndrome. Such patients may have an absent thymus and susceptibility to graft-versus-host disease following transfusion.

ANESTHETIC INDUCTION AND MAINTENANCE

What Monitors Are Needed Before Induction?

No absolute rule exists for determining the amount of monitoring necessary before induction. In some patients, particularly if a "steal" induction is ideal, anesthesia can be started with just a pulse oximeter and a precordial stethoscope. Then, as the patient is induced, electrocardiography and blood pres-

TABLE 66–5. Nonanesthetic Drugs and Dosages*

	Drug	Dose
Inotropic infusions	Epinephrine	$0.01-0.1\ \mu g \cdot kg^{-1} \cdot min^{-1}$
	Isoproterenol	$0.01-0.1\ \mu g \cdot kg^{-1} \cdot min^{-1}$
	Norepinephrine	$0.01-0.1\ \mu g \cdot kg^{-1} \cdot min^{-1}$
	Dopamine	$2-10\ \mu g \cdot kg^{-1} \cdot min^{-1}$
	Dobutamine	$2-10\ \mu g \cdot kg^{-1} \cdot min^{-1}$
	Amrinone†	$2-2.5$-$mg \cdot kg^{-1}$ bolus divided over 30–60 min, followed by $5-20$-$\mu g \cdot kg^{-1} \cdot min^{-1}$ infusion
Vasodilator infusions	Nitroglycerin	$1-2\ \mu g \cdot kg^{-1} \cdot min^{-1}$
	Nitroprusside	$1-5\ \mu g \cdot kg^{-1} \cdot min^{-1}$
	Aminophylline	$0.5\ mg \cdot kg^{-1}$ slowly, followed by $0.5-1$-$mg \cdot kg^{-1} \cdot h^{-1}$ infusion‡
	Prostaglandin E_1	$0.05-0.1\ \mu g \cdot kg^{-1} \cdot min^{-1}$
	Labetalol	$10-100\ mg \cdot h^{-1}$
Antiarrhythmic drugs	Lidocaine	1-$mg \cdot kg^{-1}$ bolus
		0.03-$mg \cdot kg^{-1} \cdot min^{-1}$ infusion
	Adenosine	0.15-$mg \cdot kg^{-1}$ bolus
	Procainamide	$2\ mg \cdot kg^{-1}$ over 5 min
	Dilantin	$2-4\ mg \cdot kg^{-1}$ over 5 min
	Bretylium	5-$mg \cdot kg^{-1}$ bolus
β-blocking drugs	Propranolol	$0.01-0.1\ mg \cdot kg^{-1}$
	Esmolol	$0.5-1$-$mg \cdot kg^{-1}$ bolus
		$100-300$-$\mu g \cdot kg^{-1} \cdot min^{-1}$ infusion
Others	Calcium chloride	$10-20\ mg \cdot kg^{-1}$
	Sodium bicarbonate	$1\ mEq \cdot kg^{-1}$ (or as determined by base deficit)
	Phenylephrine	$1-10\ \mu g \cdot kg^{-1}$
	Ephedrine	$0.05-0.2\ mg \cdot kg^{-1}$
	Heparin	$\geq 3\ mg \cdot kg^{-1}$ ($300\ U \cdot kg^{-1}$)
	Protamine	$\geq 3\ mg \cdot kg^{-1}$

*The dose of each drug varies with the clinical context.
†Cannot be mixed in dextrose-containing solutions.
‡Maintenance rate determined by plasma levels.

TABLE 66–6. Bolus Drugs Available in Syringes

Drug	Syringe Concentrations	Bolus Dose
Calcium chloride	$100\ mg \cdot mL^{-1}$	$10-20\ mg \cdot kg^{-1}$
Epinephrine	$10\ \mu g \cdot mL^{-1}$	$0.2-1\ \mu g \cdot kg^{-1}$ (inotropy)
	$100\ \mu g \cdot mL^{-1}$	$10-100\ \mu g \cdot kg^{-1}$ (cardiac arrest)
Isoproterenol	$20\ \mu g \cdot mL^{-1}$	$1-10\ \mu g$
Phenylephrine	$100\ \mu g \cdot mL^{-1}$	$1-10\ \mu g \cdot kg^{-1}$
Lidocaine	$20\ mg \cdot mL^{-1}$	$1\ mg \cdot kg^{-1}$
Esmolol*	$10\ mg \cdot mL^{-1}$	$0.5-1\ mg \cdot kg^{-1}$
Heparin	$1000\ U \cdot mL^{-1}$	$300\ U \cdot kg^{-1}$ (cardiopulmonary bypass)
		$100\ U \cdot kg^{-1}$ (vascular nonpump)
Atropine	$0.4\ mg \cdot mL^{-1}$	$0.01-0.02\ mg \cdot kg^{-1}$
Succinylcholine	$20\ mg \cdot mL^{-1}$	$1-2\ mg \cdot kg^{-1}$
Ephedrine	$5\ mg \cdot mL^{-1}$	$0.05-0.2\ mg \cdot kg^{-1}$
Sodium thiopental	$25\ mg \cdot mL^{-1}$	$3-5\ mg \cdot kg^{-1}$
Pancuronium	$1\ mg \cdot mL^{-1}$	$0.1-0.15\ mg \cdot kg^{-1}$ (intubation)

*Available for treatment of patients with tetralogy of Fallot.

sure monitoring can be quickly established. In others, it may be preferable to begin with all monitors (even invasive ones) in place. Generally, arterial and central venous catheters are placed postinduction, although occasionally they may need to be placed before the procedure.

When Does a Patient Need Intravenous Access Preinduction?

The timing of intravenous access, as noted previously, is often a matter of personal preference. However, polycythemic patients must be well hydrated either by mouth or intravenously. Children with extremely poor cardiac function and who require inotropes may not tolerate an inhalation induction; thus an intravenous induction is preferred. Most other pediatric patients tolerate a judicious inhalation induction with subsequent placement of intravenous catheters.

If myocardial reserve is impaired, a high-dose inhalation technique cannot be used for long; once catheters are placed, a transition is made to either a completely intravenous narcotic technique or to combination of intravenous and inhalation techniques. If the anesthesiologist is uncertain about his or her ability to place an intravenous catheter rapidly during an inhalation induction, it should be inserted prior to induction.

How Does Cardiac Disease Affect the Rate of Induction?

Inhalation Agents

Intracardiac shunting can alter the uptake of inhalation anesthetics.[36] The final effect on rate of induction depends on the size and direction of the shunt and the patient's cardiac output. A right-to-left intracardiac shunt prolongs induction, since the uptake of anesthetic into the blood occurs more slowly. If high concentrations of agents are used to speed induction and a relative anesthetic overdose occurs, it is difficult to remedy, since the inhalation agents are also slow to be eliminated. A left-to-right shunt generally has a negligible effect on the speed of induction if the systemic perfusion is preserved at a normal level. A left-to-right shunt may speed induction when it coexists with a large right-to-left shunt.

Intravenous Agents

Response to intravenously administered drugs is faster with a right-to-left shunt because the dilution effect and the pulmonary transmit time are reduced in proportion to the magnitude of the shunt. A left-to-right shunt has a minimal effect on the response to intravenous drugs if systemic perfusion is preserved.

What Problems Are Likely to Occur During Induction?

Any number of untoward events can occur during induction of anesthesia in pediatric patients with heart disease.

Airway Obstruction

Airway obstruction is poorly tolerated in these patients, especially small infants or those with cyanotic heart disease.

The margin for error is extremely small because minor problems can quickly become life-threatening. Airway obstruction that causes hypoxemia or hypercarbia increases pulmonary vascular resistance. A reversal of a left-to-right intracardiac shunt or aggravation of a right-to-left shunt may result, exacerbating the problem and creating a vicious cycle.

Dysrhythmias

The patient may become bradycardic or develop a nodal rhythm with induction. Since stroke volume is relatively fixed, cardiac output suffers in this context. Acidosis can occur quickly when perfusion is marginal; this further depresses myocardial contractility, increasing pulmonary and decreasing systemic vascular resistances.

Dysrhythmias can result from many causes, including light anesthesia, hypoxemia, hypercarbia, drugs, and electrolyte abnormalities.

Significant potential problems may occur during central venous access acquisition. The drapes or patient position may serve to kink the endotracheal tube as it warms to body temperature. Dysrhythmias during this phase are generally induced mechanically from the catheter or guidewire. Familiarity with the lengths of the catheter kit components makes insertion to excessive depth less likely. Mechanically induced dysrhythmias respond better to removal of the stimulus than to pharmacologic therapy.

What Anesthetic Technique Should the Anesthesiologist Use?

The choice of drug or drugs is not as important as is an understanding of the lesion's pathophysiology. Of help is the development of hemodynamic goals for each patient in terms of heart rate, contractility, preload, systemic vascular resistance, and pulmonary vascular resistance (Table 66–7).[37] In several lesions, overriding considerations dominate. An appropriate approach for a patient with aortic insufficiency may be completely different than that for a patient with tetralogy of Fallot. Once the goals are defined, appropriate agents, dosages, and routes of administration can be selected. Many agents can be used so long as they are administered in a thoughtful fashion.

How Should the Patient Be Positioned?

Data are scarce regarding the safest way to position a patient for heart surgery. The major issues are prevention of brachial plexus injury and optimal patient access. I find it useful to place the patient in a supine position on a heating blanket covered with a thin sheet and to abduct the upper arms 90° with the hands above the head to allow easy access to and inspection of arterial and venous cannulation sites. The shoulders and elbows are supported at an angle of about 30° above the table by a "wedge" cushion in order to lessen the danger of any stretch on the brachial plexus. A recent study[38] suggests that bilateral somatosensory evoked monitoring of the median and ulnar nerves may be useful to predict (and perhaps to help to prevent) such injuries during cardiac surgery. The applicability of this technique in children is unknown at this time.

TABLE 66–7. Cardiac Grid for Common Congenital Heart Diseases (Desired Hemodynamic Changes)

	Preload	PVR	SVR	HR	Contractility
ASD	↑	↑	↓	N	N
VSD (right-to-left)	N	↓	↑	N	N
VSD (left-to-right)	↑	↑	↓	N	N
Idiopathic hypertrophic subaortic stenosis	↑	N	N–↑	*↓	*↓
PDA	↑	↑	↓	N	N
Coarctation	↑	N	↓	N	N
Valvular pulmonic stenosis	↑	↓	N	↓	↑
Infundibular pulmonary stenosis	↑	↓	N	↓	*↓
Aortic stenosis	↑	N	*↑	*↓	N–↑
Mitral stenosis	↑	N–↓	N	*↓	N–↑
Aortic regurgitation	↑	N	↓	N–↑	N–↑
Mitral regurgitation	↑	N–↓	↓	N–↑	N–↑

(From Moore RA: Anesthesia for the pediatric congenital heart patient for noncardiac surgery. Anesthesiol Rev 1981; 8:27.)
*An overriding consideration.
Abbreviations: PVR = pulmonary vascular resistance; SVR = systemic vascular resistance; HR = heart rate; N = normal or no change.

Access to the patient's head is crucial for visual inspection to rule out superior vena cava syndrome, for pupil evaluation, and for airway manipulation. A piece of eggcrate foam can be placed under the patient's head to minimize the chance of pressure necrosis; many heart surgery cases are lengthy, and low perfusion pressure occurs during cardiopulmonary bypass. Since infants have such large occiputs, elevation of the head in this way may occasionally result in encroachment on the surgical field.

MONITORING

Anesthetic induction generally proceeds with noninvasive monitors. A five-lead electrocardiograph is used to facilitate detection of rhythm disturbances and myocardial ischemia. An esophageal lead can also be used to more easily diagnose dysrhythmias, especially when tachycardia is present.[39] Lead V_5 can be placed in its normal position and covered with an adhesive drape to protect it from the surgical scrub solutions. The monitor mode of the electrocardiograph will minimize

baseline drift, whereas the diagnostic mode allows better resolution of the P and T waves.

When Is an Arterial Catheter Indicated?

An indwelling arterial catheter is required whenever continuous monitoring of arterial pressure or frequent blood sampling is necessary. All procedures utilizing cardiopulmonary bypass require placement of an arterial catheter, since noninvasive methods are not useful if no pulsatile flow is present. Most closed-heart procedures also benefit from beat-to-beat monitoring of arterial pressure.

The arterial catheter is placed after intubation, preferably percutaneously in the nondominant radial artery. Other sites commonly used include the dorsalis pedis, posterior tibial, femoral, and, occasionally, temporal arteries. A surgical cutdown is used only as a last resort because of the disproportionately high incidence of thrombosis and infection. For coarctation repairs the arterial catheter must be placed in the right radial artery; if this is unsuccessful, the catheter can be placed in a temporal artery. In patients with a Blalock-Taussig shunt,

TABLE 66–8. Monitors and Infusions

Cardiac Lesion	ART	Multilumen CVP*	PA*	LA	Foley	Drug Infusions Anticipated
ASD	+	+			+	None
VSD	+		+	+	+	SNP, ±Epi, Isuprel, Amrinone
Transposition (Jatene)	+	+	±	+	+	NTG, SNP, ± Epi
Tetralogy of Fallot	+		+	±	+	SNP, ± Epi
Atrioventricular canal	+		+	+	+	SNP, Epi, ± Isuprel, Amrinone
Total anomalous pulmonary venous return	+	+	+	+	+	SNP, ± Epi, Isuprel, Amrinone
Aortic stenosis	+	+		+	+	NTG, ± Dopamine, Epi
Truncus arteriosus	+	+	+	+	+	SNP, Epi, Isuprel, Amrinone
Tricuspid atresia (Fontan)	+	+		+	+	SNP, Epi, Isuprel
Patent ductus arteriosus						None
Coarctation (right radial)	+ (right radial)	+			±	SNP, Labetalol
Blalock-Taussig shunt	+ †	+			±	None

*Choice of CVP versus PA line is often made on basis of patient size.
†Arterial line must be opposite to the surgical site.
Abbreviations: ART = arterial catheter; CVP = central venous pressure (catheter); PA = pulmonary artery catheter; LA = left atrial catheter; SNP = sodium nitroprusside; Epi = epinephrine; NTG = nitroglycerine.

the catheter must be placed on the side opposite the Blalock-Taussig shunt or in a lower extremity artery (Table 66–8). A 22- or 24-gauge catheter is used, depending on the child's size.

When Is Central Venous Access Needed?

Central Venous Catheters

Central venous access is established routinely when a knowledge of right-sided heart filling pressure trends or the need to administer vasoactive drugs rapidly is desirable. Access to the central circulation also allows placement of pulmonary artery or pacing catheters. The decision as to which type and size of catheter should be used depends on the type of operation performed and on the size and clinical status of the patient.

A central venous catheter is routine in patients undergoing cardiopulmonary bypass. Monitoring superior vena cava pressure during extracorporeal circulation is useful in assessing adequacy of venous drainage, particularly when two venous cannulas are used. A central catheter with at least two lumens allows drug and fluid delivery via one lumen and uninterrupted central venous pressure measurements via the other.

My guidelines for catheter length and size are shown in Table 66–9. Follow-up verification of appropriate catheter position occurs on review of the postoperative chest film.

Pulmonary Artery Catheters

Monitoring of pulmonary artery (PA) pressure is helpful when pulmonary vascular resistance is problematic. Placement of the PA catheter can be accomplished percutaneously or by the surgeon using a direct transthoracic approach. If the patient is too small to accept a balloon flotation catheter, a combined percutaneous and direct intraoperative approach can be employed. In this scenario, the catheter is placed through a sterility sheath into the introducer and advanced into the superior vena cava. When the chest and heart are open, the surgeon can then advance it into the proximal PA. In complex cardiac anomalies with shunts, the surgeon generally will thread the percutaneously placed PA catheter into position at the end of the surgical procedure, since the catheter is often in the field of repair.

Continuous mixed venous oximetry is also available with selected PA catheters and may be helpful in titrating vasoactive infusions, in providing an early warning of deteriorating cardiac output, and in assessing residual shunts. The patient's size must be large enough to accommodate a 5 to 6 French introducer to facilitate percutaneous placement of a PA catheter.

Smaller infants requiring PA pressure monitoring will have transthoracic PA catheters placed at the close of surgery. The PA catheter is also useful postoperatively to assess pressure gradients by carefully measuring pull-back pressures upon its removal. Some PA catheters allow measurement of cardiac output by thermodilution; however, this method is not often used because of the significant fluid load it imposes on the patient.

Left Atrial Catheters

Left atrial pressure monitoring is often used in patients with CHD because disparities in left- and right-sided heart function are often present. This catheter is inserted by the surgeon at the end of repair, usually via the right superior pulmonary vein. One must be very careful in its use; since the catheter is in the left side of the heart, the risk of systemic embolization of clot or air is very real. A risk of bleeding and cardiac tamponade is present when it is removed.

Where Should Temperature Be Measured?

The optimal site for temperature monitoring during cardiac cases is controversial; remember that gradients exist between various sites (Fig. 66–4).[40] Commonly used are the esophagus, nasopharynx, rectum, tympanic membrane, blood, and bladder. Temperature monitoring is important because the rate of cooling and rewarming appears to be important in the production of brain injury. Wide gradients (>10 °C) between body and perfusate temperature in dogs correlated with brain cell necrosis and death.[41] Monitoring in at least two sites is advisable to ensure that the temperature gradient between inflow (blood temperature) and core (bladder or rectal temperature) does not exceed 10 °C and that uniform cooling and warming has occurred.

How Do End-Tidal and Arterial Carbon Dioxide Pressures Correlate?

Monitoring of end-tidal carbon dioxide partial pressure ($P_{ET}CO_2$) is useful to corroborate tracheal intubation. The arterial to end-tidal carbon dioxide partial pressure difference ($P(a-ET)CO_2$) can be increased in patients with cardiopulmonary disease. It also may be increased in small children, depending on the sampling site and ventilatory pattern. Patients with CHD have altered ventilation/perfusion ratios; this produces abnormalities of both the physiologic dead space to tidal volume ratio (V_{DS}/V_T) and venous admixture ($\dot{Q}s/\dot{Q}t$).

In patients with cyanotic heart disease, in which $\dot{Q}s/\dot{Q}t$ can be large, $P_{ET}CO_2$ significantly underestimates $PaCO_2$.[42] Since intracardiac shunting is often dynamic, the $P(a-ET)CO_2$ is ever-changing; thus, even $P_{ET}CO_2$ trends are not reliable in these patients. Periodic measurement of $PaCO_2$ is necessary to document adequate ventilation. $P_{ET}CO_2$ monitoring during pulmonary artery banding reflects the decrease in pulmonary

TABLE 66–9. Guidelines for Central Venous Pressure Catheter Size and Length in Relationship to Patient Size

Patient Weight	Internal Jugular Catheter Size*	CVP Catheter Length
<2.5 kg	3 Fr SL or 4 Fr DL	5 cm
2.5–5.0 kg	4 Fr DL or 5 Fr SL	5 cm
5–10 kg	5 Fr DL or 5 Fr introducer	8 cm
10–20 kg	5 Fr DL or 6 Fr intoducer	8–12 cm
>20 kg	5–7 Fr DL or 6 Fr introducer	12–15 cm

*Catheter size is also influenced by operative procedure. If significant blood loss is anticipated and peripheral venous access is limited, a larger size CVP catheter may be preferred.

Abbreviations: SL = single-lumen; DL = double-lumen; Fr = French.

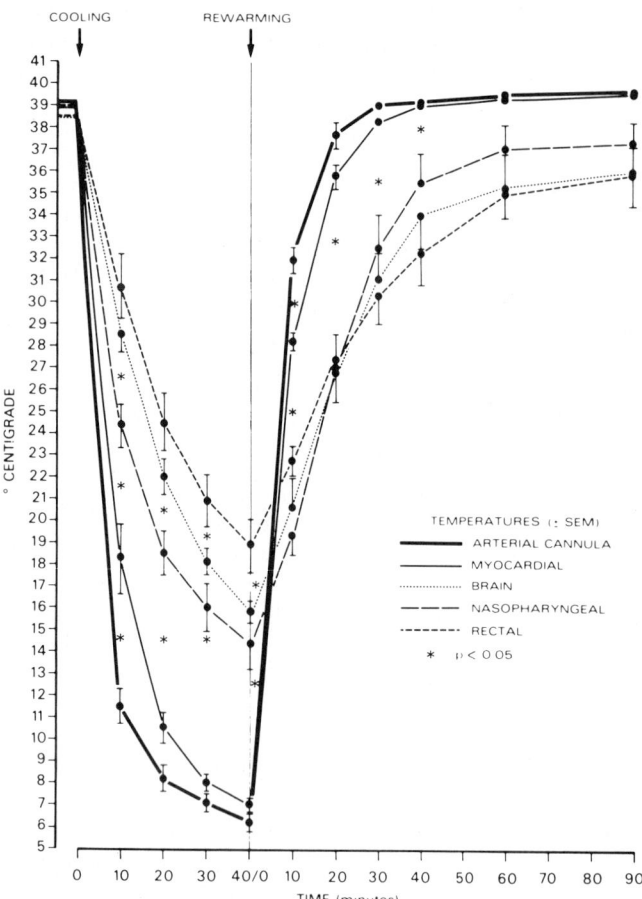

FIGURE 66–4. Average temperature (± SEM) of arterial cannula, myocardium, cerebral cortex, nasopharynx, and rectum during 40 minutes of cooling and 90 minutes of rewarming during cardiopulmonary bypass in six pigs. (From Stefaniszyn HJ, Novick RJ, Keith FM, Salerno TA: Is the brain adequately cooled during deep hypothermic cardiopulmonary bypass? Curr Surg 1983; 40:294.)

blood flow. As the band is tightened, the $P(a-ET)CO_2$ gradient increases.

Is Electroencephalography Necessary?

Central nervous system insults associated with cardiac surgery remain an unsolved problem. Brain damage can occur as a result of global ischemia or focal emboli. Electroencephalography has been used to try to provide a measure of cerebral ischemia during cardiac surgery. Unfortunately, the electroencephalogram has not proven reliable in predicting or preventing brain ischemia during cardiopulmonary bypass because of the effects of hypothermia and anesthetic agents and because of the likelihood of focal embolic injury.

Newer computerized, processed electroencephalographic monitors are less cumbersome and allow easier recognition of trends and abrupt changes. Recent data from adults suggest an improvement in neurologic outcome following interventions in response to a decrease in the power index during cardiopulmonary bypass.[43] Included were measures to increase cerebral blood flow (e.g., increasing pump flow, increasing mean arterial pressure, improving venous return). The incidence of global neurologic deficit was 44% in the control group versus 5% in the intervention group.

Whether these results also hold true for children remains to be seen. However, it is clear that the electroencephalogram can be obtained in patients of any age or size with no risk and can be effective in detecting catastrophic events such as a misplaced arterial or venous cardiopulmonary bypass circuit cannula.

What Is the Role of Echocardiography?

Perioperative echocardiography is increasingly utilized in many centers for pediatric cardiac surgery. Both epicardial and, more recently, transesophageal studies have been performed to better define cardiac anatomy and assess surgical repair. Technologic improvements allow better imaging, smaller probe size, and multiplane capability, thereby substantially increasing the information provided by this modality. The ultimate role of echocardiography in the operating room and intensive care unit is still evolving and will hinge on demonstration of improvement in outcome in these patients.

In one study of congenital heart repairs, epicardial echocardiographic Doppler color flow imaging demonstrated previously unappreciated anatomic details in 18% of patients before bypass.[44] After repair, the color flow imaging proved to be a much more sensitive method to assess quality of repair than was the surgeon's subjective impression. In 15% of cases in which the surgeon was satisfied, epicardial echocardiography after repair revealed persistent problems that required attention. If the unacceptable result determined by color flow imaging was not successfully revised before the patients left the operating room, only 21% had favorable outcomes compared with 83% of those whose results were successfully revised. When ventricular dysfunction was indicated, an unfavorable outcome was also predictable.

CARDIOPULMONARY BYPASS

How Does It Differ in Children?

The physiology of extracorporeal circulation is similar in adults and children. The details of cardiopulmonary bypass are covered in Chapter 18 and are not repeated here. However, significant differences in technique are applied to infants and small children (Table 66–10).[45] Smaller cannulas are used in children, but proportionally they may be so large that they obstruct venous drainage into the heart or arterial outflow from it before institution of bypass or after its discontinuation. Almost all cardiac repairs in children necessitate the use of dual venous cannulas so that all venous blood can be diverted to the bypass circuit and the heart can be opened to allow repair of the intracardiac defect.

TABLE 66–10. Differences in Pediatric Versus Adult Cardiopulmonary Bypass

Venous drainage problems
Necessity of occluding systemic to pulmonary shunts
Higher flow rate (70–80 mL · kg · min⁻¹)
Lower perfusion pressures (20–50 mm Hg)
Greater dilution of drugs and clotting factors (in small infants)

(Modified from Lake CL, Schwartz AJ, Campbell FW: Extracorporeal circulation. *In* Pediatric Cardiac Anesthesia. Lake CL (ed). Norwalk, CT, Appleton & Lange, 1988, p 168.)

Profound Hypothermia and Total Circulatory Arrest

An alternative method employed in very small children with complex heart disease is profound hypothermia and total circulatory arrest. This technique employs a single venous drainage cannula during the period of cooling. When a core temperature of about 15 to 20 °C is reached, the pump is stopped and the venous cannula removed. The major advantage of this technique is that it provides excellent exposure without cannulas or blood in the operative field. Deep hypothermia also enhances myocardial protection, decreases cardiopulmonary bypass time, and decreases blood trauma. Whether the method adversely affects long-term neurologic outcome is unclear.

Venous Drainage

Venous drainage problems are more common in children than in adults. The inferior vena cava is quite short, and inadvertent cannulation of the hepatic veins is possible. If this occurs, marked engorgement of the splanchnic vessels can result in mesenteric ischemia. Problems with superior vena cava drainage are also possible, especially if a left superior vena cava is present. Occlusion of this vessel causes significant venous hypertension; it must be cannulated or cerebral ischemia may result. Careful attention should be paid to superior vena cava pressure by frequent inspection of the head. The upper venous cannula can easily be kinked or drainage otherwise impaired with retraction of the heart.

Systemic to Pulmonary Artery Shunt Occlusion

When cardiopulmonary bypass is first initiated, the surgeon must quickly occlude any systemic to pulmonary artery shunts (e.g., PDA or Blalock-Taussig shunt). Otherwise, continued perfusion of these shunts will lead to underperfusion of the systemic circulation, possible hemorrhagic edema of the lungs, and continued pulmonary venous return with possible overdistention of the left side of the heart.

Perfusion Flow and Pressure

Cardiopulmonary bypass flow rates are proportionately higher in infants and children than in adults, ranging from 80 to 150 mL · kg⁻¹ · min⁻¹. Adult rates usually range from about 1.8 to 2.2 L · min⁻¹ · m²⁻¹, or about 50 mL · kg⁻¹ · min⁻¹. Perfusion pressures tend to be lower in children (20–50 mm Hg) when adequate oxygenation and perfusion are apparent. The optimal pressure or flow is unclear, and significant interinstitutional variation exists.

Moderate Hypothermia and Ventricular Fibrillation

Moderate hypothermia combined with ventricular fibrillation is used often in pediatric cardiac repair. With this technique, the patient is cooled to about 28 to 30 °C, and the heart is fibrillated but continues to be perfused because an aortic cross-clamp is not placed. The surgeon can then open the cardiac chambers without risking the entrainment of air into the left side of the heart and subsequent ejection into the arterial circulation.

Deliberate fibrillation is often used during work on the right side of the heart or for relatively simple repairs such as ASD closure. The advantages of deliberate fibrillation with moderate hypothermia include a favorable myocardial supply/demand ratio, decreased risk of air embolus to the brain, and avoidance of aortic cross-clamping and cardioplegia. However, surgical exposure is limited because of the significant amount of blood in and continued motion of the heart. Therefore, aortic cross-clamping and cardioplegic protection of the heart are necessary for more complex intracardiac repairs, especially in small children.

Bypass Circuit Volume

The bypass circuit volume is very large relative to the blood volume in infants. In pediatric cardiopulmonary bypass circuits, the priming volume is about 700 mL, whereas the estimated blood volume of a 3-kg neonate is 250 to 300 mL. The hematocrit, accordingly, is reduced by approximately 70%. In contrast, an adult cardiopulmonary bypass circuit is primed with 1500 mL for a patient with an estimated blood volume of 5 L; a less than 25% drop in hematocrit results. Small infants undergoing complex repairs often require transfusion of red blood cells, platelets, and fresh frozen plasma to offset the dilutional reduction of hematocrit and clotting factors.

When Should Blood Be Added to the Bypass Circuit?

In general, hemodilution during bypass is desirable and tolerated, since microcirculatory perfusion is improved and since metabolic needs are reduced by hypothermia. However, if the hematocrit is lowered too far, oxygen-carrying capacity is diminished, and anaerobic metabolism results. For most complex repairs, a hematocrit of 20% to 25% during cardiopulmonary bypass is ideal.

The cardiopulmonary bypass circuit must be primed. Each circuit has an obligatory volume that is required to fill the tubing, filters, pumps, and oxygenator. Even in small infants, who require the smallest tubing possible, the obligatory prime, as has already been mentioned, is about 700 to 750 mL. Therefore, red blood cells commonly are added to the priming solution to reach the desired hematocrit. Calculation of the hematocrit on bypass is quite simple:

1. Determine the patient's estimated blood volume.
2. Multiply the estimated blood volume by the measured hematocrit to yield the patient's red blood cell mass (RBCM).
3. Ask the perfusionist what the circuit priming volume is.
4. Add the estimated blood volume to the priming volume to obtain the total volume on bypass (CPBV).
5. If the predicted hematocrit on bypass is less than desired, the quantity of red blood cells that must be added is calculated as follows:

> CPBV × Desired Hematocrit = Required RBCM
>
> Required RBCM − patient's RBCM = RBCM to be added

How Is Anticoagulation Managed?

Heparin is given to prevent initiation of the coagulation cascade by contact of blood with the bypass circuit. A dose of

300 U · kg^{-1} is generally sufficient, although 400 U · kg^{-1} are sometimes recommended for neonates. This dose is given through a central catheter after aspiration to verify blood return.

Activated Clotting Time

Documentation of heparin effect can be made by measuring activated clotting time about 3 to 5 minutes later. A value of 300 to 400 seconds appears adequate to prevent clotting on bypass.

Activated clotting time is relatively simple to determine and is reasonable to monitor, since an occasional patient does exhibit marked heparin resistance. The activated clotting time can also signal a potentially catastrophic drug administration error when a substance other than heparin is injected. If the patient remains normothermic, the activated clotting time is generally rechecked every 20 to 30 minutes. With significant hypothermia, heparin effect is prolonged.

How Are Patients Weaned?

Success in weaning from bypass is critically dependent on the surgeon's ability to completely repair the defect. Residual shunts, obstruction, or valvular dysfunction are tolerated poorly following bypass.

Preparation

Be certain the patient is optimally prepared before attempting discontinuation of bypass (Table 66–11). Near the end of the surgical repair, rewarming is begun. Temperature gradients are common; be sure that the patient is thoroughly and evenly rewarmed. Infusion of afterload-reducing agents such as sodium nitroprusside during rewarming may be helpful to dilate the vascular bed and promote uniform rewarming. Allowing time for reperfusion of the heart after the cross-clamp is removed makes possible dissipation of "evil humors" (cardioplegia) and re-establishment of aerobic metabolism.

Heart Rate and Rhythm

Sinus rhythm is essential, since ventricular function is typically impaired following bypass and ischemia. Optimal heart rate is also important in improving cardiac output, since stroke volume may be less than ideal. A heart rate of 120 to 160 beats per minute is desirable. The atrium may be paced if the patient has a slower sinus rate, or sequential atrioventricular pacing may be required if a rhythm other than sinus exists. New electrocardiographic ST changes may indicate the pres-

TABLE 66–11. Checklist for Discontinuation of Bypass

1. Complete rewarming (core temperature ≥35°C)
2. Complete reperfusion of heart after cardioplegia
3. Sinus rhythm with appropriate heart rate
4. Evaluate ST changes
5. Check electrolytes, blood gases, and hematocrit
6. Optimize pulmonary function
7. Check hemodynamic monitors
8. Prepare vasodilator or inotropic drugs, if indicated
9. Prepare platelets and fresh frozen plasma, if indicated

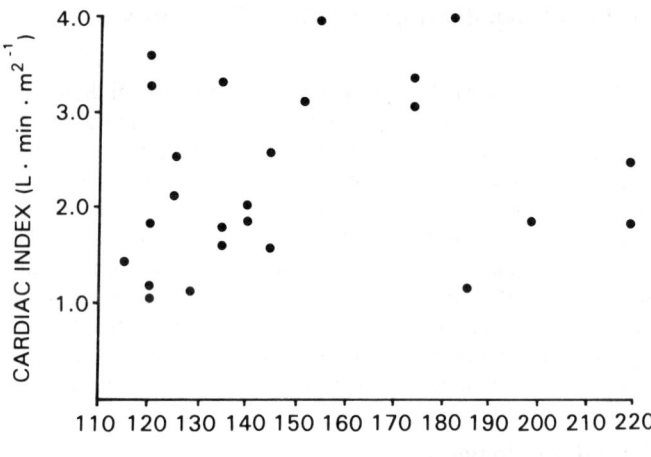

FIGURE 66–5. Comparison of cardiac index and peak systolic pressure in 25 adult patients during the first 4 hours after open intracardiac operations. (From Kouchoukos NT, Karp RB: Management of the postoperative cardiovascular surgical patient. Am Heart J 1976; 92:517.)

ence of air in the coronary arteries or ongoing myocardial ischemia. A transient increase in coronary perfusion pressure (as occurs with application of a partial occlusion clamp to the aorta distal to the aortic cannula) promotes clearance of this air.

Other Monitored Parameters

Hemodynamic monitors should be rechecked and transducers rezeroed. The surgeon may elect to insert a left atrial pressure catheter to assess ventricular filling and function. Laboratory values, including hematocrit, potassium, ionized calcium, arterial blood gas partial pressures, and pH, should be rechecked after aortic cross-clamp release and before discontinuation of bypass is attempted.

Vasoactive Drugs

Vasodilator and inotropic drugs should be available for infusion by calibrated pumps, especially after intracardiac repair. Significant hemodynamic compromise may result from edema and ischemia that are superimposed on marginal baseline ventricular function. Ventricular performance usually is readily improved by inotrope or combined inotrope and vasodilator support. Impaired postoperative cardiac performance is clearly associated with higher morbidity and mortality. In one study, acute cardiac failure accounted for over 59% of postoperative deaths in children younger than 2 years of age.[46]

Cardiovascular Changes

Arterial pressure may be normal or above normal when cardiac output is high, normal, or low; thus, knowledge of it is not helpful with regard to diagnosis of cardiac dysfunction (Fig. 66–5).[47] Following cardiopulmonary bypass, systemic vascular resistance is generally high in both adults and children because of circulating catecholamines and antidiuretic hormone as well as other influences.[48] In the neonate, this response may be amplified, leading to uninhibited vasoconstriction.

Afterload Reduction

Children tolerate an increased pressure workload poorly. Therefore, afterload reduction (generally with sodium nitroprusside) may be useful to improve cardiac output. Cardiac index increased 20% after infusion of sodium nitroprusside in 16 infants after intracardiac surgery.[49] A further 20% increase was achieved by restoration of left atrial pressure to baseline values. When cardiac output is still impaired after vasodilator therapy, a combination of afterload reduction, volume expansion, and inotropic support is warranted.

Measurement of Blood Pressure

If the blood pressure is low during attempted weaning from bypass, another method of blood pressure measurement must be available to check the accuracy of the peripheral data. The surgeon can easily place an exploring needle into the ascending aorta (often at the site of the previous cardioplegia infusion) and connect it to a pressure transducer. A noninvasive (cuff) blood pressure measurement also can be obtained.

In small children, a significant difference in blood pressure measurements is often present between central aortic and peripheral arterial sites. The reason for this discrepancy is not clear, but it usually resolves over time. Before starting administration of inotropes or vasopressors, be certain that the pressure measurement is accurate. If the discrepancy persists, placement of a femoral arterial catheter helps to guide therapy.

How Is Increased Pulmonary Vascular Resistance Managed?

Pulmonary function must be optimized before discontinuation of bypass is attempted. Increased pulmonary vascular resistance results from increased lung water, complement activation, catecholamines, and atelectasis.

Lung Expansion and Oxygenation

The lungs must be vigorously re-expanded to increase functional residual capacity (Fig. 66–6).[50] The endotracheal tube is not routinely suctioned, as suctioning may precipitate bleeding in anticoagulated patients. Any wheezing is vigorously treated with inhaled bronchodilators. I prefer albuterol, 2.5 mg, administered via a nebulizer attached between the endotracheal tube and the circle system. If secretions prevent appropriate deflation of the lungs, careful suctioning with a soft red rubber catheter is indicated.

Vigorous hyperventilation without positive end-expiratory pressure is one of the most powerful tools available to decrease pulmonary vascular resistance.[51] The pulmonary vascular responsiveness to hypercarbia is accentuated in the postbypass period; thus, even small increases in $PaCO_2$ are associated with significant increases in resistance. High inspired oxygen concentrations should be used, and metabolic acidosis should be avoided.

Pharmacologic Interventions

Alpha-stimulation causes pulmonary vasoconstriction, whereas β-stimulation causes vasodilation. Many pharmacologic

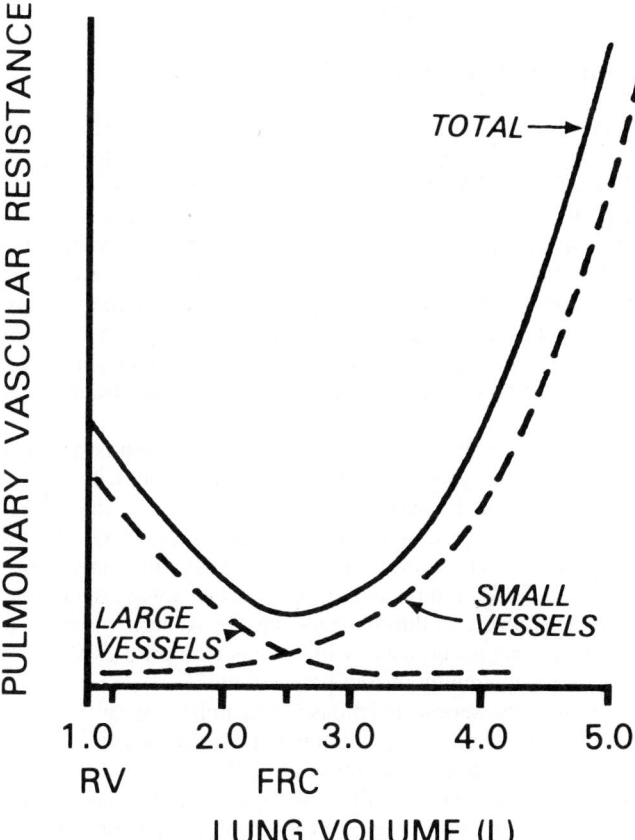

FIGURE 66–6. An asymmetric U-shaped curve relates total pulmonary vascular resistance to lung volume. The trough of the curve occurs when lung volume equals functional residual capacity (FRC). Total pulmonary resistance is the sum of resistance in small vessels (increased by decreasing lung volume) and in large vessels (increased by decreasing lung volume). RV = residual volume. (From Benumof JL: Respiratory physiology and respiratory function during anesthesia. *In* Anesthesia. 2nd ed. Miller RD (ed). New York, Churchill Livingstone, 1986, p 1122.)

agents have been used with only marginal success in the attempt to selectively decrease pulmonary vascular resistance. The ones most commonly used include sodium nitroprusside, nitroglycerin, isoproterenol, aminophylline, amrinone, and prostaglandin E_1 and perhaps adenosine. Inhaled nitric oxide offers promise as a truly selective pulmonary vasodilator but is not yet readily available.[52]

Factors that increase or decrease pulmonary vascular resistance are summarized in Table 66–12.

TABLE 66–12. Alteration of Pulmonary Vascular Resistance

Increase Resistance	Decrease Resistance
Hypoxia	Oxygen
Hypercarbia	Hypocarbia
Acidosis	Alkalosis
Hyperinflation	Normal functional residual capacity
Atelectasis	Blocking sympathetic stimulation
Sympathetic stimulation	Low hematocrit
Surgical constriction	
High hematocrit	

(From Hickey PR, Wessel DL: Anesthesia for treatment of congenital heart disease. *In* Cardiac Anesthesia. 2nd ed. Kaplan JA (ed). Orlando, Grune & Stratton, 1987, p 656.)

POSTBYPASS ISSUES

How Should Protamine Be Administered?

Protamine is given following termination of cardiopulmonary bypass to neutralize the effects of heparin. Generally, a dose of 3 to 4.5 mg · kg^{-1} (1–1.5 mg for every 100 U of heparin) is given. Satisfactory reversal of heparin is suggested by return of the activated clotting time to baseline value. Protamine can cause serious adverse reactions in some patients. These reactions include systemic hypotension, pulmonary hypertension, and allergic reactions. The mechanism for these events is not entirely clear, but may involve antibody-mediated immune responses, complement activation, and histamine release.

Histamine release is provoked by rapid administration of large doses of protamine. Slow administration with a controlled infusion is effective in ameliorating this side effect. Pretreatment with antihistamine or administration into the left atrium also has been proposed. Catastrophic pulmonary hypertension is less common and probably occurs owing to complement activation and thromboxane release. Allergic reactions to protamine can occur, usually in patients with prior exposure to protamine-containing insulin preparations.

Fortunately, serious reactions to protamine appear to be less common in neonates and children than in adults. If the drug is slowly administered after removal of the venous cannula but with the aortic cannula still in place, cardiopulmonary bypass can be quickly reinstituted if a catastrophic reaction occurs.

What Are the Causes of Low Cardiac Output?

Low cardiac output can have many causes but is categorized according to its major determinants: heart rate, rhythm, contractility, preload, and afterload.

Heart Rate

Infants and children have a relatively fixed cardiac stroke volume and therefore modify cardiac output by heart rate changes. Therefore, cardiac output is considered to be rate-dependent. Heart rates ≥120 beats per minute virtually eliminate inadequate heart rate as a gauge of low cardiac output. A lower heart rate should be treated either pharmacologically or by pacing.

Dysrhythmias

Dysrhythmias following cardiopulmonary bypass are often tolerated poorly and may require electrical conversion. Sinus rhythm at a reasonable rate is crucial to maximize cardiac output. Do not hesitate to use electrical pacing to optimize myocardial performance.

Decreased Contractility

Poor contractility can occur due to surgical trauma (as from a ventriculotomy incision), pre-existing volume or pressure overload condition, injury to a coronary artery, residual effects of myocardial preservation, metabolic and acid-base derangements, hypoxemia, and drug effects.

Decreased Preload

Decreased preload may occur from hypovolemia, cardiac tamponade, positive airway pressure, and increased pulmonary vascular resistance that causes diminished return to the left side of the heart.

Increased Afterload

Increased afterload can be a major problem for both the left and right sides of the heart. Many congenital lesions are associated with pulmonary vascular changes and pulmonary hypertension. Thus, control of right ventricular function and afterload is crucial to maintain adequate cardiac output.

What Are the Causes and Treatment of Excessive Bleeding?

Causes

Most commonly, patients bleed postoperatively as a result of inadequate surgical hemostasis. Inadequate heparin neutralization can also be a factor. Thrombocytopenia or platelet dysfunction is the next most common cause. Platelets are sequestered in the bypass circuit and become dysfunctional because of surface exposure and hypothermia.

Patients with cyanotic heart disease and significant polycythemia have a baseline abnormality of platelet function and clotting factors. They often demonstrate a decrease in Factors II, V, VII, VIII, and IX; hypofibrinogenemia; and an increase of fibrin split products, all of which may lead to excessive bleeding.[53] The use of positive end-expiratory pressure to "tamponade" the bleeding and decrease mediastinal drainage has been recommended.[54] Another study failed to confirm this effect.[55]

Treatment

While a source of bleeding is sought, the patient must be aggressively treated with volume replacement. Crystalloid solutions are the mainstay of therapy, but their administration should be tempered by the knowledge that a total body inflammatory response after bypass leads to problems with increased vascular permeability and edema. Decreased colloid oncotic pressure can be a problem following cardiopulmonary bypass because of hemodilution and destruction of serum proteins; judicious use of albumin-containing solutions may be warranted.

If continuing red blood cell loss is a problem, packed red blood cell transfusion is indicated. Typically, a hematocrit of 25% to 30% in acyanotic and 30% to 40% in cyanotic children seems reasonable. In children with good cardiac reserve following simple repairs, an even lower hematocrit of 18% to 20% may be well tolerated. If no surgical source is found and the activated clotting time is normal, an empiric platelet transfusion is often used. Only following prolonged, deep hypothermic cases in small infants should transfusion with fresh frozen plasma be necessary.

What Metabolic Problems Are Likely?

Potassium Disorders

Metabolic derangements are relatively common. Hyperkalemia and hypokalemia are the most common electrolyte abnormalities. Hyperkalemia is commonly seen immediately after the cross-clamp is removed if large amounts of cardioplegic solution have been used. If cardiac output is poor, hyperkalemia may remain problematic. Typically, hypokalemia evolves because patients exhibit a marked kaliuresis after bypass. Unless the serum potassium value is ≥ 4.5 mEq $\cdot$ L^{-1} or renal function is impaired, I almost routinely begin a potassium chloride infusion of 1 to 4 mEq $\cdot$ h^{-1} upon patient arrival in the intensive care unit. Remember that dysrhythmias associated with digitalis toxicity are enhanced by hypokalemia.

Calcium Abnormalities

Hypocalcemia occurs frequently, especially following rapid transfusion of blood products. A decrease in the ionized fraction can lead to decreased myocardial contractility and decreased vascular smooth muscle tone.

Miscellaneous Problems

Hypomagnesemia can occur and can enhance ventricular irritability. Hyperglycemia is very common following cardiopulmonary bypass and is relatively resistant to treatment with insulin. Sodium changes typically do not present a major problem after bypass, although hypernatremia can occur if large quantities of sodium bicarbonate have been given.

When Should the Patient Be Extubated?

Most patients undergoing complex repairs remain intubated and mechanically ventilated for several hours to days after surgery. This approach allows heavy sedation, recovery of myocardial function, and stabilization of hemodynamic status. For simple repairs (e.g., of ASD, simple VSD, and coarctation), extubation may be considered at the end of the procedure if the patient is stable and awake and if bleeding is controlled. Obviously, all normal criteria for extubation, including reversal of muscle relaxation, good spontaneous ventilation, and the ability to maintain and protect the airway, should be present.

References

1. Daniels SR: Epidemiology. *In* Fetal and Neonatal Cardiology. Long WA (ed). Philadelphia, WB Saunders, 1990, pp 425–438.
2. Fyler DC: Report of the New England Regional Cardiac Program. Pediatrics 1980; 65(Suppl):375.
3. Ferencz C, Rubin JD, McCarter RJ, et al: Congenital heart disease: prevalence at livebirth: the Washington-Baltimore Infant Study. Am J Epidemiol 1985; 121:31.
4. Levy RJ, Rosenthal A, Fyler DC, et al: Birth weight of infants with congenital heart disease. Am J Dis Child 1978; 132:249.
5. Rowland TW, Hubbell JP, Nadas AS: Congenital heart disease in infants of diabetic mothers. J Pediatr 1973; 83:815.
6. Warkany J, Passarge E, Smith LB: Congenital malformations in autosomal trisomy syndromes. Am J Dis Child 1966; 112:502.
7. Keith JD: Prevalence, incidence and epidemiology. *In* Heart Disease in Infancy and Childhood. Keith JD, Rowe RD, Vlad P (eds). New York, Macmillan Publishing Co, 1978, pp 3–13.
8. Rudolph AM: The changes in the circulation after birth. Circulation 1970; 41:343.
9. Lake CL: Cardiac embryology, growth and development. *In* Pediatric Cardiac Anesthesia. Lake CL (ed). Norwalk, Appleton & Lange, 1988, pp 27–41.
10. Ho SY, Angelini A, Moscoso G: Developmental cardiac anatomy. *In* Fetal and Neonatal Cardiology. Long WA (ed). Philadelphia, WB Saunders, 1990, pp 3–16.
11. Davies LK, Davis RF: Cardiothoracic anesthesia. *In* Risk and Outcome in Anesthesia. Brown DL (ed). Philadelphia, WB Saunders, 1992, pp 258–282.
12. Hickey PR, Crone RK: Cardiovascular physiology and pharmacology in children: normal and diseased pediatric cardiovascular systems. *In* A Practice of Anesthesia for Infants and Children. Ryan JF, Todres ID, Cote CJ, et al (eds). Orlando, Grune & Stratton, 1986, pp 176–180.
13. Gessner IH, Klovetz LJ, Hensen RW, et al: Hemodynamic adaptations in the newborn infant. Pediatrics 1965; 36:752.
14. Clyman RI, Heymann MA, Rudolph AM: Ductus arteriosus responses to prostaglandin E$_1$ at high and low oxygen concentrations. Prostaglandins 1977; 13:219.
15. Hagen PT, Scholz DG, Edwards WD: Incidence and size of patent foramen ovale during the first ten decades: a necropsy study of 965 normal hearts. Mayo Clin Proc 1984; 59:17.
16. Emmanouilides GC, Moss AJ, Duffie ER, et al: Pulmonary arterial pressure changes in human newborn infants from birth to three days of age. J Pediatr 1964; 65:327.
17. Rudolph AM: Congenital Disease of the Heart: Clinical-Physiologic Considerations in Diagnosis and Management. Chicago, Yearbook Medical Publishers, 1974, p 29.
18. Keen EN: The postnatal development of the human cardiac ventricles. J Anat 1955; 89:484.
19. Friedman WF: Intrinsic physiological properties of the developing heart. Prog Cardiovasc Dis 1972; 15:87.
20. Friedman WF, Pool PE, Jacobowitz D, et al: Sympathetic innervation of the developing rabbit heart: biochemical and histochemical comparisons of fetal, neonatal, and adult myocardium. Circ Res 1968; 23:25.
21. Sinha SN, Armour JA, Randall WC: Development of autonomic innervation of the heart. Circulation 1973; 48(Suppl 4):37.
22. Schwartz AJ, Campbell FW. Pathophysiological approach to congenital heart disease. *In* Pediatric Cardiac Anesthesia. Lake CL (ed). Norwalk, Appleton & Lange, 1988, pp 7–25.
23. Lees MH, King DH: Heart Disease in the Newborn. *In* Heart Disease in Infants, Children and Adolescents. Adams FH, Emmanouilides GC, Riemenschneider TA (eds). Baltimore, Williams & Wilkins, 1989, pp 842–855.
24. Paul MH, Currimbhoy Z, Miller RA, et al: Thrombocytopenia in cyanotic congenital heart disease. Circulation 1961; 24:1013.
25. Kontras SB, Sirak HD, Newton WA Jr: Hematologic abnormalities in children with congenital heart disease. JAMA 1966; 195:611.
26. Edelman NH, Lahiri S, Braudol L, et al: The blunted ventilatory response to hypoxia in cyanotic congenital heart disease. N Engl J Med 1970; 282:405.
27. Amatayakul O, Cumming GR, Haworth JC: Association of hypoglycemia with cardiac enlargement and heart failure in newborn infants. Arch Dis Child 1970; 45:717.
28. Morrison J, Killip T: Serum digitalis and arrhythmia in patients undergoing cardiopulmonary bypass. Circulation 1973; 47:341.
29. Tharion J, Johnson DC, Celermajer JM, et al: Profound hypothermia with circulatory arrest. J Thorac Cardiovasc Surg 1982; 84:66.
30. Coles JG, Taylor MJ, Pearce JM, et al: Cerebral monitoring of somatosensory evoked potentials during profoundly hypothermic circulatory arrest. Circulation 1984; 70:I96.
31. Ehyai A, Fenichel GM, Bender HW Jr: Incidence and prognosis of seizures in infants after cardiac surgery with profound hypothermia and circulatory arrest. JAMA 1984; 252:3165.
32. O'Dougherty M, Wright FS, Garmezy N, et al: Later competence and adaptation in infants who survive severe heart defects. Child Dev 1983; 54:129.
33. Hickey PR, Hansen DD, Norwood WI, et al: Anesthetic complications in surgery for congenital heart disease. Anesth Analg 1984; 63:657.
34. Strafford MA, Henderson KH: Anesthetic morbidity in congenital heart disease patients undergoing noncardiac surgery (abstract). Anesthesiology 1991; 75:A1056.
35. Nicolson SC, Dorsey AT, Schreiner MS: Shortened preanesthetic fasting interval in pediatric cardiac surgical patients. Anesth Analg 1992; 74:694.
36. Tanner GE, Angers DG, Barash PG, et al: Effect of left-to-right, mixed

left-to-right, and right-to-left shunts on inhalational anesthetic induction in children: a computer model. Anesth Analg 1985; 64:101.

37. Moore RA: Anesthesia for the pediatric congenital heart patient for noncardiac surgery. Anesthesiol Rev 1981; 8:23.

38. Hickey C, Gugino LD, Aglio LS, et al: Intraoperative somatosensory evoked potential monitoring predicts peripheral nerve injury during cardiac surgery. Anesthesiology 1993; 78:29.

39. Greeley WJ, Kates RA, Bushman GA, et al: Intraoperative esophageal electrocardiography for dysrhythmia analysis and therapy in pediatric cardiac surgical patients. Anesthesiology 1986; 65:669.

40. Stefaniszyn HJ, Novick RJ, Keith FM, Salerno TA: Is the brain adequately cooled during deep hypothermic cardiopulmonary bypass? Curr Surg 1983; 40:294.

41. Almond CH, Jones JC, Snyder HM, et al: Cooling gradients and brain damage with deep hypothermia. J Thorac Cardiovasc Surg 1964; 48:890.

42. Burrows FA: Physiologic dead space, venous admixture, and the arterial to end-tidal carbon dioxide difference in infants and children undergoing cardiac surgery. Anesthesiology 1989; 70:219.

43. Arom KV, Cohen DE, Strobl FT: Effect of intraoperative intervention on neurological outcome based on electroencephalographic monitoring during cardiopulmonary bypass. Ann Thorac Surg 1989; 48:476.

44. Ungerleider RM, Greeley WJ, Sheikh KH, et al: Routine use of intraoperative epicardial echocardiography and Doppler color flow imaging to guide and evaluate repair of congenital heart lesions. J Thorac Cardiovasc Surg 1990; 100:297.

45. Lake CL, Schwartz AJ, Campbell FW: Extracorporeal circulation. *In* Pediatric Cardiac Anesthesia. Lake CL (ed). Norwalk, CT, Appleton & Lange, 1988, pp 155–179.

46. Parr CVS, Blackstone EH, Kirklin JW: Cardiac performance and mortality early after intracardiac surgery in infants and young children. Circulation 1975; 51:867.

47. Kouchoukos NT, Karp RB: Management of the postoperative cardiovascular surgical patient. Am Heart J 1976; 92:513.

48. Gall WE, Clarke WR, Doty DB: Vasomotor dynamics associated with cardiac operations. J Thorac Cardiovasc Surg 1982; 83:724.

49. Appelbaum A, Blackstone EH, Kouchoukos NT, et al: Effect of afterload reduction on cardiac output in infants after intracardiac surgery (abstract). Circulation 1975; 51, 52(Suppl II):II151.

50. Benumof JL: Respiratory physiology and respiratory function during anesthesia. *In* Anesthesia. 2nd ed. Miller RD (ed). New York, Churchill Livingstone, 1986, p 1122.

51. Hickey PR, Wessel DL: Anesthesia for treatment of congenital heart disease. *In* Cardiac Anesthesia. 2nd ed. Kaplan JA (ed). Orlando, Grune & Stratton, 1987, pp 635–723.

52. Fratacci M, Frostell CG, Chen T, et al: Inhaled nitric oxide: a selective pulmonary vasodilator of heparin-protamine vasoconstriction in sheep. Anesthesiology 1991; 75:990.

53. Ekert H, Gilchrist GS, Stanton R, et al: Hemostasis in cyanotic heart disease. J Pediatr 1970; 76:221.

54. Hoffman WS, Tomasello DN, MacVaugh H: Control of postcardiotomy bleeding with PEEP. Ann Thorac Surg 1982; 34:71.

55. Murphy DA, Finlayson DC, Craver JM, et al: Effect of positive end-expiratory pressure on excessive mediastinal bleeding after cardiac operations: controlled study. J Thorac Cardiovasc Surg 1983; 85:864.

67

Anesthesia for Adult Cardiovascular Surgery

THOMAS J. MARTIN, M.D.

Approximately 250,000 cardiac surgery procedures are carried out annually in the United States. Anesthesia for patients undergoing cardiac surgery involves some of the greatest challenges in our specialty. Not only are the cases complicated in terms of patients' pathophysiology, but the procedures themselves are extremely invasive and technically demanding. Concentrated efforts have led to technologic and pharmacologic advances in anesthesia for cardiac procedures that are unparalleled in anesthesia for other types of surgery.

The practice of cardiac anesthesia requires an anesthesiologist to use invasive and noninvasive monitoring techniques. The information obtained through monitoring is integrated with knowledge of a patient's pathophysiology in order to directly apply basic cardiovascular physiology and pharmacology in the care of the patient. Although challenging, cardiac anesthesia provides tremendous intellectual and emotional rewards.

This chapter discusses the evaluation and anesthetic management of patients undergoing cardiovascular surgery procedures in the treatment of coronary artery disease, valvular heart disease, thoracic aortic disease, and cardiac electrophysiologic disorders.

PREOPERATIVE EVALUATION

As in all areas of anesthesia, the preoperative evaluation is the foundation for sound anesthetic management. Only with a thorough understanding of a patient's pathophysiology and severity of illness can a specific anesthetic plan be made. Clinical signs and symptoms of cardiovascular disease provide a wealth of information about the manner and degree to which a patient is affected.

What Are the Goals?

Information should be obtained about a patient's cardiovascular status and about the presence of any coexisting medical conditions. The history continues to be the most important source of information despite the availability of numerous invasive and noninvasive tests of cardiovascular function. Specifically, information should be sought about a patient's functional reserve, with particular reference to the manifestations of myocardial ischemia and congestive heart failure (CHF).

What Are the Clinical Signs and Symptoms of Myocardial Ischemia?

Myocardial ischemia is the state of inadequate oxygen (O_2) delivery to the myocardium and inadequate removal of metabolites from the myocardium as a result of an imbalance between myocardial O_2 supply and demand. The quantity of coronary blood flow and O_2 delivery required is extremely variable, depending on the circulatory and metabolic state of the heart at any given time.

Angina Pectoris

Angina pectoris is the most common symptom of myocardial ischemia but not the only one. Angina may more aptly be described as chest discomfort rather than chest pain, and it has various presentations. Patients may describe it as "tightness," "squeezing," "pressure," "heaviness," or "burning." Its location may be difficult to pinpoint, and it may radiate to the left shoulder or arm, neck, jaw, or teeth. Angina may be accompanied by dyspnea, nausea, and diaphoresis. It may be associated with exertion or may occur at rest. It may occur after eating, with exposure to cold weather, with emotional excitement or stress, or with sexual intercourse. Patients should be questioned about its frequency, duration, and severity. Angina typically lasts 2 to 10 minutes and is relieved by rest. It may last longer and be more difficult to control in patients with unstable angina or myocardial infarction. Patients should be questioned about the need to use nitroglycerin (NTG) to relieve angina.

Categorization

Angina may be categorized into four types:

I. Stable angina: Usually occurs with exertion in a stable and predictable pattern.
II. Unstable angina: Defined by the presence of one or more of the following historical features, accompanied by electrocardiographic (ECG) changes:
1. Crescendo angina (more severe, prolonged, or frequent) superimposed on a pre-existing pattern of relatively stable, exertion-related angina
2. Angina at rest as well as with minimal exertion
3. Angina of new onset (usually within 1 mo), which is brought on by minimal exertion[1]
III. Variant (Prinzmetal's) angina: Characteristically occurs at rest, although it may also occur with exercise[2]; caused by coronary artery spasm
IV. Silent ischemia: Does not manifest as angina or other symptoms, occurs quite commonly in patients with coronary artery disease. It may be more common in diabetic patients, perhaps as a result of a sensory neuropathy, but also occurs in patients who have symptomatic episodes of myocardial ischemia. It is of particular interest in the perioperative period because the majority of postoperative myocardial infarctions are silent.

What Are the Clinical Signs and Symptoms of Congestive Heart Failure?

CHF has numerous causes, either acute or chronic, that result in inadequate cardiac output to meet the metabolic needs of the tissues. The clinical manifestations result from the accumulation of fluid upstream from one or both ventricles. Symptoms of left-sided heart failure include dyspnea, orthopnea, and paroxysmal nocturnal dyspnea. Right-sided heart failure is manifested by jugular venous distention, hepatomegaly, and peripheral edema.

Dyspnea

Although dyspnea is associated with a wide variety of cardiac and pulmonary disorders, in CHF, it is an expression of pulmonary venous and pulmonary capillary hypertension, which may lead to pulmonary edema. Patients should be questioned about the amount of exertion necessary to bring on dyspnea. Dyspnea most commonly occurs with exertion but may also develop in poorly compensated patients when they are in the recumbent position. It may improve with rest or by assuming an upright position (orthopnea). In some patients with ischemic heart disease, dyspnea is an "anginal equivalent," and classic anginal symptoms may not be experienced. Dyspnea is commonly quantified by asking how many flights of stairs one can climb, how far one can walk on flat ground, and what is the most strenuous or vigorous activity one can perform.

Paroxysmal Nocturnal Dyspnea

Paroxysmal nocturnal dyspnea is a manifestation of pulmonary edema that awakens a patient from sleep. Over several hours, the redistribution of fluid in the recumbent position leads to the development of pulmonary edema. It may be associated with coughing, wheezing, and diaphoresis. Paroxysmal nocturnal dyspnea is relieved by sitting, but it may take nitroglycerin or 20 to 30 minutes for enough fluid redistribution to occur before alleviation.

Edema/Nocturia

Patients should be questioned about ankle edema that worsens over the course of the day. Also, nocturia may be caused by redistribution of peripheral edema fluid to the intravascular volume and subsequent renal excretion of excess water.

How Is the Preoperative Electrocardiogram Helpful?

The rate and rhythm may indicate the adequacy of therapy with antidysrhythmic and rate-controlling agents (digoxin, β-adrenergic blockers). Measurement of the PR, QRS, and QT intervals provides information about the conduction system. The ECG may show evidence of ischemia or previous myocardial infarction. The leads in which evidence of infarction is seen may provide information about the location of coronary artery stenoses (Table 67–1). The ECG frequently appears normal, even in the presence of severe coronary artery disease.[3]

How Is the Chest Radiograph Helpful?

Radiographic signs of CHF are correlated with poor ventricular function. Specifically, four radiographic indices are important indicators[4]: (1) the cardiothoracic ratio, (2) total heart volume, (3) left ventricular (LV) volume, and (4) signs of CHF. The latter are specific indicators of abnormal ejection fraction, end-systolic volume, cardiac index, stroke work index, end-diastolic volume, and end-diastolic pressure. The chest radiograph can also appear normal, however, in patients with significant ventricular dysfunction.

What Is the Role of Noninvasive Cardiac Studies?

Patients who present with new-onset angina or who undergo cardiac evaluation before noncardiac surgery may undergo various noninvasive cardiac studies.

Exercise Treadmill Testing

Exercise treadmill testing provides an important assessment of functional capabilities.

Patients are progressively exercised to a target heart rate. They are monitored for symptomatic and ECG evidence of myocardial ischemia (Fig. 67–1). This test is particularly helpful in that it can suggest which lead to monitor for intraoperative ischemia detection.

Thallium-201 Perfusion Scan

A ^{201}Tl perfusion study may be performed in conjunction with exercise treadmill testing. Thallium-201 is a radioactive

TABLE 67–1. Relationship Between Electrocardiographic Findings Reflecting Myocardial Ischemia and Area of Myocardium Involved

Electrocardiogram Lead	Coronary Artery Responsible for Myocardial Ischemia	Area of Myocardium That May Be Involved
II, III, aVF	Right coronary artery	Right atrium Interatrial septum Right ventricle Sinoatrial node Atrioventricular node Posterior fascicle of left bundle Posterior one-third of interventricular septum Posterior papillary muscle
V₃–V₅	Left anterior descending coronary artery	Anterolateral aspects of left ventricle Right bundle branch Anterior fascicle of left bundle Posterior fascicle of left bundle Anterior two-thirds of interventricular septum Anterior papillary muscle Posterior papillary muscle
I, aVL	Left circumflex coronary artery	Lateral aspects of left ventricle Sinoatrial node Atrioventricular node Posterior fascicle of left bundle

(From McCammon RL: Coronary artery disease. *In* Anesthesia and Coexisting Disease. 2nd ed. Stoelting RK, Dierdoirf SF, McCammon RL (eds). New York, Churchill Livingstone, 1988, pp 1–36.)

potassium analogue that is taken up by areas of myocardium that are perfused. It is injected during peak exercise, and areas of ischemia or previous infarction appear as cold spots on the imaging. With rest, 2 to 4 hours after exercise, imaging is repeated. Areas that were ischemic but still viable become perfused, and the defect on the image disappears (reversible defect). Areas of previous infarction remain as cold spots (fixed defect).

Dipyridamole-Thallium Imaging

Dipyridamole-thallium imaging can be performed in patients who cannot exercise (owing to musculoskeletal disorders, claudication, other reasons). Dipyridamole simulates ex-

ECG PATTERNS INDICATIVE OF MYOCARDIAL ISCHEMIA

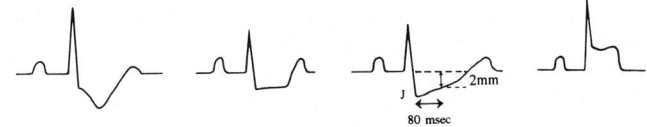

ECG PATTERNS NOT INDICATIVE OF MYOCARDIAL ISCHEMIA

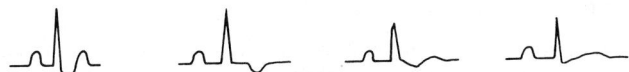

FIGURE 67–1. ECG criteria for myocardial ischemia during exercise treadmill testing: at least 1 mm of J point depression with downsloping or horizontal ST segments; slowly upsloping ST segment depression with 2 mm of ST segment depression measured at 80 ms after the J point; and ST segment elevation. ST segment depression usually indicates nontransmural ischemia, whereas ST segment elevation connotes transmural injury. Downsloping S depression more often indicates severe two- and three-vessel coronary artery disease than does horizontal or slowly upsloping ST segment depression. ST segment elevation indicates high-grade, usually proximal, coronary artery stenosis in patients without previous myocardial infarction. (Reproduced with permission, from Goldschlager N: Use of the treadmill test in the diagnosis of coronary artery disease in patients with chest pain. Ann Intern Med 1982; 97:383.)

ercise by inducing dilation of coronary arteries. Stenotic vessels cannot dilate normally, so less thallium is taken up in areas supplied by them than in areas supplied by normal coronary arteries. On images taken later, thallium redistributes into these areas of relative ischemia.

Echocardiography

Echocardiography can be used preoperatively to assess regional wall motion, ventricular function, valvular function, and the presence of intracardiac shunts. Although echocardiography may be a very useful test to diagnose ventricular dysfunction, a resting echocardiogram tells little about the potential for ischemia in a patient with severe coronary artery disease but no history of myocardial infarction. The echocardiographic detection of new wall motion abnormalities after peak exercise correlates well with the severity of coronary artery stenoses found on angiography.[5] The use of contrast echocardiography to identify coronary stenoses may have a more significant role in the future as the technology evolves.

Radionuclide Angiography

Radionuclide angiography plays a less important part now than in the past. It can provide an assessment of ventricular dysfunction due to coronary artery disease or other causes of cardiomyopathy by measurement of ejection fraction and observation of wall motion. Ejection fraction normally should increase by 5% or more after exercise.

How Are Cardiac Catheterization Data Used?

Most patients presenting for cardiac surgery have undergone diagnostic cardiac catheterization. Cardiac catheterization provides the most precise information about the location and severity of coronary stenoses, LV and right ventricular (RV) function, pulmonary and systemic vascular resistance (SVR), valvular function, and the presence of intracardiac shunts.

TABLE 67–2. Normal Hemodynamic Values Measured at Cardiac Catheterization

		a Wave	v Wave	Systolic	End-Diastolic	Mean
Pressures (mm Hg)	Right atrium	2–10	2–10			0–8
	Right ventricle			15–30	0–8	
	Pulmonary artery			15–30	3–12	9–16
	Pulmonary capillary wedge	3–15	3–12			1–10
	Left atrium	3–15	3–12			1–10
	Left ventricle			100–140	3–12	
	Aorta			100–140	60–90	70–105
Oxygen consumption index ($mL \cdot min^{-1} \cdot m^{2-1}$)		110–150				
Arteriovenous O_2 difference ($mL \cdot dL^{-1}$)		3–5				
Cardiac index ($L \cdot min \cdot m^{2-1}$)		2.6–4.2				

(From Grossman W: Cardiac catheterization. *In* Heart Disease: A Textbook of Cardiovascular Medicine. 4th ed. Braunwald E (ed). Philadelphia, WB Saunders, 1992, pp 180–203.)

Although the hemodynamic data obtained at cardiac catheterization can be extremely helpful in understanding a patient's pathophysiology, keep in mind that these data are dependent on multiple factors, including filling conditions, autonomic activity, and the presence or absence of ischemia at the time of measurement. It is not surprising, therefore, that the correlation of cardiac catheterization data with preinduction data is unreliable.[6]

Pressure Measurement

The reported hemodynamic measurements should include baseline data such as a patient's heart rate, rhythm, and blood pressure. Chamber pressures are reported as systolic and end-diastolic pressures for the ventricles and mean pressure for the atria. Normal values are shown in Table 67–2. Pressure measurements are also used to calculate SVR and pulmonary vascular resistances (PVR). If stenotic valvular lesions are present, valve areas and pressure gradients are reported. The orifice areas of stenotic valves are calculated from the pressure gradient and flow across a valve by Gorlin's formulas (Table 67–3).

Cardiac Output

Cardiac output can be determined by Fick's O_2 method or by an indicator-dilution technique (dye dilution or thermodi-

lution). There is generally good correlation between the two types of techniques. Fick's O_2 method requires estimation of O_2 consumption by collection of expired air during a 3-minute period. Cardiac output is then calculated as follows:

$$\text{Cardiac output } (L \cdot min^{-1}) = \frac{O_2 \text{ consumption } (mL \cdot min)^{-1}}{C (a - \bar{v}) O_2 (mL \cdot L^{-1})}$$

Equation 1

Thermodilution cardiac output is considerably easier to perform, but Fick's method is more accurate in patients with low cardiac output, regurgitant valvular lesions, and intracardiac shunts.

Ventricular Function

The angiography portion of the cardiac catheterization report provides information about ventricular function, coronary anatomy, and the presence of regurgitant valvular lesions. The ventriculogram may be omitted in patients with very poor ventricular function for fear that they may decompensate with injection of a large bolus of contrast material. It may also be omitted in patients with significant renal dysfunction. The report of ventriculography contains information about global LV function, as assessed by wall motion and ejection fraction, and specific information about areas with abnormal wall motion. Wall motion abnormalities may be described as hypokinesis (decreased contractility), akinesis (no contractile motion), or dyskinesis (paradoxical wall motion). A ventricular aneurysm or thrombus may be noted as well.

Coronary Vessels

The report of coronary angiography describes the coronary anatomy, including details about the sizes of vessels, the location of any anatomic variations, and the presence of calcifications and stenoses. Stenoses are characterized according to their length, the degree of diameter narrowing, and the presence of collateral filling. Narrowing of luminal diameter by 50% corresponds to a 75% reduction in cross-sectional area, and this is regarded as hemodynamically significant. The occurrence of coronary spasm may be noted by including ergonovine in the study to stimulate spasm or the use of NTG to relieve it. Normal coronary artery anatomy is depicted in Figure 67–2.

TABLE 67–3. Gorlin's Formulas for Calculation of Stenotic Valve Areas

$$\text{Aortic valve area } (cm^2) = \frac{F}{44.5 \sqrt{\Delta}}$$

$$\text{Mitral valve area } (cm^2) = \frac{F}{38.0 \sqrt{\Delta P}}$$

$$\text{Flow } (mL \cdot s^{-1}) = \frac{\text{Cardiac output } (mL \cdot min^{-1})}{\text{DFP } (s \cdot min^{-1}) \text{ or SEP } (s \cdot min^{-2})}$$

Abbreviations: DFP = diastolic filling period; SEP = systolic ejection period. These are calculated by measuring the diastolic filling time or systolic ejection time per beat and multiplying by heart rate. F = Flow across the valve ($mL \cdot s^{-1}$); ΔP = the mean pressure gradient across the valve (mm Hg).

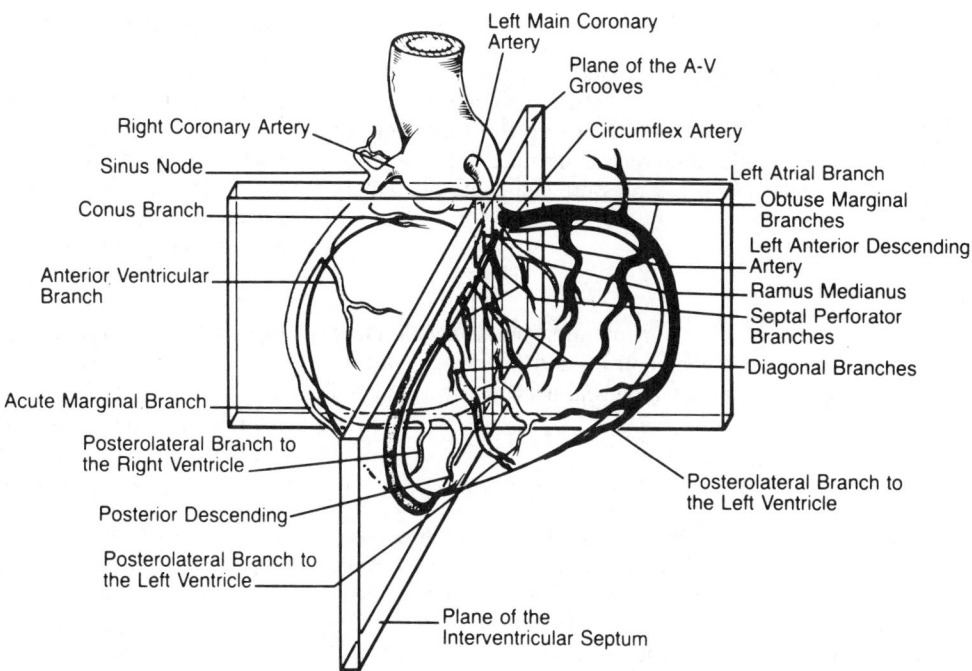

FIGURE 67–2. Normal anatomy of the coronary arteries. The right coronary artery and the left circumflex coronary artery lie in the same plane, whereas the left anterior descending coronary artery travels perpendicular to that plane. Each gives rise to branches as shown. The left circumflex artery is shown in black, the left anterior descending artery in gray, and the right coronary artery in white. (From Bashore TM, Chapman MJ: Basic anatomy and physiology of the heart. *In* Invasive Cardiology: Principles and Techniques. 1st ed. Toronto, BC Decker, 1990, pp 79–107.)

What Are the Clinical Signs and Symptoms of Valvular Disease?

Symptoms of CHF are the most important to elicit. They may reflect ventricular function but more commonly are related to preload and afterload conditions, depending on the particular valvular lesion.

Aortic Stenosis

Ventricular Hypertrophy

In aortic stenosis, the primary pathophysiology is LV pressure overload as the ventricle pumps against its obstruction to outflow. The obstruction to LV outflow leads to compensatory ventricular hypertrophy in order to generate higher systolic pressure and maintain cardiac output. The hypertrophy is said to be concentric because although the wall thickens, the LV chamber size (radius) is essentially unchanged. Therefore, as indicated by Laplace's law,

$$\text{Wall tension} = \frac{\text{Pressure} \times \text{radius}}{2 \times \text{wall thickness}} \qquad \text{Equation 2}$$

wall tension remains essentially normal in well-compensated patients with aortic stenosis. In later stages, when hypertrophy no longer matches the degree of obstruction, ventricular dysfunction is evident.

Angina

As ventricular mass increases, myocardial O_2 consumption ($M\dot{V}O_2$) increases. Systolic function is well maintained until very late in the disease process, but diastolic compliance is reduced. The loss of diastolic compliance has an important role in myocardial O_2 balance. Increased LV end-diastolic pressure (LVEDP) decreases coronary perfusion pressure (CPP). Also, the systolic ejection time becomes more prolonged at the expense of diastolic (perfusion) time. A vicious cycle of decreasing compliance and worsening ischemia may result. Consequently, even in the absence of angiographically demonstrable epicardial coronary artery disease, myocardial ischemia is a major threat and angina is common. Angina is an ominous sign, signaling either significant coronary artery disease and mild aortic stenosis or severe aortic stenosis and mild coronary artery disease. In either case, it suggests that the compensatory reserve is virtually exhausted.

Syncope and Congestive Heart Failure

Two other symptoms that, along with chest pain, make up a classic triad in patients with aortic stenosis are syncope and CHF. Syncope is due to inadequate cardiac output. It may occur during exercise when heart rate increases and the systemic vasculature dilates, resulting in inadequate preload to maintain cardiac output. CHF may occur as a result of volume overload or more commonly as a result of loss of sinus rhythm. It is particularly likely to accompany the acute onset of atrial fibrillation.

Mitral Stenosis

Dyspnea

The main symptom of mitral stenosis is dyspnea. With progressive narrowing of the mitral valve orifice, flow from the left atrium (LA) to the LV can only be maintained by increasing the transvalvular pressure gradient. Elevation of LA pressure eventually leads to elevation of pulmonary venous pressure and pulmonary artery occlusion pressure (PAOP). Dyspnea is the clinical presentation of this increase in pressures and congestion of the pulmonary vascular bed.

Patients are most likely to be symptomatic during conditions or activities that require increased heart rate and cardiac output. Examples include exercise, anemia, pregnancy, infection, emotional distress, and thyrotoxicosis.

Atrial Fibrillation

The development of atrial fibrillation is particularly deleterious because of the loss of the atrial contraction ("atrial kick") component of LA to LV flow and the shortening of diastole associated with rapid ventricular rate. This condition leads to large increases in LA pressure and acute pulmonary edema.

Miscellaneous

Other signs and symptoms of mitral stenosis include chest pain, hemoptysis, thromboembolism, and hoarseness due to compression of the recurrent laryngeal nerve by the enlarged LA.

Aortic Insufficiency

Aortic insufficiency is characterized by LV volume overload. Patients are usually asymptomatic as a result of chronic aortic insufficiency for many years until the insidious development of LV dysfunction results in symptoms of CHF. Patients may develop angina with increases in LV mass and $M\dot{V}O_2$, but this symptom is less common than in aortic stenosis. Acute aortic insufficiency may develop as a result of endocarditis, aortic dissection, or aortic trauma. Fulminant pulmonary edema is likely because the LV has not had time to dilate and hypertrophy in a controlled fashion. Acute mitral regurgitation and pulmonary edema usually follow.

Mitral Regurgitation

Patients with mitral regurgitation develop symptoms of inadequate cardiac output—weakness and fatigue. The LV chronically dilates to accommodate increased preload in order to maintain adequate cardiac output, despite an increasing proportion of the stroke volume flowing "backward" into the LA. The LA dilates to accommodate the increased volume without large increases in LA pressure.

Progression of severity of chronic mitral regurgitation is slow, but acute mitral regurgitation is much more poorly tolerated. Acute mitral regurgitation may be caused by ischemic papillary muscle dysfunction, rupture of a papillary muscle or chordae tendineae, or endocarditis. Because the LA has not progressively dilated to accommodate the regurgitant volume, abrupt onset of biventricular failure and pulmonary edema occur.

What Information Should Be Obtained from Patients with Thoracic Aortic Disease?

Repair of a thoracic aortic aneurysm, dissection, and traumatic rupture involve the same basic principles, but the emergent nature of the procedure and a patient's signs and symptoms differ according to the chronicity of the problem.

Aortic Aneurysm

A thoracic aortic aneurysm may produce pain as a result of expansion of the aneurysm or erosion of bony structures. Compression of the recurrent laryngeal nerve may be responsible for hoarseness. Airway structures, especially the left mainstem bronchus, may be compressed as well.

Aortic Dissection

Dissection of the thoracic aorta most commonly presents as severe chest or back pain with a tearing quality. Depending on its location and extent, various signs and symptoms may be noted. If one considers the course of the aorta and its branches, these signs and symptoms are logical. Dissection may involve the aortic valve and cause acute aortic insufficiency. One or both coronary ostia may be involved, producing myocardial ischemia or infarction.

Obstruction of the brachiocephalic artery, left carotid artery, or vertebral arteries may produce neurologic symptoms. Obstruction of the brachiocephalic artery or left subclavian artery may produce pulselessness of the corresponding upper extremity. Obstruction of segmental arteries may produce spinal cord ischemia and paraplegia. Involvement of the mesenteric arteries may cause bowel ischemia. Obstruction of the renal arteries produces renal hypoperfusion and resultant oliguria.

Leakage or rupture into the pericardium or pleural cavity may produce pericardial tamponade or hemothorax, respectively. It is essential that the surgeon and anesthesiologist communicate clearly about the location and extent of the dissection as determined by aortography, computed tomographic scan, or echocardiography. Two classification systems have been described (Fig. 67–3). Depending on the surgical approach, decisions are then made about monitoring and the possibility of bypass shunts.

Aortic Rupture

Traumatic aortic rupture most commonly occurs near the ligamentum arteriosum, just distal to the left subclavian artery. It may also occur just cephalad to the aortic valve. Accompanying injuries to the head and neck, chest, abdomen, and extremities are common.

What Electrophysiologic Disorders Are Important?

Patients with re-entry atrial and ventricular tachydysrhythmias are commonly treated by catheter ablation techniques in the cardiac catheterization laboratory,[7] but some still require

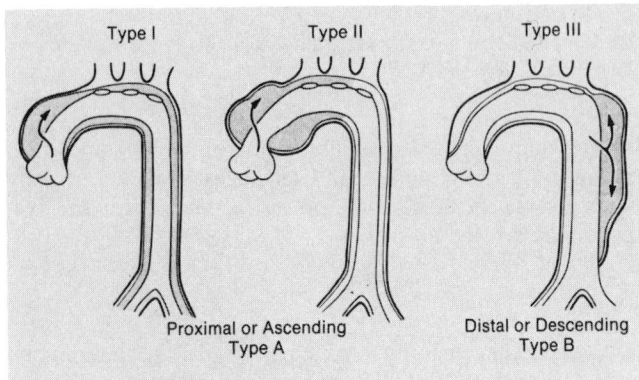

FIGURE 67–3. The anatomic classification of thoracic aortic dissections. DeBakey types I and II and Stanford type A involve the ascending aorta and arch. DeBakey type III and Stanford type B originate distal to the left subclavian artery. (From Benumof JL: Anesthesia for emergency thoracic surgery. *In* Anesthesia for Thoracic Surgery. 1st ed. Benumof JL (ed). Philadelphia, WB Saunders, 1987, pp 375–404.)

ablation of re-entry pathways or ventricular aneurysmectomy. Others with a history of recurrent ventricular tachycardia or ventricular fibrillation undergo placement of an automatic internal cardioverter-defibrillator (AICD).

The nature of the dysrhythmias and their associated symptoms, the status of antidysrhythmic therapy, and the apparent success or lack of success in controlling the problem should be determined by history, report of Holter monitoring, and electrophysiologic studies. Ventricular dysfunction and CHF should be ascertained if present. Patients with precipitation atrial re-entrant tachydysrhythmias, such as the Wolff-Parkinson-White syndrome, may have normal ventricular function and be in otherwise good health. Others may have severe ventricular dysfunction due to ischemic cardiomyopathy or idiopathic cardiomyopathy.

Pulmonary Function

Preoperative pulmonary function tests should be considered in patients scheduled for AICD implantation. Patients treated with amiodarone may develop interstitial lung fibrosis as a toxic side effect of the drug. They tend to have reduced total lung capacity and diffusion capacity.[8] Chronic obstructive pulmonary disease (COPD) should also be ruled out.

Depending on the surgical approach, one-lung ventilation may be used intraoperatively; thus, optimization of pulmonary function is especially important. If a patient may not be able to tolerate such an approach, an alternative (e.g., subxiphoid or median sternotomy) can be suggested.

THE PREOPERATIVE PERIOD

After preoperative evaluation, the anesthetic plan is constructed. It involves decisions about continuation of long-term medications, administration of preoperative sedation, the choice of monitors, and the intraoperative anesthetic management.

What Medications Should Be Continued in Patients with Coronary Artery Disease?

Patients with coronary artery disease are usually treated with one or more antianginals, including nitrates, β-adrenergic blockers, and calcium channel blockers. Antihypertensive medications, such as angiotensin-converting enzyme inhibitors or the centrally acting α_2-adrenergic agonist clonidine, may also be part of the long-term treatment regimen. Other commonly prescribed medications include diuretics, digoxin, potassium supplementation, insulin, oral hypoglycemic agents, and aspirin.

Nitrates

Oral, sublingual, or topical nitrates (NTG, isosorbide dinitrate) exert antianginal effects primarily by their systemic vasodilating effects.[9] They reduce preload by dilating capacitance veins, thereby decreasing $M\dot{V}O_2$. They also reduce afterload by dilating systemic arteries and arterioles, further decreasing $M\dot{V}O_2$. Direct vasodilation in the coronary circulation primarily involves large conductive vessels.[10]

Because nitrate therapy may contribute to stable hemodynamic function and help to prevent myocardial ischemia, it should be continued in the perioperative period. If a patient uses sublingual NTG for episodes of chest pain, the anesthesiologist should include a preoperative order that it be sent to the operating room for use as needed. Patients receiving intravenous NTG should continue to receive it during transport to the operating room.

Beta-Blockers

Patients receiving β-adrenergic blockers should continue to receive them perioperatively. These agents have beneficial effects in ischemic heart disease, primarily through their β_1-antagonist effects: reduction in heart rate, decrease in force of contraction, and decrease in renin production. The cardiac effects of β-adrenergic blockade are more marked under conditions of increased myocardial demand and increased sympathetic tone, such as during exercise. For this reason, β-blockers are particularly effective in patients with exercise-induced angina. This fact may also explain their benefit in the perioperative period, because they may blunt the tachycardiac, hypertensive response to tracheal intubation and surgical stimuli. Tachycardia is the hemodynamic response most commonly associated with perioperative ischemia that is attributed to a change in hemodynamics.[11, 12]

In the past, discontinuation of β-adrenergic blockade was recommended before surgery for fear of dangerous interaction with general anesthetic agents.[13] This concern is unfounded.[14, 15] Hemodynamic management is not complicated by the continuation of β-blockers. Discontinuation of β-adrenergic blockade not only deprives patients of its beneficial effects but also may lead to rebound phenomena. Nervousness, sweating, and tachycardia may be followed by life-threatening hypertension, myocardial ischemia, and infarction.[16]

One possible exception involves a long-acting β-blocker, nadolol, which some investigators suggest should be converted to a shorter-acting drug on the day of surgery to avoid prolonged bradycardia and myocardial depression after cardiopulmonary bypass (CPB).

Calcium Channel Blockers

Calcium channel blockers are a common part of the therapy of ischemic heart disease. The various agents exert different hemodynamic effects, including systemic vasodilation, slowing of atrioventricular conduction, depression of myocardial contractility, and prevention of coronary spasm. Interestingly, evidence that calcium channel blockers have a significant role in preventing perioperative myocardial ischemia is lacking.[18, 19]

Potential adverse side effects of continuing calcium channel blockers in cardiac surgical patients include decreased SVR, myocardial depression, and atrioventricular conduction block. However, these side effects can be overcome with vasoconstrictors, inotropes, and atrioventricular sequential pacing. Because calcium channel blockers in particular patients may play a part in control of hypertension, prevention of supraventricular tachydysrhythmias, and relief of Prinzmetal's angina, logic suggests they provide similar benefit in the perioperative period and should therefore be continued.

Clonidine

Clonidine is an α_2-adrenergic agonist commonly used to treat hypertension. Clonidine must be continued perioperatively to avoid the rebound hypertensive crisis associated with withdrawal as early as 8 hours after the last dose. Alternate routes of administration should be considered in the early postoperative period, before patients are able to receive it orally. The transdermal route is an option that must be anticipated in that it requires 24 to 48 hours to reach peak effect. Rectal administration requires 45 minutes.[20]

Aspirin

Prophylactic aspirin should be discontinued 1 week before scheduled cardiac surgery. Continuation of aspirin in the preoperative period significantly increases blood loss and transfusion requirements.[21]

Should Antidysrhythmics Be Continued for Implantation of an Automatic Internal Cardioverter-Defibrillator?

The cardiologist who treats a patient preoperatively and postoperatively should make the decision about continuation of antidysrhythmic medications. However, the anesthesiologist and surgeon should be aware of the decision and understand its implications, because the issue is somewhat controversial.

Some antiarrhythmic medications affect the testing and function of an AICD. The defibrillation threshold may be elevated by antidysrhythmic medications.[22] Class I antiarrhythmic agents would be expected to increase defibrillation threshold by depression of sodium conductance, and class III agents would be expected to lower depolarization threshold by decreasing potassium conductance.[23] In doses used clinically, however, this is not necessarily true. Class IC agents, such as encainide and flecainide, reliably increase the defibrillation threshold in animal models.[24, 25] Chronic oral administration of amiodarone has been shown to raise energy requirements for defibrillation in patients at the time of AICD implantation.[26–28] Other antidysrhythmic agents appear to be clinically less significant in altering defibrillation threshold. Slowing of conduction by class I agents and amiodarone may also cause slowing of ventricular tachycardia and may interfere with tachycardia detection by the AICD.

The best solution is to maintain patients on a stable antidysrhythmic regimen through the perioperative period. If a patient will not be maintained on such medications postoperatively, they should be stopped 1 to 2 days before surgery and the patient kept on continuous ECG monitoring.[29] A much longer period is necessary for amiodarone, because it has a mean elimination half-life of 52 days.[30]

If a patient is to be maintained on antidysrhythmic medications postoperatively, they should be continued perioperatively so that the AICD can be tested under the same pharmacologic conditions that will be present thereafter.

How Should Preoperative Sedation Be Managed Before Cardiac Surgery?

General Considerations

Preoperative medication should help to allay a patient's anxiety, suppress the pain that may be associated with the placement of intravascular catheters, and provide amnesia. The preoperative discussion should make clear to patients that you

are sensitive to their concerns and should provide enough information that none of the invasive procedures are complete surprises.

Anxiolytic treatment helps to reduce the chance that ischemia may result from a patient's sympathetic response to apprehension. Appropriate use of local anesthesia limits the pain associated with placement of invasive monitors but does not completely prevent it. Preoperative medications that provide amnesia are important for two reasons. Most patients do not want to remember the immediate preoperative period. Preoperative medication may also prevent awareness and recall of intraoperative events, particularly when the planned anesthetic is primarily opioid based.

Functional Status

Although all of these characteristics are desirable, the dosing of preoperative medication should be based on a patient's functional status. Not all patients want or need preoperative sedation. Many times, all that is needed is telling patients that such medication is available at any time they feel that it might be helpful.

If a desire for sedation is articulated, decreased amounts of sedative are administered to patients who are elderly, who have poor ventricular function, who appear to be especially susceptible to soft tissue airway obstruction, and who have known or suspected pulmonary hypertension (especially patients with valvular disease). Such patients are more safely managed by administration of a small dose of a benzodiazepine before transfer to the operating room. Additional sedation with intravenously administered opioids or benzodiazepines can be titrated for placement of intravascular catheters in the operating room, where closer observation and monitoring can be performed. Patients who are anticoagulated receive either orally or intravenously administered premedications only.

The author's opinion is that all cardiac surgery patients who have received a sedative premedication should be transported to the operating room with supplemental O_2, to provide a margin of safety. This practice is especially important for patients with pulmonary hypertension, which may be significantly worsened by hypoxemia. No matter what degree of sedation is chosen, patients about to undergo cardiac surgery should not be left unattended for long periods after receiving preoperative medication. Ideally, they should be observed by experienced nursing personnel in a preoperative holding area. Pulse oximetry may provide added safety by identifying desaturation and extremes of heart rate. Table 67–4 lists some suggested preoperative medication regimens.

TABLE 67–4. Suggested Preoperative Medications

Good LV function	Diazepam, 0.1–0.15 mg · kg⁻¹ PO
	Morphine, 0.1 mg · kg⁻¹ IM
	Scopolamine, 0.005 mg · kg⁻¹ IM
Good LV function	Diazepam, 0.1–0.15 mg · kg⁻¹ PO
Anticoagulated	Methadone, 0.1 mg · kg⁻¹ PO
Poor LV function	Diazepam, 0.07–0.1 mg · kg⁻¹ PO, or
Advanced age	midazolam, 0.02–0.04 IM
	Morphine 0.05 mg · kg⁻¹ IM
Poor LV function	Diazepam, 0.07–0.1 mg · kg⁻¹ PO, or
Pulmonary hypertension	midazolam, 0.02–0.04 mg · kg⁻¹ IM

Abbreviations: LV = left ventricular; PO = orally; IM = intramuscularly.

Should Sedation Be Administered Before Undergoing Thoracic Aortic Surgery?

The decision about whether to give sedation to a patient undergoing thoracic aortic surgery depends on whether the reason for the procedure is a chronic, stable process (aneurysm) or an acute, evolving process (dissection or traumatic rupture) and whether the patient is hemodynamically stable. A patient with a stable thoracic aneurysm that is not apparently expanding may receive a moderate amount of preoperative sedation. Sedation that leaves a patient obtunded is inappropriate in any case because it makes it impossible to monitor the neurologic findings as an indication of progression of the disease.

Patients with a dissection or rupture must be alert enough to describe the location and quality of pain, which may indicate progression of the process. If a patient is hemodynamically stable, slowly and carefully administered analgesics can be beneficial. They may prevent pain-induced hypertension and tachycardia, which could contribute to evolution of dissection or rupture.

Is Single-Dose β-Adrenergic Blockade or Clonidine Beneficial?

Beta-Adrenergic Blockade

Given the evidence that continued β-adrenergic blockade appears to reduce the incidence of perioperative myocardial ischemia, administration of a single dose of β-blocker seems to offer potential benefit even in patients not already treated with such a medication. In hypertensive patients who do not have documented coronary artery disease and are undergoing noncardiac surgery, a single dose of a β-adrenergic blocking agent appears to reduce significantly the incidence of perioperative myocardial ischemia, tachycardia, and other dysrhythmias.[31]

Clonidine

0.3 – 0.6 mg clonidine

A single preoperative dose of clonidine administered to patients undergoing coronary artery bypass graft (CABG) improves hemodynamic stability, reduces plasma catecholamine levels, reduces opioid anesthetic requirement, allows earlier extubation, and reduces postoperative shivering.[32, 33] Whether it also affects the incidence of myocardial ischemia has not been reported. The hyperdynamic state associated with withdrawal of chronic clonidine therapy does not occur after a single dose; thus, it appears to be a safe and potentially beneficial treatment option.

What Monitors Are Required?

The basic intraoperative monitors for any anesthetic as outlined by the American Society of Anesthesiologists apply to cardiac anesthesia as well. They include an inspired O_2 analyzer, pulse oximeter, electrocardiograph, blood pressure cuff, precordial (before intubation) or esophageal stethoscope, temperature probe, and qualified anesthesia personnel in the room throughout the procedure. Beyond these basic monitors, cardiac anesthesia requires additional devices or techniques that

should be considered "standard" because of the severity of illness of the patients and the invasive nature of the surgical procedure.

Electrocardiogram

Electrocardiography is an important monitor of heart rate and rhythm, atrioventricular conduction, and myocardial ischemia. Changes occur suddenly in cardiac procedures. Conduction disturbances commonly result from anesthetic agents, electrolyte and temperature changes, and surgical disruption of conduction pathways. V_5 is the preferred lead.

Blood Pressure

Arterial blood pressure must be monitored by an intra-arterial catheter in addition to a blood pressure cuff. Intra-arterial pressure monitoring provides continuous beat-to-beat measurement. Blood pressure is subject to sudden and dramatic change during cardiac surgery owing to patients' cardiovascular disease, changes in heart rhythm, the effects of anesthetic agents and airway manipulation, surgical stimulation, and direct manipulation of the heart and great vessels. During CPB, only an intra-arterial catheter can reliably measure the nonpulsatile arterial pressure.

Catheter Location

The specific location of the catheter is determined by the preference of the anesthesiologist and the requirements of the procedure. Aortic arch pressure is the measurement that is most closely related to LV stroke volume, LV contractility, and SVR.[34] Direct arterial blood pressure measurement is obtained at more distal sites, with consequent attenuation of the aortic pressure waveform. Although mean arterial pressure (MAP) may be fairly consistent throughout the arterial tree, systolic pressure, flow, and waveform characteristics in peripheral arteries are often quite divergent from those of the aorta (Fig. 67–4). Radial or femoral arterial catheters are most commonly used for cardiac surgery because of their easy accessibility and relative safety.

During CABG surgery in which a left internal mammary artery (IMA) graft is used, a right radial arterial catheter may be preferred. To facilitate surgical dissection of the left IMA, the operating table is often tilted to the left. This maneuver compresses the left arm and brachial artery between the patient's trunk and the supports of the Favoloro retractor unless the arms are positioned on wedges with the patient's hands next to his or her head. Also, traction of the Favoloro retractor on the sternum and left chest wall may cause "tenting" of the left subclavian artery. Both conditions might lead to dampening or loss of a left radial arterial pressure tracing.

If a right radial catheter cannot be placed, a femoral catheter may be inserted. Alternatively, a left radial catheter may be used and arterial pressure monitored by a blood pressure cuff on the right arm. This method can be accomplished with safety because the period of dissection of the IMA is not particularly stimulating and tends to be associated with hemodynamic stability.

Insertion of a second intra-arterial catheter may be necessary for thoracic aortic aneurysm repair. The locations of the catheters are determined by the type of aneurysm and the planned location of aortic cross-clamps and are discussed later.

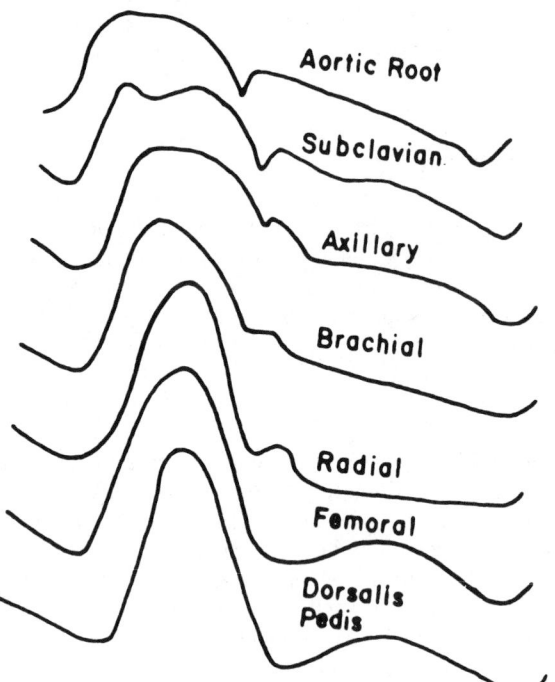

FIGURE 67-4. The arterial pressure wave undergoes considerable attenuation as it passes from the aorta to distal arterial sites. Although the measured mean pressure is fairly constant, there is considerable disparity among systolic pressures measured at various sites. (From Bedford RF: Invasive blood pressure monitoring. *In* Monitoring in Anesthesia and Critical Care Medicine. 2nd ed. Blitt CD (ed). New York, Churchill Livingstone, 1990, pp 93-134.)

Intravascular Volume

Intravascular volume is assessed by central venous pressure (CVP), pulmonary artery pressure (PAP), and PAOP or by direct measurement of LA pressure through a catheter placed by the surgeon. Such assessment is essential to maintain hemodynamic stability in cardiac surgical patients. It is especially important during weaning from CPB, when intravascular volume (preload) is optimized by delivering blood from the CPB circuit reservoir.

Central Venous Catheter

The CVP indicates right atrial (RA) and some insight into right ventricular (RV) pressure. During CPB, it should also be monitored to assess the adequacy of superior vena caval drainage and, indirectly, cerebral venous drainage. In some cases, the CVP may be the only intravascular volume monitor necessary—for example, atrial septal defect repair or CABG surgery in a patient with well-preserved ventricular function.

Pulmonary Artery Catheter

Pressure Monitoring. A pulmonary artery (PA) catheter is commonly used during cardiac surgery to measure LA and LV pressures. In addition to providing the CVP and valuable hemodynamic information, it can help to detect myocardial ischemia.

The indications for use of a PA catheter are outlined in Table 67-5. Although the use of a PA catheter with aggressive treatment of hemodynamic aberrations in patients with coronary artery disease may decrease perioperative myocardial in-

farction and mortality,[35, 36] a prospective study has shown no difference in outcome whether a PA catheter or CVP catheter was used.[37] The decision about which to use should be based on the severity of cardiac disease, the nature of the procedure, and the anesthesiologist's and surgeon's preferences for completeness of hemodynamic information.

Cardiac Output. Measurement of cardiac output is a more reliable means to assess cardiac performance than is blood pressure. In order to standardize for body size differences, it is often expressed as cardiac index (Table 67-6). Cardiac output is most easily measured using a thermodilution PA catheter. The injectate is a crystalloid solution at a temperature lower than the patient's blood temperature. Iced injectate is not necessary for accuracy or reproducibility,[38] and the solution may be saline, 5% dextrose, or lactated Ringer's, all of which have similar specific gravity and specific heat.[39] The injection should be made in triplicate at end-expiration.

Cardiac output measurements can be erroneous in patients with intracardiac shunts or right-sided valvular lesions. Thermodilution techniques measure right-sided cardiac output, which normally is the same as left-sided output. Left-to-right blood flow across an atrial septal or ventricular septal defect, however, causes the measured cardiac output to be greater than actual left-sided cardiac output and is of little or no value. Similarly, regurgitation through or stenosis of either the tricuspid valve or pulmonic valve leads to erroneous cardiac output measurements because of the altered blood flow and, therefore, thermodilution. Hence, although a PA catheter may still provide useful information about PAP, PAOP, and CVP, it should not be placed for the purpose of measuring cardiac output in patients with intracardiac shunts or right-sided valvular lesions.

Once the cardiac output and filling pressures have been measured, other hemodynamic variables can be calculated (see Table 67-6). Although these parameters can aid in the understanding of a patient's hemodynamic status, undue emphasis should not be placed on them. They are derived rather than directly measured values like heart rate, cardiac output, and blood pressure. Consequently, they are affected by small changes in each of the measured parameters, as well as by technical inaccuracies in measurement.

TABLE 67-5. Indications of a Pulmonary Artery Catheter During Cardiac Surgery

---

- Patients for CABG surgery with:
  Poor LV function (EF <0.4 or LVEDP >18 mm Hg)
  LV wall motion abnormalities
  Recent MI (<6 mo)
  Complications of recent MI (acute mitral insufficiency, ventricular septal rupture, ventricular aneurysm)
  Unstable angina requiring intravenous nitroglycerin or intra-aortic balloon counterpulsation
- Valvular disease
- Combined coronary and valvular disease
- Pulmonary hypertension
- Complex cardiac lesions
- Thoracic aortic surgery requiring cross-clamping
- Patients with significant systemic disease (e.g., renal, hepatic)

(Modified from Kaplan JA: Hemodynamic monitoring. *In* Cardiac Anesthesia. 2nd ed. Kaplan JA (ed). Orlando, FL, Grune & Stratton, 1987, pp 179-225.)
Abbreviations: CABG = coronary artery bypass graft; LV = left ventricular; EF = ejection fraction; LVEDP = left ventricular end-diastolic pressure; MI = myocardial infarction.

TABLE 67–6. Derived Hemodynamic Parameters from Pulmonary Artery Catheter Data

Formula	Units	Normal Range
$CI = \dfrac{CO}{BSA}$	$1 \cdot min \cdot m^{2^{-1}}$	2–5
$SV = \dfrac{CO}{HR}$	$mL \cdot beat^{-1}$	60–90
$SI = \dfrac{SV}{BSA}$	$mL \cdot beat \cdot m^{2^{-1}}$	40–60
$LVSWI = \dfrac{1.36\,(MAP - PCWP)}{100} \times SI$	$g \cdot m \cdot m^{2^{-1}}$	45–60
$RVSWI = \dfrac{1.36\,(PAP - CVP)}{100} \times SI$	$g \cdot m \cdot m^{2^{-1}}$	5–10
$SVR = \dfrac{(MAP - CVP)}{CO} \times 80$	$dynes \cdot s \cdot cm^{-5}$	900–1500

(From Kaplan JA: Hemodynamic monitoring. *In* Cardiac Anesthesia. 2nd ed. Kaplan JA (ed). Orlando, FL, Grune & Stratton, 1987, pp 179–225.)
Abbreviations: CI = Cardiac index; CO = cardiac output; BSA = body surface area; SV = stroke volume; HR = heart rate; SI = stroke index; LVSWI = left ventricular stroke work index; PCWP = pulmonary capillary wedge pressure; PAP = mean pulmonary artery pressure; RVSWI = right ventricular stroke work index; CVP = central venous pressure; SVR = systemic vascular resistance; PVR = pulmonary vascular resistance.

As an example, SVR is the parameter most commonly used in the clinical setting to assess LV afterload—that is, defined as the force opposing ventricular fiber shortening during LV ejection. However, during the pharmacologic manipulations commonly required for cardiac anesthesia, the SVR does not reflect true LV afterload, which depends on a multitude of factors both internal and external to the myocardium.[40] These factors include the myocardial contractile state, intraventricular pressure, geometric characteristics of the LV, elasticity and geometry of blood vessels, inertial properties of blood, and viscosity of blood.

Continuous Mixed Venous Oxygen Saturation. Continuous mixed venous O_2 saturation ($S\bar{v}O_2$) can be monitored with specially designed PA catheters. The $S\bar{v}O_2$ should reflect the global adequacy of body tissue perfusion (i.e., the balance between tissue O_2 demand and delivery). When a patient's temperature is relatively stable, a decrease in $S\bar{v}O_2$ most likely indicates decreased O_2 delivery to the tissues. Cardiac output, arterial O_2 saturation (SaO_2), and hematocrit are assessed to determine the cause, if it is unclear, and appropriate treatment is begun. Several factors can be responsible for changes in $S\bar{v}O_2$ (Table 67–7).

Left Atrial Pressure

LA pressure can be measured directly with a catheter placed by the surgeon. This procedure minimizes the effect of airway

TABLE 67–7. Factors That Influence $S\bar{v}O_2$

Causes of decreased $S\bar{v}O_2$	Decreasing or low cardiac output
	Low SaO_2
	Anemia
	Increased oxygen consumption (hyperthermia, shivering)
Causes of increased $S\bar{v}O_2$	High cardiac output (sepsis, liver failure)
	Decreased oxygen consumption (hypothermia, sepsis, liver failure)
	Cyanide toxicity
	Falsely elevated $S\bar{v}O_2$ by wedging of the catheter in a pulmonary capillary bed

pressure that may alter PAOP accuracy, but it does not accurately indicate LV pressure in the presence of mitral valvular disease. An LA catheter also introduces the risk of bleeding and air or thrombus embolization directly into the left-sided vasculature.

Urine Output

Urine output is routinely monitored during cardiac surgery. It provides an indication of the adequacy of renal perfusion and function. Renal perfusion may be altered by inadequate intravascular volume as a result of diuretic and vasodilator therapy, inadequate perfusion pressure as a result of poor cardiac output or vasodilator therapy, impairment of renal blood flow by vasoconstrictors and CPB, and various other factors.

Renal function during cardiac surgery must be maintained to prevent acute renal failure. This goal is best accomplished by ensuring adequate intravascular volume and cardiac output before and after CPB and adequate perfusion during CPB. Hemoglobinuria may be seen during cardiac surgery, most commonly as a result of hemolysis but occasionally from a transfusion reaction during CPB. Treatment with diuretics such as mannitol or furosemide is frequently recommended but remains controversial.

Temperature

Temperature must be monitored to ensure adequate, even cooling and rewarming during CPB. It can be measured at various sites. Tympanic membrane temperature is the best indication of brain temperature but has been associated with traumatic perforation.[41] Other sites are compared with tympanic membrane temperature as a standard, with rectal, bladder, esophageal, and nasopharyngeal temperatures correlating most closely.[42]

Core cooling during CPB, however, induces significant differences in temperature measured at various sites (Fig. 67–5). Esophageal and nasopharyngeal temperatures decrease most rapidly with cooling and increase most rapidly with rewarming.[43] Conversely, temperature changes most slowly in the rectum. Bladder temperature is intermediate in rate of cooling

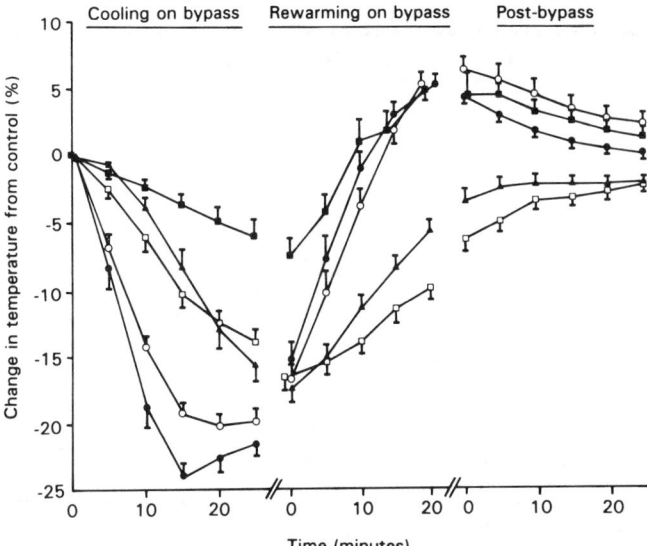

FIGURE 67–5. Changes in temperature measured at various sites during active cooling on cardiopulmonary bypass, rewarming on bypass, and post-bypass. The changes are expressed as percentage change from control. Sites are esophageal *(solid circles)*, nasopharyngeal *(open circles)*, bladder *(solid triangles)*, rectal *(open squares)*, and thumb *(solid squares)*. *Bars* indicate SEM. (From Bone ME, Feneck RO: Bladder temperature as an estimate of body temperature during cardiopulmonary bypass. Anaesthesia 1988; 43:181.)

and rewarming[43] but at the conclusion of bypass most closely indicates the temperature afterdrop that occurs postoperatively.[44]

Coagulation

Intraoperative coagulation monitoring is essential for management of the anticoagulation necessary for CPB and for assessment of post-CPB coagulation. The activated clotting time (ACT) is a simple but very useful test of heparin activity. Measurement of heparin concentration may also be of value. The viscoelastic coagulation monitors thromboelastography, and Sonoclot, although perhaps not routine in this setting, offer additional help in diagnosing and targeting treatment of post-CPB coagulation problems.

Electroencephalogram

Electroencephalography (EEG) offers potential benefits in cardiac anesthesia. The depth of anesthesia during high-dose opioid anesthesia with muscle relaxation is difficult to assess clinically. Induction of anesthesia with opioids produces progressive slowing of EEG activity. Processed EEG monitoring has made assessment more manageable in the operating room.[45] Whether EEG improves anesthetic management by indicating the need for additional agents is uncertain. EEG slowing may correlate with unresponsiveness, but whether it correlates with unconsciousness and amnesia is uncertain. The EEG is useful to assess adequate dosing of barbiturates to induce electrical silence during CPB or deep hypothermic circulatory arrest.

Which Monitors Are Most Useful to Detect Myocardial Ischemia?

One of the most important goals in the management of patients undergoing cardiac surgery, particularly CABG sur-

gery, is the prevention or timely detection of myocardial ischemia. If all ischemia were related to hemodynamic aberrations such as tachycardia, hypertension, or hypotension, sophisticated ischemia monitoring might not be necessary. Despite maintenance of stable hemodynamic parameters, however, ischemia still occurs.[11] Therefore, detection is extremely important so that treatment can be initiated before harmful consequences occur.

Electrocardiogram

Lead Selection

The ECG continues to be the mainstay of intraoperative ischemia monitoring. Most commonly, leads II and V_5 are monitored in the operating room. Lead II is important for dysrhythmia detection, and V_5 is the single most sensitive (75%) lead for intraoperative ischemia detection.[46] The combination of leads II and V_5 is 80% sensitive in the detection of myocardial ischemia.[46] The combinations of V_4/V_5 or II/V_4/V_5 are 90% and 96% sensitive, respectively.[46] These two lead combinations are not readily available on most conventional operating room ECG monitors.

Particularly in the cardiac surgical operating room, the capability of recording the ECG on paper should be available. This allows comparison of tracings from different times during the procedure. Automated ST analysis has also improved anesthesiologists' ability to detect and treat ischemic changes that might otherwise be overlooked.

Limitations

Although the ECG remains the most commonly used ischemia monitor in the operating room, questions have arisen about its sensitivity and specificity. ECG evidence of myocardial ischemia exists as one point along a continuum of manifestations of the imbalance between myocardial O_2 supply and demand. Earlier manifestations include regional lactate production, a decrease in LV compliance, and the development of regional wall motion abnormalities (RWMAs).

Myocardial lactate production cannot be readily measured in the clinical setting, but changes in LV compliance may be reflected in the PAP and PAOP tracings. RWMAs can be detected by echocardiography, a monitoring modality that is finding widespread application in cardiac anesthesia. A study of patients undergoing percutaneous transluminal coronary angioplasty has demonstrated the time course of ischemic manifestations in awake patients[47] (Table 67–8).

Ischemia is difficult to diagnose in patients who have LV hypertrophy or who are receiving digoxin therapy, because of abnormal ST segments that are present even without ischemia.

TABLE 67–8. Time Course of Ischemic Manifestations in Patients Undergoing Percutaneous Transluminal Coronary Angioplasty

Ischemic Manifestation	Time to Onset
Regional wall motion abnormalities	19 ± 8 s
Electrocardiographic ST segment changes	30 ± 5 s
Angina pectoris	39 ± 10 s

(From Hauser AM, Gangadharan V, Ramos RG, et al: Sequence of mechanical, electro-cardiographic, and clinical effects of repeated coronary artery occlusion in human beings: echocardiographic observations during coronary angioplasty. J Am Coll Cardiol 1985; 5:193.)

TABLE 67–9. Conditions Associated with ST Segment Depression

Myocardial ischemia
Digitalis treatment
Quinidine treatment
Left bundle branch block
Ventricular pacing
Acute cor pulmonale (e.g., pulmonary embolism)
Athletic heart syndrome
Prolonged QT syndromes
Mitral valve prolapse
Increased intracranial pressure
Pheochromocytoma

Ischemic changes cannot be diagnosed in patients with left bundle branch block or a paced rhythm. Subendocardial ischemia does not always cause ECG changes. Finally, even when ST changes are present on an ECG, they are not always specific for ischemia but may be caused by other conditions (Table 67–9).

Pulmonary Artery Catheter

PA catheters may also have a role in ischemia monitoring. Kaplan and Wells reported that an increase in PAOP and the development of abnormal a-c and v waves preceded ECG changes suggestive of ischemia.[48] This finding may reflect increased LV diastolic wall tension and reduced LV compliance as a result of the development of subendocardial ischemia.

Subsequent studies comparing changes in PAOP with RWMAs suggest that PAOP changes are less sensitive.[49, 50] Although such changes can be associated with ischemia, it appears that neither they nor the development of abnormal waveforms is a sensitive or reliable early indicator of myocardial ischemia.

Transesophageal Echocardiography

Transesophageal echocardiography (TEE) appears to be a sensitive monitor of myocardial ischemia. Smith and colleagues studied 50 patients undergoing myocardial revascularization or other vascular surgery.[51] New-onset RWMAs detected by TEE were seen more frequently than ST segment changes. No patients developed new ECG changes without new RWMAs. In patients who developed both RWMAs and ST segment changes, the RWMAs tended to occur earlier. Of four patients who suffered perioperative myocardial infarction, one had persistent RWMAs and ST segment changes, two had persistent RWMAs without ST segment changes, and one had only transient RWMAs without ST segment changes.

Leung and colleagues studied 50 patients undergoing myocardial revascularization.[52] Similarly, RWMAs were detected more frequently than ST segment changes, and echocardiographic evidence of postbypass ischemia was correlated with adverse cardiac outcome. Of the ischemic episodes, 73% were not associated with even a 20% change in heart rate, blood pressure, or PA pressure.

TEE appears to be a sensitive monitor for ischemia even in patients with left bundle branch block, paced rhythm, LV hypertrophy, digoxin therapy, or subendocardial ischemia. The ECG is considerably less sensitive under these circumstances.

In both of the previously quoted studies, many patients with new RWMAs did not have adverse cardiac outcomes. Thus, the specificity of TEE as a monitor of ischemia has been questioned. Causes of RWMAs other than myocardial ischemia or infarction may include nonuniform contractility in various regions of the LV,[53] myocardial "stunning" (prolonged postischemic myocardial dysfunction),[54] altered loading conditions, tethering of normally perfused myocardium adjacent to ischemic tissue,[55] or an abnormal sequence of septal depolarization (left bundle branch block, ventricular pacing). Despite questions about its specificity, TEE appears to be a valuable monitor of myocardial ischemia.

ANESTHETIC MANAGEMENT BEFORE CARDIOPULMONARY BYPASS

Before induction of anesthesia, appropriate hemodynamic goals should be determined for each patient, depending on the particular cardiovascular pathophysiology. The anesthetic plan can then be tailored with specific objectives in mind, and responses to deviations from planned limits in hemodynamic parameters will be logically implemented as they occur.

What Are the Hemodynamic Goals in Coronary Artery Disease?

The prevention of myocardial ischemia depends on balancing myocardial O_2 supply and demand. Hemodynamic goals should be chosen with this goal in mind. Myocardial O_2 supply is determined by the arterial O_2 content (CaO_2) of blood and coronary blood flow. Myocardial O_2 demand is determined by heart rate, contractility, preload, and afterload (Table 67–10).

Myocardial Oxygen Supply

Arterial Oxygen Content

CaO_2 can be calculated from the following equation:

$$CaO_2 \ (mL \cdot dL^{-1}) = (1.39) \ (Hb) \ (\% \ saturation) + (0.003) \ (PO_2) \qquad \text{Equation 3}$$

The lowest safe hemoglobin concentration for any particular patient with coronary artery disease is difficult to determine but probably lies in the range of 8 to 10 g $\cdot$ 100 mL^{-1}. Patients should receive a fraction of inspired O_2 (FIO_2) that maintains the SaO_2 >95%. Any leftward shift of the oxyhemoglobin dissociation curve (hypothermia, alkalosis, or decreased con-

TABLE 67–10. Determinants of Myocardial Oxygen Balance

Myocardial O$_2$ Supply	Myocardial O$_2$ Demand
Arterial O$_2$ content	Heart rate
Coronary blood flow	Myocardial contractility
Perfusion pressure	Wall tension
Mechanical effects	Afterload
Metabolic effects	Preload
Neural effects	
Stenoses	
Collaterals	

centration of 2,3-diphosphoglycerate) can contribute to decreased availability of O_2 at the tissues.

Coronary Blood Flow

Coronary blood flow is determined by a number of mechanical, metabolic, hormonal, and anatomic factors. The coronary arteries arise from the root of the aorta and give rise to numerous branches over the epicardial surface (see Fig. 67–2). These vessels subdivide into additional branches that course through the myocardium to form a subendocardial plexus.

Isovolemic contraction of the LV generates high tension within the myocardium, causing abrupt cessation in blood flow of the left coronary artery (Fig. 67–6). Left coronary flow begins to rise gradually during systole but occurs primarily during diastole. The phasic changes in blood flow may be even greater in intramural arteries. Approximately 85% of coronary blood flow to the LV occurs during diastole. The 15% that occurs during systole is primarily epicardial. Intracavitary systolic pressures of the RV are much lower. The majority of coronary blood flow to the RV occurs during systole.

When coronary autoregulation is normal, diastolic flow to the subendocardium is augmented by vasodilation and the presence of an anatomically greater density of subendocardial vasculature compared with the subepicardium. Nevertheless, the subendocardium is particularly susceptible to ischemia during tachycardia, because it is primarily the diastolic portion of the cardiac cycle that is shortened by increasing heart rate.

Coronary Perfusion Pressure

Perfusion pressure of most organs is calculated from the MAP minus the venous pressure of the organ. The driving pressure for blood perfusing the subendocardium is the aortic diastolic pressure. Because most of the subendocardial venous drainage is via the thebesian veins into the LV cavity, the "venous pressure" for subendocardial perfusion is the LVEDP. Thus the equation that determines CPP is as follows:

$$CPP = Diastolic\ blood\ pressure - LVEDP$$

Equation 4

For this reason, any increase in LVEDP places the subendocardium at risk of ischemia (i.e., CHF due to fluid overload, or decreased ventricular compliance due to the onset of myocardial ischemia).

Metabolic Factors

Metabolic factors have an important regulatory role in coronary blood flow, which is closely coupled to $M\dot{V}o_2$. Coronary vascular resistance is varied on a beat-to-beat basis. Factors of importance in mediating this control of vascular resistance include adenosine, hydrogen ion, carbon dioxide, lactic acid, and endothelium-derived relaxant factor (nitric oxide and possibly other compounds).

Autonomic Innervation

Coronary arteries have sympathetic adrenergic and muscarinic cholinergic receptors. Their roles in determining coronary blood flow are unclear, but they appear to be less important than metabolic factors.

Anatomic Characteristics

Anatomic characteristics of coronary artery disease influence coronary blood flow. Stenoses decrease blood flow by increasing resistance. In atherosclerotic coronary artery disease, the stenoses are fixed. In Prinzmetal's angina, they are dynamic as a result of vasospasm. The degree of stenosis and the compensatory development of collateral vessels determine the susceptibility of the myocardium to ischemia.

Myocardial Oxygen Demand

Increased heart rate increases $M\dot{V}o_2$. The increase is related not only to the increased work of more beats per minute but also to an associated increase in contractility with increasing heart rate. At the same time, tachycardia decreases myocardial O_2 supply by shortening the diastolic perfusion time. An increase in contractility also increases the work of the heart and therefore increases $M\dot{V}o_2$.

The $M\dot{V}o_2$ is closely related to ventricular wall tension. Wall tension is determined by both intracavitary pressure and

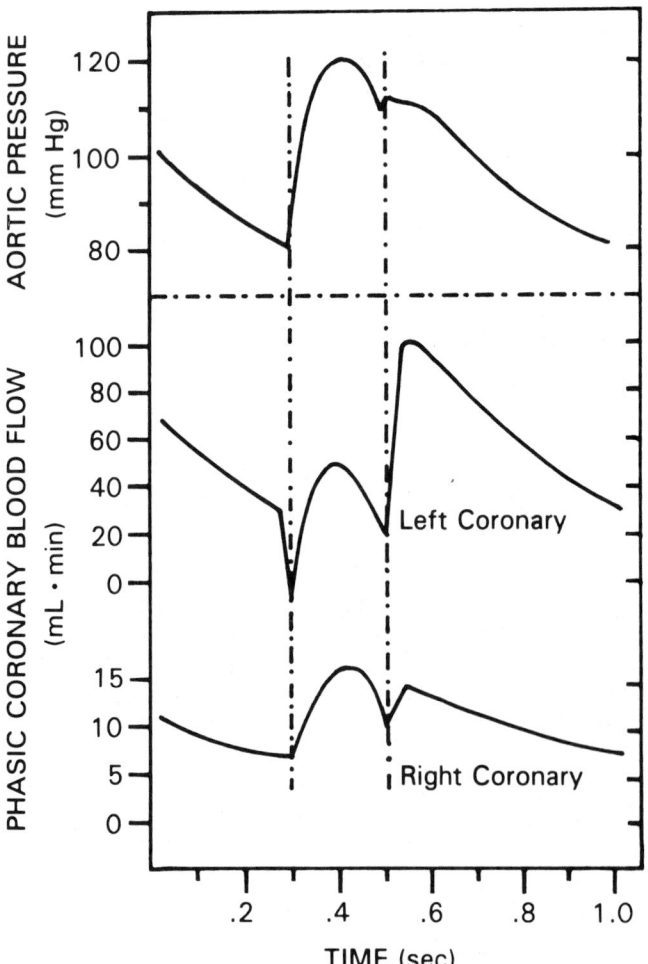

FIGURE 67–6. Comparison of phasic coronary blood flow in the left and right coronary arteries in relation to aortic pressure. Left coronary artery blood flow peaks during diastole. Right coronary artery blood flow peaks during systole. (From Berne RM, Levy MD: Cardiovascular Physiology. 2nd ed. St Louis, CV Mosby, 1972.)

TABLE 67–11. Hemodynamic Goals for Coronary Artery Disease

Heart rate	<70 to control $M\dot{V}O_2$ and allow time for diastolic coronary perfusion
Rhythm	Sinus is preferred
Preload	Decrease in order to decrease wall tension and increase coronary perfusion pressure
Afterload	Decrease slightly to decrease wall tension, but maintain adequate pressure for coronary perfusion
Contractility	Decrease to reduce $M\dot{V}O_2$ as long as adequate cardiac output is maintained

volume as was noted previously, by Laplace's law (see Equation 2).

Increased intraventricular pressure at the end of systole (afterload) and increased intraventricular volume at the end of diastole (preload) increase both wall tension and $M\dot{V}O_2$. Increased wall thickness, as occurs in LV hypertrophy, tends to decrease wall tension and $M\dot{V}O_2$ for a given area of the heart, but the increase in myocardial mass increases overall myocardial O_2 demand.

The hemodynamic goals for patients with coronary artery disease are outlined in Table 67–11. Avoidance of tachycardia appears to be the most important goal. Although most ischemia is not associated with hemodynamic abnormalities, they constitute the most easily prevented subset. Even with close adherence to these hemodynamic goals, careful ischemia monitoring should be carried out and treatment of ischemia planned.

Is Routine Use of Intravenous Nitroglycerin Effective?

Prophylactic intraoperative use of NTG infusion has been suggested as a potentially beneficial therapy for patients with coronary artery disease.[56] NTG might prevent ischemia by decreasing $M\dot{V}O_2$ via decreases in preload and afterload. It may also improve myocardial perfusion by direct effects on coronary arteries. However, a controlled study using a prophylactic infusion of $0.5~\mu g \cdot kg \cdot min^{-1}$ demonstrated no more efficacy in the prevention of myocardial ischemia than did placebo.[58] Higher doses of $1~\mu g \cdot kg \cdot min^{-1}$ also have not been shown to change outcome.

A potential adverse effect of prophylactic NTG infusion is unnecessary venodilation, leading to increased fluid requirements. Although this therapy may have no deleterious hemodynamic effect, it can lead to hemodilution and increased blood product transfusion requirements later in the procedure.[58] A more prudent approach may be to use NTG when it is specifically indicated by hypertension, increased filling pressures, or any sign of myocardial ischemia.

What Are the Hemodynamic Goals for Aortic Stenosis?

Oxygen Supply and Demand

Aortic stenosis causes LV pressure overload. The $M\dot{V}O_2$ is increased by the increased LV mass and its pressure work. O_2 supply, particularly to the subendocardium, is decreased by the reduced ventricular diastolic compliance. Therefore, even in the absence of significant coronary artery stenoses, patients with aortic stenosis may experience angina-like chest pain.

Dysrhythmias

Poor diastolic compliance also increases the importance of sinus rhythm and the atrial kick component of ventricular filling. Loss of sinus rhythm in a patient with aortic stenosis can lead to a 40% reduction in cardiac output. Sinus tachycardia is extremely damaging because it decreases diastolic filling time and increases $M\dot{V}O_2$.

Preload and Afterload

Stroke volume is relatively fixed in patients with aortic stenosis. Therefore, preload must be maintained or augmented to maintain cardiac output. Afterload reduction does not significantly increase "forward flow" but does decrease CPP. Contractility must be maintained to support adequate cardiac output. Goals are summarized in Table 67–12.

Risks

These patients are at particular risk for hemodynamic decompensation during placement of a PA catheter, induction of anesthesia, and atrial cannulation. A PA catheter is a valuable monitor in aortic stenosis, but its placement carries greater potential risk than in other patients because of these patients' poor tolerance for dysrhythmias. Atrial dysrhythmias severely decrease cardiac output. Ventricular dysrhythmias must be treated immediately with cardioversion or defibrillation because chest compressions are much less successful in maintaining cardiac output.

Induction of anesthesia is treacherous because heart rate, sinus rhythm, preload, afterload, and contractility all must be closely maintained to provide adequate coronary perfusion and cardiac output. Atrial cannulation frequently induces atrial dysrhythmias, particularly atrial fibrillation, which severely decreases ventricular filling and cardiac output.

What Are the Hemodynamic Goals for Mitral Stenosis?

Decreased flow across a stenotic mitral valve results in chronic LV underfilling. By increasing the LA pressure, diastolic LV filling can be maintained; however, this increase in LA pressure makes pulmonary vascular congestion likely. Maintenance of sinus rhythm is extremely important to pro-

TABLE 67–12. Hemodynamic Goals for Aortic Stenosis

Heart rate	● Low heart rate (50–70 bpm) is best to control $M\dot{V}O_2$ and prevent ischemia. Severe bradycardia is associated with decreased cardiac output because stroke volume is relatively fixed.
Rhythm	● Sinus rhythm is very important.
Preload	● Must be maintained or increased to maintain ventricular filling in a poorly compliant ventricle in order to maintain cardiac output.
Afterload	● Must be maintained or increased to avoid reductions in coronary perfusion pressure.
Contractility	● Maintain.

TABLE 67–13. Hemodynamic Goals for Mitral Stenosis

Heart rate	• Slow to allow more diastolic time for flow across mitral valve.
Rhythm	• Sinus rhythm is very important. If atrial fibrillation is present, control ventricular rate.
Preload	• Must be maintained or slightly increased to provide adequate flow across the mitral valve for left ventricular filling. Excessive preload may cause pulmonary edema.
Afterload	• Systemic vascular resistance should be maintained. Decreases do not improve cardiac output. Increases in pulmonary vascular resistance should be avoided.
Contractility	• Maintain to provide adequate cardiac output.

vide adequate LV filling. The heart rate must be relatively low to allow sufficient diastolic duration.

Factors that increase the PVR should be avoided (hypoxemia, hypercarbia, acidosis, hypothermia, and perhaps the use of nitrous oxide). SVR must be maintained because stroke volume is unlikely to increase with afterload reduction. Therefore, reductions in SVR only result in decreased perfusion pressure. These hemodynamic goals are summarized in Table 67–13.

What Are the Hemodynamic Goals for Aortic Insufficiency?

Regurgitant Flow

The primary hemodynamic problem in aortic insufficiency is LV volume overload, caused by filling of the LV by both LA forward flow and regurgitant flow. The amount of regurgitant flow is increased by the increasing size of the aortic valve orifice, increased pressure gradient between the LV and the aorta, and prolongation of the diastolic portion of the cardiac cycle (i.e., bradycardia).

Heart Rate and Systemic Vascular Resistance

Characteristic adaptation to chronic aortic insufficiency is a tremendous increase in concentric LV hypertrophy. The sarcomeres replicate in a fashion that allows both expansion of the chamber size and increased wall thickness. The dilated LV has a much larger end-diastolic volume with little or no increase in pressure. LV volume work consumes less energy than pressure work; thus, the stroke volume can be very large without greatly increasing $M\dot{V}O_2$. Forward flow is also aided by low SVR; further benefit may be obtained through the use of vasodilators.

Because LV regurgitant flow occurs during diastole, patients with aortic insufficiency may benefit from mild tachycardia (perhaps up to 110 beats per minute [bpm]). This rate shortens the diastolic portion of the cardiac cycle, but it may not be well tolerated in patients who have coexisting coronary artery disease. The hemodynamic goals for aortic insufficiency are listed in Table 67–14.

Acute Aortic Insufficiency

Acute aortic insufficiency presents as CHF due to sudden LV volume overload in a heart without the chronic compensatory changes. Compensatory increases of stroke volume and heart rate occur. Systemic vascular tone rises to maintain per-

TABLE 67–14. Hemodynamic Goals for Aortic Insufficiency

Heart rate	• Increase causes shortening of diastolic, which decreases the regurgitant fraction and increases cardiac output.
Rhythm	• Sinus is preferred but less important than in other valvular lesions.
Preload	• Increase to maximize forward cardiac output.
Afterload	• It is very important to decrease afterload to favor forward cardiac output.
Contractility	• Maintain.

fusion pressure but may be detrimental to forward flow. The acute increase in LV volume and pressure may cause mitral regurgitation, by distorting the mitral valve, and myocardial ischemia, by decreasing CPP. If acute afterload reduction is ineffective, emergency aortic valve replacement is the only effective treatment.

What Are the Hemodynamic Goals for Mitral Regurgitation?

Regurgitant Flow

In mitral regurgitation, a dilated LV empties by forward pumping of blood and by LA regurgitation. The degree of mitral regurgitation usually correlates with LV size. Therefore, any maneuver that decreases LV size tends to lessen the degree of mitral regurgitation. Preload reduction with vasodilators and diuretics may be beneficial, as long as it is not excessive, because adequate volume to maintain forward stroke volume is essential.

Forward Flow

Inotropes improve LV emptying. Vasodilators reduce afterload, thereby favorably changing the pressure relationship between the aorta and LA and favoring forward flow into the aorta. A mild increase in heart rate also helps to prevent increases in LV size. Sinus rhythm is important, but atrial fibrillation is not as deleterious as in a patient with mitral stenosis because the increased ventricular rate is better tolerated. The hemodynamic goals are listed in Table 67–15.

Acute Mitral Regurgitation

Acute mitral regurgitation is not as well tolerated as that which develops slowly. Sudden LA overload without compliance adaptations results in increased LA pressure and pulmonary edema. The compensatory response is increased heart rate and peripheral vasoconstriction. These changes are particularly troublesome in a patient who has coronary artery disease, a

TABLE 67–15. Hemodynamic Goals for Mitral Regurgitation

Heart rate	• Maintain or increase. Bradycardia worsens regurgitant flow.
Rhythm	• Sinus is preferred, although it is less crucial than in mitral stenosis.
Preload	• Maintain or slightly increase. Avoid extremes of high (increases regurgitant flow) or low (inadequate cardiac output) preload conditions.
Afterload	• Decrease to improve forward cardiac output.
Contractility	• Maintain or increase to decrease left ventricular volume.

common setting for acute mitral regurgitation. Acute afterload reduction is implemented; however, if this reduction, in conjunction with continuous positive airway pressure, does not control the pulmonary edema, emergency mitral valve replacement may be necessary.

What Are the Hemodynamic Goals for Thoracic Aortic Disease?

Whether a patient presents with acute aortic dissection, traumatic rupture, or chronic aneurysm, the goals of management are intended to limit the development or progression of aortic dissection and rupture. Hemodynamic control is extremely important, primarily through limitation of blood pressure and ejection force of LV blood into the aorta. Control of heart rate prevents rate-related increases in LV contractility. Systolic blood pressure should be maintained in a range of 100 to 110 mm Hg, and heart rate should be maintained in a range of 60 to 80 bpm.

In an acute dissection or rupture, these goals should be initiated on suspicion of diagnosis. The agents that may be most beneficial at this time are sodium nitroprusside (SNP) and esmolol. They are both short acting and easily titratable (Table 67–16). Patients with stable aneurysms should be considered at risk for dissection and rupture, even though tight hemodynamic control may not be quite as crucial.

ANESTHETIC TECHNIQUES

Why Are High-Dose Opioids Commonly Used?

High-dose opioid anesthesia has proved to be associated with stable hemodynamics. Initially, morphine (0.5–3.0 mg · kg^{-1}) was used and was found to produce minimally adverse effects. However, large fluid requirements and, occasionally, hypotension were noted. More recently, fentanyl (50–100 μg · kg^{-1})[59] and sufentanil (10–30 μg · kg^{-1})[60] have been shown to maintain hemodynamic stability. These opioids are commonly used for induction and maintenance in cardiac anesthesia. Compared with morphine, they are less likely to be associated with hypotension because they do not cause histamine release and venodilation. In addition to maintaining hemodynamic stability, these agents provide profound analgesia and permit the use of 100% O_2. These characteristics are particularly advantageous in patients with ventricular dysfunction and in those with severe valvular disease.

High-dose opioid techniques also reduce the hormonal response to surgical stimulation. They have been shown to prevent increases of cortisol, epinephrine, norepinephrine, and glucose, effectively reducing the stress response.[61, 62]

What Are the Disadvantages of High-Dose Opioid Anesthesia?

Stress Response

In patients with good ventricular function, an anesthetic technique using solely fentanyl or sufentanil may be only partially effective at preventing hemodynamic and hormonal responses to intubation and surgical stimulation.[63] Even very large boluses and continuous infusions of these potent opioids, despite high plasma concentrations, do not predictably and reliably prevent responses to stimulation in all patients. Rather than administer tremendously large doses of opioids, an anesthesiologist may effectively block stimulation by the concurrent use of other anesthetic agents or vasoactive adjuncts.

Inadequate Amnesia

Even very large doses of opioids are not effective in ensuring amnesia. When opioids are used alone with a muscle relaxant and O_2, this problem is compounded by difficulty in assessing the level of anesthesia. Amnesia is more likely to be achieved with the use of other anesthetic agents. Preoperative administration of scopolamine and a benzodiazepine may be beneficial.

Intraoperative administration of a benzodiazepine or a volatile anesthetic is also advised, if it can be tolerated. The interaction of a benzodiazepine and a potent opioid administered within minutes of each other may lead to significant hypotension due to a decrease in SVR.[64] However, in reduced doses with titrated administration, the combination is very well tolerated.[65]

Chest Wall Rigidity

Induction of anesthesia with high doses of opioids, particularly fentanyl, sufentanil, and alfentanil, may be associated with chest wall rigidity. This decrease in compliance makes ventilation difficult or impossible. The resultant increase in arterial partial pressure of carbon dioxide ($PaCO_2$) leads to an increase in circulating catecholamines that may cause systemic and pulmonary hypertension, tachycardia, and myocardial ischemia.

Many pharmacologic adjuncts have been suggested to prevent this rigidity, including benzodiazepines, α_2-adrenergic agonists, serotonin antagonists, and dopaminergic agonists. The most effective preventive measure—and the most effective treatment once chest wall rigidity occurs—is muscle relaxation. A small dose of nondepolarizing muscle relaxant before induction is not as effective as administration of a paralyzing dose simultaneously with the opioid[66] (Fig. 67–7).

Respiratory Depression

High-dose opioid anesthesia produces prolonged respiratory depression. Patients require mechanical ventilation for several hours postoperatively and may not be extubated until the day after surgery. Although this effect may not adversely affect a patient's outcome, it does prolong the stay in the intensive care unit and increases the cost of hospitalization.

TABLE 67–16. Hemodynamic Goals for Thoracic Aortic Dissection or Rupture

Heart rate	• Control in range of about 60–80 bpm.
Rhythm	• Sinus is preferred, but its importance depends on the individual patient.
Preload	• Maintain enough to provide adequate cardiac output for tissue perfusion.
Afterload	• Decrease to keep systolic blood pressure at 100–110 mm Hg.
Contractility	• Decrease to limit force of ejection.

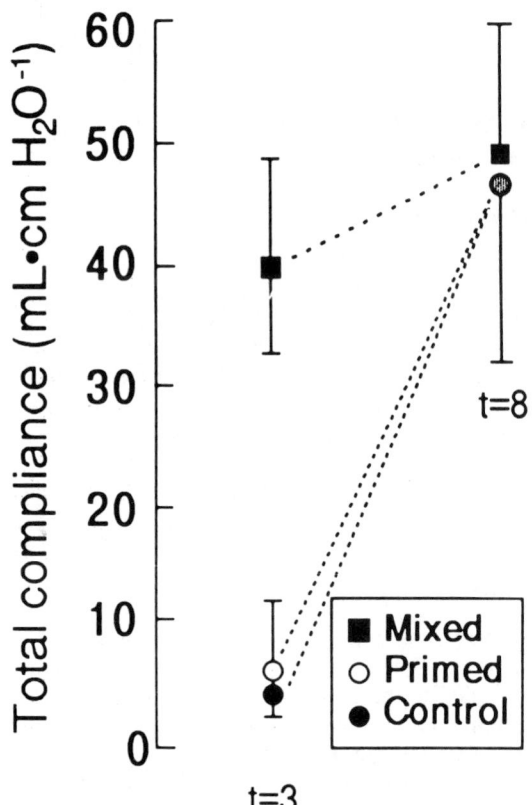

FIGURE 67–7. Ventilatory compliance during three different induction sequences. The control group received a placebo at time = 0, followed by a 2-minute infusion of sufentanil, 3 μg/kg, from time = 1 minute to time = 3 minutes, and pancuronium, 0.1 mg/kg, at time = 4 minutes. The primed group received 1 mg of pancuronium at time = 0, a 2-minute infusion of sufentanil, 3 μg/kg, from time = 1 minute to time = 3 minutes, and the balance of pancuronium, 0.1 mg/kg, at time = 4 minutes. The mixed group received a placebo at time = 0, a 2-minute infusion of sufentanil, 3 μg/kg, and pancuronium, 0.1 mg/kg, from time = 1 minute to time = 3 minutes, and a placebo at time = 4 minutes. Ventilatory compliance was significantly greater for the mixed group at time = 3 minutes compared with the control and primed groups. At time = 8 minutes, there was no difference in ventilatory compliance among the three groups. (From Horrow JC, Abrams JT, Van Riper DF, et al: Ventilatory compliance after three sufentanil-pancuronium induction sequences. Anesthesiology 1991; 75:969.)

Summary

Although high-dose opioid anesthesia may offer hemodynamic stability in high-risk patients with poor ventricular function and may be the best technique with which to minimize the stress response to surgical stimulation, shortcomings must be recognized. Combined use with other anesthetic agents provides the amnesia that may otherwise be lacking and, in many patients, may allow significant reductions in opioid doses and attendant problems.

What Are the Advantages of Other Techniques?

The realization that high-dose opioid techniques do not consistently provide unconsciousness, amnesia, and hemodynamic stability in response to noxious stimuli has led to an increased interest in alternative techniques in cardiac anesthesia. One approach is to administer opioids in a moderate loading dose (e.g., fentanyl, 25 μg · kg^{-1}), followed by a continuous infu-

sion. Intermittent small boluses may be given to precede the particularly stimulating events—intubation, incision, sternotomy—to increase plasma opioid concentration at times when it is most beneficial.

Balanced Anesthesia

The selection of a combination of agents, each with a desired effect, allows the provision of a more "complete" anesthetic, which is chosen based on a particular patient's pathophysiology. Because interactions may occur between various anesthetic agents, vasoactive agents must be immediately available to increase or decrease heart rate, blood pressure, and myocardial contractility. These combinations may decrease the total doses of anesthetic agents and their duration of action. With increasing evidence that ischemia in the early postoperative period is common and that it is predictive of poor outcome, consideration should be given to continuing opioids or other anesthetic agents for a short time postoperatively, rather than discontinuing administration at the conclusion of surgery.[52, 67]

Some suggested combinations of anesthetic agents are listed in Table 67–17. They are not meant to serve as a "cookbook" but to provide guidelines in dosing that are then adjusted according to a patient's response. Other combinations not listed may also be efficacious. Extensive reviews of the hemodynamic effects of anesthetic agents in patients undergoing cardiac surgery have been published.[68–70]

Inhalation Agents

The inhalation anesthetics can be valuable additions to a moderate dose of opioids. These agents can be used effectively to lower blood pressure and decrease myocardial contractility, thereby decreasing M$\dot{V}O_2$. The combination of an inhalation agent with a moderate dose of an opioid more effectively controls hemodynamic function than either agent alone.[71] Controversy about the possibility of "coronary steal" induced by isoflurane is discussed later.

Benzodiazepines

Induction of anesthesia with a benzodiazepine is associated with relative hemodynamic stability and profound amnesia. Diazepam may provide smoother hemodynamic conditions than midazolam by causing a smaller increase in heart rate and a smaller decrease in MAP.[72] Additional anesthesia with opioids, inhalation agents, or other intravenous agents is necessary to blunt the response to noxious stimuli.

Ketamine

Ketamine, when administered alone, often produces unwanted increases in heart rate and blood pressure. When it is administered with a benzodiazepine or an opioid, however, these detrimental effects generally are not encountered, and hemodynamic stability is maintained.[73–76] When ketamine is used in combination with opioids, benzodiazepines, or other sedatives, hallucinations and emergence delirium are unlikely.

Whether ketamine increases cerebral blood flow and intracranial pressure, thereby increasing the risk of neurologic complications during cardiac surgery, is uncertain. However, ketamine-based techniques compare favorably with various other

TABLE 67–17. Suggested Cardiac Anesthesia Technique

	Induction	Maintenance	Comments
High-dose opioid	Fentanyl, 50–100 μg · kg⁻¹	Additional boluses or infusion: fentanyl, 1–5 μg · kg · h⁻¹	Benzodiazepine or volatile agent for amnesia. Volatile agent or vasoactive agents for breakthrough tachycardia and hypertension.
	Sufentanil, 10–25 μg · kg⁻¹	Sufentanil, 0.3–2 μg · kg · h⁻¹	Preferred technique in patients with poor ventricular function.
Moderate-dose opioid	Fentanyl, 10–50 μg · kg⁻¹ Sufentanil, 3–10 μg · kg⁻¹	Benzodiazepine, volatile agent, and additional opioid boluses or infusion: Fentanyl, 0.2–2 μg · kg · h⁻¹ Sufentanil, 0.1–1 μg · kg · h⁻¹	Well tolerated by patients with preserved ventricular function who can benefit from decreased contractility associated with higher concentrations of volatile agents.
Opioid-benzodiazepine	Sufentanil, 1–2.5 μg · kg⁻¹ Midazolam, 0.1 mg · kg⁻¹	Volatile agent or infusion: Sufentanil, 0.7–1.5 μg · kg · h⁻¹ Midazolam, 0.07–0.15 mg · kg · h⁻¹	Give induction doses over at least 5 min. Treat breakthrough by increasing the infusion rate, adding volatile agent or vasoactive agent.
Benzodiazepine	Diazepam, 0.2–0.6 mg · kg⁻¹ Midazolam, 0.1–0.3 mg · kg⁻¹	Opioids and volatile agents	Induction produces mild hypotension. Other anesthetic agents are necessary to prevent tachycardia and hypertension in response to noxious stimuli. Opioids must be carefully and slowly titrated to prevent hypotensive interaction. (Avoid large doses of benzodiazepines in elderly patients and patients with hepatic dysfunction.)
Diazepam-ketamine	Diazepam, 0.3–0.4 mg · kg⁻¹ Ketamine, 2 mg · kg⁻¹	Volatile agent, opioids, or an infusion of ketamine, 1 mg · kg · h⁻¹	Minimal hemodynamic effects, even with poor ventricular function.
Midazolam-ketamine	Midazolam, 0.5 mg · kg⁻¹ Ketamine, 2 mg · kg⁻¹	Volatile agent, opioids, or vasoactive agents and an infusion of midazolam, 0.04 mg · kg · h⁻¹, ketamine, 1 mg · kg · h⁻¹	Minimal hemodynamic effects, even with poor ventricular function.
Opioid-ketamine	Ketamine, 1–2 mg · kg⁻¹ and fentanyl, 10 μg · kg⁻¹ or sufentanil, 1–2 μg · kg⁻¹	Volatile agent, opioid, or vasoactive agent and an infusion of ketamine, 1 mg · kg · h⁻¹ and fentanyl, 0.5–2 μg · kg · h⁻¹ or sufentanil, 0.2–1 μg · kg · h⁻¹	Minimal hemodynamic effects, even with poor ventricular function.

anesthetic regimens in outcome studies of patients undergoing cardiac surgery.[77, 78] In addition, ketamine and diazepam were shown to be associated with lower fluid requirements and shorter postoperative stays in intensive care than a high-dose opioid technique.[78]

What Is the Risk of Isoflurane-Induced Coronary Steal?

When an area of myocardium is dependent on perfusion through a stenotic coronary artery, any arteriolar dilator can potentially induce coronary steal by dilating normal vessels and diverting flow from the stenotic artery, which is unable to dilate. This sequence may occur after the administration of adenosine, dipyridamole, or SNP.

Isoflurane also may produce this effect, whereas enflurane and halothane do not. Reiz and colleagues demonstrated that 1% isoflurane anesthesia produced new ST-T segment depressions or decreased myocardial lactate extraction in 10 of 21 patients with coronary artery disease.[79] This finding was associated with a 40% decrease in MAP. Even when phenylephrine and NTG were used to return hemodynamic status to preanesthetic levels, these ischemic changes persisted.

In an elaborate dog experiment by Buffington and associates, during which total coronary blood flow was maintained constant, the addition of 1 minimum alveolar concentration (MAC) isoflurane led to a decrease in the ratio of flow to a collateral-dependent zone of myocardium compared with flow to a zone supplied by normal coronary arteries.[80] Although coronary flow was maintained constant in this experiment, CPP was decreased by a greater extent during isoflurane than during an equianesthetic concentration of halothane adminis-

tration, which may have affected the results. Nevertheless, these studies demonstrated that isoflurane-induced coronary steal is at least possible.

Clinical Significance

Analysis of angiographic data from the Coronary Artery Surgery Study registry reveals that 23% of patients in the registry have "steal-prone" coronary anatomy.[81] However, isoflurane is commonly used in patients with coronary artery disease and very few apparent signs of myocardial ischemia. Retrospective[82] and prospective[83] clinical studies of patients with steal-prone coronary anatomy have failed to show an increased incidence of ischemia during isoflurane anesthesia compared with other agents. Isoflurane's ability to decrease blood pressure by decreasing SVR and depressing myocardial contractility enables cardiac output to be maintained, which is an attractive feature in the management of coronary artery disease. For many anesthesiologists, the clinical significance of isoflurane-induced coronary steal is not convincing, and therefore, it is still commonly used in this setting.

Protective Effects

One clinical study suggests that isoflurane may even offer protection against ischemia. Patients with coronary artery disease were observed for signs and symptoms of ischemia at rest, during rapid atrial pacing while they were awake, and during rapid atrial pacing with isoflurane/nitrous oxide anesthesia. The rate at which signs of ischemia (ST segment changes, angina in awake patients, increases in PAOP, or onset of v waves) developed was less during isoflurane anesthesia than in awake patients.[84]

It has been suggested that isoflurane does not often cause ischemia despite its vasodilating property because, unlike a pure vasodilator such as adenosine, it also possesses a negative inotropic effect.[85] It may decrease $M\dot{V}O_2$ enough by depressing the contractility to such a degree that coronary blood flow redistribution is less harmful than expected.

Tight hemodynamic control and aggressive monitoring for ischemia may be more important than the agent chosen. One should be aware of the potential for ischemia as a result of isoflurane-induced coronary steal, but isoflurane should not be considered contraindicated for use in patients with coronary artery disease. If signs of ischemia develop during isoflurane anesthesia despite favorable hemodynamic parameters, the presence of coronary steal should be considered, and substitution of another inhalation anesthetic or conversion to an opioid technique may be effective.[79, 86]

Does the Choice of Anesthetic Influence Outcome?

The fact that so many different anesthetic techniques are used in cardiac anesthesia makes one wonder if the specific method chosen really makes a difference. Primary anesthetic techniques for CABG surgery have been examined in two studies, each with more than 1000 patients.[77, 87] Compared with patients receiving sufentanil, those receiving halothane, enflurane, or isoflurane were more likely to have episodes of intraoperative hypotension, less likely to have hypertension both intraoperatively and postoperatively, and required a shorter period of tracheal intubation.[87] The incidences of ischemia, tachycardia, and adverse outcome did not differ among the various techniques. A comparison of high-dose fentanyl, moderate-dose fentanyl, sufentanil, diazepam-ketamine, and halothane likewise showed no difference in morbidity or mortality.[77] Diazepam-ketamine–anesthetized patients had a lower incidence of hypotensive episodes.

Physiologic Effects

Hemodynamic and other physiologic effects differ greatly among anesthetic agents. The different effects do not, however, correlate well with outcome variables. Other factors, including preoperative cardiac status, perioperative hemodynamic stability, the incidence of perioperative myocardial ischemia, and the technical quality of coronary bypass grafts are more important than the choice of anesthetic agents. As long as an anesthesiologist is fully aware of a patient's pathophysiology and the pharmacology of the agents chosen and promptly treats hemodynamic aberrations and myocardial ischemia, the anesthetic agents themselves are of secondary importance.

MANAGEMENT OF SURGICAL EVENTS IN CARDIAC SURGERY

Certain surgical events are of particular importance to anesthesiologists, either because of their physiologic impact or because of the participatory role an anesthesiologist must have.

What Should Be Anticipated After Induction and Intubation?

After these events follows a period of minimum stimulation, during which antiseptic preparation and draping take place. Raising the legs to scrub for saphenous vein dissection leads to an increase in drainage from lower extremity veins, producing an increase in filling and systemic pressures. These changes revert when the legs are returned to table level. During this period, the anesthesiologist records postinduction hemodynamic data, places the TEE probe if one is used, ensures that the patient is safely positioned with all intravenous catheters and invasive monitors functioning, and prepares for the next noxious stimuli—incision and sternotomy. The depth of anesthesia should be increased in anticipation of these events to treat hypertensive/tachycardiac breakthrough and myocardial ischemia. When intraoperative ischemia occurs, it is most commonly associated with induction, intubation, skin incision, sternotomy, and cannulation for CPB.[11]

Sternotomy

At the time of sternotomy, a patient's lungs should be deflated to decrease the risk of laceration of the pleura or lung parenchyma by the sternal saw. The lungs may be immediately substernal during full inflation. Deflation is most reliably accomplished by detaching one limb of the breathing circuit until sternotomy is complete.

In a patient who has previously undergone cardiac surgery, close attention during sternotomy is especially important. The heart or coronary bypass grafts may be adherent to the sternum. An oscillating saw, which resembles a cast cutter, is used to cut slowly through the sternum. Ventilation may be continued until sternotomy is nearly complete. Blood should be available in the operating room and already cross-checked with the patient's identification so that it can be rapidly transfused if the heart or great vessels are injured.

The surgeon should prepare the femoral area for potential femoral artery cannulation. The cardiotomy suction can be placed in the chest to serve as a venous return line, and the aortic line can be attached to the femoral arterial cannula to initiate "sucker bypass." Alternatively, femoral artery–femoral vein bypass can be established before sternotomy or in the event of major bleeding.

Should Autologous Blood Be Drawn Before and Infused After Cardiopulmonary Bypass?

Intraoperative withdrawal of blood before CPB for infusion afterward is done in many institutions as a blood conservation measure. The theoretic benefit is that fresh autologous whole blood that has not been exposed to the adverse effects of CPB on platelets is then available for transfusion after discontinuation of CPB.

Blood is withdrawn through an arterial or venous catheter and collected in a bag containing heparin or citrate. Alternatively, the perfusionist can withdraw blood through the venous cannula after heparinization. This should provide a safe source of red blood cells, coagulation factors, and platelets.

Risks

Potential risks are present. An equal volume of colloid or three times the volume of blood in crystalloid must be infused during collection to preserve hemodynamic stability. Patients with a preoperative hematocrit of <33% to 35% probably do not benefit very much, because after withdrawal of blood the initiation of CPB may cause hemodilution to a hematocrit <20%. Withdrawal of blood through an arterial or intravenous catheter can be time-consuming and distracting to the anesthesiologist. Inadequate mixing of the blood with an anticoagulant or blood withdrawal in excess of the citrate anticoagulation capacity (~450 mL) can allow coagulation. Strict aseptic technique is another consideration, because the withdrawn blood is a perfect culture medium and is usually stored at room temperature.

Outcome Analysis

The most important questions are whether or not intraoperative harvesting and reinfusion improves coagulation, decreases post-CPB bleeding, and ultimately decreases transfusion requirement. Unfortunately, the literature does not provide clear answers. Some reviews suggest equivocal results.[88, 89] Other factors related to surgical technique (intraoperative blood salvage from the surgical site, limitation of pre-CPB fluid administration, collection and autotransfusion of chest tube drainage, and a willingness to accept normovolemic anemia) are probably more important in determining perioperative blood use.[88] Withdrawal of heparinized blood through the venous cannula is simpler, less time-consuming, and less distracting than withdrawal of nonheparinized blood through an arterial or venous catheter if this approach is chosen.[89]

What Are the Concerns During Internal Mammary Artery Dissection?

If the IMA is to be used as a bypass graft, the surgeon dissects it out after sternotomy. The left IMA is usually grafted to the left anterior descending coronary artery. In patients with previous saphenous vein grafting or vein stripping procedures, the right IMA may also be used.

The IMA lies along the anterior chest wall posterior to the cartilages of the first six ribs, about 1.25 cm from the lateral margin of the sternum. A Favoloro retractor is placed to lift the sternum, and the operating table is tilted away from the surgeon. While tilting the table, the anesthesiologist should ensure that tension on the endotracheal tube does not displace it. The effect of this position change on the transducers' zero reference levels must also be considered. If a radial arterial catheter has been placed on the side to which the table is tilted, the tracing may be lost, as discussed earlier. Alternative blood pressure monitoring must be available. Finally, the arm may be compressed between the patient's chest and the retractor post, causing neurologic damage (particularly by compression of the radial nerve in the spiral groove of the humerus) or ischemia to the hand.

Mechanical ventilation of the lungs during IMA dissection may obscure the surgical field. Reduction of tidal volume and increase of respiratory rate to maintain constant alveolar ventilation are often helpful.

The surgeon may occasionally use papaverine or another vasodilator to maximally dilate the IMA. It may be injected into the IMA and tissue surrounding it, or a sponge soaked with the vasodilator may be applied. Transient systemic hypotension may ensue.

How Is Heparin Administered in Preparation for Cardiopulmonary Bypass?

Heparin is administered before the initiation of CPB. Contact between blood and the materials of the CPB circuit activates the coagulation and the fibrinolytic systems; enough heparin must be administered to prevent gross and microscopic coagulation. Its effect is most commonly monitored by assessing the activated coagulation time (ACT).

At the beginning of the procedure, preferably after skin incision, a blood sample is withdrawn for determination of a baseline ACT. Before cannulation of the aorta and right atrium, heparin is administered in a dose of 300 to 400 units · kg^{-1}. The ACT is measured again before initiation of CPB. An ACT <400 seconds is the minimum safe degree of anticoagulation for CPB.[90] If the priming solution contains 5000 to 10,000 units of heparin, CPB may be initiated when the ACT after the dose of heparin is very close to 400 seconds. The ACT should again be measured immediately after the initiation of CPB.

Heparin should be administered through a central venous catheter after aspiration to ensure blood return. Some surgeons prefer to inject heparin directly into the RA to be certain that it is delivered to the central circulation.

Heparin Resistance

Adequate anticoagulation after a standard dose of heparin cannot be assumed. If the ACT is inadequate for CPB, additional heparin should be given in doses of 5000 to 10,000 units. If additional doses do not result in an adequate ACT, reasons for heparin resistance should be considered (Table 67–18).

One cause of heparin resistance that does not respond well to even large doses of heparin is antithrombin III deficiency.

TABLE 67–18. Conditions and Situations Causing Real or Apparent Heparin Resistance

Technical reasons	Mislabeled heparin syringe
	Heparin not injected intravascularly (extravasation, tubing disconnected, other)
Heparin resistance	Previous or ongoing administration of heparin
	Heparin-induced thrombocytopenia
	Pregnancy
	Use of oral contraceptives
	Intra-aortic balloon counterpulsation
	Shock
	Previous administration of streptokinase
	Antithrombin III deficiency
	Low-grade disseminated intravascular coagulation
	Infective endocarditis
	Presence of a clot within the body (intracardiac thrombus)
	Increased platelet count

(Data from Anderson EF: Heparin resistance prior to cardiopulmonary bypass. Anesthesiology 1986; 64:504, *and* Romanoff ME, Rung GW: Anesthetic management in the precardiopulmonary bypass period. *In* The Practice of Cardiac Anesthesia. Hensley FA Jr, Martin DE (eds). Boston, Little, Brown & Co, 1990, pp 202–222.)

Antithrombin III is a plasma protein that acts as an inhibitor of thrombin and the serine proteases. Heparin acts by binding to antithrombin III, speeding up the relatively slow inhibitory action of antithrombin III on thrombin. Patients with antithrombin III deficiency have a tendency to thrombosis and a resistance to the anticoagulant effect of heparin. Transfusion of two units of fresh-frozen plasma provides enough antithrombin III to overcome heparin resistance.

What Are the Concerns During Cannulation for Cardiopulmonary Bypass?

After the pericardium is opened, the surgeon prepares for aortic and RA cannulation. The aorta is cannulated first so that if a problem develops with atrial cannulation, such as significant dysrhythmia or hemorrhage, bypass can be immediately instituted or volume infusion from the CPB pump through the aortic cannula can be established, respectively. If difficulty is encountered with atrial cannulation and hemodynamic instability results, CPB can be initiated by sucker bypass, in which the cardiotomy suckers substitute for the atrial cannula.

Aortic

In preparation for aortic cannulation, the systolic blood pressure should be reduced to about 100 to 110 mm Hg to decrease the risk of aortic dissection. Aortic cannulation frequently is associated with a hypertensive response despite deep anesthesia because it is more stimulating than the events preceding it or because of direct stimulation of sympathetic nerves in the aortic arch.

Blood pressure control may be achieved by increasing the concentration of the volatile agent or by administering short-acting vasoactive agents such as NTG, SNP, or esmolol. After the aortic cannula is placed and the CPB tubing is connected, the surgeon and anesthesiologist should visually inspect the tubing and cannula for the presence of air bubbles before any volume is infused to the patient.

Atrial

RA cannulation may involve a single two-stage cannula or two separate cannulas to drain the superior and inferior vena cavas. A two-stage cannula is used most often for CABG and aortic valve procedures. RA cannulation may be complicated by supraventricular dysrhythmias, including atrial fibrillation, which may lead to decreased cardiac output and hypotension. This problem is particularly troublesome in a patient with a poorly compliant LV whose LV filling and cardiac output are dependent on the atrial kick. Cardioversion is the treatment of choice in this situation. If it is unsuccessful and hemodynamic instability results, expedient initiation of CPB may be necessary.

Cardioplegia Catheters

The surgeon also places one or more cardioplegia catheters for anterograde, retrograde, or both types of cardioplegia delivery.

How Must the Anesthesiologist Prepare for Cardiopulmonary Bypass?

Before the initiation of CPB, anticoagulation must be adequate as assessed by an ACT >400 seconds. The intravenous infusions may be turned off except for one central venous catheter, into which medications may be administered and through which the CVP is monitored.

Physical Examination

The patient's neck and eyes should be examined before and immediately after initiation of CPB in order to detect improper placement of aortic and venous cannulas. Sudden distention of the jugular veins and the development of facial edema may indicate obstruction to cerebral venous drainage. Palpation of a thrill on one side of the neck or a temperature difference between left and right sides of the neck suggests misplacement of the aortic cannula such that the majority of flow is being directed to only half of the cerebral circulation. The pupils should be small and equal before CPB. A sudden change may occur with a misplaced aortic or venous cannula.

Hemodilution and Drug Concentrations

With the initiation of CPB, significant hemodilution occurs, with resultant decreases in the plasma concentrations of most drugs. Consideration should be given to administration of additional opioids and amnestic agents around the time of initiation of CPB to counteract this effect.

Blood Pressure Control

Blood pressure commonly drops with the initiation of CPB. This observation has been attributed to one or more of various causes. Hemodilution reduces the hematocrit and concentrations of plasma proteins, thus reducing the viscosity of blood. Vasodilation may occur in response to hemodilution or to the loss of pulsatile flow. Acute dilution of circulating catecholamines may also produce vasodilation. This sudden decrease in MAP may not be clinically important if a patient's temperature is rapidly lowered with the initiation of CPB. If normothermia is maintained, however, restoration of perfusion pressure (60–80 mm Hg) is more important. Therefore, phenylephrine should be immediately available for bolus injection (40–200-μg doses) or continuous infusion.

Aortic Dissection

Hypotension associated with markedly elevated aortic line pressure from the CPB pump and decreased venous drainage to the reservoir can occur with an aortic dissection at the cannulation site. A hematoma may be seen within the wall of the aorta. This finding necessitates discontinuation of CPB to reposition the aortic cannula and repair the dissection.

Pulmonary Artery Catheter Positioning

The PA catheter should be withdrawn to the main PA (usually ~5 cm) during CPB to decrease the risk of arterial rupture. The catheter becomes quite stiff when the patient is cooled, and emptying and manipulating the heart cause it to advance as well. With rewarming, the catheter length may straighten out, also causing the tip to advance. The PA pressure tracing should be observed throughout CPB and should be 15 mm Hg or less. Higher pressures may be a sign that the catheter is "overwedging," and it should be withdrawn farther. With adequate venous drainage, the RA should be relatively empty and the CVP should be <5 mm Hg.

"Inspired" Gas

Once adequate CPB flow is reached, the inspired gas mixture is changed to air, the anesthetic vaporizer is turned off, and the ventilator may be turned off. This switch to air is thought to decrease the degree of post-CPB intrapulmonary shunt by decreasing both the direct toxic effects of a high FIO_2 and absorption atelectasis. No advantage in regard to postoperative pulmonary function results from continuing ventilation. The pulse oximeter, mass spectrometer, and capnograph may also be turned off, because they do not provide useful information during CPB.

WEANING AND SEPARATING FROM CARDIOPULMONARY BYPASS

The process of weaning and separating from CPB is the climax of cardiac surgical procedures. It tests the success of surgical interventions and provides a challenge to the anesthesiologist to optimize hemodynamic variables through this very important transitional period.

What Preparations Should Be Made During Cardiopulmonary Bypass?

Toward the end of CPB, the anesthesiologist formulates a plan for hemodynamic management based on an assessment of ventricular function. This assessment is drawn from preoperative information (history and physical examination, cardiac catheterization data); pre-CPB information (e.g., response to anesthetic and surgical manipulations, hemodynamic parameters, transesophageal echocardiography); the apparent status of ventricular function during CPB as seen by visual inspection and TEE; and the surgeon's impression of the adequacy of the surgery (quality of coronary bypass grafts, valve replacement/repair, and so on).

Depending on this assessment, inotropes, vasodilators, and vasoconstrictors are selected and prepared. NTG, SNP, and an inotrope such as dopamine or dobutamine should be available in all procedures. If it is believed that an inotrope will be necessary, the infusion should be started about 5 minutes before weaning to allow time for the drug to circulate and begin to have its effects. Starting an inotrope earlier than necessary may worsen ischemic injury and reperfusion injury by raising $M\dot{V}O_2$.[91, 92]

Venting of Air

After an open cardiac procedure, air remains in the left side of the heart. Before weaning from CPB and before the heart is

allowed to eject blood, efforts must be made to remove the air to avoid embolization to the coronary and cerebral vasculature. With the head lowered (Trendelenburg position), the patient is manually ventilated to force air and blood back to the left side of the heart from the pulmonary vasculature. While the heart is tilted back and forth, air is aspirated through a needle at the apex. TEE can be used to assess the presence of residual intracardiac air. The surgeon may insert a 25-gauge needle into the coronary grafts to allow air and blood to exit. This procedure also confirms blood flow in the grafts.

Cardiac Pacing

A pacemaker must be available. Function of the pacemaker may be confirmed during CPB after the surgeon places epicardial leads. Pacing facilitates weaning from CPB by optimizing heart rate (70–90 bpm) and providing synchronous atrioventricular contraction (atrial pacing or atrioventricular sequential pacing).

Rewarming

Patients must be adequately rewarmed. Although esophageal and nasopharyngeal temperatures rise quite rapidly with rewarming, the temperature of peripheral tissues rises more slowly. Rectal temperature should be >35 °C before separation from CPB. Otherwise, the SVR may remain high, and hypothermia will recur.

Metabolic Status

Electrolyte concentrations and acid-base status should be investigated. Potassium concentration may be slightly elevated at the end of CPB owing to absorption of cardioplegia solution, but it usually decreases soon afterward as long as renal function is adequate. Severe hyperkalemia may induce conduction disturbances and depress contractility. Hypokalemia in this setting ($K^+ <4$ mEq · L^{-1}) predisposes to ventricular irritability and should be corrected before weaning from CPB. Mild hypocalcemia at the end of CPB is very common and probably does not warrant treatment. Severe hypocalcemia may develop, particularly in patients who require transfusion of citrate-preserved blood products during CPB, and may induce myocardial depression and systemic vasodilation.[93] Severe hypocalcemia (<0.80 mmol · L^{-1}) should be treated with calcium salts after separation from CPB (see later discussion).

Fluids and Blood

Intravenous fluids should be available for infusion after weaning from CPB. Packed red blood cells are indicated if the hemoglobin concentration is <7.0 g · 100 mL^{-1} or if it is suspected that O_2 delivery after CPB may be marginal owing to low cardiac output. Otherwise, crystalloid solutions and colloids such as hydroxyethyl starch, purified protein fraction, or albumin should be available.

Anesthetic Requirements

During the rewarming phase of CPB, metabolism of drugs increases and cerebral function increases. Therefore, anesthetic

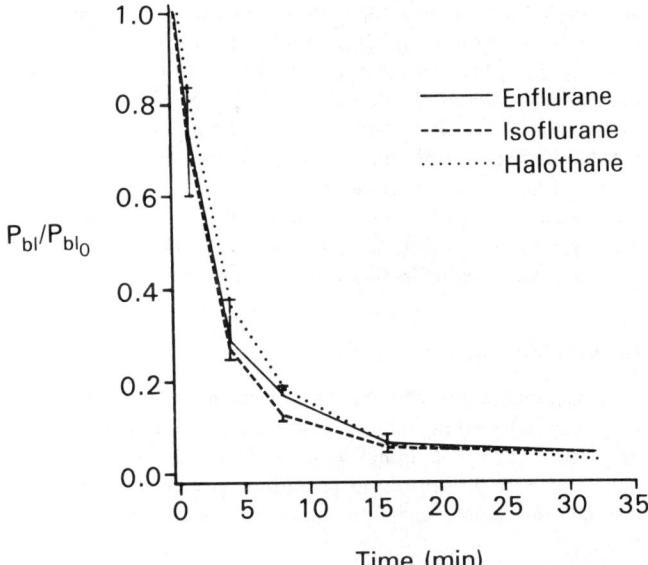

FIGURE 67–8. Washout of inhaled anesthetics using an in vitro model of cardiopulmonary bypass at 24° C to 26° C. The partial pressures of anesthetics are expressed as the ratio of the partial pressure of anesthetic in blood at a given time, divided by the partial pressure of anesthetic in blood just prior to discontinuation of administration. Washout of anesthetics during rewarming may be more rapid because of decreased solubility of gases in blood with increasing temperatures. (From Nussmeier NA, Moskowitz GJ, Weiskopf RB, et al: In vitro anesthetic washing and washout via bubble oxygenators: influence of anesthetic solubility and rates of carrier gas inflow and pump blood flow. Anesth Analg 1988; 67:982.)

requirements likewise increase. At this time, additional opioids, amnestic agents, and muscle relaxants may be required. Some prefer not to administer additional muscle relaxants because they are not necessary for completion of the operation and their use prevents patients' movement indicating awareness.

Choice of a "landmark" temperature at which additional anesthetic is administered may help an anesthesiologist to develop a routine so that this factor is not overlooked. For example, at a blood (not rectal) temperature of 35 °C, additional intravenous agents may be given and any inhaled agent administered into the pump may be discontinued. This process allows adequate time for inhaled anesthetics to wash out, so that residual myocardial depressant effects will be dissipated at the time of weaning from CPB. Greater than 90% washout of inhaled anesthetics requires approximately 15 minutes[94] (Fig. 67–8).

Monitoring and Ventilation

The pressure transducers must be recalibrated and the other monitors (pulse oximeter, capnograph, mass spectrometer, and so on) turned on before weaning from CPB. The lungs are gently re-expanded by manually delivering first a few small-volume then a few large-volume breaths and sustaining airway pressure at approximately 20 cm H_2O for a few seconds. Then mechanical ventilation is resumed with 100% O_2. Administration of a few small breaths first is especially important after the left IMA has been used as a graft, because the inflated lung may apply tension on it. If this occurs, the surgeon can revise the IMA path.

When all of these preparations have been made and there is agreement among the surgeon, anesthesiologist, and perfusion-

ist that conditions are optimum, the patient is weaned from CPB.

How Is Weaning and Separation Accomplished?

Technique

Weaning from CPB involves a gradual transition from complete support of perfusion and oxygenation by the CPB pump to resumption of these functions by the heart and lungs. The venous line is partially occluded by the surgeon or perfusionist to allow gradual filling of the right side of the heart, ejection into the pulmonary vasculature, and return of blood to the left side of the heart for distribution to the systemic vasculature. As this process increases left-sided preload, the inflow from the pump to the aorta is gradually decreased by increments of 0.5 to 1.0 L · min^{-1}, while hemodynamic parameters are observed.

With partial occlusion of the venous line, some blood is still returned to the pump while the remainder returns to the right side of the heart. Preload is adjusted according to the hemodynamic response by altering the amount of venous line occlusion to provide enough blood for adequate cardiac output without overdistending the heart. Distention must be avoided because it increases M$\dot{V}O_2$ while reducing coronary perfusion pressure.

Assessment

Preload is estimated by the appearance of the heart, the measurements of CVP, PA diastolic pressure, PAOP, LA pressure (as available), and the TEE assessment of LV volume. LV compliance may change significantly compared with pre-CPB values, so pressure readings can be misleading. The gradient between PA diastolic pressure and PAOP also may change significantly.[95] Thus, if PA diastolic pressure is chosen as a measure of preload, frequent correlations between it and PAOP should be measured after CPB. This change in compliance persists for at least the first few hours postoperatively.[96] The PA diastolic pressure and PAOP, therefore, may need to be higher than before CPB to obtain a similar filling volume.

As pump flow is decreased to approximately 1 L · min^{-1}, if the heart is able to generate adequate systemic pressure (>90 mm Hg systolic) at the desired preload, CPB may be terminated. Pump flow is stopped, and both the venous and aortic lines are clamped, but connections are left intact while the hemodynamic status is monitored. Preload may still be augmented by transfusing volume from the CPB through the aortic cannula in increments of 50 to 100 mL.

This sequence of events may be accomplished quickly in patients with adequate ventricular function. Patients with poor ventricular function, at higher risk for ventricular distention and failure, may benefit from slower weaning with more careful adjustment of preload and inotropic support.

What Are the Hemodynamic Goals?

The hemodynamic goals for all post-CPB patients are similar unless residual valvular lesions are present. The means of attaining those goals differ according to a patient's ventricular function and afterload condition (Table 67–19).

TABLE 67–19. Hemodynamic Goals After
Cardiopulmonary Bypass

Heart rate	Moderate heart rate (70–90 bpm) is best to maintain adequate cardiac output without increasing M$\dot{V}O_2$ excessively.
Rhythm	Sinus rhythm is preferred. Atrioventricular sequential pacing is equally beneficial.
Preload	Preload must be enough to support adequate cardiac output without overdistending.
Afterload	Reduced afterload decreases wall tension and M$\dot{V}O_2$ and increases cardiac output. Afterload must be high enough to allow adequate systemic and coronary perfusion pressures.
Contractility	Contractility should be increased to maintain adequate cardiac output without excessively increasing M$\dot{V}O_2$ and inducing ischemia.

Heart Rate

The heart rate must be adequate to provide sufficient cardiac output (usually 70–90 bpm). In many patients, lower heart rates may be inadequate because of the altered ventricular compliance discussed earlier. Higher heart rates also may be detrimental by shortening the diastolic period, decreasing stroke volume through insufficient diastolic filling, and decreasing coronary perfusion. At the same time, increased heart rate increases M$\dot{V}O_2$. Bradycardia is most easily overcome by pacing. The treatment options for tachycardia are discussed later.

Heart rhythm should be sinus. Atrioventricular sequential pacing may be used to overcome heart block. Dysrhythmias should be treated pharmacologically and electrically as indicated.

Preload

Preload should be optimized as outlined previously. Additional volume may be transfused from the CPB reservoir via the aortic cannula, or volume may be infused intravenously. It is most convenient to administer volume from the reservoir until the time of aortic decannulation. This process takes full advantage of a patient's autologous blood contained in the pump before transfusing homologous blood or infusing crystalloids and colloids, which lead to further hemodilution. Excessive preload may be relieved by infusion of intravenous NTG or administration of a diuretic. Severe overload can be relieved by reopening the venous line or atriotomy site and phlebotomizing blood to the CPB reservoir.

Afterload

Reduction of afterload is advantageous to a post-CPB heart. Decreased wall stress lowers M$\dot{V}O_2$, which lessens the risk of ischemia. Afterload reduction favors forward flow from the LV. This relationship is especially important in patients with mild residual mitral regurgitation and in patients with a poorly compliant LV. In patients who are post-CPB after mitral valve replacement for either mitral insufficiency or mitral stenosis, afterload reduction is especially important.

Mitral Insufficiency

The LV in mitral insufficiency has dilated to accommodate additional preload to maintain cardiac output despite regurgitant flow. Loss of this pressure relief after mitral valve replace-

ment increases the effective afterload. Afterload reduction with a vasodilator may improve cardiac output.

Mitral Stenosis

Patients with mitral stenosis have a relatively underloaded LV before mitral valve replacement. After replacement, afterload reduction may help to increase cardiac output while the ventricle accepts more preload. Reduction is best accomplished by administration of SNP. If both afterload reduction and inotropic support are needed, dobutamine or amrinone may be indicated.

Afterload may sometimes be too low to allow adequate coronary and systemic perfusion pressures. Blood pressure may be raised by adding inotropes and augmenting preload, but these maneuvers may be unnecessary and can worsen ischemia. Addition of a vasoconstrictor, such as phenylephrine, may be done cautiously. Raising perfusion pressure may improve coronary perfusion and improve ventricular function. Remember, however, that a vasoconstrictor may decrease output and induce coronary spasm.

Contractility

Myocardial contractility should be optimum in order to maintain adequate cardiac output. Contractility may be assessed by TEE, visual inspection, and cardiac output measurement in relationship to other hemodynamic parameters. The choice of inotropic support depends on the severity of ventricular dysfunction, the heart rate, the afterload conditions, and personal preference. Currently available inotropes, dosages, and effects are listed in Table 67–20.

The efficacy of one's choice of inotrope must be repeatedly reassessed so that alternative or additional choices may be made rapidly. If aggressive inotropic support fails to improve hemodynamic status, a return to CPB may be indicated. The heart is "rested," correctable causes of myocardial dysfunction are sought, additional drug combinations are tried, and consideration is given to mechanical support.

PROBLEMS AFTER BYPASS

After separation from CPB, close monitoring of patients continues because this period may be fraught with various complicating circumstances (Table 67–21).

What Are the Causes and Treatment of Left Ventricular Failure?

LV failure after CPB has many causes (Table 67–22). Rapid identification is important to determine therapy. If the cause is surgically correctable, the patient is returned to CPB and the repair is made. Otherwise, LV failure may be treated by pharmacologic means, by intravenous fluid administration, and by ensuring adequate ventilation and oxygenation.

Ischemia

Myocardial ischemia is treated by administration of NTG to decrease preload and improve coronary collateral blood flow. CPP is raised by improving cardiac output with inotropes,

TABLE 67–20. Inotropic Medications

Drug	Dosing		Benefits	Risks
	Bolus	*Infusion*		
Dopamine	—	2–20 µg · kg^{-1} · min^{-1}	Increased renal blood flow at low doses Mild vasoconstriction at moderate doses	Tachycardia Dysrhythmias Vasoconstriction at high doses
Dobutamine	—	2–20 µg · kg^{-1} · min^{-1}	Vasodilation Little tachycardia at low doses	Tachycardia at high doses Dysrhythmias at high doses Nonselective vasodilator
Epinephrine	5–10 µg	0.02–0.50 µg · kg^{-1} · min^{-1}	Most potent inotrope Bronchodilation	Tachycardia Dysrhythmias Vasoconstriction
Norepinephrine	—	0.03–0.30 µg · kg^{-1} · min^{-1}	Most potent vasoconstrictor	Vasoconstriction Tachycardia Dysrhythmias
Isoproterenol	—	0.02–0.50 µg · kg^{-1} · min^{-1}	Most potent β-agonist Bronchodilation Increases heart rate Vasodilator	Tachycardia Dysrhythmias Hypotension
Amrinone	0.75–3.0 mg · kg^{-1} (over 10 min)	5–20 µg · kg^{-1} · min^{-1}	Vasodilator No tachycardia	Hypotension with rapid bolus

administering fluids to increase preload if necessary, and administering phenylephrine to increase peripheral vascular tone. If a patient is anemic, blood transfusion may improve ischemia by raising O_2 delivery. Tachycardia may be controlled by administering additional anesthetic agents, a β-blocker, digoxin, or a calcium channel blocker.

Ventricular Failure

Ventricular dysfunction that is not related to ongoing ischemia is treated with inotropes and, as long as perfusion pressure is adequate, vasodilators. A less potent inotrope such as dobutamine or dopamine is most commonly attempted first. If these are unsuccessful, epinephrine may be more effective. The phosphodiesterase inhibitor amrinone offers the advantages of inotropy and vasodilation without tachycardia and dysrhythmias.

Acid-Base Status

Acid-base and electrolyte abnormalities must be promptly identified and corrected to avoid dysrhythmias and to allow maximum benefits of inotropes.

TABLE 67–21. Postcardiotomy Bypass Problems

Left ventricular failure
Right ventricular failure
Myocardial ischemia
Dysrhythmias
Pulmonary hypertension
Prosthetic valve failure
Protamine reactions
Coagulopathy
Acid-base abnormalities
Electrolyte abnormalities
Bronchospasm
Pulmonary edema
Hypothermia
Pacemaker failure

Artifact

Monitoring artifacts should also be considered. The arterial pressure measured in a radial artery after CPB is often significantly lower than the aortic pressure either because of decreased forearm vascular resistance with rewarming[97] or because of hypovolemia and vasoconstriction.[98] If doubt exists concerning the accuracy of pressure measured from a radial arterial catheter after CPB, a more central arterial pressure should be measured (blood pressure cuff, aortic cannula, needle placed in the aortic root, femoral arterial catheter).

When these measures are unsuccessful, mechanical support (intra-aortic balloon pump [IABP] or LV assist device [LVAD]) may become necessary.

What Are the Causes and Treatment of Right Ventricular Failure?

Many of the factors responsible for LV failure also may cause RV failure. Additional possibilities are listed in Table 67–23. The RV, because of its thinner wall, is affected more by increases in afterload. Therefore, any factors that result in increased PVR place a patient at risk for RV failure.

Ischemia

Ischemic RV failure is treated similarly to ischemic LV failure. Although the emphasis has been placed on the LV in considerations of myocardial ischemia, the RV is also susceptible to ischemia, and the effects are detrimental to overall cardiac function. Also, ischemia may develop secondarily in right-sided heart failure. In response to pulmonary hypertension, the cavitary diameter of the RV increases, thereby increasing wall stress and restricting subendocardial blood flow, which in turn leads to depression of RV contractility.[99]

Control of Preload

Maintaining preload is important to provide adequate RV stroke volume and LV function. When RV failure is caused

TABLE 67–22. Causes of Left Ventricular Failure

Ischemia	Coronary graft failure	Thrombosis
		Constriction by suture at proximal or distal anastomosis
		Kinking of graft
		Air in graft
		Vein graft sewn in backward (no flow across valves)
		Inadequate internal mammary artery graft flow
	Inadequate coronary blood flow	Incomplete revascularization
		Inadequate coronary perfusion pressure
		Coronary embolism (air, clot, plaque)
		Coronary spasm
		Tachycardia (shortening of diastole)
		Increased myocardial O_2 demand
	Ischemic myocardial damage	Incomplete myocardial protection during cardiopulmonary bypass
		Myocardial infarction
Valve failure	Prosthetic valve	Sewn in backward
		Perivalvular leak
		Mechanical failure (immobile disk)
	Native valve	Ischemic papillary muscle dysfunction or rupture
Gas exchange problems	Hypoxemia	Inadequate F_{IO_2}
		Mechanical ventilator failure
		Bronchospasm
		Pulmonary edema
	Hypoventilation	
Inadequate preload		
Volume overload		
Reperfusion injury		
Miscellaneous causes of decreased contractility	Pre-existing left ventricular failure	
	Medications	Blockade
		Calcium channel blockers
		Inhalation anesthetics
		Antiarrhythmics
	Acidemia	
	Electrolyte abnormalities	Hypocalcemia
		Hyperkalemia

(From Romanoff ME, Larach DR: Weaning from cardiopulmonary bypass. *In* The Practice of Cardiac Anesthesia. Hensley FA Jr, Martin DE (eds). Boston, Little, Brown & Co, 1990, pp 252–266.)

solely by pump failure (e.g., RV infarction), simply augmenting preload may be sufficient to overcome the poor contractility and low cardiac output. However, excessive RV preload can induce a leftward septal shift and thereby impair LV diastolic filling. Inotropic support in this situation may be more beneficial.[100]

Pulmonary Vascular Resistance

Prostaglandin E₁ and Norepinephrine

When RV failure is caused more by high afterload than pump failure alone, the combination of inotropic support and

TABLE 67–23. Causes of Right Ventricular Failure

Right ventricular ischemia or infarction
Pre-existing pulmonary hypertension
    Chronic mitral stenosis or insufficiency
    Septal defect (atrial or ventricular)
Respiratory disease
    Chronic obstructive pulmonary disease
    Adult respiratory distress syndrome
Effects of mechanical ventilation
    Positive pressure ventilation
    Positive end-expiratory pressure
Protamine reaction (pulmonary vasoconstriction)
Pulmonary embolism (air, thrombus)

pulmonary vasodilation, along with augmentation of preload, may be most effective. One successful technique that has been described is administration of prostaglandin E_1 (PGE_1) and norepinephrine through RA and LA catheters, respectively.[101]

PGE_1 is a potent pulmonary vasodilator that is metabolized in the pulmonary vasculature. Incomplete metabolism and shunting to the systemic circulation lead to systemic vasodilation as well. Norepinephrine infusion via an LA catheter provides some compensatory systemic vasoconstriction and inotropic stimulation. Central venous infusions of ultra–short-lived substances like adenosine ultimately may be useful to provide selective pulmonary vasodilation.

Nitric Oxide

Another drug still in investigational stages, inhaled nitric oxide, may someday be available clinically as a selective pulmonary vasodilator.[102] It is devoid of systemic hypotensive effects because it is rapidly inactivated by binding to hemoglobin in the pulmonary vasculature.

Amrinone

The combined inotropic and vasodilating effects of amrinone make it an attractive alternative in RV failure. It has been shown to be effective in this situation, more by reduction of RV afterload than by direct inotropic effects.[103]

What Mechanical Devices Can Be Used?

When pharmacologic treatment is inadequate for a patient with post-CPB heart failure, mechanical assist devices may become necessary. They include the IABP, ventricular assist devices (VADs), and the total artificial heart.

Intra-Aortic Balloon Pump

The IABP is the most commonly used circulatory assist device. The indications for IABP use are (1) intractable cardiac failure after CPB, (2) preoperative stabilization of refractory angina or LV failure, and (3) complications of myocardial infarction refractory to pharmacologic therapy.[104] Its function increases coronary artery perfusion and decreases LV afterload.

Mechanism of Action

The IABP is placed percutaneously or by surgical cutdown via a femoral artery or the aorta. It is advanced to the descending aorta so that the balloon lies distal to the left subclavian artery and proximal to the renal arteries (Fig. 67–9). The balloon inflates at the beginning of diastole (closure of the aortic valve), forcing blood into the coronary ostia, thereby augmenting coronary artery perfusion. With the beginning of systole, it deflates, causing a sudden decrease in afterload and favoring increased ejection of blood from the LV. The IABP is triggered automatically by either the ECG or arterial pressure waveform. The timing of inflation and deflation is critical to provide maximum benefit.

Effectiveness

The IABP is effective only if a patient has some ventricular function and a fairly regular rhythm. It is meant to assist LV output and is ineffective in the presence of extremely severe ventricular dysfunction, asystole, severe ventricular dysrhythmias, and rapid or irregular atrial or ventricular rhythms. Irregular rhythms make IABP timing difficult. Rapid rates allow insufficient time for ventricular filling. If these problems cannot be corrected by pharmacologic means or pacing, a VAD may be more appropriate.

Contraindicators

The IABP is contraindicated in patients with significant aortic insufficiency. Diastolic inflation increases regurgitant flow and worsens LV failure. Placement may be difficult or impossible in patients with peripheral vascular disease. The device is relatively contraindicated in patients with thoracic or abdominal aortic aneurysms.

Ventricular Assist Devices

VADs may be used to augment LV or RV function and for short or extended periods in the intensive care unit. Indications and contraindications are listed in Table 67–24.

An LVAD takes over the work of the LV. The ventricle is unloaded through an LA or LV cannula, and blood is returned to the aorta via the LVAD. When the LVAD is placed only temporarily, LA access is preferred. When isolated RV failure is present or when an LVAD cannot function properly, a RVAD may be implanted. The RV is unloaded with a cannula placed in the RA appendage, and blood is returned to the PA.

The goal of mechanical circulatory assistance is to decrease $M\dot{V}O_2$ while allowing time for metabolic recovery of the myocardium. If sufficient ventricular recovery to allow weaning from mechanical assistance does not occur, consideration is given to the use of such a device as a bridge to transplantation.

TABLE 67–24. Ventricular Assist Devices: Indications and Contraindications

Indications for left ventricular assist devices	• Post-CPB cardiogenic shock with inadequate response to pharmacologic support and intra-aortic balloon counterpulsation • Bridge to heart transplantation • Cardiogenic shock after myocardial infarction
Indications for right ventricular assist devices	• Isolated post-CPB right ventricular failure
Indications for biventricular assist devices	• Severe post-CPB biventricular failure • Severe biventricular failure after myocardial infarction • Failure of left ventricular assist device to adequately improve hemodynamics as a result of right ventricular failure • Bridge to transplantation
Contraindications to ventricular assist devices	• No reasonable expectation of ventricular recovery in a patient not considered a candidate for heart transplantation • Sepsis

Abbreviation: CPB = cardiopulmonary bypass.

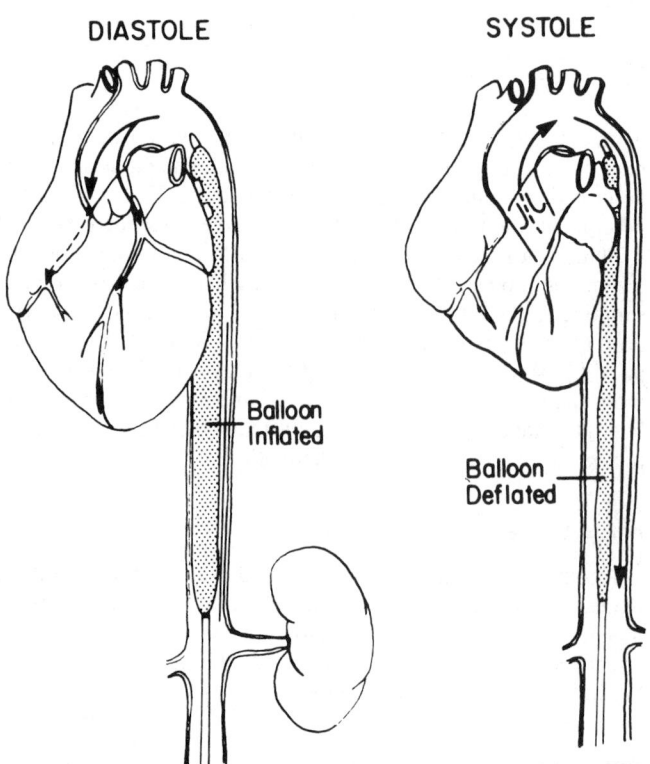

FIGURE 67–9. Proper positioning of the intra-aortic balloon pump below the left subclavian artery and above the renal arteries. The balloon inflates during diastole, forcing blood into the coronary arteries. It deflates during systole, creating a void that decreases impedance to left ventricular ejection. (From Maccioli GA, Lucas WJ, Norfleet EA: The intraaortic balloon pump: a review. J Cardiothorac Anesth 1988; 2:365.)

Types

Three types of VADs are currently available: (1) roller pumps, (2) centrifugal pumps, and (3) pneumatic pulsatile pumps. Roller pumps are readily available, simple, and inexpensive, but they require systemic anticoagulation, produce nonpulsatile flow, and induce significant blood trauma.

The advantages of centrifugal pumps are that they are readily available, simple, and relatively inexpensive. They do not require full heparinization, but if no heparin is used, the pump head must be changed every 48 to 72 hours.[105]

Pneumatic assist pumps provide pulsatile flow. They are designed to minimize blood trauma and to operate without systemic heparinization, so complete reversal of heparin may be accomplished. The disadvantages of pneumatic VADs are that they are very expensive and available at only a few centers with approval of the Food and Drug Administration.

Management Goals

The management goal of VAD therapy is to maintain adequate perfusion to all tissues. Assessment includes evaluation of acid-base status, arterial and venous O_2 saturation, and urine output. Appropriate hemodynamic goals are to maintain an MAP of 60 to 70 mm Hg, an LA pressure of about 10 mm Hg, and a cardiac index of $2.4 \text{ L} \cdot \text{min}^{-1} \cdot \text{m}^{-2}$.[106] The unassisted ventricle may benefit from inotropes or vasodilators. Most patients require 3 to 7 days of support with a VAD and can then be successfully weaned to pharmacologic support. Ventricular recovery and successful discharge from the hospital have been reported in as many as 40% of patients who require VAD support for cardiogenic shock following cardiac surgery.[106] Without VAD support, these patients would die.

Total Artificial Heart

In a few centers, a total artificial heart is available as a bridge to heart transplantation. Disadvantages include its irreversibility and a high incidence of complications including bleeding, thrombosis, and multiple organ failure.

What Are the Causes and Treatment for Dysrhythmias?

Ventricular

Dysrhythmias in post-CPB patients are a common problem (Table 67–25). Rapid search for the cause and prompt treatment are essential. Ventricular tachycardia and ventricular fibrillation should be immediately treated with internal defibrillation. Table 67–26 lists agents used in the treatment of ventricular tachydysrhythmias.

Supraventricular

Supraventricular tachydysrhythmias, such as atrial fibrillation and tachycardia, should be treated with synchronized internal cardioversion. While arterial blood is drawn for evaluation of blood gases, acid-base status, and electrolyte concentrations, efforts should be made to optimize preload and afterload. Because ischemia is such an important cause of post-CPB dysrhythmias, its presence should be assumed and coronary perfusion optimized by raising perfusion pressure and

administering NTG. Antidysrhythmic therapy should then be added as indicated.

Supraventricular tachycardia can be difficult to treat. Various medications are available, but each has undesirable side effects (Table 67–27). Digitalis is unlikely to be effective acutely and carries the risk of inducing toxic ventricular and supraventricular dysrhythmias. Verapamil, procainamide, and β-blockers all may cause myocardial depression. Procainamide may induce a long QT interval and predispose to ventricular dysrhythmias.

Edrophonium may exert undesirable cholinergic side effects, most notably bronchospasm, and also requires additional dosing of muscle relaxation to prevent patients' movement. Adenosine can be used, but early experience in post-CPB patients with coronary artery disease indicates that it may cause ischemia by inducing coronary steal.[107]

How Is Valvular Function Assessed?

Until the introduction of TEE, assessment of valvular function after CPB was based on observation of overall cardiac function and observation of the PAP, PAOP, and CVP waveforms. TEE has made evaluation of valvular function much more straightforward.

The mitral valve, in particular, is well visualized with TEE. Mitral regurgitation after mitral valve repair or replacement or due to ischemic dysfunction of papillary muscles can be assessed during weaning from CPB. In patients undergoing mitral valve replacement, detection of valvular dysfunction after CPB may prompt a return to CPB for correction and is predictive of postoperative cardiac morbidity and mortality if left uncorrected.[108]

Even in centers where TEE is not available for all procedures, it is often brought to the operating room and used for assessment of valve function after mitral valve replacement. The development of biplane probes has made the other cardiac valves accessible to high-quality imaging.

How Is the Dose of Protamine Determined?

Standard Doses

The proper dose of protamine depends on the remaining heparin activity after CPB. It may be given as a standard dose based on the original dose of heparin or the total dose of heparin during CPB (e.g., 1 mg protamine per 100 units of heparin).

Heparin Versus Activated Clotting Time Dose-Response Curve

The protamine dose may also be determined from the dose-response curve of heparin dose versus ACT constructed before CPB (Fig. 67–10). This curve is easily generated using a graph in which ACT is on the x-axis and heparin dose (in milligrams per kilogram) on the y-axis. The baseline ACT determines the point corresponding to no heparin, and the postheparin ACT the second point, corresponding to the administered heparin dose. Because the relationship is linear, these two points are all that is needed.

The ACT after bypass is then plotted on the line, the effective remaining heparin dose is read off the axis, and the appro-

TABLE 67–25. Causes of Dysrhythmias After Cardiopulmonary Bypass

Cardiac dysfunction	Impaired myocardial O_2 supply	Low Pao_2
		Low blood O_2-carrying capacity
		Impaired coronary perfusion (residual coronary stenoses, emboli, low perfusion pressure)
		Impaired cellular O_2 use (nitroprusside-induced cyanide toxicity)
	Cell death, trauma	Myocardial infarction
		Inadequate myocardial protection during cardiopulmonary bypass
		Reperfusion injury
		Surgical trauma
	Specific cardiac abnormalities	Congenital
		Valvular disease (mitral valve prolapse, mitral insufficiency related to papillary muscle dysfunction or rupture)
		Cardiomyopathy
		Long QT syndrome (congenital; electrolyte, metabolic, or drug induced)
Acid-base and electrolyte disorders	Hyperkalemia	Renal dysfunction, residual cardioplegia, rapid transfusion of stored blood, rapid administration of potassium chloride
	Hypokalemia	
	Hypermagnesemia, hypomagnesemia	
	Hypercalcemia, hypocalcemia	
	Acidosis, alkalosis	
	Hypercarbia, hypocarbia	
Electromechanical cardiac stimulation	Surgical manipulation	
	Intravascular catheter or wire (pulmonary artery catheter, pacing wire)	
	Overdistention of atrium or ventricle	
	Macroshock, microshock	
	Pacemaker induced	Malfunction
		Inappropriate discharge
		Inappropriate settings
	R-on-T phenomena	
Autonomic imbalance	Inadequate anesthesia for surgical stimulation	
	Reflex activation with hypotension	
	Myocardial ischemia	
Drugs	Drug overdose	
	Idiosyncratic or allergic drug reaction	
	Pharmacokinetic or pharmacodynamic drug interactions	
	Specific drugs	Anesthetics and muscle relaxants
		Proarrhythmic effects of antiarrhythmics (long QT)
		Digitalis toxicity
		Catecholamines or sympathomimetics
		Calcium channel blockers
		Beta-blockers
		Cholinergic or anticholinergic drugs
		Respiratory drugs (aminophylline, β-agonists)
	Hypothermia	
	Pseudodysrhythmias	Incorrect electrocardiogram interpretation
		Electrocardiographic artifacts (extracardiac electrical signals, electrical interference)

(Modified from Springman SR, Atlee JL: The etiology of intraoperative arrhythmias. Anesth Clin North Am 1989; 7:293.)

TABLE 67–26. Antiarrhythmic Drugs Used in the Treatment of Ventricular Tachydysrhythmias

Drug	Intravenous Loading Dose	Infusion
Lidocaine	1.5 mg · kg^{-1} × 2 doses	1–4 mg · min^{-1} (15–50 μg · kg^{-1} · min^{-1})
Procainamide	20–50 mg · min^{-1} up to 1000 mg, control of dysrhythmia, hypotension, or >50% increase in QRS duration	2 mg · kg^{-1} · h^{-1}
Bretylium	5–10 mg · kg^{-1} over 10 min	5–10 mg · kg^{-1} over 10 min every 6 h or 1–2 mg · min^{-1}
Esmolol	0.5 mg · kg^{-1}	50 μg · kg^{-1} · min^{-1}
Magnesium	2 g over 6 min	1–2 g · h^{-1} for 5 h

TABLE 67–27. Antiarrhythmic Drugs Used in the Treatment of Supraventricular Tachycardia After Cardiopulmonary Bypass

Drug/Treatment	Intravenous Dose
Synchronized internal cardioversion	Start at 10–20 J
Overdrive pacing	
Digoxin	0.5–1.0 mg
Esmolol	0.5 mg · kg^{-1} (if effective, consider infusion)
Verapamil	0.075–0.15 mg · kg^{-1}
Edrophonium	5–10 mg
Procainamide	20–50 mg · min^{-1} to effect, up to 1000 mg or toxic effect (hypotension, QRS prolonged by 50%)
Adenosine	6–12 mg

priate protamine dose (1 mg per 100 units of remaining heparin activity) is then based on the heparin dose predicted to give that ACT value.[109]

Protamine Titration

A third technique for determining the appropriate dose of protamine is the protamine titration technique. It may be accomplished manually by adding variable amounts of protamine to tubes of blood, determining which clots first, and then calculating a proportional dose of protamine based on the patient's estimated blood volume. Protamine titration may also be performed mechanically with an automated heparin-protamine titration system.

Heparin Concentration

Heparin and protamine management may also be carried out based on measurement of heparin concentration. One study

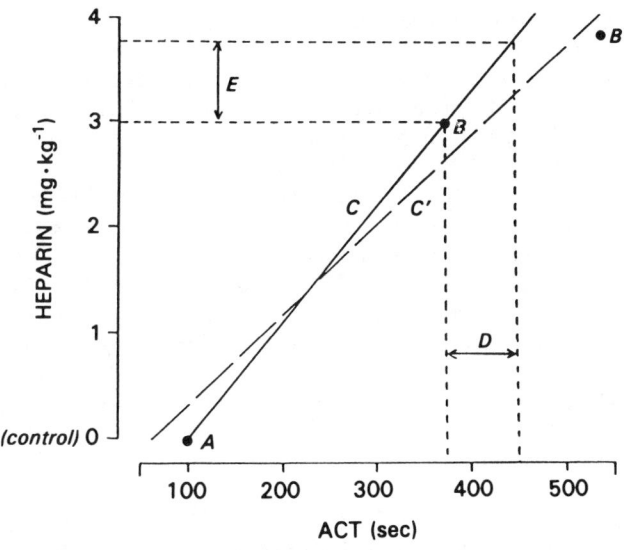

FIGURE 67–10. Construction and use of the heparin dose-activated coagulation time (ACT) response curve. A = Plot ACT control versus no heparin. B = Plot ACT response versus initial heparin dose. C = Draw dose-response curve. D = Locate desired ACT increase. E = Locate corresponding change in circulating heparin and administer this dose. B′ = Plot new ACT response versus expected circulating heparin. C′ = Revise dose-response curve. Repeat D–C′ as needed. (From Cohen JA: Activated coagulation time method for control of heparin is reliable during cardiopulmonary bypass. Anesthesiology 1984; 60:122.)

demonstrated that when anticoagulation was based on heparin concentration rather than ACT, higher heparin concentrations were maintained during CPB with less activation of the coagulation system but with greater post-CPB blood loss.[110] The same investigators found that heparin rebound after CPB was more common when management was based on heparin concentration rather than on ACT.[111] As long as patients were closely monitored postoperatively by measuring ACT and treating with additional doses of protamine, heparin rebound did not lead to excessive postoperative bleeding. The additional measurement of heparin concentration appears to be neither detrimental nor beneficial. Its clinical role has yet to be fully elucidated.

Whatever technique is chosen to determine protamine dose, the ACT should be measured 5 to 10 minutes after protamine administration. Additional protamine may be given to return the ACT to the baseline range or, if the patient was receiving heparin preoperatively, to the normal range (~100–160 s).

What Are the Manifestations and Risks of Protamine Toxicity?

Protamine is known to cause various degrees of adverse cardiovascular responses, some of which are predictable and some of which are not. Protamine reactions have been classified into three types.[112]

Hypotensive (Type I)

Transient hypotension with rapid injection is a predictable adverse effect, so protamine should be administered slowly (e.g., through a minidripper diluted in 100 mL saline). The calculated dose should be given over 10 minutes or more. Injection through a peripheral rather than central venous catheter may be preferable to allow more dilution of protamine before its delivery to the pulmonary vasculature. Administration of protamine via the left atrium or aorta does not appear to offer any advantage over peripheral administration. The hypotension associated with rapid injection results from systemic vasodilation and may be treated with a vasoconstrictor such as phenylephrine and volume as needed.

Anaphylactic/Anaphylactoid (Type II)

An adverse response to protamine may be a true allergic reaction (anaphylaxis) or a reaction due to the release of vasoactive mediators or the activation of complement (anaphylactoid reaction).

Patients who are allergic to fish may develop an allergic reaction to protamine because it is prepared from salmon gonads. Patients who have had a vasectomy commonly develop an antibody to their own sperm, which theoretically may cross-react with protamine. However, the clinical significance of this relationship is doubtful.

Diabetic patients who have been treated with NPH insulin or PZI insulin commonly develop antibodies to protamine, which is an ingredient in these preparations. However, no prospective data document an increased incidence of these reactions in diabetic compared with nondiabetic patients.

Catastrophic Pulmonary Vasoconstriction (Type III)

This reaction is characterized by systemic hypotension in the presence of severe pulmonary vasoconstriction and elevated PAP. (A type I or type II reaction is characterized by systemic hypotension and decreased PAP.) The postulated mechanism involves activation of the complement system in the pulmonary vasculature by heparin-protamine complexes. Release of lysosomal enzymes causes additional activation of the arachidonic acid pathways to form thromboxane, a potent vasoconstrictor.[112] This type of reaction may result in RV failure and must be treated as such.

Should Calcium Salts Be Administered Routinely?

Once thought to be valuable inotropes, calcium salts have now been recognized as potentially harmful medications. Calcium plays an important part in ischemia and reperfusion injury.[113]

Ionized Hypocalcemia

Serum ionized calcium is commonly measured during cardiac surgery. Mild ionized hypocalcemia (0.80–1.00 mmol · L^{-1}) is common during CPB. Animal studies have demonstrated that administration of calcium to treat severe hypocalcemia (<0.60 mmol · L^{-1}) results in significant improvement in ventricular function, but administration of calcium at a normal baseline calcium concentration causes little improvement.[114] Although blood pressure may increase after administration of calcium under normocalcemic conditions, it is a result of increased SVR and is not associated with increases in cardiac output or stroke volume.[115]

To test the efficacy of calcium administration in post-CPB patients with mild hypocalcemia, a randomized, controlled study was conducted.[116] Calcium chloride or a placebo was administered on separation from CPB. Although administration of calcium raised ionized calcium concentration and MAP significantly, no difference in cardiac index was detected between the calcium and placebo groups in the first few minutes after separation. Increased MAP without an increase in cardiac output results from an increase in afterload, which implies increased $M\dot{V}O_2$.

Although administration of calcium salts may be indicated in patients with significant hypocalcemia, it does not appear to be beneficial in patients with the slightly decreased ionized calcium concentrations commonly noted during cardiac surgery. Furthermore, ionized calcium concentration returns to normal levels in the post-CPB period even without administration of calcium salts.[117]

Detrimental Effects

The potential detrimental effects of calcium on the post-CPB heart relate to the role of intracellular calcium in ischemic damage. During reperfusion of ischemic myocardium, large amounts of intracellular calcium accumulate.[118–120] An increase in intracellular calcium activates various enzymes (phospholipases, proteases, and nucleases) that may contribute to ischemic damage. Activation of calcium-adenosine triphosphatase may increase the use of adenosine triphosphate, which is already in short supply in the ischemic cells. Mitochondrial oxidative phosphorylation may become uncoupled.[121] Other potential problems include coronary spasm and dysrhythmias[122] and an increased risk of pancreatitis.[123]

Indications

Despite these concerns, the issue of calcium administration after CPB remains controversial because of its widespread use and apparent safety, at least when measured ionized calcium concentration is low.[124] Also, the relationship of intracellular to extracellular concentrations of calcium after its administration remains unknown. Situations in which administration of calcium is clearly indicated include treatment of severe hypocalcemia associated with transfusion of citrate-containing blood products and treatment of severe hyperkalemia.

Why Do Pulmonary Problems Occur?

Pump Lung

Postreperfusion lung, also known as "pump lung," was first described in 1960.[125] Although its incidence has decreased with the development of improvements in the CPB apparatus, it is still occasionally encountered. The problem represents a form of noncardiogenic pulmonary edema, characterized by hypoxemia due to intrapulmonary shunting, diffuse pulmonary infiltrates on a chest radiograph, increased pulmonary capillary permeability, decreased lung compliance, and atelectasis.

The mechanism is not clearly understood, but several possible explanations exist. The severity of pulmonary edema seems to be related to the duration of CPB. It may be related to hypoperfusion of the alveolar epithelium during CPB, depletion of surfactant, activation of the complement system by the CPB circuit or by heparin-protamine interaction, or neutrophil activation with release of proteolytic enzymes within the lungs during CPB. Cardiogenic pulmonary edema may also result from LV failure of any cause (see Table 67–22) or valvular dysfunction.

Bronchospasm

Post-CPB bronchospasm may occur, particularly in patients with COPD. Observation of the chest reveals that the lungs expand with inspiration but fail to empty with expiration. The treatment of bronchospasm after CPB is complicated by the dysrhythmogenic potential of the available treatments in patients already at risk for dysrhythmias.

Treatment with a nebulized β_2-adrenergic agonist should be attempted first and is quite effective in many patients. When bronchospasm is extremely severe, however, nebulized medications may not be effectively delivered to areas of air trapping. Other treatments that may be considered include intravenous lidocaine, glycopyrrolate, epinephrine, or aminophylline. If ventricular function is adequate, inhaled anesthetics may provide some bronchodilation. The use of mechanical expiratory retardation, similar to that used in COPD, may also be effective.[126]

Why Does Coagulopathy Occur?

Coagulopathy after CPB may have many causes (Table 67–28). Pre-existing coagulation problems should be carefully sought in the preoperative evaluation. Adequate surgical hemostasis is extremely important. The sites most likely to be responsible for postoperative bleeding are the IMA harvest site and its coronary anastomosis, the proximal and distal anasto-

TABLE 67–28. Causes of Postcardiopulmonary
Bypass Coagulopathy

- Inadequate surgical hemostasis
- Residual heparin effect
  Inadequate reversal with protamine
  Heparin rebound
- Thrombocytopenia
- Platelet dysfunction
  Aspirin induced
  Related to activation during cardiopulmonary bypass
  Hypothermia induced
- Pre-existing coagulopathy
  Congenital
  Acquired disorders
    Liver disease, uremia, hematologic diseases
  Induced by medications
    Warfarin, heparin, antiplatelet drugs, tissue plasminogen activator,
    streptokinase
- Decreased coagulation factors
- Primary fibrinolysis
- Disseminated intravascular coagulation

moses of vein grafts, side branches of vein grafts, sites of cannulation (especially aortic cannulation), and the sternum.

Heparin and Protamine

Inadequate reversal of heparin should be diagnosed by measuring the ACT. Postoperatively, heparin rebound may occur. This is a return of heparin effect despite initially adequate reversal. If suspected, the blood should be tested for prolongation of the ACT. Administration of a small excess of protamine appears unlikely to induce a coagulopathy.[127]

Platelets and Platelet Function

The most common causes of abnormal coagulation caused by CPB are thrombocytopenia and qualitative platelet dysfunction. Thrombocytopenia is due in part to hemodilution but also results from destruction at blood-gas interfaces, such as in the cardiotomy suction and bubble oxygenator.

Qualitative platelet dysfunction may be more important and occurs whether a membrane oxygenator or bubble oxygenator is used. Contact between platelets and the artificial surfaces of the CPB circuit leads to platelet activation, manifested by release of α-granules, platelet factor 4, and β-thromboglobulin.[128, 129] These activated platelets continue to circulate and exhibit abnormal aggregation and adhesion.[129, 130] Platelet function improves over a few hours after CPB. Another potential cause of platelet dysfunction after CPB and in the postoperative period is hypothermia.[131]

Coagulation Factors

Concentrations of coagulation factors decrease during CPB by about 50% owing to hemodilution, but abnormal coagulation should not be noted until concentrations of coagulation factors are reduced to 30% or less of normal (10–15% for Factor V).[128] These decreases may occur in procedures requiring unusually large amounts of fluids, including transfusion of packed red blood cells and washed blood.

Fibrinolysis

Although anticoagulation with heparin also limits fibrinolytic activity, fibrinolysis is known to occur during CPB.[132]

Fibrinolytic activity seems to return to baseline rapidly after CPB, so the significance of this ablation is uncertain. Inhibition of fibrinolysis by antifibrinolytic agents during CPB may reduce blood loss, however, as discussed later.

Disseminated Intravascular Coagulation

Disseminated intravascular coagulation (DIC) may occur during cardiac surgery, but as in other surgical settings, it is extremely rare. When coagulation studies demonstrate thrombocytopenia, prolonged prothrombin time (PT) and partial thromboplastin time (PTT), hypofibrinogenemia, and the presence of fibrin degradation products (FDPs), the coagulopathy is more likely a result of severe hemodilution and the FDPs are related to low-grade fibrinolysis during CPB. However, DIC can be noted in the presence of sepsis, hemolytic transfusion reactions, and allergic reactions.

How Are Coagulation Problems Diagnosed and Treated?

The diagnosis of post-CPB coagulopathy is problematic. If pre-existing coagulation problems are known, therapy may be guided by preoperative plans. If residual heparin activity is the only problem, it should be readily diagnosed by measuring the ACT (and perhaps the heparin concentration) and treating with additional protamine. Diagnosis and treatment of other coagulation problems depend on three possible approaches: (1) empirical treatment, (2) standard coagulation tests, or (3) viscoelastic coagulation testing.

Empirical Treatment

Empirical treatment is often used to treat "nonsurgical bleeding" because standard coagulation tests may take too long to be helpful in a patient with clinically significant bleeding. Because platelet dysfunction is the most likely coagulation defect, treatment with desmopressin (DDAVP) or transfusion of platelets may be indicated while awaiting results of standard coagulation tests.

If these measures do not correct the apparent coagulopathy, no other cause is identified, and test results have not yet returned, transfusion of fresh-frozen plasma may be the next logical step. Although this approach is not particularly scientific, the wide range of transfusion practice in the United States suggests that some variation of this approach is commonly used.[133] However, "prophylactic" transfusion of platelets or fresh-frozen plasma, even in patients with preoperative risk factors for platelet dysfunction, is not beneficial.[134, 135]

Standard Coagulation Tests

In some centers, results are returned very rapidly from the coagulation laboratory. Standard coagulation tests are also helpful in the postoperative period. Blood products must only be transfused to treat documented bleeding and should not be used to "correct the numbers." This admonition is illustrated by the finding in one study that 80% of patients had a prolonged PT that was a very poor predictor of postoperative bleeding.[136]

If bleeding is present, useful goals of therapy include platelet count >100,000 · mm^{-1}, PT and PTT <1.2 times the control value, and fibrinogen >100 mg · dL^{-1}. A postoperative bleeding time <10 minutes precludes platelet dysfunction. Unfortunately, the bleeding time is not generally available intraoperatively because it requires time and attention, access to an extremity, and familiarity with the technique.

Viscoelastic Tests

Viscoelastic coagulation monitors, namely thromboelastography and Sonoclot, may also be beneficial in guiding coagulation therapy. The advantages of these techniques are that (1) they require very small specimens of blood, (2) they can be performed in the operating room without sending specimens to a laboratory, (3) results are usually obtained more rapidly than with standard coagulation tests, and (4) they provide more information about platelet function and fibrinolysis than can be obtained with standard coagulation tests. Both are better predictors of post-CPB bleeding than standard coagulation tests.[137, 138]

Is Desmopressin Efficacious After Cardiopulmonary Bypass?

Initial experience with DDAVP suggested that it may decrease blood loss in complex cardiac procedures.[139, 140] The mechanism of action of DDAVP appears to be a release of von Willebrand's factor, which is involved in the interaction of platelets with subendothelial tissue. Subsequent studies have not confirmed significant benefits of DDAVP after CPB.[141, 142]

DDAVP may improve platelet function in some patients (e.g., patients with uremia or patients taking antiplatelet drugs preoperatively), but its routine use does not appear warranted. When administered, the intravenous dose is 0.3 μg · kg^{-1} over 15 to 20 minutes to avoid hypotension.

Do Antifibrinolytic Agents Reduce Blood Loss?

Three antifibrinolytic agents have been studied in the setting of cardiac surgery to determine whether clinically significant reductions in blood loss and transfusion requirements may be obtained. The agents studied are ε-aminocaproic acid, tranexamic acid, and aprotinin. Randomized trials of ε-aminocaproic acid[143] and tranexamic acid[144] have been shown to decrease blood loss by about 10% to 20% without apparent increased risk of thrombotic complications.

Aprotinin

Aprotinin has been extensively studied and is in widespread use outside the United States. Its efficacy in markedly reducing blood loss and transfusion requirements in cardiac surgery has been well documented.[145, 146] Aprotinin is an antifibrinolytic agent, but it may also prevent activation of platelets during CPB without impairment of platelet function at sites of bleeding.[147] Its mechanism of action has not been completely determined but may include inhibition of kallikrein-activated fibrinolysis, inhibition of fibrinogenolysis, and inhibition of release of endothelial plasminogen activator. The platelet-sparing ef-

fect may reflect a direct effect on platelets[147] or may involve an indirect effect due to inhibition of the activation of platelets through the fibrinolytic system.[148]

Although antifibrinolytic agents, particularly aprotinin, appear to offer benefit to patients undergoing CPB procedures, larger studies need to be carried out to document their safety, especially with regard to the risk of thrombotic complications.

ANESTHESIA FOR THORACIC AORTIC PROCEDURES

The preoperative evaluation, hemodynamic goals, and role of preoperative sedation of patients undergoing thoracic aortic surgery were discussed previously. The anatomic location of the aortic lesion (see Fig. 67–3) and the planned surgical approach are important considerations in determining the placement of arterial catheters for pressure monitoring, the need for CPB or other bypass shunt apparatus, and the need for brain or spinal cord protection.

What Are the Major Considerations in Ascending Aortic Operations?

Patients are placed in the supine position, and surgery is carried out through a median sternotomy. Full CPB is necessary, usually involving cannulation of the RA and femoral artery for retrograde aortic perfusion. If the coronary ostia and aortic valve are involved, a composite graft consisting of a synthetic tube graft sewn to a prosthetic valve is most often used.

Coronary perfusion must be re-established by anastomosis of the native coronary ostia to the tube graft or by the use of vein grafts or an additional synthetic graft from the tube graft to the native coronary arteries. If the lesion does not involve the aortic valve or coronary arteries and does not extend into the transverse aortic arch, a simple tube graft may be interposed.

As with all aortic lesions, the hemodynamic goals should include maintaining low-normal heart rate and blood pressure. The anesthetic technique should be chosen with these goals in mind. Particularly with disease of the ascending aorta, the hemodynamic status may be further complicated at any time by proximal dissection of the aneurysm, causing myocardial ischemia, acute aortic insufficiency, or pericardial tamponade. If these complications develop, the hemodynamic goals must be adjusted accordingly.

Intravenous and Arterial Catheters

To improve surgical exposure, the innominate vein may have to be ligated. Therefore, intravenous access in the right arm may be lost. Because the ascending aortic lesion may extend to involve the brachiocephalic artery, a right arm arterial catheter should also be avoided. If the aortic arch might possibly be involved and a cross-clamp may need to be applied near or distal to the left subclavian artery, a lower extremity arterial catheter should be placed in addition to a left arm arterial catheter.

What Are the Major Considerations in Aortic Arch Procedures?

Cerebral Perfusion

Aortic arch procedures are complicated by the likelihood of interruption of cerebral perfusion and the need for methods of cerebral protection. A median sternotomy is performed, and full CPB is required through RA and femoral artery cannulation. An arterial catheter should be placed in a lower extremity and perhaps the left arm, although the left subclavian artery may be within the clamped portion of the aorta if the entire arch is involved.

Proximal Aortic Arch Lesions

If the lesion involves only the proximal aortic arch, the surgeon may place an aortic cross-clamp between the takeoffs of the brachiocephalic and left carotid arteries. Cerebral perfusion would thus be provided during CPB by retrograde aortic flow to the left carotid artery and to both sides of the brain via collateral flow through the circle of Willis.

Complete Arch Involvement

If the entire arch is involved, cerebral perfusion must be completely interrupted during the repair. The introduction of deep hypothermic circulatory arrest (DHCA) by Griepp and colleagues has allowed this procedure to be performed with acceptable morbidity and mortality.[149] After CPB is initiated, the body is cooled to 16 °C to 20 °C and the head is packed in ice. Before cross-clamping, sodium thiopental is administered intravenously, either by titration to electrical EEG silence (ideally) or by an arbitrary dose of as much as 30 to 40 mg · kg^{-1}. Other frequently used pharmacologic adjuncts for cerebral protection include steroids (methylprednisolone, 1–2 g), mannitol, calcium channel blockers (nimodipine), superoxide dismutase, and isoflurane.

DHCA provides cerebral protection by temperature-related reductions in cerebral metabolism and therefore prolongs the safe period of ischemia. Additional factors that are important during DHCA include preservation of high-energy phosphate stores and maintenance of electrochemical neutrality across cell membranes, both of which may be related to hypothermia-induced increases in pH.[150] The safe time limits of DHCA in adults are unknown, but children have undergone 60 minutes or more of DHCA at 20 °C without neurologic complications.[151, 152]

Bypass flow is arrested, and the head is lowered to minimize air entry when the aortic arch is clamped and opened. The distal anastomosis is completed first, usually by suturing a synthetic graft to an island of aorta that includes the takeoffs of the arch vessels. When the distal anastomosis is complete, the proximal end of the graft is clamped. The distal clamp is released, allowing blood to flow back into the arch and air to escape through the proximal end of the graft. The proximal end of the graft then is clamped again, and CPB flow is resumed to restore cerebral perfusion via retrograde flow. Rewarming is carried out while the proximal anastomosis is completed.

What Are the Major Considerations in Descending Aortic Procedures?

Just as cerebral protection is a primary concern in aortic arch surgery because of interruption of cerebral perfusion, spinal cord protection is a primary concern in descending aortic procedures because of the likelihood of interruption of spinal cord perfusion. The surgical approach is through a left thoracotomy. Full CPB is not used for these procedures. One-lung ventilation is usually used to improve surgical exposure and to limit trauma to the lung parenchyma. A right arm arterial catheter should be placed. If a shunt or partial bypass is used to perfuse the distal aorta, a lower extremity arterial catheter should also be placed. If simple clamping is used, a lower extremity arterial catheter is of little value, demonstrating a pressure of 20 to 40 mm Hg without pulsation.

Morbidity and Mortality

The largest experience with descending aortic procedures is by Crawford and colleagues, who reported 8.9% 30-day mortality.[153] The factors most predictive of mortality were advanced age, cross-clamp time >60 minutes (indicative of more complex repairs), and coexisting illnesses, including COPD, renal artery stenosis, coronary artery disease, and renal insufficiency. The incidence of lower extremity neurologic complications was 11%, including a 6% incidence of paraplegia.

The most important risk factors predictive of lower extremity neurologic complications were aortic dissection and the extent of the lesion. These factors were responsible for the significance of other risk factors: the extent of the aorta replaced, the cross-clamp time, and attempts at spinal artery reattachment. Rupture and advanced age were also predictive.

Spinal Cord Perfusion

Clearly, the occurrence of paraplegia is dependent on multiple factors. Spinal cord perfusion is provided by a pair of posterior spinal arteries and a single anterior spinal artery. Neurologic complications after descending aortic surgery are consistent with insufficient anterior spinal artery perfusion.[154] The number and distribution of anterior radicular arteries determine the blood supply to the anterior spinal artery.

The largest of these arteries supplying the anterior spinal artery is Adamkiewicz's artery, which has a variable anatomic location. It originates from the aorta between the T-5 to T-8 levels of the spinal cord in 12% to 15% of individuals, between the T-9 to T-12 levels of the spinal cord in 60%, at L-1 in 14%, at L-2 in 10%, and between L-3 and L-5 in the remainder.[155] Thus, during descending aortic surgery, Adamkiewicz's artery and other important radicular arteries can very well be located within the clamped portion of the aorta.

Preoperative angiographic identification of critical arteries may guide the surgeon to reimplant those vessels, but in practice, it is often difficult to locate them, and the attempt may add to the duration of cross-clamping. Intraoperative localization of critical arteries by monitoring somatosensory evoked potentials has been disappointing because of a high incidence of false positives and false negatives, and it has not improved neurologic outcome.[156] Technical (spinal fluid drains) and pharmacologic (steroid, naloxone) attempts at preservation of spinal cord perfusion also have been unsuccessful for the most part.

Does a Shunt or Partial Bypass Provide Any Benefit?

Placement of a shunt from the heart or proximal aorta to the distal aorta offers hemodynamic benefits and theoretic improvement in spinal cord perfusion. Cross-clamping the thoracic aorta causes a 40% increase in MAP, with significant increases in PAOP and CVP and a 30% decrease in cardiac index.[157] In some patients, thoracic cross-clamping precipitates acute CHF. A shunt minimizes changes in MAP and filling pressures and lessens the decrease in cardiac index.[157]

Shunting Without Bypass

Several options are available. The simplest technique involves placement of a heparin-bonded shunt from the proximal to the distal aorta (Fig. 67–11). Perfusion pressure to the distal aorta is determined by the pressure generated in the LV.

Partial Bypass

Partial bypass may be used in several ways. A cannula from the LA, LV, or proximal aorta delivers blood to a centrifugal pump, which then pumps it to the distal aorta (Fig. 67–12). Because the blood has already been oxygenated, an oxygenator is unnecessary, and systemic heparinization is avoided.

Alternatively, venous blood may be withdrawn through a femoral vein cannula to a CPB machine with an oxygenator and returned to the distal aorta. This technique decreases proximal hypertension during cross-clamping by decreasing venous return to the left side of the heart. A potential danger is that if

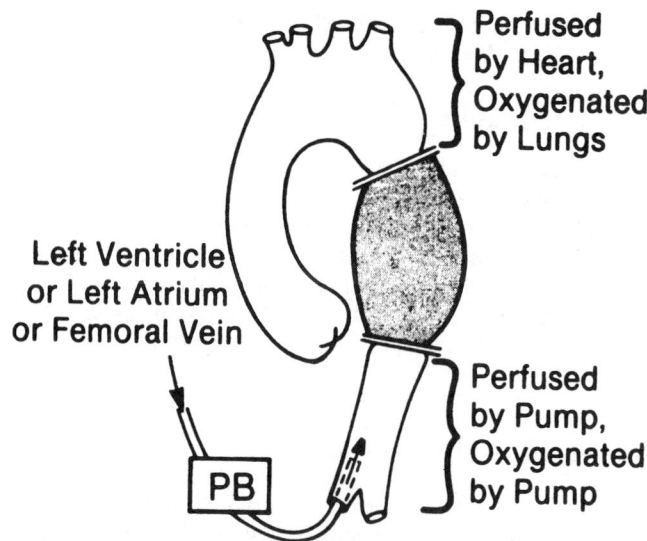

FIGURE 67–12. The partial bypass method during descending aortic surgery drains oxygenated blood from the left atrium, left ventricle, or proximal aorta to a centrifugal pump for distal aortic perfusion. Venous blood may be drained through a femoral vein cannula, oxygenated by a cardiopulmonary bypass machine, and pumped to the distal aorta. (From Benumof JL: Anesthesia for emergency thoracic surgery. *In* Anesthesia for Thoracic Surgery. 1st ed. Benumof JL (ed). Philadelphia, WB Saunders, 1987, pp 375–404.)

too much venous blood is withdrawn to the CPB pump and too little venous return is provided to the left side of the heart, coronary and cerebral perfusion will decrease.

Filling pressures must be closely monitored with a PA catheter, and volume replaced if necessary. Pump flow must be adjusted to maintain adequate perfusion pressure in both the proximal and distal aorta. Inclusion of an oxygenator requires complete heparinization, which may contribute to bleeding problems.

Outcome Analysis

The theoretic advantage of shunting or partial bypass with regard to spinal cord protection is that distal aortic pressure can be maintained at a mean value of 60 to 70 mm Hg. However, the use of a shunt or partial bypass has not been shown to decrease the incidence of lower extremity neurologic complications.[158] Perhaps the theoretic benefits of these techniques are outweighed by more important (and less well understood) factors in determining the occurrence of neurologic complications. The primary benefit of shunts and partial bypass is that the hemodynamic management is less complicated and there is less need for vasodilator therapy.

Does Cerebrospinal Fluid Drainage Decrease Neurologic Complications?

Spinal cord perfusion pressure (SCPP) is determined by MAP and cerebrospinal fluid pressure (CSFP):

$$SCPP = MAP - CSFP$$

Equation 5

Thoracic aortic clamping leads to proximal aortic hypertension, distal aortic hypotension, and an increase in CSFP.[159] The elevation of CSFP may be due to proximal arterial pressures exceeding the limits of cerebral autoregulation and there-

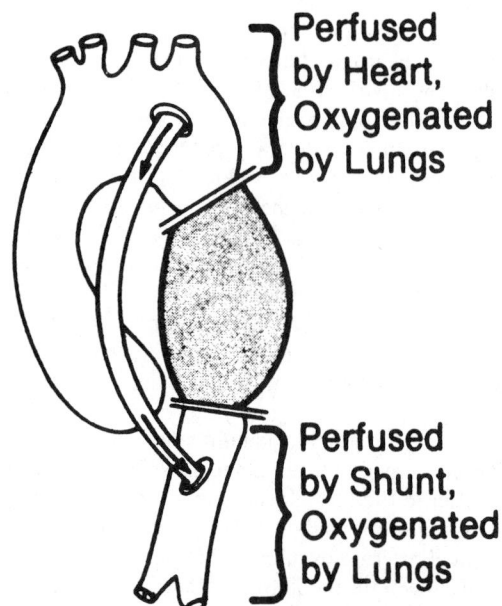

FIGURE 67–11. A heparin-bonded shunt may be placed in the proximal aorta to deliver oxygenated blood to the distal aorta. (From Benumof JL: Anesthesia for emergency thoracic surgery. *In* Anesthesia for Thoracic Surgery. 1st ed. Benumof JL (ed). Philadelphia, WB Saunders, 1987, pp 375–404.)

fore increasing cerebral blood flow, cerebral blood volume, intracranial pressure, and CSFP, which is transmitted through the CSF to the spinal cord.

More than 30 years ago, CSF drainage was thought possibly to improve spinal cord perfusion by decreasing CSFP.[160] CSF drainage has been shown to increase SCPP,[161] but a randomized prospective study failed to show a decrease in neurologic complications compared with controls.[162] Partial bypass was used in some patients, but its use with and without CSF drainage was not randomized. Although patients may benefit from CSF drainage, its indications have not been established.

Does Sodium Nitroprusside Increase the Risk of Spinal Cord Ischemia?

SNP is commonly used to treat the proximal hypertension associated with aortic cross-clamping, particularly when shunting or partial bypass techniques are not used.[163] Nitroprusside acts as a cerebral vasodilator and causes increases in cerebral blood volume, which lead to increased intracranial pressure and CSFP. In addition to increasing CSFP, SNP decreases MAP; both of these effects decrease SCPP. CSF drainage did not completely counteract the rise in CSFP due to aortic cross-clamping and administration of SNP in an animal model.[164] After 10 minutes, it became impossible to drain CSF despite continued increases in CSFP. The investigators suggested that this finding was due to progressive spinal cord edema, to which SNP may have contributed.

When simple aortic clamping is used, a vasodilator such as SNP is necessary to prevent proximal hypertension and decrease cardiac work. The potentially deleterious effects of SNP on spinal cord perfusion appear to support the argument for shunting or partial bypass techniques that decrease or eliminate the need for SNP.

Do Any Measures Decrease Spinal Cord Ischemia?

Hypothermia

Animal models suggest that tolerance to central nervous system ischemia is increased by hypothermia. Although deep hypothermia may complicate the procedure beyond its benefits, mild hypothermia to 34 °C during ischemia may increase the tolerated time of ischemia.[165]

Avoidance of Dextrose

Administration of dextrose before spinal cord ischemia may worsen neurologic outcome.[166] Avoidance of dextrose-containing solutions during descending aortic surgery may offer some benefit as long as hypoglycemia is not allowed to develop.

PROCEDURES NOT REQUIRING CARDIOPULMONARY BYPASS: PACEMAKER IMPLANTATION

What Are the Anesthetic Considerations?

Implantation of a permanent transvenous pacemaker may be carried out in a cardiac catheterization laboratory or an oper-

ating room. Most commonly, access to a subclavian vein is obtained, and pacemaker leads are inserted under fluoroscopic guidance. A subcutaneous pocket is then created for the pulse generator.

A permanent pacemaker is indicated for conduction defects or bradydysrhythmias that result in symptoms of inadequate cardiac output, such as lightheadedness, syncope, or CHF. Pacemakers may also be used to suppress ventricular and supraventricular tachydysrhythmias.

Some patients will already have a temporary transvenous pacemaker in place. If not, alternative pacing equipment must be available. A transcutaneous pacemaker provides rapid, noninvasive pacing capability if the need arises. The equipment necessary to insert a transvenous pacing wire via the right or left internal jugular vein should be available. Resuscitation drugs such as atropine, isoproterenol, and epinephrine should be available to treat bradycardia. Stimulation of the endocardium with a pacemaker electrode can induce dysrhythmias. These most often resolve spontaneously with removal of the mechanical stimulus, but antidysrhythmic agents should be readily available as well.

Local Infiltration and Regional Block

Pacemaker implantation should be performed with infiltration of local anesthesia if at all possible. Intravenous sedation should be administered judiciously. To provide adequate anesthesia without oversedation of patients who are often critically ill, a technique of regional anesthesia has been described.[167] The technique involves the combination of a cervical plexus block and blocks of the second, third, and fourth intercostal nerves. An interscalene cervical plexus block is performed with 15 mL of a local anesthetic mixture consisting of 1% mepivacaine, 0.2% tetracaine, and 1:200,000 epinephrine. Blocks of T-2, T-3, and T-4 are performed with 3 mL for each nerve. Safe and effective anesthesia is obtained without the need for supplemental analgesics.

General Anesthesia

If general anesthesia is required, temporary pacing with a transcutaneous or transvenous pacemaker should be established before induction. The specific technique should be chosen with consideration of a patient's ventricular function. Otherwise, no specific anesthetic agents are contraindicated for pacemaker implantation.

AUTOMATIC INTERNAL CARDIOVERTER-DEFIBRILLATOR IMPLANTATION

What Are the Indications?

Indications for AICD implantation are listed in Table 67–29. An AICD improves survival of patients at high risk for sudden death. Pharmacologic treatment of recurrent ventricular tachydysrhythmias has been disappointing.[168, 169] Patients who meet the criteria in Table 67–29 are considered for AICD implantation if the dysrhythmia is life threatening, causing sudden death, syncope, or severe hemodynamic compromise. It must not be related to acute myocardial infarction, myocardial ischemia, electrolyte abnormalities, or drug toxicity. The device is contraindicated in incessant ventricular tachycardia

TABLE 67–29. Indications for Implantation of Automatic Internal Cardioverter-Defibrillator

Conditions for which there is general agreement	• One or more documented episodes of hemodynamically significant ventricular tachycardia or ventricular fibrillation in a patient in whom electrophysiologic testing and ambulatory monitoring cannot be used to accurately predict efficacy of therapy.
	• One or more documented episodes of hemodynamically significant ventricular tachycardia or ventricular fibrillation in a patient in whom no drug was found to be effective or no drug currently available and appropriate was tolerated.
	• Continued inducibility at electrophysiologic study of hemodynamically significant ventricular tachycardia or ventricular fibrillation despite the best available drug therapy or despite surgery or catheter ablation if drug therapy has failed.
Conditions for which use is frequent but there is divergence of opinion about their necessity	• One or more documented episodes of hemodynamically significant ventricular tachycardia or ventricular fibrillation in a patient in whom drug efficacy testing is possible.
	• Recurrent syncope of undetermined origin in a patient with hemodynamically significant ventricular tachycardia or ventricular fibrillation induced at electrophysiologic study in whom no effective or no tolerated drug is available or appropriate.

(Modified from Guidelines for implantation of cardiac pacemakers and antiarrhythmia devices: A report of the American College of Cardiology/American Heart Association Task Force on Assessment of Diagnostic and Therapeutic Cardiovascular Procedures (Committee on Pacemaker Implantation). J Am Coll Cardiol 1991; 18:1.)

or fibrillation (i.e., one or more episodes daily) because the AICD battery would be rapidly depleted.

What Are the Components?

An AICD device consists of two defibrillating electrodes, one or two rate-sensing electrodes, and a pulse generator (Figs. 67–13 and 67–14). The first defibrillating electrode is either an intravascular spring electrode placed in the superior vena cava near the RA or a wire mesh patch sewn to the RA or RV. The second defibrillating electrode is a wire mesh patch sewn to the apex of the LV.

The rate-sensing electrode system is either a pair of screw-in electrodes placed in normal epicardium or a single transvenous electrode attached to the RV endocardium like a pacemaker lead. The ends of the electrodes are tunneled sub-

cutaneously to a left upper quadrant pouch, where the pulse generator is placed.

How Does the Device Function?

The sensing electrode system of an AICD determines heart rate and characteristics of the ECG waveform. Specifically, a probability density function analyzes the amount of time the QRS complex spends away from the isoelectric baseline. During ventricular tachycardia or coarse ventricular fibrillation, the waveform deviates from the isoelectric baseline much more than during sinus rhythm. The sensing of rapid heart rate or a rapid heart rate and altered ECG morphology leads to activation of the countershock sequence.

Five to 15 seconds is required for the AICD to determine that a malignant dysrhythmia is in progress. An additional 5 to 15 seconds is required to charge the energy-storage capaci-

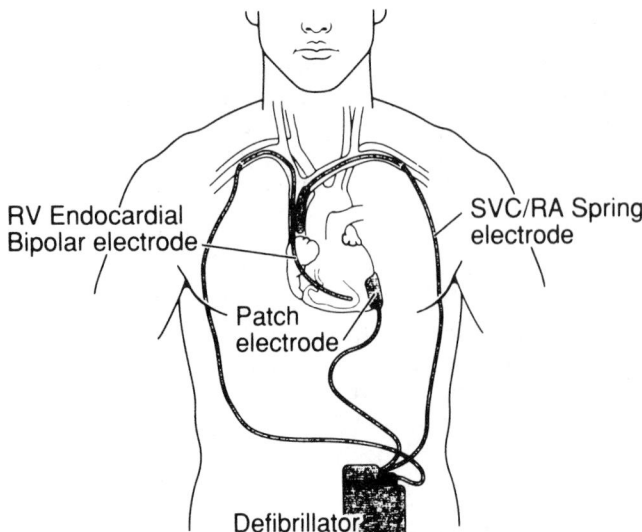

FIGURE 67–13. Automatic internal cardioverter-defibrillator with an electrode configuration consisting of a transvenous rate-sensing bipolar electrode, a transvenous defibrillating spring electrode, and a single epicardial defibrillating patch electrode. (From Deutsch N, Hantler CB, Morady F, et al: Perioperative management of the patient undergoing automatic internal cardioverter-defibrillator implantation. J Cardiothorac Anesth 1990; 4:236.)

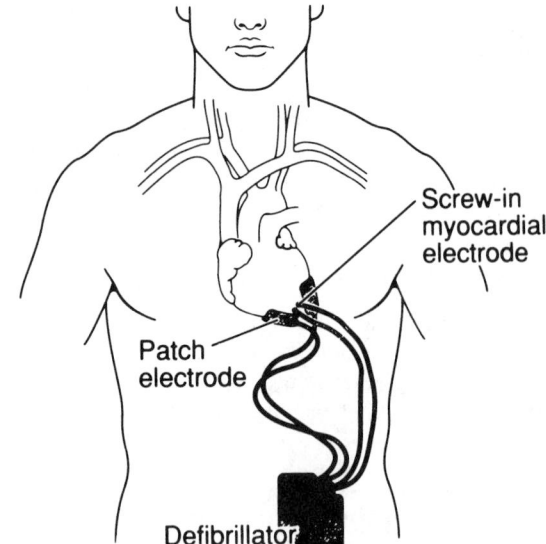

FIGURE 67–14. Automatic internal cardioverter-defibrillator with electrode configuration consisting of a screw-in rate-sensing electrode and two epicardial defibrillating patch electrodes. (From Deutsch N, Hantler CB, Morady F, et al: Perioperative management of the patient undergoing automatic internal cardioverter-defibrillator implantation. J Cardiothorac Anesth 1990; 4:236.)

tors. A 25-J pulse is then delivered. The sensing and charging cycles are repeated, if necessary, and up to three more shocks of 30 J each may be delivered.

What Is the Surgical Approach?

The possible surgical approaches for AICD implantation are median sternotomy, left subxiphoid, left subcostal, and left anterior thoracotomy.

Median Sternotomy

If a patient is undergoing a concurrent cardiac surgical procedure, the AICD is placed via median sternotomy at the completion of the primary procedure. Some surgeons prefer this approach even if a patient is not undergoing another cardiac operation. It affords the best exposure for placement of the AICD components, allows rapid cannulation for CPB if complications develop, and is associated with less postoperative pain than a thoracotomy or subcostal approach.[170, 171]

Subxiphoid

The subxiphoid approach is less invasive and may be the preferred technique for AICD implantation in patients without previous or concurrent cardiac surgery.[172] Through a subxiphoid incision, the pericardium is opened for placement of electrodes. Alternatively, the patches may be placed extrapericardially.

Anterior Thoracotomy

Anterior thoracotomy is most useful in patients with previous median sternotomy. This approach minimizes the dissection required for placement of patches and decreases the risk of injury to bypass grafts. A subcostal approach has also been used. In all of these approaches, a subcutaneous pocket is created in the left upper quadrant or left paraumbilical area in order to house the pulse generator.

What Are the Intraoperative Anesthetic Considerations?

Monitoring

Patients undergoing AICD implantation should be monitored according to the degree of myocardial dysfunction. All patients should have intra-arterial blood pressure monitoring. A PA catheter is frequently placed to assist in the intraoperative and postoperative hemodynamic management. Alternatively, a CVP catheter may be sufficient if ventricular function is well preserved.

Dysrhythmia Control

An external defibrillator should be immediately available at all times in case ventricular tachycardia or ventricular fibrillation develops. Such dysrhythmias preferably should not be treated with antidysrhythmics before AICD implantation, because they are unlikely to be successful and may alter fibrillation and defibrillation thresholds during testing. If external

defibrillation alone does not halt malignant ventricular dysrhythmias, however, the combination of external defibrillation with lidocaine, procainamide, and bretylium may be necessary in a life-threatening situation.

Other emergency medications to have immediately available include ephedrine, atropine, and epinephrine (in both 100 μg · mL^{-1} and 10 μg · mL^{-1} concentrations). Isoproterenol is sometimes used to facilitate dysrhythmia induction.

General Anesthesia

A general anesthetic technique is used. Consideration should be given to epidural or intrathecal narcotics for postoperative pain management, particularly when a thoracotomy or subcostal approach is used. The choice of anesthetic agents depends on a patient's ventricular function and whether or not a concurrent cardiac surgical procedure is planned. For isolated AICD implantation, extubation at the end of the procedure or in the early postoperative period is usually possible.

Placement of a double-lumen tube for one-lung ventilation facilitates surgical exposure and may protect against trauma to the lung when the thoracotomy approach is used.

Intraoperatively, after placement of the electrodes, a series of tests are performed to ensure that the sensing and defibrillating components function adequately. Testing involves induction of ventricular tachycardia and ventricular fibrillation several times to determine adequate sensing and the defibrillation threshold for each dysrhythmia. Hypotension develops as the dysrhythmia is induced but resolves after each defibrillation. In some patients, treatment with ephedrine, 5 mg, or epinephrine, 10 μg, may be necessary to assist recovery of blood pressure and contractility.

External defibrillator pads or paddles must be in place, and internal paddles must be available in case defibrillation is unsuccessful with the AICD electrodes. Despite the fact that many of these patients have marginal myocardial function, electrophysiologic testing both intraoperatively and postoperatively has not been shown to further depress LV function.[173, 174]

PERICARDIOTOMY

What Are the Indications?

Pericardiotomy is used to drain a pericardial effusion or to relieve pericardial tamponade. It is performed emergently after cardiac surgery, thoracic surgery, or chest trauma when hemodynamic measurements suggest pericardial tamponade. Semi-elective pericardiotomy is indicated in patients with chronic pericardial effusions due to malignancy, renal disease, connective tissue disorders, and so on. When pericardial tamponade develops as a result of nonsurgical, nontraumatic etiologies, immediate pericardiocentesis is the treatment of choice.

What Are the Signs and Symptoms of Pericardial Tamponade?

Fluid accumulation in the pericardial space causes increased intrapericardial pressure and impairment of venous return, and it ultimately leads to decreased stroke volume and cardiac output. Reflex tachycardia and vasoconstriction develop to maintain cardiac output and blood pressure. Systemic hypotension results as filling pressures (mean RA, LA, PAOP, and LV and RV diastolic pressures) tend to equalize.[175] Other clinical findings include jugular venous distention, pulsus paradoxus, and muffled heart sounds. The chest radiograph may show mediastinal widening.

What Are the Anesthetic Considerations?

Pericardial Tamponade

The hemodynamic goals in a patient with tamponade physiology are to prevent decreases in preload, afterload, heart rate, and contractility in order to maximize cardiac output. Monitoring should include an arterial catheter and, in most cases, a central venous catheter.

For a patient who develops pericardial tamponade in the early postoperative period after cardiac or thoracic surgery while still intubated, administration of an opioid and a muscle relaxant may provide sufficient anesthesia. In other patients who are hemodynamically unstable, pericardiocentesis or subxiphoid pericardiotomy should be performed with local anesthesia only. If a patient is stable enough to receive sedation, small doses of ketamine are a good choice.[176]

Chronic Pericardial Effusion

Patients with chronic pericardial effusions may be well compensated enough to receive a general anesthetic, but the same hemodynamic goals as for pericardial tamponade should be kept in mind until pericardial fluid has been removed. Until that has been accomplished, spontaneous ventilation, perhaps including awake intubation, should be maintained to avoid reductions in venous return due to positive-pressure ventilation.

References

1. Rutherford JD, Braunwald E: Chronic ischemic heart disease. *In* Heart Disease: A Textbook of Cardiovascular Medicine. 4th ed. Braunwald E (ed). Philadelphia, WB Saunders, 1992, pp 1292–1364.
2. Prinzmetal M, Kennamer R, Merliss R, et al: A variant form of angina pectoris. Am J Med 1959; 27:375.
3. Benchimol A, Harris CL, Desser KB, et al: Resting electrocardiogram in major coronary artery disease. JAMA 1973; 224:1489.
4. Mangano DT: Preoperative assessment of the patient with ischemic heart disease. *In* Preoperative Cardiac Assessment. Mangano DT (ed). Philadelphia, JB Lippincott, 1990, pp 1–55.
5. Sheikh KH, Bengston JR, Helmy S, et al: Relation of quantitative coronary lesion measurements to the development of exercise-induced ischemia assessed by exercise echocardiography. J Am Coll Cardiol 1990; 15:1043.
6. Kressin N, Laravuso RB: Hemodynamic measurements in patients for coronary artery surgery: cath lab vs. operating room (Abstract). Anesthesiology 1983; 59:A6.
7. Newman MF, Martin TJ: Anesthesia for interventional cardiac catheterization. *In* Probl Anesth (in press).
8. Kudenchuk PJ, Pierson DJ, Greene HL, et al: Prospective evaluation of amiodarone pulmonary toxicity. Chest 1984; 86:541.
9. Parker JO: Nitrate therapy in stable angina pectoris. N Engl J Med 1987; 316:1635.
10. Fam WM, McGregor M: Effect of coronary dilator drugs on retrograde flow in areas of myocardial ischemia. Circ Res 1964; 15:355.
11. Slogoff S, Keats AS: Does perioperative myocardial ischemia lead to postoperative myocardial infarction? Anesthesiology 1985; 62:107.
12. Slogoff S, Keats AS: Further observations on perioperative myocardial ischemia. Anesthesiology 1986; 65:539.
13. Viljoen JF, Estafanous FG, Kellner GA: Propranolol and cardiac surgery. J Thorac Cardiovasc Surg 1972; 64:826.
14. Slogoff S, Keats AS, Hibbs CW, et al: Failure of general anesthesia to potentiate propranolol activity. Anesthesiology 1977; 47:504.
15. Kopriva CJ, Brown ACD, Pappas G: Hemodynamics during general anesthesia in patients receiving propranolol. Anesthesiology 1978; 48:28.
16. Weiner N: Drugs that inhibit adrenergic nerves and block adrenergic receptors. *In* Goodman and Gilman's The Pharmacological Basis of Therapeutics. 7th ed. Gilman AG, Goodman LS, Rall TW, Murad F (eds). New York, MacMillan Publishing Co, 1985, pp 181–214.
17. Martin DE, Hensley FA Jr, Luck JC: The cardiac patient. *In* The Practice of Cardiac Anesthesia. Hensley FA Jr, Martin DE (eds). Boston, Little, Brown & Company, 1990, pp 3–37.
18. Slogoff S, Keats AS: Does chronic treatment with calcium entry blocking drugs reduce perioperative myocardial ischemia? Anesthesiology 1988; 68:676.
19. Chung F, Houston PL, Cheng DCH, et al: Calcium channel blockade does not offer adequate protection from perioperative myocardial ischemia. Anesthesiology 1988; 69:343.
20. Berge KH, Lanier WL: Myocardial infarction accompanying acute clonidine withdrawal in a patient without history of ischemic coronary artery disease. Anesth Analg 1991; 72:259.
21. Taggart DP, Siddiqui A, Wheatley DJ: Low-dose preoperative aspirin therapy, postoperative blood loss, and transfusion requirements. Ann Thorac Surg 1990; 50:425.
22. Babbs CF: Alteration of defibrillation threshold by antiarrhythmic drugs: a theoretical framework. Crit Care Med 1981; 9:362.
23. Gottlieb CG, Horowitz LN: Potential interactions between antiarrhythmic medication and the automatic implantable cardioverter defibrillator. PACE 1991; 14:898.
24. Fain ES, Dorian P, Davy J-M et al: Effects of encainide and its metabolites on energy requirements for defibrillation. Circulation 1986; 73:1334.
25. Reiffel JA, Coromilas JM, Zimmerman JM: Drug-device interactions: clinical considerations. PACE 1985; 8:369.
26. Fogoros RN: Amiodarone-induced refractoriness to cardioversion. Ann Intern Med 1984; 100:699.
27. Troup PJ, Chapman PD, Olinger GN, et al: The implanted defibrillator: relation of defibrillating lead configuration and clinical variables to defibrillation threshold. J Am Coll Cardiol 1985; 6:1315.
28. Guarnieri T, Levine JH, Veltri EP, et al: Success of chronic defibrillation and the role of antiarrhythmic drugs with the automatic implantable cardioverter/defibrillator. Am J Cardiol 1987; 60:1061.
29. Gaba DM, Wyner J, Fish KJ: Anesthesia and the automatic implantable cardioverter/defibrillator. Anesthesiology 1985; 62:786.
30. Holt DW, Tucker GT, Jackson PR, et al: Amiodarone pharmacokinetics. Am Heart J 1983; 106:840.
31. Stone JG, Foex P, Sear JW, et al: Myocardial ischemia in untreated hypertensive patients: effect of a single small oral dose of a beta-adrenergic blocking agent. Anesthesiology 1988; 68:495.
32. Ghignone M, Quintin L, Duke PC, et al: Effects of clonidine on narcotic requirements and hemodynamic response during induction of fentanyl anesthesia and endotracheal intubation. Anesthesiology 1986; 64:36.
33. Flacke JW, Bloor BC, Flacke WE, et al: Reduced narcotic requirement by clonidine with improved hemodynamic and adrenergic stability in patients undergoing coronary bypass surgery. Anesthesiology 1987; 67:11.
34. Bedford RF: Invasive blood pressure monitoring. *In* Monitoring in Anesthesia and Critical Care Medicine. 2nd ed. Blitt CD (ed). New York, Churchill Livingstone, 1990, pp 93–134.
35. Moore CH, Lombardo TR, Allums JA, et al: Left main coronary artery stenosis: hemodynamic monitoring to reduce mortality. Ann Thorac Surg 1978; 26:445.
36. Rao TLK, Jacobs KH, El-Etr AA: Reinfarction following anesthesia in patients with myocardial infarction. Anesthesiology 1983; 59:499.
37. Tuman KJ, McCarthy RJ, Spiess BD, et al: Effect of pulmonary artery catheterization on outcome in patients undergoing coronary artery surgery. Anesthesiology 1989; 70:199.
38. Nelson LD, Anderson HB: Patient selection for iced versus room temperature injectate for thermodilution cardiac output determination. Crit Care Med 1986; 13:182.
39. Wolman RL, Shah J, Shapiro JH: Does the type of injectate solution alter the result of thermodilution cardiac output measurements? Annual Meeting of the Society of Cardiovascular Anesthesiologists, 1991.
40. Lang RM, Borow KM, Neumann A, et al: Systemic vascular resistance:

an unreliable index of left ventricular afterload. Circulation 1986; 74:1114.

41. Wallace CT, Marks WE, Adkins WY, et al: Perforation of the tympanic membrane: a complication of tympanic thermometry during anesthesia. Anesthesiology 1974; 41:290.

42. Cork RC, Vaughan RW, Humphrey LS: Precision and accuracy of intraoperative temperature monitoring. Anesth Analg 1983; 62:211.

43. Bone ME, Feneck RO: Bladder temperature as an estimate of body temperature during cardiopulmonary bypass. Anaesthesia 1988; 3:181.

44. Ramsay JG, Ralley FE, Whalley DG, et al: Site of temperature monitoring and prediction of afterdrop after open heart surgery. Can Anaesth Soc J 1985; 32:607.

45. Scott JC, Ponganis KV, Stanski DR: EEG quantitation of narcotic effect: the comparative pharmacodynamics of fentanyl and sufentanil. Anesthesiology 1985; 62:234.

46. London MJ, Hollenberg M, Wong MG, et al: Intraoperative myocardial ischemia: localization by continuous 12-lead electrocardiography. Anesthesiology 1988; 69:232.

47. Hauser AM, Gangadharan V, Ramos RG, et al: Sequence of mechanical, electrocardiographic and clinical effects of repeated coronary artery occlusion in human beings: echocardiographic observations during coronary angioplasty. J Am Coll Cardiol 1985; 5:193.

48. Kaplan JA, Wells PH: Early diagnosis of myocardial ischemia using the pulmonary artery catheter. Anesth Analg 1981; 60:789.

49. Haggmark S, Hohner P, Ostman M, et al: Comparison of hemodynamic, electrocardiographic, mechanical, and metabolic indicators of intraoperative myocardial ischemia in vascular surgical patients with coronary artery disease. Anesthesiology 1989; 70:19.

50. van Daele MERM, Sutherland GR, Mitchell MM, et al: Do changes in pulmonary capillary wedge pressure adequately reflect myocardial ischemia during anesthesia? A correlative preoperative hemodynamic, electrocardiographic, and transesophageal echocardiographic study. Circulation 1990; 81:865.

51. Smith JS, Cahalan MK, Benefiel DJ, et al: Intraoperative detection of myocardial ischemia in high-risk patients: electrocardiography versus two-dimensional transesophageal echocardiography. Circulation 1985; 72:1015.

52. Leung JM, O'Kelly B, Browner WS, et al: Prognostic importance of postbypass regional wall-motion abnormalities in patients undergoing coronary artery bypass graft surgery. Anesthesiology 1989; 71:16.

53. Haendchen RV, Wyatt HL, Maurer J, et al: Quantitation of regional cardiac function by two-dimensional echocardiography. I. Patterns of contraction in the normal left ventricle. Circulation 1983; 67:1234.

54. Braunwald E, Kloner RA: The stunned myocardium; prolonged postischemic ventricular dysfunction. Circulation 1982; 66:1146.

55. Force T, Kemper A, Perkins L, et al: Overestimation of infarct size by quantitative two-dimensional echocardiography: the role of tethering and of analytic procedures. Circulation 1986; 73:1360.

56. Coriat P, Daloz M, Bousseau D, et al: Prevention of intraoperative myocardial ischemia during noncardiac surgery with intravenous nitroglycerin. Anesthesiology 1984; 61:193.

57. Thomson IR, Mutch WAC, Culligan JD: Failure of intravenous nitroglycerin to prevent intraoperative myocardial ischemia during fentanyl-pancuronium anesthesia. Anesthesiology 1984; 61:385.

58. Lowenstein E, Hallowell P, Levine FH, et al: Cardiovascular response to large doses of intravenous morphine in man. N Engl J Med 1969; 28:1389.

59. Stanley TH, Webster LR: Anesthetic requirements and cardiovascular effects of fentanyl-oxygen and fentanyl-diazepam-oxygen anesthesia in man. Anesth Analg 1978; 57:411.

60. Sebel PS, Bovill JG: Cardiovascular effects of sufentanil anesthesia: a study in patients undergoing cardiac surgery. Anesth Analg 1982; 61:115.

61. Stanley TH, Berman L, Green O, et al: Plasma catecholamine and cortisol responses to fentanyl-oxygen anesthesia for coronary artery operations. Anesthesiology 1980; 53:250.

62. Sebel PS, Bovill JG, Schellekens APM, et al: Hormonal responses to high-dose fentanyl anaesthesia: a study in patients undergoing cardiac surgery. Br J Anaesth 1981; 53:941.

63. Philbin DM, Rosow CE, Schneider RC, et al: Fentanyl and sufentanil anesthesia revisited: how much is enough? Anesthesiology 1990; 73:5.

64. Tomicheck RC, Rosow CE, Philbin DM, et al: Diazepam-fentanyl interaction—hemodynamic and hormonal effects in coronary artery surgery. Anesth Analg 1983; 62:881.

65. Tuman KJ, McCarthy RJ, El-Ganzouri AR, et al: Sufentanil-midazolam anesthesia for coronary artery surgery. J Cardiothorac Vasc Anesth 1990; 4:308.

66. Horrow JC, Abrams JT, Van Riper DF, et al: Ventilatory compliance after three sufentanil-pancuronium induction sequences. Anesthesiology 1991; 75:969.

67. Mangano DT, Browner WS, Hollenberg M, et al: Association of perioperative ischemia with cardiac morbidity and mortality in men undergoing noncardiac surgery. N Engl J Med 1990; 323:1781.

68. Sebel PS, Bovill JG: Opioid analgesics in cardiac anesthesia. In Cardiac Anesthesia. 2nd ed. Kaplan JA (ed). Orlando, FL, Grune & Stratton, 1987, pp 67–123.

69. Reves JG, Flezzani P, Kissin I: Pharmacology of intravenous anesthetic induction drugs. In Cardiac Anesthesia. 2nd ed. Kaplan JA (ed). Orlando, FL, Grune & Stratton, 1987, pp 125–150.

70. Lowenstein E, Reiz S: Effects of inhalation anesthetics on systemic hemodynamics and the coronary circulation. In Cardiac Anesthesia. 2nd ed. Kaplan JA (ed). Orlando, FL, Grune & Stratton, 1987, pp 3–35.

71. Moffit EA, Sethna DH: The coronary circulation and myocardial oxygenation in coronary artery disease: effects of anesthesia. Anesth Analg 1986; 65:395.

72. Samuelson PN, Reves JG, Kouchoukos NT, et al: Hemodynamic responses to anesthetic induction with midazolam or diazepam in patients with ischemic heart disease. Anesth Analg 1981; 60:802.

73. Kumar SM, Kothary SP, Zsigmond EK: Plasma free norepinephrine and epinephrine concentrations following diazepam-ketamine induction in patients undergoing cardiac surgery. Acta Anaesthesiol Scand 1978; 22:593.

74. Jackson APF, Dhadphale PR, Callaghan ML, et al: Haemodynamic studies during induction of anaesthesia for open-heart surgery using diazepam and ketamine. Br J Anaesth 1978; 50:375.

75. Tuman KJ, McCarthy RJ, Ivankovich AD: Perioperative hemodynamics using midazolam-ketamine for cardiac surgery (Abstract). Anesth Analg 1988; 67:S238.

76. Newsome LR, Moldenhauer CC, Hug CC Jr, et al: Hemodynamic interactions of moderate doses of fentanyl with etomidate and ketamine. Anesth Analg 1985; 64:260.

77. Tuman KJ, McCarthy RJ, Spiess BD, et al: Does choice of anesthetic agent significantly affect outcome after coronary artery surgery? Anesthesiology 1989; 70:189.

78. Tuman KJ, Keane DM, Spiess BD, et al: Effects of high-dose fentanyl on fluid and vasopressor requirements after cardiac surgery. J Cardiothorac Anesth 1988; 2:419.

79. Reiz S, Balfors E, Sorensen MB, et al: Isoflurane—a powerful coronary vasodilator in patients with coronary artery disease. Anesthesiology 1983; 59:91.

80. Buffington CW, Romson JL, Levine A, et al: Isoflurane induces coronary steal in a canine model of chronic coronary occlusion. Anesthesiology 1987; 66:280.

81. Buffington CW, Davis KB, Gillespie S, et al: The prevalence of steal-prone coronary anatomy in patients with coronary artery disease: an analysis of the Coronary Artery Surgery Study registry. Anesthesiology 1988; 69:721.

82. Slogoff S, Keats AS, Dear WE, et al: Steal-prone coronary anatomy and myocardial ischemia associated with four primary anesthetic agents in humans. Anesth Analg 1991; 72:22.

83. Pulley DD, Kervassilis GV, Kelermenos N, et al: Regional and global myocardial circulatory and metabolic effects of isoflurane and halothane in patients with steal-prone coronary anatomy. Anesthesiology 1991; 75:756.

84. Tarnow J, Markschies-Hornung A, Schulte-Sasse U: Isoflurane improves the tolerance to pacing-induced myocardial ischemia. Anesthesiology 1986; 64:147.

85. Lillehaug SL, Tinker JH: Why do "pure" vasodilators cause coronary steal when anesthetics don't (or seldom do)? Anesth Analg 1991; 73:681.

86. Gross JB: Myocardial ischemia during isoflurane anesthesia: the effect of substituting halothane. Anesthesiology 1989; 70:1012.

87. Slogoff S, Keats AS: Randomized trial of primary anesthetic agents on outcome of coronary artery bypass operations. Anesthesiology 1989; 70:179.

88. Robblee JA: Pro: blood should be harvested immediately before cardiopulmonary bypass and infused after protamine reversal to decrease blood loss following cardiopulmonary bypass. J Cardiothorac Anesth 1990; 4:519.

89. Starr NJ: Con: blood should not be harvested immediately before cardiopulmonary bypass and infused after protamine reversal to decrease blood loss following cardiopulmonary bypass. J Cardiothorac Anesth 1990; 4:522.

90. Young JA, Kisker CT, Doty DB: Adequate anticoagulation during car-

diopulmonary bypass determined by activated clotting time and the appearance of fibrin monomer. Ann Thorac Surg 1978; 26:231.

91. Ward HB, Einzig S, Wang T, et al: Comparison of catecholamine effects on canine myocardial metabolism and regional blood flow during and after cardiopulmonary bypass. J Thorac Cardiovasc Surg 1984; 87:452.

92. Lazar HL, Buckberg GD, Foglia RP, et al: Detrimental effects of premature use of inotropic drugs to discontinue cardiopulmonary bypass. J Thorac Cardiovasc Surg 1981; 82:18.

93. Drop LJ: Ionized calcium, the heart, and hemodynamic function. Anesth Analg 1985; 64:432.

94. Nussmeier NA, Moskowitz GJ, Weiskopf RB, et al: In vitro anesthetic washin and washout via bubble oxygenators: influence of anesthetic solubility and rates of carrier gas inflow and pump blood flow. Anesth Analg 1988; 67:982.

95. Heinonen J, Salmanpera M, Takkunen O: Increased pulmonary artery diastolic-pulmonary wedge pressure gradient after cardiopulmonary bypass. Can Anaesth Soc J 1985; 32:165.

96. Hansen RM, Viquerat CE, Matthay MA, et al: Poor correlation between pulmonary arterial wedge pressure and left ventricular end-diastolic volume after coronary artery bypass graft surgery. Anesthesiology 1986; 64:764.

97. Stern DH, Gerson GI, Allen FB, et al: Can we trust the direct radial artery pressure immediately following cardiopulmonary bypass? Anesthesiology 1985; 62:557.

98. Mohr R, Lavee J, Goor DA: Inaccuracy of radial artery pressure measurement after cardiac operations. J Thorac Cardiovasc Surg 1987; 94:286.

99. Lavr MB, Strauss HW, Pohost GM: Right and left ventricular geometry: adjustments during acute respiratory failure. Crit Care Med 1979; 7:509.

100. Swerdlow CD, Winkle RA, Mason JW: Determinants of survival in patients with ventricular tachyarrythmias. N Engl J Med 1983; 308:1436.

101. Wilber DJ, Garan H, Finkelstein D, et al: Out-of-hospital cardiac arrest: use of electrophysiologic testing in the prediction of long-term outcome. N Engl J Med 1988; 318:19.

102. Blakeman BM, Wilber D, Pifarre R: Median sternotomy for implantable cardioverter/defibrillator. Arch Surg 1989; 124:1065.

103. Gartman DM, Bardy GH, Allen MD, et al: Short-term morbidity and mortality of implantation of automatic implantable cardioverter-defibrillator. J Thorac Cardiovasc Surg 1990; 100:353.

104. Watkins L Jr, Taylor E Jr: The surgical aspects of automatic implantable cardioverter-defibrillator implantation. PACE 1991; 14:953.

105. Antunes ML, Spotnitz HM, Livelli FD Jr, et al: Effect of electrophysiological testing on ejection fraction during cardioverter/defibrillator implantation. Ann Thorac Surg 1988; 45:315.

106. Stoddard MF, Redd RR, Buckingham TA, et al: Effects of electrophysiologic testing of the automatic implantable cardioverter-defibrillator on left ventricular systolic function and diastolic function. Am Heart J 1991; 122:714.

107. Reddy S, Curtiss EI, O'Toole JD, et al: Cardiac tamponade: hemodynamic observations in man. Circulation 1978; 58:265.

108. Kaplan JA, Bland JW Jr, Dunbar RW: The perioperative management of pericardial tamponade. South Med J 1976; 69:417.

109. Bull BS, Huse WM, Brauer FS, et al: Heparin therapy during extracorporeal circulation. II. The use of a dose-response curve to individualize heparin and protamine dosage. J Thorac Cardiovasc Surg 1975; 69:685.

110. Gravlee GP, Haddon WS, Rothberger HK, et al: Heparin dosing and monitoring for cardiopulmonary bypass: a comparison of techniques with measurement of subclinical plasma coagulation. J Thorac Cardiovasc Surg 1990; 99:518.

111. Gravlee GP, Rogers AT, Dudas LM, et al: Heparin management protocol for cardiopulmonary bypass influences postoperative heparin rebound but not bleeding. Anesthesiology 1992; 76:393.

112. Horrow JC: Protamine allergy. J Cardiothorac Anesth 1988; 2:225.

113. Cheung JY, Bonventre JV, Malis CD, et al: Calcium and ischemic injury. N Engl J Med 1986; 314:1670.

114. Drop LJ, Geffin GA, O'Keefe DD, et al: Relation between ionized calcium concentration and ventricular pump performance in the dog under hemodynamically controlled conditions. Am J Cardiol 1981; 47:1041.

115. Drop LJ, Scheidegger D: Plasma ionized calcium concentration: important determination of the hemodynamic response to calcium infusion. J Thorac Cardiovasc Surg 1980; 79:425.

116. Royster RL, Butterworth JF IV, Prielipp RC, et al: A randomized, blinded, placebo-controlled evaluation of calcium chloride and epinephrine for inotropic support after emergence from cardiopulmonary bypass. Anesth Analg 1992; 74:3.

117. Robertie PG, Butterworth JF IV, Royster RL, et al: Normal parathyroid hormone responses to hypocalcemia during cardiopulmonary bypass. Anesthesiology 1991; 75:43.

118. Zimmerman ANE, Daems W, Hulsmann WC, et al: Morphologic changes of heart muscle caused by successive perfusion with calcium-free and calcium-containing solutions (calcium paradox). Cardiovasc Res 1967; 1:201.

119. Shen AC, Jennings RB: Myocardial calcium and magnesium in acute ischemic injury. Am J Pathol 1972; 67:417.

120. Henry PD, Schuchlieb R, Davis J, et al: Myocardial contracture and accumulation of mitochondrial calcium in ischemic rabbit heart. Am J Physiol 1977; 233:H677.

121. Jennings RB, Ganote CE: Mitochondrial structure and function in acute myocardial ischemic injury. Circ Res 1976; 38:I–80.

122. Moffit EA, Sethna DH, Gray RJ, et al: Effects of calcium on the coronary and systemic circulation in patients after coronary surgery. Can Anaesth Soc J 1982; 29:313.

123. Fernandez-Del Castillo C, Harringer W, Warshaw AL, et al: Risk factors for pancreatic cellular injury after cardiopulmonary bypass. N Engl J Med 1991; 325:382.

124. Koski G: Con: calcium salts are contraindicated in weaning of patients from cardiopulmonary bypass after coronary artery surgery. J Cardiothorac Anesth 1988; 2:570.

125. Baer DM, Osborn JJ: The post perfusion pulmonary congestion syndrome. Am J Clin Pathol 1960; 34:442.

126. Weng JT, Smith D, Graybar G, et al: Hypotension secondary to air trapping treated with expiratory flow retard. Anesthesiology 1984; 60:82.

127. Ellison N, Ominsky AJ, Wollman H: Is protamine a clinically important anticoagulant? a negative answer. Anesthesiology 1971; 35:621.

128. Harker LA, Malpass TW, Branson HE, et al: Mechanism of abnormal bleeding in patients undergoing cardiopulmonary bypass: acquired transient platelet dysfunction associated with selective α-granule release. Blood 1980; 56:824.

129. Rinder CS, Bohnert J, Rinder HM, et al: Platelet activation and aggregation during cardiopulmonary bypass. Anesthesiology 1991; 75:388.

130. Rinder CS, Mathew JP, Rinder HM, et al: Modulation of platelet surface adhesion receptors during cardiopulmonary bypass. Anesthesiology 1991; 75:563.

131. Valeri ACR, Cassidy G, Khuri S, et al: Hypothermia-induced reversible platelet dysfunction. Ann Surg 1987; 205:175.

132. Kucuk O, Kwaan HC, Frederickson J, et al: Increased fibrinolytic activity in patients undergoing cardiopulmonary bypass operation. Am J Hematol 1986; 23:223.

133. Goodnough LT, Johnston MFM, Toy PTCY: The variability of transfusion practice in coronary artery bypass surgery. JAMA 1991; 265:86.

134. National Institutes of Health Consensus Conference: platelet transfusion therapy. JAMA 1987; 257:1777.

135. National Institutes of Health Consensus Conference: Fresh-frozen plasma: indications and risks. JAMA 1985; 253:551.

136. Bachmann F, McKenna R, Cole ER, et al: The hemostatic mechanism after open-heart surgery. I. Studies on plasma coagulation factors and fibrinolysis in 512 patients after extracorporeal circulation. J Thorac Cardiovasc Surg 1975; 70:76.

137. Spiess BD, Tuman KJ, McCarthy AJ, et al: Thromboelastography as an indicator of postcardiopulmonary bypass coagulopathies. J Clin Monit 1987; 3:25.

138. Tuman KJ, Spiess BD, McCarthy RJ, et al: Comparison of viscoelastic measures of coagulation after cardiopulmonary bypass. Anesth Analg 1989; 69:69.

139. Salzman EW, Weinstein MJ, Weintraub RM, et al: Treatment with desmopressin acetate to reduce blood loss after cardiac surgery: a double-blind randomized trial. N Engl J Med 1986; 314:1402.

140. Czer LSC, Bateman ATM, Gray RJ, et al: Treatment of severe platelet dysfunction and hemorrhage after cardiopulmonary bypass: reduction in blood product usage with desmopressin. J Am Coll Cardiol 1987; 9:1139.

141. Rocha E, Llorens R, Paramo JA, et al: Does desmopressin acetate reduce blood loss after surgery in patients on cardiopulmonary bypass? Circulation 1988; 77:1319.

142. Hackmann T, Gascoyne RD, Naiman SC, et al: A trial of desmopressin (1-desamino-8-D-arginine vasopressin) to reduce blood loss in uncomplicated cardiac surgery. N Engl J Med 1989; 321:1437.

143. Vander Salm TJ, Ansell JE, Okike ON, et al: The role of epsilon-aminocaproic acid in reducing bleeding after cardiac operation: a double-blind randomized study. J Thorac Cardiovasc Surg 1988; 95:538.

144. Horrow JC, Hlaavacek J, Strong MD, et al: Prophylactic tranexamic acid decreases bleeding after cardiac operations. J Thorac Cardiovasc Surg 1990; 99:70.

145. Royston D, Bidstrup BP, Taylor KM, et al: Effect of aprotinin on need for blood transfusion after repeat open-heart surgery. Lancet 1987; 2:1289.

146. Bidstrup BP, Royston D, Sapsford RN, et al: Reduction in blood loss and blood use after cardiopulmonary bypass with high dose aprotinin (Trasylol). J Thorac Cardiovasc Surg 1989; 97:364.

147. van Oeveren W, Jansen NJG, Bidstrup BP, et al: Effects of aprotinin on hemostatic mechanisms during cardiopulmonary bypass. Ann Thorac Surg 1987; 44:640.

148. Marx G, Pokar H, Reuter H, et al: The effects of aprotinin on hemostatic function during cardiac surgery. J Cardiothorac Vasc Anesth 1991; 5:467.

149. Griepp RB, Stinson EB, Hollingsworth JF, et al: Prosthetic replacement of the aortic arch. J Thorac Cardiovasc Surg 1975; 70:1051.

150. Hickey PR, Andersen NP: Deep hypothermic circulatory arrest: a review of pathophysiology and clinical experience as a basis for anesthetic management. J Cardiothorac Anesth 1987; 1:137.

151. Dickinson DF, Sambrooks JE: Intellectual performance in children after circulatory arrest with profound hypothermia in infancy. Arch Dis Child 1979; 54:1.

152. Clarkson PM, MacArthur BA, Barratt-Boyes BG, et al: Developmental progress after cardiac surgery in infancy using hypothermia and circulatory arrest. Circulation 1980; 62:85.

153. Crawford ES, Crawford JL, Safi HJ, et al: Thoracoabdominal aortic aneurysms: preoperative and intraoperative factors determining immediate and long-term results of operations in 605 patients. J Vasc Surg 1986; 3:389.

154. Costello TG, Fisher A: Neurologic complications following aortic surgery: case reports and review of the literature. Anaesthesia 1983; 38:230.

155. Wadouh F, Lindemann E, Arndt CF, et al: The arteria radicularis anterior as a decisive factor influencing spinal cord damage during aortic occlusion. J Thorac Cardiovasc Surg 1984; 88:1.

156. Crawford ES, Mizrahi EM, Hess KR, et al: The impact of distal aortic perfusion and somatosensory evoked potential monitoring on prevention of paraplegia after aortic aneurysm operation. J Thorac Cardiovasc Surg 1988; 95:357.

157. Kouchoukos NT, Lell WA, Karp RB, et al: Hemodynamic effects of clamping and decompression with a temporary shunt for resection of the descending thoracic aorta. Surgery 1979; 85:25.

158. Najafi H, Javid H, Hunter J, et al: Descending aortic aneurysmectomy without adjuncts to avoid ischemia. Ann Thorac Surg 1980; 30:326.

159. Berendes JN, Bredee JJ, Schipperheyn JJ, et al: Mechanisms of spinal cord injury after crossclamping the descending thoracic aorta. Circulation 1982; 66:I–112.

160. Miyamoto K, Ueno A, Wada T, et al: A new and simple method of preventing spinal cord damage following temporary occlusion of the thoracic aorta by draining the cerebrospinal fluid. J Cardiovasc Surg 1960; 16:188.

161. McCullough JL, Hollier LH, Nugent M: Paraplegia after thoracic aortic occlusion: influence of cerebrospinal fluid drainage. J Vasc Surg 1988; 7:153.

162. Crawford ES, Svensson LG, Hess KR, et al: A prospective randomized study of cerebrospinal fluid drainage to prevent paraplegia after high-risk surgery on the thoracoabdominal aorta. J Vasc Surg 1990; 13:36.

163. Marini CP, Grubbs PE, Toporoff B, et al: Effect of sodium nitroprusside on spinal cord perfusion and paraplegia during aortic cross-clamping. Ann Thorac Surg 1989; 47:379.

164. Woloszyn TT, Marini CP, Coons MS, et al: Cerebrospinal fluid drainage does not counteract the negative effect of sodium nitroprusside on spinal cord perfusion pressure during aortic cross-clamping. Curr Surg 1989; 46:489.

165. Vacanti FX, Ames A III: Mild hypothermia and magnesium protect against irreversible damage during CNS ischemia. Stroke 1984; 15:695.

166. Drummond JC, Moore SS: The influence of dextrose administration on neurologic outcome after temporary spinal cord ischemia in the rabbit. Anesthesiology 1989; 70:64.

167. Raza SM, Vasireddy AR, Candido KD, et al: A complete regional anesthesia technique for cardiac pacemaker insertion. J Cardiothorac Vasc Anesth 1991; 5:54.

168. Swerdlow CD, Winkle RA, Mason JW: Determinants of survival in patients with ventricular tachyarrhythmias. N Engl J Med 1983; 308:1436.

169. Wilber DJ, Garan H, Finkelstein D, et al: Out-of-hospital cardiac arrest: use of electrophysiologic testing in the prediction of long-term outcome. N Engl J Med 1988; 318:19.

170. Blakeman BM, Wilber D, Pifarre R: Median sternotomy for implantable cardioverter/defibrillator. Arch Surg 1989; 124:1065.

171. Gartmann DM, Bardy GH, Allen MD, et al: Short-term morbidity and mortality of implantation of automatic implantable cardioverter-defibrillator. J Thorac Cardiovasc Surg 1990; 100:353.

172. Watkins L Jr, Taylor E Jr: The surgical aspects of automatic implantable cardioverter-defibrillator implantation. PACE 1991; 14:953.

173. Antunes ML, Spotnitz HM, Livelli FD Jr, et al: Effect of electrophysiological testing on ejection fraction during cardioverter/defibrillator implantation. Ann Thorac Surg 1988; 45:315.

174. Stoddard MF, Redd RR, Buckingham TA, et al: Effects of electrophysiologic testing of the automatic implantable cardioverter-defibrillator on left ventricular systolic function and diastolic function. Am Heart J 1991; 122:714.

175. Reddy S, Curtiss EI, O'Toole JD, et al: Cardiac tamponade: hemodynamic observations in man. Circulation 1978; 58:265.

176. Kaplan JA, Bland JW Jr, Dunbar RW: The perioperative management of pericardial tamponade. South Med J 1976; 69:417.

CHAPTER 68

Anesthetic Considerations for Thoracic Surgery

PHILIP G. BOYSEN, M.D., F.A.C.P., F.C.C.P.

Preoperative assessment of the patient being considered for resection of lung tissue is unique. It includes delineation of the degree of underlying pulmonary compromise. Of equal importance are the determinations of (1) resectability of the intrapulmonary lesion and (2) operability as ascertained using physiologic function studies. With respect to the former, the preoperative search is for anatomic evidence of contiguous spread of the cancer or metastatic disease. Unfortunately, the imaging studies currently available often do not yield the necessary information to make this determination. For this reason, a stepwise procedural effort is made intraoperatively to define anatomic variation. This sequence usually begins with flexible fiberoptic or rigid bronchoscopy to examine the conducting airways and is followed by either mediastinoscopy or limited thoracotomy (Chamberlain's procedure) to further examine the mediastinum. The surgical procedure may be terminated following either of these examinations if contralateral disease or evidence of spread to lymph nodes is discovered. Prior to the surgical procedure, examination of the bones, brain, liver, and skin is extensive in an effort to identify metastatic disease.

Operability relates to the physiologic condition of the lungs and to the physiologic function that will remain following resection. As with any other form of cancer surgery, extirpation of the tumor depends not only on demonstration of the absence of metastatic disease but also on the sacrifice of a certain amount of functional tissue with the operation. Each patient is evaluated as if the most extensive form of surgery (i.e., pneumonectomy) will take place. The ultimate extent of the surgical procedure necessary to remove a tumor may not actually be known until the surgeon examines the open chest.

PULMONARY FUNCTION TESTING

What Is the Role of Spirometry?

Physiologic function begins with pulmonary function testing, including spirometry before and after the administration of nebulized bronchodilators, determination of lung volumes, and calculation of diffusing capacity. "Cutoff" values that indicate a poor prognosis are presented in Table 9–3.

Forced Vital Capacity

A decreased forced vital capacity (FVC) <50% of predicted or an absolute value <1.75 to 2.0 L predicts an increased risk of complications postoperatively.[1–3] This measurement defines restrictive components of lung disease.

Forced Expired Volume in One Second

Lower than normal values are associated with obstructive abnormalities. The absolute value of the forced expiratory volume in 1 second (FEV_1) and the maximal voluntary ventilation (MVV) seem to be particularly sensitive indicators of poor prognosis. An FEV_1 <800 mL generally precludes thoracic resection.[4, 5] Values <2 L are predictive of a perioperative mortality of 20% to 45%.[6, 7]

Maximum Voluntary Ventilation

The test of MVV requires sustained patient cooperation. A value >50% of predicted was associated with zero to 5% mortality in some studies.[1, 3] In another study,[7] if it was <60% of predicted, mortality was 32%.

Midflow Measurements

Midflow measurements can also be derived from a spirogram. These include measurement of the maximum midexpiratory flow rate and the forced expiratory flow between 25% and 75% of the exhaled volume ($FEF_{25\%-75\%}$) (see Fig. 9–1). These tests are sensitive indicators of small airway dysfunction.[8, 9] In chronic obstructive lung disease (COLD), midexpiratory flow measurements are always abnormal. A value that is less than predicted indicates a higher risk of pulmonary dysfunction after either thoracic or abdominal surgical procedures.[9] The $FEF_{25\%-75\%}$ is a highly specific indicator of postoperative complications.[6]

In patients with COLD, the immediate response to nebulized bronchodilators is assessed as a part of routine testing (see Fig. 56–1). This response has both diagnostic and prognostic importance, since improvement in airflow obstruction may indicate a better postoperative prognosis. In addition, some patients who show little or no response to nebulized bronchodilators eventually improve after an intensive regimen that includes bronchodilator use, hydration, antibiotic therapy, and cessation of smoking. Using the best values for FEV_1 and FVC that can be obtained is advisable; testing can be done immediately or after bronchodilator therapy has been optimized. Patients whose $FEF_{25\%-75\%}$ or MMV does not improve after such a therapeutic regimen have a higher incidence of postoperative pulmonary complications.[9]

In general, midflow measurements refine the clinical impression of obstructive airway disease, although restrictive diseases also can decrease midflow measurements. The combination of all available spirometric data enhances the clinical assessment.[10, 11]

Assessment

In assessing spirometry, the accepted routine is to perform three spirometric evaluations before and after the administration of nebulized bronchodilator. These may vary somewhat, but the patient's best effort is used to make all necessary calculations. This approach implies that a decrease in performance due to fatigue or that an improvement in performance due to bronchodilation may be acceptable in the choice of ''best function.'' Preparation for surgery should include adequate bronchodilation as well as assessment of lung drainage, stasis, and the presence of intercurrent infection. With such preparation, lung function can be optimized before the patient undergoes the operation.

What Is Diffusing Capacity?

Diffusing capacity can be low whether restrictive or obstructive physiology is present. With restricted physiology, a lower diffusing capacity suggests an impediment to gas transfer, specifically to the transfer of oxygen at the alveolo-capillary membrane. With obstructive physiology, a low diffusing capacity reflects less effective area for gas transfer. A diffusing capacity <15 mL $\cdot$ min^{-1} $\cdot$ mm Hg^{-1} is associated with an 18% mortality rate as opposed to a 7% mortality rate when the value is greater. However, the test's results are not always a good indicator of either the presence of obstructive airway disease or of postoperative morbidity and mortality.[12]

When Are Split Function Lung Studies Helpful?

Failure of a patient to achieve or exceed any one of the parameters in Table 9–3 indicates the necessity for split function lung testing. In this case, the goal is to demonstrate the worst-case remaining physiologic function (i.e., the patient loses the entire lung on the affected side). Predictive formulas have been combined with various split function assessment techniques to predict the postoperative level of function, particularly the postoperative FEV_1.

Bronchospirometry

Split function testing can be accomplished using a variety of techniques. The first of these is bronchospirometry.[13, 14] A double-lumen tube is introduced into the airway of an awake patient, and the right lung and left lung are isolated from one another by the inflation of tracheal and endobronchial cuffs.[12, 13] Each of these channels is then connected to a spirometer, and the patient is asked to perform a vital capacity test (maximum exhalation following maximum inhalation). Knowledge of the preoperative vital capacity with both lungs intact allows the subsequent determination of how much function is attributable to each lung. This assessment is of considerable consequence for the patient whose overall function is not compatible with pneumonectomy because of the often markedly diminished contribution of the diseased side to total function. A pneumonectomy does not necessarily cause the expected 50% decrease in pulmonary function in such cases.

Flow studies, such as those that assess FEV_1 and MVV, underestimate flow owing to the presence of a narrowed airway in the double-lumen tube; however, bronchospirometry has been used to predict postoperative FEV_1 and MVV.[15-17] Other techniques have been developed in an effort to gain the same information with less trauma and discomfort.

Ventilation and Perfusion Scanning

Ventilation and perfusion lung scanning have come to the forefront in this regard. In particular, perfusion lung scanning appears to be a useful and widely accepted technique. Most hospitals have the isotopes necessary to perform this procedure. These isotopes are stable, and the expense of the technique is minimal when it is compared with the cost for complete ventilation/perfusion ($\dot{V}/\dot{Q}$) scanning. A radioisotope such as ^{99}Tc combined with telemeter lung scanning and a split function crystal centered on the mediastinum allows relatively easy calculation of the per cent of perfusion to the right and left lungs.

Although patients with lung cancer often have a history of cigarette use and, thus, COPD with abnormal $\dot{V}/\dot{Q}$ relationships for the lungs as a whole, the information obtained from the perfusion scan of these patients correlates well with information from the ventilation scan. Because of this, one may take the percentage of perfusion to the uninvolved lung and multiply it by the values of other ventilatory function studies to obtain a predicted postoperative value.

For example, if a patient has a preoperative FEV_1 of 2.0 L and the uninvolved side accepts 55% of the blood flow, the predicted postoperative FEV_1 is 1.10 L. Patients studied in this way are also recommended for surgery, including pneumonectomy, if the predicted postoperative FEV_1 is >800 mL. This technique has been prospectively tested several times and is remarkably accurate.[4, 5]

Unilateral Pulmonary Artery Occlusion

Should the patient fail this secondary line of examination, surgery may still be possible. Hemodynamic assessment has been useful in the past to delineate postoperative morbidity and mortality. The technique used is temporary unilateral pulmonary artery occlusion with a balloon-fitted catheter that is much like the Swan-Ganz catheter. Under fluoroscopic guidance, the catheter is passed into the affected lung; the balloon is inflated so that all flow to the cancerous side is occluded. Since ventilation rapidly shifts away from that lung when perfusion is interrupted, a temporary, unilateral ''functional pneumonectomy'' is performed that allows the collection of both ventilation and hemodynamic data.

Should the mean pulmonary artery pressure exceed 35 mm Hg or should the arterial oxygen partial pressure fall to <45

mm Hg, the patient will not tolerate pneumonectomy.[18] Even in the supine position, low levels of exercise (100 J) can be performed using a bicycle ergometer to assess the effect on hemodynamic data. This testing identifies the patient in whom postoperative pulmonary vascular hypertension and right-sided heart failure may occur, resulting in respiratory invalidity.

To define postoperative function for the lobectomy patient, a formula can be constructed to predict postoperative function:

$$\text{Functional loss} = \text{Preoperative FEV}_1 \times \% \text{ Perfusion of cancerous lung} \times \frac{\text{Segments resected}}{\text{Total segments of affected side}}$$

If the right upper lobe is to be removed, 3 of 10 bronchopulmonary segments in the right lung will be resected; hence, 30% of the right-sided function will be eliminated following resection. Remember, however, that the remaining lung on the operative side may actually be edematous and atelectatic. In the early postoperative period, hypoxemia and shunt may follow until the remaining lung has recovered function.

INTRAOPERATIVE ANESTHETIC MANAGEMENT

What General Considerations Are Important?

Induction

Anesthetic induction can be accomplished by using a variety of techniques. Other than those incorporated in the preoperative pulmonary preparation discussed earlier, medications are not usually necessary. Depending on the speed of the surgeon and the degree of compromise, the choice of monitors may also vary. In addition to "routine" monitors, an intra-arterial catheter to measure blood pressure and to obtain arterial spec-

TABLE 68–1. Indications for Separation of the Two Lungs (Double-Lumen Tube Intubation) and One-Lung Ventilation

Absolute	Isolation of one lung from the other to avoid spillage or contamination
	Infection
	Massive hemorrhage
	Control of the distribution of ventilation
	Bronchopleural fistula
	Bronchopleural cutaneous fistula
	Surgical unilateral lung cyst or bulla
	Tracheobronchial tree disruption
	Unilateral bronchopulmonary lavage
	Pulmonary alveolar proteinosis
Relative	Surgical exposure—High priority
	Thoracoscopy
	Thoracic aortic aneurysm
	Pneumonectomy
	Upper lobectomy
	Surgical exposure—Low priority
	Middle and lower lobectomies and subsegmental resections
	Esophageal resection
	Thoracoscopy
	Procedures on the thoracic spine
	Postcardiopulmonary bypass status after removal of totally occluding chronic unilateral pulmonary emboli

(Modified from Benumof JL (ed): Anesthesia for Thoracic Surgery. Philadelphia, WB Saunders, 1987, p 224.)

imens for blood gas analysis is generally useful. Central venous access may not be as useful during the course of the anesthetic and surgical procedure as it is during the immediate postoperative period. If a subclavian central venous access route is chosen, it is prudent to use the operative side, since pneumothorax is then less of a problem than if it were to occur on the nonoperated side.

If bronchoscopy is employed and if mediastinoscopy or Chamberlain's techniques are then used to examine the airways and mediastinum, some degree of narcotic administration is usually beneficial. During this stepwise process, a large, single-lumen endotracheal tube is introduced into the airway so that the examination can be carried out while the patient is anesthetized and paralyzed. A laryngotracheal spray that contains a local anesthetic such as lidocaine facilitates anesthesia and makes bronchoscopic examination easier. Since narcotics predispose to alveolar hypoventilation, they are best used at the beginning of the procedure. The rest of the anesthetic maintenance relies more heavily on volatile anesthetic agents.

Why and How Is a Double-Lumen Tube Placed?

Indications

The double-lumen tube is most useful during thoracotomy and thoracoscopy. It enhances the surgeon's ability to work on the operative side (with the lung partially or completely collapsed) while ventilation to the unaffected lung is maintained. Absolute and relative indications for double-lumen tube insertion are listed in Table 68–1.

Because the tube contains two lumens and since part of its internal diameter is taken up by a septum, a larger outside-diameter tube is usually placed. In a woman, a 35 or 37 French tube typically is used, whereas in a man a 39 or 41 French tube usually is chosen. If the right lung is to be operated on, a left bronchial intubation generally is preferred. If the left lung is the operative one, either a right-sided or a left-sided tube may be used.

Some physicians use a left-sided tube in either event because of the greater difficulty in maintaining ventilation with the right-sided tube. Because of the proximal take-off of the right upper lobe bronchus (Fig. 68–1), a separate orifice in the wall of the endobronchial portion is provided so that ventilation to that area can be maintained (Fig. 68–2). Unless the right upper lobe orifice is in perfect apposition to the endobronchial tube aperture, ventilation of this portion of the lung may be difficult or impossible.

Since the tube is easily moved during positioning or the surgical procedure, the left-sided double-lumen tube is often preferred because it allows a greater range for tube position changes. If a left endobronchial tube is used during a left pneumonectomy, simply withdraw it into the trachea before the left mainstem bronchus is resected and leave it there for the remainder of the procedure.

Technique

When the tube is passed, it is introduced into the airway with the curvature of the endobronchial lumen (i.e., the tip) in the anterior position to facilitate entry into the larynx. Care should be taken to avoid laceration of the tracheal cuff on the teeth because this cuff is much farther from the tip than it is

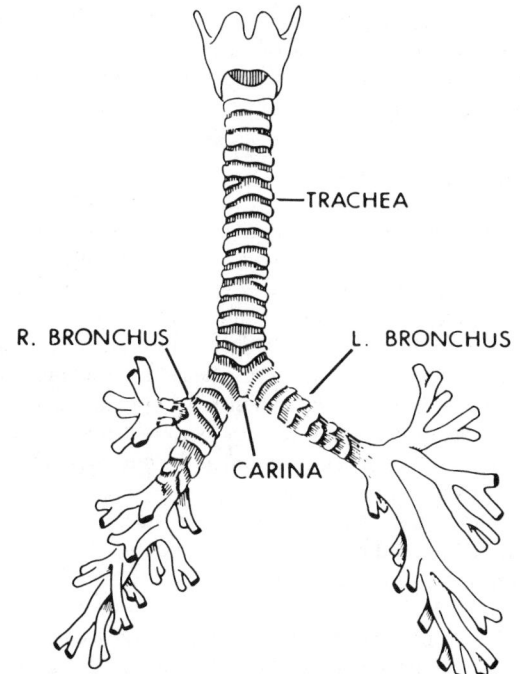

FIGURE 68–1. Normal anatomy of the tracheobronchial tree. Note the close proximity of the right upper lobe bronchus to the carina. This distance may be as little as 1 cm in adults. (From Kirby RR: Respiratory system. *In* Manual of Complications During Anesthesia. Gravenstein N (ed). Philadelphia, JB Lippincott, 1991, p 318.)

on a conventional tube. Once past the vocal cords, the tube is rotated 90° so that the endobronchial tip is aimed to the appropriate side. The tube is then gently advanced until resistance is met, indicating lodgment in the designated airway. At this point, both cuffs are inflated, and the right and left sides are ventilated to verify intratracheal placement.

Verification of Position: Physical Signs

With a single side clamped and both cuffs inflated, unilateral breath sounds should be present over the contralateral side. The relatively compliant hemithorax should rise and fall smoothly as the single side is ventilated. Unclamping the first side and clamping the other side should result in similar findings but on the opposite side. In addition, if the clamped, nonventilated side is opened to air, the open port can be auscultated to verify that no leak is present (i.e., that the

endobronchial cuff has occluded the mainstem bronchus). This maneuver is also useful to adjust endobronchial cuff inflation volume just to the point at which an air seal is obtained. As one observes the chest, the "rocking boat" phenomenon should be noted as one lung is ventilated and the other lung is not.

Possible malpositions of the double-lumen tube include its placement in the wrong mainstem bronchus; too deep a placement on one or the other side; or too shallow a placement (not in the mainstem bronchus) (Fig. 68–3). A smooth exhalation is crucial. If it does not occur, the tube is likely inserted either too far, with resultant partial obstruction of the tracheal lumen by the carina, or not far enough, with resultant obstruction of the trachea by the endobronchial cuff. Fiberoptic bronchoscopy can be used to resolve all questions regarding tube position.

Verification of Placement: Fiberoptic Bronchoscopy

Indications

Often, tube placement is questionable despite favorable visible and auscultatory findings on examination of the chest. Such examination may be insensitive, or the patient may be moved, prepared, or draped, with subsequent movement of the tube from the original position. Turning the patient from the prone to decubitus position may be associated with head and tube movement sufficient either to pull the endobronchial tube back into the trachea or to pull it back into the trachea and then readvance it such that it ends up in the opposite mainstem bronchus when positioning is completed.

For these reasons, a flexible fiberoptic bronchoscope (FFB) is recommended to ascertain initial tube placement. Re-examination is routinely performed once the patient is placed in the final position. A stepwise procedure is used to examine the airways.

Technique

A pediatric FFB is required. A scope with an outside diameter of <4 mm can be easily passed down each lumen of a 35-French or larger double-lumen tube. First, the FFB is introduced into the tracheal lumen, whereupon one should see a sharp carina as the scope emerges from the tube and a clear, right mainstem bronchus. The left mainstem bronchus should be occluded by the endobronchial stem of the tube, and the

Double-Lumen Tubes

FIGURE 68–2. This schematic diagram depicts the essential features and parts of right-sided and left-sided double-lumen tubes. RUL = right upper lobe; LUL = left upper lobe. (From Benumof JL: Anesthesia for Thoracic Surgery. Philadelphia, WB Saunders, 1987, p 227.)

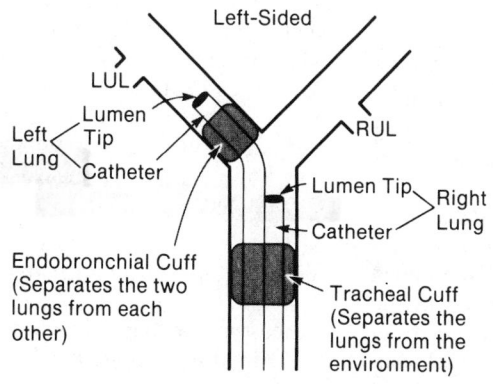

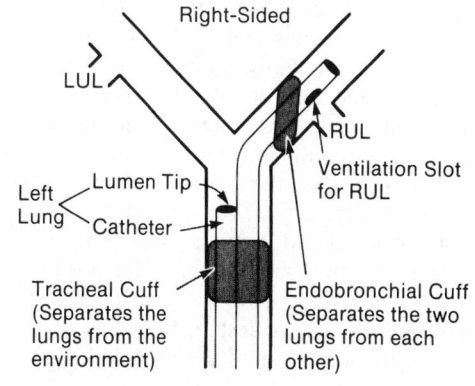

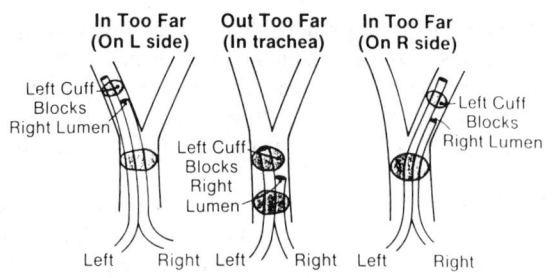

Procedure	Breath Sounds Heard		
Clamp Right Lumen Both Cuffs Inflated	Left	Left and Right	Right
Clamp Left Lumen Both Cuffs Inflated	None or Very ↓↓	None or Very ↓↓	None or Very ↓↓
Clamp Left Lumen Deflate Left Cuff	Left	Left and Right	Right

FIGURE 68–3. Three major whole-lung malpositions of a left-sided double-lumen endotracheal tube can also occur. The tube can be in too far on the left (both lumens in the left mainstem bronchus), out too far (both lumens in the trachea), or down the right mainstem bronchus (at least the left lumen is in the right mainstem bronchus). In each malpositioning, the left cuff, when fully inflated, can completely block the right lumen. Inflation and deflation of the left cuff while the left lumen is clamped creates a breath sound differential diagnosis of tube malposition. L = left; R = right; ↓ = decreased. (From Benumof JL: Intraoperative considerations for all thoracic surgery. *In* Anesthesia for Thoracic Surgery. Benumof JL (ed). Philadelphia, WB Saunders, 1987, p 236.)

endobronchial cuff should be just visible at the carina, with the marker line clearly visible above the carina.

My preference is to inflate and deflate the endobronchial cuff under direct examination of the airways. This maneuver shows that the bronchial lumen can indeed be occluded with minimal volume placed into the cuff and that the cuff does not herniate over the carina into the other mainstem bronchus. If it does so on inflation, airflow into the other lung will be occluded.

Once correct endobronchial cuff placement is confirmed and no obstruction to the contralateral bronchus is demonstrated, the FFB is removed and introduced into the endobronchial port. The tube should not be impacted into the tracheobronchial mucosa, and, in the case of a left-sided tube, the left upper lobe, lingula, and left lower lobe orifices should be visible. If such is the case, the endobronchial cuff is adequately positioned either to ventilate that particular lung or to allow the lung to be collapsed if the endobronchial lumen is opened to air.

A right-sided endobronchial tube is examined in analogous fashion. However, during the endobronchial lumen examination, the right upper lobe ventilation orifice is verified to be opposite the right upper lobe bronchial orifice. This position must be preserved during cuff inflation and deflation. The right upper lobe bronchus has a characteristic trifurcated appearance that distinguishes it from other bronchi.

These techniques and FFB availability for subsequent re-examination should the patient be moved obviate many of the problems that tend to occur during the course of one-lung ventilation and anesthesia. Should the "feel" of the lung change, in 90% of cases FFB re-examination quickly identifies the problem (e.g., the presence of secretions, tube migration, or airway obstruction). In my experience, the most common problem is migration of the tube position. Benumof has described the "margin of safety" for positioning double-lumen tubes; in the description, a left-sided tube is defined as the length of the left mainstem bronchus minus the length from the proximal margin of the bronchial cuff to the left lumen

tip.[19] With an average carina–to–left upper lobe distance of 45 mm, the positioning margin of safety is <2 cm. This much movement readily occurs with neck flexion or extension and thus must be anticipated.

Bronchial Blocker Tube

Another approach to one-lung ventilation is to insert a tube fitted with an inflatable bronchial blocker. The tube's exterior dimensions are similar to those of a conventional endotracheal tube. It includes an accessory channel that contains a moveable stylet with an inflatable bronchial blocker (cuff) attached to it. Once the tube is placed in the trachea, the bronchial blocker can be advanced into either mainstem bronchus under fiberoptic guidance in a fashion analogous to that for positioning a double-lumen tube. When positioned, the cuff is incrementally inflated until a seal is obtained.

The volume necessary to inflate the blocker cuff is larger than the corresponding volume for a double-lumen tube. At times, up to 8 mL of air are needed to effect a "just sealed" condition.[20] The greater cuff inflation volume required with the blocker as compared with that needed for a double-lumen tube is a consequence of the cuff's need to fill the entire lumen of the bronchus because it is not supported by a ventilating lumen. Also, the blocker acts as a high-pressure cuff; thus, gas volume is lost to compression. When the need for one-lung ventilation is no longer present, the blocker is deflated and withdrawn into the lumen of the main tube.

What Are the Considerations During One-Lung Ventilation?

Successful ventilation of one lung depends on precise positioning of the double-lumen tube and isolation of the two airways. The consequences of one-lung ventilation also depend on patient position, which most often is lateral decubitus (operative side "up-lung," and nonoperative side "down-lung"). In normal individuals in the supine position, an average of 55% of the perfusion fraction goes to the right lung and 45% to the left lung.

When the patient is placed in the lateral decubitus position, the changes that occur are a consequence of gravitational forces. If the left lung is the up-lung and the right side is the down-lung, 35% of the perfusion goes to the left lung and 65% of total perfusion goes to the right lung. Conversely, if the right lung is the operative lung and the patient is in the left lateral decubitus position, 45% of perfusion goes to the right lung and 55% to the left.

The normal shunt fraction of 0.05 increases to about 0.25 on changeover from spontaneous ventilation to mechanical ventilation in the lateral position. It increases to almost 0.4 when the chest is open and when one-lung ventilation is begun without end-expiratory pressure on either lung. With collapse of the operative side, a decrease in perfusion takes place (some perfusion still occurs). In general, roughly 80% of perfusion now flows to the down-lung, whereas 20% flows to the poorly inflated operative lung.

Shunt Change Mechanisms

Reasons for these alterations in blood flow are multifactorial. Blood flow to the nondependent lung is altered, and flow is diverted to atelectatic areas of the down-lung with an increase in pulmonary vascular resistance. Hypoxic pulmonary vasoconstriction (HPV) is a physiologic response to these changes (i.e., the lack of ventilation to the nondependent lung) and autoregulates flow to a certain extent. Its effect is to divert blood away from the collapsed lung and to lessen the shunt.

Drugs

Many drugs inhibit HPV and interfere with this flow diversion. Drugs that have this effect are vasodilators such as nitroglycerin, sodium nitroprusside, dobutamine, calcium channel blockers, and β_2-agonists.

Vasoconstrictors can increase pulmonary pressure and vascular resistance and, thus, also reverse HPV and divert blood back into the atelectatic lung with the attendant consequences. Halogenated anesthetics also alter HPV but usually not to a degree that is clinically significant. Generally, these agents are beneficial because of the bronchodilation they effect and of their administration with high inspired oxygen partial pressures. Anesthesia at 1 minimum alveolar concentration appears to be safe with respect to major changes in HPV. Intravenous anesthetics do not alter HPV, and their use is therefore often a part of the anesthetic management.

Physical Factors

Blood flow to the dependent lung is also affected by gravitational changes. The nondependent lung may have increased pulmonary vascular resistance. This change results from a variety of circumstances, including anesthetic induction with a loss of lung volume; the weight of the mediastinum on the dependent lung, which causes a decrease in lung volume and increased pulmonary vascular resistance, or cephalad displacement of the diaphragm.

Positional changes are also important, particularly because the patient is often draped over a kidney rest so that his or her ribs can be spread on the operative side. This combination of forces results in a loss of lung volume, a decrease in functional residual capacity, a change in the caliber of blood vessels that go to that lung, and an increase in pulmonary vascular resistance. Secondly, some degree of absorption atelectasis also contributes to shunt in the dependent lung; this is compounded by the fact that secretion removal may be more difficult with the loss of lung volume.

How Is One-Lung Anesthesia Performed?

Ventilation

Several principles and guidelines are useful for intraoperative management. First, the fraction of inspired oxygen is usually maintained at 1.0 during one-lung ventilation and anesthesia. Despite the possibility of absorption atelectasis and oxygen toxicity, neither of these risks exceed the benefits of the administration of 100% oxygen. The cases are generally too short to cause oxygen toxicity, and the consequences of atelectasis, if they occur, can be managed during the course of the surgical procedure.

Tidal volume is usually adjusted to 10 mL · kg^{-1} for the dependent lung. This value allows adequate inflation without producing high inflation pressures that might cause barotrauma

or excessively alter blood flow to the dependent lung. The respiratory rate usually must be increased by approximately 20% with the goal of maintaining an arterial carbon dioxide partial pressure of about 44 mm Hg. An inspiratory flow pattern that minimizes mean airway pressure should be selected.

Cardiovascular Function

In addition to the onset of HPV, which is a protective mechanism, cardiac output during one-lung anesthesia is increased in a significant number of patients. With a certain degree of shunt and blood flow, the increase in cardiac output "protects" the arterial oxygen partial pressure. This change may also be reflected by increased mixed venous oxygen partial pressure and saturation.

Anesthetic Maintenance

After anesthetic induction with intravenous narcotics and an intermediate or long-acting neuromuscular blocker, a switch to volatile agents for anesthetic maintenance follows. With the use of volatile anesthetic agents, a high fraction of inspired oxygen can be maintained. Volatile agents provide good bronchodilation, a property beneficial to patients with COPD and a tendency toward bronchospasm. If necessary, further bronchodilatation can be achieved with the administration of nebulized β_2-agonists, atropine, or atropine analogues into the anesthetic circuit (see Table 9–2).

How Should Intraoperative Hypoxia Be Managed?

Despite redirection of blood flow, increased cardiac output, and appropriate placement of the double-lumen tube, significant hypoxia may occur in some patients. Several methods can be used to manage this problem (Table 68–2).[21, 22] First, one can intermittently inflate the operative lung with 100% oxygen and ventilate it briefly to re-establish more normal V̇/Q̇ relationships, minimize shunt, and raise alveolar oxygen partial pressure in that lung. Enough residual oxygen should remain in the alveoli to allow another 10 to 15 minutes of operating time without reoccurrence of hypoxia.

Positive Airway Pressure

Theoretically, positive end-expiratory pressure (PEEP) applied to the dependent lung should increase functional residual

TABLE 68–2. Approaches to Independent Lung Ventilation in Lateral Decubitus Position

"Up" Lung	"Dependent" Lung
CPAP (5–10 cm H$_2$O) (apneic concentration)	Ventilate
Constant CPAP, apneic oxygenation, periodic ventilation	Ventilate
No ventilation	Ventilate with CPAP (5–10 cm H$_2$O)
HFV	Ventilate with or without CPAP

(From Kirby RR: Respiratory system. *In* Manual of Complications During Anesthesia. Gravenstein N (ed). Philadelphia, JB Lippincott, 1991, p 319.)
Abbreviations: CPAP = continuous positive airway pressure; HFV = high-frequency ventilation.

capacity; however, it also results in a further increase in pulmonary vascular resistance and diversion of blood flow into the operative lung, which worsens the degree of shunt. The more appropriate intervention is, in fact, to first administer low-level (5 cm H_2O) continuous positive airway pressure (CPAP) with 100% oxygen to the nondependent or operative lung.

The algorithm for intraoperative hypoxemia should always begin with a check of tube placement to make sure that no mechanical problem is related to this device. If tube placement is appropriate, 5- to 7-cm H_2O CPAP is administered *after* adequate inflation of the lung. Be sure to re-establish the functional residual capacity of the operative lung before making the transition to CPAP alone; otherwise, CPAP is likely to be ineffective. A method to provide one-lung CPAP is presented in Figure 68–4.[21, 22]

A further step that may be taken is to give differential lung PEEP/CPAP. With this technique, an alveolar concentration of oxygen is re-established in the operative lung, and the small amount of PEEP that is given to the dependent lung does not result in a redistribution of blood flow and a worsening of the shunt.

In 90% of cases, hypoxemia can be alleviated within several minutes. Administration of PEEP to the dependent lung is rarely necessary. High frequency jet ventilation and apneic oxygenation by tracheal insufflation of oxygen also have been recommended as adjunctive techniques. Whereas they may be useful, they are rarely necessary. If the patient is to have a pneumonectomy and hypoxia persists despite the application of the interventions described, the pulmonary artery to the operative lung can be clamped so that V̇/Q̇ relationships in the remaining lung are restored to nearly normal.

If a bronchial blocker is in place, intermittent ventilation or application of apneic CPAP to the up-lung (i.e., the nonventilated lung) is possible but more difficult to apply.

Manual Ventilation

Manual ventilation during one-lung anesthesia should be performed intermittently, since changes in resistance or compliance of the ventilated lung may be perceived. In addition to difficulty with insufflating gas into the airway, hyperinflation and overdistention of the ventilated lung may occur, effecting an increase in trapped gas, changes in pulmonary vascular resistance, and a subsequent decrease in cardiac output and gas exchange.

How Is Fluid Volume Managed During Lung Surgery?

As a case proceeds, an increase in extravascular lung water occurs in the dependent lung. Formation of a transudate further compromises compliance, lung volume, and pulmonary vascular resistance. For this reason, restriction of fluid volume is recommended during thoracotomy. For the adult male, an intraoperative fluid volume of <1800 mL is often provided.

Such fluid restriction may be problematic for two reasons. First, lung surgery patients are often dehydrated prior to surgery and have a low intravascular volume; thus, maintenance of blood pressure and cardiac output may be difficult without the administration of fluids. Second, transudation of fluid probably is more closely related to surgical trauma to the lung and to the duration of the procedure than to the administered fluid volume. Despite the absence of a correlation between intraoperative fluid administration and postoperative pulmonary edema or atelectasis, fluid restriction is generally employed. There is no proven advantage of colloid solutions over crystalloid solutions when fluids are to be given.

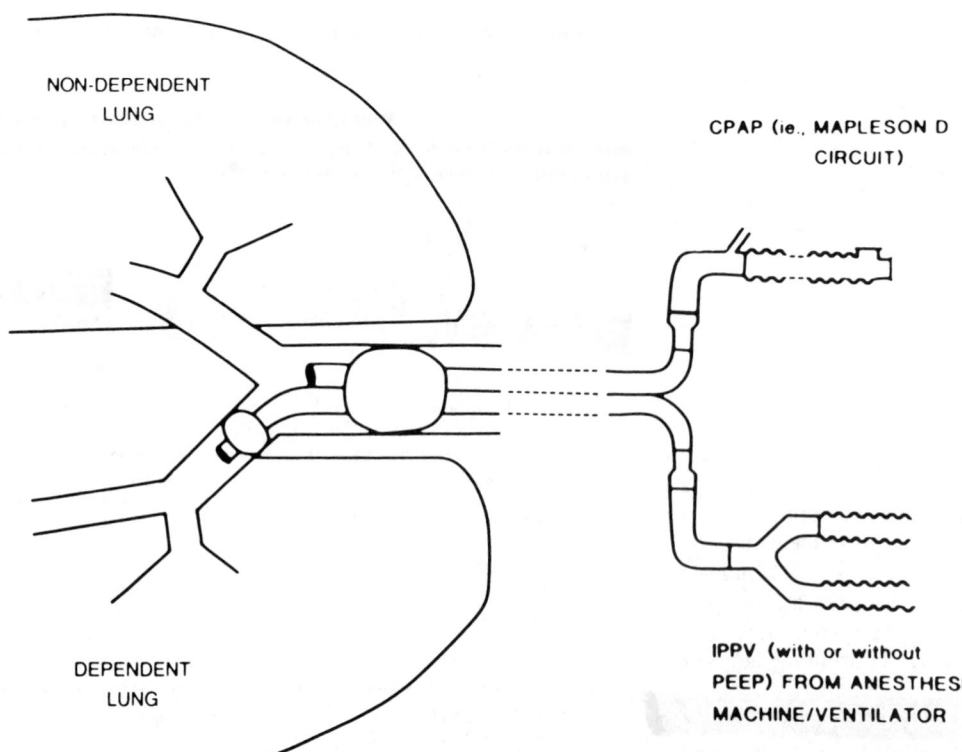

NON-DEPENDENT LUNG

DEPENDENT LUNG

CPAP (ie., MAPLESON D CIRCUIT)

IPPV (with or without PEEP) FROM ANESTHESIA MACHINE/VENTILATOR

FIGURE 68–4. One method to improve oxygenation during thoracic surgical procedures is to ventilate the dependent lung normally, with or without PEEP, using a double-lumen tube. CPAP and oxygen are provided to the nondependent lung. A Mapleson D apparatus with the pop-off valve closed and a PEEP valve replacing the breathing bag is satisfactory with 2 to 3 L · min⁻¹ of O_2 from an E cylinder. (From Kirby RR: Respiratory system. *In* Manual of Complications During Anesthesia. Gravenstein N (ed). Philadelphia, JB Lippincott, 1991, p 320.)

MEDIASTINAL LESIONS

How Are Flow-Volume Loops Used?

Mediastinal lesions may pose a particular problem because of the airway compromise that can occur with changes in patient position. If a mediastinal lesion is present, flow-volume loops obtained with the patient in both the erect and supine positions should be examined. Anterior mediastinal masses may only manifest when the patient is supine; hence, multi-position (dynamic) determinations are needed.

The types and positions of lesions within the trachea change during inspiration and expiration, depending on the severity and degree of anatomic compromise. An intrathoracic mediastinal lesion that occludes the trachea is associated with an alteration of gas flow during exhalation. Conversely, an extrathoracic tracheal or laryngeal lesion promotes airway occlusion during forced inspiration. Again, the compromise may be positional, and the patient should repeat these maneuvers in the proposed operative position. Flow-volume loop testing with the patient in the sitting, supine, and right or left lateral decubitus positions can cause not only patient distress but also indicate the presence of physiologic problems.

How Is Ventilation Supported?

Should the patient have a mediastinal or tracheal lesion, positive-pressure ventilation may be easily accomplished after the trachea has been intubated *if* the lesion does not affect the trachea below the tip of the endotracheal tube. If the tumor is more distally located, difficulty may be observed during exhalation. Air introduced into the tracheobronchial tree may forcibly separate and, thus, alleviate tracheal occlusion. However, the gravitational effects of the mediastinal mass may occlude exhaled gas flow.

Because of the disastrous consequences that have been described with airway obstruction following induction of general anesthesia in patients with anterior mediastinal masses, a conservative approach is recommended (Fig. 68–5).[23] Local anesthesia should be used for a diagnostic mediastinoscopy; general anesthesia with preservation of spontaneous ventilation can be employed if local anesthesia is not an option. Another—albeit rarely employed—option is femoral-femoral cardiopulmonary bypass. Even though it is rarely employed, it is wise to recognize it as an alternative when needed. A large number of these tumors are radiosensitive, and preoperative irradiation is associated with improvement in dynamic pulmonary function and decreased risk to the patient. Preoperative irradiation does not usually interfere with subsequent tissue diagnosis.

POSTOPERATIVE PAIN MANAGEMENT

What Is the Effect on Postoperative Pulmonary Function?

In order to provide for a smooth postoperative course, a sophisticated and intensive pain management plan should be provided to most thoracotomy patients. Three major options may be utilized to advantage postoperatively.

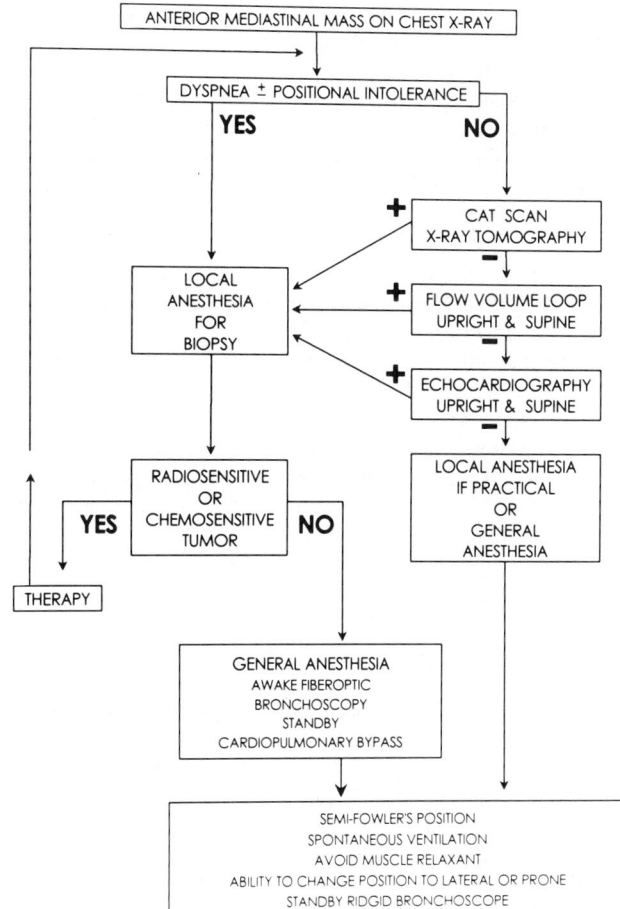

FIGURE 68–5. Flow chart describing the preoperative evaluation of the patient with an anterior mediastinal mass. Plus sign (+) indicates positive finding; minus sign (−) indicates negative work-up. (From Neuman GG, Weingarten AE, Abramowitz RM, et al: The anesthetic management of the patient with an anterior mediastinal mass. Anesthesiology 1984; 60:146.)

Patient-Controlled Analgesia

Patient-controlled analgesia provides small intermittent doses of narcotic according to a specific programmed regimen that is maintained by a computer. The advantage is that administration of smaller doses of narcotics may provide adequate pain relief and avoid subtherapeutic blood levels. With this technique, administration of high blood levels of narcotic, which suppress ventilation, occurs less frequently than with other methods.

The goal of any pain relief technique for the thoracotomy patient is to provide satisfactory analgesia for early ambulation and to achieve deep lung inflation that reverses postoperative atelectasis in the operative lung. Additionally, early ambulation and deep breathing facilitate removal of secretions because they enable the patient to produce an adequate productive cough.

Epidural Analgesia

The second useful and, in most cases, preferred technique is epidural analgesia. It can be provided using a variety of mechanisms that vary according to the practice setting. Thoracic epidural catheter placement preferentially provides analgesia to the dermatomes involved in the operative incision. This catheter is more difficult to place than is its lumbar counterpart but provides more precise analgesic delivery with the least amount of narcotic (if fentanyl or sufentanil is used).

As an alternative, many clinicians choose to use the more familiar lumbar epidural approach but administer either a large volume of a relatively lipid-soluble agent (fentanyl or sufentanil) or use the less lipid-soluble drug morphine. Instead of intermittent bolus dosing, one can also provide adequate analgesia by continuous infusion with shorter-acting agents. I use a thoracic epidural catheter with 5 to 7.5 $\mu g \cdot mL^{-1}$ fentanyl as an infusion with the addition of a very dilute dose of local anesthetic (1/16% bupivacaine) to optimize pain relief. With a background infusion, the epidural system can be connected to a patient-controlled analgesia unit so that the patient can actually administer the dose of the epidural agent in addition to the maintenance infusion.

With epidural analgesia, an improved breathing pattern that may be due to effects other than pain relief has been noted. Postoperative diaphragmatic dysfunction is thought to be caused by an inhibitory reflex that is mediated at the spinal cord; epidural analgesia has a salutary affect on postoperative diaphragmatic dysfunction.

Intrathecal Morphine

Intrathecal morphine is generally administered as a single dose, since one dose can provide adequate analgesia for 24 to 48 hours. Approximately 0.5 mg of preservative-free morphine is introduced into the lumbar cerebrospinal fluid.

Like epidural analgesia, this technique is associated with several complications that occur frequently, including urinary retention and pruritus. Most patients receiving epidural analgesia have a urinary catheter, thus the former problem is avoided. If pruritus is intense and does not respond to small (12.5-mg intravenous) intermittent doses of diphenhydramine, naloxone, 20 to 40 μg intravenously, is administered repeatedly until relief occurs.

The last complication of importance is respiratory depression. It probably results from rostral spread of the narcotic agent, regardless of whether it is in the intrathecal or the epidural space. This problem responds predictably to naloxone, which is again given in small 20- to 40-μg boluses until the desired response is elicited. A dilute infusion of naloxone (e.g., 100 $\mu g \cdot h^{-1}$) may be started prophylactically or begun if respiratory depression is observed.

Optimal monitoring for patients undergoing lung surgery has not been standardized. Whereas arterial oxygen saturation by oximetry has become widely available, the effects of narcotics on ventilation suggest that capnography or inductance plethysmography (i.e., assessment of respiratory motion) may be more appropriate.

Why Is Pre-Emptive Analgesia Important?

Perhaps the most important thing anesthesiologists have learned in the last several years with respect to optimizing analgesia after thoracotomy is that it should be provided preemptively. Very simply stated, injury and its perception influence the central nervous system's response to subsequent input. If the operative pain is modulated locally, such as at the cutaneous or spinal cord level, subsequent analgesic requirement is reduced.[24] If it is not, the pain perception may persist even after healing has occurred. An extreme example of this phenomenon is phantom limb pain.

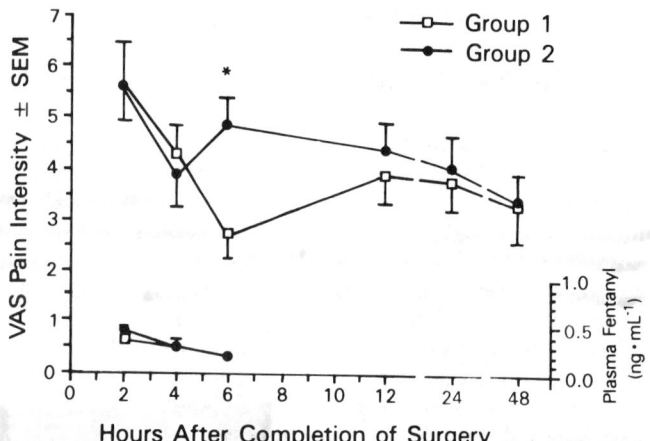

FIGURE 68–6. Postoperative visual analogue scale (VAS) pain intensity scores and plasma fentanyl levels for thoracotomy patients receiving epidural fentanyl before incision (Group 1) versus after incision (Group 2). Zero hours refers to the time that patients were admitted to the recovery room. (*$P >$ 0.05.) (From Katz J, Kavanagh BP, Sandler AN, et al: Preemptive analgesia: clinical evidence of neuroplasticity contributing to postoperative pain. Anesthesiology 1992; 77:443.)

Pretreatment with local anesthetic or opioid receptor agonists prior to skin incision reduces postoperative pain intensity and duration. This finding occurs even in the presence of an otherwise adequate general anesthetic and thus is almost counterintuitive. The effect has been strikingly demonstrated in thoracotomy patients who were administered epidural fentanyl either before incision or 15 minutes after incision (see Fig. 68–6).[24] Despite identical plasma fentanyl levels, postoperative pain scores were significantly higher and the supplemental analgesic requirement significantly greater at up to 24 hours postoperatively in the postincision fentanyl administration group than in the preincision group. We now routinely place all epidural catheters for thoracotomy patients before induction of general anesthesia and administer narcotic boluses prior to incision. Patients are then given a continuous narcotic infusion that is supplemented with local anesthetic during the case, followed by a narcotic infusion with or without dilute local anesthetic into the postoperative period.

Each of the analgesic techniques described has been associated with improved postoperative pulmonary function and is thought to influence outcome by decreasing morbidity. A *tendency* for reduced postoperative complications, such as atelectasis, stasis of secretions, tracheal bronchitis, and pneumonia, as well as the necessity for reintubation and mechanical ventilation, has been noted. The obvious goal, therefore, is to return all patients to spontaneous breathing at the end of the procedure. A delicate balance must be struck between preservation of central stimulation to alveolar ventilation and respiratory muscle function. Resultant changes in physiologic function in addition to breathing pattern include improved FVC, FEV_1, and peak expiratory flow rate. As always, the hope is that improved physiology leads to better outcome. For pulmonary surgery patients, improved comfort alone is reason enough to initiate these postoperative techniques.

References

1. Mittman C: Assessment of operative risk in thoracic surgery. Am Rev Respir Dis 1961; 84:197.
2. van Nostrand D, Kjeisberg MO, Humphrey EW: Preresectional evaluation of risk from pneumonectomy. Surg Gynecol Obstet 1968; 127:306.

3. Gaensler EA, Cugell DW, Lindgren I, et al: The role of pulmonary insufficiency in mortality and invalidism following surgery for pulmonary tuberculosis. Thorac Surg 1955; 29:163.

4. Kristersson S, Lindell SE, Svanberg L: Prediction of pulmonary function loss due to pneumonectomy using ^{133}Xe-radiospirometry. Chest 1972; 62:294.

5. Olsen GN, Block AJ, Swenson EW, et al: Pulmonary function evaluation of the lung resection candidate: a prospective study. Am Rev Respir Dis 1975; 111:379.

6. Boushy SF, Billig DM, North LB, et al: Clinical course related to preoperative and postoperative pulmonary function in patients with bronchogenic carcinoma. Chest 1971; 59:383.

7. Didolkar MS, Moore RH, Takita H: Evaluation of the risk of pulmonary resection for bronchogenic carcinoma. Am J Surg 1974; 127:700.

8. McFadden ER Jr, Kiker R, Holmes B, et al: Small airway disease: an assessment of the tests of peripheral airway function. Am J Med 1974; 57:171.

9. Gracey DR, Divertie MR, Didier EP: Preoperative pulmonary preparation of patients with chronic obstructive pulmonary disease: a prospective study. Chest 1979; 76:123.

10. Miller WF, Wu N, Johnson RL: Convenient method of evaluating pulmonary ventilatory function with a single breath test. Anesthesiology 1956; 17:480.

11. Redding JS, Yakaitis RW: Predicting the need for ventilatory assistance. Md State Med J 1970; 19:53.

12. Karliner JS, Coomaraswamy R, Williams MH Jr: Relationship between preoperative pulmonary function studies and prognosis of patients undergoing pneumonectomy for carcinoma of the lung. Dis Chest 1968; 54:112.

13. Olsen GN: The evolving role of exercise testing prior to lung resection. Chest 1989; 95:218.

14. Uggla LG: Indications for and results of thoracic surgery with regard to respiratory and circulatory function tests. Acta Chir Scand 1956; 11:197.

15. Svanberg L: Bronchospirometry in the study of regional lung function. Scand J Respir Dis 1966; 62(Suppl):91.

16. Svanberg L: Regional functional decrease in bronchial carcinoma. Ann Thorac Surg 1972; 13:170.

17. Neuhaus H, Cherniack NS: A bronchospirometric method of estimating the effect of pneumonectomy on the maximum breathing capacity. J Thorac Cardiovasc Surg 1968; 55:144.

18. Boysen PG, Clark CA, Block AJ: Graded exercise testing and post thoracotomy complications. J Cardiothorac Anesth 1990; 4:68.

19. Benumof JL, Partridge BL: Margin of safety in positioning modern double-lumen endotracheal tubes. Anesthesiology 1987; 67:729.

20. Gayes JM: Pro and con: the Univent tube is the best technique for providing one-lung ventilation: pro. J Cardiothorac Vasc Anesth 1993; 7:103.

21. Benumof JL: Separation of the two lungs (double-lumen tube intubation). *In* Anesthesia for Thoracic Surgery. Benumof JL (ed). Philadelphia, WB Saunders, 1987, pp 223–259.

22. Kirby RR: Respiratory system. *In* Manual of Complications During Anesthesia. Gravenstein N (ed). Philadelphia, JB Lippincott, 1991, pp 303–352.

23. Neuman GG, Weingarten AE, Abramowitz RM, et al: The anesthetic management of the patient with an anterior mediastinal mass. Anesthesiology 1984; 60:144.

24. Katz J, Kavanagh BP, Sandler AN, et al: Preemptive analgesia: clinical evidence of neuroplasticity contributing to postoperative pain. Anesthesiology 1992; 77:439.

CHAPTER 69

Anesthesia for Aortic Vascular Surgery

DONN M. DENNIS, M.D.

Patients undergoing operations on the aorta and its major branches present a formidable anesthetic challenge. The high incidence of severe coexisting disease and patients' advanced age combined with the abrupt and severe physiologic trespasses of the operations impose a significant burden on these patients. In perhaps no other area of surgery have anesthesiologists made such key contributions during the past 30 years. The 6-day mortality rate of major vascular surgery in the mid-1960s was 25% to 30% for patients undergoing major aortic reconstruction; it has decreased to <3% today.

The reasons for this impressive reduction in the death rate are multifactorial. Refined surgical techniques and graft materials, better preoperative assessment, more thoughtful selection of patients and perioperative care, improved monitoring techniques, and better anesthetics have had an important role.[1] In addition, an improved understanding of the pathologic homeostatic mechanisms that are operative in patients suffering from vascular disease has been critical.

The discussion here is limited to those issues directly related to the anesthetic care of patients undergoing major vascular operations. Preoperative, intraoperative, and postoperative concerns are discussed with special emphasis on the care of patients scheduled for repair of thoracoabdominal aortic aneurysms, abdominal aortic aneurysms, and aortoiliac occlusive disease.

AORTIC DISEASE

Major disease processes that damage the aorta are atherosclerosis, medial degeneration, aortitis, and trauma. These entities, in turn, render the aorta susceptible to additional disease processes, such as formation of aneurysms, medial dissection, and aorto-occlusive disease. Certain areas of the aorta may be especially sensitive to a particular form of injury. For example, dissection is most likely to occur in the ascending aorta because the shear forces from blood flow are greatest here, whereas aneurysmal formation is most likely to occur in the infrarenal abdominal aorta.

What Is Atherosclerosis?

Natural History and Evolution

Arteriosclerosis is a generic term that indicates thickening and hardening of the arterial wall. One form of arteriosclerosis is *atherosclerosis*. This process involves larger vessels such as the aorta, coronary arteries, carotid arteries, and the major arteries of the lower extremities. Atherosclerosis is a disease that initially attacks the intima but later in its natural history also involves the underlying media. It is by far the most common cause of aortic disease and death in the United States and is present to some extent in virtually every American.

Intimal deposits of lipid and fatty streaks are typically found in children younger than 10 years. By the time young adulthood has been reached, these lesions have progressed to elevated gray-yellow intimal plaques containing soft, lipid-rich material. During later years, hemorrhage into the plaque occurs, followed by calcification, ulceration, and superimposed thrombus formation.[2] These events complete a typical atherosclerotic lesion. The media underlying severely affected segments of intima may weaken, and the process of aneurysmal formation or predisposition to dissection commences (Fig. 69–1).

Risk Factors

Certain behavioral and metabolic risk factors are independent predictors of significant atherosclerotic development. Hypertension, fatty diet, male sex, diabetes mellitus, smoking, and hyperlipidemias dramatically increase the incidence and severity.[3] Data implicating a sedentary lifestyle, aggressive personality (type A behavior), and alcohol consumption are less clear.

Progressive atherosclerosis produces luminal narrowing of blood vessels, damage to the vessel wall, thrombosis, and ultimately aneurysm formation, dissection, or occlusion. Aortic atherosclerosis typically is most severe at the terminal end of the abdominal aorta and may extend into the iliac arteries (i.e., aortoiliac disease). Because the majority of aneurysms

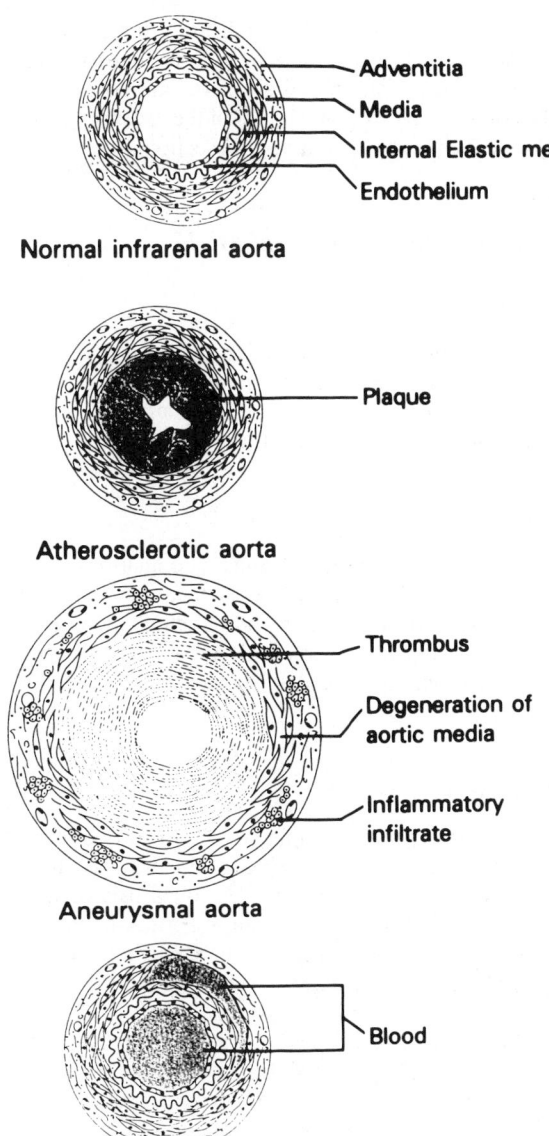

FIGURE 69–1. Schematic representation of the normal aorta with its three distinct layers: the intima, the media, and the adventitia. Atherosclerosis results in intimal thickening secondary to the formation of plaque. An aneurysm is a dilation of an artery with degeneration of the media. The inner lining is a layer of thrombus. Aortic dissection results from an intimal tear and a consequent plane of blood cleaving the media. (From Tilson MD III, Brophy CM: Pathogenesis of aneurysms. *In* Surgery: Scientific Principles and Practice. Greenfield, et al (eds). Philadelphia, JB Lippincott, 1993, p 1676.)

require atherosclerotic lesions as a nidus for their growth, the incidence of aortic disease cannot be expected to decrease significantly unless the incidence of atherosclerosis is reduced. Sadly, despite intensive public education about proper diet and exercise, the incidence of abdominal aortic aneurysms in population-based studies has increased 11-fold since 1951.[4] Part of this increase, however, can be attributed to prolonged life expectancy and improved methods of aneurysm detection. Anesthesiologists will continue to treat these patients into the foreseeable future.

How Do Aortic Aneurysms and Dissections Differ?

Aneurysms

A true aortic aneurysm is defined as an abnormal widening with a minimum 50% increase of all layers (i.e., tunica intima, media, adventitia) of the vessel wall.[5] The most common cause of aortic aneurysms is hypertension-induced arteriosclerosis or degenerative disease of the aortic wall. The second most common defect predisposing to aneurysm formation is chronic aortic dissection. In this situation, the basic defect lies in the media. Destruction of elastin fibers causes an abnormal dilatation of the remaining fibrous tissue. The resultant increase in vessel diameter directly increases wall tension (Laplace's law). As the aneurysm becomes progressively larger, the tension correspondingly rises, the risk of encroachment on other organs increases, and rupture becomes more likely.

Dissections

Unlike aortic aneurysm formation, which is a *chronic* process unless rupture or leakage occurs, aortic dissection is the most important *acute* disease. Acute dissections of the thoracic portion are frequent, lethal aortic catastrophes, occurring twice as often as ruptured abdominal aortic aneurysms. Acute dissections of the ascending aorta are true emergencies, with a mortality rate of 1% to 2% per hour during the first 48 hours. A dissection is termed *chronic* when it is has been present for at least 14 days.

Pathogenesis

The underlying lesion in all cases of dissection is a disruption of the intimal layer by excessive hemodynamic shear forces that ultimately cause medial dissection. Stretching of the aorta increases its diameter, in turn placing supranormal levels of stress on the aortic vessel wall. Hypertension or evidence thereof is found in approximately 80% of patients.

Additional disease processes such as cystic medial necrosis, found in Marfan's syndrome, are a common precursor to this initial stress. A true dissection is characterized by separation of layers of the media wall by a column of circulating blood that creates a *false lumen.* The false lumen can easily occlude 50% to 75% of the true luminal cross-sectional area. External rupture is the most frequent cause of death. The rupture tends to occur through the false lumen opposite to the intimal tear.

Note that a dissection of the aorta is not an aneurysm. The term *dissecting aneurysm* is best reserved for a chronic aortic dissection with aneurysmal dilatation of a false lumen. Medial dissection most commonly occurs in the fifth to seventh decade of life and occurs twice as often in men as in women. It is also associated with coarctation of the aorta, bicuspid aortic valve, and Marfan's syndrome.

What Are Fusiform and Saccular Aneurysms?

The morphology of an aneurysm is related to the risk of rupture. A fusiform aneurysm is a spindle-shaped dilatation that symmetrically encompasses the circumference of the aorta. A saccular aneurysm is a pouchlike dilatation that begins at a narrow neck (i.e., a protruding segment from the aortic wall). The large majority of aneurysms, particularly abdominal aortic aneurysms caused by atherosclerosis, are fusiform. Many aneurysms are not pure examples of either type.

Saccular aneurysms have a higher rate of rupture and may be treated surgically regardless of size. On the other hand, the type of aneurysm may influence the surgical approach and the consequent hemodynamic changes associated with repair. If the aneurysm is saccular and the diameter is less than half the circumference of the aorta, a surgeon may be able to repair it by using a partial aortic cross-clamp technique. This factor is important, particularly for a thoracic aortic aneurysm, because the hemodynamic effects of partial aortic cross-clamping are significantly reduced compared with complete occlusion.

What Areas Are Particularly Sensitive to Shearing Injury?

The aortic root and the area just distal to the takeoff of the left subclavian artery (aortic isthmus) are most sensitive to shearing injuries (Fig. 69–2). Because the aortic arch is secured by the great arteries, aortic root, and ligamentum arteriosum, and the descending aorta is relatively free of attachment, sudden anteroposterior deceleration can rupture the aortic segment at the isthmus. Indeed, the isthmus (the area of the aorta just distal to the ligamentum arteriosum) is the most common site of traumatic aortic disruption.[6] Similarly, each cardiac

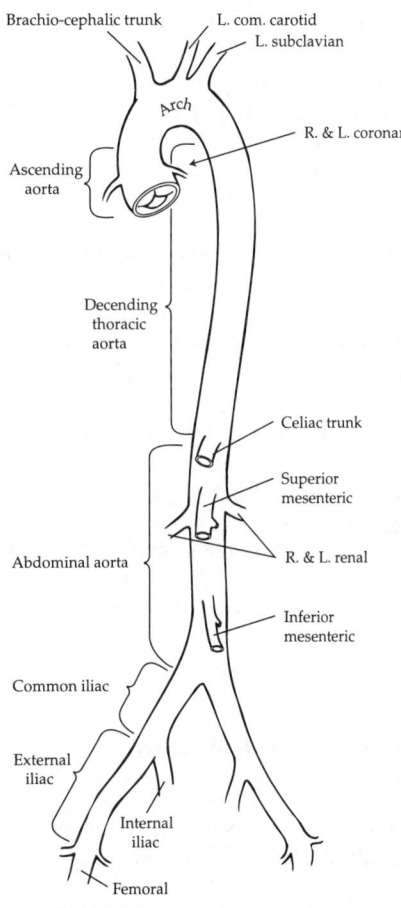

FIGURE 69–2. Anatomy of the aorta.

contraction produces a systolic thrust (shearing force) that can produce or aggravate intimal injury. Thus, standard management is to reduce heart rate, blood pressure, and contractility. Because the force intensity is maximum in the ascending aorta, this is the most common site of aortic dissection.

How Are These Disorders Diagnosed?

Diagnostic Imaging

An aortic dissection or aneurysm can be *suspected* on the basis of a history and physical examination. However, only radiographic studies can lead to a definitive diagnosis. A wide variety of techniques have been used for this purpose.

Chest Radiographs

Chest radiographs are useful screening examinations.[7] Findings are abnormal in 80% of patients with dissection of the thoracic aorta. The most common radiographic findings are widening of the mediastinum, tracheal deviation to the right, blurring of aortic contours, and displacement of intimal calcifications.

Echocardiography

Echocardiography often is the diagnostic modality of choice (Table 69–1). It is particularly valuable for diagnosis of dissection or aneurysm of the aortic root. The diagnosis of aortic dissection requires demonstration of an abnormal linear echo (i.e., the intimal flap) in the aortic lumen. Transthoracic echocardiography alone is not sufficient because the entire thoracic aorta cannot be visualized in approximately one third of patients; therefore, it is combined with transesophageal examination. Biplane and omniplane probes are especially effective for evaluating extension into the aortic arch vessels.[8]

Computed Tomography

Contrast-enhanced computed tomographic (CT) scanning is highly accurate. However, because angiographic studies may be required for definitive diagnosis of dissection, the requirement for contrast in CT studies to demonstrate the intimal flap makes this diagnostic modality less attractive in the initial evaluation.

Aortography

Although aortography has long been considered the gold standard for diagnosing aortic dissections and still remains the most accurate method, newer diagnostic modalities have supplanted its routine use. Aortography is a valuable tool with which to plan the approach to surgical repair. It clearly identifies associated visceral artery obstruction or stenosis and the presence and location of accessory renal arteries.

Angiographic diagnosis of aortic dissection is based on demonstrating an intimal flap separating the true and false lumina. In aortic aneurysms, aortography only shows the luminal size of the aneurysm and cannot be relied on to determine its overall size.

None of these modalities provides all of the information

TABLE 69–1. Diagnosis Using Transesophageal Echocardiography, Computed Tomography, and Aortography in Patients with Aortic Dissection

Results for Patient Groups		Transesophageal Echocardiography (%)	Computed Tomography (%)	Angiography (%)
Surgery/autopsy	Sensitivity	98	77	89
	Specificity	88	100	87
	Positive predictive accuracy	97	100	96
	Negative predictable accuracy	93	33	68
Without surgery	Sensitivity	100	93	95
	Specificity	100	100	97
	Positive predictive accuracy	100	100	94
	Negative predictive accuracy	100	98	92
Total study group	Sensitivity	99	83	88
	Specificity	98	100	94
	Positive predictive accuracy	98	100	96
	Negative predictive accuracy	99	86	84

(From Rennollet R, Engberding R, Visser CA, et al: Transesophageal imaging of the thoracic aorta in aortic dissection. *In* Transesophageal Echocardiography. A New Window to the Heart. Erbel R, Khandheria BK, Brennecke R, et al (eds): Berlin, Springer-Verlag, 1989, p 140.)

needed to formulate rational therapy. Hemodynamically unstable patients with aortic dissection diagnosed by echocardiography probably are best served by transport to the operating room (or) without additional diagnostic studies.

What Is the Distribution?

Aneurysms

Seventy-five per cent of all aortic aneurysms are located in the infrarenal abdominal aortic area. The approximate location of thoracic aneurysms is as follows: ascending aorta, 25%; aortic arch, 30%; descending thoracic aorta, 45%.[9]

Dissections

The vast majority of all aortic intimal tears are located in the thoracic aorta. The site of the primary tear in aortic dissection is as follows: ascending aorta, 70%; aortic arch, 8%; aortic isthmus and descending thoracic aorta, 21%; abdominal aorta, 1%.[10]

Why Is Laplace's Law Relevant?

Laplace's law directly relates wall tension to internal pressure and radius according to the following equation:

$$T = \frac{P \times R}{\delta}$$

Equation 1

where T, P, R and δ denote the circumferential wall tension, internal pressure, internal radius, and wall thickness, respectively. An increase in arterial blood pressure and aneurysm size increases wall tension and the risk of rupture. The thickness of the aneurysmal wall, however, varies inversely with wall tension; thinner aneurysms are more likely to rupture than thicker ones. Rupture occurs when the circumferential wall tension exceeds the wall tensile strength. The relationships described in this equation have been confirmed by clinical findings.[11] Hypertension and large aneurysm sizes are definite risk factors for rupture.

The diameter of a normal aorta is 2.5 to 3 cm. This large conducting blood vessel must withstand tremendous shearing forces with each systolic thrust. Because the aorta has the largest diameter of any blood vessel in the body, it also must endure the greatest wall stress of any vessel.

What Coexisting Diseases Are Common?

Atherosclerotic vascular disease is protean in manifestations and can involve virtually every organ system. Patients who undergo major vascular surgery are often elderly and have multiorgan dysfunction (e.g., cardiac, brain, renal, or pulmonary disease) (Table 69–2). A substantial number of these patients have a greater than 100 pack-year smoking history that is associated with atherogenesis and chronic obstructive lung disease (COLD). However, the most frequently and significantly involved organ is the heart. Hertzer and colleagues, in their landmark study, showed that only 8% of patients undergoing vascular surgery had normal coronary arteries as determined by angiography.[12] Thirty-one per cent (25% correctable and 6% inoperable) had severe coronary artery disease.

What Are the Major Causes of Perioperative Morbidity and Mortality?

Hollier found that the dominant primary risk factors for morbidity and mortality in 100 patients scheduled for abdom-

TABLE 69–2. Prevalence of Coexisting Disease in Patients Scheduled for Vascular Surgery

Hypertension	40–60%
Heart disease	50–70%
Angina	10–20%
Previous myocardial infarction	40–60%
Congestive heart failure	5–15%
Diabetes mellitus	8–12%
Chronic obstructive lung disease	25–50%
Renal disease	5–25%

(Adapted from Clark NJ, Stanley TH: Anesthesia for vascular surgery. *In* Anesthesia. 3rd ed. Miller RD (ed). New York, Churchill Livingstone, 1990, p 1694.)

inal aortic aneurysmectomy were cardiac (47%), pulmonary (31%), age >85 years (17%), renal failure (2%), retroperitoneal fibrosis (2%), and cirrhosis with ascites (1%).[13] Although morbid obesity, stroke with residual hemiplegia, and multiple previous abdominal operations added some operative risk, these problems were not sufficient to place patients in the high-risk category.[13] Thus, a preoperative assessment that emphasizes evaluation of cardiac function is appropriate. The second most common cause of death is postoperative renal failure, except in patients undergoing carotid endarterectomy, in whom the second most common cause of death is stroke.

How Are Specific Risks Managed?

An aneurysm of the aorta is a potentially lethal disease. The repair of major vascular disease such as abdominal aortic aneurysms prolongs life expectancy and improves its quality.[14] As a result, most vascular surgeons believe that even high-risk patients with asymptomatic aneurysms should undergo elective aneurysmorrhaphy. Nearly one in three high-risk patients dies of aneurysmal rupture without elective repair. Selection of patients for repair should be relatively liberal, with very few absolute contraindications. Nevertheless, a thorough preoperative assessment that recognizes those patients at increased risk, along with optimal medical treatment preoperatively, can lessen morbidity and mortality.

Cardiac Disease

Coronary arterial disease is the single most important risk factor in patients scheduled for aortic surgery. A history of congestive heart failure (CHF), particularly if it is recurrent despite medical treatment; an ejection fraction <30%; prior myocardial infarction, especially within the past 6 months; angina; or abnormal findings on an electrocardiogram (ECG) are important risk factors and are associated with a threefold increase in operative mortality.[15] Patients with class 3 or 4 angina should undergo coronary angiography to stratify their risk and assess their suitability for aortocoronary bypass before aneurysm resection. Aortocoronary bypass before resection lowers the mortality rate.[16] Even in those patients who are not suitable candidates for coronary revascularization, knowledge of myocardial function and the extent and location of coronary disease can help the anesthesiologist plan the anesthetic technique.

Hemodynamic Monitoring

The type of hemodynamic monitoring used during aortic vascular surgery is dependent on the type of operation (location of aortic disease) and the degree of pre-existing left ventricular dysfunction (group 1 versus group 2 patients (Table 69–3). In all major vascular operations, arterial blood pressure should be measured directly. Cannulation of an artery provides beat-to-beat arterial pressure readings and allows easy access to arterial blood for analyses.

At a minimum, central venous pressure (CVP) should be measured in all patients undergoing abdominal aortic aneurysmorrhaphy or bypass procedures. If a patient has poor left ventricular function (i.e., a group 2 patient), I insert a pulmonary artery catheter and often use transesophageal echocardiography (TEE) during operations on the abdominal aorta. For

TABLE 69–3. Classification of Left Ventricular Function in Patients with Atherosclerotic Heart Disease

Group 1: Well-Preserved Left Ventricular Function in the Presence of Coronary Artery Disease	Group 2: Poor Left Ventricular Function in the Presence of Coronary Artery Disease
• Occult coronary artery disease	• Overt coronary artery disease
• No historical, physical, laboratory, or hemodynamic evidence of heart disease	• Historical, physical, laboratory, or hemodynamic evidence of heart disease
• Ejection fraction >0.55–0.60	• Ejection fraction <0.40
• Cardiac index >2.5 L · min · m$^{2-1}$	• Cardiac index <2.0 L · min · m$^{2-1}$
• No prior history of myocardial infarction	• History of myocardial infarction(s)
• Normal ventricular wall motion	• Global hypokinesis and/or dyskinetic wall motion abnormalities
• Pulmonary capillary wedge pressures <12 mm Hg	• Pulmonary capillary wedge pressures >15–18 mm Hg

(Adapted from Attia RR, Murphy JD, Snider M, et al: Myocardial ischemia due to infrarenal aortic cross-clamping during aortic surgery in patients with severe coronary artery disease. Circulation 1976; 53:961.)

operations on the thoracic aorta (thoracic dissection or thoracoabdominal aortic aneurysm repair), hemodynamic monitoring includes an arterial catheter located in the right upper extremity, a pulmonary artery catheter, and TEE.

Pulmonary Disease

A forced expired volume in 1 second (FEV$_1$) <1 L, dyspnea at rest, or an oxygen (O$_2$) partial pressure (PaO$_2$) <50 mm Hg when a patient breathes room air indicates severe pulmonary insufficiency. These factors, alone or in combination, identify those patients at highest risk for perioperative pulmonary complications. The majority of patients with COLD can safely undergo operation if aggressive perioperative pulmonary toilet therapy is provided. I initiate bronchodilator and oral antibiotic therapy (if indicated) 2 days before the scheduled operation.

Patients with severe preoperative pulmonary dysfunction may benefit from postoperative epidural analgesia. This treatment perhaps minimizes the morbidity and mortality associated with postoperative pulmonary complications by allowing earlier ambulation, deep breathing, and coughing.

Smoking

Although many physicians advocate the cessation of smoking 2 to 3 weeks in advance of the operation, this recommendation may be potentially deleterious to patients who smoke heavily and is unlikely to be of much help. The majority of these patients are addicted to nicotine. To discontinue this habit suddenly may be counterproductive. Because only 8% of patients with aneurysm have normal coronary arteries, myocardial ischemia may actually be increased by the stress of acute discontinuation of smoking.

Renal Disease

Patients undergoing aortic vascular surgery are predisposed to postoperative renal dysfunction. In addition to the operative insult, renal vessels frequently show extensive atherosclerosis

TABLE 69–4. Anatomic Divisions of the Aorta

Aortic Division	Mediastinal Division	Anatomic Origin	Anatomic Termination
Ascending aorta	Middle	Aortic valve	Innominate artery (T-4)
Aortic arch	Superior	Innominate artery (T-4)	Ligamentum arteriosum (T-4)
Descending aorta	Posterior	Ligamentum arteriosum (T-4)	Diaphragm (T-12)
Abdominal aorta	—	Diaphragm (T-12)	Common iliac arteries (L-4)

Parentheses indicate the corresponding vertebral level of the anatomic structure.

or may be directly involved with the aneurysmal/dissection process. Patients with creatinine values >3 mg · dL⁻¹ or a creatinine clearance <20 mL · min⁻¹ are particularly at risk. Many of these patients receive contrast material for angiographic studies and may suffer nephrotoxicity on this basis. Although hydration can ameliorate the contrast effects, elective surgery probably should be delayed 48 hours after the dye load. For those patients who develop contrast-induced renal failure, elective surgery should be delayed 2 weeks.[13]

Prophylaxis

To minimize the incidence of perioperative renal failure, especially with suprarenal aortic cross-clamping, liberal hydration (preservation of adequate intravascular volume) and the avoidance of hypotension are the most important factors. I routinely administer mannitol (0.5–0.75 g · kg⁻¹) at least 30 minutes before aortic cross-clamping. In addition, administration of dopamine (at approximately 2 μg · kg⁻¹ · min⁻¹) is considered in two situations: (1) if pre-existing renal disease (creatinine level >2 mg · dL⁻¹) is present and (2) for those operations in which renal blood flow is reduced the most (i.e., supraceliac and suprarenal aortic cross-clamping).

Advanced Age

Advanced age (i.e., >80 y) is not a contraindication to major vascular surgery. The once widespread belief that such a patient is too old and at too great a risk to be operated on is being invalidated. Surgeons now routinely perform aortic surgery on octogenarians, with excellent results.[17]

ANATOMIC CONSIDERATIONS

The thoracic and abdominal divisions are the major components of the aorta (see Fig. 69–2). The thoracic division is confined entirely within the mediastinum, and the abdominal division starts at the level of the diaphragm and bifurcates at vertebral level T-4 into the common iliac arteries (Table 69–4). The thoracic aorta is subdivided into the ascending aorta, aortic arch, and descending aorta.

How Are Aortic Dissections Classified?

Multiple classifications systems based on the location of the dissection have been proposed. However, DeBakey's[18] and

Dailey's (or Stanford)[19] classifications are most commonly used.[18, 19] These are listed in Table 69–5 and illustrated in Figures 69–3 and 69–4. Involvement of the ascending aorta is the single most important predictor of clinical outcome. Neither the exact site of intimal dissection nor the extent of distal extension of the dissection significantly influences subsequent clinical presentation. Types I, II, and A indicate involvement of the ascending aorta, and types III and B denote dissections starting at the aortic isthmus and not involving the ascending aorta (see Table 69–5). Although a type B dissection may be restricted to the thoracic aorta, it usually extends into the abdominal aorta. In contrast to type A dissections, type B dissections have no retrograde component.

When Are Aneurysms and Dissections Repaired?

Abdominal Aneurysms

Abdominal aortic aneurysms of any size are repaired if they are symptomatic or rapidly growing; early rupture of these aneurysms is the rule. If an aneurysmal diameter is ≥5 cm, it is repaired promptly even if asymptomatic; at this diameter, the mortality rate from rupture equals or exceeds the operative mortality.

Risk of Rupture

The rationale for operating on aneurysms ≥5 cm in diameter is based on the following line of reasoning: If left untreated, the yearly risk of rupture is about 10% for aneurysms that are 5 cm in diameter and almost 40% for aneurysms that are 7 cm in diameter.[20] A sharp rise in the rate of aneurysmal rupture occurs at a diameter of 6 cm. Autopsy studies show that rupture occurs in 60% of aneurysms >10.1 cm in diameter, 45% of aneurysms between 7.1 and 10 cm in diameter, 25% of aneurysms between 4.1 and 7 cm in diameter, and 8% of aneurysms <4 cm in diameter. Hence, even the 6-cm value should not be taken as an absolute minimum indication for surgery.[21] Clearly, even small anuerysms can rupture at any time. The rate of aneurysmal expansion is approximately 0.4 cm · y⁻¹.[11]

Mortality Rates

The mortality rate for elective aortic aneurysmal resection is about 3%[13] and for emergency repair of a ruptured abdominal aortic aneurysm ranges from 15% to 78% (average of about 50%).[22] The most common judgmental error associated with mortality of ruptured abdominal aortic aneurysms is fail-

TABLE 69–5. Classification of Aortic Dissections

DeBakey's Classification (Modified Form)

Type I	Dissection starts in the ascending aorta and involves entire length of aorta
Type II	Dissection limited to the ascending aorta
Type III	Dissection starts distal to the left subclavian artery but spares the ascending aorta and aortic arch

Dailey's Classification (Stanford Classification)

Type A	Dissection involves any portion of the ascending aorta
Type B	Dissection starts distal to the left subclavian artery

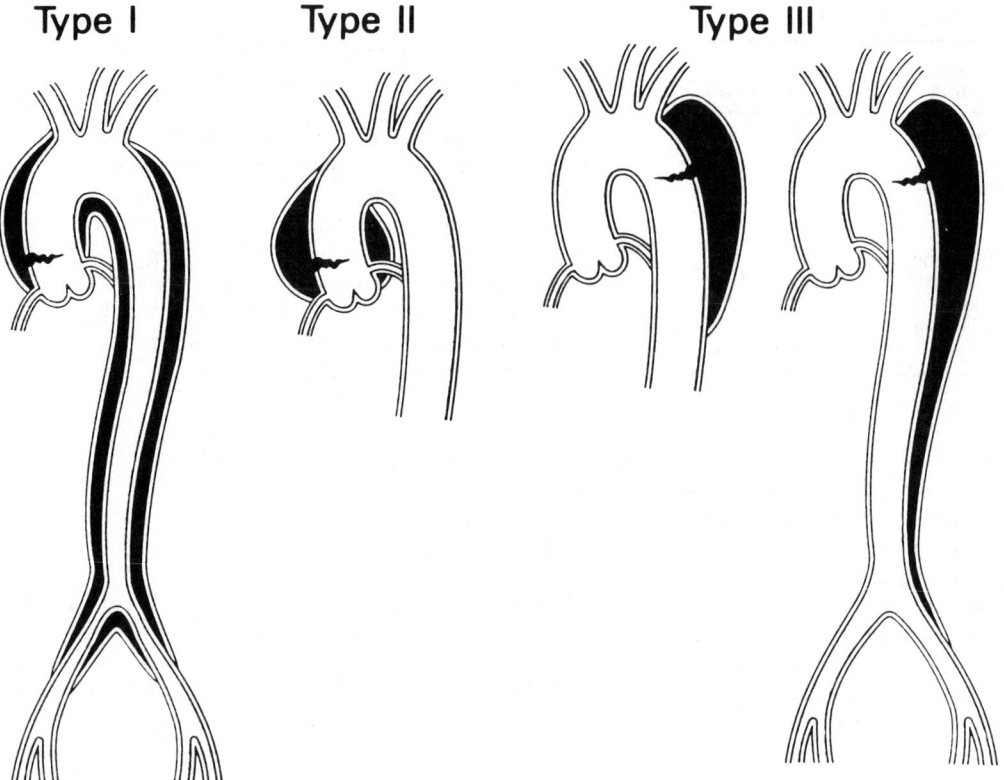

Type I   **Type II**   **Type III**

FIGURE 69–3. DeBakey's classification of aortic dissections. (Adapted from DeBakey ME, McCollum CH, Crawford ES, et al: Dissection and dissecting aneurysms of the aorta: twenty-year follow-up of five hundred twenty-seven patients treated surgically. Surgery 1982; 92:1118.)

ure to repair the aneurysm electively. Some surgeons believe that the benefit-risk ratio is so favorable with elective aneurysmectomy that they advocate surgical repair of abdominal aortic aneurysms ≥4 cm in diameter.[13]

Others advocate serial ultrasonographic studies to monitor the size of aneurysms <5 cm in diameter. The rationale behind this recommendation is that the risk of rupture for an aneurysm <5 cm approximates the 3% to 5% surgical mortality. Given the lack of predictability of aneurysmal rupture, this approach may not be a prudent option for patients who live where 24-hour in-house coverage by anesthesiologists and surgeons is

not available. For these patients, elective repair probably is suitable regardless of size. The *presence*, not the *size*, is the important consideration.

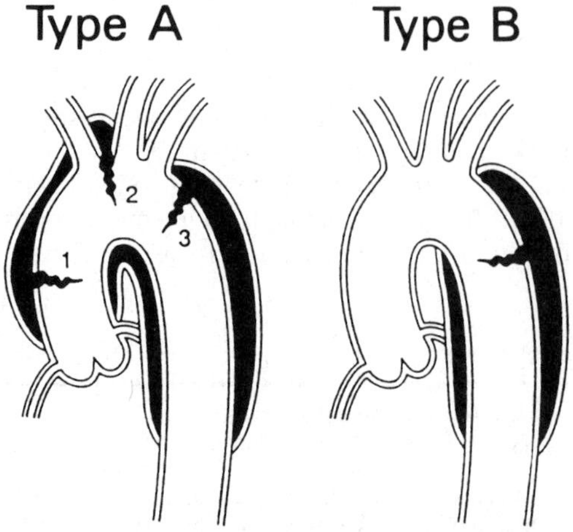

Thoracoabdominal Aneurysms

Large thoracoabdominal aortic aneurysms in low-risk patients should be surgically repaired. Elective repair is generally indicated when the diameter of the aneurysm is at least twice the diameter of the uninvolved or predicted aortic diameter (6–7 cm). In higher-risk patients with associated medical diseases, elective repair should be delayed unless predicted life expectancy exceeds 2 years. In those patients with prohibitive risks, repair is not indicated until complications of the aneurysm mandate surgical intervention.

Aortic Dissections

With regard to acute aortic dissections, initial treatment depends on the location of the dissection (type A versus type B) (see Table 69–5) and a patient's symptoms.[23–25] Dissections that begin in the ascending aorta are the most lethal (e.g., extend retrograde into the intracardiac portion of the aorta causing cardiac tamponade, acute aortic insufficiency, or coronary artery occlusion). Thus, all patients with type A dissection are surgical candidates, except possibly those with evolving central nervous system (CNS) signs. Heparinization that is necessary to initiate cardiopulmonary bypass required for repair of type A dissections, followed by restoration of normal or increased blood flow to the brain, can produce massive intracranial hemorrhage in patients with pre-existing ischemic stroke. Nevertheless, no absolute contraindications to surgical repair of acute type A aortic dissections exist. The appropriate-

Type A   **Type B**

FIGURE 69–4. Dailey's (Stanford's) classification of aortic dissections. Numbers indicate potential locations of the site of primary intimal tear. (Adapted with permission from Miller DC, Stinson EB, Oyer PE, et al: Operative treatment of aortic dissections: experience with 125 patients over a sixteen-year period. J Thorac Cardiovasc Surg 1979; 78:365.)

ness of surgical intervention must be considered for each patient.

In contrast, type B dissections do not require urgent or early operation and are best treated medically unless they are complicated. The latter dissections show evidence of vascular obstruction, compromise of a major aortic branch, or continued expansion of the dissection despite intensive medical therapy (e.g., pain relief and blood pressure control using β-adrenergic blockers and sodium nitroprusside [SNP]). Because the mortality rate for surgical repair of uncomplicated type B dissections is greater than the mortality rate of medical therapy, surgical intervention should be temporized.

ANESTHESIA FOR CENTRAL AORTIC SURGERY

Is a Documented Preferred Technique Available?

No single *best* anesthetic technique exists. Anesthetic technique, per se, probably is not a key factor in a patient's outcome. The surgeon's skill and speed and the anesthesiologist's ability to maintain homeostasis during the physiologically stressful perioperative period are key elements to success. Major anesthetic goals during vascular surgery are outlined in Table 69–6.

The anesthesiologist must attempt to preserve the integrity and function of the myocardium, brain, kidneys, lungs, and visceral systems. Some investigators have concluded that dextrose-containing solutions worsen neurologic outcome.[26, 27] Because glucose supplementation is rarely necessary in adults patients anyway, I routinely avoid these solutions during major vascular surgery. Experimental evidence suggests that insulin protects the spinal cord from ischemic injury.[28] For this reason, treatment of glucose levels >200 mg · dL^{-1} with low-dose insulin may be prudent.

The anesthetic technique and extent of hemodynamic monitoring are best determined by the location of the aortic cross-clamp and the degree of preoperative left ventricular dysfunction, both of which were discussed earlier. Other factors such as preoperative renal function and pulmonary status play a part, but not to the same extent.

Left Ventricular Function

As illustrated in Table 69–3, patients undergoing major vascular operations are divided into two groups.[29] Group 1 consists of patients with "well-preserved" or normal left ventricular function, whereas patients in group 2 have poor left ventricular function.

TABLE 69–6. Major Anesthetic Goals During Vascular Surgery

- Maintain stable cardiodynamics by aggressive hemodynamic monitoring and judicious use of vasoactive drugs.
- Maintain adequate urine output by proper hydration and the use of mannitol and/or dopamine (particularly for thoracic and suprarenal aortic cross-clamping).
- Maintain adequate oxygen-carrying capacity by using volume replacement and blood products.
- Maintain body temperature.
- Maintain acid-base status.

The exact anesthetic plan is of less concern to group 1 patients, who generally can tolerate primarily volatile-based anesthesia. I am reluctant to use this technique with group 2 patients. Volatile anesthetics in vitro produce a state of uncompensated CHF (i.e., they profoundly depress myocardial contractile function). However, this impairment of contractility (and hence cardiac function) is offset by a reflex increase in medullary sympathetic tone. Patients exhibiting severe cardiac dysfunction (i.e., borderline CHF) may not be able to compensate. A balanced technique consisting of narcotics, muscle paralysis, and isoflurane at low end-tidal concentrations (approximately 0.5%) is preferred for patients in groups 1 and 2.

Isoflurane and Coronary Steal

Isoflurane, more than halothane or enflurane, is a potent dilator of resistance vessels located within the myocardial wall and is associated with *coronary steal* in animal models.[30–32] Application of these findings to humans remains controversial. Although some investigators have demonstrated an isoflurane-induced coronary steal phenomenon in humans, even in the absence of significant hemodynamic changes, others have found no clinically significant effect.[33–36] At higher concentrations, isoflurane appears to attenuate autoregulation of myocardial blood flow, produce a functional uncoupling of cardiac perfusion to metabolism, and worsen myocardial ischemia in a dose-dependent fashion. However, at concentrations <0.75%, its effect on autoregulation of myocardial blood flow is not apparent.[34]

In order for patients to be susceptible to coronary steal, a specific anatomic arrangement of coronary occlusion, collateral vessels, and stenosis of the artery supplying the vessels is required.[37] Buffington and colleagues showed that 23% of 16,249 patients in the Coronary Artery Surgery Study (CASS) Registry had steal-prone coronary anatomy.[37] Opinions vary widely on the appropriateness of isoflurane in patients with coronary arterial disease. Although Becker stated that "isoflurane may be dangerous" in these patients, Tinker disagrees.[38, 39] Pending a large prospective study, this question may never be answered conclusively.

Narcotic-Based Techniques

In a number of investigations, a narcotic-based anesthetic technique (e.g., sufentanil or fentanyl) was associated with a lower incidence of postoperative myocardial and renal morbidity following aortic vascular surgery than was a volatile agent, nitrous oxide–based technique.[34, 40] A potential drawback to high-dose narcotic anesthesia is prolonged postoperative ventilator dependence. Because aortic vascular surgery is a stressful event associated with the sometimes massive administration of fluids and blood, this *drawback* is often beneficial. Fluid given intraoperatively can be mobilized, and hypothermia that may have developed can be slowly corrected without shivering. Narcotics alone often are not effective in attenuating the hypertension and tachycardia associated with major vascular surgery. Volatile anesthetics, nitrous oxide, vasodilators (nitroglycerin and SNP), adrenergic blockers (esmolol, labetalol, or propranolol), and benzodiazepines (midazolam) can be useful adjuncts.

What Are the Management Guidelines for Thoracoabdominal Aortic Aneurysms?

Preoperative Assessment and Planning

To optimize the surgical outcome of these patients, a number of anesthetic- and institution-related resources must be in place and functioning efficiently during the preoperative and intraoperative phases. A benefit-risk assessment must be made for every patient.

Consultation

To evaluate these high-risk surgical patients comprehensively, good communication between the anesthesiologist, vascular surgeon, and other medical specialists (e.g., cardiologist, nephrologist, and pulmonologist) is essential. Through these discussions, a patient's risks during the procedure can be stratified, medical therapy can be optimized, and a decision about the advisability of operation can be rendered.

A thorough medical work-up that emphasizes examination of those organ systems most often targeted by or associated with atherosclerotic disease (e.g., cardiovascular, pulmonary, renal, CNS) is necessary to detect end-organ vascular disease.

Blood and Blood Products

Preoperatively, all patients scheduled for elective aortic repairs are encouraged to donate autologous blood if their medical condition permits. A blood bank that promptly provides large quantities of blood products, a pathology laboratory that reliably performs immediate chemistry studies, and a cell-saver team that keeps pace and immediately provides washed salvaged blood are key components in a favorable outcome.

With regard to anesthetic care, the following general guidelines apply: (1) insertion of large-bore intravenous access catheters (a minimum of two large peripheral venous catheters), (2) use of comprehensive hemodynamic monitoring (e.g., right arm arterial catheter, pulmonary artery catheter, and possibly TEE), and (3) use of one-lung ventilation (see Chapter 68).

One-Lung Ventilation

One-lung ventilation should be used in the repair of thoracoabdominal aortic aneurysms. It dramatically improves surgical exposure, prevents traction on the left lung, and averts potential contamination of the contralateral lung. Thus, placement of a double-lumen endotracheal tube, usually on the left side, is a high priority under general anesthesia.

Because this aneurysm often encroaches on the left mainstem bronchus, great care must be exercised not to rupture it during endobronchial tube placement. Preoperative diagnostic imaging studies can be of great assistance in localization. Many aneurysms are friable, and even gentle impingement may produce a catastrophic event. For this reason, the bronchial tip is inserted into the trachea and the tube initially used as though it contained a single lumen. Fiberoptic bronchoscopic visualization is then used to rule out encroachment of the left mainstem bronchus by the aneurysm. The bronchial tip is then advanced into the left mainstem bronchus, and the cuff inflated under direct vision.

Left-Sided Versus Right-Sided Tubes

Despite the potential problem of aneurysmal rupture associated with left-sided double-lumen endotracheal tubes, they are believed to be preferable to right-sided tubes. Although the risk of rupture probably is reduced with a right-sided tube, the likelihood of dislodging the tip or blocking the right upper lobe bronchus during surgery is high. In this complex operation, loss of surgical exposure during the critical period of cross-clamping may be disastrous. A right-sided double lumen endotracheal tube is resorted to only if a left-sided tube cannot be safely or easily placed. Alternatively, a bronchial blocker can be used to provide one-lung anesthesia. However, only a double-lumen tube can be used for *differential* lung ventilation.

Oxygenation

One-lung ventilation impairs the lungs' ability to oxygenate blood. Severe hypoxemia is common in patients with marginal preoperative pulmonary function. Most operations that use this technique are performed in patients who have pre-existing lung disease and who require lateral decubitus positioning. Such positioning is associated with reductions in functional residual capacity (FRC), altered lung compliance, loss of active diaphragmatic movement, and suboptimal positioning with rolls and packings, all of which can produce ventilation/perfusion ($\dot{V}A/\dot{Q}$) mismatch.

Hypoxic Pulmonary Vasoconstriction

With one-lung ventilation, pulmonary blood flow to the nondependent, nonventilated *(up)* lung constitutes an obligatory right-to-left transpulmonary shunt. Hypoxic pulmonary vasoconstriction (HPV) causes a rise in pulmonary vascular resistance (PVR) in the nondependent lung that typically decreases pulmonary blood flow by 50% (from 40% of total flow during two-lung ventilation to 20% of total flow during one-lung ventilation).

Although intravenous anesthetic agents (narcotics, barbiturates, and benzodiazepines) do not alter HPV, volatile anesthetics appear to cause dose-dependent reductions. Potent vasodilators such as SNP, nitroglycerin, calcium channel blockers, and minoxidil also attenuate HPV.[41, 42] If hypoxemia occurs during one-lung ventilation and the patient is hemodynamically stable, the protocol outlined in Table 69–7 should be initiated. (See also Table 68–2 and Fig. 68–4.)

The most important single step in correcting hypoxemia is the use of continuous positive airway pressure (CPAP) in the nonventilated lung.[43] This approach corrects the majority of

TABLE 69–7. Diagnostic and Therapeutic Protocol for Hypoxemia Occurring During One-Lung Ventilation

1. Check ventilation using 100% inspired O_2; keep tidal volumes $\geq$ 20 mL · kg^{-1}.
2. Confirm position of the double-lumen tube with fiberoptic bronchoscopy.
3. Add nondependent lung continuous positive airway pressure with 100% O_2 at 5–10 cm H_2).
4. Add dependent lung positive end-expiratory pressure at 5–10 cm H_2).
5. Institute intermittent positive-pressure ventilation of the nondependent lung with 100% O_2.
6. *If none of the previous five maneuvers are successful*, ask the surgeon to clamp the pulmonary artery supplying the nondependent lung.

hypoxemic episodes by maintaining airway patency and decreasing blood flow to the nondependent lung. However, application of CPAP to this lung may interfere with surgical exposure. Positive end-expiratory pressure (PEEP) in combination with manual or mechanical inflation of the dependent lung produces unpredictable results. Although oxygenation may be improved by increasing the FRC in the dependent lung, it can be decreased by forcing blood flow into the nonventilated, nondependent lung.

Positioning

After placement of intravenous, intra-arterial, and urinary catheters and a nasogastric tube, the patient is turned into a partial right lateral decubitus position with the left side of the chest elevated 60° to 75°. Depending on the type of repair, a posterolateral thoracoabdominal incision can be made anywhere from the sixth to ninth interspace.

After change to the operative position, correct placement of the double-lumen tube should be reverified. Care must be taken while turning a patient to prevent unnecessary tube movement, which could lead to erosion into the aneurysm. A chest roll usually is not required. However, be sure to avoid stretching the left brachial plexus.

Monitoring

Hemodynamic

Because of the complexity of the operation and its associated physiologic stresses, all patients benefit from placement of a pulmonary artery flow-directed balloon catheter. Arterial blood pressures must be measured directly with a right arm arterial catheter. Because the left subclavian artery is commonly occluded during repair, an arterial catheter placed in the left arm does not function during cross-clamping. Intraoperative TEE imaging is valuable. It provides beat-to-beat assessment of left ventricular function and volume and is most helpful during clamping/unclamping when the incidence of myocardial ischemia (appearance of systolic wall motion and systolic wall thickening abnormalities) increases and the largest shifts in intravascular volume occur.

Cerebrospinal Fluid

Although cerebrospinal spinal fluid (CSF) drainage is controversial, I believe it is warranted. Pressure measurement and drainage offer a relatively safe treatment adjunct that may provide tremendous benefit at little risk.[44, 45] A lumbar epidural catheter or preferably a Silastic spinal drain catheter is inserted into the subarachnoid space before operative positioning. The larger bore diameter of the Silastic spinal drain appears more efficacious in removing fluid and monitoring CSF pressures.

Evoked Potentials

Somatosensory evoked potentials (SSEPs) have been advocated as a monitoring tool to detect spinal cord ischemia during thoracoabdominal aortic aneurysm repair.[45–48] However, the utility of SSEPs for this purpose is both controversial and equivocal. In addition to spinal ischemia, a number of other factors can cause changes in the SSEPs, including volatile anesthetics, peripheral neuropathies, hypoxia, hypotension, and temperature.

Applicability. What is known with certainty is that unless the surgeon or anesthesiologist is willing to alter the technique based on intraoperative changes in SSEPs, such monitoring is of no value. Specifically, the disappearance of SSEPs might prompt a surgeon to insert an arterial-arterial shunt from the left ventricular apex to the femoral artery or to reimplant critical intercostal/lumbar arteries into the graft. An anesthesiologist might induce proximal hypertension, drain additional CSF to increase spinal cord perfusion pressure, or both. However, these surgical maneuvers take time, and the incidence of paraplegia rises rapidly after 30 minutes of cross-clamp time has elapsed.[49, 50] This observation is consistent with a warm ischemic time for the spinal cord of about 30 minutes.[51]

Outcome. Patients whose SSEPs never change during repair uniformly have normal postoperative neurologic findings. In the event that SSEPs disappear during repair, the critical factor that determines whether paraplegia results is the period of time they are absent. When SSEPs disappear for <14 minutes, no postoperative neurologic deficits are found.[48] However, if they disappear for >14 minutes, patients may be paraplegic even if the SSEPs return to baseline values during the repair.

Because the pathways that mediate conduction of SSEPs are located predominantly in the posterior third of the spinal cord (dorsal column–medial lemniscus), some investigators argue that SSEPs may not adequately monitor the integrity of the anterior two thirds of the spinal cord (motor function). Blood supply to the dorsal column in the midthoracic region of the spinal cord is more generous than that to the anterior spinal cord. Thus, changes suggestive of spinal cord ischemia (prolonged latency and decreased amplitude) or the disappearance of SSEPs after cross-clamping probably indicates that such ischemia has been present longer and to a greater degree in the motor than dorsal column areas of the spinal cord. Refer to Chapter 22 for a detailed treatise on SSEP monitoring.

Urine

During all major vascular operations, the quantity of urine produced is closely monitored. The rationale is that urine production presuably is an index of the adequacy of renal blood flow. The kidneys are resilient to ischemia, and in general, if suprarenal and infrarenal aortic cross-clamp times are kept to 40 minutes or less, no impairment of renal function (e.g., rise in creatinine levels) occurs postoperatively.[52] Interestingly, however, in one investigation the volume of urine measured intraoperatively during supraceliac and infrarenal aortic aneurysmectomies was not predictive of postoperative renal function.[52]

More important to the preservation of renal integrity than urine output is the maintenance of normovolemia. Mannitol, dopamine, and under certain circumstances furosemide can be used to minimize the risk of ischemic renal injury. Other pharmacologic agents that have been studied as renal protective drugs, such as allopurinol and calcium channel blockers, currently are not given routinely to these patients.

What Can Be Done to Preserve Renal Function?

Mechanisms of Injury

Mechanisms by which the kidneys are injured during major vascular operations are multifactorial. The extent that renal blood flow is reduced depends primarily on the level of cross-clamping. In general, infrarenal aneurysm repairs are rarely associated with perioperative renal failure (<5% of cases). Infrarenal cross-clamp and repair reduces renal blood flow by about 40%, whereas a supraceliac approach decreases it by almost 90%.[53, 54] Cross-clamping the aorta at levels above the renal arteries causes urine production to cease.

Potent vasodilators such as SNP are potentially deleterious because they aggravate the reduction in renal blood flow. Other factors such as general anesthetics, intraoperative hypotension due to central hypovolemia or cardiac depression, atheromatous embolization from manipulation of atherosclerotic aneurysms, the proximity of the kidneys to the operative field (direct surgical trauma), reperfusion injury secondary to free radicals (reactive hyperemia), and an increase in plasma renin activity also contribute to perioperative impairment of renal function.[55–57]

Mortality

Various approaches have been taken to preserve renal function during aortic surgery, especially for those operations that require suprarenal aortic cross-clamping. Prevention of renal failure in this setting is important; when it occurs, the mortality rate exceeds 30%.[57] Attempts generally have been successful. In the 1960s, renal failure caused 25% of all postoperative deaths. It is currently responsible for 1% to 2% of such deaths.

Therapeutic Approaches

Five basic approaches have been used (Table 69–8). The most important predictors of postoperative renal failure are preoperative renal function, maintenance of intravascular volume, and avoidance of intraoperative hypotension. Optimal volume administration and adequate O_2 delivery ameliorate or even prevent renal injury associated with aortic cross-clamping.[58]

Mannitol

I routinely administer mannitol at a dose of 0.5 to 0.75 g · kg^{-1} at least 30 minutes before suprarenal or infrarenal cross-clamping. It is preferable for osmotic diuresis to commence before cross-clamping of the aorta. Mannitol has two major renal protective actions: (1) It scavenges free radicals and thus attenuates reperfusion injury, and (2) it tends to reverse cortical ischemia.[59, 60] With thoracic aorta cross-clamping, mannitol has another beneficial effect. It decreases CSF pressure and may protect the spinal cord from ischemia by increasing the distal cord perfusion pressure.

The pathogenesis of renal injury, which can occur secondary to cross-clamping, is associated with a shift in the intrarenal distribution of blood flow. Blood tends to be drawn from cortical to juxtamedullary nephrons. The net result is salt retention and a reduction in urine output. Mannitol can reverse this shift, cause an osmotic diuresis, and prevent cortical ischemia. Nevertheless, mannitol has not been conclusively proved to improve outcome after major vascular surgery.

Dopamine and Furosemide

The renovasodilating effects of low-dose dopamine (2 μg · kg^{-1} · min^{-1}) may be protective. In addition to mannitol, the use of dopamine is considered in patients with pre-existing renal dysfunction (creatinine level >2 mg · dL^{-1}) or in those patients undergoing aortic aneurysmorrhaphies that require suprarenal cross-clamping. I use furosemide only if oliguria is present (urine output <0.5 mL · kg^{-1} · h^{-1}), the patient is normovolemic, and mechanical obstruction to urine flow has been ruled out. Under these circumstances, small doses of furosemide (0.15 mg · kg^{-1}) are given to augment urine output. Recall that urine output is not a reliable predictor of perioperative renal failure. Furosemide can also reduce preload and induce a diuresis that makes regulation of intravascular volume problematic. For these reasons, it has a limited role in routine intraoperative management.

Renoplegia

Renoplegia can protect the kidneys from ischemic damage. In a manner analogous to cardioplegia, renoplegia requires the infusion of cold (4°C) crystalloid solution through the renal arteries at the time of aneurysm excision. Injection is repeated periodically. Although this technique confers renal protection, it frequently causes hypothermia and fluid overload.

Shunts

Aortic shunts are yet another approach to protecting the kidneys. However, shunts are associated with increased perioperative bleeding and morbidity. Thus, their use for renal protection is not justified, particularly when other effective means are available.

Ancillary Measures

The efficacy of a number of other treatment adjuncts has been evaluated in experimental animal models. Drugs of even less proven value than mannitol, dopamine, or furosemide include free radical scavengers (e.g., allopurinol), calcium channel blockers, and renin antagonists.

Does Transesophageal Echocardiography Reliably Detect Myocardial Ischemia?

Unlike its role in assessing volume status and cardiac valvular function, the use of TEE to detect myocardial ischemia is unclear. Although electrocardiography appears to be the most *specific* indicator of ischemia, TEE may be the most *sensitive* indicator.[61–63] In thoracoabdominal aortic aneurysmal repair, whether TEE is a sensitive and specific indicator of myocardial ischemia is particularly important. Because repair requires a left posterolateral thoracotomy incision, the lateral ECG chests leads, V_4 and V_5, cannot be used.

TABLE 69–8. Methods to Prevent Renal Failure During Aortic Surgery

- Optimization of intravascular volume pre-, intra-, and postoperatively
- Minimization of aortic cross-clamp time
- Institution of drug therapy (e.g., mannitol, dopamine, furosemide, allopurinol, calcium channel blockers)
- Use of distal shunts to increase renal blood flow
- Selective renal hypothermia (renoplegia)

Systolic and Regional Wall Motion Abnormalities

Ischemic areas of the myocardium typically are associated with systolic or regional wall motion abnormalities and systolic wall thickening abnormalities. Although many investigators believe that TEE is optimum to detect myocardial ischemia, others disagree.[61-65] Not every regional wall motion abnormality is caused by myocardial ischemia. Well-known regional differences in contractile function of normal myocardium can manifest as such abnormalities.

On balance, the role of TEE as a reliable indicator of myocardial O_2 supply-and-demand relationships shows tremendous promise but needs additional validation and further study. No definitive evidence associates intraoperative systolic wall motion abnormalities with postoperative cardiac complications.[65] These abnormalities tend to overestimate the actual ischemic myocardial mass. Nevertheless, they warn anesthesiologists of possible myocardial hypoperfusion and the potential need for early, aggressive treatment.

Electrocardiographic Correlation

Mechanical changes associated with episodes of myocardial ischemia can be detected with TEE before the changes observed with electrocardiography. London and colleagues demonstrated a discordance between TEE and ECG changes and concluded that careful monitoring of the ECG is necessary with TEE.[65] Regional wall motion abnormalities may be particularly ominous in the setting of thoracic aortic cross-clamping (or declamping); myocardial ischemia must be high on the differential diagnosis list. The anesthesiologist must closely scrutinize other available information for evidence of myocardial injury.

Left Ventricular Volume

Perhaps a more important use of TEE is to prevent rather than detect myocardial ischemia by providing real-time estimates of left ventricular volume. TEE is unrivaled for its rapidity in assessing the heart's functional status. It can readily detect two conditions that are common precursors to myocardial ischemia: (1) inadequate left ventricular preload secondary to hypovolemia and (2) excess left ventricular volume secondary to fluid overload. In addition, TEE might be useful to evaluate the efficacy of surgical and pharmacologic treatment of documented myocardial ischemia.

How Are Other Indicators of Myocardial Ischemia Assessed?

Electrocardiography

Lead Selection

The primary means for detecting myocardial ischemia is an ECG. If a patient had preoperative cardiac catheterization, the coronary artery anatomy is known; special care should be taken to scrutinize an ECG lead that covers the affected area if one is present. However, anatomic obstruction (e.g., right coronary artery) and ischemic changes on the ECG (inferior wall lead 2) do not reliably correlate. Thus, to guide intraoperative ECG lead selection, any preoperative association be-

tween ischemic events and the location of ECG changes (i.e., what leads were affected) should be documented.

ST Segment Changes

ST segment changes are the most reliable ECG indicators of myocardial ischemia and are believed to be secondary to the loss of intracellular potassium from cardiomyocytes during the ischemic epoch. The depth of ST depression correlates with both the mass of myocardium involved and the severity of the ischemic insult.

A diagnosis of myocardial ischemia using ECG criteria should be made by computed ST segmenting trending (if available). Diagnosis is dependent on the morphology of the ST segment depression. For example, an upsloping ST segment depression requires that the depression be at least 2 mm below the PR segment baseline 80 msec after the J point (the junction between the S wave and the ST segment). A pattern that is particularly indicative of myocardial ischemia is a horizontal ST depression of 1 mm 60 msec from the J point.

The morphology of ST segment depression can also be predictive of outcome. Downsloping ST segments, compared with horizontal ones, typically portend a worse prognosis and higher mortality and may indicate transmural myocardial ischemia. Other ECG evidence of myocardial injury such as symmetric T wave inversion is also indicative of ischemia.

Pulmonary Artery Catheterization

Observation of hemodynamic waveforms also can provide evidence of myocardial ischemia. The presence of a-c waves >15 mm Hg or v waves >20 mm Hg in the setting of an acute increase in the pulmonary artery occlusion pressure (PAOP) is thought to represent intraoperative ischemia. These findings may indicate a sudden decrease in left ventricular compliance secondary to myocardial ischemia, mitral regurgitation, or both.[66] However, others have found that the PAOP was not helpful in the diagnosis of early myocardial ischemia and poorly predicted the onset of myocardial ischemia.[67, 68] Thus, use of a pulmonary artery catheter as an independent means to detect myocardial ischemia has serious limitations and cannot be recommended routinely for this purpose.

Despite problems of diagnostic sensitivity and specificity, the sudden appearance of increased a-c or v waves, particularly in the setting of ST segment changes, in patients known to have a high incidence of coronary arterial disease (e.g., vascular surgical patients) should cause a clinician to search for evidence of myocardial ischemia using other complementary diagnostic modalities.

Why Should the Hematocrit Be Greater Than 30%?

Myocardial Oxygen Delivery

Patients suffering from aorto-occlusive vascular disease, aneurysms, or dissections usually have significant atherosclerotic disease of the vessel-rich organs (brain, myocardium, and kidneys). Because the single most important factor in patients' survival after major vascular surgery is cardiac function, strict attention must be paid to those factors that regulate cardiac O_2 supply-and-demand balance. The rationale for keeping a hematocrit >30% in patients undergoing major vascular surgery is best illustrated by the following equations:

$$So_2 = Cao_2 \times CoBF \qquad \text{Equation 2}$$

$$Cao_2 = 1.34 \, [Hb] \, [\%HbO_2 \, Sat] \qquad \text{Equation 3}$$
$$+ \, 0.0031 \, Pao_2$$

So_2, Cao_2, CoBF, [Hb], and $\%HbO_2$ Sat denote the rate of O_2 transport to the heart (mL $\cdot$ min^{-1}), content of O_2 in arterial blood (mL $\cdot$ dL^{-1}), coronary arterial blood flow (mL $\cdot$ min^{-1}), concentration of hemoglobin in blood (g $\cdot$ dL^{-1}), and the percentage of hemoglobin saturated with O_2, respectively. The value of 1.34 indicates the maximum binding of O_2 (mL) by 1 g hemoglobin.

As shown in Equation 2, the rate of O_2 delivery to the myocardium (So_2) is governed by the product of Cao_2 and CoBF. Cao_2 is determined by [Hb], $\%HbO_2$ Sat, and Pao_2 (Equation 3). Because the $\%HbO_2$ Sat is normally >93% in humans under either room air breathing or anesthetic conditions, the Cao_2 is essentially fixed.

Coronary Artery Blood Flow

Because the heart is primarily an aerobic organ and already extracts a large fraction of O_2 from its blood supply (myocardial O_2 extraction ratio [MOER] $\approx$ 67%) under normal conditions, an increase in the MOER cannot be an important physiologic mechanism to maintain oxygenation under stressful conditions (e.g., exercise). In fact, the MOER of the heart *at rest* is similar to the *maximum* O_2 extraction ratio observed in skeletal muscle under the most severe metabolic conditions.

Clearly, the only way the myocardium can increase its O_2 supply is by increasing CoBF. Indeed, under conditions of maximum exercise, increases four- to fivefold above baseline values occur. Stenotic atherosclerotic lesions in the coronary arteries, particularly those that occlude 70% of the vessel cross-sectional area, dramatically reduce this *coronary vascular reserve*. If the myocardial O_2 demand cannot be met by an increase in CoBF, myocardial ischemia ensues.

The ability of the heart to regulate its O_2 supply in the setting of significant coronary arterial disease is decreased secondary to a diminished coronary vascular reserve. Hence its integrity is dependent on the blood O_2 content. Accordingly, it seems unwise to let the hematocrit decrease to values that would be easily tolerated by most normal patients (<30%).

Blood Rheology

Would even higher hematocrit values lead to further increases in myocardial O_2 supply? The answer to this question necessitates consideration of the rheologic properties of blood. The flow of blood is non-newtonian (i.e., blood viscosity is dependent on shear rate). As the concentration of hemoglobin increases and flow rate slows, the viscosity of blood increases. Thus, the enhanced O_2-carrying capacity associated with higher levels of hemoglobin is offset by a reduction in CoBF secondary to increases in blood viscosity.

For these reasons, blood losses incurred during major vascular surgery are aggressively treated with crystalloid, colloid, or both until the hematocrit approaches 30%. At this point, additional blood losses ideally would be replaced with whole blood, which generally is unavailable. Thus, I use packed red blood cells diluted with normal saline.

ANESTHETIC INDUCTION AND MAINTENANCE

How Important Is the Choice of Drugs?

Induction

In almost every investigative series, the major cause of short- and long-term morbidity and mortality in patients undergoing major vascular surgery is cardiac dysfunction (e.g., myocardial infarction, CHF). Accordingly, the drugs used during the induction and maintenance phases of anesthetics are selected with concern for cardioprotection.

Group 1 Patients

Selection is less important for patients with well-preserved left ventricular function (group 1 patients, see Table 69–3). As has been noted, patients in group 1 can easily tolerate a volatile anesthetic-based technique. The myocardial depression produced by volatile anesthetics may actually exert a beneficial effect on the myocardial O_2 supply-and-demand quotient by depressing left ventricular contractility. Little is to be gained, however, with a volatile anesthetic-based technique in patients with compromised left ventricular function (group 2 patients, see Table 69–3).

Group 2 Patients

These patients are treated in much the same way as patients scheduled for aortocoronary bypass. If the procedure is not emergent, a slow, methodic, narcotic-based anesthetic induction in conjunction with a nondepolarizing muscle relaxant is preferable. A continuous infusion of nitroglycerin runs at 1 to 2 μg $\cdot$ kg^{-1} $\cdot$ min^{-1} during the entire induction sequence. Midazolam, 0.05 to 0.10 mg $\cdot$ kg^{-1}; vecuronium, 0.15 to 0.20 mg $\cdot$ kg^{-1}; and incremental doses of fentanyl, to a total dose of 20 to 40 μg $\cdot$ kg^{-1} (or alternatively sufentanil 2–4 μg $\cdot$ kg^{-1}) are administered. If a patient's heart rate is <60 beats per minute (bpm), pancuronium is substituted for vecuronium. Excessive bradycardia and subsequent left ventricular distention can be prevented by using the mild anticholinergic effect of pancuronium to offset narcotic-induced heart rate slowing.

Midazolam is administered *up front* for two reasons. First, not only does it produce anxiolysis and amnesia, but also it may reduce the incidence of narcotic-induced chest wall rigidity. Second, in my experience, the incidence of hypotension during induction is lower when narcotics are titrated *on top* of a benzodiazepine. A stable induction is more difficult to achieve when comparable doses of midazolam are given *after* a large dose of narcotic. If vital signs are stable, the patient is intubated.

Maintenance

Anesthesia is maintained by incremental doses of narcotic or, preferably, by infusing fentanyl, 2 to 5 μg $\cdot$ kg^{-1} $\cdot$ hr^{-1}, or sufentanil, 0.2 to 0.5 μg $\cdot$ kg^{-1} $\cdot$ hr^{-1}, in conjunction with isoflurane at an end-tidal concentration of about 0.5%. Muscle relaxation is used as necessary. Nitroglycerin is infused at a rate of 1 to 2 $\mu g \cdot kg^{-1} \cdot min^{-1}$ throughout the case, and its concentration varied depending on the hemodynamic changes. During thoracic aortic cross-clamping, nitroglycerin has the potential to further decrease blood flow to those organs distal to the cross-clamp (e.g., spinal cord). However, for reasons discussed later, its use seems warranted.

A vasodilator drug, whether it be isoflurane, SNP, nitroglycerin, or some combination of these, ultimately must be administered in virtually all cases of thoracic aortic cross-clamping to attenuate the large increase in proximal blood pressure that can cause myocardial infarction or stroke. Even with aggressive treatment of proximal hypertension, myocardial infarction still remains the major cause of death in these patients.

What Is the Role of Adjunctive Epidural Anesthesia?

Epidural anesthesia as an adjunct during major vascular surgery also involves tradeoffs. Some investigators have reported significant complications with this technique in the setting of major vascular surgery; others have touted its many benefits.[69-76] Many patients with vascular disease come to the OR with heparin infusions (in the setting of acute thrombosis), are administered heparin, or develop bleeding dyscrasias during the course of an operation. One of the most feared complications in these patients is the development of an epidural hematoma with a subsequent neurologic deficit.[69] Another potential drawback is fluid overload in the perioperative time period as autonomic blockade recedes.

Potential Benefits

Epidural anesthesia can provide significant benefits. It reduces the incidence of myocardial ischemia, provides excellent muscle relaxation, decreases bowel size (improves operating conditions), and allows deep breathing and earlier ambulation.

Potential Problems

Three problems are of concern with respect to epidural anesthesia as an adjunct for *supraceliac* aortic surgery.

Epidural Hematoma

Patients undergoing thoracoabdominal repairs almost invariably are anticoagulated when they leave the OR. The massive volume shifts and dilutional thrombocytopenia commonly occurring with this procedure may render them especially susceptible to an epidural hematoma. One might argue that placement of an intrathecal catheter for CSF drainage is associated with similar problems. However, insertion of an epidural catheter essentially doubles the risk of hematoma formation.

These concerns, admittedly, may be more theoretic than clinical. Rao and El-Etr placed epidural catheters in patients scheduled for aortocoronary bypass.[70] They found that epidural catheters in the setting of full heparinization did not increase the complication rate. Atraumatic placement of the epidural catheter (or CSF drain) obviously is important in preventing this complication. If blood is observed in the epidural needle during placement of either catheter, delay of surgery for 24 hours to allow clot formation may be prudent.

Blood Loss

Blood loss can be massive. If an epidural catheter is dosed with local anesthetic and a total sympathectomy (T-1–L-1 spinal segment blockade) results, cardiodynamic control is much more difficult. This problem can be minimized but not eliminated; be careful and deliberate about dose titration.

Motor Weakness

After supraceliac aortic cross-clamping, residual postoperative motor weakness from local anesthetics administered through an epidural route can confound the diagnosis and treatment of epidural hematoma. As was mentioned previously, high levels of aortic cross-clamping can produce postoperative paraplegia.

In summary, I am more likely to use an epidural as an anesthetic adjunct in the setting of peripheral vascular operations or in those aortic procedures in which blood loss and hemodynamic perturbations are less frequent (i.e., infrarenal aortic procedures). Indeed, Yeager and colleagues have shown that epidural anesthesia and postoperative analgesia, when compared with general anesthesia, had fewer cardiovascular and infectious complications.[74]

What Precautions Should Be Taken for Thoracic Aortic Cross-Clamping?

General Considerations

Aortic cross-clamping is required to isolate the diseased section of the aorta. Cross-clamping of the descending thoracic aorta during repair of a thoracoabdominal aortic aneurysm is among the greatest physiologic stresses a human can endure. To minimize the morbidity and mortality associated with this repair, an anesthesiologist should strive to achieve two major therapeutic goals during the period of cross-clamping: (1) Prevent *hypertensive* injury to those organs located proximal to cross-clamp (heart and brain) and (2) prevent *hypotensive* injury to those organs distal to the cross-clamp (segments of the spinal cord, kidneys, and gut). Although these goals are easily promulgated, their achievement often is difficult.

Therapeutic Conundrums

Treatment to attain one goal is often deleterious to that of another. For example, although liberal use of potent vasodilators such as SNP can effectively blunt the large increase in proximal hypertension associated with cross-clamping, it may concomitantly cause ischemic injury to those organs distal to the clamp by reducing blood flow.[77, 78]

Spinal Cord Blood Flow

To illustrate this concept, let us examine the effect of SNP on spinal cord blood flow during cross-clamping. Spinal cord perfusion pressure is the difference between distal mean arterial pressure (MAP) and CSF pressure. By increasing CSF pressure and decreasing distal MAP, SNP may cause a large reduction in spinal cord perfusion pressure and blood flow. For this and similar other reasons, the implications of using potent vasodilators to treat proximal hypertension should be carefully and judiciously considered.

Myocardial Preservation

Whereas large increases in MAP proximal to the cross-clamp promote blood flow to those organs located distal to the clamp, proximal hypertension, especially when it exceeds the limits of autoregulation, can also lead to cerebral hemorrhage or myocardial infarction. Because of the previously discussed short- and long-term effects of perioperative myocardial dysfunction, attempts are made to preserve the myocardium without unduly jeopardizing the integrity of those organs located distal to the cross-clamp.

As an alternative to drug therapy and a potential way to bypass the deleterious effects of vasodilators on distal blood flow, mechanical unloading of the left ventricle using shunts or partial cardiopulmonary bypass has been proposed. However, these approaches appear to have no great benefit over *clamp-and-sew* techniques and offer their own set of complications (increased heparin use and increased bleeding).

Before Cross-Clamping

About 30 minutes before cross-clamping the thoracic aorta, slowly remove CSF (10–20 mL) from the subarachnoid space until the lumbar CSF pressure is >0 but <10 mm Hg. Infuse mannitol (0.5–0.75 g · kg^{-1}) to establish an osmotic diuresis and to further reduce CSF pressure before application of the aortic cross-clamp. Approximately 1 to 2 minutes before cross-clamping, measures are taken to achieve two goals: (1) Blunt the rise in proximal blood pressure by using drugs having different pharmacologic mechanisms while concomitantly attempting to preserve adequate distal blood flow and (2) ameliorate the rise in proximal MAP by using drugs that are easily titratable (with short half-lives), thus allowing rapid changes to be made immediately based on a patient's condition (e.g., isoflurane, nitroglycerin, SNP, esmolol).

Nitroglycerin

While anesthesia is administered to patients with a risk of coronary artery disease, nitroglycerin is used ubiquitously. No definitive evidence shows that prophylactic nitroglycerin infused during anesthetic induction or maintenance improves outcome. However, it may reduce the incidence of perioperative myocardial ischemia, and it is of tremendous assistance in maintaining stable cardiodynamics during the operation.

After communicating with the surgeon, I typically double the baseline infusion rate of nitroglycerin to 2 to 4 μg · kg^{-1} · min^{-1} 1 to 1.5 minutes before application of the thoracic aortic cross-clamp. In almost all cases, additional vasodilator therapy is required to ameliorate the hemodynamic effects. The choice of vasodilator is controversial and is to some extent dependent on a patient's pre-existing left ventricular function.

Isoflurane and Sodium Nitroprusside

Although patients in group 1 (see Table 69–3) probably can tolerate large increases in the concentration of isoflurane, this same intervention in patients in group 2 may cause CHF. A more rational approach for group 2 patients is to use SNP as the additional vasodilator and to avoid large increases in the concentration of isoflurane.

Although isoflurane may confer a similar neuroprotective effect on the spinal cord as it does on the brain during cerebral ischemia,[79] this duality of action is not documented. Isoflurane

used to control proximal hypertension reduces spinal cord perfusion pressure even more than SNP.[80] For these reasons, I tend to keep isoflurane at the same concentrations used for maintenance and resort to nitroglycerin, SNP, or both, plus β-blocker therapy to control proximal hypertension.

After Cross-Clamping

Hemodynamic Goals

Perhaps more important to good neurologic outcome, rather than the use of a particular vasodilator, is strict attention to those factors that control distal blood flow. The proximal MAP probably should be allowed to rise to the upper limit of myocardial blood flow regulation (120 mm Hg) or to a MAP at which signs of cardiac ischemia occur (whichever value is lower). Sodium nitroprusside, 1 to 3 μg · kg^{-1} · min^{-1}, is added to the already infusing baseline nitroglycerin, 1 to 3 μg · kg^{-1} · min^{-1}.

If a patient has reasonable left ventricular function and the heart rate is >80 bpm, a short-acting β-blocker such as esmolol is infused at a starting dose of 50 to 75 μg · kg^{-1} · min^{-1} until a heart rate of approximately 65 bpm is achieved. Beta-adrenergic blockers are particularly important in acute dissections of the thoracic aorta. Reduction in cardiac contractility may slow the progression of the dissection significantly and is a mainstay of medical therapy for this condition. This pharmacologic regimen is rapidly titratable and allows quick changes based on a patient's response to cross-clamping. For those vascular procedures in which renal function is most jeopardized (thoracic and supraceliac cross-clamps), *renal dose* dopamine is infused at a rate of 2 μg · kg^{-1} · min^{-1}. This dose selectively activates the dopaminergic (renal vasodilation) but not the α-adrenergic (vasoconstriction) receptors in the renal vasculature. Dopamine is not routinely used for infrarenal aneurysm resection unless renal function is already comprised preoperatively (creatinine level >2 mg · dL^{-1}).

Carbon Dioxide Control

With regard to the partial pressure of arterial carbon dioxide (Paco$_2$), normocapnia is preferable. Regulation of spinal cord blood flow is similar to that of the cerebral vasculature.[78, 81] Thus, although hypocapnia might ameliorate the increase in intracranial and CSF pressures observed after application of the thoracic cross-clamp, it may concomitantly reduce spinal cord blood flow distal to the cross-clamp.[81]

Control of Spinal Cord Perfusion

If the CSF pressure rises above 10 mm Hg after thoracic aortic cross-clamping, additional CSF, up to a total of 50 mL, should be removed until the CSF pressure is again in the range of 0 to 10 mm Hg. Monitoring of CSF pressure should extend into the postoperative period as well. Potential side effects of CSF drainage are headache and, very rarely, intrathecal hemorrhage or transtentorial herniation. In cases of potential head injury, CSF drainage must be used very cautiously. Because of the increased risk of herniation, a more conservative approach uses an osmotic agent such as mannitol to reduce CSF pressure.

Although perfusion pressures that protect the spinal cord against ischemic injury have been determined in a dog model during supraceliac aortic cross-clamping, no corresponding critical level has been established in humans. Differences in the anatomic spinal cord blood supply between humans and dogs probably make comparisons between the two species inappropriate. Recall that the spinal cord perfusion pressure is the difference between distal MAP and CSF pressures. Although some anesthesiologists routinely measure femoral pressure, because the threshold value for cord perfusion is unknown in humans, I do not insert a femoral arterial catheter but instead use routine measures that are designed empirically to maximize perfusion (e.g., CSF drainage, mannitol). Proximal MAP following cross-clamping is not aggressively treated unless evidence of proximal organ injury appears.

Intraoperative Monitoring

Changes in a vasodilator, β-blocker, or both are best guided by the pulmonary artery catheter, ECG, and TEE. These tools allow the titration of proximal MAP. For example, if on application of the aortic cross-clamp the proximal MAP increases significantly, the heart rate decreases to <60 bpm, and the left ventricle does not appear distended, the esmolol infusion rate is decreased and SNP is increased. On the other hand, if the left ventricle is distended, an increase in both nitroglycerin and nitroprusside is warranted.

Roizen and colleagues found that despite a 93% incidence of ischemic changes on TEE (presence of regional wall motion abnormalities after application of the thoracic aortic cross-clamp), only 8% of these patients actually were shown to have a perioperative myocardial infarction.[82] They attributed this low incidence of infarction to intensive vasodilator therapy that kept vital signs within a predetermined range based on their preoperative values.

Shunts or Bypass

To monitor pressures distal to the thoracic aortic cross-clamp, some anesthesiologists routinely insert femoral arterial catheters. Surgeons sometimes place an arterial-arterial shunt (Gott's shunt: a heparin-bonded shunt from the apex of the left ventricle to the femoral artery) or institute femoral artery–femoral vein bypass, venoarterial bypass, or left atrial–femoral artery bypass to enhance distal blood flow.

Although distal blood flow is improved, a number of potentially serious limitations may complicate bypass or shunt use. Both procedures require cannulation of major blood vessels (potential sites of bleeding postoperatively) and may require full systemic heparinization. In addition, limitations in the size of shunts, large regurgitant blood fractions, and possible kinking of the shunt can seriously limit blood flow.

The largest Gott's shunt is 9 mm in diameter, which corresponds to only 7% of the cross-sectional area of the descending aorta. Because these shunts are not equipped with flow monitors, their presence does not guarantee adequate distal blood flow. Most surgeons and anesthesiologists believe that the coagulation problems associated with thoracoabdominal aneurysm repair are already severe enough and that the risk of these interventions exceeds their potential benefit.

Hypothermia

Hypothermia is protective against spinal cord ischemic injury in a number of experimental animal models. During cir-

culatory interruption of aortic blood flow, a reduction in body temperature of 3 °C in rabbits caused a doubling of the duration of ischemia that could be reversibly sustained.[83] Berguer and colleagues found that selective deep hypothermia (12–19 °C) of the spinal cord in dogs avoided the ischemic injury associated with aortic cross-clamping.[84] However, the benefits shown in animal models have yet to be clearly translated to humans. Reduction of body temperature to a level of 35 °C in a highly controllable manner is difficult. Thus, intentional hypothermia is not recommended routinely to protect the spinal cord from ischemic injury.

Problems of induced hypothermia include "overshoot" when patients become too cold; offsetting of cooling by the transfusion of massive quantities of warmed blood and fluids; and aggravation of coagulation abnormalities by induced platelet dysfunction. Nevertheless, if the body temperature drifts down to 35 °C during the course of a thoracic aneurysm repair, this change may be advantageous and confer some protection to the spinal cord. Further reductions should be prevented. In contrast, hyperthermia renders the heart, spinal cord, and brain more susceptible to ischemic damage.

What Are the Hemodynamic Effects of Aortic Cross-Clamping?

The degree and direction of change in cardiodynamics are directly related to the proximity of the aortic cross-clamp to the heart and pre-existing left ventricular function[85–89] (Table 69–9). As expected, aortic cross-clamping at a suprarenal but infraceliac location causes intermediate changes in cardiovascular parameters. Similarly, the greatest increases in CSF pressure are observed after proximal occlusion of the thoracic aorta (aortic isthmus).

Group 1 Versus Group 2 Patients

Attia and colleagues showed that preoperative left ventricular function (see Table 69–3) dramatically changes the effects of aortic cross-clamping on hemodynamic parameters.[29] Infrarenal cross-clamping caused a decrease in CVP, pulmonary arterial pressures, and PAOP patients in group 1; the opposite

TABLE 69–9. Effect of Aortic Cross-Clamp Level on Myocardial Variables (% Change from Baseline Values)

Cardiovascular Parameter	Supraceliac	Suprarenal-Infrarenal	Infrarenal
Mean arterial pressure (mm Hg)	54	5*	2*
Pulmonary capillary wedge pressure (mm Hg)	38	10*	0*
End-diastolic area (cm²)	28	2*	9*
End-systolic area (cm²)	69	10*	11*
Ejection fraction (%)	−38	−10*	−3*
Abnormal motion of wall (% of patients)	92	33	0
New myocardial infarctions (% of patients)	8	0	0

(Adapted from Roizen MF, Beaupre PN, Alpert RA, et al: Monitoring with two-dimensional transesophageal echocardiography: comparison of myocardial function in patients undergoing supraceliac, suprarenal-infraceliac, or infrarenal aortic occlusion. J Vasc Surg 1984; 1:300.)
*Statistically different from group undergoing supraceliac aortic occlusion (P < .05).

changes were noted in group 2 patients (Fig. 69–5). This study clearly demonstrated that patients with pre-existing left ventricular dysfunction do not tolerate the stress of infrarenal aortic cross-clamping nearly as well as those with well-preserved myocardial function. With pressure, ECG, TEE, and urine output monitoring, the consequences of aortic clamping (and unclamping) can be mitigated or avoided by judicious use of intravascular volume expansion and vasodilator therapy.[90]

Modulation of Hemodynamic Effects

Control of Preload

Various factors modulate the hemodynamic effects of cross-clamping in addition to the site chosen. To give compensatory mechanisms an adequate amount of time to be operative, surgeons should be encouraged to occlude the aorta slowly. Patients who are hypervolemic tend to have greater perturbations in cardiodynamics than those who are euvolemic or slightly hypovolemic at the time of clamp application. For this reason, I try to reduce left ventricular preload before clamping using TEE and invasive hemodynamic monitors as guidelines.

Anesthetic Management

The anesthetic technique can have a modulating role. An isoflurane-based technique attenuates the hemodynamic effects of cross-clamping more than a narcotic-based approach.

Vessel Collateralization

Increased collateralization significantly reduces the cardiodynamic impact. Chronic aortic obstruction (e.g., atherosclerosis-induced aortoiliac obstructive disease) allows time for collateral blood flow development. The cardiovascular effects of cross-clamping in aortic coarctation or aortoiliac obstruction are less than those observed for aneurysmal disease of the abdominal or thoracic aorta.

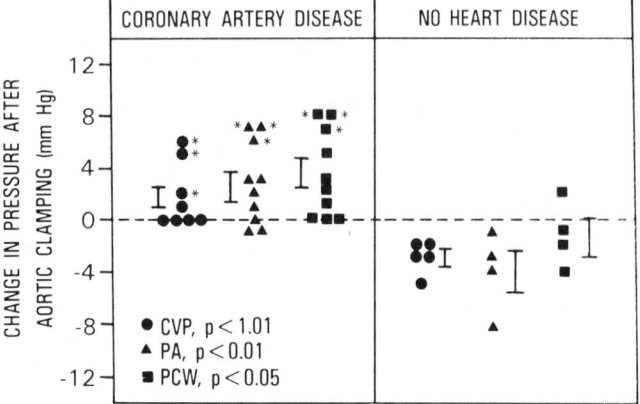

FIGURE 69–5. Comparison of changes in central venous pressure (CVP), pulmonary artery pressure (PA), and pulmonary capillary wedge pressure (PCWP) in patients with and without coronary artery disease. *Asterisks* indicate patients that developed myocardial ischemia during infrarenal aortic cross-clamping. (From Attia RR, Murphy JD, Snider M, et al: Myocardial ischemia due to infrarenal aortic cross-clamping during aortic surgery in patients with severe coronary artery disease. Circulation 1976; 53:961.)

What Is the Effect of Cross-Clamping on Carbon Dioxide?

The equation relating the $Paco_2$ to alveolar ventilation ($\dot{V}A$) and CO_2 production ($\dot{V}co_2$) is as follows:

$$Paco_2 = \frac{K \times \dot{V}co_2}{\dot{V}A}$$

Equation 4

K is a proportionality constant.

Organs and tissues perfused by arteries located distal to the aortic cross-clamp are, barring extensive collateral blood flow, essentially excluded from the central circulation. Thus, CO_2 produced in these regions is not carried to the heart, and the apparent $\dot{V}co_2$ is reduced. The effect is a decrease in $Paco_2$ and the partial pressure of end-tidal carbon dioxide ($Petco_2$). The location of aortic cross-clamping and existence of collateral circulation around the aortic cross-clamp modulate this effect. A more proximal application causes a larger reduction in $Paco_2$, all other factors remaining equal.

Why Does Paraplegia Occur?

Anterior Spinal Artery Syndrome

Unlike the posterior third of the spinal cord, the anterior two thirds of the cord has poor collateral blood flow. Aortic cross-clamping at higher levels renders perfusion of the anterior spinal cord tenuous, particularly in the midthoracic regions (T-4–T-6). Indeed, prolonged ischemia can result in well-known clinical findings referred to as the *anterior spinal artery syndrome*. Its clinical presentation of paraplegia, rectal and urinary incontinence, or both and loss of pain and temperature sensation is explained by disruption of corticospinal and spinothalamic pathways in the anterior spinal cord. Vibration and proprioception are characteristically spared because their pathways, the fasciculus cuneatus and gracilis, are located in the posterior spinal cord.

Blood Flow Distribution

Susceptibility to ischemia of the anterior two thirds of the spinal cord is explained by the anatomy of spinal cord blood flow in humans (Figs. 69–6 and 69–7). The blood supply is quite variable and has not been well delineated until recently.[91, 92] It can be most readily understood by dividing it into three distinct divisions: (1) a primary or proximal (in relation to the aorta) division, (2) an intermediate division, and (3) a terminal division. Lack of intermediate division development renders the spinal cord susceptible to ischemic injury.

Primary and Intermediate Divisions

The primary system consists of the vertebral, costocervical, thyrocervical, intercostal, and lumbar arteries. The intermediate division contains the radicular branches of arterial trunks of the primary system. Each vertebral segment in the embryonic stage receives a pair of radicular arteries. However, during embryonic development or the early neonatal period, several of these radicular branches disappear. In adult life, only a few of the original radicular branches remain functional: one

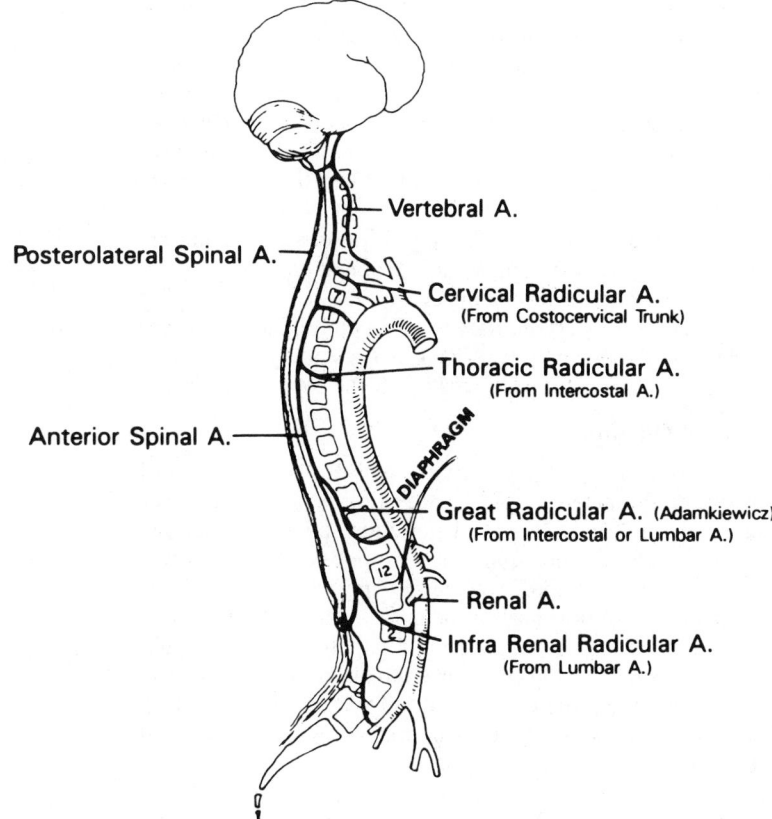

FIGURE 69–6. Spinal cord blood supply. (Adapted from Szilagyi DE, Hageman JH, Smith RF, Elliott JP: Spinal cord damage in surgery of the abdominal aorta. Surgery 1978; 83:38.)

1. Lumbar (Intercostal) A.
2. Anterior Ramus Lumbar (Intercostal) A.
3. Posterior Ramus Lumbar (Intercostal) A.
4. Spinal A.
5. Anterior Radicular A.
6. Anterior Spinal A.
7. Posterior Radicular A.
8. Posterolateral Spinal A.
9. Muscular Branches

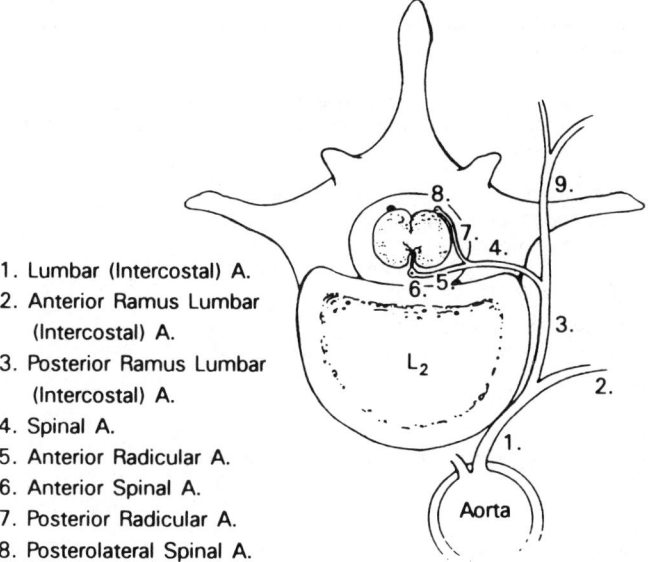

FIGURE 69–7. Spinal cord blood supply. (Adapted from Szilagyi DE, Hageman JH, Smith RF, Elliott JP: Spinal cord damage in surgery of the abdominal aorta. Surgery 1978; 83:38.)

to two branches in the cervical spinal cord, two to three branches in the thoracic spinal cord, and one to two branches in the lumbar spinal cord.

The most important and largest of the radicular arterial branches arises from the lower thoracic and upper lumbar regions and is called *Adamkiewicz's artery*, the *great radicular artery*, or the *arteria radicularis magna*. Wadouh and colleagues have shown that Adamkiewicz's artery arises from the aorta between T-5 and T-8 in 12% to 15% of the population, between T-9 and T-12 in 60%; at L-1 in 14%; at L-2 in 10%; at L-3 in 1%; and between L-4 and L-5 in 0.2%.[91] It arises from the left side of the aorta about 75% of the time.[92]

Unless an unusually well-developed infrarenal radicular artery is present, ischemic injury to the spinal cord is typically caused by trauma to Adamkiewicz's artery or cross-clamping on both sides of its origin. Rarely, spinal cord injury can occur if collateral blood supply to Adamkiewicz's artery is poor and the takeoff of this artery is located below the cross-clamp level.

Terminal Division

The terminal division of blood supply to the spinal cord consists of the anterior spinal artery, located in the anterior median fissure, and the paired posterior spinal arteries (see Fig. 69–7). The anterior spinal artery supplies the anterior two thirds of the spinal cord, whereas the posterior spinal artery supplies the posterior third of the cord. Although the anterior spinal artery is the largest, its blood supply is the most tenuous. The vertical pathway of the spinal arteries is long and extends from the proximal to the distal end of the spinal cord. The anterior spinal artery relies on reinforcement of its blood supply by feeding radicular branches.

As shown in Figure 69–6, large areas (multiple levels) of the spinal cord do not receive feeding radicular branches. These wide separations leave watershed areas of the spinal cord that are particularly susceptible to ischemic injury. Interruption of the feeding radicular vessels may cause neurologic damage. The posterior spinal arteries have well-developed vertical communications and are thus less dependent on the integrity of feeding radicular vessels.

Do Preventive Measures Decrease Paraplegia?

Shunt Placement

The majority of vascular surgeons believe that if the duration of clamp time is 30 minutes or less, placement of a shunt is not warranted. For cross-clamp times >30 minutes, the need for shunts becomes more controversial. The risk of postoperative paraplegia rises rapidly after 30 minutes of thoracic aortic cross-clamp time.[49, 50] These repairs are complex operations that require significant volume and blood replacement. Patients uniformly leave the OR with a coagulopathy that is most likely due to massive blood transfusion (dilutional thrombocytopenia is most common). In the majority of cases, the bleeding is not attributable to disruption of suture lines but rather to a dysfunctional coagulation cascade.

In the experience of Hollier and colleagues[93] and Crawford and associates,[94, 95] no significant benefit was attributable to shunts or bypass procedures compared with direct aortic clamping with vasodilators to control proximal hypertension. These investigators previously recommended left atrial-to-femoral bypass, femoral-femoral partial cardiopulmonary bypass, hypothermia, or temporary shunts during the period of

aortic occlusion. More recently, they discontinued these treatment adjuncts because in their large series they found no reduction in postoperative paraplegia (which occurs in 3–4% of patients regardless of what is done) and frequently encountered the complications associated with shunts or bypass.

Exceptions to this recommendation are patients who have aortic valvular regurgitation and cannot tolerate thoracic cross-clamping because of large increases in left ventricular end-diastolic pressure. In this situation, the prudent approach is femorofemoral bypass or atriofemoral bypass.

Cerebrospinal Fluid Drainage

CSF drainage may decrease the incidence of postoperative neurologic deficit.[44, 45] To understand why, consider the relationship that illustrates the physiologic factors controlling spinal cord blood flow during aortic cross-clamping:

$$SCBF = \frac{\text{Distal SCPP}}{\text{Distal SCVR}}$$

$$= \frac{\text{Distal MAP} - \text{CSF pressure}}{\text{Distal SCVR}} \qquad \text{Equation 5}$$

in which SCBF, SCPP, and SCVR denote spinal cord blood flow, spinal cord perfusion pressure, and spinal cord vascular resistance, respectively.

This equation provides the rationale for various therapeutic interventions (Table 69–10). Withdrawal of CSF increases SCPP by decreasing CSF pressure and thus may increase blood flow to the spinal cord. However, in the only randomized prospective study in humans that examined the role of CSF drainage, postoperative paraplegia or paresis was not prevented.[96]

TABLE 69–10. Potential Treatment Adjuncts to Increase Spinal Cord Blood Flow During Thoracic Aortic Cross-Clamping

↑ **Spinal Cord Perfusion Pressure**
↑ Distal aortic pressure
  Partial cardiopulmonary bypass (venovenous, venoarterial bypass)
    Left atrium, pulmonary artery, or right atrium to distal aorta or femoral artery shunt
  Simple shunts
    Arterial-arterial shunt (e.g., Gott's shunt)
    Thoracic aortic–aortic shunt
    ↓ Cerebrospinal fluid pressure
  Direct removal (e.g., cerebrospinal fluid drainage)
  Osmotic action (e.g., mannitol)

↓ **Spinal Cord Vascular Resistance**
Intrathecal papaverine (dilates anterior spinal artery)

Biochemical
Methylprednisolone
Magnesium
Calcium channel blockers (e.g., flunarizine, verapamil)
Allopurinol
Superoxide dismutase
Naloxone
Barbiturates (e.g., thiopental)
Calmodulin
Thyroid-releasing hormone
Desferoxamine

Other
Hypothermia

Although the effectiveness of CSF drainage remains unproven in humans, it is a relatively safe procedure and may allow a few extra minutes before irreversible neurologic damage occurs. Conversely, pharmacologically (nitrates) or mechanically (cross-clamping) induced increases in CSF pressure have the opposite effect. The price paid for overly aggressive treatment of proximal hypertension may be postoperative paraplegia.

Corticosteroids

During the National Acute Spinal Cord Injury Study (NASCIS), a multicenter prospective randomized placebo-controlled trial, patients with acute spinal cord injury received either a 30 mg $\cdot$ kg^{-1} dose of methylprednisolone followed by an infusion at 5.4 mg $\cdot$ kg^{-1} $\cdot$ hr^{-1} for the next 23 hours; 5.4 mg $\cdot$ kg^{-1} naloxone, followed by an infusion at 4 mg $\cdot$ kg^{-1} $\cdot$ hr^{-1} for the next 23 hours; or placebo. Significant improvement in both motor and sensory function at 6 weeks, 6 months, and 1 year occurred with incomplete and complete spinal cord lesions in patients receiving methylprednisolone; no benefit was found with naloxone.[97]

A key factor to improved outcome is early administration of the steroid. To have any beneficial effect, methylprednisolone must be given within 8 hours of the injury. Although the improvement was not dramatic, the differences found were significant. For this reason, many experts believe that methylprednisolone should be administered according to the NASCIS protocol to *all* patients considered at risk of spinal cord ischemia, including those undergoing aneurysm resection and repair. To avoid the potentially deleterious effects of methylprednisolone-induced hyperglycemia on neuronal injury (via its glucocorticoid effect), newer steroids such as tirilazid that have minimum to no glucocorticoid effect are being used.

Papaverine

Papaverine has been administered intrathecally to enhance distal spinal cord blood flow by anterior spinal artery dilatation.[98–100] Most investigators administer papaverine in the following manner: (1) Remove 20 mL of CSF approximately 30 minutes before aortic cross-clamp; (2) instill 3 mL of 1% papaverine in 10% dextrose warmed to 37 °C 10 minutes before aortic cross-clamping. (Papaverine must be warmed to body temperature to prevent hypotension.) During the period of aortic cross-clamp, 10- to 15-mL aliquots of CSF (maximum of 50 mL) are withdrawn every 15 minutes to keep CSF pressures <10 mm Hg. Additional CSF drainage may cause herniation. In addition to inducing smooth muscle relaxation, papaverine may also block calcium channels and indirectly scavenge free radicals.

Miscellaneous Therapy

Other treatment adjuncts such as magnesium, thyrotropin-releasing hormone, sodium bicarbonate infusion during aortic cross-clamping, local anesthetics, dantrolene, and benzodiazepines have been proposed. Each has its proponents, but most have given equivocal results.

Summary

No treatment adjunct decreases the incidence of postoperative paraplegia following thoracic aortic cross-clamping to zero. However, judicious use of some agents can reduce the incidence of this devastating complication. I recommend CSF drainage, methylprednisolone, maintenance of proximal hypertension (as tolerated by the myocardium and brain), correction of metabolic acidosis during cross-clamp, and possibly intrathecal papaverine. Hypothermia to 35 °C probably is beneficial.

Does Paraplegia Occur in Patients Having Abdominal Aortic Surgery?

Yes, but the incidence is very low. In a series of 3164 patients, the overall incidence of spinal cord damage following abdominal aortic surgery was only 0.25%.[92] All cases of paraplegia occurred after aneurysmal aortic surgery; none followed surgery for occlusive aortic disease. The incidence of postoperative paraplegia in patients having emergency surgery for ruptured abdominal aortic aneurysms was 10 times higher than in patients having surgery on unruptured aneurysms. The investigators concluded that (1) postoperative spinal cord damage following abdominal aortic operations was caused by interruption of a critical radicular artery at the lower thoracic or high lumbar vertebral levels (in the presence of anomalous greater radicular or infrarenal radicular arteries); and (2) the higher incidence of paraplegia following emergency repair was attributed to higher levels (T-10–L-1) of aortic cross-clamping.[92]

Thus, the probability of spinal cord ischemia is markedly increased if cross-clamping of the aorta proximal to the takeoff of Adamkiewicz's artery occurs in patients who do not have a very large, well-developed infrarenal lumbar articular artery. The extent of the ischemia is dependent on collateral blood flow and is modulated by such factors as hypotension, atherosclerotic disease, or thrombosis.[92] These secondary factors are probably critical in explaining postoperative paraplegia following aortic cross-clamping.

Before Aortic Cross-Clamp Removal, What Preparations Are Necessary?

Blood Replacement

Preparation for aortic declamping should begin at the time of cross-clamping. Blood losses are aggressively replaced with warmed packed red blood cells and crystalloid to keep the hematocrit at 30%. If blood losses are replaced with crystalloid in a 3:1 ratio, the acceptable blood loss (ABL) can be estimated by the following equation:

$$ABL = 3\ EBV\left(\frac{Hct - 30}{100}\right)$$

Equation 6

where EBV, Hct, and ABL denote the estimated blood volume, hematocrit, and allowable blood loss, respectively. The EBV in adults is 60 to 75 mL $\cdot$ kg^{-1} for men and 55 to 65 mL $\cdot$ kg^{-1} for women.

Sodium Bicarbonate

During cross-clamping, nitroglycerin and SNP are administered together with additional blood and fluids. Unless a patient is significantly acidemic, sodium bicarbonate is not administered. In contrast, if a significant metabolic acidosis (pH <7.25) develops, sodium bicarbonate is infused at a rate of $0.05 \text{ mEq} \cdot \text{kg}^{-1} \cdot \text{min}^{-1}$. Infusion is preferable to bolus administration. Saleh and colleagues showed that sodium bicarbonate infusion at a rate of $0.05 \text{ mEq} \cdot \text{kg}^{-1} \cdot \text{min}^{-1}$ was not associated with sudden shifts in pH, P_{CO_2}, potassium, or serious cardiac dysrhythmias.[101]

Rather than administer bicarbonate empirically, I prefer to calculate the total dose according to the following equation:

$$\text{Dose (mEq)} = 0.3 \left(\frac{\text{BW (kg)} \times \text{BD (mEq} \cdot \text{kg}^{-1})}{2} \right) \quad \text{Equation 7}$$

in which BW and BD denote body weight and base deficit, respectively. Sodium bicarbonate is rarely needed for abdominal aneurysm repairs.

Fresh-Frozen Plasma and Platelets

Fresh-frozen plasma (FFP), platelets, or both are useful in the setting of massive blood losses. Blood component therapy should be guided by laboratory measurements (hemoglobin, prothrombin time, partial thromboplastin time, platelet count). However, during a thoracoabdominal repair, blood often is lost at a rate that makes laboratory measurements impractical. In this situation, administration of FFP after the 10th unit of packed red blood cells is reasonable. I do not administer platelets unless the count is $<100,000 \cdot \text{mm}^{3-1}$, more than 10 units of washed cell-saver red blood cells have been administered, or clinical evidence of coagulopathy is present.

Attention to detail is important to prepare patients for removal of the aortic cross-clamp.[90] Blood diluted with normal saline and crystalloid is pressurized and ready to be administered rapidly through a blood warmer if the need arises after the cross-clamp is removed. The surgeon can reduce the hemodynamic effects by removing the clamp slowly. Although large volumes typically are administered to patients undergoing a thoracic aneurysm repair, be sure not to cause myocardial ischemia by administering too much volume and blood. Dilatation of the left ventricle can be prevented by closely scrutinizing the TEE and pulmonary artery catheter data during this critical period.

What Factors Cause Declamping Hypotension?

For the most part, the hemodynamic changes associated with declamping are the opposite of those observed with clamping. A rapid decrease in systemic vascular resistance leads to a decrease in MAP. Stable cardiodynamics necessitate adequate left ventricular preload to ensure maintenance of stroke volume and cardiac output; otherwise, precipitous hypotension can result. Mechanisms that contribute to the decrease in blood pressure are thought to include (1) reactive hyperemia secondary to free radicals, (2) redistribution of blood from the upper to lower body, (3) decrease in peripheral vasomotor tone (vasomotor paralysis), and (4) systemic effects of acidosis and metabolites (e.g., lactic acid, adenosine, endothelium-derived relaxing factor, myocardial depressant factor).[102-104] Reactive hyperemia and relative hypovolemia probably are the major causes. The severity is related to the

location of the cross-clamp. Severe hypotension following release of an infrarenal abdominal aortic cross-clamp is unusual but is common after release of a thoracic cross-clamp.

Should Patients Be Extubated in the Operating Room?

All patients are kept intubated after thoracic aneurysm repair. At the end of the operation, the double-lumen endotracheal tube is typically changed to a single-lumen endotracheal tube. However, because of the nature of these repairs and the associated massive volumes shifts, significant neck or airway edema often is present. In these patients, direct laryngoscopy is performed; if the vocal cords are easily visualized, the double-lumen tube is exchanged for a single-lumen tube. If the vocal cords cannot be visualized and the airway appears edematous, the double-lumen tube is converted to a single one by pulling the bronchial tip into the trachea. At a later time, the double-lumen tube can be changed when swelling subsides, or it can be left in place until the patient is extubated. Newer endotracheal tubes that contain a bronchial blocker obviate changing the tube at the end of the procedure.

CONCLUSION

An anesthesiologist rarely encounters situations with a greater sense of urgency than a ruptured abdominal aortic aneurysm. Survival is critically dependent on the surgeon's gaining prompt proximal control of the aorta. This fact must take precedence in the overall anesthetic management. Accordingly, these patients are best resuscitated by the anesthesiologist and the surgical team in the OR. Valuable time must not be wasted attempting to place an arterial, central venous, or pulmonary artery catheter or a transesophageal probe. Only the minimum preparations necessary to allow the operation to commence should be undertaken. These include placing two large-bore intravenous catheters; obtaining specimens of blood

TABLE 69–11. Mortality Rates from Ruptured Aortic Aneurysm

	Intraoperative (%)	Overall (%)
Preoperative Factors		
History of heart disease	29	—
History of hypertension	30	—
Frank ecchymosis	57	—
Pulsatile abdominal mass	24	—
Preoperative hypotension	39	78
Blood urea nitrogen >30 mg · dL^{-1}	47	82
Creatinine >3 mg · dL^{-1}	—	71
Hematocrit 30–32.5%	—	75
Intraoperative Factors		
Operation time >400 min	—	100
Hypotension >100 min	—	88
Blood loss >11,000 mL	—	75
Blood transfusions >17 units	—	68
Fluid >7000 mL	—	70
Blood pressure <100 mm Hg at conclusion of operation	—	88
Cardiac arrest	77	82

(From Wakefield TW, Whitehouse WM Jr, Wu S-C, et al: Abdominal aortic aneurysm rupture: statistical analysis of factors affecting outcome of surgical treatment. Surgery 1982; 91:586.)

to type and crossmatch (if not obtained previously) 12 units of blood; infusion of sufficient quantities of crystalloid to raise the systolic blood pressure to 80 to 90 mm Hg; and procurement of a cell-saver to salvage shed blood.

Because typed and crossmatched blood may not arrive at the OR in a timely manner, five to seven units of type O-negative blood are also ordered. Most ruptures occur in the retroperitoneal space, where bleeding may be tamponaded. However, 25% of all infrarenal aneurysms rupture into the peritoneal cavity.[105] Patients with a free peritoneal rupture hemorrhage more and have higher mortality rates. The most frequent cause of early death is hemorrhage, whereas the most important cause of late death is myocardial infarction.

As illustrated in Table 69–11, various preoperative and intraoperative factors are predictive of mortality. Although the single most important factor in this study was an operation time >400 minutes, many other studies show that sustained preoperative hypotension is the most significant factor. However, these studies generally did *not* analyze the role of operation length on patients' survival.

Chronic aortoiliac obstruction typically is caused by longstanding atherosclerosis. Obstruction of the aortic bifurcation with superimposed thrombosis of the stenotic area is usually found. The end-to-side bypass with a flexible knitted, albumin-coated Dacron bifurcation graft is the preferable method of treatment. Typically, the observed hemodynamic effects following cross-clamping of the abdominal aorta are significantly less in aortoiliac obstructive disease compared with those observed in the setting of aneurysm repair. This observation is at least partly attributable to the chronicity of obstruction in which significant vessel collateralization forms, a phenomenon also encountered with aortic coarctation. In contrast, release of the cross-clamp is still associated with declamping hypotension.

References

1. Crawford ES, Saleh SA, Babb JW III, et al: Infrarenal abdominal aortic aneurysm. Factors influencing survival after operation performed over a 25-year period. Ann Surg 1981; 193:699.
2. Ross R: The pathogenesis of atherosclerosis—an update. N Engl J Med 1986; 314:488.
3. Ross R: Pathophysiology of atherosclerosis. *In* Vascular Surgery Principles and Practice. Wilson SF, Veith FJ, Hobson RW, et al (eds) McGraw-Hill, New York, 1987, p 11.
4. Melton LJ, Bickerstaff LK, Hollier LH, et al: Changing incidence of abdominal aortic aneurysms: a population based study. Am J Epidemiol 1984; 120:379.
5. Johnston KW, Rutherford RB, Tilson MD, et al: Standards for reporting on aneurysms. J Vasc Surg 1991; 12:440.
6. Parmley LF, Mattingly TW, Manion WC, et al: Non-penetrating traumatic injury of the aorta. Circulation 1958; 17:1086.
7. Itzchak Y, Rosenthal T, Adar R, et al: Dissecting aneurysm of the thoracic aorta: reappraisal of radiologic diagnosis. AJR 1975; 125:559.
8. Rennollet R, Engberding R, Visser CA, et al: Transesophageal imaging of the thoracic aorta in aortic dissection. *In* Transesophageal Echocardiography. A New Window to the Heart. Erbel R, Khandheria BK, Brennecke R, et al (eds). Springer-Verlag, Berlin, 1989, p 140.
9. Joyce JW, Fairburn JF II, Kincaid OW, et al: Aneurysms of the thoracic aorta, a clinical study with special reference to prognosis. Circulation 1964; 29:176.
10. Roberts WC: Aortic dissection: anatomy, consequences, and causes. Am Heart J 1981; 101:195.
11. Cronenwett JL, Sargent SK, Wall MH, et al: Variables that affect the expansion rate and outcome of small abdominal aortic aneurysms. J Vasc Surg 1990; 11:260.
12. Hertzer NR, Beven EG, Young JR, et al: Coronary artery disease in peripheral vascular patients. Ann Surg 1984; 199:223.
13. Hollier LH: Surgical management of abdominal aortic aneurysms in the high risk patient. Surg Clin North Am 1986; 66:269.
14. Szilagyi DE, Smith RF, DeRusso FI, et al: Contribution of abdominal aortic aneurysmectomy to prolongation of life. Ann Surg 1966; 164:678.
15. Brown OW, Hollier LH, Pairolero PC, et al: Abdominal aortic aneurysms and coronary artery disease. Arch Surg 1981; 116:1484.
16. Hertzer NR, Young JR, Kramer JR, et al: Routine coronary angiography prior to elective aortic reconstruction: results of selective myocardial revascularization in patients with peripheral vascular disease. Arch Surg 1979; 114:1336.
17. O'Donnell TF Jr, Darling RC, Linton RR: Is 80 years too old for aneurysmectomy? Arch Surg 1976; 111:1250.
18. DeBakey ME, Cooley DA, Creech O Jr: Surgical considerations of dissecting aneurysms of the aorta. Ann Surg 1955; 142:586.
19. Dailey PO, Trueblood HN, Stinson EB, et al: Management of acute aortic dissections. Ann Thorac Surg 1970; 10:237.
20. Rutherford RB: Infrarenal aortic aneurysms: *In* Vascular Surgery. Rutherford RB (ed). Philadelphia, WB Saunders, 1984, p 755–771.
21. Darling RC, Messina CR, Brewster DC, et al: Autopsy study of unoperated abdominal aneurysms. The case for early resection. Cardiovasc Surg 1977; 56:161.
22. Wakefield TW, Whitehouse TW Jr, Wu S-C, et al: Abdominal aortic aneurysm rupture: statistical analysis of factors affecting outcome of surgical treatment. Surgery 1982; 91:586.
23. Ergin MA, Galla JD, Lansman S, et al: Acute dissections of the aorta: current surgical treatment. Surg Clin North Am 1985; 65:721.
24. Miller DC, Mitchell RS, Oyer PE, et al: Independent determinants of operative mortality for patients with aortic dissection. Circulation 1984; 70:I153.
25. Wolfe WG, Moran JF: The evolution of medical and surgical management of acute aortic dissection. Circulation 1977; 56:503.
26. Drummond JC, Moore SS: The influence of dextrose administration on neurologic outcome after temporary spinal cord ischemia in the rabbit. Anesthesiology 1989; 70:64.
27. Lundy EF, Ball TD, Mandell MA, et al: Dextrose administration increases sensory/motor impairment and paraplegia after infrarenal aortic occlusion in the rabbit. Surgery 1987; 102:737.
28. Robertson CS, Grossman RG: Protection against spinal cord ischemia with insulin-induced hypoglycemia. J Neurosurg 1987; 67:739.
29. Attia RR, Murphy JD, Snider M, et al: Myocardial ischemia due to infrarenal aortic cross-clamping during aortic surgery in patients with severe coronary artery disease. Circulation 1976; 53:961.
30. Still JC, Bove AA, Nugent M, et al: Effects of isoflurane on coronary arteries and coronary arterioles in the intact dog. Anesthesiology 1987; 66:273.
31. Buffington CW, Romson JL, Levine A, et al: Isoflurane induces coronary steal in a canine model of chronic coronary occlusion. Anesthesiology 1987; 66:280.
32. Hickey RF, Sybert PE, Verrier ED, et al: Effects of halothane, enflurane, and isoflurane on coronary blood flow regulation and coronary vascular reserve in the canine heart. Anesthesiology 1988; 68:21.
33. Moffitt ET, Barker RA, Glenn JJ, et al: Myocardial metabolism and hemodynamic responses with isoflurane anesthesia for coronary arterial surgery. Anesth Analg 1986; 65:53.
34. Reiz S: Myocardial ischaemia associated with general anaesthesia. Br J Anaesth 1987; 61:68.
35. Reiz S, Balfors E, Haggmark S, et al: Isoflurane—a powerful coronary vasodilator in patients with coronary artery disease. Anesthesiology 1983; 59:91.
36. Carson BA, Verrier ED, London MJ, et al: Effects of isoflurane and halothane on coronary vascular resistance and collateral myocardial blood flow: their capacity to induce coronary steal. Anesthesiology 1987; 67:665.
37. Buffington CW, Davis KB, Gillispie S, et al: The prevalence of steal-prone coronary anatomy in patients with coronary artery disease: an analysis of the coronary artery surgery study registry. Anesthesiology 1988; 69:721.
38. Becker LC: Is isoflurane dangerous for the patient with coronary artery disease? Anesthesiology 1987; 66:259.
39. Tinker JH: Anaesthesia for the patient with cardiac disease. Can J Anaesth 1988; 35:S9.
40. Benefiel DJ, Roizen MF, Lampe GH, et al: Morbidity after aortic surgery with sufentanil vs isoflurane. Anesthesiology 1986; 65:A516.
41. Benumof JL: Hypoxic pulmonary vasoconstriction and sodium nitroprusside infusion. Anesthesiology 1979; 50:481.
42. Bishop MJ, Cheney FW: Minoxidil and nifedipine inhibit hypoxic pulmonary vasoconstriction. J Cardiovasc Pharmacol 1983; 5:184.
43. Benumof JL: One-lung ventilation: which lung should be PEEPed? Anesthesiology 1982; 56:161.

44. McCullough JL, Hollier LH, Nugent M: Paraplegia after thoracic aortic occlusion: influence of cerebrospinal fluid drainage. J Vasc Surg 1988; 7:153.

45. Grubbs P, Marini CP, Toporoff B, et al: Somatosensory evoked potentials and spinal cord perfusion pressure are significant predictors of postoperative neurologic dysfunction. Surgery 1988; 104:216.

46. Cunningham JN Jr, Laschinger JC, Merkin HA, et al: Measurement of spinal cord ischemia during operations upon the thoracic aorta. Ann Surg 1982; 196:285.

47. Ginsburg HH, Shetter AG, Ruadzens PA: Postoperative paraplegia with preserved intraoperative somatosensory evoked potentials. J Neurosurg 1985; 63:296.

48. Kaplan BJ, Friedman WA, Alexander JA, Hampson SR: Somatosensory evoked potential monitoring of spinal cord ischemia during aortic operations. Neurosurgery 1986; 19:82.

49. Livesay JJ, Cooley DA, Ventemiglia RA, et al: Surgical experience in descending thoracic aneurysmectomy with and without adjuncts to avoid ischemia. Ann Thorac Surg 1984; 37:37.

50. Katz NW, Blackstone EH, Kirklin JW, et al: Incremental risk factors for spinal cord injury following operation for acute traumatic aortic transection. J Thorac Cardiovasc Surg 1981; 81:669.

51. Diehl JT, Cali RF, Hertzer NR, et al: Complications of abdominal aortic reconstruction: an analysis of perioperative risk factors in 557 patients. Ann Surg 1983; 197:49.

52. Alpert RA, Roizen MF, Hamilton, et al: Intraoperative urinary output does not predict postoperative renal function in patients undergoing abdominal aortic revascularization. Surgery 1984; 95:707.

53. Gamulin Z, Forster A, Morel D, et al: Effects of infrarenal aortic cross-clamping on renal hemodynamics in humans. Anesthesiology 1984; 61:394.

54. Gelman S, Reves JG, Fowler K, et al: Regional blood flow during cross-clamping of the thoracic aorta and infusion of sodium nitroprusside. Thorac Cardiovasc Surg 1983; 85:287.

55. Bush HL: Renal failure following abdominal aortic reconstruction. Surgery 1983; 93:107.

56. Myers BD, Miller DC, Mehigan JT, et al: Nature of the renal injury following total renal ischemia in man. J Clin Invest 1984; 73:329.

57. Miller DC, Myers BD: Pathophysiology and prevention of acute renal failure associated with thoracoabdominal or abdominal aortic surgery. J Vasc Surg 1987; 5:518.

58. Bush HL, Huse JB, Johnson WC, et al: Prevention of renal insufficiency after abdominal aortic aneurysm resection by optimal volume loading. Arch Surg 1981; 116:1517.

59. Abbott WM, Austen WG: The reversal of renal cortical ischemia during aortic occlusion by mannitol. J Surg Res 1974; 16:482.

60. Barry KG, Cohen A, Knochel JP: Mannitol infusion II. The prevention of acute functional renal failure during resection of an aneurysm of the abdominal aorta. N Engl J Med 1961; 264:967.

61. Smith JS, Cahalan MK, Benefiel DR, et al: Intraoperative detection of myocardial ischemia in high-risk patients: electrocardiography versus two-dimensional transesophageal echocardiography. Circulation 1985; 72:1015.

62. Cahalan MK: Pro: transesophageal echocardiography is the "gold standard" for detection of intraoperative myocardial ischemia. J Cardiothorac Anesth 1989; 3:369.

63. Mitchell MM, Sutherland GR, Gussenhoven EJ, et al: Transesophageal echocardiography. J Am Soc Echocardiogr 1988; 1:362.

64. McCloskey G, Barash PG: Con: transesophageal echocardiography is not the "gold standard" for detection of myocardial ischemia. J Cardiothorac Anesth 1989; 3:372.

65. London MJ, Tubau JF, Wong MG, et al: The "natural history" of segmental wall motion abnormalities in patients undergoing noncardiac surgery. Anesthesiology 1990; 73:644.

66. Kaplan JA, Wells PH: Early diagnosis of myocardial ischemia using the pulmonary arterial catheter. Anesth Analg 1981; 60:789.

67. van-Daele ME, Sutherland GR, Mitchell MM, et al: Do changes in pulmonary capillary wedge pressure adequately reflect myocardial ischemia during anesthesia? A correlative preoperative hemodynamic, electrocardiographic and transesophageal echocardiographic study. Circulation 1990; 81:865.

68. Oshita S, Masuda N, Kunil T, et al: Evaluation of pulmonary capillary wedge pressure tracing for the detection of intraoperative myocardial ischemia. Masui 1991; 40:1052.

69. Spurny OM, Rubin S, Wolf JW, et al: Spinal epidural hematoma during anticoagulant therapy: report of two cases. Arch Intern Med 1964; 114:103.

70. Rao TLK, El-Etr AA: Anticoagulation following placement of epidural and subarachnoid catheters: an evaluation of neurological sequelae. Anesthesiology 1981; 55:618.

71. Barron HC, LaRaja RD, Rossi G, et al: Continuous epidural analgesia in the heparinized vascular surgical patient: a retrospective review of 912 patients. J Vasc Surg 1987; 6:144.

72. Baron J-F, Bertrand M, Barre E, et al: Combined epidural and general anesthesia versus general anesthesia for abdominal aortic surgery. Anesthesiology 1991; 75:611.

73. Tuman KJ, McCarthy RJ, March RJ, et al: Effects of epidural anesthesia and analgesia on coagulation and outcome after major vascular surgery. Anesth Analg 1991; 71:696.

74. Yeager MP, Glass DD, Neff RK, et al: Epidural anesthesia and analgesia in high-risk patients. Anesthesiology 1987; 66:729.

75. Bunt TJ, Manczuk M, Varley K: Continuous epidural anesthesia for aortic surgery: thoughts on peer review and safety. Surgery 1987; 101:706.

76. Mason RA, Newton GB, Cassel W: Combined epidural and general anesthesia in aortic surgery. J Cardiovasc Surg 1989; 31:442.

77. Marini CP, Grubbs P, Toporoff B, et al: Effect of sodium nitroprusside on spinal cord perfusion pressure and paraplegia during aortic cross-clamping. Ann Thorac Surg 1989; 47:379.

78. Hickey R, Albin M, Bunegin L, et al: Autoregulation of spinal cord blood flow: is the cord a microcosm of the brain? Stroke 1988; 7:153.

79. Newberg LA, Michenfelder JD: Cerebral protection by isoflurane during hypoxemia and ischemia. Anesthesiology 1983; 59:29.

80. Grum DF, Svensson LG: Changes in cerebrospinal fluid pressure and spinal cord perfusion pressure prior to cross-clamping of the thoracic aorta in humans. J Cardiothorac Vasc Anesth 1991; 5:331.

81. Messick JM Jr, Newberg LA, Nugent M, et al: Principles of neuroanesthesia for the non-neurosurgical patient with central nervous system pathophysiology. Anesth Analg 1985; 64:143.

82. Roizen MG, Beaupre PN, Alpert RA, et al: Monitoring with two-dimensional transesophageal echocardiography: comparison of myocardial function in patients undergoing supraceliac, suprarenal-infraceliac, or infrarenal aortic occlusion. J Vasc Surg 1984; 1:300.

83. Vacanti FX, Ames A: Mild hypothermia and Mg^{++} protect against irreversible damage during CNS ischemia. Stroke 1984; 15:695.

84. Berguer R, Porto J, Fedoronko B, et al: Selective deep hypothermia of the spinal cord prevents paraplegia after aortic cross-clamping in the dog model. J Vasc Surg 1992; 15:62.

85. Dunn E, Prager RL, Fry W, et al: The effect of abdominal aortic cross-clamping on myocardial function. J Surg Res 1977; 22:463.

86. Gooding JM, Archie JP, McDowel H: Hemodynamic response to infrarenal aortic crossclamping in patients with and without coronary artery disease. Crit Care Med 1980; 8:382.

87. Huval WV, Lelcuk S, Allen PD, et al: Determinants of cardiovascular stability during abdominal aortic aneurysmectomy (AAA). Ann Surg 1984; 199:216.

88. Meloche R, Pottecher T, Audet J, et al: Hemodynamic changes during clamping of the abdominal aorta. Can Anaesth Soc J 1977; 24:20.

89. Svensson LG, Von Ritter CM, Groeneveld HT, et al: Cross-clamping of the thoracic aorta. Ann Surg 1986; 204:38.

90. Silverstein PR, Caldera DL, Cullen DJ, et al: Avoiding the hemodynamic consequences of aortic cross-clamping and unclamping. Anesthesiology 1979; 50:462.

91. Wadouh F, Lindemann E, Arndt CF, et al: The arteria radicularis magna anterior as a decisive factor influencing spinal cord damage during aortic occlusion. J Thorac Cardiovasc Surg 1984; 88:1.

92. Szilagyi DE, Hageman JH, Smith RF, et al: Spinal cord damage in surgery of the abdominal aorta. Surgery 1978; 83:38.

93. Hollier LH, Symmonds JB, Pairolero PC, et al: Thoracoabdominal aortic aneurysm repair: analysis of postoperative morbidity. Arch Surg 1988; 123:871.

94. Crawford ES, Walker HS, Saleh SA, et al: Graft replacement of aneurysm in descending thoracic aorta: results without bypass or shunting. Surgery 1981; 89:73.

95. Crawford ES, Crawford JL, Safi JH. et al: Thoracoabdominal aortic aneurysms: preoperative and intraoperative factors determining immediate and long-term results of operations in 605 patients. J Vasc Surg 1986; 3:389.

96. Crawford ES, Svensson LG, Hess KR, et al: A prospective randomized study of cerebrospinal fluid drainage to prevent paraplegia after high-risk surgery on the thoracoabdominal aorta. J Vasc Surg 1991; 13:36.

97. Bracken MB, Shepard MJ, Collins WF, et al: A randomized, controlled trial of methylprednisolone or naloxone in the treatment of acute spinal-cord injury. N Engl J Med 1990; 322:1405.

98. Svennson LG, Von-Ritter CM, Groeneveld HT, et al: Cross-clamping of the thoracic aorta: influence of aortic shunts, laminectomy, papaverine, calcium channel blocker, allopurinol, and superoxide dismutase on spinal cord blood flow and paraplegia in baboons. Ann Surg 1986; 204:38.

99. Svensson LG, Grum DF, Bednarski M: Appraisal of CSF alterations during aortic surgery with intrathecal papaverine administration and CSF drainage. J Vasc Surg 1990; 11:423.

100. Svensson LG, Stewart RW, Cosgrove DM, et al: Intrathecal papaverine for the prevention of paraplegia after operation on the thoracic or thoracoabdominal aorta. J Thorac Cardiovasc Surg 1988; 96:823.

101. Saleh SA, Crawford ES, Bomberger RA, et al: Intraoperative acid-base management for the resection of thoracoabdominal aneurysms: a comparison of continuous infusion of sodium bicarbonate versus the bolus. Anesth Analg 1982; 61:213.

102. Damask MC, Weissman C, Rodriguez J, et al: Abdominal aortic cross-clamping. Metabolic and hemodynamic consequences. Arch Surg 1984; 119:1332.

103. Vetto RM, Brant B: Control of declamping shock. Am J Surg 1968; 116:273.

104. Eklof B, Neglen P, Thomson D: Temporary incomplete ischemia of the legs induced by aortic clamping in man. Effects on central hemodynamics and skeletal muscle metabolism by adrenergic blockade. Ann Surg 1981; 193:89.

CHAPTER 70

Genitourinary Surgery

JERRY J. BERGER, M.D.

Genitourinary surgery encompasses renal, ureteral, bladder, and prostate procedures. Because of the dermatomes involved, regional anesthesia and local anesthesia are options to be considered in many cases. Many of the general considerations that relate to abdominal surgery are applicable to urogenital surgery as well. In addition, special problems occur in selected operations such as transurethral resection of the prostate (TURP). These problems receive emphasis in this chapter. Anesthesic considerations for renal transplantation and extracorporeal shock wave lithotripsy are discussed in Chapters 77 and 79, respectively.

ANATOMIC CONSIDERATIONS

What Is the Celiac Plexus?

The celiac plexus comprises visceral afferent and efferent fibers from T-5 to T-12[1] and parasympathetic fibers that originate in the cranial and sacral areas. It innervates the kidneys, ureters, and adrenal glands. Innervation of the kidneys is thoracolumbar in origin (from T-12 to L-2).

Splanchnic Nerves

All three splanchnic nerves, which are preganglionic, synapse in the celiac plexus; the postganglionic fibers travel to the aortic, renal, and hypogastric plexuses that provide innervation to the viscera. The lumbar sympathetic ganglia lie at the anterolateral border of the vertebral bodies. The lumbar sympathetic chain innervates the urogenital organs, colon, and rectum.[2]

Celiac plexus and lumbar sympathetic blocks are not used alone for surgical procedures, since they provide exclusively autonomic blockade. Thus, they must be combined with other somatic nerve blocks. Because of their technical ease, epidural or spinal anesthetics that block both autonomic and somatic nerves usually are chosen when a regional anesthetic technique is desired.

What Is the Lumbar Plexus?

The lumbar plexus (Fig. 70–1) derives its innervation from the L-1, L-2, L-3, L-4, and L-5 somatic nerve roots. Together

with the T-11 and T-12 somatic nerve roots, it innervates the inguinal region and canal, including the spermatic cord. After traveling between the transverse and internal oblique muscles, the 11th and 12th thoracic nerves pass through the rectus sheath. Their roots innervate the rectus muscle and sheath and the internal, external, and transverse oblique muscles.

Ilioinguinal and Iliohypogastric Nerves

The T-12 and L-1 roots form the ilioinguinal and iliohypogastric nerves, which are retroperitoneal until they penetrate the transverse oblique muscle. The internal oblique muscle is penetrated more medially, and the nerves enter the inguinal canal on the anterior surface of the spermatic cord.

Genitofemoral Nerve

The genitofemoral nerve is derived from the L-1 and L-2 nerve roots and is located on the posterior surface of the spermatic cord. The genital branch supplies sensation to the cremaster muscle and the scrotum. The femoral branch innervates Scarpa's fascia and a small area on the anterior thigh.[3]

Pudendal Nerves

The pudendal nerves are derived from the somatic roots of S-2, S-3, and S-4 from the sacral plexus. The nerves branch under the pubic bone to produce the left and right dorsal nerves of the penis, which supply all innervation to the penis.[4]

How Is Regional Anesthesia of the Inguinal Region Performed?

Regional anesthesia of the inguinal region may be advantageous for several reasons. Earlier ambulation, discharge, and lower morbidity occur in patients receiving this anesthetic compared with those who are administered a general anesthetic. It may be the technique of choice in patients with severe systemic illnesses, especially those that involve the pulmonary and cardiac systems.[4] Blockade of the inguinal region requires several injections. Landmark identification is imperative (Fig. 70–2). Regional blockade of this area should provide signifi-

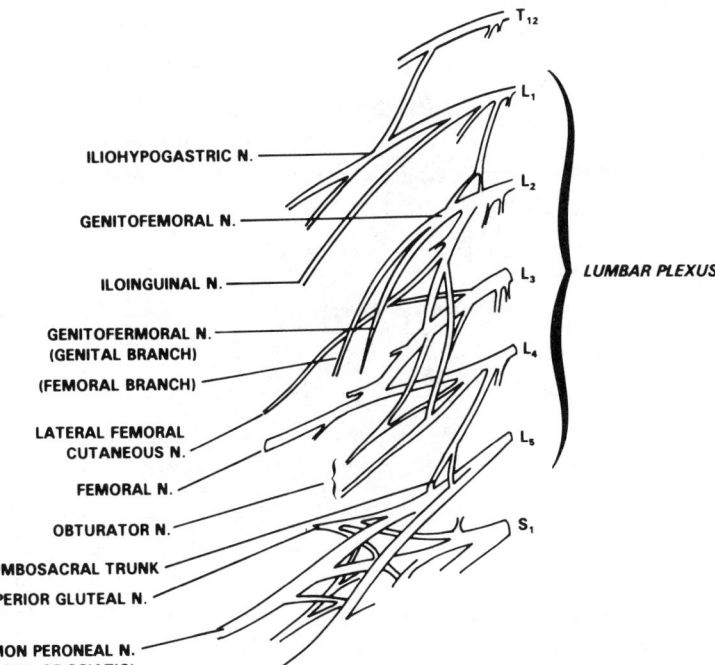

FIGURE 70–1. View of the lumbar plexus forming the nerves of the inguinal region.

cant postoperative analgesia in patients undergoing surgical manipulation of the inguinal canal, spermatic cord, and testes.

Technique

A line is drawn from the anterosuperior iliac spine to the umbilicus. A second line is drawn from the anterosuperior iliac spine to the pubic tubercle along the course of the inguinal ligament. The initial injection is performed along the first line, 1 inch from the anterosuperior iliac spine, and anesthetizes the ilioinguinal and iliohypogastric nerves. A 22- or 25-gauge 1½-inch or 2-inch needle is inserted through a skin wheal and advanced downward and lateral to the iliac crest. Five to 10 mL of 1% lidocaine with epinephrine are injected along the medial aspect of the iliac bone. The needle is then withdrawn

and reinserted slightly more medially so that the infiltration is fanned out, and another 4 to 5 mL of the solution are injected deep into the transversalis fascia. The injection is continued as the needle is withdrawn. The procedure is repeated several times as the needle is advanced more medially (Fig. 70–3).

Twenty milliliters of a 0.5% lidocaine solution with epinephrine (1:200,000) are injected subcutaneously along the two lines that were drawn previously. The index finger should palpate the femoral artery during injection to prevent puncture and intravascular injections. After infiltration, the needle is inserted perpendicular to the skin above and lateral to the superior ramus of the pubic bone. Additional injections of the same solution (15 mL total) are made on each side of the spermatic cord, into the rectus muscle attachments to the pubis, along the superior ramus of the pubic bone, and into

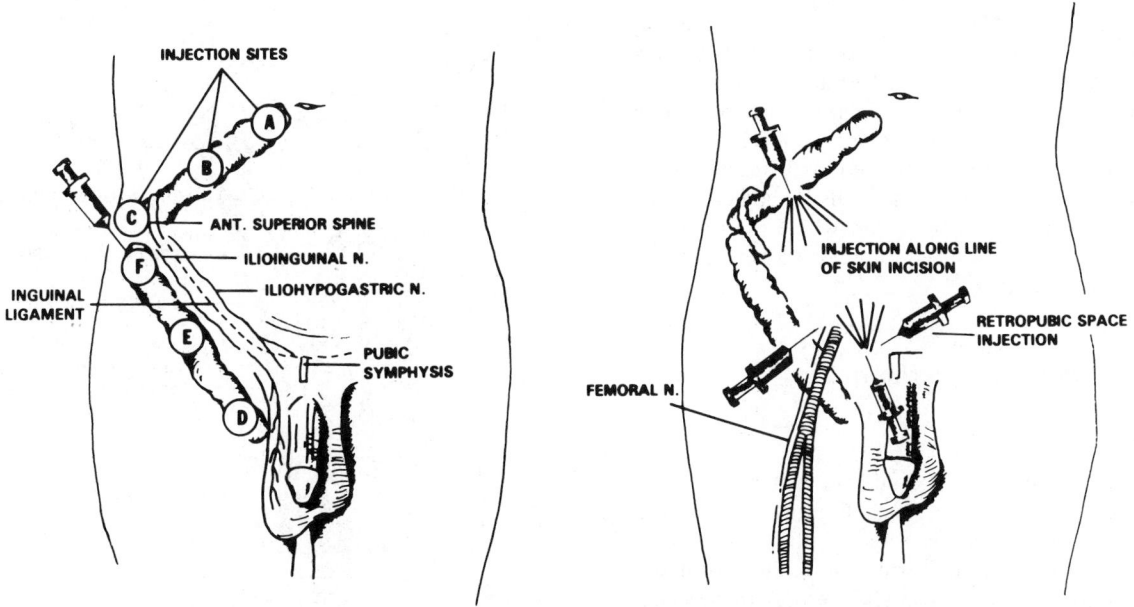

FIGURE 70–2. Overall view of the injection sites for complete ilioinguinal anesthesia.

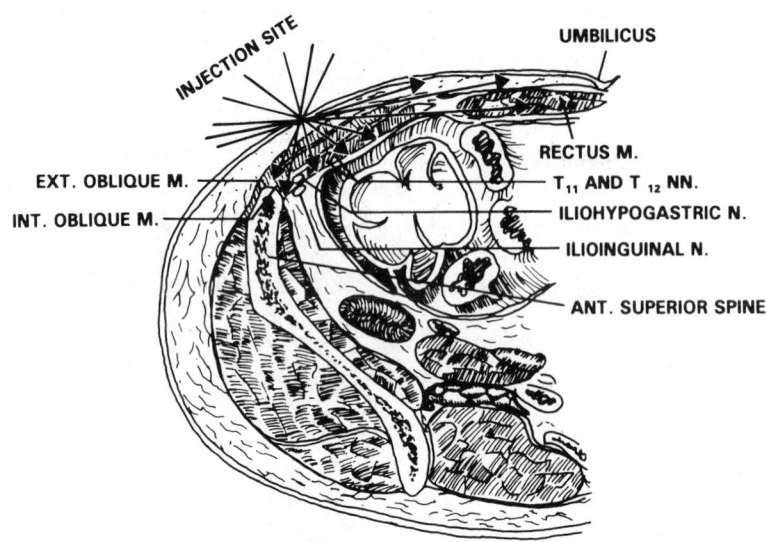

FIGURE 70–3. Sagittal view of the abdominal wall at the level of the umbilicus. Injection of local anesthetic and the fanning technique are shown.

the space between the bladder and the pubic bone (the space of Retzius). The final local infiltration should be made along the anticipated line of the skin incision using the same solution.[3]

Potential Complications

A large volume of local anesthetic is required for block of the inguinal region. Remember that the toxic dose of lidocaine with epinephrine is 7 mg · kg^{-1}; dosages need to be adjusted according to the patient's body weight. Bilateral procedures should not be performed simultaneously using this technique, since local anesthetic dosages will be excessive.[4] In addition to local anesthetic toxicity, inadvertent motor weakness of the quadriceps femoris accompanied by sensory loss over the distribution of the femoral nerve in the anterior thigh may occur.

How Is the Spermatic Cord Blocked?

Regional nerve block involving the spermatic cord may be used for surgical procedures of the scrotum, including orchiectomy, vasovasostomy, spermatocelectomy, and hydrocelectomy.[5, 6] A 25-gauge 1½-inch needle must be used to inject 10 mL of 1% lidocaine (without epinephrine) into each spermatic cord just below the superficial inguinal ring. The entire cross-sectional area of the cord is infiltrated, with special care being taken in the region of the vas deferens.[4] Another injection is made along the anterior scrotal skin where the incision is to be made. Care should be taken to prevent a hematoma in this sensitive area (Fig. 70–4).

How Is a Penile Block Performed?

Innervation

Regional anesthesia may be utilized for operations on the penis and all of its structures, including the prepuce, urethra, glans, and corpora cavernosa. Although the most frequent indication is circumcision, placement of penile prostheses and manipulation of the urethra can also be performed satisfactorily. The left and right dorsal nerves of the penis, which are

branches of the pudendal nerves, are formed by the S-2, S-3, and S-4 roots. The dorsal nerve of the penis branches into anterior and posterior components after it passes underneath the pubic bone. The anterior branches supply sensation to the dorsum of the penis and the glans. The smaller posterior branches innervate the underside of the penis and frenulum. Skin at the base of the penis is innervated by the ilioinguinal nerve and occasionally a branch of the genitofemoral nerve (see Fig. 70–4).[3]

Technique

Block of the penis is performed using a 25- or 27-gauge ¾-inch needle. Intradermal skin wheals are raised ½ inch caudal and ½ inch medial to each pubic tubercle (Figs. 70–5 and 70–6). The intradermal wheals are connected by intradermal and subcutaneous infiltration of 10 mL of 1% lidocaine, with or without epinephrine (1:200,000). A skin wheal also is raised on the median raphe of the scrotum at the base of the penis, and the intradermal and subcutaneous infiltrations are extended bilaterally to this point. Twenty milliliters of the anesthetic

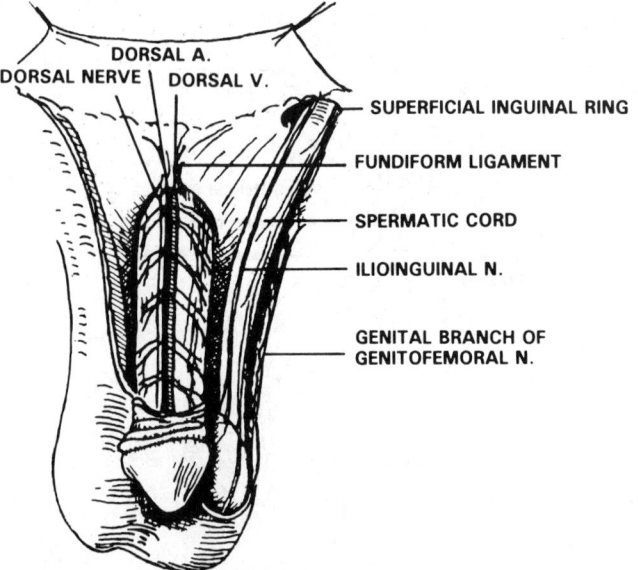

FIGURE 70–4. Relevant neuroanatomy of the penis.

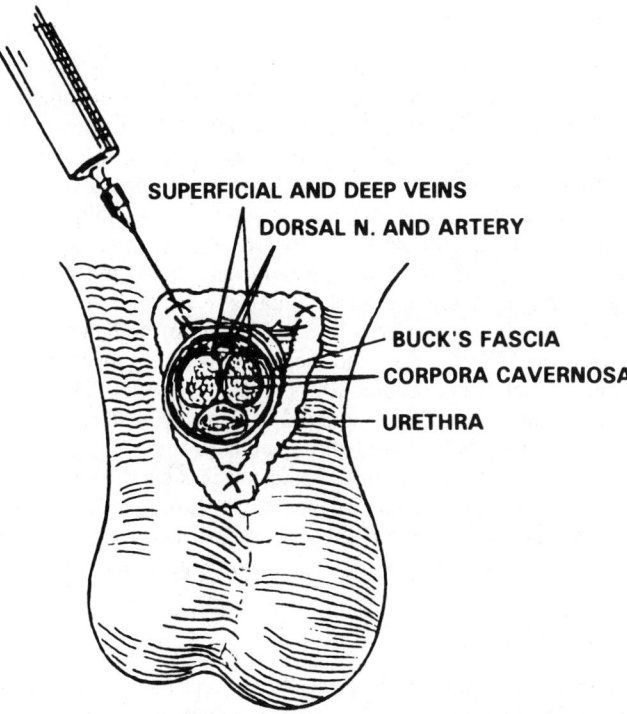

FIGURE 70–5. Injection points for penile block.

SUPERFICIAL AND DEEP VEINS
DORSAL N. AND ARTERY
BUCK'S FASCIA
CORPORA CAVERNOSA
URETHRA

solution are used.[3] Care must be taken not to inject intravascularly.

Duration of analgesia is for 1¼ to 3 hours; the longer duration follows injection of epinephrine-containing solutions. Impotence following penile block apparently has followed placement of the local anesthetic under the penile fascia.

INTERPLEURAL ANESTHESIA

Interpleural anesthesia has been advocated for patients undergoing a variety of procedures from cholecystectomies to renal surgery. Trivedi and coworkers described interpleural block with 30 mL of 0.5% bupivacaine for patients undergoing percutaneous nephrostomy and nephrolithotomy.[7] The ultimate role of interpleural block in regional anesthesia remains to be defined, but advantages over segmental epidural or subarachnoid block are not obvious.

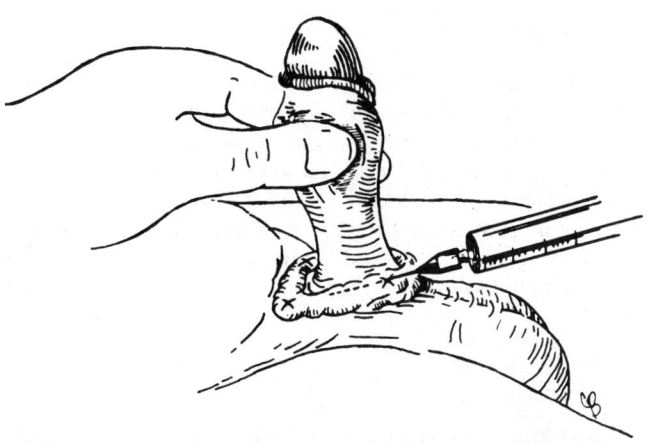

FIGURE 70–6. Intradermal skin wheals for penile block.

How Is It Performed?

Interpleural catheters are placed using 16- or 18-gauge Tuohy needles that are inserted along the superior border of the eighth rib, 8 to 10 cm from the posterior midline. The needle is advancing using either a loss of resistance technique with a glass syringe or a hanging drop method. When the pleural cavity is identified, a catheter is placed 5 to 6 cm past the end of the needle. A test dose of 0.5% bupivacaine with epinephrine (1:200,000) is injected; this is followed by a loading dose of 20 mL.

Advocates of this block point to its maintenance of hemodynamic stability as a distinct advantage. The duration of effect is claimed to be 9 to 10 hours.[8] Reverse diffusion of local anesthetic from the parietal pleura to the intercostal muscles and also to the intercostal nerves is thought to provide analgesia.

What Problems May Occur?

Local Anesthetic Toxicity

Questions arise as to whether local anesthetic toxicity is a major concern when using this route of injection.[9] Seltzer and colleagues measured blood levels at different time intervals following administration of a 30-mL dose of 0.5% bupivacaine with epinephrine (1:100,000) and found absorption from the pleural space similar to that in other areas of the body. Maximum bupivacaine plasma concentrations were reached in between 10 and 30 minutes and ranged from 1.1 to 3.3 $\mu g \cdot mL^{-1}$.[10] Plasma levels of bupivacaine ≥ 4 $\mu g \cdot mL^{-1}$ are associated with central nervous system toxicity. Lower concentrations of bupivacaine in the injectate were correlated with poor pain relief.[10]

Other Complications

Possible complications include pneumothorax, hemothorax, empyema, systemic local anesthetic toxicity, intravascular injection, and Horner's syndrome. Contraindications to interpleural block include pleural fibrosis, pleural effusion, pleural infections, pneumothorax, and severely compromised cardiorespiratory function.[7]

PROSTATIC SURGERY

Benign prostatic hyperplasia generally begins in the fourth decade of life. When hyperplasia becomes symptomatic, patients usually require surgery to alleviate their symptoms.

What Is the Purpose of Balloon Dilatation?

Balloon dilatation of the prostate initially was used as an alternative to more invasive TURP surgery in high-risk patients. The procedure involves dilation of the prostatic urethra with a balloon catheter of up to size 90 French that is inflated for 10 minutes.[11] The incidence of complications from the procedure is extremely low, and it now is offered to an increasing number of patients with symptomatic benign prostatic hyperplasia.[12]

Anesthesia

Initially, the procedure was performed using general or regional anesthesia, since dilation is painful. This approach necessitated long postanesthesia care unit stays for monitoring. However, it is increasingly performed with local anesthesia or with a combination of local anesthesia and intravenous sedation.

Technique

The technique involves placement of the patient in a dorsal lithotomy position. Reddy performs anesthesia of the perineum using a 25-gauge needle to infiltrate 1% lidocaine bilaterally into the skin 1 cm above and lateral to the anal orifice.[11] While a finger is placed in the rectum, a 20-gauge, 5-inch spinal needle is advanced, and 5 mL of 1% lidocaine is infiltrated along the left lateral border of the prostate to the junction of the prostate and left seminal vesicle. Ten to 15 mL of 1% lidocaine is deposited in this area. The same procedure is then performed on the right side. If the needle is placed too far anteriorly or laterally, it will hit the pubic ramus and must be redirected. The dilatation can then be performed usually without any additional sedative or analgesic supplement.

Sedoanalgesia

Alternatively, local anesthetic instillation or infiltration techniques have been used. The urethra can be anesthetized by instillation of 2% lidocaine jelly. Concurrent intravenous sedation is achieved with short-acting narcotics, alone or combined with a benzodiazepine such as midazolam or diazepam or with a propofol infusion, 30 to 50 $\mu g \cdot kg^{-1} \cdot min^{-1}$. The combination of local anesthesia and sedation is referred to as *sedoanalgesia* and has been used with great success in urology.[13] Advantages of these local techniques are shorter stays in postanesthesia care units and improved outpatient performance on discharge.

How Is Prostatic Resection Accomplished?

The prostate gland can be excised by transurethral resection or using an open approach. Large prostate glands ($\geq$80 g) are generally best resected by open prostatectomy. Prostate procedures generally are performed with the patient in a lithotomy position and with the operating table adjusted to some degree of the Trendelenburg tilt. Padding under the hips to provide better exposure of the prostate is often used. The prostate is a very vascular structure; thus, bleeding may be significant and at times difficult to control regardless of the surgical approach employed.

TABLE 70–1. Transurethral Resection of the Prostate and Coexisting Disease

Disease	%
Pulmonary	14.1
Gastrointestinal	13.2
Hypertension	43
Previous myocardial infarction	12.3
Dysrhythmias	12.4
Renal insufficiency	9.8
Diabetes	9.8

(From Mebust WK, Holtgrewe HL, Cockett ATK, et al: Transurethral prostatectomy: immediate and postoperative complications: a cooperative study of 13 participating institutions evaluating 3885 patients. J Urol 1989; 14:243. © American Urological Association, Inc., 1989.)

Open Prostatectomy

This procedure can be safely and effectively accomplished using a general, regional, or combined anesthetic technique. The head-down position, the use of retractors, and the length of the procedure normally indicate the need for a general anesthetic, either alone or in combination with epidural anesthesia. Benefits of regional and combination techniques include decreased intraoperative blood loss (37%), lowered incidence of pelvic deep vein thrombosis (77%), and postoperative analgesia with epidural narcotics.[14]

A lowered mean arterial pressure (inflow) and decreased venous tone (outflow) are the mechanisms likely to influence the beneficial effect on blood loss and thrombosis. Placement of and dosing through the epidural catheter prior to induction of general anesthesia avoid most hemodynamic changes and allow the patient to identify a paresthesia should one occur. Use of a central venous catheter is also frequently recommended; the bladder is open during the procedure, thus, urine output is not available to help guide fluid management.

Venous Air Embolism

Venous air embolism is a possibility, and its occurrence in this setting has been described.[15] The actual incidence of this complication during open prostatectomy is unknown. However, the hydrostatic pressure gradient between the prostatic fossa and the right side of the heart when the patient is in a head-down position, the extensive venous plexus, the use of retractors, and significant blood loss in combination predispose patients to such embolism. This complication merits inclusion in the differential diagnosis of hypotension.

Transurethral Resection

TURP still is the primary method used to relieve bladder outlet obstruction from prostatic hyperplasia. In a cooperative study that evaluated 3885 patients, Mebust and associates reviewed patient demographics: the average patient age was 69 years; also, 81% of patients were white, 10% were black, 0.3% were Asian, and 5% were Hispanic (the ethnic affiliation of 3% of patients was not recorded). The age distribution of patients was as follows: 15% were younger than 60 years; 38% were aged from 60 to 69 years; 35% were aged from 70 to 79 years; and 12% were older than 80 years.[16] Only 24.3% had no other recorded medical problems (Table 70–1).

Anesthesia

In the study of Mebust and associates, 77% of surgeries were performed with spinal anesthesia; 20% were performed with general anesthesia; and the remaining 3% used either epidural or local anesthesia. In some areas, local anesthesia with sedation is growing in popularity; for example, small glands can be resected using this approach.[13] Regional anesthesia is the preferred method for patients undergoing TURP, since it facilitates early recognition of complications (Table 70–2).

Complications

Morbidity and Mortality. Mebust and associates noted 9 postoperative deaths (0.23%). In patients with benign disease,

TABLE 70–2. Signs and Symptoms of Complications of
Transurethral Resection of the Prostate

Fluid Overload	Tachypnea; ↓ Spo₂
Hyponatremia	Restlessness; confusion; nausea; seizures
Glycine Toxicity	Encephalopathy; transient blindness (rarely)
Bladder Perforation	
Extraperitoneal	Decreased irrigating fluid return; abdominal pain and distention; nausea; sweating
Intraperitoneal	Rapid onset of extraperitoneal symptoms as well as shoulder pain

mortality was 0.1%.[16] Causes of death were sepsis in 5 patients, myocardial infarction in 1 patient, and other nonspecific conditions in 3 patients. No intraoperative deaths occurred. A total of 272 complications (6.9%) occurred intraoperatively.[16]

Bleeding. The most common complication was bleeding sufficient to require transfusion in 2.5% of patients. When resection time is >90 minutes, the incidence of intraoperative bleeding is 7.3% (compared with 0.9% when resection time is <90 minutes).[16] The near constant flow of irrigating solution makes assessment of blood loss difficult. Additionally, the absorption—or more correctly stated, the infusion—of irrigating solution through the opened prostatic venous channels, combined with the absorption of fluid from retroperitoneal and perivesical spaces, masks the usual hemodynamic changes associated with blood loss.

Transurethral resection of larger glands (i.e., those >50 g) and procedures that are of long duration (i.e., >1 hour) are associated with increased blood loss. A blood loss of 15 mL per gram of resected tissue should be anticipated.[17, 18] A predictable decrease in blood loss with regional compared with general anesthesia has not been documented.

Resections of prostate glands >45 g in weight have a statistically greater incidence of intraoperative bleeding (10%) than do those of smaller glands (0.9%) and require a greater amount of time to perform. The incidence of the TURP syndrome is also higher (1.5% compared with 0.8% for smaller glands).

Hypothermia. Hypothermia results from reduced temperatures in the operating room environment and the use of room-temperature irrigating solutions. Routine use of irrigating solutions that are warmed to body temperature prevents this complication. If room-temperature irrigating fluids are used, the average decrease in body temperature is 1.8 °C for a 70-minute TURP.[19]

Sepsis. Sudden cardiovascular collapse, rigors, or tachycardia suggest the presence of bacteremia. Treatment is symptomatic and includes broad-spectrum antibiotic coverage. Procedures on the very vascular genitourinary system predispose the patient to intravascular inoculation and bacteremia if an infection is present. Thus, prostate or urinary tract infections should be treated preoperatively.

Obturator Nerve Stimulation. Stimulation of the obturator nerve by the electric resectoscope sometimes occurs. The obturator nerve traverses the pelvis adjacent to the inferolateral wall of the bladder, the bladder neck, and the lateral prostatic urethra. It is a branch of the lumbar plexus (L2-4). As it emerges from the obturator canal, it divides into the superficial and profunda branches. The superficial branch innervates the short, long, and gracilis adductor muscles. The profunda branch innervates the adductor magnus and internus muscles.

Adductor contraction results from direct stimulation of the motor neurons within the obturator nerve by the electrical

current from the resectoscope.[20] Jerking of the legs may be so violent as to cause inadvertent bladder perforation or inability of the urologist to resect the prostate adequately. Neuromuscular blocking agents prevent adductor contraction.[21] Although nondepolarizing and depolarizing agents accomplish neuromuscular blockade, direct muscle stimulation from the current can best be prevented by using a depolarizing agent. If repetitive adductor muscle contraction is a problem during general anesthesia, a succinylcholine infusion should be considered.

The obturator nerve can be blocked. In one series, an obturator block obtained with 30 mL of 2% lidocaine with epinephrine produced complete ablation of adductor spasm in 11 of 13 patients; the remaining 2 patients had 80% reduction of the spasm.[22]

To perform the block, the adductor longus tendon is palpated where it inserts into the pubic tubercle. A 22-gauge spinal needle is placed 2 cm lateral and caudad to the pubic tubercle (Fig. 70–7). The needle is aimed slightly lateral (15–20°) and cephalad (10–30°) and is advanced to the superior pubic ramus. It is then *walked* off the inferior margin of the superior pubic ramus and advanced 1.5 to 2 cm in a posterior, superior, and lateral direction (Fig. 70–8). One-half of the volume is injected, the needle is withdrawn and repositioned 1 cm laterally, and one-half of the remaining lidocaine is injected. The needle is again repositioned 1 cm medial to the original site, and the remainder of the anesthetic is injected[22] (Fig. 70–9).

Venous Thrombosis. A potentially devastating complication after prostatic surgery is deep vein thrombosis with resultant pulmonary embolus. Nicolaides and coworkers studied 50 patients who underwent TURP or retropubic prostatic resec-

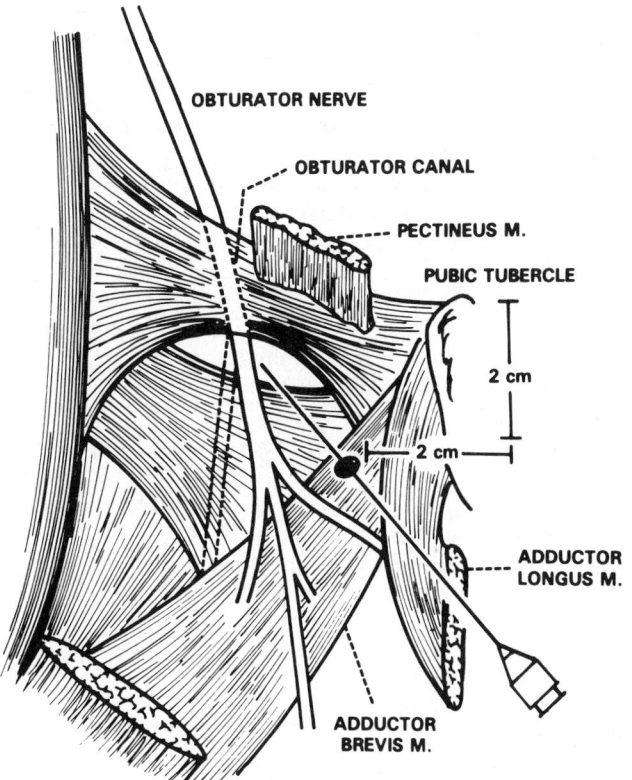

FIGURE 70–7. View of the obturator nerve as it passes through the obturator canal. (Redrawn from Augspurger RR, Donohue RE: Prevention of obturator nerve stimulation during transurethral surgery. J Urol 1980; 123:170. © American Urological Association, Inc., 1980.)

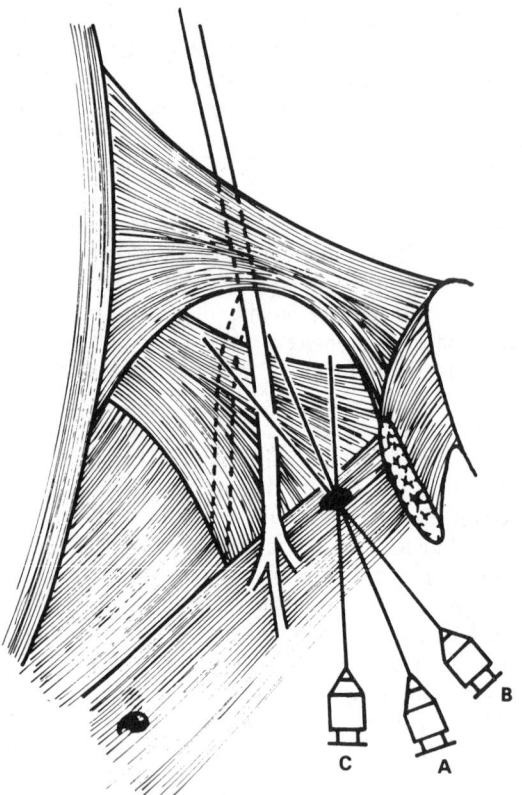

FIGURE 70–8. Site of local anesthetic infiltration for obturator nerve block. *A,* Midobturator canal. *B,* One centimeter lateral. *C,* One centimeter medial.

tion.[23] They found that the incidence of deep vein thrombosis was 47.6% following retropubic prostatectomy and only 6.8% following TURP. In a study by Mayo and associates, the incidence of deep vein thrombosis was 51% for retropubic prostatectomy and 10% for TURP.[24] These authors believed that the incidence was less for TURP because a patient's legs are elevated during this procedure.[24]

The relative absence of pain following TURP compared with open procedures allows patients to ambulate sooner and be more active in the early postoperative period. Ljunger and colleagues studied the difference in plasminogen activator content in 56 patients who underwent either transvesical prostatectomy or TURP.[25] A decrease in plasminogen activator content by more than 0.5 unit was found in 75% of the patients who had transvesical surgery compared with only 30% of the patients in the TURP group on the first postoperative day. No difference in the activity decrease was noted between general versus regional anesthesia patients. These authors concluded that the plasminogen activator difference may in part be responsible for the increased incidence of deep venous thrombosis in open versus transurethral resection of the prostate.

THE TURP SYNDROME

What Is It?

The TURP syndrome is a complication that can occur during or after TURP in up to 10% of patients.[26] A disproportionately higher mortality is noted in those patients who develop

it compared with those who do not. Acute intravascular volume shifts and acute changes in plasma solute concentrations are responsible. The latter include hyponatremia, decreased serum osmolarity, and increased glycine and ammonia concentrations. Manifestations of this syndrome as well as the systems that are affected are varied (Table 70–3).

What Causes It?

Osmolality Changes

The most serious derangement in the TURP syndrome is not hyponatremia per se but rather the acute hypo-osmolality that it causes; this hypo-osmolality in turn results in cerebral and pulmonary edema.[26] Therefore, serum sodium determination is not always a reliable indicator of serum osmolality or of the TURP syndrome.

Irrigating Fluid Absorption

Ten to 30 mL of irrigant is absorbed per minute of resection time, yielding an average irrigant absorption of approximately 1000 mL in the course of an operation.[27] The rate of irrigating fluid absorption is also related to the height of the irrigating fluid reservoir above the bladder. Ideally, the fluid reservoir irrigating pressure should not exceed venous pressure, but it should be sufficiently great to maintain visibility and to wash away blood and tissue.

The most commonly used system is one in which the resectoscope simultaneously irrigates and drains irrigating fluid. This method keeps the irrigating fluid pressure relatively low unless the hydrostatic pressure of the fluid reservoir exceeds the low resistance drainage capacity of the resectoscope or unless the drainage channel becomes obstructed.

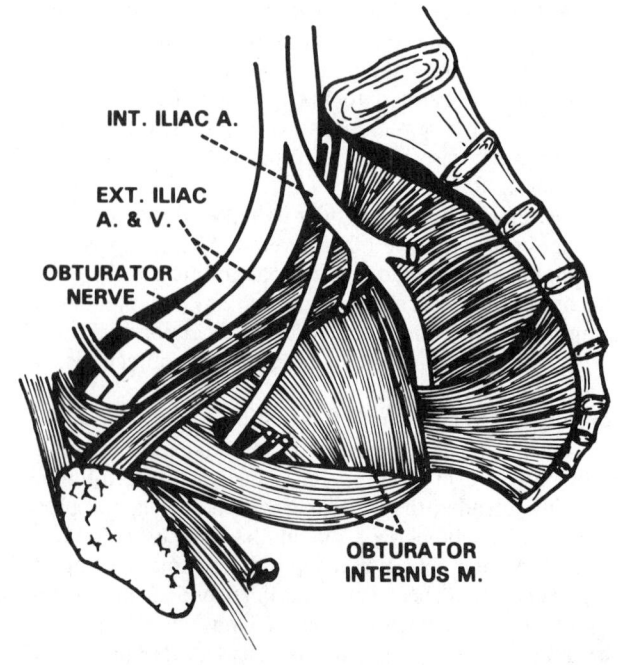

FIGURE 70–9. View of the obturator nerve as it passes through the pelvis.

TABLE 70–3. Signs and Symptoms Attributed to TURP Syndrome

Cardiopulmonary	Hematologic and Renal	Central Nervous System
Respiratory distress	Hemolysis	Nausea/vomiting
Cyanosis	Acute renal failure	Confusion
Hypertension	Hyponatremia	Twitches
Widened QRS or elevated ST segment	Hypo-osmolality	Visual disturbance
Dysrhythmia	Hyperglycinemia	Seizures
Bradycardia	Hyperammonemia	Paralysis
Hypotension		Coma
Shock		

What Irrigating Fluids Are Available?

A TURP requires a solution that does not conduct electricity and that provides a clear visual field. It has evolved from plain water in the past to 1.5% glycine and Cytal (2.7% sorbitol and 0.54% mannitol). Plain water irrigation has been virtually abandoned because it causes unacceptable degrees of hemolysis, hyponatremia, and renal failure.

Nonelectrolyte 1.5% glycine solution is slightly hypo-osmolar (230 mOsm) but is inexpensive when compared with Cytal, which is isotonic. An additional consequence is that glycine has ammonia as a metabolic by-product and, thus, predisposes the patient to sequelae of hyperglycemia and hyperammonemia, which can lead to encephalopathy and transient blindness. Other irrigating fluids that are used include solutions of 1.2% glycine, 2.5% glycine, 5% mannitol, and 5% sorbitol.

How Is It Diagnosed?

The occurrence of any of the signs or symptoms listed in Table 70–3, the presence of any of the electrocardiographic changes listed in Table 70–4, or a resection that lasts longer than 60 minutes suggests the urgent need for serum sodium measurement and, if available, a serum osmolality determination. One per cent ethanol in the irrigating solution has also been used as a marker for early detection of both irrigating fluid absorption and hyponatremia (Figs. 70–10 and 70–11).[28] This assessment is an alternative to repetitive serum sodium and osmolality determinations and measures the ethanol content of the expired breath with a Breathalyzer.

TABLE 70–4. Acute Changes in Serum Sodium

Serum Sodium	Electrocardiographic Changes	Irritability
120 mEq · L^{-1}	May see widened QRS	Restlessness; confusion
115 mEq · L^{-1}	Widened QRS; elevated ST segment	Nausea; vomiting; semicoma
100 mEq · L^{-1}	Ventricular tachycardia or fibrillation	Seizures

(From Berger JJ: Transurethral resection of the prostate. Lesson 20. Curr Rev Clin Anesth 1981; 1:165.)

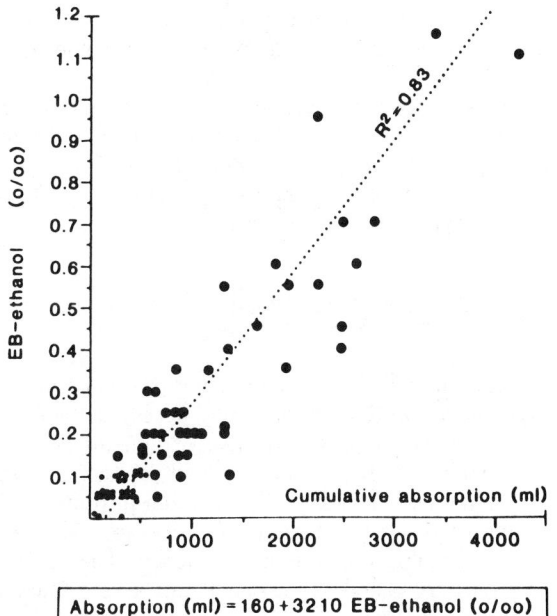

$$\text{Absorption (ml)} = 160 + 3210 \text{ EB-ethanol (o/oo)}$$

FIGURE 70–10. The relationship between the ethanol concentration in the expired breath (EB-ethanol) and the cumulative absorption of irrigant measured for 10-minute periods during transurethral resection. (From Hahn RG: Early detection of the TUR syndrome by marking the irrigating fluid with 1% ethanol. Acta Anaesthesiol Scand 1989; 33:147.)

When Is the Syndrome Treated?

This syndrome probably should be treated only if it is symptomatic—that is, a patient should not be treated just because his serum sodium level is decreased.[29] If TURP syndrome occurs intraoperatively, the operation should be concluded as quickly as possible using the minimum acceptable irrigating

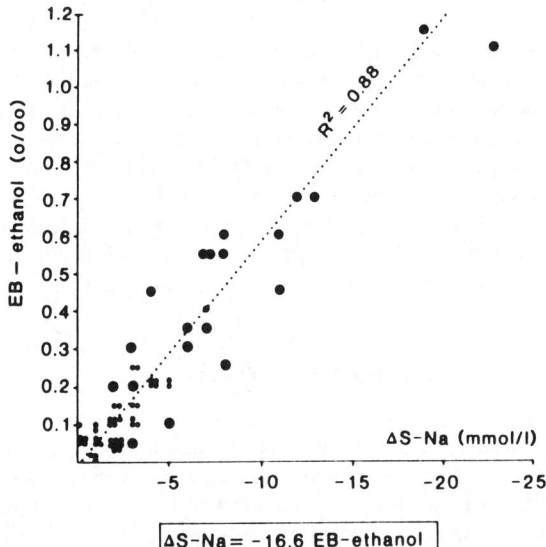

$$\Delta S\text{-Na} = -16.6 \text{ EB-ethanol}$$

FIGURE 70–11. The relationship between the ethanol concentration in the expired breath (EB-ethanol) and the change in the serum sodium concentration since the commencement of the operation. The data relate to the end of the 10-minute period during resections when the EB-ethanol concentration indicated that irrigant was being absorbed. (From Hahn RG: Early detection of the TUR syndrome by marking the irrigating fluid with 1% ethanol. Acta Anaesthesiol Scand 1989; 33:147.)

fluid pressure. The acute treatment end point should be resolution of symptoms rather than complete correction of hyponatremia.[29]

This conservative approach minimizes the risk of central pontine myelinolysis from overly rapid correction of hyponatremia (hypo-osmolality).[30] Myelinolysis is rare and is more commonly seen in cases of chronic hypo-osmolality. Its association with hyponatremia is unclear.[31]

How Is It Treated?

In addition to rapid conclusion of the procedure, treatment of symptomatic TURP syndrome may necessitate administration of 3% saline. Seizures are treated with thiopental or a benzodiazepine, whereas fluid overload is treated with diuresis. The diuresis should be initiated with furosemide, 20 to 40 mg intravenously, since the aberration is free water excess rather than an absolute sodium deficiency. The amount of sodium necessary to correct the deficit can be calculated using the following equation:

$$\text{mEq of Sodium Deficit}$$
$$= \text{Desired Sodium (mEq} \cdot \text{L}^{-1})$$
$$- [\text{Normal Sodium (mEq} \cdot \text{L}^{-1}) \times \text{TBW (L)}]$$

Equation 1

in which TBW is total body water.

Since 3% saline contains 513 mEq $\cdot$ L^{-1} of sodium, the volume required is calculated as follows:

$$\text{mL Required} = \frac{\text{mEq of Sodium Deficit}}{513 \text{ mEq} \cdot \text{L}^{-1}} \times 100$$

Equation 2

(For 5% saline, substitute 855 mEq $\cdot$ L^{-1} for 513 mEq $\cdot$ L^{-1}).

Only one-quarter to one-half of the fluid should be administered unless symptoms resolve earlier; if this occurs, administration is stopped. After this partial calculated deficit correction, serum sodium measurement is repeated. Measurement of serum sodium or osmolality, or both, is a key factor in the early diagnosis and treatment of TURP syndrome. Some clinicians determine these values as often as every 15 to 30 minutes. Be sure that the baseline and subsequent determinations are made with the same analyzer, as significant differences can occur with the use of different analyzers.

NEPHRECTOMY

This procedure is performed on the donor for living-related kidney transplantation and is the operation of choice for the treatment of renal cell carcinoma. Depending on the surgeon's preference and on the extent of the tumor (e.g., possible invasion of inferior vena cava), the affected kidney may be removed via a transabdominal, flank, or thoracoabdominal incision. In all cases, the table is adjusted so as to provide maximum exposure of the kidney, which is otherwise partially obscured by the lower rib cage. One or two ribs may be removed.

How Should Anesthesia Be Administered?

Intraoperative management of a patient includes placement of intra-arterial and central venous catheters. If the tumor extends into the inferior vena cava or the right atrium, transesophageal echocardiography is helpful to identify tumor embolus if it occurs and provides another monitor of cardiac function and volume status.

Pre-emptive and Postoperative Analgesia

A combined technique using epidural and general anesthesia not only facilitates muscle relaxation and decreases the requirement for volatile anesthetics and narcotics but also provides a route for pre-emptive and postoperative analgesia. The average length of hospitalization was almost 2 days shorter for donor nephrectomy patients who received postoperative pain management by epidural fentanyl infusion compared with those who received morphine with a patient-controlled analgesia device.[32]

What Problems Should Be Anticipated?

Pneumothorax

Because the kidney lies in the posterior upper abdomen adjacent to the posterior diaphragmatic attachment, the possibility of an intraoperative pneumothorax exists. This complication may first manifest as unexplained hypotension on closure of the abdomen. When it occurs, it is ipsilateral to the surgery and is readily treated by simple aspiration and tube thoracostomy.

Inferior Vena Caval Obstruction

A second special consideration is inferior vena caval obstruction from retractor placement. This problem is most likely to occur during right nephrectomy and radical nephrectomy for tumor. The diagnosis of both pneumothroax and inferior vena caval obstruction is facilitated by the presence of an intra-arterial catheter.

CYSTECTOMY

Total cystectomy is performed on patients with deeply infiltrating cancer of the bladder. It requires removal of the bladder and its replacement with an ileal conduit. Bladder extirpation with the prostatic urethra and, frequently, the pelvic lymph nodes is associated with a great deal of blood loss. The ileal conduit urinary diversion usually incurs little additional blood loss.

How Should Anesthesia Be Administered?

Ryan compared two anesthetic regimes for this procedure: epidural anesthesia utilizing bupivacaine, 0.5% plain, supplemented with nitrous oxide–oxygen–enflurane versus general anesthetic–relaxant using nitrous oxide–oxygen–fentanyl and pancuronium.[33] The epidural group had a significantly lower mean systolic blood pressure (80 mm Hg compared with 115 mm Hg for the second group) and a markedly lower mean blood loss (2075 mL compared with a 2708 mL for the second group). However, a wide variation in blood loss occurred within each group. All patients had similar cardiovascular changes during the first 12 hours postoperatively.[33]

Controlled Hypotension

Ahlering and coworkers studied controlled hypotension to reduce blood loss during radical cystectomy.[34] Hypotension was induced with enflurane or trimethaphan to maintain blood pressure at 90/60 mm Hg. The mean operative blood loss was reduced significantly in the hypotensive group compared with the normotensive group (740 ± 14 mL versus 821 ± 78 mL, respectively). Ninety per cent of the normotensive patients received blood transfusions compared with only 69% of the hypotensive patients.

NONCHROMAFFIN PARAGANGLIOMAS

Nonchromaffin paragangliomas of the bladder do occur, but most are inactive. However, Splinter and associates reported a tumor that released catecholamines.[35] Such a tumor occasionally is malignant. A patient may present with the classic symptoms of a pheochromocytoma (hypertension, tremulousness, anxiety, and a pounding sensation in the head and chest).

How Should Anesthesia Be Managed?

Preoperative treatment should be similar to that for patients with pheochromocytomas. Alpha-blockers followed by β-blockers, calcium channel blockers, and inhibitors of catecholamine synthesis are administered with magnesium sulfate as needed. In the reported case, prazosin and propranolol were used. Additional nifedipine was added to control blood pressure.[35]

Several anesthetic techniques have been used during resection of catecholamine-producing tumors, and no one method was proved to be superior. Splinter and associates employed arterial and pulmonary artery catheterization.[35] Anesthesia was induced with fentanyl, thiopental, and vecuronium, and it was maintained with isoflurane, nitrous oxide, fentanyl, and vecuronium. A continuous infusion of sodium nitroprusside was necessary to maintain an acceptable blood pressure as well as bolus doses of phentolamine.

LASER SURGERY

What Are the Applications?

In addition to radical surgery for bladder carcinomas, laser treatment in outpatient settings is utilized for these tumors and for genital condylomata. Carbon dioxide, argon, and neodymium-yttrium-aluminum-garnet (Nd.YAG) lasers are most frequently utilized in urologic surgery.

Carbon Dioxide Laser

The carbon dioxide laser can be used in relatively inaccessible areas. Its advantage is that it can cut and coagulate tissue to maintain a bloodless field. A major disadvantage is that it cannot penetrate a quantity of water >0.1 mm in depth; therefore, it cannot be used in water or urine-filled organs. Its role in urology is in the treatment of cutaneous lesions such as condylomata acuminata and of premalignant and malignant cutaneous lesions of the penis.

Argon Laser

The argon laser can be used with a fiberoptic guide. Water does not prevent its penetration; thus, it can be used to treat lesions within the bladder. Argon laser use combined with concomitant administration of intravenous hematoporphyrin derivatives produces tumoricidal effects on bladder cancer. Urethral strictures also can be removed. With increasing power settings, large defects in the tissue occur; these defects can lead to bladder perforation. Therefore, the argon laser is limited in use to the treatment of superficial bladder cancers.

Neodymium-Yttrium-Aluminum-Garnet Laser

The Nd.YAG laser is most useful for urologic surgery. Its tissue-penetrating ability is the highest of the three available lasers. It can be used in water or urine without loss of power and can be adapted to a fiberoptic light source. Bloodless destruction of cancer cells and a small risk of bladder perforation are advantages of the Nd.YAG laser. Contraindications to its use are very large or extensive tumors that require increased photoradiation. Patients with potential bladder outlet obstruction must be observed for urinary retention postoperatively.

How Is Anesthesia Administered?

Bladder Cancer

Male and female patients with bladder cancer can undergo Nd.YAG laser surgery with intravenous sedation and an instillation of 2% lidocaine hydrochloride jelly into the urethra. If extensive or numerous tumors are present, the patient may require a general or regional anesthetic. The postanesthesia care unit stay may be prolonged following a regional anesthetic case. Evaluation of the abdomen is done prior to discharge to verify that no laser-induced intraperitoneal perforations have occurred.

Condylomata Acuminata

When the laser is utilized for the treatment of condylomata acuminata, more than 90% of patients receive local anesthesia. Lidocaine 1% is infiltrated at the base of each lesion. If the warts involve the penis, a penile block is performed. For urethral condylomata, a general or regional anesthetic is usually administered because local anesthetic alone is not sufficient to prevent pain caused by the laser phototherapy.[36]

NONINVASIVE UROLOGIC SURGERY

Since the early 1980s, a large proportion of open urologic surgical procedures have been eliminated by technology that allows intervention with minimally invasive techniques.

What Are Percutaneous Nephrostomy and Urethroscopy?

Percutaneous nephrostomy and urethroscopy enable 90% of procedures that involve calculi of the upper urinary tract to be performed endoscopically. Patients who previously had to stay in the hospital 1 to 2 weeks after an open surgical procedure and could not go back to work for weeks can now be discharged within 24 hours and can return to work within a few days. Virtually the only remaining indication for open surgery is the combination of a stone and stenosis at the ureteropelvic junction (see Chapter 54).

What Are the Anesthetic Requirements?

Because nephrostomy and urethroscopy are performed without a scalpel, minimal tissue trauma occurs; thus, the need for general anesthesia is greatly reduced. For elderly or high-risk patients who require urologic procedures, a local anesthetic frequently is the technique of choice.

Sedoanalgesia

Many urologic procedures, both endoscopic and open, can be performed following regional anesthesia. Owing to the patient's embarrassment or anxiety or to the extent of the procedure, local anesthesia may not provide an acceptable alternative. If the limiting factor is the extent of the procedure, regional or general anesthetia is performed. If it is anxiety, administration of an anxiolytic agent can improve the conditions of surgery considerably. Sedoanalgesia, as was noted earlier, places equal emphasis on sedation and analgesia.

Birch and colleagues reported the results of this technique for 1020 patients. The short-acting benzodiazepine midazolam provided the hypnosedation and amnesia, whereas intramuscular meperidine and topical lidocaine gel provided the analgesia.[13] Midazolam was administered 20 to 30 minutes before surgery in a dose of 0.1 to 0.12 mg · kg^{-1} intramuscularly. In elderly, unfit patients, the dosage was reduced 30% to 60%. The urethra was anesthetized with 2% lidocaine gel 10 to 15 minutes after premedication was given. Monitoring included electrocardiography, automatic blood pressure measurement, and pulse oximetry.

If a patient was still anxious before the procedure began, midazolam was titrated intravenously in 1-mg increments. Cystoscopies required no further anesthetic supplementation. However, for biopsies, diathermy, and incisions, 1% lidocaine with epinephrine (1:200,000) was injected into the area. The investigators concluded that sedoanalgesia greatly increased the efficiency of outpatient surgeries. Eighty per cent of their patients were fit for discharge 1 hour postoperatively.[13, 37]

References

1. Thompson G, Moore D: Celiac plexus intercostal and minor peripheral blocks. *In* Clinical Anesthesia and Management of Pain. 2nd ed. Cousins MJ, Bridenbaugh PO (eds). Philadelphia, JB Lippincott, 1988, pp 503–530.
2. Lofstrom JB, Cousins M: Sympathetic neural blockade of upper and lower extremities. *In* Clinical Anesthesia and Management of Pain. 2nd ed. Cousins MJ, Bridenbaugh PO (eds). Philadelphia, JB Lippincott, 1988, pp 483–492.
3. Moore D: Block of the inguinal region. *In* Regional Blockade. 4th ed. Moore D (ed). Springfield, IL, Charles C Thomas, 1981, pp 167–173.
4. Cassady JJI: Regional anesthesia for urologic procedures. Urol Clin North Am 1987; 14:43.
5. Fuchs GF: Cord block anesthesia for scrotal surgery. J Urol 1982; 128:718.
6. Kaye KW, Lange PH, Fraley EE: Spermatic cord block in urologic surgery. J Urol 1982; 128:720.
7. Trivedi NS, Robalino J, Shevde K: Intrapleural block: a new technique for regional anesthesia during percutaneous nephrostomy and nephrolithotomy. Can J Anaesth 1990; 37:479.
8. Perestad F, Stromskag KE: Interpleural catheter in the management of postoperative pain: a preliminary report. Reg Anesth 1986; 11:89.
9. Covino BG: Interpleural regional analgesia (Editorial). Anesth Analg 1988; 67:427.
10. Seltzer JL, Larijani GE, Goldberg ME, et al: Intrapleural bupivacaine: a kinetic and dynamic evaluation. Anesthesiology 1987; 67:798.
11. Reddy PK: New technique to anesthetize the prostate for transurethral balloon dilation. Urol Clin North Am 1990; 17:55.
12. Reddy PK, Wasserman W, Castaneda F, et al: Balloon dilatation of the prostate for treatment of benign hyperplasia. Urol Clin North Am 1988; 15:529.
13. Birch BRP, Anson KM, Miller RA: Sedoanalgesia in urology: a safe, cost-effective alternative to general anesthesia: a review of 1020 cases. Br J Urol 1990; 66:342.
14. Hendolin H, Mattila MAK, Poikolainen E: The effect of lumbar epidural analgesia on the development of deep vein thrombosis of the legs after open prostatectomy. Acta Chir Scand 1981; 147:425.
15. Albin MS, Ritter RR, Reinhart R, et al: Venous air embolism during radical retropubic prostatectomy. Anesth Analg 1992; 74:191.
16. Mebust WK, Holtgrewe HL, Cockett ATK, et al: Transurethral prostatectomy: immediate and postoperative complications: a cooperative study of 13 participating institutions evaluating 3,885 patients. J Urol 1989; 14:243.
17. Levin K, Nyren O, Pompeius R: Blood loss, tissue weight, and operating time in transurethral prostatectomy. Scand J Urol Nephrol 1981; 15:197.
18. Nielson KK, Andersen K, Asbjorn VF, et al: Blood loss in transurethral prostatectomy: epidural vs. general anesthesia. Int Urol Nephrol 1987; 19:287.
19. Rabke HB, Jenicek JA, Khouri E: Hypothermia associated with transurethral resection of the prostate. J Urol 1962; 87:447.
20. Augspurger RR, Donohue RE: Prevention of obturator nerve stimulation during transurethral surgery. J Urol 1980; 123:170.
21. Narins L, Lief PA: Abolition of mass femoral muscular contractions during transurethral resection. J Mt Sinai Hosp 1957; 24:23.
22. Hradec E, Soukup F, Novah J, et al: The obturator nerve block: preventing damage of the bladder wall during transurethral surgery. Int Urol Nephrology 1983; 15:149.
23. Nicolaides AN, Field ES, Kakkar VV, et al: Prostatectomy and deep vein thrombosis. Br J Surg 1972; 59:487.
24. Mayo ME, Halil T, Browse NL: The incidence of deep vein thrombosis after prostatectomy. Br J Urol 1971; 43:738.
25. Ljunger H, Bergquist D, Isacson S: Plasminogen activator activity in patients undergoing transvesical and transurethral prostatectomy. Eur Urol 1983; 9:24.
26. Ghanem AN, Ward JP: Osmotic and metabolic sequelae of volumetric overload in relation to the TUR syndrome. Br J Urol 1990; 66:71.
27. Hahn RG: Relations between irrigant absorption rate and hyponatremia during transurethral resection of the prostate. Acta Anaesthesiol Scand 1987; 32:53.
28. Hahn RG: Early detection of the TUR syndrome by marking the irrigating fluid with 1% ethanol. Acta Anaesthesiol Scand 1989; 33:149.
29. Norenberg MD, Papendick RE: Chronicity of hyponatremia as a factor in experimental myelinolysis. Ann Neurol 1984; 15:544.
30. Brunner JE, Redmond AM, Haggar AM, et al: Central pontine myelinolysis and pontine lesions after rapid correction of hyponatremia: a prospective magnetic resonance imaging study. Ann Neurol 1990; 27:61.
31. Layon AJ, Bernards WC, Kirby RR: Fluids and electrolytes in the critically ill. *In* Critical Care. 2nd ed. Civetta JM, Kirby RR, Taylor RW (eds). Philadelphia, JB Lippincott, 1992, pp 457–480.

32. Dixon CL, Sefton W, Gravenstein N: Epidural analgesia after donor nephrectomy decreases duration of hospitalization (Abstract). Reg Anesth 17:75,1992.

33. Ryan DW: Anaesthesia for cystectomy: a comparison of two anaesthetic techniques. Anaesthesia 1982; 37:554.

34. Ahlering TE, Henderson JB, Skinner DG: Controlled hypotensive anesthesia to reduce blood loss in radical cystectomy for bladder cancer. J Urol 1983; 129:953.

35. Splinter WM, Milne B, Nickel C, et al: Perioperative management for resection of a malignant nonchromaffin paraganglioma of the bladder. Can J Anaesth 1989; 36:215.

36. Malloy TR, Wein AJ: Laser treatment of bladder carcinoma and genital condylomata. Outpatient Urol Surg 1987; 14:121.

37. Miller RA, Birch BRP, Anson KU, et al: The impact of minimally invasive surgery and sedoanalgesia on urological practice. Postgrad Med 1990; 66(Suppl):572.

CHAPTER 71

Anesthesia for Orthopedic Surgery

F. KAYSER ENNEKING, M.D.

MARK T. SCARBOROUGH, M.D.

Orthopedic surgery encompasses a broad spectrum of procedures, from simple closed reductions of a dislocated joint to complicated excision and reconstruction of a cancerous extremity. Patients of all ages undergo orthopedic procedures and have a wide range of associated illnesses. Anesthesiologists should be aware of the spectrum of disease states and of specific perioperative considerations frequently encountered during orthopedic procedures. This chapter approaches this broad topic by category, addressing in turn the topics of trauma, total joint replacement, rheumatoid arthritis, orthopedic oncology, scoliosis, amputation, and ambulatory procedures. In addition, some specific considerations that are the source of frequent questions from anesthesiologists are addressed to help bridge the gulf that exists across the surgical drapes.

ORTHOPEDIC TRAUMA

What Factors Are Important in Evaluation?

Patient Profiles

Although trauma can occur in any age group, high-speed motor vehicle accidents frequently involve patients under the age of 30 years. Alcohol and illegal drug use are common among victims. Blood and urine samples for toxicologic screening should be obtained as part of the preoperative workup. Acute intoxication might change the anesthetic management by altering the patient's responses to certain drug therapies, by rendering the patient unable to cooperate for a regional technique, or by slowing arousal following general anesthesia. Health care workers should be extremely cautious because the rate of human immunodeficiency virus and hepatitis B infection is higher among these patients than it is in the general population.

What Is the Significance of an Open Fracture in Multiple Trauma?

Multiple trauma resulting from high-velocity motor vehicle accidents is one of the most common causes of orthopedic

injuries (Table 71–1). Patients may have dramatic and obvious extremity trauma without other readily apparent injury. However, the magnitude of force required to cause an open fracture is such that the patient must be systematically evaluated for other less apparent associated injuries. Enormous external forces are required to disrupt the bone of the pelvis; consequently, associated injuries are common. The reported mortality rate is 5% to 20%, and each patient has an average of 2.7 other associated major injuries.[1]

Associated Injuries

Typical injuries resulting from rapid acceleration and deceleration include flexion and extension injuries to the spine; pulmonary and cardiac contusions caused by the seat belt or steering wheel; shearing of organ pedicles that are anatomically fixed, including the ascending aorta and mesentery; femoral fractures; and ligamentous knee injuries.

If the patient is ejected from a vehicle or sustains a fall from height, the injury pattern differs. A systematic evaluation from head to toes should be undertaken. Closed head injuries and cervical spine trauma should be searched for, especially in motorcycle accident victims. Flail chest and pneumothorax are common thoracic injuries in these patients. Laparotomy is frequently required for abdominal injuries (see Chapter 59).

Urethral and bladder injuries require early urologic consultation. Catheterization of the bladder with a Foley or suprapubic catheter should be performed upon the patient's arrival at the hospital. Rectal lacerations and small and large bowel perforations are commonly associated with pelvic fractures. These injuries require primary repair or diverting colostomy, or both.

Traction injuries to the lumbosacral plexus are not unusual and are usually treated by stabilization of the pelvis by external or internal fixation. Lower extremity denervation or loss of bowel, bladder, or sexual function may occur from injury to sacral nerve roots. Falls from a height of 6 feet or greater commonly cause foot (especially calcaneal) fractures in addition to pelvic and spinal injuries.

TABLE 71–1. Common Orthopedic Injuries

Injury	Imaging	Treatment	Emergent Fixation Required
Cervical spine	Cross-table lateral x-ray; cervical spine series; CT; MRI	Halo cast versus cervical instrumentation versus cervical fusion	Not unless progressive neurologic compromise occurs
Thoracic spine; lumbar spine	AP, lateral x-ray; CT	Cast versus instrumentation and fusion	Not unless progressive neurologic compromise occurs
Pelvic fracture	CT; AP x-ray	ORIF versus external fixation	If patient hemodynamically stable, wait at least 72 h; if patient hemodynamically unstable, fixation ASAP
Femur fractures	AP; lateral x-ray	ORIF versus external fixation	Yes, within 24 h
Open fracture	X-ray	Irrigation and débridement ORIF versus external fixation	Yes, within 6–8 h
Open fracture with arterial injury	X-ray; angiography	Irrigation and débridement; arterial repair ORIF versus amputation	Yes, ASAP
Knee dislocation	X-ray; angiography	Repair ligaments and popliteal vessels	Yes, ASAP
Hip dislocation	X-ray; CT	May require muscle relaxation for closed reduction versus open reduction	Yes, ASAP
Shoulder dislocation	X-ray	May require muscle relaxation for closed reduction versus open reduction	Yes, ASAP
Supracondylar elbow fracture; no vascular compromise; vascular compromise	X-ray	Closed reduction percutaneous pinning versus ORIF	Yes, within 6–8 h
Compartment syndromes	Compartment pressure measurement	Fasciotomy	Yes, ASAP
Hip fracture	X-ray; CT	ORIF versus hip replacement	Yes, within 24 h Yes, within 48 h
Septic joint	Joint aspiration	Irrigation and débridement	Yes, ASAP
Other closed fractures	X-ray; CT	Closed reduction versus percutaneous pinning versus ORIF	Yes, within 24 h or 2–5 d later, when swelling has reduced

Abbreviations: CT = computed tomography; MRI = magnetic resonance imaging; AP = anteroposterior; ORIF = open reduction, internal fixation; ASAP = as soon as possible.

How Much Bleeding Can Occur from Femur and Pelvic Fractures?

Closed femoral fractures cause damage to the thigh musculature that can result in the loss of up to 2 units of blood into the thigh before tamponade occurs. Compartment syndromes of the thigh have been reported in association with this type of injury, but they are not common.[2]

Pelvic fractures may result in uncontrollable retroperitoneal bleeding. Patients with such fractures that disrupt the pubic symphysis (open book–type fractures) are at high risk for massive blood loss. The average blood loss associated with closed fractures of the pelvis is 6 units in contrast to 18 units for open pelvic fractures.

Methods to control blood loss associated with pelvic fractures include external fixation, angiographic techniques, wound packing, military antishock trouser placement, ligation of ruptured vessels, and, rarely, hemipelvectomy. The most desirable approach is pelvic external fixation, which involves placing metal pins in both iliac wings and connecting the pins with an external frame. The iliac wings are then compressed, and the fixator is tightened; this stabilizes the pelvis. External fixation is a quick, reliable method to control hemorrhage and does not interfere with general surgical or urologic access to the patient for other procedures.

When Should the Military Antishock Trousers Be Released?

Military antishock trousers may be applied by paramedical personnel prior to hospital transfer to support blood pressure and to stabilize lower extremity fractures. If they are placed for blood pressure support, they should be released incrementally after hemodynamic stability has been achieved with concurrent volume replacement. If they are placed only for fracture stabilization and the patient is hemodynamically stable, they should be released as quickly as possible. Multiple case reports exist of compartment syndromes that develop when military antishock trousers are inflated for longer than 120 minutes.[3–5]

What Studies Should Be Performed to Evaluate the Cervical Spine?

If the patient arrives in extremis, intubation with direct visualization by the anesthesiologist (with the assistance of the surgeon, who holds the head and neck in rigid traction) should be performed without delay. The neck must be held firmly in the neutral position until the cervical spine has been examined radiographically.

Screening lateral radiographs of the cervical spine from the occiput to the first thoracic vertebra must be obtained in any patient admitted with a history of major skeletal trauma, a fall, head or facial injury, neurologic symptoms, or loss of consciousness. The bone architecture and alignment of the cervical spine should be evaluated, and the adjacent soft tissues should be examined for swelling. Cervical neutrality should be maintained in patients with a possible cervical neck injury (those with neck pain, paresthesias, or momentary paralysis at the scene) until a formal neurosurgical evaluation has been performed, even if findings on screening cross-table lateral radiography are negative.

Which Orthopedic Injuries Require Emergency Surgery?

Table 71–1 outlines the urgency of many common orthopedic injuries. In general, emergent surgery (i.e., in the next available operating room [OR]) should be carried out whenever a limb is at risk for disruption of its blood supply. This problem may result from direct trauma to the vessels or from joint dislocation. Open fractures require urgent irrigation and débridement at a maximum of 6 to 8 hours from the time of injury to prevent deep-seated bone infections. Closed fractures requiring open repair need surgical attention prior to the development of skin breakdown from edema formation (fracture blisters). These blisters can develop within 12 hours if the extremity is not properly elevated.

Why Do Closed Femur Fractures Require Early Stabilization?

Early stabilization of femur fractures in multiple trauma patients decreases the incidence of complications.[6] Rigid internal fixation allows early mobility and improved respiratory care. The result is a decrease in the incidence of acute respiratory failure, fat emboli, and pneumonia. When fracture stabilization is delayed for longer than 24 hours, the length of the intensive care unit [ICU] stay and the overall duration of hospitalization are increased. Hospital costs are nearly 50% greater for these patients than for patients whose fractures were stabilized.[7] The greatest improvement in outcome has been shown in patients with the highest injury severity scores.[8] Such patients should be brought to the OR as soon as their diagnostic work-up is completed.

What Common Orthopedic Injuries Require Urgent Operations?

Dislocations of the hip should be relocated within 6 to 12 hours to restore blood supply to the femoral head and prevent avascular necrosis. Knee dislocations require urgent operative intervention because they are frequently associated with vascular injury.

Compartment syndromes are diagnosed by measuring pressures within an anatomic compartment, such as the volar aspect of the forearm (Fig. 71–1). The extremity is usually tense, and capillary refill may be delayed. The quality of the pulse is not a reliable indicator of compartment pressures. Compartment syndromes of soft tissue or from bone injuries can develop intraoperatively if vascular access catheters infiltrate or

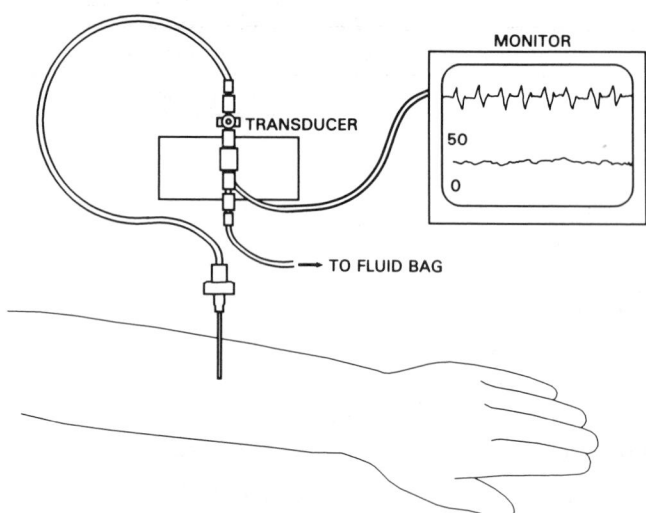

FIGURE 71–1. Measurement of tissue (compartment) pressure following orthopedic extremity trauma.

in the presence of poor extremity positioning. The problem should be brought to the immediate attention of the surgical team. Treatment of compartment syndromes includes mandatory emergent surgical fasciotomy.

What Is the Prognosis for Elderly Patients Who Sustain a Hip Fracture?

The mortality rate for American Society of Anesthesiologists' (ASA) class 3 and 4 patients is sixfold that for age-matched controls during the first year following the fracture.[9] Many studies have attempted to assess the cause of the high rates of morbidity and mortality in the elderly population. The single best predictor of mortality is preoperative mental status.[10]

TOTAL JOINT REPLACEMENT

Replacement of diseased joints with implantable prosthetic devices is one of the major advances of orthopedic surgery since the early 1960s. The vast majority of patients who undergo replacement surgery are over 60 years of age and are generally in good health. Of concern, however, is that patients with arthritis may not report symptoms of cardiac or respiratory insufficiency because adaptive changes that they have made in their lifestyle severely restrict their activity level. In addition, certain patients require special consideration, including those with rheumatoid arthritis, avascular necrosis of the femoral head, congenital hip deformities, and infection as well as those undergoing revision of a previous arthroplasty.

What Are the Fluid Requirements?

Primary total joint replacements usually do not involve tremendous fluid shifts. A transient decrease in blood pressure occurs at predictable times during total hip (cementing) and total knee (tourniquet release) arthroplasties and should be

TABLE 71–2. Procedures Likely to Have an Estimated Blood Loss of >1 L

- Revision total hip arthroplasty
- Arthroplasty for congenital hip deformity
- Removal of infected prosthesis
- Intramedullary rodding of a femur fracture
- Resection and reconstruction of bone lesions
- Bilateral total knee arthroplasties
- Biopsy of any sacral lesion
- Spinal fusion at more than three levels

anticipated with an appropriate volume replacement strategy. Fluids should be administered based on preoperative deficit, maintenance requirements, estimated blood loss, and third space losses. The fluid replacement requirement for primary total hip arthroplasty is approximately $5 \ mL \cdot kg^{-1} \cdot h^{-1}$ and that for total knee and shoulder replacements is approximately $4 \ mL \cdot kg^{-1} \cdot h^{-1}$.

What Is the Anticipated Blood Loss?

Total Hip Arthroplasty

Intraoperative blood loss during an uncomplicated primary total hip arthroplasty for arthritis is usually between 400 and 800 mL when cemented prostheses are placed. If, on the other hand, a noncemented prosthesis is placed, higher blood losses can be expected both intraoperatively and postoperatively.

Anticipated blood loss during total hip arthroplasty for congenital deformities, for cancerous bone lesions, or for revision of a previous joint replacement is much less predictable. Frequently, these operations are technically difficult to perform, and blood loss of more than 1500 mL is not uncommon (Table 71–2).

Total Knee Replacement

Because a total knee replacement is performed below the point where the tourniquet is placed, blood loss does not begin until the tourniquet is deflated. Some orthopedists close the wound and apply the dressing before they release the tourniquet, thereby minimizing intraoperative blood loss. The average blood loss for a knee replacement is 200 to 600 mL, regardless of when the tourniquet is deflated.

Total Shoulder Replacement

Total shoulder replacements are frequently technically difficult, and average blood losses vary from 300 to 1000 mL. Preoperative consultation with the surgeon is particularly helpful, since patients who require shoulder replacement are frequently afflicted with severe rheumatoid arthritis.

Removal of an Infected Prosthesis

During removal of an infected prosthesis, major blood loss can be anticipated as the surgeon attempts a deep débridement. Unless the ''infection'' is thought to be sterile, use of a cell saver is contraindicated.

When Should Invasive Monitors Be Utilized?

The decision to place invasive monitors should always be made on a case by case basis, depending on the patient's physical status and on the type of operation to be performed. Certain procedures present the potential for tremendous blood loss. Patients who are to have such procedures should undergo invasive monitoring of their arterial and central venous pressures.

Routine pulmonary artery pressure monitoring has been advocated by some investigators to detect fat embolization in bilateral knee arthroplasties.[11] As with any anesthetic, invasive monitoring should be considered for any patient with impaired cardiopulmonary reserve.

Routine intraoperative transesophageal echocardiography during complicated joint arthroplasties may soon be commonplace. However, the technical problem of visualizing the heart when the patient is in the right lateral decubitus position must be resolved first.

Why Does Hypotension Occur During Lower Extremity Joint Replacement?

Immediately after the femoral prosthesis has been cemented, the majority of patients who undergo hip replacement surgery experience a decrease in blood pressure for several minutes. Two mechanisms probably are responsible. First, emboli of fat, marrow, and air are extruded from the femoral canal into the pulmonary circulation, resulting in transient pulmonary arteriolar obstruction. Second, direct vasodilation is caused by the methylmethacrylate monomer.

If a tourniquet is not utilized for a total knee replacement, hypotension from the same mechanism may occur when the femoral component is seated. The degree of hypotension is usually not as great as that associated with tourniquet use, probably because a smaller volume of marrow is displaced. However, total knee arthroplasty is usually performed with a tourniquet, and hypotension is most likely to occur immediately after tourniquet release. Although hypotension is thought to be related to the presence of small emboli, other factors related to ischemia of the extremity, including reactive hyperemia and the release of adenosine, may also play a role.

What Factors Predispose to Osteonecrosis of the Femoral Head?

Osteonecrosis of the femoral head is the result of impaired circulation. The most common causes of this syndrome are

TABLE 71–3. Conditions Associated with Avascular Necrosis of the Hip

Corticosteroid use
Alcoholism
Pancreatitis
Sickle cell anemia
Polycythemia
Dysbaric ischemia
Obesity
Diabetes mellitus
Fat embolism
Trauma to the hip

alcoholism or steroid use, or they are idiopathic (Table 71–3). Trauma is frequently the culprit in young patients. However, these patients may have serious systemic diseases that lead to osteonecrosis. In general, the technical difficulty of the surgery and the operative blood loss are similar to those for a primary arthroplasty for osteoarthritis.

Why Are Some Total Joints Placed Without Cement?

Fixation of total joint prosthesis can be accomplished with acrylic cement or using a "press fit" technique. The indications for choosing one technique over another is an area of great controversy among orthopedic surgeons. In theory, the noncemented joints should have increased longevity because the prosthesis becomes biologically incorporated into the native bone. Noncemented prostheses are usually placed in young patients and in more active older patients.

Whether noncemented prostheses actually last longer than cemented ones is debatable. The noncemented joints require a prolonged period of nonweight-bearing ambulation and thus are not recommended in debilitated patients. Press fit prostheses are easier to revise than are cemented ones; this feature is a distinct advantage in young patients who can anticipate revision every 5 to 10 years, depending on their activity level.

Why Is Muscle Relaxation Necessary During Total Hip Replacement?

During total hip arthroplasty, the head of the femur is dislocated from its position in the acetabulum. This maneuver does not require flaccid paralysis. However, the powerful quadriceps and hip flexor muscles will hamper this action if some degree of muscle relaxation is not used. Application of regional techniques or administration of a muscle relaxant during general anesthesia is suitable. The combination of muscle relaxation and surgical tugging results in postoperative lower back discomfort in almost all hip replacement patients, regardless of the anesthetic technique chosen.

RHEUMATOID ARTHRITIS

Rheumatoid arthritis is an autoimmune system–mediated inflammatory process that affects connective tissue. Joint instability and destruction are the primary manifestations of this disease. Typically, patients have morning stiffness, pain on motion, swelling, and tenderness of multiple joints. The incidence of rheumatoid arthritis is about 0.5%, and the disease occurs most frequently in females between the ages of 30 and 60 years. The natural history of the disease is characterized by spontaneous exacerbations and remissions over a patient's lifetime. Patients frequently require multiple orthopedic interventions.

Why Do These Patients Have Difficult Airways?

Cervical instability, micrognathia, and limited mobility of the temporomandibular joints and cervical spine are common

findings. Radiographic evidence of cervical spine involvement can be found in ≤90% of patients.[12] The most common form of cervical spine involvement is atlantoaxial instability. This condition allows excessive motion between C-1 and C-2 and can result in cervical spinal cord impingement.

A subset of patients develop triplanar deviation of the larynx in which the larynx is displaced caudally, deviated to the left, rotated to the right, and anteriorly angulated (Fig. 71–2).[13] Involvement of the cricoarytenoid joints decreases the diameter of the airway such that smaller than anticipated endotracheal tubes must be used for intubation.

A detailed airway examination should be performed to assess for possible paresthesias or dizziness with neck motion in all planes, tracheal deviation, and hoarseness. Physical examination and flexion-extension lateral cervical spine films usually identify those patients who require awake fiberoptic intubation and positioning.

What Other Systemic Involvement Is Important?

The incidence of heart disease is increased in patients with rheumatoid arthritis compared with age-matched controls.[14] Coronary arteritis, conduction defects, valvular heart disease, and pericarditis have been attributed to rheumatoid disease and should be sought. Extrinsic and intrinsic restrictive lung disease can occur. Pulmonary function tests should be performed preoperatively if the rheumatoid patient has complaints of dyspnea. Anemia is frequently present as well.

Review of the drug history is essential. These patients frequently take large doses of nonsteroidal anti-inflammatory drugs. Platelet dysfunction and renal impairment as a result of this therapy should be evaluated preoperatively. Steroid therapy is commonly employed clinically during exacerbations of the disease. Perioperative stress steroid coverage is most commonly achieved by administering a large dose of a corticosteroid drug (i.e., 100 mg of hydrocortisone) before, during, and after the operation if the patient has received exogenous steroids within the previous 6 months. No controlled studies have confirmed the necessity for these large doses.

Gold salts, hydroxychloroquine (Plaquenil), penicillamine, and methotrexate are used to induce remission of rheumatoid arthritis. The most common adverse side effect of these drugs is suppression of the hematopoietic system, but renal and hepatic damage can also occur. In addition, gold salts rarely can cause interstitial lung disease.

Is Regional Anesthesia Advantageous?

Patients with severe disease often have progression of joint dysfunction and airway involvement throughout their lifetimes. Intubation can be a harrowing experience for the patient and the anesthesiologist. Severe hypoxia may occur during a difficult intubation, even in the conscious but sedated patient during fiberoptic bronchoscopy.

Extubation may also be problematic. Airway edema, especially after a traumatic intubation, causes critical narrowing of an already compromised airway and thus makes extubation

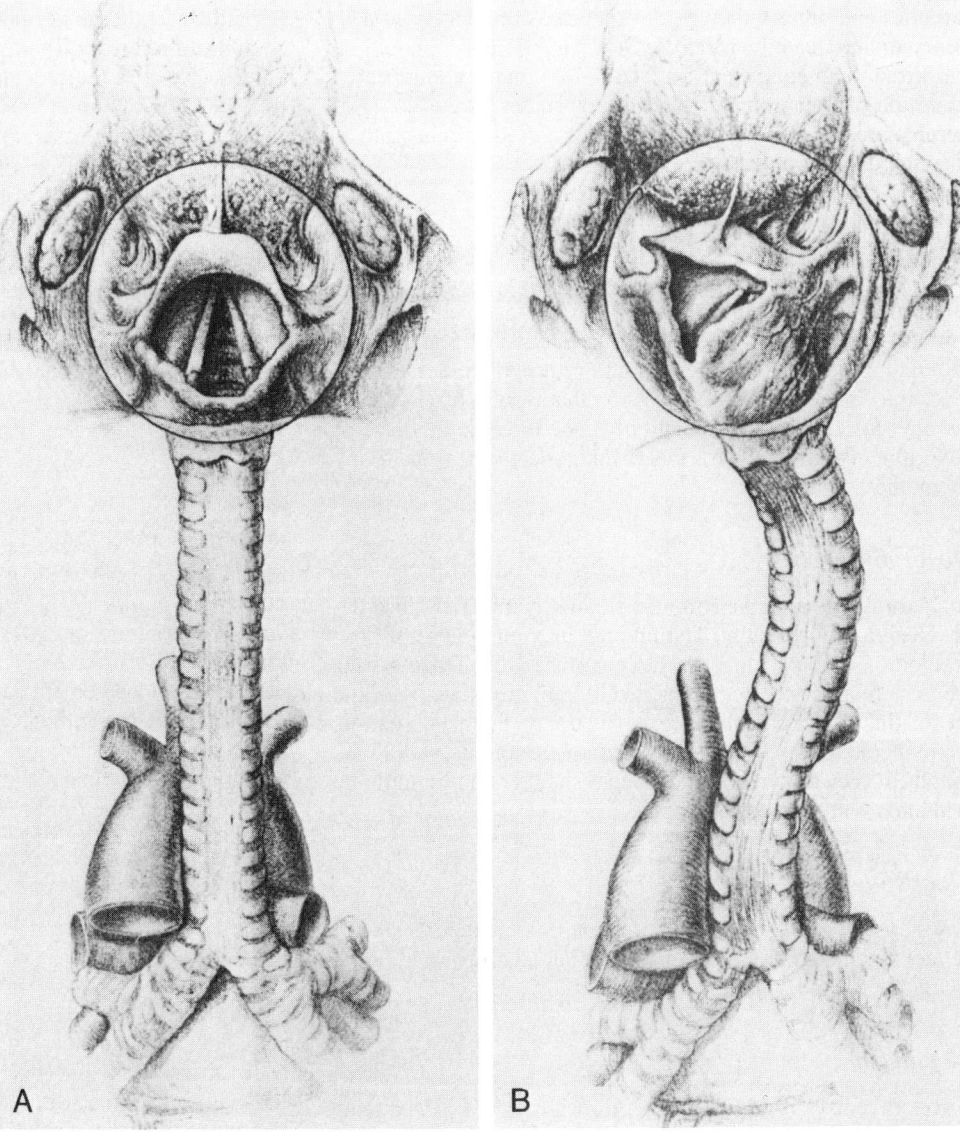

FIGURE 71–2. *A,* Normal position of the trachea and larynx. Circled area represents view through a fiberoptic bronchoscope. *B,* Deviated position of the trachea and larynx associated with severe rheumatoid arthritis. Note the triaxial deviation of the airway and the small glottic opening. (From Keenen MA, Siles CM, Kaufman RL: Acquired laryngeal deviation associated with the cervical spine disease in erosive polyarticular arthritis. Anesthesiology 1983; 58:441.)

unwise. Thus, selecting a regional technique that avoids airway manipulation may be prudent. However, it must be conducted with recognition that emergency intubation may not be possible.

Positioning during a regional anesthetic procedure is almost an art form. Rheumatoid arthritis patients often have other joint involvement that makes it difficult for them to be maintained in the same position for many hours regardless of how well padded they are. Finally, these patients will return to the OR for future surgery; therefore, frank discussion of their disease and anesthetic options is essential to gain their cooperation and understanding. Unless they are exceptionally motivated, no significant advantage is gained with regional anesthesia during major joint replacement procedures.

ORTHOPEDIC ONCOLOGY

Orthopedic oncology encompasses a wide range of diagnostic, therapeutic, and reconstructive procedures in patients of all age groups. Although primary bone tumors are exceedingly rare, soft tissue sarcomas and metastatic bone disease are frequently encountered. Anesthesiologists should be aware of

specific concerns that are applicable to almost any oncology patient.

Why Should Impending Pathologic Fractures Be Stabilized?

"Patients treated prophylactically for impending fractures have a lower surgical mortality, fewer complications, fewer stabilization failures, and more successful rehabilitation than those who suffer pathologic fractures."[15] All pathologic fractures should undergo stabilization if the patient's quality of life will be improved by the procedure (i.e., if the procedure will provide pain relief or improved mobility).

What Problems Are Common to Patients with Bone Cancers?

Pain

Bone lesions frequently are very painful. Patients commonly take large doses of analgesics and may have a tolerance to narcotics and other sedatives. An accurate drug history is necessary to anticipate their needs. Oral narcotic doses should be converted to an equivalent parenteral dose that is administered while the patients remain in nil per os status. Stress doses of steroids are *not* indicated if steroids were used for chemotherapeutic purposes only.

Chemotherapy

Frequently, oncology patients receive chemotherapy that results in anemia, granulocytopenia, thrombocytopenia, or any combination of these. The recent introduction of granulocyte-stimulating factors and recombinant erythropoietin lessens the severity of bone marrow suppression that results from chemotherapy. Specific inquiry should be made regarding the use of doxorubicin (Adriamycin), vincristine, and bleomycin in any chemotherapy regimen.

Doxorubicin

Doxorubicin can cause immediate and cumulative dose-dependent cardiomyopathy. The lifetime maximum dose of doxorubicin is 450 mg $\cdot$ m$^{2-1}$ of body surface area. Toxic effects are dose related and are potentiated by radiation therapy of the mediastinum. If a patient has received doxorubicin at any time, a preoperative assessment for cardiac symptoms should be sought; if they are present, the patient should at a minimum be evaluated with echocardiography.

Vincristine

Vincristine can be neurotoxic; any neurologic defects should be documented preoperatively, especially before a regional technique is used.

Bleomycin

Bleomycin causes pulmonary fibrosis in 10% of patients who receive a full course of this drug (300 U). The extent of involvement can be followed with measurements of carbon monoxide diffusing capacity. Because the severity of fibrosis can possibly be potentiated by the administration of oxygen (O_2)–enriched gases, any patient with a decreased carbon monoxide diffusing capacity should not receive a fraction of inspired O_2 >30%, if possible.

Metastatic Disease

Tumors metastatic to bone commonly have associated pulmonary involvement; conversely, the lungs are the most common site of metastatic primary sarcomas. Therefore, bone cancer patients require a preoperative chest radiograph that can be used to search for pulmonary metastases and malignant pleural effusions.

Which Procedures Have a Potential for Massive Blood Loss?

Large Resections

The most common orthopedic oncology procedures that result in large volumes of blood loss are large bone tumor resections in the spine, pelvis, sacrum, proximal femur, and shoulder girdle (see Table 71–2). Surgery in these areas precludes use of a tourniquet, and control of bleeding may be difficult. Sacral tumor resections are renowned for massive blood loss. The rich sacral venous plexus is often violated, and blood loss is difficult to control. Whole blood volume losses are not uncommon.

Sacral resections may be performed for sacral tumors or in conjunction with pelvic resections. In cases in which the tumor is in such a location that a tourniquet can be used, resection is usually done with the tourniquet inflated. Blood loss in these cases follows deflation of the tourniquet during the complex bone reconstruction, and the volume lost commonly exceeds 1 L.

Biopsies

Most biopsies of orthopedic tumors do not result in massive blood loss. Exceptions do occur and may be unpredictable. Sacral tumors, metastatic hypernephroma, and some other primary bone tumors may result in blood loss of >1 L from a small biopsy incision. After tissue is obtained, bleeding from the biopsy site frequently is controlled by packing the bone defect with bone cement (polymethylmethacrylate).

Preoperative communication with the surgeon about the procedure, the positioning, and the potential for blood loss is essential to anticipate each patient's needs. Venous access must be established prior to the start of these procedures because the blood loss that occurs frequently is "fast and furious."

SCOLIOSIS

Surgical correction of scoliosis is considered in patients with spinal curves that exceed 45° or with smaller curves that have been observed to progress on sequential radiographs. Other indications include trunk deformity, pain, decreasing cardiopulmonary status, familial history of severe scoliosis, and loss of function.

Does the Underlying Cause of Scoliosis Have Anesthetic Implications?

Idiopathic scoliosis accounts for approximately 70% of all cases. Patients are most commonly adolescent females who have no other systemic diseases. Congenital scoliosis can result from vertebral anomalies (e.g., spina bifida) and may be associated with neurologic deficits. These patients commonly have tethered spinal cords, which increase the risk of neurologic damage and paraplegia during corrective surgery.[16] In addition, a high incidence of cardiovascular, gastrointestinal, and urologic anomalies is associated with congenital scoliosis (VATER syndrome [vertebral defects, imperforate anus, tracheoesophageal fistula, and radial and renal dysplasia]).

Neuromuscular scoliosis can be classified as neuropathic or myopathic. With the eradication of polio, neuropathic scoliosis is most commonly the result of cerebral palsy. The muscular dystrophies are the cause of most myopathic scoliosis. Curvature worsens as muscular weakness progresses. Respiratory impairment from muscular weakness can be a significant problem for these patients postoperatively; thus, screening pulmonary function tests are essential.[17] Neurofibromatosis is another common cause of neuromuscular scoliosis. Anesthetic considerations associated with neurofibromatosis include paying strict attention to the possibility of airway neurofibromas.

What Are the Respiratory Effects?

Patients with idiopathic scoliosis have a restrictive lung defect that is the result of rib cage deformity. This deformity impairs development of the number of vascular units per volume of lung.[18] The lungs, being compressed by the rib cage deformity, have reduced compliance and abnormal ventilation/perfusion characteristics. These create increases in the ratio of dead space to tidal volume and in the alveolar-arterial O_2 partial pressure difference. Hypercapnia, arterial hypoxemia, and pulmonary hypertension often result. The severity of these derangements is directly related to the degree of curvature. The vital capacity is not severely impaired until the curve progresses to >60° (Fig. 71–3).

The rib cage abnormality in idiopathic scoliosis is usually not as severe as it is in patients with neuromuscular scoliosis, but the same mechanisms of respiratory impairment can be present. In addition, these patients have muscle weakness that impairs their ability to sigh and cough. Frequently, they have abnormal airway reflexes and are prone to aspiration.

Why Do Curves Greater Than 65° Need to Be Corrected?

If the spinal deformity is <65°, lung function can be considered normal.[19] Patients with greater curves should be thoroughly evaluated for pulmonary and cardiac dysfunction preoperatively. Surgical correction will not restore normal pulmonary function, but it will arrest further progression and preserve a patient's mobility.

How Should Spinal Cord Function Be Monitored Intraoperatively?

Wake-Up Test

The wake-up test, as the name implies, involves discontinuation of the anesthetic and reversal of neuromuscular blockade after distraction of the spine. The patient is asked to move an arm to confirm cooperation; then, he or she is asked to move the legs to confirm motor function. The anesthetic is then readministered, and the operation is continued.

A narcotic-based anesthetic is most often administered because it can be reversed with a narcotic antagonist; however, an inhalation technique using isoflurane with nitrous oxide also has been used. Regardless of the technique, few patients have any recall of the test. If they are informed preoperatively of the test, emergence is smoother and usually more rapid. The major limitation of the wake-up test is that it only gives information at a single time during the operation (see Chapter 22).

Somatosensory Evoked Potentials

Somatosensory evoked potentials (SSEPs) provide a continuous monitor of neural integrity. They are widely accepted as the standard of care for any procedure in which spinal cord integrity might be compromised. SSEPs are gathered using electroencephalographic monitoring during the presentation of a repetitive peripheral stimulus. Neural impulses travel from the site of stimulus to the brain. Because these impulses are not discernible in the raw electroencephalographic data, the stimulus is repeated thousands of times. When these impulses are collated, random impulses in the raw electroencephalogram are cancelled out, and a distinctive series of waves emerges.

Baseline tracings are recorded for continuous comparison throughout the perioperative period. If a significant change in the amplitude (height) or latency (time from impulse to detection at the brain) from baseline occurs, neural integrity must be verified, and a wake-up test should be performed.

No true false-negative results (abnormal sensory function with no change in the SSEP observed) have occurred with properly conducted SSEP monitoring. This technique does not monitor motor function; however, in scoliosis surgery, SSEP changes correlate reliably with motor changes. False-positive results (normal sensory function with a significant change in SSEP) can occur for a variety of reasons. Abrupt changes in temperature, blood pressure, and depth of anesthesia produce dramatic changes. Anesthetic techniques also influence the SSEP trace quality. A continuous infusion of narcotics complemented with low dose isoflurane and avoidance of nitrous

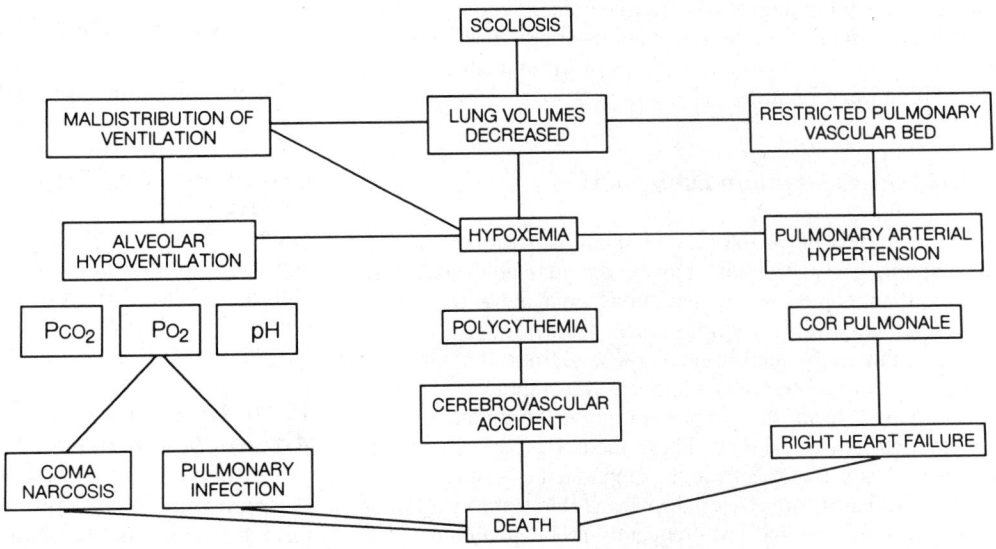

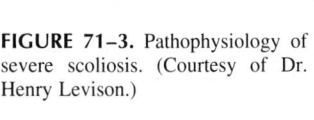

FIGURE 71–3. Pathophysiology of severe scoliosis. (Courtesy of Dr. Henry Levison.)

oxide is the preferred technique to maximize the quality of SSEP monitoring during spine surgery (see Chapter 22).

When Are Anterior Approaches to the Spine Used?

Anterior approaches are used when the anterior elements of the spine must be accessed for release of soft tissues, removal of tumor, bone grafting, and internal fixation. These approaches typically are used for severe forms of scoliosis, some cases of congenital scoliosis, spinal trauma, tumors, or severe kyphotic deformities.

What Is Important About Instrumentation for Spinal Surgery?

The range of instrumentation used in spinal surgery has grown over the past decade from a few simple rod and hook components to innumerable complex systems (e.g., the Harrington, Cotrel-Dubousset, Scottish-Rite, and Luque systems). The system is not as important as the technique used for securing the hardware to the spinal column and the susceptibility of the spinal cord tissue to injury. Traction, compression, or direct trauma to the spinal cord can cause neural injury. When an instrumentation system is tensed or compressed, neural injury also can occur. Following such cord manipulation, evaluation of neural function is critical.[20]

Sublaminar wires are used with a variety of instrumentation systems for rigid spinal fixation (e.g., Luque rods, Cotrel-Dubousset, and, occasionally, Harrington rods). They require the passage of a wire beneath the lamina immediately adjacent to the neural elements, exposing the neural structures to the potential for direct injury. In up to 25% of cases in which sublaminar wires are used, slight changes in the monitored SSEP have been reported.[21, 22]

AMPUTATIONS AND PHANTOM LIMB PAIN

Unfortunately, amputations are neither unique to orthopedics nor are they likely to become obsolete in the near future. The most common indications are ischemia, infection, trauma, and cancer. Frequently, these operations are the best option to restore a patient's mobility and function (provided that he or she will be free of pain).

What Causes Phantom Limb Pain?

The etiology of phantom limb pain is still not entirely understood, but prevention may be an attainable goal. Virtually all amputees report sensations emanating from their amputated extremity. Position, touch, temperature, and nociceptive input are frequently cited. These sensations are thought to be the result of centrally imprinted remembrances.[23] Afferent impulses from the amputated nerve stimulate cortical "memories" of sensations. These memories are cognitively interpreted as sensations from the amputated extremity.

This mechanism may explain why children rarely develop phantom limb pain and less frequently report phantom sensa-

tions. They have not developed as many phantom memories as have adults. This may explain why patients with a very painful extremity prior to amputation have a higher incidence of significant phantom pain.

How Can Phantom Limb Pain Be Prevented?

Epidural Analgesia

Bach and coworkers reported 11 patients with painful extremities that required amputation.[24] In all cases, epidural analgesia was provided for 3 days preoperatively to render the extremity pain-free prior to amputation. Postoperative pain was managed with intravenous and oral narcotics. At the 12-month follow-up examination, none of these patients developed phantom limb pain. In the control group of 15 patients whose preoperative pain was controlled with intravenous and oral narcotics only, a 27% incidence of phantom pain was present at 1 year.

Local Anesthetic Bathing

Fisher and Meller also reported 11 patients requiring amputation. A catheter was placed intraoperatively into the exposed nerve sheaths of these patients. The nerve sheath was then bathed in a local anesthetic solution via a continuous infusion system for 3 days postoperatively. Patients had minimal pain. At the 12-month follow-up, none of the patients had phantom limb pain.[25]

Malawer and associates used the nerve sheath catheter technique to provide postoperative analgesia to patients after amputations and major limb salvage reconstructions because these patients frequently have debilitating deafferentation pain. Again, no phantom pain was reported by any of the patients, and significant reductions in postoperative narcotic usage were noted.[26]

The latest follow-up in any of these reports is at 2 years (personal communication); however, these initial reports are very encouraging. The best time to initiate local anesthetic blockade is unclear. However, if the prevention of the formation of painful "memories" is the goal, the patient should emerge from anesthesia with a pain-free extremity.

AMBULATORY ORTHOPEDIC SURGERY

Minor orthopedic surgery involves an array of procedures that includes arthroscopies of the knee, ankle, shoulder, elbow, and wrist as well as soft tissue procedures such as tendon transfers, rotator cuff repairs, and ligamentous reconstruction. All procedures of the hands, ankles, and feet are considered minor. The advent of arthroscopic equipment and procedures and improvements in postoperative pain control allow the vast majority of these procedures to be done in the outpatient setting.

What Are the Causes of Pain During Arthroscopic Procedures?

Arthroscopic procedures require several small incisions for the introduction of the scope and instruments; these can be performed with local anesthetic infiltration at the portals. Pain during the procedure results from distention of the capsule that surrounds the joint with fluid (usually normal saline). Stretch receptors in the capsule cause a throbbing pain. Some centers report adequate analgesia when a local anesthetic is added to the irrigating solution and intravenous sedatives. A femoral nerve block alone is not sufficient to provide reliable anesthesia for this procedure because the sciatic nerve serves the distal portion of the knee. Postoperatively, edema from the extravasated irrigating solution is the major source of pain for most patients (if no bone work has been performed).

When Are Tourniquets Required?

Tourniquets are applied routinely except for shoulder procedures. If bleeding from synovial vessels obscures the surgical field, the tourniquet is inflated or the inflow pressure of irrigant is increased. Obviously, a tourniquet cannot be applied to the shoulder; hence, epinephrine routinely is added to the irrigant solution (1 mg epinephrine to each 3-L bag). Epinephrine increases the patient's blood pressure as it is systemically absorbed. Many orthopedic surgeons may not be aware of this systemic absorption and of its consequent effect on hemodynamics.

What Problems Occur With Shoulder Operations?

Muscle Relaxation

An important aspect of surgery for shoulder instability, as opposed to that for rotator cuff repair, is the examination conducted at the start of the case while the patient is under anesthesia. Frequently, the surgeon compares one shoulder to the other to assess the degree of laxity intrinsic to that patient. Complete abolition of muscle tone is unnecessary, but some relaxation is required to overcome the powerful shoulder girdle.

Monitoring

In the beach-chair or semirecumbent position, the entrainment of air is a theoretic risk because the operative field is above the heart. However, no case of such entrainment has been reported. Monitoring of end-tidal gases is probably sufficient to provide data in the event of the unlikely occurrence of this phenomenon.

Electrocardiographic leads require unique placement. The arm lead for the operative side should be placed medial to the scapula on that side so that it is out of the surgical field. If the patient is at risk for ischemia, a V_5 or V_4 lead is readily preserved. If blood pressure is to be measured noninvasively, the lower extremity should be used so as not to interfere with pulse oximetry monitoring and vascular access. However, one should remember to compensate for the hydrostatic effect of measuring blood pressure at a point significantly below the level of the head.

Nerve Damage

The entire brachial plexus can be stretched during shoulder surgery if the upper extremity is not supported adequately. This complication can occur if the patient is pulled off the edge of the operating table to promote exposure of both sides of the shoulder. In addition, the axillary and radial nerves may be compressed during the dissections of the shoulder.

REGIONAL ANESTHESIA

By virtue of its concentration on the extremities, orthopedic surgery lends itself to the use of regional anesthetics. Whether a real advantage accrues to such techniques is a constant source of debate among anesthesiologists worldwide. Conflicting studies have attempted to distinguish a difference in outcome for orthopedic patients as a result of the anesthetic techniques employed. However, in the final analysis, patient satisfaction will dictate your practice in most cases.

What Are the Important Factors in Upper Extremity Blocks?

As in real estate, the most important consideration is "location, location, and location." After location, one must consider the potential complications as well as the unique advantages of each of the upper extremity blocks.

Intravenous Regional Techniques

Intravenous regional blocks of the upper extremity are technical "no-brainers" that require an intravenous catheter, an Esmarch bandage, and a tourniquet. This simplicity has allowed surgeons to perform these blocks in emergency department settings for years without much guidance from anesthesiologists. They have a reliable, rapid onset and are safe when used with the proper equipment and drugs. Unfortunately, they are effective only for distal procedures of short duration.

A double-cuff tourniquet that has been checked and calibrated prior to placement on the patient should be used. Tourniquet failure is the most common cause of complications. Bupivacaine should not be used for an intravenous regional anesthetic because of possible cardiotoxicity should tourniquet failure occur. Lidocaine and prilocaine are the safest agents available because of their rapid clearance and low toxicity.

Brachial Plexus Blocks

Axillary, interscalene, and subclavian perivascular blocks are the three most commonly used brachial plexus blocks. Figure 71–4 shows the upper extremity peripheral innervation.

Axillary

Axillary blocks are very safe and have a low risk of complications. The incidence of postoperative paresthesias is no different with the transarterial approach than it is with the eliciting of paresthesias.[27] With a transarterial approach, one must be vigilant when searching for signs and symptoms of local anesthetic toxicity because of the possibility of intravascular injection. Bupivacaine should probably not be used for this block because of this risk. If a longer block is required, the clinician should consider an alternative site for the block.

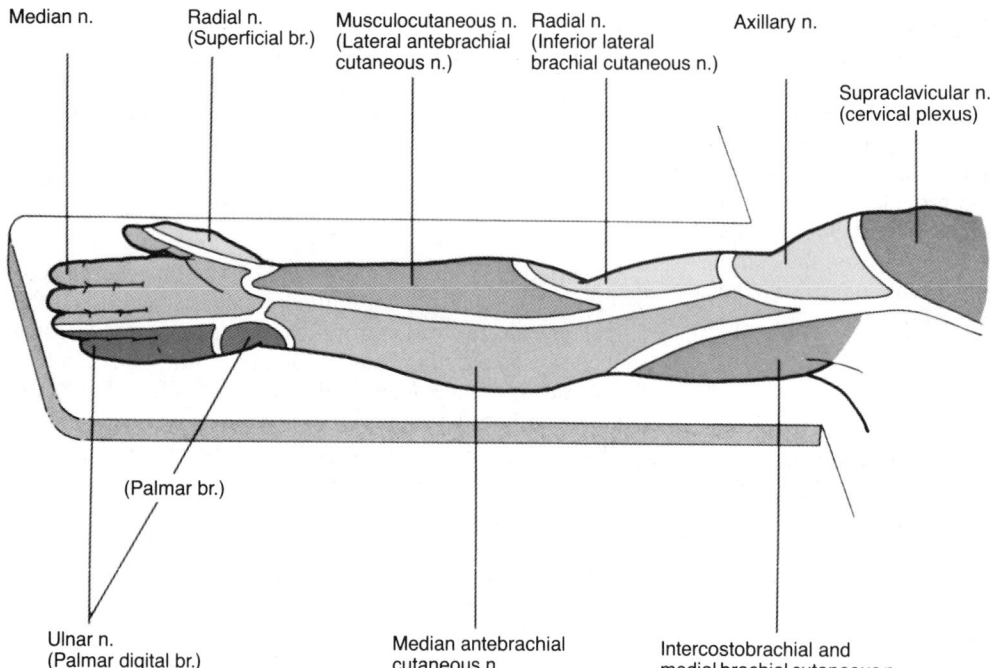

FIGURE 71–4. Upper extremity peripheral innervation with arm supinated on arm board. (From Brown DL: Atlas of Regional Anesthesia. Philadelphia, W. B. Saunders, 1992, p 16.)

An axillary block usually has the most easily locatable landmarks, even in an obese patient. Because this block can be done reliably with a paresthesia technique or with a transarterial approach, it is often the easiest brachial plexus block to perform. If the artery is not palpable, a Doppler probe can be used to direct the needle to the neurovascular bundle. An axillary block does not provide adequate sensory anesthesia for procedures above the elbow. Supplementation with separate musculocutaneous and intercostal brachialis injections improves the success of this block in most patients.

Interscalene

For shoulder surgery, an interscalene block is the only technique that predictably provides shoulder relaxation.[28] However, it does not reliably provide a complete sensory block of the hand and is a poor choice for hand surgery and in particular for any surgery that is performed in the field of the ulnar nerve distribution.

Complications of interscalene blocks include vertebral artery and subarachnoid injection and the spread of the local anesthetic solution into the epidural space, which results in a high cervical epidural blockade. One should expect a phrenic nerve paralysis from blockade of C-3, C-4, and C-5 fibers. Bilateral interscalene blocks should never be performed, and the performance of these blocks in patients with limited respiratory reserve should be carefully considered.

The interscalene block is unique in its ability to provide shoulder relaxation. Traditionally, a paresthesia below the elbow is required for reliable brachial plexus blockade. Recently, Roch and colleagues reported on the use of shoulder paresthesia for patients who had an interscalene brachial plexus block for shoulder surgery.[28] In 45% of these patients, the initial elicited paresthesia was to the shoulder, whereas in 55% of patients, a paresthesia was distal to the shoulder. All of the patients developed a brachial plexus block adequate for shoulder surgery.

Subclavian Perivascular

The subclavian perivascular block provides excellent anesthesia of the entire upper extremity from the shoulder downward. This approach to the brachial plexus results in the most profound neural blockade and requires the smallest amount of local anesthetic because of the tight fascial investment of the neurovascular bundle at this level.[29] Therefore, it is an excellent choice for patients who require prolonged neural blockade of the upper extremity with a single-shot technique.

The most worrisome complication of the subclavian perivascular technique is pneumothorax. Among experienced anesthesiologists, this occurs with a frequency of ≤6%.[29] The manifestation of pneumothorax can be delayed for up to 12 hours after performance of the block. Therefore, outpatients should be counseled about the possibilities of breathing difficulties postoperatively and must be able to reach a medical facility within a reasonable amount of time.

If a pneumothorax develops from a needle puncture of the pleura, aspiration through an 8-French Teflon catheter may be the only treatment necessary. An algorithm for the treatment of needle-induced pneumothoraces is outlined in Figure 71–5.

What Are the Important Considerations in Lower Extremity Blocks?

Options

Again, the site of the surgical incision is the most important determinant. Subarachnoid block provides adequate anesthesia for all operations of the lower extremity. Epidural blockade, however, is occasionally inadequate for operations on the foot or ankle. Ankle blocks work well if placed 20 to 40 minutes prior to surgery and if an Esmarch tourniquet is used at the ankle. However, if a thigh tourniquet is used, pain from its application may make the patient uncomfortable.

Femoral sciatic block provides excellent anesthesia for pro-

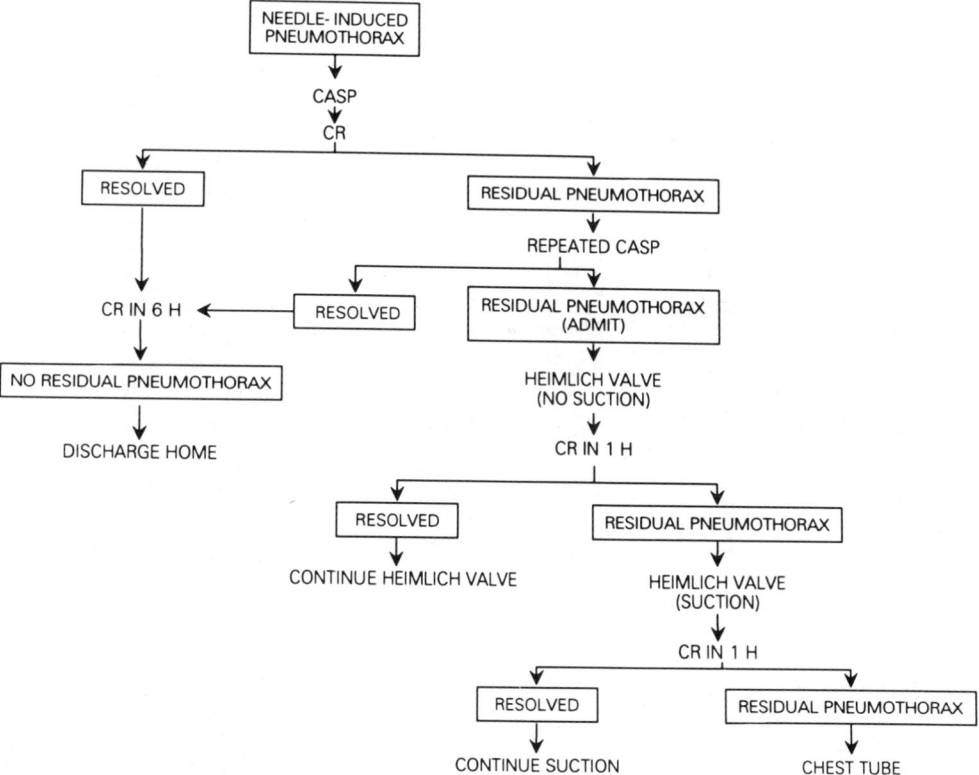

FIGURE 71–5. Algorithm for the treatment of needle-induced pneumothoraces. CASP = 8F-16G simple catheter aspiration of pneumothorax; CXR = chest x-ray; Heimlich valve: one-way flapper valve attached to catheter. (Modified from Delius RE, Obeid FN, Horst M, et al: Catheter aspiration for simple pneumothorax experience with 114 patients. Arch Surg 1989; 124:833–836. Copyright 1989, American Medical Association.)

cedures on the distal extremity but is technically more difficult to perform than other approaches. Intravenous regional blocks in the lower extremity frequently are inadequate because of the bulky muscles. They make complete exsanguination of the lower extremity difficult and tourniquet occlusion of the deep vessels less than complete. Hence, intravenous regional techniques are a poor choice for lower extremity surgery.

Positioning

Lateral or prone positioning is often required to adequately expose the operative field, and such positioning may influence the anesthetic choice. Many practitioners prefer to combine a regional technique with general anesthesia for patients in non-supine positions.

Body Habitus

A patient's body habitus has a greater role in lower extremity block selection than it does in choosing blocks to be performed elsewhere. As noted, lower extremity intravenous regional techniques are difficult even in thin patients because of the bulk of calf and thigh musculature. Sciatic nerve blocks are difficult in obese individuals because of the great distance the needle must cross to get close to the nerve.

Does Regional Anesthesia Reduce Morbidity or Mortality for Hip Fractures?

McKenzie and associates reported on mortality at 2 weeks following hip fracture repair in a comparison of spinal and general anesthesia. Patients in the spinal group had a mortality of 5% compared with 15% for those who received general anesthesia at that time.[30] However, at 2 months, the cumulative

mortality in each group reportedly was the same. A recent meta-analysis by Sorenson and Pace combined 13 studies that compared regional anesthesia with general anesthesia for surgical repair of femoral neck fractures.[31] With a database that included 2000 patients, they found the difference in mortality to be insignificant (2.7% less following regional anesthesia).

What Are the Advantages of Regional Anesthesia?

Blood Loss

Modig showed a clear reduction in blood loss during total hip replacement procedures performed under epidural anesthesia compared with those performed under general anesthesia.[32] This difference extends into the postoperative period and should be considered a real advantage (Fig. 71–6). The mechanism is thought to be related to decreases in venous pressures. Allowing the patient to ventilate spontaneously reduces transmitted thoracic pressure caused by positive-pressure ventilation. This effect, coupled with reduced venous tone from the sympathectomy, makes a difference in the amount of oozing that occurs from open bone interstices.

Pulmonary Thromboembolism

The influence of regional anesthesia on the incidence of postoperative thromboembolism is real but perhaps less important today than it was in the past. Evidence suggests a lower incidence of deep venous thrombosis in patients undergoing total hip replacement with regional anesthesia (spinal or epidural) than with general anesthesia.[33, 34] However if the patients in the general anesthesia group are given antithrombotic pro-

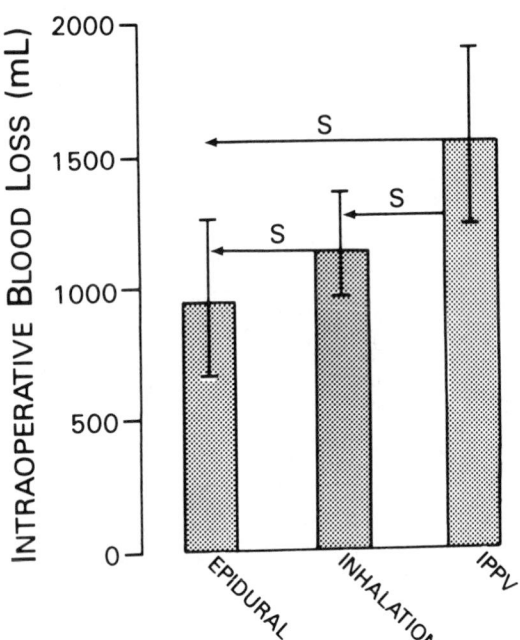

FIGURE 71–6. Intraoperative blood loss during total hip arthroplasty. Epidural: Spontaneous ventilation without intubation; Inhalation: General endotracheal anesthesia (GETA) with spontaneous ventilation; IPPV: GETA with controlled intermittent positive-pressure ventilation; S = significant difference. (From Modig J: Regional anesthesia and blood loss. Acta Anaesthesiol Scand 1988; 32:45.)

phylaxis, no difference occurs.[35, 36] Since new techniques have been developed to prevent deep venous thrombosis (low-dose sodium warfarin (Coumadin) administration, use of pneumatic intermittent compression stockings), the advantage of the intraoperative technique may be less important.[37]

Tourniquet Pain

Tourniquet pain, the nemesis of all orthopedic anesthesiologists, is diminished with regional techniques. This fact should be kept in mind when planning an anesthetic for a patient in whom swings in hemodynamic variables are undesirable.[37]

Postoperative Pain Management

The major advantage of regional anesthesia for patients undergoing orthopedic procedures is the extension of analgesia into the postoperative period. As physicians become more knowledgeable about the detrimental effects of postoperative pain, patients come to expect a pain-free recovery from surgery. Regional analgesia is eminently suited to the orthopedic patient, and its use will continue to spread as its long-term benefits become apparent.

ANTIBIOTICS

When Are Prophylactic Antibiotics Indicated?

Prophylactic antibiotics are indicated for all clean orthopedic operative procedures that involve implantation of foreign materials, including prostheses, plates, and screws, or the

transplantation of tissues (whether autologous or allograft). Appropriate antibiotic prophylaxis for soft tissue procedures, particularly those of short duration, is less clear.

The timing of the administration of the antibiotics is critical and should be done at least 5 minutes prior to the inflation of a tourniquet or prior to the incision in order that prophylactic soft tissue and bone antibiotic drug levels are achieved at the operative site. The recommended duration of prophylactic antibiotic administration is 24 to 48 hours postoperatively (e.g., cefazolin, 1 g intravenously, every 8 hours for 24–48 hours in a healthy adult patient).

Prophylaxis for open fractures typically consists of administration of a first-generation cephalosporin (e.g., cefazolin) and an aminoglycoside (e.g., gentamicin or tobramycin). Penicillin may be added for severely contaminated wounds. Appropriate tetanus coverage is also important in patients who have open fractures.

Which Antibiotics Are Most Effective?

Cefazolin (Kefzol or Ancef) is the most commonly used prophylactic antibiotic. This antibiotic has good bone penetration characteristics, provides broad spectrum microbial coverage of the most commonly encountered orthopedic pathogens (staphylococcal and streptococcal), is relatively inexpensive, and has been used successfully for many years.

In penicillin-allergic patients, vancomycin is most frequently used as an alternative prophylactic antibiotic agent. However, vancomycin requires approximately 1 hour for its complete administration if the "red man syndrome" is to be avoided; furthermore, this drug is very expensive. Clindamycin is an attractive alternative for penicillin-allergic patients. It can be given as a bolus, has relatively few side effects, and is inexpensive.

Why Is Antibiotic Coverage Crucial?

Many orthopedic procedures involve implantation of synthetic materials such as rods, prostheses, plates, and allografts. Some bacteria readily bind to such materials by elaborating glycocalyx. Once bound, infection can be established by proliferation of implant-bound bacteria. Prophylactic antibiotic therapy dramatically reduces the incidence of infection in hip replacement surgery from 2% to 3% to <1% in most series.[38–40] Patzakis and coworkers reported a decrease in infection rate for open fractures from 13% to 2.3% when prophylactic antibiotics were administered.[40]

The potential for wound contamination is high in orthopedic procedures for several reasons. For example, many procedures are relatively long and frequently performed under ischemic conditions. If antibiotics have not been administered prior to tourniquet inflation, the wound provides an ideal media for bacterial growth. Also, preparation of the bone for implantation by drilling and reaming causes local bone necrosis and thus provides another site for bacterial proliferation and glycocalyx production.

Once the presence of a bone infection has been established, it is very difficult to eradicate. Frequently, extensive bone débridement and prolonged antibiotic therapy are required. Reconstruction can only take place after the infection is cleared and frequently is technically difficult. Because of the potential risk of blood-borne microorganisms seeding implanted synthetic material, some practitioners recommend the use of prophylactic antibiotics for any procedure that might lead to septicemia. The recommendations are similar to those for subacute bacterial endocarditis prophylaxis.

BLOOD LOSS

The unique anatomy of bone, which is characterized by movement of the blood supply through solid interstices, often impairs hemostasis during operative procedures. No vessels can be ligated on raw bone surfaces. Bone wax is effective at plugging bleeding surfaces but inhibits bone union and therefore is infrequently used by orthopedic surgeons. Thus, patients undergoing orthopedic surgery are predisposed to continuous blood loss intraoperatively and often into the postoperative period. Any mechanism to decrease the mass of red blood cell loss intraoperatively should be aggressively pursued.

When Should Preoperative Autologous Blood Donation Be Recommended?

The following factors should be considered before surgery: probable estimated blood loss, preoperative hematocrit, and general patient condition. If the estimated blood loss is projected to be greater than 500 mL, preoperative blood donation should be considered.

The minimum criteria that a patient must satisfy for autologous blood donation to be an option are a hemoglobin level of $11.0 \text{ g} \cdot \text{dL}^{-1}$ and a weight of 100 lbs (personal communication, Civitan Regional Blood Bank, Gainesville, FL). Patients can donate every 72 hours up to the time of surgery. No age limitations exist for autologous blood donations, and all units are tested for blood-borne disease markers.

Contraindications are few but may include the presence of serious cardiac disease or anemia as well as the use of home O_2 therapy. Thus, autologous blood donation has become the preferred method for obtaining blood products for elective surgery since 1988.

Human erythropoietin produced using recombinant deoxyribonucleic acid techniques is available for clinical use. If used in conjunction with iron sulfate therapy, it allows a greater number of autologous units to be harvested prior to surgery.[41] Although still quite expensive, this alternative should be considered for any patient likely to require more than 2 units of blood, especially if other means of scavenging blood are not available because of the presence of malignancy or infection.

How Can Intraoperative Blood Loss Be Decreased?

Induced Hypotension

Hypotensive anesthesia decreases blood loss in hip replacement surgery, spinal surgery, and orthognathic surgery.[42–46] Hypotension has been accomplished with a variety of agents and techniques, including the use of sodium nitroprusside, trimethaphan, deep inhalation anesthesia, and regional anesthesia, with varying degrees of success.

Because most blood loss during orthopedic procedures

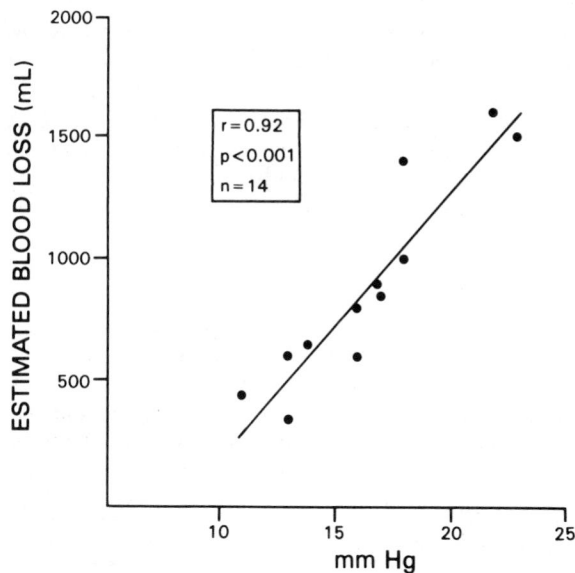

FIGURE 71–7. Relationship between mean venous pressure and intraoperative blood loss during total hip arthroplasty. (From Modig J: Regional anesthesia and blood loss. Acta Anaesthesiol Scand 1988; 32:46.)

comes from continual bone oozing, any technique that decreases peripheral venous pressure might be expected to decrease intraoperative blood loss (Fig. 71–7). A direct correlation exists between peripheral venous pressure measured in the wound and intraoperative blood loss.[32] Therefore, spontaneous ventilation, regional anesthesia, and vasodilator-induced hypotension with a drug such as nitroglycerin should decrease intraoperative blood loss.

Another benefit of induced hypotension is the vast improvement it brings about in the quality of the operating field. Even modest reductions in mean arterial pressure provide a clearer, drier operating field. Lessard and associates documented this improvement using a five-point scale to rate the quality of the operative field (Fig. 71–8) during induced hypotension.[44]

Hemodilution

Intraoperative hemodilution should be considered for patients who arrive in the OR with a hemoglobin level of

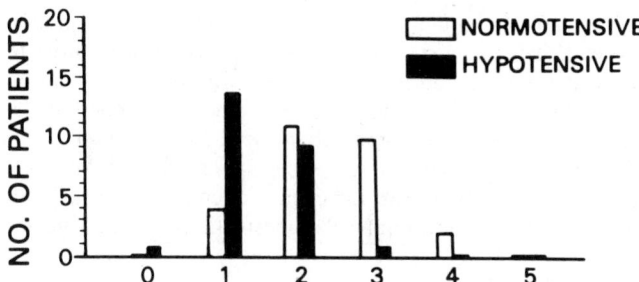

FIGURE 71–8. Quality of surgical field in normotensive and hypotensive conditions. 0 = No bleeding, virtually bloodless field; 1 = bleeding so mild that it is not a surgical nuisance; 2 = moderate bleeding that is a nuisance but that does not interfere with accurate dissection; 3 = moderate bleeding that moderately compromises surgical dissection; 4 = heavy but controllable bleeding that significantly interferes with dissection; 5 = massive uncontrollable bleeding. (Graph from Lessard MR, Trepanier CA, Baribault JP, et al: Isoflurane-induced hypotension in orthognathic surgery. Anesth Analg 1989; 69:379. Scale from Fromme GA, MacKenzie RA, Gould AB, et al: Controlled hypotension for orthognathic surgery. Anesth Analg 1986; 42:356.)

12 g · dL^{-1} or greater and in whom the blood loss can be projected to be at least 1 L. The actual red blood cell mass that is saved may be inconsequential, but the reinfusion of autologous fresh whole blood at the end of a long procedure frequently dries the field substantially. This approach has been utilized with great success in cardiac patients following bypass but is applicable to many types of surgery.

Blood Salvage

Blood salvaging devices have been used for many years with great success. Few contraindications to the reinfusion of wasted scavenged blood exist (among them are sickled red blood cells, active infection, and cancerous contamination). These devices are employed for any procedure in which the blood loss can be predicted to be >500 mL.

Desmopressin

Desmopressin acetate use created a great deal of excitement when it was reported to decrease the intraoperative blood loss during scoliosis surgery.[45] The mechanism of decreased blood loss was thought to be increased platelet adherence. Unfortunately, no other studies have supported these findings, and enthusiasm for this treatment has diminished.[46]

How Much Postoperative Blood Loss Can Be Expected?

In most major orthopedic operations, continued oozing and drainage is expected for 24 to 48 hours postoperatively. Up to 1 L of drainage in the first hours after spinal surgery, total joint replacements, and large tumor resections is common. This volume must be carefully monitored and replaced as needed.

Several systems have been developed to scavenge the initial drainage for reinfusion. Most commonly, a small amount of anticoagulant is added to the system to prevent drain clotting. The drainage is then collected for 3 to 4 hours postoperatively and reinfused.

POSITIONING

The most important goals of positioning for any operation are patient safety and optimal surgical conditions. In order to meet these goals during orthopedic procedures, discussion about the desired positioning should occur preoperatively. Many of the positions commonly utilized (prone, lateral decubitus, and beach-chair) do not allow the anesthesiologist easy access to the airway or to the central circulation. This should be considered in developing the anesthetic plan (see Chapter 30).

Why Are Chest Rolls Used in the Prone Position?

Chest rolls allow the abdominal contents to hang freely without being compressed by the operating table. Cephalic displacement of the diaphragm by the abdominal contents is thus prevented, and ventilation is aided. In addition, increased abdominal pressure impedes venous circulation. The result is increased venous volume and pressure in the epidural venous plexus and poor operating conditions for spinal surgery. A variety of frames and tables are utilized to free the abdominal contents for procedures that are performed in the prone position. The multitude of available devices attests to the difficulty associated with achieving the ideal prone position.

What Is the Correct Position for Longitudinal Chest Rolls?

The cephalic end of longitudinal chest rolls should extend to just below the clavicle so that they avoid clavicular impingement on the brachial plexus. The breasts should be directed medially if possible; they should not be brought out laterally. Nipples should not be compressed by the chest rolls. The abdomen should hang freely between the rolls, which should extend to the iliac crests. Male genitalia should be in a neutral position and free of compression. The knees should be padded and the feet supported by pillows. The arms should be carefully padded and tucked or abducted but not by >90° from the sides and anterior to the plane of the thorax.

What Are Important Considerations When Using the Beach-Chair Position?

When using the upright, semirecumbent, beach-chair position, several important considerations must be kept in mind. As the patient is changing position from supine to partially seated and upright, attention must be directed to hemodynamic stability. Hypotension is frequently encountered during this maneuver. Hypovolemia, myocardial depression, vasodilation from the anesthetic, and slow sympathetic response can all play a role.[47]

To avoid hypotension, the patient should assume an upright position gradually, and careful monitoring of the blood pressure should be paramount. In addition, sequential inflation of stockings wrapped around the lower extremities counteracts the venous pooling that occurs when the patient is in this position.

If the anesthetic plan calls for intubation, the endotracheal tube should be secured on the side opposite to the operative site. The head must be firmly secured to the frame of the bed in a forward-facing direction. This prevents the head from turning opposite to the surgical field and stretching the brachial plexus. It also helps to prevent accidental extubation during exuberant surgical manipulation of the extremity.

What Are Potential Complications of the Lateral Decubitus Position?

Careful attention must be directed toward the dependent extremities when the patient is positioned in the lateral decubitus position. Compression of the neurovascular bundle in the axilla can occur if the weight of the torso is not supported by a chest roll. This problem may result in nerve palsies or compartment syndromes, or both.

Complications in the dependent leg during hip surgery performed in the lateral decubitus position rarely occur. Lachiewicz and Latimer reported six cases of swelling of the gluteal muscle compartments, rhabdomyolysis, myoglobinuria, and

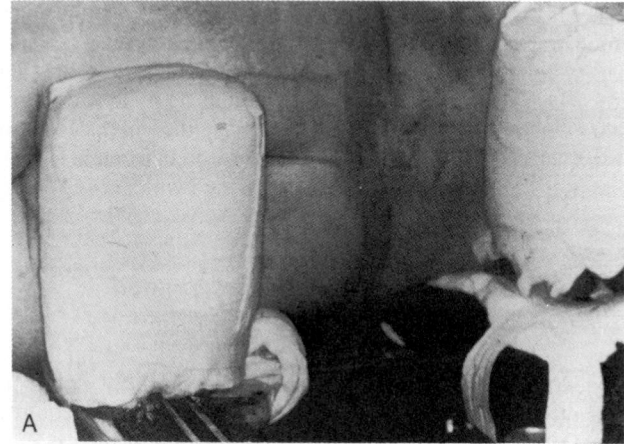

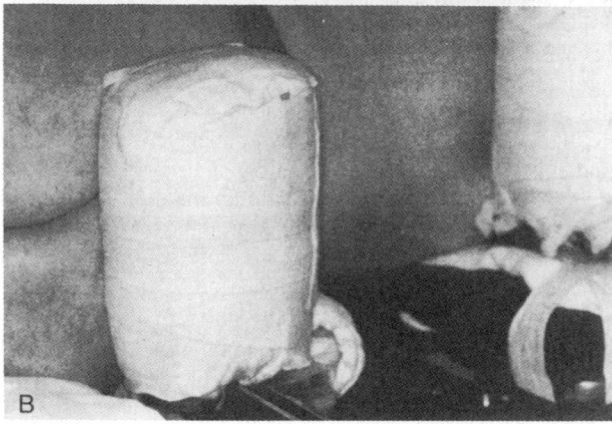

FIGURE 71–9. Placement of buttock supports for the lateral decubitus position. *A,* Incorrect placement of the posterior pad on the gluteal muscles can cause gluteal crush injury. *B,* Correct placement of the posterior pad on the sacrum frees the gluteal muscles. (From Lachiewicz PF, Latimer HA: Rhabdomyolysis following total hip arthroplasty. J Bone Joint Surg [Br] 1991; 73B:578.)

sciatic nerve palsy.[48] Risk factors for these complications included obesity, prolonged operating time, and use of the lateral decubitus position. Complications ranging from nerve palsies to ischemia of the dependent leg that resulted in acute renal failure and death have been reported during total hip arthroplasty.[49] These problems also can be minimized by careful padding and gentle flexion of the hip, buttocks, and knee of the dependent extremity. Figure 71–9 demonstrates the correct placement of the buttock support for the lateral decubitus position.

TOURNIQUETS

Tourniquets are frequently applied during extremity surgery to limit blood loss, to provide a bloodless surgical field, and to perform intravenous regional blockade. Anesthesiologists and surgeons are jointly responsible for their proper application and use in the OR.

What Are the Potential Complications?

Neural damage, muscle necrosis, arterial and deep venous thrombosis, and skin injury are reported complications of tourniquet use. The incidence of the complications is very low when properly calibrated equipment is used and a schedule of inflation/deflation times is followed. In 21 of 25 cases in which the tourniquet was checked after a tourniquet-induced injury occurred, patients had been exposed to excessive pressure caused by tourniquet malfunction.[50] Proper tourniquet calibration should be verified before each use.

Nerve Damage

Nerve damage is the result of direct axonal compression of the nerve, usually at the edge of the cuff. Excessive cuff pressure appears to be the major factor leading to nerve injury, with duration of application as a secondary influence.[50] Symptoms of tourniquet-induced nerve injury range from transient mild paresthesias to permanent paralysis of the nerves involved. The radial nerve is most frequently involved in tourniquet-induced palsies. Its location adjacent to the humerus allows it to be easily compressed against the bone by the tourniquet. Lower extremity nerve injuries are much less common because their greater muscle mass protects the nerves and because in the lower extremity the peroneal nerve is the only nerve closely approximated to a bone.

Muscle Damage

Muscle damage from tourniquet-induced ischemia is less dramatic than nerve damage in its presentation but probably occurs with a greater frequency. Saunders and associates reported on 48 patients who underwent knee surgery with the use of a thigh tourniquet. Eighty-five per cent of the patients with thigh tourniquets inflated for 60 minutes or longer demonstrated abnormal electromyographic data and muscle weakness. The incidence of abnormal electromyograms in this study directly correlated with the length of tourniquet inflation (Table 71–4). In all patients, the electromyographic abnormalities resolved over varying amounts of time up to 5 months postoperatively.[51]

Edema associated with reperfusion hyperemia develops immediately upon tourniquet deflation. The post-tourniquet syndrome is characterized by tissue edema, pallor, stiffness, weakness without paralysis, and subjective numbness of the extremity. This syndrome is probably the result of the edema's compressing vessels, joint capsules, and nerve endings. The symptoms usually resolve within a week of the insult, although the edema may take longer to disappear.

TABLE 71–4. Effect of Tourniquet Time on Quadriceps Function After Knee Arthroscopy*

| | | Abnormal Electromyogram | |
No. of Patients	Tourniquet Time (min)	*No.*	*%*
13	≥60	11	85
14	30–60	10	71
12	15–30	7	58
9	<15	2	22

(From Saunders KC, Louis DL, Weingarden SI, et al: Effect on tourniquet time on postoperative quadriceps function. Clin Orthop 1979; 143:194.)
*Tourniquet inflation may cause significant electromyographic abnormalities postoperatively.

What Is the Optimal Tourniquet Inflation and Release Scheme?

Sapega and colleagues performed histologic canine muscle studies following a variety of inflation/deflation schemes.[52] They demonstrated a direct relationship between the time of continuous tourniquet inflation and the degree of muscle damage. By limiting the initial period of ischemia to 90 minutes, they found that recovery prior to reinflation of the tourniquet could be achieved in 5 minutes.[53] Thus, for procedures likely to exceed 2 hours, surgeons should be encouraged to deflate the tourniquet after 90 minutes to allow a 5-minute reperfusion period.

Why Are Surgeons Reluctant to Deflate a Tourniquet Intraoperatively?

Edema formation begins immediately upon tourniquet deflation. Visualization of anatomic structures is often difficult after even short periods of tourniquet inflation, not because blood is present in the field but because edema occludes the structures. If the tourniquet is released after the application of dressings and splinting devices, many surgeons believe the amount of edema formation is reduced. In addition, they believe that blood loss is decreased if a pressure dressing is applied prior to tourniquet release. Therefore, if an entire procedure is anticipated to be accomplished in <150 minutes, most surgeons prefer not to deflate the tourniquet for reperfusion.

In defense of this practice, data from human studies have demonstrated that the rate of metabolite accumulation and high-energy phosphate depletion decreased with increasing tourniquet time.[53] This observation is thought to be the result of decreased metabolic needs that occur with cooling of the unperfused extremity. However, surgeons should be informed of the amount of ischemic time (which should be charted) that has elapsed at hourly intervals for the first 2 hours, again at 2.5 hours, and at 15-minute intervals thereafter.

What Is the Optimal Tourniquet Pressure?

Tourniquet inflation pressure frequently is chosen arbitrarily to be 250 mm Hg for the upper extremities and 350 mm Hg for the lower extremities. These values may be satisfactory for normally shaped extremities in nonhypertensive patients who require short periods of tourniquet inflation. However, in patients requiring long tourniquet inflation times, in hypertensive patients, and in extremely thin or obese patients, a more scientific approach should be used. The inflation pressure required to eliminate the pulse detected by an ultrasonic Doppler flow meter can be determined prior to tourniquet inflation. For upper extremity operations, 50 mm Hg should be added to the Doppler occlusion pressure; for lower extremity operations, 75 mm Hg should be added. Using this scheme, Reid achieved adequate hemostasis in a series of 84 patients with tourniquet inflation pressures of 135 to 255 mm Hg for the upper extremities and with pressures of 175 to 305 mm Hg for the lower extremities.[54]

The width of the tourniquet is another important factor to consider in choosing a tourniquet inflation pressure. Standard 8.5-cm pneumatic tourniquets exert the highest pressure at the midcuff subcutaneous level. The pressure diminishes at deeper tissue planes and toward the cuff edges. Moore and colleagues demonstrated Doppler occlusion pressures that were lower than systolic blood pressures using a tourniquet 15 cm in width. They theorized that "an accumulation of frictional resistance along the compressed length" of the cuff accounted for the subsystolic pressures required to stop detectable flow.[56] Perhaps 15-cm cuffs should always be used when possible.

What Causes Bleeding Distal to an Inflated Tourniquet?

Inadequate extremity exsanguination is the most common cause of bleeding distal to a tourniquet. This problem requires release of the tourniquet and re-exsanguination of the extremity. During an intravenous regional anesthetic case, this approach is unacceptable. Thus, one must be meticulous in exsanguination during preparation for this block.

Insufficient hemostasis from inadequate inflation pressure is most likely to occur in hypertensive patients. Wide swings in blood pressure may allow arterial breakthrough, a fact that should be considered when choosing an inflation pressure for hypertensive patients. Arterial breakthrough can be treated by increasing the tourniquet inflation pressure so long as the extremity does not require re-exsanguination.

Tourniquet "ooze" is due to the entry of blood into the bone medulla through nutrient arteries proximal to the tourniquet. This problem cannot be treated by increasing the tourniquet inflation pressure.[50]

What Is Tourniquet Pain?

Characteristics

Tourniquet pain is an ill-defined, dull, aching pain described by patients who undergo operations that require tourniquet inflation. It usually occurs 45 to 60 minutes after inflation of the tourniquet, even when otherwise adequate surgical levels of general and regional anesthesia are provided. During general anesthesia, it is manifested by hypertension, which has been reported to occur in as many as 66% of patients. During regional anesthesia, the patient may complain of an annoying ache that is accompanied by restlessness and agitation; interestingly, however, hypertension is much less common[56] (Table 71–5). In either case, release of the tourniquet provides instant relief. With reinflation, the pain usually occurs earlier than it did initially.

Cause

The pathologic basis of tourniquet pain is not entirely understood. Because unmyelinated C fibers transmit impulses associated with dull, persistent, poorly localized pain, it is these fibers that are probably responsible.[57–59] In an in vitro model, Gissen and coworkers showed that C fibers are more resistant to local anesthetic-induced conduction blockade than are the larger A fibers.[58] In addition, they found that as tetracaine concentrations decreased, C fiber action potential amplitudes returned to normal levels, whereas A fiber action potentials were still suppressed. Bupivacaine did not exhibit this differential effect to the same degree.

TABLE 71–5. Occurrence of Hypertension in Patients Requiring Tourniquet Inflation for Extremity Surgery As a Function of Anesthetic Type

Type of Anesthesia	Patient No.	Hypertension	
		No.	*%*
General	240	160	66.7
Spinal	335	9	2.7
Plexus	40	1	2.5
Intravenous regional	59	11	18.6
Combination	25	4	16.0
Total	**699**	**185**	**26.5**

(From Valli H, Rosenberg PH, Kytta J, et al: Arterial hypertension associated with the use of a tourniquet with either general or regional anaesthesia. Acta Anaesthesiol Scand 1987; 31:279.)

This theory of tourniquet pain is well supported by the findings of Concepcion and associates, who reported significantly less tourniquet pain in patients anesthetized with intrathecal bupivacaine than in those given tetracaine for lower extremity procedures, despite the presence of longer tourniquet times in the bupivacaine group.[57]

What Physiologic Effects Occur with Tourniquet Deflation?

Following deflation of a lower extremity tourniquet, the most obvious clinical effects are hypotension, a transient increase in end-tidal carbon dioxide tension, and a small decrease in patient temperature. These changes can also be seen with deflation of upper extremity tourniquets, but the degree of change usually is not as significant. Presumably, postischemic reactive hyperemia induced by tissue anoxia is responsible.

The exact mediators of postischemic reactive hyperemia have not been identified, but clinicians frequently refer to them as "evil humors." Leading candidates are bradykinin, lactate, adenosine, and inorganic phosphate. After tourniquet deflation, increased blood flow to the extremity rapidly washes out the products of anaerobic metabolism. End-tidal carbon dioxide may increase as much as 18 mm Hg during this washout phase.[60]

Transient temperature drops of as much as 1.5 °C may be seen at this time. Significant convective heat loss can occur in the unperfused extremity during prolonged tourniquet inflation. The vasodilation associated with postischemic reactive hyperthermia may make it difficult to regain the pretourniquet deflation temperature.

Hypotension frequently occurs in the immediate postdeflation period and probably has a variety of causes. Central blood volume is acutely decreased as blood returns to the postischemic vasodilated extremity. This factor, coupled with the dramatic relief of tourniquet pain, may result in transient moderate systolic hypotension. Adequate volume replacement prior to tourniquet deflation attenuates this effect.

SPLINTING

Why Is the Timing of the Wake-Up Important in Orthopedic Cases?

Orthopedic cases that involve reduction and fixation of fractures, ligament repair, or other fixation of anatomic structures require postoperative immobilization for adequate healing. The first step in postoperative immobilization is the application of a splint that provides rigid immobilization and accommodates postoperative swelling. In such cases, the patient must remain immobile. Splints using plaster of Paris require roughly 10 minutes to become rigid following application. Premature cessation of the anesthetic can have dire consequences, including loss of fracture reduction or failure of the repair. Some splints are placed for patient comfort and do not require patient immobility during application. Querying the surgeon as to the appropriate time for patient wake-up is appreciated and recommended.

What Are the Dangers Associated with Plaster Splints?

Plaster of Paris splinting material hardens with an exothermic chemical reaction. Burns can result from this reaction. Adequate ventilation of the plaster material is important to prevent excessive heat accumulation. The splint should not be covered with blankets or be in contact with plastic-covered pillows during the exothermic phase (in the operative setting, this phase usually lasts until after the patient reaches the postanesthesia care unit).

VENOUS THROMBOEMBOLISM

Venous thrombosis is a serious complication of lower extremity orthopedic surgery. Fatal pulmonary embolism is reported in 1% to 3% of patients who did not receive prophylaxis against thrombosis after total hip replacement.[61] With prophylaxis, the incidence of deep venous thrombosis can be reduced to as low as 20%, and fatal pulmonary emboli can be nearly eliminated.[62, 63]

Which Patients Are at Risk for Thromboembolic Disease?

Deep venous thromboses and pulmonary emboli occur most often in orthopedic patients following hip and knee surgery. The cited incidence of deep venous thromboses depends on the mechanism for documentation of embolism (i.e., venography, pulmonary angiography, Doppler or ultrasonographic studies) and can be as high as about 75%. Risk factors include hip surgery, advanced age, female gender, previous thromboembolic disease, malignant disease, and prolonged bed rest. General anesthesia, as noted earlier, is associated with a higher rate of intraoperative thrombosis formation than is regional anesthesia.[33, 34] However, in patients receiving low-dose sodium warfarin prophylaxis following hip surgery under general anesthesia, the incidence of symptomatic thrombotic events is no different.[35, 36]

What Can Be Done to Prevent Thromboembolism in Orthopedic Patients?

Strategies to prevent thromboembolic disease in orthopedic patients include use of regional anesthesia, early patient mobilization, use of mechanical devices (e.g., pneumatic compression stockings), prophylactic drug therapy, and application of vascular filters. Multiple studies have confirmed that prophylactic drug therapy is the most effective means to prevent thromboembolic disease.[35–39, 62] Prophylactic agents that have been studied include aspirin, dextran, low-dose heparin, low-dose heparin with antithrombin III, adjusted-dose heparin, warfarin, and low-molecular-weight heparin. The most effective agent is warfarin. Bleeding can be minimized by using low-dose warfarin, by carefully monitoring the prothrombin time and partial thromboplastin time, and by screening high-risk patients. Aspirin, dextran, and low-dose heparin are not effective and should not be used in this patient population.

PAIN CONTROL

We are entering a new era in surgical progress in which strategies to prevent postoperative pain, and not just alleviate it, are developing. These strategies are particularly applicable to orthopedic patients who frequently have intense postoperative pain and require postoperative physical therapy as soon as it can be tolerated.

Which Orthopedic Procedures Are Particularly Painful?

Pain following orthopedic procedures is the result of inflammation and edema, which cause compression and deformation of the exquisitely sensitive periosteum. The bone itself is insensate. From this knowledge, it follows that surgery in an area of well-defined fascial compartments that produces edema and hemorrhage is very painful. Thus, patients who undergo total knee replacements may have much more pain postoperatively than do patients who undergo total hip replacement. During total knee replacement operations, the edema, inflammation, and hemorrhage are enclosed by the tight fascial investments around the musculature of the knee. Following total hip replacements, edema fluid oozes into the loose areolar tissue about the hip.

Ankle and wrist fractures are particularly painful, perhaps because the edema is confined by tight ligamentous attachments. This phenomenon also explains why fracture blisters occur rapidly if an ankle fracture is not promptly elevated.

Preble and colleagues recorded average patient-controlled analgesia (PCA) narcotic use after different orthopedic procedures. Although wide variations in the reported pain scores occurred, most were consistently in the 5 to 7 range. Narcotic use is high (2–5 mg of morphine per hour) (Table 71–6).[64]

What Strategies for Postoperative Pain Control Can Be Applied?

The acute pain cycle can and should be aggressively attacked at multiple sites to prevent postoperative pain (Fig. 71–10). Local infiltration of the operative site prior to incision has been shown to reduce postoperative pain in hernia repair and cholecystectomy.[65–67] Preincisional infiltration with local anesthetics may prevent activation of nociceptor afferent impulses from reaching the spinal cord. Ketorolac, an intravenous nonsteroidal anti-inflammatory drug, may inhibit prostaglandin release and diminish the local inflammatory reaction. Theoretically, it should be given prior to incision to prevent the initiation of the arachidonic cascade.

Intra-Articular Injection

For patients having arthroscopic surgery of the knee, intra-articular injection of bupivacaine is routine. Joshi and coworkers reported near complete analgesia for the entire postoperative period in patients given 5 mg of intra-articular morphine sulfate alone or in combination with bupivacaine[68] (Fig. 71–11). The significance of peripheral opioid receptors in the knee is currently the subject of some debate.[69]

The Cryocuff

Another nonpharmacologic intervention that should be considered for the prevention of postoperative pain in the orthopedic patient is the cryocuff (Aircast, Aircast, Inc., Summit, NJ). This device provides cold therapy in combination with compression to prevent edema formation. It has a high satisfaction rating among patients, perhaps because it gives them an active role in their own pain prevention.

Continuous Local Anesthetic Infusions

Continuous infusions of local anesthetics through catheters placed in the wound or directly on nerve sheaths has been used for postoperative pain control with great success.[24, 25, 70] Significant reductions in postoperative narcotic use occurred in patients who required iliac bone graft harvesting. A continuous infusion of 0.25 bupivacaine at 5 mL · h^{-1} was used to bathe the harvest site as long as a drain remained in place.[70]

TABLE 71–6. Pain Scores and Average Narcotic Consumption After Various Orthopedic Procedures

	VAS Pain Score (Mean ± SD)	Range	PCA Morphine (mg · h^{-1}, Mean ± SD)	Patient Age (Mean ± SD)
ACL repair	5.0 ± 1.4	4–7	4.6 ± 1.6	26.0 ± 7.1
Ankle	6.3 ± 1.9	4–10	3.4 ± 1.6	48.4 ± 17.5
Femur	5.9 ± 2.5	2–10	3.6 ± 2.8	34.2 ± 16.1
Back fusion	6.2 ± 2.0	3–9	5.4 ± 4.8	33.6 ± 8.9
Total hip	2.6 ± 1.9	0–6	1.2 ± 1.0	67.0 ± 12.3
Tibia	4.8 ± 1.9	2–6	3.0 ± 0.4	22.8 ± 1.6
Laminectomy	4.4 ± 2.3	3–10	2.8 ± 2.0	49.6 ± 13.7
Total knee	5.3 ± 3.0	3–10	2.1 ± 0.8	61.7 ± 16.4

(From Preble L, Paige D, Sinatra R, et al: Varying narcotic requirements among orthopedic patients. Anesthesiology 1990; 73:A813.)
Abbreviation: ACL = anterior cruciate ligament.

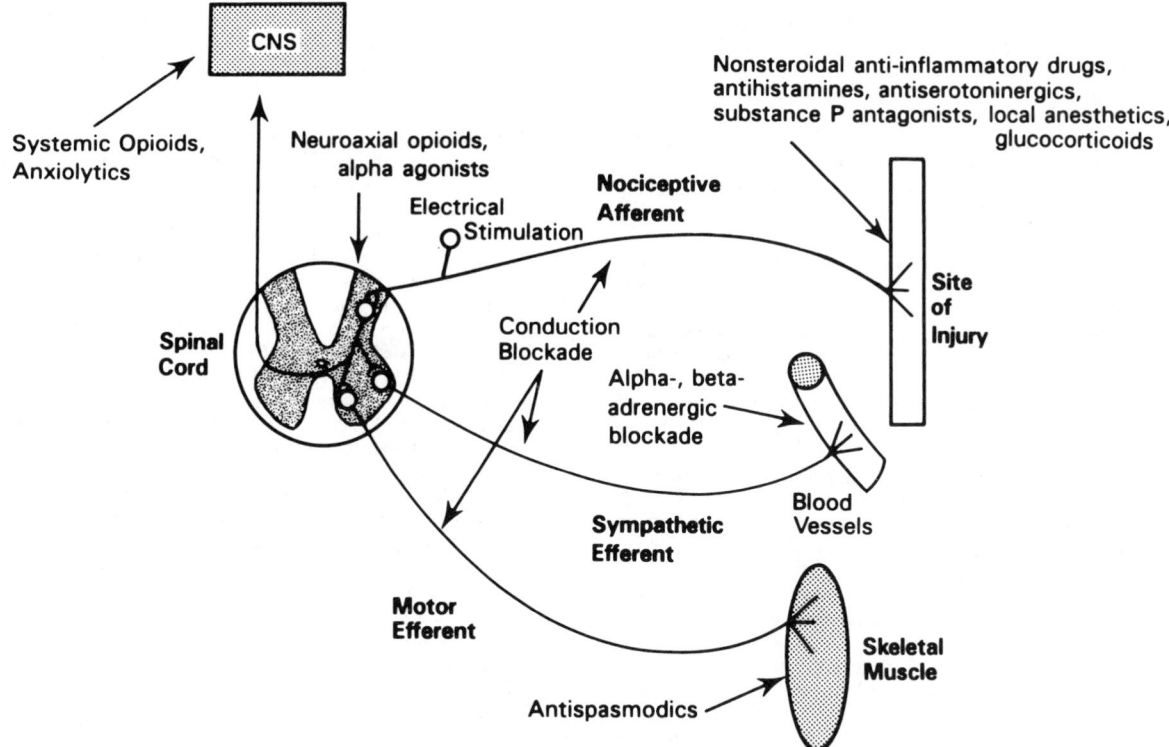

FIGURE 71–10. Potential sites for modulation of the acute pain cycle. (Modified from Sinatra RS: Pathophysiology of acute pain. *In* Acute Pain: Mechanisms and Management. Sinatra RS, Hord AH, Ginsberg B (eds). Chicago, Mosby–Year Book, 1992, p 55.)

Malawer and associates reported a decrease of up to 90% in narcotic requirements following major amputations when catheters were surgically placed directly on the nerve sheaths. Local anesthetic infusions were started intraoperatively and the patients were essentially free of pain in the postoperative period. At 2-year follow-up, none of the 23 patients had phantom limb pain.[26]

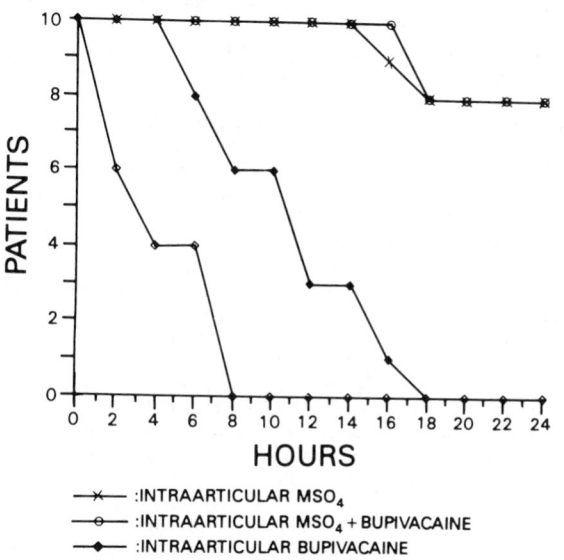

FIGURE 71–11. Number of patients not requiring analgesics for 24 hours after knee arthroscopy. (From Joshi GP, McCarroll SM, O'Brien TM, et al: Intraarticular analgesia following knee arthroscopy. Anesth Analg 1993; 76:333, © International Anesthesia Research, Inc.)

How Can Postoperative Management Affect Pain Therapy?

Specific aspects of the postoperative management should be discussed preoperatively with the surgeon. The decision to maintain an epidural catheter may affect planned anticoagulation. If ambulation and immediate physical therapy are anticipated, local anesthetic infusions might be a hindrance. On the other hand, a significant motor block is the desired end point in some patients with extremity manipulations; alternatively, a continuous passive motion device can be used. Perioperative pain management has turned the corner from art to science. We can look forward to continued advances in our approach to caring for patients postoperatively.

References

1. Perry JF: Pelvic open fractures. Clin Orthop 1980; 151:41.
2. Viegas S, Rimoldi R, Scarborough M, et al: Acute compartment syndrome in the thigh: a case report and review of the literature. Clin Orthop 1988; 234:232.
3. Taylor DC, Salvian AJ, Shackleton CR: Crush syndrome complicating pneumatic antishock garment (PASG) use. Injury 1988; 19:43.
4. Bass RR, Allison EJ, Reines HD, et al: Thigh compartment syndrome without lower extremity trauma following application of pneumatic antishock trousers. Ann Emerg Med 1983; 12:382.
5. Johnson BE: Anterior tibial compartment syndrome following use of MAST suit. Ann Emerg Med 1981; 10:209.
6. Seibel R, LaDuca J, Hassett JM, et al: Blunt multiple trauma (ISS 36), femur traction, and the pulmonary failure-septic state. Ann Surg 1985; 202:283.
7. Bone LB, Johnson KD, Weigelt J, et al: Early versus delayed stabilization of femoral fractures: a prospective randomized study. J Bone Joint Surg [Am] 1989; 71A:336.
8. Johnson KD, Cadambi A, Seibert GB: Incidence of adult respiratory

distress syndrome in patients with multiple musculoskeletal injuries: effect of early operative stabilization of fractures. J Trauma 1985; 25:375.

9. White BL, Fisher WD, Laurin CA: Rate of mortality for elderly patients after fracture of the hip in the 1980s. J Bone Joint Surg [Am] 1987; 69A:1335.

10. Ions GK, Stevens J: Prediction of survival in patients with femoral neck fractures. J Bone Joint Surg [Br] 1987; 69B:384.

11. Dorr LD, Merkel C, Mellman MF, et al: Fat emboli in bilateral total knee arthroplasty: predictive factors for neurologic manifestations. Clin Orthop 1989; 248:112.

12. Pellicci PM, Ranawat CS, Tsairis P: A prospective study of the progression of rheumatoid arthritis of the cervical spine. J Bone Joint Surg [Am] 1981; 63A:342.

13. Keenen MA, Siles CM, Kaufman RL: Acquired laryngeal deviation associated with the cervical spine disease in erosive polyarticular arthritis. Anesthesiology 1983; 58:441.

14. Cathcart ES, Spodick DH: Rheumatoid heart disease: a study of the incidence and nature of cardiac lesions in rheumatoid arthritis. N Engl J Med 1962; 266:959.

15. Orthopedic Knowledge Update 3: Hip trauma. Zuckerman JD (ed). American Academy of Orthopedic Surgeons, 1990, p 499.

16. MacEwen GD, Bunnell WP, Sriram K: Acute neurological complications in the treatment of scoliosis: a report of the Scoliosis Research Society. J Bone Joint Surg [Am] 1975; 57A:404.

17. Millne B, Rosales JK: Anesthetic consideration in patients with muscular dystrophy undergoing spinal fusion and Harrington rod instrumentation. Can Anaesth Soc J 1982; 29:750.

18. Kafer ER: Idiopathic scoliosis: mechanical properties of the respiratory system and the ventilatory response to carbon dioxide. J Clin Invest 1975; 55:1153.

19. Holtby HM, Relton JES: Orthopedic diseases. In Orthopedic Diseases. Katz J (ed). Philadelphia, WB Saunders, 1987, p 370.

20. Bieber E, Tolo V, Uematsu S: Spinal cord monitoring during posterior spinal instrumentation and fusion. Clin Orthop 1988; 229:121.

21. Luque ER: Sequential spinal instrumentation of the lumbar spine. Clin Orthop 1986; 203:126.

22. Rossier AB, Cochran TP: The treatment of spinal fusion with Harrington compression rods and sequential sublaminar wiring: a dangerous combination. Spine 1984; 9:796.

23. Katz J, Melzack R: Pain ''memories'' in phantom limbs: review and clinical observations. Pain 1990; 43:319.

24. Bach S, Noreng MF, Tjelden NU: Phantom limb pain in amputees during the first 12 months following limb amputation, after preoperative lumbar epidural blockade. Pain 1988; 33:297.

25. Fisher A, Meller Y: Continuous postoperative regional analgesia by nerve sheath block for amputation surgery: a pilot study. Anesth Analg 1991; 72:300.

26. Malawer MM, Buch R, Khurana JS, et al: Postoperative infusional continuous regional analgesia: a technique for relief of postoperative pain following major extremity surgery. Clin Orthop 1991; 266:227.

27. Goldberg ME, Gregg C, Larijan GE, et al: A comparison of three methods of axillary approach to brachial plexus blockade for upper extremity surgery. Anesthesiology 1987; 66:814.

28. Roch JJ, Sharrock NE, Neudachin L: Interscalene brachial plexus block for shoulder surgery: a proximal paresthesia is effective. Anesth Analg 1992; 75:386.

29. Hickey R, Garland TA, Ramamurthy S: Subclavian perivascular block: influence of locations of paresthesia. Anesth Analg 1989; 68:767.

30. McKenzie PJ, Wishart HY, Smith G: Long-term outcome after repair of fractured neck of femur: comparison of subarachnoid and general anesthesia. Br J Anaesth 1984; 56:581.

31. Sorenson RM, Pace NL: Anesthetic techniques during surgical repair of femoral neck fractures: a meta-analysis. Anesthesiology 1992; 77:1095.

32. Modig J: Regional anaesthesia and blood loss. Acta Anaesth Scand Suppl 1988; 89:44.

33. Modig J, Borg T, Karlstrom G, et al: Thromboembolism after total hip replacement: role of epidural and general anesthesia. Anesth Analg 1983; 62:174.

34. Thorburn J, Loudon JR, Vallance R: Spinal and general anesthesia in total hip replacement: frequency of deep vein thrombosis. Br J Anaesth 1980; 52:1117.

35. Francis CW, Pellegrini VD, Marder VJ, et al: Comparison of warfarin and external pneumatic compression in prevention of venous thrombosis after total hip replacement. JAMA 1992; 267:2911.

36. Vresilovic EJ, Hozack WJ, Booth RE, et al: Incidence of pulmonary embolism after total knee arthroplasty with low-dose coumadin prophylaxis. Clin Orthop 1993; 286:27.

37. Hodge WA: Prevention of deep vein thrombosis after total knee arthroplasty: coumadin versus pneumatic calf compression. Clin Orthop 1991; 271:101.

38. Hull RD, Raskob GE: Current concepts review: prophylaxis of venous thromboembolic disease following hip and knee surgery. J Bone Joint Surg [Am] 1986; 68A:146.

39. Lotke PA: Indications for the treatment of deep venous thrombosis following total knee replacement. J Bone Joint Surg [Am] 1984; 66A:202.

40. Patzakis MJ, Harvey JP, Ivler D: The role of antibiotics in the management of open fractures. J Bone Joint Surg [Am] 1974; 56A:432.

41. Goodnough LT, Rudnick S, Price TH, et al: Increased preoperative collection of autologous blood with recombinant human erythropoietin therapy. N Engl J Med 1989; 17:1163.

42. McNeil TW, DeWald RL, Kuo KN, et al: Controlled hypotensive anesthesia in scoliosis surgery. J Bone Joint Surg [Am] 1974; 56A:1167.

43. Barbier-Bohm G, Desmonts JM, Couderc E, et al: Comparative effects of induced hypotension and normovolaemic hemodilution on blood loss in total hip arthroplasty. Br J Anaesth 1980; 52:1039.

44. Lessard MR, Trepanier CA, Baribault JP, et al: Isoflurane-induced hypotension in orthognathic surgery. Anesth Analg 1989; 69:379.

45. Kobrinsky NL, Letts RM, Patel LR, et al: 1-Desamino-8-D-arginine (desmopressin) decreases operative blood loss in patients having Harrington rod spinal fusion surgery. Ann Intern Med 1987; 107:446.

46. Guay J, Reinberg C, Poitras B, et al: A trial of desmopressin to reduce blood loss in patients undergoing spinal fusion for idiopathic scoliosis. Anesth Analg 1992; 75:405.

47. Elliott BA: Positioning and monitoring. In Orthopedic Anesthesia. Wedel DJ (ed). New York, Churchill Livingstone, 1993, pp 101–102.

48. Lachiewicz PF, Latimer HA: Rhabdomyolysis following total hip arthroplasty. J Bone Joint Surg [Br] 1991; 73B:576.

49. Smith JW, Pellicci PM, Sharrock NE: Complications after total hip replacement. J Bone Joint Surg [Am] 1989; 71A:528.

50. Monroe MC: The arterial tourniquet. In Manual of Complications During Anesthesia. Gravenstein N (ed). Philadelphia, JB Lippincott, 1991, p 683.

51. Saunders KC, Louis DL, Weingarden SI, et al: Effect of tourniquet time on postoperative quadriceps function. Clin Orthop 1979; 143:194.

52. Sapega AA, Heppenstall RB, Chance B, et al: Optimizing tourniquet application and release times in extremity surgery: a biochemical and ultrastructural study. J Bone Joint Surg [Am] 1985; 67A:303.

53. Haljamae H, Enger E: Human skeletal muscle energy metabolism during and after complete tourniquet ischemia. Ann Surg 1975; 182:9.

54. Reid HS, Camp RA, Jacob WH: Tourniquet hemostasis: a clinical study. Clin Orthop 1983; 177:230.

55. Moore MR, Garfin SR, Hargens AR: Wide tourniquets eliminate blood flow at low inflation pressures. J Hand Surg 1987; 12A:1006.

56. Valli H, Rosenberg DH, Kytta J, et al: Arterial hypertension associated with the use of a tourniquet with either general or regional anesthesia. Acta Anaesth Scand 1987; 31:279.

57. Concepcion MA, Lambert DH, Welch KA, et al: Tourniquet pain during spinal anesthesia: a comparison of plain solutions of tetracaine and bupivacaine. Anesth Analg 1988; 67:828.

58. Gissen AJ, Covino BG, Gregus J: Differential sensitivities of mammalian nerve fibers to local anesthetic agents. Anesthesiology 1980; 53:467.

59. Stewart A, Lambert DH, Concepcion MA: Decreased incidence of tourniquet pain during spinal anesthesia with bupivacaine: a possible explanation. Anesth Analg 1988; 67:833.

60. Dickson M, White H, Kinney W, et al: Extremity tourniquet deflation increases end-tidal P_{CO_2}. Anesth Analg 1990; 70:457.

61. Collins R, Scrimgeour A, Yusef S, et al: Reduction in fatal pulmonary embolism and venous thrombosis by perioperative administration of subcutaneous heparin. N Engl J Med 1988; 318:1162.

62. Kaempffe FA, Lifeso RM, Meinking C: Intermittent pneumatic compression versus coumadin: prevention of deep venous thrombosis in lower extremity total joint arthroplasty. Clin Orthop 1991; 269:89.

63. Hull RD, Raskob GE, Gent M, et al: Effectiveness of intermittent pneumatic leg compression for preventing deep vein thrombosis after total hip replacement. JAMA 1990; 263:2313.

64. Preble L, Paige D, Sinatra R, et al: Varying narcotic requirements among orthopedic patients. Anesthesiology 1990; 73:A813.

65. Ejlersen E, Andersen HB, Eliasen K, et al: A comparison between preincisional and postincisional lidocaine infiltration and postoperative pain. Anesth Analg 1992; 74:495.

66. Tverskoy M, Cozacov C, Ayache M, et al: Postoperative pain after in-

guinal herniorrhaphy with different types of anesthesia. Anesth Analg 1990; 70:29.

67. Moss G, Regal ME, Lichtig L: Reducing postoperative pain, narcotics, and length of hospitalization. Surgery 1986; 99:206.

68. Joshi GP, McCarroll SM, O'Brien TM, et al: Intraarticular analgesia following knee arthroscopy. Anesth Analg 1993; 76:33.

69. Stein C: Peripheral mechanisms of opioid analgesia. Anesth Analg 1993; 76:182.

70. Brull SJ, Lieoponis JV, Murphy MJ, et al: Acute and long-term benefits of iliac crest donor site perfusion with local anesthetics. Anesth Analg 1992; 74:145.

CHAPTER 72

Otolaryngologic and Maxillofacial Surgery

ALEXANDER W. GOTTA, M.D.

MICHAEL J. FEFFER, M.D.

COLLEEN A. SULLIVAN, M.B., Ch.B.

The type and magnitude of surgery about the head and neck vary greatly and present a number of problems in terms of clinical anesthetic management. Despite the variety and complexity, a common theme is present almost without exception: how to secure and to maintain the airway (Fig. 72–1). In few areas of surgical and anesthetic care do the principals have to vie for this common ground to the same extent. Similarly, in almost no other area is securing the airway so difficult nor the margin for error so small. Specific considerations involving anesthesia for surgery of the face, head, and neck are dealt with here.

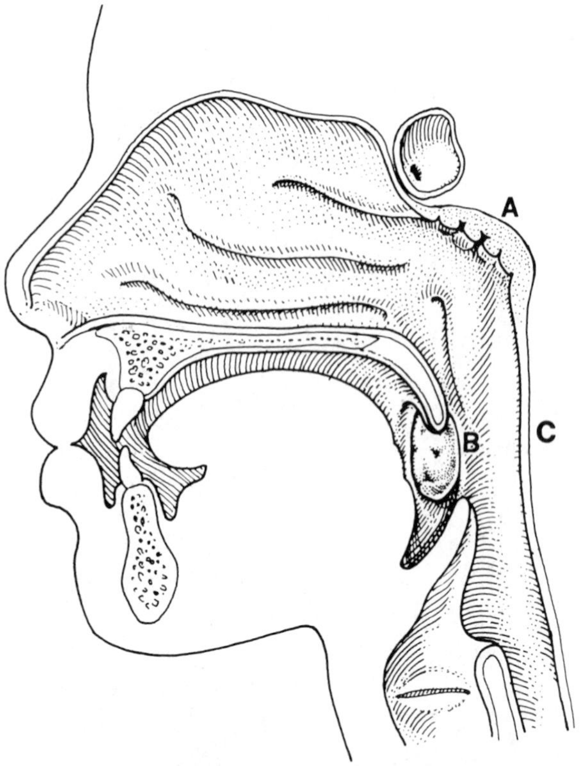

MYRINGOTOMY

What Are the Indications?

Chronic or recurrent otitis media is a highly prevalent pediatric disorder. Untreated, this condition may lead to middle ear damage and permanent hearing impairment. Consequently, elective myringotomy with insertion of tympanotomy tubes is currently among the most commonly performed pediatric surgical procedures.

Nonpurulent effusions appear to be related to abnormal eustachian tube function, which results in impaired venting of the middle ear. Bacterial infection is frequently superimposed and is treated with appropriate antibiotics before myringotomy.

Which Technique Is Preferred?

Bilateral myringotomies with tube insertions are typically very short operations. Sedative premedication may outlast the procedure and is usually not necessary. Mask induction and maintenance using oxygen, nitrous oxide (N_2O), and halothane is routine. Intubation is performed only if airway difficulties are anticipated, if halothane is contraindicated, or if the procedure is to be combined with adenotonsillectomy.

Is Intravenous Access Required?

Because the procedure is short, without risk of significant bleeding, fluid replacement is not required. Some clinicians argue that access should be obtained in case airway obstruction

FIGURE 72–1. Sagittal view of the relevant anatomic relationships of the upper airway. A = adenoids; B = palatine tonsil; C = posterior wall of pharynx.

(especially laryngospasm) occurs. In training programs, this approach may be justified. We believe, however, that skillful airway management and provision of an adequate depth of inhalation anesthesia effectively minimize this risk. Furthermore, intramuscular succinylcholine has been used effectively at a dose of 5 mg · kg⁻¹ in infants and 4 mg · kg⁻¹ in children and adults to treat laryngospasm.[1, 2] Intramuscular administration of succinylcholine results in a delayed onset and longer duration of action than seen with the intravenous route.

ADENOTONSILLECTOMY

What Are the Indications?

Indications for adenotonsillectomy as well as timing and risks versus benefits are topics of considerable debate among pediatricians and otolaryngologists.[3] Absolute indications include unilateral enlargement (suggesting neoplasm) and airway obstruction or sleep apnea (Table 72–1).

Obstructive sleep apnea occurs in children, either alone or in association with congenital neuromuscular or craniofacial anomalies. Some of these (e.g., Pierre Robin and Treacher Collins syndromes) may make airway management extremely difficult. Fortunately, mere tonsillar hypertrophy is seldom very problematic.

Adults with sleep apnea are typically obese and may present serious airway problems. Chronic hypoxemia may cause cor pulmonale; cardiac status must be expertly assessed and optimized preoperatively in these patients. In either age group, a history of snoring, somnolence, or recurrent respiratory infections suggests the diagnosis, which is confirmed by polysomnography. Sedative premedication is strictly avoided in patients with such a history.

How Are Patients Assessed?

Preoperative evaluation always begins with a carefully taken history. Airway obstruction and bleeding are the major perioperative risks, and emphasis is placed on these considerations.

Coagulation Profile

A history of liver disease in the patient or in his or her family or a bleeding tendency obviously indicates that a full coagulation profile be obtained. History of recent medications should be elicited; remember that aspirin is found in numerous nonprescription concoctions. Aspirin impedes platelet aggregation and should be discontinued at least 1 week before surgery. More recent ingestion indicates that surgery should be deferred. Without a specific indication, the value of routine

coagulation testing has been questioned.[4, 5] One study however, has described an association between prolonged clotting times and post-tonsillectomy bleeding in patients without a history of bleeding.[6] Because this issue remains unresolved, widespread routine use of these tests continues.

How Is Anesthesia Managed?

Induction

Pediatric patients without airway obstruction may be premedicated if necessary. After mask induction using oxygen, N₂O, and halothane, intravenous access is obtained. Intubation is then performed using a nondepolarizing muscle relaxant. An oral (RAE) tube commonly is chosen, although a conventional tube with a 60° or flexible connector is also convenient.[7]

Recall that a properly sized pediatric endotracheal tube should allow a leak at 20 cm H₂O airway pressure to reduce the likelihood of postoperative croup. The tube is taped to the midline of the lower lip, where it is grasped by the tongue blade of a Crowe-Davis gag (Fig. 72–2). Continuous capnography and auscultation of breath sounds are essential because kinking, extubation, or bronchial intubation may occur. In obese adults with sleep apnea, we routinely perform awake fiberoptic intubation.

Maintenance

Anesthesia is maintained by continuing inhalation agents. Because tonsillectomy is severely painful, a small dose of narcotic allows for a smoother emergence and recovery. Alternatively, local anesthetic (e.g., bupivacaine 0.25%) may be instilled into the tonsillar fossa. Topical anesthetics should be avoided because spread through the hypopharynx could impair

TABLE 72–1. Indications for Adenotonsillectomy

Recurrent tonsillitis
Recurrent otitis media
Peritonsillar abscess
Airway obstruction/sleep apnea*
Unilateral enlargement*

*Absolute indications.

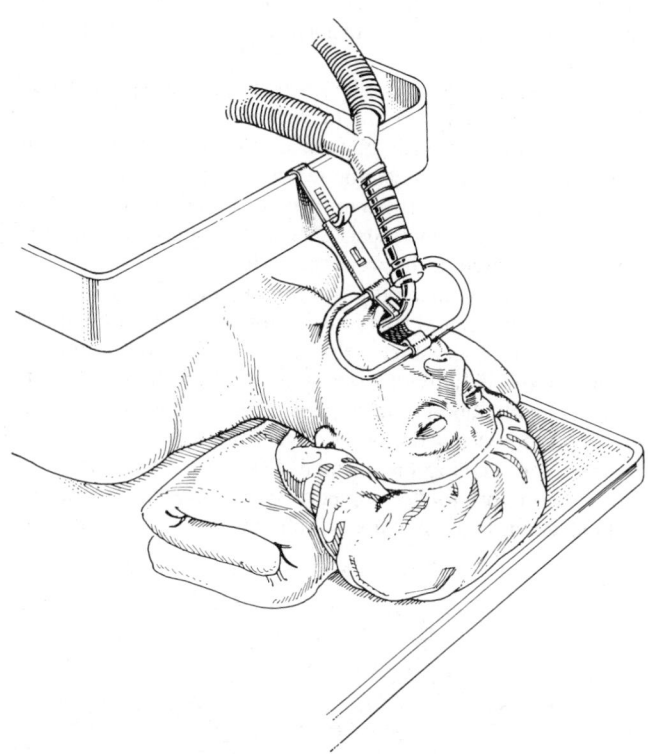

FIGURE 72–2. Crowe-Davis mouth gag.

essential postoperative airway reflexes. Although ketorolac has been used in ambulatory anesthesia, it theoretically may impair platelet function and increase the risk of post-tonsillectomy bleeding.

Blood Loss

Blood loss is difficult to measure owing to drainage into the stomach but probably averages 50 to 100 mL. Hence, a small child can easily lose 10% or more of his or her blood volume. Topical or infiltrated epinephrine reduces bleeding but may cause or aggravate dysrhythmias, particularly in the presence of halothane, hypercarbia, or hypoxia. Children are less sensitive to the dysrhythmogenic effects of epinephrine than adults and have been found to tolerate up to 10 $\mu g \cdot kg^{-1}$ without ectopy under halothane anesthesia.[8] Alternatively, phenylephrine (1:100,000) can be substituted and is not dysrhythmogenic.

Interestingly, saline injection also reduces bleeding, presumably by vascular compression. Local anesthetic injection has an additional benefit in that it provides effective postoperative analgesia. Topical anesthetics, as noted previously, should still be avoided because spread through the hypopharynx impairs essential postoperative airway reflexes.

Emergence and Extubation

After completion of surgery, the pharynx is gently cleared using a soft catheter. Suctioning the stomach is also attempted, although it is doubtful that it is ever completely emptied. Ideally, the surgeon suctions the stomach in an attempt to remove swallowed blood and to decrease subsequent nausea and vomiting. The surgeon can better direct the suction catheter to avoid stirring up bleeding from the operated site. On verification of hemostasis, anesthesia is discontinued and muscle relaxants are reversed. Lidocaine (1.5 mg $\cdot$ kg^{-1}) given intravenously reduces the incidence of postextubation laryngospasm.[9]

When the patient is awake, responsive, and spontaneously breathing 100% oxygen, the trachea is extubated. The "tonsil position" (Fig. 72–3) is maintained during recovery, so that blood and secretions cannot reach the glottis and provoke laryngospasm. Our tonsillectomy patients spend a minimum of 2 hours in the postanesthesia care unit. Continuous pulse oximetry is required in the recovery period.

Although adenoidectomy is routinely an ambulatory procedure, in many centers post-tonsillectomy patients are admitted for overnight observation. Selection of patients for ambulatory tonsillectomy is individualized and based on the needs of the patient, family, and referring physician.[10] Ambulatory patients are observed on a pediatric or otolaryngology ward for 6 to 8 hours before leaving the hospital. Discharged patients are instructed to return to the hospital in case of bleeding, vomiting, lightheadedness or dizziness, palpitations, or mental status changes. A history of coagulopathy or sleep apnea clearly contraindicates same-day discharge.

How Is Post-Tonsillectomy Bleeding Managed?

The reported incidence of post-tonsillectomy bleeding varies considerably (0.6–8.1%).[11–15] The vast majority of patients who bleed significantly do so within 4 to 8 hours after surgery. The reoperation rates are in the range of 0.3% to 0.6%. Criteria for having discharged patients return to the hospital for evaluation of post-tonsillectomy bleeding are listed in Table 72–2.

Presenting Signs

A slow, persistent "ooze" is far more common than profuse bleeding. If a patient is kept in the tonsil position during recovery, blood may be seen draining from the mouth. Pharyngeal blood is frequently swallowed, however; hematemesis and signs of hypovolemia are the presenting features. Airway obstruction or aspiration of clots may also occur; signs of hypoxia such as agitation or obtundation must be viewed with a high index of suspicion in these patients.

Treatment

In some instances, attempts can be made to achieve hemostasis using electrocautery, silver nitrate, packing, or topical vasoconstrictors. Note that mortality in these cases is often attributed to underestimating blood loss and delaying definitive treatment.[11]

A hurried approach to reoperation of a bleeding tonsil can lead to disaster. Volume replacement must be completed, as judged by improvement in vital signs, including correction of orthostatic hypotension. Two units of crossmatched packed red blood cells, the hematocrit, and a coagulation profile should be obtained. The short time required to accomplish these steps is justified, except in the most unusual case of impending exsanguination.

Anesthesia Induction

The precarious nature of this situation has yielded controversy about anesthetic induction. The various recommendations include (1) awake intubation, (2) rapid-sequence induction, and (3) mask induction in the tonsil position and intubation using succinylcholine after visualization of the cords.

We believe that a rapid-sequence induction with cricoid pressure is acceptable in the vast majority of cases. The mouth and nasopharynx are cleared of clots before induction. Ideally,

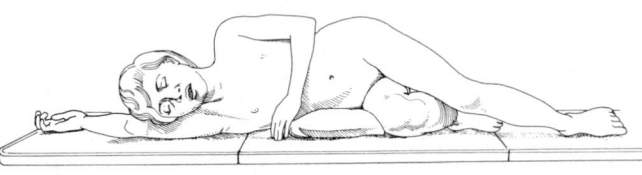

FIGURE 72–3. Tonsil position.

TABLE 72–2. Condition of Patients Who Should Remain in or Return to the Hospital After Tonsillectomy

Persistent hematemesis
Tachycardia
Obtundation
Agitation
Orthostatic hypotension

two large-bore suckers are prepared, as are duplicate laryngoscopes and endotracheal tubes. After thorough denitrogenation, thiopental (in modest doses), ketamine, or etomidate is an appropriate agent.

Whatever technique is chosen, an experienced surgeon must be prepared to perform immediate cricothyrotomy should intubation fail. Maintenance and emergence are conducted as described previously, with patients fully awake and protective airway reflexes intact before extubation.

MIDDLE EAR SURGERY

What Are the Implications of Patient Positioning?

Typically, the table is turned 90° from the induction position, with the patient's head turned toward the anesthetic machine. Three likely problems can occur: (1) circuit disconnection under the drapes, (2) mainstem intubation resulting from caudal movement of the tube when the head is turned or if the neck is flexed, and (3) extubation due to either traction on the endotracheal tube or extension of the neck with rostral movement of the endotracheal tube.

The risk of disconnection is minimized by removing strain from all of the slip-fit connections, by the use of a long breathing circuit, and by the use of a tube holder. Mainstem intubation is not so much avoided as it is identified by auscultation of both hemithoraces after the bed and patient are in their final position. Accidental extubation is guarded against in similar fashion to disconnection. Ventilation must be continuously monitored during surgery using a stethoscope and capnometry so that any problems can be immediately identified and corrected.

Is Nitrous Oxide Contraindicated?

N_2O diffuses into air-filled spaces much faster than nitrogen diffuses out. An increased gaseous pressure or volume (or both) occurs within the space, depending on its compliance. The intact middle ear is a noncompliant air-filled space that is intermittently vented to the oropharynx via the eustachian tube. This venting occurs both actively (as during swallowing) and passively (when middle ear pressure exceeds 20–40 cm H_2O in normal individuals).[16]

Middle ear pressure (MEP) rises at a rate of approximately 1 cm H_2O per minute under 67% N_2O anesthesia (Fig. 72–4). Hence, MEP peaks and is passively vented after 30 to 40 minutes in normal patients. However, passive or even active venting may be impaired in the presence of sinusitis, pharyngitis, or otitis or after adenoidectomy.[17] Tympanic membrane rupture has occurred under such conditions and is generally a risk when MEP exceeds 100 cm H_2O.[18]

Discontinuation

Tympanic membrane perforation or mastoidectomy opens the middle ear cavity; hence, MEP equilibrates with atmospheric pressure. When the cavity is then closed, as in placement of a tympanic membrane graft, blood-borne N_2O diffuses into the space and increases MEP. If it cannot be vented via the eustachian tube, the graft is often dislodged.

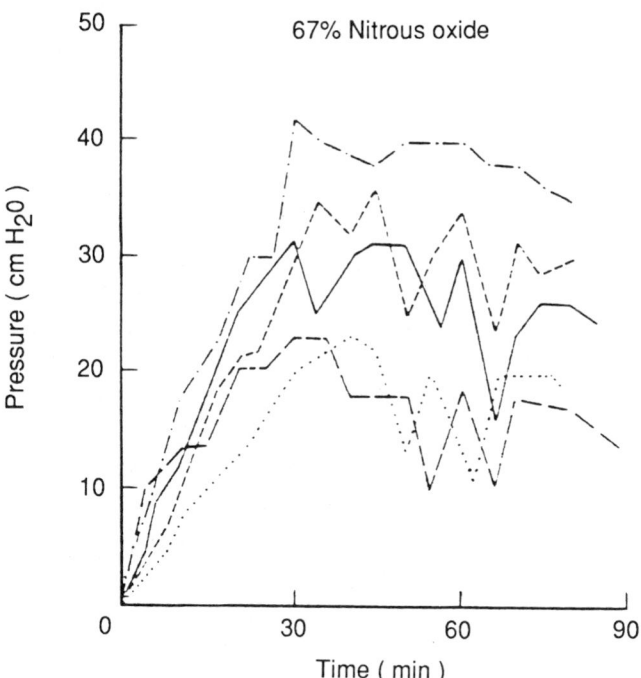

FIGURE 72–4. Middle ear pressure over time during inhalation of 67% nitrous oxide.

Discontinuation of N_2O has the opposite effect: Diffusion out of the space causes reductions in pressure. Preanesthetic levels of MEP are usually reached within an hour after discontinuation, and in some cases, considerable subatmospheric pressure may result. Because the eustachian tube functions as a one-way valve, passive venting of negative MEP does not normally occur. When equilibration is not achieved by active measures such as yawning or swallowing, negative MEPs may result in nausea, vomiting, serous otitis media, hemotympanum, and stapes disarticulation with resultant hearing loss.[19, 20]

Obviously, the use of N_2O should be restricted not only in middle ear surgery but in all patients with a history of otolaryngologic disease. Recommendations include limiting concentrations and discontinuing the agent before middle ear closure. However, increasing MEPs have been observed even 10 to 20 minutes after discontinuation.[19, 20] Based on the foregoing considerations, we prefer to avoid N_2O, particularly because anesthesia can easily be maintained with other agents.

OTOLOGIC AND PAROTID SURGERY

Should Muscle Relaxants Be Used?

The facial nerve courses through a periosteal sheath within the medial wall of the tympanic cavity. After it emerges from the stylohyoid foramen, ramifications of the nerve traverse and envelop the substance of the parotid gland (Fig. 72–5). Thus, it is susceptible to injury during otologic and parotid surgery. Direct electrical stimulation is used to facilitate nerve identification and thereby prevent facial nerve palsy. Although considerable degrees of neuromuscular blockage allow response to direct stimulation, many surgeons prefer that nondepolarizing muscle relaxants be completely avoided.

Intermediate-acting drugs are acceptable in judicious doses, provided that careful monitoring of the neuromuscular junction

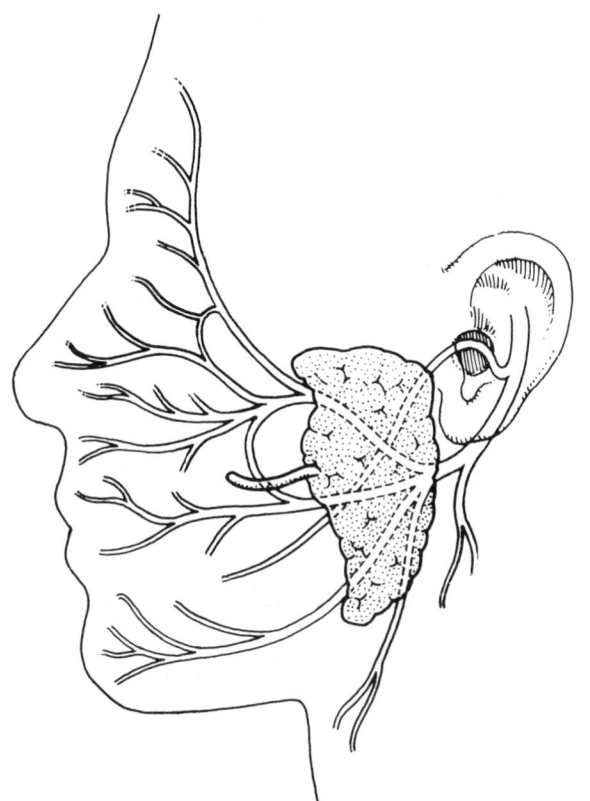

FIGURE 72–5. Facial nerve distribution.

is maintained and precisely documented. Communication with the surgeon allows spontaneous recovery of neuromuscular transmission when use of the nerve stimulator is anticipated. A long-acting relaxant should not be used for intubation or anesthetic management. Surgeons who disclaim the need for a nerve stimulator often change their minds during surgery, thus necessitating a change in the anesthetic plan, which may be difficult to carry out. Because neuromuscular blockade is not otherwise necessary for this surgery, we believe that these drugs are best avoided whenever possible, if only for medicolegal reasons. If they have been used, documentation of recovery of neuromuscular function in the record before the at-risk portion of the operation is wise.

Is Induced Hypotension Useful?

Successful use of an operating microscope requires a virtually bloodless surgical field. In the past, some have advocated profound degrees of deliberate hypotension to achieve this results.[21] In fact, one blinded study found no correlation between blood pressure and the surgeon's assessment of operative conditions.[22] Although most patients tolerate modest reductions in blood pressure, the safety and benefit of extreme levels of hypotension are not documented. In most instances, a modest (10–15°) head-up position, topical and injected vasoconstrictors, and systolic blood pressure reduction to 75% of awake level are satisfactory.

In summary, during otologic surgery, general anesthesia using a potent volatile agent allows avoidance of N_2O, avoidance of longer-acting muscle relaxants, and easy titration to the desired blood pressure.

CLEFT LIP AND PALATE

How Is the Airway Secured?

Cleft Lip

Management of unilateral cleft lip repair consists of routine induction, followed by oral intubation using an oral RAE tube.[14] Tincture of benzoin and tape are used to secure the tube to the lower lip in the midline. After the surgery, a Logan bow (Fig. 72–6) may be placed across the lip to decrease tension on the sutures. This approach impairs mask ventilation; extubation is performed when patients are awake.

Cleft Palate

Cleft palate repair may be performed in stages, depending on the extent of the defect. Initial surgery is indicated when a child is 10 weeks old, weighs 10 pounds, and has a hemoglobin of 10 g · dL^{-1} and a white blood cell count <10,000 · mm$^{3-1}$.[23] The first operation repairs the lip and anterior portion of the hard palate. The soft palate and any other deformities are corrected later, usually after 6 months of age.

During cleft palate surgery, a specialized mouth gag (Millard-Dingman retractor) is used to hold the mouth open and an endotracheal tube in place (Fig. 72–7). An oral RAE tube is secured at the lower lip in the midline. Before emergence, a suture is placed through the tongue to eliminate the need for an oral airway, because the latter would risk damaging the palatal repair. If soft tissue–related obstruction occurs during emergence or recovery, traction on the suture usually alleviates the problem.

CALDWELL-LUC PROCEDURE

What Are the Indications?

The Caldwell-Luc procedure is performed to gain access to the maxillary sinus. The operation consists of an incision and osteotomy above the ipsilateral premolars. Usually indicated

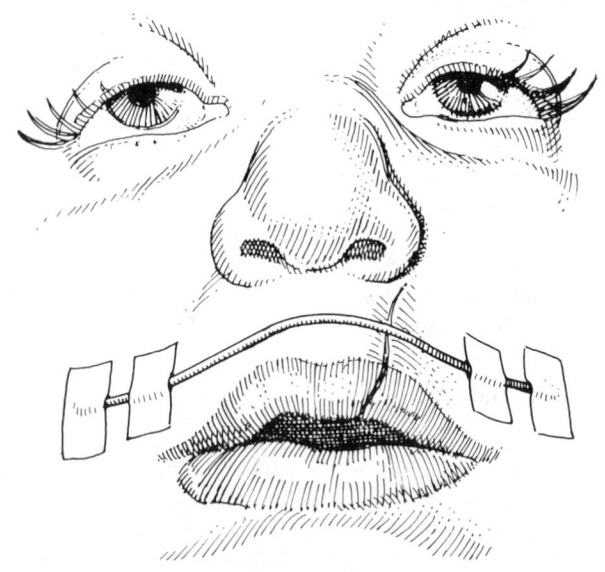

FIGURE 72–6. Logan bow.

for the drainage of chronic infection, the approach is also used for biopsies and for reduction and fixation of inferior orbital fractures.

What Are the Anesthetic Concerns?

Although an antrostomy can be performed using local anesthesia, general anesthesia is usually chosen and is often necessary for additional work within the antrum. Orotracheal intubation and fixation of the tube in the contralateral corner of the mouth are routine.

Injection of epinephrine-containing solutions is common, and concomitant use of halogenated anesthetics increases the risk of ventricular dysrhythmias. The anesthesiologist is obliged to monitor the dose of epinephrine injected and to observe for any systemic signs of absorption. Note that dysrhythmias may occur in the absence of hypertension. Limitation of epinephrine dose, provision of adequate anesthetic depth, and avoidance of hypoxia, hypercarbia, and halothane minimize the risk of ventricular ectopy (Table 72–3).[24–27]

PHARYNGEAL ABSCESS

What Is It?

The site and size of the collection affect the decision about how to secure the airway. Abscess formation tends to occur either adjacent to an infected tonsil, where it is called *quinsy,* or within the posterior pharyngeal wall. Quinsy causes severe pain and trismus, and it occasionally may obstruct the airway. Risks of general anesthesia include difficult intubation and aspiration. In particular, right-sided quinsy may interfere with glottic visualization; therefore, drainage under local anesthesia is preferred when possible. In most cases, however, the high and lateral location does not impair glottic visualization. Nevertheless, retropharyngeal collections may obliterate the hypopharynx and must be managed with extreme caution. Preoperative discussion with the surgeon is thus important to identify the abscess site because of the obvious implications for airway management.

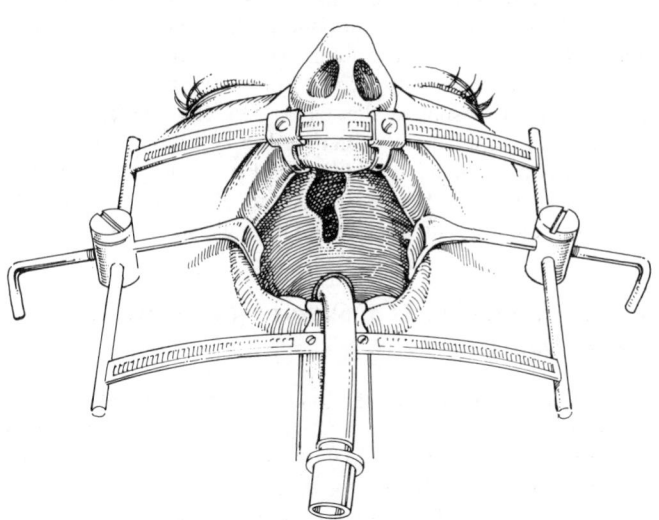

FIGURE 72–7. Millard-Dingman retractor.

TABLE 72–3. Minimizing Epineprhine-Induced Ventricular Irritability Under General Anesthesia

Isoflurane is the potent volatile agent of choice when epinephrine injection is anticipated.

Agent (1.25 MAC)	Maximum recommended dose (in 0.5% lidocaine)
Halothane	$2.1\ \mu \cdot kg^{-1}$
Enflurane	$3.4\ \mu \cdot kg^{-1}$
Isoflurane	$6.7\ \mu \cdot kg^{-1}$

Incidence of arrhythmias is not related to dose of inhaled agent.
Nitrous oxide does not enhance epinephrine-induced irritability.
Use of lidocaine as a vehicle increases the arrhythmogenic dose of epinephrine.
Epinephrine concentrations stronger than 1:100,000 increase risk of ectopy without increasing hemostasis.
In adults, do not exceed 10 mL in 10 minutes or 30 mL in 1 hour using epinephrine 1:100,000.
Avoid hypoxia, hypercarbia, and light anesthesia.
Presence of sympathetic-modifying drugs increases the risk of arrhythmias (e.g., β-agonists, tricyclic antidepressants, monoamine oxidase inhibitors, methyldopa, cocaine, aminophylline, reserpine, guanethidine).
Ephedrine (1:1000) or phenylephrine (1:10,000) may be substituted for infiltration and is far less arrhythmogenic.
Intravenous lidocaine or β-blockers or both are effective therapies when treatment is necessary.

Abbreviations: MAC = minimum alveolar concentration.

How Is the Airway Secured?

Awake Intubation

A large or tense and fluctuant abscess presents a formidable dilemma. Rupture after induction can result in disastrous aspiration of purulent material. Severe infections are accompanied by generalized edema and hyperemia of all pharyngeal mucosa that may further complicate both ventilation and laryngoscopy. Hence, drainage under local anesthesia or awake intubation may be attempted.

Tracheotomy

These approaches usually require sedation, which, when combined with topical and local anesthesia, impairs protective reflexes. In some cases, tracheotomy may be necessary either to relieve airway obstruction or to protect the trachea from purulent drainage, because the infection is surgically drained into the pharynx. A plan for airway management must be discussed and agreed on with the surgeon before the operation.

LUDWIG'S ANGINA

What Is It?

Ludwig's angina is cellulitis of the floor of the mouth caused by bacterial infection of the sublingual and submandibular spaces (Table 72–4). If untreated, it progresses to stridor, asphyxia, and death. Antibiotic therapy may be unsuccessful because of a mixed bacterial flora and poor penetration into

TABLE 72–4. Characteristics of Ludwig's Angina

Induration of the neck
Trismus
Dysphonia
Drooling
Edema and elevation of the tongue
Dyspnea
Stridor

the abscess. Ludwig's angina usually follows dental therapy but is not necessarily associated with tooth extraction.

How Is the Airway Secured?

A patient with Ludwig's angina should not be anesthetized before the airway is secured. Increasing dyspnea, arterial oxyhemoglobin desaturation, and hypercarbia are indications for surgical drainage. The airway must be secured by awake tracheal intubation or tracheotomy. Attempted fiberoptic intubation is often fruitless because of anatomic distortion, edema, and erythema.

If the airway cannot be obtained via awake intubation and symptoms progress, tracheotomy is mandated. This surgical maneuver may also be difficult to perform in this setting because of the dense edema and cellulitis of the neck. Planning for possible emergency cricothyroid puncture and catheter placement is part of the preparation before attempting to secure the airway, regardless of the route.

AIRWAY NEOPLASIA

How Is the Airway Evaluated?

Neoplasia can so distort the anatomy of the airway that tracheal intubation is difficult, if not impossible.

Historical Facts

Any intraoral mass can become so large that it makes direct visualization of the larynx impossible. Lesions within the airway may lead to hypoventilation and even asphyxiation if neglected. Prior treatment of an airway lesion often causes significant problems. Radiation therapy can stiffen normally pliable tissues and make laryngoscopy difficult. If one or both temporomandibular joints (TMJs) have been included in the radiation field, the mouth may be impossible to open. Friable or vascular lesions may bleed quite severely if manipulated during intubation. Prior surgery, especially mandibulectomy (partial or complete), may also distort the anatomy and make intubation impossible. Specifically seek a history of respiratory distress. Dysphagia indicates an expanding mass growing out of the airway and impinging on the esophagus.

Physical Findings

Patients' ability to open their mouth must be evaluated. If the intraoral lesion is readily apparent, it must be evaluated for size and texture (using a gloved finger). Is the tongue mobile? Is the lesion friable? Does it bleed on gentle manipulation? Direct or mirror laryngoscopy may also aid in evaluating the tumor and will have been performed by the surgeon preoperatively. The surgeon's findings should be reviewed or discussed before anesthetizing a patient.

Radiographic and Laboratory Studies

Advanced radiographic techniques such as computed tomography (CT) scanning or magnetic resonance imaging can give a very clear assessment of tumor location, size, invasion of adjacent tissue, degree of encroachment, and airway compromise. Measurements made during review of these studies can also identify if a smaller endotracheal tube than usual is needed. Pulmonary function tests may help to determine the extent of airway obstruction. Arterial blood gas values may assist in assessing total ventilatory adequacy.

How Is Intubation Performed?

If there is any doubt about the ability to intubate an anesthetized patient, awake intubation is mandated. Fiberoptic intubation may be unsuccessful in the presence of a severely altered airway and risks serious hemorrhage if a friable tumor is traumatized by the bronchoscope. Above all, do not put a compromised airway at greater risk by attempting to intubate a paralyzed patient because a surgeon gives assurance that he or she can rapidly perform a tracheotomy. Even in the best circumstances, a tracheotomy requires more than 5 minutes to complete.

RADICAL HEAD AND NECK SURGERY

The most important and vulnerable nerves during radical head and neck surgery are the recurrent laryngeal, superior laryngeal, and phrenic. Damage may occur to any or all of these structures. The resultant functional loss may be complete or incomplete and permanent or temporary, depending on whether the nerve is completely or partially severed or is trapped by surrounding edematous tissue in a closed fascial plane.

What Are the Effects of Recurrent Laryngeal Nerve Damage?

If both recurrent laryngeal nerves are partially damaged, the glottis closes when the endotracheal tube is removed (Fig. 72–8, Part III [a]). This situation is an obviously acute emergency and demands immediate recognition and reintubation. Following total section of both nerves, the vocal cords are fixed in midposition (see Fig. 72–8, Part III [b]).

The problem is much more difficult to recognize if only one recurrent laryngeal nerve has been sectioned, because the glottis does not close completely and the vocal cord on the injured side is drawn (adducted) immobile to the center of the glottic chink (see Fig. 72–8). The diagnosis is suggested by postoperative hoarseness and confirmed by laryngoscopy.

Attempts to visualize the larynx directly at the time of extubation or immediately afterward to determine mobility of both cords are usually unavailing and prone to giving a false sense of security. The denervated cord often moves passively in the turbulent air stream passing through the larynx.

What Are the Effects of Superior Laryngeal Nerve Damage?

Section of the superior laryngeal nerve denervates the cricothyroid muscle, a tensor of the vocal cords. Permanent loss of function of this nerve does not close the larynx, but the patient may not be able to vocalize high-pitched tones. More importantly, loss of function of the internal branch of the superior laryngeal nerve causes loss of sensation within the

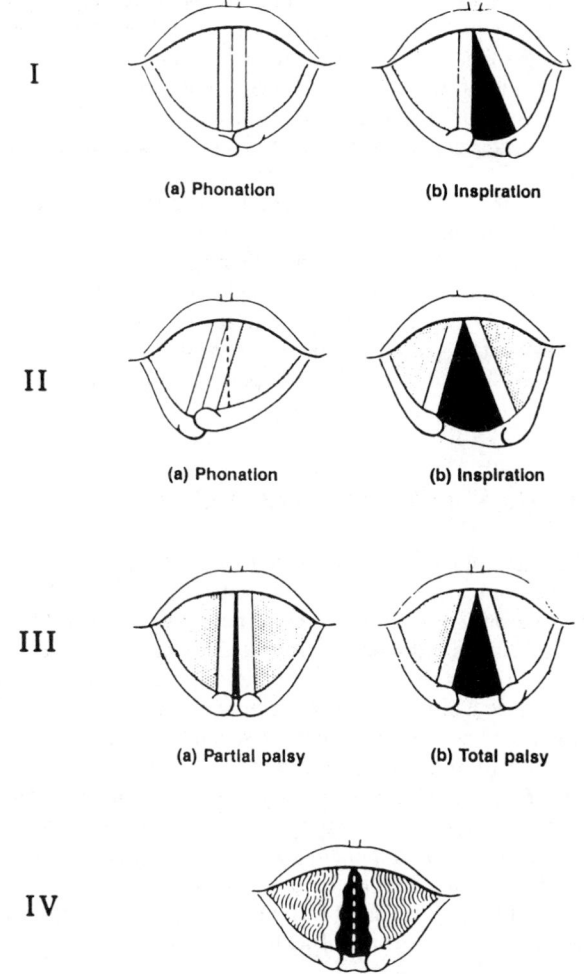

I
(a) Phonation   (b) Inspiration

II
(a) Phonation   (b) Inspiration

III
(a) Partial palsy   (b) Total palsy

IV

FIGURE 72–8. (I) Pure abductor palsy. (II) Abductor and adductor palsy. (III) Bilateral damage to the recurrent laryngeal nerves. (IV) Bilateral palsy of the recurrent laryngeal nerves with palsy of the external branch of the superior laryngeal nerve. (From Churchill-Davidson HC: A Practice of Anesthesia. 4th ed. Chicago, Year Book Medical Publishers, 1978, p 18. Reproduced by permission of Edward Arnold (Publishers) Limited.)

larynx. The laryngeal protective reflexes are thus ablated, making the patient vulnerable to aspiration of oral secretions and food.

What Are the Effects of Phrenic Nerve Damage?

The phrenic nerve lies deep within the neck and is well protected. Section of this nerve leads to loss of motor activity in the ipsilateral diaphragmatic leaf. This loss of function is usually of little consequence in a patient without significant respiratory disease and often remains unrecognized—witness interscalene block after which the ipsilateral phrenic nerve is temporarily paralyzed more than 80% of the time.

Bilateral loss of phrenic nerve function, however, denervates the diaphragm, making it useless as a muscle of respiration and imposing an increased burden on the intercostal muscles. Furthermore, the flaccid diaphragm tends to rise into the thoracic cavity, decreasing the functional residual capacity and dramatically altering ventilation/perfusion relationships.

AIRWAY EDEMA

How Does It Present?

Airway edema may occur as a result of trauma or traumatic intubation, venous stasis, or fluid resuscitation. As a patient struggles to breathe, the alae nasi flare and the accessory muscles of respiration are called into use. A paradoxical "rocking boat" type of respiration frequently is present as the powerful diaphragm sucks the thoracic cage inward in the struggle to pull air through the narrowed airway. Patients often are diaphoretic, cyanotic, and anxious.

Normal conversation is impossible because of the resulting dyspnea. If the process develops more insidiously, the work of breathing progressively increases and is associated with inspiratory stridor. Auscultation of the larynx with a stethoscope helps to detect the sounds of turbulent airflow. Subglottic airway edema related to tracheal intubation typically manifests within the first 4 hours after extubation.

How Is It Treated?

With severe airway edema, restoration of the airway via tracheal intubation, translaryngeal ventilation, or tracheotomy is indicated, the route determined by clinical assessment and relative immediacy of the problem. Steroid administration (e.g., dexamethasone, 4–12 mg intravenously) either as prophylaxis or treatment is common, but with little scientific evidence of efficacy. Humidified air/oxygen while the patient is kept in a head-elevated position is adequate therapy in mild cases. Racemic epinephrine (0.5–1 mL of a 2% solution diluted to a volume of 3–5 mL) nebulized through a facemask or mouthpiece, acting as a topical vasoconstrictor, has been efficacious in treating upper airway edema.[28]

DENTAL REPAIRS IN RETARDED AND UNCOOPERATIVE PATIENTS

What Problems Should Be Anticipated?

Because of the care and attention needed to maintain good dental hygiene, retarded patients, both children and adults, often suffer marked deterioration in tooth and gum health and require operative dental repair. Patients may have significant congenital malformations not as readily apparent as the retardation and, of course, may have acquired any disease common to their more fortunate peers. Because retarded patients usually cannot give a satisfactory history, discovery and evaluation of significant alterations in cardiac or pulmonary function that may affect anesthetic management can be difficult and challenging.

How Is Anesthesia Managed?

If a patient is placid, anesthetic management does not differ markedly from that of a normal child or adult. Unfortunately, retarded patients may be disruptive and even violent and represent a danger to themselves and to those who care for them. The sedative medication that a patient takes regularly must be continued into the perioperative period and started again as soon as possible after anesthesia and surgery are completed.

Retarded patients frequently develop a close personal relationship with a parent, friend, or health care worker. This personal associate should be allowed to accompany the patient to the operating room, where his or her presence may have a calming effect that transforms a potentially stormy induction into a more pleasant entry to the anesthetized state.

Induction Technique

Whenever possible, an intravenous infusion should be initiated before any attempts at anesthetic induction, because intravenous agents are usually much better tolerated than attempts at mask induction. Do not adhere rigidly to definite drugs and dosages for premedication, because patients vary considerably in their states of agitation, maintenance medication, and increased metabolic activity secondary to enzyme induction.

Rectal instillation of a barbiturate (e.g., thiopental) or short-acting benzodiazepine (e.g., midazolam) may have superficial appeal. However, inserting a tube in the rectum is often more difficult and presents greater hazards to the physician or nurse than starting an intravenous infusion.

Oral midazolam is very effective to sedate retarded children. We use 0.5 mg · kg^{-1} orally in apple juice in the preoperative holding area. Patients are continuously observed and monitored with a pulse oximeter after this premedication.

A further cautionary note is to be aware of gingival hyperplasia. Many of these patients receive phenytoin (Dilantin) to control seizures. Because the gingiva is highly vascular, surgical manipulation may lead to greater than anticipated blood loss.

CRANIOFACIAL TRAUMA

The facial skeleton is in contact with the cranial skeleton. Because great forces are generated in the mouth during the normal process of mastication, bony buttresses and arches prevent displacement of one skeleton against the other.

Horizontal posterior displacement is limited by the zygomatic process of the temporal bone; oblique posterior displacement, by the pterygoid process of the sphenoid bone; and vertical posterior displacement, by the greater wing of the sphenoid bone. Upward displacement is checked by the zygomatic process of the frontal bone, the nasal part of the frontal bone, and the roof of the mandibular fossa.

In addition to the bony buttresses, a series of arches is present in the craniofacial skeleton. The arch created by the zygomatic process of the temporal bone extends via the zygoma to the zygomaticomaxillary suture. Another extends between the head and neck of the mandibular condyle, to the coronoid process.

What Anatomic Structures Determine the Sites of Fracture?

Dispersal of Forces

The buttresses and arches of the craniofacial skeleton redistribute and disperse the forces generated within the oral cavity during chewing and protect the skeleton from displacement or fracture by these forces. A normal vector of force dispersion redistributes physiologic forces and forces resulting from a blow to the face. A blow to the mandible may fracture the jaw at the point of impact or at other points in the bone. The fracture very rarely extends into the cranium because the force follows a normal dispersion vector and is redistributed (Fig. 72–9).

A blow to the face from the front, however, and especially from the front and above, does not follow a normal vector of force dispersion. An abnormal shearing force that may be generated tends to tear the facial skeleton away from the cranium and may extend a fracture into the base of the skull (see Fig. 72–9). The possibility of basal skull fracture, therefore, must always be considered in the patient with severe midface trauma.

When Do Mandibular Fractures Occur?

The mandible is a tubular bone and derives its strength from the bony cortex. It is strongest and least vulnerable to fracture at its anteroinferior border, where the cortex is thickest. The cortex thins, and vulnerability to fracture increases posteriorly. Thus, most fractures of the mandible occur in the ramus. The second most common site of fracture is in the body of the mandible at the level of the first or second molar.

The site of fracture is determined to some extent by the nature of the traumatic blow. High-velocity and high-impact types of injuries, such as those produced in an automobile accident, create a high incidence of condylar, subcondylar, and angle of the ramus fractures. Low-velocity, low-impact forces, such as a blow by a fist or fall, tend to produce symphyseal, parasymphyseal, and body fractures. Because of the mandi-

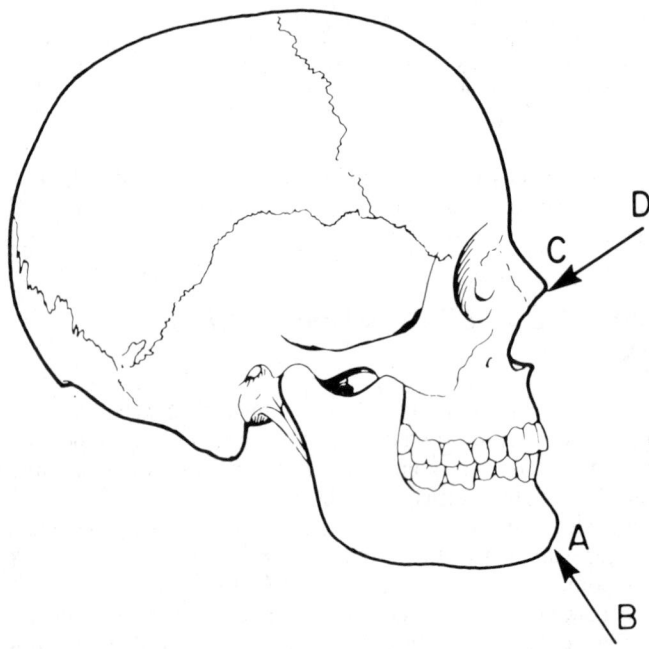

FIGURE 72–9. Dispersion of forces in craniofacial trauma. A blow along the line *AB* follows a normal vector of force dispersion and distribution. The mandible may be fractured, but the fracture line will not extend into the skull. A blow along the line *CD* does not follow a normal vector of force dispersion and distribution and will generate an abnormal shearing force that may tear the facial skeleton and cranial skeleton.

ble's unique horseshoe shape, any blow creates shearing forces that tend to fracture it at its weakest points, no matter where the point of impact may be.

How Are Facial Fractures Classified?

Early in this century, Rene Le Fort of Lille, France, published the results of a series of interesting and even bizarre experiments on cadavers and cadaver skulls.[29] Intact cadavers were dropped from a height onto a stone floor, or severed heads were ground in a vise. The soft tissue was then carefully dissected away to reveal underlying structural damage. Le Fort had two goals: (1) to determine the relationship between soft tissue trauma and fractures of the facial bones and (2) to ascertain the common lines of fracture of the midface. He noted no pathognomonic soft tissue representation of facial features and delineated the midfacial fractures that bear his name—Le Fort I, Le Fort II, and Le Fort III.

Le Fort I Fracture

The Le Fort I fracture (also known as Guerin's fracture) is a horizontal fracture of the maxilla, passing above the floor of the nose, involving the lower third of the septum, and mobilizing the palate, maxillary alveolar process, the lower third of the pterygoid plates, and parts of the palatine bones (Fig. 72–10A). The fracture segment may be displaced posteriorly or laterally or rotated about a vertical axis, or it may involve a combination of any of these variations.

Le Fort II Fracture

The Le Fort II fracture is pyramidal, beginning at the junction of the thick upper part of the nasal bone and the thinner portion forming the upper margin of the anterior nasal aperture (see Fig. 72–10B). The fracture crosses the medial wall of the orbit, including the lacrimal bone, then passes beneath the zygomaticomaxillary suture, crosses the lateral wall of the antrum, and traverses posteriorly through the pterygoid plates.

Le Fort III Fracture

In a Le Fort III fracture, the midface is separated from the cranium (see Fig. 72–10C). The fracture line extends through the base of the nose and the ethmoid in its depth and through the orbital plates in proximity to the cribriform plate, which may also be fractured. It crosses the lesser wing of the sphenoid, then passes downward to the pterygomaxillary fissure and sphenopalatine fossa. From the base of the inferior orbital fissure, it extends laterally and upward to the frontozygomatic suture and downward and backward to the root of the pterygoid plates. The zygomatic arch of the temporal bone also is fractured bilaterally.

How Do Le Fort Fractures Influence Anesthetic Management?

Le Fort I

A Le Fort I fracture generally affords little difficulty for an anesthesiologist. Patients may be intubated orally or nasally, and the airway usually is secured without problem.

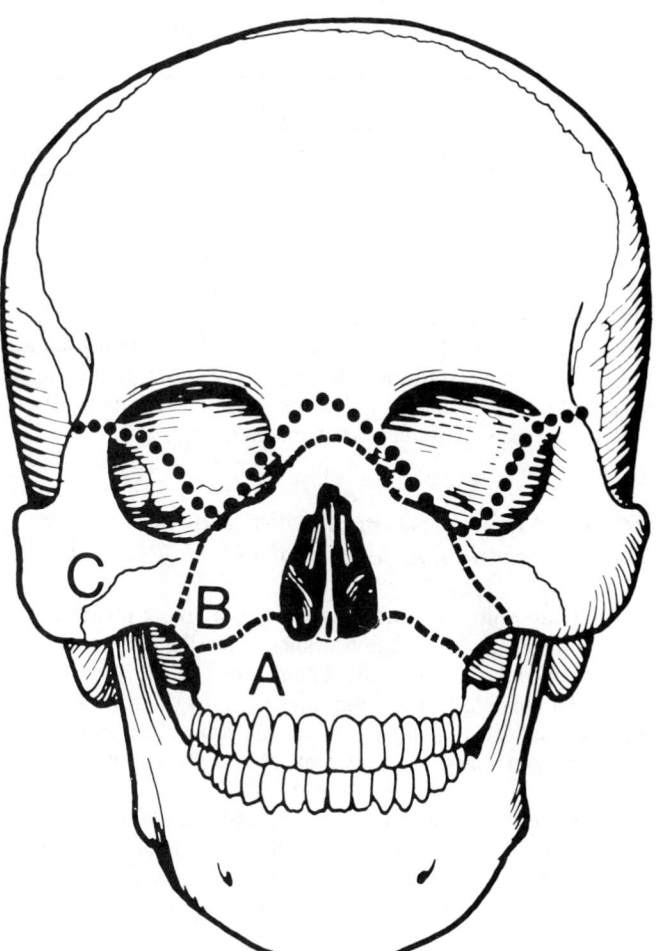

FIGURE 72–10. A Le Fort I fracture (A) is a horizontal fracture of the maxilla. A Le Fort II fracture (B) is a pyramidal fracture of the midface, whereas a Le Fort III fracture (C) separates the facial and cranial skeletons.

Le Fort II

A Le Fort II fracture involves fracture of the nose and is thus a relative but not absolute contraindication to nasal intubation. Because the force of the blow to the midface necessary to create this type of fracture is substantial, one must always consider the possibility of a concomitant fracture of the base of the skull. Unless this is definitively ruled out by a radiograph or CT scan, nasal intubation of any type should be avoided.

Le Fort III

Basal skull fracture is much more likely with a Le Fort III fracture, because the ethmoid bone is involved in the fracture line. Although fracture of the cribriform plate of the ethmoid is not per se part of the definition of a Le Fort III fracture, it *may* be involved. In such cases, the intracranial subarachnoid space may be open and communicating with a nasal cavity, rendering it vulnerable to false passage of a nasally placed tube (endotracheal or gastric) and infection.

Attempted nasotracheal intubation of a patient with a basal skull fracture involves the very serious risks of introducing the tube into the skull, dragging contaminated foreign material into the subarachnoid space and causing meningitis. The tube may also inflict severe damage on the brain itself. Even posi-

TABLE 72–5. Clinical Signs/Findings Suggestive of Basilar Skull Fracture

Blood behind a tympanic membrane
Periocular ecchymosis (raccoon eyes)
Predisposing facial fracture (Le Fort II or III)

TABLE 72–6. Incidence of Other Injuries Associated with Maxillofacial Trauma

Injury	High Velocity (Vehicular)	Low Velocity (Personal)
Major (life threatening)	32%	4%
Minor	31%	10.5%

(From Luce EA: Review of 1,000 major facial fractures and associated injuries. Plast Reconstruct Surg 1979; 63:26.)

tive-pressure ventilation with bag and mask predisposes to introduction of foreign material into the subarachnoid space.[30]

Clinical signs and findings suggestive of basilar skull fracture are listed in Table 72–5. Whenever a basal skull fracture is suspected or is confirmed radiologically, nasal intubation is absolutely contraindicated unless radiographic evidence establishes that basal skull integrity is maintained.

What Are the Effects and Implications of Temporomandibular Joint Injuries?

The temporomandibular articulation is a ginglymoarthrodial joint, with a hingelike action allowing flexion and extension in only one plane. Two articulations are present: One is between the condyle and articular disk, and the other is between the disk and the mandibular fossa. Motion of the joint takes place in both parts. As the joint opens, the condyle glides forward.

Function of the joint may be limited by fracture segments interposed directly into the articulation. A fracture of the zygoma with posteroinferior depression impinges on the coronoid process, thus limiting the forward gliding action of the mandible as a whole.

Technique of Intubation

Patients with maxillofacial trauma may be unable to open the mouth, thus presenting special problems for an anesthesiologist who must intubate the trachea. The most common causes of jaw immobility are pain, trismus, and edema.

Pain responds to anesthetics and muscle relaxants and presents no serious problem. Trismus is spasm of the masseter muscles and also responds similarly. However, the time of fracture, duration of trismus, and prior imposed immobility deserve consideration. If the fracture is more than 2 weeks old, fibrosis is present in the masseter muscles; fibrotic muscles do *not* respond to an anesthetic and muscle relaxant. Edema is rarely so severe that it presents a major challenge. However, awake intubation *must* be considered.

Functional Impairment

Several fractures may directly cause impairment of the TMJ. Mechanical dysfunction of the joint does not respond to anesthetics and relaxants, and proven or suspected mechanical impairment necessitates awake intubation.

If the condyle is fractured, TMJ function may be disrupted by bony fragments within the joint. A fracture of the zygomatic arch of the temporal bone may drive the proximal (temporal) fragment posteroinferiorly into the TMJ, thus locking it closed. Such fractures are rare, because the bone is enveloped in the thick, strong temporal fascia. However, a blow to the side of the head from above may be powerful enough to rupture this membrane and fracture the bone. TMJ dysfunction

must be considered in any displaced fracture of the zygomatic arch.

A fracture of the zygoma may cause posteroinferior displacement of the fracture segment, impinging it on the coronoid process. Forward motion of the mandible is limited as it opens, thereby effectively locking it closed. This is a rare event that we have never personally witnessed. Nevertheless, it merits consideration.

What Are the Most Frequent Associated Injuries?

The nature and incidence of associated injuries in patients with maxillofacial trauma depend on the nature of the inciting force. In one study that compared high-velocity–high-impact forces with low-velocity–low-impact forces, both major and minor associated injuries were significantly higher in high-velocity injuries (Table 72–6).

Cervical Spine

Perhaps most vexing to anesthesiologists is trauma to the cervical spine that injures the spinal cord or puts it at risk during the perioperative period. Radiographs of the cervical spine are indicated for any suspicion of cervical spine injury (pain or tenderness in the neck, loss of consciousness, or neurologic signs and symptoms indicative of spinal injury). Always err on the conservative side and order too many "negative" radiographs rather than miss a cervical spine injury.

Tracheal intubation of patients with cervical spine injury risks further and often irreparable damage to the spinal cord. In one study of 2555 patients with facial skeletal trauma, 32 patients (1.3%) sustained cervical spine injury. Of these, 11 (34%) were unstable.[31] In patients with mandibular fracture, associated injuries were varied (Table 72–7).[32]

TABLE 72–7. Mandibular Fractures: Associated Injuries

Type of Injury	Number	%
Facial fracture	70	35
Intracranial	30	15
Cervical spine (Fracture/dislocation)	12	6
Extremity	42	21
Chest	27	14
Abdominal	6	3
Airway problem	13	6

(From Busuito MJ, Smith DJ, Robson MC: Mandibular fractures in an urban trauma center. J Trauma 1986; 26:826. © Williams & Wilkins, 1986.)

AWAKE TRACHEAL INTUBATION

What General Concepts Are Applicable?

Nasotracheal intubation is relatively (but not absolutely) contraindicated in patients with a nasal fracture. The greater the degree of deformity, the greater is the contraindication. Basal skull fracture is an absolute contraindication to nasotracheal intubation. In instances of severe fracture-deformity of the nose or basal skull fracture, the route of choice is oral intubation or, if this approach is not feasible, tracheotomy.

Nasotracheal intubation is the preferred technique with mandibular fractures requiring internal fixation, because the fixation apparatus cannot be closed over an oral tube. If nasal intubation is not feasible and tracheotomy is undesirable, the fixation apparatus can be placed but not closed with wires until the patient is awake and the oral tube is removed.

How Is the Patient Prepared?

Placement of a rather large plastic endotracheal tube into an awake patient's airway is a formidable and unpleasant task. The larynx is designed to prevent entry of foreign material, and the protective reflexes are acute and potent.

Topical Anesthesia

The nose, mouth, and oropharynx can be anesthetized with topically applied local anesthetics. The first step is to administer atropine or glycopyrrolate. If the oropharyngeal mucosa is not relatively dry, topical anesthesia is impaired by dilution and diffusion across the saliva to the tissues. Inhalation of vaporized lidocaine has been recommended as an effective technique to anesthetize the airway. Our experience suggests that this method is not as dependable nor as effective as direct topical application coupled with bilateral superior laryngeal nerve block.

Cocaine

Local anesthetics may be applied via anesthetic-soaked cotton pledgets in the nose. Cocaine is an especially useful agent because it is a potent topical anesthetic and the only one that, in conventional concentrations (2–4%), is also a vasoconstrictor.[33] However, cocaine has an illicit value that makes its storage hazardous. Also, cocaine is toxic. Although the toxic dose is generally calculated at about 200 mg in an adult, serious toxicity has resulted from as little as 50 mg.

Lidocaine

We favor lidocaine, 2% to 4%, to which is added a few drops of phenylephrine hydrochloride (0.25%) for vasoconstriction. This combination of drugs has neither the street value nor the toxicity of cocaine. Atomizers are unreliable and do not produce a uniform dose. We suggest drawing the anesthetic into a syringe and squirting it into the nose and mouth. Anesthesiologists commonly forgo application of local anesthetic in the mouth, especially if the jaw is wired shut, but local anesthetic can be injected past the wires through an intravenous catheter without difficulty.

What Is the Sensory Innervation of the Larynx?

Innervation of the larynx is provided by the superior laryngeal nerve, a branch of the vagus nerve derived from the nodose ganglion. It travels with the main trunk of the nerve to the level of the larynx, where it angles forward and terminates in internal (sensory) and external (motor) branches.

The external branch penetrates and innervates the cricothyroid muscle, a tensor of the vocal cords. The internal branch penetrates the thyrohyoid membrane and ramifies immediately, providing sensory innervation from the base of the tongue to the vocal cords. After penetrating the thyrohyoid membrane, the nerve rests in a closed space bounded superiorly by the inferior surface of the hyoid bone, inferiorly by the superior edge of the thyroid cartilage, medially by the laryngeal mucosa, and laterally by the thyrohyoid membrane (Fig. 72–11).

How Is the Superior Laryngeal Nerve Blocked?

The nerve can be blocked by placing a needle in the closed space and depositing a local anesthetic. The landmarks are as follows:

1. The hyoid bone, a freely movable bone in the upper neck that articulates with no other bone (see Fig. 72–11)
2. The thyroid cartilage
3. The thyrohyoid membrane, which binds the two together

A patient's head should be extended to maximize the distance between the hyoid and thyroid cartilages. A 22- or 23-gauge needle attached to a syringe containing 2 mL of 2% lidocaine is directed at the hyoid, parallel to the coronal plane. When the needle strikes the bone, a characteristic gritty feeling may be appreciated. The sensation is like that felt during an intercostal block when the rib is struck. The needle is then "walked" caudad, until it slips off the bone and through the thyrohyoid membrane. Aspiration should yield nothing, at which point the anesthetic may be injected and the block repeated on the opposite side. If air is aspirated, the needle is in the larynx; blood indicates penetration of a blood vessel (i.e., one of the major structures within the carotid sheath).

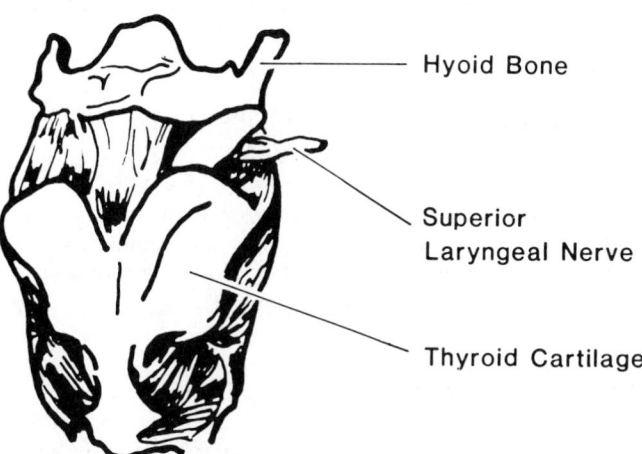

Hyoid Bone

Superior Laryngeal Nerve

Thyroid Cartilage

FIGURE 72–11. Anatomic relationship of the superior laryngeal nerve, hyoid bone, and thyroid cartilage.

Contraindications

Contraindications to a superior laryngeal nerve block include (1) a full stomach because the block will ablate protective laryngeal reflexes, (2) infection at the site of the block, and (3) tumor at the site of the block.

We consider these to be relative, not absolute, contraindications that necessitate careful, individual, case-by-case assessment of risk versus benefit.

Complications

Complications of the block include intravascular injection of local anesthetic with subsequent seizure. The only other complication we have personally witnessed is one instance of a small, easily contained hematoma.

Why Not Block the Recurrent Laryngeal Nerves?

Sensory innervation of the trachea is provided by the recurrent laryngeal nerves. Because these nerves also provide motor innervation of the intrinsic muscle of the larynx, their block risks acute airway closure and is contraindicated.

How Is Translaryngeal Analgesia Obtained?

Sensory analgesia can be provided by translaryngeal application of local anesthetic. The cricothyroid membrane is identified in the midline. Major neural or vascular structures are absent in this area, and penetration of the membrane entails no great risk.

A 22-gauge needle attached to a syringe containing 4 mL of 2% lidocaine is thrust through the membrane until air is freely aspirated. The bevel of the needle may be turned caudad, facing the carina. The patient is instructed to inhale deeply, then exhale maximally. At the end of expiration, the lidocaine is rapidly injected, and the needle removed from the neck. Local anesthetic striking the carina stimulates a vigorous cough that sprays droplets along the trachea and the inferior surface of the vocal cords.

The procedure should be done using both hands to steady the syringe and needle. When the inevitable cough occurs, the needle can be rapidly withdrawn so that it does not lacerate or puncture the posterior tracheal wall.

ALTERNATIVE TECHNIQUES TO SECURE THE AIRWAY

Occasionally, the airway must be secured quickly, often under suboptimal conditions. This situation is most likely to occur with severe crush injury of the face or massive destruction such as that caused by a shotgun blast.

What Is an Andy Gump Fracture?

Particularly dangerous is a bimandibular fracture, in which the body of the mandible has been fractured on both sides. If the distal fracture segment is mobilized, it may be distracted posteroinferiorly by the muscles of the floor of the mouth (genioglossus, mylohyoid, and digastric). As the fracture segment is distracted, it brings with it the tongue and paraglottic soft tissues, impacting them into the upper airway and causing severe and even complete airway obstruction.

Because of the characteristic foreshortening of the mandible associated with this injury, it is sometimes known as an *Andy Gump fracture* after the popular comic strip character with a hypoplastic mandible. Attempted tracheal intubation of a patient with an Andy Gump fracture probably will prove fruitless. Initially, it is worth an attempt to restore the airway by gentle forward traction on the mandible, thereby reducing the fracture and disimpacting the tongue and associated soft tissues.

What Problems Are Associated with Emergency Airway Management?

In any instance of acute upper airway closure, when oral or nasal intubation is either contraindicated or has failed, the airway must be secured via tracheotomy, cricothyroidotomy, or translaryngeal ventilation. Emergency tracheotomy in a patient struggling furiously for every breath is harrowing, difficult, and sometimes impossible. Operative or percutaneous cricothyroidotomy through the cricothyroid membrane may be performed more quickly but should be converted to a tracheotomy within 24 to 48 hours.

How Is Translaryngeal Jet Ventilation Accomplished?

The airway may be quickly secured by passing a 14-gauge catheter-over-needle through the cricothyroid membrane. The needle is then removed, leaving the catheter behind. To the catheter one connects (previously prepared) a small (e.g., tuberculin) syringe attached to high-pressure oxygen tubing, coupled to the common gas outlet of an anesthesia machine (Fig. 72–12).

Ventilation via the anesthesia breathing circuit is inadequate because it is too compliant to allow sufficient pressures for adequate tidal volume delivery. Patients can be oxygenated and ventilated with this system with short, intermittent, rapid bursts of oxygen via the machine flush valve and maintained if they are able to exhale via the oropharynx while other plans for establishing the airway are considered.

A more sophisticated technique uses a Sanders valve, which has a Luer-Lok, obviating the ''jury-rigged'' system described earlier. When translaryngeal jet ventilation is used, the airway must be at least partially open above the cricothyroid membrane. If not, gas under pressure accumulates within the lungs, and pneumothorax is a likely result.

When Are Fiberoptic Techniques Indicated?

Fiberoptic intubation techniques should be considered whenever a patient must be intubated awake. The indication is relative, not absolute, because awake intubation may be effected under direct vision or even blindly. However, fiberoptic techniques are difficult after failed attempts at awake blind

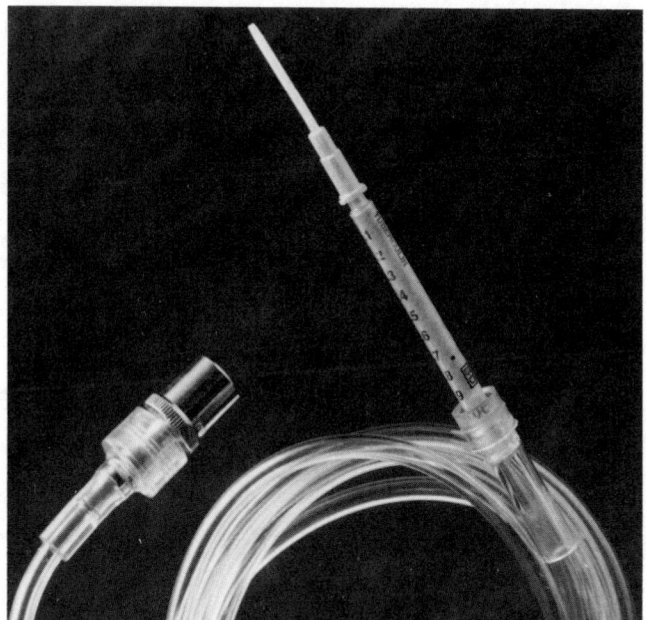

FIGURE 72–12. Translaryngeal jet ventilation may be accomplished by placing a 14-gauge catheter through the cricothyroid membrane and by attaching it to high-pressure tubing that is directly connected to the common gas outlet of an anesthesia machine.

nasal intubation because of nasopharyngeal trauma, coupled with epistaxis, erythema, edema, and secretions.

If serious doubt exists about the feasibility of awake intubation under direct vision, fiberoptic visualization and intubation are indicated and should be tried first. Awake intubation is mandated with dysfunction of the TMJ that locks the jaw shut, fibrosis of the masseter muscles following prolonged trismus, or immobilization of the jaw and Ludwig's angina. Extensive facial trauma with anatomic distortion, hemorrhage, erythema, and edema often makes fiberoptic techniques impossible.

Failed fiberoptic techniques should never be followed by administration of anesthetic agents and muscle relaxants in an attempt to visualize the airway. To do so entails the very serious risks of failure to intubate and ventilate. Failed fiberoptic techniques mandate awake intubation under direct visualization, if possible, or tracheotomy, if necessary.

What Are the Indications for Tracheotomy?

Tracheotomy is occasionally necessary in cases of severe maxillofacial trauma. In most instances of Le Fort III fractures, tracheotomy is performed. Indications include (1) severe anatomic distortion that makes oral or nasotracheal intubation impossible, (2) airway obstruction when oral or nasotracheal intubation is impossible, and (3) basilar skull fracture when oral intubation is not feasible because of the surgical technique or approach.

Basilar skull fracture is an absolute contraindication to nasotracheal intubation. If, in the presence of basal skull fracture, the surgeon cannot work with an oral tube in place, tracheotomy is the most prudent choice.

How Should a Patient Whose Jaw Is Wired Be Extubated?

Extubation of a patient whose jaw is wired demands judgment about timing, available equipment, and a suitable plan for reintubation or securing the airway in another manner, on an emergent basis. An oral surgeon or otolaryngologist should be immediately available to cut the wires if necessary. In addition, equipment to perform translaryngeal jet ventilation should be at the bedside. A tracheotomy set should also be readily available.

If extensive edema is present, particularly near the angle of the jaw, extubation should be deferred for at least 24 hours. One useful technique is to insert a fiberoptic bronchoscope through the endotracheal tube and then to remove the tube over the bronchoscope, leaving the bronchoscope in the larynx and trachea. Should intubation become necessary, the bronchoscope is already in place and the tube can be reinserted expeditiously.

Before extubation, be sure that patients are awake, reactive, and responsive to verbal commands and that they meet all criteria for removal of ventilatory support.

References

1. Liu LMP, DeCook CH, Goudsouzian NG, et al: Dose response to intramuscular succinylcholine in children. Anesthesiology 1981; 55:599.
2. Goudsouzian NG: Relaxants in pediatric anesthesia. Clin Anesthesiol 1985; 3:539.
3. McGoldrick K: Anesthesia for elective ENT surgery. *In* Anesthesia for Ophthalmic and Otolaryngologic Surgery. McGoldrick K (ed). Philadelphia, WB Saunders, 1992, pp 97–111.
4. Eisenberg JM, Clarke JR, Sussman SA: Prothrombin and partial thromboplastin times as preoperative screening tests. Arch Surg 1982; 117:48.
5. Rohrer JM, Michelotti MC, Nahrwold DL: Prospective evaluation of the efficacy of preoperative coagulation testing. Ann Surg 1988; 208:554.
6. Tami TA, Parker GS, Taylor RE: Post-tonsillectomy bleeding: an evaluation of risk factors. Laryngoscope 1987; 97:1307.
7. Ring WH, Adair JC, Elwyn RA: A new pediatric endotracheal tube. Anesth Analg 1975; 54:273.
8. Karl HW, Swedlow DB, Lee KW, et al: Epinephrine-halothane interactions in children. Anesthesiology 1983; 58:142.
9. Gefke K, Andersen LW, Friesel E: Intravenous lidocaine as a suppressant of cough and laryngospasm with extubation after tonsillectomy. Acta Anaesthesiol Scand 1983; 27:112.
10. Guida RA, Mattucci KF: Tonsillectomy and adenoidectomy: an inpatient or outpatient procedure? Laryngoscope 1990; 100:491.
11. Tate N: Deaths from tonsillectomy. Lancet 1963; 2:1090.
12. Carithers JS, Gebhart DE, Williams JA: Postoperative risk of pediatric tonsilloadenectomy. Laryngoscope 1987; 97:422.
13. Colclasure JB, Graham SS: Complications of outpatient tonsillectomy and adenoidectomy: a review of 3340 cases. Ear Nose Throat J 1968; 69:155.
14. Chaing TM, Sukis AE, Ross DE: Tonsillectomy performed on an outpatient basis: report of a series of 40,000 cases without a death. Acta Otolaryngol 1968; 88:105.
15. Crysdale WS, Russel D: Complications of tonsillectomy and adenoidectomy in 9409 children observed overnight. Can Med Assoc J 1986; 135:1139.
16. Davis I, Moore JRM, Lahiri SK: Nitrous oxide and the middle ear. Anaesthesia 1979; 34:147.
17. Owens WD, Gustave F, Sclaroff A: Tympanic membrane rupture with nitrous oxide anesthesia. Anesth Analg 1978; 57:283.
18. Armstrong HG, Hein JW: The effect of flight on the middle ear. JAMA 1937; 109:417.
19. Patterson ME, Bartlett PC: Hearing impairment caused by intratympanic pressure changes during general anesthesia. Laryngoscope 1976; 86:399.
20. Waun NE, Sweitzer RS, Hamilton WK: Effect of nitrous oxide on middle ear mechanics and hearing acuity. Anesthesiology 1967; 28:846.
21. Kerr AR: Anesthesia with profound hypotension for middle ear surgery. Br J Anaesth 1977; 49:477.

22. Eltringham RJ, Young PN, Fairburn MD, et al: Hypotensive anesthesia for microsurgery of the middle ear: a comparison between enflurane and halothane. Anaesthesia 1982; 37:1028.

23. Goudsouzian N, Miler V: Anesthesia for plastic surgery in children. *In* Anesthesia for Plastic and Reconstructive Surgery. Abadir AR, Humayun SG (eds). St Louis, Mosby–Year Book, 1991, p 211.

24. Johnston RR, Eger EI, Wilson C: A comparative interaction of epinephrine with enflurane, isoflurane, and halothane in man. Anesth Analg 1976; 55:709.

25. Metz S, Maze M: Halothane concentration does not alter the threshold for epinephrine-induced arrhythmias in dogs. Anesthesiology 1985; 62:470.

26. Katz RL, Katz GJ: Surgical infiltrations of pressor drugs and their interaction with volatile anesthetics. Br J Anaesth 1966; 38:712.

27. Tucker WK, Packstein AD, Munson ES: Comparison of arrhythmic doses of adrenaline, metaraminol, ephedrine, and phenylephrine during isoflurane and halothane anesthesia in dogs. Br J Anaesth 1974; 46:392.

28. Jordan WS, Graves CL, Elwyn RA: A new therapy for postintubation laryngeal edema and tracheitis (croup) in children. JAMA 1970; 212:585.

29. LeFort R: Etude experimentale sur les fractures de la machoire superirure. Rev Chir 1901; 23:208, 360, 479.

30. Kitahata LM, Collins WF: Meningitis as a complication of anesthesia in a patient with a basal skull fracture. Anesthesiology 1970; 32:282.

31. Davidson JSD, Birdsell DC: Cervical spine injury in patients with facial skeletal trauma. J Trauma 1989; 29:1276.

32. Busuito MJ, Smith DJ, Robson MC: Mandibular fractures in an urban trauma center. J Trauma 1986; 26:826.

33. Ritchie JM, Cohen PJ: Cocaine, procaine, and other synthetic local anesthetics. *In* The Pharmacological Basis of Therapeutics. 5th ed. Goodman LS, Gilman A (eds). New York, Macmillan, 1975, pp 338–393.

CHAPTER 73

Neurologic Surgery

MICHAEL E. MAHLA, M.D.

In neuroanesthesia, unlike other subspecialties of anesthesiology, the organ system involved with the surgical procedure is also the primary site of action of the hypnotic, analgesic, and amnestic effects of anesthetic drugs. This distinction is important for two reasons. First, anesthetic drugs have profound effects on central nervous system (CNS) function and may alter homeostatic mechanisms such as autoregulation or the vascular response to carbon dioxide (CO_2). In addition, measurable parameters such as CNS blood flow (CBF), CNS blood volume (CBV), and CNS metabolism ($CMRo_2$) may be changed. Because of these effects, anesthetic drugs have the potential to unfavorably alter blood flow and intracranial pressure (ICP). If CNS pathology already has altered ICP and CBF, further drug-induced changes may cause permanent damage independently of the surgical procedure.

Second, the normal effects of drugs that we use may be difficult to distinguish from the signs and symptoms produced by many different types of CNS pathology. For example, distinguishing between unresponsiveness produced by residual levels of isoflurane, fentanyl, and pancuronium and the unresponsiveness produced by inadvertent interruption of the middle cerebral artery following aneurysm clipping can be difficult but is vitally important. The effects of anesthetic drugs eventually dissipate without harm. Loss of blood supply to the frontal, parietal, and temporal lobes, however, has long-term devastating effects that often are not reversible. Thus, an important goal of neuroanesthesia is that the hypnotic effects of anesthetic drugs should dissipate rapidly at the conclusion of the operation to allow early assessment of neurologic function and rapid detection of potentially reversible surgical problems.

NEUROPHYSIOLOGY AND NEUROPHARMACOLOGY

Do Anesthetics or Adjunctive Drugs Influence Outcome?

No prospective randomized or retrospective study in neurosurgical patients has shown a superior patient outcome with one anesthetic technique compared with another. Clinicians are presented with a wide array of frequently conflicting laboratory and clinical data from studies that elucidate the primary CNS properties and side effects of most anesthetic and adjunctive therapeutic drugs (e.g., vasodilators and vasopressors). Major conclusions regarding the appropriateness of these drugs during neurologic surgery often are made without any evidence that they affect ultimate outcome or influence intraoperative surgical conditions.[1-3] Authors of these studies emphasize, however, that clinicians must be aware of the CNS effects of the drugs they use in order to use each drug *appropriately*. For example, a drug that increases CBV is inappropriate for a patient with increased ICP unless some therapeutic intervention such as hyperventilation or mannitol diuresis is employed to prevent a further rise in ICP.

What Homeostatic Mechanisms Are Important During Neurologic Surgery?

Both anesthetic and adjunctive medications affect normal CNS function and important homeostatic regulatory mechanisms. Many of these parameters are measurable, including autoregulation of blood flow, vascular responsiveness to CO_2, $CMRo_2$, CBF, CBV, and ICP.

Autoregulation of Cerebral or Spinal Cord Blood Flow

If an organ is able to autoregulate, blood flow is maintained at a constant value over a range of perfusion pressures. CBF is constant and normal at mean perfusion pressures that range from 50 to 130 mm Hg (Fig. 73–1A). If a pathologic condition or drug causes loss of autoregulation, blood flow varies directly with perfusion pressure (see Fig. 73–1B). Perfusion pressures that would produce normal blood flows with intact autoregulation often produce abnormal flows when autoregulation is impaired. Low flows may produce ischemia, and high flows may cause edema and hemorrhage. Thus, more rigid control of blood pressure to maintain normal CBF seems to be important in such patients whether autoregulation is impaired by drugs or by pathologic change.

Responsiveness to Carbon Dioxide

Carbon dioxide is a potent cerebral vasodilator. Decreases in CO_2 cause cerebral vasoconstriction and reductions in CBF

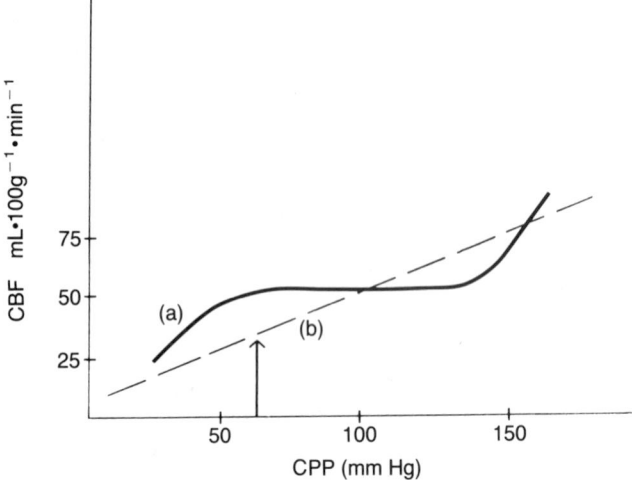

FIGURE 73–1. Normal autoregulation (a) and failure of autoregulation (b). *Arrow* shows a mean cerebral perfusion pressure that would produce a normal CBF if autoregulation were intact and a low CBF if autoregulation had failed.

and CBV. This normal cerebrovascular response enables the clinician to reduce brain bulk during surgery by hyperventilating the patient and is the basis of the most important first-line treatment directed at reduction of elevated ICP. If vascular responsiveness to CO_2 is impaired or lost, however, hyperventilation no longer is effective in reducing brain bulk or in lowering ICP. Since hyperventilation may have undesirable effects, such as reduction of perfusion to other organs or elevation of mean airway pressures with decreased venous return to the heart, the loss of vascular responsiveness to CO_2 is important to ascertain.

Cerebral Oxygen Demand

Oxygen (O_2) is used equally by the brain to maintain both function and cellular integrity. As the O_2 supply decreases, the brain first sacrifices function and devotes all available O_2 to the maintenance of cellular integrity. Further reduction in O_2 may result in cell damage or cell death. When the O_2 supply is restored, function returns to normal, provided that cellular damage has not occurred. The $CMRO_2$ is important for several reasons. It may determine the relative risk to the brain of an ischemic insult. Further, the relationship between $CMRO_2$ and CBF forms the basis of pharmacologically induced reduction of ICP.

Brain Tolerance to Ischemic Insults

Until recently, most clinicians believed that reduction of $CMRO_2$ was the most important factor during attempts to increase brain tolerance to an ischemic insult. Therefore, drugs that lowered $CMRO_2$ were thought to protect the brain from intraoperative ischemia. However, studies have suggested that reduction of $CMRO_2$ is not always associated with ischemic cerebral protection. In addition, some drugs that do not decrease $CMRO_2$ appear to be protective in animal experiments.[4, 5] Available data suggest that $CMRO_2$ is an important factor in determining CNS tolerance to ischemia, but this is clearly only part of the story.

The $CMRO_2$ normally is coupled to CBF. Unless the relationship between demand and flow is uncoupled (e.g., by potent inhalation agents), drugs or conditions that increase O_2

demand also increase CBF and CBV. Conversely, a decreased O_2 demand is associated with decreases of CBF and CBV. This relationship is the basis for the pharmacologic reduction of ICP with barbiturates. Barbiturates suppress the electroencephalogram (EEG) in a dose-related fashion, reducing O_2 demand associated with electrical function ultimately to zero. A corresponding reduction in CBF, CBV, and ICP follows.

Cerebral Blood Flow and Cerebral Blood Volume

CBF provides the brain with O_2 for function and maintenance of cellular integrity. Reductions in CBF <10 to 20 mL · 100 g^{-1} · min^{-1} under anesthesia are associated with a loss of function; reductions <5 to 10 mL · 100 g^{-1} · min^{-1} result in loss of cellular integrity and death.[6, 7]

Changes in CBV normally are directly related to changes in CBF. How much CBV changes with a change in CBF is unknown and probably depends on the mechanism by which the change occurs. Cerebral blood volume may also change without a change in CBF as, for example, during a change in head position from elevated to supine. Changes in CBV normally are not clinically significant. However, in patients with poor intracranial elastance (i.e., in whom large changes in ICP occur with small changes in intracranial volume), increases or decreases in CBV can produce similar changes in ICP.

Intracranial Pressure

The ICP is important for two reasons. First, it is a primary determinant of cerebral perfusion pressure (CPP), which is defined as mean arterial pressure (MAP) minus ICP or central venous pressure (CVP), whichever is greater:

$$CPP = MAP - ICP \text{ (or CVP)} \qquad \text{Equation 1}$$

If MAP remains constant and ICP increases, CPP decreases. This decrease becomes important once CPP falls below the lower limits for cerebral autoregulation. In patients with impaired autoregulation, blood flow may fall substantially with increases in ICP that do not cause CPP to drop below the lower limits for autoregulation (see Fig. 73–1). If the fall in blood flow is significant enough, loss of function and cellular death may ensue.

The numerical value of the ICP is less important than that for the CPP. Moderate elevations in ICP may actually be beneficial. Following subarachnoid hemorrhage (SAH), an increase in ICP (while CPP is still within the autoregulatory range) reduces the transmural wall pressure of the aneurysm and the risk of rebleeding without reducing CBF.

ICP may vary between the cerebral and spinal compartments. Significant regional elevations in pressure can produce a pressure gradient sufficient to cause herniation of the contents of one compartment into another. This finding is fairly common when significant elevation of supratentorial ICP causes the temporal lobe or lobes to herniate through the tentorium cerebri. The resulting compromise of blood flow to the herniated brain tissue causes loss of function and cell death.

What Drug Effects Are Important?

Table 73–1 summarizes much of the animal and human data available on many drugs that are commonly used during an-

TABLE 73–1. Anesthetic Effects on Physiologic Variables

Drug or Drug Class*	CMRo$_2$	CBF	CBF/CMRo$_2$	CBV	AR	CO$_2$	BP	ICP	CPP
Barbiturates (includes etomidate)	↓	↓	0	↓	N	↓	↓	↓	↑,↓,0*
Propofol	↓	↓	0,?↓	↓	N	N	↓	↓	↑,↓,0
Benzodiazepines	↓	↓	0	↓	N	N	↓	↓	↑,↓,0*
Opiates	0	↓,?↑	0	0	N	N	0,↓	0,?↑	0,↓
Ketamine	↑	↑	0,↑	↑	?	N	↑	↑	↑,↓,0*
Nitrous oxide†	↑	↑	0	↑	N	N	0,↓	0,↑	0,↓
Halothane	↓	↑	↑		↓	N	↓	0,↑	↓
Enflurane	↓,↑‡	↑	↑		↓	N	↓	0,↑	↓
Isoflurane, desflurane	↓	↑	↑		↓	N	↓	↑	↓
Succinylcholine	0	0,↑	0,↑	0,↑	N	N	0	0,↑	0,↓
Pancuronium	0	0	0	0	N	N	0,↑	0	0
Doxacurium, pipecuronium, vecuronium	0	0	0	0	N	N	0	0	0
Atracurium	0	0	0	0	N	N	0,↓	0	0,↓
α- and β-blocking agents	0	0	0	0	N	N	↓	0	↓
Sodium nitroprusside	0	↑	↑	↑	↓	↓	↓	↑	↓
Nitroglycerine	0	↑	↑	↑	↓	↓	↓	↑	↓
Trimethaphan	0	0	0	0	N	↓	↓	0	↓
Calcium channel blocking agents	0	↑	↑		N,↓	N	↓	0	0
Phenylephrine	0	0,↑	0,↑		N	N	↑	0,↑	0,↑
Ephedrine	0,↑	0,↑	0,↑		N	N	↑	0,↑	0,↑

*Overall effect depends on what changes more—blood pressure or ICP.
†In anesthetized patients or animals (i.e., when N$_2$O is added to another agent, such as a barbiturate, the value will not exceed that in an awake subject).
‡High dose, during seizure.
Key: AR = cerebral autoregulation; BP = blood pressure; CO$_2$ = vascular response to carbon dioxide; CPP = cerebral perfusion pressure; 0 = no clinically important effect; ↑ = increases parameter; ↓ = decreases parameter; N = preserves normal function. If more than one effect is shown, effect varies, depending on patient pathology or if unresolved controversy exists.

esthesia for craniotomies.[5, 8–64] The effects shown represent a synthesis of frequently conflicting animal and human studies as well as my opinion regarding the clinical importance of the reported effects. Thus, the table shows no important effect of a given drug—even when the literature reports an effect—if in my opinion the effect is not *clinically* important.

When planning to use any drug during neurologic surgery, the anesthesiologist needs to consider its effects on CPP, CBF, and CBV. Provided that each of these interdependent values can be kept within acceptable limits, use of a particular drug or drug combination is unlikely to affect outcome in any fashion that can be currently measured.

The importance of each of these parameters varies from operation to operation (Table 73–2). Sodium nitroprusside ad-ministered to reduce blood pressure in a patient with a large intracranial mass may increase ICP because of its effects on CBV. This drug, therefore, generally is not chosen to lower blood pressure in such patients. On the other hand, because sodium nitroprusside increases CBF, it is a drug of choice for induced hypotension during aneurysm clippings, since CBF is preserved even at low CPP.

Clearly, an understanding of the pathophysiology of the disease state involved and the nature of the planned operation is necessary before anesthetic or associated drugs are chosen for use during surgery. Drugs and adjunctive measures (such as hyperventilation or mannitol administration) can be chosen that minimally affect, or even improve, pre-existing physiologic disturbances.

TABLE 73–2. Examples of the Changing Relative Importance of Physiologic Parameters with Different Types of Neurosurgical Operations

Type of Operation	CBF	CBV	CPP	Rationale
Craniotomy for large intracranial mass	3	3	3	Increased CBF increases CBV, which in turn increases ICP and decreases CPP.
Craniotomy for clipping of intracranial aneurysm	3	2	3	Preservation of CBF is very important. ICP is usually not elevated to dangerous levels. Hyperventilation may lower CBF, CBV, and ICP and increase the risk of rebleeding.
Craniotomy following head trauma	3	3	3	Maintenance of CPP is critical to survival.
Transsphenoidal resection of pituitary mass	1	1	1	Poor intracranial elastance is rare. Hyperventilation-induced decreases in ICP may impair tumor delivery through the sphenoid sinus.
Vertebrectomy and posterior spinal fusion	3	1	3	Preservation of cerebral and spinal cord blood flow during induced hypotension is important.
Ventriculoperitoneal shunt	3	3	3	Intracranial elastance is often poor. Same considerations apply as for craniotomy for mass.
Microvascular decompression of cranial nerves V or VIII	1	1	1	Patient has a normal brain. Technique should help minimize retraction.

Key: 1 = parameters may vary greatly without changing operating conditions; 2 = moderately important—large changes may produce significant changes in operating conditions; 3 = critically important—small changes in these parameters may greatly change operating conditions.

TABLE 73–3. Most Common Positions for Neurosurgical Procedures

Operation	Position
Lumbar laminectomy or disk surgery, thoracic or lumbar spinal cord surgery	Prone, lateral decubitus
Cervical laminectomy, disk, or spinal cord surgery	Supine (anterior approach) Sitting (posterior approach) Prone (posterior approach)
Craniotomy for aneurysm	Anterior circulation: Supine with head turned Basilar apex: Supine with head turned, or lateral decubitus Posterior circulation: Three-quarter prone or prone
Craniotomy for mass resection	Frontal: Supine Temporal: Supine with head turned, or lateral decubitus Parietal: Supine with head turned, or lateral decubitus Occipital: Three-quarter prone, or sitting Posterior fossa: Three-quarter prone, or sitting
Transsphenoidal resection	Supine, head elevated (beach-chair)
Microvascular decompression	Three-quarter prone, or sitting

POSITIONING

The most common patient positions during neurosurgical procedures are the supine, prone, three-quarter prone, and sitting positions. Table 73–3 lists those positions used during specific types of neurosurgical procedures.

Why Do Neurosurgeons Choose One Position Over Another?

General Considerations

Perhaps the most important reason for choosing a surgical position is familiarity. Surgeons trained to perform acoustic tumor resections with patients in the sitting position are likely to continue using that position in practice. Next is a desire to provide optimum operating conditions. Intracranial neurosurgical procedures generally involve removal of a neoplasm or require retraction of brain in order to gain access to a neoplasm, blood vessel, or cranial nerve. Neoplasms may elevate ICP, reduce intracranial elastance, or both. Correct positioning can lessen ICP or reduce the amount of retractor pressure necessary for exposure by facilitating venous drainage (head-up position) and by reducing CBV. Incorrect positioning (e.g., with the head down or turned so far as to occlude jugular venous drainage) can increase ICP or the need for retraction because of increased brain bulk. Similar positioning considerations apply for spinal surgery. Table 73–4 identifies common positioning errors that impact directly on the surgical procedure and their consequences.

Gravitational Effects

Positioning may help to improve exposure by taking advantage of gravitational effects. When a patient is in the three-quarter prone position, the cerebellum may be positioned so that the amount of retraction necessary to move it out of the

TABLE 73–4. Common Positioning Errors in Neuroanesthesia

Error	Consequence
Head rotated too far	Venous drainage obstructed Increased CBV Increased ICP or increased brain bulk
Head flexed too far	Decreased upper cervical spinal cord and medullary blood flow → quadriplegia
Head not elevated	Decreased venous drainage Increased CBV Increased ICP or increased brain bulk
Abdomen not free in prone position	Increased venous bleeding Increased difficulty with ventilation

way during microvascular decompression of the fifth or seventh cranial nerve is decreased. The sitting position allows blood and cerebrospinal fluid (CSF) to drain out of the incision without the need for constant suctioning and thereby improves visibility. Positioning also helps with the incision and makes the surgeon comfortable during these frequently very long operations.

How Is Anesthesia Affected?

Venous Air Embolism

Positioning may create special monitoring needs. Any time the incision is above the level of the heart, the patient is at risk for venous air embolism. The size of the incision also is important. A posterior fossa exploration with a patient in the sitting position is associated with a much higher incidence of venous air embolism than is a posterior cervical laminectomy with a patient in the same position. Air embolism also has been reported during lumbar surgery.[65]

My practice is to monitor all patients with head-elevated positions for venous air embolism. If the risk is significant (e.g., as with posterior fossa explorations in the sitting position), a right atrial catheter is placed at the superior vena cava–right atrial junction for aspiration of large, hemodynamically significant air emboli.[66–68] Although air embolism can occur in any neurosurgical procedure, Table 73–5 lists the procedures that I consider to be associated with the highest risk.

IMPACT OF NEUROLOGIC DISEASE ON ANESTHETIC MANAGEMENT

What Aspects Are Important?

Eight specific areas should be addressed (Table 73–6). I consider relevant neuroanatomy, physiology, pathology, and the nature of the planned surgical procedure to be particularly important.

TABLE 73–5. Neurosurgical Procedures in Which Air Embolism Risk is Greatest

- Sitting posterior fossa exploration
- Sitting cervical laminectomies
- Craniofacial reconstructions, especially for cranial synostosis

TABLE 73–6. Approach to the Neurosurgical Patient

Special Areas for Consideration Include:
- Neuroanatomy, physiology, and pathology related to the disease process and the planned surgical procedure
- Nature of the planned surgical procedure
- Preoperative functional level of the nervous system
- Other systemic illnesses
- Premedication
- Intraoperative monitoring
- Induction and maintenance of anesthesia (special techniques)
- Emergence from anesthesia

Neuroanatomy, Physiology, and Pathology

In planning the anesthetic for a patient with a large brain tumor, such as a glioblastoma multiforme, the size of the mass and whether significant mass effect and surrounding edema are present must be known. In patients with large mass effect, small changes in CBV likely will produce a marked rise in ICP. In addition, large areas of the brain may not autoregulate blood flow normally; increases or decreases in blood pressure that normally would not cause concern may have disastrous consequences.

Surgical Procedure

The nature of the surgical procedure often has a major impact on management. Resection of a large tumor in the posterior fossa that involves multiple cranial nerves makes intraoperative bradycardic episodes more likely. It also may seriously impair postoperative airway reflexes, thus necessitating prolonged tracheal intubation. If temporary occlusion of major cerebral vessels during aneurysm clipping is planned, preoperative anticipation of moderate hypothermia and possible barbiturate cerebral protection is helpful. The nature of the planned procedure and the location of the lesion also help determine the intraoperative position.

Functional Status

Functional status of the nervous system is a major concern. Patients with pre-existing neurologic compromise likely will suffer at least transient worsening of neurologic function postoperatively. This finding is particularly true of patients with depressed mental status. Transient neurologic deterioration also may necessitate at least brief postoperative retention of the endotracheal tube. Whether a postoperative deficit was, in fact, also present preoperatively is essential to know. If the deficit was *not* present preoperatively, its presence may represent a complication of the surgical procedure that is partially or fully correctable if it is recognized promptly.

Coexisting Disease

Neurosurgical procedures often are conducted on patients with other systemic illnesses. These illnesses sometimes make special techniques or even something as basic as positioning very risky. For a patient with severe chronic obstructive lung disease and a large posterior fossa brain tumor, the prone position can make deliberate hyperventilation difficult or impossible. If the same patient instead requires surgery for removal of a thoracic vertebral body, deliberate hypotension to reduce blood loss may cause severe hypoxemia because of vasodilator-induced loss of hypoxic pulmonary vasoconstriction.

Premedication

Since the target organ is the CNS, premedication is sometimes hazardous in patients with neurologic disease. The effect of a benzodiazepine may be greatly exaggerated and lead to coma in a patient with a frontal mass. Respiratory depression associated with many premedicants can increase arterial partial pressure of CO_2, CBF, CBV, and ICP. Premedications should *never* be given routinely. The risks of hypoventilation, an exaggerated preoperative effect, and persistent postoperative influence must be carefully balanced against the anticipated benefits of reduced patient anxiety and blood pressure and of increased patient comfort.

When no special risk factors are present, as for a patient about to undergo lumbar disk surgery or transsphenoidal resection of a small pituitary tumor, premedication may be given as needed or desired. When significant risk is involved but premedication is felt to be necessary, the premedication should be given only in carefully monitored environments with pulse oximetry available.

Monitoring

Intraoperative monitoring during neurosurgical procedures is determined by multiple factors, including the anticipated blood loss; special techniques such as induced hypotension or barbiturate coma; positioning; the nature of the planned procedure; and the patient's overall medical condition.

Consider a microvascular decompression of the trigeminal nerve. In this procedure, a sponge is placed between the trigeminal nerve and a nearby blood vessel that is compressing the nerve. The procedure generally is not associated with a large blood loss and does not require any special anesthetic techniques. It usually is conducted with the patient in the three-quarter prone position, which does not create any special monitoring needs. However, the cerebellum must be retracted medially, and this stretches the eighth cranial nerve. Large blood pressure variations during the time of sponge placement as well as postdecompression hypertension that requires vasodilator treatment are common.

Assuming the patient is otherwise healthy, monitoring should consist of continuous electrocardiography; blood pressure monitoring with the cuff on the *nondependent* arm so the patient does not lie on the cuff during the case; pulse oximetry using the *dependent* hand to assess perfusion (grossly) of the dependent arm as well as oxyhemoglobin saturation; end-tidal CO_2 monitoring to assess the adequacy of hyperventilation; intra-arterial catheter placement after induction to assist with blood pressure management; and recording of auditory evoked potentials (not usually performed by the anesthesiologist) to help detect damage to the eighth cranial nerve caused by cerebellar retraction (see Chapter 22).

Induction and Maintenance

Induction and maintenance techniques are most likely selected based on familiarity. Many laboratory studies show *theoretic* advantages or disadvantages to various anesthetic and adjunctive drugs. The data in Table 73–1 combined with the relative goals in Table 73–2 allow development of a strat-

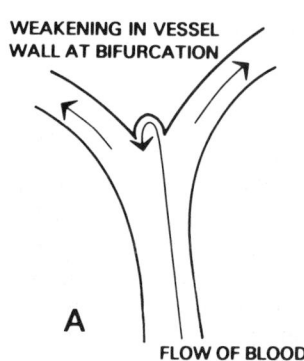 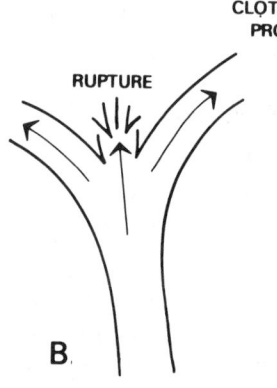 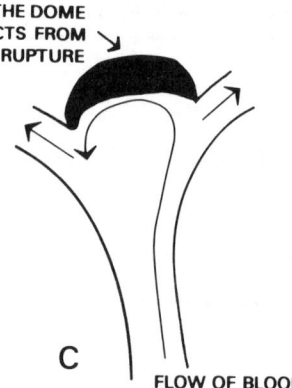

FIGURE 73–2. Schematic representation of aneurysm development. *A*, Asymptomatic small intracranial aneurysm. *B*, Aneurysmal rupture. *C*, Formation of giant aneurysm with wall reinforced by clot that may be calcified.

egy for most neurosurgical procedures. Preoperative planning for special anesthetic and adjunctive procedures such as induced hypotension or barbiturate cerebral protection obviously is of great importance.

Emergence

Finally, as has been stated previously, the target organ of both the operation and the anesthetic is the same. Anesthetic drugs routinely cause impairment of CNS function that often is indistinguishable from surgically induced damage. Anesthetic-induced problems improve as drug levels fall; surgical problems do not. A very short time may be available before potentially reversible problems become irreversible. Thus, the effects of anesthetic drugs must be minimized at the conclusion of surgery so that the neurosurgeon can assess the level of function and be reasonably sure that any problems detected are not anesthetic-induced. Preoperative planning to ensure reversibility is thus an important goal for all neurologic surgery. Sometimes, of course, such reversibility is impossible, as in the case of the patient who is given large doses of sodium thiopental during surgery for cerebral protection.

NEUROVASCULAR SURGERY

What Is an Intracranial Aneurysm?

Pathogenesis

An intracranial aneurysm is produced by a weakening in the wall of a blood vessel usually at a bifurcation (Fig. 73–2). Turbulent flow of blood at the bifurcation predisposes that area to aneurysmal dilatation. As the aneurysm enlarges, the elastance of the wall decreases. Wall tension rises, and the risk of rupture and SAH increases. If the aneurysm does not rupture, it may continue to grow and become a giant aneurysm (i.e., >2 cm in diameter). Table 73–7 shows those anatomic and physiologic characteristics of a patient's intracranial aneurysm and SAH that likely impact on anesthetic management.

Morbidity and Mortality

Approximately 11 in 100,000 individuals experience an SAH. About 28,000 patients with aneurysmal hemorrhages reach hospitals for treatment annually in the United States. Despite improvements in the surgical, anesthetic, and medical management of these patients, the overall mortality remains about 50%.

The most common causes of mortality include rebleeding and vasospasm (delayed ischemic encephalopathy). Of those who survive the initial hemorrhage, 19% whose aneurysms are not surgically clipped rebleed in the first 2 weeks; one-half of these die.[69] Roughly 60% of patients with SAH, whether clipped or unclipped, develop vasospasm. Approximately one-half of these patients are symptomatic, with signs ranging from focal neurologic deficit to massive stroke and death.[70] Many neurosurgeons now believe that vasospasm following SAH produces more morbidity than rebleeding.

When Should Surgery Be Performed Following Hemorrhage?

Aneurysmal SAH is a condition that requires surgical repair to prevent rebleeding. No reliably effective medical management is available. Timing of aneurysm surgery after SAH, however, remains controversial. Because SAH may produce cerebral edema, aneurysm exposure during surgery early after SAH sometimes is technically more difficult and associated with increased need for brain retraction to expose the aneurysm. This retraction will subject the neural tissue to increased pressures at a time when it may already be ischemic. On the other hand, early operation limits further morbidity and mortality from aneurysm rebleeding. Finally, early clipping of the aneurysm increases the safety of hypervolemic, hypertensive therapy, a promising approach to the treatment and prevention of vasospasm.

A multicenter, prospective, international cooperative study on the timing of aneurysm surgery demonstrated that many patients whose surgery was delayed had major complications or died prior to surgery.[71–73] However, patients who survived had better postoperative results if surgery was delayed until the second week after SAH. Overall morbidity and mortality was nearly identical for both the early and delayed surgery groups.

TABLE 73–7. Important Anatomic and Physiologic Factors for Patients Undergoing Aneurysm Surgery

Location
Size
Rupture?
Vasospasm?
Systemic manifestations
Pre-existing medical illness

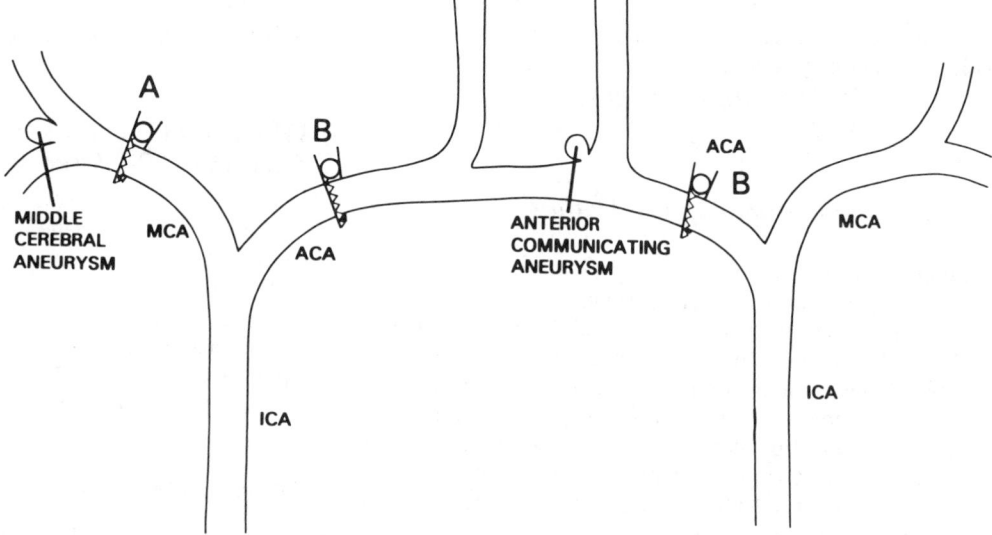

FIGURE 73–3. Planning for rupture. *A,* A temporary clip on the middle cerebral artery (MCA) that stops bleeding from a ruptured MCA aneurysm. *B,* Rupture of an anterior communicating artery aneurysm may require clips on both anterior cerebral arteries (ACA) to control intraoperative hemorrhage. ICA = internal carotid artery.

Why Is Location of the Aneurysm Important?

Positioning

The location of the aneurysm determines the patient's position. In general, anterior circulation aneurysms may be approached with the patient supine and the head slightly turned. Basilar aneurysms are approached either with the patient in the full lateral position or supine and the head turned to a greater extent. Posterior fossa aneurysms are usually approached with the patient in the three-quarter prone or prone position.

Treatment of Catastrophic Rupture

The location of the aneurysm also affects planning for intraoperative catastrophic rupture. Hemorrhage from aneurysms located at bifurcations of terminal arteries (such as the middle cerebral artery) may be readily controlled with a temporary clip on the parent vessel (Fig. 73–3). Those located on vessels

with multiple points of inflow and outflow are more problematic. For example, an aneurysm on the anterior communicating artery may require temporary clips on both anterior cerebral arteries to control intraoperative hemorrhage. Although good intravenous access is needed in all cases, even better access is needed in cases where hemorrhage cannot be as easily controlled.

How Does Aneurysmal Size Affect Anesthetic Management?

The size of an aneurysm may create special problems. As an aneurysm enlarges, major outflow vessels and perforating vessels are more likely to be involved in the aneurysm's dome (Fig. 73–4). Repair sometimes necessitates temporary occlusion of the vessels supplying the aneurysm (see Fig. 73–4). In such a case, tolerance to focal ischemia may be increased by lowering the $CMRo_2$ with barbiturates or, perhaps more importantly, by decreasing the patient's temperature. Review of

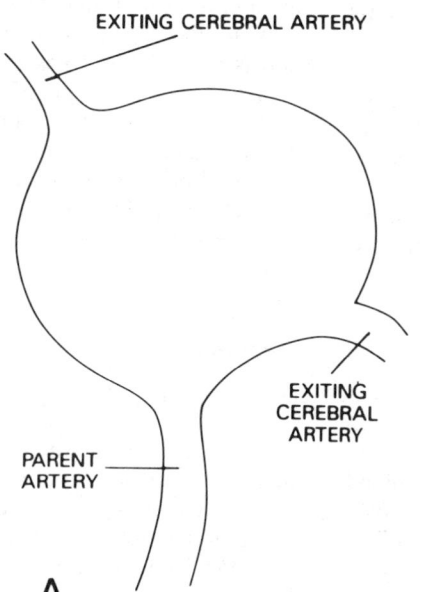

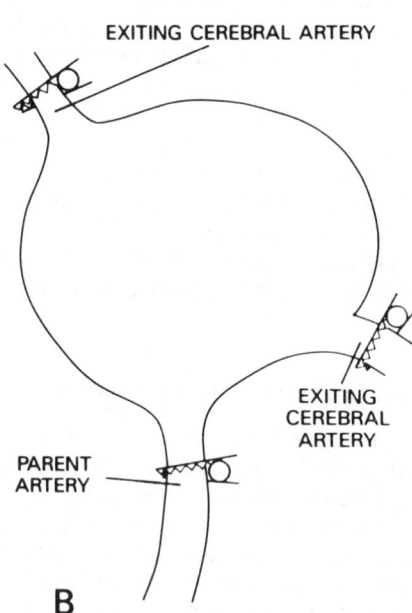

FIGURE 73–4. Schematic representation of giant aneurysms. *A,* As aneurysms enlarge, they may involve other vessels in addition to the parent vessel. Shown here, an aneurysm enlarges to involve two exiting cerebral arteries. *B,* Operative repair (if possible) may involve temporary or permanent occlusion of major cerebral vessels.

the angiogram and discussion with the surgeon preoperatively can help the anesthesiologist to anticipate the need for such therapy. I routinely reduce the patient's temperature to 33 °C in the event that the surgeon unexpectedly and temporarily must place a clip on a major cerebral vessel.

Why Does Aneurysm Rupture Matter?

Ruptured aneurysms are at high risk for rebleeding. This risk can be minimized by careful control of blood pressure. Preoperative insertion of invasive arterial monitoring catheters facilitates this control, but insertion must be as painless as possible, since noxious stimuli may cause hypertension. Patients with preoperative hypertension who need sodium nitroprusside for control of blood pressure *require* invasive monitoring. Patients who are normotensive and stable may have the arterial catheter placed after induction but preferably before strong stimuli such as laryngoscopy occur.

A study conducted in humans undergoing aneurysm clipping showed that the pressure inside the aneurysm lumen and the artery supplying it are equal unless the aneurysm is thrombosed.[74] Aneurysmal wall tension is related directly to the radius of the aneurysm, which in turn is related to the pressure inside the aneurysmal lumen. Sudden increases or decreases in blood pressure, unless the aneurysm is partially thrombosed, are fully transmitted to the aneurysm wall, alter wall tension, and may cause rupture.

Increased Intracranial Pressure

Aneurysmal rupture causes a rapid increase in ICP immediately after SAH. This increase in ICP helps to tamponade the aneurysm and stop bleeding. The ICP usually returns to mildly elevated levels in a matter of minutes to hours. However, blood in the CSF interferes with CSF reabsorption and may cause hydrocephalus. In addition, hemorrhage into the parenchyma of the brain produces an intracerebral hematoma. In either of these cases, ICP may remain elevated at the time the patient arrives in the operating room.

For patients with altered mental status and hydrocephalus, a ventriculostomy catheter often is inserted preoperatively. Cerebrospinal fluid pressure is then gradually reduced over several hours to improve cerebral perfusion (but generally is not reduced to <20 mm Hg). Sometimes dramatic improvements in neurologic status may be seen after this intervention. Although a decrease in ICP improves cerebral perfusion and CBF, aneurysmal transmural wall pressure increases and makes rebleeding more likely. Any reduction in CSF pressure, therefore, must be very gradual. The ICP may be very high in patients with giant aneurysms, large intracerebral hematomas, or massive hydrocephalus. Immediate treatment to reduce ICP is often necessary.

Loss of Cerebral Autoregulation

Aneurysmal rupture can result in loss of cerebral autoregulation, which may be diffuse or restricted mainly to the vascular bed involved with the hemorrhage. Reductions in blood pressure that normally do not cause a decrease in CBF may cause marked decreases in such cases (see Fig. 73–1). When induced hypotension is deemed necessary, the adequacy of cerebral perfusion should be monitored with an electroenceph-

alogram or somatosensory evoked potentials (SSEPs), if possible (see Chapter 22).

Why Does Cerebral Vasospasm Follow Aneurysmal Rupture?

Vasospasm is a potentially devastating physiologic disturbance that occurs in some patients 72 hours or more following SAH. It is not seen in a patient with aneurysms that have not ruptured. Manifestations are highly variable, ranging from an asymptomatic condition that is seen only on cerebral angiography to severe cerebral ischemia with focal or global neurologic deficits and massive stroke.

Pathophysiology and Diagnosis

Vasospasm is thought to be caused by the breakdown of red blood cells in CSF; the risk increases with increased amounts of blood. The condition initially is diagnosed by a typically gradual deterioration of the level of consciousness and the development of focal neurologic findings. Headache is common, and blood pressure frequently increases. Such clinical findings also can be caused by other treatable lesions such as rebleeding, hematoma, hydrocephalus, or metabolic abnormalities (commonly hyponatremia). Once these other lesions are ruled out, the diagnosis of vasospasm may be confirmed angiographically. Noninvasive transcranial Doppler ultrasound measurements of blood flow velocities in the basal arteries of the brain also can detect and document the severity of vasospasm (see Chapter 22).

Clinical Implications

Detection of vasospasm is critical, since patients are at particular risk if they become hypotensive. Vessels distal to the vasospastic site are no longer able to autoregulate, and critical reductions in CBF may occur with decreases in blood pressure even to the "normal" range (see Fig. 73–1). In the awake patient, such a reduction in flow usually is detectable by the onset of a focal or global neurologic deficit.

While the patient is anesthetized, the neurologic examination is unavailable; electrophysiologic brain monitoring may be used to determine the lower limits of blood pressure tolerated in areas supplied by the vasospastic vessels. With such monitoring, the clinician may properly balance the need for decreased blood pressure to prevent aneurysm rupture and to facilitate clipping against the requirement for higher blood pressure to ensure adequate perfusion through vasospastic vessels.

Treatment

Hypervolemic, Hypertensive Therapy

No reliably effective treatment exists for vasospasm. Increases of cardiac output and MAP are thought to overcome the vessel narrowing produced by vasospasm and to restore normal blood flow. A prospective study examining the effects of prophylactic hypervolemic, hypertensive therapy (HHT) demonstrated a marked reduction in morbidity and mortality

TABLE 73–8. Hypervolemic Hypertensive Therapy for Cerebral Vasospasm

- MAP >110 mm Hg
- Pulmonary capillary wedge pressure 18–20 mm Hg
- Hematocrit 30–33%
- Cardiac index >3.0 (use inotrope if increased filling pressures are not enough to accomplish this)

in patients with post-SAH vasospasm (Table 73–8).[17] Treatment of established vasospasm with HHT was also shown to be effective in a series of 118 consecutive SAH patients.[76] Overall, the rate of death and major neurologic deficit in this series was an impressively low 7%.

HHT produces a hyperdynamic circulation and may increase the risk of aneurysm rupture if it is initiated prior to clipping. Early aneurysm clipping allows HHT to be undertaken without fear of rupture or cerebral swelling, which would impede surgical aneurysm exposure. Further studies involving larger numbers of patients are needed before this therapy becomes a standard of care. Early results, however, are promising, and it has found widespread clinical use.

Calcium Channel Blockers

Calcium channel blocker therapy for prophylaxis and treatment of established vasospasm appears promising and can be used safely whether or not the aneurysm is clipped.[77, 78] Enterally administered nimodipine is most commonly used.

Clot Removal

Since the risk of cerebral vasospasm increases with the increase in the amount of blood in the subarachnoid space, removal of clot theoretically might lessen vasospasm. Early trials using surgical irrigation to remove blood had promising results, but clot removal takes time, may be difficult, and may itself produce brain damage. Recently, a phase I trial using recombinant tissue plasminogen activator instilled via ventriculostomy to facilitate clot removal was completed.[79] Ten patients with grade 3 or 4 SAH were enrolled in the study. Six of these patients showed good outcome at 3 months post-SAH. These results, although promising, must be duplicated in trials with larger numbers of patients.

Cerebral Angioplasty

Patients who fail medical treatment may respond to cerebral angioplasty. A small number of patients have been reported to have good results following forced balloon dilation of vasospastic vessels following aneurysm clipping.[80] A risk of arterial rupture or dissection follows this procedure; therefore, it is used only on patients with severely narrowed vessels who are not responsive to medical management.

Does Preoperative Vasospasm Treatment Affect Anesthetic Management?

When HHT is used preoperatively, the patient must be examined carefully for evidence of pulmonary edema. Increased concentrations of O_2 and expiratory positive airway pressure

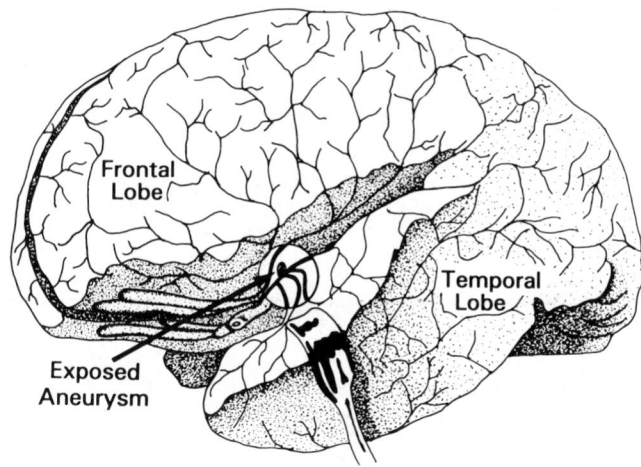

FIGURE 73–5. Aneurysms are generally accessible only by retracting brain tissue. In this case, the sylvian fissure is split and retracted, revealing a middle cerebral artery aneurysm.

may be needed intraoperatively to obtain adequate oxygenation. Some of the calcium channel antagonists, particularly nimodipine, may reduce systemic vascular resistance. If calcium channel blockers are used preoperatively, this effect may necessitate greater amounts of intravenous fluids, vasopressors, or both to maintain adequate blood pressure while the patient is anesthetized.

How Does Aneurysm Clipping Differ from Other Neurosurgical Operations?

Aneurysms are rarely superficial, and access to them generally can only be obtained by spreading anatomic fissures or by retraction on a lobe of the brain (Fig. 73–5). Anterior circulation aneurysms usually are approached via a pterional craniotomy. The sylvian fissure is split, and the frontal and temporal lobes are retracted to reveal the aneurysm. Basilar apex aneurysms usually require a temporal craniotomy and retraction of the temporal lobe superiorly.

Retractor pressure reduces perfusion to the underlying brain and may produce neurologic damage, particularly if perfusion is already reduced by vasospasm or induced hypotension. Therapy directed at decreasing brain bulk is useful in decreasing the amount of retractor pressure necessary to expose the aneurysm (Table 73–9). Methods of reducing brain bulk include mannitol infusion, CSF removal by spinal drain or ventriculostomy, and hyperventilation.

Hyperventilation may be deleterious. A rapid lowering of ICP, as has been discussed previously, can increase transmural aneurysmal pressure, predisposing to rupture. It also may produce further reduction in blood flow to areas of the brain already at risk for ischemia. However, hyperventilation may

TABLE 73–9. Methods to Minimize Retractor Pressure Needed for Exposure

Hyperventilation
Mannitol infusion
CSF drainage (spinal drain, ventriculostomy)
Pharmacologic
Positioning (enhanced venous drainage)

TABLE 73–10. Classification System for Aneurysmal Subarachnoid Hemorrhage

Grade	Description
0	Asymptomatic, never ruptured
1	Headache only, no other symptoms
2	Severe headache, nuchal rigidity, cranial nerve deficit
3	Global alteration of consciousness, major focal neurologic deficit (e.g., hemiparesis)
4	Deep coma
5	Moribund

be necessary to reduce retractor pressure if the other methods are inadequate. It should only be instituted after dural opening unless ICP is very high.

What Is the Impact of Preoperative Central Nervous System Function?

Central nervous system function following SAH is usually determined by four primary factors: brain injury produced by the subarachnoid hemorrhage; cerebral vasospasm; loss of cerebral autoregulation; and hydrocephalus. Patients with focal or global alterations of CNS function and high-grade SAHs (Table 73–10) are likely to have a problem in at least one of these areas. Maintenance of adequate cerebral perfusion during surgery is particularly important in these patients who have lost the ability to maintain and control CBF.

How Does Subarachnoid Hemorrhage Alter Other Organ Systems?

Marked abnormalities can occur in other organ systems following SAH. The most overt problems are cardiopulmonary in origin.

Cardiovascular

New-onset hypertension or exacerbation of previously existing hypertension is common and frequently requires administration of intravenous antihypertensives such as nitroprusside, nitroglycerin, esmolol, or labetalol. Cardiac ischemia also may be produced. Numerous case reports describe electrocardiographic changes with SAH. Early articles suggested that these changes did not correlate with significant myocardial damage or dysfunction.[81, 82] One study supports the view that true myocardial dysfunction following SAH may occur and should be investigated in patients who show significant electrocardiogram abnormalities.[83] The exact mechanism that produces cardiac damage is not clear. Also unclear is how often cardiac dysfunction occurs after SAH and how it should affect management. Usually, electrocardiographic changes and functional changes, such as wall motion abnormalities, resolve within a few days following SAH.[83]

Pulmonary

Cardiogenic and noncardiogenic pulmonary edema also has been reported after SAH. Treatment with increased inspired O_2, positive-pressure ventilation, or continuous positive airway pressure may be required perioperatively. Hypervolemic hypertensive therapy frequently makes this problem worse and may necessitate prolonged intubation and ventilatory support.

How Does Pre-Existing Disease Impact Anesthetic Management?

As just noted, SAH has the potential to cause ischemic myocardial damage in patients without coronary disease. The impact of such damage may be even greater on patients with pre-existing ischemic cardiac disease. Reductions in diastolic blood pressure and increases in heart rate accompanying induced hypotension needed for aneurysm clipping may not be tolerated. Patients with pre-existing pulmonary disease sometimes experience marked decreases in arterial partial pressure of O_2 (PaO_2) if induced hypotension is required, and inhibition of hypoxic pulmonary vasoconstriction leads to worsening of intrapulmonary shunt. Worsening of renal function following induced hypotension may occur in patients with pre-existing disease. Mannitol administration may obscure decreases in urine output that would otherwise occur.

Should Preoperative Medication Be Used?

Sedatives

Patients undergoing cerebral aneurysm clipping following SAH are often heavily premedicated to prevent anxiety- or pain-induced fluctuations in blood pressure. The preoperative neurologic condition of the patient, however, makes *unmonitored* premedication dangerous. Increased ICP from hydrocephalus or intracranial hematoma worsens with respiratory depression and increased arterial partial pressure of CO_2. Preoperative global depression of mental status caused by the hemorrhage or by subsequent vasospasm often leads to inordinate sensitivity from any premedication.

Premedication may result in somnolence, which may simulate neurologic changes that could occur with rebleeding or worsening vasospasm. Rebleeding and vasospasm may preclude operation; therefore, the ability to distinguish between premedication effects and rebleeding is vitally important. My practice is to avoid any CNS-active premedicants until I can be with the patient continuously.

Anticonvulsants

Patients with SAH are at high risk for seizures. They are usually given phenytoin (Dilantin) or phenobarbital on admission to the hospital. Anticonvulsant blood levels should be checked if possible, and the anticonvulsant should be continued preoperatively and throughout surgery into the postoperative period.

Patients Without Hemorrhage or Mass Effect

Patients presenting for elective aneurysm clipping (i.e., they have had no recent SAH) who do not have a giant aneurysm that causes significant mass effect may be safely premedicated. Short-acting agents should be used, however, so that *postoperative* somnolence does not result. Somnolence also could result from clip misplacement, retraction, or a postsurgical hematoma. A long-acting premedicant drug might create difficulties in the differential diagnosis of postoperative somnolence.

What Monitoring Should Be Used?

Urgent or Emergent Clipping

Invasive arterial blood pressure monitoring should be started before induction, if possible, for any hypertensive patient with SAH. Many patients with SAH require intravenous antihypertensive agents and already have an arterial catheter in place. Normotensive, otherwise healthy patients with SAH may have the arterial catheter placed after induction but before such a potent stimulus as intubation.

Some patients with SAH who are felt to be at high risk for vasospasm may already have a pulmonary artery or central venous catheter in place to monitor HHT therapy prior to surgery. Patients with significant symptomatic coronary artery disease or SAH-induced cardiovascular dysfunction may benefit from continuous ST segment analysis, pulmonary artery pressure monitoring, two-dimensional transesophageal echocardiography, or all three. These monitors improve the detection of myocardial ischemia or left ventricular failure induced by HHT or by special techniques such as deliberate hypotension or attempted barbiturate cerebral protection. If these techniques cause serious cardiovascular compromise, appropriate therapy (e.g., volume therapy, inotropic agent administration, or β-blockade) is instituted.

Elective Clipping

Patients undergoing elective aneurysm clipping may have invasive monitors placed following induction. I also place a central venous catheter for the administration of vasoactive drugs when an immediate effect is desired (such as rapidly induced hypotension following inadvertent rupture). I routinely employ a long-arm catheter; this approach avoids the potential complications of pneumothorax or carotid puncture. More invasive monitoring is utilized if pre-existing disease or special techniques such as barbiturate cerebral protection are anticipated.

Electrophysiologic Monitoring

Cortical SSEPs may be used to monitor cerebral function during aneurysm clippings.[84, 85] The best results are seen with anterior circulation aneurysms. If blood flow through the anterior or middle cerebral arteries is reduced, the SSEPs are attenuated or lost. Since most aneurysms are proximally located, all sections of cortex supplied by the artery are equally affected; hence, loss of SSEPs correlates with loss of motor functions as well.

The posterior circulation provides blood via perforating vessels to the somatosensory pathway as it ascends through the brainstem to the thalamus. However, this circulation also supplies blood to large portions of the brainstem that are not involved with the somatosensory pathway. Thus, damage can occur to motor pathways and to the reticular formation, resulting in motor deficit or global depression of consciousness, or both, without any change in SSEPs.[86]

In summary, anterior circulation aneurysms should be monitored with SSEPs whenever possible. Evoked potentials are particularly useful for determining the adequacy of CBF during vasospasm; induced hypotension or hyperventilation; after placement of the aneurysm clip; and during temporary occlusion of major cerebral vessels, even if barbiturates are given. Evoked potentials may also be useful for monitoring the brain during clipping of posterior circulation aneurysms. However, correlation with outcome in this area is not as good.

How Is Anesthesia Managed?

Multiple anesthetic regimens can be used for aneurysm clipping. Common goals of these techniques are listed in Table 73–11. Which drug regimen is used is not particularly important provided that it meets as many of the goals as possible. After induction of anesthesia, good intravenous access should be obtained. Particular care should be taken with patient positioning, as these operations usually are very long. Padding of pressure points is even more important if induced hypotension is planned, since perfusion of compressed skin will be further reduced.

Control of Intracranial Pressure

Patients with SAH rarely have very high ICPs. However, as was discussed previously, therapy directed at decreasing brain bulk is useful to reduce the amount of retractor pressure necessary to expose the aneurysm (see Table 73–9). If possible, anesthetic and adjunctive therapeutic drugs that do not increase brain bulk significantly should be chosen (see Table 73–1). Such choices are not always possible, but the therapeutic maneuvers listed in Table 73–9 often compensate for anesthetic drug–induced increases in brain bulk.

Normocapnia as determined by preoperative blood gas partial pressure measurements should be maintained throughout surgery. The need for and risk of hyperventilation have been discussed in detail previously. Mannitol should be withheld until just before the removal of the bone flap. This regimen produces a maximum decrease in brain bulk at a time when retraction is needed to expose the aneurysm. Spinal fluid drainage via a ventriculostomy or by a spinal drain may be used during some aneurysm clippings. No more than 25 mL of fluid should be drained slowly at one time over 10 to 20 minutes. Fluid should *never* be aspirated. Rapid drainage of CSF produces hypertension, a sharp decrease in ICP, and a predisposition to aneurysmal rupture.

TABLE 73–11. Anesthetic Goals During Aneurysm Surgery

1. Prevention of rapid changes in blood pressure
2. Prevention of rapid changes in ICP
3. Reduction of brain oxygen consumption
4. Maintenance of adequate CBF
5. Reduction in brain bulk to minimize retraction needed just before removal of bone flap
6. Minimal suppression of evoked potentials/electroencephalogram, if employed (see Tables 22–13 and 22–14)
7. Prevention of position-related injuries in these lengthy operations
8. Rapid emergence

Fluid Therapy

The patient should be kept at least normovolemic during surgery in order to maintain adequate blood pressure and cardiac output and to minimize the effects of pre-existing vasospasm on CBF. Hypervolemia associated with HHT may increase cerebral edema and the degree of retractor pressure needed for exposure. I do not recommend instituting hypervolemia until after the aneurysm is clipped. After clipping, particularly if the patient is at risk for vasospasm, moderate hypervolemia is indicated.

The type of fluid used for this therapy is somewhat controversial. Most clinicians employ a mixture of crystalloid, colloid, and blood to produce hypervolemia and maintain a hematocrit at around 30%.[75] Maintenance of at least normal plasma osmolality appears to be very important in the prevention of postoperative cerebral edema.

Animal data suggest that glucose-containing fluids worsen outcome following global cerebral ischemia. In the absence of documented hypoglycemia, such fluids should be avoided, since these patients are at significant risk for intraoperative cerebral ischemia.

Induced Hypotension

Pressure inside an aneurysm is about the same as arterial pressure.[16] The radius of the aneurysm changes in direct proportion to this pressure, and aneurysmal wall tension changes proportionately to the aneurysmal radius. Induced hypotension, therefore, greatly decreases wall tension and the risk of intraoperative rupture. It also decreases aneurysmal bulk, thereby facilitating placement of a clip on the neck, which otherwise would be obscured by the dome.

Risks

Induced hypotension is associated with substantial risk. CBF may be critically reduced, resulting in ischemia. This problem is most likely in the patient with pre-existing vasospasm or longstanding arterial hypertension, or both. Hypotension should be used only with caution in these patients. Electroencephalography or cortical SSEPs are helpful to determine the limits of hypotension when it is needed. Hypotension also may be harmful to other organ systems as has been discussed previously. Many neurosurgeons request hypotension only when catastrophic rupture is imminent or has occurred.

Agents

Certain hypotensive drugs preserve CBF better than do others. Sodium nitroprusside and isoflurane appear to be the current agents of choice. The former agent is easy to titrate and preserves adequate CBF even in the face of severe hypotension (MAP = 40 mm Hg).[87] Thus, sodium nitroprusside is very useful if intraoperative rupture of the aneurysm occurs.

Rapid adjustments of blood pressure are more difficult with isoflurane. However, this drug has a potential advantage over sodium nitroprusside because it maintains CBF *and* reduces brain O_2 consumption.[88] Unfortunately, isoflurane, in the high concentrations sometimes necessary for hypotension, suppresses both the electroencephalogram and cortical evoked potentials. Thus, although CBF may supply the brain with sufficient O_2, documentation of the adequacy of perfusion is not possible. In addition, evidence suggests that despite reductions of $CMRO_2$, isoflurane may not protect the brain from focal ischemia.[4]

Hyperventilation

Since hyperventilation normally reduces CBF, it should be employed with caution when induced hypotension (which may also reduce CBF) is used. One study[89] demonstrated that moderate hypocarbia (arterial partial pressure of CO_2 = 30 mm Hg) and induced hypotension within the autoregulatory range (MAP >50 mm Hg) usually are associated with adequate CBF. Other studies have shown that vasodilators used to induce hypotension impair the brain's vascular response to CO_2. Monitoring with electroencephalography or SSEPs may be helpful to guide therapy.

Cerebral Protection

Hypothermia

The only widely accepted method of producing brain protection is reduction in $CMRO_2$. This reduction may be accomplished by active or passive cooling. Cerebral O_2 demand is reduced approximately 7% per 1 °C decrease in temperature.[90] The temperature should be kept above 33 °C, as the incidence of serious ventricular dysrhythmias begins to increase below this level.

Electroencephalographic Suppression

The O_2 consumed during generation of the cortical spontaneous electroencephalogram may be reduced by several drugs, including barbiturates, etomidate, propofol, and isoflurane (see Table 73–1). The only drugs that nearly all experts agree produce protection from focal ischemia are the barbiturates. Complete suppression of the spontaneous electroencephalogram with barbiturates reduces brain O_2 requirements by about 50%.[91]

This level of suppression may require large doses of barbiturate (e.g., a loading dose of 15 mg $\cdot$ kg^{-1} of thiopental followed by an infusion of 10–30 mg $\cdot$ kg^{-1} $\cdot$ h^{-1}). Additional barbiturate produces no further reduction in cerebral O_2 demand. Since high-dose barbiturate administration is accompanied by marked cardiovascular depression, inotropic support is often required. Phenylephrine, dopamine, dobutamine, epinephrine, and other inotropes have been used successfully in this setting. Interestingly, cortical SSEPs may still be monitored even with total barbiturate suppression of the electroencephalogram.

What Factors Are Important During Emergence?

Most patients who were not neurologically impaired preoperatively may be extubated immediately postoperatively once normal neurologic function has been documented. Patients who do not promptly return to normal function should remain intubated until a cause is determined. Usually, a computed tomography (CT) scan or angiography is needed. Blood pressure should be maintained at normal to moderately elevated levels. This approach is particularly important in patients with vasospasm.

TABLE 73–12. Common Mechanisms of Neural Compression in Patients with Disease of the Spinal Column or Spinal Cord*

Pathology		Symptoms
Disk herniation (D, T)	Posterolateral†	Radicular pain, paresthesias, weakness (radiculopathy)
	Posterior†	Pain, paresthesias or weakness in spinal cord (or cauda equina distribution caudal to disk herniation [myelopathy])
Bone compression (D, T)	Lateral†	Radicular pain, paresthesias
	Anterior†	Pain, paresthesias, or weakness in spinal cord, or cauda equina distribution caudal to bone compression
	Spinal canal stenosis	Radiculopathy or myelopathy, or both, depending on where stenosis occurs and whether there is concomitant disk or bone compression
Instability (C, D, T)		Radiculopathy or myelopathy, or both, depending on where the instability produces compression
Neoplasm	Intramedullary	Sensory, motor, or cerebellar symptoms in distribution of spinal cord distal to lesion
	Extramedullary	Radiculopathy or myelopathy, or both
Syrinx (intramedullary fluid collection)		Sensory, motor, or cerebellar symptoms in distribution of spinal cord distal to lesion

*See also Figure 73–7.
†Denotes direction of herniation or location of bone compression.
Abbreviations: T = trauma-induced; C = congenital; D = degenerative.

Patients who were obtunded preoperatively usually do not improve in the immediate postoperative period. They should not be extubated nor should those with vasospasm undergoing vigorous HHT who may need continued postoperative positive-pressure ventilation. When postoperative maintenance of intubation is planned, frequent assessment of the patient's neurologic status is critical. After initial neurologic assessment, a propofol infusion may be useful. Rapid return to normal mental status occurs after the infusion is discontinued, even if it has been used for a prolonged period.[92]

What Is an Arteriovenous Malformation?

Cerebral arteriovenous malformations (AVMs) are composed of thin-walled vessels that provide varying degrees of direct arteriovenous shunt, depending on their size and flow. These malformations cause preoperative symptoms by a number of mechanisms, including hemorrhage, mass effect, and ''steal'' of blood flow from the surrounding normal brain. Common presenting symptoms include seizures and headaches of varying severity. Hemorrhage produces symptoms similar to those following aneurysmal hemorrhage.

Most AVMs now are treated preoperatively by neuroradiologic embolization. Thrombogenic material is injected into the major arterial feeders of the malformation, lodges in the smaller vessels, and reduces flow through the malformation. This technique helps to reduce intraoperative blood loss and the likelihood of ''breakthrough'' bleeding or edema after the arterial inflow to a high-flow AVM is occluded.

AVMs should not be confused with cavernous malformations or venous malformations, which also are associated commonly with seizures and headache. Unlike AVMs, these lesions only rarely present with hemorrhage; since they lack an arterial component, significant intraoperative bleeding is rare.

Breakthrough Bleeding and Edema

If flow through an AVM is sufficiently high, the surrounding normal brain receives inadequate blood flow. In response, the vessels supplying the normal brain dilate to better ''compete'' with the AVM for blood flow. When the arterial inflow to a high-flow AVM is abruptly stopped during surgery, the surrounding brain receives a much higher blood flow than it did prior to AVM interruption. Vessels leading to the surrounding brain, which have been chronically vasodilated, are initially unable to constrict to reduce flow. The resultant very high blood flow can lead to cerebral edema and frank hemorrhage in the normal brain.

Following AVM inflow occlusion, I routinely lower blood pressure to a mean of 50 to 60 mm Hg in patients with high-flow AVMs provided that other organ systems will tolerate hypotension. Even if intraoperative breakthrough bleeding or edema is absent, either condition may develop after dural closure. This reduction in blood pressure sometimes is necessary for several days before restoration of normal autoregulation occurs. In extreme cases not controlled by these measures, high-dose barbiturates can be used to reduce blood flow and cerebral edema.

SPINAL COLUMN AND SPINAL CORD SURGERY

What Are the Indications?

Generally, patients undergo surgery on the spinal cord or spinal column because they have symptoms related to compression of neural tissue. Common etiologic factors include congenital abnormalities, trauma, degenerative disease, and neoplasms—both intrinsic and extrinsic to the CNS.

Mechanisms of neural compression are shown in Table 73–12 and Figure 73–6. Herniation of disk tissue or abnormal bone compression posterolaterally compresses nerve roots at their exit from the spinal column and produces radiculopathy at the involved level (Table 73–13). Above L1-L2, such changes may compress the spinal cord and produce myelopathy (see Table 73–13). Stenosis of the spinal canal also can produce radiculopathy or myelopathy. More commonly, stenosis worsens the degree of neural compression produced by disk herniation or bone prominences.

Instability that results from trauma, degenerative diseases (e.g., rheumatoid arthritis), or congenital abnormalities (e.g., trisomy 21, Klippel-Feil syndrome) can also produce radiculopathy or myelopathy. Associated neural compression is variable in severity, depending on a patient's position or motion. Symptoms and signs of radiculopathy or myelopathy (see Table 73–13) may be severe under baseline conditions or only occur at extremes of rotation, flexion, or extension. Patients may be asymptomatic, as is frequently the case with patients who have rheumatoid arthritis and atlantoaxial instability.[93]

Nerve root neoplasms can produce radiculopathy in the associated dermatome as the nerve root is progressively stretched by the growing tumor. This neoplasm also can compress the adjacent spinal cord by encroaching upon the limited confines of the spinal column. Intramedullary tumors (arising from the spinal cord) produce myelopathy by stretching white matter pathways and displacing gray matter. Metastatic tumors may involve the bone support structures of the spinal cord and invade the epidural space. Radiculopathy or myelopathy, or both, often result.

Finally, when the normal circulation of CSF is disrupted by tumor or trauma, dissection of fluid into the spinal cord may occur. An intramedullary fluid collection known as *syrinx* displaces and stretches white matter pathways and compresses gray matter.

Why Are Radiculopathy and Myelopathy Important?

These syndromes have significance in four main areas: the method of intubation, positioning, the choice of muscle relaxants during surgery (if used), and blood pressure control.

Intubation and Postioning

Cervical Radiculopathy

Intubation and positioning are particularly important in patients with cervical spine pathology, since the cervical spine is considerably more mobile than is the thoracic or lumbar spine. Thus, positioning changes are more likely to cause exacerbations of pre-existing neural compression.

Patients with cervical radiculopathy have one or more compressed nerve roots. Changes in neck alignment associated with intubation are unlikely to cause nerve root damage, since the roots are relatively resistant to brief periods of worsened compression or ischemia. Most patients with cervical radiculopathy can be intubated following general anesthesia unless

TABLE 73–13. Radiculopathy versus Myelopathy

Syndrome	Motor Function	Sensory Function	Reflexes
Radiculopathy (Signs/symptoms restricted to dermatome)	Normal or weak	Pain or numbness	Decreased
Myelopathy (Signs/symptoms caudal to lesion)	Normal or weak; spasticity common	Pain or numbness	Increased

the preoperative cervical range of motion is also severely compromised.

Prolonged nerve root compression associated with positioning, however, can produce permanent damage. Patients with radiculopathy should be tested preoperatively for the development of symptoms by placing them in the planned surgical position for at least 5 minutes. A 5-minute test is used because such symptoms may take time to develop; shorter exposure of a patient to a surgical position may not demonstrate more slowly developing symptoms.

Cervical Myelopathy

Patients with cervical myelopathy have spinal cord compression at one or more levels. The spinal cord is more sensitive to ischemic damage from compression than are the nerve roots. Position changes that result from intubation may cause increased spinal cord compression. More importantly, worsened compression can result from surgical positioning. Extreme care must be taken with intubation and positioning.

I recommend awake intubation and positioning for any patient with cervical myelopathy so that the patient can warn the anesthesiologist when symptoms are produced by neck movement. In the absence of instability, permanent neurologic damage from intubation and positioning is unlikely to occur in patients with cervical myelopathy. Nevertheless, the consequences of damage to the cervical spinal cord are so great that I consider awake intubation and positioning worthwhile. The actual injury rate is unknown, but isolated case reports of sudden, unexpected perioperative death of myelopathic patients have been reported.[94]

Thoracic and Lumbar Radiculopathy and Myelopathy

Radiculopathy and myelopathy in the thoracic or lumbar spine are unlikely to be affected by intubation and positioning. Only in patients with gross instability does positioning cause worsening of spinal cord compression in these areas. In these rare cases, awake intubation and positioning may be helpful.

Muscle Relaxants

Patients with myelopathy and even radiculopathy are at increased risk for hyperkalemia following succinylcholine administration.[95] In almost all cases, the deficit that results from the radiculopathy and myelopathy is not stable or long-term (i.e., unchanged for 6 months or longer). Thus, succinylcholine use generally should be avoided in such patients.

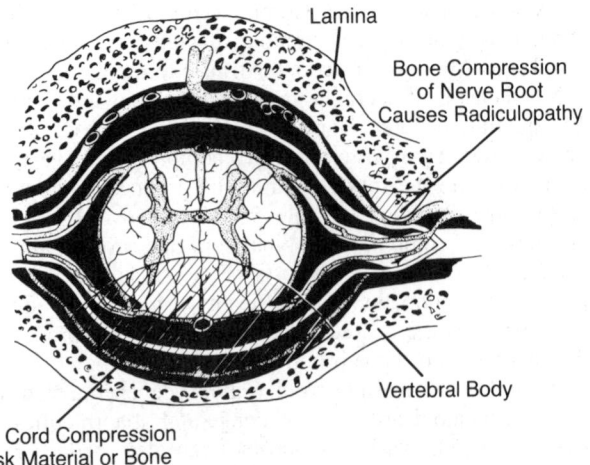

FIGURE 73–6. Schematic of myelopathy versus radiculopathy. Compression of the nerve root produces radiculopathy. Compression of the spinal cord produces myelopathy.

Blood Pressure Control

Blood pressure control is critically important in myelopathic patients. Spinal cord perfusion pressure is defined as MAP minus CSF pressure. In patients with spinal cord compression, however, the perfusion pressure is actually MAP minus the compression pressure. Decreases in blood pressure that normally would cause no concern may cause spinal cord ischemia. Electrophysiologic monitoring may be helpful to decide what level of hypotension needs to be treated (Chapter 22). In the absence of such monitoring, however, blood pressure should be maintained at or above the patient's normal range.

What Operations Are Performed to Relieve Neural Compression?

Diskectomy

Diskectomy is the procedure of choice for disk herniations. In the lumbar spine, this procedure is usually performed through a small, posterior laminotomy. The herniated disk is removed, often with the aid of an operating microscope. In the thoracic spine, a herniated disk may be removed using a posterior approach similar to that used for lumbar surgery or, in some cases, anteriorly through a lateral thoracotomy. In the latter situation, the lung is retracted or deflated using one-lung ventilation.

A lateral extracavitary approach may largely replace thoracotomy to approach disks that cannot be removed posteriorly.[96] With this technique, a small segment of the proximal portion of several ribs is removed. The lung is retracted laterally, exposing the vertebral bodies and the intervertebral disk (Fig. 73–7).

In the cervical spine, disk herniations are most commonly removed using an anterior approach. A small transverse incision is made adjacent to the trachea. Vascular structures are retracted laterally (the trachea may be retracted medially), exposing the vertebral column, and the disk is removed.

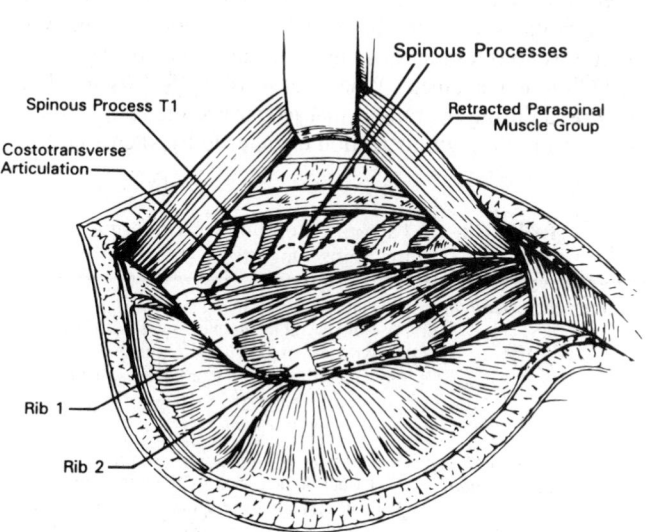

FIGURE 73–7. Schematic of lateral extracavitary approach to the thoracic spine. Removal of the proximal portion of two ribs and retraction of the lung allows access to the spinal column.

Labels on figure: Spinous Process T1; Costotransverse Articulation; Spinous Processes; Retracted Paraspinal Muscle Group; Rib 1; Rib 2

Decompression

Laminectomy, Foramenotomy

In cases of bone compression, the approach depends on whether the compression is caused by posterior, lateral, or anterior elements or by a combination of spinal column components. Global compression is usually treated with laminectomy. If bone decompression of nerve roots is necessary, the nerve root foramen may be widened (foramenotomy). Anterior compression is more difficult to treat. Sometimes, it may be relieved by widening the spinal canal with a posterior laminectomy.

Vertebrectomy

Alternatively, anterior compression is relieved by removing all or a portion of the vertebral body. In the lumbar region, vertebrectomy may be performed using a lateral extracaitary approach while the patient is in a prone position or using a retroperitoneal, thoracoabdominal approach while the patient is in a lateral position. Thoracic vertebrectomy also may be done in the lateral position with a thoracotomy or in the prone position through a lateral extracavitary approach (see Fig. 73–7). In the cervical region, vertebrectomy is performed in the supine position from an anterior approach with retraction on the trachea and vascular structures (as for diskectomy).

Stabilizations and Fusions

Instability may be congenital or result from trauma, other spine surgery (e.g., vertebrectomy), or degenerative disease. It usually is corrected with some form of posterior spinal fusion. Most commonly, fusion is accomplished with both hardware and autologous or homologous bone grafting.

Tumor Excision

The surgical approach to intrinsic spinal neoplasms or spinal cord syrinx is usually posterior laminectomy, the extent of which is determined by the size of the lesion. Extrinsic or metastatic neoplasms that involve the vertebral bodies are approached in the same fashion as anterior bone compression. Those in the epidural space are usually approached posteriorly.

Why Is Preoperative Functional Status Important?

Acute Versus Chronic Changes

Patients with rapidly deteriorating neurologic function must have expedient correction of neural compression if return of function is to occur. If these patients have coexisting disease that can have a potential impact on anesthetic management, work-up and treatment must occur quickly before CNS deterioration becomes irreversible. The outcome of patients with acute traumatic myelopathy may be improved by the administration of high-dose methylprednisolone given within 8 hours of the injury (30-mg · kg^{-1} bolus followed by a 23-hour infusion at 5.4 mg · kg^{-1} · h^{-1}).[97, 98]

Patients with chronic loss of function or pain may be treated more electively; coexisting disease can be adequately evaluated and appropriate treatment started. Knowledge of the level of neurologic function helps to determine whether radiculopathy or myelopathy will affect the methods of intubation and positioning, blood pressure control, and the choice of relaxants.

Blood Pressure Aberrations

Autonomic control of blood pressure often is deranged in acutely or chronically myelopathic patients. Acute, high spinal cord injury may produce spinal shock. The patient loses sympathetic control of heart rate and blood pressure and becomes hypotensive and bradycardic. Compensation for anesthetic-induced cardiovascular depression or hemorrhage with increases in heart rate and peripheral vascular resistance cannot occur. Direct-acting vasopressors and positive chronotropic agents often are necessary to prevent further spinal cord injury from hypotension. Patients with chronic injury may show a similar failure of autonomic dysfunction but in addition can develop autonomic hyperreflexia.

Autonomic Hyperreflexia

When noxious sensations reach the spinal cord, a normal, sympathetically induced spinal reflex causes vasoconstriction in the region of the injury. Generalized vasoconstriction is modulated or prevented by supraspinal sympathetic control. Patients with chronic myelopathy from any mechanism, but most commonly following complete spinal cord injury, permanently lose supraspinal control of the sympathetic nervous system. Thus, local vasoconstriction following noxious stimuli may become generalized. If the level of spinal cord injury is at T-6 or higher, vasodilation above the lesion is insufficient to compensate for generalized vasoconstriction below the lesion. Severe hypertension frequently results. This syndrome is known as autonomic hyperreflexia. It should be anticipated and prevented with spinal blockade or deep anesthesia or rapidly treated with vasodilators.

How Does Pre-Existing Disease Affect Anesthetic Management?

Operative trauma associated with spine surgery varies greatly among the different procedures. A lumbar diskectomy does not usually involve major blood loss or fluid shifts. A thoracic vertebrectomy, however, may be associated with major retraction on the lung as well as large blood loss and third space fluid requirements. Impact of pre-existing disease increases with operative trauma.

Cardiovascular Function

Pre-existing cardiac disease presents problems in any of these operations but has a larger impact during procedures associated with large blood loss or significant third space fluid requirements. In addition, these operations often are conducted with a patient in the prone position. Patients with poor ventricular function may not tolerate the decreased venous return that sometimes occurs. Since these operations frequently are associated with large blood loss, induced hypotension is often used. Reductions in diastolic pressure and increases in heart rate may be poorly tolerated.

Some neurosurgeons prefer that patients undergoing certain spinal operations not be given muscle relaxants so that inadvertent manipulation of neural tissue can be detected by patient movement. An amount of anesthetic agent sufficient to ensure immobility of a patient with poor ventricular function may result in significant undesired hypotension, particularly during periods of reduced stimulation. These patients usually require at least partial neuromuscular blockade to prevent movement-induced injury during microsurgery or pin fixation of the head.

Pulmonary Fixation

Patients with pre-existing pulmonary disease often experience marked decreases in PaO_2 during induced hypotension. Vasodilator-induced inhibition of hypoxic pulmonary vasoconstriction is in large part responsible, as has been discussed previously. The weight of the body on the thorax and cephalic movement of the diaphragm, which are associated with the prone position, reduce functional residual capacity and worsen shunt.

Should Patients Be Premedicated?

Unlike patients undergoing some intracranial procedures, patients scheduled for spine surgery are not at increased risk for premedication compared with the general population unless they have a high cervical lesion and impaired ventilation. Premedication generally may be given as indicated.

What Monitoring Is Needed?

General Considerations

Monitoring for spine surgery should be determined by the factors shown in Table 73–14. Otherwise, healthy patients having disk surgery for radiculopathy can be monitored noninvasively. Those undergoing major spine operations associated with significant blood loss and fluid shifts benefit from invasive arterial blood pressure monitoring, particularly if induced hypotension is planned. Invasive arterial monitoring also facilitates frequent blood gas and laboratory analyses. Central venous pressure monitoring also may be helpful to guide fluid management. Whenever possible, SSEPs should be monitored during operations that jeopardize the spinal cord or its perfusion through distraction or induced hypotension.

TABLE 73–14. Factors Determining Monitoring During Spine Operations

Nature of the Operation	Anticipated blood loss
	Use of special techniques, such as induced hypotension, one-lung ventilation
	Spinal cord blood flow or neural structures at risk from surgery
	Positioning of patient
Preoperative Level of Neurologic Function	Patient with myelopathy at risk for aggravation of neurologic deficit by hypertension
	Patient with complete spinal cord injury at T-6 or higher at risk for autonomic hyperreflexia
Coexisting Disease	Pre-existing cardiac, pulmonary, or renal disease

Preoperative Neurologic Function and Coexisting Disease

Patients undergoing spine operations who are myelopathic require close monitoring of blood pressure to prevent hypotension-induced worsening of neurologic function. Even minor reductions in blood pressure from baseline should be quickly corrected. Patients with serious cardiopulmonary disease may benefit from invasive monitoring even for relatively minor spine procedures.

How Is Anesthesia Induced and Maintained?

Many reasonable anesthetic regimens can be used for patients undergoing spine operations, the common goals of which are listed in Table 73–15. Provided that the regimen chosen meets as many of these goals as possible, the choice of drug or drugs is relatively unimportant. Positioning, however, is extremely important.

Positioning

With the exception of some cervical operations, these procedures are conducted with patients in the prone or lateral position. Careful positioning that avoids stretching or compression of nerves helps to prevent injury during these frequently lengthy operations. Meticulous padding helps to prevent skin breakdown. The prone patient should be placed on chest rolls or a frame that allows the abdomen to be suspended above the table; this minimizes intra-abdominal pressure. Increases in intra-abdominal pressure also are undesirable from a pulmonary standpoint, since higher airway pressures will be necessary for ventilation, the functional residual capacity will decrease, and ventilation-perfusion mismatch will increase. Intra-abdominal pressure increases also impede inferior vena caval venous return to the heart, diverting blood to the epidural venous plexus and the azygos system. Distention of these veins increases surgical bleeding (see Chapter 30).

Head Position in Lumbar and Thoracic Spine Operations

In lumbar and lower thoracic operations, head position is unimportant to the surgeon. Usually, the head is turned to the side and placed on a padded "donut" (Fig. 73–8A). The dependent eye and ear must be absolutely free of pressure to prevent blindness and external ear necrosis, respectively. Turning the head to the side, however, may impede its venous drainage. Because large amounts of intravenous fluids are frequently needed during these operations, severe swelling of the face, tongue, pharynx, and larynx often occurs.

Several foam headrests are available that allow the patient

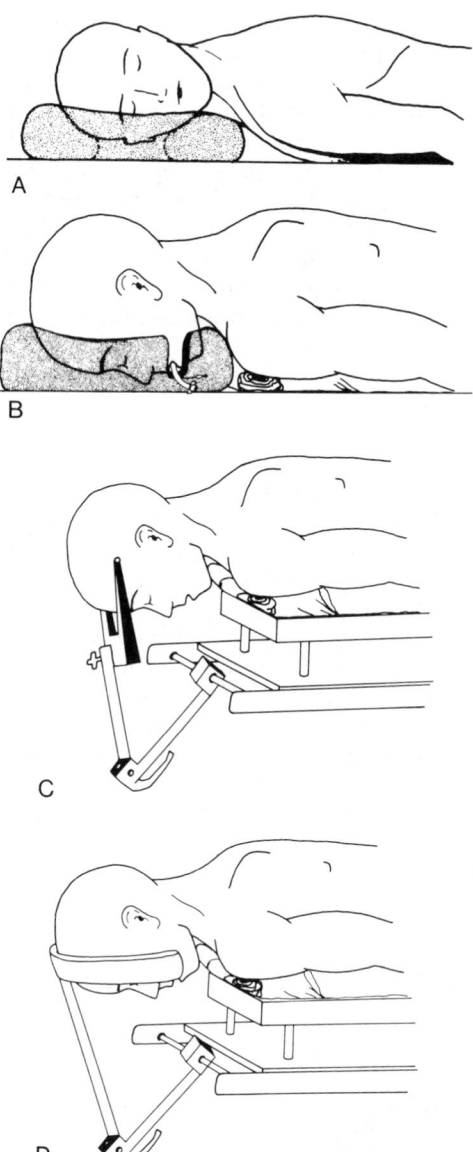

FIGURE 73–8. Positioning the head in the prone position. *A,* The head is rotated to the side and placed on a soft foam donut. Eyes and ears are free of pressure. *B,* The head in the neutral position. The head rests on a foam cushion with a cutout for eyes, nose, and endotracheal tube. *C,* The head in the neutral position. The head is supported by a pinion and is suspended. *D,* The head in the neutral position. The head rests on a horseshoe-shaped headrest that leaves the eyes and nose free of pressure.

to be positioned face-down with the head in the neutral position (see Fig. 73–8B). This position allows unimpeded venous drainage from the head and minimizes soft tissue swelling. These headrests also have cutout sections that prevent pressure on the eyes. Even with the best precautions, however, pressure-related injury to the head may occur during these very lengthy operations. The only reliable way to prevent pressure-related injury to the head is to attach a pinion that suspends the head (see Fig. 73–8C).

Head Position in Cervical Spine Operations

During operations on the cervical spine, the head *must* be kept midline, with the amount of flexion or extension adjustable, depending on the type and level of the operation. Most

TABLE 73–15. Anesthetic Goals During Spine Surgery

1	Preserve spinal cord perfusion
2	Protect patient from position-related injury
3	Minimize blood loss
4	Provide good exposure for surgeons
5	Minimal effect on electrophysiologic monitoring if used (Chapter 22)
6	Rapidly reversible to assess neurologic examination

surgeons utilize a head pinion to hold the head absolutely immobile. If head flexion is desired, I limit the amount so that at least two fingerbreadths of space remain between the mentum and manubrium. A head pinion allows great flexibility in flexing or extending the neck during initial positioning.

Alternatively, the patient may be placed on a foam horseshoe-shaped headrest. The eyes, nose, and mouth are in the open area of the horseshoe, and the forehead and malar eminence are in contact with the foam (see Fig. 73–8D). In my opinion, this headrest should be used only for operations expected to last less than 3 hours. Despite the best precautions, it may cause pressure injuries to the forehead and cheeks if surgery is prolonged or if induced hypotension is used.

Bite Block Insertion

Some type of bite block should be used in all patients undergoing surgery in the prone position to prevent occlusion of the endotracheal tube if the patient's mouth clamps shut during periods of light anesthesia. This complication is much more difficult to treat in the prone position. Oral airways commonly have been used for this purpose. With head flexion, however, this airway may compress the hard and soft palates, producing mucosal necrosis.[99] In addition, it may impair venous drainage from the tongue, resulting in swelling. Because of these problems, I use a hard plastic sleeve that fits over the endotracheal tube and prevents bite occlusion (Fig. 73–9). These sleeves frequently are used for intubated intensive care unit patients. They do not impair tongue drainage, and the potential for palatal pressure injury is minimal.

Fluid Therapy

No data show that one fluid strategy is superior to another during spine surgery. Most clinicians use a mixture of crystalloid and colloid solutions. Blood products are given based on intraoperative losses and the presence of coexisting diseases. I have found that an infusion of up to 1 L of 3% saline solution substantially reduces the total intravenous fluid requirements and appears to reduce postoperative peripheral edema. Although glucose-containing solutions administered during spinal cord ischemia have not been studied in an animal model, I do not use them unless hypoglycemia is documented.

Do Anesthetic Considerations Vary with the Operation?

Lumbar Microdiskectomy

This procedure usually is not associated with major blood loss. However, the aortic bifurcation and iliac arteries are just ventral to the anterior longitudinal ligament in the lumbosacral area; inadvertent laceration of a major artery may occur with resultant massive blood loss. This loss usually is occult, since the retroperitoneal hemorrhage does not escape through the small hole in the anterior longitudinal ligament. The diagnosis should be considered early if unexplained, intractable hypotension occurs during lumbar disk surgery. Failure to diagnose and treat usually almost immediately results in a lethal outcome.

Anterior Cervical Diskectomy, Corpectomy, or Fusion

Exposure during these operations is obtained by lateral retraction of vascular structures and medial retraction of the trachea. The former action may cause compression of the common carotid artery and cerebral ischemia in some patients. Monitoring the superficial temporal pulse during these operations will detect occlusion of the common carotid artery, allowing prompt adjustment of the retractor.

Retraction of the trachea potentially reduces mucosal perfusion by two mechanisms: direct pressure and an increase in endotracheal tube cuff pressure. Restoration of perfusion may predispose to significant postoperative edema. Cuff pressure should be retested after retractor positioning or repositioning and adjusted to produce a minimal seal. If prolonged, significant tracheal retraction is necessary, consideration should be given to leaving the patient intubated postoperatively. However, major retraction usually is unnecessary during diskectomy, and most patients can be extubated immediately following the procedure. The bone plug placed in the empty disk space may become dislodged with coughing and bucking against the tube. A technique that avoids these problems during and prior to extubation is desirable.

During multiple-level corpectomies, particularly at higher levels (C3-5), extensive retraction is often needed. In addition, these operations are sometimes associated with large blood loss. The combination of tracheal retraction with the administration of large amounts of intravenous fluids may cause severe edema of the larynx and upper trachea.

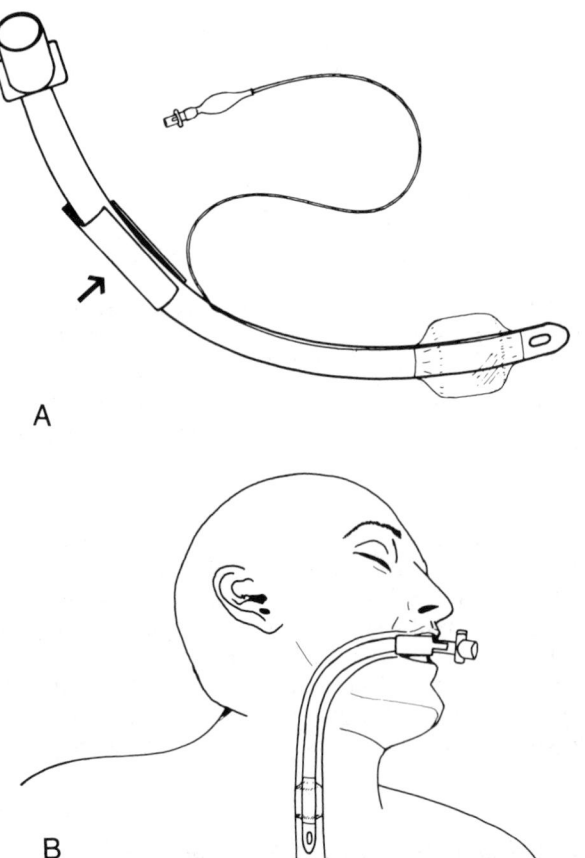

FIGURE 73–9. Bite block protection of the endotracheal tube. *A,* A hard plastic sleeve around the endotracheal tube fits between the teeth. *B,* There is no pressure on the palate, and venous drainage from the tongue is not impaired.

In my opinion, patients who have undergone cervical corpectomy at two or more levels that was associated with significant blood loss should remain intubated postoperatively until the head can be elevated at least overnight to allow swelling to resolve. Serious problems admittedly are uncommon, but when airway obstruction occurs after these operations, reintubation is sometimes impossible, necessitating emergency cricothyroidotomy or tracheotomy. As with diskectomies, coughing and bucking should be prevented.

Spinal Fusions with Instrumentation and Distraction

Many forms of spinal instrumentation place neural tissue at risk, particularly if instruments invade the spinal canal or if distraction of the spinal column is planned to correct scoliosis or kyphosis. Blood loss may be extensive, and induced hypotension is often used.[100] The combination of induced hypotension and distraction of the spinal column may produce critical reductions in spinal cord blood flow. Monitoring of sensory or motor evoked potentials is recommended for early detection of reduced spinal cord blood flow or of instrumentation-related problems during posterior spinal fusions. The wake-up test also is used to assess motor function after distraction and instrumentation are complete. Both of these techniques have special requirements for anesthesia (see Chapter 22).

No large-scale prospective randomized studies demonstrate reduction in blood loss with induced hypotension during these operations. The practice is nonetheless widespread. Agents and techniques include sodium nitroprusside, nitroglycerin, trimethaphan, hydralazine, α- and β-blocking agents, and deep inhalation anesthesia. Deep inhalation anesthesia has the advantage of easy control of blood pressure without invasive monitoring. However, it often makes SSEP monitoring difficult and motor evoked potential monitoring impossible. I prefer nitroglycerin or sodium nitroprusside in combination with a β-blocker such as esmolol, propranolol, or labetalol to reduce the vasodilator dose.

Lateral Extracavitary and Anterior Thoracic Corpectomy or Diskectomy

These procedures, particularly when performed in the upper thoracic spine, require retraction of the lung in order to gain exposure. In such cases, one-lung ventilation may be helpful to the surgeon. Two cautionary notes are important. First, induced hypotension to reduce blood loss combined with one-lung ventilation create potential major problems with oxygenation. Second, if the procedure is associated with major blood loss, changeover from a double-lumen endotracheal tube to a single-lumen tube at the end of the operation may be extremely hazardous because of airway edema. I have found endotracheal tubes with a built-in bronchial blocker to be extremely useful in these cases. The bronchial blocker may be withdrawn at the end of the operation, thus making an endotracheal tube change unnecessary (see Chapter 68).

Neoplasms

Spinal neoplasms necessitate special anesthetic considerations because of the potential for bleeding and because of the need to monitor spinal cord function. The greatest blood loss may be expected from tumors that involve the skeleton. Con-

trol of hemorrhage from these lesions is difficult until resection is complete, and the potential for massive blood loss is high. Preoperative embolization of the tumor may help to reduce intraoperative blood loss.

Patients with neoplasms frequently have myelopathy. Thus, avoiding even minor degrees of hypotension is a major goal. Induced hypotension to reduce blood loss should not be used, in my opinion, despite the risks associated with transfusion. If myelopathy is not present, deliberate hypotension may be useful.

Trauma

Spine trauma creates special anesthetic considerations because of instability, spinal cord injury, the potential for bleeding, and the need to monitor spinal cord function.

Instability

The impact of spinal instability is greatest in the cervical region. Movement of the head and neck during intubation and positioning may cause injury or exacerbate pre-existing injury. Patients with an unstable cervical spine should be intubated and positioned while awake, if possible, so that the neurologic function can be carefully monitored. Alternatively, if a patient cannot tolerate awake intubation and positioning, SSEPs may be monitored and then continued during the stabilization procedure. Such monitoring helps to ensure that proper spinal alignment is maintained and that the instrumentation used for stabilization does not injure the spinal cord.

Because of support from surrounding tissues, movement has much less impact on thoracic and lumbar spinal alignment. Most patients with instability in these regions can be intubated and positioned after induction of anesthesia with little risk of damage to the spinal cord. However, if the patient has severe instability with bone or disk material in the spinal canal, I recommend awake positioning or SSEP monitoring.

Injury

Spinal cord injury associated with trauma impacts on anesthetic management in four areas: sympathetic nervous system function; choice of muscle relaxants; control of blood pressure; and use of steroids to improve outcome.

Sympathetic Dysfunction. As was discussed earlier, both acute and chronic spinal cord injury may affect sympathetic nervous system function. Spinal shock often occurs in the acute setting and produces hypotension and bradycardia; autonomic hyperreflexia may occur in the chronically injured patient. The latter condition does not occur until after spinal shock has resolved. Direct-acting vasopressors and vasodilators should be readily available to control blood pressure in both the acute and chronically injured patient.

Succinylcholine-Induced Hyperkalemia. After loss of innervation following nerve, spinal cord, or brain injury, rapid up-regulation of acetylcholine receptors on the muscle membranes occurs and becomes significant 48 hours after the injury. After that time, succinylcholine administration may produce a massive release of potassium, particularly if the denervated muscle mass is large. Thus, succinylcholine may be used safely if needed for an acute injury situation but should be avoided if the injury is more than 48 hours old. Chronically denervated muscle will atrophy, and succinylcholine is unlikely to produce hyperkalemia if stable denervation injuries are older than 6 months. However, I still avoid this drug, even in chronically denervated patients, unless a rapid sequence induction is absolutely necessary.

High-Dose Methylprednisolone. High-dose methylprednisolone, begun within 8 hours of the spinal cord injury with a bolus dose of 30 mg · kg^{-1}, followed by a 23-hour infusion of 5.4 mg · kg^{-1} · h^{-1} significantly improved outcome in a prospective, randomized, placebo-controlled study.[97, 98] This therapy should be initiated in any patient presenting for surgery acutely following spinal cord injury or when spinal cord injury occurs or is suspected intraoperatively.

Blood Pressure Control. Blood pressure control is important for patients with spinal cord injury. Spinal cord blood flow falls following injury when the injured spinal cord cannot autoregulate its blood flow. Decreases in blood pressure reduce blood flow and potentially aggravate the injury. Induced hypotension, as noted previously, should not be used to reduce blood loss.

INTRACRANIAL NEOPLASM

What Are Intracranial Neoplasms?

Intracranial neoplasms may arise from any intracranial tissue or may be metastatic. An estimated 24,000 primary brain tumors and an equal number of metastatic brain tumors are diagnosed each year in the United States, resulting in an overall incidence of 8 to 10 per 100,000 population.[101] Tumors that arise from glial cells are the most common, followed by those that arise from the meninges. Characteristics vary according to the type of neoplasm. Those that are important to anesthetic management are listed in Table 73–16, whereas some of the more common types of intracranial tumors and their important characteristics are categorized in Table 73–17.

Why Are Tumor Size and Rate of Growth Important?

Size of a tumor would seem, a priori, to be the most important factor determining ICP. The ICP–volume curve (Fig. 73–10) demonstrates that pressure changes very little until a *significant* volume is added. Most figures similar to this one do not specify numerical values on the x-axis because the point at which ICP increases varies with the rate at which the volume is added. For example, a rapidly growing mass such as an epidural hematoma (which expands over minutes) or a glioblastoma multiforme (Fig. 73–11*A*) with edema (which expands over weeks or months) produces a much higher ICP than a very slowly growing meningioma (which expands over years) (see Fig. 73–11*B*) that is actually twice as large.

TABLE 73–16. What Properties of Brain Tumors Are Important?

Size
Growth rate → ICP and cerebral elastance
Location
Surrounding edema
Vascularity
Effects of neurologic function
Seizures?

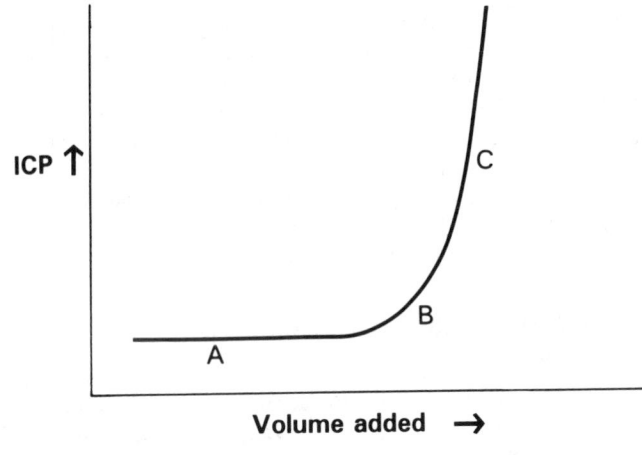

FIGURE 73–10. Intracranial elastance curve. *A*, Normal elastance. *B*, Reduced elastance (small ICP increase with increasing intracranial volume). *C*, Poor elastance (large ICP increase with minimal increase in cerebral volume).

As a rapidly growing tumor or hematoma increases in size, compensatory mechanisms act immediately to prevent rises in ICP: CSF is displaced to spinal levels, and CBV (mainly venous) is decreased. Neural tissue, however, is not acutely compressible; once CSF and blood mechanisms have been exhausted, pressure begins to rise rapidly (see Fig. 73–10*B* and *C*). A global rise in ICP is accompanied by direct pressure of the expanding mass on adjacent neural tissue; this causes loss of function.

Chronic, gradual compression of neural tissue also can occur. The slowly growing tumor may reach a very large size, producing slow displacement and compression of neural tissue without any increase in ICP. Displacement of CSF or blood may not even occur, and structures such as the falx cerebri or the ventricles may not show any shift from normal position (see Fig. 73–11*B*). Computed tomographic and magnetic resonance imaging scans may provide clues as to whether a mass has caused an increase in ICP (Table 73–18). These signs are by no means quantitative and do not substitute for pressure measurements. Thus, size and rate of growth must be considered together when one tries to determine whether a patient has elevated ICP or decreased intracranial elastance, or both.

Why Is Treatment of Cerebral Edema Important?

Some tumors cause the surrounding brain to develop edema (see Table 73–17). Brain edema surrounding a tumor is indicative of the failure of normal capillary endothelial blood-brain barrier function. Sodium, which normally does not cross the blood-brain barrier, crosses freely and brings water with it, producing cerebral edema located mainly in the white matter extracellular space. This edema is termed *vasogenic edema*. When edema is limited to a small area or is mild in degree, it is of little clinical significance. When more generalized or severe, however, edema leads to loss of neural function. The increase in brain water surrounding a mass further aggravates any increase in ICP caused by tumor size and rate of growth. Reduction of this edema with preoperative steroid treatment often substantially lowers ICP and improves cerebral elastance. Steroids are thought to restore normal capillary permea-

TABLE 73–17. Important Properties of Common Intracranial Neoplasms

Skull	ICP rarely elevated May be very vascular
Meninges (Meningioma)	Cause symptoms by compressing neural tissue Slow growth, may attain very large size with relatively few symptoms ICP varies, but in general is not frankly elevated because of slow growth; elastance may be poor Supratentorial or infratentorial in location Often hypervascular; blood loss may be great Variable edema Seizures common
Glial Cells (Glioma, oligodendroglioma, optic nerve glioma, medulloblastoma, ependymoma)	Cause symptoms by compressing neural tissue Highly malignant gliomas grow rapidly, whereas less malignant gliomas grow slowly ICP varies, may be very high with rapidly growing tumors Supratentorial or infratentorial in location Variable vascularity, frequently hypovascular Variable edema Seizures common
Pituitary Gland (Pituitary adenoma)	Cause symptoms secondary to endocrine dysfunction and compression of surrounding tissue (optic nerve, cranial nerves III, IV, and VI, hypothalamus) Growth slow ICP usually normal Usually not hypervascular Edema uncommon
Hypophyseal Duct (Craniopharyngioma)	Cause symptoms by compressing pituitary gland (panhypopituitarism, diabetes insipidus) and optic chiasm Growth rate slow ICP may be elevated, especially if tumor invades third ventricle and causes hydrocephalus Not hypervascular Edema uncommon
Blood Vessel (Hemangioblastoma)	Cause symptoms by cerebellar compression Growth rate variable Posterior fossa hypertension possible Occurs only in posterior fossa or spinal cord; most commonly in cerebellum, occasionally arise from brainstem Brainstem compression possible Very hypervascular, massive hemorrhage possible Hematocrit frequently high on presentation
Cranial Nerve (Acoustic schwanomma, other cranial nerve schwannomas rare)	Cause symptoms by stretching eighth cranial nerve (deafness, tinnitus), adjacent cranial nerves (VII, V, IX, X), and with large tumors, compression of cerebellum (ataxia), brainstem, and fourth ventricle (hydrocephalus) Growth rate slow Posterior fossa hypertension with larger tumors; supratentorial ICP elevated when hydrocephalus occurs Ninth and tenth cranial nerve involvement may depress airway reflexes Vascularity variable Edema uncommon
Metastatic (Lung, melanoma, breast, renal, gastrointestinal)	Cause symptoms by compressing neural tissue Growth rate variable, but usually rapid ICP varies, may be very high with rapidly growing tumors Supratentorial or infratentorial in location Variable vascularity Variable edema Seizures common

bility. Their effect is rapid, with improvement of symptoms noted in hours.

How Does Tumor Location Influence Management?

Positioning

Location of a tumor affects many aspects of anesthetic management. First, it determines the position chosen for surgery. In general, all positions used for craniotomy have some degree of head elevation, the details of which were discussed earlier.

Retraction and Brain Bulk Reduction

Location also determines the need for surgical retraction and affects the requirement for brain bulk reduction (hyperventilation, mannitol, spinal fluid drainage). If the tumor is located on the cortical surface, retraction is minimal. In this case, if ICP is not elevated, mannitol and hyperventilation usually are unnecessary and sometimes are deleterious. For example, if mannitol is given during resection of a small, superficial meningioma, the distance between the dura and cortical surface at the conclusion of surgery can be increased greatly, allowing a postoperative collection of blood and CSF. On the other hand, if this same small meningioma is located on the sphenoid wing, retraction of the frontal and temporal lobes is needed to reach the tumor. Mannitol and hyperventi-

TABLE 73–18. Computed Tomographic and Magnetic Resonance Imaging Scan Signs of Increased Intracranial Pressure*

- Shift of structures from normal anatomic position
- Small or absent ventricles
- Loss of cortical folds
- Loss of CSF in prepontine and mesencephalic cisterns
- Cerebral edema (white matter)
- Hydrocephalus with loss of cortical folds

*See also Figure 73–11A.

lation in this case are beneficial as these reduce the amount of retractor pressure necessary for tumor exposure.

Nearby Structures

Tumor location near or involving important intracranial structures can be a critical factor. A large sphenoid wing meningioma frequently envelops the carotid artery or middle cerebral artery, or both. In this case, large-bore venous access is needed in the event that major hemorrhage occurs. Electrophysiologic monitoring and barbiturate cerebral protection are useful if temporary vessel occlusion is necessary for tumor resection.

Why Is Vascularity Important?

Tumors have widely varying vascularity (see Table 73–17). Meningiomas, hemangioblastomas, and some metastatic lesions carry a significant risk of serious intraoperative hemorrhage. These tumors may be embolized preoperatively to help reduce intraoperative blood loss. Resection of vascular tumors necessitates large-bore intravenous access. Measurement of central venous or pulmonary artery pressures helps to guide fluid replacement.

What Operations Are Performed?

Craniotomy

Surgical procedures for intracranial neoplasms are performed for several reasons, including definitive, curative re-

moval, debulking of tumor mass in nonsurgically curable lesions, and tissue biopsy for pathologic diagnosis. For curative removal and debulking operations, a formal craniotomy is performed, and the lesion is completely removed. Lesions in the frontal, temporal, parietal, and occipital regions are approached by removing a plate of bone (i.e., craniotomy), opening the dura, and excising the tumor.

If the tumor is not on the surface, retraction of neural tissue or an incision in the cortex is necessary to gain access for tumor removal or debulking. The bone plate is usually replaced after surgery. Because of the thickness of the bone in the suboccipital region, craniotomy with removal of a bone plate often is not possible. Instead, burr holes are made and then widened by removing small bites of bone at a time (craniectomy). This bone usually is not replaced.

Stereotactic Surgery

Local Anesthetics

For patients in whom surgical cure is either impossible or associated with major morbidity, tissue diagnosis may be obtained using stereotactic neurosurgical techniques performed with local anesthetics. These techniques greatly decrease surgical trauma and hospital stay. Prior to stereotactic neurosurgery, the patient's head is secured in a radiopaque frame using local anesthesia for pin fixation. A CT scan is then made (Fig. 73–12A). The radiopaque frame places reference points on the CT scan. Using these reference points, computer calculations are made to localize the tumor with reference to the frame.

Upon completion, the patient is taken to the operating room, and the scalp is prepared. A sterile operating frame is attached to the stereotactic frame (see Fig. 73–12B). Using coordinates determined from the CT scan, the surgeon drills a small burr hole using local anesthesia. A biopsy needle is placed to a calculated depth, and the tissue sample is sent to the lab. Once the adequacy of the sample is confirmed by frozen section, the incision is closed, and the patient is again taken to the CT scanner to make certain that hemorrhage has not occurred. The patient is discharged home the next day.

General Anesthesia

When the patient is not cooperative, stereotactic biopsy may also be done under general anesthesia. If the stereotactic frame

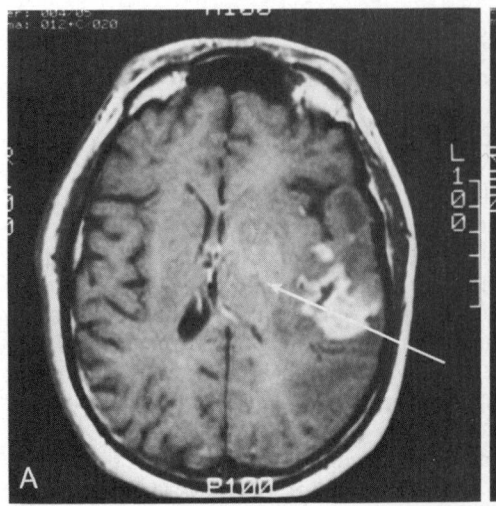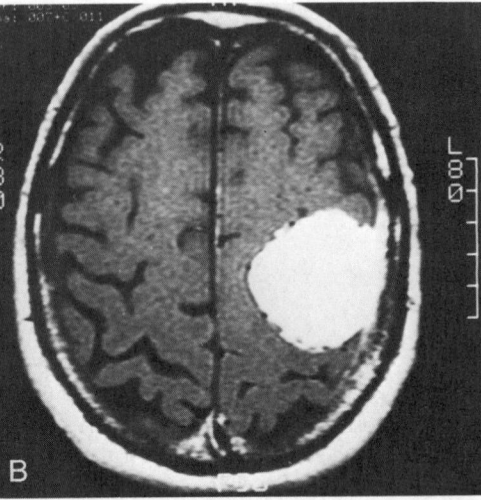

FIGURE 73–11. *A,* Magnetic resonance scan of a patient with glioblastoma multiforme. Note the shift of structures *(arrow)* and loss of cortical folds. *B,* Magnetic resonance scan of a patient with a meningioma. Note the absence of shift in structures and the preservation of cortical folds despite the presence of a very large tumor.

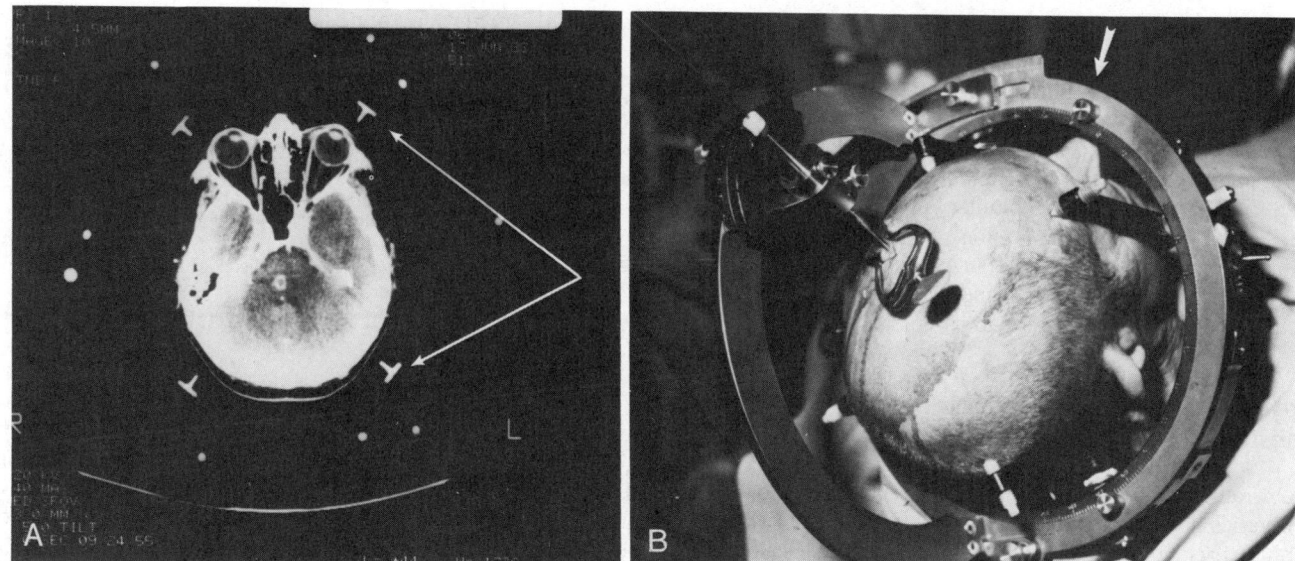

FIGURE 73–12. *A,* Computed tomography scan of a patient with a stereotactic frame in place. Note the coordinates placed by the frame on the scan *(arrow).* *B,* A patient in the operating room with a stereotactic frame in place. Note that this frame interferes with access to the airway *(arrow).*

is placed on the patient's head prior to the induction of anesthesia, airway management may be extremely difficult, since the inferior portion of the frame crosses in front of the mouth and nose and interferes with both mask ventilation and intubation (see Fig. 73–12). If possible, the patient should be anesthetized and intubated prior to placement of the frame.

Alternatively, the frame may be placed under local anesthesia in the CT scanner as was described previously. The patient is then taken to the operating room, and an awake, fiberoptic tracheal intubation is performed. When the airway is secured, induction of general anesthesia follows. Some newer stereotactic devices allow removal of the portion of the frame in front of the airway, thus avoiding these problems.

How Does Preoperative Neurologic Function Influence Management?

General Considerations

Tumors have a variety of effects on preoperative neurologic function. Faster growing tumors with surrounding edema and tumors located near eloquent areas of the brain (i.e., areas whose function may be tested by clinical examination) have the greatest effects. Vasogenic edema also may produce loss of function. In contrast, slowly growing tumors may reach a very large size without changing neurologic function at all.

Seizures

New onset of seizures is a common presentation of an intracranial mass. Seizures can occur with tumors of any size. They are most common with those located in the cerebral cortex. Tumors in subcortical regions or in the posterior fossa usually are not accompanied by seizure activity. Therapeutic anticonvulsant levels should be attained preoperatively in patients with seizures. Unless intraoperative electrocorticography for seizure localization is planned, therapy should be continued during surgery, and levels should be checked again postoperatively.

Patients with cortical tumors who do not have seizures usually are started on prophylactic anticonvulsants either preoperatively or during surgery. This therapy helps to prevent postoperative seizures, which are common following manipulation of the cerebral cortex. Patients with subcortical tumors (e.g., pituitary adenoma) or with tumors in the posterior fossa (e.g., acoustic neuroma) usually do not require seizure prophylaxis.

Many anticonvulsants induce hepatic microsomal enzymes. Thus, another consequence of anticonvulsant therapy is that hepatically metabolized anesthetic drugs (e.g., muscle relaxants and narcotics) can have a remarkably reduced duration of clinical effect.

Homeostatic Mechanisms

Laboratory studies of experimental brain tumors and clinical data suggest that autoregulation and CO_2 responses are impaired or absent.[102, 103] Tumors may also influence homeostatic mechanisms in the surrounding brain. If function of an area of the brain remains normal, autoregulation and response to CO_2 likely are intact. If function is lost, either from direct compression of neural tissue or from the development of edema, both autoregulation and response to CO_2 are likely impaired or lost in that region. If autoregulation is lost (see Fig. 73–1*B*), slight decreases in blood pressure within the normal range may produce a significant reduction in CBF, whereas increases augment CBF and CBV.

When intracranial elastance is poor, even small changes in CBV produce large changes in ICP. Thus, careful control of blood pressure is extremely important in the patient with an intracranial mass and impaired autoregulation. If the response to CO_2 is also lost, hyperventilation does not decrease CBF or CBV in the affected area. Other methods of ICP control or brain bulk reduction, such as mannitol infusion and drainage of CSF through a ventriculostomy catheter, must be used in these patients.

Rapidity of Deterioration

Patients with intracranial mass, severe headache, and rapidly deteriorating level of consciousness likely have significantly elevated ICP and may be close to herniation. When coexisting disease impacts on anesthetic management, work-up and treatment must take place quickly. No medical conditions take priority over surgical decompression of a patient with impending cerebral herniation.

Patients with preoperative *focal* abnormalities may also need urgent surgery. A large pituitary tumor may be associated with rapidly deteriorating vision. Urgent optic nerve decompression is needed to prevent permanent blindness. Preoperative communication with the neurosurgeon helps to determine the urgency of an individual operation.

How Does Pre-Existing Disease Affect Anesthetic Management?

Operative trauma associated with intracranial tumor resection varies greatly. Removal of a small, superficial, low-grade glioma does not usually involve major blood loss or fluid shifts. Mannitol is unnecessary to reduce ICP. Removal of a large meningioma or glioblastoma multiforme, however, may be associated with a significant blood loss. In this situation, mannitol may be necessary to reduce brain bulk and lower ICP.

Cardiovascular Function

Pre-existing cardiac disease may present problems in any of these operations but has a greater impact during procedures that are associated with large blood loss or that require mannitol administration to lower ICP. Acutely, mannitol increases preload and may precipitate congestive heart failure. Later, mannitol-induced reduction of ventricular preload is not well tolerated by patients with poor ventricular function and can result in significant hypotension unless preload is maintained. Many of these operations are conducted with patients in positions other than the supine. Patients with poor ventricular function, as has been noted repeatedly, may not tolerate decreased venous return that is sometimes associated with the sitting, prone, or three-quarter prone positions.

Pulmonary Function

Nearly all neurosurgical positions, with the exception of the sitting position, are associated with a marked reduction in functional residual capacity. Patients with pre-existing pulmonary disease may experience worsening of ventilation/perfusion mismatch after positioning, particularly in the prone, three-quarter prone, or lateral position. Unless the patient is obese, the sitting position generally is well tolerated.

Can Patients with Intracranial Masses Be Safely Premedicated?

Patients with intracranial masses may be very sensitive to premedication for two reasons. First, many premedications produce respiratory depression. Increases in arterial partial pressure of CO_2 cause increases in CBF and CBV and may result in a dangerous increase in ICP. Second, some brain tumors, particularly those located in the frontal lobes or in the posterior fossa, seem to cause increased sensitivity to the sedating and respiratory depressant properties of premedicant drugs.

TABLE 73–19. Premedication for Patients with Intracranial Masses

- After the preoperative interview, if the patient appears calm, a premedication is usually not needed.
- If the patient appears very anxious, the patient is brought to the preoperative holding area, and premedication is given. Pulse oximetry with the patient breathing room air is monitored to facilitate early detection of respiratory depression. Neurologic function is monitored by the preoperative nursing personnel.
- Do not give premedication or sleeping medications to patients with brain tumors who are in unmonitored environments.

Therefore, the simplest and safest answer to the question posed by this section is "No." However, many of these patients are appropriately anxious and benefit from anxiolysis. Patients with intracranial masses but normal intracranial elastance readily tolerate mild to moderate respiratory depression and exhibit normal sensitivity to premedication. Several sedative medications such as diphenhydramine and hydroxyzine are not associated with respiratory depression. Some premedications such as barbiturates, although producing respiratory depression, may be associated with a smaller increase in CBV because of their own cerebral vasoconstricting properties.

My premedication practice for these patients is shown in Table 73–19. This policy clearly is very conservative. However, since most of these patients are admitted to the hospital *after* surgery, no other method is both feasible *and* safe.

What Monitoring Is Necessary?

Monitoring needs for intracranial mass resections are determined by several factors (Table 73–20). As with other neurosurgical procedures, coexisting cardiac, pulmonary, or renal disease may impose requirements independent of the operation.

Type of Operation

The first consideration, obviously, is the nature of the operation. A limited stereotactic procedure conducted under local anesthesia needs only routine, noninvasive monitoring. Definitive resection of a highly vascular large meningioma that may involve major blood loss necessitates invasive arterial pressure monitoring.

Resection of mass lesions located next to eloquent CNS structures may require special monitoring to prevent neurologic damage. Consider the patient with a left temporal lobe mass located near the speech center. In order to localize the

TABLE 73–20. Factors Influencing Monitoring for Removal of an Intracranial Mass

Nature of the operation
    Limited procedure for tissue diagnosis versus definitive removal
    Anticipated blood loss
    Location of the lesion, adjacent neural structures at risk from surgery
    Sudden vital sign changes likely during manipulation of neural structures
    Positioning of the patient
Preoperative intracranial elastance and ICP
Coexisting disease
    Pre-existing cardiac, pulmonary, or renal disease

speech center precisely and thus prevent inadvertent resection of eloquent tissue, resection is best performed using local anesthesia. The function of the neural tissue can then be tested while the patient is awake and can talk (see Chapter 22).

Localization within the motor cortex is possible by using direct intraoperative electrical stimulation of the cortex and by observing a peripheral motor response. In similar fashion, the sensory cortex may be localized by electrical stimulation of peripheral nerves and by recording the response directly from the cortex.

Occasionally, tumors are located near or involve structures that when manipulated may cause large changes in blood pressure or heart rate. For example, some posterior fossa tumors involve the vagus nerve. Resection of these tumors may be associated with sudden severe bradycardia or asystole. Central venous access in these cases is helpful to administer drugs for correction of life-threatening, surgically induced hemodynamic instability.

Positioning

Resections, particularly when tumors are located in the posterior fossa, may be conducted with the patient in the sitting position. As discussed previously, the precordial Doppler and central venous catheter are helpful in the diagnosis and treatment of venous air embolism. Many posterior fossa explorations are conducted with the patient in the three-quarter prone position; they also are associated with a significant incidence of air embolism.[104] In my experience, craniofacial repairs in children and bifrontal craniotomies in adults also are associated with a high incidence of venous air emboli. Precordial Doppler monitoring is noninvasive and inexpensive. I use it routinely when the head is elevated >30°.

Increased Intracranial Pressure and Decreased Elastance

Preoperative intracranial elastance and ICP also influence monitoring. Patients with high ICP or poor intracranial elastance are at high risk for hypotension-related decreases in cerebral perfusion. If possible, invasive arterial monitoring should be started before induction of anesthesia to enable rapid detection and correction of hypotension.

How Should Anesthesia Be Managed?

Anesthetic planning for removal of intracranial masses centers on three factors: the type of operation, the type of tumor (see Table 73–17), and the patient's position (see Tables 73–3 and 73–4). Multiple anesthetic regimens can be used (see Table 73–1). Common goals are listed in Table 73–21. As always, provided that the anesthetic regimen chosen meets as many of these goals as possible, the choice of drug and technique are relatively unimportant to the operation's success. Outcome studies examining intraoperative conditions and postoperative parameters such as rapidity of emergence and use of antihypertensive agents fail to demonstrate a difference between drug regimens when all drugs are used appropriately.[1–3]

Positioning

Careful positioning that avoids nerve stretching or compression and application of padding to avoid pressure on the skin

TABLE 73–21. Anesthetic Goals During Intracranial Tumor Surgery

1	Prevention of decreases in cerebral perfusion and CBF
	   Prevent decreases in blood pressure
	   Prevent increases in ICP

2	Reduction in brain bulk *if needed* to decrease ICP and minimize retraction needed for tumor exposure
3	Protection of patient from position-related injury, including air embolism
4	Rapid emergence to allow neurologic assessment at the conclusion of surgery

help to avoid position-related injury in these frequently very lengthy operations.

Head Position

Elevation of the head above the level of the heart facilitates venous drainage and minimizes the effect of intracranial venous blood volume on intracranial elastance and ICP. A balance assessment between the beneficial ICP and elastance effects of head elevation and the harmful risk of air embolism must be made.

No studies determining the degree of head elevation that produces an ideal balance have been performed. The normal CVP of most patients is between 5 and 15 cm H_2O. I speculate that for a normovolemic patient, a head elevation of ≤20° probably is not associated with greatly subatmospheric cerebral venous pressures and high risk of venous air embolism. This degree of elevation still provides excellent venous drainage and minimizes venous blood volume. Rotation of the head away from midline may impede venous drainage and increase cerebral venous blood volume. Significant rotation may also impede vertebral artery flow.[105]

If surgical exposure requires a head rotation of >30°, I turn the body until neck rotation is <30° while keeping the head fixed in position. This goal may require that the patient be placed nearly lateral, lateral, or even beyond lateral into the three-quarter prone or prone position. When the surgeon requests head flexion, I limit it so that at least 2 fingerbreadths of distance remain between the mentum and the manubrium.

Bite Block Insertion

Some type of bite block is desirable to prevent occlusion of the endotracheal tube if the patient's mouth clamps shut during periods of light anesthesia. Since craniotomies are frequently associated with some degree of head flexion, the oral airway, as discussed previously, may compress the hard and soft palates, producing mucosal necrosis.[99] A hard plastic sleeve that is fitted over the endotracheal tube effectively prevents bite occlusion (see Fig. 73–9) without causing oropharyngeal injury.

How Should Fluids Be Managed?

Classical teaching recommends that patients undergoing resection of an intracranial tumor should be kept relatively hypovolemic, presumably to prevent edema related increases in brain bulk and ICP. As our understanding of the blood-brain barrier has improved, several investigators have questioned the wisdom of this management. Three concepts—osmolality, tissue elastance, and colloid oncotic pressure—must be understood.

Plasma Osmolality

Osmolality is the number of osmotically active particles per kilogram of solvent (Osm $\cdot$ kg^{-1}). Osmolality is determined by a measurement technique known as *freezing point depression*. A solution with more osmotically active particles than another shows greater depression of its freezing point. Solution osmolality (a measured parameter) may be roughly estimated by calculation of its osmolarity. The calculation assumes that all dissolved molecules completely dissociate in solution. For example, normal saline has a sodium chloride concentration of 154 mmol $\cdot$ L^{-1}. Completely dissociated, this solution would have a concentration of 154 mEq $\cdot$ L^{-1} of sodium and 154 mEq $\cdot$ L^{-1} of chloride. The calculated osmolarity is 154 $\times$ 2 = 308 mOsm $\cdot$ L^{-1}. Sodium chloride molecules, however, are not completely dissociated in solution. This observation is important, since a nondissociated molecule of sodium chloride is only one osmotically active particle, whereas a dissociated molecule generates two osmotically active particles. Thus, fewer than predicted osmotically active particles are present, and normal saline has a measured osmolality of only 280 mOsm $\cdot$ kg^{-1}. See Table 73–22 for the osmolarities and osmolalities of other intravenous fluids.

Osmotically active particles draw water across a semipermeable biologic membrane (such as the capillary wall or cell membrane) until the same osmolality is present on both sides of the membrane. Osmotic activity may also be described in terms of osmotic pressure, estimated by the equation:

Osmotic pressure (mm Hg)
= 19.3 $\times$ osmolality (mOsm $\cdot$ kg^{-1} solution)   Equation 2

For plasma with a normal osmolality of 280 mOsm $\cdot$ kg^{-1}, the osmotic pressure is >5400 mm Hg. Sodium chloride accounts for most of the plasma osmolality and, thus, osmotic pressure. Plasma proteins account for slightly more than 1 mOsm $\cdot$ kg^{-1} or 24 mm Hg of osmotic pressure.

TABLE 73–22. Osmolarity and Osmolality of Common Intravenous Fluids

Fluid	Osmolarity	Osmolality
Water	0	0
D5W	252	259
D5 .2NS	325	321
NS	308	282
LR	273	250
D5LR	525	524
3% Saline	1027	921
6% Hetastarch	310	307
20% Mannitol	1098	1280
Plasma protein fraction	—	261

Abbreviations: D5W = 5% dextrose in water; D5 .2NS = 5% dextrose in 0.2 normal saline; D5NS = 5% dextrose in normal saline; D5LR = 5% dextrose in lactated Ringer's solution.

Hypo-Osmotic Fluids

If hypo-osmotic intravenous fluids are given (e.g., 5% dextrose in water, 0.45% sodium chloride, or lactated Ringer's solution [250 mOsm $\cdot$ kg^{-1}]), plasma osmolality falls. Osmotic pressure changes cause water to pass from the capillaries into the interstitial space throughout the body, including the brain. As an example, an acute drop in plasma osmolarity of 20 mOsm $\cdot$ L^{-1} (decrease in sodium from 140 to 130 mEq $\cdot$ L^{-1}) results in a net osmotic pressure change of nearly 400 mm Hg, drives water into the interstitium, and produces edema.

The Blood-Brain Barrier

Outside the CNS, sodium normally crosses the capillary endothelial barrier into the interstitial space, drawing water with it. Administration of a large isosmotic fluid load that causes an increase in capillary hydrostatic pressure, therefore, may produce peripheral edema even in a normal patient until lymphatic and excretory mechanisms eliminate the excess solute and water. However, the blood-brain barrier normally does not allow sodium to cross. Administration of a large isosmotic fluid load does *not* produce interstitial cerebral edema, even though edema elsewhere may occur. Most experts now agree that the *osmolality* of administered fluid has a much greater impact on cerebral edema formation than does the absolute *amount* of intravenous fluid.

Tissue Elastance

Tissue elastance is defined as the change in interstitial pressure per milliliter of volume added. It can be considered a measure of the tendency of a tissue to develop edema. A highly elastic tissue, such as the bowel wall, readily forms edema. Interstitial hydrostatic pressure does not increase until a very large amount of edema is present. The brain, however, with its dense network of glial cells, is inelastic. Interstitial hydrostatic pressure begins to rise rapidly even with minimal edema. Thus, usual capillary hydrostatic pressure changes are insufficient to cause significant edema. A drop in serum osmolality, however, produces a significant driving force for edema formation in the brain and the rest of the body.

Colloid Oncotic Pressures

The osmotic (oncotic) pressure exerted by plasma proteins (24 mm Hg) is very small when compared with the total osmotic pressure (>5400 mm Hg). However, osmotic pressure exerted by sodium chloride is nearly the same on both sides of the capillary membrane, whereas proteins are predominantly intravascular. The colloid oncotic pressure, therefore, plays a very important role in helping to keep fluids intravascular.

Since the colloid oncotic pressure normally is only about 24 mm Hg, a fall in this value cannot produce much interstitial edema. That which forms is primarily in elastic tissues, such as the bowel wall or the lungs, that can increase water content without immediately increasing tissue hydrostatic pressure. In the inelastic brain, however, an increase in brain water caused by decreased colloic oncotic pressure results in an immediate increase in tissue hydrostatic pressure that opposes further edema formation. Even large decreases in colloid oncotic pressure are unlikely to cause significant cerebral edema.

The Bottom Line

The preceding discussion is somewhat theoretic and assumes normal blood-brain barrier function. In many patients with brain tumors, however, this normal function is lost, and sodium may readily cross into the interstitial space. However, at least in brain trauma, experimental evidence suggest that increases in cerebral edema associated with decreases in plasma osmolality occur primarily in areas of normal brain (i.e., the blood-brain barrier is intact). In my opinion, the most important goals of intraoperative fluid management during surgery for removal of brain tumors (and in fact for all intracranial neurologic surgery) are maintenance of at least normal plasma osmolality, adequate cardiac output, and cerebral perfusion.

Fluids of Choice

Maintenance of normal (290 mOsm $\cdot$ kg^{-1}) osmolality can be readily accomplished using isosmotic fluids. I generally use 0.9% sodium chloride solution. Lactated Ringer's solution, although generally thought to be isosmotic, actually has an osmolality of only 250 mOsm $\cdot$ kg^{-1} and should, in my opinion, not be used during intracranial surgery. I avoid the administration of dextrose during intracranial surgery unless hypoglycemia is documented.

Syndrome of Inappropriate Antidiuretic Hormone Secretion

Some patients with intracranial masses develop the syndrome of inappropriate antidiuretic hormone secretion and come to the operating room with an already decreased serum osmolality. In these patients, I gradually return the sodium level to normal values at a rate of 1 to 2 mEq $\cdot$ L^{-1} $\cdot$ h^{-1} using mannitol (free water diuresis) and isosmotic 0.9% sodium chloride. Occasionally, a slow infusion of hypertonic saline is needed.

Summary

Prevention of cerebral edema by fluid restriction makes no sense if this goal is accomplished at the cost of decreased cardiac output, blood pressure, and CBF. If the patient has excellent cardiovascular function and maintains blood pressure and cardiac output even with decreased preload, fluid restriction may not be harmful. A patient with poor ventricular function, however, may require restoration of normal preload after mannitol administration if hypotension develops. I emphasize again that *the amount of fluid administered is a much less important factor driving the formation of cerebral edema than is the plasma osmolality.*

What Factors Are Particularly Important During Emergence?

Blood Pressure Control

Control of blood pressure during emergence is very important. Bleeding may readily occur from incompletely resected tumors or from the tumor bed. I aggressively treat elevations >20% above the blood pressure just prior to dural closure and prefer short-acting drugs such as sodium nitroprusside and esmolol during this very labile period. Once extubation and transport to the intensive care unit have been completed, the magnitude of blood pressure changes usually decreases. In this

more stable period, weaning from sodium nitroprusside with substitution of longer-acting drugs such as labetalol as needed is appropriate.

Neurologic Assessment

Quick emergence from anesthesia at the conclusion of the operation is needed to allow assessment of neurologic status. If the patient does not promptly return to baseline status, a computed tomography scan is needed to rule out a postoperative hematoma.

Maintenance of Intubation

Patients with preoperative severe global neurologic impairment should remain intubated at the conclusion of surgery. Continued intubation allows careful control of arterial partial pressures of O_2 and CO_2 during this critical period. Muscle relaxation and sedation should be minimized.

CONCLUSIONS

Neuroanesthetic management, including choice of drugs, special techniques, positioning, and fluid management, directly affects normal and pathologic neurologic function. Unlike many other organ systems, neural tissue has only a very limited capacity for repair or regeneration. Surgically induced or anesthetic-induced damage thus may produce permanent change in function. As our understanding of anesthetic effects has improved and new monitoring techniques have become available, appropriate anesthetic management has made major contributions to the ease and success of increasingly complex neurosurgical procedures.

This chapter provides a framework to organize large amounts of data concerning anesthetic drugs and special techniques, neurophysiology and neuroanatomy, neuropathology and neurosurgical procedures into a coherent, logical approach to the neurosurgical patient. Although the scope is necessarily limited, the approaches discussed for vascular neurosurgery, spine surgery, and tumor surgery are equally applicable to patients with any neurosurgical problem.

References

1. Grundy BL, Pashayan AG, Mahla ME, et al: Three balanced anesthetic techniques for neuroanesthesia: infusion of thiopental sodium with sufentanil or fentanyl compared with inhalation of isoflurane. J Clin Anesth 1992; 4:372.
2. From RP, Warner DS, Todd MM, et al: Anesthesia for craniotomy: a double-blind comparison of alfentanil, fentanyl and sufentanil. Anesthesiology 1990; 73:896.
3. Todd MM, Warner DS, Sokoll M et al: A prospective, comparative trial of three anesthetics for elective supratentorial craniotomy: propofol/fentanyl, isoflurane/nitrous oxide, and fentanyl/nitrous oxide. Anesthesiology 1993; 78:1005.
4. Nehls DG, Todd MM, Spetzler RF, et al: A comparison of the cerebral protective effects of isoflurane and barbiturates during temporary focal ischemia in primates. Anesthesiology 1987; 66:453.
5. Hoffman WE, Pelligrino D, Werner C, et al: Ketamine decreases plasma catecholamines and improves outcome from incomplete cerebral ischemia in rats. Anesthesiology 1992; 76:755.
6. Messick JM, Casement B, Sharbrough FW, et al: Correlation of regional cerebral blood flow (rCBF) with EEG changes during isoflurane anesthesia for carotid endarterectomy: critical rCBF. Anesthesiology 1987; 66:344.
7. Sundt TW, Sharbrough FW, Piepgras DG, et al: Correlation of cerebral

blood flow and electroencephalographic changes during carotid endarterectomy: with results of surgery and hemodynamics of cerebral ischemia. Mayo Clin Proc 1981; 56:533.

8. Kassel NF, Hitchon PW, Gerk MK, et al: Influence of changes in arterial pCO_2 on cerebral blood flow and metabolism during high-dose barbiturate therapy in dogs. J Neurosurg 1981; 54:615.

9. Cold GE, Eskesen V, Eriksen H, et al: CBF and $CMRo_2$ during continuous etomidate infusion supplemented with N_2O and fentanyl in patients with supratentorial tumour: a dose response study. Acta Anaesthesiol Scand 1985; 29:490.

10. Pinaud M, Lelausque JN, Chetanneau A, et al: Effects of propofol on cerebral hemodynamics and metabolism in patients with brain trauma. Anesthesiology 1990; 73:404.

11. Weinstabl C, Mayer N, Jammerle AF, et al: The effects of propofol bolus administration on the intracranial pressure in craniocerebral trauma. Anaesthetist 1990; 39:521.

12. Eng C, Lam AM, Mayberg TS, et al: The influence of propofol with and without nitrous oxide on cerebral blood flow velocity and CO_2 reactivity in humans. Anesthesiology 1992; 77:872.

13. Fox J, Gelb AW, Enns J, et al: The responsiveness of cerebral blood flow to changes in arterial carbon dioxide is maintained during propofol–nitrous oxide anesthesia in humans. Anesthesiology 1992; 77:453.

14. Van Hemelrijck J, Fitch W, Mattheussen M, et al: Effect of propofol on cerebral circulation in the baboon. Anesth Analg 1990; 71:49.

15. Larsen R, Hilfiker O, Radke J, et al: The effects of midazolam on the general circulation, cerebral blood flow and cerebral oxygen consumption in man. Anaesthetist 1981; 30:18.

16. Forster A, Juge O, Morel D: Effects of midazolam on cerebral hemodynamics and cerebral vasomotor responsiveness to carbon dioxide. J Cereb Blood Flow Metab 1983; 3:246.

17. Forster A, Juge O, Morel D: Effects of midazolam on cerebral blood flow in human volunteers. Anesthesiology 1982; 56:453.

18. Jobes DR, Kennell E, Bitner R, et al: Effects of morphine–nitrous oxide anesthesia on cerebral autoregulation. Anesthesiology 1975; 42:30.

19. McPherson RW, Traystman RJ: Fentanyl and cerebral vascular responsitivity in dogs. Anesthesiology 1984; 60:180.

20. McPherson RW, Krempansanka E, Eimerl D: Effects of alfentanil on cerebral vascular reactivity in dogs. Br J Anaesth 1985; 57:1232.

21. Sperry RJ, Bailey PL, Reichman MV, et al: Fentanyl and sufentanil increase intracranial pressure in head trauma patients. Anesthesiology 1992; 77:416.

22. Weinstabl C, Mayer N, Richling B, et al: Effect of sufentanil on intracranial pressure in neurosurgical patients. Anaesthesia 1991; 46:837.

23. Shupak RC, Harp JR: Comparison between high-dose sufentanil-oxygen and high-dose fentanyl-oxygen for neuroanesthesia. Br J Anaesth 1985; 57:375.

24. Marx W, Shah N, Long C, et al: Sufentanil, alfentanil and fentanyl: impact on cerebrospinal fluid pressure in patients with brain tumors. J Neurosurg Anesthesiol 1989; 1:3.

25. Turner DM, Kassell NF, Sasaki T, et al: Cerebral and systemic vascular effects of naloxone in pentobarbital-anesthetized normal dogs. Neurosurgery 1984; 14:276.

26. Thiel A, Adams HA, Fengler G, et al: Studies using S(+)ketamine on probands: computerized EEG-analysis and transcranial Doppler ultrasonography. Anaesthetist 1992; 41:604.

27. Cavazzuti M, Porro CA, Biral GP, et al: Ketamine effects on local cerebral blood flow and metabolism in the rat. J Cereb Blood Flow Metab 1987; 7:806.

28. Young WL, Prohovnik I, Correll JW, et al: Cerebral blood flow and metabolism in patients undergoing anesthesia for carotid endarterectomy: a comparison of isoflurane, halothane, and fentanyl. Anesth Analg 1989; 68:712.

29. Miletich DJ, Ivankovich AD, Albrecht RF, et al: Absence of autoregulation of cerebral blood flow during halothane and enflurane anesthesia. Anesth Analg 1976; 55:100.

30. Algotsson L, Messeter K, Nordstrom CH, et al: Cerebral blood flow and oxygen consumption during isoflurane and halothane anesthesia in man. Acta Anaesthesiol Scand 1988; 32:15.

31. Madsen JB, Cold GE, Hansen ES, et al: The effect of isoflurane on cerebral blood flow and metabolism in humans during craniotomy for small supratentorial cerebral tumors. Anesthesiology 1987; 66:332.

32. Madsen JB, Cold GE, Eriksen HO, et al: CBF and $CMRo_2$ during craniotomy for small supratentorial cerebral tumours in enflurane anesthesia: a dose-response study. Acta Anaesthesiol Scand 1986; 30:633.

33. Muzzi D, Losasso T, Dietz N, et al: The effect of desflurane and isoflurane on cerebrospinal fluid pressure in humans with supratentorial mass lesions. Anesthesiology 1992; 76:720.

34. Archer DP, Labrecque P, Tyler JL, et al: Cerebral blood volume is

increased in dogs during administration of nitrous oxide or isoflurane. Anesthesiology 1987; 67:642.

35. Algotsson L, Messeter K, Rosen I, et al: Effects of nitrous oxide on cerebral haemodynamics and metabolism during isoflurane anaesthesia in man. Acta Anaesthesiol Scand 1992; 36:46.

36. Roald OK, Forsman M, Heier MS, et al: Cerebral effects of nitrous oxide when added to low and high concentrations of isoflurane in the dog. Anesth Analg 1991; 72:75.

37. Baughman VL, Hoffman WE, Miletich DH, et al: Cerebrovascular and cerebral metabolic effects of N_2O in unrestrained rats. Anesthesiology 1990; 73:269.

38. Kaieda R, Todd MM, Warner DS: The effects of anesthetics and $PaCO_2$ on the cerebrovascular, metabolic, and electroencephalographic responses to nitrous oxide in the rabbit. Anesth Analg 1989; 68:135.

39. Baughman VL, Hoffman WE, Thomas C, et al: The interaction of nitrous oxide and isoflurane with incomplete cerebral ischemia in the rat. Anesthesiology 1989; 70:767.

40. McPherson RW, Briar JE, Traystman RJ: Cerebrovascular responsiveness to carbon dioxide in dogs with 1.4% and 2.8% isoflurane. Anesthesiology 1989; 70:843.

41. Archer DP, Labrecque P, Tyler JL, et al: Measurement of cerebral blood flow and volume with positron emission tomography during isoflurane administration in the hypocapnic baboon. Anesthesiology 1990; 72:1031.

42. Artru AA: Partial preservation of cerebral vascular responsiveness to hypocapnia during isoflurane-induced hypotension in dogs. Anesth Analg 1986; 65:660.

43. McPherson RW, Traystman RJ: Effects of isoflurane on cerebral autoregulation in dogs. Anesthesiology 1988; 69:493.

44. Young WL, Prohovnik I, Correll JW, et al: A comparison of cerebral blood flow reactivity to CO_2 during halothane versus isoflurane anesthesia for carotid endarterectomy. Anesth Analg 1991; 73:416.

45. Leon LE, Bissonnette B: Cerebrovascular responses to carbon dioxide in children anesthetized with halothane and isoflurane. Can J Anaesth 1991; 38:817.

46. Lutz LJ, Milde JH, Milde LN: The response of the canine cerebral circulation to hyperventilation during anesthesia with desflurane. Anesthesiology 1991; 74:504.

47. Lanier WL, Milde JH, Michenfelder JD: Cerebral stimulation following succinylcholine in dogs. Anesthesiology 1986; 64:551.

48. Lanier WL, Milde JH, Michenfelder JD: The cerebral effects of pancuronium and atracurium in halothane-anesthetized dogs. Anesthesiology 1985; 63:589.

49. Grubb RL, Raichle ME: Effects of hemorrhagic and pharmacologic hypotension on cerebral oxygen utilization and blood flow. Anesthesiology 1982; 56:3.

50. Larsen R, Drobnik L, Teichmann J, et al: The effects of halothane-, nitroprusside-, and trimethaphan-induced hypotension on cerebral blood flow and intracranial pressure. Anaesthetist 1979; 28:494.

51. Weiss MH, Spence J, Apuzzo ML, et al: Influence of nitroprusside on cerebral pressure autoregulation. Neurosurgery 1979; 4:56.

52. Stange K, Lagerkranser M, Sollevi A: Nitroprusside-induced hypotension and cerebrovascular autoregulation in the anesthetized pig. Anesth Analg 1991; 73:745.

53. Candia GJ, Heros RC, Lavyne MH, et al: Effect of intravenous sodium nitroprusside on cerebral blood flow and intracranial pressure. Neurosurgery 1978; 3:50.

54. Artru AA: Cerebral vascular responses to hypocapnia during nitroglycerine-induced hypotension. Neurosurgery 1985; 16:468.

55. Burt DE, Verniquet AJ, Homi J: The response of the canine intracranial pressure to systemic hypotension induced with nitroglycerine. Br J Anaesth 1982; 54:665.

56. Ishikawa T, Funatsu N, Okamoto K, et al: Cerebral and systemic effects of hypotension induced by trimethaphan or nitroprusside in dogs. Acta Anaesthesiol Scand 1982; 26:643.

57. Ulrich K, Kuschinsky W: In vivo effects of alpha-adrenoreceptor agonists and antagonists on pial veins of cats. Stroke 1985; 16:880.

58. Davis DH, Sundt TM Jr: Relationship of cerebral blood flow to cardiac output, mean arterial pressure, blood volume and alpha and beta blockade in cats. J Neurosurg 1980; 52:745.

59. Madsen PL, Vorstrup S, Schmidt JF, et al: Effect of acute and prolonged treatment with propranolol on cerebral blood flow and cerebral oxygen metabolism in healthy volunteers. Eur J Clin Pharmacol 1990; 39:295.

60. Dahlgren N, Ingvar M, Siesjo BK: Effect of propranolol on local cerebral blood flow under normocapnic and hypercapnic conditions. J Cereb Blood Flow Metab 1981; 1:429.

61. Gaab MR, Hollerhage HG, Walter GF, et al: Brain edema, autoregulation, and calcium antagonism: an experimental study with nimodipine. Adv Neurol 1990; 52:391.

62. Hill AC, Schecter WP, Mori H, et al: The effect of verapamil on cerebral cortical and spinal cord blood flow during proximal descending aortic occlusion. J Trauma 1988; 28:1214.

63. Pearce WJ, Bevan JA: Diltiazem and autoregulation of canine cerebral blood flow. J Pharmacol Exp Ther 1987; 242:812.

64. Brooks DJ, Redmond S, Mathias CJ, et al: The effect of orthostatic hypotension on cerebral blood flow and middle cerebral artery velocity in autonomic failure, with observations on the action of ephedrine. J Neurol Neurosurg Psychiatry 1989; 52:962.

65. Albin MS, Ritter RR, Pruett CE, et al: Venous air embolism during lumbar laminectomy in the prone position: report of three cases. Anesth Analg 1992; 75:152.

66. Bunegin L, Albin MS, Helsel PE, et al: Positioning the right atrial catheter: a model for reappraisal. Anesthesiology 1981; 55:343.

67. Hanna PG, Gravenstein N, Pashayan AG: In vitro comparison of central venous catheters for aspiration of air embolism: effect of catheter type, catheter tip position, and cardiac inclination. J Clin Anesth 1991; 3:290.

68. Colley PS, Artru AA: Bunegin-Albin catheter improves air retrieval and resuscitation from lethal venous air embolism in upright dogs. Anesth Analg 1989; 68:298.

69. Philips LH, Whisnant JP, O'Fallon WM, et al: The unchanging pattern of subarachnoid hemorrhage in a community. Neurology 1980; 30:1034.

70. Weir B: Medical aspects of the preoperative management of aneurysms: a review. Can J Neurol Sci 1981; 8:21.

71. Flamm ES: The timing of aneurysm surgery. Clin Neurosurg 1986; 33:147.

72. Adams HP: Early management of the patient with recent aneurysmal subarachnoid hemorrhage. Stroke 1986; 17:1068.

73. Disney L, Weir B, Petruk K: Effect on management and mortality of a deliberate policy of early operation on supratentorial aneurysms. Neurosurgery 1987; 20:695.

74. Ferguson GG: Direct measurement of mean and pulsatile blood pressure at operation in human intracranial saccular aneurysms. J Neurosurg 1972; 36:560.

75. Solomon RA, Fink M, Lennihan L: Early aneurysm surgery and prophylactic hypervolemic hypertensive therapy for the treatment of subarachnoid hemorrhage. Neurosurgery 1988; 23:699.

76. Awad IA: Clinical vasospasm after subarachnoid hemorrhage: response to hypervolemic hemodilution and arterial hypertension. Stroke 1987; 18:365.

77. Tettenborn D, Porto L, Ryman T, et al: Survey of clinical experience with nimodipine in patients with subarachnoid hemorrhage. Neurosurg Rev 1987; 10:77.

78. Allen GS, Ahn HS, Preziosi TJ, et al: Cerebral arterial spasm: a controlled trial of nimodipine in patients with subarachnoid hemorrhage. N Engl J Med 1983; 309:308.

79. Zabramski JM, Spetzler RF, Lee KS, et al: Phase I trial of tissue plasminogen activator for the prevention of vasospasm in patients with subarachnoid hemorrhage. J Neurosurg 1991; 75:189.

80. Zubrov YLN, Nikiforov BM, Shustin VA: Balloon catheter techniques for dilation of constricted cerebral arteries after aneurysmal subarachnoid hemorrhage. Acta Neurochir 1984; 70:65.

81. Beard EF, Robertson JW, Robertson RCL: Spontaneous subarachnoid hemorrhage simulating acute myocardial infarction. Am Heart J 1959; 58:755.

82. Diamond T, Segal F: Subarachnoid hemorrhage masquerading electrocardiographically as acute myocardial infarction. Heart Lung 1984; 13:451.

83. Pollick C, Cujec B, Parker S, et al: Left ventricular wall motion abnormalities in subarachnoid hemorrhage: an echocardiographic study. J Am Coll Cardiol 1988; 12:600.

84. Friedman WA, Chadwick GM, Verhoeven FJS, et al: Monitoring of somatosensory evoked potentials during surgery for middle cerebral artery aneurysms. Neurosurgery 1991; 29:83.

85. Friedman WA, Kaplan BL, Day AL, et al: Evoked potential monitoring during aneurysm operation: observations after fifty cases. Neurosurgery 1987; 20:678.

86. Little JR, Lesser RP, Lüders H: Electrophysiologic monitoring during basilar aneurysm operation. Neurosurgery 1987; 20:421.

87. Pinaud M, Souron R, Lelausque JN, et al: Cerebral blood flow and oxygen consumption during nitroprusside-induced hypotension to less than 50 mm Hg. Anesthesiology 1989; 70:255.

88. Newberg LA, Milde JH, Michenfelder JD: The cerebral metabolic effects of isoflurane at and above concentrations that suppress cortical electrical activity. Anesthesiology 1983; 59:23.

89. Artru AA, Katz RA, Colley PS: Autoregulation of cerebral blood flow during normocapnia and hypocapnia in dogs. Anesthesiology 1989; 70:288.

90. Michenfelder JD, Theye RA: Hypothermia: effect on canine brain and whole body metabolism. Anesthesiology 1968; 29:1107.

91. Michenfelder JD: The in vivo effects of massive concentrations of anesthetics on canine cerebral metabolism. *In* Molecular Mechanisms of Anesthesia. Fink BR (ed). New York, Raven Press, 1975, p 537.

92. Carrasco G, Molina R, Costa J: Propofol versus midazolam in short-, medium-, and long-term sedation of critically ill patients. Chest 1993; 103:557.

93. Halla JT, Hardin JG, Vitek J, et al: Involvement of the cervical spine in rheumatoid arthritis (Review). Arthritis Rheum 1989; 32:652.

94. Yaszemski MJ, Shepler TR: Sudden death from cord compression associated with atlanto-axial instability in rheumatoid arthritis. Spine 1990; 15:338.

95. Kay NH, Blogg CE: Rises in serum potassium after suxamethonium following a brachial plexus injury. Anaesthesia 1982; 37:1217.

96. Fessler RG, Dietze DD Jr, MacMillan MM, et al: Lateral parascapular extrapleural approach to the upper thoracic spine. J Neurosurg 1991; 75:349.

97. Bracken MB, Shepard MJ, Collins WF, et al: A randomized, controlled trial of methylprednisolone or naloxone in the treatment of acute spinal-cord injury: results of the Second National Acute Spinal Cord Injury Study. N Engl J Med 1990; 322:1405.

98. Bracken MB, Shepard MJ, Collins WF Jr, et al: Methylprednisolone or naloxone treatment after acute spinal cord injury: 1-year follow-up data: results of the second national acute spinal cord injury study. J Neurosurg 1992; 76:23.

99. Stauffer JL, Petty TL: Cleft tongue and ulceration of hard palate: complications of oral intubation. Chest 1978; 74:317.

100. Lennon RL, Hosking MP, Gray JR, et al: The effects of intraoperative blood salvage and induced hypotension on transfusion requirements during spinal surgical procedures. Mayo Clin Proc 1987; 62:1090.

101. Walker AE, Robins M, Weinfeld FD: Epidemiology of brain tumors: the national survey of intracranial neoplasms. Neurology 1985; 35:219.

102. Kato A, Sako K, Diksic M, et al: Regional glucose utilization and blood flow in experimental brain tumors studied by double tracer autoradiography. J Neurooncol 1985; 3:271.

103. Panther LA, Baumbach GL, Bigner DD, et al: Vasoactive drugs produce selective changes in flow to experimental brain tumors. Ann Neurol 1985; 18:712.

104. Black S, Ockert DB, Oliver WC, et al: Outcome following posterior fossa craniectomy in patients in the sitting or horizontal positions. Anesthesiology 1988; 69:49.

105. Hanakita J, Miyake H, Nagayasu S, et al: Angiographic examination and surgical treatment for bow hunter's stroke. Neurosurgery 1988; 23:228.

CHAPTER 74

Surgery of the Endocrine System

EDWARD D. MILLER, Jr., M.D.

Some surgical procedures are designed to treat the metabolic or structural consequences of an endocrinopathy. Generally, the problem results from overproduction or underproduction of a specific organ's hormones and is associated with changes of the hormone-producing or responding organ. This chapter describes the intraoperative management of patients with insulinoma and with pituitary, parathyroid, thyroid, pancreatic, and adrenal abnormalities that are surgically treated. A screening evaluation for global assessment of endocrine function is shown in Table 74–1. If the criteria are met, a significant endocrine abnormality is unlikely (see Chapter 12).

PITUITARY GLAND

What Are the Components?

Anterior Pituitary

The pituitary gland is divided into anterior and posterior portions. The anterior pituitary gland secretes prolactin, growth hormone, gonadotropins, thyroid-stimulating hormone (TSH), and adrenocorticotropic hormone (ACTH). Only about 10% of intracranial neoplasms are found in the pituitary. They usually are detected because of a mass effect or hypersecretion of certain hormones. The tumors are rarely metastatic. They produce local symptoms by bony invasion, by compression of a cranial nerve, especially the optic nerve, or secondary to hydrocephalus. Almost 50% of the lesions in this area are nonsecretory and are called *chromophobe adenomas.*

In general, anterior pituitary abnormalities follow a sequence in which gonadal dysfunction precedes growth dysfunction, which occurs before adrenal cortical dysfunction. Rarely is TSH activity lost.

Posterior Pituitary

The posterior pituitary gland is composed of terminal nerve endings that extend from the ventral hypothalamus. Vasopressin (ADH) and oxytocin are the two principal hormones secreted by this structure. Both hormones are synthesized in the supraoptic and paraventricular nuclei of the hypothalamus and are transported to the posterior pituitary by a portal system that extends from the hypothalamus.

ADH is responsible for regulation of extracellular fluid volume and plasma osmolality. Oxytocin causes uterine contraction and promotes milk secretion. Diseases of the posterior pituitary or the neural axis are responsible for diabetes insipidus.

Why Is Transsphenoidal Hypophysectomy Preferred?

The transsphenoidal approach has gained popularity for several reasons. Antibiotic therapy makes postoperative meningitis extremely uncommon. The operating microscope allows excellent visualization of the deeply situated operative site. Unlike a subfrontal craniotomy, no frontal lobe retraction is necessary, and the adenoma can be selectively removed, thus sparing the normal tissue. The transsphenoidal approach is most commonly used when the lesion remains within the confines of the sella turcica.

Special Concerns

The Airway

A number of potential problems must be considered (Table 74–2). If a patient is acromegalic, an important question involves adequacy of the airway.[1] Mandibular and soft tissue enlargement in advanced acromegaly can make conventional oral intubation impossible. Subglottic abnormalities are occasionally present as well.[2] Pharyngeal soft tissue and epiglottic enlargement predispose patients to airway obstruction after induction of anesthesia. One should have a particularly high index of suspicion for this problem if a patient snores while sleeping. Hoarseness suggests laryngeal or vocal cord involvement; the requirement for a smaller endotracheal tube should

TABLE 74–1. History Suggesting Normal Endocrine Function

Absence of glucosuria
Blood pressure and heart rate normal
Body weight unchanged
Sexual function normal
No history of recent medication

TABLE 74–2. Transsphenoidal Surgery Considerations

Airway obstruction
Hypertension/dysrhythmias
Swelling of tongue
Air embolism

be anticipated. If any question concerning airway adequacy remains unanswered, awake intubation is preferred. If a patient is to be anesthetized for transsphenoidal surgery, then the oral route must be used because the nose is the operative field.

Local Anesthetic/Epinephrine Infiltration

A second major issue is the generous infiltration of the mucosa with a mixture of local anesthetic and epinephrine to minimize bleeding. Because this is a highly vascular region, the amount of epinephrine must be limited and ventricular dysrhythmias and hypertension treated if they occur (Fig. 74–1). An alternative drug, phenylephrine, results only in hypertension from systemic absorption. This hypertension readily responds to phentolamine, 1 to 4 mg as an intravenous bolus.

Arterial Collateral Flow

If an arterial catheter is placed, care should be taken to verify adequate collateral ulnar artery circulation. This is an important issue, because the vessel can be occluded as a result of tissue growth and compression in as many as half of acromegalic patients, even in the absence of carpal tunnel symptoms.[3]

Air Embolism

Air embolism during the procedure is a potential although extremely uncommon problem. Because the head is above the level of the heart for this procedure, it should be considered in

the differential diagnosis if an unexpected drop in end-tidal carbon dioxide or blood pressure occurs.

Postextubation Airway Obstruction

Before extubation, consideration is given to intraoperative swelling of the tongue or posterior pharynx. This problem is of particular concern because the nose is packed; hence, a nasopharyngeal airway cannot be used. Inspect the pharynx to make sure that the packs have been removed and that excess swelling or bleeding is not present.

PARATHYROID GLANDS

Four parathyroid glands usually are present. The superior parathyroids lie in the midportion of the posterior aspect of the thyroid gland; the two inferior parathyroid glands are usually in the lateral or posterior surface of the lower poles of the thyroid gland. The inferior glands are much more variable in their location, however, and sometimes are found in the mediastinum.

The major function of parathyroid hormone (parathormone) is to regulate calcium homeostasis. Parathormone increases serum calcium by promoting bone reabsorption, limits renal excretion of calcium, and indirectly enhances gastrointestinal calcium absorption by its effect on vitamin D metabolism. It also increases the renal excretion of phosphate. The effects of parathormone on serum calcium levels are countered by calcitonin, a hormone excreted by the thyroid gland.[4]

How Is Calcium Fractionated?

Serum calcium is divided into three fractions: protein bound, approximately 40%; a diffusible but un-ionized fraction component chelated with bicarbonate, phosphate, and citrate, approximately 10%; and an ionized fraction, approximately 50%. The ionized fraction is physiologically active and homeostatically regulated (Fig. 74–2).

How Is Serum Calcium Altered?

Protein Concentration

Changes in serum albumin or protein concentrations are associated with changes in total serum calcium concentrations. Albumin binds about 90% of protein-bound calcium on its carboxyl groups. A rough rule of thumb is that for every increment or decrement in albumin of $1 \text{ g} \cdot \text{dL}^{-1}$, a similar directional change of about $0.8 \text{ mg} \cdot \text{dL}^{-1}$ in total serum calcium occurs.

Acid-Base Changes

The binding of calcium to protein carboxyl groups is altered by blood pH (Fig. 74–3). Acute acidosis decreases protein binding and thereby increases ionized calcium, whereas acute alkalosis increases protein binding and decreases ionized calcium. The concentration of ionized calcium decreases by approximately 10% with every 0.1 unit increase in arterial pH.

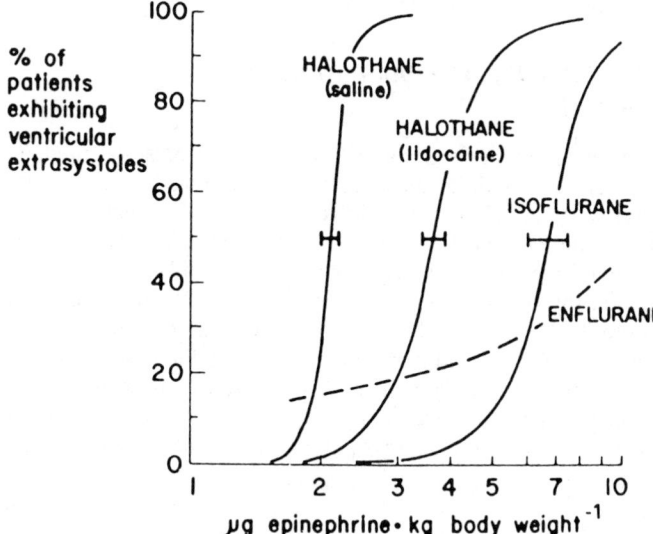

FIGURE 74–1. Per cent of patients exhibiting three or more ventricular extrasystoles in response to a subcutaneous injection of epinephrine. (From Johnston RR, Eger EI, Wilson C: A comparative interaction of epinephrine with enflurane, isoflurane, and halothane in man. Anesth Analg 1976; 44:709. © Williams & Wilkins, 1976.)

When Is Hypercalcemia a Problem?

If serum calcium level is <14 mg $\cdot$ dL^{-1}, few calcium-related problems occur intraoperatively. However, if higher levels are present, hydration with normal saline to dilute the serum calcium and inhibit tubular reabsorption, as well as diuresis with furosemide to increase excretion, should be instituted before the surgical procedure. If surgery is indicated for severe hypercalcemia, hypoventilation should be avoided, because acidosis increases the ionized fraction (see Fig. 74–3). Acute elevations in calcium level can cause cardiac dysrhythmias. The response to muscle relaxants may be exaggerated in patients with pre-existing weakness because of the effects of calcium on the neuromuscular junction.[5]

A hypercalcemic patient who is delirious, psychotic, or comatose is in extremis. If the QT interval is prolonged, the serum calcium level is >16 mg $\cdot$ dL^{-1}.[6] These patients are predisposed to bone fractures when they are moved and vertebral compression fractures during laryngoscopy because of severe osteoporosis.

What Are the Postoperative Considerations After Parathyroidectomy?

Special problems to be considered include hemorrhage into the neck or damage to the recurrent laryngeal nerve. Recurrent laryngeal nerve injury is neither sufficiently common nor serious enough to warrant routine intraoperative evaluation of function. Postoperative examination is only required if the

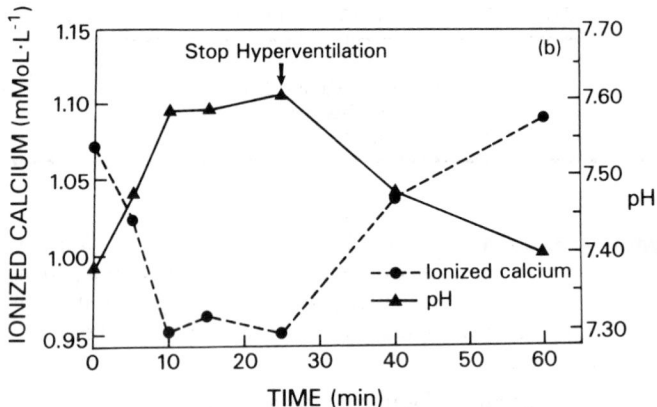

FIGURE 74–3. Effects of changes in acid-base status (pH) on level of ionized calcium. (From Scamonda B, Towfighi J, Arvan DA: Determination of ionized calcium in serum by use of an ion-selective electrode. Clin Chem 1972; 18:155.)

patient or surgeon believes that a voice or functional change has occurred or if the surgeon thinks he or she may have injured the nerve.[7]

Hypocalcemia may be a problem. Severe hypocalcemia, although rare, should be recognized by measuring serum calcium level and by noting greatly increased neuromuscular excitability brought about by a decrease in plasma ionized calcium. The most striking manifestation of this deficiency is tetany. Carpal pedal spasm and Chvostek's sign can be present.

THYROID GLAND

Thyroid hormone increases carbohydrate and fat metabolism by activating adenyl cyclase. The result is an increase in heart rate, contractility, metabolic rate, oxygen consumption, and carbon dioxide production. Thyroid hormone is important to many aspects of growth and function, but for those engaged in the perioperative care of patients with thyroid hormone or gland disease, the concerns focus on the cardiovascular and airway manifestations of disease.

What Are the Metabolic Pathways of Interest?

Dietary iodine is absorbed by the gastrointestinal tract, is converted to iodide ion, and is actively transported into the thyroid gland. Here, it is oxidized back to iodine that is bound to the amino acid tyrosine. Two hormones are formed: triiodothyronine (T_3) and thyroxine (T_4) (Fig. 74–4). The more potent thyroid hormone is T_3, even though the gland releases more T_4. T_3 is formed peripherally from the partial deiodinization of T_4. Thyroid hormone synthesis and release are under the control of the hypothalamus via thyrotropin-releasing hormone; of the anterior pituitary by TSH; and by autoregulation within the gland secondary to thyroid iodine concentration (see Fig. 74–4).

What Thyroid Function Test Is Most Helpful?

Serum T_4 determination is the standard screening test for evaluation of thyroid gland function. Levels are elevated in

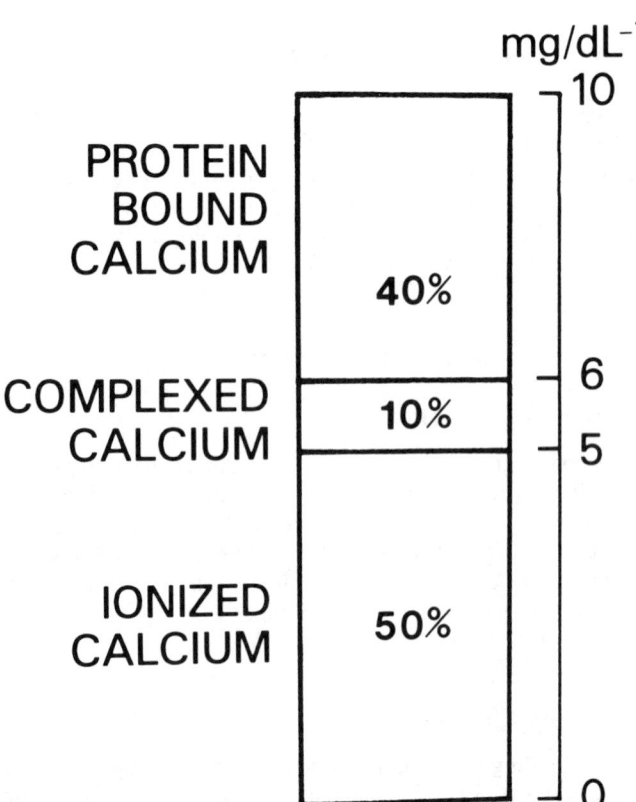

FIGURE 74–2. Distribution of serum calcium. (From Chernow B, Zaloga GP: Ions or society members. *In* Critical Care: State of the Art. Vol 5. Fullerton, CA, Society of Critical Care Medicine, 1984. © Williams & Wilkins, 1984.)

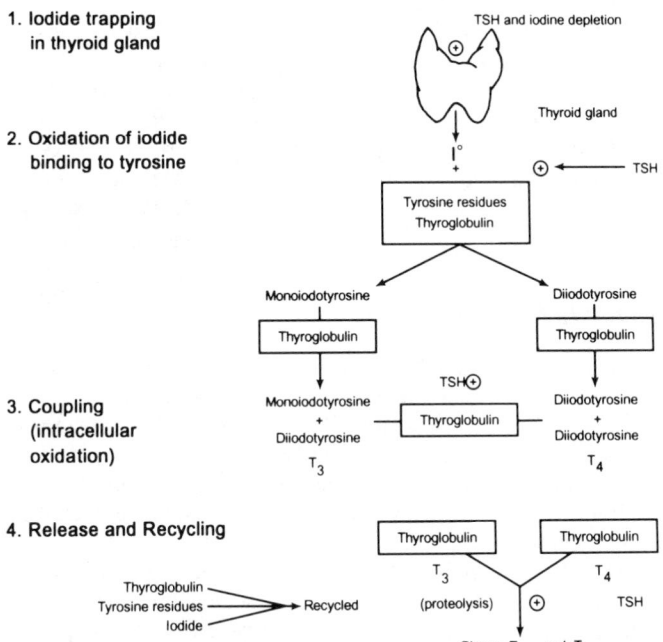

1. Iodide trapping in thyroid gland

2. Oxidation of iodide binding to tyrosine

3. Coupling (intracellular oxidation)

4. Release and Recycling

FIGURE 74–4. Thyroid hormone biosynthesis consists of four stages: (1) organization; (2) binding; (3) coupling; and (4) release. (From Barash PG, Cullen BF, Stoelting RK: Clinical Anesthesia. Philadelphia, JB Lippincott, 1989, p 1189.)

approximately 90% of patients with hyperthyroidism and are low in 85% of those who are hypothyroid (Table 74–3). Of note is that thyroid function tests may incorrectly indicate hypothyroidism after anesthesia or surgery; thus they should be performed preoperatively.[8]

What Is Hyperthyroidism?

Hyperthyroidism results from excessive thyroid hormone. Signs and symptoms of hyperthyroidism are listed in Table 74–4. Most patients with hyperthyroidism are middle-aged women.

Thyroid Storm

Thyroid storm is a life-threatening exacerbation of hyperthyroidism. Manifestations reflect increased circulating thyroid hormone or increased responsiveness to hormone (Table 74–5). Therapy is aimed at decreasing sympathetic hyperactivity and decreasing both thyroid hormone synthesis and release of preformed hormone (Table 74–6). This syndrome can mimic malignant hyperthermia but is not associated with muscle rigidity, severe hypercarbia, or elevated levels of lactate, potassium, and creatine kinase.

TABLE 74–3. Test of Thyroid Function

	T_4	T_3	Thyroid-Stimulating Hormone
Hyperthyroidism	Elevated	Elevated	Normal or low
Primary hyperthyroidism	Low	Low or normal	Elevated

TABLE 74–4. Signs and Symptoms of Hyperthyroidism

Heat intolerance
Nervousness
Warm, moist skin
Neck mass
Resting sinus tachycardia
Atrial fibrillation
Weight loss
Exophthalmos

Treatment

Inhibition of the peripheral conversion of T_4 to T_3 is achieved with propythlthiouracil. The addition of iodine causes a decrease in the size of the gland.[9] Treatment of excess sympathetic activity is based on the empirical use of β-adrenergic antagonists or diltiazem. Propranolol is frequently used preoperatively in order to decrease heart rate and ameliorate the other symptoms of hyperthyroidism. Remember, however, that in older patients, long-standing hyperthyroidism may result in cardiomyopathy; β-adrenergic antagonists in such individuals should be carefully titrated.[10, 11] A useful end point is a heart rate of approximately 85 beats per minute (bpm) (Fig. 74–5).

Special Concerns

Elective Surgery

Hyperthyroid patients who are scheduled for elective thyroidectomy should be clinically euthyroid before the surgical procedure. The heart rate should be <85 bpm at rest, and the symptoms of hyperthyroidism should have been diminished markedly by preoperative therapy. If a patient is tachycardiac and hyperthermic, an elective procedure should be postponed.

No evidence supports the view that a hyperthyroid patient needs an emergency procedure to remove the thyroid gland. The half-life of T_3 is 24 to 30 hours; therefore, symptoms persist despite total removal of the gland. Appropriate medical therapy before the surgical procedure is needed. The old concept of "stealing" a patient to the operating room is no longer viable.

Emergency Surgery

Occasionally, a hyperthyroid patient is unrecognized before a surgical emergency or only recently has started therapy. In these circumstances, the extent of underlying cardiac disease secondary to hyperthyroidism is often impossible to discern. Invasive blood pressure monitoring is indicated. Tachycardia should be controlled with β-blockade; an esmolol infusion is a practical approach to this problem. Postoperative management should include observation in an acute care unit because the half-life of T_3 is so long.

TABLE 74–5. Manifestations of Thyroid Storm

Hyperpyrexia
Tachycardia
Hyperventilation
Extreme anxiety
Cardiovascular instability

TABLE 74–6. Acute Therapy of Thyrotoxicosis

1. Control heart rate and blood pressure with β-blockers. Digitalis or verapamil may be indicated if there is atrial fibrillation with a fast ventricular response. Supplemental oxygen should be administered if there is a possibility of myocardial ischemia.
2. Treat hyperthermia with cooling blankets, cold intravenous fluids, and gastric and colonic lavage.
3. Prevent further release of thyroid hormone with iodine, propylthiouracil, and adrenocortical steroids.
4. Administer sympatholytic agents (e.g., propranolol)

(From Merrell WJ, Bingham HL: Endocrine/renal system. *In* Manual of Complications in Anesthesia. Gravenstein N (ed). Philadelphia, JB Lippincott, 1991, p 508.)

Recurrent Laryngeal Nerve Injury

Unilateral damage causes hoarseness, and bilateral damage may cause aphonia and stridor. The latter condition is rare. Protective airway reflexes are lost as well. I do not perform direct laryngoscopy at the end of a surgical thyroidectomy unless the surgeon believes that the recurrent laryngeal nerve has been injured. In that case, deep extubation and cord visualization can be performed directly or with a fiberoptic bronchoscope.

Better still is preoperative assessment by having the patient say "eee" and then repeating the procedure in the postanesthesia care unit (PACU) when the patient is awake. A difference between the preoperative and postoperative response suggests the need for fiberoptic examination in the PACU so that the surgeon can make the decision about whether to re-explore the wound.

Other Considerations

Exophthalmos, if present, predisposes patients to corneal ulceration; thus, their eyes should be lubricated and the lids carefully secured and shielded. Hematoma formation may cause the airway to be compromised. If the gland has invaded the trachea, tracheomalacia may be present. This condition

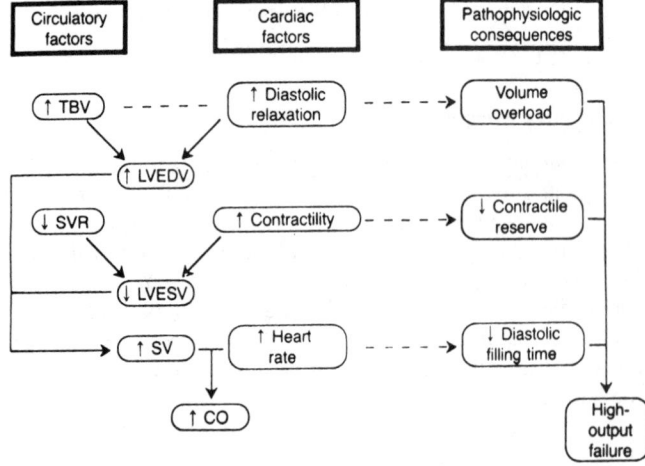

FIGURE 74–5. Factors that produce the cardiovascular effects of thyrotoxicosis. TBV = Total blood volume; LVEDV = left ventricular end-diastolic volume; SVR = systemic vascular resistance; LVESV = left ventricular end-systolic volume; SV = stroke volume; CO = cardiac output. *Solid arrows* indicate direct effects, and *dashed arrows* show potential consequences. (Adapted from information appearing in Woeber K: Thyrotoxicosis and the heart. N Engl J Med 1992; 327:94. By permisson of the New England Journal of Medicine.)

may be evidenced by inspiratory stridor and must be considered in concert with the surgeon before extubation.[12, 13]

Hypoparathyroidism secondary to inadvertent surgical removal of the parathyroid glands is most frequently encountered after total thyroidectomy. The symptoms of hypocalcemia develop within 24 to 48 hours; laryngeal stridor may be one of the first indications of hypocalcemic tetany. Treatment is accomplished with calcium gluconate or chloride.[14, 15]

What Is Hypothyroidism?

Nearly 1% of the adult population is hypothyroid. Hypothyroidism can be caused by autoimmune disease, treatment with radioactive iodine, or various other factors. Clinical manifestations in adults are usually subtle and include weight gain, cold intolerance, muscle fatigue, dull facial expressions, and depression. Heart rate, myocardial contractility, and cardiac output all are decreased.

The diagnosis may be confirmed by an elevated TSH level. T_4 level may be low or normal. Myxedema coma results from extreme hypothyroidism and is characterized by impaired mentation, congestive heart failure, hypothermia, and hypoventilation. Treatment with T_3 or T_4 and steroid replacement to offset the adrenal suppression is effective. Clinically euthyroid (asymptomatic) hypothyroid patients are not at increased risk of perioperative complications.

Diagnosis

The diagnosis should be entertained whenever patients awaken unusually slowly from general anesthesia or are unable to maintain their body temperature. It is often made after a patient has a prolonged stay in the PACU or intensive care unit with a delayed awakening that is not anticipated.

The decreased metabolic rate and reduced demands on the heart can mask or moderate significant coronary artery disease. Because therapy of hypothyroidism with thyroid hormone may aggravate myocardial ischemia in this subset of patients, coronary angioplasty or coronary revascularization should be performed before therapy.[17]

Airway Obstruction

Many causes of airway distress are associated with thyroid disease (Table 74–7).[18] Most common is upper airway obstruction due to goiter. Symptoms include shortness of breath, difficulty swallowing, and pressure or sensation of fullness in the neck. Approximately one-third of patients with benign goiter have evidence of tracheal or esophageal compression. Almost one-third of the patients who had symptoms of airway obstruction and who underwent pulmonary function testing with flow-volume loop recordings were found to have upper airway obstruction; two-thirds had normal flow-volume loops; and 4% had intrapulmonary airflow limitation.[19] The investigators recommend a flow-volume loop study in any symptomatic patient with goiter based on a sensitivity of 100%, specificity of 78%, and accuracy of 91%.[19]

INSULINOMA

Hypoglycemia can be caused by various entities, but one that is surgically correctable is an insulinoma. In patients with insulinoma, the serum insulin level does not decrease appro-

TABLE 74–7. Causes of Airway Distress Due to Thyroid Disease

Preoperative	Tracheal deviation and compression with large goiter
	Substernal goiter
	Hemorrhage in thyroid causing tracheal compression
	Associated with upper respiratory tract infection
	Tracheal invasion by tumor (commonly anaplastic tumor)
	Bleeding inside trachea
	Respiratory insufficiency (metastasis, pulmonary disease)
Intraoperative	Intubation problem
	Anesthetic causes (e.g., kink of tube, mucous plug, other)
Postoperative	Wound hematoma
	Postintubation laryngeal edema
	Bilateral vocal cord paralysis
	Tracheomalacia

(From Shaha A, Alfonso A, Jaffe BM: Acute airway distress due to thyroid pathology. Surgery 1987; 102:1068.)

priately with decreasing serum glucose. The symptoms of hypoglycemia are characterized by tachycardia, diaphoresis, tremulousness, and neuroglycopenia resulting in headaches, confusion, and even coma.

What Is the Intraoperative Concern?

Because manipulation of the tumor may cause massive releases of insulin, severe hypoglycemia can result while a patient is anesthetized and unable to manifest any symptoms. Some would suggest that insulinoma should only be operated on in centers that have a mechanical pancreas so that on-line blood glucose level can be analyzed and glucose administered appropriately. Very frequent intraoperative measurement of blood glucose levels, at least every 30 minutes, is the minimum that should be done. Because hyperglycemia is generally benign whereas even transient hypoglycemia can be catastrophic, administration of glucose-containing solutions is mandatory. These patients also benefit from a maintenance infusion of 5% dextrose in water when they begin their preoperative nil per os status. Although it is not a particularly reliable test, some suggest that a postoperative rebound hyperglycemia of more than $400 \text{ mg} \cdot \text{dL}^{-1}$ is consistent with complete tumor removal.[20]

ADRENAL GLANDS

The adrenal glands are composed of the cortex and the medulla. The cortical region synthesizes and secretes three types of hormones (Table 74–8). Endogenous and dietary cholesterol is used in the adrenal glands to synthesize glucocorticoids, mineralocorticoids, and androgens. The major biologic effects of adrenocortical hyperfunction or hypofunction occur as a result of cortisol or aldosterone excess or deficiency.

The adrenal medulla is derived from neuroectodermal cells and is actually a specialized part of the sympathetic nervous system. It should be considered separate and distinct from the adrenal cortex. The adrenal medulla synthesizes and secretes catecholamines, approximately 80% epinephrine and 20% norepinephrine. Disorders of the adrenal glands produce profound symptoms in surgical patients, including severe and sometimes life-threatening hypertension and dysrhythmias.

What Is Pheochromocytoma?

A tumor of the medullary portion of the adrenal gland producing catecholamines is called a *pheochromocytoma* because it is yellow when cut open. Extremely high serum catecholamine levels may result when the tumor is manipulated. Perioperative preparation and management of these patients are designed to minimize fluctuations in catecholamine release and their effects (see Chapter 12).

Signs and Symptoms

Pheochromocytomas may occur at any age, but they are most common in young persons and middle-aged adults. Therefore, young patients who have unexpected hypertension should be questioned closely. Although hypertension is frequently noted in these patients, it is not always present. Forty per cent of patients have only paroxysmal hypertension. However, patients who are hypertensive and have weight loss, constipation, and palpitations should be carefully screened. The triad of paroxysmal sweating, hypertension, and headache is more sensitive and specific than any laboratory test for the diagnosis of pheochromocytoma.[21]

Screening Tests

If the diagnosis of pheochromocytoma is suspected, elective surgery should be postponed until it can be ruled in or out. Anesthetic mortality in a patient with unrecognized pheochromocytoma is extremely high. Normal screening tests include measurement of a 24-hour urinary excretion of catecholamine metabolites (vanillylmandelic acid and metanephrines). If these values are elevated, plasma catecholamine levels are measured. Subsequent work-up includes a computed tomographic scan of the adrenal area, because most pheochromocytomas are found in one or the other adrenal gland.

Preoperative Preparation

Preoperative treatment is the major reason for the decrease in mortality from as high as 70% to virtually zero. Anesthesiologists must consider volume status, the degree of α- and β-blockade, and myocardial function.

Patients with pheochromocytoma may have underlying cardiac disease or a cardiomyopathy secondary to chronic stimulation of the myocardium due to excessive catecholamine secretion. This problem may be evidenced by myocardial necrosis and congestive heart failure. Electrocardiography and echocardiography (if suspicion of cardiac dysfunction exists) should be performed before the surgical procedure.[22, 23]

Treatment of patients with α-blockers and, if tachycardiac, β-blockers is mandatory before the surgical procedure, even if the blood pressure is not elevated. Small doses of phenoxybenzamine, 10 mg twice daily, titrated up to 60 mg per day as

TABLE 74–8. Hormones Secreted by the Adrenal Glands

Cortex	Glucocorticoids (cortisol)
	Mineralocorticoids (aldosterone)
	Androgens
Medulla	Epinephrine (80%)
	Norepinephrine (20%)

tolerated, are advocated. The goal is to produce at least a 10 mm Hg orthostatic blood pressure drop and to establish a degree of α-blockade such that the patient does not have blood pressure any higher than 160/90 mm Hg preoperatively. Propranolol administration to decrease heart rate to <100 bpm is also indicated after α-blockade has been initiated.

Because of their long-standing secretion of catecholamines, these patients have decreased plasma volumes. Treatment for 2 to 3 weeks with α- and β-blockers allows restitution of volume and a marked diminution in symptoms. Whether a shorter course of α-blockade is equally effective is unknown. Patients are premedicated with one-half the current dose of phenoxybenzamine and a sedative. Note that hematocrit may fall as a result of increased plasma volume; signs of constipation, palpitations, and flushing will cease.

Anesthetic Choice

The major issue in pheochromocytoma is intraoperative treatment of hypertension and tachycardia. Various methods have been advanced. No one method has been shown to be superior to others (Table 74–9). I personally believe that sodium nitroprusside and esmolol or propranolol, against the background of an inhalation anesthetic such as isoflurane, are acceptable. Probably most important is anticipation and prevention or control of hypertension at the time of tumor manipulation. Dysrhythmias often do not occur if the blood pressure is well controlled. If they occur despite blood pressure control, they appear to respond predictably to β-blockers and lidocaine.

Hypotension Following Tumor Removal

Total excision of the tumor and the loss of excess catecholamines may result in profound hypotension. This problem can best be prevented by making sure that adequate volume replacement has occurred preoperatively. A central venous catheter can be helpful in the assessment of intraoperative volume

TABLE 74–9. Incidence of Complications During Removal of Pheochromocytoma Using Various Anesthetics

	Enflurane	Halothane	Innovar	Regional
n =	6	6	7	5
Ventricular tachycardia	5	6	6	5
Treated ventricular tachycardia	0	1	1	0
Intraoperative vasodilator required	6	6	7	5
Intraoperative vasopressor required	0	1	1	0
Postoperative vasodilator required	0	1*	1*	0
Perioperative vasopressor required	0	0	0	0
Perioperative myocardial infarction	0	0	0	0
Perioperative renal failure	0	0	0	0
Perioperative congestive heart failure	0	1	1	1
Perioperative stroke	0	0	0	0
Perioperative mortality	0	0	0	0

(From Roizen MF, Horrigan RW, Koike M, et al: A prospective randomized trial of four anesthetic techniques for resection of pheochromocytoma. Anesthesiology 1982; 57:A43.)
*No abnormally secreting tumor tissue removed from patient.

status. An infusion of phenylephrine hydrochloride (Neo-Synephrine) or norepinephrine should be available to support blood pressure as necessary.

What Is Adrenocortical Insufficiency?

Patients with glucocorticoid deficiency have symptoms that are often vague. They complain of weakness, fatigue, hypoglycemia, hypotension, and weight loss. These deficiencies may represent primary disease of the adrenal glands (Addison's disease) or inadequate ACTH secretion by the pituitary gland. The most common cause of secondary adrenal insufficiency is current or recent (within 1 y) iatrogenic administration of exogenous glucocorticoids.

Steroid Replacement

Adults normally secrete about 20 mg of cortisol daily, but during the perioperative period this value may increase to >300 mg per day (Fig. 74–6). Administration of 100 mg of hydrocortisone phosphate every 8 hours, beginning the evening before and on the morning of surgery, is common for replacement. Other regimens are equally effective, but short-term use in this manner has minimal side effects and therefore is appropriate.

Glucocorticoid Excess

Glucocorticoid excess may be due to exogenous administration of steroid hormones; intrinsic hyperfunction of the adrenal cortex, such as an adrenocortical adenoma; ACTH production by a nonpituitary tumor; or hypersecretion by a pituitary adenoma (Cushing's disease). Regardless of the cause, an excess of cortical steroids produces Cushing's syndrome, characterized by muscle weakness and wasting, osteoporosis, central obesity, abdominal striae, glucose intolerance, hypertension, and mental changes.[24] These patients tend to have intravascular volume overload and fragile, paper-thin skin and veins.

Special Concerns

If a patient is scheduled for bilateral adrenalectomy, several concerns need to be addressed. The degree of osteoporosis and inability to extend the neck may result in difficult airway management. The characteristic buffalo hump and excess central fat also can make intubation difficult. Metabolic alkalosis may be severe. Close attention to perioperative glucose monitoring is crucial.[25]

Mineralocorticoid Excess

In patients with an adenoma that produces excess aldosterone, several important clinical concerns should be addressed. These patients retain excess amounts of sodium and excrete large amounts of potassium. They are hypertensive and severely potassium depleted (Table 74–10).[26] If a patient has a serum potassium level <3 mEq · L^{-1} and is hypertensive, the diagnosis of primary aldosterone-producing tumor (Conn's syndrome) should be suspected.

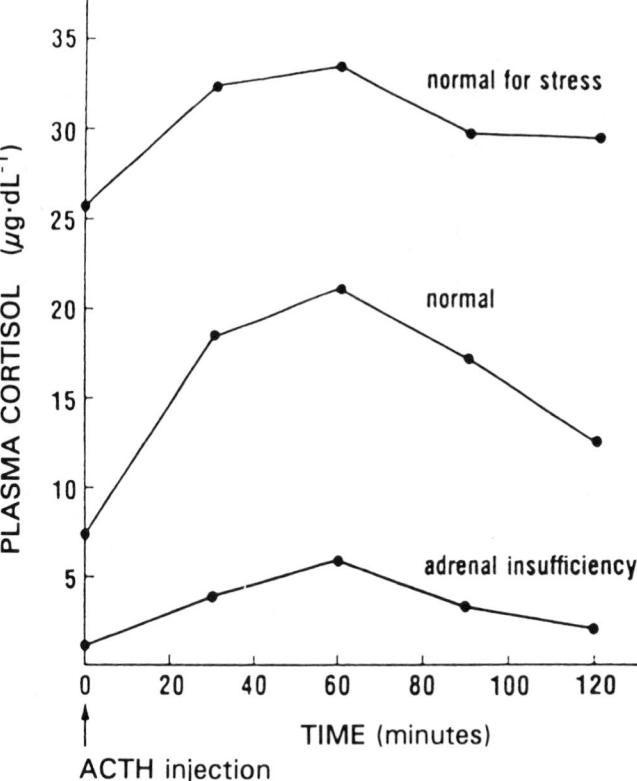

FIGURE 74–6. Change in plasma cortisol in response to ACTH administration in normal, adrenal insufficiency, and stress states. (From Thompson WL, Shoemaker W: Hormonal and metabolic considerations in critical care medicine. *In* Critical Care: State of the Art. Vol 3. Fullerton, CA, Society of Critical Care Medicine, 1982.)

Preoperative Preparation

Control of hypertension before the procedure is an important step. Treatment with an aldosterone-blocking agent such as spironolactone is effective in controlling the blood pressure and, more importantly, allowing total potassium stores to be replaced. Several weeks should be allowed for correction. The diuresis induced by spironolactone occasionally causes volume depletion. This possibility should be anticipated and offset with fluid replacement if orthostatic blood pressure changes follow the preoperative preparation.

Intraoperative Management

Intraoperative care of patients with Conn's syndrome is straightforward. Intra-arterial blood pressure monitoring is generally believed to be indicated because of the history of hypertension and the frequent coexistence of ischemic heart disease. However, large swings in blood pressure are not common because "volume overload" is present.

Appropriate anesthetic techniques minimize the effect of noxious stimuli and severe hypertension. Adequate serum potassium levels should be present before the surgical procedure. A computed tomography scan usually has localized the tumor.[27] If bilateral adrenal mobilization occurs, a patient may become transiently or permanently addisonian. Acute cortisol

supplementation should then be considered. Large swings in blood pressure at the time of tumor manipulation are not expected, because aldosterone has minimum cardiovascular effects by itself.

References

1. Southwick JP, Katz J: Unusual airway difficulty in the acromegalic patient: indications for tracheostomy. Anesthesiology 1979; 51:72.
2. Hassan SZ, Matz G, Lawrence AM, et al: Laryngeal stenosis in acromegaly: a possible cause of airway difficulties associated with anesthesia. Anesth Analg 1976; 55:57.
3. Compkin TV: Radial artery cannulation, potential hazard in patients with acromegaly. Anesthesia 1980; 35:1008.
4. Bone HG, III, Snyder WH, Pak CYC: Diagnosis of hyperparathyroidism. Annu Rev Med 1977; 28:111.
5. Hensel P, Roizen MF: Patients with disorders of parathyroid function. Anesthesiol Clin North Am 1987; 5:287.
6. Rumancik WM, Denlinger JK, Nahrwold ML, et al: The QT interval and serum ionized calcium. JAMA 1978; 240:366.
7. Jarjult J, Lindestad P-A, Nordenstrom J, et al: Routine examination of the vocal cords before and after thyroid and parathyroid surgery. Br J Surg 1991; 78:1116.
8. Chopra LJ, Hershman JM, Pardridge WM, et al: Thyroid function in nonthyroidal illnesses. Ann Intern Med 1983; 98:946.
9. Mackin JE, Canary JJ, Pittman CS: Thyroid storm and its management. N Engl J Med 1974; 291:1396.
10. Woeber K: Thyrotoxicosis and the heart. N Engl J Med 1992; 327:94.
11. Stehling LC: Anesthetic management of the patient with hyperthyroidism. Anesthesiology 1974; 41:585.
12. Wade JSH: Respiratory obstruction in thyroid surgery. Ann R Coll Surg Engl 1980; 62:15.
13. Green WER, Sheppard HWH: Tracheal collapse after thyroidectomy. Br J Surg 1979; 66:544.
14. Capiferri R, Evered D: Investigation and treatment of hypothyroidism. Clin Endocrinol Metab 1979; 8:39.
15. Hall R, Scanlon MF: Hypothyroidism: clinical features and complications. Clin Endocrinol Metab 1979; 8:29.
16. Cooper DS: Subclinical hypothyroidism. JAMA 1987; 258:246.
17. Becker C: Hypothyroidism and atherosclerotic heart disease: pathogene-

TABLE 74–10. Manifestations of Primary Aldosteronism

Hypertension
Low serum and total body potassium
Low renin activity
Metabolic alkalosis
Skeletal muscle weakness

sis, medical management and the role of coronary artery bypass surgery. Endocrinol Rev 1985; 6:432.

18. Smallridge RC: Metabolic and thyroid emergencies: a review. Crit Care Med 1992; 20:276.
19. Miller MR, Pincock AC, Oates GD, et al: Upper airway obstruction due to goiter: detection, prevalence, and results of surgical management. Q J Med 1990; 274:177.
20. Schell N, Molnar GD, Ferris DO, et al: Circulating glucose and insulin in surgery for insulinomas. JAMA 1971; 217:1072.
21. Roizen MF: Diseases of the endocrine system. *In* Anesthesia and Uncommon Diseases. 3rd ed. Katz J, Benumof JL, Kadis LB (eds). Philadelphia, WB Saunders, 1990, p 276.
22. Schaffer MS, Zuberbuhler P, Wilson G, et al: Catecholamine cardiomyopathy: an unusual presentation of pheochromocytoma in children. J Pediatr 1981; 99:276.
23. Roizen MF, Horrigan RW, Koike M, et al: A prospective randomized trial of four anesthetic techniques for resection of pheochromocytoma. Anesthesiology 1982; 57:A43.
24. Kaplan SA: Diseases of the adrenal cortex. II. Congenital adrenal hyperplasia. Pediatr Clin North Am 1989; 26:77.
25. Gold EM: The Cushing syndromes: changing views of diagnosis and treatment. Ann Intern Med 1979; 90:829.
26. Weinberger MH, Grim CE, Hollifield JW, et al: Primary aldosteronism: diagnosis, localization and treatment. Ann Intern Med 1979; 90:386.
27. White EA, Schambelan M, Rost CR, et al: The use of computed tomography in diagnosing the cause of primary aldosteronism. N Engl J Med 1980; 303:1503.

CHAPTER 75

Anesthetic Management for Heart Transplantation

MARK C. MONROE, M.D.

Great advances have been made in the field of heart transplantation. Recipient selection criteria, immunosuppressive therapy, and immune surveillance by endomyocardial biopsy have resulted in a 5-year survival of >70%. In addition, 90% of recipients have New York Heart Association Class I functional status and resume an active lifestyle.[1]

Because of improved survival, an increase in the number of patients undergoing transplantation and in the number of medical centers active in this area has occurred (Fig. 75–1). At least 148 centers in the United States currently perform heart transplantation, and more than 12,000 orthotopic heart transplantation procedures were done in the 1980s.[1]

With improvements in survival, many transplant recipients undergo other operations subsequent to their transplant procedure. As many as one in three heart transplantation recipients apparently will present subsequently for noncardiac operations.[2-10] Although the anesthesiologist providing anesthesia care for heart transplantation is most likely be a specialist in this area, any anesthesiologist in practice may be asked to provide anesthesia for surgery done after transplantation.

SELECTION CRITERIA

Why Are They Critical?

The number of potential heart transplantation recipients exceeds the number of available donor hearts. Thus, heart transplantation must be restricted to those patients who would predictably benefit from the procedure and who also have a high probability of survival. Most cardiac transplantation programs have established specific recipient selection criteria. The indications and relative contraindications for heart transplantation are summarized in Tables 75–1 and 75–2.[11-16] These are not absolute criteria, and they vary slightly among different transplantation centers.

Cardiac transplantation usually is restricted to patients with end-stage heart disease that is refractory to medical or other surgical therapy. In 90% of patients, the indication is coronary artery disease that is not amenable to surgical correction or idiopathic cardiomyopathy. Patients are usually in New York

Heart Association Class III or IV functional status and have a limited life expectancy.

Contraindications

Irreversible pulmonary hypertension is a contraindication to orthotopic cardiac transplantation because the increased afterload it places on the right ventricle of the new heart predisposes the patient to acute right ventricular failure and inability to separate from cardiopulmonary bypass (CPB). The criterion generally used to exclude patients is a calculated pulmonary vascular resistance of <6 to 8 Wood units that is unresponsive to pulmonary vasodilators.[11, 12] Wood units are calculated by subtracting the pulmonary artery (PA) occlusion pressure from the mean PA pressure and dividing the difference by the cardiac output. In this situation, combined heart-lung transplantation is generally indicated. Other contraindications to heart transplantation include an active systemic infection that likely would be uncontrollable during immunosuppressive therapy. A separate systemic disease, such as a malignancy, or one that

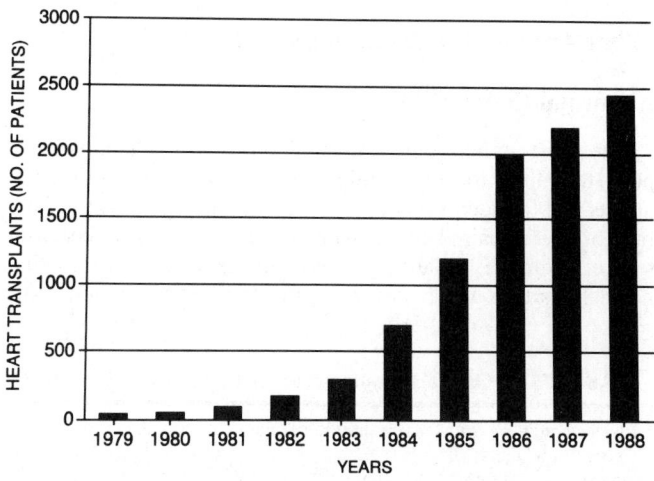

FIGURE 75–1. Number of heart transplantations performed by year. (From Heck CF, Shumway SJ, Kaye MP: The Registry of the International Society for Heart Transplantation: Sixth Official Report—1989. J Heart Transplant 1989; 8:271–276.)

TABLE 75–1. Indications for Cardiac Transplantation

- End-stage heart disease refractory to other medical or surgical treatment
- Prognosis for 1 y survival <75%
- New York Heart Association Class III–IV symptoms with maximum medical therapy
- Age younger than 60 y (exceptions occur)
- No other major systemic diseases likely to independently limit survival
- Patient emotionally stable, well motivated, and medically compliant
- Supportive family

would independently limit survival, such as end-stage emphysema or cirrhosis, is also a contraindication.

END-STAGE HEART DISEASE

What Is the Underlying Pathophysiology?

Optimal management of the cardiac transplantation patient requires the anesthesiologist to have a sound appreciation of the pathophysiology of severe end-stage heart disease. Once the pathophysiology is understood, appropriate management principles become almost intuitively obvious. The basic pathophysiology is that of any patient with severe end-stage congestive heart failure.

Progression of end-stage heart disease results in a deterioration of systolic pump function, which leads to severe congestive heart failure, and in maximum utilization of all available physiologic mechanisms to maintain cardiac output.[17–19] Congestive heart failure results in increased interstitial lung water, reduced lung compliance, and, in the preterminal stages, pulmonary hypertension.

As cardiac output falls, tissue oxygen (O_2) delivery becomes inadequate, and vital organ function is compromised. At this stage, the left ventricle functions with abnormal contractility, preload dependence, and afterload sensitivity.[20] Patients with ischemic cardiomyopathies or intractable angina unresponsive to medical therapy are additionally at risk for myocardial infarction.

What Are the Anesthetic Implications?

Abnormal Contractility

The heart with severely impaired *contractility* demonstrates poor tolerance for the administration of negative inotropic agents and for agents that decrease heart rate significantly. The rate of the impaired heart maintains cardiac output because stroke volume is relatively fixed; this is in contrast to the normal heart, in which stroke volume changes as a function of

TABLE 75–2. Contraindicatiaons to Cardiac Transplantation

- Elevated pulmonary vascular resistance refractory to vasodilatory therapy (>6–8 Wood units)
- Separate major disease that would independently limit survival (e.g., emphysema, cirrhosis, malignancy, severe cerebral or peripheral vascular disease)
- Active systemic infection
- Unresolved pulmonary embolus or infarction, or both
- Psychiatric disease or substance abuse

preload and contractility. If the impaired heart is unable to increase contractility, it will be unable to maintain or increase cardiac output in response to surgical or anesthetic stresses that increase afterload.

A hypertensive response to light anesthesia probably will not occur. In fact, the heart may respond to stress with rapid decompensation.[20] Impaired contractility is associated with a decrease in myocardial catecholamines and in myocardial β-receptor density.[21] This deficit has important implications for anesthetic management. One can expect decreased effectiveness of inotropic agents that act via β-receptor stimulation. This response is particularly common in intensive care unit (ICU) patients who require inotropic support preoperatively. Much higher doses of inotropic agents may be required during anesthesia and surgery; alternatively, inotropes that bypass the β-receptor (such as amrinone) may be useful.

Preload Dependence

As heart failure supervenes, the principal compensatory mechanism is an increase in left ventricular end-diastolic volume. The heart functions on the flat portion of the Starling curve and is *preload-dependent,* that is, it requires a higher than normal preload to maintain cardiac output and systemic perfusion.[20] Decreased preload can result in sudden decompensation and circulatory collapse. Intravascular volume augmentation (increased preload) does not predictably increase stroke volume and can lead to decreased cardiac output. The maximum stroke volume is fixed, and cardiac output is again heart rate–dependent.

Anesthetic agents can result in venodilatation and decreased preload, surgery results in volume loss through multiple mechanisms, and positive-pressure ventilation can impede venous return to the heart. The importance of closely monitoring intravascular volume status and careful volume replacement is obvious.

Afterload Sensitivity

The third abnormality of importance in understanding the delicate cardiovascular state of these patients is *afterload sensitivity.* Any increase in afterload or systemic vascular resistance without a corresponding increase in myocardial contractility can result in a rapid decrease in stroke volume, cardiac output, and systemic perfusion.[20] In addition, because of the fixed stroke volume, rapid decreases in afterload are poorly tolerated and often result in hypotension.

Summary

The cardiovascular state of the heart transplant patient is usually that of marginal compensation at best. Any physiologic insult such as decreased preload, increased afterload, drug-induced myocardial depression, or decreased heart rate can easily result in rapid decompensation.

PREANESTHETIC MANAGEMENT

The major anesthetic considerations in the patient undergoing heart transplantation are similar to those of any patient with severe congestive heart failure. However, several factors are different in heart transplant patients.

What Is the Impact of Coexisting Disease?

Transplant centers designate a transplant coordinator who is responsible for maintaining communication between the organ harvest and transplant teams.[22, 23] The anesthesiologist must be in close touch with this coordinator. Patients will already have undergone an extensive evaluation by transplant surgeons, cardiologists, and other specialists in order to be listed as a potential recipient. This information is up-to-date and readily available in the patient's chart or from the transplant coordinator. Thus, an additional detailed history of present illness beyond an interval history for the period between the pretransplant work-up and the transplant date is seldom beneficial.

Heart transplantation is not an elective procedure but rather a life-saving operation; rarely is it appropriate for the anesthesiologist to cancel or delay the surgery for medical optimization. Because of the urgency of the procedure and the time constraints related to harvesting the donor heart, the anesthesiologist often has limited time for preanesthetic evaluation. The patient will have manifestations of severe cardiac failure and usually some *reversible* compromise of renal, hepatic, or pulmonary function. In one series, 42% of patients were orthopneic on the day of surgery, 27% had peripheral edema, 12% were receiving inotropic support, 2% had an intra-aortic balloon pump in place, 41% had renal dysfunction, 52% had liver dysfunction, and 12% had cardiac dysrhythmias.[24]

History

Taking these considerations into account, the preoperative assessment should concentrate on the cardiovascular system and on the degree of impairment of other major organ systems. Review of a patient's chart reveals the recent clinical course. The anesthesiologist should review the technical cardiovascular evaluation date (e.g., echocardiogram, cardiac catheterization) to get an idea of how severe the patient's state is and to predict the degree of cardiovascular support that will be required during the prebypass period. The history should concentrate on previous anesthetic experiences, current medication regimen, allergies, and a brief review of systems.

Physical Examination

The physical examination should concentrate on a patient's vital signs and weight, airway status, neurologic function, and cardiopulmonary system status. Simple observation provides the answers to obvious and important questions: Is the patient ambulatory and thus stable or reasonably compensated, or is he or she moribund in the ICU and dependent on mechanical circulatory support? What catheters are in place and can be used, and which need to be replaced to minimize the risk of infection? Examination of the cardiopulmonary system helps to predict if the Trendelenburg position will be tolerated for awake central venous catheter insertion and also to anticipate the cardiovascular response to anesthetic induction.

Laboratory Tests

The laboratory data should be reviewed for evidence of renal and hepatic dysfunction, which often occur secondary to low perfusion or chronic passive congestion. Coagulation abnormalities are not uncommon in the presence of hepatic dysfunction; also, transplant candidates are often anticoagulated

with warfarin as prophylaxis for intracardiac thrombi that can occur secondary to low cardiac output or atrial fibrillation, or both.

If patients come to the operating room (OR) from the ICU, their blood gases and pH should be analyzed for evidence of pulmonary insufficiency and metabolic acidosis. If time permits, the chest radiograph should be reviewed for evidence of congestive heart failure and pleural effusions. If effusions are noted, the pulmonary status is improved by having them drained through the surgical field intraoperatively. The chest radiograph typically shows four-chambered cardiomegaly. Finally, the electrocardiogram and rhythm strips should be reviewed for evidence of cardiac ischemia and dysrhythmias.

Should Premedication Be Given?

Heavy premedication in marginally compensated patients is not without risk. Even slight sympatholysis, especially from benzodiazepines, can result in hemodynamic decompensation. For stable ambulatory patients, light sedation may be appropriate prior to transport to the OR; it can then be augmented when the patient is monitored continuously in the OR.

Should Transplant Patients Be Considered to Have Full Stomachs?

Although transplant coordinators instruct ambulatory patients to stop oral intake, several factors suggest that these patients should be considered to have full stomachs. Although many hours of fasting usually occur prior to the induction of anesthesia, most patients are anxious about the procedure and are unlikely to have normal gastric motility. Also, most heart transplantation immunosuppression protocols include the *oral* administration of cyclosporin A preoperatively, usually with milk or orange juice, neither of which is a clear liquid. Thus, premedication to minimize the risk of serious aspiration is appropriate. Metoclopramide, histamine$_2$ blockers, a nonparticulate antacid, or a combination of these, can be utilized. If a nasogastric tube is placed, it should not be drained lest the immunosuppressant drug be removed.

Does Anesthesia Equipment Differ from That for Other Open Heart Procedures?

Preparation of anesthesia equipment for heart transplantation differs somewhat from that for routine open heart cases because of the former's requirement for maximum sterile conditions. The anesthesia machine should be set up with a sterile, disposable anesthetia bag and circuit.[13, 20, 25, 26] In addition, some centers routinely use bacterial filters on the breathing circuit,[13] although this practice is not universal.[25] In many centers, a sterile intubation tray is employed (Table 75–3).

What Monitors Should Be Utilized?

The intraoperative monitoring of the patient undergoing cardiac transplantation is similar to that used for other cardiac procedures. Noninvasive monitors include a multilead electro-

TABLE 75–3. Sterile Intubation Tray for Heart Transplantation

Oral airways
Tongue blades
Cloth towels for draping
Laryngoscope handle (without batteries)
Laryngoscope batteries (taped to outside of sterile tray)
Laryngoscope blades
Endotracheal tubes
Endotracheal tube stylet
Syringe (10-mL)
Magill forceps
Disposal esophageal stethoscope and temperature probe
Nasogastric tubes

cardiograph, blood pressure cuff, pulse oximeter, capnograph, esophageal stethoscope, urinary catheter, and two temperature probes (usually esophageal and bladder).[24, 27–29] Invasive monitors include a radial or femoral arterial catheter and a central venous or PA catheter.

Pulmonary Artery Catheters

Whether PA catheterization should be performed in heart transplantation is a subject of controversy. A survey of heart transplantation centers in North America indicated that 32% utilized the PA catheter before bypass and that 44% used it after bypass.[30, 31] Advocates claim that rational anesthetic management is possible only with such monitoring.[30] Other authorities claim that PA catheters are unnecessary for patients who do not have pulmonary hypertension. Their use increases the risk of infection, and they must be pulled back into the sterility sheath prior to removal of the recipient's heart.[14, 24, 26, 27] Still others claim that PA catheters are contraindicated.[28]

A reasonable approach is to use a central venous pressure (CVP) catheter in patients without pulmonary hypertension; a multilumen polyurethane catheter permits simultaneous drug infusion and CVP monitoring and also minimizes the risk of superior vena caval or right atrial perforation.[32, 33] A PA catheter is most useful in patients with pulmonary hypertension. Initially, it is advanced only 15 to 20 cm and used to measure CVP, with the sterility sheath fully extended over the catheter. It is then advanced into the PA after separation from CPB.

With the catheter only partially inserted, the CVP port and possibly the venous infusion ports may be outside the sheath; therefore, medications given via these routes do not reach the circulation.

Several factors can make placement of a PA catheter difficult in heart transplantation patients, including cardiac dysrhythmias, a large dilated heart with poor ejection, tricuspid regurgitation, and poor tolerance of the head-down position by awake patients.

Internal Jugular Access

Because the right internal jugular vein is used postoperatively for transvenous endomyocardial biopsy, many authorities recommend that the left internal jugular vein be preferentially used for intraoperative invasive cardiac monitoring. However, owing to the anatomic relationship of the brachiocephalic vein to the superior vena cava, and to the tortuous course pursued by the catheter, the left-sided approach for invasive monitoring increases the risk of vascular perforation by the catheter.[32, 33] The catheter must be long enough for its

tip to reach beyond the junction of the brachiocephalic and internal jugular veins. Polyurethane or, preferably, pigtail catheters are recommended because they are less likely to perforate the vessel wall.[33] A follow-up chest radiograph should verify that the catheter tip and superior vena cava are parallel or, at worst, not at more than a 40° angle with respect to one another.

Infection Control

Infection is a leading cause of morbidity and mortality in heart transplant recipients.[15, 34] Thus, all invasive catheters must be placed with sterile technique. For intravenous catheters, the site should be prepped with povidone-iodine and draped with sterile towels; sterile gloves should be worn during insertion. Although suprapubic catheters sometimes are used to minimize the risk of bladder infection, this problem has not proved to be significant; most surgeons use Foley catheters.

PREINDUCTION PERIOD

What Other Factors Are Important?

Blood

The immunosuppressed heart transplantation patient is at risk for cytomegalovirus sepsis; thus, the blood bank should obtain cytomegalovirus-free blood products for those patients who lack cytomegalovirus antibodies.

Drugs

Because transplant patients have poor baseline ventricular function, a variety of inotropic and vasoactive agents should be premixed and immediately available during induction; direct-acting agents such as dobutamine, epinephrine, phenylephrine, isoproterenol, and sodium nitroprusside are most useful.

Placement of Monitoring Devices

Transplant patients who have previously undergone heart surgery are likely to require more time for placement of invasive monitors, chest opening, and cannulation for CPB than patients who have not. This factor must be considered preoperatively so that donor organ ischemic times are not prolonged unnecessarily. Intravenous catheters and invasive monitors can be placed conveniently under local anesthesia in the ICU prior to transport to the OR. This approach is inherently less sterile. Alternatively, the patient can be transported to the OR early enough to allow sufficient time for catheter placements.

Transport and Timing of Induction

If the patient is in the ICU and, in particular, if he or she is receiving mechanical cardiac support, a plan for organized transport to the OR is mandatory; early communication with ICU nurses and personnel responsible for operating the support devices facilitates transport in an expeditious and safe manner. Also, the timing of anesthesia induction must take into account arrival of the donor heart. Donor heart ischemic time should not be prolonged by allowing the heart to arrive before the recipient is ready. Finally, induction should be planned so as to avoid prolonging the prebypass period (or CPB if the patient becomes unstable). Frequent communication among all involved is necessary to achieve this goal.

ANESTHETIC INDUCTION

Induction of anesthesia is perhaps the most critical period of anesthetic care. The combination of negative inotropic anesthetic agents, ablation of sympathetic tone, venous dilatation, anesthetic-induced decreases in heart rate, and positive-pressure ventilation in a patient with no or little cardiac reserve can result in sudden cardiovascular collapse. Primary goals are to monitor hemodynamic function closely, minimize the administration of negative inotropic agents, maintain heart rate and intravascular volume, avoid arterial and venous dilatation, and minimize the risk of aspiration.

What Are the Options?

Anesthetic techniques used for other cardiac surgical patients who have poor ventricular function are appropriate for the transplant recipient and many have been used successfully.[14, 20, 24, 25, 28–30, 35, 36] The risk of aspiration must be considered. In the anesthetic management survey of Hensley and coworkers, aspiration precautions were taken in 88% of cases; rapid-sequence induction was employed in 11 of 30; and modified rapid-sequence induction was used in 15 of 30.[30] Baum, however, did not consider the small amount of oral cyclosporine A to be an indication for a rapid-sequence induction.[25]

Rapid-Sequence Induction

Generally, one of three approaches is taken. A classic rapid-sequence induction of anesthesia with cricoid pressure is frequently recommended.[24, 29, 30] The induction agents most commonly used for this technique are ketamine and etomidate. Ketamine may seem to be the best agent. However, its indirect sympathomimetic effects may not manifest in these catecholamine-depleted patients, and its direct negative inotropic effects may result in significant hypotension.

Routine Induction

Some authorities prefer a slow, titrated anesthetic induction technique.[14, 28] The agents most often used are the potent synthetic narcotics, fentanyl or sufentanil, along with benzodiazepines, low-dose inhaled agents, or scopolamine. These drugs can be titrated slowly or administered by slow infusion.

Care must be taken when inducing anesthesia with high-dose potent synthetic narcotics (especially sufentanil) to avoid slowing of the heart rate from central narcotic-induced vagotonia. Hemodynamic decompensation can be precipitated in patients with rate-dependent cardiac output. This problem usually can be minimized by the simultaneous administration of incremental doses of pancuronium. This drug's vagolytic effects minimize slowing of heart rate.

Modified Rapid-Sequence Induction

A third commonly used approach is a modified rapid-sequence induction in which potent synthetic narcotics, muscle relaxants, and benzodiazepines or low-dose inhaled agents are administered slowly with continuous application of cricoid pressure and assisted or controlled ventilation.[25]

Summary

For patients coming from home who have compensated ventricular function and full stomachs, premedication with histamine$_2$ blockers and metoclopramide and a rapid-sequence induction with etomidate or ketamine and succinylcholine are reasonable. Potent narcotics can be slowly titrated before and after induction as needed.

For the hospitalized patient who is uncompensated, is receiving inotropic support, and is in nil per os status (except for oral cyclosporine A administration), a slow, gentle, modified rapid-sequence induction technique with cricoid pressure is reasonable. No matter what induction technique is used, the hemodynamic status must be monitored closely; fluids, anesthetics, and vasoactive agents are administered as clinically indicated.

Can Sterile Intubation Be Performed?

Although the trachea cannot be intubated in a sterile fashion, anesthesiologists should attempt to perform the intubation in as clean a manner as possible in order to minimize the risk of pulmonary infection. A sterile intubation tray can be used (see Table 75–3). Sometimes a designated intubator (a second anesthesiologist) drapes the patient's face with sterile towels and performs the intubation with a sterile laryngoscope and endotracheal tube.[14, 26] A nasal intubation should be avoided if at all possible, since it predisposes the patient to bacteremia and subsequent sinus infection.

ANESTHETIC MAINTENANCE

What Are the Best Agents?

A variety of anesthetic agents have been used successfully for anesthetic maintenance; no correlation can be found between anesthetic techniques and operative outcome.[24] A survey of anesthetic practices at 34 centers indicated that narcotic-based anesthesia, which causes minimal cardiac depression, was used in the majority of 1273 heart transplantations.[30] Potent inhaled agents are rarely used as the primary maintenance anesthetic for heart transplantation.[30] Such use has been complicated by hypotension.[24, 36]

Precautions

The success with which a variety of agents have been used for maintenance of anesthesia during cardiac transplantation suggests that the skill and care with which the anesthetic is administered are probably of greater importance than the particular agent or agents that are used. However, several points merit discussion. Benzodiazepines are often used to supplement narcotic anesthesia for heart transplantation. These agents can lower systemic vascular resistance and produce myocardial depression when combined with narcotic agents. Nitrous oxide is not recommended because it can further depress myocardial contractility, and any air emboli incurred during the open heart procedure may undergo expansion. Excessive doses of narcotics should be avoided, if possible, because prolonged mechanical ventilatory support increases the risk of pulmonary infection in these immunocompromised patients.

Goals

Regardless of the technique used, several anesthetic goals are worth reviewing. Prior to CPB, maintenance of the patient's baseline hemodynamic state is a primary consideration. Efforts to make a stable patient "better" before CPB are as likely to create problems as they are to prevent them. Be prepared to administer pharmacologic cardiovascular support. Inotropic support was increased postinduction in 44% of cases according to Hensley and coworkers.[30] During mobilization and exposure of the heart, hemodynamic instability and cardiac dysrhythmias are common, especially with dissection of adhesions and placement of the vena cava–encircling snares. Constant vigilance and interaction with the surgical team are essential.

When mobilization and exposure of the heart have been completed, heparin is administered in preparation for cannulation of the great vessels. After adequate anticoagulation is verified and the great vessels are cannulated, a dose of intravenous steroid is administered per the transplant protocol upon arrival of the donor heart, and CPB is initiated.

THE ANESTHESIOLOGIST'S RESPONSIBILITIES DURING CARDIOPULMONARY BYPASS

How Do They Differ from Those During Other Cardiac Procedures?

Most anesthesiologists treat this period similarly in transplantation and in other cardiac procedures. However, several considerations are different for heart transplantation. If a PA catheter is in place, it is withdrawn into the proximal superior vena cava prior to the sealing off of the vena cava around the venous cannula. Early in the CPB period, blood gas measurements often reveal metabolic acidosis; this reflects the large O_2 debt in the peripheral tissues of patients with severe heart failure. The anesthesiologist and perfusionist should make sure that these abnormalities are corrected before separation from CPB is attempted. In addition to myocardial depression, metabolic acidosis may exacerbate pulmonary hypertension.

What Drugs Should Be Available?

During CPB, ensure that appropriate inotropic agents are available for weaning from CPB. These include isoproterenol or dobutamine and nitroglycerin. Prostaglandin E_1 should also be readily available, since it has been demonstrated to be useful in managing pulmonary hypertension during separation from CPB.[37, 38] Be prepared to administer immunosuppressive agents prior to removal of the aortic cross-clamp and during reperfusion of the transplanted heart. As with other cardiac procedures performed under CPB, additional narcotic, anesthetic, muscle relaxant, or benzodiazepine is administered during rewarming, as clinically indicated.

THE OPERATIVE PROCEDURE

How Is It Performed?

Donor Heart

A brief description of the transplantation procedure helps one to understand the unique cardiac physiology and pharmacology.[39] The donor heart is resected so that the posterior atrial walls (including the sinoatrial node), pulmonary veins, and vena cava are intact. The great vessels are divided above the semilunar valves.

Recipient Heart

The recipient's heart is exposed using midline sternotomy. Heparin is given in the usual manner prior to CPB. Ideally, CPB is initiated just before arrival of the donor heart. The aorta is cross-clamped, and *after* the donor heart is in the room and is determined to be suitable, the recipient's heart is removed. The atria are transected above the atrioventricular grooves, leaving the posterior atrial walls and the sinoatrial node intact, and the great vessels are divided above the valves.

Anastomoses

The operation requires the completion of four major anastomoses. First, the left and right atrial anastomoses are completed, and then the aortic and pulmonary artery anastomoses are performed. Subsequently, air is evacuated, a second dose of steroid is administered, the cross-clamp is removed, and rewarming is completed. The result is an implanted heart that is totally devoid of autonomic innervation and one that contains two sinoatrial nodes.

The patient is weaned from CPB in the usual manner, except that an infusion (e.g., isoproterenol, usually at 0.01 $\mu g \cdot kg^{-1} \cdot min^{-1}$) is used to maintain the heart rate at about 100 beats per minute. Temporary pacing wires are also placed.

DENERVATED HEART FUNCTION

The transplanted heart is excluded from all normal autonomic innervation. Thus, its physiology and pharmacologic response to drugs are altered. These effects impact on postbypass anesthetic management.

Denervation does not impair the heart's intrinsic impulse formation and conduction system. The heart rate is controlled by the donor sinoatrial node, which does not respond to direct autonomic nervous system stimulation. The basal heart rate is usually 90 to 100 beats per minute, the intrinsic rate of a denervated heart.[40]

What Physiologic Alterations Occur?

Exercise

Studies of heart transplantation patients demonstrate that they have an altered hemodynamic response to stress and exercise.[41–46] The rate response of the denervated heart is delayed, gradual, and reduced.[42, 43, 45] Increase in cardiac output induced by exercise or stress is almost entirely mediated through an increase in stroke volume as a result of increased venous return and the Frank-Starling mechanism.[42, 43] Thus, cardiac output is preload-dependent.

Later, and with more severe exercise, heart rate and contractility increase in response to circulating catecholamines. The result is an even greater cardiac output.[43] With cessation of exercise or stress, a more gradual return to baseline hemodynamic values than in normal subjects occurs. This gradual return to baseline correlates with decreasing circulating catecholamine levels.[43]

Reflex Changes

Denervation also removes the heart from physiologic control loops that require intact autonomic innervation. Thus, reflex increases in heart rate to augment cardiac output cannot occur immediately in response to vasodilation or sudden blood loss. Also, the heart rate will not respond immediately to inadequate anesthesia; any response in heart rate that results will also lag in onset, be minor in magnitude, and lag in termination.

How Are Pharmacologic Responses Altered?

The second major consequence of cardiac denervation is the altered response to various cardiovascular drugs. Since the heart is denervated, medications that act via the autonomic nervous system do not elicit the expected response. For example, atropine normally accelerates heart rate by blocking vagal tone. This effect is not seen in the denervated heart; thus, atropine is totally ineffective in treating bradycardia or conduction system defects.[47, 48]

Although adrenergic neurotransmission has been permanently disrupted, the adrenergic receptors are intact, and the response of the denervated heart to direct adrenergic agonists, isoproterenol, epinephrine, dobutamine, norepinephrine, and phenylephrine is preserved.[48–50] Bradydysrhythmias can be treated with direct β-adrenergic stimulating agents. However, reflex changes associated with direct-acting agents are absent. As an example, the reflex bradycardia normally seen in response to phenylephrine hydrochloride (Neo-Synephrine) administration does not occur.

Drugs that act both directly and indirectly (dopamine, ephedrine) have diminished effects. Although these drugs have not been carefully studied, several reports indicate that they are useful in cardiac transplantation patients.[27–30] Since most clinicians probably are more familiar with ephedrine than epinephrine for vasopressor support, initial support with ephedrine is reasonable.

How Effective Are Antidysrhythmic Agents?

Digoxin

Digoxin produces little acute change in sinus node activity and atrioventricular conduction because these functions are primarily indirect and autonomically mediated. It has a positive inotropic action (direct effect) in heart transplant patients.[40, 48, 51] Thus, digoxin is not useful for acute control of the ventricular rate in atrial fibrillation. Chronic oral administration, however, effectively depresses atrioventricular conduction, making digoxin useful for long-term rate control in atrial fibrillation.[52]

β-Blockers

As expected, β-blockers decrease heart rate in the denervated heart.[53, 54] Few studies concerning the effects of β-blockers on cardiac output, ejection fraction, or any other measure of ventricular systolic function have been performed. However, studies have demonstrated that β-blockers can significantly reduce exercise tolerance in these patients.[53, 54] As was noted earlier, the denervated heart's peak cardiac output is highly dependent on elevated catecholamine levels. Heart transplant patients should be considered extremely sensitive to the effects of β-blockers.

Verapamil

Verapamil is effective in its direct action on the calcium channels of the transplanted heart and decreases atrial rate and atrioventricular conduction. Thus, it can be used in supraventricular tachydysrhythmias.[55]

Quinidine and Procainamide

The electrophysiologic effects of quinidine and procainamide are very similar in that they exert both direct and autonomically mediated effects on the heart. The increase in heart rate is due to an atropine-like effect on the sinoatrial and atrioventricular nodes and is absent in the denervated heart.[56] The direct effects of these agents—suppression of the sinoatrial and atrioventricular nodes and of the His-Purkinje conduction—are present, and they appear useful to suppress supraventricular dysrhythmias in the denervated heart.[56]

Lidocaine

The effects of lidocaine are almost completely independent of the autonomic nervous system. Lidocaine is useful for control of ventricular dysrhythmias in these patients.

WEANING FROM CARDIOPULMONARY BYPASS

How Does It Differ in the Transplant Patient?

Before Separation from Bypass

The postbypass period of cardiac transplantation presents the obvious requirement for maintenance of anesthesia and management of the acutely denervated and transplanted heart. The newly transplanted heart does not function normally as a result of the typically more prolonged ischemia (often 2.5 hours or longer) and cardioplegia that occur during donor cardiectomy and recipient implantation.

Inotropic Support

Contractility and stroke volume are often decreased, and cardiac output becomes volume-dependent and rate-dependent. Therefore, use of an isoproterenol infusion is common. Volume status is gauged by left atrial pressure or PA occlusion pressure, except in the recipient with normal pulmonary vascular resistance in whom CVP measurement often suffices. Transesophageal echocardiography has a role here as well. It allows verification that the therapeutic interventions are adequate and provides a direct, objective assessment of left ventricular volume. This benefit is particularly relevant when left ventricular compliance is decreased, since left atrial pressure and PA occlusion pressure do not provide an accurate assessment of volume status or compliance.

After Release of the Aortic Cross-Clamp

After release of the aortic cross-clamp, a sinus or slow junctional rhythm usually develops. If spontaneous defibrillation has not occurred when core temperature reaches 34°C to 36°C, electrical defibrillation should be undertaken. The intrinsic rate of the denervated heart initially may be quite slow.

Maintenance of Heart Rate and Contractility

To ensure an adequate heart rate and to enhance contractility, an infusion of isoproterenol, 0.005 to 0.05 $\mu g \cdot kg^{-1} \cdot min^{-1}$, is begun during the final stages of CPB and is titrated to achieve a heart rate of 90 to 100 beats per minute. Isoproterenol also decreases pulmonary vascular resistance, enhances diastolic relaxation, and improves cardiac filling. Dobutamine, which has effects similar to those of isoproterenol, is used in some centers.[14] Pacing is occasionally required. Low-dose dopamine is also frequently employed to augment urine output. It may also produce a slight increase in systemic vascular resistance, offsetting peripheral isoproterenol-induced vasodilatation.

Volume Sensitivity

The newly transplanted ischemic heart is volume-sensitive and usually functions best when CVP is 10 to 15 cm H_2O. Higher filling pressures are required in cases of graft dysfunction. With adequate heart rate and preload, weaning from CPB is usually straightforward. Occasionally, high doses of isoproterenol or dobutamine and epinephrine, norepinephrine, or amrinone are necessary. This requirement occurs in the setting of pulmonary hypertension and prolonged ischemic times. Only rarely is an intra-aortic balloon pump or ventricular assist device support required. Hensley and coworkers reported the use of an intra-aortic balloon pump to separate patients from CPB in only 2% of cases.[30]

After Separation from Bypass

After separation from bypass, anesthetic management is similar to that for most open heart procedures with a few special considerations. Postoperative function of the graft is subnormal for several days.[57] For this reason, most authorities recommend that isoproterenol not be completely discontinued in the operative and immediate postoperative periods, even if the heart is functioning well.[28]

Transplanted patients typically do well and are good candidates for early extubation. Since prolonged intubation may present a significant infectious disease risk, anesthetic management (narcotic dosing) should be tailored to allow early extubation, if possible. Also, blood products should be avoided, if possible, in these patients with compromised immunity to minimize the risk of transmission of unscreened viral agents.

What Are the Options When Failure to Wean Occurs?

In approximately 1% of cases, the donor heart does not function adequately despite aggressive inotropic and intra-aortic and balloon pump support.[30] The most common cause for failure to wean (45%) is right ventricular dysfunction.[30] Post-ischemic ventricular dysfunction and, rarely, acute rejection are other causes. In the event of the occurrence of these phenomena, only retransplantation, with temporary mechanical support using a ventricular assist device or total artificial heart as a bridge, will suffice until a suitable donor for retransplantation can be located.

Right Ventricular Failure and Pulmonary Hypertension

If right ventricular failure from pulmonary hypertension is the reason for inability to wean, retransplantation is unlikely to be a cure, and mechanical support with further aggressive pharmacologic and respiratory therapy is recommended.

In the setting of cardiac transplantation, right ventricular failure is almost always secondary to excessive right ventricular afterload. It is imminent when the mean pulmonary artery pressure ($\overline{PAP}$) exceeds 30 mm Hg.[57] Patients with pre-existing pulmonary hypertension are at the greatest risk. Even with mild pre-existing disease, severe acute pulmonary hypertension can be seen after CPB. Treatment modalities are summarized in Table 75–4. The most effective are pulmonary vasodilatation and inotropic support, along with maintenance of normocarbia or hypocarbia.

Prostaglandin E₁

Prostaglandin E_1 is the best pulmonary vasodilator. In doses of 30 to 150 $\mu g \cdot kg \cdot min^{-1}$, it usually lowers pulmonary vascular resistance when other agents have failed.[37, 38] Nitroprusside, nitroglycerin, and priscoline are nonspecific vasodilators that have been used with limited success.

Inotropic Support

Inotropic agents with vasodilatory properties, such as isoproterenol, amrinone, and dobutamine, should be the primary agents selected.

TABLE 75–4. Treatment of Right Ventricular Failure

Inotropic Support	Isoproterenol
	Dobutamine
	Amrinone
Pulmonary Vasodilators	Prostaglandin E₁
	Sodium nitroprusside
	Nitroglycerin
	Priscoline
Mechanical Right Ventricular Support	Right ventricular assist device
	Total artificial heart
Other	Hyperventilation
	Correction of hypoxemia
	Correction of acidosis
	Minimal positive end-expiratory pressure/continuous positive airway pressure

Hyperventilation

Hyperventilation with minimal positive end-expiratory pressure and correction of acidosis are also important measures to minimize pulmonary vasoconstriction. The effect of hypoventilation or hyperventilation on pulmonary vascular resistance should not be underestimated. An increase in arterial carbon dioxide partial pressure from only 38 to 49 mm Hg has been shown to cause a 54% increase in pulmonary vascular resistance, a 34% increase in $\overline{PAP}$, and an increase in right ventricular volume.[58]

Nitric Oxide

Nitric oxide soon may become part of our armamentarium as it shows exceptional promise as a selective pulmonary vasodilator.

If the measures discussed fail, institution of mechanical right ventricular support may be the only way to avoid a fatal outcome.[38]

How Common Are Cardiac Dysrhythmias?

The denervated heart often exhibits sinus bradycardia or low-grade atrioventricular block in the early post-CPB period and thus requires the institution of either chronotropic or pacemaker support. Approximately 5% to 10% of transplant patients have persistence of bradydysrhythmias and require placement of a permanent pacemaker. Patients can develop any of the wide variety of dysrhythmias seen in other cardiac surgical patients; these dysrhythmias may be more common in the denervated heart.[40, 59] When treating them, remember that antidysrhythmic and chronotropic agents that act via the autonomic nervous system will not be effective.

How Common Is Bleeding?

Bleeding is more likely to be a problem in the cardiac transplantation patient than in the average open heart surgery patient. It can be multifactorial in origin (Table 75–5). Many potential cardiac transplantation patients are chronically anticoagulated with warfarin to reduce the risk of thrombotic complications associated with low cardiac output. Some cardiac transplantation patients have decreased levels of coagulation factors secondary to preoperative liver dysfunction. Although efforts are usually made to correct the coagulopathy preoperatively, most patients are still anticoagulated to some degree at the time of transplantation.

TABLE 75–5. Potential Causes of Bleeding in the Cardiac Transplantation Patient

Anticoagulation therapy
Coagulation factor deficiency from hepatic dysfunction
Dilutional coagulopathy
Thrombocytopenia
    Secondary to preoperative heparin therapy
    Dilutional
    Damage secondary to CPB
Suture line

TABLE 75–6. Common Surgical Procedures Performed After Cardiac Transplantation

- Emergency exploration for mediastinal bleeding
- Thoracotomy for repair of perforated endomyocardial biopsy site
- Retransplantation
- Complications caused by infection
    Laparotomy
    Craniotomy
    Bronchoscopy
    Mediastinoscopy or thoracostomy
    Extremity abscess drainage
- Complications caused by steroid treatment
    Repair of hip fracture/total hip replacement
    Laparotomy for perforated viscous cataract excision
- Vascular surgery
    Aortic
    Peripheral
    Amputations
- Cardioversion
- Other procedures
    Elective
    Trauma
    Obstetric

Treatment of Coagulopathy

Vitamin K administered prior to surgery is not effective for at least 24 to 48 hours. In addition, since most transplantation patients have some degree of impaired hepatic function, and since vitamin K effects depend on the hepatic synthesis of water-soluble factors, vitamin K should not be expected to have maximum effectiveness in these patients.

Correction of the coagulopathy preoperatively is not without risk; 2 units of fresh-frozen plasma (FFP) may be enough to precipitate acute heart failure. If correction is necessary preoperatively, careful monitoring and even concomitant administration of a diuretic should be considered. Most patients need fresh-frozen plasma or platelets, or both, to correct their bleeding diathesis. This need should be anticipated well in advance so that cytomegalovirus-free and irradiated blood products can be procured. Do not forget surgical causes of bleeding that are related to the four major anastomoses between the donor heart and the recipient.

ANESTHESIA AFTER CARDIAC TRANSPLANTATION

Why Is Additional Surgery Necessary?

Up to 30% of heart transplantation recipients require surgery at a later date. Surgery may be necessary as a result of complications of the transplantation procedure, progression of an underlying disease process, or complications of immunosuppressive therapy or for reasons completely unrelated to the transplantation procedure (Table 75–6). These patients provide an anesthetic challenge because the additional surgery often is emergent, patients often are seriously ill, their hearts remain denervated, and several complications may have developed. A complete preanesthetic evaluation with emphasis in a few areas identifies the significant problems (Table 75–7).

What Problems Must Be Addressed?

Infection

Infection is still the number one cause of death in transplant patients. Pulmonary infections are most common (65%), the

TABLE 75–7. Important Anesthetic Considerations in Patients Who Are to Undergo Surgery After Cardiac Transplantation

- Physiology and pharmacology of the denervated heart
- Risk of infection
- Common complications
  - Acute rejection
  - Chronic rejection/graft arteritis (vasculitis)
  - Complications of immunosuppressive therapy
- Perioperative maintenance of immunosuppression
- Perioperative steroid coverage

most serious of which are bacterial and fungal.[15] Optimization of preoperative pulmonary function, extubation as early as possible, and plans for aggressive postoperative respiratory therapy should be made. Meticulous aseptic technique is mandatory in the management of transplant patients.

Acute Rejection

Acute rejection is the second most common cause of death in the first 2 years after transplantation. Clinical signs of acute rejection include tachycardia, fever, dysrhythmias,[60] and heart failure. The undertaking of surgery and anesthesia during a period of acute rejection places the patient at high risk for morbidity and mortality. In many centers, cardiac catheterization and endomyocardial biopsy are recommended prior to elective surgery.

The immunologist managing the patient should be consulted so that appropriate plans are made for perioperative immunosuppressive therapy. Patients continue to receive appropriate immunosuppressive therapy. Elective surgery is generally postponed until after the first year following transplantation, at which time immunosuppressant use will have been reduced to maintenance doses and acute rejection becomes unlikely.

Cardiovascular Function

Although heart transplant patients may be functioning very well, they do not have a normal cardiovascular system. As was discussed earlier, they have altered cardiovascular physiologic and pharmacologic responses. In addition, left ventricular dysfunction secondary to chronic rejection, graft arteritis/vasculitis, or both, may be present.

Chronic Rejection

Chronic rejection, which is manifested as diffuse coronary arteritis, is a complication of heart transplantation. Its prevalence rises progressively with time: 18% at 1 year, 27% at 2 years, and 44% at 3 years after transplantation.[61, 62] This arteritis tends to be much different from atherosclerosis in that it is diffuse, concentric, and obliterative. Thus, little collateral vessel flow is present, and the lesion is not amenable to angioplasty. Clinical manifestations of chronic rejection do not include angina because the heart is denervated. Instead, the patient usually presents with angina equivalents such as dysrhythmias, heart failure, or sudden death.

Chronic Immunosuppression

Chronic immunosuppression is necessary for survival of heart transplantation patients; however, many side effects and

complications may result (Table 75–8). The anesthesiologist should review the immunosuppressive regimen and look for the development of these complications, especially renal insufficiency and hypertension. Serum creatinine typically is >2 mg · dL^{-1}. The implications for drugs that undergo renal clearance are obvious. Patients usually are treated with chronic administration of corticosteroids; thus, supplemental steroids should be considered.

Miscellaneous Considerations

Since most of these patients have been previously exposed to blood products, they will be more difficult to cross-match. The need for blood products must be considered preoperatively. Cytomegalovirus infection is devastating; cytomegalovirus-negative blood should be requested.

The direct-acting vasoactive agents that were used for cardiac transplantation should also be prepared prior to the induction of anesthesia. A transvenous or transcutaneous pacemaker should be readily available for the treatment of bradydysrhythmias if pharmacologic agents are ineffective.

Monitoring

The need for invasive monitoring is dictated by the function of the transplanted heart and by the operative procedure. Since the risk of infection associated with invasive monitoring is increased, the anesthesiologist must carefully weigh the advantages and disadvantages of invasive monitoring. Ream and associates have written that "a pulmonary artery catheter is contraindicated, unless severe pulmonary hypertension exists."[28] Although I agree that a PA catheter should not be used in a cavalier fashion, I do not accept the exclusion of such monitoring that is implicitly suggested in the directive of these authors.

Does the Anesthetic Technique Matter?

A multitude of reports have recommended a variety of anesthetic agents and techniques; general and regional methods have been used without significant problems.[63–69] No evidence

TABLE 75–8. Complications of Immunosuppressive Therapy

General		Infection
		Malignancy
		Pancytopenia
Agent Specific	*Cyclosporin A*	Renal insufficiency
		Hypertension
	Prednisone	Adrenal suppression
		Glucose intolerance
		Hypertension
		Osteoporosis
		Aseptic necrosis
		Gastrointestinal bleeding
		Electrolyte disturbances
		Fragile skin
	Azathioprine	Pancytopenia
		Liver dysfunction
	T Cell Agents	Hypotension
		Nausea and vomiting
		Pulmonary edema
		Serum sickness–like syndrome
		Aseptic meningitis

TABLE 75–9. Conditions During Anesthesia for the Patient with a Transplanted Heart

---

Avoid:
   Rapid decreases in filling pressure
   Rapid fall in heart rate
   Significant decrease in systemic vascular resistance
Maintain high-normal filling pressures
Use direct-acting vasoactive drugs
Avoid hypercarbia, which increases pulmonary vascular resistance

---

shows that regional anesthesia is safer than general anesthesia. Recommendation for a specific technique to the exclusion of others cannot and should not be made. As long as the pharmacologic and physiologic changes discussed earlier are appreciated, the anesthetic technique selected does not appear to be critical.[70]

Several points deserve special emphasis (Table 75–9). Avoid any maneuver that rapidly reduces filling pressures, heart rate, or systemic vascular resistance because transplant patients cannot immediately compensate for these physiologic stresses. They function best with high-normal filling pressures. This admonition is especially important to keep in mind if spinal or epidural anesthesia is utilized. Changes in heart rate are poor indicators of the adequacy of anesthesia and intravascular volume. Again, drugs that stimulate receptors directly have the most reliable effect in the denervated heart.

References

1. Heck CF, Shumway SJ, Kaye MP: The Registry of the International Society for Heart Transplantation: Sixth Official Report—1989. J Heart Transplant 1989; 8:271.
2. Shaw IH, Kirk AJ, Conacher ID: Anesthesia for patients with transplanted hearts and lungs undergoing non-cardiac surgery. Br J Anaesth 1991; 67:772.
3. Jones MT, Menkis AH, Kostuk WJ, et al: Management of general surgical problems after cardiac transplantation. Can J Surg 1988; 31:259.
4. Isono SS, Woolson ST, Schurman DJ: Total joint arthroplasty for steroid-induced osteonecrosis in cardiac transplant patients. Clin Orthop 1987; 217:201.
5. Merrel SW, Ames SA, Nelson EW, et al: Major abdominal complications following cardiac transplantation. Arch Surg 1989; 124:889.
6. Disea VJ, Kirkman RL, Tilney NL, et al: Management of general surgical complications following cardiac transplantation. Arch Surg 1989; 124:539.
7. Steed DL, Brown B, Reilly JJ, et al: General surgical complications in heart and heart-lung transplantation. Surgery 1985; 98:739.
8. Colon R, Frazier OH, Kahan BD, et al: Complications in cardiac transplant patients requiring general surgery. Surgery 1988; 103:32.
9. Burton DS, Mochizuki RM, Halpern AA: Total hip arthroplasty in the cardiac transplant patient. Clin Orthop 1978; 130:186.
10. Reitz BA, Baumgartner WA, Oyer PE, et al: Abdominal aortic aneurysmectomy in long-term cardiac transplant survivors. Arch Surg 1977; 112:1057.
11. Renlund DG, Bristow MR, Lee HR, et al: Medical aspects of cardiac transplantation. J Cardiothorac Anesth 1988; 2:500.
12. Copeland JG, Emery RW, Levinson MM, et al: Selection of patients for cardiac transplantation. Circulation 1987; 75:2.
13. Firestone L: Heart transplantation. Int Anesthesiol Clin 1991; 29:41.
14. Gallo JA, Cork RC: Anesthesia for cardiac transplantation. Contemp Anesth Pract 1987; 10:47.
15. Pennock JL, Oyer PE, Reitz BA, et al: Cardiac transplantation in perspective for the future: survival, complications, rehabilitation, and cost. J Cardiovasc Surg 1982; 83:168.
16. Achuff SC: Clinical evaluation of potential heart transplantation recipients. In Heart and Heart-Lung Transplantation. Baumgartner WA, Reitz BA, Achuff SC (eds). Philadelphia, WB Saunders, 1990, pp 51–57.
17. Weber KT, Janicki JS, Maskin CS: Pathophysiology of cardiac failure. Am J Cardiol 1985; 56:3B.
18. Parmley WW: Pathophysiology of congestive heart failure. Am J Cardiol 1985; 56:7A.
19. Braunwald E: Heart failure: pathophysiology and treatment. Am Heart J 1981; 102:486.
20. Clark NJ, Martin RD: Anesthetic considerations for patients undergoing cardiac transplantation. J Cardiothorac Anesth 1988; 2:519.
21. Fowler MB, Laser JA, Hopkins GL, et al: Assessment of the β-adrenergic receptor pathway in the intact failing human heart: progressive receptor down-regulation and subsensitivity to agonist response. Circulation 1986; 74:1290.
22. Davis FD: Coordination of cardiac transplantation: patient processing and donor organ procurement. Circulation 1987; 75:29.
23. Baumgartner WA, Borkon AM, Achuff SC, et al: Organization, development and early results of a heart transplant program: the Johns Hopkins experience. Chest 1986; 89:836.
24. Demas K, Wyner J, Mihm FG, et al: Anesthesia for heart transplantation: a retrospective study and review. Br J Anaesth 1986; 58:1357.
25. Baum VC: Anesthesia for heart transplantation recipients. Semin Anesth 1990; 9:298.
26. Humphrey LS, Blanck TJ: Anesthetic management of the heart or heart-lung transplant patient. In Heart and Heart-Lung Transplantation. Baumgartner WA, Reitz BA, Achuff SC (eds). Philadelphia, WB Saunders, 1990, pp 103–112.
27. Grebenik CR, Robinson PN: Cardiac transplantation at Harefield: a review from the anesthetist's standpoint. Anaesthesia 1985; 40:131.
28. Ream AK, Fowles RE, Jamieson S: Cardiac Transplantation, Cardiac Anesthesia. Vol. II. Kaplan JA (ed). Philadelphia, WB Saunders, 1987, pp 881–891.
29. Wyner J, Finch E: Heart and heart lung transplantation. In Anesthesia and Organ Transplantation. Gelman S (ed). Philadelphia, WB Saunders, 1987, pp 111–135.
30. Hensley FA, Martin DE, Larach DR, et al: Anesthetic management for cardiac transplantation in North America—1986 survey. J Cardiothorac Anesth 1987; 1:429.
31. Curling PE, Zaidan JR, Murphy DA, et al: Treatment of pulmonary hypertension after human orthotopic heart transplantation. Anesth Analg 1987; 66:S37.
32. Ellis L: Hydrothorax as a late complication of central venous indwelling catheters. Surgery 1983; 94:842.
33. Gravenstein N, Blackshear RH: In vitro evaluation of relative perforating potential of central venous catheters: comparison of materials, selected models, number of lumens, and angles of incidence to simulated membrane. J Clin Monit 1991; 7:1.
34. Kaye MP: The Registry of the International Society for Heart Transplantation: Fourth Official Report—1987. J Heart Transplant 1987; 6:63.
35. Berberich JJ, Fabian JA: A retrospective analysis of fentanyl and sufentanil for cardiac transplantation. J Cardiothorac Anesth 1987; 1:200.
36. Keats AS, Strong MJ, Girgis KZ, et al: Observations during anesthesia for cardiac homotransplantation in ten patients. Anesthesiology 1969; 30:192.
37. Armitage JM, Hardesty RL, Griffith BP: Prostaglandin E1: an effective treatment of right heart failure after orthotopic heart transplantation. J Heart Transplant 1987; 6:348.
38. Fonger JD, Borkon AM, Baumgartner WA, et al: Acute right heart failure following heart transplantation: improvement with prostaglandin E1 and right ventricular assist. J Heart Transplant 1986; 5:317.
39. Gay WA: Cardiac transplantation: a surgical perspective. J Cardiothorac Anesth 1988; 2:513.
40. Mason JW, Stinson EB, Harrison DC: Autonomic nervous system and arrhythmias: studies in the transplanted denervated human heart. Cardiology 1976; 61:75.
41. Verani MS, George SE, Leon CA, et al: Performance at rest and during exercise in heart transplant recipients. J Heart Transplant 1988; 7:145.
42. Stinson EB, Griepp RB, Schroeder JS, et al: Hemodynamic observations one and two years after cardiac transplantation in man. Circulation 1972; 45:1183.
43. Pope SE, Stinson EB, Daughters GT, et al: Exercise response of the denervated heart in long-term cardiac transplant recipients. Am J Cardiol 1980; 46:213.
44. McLauglin PR, Klieman JH, Martin RP, et al: The effect of exercise and atrial pacing on left ventricular volume and contractility in patients with innervated and denervated hearts. Circulation 1978; 58:476.
45. Pflugfelder PW, Purves PD, McKenzie FN, et al: Cardiac dynamics during supine exercise in cyclosporine-treated orthotopic heart transplant recipients: assessment by radionuclide angiography. J Am Coll Cardiol 1987; 10:336.
46. Wielhorski WA, Paiement B, Dyrda I, et al: The performance of nine human hearts before, during, and after transplantation. Can Anaesth Soc J 1970; 17:97.

47. Cannom DS, Graham AF, Harrison DC: Electrophysiologic studies in the denervated transplanted human heart: response to atrial pacing and atropine. Circ Res 1973; 32:268.

48. Leachman RD, Cokkinos DV, Cabrera R, et al: Response of the transplanted, denervated human heart to cardiovascular drugs. Am J Cardiol 1971; 27:272.

49. Cannom DS, Rider AK, Stinson EB, et al: Electrophysiologic studies in the denervated human heart: II. Response to norepinephrine, isoproterenol and propranolol. Am J Cardiol 1975; 36:859.

50. Borow KM, Neumann A, Arensman PW, et al: Left ventricular contractility and contractile reserve in humans after cardiac transplantation. Circulation 1985; 71:866.

51. Goodman DJ, Rossen RM, Ingham R, et al: Sinus node function in the denervated heart: effect of digitalis. Br Heart J 1975; 37:612.

52. Ricci DR, Orlick AE, Reitz BA, et al: Depressant effect of digoxin on atrioventricular conduction in man. Circulation 1978; 57:898.

53. Bexton RS, Milne JR, Cory-Pearce R, et al: Effect of beta blockade on exercise response after cardiac transplantation. Br Heart J 1983; 49:584.

54. Yusuf S, Theooropoulus S, Dhalla N, et al: Effect of beta blockade on dynamic exercise in human heart transplant recipients. J Heart Transplant 1985; 4:312.

55. Bexton RS, Cory-Pearce R, Spurrel RA, et al: Electrophysiologic effects of nifedipine and verapamil in the transplanted human heart. J Heart Transplant 1984; 3:97.

56. Mason JW, Winkle RA, Rider AK, et al: The electrophysiological effects of quinidine in the transplanted human heart. J Clin Invest 1977; 59:481.

57. Sibbald WJ, Driedger AA: Right ventricular function in acute disease states: pathophysiologic considerations. Crit Care Med 1983; 11:339.

58. Vijtanen A, Salmenperä M, Heinonen J: Right ventricular response to hypercarbia after cardiac surgery. Anesthesiology 1990; 73:393.

59. Stinson EB, Caves PK, Griepp RB, et al: Hemodynamic observations in the early period after human heart transplantation. J Thorac Cardiovasc Surg 1975; 69:264.

60. Schroeder JS, Berke DK, Graham AF, et al: Arrhythmias after cardiac transplantation. Am J Cardiol 1974; 33:604.

61. Uretsky BF, Murali S, Reddy S, et al: Development of coronary artery disease in cardiac transplant patients receiving immunosuppressive therapy with cyclosporine and prednisone. Circulation 1987; 76:827.

62. Chomette G, Auriol M, Cabrol C: Chronic rejection in human heart transplantation. J Heart Transplant 1988; 7:292.

63. Camann WR, Goldman GA, Johnson MD, et al: Cesarean delivery in a patient with a transplanted heart. Anesthesiology 1989; 71:618.

64. Eisenkraft JB, Dimich I, Sachdev VP: Anesthesia for major noncardiac surgery in a patient with a transplanted heart. Mt Sinai J Med 1981; 48:116.

65. Bricker SRW, Sugden JC: Anesthesia for surgery in a patient with a transplanted heart. Br J Anaesth 1985; 40:210.

66. Samuels SI, Wyner J: Anesthesia for surgery in a patient with a transplanted heart. Br J Anaesth 1986; 58:1199.

67. McKeown DW, Armstrong IR: Anesthesia for surgery in a patient with a transplanted heart. Br J Anaesth 1986; 58:1200.

68. Kanter SF, Samuels SI: Anesthesia for major operations on patients who have transplanted hearts: a review of 29 cases. Anesthesiology 1977; 46:65.

69. Cooper DKC, Becerra EA, Novitsky D, et al: Surgery in patients with heart transplants: anesthetic and operative considerations. S Afr Med J 1986; 70:137.

70. Samuels SI, Kanter SF: Anesthesia for major surgery in a patient with a transplanted heart. Br J Anaesth 1977; 49:265.

CHAPTER **76**

Orthotopic Liver Transplantation

AVNER SIDI, M.D.

Orthotopic liver transplantation (OLT) is the most common liver transplant procedure and is performed by transplanting the donor liver to the same site after hepatectomy (Fig. 76–1). In heterotopic (auxiliary) liver transplantation, the donor liver is placed in the paravertebral gutter or in the pelvis without removal of the diseased liver.[1] The latter technique is frequently complicated by atrophy of the grafted liver (because of low portal and hepatic arterial blood flow). Therefore, it is only recommended for high-risk surgical patients or those who have reversible liver disease.

GENERAL CONSIDERATIONS

What Is the Impact of Timing?

Timing of transplantation is crucial; poor timing may convert an otherwise acceptable candidate for OLT into an unacceptable one, because a patient's general neurologic condition, coagulopathy, acidosis, sepsis, and cardiovascular instability are important prognostic determinants (discussed later). Although preoperative severe hypoxemia may be a contraindication to OLT, the adult respiratory distress syndrome (ARDS) associated with hepatic failure improves dramatically with liver transplantation.

Pulmonary infection must be treated before surgery, as must other sources of infection and sepsis. The semi-emergent nature of this surgery allows time for the treating physician to correct preoperative abnormalities indicated by a patient's laboratory values. When a patient has grade 4 encephalopathy (discussed later) and is dependent on mechanical ventilation, OLT usually is too late. However, to allow a patient's condition to deteriorate to a point that necessitates life-support systems before consideration of the transplantation option is unacceptable.

Who Are Adult Candidates?

OLT is considered as a last resort for virtually every patient with lethal hepatic disease.[2] The list of liver diseases is huge (Table 76–1), and selection of appropriate recipients from such a large pool requires individual assessment. In 1982, the annual need for OLT was estimated at 15 per million popula-

tion.[3] Today's need is even greater because of fewer restrictions on candidacy.

Nonmalignant End-Stage Liver Disease

From a purely medical standpoint, candidacy for OLT is relatively clear: nonmalignant end-stage liver disease that will not recur in the hepatic graft. Little debate focuses on this rationale for transplantation.

Other Causes of End-Stage Liver Disease

Any other cause of end-stage liver disease is not considered to be a complete contraindication. The most common diagnoses are chronic active hepatitis (non-A, non-B), cryptogenic

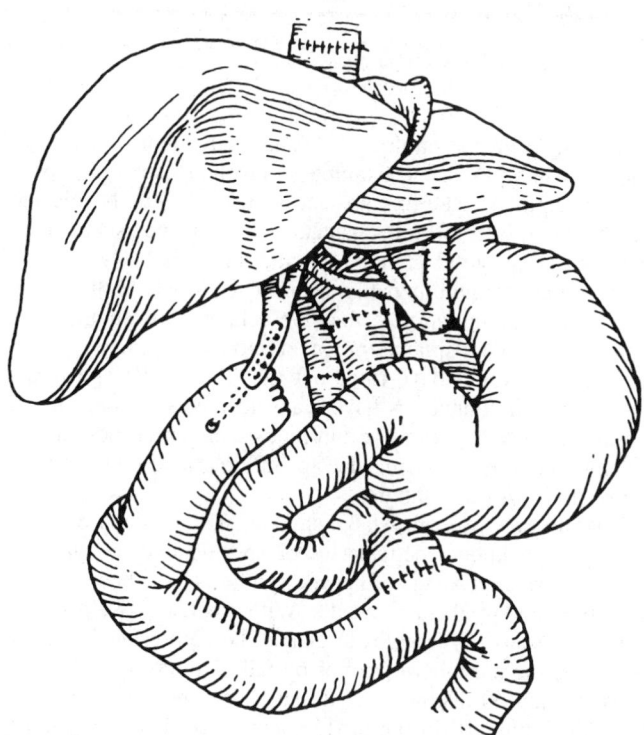

FIGURE 76–1. Orthotopic liver transplantation. (Modified from Starzl TE, Demetris AJ, Van Thiel D: Liver transplantation (first of two parts). N Engl J Med 1989; 321:1014, by permission of the New England Journal of Medicine.)

TABLE 76–1. Classification of Liver Diseases

I. Disorders of circulation
  A. Passive congestion due to heart failure and cardiac cirrhosis
  B. Hepatic vein thrombosis (Budd-Chiari syndrome)
  C. Portal vein thrombosis
  D. Disorders of the hepatic artery (e.g., polyarteritis nodosa, hepatic artery aneurysms)
  E. Hepatic infarction
II. Disorders secondary to biliary obstruction
  A. Extrahepatic biliary obstruction
    1. Tumors of the bile duct, gallbladder, pancreas, ampulla of Vater, duodenum, congenital biliary atresia
    2. Choledocholithiasis
    3. Bile duct strictures, diverticula, and so on
    4. Sclerosing cholangitis
  B. Intrahepatic biliary obstruction
    1. Intrahepatic bile duct stone or tumor
    2. Cholangitis
    3. Intrahepatic cholestasis (e.g., drugs)
    4. Primary biliary cirrhosis
III. Parenchymal disorders
  A. Focal liver disease
    1. Abscess (pyogenic, amebic); other suppurative processes (e.g., actinomycosis)
    2. Neoplasms (primary and secondary), benign and malignant
    3. Cysts (e.g., echinococcal, congenital), gummas
    4. Granulomas (sarcoidosis, tuberculosis, berylliosis, histoplasmosis, other)
  B. Diffuse liver disorders
    1. Inborn errors of bilirubin metabolism
      a) Gilbert's syndrome
      b) Dubin-Johnson and Rotor's syndromes
    2. Hepatitis
      a) Viral (Epstein-Barr virus, cytomegalovirus, herpesvirus), hepatitis A and hepatitis B, non-A, non-B virus
      b) Parasitic leptospirosis
      c) Bacterial
      d) Drug-induced hepatitis
      e) Chronic active hepatitis

III. Parenchymal disorders *(Continued)*
  B. Diffuse liver disorders *(Continued)*
    3. Causes of cirrhosis
      a) Acquired
        (1) Alcohol
        (2) Hepatitis virus(es)
        (3) Hepatotoxins (e.g., phosphorus)
        (4) Drug hypersensitivity reactions (e.g., halothane)
        (5) Biliary cirrhosis
          (a) Primary biliary cirrhosis
          (b) Secondary
            i) Gallstones
            ii) Bile duct stricture
        (6) Cardiac cirrhosis
        (7) Infiltrative diseases—sarcoidosis (rare)
        (8) Infectious diseases
        (9) Nutritional
      b) Genetically determined
        (1) Hepatolenticular degeneration (Wilson's disease)
        (2) Hemochromatosis
        (3) Galactosemia
        (4) Cystic fibrosis
        (5) Alpha$_1$-antitrypsin deficiency
      c) Cryptogenic
    4. Infiltrative diseases
      a) Fatty liver
      b) Amyloidosis, Gaucher's disease, Neimann-Pick disease
      c) Leukemia, lymphoma
    5. Metabolic
      a) Alpha$_1$-antitrypsin deficiency
      b) Fibrocystic disease
      c) Fatty liver of pregnancy
      d) Reye's syndrome
IV. Traumatic
  A. Penetrating
  B. Nonpenetrating

(Modified from Maddrey W (section ed): Disease of the liver (Section 10). *In* The Principles and Practice of Medicine. 19th ed. Harvey AM, Johns RJ, Owens AH Jr, et al (eds). New York, Appleton-Century-Crofts, 1979, pp 865–922.)

cirrhosis, primary biliary cirrhosis, and inborn errors of metabolism.[2, 4] A prime example is alcoholic cirrhosis. With multidisciplinary care for substance abuse in properly selected cases, the results of transplantation for Laennec's alcoholic cirrhosis are as good as those for other diseases.

Even patients with hepatitis B cirrhosis, in whom the recurrence of viral infection cannot be reliably prevented, have benefited from transplantation. In addition to disease states that at one time would have ruled out OLT, inflexible age limits have been eliminated, as have many technical or mechanical obstacles such as extensive thrombosis of portal-mesenteric-splenic veins and scarring due to multiple abdominal operations (portosystemic shunts).

The inborn errors of metabolism that result partially or completely from known deficiencies of specific liver enzyme or from abnormal products of hepatic synthesis have been treated with the most predictable results. With other, less well-understood disorders, OLT helps to clarify the pathogenesis, either by correcting the inborn error or by failing to do so.

More than 60 distinct liver diseases have been treated with OLT, including 16 in the broad category of inborn errors of metabolism and 14 in the category of cholestatic disease.

Hepatic Cancer and HIV Infection

The major controversial issues are whether patients with hepatic cancers and those with antibodies for human immuno-deficiency virus (HIV) should be excluded from candidacy. The percentage of patients with a tumor in large transplantation programs ranges from 4% to 34%[2, 5]; a crucial requirement for candidacy in this group is that the tumor not have spread beyond the liver. A relatively high percentage of patients can have prolonged benefit from OLT despite a positive HIV test result.[2]

Who Are Pediatric Candidates?

Half of the pediatric recipients have biliary atresia, making it the leading reason for OLT in this age group[2, 4, 5] and accounting for 17% of all OLT recipients. Inborn errors of metabolism are a distant second (Tables 76–2 and 76–3). Cholestatic (obstructive) diseases, including biliary atresia, account for 55% of all pediatric recipients (see Table 76–3).

Is the Severity of Liver Disease Important to the Prognosis?

The cause of the disease may be, by itself, an important prognostic determinant.[6] Features that even before surgery predict imminent death include relentless progression, grade 3 or 4 encephalopathy, severe coagulopathy, rapid shrinkage of the

TABLE 76–2. Native Liver Disease in 400 Pediatric and 858 Adult Recipients of Liver Transplants at the University of Pittsburgh, 1981–1988

Disease	Number of Cases
Parenchymal	*522*
Postnecrotic cirrhosis	348
Alcoholic cirrhosis	76
Acute liver failure	54
Budd-Chiari syndrome	18
Congenital hepatic fibrosis	9
Cystic fibrosis	6
Neonatal hepatitis	8
Hepatic trauma	3
Cholestatic	*544*
Biliary atresia	217
Primary biliary cirrhosis	186
Sclerosing cholangitis	100
Secondary biliary cirrhosis	25
Familial cholestasis	16
Inborn errors of metabolism	*114*
Tumors	*78*
Benign	10
Primary malignant	60
Metastatic	8
Total	*1258*

(Reprinted from Starzl TE, Demetris AJ, Van Thiel D: Liver transplantation (first of two parts). N Engl J Med 1989; 321:1014, by permission of the New England Journal of Medicine.)

liver, metabolic acidosis, cardiovascular instability, and sepsis.[2] Pulmonary infection contraindicates surgery, because of the high incidence of life-threatening postoperative pneumonia that occurs in immunosuppressed patients.

Any surgical procedure poses a risk proportional to the severity of hepatic disease, but the magnitude of surgery also contributes to the outcome and influences it. When reviewing the risk factors in cirrhotic patients (Table 76–4), one should note that (1) only five variables are included before considering the surgical procedure; (2) transaminases are not included; and (3) prothrombin time (PT) represents an extremely valuable laboratory test for prognosis and surgical risk assessment.

TABLE 76–3. Indications for Liver Transplantation in 216 Pediatric Patients

		Number of Cases	%
Obstructive	Biliary atresia	106	55
	Byler's disease	2	
	Alagilles syndrome	16	
	Alpha$_1$-antitrypsin deficiency	29	
Failed liver transplant		65	23
Miscellaneous	Wilson's disease	5	22
	Chronic active hepatitis	6	
	Tyrosinemia	4	
	Neonatal hepatitis	5	
	Glycogen storage disease	5	
	Familial cholestasis	5	
	End-stage liver failure	30	
	Hepatic tumor	3	
Total		281	100

(From Borland LM, Martin DJ: Anesthesia consideration for orthotopic liver transplantation. Contemp Anesth Pract 1987; 10:157.)

TABLE 76–4. Surgical Risk Factors in Cirrhotic Patients

Variable	Points		
	1	*2*	*3*
Ascites	None	Moderate	Severe
Encephalopathy grade	None	1–2	>2
Bilirubin (mg · dL^{-1})	1.5	1.5–2.0	>2.0
Albumin (mg · dL^{-1})	3.5	2.0–3.5	<2.0
Prothrombin time (seconds of control)	1–4	4–6>	1>6
Legend:	*Good risk* (5% mortality)	5–6 points	
	Moderate risk (10–20% mortality)	7–9 points	
	Poor risk (>50% mortality)	>10 points	

(Data from Pugh RNH, Murray-Lyon M, Dawson JL, et al: Transection of the esophagus for bleeding varices. Br J Surg 1973; 60:646.)

What Is the Expected Survival?

Patients requiring fewer than 30 units of red blood cells (RBCs) have a survival rate >75%, whereas for those needing more than 70 units, survival is <15%.[7]

The overall survival in different series of patients after introduction of the new immunosuppressive drugs is 70% to 80% (Figs. 76–2 and 76–3). Survival remains unchanged for 12 to 18 months after OLT and varies from 75% to 85% according to clinical severity at the time of transplantation.

PREANESTHETIC EVALUATION

How Does It Differ?

Preoperative evaluation is performed in two stages. In the "early" first stage, all OLT candidates are examined by anesthesiologists. This assessment is to rule out any condition contraindicating surgery and to determine physical aspects that can be improved or tests that should be performed to prepare patients optimally. Similar evaluation by hepatologists, surgeons, intensivists, and nurses can take place in a parallel manner or in a joint meeting with the anesthesiologists. The patient and the family are briefed, and the preoperative care and possible risks explained. A later, second-stage evaluation is performed immediately before surgery.

What Are the Signs and Symptoms of Hepatic Failure?

Failure of hepatic cell function produces generalized manifestations that are constitutional, cutaneous, endocrine, and hematologic (Table 76–5). They reflect the liver's central role in metabolism and homeostasis. The more dramatic include jaundice, ascites, bleeding from varices due to portal hypertension, and mental changes associated with hepatic encephalopathy. Hypoxemia, anemia, and coagulopathy often accompany hepatic disease. Encephalopathy, renal dysfunction, and ascites are also common.

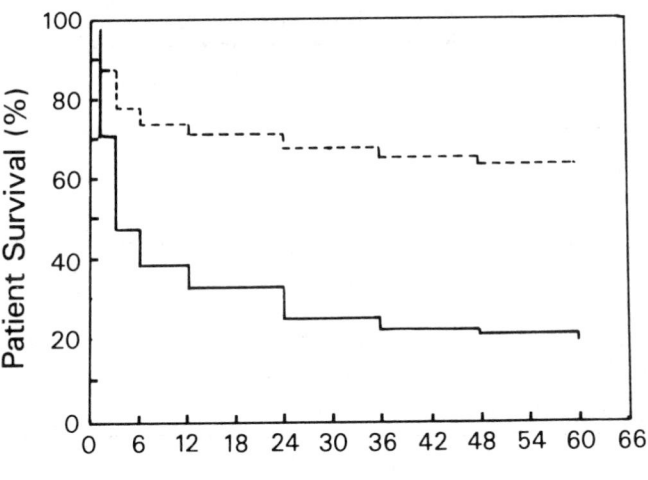

FIGURE 76–2. Survival of 170 liver transplant recipients treated before cyclosporine became available (1963–1979) as compared with the survival of 1258 recipients treated between 1980 and mid-1988. The patients were treated by a single team at the University of Colorado through 1980 and at the University of Pittsburgh thereafter. The *solid line* denotes patients who received azathioprine (n = 170), and the *broken line* indicates those who received cyclosporine (n = 1258). Survival is calculated with use of the life-table method. (Reprinted from Starzl TE, Demetris AJ, Van Thiel D: Liver transplantation (second of two parts). N Engl J Med 1989; 321:1092, by permission of the New England Journal of Medicine.)

For clinical purposes, patients with liver diseases can be divided into two main groups:

1. Parenchymal disease is usually associated with a hyperdynamic circulatory state. It is characterized by decreased vascular resistance (peripheral vasodilation, increased arteriovenous shunting); increased circulating blood volume and cardiac output; and increased splanchnic (except the liver), pulmonary, and skin blood flow. Systemic and cardiac filling pressures, heart rate, hepatic arterial (but not portal) blood flow, and renal blood flow are maintained.

2. Cholestasis with jaundice as the primary manifestation.

What Associated Problems May Be Present?

Cardiovascular

The *hyperkinetic circulation* observed in patients with chronic liver disease is thought to be caused by pulmonary and portosystemic shunts and circulating vasoactive substances (glucagon, ferritin, atrial natriuretic factor, vasodilating prostaglandin E_1, vasointestinal polypeptide) that have not been detoxified by cirrhotic patients. Plasma volume expansion is probably not a major factor.

A vasodilation-induced decrease in systemic pressure and stimulation of baroreceptors provoke a subsequent increase in sympathetic tone and an increase in arginine vasopressin and renin release. A high cardiac output results, as do splanchnic vasoconstriction and increased preload.

Paradoxically, many cirrhotic patients have impaired contractile function and cardiomyopathy. The production of false neurotransmitters with norepinephrine depletion and low myocardial β-adrenergic receptor density correlates with catecholamine hyposensitivity. Overall, a cirrhotic patient's heart has a very limited ability to respond to stress.

Pulmonary

Hypoxemia is often associated with severe hepatic disease and results from ventilation/perfusion ($\dot{V}/\dot{Q}$) abnormalities, including impaired hypoxic pulmonary vasoconstriction; rightward shift of the oxyhemoglobin dissociation curve; hypoventilation due to ascites; decrease in pulmonary diffusing capacity resulting from an increase in extracellular fluid; and right-to-left shunts across the lungs. The latter are due to lung spider angiomas, portopulmonary communications, and humoral factors. Tidal volume, vital capacity, and functional residual capacity are decreased, yet compensatory tachypnea can result in respiratory alkalosis. Acute respiratory failure sometimes develops in patients with severe hepatocellular dysfunction, possibly secondary to the decreased hepatic clearance of endotoxin.

Hematologic

Anemia, which may be hypochromic, microcytic, or macrocytic, invariably develops in cirrhotic patients as a result of malabsorption of iron and folic acid, frequent variceal bleeding, and hypersplenism. Furthermore, changes in lipid metabolism of cell membranes shorten RBC survival. In severe hepatocellular disease, a coagulopathy is also evident.

TABLE 76–5. Systemic Signs and Symptoms in Hepatic Disease

Manifestation	Possible Mechanisms
	Constitutional
Anorexia	Overall hepatic failure
Weight loss	
Weakness, fatigue	
Nausea	Splanchnic congestion
	Ascites
Flatulence	
Fever	Hepatic inflammation
	Reduced resistance to infection
Fetor hepaticus	Abnormal methionine metabolism
	Cardiovascular
Hyperdynamic circulation	Hormone-induced general vasodilation
Bounding pulses—wide pulse pressure	
Increased cardiac output	
Tachycardia	
Increased plasma volume	Associated with portal hypertension
Cyanosis	Arteriovenous anastomoses (lung, liver, systemic)
Clubbing	Arterial oxygen saturation
	Cutaneous and Endocrine
Spider telangiectases	Abnormal metabolism of estrogens and androgens
Palmar erythema	
Menstrual irregularities	
Impotence	
Gynecomastia	
	Hematologic
Petechiae	Decreased platelet count often associated with leukopenia and anemia
Ecchymoses	Impaired production of coagulation proteins
Generalized bleeding tendency	Both of above

(Modified from Maddrey W (section ed): Disease of the liver (Section 10). *In* The Principles and Practice of Medicine. 19th ed. Harvey AM, Johns RJ, Owens AH Jr, et al (eds). New York, Appleton-Century-Crofts, 1979, pp 865–922.)

Central Nervous System

Patients may exhibit minimal confusion (stage 1), gross mental confusion (stage 2), somnolence and stupor (stage 3), or deep coma with response only to pain (stage 4 encephalopathy). Hepatic encephalopathy is considered to be associated with increased blood ammonia level and accumulations of other substances (mercaptans, short-chain fatty acids, false neurotransmitter, and γ-aminobutyric acid). Several factors may worsen encephalopathy, including diuretics, gastrointestinal bleeding, infection, and further hepatic damage. Brain edema formation appears with fulminant hepatic failure, and intracranial hemorrhage may develop with severe coagulopathy.

Renal Fluids and Electrolytes

Three types of *renal dysfunction* are encountered: (1) hepatorenal syndrome, characterized by low urine sodium (U_{Na^+} <10 mEq · L^{-1}); (2) tubular necrosis, characterized by high U_{Na^+} excretion with casts; and (3) prerenal azotemia with low U_{Na^+} (Table 76–6). Patients may recover from the last two complications, but hepatorenal syndrome is frequently lethal. It may improve after transplantation.[1]

Differentiation of the syndrome from other renal diseases is very difficult because of the frequent use of complex diuretic therapy. Kidney dysfunction is associated with enhanced renin-angiotensin activity, hyperaldosteronism, increased sympathetic tone, increased antidiuretic hormone activity, increased conjugated bilirubin levels, and altered activity of the renal prostaglandins or kallikrein-kinin systems. Inadequate intravascular volume and cyclosporine-induced nephrotoxicity further impair renal function.

Blood Volume

Blood volume increases by 10% to 20% above normal levels. However, intravascular volume can be depleted owing to continuous formation of ascites or diuretic therapy to treat ascites. Caution must be exercised during repletion because rapid administration of volume, including blood and its products, may cause intravascular overloading, especially if myocardial dysfunction is evident.

Hyponatremia

Hyponatremia is a common finding because of water retention due to antidiuretic hormone activity, impaired renal water excretion, or true sodium deficiency (therapeutically produced). This multifactorial combination may explain why preoperative correction of hyponatremia is very difficult and therefore is best accomplished with the aid of hemodynamic and laboratory monitoring.

Hypokalemia

Hypokalemia is a chronic finding because depletion of total body potassium frequently follows diuretic therapy, inadequate intake, and continuous loss (vomiting and diarrhea). Aggressive and complete correction of acute hypokalemia should be avoided because of the preoperative difficulties in treatment and because the situation usually reverses to hyperkalemia after reperfusion of the new liver (discussed later). Hyperkalemia may be observed in patients with moderate to severe renal dysfunction.

Acid-Base Derangements

Metabolic alkalosis in patients with chronic liver disease is associated with hyperaldosteronism, vomiting, and diarrhea. It is frequently complicated by hypoxia-induced respiratory alkalosis. On the other hand, metabolic acidosis often is found in patients with acute fulminant hepatitis, rapidly progressive hepatic failure, or unrecognized infection.

Why Does Coagulopathy Occur in Chronic Liver Disease?

Coagulopathy in hepatic disease results from

1. Malabsorption of substrates.
2. Thrombocytopenia—occurs in 70% of cases owing to hypersplenism.
3. Impaired platelet function resulting from small, hypofunctional platelets.
4. Increased fibrinolytic activity, with decreased production of antiplasmin and inadequate clearance of tissue plasminogen activators.
5. Decreased hepatic synthesis of plasma clotting factors. All coagulation factors decrease except fibrinogen and Factor VIII (the latter mostly produced in vascular endothelium). Dysfibrinogenemia may follow the formation of abnormally structured fibrinogen.
6. Shortened half-lives of plasma clotting factors because of defective hepatic synthetic function.
7. Formation of abnormal coagulation products.

How Much Bleeding Is Expected in Orthotopic Liver Transplantation?

The amount of bleeding expected during OLT is highly variable, ranging in different series from 1 to more than 100 units of RBCs and fresh-frozen plasma (FFP).[1, 5, 7] Estimated blood loss ranges from 10 to 1000 mL · kg^{-1}, with an average of >100 mL · kg^{-1}.[8] The clinical significance of coagulopathy

TABLE 76–6. Urinary Composition in Oliguria

Component	Hepatorenal Syndrome	Prerenal Failure	Acute Tubular Necrosis	Hepatorenal Failure
Urinary sodium	<10 mEq · L^{-1}	<25 mEq · L^{-1}	>25 mEq · L^{-1}	<10–20 mEq · L^{-1}
Urinary specific gravity	>1.024	>1.015	1.010–1.015	>1.015
Urinary:plasma osmolality	>2.5:1	>1.8:1	≤1.1:1	>1.2:1
Urinary:plasma urea	>100:1	>20:1	3:1, rarely >10:1	>10:1
Urinary:plasma creatinine	>60:1	>30:1, rarely <10:1	<10:1	>40:1

(Compiled from Mazze RI: Critical care of the patient with acute renal failure. Anesthesiology 1977; 47:138, *and* Miller TR, Anderson RJ, Linas SL, et al: Urinary diagnostic indices in acute renal failure: a prospective study. Ann Intern Med 1978; 89:47.)

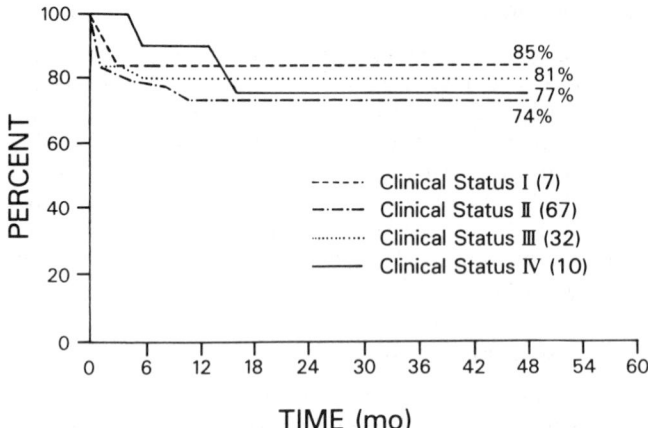

FIGURE 76–3. Survival of pediatric patients undergoing liver transplantation. Patients were grouped by clinical status at the time of transplantation. Group I—children who received no medical therapy for liver disease or its complications; Group II—children living at home and receiving outpatient medical management; Group III—children with accelerating decompensation of their disease; and Group IV—children confined to the intensive care unit because of their liver disease or complications. (From Davis PJ, Cook DR: Anesthetic problems in pediatric liver transplantation. Transplant Proc 1989; 21:3493. © 1989. Reprinted by permission of Appleton & Lange, Inc.)

is confirmed by the correlation between its preoperative severity and intraoperative blood product requirements. Patients with hepatocellular disease and poor preoperative coagulation profile require more blood products.[7]

Type of Liver Disease

Statistically significant differences for RBC replacement according to the diagnostic group have been reported. Patients with chronic active hepatitis tend to require more blood and blood products than do patients with perisclerosing cholangitis (Table 76–7), although the latter patients tend to require more blood than do those with primary biliary cirrhosis. Patients in the last two categories are usually diagnosed earlier, treated earlier, and suffer less parenchymal damage with less severe subsequent clotting abnormalities.

When patients are classified into risk categories for likelihood of bleeding, according to age, weight, diagnosis, coagulation status, previous operation, and so on (similar to Table 76–4), a significant difference has been noted between high-risk and low-risk cases in adults (Table 76–8). *Median* requirement for RBCs and FFP by those classified as high-risk cases was almost twice the amount needed in low-risk cases, al-

though the *average* use was similar. This observation probably reflects that a few low-risk patients had substantial bleeding that necessitated a large number of blood units.

A more specific isolation of the relationship between blood and blood components consumed intraoperatively and the extent of liver disease was found with elevated PT (>15.0 s) and presence of ascites (Tables 76–9 and 76–10). Pediatric patients have a tendency toward a lower estimated blood loss (see Table 76–8), but mean loss in milliliters per kilogram is similar.[8]

What Should Be Known About Organ Preservation Techniques?

Simple Hypothermia

Simple hypothermia is frequently used for preservation of the donor liver. It consists of irrigation of the hepatic vascular tree and bathing the liver in iced preservation solution. Continuous perfusion is used rarely, because complex equipment is required, vascular resistance may increase gradually, and the outcome is not superior to that of simple hypothermia.

Preservation Solution

The preservation solution has an electrolyte composition similar to intracellular fluid (high potassium and low sodium concentrations). Collins's solution provides a clinically satisfactory cold ischemia time of 10 hours. The Wisconsin solution allows a cold ischemia time of 24 hours.[9] This long ischemia time permits the liver team to plan ahead for daytime operation on a semi-emergency basis.

All preservation methods can affect recipient homeostasis. Rapid influx of acidic and metabolite-rich solution, flushed into the systemic circulation when the grafted liver is perfused, may cause hemodynamic instability, requiring therapy with epinephrine or phenylephrine (discussed later), especially if chlorpromazine is added in an attempt to maintain hepatocyte membrane integrity (Table 76–11).

Timing

Recall that most donors are declared brain-dead and eligible for organ donation during usual working hours. Additional time is needed to coordinate the different organ harvest teams, travel and harvest time, and selection and preparation of the OLT candidate. When the preservation time of the donor liver was short,[10] 85% of liver transplantations began outside usual working hours (Fig. 76–4).

TABLE 76–7. Intraoperative Blood and Blood Component Use (in Units) for 66 First-Transplant Patients, Shown by Major Diagnostic Group

Type of Transfusion	CAH (n = 24)		PSC (n = 22)		PBC (n = 20)		P*
	Mean	*Median*	*Mean*	*Median*	*Mean*	*Median*	
Erythrocytes	23.7	16.9	20.7	13.7	13.5	9.4	.17
Fresh-frozen plasma	18.3	15.0	12.4	7.5	10.3	8.5	.04
Cryoprecipitate	23.3	20.0	15.3	10.0	10.1	10.0	.02
Platelets	21.9	14.5	17.0	12.0	10.7	12.0	.02

(From Motschman TL, Taswell HF, Brecher ME, et al: Intraoperative blood loss and patient and graft survival in orthotopic liver transplantation: their relationship to clinical and laboratory data. Mayo Clin Proc 1989; 64:346. By permission.)
*Kruskal-Wallis one-way analysis of variance of ranks of median usage for three groups.
Abbreviations: CAH = chronic active hepatitis; PSC = primary sclerosing cholangitis; PBC = primary biliary cirrhosis; 17 patients had other diagnoses.

TABLE 76–8. Intraoperative Blood and Blood Component Use (in Units) in the First 100 Liver Transplantations at the Mayo Clinic, Shown by Risk Category

| | Adult | | | | Child | | |
| | High-Risk (n = 68) | | Low-Risk (n = 27) | | (n = 5) | | |
Type of Transfusion	Mean	Median	Mean	Median	Mean	Median	P*
Erythrocytes	19.2	14.8	19.0	8.4	5.2	4.7	.02
Fresh-frozen plasma	15.3	12.0	11.9	7.0	4.6	3.0	.03
Cryoprecipitate	19.6	17.0	13.4	10.0	9.0	10.0	.11
Platelets	18.9	12.0	13.6	12.0	6.8	6.0	.06

(From Motschman TL, Taswell HF, Brecher ME, et al: Intraoperative blood loss and patient and graft survival in orthotopic liver transplantation: their relationship to clinical and laboratory data. Mayo Clin Proc 1989; 64:346. By permission.)
*Rank sum test, adult high-risk versus adult low-risk median usage.

TABLE 76–9. Comparison of Intraoperative Blood Use (in Units) in Relationship to Prothrombin Time in the First 100 Liver Transplantations at the Mayo Clinic

| | PT > 15.0 (n = 28) | | PT ≤ 15.0 (n = 72) | | |
Type of Transfusion	Mean	Median	Mean	Median	P*
Erythrocytes	25.2	20.4	15.8	10.8	.007
Fresh-frozen plasma	18.8	20.5	11.9	10.0	.004
Cryoprecipitate	25.9	20.0	14.1	10.0	.005
Platelets	22.1	19.0	14.8	12.0	.001

(From Motschman TL, Taswell HF, Brecher ME, et al: Intraoperative blood loss and patient and graft survival in orthotopic liver transplantation: their relationship to clinical and laboratory data. Mayo Clin Proc 1989; 64:346. By permission.)
*Rank sum test, comparison of median values.
Abbreviation: PT = prothrombin time.

TABLE 76–10. Comparison of Intraoperative Blood Use (in Units) in Relationship to Presence of Ascites in the First 100 Liver Transplantations at the Mayo Clinic

| | Ascites (n = 37) | | No Ascites (n = 63) | | |
Type of Transfusion	Mean	Median	Mean	Median	P*
Erythrocytes	26.4	22.3	13.7	9.7	<.0001
Fresh-frozen plasma	19.2	18.0	10.7	8.0	<.001
Cryoprecipitate	21.5	20.0	15.0	10.0	.001
Platelets	20.9	18.0	14.5	12.0	.001

*Rank sum test, adult high-risk versus adult low-risk median usage.

TABLE 76–11. Circulatory Effects of Preservation Solution During the Neohepatic Stage

	Collins's Solution	Collins's with Chlorpromazine	Wisconsin Solution
SBP (stage III + 5 min; mm Hg)	102.5 ± 3.6	94.2 ± 7.9	95.0 ± 4.2
SBP < 100 (min)	81.5 ± 16.9	127.0 ± 15.5*	65.0 ± 11.4
SBP < 80 (min)	6.5 ± 1.8	24.0 ± 5.1	10.5 ± 2.5*
Epinephrine (% of patients requiring)	10.4	49.0*	18.3
Phenylephrine (% of patients requiring)†	8.2	19.0*	7.3

(From Kang YG, Freeman JA, Aggarwal S, et al: Hemodynamic instability during liver transplantation. Transplant Proc 1989; 21:3489.)
*Values are mean ± standard error of the mean.
†P < .05 compared with Collins's group. Retrospective study; end point to keep hemodynamic baseline level. No specific order.
Abbreviation: SBP = systemic blood pressure.

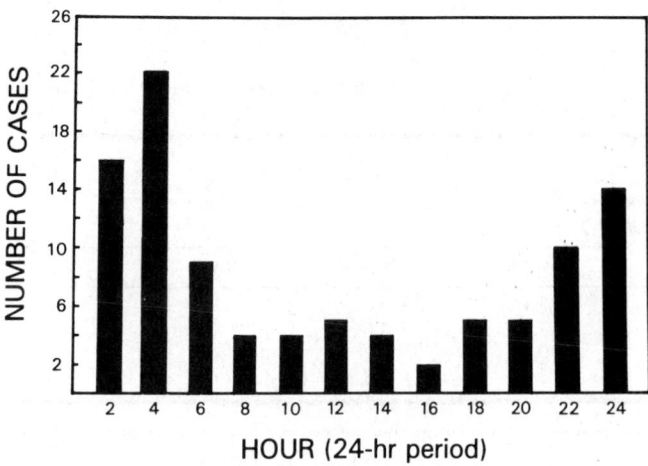

FIGURE 76–4. Comparison between time of day and number of liver transplantations begun (an analysis of the *first* 100 procedures at the Mayo Clinic). (By permission from Rettke SR, Chantigian RC, Janossy TA, et al: Anesthesia approach to hepatic transplantation. Mayo Clin Proc 1989; 64:224.)

How Is the Preparation Phase Organized?

Use of resources is the prime consideration during preparation for OLT. One should plan for an operating room time of 8 to 20 hours,[8] with an average total time of 8.5 hours for anesthesia, of which 7 hours is devoted to surgery (Table 76–12).

The minimum anesthesia staff should be a 3:2 ratio of physicians to Certified Registered Nurse Anesthetists or technicians to deal with simultaneous administration of anesthesia and operation of the rapid-infusion device and the thromboelastograph (TEG). A courier, responsible solely for the transport of specimens and blood products, is indispensable.

The Liver Team Approach

The liver team is a multidisciplinary team of administrators, hepatologists, surgeons, anesthesiologists, internists, technicians (including perfusionist), and nurses. Among the administrators should be a central role coordinator who assembles the different services involved in the OLT and notifies laboratory and support personnel about expected candidates and donors.

Anesthesia personnel should see the patient, assemble medications and supplies, and set up the operating room. The liver team should meet for preoperative evaluations/discussions and postoperative analysis of complications or follow-up.

What Should Be Accomplished During the Second-Stage Evaluation?

A brief second examination is performed immediately before surgery when a donor organ has been identified. Attention should be directed to evaluating any neurologic deterioration since the initial first-stage evaluation. Signs of progressive metabolic acidosis, infection, or sepsis should be sought. Correct and treat cardiovascular instability, pulmonary infection, and severe coagulopathy.

The internist should ensure that a patient is in the best condition for surgery. Ideally, ascites should be controlled and nutrition improved, with PT showing a return toward normal. Parenteral vitamin K should have been given at least 3 days preoperatively if possible. It corrects coagulation defects within 24 to 36 hours, unless liver function is so poor that vitamin K–dependent proteins such as Factor V and prothrombin cannot be synthesized. Albumin, FFP, and cryoprecipitate can be given immediately before surgery; platelets can be infused (if the count is $<50,000 \cdot mn^{3-1}$) immediately after induction or cannulation. Urine output and creatinine levels should be determined.

Premedication

Because coagulation may be abnormal preoperatively, intramuscular premedication is ill advised. Hepatic encephalopathy is another contraindication. If coagulation and level of consciousness are normal, standard medications are not contraindicated. The dose is usually adjusted downward because of reduced hepatic function, including drug elimination. Premedication is frequently eliminated. Preoperative counseling often suffices for patients' preparation and allows family interaction with an alert individual before surgery. However, if a patient so desires, short-acting benzodiazepines are often appropriate.

How Should the Operating Room Be Set Up?

The anesthesiologist should have access to the patient's head, neck (including insertion sites for left and right central catheters), and arms (including locations for a radial arterial catheter and the antecubital vein of the side opposite to the venovenous bypass [VVB]). Adequate space must be available at the anesthesia end/side of the room for the rapid-infusion system (RIS), TEG machine, monitors, infusion pumps, drug cart, and the anesthesia machine (Fig. 76–5).

TABLE 76–12. Mean Operating Room Times During Various Periods of Orthotopic Liver Transplantation at the Mayo Clinic

Group	Total Time (min)		
	Anesthesia	*Surgical*	*Anhepatic*
First 100 procedures	510.1 ± 98.4	413.2 ± 87.5	130.4 ± 39.9
By diagnosis:			
CAH (n = 24)	541.0 ± 76.4	433.0 ± 76.5	145.1 ± 76.5
PSC (n = 22)	558.9 ± 75.7	459.2 ± 75.7	125.0 ± 75.7*
PBC (n = 20)	444.0 ± 73.0†	357.1 ± 73.0†	114.0 ± 73.0*
Retransplant (n = 17)	471.8 ± 90.3	378.3 ± 77.4	134.3 ± 48.1

(From Rettke SR, Chantigian RC, Janossy TA, et al: Anesthesia approach to hepatic transplantation. Mayo Clin Proc 1989; 64:224. By permission.)
*Significantly lower than for CAH ($P < .05$).
†Significantly lower than for CAH and PSC ($P < .05$).
Abbreviations: CAH = chronic active hepatitis; PBC = primary biliary cirrhosis; PSC = primary sclerosing cholangitis.

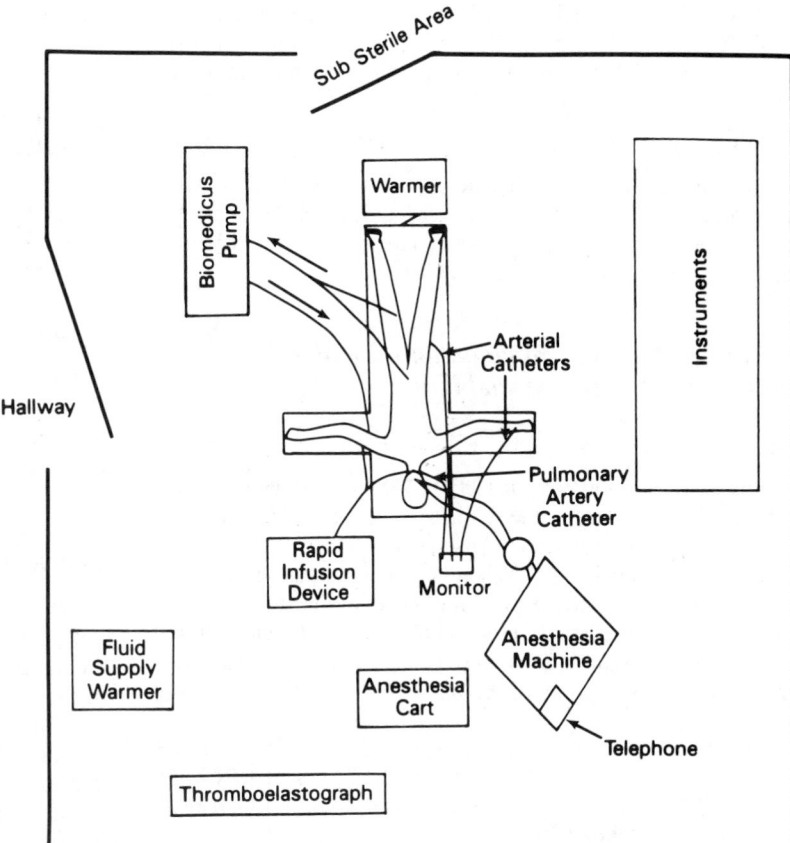

FIGURE 76–5. Suggested room layout for anesthesia and surgery of OLT.

At the foot end of the operating room table and on both sides, space must be available for the VVB pump (reaching up to the patient's axilla), surgical instruments (including an area to work on the donor liver), blanket warmer, blood and blood product warmer, and fluid storage.

What Equipment Is Needed by Anesthesia Personnel?

Equipment used by anesthesia personnel can be divided into three categories:

1. That which is used for "regular" major abdominal surgery cases, including anesthesia gas machine, ventilator, positive end-expiratory pressure (PEEP) valves, humidifier, multiple-channel vital sign monitor, urinary catheter, automated record keeper (desirable, not routine), pulse oximeter, esophageal stethoscope, respiratory gas analyzer, nasogastric tube, warming blanket, medication infusion sets, supply cart, and telephone.

2. That which is used for a major vascular surgery case with the potential for significant blood or contractility loss: invasive blood pressure monitoring capabilities (radial *and* femoral, because of frequent blood sampling from a nonheparinized line in a vasoconstricted, cold patient), cardiac output monitor, on-line mixed venous oximetry, cardiac defibrillator, blood pump and blood warmer, nonautologous infusion system, and autotransfusion system. The latter device may be advantageous even with an RIS,[11] although most centers eliminate it if the RIS is present.

3. That which is somewhat unique to OLT: two invasive arterial pressure monitors, the RIS, TEG, and VVB device.

What Is the Recommendation for Venous Access?

Adults

Venous access entails a large 10- to 12-gauge or 8 to 8.5 French catheter in the antecubital vein opposite to the VVB side and a 9 French catheter in the left internal or external jugular vein or subclavian vein. The right internal jugular vein is used for placement of an oximetric pulmonary artery (PA) catheter. Possible impediment of cerebral venous return because of bilateral jugular cannulation has not been observed to be a problem. The large-bore access with warmed fluids infused may affect cardiac output measurement, making cardiac output readings falsely high.

Children

For pediatric patients, smaller catheters are used for central venous pressure (CVP) monitoring. A 5.5 or 4 French introducer for oximetric PA catheter placement is inserted. The oximeter catheter is placed just beyond the introducer tip because it does not have balloon flotation capabilities. Peripheral catheters are similar in number and location but smaller in dimension (14- to 20-gauge catheters) according to a patient's size.

How Is Arterial Pressure Monitored?

Arterial pressure monitoring and blood sampling are carried out after insertion of a 20-gauge, 18-gauge, or 5 French cannula into the femoral artery (the side opposite the VVB), as well as a 20-gauge radial arterial catheter for backup. In pediatric patients, smaller catheters, 24-gauge or 3 French, are used femorally and 22- or 24-gauge for the radial arterial catheter.

Flush Solutions

Catheter flushing solutions are heparin free in order to avoid additional, unnecessary disturbances in the clotting mechanism. All arterial catheters should have continuous (3 mL · h^{-1}), pressure-driven flush devices attached.

What Are the Recommendations for Blood and Blood Product Availability?

Adults

Preliminary reports of the 1981 to 1983 experience from the largest OLT center in the United States cited median and maximum intraoperative RBC use in adult patients of 28.5 and 251 units, respectively.[12] When the blood bank initiates an OLT program, it should plan for the extreme possibility of blood loss, even though later reports,[7, 11] with and without autotransfusion (autologous) systems, claim lower median and maximum consumption of blood and blood products from 1985 to 1989.

Based on these data, we set aside blood products in two locations: the operating room (20 units of packed RBCs, 20 units of FFP, 20 units of cryoprecipitate) and the blood bank (200 units of packed RBCs).

Children

For pediatric patients, we prepare half of the adult blood unit number in the operating room (10 units of each) and a quarter (50 units) in the blood bank.

How and When Is the Rapid-Infusion System Used?

Adults

The RIS should be used in any adult OLT. Massive transfusion up to 500 to 700 mL · min^{-1} is common. Even in cases that require less than 10 RBC units, rapid transfusion is necessary to maintain normovolemia[1] for short periods of time. The RIS is designed to deliver prewarmed (>35 °C), premixed, air-free blood or fluid at low pressure (<300 mm Hg) through 170-μm and 40-μm filters at controlled and rapid rates up to 1500 mL · min^{-1}. The RIS should be ready for use before the first stage of surgery (discussed later).

Children

For pediatric patients, in whom total blood loss and rate of maximum transfusion are expected to be lower than in adults, the potential for RIS overtransfusion is higher, and catheter size is relatively small for the low pressure and adequate flow requirements of the RIS. Thus, I use two to four pneumatic pressure devices (Alton-Dean) instead. Regular pressure bags can also serve this function if they are attached to a tourniquet box. When the RIS system is not used, no air detector is in the system, and scrupulous care must be taken to avoid pressurized air infusion and embolization.

Priming

Preparation of the RIS to deliver fluid, including loading of the reservoir and elimination of all air in the system, is called *priming*. Before this stage is complete, the system is not operable. The fluid used is saline or Plasmalyte A, which is compatible with blood administration. I usually do not prime with a blood product, because debubbling is very difficult. Furthermore, not every patient needs blood or blood products as the first fluid dose at the initial stage of surgery.

Plasmalyte A

Plasmalyte A (Table 76–13) is calcium and glucose free. It has a minimum amount of gluconate (23 mEq · L^{-1}) without any lactate or citrate components. This feature is important because of a diseased liver's inability to handle acid metabolites.

Red Blood Cells and Fresh-Frozen Plasma

When blood is added to the solutions, the resultant hematocrit should be 26% to 28% to reduce RBC loss and improve circulatory rheology. The low colloid oncotic pressure typical in these patients necessitates colloid or FFP. Fluid containing FFP, platelets, and cryoprecipitate is used to replace factors lost or reduced owing to bleeding or existing coagulopathies and to prevent dilution-induced coagulopathies.

These multiple goals are achieved by using a fixed ratio of RBCs, FFP, and Plasmalyte A. If the RIS is primed with blood, a combination of 300 mL (one unit) of RBCs, 250 mL (one unit) of FFP, and 250 mL of Plasmalyte A is used. The composition of the solution can be modified intraoperatively based on a patient's laboratory data (hematocrit, platelet count, and coagulation profile).

ANESTHETIC INDUCTION

What Drugs Should Be Used?

Rapid-sequence induction is performed because many of these patients have ascites and, perhaps, the equivalent of a full stomach. Delayed gastric emptying often exists in patients taking cyclosporine orally. Thiopental, 4 mg · kg^{-1}, ketamine, 1 to 2 mg · kg^{-1}, or etomidate, 0.3 to 0.5 mg · kg^{-1}, is used. Succinylcholine, 1 to 2 mg · kg^{-1}, is added to facilitate tracheal intubation while cricoid pressure is maintained. The induction agents are protein bound, and the free drug fraction is increased in liver disease when serum albumin is low, leading to an enhanced effect. Thiopental and etomidate are metabolized in the liver, but their activity is terminated by redistribution. Hence, their duration of action is normal unless the doses are large or repeated.

TABLE 76–13. Composition of Plasmalyte A

Na$^+$	140 mEq · L^{-1}
K	5 mEq · L^{-1}
Mg^{2+}	3 mEq · L^{-1}
Acetate	27 mEq · L^{-1}
Gluconate	23 mEq · L^{-1}
Osmolality	294 Osm
pH	7.4

Should Nasotracheal and Nasogastric Tubes Be Inserted?

Nasotracheal intubation, as a rule, is not performed out of consideration for the likelihood of preoperative as well as subsequent intraoperative abnormal coagulation function.

Similar concerns exist about insertion of nasogastric tubes. However, careful insertion after tracheal intubation and the application of topical vasoconstrictors provides the necessary gastric decompression during the case. If an incompletely corrected preoperative coagulopathy exists, an alternative approach is to place an orogastric tube, which can be converted to a nasogastric tube at a later time.

How Is a Patient Positioned?

The recipient is placed on a gel pad–covered operating table with both arms abducted and resting on egg crate foam–padded arm boards (see Fig. 76–5). The occiput and heels are also placed on egg crate foam pads to prevent any pressure injury. Because the VVB involves axillary dissection, care should be taken to avoid extreme extension and brachial plexus injury.

The operating time is long, and the viscera are exposed. Thus, heat loss is significant, and the operating room table should have a warming blanket. After catheters are placed, the upper extremities and head are wrapped with vinyl covers to minimize heat loss. Other measures may be applicable (see Chapter 49).

How Are Drugs Handled by Liver Transplant Recipients?

Factors in Drug Tolerance/Intolerance

Patients with parenchymal liver disease represent a spectrum from mild to severe hepatic derangement (see Table 76–1). Although in early liver disease, particularly alcoholic, drug tolerance may be present, this is not the case in more severe forms. Drug tolerance/intolerance results from a multitude of factors:

1. Central nervous system changes. The blood-brain barrier in cirrhotic patients is abnormal, as are neural receptors.
2. Increased volume of distribution (V_D) (suggests the need to increase the first dose of the drug).
3. Reduced synthesis of albumin reduces plasma-binding sites for the drug and increases the free active drug fraction (suggests the need to decrease the first drug dose).
4. Decreased hepatic blood flow.
5. Decreased biotransformation enzyme content and activity. Enzymes of phase 1 biotransformation (e.g., oxidation) are impaired at an earlier stage than phase 2 (e.g., conjugation).
6. Portacaval shunting may increase the bioavailability of orally administered drug by reducing first-pass metabolism.
7. Coexisting impaired renal function decreases drug clearance.

Depending on which of these factors predominates, a drug may produce a more or less profound and prolonged or shortened effect than normal. The initial dose should be titrated against response. The effect of centrally acting agents may be particularly pronounced (e.g., barbiturates, narcotics, and benzodiazepines).

Evidence shows that the benzodiazepine antagonist flumazenil can temporarily worsen hepatic encephalopathy. This observation may suggest a gabaminergic mechanism in the brains of patients with hepatic encephalopathy.[13] The effects of liver disease on some commonly used anesthetic agents are listed in Table 76–14.

Biotransformation

Although the liver is the major site of drug biotransformation, the effects of hepatic dysfunction on drug handling are inconsistent. Such inconsistency may reflect the heterogeneous pathophysiology of liver disease with respect to hepatocellular function, protein binding, and hepatic blood flow.

For hepatic diseases with preserved hepatic blood flow but impaired hepatocellular function, the pharmacokinetic profile of a drug with high hepatic extraction dependency is relatively unaffected. On the other hand, a drug with a low extraction dependency has a pronounced alteration in its disposition and elimination.[14]

Some reports suggest that pharmacokinetic differences between children and adults in terms of anesthetic agents (e.g., alfentanil) are a result of differences in the underlying pathophysiology of cholestatic versus hepatocellular dysfunction; the latter is associated with lower clearance and longer elimination half-life.[15]

Muscle Relaxants

The pharmacokinetics of muscle relaxants in adults with hepatic dysfunction has been studied extensively[16] (see Table 76–14). Vecuronium is less affected, although dose-dependent alterations have been observed. The pharmacokinetics of atricurium are unaffected by liver disease. However, the V_D is larger for all relaxants; accordingly, the distribution half-lives are shorter in patients with severe hepatorenal dysfunction.

Any muscle relaxant can be used in patients with advanced liver disease; however, titration using nerve stimulation monitoring is recommended in order to avoid inadequate or prolonged effects. For OLT surgery that lasts 8 to 12 hours and with the significant time of postoperative intubation and ventilation, the clinical importance of the latter effect is generally minor. Even doxacurium, a long-acting relaxant, is satisfactory.[1] Finally, although the synthesis of pseudocholinesterase is reduced, the clinical effect on succinylcholine duration of action is insignificant.

ANESTHETIC MANAGEMENT

Does It Differ from Typical Major Abdominal Cases?

Narcotics

Anesthetic maintenance is in many ways similar to that in other major abdominal surgery. A narcotic can be successfully used in patients with hepatic disease despite the pharmacologic consequences of decreased clearance and prolonged half-life (see Table 76–14). Fentanyl, sufentanil, and alfentanil all are suitable opioid analgesic agents because they have short half-lives and inactive metabolites. Interestingly, fentanyl does not decrease hepatic oxygen and blood supply or prevent increases

TABLE 76–14. Anesthetic Drugs In Liver Disease

Class of Drug	Drug	Effect of Decreased Serum Albumin	Effect of Decreased Hepatic Metabolism	Other Effects
Induction agents	Thiopental	Increased free drug	Increased elimination half-life	
	Ketamine		Prolonged action, decreased clearance	Phase 1 metabolism affected
	Etomidate	Increased free drug	Increased elimination half-life	
Opioid analgesic agents	Meperidine		Prolonged effect	Decreased first-pass metabolism
	Phenoperidine			
	Fentanyl			
	Sufentanil	Increased free drug	Prolonged effect	Decreased first-pass metabolism
	Morphine			Narcotic effect terminated by redistribution and extrahepatic glucuronidation
Benzodiazepines	Diazepam	Increased free drug	Prolonged action, decreased clearance	Phase 1 metabolism affected
	Chlordiazepoxide			
	Midazolam			
	Oxazepam		Normal clearance and duration of action	Phase 2 metabolism spared
	Lorazepam			
Beta-adrenergic blocking agents	Propranolol	Increased free drug	Increased oral bioavailability, decreased clearance	Decreased first-pass metabolism, reduced dose for treatment of portal hypertension
Local anesthetic agents	Lidocaine		Decreased clearance, increased elimination half-life	
Neuromuscular blocking agents	Succinylcholine			Decreased plasma cholinesterase, slightly prolonged apnea
Nondepolarizing muscle relaxants	Pancuronium	Bound to hemoglobin	Prolonged elimination half-life	Significantly metabolized. Altered pharmacokinetics in patients with hepatic or biliary disease
	d-Tubocurarine	No effect	Prolonged elimination half-life	Significantly metabolized
	Vecuronium	No effect	Prolonged effect in large doses	Significantly metabolized. Altered pharmacokinetics in patients with hepatic or biliary disease. Metabolized to 3-acetyl derivative
	Atracurium	No effect	Action unaffected by hepatic and renal disease	Significantly metabolized. Elimination by Hoffman degradation and ester hydrolysis

(Modified from McEvedy BA, Shelley MP, Park GR: Anesthesia and liver disease. Br J Hosp Med 1986; 36:26.)

in demand when used in moderate doses (50 μg · kg^{-1} bolus and 0.5 μg · kg^{-1} · min^{-1} infusions).[17] Studies comparing fentanyl and morphine pharmacokinetics in adult patients with normal or abnormal liver function have not shown a different effect on disposition and elimination in adults, or of alfentanil in children.[15]

Inhalation Agents

Anesthesia can be maintained with an inhalation agent, as well as with tranquilizers or narcotics or any combination thereof. The effect of anesthetic drugs on hepatic function is as important as the effect of hepatic disease on the pharmacokinetics of the anesthetic agents. Halothane is avoided in favor of isoflurane for OLT.

Halothane, enflurane, and isoflurane all reduce liver blood flow, but halothane produces a proportionately larger decrement because it reduces hepatic arterial flow to a greater extent. Thus, hepatic oxygen supply is well maintained.[17]

Nitrous oxide has been used for many years without increased anesthesia-related postoperative hepatic complications. However, its sympathomimetic effect and accumulation in the intestinal lumen, with the potential for subsequent distention in protracted cases, make it counterproductive in many peoples' minds.

Why Is Hourly Laboratory (Blood Sampling) Monitoring Recommended?

Tight control of physiologic parameters is essential to maintain homeostasis during OLT. Therefore, a system for rapid assessment of coagulation profile (hematocrit, PT, partial thromboplastin time [PTT], platelets), blood gas partial pressures (of oxygen and carbon dioxide [CO_2]), acid-base status (pH/bicarbonate/base excess), electrolytes (sodium, potassium, serum ionized calcium), blood glucose values, and lactate levels should be used at least hourly. In the operating room, TEG monitoring of the coagulation profile can be performed even more frequently. Fibrinogen or fibrin degradation product (FDP) measurement, serum osmolality, and urinary sodium determinations are desirable perioperatively but are not essential hourly.

What Immunosuppressive Drugs Are Used?

Cyclosporine is the most commonly used maintenance immunosuppressive drug. Steroids are almost invariably added.[18] Azathioprine may be used as a third agent to reduce the dose of cyclosporine and, in some cases, may replace cyclosporine altogether when the latter is contraindicated or can no longer be used because of adverse side effects.

Antilymphocyte globulin preparations, including the monoclonal antibody OKT-3,[19] have been given prophylactically and for specific indications to prevent rejection. OKT-3 reacts against all mature T lymphocytes.

Cyclosporine is given before surgery (orally or intravenously) as part of the premedication. It is not repeated intraoperatively because of the impracticality of controlling or monitoring effective or toxic blood levels and is only repeated postoperatively with dose adjustments on the basis of drug levels and creatinine clearance. Methylprednisolone, 500 mg, is given before surgery and repeated every 6 hours.

SURGICAL STAGES IN ORTHOTOPIC LIVER TRANSPLANTATION

What Is the Preanhepatic Phase?

The first stage in OLT is the *preanhepatic phase.* It lasts from skin incision to the point at which the native liver is freed to its vascular pedicle. The skin incision is wide, bilateral, and subcostal, with cephalic extension to the xiphoid. The xiphoid process is removed without entering the thorax.

What Is the Anhepatic Phase?

The second stage is referred to as the *anhepatic phase.* It begins with clamping of the suprahepatic and infrahepatic inferior vena cava (IVC), portal vein, and hepatic artery, after which the diseased liver is removed. This stage includes the hepatectomy and ends when vascular anastomosis of the IVC and portal vein is complete; the infrahepatic IVC anastomosis is prepared but not completed until late in this stage.

Three separate or combined techniques are used during this stage: (1) simple cross-clamping; (2) VVB (femoral-axillary) to avoid physiologic stress; and (3) either 1 or 2 combined with flushing of the donor liver with lactated Ringer's solution via the portal vein (100 mL in children, 200–300 mL in adults) to remove transport infusate and to clear the donor liver vasculature of air. The infrahepatic IVC and portal vein repairs are then completed.

What Is the Neohepatic Phase?

The third stage is called the *neohepatic* or *postanhepatic phase.* Here, the donor liver is incorporated into the recipient's circulatory system by releasing, in sequence, clamps from the portal vein, the infrahepatic IVC, and the suprahepatic IVC. Subsequently, the portal artery anastomosis is performed, and after adequate hemostasis, the bile duct is reconstructed. If a patient has a normal extrahepatic bile duct system, duct-to-duct anastomosis is performed; if it is abnormal (biliary atresia, biliary cirrhosis, perisclerosing cholangitis), a Roux-en-Y choledochojejunostomy is performed. Finally, an intraoperative cholangiogram is obtained to assess patency of the biliary system and biliary drainage.

The average total surgical time (see Table 76–12) is >6 hours (range 4–12 h), and the average anhepatic phase is >2 hours (range 1½–5 h). The anhepatic time for patients with chronic active hepatitis is longer than for patients with primary biliary cirrhosis. This difference is attributable to more difficult surgical techniques and hemostatic conditions. Total surgical time for patients with primary biliary cirrhosis is significantly less than for those with chronic active hepatitis or perisclerosing cholangitis. Dissection to free the diseased liver is more difficult in the presence of portal hypertension, and hepatojejunostomy with Roux-en-Y loop takes longer than end-to-end choledochocholedochostomy.

What Does the Anesthetist Need to Know About Venovenous Bypass?

Indications

During the anhepatic phase, cross-clamping of the IVC and portal vein for hepatectomy reduces venous return to the heart and cardiac output by about 50%, creating congestion of the IVC and portal system. VVB is suggested for venous decompression, improved hemodynamic stability, and decreased intraoperative blood loss.[20] In addition, VVB has been reported to improve renal function, eliminate gastrointestinal hemorrhage, decrease operative mortality from 10% to 1%, and provide additional time for completion of the vascular anastomoses.

Technique

Figure 76–6 illustrates the routine connection of the extracorporeal bypass circuit. Blood is pumped from the portal and femoral veins by a centripetal pump without heparin, although the tubing may be heparin bonded. A small dose of heparin, 1000 to 2000 units, may be added to the bypass cannula. The VVB flow rate is up to 40% of cardiac output; hemodynamic changes usually do not occur if adequate flow is maintained.

During VVB, a patient's intravascular volume serves as a bypass reservoir. Bypass flow depends on inflow. It decreases when cannulas are obstructed by the vessel wall, kinked tubing, excessive centripetal force (suction), or low cardiac output. Hemodynamic stability depends on flow exceeding $2.5\ L \cdot min^{-1}$. Patients may suffer protracted hypotension when fluctuations in VVB flow are $>500\ mL \cdot min^{-1}$ (Table 76–15).

Routine Use

Routine use of VVB during the anhepatic phase is somewhat controversial.[20] It is not recommended in younger patients or those who are in reasonably good physiologic condi-

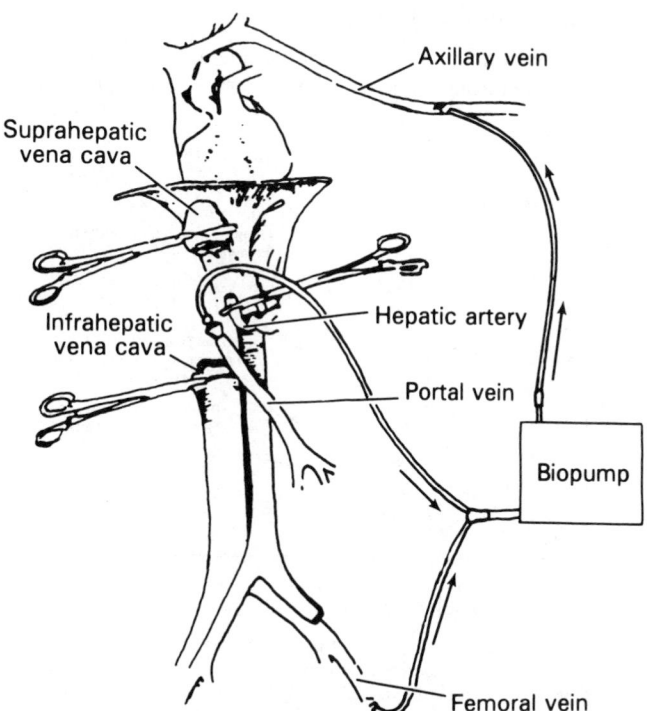

FIGURE 76–6. Diagram depicting the routine implementation of venovenous bypass in the adult patient. (From Paulsen AW, Whitten CW, Ramsay MAE, et al: Considerations for anesthetic management during veno-venous bypass in adult hepatic transplantation. Anesth Analg 1989; 58:489. © Williams & Wilkins, 1989.)

TABLE 76–15. Venovenous Bypass Flow Fluctuations and Hypotension

	Duration of Hypotension (min)	
Flow Changes*	SBP <100 mm Hg	SBP <80 mm Hg
≤500 mL · min⁻¹	27.5 ± 2.7	4.5 ± 0.7
500 to 1000 mL · min⁻¹	35 ± 3.1†	14.5 ± 2.6†
>1000 mL · min⁻¹	49.5 ± 3.6†	23.5 ± 3.2†

(From Kang YG, Freeman JA, Aggarwal S, et al: Hemodynamic instability during liver transplantation. Transplant Proc 1989; 21:3489. © 1989. Reprinted by permission of Appleton & Lange, Inc.)
*Values are mean ± standard error of the mean.
†$P < .05$ compared with minimum flow change group (<500 mL).
Abbreviation: SBP = systemic blood pressure.

tion and who are able to respond to the sudden loss of venous return with vasoconstriction and tachycardia. Vigorous volume infusion often results in some improvement, yet a penalty of fluid overload is paid when the liver is revascularized and venous return is restored. Some transplant centers use VVB routinely, whereas others use various bypass techniques only for specific diagnoses or when suprahepatic IVC occlusion is not tolerated.[20] Few centers do not use it at all.

Hypothermia

Hypothermia during VVB may pose another significant problem, because it is potentiated by an extracorporeal circuit that does not contain a heat exchanger. A heat exchanger is avoided because of its large, potentially thrombogenic surface area. Heat loss from the bypass circuit can decrease core temperature three times more rapidly (0.9 °C · h⁻¹) during bypass than at any other time during OLT. It is directly related to VVB flow (Fig. 76–7).

Miscellaneous Problems

Other complications of bypass include air emboli from the cannulation site, laceration of the portal vein, and pulmonary

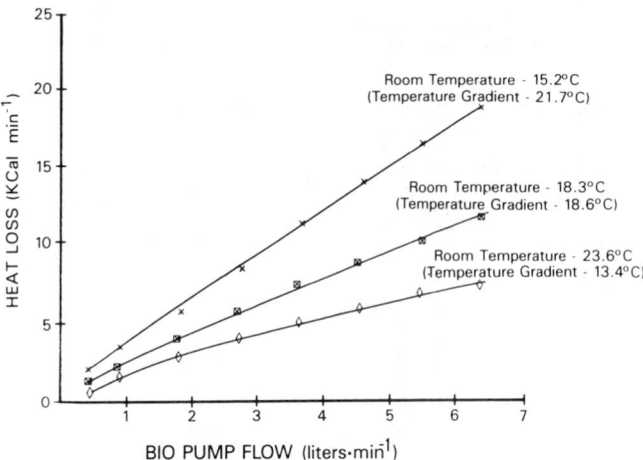

FIGURE 76–7. Calculated heat loss from the bypass circuit as a function of pump flow and room temperature, or temperature gradient between the circulating fluid and the room. Estimated heat loss for blood flowing through the bypass circuit was computed by substituting the specific gravity and specific heat of blood for those of distilled water. Since no consideration was given to the possibility that red blood cell motion may disturb the unstirred layer at the inner wall of the tubing, the heat loss may actually be underestimated. (From Paulsen AW, Whitten CW, Ramsay MAE, et al: Considerations for anesthetic management during veno-venous bypass in adult hepatic transplantation. Anesth Analg 1989; 58:489. © International Anesthesia Research Society.)

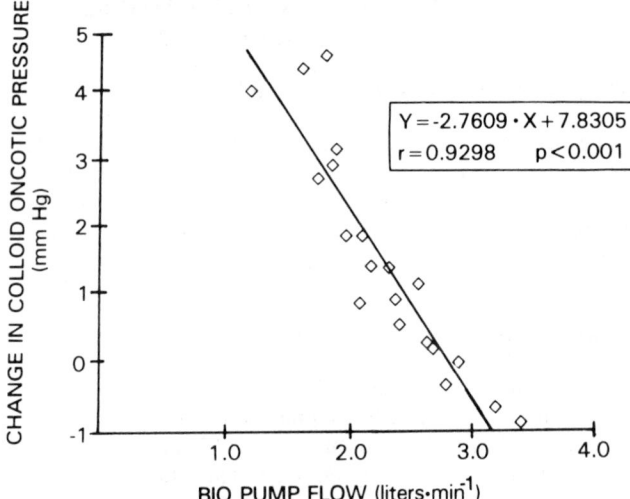

FIGURE 76–8. Changes in colloid oncotic pressure of the plasma as a function of the flow through the extracorporeal circuit. (From Paulsen AW, Whitten CW, Ramsay MAE, et al: Considerations for anesthetic management during veno-venous bypass in adult hepatic transplantation. Anesth Analg 1989; 58:489. © International Anesthesia Research Society.)

thromboembolism from migration of pre-existing thrombi in the portal or deep venous systems via the low-resistance VVB circuit.[21] Plasma colloid oncotic pressure is decreased during VVB as a function of the flow (Fig. 76–8).

What Physiologic Changes Should Be Expected During the Preanhepatic Phase?

Intraoperative changes in physiologic variables are listed in Table 76–16.

Cardiovascular/Hemodynamic

At the beginning of surgery, high filling pressure due to fluid overload, ascites, pleural effusion, pulmonary hypertension, and a hyperdynamic cardiovascular state persists as long as volume loss secondary to surgical bleeding and continuous formation of ascites is adequately replaced.

Surgical manipulation of major vessels reduces venous return, and prolonged hypotension may require adjustments of

TABLE 76–16. Characteristic Intraoperative Changes in Physiologic Variables

Variable	Preanhepatic Stage	Anhepatic Stage	Neohepatic Stage	
			Early	Late
Cardiac output	High	Low	High	High
Heart rate	High	High	Low	High
Mean arterial pressure	Normal	Low	Very low	Normal
Filling pressure	Normal	Low	High	Normal
Vascular resistance	Low	High	Very low	Low
Pao_2	Normal	Normal	Normal	Normal
Pco_2	Normal	Low	Normal	Normal
Base deficit	Normal	High	Very high	Normal
Serum Na⁺	Low	Normal	Normal	Normal
Serum K⁺	Low	Normal	Very high	Low
Serum Ca²⁺	Normal	Very low	Low	Normal
Serum citrate	Normal	High	High	Low

(From Kang YG, Freeman JA, Aggarwal S, et al.: Hemodynamic instability during liver transplantation. Transplant Proc 1989; 21:3489–3492. © 1989. Reprinted by permission of Appleton & Lange, Inc.)

surgical technique. At the end of the preanhepatic phase, caudad traction on the liver to isolate the suprahepatic IVC may cause transient dysrhythmias and hypotension. Marginal cardiac performance necessitates a vasopressor (e.g., dopamine, 2–5 μg $\cdot$ kg^{-1} $\cdot$ min^{-1} as a starting dose). End-stage liver disease may increase catecholamine resistance, necessitating a higher dose.

Alpha-agonists are of questionable value because they increase peripheral and coronary resistance. At the same time, they may decrease shunt fraction and improve tissue perfusion. Continuous monitoring of mixed venous oxygen saturation (S$\bar{v}$O$_2$) helps to assess preload and cardiac output, assuming oxygen-carrying capacity, oxygen consumption, and myocardial contractility remain constant. Because of arteriovenous shunting, S$\bar{v}$O$_2$ and cardiac output are expected to be falsely high; thus S$\bar{v}$O$_2$ serves more as a trend monitor. A more reliable sign of inadequate tissue perfusion is metabolic acidosis.

Coagulation

During the preanhepatic phase, a dilutional coagulopathy is superimposed on the underlying disease-induced coagulopathy. FFP (given via the RIS) corrects low coagulation factors, and platelet transfusion (not through the RIS) increases platelet count (40,000–50,000 per 10-unit transfusion). Cryoprecipitate, which contains fibrinogen, Factor VIII, and Factor XIII, is rarely necessary during this period. Attempts should be made to correct coagulation problems during this stage.

Temperature

Body temperature gradually decreases from the effects of anesthetics, muscle relaxants, cold environment, and insufficient energy production by the liver.

Hypoglycemia

Hypoglycemia due to loss of liver gluconeogenic capacity may be a concern but has not been observed frequently. Transfusion of blood can maintain blood glucose at a normal level because each unit of whole blood contains 0.5 g of glucose before processing. When blood replacement is minimum, small intravenous doses of glucose avoid hypoglycemia.

Hypocalcemia

Transient citrate-induced hypocalcemia from the banked blood may follow rapid transfusion. A 500-mL unit of whole blood contains 1.7 g of hydrated trisodium citrate. The amount of citrate in a unit of packed RBCs is variable. The volume and rate of transfusion correlate with a decrease of ionized calcium, but total calcium levels do not correlate with serum ionized calcium.

What Physiologic Changes Should Be Expected During the Anhepatic Phase?

Cardiovascular/Hemodynamic

Cross-clamping of the IVC, which heralds the beginning of the anhepatic phase, causes significant hypotension due to reduced venous return. The loss of portal blood flow has little effect on total venous return, especially in patients with signif-

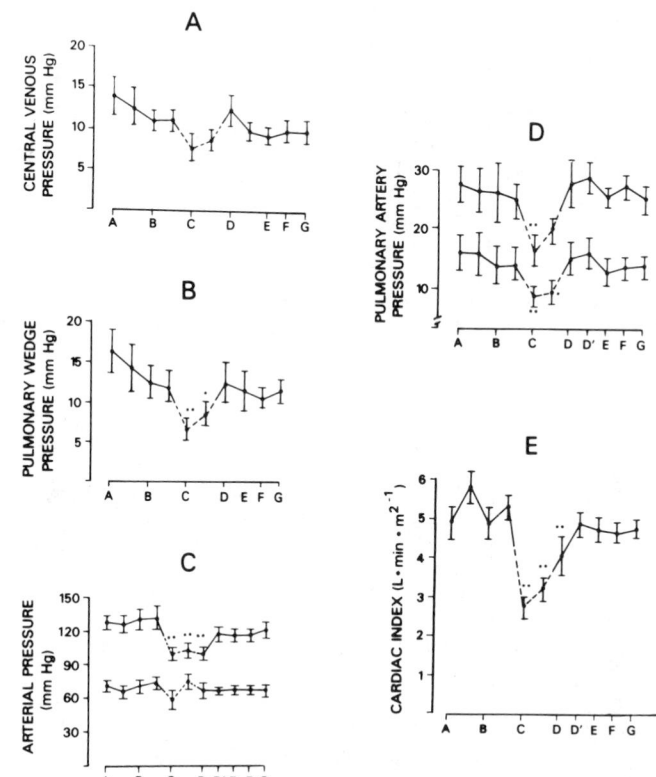

FIGURE 76–9. *A–E,* Changes in measured hemodynamic parameters during liver transplantation. Mean $\pm$ SEM for nine patients. Phase: A = Induction; B = dissection; C = anhepatic; D = partial anhepatic; E = gallbladder anastomosis; F = skin closure; G = end of procedure; * = different from preclamping values ($P < .05$); ** = different from preclamping values ($P < .01$). (From Carmichael FJ, Lindop MJ, Farman JV: Anesthesia for hepatic transplantation: cardiovascular and metabolic alterations and their management. Anesth Analg 1985; 64:108. © Williams & Wilkins, 1985.)

icant collateral flow. Reduced right- and left-sided filling pressures, systemic and pulmonary pressures, and cardiac index (Fig. 76–9) and increased heart rate, systemic resistance, and pulmonary resistance (Fig. 76–10) all are related to reduced venous return. Changes in systemic vascular resistance and afterload are less with this venous inflow occlusion than with major arterial occlusion, in which reduced cardiac output is, in part, related to extreme afterload and hypertension.

Volume expansion and administration of inotropic agents can ameliorate the negative hemodynamic changes associated with IVC clamping. However, as was noted earlier, with volume expansion comes the possibility of fluid overload during this stage (using the RIS) and later during stage 3 reperfusion. Vessel occlusion also promotes surgical bleeding, hematuria, and congestive ischemia of the bowel. All of these problems can be avoided by VVB.

Venovenous Bypass

Initiation of VVB restores venous return but may produce transient bradycardia and peaked T waves, owing to rapid influx of room temperature priming solution. Hypothermia due to heat loss and thromboembolism may be encountered, as also was noted previously.

By the end of the anhepatic phase, portal vein anastomosis is completed. VVB then carries only systemic venous blood (partial bypass); the resulting hypovolemic state, lasting 10 to

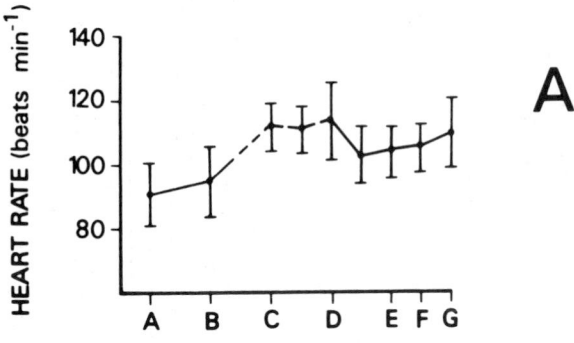

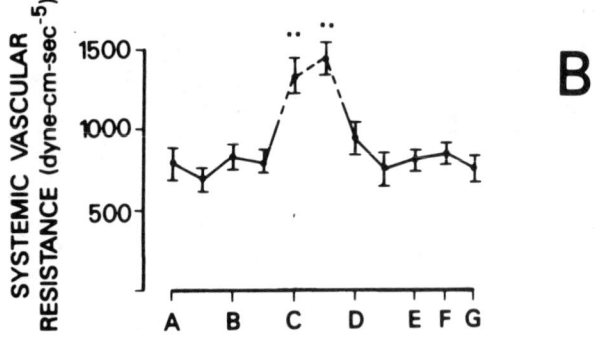

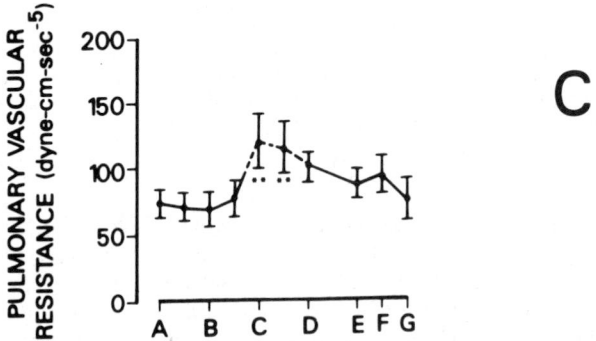

FIGURE 76–10. *A–C,* Changes in heart rate, systemic vascular resistance, and pulmonary vascular resistance during liver transplantation. Mean ± SEM for nine patients. Phase: A = Induction; B = dissection; C = anhepatic; D = partial anhepatic; E = gallbladder anastomosis; F = skin closure; G = end of procedure; ** = different from preclamping values (*P* < .01). (From Carmichael FJ, Lindop MJ, Farman JV: Anesthesia for hepatic transplantation: cardiovascular and metabolic alterations and their management. Anesth Analg 1985; 64:108. © Williams & Wilkins, 1985.)

15 minutes, may require additional fluids, with similar concerns about overloading.

Coagulation

At the onset of VVB, heparin effect may be detected by the TEG because a small dose of heparin may be added in the bypass cannula. This effect lasts for only 30 to 60 minutes. Dilutional coagulopathy may continue, although surgical bleeding is less severe owing to bypass decompression. Marked fibrinolysis related to progressively increased levels of plasminogen activators, which do not undergo hepatic clearance, can occur during the anhepatic phase. Administration of platelets and ε-aminocaproic acid during this stage should be reserved for severe cases of bleeding due to thrombocytopenia or fibrinolysis in order to avoid thromboembolism in the unheparinized VVB system.

Temperature

Further decreases in body temperature take place secondary to the absence of hepatic energy production, heat loss from the exposed viscera, and heat loss from the VVB.

Hypoglycemia/Hypocalcemia

Hypoglycemia and hypocalcemia occur maximally, and severe ionized hypocalcemia (<0.6 mmol $\cdot$ L^{-1}) is sometimes unavoidable during the anhepatic phase or during rapid blood transfusion. This change can produce myocardial depression if not treated with calcium.

Electrolytes

Preoperative hyponatremia and hypokalemia subside during surgery (see Table 76–16). Sodium and potassium are normalized by the large volume of FFP and Plasmalyte solution (5 mEq $\cdot$ L^{-1} of potassium in Plasmalyte). Hypernatremia can emerge secondary to repeated sodium bicarbonate administration to correct metabolic acidosis. Progressive hyperkalemia may result from inadequate renal function and large volumes of transfused banked blood.

Renal

Urine output should be maintained because hemolysis often occurs after massive transfusions; cyclosporine may damage renal function (usually postoperatively); and IVC clamping can lead to renal venous congestion with hematuria. The latter usually resolves gradually at the end of surgery. Mannitol and low-dose dopamine (2–3 μg $\cdot$ kg^{-1} $\cdot$ min^{-1}) have been shown to improve postoperative renal function in this setting.[22]

Acid-Base

Progressive metabolic acidosis (Fig. 76–11) and increased lactate levels during the anhepatic phase result from rapid transfusion of blood with acid metabolites, deficient hepatic clearance of acidic substances, and stagnation of blood flow below the diaphragm. Reduced perfusion leads to anaerobic metabolism. The acidosis becomes persistent in patients with unstable cardiovascular function, and further compromise of tissue perfusion follows.

Metabolic acidosis is treated with sodium bicarbonate in order to maintain a base excess no lower than -5 mEq $\cdot$ L^{-1}, particularly at the end of the anhepatic phase and start of the neohepatic phase. Although this treatment may promote hypernatremia, hyperosmolarity, and postoperative alkalemia, these conditions are believed by many to be benign compared with the hemodynamic deterioration induced by severe metabolic acidosis. Keep in mind, however, that severe myocardial depression and long-standing lactic acidosis are thought by many investigators to be worsened by the administration of bicarbonate.

Complex changes in CO_2 homeostasis take place during OLT.[23] Patients may be hyperventilated to a mild degree of

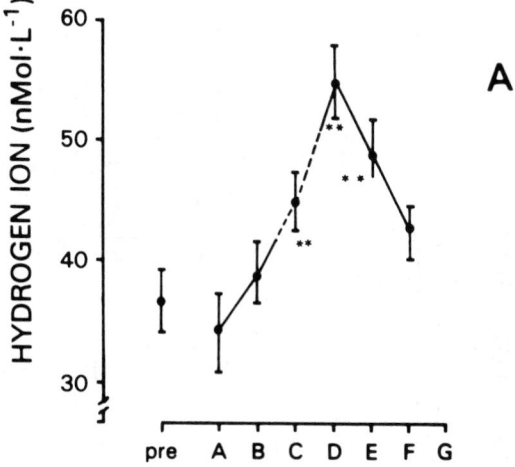

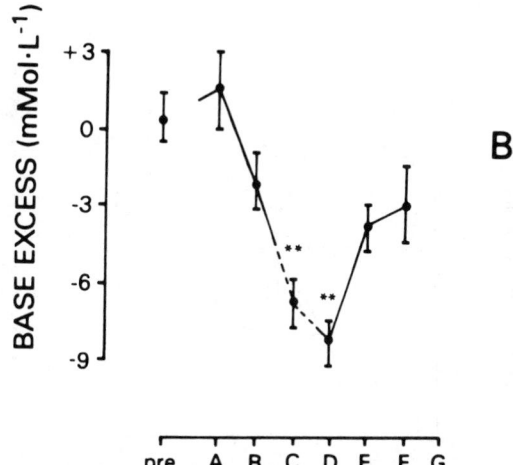

FIGURE 76–11. *A and B,* Changes in arterial plasma hydrogen ion concentrations and base deficit during liver transplantation. Mean ± SEM for nine patients. Phase: A = Induction; B = dissection; C = anhepatic; D = partial anhepatic; E = gallbladder anastomosis; F = skin closure; G = end of procedure; ** = different from preclamping values (*P* < .01). (From Carmichael FJ, Lindop MJ, Farman JV: Anesthesia for hepatic transplantation: cardiovascular and metabolic alterations and their management. Anesth Analg 1985; 64:108. © Williams & Wilkins, 1985.)

crease is followed by restoration of venous return on unclamping of the suprahepatic IVC. At this point (within a few minutes), the picture of *postperfusion syndrome* (similar to postacute arterial occlusion) appears. It consists of progressive bradycardia, hypotension, high filling pressures, and decreased systemic vascular resistance.

Cardiac Output

During the early reperfusion period, thermodilution measurements of cardiac output are unreliable (falsely low) owing to rapid influx of cold preservation solution. In contrast, dye dilution technique cardiac output studies show a real increase in comparison with the anhepatic phase, although output values remain lower than baseline levels.[23] In 30% of the cases in which extreme postperfusion hypotension (<70% of baseline) occurs, it is likely related to vasoactive substances released from the grafted liver. It does not correlate with the degree of

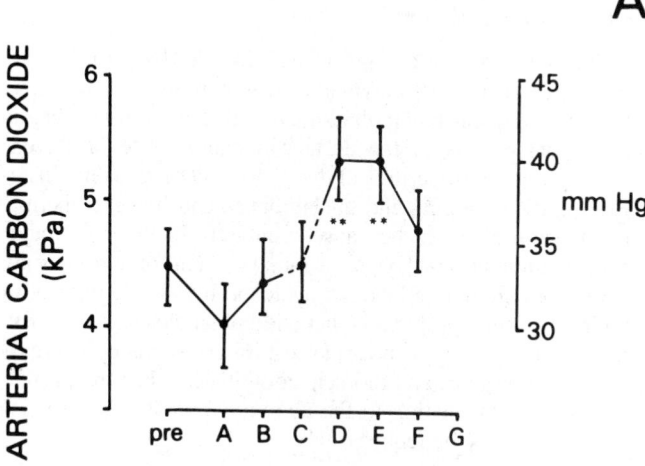

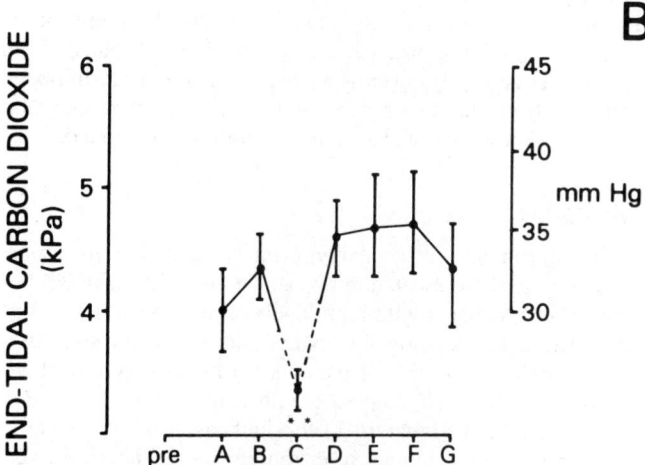

FIGURE 76–12. *A and B,* Changes in arterial and end-tidal CO_2 during liver transplantation. Mean ± SEM for nine patients. Phase: A = Induction; B = dissection; C = anhepatic; D = partial anhepatic; E = gallbladder anastomosis; F = skin closure; G = end of procedure; ** = different from preclamping values (*P* < .01). (From Carmichael FJ, Lindop MJ, Farman JV: Anesthesia for hepatic transplantation: cardiovascular and metabolic alterations and their management. Anesth Analg 1985; 64:108. © Williams & Wilkins, 1985.)

alkalemia in order to compensate partially for the metabolic acidosis. With hypothermia, the CO_2 production rate is expected to decrease; however, rapid transfusion of blood transiently increases the CO_2 load. A reduction of pulmonary gas exchange with arterial hypotension or reduced lung perfusion results in a progressive buildup of body stores of CO_2, increase in arterial CO_2 partial pressure (Pa_{CO_2}), and decrease in end-tidal CO_2 (Fig. 76–12).

What Physiologic Changes Should Be Expected in the Neohepatic Phase?

Cardiovascular/Hemodynamic

Abrupt hemodynamic changes occur on reperfusion of a grafted liver. Subsequent unclamping of the portal vein and infrahepatic IVC decreases preload into the VVB. This de-

hypokalemia, and symptoms persist even after core temperature returns to >34 °C. The syndrome is treated with epinephrine (5–10-µg boluses) to restore heart rate and contractility.

Calcium chloride and bicarbonate are administered to treat hyperkalemia and acidosis. Calcium used prophylactically maintains cardiac output but does not prevent bradycardia and hypotension. Aggressive treatment of hyperkalemia usually is unnecessary because it disappears within minutes (Fig. 76–13A).

The acute reperfusion hemodynamic insult lasts 5 to 30 minutes; however, filling pressures stay high longer (30–120 min), whereas systemic vascular resistance remains low.

Air Emboli

The high filling pressures are probably related to increased preload, myocardial depression, and air emboli. Air emboli originating from the donor liver can be detected immediately after reperfusion using echocardiography.

Surgical Manipulation

The late neohepatic stage (see Table 76–16) is relatively uneventful as the hemodynamic profile returns to baseline. However, surgical manipulation can still have a role: hepatic artery anastomosis to the aorta can cause acute or diffuse bleeding (e.g., retroperitoneal dissection), hemodynamic instability (aortic clamping and unclamping), and bowel ischemia. Hypotension also can be caused suddenly by liver or major vessel manipulations. Hypertension at the end of surgery may result from fluid overload or cyclosporine (most typical in children). A final problem is that abdominal closure may interfere with the hemodynamic and respiratory status by decreasing filling pressures and thoracic compliance when the grafted liver is large in relation to the abdominal cavity size; secondary closure may be required.

Coagulation

Reperfusion of the new liver often induces a severe coagulopathy for several reasons: (1) dilution by the preservation solution, (2) release of heparin or heparinlike substances from donor liver cells, (3) fibrinolysis due to release of plasminogen activator from the donor liver, and (4) inhibition of coagulation by unknown substances other than those mentioned.[24]

Fibrinolysis

The fibrinolysis is probably primary, although it can be secondary to disseminated intravascular coagulation (DIC) because it is associated with high levels of fibrinogen, Factors V and VIII, and plasminogen activator and *not* Factor consumption. Indeed, about 30% of patients before surgery have high levels of FDPs, which suggest the presence of DIC.[5]

The "explosive" nature of fibrinolysis in early stage 3, occurring within 5 minutes after reperfusion of the graft liver, makes sudden quantitative changes in coagulation factors and fibrinolytic proteins an unlikely cause. Qualitative changes probably account for the acute development of primary fibrinolysis. They may result from changes in cellular membrane permeability (even though the graft is preserved hypothermically in a solution with simulated intracellular composition).

Diagnosis. The differential diagnosis can be made by as-

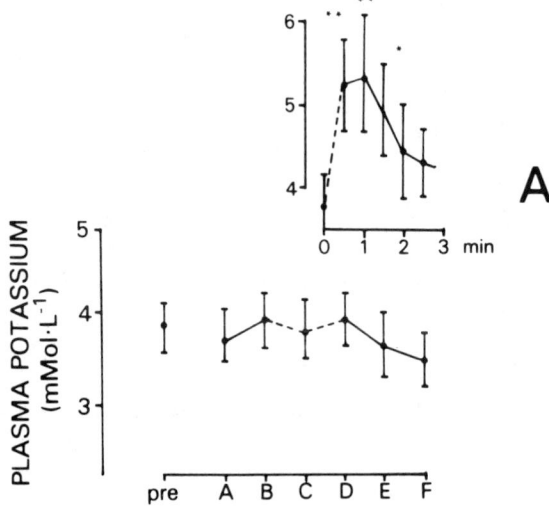

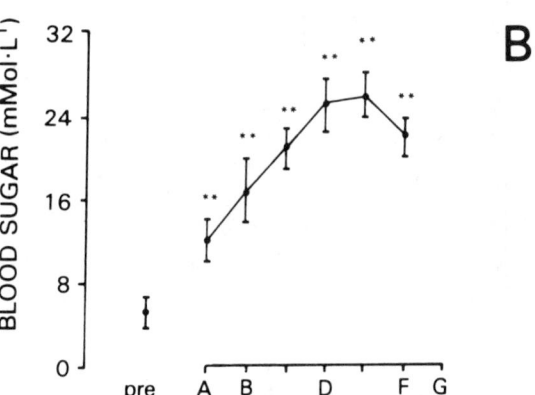

FIGURE 76–13. *A and B,* Changes in plasma potassium and blood sugar concentrations during liver transplantation. Mean ± SEM for nine patients. Phase: A = Induction; B = dissection; C = anhepatic; D = partial anhepatic; E = gallbladder anastomosis; F = skin closure; G = end of procedure; ** = different from preclamping values (P < .05 or .01). *Inset,* Plasma potassium samples taken from the pulmonary artery catheter over 30-s periods after the release of clamps from the portal vein and suprahepatic artery in eight patients. ** = Different from preclamping values (P < .05); ** = different from preclamping values (P < .01). (From Carmichael FJ, Lindop MJ, Farman JV: Anesthesia for hepatic transplantation: cardiovascular and metabolic alterations and their management. Anesth Analg 1985; 64:108. © Williams & Wilkins, 1985.)

sessing the effect of different replacement therapies on the TEG. Protamine sulfate, 50 mg, reverses persistent (>30 min postreperfusion) heparin effect. Epsilon-aminocaproic acid, 1 g, treats severe fibrinolysis (<60 min TEG lysis time). Effectiveness of the latter agent without thrombotic complications also points to a primary fibrinolysis.

Treatment. The severe coagulopathy typically improves during the neohepatic phase unless the grafted liver does not function adequately or major surgical bleeding occurs. If bleeding is not severe, the coagulopathy should be treated aggressively, even if the TEG looks abnormal.

Perioperative graft failures due to technical complications occur in 10% of adults and 30% of children.[2] Iatrogenic problems, such as overzealous correction of clotting defects and polycythemia caused by overtransfusion, may contribute to hepatic artery or portal vein thrombosis. The risk in infants is inversely related to the patient's size, and complications are mainly attributed to vascular thrombosis.[25]

A hypercoagulable state sometimes occurs in patients with hepatic tumors or Budd-Chiari syndrome before surgery. With surgical bleeding, this situation probably will reverse. When surgical bleeding is minimal, low-dose heparin, 1000 to 2000 units, should be considered during VVB.

Acid-Base

The acidosis and rise in $Paco_2$ at revascularization are the result of metabolites flushed out of the donor liver. Treatment of some patients with bicarbonate at this stage contributes to further $Paco_2$ elevation but also minimizes the fall in bicarbonate and pH levels. In any case, metabolic acidosis should be treated conservatively based on blood gas determinations; moderate to severe metabolic alkalosis is observed soon after OLT and may persist for days. This late alkalosis is a result of citrate metabolism and diuretic administration.

Electrolytes

Acute hyperkalemia (*potassium cardioplegia*-like effect) with levels up to 11 mEq $\cdot$ L^{-1} may be detected.[5] The early rise in potassium seen 1 minute after revascularization (see Fig. 76–13A) is probably a result of incomplete flushing of the liver preservation solution before revascularization. This solution is rich in potassium, which has been lost from cells during preservation (preservation solution itself has initially low potassium). During the later neohepatic phase, potassium is taken up by the donor liver and by all cells of the body because of the alkalosis-induced intracellular shift. Supplemental potassium is usually required but may potentiate hyperkalemia in those cases of postoperative renal or liver donor dysfunction; it should be undertaken carefully.

Hyperglycemia

On reperfusion, sudden severe hyperglycemia may also occur, secondary to massive release of glucose from the donor liver. Glucose levels remain high during the third stage (see Fig. 76–13B) and slowly return to normal levels within 24 hours. Persistent hyperglycemia relates to impaired glucose reuptake and glycogenolysis by the new liver; low insulin levels during stages 2 and 3; and increased glucagon levels on reperfusion.

When Does the New Liver Begin to Function?

Function of the grafted liver is detectable about 2 hours after reperfusion or occasionally at the end of the operation: Citrate, lactate, and glucose levels decrease gradually; coagulopathy improves; bile is produced; and urine bilirubin is minimal. Liver enzymes, however, may still be very high, with serum levels of glutamic-oxaloacetic transaminase and glutamic-pyruvic transaminase >100 IU $\cdot$ L^{-1} owing to preservation injury. Persistent citrate intoxication, lactic acidosis, hyperglycemia, and coagulopathy augur a poor prognosis for new liver function.

What Factors Cause Intraoperative Hypotension?

Intraoperative hypotension occurs because of one or more factors:

1. Inadequate replacement of the massive amounts of fluid and blood lost during the procedure
2. Cardiac dysfunction secondary to decreased serum concentration of ionized calcium
3. Surgical manipulations that disturb preload (including IVC occlusion)
4. Dysrhythmias caused by metabolic disorders—hypokalemia and hyperkalemia, acidosis
5. Pre-existing myocardial disease
6. Emboli from the VVB or the donor liver
7. Myocardial ischemia secondary to hypotension, right ventricular overload due to overtransfusion, and paradoxical air emboli

How Are the Metabolic Changes Treated?

Hyperkalemia

Hyperkalemia may be treated by glucose and insulin: 1 to 2 g $\cdot$ kg^{-1} glucose (2–4 mL $\cdot$ kg^{-1} of 50% glucose) with 0.2 units of regular insulin per gram of glucose (5 g glucose per unit of insulin). Its effectiveness is unknown in patients with insulin resistance. Severe hyperkalemia (7–10 mEq $\cdot$ L^{-1}), which can occur during reperfusion and lead to electrocardiographic and heart rate changes, is treated by intravenous calcium chloride ($CaCl_2$, adults 500 mg–1 g; children, 10–30 mg $\cdot$ kg^{-1}) and bicarbonate, 1 to 2 mEq $\cdot$ kg^{-1}, as symptomatic therapy in addition to glucose and insulin.

Hypocalcemia

The treatment of hypocalcemia, which can produce myocardial ischemia, mandates frequent measurements and normalization of ionized calcium. Because calcium gluconate requires hepatic metabolism in order to liberate ionized calcium, the $CaCl_2$ preparation is preferred. However, equimolar doses of $CaCl_2$ and calcium gluconate have been shown to correct ionized hypocalcemia in patients undergoing OLT.[26] In any case, calcium is given via a central catheter as a bolus, 15 mg $\cdot$ kg^{-1}.

Hyperglycemia

Hyperglycemia (glucose levels >250 mg $\cdot$ dL^{-1}) should be treated with small insulin doses (5–10 units) after hourly blood glucose determination.

Metabolic Acidosis

Progressive *acidosis* (BE > −7 mEq $\cdot$ L^{-1}) is treated with bicarbonate according to the following formula:

$$HCO_3^- \text{ (mEq)} = \frac{BE \times \text{weight (kg)} \times 0.3}{2}$$

Aggressive treatment is not suggested if the donor liver is functional and urine formation is adequate.

SPECIALIZED EQUIPMENT

Throughout this chapter, references have repeatedly been made to the RIS and TEG. A more detailed discussion of their function and use follows.

How Does the Rapid-Infusion System Work?

The RIS is designed to deliver low-pressure, prewarmed, filtered, premixed, and air-free blood at a controlled and rapid rate. The Haemonetics RIS is a total fluid management system that can mix blood, FFP, Plasmalyte, saline, and other solutions with the same osmolality of blood in a 3-L reservoir. It offers a faster alternative to all conventional fluid and blood replacement techniques and is capable of fluid infusion in a controlled manner at a rate up to 1500 mL · min^{-1}.

Avoidance of high pressure (>300 mm Hg), low temperature (<35 °C), and infusion of aggregates or air during rapid fluid delivery is ensured through the use of infusate temperature monitoring, ultrasonic air detectors, and pressure sensors in the fluid line. The infusate is warmed by an in-line heat exchanger and filtered through high-capacity macroaggregate and microaggregate filters (Fig. 76–14).

Total fluid therapy can be managed by a single person. Simple, easy-to-use features give operators finger tip control (Fig. 76–15) of (1) flow rates as required (milliliters per minute or per hour), (2) continuous or bolus delivery of infusate, (3) fluid temperature, even when not in the infuse mode, and (4) uninterrupted fluid delivery during transport of patients or electrical failure by switchover to the battery mode.

The RIS has five modes of operation.

Prime

This mode ensures that the disposable set is filled with fluid, thus getting rid of all air in the system. The RIS operates in this mode only when power is on. "Load" opens the valves so that the disposable tubing may be installed. To prime the RIS, tubings should be connected as shown in Figure 76–14, not to the patient. Once priming is finished, the lower set of buttons in the bottom of the control panel should be shielded from further manipulation and covered, and infusion lines should be separated from the reservoir and connected to the patient.

Infuse

This is the normal operating mode. Only after the infuse mode is set does the RIS infuse fluid automatically at the rate that is selected on the infuse dial.

Stop

The machine may be placed in this mode before fluid challenge or will enter it automatically under certain circumstances, when the operation must be stopped. Whenever the system detects a condition requiring attention, such as low reservoir volume (200 mL), in-line air, high temperature (>41 °C), or high pressure (>500 mm Hg), it stops the pump, sounds an alarm, and lights a display warning.

Fluid Challenge

The fluid challenge mode initiates a fluid bolus of 100 mL or 1000 mL.

Recirculate

This mode is used to warm fluid in the reservoir, to maintain the temperature >35 °C, and to clear the filter of air bubbles by connecting it directly back to the reservoir.

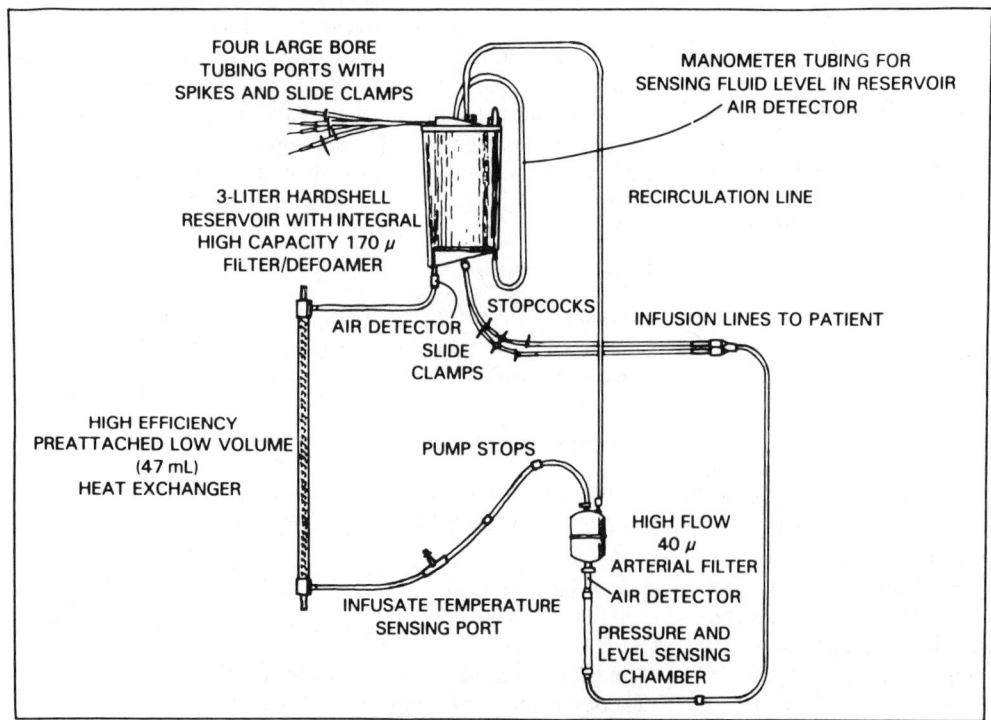

FIGURE 76–14. The rapid infusion system. (From Directions for Use RIS: Disposal Set List No. 400. MA, Haemonetics, Surgical Products Division.)

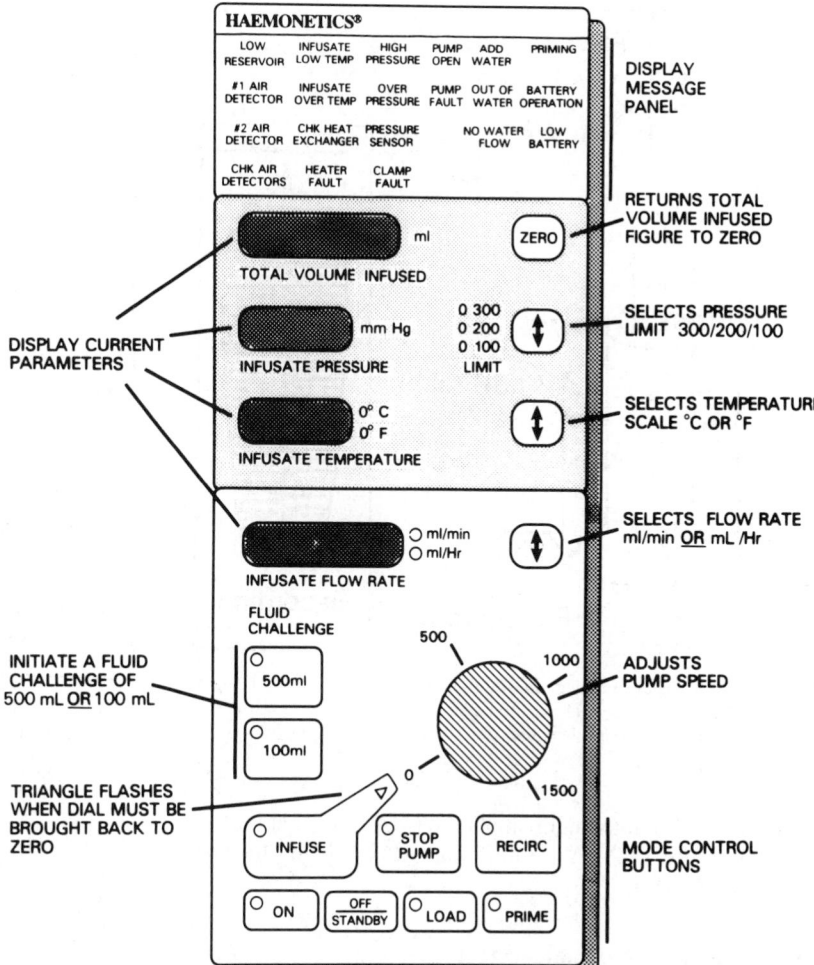

FIGURE 76–15. Rapid infusion system, control panel. (From Directions for Use RIS: MA, Haemonetics, Surgical Products Division.)

Safety Features

Safety features in the RIS include (1) temperature probe control of the heater power (below 34 °C, the RIS pump is automatically slowed but not stopped), (2) pressure sensor slowing of the RIS pump at a chosen level (100, 200, 300 mm Hg) and stopping (540 mm Hg), and (3) system air detection by three ultrasonic air detectors: reservoir, fluid line as it leaves the reservoir, and in-line as fluid leaves the machine to be infused.

How Does the Thromboelastograph Work?

Because of the possibility of severe coagulopathy, aggressive monitoring and proper treatment are essential. A simple coagulation profile (PT, PTT), platelet count, FDP, euglobulin lysis time, and fibrinogen level can be used but have drawbacks. The PT is already prolonged in many patients, because it depends on hepatic function. The PTT may be clinically helpful, but heparin is not always a major cause of coagulopathy. Platelet counts provide quantitative but not qualitative information. FDPs are usually positive during major surgery owing to reabsorption after extravascular fibrinolysis. The euglobulin lysis time measures plasminogen activity but ignores antiplasmin activity, which may play a part in fibrinolysis. Fibrinogen levels give information about consumption during

DIC, which may be primary or secondary in the complex picture of coagulopathy during OLT. Finally, this profile requires time for completion (>30 min), and interpretation of results may be difficult in this *dynamic* situation.

As an alternative, the TEG has proved to be extremely valuable for relatively fast interpretation and understanding of the dynamic and complex coagulopathy pattern that is part of this procedure, thus guiding effective clinical therapy. Clinically useful information is available *within* 30 minutes.[1]

Principles of Operation

The TEG device consists of a highly polished stainless steel cup that contains 0.36 mL of whole blood and a pin freely suspended by a torsion wire (Fig. 76–16). The temperature in the cup is kept at 37 °C, and the cup oscillates 4.45 degrees on its vertical axis every 9 seconds. As long as the blood in the cup remains fluid, the cup's oscillation is not transmitted to the pin. However, as soon as fibrin strands are formed between the cup surface and the pin, the cup's motion is transmitted to the pin, and the pin's motion is transmitted to the torsion wire and recorded on thermal paper.

The TEG monitors and records the entire coagulation process, including the initial fluid state, graded increase in the strength of fibrin strands, and resolution (fibrinolysis) of those strands. The variables measured are reaction time (r [min]); coagulation process-starting time (r + k [min]); rate of clot

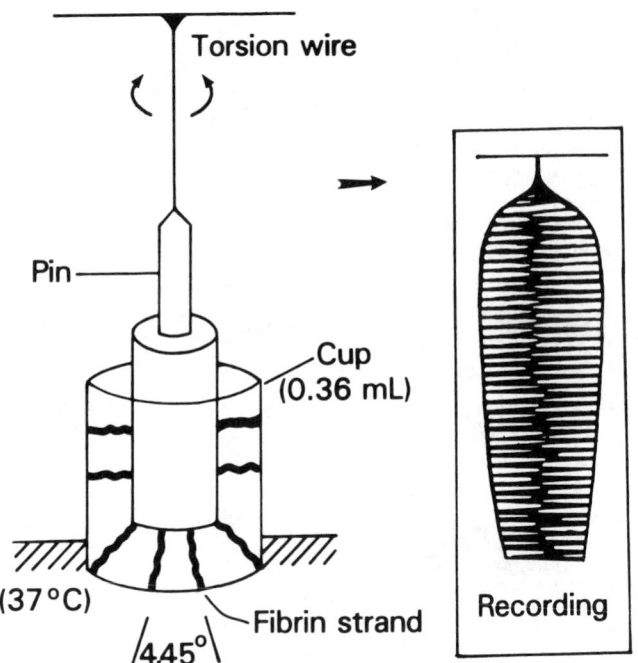

FIGURE 76–16. Schematic diagram of thromboelastography. (From Kang Y, Lewis JH, Navalgund A, et al: Epsilon-aminocaproic acid for treatment of fibrinolysis during liver transplantation. Anesthesiology 1987; 66:766.)

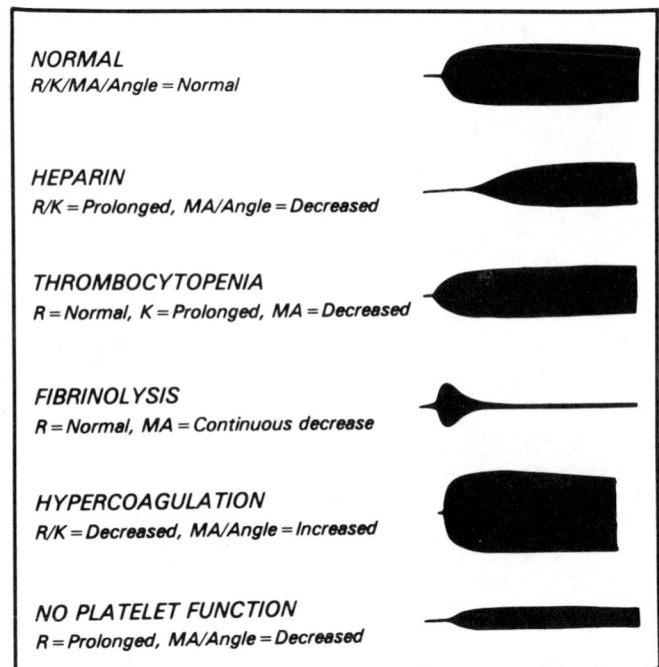

FIGURE 76–18. Qualitative analysis from the TEG coagulation analyzer. (From Overview of Thromboelastograph Coagulation Analyzer: A Unique Analytical Device. Morton Grove, IL, Haemoscope Corporation, p 8.)

formation (α [°]); maximum amplitude (MA [mm]); amplitude 60 minutes after MA (Λ_{60} [mm]); and whole blood clot lysis time (F [min]) (Fig. 76–17).

Variations from Normal

The TEG output may be varied from normal (Fig. 76–18) to produce information on the following aspects of coagulation.

Clotting Time

The onset of clotting on the TEG (r or r + k) correlates with whole blood clotting time. A normal r time is 6 to 8 minutes. In the presence of heparin, r + k is prolonged (see heparin profile, Fig. 76–18). This change suggests that protamine could be titrated to neutralize the heparin anticoagulant effects. A loss of clotting factors gives a similar TEG plotting deformity (r + k prolonged), but the MA angle α is decreased

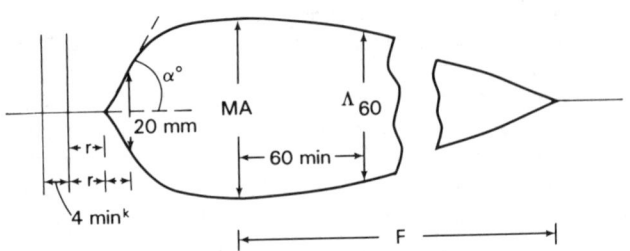

FIGURE 76–17. Variables measured by thromboelastography and their normal values. r = Reaction time (min); r + k = coagulation time (min); α = clot formation rate (°); MA = maximum amplitude (mm); Λ_{60} = amplitude 60 min after maximum amplitude (mm); F = whole blood clot lysis time (min). (Modified from Kang Y, Lewis JH, Navalgund A, et al: Epsilon-aminocaproic acid for treatment of fibrinolysis during liver transplantation. Anesthesiology 1987; 66:766.)

as well. This abnormality may be treated with FFP and cryoprecipitate.

Any clotting times shorter than these are hypercoagulable (see hypercoagulation, Fig. 76–18). This generalization, based on the onset of clotting and the MA angle α, is prone to error because clot structure and stability are not considered.

Clot Strength

The strength of a clot determines its ability to perform hemostasis and can be determined from MA of the TEG. The strength is a direct result of platelet function and plasma factors (e.g., fibrinogen) and their interaction. A normal MA is 50 to 70 mm. Thus a clot with a low MA but normal r is missing platelet function (see thrombocytopenia, Fig. 76–18), and a clot with similar low MA but prolonged r is missing plasma factors *and* platelets.

Because platelets concentrate plasma factors and make clotting kinetics more effective, they should be the primary choice in therapy when MA is small (see no platelet function, Fig. 76–18). Hypercoagulable conditions can be identified as a result of either excess platelet function *or* elevated fibrinogen. The condition produces clots with MA >70 mm and usually with short r. Such patients usually require anticoagulation. However, before any treatment is initiated, determine if the clot is stable or unstable.

Clot Stability

Clot stability refers to its potential to redissolve because of circulating fibrinolytic components that activate plasminogen in the clot. The TEG identifies this condition by showing early diminution of MA (see fibrinolysis profile, Fig. 76–18), with several low indices (Λ_{60}, F) (see Fig. 76–17) showing the degree of dissolution over time. Patients with DIC or fibrinolytic conditions can be identified during early stages of this condition using TEG analysis even before clinical bleeding is evident. Possible correction of this condition can even be tested on the TEG by using EACA added to the specimen in vitro before it is given to a patient.[27]

Clot Growth Kinetics

The TEG presents the rate of clot growth and formation as the angle α and K time (see Fig. 76–17). These parameters correlate with polymerization in clotting. Several aspects pertain to determining those factors missing according to clot growth rate. In untreated individuals, this rate is a function of platelets and plasma components (complexes) residing on the platelet surface. Variation in growth rate results from decreased platelet function or plasma factors (e.g., fibrinogen or specific enzyme-complex proteins) or anticoagulants (e.g., warfarin, heparin, FDP). Heparin has the most characteristic shape and resembles a needle nose with angles of 5° to 15° (a normal α angle is >50°).

Guidelines for Coagulation Therapy According to Thromboelastograph Monitoring

Clot Formation

The most important consideration in TEG analysis is the fact that all aspects (clotting time, strength, stability, and kinetics) and overall pattern of the TEG profile provide a more comprehensive clinical assessment of a patient's hemostasis than does any one variable of the TEG or coagulation test profile. A patient can have abnormal onset and growth kinetics but still form a normal, stable clot. Thus, although bleeding time can be prolonged, it may not represent a significant clinical problem. On the other hand, a short onset with rapid growth, good strength, and rapid lysis may predict or represent a dangerous clinical condition of consumption coagulopathy.

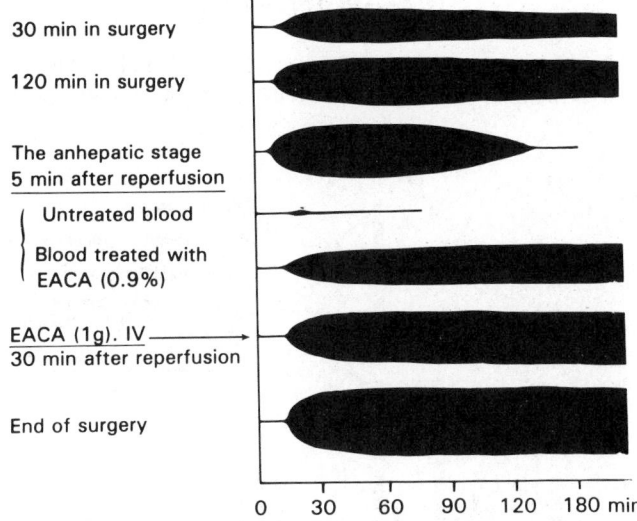

FIGURE 76–19. Thromboelastographic patterns in a patient undergoing liver transplantation. Epsilon-aminocaproic acid (EACA, 1 g) was administered intravenously when severe fibrinolysis was observed on thromboelastography; generalized oozing occurred in a previously dry surgical field and EACA-treated fibrinolysis in vitro. (From Kang Y, Lewis JH, Navalgund A, et al: Epsilon-aminocaproic acid for treatment of fibrinolysis during liver transplantation. Anesthesiology 1987; 66:766.)

The clinical picture and evolution/resolution of the coagulation status have to be considered as well before treating coagulopathy according to TEG monitoring. This goal is accomplished hourly (or even half-hourly) during massive transfusion or early in the neohepatic phase.

Fibrinolysis

Fibrinolysis occurring during OLT usually is primary in origin.[27] Although fibrinolysis is more dramatic on reperfusion of the graft liver, it may also occur during the preanhepatic and anhepatic phases. In these early stages, it may be caused by decreased clearance of plasminogen, release of plasminogen activator, and decreased synthesis of inhibitor. The previously discussed explosive fibrinolysis that occurs in the early neohepatic phase is probably caused by substances originating from the donor liver.

Although fibrinolysis increases progressively during OLT in >80% of patients, it is severe on reperfusion in only 34%.[27] A high incidence of hypercoagulable states and pulmonary emboli in OLT patients, both with and without EACA treatment, has led to the suggestion that because fibrinolysis during OLT is a self-limiting process, pharmacologic intervention is not necessary and might be harmful.[28]

Epsilon-Aminocaproic Acid Administration

The controversy surrounding EACA administration stems from evaluating unique patient populations (neoplasms with hypercoagulable state), overdose treatment (EACA up to 100 mg · kg^{-1}), poor indications for treatment, and inadequate lysis monitoring. With the characteristic TEG tracing showing fibrinolysis, Kang and colleagues demonstrated the effectiveness of in vitro doses of EACA (0.03 mL of 1% EACA) (Fig. 76–19). When this in vitro test showed effectiveness and reversed the TEG configuration to normal, 1 g of EACA (single intravenous dose) then was administered in vivo with good results and no hemorrhagic or thrombotic complications.[27] Thus, for patients undergoing OLT, judicious use of small doses of EACA only after its effectiveness is confirmed in vitro is recommended.

PEDIATRIC ORTHOTOPIC LIVER TRANSPLANTATION

Some aspects of pediatric OLT have been discussed. More detailed information follows.

How Does It Differ?

Type of Disease

Pediatric candidates for OLT most often suffer from cholestatic disease or an inborn error of metabolism. This fact may be significant regarding the extent of hepatocellular damage, drug handling, bleeding tendencies, and survival.

Monitoring

PA catheterization does not appear to be necessary in many children because of their relatively healthy myocardium and difficult access. A CVP oximeter catheter can be used to monitor the trend in cardiac output.

Blood and Fluid Management

Although blood transfusion requirements are proportional to those in adults (considering milliliters per kilogram consumption), the RIS may not be necessary because of the smaller total transfusion volumes. I use pneumatic pressure bags instead of an RIS.

Hemodynamic Changes

Children appear to tolerate cross-clamping of major vessels with less hemodynamic instability. VVB is used only for children >20 kg body weight or older than 12 years, primarily out of consideration for difficulties in achieving safe, minimum bypass flow. In marginal cases, the effect of cross-clamping on hemodynamic function can be tested with some fluid load; the use of VVB then is decided according to the degree of hemodynamic instability.

Other Changes

Children and adults have similar metabolic changes, reperfusion syndrome, and intraoperative coagulopathy. In adults, however, coagulation problems occur to a lesser degree because cholestatic disease is more prevalent in children.[29] The chance for hepatic vessel thrombosis postoperatively is higher in children. This observation may influence the aggressiveness of treating coagulopathy in the neohepatic phase. In general, children tend to develop hypertension and metabolic alkalosis earlier than adults.

Donor Liver Size

Donor liver size may pose problems in pediatric patients in terms of dissection and surface bleeding of the liver or decreased filling pressures and hemodynamic problems during abdominal closure when it must adapt to the smaller abdominal cavity.

RECOVERY AFTER ORTHOTOPIC LIVER TRANSPLANTATION

How Long Is the Hospitalization Period?

The hospitalization period can vary between 0.5 and 3 months (mean 47 ± 25 days).[8] The average duration in the intensive care unit (ICU) is 1 to 2 weeks (mean 5.9 ± 9 or 12.7 ± 12.6 days after OLT and 6.15 ± 7.0 days for readmission) according to several series.[8, 30] A 10% death rate occurs in the ICU, and an additional 5% after OLT outside the ICU.[30] Considering the overall survival rate of 70% to 80%, mortality in the ICU is relatively high.

What Problems Occur in the Intensive Care Unit?

During the immediate postoperative period, hypothermia and hyperglycemia invariably occur. Later during the initial

admission or on readmission, multiple problems are expected, but most significant are infections and renal insufficiency. Prompt diagnosis and treatment are also necessary for signs and symptoms of hypertension, hypokalemia, severe metabolic alkalosis (as citrate is metabolized), fever, altered mental status, oliguria, and signs of graft failure.

Repeated procedures, tests, and studies are needed to ensure graft function. These tests include liver biopsy, angiography, computed tomographic scan, and exploratory laparotomy. Selective bowel decontamination minimizes the occurrence of gram-negative and fungal sepsis, and the use of antihypertensive agents and correction of coagulopathies may decrease the risk of intracranial bleeding.

ANESTHESIA FOR RETRANSPLANTATION

How Does It Differ?

Retransplantation rates vary from center to center, but the overall incidence is <15% in adult patients.[1] The reasons for retransplantation are a poorly functioning donor liver, vascular complications (e.g., hepatic arterial or portal venous thrombosis), and development of hyperacute rejection. These patients may have other problems active at the same time (e.g., ARDS, metabolic alkalosis) and require aggressive supportive therapy.

When severe liver necrosis develops, early removal of a dying graft minimizes its toxic effects. In these patients, retransplantation is relatively simple from a technical standpoint; all dissections have been performed, and all monitoring and infusion cannulas are in situ. Otherwise, anesthetic considerations are similar, but anesthetic and surgical times are expected to be significantly lower, and the physiologic effects (hemodynamic, blood loss) during the preanephatic phase are less severe.

ASSOCIATED PROCEDURES IMMEDIATELY AFTER ORTHOTOPIC LIVER TRANSPLANTATION

Postoperatively, patients are routinely kept intubated for the first 24 hours and are usually extubated on the second postop-

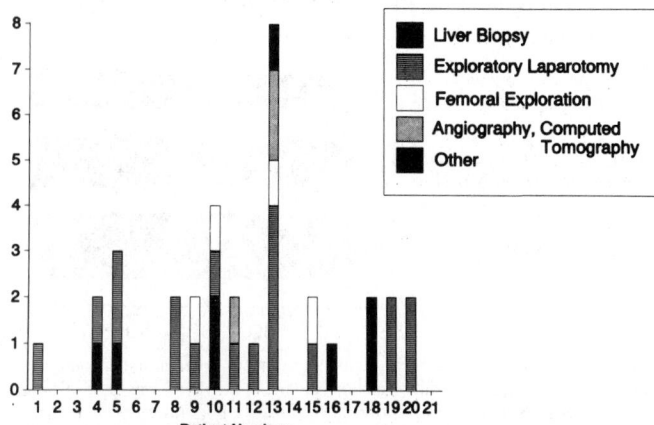

FIGURE 76–20. Additional procedures requiring general anesthesia (after OLT surgery) performed at the University of Florida in 1990 and 1991 in 21 patients during hospital stay.

erative day.[5] However, because of the multiple physiologic (hemodynamic, metabolic) problems expected in this stage, a longer period of intubation may be necessary.

During the ICU stay, additional procedures may be needed to identify and treat sources of infection, bleeding, or graft failure, many of which require general anesthesia (Fig. 76–20). Such procedures are performed in up to 50% of post-OLT patients, and in 50% of these patients more than one procedure may be required.[8] Because the procedures are relatively short and patients are already intubated or expected to stay that way, major issues concerning anesthesia are few. However, bleeding or hemodynamic stability is, as always, a concern.

References

1. Kang Y: Anesthesia for liver transplantation. Anesthesiol Clin North Am 1989; 7:551.
2. Starzl TE, Demetris AJ, Van Thiel D: Liver transplantation (first of two parts). N Engl J Med 1989; 321:1014.
3. Starzl E, Iwatsuki S, Van Thiel DH, et al: Evolution of liver transplantation. Hepatology 1982; 2:614.
4. Borland LM, Martin DJ: Anesthesia considerations for orthotopic liver transplantation. Contemp Anesth Pract 1987; 10:157.
5. Samuel D, Benhamou JP, Bismuth H, et al: Criteria of selection for liver transplantation. Transplant Proc 1987; 19:2383.
6. O'Grady JG, Alexander GJM, Hayllar KM, et al: Early indicators of prognosis in fulminant hepatic failure. Gastroenterology 1989; 97:439.
7. Motschman TL, Taswell HF, Brecher ME, et al: Intraoperative blood loss and patient and graft survival in orthotopic liver transplantation: their relationship to clinical and laboratory data. Mayo Clin Proc 1989; 64:346.
8. Sidi AS: Anesthesia for orthotopic liver transplantation (OLT): University of Florida data. Refresher Course, 16th International Congress of the Israeli Society of Anesthesiologists, 1992, pp 233–234.
9. Kalayoglu M, Sollinger HW, Stratta RJ, et al: Extended preservation of the liver for clinical transplantation. Lancet 1988; 1:617.
10. Rettke SR, Chantigian RC, Janossy TA, et al: Anesthesia approach to hepatic transplantation. Mayo Clin Proc 1989; 64:224.
11. Williamson KR, Taswell HF, Rettke SR, et al: Intraoperative autologous transfusion: its role in orthotopic liver transplantation. Mayo Clin Proc 1989; 64:340.
12. Butler P, Israel L, Jenkins DE, et al: Blood transfusion during liver transplantation (Abstract). Transfusion 1983; 23:433.
13. Brown BR: Anesthetizing the patient with abnormal liver function. ASA 1990 Annual Refresher Course Lecture 32. Park Ridge, IL.
14. Williams R: Drug administration in hepatic disease. N Engl J Med 1984; 309:1616.
15. Davis PJ, Cook DR: Anesthetic problems in pediatric liver transplantation. Transplant Proc 1989; 21:3493.
16. McEvedy BA, Shelley MP, Park GR: Anesthesia and liver disease. Br J Hosp Med 1986; 36:26.
17. Gelman S: Anesthesia for the patient with liver disease. ASA 1990 Annual Refresher Course Lecture 143. Park Ridge, IL.
18. Starzl TE, Demetris AJ, Van Thiel D: Liver transplantation (second of two parts). N Engl J Med 1989; 321:1092.
19. Cosimi AB, Cho SI, Delmonico FL, et al: A randomized clinical trial comparing OKT3 and steroids for treatment of hepatic allograft rejection. Transplantation 1987; 43:91.
20. Paulsen AW, Whitten CW, Ramsay MAE, et al: Considerations for anesthetic management during veno-venous bypass in adult hepatic transplantation. Anesth Analg 1989; 58:489.
21. Kang Y, Aggarwal S, Freeman JA: Intraoperative mortality during liver transplantation. Transplant Proc 1988; 20(Suppl 1):600.
22. Polson RJ, Parks GR, Lindop MJ, et al: The prevention of renal impairment in patients undergoing orthotopic liver transplantation by infusion of low dose of dopamine. Anesthesiology 1987; 42:15.
23. Carmichael FJ, Lindop MJ, Farman JV: Anesthesia for hepatic transplantation: cardiovascular and metabolic alterations and their management. Anesth Analg 1985; 64:108.
24. Groth CG, Pechet L, Starzl TE: Coagulation during and after orthotopic transplantation of the human liver. Arch Surg 1969; 98:31.
25. Esquivel CO, Koneru B, Karrer F, et al: Liver transplantation before 1 year of age. J Pediatr 1987; 110:545.
26. Martin T, Kang Y, Marquez JM, et al: Pharmacokinetics and hemodynamic effects of calcium chloride and calcium gluconate during liver transplantation. Anesthesiology 1988; 69:A451.
27. Kang Y, Lewis JH, Navalgund A, et al: Epsilon-aminocaproic acid for treatment of fibrinolysis during liver transplantation. Anesthesiology 1987; 66:766.
28. Von Kaulla KN, Kaye H, Von Kaulla E, et al: Changes in blood coagulation before and after hepatectomy or transplantation in dogs and man. Arch Surg 1966; 92:71.
29. Kang Y, Borland LM, Picone J, et al: Intraoperative changes in coagulation during liver transplantation in children. Anesthesiology 1987; 65:A525.
30. Plevak DJ, Southorn PA, Narr BJ, et al: Intensive-care unit experience in the Mayo liver transplantation program: the first 100 cases. Mayo Clin Proc 1989; 64:433.

CHAPTER 77

Renal Transplantation

AVNER SIDI, M.D.

As with many other types of surgery, clinical experience and development of new techniques and drugs make the complex task of transplantation and, in particular, provision of anesthesia for renal transplantation more simple and successful. Today, the task seems fairly routine and has a low complication rate. During the 1980s, well over 60,000 renal homografts were performed throughout the world; half were still alive with their grafted kidney in place.[1] Approximately 10,000 renal transplants are performed annually in the United States.[2] Advances in organ preservation, histocompatibility testing, and immunosuppression have enabled prolonged survival of both cadaveric allograft and living-related donor renal transplants. The actual technique of transplantation has changed little through the years (Fig. 77–1).

GENERAL CONSIDERATIONS

How Long Can Donor Kidneys Be Preserved?

Kidney preservation allows time for transportation and evaluation of potential recipients for cytotoxic antibody tests. Preservation techniques include simple hypothermic storage, which preserves tissue for up to 48 hours. A more expensive and difficult option is pulsatile preservation, in which the organ's vascular system is flushed and supplied with preservation solutions delivered by a pulsatile pump. This method preserves tissue up to 60 hours. The preservation solution is cold (4 °C), contains potassium, and is hyperosmolar.

What Is Tissue Matching?

Tissue typing (HLA typing), or histocompatibility testing, consists of two main components: (1) antigen matching—with a match of six major histocompatibility antigens, outcome of cadaveric allograft is improved by 20%[3]; (2) detection of cytotoxic antibodies—cytotoxic antibodies in the potential recipient against donor antigen are predictive of a poor outcome; transplantation should be avoided in such a patient.

What Universal Immunosuppression Protocols Are Used?

Immunosuppression of the recipient often follows a different protocol in each transplant center. Most centers include a protocol consisting of cyclosporin A and steroid administration. In certain types of patients (e.g., those undergoing retransplantation or those who cannot tolerate cyclosporine), the protocol may include azathioprine, antithymocyte, antilymphocyte globulin, or monoclonal antibodies, or a combination of these (Table 77–1).

PREOPERATIVE CONCERNS

Kidney failure is associated with and induces systemic abnormalities, including behavioral, cardiovascular, pulmonary,

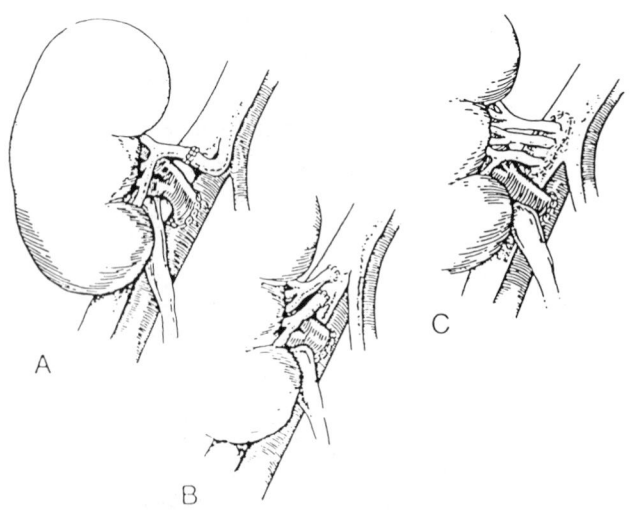

FIGURE 77–1. Techniques of re-establishing the allograft's vascular supply. *A,* Renal artery to internal iliac artery. *B,* Anastomosis of multiple renal arteries to the external iliac artery. *C,* Carrel patch anastomosis to external iliac artery. (From Whelchel JD: Surgical aspects of renal transplantations. *In* Anesthesia for Renal Transplantation. Graybar GB, Bready LL (eds). Boston, Martinus Nijhoff, 1987, p 90.)

TABLE 77–1. Intraoperative Drug Immunosuppression, Antibiotics, and Diuresis in a Protocol for Renal Transplantation

- Cephazolin, 1 g IV, just after induction of anesthesia; gentamicin, 2 mg · kg^{-1}, should be substituted if patient allergic to cephalosporins
- Continue cyclosporine, 1.5 mg · kg^{-1} in 120 mL of DW at 10 mL · h^{-1} b.i.d.; cyclosporine is not compatible with other IV medications. Should be started preoperatively if not already with patient coming from floor at 3 mg · kg^{-1}
- Methylprednisolone, 1 g IV (for peds use 20 mg · kg^{-1} if weight is <50 kg), slow IV push; drip is continued
- Azathioprine, 3 mg · kg^{-1} (maximum: 250 mg) IV
- Furosemide, 60 mg IV
- Mannitol, 25 mg, at start of anastomosis (with methylprednisolone sodium succinate [Solu-Medrol] bolus, azathioprine [Imuran], and furosemide [Lasix])

Abbreviations: IV = intravenous(ly); DW = dextrose in water.

hematologic, metabolic, neurologic, endocrine, gastrointestinal, and immunologic changes (Table 77–2).

What Abnormalities Are Likely?

Cardiopulmonary

As the kidneys' ability to excrete water becomes impaired, peripheral and dependent edema, hypertension, and a hyperdynamic state often evolve. Pulmonary edema and pericardial effusion may be present. Congestive heart failure, left ventricular hypertrophy, and cardiac tamponade are possible complications. A chest radiograph and electrocardiogram are obligatory.

The patient's usual blood pressure range and the medications that he or she is taking should be recorded, and antihypertensive drugs should be continued perioperatively. Hypertension may correlate with sodium and water loading or with renin levels; therefore, treatment should be directed toward controlling these factors. Blood volume should be normal or even slightly high prior to induction and maintenance of anesthesia if hypotension is to be avoided. At the end of the last preoperative dialysis or prior to induction, the patient's weight should be 1 to 2 kg above *dry* weight. Patients usually know their dry weight and how much fluid is taken off during each dialysis.

Hematologic

Anemia of chronic renal disease is common, may be severe, and is often associated with a hematocrit that is less than one-half of normal. The cause is a decrease in the production and survival of red blood cells. The effects of anemia are compensated by increased cardiac output and a rightward shift of the oxyhemoglobin dissociation curve. Preoperative hemoglobin and hematocrit levels should be compared with the patient's usual values.

Anemia is usually well tolerated because of normovolemic or even hypervolemic compensation and because of its gradual onset and chronic nature. However, at some level, decompensation at rest or during stress occurs. This point varies and is a function of age, sympathetic activity, flow and volume in shunts and fistulas, and the presence of vascular disease.

A patient's ability to tolerate moderate activity without becoming symptomatic suggests that decompensation is not

present and that a transfusion is unnecessary. Transfusion in these patients predisposes to fluid overload and congestive heart failure, along with the usual risk of disease transmission. However, in the presence of severe anemia (hemoglobin <6 g · dL^{-1}), hypovolemia, or signs and symptoms of myocardial or cerebral hypoxia, blood should be administered. Severe anemia may decrease the blood-gas partition coefficient for inhalation agents by as much as 25%, increasing the rates of induction and emergence.

Coagulation

Platelet function may be abnormal as a consequence of decreased platelet factor 3, decreased adhesiveness, and decreased aggregation; bleeding times should be evaluated. The prothrombin time (PT) and partial thromboplastin time (PTT) are usually less affected. Platelet dysfunction can be treated and corrected by platelet transfusion or by the administration of desmopressin or even conjugated estrogens.[4] Although theoretic objection exists to perioperative blood transfusions, some clinicians transfuse preoperatively because of possible improvement in graft survival when a recipient shares at least one HLA-DR antigen with the donor.[5]

Metabolic

Abnormalities of water balance, acid-base regulation, and electrolytes (sodium, potassium, chloride, phosphate, calcium, and magnesium) become more common as the degree of renal failure increases. Osteomalacia and osteosclerosis occur during renal failure and uremia. Glucose intolerance with insulin resistance is common. Hypoalbuminemia results from poor nutrition and urinary losses and leads to hypovolemia and extravascular edema.

Neurologic

Encephalopathy, peripheral neuropathy, and autonomic dysfunction occur in uremic patients.[7] Patients with peripheral neuropathy often have autonomic neuropathy as well that is best detected by a tilt test. Such patients may respond abnormally to stress produced by surgery and anesthesia. Hypertensive encephalopathy may occur in these patients.

Endocrine

Hyperparathyroidism due to hypocalcemia and adrenal insufficiency due to steroid use may be present and should be considered.

Gastrointestinal

Hepatitis antigen status, PT, PTT, and fibrinogen levels should be checked in patients with renal failure or uremia. Parotitis, oral ulcers, delayed gastric emptying, hyperacidity, increased gastric volume, and gastroduodenal ulcers occur with increased frequency as renal function declines.[7] The most common gastrointestinal symptoms of uremia are anorexia, nausea, vomiting, bleeding, diarrhea, and hiccups. The last of these may be relieved by phenothiazines or may require mechanical stimulation of the nasopharynx with a soft rubber catheter (the tendency for bleeding should be borne in mind).

TABLE 77–2. Signs and Symptoms of Uremia

Behavioral, Mental, or Neurologic	Depressive: Fatigue, asthenia, malaise, shortening of concentration, memory defects, anorexia, drowsiness, suicidal thoughts, stupor, precoma, coma Irritative: Anxiety, fasciculations, twitching, headache, ataxia, asterixis, abnormal gait, vertigo, nausea, convulsions Psychiatric: Personality change, bizarre behavior, phobias, organic psychosis, selective amnesia, denial, kleptomania Peripheral: Pruritus, paresthesias, restless leg syndrome, monoplegia, paraplegia, sensory and motor defects, bladder atony, dysfunction Ophthalmic: Nystagmus, miosis, anisocoria, band keratopathy
Gastrointestinal	Membrane problems: Glossitis, stomatitis, esophagitis, enteritis, pancreatitis, colitis, ileus Functional problems: Anorexia, dysgeusia, nausea, vomiting, hematemesis, constipation, diarrhea, abdominal distention Structural problems: Peptic and colonic ulceration
Cardiovascular-Pulmonary	Pericarditis, acute and constrictive Pleuritis Congestive heart failure Change in blood pressure Dysrhythmias Vascular calcification Accelerated atherosclerosis Cheyne-Stokes or Kussmaul's breathing, or both
Hematologic	Anemia: Normochromic, normocytic Bleeding abnormalities: Prolonged bleeding time, abnormal platelet aggregation Lymphopenia, mild thrombocytopenia

Metabolic	Hyperkalemia
	Metabolic acidosis
	Hypermagnesemia
	Hyperphosphatemia
	Hypocalcemia
	Metastatic calcification
	   Medium sized arteries: arterial insufficiency, ischemia, skin ulceration, gangrene
	   Joints, sites of pressure: arthritis, decreased range of motion
	   Myocardium, skeletal muscle, lung
	Musculoskeletal muscle pain and weakness, proximal myopathy, bone pain, bone fractures
	Aseptic necrosis of bone
	Disturbances in multiple endocrine system
	Carbohydrate intolerance
	Hyperlipidemia
	Gout and pseudogout
	Wasting and abnormalities in protein metabolism

Immunologic	Reduced T cell–mediated immune function Impaired phagocytosis and chemotaxis Atrophy of the lymphoid system, including the thymus Reduced immune surveillance of neoplasia
Miscellaneous	Reduced wound healing Hypothermia Impaired response to pyrogen

(From Schreiner GE: Uremia. *In* Textbook of Nephrology. Massry SG, Glassock RJ [eds]. Baltimore, Williams & Wilkins, 1983, p 452. © Williams & Wilkins, 1983.)

Immunologic

Infections are common owing to defects in immunity and white blood cell function, specifically, reduced T cell–mediated immune function caused by uremia, immunosuppressive therapy, and increased exposure to invasive procedures. Hepatitis, urinary tract infection, peritonitis with peritoneal dialysis, atrioventricular fistula infection, and pneumonia must all be considered. Strict sterile techniques should be adhered to for invasive procedures.

What Are the Pertinent Laboratory Data?

Patients with end-stage renal disease (ESRD) often sustain metabolic acidosis, anemia, electrolyte abnormalities, cardiovascular disturbances, platelet dysfunction, residual heparin effect after dialysis, and a high incidence of serum hepatitis (40% of kidney recipients are positive for Australia antigen).[8]

Laboratory data that should be monitored in the preoperative and perioperative period are hemoglobin/hematocrit, measurements of serum sodium, potassium, and calcium, platelets, bleeding time, and, less frequently, PT and PTT and bicarbonate or base excess.

Hyperkalemia

Hyperkalemia usually is not a problem until late in the course of the disease; uremic patients tolerate moderate degrees of hyperkalemia well. The current practice of dialysis just before transplantation, together with better dialysis techniques, have almost eliminated this problem.

Little evidence supports the concept that patients with a serum potassium level that is >5.5 mEq · L^{-1} should not be anesthetized; even higher levels probably are acceptable, providing that electrocardiogram changes are not present. In any case, when hyperkalemia is present, situations that elevate the serum potassium level further (e.g., hypoventilation and succinylcholine administration) should be avoided.

The membrane effects of hyperkalemia can be reversed by calcium administration. Serum levels can also be reduced by hyperventilation or sodium bicarbonate administration, or by producing "internal shifts" of potassium with glucose and insulin infusions.

What Is the Role of Preoperative Dialysis?

All problems related to fluid and electrolyte disturbances can be reversed by adequate hemodialysis and ultrafiltration. Routine hemodialysis markedly decreases electrolyte abnormalities and the need for antihypertensive medications preoperatively. However, even in its absence, the metabolic and hemodynamic changes during induction and maintenance of anesthesia are manageable.

Problems related to uremia, for the most part, are partially, if not totally, reversible by adequate dialysis. Some abnormalities, however, are not significantly improved by dialysis. These include susceptibility to infection, refractory (renin-dependent) hypertension, and anemia.

Dialysis also may cause problems. Regionally administered heparin (i.e., that within the dialysis machine) may *spill over* into the patient. Rebound heparinization may occur up to 2 hours after dialysis and present as a bleeding diathesis. It is reversible with protamine.

What Abnormal Drug Responses Occur?

Patients with uremia may have unusual responses to drugs for several reasons (Table 77–3). Accordingly, narcotics and sedatives, including tranquilizers and antiemetic drugs, should be avoided or used very carefully and in minimal doses.

Narcotics

Morphine has a prolonged effect in anephric patients owing to longer-lasting plasma concentration and accumulation of its active metabolite (morphine-3-glucuronide).[9] The newer, synthetic narcotics (fentanyl, sufentanil, and alfentanil) also are reported to have a prolonged and more pronounced effect and to cause respiratory depression with elevated blood levels or increased unbound levels in renal failure.[10, 11]

Tranquilizers

Diazepam is metabolized by the liver, but the active metabolites are renally excreted, causing variable prolongation of the sedative effect in ESRD. Midazolam can delay emergence after induction.[12]

Antiemetics

Metoclopramide kinetics correlate with creatinine clearance; its clearance is not improved by dialysis. Plasma concentrations of several histamine₂ blockers, including ranitidine, are reduced by dialysis.[11] Cimetidine should be of concern because of its significant clinical effect as an immunostimulating agent.[11]

TABLE 77–3. Reasons for Abnormal Drug Responses in Patients with Chronic Renal Failure

- Protein binding is decreased; thus, highly protein-bound drugs may cause exaggerated responses (barbiturates, diazepam)
- Pseudocholinesterase level is low (rarely significant clinically)
- Electrolyte/acid-base abnormalities (acidosis prolongs effects of muscle relaxants)
- Drug clearance reduced by decreased renal excretion; smaller than usual doses, increased interval between doses may be necessary. Use of drugs not dependent on renal excretion is preferable when possible (e.g., vecuronium instead of pancuronium)
- Total body water and volume of distribution usually increased (however, may be decreased in recently dialyzed patients)

Diuretics

Pharmacokinetic studies with furosemide in ESRD reveal marked reduction in its clearance.[13] Furosemide has a direct depressant effect on the neuromuscular junction. However, when it is used in the treatment of congestive heart failure or for blood pressure control, it should be continued in the preoperative period.

Antihypertensives

Beta-blockers and clonidine are frequently used to treat hypertension in ESRD patients. They should be continued without interruption to prevent rebound hypertension, even though the usual dose of propranolol can result in higher peak blood concentrations because of reduced plasma clearance. Propranolol is not cleared by dialysis.[40] Verapamil and nifedipine enhance the neuromuscular blockade of nondepolarizing relaxants. Thus, when they are administered, careful neuromuscular junction monitoring is indicated.

Antidysrhythmics

Dysrhythmias in ESRD compromise the cardiovascular system even further. Electrolyte and metabolic imbalance (e.g., acidosis, alkalosis, hyperkalemia, hypokalemia) and untreated hypertension should be corrected as part of the antidysrhythmic regimen.

Lidocaine pharmacokinetics and metabolism are not significantly impaired in ESRD; however, active metabolites may accumulate. Procainamide urinary excretion is proportional to creatinine clearance. Quinidine, which undergoes hepatic oxidation, is 80% protein-bound, but its therapeutic concentration does not exceed normal ranges in ESRD.[14]

Does Immunosuppressive Treatment Influence Anesthesia?

Preoperative oral administration of cyclosporine creates "full stomach" conditions. When it is used, induction is performed with thiopental and succinylcholine (unless the patient is hyperkalemic) and the Sellick maneuver.

Cyclosporine has been implicated as a cause of respiratory failure in anephric renal transplant recipients who received atracurium or vecuronium. This effect probably was caused by its solvent potentiating neuromuscular blockade.[15] Azathioprine may have similar effects on neuromuscular transmission.[16]

Antilymphocytic or antithymocytic globulin, which is administered for immunosuppression, may produce fever owing to an allergic (anaphylactic-type) reaction. High-dose steroid use may produce hyperglycemia as a side effect.

ANESTHETIC INDUCTION

Hemodynamic control should be achieved by antihypertensive treatment prior to surgery or even during the preinduction period. The latter approach, however, prolongs induction. The combination of a short-acting β-blocker (e.g., esmolol in 0.5 mg · kg⁻¹ increments) and a vasodilator (e.g., hydralazine, 5–10 mg, or labetalol in 0.1–0.2 mg · kg⁻¹ increments) brings the blood pressure of most patients into a reasonable range. Invasive monitoring of blood pressure is helpful in those patients who are labile or unusually sensitive to these drugs.

Sodium nitroprusside toxicity has been reported in renal transplant patients; this is probably a result of the lack of detoxification, impaired excretion of cyanide, and the use of the high doses necessary to control hypertension as well as other unclear causes of metabolic acidosis (renal failure versus cyanide toxicity).

What Drugs Should Be Used for Premedication?

Premedication, induction, and maintenance can vary according to the anesthesiologist's preference as long as the appropriate doses and their redosing frequency are taken into account (see discussion of abnormal drug response earlier in this chapter). Patients can be premedicated with diazepam, midazolam, or phenergan along with ranitidine or sodium citrate, or both.

What Monitoring Is Advisable?

Monitors routinely used for renal transplantation (Table 77–4) generally are similar to those used for a typical abdominal surgery case. Invasive monitoring (if needed) and vascular access must be conducted with a sterile technique because of the immunosuppression related to the underlying disease and the treatment. The *relatively* healthy ESRD patient (one without major cardiovascular and respiratory complications) who has a short history of dialysis should not routinely require invasive monitoring.

Central Venous Catheters

The renal transplant patient who is medically compromised may need invasive perioperative monitoring. A central venous pressure catheter provides measurement of right-sided filling pressures, potentially large-bore venous access, a blood sampling site, and a route for administration of vasoactive drugs. Such monitoring, however, is not undertaken casually because of the possibility of bleeding abnormalities, the potential for infection, and the desire to preserve veins for dialysis access

TABLE 77–4. Monitors Needed for Anesthesia in a "Routine" Renal Transplantation Case*

- Stethoscope (precordial or esophageal, or both)
- Electrocardiogram, preferably with printer
- Arterial blood pressure monitor (indirect or direct, or both)
- Monitor of inspired oxygen concentration
- Anesthetic circuit pressure monitor
- Pulse oximeter (to measure oxygen saturation)
- Monitor of end-tidal carbon dioxide
- Urinary catheter
- Thermometer
- Peripheral nerve stimulator (general anesthesia)

(From Schreiner GE: Uremia. *In* Textbook of Nephrology. Massry SG, Glasscock RJ (eds). Baltimore, Williams & Wilkins, 1983, p 452.)
*Other monitors may be employed if indicated by patient's medical condition.

in these patients. It is indicated when fluid balance cannot be clarified, when the surgical procedure is complicated, or when the expected blood loss exceeds 20% of the blood volume. It provides valuable hemodynamic information when colloids, crystalloids, and osmotic diuretics are given as part of the renal transplant "protocol."

Pulmonary Artery Catheters

Pulmonary artery pressure monitoring is performed even less routinely than central venous monitoring. The relationship among risk, benefit, and expense of this procedure is difficult to describe. However, the maintenance of a mean pulmonary artery pressure at >20 mm Hg is purported to prevent acute tubular necrosis and to improve postoperative function of cadaveric grafts.[17] In most transplant centers, pulmonary artery catheters are not inserted unless left ventricular function is poor, fluid balance status cannot be clarified by other means, or disparity between left and right ventricular function is strongly suspected.[12]

Arterial Catheters

Invasive blood pressure monitoring with a radial or other arterial catheter is not routine. In addition to the ordinary risks of arterial catheterization, radial artery damage can make this site unsuitable for vascular access later—a major consideration in these patients. The benefit of such monitoring is tighter hemodynamic control during volume infusion and regulation of hypertension and of autonomic insufficiency intraoperatively and postoperatively.

Placement Sites

Placement of a 20- to 22-gauge radial artery catheter is associated with a low incidence of complications[18]; however, in the patient with ESRD, the placement site should be selected individually and carefully. When a vascular access for dialysis is present in one extremity, the radial artery of the opposite side should be cannulated. If both upper extremities have a vascular access, alternative sites in the lower extremities should be used. An arterial catheter placed at a location proximal or distal to an arteriovenous fistula underestimates central arterial pressure. If a lower extremity artery is cannulated, the limb contralateral to the transplant site should be used, since the ipsilateral iliac artery is occluded during vascular anastomosis.

Arterial or venous catheters should not be inserted electively into the limb containing an arteriovenous fistula because of the risk of thrombosis or infection. However, in acute situations in which large vessels are required for fluid resuscitation, this large, peripheral, easily identified venous access site should not be forgotten, denied, or contraindicated, especially in view of the fact that during each dialysis, larger bore cannulas are inserted into it. In the case of a nonfunctioning arteriovenous fistula, retrograde flow from the ulnar artery may produce a palpable and usable radial artery. Catheterization is unlikely to succeed if the radial artery is permanently occluded above the pulse.

Is Regional Anesthesia an Option?

A regional technique (spinal or epidural) may be considered. The pros and cons of this technique are listed in Table 77–5. With improved preoperative patient preparation, the use of newer anesthetic drugs that have reduced dependence on renal extraction, and improved monitoring, general anesthesia can be applied with great safety. Either regional or general anesthesia can be chosen in order to meet the individual needs of the patient, anesthesiologist, and surgeon. Because of the relative contraindications to regional anesthesia (see Table 77–5), we prefer general anesthesia for most transplant recipients.

If a regional technique is chosen, a bleeding time should be measured in addition to a platelet count, fibrinogen level, prothrombin time, and partial thromboplastin time. The amount of local anesthetic used and the frequency of its administration should be conservative; the anesthesiologist should take into account the increased potential for local anesthetic toxicity and the possibly higher regional anesthetic block level and its shorter duration in these patients.[19]

What Muscle Relaxants Are Suitable?

Succinylcholine

Succinylcholine is commonly used because it provides rapid-sequence anesthetic induction and is generally safe if

TABLE 77–5. Pros and Cons of Regional Anesthesia for Renal Transplantation

Pros	• Avoids tracheal intubation
	• Avoids pharmacokinetic and pharmacodynamic problems of intravenous and inhalation agents
	• Induces peripheral vasodilatation; decreases myocardial work, preload, and afterload
Cons	• Coagulation problems may contraindicate
	• Peripheral neuropathies may be present
	• Intravascular volume estimates are difficult
	• Risk of infection (minimal)
	• Psychologic factors (needle intolerance, awareness during procedure)
	• Unpredictable duration of surgery
	• Hypotension because of dialysis- and anesthetic-induced ''hypovolemia''
	• Volume overload as block recedes and central circulation becomes plethoric
	• Local anesthetic toxicity increased with acidosis (minimal)

serum potassium is <5.5 mEq · L^{-1}. It will cause a predictable increase in potassium of about 0.5 mEq · L^{-1} in both normal and renal failure patients. Cholinesterase levels are depressed by dialysis with cellophane membranes; this leads to a clinically increased but generally insignificantly longer duration of action when viewed in the context of the relatively lengthy operation time.

When succinylcholine is given after anticholinesterase administration to patients with ESRD, its duration of action is prolonged because of the prolonged duration of action of the anticholinesterase.[20] When infused for >2 hours, succinylcholine can produce a phase II (desensitization) block, even in normal patients. Many patients with chronic renal failure have decreased muscle mass; a reduced dose of muscle relaxant suffices in these patients.

Atracurium

Atracurium's volume of distribution, elimination half-life, and clearance are not influenced by renal failure. Hence, its onset and duration of action are not different from that in normal patients. Metabolism produces levels of laudanosine (a central nervous system excitant) that are somewhat higher in patients with renal failure.[21]

Vecuronium

The volume of distribution of this drug is also not affected by renal failure. Approximately 20% is excreted unchanged in urine. Most of its excretion is biliary, so clearance and elimination half-life may be slightly prolonged. Despite the pharmacokinetic changes, time to onset and duration of action of vecuronium are little different in ESRD than in other disease.[21] Although some accumulation has been reported, it has not been associated with major clinical problems.

In the patient with normal liver function, atracurium or vecuronium is probably indicated for ESRD patients. However, other relaxant use is also possible as long as one takes into consideration (1) autonomic side effects, (2) duration of action (the dose should be decreased appropriately, e.g., one-half the dose should be used with pancuronium), and (3) monitoring of neuromuscular function. Metubine use is not recommended, as it is largely excreted by the kidney.

Curare

In renal failure, clearance and half-life of curare are prolonged, but its biliary excretion increases fourfold. Protein binding is unchanged. Undesired drug effects include ganglionic blockade with hypotension and possible ''recurarization.''[22]

Pancuronium

Volume of distribution of pancuronium is probably not significantly changed in renal failure. Its half-life and clearance are prolonged, and its duration of action is increased.[23]

Anticholinesterases

Neostigmine clearance is dependent on renal excretion for 50% of the dose; therefore, the duration of action is increased in ESRD. Both relaxants and anticholinesterases appear to be similarly affected, providing some safety against recurarization.

What Drugs Should Be Used for Induction?

Induction can be carried out with thiopental, fentanyl, and lidocaine. With thiopental, the volume of distribution is increased, elimination half-life and clearance are only slightly prolonged, and the percentage of free drug state is increased. Nevertheless, it is generally considered the induction agent of choice.

ANESTHETIC MAINTENANCE

The current choice for maintenance of general anesthesia is isoflurane with or without a supplemental narcotic (e.g., fentanyl) and air/oxygen or nitrous oxide/oxygen. Although kidney recipients are anemic, they are typically tolerant to the cardiovascular effect of inhalation anesthetics as long as they are at least euvolemic.

What Is the Role for Other Inhalation Agents?

Halothane is considered in some centers as a second-choice drug because it brings about more pronounced myocardial depression and it has the potential for causing hepatitis.

At about the same time that renal transplantation became common, methoxyflurane was found to be nephrotoxic because of the fluoride ion metabolite that it produces. It never became popular for kidney transplantation.

Enflurane may also lead to slightly elevated fluoride levels (up to 20 mmol $\cdot$ L^{-1}), even though in large series it was reported to have been used without problem.[11]

How Much Neuromuscular Blockade Is Needed?

Profound muscle relaxation is not a major consideration for this surgical procedure because the operative site is easily accessible. In adults, the lower abdominal extraperitoneal approach is used, and the donor kidney is placed in the iliac fossa. In children, the donor kidney is usually placed in the retroperitoneal space and only occasionally intra-abdominally.

How Should Volume and Pressure Be Managed During Revascularization?

Fluids

The renal vein is anastomosed to the iliac vein or vena cava, and the renal artery is connected to the iliac artery, hypogastric artery, or aorta (see Fig. 77–1). Circulating blood volume and systemic pressure should be normal or slightly elevated at the time of revascularization to ensure adequate graft perfusion. Expansion of blood volume using crystalloids or colloids mandates careful assessment. For patients with marginal cardiac function, central venous pressure monitoring should be considered at a minimum. When in doubt, err on the side of excess volume replacement; if renal function is maintained, excess fluid can be removed by pharmacologic translocation (nitroglycerin) or diuresis as needed.

Mannitol

Mannitol is used as both a blood volume expander and a diuretic; its diuretic effect is important following revascularization, during and after ureter reimplantation. Relatively large doses of mannitol (1.5–2.5 g $\cdot$ kg^{-1}) sometimes are administered to patients in renal failure. A dilutional hyponatremia may result as water is drawn from the extracellular space.[24] I recommend moderate doses of mannitol (0.25–0.5 g $\cdot$ kg^{-1}), depending on the patient's state of hydration. Mannitol usually decreases serum potassium level. Occasionally, however, potassium increases as a result of water extraction and diuresis.[25]

Pharmacologic Interventions

Various pharmacologic agents may also be infused during revascularization and immediately before unclamping. The routes of administration and the drugs used vary from direct papaverine injection into the renal artery to intravenous injection of hydrocortisone, procaine, furosemide, or dopamine (5–10 µg $\cdot$ kg^{-1} $\cdot$ min^{-1}). The common goal underlying the pharmacologic therapy at this stage is to maintain and promote graft vasodilation, kidney perfusion, and forced diuresis. The doses and timing of drug administration can differ according to the protocol used by the transplant team (see Table 77–1).

What Happens with Unclamping?

Unclamping increases the blood volume by up to 300 mL and releases various endogenous vasodilating agents. Significant myocardial depression is not associated with these substances. Hypotension can be treated either with volume expanders or vasoactive agents, or both (e.g., 10 µg $\cdot$ kg^{-1} $\cdot$ min^{-1} of dopamine). Vasoactive drugs with α-adrenergic effects constrict renal vessels and should be avoided. In rare cases of transplantation with an intact adrenal gland (cadaveric donor), a hypertensive crisis can result (including ventricular tachycardia or sinus bradycardia); this crisis should be treated with β-blockers.[26]

How Are Fluids Managed?

Fluid replacement for patients with renal dysfunction is based on *conventional* principles. First, the preanesthetic deficit is determined (compare current weight to dry weight). Which fluids to administer intravenously is widely debated.[8] Lactated Ringer's solution probably should not be used in anuric patients. Dextrose, 5% and 0.2% saline, is the preferred maintenance fluid and should be used in amounts appropriate for the fluid requirements of anuric patients (400 mL $\cdot$ m$^{2-1}$ $\cdot$ d^{-1}). Second, intraoperative fluid and blood losses and third space losses are determined, with the understanding that the patient's ability to compensate for fluid load via urine formation is gone. Deficits should be replaced preoperatively. If these are estimated to exceed 15% of blood volume, invasive monitoring should be considered. Anemia should be corrected only if hemoglobin is <6 g $\cdot$ dL^{-1}.

Preanesthetic Deficit

Fluid requirement is related to metabolic rate (protein and electrolyte intake): 1 mL of water is required for each kilocalorie consumed, and 0.7 mL $\cdot$ kcal^{-1} is utilized for renal excretion of metabolites and electrolytes; the remainder, 0.3 mL $\cdot$ kcal^{-1}, represents insensible loss.

Each 1 g of protein catabolized produces approximately 6 mOsm of urea; the daily production is approximately 6 mOsm $\cdot$ kg^{-1}. Each milliequivalent of sodium or potassium administered is equivalent to approximately 2 mOsm (because of the accompanying anion); this amounts to approximately 6 mOsm $\cdot$ kg^{-1} $\cdot$ d^{-1}. Other metabolites account for an additional 2 to 3 mOsm $\cdot$ kg^{-1} $\cdot$ d^{-1}. The ideal time for dialysis is probably the day before anesthesia and surgery; this allows time for equilibration of dialysis-induced fluid and electrolyte shifts.

Intraoperative Requirements

Intraoperative losses of $>15\%$ of blood volume should be replaced with colloid solution on a 1:1 or 1:2 ratio after red blood cell losses are corrected. Small losses can be replaced with the usual 3:1 ratio of crystalloid solution to blood loss. Crystalloid replacement of blood loss is usually with normal saline. Insufficient information is available to recommend 3% saline for volume replacement or expansion in ESRD. It may promote diuresis and decrease total water load. However, its clearance may be reduced, causing intravascular volume overload and electrolyte imbalance.

Third Space Losses

I routinely have 2 units of RBCs available perioperatively. Third space losses should be replaced initially by isotonic crystalloid solution *without* potassium and excess chloride or lactate. Bicarbonate salts can be used to decrease chloride concentration in fluid to about 100 mEq $\cdot$ L^{-1} and to correct existing metabolic acidosis. Since the critical goal is to maintain blood volume, initial third space fluid replacement is 2 to 3 mL $\cdot$ kg^{-1} $\cdot$ h^{-1}; further titration is guided by monitored variables. The choice between crystalloid and colloid solutions can be guided by colloid oncotic pressure and hemoglobin/hematocrit monitoring. Generally speaking, if both values increase, crystalloid solutions are indicated, and if both fall, crystalloid solutions probably are in excess, and colloid solutions should be given. This interpretation obviously depends also on an analysis of blood loss.

Urine output usually is monitored only after ureter anastomosis, which can be done by one of three different procedures: donor-to-recipient anastomosis, ureteral implant, or, rarely, urinary diversion. Urine output is the only real-time monitor of renal function. I sustain normal systemic pressure, intravascular volume, and renal perfusion in order to maintain and even to force diuresis.

TABLE 77–6. Causes of Intraoperative Hyperkalemia

- Pre-existing hyperkalemia not treated or corrected by dialysis
- Succinylcholine administration (average increase: 0.5–0.7 mEq $\cdot$ L^{-1})
- Metabolic acidosis due to renal insufficiency
  Lactic acid following hypotension/hypoperfusion
  Acid metabolites accumulating during vascular occlusion
  Ketoacidosis
- Washout acidosis following declamping of grafted vessels
- Red blood cell transfusion (a minor problem in most cases, but bank blood generally should be <3 d old[8])

What Electrolyte and Acid-Base Changes Are Important?

Hyperkalemia

Hyperkalemia may complicate intraoperative management of renal transplant patients,[27] particularly in diabetics. Numerous intraoperative events may cause an increase in serum potassium concentration (Table 77–6).

Acidosis

Acidosis is a potential intraoperative complication (see Table 77–6). Treatment of metabolic acidosis with bicarbonate should be started if the base excess exceeds -7 mEq $\cdot$ L^{-1}. A functioning renal graft with appropriate diuresis should be sufficient to handle pre-existing acidosis and hyperkalemia. Additional respiratory acidosis may be hazardous. A poorly prepared, acidotic patient may spontaneously hyperventilate preoperatively to compensate. Failure to maintain a similar degree of hyperventilation may result in further decrease in pH with potentially significant increases in serum potassium and myocardial depression.

How Is the Renal Transplant Patient Positioned?

Handling and protection of an arteriovenous fistula in ESRD are important to avoid clotting, thrombosis, or infection. Continuous protection of the vascular access and periodic evaluation for a palpable thrill over the fistula are recommended. If the arm with vascular access is tucked at the patient's side, a cushioned rigid protector is helpful.

POSTOPERATIVE CARE

When Is Intensive Care Unit Admission Advisable?

Postoperatively, these patients should be observed in the postanesthesia care unit or special transplant recovery unit. Special attention is directed to strict monitoring of fluid intake and output, since massive, dilute urine output may be present immediately after transplantation and can lead to hypotension or electrolyte depletion, or both. Blood pressure monitoring should be done on the arm without the arteriovenous fistula. Fluid and electrolyte administration should be adjusted according to electrolyte and hemodynamic values, since optimal hydration has been shown to improve the function of a new graft.[17]

This care can be provided in the postanesthesia care unit or in an intermediate care unit, even though hemodynamic and physiologic and pharmacologic alterations make the recipient different from the routine postoperative patient. The prerequisite is that the patient be at *low risk* (i.e., relatively young and otherwise healthy).

High-risk patients include those individuals with other systemic diseases such as diabetes, pancreatitis, hypertension, and uremia, a history of gastrointestinal bleeding, coronary artery disease, and age >50 years.[28] These patients are more likely to require and benefit from intensive care unit management postoperatively.

CADAVERIC DONOR HARVESTING

What Factors Are Important?

General Criteria

Most transplanted kidneys are cadaveric in origin. The donors should be "heart-beating," with stable hemodynamic function and adequate respiratory support. Organs harvested after cardiopulmonary arrest and longer warm ischemia time are associated with a high incidence of graft failure. Brain-dead donors must satisfy the additional requirements listed in Table 77–7.

"Minimum Hundred Criteria"

I try to keep the donor normovolemic to hypervolemic before harvesting. Fluid infusion and blood pressure support mandate additional intravenous catheters for vascular access and possibly invasive monitoring. A guideline for care of the adult donor is satisfaction of the "minimum hundred criteria": maintenance of systolic blood pressure at >100 mm Hg; PaO_2 at >100 mm Hg; and urine output at >100 mL · h^{-1}. Fluids may include crystalloids, colloids, and blood. Diuretics (mannitol, furosemide) can be used according to protocol. Blood pressure support and urine production can be achieved with dopamine (5–10 μg · kg^{-1} · min^{-1}). However, vasopressors with α-agonist effects may constrict renal vessels, compromise the graft, and adversely affect the function of a concurrently donated heart.

Respiratory support, mechanical ventilation, fraction of inspired oxygen, and positive end-expiratory pressure are provided in order to maintain normocarbia, normoxia, and normal pH. Following heparin administration and after removal of the organs, ventilation is discontinued, and anesthetic support

TABLE 77–7. Additional Requirements for Brain-Dead Cadaveric Donors

- Age <65 y
- Normal renal function
- No hypertension
- No insulin-dependent diabetes mellitus
- No active infection
- No malignancy

ceases. Other organ tissues can still be harvested at this point (skin, bone, cornea). Although no anesthetic agents are used, muscle relaxation may be required.

LIVING-RELATED DONOR HARVESTING

How Is It Different from Cadaveric Renal Transplant?

With living-related donor transplantation, anesthesia and surgery are scheduled electively, enabling complete preparation of both recipient and donor. The donor should be in good health and free of systemic and chronic disease, renal disease, or hypertension. The exclusion criteria are similar to those described for the cadaveric donor.

The allograft is a normal kidney with a minimal warm and cold ischemia time because it is removed under optimal conditions in a setting adjacent to the transplant recipient who is prepared simultaneously.

What Are the Effects of Positioning for a Flank Nephrectomy?

Donor nephrectomy is usually performed through a subcostal flank incision, with the patient positioned in a flank (nephrectomy, kidney) position or the prone position (Fig. 77–2). The flank position often impairs venous return. Several quick blood pressure checks immediately after positioning identify position-related impairment of venous return. Wrapping the legs minimizes venous pooling. Extreme flexion should be avoided, since it may injure the lower spine, compresses the abdominal aorta, and reduces cardiac output. Padding of the head, face, thorax, and bone prominences as well as protection of the peripheral nerves are essential to prevent compression injury, particularly in arthritic patients or in those with back problems. The flank position can produce adverse respiratory effects, which can lead to ventilation/perfusion mismatch. Decreased oxygenation may result from hyperperfusion and hypoventilation of the down-lung and hyperventilation and relative ischemia of the up-lung. Additionally, thoracic compliance is reduced by this position.

How Should Anesthesia Be Administered?

Agents

General anesthesia is preferred because of the awkwardness of the position and the length of the procedure. Induction and maintenance agents and muscle relaxants are titrated according to the patient's need and the anesthesiologist's preference. The main considerations are hemodynamic stability and maintenance of renal perfusion. Inhalation agents are widely used.[30] Potentially nephrotoxic inhalation agents (e.g., methoxyflurane) obviously should not be used. High doses of drugs that are renally excreted should be avoided when possible, since postnephrectomy renal reserve may decrease. Suggested simple, safe, and effective techniques include the use of nitrous oxide, oxygen, narcotics, and relaxants.

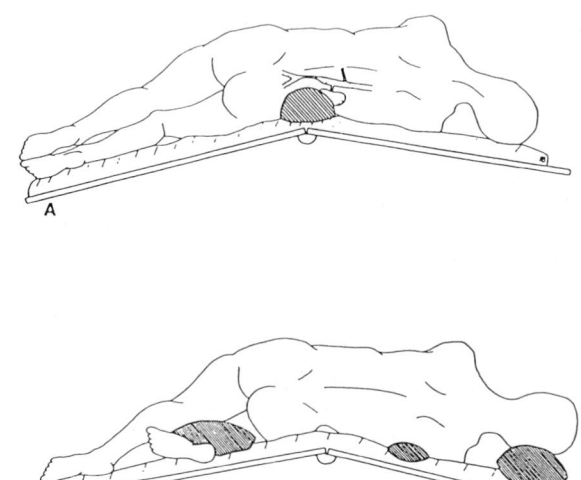

FIGURE 77–2. *A*, Incorrect lateral nephrectomy position. The top leg lies directly over the bottom leg, so that bone prominences are directly opposing each other, with inadequate padding between them. Inadequate support under the head permits excessive lateral flexion of the head. A lack of padding behind the rib cage leaves the head of the humerus directly under the thorax. Exaggerated kidney rest constricts the inferior vena cava. The brachial plexus is consequently compressed. *B*, Correct lateral nephrectomy position. The bottom leg is flexed more than the top leg is, so that bone prominences are opposed by soft muscles. Padding between the legs is ample. A pillow prevents excessive lateral flexion of the head. Padding behind the lower rib cage permits slight posterior tilting of the upper part of the rib cage; as a result, the humeral head is anterior to the thorax, preventing compression of the brachial plexus. A small or no kidney rest ensures free flow of blood through the inferior vena cava. (From Britt BA, Joy N, Mackay MB: Positioning trauma. *In* Complications in Anesthesiology. Orkin FK, Cooperman LH (eds). Philadelphia, JB Lippincott, 1983, p 646.)

Combined Techniques

A technique that combines epidural and general anesthesia has merit and allows an easy transition to postoperative pain management with peridural narcotics. This approach has been shown in a preliminary report to decrease the length of hospitalization when compared with conventional narcotic analgesic administration.[31]

Regardless of the agents chosen, mechanical ventilation should maintain normocapnia, since hyperventilation or hypoventilation may cause renal artery constriction or venous pooling, respectively. The interaction between ventilation and renal function is complex. Mechanical ventilation has direct (renal) and indirect (cardiovascular, neural, humoral) effects, all of which decrease renal blood flow.

How Should Ventilatory Support Be Provided?

Direct Renal Effects

Direct renal effects of different modes of ventilatory support have been studied.[32] Intermittent positive-pressure ventilation and continuous positive airway pressure may reduce renal blood flow, glomerular filtration rate, and urine output. Continuous positive-pressure ventilation has the most adverse effects on these parameters and on urinary sodium excretion and osmolar clearance. Other coexisting variables such as temperature, hematocrit, intravascular volume, and acid-base status may also affect renal function, directly or indirectly, by modifying the cardiovascular response to ventilation. Thus, the renal effects of ventilation in an individual patient are impossible to predict.

Hemodynamic Changes

Renal function is largely determined by hemodynamic alterations, which, in turn, may depend on the mode of ventilation, lung compliance, blood volume, and cardiac function. Mechanical ventilation, particularly continuous positive-pressure ventilation, impairs renal function primarily by having an adverse effect on the effective intravascular volume and renal perfusion pressure rather than by directly decreasing cardiac output. The increase in intrathoracic pressure with continuous positive-pressure ventilation results in an increase in inferior vena cava, hepatic, and renal venous pressures, all of which may further impede renal perfusion if systemic arterial pressure decreases. Careful fluid infusion often minimizes these changes.

Baroreceptor and Humoral Changes

The relative importance of cardiac low-pressure receptors and renal high-pressure receptors in modulating renal function and intrarenal hemodynamics during mechanical ventilation is not yet established. Systemic baroreceptors (aortic arch, carotid sinus) may play a role in initiating renal dysfunction during continuous positive-pressure ventilation.[5] The primary role of antidiuretic hormone in the pathogenesis of reduced urine output also is not clear. However, plasma renin activity and aldosterone level may increase during continuous positive-pressure ventilation[33]; this increase is probably related to reduction in renal perfusion pressure and glomerular filtration rate.

Pharmacologic Support

Renal dysfunction during ventilation may resemble prerenal failure and should be treated as such. Adequate hydration to maintain filling pressures, cardiac output, and perfusion pressure is essential. A clinical dilemma may arise because what is therapeutically optimal for the kidney (i.e., volume infusion) is not necessarily optimal for other organs (i.e., the lungs and heart). Prophylaxis starts with choosing the ventilation mode that is least likely to depress cardiac performance. Also, pharmacologic agents (e.g., dopamine) can be incorporated for prevention or treatment to improve renal function or cardiac performance, or both. The adverse effect of continuous positive-pressure ventilation on renal function can be corrected by the administration of dopamine in a mean dose of 5 $\mu g \cdot kg^{-1} \cdot min^{-1}$.[34]

Pneumothorax

Pneumothorax may develop during nephrectomy or in the immediate postoperative period. This is perhaps the most frequent serious acute perioperative complication after donor nephrectomy. Early recognition is critical. Hypotension following closure should provoke an examination to rule out pneumothorax. Nitrous oxide administration should be discontinued to avoid pneumothorax expansion; this should be followed by the institution of mechanical maneuvers (either tube drainage or needle aspiration) to ensure lung inflation. Regardless of whether a pneumothorax occurs or is suspected, a chest radiograph should be obtained immediately after nephrectomy.

How Are the Kidneys Protected During Transplantation?

Maintenance of optimum circulating blood volume is essential. If hypotension occurs, volume expansion is preferred to vasopressor administration. However, dopamine is also used (5–10 $\mu g \cdot kg^{-1} \cdot min^{-1}$) to promote renal blood flow and as a β-agonist. Use of α-agonists should be avoided.

Low urine output necessitates fluid administration with loop (e.g., furosemide) or osmotic (e.g., mannitol) diuretics. Most protocols incorporate mannitol, 12.5 to 25 g intravenously, when surgical manipulation of the kidney begins and if urine output decreases.

Local anesthetics may be applied to the renal vessels after dissection to minimize vascular spasm. Many protocols also use heparinization. Different agents may be used to prevent renal vasoconstriction during anesthesia that is associated with sympathetic stimulation; these agents include vasodilators, calcium channel blockers, and prostaglandins D_2, E_2, and I_2. These substances oppose the effects of endogenous norepinephrine, angiotensin, antidiuretic hormones, and atrial natriuretic factor. At the same time, systemic venodilation with hypotension should absolutely be avoided.

How Much Blood Loss Is Expected?

Imperfect hemostasis during nephrectomy can be associated with considerable blood loss. The use of two large-bore intravenous catheters is indicated, since operative blood loss exceeds 500 mL in 25% of patients and transfusion is performed in 75%.[35] The need for transfusion may be less in the future as we continue to redefine and lower our "transfusion trigger"; however, this approach serves to increase other fluids and replace the blood loss.

References

1. Terasaki PI, Perdue ST, Sasaki N, et al: Improving success rates of kidney transplantation. JAMA 1983; 250:1065.
2. McDonald JC: The National Organ Procurement and Transplantation Network. JAMA 1988; 259:725.
3. Opelz G: Correlation of HLA matching with kidney graft survival in patients with or without cyclosporine treatment. Transplantation 1985; 40:240.
4. Sladen RN: Perioperative renal protection. ASA Annual Refresher Course #255. 1991 Annual ASA meeting. Park Ridge, IL, American Society of Anesthesiologists, 1991.
5. Schrier RW: Effects of adrenergic nervous system and catecholamines on systemic and renal hemodynamics, sodium, and water excretion and renin excretion. Kidney Int 1974; 6:291.
6. Livio M, Mannucci PM, Vigano G, et al: Conjugated estrogens for the management of bleeding associated with renal failure. N Engl J Med 1986; 315:86.
7. Weir PHC, Chung FF: Anaesthesia for patients with chronic renal disease. Can Anaesth Soc J 1984; 31:468.
8. Cook DR: Anesthetic considerations for organ transplantation. ASA Annual Refresher Course #255. 1989 Annual ASA meeting. Park Ridge, IL, American Society of Anesthesiologists, 1991.
9. Don HF, Dieppa RA, Taylor P: Narcotic analgesics in anuric patients. Anesthesiology 1975; 42:745.
10. Wiggum DC, Cork RC, Weldon ST, et al: Postoperative respiratory depression and elevated sufentanil levels in a patient with chronic renal failure. Anesthesiology 1985; 63:708.
11. Smith BE: Renal failure, renal transplantation, and anesthesia. ASA Annual Refresher Course #241. 1990 Annual ASA meeting. Park Ridge, IL, American Society of Anesthesiologists, 1990.
12. Bready LL: Kidney transplantation. Anesth Clin North Am 1989; 7:487.
13. Tilstone WJ, Fine A: Furosemide kinetics in renal failure. Clin Pharmacol Ther 1978; 23:644.
14. Lowenthal DT: Pharmacokinetics of propranolol, quinidine, procainamide, and lidocaine in chronic renal disease. Am J Med 1977; 62:532.
15. Sidi A, Kaplan RF, Davis RF: Prolonged neuromuscular blockade and ventilatory failure after renal transplantation and cyclosporine. Can J Anaesth 1990; 37:543.
16. Dretchen KL, Morgenroth VH, Standaert FG, et al: Azathioprine: effects on neuromuscular transmission. Anesthesiology 1976; 45:604.
17. Carlier M, Squifflet JP, Pirson Y, et al: Maximal hydration during anesthesia increases pulmonary artery pressures and improves early function of human renal transplant. Transplantation 1982; 34:201.
18. Slogoff S, Keats AS, Arlund C: On the safety of radial artery cannulation. Anesthesiology 1983; 59:42.
19. Orko R, Pitkanen M, Rosenberg PH: Subarachnoid anaesthesia with 0.75% bupivacaine in patients with chronic renal failure. Br J Anaesth 1985; 58:605.
20. Bishop MJ, Hornbein TF: Prolonged effect of succinylcholine after neostigmine and pyridostigmine administration in patients with renal failure. Anesthesiology 1983; 58:384.
21. Miller RD: Pharmacokinetics of atracurium and other nondepolarizing neuromuscular blocking agents in normal patients and those with renal or hepatic dysfunction. Br J Anaesth 1986; 58:11S.
22. Miller RD, Cullen DJ: Renal failure and postoperative respiratory failure: recurarization? Br J Anaesth 1976; 48:253.
23. McLeod K, Watson MJ, Rawlings MD: Pharmacokinetics of pancuronium in patients with normal and impaired renal function. Br J Anaesth 1976; 48:341.
24. Borges HF, Hocks J, Kjellstrand CM: Mannitol intoxication in patients with renal failure. Arch Intern Med 1982; 142:63.
25. Charters P: Mannitol, osmolality and steroids during renal transplantation. Anaesthesia 1983; 38:327.
26. Freilich JD, Waterman PM, Rosenthal JT: Acute hemodynamic changes during renal transplantation. Anesth Analg 1984; 63:158.
27. Hirshman CA, Leon D, Edelstein G, et al: Risk of hyperkalemia in recipients of kidneys preserved with an intracellular electrolyte solution. Anesth Analg 1980; 59:283.
28. Ivey GL, Richie RE, Niblack GD, et al: Renal transplantation: a twenty-year experience in a Veterans Administration Medical Center. Arch Surg 1985; 120:1021.
29. Phillips MG: Cadaver-donor nephrectomy. *In* Urologic Surgery. Glenn JF (ed). Philadelphia, JB Lippincott, 1983, p 329.
30. Aldrete JA, Swanson JT, Penn I, et al: Anesthesia experience with living renal transplant donors. Anesth Analg 1971; 50:169.
31. Dixon C, Sefton W, Gravenstein N: Epidural analgesia after donor nephrectomy decreases duration of hospitalization (Abstract). Regional An-

esthesia. J Neural Blockade in Obstetrics, Surgery, and Pain Control 1992; 17(3S):75.

32. Priebe HJ, Hedley-Whyte J: Respiratory support and renal function. Int Anesth Clin 1984; 22:203.

33. Annat G, Viale JP, Xuan BB, et al: Effect of PEEP ventilation on renal function, plasma renin, aldosterone, neurophysins and urinary ADH, and prostaglandins. Anesthesiology 1983; 58:136.

34. Lindner A, Cutler RE, Goodman G: Synergism of dopamine plus furosemide in preventing acute renal failure in the dog. Kidney Int 1979; 16:158.

35. Weiland D, Sutherland DER, Chavers B, et al: Information on 628 living-related kidney donors at a single institution, with long-term follow-up in 472 cases. Transplant Proc 1984; 16:5.

CHAPTER 78

Lasers and Laser Safety

ANNETTE G. PASHAYAN, M.D.

The possibility of laser energy was proposed by Albert Einstein in 1917. It was not until the early 1950s, however, that the first prototype laser was developed. Since then, lasers have been applied throughout medicine and surgery and are now considered a common treatment modality in most medical communities in the United States. Although lasers offer therapeutic advantages, they also present risks—not only to the patient but also to health care providers who work with them.

Most anesthesiologists care for patients receiving laser surgery of one sort or another and must be acquainted with basic laser safety. Those anesthesiologists whose practice includes patients with laryngeal and tracheal lesions have special concerns regarding the use of lasers in the airway. The objective of this chapter is to review the basic principles of lasers and laser safety as well as to discuss airway management during airway laser applications.

BASIC PRINCIPLES

What Is a Laser?

The word *laser* is an acronym for *light amplification of the stimulated emission of radiation.* A laser is an instrument that produces a form of light known as *coherent radiation.* Coherent radiation has three characteristics that differentiate it from other forms of electromagnetic energy:

1. *Monochromaticity:* All waves are of exactly the same wavelength or color.
2. *Collimation:* All waves are parallel to each other and do not diverge.
3. *Coherence:* All waves travel in phase in the same direction.

Coherent radiation can be focused to a spot size of energy density that is great enough to vaporize tissue.

How Is Coherent Radiation Produced?

Coherent radiation is produced by an internal atomic action known as *stimulated emission.* Electrons normally occupy a ground state energy level (E_1; Fig. 78–1) but can jump to a higher energy level (E_2) by absorbing outside energy from either an external light source or electrical discharges. Owing to the quantum nature of atoms, only the exact amount of energy that will move the electron to E_2 is absorbed; after this has occurred, the atom is now said to be "excited."

A group of molecules that have absorbed external energy in this manner is said to have undergone "population inversion." Excited atoms tend to revert to the lowest energy state; in the process, they emit photons with energy equal to the difference between the excited and the lower energy levels (ΔE [in joules]). The ΔE is responsible for the frequency (f) of the emitted photons; ΔE and f are related by Planck's constant (h):

$$\Delta E = hf \qquad \text{Equation 1}$$

The frequency of the photons is inversely related to the wavelength of the emitted light:

$$f = c / \lambda \qquad \text{Equation 2}$$

where c is the speed of light and λ is the wavelength. The emitted photon, with its specific frequency and wavelength, can then interact with another similarly stimulated atom, resulting in the release of a second photon. If the population of molecules is uniform, the frequency, energy, direction, and phase of the second photon will be the same as that of the first photon. These two photons continue to release similar photons from other excited atoms in the process of stimulated emission.

What Are the Main Components of a Laser?

Three main components constitute a laser: an energy source, a lasing medium, and an optical cavity (Fig. 78–2).

Energy Source

The energy source, or "pump," can be an electrical or chemical source, flash lamps, or other laser systems. It induces population inversion of the molecules in the lasing medium, initiating the process of stimulated emission.

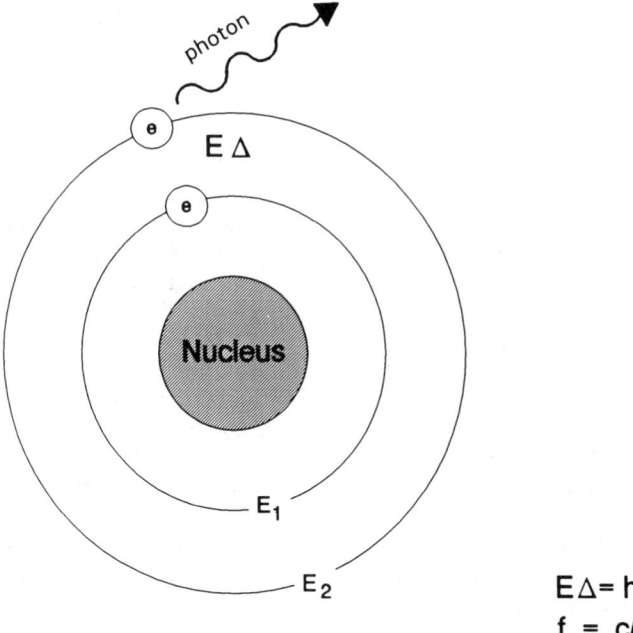

FIGURE 78–1. Electron (e) transition from a higher energy level (E_2) to a lower energy level (E_1), producing a photon of light. The frequency (f) of the photon is related to the energy change (ΔE) by Planck's constant (h), and f is related to wavelength (λ) by the speed of light (c).

$$E\Delta = hf$$
$$f = c/\lambda$$

Lasing Medium

The lasing or active medium is the population of molecules used to produce the photons. Lasers are named after the lasing media that they employ. For instance, the carbon dioxide (CO_2) laser uses CO_2 molecules to produce its coherent radiation. The lasing medium is also responsible for the wavelength that the laser emits, since the frequency of the emitted photon is related to the specific electron energy levels of that molecule. Lasing media may consist of gas, such as CO_2, or of a solid or liquid material.

Optical Cavity

Population inversion of the lasing medium takes place inside an optical cavity. Mirrors placed at either end of the optical cavity reflect the photons back and forth; this continues the process of stimulated emission and causes the beam to grow in strength. The mirror at one end of the cavity is totally

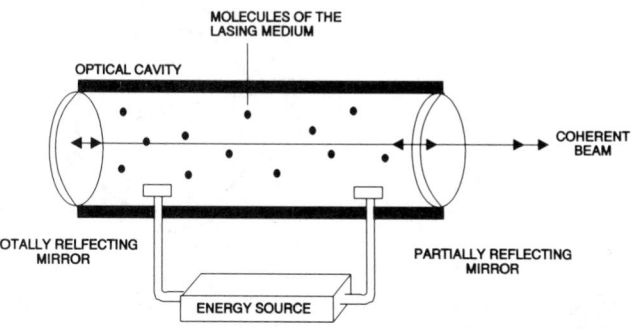

FIGURE 78–2. The three principal parts of a laser: the energy source; the lasing medium; and the optical cavity.

reflective, but the opposite mirror is only partially reflective, allowing beam transmission when a shutter is opened.

MEDICAL APPLICATIONS

How Is Coherent Radiation Used?

Laser beams are applied for their thermal effect and can be used to cut, coagulate, or vaporize tissues. The exact tissue interaction of a laser is dependent on several variables, including the wavelength of the emitted beam, the tissue being irradiated, and the beam's power density. Commonly used wavelengths, their respective lasing media, and their general characteristics are listed in Table 78–1.

Tissue Effects

When a laser beam strikes a tissue, it may be reflected, scattered, transmitted, or absorbed. If the beam is reflected off a surface, there is, in essence, no effect on the surface from which it is reflected. If a beam is scattered, the laser energy is spread over an area wider than the beam's spot size so that the energy is diffused. A transmitted beam is one that passes through a tissue with little or no thermal effect on that tissue. Therefore, the thermal effect of a laser beam is primarily caused by beam absorption.

Various wavelengths are absorbed differently by tissue. For

TABLE 78–1. Lasers Commonly Used in the Operating Room

Laser	Wavelength (nm)	General Characteristics
Argon	488/515 (blue/green)	Absorbed selectively by hemoglobin and melanin or other similar pigments Transmitted through clear substances Tissue penetration: 0.5 to 2 mm
Potassium titanyl phosphate (frequency-doubled YAG)	532 (green)	Strongly absorbed by hemoglobin, melanin, and similar pigments Transmitted through clear substances Tissue penetration: 0.5 to 2 mm
Nd.YAG	1065 (near-infrared)	More readily absorbed by dark tissue Transmitted through clear fluids Tissue penetration: 2 to 6 mm
CO_2	10,600 (far-infrared)	Strongly absorbed by water and, thus, by all tissue (pigmented or not)
Helium-neon	632 (red)	Used as a low-power coaxial aiming beam for nonvisible lasers (CO_2 and Nd.YAG) Has no significant tissue interaction

Abbreviation: Nd.YAG = neodymium-yttrium-aluminum-garnet.

example, the far-infrared wavelength of the CO_2 laser is absorbed by all tissues whether they be clear or pigmented; hence, the CO_2 laser beam exerts its effect on whatever surface it strikes first. The green beam of the potassium titanyl phosphate laser, on the other hand, is transmitted through clear tissues but is highly absorbed by pigments such as hemoglobin and melanin.

Thermal Damage

The extent of thermal damage caused by a laser is highly dependent on the beam's power density. The power density is calculated as follows:

$$\text{Power density} = \frac{\text{Watts}}{\text{Spot size (cm}^2)}$$

Equation 3

The power density is also known as the "irradiance." For a given laser output, a small spot size concentrates the power, making the beam more intense, and a large spot size diffuses the power, making the beam less intense. The extent of thermal damage is modified by heat dissipation, which depends on tissue density and blood flow.

What Risks Are Associated with Laser Procedures?

Accidental or inappropriate direction or reflection of a laser beam can result in thermal damage to normal tissues. Lasers have other associated hazards; for example, they can produce airborne contaminants and can cause fires and explosions. The American National Standards Institute has classified the potential hazards of lasers based on their optical emissions (Table 78–2) such that the higher the class of laser, the greater the

hazard that is presented.[1] Class 4 lasers are thus the most hazardous; most lasers used in the operating room are class 4 lasers.

Eye Injury

The eyes of patients and of the medical personnel caring for them are at risk for injury by laser beams. The nature and extent of eye injury depends on the wavelength of the laser that is encountered as well as on the manner in which the exposure occurs. Since far-infrared wavelengths are absorbed by whatever surface is first encountered, the CO_2 laser causes corneal ulcerations and scars (Fig. 78–3). Visible and near-infrared wavelengths (400–1400 nm), on the other hand, are transmitted through the clear structures in the anterior chamber of the eye and are then absorbed in the pigmented retina (see Fig. 78–3). As such beams are transmitted through the anterior chamber, the light is focused by the eye's lens; this produces a small spot of high power density and thus presents considerable danger to the retina. Direct intrabeam viewing of a laser beam is more likely to result in eye injury than is viewing of a diffusely reflected beam (Fig. 78–4).

Skin Injury

Although human skin is less vulnerable to laser injury than is the eye, direct, high-intensity exposure can result in skin burns. The patient's skin in the area of the operative site is at particular risk because of its proximity to the targeted tissue. As with other forms of electromagnetic radiation, laser light can be mutagenic. Even if the laser intensity is low and a burn is unlikely, direct skin exposure should be avoided.

Smoke Inhalation

Tissue vaporization by a laser beam produces a smoke known as "laser plume." Laser plume may contain infectious

TABLE 78–2. Classification Established by the American National Standards Institute for Lasers and Laser Hazards

Class	Description	Examples	Control Measures
1	Beam is totally contained, and device cannot emit accessible laser radiation	Lasers used in laboratories for diagnostic work	No
2	Low-power visible lasers that are not intended for prolonged viewing; the normal blink reflex protects the eye	Helium-neon aiming beam for CO_2 and Nd.YAG	Yes
3a	Normally would not pose a hazard if viewed momentarily with the unaided eye	Some ophthalmologic lasers are higher class 3	Yes
3b	May produce a hazard if viewed directly (intrabeam viewing and specular reflection)		
4	Hazardous if viewed directly or from diffuse reflection; also produces fire hazards and skin hazards	Most medical lasers, including CO_2, Nd.YAG, argon, and potassium titanyl phosphate	Yes

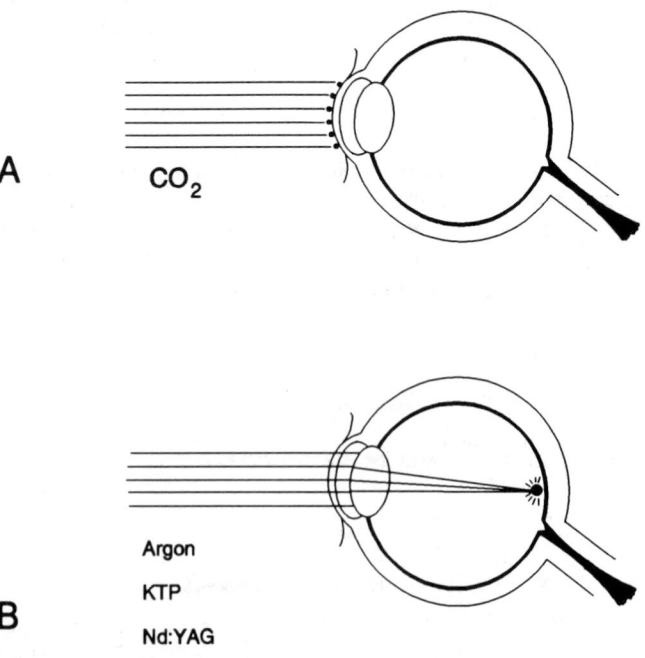

FIGURE 78–3. Lasers that emit wavelengths in the infrared portion of the spectrum *(A)* are absorbed by the cornea, whereas wavelengths in the range of 400–1400 nm pass through the cornea and are absorbed by pigmented retina *(B)*.

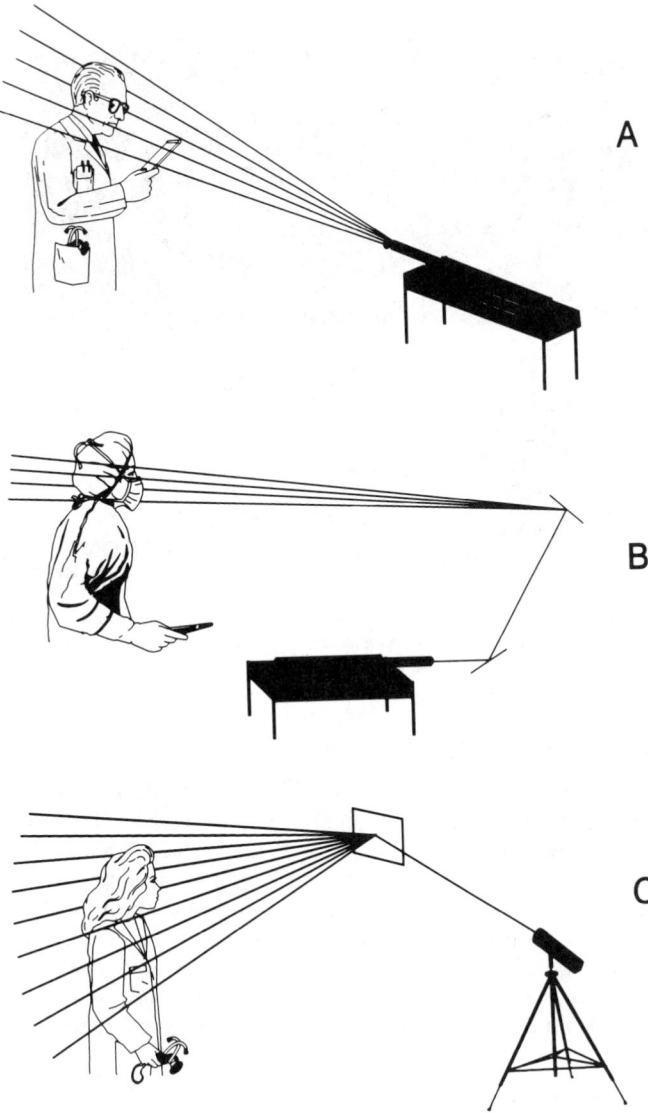

FIGURE 78–4. The risk of eye injury depends on how the laser beam is viewed. Direct intrabeam viewing *(A)* is most hazardous, followed by specular reflection *(B)* and diffuse reflection *(C)*. *Specular reflection* means that the angle of incidence equals or nearly equals the angle of reflection, and *diffuse reflection* means that the radiation is reflected over a wide range of angles. (Reproduced with permission from Pashayan AG: Lasers and electrical safety in the operating room. Part I: Lasers. *In* Ehrenwerth J, Eisenkraft JB (eds): Anesthesia Equipment. Principles and Applications. St Louis, Mosby–Year Book, 1993, p 436.)

particles, such as viral DNA,[2, 3] and may be mutagenic[4, 5] in much the same way as cigarette smoke is. Tracheal and bronchial irritation and pneumonitis have been produced in animal models of laser plume inhalation.[6, 7] Other potential reactions to laser plume include lacrimation, nausea, and vomiting.

Fire

Fires and explosions can occur if the laser beam contacts combustible material in the operating room. The ignition of surgical drapes[8, 9] by a laser can result in severe and extensive burns to the patient as well as in inhalation injury to surrounding personnel.

Of particular concern to anesthesiologists is the problem of fire that can occur if the laser ignites flammable tracheal tubes or tracheal tube components.[10, 11] This problem can arise directly from laser beam contact or indirectly from burned tissue that comes in contact with a tracheal tube or a fiberoptic bronchoscope.

The risk of tracheal tube fire is particularly great when a laser is used for resection of lesions in the laryngotracheal region because the ignition source (the laser beam) is so close to the fuel (the flammable tube) and to an oxidizer (the oxygen or nitrous oxide inside the tracheal tube).

Miscellaneous Problems

Besides the risks associated with the laser beam itself, other hazards have been reported to be associated with the use of lasers and their delivery systems. Fatal gas embolization has occurred during laser hysteroscopy owing to the use of gas-cooled delivery probes.[13] This complication has led to the recommendation that only liquid-cooled laser probes be used for laser hysteroscopy. Electrocutions have been reported among personnel who service high-voltage laser equipment; this has resulted in the implementation of strict safety guidelines for laser service personnel.[14]

How Can Laser Injury Risk Be Minimized?

Laser Safety Committee

The risk of laser accidents can be reduced through the implementation of a formal laser safety program in the hospital or health care facility in which the laser is used. The safety program is overseen by a laser safety committee consisting of administrators, nurses, operating room technicians, biomedical engineers, and physicians who work with lasers.

The committee should have physician representation from each surgical service that performs laser operations. An anesthesiologist should participate in this committee, especially in an institution where laser airway endoscopy under general anesthesia is performed. Responsibilities of the laser safety committee include strategic planning, physician credentialing, formulation of safety policies and protocols, and in-service education of health care personnel.[15]

Laser Safety Officer

A laser safety officer (LSO) should head the laser safety committee. The LSO is usually a technician, nurse, or biomedical engineer who has special training in laser safety and maintenance and who has "the authority and responsibility to monitor and enforce the control of laser hazards, and to effect the

TABLE 78–3. Responsibilities of the Laser Safety Officer

- Classification of laser systems in the hospital according to standards of the American National Standards Institute
- Hazard evaluation of laser treatment areas
- Prescription and documentation of use of control measures
- Approval and documentation of procedures and protocols
- Recommendation, approval, and inspection of protective equipment
- Approval of equipment installation and authorization of laser technicians
- Assurance of safety training for all personnel working with laser
- Determination of need for medical surveillance of personnel working with laser
- Investigation of alleged laser accidents
- Approval of warning signs and equipment labels

knowledgeable evaluation and control of laser hazards.''[1] The LSO is knowledgeable about practical procedures and equipment and understands the requirements of local, state, and federal regulations. In small health care facilities, the LSO may personally participate in each laser procedure to ensure compliance with laser safety committee protocols. In most hospitals, however, the LSO designates laser nurses to monitor and document compliance with approved protocols. Responsibilities of the LSO are listed in Table 78–3.

Specific Safety Measures

Credentialing

One of the most important steps in avoiding laser injuries is to prevent medical personnel who are not properly trained in laser surgery from using laser instruments. Surgeons and physicians such as otolaryngologists, gastroenterologists, and pulmonologists who actually operate lasers should be credentialed in laser use by their hospitals' governing boards. The credentialing procedure usually consists of attendance at a training course and a subsequent preceptorship with a physician who has already been approved to use a laser of the specific wavelengths.[15]

Physicians whose residency training included laser operation may forego such a course and preceptorship, provided that their training in laser use is documented by the residency training director. Physicians must be credentialed separately for each wavelength of laser that they wish to use. Formal credentialing of anesthesiologists who participate in laser cases is not generally required by hospital boards. However, laser safety committees may require education programs for their anesthesiologists as well as for the operating room technicians and nurses participating in laser surgery.

Identification of Laser Procedures

Another key component to avoid laser injuries is to identify clearly those operating rooms in which laser operations take place so that unprotected personnel do not accidentally stray into the path of a laser beam. The laser surgery nurse or operating room technician should post warning signs at all entrances to these rooms before each laser case commences. These signs must specify the class and wavelength of the laser being used as well as the appropriate protective measures that must be implemented when this wavelength is being used (Fig. 78–5).

Wearing of Goggles

Personnel in the operating room must protect their eyes by wearing goggles that are appropriate for the wavelength in use while the laser is in operation. For the CO_2 laser, any type of glass or plastic is protective because the far-infrared beam is absorbed by any surface that it hits. Since prescription eyeglasses generally lack side protectors, plastic goggles are usually worn over them.

For all short-wavelength lasers, goggles that specifically filter out the wavelengths in use must be available. Such goggles should be labeled with the wavelength for which they are protective. Protective eyewear can be tinted and thus can distort the anesthesiologist's color perception so that cyanosis may be even more difficult to detect than usual.

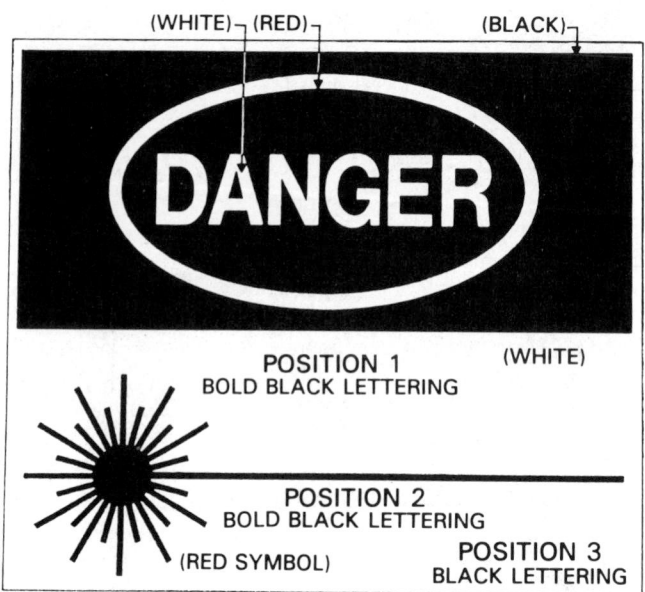

FIGURE 78–5. A warning sign should be posted at each entrance to a room in which a laser operation is taking place. The numbered positions correspond to specifications for wavelength of laser, class of laser, and the need for eyewear or other protection.

Prevention of Beam Reflection

Preventing specular reflection of the laser beam from surgical instruments such as scalpels, forceps, and bronchoscopes also decreases the risk of ocular damage. Standard metallic surgical instruments have a polished surface that reflects light in a specular manner. Matte-finish instruments reflect the laser beam in a diffuse, less harmful manner. The patient's eyes should be lubricated with a water-based, nonflammable solution and then closed and covered with wet gauze to protect them from the laser during nonophthalmologic procedures.

Skin Protection

Skin damage from direct laser contact is usually of secondary concern, but the patient's skin immediately surrounding the surgical field should be protected with wet towels and drapes, since it is in close vicinity to the focused laser beam. This procedure not only protects the skin from direct laser contact but may also prevent a drape fire, which could result in more severe burns.

Flame-Retardant Drapes

Flame-retardant drapes that also can reduce the risk of drape fires are available. Fires of the tracheal tube and airway circuit are also of major concern to the anesthesiologist, especially during laser operations on the airway.

SPECIAL CONCERNS DURING LARYNGEAL LASER OPERATIONS

Because they enable very precise excision that produces minimal edema, lasers are favored by many surgeons for resection of tumors and other obstructions in the airway. Since the laser is an intense light that provides an ignition source, laser surgery risks fire when flammable materials are present, especially in the oxygen (O_2)–enriched atmosphere that is often present during general anesthesia.[10, 11, 16] Such fire can cause severe, life-threatening burns of the larynx and trachea and can also spread throughout the anesthesia circuit and into the operating room.

While no method absolutely prevents fire when a laser is used for airway surgery, appropriate selection of airway appliances (e.g., tracheal tubes) and adherence to fire safety protocols minimize the risk. The upper airway is considered separately from the trachea and bronchi because the latter two areas require different management approaches.

For operations in and around the larynx, the CO_2 laser is most often used because of its shallow depth of burn and extreme precision (see Table 78–1). Occasionally, the neodymium-yttrium-aluminum-garnet (Nd.YAG) or potassium titanyl phosphate laser may also be used. The CO_2 laser beam can be delivered via an operating microscope positioned at the lens focal length from the larynx. The beam is positioned with a micromanipulator using a coaxial, visible helium-neon beam.

For many laryngeal operations, such as vocal cord papilloma or polyp resections, the beam is aimed at tissue that is in immediate contact with the tracheal tube; thus, the risk of fire is quite high. Approaches to airway management during such procedures include the use of a small endotracheal tube or no endotracheal tube at all.

What Are the Alternatives to Tracheal Intubation?

Jet Ventilation

When a tracheal tube is not used for laser laryngoscopies, a metal needle mounted in the operating laryngoscope can be used for jet ventilation.[17] With the tip of the needle either above or below the glottis, a high-velocity jet of O_2 is directed into the airway lumen by the surgeon so that the lungs are ventilated with a mixture of jet-injected O_2 and entrained room air. Since no flammable material is in the airway, a fire is unlikely.

Potential Complications

Jet ventilation is favored by many surgeons because it allows excellent visualization of the surgical field. The airway, however, is not protected from other risks. Hypoventilation can be a problem with jet ventilation, particularly in patients with a highly obstructive airway lesion, in whom it may be difficult for the surgeon to aim the jet into the airway lumen. If the jet is not accurately aimed, gastric distention or barotrauma, including pneumothorax and pneumomediastinum, can also result.

Patients with decreased pulmonary compliance or increased airway resistance from bronchospasm, obesity, or chronic obstructive pulmonary disease are at high risk of hypoventilation with jet techniques. Spirometry is not possible, and capnography is difficult and inaccurate in unintubated patients; thus, hypoventilation may go undetected.

Other risks to the unprotected airway include aspiration of gastric contents, surgical debris, and laser plume as well as inadvertent laser perforation of the trachea or carina distal to the area of resection.[18] Although unlikely, airway fire can still

occur because a high O_2 concentration is present and because combustible material near the airway can ignite.[19]

Insufflation

Another method of airway management that does not require intubation is insufflation.[20] While the patient is breathing spontaneously, a potent inhalation agent is insufflated through a side port of the operating laryngoscope, a metal hook, or a catheter. As with jet ventilation, absence of flammable material in the airway minimizes the risk of fire and allows excellent visualization of the surgical field.

Potential Complications

Again, as with any nonintubation technique, aspiration is a risk and hypoventilation can occur and go undetected because capnography is difficult to perform and inaccurate without a tracheal tube.

Ventilation cannot be assisted or controlled with the insufflation technique. The depth of anesthesia may fluctuate, and because muscle relaxants may not be used for spontaneously breathing patients, patient movement may result in inadvertent contact of healthy tissue or flammable materials, such as drapes and catheters, by the laser beam. Insufflation also contaminates the ambient air with inhalation anesthetic agents and thus exposes operating room personnel to associated risks. If a catheter is used as the insufflation device, the risk of fire is substantially increased.

How Is Tracheal Intubation Utilized?

Tracheal intubation secures the airway and, thus, protects it from aspiration of gastric contents, laser plume, and inadvertent laser burn to the trachea. It also provides a means of controlling and monitoring ventilation. With intubation, both inhalation and intravenous agents as well as muscle relaxants can be safely administered. However, all conventional tracheal tubes are composed of materials that are readily ignitable and flammable[21] (Table 78–4); thus, special precautions must be taken when using these tubes. A variety of tracheal tubes are available.

TABLE 78–4. Combustion Properties of Materials Composing Conventional Tracheal Tubes

Material	Times with a 10-W Laser Beam and 50% Oxygen and 50% Nitrogen		
	Oxygen Index of Flammability*†	Penetration Time (s)‡	Mean Time to Ignition (s)‡
Polyvinylchloride	0.263 ± 0.004	0.77	3.06 ± 0.79
Silicone	0.189 ± 0.009	Not tested	Not tested
Red rubber	0.176 ± 0.003	41.48	33 ± 1.01

*Concentration of O_2 that sustains a candlelike flame.
†Data from Wolf GL, Simpson JL: Flammability of endotracheal tubes in oxygen- and nitrous oxide–enriched atmosphere. Anesthesiology 1987; 67:236–239.
‡Data from Ossoff RG: Laser safety in otolaryngology—head and neck surgery: anesthetic and educational considerations for laryngeal surgery. Laryngoscope 1989; 99(Suppl 48):1–26.

TABLE 78-5. Helium Protocol for Laryngotracheal Carbon Dioxide Laser Operations

	Protocol Consideration	Limitations
Gases	Helium	Fraction of inspired helium >0.6
	O_2	Fraction of inspired $O_2 \leq 0.4$
	Inhalation anesthetics	Enflurane, halothane, or isoflurane
	Nitrous oxide	Cannot be used for anesthetic maintenance
Endotracheal Tube	CO_2 laser	Unmarked, unwrapped PVC without barium stripe
	Power density	≤ 10 W at 0.8 mm spot size (1992 $W \cdot cm^{2-1}$)
	Exposure	Repeated bursts (<10 s of 0.5-s pulsed beam)
Monitors		Standard monitors, O_2 analyzer, and pulse oximeter

(Reproduced from Pashayan AG, Gravenstein JS, Cassisi NJ, et al: The helium protocol for laryngotracheal operations with CO_2 laser: a retrospective review of 523 cases. Anesthesiology 1988; 68:801–804.)

Polyvinyl Chloride Tubes

Polyvinyl chloride (PVC) tracheal tubes, which are the tubes most commonly used in operating rooms, are favored for non-laser operations because they are clear and soft, retain a patent lumen and a shape that conforms to the natural curves of the airway anatomy, and are nontraumatic. Under well-controlled conditions, such as during strict adherence to the helium protocol (Table 78–5), PVC does not ignite when it is in contact with the laser beam.[22, 23] Such contact between laser beam and endotracheal tube is extremely common, occurring in about 50% of all upper airway laser cases.[23]

PVC tracheal tubes do not reflect laser light nor retain and transfer heat, and thus they are not associated with injury to nontargeted tissue. Since PVC is transparent, condensation of airway vapor, as well as evidence of combustion within the lumen, can be monitored visually.

PVC tubes have a higher O_2 index of flammability (see Table 78–4) and thus require a higher concentration of O_2 to sustain a flame than do other conventional tracheal tubes that burn in room air. Despite the advantages of PVC tubes, they can ignite if excess laser exposure or power density occurs and, once ignited, can sustain a torchlike flame. Hence, the use of plain PVC tubes during airway laser surgery is still very controversial.[24, 25] PVC may be the tube material of choice in selected patients (e.g., those with highly stenotic, friable airway lesions). In such patients, PVC tubes can be used if strict adherence to a protective protocol is followed.

Red Rubber Tubes

Red rubber tubes sustain combustion in room air more readily than do PVC tubes (see Table 78–4).[21] Thus, red rubber is susceptible to extraluminal fires; however, because it is more resistant to puncture by CO_2 laser energy than is PVC, intraluminal fires are less likely to occur.[26, 27] The surgeon and anesthesiologist may have more time to extinguish an extraluminal fire before it spreads to the O_2-rich environment inside the tube.

A disadvantage of red rubber tubes is their opacity. Should an intraluminal fire develop, it could go undetected for a longer period of time than it would if a PVC tube were used and, therefore, could cause more extensive damage. An advantage to red rubber tubes is that, if ignited, they are less likely than PVC tubes to soften, deform, or fragment into the tracheobronchial tree.

Silicone Tubes

Silicone, much like red rubber, can ignite in room air.[21] If ignited, it rapidly becomes a brittle ash that easily crumbles,[26]

resulting in retention of tube segments and debris in the tracheobronchial tree.

What Types of Injury Occur?

Combustion by-products of PVC, red rubber, and silicone can be highly toxic to the respiratory tract and are of obvious concern in this clinical setting.[26] However, thermal injury from a tracheal tube fire is of greater immediate concern and significance to a patient's outcome than is the inhalation of toxic by-products.[28]

Each of the three available conventional tracheal tube materials has its own advantages and disadvantages. Red rubber is perhaps the most popular material, followed by PVC; silicone is rarely used.

What Are Laser-Resistant Wraps?

Metallic Tape

In order to decrease the risk of fire, some practitioners wrap conventional tracheal tubes with metallic tape or metallic material–backed surgical sponges to shield the flammable tube from the laser beam. Laser-resistant wraps can prevent the laser from igniting the tracheal tube. However, metallic tape has not been specially made for this use; therefore, clinicians must employ tapes designed for nonmedical use. Metallic tape may reflect the laser beam toward nontargeted tissues, may have rough edges that can abrade mucosa, may cause the tube to kink, or may become dislodged and thus occlude the airway. When wrapping a tube, care must be taken to avoid gaps that can leave part of the tube exposed.

Tubes cannot be wrapped at or below the cuff, a region that is at high risk for laser contact[23]; thus, this area always remains exposed. The adhesive backing or surface coating of some tapes can be ignited by the laser. Not all metallic tapes protect all types of tubes from all types of lasers at every power setting (Table 78–6).[29–32] Of the commonly employed tapes, copper foil (Venture) and aluminum tape (3M 425) are the most widely applicable.

Metallic Sponge

A metallic material–based surgical sponge (Merocel) has been specially designed to wrap tracheal tubes for airway laser surgery. This preparation is preferred to metallic tape as it provides a smoother surface against the tracheal mucosa and is less likely to allow gaps in coverage. Since the sponge is

TABLE 78–6. Commonly Available Laser-Resistant Wrapping for Conventional Tracheal Tubes

Laser-Resistant Wrapping (Manufacturer)	Applicable Laser
Copper (3M)	CO_2, Nd.YAG, KTP
Aluminum (3M)	CO_2, Nd.YAG, KTP
Sensing foil (Radio Shack)	CO_2
Metal-backed sponge (Merocel)	CO_2, KTP

Abbreviation: KTP = potassium titanyl phosphate.

wetted with saline when in use, it absorbs the beam; the likelihood of reflection and damage to nontargeted tissue is thus minimized. The wetted sponge, however, swells and thickens the tube, making it less useful than metallic wrapping for small children and patients with highly stenotic airways. The sponge must be kept wet throughout the operation to prevent thermal injury, fire, and tissue abrasion. Like tape wrapping, the sponge wrapping may occlude the airway should it become dislodged, may cause tube kinking, and does not protect the distal portion of the tracheal tube, including the tracheal tube cuff.

Should Laser-Resistant Endotracheal Tubes Be Used?

All tube wrappings require tracheal tube preparation prior to clinical use. Thus, quality consistency depends on the anesthesiologist. In order to ensure a consistent level of laser resistance and general safety, anesthesiologists may prefer to purchase one of a number of commercially prepared laser-resistant tracheal tubes (Table 78–7). These products are specifically designed to resist damage from laser energy; yet, most of the tubes contain flammable components, and airway fires with their use have been reported.[33] Strict adherence to manufacturer warnings, precautions, and directions is highly advisable.

Laser-resistant tubes have properties that are quite different from those of standard PVC tubes,[29, 34] including decreased flexibility and ease of intubation, increased likelihood of kinking, and more difficult cuff inflation and deflation properties. Tubes composed in part or entirely of metal can be abrasive to the tracheal mucosa and may cause bleeding of friable lesions.

Metal tubes are thicker than standard tubes with the same outer diameter and, therefore, produce more resistance to ventilation. These tubes are 10- to 50-fold more expensive than PVC or red rubber tubes; thus, many practitioners still prefer to wrap their own tubes.

What Additional Protective Measures Should Be Taken?

Additional protective measures should be taken to prevent fire when flammable material is in the surgical field during airway laser operations.

Oxygen and Nitrous Oxide

Oxidizers should be strictly limited to the minimum concentration of O_2 needed to support a clinically acceptable arterial O_2 saturation. The balance of fresh gas flow should be helium or nitrogen, with potent nonflammable inhalation agents added as clinically indicated. Nitrous oxide should not be used because it is an oxidizer and, thus, can support ignition and sustain combustion.[21]

Helium

Helium reduces the risk of ignition of tracheal tubes that are made with either PVC or red rubber [27, 35] and has the additional advantage of facilitating gas flow through an area of obstruction in the airway. Even if helium is used, the fraction of inspired oxygen (FIO_2) should not exceed 0.4. With nitrogen, it should be <0.3 whenever feasible.[35] If a higher FIO_2 is needed to raise the arterial O_2 saturation, laser resection should be temporarily stopped while the patient is ventilated with O_2. When the saturation rises, the O_2 should be lowered and confirmed to be below the stated limits before laser resection is resumed.

Positive Airway Pressure

Positive pressure in the airway further reduces the risk of fire[36]; thus, positive end-expiratory pressure may be added to the respiratory circuit.

TABLE 78–7. Advantages and Disadvantages of Commonly Available Laser-Resistant Tracheal Tubes

Description of Resistant Tube (Manufacturer)	Applicable Laser	Advantages	Disadvantages
Aluminum/silicone spiral with self-inflating foam cuff (Bivona)	CO_2	Atraumatic external surface; cuff maintains seal even if punctured by laser; nonflammable inner surface	Contains flammable material (silicone); cuff difficult to deflate if punctured
Airtight, stainless steel, corrugated spiral with PVC tip and double cuff (Mallinckrodt)	CO_2, KTP	Tube maintains shape well; double cuff maintains seal after proximal cuff puncture; body of tube is nonflammable; noncuffed version available	Cuffed version contains flammable material (PVC); tubes are thick-walled; metal may reflect beam onto nontargeted tissue
Silicone tubes wrapped with aluminum and Teflon, with methylene blue in cuff (Xomed)	CO_2, KTP	Wrapping protects flammable material and is smoother than manual tape wrapping; methylene blue aids in detection of cuff perforation	Contains flammable material (silicone); single cuff is vulnerable to laser damage
Silicone elastomer with ceramic powder suspension (Fuji Systems)	CO_2, Nd.YAG	Atraumatic surfaces with general characteristics comparable with those of standard tubes	Ignites on exposure to laser energy in O_2-enriched environment; easily fragments and produces ash if burned

Power Density

Limitation of the laser to the lowest clinically acceptable power density also helps to prevent airway fires[27, 35] and limits the depth of burn and extent of tissue damage.

Tracheal Tube Cuff

Filling a tracheal tube cuff with saline instead of air is another precautionary measure[37]; addition of methylene blue or some other biocompatible dye to the saline may be useful to detect cuff perforation. To further protect the cuff, saline-soaked pledgets can be applied above it. The pledgets should be layered and carefully placed to reduce the possibility of laser penetration. If not kept wet, pledgets may ignite. Strings attached to a pledget, if nonmetallic, can be severed and ignited by a laser.

SPECIAL CONCERNS REGARDING THE LOWER RESPIRATORY TRACT DURING LASER SURGERY

For lesions below the larynx but above the carina, CO_2, Nd.YAG, or potassium-titanyl-phosphate wavelengths may be used. The longer CO_2 wavelength is usually preferred because tracheal perforation is less likely to occur than with the more penetrating shorter wavelengths. A bronchoscope commonly is employed.

Which Bronchoscope Should Be Used?

Rigid Metal

With any of these lasers, surgical access may be obtained with a rigid, metal bronchoscope, and ventilation may be maintained through the side arm of the bronchoscope. The risk of fire is low with a metal bronchoscope as long as a flammable cuff is not used to seal the airway. Saline-soaked gauze applied around the bronchoscope in the upper airway may be used instead of a cuff to maintain a seal during ventilation.

The FIO_2 is not of great concern if only metal is in the airway; however, in rare cases, a high FIO_2 may cause desiccated tissues to spark as they are resected, possibly leading to a fire. Helium added to the inspired gases not only decreases the risk of fire but also improves gas flow through the bronchoscope or past the obstructive airway lesion, or both. Special metal bronchoscopes with a matte finish are available for laser bronchoscopy; with these bronchoscopes, a reflected beam is diffused and less likely to injure nontargeted tissue.

Although it is difficult to keep the patient from inhaling smoke generated by laser resection during bronchoscopy, induced apnea during laser firing minimizes this possibility. After brief periods of resection, the field should be suctioned, the airway sealed, and the lungs ventilated. The effect of apnea on arterial O_2 saturation during such intermittent ventilation can be monitored by pulse oximetry. If the pulse oximeter response time is adjustable, use of the rapid response mode is recommended. This mode allows the earliest detection of desaturation and also heralds the desired response to ventilation faster than if the instrument default response time setting were used.

For lesions below the carina, the Nd.YAG beam is most often used because it can be transmitted by fiberoptic cable. The surgeon can, therefore, access the field with either a rigid (metal) or flexible bronchoscope. A metal bronchoscope is preferred by most bronchoscopists during general anesthesia because its rigidity provides better access for biopsy, suctioning, and ventilation.[38, 39] Ventilation may be maintained by any of several techniques, including side arm–bag ventilation or jet ventilation through either the side arm or a tracheal catheter.[38]

A metal bronchoscope reduces the risk of fire, but suction catheters and the fiberoptic cable carrying the laser beam are potential sources of ignition.[12] The risk of fire is increased as the cable becomes soiled with darkened, charred tissue because the Nd.YAG's wavelength is highly absorbed by these darkly pigmented materials. Thus, care must be taken to keep the fiberoptic tip clean throughout the laser procedure.

Flexible Fiberoptic

Small, distal airway lesions may be inaccessible with a rigid bronchoscope; in such cases, a fiberoptic bronchoscope may be used for Nd.YAG laser resection. When a fiberoptic endoscope is used, anesthesia may consist of a topical agent with intravenous sedation. This approach requires a very cooperative patient because bronchial perforation may easily occur if the patient moves and displaces the targeted tissue. Ventilation and oxygenation may be difficult to control without tracheal intubation, and smoke inhalation is highly likely in a conscious, spontaneously breathing patient.

When general anesthesia is used, the fiberoptic bronchoscope can be inserted through a large-diameter tracheal tube. Clear plastic tracheal tubes with no markings are less vulnerable to damage by the Nd.YAG laser than are standard PVC tubes with markings and radiopaque stripe or red rubber tubes.[40] If the PVC tube is soiled with blood or mucus, however, ignitability is greatly increased.[41] Since the beam is delivered either through the tube or distal to its tip, wrapping the outer surface with metallic tape does not protect it during distal laser bronchoscopy. Activating the laser during an end-inhalation pause and suctioning laser plume in the proximal airway during exhalation minimize the volume of inhaled smoke and debris.

In addition to the tracheal tube, the flexible endoscope may also ignite.[12] Ventilation with the lowest clinically acceptable FIO_2 in helium is likely to further decrease the risk of fire, but safe limits for FIO_2 and power density have not been determined for this system. Therefore, metal bronchoscopes are preferred over flexible bronchoscopes (whenever possible) for lower airway laser operations.

MANAGEMENT OF AIRWAY FIRE

Because the risk of fire cannot be completely eliminated when a laser is used in the airway, the operating room team should prepare and rehearse for airway fire and must be constantly on the alert.[42] If immediate steps are followed to prevent fire from extending down the tracheobronchial tree (Table 78–8) and if appropriate secondary steps are taken in evaluation and treatment, the morbidity from a laser fire is minimized.

If a fire occurs, disconnecting the breathing circuit from the tracheal tube is the quickest method of stopping the gas flow;

TABLE 78–8. Response Algorithm for Airway Fire During Laser Operations on the Airway

	Steps	Measures
Immediate	1.	Disconnect O_2 source at Y-piece and remove burning objects from the airway
	2.	Irrigate site with water if fire is still smoldering
	3.	Ventilate the patient by mask or reintubate the patient and ventilate with as low a fraction of inspired O_2 as possible
Secondary	4.	Evaluate extent of injury using bronchoscopy and laryngoscopy
	5.	Reintubate the patient or perform a tracheostomy if needed
	6.	Monitor with oximetry and arterial blood gas analysis and serial chest radiographs
	7.	Use ventilatory support, steroids, and antibiotics as needed

the fire intensity is reduced by cutting off the O_2 supply. Since the intense heat from the fire lingers in the tracheal tube, it should be simultaneously removed to minimize thermal and chemical damage to the airway. Any smoldering materials should be irrigated with water immediately.

If no obvious tube fragments or other foreign material are present in the airway, the patient may be reintubated or ventilated by mask. Ventilation should initially be resumed with as low an FIO_2 as clinically feasible to avoid rekindling of undetected smoldering material.

After these immediate steps have been taken, the airway must be evaluated more thoroughly by bronchoscopy and laryngoscopy to assess the extent and severity of injury (see Table 78–8). The duration of monitoring and the need for respiratory support and treatment are based on this evaluation. Steroids and antibiotics are generally not recommended for prophylactic use in this setting.

References

1. American National Standards Institute: American national standard for the safe use of lasers. ANSI Z136.1, 1986.
2. Garden JM, O'Banion MK, Shelnitz LS, et al: Papillomavirus in the vapor of carbon dioxide–treated verrucae. JAMA 1988; 259:1199.
3. Ferenczy A, Bergeron C, Richart RM: Carbon dioxide laser energy disperses human papillomavirus deoxyribonucleic acid onto treatment fields. Am J Obstet Gynecol 1990; 163:1271.
4. Tomita Y, Mihashi S, Nagata K, et al: Mutagenicity of smoke condensates induced by CO_2 laser irradiation and electrocauterization. Mutat Res 1981; 89:145.
5. Kokosa J, Eugene J: Chemical composition of laser-tissue interaction smoke plume. J Laser Appl 1989; 2:59.
6. Freitag L, Chapman G, Sielczak M, et al: Laser smoke effect on the bronchial system. Lasers Surg Med 1987; 7:283.
7. Baggish MS, Elbakry M: The effects of laser smoke on the lungs of rats. Am J Obstet Gynecol 1987; 156:1260.
8. ECRI: The devastation of patient fires. Health Dev 1992; 21:3.
9. Bauman N: Laser drape fires: how much of a risk? Laser Med Surg News Adv 1989; 7:2.
10. Snow JC, Norton ML, Saluja TS, et al: Fire hazard during CO_2 laser microsurgery on the larynx and trachea. Anesth Analg 1976; 55:146.
11. Hirshman CA, Smith J: Indirect ignition of the endotracheal tube during carbon dioxide laser surgery. Arch Otolaryngol 1980; 106:639.
12. Casey KR, Fairfax WR, Smith SJ, et al: Intratracheal fire ignited by the Nd-YAG laser during treatment of tracheal stenosis. Chest 1983; 84:295.
13. Challener RC, Kaufman B: Fatal venous air embolism following sequen-

tial unsheathed (bare) and sheathed quartz fiber Nd:YAG laser endometrial ablation. Anesthesiology 1990; 73:548.
14. Mallow A, Chabot L: Laser Safety Handbook. New York, Van Nostrand Reinhold, 1978, pp 133–138.
15. Ball K: Lasers: the perioperative challenge. Philadelphia, CV Mosby, 1990, pp 185–196.
16. Fried M: Complications of CO_2 laser surgery of the larynx. Laryngoscope 1983; 93:275.
17. Rontal E, Rontal M, Wenokur ME: Jet insufflation anesthesia for endolaryngeal laser surgery: a review of 318 consecutive cases. Laryngoscope 1985; 95:990.
18. Ganfield RA, Chapin JW: Pneumothorax with upper airway laser surgery. Anesthesiology 1982; 56:398.
19. Wegrzynowicz ES, Jensen JF, Pearson KS, et al: Airway fire during jet ventilation for laser excision of vocal cord papillomata. Anesthesiology 1992; 76:468.
20. Johan TG, Reichart TJ: An insufflation device for anesthesia during subglottic carbon dioxide laser microsurgery in children. Anesth Analg 1984; 63:368.
21. Wolf GL, Simpson JI: Flammability of endotracheal tubes in oxygen and nitrous oxide–enriched atmosphere. Anesthesiology 1987; 67:236.
22. Pashayan AG, Gravenstein JS, Cassisi NJ, et al: The helium protocol for laryngotracheal operations with CO_2 laser: a retrospective review of 523 cases. Anesthesiology 1988; 68:801.
23. Pashayan AG, Gravenstein N: High incidence of CO_2 laser beam contact with the tracheal tube during operations on the upper airway. J Clin Anesth 1989; 1:354.
24. Sosis M: Polyvinylchloride endotracheal tubes are hazardous for CO_2 laser surgery (Letter to the editor). Anesthesiology 1988; 69:801.
25. Pashayan AG, Gravenstein JS, Cassisi NJ, et al: Polyvinylchloride endotracheal tubes are hazardous for CO_2 laser surgery (Reply). Anesthesiology 1988; 69:801.
26. Ossoff RH, Eisenmann TS, Duncavage JA, et al: Comparison of tracheal damage from laser-ignited endotracheal tube fires. Ann Otol Rhinol Laryngol 1983; 92:333.
27. Ossoff ARG: Laser safety in otolaryngology—head and neck surgery: anesthetic and educational considerations for laryngeal surgery. Laryngoscope 1989; 99(Suppl 48):1–26.
28. Bingham HG, Gallagher TJ, Singleton GT, et al: Carbon dioxide laser burn of laryngotracheobronchial mucosa. J Burn Care Rehab 1990; 11:64.
29. ECRI: Laser-resistant endotracheal tubes and wraps. Health Dev 1990; 19:107.
30. Sosis MB: Evaluation of five metallic tapes for protection of endotracheal tubes during CO_2 laser surgery. Anesth Analg 1989; 68:392.
31. Sosis M, Dillon F: What is the safest foil tape for endotracheal tube protection during Nd-YAG laser surgery?: a comparative study. Anesthesiology 1990; 72:553.
32. Sosis M, Braverman B, Ivankovich AD: Evaluation of foil coverings for protecting endotracheal tubes from KTP laser (Abstract). Anesthesiology 1991; 75:A501.
33. Sosis MB: Airway fire during CO_2 laser surgery using a Xomed Laser endotracheal tube. Anesthesiology 1990; 72:747.
34. ECRI: Laser-resistant tracheal tubes. Health Dev 1992; 21:4.
35. Pashayan AG, Gravenstein JS: Helium retards endotracheal tube fires from carbon dioxide lasers. Anesthesiology 1985; 62:274.
36. SanGiovanni CM, Pashayan AG, Gater RA, et al: Intraluminal gauge pressure of tracheal tubes and risk of fire from CO_2 lasers: clinical model (Abstract). Anesthesiology 1991; 75:A399.
37. Sosis M, Dillon FX: Saline-filled cuffs help prevent CO_2 laser–induced PVC endotracheal tube fires. Anesth Analg 1991; 72:187.
38. Van der Spek AFL, Spargo PM, Norton ML: The physics of lasers and implications for their use during airway surgery. Br J Anaesth 1988; 60:709.
39. Brutinel WM, Cortese DA, Edell LES, et al: Complications of Nd:YAG laser surgery (Editorial). Chest 1988; 94:902.
40. Geffin B, Shapshay SM, Bellack GS, et al: Flammability of endotracheal tubes during Nd-YAG laser application in the airway. Anesthesiology 1986; 65:511.
41. Sosis M, Dillon FX: Hazards of a new, clear unmarked polyvinylchloride tracheal tube designed for use with the Nd-YAG laser. J Clin Anesth 1991; 3:358.
42. Schramm VL Jr, Mattox DE, Stool SE: Acute management of laser-ignited intratracheal explosion. Laryngoscope 1981; 91:1417.

CHAPTER 79

Extracorporeal Shock Wave Lithotripsy

VINOD MALHOTRA, M.D.

Extracorporeal shock wave lithotripsy (ESWL) is a technique in which shock waves are used to break kidney stones. First introduced in the United States in 1984, ESWL has been aptly described as a well-engineered, highly selective application of brute force. The first clinical model of the lithotripter in the United States was the Dornier HM3. This lithotripter employed a water bath into which the patient was immersed; the shock waves were produced at the base of the tub.[1, 2] This clinical model is still in common use. More recent lithotripter designs do not employ a water bath. However, the technical aspects of shock wave production and its application to kidney stone disintegration remain similar among most lithotripters.

TECHNICAL ASPECTS

What Are the Anesthesiologist's Concerns?

The Dornier HM3 lithotripter requires that the patient be immersed in a water bath and secured in a gantry chair in a semi-reclining position during treatment (Fig. 79–1). The gantry chair and its metal frame are hydraulically elevated close to the ceiling and then transferred along rails until they are above the water bath; it is then lowered into the bath. The patient can be immersed up to his or her clavicles.

The shock wave is produced at the base of the tub by an electrode to which 18 to 24 kV of electricity is applied. This electrical energy produces a spark across the gap of the electrode, with resultant explosive vaporization of water and the generation of a mechanical pressure wave (the so-called "shock wave"). The shock wave is generated in the first of two focal points (F_1) in an ellipsoid reflector; it is then reflected to the second focal point (F_2) (Fig. 79–2).

The position of the patient and the gantry chair is adjusted with the aid of biplanar fluoroscopy to bring the kidney stone into F_2. Shock waves travel through the water and through body tissue without causing much tissue injury and with little loss of energy because the acoustic impedance of water and of body tissues is approximately the same. However, when the focused shock waves encounter the kidney stone, they come across a change of medium with an interphase of water and the solid stone. The physical properties of the shock wave are such that when it encounters a different substance (kidney stone), energy dissipation on the order of several hundred atmospheres occurs at the interface. This energy is ultimately responsible for stone disintegration. If it encounters other interfaces (e.g., lung, pacemaker, bone, or orthopedic hardware), complications may result.

For the shock wave to be effective, the stone must remain in focus (i.e., at F_2), since the shock wave energy decreases rapidly along the blast path on either side of this focal point.[3] The anesthesiologist must consider and plan to minimize movement of the diaphragm, which causes movement of the kidney.

PREOPERATIVE CONSIDERATIONS

What Factors Must Be Assessed?

Special considerations include the patient's size, weight, body habitus, stone burden, and pregnancy status as well as the possible presence of a pacemaker, bleeding disorders, urosepsis, and chronic obstructive lung disease (Table 79–1).

Body Habitus

The patient's size is occasionally a limiting factor in ESWL, since the gantry chair is designed to be used with adults who are not taller than 6 ft 3 inches. The weight limitation on the Dornier HM3 lithotripter is 135 kg. Body habitus is important in extremely obese individuals. Once an obese patient is positioned in the gantry chair and lowered into the tub, the urologist may be unable to bring the kidney stone into F_2 either because the patient's back hits the bottom of the ellipsoid reflector or because his or her abdomen strikes the image intensifiers.

Generally, this group of patients tends to be at increased risk for anesthesia and airway management problems. Hence, the possibility of successful lithotripsy must be carefully determined prior to the administration of anesthesia. Trial positioning in the lithotripter without anesthesia can be attempted to ascertain whether the kidney stone can be visualized and brought into the treatment zone. If positioning is successful, anesthesia can be induced.

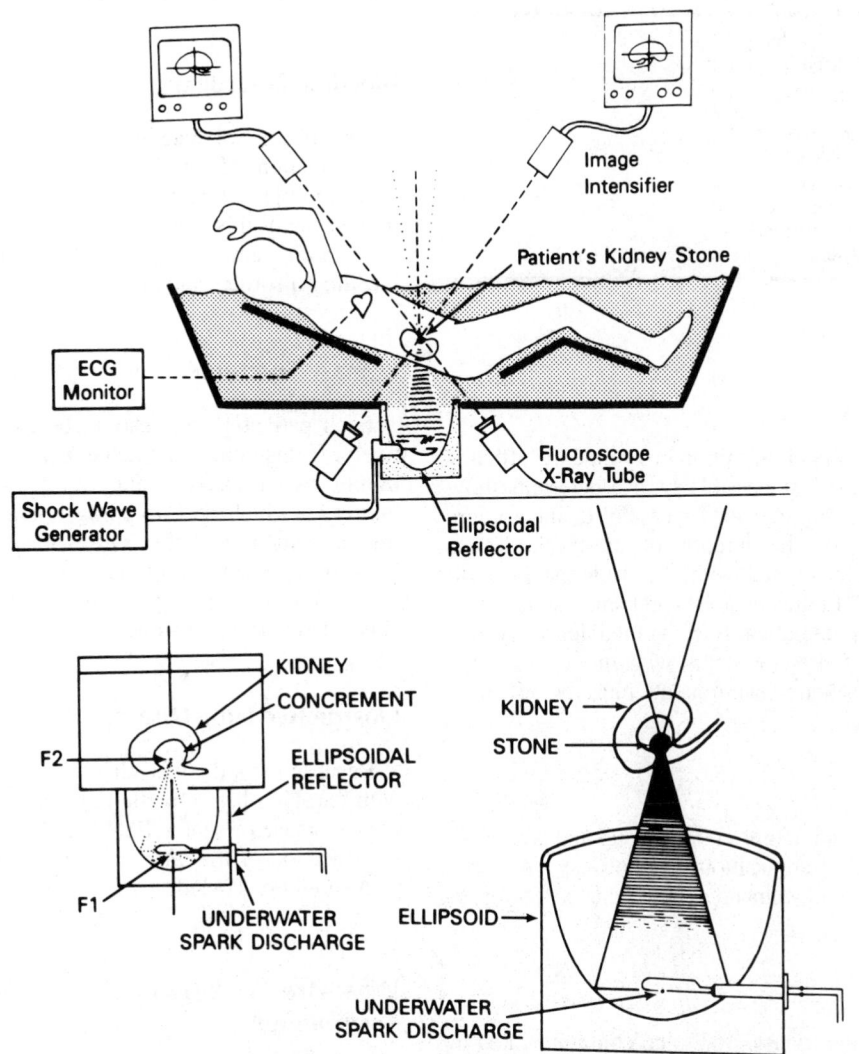

FIGURE 79–1. Patient secured in a gantry chair in a semi-reclining position. (From Hunter PT II: The physics and geometry pertinent to ESWL. *In* Principles of Extracorporeal Shock Wave Lithotripsy. Riehle RA Jr, Newman RC (eds). New York, Churchill Livingstone, 1987, p 14.)

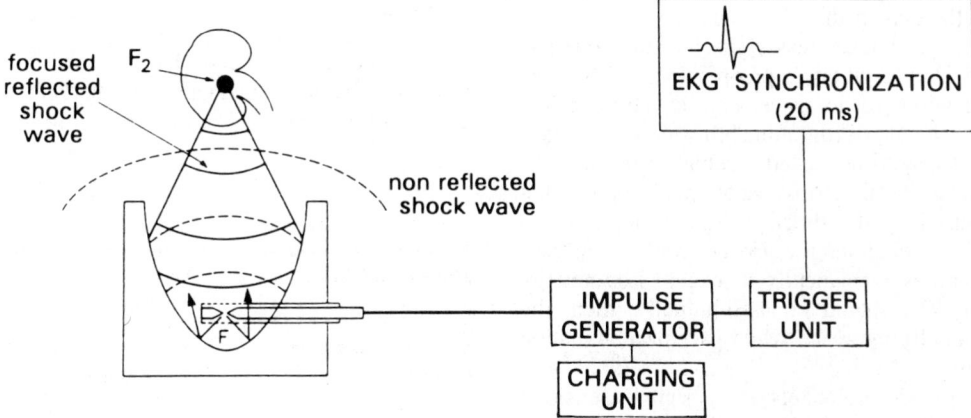

FIGURE 79–2. Technical aspects of ESWL.

TABLE 79–1. Preoperative Considerations of Special Interest for Lithotripsy

- Patient size, weight, body habitus
- Stone size, location, visibility
- Pregnancy (contraindication)
- Pacemakers
    Pectoral: Special precaution
    Abdominal: Contraindication
    Pacemaker wire location
- Bleeding disorders (contraindication)
- Urinary tract infection, septic shower
- Chronic obstructive pulmonary disease (location of lung base)

Stone Characteristics

Stone size, location, and composition determine the efficacy of the procedure in most instances. They also determine how many shock waves are required for successful disintegration, which in turn impacts on the duration of anesthesia. These parameters should be discussed with the urologist prior to anesthetic induction. Radiolucent stones and small stones may not be visualized when the patient is in the tub. Hence, cystoscopy and placement of ureteral stents with injection of dye may be required. Anesthetic requirements must be modified accordingly.

Pregnancy

Pregnancy testing in women of child-bearing age is a must, since pregnancy is a contraindication to lithotripsy.[4] A negative test result must be documented in the record prior to lithotripsy.

Pacemakers

Lithotripsy is no longer considered to be contraindicated in patients with pacemakers. The only exception to this general statement concerns patients with abdominally placed pacemaker generators that are used for epicardial pacing. Since this generator is in the blast path of the shock wave, such patients should not be treated with lithotripsy. However, most pacemaker generators are in a pectoral location and, thus, are at a safe distance from the blast path.

A patient with a pacemaker needs special attention, and special precautions should be taken preoperatively. The type of pacemaker, indications for its placement, degree of patient dependence, and pacemaker programmability must be determined prior to lithotripsy. A dedicated pacemaker programmer should be available in the lithotripsy suite should pacemaker malfunction be caused by the shock waves. In addition, an alternative means of pacing should also be available in case the pacemaker becomes permanently damaged. Low-energy shock waves (<16 kV) should be used initially; then, the energy level is gradually increased while pacemaker function is monitored carefully.

Dual-chamber demand pacemakers are especially sensitive to shock waves. They may need to be programmed to a ventricular pacing mode or switched from demand to nondemand pacing so that lithotripsy can be conducted safely. If all of the

discussed precautions are observed, patients with pacemakers can be treated safely with ESWL.[5–7]

Bleeding Disorders

Any history of bleeding disorder should be obtained, and determination of prothrombin time, partial thromboplastin time, and platelet count should be ordered. Almost all patients treated with lithotripsy develop hematuria; occasionally, a perinephric hematoma occurs. For these reasons, patients with bleeding disorders should not undergo lithotripsy.[4]

Urinary Tract Infection

Each patient's urine should be free of infection preoperatively. If this goal is not achievable because the stone is functioning as an abscess nidus, the patient should receive antibiotics to which the offending organism is sensitive. ESWL trauma, which inevitably causes bleeding, predisposes the patient to bacteremia; a septic shower can result. This problem may occur in a patient with sterile urine if an abscess is concealed within the stone.

Obstructive Lung Disease

Because the kidney is adjacent to the diaphragm, the patient with chronic obstructive lung disease and hyperinflated lungs is at increased risk for ESWL-induced pulmonary contusion. The location of the lung bases in relation to the ESWL blast path should be considered.

What Are the Risks of Gantry Chair Positioning?

Positioning in the gantry chair presents risks of mechanical trauma, brachial plexus injury, and postural hypotension (Table 79–2).

Trauma

Even though the metal chair is padded, trauma can result from pressure, scraping against metal, and hitting hard surfaces during patient transfer from a stretcher to the chair. In the tub,

TABLE 79–2. Risks of Positioning During Lithotripsy

Mechanical Trauma	Pressure injury
	Scraping
	Hitting the metal frame
Brachial Plexus Injury	Due to outstretched arms
Hypotension	Sitting position with sympathetic block
	Incidence
	Spinal: 27%
	Epidural: 18%
	General: 13%

the patient is placed with his or her arms spread around the imaging intensifiers in the water bath. This position predisposes to brachial plexus stretch injury, especially in lean subjects undergoing general anesthesia. Inflatable flotation sleeves on the forearms appear to eliminate these injuries.

Postural Hypotension

Sympathetic block and vasodilatation with venous pooling during general anesthesia and high epidural or spinal anesthesia frequently result in postural hypotension as a patient is changed from a supine position to the beach-chair position. A $\geq 20\%$ decrease in blood pressure following repositioning is common.

In my experience, the incidence of hypotension in patients undergoing general anesthesia is 13% compared with 18% in patients undergoing epidural anesthesia and 27% in those undergoing spinal anesthesia.[8] Adequate hydration and prudent use of vasopressors help to minimize these changes. If hypotension occurs, one available solution is to immerse the patient in the bath up to the midthoracic level.

PHYSIOLOGIC EFFECTS OF IMMERSION

The physiologic effects of immersion in water are quite important for patient management during ESWL. The most important changes are in cardiopulmonary function (see Table 79–3).

What Cardiovascular Changes Occur?

Filling Pressures

Cardiovascular changes that occur as a result of immersion up to the clavicles increase central blood volume, central venous pressure, and pulmonary artery pressures (Fig. 79–3).[9–14] Weber and coworkers demonstrated that the increases in central venous and pulmonary artery pressures closely correlate with the level of immersion.[9] With immersion to the clavicles, the central venous pressure may increase by as much as 10 to

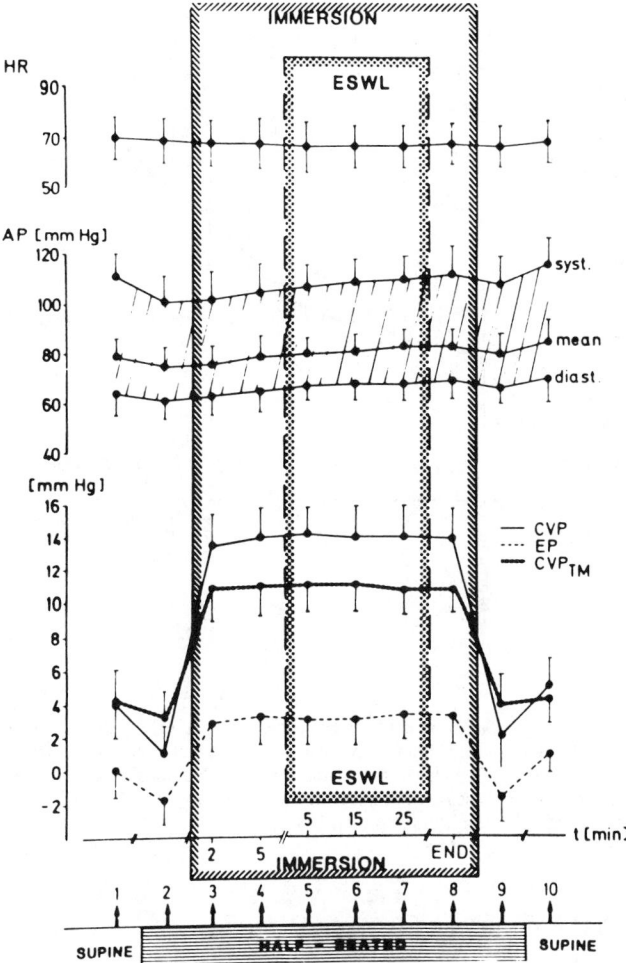

FIGURE 79–3. Effects of positioning, immersion, and emersion on heart rate (HR) (beats per minute); systolic (syst.), mean, and diastolic (diast.) arterial pressures (AP); and central venous (CVP) and esophageal (EP) pressures and transmural CVP (CVP$_{TM}$) in 25 patients during treatment with ESWL. The numbers along the bottom of the graph refer to the number of measurements. Mean and standard deviations are shown. (From Weber W, Madler C, Kerl B, et al: Cardiovascular effects of ESWL. *In* ESWL for Renal Stone Disease: Technical and Clinical Aspects. Gravenstein JS, Peter K (eds). Boston, Butterworth's, 1986, p 104.)

14 cm H$_2$O (Fig. 79–4). Pulmonary artery pressures increase accordingly.[9] Immersion to the umbilicus raises central venous pressure to its level when the patient is supine. Immersion to the xiphoid process increases central venous pressure by only half as much as does immersion to the clavicles.

Cardiac Output and Systemic Vascular Resistance

A recent study revealed a decrease in cardiac output and an increase in mean arterial pressure and systemic vascular resistance during ESWL performed with general anesthesia.[15] These hemodynamic changes are a source of serious concern for patients with advanced cardiovascular disease. Patients at risk for cardiac decompensation (i.e., those with congestive heart failure) are treated with minimal immersion so that only the shock wave entry site is covered by water. The exit site is left uncovered or covered with a wet towel.

TABLE 79–3. Immersion Effects During Lithotripsy

Cardiovascular	Increased stroke volume
	Increased central blood volume
	Increased cardiac output
	Increased central venous pressure
	Increased pulmonary arterial pressure
Respiratory Effects	Decreased functional residual capacity
	Decreased vital capacity
	Increased respiratory rate
	Decreased tidal volume
	Increased pulmonary capillary blood flow
Renal Effects	Decrease in antidiuretic hormone
	Natriuresis
	Diuresis
	Kaliuresis
	Decrease in prostaglandins
Body Temperature	Rapid change with bath temperature
	Hypothermia
	Hyperthermia

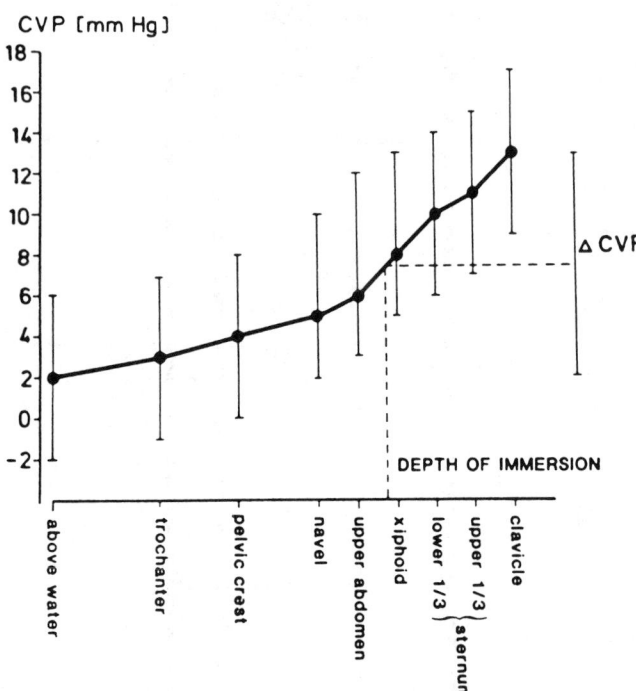

FIGURE 79–4. Change in central venous pressure (ΔCVP) of 21 patients as correlated to depth of immersion. Median values and ranges are shown. (From Weber W, Madler C, Kerl B, et al: Cardiovascular effects of ESWL. *In* ESWL for Renal Stone Disease: Technical and Clinical Aspects. Gravenstein JS, Peter K (eds). Boston, Butterworth's, 1986, p 105.)

What Pulmonary Changes Occur?

Pulmonary changes notable with immersion include a decrease in both functional residual capacity and vital capacity. The functional residual capacity may be decreased by 25% to 30%, and the vital capacity may be reduced by 20% to 30%.[13] In addition, since patients are strapped in the gantry chair and the straps across the abdomen are relatively tight, they tend to breathe with shallow, rapid respirations.[16] Pulmonary blood flow increases. These contrasting changes promote a mismatch of ventilation and perfusion, which, when combined with the altered breathing patterns, predisposes patients to hypoxemia if they are oversedated.

How Is Renal Function Altered?

The renal effects of immersion include a decrease in antidiuretic hormone and prostaglandins. The result is diuresis, natriuresis, and kaliuresis. These effects, however, do not acutely impact on anesthetic management.

Why Is Water Temperature Important?

Another important consideration is the effect of the temperature of the water in the bath on body temperature and on systemic vascular resistance. Since general and epidural anesthesia produce vasodilatation and reduce the patient's ability to compensate for temperature changes, any change in bath temperature rapidly affects body temperature. Hypothermia and hyperthermia have been reported.[17, 18] The bath temperature is continuously displayed on the control console and should be inspected frequently. The thermoneutral temperature is from 35.5 °C to 36 °C. Higher temperatures increase vasodilatation and decrease systemic vascular resistance and blood pressure.

PATIENT SAFETY

What Are the Monitoring Requirements?

ESWL requires the dimming of room lights so that fluoroscopy can be conducted. Standard guidelines for monitoring should be followed. However, certain special considerations are important. Because of the patient's remote location and the darkness, all monitors should be well lit, and all monitoring cables should be sufficiently long.

If general anesthesia is used, extra-long or double-length breathing circuits are required to cover the distances between the stretcher, the gantry chair, and the tub. Electrocardiographic electrodes are attached to the shoulder in the V_5 position and covered with an occlusive drape. Pulse oximetry is performed with an ear probe that is kept dry. Noninvasive blood pressure and respiratory gas monitoring is unaffected by the ESWL environment.

How Does Lithotripter Grounding Ensure Patient Safety?

Consider that a patient is immersed in a tub of water with an electrode to which 18 to 24 kV of electrical energy is applied. These facts underscore the importance of understanding lithotripter grounding. An intricate grounding system for the bath tub and ellipse is in place to ensure that leakage currents, including electrostatic and electromagnetic currents, do not reach the patient. The electrode is surrounded by a cage of six copper wires that quench any build-up of electrostatic or electromagnetic energy during the so-called "jitter period."[19]

Does the Electrode Cause Cardiac Dysrhythmias?

The electrical energy generated by the electrode is rapidly attenuated by the lithotripter and ellipse grounding. The attenuation ratio between F_1 (the tip of the electrode) and the rim of the ellipse (which might come in contact with the patient's body) is on the order of 1:10,000. Thus, electrical energy reaching the rim may be as low as 20 V. Based on this data, the current density that reaches the myocardium if the patient's back is in direct contact with the ellipse rim is 5×10 mA · cm^{2-1}. This value is $\frac{1}{100}$ of the current density delivered by a pacemaker that is connected directly to the myocardium. Furthermore, the duration of the ESWL current (6–10 μs) is also $\frac{1}{100}$ of that delivered by a pacemaker that is directly applied to the heart. Hence, escape currents from the electrode are unlikely to produce cardiac dysrhythmias during lithotripsy.[19]

Why Do Cardiac Dysrhythmias Occur?

Cardiac dysrhythmias do occur during lithotripsy. They are thought to be caused by the mechanical forces of the shock

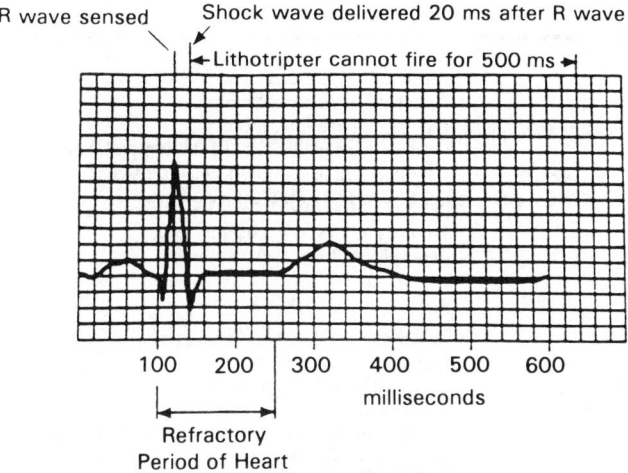

R wave sensed

Shock wave delivered 20 ms after R wave

Lithotripter cannot fire for 500 ms

100   200   300   400   500   600

milliseconds

Refractory
Period of Heart

FIGURE 79–5. Timing of the delivered shock wave in relation to the R wave and refractory period. (From Weber W, Bach P, Wildgans H, et al: Anesthetic considerations in patients with cardiac pacemakers undergoing ESWL. Anesth Analg 1988; 67:S251. © Williams & Wilkins, 1988.)

waves that pass through the conduction system of the heart. To reduce the incidence of these dysrhythmias, the shock wave is synchronized with a patient's electrocardiogram at 20 ms following the R wave. This technique ensures that the shock wave is delivered during and is followed by a 300- to 500-ms refractory period (Fig. 79–5). Despite this, 10% to 14% of patients experience dysrhythmias; these dysrhythmias commonly include premature atrial contractions or premature ventricular complexes.[20] Occasionally, supraventricular tachycardia occurs but this typically reverts as soon as the shock wave treatment is stopped.[21]

The timing and refractory period of the firing mechanism effectively limit the treatment rate to 120 to 130 shocks per minute. At rapid heart rates, the lithotripter blocks down and treats at one-half the heart rate. The lithotripter should never be fired by hand. Also, one must take care not to allow extraneous artifact (e.g., patient shivering or twitch monitor use) to create an electrocardiographic artifact that the lithotripter might use as a trigger.

STONE MOVEMENT

What Is Its Significance?

For the shock wave to be effective, the stone must lie in the second focus, since maximum pressure energy is delivered at this point. Beyond this point, the pressure energy decreases in an exponential fashion.[3] As the diaphragm moves up and down, so do the kidney and the kidney stone. Hence, the patient's respiration must be such that the kidney stone remains in the second focus during respiratory excursions. Investigators have employed innovative techniques to control the respiratory excursions.[22–27]

High-Frequency Ventilation

High-frequency jet ventilation and high-frequency conventional ventilation have been studied. With the high-frequency jet ventilation, kidney stone movement can be significantly decreased, thereby increasing the efficacy of the shock wave treatment.[22] Some have claimed that a smaller number of shock

waves are needed for effective treatment.[23] However, several previously discussed variables come into play when one determines the efficacy of shock wave treatment. Most important, perhaps, is the personal preference of the urologist.

High-frequency, small-tidal-volume, conventional ventilation has also been used effectively to reduce the respiration-related excursion. However, the need for high-frequency techniques has been questioned.[27] Most anesthesiologists do not employ jet ventilation or high-frequency conventional ventilation in their practices and no data prove that shock wave treatment in their centers is any less effective than elsewhere. My approach is to use conventional ventilation and to ask the surgeon, who observes ventilation-induced stone movement during fluoroscopy, if the stone movement is a problem. If keeping the stone positioned in the F_2 zone is difficult, I institute high-frequency ventilation with the anesthesia ventilator.

Regional Anesthesia

In properly sedated patients receiving regional anesthesia, respiration-related stone movement is usually restricted to the F_2 zone.[28] The tidal volume can be reduced by coaching the patient or by carefully sedating him or her, or both.

What Is the Risk of Lung Injury?

Shock waves pass through most body tissues without causing significant tissue injury; however, air-filled lungs are exquisitely vulnerable.[29] If lung tissue is in the blast path, the shock wave travels through water and body tissues virtually unattenuated until it encounters the air in the lung. This water-to-air interface results in a dissipation of shock wave energy, resulting in trauma to the lung tissue. The usual injury includes alveolar rupture, hemorrhage, and hemoptysis. In animal experiments, even one shock wave has been shown to cause significant pulmonary damage and death.[29]

Lung injury has been reported in both adults and children.[30, 31] In pediatric patients, the distance between the kidney and the pulmonary bases is shorter than that in adults; this places their lungs at an increased risk of injury. It has been recommended that the lung bases in children be protected through the use of Styrofoam boards or Styrofoam tapes attached to their backs, as these materials can attenuate the shock waves.[32] In the child or chronic obstructive lung disease patient, the lung bases should be percussed at end-inspiration, and an electrocardiogram wire should be taped across the back at that level. The wire is readily visible during fluoroscopy, and its location can be compared with the blast path to ensure that the lung is not injured.

ANESTHETIC TECHNIQUE

What Are the Considerations in Selection?

Many anesthetic techniques have been employed successfully for lithotripsy.[33–38] Major determining factors include the anesthesiologist's preference and familiarity with the technique; the patient's preference; the surgeon's preference; and local conditions such as the location of the lithotripsy suite, the requirements for transport between the lithotripsy suite and

TABLE 79–4. Anesthetic Techniques: Advantages and Disadvantages Specific to Lithotripsy

Technique	Advantages	Disadvantages
General Anesthesia	Control of ventilation Control of patient movement High-frequency ventilation may be used Rapid induction time	Likelihood of positional injury Hypotension in sitting position Potential dangers associated with transporting an anesthetized patient if attendant procedures required Side effects and complications of general anesthesia
Epidural Anesthesia	Less likely to involve positional injury Attendant procedures can be done with the same anesthetic Can be reinforced as needed	Hypotension in sitting position Motor block of lower extremity Slow onset Side effects and complications of spinal anesthesia
Spinal Anesthesia	Fast onset More profound block Attendant procedures can be done	Cannot be reinforced Higher incidence of hypotension Spinal headache Side effects and complications of spinal anesthesia
Intercostal Block with Local Infiltration	Least likely to involve positional injury Attendant procedures can be done Hemodynamic stability Rapid recovery	May not be suitable for all patients Side effects and complications of intercostal block and local anesthetics Respiratory depression with decrease in hemoglobin saturation Patient movement
Sedoanalgesia (Maximum Alveolar Concentration)	Positional injury least likely Hemodynamic stability Simplicity Rapid recovery Best suited for lithotripters that do not use a water bath	Patient discomfort

the cystoscopy area, and the requirements for transport between the lithotripsy suite and the recovery room. Specific advantages and disadvantages of various techniques are listed in Table 79–4.

General Anesthesia

General anesthesia offers the advantages of rapid onset, controllability of respiration, and lack of patient movement during the procedure. Disadvantages include having to lift and transport a patient to and from the gantry chair, which contributes additional strain to the personnel and increases the possibility of positioning injury to the patient.

If general anesthesia is employed, extra-long anesthesia circuit tubing is required. Circuit disconnect is a possibility. Hypotension is also a concern, since the patient is placed in a sitting position. General anesthesia may also lead to difficulty in transporting patients between the cystoscopy and lithotripsy suites if these two areas are not adjacent, as well as to problems in transporting patients to the postanesthesia care unit, which may be far from the lithotripter.

Epidural Anesthesia

Epidural anesthesia offers the advantage of ease of transport. Since the upper torso and extremities are not anesthetized, a patient can help with positioning in the gantry chair; therefore, the likelihood of injury is decreased compared with that with general anesthesia. The same anesthetic can be used for additional procedures such as cystoscopy, placement of stents, and stone manipulation.

Disadvantages include slow anesthesia onset and a high incidence of hypotension when patients are in the sitting position[8]; epidural block must reach from the T-4 to the T-6 level to be adequate.

Patient movement in the tub usually is not a problem. Control of respiration-related stone movement must be modified with the use of intravenous sedatives in the very anxious patient.

Special precautions should be observed when identifying the epidural space. Air injected into the epidural space may account for some epidural tissue damage, since bubbles present an interface to the shock wave.[39] I place epidurals using normal saline or local anesthetic solution rather than air for loss-of-resistance epidural space identification. Korbon and associates reported changes in epidural compliance and pain on injection in repeat epidural anesthesia for multiple lithotripsy.[40] If air is used, its volume should be kept as small as possible.

Epidural catheters should be taped to the side opposite that being treated. Tape entraps some air bubbles, causing ecchymoses and attentuation of shock wave energy at the skin and reducing the efficacy of the shock waves that reach the kidney stone.[41]

Spinal Anesthesia

Spinal anesthesia offers an alternative to epidural anesthesia. It has the advantage of a more rapid onset, but it is associated with a higher incidence of hypotension when the patient is in the sitting position.[8] Since most patients are treated on an ambulatory basis, the likelihood of spinal headaches should also be considered.

Local Infiltration and Intercostal Block

Regional anesthesia (local infiltration of the flank and intercostal block) has been successfully used in ESWL.[34] It is the mainstay of anesthesia for lithotripsy at our institution, and we have successfully completed nearly 2000 treatments with its use. Advantages include minimal physiologic trespass and avoidance of hypotension. The patient can help himself or herself in and out of the gantry chair so that the likelihood of positional injury is reduced. For ambulatory patients, the time spent in the postanesthesia care unit is decreased. However, as with any regional technique, it may not be suitable for all patients. Some sedation is necessary to provide analgesia for the deep visceral discomfort, since the local anesthetic provides anesthesia for only the skin and the subcutaneous tissues.

Intravenous Techniques

Intravenous techniques of sedoanalgesia also have been successfully used.[36–38] Commonly employed regimens include combinations of midazolam and alfentanil, fentanyl and propofol, and midazolam and ketamine.[36, 37] Advantages include simplicity, hemodynamic stability, and a shorter recovery time. Disadvantages are occasional patient discomfort, patient movement, and respiratory depression.

Newer lithotripters do not employ a water bath and have a smaller focal zone and a lower induced pain intensity. These are especially conducive to the use of intravenous sedoanalgesia, with or without local infiltration anesthesia. Lithotripsy usually can be accomplished without sedation or field block.[38]

Miscellaneous Techniques

Other techniques have been tried with limited success and include the use of epidural opiates and interpleural anesthesia. The former, when used alone, have mixed success.[41–44] However, the addition of opiates to local anesthetics in the epidural space allows the use of a lower concentration of the local anesthetic, thereby decreasing the incidence of motor block. Interpleural anesthesia provides inadequate analgesia for ESWL.[45]

How Is the Anesthetic Choice Affected by Attendant Procedures?

Attendant procedures that are frequently associated with lithotripsy include cystoscopy, ureteroscopy, placement of stents, stone manipulation, and, in some cases, laser lithotripsy of lower ureteral stones. These procedures require anesthesia in addition to that necessary for ESWL and frequently modify the choice of anesthetic technique. In some cases, general anesthesia may be required for the attendant procedure more so than for the lithotripsy. If the patient needs to be transported from the lithotripsy suite to and then from a cystoscopy suite that is not adjacent to the lithotripsy suite, a regional anesthetic is preferable. If the location of the lithotripsy suite is quite far from the postanesthesia care unit (e.g., in a mobile unit), a regional anesthetic also may be preferable.

MISCELLANEOUS CONSIDERATIONS

How Is Postoperative Pain Managed?

Postoperatively, pain occurs mostly at the shock wave entry site; patients usually complain of flank discomfort. Most severe pain is caused by the passage of stone fragments, which occasionally results in ureteral obstruction and colic. However, the incidence of severe pain that requires parenteral narcotics is low enough that aggressive pain management with patient-controlled analgesia, epidural opioid analgesia, or other such modalities is unnecessary.[34] The majority of lithotripsy cases are done as outpatient procedures, making implementation of the aforementioned pain management techniques difficult. Parenteral and oral opioids and nonopioid analgesics usually suffice.

Are Occupational Hazards Associated with Lithotripsy?

Several occupational hazards unique to the lithotripsy suite are a concern to those who work regularly in these areas. Most notable are noise and radiation hazards. Shock wave noise levels as high as 110 dB have been recorded. Old electrodes make louder sounds when fired than do newer ones. The Occupational Safety and Health Administration (OSHA) recommends a maximum noise exposure of 90 dB for no longer than 8 hours.

Since shock waves are emitted intermittently and the noise with each shock wave lasts only a few milliseconds, the total exposure to personnel during any given day is far below the maximum in the government's recommendations. One must realize, however, that with intermittent noise, the protective stapedius reflex in the inner ear comes into play only after the exposure to sound; hence, the protection afforded by this reflex is not as effective as it is in the presence of continuous noise. Thus, personnel should use ear plugs or ear cups as a protective measure.[46, 47]

Radiation precautions are also necessary, since fluoroscopy is used with ESWL. The anesthesiologist should wear lead shielding because of his or her proximity to the fluoroscopy unit and to x-rays that are used intermittently throughout the procedure to verify that the stone target is still in the proper position.

SUMMARY

The newest generation of lithotripters requires little, if any, anesthesia or analgesia. The water bath has been eliminated, and the shock waves are instead generated within an enclosed water casing that comes in contact with the patient's flank via a plastic membrane. The absence of the water bath and of all of the physiologic consequences of anesthesia and immersion markedly simplify this form of therapy.

References

1. Chaussy CG, Fuchs GJ: World experience with ESWL for the removal of urinary stones: an assessment of its role after 5 years of clinical use. Endourology 1986; 1:7.
2. Drach DW, Dretler S, Fair W, et al: Report of the United States cooperative study of ESWL. J Urol 1986; 135:1127.
3. Gravenstein JS, Peter K (eds): ESWL for Renal Stone Disease: Technical and Clinical Aspects. Boston, Butterworth's, 1986, pp 9–28.
4. Gravenstein JS, Peter K (eds): ESWL for Renal Stone Disease: Technical and Clinical Aspects. Boston, Butterworth's, 1986, p 68.
5. Weber W, Bach P, Wildgans H, et al: Anesthetic considerations in patients with cardiac pacemakers undergoing ESWL. Anesth Analg 1988; 67:S251.
6. Markewitz A, Weber W, Wildgans H: Does ESWL affect pacemaker function? Pace 1987; 10(3/II):711.

7. Garza J, Tansey M, Florio J: The effect of ESWL on implantable cardiac pacemakers. Pace 1987; 10:675.
8. London RA, Kudlak T, Riehle RA: Immersion anesthesia for ESWL: review of two hundred twenty treatments. Urology 1986; 28:86–93.
9. Weber W, Chaussy C, Madler C, et al: Cardiocirculatory changes during anesthesia for ESWL. J Urol 1984; 4:246A.
10. Arborelius M Jr, Balldin UI, et al: Hemodynamic changes in man during immersion with head above water. Aerospace Med 1972; 43:592.
11. Begin R, Epstein M, Sackner MA, et al: Effects of water immersion to the neck on pulmonary circulation and tissue volume in man. J Appl Physiol 1976; 40:293.
12. Farhi LE, Linnarsson D: Cardiopulmonary readjustments during graded immersion in water at 35 degrees C. Respir Physiol 1977; 30:35.
13. Loellgen H, Von Neiding G, Howes R: Respiratory and hemodynamic adjustment during head out of water immersion. Int J Sports Med 1980; 1:25.
14. Risch WD, Koubenec HJ, Beckmann U, et al: The effect of graded immersion on heart volume, central venous pressure, pulmonary blood distribution, and heart rate in man. Pflugers Arch 1978; 374:115.
15. Behnia R, Shanks CA, Ovassapian A, et al: Hemodynamic responses associated with lithotripsy. Anesth Analg 1987; 66:354.
16. Bromage PR, Bonsu AK, el-Faqih SR, et al: Influence of Dornier HM3 system on respiration during extracorporeal shock-wave lithotripsy. Anesth Analg 1989; 68:363.
17. Higgins TL, Miller EV, Roberts J: Accidental hyperthermia as a complication of ESWL under general anesthesia. Anesth Analg 1987; 66:389.
18. Malhotra V: Hyperthermia and hypothermia as complications of ESWL. Anesthesiology 1987; 67:448.
19. Gravenstein JS, Peter K (eds): ESWL for Renal Stone Disease: Technical and Clinical Aspects. Boston, Butterworth's, 1986, pp 29–32.
20. Simon CA, LeHenzey NY, Baras E, et al: Cardiac arrhythmias during ESWL under general anesthesia. Anesthesiology 1986; 65:A147.
21. Walts LF, Atlee JL: Supraventricular tachycardia associated with ESWL. Anesthesiology 1986; 65:521.
22. Carlson CA, Boysen PG, Banner MJ, et al: Conventional vs HFJV for ESWL. Anesthesiology 1985; 63:A530.
23. Esch JS, Kochs E, Meyer WH: Improved efficiency of ESWL during HFJV. Anesthesiology 1985; 63:A177.
24. Carlson CA, Gravenstein JS, Banner MJ, et al: Monitoring techniques during anesthesia and HFJV for ESWL. Anesthesiology 1985; 63:A178.
25. Berger JJ, Boysen PG, Gravenstein J, et al: Failure of HFJV to ventilate patients adequately during ESWL. Anesth Analg 1987; 66:262.
26. Berger JJ, Boysen PG, Gravenstein JS, et al: Optimal settings for tidal volume with high frequency ventilation for ESWL. Anesthesiology 1986; 65:A485.
27. Perel A, Hoffman B, Podeh D, et al: High frequency conventional ventilation also minimizes respiratory-related movement of kidney stone during ESWL; is it, however, indicated? Anesthesiology 1986; 65:A160.
28. Malhotra V, Benetos F: Kidney stone movement with spontaneous respiration during ESWL with intercostal blocks and local infiltration anesthesia. Reg Anesth 1989; 14:39.
29. Chaussy CG: ESWL: New Aspects in the Treatment of Kidney Stone Disease. Munich, Karger, 1982, pp 24–35.
30. Malhotra V, Gomillion GC, Artusio JF: Hemoptysis in a child during ESWL. Anesth Analg 1989; 69:526.
31. Malhotra V, Rosen RJ, Slepian RL: Life-threatening hypoxemia in an adult due to shock-wave–induced pulmonary contusion. Anesthesiology 1991; 75:529.
32. Tredrea CR, Pathak D, From RP, et al: Lung protection in children during ESWL. Anesth Analg 1987; 66:S178.
33. Duvall JO, Griffith DP: Epidural anesthesia for ESWL. Anesth Analg 1985; 64:544.
34. Malhotra V, Long CW, Meister MJ: Intercostal blocks with local infiltration anesthesia for ESWL. Anesth Analg 1987; 66:85.
35. Abbott MA, Samuel JR, Webb DR: Anaesthesia for ESWL. Anaesthesia 1985; 40:1065.
36. Monk TG, Rater JM, White PF: Comparison of alfentanil and ketamine infusions in combination with midazolam for outpatient lithotripsy. Anesthesiology 1991; 74:1023.
37. Monk TG, Boure B, White PF, et al: Comparison of intravenous sedative-analgesic techniques for outpatient immersion lithotripsy. Anesth Analg 1991; 72:626.
38. Freilich JD, Brull SJ, Schiff S, et al: Anesthesia for lithotripsy: efficacy of monitored anesthesia care with alfentanil. Anesth Analg 1990; 70:S115.
39. Lander CJ, Korbon GA, Monk CR, et al: Epidural anesthesia and ESWL: pathologic effects on the epidural space. Anesthesiology 1987; 67:A227.
40. Korbon GA, Lunch C, Arnold WP, et al: Repeated epidural anesthesia for ESWL is unreliable. Anesth Analg 1987; 66:669.
41. Pandit SK, Powell RB, Crider B, et al: Epidural fentanyl is not effective for analgesia for ESWL. Anesthesiology 1988; 68:176.
42. Pandit SK, Powell RB, Crider B, et al: Epidural fentanyl: a simple and novel approach to anesthetic management for ESWL (Abstract). Anesthesiology 1987; 67:A225.
43. Bromage PR, Al-Faqih S, Kadiwal GH, et al: Evaluation of bupivacaine and fentanyl analgesia for ESWL. Anesthesiology 1987; 67:A226.
44. Gissen D, Naroll M, Katz RL: Epidural fentanyl for ESWL. Reg Anesth 1988; 13:40.
45. Stromskag KE, Steen PE: Comparison of interpleural and epidural anesthesia for ESWL. Anesth Analg 1988; 67:1181.
46. Arnold WP, Ruth RA, Ross WT, et al: The lithotripter as a sound hazard. Anesthesiology 1985; 63:A179.
47. Lusk RP, Tyler RS: Hazardous sound levels produced by ESWL. J Urol 1987; 137:1112.

CHAPTER 80

Outpatient Surgery

BURTON S. EPSTEIN, M.D.
RAAFAT S. HANNALLAH, M.D.

Spending a night in a hospital prior to the day of surgery is increasingly unusual for patients. Admission to a facility on the day of surgery should not result in a greater rate of complications or mortality than would occur with admission on the previous day; however, other issues are important to address. Approach to the patient, facility organization, and the goals of treatment have similarities and differences in both scenarios.

SCREENING

What Roles Must Be Fulfilled Before Surgery?

The Anesthesiologist

The anesthesiologist must ensure that the patient is aware of the anesthetic plan, agrees to it, and is adequately evaluated and that any problems are identified, corrected, or suitably controlled.

The Facility Personnel

The personnel of the facility in which the surgery will be performed must provide information in advance so that the admitting process is conducted expeditiously, accurately, and cordially.

The Surgeon and Referring Physician

Ideally, the primary physician refers the patient to a surgeon, and the results of the examination are conveyed not only to the patient but also back to the primary physician. Unfortunately, the primary physician may be notified that a surgical procedure is required but not be given the date and time of this event.

This omission may result in a series of misunderstandings. The patient and anesthesiologist assume that the surgeon has informed the primary physician. At the same time, the anesthesiologist may have been told little or nothing by either physi-

cian. Finally, the patient may know little or nothing about the nature of any comorbid condition, the adequacy of its control, or the drugs used to treat it. Clearly, the communication link between the patient and the three caregivers may not be ideal. Furthermore, in outpatient surgery, a place for sorting out problems and convening the group on the day of surgery usually is not available.

What Is the Purpose of a Preoperative Screening Clinic?

The clinic should be identified as the facility in which administrative and medical information is received, collected, and made readily available in an organized form for easy access and efficient use. Administrative information includes patient identification (facility/medical record number), insurance coverage, and the name of the closest relative or significant other. Medical information includes the results of any laboratory evaluation, data from the physician consultation, a list of current medications, and identification of allergies, if any.

Do All Facilities Need a Screening Clinic?

All facilities need to identify an area to which all relevant patient data are to be directed. Some individual must assume responsibility for this service. In a small urban or rural area in which the anesthesiologist, surgeon, and referring physician communicate about patient management problems routinely, it is not usually essential to require that a clinic be set up or that the patient visit the facility before the day of surgery. However, contact between the patient and a member of the anesthesia care team should be made before the day of surgery. A telephone call may suffice. The intent is to introduce the patient to the caregiver and to create an atmosphere in which questions may be asked by both and in which a satisfactory plan can be devised. If a special visit to meet with the anesthesiologist is recommended, it can be arranged at that time.

Must All Patients Visit an Existing Clinic?

Telephone Screening

In addition to the anesthesiologist's informal interview with the patient, some facilities have designed a formal telephone screening process.[1] In this process, a member of the anesthesia care team or a designee (e.g., physician's assistant, nurse practitioner, or registered nurse) telephones the patient using a predetermined problem checklist. An example of one checklist used at Childrens' National Medical Center (CNMC) in Washington, D.C., is shown in Figure 80–1.

When certain risk factors are identified during the telephone call, a determination is made whether to have the patient come to the hospital for a special visit or whether additional information needs to be obtained from the attending physician.

Clinic Visits

In other screening clinic models, all or some patients are required to visit the facility before the day of the scheduled surgery. When all patients visit, interviews are scheduled with anesthesia personnel, appropriate laboratory tests are performed, and administrative processing is done. When only some patients are required to visit, the decision whether a preoperative visit is necessary is usually based on perceived risk factors (Table 80–1). A visit may also be required to expedite the admission process (e.g., in the case of a patient scheduled as the first case of the day).

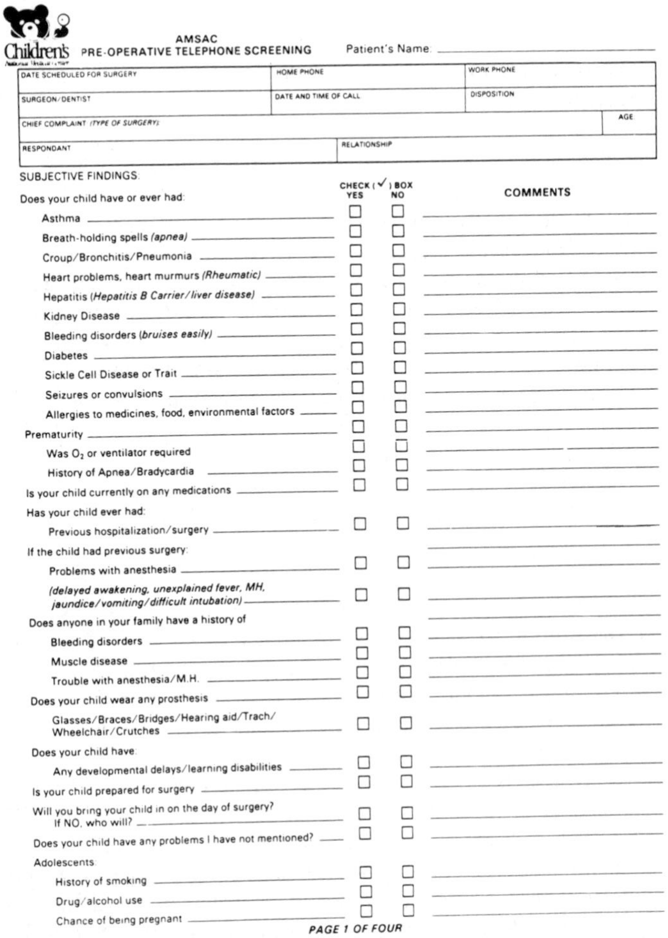
Children's
AMSAC
PRE-OPERATIVE TELEPHONE SCREENING   Patient's Name: ______

DATE SCHEDULED FOR SURGERY	HOME PHONE	WORK PHONE
SURGEON/DENTIST	DATE AND TIME OF CALL	DISPOSITION
CHIEF COMPLAINT (TYPE OF SURGERY)		AGE
RESPONDANT	RELATIONSHIP	

SUBJECTIVE FINDINGS:

	CHECK (✓) BOX YES	NO	COMMENTS
Does your child have or ever had:			
Asthma	☐	☐	
Breath-holding spells *(apnea)*	☐	☐	
Croup/Bronchitis/Pneumonia	☐	☐	
Heart problems, heart murmurs *(Rheumatic)*	☐	☐	
Hepatitis *(Hepatitis B Carrier/liver disease)*	☐	☐	
Kidney Disease	☐	☐	
Bleeding disorders *(bruises easily)*	☐	☐	
Diabetes	☐	☐	
Sickle Cell Disease or Trait	☐	☐	
Seizures or convulsions	☐	☐	
Allergies to medicines, food, environmental factors	☐	☐	
Prematurity	☐	☐	
Was O_2 or ventilator required	☐	☐	
History of Apnea/Bradycardia	☐	☐	
Is your child currently on any medications	☐	☐	
Has your child ever had:			
Previous hospitalization/surgery	☐	☐	
If the child had previous surgery:			
Problems with anesthesia	☐	☐	
(delayed awakening, unexplained fever, MH, jaundice/vomiting/difficult intubation)	☐	☐	
Does anyone in your family have a history of			
Bleeding disorders	☐	☐	
Muscle disease	☐	☐	
Trouble with anesthesia/M.H.	☐	☐	
Does your child wear any prosthesis	☐	☐	
Glasses/Braces/Bridges/Hearing aid/Trach/ Wheelchair/Crutches	☐	☐	
Does your child have:			
Any developmental delays/learning disabilities	☐	☐	
Is your child prepared for surgery	☐	☐	
Will you bring your child in on the day of surgery? If NO, who will?	☐	☐	
Does your child have any problems I have not mentioned?	☐	☐	
Adolescents:			
History of smoking	☐	☐	
Drug/alcohol use	☐	☐	
Chance of being pregnant	☐	☐	

PAGE 1 OF FOUR

FIGURE 80–1. Children's National Medical Center predetermined problem checklist for telephone screening. (Courtesy of Children's National Medical Center, Washington, DC.)

TABLE 80–1. Perceived Risk Factors for Outpatient Surgery

- Age over 65 y
- Major organ system involvement
- ASA physical status class 3 or 4
- "Major" surgical procedure in conjunction with one or more of the preceding factors

Is Anesthesia Outcome Influenced by Advance Screening?

Major morbidity and mortality after outpatient surgery and anesthesia are so low that statistical evidence of improving outcome by screening is lacking. Screening, however, may result in a reduction in the rate of cancellation of surgery; without it, inadequate evaluation and patient preparation may occur.[1, 2] Although screening avoids or minimizes delays and postponements, at least one report suggests that the information obtained does not always change the risk for adverse events in the perioperative period.[3] In addition, discharge planning and the need to consult with social services representatives are best managed before the day of surgery. Issues that can be addressed are noted on a patient discharge planning questionnaire such as that shown in Figure 80–2.

What Laboratory Tests Are Required or Indicated?

Institutions, facilities, and local and state governments are attempting to define laboratory tests that can be used to identify patient risk factors and improve outcome. This approach is intended to reduce unnecessary testing and the cost of health care. The Joint Commission on the Accreditation of Healthcare Organizations (JCAHO) does not require any specific testing but it does depend on each facility to define those tests that are needed. The American Society of Anesthesiologists (ASA) has issued the *Statement on Routine Preoperative Laboratory and Diagnostic Screening* (Table 80–2).[4] As a result of the publication of this and other such documents, some facilities do not require any laboratory testing on healthy young individuals.

Most authorities agree that the best source for determining which test or tests are needed is an accurate patient history. Roizen has developed a standardized evaluation known as the "Health Quiz." From the results of this quiz, he derives a "Simplified Strategy for Preoperative Testing" (Table 80–3).[5] This strategy requires that an accurate history be obtained on every patient.

Which Patients Are Unacceptable Candidates?

When modern outpatient surgery was evolving in the late 1960s and early 1970s, the list of unacceptable candidates was lengthy. As more and more experience has been gained in judging outcome and as the age and risk of a patient have

THE GEORGE WASHINGTON UNIVERSITY HOSPITAL

PATIENT DISCHARGE PLANNING

PRE-ADMISSION SCREENING SERVICES (PASS)

Instructions:

Please fill this out while in your Doctor's office. If you have any questions ask for assistance or call the PASS Unit Staff at 994-7277.

BRING THIS FORM WITH YOU WHEN YOU COME TO THE HOSPITAL.

_____ _____ _____
(DATE)   (YOUR NAME)   (TELEPHONE)

1. Do you live alone?   [ ] Yes   [ ] No

2. Do you have a responsible adult to transport you home following your surgery?   [ ] Yes   [ ] No

3. Will there be someone, for example a spouse or friend, to help you when you get home after surgery (24 - 48 hours)?

                                         [ ] Yes   [ ] No

4. Place a check in the box that best describes the area(s) you may need help with after your surgery. (check all that apply)

   [ ] Meals at home   [ ] Equipment, i.e., cane,
   [ ] Transportation home or to   wheelchair, etc.
       return for follow-up Doctor's [ ] Getting up the stairs
       visit   [ ] Physical Care
   [ ] Money for food, housing or   (bathing,dressing,etc)
       medication   [ ] Other types of help
   [ ] Nursing care, i.e., assistance
       with bandages, medications, etc. _____

5. Were you receiving help from a community agency for any of the things listed above?   [ ] Yes   [ ] No

   If yes, please check which of the following:

   [ ] Home Health Agency   [ ] Church Group
   [ ] Meals on Wheels or other [ ] Senior Citizen Center
       nutrition program   [ ] Other

If after answering these questions you think you may need some type of help after your surgery, please alert your Doctor's office or call us at 994-7277 (PASS).

FIGURE 80–2. George Washington University Hospital patient discharge planning questionnaire. (Courtesy of George Washington University Hospital, Washington, DC.)

been more carefully matched to the complexity and severity of a given procedure, outpatient surgery is considered undesirable or unacceptable for only a few patients. These include but are not limited to formerly premature infants, morbidly obese adults, and possibly malignant hyperthermia–susceptible patients.

TABLE 80–2. American Society of Anesthesiologists' Statement on Routine Preoperative Laboratory and Diagnostic Screening*

Preanesthetic laboratory and diagnostic testing is often essential; however, no routine† laboratory or diagnostic screening‡ test is necessary for the preanesthetic evaluation of patients. Appropriate indications for ordering tests include the identification of specific clinical indicators or risk factors (e.g., age, pre-existing disease, magnitude of the surgical procedure). Anesthesiologists, anesthesiology departments, or health care facilities should develop appropriate guidelines for preanesthetic screening tests in selected populations after considering the probable contribution of each test to patient outcome. Individual anesthesiologists should order test(s) when, in their judgment, the results may influence decisions regarding risks and management of the anesthesia and surgery. Legal requirements for laboratory testing where they exist should be observed.

*Approved by House of Delegates on October 14, 1987.
†"Routine" refers to a policy of performing a test or tests without regard to clinical indications in an individual patient.
‡Screening means efforts to detect disease in unselected populations of asymptomatic patients.

The Former Preterm Infant (the Ex-Premie)

Infants born prematurely (at ≤37 weeks of gestation) are at an increased risk for postoperative apnea, periodic breathing, oxygen desaturation, or any combination of these.[6–9] The risk of apnea is highest in the immediate postoperative period but can persist for 12 to 24 hours, especially in the extremely premature infant. Factors other than the degree of prematurity that increase the likelihood of postoperative apnea include anemia, a history of apnea, gastroesophageal reflux, chronic lung disease, and intraventricular hemorrhage.

Most authors agree that the risk of apnea inversely correlates with the infant's postconceptual (gestational plus postnatal) age (PCA) at the time of surgery. Reported episodes of apnea following minor surgical interventions (e.g., hernia repair) usually were seen in infants whose PCA was <44 to 46 weeks.[6, 7, 9] Some authors, however, have reported apnea in infants as old as 60 weeks PCA.[8]

Recommendations

At CNMC, otherwise healthy former preterm infants are accepted as outpatients for minor surgical procedures when they reach 46 weeks PCA. The decision to discharge these patients is individualized and is guided by the response of the infant to anesthesia and surgery, the speed and course of recovery, the response to feeding, and the absence of any perioperative complications. These are only guidelines. The anesthesiologist may decide to admit the patient to the hospital for overnight postoperative monitoring (apnea and pulse oximetry) if any concerns exist about the promptness of recovery. Other institutions use guidelines that require infants to reach a PCA of ≥50 weeks before they are acceptable for minor outpatient surgery.

Contraindications

Former preterm infants who had a complicated postnatal course (e.g., those who required oxygen therapy or mechanical ventilation, suffered intracranial hemorrhage, experienced repeated episodes of neonatal apnea, or developed bronchopulmonary dysplasia) should be considered high-risk infants for at least the first 6 months of life and are best cared for in an inpatient facility where postoperative monitoring can be instituted.

Postponement of Elective Procedures

Truly elective outpatient procedures in the former preterm infant (e.g., cosmetic surgery) can and probably should be postponed. This minimizes the concern over postoperative apnea and eliminates the expense and the inconvenience of the hospitalization that would be required for postoperative monitoring.

Inguinal hernia, in contrast, is an example of a condition that is fairly common in former preterm infants. Because of the high risk of incarceration, prompt surgical repair is usually recommended, often while the infant is still considered at risk for postoperative apnea. In addition, many pediatric ophthalmologists believe that surgery for the repair of congenital cataract is best performed during the first months of life.

TABLE 80–3. Simplified Strategy for Preoperative Testing*

Preoperative Conditions	Male	Female	White Blood Cell Count	Prothrombin Time/Partial Thromboplastin Time	Platelet Count, Bleeding Time	Electrolytes	Creatine, Blood Urea Nitrogen	Blood Glucose	Serum Glutamic-Oxaloacetic Transaminase/ Alkaline Phosphatase	X-Ray	Electrocardiogram	Pregnancy
Procedure with blood loss	X	X										X
Procedure without blood loss												
Neonates	X	X										
Age <40 y		X										
Age 40–49 y	X	X								±	m	
Age 50–64 y	X	X								X	X	
Age ≥65	X	X								X	X	
Cardiovascular disease							X					
Pulmonary disease										X		
Malignancy	X	X	†	†						X		
Radiation therapy			X							X	X	
Hepatic disease				X					X			
Exposure to hepatitis									X			
Renal disease	X	X		X		X	X					
Bleeding disorder				X	X							
Diabetes						X	X	X			X	
Smoking ≥20 pack years	X	X								X		
Possible pregnancy												X
Diuretic use						X	X				X	
Digoxin use						X	X				X	
Steroid use						X		X	X			
Anticoagulant use	X	X		X								
Central nervous system disease			X			X	X	X			X	

*Not all diseases are included in this table. The physician's own judgment is called upon regarding patients with diseases that are not listed. These recommendations are modified so that fewer tests are ordered for individuals undergoing surgery with a very low complication rate (carpal tunnel surgery, transurethral resection of the prostate, and cataract surgery) as long as a careful history and the physician's judgment are documented (Roizen, 1992, personal communication).
Symbols: ± = perhaps obtain; † = obtain for leukemias only; X = obtain; m = obtain in men only; T/S = blood typing and screen for unexpected antibodies.

Anesthetic Technique

Welborn and coworkers at CNMC prospectively examined the incidence of postoperative apnea in formerly preterm infants who underwent hernia repair under general (halothane) versus spinal (tetracaine) anesthesia.[10] No episodes of apnea in the infants who received unsupplemented spinal anesthesia were reported; in contrast, a 31% incidence of apnea was noted following halothane use. However, infants who received ketamine ($1-2$ mg $\cdot$ kg^{-1}) for sedation during spinal anesthesia had an even higher (98%) incidence of apnea.[10] The same investigators also reported that the intravenous administration of caffeine (10 mg $\cdot$ kg^{-1}) during surgery for repair of inguinal hernia under halothane anesthesia in formerly preterm infants was effective in suppressing postoperative apnea.[11]

Based on these findings, at CNMC, where suitably trained pediatric anesthesiologists are available, unsupplemented spinal anesthesia is frequently used in at-risk infants who must undergo hernia repair. Caffeine is routinely used if general anesthesia is chosen. However, until a large number of patients are studied, these infants will continue to be admitted to the hospital for postoperative apnea monitoring regardless of the anesthetic technique used.

The Full-Term Infant

No prospective studies have been published on the postoperative course of recovery in full-term infants following routine minor outpatient procedures. However, anecdotal stories and case reports describe apneic episodes or even unexpected death in otherwise healthy full-term infants who have undergone uncomplicated minor surgery.[12] The possible occurrence of sudden infant death syndrome in patients of this age group cannot be completely ruled out, although the possible association of sudden infant death syndrome and surgery is thought to be extremely unlikely.[13]

At CNMC, otherwise healthy full-term infants can be scheduled as outpatients any time after the age of 2 weeks. This guideline is arbitrary. It varies among institutions, and in some centers, the required minimum age can be as great as 6 months.

The Morbidly Obese Adult

Morbidly obese adults frequently have severe disease of many organ systems, including the cardiovascular and respiratory systems. Hypoxia, hypercarbia, and pulmonary hypertension may exist. In addition, sleep apnea may result in respiratory insufficiency in the postoperative phase, whether in the health care facility or at home.

The Malignant Hyperthermia–Susceptible Patient

A patient susceptible to malignant hyperthermia may be an acceptable candidate for outpatient surgery, depending on the choice of anesthetics, the nature of the procedure, and the perioperative course.[14] A facility that accepts such a patient for outpatient surgery must have dantrolene on the premises, be able to perform continuous capnography and temperature monitoring in the operating room, and have ready access to the results of analysis of arterial blood gases and pH. The last of these may be the limiting factor in a freestanding facility.

Uncooperative Patients

Such patients may include substance abusers, those with major psychologic problems, or individuals who live alone and are incapable of caring for themselves. With regard to the last of these, the use of social services may be required.

American Society of Anesthesiologists' Class 3 or 4 Patients Who Require Acute Care

Patients with bronchial asthma who require therapy with aminophylline as well as brittle diabetics who require repeated analysis of blood sugar and electrolytes with adjustment in therapy are examples of ASA class 3 and 4 patients. Therapy must be required and administered in advance of the day of surgery if an overnight stay is planned. Otherwise, insurance companies may not agree to pay for this service.

Patients Who Require Invasive Monitoring

Occasionally, even in an outpatient facility, pulmonary artery catheter monitoring may be indicated. An example is the elderly patient with two-pillow orthopnea who has chronic, borderline, stable congestive heart failure and is scheduled for cataract surgery under retrobulbar block anesthesia and monitored anesthesia care. Many would argue that this patient should be hospitalized. Most, if not all, freestanding ambulatory surgery centers are unable to provide this type of monitoring.

PROCEDURES

What Procedures Generally Are Acceptable?

The list of these procedures is lengthy but fairly well defined. Table 80–4 is an example of such a list.

What Procedures Are Debatable?

Tonsillectomy

Procedures such as tonsillectomy are acceptable to some and undesirable or unacceptable to others. Two major problems are bleeding and apnea or obstruction.

Bleeding

The controversy centers on whether bleeding is likely to occur and when it may take place. Bleeding that occurs in the postanesthesia care unit can be managed in the same manner as a similar event that occurs after any surgical procedure. Hospitalizing the patient overnight may provide the means to facilitate the recognition of bleeding that takes place after the postanesthesia care unit stay and to deal with it immediately, even if surgery is required. The controversy, however, is that many episodes of bleeding after tonsillectomy are delayed and occur days after the procedure. One night in the hospital does not protect against this eventuality.

Apnea or Obstruction

Reports of postoperative apnea or obstruction, or both, in children following tonsillectomy have appeared.[15, 16] Many of

TABLE 80–4. Operative Procedures Routinely Performed on an Outpatient Basis

Surgical Specialty	Types of Procedures
Dental	Extraction, restoration
Dermatology	Excision of skin lesion
Otorhinolaryngology	Adenoidectomy, antrostomy, microlaryngoscopy, myringotomy, nasal polypectomy, tonsillectomy
Ophthalmology	Cataract extraction, chalazion excision, examination under anesthesia, nasolacrimal duct probing, ptosis repair, strabismus correction, tonometry
General practice	Biopsy, endoscopy, excisions of masses (e.g., lipomas or lymph nodes), fissurectomy, hemorrhoidectomy, herniorrhaphy, incision and drainage of abscesses, varicose vein stripping
Gynecology	Biopsy, dilatation and curettage/extraction, marsupialization of Bartholin's cyst, laparoscopy
Internal medicine, orthopedics	Bronchoscopy, endoscopy, sigmoidoscopy, carpal tunnel decompression, exostectomy, ganglionectomy, hand/foot procedure, manipulation under anesthesia, arthroscopy
Pain management	Chemical sympathectomy, intrathecal/epidural injection, nerve block
Pediatrics	Biopsy, circumcision, endoscopy, herniorrhaphy, release of adhesions, suture removal
Plastic surgery	Cosmetic procedure (e.g., scar removal, blepharoplasty, or otoplasty), septorhinoplasty
Urology	Circumcision, cystoscopy, frenulectomy, meatotomy, orchiopexy, vasectomy

(Adapted from McTaggart RA: Selection of patients for day care surgery. Can Anaesth Soc J 1983; 30:543, as appearing in White PF: Outpatient anesthesia. *In* Anesthesia. 2nd ed. Vol. 3. Miller RD (ed). New York, Churchill Livingstone, 1986, p 1898.)

the patients are young (under the age of 3 years) and have a documented history of preoperative sleep apnea or other obstructive phenomena during sleep. In extreme cases, airway obstruction can result in pulmonary hypertension and cor pulmonale. Thus, the indication for tonsillectomy (severity of repeated infections versus that of obstructive symptoms) must be reviewed carefully, especially in young patients. Postoperative observation or even intensive care unit admission for airway support may be indicated in young patients.

What Procedures Are Unsatisfactory or Unacceptable?

Surgical procedures associated with major intraoperative physiologic derangements (fluid shifts, bleeding), excessive pain, or frequent postoperative complications should not be performed in an outpatient setting.

Liposuction of a Volume Greater Than 1500 Millimeters

An example of a potentially inappropriate procedure is extraction of >1500 mL during liposuction. Red blood cell mass and albumin are reduced in proportion to the volume of fluid extracted. Autologous blood and plasma expanders are recommended when extractions >1500 mL are performed.[17] Because of possible increased morbidity in the form of syncope, pounding headache, debility, and debilitating fatigue, overnight admission may be judicious.

Excessive or Difficult to Manage Pain

Postoperative pain should be managed satisfactorily with customary analgesic medications, with or without local anes-

thesia. If more aggressive treatment is necessary, the patient should be admitted on the day prior to surgery.

Unexpected Complications

Unexpected complications that require extensive management may result in an unplanned hospitalization. Most facilities attempt to keep the admission rate below 0.5% to 2% and maintain a record of the procedures, surgeons, and events necessitating admission. A review of the data becomes part of the continuous quality improvement process and allows adaptation of institutional guidelines to achieve an admission rate that is below this reference range.

THE PERIOPERATIVE PERIOD

Should Patients Be Nil Per Os After Midnight?

Many studies, several editorials, and a review article[18] have been devoted to this subject. The major issue centers on the relative risk to benefit of allowing children and adults to ingest clear liquids after midnight. Clear liquids (water, non–pulp-containing juices, tea, coffee) do not require a breakdown in size and, on the average, pass through the stomach in 2 hours.

Little to no debate involves the subject of the ingestion of solid food. Most authorities recommend that solid food, milk, and pulp-containing liquids be restricted prior to midnight. Active contraction of the stomach is required to break down the particles of such material, particularly solid food, to a size sufficient for movement beyond the stomach.[19]

Can Liquid Aspiration Occur Beyond 2 Hours?

The risk of a patient's developing aspiration pneumonitis depends on the pH of the fluid and its volume. Even if no fluids are ingested, the stomach secretes acid at the rate of 0.6 mL · kg^{-1} · h^{-1}. With a prolonged fast, the classic requirements for Mendelson's syndrome (volume = 0.3–0.4 mL · kg^{-1}; pH <2.5) are met or exceeded.

Current Recommendations

Most authorities believe that one can never assume that a patient has an empty stomach. In an otherwise healthy patient who presents for elective surgery and who is without additional risk factors, the following guidelines are recommended by Goresky and Maltby[20]:

1. No consumption of solids on the day of surgery
2. Unrestricted consumption of clear liquids until 3 hours before the scheduled time of surgery
3. Administration of oral medications with 30 mL of water up to 1 hour before surgery
4. Consideration of administration of a histamine$_2$-receptor blocker for patients who may be at increased risk of regurgitation and aspiration of gastric contents

What Is the Risk of Aspiration of Vomitus?

Studies have been performed in which the factors that increase the risk of aspiration of vomitus (increased gastric volume, lowered gastric pH) are minimized, neutralized, or eliminated.[18] Studies have not been performed on large-scale populations to determine whether the actual frequency of aspiration pneumonitis has been reduced accordingly. In a large retrospective study in which aspiration of vomitus was correlated with risk factors, the following points were noted[21]:

1. In 83% of the patients, one or more preoperative risk factors were present.
2. In the 185,000 patients studied, 15 who aspirated were identified as healthy; however, in 10 of these, airway management difficulty was noted.
3. Other frequent factors were emergent versus elective surgery; abdominal or obstetric surgery; recent food and fluid intake; trauma; and the use of narcotics. Most of these conditions are not present in the patient scheduled for ambulatory surgery. Furthermore, in a survey of 500,000 outpatient anesthetics at 181 centers, the overall risk of aspiration was 1.7 per 10,000.[22]

Identified risk factors include pregnancy, gastrointestinal reflux, obesity, hiatal hernia, and diabetic neuropathy. Other suggested factors are difficulty in airway management, previous aspiration, esophageal or gastric pathology, outpatient status, anxiety (stress factors), smoking, advanced age, infancy, and mask anesthesia. Whether a patient scheduled for outpatient surgery truly represents a special risk remains controversial.

What Precautions Should Be Taken for the Patient at Risk?

Although no controlled studies have been performed, a patient identified as at risk probably should be restricted from ingesting food and fluids after midnight. Many prophylactic regimens have been studied and have been well summarized by White (Table 80–5).[23] Therapy should include administration of sodium citrate and citric acid solution (Bicitra), a histamine₂-receptor blocker, and metoclopramide.

THE PREINDUCTION PERIOD

When Is Premedication Useful?

Many patients scheduled for outpatient surgery are anxious[24] because of the proposed operation, lack of familiarity with the facility, and the emphasis on speed rather than personalized care. Although premedication with sedative or anxiolytic drugs does not necessarily delay recovery, most facilities reserve their use for those who need them most (e.g., children).

The paucity of premedicant use in adults often is related to the logistics of the process as well as the structure of the facility. Frequently, neither adequate time nor space allows an adult to rest comfortably after the medication has been given. Obviously, when a patient is especially apprehensive or has a problem that may impede cooperation (e.g., mental retardation), special arrangements are made and the necessary drugs are given.

Do All Children Need Premedication?

The use of premedication in children may be increasing. The 80:20 rule applies here—that is, approximately 80% of pediatric outpatients do well during anesthesia induction with or without premedication. In the past, most anesthesiologists elected to avoid routine premedication in pediatric ambulatory patients. One of the most important reasons for that trend was the concern over prolonging recovery and discharge times when long-acting drugs such as morphine or pentobarbital were used. Their effect was unpredictable, and most patients required an intramuscular injection. Trauma associated with their administration was often worse than was the struggle during induction.

TABLE 80–5. Prophylactic Regimens Used to Decrease the Risk of Aspiration Pneumonitis in Outpatients

Medication and Its Dose	Dosing Interval (min)*	Gastric Volume (mL)*	Gastric pH*	Patients with a pH <2.5 and Volume >25 mL (%)	Untreated "Controls" with a pH <2.5 and Volume >25 mL (%)†
Ranitidine, 1.5 mg · kg⁻¹ IV	83 (±6.4)	11 (±2)	6.8 (±18)	0	36
Ranitidine, 150 mg PO	113 (±8.4)	1 (±2)	5.2 (±0.3)	0	35
	154 (±13)	10 (±2)	6.4 (±0.41)	5	60
with 150 mL water	159 (±37)	10 (±13)	6.2 (±1.5)	0	48
with 150 mL coffee	160 (±34)	14 (±15)	5.7 (±2.1)	6	38
with 150 mL juice	142 (±37)	15 (±17)	5.4 (±2.1)	8	42
Cimetidine, 300 mg PO	146 (±9.9)	13 (±2)	5.0 (±0.44)	4	48
Bicitra, 15 mL PO, and metoclopramide, 10 mg IV	50 (±3.5)	22 (±4)	3.4 (±0.29)	4	36
Bicitra, 30 mL PO, and metoclopramide, 10 mg IV	50 (±3.6)	26 (±6)	3.7 (±0.30)	8	36
Bicitra, 15 mL PO	45 (±3.5)	32 (±6)	3.2 (±0.21)	12	36
Bicitra, 30 mL PO	46 (±3.5)	58 (±9)	3.7 (±0.17)	12	36
Cimetidine, 400 mg PO	105 (±6.1)	13 (±2)	5.0 (±0.4)	12	35

(Modified from White PF: Outpatient anesthesia—an overview. *In* Outpatient Anesthesia. White PF (ed). New York, Churchill Livingstone, 1990, p 12.)
*Mean values ±SD.
†Average duration of fasting, 12–14 h.
Abbreviations: IV = intravenous; PO = peroral.

What Are the Advantages of Oral Drugs?

The finding that some sedative drugs can be effective when administered orally opened the door for the increased use of premedication in pediatric outpatients. Although many drugs or drug combinations have been investigated, oral midazolam (0.5–0.75 mg · kg^{-1}) is the current favorite and is so efficacious that it has revolutionized pediatric premedication practice.[25] The drug is usually effective in producing adequate preoperative sedation in 15 to 30 minutes following oral ingestion. Separation from the parents is more likely to be peaceful than if the drug is not given, and mask induction usually is acceptable without significant prolongation of recovery and discharge times.

Unfortunately, oral midazolam preparations are currently unavailable in the United States. Most practitioners, therefore, administer the parenteral preparation orally. The extremely bitter taste of the drug can be more or less neutralized by mixing it with a strong-tasting liquid (e.g., cola drink, Tylenol cherry-flavored syrup, or melted popsicle).

How Do Preinduction Drugs Differ from Premedication Drugs?

Premedication drugs frequently must be administered well before (30–60 minutes) the time of induction. They usually are given routinely to all children regardless of need or otherwise not at all. Preinduction drugs, in contrast, are used selectively in children who refuse to separate from their parents or who, at the last minute, struggle against a planned mask induction. To be useful, they should have a quick onset of sedation (3–5 minutes) so as not to interfere with the efficient function of the outpatient facility. Ideally, the effects on recovery and discharge should also be minimal. The route of administration should not be painful or threatening (e.g., no injections should be given). Unfortunately, the ideal preinduction drug or technique remains to be discovered.

Ketamine

At CNMC, low-dose intramuscular ketamine (2 mg · kg^{-1}) is used most often in small, unpremedicatable children who refuse mask induction and who have no visible veins that allow quick intravenous access.[26] The onset time is short (2–3 minutes), and subsequent mask acceptance ranges from good to excellent in most cases *as long as the mask is not allowed to touch the child's face*. If the rest of the anesthetic is conducted with mask-administered halothane, recovery and discharge times are not significantly delayed.

Patients who require tracheal intubation may take longer to meet extubation criteria unless the anesthetic maintenance is modified to ensure the lightest possible supplementation to the analgesic effects of ketamine. When this small dose of ketamine is combined with the hypnotic effect of halothane or other sedatives, postoperative hallucinations and bad dreams are not observed.

What Are Transmucosal Approaches to Premedication?

At least three routes are recognized for the transmucosal administration of preoperative sedation. No transmucosal technique has proved to be totally satisfactory, and thus each has been largely replaced by the oral administration of midazolam.

Rectal

Methohexital

Presently, methohexital is the most frequently administered rectal preinduction drug. Methohexital in a dose of 25 mg · kg^{-1} (10% solution) induces sedation usually in 10 to 15 minutes.[27] This rather long onset time mandates careful and early screening of potential candidates to allow early administration. Defecation follows in up to 10% of children and may result in the loss of drug and the soiling of the parent's clothing. Since airway obstruction or desaturation, or both, can result, the child must be continuously observed during the onset of sedation.

Midazolam

Midazolam (1 mg · kg^{-1}) has been used rectally by a few clinicians with apparently good results.[28] Recovery and discharge times are not greatly prolonged as long as the agents used for anesthetic maintenance are appropriately reduced.

Nasal

The nasal mucosa has a rich blood supply that allows rapid absorption of many topically applied drugs. Nasally applied midazolam (0.2 mg · kg^{-1}) or sufentanil (2 μg · kg^{-1}) results in quick onset of sedation, allows easy separation from parents in <10 minutes, and leads to better cooperation with mask or intravenous induction.[29]

Unfortunately, nasal midazolam is not well accepted by most children because of its extremely irritating effect on the nasal mucosa. Nasal sufentanil, on the other hand, is less irritating but results in an unacceptably high incidence of serious side effects such as chest wall rigidity and arterial oxygen desaturation.

Oral

Although narcotics for preoperative sedation in children are not desirable, some investigators have found that oral, transmucosal fentanyl citrate (15–25 μg · kg^{-1}) results in effective sedation in 20 to 25 minutes.[30] The long onset time means that this approach may be more suitable for premedication than for preinduction.

Although the gastric volume is increased with this technique, the difference is not statistically significant when compared with the gastric volume in fasted children. Hypoventilation, oxygen desaturation, nausea, and vomiting as well as prolonged recovery are other drawbacks of this technique. The ultimate role of this approach in pediatric anesthesia practice remains to be established; however, it probably will not be used frequently in ambulatory patients.

GENERAL ANESTHESIA

The ideal induction agent and technique for pediatric outpatients should allow, among other things, a rapid and pleasant onset of sleep in the absence of premedication. This goal should be achieved without excessive drowsiness or excessive nausea and vomiting postoperatively; otherwise, recovery and discharge can be prolonged. Although the ideal agent is yet to be developed, many of the currently available drugs come fairly close.

What Is the Value of Inhalation Induction?

When given a choice, young children usually select inhalation induction. Going to sleep blowing a balloon is certainly less threatening than having an injection. From the anesthesiologist's point of view, inhalation induction is technically easier to perform than attempting intravenous cannulation in small and often uncooperative young children.

Halothane

Modern inhalation anesthetics (e.g., halothane) result in rapid onset of sleep and prompt recovery. Halothane has a pleasant smell and is readily accepted by most children (75–80%), even in the absence of premedication. Anesthesiologists can encourage a child's cooperation by telling stories, by allowing the child to hold the mask and to sit up during induction, and by painting the inside of the mask with a flavor of the child's choice.

Isoflurane

Other inhalation anesthetics have been used for induction in unpremedicated children. Isoflurane produces more airway irritation than does halothane. The recovery following short outpatient procedures is not significantly different than that for halothane.

Desflurane

The newer inhalation agent desflurane results in severe airway irritation and an unacceptably high incidence of laryngospasm and oxygen desaturation during induction. The very low solubility of desflurane, however, results in very rapid recovery, even when halothane has been used for the initial induction.

Sevoflurane

Early experience with sevoflurane indicates that induction is smooth and that recovery is fast.[31]

What Should Be Done with Resistant Children?

Up to 20% of unpremedicated children do not cooperate with any attempts at mask induction. Some of them have had a bad experience with a previous anesthetic induction or have a specific fear of having a mask on their face. If this history is available in advance of surgery, premedication or a preinduction technique is strongly indicated. For children who declare their displeasure with the smell of the anesthetic and resist attempts at mask induction, an intravenous induction technique can be utilized.

How Is Intravenous Induction Managed?

The willingness of the child or the anesthesiologist, or both, to accept an intravenous technique as a first choice for anesthetic induction varies tremendously. It depends to a great degree on the cultural and socioeconomic background of the child and, more importantly, on the attitude and technical skill of the anesthesiologist.

An intravenous induction can be made more appealing to children by the use of a local anesthetic (e.g., EMLA cream) on the skin or by performing the venipuncture under nitrous oxide analgesia. A supportive attitude by an anesthesiologist who is skilled in performing venous cannulation in children is very important.

Sodium thiopental is the traditional induction drug when an intravenous technique is used. Propofol is safe and effective in children and, unlike thiopental, does not delay recovery when compared with a halothane inhalation technique.[32, 33] Pain on injection is relatively common with propofol but can be minimized by using a large antecubital vein or by adding lidocaine $(1 \text{ mg} \cdot \text{mL}^{-1})$ immediately before injection.

Which Maintenance Agents or Techniques Are Preferred?

Rapid induction and emergence are desirable features. The induction should be associated with minimal side effects such as coughing, breath-holding, laryngospasm, and extraneous involuntary movements. Emergence should be associated with rapid return of airway reflexes, early return of cognitive and psychomotor function, and minimal nausea and vomiting.

Propofol

If all of the desirable attributes are considered, propofol appears to most closely resemble the ideal agent. The drug is particularly suitable for induction of anesthesia. Psychomotor performance recovers more rapidly than following the administration of thiopental.[34] Propofol administration can then be continued for maintenance as a total intravenous anesthetic and is particularly useful in short procedures. Another technique or agent may be better suited to the patient with cardiovascular disease, in whom hypotension is unacceptable or undesirable, or in a patient who is undergoing a procedure in which profound analgesia is desirable.

Nausea and Vomiting

Propofol is particularly useful in patients who have a high predisposition to vomiting[35, 36] and for procedures in which a high percentage of vomiting is anticipated. These include strabismus surgery, ear surgery, and laparoscopy. In two separate controlled studies of patients undergoing strabismus surgery,[37, 38] the frequency of vomiting was reduced markedly when propofol was used compared with a standard nitrous oxide–oxygen–halothane anesthetic. In preliminary work at CNMC, Hannallah and associates reported a vomiting rate of 11% compared with a 59% rate with a standard technique.[38]

TABLE 80–6. Recovery Times (in minutes) Following Propofol Versus Thiopental/Isoflurane Anesthesia[39]

Nitrous Oxide Off To:	Propofol	Thiopental/Isoflurane
Orientation	5.7	10
Standing	66*	92
Tolerates PO fluids	61*	129
Voiding	103*	184
Ready to go home	136*	204

*$P < .05$.

Recovery Time

In work at the University of Chicago, Kortilla and coworkers[39] compared a propofol anesthetic added to nitrous oxide–oxygen–fentanyl muscle relaxant with thiopental–nitrous oxide–oxygen–fentanyl–isoflurane muscle relaxant. Recovery times (in minutes) are noted in Table 80–6.

Applicability for Pediatric Outpatient Procedures

A limited number of studies show that propofol infusion is safe and effective for anesthesia maintenance in pediatric outpatients. The infusion can be started either following an induction bolus of propofol in children for whom an intravenous induction is selected[32] or following mask induction with halothane.[37]

When propofol is not supplemented with opioids or other systemic analgesics, the infusion requirements in children are higher than those in adults. Recovery is very prompt and associated with an extremely low incidence of vomiting even following surgical procedures that are known to result in a high incidence of vomiting when other agents are used.[36–38]

Desflurane

Desflurane has been studied extensively in outpatient surgery. Its blood/gas solubility coefficient (0.42) is lower than that of other inhalation anesthetics, including nitrous oxide. Uptake and elimination are very rapid. Rapid induction occurs in adults if desflurane is administered following an intravenous induction. An inhalation induction is associated with an unacceptably high frequency of coughing and laryngospasm in children.[40] Special heated and pressurized vaporizers are required for its administration. The cost of this conversion and of the anesthetic is unknown at this time.

Desflurane could be particularly useful in outpatient surgery when an inhalation agent is indicated, largely because of the rapid awakening and minimal nausea and vomiting associated with its use. It may play an important role in expediting awakening and early return of airway reflexes when it is difficult or impossible to judge the termination of the surgical procedure (e.g., laparoscopy, arthroscopy, or application of casts).

Nitrous Oxide

The use of nitrous oxide remains controversial. It reduces the minimum alveolar concentration requirements for other agents, including narcotics. Narcotics use is particularly associated with vomiting, but nitrous oxide use has been implicated also. Recent work pertaining to strabismus surgery suggests a reduction in vomiting when propofol is used as a total intravenous anesthetic without nitrous oxide compared with when it is given with nitrous oxide.[37] Nitrous oxide does not appear to be associated with a significant increase in bowel gas during laparoscopic cholecystectomy.[41]

AIRWAY MANAGEMENT

Is Tracheal Intubation Required for Laparoscopy?

This debate has been ongoing since laparoscopy became an established procedure. We feel that many factors influence the rate and magnitude of complications associated with abdominal laparoscopy (Table 80–7).

Factors promoting regurgitation of gastric contents are obstructed airway, Trendelenburg's position, and a distended abdomen. Perforation of a distended stomach, hemorrhage, and gas emboli have been reported. The last of these was detected by the use of capnography in conjunction with tracheal intubation.[42]

A skilled anesthesiologist and surgeon working as a team under the right operating conditions on a small, otherwise healthy patient might make conditions favorable for the use of a mask-administered general anesthetic. However, in most situations, tracheal intubation appears to present maximum benefit and minimum risk.

Should Tracheal Intubation Be Used in Pediatric Outpatients?

When indicated, tracheal intubation can be safely performed in pediatric outpatients. Modern endotracheal tube design, coupled with the awareness that tight fit should be avoided, minimizes the chance that postintubation croup will ensue. Children under 4 years of age whose tracheas are intubated should be observed for any symptoms or signs of croup for 1 to 2 hours postoperatively. If no symptoms of croup develop during that time, they are unlikely to start de novo at a later time.

Contraindications

Sometimes, elective intubation is undesirable or not indicated. Children with symptoms of upper respiratory tract infections have been reported to have a much higher incidence of adverse respiratory events during anesthesia when an endotracheal tube is used as opposed to when an anesthetic is delivered using a facemask.[43]

TABLE 80–7. Factors Influencing Complications in Laparoscopy

The patient: Size, weight, airway, associated comorbid conditions
The procedure: Extent, duration; position of the operating table; amount of distending gas
The surgeon: Skill, experience

Many pediatric outpatient procedures are of very short duration (e.g., myringotomy and tube insertion) or do not require intense muscle relaxation (e.g., hernia repair in children older than 1 year of age). Anesthesia induced by mask is usually satisfactory, especially when the inhalation technique is supplemented with a regional block (caudal or ilioinguinal/iliohypogastric nerve block). Avoiding tracheal intubation under these circumstances does not compromise the surgical conditions, prevents even the minimal postintubation sequelae (e.g., sore throat), and speeds the recovery and turnaround time between cases.

INTRAVENOUS INFUSIONS

Does Every Pediatric Outpatient Need One?

The reasons for establishing an intravenous infusion during pediatric outpatient anesthesia include the need to ensure proper fluid replacement and to have ready access for the administration of adjunctive or emergency drugs. Since the current trend minimizes preoperative fasting times, most children arrive at day surgery units well hydrated. If surgery is of short duration (e.g., shorter than 30 minutes), and is not expected to be associated with postoperative nausea and vomiting, and if someone is immediately available to establish intravenous access if it is needed emergently, some anesthesiologists feel that an infusion is unnecessary.[44] Many, however, insist that such access is an integral part of all anesthetics.

What Is "Routine" Intravenous Fluid Therapy?

The volume and composition of intraoperative fluid therapy must be tailored to the needs and response of each individual child. "Cookbook" formulas are meant to serve only as guidelines.

Calculations

When estimating the intravenous infusion rate, calculate the total volume that needs to be infused until the child is released from the hospital before determining an hourly rate for infusion. The total volume should include replacement of any existing preoperative deficits, normal fluid maintenance needs, and replacement of any intraoperative losses as well as an allowance for possible inability to tolerate oral fluid following surgery.

For example, in a 6-year-old (30-kg) child who is scheduled for strabismus surgery, the fluid needs can be determined as in Table 80–8. The numbers are estimated by using the maintenance fluid replacement guidelines of 4 mL · kg^{-1} · h^{-1} for the first 10 kg of body weight, 2 mL · kg^{-1} · h^{-1} for the next 10 kg of body weight, and 1 mL · kg^{-1} · h^{-1} for each additional kilogram of body weight. In this example, the hydrating infusion should be administered over several hours rather than given as a massive bolus in the operating room or just prior to discharge from the facility in order to "catch up."

TABLE 80–8. Example of Pediatric Fluid Requirement Calculation*

Last oral fluid intake	6:00 AM
Anesthesia induction	10:00 AM
Expected duration of surgery	1 h
Expected total recovery time	4 h
Total time IV catheter in place	5 h
Normal IV maintenance rate	70 mL · h^{-1}
Preoperative deficit	Negligible
Intraoperative losses	Negligible

*Assume that the child will be discharged nil per os and will remain so until bedtime (approximately 7 h); total IV requirements for the day (intraoperative and postoperative nil per os time) = 12 h; total IV volume goal: 12 × 70 = 840 mL; required average IV rate = 840/5 = 168 mL · h^{-1}.

What Fluids Are Appropriate?

Although one-third normal saline (⅓ NS) solution (usually 5% dextrose in water–⅓ NS) is a rational choice for intravenous *maintenance* therapy in most pediatric patients, its routine use in pediatric outpatients is not recommended. As illustrated in the previous example, perioperative fluid administration combines both maintenance and replacement components.

An "isotonic" solution such as normal saline or lactated Ringer's solution is preferable for replacement therapy. Hypotonic solutions (e.g., ⅓ NS) used to replace fluid lost through vomiting can lead to serious hyponatremia, cerebral edema, and even convulsions.

Since two separate infusions, one for maintenance (e.g., ⅓ NS) and another for replacement (Ringer's solution), are not practical, most pediatric anesthesiologists simply choose Ringer's solution (or an equivalent) to supply both maintenance and replacement needs. The extra sodium load is easily handled by the kidneys in otherwise healthy children.

Should Routine Intravenous Fluid Contain Glucose?

This question has caused more controversy during the last few years than any other fluid management issue. Infants need sugar to make up for their limited glycogen stores. Most older children who fast for a reasonable period of time before surgery (6–8 hours) have a normal blood glucose level at the time of induction. Recent studies, however, have shown that children who are subjected to a prolonged fast (>12 hours) may have low blood glucose levels (<50 mg · dL^{-1}) at the time of induction.[45] Moreover, the "stress-induced" intraoperative increase in blood glucose level was not a consistent response in pediatric outpatients. In fact, 13% to 15% of children exhibited no change or even a further decrease in blood glucose level at the end of surgery compared with at induction.

Administration

Children who routinely receive a maintenance solution containing 5% glucose become hyperglycemic at the end of surgery.[45] Welborn and colleagues suggest that when glucose is indicated, infusion of lactated Ringer's solution containing 2.5% dextrose and at the infusion rates normally required may be appropriate.[46] Recent studies have shown that the new guidelines, which limit preoperative fasting (liquids) to 3 hours before surgery, have minimal effects on perioperative glucose homeostasis.[47] Although hypoglycemia is less likely at the time of induction, the actual change in blood glucose during surgery (increase, decrease, or no change) is not affected.

Intraoperative

Our current practice is to administer lactated Ringer's solution as the only solution for both maintenance and replacement to children who have not fasted for more than 4 to 8 hours. Children who, for whatever reason, have fasted for a prolonged period (>10–12 hours) either receive a 2.5% dextrose–lactated Ringer's solution or have their blood glucose monitored at the time of induction.

Postoperative

The glucose need of children in the postoperative period also must be considered. Children who cannot tolerate or are not offered oral fluids before discharge home must have the total period of glucose deprivation determined since their last oral intake. If the period is prolonged, glucose can be added to the infused solution.

REGIONAL ANESTHESIA

What Is Its Role in Outpatient Surgery?

Two features of regional anesthesia are particularly useful: operative anesthesia and relief of postoperative pain. The use of local anesthetics in regional blocks during circumcision and hernia repair is increasingly widespread in adults and children. Spinal and epidural anesthesia are becoming more popular but have limitations. In both, prolonged autonomic blockade impedes early ambulation and voiding and potentially delays discharge. Several concepts should be addressed:

1. Local anesthetics such as tetracaine and bupivacaine are especially long acting and probably have little or no role in outpatient spinal anesthesia; discharge criteria may not be met for up to 8 to 12 hours following injection of these agents.
2. In a relatively short operation (60–90 minutes), a *single-shot* spinal anesthetic using lidocaine with epinephrine is particularly useful.
3. In a procedure that lasts longer than 60 to 90 minutes or in one of unknown length, select an epidural anesthetic so that a catheter can be inserted. Intermittent injection through the catheter for a short-acting agent, such as lidocaine, is recommended to allow titration of the anesthetic to the length of the procedure.[48]
4. Postdural puncture headache is annoying in the ambulatory surgical patient and is best avoided by the use of the smallest possible needle (26- or 27-gauge) with a blunt tip (Sprotte, Whitaker) and with a single-injection technique.
5. A patient's ability to void is impaired after spinal or epidural anesthesia because of reflex urethral spasm and inhibition of normal bladder detrusor muscle activity. Normal bladder capacity in an adult is 400 to 500 mL. During spinal anesthesia with a *routine* intravenous fluid administration of 300 mL · h⁻¹, mean urine production was found to be 950 mL in 6 hours. After the use of bupivacaine and tetracaine, com-

plete recovery of the detrusor muscle took 7 to 8 hours.[49] When the bladder capacity is exceeded, it becomes overdistended and its function is reduced. Catheterization then becomes essential.

In order to reduce the duration of autonomic blockade and overdistention of the bladder following spinal or epidural anesthesia, short-acting local anesthetics should be used, and administration of intravenous fluids should be minimized.

MONITORED ANESTHESIA CARE

Monitored anesthesia care is popular in a variety of outpatient procedures largely because of the availability of newer intravenous sedatives and analgesics.

What Agents Are Useful?

Midazolam may provide sedation, anxiolysis, and amnesia. Fentanyl or alfentanil are rapid-acting, short-duration, potent narcotics that provide profound analgesia. Propofol may be used alone or in combination with other agents to produce sedation.

What Is Its Optimum Role?

This technique is most effective when analgesia is adequate with local anesthesia. Supplementation with adjunctive drugs can then be provided to relax the patient and to provide sedation and amnesia, if desired.

What Should Be Done If Pain Relief Is Inadequate?

When monitored anesthesia care is used to provide analgesia, the requirement for narcotics is increased. Respiratory depression, reduced respiratory rate, shift of the carbon dioxide response curve to the right, periodic breathing, and apnea may result. Respiratory depression is far more likely to occur when an agent such as midazolam is used in conjunction with the narcotic.[50]

Respiratory depression may produce hypoxemia unless oxygen supplementation is successful. Sleep also shifts the carbon dioxide response curve to the right. Elderly patients and those with chronic obstructive lung disease are particularly vulnerable to the respiratory depressant effects of intravenous sedative and narcotic agents. Monitored anesthesia care is a particularly dangerous technique when undesirable respiratory effects are produced because the airway may be unprotected, not easily established, or inaccessible (e.g., as in cataract surgery).

What Is the Role of the Reversal Agents?

Naloxone

The respiratory depressant effect of narcotics may be reversed by a narcotic antagonist like naloxone. However, naloxone may be associated with major side effects such as overwhelming sympathetic response, pulmonary hypertension, pulmonary edema, or death. Thus, it should always be titrated to effect (e.g., 0.5 $\mu g \cdot kg^{-1}$ repeatedly until the desired degree of reversal has occurred).

Flumazenil

Flumazenil is a benzodiazepine antagonist that has little or no intrinsic toxicity. It effectively reverses the sedation and some respiratory depressant effects of the benzodiazepines, but the duration of its effect may even be shorter than that of midazolam. The manufacturer recommends monitoring for resedation, respiratory depression, or other residual benzodiazepine effects for up to 120 minutes following its use.[51] This approach can delay discharge, even though the patient is awake and breathing adequately.

THE RECOVERY PERIOD

Unlike the patient who will undergo surveillance within a hospital or similar facility, the patient who has undergone outpatient surgery is discharged home. Criteria for discharge must be available so that the care provided is uniform for all patients and so that the risks are minimized.

What Are the Traditional Guidelines for Safe Discharge?

An example of guidelines for safe discharge after ambulatory surgery is shown in Table 80–9.[23] Of note is that discharge criteria generally do not include any psychomotor tests beyond the requirement that the patient be able to stand and walk unassisted. As the practice of outpatient anesthesia evolves, administering more sensitive and sophisticated tests of psychomotor impairment, the Trieger dot test, or the modified Bender Visual-Motor Gestalt Solid Line test may become routine. Despite having been available for many years, to date these tests are still only rarely used, perhaps reflecting that we all expect and assume all patients to have residual psychomotor impairment for 24 hours after a procedure.

TABLE 80–9. Guidelines for Safe Discharge After Ambulatory Surgery

- Patient's vital signs must have been stable for at least 1 h
- Patient must have no evidence of respiratory depression
- Patient must be
  Oriented to person, place, and time
  Able to maintain orally administered fluids*
  Able to dress himself or herself
  Able to walk without assistance
  Able to void*
- Patient must not have
  More than minimal nausea or vomiting
  Excessive pain
  Bleeding
- Patient must be discharged by both the person who administered anesthesia and the person who performed surgery, or by their designees. Written instructions for the postoperative period at home, including a contact place and person, need to be reinforced.
- Patient must have responsible adult escort him or her home and stay with him or her.

*The role of these variables as criteria for discharge remains to be established.

Should Children Be Required to Drink Before Discharge?

The ability to drink and retain clear liquids as a prerequisite for discharge has been questioned. Many children vomit and eventually require antiemetic therapy, overnight admission to a hospital, or both, as a result of being forced to drink. Schreiner and coworkers found that children who were not forced to drink had less vomiting and had a shorter stay in the day surgery unit than those who were required to drink.[52] He concluded that, as long as hydration is adequate, drinking is an unnecessary prerequisite for discharge.

Must the Patient Void?

Adults

In order to reduce or eliminate the possibility of overdistention of the bladder in adults, voiding is usually required before discharge, especially after regional anesthesia. In the absence of regional anesthesia, the patient may be discharged, even though voiding has not occurred. The surgeon must carefully instruct the patient what to do (where to go, whom to call) should voiding not commence by a given time.

Children

The ability to void is not considered a requirement for discharge, even following genitourinary procedures or when caudal blocks are performed, or both. Overdistention of the bladder is unlikely to occur in children. Voiding may be useful, however, to help assess the hydration status of some children before they are released from the facility.

Is Croup a Contraindication to Discharge?

With careful selection of endotracheal tube sizes to avoid a tight fit, the incidence of postextubation croup should be low (<1%).[53] Subglottic swelling that may develop in these patients occurs relatively early (at 1–2 hours) following extubation. If hoarseness, croupy cough, chest retractions, or any combination of these, are not present during that time, they usually will not occur later. Many anesthesiologists, therefore, feel comfortable discharging children whose tracheas were intubated if they are symptom-free for 1 to 2 hours after extubation.

Most children who develop minimal croup symptoms (e.g., hoarseness) respond well to cool mist and can be discharged home if the symptoms improve and the parents are comfortable and reassured as well as capable of understanding the instructions to continue mist therapy at home.

Racemic Epinephrine

Children who require racemic epinephrine inhalation to control croup present a problem. Although racemic epinephrine is effective, its duration is short-lived, and rebound edema may recur in 2 to 3 hours. Therefore, children who receive this treatment should be observed for at least this long to ensure that symptoms have subsided and do not recur. If they do, repeated treatment or overnight hospital admission, or both, may be required.

How Are Discharge Orders and Instructions Provided?

A uniform format for orders and instructions should be provided, and a sample physician order sheet is shown in Figure 80–3. It incorporates the initial recovery room care with the orders at the time of discharge.

What Instruction Should Be Given?

Sample forms incorporating discharge instructions are shown in Figures 80–4 and 80–5. These instructions are given to the patient on behalf of the departments of surgery and anesthesiology at the time of discharge from the facility. The recovery room nurse explains the instructions to the patient and reinforces them, and the patient and anesthesiologist attest to this act with their signatures. This same process is also followed by the surgeon. Written instructions are essential, since a patient may not recall instructions because of stress or the lingering amnestic effects of the administered drugs despite otherwise appearing to be completely recovered.

Who Determines Suitability for Discharge?

Ideally, a physician should evaluate the patient at the time of anticipated discharge from the facility. This is a requirement with one accrediting body, the American Association of Ambulatory Health Care. The JCAHO allows another option (Table 80–10).[54]

This process is designed to ensure that uniform discharge criteria are employed, regardless of who is present to make the assessment. A nurse acts as an observer and records all criteria for discharge. The criteria are set by one of the "licensed independent practitioners" on staff. One of the latter must assume responsibility for the patient's discharge.

Who Is Considered a Responsible Adult?

A responsible adult is one who is mentally and physically able to assist the patient and his needs. According to the intent of the *Scoring Guidelines of the JCAHO*, "a minor, taxi driver, or 'courtesy' driver" does not qualify as a designated or responsible adult.[55]

UNPLANNED HOSPITALIZATION

One of the goals of outpatient surgery is to minimize the rate of unplanned hospitalization. Most of the causes are well known. Some can be avoided or reduced in frequency.

CHILDREN'S HOSPITAL NATIONAL MEDICAL CENTER
Washington, D. C. 20010

PHYSICIAN'S ORDER SHEET

(Do not write orders unless patient information is complete.)

1. All orders for drugs that require by law a prescription (legend drugs) shall be automatically discontinued after 7 days, unless
   (A) The order indicates an exact number of doses to be administered.
   (B) An exact period of time that the medication is to be administered is specified, or
   (C) The physician reorders the medication
   Exceptions are narcotics, other Schedule II drugs and I.V. fluids which have an automatic stop order period of 24 hours.
2. Authorization is hereby given for dispensing an equivalent drug by generic name unless the drug name prescribed is followed by the designation Medical Necessity.

ORDERED		PHYSICIAN'S ORDERS	CARRIED OUT	
DATE	HOUR		HOUR	INITIAL
		PATIENT AGE ☐ CBC ☐		
		PATIENT WEIGHT ☐ URINALYSIS ☐		
		TINE TEST ☐ SSRU/I & O		
	1.	Vital signs q15 x 4:q30 min x 2, q 1 hr x 4 - q 4 hrs		
	2.	Diet clear liquids advance as tolerated		
	3.	Activity: up ad lib with assistance (age appropriate)		
	4.	IV solution, specify ______		
		at ____ cc/hr. Discontinue when tolerating po fluids		
	5.	Medications.		
		Pain: Tylenol ____ mg po q ____ hrs PRN when tolerating po fluids		
		Other: Specify drug, dosage, route, frequency		
	6.	Dressing Care (specify)		
	7.	Home Care Instructions (specify)		
	8.	Discharge (specify by checking appropriate box(es)		
		☐ Discharge when criteria met (Required for SSRU)		
		☐ Discharge when criteria met, but not before ____ AM/PM		
		☐ Discharge when criteria met after checked by ____ M.D.		
		☐ Discharge when criteria met, but not before ____ AM/PM and		
		seen by ____ M.D.		
		____ M.D.		

HAVE YOU RENEWED THE "STOP ORDER" MEDICATIONS?

FIGURE 80–3. Discharge order and instruction format. (Courtesy of Children's National Medical Center, Washington, DC.)

BRIGHTON FORMS & PRINTING INC

THE GEORGE WASHINGTON UNIVERSITY MEDICAL CENTER

IN AND OUT SURGERY
POST-ANESTHESIA INSTRUCTIONS

(PATIENT IDENTIFICATION)

IF YOU HAD GENERAL ANESTHESIA OR SEDATION, PLEASE PAY ATTENTION TO THE FOLLOWING INSTRUCTIONS:

1. DO NOT DRINK ALCOHOLIC BEVERAGES FOR 24 HOURS. ALCOHOL MAY INCREASE THE EFFECTS OF ANESTHESIA AND SEDATION.
2. DO NOT DRIVE A MOTOR VEHICLE, OPERATE MACHINERY OR POWER TOOLS FOR 24-48 HOURS.
3. DO NOT MAKE ANY IMPORTANT DECISIONS OR SIGN IMPORTANT PAPERS FOR 24-48 HOURS. YOU MAY BE FORGETFUL DUE TO THE MEDICATIONS ADMINISTERED.
4. YOU MAY EXPERIENCE LIGHTHEADEDNESS, DIZZINESS OR SLEEPINESS FOLLOWING SURGERY. PLEASE DO NOT STAY ALONE.
5. REST AT HOME WITH MODERATE ACTIVITY AS TOLERATED. IT MAY NOT BE NECESSARY TO GO TO BED, BUT IT IS IMPORTANT TO REST FOR 24 HOURS FOLLOWING GENERAL ANESTHESIA.
6. PROGRESS SLOWLY TO A REGULAR DIET UNLESS OTHERWISE INSTRUCTED. START WITH LIQUIDS, THEN SOUP AND CRACKERS GRADUALLY WORKING UP TO SOLID FOODS.
7. CERTAIN ANESTHETICS AND PAIN MEDICATIONS MAY PRODUCE NAUSEA AND VOMITING. IF NAUSEA OR VOMITING BECOMES A PROBLEM AT HOME, CALL YOUR PHYSICIAN DR. ____________ AT ____________ OR THE ANESTHESIA DEPARTMENT AT G.W.U.H. AT 994-3134 OR THE PAGE OPERATOR AT 994-3321 AND ASK FOR THE ANESTHESIOLOGIST ON CALL.

SPECIAL INSTRUCTIONS FOLLOWING REGIONAL ANESTHESIA:

OTHER INSTRUCTIONS: ____________

IF YOU SHOULD EXPERIENCE DIFFICULTY IN BREATHING, BLEEDING THAT YOU FEEL IS EXCESSIVE, PERSISTENT NAUSEA AND VOMITING, PAIN THAT IS UNUSUAL, SWELLING OR FEVER, PLEASE CALL YOUR PHYSICIAN OR THE ANESTHESIA DEPARTMENT. AN ANESTHESIOLOGIST CAN BE REACHED 24 HOURS A DAY.

DATE ________ TIME ________ ANESTHESIOLOGIST'S SIGNATURE ____________

I HAVE RECEIVED AND UNDERSTAND THE POST-ANESTHESIA INSTRUCTIONS GIVEN TO ME.

DATE ________ TIME ________ PATIENT'S SIGNATURE ____________
OR
RESPONSIBLE PARTY'S SIGNATURE ____________

7540-75-090 (8-88)

FIGURE 80–4. Post-anesthesia instructions. (Courtesy of George Washington University Hospital, Washington, DC.)

THE GEORGE WASHINGTON UNIVERSITY MEDICAL CENTER

The George Washington University WASHINGTON DC

IN AND OUT SURGERY
POST-OPERATIVE INSTRUCTIONS

(PATIENT IDENTIFICATION)

1. WOUND OR INCISION CARE? ☐ YES ☐ NO (IF NOT APPLICABLE)

2. PHYSICAL ACTIVITIES: ____________

3. DIET: RESUME NORMAL DIET? ☐ YES ☐ NO (IF NO, SPECIFY)

4. MEDICATIONS: PRESCRIPTIONS GIVEN ☐ YES ☐ NO (IF YES, LIST & INCLUDE STRENGTH, DOSAGE, SCHEDULE & ROUTE)

5. FOLLOW UP VISIT TO PHYSICIAN'S OFFICE:

IN ________ DAYS. CALL OFFICE FOR APPOINTMENT.

6. OTHER: ____________

If you experience either pain (not relieved by the prescribed medication) or bleeding that is greater than what your attending surgeon explained to you that you might experience without concern, please call your surgeon.

DOCTOR	TELEPHONE NO.

DATE ________ TIME ________ PHYSICIAN'S SIGNATURE ____________

I HAVE GIVEN THE POST-OPERATIVE INSTRUCTIONS FORM TO THE PATIENT.

R.N.'S SIGNATURE ____________

I HAVE RECEIVED AND UNDERSTAND THE POST-OPERATIVE INSTRUCTIONS GIVEN TO ME.

PATIENT'S SIGNATURE ____________

76-090 (11/90) (344)

FIGURE 80–5. Post-surgical instructions. (Courtesy of George Washington University Hospital, Washington, DC.)

TABLE 80–10. Discharge Requirements (Joint Commission on the Accreditation of Health Care Organizations)

SA.1.6.6	A licensed independent practitioner who has appropriate clinical privileges and who is familiar with the patient is responsible for the decision to discharge a patient from a postanesthesia recovery area or, when the surgical or anesthesia services are provided on an ambulatory basis, from the hospital.
SA.1.6.6.1	When the responsible licensed independent practitioner is not personally present to make the decision to discharge or does not sign the discharge order, then
SA.1.6.6.1.1	The name of the licensed independent practitioner responsible for the discharge is recorded in the patient's medical record; and
SA.1.6.6.1.2	Relevant discharge criteria that are approved by the medical staff are rigorously applied to determine the readiness of the patient for discharge.

(From Surgical and Anesthesia Services, Accreditation Manual for Ambulatory Health Care. JCAHO, 1992.)

What Are the Main Causes?

Four categories predominate and are listed in Table 80–11. Most causes linked to the anesthetic management may also be related to the procedure, for example, vomiting after strabismus surgery or pain following hernia repair.[56–59] According to Gold and associates,[58] the factors shown in Table 80–12 were independently related to unexpected admission. When age is separated from physical status, pre-existing disease is not an independent variable.

Postoperative Vomiting

Reduction in vomiting postoperatively may begin with the assessment of the patient preoperatively and end with the safe discharge home free of emesis. In 1992, an entire issue of the *British Journal of Anaesthesia* was devoted to the subject of vomiting; this issue is highly recommended to those who are particularly interested in a comprehensive review of the subject.[59] The steps outlined in Table 80–13 should be considered when designing a management plan. If vomiting or severe nausea occurs during the recovery period, the steps outlined in Table 80–14 should be considered.[60, 61]

Minimization of Postoperative Pain

Three approaches have been used:

1. Use of narcotic agents
2. Administration of nonsteroidal anti-inflammatory or analgesic drugs
3. Application of regional blocks

TABLE 80–11. Primary Causes of Unplanned Hospitalization

Surgical	Bleeding, perforation of a viscus
Medical	Myocardial infarction, chest pain
Anesthetic	Vomiting, pain
Social	Absence of a responsible adult who can provide transportation and care

TABLE 80–12. Multivariate Logistic Regression Analysis of Factors Associated with Unanticipated Admission

Factors	Odds Ratio	95% Confidence Interval
General anesthesia	5.18*	2.60–10.30
Emesis	3.03*	1.35–6.81
Abdominal surgery	2.89*	1.07–7.79
Operating room time >1 h	2.72*	1.46–5.08
Age (30-y intervals)	2.56*	1.32–4.22
Laparoscopy	1.71	0.69–4.22
Drive >1 h	1.49	0.79–2.80

(From Welborn LG, Hannallah RS, McGill WA, et al: Choosing a glucose concentration for routine infusion in pediatric outpatient surgery. Anesthesiology 1987; 67:427.)
*$P < .05$.

Narcotic agents may produce respiratory and circulatory depression and vomiting. Nonsteroidal anti-inflammatory drugs do not produce the side effects associated with narcotics and have been very effective in the prophylaxis and treatment of pain associated with laparoscopy.[62] In some centers, ketorolac (Toradol), 30 to 60 mg, is given intramuscularly 60 minutes before the termination of surgery. If given in the postanesthesia care unit for the first time, 60 minutes may be required for peak effect to be achieved. This drug can be continued every 6 hours in the postoperative period, administered either parenterally by a home health care service in its oral form, or it can be replaced by some other oral nonsteroidal anti-inflammatory drug unless a contraindication is present.

Regional anesthesia is particularly helpful in several circumstances (Table 80–15).[63–66] If local anesthesia has been found to be effective, be sure to use it as a supplement to general or regional anesthesia so that the patient can obtain prolonged relief after the effect of the primary anesthetic has dissipated.

MORBIDITY AND MORTALITY

In comparison with the early years of modern outpatient surgery, patients are now older and sicker and undergo more complex procedures. Major morbidity and mortality are uncommon but do occur. Aspiration pneumonitis, pulmonary edema, myocardial infarction, and death have been reported.[67] Not all of these complications are related to the age of the

TABLE 80–13. Preoperative Assessment for Vomiting

Preoperative	• Is there a history of motion sickness? vomiting with previous anesthesia? • What is the surgical procedure? • Is the procedure likely to be associated with nausea and vomiting (e.g., strabismus, laparoscopy, orchiopexy, therapeutic abortion, or varicocelectomy)?
Premedication	• Should an antiemetic be administered before vomiting occurs (e.g., metoclopramide, 25 mg · kg⁻¹ IV, or droperidol, 10–20 mg · kg⁻¹ IV or greater, with strabismus surgery)?
Induction and Maintenance	• Should (can) narcotic agents be avoided? • Can total IV anesthesia with propofol be considered? • Can regional anesthesia be used instead of general anesthesia?

TABLE 80–14. Treatment of Severe Postoperative Nausea and Vomiting

- Salt-containing solutions should be administered intravenously
- Oral fluids should not be administered
- If moderate to severe pain persists, it should be treated
- An antiemetic agent should be administered (metoclopramide, 0.15 mg · kg⁻¹ IV, or droperidol, 10–20 μg · kg⁻¹ IV or greater, after strabismus surgery)
- If vomiting occurs primarily or exclusively after patient movement to the upright position, ephedrine, 0.5 μg · kg⁻¹, may be administered intramuscularly or in a small dose, 5–15 mg IV
- Ondansetron (Zofran), 4 mg, may be effective and has no sedative or extrapyramidal effects

TABLE 80–16. Useful Clinical Indicators in the Hospital-Integrated Ambulatory Surgery Unit

- Patient satisfaction
- Postoperative occurrence in the ambulatory surgery unit
- Problems encountered on patient follow-up
- Prolonged stay in postanesthesia care unit
- Unanticipated admissions
- Cancellation on the day of surgery
- Medical record review

patient, the existence of comorbid conditions, or the surgical procedure.

The factors that lead to aspiration pneumonitis have been discussed previously. Noncardiac pulmonary edema may follow postextubation airway obstruction. Carbon dioxide embolus and cardiac arrest have occurred during laparoscopy.[68, 69] The degree of vigilance, monitoring, or overall quality of care required for outpatient anesthesia is no different than it is for inpatient anesthesia.

A new consideration is the November 1993 letter to anesthesia practitioners from a manufacturer of succinylcholine (Burroughs Wellcome Co., Research Triangle Park, NC). This letter details new warnings and contraindications to the routine use of succinylcholine currently popular in many outpatient anesthesia practices. Specifically, the package insert now includes new warnings and contraindications, including the following: "Except when used for emergency tracheal intubation or in instances where immediate securing of the airway is necessary, succinylcholine is contraindicated in children and adolescent patients;" and "it is also contraindicated after the acute phase of injury following major burns, multiple trauma, extensive denervation of skeletal muscle, or upper motor neuron injury."[70]

The manufacturer, in collaboration with the Food and Drug Administration (FDA) and the FDA Anesthetic and Life Support Drugs Advisory Committee, made these changes out of concern for the very small but confirmed incidence of hyperkalemia-induced cardiac arrest in children and adolescent patients receiving succinylcholine as well as out of concern for the risk of succinylcholine-induced hyperkalemia following the acute phase of certain injuries. They suggest that the poten-

tial for hyperkalemia and rhabdomyolysis in children occurs in those with previously undiagnosed myopathy (e.g., muscular dystrophy). This situation would be unlikely in an adult.

Indications for use in adult patients are as before, but with the proviso that succinylcholine not be used after the acute phase of the injuries described. These recommendations, especially as they pertain to children and adolescents, represent a substantial departure from current practice and are, of course, applicable to inpatient as well as outpatient practice.

QUALITY IMPROVEMENT PROGRAMS

Interest in the quality of health care services has increased substantially, and efforts to develop feasible and acceptable methods to assess and ensure high-quality care and services have intensified.[71] Each facility must not only establish clinical indicators but also, if possible, establish thresholds for each of the indicators used. Examples of useful clinical indicators in the hospital-integrated ambulatory surgery unit are summarized in Table 80–16.

The success of contacting patients at home with a telephone follow-up is less than 50%; thus, the usefulness of a survey of this type is limited. Data that have been collected show that many patients report residual problems at home such as sore throat, nausea, headache, and backache.[2] Analysis of results such as these are imperative if improvement in care is desired.

TABLE 80–15. Regional Anesthesia for Postoperative Pain Relief

Circumcision
    Dorsal nerve block of penis
    Ring block
    Topical anesthesia
    Caudal
Herniorrhaphy
    Ilioinguinal–iliohypogastric nerve block
    Infiltration of incision
    "Splash"[50]
Orchiopexy
    Ilioinguinal–iliohypogastric nerve block
    Caudal
Arthroscopy
    Intra-articular administration of bupivacaine has been associated with mixed success[51] but is still widely used. One report describes the successful use of intra-articular morphine.[52]

References

1. Patel RI, Hannallah RS: Preoperative screening for pediatric ambulatory surgery: evaluation of a telephone questionnaire method. Anesth Analg 1992; 76:258.
2. Conway JB, Goldberg J, Chung F: Preadmission anaesthesia consultation clinic. Can J Anaesth 1992; 39:1051.
3. Duncan PG, Cohen MM, Tweed WA, et al: The Canadian Four-Centre Study of Anaesthetic Outcomes: III. Are anaesthetic complications predictable in day surgical practice? Can J Anaesth 1992; 39:440.
4. American Society of Anesthesiologists' 1993 Directory of Members, p 739.
5. Roizen M: Preoperative evaluation. In Anesthesia. 3rd ed. Miller RD (ed). New York, Churchill Livingstone, 1990, p 763.
6. Liu LMP, Coté CJ, Goudsouzian NG, et al: Life-threatening apnea in infants recovering from anesthesia. Anesthesiology 1983; 59:506.
7. Welborn LG, Ramirez N, Oh TH, et al: Postanesthetic apnea and periodic breathing in infants. Anesthesiology 1986; 65:656.
8. Kurth CD, Spitzer AR, Broennle AM, et al: Postoperative apnea in preterm infants. Anesthesiology 1987; 66:483.
9. Malviya S, Swartz J, Lerman J: Are all preterm infants younger than 60 weeks postconceptual age at risk for postanesthetic apnea? Anesthesiology 1993; 78:1076.
10. Welborn LG, Rice LJ, Hannallah RS, et al: Postoperative apnea in former preterm infants: prospective comparison of spinal and general anesthesia. Anesthesiology 1990; 72:838.
11. Welborn LG, Hannallah ARS, Fink R, et al: High dose caffeine prevents postoperative apnea in former preterm infants. Anesthesiology 1989; 71:342.

12. Tetzlaff JE, Annand DW, Pudimant MA, et al: Postoperative apnea in a full-term infant. Anesthesiology 1988; 69:426.

13. Steward DJ: Is there a risk of general anesthesia triggering SIDS? Possibly not. Anesthesiology 1985; 63:326.

14. Yentis SM, Levine MF, Hartley EJ: Should all children with suspected or confirmed malignant hyperpyrexia susceptibility be admitted after surgery?: a 10-year review. Anesth Analg 1992; 75:345.

15. Berkowitz RG, Zalzal GH: Tonsillectomy in children under 3 years of age. Arch Otolaryngol Head Neck Surg 1990; 116:685.

16. Tom LWC, DeDio RM, Cohen D, et al: Is outpatient tonsillectomy appropriate for young children? Laryngoscope 1992; 102:277.

17. Hetter GP: Blood and fluid replacement for lipoplasty procedures. Clin Plast Surg 1989; 16:245.

18. Kallar SK, Everett L: Potential risks and preventive measures for pulmonary aspiration: new concepts in preoperative fasting guidelines. Anesth Analg 1993; 77:171.

19. Minami H, McCallum RW: The physiology and pathophysiology of gastric emptying in humans. Gastroenterology 1986; 86:1592.

20. Goresky GV, Maltby JR: Fasting guidelines for elective surgical patients (Editorial). Can J Anaesth 1990; 37:493.

21. Olson GL, Hallen B, Hambraeus-Jonzon K: Aspiration during anesthesia: a computer-aided study of 188,358 anesthetics. Acta Anaesth Scand 1986; 30:84.

22. Kallar SK: Aspiration pneumonitis: fact or fiction? Probl Anesth 1988; 2:29.

23. White PF: Outpatient anesthesia: an overview. *In* Outpatient Anesthesia. White PF (ed). New York, Churchill Livingstone, 1990, pp 12 *and* 370.

24. Vetter TR: The epidemiology and selective identification of children at risk for preoperative anxiety reactions. Anesth Analg 1993; 77:96.

25. Feld LH, Negus JB, White PF: Oral midazolam preanesthetic medication in pediatric outpatients. Anesthesiology 1990; 73:831.

26. Hannallah RS, Patel RI: Low-dose intramuscular ketamine for anesthesia pre-induction in young children undergoing brief outpatient procedures. Anesthesiology 1989; 70:598.

27. Goresky GV, Stewart DJ: Rectal methohexitone for induction of anaesthesia in children. Can Anaesth Soc J 1979; 26:213.

28. Spear RM, Yaster M, Berkowitz ID, et al: Preinduction of anesthesia in children with rectally administered midazolam. Anesthesiology 1991; 74:670.

29. Karl HW, Keifer AT, Rosenberg JL, et al: Comparison of safety and efficacy of intra-nasal midazolam or sufentanil for preinduction of anesthesia in pediatric patients. Anesthesiology 1992; 76:209.

30. Nelson PS, Streisand JB, Mulder SM, et al: Comparison of oral transmucosal fentanyl citrate and an oral solution of meperidine, diazepam, and atropine for premedication in children. Anesthesiology 1989; 70:616.

31. Tamai YN, Shinguk K, Fujimori R, et al: Comparison between sevoflurane and halothane for paediatric ambulatory anaesthesia. Br J Anaesth 1991; 67:387.

32. Hannallah R, Schafer P, Britton J, et al: Recovery and discharge times following propofol, thiopental, and halothane anesthesia in pediatric outpatients. Anesthesiology 1991; 75:A25.

33. Hannallah RS, Baker SB, Casey W, et al: Propofol: effective dose and induction characteristics in unpremedicated children. Anesthesiology 1991; 74:217.

34. Kortilla K, Nuotto E, Lichtor J, et al: Clinical recovery and psychomotor function after brief anesthesia with propofol or thiopental. Anesthesiology 1993; 76:676.

35. Martin TM, Nicolson SC, Bargas MS: Propofol anesthesia reduces emesis and airway obstruction in pediatric outpatients. Anesth Analg 1993; 76:144.

36. Weir PM, Munro HM, Reynolds PI, et al: Propofol infusion and the incidence of emesis in pediatric outpatient strabismus surgery. Anesth Analg 1993; 76:760.

37. Watcha MF, Simeon RM, White PF, et al: Effect of propofol on the incidence of postoperative vomiting after strabismus surgery in pediatric outpatients. Anesthesiology 1991; 75:204.

38. Hannallah R, Britton J, Schafer P, et al: Effects of propofol anesthesia on the incidence of vomiting after strabismus surgery in children (Abstract). Anesth Analg 1992; 74:S131.

39. Kortilla K, Ostman P, Faure E, et al: Randomized comparison of recovery after propofol–nitrous oxide versus thiopentone–insoflurane–nitrous oxide anaesthesia in patients undergoing ambulatory surgery. Acta Anaesthesiol Scand 1990; 34:400.

40. Kwass MS, Fisher DM, Welborn LG, et al: Induction and maintenance characteristics of anesthesia with desflurane and nitrous oxide in infants and children. Anesthesiology 1992; 76:373.

41. Taylor E, Feinstein R, White PF, et al: Anesthesia for laparoscopic cho-

lecystectomy: is nitrous oxide contraindicated? Anesthesiology 1992; 76:541.

42. McGrath BJ, Zimmerman JE, Williams JF, et al: Carbon dioxide embolism treated with hyperbaric oxygen. Can J Anaesth 1989; 36:586.

43. Cohen MM, Cameron CB: Should you cancel the operation when a child has an upper respiratory tract infection? Anesth Analg 1991; 72:282.

44. American Academy of Pediatrics Committee on Drugs: Guidelines for monitoring and management of pediatric patients during and after sedation for diagnostic and therapeutic procedures. Pediatrics 1992; 89:1110.

45. Welborn LG, McGill WA, Hannallah RS, et al: Perioperative blood glucose concentrations in pediatric outpatients. Anesthesiology 1986; 65:543.

46. Welborn LG, Hannallah RS, McGill WA, et al: Choosing a glucose concentration for routine infusion in pediatric outpatient surgery. Anesthesiology 1987; 67:427.

47. Welborn L, Norden J, Seiden N, et al: Effect of minimizing preoperative fasting on perioperative blood glucose homeostasis in children. Paediatr Anaesth 1993; 3:167.

48. Kopacz DJ, Mulroy MF: Chloroprocaine and lidocaine decrease hospital stay and admission rate after outpatient epidural anesthesia. Reg Anesth 1990; 15:19.

49. Axelsson K, Mollefors K, Olsson JO, et al: Bladder function in spinal anesthesia. Acta Anaesthesiol Scand 1985; 29:315.

50. Bailey PL, Pace NL, Ashburn MA, et al: Frequent hypoxemia and apnea after sedation with midazolam and fentanyl. Anesthesiology 1990; 73:826.

51. Mazicon (Flumazenil/Roche) Product Monograph. Hoffman-LaRoche, 1992, p 57.

52. Schreiner MS, Nicolson SC, Martin T, et al: Should children drink before discharge from day surgery? Anesthesiology 1992; 76:528.

53. Koka BV, Jeon IS, Andre JM, et al: Postintubation croup in children. Anesth Analg 1977; 56:501.

54. Surgical and Anesthesia Services, Accreditation Manual for Ambulatory Health Care. JCAHO, 1993, p 168.

55. Surgical and Anesthesia Services, Accreditation Manual for Hospitals. Vol. II. Scoring Guidelines. SA 2.2, p 25.

56. Patel RI, Hannallah RS: Anesthetic complications following pediatric ambulatory surgery: a 3-year study. Anesthesiology 1988; 69:1009.

57. Patel RI, Hannallah RS: Complications following pediatric ambulatory surgery: less of the same? Anesthesiology 1993; 79:A22.

58. Gold BS, Kitz DS, Lecky JH, et al: Unanticipated admission to the hospital following ambulatory surgery. JAMA 1989; 262:3008.

59. Supplement on postoperative nausea and vomiting. Br J Anaesth 1992; 69(Suppl 1):1S.

60. Broadman LM, Cerruzi W, Patane PS, et al: Metoclopramide reduces the incidence of vomiting following strabismus surgery in children. Anesthesiology 1990; 72:245.

61. Rothenberg DM, Parness SM, Litwack K, et al: Efficacy of ephedrine in the prevention of postoperative nausea and vomiting. Anesth Analg 1991; 72:58.

62. Rosenblum M, Weller RS, Conard PL, et al: Ibuprofen provides longer lasting analgesia than fentanyl after laparoscopic surgery. Anesth Analg 1991; 73:255.

63. Casey WF, Rice LJ, Hannallah RS, et al: A comparison between bupivacaine instillation versus ilioinguinal/ilio-hypogastric nerve block for postoperative analgesia following inguinal herniorrhaphy in children. Anesthesiology 1990; 72:637.

64. Milligan KA, Mowbray MJ, Mulrooney L: Intra-articular bupivacaine for pain relief after arthroscopic surgery of the knee joint in day case patients. Anaesthesia 1988; 43:563.

65. Stein C, Comisel K, Haimerl E, et al: Analgesic effect of intraarticular morphine after arthroscopic knee surgery. N Engl J Med 1991; 325:1123.

66. Joshi GP, McCarroll SM, O'Brien TM, et al: Intra-articular analgesia following knee arthroscopy. Anesth Analg 1993; 76:333.

67. Levy ML: Outcome after outpatient anesthesia. *In* Clinical Anaesthesia. Desmonts J (ed). London, Bailliere, 1992.

68. Cunningham AJ, Brull SJ: Laparoscopic cholecystectomy: anesthetic implications. Anesth Analg 1993; 76:1120.

69. Hasel R, Arora SK, Hickey D: Intraoperative complications of laparoscopic cholecystectomy. Can J Anaesth 1993; 40:459.

70. Burroughs Wellcome Co.: Cardiac arrest in children and adolescent patients receiving succinylcholine and succinylcholine-induced hyperkalemia. Burroughs Wellcome Co., Research Triangle Park, NC, November 1993.

71. Twersky RS, Barlow JC: Quality assurance in ambulatory surgery hospital and freestanding facilities. ASA Newsletter 1991; 55:16.

Index

Note: Page numbers in *italics* refer to illustrations; numbers followed by (t) indicate tables.

a wave, 373
AARKs. See *Automated anesthesia recordkeepers (AARKs)*.
AAS (atlantoaxial subluxation), causes of, 224, 226
  in rheumatoid arthritis, 464, *465*
  radiographic findings in, 224, 226, *227*, *228*
Abbreviated Injury Scale (AIS), 985
Abdomen, distention of, and alveolar hypoventilation, 805
  injuries of, traumatic, assessment of, 997, 998
    thoracic injuries with, 1005
  lower, surgery of, in children, epidural analgesia for, 269
  pain in, in children, treatment of, 272, 273
  position of, in prone position, 508
  radiography of, 226, *229–232*
  wall of, defects of, congenital, 1027, *1027*, 1028, *1028*
    hernias of, 1133, 1134
    relaxation of, 1109
    surgery of, 1133, 1134
Abdominal aorta, surgery of, and paraplegia, 1229
Abdominal aortic aneurysm, repair of, 1215, 1216
  mortality rate in, 126
Abdominal surgery, 1109–1134
  complications of, pulmonary, 149(t), 1132, 1133
    classification of, 148(t)
  effects of, on pulmonary function, 1130–1132, *1130*, *1131*, 1131(t)
  emergency, rapid-sequence induction in, 1118, 1119
  epidural anesthesia for, 1113, 1114
  fluid management in, 1119–1121
    with acute intra-abdominal disease, 1120
  general anesthesia for, 1109, 1110
    regional anesthesia with, 1114
  hypotension during, 1114, 1115, *1115*, 1115(t)
    treatment of, 1114
  in ascites, 1124, *1124*, 1125, *1125*
  intestinal motility after, 1133
  lower, sensory block for, 1114
  muscle relaxation for, 1110–1113, *1112*, 1112(t)
    choice of, 1110
    clinical criteria for, 1111
    duration of, factors in, 1110, 1111
    hiccups effects on, 1112

Abdominal surgery *(Continued)*
    inadequate, during peritoneal closure, 1112, 1113
    reversal of, re-establishment after, 1113
  nasogastric tubes for, 1117, 1118, *1118*
    in esophageal varices, 1117
    insertion of, 1117, *1118*
      failure of, 1118
    types of, 1117
  oxygen after, need for, 1132
  pain after, effects of, on pulmonary function, 1131, 1131(t)
  spinal anesthesia for, 1113, 1114
  upper, elective, delay of, pulmonary considerations in, 147, 147(t), 148, 148(t)
    pulmonary consultation before, 143
    risk of, chronic obstructive pulmonary disease in, 966, 966(t)
    sensory block for, 1113, 1114
Abdominal viscera, puncture of, during sympathetic nerve block, 491, 492
ABGs. See *Arterial blood gases (ABGs)*.
Abortion, spontaneous, anesthesia and, 1101, 1102
Abscess, pharyngeal, 1273
  airway management in, 1273
Accelerometry, in neuromuscular blockade assessment, 419
Accountability, determination of, 59
Accreditation Manual for Hospitals (AMH), 35
ACE (angiotensin-converting enzyme) inhibitors, drug interactions with, 655(t)
  for shock, 665, 666
  perioperative continuation of, 139
Acetaminophen, for pain, acute, 240(t)
  in children, 264, 264(t)
    with cancer, 272
Acetazolamide, drug interactions with, 647(t)
  in ester metabolism, 625, 625(t)
Acetylation, genetic factors in, 569
Acetylcholine esterase inhibitors, drug interactions with, 646(t)
Acetylsalicylic acid, perioperative use of, 7, 8
Acid, definition of, 732
α_1-Acid glycoprotein, in drug distribution, 648
  in local anesthetic toxicity prevention, 634
Acid-base balance, 732–741
  analysis of, arterial blood gases in, 343
  changes in, assessment of, 735
    during renal transplantation, 1365
    effects of, on serum calcium, 1313, *1314*
    in chronic liver disease, 1337
  disturbances of, 737–740

Acid-base balance *(Continued)*
    and left ventricular failure, after cardiopulmonary bypass, 1182
  effects of, 740, 741
  management of, during cardiopulmonary bypass, 327, 328
  postoperative, 101, 102
  renal response to, 735, 736, *736*
  effects on, of metabolism, 738–740, 738(t), 739(t), *740*
    of orthotopic liver transplantation, during anhepatic phase, 1348, 1349, *1349*
      during neohepatic phase, 1351
    of ventilation, 734, *734*, 735, *735*, 737, *737*, 738
  in drug transport, 565, 566
  in pyloric stenosis, 1026, 1027
  liver in, 736, 737
  physiology of, 732–734
Acidemia, definition of, 732
  metabolic, postoperative, effects of, 101
    factors in, 101
    treatment of, 101, 102
  respiratory, postoperative, effects of, 101
    factors in, 101
    treatment of, 101
Acidity, measurement of, 733, 733(t)
Acidosis, during renal transplantation, 1365
  in alveolar hyperventilation, 809
  lactic. See *Lactic acidosis*.
  local anesthetic overdose and, treatment of, 635
  metabolic. See *Metabolic acidosis*.
  respiratory. See *Respiratory acidosis*.
Acoustic schwannoma, properties of, 1303(t)
Acquired immunodeficiency syndrome (AIDS). See also *Human immunodeficiency virus (HIV) infection*.
  pediatric, epidemiology of, 853, 854
Acromegaly, clinical features of, 185
  complications of, 186(t)
  definition of, 185
  diagnosis of, 185
  management of, 185, 186
    perioperative, 186, 186(t)
ACT (activated clotting time), monitoring of, in cardiovascular surgery, 1168
  pediatric, 1152
ACTH. See *Adrenocorticotropic hormone (ACTH)*.
Action potential, local anesthetic effect on, 622, *622*

Activated clotting time (ACT), monitoring of, in cardiovascular surgery, 1168
  pediatric, 1152
Active electrode, 416
Acute tubular necrosis (ATN), 694
Acute ventilatory failure, after abdominal surgery, 1132
AD. See *Autonomic dysreflexia (AD)*.
Addison's disease, clinical features of, 190(t)
  complications of, perioperative, 194
  definition of, 189
  diagnosis of, 191, 192
  evaluation of, preoperative, 193
  management of, perioperative, 193
  preoperative, 191, 192, 193
Adenoma, chromophobe, 1312
Adenoreceptors, for intraoperative hemodynamic stabilization, in shock, 690, 690
Adenosine, action of, mechanism of, 849
  for life-threatening dysrhythmias, 850
  for supraventricular tachycardia, after cardiopulmonary bypass, 1187(t)
  in cardiopulmonary resuscitation, 849
    complications of, 849
    dosage of, 849
    indications for, 849
  in pediatric cardiovascular surgery, 1146(t)
Adenotonsillectomy, 1269–1271, *1269*, 1269(t), *1270*, 1270(t)
  anesthesia for, emergence from, 1270, *1270*
    induction of, 1269, *1269*
    management of, 1269, *1269*, 1270
  bleeding after, management of, 1270, 1270(t), 1271
  extubation after, 1270
  indications for, 1269, 1269(t)
  preoperative evaluation in, 1269
ADH (antidiuretic hormone), deficiency of, in diabetes insipidus, 186
  in urine output, 385
Adjustable pressure-limiting (APL) valve, 280, 281
  of anesthesia machine, isolation of, 296
Adrenal glands, diseases of, 189–196, 190(t), 192(t), 195(t)
  dysfunction of, clinical features of, 190(t)
  failure of, primary, 189
    secondary, 189
  function of, in acromegaly, 186
  hormones secreted by, 1317(t)
  surgery of, 1317–1319, 1317(t)–1319(t), *1319*
  tumors of, surgical treatment of, 191
Adrenal insufficiency, delayed emergence in, 164(t)
  in hypothyroidism, 200
Adrenal suppression, history of, 4, *4*
Adrenalectomy, bilateral, 1318
Adrenergic receptors, for perioperative myocardial dysfunction, 765, 765(t)
Adrenocortical insufficiency, 1318, 1319, *1319*, 1319(t)
  management of, intraoperative, 1319
  surgery for, preoperative preparation in, 1319
Adrenocorticosteroids, for bronchial asthma, 958, 958(t)
Adrenocorticotropic hormone (ACTH), 189
  in Addison's disease diagnosis, 191
  in Cushing's syndrome diagnosis, 190
  perioperative use of, 7
  production of, pituitary vs. ectopic, 190
Adult(s), morbidly obese, outpatient surgery in, 1393
  pain management consultation in, 233–257
  tracheal intubation in, tube size for, 308

Adult respiratory distress syndrome (ARDS), after trauma surgery, 1008
  pulmonary edema with, intraoperative management of, 976
  radiographic findings in, 216, *220*
  shock and, 695, *695*, 695(t)
Advanced life support (ALS), 835
Advanced Trauma Life Support (ATLS), 990
"Adverse events," 57
Adverse patient outcomes (APOs), 38
Affinity, definition of, 569
Afterload, after cardiopulmonary bypass, goal for, 1181
  in aortic stenosis, 1171
  of right ventricle, reduction of, for right ventricular infarction, 678, 679, *679*
  quantification of, 763
  stroke volume, 757, *758*
Afterload sensitivity, in end-stage heart disease, 1322
Age, advanced. See also *Geriatric patients*.
  in perioperative risk, 64, 64(t)
  cervical spine changes with, 463, 463(t)
Agenda for Change, 32, 40
Aging, effects of, 1067, 1068
  on cervical spine motion, 464
  on circulation, 1071
  on lumbar spine, 473
  on postoperative functional residual capacity, 79
  on ventilation, 1071, 1072, 1072(t)
Agonists, 570
AICD. See *Automatic internal cardioverter-defibrillator (AICD)*.
AIDS (acquired immunodeficiency syndrome). See also *Human immunodeficiency virus (HIV) infection*.
  pediatric, epidemiology of, 853, 854
Air embolism, and delayed awakening, 165
  and pulmonary edema, 977
  head-up position and, 509
  in anesthetic agent monitoring, 350
  in burn surgery, 709
  in congenital heart disease, 1044
  in neurologic surgery, 1286, 1286(t)
  in orthotopic liver transplantation, during neohepatic phase, 1350
  in persistent postoperative unconsciousness, 97
  in transsphenoidal hypophysectomy, 1313
  venous, open prostatectomy and, 1238
Air transportable hospital (ATH), 879
Airway(s), adjuncts to, for cardiopulmonary resuscitation, 837, *837*, 838, *838*
  anatomy of, functional, 439–456
    normal, on chest radiography, 213
    phylogenetic considerations in, 439
    topical, 439–442, *440*, 440(t), *441*
  closure of, reflex, larynx in, 449, 450
  cross-sectional area of, reduction in, with facemask ventilation, 924
  difficult, anesthetic technique for, 585(t)
    management of, 921–952
  disorders of, in rheumatoid arthritis, 1250, *1250*
  edema of, 1275
    presentation of, 1275
    treatment of, 1275
  establishment of, alternative methods of, 316, 317
    devices for, application of, 298–317
    for cesarean section, 1093
  evaluation of, in anaphylaxis, 748
    in trauma, 991, 992
    preanesthetic, 10, *10*
    problems in, 440(t)
  for facemask airway obstruction, 927

Airway(s) *(Continued)*
  hyperreactivity of, causes of, 955
    in children, 1004
    in neonates, 1014, 1015
  laser surgery of, fire caused by, management of, 1378, 1379, 1379(t)
  management of, documentation of, 23
    in alveolar hypoventilation, 806, *806*, 807, *807*
    in cardiopulmonary resuscitation, 835, 836, *836*
    in children, conditions associated with, 1054(t)
    for anesthesia induction, 1049, 1050, *1050*
    in neonates, 1022, 1023
    in otolaryngologic/maxillofacial surgery, 1280, 1281, *1281*
      emergency, 1280
    in outpatient surgery, 1398, 1398(t), 1399
    in pharyngeal abscess, 1273
    in postextubation airway obstruction, 950
    in pregnant patient, during nonobstetric surgery, 1100
    in radiation therapy anesthesia, 917, *917*
    in spinal cord shock, 685
    in transsphenoidal hypophysectomy, 1312, 1313, 1313(t)
  principles of, 921, 922, 922(t)
  maneuvering of, with injured neck, 468
  nasal, 298, 299, *299*
    applications of, 298
    for facemask airway obstruction, 926
    insertion of, 299, *299*
    problems in, 299
  neoplasia of, 1274
    intubation with, 1274
  oral, 298, 299, *299*
    applications of, 298
    insertion of, 298, 299, *299*
    problems in, 299
  reactive, difficult intubation with, 942, 942(t)
  upper, anatomy of, *1268*
    of children, preanesthetic assessment of, 1040, 1041
    of geriatric patients, 1070
Airway obstruction, and postoperative hypoxemia, 78
  assessment of, in trauma, 991
  during intravenous induction, management of, 589, 590
  effects of, on ventilatory work, 812, *812*, 813
  facemask, 923, 924
    avoidance of, 925
    causes of, 927
    management of, 926, 927
    recognition of, 924, 924(t), 925
    refractory, management of, 928
  in children, intraoperative, 1059
    during cardiovascular surgery, 1147
    postanesthesia, 1062
  in hyperthyroidism, 201
  in hypothyroidism, 201, 1316
  in outpatient tonsillectomy, 1393, 1394
  laryngeal cartilages in, 445, 446
  postextubation, in transsphenoidal hypophysectomy, 1313
    management of, 950, 951
  proximal, emergency treatment of, 82, *82*
  relief of, in alveolar hypoventilation, 807
  pulmonary edema after, 978, 979
Airway pressure, changes in, in postoperative pulmonary blood flow, 80
  increased, intraoperative, treatment of, 967, 967(t)
  monitoring of, 344, 345, *347*
    intraoperative, value of, 344

Airway pressure *(Continued)*
 manometer in, 344, 345, *347*
Airway pressure gauge, of breathing system, 288, *289*
Airways resistance, distal, 82, 83
 in work of breathing, 957
 increased, facemask ventilation in, 924, 924(t)
 in spontaneous breathing, during inhalation anesthesia, 611, *611*
 upper, increase in, causes of, 82, 82(t)
 diagnosis of, 83
 effects of, 82, *82*, 82(t)
 treatment of, 83
 emergency, 82, *82*
AIS (Abbreviated Injury Scale), 985
Alarm, of monitoring device, activation of, 339
Albumin, in drug distribution, 648
 in hemostasis, 728
Albuterol, 145(t)
 for bronchial asthma, 957(t), 958(t)
Alcohol, ingestion of, preanesthetic evaluation of, 9
Alcohol intoxication, 999, 1000
Alcohol withdrawal syndrome, 1000
Alcoholism, delayed emergence in, 164(t)
Aldosterone, measurement of, in Addison's disease diagnosis, 192
Aldosteronism, primary, manifestations of, 1318, 1319(t)
Alfentanil, dose of, equieffective, 658(t)
 drug interactions with, 652(t), 654(t)
 for acute pain, 241(t)
 intraspinal, for acute pain, 248(t)
 intravenous, patient-controlled, guidelines for, 245(t)
 properties of, 598(t), 600(t)
Aliphatic, adverse effects of, 656(t)
Alkalemia, definition of, 732
 metabolic, postoperative, effects of, 102
 factors in, 102
 treatment of, 102
 respiratory, postoperative, effects of, 102
 factors in, 102
 treatment of, 102
Alkalinization, of local anesthetics, 629
Alkalosis, metabolic. See *Metabolic alkalosis.*
 respiratory. See *Respiratory alkalosis.*
Allen's test, 11, 11(t)
Allergic reaction, characteristics of, 743, 743(t)
Allergy(ies), 743–750
 preanesthetic evaluation of, 9
 to contrast agents, 902
 to local anesthetics, 635, 636, *636*, 636(t)
Alpha rhythm, in electroencephalography, 400, *400*
Alpha stat method, of arterial blood gas analysis, 342
Alpha-adrenergic receptors, stimulation of, in postoperative hypertension, 91, 92
Alpha-methylparatyrosine, for blood pressure control, in pheochromocytoma, 195, 195(t)
ALS (advanced life support), 835
Alternating current, 886
Alveolar air equation, 342, 800, 801, 921
Alveolar epithelium, in pulmonary edema, 969, *970*
Alveolar hyperventilation, 807–809
 causes of, 808, 808(t), 809
 effects of, 807, 808
Alveolar hypoventilation. See *Hypoventilation, alveolar.*
Alveolar oxygen tension, formula for, 692(t)
Alveolar recruitment, 795
Alveolar ventilation, larynx in, 449
Alzheimer's disease, 1079
Ambulatory surgery. See *Outpatient surgery.*

American Society for Testing and Materials (ASTM), 296
American Society of Anesthesiologists (ASA), physical status classification of, 14, 15, 15(t), 127, 127(t)
AMH (Accreditation Manual for Hospitals), 35
Amides, metabolism of, 625
 properties of, clinical, 627(t)
 use of, in malignant hyperthermia, 827(t)
Aminoglycosides, drug interactions with, 652(t), 654(t)
Aminophylline, for anaphylactic shock, 683(t)
 for anaphylaxis, 748
 for bronchial asthma, 958(t)
 in pediatric cardiovascular surgery, 1146(t)
 perioperative use of, 6, 7
 with halothane, 6
Amiodarone, drug interactions with, 645(t)
 perioperative use of, 6
Amitriptyline, for pain, 242(t)
Ammonium salts, in acid-base balance, 736
Amnesia, inadequate, with high-dose opioids, for cardiovascular surgery, 1173
Amniotic fluid embolism, during cesarean section, 1093
Amoxapine, drug interactions with, 651(t)
Amoxicillin, in bacterial endocarditis prophylaxis, 15(t)
Amphetamines, abuse of, diagnostic features of, 1000(t)
 use of, and hyperthermia, 826
Ampicillin, in bacterial endocarditis prophylaxis, 15(t)
AMPLE history, 990, 991(t)
Amputation, 1254
Amrinone, 1182(t)
 for anaphylaxis, 748
 for perioperative myocardial dysfunction, 766(t)
 for right ventricular failure, after cardiopulmonary bypass, 1183
 in pediatric cardiovascular surgery, 1146(t)
Amyl nitrate, in heart murmur evaluation, 11(t)
Analgesia, administration of, in children, techniques of, 265–267, 265(t)
 after battlefield surgery, 881
 after general anesthesia, indications for, 594
 after nephrectomy, 1242
 epidural, after thoracic surgery, 1207, 1208
 for awake neurologic monitoring, 392
 for burns, in children, 271
 for labor, 1085–1087, 1085(t), *1086*
 choice of, 1087
 for postoperative hypoxemia, 79
 for potentially difficult intubation, 936
 for vascular access, 544
 inhalation, in obstetric patients, 1089
 narcotics for, alternatives to, 605
 non-narcotic, use of, in postanesthesia care unit, 76
 nonopioid, for acute pain, 240(t)
 patient-controlled. See *Patient-controlled analgesia (PCA).*
 peridural, in adults, 246, *246*
 in cancer, 250, *252*
 in chronic pain, 250, 252(t)
 postoperative, 70, 71
 advantages of, 70
 costs of, 71
 regional anesthesia in, 69
 risks of, 70, 70(t)
 pre-emptive, after thoracic surgery, 1208, *1208*
 regional, in children, 267–270
 contraindications to, 267
 pharmacology of, 267

Analgesia *(Continued)*
 translaryngeal, for awake tracheal intubation, 1280
Anaphylactic reactions, definition of, 680, 681
 treatment of, 747(t)
Anaphylactic shock, 680–682, 681(t)–683(t)
 mechanisms of, 681, 681(t)
 pathophysiologic end point of, 681
 signs and symptoms of, 681
 treatment of, 681, 683(t)
Anaphylactoid reactions, 744
 definition of, 681
 treatment of, 747(t)
Anaphylatoxins, 681
Anaphylaxis, 744–746
 chemical mediators in, cardiopulmonary effects of, 744, 745
 chemotactic factors of, cardiopulmonary effects of, 744, 745
 complement activation in, 746
 non–IgE-mediated, 746
 pathophysiology of, 744, *745*
 perioperative, 748–750, 749(t)
 drugs causing, 748, 749, 749(t)
 evaluation of, 749, 749(t), 750
 recognition of, 749, 749(t)
 recognition of, 745, 746
 treatment of, 746–748, 747(t)
Andy Gump fracture, 1280
Anemia, dilutional, effects on, of hypocapnia, 671
 in shock, 668
 effects of, on myocardial oxygen consumption, 669
 hypovolemic, 669
 in chronic liver disease, 1336
 in dialysis patient, 183
 in hypoxemia, 785
 in intraventricular hemorrhage, 1019
 normovolemic, 669
 effects of, on myocardium, 671, *671*, 672
Anesthesia, adult vs. neonate, 1014(t)
 caudal. See *Caudal anesthesia.*
 complications of, assessment of, 62
 definition of, 62
 costs of, 109–123
 during pregnancy, 1099, 1100, 1100(t)
 effects of, nonmedical, 114
 on electroencephalography, 401, 402
 on evoked potentials, 404(t)
 minimization of, 404(t)
 on intracranial pressure, 774–781
 emergence from, after neurologic surgery, 1287, 1288, 1309
 after neurovascular surgery, 1294, 1295
 delayed, 163–165, 164(t)
 drugs in, 163, 164
 overdose in, 164
 rare events in, 165
 surgical procedure in, 164
 intracranial pressure control during, 780, 780(t)
 negligence in, 55, 56
 thermoregulation during, 821, 821(t)
 epidural. See *Epidural anesthesia.*
 equipment for, funding of, 118–120, *119*
 for potentially difficult intubation, 934, 935
 for vascular access, 544
 general. See *General anesthesia.*
 hypotensive, in pregnant patient, for nonobstetric surgery, 1106
 hypoxemia during, causes of, 796
 in battlefield surgery, 874–883
 in children, maintenance of, 1054–1056, 1054(t), *1055*, 1056(t)
 procedures requiring, 1062–1064, *1063*

Anesthesia *(Continued)*
  in geriatric patients, management of, factors
    in, 1070–1073, 1070(t), 1072(t)
  in obstetric patients, fetal effects of, 1101,
    1101(t)
    guidelines for, 1082(t)
  induction of, for acute gastrointestinal bleed-
    ing, 1122
    for adenotonsillectomy, 1269, *1269*
    for aortic vascular surgery, 1222
    for cardiovascular surgery, pediatric,
      1145–1148
      problems in, 1147
    for heart transplantation, 1325
    for neurologic surgery, 1287, 1288
    for orthotopic liver transplantation, 1342,
      1343
      intubation in, nasogastric, 1343
        nasotracheal, 1343
      positioning in, 1343
    for renal transplantation, 1362–1364,
      1362(t), 1363(t)
      muscle relaxation in, 1363, 1364
    for spinal surgery, 1299
    for thoracic surgery, 1202
    in children, 1049–1054, *1050*, 1052(t),
      1053, 1053(t)
      airway management in, 1049, 1050,
        1050
      equipment for, 1052–1054, 1053(t)
      intramuscular, 1052
      intravenous, 1051, 1052, 1052(t)
      parent presence during, 1050, 1051
      rectal, 1052
    in chronic obstructive pulmonary disease,
      966
    in obstetric patient, 1091
    in shock, intraoperative, 688
      spinal cord, 686
    intracranial pressure control during, 777,
      778, 778(t)
    intubation after, 938–942
    narcotics in, 604
    negligence in, 55
    rapid-sequence, in emergency abdominal
      surgery, 1118, 1119
      risks of, 941, 942
    rate of, 571
      cardiac disease in, 1147
    time to, 649
  inhalation. See *Inhalation anesthesia.*
  intravenous, and postoperative nausea, 99
  laryngotracheal, stylet for, function of, 316
  mask, in children, 1054, 1055
    indications for, 588
    with intravenous induction, 589
  one-lung, technique of, 1205
  outpatient, in geriatric patients, 1079, 1080
  prior adverse reaction to, 2
  regional. See *Regional anesthesia.*
  response to, genetic factors in, 569
  risk of, calculation of, 14, 15, 15(t)
    to fetus, 1101–1104, *1102*, 1102(t)
  spinal. See *Spinal anesthesia.*
  thermoregulation during, 817, 818, *818*,
    818(t)
  topical, for tracheal intubation, in conscious
    patients, 453
    to nose, 441
  with abnormal intracranial pressure, 772
Anesthesia Apparatus Checkout
  Recommendations, 292, 293(t)
Anesthesia machine, 276–297
  breathing system of, 276
  components of, 276, *277*
  design of, changes in, 296
    standards for, 296

Anesthesia machine *(Continued)*
  gas delivery system of, troubleshooting for,
    291–294
  high-pressure system of, 276–281, 277(t),
    278–281
    pressure gauges of, checking of, 279
    safety features of, 277–279, *278–280*
    structural components of, 276–279, 277(t)
  in patient injury, 294
  low-pressure system of, 276, 281–285
    components of, 281, 281(t), *282*
  malfunction of, management of, 295, 296
  monitoring instruments of, 276
  monitoring of, 294–296, 294(t)
  obsolescence of, 296, 297
  scavenging system of, 276
Anesthesia vaporizer, in cardiopulmonary
  bypass, 322
Anesthesia ventilator, 276–297
Anesthesiologist, as expert witness, 59, 60
Anesthetic agent(s), allergic reaction to, 9
  and perioperative oliguria, 386
  characteristics of, 570, 571
  concentration of, monitoring of, 348
  cost of, 120
  effects of, on brainstem evoked potentials,
    406(t)
    motor, 408, 408(t)
    somatosensory, 406(t)
  elimination of, drug interactions in, 648
  for general anesthesia, 591, 592, *592*, *593*,
    593(t)
  in malignant hyperthermia, 827, 827(t)
  inappropriate dose of, consequences of, 295
    management of, 295
  intravenous, 597–605
    and postoperative nausea, 99
    clearance of, factors in, 599, 600, 600(t)
    distribution of, factors in, 597, 598, *598*,
      598(t)
      volume of, 597, 597(t)
    facemask ventilation with, 925
    for battlefield surgery, 880, 881
    for burn surgery, 710, 711(t)
    for radiation therapy, 917, 918
    infusion of, continuous, effects of, 598,
      599
      indications for, 598, 599, 599(t)
      rate of, 599, 600(t)
    overdose of, 600, 601, 601(t)
    properties of, 598(t)
      pharmacokinetic, 597–601
    reversal of, agents for, 601
    types of, 601–605, *602*, 603(t)
    volume of, factors in, 600
  monitoring of, 348–350
    potential errors in, 348–350
  rectal, for radiation therapy, 918
  scavenging of, 869, 870, *870*
  selection of, 571–574
    for burn surgery, 711
    in pheochromocytoma, 196
  volatile, in chronic obstructive pulmonary
    disease, 967
    in intraoperative intracranial pressure con-
      trol, 779
    metabolism of, 648, 649
    use of, with catecholamines, 613
Anesthetic prescription, 67–70, 68(t), 70(t)
  "default mode" of, 64
  monitoring devices in, 67, 67(t)
Anesthetic record, 20–30, *20*
  creation of, 24–28, *25–27*
  handwritten, accuracy of, 26, *26*
    in blood pressure recording, 26
    advantages of, 25
    completeness of, 26

Anesthetic record *(Continued)*
  legibility of, 27, *27*
  vs. automated anesthesia recordkeepers,
    25, *25*, 26
  in liability exposure, 20
  in medicolegal issues, 22, 56, 57
  inaccuracy of, penalties for, 24
  inclusiveness of, limitations on, 24
  information in, 22, 23, *23*
    billing use of, 24
    interpretation of, 24
    on airway management, 23
    on equipment checks, 23
    on potential postoperative problems, 23
    presentation of, 24
  meaningful, definition of, 22
  purposes of, 21–24, 21(t), *23*
  uses of, 21, 21(t), 22
    as log book, 21, 22
    in administration, 22
    in auditing, 24
    in clinical management, 22
    in patient care, 21, 22
    in research and education, 22
    in trend plotting, 24
Aneurysm(s), aortic. See *Aortic aneurysm(s).*
  fusiform, 1211, 1212
  intracranial. See *Intracranial aneurysm(s).*
  saccular, 1211, 1212
  thoracoabdominal, management of, 1218,
    1218(t), 1219
  repair of, 1216
Angina, Ludwig's, 1273, 1273(t), 1274
  tracheotomy in, 1274
Angina pectoris, 1157, 1158
  history of, 2
  in aortic stenosis, 1161
  in coronary artery disease, 754
  preoperative, in cardiac risk assessment, 129
  types of, 1158
Angiography, cerebral, risks of, 905
  radionuclide, before cardiovascular surgery,
    1159
    gated, in preanesthetic evaluation, of coro-
      nary artery disease, 13
  spinal, risks of, 905
Angioplasty, balloon, laser, in cardiogenic
    shock, 674
  cerebral, for cerebral vasospasm, after intra-
    cranial aneurysm rupture, 1291
  coronary, before noncardiac surgery, 134,
    135
  in cardiogenic shock, 673
Angiotensin-converting enzyme (ACE)
  inhibitors, drug interactions with, 655(t)
  for shock, 665, 666
  perioperative continuation of, 139
Anhepatic phase, of orthotopic liver
    transplantation, 1345
  physiologic changes in, 1347–1349, *1347*,
    1348
Anion gap, 734
  in metabolic acidosis, 738, 738(t)
Ankle block, 533, 534, *534*
  drug choice for, 533
  needle placement for, 533, *534*
  patient selection for, 533
  potential problems with, 534
Ankylosing spondylitis, cervical spine anatomy
    in, 465, *466*
Anomalies, congenital, anesthesia and, 1101,
    1102
ANS. See *Autonomic nervous system (ANS).*
Antacids, nonparticulate, in pulmonary
    aspiration prevention, 86
  selection of, factors in, 573
Antagonists, 570, *570*

Anterior epidural space, in lumbar spine, 472, *473*
Anterior pituitary gland, 1312
Anterior spinal artery syndrome, 1226
Anterior thoracic corpectomy/diskectomy, anesthetic considerations in, 1301
Antianginal medication, perioperative use of, 6
Antibiotics, use of, drug interactions with, 658, 658(t)
    perioperative, 8, 9(t)
    preoperative, indications for, 15, 15(t), *16*
    prophylactic, for orthopedic surgery, 1258, 1259
Antibodies, 743, 744, *744*
Anticholinergic agents, drug interactions with, 646(t)
    for bronchial asthma, 958
    for contrast agent reactions, 904
    in premedication, 583
        pediatric, 1047
    overdose of, physostigmine for, 164
Anticholinesterases, drug interactions with, 647(t)
    for myasthenia gravis, 153
    in renal transplantation, 1363, 1364
Anticoagulants, discontinuation of, preoperative, guidelines for, 155
    drug interactions with, 644(t)–646(t)
    perioperative use of, 8
Anticoagulation, epidural anesthesia with, 253
    in peridural hematoma formation, 253
    management of, in pediatric cardiopulmonary bypass, 1151, 1152
        perioperative, with prosthetic heart valve, 138
Anticonvulsants, drug interactions with, 644(t), 645(t)
    use of, before neurovascular surgery, 1292
        perioperative, 7, 159, 159(t)
Antidepressants, drug interactions with, 650, 651
    for pain, 242(t)
    perioperative use of, 7
    tricyclic. See *Tricyclic antidepressants.*
Antidiuretic agents, administration of, for diabetes insipidus, 187
Antidiuretic hormone (ADH), deficiency of, in diabetes insipidus, 186
    in urine output, 385
Antidysrhythmics, continuation of, for automatic internal cardioverter-defibrillator implantation, 1164
    drug interactions with, 657, 658
    perioperative use of, 6
    response to, in chronic renal failure, 1361
Antiemetics, prophylactic, 245(t)
    response to, in chronic renal failure, 1361
Antifibrinolytic agents, in blood loss prevention, after cardiopulmonary bypass, 1190
Antigens, 743, 743(t), 744
Antiglaucoma agents, perioperative use of, 8, *8*
Antihistamines, analgesic potential of, 244(t)
    for anaphylactic shock, 683(t)
    for anaphylaxis, 748
    for contrast agent reactions, 904
    selection of, factors in, 573
Antihypertensives, centrally acting, effects of, on minimum alveolar concentration, 656, *656*
    continuation of, perioperative, 139, 140
    discontinuation of, preoperative, 651
    efficacy of, assessment of, preoperative, 170
    in postoperative pulmonary blood flow, 80
    response to, in chronic renal failure, 1361
    use of, perioperative, 5

Anti-inflammatory drugs, perioperative use of, 7, 8
Antineoplastic agents, perioperative use of, 8
Antiplatelet agents, discontinuation of, preoperative, guidelines for, 155
Antipsychotic medications, drug interactions with, 650, 656(t)
    perioperative use of, 7
Anxiety, and postoperative pain, 76
    in alveolar hyperventilation, 808
Anxiolytics, abuse of, diagnostic features of, 1000(t)
    pharmacologic, indications for, 578, 579, 579(t)
AOG (atlanto-occipital gap), effects of, on tracheal intubation, 464
Aorta, anatomy of, *1212*
    ascending, surgery of, 1190
    cross-clamping of, and paraplegia, 1226–1228
        prevention of, 1228, 1228(t), 1229
    and pulmonary edema, 980
    discontinuation of, 1229, 1230, 1230(t)
        in heart transplantation, 1328
    hemodynamic effects of, 1225, 1225(t), 1226, *1226*
    descending, surgery of, 1190–1192
    disease of, 1210–1215
        diagnosis of, 1212, 1213, 1213(t)
        diseases coexisting with, 1213, 1213(t)
        distribution of, 1213
    disruption of, traumatic, assessment of, 996, *996*
    shearing of, 1212
    thoracic. See *Thoracic aorta.*
Aortic aneurysm(s), abdominal, repair of, 1215, 1216
        mortality rate in, 126
    differential diagnosis of, 1211
    distribution of, 1213
    rupture of, mortality of, 1230(t)
    thoracic, 1162
Aortic arch, surgery of, 1191
Aortic cannulation, for cardiopulmonary bypass, concerns during, 1178
Aortic dissection, before cardiopulmonary bypass, 1178
    classification of, 1215, 1215(t), *1216*
    differential diagnosis of, 1211
    distribution of, 1213
    pathogenesis of, 1211
    repair of, 1216, 1217
    thoracic, 1162, *1162*
Aortic insufficiency, hemodynamic goals in, 1172, 1172(t)
    operative risks in, 1172
    signs and symptoms of, 1162
Aortic regurgitation, preoperative assessment of, 138
Aortic stenosis, hemodynamic goals in, 1171, 1171(t)
    operative risks in, 1171
    preoperative assessment of, 137, 138
    regional anesthesia in, 514
    signs and symptoms of, 1161
Aortic vascular surgery, 1210–1231
    anatomic considerations in, 1215–1217, 1215(t), *1216*
    anesthesia for, induction/maintenance of, 1222–1230
    central, anesthesia for, 1217–1222, 1217(t)
    extubation after, 1230
    hematocrit in, 1221, 1222
    myocardial ischemia in, detection of, 1220, 1221
    perioperative morbidity and mortality in, 1213, 1214

Aortic vascular surgery *(Continued)*
    renal function preservation in, 1219, 1220, 1220(t)
    risks of, 1210–1211
        management of, 1214, 1215
Aortocaval compression syndrome, 1099, 1100
Aortography, in aortic disease diagnosis, 1212, 1213
    in multiple trauma, 1005
APCs (atrial premature contractions), origination of, 92
APL (adjustable pressure-limiting) valve, 280, 281
    of anesthesia machine, isolation of, 296
Apnea, hypoxemia prevention in, 795, 796(t)
    management of, in cardiopulmonary resuscitation, 836, 837
    in outpatient tonsillectomy, 1393, 1394
    perioperative, in former premature infants, 1021
    sleep, obstructive, 161
Apnea of prematurity, 81, 82
APOs (adverse patient outcomes), 38
Apparent volume of distribution, definition of, 563, *563*
Argon laser, 1371(t)
    for genitourinary surgery, 1243
Arm(s). See also *Upper extremity* entries.
    dependent, positioning of, in lateral decubitus position, 508
    positioning of, in prone position, 508
        in supine position, 506
Arousal, after battlefield surgery, 881
Arterial blood gases (ABGs), analysis of, 341–343, *343*, 786
    importance of, 341
    in chronic obstructive pulmonary disease, 966
    pH-stat method of, 342
    preanesthetic, 14
    preoperative, 150
    α-stat method of, 342
    timing of, 342
    transcutaneous, 786, *786*, 787
    units for, 342
    changes in, postoperative, 149
    in acid-base balance analysis, 343
    values for, noncorrected, 342
    temperature-corrected, 342
Arterial blood pressure. See *Blood pressure.*
Arterial cannula, in cardiopulmonary bypass, 322
Arterial catheterization, 496–498, *497*, *498*
    advantages of, 545, 548(t)
    complications of, 549, 549(t), 550
        factors predisposing to, 549, 549(t), 550
        prevention of, 372, 373
    contraindications to, 547(t)
    disadvantages of, 545, 548(t)
    equipment for, 543, 543(t)
    in ascending aorta surgery, 1190
    in blood pressure measurement, 372, 373, 373(t)
    in pediatric cardiovascular surgery, 1148, 1148(t), 1149
    in renal transplantation, 1362, 1363
    indications for, 545, 547(t)
    techniques of, 547–550
Arterial collateral flow, in transsphenoidal hypophysectomy, 1313
Arterial oxygen content, formula for, 692(t)
Arterial pressure, monitoring of, devices for, cost of, 117, 117(t)

Arterial pressure *(Continued)*
　in orthotopic liver transplantation, 1341,
　　1342
Arterial pressure wave, characteristics of, 367,
　369, 369(t)
Arterial venous mixing, effect of, on
　transcutaneous blood gas measurement,
　786, *786*
Arterial-venous oxygen content difference,
　formula for, 692(t)
Arteriovenous fistula, for dialysis, management
　of, 183
Arteriovenous malformation (AVM), cerebral,
　1295
Arthritis, rheumatoid. See *Rheumatoid arthritis.*
Arthropathy, inflammatory, cervical spine
　anatomy in, 464, 465, *465, 466*
Arthroplasty, of hip, pain after, local
　anesthetics for, 247
　total, blood loss in, 1249, 1249(t)
　　muscle relaxation during, 1250
Arthroscopy, pain during, causes of, 1254,
　1255
　tourniquet use in, 1255
Articular processes, of spine, 459
Artifact(s), monitoring, in left ventricular
　failure, after cardiopulmonary bypass,
　1182
　recording of, by automated anesthesia
　　recordkeepers, 26
Artificial nose, in intraoperative hypothermia
　prevention, 434
Arytenoid cartilage, 445, *445*
　attachments of, 445
ASA (American Society of Anesthesiologists),
　physical status classification of, 14, 15,
　15(t), 127, 127(t)
Ascites, abdominal surgery in, 1124, *1124,*
　1125, *1125*
　fluid in, drainage of, effects of, 1124, *1124,*
　　1125
　replacement of, intraoperative, 1125
Aspiration, after extubation, prevention of, 951
　after rapid-sequence induction and intuba-
　　tion, 942
　full stomach and, 1000, 1001
　in facemask airway obstruction, management
　　of, 926
　incidence of, *582*
　mortality of, *581*
　of foreign body, radiographic findings in,
　　224
　of vomitus, during outpatient surgery, 1395
　perioperative, antibiotic prophylaxis for, 15
　prevention of, airway management in, 922
　　in children, 1048, 1049, *1049*
　　indications for, 582(t)
　pulmonary, 85–87, 85(t)
　　documentation of, 87
　　in postanesthesia care unit, risk of, 87
　　of blood, 86
　　of clear oral secretions, 86
　　of foreign bodies, 86
　　of gastric contents, 86
　　　and postoperative pulmonary edema,
　　　　979, *979,* 979(t)
　　　during tracheal intubation, 456
　　　intraoperative, in pulmonary patient,
　　　　145
　　　prevention of, rapid-sequence induction
　　　　in, 590, 590(t)
　　　risk factors for, 590, 590(t)
　　prevention of, 86, 87
　　risk of, factors in, 86
　risk of, in children, 1040, 1040(t)
　types of, 590, 591(t)
Aspiration pneumonitis, 3, *3*

Aspiration pneumonitis *(Continued)*
　during outpatient surgery, prevention of,
　　1395, 1395(t)
Aspirin, discontinuation of, preoperative,
　guidelines for, 155
　for acute pain, 240(t)
　perioperative use of, 7, 8, 1164
Asthma, bronchial, 955–961
　anesthesia in, 959, 959(t), 960
　assessment of, preanesthetic, 959
　characteristics of, 956, *956,* 957, 963(t),
　　964
　conditions aggravating, 957
　management of, 957, 957(t), 958, 958(t)
　　perioperative, 958, 959
　　postoperative, 961
　pathophysiology of, 955, 956, 956(t)
　types of, 955, 956, 956(t)
　effects of, on anesthetic technique, 585(t)
　in anesthetic risk, 66
　in children, 1042, 1043
　in obstetric patient, 1094
ASTM (American Society for Testing and
　Materials), 296
ASTM F1161, 296
Asystole, ventricular, treatment of, emergency,
　850, 851
Atarax, analgesic potential of, 244(t)
Atelectasis, denitrogenation, 792, *792*
　resorption, postoperative, 78
ATH (air transportable hospital), 879
Atherosclerosis, left ventricular function in,
　classification of, 1214(t)
　natural history of, 1210, *1211*
　risk factors for, 1210
Ativan, for acute pain, 242(t)
Atlantoaxial joint, 460, *461*
Atlantoaxial subluxation (AAS), causes of, 224,
　226
　in rheumatoid arthritis, 464, *465*
　radiographic findings in, 224, 226, *227, 228*
Atlanto-occipital gap (AOG), effects of, on
　tracheal intubation, 464
Atlas, anatomy of, 460, *461*
ATLS (Advanced Trauma Life Support), 990
ATN (acute tubular necrosis), 694
Atracurium, dose of, in children, 1056(t)
　effects of, physiologic, 1285(t)
　for abdominal surgery, 1113
　for liver disease, 1344(t)
　for renal transplantation, 1363
　selection of, factors in, 573
Atrial depolarization, 362
Atrial dysrhythmias, electrocardiographic
　characteristics of, 365, 366
Atrial fibrillation, electrocardiographic
　characteristics of, 366
　in mitral stenosis, 1162
　postoperative, 94
　　management of, 139
　treatment of, emergency, 850
　　in intraoperative stroke prevention, 154,
　　　155
Atrial flutter, electrocardiographic
　characteristics of, 366
　postoperative, 94
　　management of, 139
Atrial premature contractions (APCs),
　origination of, 92
Atrioventricular (AV) block,
　electrocardiographic characteristics of,
　366, 367
　second-degree, treatment of, emergency, 851
　third-degree, treatment of, emergency, 851
Atrioventricular dysrhythmias,
　electrocardiographic characteristics of, 366
Atropine, action of, mechanism of, 846

Atropine *(Continued)*
　for imaging studies, 911(t)
　in cardiopulmonary resuscitation, 846
　　complications of, 846
　　dosage of, 846
　　indications for, 846
　in pediatric cardiovascular surgery, 1146(t)
　use of, intraoperative, 145
Auditing, anesthetic record use in, 24
Auscultation, in circulation monitoring, in
　anesthetized patient, 337
Auto Vent 2000 ventilator, 427(t)
Autologous blood donation, preoperative,
　erythropoietin use with, 5, *6*
Automated anesthesia recordkeepers (AARKs),
　25, 28, 29
　access to, 29
　accuracy of, in blood pressure recording, 26
　artifact recording by, 26
　completeness of, 26, 27
　cost-effectiveness of, 28
　effects of, on liability exposure, 29
　　on patient care, 28
　　on physician workload, 28
　　on vigilance, 27, 28
　in billing and collection, 28
　in quality assurance, 28, 29
　in research activities, 29
　legibility of, 27, *27*
　magnetic recording of, 27
　vs. handwritten recordkeeping, 25, *25,* 26
Automatic internal cardioverter-defibrillator
　(AICD), 1163
　components of, 1194, *1194*
　function of, 1194, 1195
　implantation of, anesthetic considerations in,
　　1195
　　antidysrhythmic agent continuation for,
　　　1164
　　approach to, 1195
　indications for, 1193, 1194, 1194(t)
Automaticity, in dysrhythmia genesis, 365
Autonomic dysreflexia (AD), 492–494, *493*
　causes of, 493
　in pregnancy, quadriplegia with, 494
　prophylaxis for, 493, 494
　risk of, factors in, 493
　signs and symptoms of, 493
Autonomic hyperreflexia, 5, 1298
Autonomic nervous system (ANS), 482–494
　activity of, 482, 483
　anatomy of, 482–485, *483, 484*
　blockade of, methods of, 485, 486
　dysfunction of, 492–494, *493*
　enteric, 482
　function of, 482–485
　monitoring of, in anesthetized patient, 337
　parasympathetic, 482, *483*
　sympathetic, 482, *483*
　vs. somatic nervous system, 482, 483
Autoregulation, cerebral, failure of, 393, 393(t)
　of glomerular filtration rate, 384
　of renal blood flow, 384
AV (atrioventricular) block,
　electrocardiographic characteristics of,
　366, 367
　second-degree, treatment of, emergency, 851
　third-degree, treatment of, emergency, 851
Avascular necrosis, of hip, conditions
　associated with, 1249(t)
AVM (arteriovenous malformation), cerebral,
　1295
AVPU survey, 994, 995(t)
Awakening, delayed, 163–165, 164(t)
　differential, 163
Axilla, in temperature monitoring, 433

Axilla *(Continued)*
  positioning of, in lateral decubitus position, 508
Axillary artery, catheterization of, 496, 497
  advantages of, 548(t)
  disadvantages of, 548(t)
  techniques of, 548
Axillary block, 529, *529*, 530, *530*
  anatomic considerations in, 529, *529*
  drug choice for, 529
  for orthopedic surgery, 1255, 1256, *1256*
  needle placement for, 530, *530*
  patient selection for, 529
  positioning for, 529
Axis, anatomy of, 460, 461, *462*
Axonotmesis, prognosis in, 162
Azathioprine, complications of, 1330(t)
  drug interactions with, 653(t)
Azygos vein, normal anatomy of, on chest radiography, *212*, 213, *214*

Bacitracin, drug interactions with, 652(t)
Back, low, pain in, causes of, 475, *476*
  pain in, chronic, anatomic factors in, 475, 476(t)
    in pregnancy, 474
    postoperative, etiology of, 477, 478
      surgical positioning in, 504
    postpartum, etiology of, 477, 478
    preanesthetic evaluation of, 11
Back pressure, fluctuating, compensation for, low-pressure anesthesia machine vaporizer in, 282, 283
Baclofen, analgesic potential of, 244(t)
BAEPs. See *Brainstem auditory evoked potentials (BAEPs).*
Bag-valve ventilation, 301, 302, *303*
Bag-valve-mask ventilation, in resuscitation, cardiopulmonary, 837
  neonatal, 1034
Bain circuit, for pediatric anesthesia, 1055, *1055*
Bainton blade, 304
Balloon dilatation, of prostate, 1237, 1238
  anesthesia for, 1237, 1238
  sedoanalgesia for, 1238
Balloon mitral valvuloplasty, 138
Baralyme, carbon dioxide reaction with, 287, 288(t)
Barbiturates, abuse of, diagnostic features of, 1000(t)
  $CMRo_2$ suppression by, detection of, electro-encephalography in, 401
  drug interactions with, 645(t), 647(t), 652(t), 653(t)
  effects of, on evoked potentials, 406(t), 408(t)
    physiologic, 1285(t)
  for cerebral protection, during cardiopulmonary bypass, 328, 329
  for malignant hyperthermia, 827(t)
  in intracranial pressure control, 776
  in intravenous anesthesia, 601, 602
Barium hydroxide, carbon dioxide absorption by, 356
Barotrauma, pulmonary, radiographic findings in, 216, 219, *221–223*
Base excess, 735, *735*
Basic life support (BLS), 835
Basilar skull fracture, signs and symptoms of, 1278, 1278(t)
Basilic vein, branches of, catheterization of, 498, *499*
Basophils, in anaphylactic shock, 681, 682(t)
Battlefield surgery, anesthesia in, 874–883

Battlefield surgery *(Continued)*
    problems in, 877, 878, 878(t)
    postoperative concerns in, 881
    problems in, 881–883, 881(t)
    ventilation in, 881
Bayesian analysis, of cardiac risk factors, in noncardiac surgery, 128, *129*
Beach-chair position, for orthopedic surgery, 1260
Beclomethasone, for bronchial asthma, 958(t)
Bellhouse blade, 304
Bellows, of breathing system, upright vs. hanging, 288, *289*
Benign intracranial hypertension, 157
Bennett blade, 304
Benzidamine, for acute pain, 240(t)
Benzocaine, properties of, clinical, 628(t)
Benzodiazepines, analgesic potential of, 244(t)
  avoidance of, in opiate dependence, 252
  drug interactions with, 644(t), 652(t)–654(t), 658
  effects of, on evoked potentials, 406(t), 408(t)
    physiologic, 1285(t)
  for acute pain, 242(t)
  for cardiovascular surgery, 1174, 1175(t)
  for eclamptic seizures, 158
  in geriatric patients, 1075, 1075(t)
  in premedication, 579–581, 579(t), *580*
  in shock, 688
  perioperative use of, 8, 9
  reversal of, flumazenil in, 164, 573
  selection of, factors in, 571, 572
Bernoulli equation, 137
Beta rhythm, in electroencephalography, 400, *400*
Beta-blockers, action of, mechanism of, 848
  continuation of, perioperative, 139, 1163
  drug interactions with, 645(t), 646(t), 652(t), 654(t)–657(t)
  effects of, cardiovascular, 760(t)
    physiologic, 1285(t)
  for dysrhythmias, during tracheal intubation, 455
  for hyperthyroidism, 200
  for intraoperative myocardial ischemia, 760, 760(t)
  for life-threatening dysrhythmias, 850
  in cardiopulmonary resuscitation, 848
    complications of, 848
    dosage of, 848
    indications for, 848
  in premedication, 583
  in preterm labor prevention, 1104
  single-dose, before cardiovascular surgery, 1165
  use of, after heart transplantation, 1327
    in cardiogenic shock, after thrombolysis, 674
    perioperative, pulmonary effects of, 151
    preoperative, in coronary artery disease, 755, 756
Bicarbonate, plasma, in alveolar hyperventilation, 809
  reabsorption of, definition of, 735, 736
Bicitra, in aspiration pneumonitis prevention, for outpatient surgery, 1395(t)
Bier's block. See *Intravenous regional anesthesia.*
Bile salts, for renal failure, in obstructive jaundice, 1123
Biliary spasm, narcotic administration and, 1116, 1117
Binasal pharyngeal airway (BNPA), 300, *300*
Bioavailability, definition of, 562
  of drugs, measurement of, 562
Biofeedback, for pain, in adults, 257

Biomed IC2A ventilator, 427(t)
Biopsy, muscle, in malignant hyperthermia, 832
  of orthopedic tumors, blood loss in, 1252
Biotransformation, definition of, 566
Bird Space Technologies Mini-TXP ventilator, 427(t)
Birth, cardiovascular system changes at, 1015, 1016
Bite block, insertion of, 1300, *1300*
  for intracranial neoplasm surgery, 1307
Bitolterol, 145(t)
Black bodies, 430
Bladder, cancer of, laser surgery for, 1243
  catheterization of, indications for, 384(t)
  in temperature monitoring, 432, *433*
Blade(s), of laryngoscope, curved, 303, *304*
  for tracheal intubation, 450
  straight, 304
Blanket, heating, in skin surface warming, 435, 436
Blast injury, 876
Blechman blade, 303
Bleeding. See also *Hemorrhage.*
  abnormal intracranial pressure in, management of, 775
  after adenotonsillectomy, management of, 1270, 1270(t), 1271
  after pediatric cardiopulmonary bypass, causes of, 1154
    treatment of, 1154
  after transurethral resection of the prostate, 1239
  arterial catheterization and, 549, 550
  distal to inflated tourniquet, 1262
  during heart transplantation, 1329, 1329(t)
  during orthotopic liver transplantation, 1337, 1338, 1338(t), 1339(t)
  during tonsillectomy, 1064
    outpatient, 1393
  gastrointestinal, acute, 1121, 1122
    anesthesia induction in, 1122
  in femoral fracture, 1247
  in pelvic fracture, 1247
  intra-abdominal, after trauma surgery, 1007
  intraoperative, fluid loss with, 716, *717*
  sympathetic nerve block and, 492
Bleeding disorders, extracorporeal shock wave lithotripsy in, 1382
Bleomycin, for bone cancer, 1252
  perioperative use of, 8
Blood, addition of, to pediatric cardiopulmonary bypass circuit, 1151
  arterial, for acid-base status analysis, 733
    oxygen content of, 782–785
      relationship of, to Pao_2, 782, *783*
  aspiration of, pulmonary, 86
  availability of, for orthotopic liver transplantation, 1342
    for pediatric cardiovascular surgery, 1145
    in thoracoabdominal aneurysm management, 1218
  disorders of, in chronic liver disease, 1336
    in renal failure, 1359, 1360(t)
  donation of, autologous, before cardiopulmonary bypass, 1176, 1177
    preoperative, 1259
      erythropoietin use with, 5, 6
  effects on, of hyperthermia, 824
  loss of, after cardiopulmonary bypass, prevention of, antifibrinolytic agents in, 1190
    in adenotonsillectomy, 270
    in liver resection, minimization of, 1123
    in neonates, replacement of, 1025
    in orthopedic oncology procedures, 1252
    in orthopedic surgery, 1259, *1259*, 1259(t), 1260

Blood *(Continued)*
  amount of, 1260
    reduction of, 1259, 1260
    with regional anesthesia, 1257, *1258*
  in renal transplantation, 1368
  in total joint replacement, 1249, 1249(t)
  intraoperative, in burns, 708
    in children, 1058, 1059
  replacement of, 723
  pulmonary, mean transit time of, 785
  replacement of, before aortic cross-clamp
      removal, 1229
    inadequate, postoperative, and absolute
        hypovolemia, 88
  supply of, to larynx, 447
  venous, for acid-base status analysis, 733
    mixed, desaturation of, in postoperative
        hypoxemia, 80
Blood flow, arterial, end point for, 369
  cerebral. See *Cerebral blood flow (CBF)*.
  coronary, factors in, 1170, *1170*
  in coronary artery, during aortic vascular sur-
      gery, 1222
  pulmonary, disorders of, in hypoxemia, 784,
      785(t)
    in postoperative oxygenation, 80
    reduced, and alveolar hypoventilation, 803
  renal, autoregulation of, 384
    effects on, of cardiopulmonary bypass,
        330
  to spinal cord, anatomy of, 1226–1228, *1227*
    autoregulation of, 1283
    during thoracic aorta cross-clamping, 1223
    surgical blockage of, somatosensory
        evoked potential monitoring in, 404
Blood pressure, 367–373
  arterial, in conscious patients, monitoring of,
      335
  assessment of, cerebral blood flow in, 393,
      393
    preanesthetic, 10, *10*
  control of, before cardiopulmonary bypass,
      1178
    before spinal surgery, 1298
    in anesthetic risk, 67
    in intraoperative myocardial ischemia,
        752, 757
    in intraoperative stroke prevention, 155
    in myelopathy/radiculopathy, 1297
    in pulsatile cardiopulmonary bypass, 330
    in spinal cord injury, 1302
    in trauma, 994, 994(t)
    preoperative, in pheochromocytoma, 195,
        195(t)
    with ruptured intracranial aneurysm, 1290
  guidelines for, 170, 171
  improvement of, in cardiopulmonary resusci-
      tation, pharmacologic therapy in, 849,
      850
  in perioperative intracranial pressure control,
      778
  intraoperative recording of, accuracy of, 26
  monitoring of, during cardiopulmonary by-
      pass weaning, in pediatric cardiovascu-
      lar surgery, 1153
    in geriatric patient, 1073
    intraoperative, 69
      in cardiovascular surgery, 1165, *1165*
    invasive, 371–373, 371(t), *372*, 373(t)
    near magnetic resonance imaging scanner,
        916
    noninvasive, 369–371, *369*, *370*, 370(t)
    pulse oximetry in, 356
  variations in, cuff placement in, 337, 338
    intraoperative, in children, 1060
Blood pressure cuff, application of, 337, 338

Blood pressure cuff *(Continued)*
  site of, blood pressure variations with, 337,
      338
Blood salvage, during orthopedic surgery, 1260
Blood substitutes, 721
  types of, 721
Blood transfusion, and hyperthermia, 825
  for intraventricular hemorrhage, 1020
  in burns, 702, 703
  in children, 1056–1059
  in cytomegalovirus transmission, 864
  in orthotopic liver transplantation, 1338,
      1338(t), 1339(t)
  in trauma, 994
    postoperative, 1008
  warming of, in intraoperative hypothermia
      prevention, 436
Blood urea nitrogen (BUN), measurement of, in
    syndrome of inappropriate antidiuretic
    hormone secretion, 188
  relationship of, to glomerular filtration rate,
      179, *179*
  significance of, 178, 179, *179*
Blood vessels, epidural anesthetic injection
    into, 522
  sympathetic nerve block injection into, 492
Blood volume, control of, in regional
    anesthesia, for obstetric patient, 1092
  in chronic liver disease, 1337
  in shock, limits for, 670, *671*
    relationship of, to central venous pressure,
        670, *671*
Blood-brain barrier, 1308
Blood:gas partition coefficient, of anesthetic
    agents, 570
BLS (basic life support), 835
"Blue bloaters," 149
B-mode echocardiography, 381, *381*
BNPA (binasal pharyngeal airway), 300, *300*
Body composition, of geriatric patients, 1070
Body habitus, in extracorporeal shock wave
    lithotripsy, 1380
Bomb blast injuries, 877
Bone(s), cancer of, chemotherapy for, 1252
    metastatic, 1252
    pain in, 1251, 1252
  effects on, of hypercalcemia, 204
Bone marrow transplantation, inhalation
    anesthesia in, 615
Bone prominences, position of, in prone
    position, 508
Bowel, effects on, of shock, 694
Bowel anastomosis, neostigmine effects on,
    1113
Bowel distention, nitrous oxide and, 1115,
    1116, *1116*
Bowel obstruction, radiographic findings in,
    226, 229, 230
Bowel preparation, preoperative, for abdominal
    surgery, 1120
  protocol for, 245(t)
BPD (bronchopulmonary dysplasia), in former
    premature infants, 1021
Brachial artery, catheterization of, 497
    advantages of, 548(t)
    disadvantages of, 548(t)
    techniques of, 548
Brachial plexus, anatomy of, 524, 525, *526*
  injury of, surgical positioning in, 504, *504*,
      512
    prevention of, 511(t)
  nerve blocks of, for orthopedic surgery,
      1255, 1256, *1256*
    in children, 268
Brachiocephalic vein, normal radiographic
    anatomy of, 213
Bradycardia, and postoperative hypotension, 91

Bradycardia *(Continued)*
  idioventricular, 94
  intraoperative, in children, 1060
  postoperative, 94
  profound, during regional anesthesia, 537
  sinus, electrocardiographic characteristics of,
      366
    treatment of, emergency, 851
  treatment of, emergency, 843, 844(t)
Brain, abnormal tissue of, resection of,
    intraoperative electrophysiologic
    monitoring during, 160
  dysfunction of, postoperative, in geriatric
    patients, 1079, *1079*
  effects on, of ischemia, 1284
    of isovolemic hemodilution, 670
  function of, analysis of, electroencephalogra-
      phy in, 400, *401*
  herniation of, intracranial hypertension and,
      771, *771*
  injury to, hypoxic, 166
    in postoperative delirium, 165
    postischemic, 166
  mass of, in geriatric patients, 1071
  oxygen demand of, 1284
  oxygenation of, disorder of, in postoperative
    delirium, 165
  protection of, in neurovascular surgery, 1294
  tumor of. See *Intracranial neoplasm(s)*.
Brain death, confirmation of, transcranial
    Doppler ultrasonography in, 397, *397*, 398
  diagnosis of, 166
Brainstem, function of, evaluation of, 773, *774*
Brainstem auditory evoked potentials (BAEPs),
    160, 406, *406*
  alterations in, factors in, 407
  anesthetic effects on, 161, 406(t)
  use of, intraoperative, 406, 407, *407*
Breath sounds, auscultation of, in tracheal tube
    placement verification, 943, 944
Breathing, assessment of, in trauma, 992, 993
  in cardiopulmonary resuscitation, 836–840,
      837–839
  management of, in inhalation anesthesia,
      610–612, 610(t), *611*, *612*
  pattern of, in conscious patients, 334, 335
  sounds of, in conscious patients, 335
  spontaneous, during general anesthesia, 592–
      594
    during inhalation anesthesia, 611, *611*
      increased airway resistance in, 611, *611*
    ventilatory work during, 811, *811*, 812
  work of, airway resistance in, 957
    reduction of, postoperative, 148
Breathing exercises, after abdominal surgery,
    1133
Breathing system, 276–297
  bellows of, upright vs. hanging, 288, *289*
  breathing hose of, compliance of, 287, 288(t)
  components of, 285–288, 285(t), *286*, *287*,
      288(t)
  disorders of, and alveolar hypoventilation,
      802, 802(t), 803
  for pediatric anesthesia, 1055, *1055*
  gas flow in, 285, 286, *287*
    resistance to, 811
  pressure gauge of, positive end-expiratory
    pressure registration on, 288, *289*
  safety features of, 285
  unidirectional valves of, incompetency of,
      286, 287
Bretylium, for ventricular tachydysrhythmia,
    1186(t)
Bretylium tosylate, action of, mechanism of,
    847
  in cardiopulmonary resuscitation, 847
  dosage of, 847

Bretylium tosylate *(Continued)*
    indications for, 847
Bronchial blocker tube, in double-lumen tube
        position verification, 1204
Bronchial intubation, 456, 948
Bronchial suctioning, 443, *443*
Bronchitis, chronic, features of, 963, 963(t),
        964
Bronchoconstriction, in geriatric patients, 1072
Bronchodilators, for bronchial asthma, 957,
        957(t), 958, 958(t)
    for chronic obstructive pulmonary disease,
        965
    inhaled, for intraoperative bronchospasm,
        961, *961*
    metered-dose, 145(t)
    use of, intraoperative, 6, 7, 145
        preoperative, 144
Bronchomotor tone, effects on, of alveolar
        hyperventilation, 808
    of alveolar hypoventilation, 801
Bronchopulmonary dysplasia (BPD), in former
        premature infants, 1021
Bronchoscope(s), 305, 306
    diagnostic, 305
    fiberoptic, components of, 305
        flexible, 305
            for potentially difficult intubation, 937
            in double-lumen tube position verifica-
                tion, 314, 1203, 1204
            in endotracheal tube changing, 952
            laser use with, 1378
        maintenance of, 305, 306
        problems with, 306
    intubating, rigid, 305
Bronchoscopy, fiberoptic, in thermal injuries,
        705
    in children, anesthetic considerations in,
        1062, 1063, *1063*
    laser use with, 1378
Bronchospasm, 450
    after cardiopulmonary bypass, 1188
    and difficult ventilation, 946, 947
    and facemask·airway obstruction, 927
    control of, preoperative, 144, 145(t)
    drugs promoting, 960, 960(t)
    fiberoptic bronchoscopy and, 306
    in asthma, mediators of, 955, 956(t)
    intraoperative, 960, 960(t), 961, *961*
        differential diagnosis of, 960
        inhaled bronchodilators for, 961, *961*
        treatment of, 960
    postoperative, treatment of, 83
Bronchospirometry, 1201
Bronchus(i), injuries of, traumatic, assessment
        of, 997
    intubation of, 443
    upper lobe, right, occlusion of, and hypox-
        emia, 948, *948*
Bruit, carotid, in anesthetic risk, 67
Bryce Smith tube, 313
Budesonide, for bronchial asthma, 958(t)
Buffer base, 735
Buffering, mechanism of, 732
Buffers, definition of, 732
    phosphate, in acid-base balance, 736
Bull neck, tracheal intubation in, 929, 930
Bullae, in emphysema, radiographic
        demonstration of, 213, *215*
Bullard fiberoptic laryngoscope, rigid, 306,
        307, *307*
Bumetanide, drug interactions with, 647(t)
BUN (blood urea nitrogen), measurement of, in
        syndrome of inappropriate antidiuretic
        hormone secretion, 188
    relationship of, to glomerular filtration rate,
        179, *179*

BUN (blood urea nitrogen) *(Continued)*
    significance of, 178, 179, *179*
Bupivacaine, 631
    action of, duration of, *516*
    alkalinization of, 629
    carbonation of, 629
    chloroprocaine with, 630
    for epidural anesthesia, 521
    for postoperative pain, dose of, determination
        of, 247, 248(t)
    for spinal anesthesia, 517
    in children, dosage of, 267, 267(t)
    in geriatric patients, 1077(t)
    intra-articular injection of, for pain control,
        in orthopedic surgery, 1264, *1265*
    lidocaine with, 630
    pharmacology of, 516(t)
    properties of, clinical, 627(t)
    toxicity of, 632, *632*, 633, *633*
Buprenex, for acute pain, 241(t)
Buprenorphine, for acute pain, 241(t)
    intravenous, patient-controlled, guidelines
        for, 245(t)
Burn(s), analgesia for, 711
    in children, 271
    classification of, 700, 701(t)
    debridement of, 708
    edema formation in, control of, 703, 704
    fluid shifts in, 703
        effects of, 703
    fluid therapy in, 730
    history of, 5
    hypothermia in, 819
    in electrosurgical unit, 893
    intraoperative monitoring in, 708, 709
    magnetic resonance imaging in, 913, 914
    operative blood loss in, 708
    severity of, assessment of, 701, 702(t)
    skin grafting in, 708
    surgery of, anesthesia for, contraindications
        to, 710
    wound of, sepsis of, 707, 708
        treatment of, 707, 708
    zones of, 699
Burn toxins, effects of, 702, 702(t), 703
Burst fracture, in cervical spine instability, 467
Burst suppression, isoflurane and, 609, *609*
Butorphanol, for acute pain, 241(t)
    intravenous, 603(t), 604
Butyrophenone, adverse effects of, 656(t)
Bypass circuit volume, in pediatric
        cardiopulmonary bypass, 1151

c wave, 373
CABG (coronary artery bypass grafting), before
        noncardiac surgery, indications for, 134,
        135
    cerebral protection during, barbiturates in,
        329
CAD. See *Coronary artery disease (CAD)*.
Cadaveric donor harvesting, in renal
        transplantation, 1366
Caffeine withdrawal, in persistent postoperative
        unconsciousness, 96
Calcium, 175, 176, 176(t)
    control of, hormonal, 202
    disorders of, 726, 726(t), 727, 727(t)
        after pediatric cardiopulmonary bypass,
        1155
    drug interactions with, 205, 658(t)
    extracellular, phases of, 175
    in anaphylactic shock, 681
    ionized, administration of, perioperative, in
        parathyroid disease, 204

Calcium *(Continued)*
    measurement of, preoperative, in parathy-
        roid function assessment, 202
    serum, alteration of, 1313
        fractionation of, 1313, *1314*
Calcium channel blockers. See also *Calcium
        entry blockers.*
    action of, mechanism of, 848
    drug interactions with, 645(t)
    effects of, on cardiovascular function, during
        anesthesia, 657
        physiologic, 1285(t)
    for cerebral vasospasm, after intracranial
        aneurysm rupture, 1291
    for life-threatening dysrhythmias, 850
    for pain, effects on, of concurrent medical
        condition, 237
    in cardiopulmonary resuscitation, 848, 849
        complications of, 849
        dosage of, 849
        indications for, 849
    preoperative continuation of, 1163
Calcium chloride, action of, mechanism of, 848
    for hypocalcemia, 176
    for perioperative myocardial dysfunction,
        765
    in cardiopulmonary resuscitation, 848
        complications of, 848
        dosage of, 848
        indications for, 848
    in pediatric cardiovascular surgery, 1146(t)
Calcium entry blockers, effects of,
        cardiovascular, 760(t)
    for intraoperative myocardial ischemia,
        760(t), 761
    preoperative use of, in coronary artery dis-
        ease, 756
Calcium gluconate, for hypocalcemia, 176
Calcium salts, administration of, after
        cardiopulmonary bypass, 1188
Caldwell-Luc procedure, 1272, 1273, 1273(t)
    anesthetic concerns in, 1273, 1273(t)
    indications for, 1272, 1273
Calibration, faulty, in oxygen monitoring, 343
    of gas monitor, for anesthetic agent monitor-
        ing, 349, 350
Canada, health care system in, 109, 110
Cancer, delayed emergence in, 164(t)
    pain in, in children, 262, 262(t), 271, 271(t),
        272
        palliative management of, 272
        peridural analgesia for, 250, *252*
        regional anesthesia for, 254
        steroids for, 244(t)
        treatment of, 240, *243*, 244(t), 245(t)
Cannula, arterial, in cardiopulmonary bypass,
        322
    venous, in cardiopulmonary bypass, 320
Cannulation. See also *Catheterization*.
    for cardiopulmonary bypass, concerns dur-
        ing, 1178
Capacitance, 885, 886
Capacitive coupling, 886
Capacitor, stray, 886
Capillaries, permeability of, in colloid
        distribution, 719
Capillary refill, monitoring of, in anesthetized
        patient, 337
Capnography, alveolar plateau cleft, 353
    carbon dioxide decrease in, 354
    elevated baseline in, 353, 354
    in abnormal ventilation, 800
    in neonates, 1026
    in shock, 680
    in tracheal tube malpositioning assessment,
        802
    inspiratory valve leak in, 354, *355*

Capnography *(Continued)*
  intraoperative, in children, 1059
  normal, 351, *351*
  oxygraphy with, in circuit valve leak detection, 344, *346*
  sidestream vs. mainstream, 353
  steep plateau in, 353, *353*
  study of, 353, *353*, 354, *355*
Capnometry, in neonates, 1026
  use of, near magnetic resonance imaging scanner, 916
Captopril, drug interactions with, 646(t), 655(t)
Carbamazepine, 159(t)
  drug interactions with, 644(t)–647(t), 652(t)
Carbicarb, for lactic acidosis, 739
Carbidopa-levodopa, in Parkinson's disease, 154
Carbon dioxide, absorption of, 356–358, *357*
  by soda lime, 356, *357*
    efficiency of, 356, 357
  arterial, partial pressure of, in general anesthesia, 593
  body, changes in, effects of, 734, *734*
  control of, before thoracic aorta cross-clamping, 1224
  effects on, of alveolar hyperventilation, 807, 808
    of aortic cross-clamping, 1226
  end-tidal, definition of, 350, *351*
    in tidal volume monitoring, 345, 346
    monitoring of, in geriatric patient, 1073, 1074
    partial pressure of, monitoring of, in pediatric cardiovascular surgery, 1149, 1150
  exhaled, analysis of, in tracheal tube placement verification, 944
  extracorporeal, removal of, for alveolar hypoventilation correction, 807
  in central nervous system homeostasis, 1283, 1284
  leak of, in capnography, 354
  monitoring of, 350–354, *353*, 353(t)
    respiratory gas drying before, 352
    techniques for, 353, 353(t)
  production of, effects of, on ventilatory work, 814
    formula for, 692(t)
    in pregnancy, *1084*
    increase in, and postoperative ventilatory failure, 85
  removal of, airway management in, 921
    from respiratory gas, in breathing system, 285–288, *287*, 288(t)
  transport of, failed, and alveolar hypoventilation, 803
Carbon dioxide laser, 1371(t)
  for genitourinary surgery, 1243
Carbon monoxide intoxication, in thermal injuries, 704
  intraoperative, 358
Carbonation, of local anesthetics, 629
Carboxyhemoglobin, effects of, on pulse oximetry, 355
Cardiac arrest, outcome of, prediction of, 166, 166(t)
Cardiac catheterization, before cardiovascular surgery, 1159, 1160, 1160(t)
  hemodynamic values measured by, 1160, 1160(t)
  in congenital heart disease assessment, 1143
  preoperative, in cardiac risk assessment, 134, 135
Cardiac compression, closed, 840, *840*, 841
  complications of, 841, 841(t)
  compression/relaxation cycle in, 840, 841
  rate of, 841

Cardiac compression *(Continued)*
  with single rescuer, 841
  with two rescuers, 841
Cardiac function, in conscious patients, monitoring of, 335
Cardiac index, in cardiogenic shock, 675, *675*
  parameters for, 691(t)
Cardiac output, 378–383
  during cardiopulmonary resuscitation, 840, 841
    pharmacologic therapy for, 849, 850
  during one-lung anesthesia, 1205
  during pregnancy, *1084*
  effects on, of immersion, for extracorporeal shock wave lithotripsy, 1383
    of orthotopic liver transplantation, during neohepatic phase, 1349, 1350, *1350*
  in congenital heart disease, 1044
  in geriatric patients, 1071
  in hypoxemia, 785, 785(t)
  low, after pediatric cardiopulmonary bypass, 1154
  measurement of, cardiac catheterization in, 1160
    continuous, 379, 380
    invasive, 379, 379(t), 380
    noninvasive, 380
    pulmonary artery catheterization in, 1166, 1167
Cardiac risk index, Goldman's, 127, 127(t)
Cardiac standstill, treatment of, epinephrine in, 844, 845(t)
Cardiac studies, noninvasive, before cardiovascular surgery, 1158, 1159
Cardiac tamponade, after trauma surgery, 1007
  traumatic, assessment of, 995
Cardioembolic stroke, and delayed awakening, 165
Cardiogenic pulmonary edema, radiographic findings in, 216
Cardiogenic shock, 672–677
  characteristics of, 672
  in myocardial ischemia, management of, 761
  intraoperative hemodynamic stabilization in, 689
  mechanical assistance in, 675–677, *676*
  mortality rate in, 672
  resuscitation in, endpoints for, 675
  treatment of, 672, 673
    complications of, 673, 674
    heparin in, 674
    thrombolytic therapy in, 674
Cardiologist, role of, in preoperative cardiac risk assessment, 135–138, 135(t)–137(t), *136*
Cardiology consultation, 125–140
  criteria for, 136(t)
  postoperative, 138–140
Cardiomediastinal silhouette, on chest radiography, 213, *214*
Cardiomegaly, diagnosis of, preoperative chest radiography in, 130, *131*
Cardiomyopathy, obstructive, hypertrophic, preoperative assessment of, 138
  treatment of, preoperative, in pheochromocytoma, 195
Cardioplegia, blood-based vs. crystalloid, 325
  during cardiopulmonary bypass, antegrade, 324
    hypothermic, 324, 324(t)
    retrograde, 324, 324(t)
  solutions for, composition of, 324, 325(t)
  warm, continuous, safety of, 325
Cardioplegia apparatus, in cardiopulmonary bypass, 323
Cardioplegia catheters, for cardiopulmonary bypass, 1178

Cardiopulmonary bypass (CPB), 320–331
  autologous blood donation before, 1176, 1177
  cannulation for, concerns during, 1178
  components of, 320–323, 320(t), *321*, *323*
  hemodynamic goals after, 1180, 1181, 1181(t), *1182*(t)
  in heart transplantation, 1326
    weaning from, 1327–1329, 1328(t), 1329(t)
  in pediatric cardiovascular surgery, 1150–1153, 1150(t), *1152*, 1152(t), *1153*, 1153(t)
    anticoagulation in, 1151, 1152
    circuit for, blood addition to, 1151
    weaning from, 1152, *1152*, 1152(t), 1153
  in pregnancy, 1106, 1107
  myocardial protection in, 323–325, *323*, 324(t), 325(t)
  neurologic outcome with, 326–328, 327(t)
  nonpulsatile, 330, 331
  pathophysiology of, 326–331, *326*, *327*, 327(t)–329(t)
  preanesthetic management of, 1169–1173, 1169(t), *1170*, 1171(t), 1172(t)
  preparation for, anesthesiologist in, 1178, 1179
    heparin in, 1177, 1177(t), 1178
  problems after, 1181–1190, 1182(t)
  pulmonary edema after, 980, 981
  pulsatile, 330, 331
  reperfusion injury in, 325, 326
  rewarming after, consequences of, 821
  stress response to, 326, *326*
  transcranial Doppler ultrasonography in, 397
  weaning from, 1179–1181, *1180*
Cardiopulmonary dysfunction, in scoliosis, 470
Cardiopulmonary resuscitation (CPR), 835–851
  airway in, 835, 836, *836*
  blood pressure control in, pharmacologic therapy for, 849, 850
  breathing in, 836–840, *837–839*
  cardiac output control in, pharmacologic therapy for, 849, 850
  circulation in, 840–843, *840*, 841(t), *842*, *843*
  efficacy of, monitoring of, 841, *842*
  goals of, 835
  in life-threatening dysrhythmias, 850, 851
  in pulseless electrical activity, 851
  pharmacologic therapy in, 843–849
Cardiopulmonary system, assessment of, during patient transport, equipment for, 426
  disorder of, in hypoxemia, 784, 785, 785(t)
    in renal failure, 1359, 1360(t)
  effects on, of chemical mediators, 744, 745
Cardiorespiratory compromise, in spinal cord shock, management of, 685
  surgical positioning in, 504
Cardiorespiratory function, formulas for, 692(t)
Cardiotomy sucker, in cardiopulmonary bypass, 320
Cardiovascular collapse, local anesthetic overdose and, treatment of, 635
Cardiovascular monitoring, 360–386
Cardiovascular surgery, 1157–1196
  anesthesia techniques for, 1173–1176, *1174*, 1175(t)
  monitoring in, 1165–1169, *1166*, 1166(t)–1169(t), *1168*
  outcome of, anesthetic choice in, 1176
  pediatric, 1138–1155
    anesthesia for, hemodynamic goals of, 1147, 1148(t)
    induction/maintenance of, 1145–1148, 1148(t)

Cardiovascular surgery *(Continued)*
  cardiopulmonary bypass in. See *Cardiopulmonary bypass (CPB), in pediatric cardiovascular surgery.*
    equipment/infusions for, 1144, 1145, 1145(t)
    postbypass concerns in, 1154, 1155
    risk of, 1143, 1143(t)
    preoperative evaluation in, 1157–1163
    preoperative period in, 1163–1169
    surgical events in, management of, 1176–1179, 1177(t)
Cardiovascular system, changes in, during cardiopulmonary bypass weaning, 1152, 1153, *1153*
    during patient transport, monitoring of, 421
    disorders of, in anaphylactic shock, 681
      in chronic liver disease, 1336
      in diabetes mellitus, 207
      in hyperthyroidism, 201
      in hypothyroidism, 200
      tracheal intubation and, 455
      Trendelenburg surgical positioning in, 510
    effects on, of alveolar hyperventilation, 807, 808
      of bronchial asthma, 957
      of burns, 703
      of electrical injury, 699, 700
      of hyperthermia, 823, 824
      of hypocalcemia, 176
      of hypothermia, 819(t), 820, *820*
      of immersion, for extracorporeal shock wave lithotripsy, 1383, *1383*
      of local anesthetic overdose, 538, 632, *632*, 633, *633*
      of orthotopic liver transplantation, during anhepatic phase, 1347, *1347*, *1348*
        during neohepatic phase, 1349
        during preanhepatic phase, 1346, 1347
      of regional anesthesia, 537
      of spinal cord shock, 686
      of subarachnoid hemorrhage, 1292
      of thyrotoxicosis, 1315, *1316*
    function of, after heart transplantation, 1330
      before spinal surgery, 1298
      during anesthesia, calcium channel blockers in, 657
      preoperative, effects of, on intracranial neoplasm surgery, 1306
      of neonates, 1015
    postoperative pain in, 246
    preanesthetic evaluation of, 2, 3
    reaction of, to contrast agent, 902
      to timolol, 8, *8*
Cardioversion, electrical, in cardiopulmonary resuscitation, 843, *844*
    for life-threatening dysrhythmias, 850
Carlens tube, 313
Carotid artery(ies), disease of, cardiopulmonary bypass in, neurologic deficit after, 329, 330
    location of, 500
    puncture of, during central venous catheterization, 374
      during internal jugular vein catheterization, 551
    surgery of, electroencephalography during, 401
Carotid bruits, in anesthetic risk, 67
Carotid endarterectomy (CEA), intraoperative electrophysiologic monitoring during, 160
    transcranial Doppler ultrasonography during, 396, 397
Cartilage(s), corniculate, 446
    functions of, 446
  cuneiform, 446

Cartilage(s) *(Continued)*
    functions of, 446
  laryngeal, 444–446, *445*
    in airway obstruction, 445, 446
CASS (Coronary Artery Surgery Study), 128
Catapres, analgesic potential of, 244(t)
Catecholamines, for anaphylaxis, 748
    for contrast agent reactions, 904
    for perioperative myocardial dysfunction, 766(t)
    in pheochromocytoma, 194, 195
    in stress response, to cardiopulmonary bypass, 326
    in urine output, 384
    volatile anesthetic use with, 613
Catheter(s), cardioplegia, for cardiopulmonary bypass, 1178
    central venous, misplaced, rewiring of, 555
      tip of, positioning of, 553–555, *555*
    cerebrospinal fluid, lumbar, in intracranial pressure measurement, 395
    cricothyroid, insertion of, 940, *940*
    insertion of, for epidural anesthesia, 522
    retrograde, placement of, for airway maintenance, 316
    sampling, leak in, in anesthetic agent monitoring, 350, *350*
    transtracheal, ventilation with, in cardiopulmonary resuscitation, 838–840, *839*
    ventricular, in intracranial pressure measurement, 394, *394*
Catheterization, arterial. See *Arterial catheterization.*
  cardiac. See *Cardiac catheterization.*
  central venous. See *Central venous catheterization.*
  intra-arterial, in cardiovascular surgery monitoring, 1165, *1165*
  intravenous, in trauma, 994
  left atrial, in pediatric cardiovascular surgery, 1149
  of axillary artery, 496, 497
  of basilic vein branches, 498, *499*
  of bladder, indications for, 384(t)
  of brachial artery, 497
  of cephalic vein branches, 498
  of corpora cavernosa, 499, 500
  of dorsal vein of penis, 499, 500
  of dorsalis pedis artery, 497, *498*
  of external jugular vein, 502
  of femoral artery, 496, *498*
  of femoral vein, 502
  of internal jugular vein, 500, *500*
    in heart transplantation, 1324
    precautions in, 501
  of median cubital vein, 498, 499
  of metacarpal veins, 498
  of radial artery, 496, *497*
  of subclavian vein, 501, *501*, 502
  of superficial temporal artery, 498
  peripheral venous. See *Peripheral venous catheterization.*
  pulmonary artery. See *Pulmonary artery catheterization.*
  umbilical, in neonates, 1024
Cations, exchange of, distal tubules in, 736, *736*
Caudal anesthesia, 523, *523*, 524, *524*
  anatomic considerations in, 523, *523*
  drug choice for, 523
  dural puncture during, 479
  for nonobstetric surgery, in pregnant patient, 1105
  in children, 1060, 1060(t), 1061, *1061*
  misplacement of, *478*, 479
  needle placement for, 523, 524, *525*
  patient selection for, 523

Caudal anesthesia *(Continued)*
  positioning for, 523, *524*
  potential problems with, 524
CBF. See *Cerebral blood flow (CBF).*
CBV (cerebral blood volume), relationship of, to cerebral blood flow, 1284
CDH (congenital diaphragmatic hernia), 1031–1033, *1032*
CEA (carotid endarterectomy), intraoperative electrophysiologic monitoring during, 160
  transcranial Doppler ultrasonography during, 396, 397
Cecal ileus, radiographic findings in, 226
Cefazolin, in antibiotic prophylaxis, for orthopedic surgery, 1258
Celiac plexus, anatomy of, 1234, *1235*
Celiac plexus block, 489
  technique of, 489, 490
Central anticholinergic syndrome, and hyperthermia, 825
Central hyperventilation, 809
Central nervous system (CNS), changes in, in pregnancy, 1085
  disease of, in altered sensorium, during emergence, 98
    in persistent postoperative unconsciousness, 97
    inhalation anesthesia in, 608–610, *609*, 610(t)
    recovery after, 610
  disorders of, in chronic liver disease, 1337
  effects on, of alveolar hyperventilation, 807
    of alveolar hypoventilation, 801, 809
    of hyperthermia, 824
    of hypocalcemia, 175, 176
    of local anesthetic overdose, 538, 632, *632*
  fever caused by, 826
  function of, in geriatric patients, 1070, 1070(t), 1071
    postoperative, 95–98, 96(t), 97(t)
  homeostasis of, mechanisms of, 1283, 1284, *1284*
  injury to, cardiopulmonary bypass in, 326–328, 327(t)
  monitoring of, in awake patient, 391, 392, 392(t)
  reaction of, to contrast agent, 902, 903
Central venous catheterization, 500–502, *500*, *501*
  catheter tip position in, 553–555, *555*
  complications of, 374, 375, 375(t), 557, 557(t)
  difficult, management of, 555, 556
  equipment for, 542, 543, 543(t)
  in cardiovascular surgery, 1166
    pediatric, 1148(t), 1149, 1149(t)
  in children, 1057
  in renal transplantation, 1362
  indications for, 545, 545(t)
  intraoperative, indications for, 373, 373(t), 374
  malpositioning in, correction of, 555
  radiographic findings with, 223, *224*, 555
  replacement of, 556, 557
  site selection for, 545, 546(t), 547(t)
  techniques of, 550–557, *552–555*, 557(t)
Central venous pressure (CVP), 373–375
  clinical relevance of, 374, 374(t)
  estimation of, clinical, 336, *337*
  factors in, 374, 374(t)
  monitoring of, intraoperative, 69
  normal, 373, *373*, 374
  relationship of, to blood volume, in shock, 670, *671*
Centroneuraxis blocks, 516–524, *518–524*
  problems with, 536, 537

Cephalic vein, branches of, catheterization of, 498

Cephalosporins, allergic reaction to, 9
drug interactions with, 645(t), 646(t)

Cerebral angiography, risks of, 905

Cerebral angioplasty, for cerebral vasospasm, after intracranial aneurysm rupture, 1291

Cerebral autoregulation, failure of, 393, 393(t)
loss of, in ruptured intracranial aneurysm, 1290

Cerebral blood flow (CBF), autoregulation of, 1283, *1284*
during cardiopulmonary bypass, perfusion pressure for, 327, *327*
pulsatile, 330
effects on, of alveolar hypoventilation, 801
of inhalation anesthesia, 609, 610
in geriatric patients, 1071
measurement of, direct, 395–398, *395–397*
monitoring of, during general anesthesia, 392–395
importance of, 392, 393, 393(t)
in blood pressure assessment, 393, *393*
planned interruption of, effects of, on inhalation anesthetic choice, 608, 609, *609*
relationship of, to cerebral blood volume, 1284
to intracranial pressure, 394

Cerebral blood volume (CBV), relationship of, to cerebral blood flow, 1284

Cerebral contusion, diffuse, abnormal intracranial pressure in, management of, 775

Cerebral cortex, function of, monitoring of, somatosensory evoked potentials in, 404, 405, *405*

Cerebral edema, during neurosurgery, fluid therapy for, 730
in intracranial neoplasm, 1302, 1303

Cerebral embolism, in persistent postoperative unconsciousness, 97

Cerebral hypoxia, in persistent postoperative unconsciousness, 97

Cerebral ischemia, detection of, electroencephalography in, 400, *401*
intracranial hypertension and, 771

Cerebral oxygen, supply/demand of, balance of, measurement of, 398–408

Cerebral perfusion, in aortic arch surgery, 1191

Cerebral perfusion pressure (CPP), 393, *393*
calculation of, 1284
decreased, 393
increased, 393
maintenance of, in traumatic head injury, 1002
relationship of, to intracranial pressure, 770

Cerebral protection, during cardiopulmonary bypass, barbiturates in, 328, 329

Cerebral vasoconstriction, alveolar hyperventilation and, 807
hypocapnia-induced, 609, 610

Cerebral vasospasm, after intracranial aneurysm rupture, 1290, 1291, 1291(t)
detection of, transcranial Doppler ultrasonography in, 397, *397*
preoperative treatment of, 1291

Cerebrospinal fluid (CSF), drainage of, in intraoperative intracranial pressure control, 779
in paraplegia prevention, after aortic cross-clamping, 1228, 1228(t), 1229
in thoracic aorta surgery, 1192, 1193
in thoracoabdominal aneurysm management, 1219
effects on, of inhalation anesthesia, 610, 610(t)
in intracranial pressure measurement, 395

Cerebrospinal fluid (CSF) *(Continued)*
regulation of, in abnormal intracranial pressure, 772

Cerebrovascular accident (CVA). See *Stroke.*

Cerebrovasodilation, anesthetic-induced, 609

Cerium nitrate, for burn wound sepsis, 707

Cervical cerclage, inhalation anesthesia for, 616

Cervical myelopathy, intubation in, 1296
positioning in, 1296

Cervical radiculopathy, intubation in, 1296
positioning in, 1296

Cervical spine, 460–468
anatomy of, 460, 461, *461*
effects on, of aging, 463, 463(t)
of inflammatory arthropathies, 464, 465, *465, 466*
in children, 461
assessment of, 1247, 1248
in trauma, 991, 992
radiographic, 995
congenital anomalies of, 461–463, 461(t), *462,* 462(t)
clinical significance of, 463
preanesthetic evaluation of, 463
fracture of, cardiopulmonary resuscitation in, 835, 836, *836*
injury of, 1001, 1247(t)
craniofacial trauma with, 1278
in children, characteristics of, 467, 468
instability of, conditions associated with, 467(t)
in prone position, management of, 508
mechanisms of, 467, 467(t), *468*
management of, in prone position, 507, 508
motion of, clinical evaluation of, 464
factors in, 464
stability of, anatomic structures in, 465, 466
surgery of, anesthetic considerations in, 1300, 1301
head position in, 1299, 1300, *1300*
vertebrae of, lower, 461

Cesarean section, 1089–1091
anesthetic options for, 1089–1091
maternal complications of, 1093
performance of, fetal distress in, 1096

Challenge tests, in bronchial asthma, 957

CHD. See *Congenital heart disease (CHD).*

Chemical inactivation, in drug incompatibility, 640

Chemical injury, effects of, 700

Chemotactic factors of anaphylaxis, cardiopulmonary effects of, 744, 745

Chemotherapy, for bone cancer, 1252

Chest, computed tomography of, in multiple trauma, 1005
flail, in postoperative hypoventilation, 84
injury to, on battlefield, causes of, 877(t)
positioning of, in prone position, 508
preanesthetic assessment of, in children, 1041

Chest compression, in neonatal resuscitation, 1034

Chest radiography, after central venous catheterization, 555
assessment of, factors in, 211
before cardiovascular surgery, 1158
in aortic disease, 1212
in congenital heart disease, 1143
in pulmonary edema, 972, 972(t), *973*
normal anatomy on, 211–213, *212, 214*
preoperative, 66
in cardiac risk assessment, 130, *131,* 131(t)

Chest rolls, for orthopedic surgery, 1260

Chest tubes, radiographic findings with, 219

Chest wall, excursion of, in tracheal tube placement verification, 943

Chest wall *(Continued)*
of neonates, 1015
rigidity of, with high-dose opioids, for cardiovascular surgery, 1173, *1174*

Chest wall compliance, decrease in, causes of, 813, 814
effects of, on ventilatory work, 813

CHF. See *Congestive heart failure (CHF).*

Chickenpox, 862–864
diagnosis of, 863
manifestations of, 862, 863
prevention of, 863, 864
prognosis in, 863

Child(ren), 1038–1064
acquired immunodeficiency syndrome in, epidemiology of, 853, 854
anesthesia in, induction of, 1049–1054, *1050,* 1052(t), *1053,* 1053(t)
equipment for, 1052–1054, 1053(t)
parent presence during, 1050, 1051
maintenance of, 1054–1056, 1054(t), *1055,* 1056(t)
problems after, 1061, 1062
procedures requiring, 1062–1064, *1063*
asthma in, 1042, 1043
blood transfusion in, 1056–1059
burns in, analgesia for, 271
cancer in, pain in, 271, 271(t), 272
palliative management of, 272
cardiovascular surgery in. See *Cardiovascular surgery, pediatric.*
cervical spine of, anatomy of, 461
injuries of, characteristics of, 467, 468
congenital heart disease in, 1043, 1044, 1044(t). See also *Congenital heart disease, in children.*
endotracheal tubes for, size of, 308, 308(t), 309
epidural analgesia in, continuous, management of, 269, 270
differences in, 269, *269*
indications for, 268, 269, 269(t)
fluid therapy in, 730, 1056–1059
glucose-in-water use in, 722
heart of, structure of, 1140, *1140*
intraoperative monitoring of, 1059, 1060
intraoperative problems in, 1059, 1060
local analgesia in, toxicity of, 267, 267(t)
local anesthesia in, 268–270, *269,* 269(t)
magnetic resonance imaging in, indications for, 911(t)
malignant hyperthermia in, 1044–1046, 1045(t), 1046(t)
orthotopic liver transplantation in, 1355, 1356
outpatient surgery in, general anesthesia for, 1397
intravenous infusions in, 1399, 1399(t), 1400
tracheal intubation for, 1398, 1399
pain in, 261–273
peripheral venous catheterization in, 500
preanesthetic assessment of, 1038–1041, 1039(t), 1040(t)
information exchange in, 1038, 1039
laboratory studies in, 1040
medical record review in, 1039
physical examination in, 1039, 1040
premedication in. See *Premedication, in children.*
preoperative fasting guidelines for, 1040, 1040(t), 1041
regional analgesia in, 267–270
contraindications to, 267
regional anesthesia in, 1060, 1060(t), 1061, *1061*
trauma in, 1003–1005, 1004(t), 1005(t)

Child(ren) *(Continued)*
  upper respiratory tract infection in, 1041, 1042
  vascular access in, 1056, 1057, *1057*
  vital signs in, in trauma, 1004, 1004(t)
Chloral hydrate, for imaging studies, 910(t)
  in pediatric premedication, 1048(t)
Chlordiazepoxide, for acute pain, 242(t)
  in liver disease, 1344(t)
Chlorfluorocarbons, environmental effects of, 114
Chloride, disorders of, 727
Chloroprocaine, 630
  action of, duration of, *516*
  bupivacaine with, 630
  neurotoxicity of, 636
  pharmacology of, 516(t)
  properties of, clinical, 628(t)
Chlorothalidone, drug interactions with, 647(t)
Chlorothiazide, drug interactions with, 647(t)
Chlorpromazine, drug interactions with, 652(t)
  for imaging studies, 911(t)
  for pain, 242(t)
Chlorprothixene, for pain, 242(t)
Cholecystotomy, percutaneous, complications of, 908
  technique of, 908, *908*
Choledochoduodenal sphincter, contraction of, narcotic administration and, 1116, 1117
Cholestasis, 1122, 1123
Choline magnesium trisalicylate, for acute pain, 240(t)
Cholinesterase, atypical, in ester metabolism, 624
Chromophobe adenoma, 1312
Chronic obstructive lung disease (COLD), 963–968
  anesthesia in, 966, 967, 967(t)
    complications of, 967, 967(t)
  extracorporeal shock wave lithotripsy in, 1382
  extubation in, 949
  history of, 3, 965
  hypoxemia in, oxygen therapy for, 795
  in anesthetic risk, 66
  in reduced postoperative functional residual capacity, 79
  management of, 965
    perioperative, 965, 966, 966(t)
    postoperative, 967, 968
  pathophysiology of, 963, 964
  physical examination in, 965
  postoperative pulmonary function tests in, 149
  respiratory center depression in, 803
  signs and symptoms of, 964, *964*, 964(t)
  types of, 963, 963(t)
Chronic obstructive pulmonary disease (COPD). See *Chronic obstructive lung disease (COLD).*
Chronotropy, in stroke volume, 757
Cimetidine, drug interactions with, 644(t)–646(t)
  in aspiration pneumonitis prevention, for outpatient surgery, 1395(t)
  in children, 1049, *1049*
Ciprofloxacin, drug interactions with, 646(t), 647(t)
Circuit breakers, in electric shock prevention, 889, 890
Circulation, assessment of, in trauma, 993, 993(t), 994, 994(t)
  instrumentation for, 338
  pulse oximetry in, 355, 356
  effects on, of acid-base disturbances, 740, 741
  of aging, 1071

Circulation *(Continued)*
  fetal, 1015, *1016*
    vs. adult circulation, 1139, *1139*
  hyperkinetic, in chronic liver disease, 1336
  in anesthetized patient, monitoring of, 336, 337, *337*, 337(t)
  in cardiopulmonary resuscitation, 840–843, *840*, 841(t), *842*, *843*
  in conscious patients, monitoring of, 335
  intraoperative, standards for, 123
  management of, in inhalation anesthesia, 612, 612(t), 613
  monitoring of, intraoperative, standards for, 68(t)
    variables in, 334(t)
  total arrest of, during cardiopulmonary bypass, for pediatric cardiovascular surgery, 1151
  transitional, definition of, 1139
Circumcision, in children, epidural analgesia for, 268
Cirrhosis, effects of, on abdominal muscle relaxation, 1111
  orthotopic liver transplantation in, risk factors in, 1335, 1335(t)
  portosystemic shunting in, outcome of, 1128, 1129(t)
Citrate, metabolism of, after liver resection, 1124
Claims-made insurance policy, 60
Cleft lip, 1272, *1272*
Cleft palate, 1272, *1273*
Clindamycin, drug interactions with, 652(t)
  in bacterial endocarditis prophylaxis, 15(t)
  perioperative use of, 9(t)
Clinoril, for acute pain, 240(t)
Clomipramine, for pain, 242(t)
Clonazepam, 159(t)
Clonic shivering, 821
Clonidine, analgesic potential of, 244(t)
  continuation of, perioperative, 139, 1163, 1164
    drug interactions with, 655(t)
    for narcotic withdrawal, 867
    in premedication, 583
  patch for, application of, preoperative, 171
  single-dose, before cardiovascular surgery, 1165
  withdrawal of, rebound hypertension after, 171
Clotting, after liver resection, 1123, 1124
Clotting factors, effects on, of hydroxyethyl starch, 728
CMRo₂, barbiturate suppression of, detection of, electroencephalography in, 401
CMV. See *Cytomegalovirus (CMV).*
CNS. See *Central nervous system (CNS).*
Coagulation, analysis of, thromboelastography in, 1353–1355, *1354*, *1355*
  disorders of, after cardiopulmonary bypass, diagnosis/treatment of, 1189, 1190
    after trauma surgery, 1008
    in renal failure, 1359
  effects on, of fluid therapy, 727, 728
    of hypothermia, 819(t), 820
    of orthotopic liver transplantation, during anhepatic phase, 1348
      during neohepatic phase, 1350, 1351
      during preanhepatic phase, 1347
  in geriatric patients, epidural anesthesia effects on, 1077
  monitoring of, in cardiovascular surgery, 1168
  zone of, in burns, 699
Coagulation factors, disorders of, after cardiopulmonary bypass, 1189

Coagulation profile, before adenotonsillectomy, 1269
  in congenital heart disease assessment, 1143
Coagulopathy, after cardiopulmonary bypass, 1188, 1189, 1189(t)
  after peritoneovenous shunting, 1126, *1126*
  in chronic liver disease, 1337
  in heart transplantation, 1329
  in portosystemic shunting, 1130
  regional anesthesia in, 514, 515
Cocaine, 630
  abuse of, diagnostic features of, 1000(t)
  for awake tracheal intubation, 1279
  properties of, clinical, 628(t)
  use of, and hyperthermia, 826
Codeine, for pain, acute, 241(t)
  in children, 264(t), 265
    with cancer, 272
Codman, E.A., 20, 32
Cognitive-behavioral therapy, for pain, in adults, 256, 257, 257(t)
Coherent radiation, 1370
  medical applications of, 1371, 1371(t), 1372
  production of, 1370, *1371*
COLD. See *Chronic obstructive lung disease (COLD).*
Colistin, perioperative use of, 9(t)
Collaborative Confidential Inquiry into Perioperative Death, 62
Collateralization, during thoracic aorta cross-clamping, 1226
Collins' solution, 1338, 1339(t)
Colloid oncotic pressure, in intracranial neoplasm surgery, 1308
  in pulmonary edema, interstitial, 971
    plasma, 971
  maintenance of, in shock, 667, 668
Colloids, 718, 719
  administration of, during abdominal surgery, 1121
    in neonates, 1025
    in shock, 668
    intravenous, for anaphylactic shock, 683(t)
    preoperative, in pulmonary edema, 974
  distribution of, 719, *719*
  for fluid resuscitation, in thermal injuries, 706, 706(t)
  in intracranial pressure control, 776
  therapeutic use of, 720
    costs of, 720, 720(t)
  vs. crystalloids, 719, *719*
Colonic ileus, radiographic findings in, 226
Coma, postoperative, assessment of, 165(t)
Common gas outlet, of low-pressure anesthesia machine, 282
Common peroneal nerve, injury to, lithotomy position in, 510
Comparative negligence, 59
Compartment syndromes, 1247(t), *1248*
  acute, assessment of, 999
  in thermal injuries, 706, 707
Complement, activation of, in anaphylaxis, 681, 746
  in burns, 702
Compliance, of breathing hose, 287, 288(t)
  of chest wall, decrease in, causes of, 813, 814
    effects of, on ventilatory work, 813
  of heart, in children, 1140, *1140*
  pulmonary. See *Pulmonary compliance.*
  ventilatory, decrease in, with high-dose opioids, for cardiovascular surgery, 1173, *1174*
  ventricular, in pulmonary artery pressure monitoring, 376, 376(t)
Compressed spectral array (CSA), 160, *160*

Compromise, cardiorespiratory, in spinal cord shock, 685

Computed tomography (CT), 897–918
anesthesia/sedation for, 910, 910(t), 911, 911(t)
complications of, 911
in aortic disease diagnosis, 1212, 1213(t)
in intracranial pressure measurement, 395, 395(t)
in pain diagnosis, in adults, 239
in trauma care, 988
in traumatic abdominal injury assessment, 998
in traumatic retroperitoneal injuries, 1001
mechanism of, 909, *909*, 910
of chest, in multiple trauma, 1005
technique of, 910

Conduction, abnormal, in geriatric patients, 1071
in heat loss, 693, 818(t), 819
nerve, physiology of, 621, 622, *622*, *623*

Conduction blocks, postoperative, management of, 139, 139(t)

Conductivity, cardiac, local anesthetic overdose effect on, 632, *632*, 633, *633*

Condylomata acuminata, laser surgery for, anesthesia administration in, 1243

Congenital diaphragmatic hernia (CDH), 1031–1033, *1032*

Congenital heart disease (CHD), characteristics of, 1140, 1141, 1141(t)
detection of, 1141
in children, 1043, 1044, 1044(t)
anesthetic effects on, 1044
classification of, 1044(t)
management of, 1044
noncardiac surgery in, 1043, 1044
in obstetric patient, 1094, *1094*
incidence of, 1138, 1139(t)
physiologic considerations in, 1139–1141, *1139*, 1139(t), *1140*, 1141(t)
preoperative assessment of, 1141–1144, *1142*, 1144(t)
prognosis in, 1138, 1139
severity of, 1138
surgery for, complications of, 1143, 1144(t)

Congestive heart failure (CHF), fluid therapy in, 729
history of, 2
in anesthetic risk, 65
in aortic stenosis, 1161
in congenital heart disease, 1141, 1142
postoperative, manifestations of, 138, 139
radiographic findings in, 216, *218*, *219*
signs and symptoms of, 1158

Connectors, ''quick,'' 277, *279*

Conn's syndrome, 1318, 1319

Consciousness, level of, definitions of, 900, 900(t)
loss of, traumatic head injury and, 1002

Consensus-2 trial, 665

Consent, informed, for anesthesia, 1
for vascular access, 543, 544(t)

Consultation, endocrine, 185–208
neurologic. See *Neurologic consultation.*
preoperative, 14, 15, 15(t)
pulmonary. See *Pulmonary consultation.*

Consumable supplies, cost of, 117, 117(t)

Contact probes, in temperature monitoring, 429, 430

Continuous positive airway pressure (CPAP), for alveolar hypoventilation, 806, *806*, *807*
for hypoxemia, 795
postoperative, 79
for hypoxia, during thoracic surgery, 1206, *1206*
preoperative, in pulmonary edema, 974

Continuous positive airway pressure (CPAP) (*Continued*)
ventilatory work in, 811, *811*, 812

Contoured supine position, for surgery, 506, *506*, 507

Contractility, cardiac, abnormal, in end-stage heart disease, 1322
goal for, after cardiopulmonary bypass, 1181, 1182(t)
local anesthetic overdose effect on, 632
in stroke volume, 757, *758*
quantification of, 763, 764

Contracture, muscle, testing of, in malignant hyperthermia, 832

Contrast agents, for magnetic resonance imaging, 914, 915, 915(t)
intravascular, chemical structure of, 901, 901(t), 902
ionic vs. non-ionic, 902
reactions to, 901–905
frequency of, 903, 903(t)
mediators in, 903
prevention of, 904, 905
risk factors for, 904
treatment of, 903, 904
types of, 902, 902(t), 903, *903*

Control, exercise of, in psychologic surgical preparation, 577

Contusion, myocardial, traumatic, assessment of, 995, 996
pulmonary, traumatic, assessment of, 995

Convection, in heat loss, 693, 818(t), 819

Cooling, during cardiopulmonary bypass, myocardial, 324, 324(t)
systemic, 323, 324

Cooperman's equation, in preoperative cardiac risk assessment, 126, 127

COPD. See *Chronic obstructive lung disease (COLD).*

Coping, mechanisms for, in psychologic surgical preparation, 577, 578

Cor pulmonale, radiographic findings in, 216, *217*

Cornea, injury to, postoperative, 103

Corniculate cartilages, 446
functions of, 446

Coronary angioplasty, before noncardiac surgery, 134, 135

Coronary artery, blood flow in, during aortic vascular surgery, 1222

Coronary artery bypass grafting (CABG), before noncardiac surgery, indications for, 134, 135
cerebral protection during, barbiturates in, 329

Coronary artery disease (CAD), blood pressure differences in, *10*
extent of, in noncardiac vascular surgery patients, 126, 126(t)
hemodynamic goals in, 1169–1171, 1169(t), *1170*, 1171(t)
history of, 2, *3*
in anesthetic risk, 65
inhalation anesthesia in, 612, 613
medications for, preoperative continuation of, 1163, 1164
myocardial ischemia in, 754, *755*
preanesthetic evaluation of, 12, 13, *13*
prevalence of, in surgical patients, 125, *125*
surgery in, decision for, 755, 756
treatment of, in intraoperative stroke prevention, 154, 155

Coronary Artery Surgery Study (CASS), 128

Coronary blood flow, factors in, 1170, *1170*

Coronary perfusion pressure, determination of, 1170
parameters for, 691(t)

Coronary revascularization, before noncardiac surgery, 134, 135

Coronary steal, 759
isoflurane and, 1175, 1176
in central aortic surgery, 1217

Coronary vessels, anatomy of, demonstration of, cardiac catheterization in, 1160, *1161*

Corpectomy, extracavitary, lateral, 1301
thoracic, anterior, 1301

Corpora cavernosa, catheterization of, 499, 500

Corticosteroids, administration of, excessive, in Addison's disease, 194
drug interactions with, 194, 645(t)
effects of, 189
for anaphylactic shock, 683(t)
for anaphylaxis, 748
for contrast agent reactions, 904
in chronic obstructive pulmonary disease, 965
in paraplegia prevention, after aortic cross-clamping, 1229
metabolism of, in Addison's disease, 194
supplementation of, perioperative, in Cushing's disease, 193
use of, history of, 4, *4*
perioperative, 7, 7(t)
pulmonary effects of, 150

Corticotropin-releasing hormone (CRH), 189
measurement of, in Addison's disease diagnosis, 191
in Cushing's syndrome diagnosis, 190

Cortisol, in adrenal replacement therapy, 192(t)
measurement of, in Addison's disease diagnosis, 191

Cortisone, in adrenal replacement therapy, 192(t)

Cortrosyn test, 191

Coughing, after intubation, treatment of, 454

CPAP. See *Continuous positive airway pressure (CPAP).*

CPB. See *Cardiopulmonary bypass (CPB).*

CPP. See *Cerebral perfusion pressure (CPP).*

CPR. See *Cardiopulmonary resuscitation (CPR).*

CPT-4, 111

Cranial nerves, neoplasm of, properties of, 1303(t)

Cranial vault, contents of, 769, *769*, 770

Craniofacial trauma, 1276–1278, *1276*, *1277*, 1278(t)
injuries associated with, 1278, 1278(t)
intubation in, 1278
site of, anatomic factors in, 1276, *1276*

Craniopharyngioma, properties of, 1303(t)

Craniotomy, for intracranial neoplasm, 1304

CRH (corticotropin-releasing hormone), 189
measurement of, in Addison's disease diagnosis, 191
in Cushing's syndrome diagnosis, 190

Cribriform plate, perforation of, nasal intubation in, 934

Cricoarytenoid joints, in rheumatoid arthritis, 445

Cricoarytenoid muscles, lateral, 448

Cricoid cartilage, 444, 445, *445*
attachments of, 444, 445

Cricoid pressure, application of, in children, *1050*
release of, for vomiting, during emergency abdominal surgery, 1119, *1119*

Cricothyroid catheter, insertion of, 940, *940*

Cricothyroidotomy, emergency, 940, *940*, 992
for proximal airways obstruction, 82, *82*
in cardiopulmonary resuscitation, 838, *838*, *839*

Cricothyrotomy, in thermal injuries, 705

Cromolyn sodium, for bronchial asthma, 958

Croup, effects of, on outpatient discharge, 1401
postintubation, 1062
Crowe-Davis mouth gag, 1269, *1269*
Crush syndrome, 876
Cryocuff, in orthopedic surgery, for pain control, 1264
Crystalloids, conventional, 717, 717(t), 718
distribution of, 718, *718*
for shock, 667, 668
in intracranial pressure control, 776
vs. colloids, 719
CSA (compressed spectral array), 160, *160*
CSF. See *Cerebrospinal fluid (CSF)*.
CT. See *Computed tomography (CT)*.
Cuff(s), blood pressure, application of, 337, 338
site of, blood pressure variations with, 337, 338
size of, 369
of endotracheal tube, high-pressure low-volume, 310, 311, *311*
inflation of, 311
minimal leak technique of, 312
no leak technique of, 312
problems in, 310–312, *311*, *312*
leak in, 951
low-pressure high-volume, 311, *311*
pressure in, measurement of, 311, 312
size of, 311, *312*
volume in, measurement of, 311, 312
of tracheal tubes, 451
Cuneiform cartilages, 446
functions of, 446
Cupola, of lung, location of, 501
Curare, in renal transplantation, 1363
Cushing's syndrome, clinical features of, 190(t)
complications of, perioperative, 193, 194
definition of, 189
diagnosis of, 190
management of, 190, 191
medical, 191
perioperative, 193
preoperative, 189, 190
surgical, 191
CVA (cerebrovascular accident). See *Stroke*.
CVP. See *Central venous pressure (CVP)*.
Cyanide intoxication, in thermal injuries, 704
Cyanosis, in congenital heart disease, 1141, 1142, *1142*
preanesthetic evaluation of, 9
Cyclophosphamide, drug interactions with, 647(t)
Cyclosporin A, complications of, 1330(t)
Cyclosporine, drug interactions with, 647(t)
in orthotopic liver transplantation, 1344
in renal transplantation, 1361, 1362
Cylinder, of high-pressure anesthesia machine, operating pressure of, 279, 280, *281*
Cystectomy, 1242, 1243
anesthesia for, administration of, 1242, 1243
Cytal, in transurethral resection of the prostate, 1240, 1241
Cytochrome P$_{450}$ enzymes, response to, genetic factors in, 569
Cytokines, in multiple system organ failure, 1010
Cytomegalovirus (CMV), 864
diagnosis of, 864
epidemiology of, 864
prevention of, 864
prognosis in, 864

Dalmane, for acute pain, 242(t)
Damping coefficient, in fluid-coupled transducing system, 372, *372*

Dantrolene, for malignant hyperthermia, 828, 829, 829(t)
Database, computerized, for quality assurance, 41, *43–45*, 45
selection of, 51, 52
DBS (double-burst stimulation), 418, *418*, 419
DCS (dorsal column stimulator), for pain, in adults, 255, 255(t)
DDAVP (1-deamino-8-D-arginine vasopressin), for diabetes insipidus, 187
Dead space, changes in, in alveolar hyperventilation, 808
increase in, effects of, on ventilatory work, 814
postoperative, 85, 85(t)
Dead space ventilation, in hypoxemia, 784
1-Deamino-8-D-arginine vasopressin (DDAVP), for diabetes insipidus, 187
Death, brain, confirmation of, transcranial Doppler ultrasonography in, 397, *397*, 398
diagnosis of, 166
of obstetric patient, general anesthesia in, 1091, 1091(t)
Decompression, for compartment syndromes, in thermal injuries, 707
surgical, of neural compression, 1297
Deep peroneal nerve, in ankle block, 533
Deep vein thrombosis, after transurethral resection of prostate, 1239, 1240
Defasciculating drug, administration of, before succinylcholine injection, 591, 591(t)
Defibrillation, ventricular, in cardiopulmonary resuscitation, 841–843, *843*
Dehydration test, in diabetes insipidus, 187
Delirium, emergence, in children, 1061
postoperative, 165, 165(t), 166
assessment of, 165(t)
causes of, 165
differential diagnosis of, 165, 166
Delivery, epidural anesthesia for, 1089
operative, inhalation anesthesia for, 616
Delta hepatitis, 860, 861
Delta rhythm, in electroencephalography, 400, *400*
Demeclocycline, for syndrome of inappropriate antidiuretic hormone secretion, 189
Deming, W. Edwards, 31
Denitrogenation, for general anesthesia, 586–588, *587*
preinduction, 344, *345*
Denitrogenation atelectasis, 792, *792*
Dental appliances, examination of, before intubation, 440
Dental repairs, in retarded/uncooperative patients, 1275, 1276
Dentition, preanesthetic evaluation of, 10
Dentures, removal of, for general anesthesia, 585
Depolarization, atrial, 362
re-entrant, postoperative, 93, *93*
ventricular, 362
Desflurane, effects of, circulatory, 612(t)
physiologic, 1285(t)
for outpatient surgery, 617, 1397, 1398
Desiccated thyroid, for hypothyroidism, 198
Desipramine, for pain, 242(t)
Desmopressin, after cardipulmonary bypass, 1190
during orthopedic surgery, for intraoperative blood loss reduction, 1260
Detsky's multifactorial index, in preoperative cardiac risk assessment, 128, 128(t), *129*
Dexamethasone, for bronchial asthma, 958(t)
for cancer pain, 244(t)
in adrenal replacement therapy, 192(t)
Dexedrine, analgesic potential of, 244(t)

Dextran, effects of, on coagulation, 728
in local anesthesia, 629
types of, 728
Dextroamphetamine, analgesic potential of, 244(t)
Dextrose, administration of, perioperative, 171, 172, 172(t)
complications of, 171, 172
indications for, 172
avoidance of, in thoracic aorta surgery, 1193
Diabetes insipidus, and perioperative oliguria, 386
and postoperative polyuria, 95
classic (central/neurogenic), 186
definition of, 186
diagnosis of, 186, 187, 187(t)
fluid therapy for, 730
permanent, 186
postoperative/post-traumatic, 186
transient, 186
treatment of, 187
triphasic, 186
Diabetes mellitus, 205–208
assessment of, 207
cardiopulmonary bypass in, neurologic dysfunction after, 329, 329(t)
characteristics of, 206, 207
complications of, assessment of, 207
delayed emergence in, 164(t)
glucose-in-water administration in, 721, 722
history of, 4
inhalation anesthesia in, 614
management of, perioperative, 207, 208, 208(t)
type I, 206
type II, 206
Diabetic ketoacidosis (DKA), 205, 206
Diagnostic peritoneal lavage (DPL), 997
Dialysis, 183, *183*, 183(t), 184
anemia in, 183
anesthetic implications of, *183*, 184
before renal transplantation, 1361
postoperative effects of, 183, 184
preoperative, timing of, 183
sequelae of, 183(t)
site of, management of, 183
tilt testing in, 183
Diameter Index Safety System (DISS), 277, *278*
Diamorphine, for acute pain, 241(t)
intraspinal, 248(t)
Diaphragm, injuries of, traumatic, assessment of, 996, 997, *997*, *998*
motion of, restriction of, after abdominal surgery, 1130, 1131, *1131*
in postoperative hypoventilation, 84
Diastolic dysfunction, 758, 759(t)
Diazepam, for acute pain, 242(t)
for cardiovascular surgery, 1164(t), 1175(t)
for imaging studies, 910(t), 911(t)
for perioperative hypertension, 171(t)
half-life of, 565, *565*
in liver disease, 1344(t)
in premedication, 579, 579(t), *580*
pediatric, 1048(t)
properties of, 598(t), 600(t)
selection of, factors in, 572
Dibenzoxazepine, adverse effects of, 656(t)
Dibenzyline, analgesic potential of, 244(t)
Dibucaine, properties of, clinical, 627(t)
DIC (disseminated intravascular coagulation), after cardiopulmonary bypass, 1189
Diclofenac, for acute pain, 240(t)
Dicumarol, drug interactions with, 644(t)
Died of wounds (DOW), 875
Differential awakening, 163

Diffuse idiopathic skeletal hyperostosis (DISH), 463, *464*

Diffusing capacity, definition of, 1201

Diffusion block, and alveolar hypoventilation, 805, 806

Diffusion hypoxia, 796
 postoperative, 78

Diflunisal, for acute pain, 240(t)

Digitalis, for life-threatening dysrhythmias, 850

Digitalis glycosides, perioperative use of, 6

Digoxin, after heart transplantation, 1327
 drug interactions with, 646(t), 647(t), 654(t)
 for supraventricular tachycardia, after cardiopulmonary bypass, 1187(t)
 perioperative use of, 6
 preoperative assessment of, in congenital heart disease, 1143

Dihydroindolone, adverse effects of, 656(t)

Dilaudid, for acute pain, 241(t)

Diltiazem, drug interactions with, 645(t), 647(t)

Dipyridamole, oral administration of, in preoperative cardiac risk assessment, 131, 132

Dipyridamole-thallium imaging, before cardiovascular surgery, 1159
 in coronary artery disease evaluation, 12, 13, *13*

Direct current, 886, *996*

Discharge, of outpatient, criteria for, 1401, 1401(t), *1402, 1403,* 1404(t)

DISH (diffuse idiopathic skeletal hyperostosis), 463, *464*

Diskectomy, 1297, *1297*
 extracavitary, lateral, 1301
 thoracic, anterior, 1301

Disopyramide, perioperative use of, 6

DISS (Diameter Index Safety System), 277, *278*

Disseminated intravascular coagulation (DIC), after cardiopulmonary bypass, 1189

Distribution, of drugs, factors in, 643, 648, 648(t)

Disulfiram, drug interactions with, 644(t)
 in drug abuse treatment, 867

Diuresis, forced, in traumatic head injury, 1002
 osmotic, and postoperative polyuria, 95
 vs. diabetes insipidus, 187, 187(t)

Diuretics, for oliguria, indications for, 181, 182
 in intracranial pressure control, 776, 777
 intraoperative, 779
 in lithium excretion, 649
 in perioperative oliguria, 386
 loop, drug interactions with, 647(t), 654(t)
 osmotic, in pregnancy, 1106
 response to, in chronic renal failure, 1361
 thiazide, drug interactions with, 647(t)
 use of, perioperative, 5, *6*

DKA (diabetic ketoacidosis), 205, 206

DLTs. See *Double-lumen tubes (DLTs).*

Dobhoff tube, positioning of, *232*

Dobutamine, 1182(t)
 for intraoperative hemodynamic stabilization, in shock, 690(t), 692
 for perioperative myocardial dysfunction, 766(t)
 in preoperative cardiac risk assessment, 132, 133

Documentation, in preoperative cardiac risk assessment, 129
 in trauma care, 988, *989*
 of surgical patient positioning, 505, *506*
 postanesthesia, 29

Dolobid, for acute pain, 240(t)

Donabedian, Avedis, 35

"Do-not-resuscitate" patient, geriatric, 1080
 preanesthetic evaluation of, 17

Dopamine, 1182(t)

Dopamine *(Continued)*
 drug interactions with, 655(t)
 for intraoperative hemodynamic stabilization, in shock, 690(t), 691
 for perioperative myocardial dysfunction, 766(t)
 in neuroleptic malignant syndrome, 158
 in pediatric cardiovascular surgery, 1146(t)
 in renal function preservation, in aortic vascular surgery, 1220

Doppler flow echocardiography, 381, 382

Doppler sphygmomanometry, 369, 370

Doppler ultrasonography, pulsed-wave, in cardiac output measurement, 380

Dornier HM3 lithotripter, 1380

Dorsal column stimulator (DCS), for pain, in adults, 255, 255(t)

Double-lumen tubes (DLTs), 312–315, *312, 314,* 315(t)
 complications of, 314, 315, 315(t)
 contraindications to, 313
 for thoracic surgery, 1202–1204
 indications for, 1202, 1202(t)
 position of, verification of, 1203, *1203,* 1204, *1204*
 indications for, 313
 insertion of, 313, 314
 fiberoptic bronchoscopy in, 314
 malpositioning of, 314, *314*
 placement of, verification of, 313, 314
 role of, 312, *312*
 types of, 313

Dorsal vein of penis, catheterization of, 499, 500

Dorsalis pedis artery, catheterization of, 497, *498*
 advantages of, 548(t)
 disadvantages of, 548(t)
 techniques of, 548

Dosing interval, 568

Double-burst stimulation (DBS), 418, *418,* 419

DOW (died of wounds), 875

"Down lung syndrome," 79

Down's syndrome, cervical spine anomalies in, 462

Doxacurium, dose of, in children, 1056(t)
 effects of, physiologic, 1285(t)

Doxapram, in intravenous anesthesia reversal, 601
 selection of, factors in, 573

Doxepin, for pain, 242(t)

Doxorubicin, for bone cancer, 1252
 perioperative use of, 8

DPL (diagnostic peritoneal lavage), 997

Dräger ventilator, 347

Draw-over vaporizer, in battlefield surgery, 879, *879*

Droperidol, in postoperative nausea prevention, 99

Drug(s). See also *Medication(s);* specific drugs and drug groups.
 absorption of, drug interactions in, 641–643, *643*
 accumulation of, 568, 569, 569(t)
 actions of, effects on, of acid-base disturbances, 741
 bioavailability of, measurement of, 562
 clearance of, 566
 organs in, 566
 perioperative, factors in, 567, 568, 568, 568(t)
 disposition of, 561–565
 effects on, of administration route, 561, 562, *562*
 distribution of, 561, *561*
 factors in, 563, *563,* 564, *564,* 643, 648, 648(t)

Drug(s) *(Continued)*
 elimination of, 561, *562,* 649
 fat-soluble, distribution of, effects on, of volume of distribution, 565, *565*
 half-life of, 563, 564, *564*
 effects of, on clearance, 568, 568(t)
 long, biologic effects of, 564, *564*
 illicit, use of, preanesthetic evaluation of, 9
 in postoperative delirium, 165
 inhibition of, 649
 intravenous, dosing regimens for, 567, *567*
 metabolism of, in drug interactions, 648, 649
 response to, characteristics of, 569, 570, *570*
 pharmacologic, 562, 563, *563*
 resuscitation, for burn surgery, 709, 709(t)
 transport of, across placenta, 566
 membrane, 565, 566
 water-soluble, distribution of, effects on, of volume of distribution, 565, *565*

Drug abuse, 865–868, 865(t)
 causes of, 865, 865(t)
 enabling behavior in, 866
 prevention of, 867, 868
 recognition of, 866
 signs and symptoms of, 865, 866, 866(t)
 treatment of, 866, 867

Drug incompatibility, 640, 641, *642*
 detection of, 641
 harmful effects of, 641
 physical, causes of, 640, 641
 types of, 640

Drug interactions, 640–659
 enteral, 643
 in geriatric patients, 1078, 1078(t)
 in intravenous anesthetic agent clearance, 600
 in local anesthetic metabolism, 625
 in local anesthetic toxicity, 633, 634
 incidence of, 640, *640*
 parenteral, 643
 pharmacodynamic, 650–659, 650(t), 652(t)–658(t), *656*
 classification of, 650, 650(t)
 pharmacokinetic, 641–649, *642,* 644(t)–647(t)

Drug intoxication, 999, 1000, 1000(t)

Dual oximetry, 790

Duchenne's muscular dystrophy, malignant hyperthermia in, 830

Ductus arteriosus, 1015, 1139
 closure of, 1139, 1140

Ductus venosus, 1015, 1139
 closure of, 1140

Dural fold, posterior, in lumbar spine, 471

Dural puncture, during caudal anesthesia, 479

Dyes, effects of, on pulse oximetry, 354, 355

Dypirone, for acute pain, 240(t)

Dyshemoglobinemias, 782

Dyspnea, in congestive heart failure, 1158
 in mitral stenosis, 1161

Dysrhythmia(s), after cardiopulmonary bypass, 1185, 1186(t)
 alveolar hyperventilation and, 808
 alveolar hypoventilation and, 801
 atrial, electrocardiographic characteristics of, 365, 366
 central venous catheterization and, 374, 375
 control of, in automatic internal cardioverter-defibrillator implantation, 1195
 preoperative, in pheochromocytoma, 195
 during anesthetic induction, in pediatric cardiovascular surgery, 1147
 during extracorporeal shock wave lithotripsy, 1384, 1385, *1385*
 heart transplantation and, 1329
 in aortic stenosis, 1171
 in postoperative hypotension, 90, 91

Dysrhythmia(s) *(Continued)*
  intraoperative, 365(t)
    factors in, 360, 360(t)
    in children, 1060
    potassium level in, 5, *6*
  life-threatening, cardiopulmonary resuscitation in, 850, 851
  origination of, 365, *365*
  postoperative, management of, 139, 139(t)
  sinus, electrocardiographic characteristics of, 366
  symptomatic, history of, 3
  tracheal intubation and, 455
  ventricular, electrocardiography in, 367

EA (esophageal atresia), in neonates, 1030, 1031, *1031*
EACA (epsilon-aminocaproic acid), administration of, in orthotopic liver transplantation, 1355
  for fibrinolysis, 1350
ECF (extracellular fluid), loss of, in abdominal surgery, 1119–1121
ECG. See *Electrocardiography (ECG).*
Echocardiography, before cardiovascular surgery, 1159
  in aortic disease, 1212, 1213(t)
  in congenital heart disease, 1143
  in coronary artery disease, 13
  in geriatric patient, 1074
  in pediatric cardiovascular surgery, 1150
  in postoperative myocardial infarction, 763, *763*
  preoperative, 65
    in cardiac risk assessment, 132, 133
  transesophageal. See *Transesophageal echocardiography (TEE).*
  types of, 381, *381*, 382
Echos, specular, 381
Echothiophate, drug interactions with, 647(t)
  in ester metabolism, 625, 625(t)
  perioperative use of, 8
Eclampsia, 157, 158
  delayed emergence in, 164(t)
  neurologic evaluation in, 157
  seizures in, management of, 157, 158
E-cylinder pressure, 279, 280
Edema, cerebral, in intracranial neoplasm, 1302, 1303
  formation of, in burns, control of, 703, 704
  laryngeal, tracheal intubation and, 456
  of airways, 1275
    presentation of, 1275
    treatment of, 1275
  pulmonary. See *Pulmonary edema.*
  vasogenic, 1302
EDRF (endothelium-derived relaxing factor), 664
Edrophonium, for supraventricular tachycardia, after cardiopulmonary bypass, 1187(t)
  in myasthenia gravis, 154
EDTA (ethylenediaminetetraacetic acid), 630
EDWS (end-diastolic wall stress), calculation of, 758
EEG. See *Electroencephalography (EEG).*
Efficacy, definition of, 569, *570*
EGTA (esophageal gastric tube airway), in cardiopulmonary resuscitation, 837, 838, *838*
Eicosanoids, effects on, of burns, 703
Einthoven triangle, *338*
Ejection fraction, in preoperative cardiac risk assessment, 133
  quantification of, 764
EJV. See *External jugular vein (EJV).*

Elastance, end-systolic, 765, *765*
  intracranial, assessment of, 773, 774
  tissue, in intracranial neoplasm, 1308
Elbow, fracture of, supracondylar, 1247(t)
Elderly. See *Geriatric patients.*
Electric shock, circuit requirements for, 888, *889*
  determinants of, 887, 888, *888*
Electrical cardioversion, in cardiopulmonary resuscitation, 843, *844*
Electrical current, flow of, 885, 886, *886*
Electrical injury, effects of, 699, 700
Electrical safety, 885–896
  in operating room, 890, *890*, 891, *891*
Electricity, loss of, sudden, 895, 896
Electrocardiography (ECG), 338, *338*, 360–367
  admission, indications for, 65
    usefulness of, 65
  ambulatory, preoperative, in cardiac risk assessment, 134
    postoperative cardiac event correlation with, 134
  before cardiovascular surgery, 1158, 1159(t)
  characteristics of, 361, 362, *362*
  deflection of, factors in, 361
  facsimile-transmitted, 130
  in atrial dysrhythmias, 365, 366
  in atrioventricular block, 366, 367
  in atrioventricular dysrhythmias, 366
  in burn surgery, 708, 709
  in congenital heart disease, 1143
  in electrolyte disorders, 367, 368(t)
  in electrosurgical unit, 893, *893*
  in geriatric patient monitoring, 1073
  in myocardial infarction, 364, 365(t)
  in myocardial injury, 364, *364*
  in myocardial ischemia detection, 363, *363*, 364, 364(t)
    in aortic vascular surgery, 1221
    intraoperative, 755(t), 1168, 1168(t), 1169, 1169(t)
  in ventricular dysrhythmias, 367
  information provided by, 362, 363(t)
  intraoperative, in cardiovascular surgery, 1165
  leads for, 361, 361(t)
    placement of, 361, 361(t)
  postoperative, abnormal findings in, 92–94, *93*, 94(t)
  preoperative, in cardiac risk assessment, 129, 130
    in cardiovascular morbidity prediction, 130
    in preanesthetic evaluation, 11, 12, *12*
  signal fidelity in, 362, *362*, 362(t)
  use of, near magnetic resonance imaging scanner, 915
  value of, 360
  vs. transesophageal echocardiography, 382
Electrocautery, 892, *892*
Electrocution, 885–890
  mechanisms of, 888, *889*
Electrode(s), active, 416
  dispersive, for electrosurgery, placement of, 892, 893
  for electrocardiography, placement of, 361, 361(t)
  for electroencephalography, placement of, 398, 399, *399*
  for nerve stimulation, built-in, 416
    placement of, 414–416, *415*
  inactive (indifferent), 416
Electroencephalographic suppression, in cerebral protection, in neurovascular surgery, 1294
Electroencephalography (EEG), 398–402
  anesthesia effects on, 401, 402

Electroencephalography (EEG) *(Continued)*
  in cardiovascular surgery, 1168
    pediatric, 1150
  in carotid surgery, 401
  in inhalation anesthesia, 610
  in shock, 680, *680*
  intraoperative, 159, 160, *160*, 160(t)
  recording of, 398, 399, *399*
    display of, 399, 400, *400*
    Ten-Twenty Electrode System in, 398, 399, *399*
  tracings of, computer processing of, 160, *160*
    interpretation of, 160, 160(t)
    patterns of, amplitude of, 400
      frequency of, 400, *400*
  usefulness of, to anesthesiology, 400, *401*
Electrolyte(s), 714–731
  administration of, in neonates, 1025
  effects on, of fluid therapy, 728, 729
    of orthotopic liver transplantation, during anhepatic phase, 1348
    during neohepatic phase, 1351
  imbalance of, alveolar hypoventilation and, 801
    during renal transplantation, 1365
    electrocardiographic changes with, 367, 368(t)
    in chronic liver disease, 1337, 1337(t)
    in uremia, 183, 183(t)
    postoperative, 102, 103
    signs and symptoms of, 178(t)
    treatment of, 178(t)
  management of, perioperative, 723–727
  measurement of, in intraoperative hemodynamic stabilization, in shock, 692
  preoperative, in congenital heart disease, 1143
  solutions of, for fluid resuscitation, in thermal injuries, 706(t)
Electromechanical dissociation (EMD), treatment of, emergency, 843, 844(t)
  epinephrine in, 844
Electromyography (EMG), in facial nerve monitoring, 408, *409*
  in intraoperative seizure monitoring, 160
  in neuromuscular blockade assessment, 419
  in pain diagnosis, in adults, 239
Electroneutrality, kidneys in, 736, *736*
Electrophysiologic disorders, evaluation of, before cardiovascular surgery, 1162, 1163
Electrophysiologic monitoring, in peripheral nerve injury evaluation, 162
  intraoperative, indications for, 160, 161
Electrostatic detection apparatus (ESDA), 57
Electrosurgery, 891–893, *892*, *893*
  grounding for, 892, *892*
Electrosurgical unit (ESU), 891, 892
  bipolar, 893
  burns in, 893
  electrocardiography in, 893, *893*
  fires in, 893
  interference of, with pacemaker function, 894, 895, 895(t)
ELISA (enzyme-linked immunosorbent assay), in human immunodeficiency virus infection diagnosis, 855
  in perioperative anaphylaxis evaluation, 750
Embolism, air. See *Air embolism.*
  amniotic fluid, during cesarean section, 1093
  cerebral, in persistent postoperative unconsciousness, 97
  fat, delayed emergence in, 164(t)
Embolization, after cardiopulmonary bypass, and neurologic deficit, 326, 327
  arterial catheterization and, 549, 550
  in geriatric patients, 1071
  in pulmonary edema, 977

Embolization *(Continued)*
vascular, materials for, 905, 906, 906(t)
EMD (electromechanical dissociation),
treatment of, emergency, 843, 844(t)
epinephrine in, 844
Emergence, from anesthesia. See *Anesthesia,
emergence from.*
Emergence delirium, in children, 1061
Emergency Department, preparation of, for
trauma care, 985–990, *986,* 987(t), 988(t),
989
role of, in thermal injury therapy, 704, 705
EMG. See *Electromyography (EMG).*
Emission, stimulated, 1370
EMLA (eutectic mixture of local anesthetics),
pediatric use of, 270
Emotional disorders, effects of, on pain
perception, 238
Emphysema, features of, 963, 963(t)
interstitial, pulmonary, radiographic findings
in, 216, 219, *221*
radiographic findings in, 213, *215,* 216, *217*
Enalapril, drug interactions with, 646(t), 655(t)
perioperative continuation of, 139
Encephalitis, and delayed awakening, 165
Endarterectomy, carotid, intraoperative
electrophysiologic monitoring during,
160
transcranial Doppler ultrasonography during, 396, 397
End-diastolic wall stress (EDWS), calculation
of, 758
Endocarditis, prophylaxis for, 15, 15(t)
contraindications to, 137(t)
in congenital heart disease, 1044, 1045(t)
indications for, 137(t)
Endocrine consultation, 185–208
Endocrine system, disorders of, in
postoperative delirium, 165
in renal failure, 1359
effects on, of hyperthermia, 824
of inhalation anesthesia, 614
function of, normal, 1312(t)
preanesthetic evaluation of, 4, *4*
response of, to thermal injury, 701
surgery of, 1312–1319
Endocrinopathy, acromegaly with, perioperative
management of, 186
hypothyroidism with, 198
Endoperoxidase inhibitors, for spinal cord
shock, 684, 685
Endorphins, intravenous, 603(t)
Endoscopy, with tracheal intubation, 930, 931
Endothelium, microvascular, in pulmonary
edema, 969, *969*
vascular, in shock, 664, 665
Endothelium-derived relaxing factor (EDRF),
664
Endotracheal intubation, in neonates, 1023
retrograde, in children, 1052, *1053*
Endotracheal tube(s), calibration of, 308
changing of, indications for, 951, 952
components of, 308
construction of, 307, 308
cuff of. See *Cuff(s), of endotracheal tube.*
dimensions of, 308
double-lumen, 312–315, *312, 314,* 315(t)
insertion of, technique of, 309, 310, 310(t)
kinking of, and difficult ventilation, 946
malfunction of, 951
management of, in prone position, 507
materials for, 307
modifications of, 308
pediatric, 1053, 1054
radiographic findings with, 219
single-lumen, 307–312, 308(t), 310(t), *311,
312*

Endotracheal tube(s) *(Continued)*
size of, importance of, 309
selection of, 308, 308(t), 309
in adults, 308
in children, 308, 308(t), 309
End-stage heart disease, 1322
anesthetic implications of, 1322
pathophysiology of, 1322
End-stage liver disease, orthotopic liver
transplantation in, 1333
End-stage renal disease (ESRD), laboratory
data in, 1360, 1361
End-systolic elastance, 765, *765*
End-systolic pressure-volume relation
(ESPVR), quantification of, 764, *764*
End-tidal carbon dioxide, definition of, 350,
351
in tidal volume monitoring, 345, 346
monitoring of, in geriatric patient, 1073,
1074
partial pressure of, monitoring of, in pediatric cardiovascular surgery, 1149, 1150
Energy, source of, for laser, 1370, *1371*
Enflurane, drug interactions with, 644(t), 654(t)
effects of, circulatory, 612(t)
on evoked potentials, 406(t), 408(t)
physiologic, 1285(t)
for pheochromocytoma surgery, 1318(t)
in intraoperative bronchodilation, 146
in low-pressure anesthesia machine vaporizer, misfilling of, 285, 285(t)
in renal disease, 613, 614
in seizure disorders, 159
selection of, factors in, 571
Enoximone, for anaphylaxis, 748
Enterocolitis, necrotizing, in neonates, 1028,
1029, *1029*
Environment, effects of, on pain perception,
238
effects on, of anesthetic agents, 114
Enzyme-linked immunosorbent assay (ELISA),
in human immunodeficiency virus
infection diagnosis, 855
in perioperative anaphylaxis evaluation, 750
Enzymes, induction of, in drug interactions,
648, 649
EOA (esophageal obturator airway), 300, *300*
in cardiopulmonary resuscitation, 837, *837,*
838
Ependymoma, properties of, 1303(t)
Ephedrine, drug interactions with, 655(t)
effects of, physiologic, 1285(t)
for anaphylactic shock, 683(t)
for bronchial asthma, 958(t)
for perioperative myocardial dysfunction,
766(t)
in pediatric cardiovascular surgery, 1146(t)
in postoperative nausea prevention, 99
Epidural analgesia, for pain, after thoracic
surgery, 1207, 1208
in children, continuous, management of, 269,
270
differences in, 269, *269*
indications for, 268, 269, 269(t)
Epidural anesthesia, anatomic considerations in,
521, *521*
and peripheral nerve injury, 511, 512
and postoperative ileus, 1133
anticoagulation with, 253
catheter insertion for, 522
complications of, 522, 523
neurologic, 163
drug choice for, 520, 521
for abdominal surgery, 1113, 1114
for aortic vascular surgery, 1223
for delivery, 1089

Epidural anesthesia *(Continued)*
for extracorporeal shock wave lithotripsy,
1386, 1386(t)
for nonobstetric surgery, in pregnant patient,
1105, 1105(t)
in children, 1060(t), 1061
in geriatric patients, 1076, 1077
effects of, on coagulation, 1077
in obstetric patients, 1087–1089, 1087(t)–
1089(t), 1092, 1093, *1093*
drug choice for, 1088, 1088(t), 1089
monitoring of, 1089
technique of, 1088
in phantom limb pain prevention, 1254
in spina bifida, 473
needle placement in, 521, 522, *522*
hanging drop technique of, 522, *522*
loss of resistance technique of, 521, 522,
522
patient selection for, 520
positioning for, 521
postsurgical, 476, 477
technical considerations in, 476, 477(t)
shivering during, 818
technique of, 520–523, *521, 522*
thermoregulation during, 817, 818
vasoconstrictor use with, 626–628
Epidural blood patch, for post–dural puncture
headache, 539
Epidural fat pad, posterior, in lumbar spine,
471
Epidural hematoma, treatment of, 1005
Epidural puncture, midline approach to, 469,
469
paramedian approach to, 469
technique of, 469, *469*
Epidural space, anatomy of, 460
anterior, in lumbar spine, 472, *473*
depth of, 473, 474, *474*
via paramedian approach, 474, 475, *476*
effects on, of spinal injury/surgery, 475–477,
477(t)
in thoracic spine, 468, 469
Epidural venous plexus, in pregnancy, 474, *475*
Epiglottis, 446
attachments of, 446
function of, 446
of neonates, 1014
Epiglottitis, radiographic findings in, 224, *225*
Epinephrine, 145(t), 1182(t)
action of, mechanism of, 843, 844
drug interactions with, 643, *643,* 654(t),
655(t)
effect of, on local anesthesia duration, 625(t)
for anaphylactic shock, 683(t)
for anaphylaxis, 747, 748
for bronchial asthma, 957(t), 958(t)
for intraoperative hemodynamic stabilization,
in shock, 690(t), 692
for perioperative myocardial dysfunction,
766(t)
in cardiopulmonary resuscitation, 843–845
administration of, route of, 845, 845(t)
dosage of, 845
indications for, 844, 845
in neonatal resuscitation, 1035(t)
in pediatric cardiovascular surgery, 1146(t)
injection of, in transsphenoidal hypophysectomy, 1313, *1313*
use of, with regional anesthesia, 537
Epistaxis, 441
nasal intubation and, 933
Epithelium, alveolar, in pulmonary edema, 969,
970
EPs. See *Evoked potentials (EPs).*

Epsilon-aminocaproic acid (EACA),
   administration of, in orthotopic liver
     transplantation, 1355
  for fibrinolysis, 1350
Equilibration, in inhalation anesthesia, rapidity
   of, 607, *608*
Erythromycin, drug interactions with, 645(t)–
   647(t)
  in bacterial endocarditis prophylaxis, 15(t)
Erythropoietin, use of, with preoperative
   autologous blood donation, 5, *6*
Escharotomy, for compartment syndromes, in
   thermal injuries, 707
ESDA (electrostatic detection apparatus), 57
Esmolol, drug interactions with, 646(t)
  for supraventricular tachycardia, after cardio-
    pulmonary bypass, 1187(t)
  for ventricular tachydysrhythmia, 1186(t)
  in pediatric cardiovascular surgery, 1146(t)
  use of, perioperative, pulmonary effects with,
    151
Esophageal atresia (EA), in neonates, 1030,
   1031, *1031*
Esophageal gastric tube airway (EGTA), in
   cardiopulmonary resuscitation, 837, 838,
   838
Esophageal intubation, 456, 944, 945
  and hypoxemia, 948
  detection of, 454
Esophageal obturator airway (EOA), 300, *300*
  in cardiopulmonary resuscitation, 837, *837*,
   838
Esophageal tracheal combitude (ETC), 300
Esophageal tubes, 299–301, *300*
  use of, method of, 299–301
Esophageal varices, abdominal surgery with,
   nasogastric tube use in, 1117
Esophageal-tracheal double-lumen airway, in
   cardiopulmonary resuscitation, 837
Esophagus, in temperature monitoring, 432,
   432
  injuries of, traumatic, assessment of, 997
  perforation of, sympathetic nerve block and,
    492
ESPVR (end-systolic pressure-volume relation),
   quantification of, 764, *764*
ESRD (end-stage renal disease), laboratory data
   in, 1360, 1361
Esters, metabolism of, 624, 625
  properties of, clinical, 628(t)
  use of, in malignant hyperthermia, 827(t)
ESU. See *Electrosurgical unit (ESU)*.
ESWL. See *Extracorporeal shock wave
   lithotripsy (ESWL)*.
ETC (esophageal tracheal combitude), 300
Ethacrynic acid, drug interactions with, 647(t)
Ethanol, concentration of, in expired breath, in
   transurethral resection of prostate
    syndrome, 1241, *1241*
  drug interactions with, 644(t)
  effects of, on anesthetic agent monitoring,
    348
  half-life of, 565, *565*
Ethosuximide, 159(t)
Ethyl violet, as carbon dioxide aborption
   indicator, 357
Ethylenediaminetetraacetic acid (EDTA), 630
Etidocaine, 631
  action of, duration of, *516*
  dosage of, in children, 267(t)
  pharmacology of, 516(t)
  properties of, clinical, 627(t)
ETOH, abuse of, diagnostic features of, 1000(t)
Etomidate, effects of, on evoked potentials,
   406(t), 408(t)
  in geriatric patients, 1075
  in liver disease, 1344(t)

Etomidate *(Continued)*
  in shock, 688
  intravenous, 602, 603
  properties of, 598(t), 600(t)
Eutectic mixture of local anesthetics (EMLA),
   pediatric use of, 270
Euthyroid hyperthyroxinemia, 197
Euthyroid sick syndrome, 198
Evaporation, in heat loss, 693, 818(t), 819
EVLW (extravascular lung water),
   measurement of, in pulmonary edema, 972
Evoked potentials (EPs), 402–408
  anesthesia effects on, 404(t)
   minimization of, 404(t)
  auditory, brainstem. See *Brainstem auditory
    evoked potentials (BAEPs)*.
  description of, 402, *402*
  during nerve stimulation, 417, *417*
  in intraoperative seizure monitoring, 160
  monitoring of, anesthetics for, 161
   in inhalation anesthesia, 610
  motor, 407, 408, *408*, 408(t)
   anesthetic agent effects on, 408, 408(t)
  recording of, location of, 402
  somatosensory. See *Somatosensory evoked
    potentials (SSEPs)*.
  types of, 160
  visual, 407
Exercise(s), breathing, after abdominal surgery,
   1133
  hemodynamic response to, after heart trans-
    plantation, 1326, 1327
  therapeutic, for pain, in adults, 256
Exercise testing, preoperative, 66, 1158, *1159*
  in cardiac risk assessment, 130, *131*
Exhalation, active, in breathing system, 286,
   287
Exhalation valve, in ventilatory work, 811, *811*,
   812
Exophthalmos, 1316
Expert witness, anesthesiologist as, 59, 60
  qualifications of, 60, 60(t)
Expiratory pause, in breathing system, 286, *287*
Exsanguination, in intravenous regional
   anesthesia, of upper extremity, 530
Extension, of thoracic spine, 468
External jugular vein (EJV), catheterization of,
   502
  advantages of, 546(t)
  difficult, management of, 555, 556
  disadvantages of, 546(t)
  technique of, 550
Extracellular fluid (ECF), loss of, in abdominal
   surgery, 1119–1121
Extracorporeal shock wave lithotripsy (ESWL),
   1380–1387
  anesthetic technique in, 1385–1387, 1386(t)
  cardiac dysrhythmias during, 1384, 1385,
   1385
  immersion in, physiologic effects of, 1383–
    1385, *1383–1385*, 1383(t)
  occupational hazards with, 1387
  pain after, 1387
  preoperative considerations in, 1380–1383,
    1382(t)
  technical aspects of, 1380, *1381*
Extraction ratio, definition of, 562
Extravascular lung water (EVLW),
   measurement of, in pulmonary edema, 972
Extremity(ies), lower. See *Lower extremity(ies)*.
  nerves of, injuries of, *505*
  preanesthetic evaluation of, 11, 11(t)
  upper. See *Upper extremity(ies)*.
Extubation, 454, 455
  after abdominal surgery, 1132
  after adenotonsillectomy, 1270

Extubation *(Continued)*
  after aortic vascular surgery, 1230
  after general anesthesia, 594–596
  after jaw wiring, 1281
  after pediatric cardiopulmonary bypass, 1155
  criteria for, 949
  difficulties in, 455
  failure of, causes of, 949, 950
  oxygen administration during, 454
  precautions in, 455
  preparation for, 454
  problems after, 949–952
   treatment of, 950–951
  technique of, 454, 455
  tracheal, in spinal cord shock, 686
   postoperative, criteria for, 149(t)
   risks of, 310(t)
Eye, injury to, lasers in, 1372, *1372, 1373*

Face, examination of, before intubation, 440
  fractures of, classification of, 1277, *1277*
  trauma to. See *Craniofacial trauma*.
Facemask, 301, 302, *302*
  application of, 301, 302
  problems with, 302
Facemask ventilation, 922–928
  contraindications to, 922, 923
  detrimental manipulations in, 925, 926
  facemask seal in, 923
  for difficult intubation, 941
  in airway obstruction, 923, 924
  indications for, 922
  preoxygenation in, 925
  risks of, 922
Facet joints, of spine, 459
Facial nerve, distribution of, 1271, *1272*
  monitoring of, 408, 409, *409*
  stimulation of, electrode placement for, 415,
   415
Famotidine, for burn surgery, 711(t)
Fast flush test, 372, *372*
FAST (Flying Ambulance Surgical Trauma)
   team, 882, 882(t)
Fasting, and pediatric fluid deficit, 1058
  guidelines for, before elective surgery, 17,
    17(t)
   preoperative, in children, 1040, 1040(t),
     1041
   in neonates, 1021, 1022
Fat, metabolism of, after trauma surgery, 1006
Fat embolism, and pulmonary edema, 977
  delayed emergence in, 164(t)
Fatigue, occupational, 868
Faucial pillars, in airway maintenance, 10, *10*
Fear, and postoperative pain, 76
  level of, preoperative, 576, 577, *577*, 578(t)
Feldene, for acute pain, 240(t)
Femoral artery, catheterization of, 496, *498*
  advantages of, 548(t)
  disadvantages of, 548(t)
  techniques of, 548
Femoral head, osteonecrosis of, factors in,
   1249, 1249(t), *1250*
Femoral hernia, repair of, anesthesia for, 1134
Femoral nerve, injury to, lithotomy position in,
   510
Femoral nerve block, 532, *532*
  anatomic considerations in, 532
  drug choice for, 532
  needle placement for, 532, *532*
  patient selection for, 532
  potential problems with, 532
Femoral vein, catheterization of, 502
  advantages of, 546(t)
  difficult, management of, 556

Femoral vein (Continued)
    disadvantages of, 546(t)
    technique of, 553, *554*
Femur, fracture of, 1247(t)
    bleeding in, 1247
    closed, early stabilization of, 1248
Fenoprofen, for acute pain, 240(t)
Fentanyl, administration of, transmucosal, in
    children, 270
    adverse outcome with, 70(t)
    drug interactions with, 653(t), 654(t)
    for acute pain, 241(t)
    for burn surgery, 711(t)
    for cardiovascular surgery, 1175(t)
    for continuous sedation, in children, 270
    for pain, in children, 264(t), 265
    for perioperative hypertension, 171(t)
    for premedication, in children, 1048, 1048(t)
    in liver disease, 1344(t)
    intraspinal, for acute pain, 248(t)
    intravenous, 603(t), 604
        patient-controlled, guidelines for, 245(t)
    perioperative requirements for, 657(t)
    properties of, 598(t), 600(t)
    selection of, factors in, 572, 573
Ferromagnetic materials, 912–913, 913t
Fetal circulation, 1015, *1016*
''Fetal distress,'' during cesarean section, 1096
Fetus, anesthesia risk to, 1101–1104, *1102,*
    1102(t)
    death of, after maternal trauma, 1003
    effects on, of inhalation anesthesia, 616
        of labor analgesia, 1085, 1085(t)
        of maternal anesthesia, 1101, 1101(t)
        of maternal diagnostic radiation, 1103,
        1104
    heart rate of, alterations in, significance of,
        1096
        patterns of, 1095, 1096, *1096*
    homeostasis of, preservation of, during labor,
        1086, *1086*
    monitoring of, 1095–1097, *1096*
        in maternal trauma, 1003, 1003(t)
    oxygen consumption by, 1083
    protection of, from transplacental drug trans-
        port, 566
    risks to, of radiation exposure, 899
FEV_1 (forced expired volume in one second), in
    thoracic surgery, 1200
Fever, causes of, central nervous system in, 826
    in alveolar hyperventilation, 809
    in hyperthyroidism, 201
    rheumatic, history of, 2
    shivering effects on, 821, 822
FFP (fresh-frozen plasma), administration of,
    before aortic cross-clamp removal, 1230
    in orthotopic liver transplantation, 1342
Fibrillation, atrial. See *Atrial fibrillation.*
    ventricular. See *Ventricular fibrillation.*
Fibrinolysis, after cardiopulmonary bypass,
    1189
    in orthotopic liver transplantation, during
        neohepatic phase, 1350, 1351
        treatment of, 1355
Fibroplasia, retrolental, 1020, 1021
Fick's law of diffusion, 566
Fink blade, 303
F_{IO_2} (fraction of inspired oxygen), alteration of,
    in hypoxemia correction, 791, *791, 792,*
    793
    increase in, equipment for, 794, 794(t)
    ratio of, to oxygen partial pressure, 790
Fire, airway laser surgery and, management of,
    1378, 1379, 1379(t)
    in electrosurgical unit, 893
Fistula, tracheoesophageal, in neonate, 1030,
    1030, 1031

Flagg blade, 304
Flail chest, assessment of, 993
    in postoperative hypoventilation, 84
Flexible lumen finder, 316
Flexion, in cervical spine instability, 467
    of thoracic spine, 468
Flexion-rotation, in cervical spine instability,
    467
Florida Comprehensive Medical Malpractice
    Reform Act, 33
Flow control valves, of low-pressure anesthesia
    machine, 281
Flow meter, of low-pressure anesthesia
    machine, 281
    arrangement of, 282, *283*
Flow-volume loop testing, in mediastinal
    lesions, 1207
Fluconazole, drug interactions with, 644(t)
Fludrocortisone, in adrenal replacement
    therapy, 192(t)
Fluid(s), 714–731
    administration of, for contrast agent reac-
        tions, 904
        for hypothyroidism, 200
        in neonates, 1024, 1025
        in pyloric stenosis, 1026
    balance of, during surgery, 715, 716
    body, composition of, regulation of, 715, *715*
    deficiency of, before abdominal surgery,
        1119
        calculation of, 173
        preoperative, 722, *722,* 723, *723*
    excess of, administration of, vs. diabetes
        insipidus, 187, 187(t)
        calculation of, 173
    intravenous, composition of, 717(t)
        for pediatric outpatient surgery, 1399,
        1399(t)
        perioperative, selection of, 171
        warming of, in intraoperative hypothermia
        prevention, 436
    irrigating, in transurethral resection of pros-
        tate, 1240, 1241
    loss of, intraoperative, in children, 1058,
        1059
        trauma-induced, 716
    maintenance of, in children, 1057, 1058
    management of, in abdominal surgery, 1119–
        1121
        with acute intra-abdominal disease,
        1120
        in general anesthesia, 592
        in intracranial neoplasm surgery, 1307–
        1309, 1308(t)
        in neurovascular surgery, 1294
        in portosystemic shunting, 1129, 1130
        in renal transplantation, 1364, 1365
        in spinal surgery, 1300
        preoperative, in pulmonary edema, 974
    replacement of, for diabetes insipidus, 187
        in children, 1056–1059
        in thermal injuries, 705
        postoperative, inadequate, and absolute
        hypovolemia, 88
    requirements for, estimation of, 722, 723,
        723
        in total joint replacement, 1248, 1249
    restriction of, for syndrome of inappropriate
        antidiuretic hormone secretion, 189
    resuscitation of, in thermal injuries, 705, 706,
        706(t)
    shifting of, in burns, 703
        effects of, 703
    volume of, expansion of, for anaphylaxis,
        747
        in syndrome of inappropriate antidiuretic
        hormone secretion, 188

Fluid(s) (Continued)
    laboratory evaluation of, 188
    management of, during lung surgery, 1206
    monitoring of, in cardiovascular surgery,
        1166, 1166(t), 1167, 1167(t)
    replacement of, in shock, 691, 692
    status of, assessment of, 89, *89*
Fluid compartments, 714, 715
    extracellular, composition of, 714, *714,* 715
    intracellular, composition of, 714, *714,* 715
Fluid therapy, and perioperative oliguria, 385,
    386
    complications of, 728, 729
    effects of, on coagulation, 727, 728
    in burns, 730
    in children, 730
    in intracranial pressure control, 776, *777*
    in liver failure, 730
    in neurosurgery, 730
    in sepsis, 730
    in shock, 667, 668
    in transurethral resection of prostate, 729,
        730
    in trauma, 994
    intraoperative, 716–720
    intravenous, for renal toxicity, 182
    nephrology consultation for, 171, 172, 172(t)
    postoperative, 716–720
Flumazenil, drug interaction with, 659
    for benzodiazepine overdose, 164
    in intravenous anesthetic agent reversal, 601
    in monitored anesthesia care, in outpatient
        surgery, 1401
    in sedation reversal, 96, 573
Flunisolide, for bronchial asthma, 958(t)
Fluoxetine, drug interactions with, 651(t)
Flupenthixol, for pain, 242(t)
Fluphenazine, for pain, 242(t)
Flurazepam, for acute pain, 242(t)
Flutter, atrial, electrocardiographic
    characteristics of, 366
    postoperative, 94
    management of, 139
Flying Ambulance Surgical Trauma (FAST)
    team, 882, 882(t)
Foramen ovale, 1015, 1139
    closure of, 1140
Foramenotomy, 1297
Forced expired volume in one second (FEV_1),
    in thoracic surgery, 1200
Forced vital capacity (FVC), after abdominal
    surgery, 1130–1132, *1130*
    in thoracic surgery, 1200
Forceps, intubating, for tracheal intubation, 451
    uses of, 315
Forehead, in temperature monitoring, 433
Foreign body(ies), aspiration of, pulmonary, 86
    radiographic findings in, 224
    in airway, removal of, in cardiopulmonary
        resuscitation, 836
Forward surgical teams, for battlefield surgery,
    882
Fracture(s). See also sites of specific fractures,
    e.g., *Face, Skull.*
    burst, in cervical spine instability, 467
    critical, complications of, 999
    open, 1247(t)
        in multiple trauma, significance of, 1246
    pathologic, impending, stabilization of, 1251
FRC (functional residual capacity), after
    abdominal surgery, 1130–1132, *1130*
    reduction of, and postoperative hypoxemia,
        79, 796
Free radicals, in oxygen therapy, protection
    against, 793
Fresh-frozen plasma (FFP), administration of,
    before aortic cross-clamp removal, 1230

Fresh-frozen plasma (FFP) *(Continued)*
in orthotopic liver transplantation, 1342
Functional residual capacity (FRC), after
abdominal surgery, 1130–1132, *1130*
reduction of, and postoperative hypoxemia,
79, 796
Furosemide, drug interactions with, 645(t),
647(t)
for oliguria, 181
in renal function preservation, in aortic vascular surgery, 1220
Fuses, in electric shock prevention, 889, 890
Fusiform aneurysm, 1211, 1212
FVC (forced vital capacity), after abdominal
surgery, 1130–1132, *1130*
in thoracic surgery, 1200

Gadolinium, for magnetic resonance imaging,
914, 915, 915(t)
Ganglion(a), cervical, inferior, anatomy of, *488*
intermediate, of sympathetic nervous system,
484, *484*
preverterbral, of sympathetic nervous system,
484, 485
Ganglionic block, 489
Ganglioside GM$_1$, for spinal cord shock, 685
Gantry chair, for extracorporeal shock wave
lithotripsy, risks of, 1382, 1382(t), 1383
Gas(es), exhaled, monitoring of, in burn
surgery, 709
flow of, impedance to, in difficult ventilation,
946
in breathing circuit, resistance to, 811
fresh, flow of, in general anesthesia, 592,
593(t)
in preoxygenation, 586–588, *587*
hypoxic, causes of, 294, 294(t)
delivery of, fail-safe mechanism with, 281
inspiration of, consequences of, 294
management of, 295
inspired, heating of, in intraoperative hypothermia prevention, 434
respiratory, drying of, before analysis, 352,
353
flow of, in breathing system, 285–288,
287, 288(t)
source of, in high-pressure anesthesia
machine, 276, 277, *277*
trace, exposure to, 868–870
effects of, 868, 869
sources of, 869, 869(t)
unusual, effects of, on anesthetic agent monitoring, 348
Gas scavenging system, of anesthesia machine,
276–297
classification of, 288–290, 289(t)
components of, 290, 290(t)
gas reservoir in, 290, 291
hoses of, 291
obstruction of, 291
in patient injury, 290
Gastric contents, aspiration of, pulmonary. See
Aspiration, pulmonary, of gastric contents.
modification of, during preoperative visit,
581–583, *581*, *582*, 582(t)
Gastric emptying, delayed, causes of, 582(t)
interference with, in pulmonary aspiration,
86
Gastrointestinal bleeding, acute, 1121, 1122
anesthesia induction in, 1122
Gastrointestinal motility, postoperative, local
anesthesia effects on, 247
Gastrointestinal tract, changes in, in pregnancy,
1084
disorders of, in diabetes mellitus, 207

Gastrointestinal tract *(Continued)*
in renal failure, 1359, 1360(t)
in spinal cord shock, 686
postoperative pain in, 246
preanesthetic evaluation of, 3, *3*, 4
Gastroschisis, 1027, *1027*
Gate control theory, of pain, 255
Gated nuclide ventriculography, in cardiac risk
assessment, 133
Gated radionuclide angiography, in coronary
artery disease evaluation, 13
Gauge, airway pressure, of breathing system,
288, *289*
General anesthesia, 585–596
advantages of, 69, 70, 70(t)
adverse outcomes with, 70(t)
analgesia after, indications for, 594
cerebral blood flow monitoring during, 392–
395
depth of, monitoring of, 592, 593
effects of, on fluid balance, 716
on postoperative cerebral dysfunction, in
geriatric patients, 1079, *1079*
emergence from, 594–596
extubation after, 594–596
facemask, for intubation, 938
for abdominal surgery, 1109, 1110
regional anesthesia with, 1114
for automatic internal cardioverter-defibrillator implantation, 1195
for cancer therapy-related pain, in children,
271, 272
for extracorporeal shock wave lithotripsy,
1386, 1386(t)
for imaging studies, 900(t), 901
for nonobstetric surgery in pregnant patient,
1105, 1105(t)
for outpatient surgery, 1396–1398
in children, 1397
for pacemaker implantation, 1193
for potentially difficult intubation, 935
for stereotactic surgery for intracranial neoplasm, 1304, 1305
heat loss during, 818(t)
in autonomic dysreflexia prevention, 494
in bronchial asthma, complications of, 960
in chronic obstructive pulmonary disease,
966, 967
in geriatric patients, 1074–1076, *1075*,
1075(t), *1076*
in obstetric patients, 1091, 1091(t), 1092
in pseudotumor cerebri, 157
in seizure disorders, 159
induction of, 586–591
inhalation, 588, 589
without halogenated drug, 590
intravenous, 589
mask with, 589
intubation/ventilation failure in, 591
patterns of, 588(t)
preoxygenation before, 586–588, *587*
rapid-sequence, 590, 590(t), 591, 591(t)
requirements for, 585, 585(t), 586
maintenance of, 591–594, *592*, *593*, 593(t)
monitoring of, devices for, evaluation of,
116, 117
maintenance/repair of, 117
standards for, 116
Genitofemoral nerve, anatomy of, 1234, *1235*
Genitourinary surgery, 1234–1244
anatomic considerations in, 1234–1237,
1235–1237
laser, 1243
anesthesia for, 1243
applications of, 1243
noninvasive, 1244
sedoanalgesia for, 1244

Genitourinary tract, disorders of, in diabetes
mellitus, 207
preanesthetic evaluation of, 4
Gentamicin, nephrotoxicity of, 182
perioperative use of, 9(t)
Geriatric patients, 1067–1080
anesthesia in, management of, 1070–1073,
1070(t), 1072(t)
outpatient, 1079, 1080
cerebral dysfunction in, postoperative, 1079,
1079
demographics of, 1067
do-not-resuscitate orders in, postoperative,
1080
drug interactions in, 1078, 1078(t)
general anesthesia in, 1074–1076, *1075*,
1075(t), *1076*
hip fracture in, prognosis in, 1248
hypothermia in, 819
monitoring of, 1073, 1073(t), 1074
muscle relaxation in, 1076
pain in, postoperative, management of, 1077,
1078
perioperative mortality in, 1068, 1068(t),
1069
systemic disease in, 1068, 1068(t), 1069
preoperative pulmonary consultation for,
143, 144
regional anesthesia in, 1076, 1077, 1077(t)
surgery in, types of, 1069, 1069(t), 1070
Germany, health care system in, 110, *111*,
111(t)
GFCIs (ground fault circuit interrupters), 890
GFR. See *Glomerular filtration rate (GFR).*
Glial cells, neoplasm of, properties of, 1303(t)
Glioblastoma multiforme, *1304*
Glioma, optic nerve, properties of, 1303(t)
Glomerular filtration rate (GFR), autoregulation
of, 384
calculation of, 179
in chronic renal failure, *180*
relationship of, to blood urea nitrogen, 179,
179
Glomerulus, development of, in neonate, 1017
Glottis, visualization of, during tracheal
intubation, factors in, 928–930, 929(t)
Glucagon, for anaphylactic shock, 683(t)
Glucocorticoids, administration of,
perioperative, in Addison's disease
management, 193
deficiency of, in Addison's disease, treatment
of, 192, 193
effects of, 189
excess of, clinical features of, 190(t)
in adrenocortical insufficiency, 1318
Glucose, administration of, in neonates, 1025
intravenous, for pediatric outpatient surgery, 1399, 1400
perioperative, 171, 172
blood, concentration of, during cardiopulmonary bypass, 329, 329(t)
control of, in diabetes mellitus, 207
regulation of, 205, *206*
disorders of, 727
in geriatric patients, 1072, 1073
postoperative, 102, 103
for fluid resuscitation, in thermal injuries,
706(t)
neonatal, 1035(t)
for neurosurgical fluid therapy, 730
management of, perioperative, 723–727
in pheochromocytoma, 196
metabolism of, after liver resection, 1124
monitoring of, perioperative, in diabetes mellitus, 207, 208
preoperative assessment of, in congenital
heart disease, 1143

Glucose *(Continued)*
requirement for, in children, 1058
solutions of, complications of, 729
Glucose in water, indications for, 721, 722
Glucose-6-phosphate dehydrogenase, deficiency
of, genetic factors in, 569
Glycine, in transurethral resection of the
prostate, 1240, 1241
Glycoprotein, α_1-acid, in drug distribution, 648
in local anesthetic toxicity prevention, 634
Glycopyrrolate, selection of, factors in, 573
Goldman's multifactorial index, in preoperative
cardiac risk assessment, 127, 127(t), 128
Gorlin's formulas, 1160, 1160(t)
Granulocytes, in complement activation, in
anaphylaxis, 746
Greenhouse effect, 114
Ground fault circuit interrupters (GFCIs), 890
Grounding, 887, *887*
for electrosurgery, 892, *892*
in electric shock prevention, 888, 889, *889*
G-suit, in cardiopulmonary resuscitation, 841
Guedel blade, 304
Guillain-Barré syndrome, 156, 157
anesthetic considerations in, 156, 157
effects of, on nervous system, 156

Halcion, for acute pain, 242(t)
Half-life, definition of, 563, 564, *564*
effects of, on clearance, 568, 568(t)
long, biologic effects of, 564, *565*
of diazepam, 565, *565*
of ethanol, 565, *565*
of midazolam, 564, *564*
of thiopental, 564, *564*
Halogenated agents, in abdominal surgery,
1110
Haloperidol, for Huntington's disease, 157
for pain, 242(t)
Halothane, administration of, postoperative
headache after, 167
adverse outcome with, 70(t)
drug interactions with, 644(t), 652(t)–654(t)
effects of, circulatory, 612(t)
on evoked potentials, 406(t), 408(t)
on myocardial dysfunction, 759
physiologic, 1285(t)
for outpatient surgery, 1397
for pheochromocytoma surgery, 1318(t)
in geriatric patients, 1076, *1076*
in hepatic insufficiency, 614
in intraoperative bronchodilation, 146
in low-pressure anesthesia machine vaporizer, concentration of, 283, *284*
misfilling of, 283–285, 285(t)
in reactive airway disease, 611
in seizure disorders, 159
selection of, factors in, 571
use of, perioperative, with aminophylline, 6
with theophylline, 150
Halothane hepatitis, 648, 649
Hamilton MAX ventilator, 427(t)
Hanging drop technique, of epidural block
needle placement, 522, *522*
Haptens, 743
Hashimoto's thyroiditis, 197
HAV (hepatitis A virus), 858, 859, *859*
HBV (hepatitis B virus), 859, *859*, 859(t), 860
HCQIA (Health Care Quality Improvement
Act), 32
HCV (hepatitis C virus), 860
HDV (hepatitis D virus), 860, 861
Head, elevation of, in intracranial pressure
control, 776

Head *(Continued)*
injuries to, and abnormal intracranial pressure, 772
blunt, 1002
and bacterial meningitis, 1002
intracranial pressure control after, 776,
777, 777(t)
monitoring of, during patient transport,
428
traumatic, 1001, 1002
position of, for intracranial neoplasm surgery, 1307
in intraoperative intracranial pressure control, 779
in lateral decubitus position, 508
in prone position, 507
surgery of, radical, 1274, 1275
turning of, for facemask airway obstruction,
926
Headache, in children, treatment of, 272
post–dural puncture. See *Post–dural puncture headache.*
postoperative, 167, 167(t)
diagnostic work-up for, 167, 167(t)
spinal anesthesia in, 167
spinal, in geriatric patients, 1077
Head-up position, for surgery, problems
associated with, 509
Health Care Quality Improvement Act
(HCQIA), 32
Health care system, in Canada, 109, 110
in Germany, 110, *111*, 111(t)
in Netherlands, 110, *111*, 111(t)
in United States, cost containment in, 112–
114
Health maintenance organization (HMO), 112,
113
Healthdyne 105 ventilator, 427(t)
Hearing, effects on, of magnetic resonance
imaging, 914
Heart, abnormalities of, in scoliosis, 471
artificial, for heart failure, after cardiopulmonary bypass, 1185
function of, denervated, in heart transplantation, 1326, 1327
of neonate, 1016
preanesthetic evaluation of, 10, 11, 11(t)
size of, normal, on chest radiography, 213
structure of, in child, 1140, *1140*
Heart disease, assessment of, preoperative, 12,
13, *13*
cardiologist in, 135–138, 135(t)–137(t),
136
congenital. See *Congenital heart disease
(CHD).*
contrast agent reaction in, 904
effects of, on anesthetic induction rate, 1147
end-stage, 1322
anesthetic implications of, 1322
pathophysiology of, 1322
in acromegaly, 186
management of, in aortic vascular surgery,
1214, 1214(t)
pulmonary edema with, preoperative management of, 975, *975*
rheumatic, in obstetric patient, 1094, *1094,
1095*
risk factors for, 126–135
assessment of, 126–128, 127(t), 128(t)
shortcomings of, 128
categorization of, 126, 126(t)
in noncardiac surgery, Bayesian analysis
of, 128, *129*
Heart failure, after cardiopulmonary bypass,
mechanical devices for, 1184, *1184*,
1184(t), 1185

Heart failure *(Continued)*
treatment of, preoperative, in pheochromocytoma, 195
Heart rate, fetal, alterations in, significance of,
1096
patterns of, 1095, 1096, *1096*
goal for, after cardiopulmonary bypass, 1181
in aortic insufficiency, 1172
in myocardial ischemia, perioperative, 752,
757
of neonate, 1016, 1016(t)
Heart transplantation, 1321–1331
additional surgery after, 1329, 1329(t)–
1331(t)
and cardiac dysrhythmias, 1329
anesthesia after, 1329–1331, 1329(t)–1331(t)
anesthesia for, equipment for, 1323, 1324(t)
induction of, 1325
maintenance of, 1325, 1326
antidysrhythmic agent use after, 1327
bleeding during, 1329, 1329(t)
cardiopulmonary bypass in, 1326
weaning from, 1327–1329, 1328(t),
1329(t)
contraindications to, 1321, 1322, 1322(t)
criteria for, 1321, *1321*, 1322, 1322(t)
denervated heart function in, 1326, 1327
laboratory tests in, 1323, 1324, 1324(t)
management of, preanesthetic, 1322, 1323
monitoring in, 1323, 1324
preinduction period in, 1324, 1325
problems after, 1329–1331, 1330(t)
procedure for, 1326
Heat, generation of, magnetic resonance
imaging in, 913, 914, 914(t)
therapeutic, for pain, in adults, 256, 256(t)
Heat and moisture exchanger (HME), 822
Heat loss, in neonates, 1017, 1017(t)
mechanisms of, 818, 818(t), 819
Heater, radiant, in skin surface warming, 435
Heating blanket, in skin surface warming, 435,
436
Helium, in laryngeal laser operations, 1377
Helium-neon laser, 1371(t)
Hemangioblastoma, properties of, 1303(t)
Hematocrit, in aortic vascular surgery, 1221,
1222
in children, intraoperative, 1059
preanesthetic, 1040
in congenital heart disease assessment, 1142
in shock, 668
values for, 669, *669–671*, 670
Hematologic system, preanesthetic evaluation
of, 5, 6
Hematoma(s), epidural, aortic vascular surgery
and, 1223
treatment of, 1005
peridural, risk of, factors in, 252, 253
subdural, treatment of, 1005
Hematopoiesis, effects on, of inhalation
anesthesia, 615
Hemidiaphragm, injuries of, traumatic,
assessment of, 996, 997, *997*, 998
Hemodilution, before cardiopulmonary bypass,
1178
during orthopedic surgery, for intraoperative
blood loss reduction, 1259, 1260
isovolemic, effects of, on brain, 670
Hemodynamic monitoring, during noncardiac
surgery, 135, 136, *136*
during patient transport, 428
invasive, indications for, 14
Hemodynamics, effects on, of orthotopic liver
transplantation, during anhepatic
phase, 1347, *1347, 1348*
during neohepatic phase, 1349
during preanhepatic phase, 1346, 1347

Hemodynamics *(Continued)*
in septic shock, 687
stabilization of, intraoperative, in shock, 689–692, *689*
Hemoglobin, abnormal, effects of, on pulse oximetry, 354, 355
in children, preanesthetic assessment of, 1040
in intraventricular hemorrhage, 1019, 1020
in shock, 668
recombinant, 670
values for, 669, 670
stroma-free, 721
synthetic, 721
Hemoglobin saturation, preanesthetic evaluation of, 10
Hemoglobin-oxygen uptake, pulmonary, 785
Hemorrhage. See also *Bleeding.*
during cesarean section, 1093
in shock, evaluation of, 666, 667(t)
subarachnoid. See *Subarachnoid hemorrhage (SAH).*
Hemostasis, albumin in, 728
Hemothorax, after trauma surgery, 1007
massive, assessment of, 993
Henderson-Hasselbalch equation, 566, 732
Heparin, administration of, before cardiopulmonary bypass, 1177, 1177(t), 1178
drug interactions with, 646(t)
for cardiogenic shock, 674
in pediatric cardiovascular surgery, 1146(t)
inadequate reversal of, after cardiopulmonary bypass, 1189
perioperative use of, 8
resistance to, causes of, 1177, 1177(t), 1178
subcutaneous, in peridural hematoma formation, 252, 253
Heparin vs. activated clotting time dose-response curve, 1185–1187, *1187*
Hepat-. See also *Liver* entries.
Hepatitis (hepatitides), 858–862
epidemiology of, 858
halothane, 648, 649
prevention of, 861, 861(t)
primary, 858–861
secondary, 861, 862
Hepatitis A virus (HAV), 858, 859, *859*
Hepatitis B virus (HBV), 859, *859*, 859(t), 860
Hepatitis C virus (HCV), 860
Hepatitis D virus (HDV), 860, 861
Hernia, hiatal, anesthetic technique for, 585(t)
in aspiration pneumonitis, 3, *3*
of abdominal wall, 1133, 1134
Herniation, of brain, intracranial hypertension and, 771, *771*
Heroin, for acute pain, 241(t)
Herpes zoster, 862–864
Herpetic whitlow, 862
HES (hydroxyethyl starch), effects of, on coagulation, 728
HHT (hypervolemic hypertensive therapy), for cerebral vasospasm, after intracranial aneurysm rupture, 1290, 1291, 1291(t)
Hiatal hernia, anesthetic technique for, 585(t)
in aspiration pneumonitis, 3, *3*
Hibernating myocardium, 756
Hiccups, effects of, on abdominal muscle relaxation, 1112
treatment of, pharmacologic, 1112, 1112(t)
Hip(s), arthroplasty of, pain after, local anesthetics for, 247
total, blood loss in, 1249, 1249(t)
muscle relaxation during, 1250
avascular necrosis of, conditions associated with, 1249(t)
dislocation of, 1247(t)

Hip(s) *(Continued)*
fracture of, 1247(t)
in geriatric patients, prognosis in, 1248
regional anesthesia for, 1077, 1077(t)
morbidity/mortality of, regional anesthesia in, 1257
positioning of, in lateral decubitus position, 508
Histamine, cardiopulmonary effects of, 744
release of, in burns, 702
nonimmunologic, 746–748, 746(t)
postoperative, and relative hypovolemia, 89
Histamine blockers, in postoperative nausea prevention, 99
in pulmonary aspiration prevention, 86, 87
History, patient, in preanesthetic evaluation, 2–5, *3–6*
in preoperative cardiac risk assessment, 128, 129
social, in preanesthetic evaluation, 9
HIV infection. See *Human immunodeficiency virus (HIV) infection.*
HIV-negative CD4+ lymphopenia, 858
HME (heat and moisture exchanger), 822
HMO (Health Maintenance Organization), 112, 113
Hoffman-Rigler sign, 213, *214*
Holter monitor, in coronary artery disease assessment, 13
Homeostasis, with intracranial neoplasm, 1305
Honey, for burn wound sepsis, 707, 708
Hormones. See also names of specific hormones.
in fluid and electrolyte balance, 715
Horner's syndrome, sympathetic nerve block and, 486
Hose, breathing, compliance of, 287, 288(t)
of gas scavenging system, of anesthesia machine, 291
obstruction of, 291
ventilator, elimination of, 296
Hospital, rate charged by, setting of, 113, 114
Hospital waste, 114–118
clinical monitoring standards for, 116
definition of, 115
handling of, 115
importance of, 114, 115
reduction of, 115, 116
Hospitalization, for thermal injuries, indications for, 704
unplanned, after outpatient surgery, 1402–1404, 1404(t)
Howland adapter handle, 305
HPA (hypothalamic-pituitary-adrenal) axis, 189
function of, during stress, 192
steroid suppression by, susceptibility to, 192
HPV (hypoxic pulmonary vasoconstriction), 79, 80, 1205
in thoracoabdominal aneurysm management, 1218, 1219
Huffman blade, 303
Human immunodeficiency virus (HIV) infection, 853–858
diagnosis of, 855
epidemiology of, 853, 853(t), 854(t)
exposure to, testing after, 857
in health care worker, patient risk with, 857, 858
injuries causing, 856
orthotopic liver transplantation in, 1334
prevention of, 854
transmission of, to health care workers, 855–857, 856(t)
treatment of, 854
virology of, 854, 855
Hungry bone syndrome, 205

Huntington's disease, 157
anesthetic considerations in, 157
Hustead needle, for epidural anesthesia, *521*
Hyaline membrane disease, 1018, 1019
Hyaluronidase, in local anesthesia, 629
Hydralazine, drug interactions with, 646(t)
for perioperative hypertension, 171(t)
Hydrocephalus, abnormal intracranial pressure in, management of, 775
Hydrochlorofluorocarbons, environmental effects of, 114
Hydrochlorothiazide, drug interactions with, 647(t)
Hydrocodone, for acute pain, 241(t)
Hydrocortisone, for bronchial asthma, 958(t)
in adrenal replacement therapy, 192(t)
Hydrogen, buffering of, 732
Hydrogen ion, concentration of, relationship of, to pH, 733, 733(t)
Hydrogen peroxide, in reperfusion injury, 326
Hydromorphone, for acute pain, 241(t)
intraspinal, 248(t)
intravenous, patient-controlled, guidelines for, 245(t)
Hydrostatic pressure, interstitial, in pulmonary edema, 971
microvascular, in pulmonary edema, 970
Hydrothorax, and alveolar hypoventilation, 806
Hydroxyethyl starch (HES), effects of, on coagulation, 728
Hydroxyzine, analgesic potential of, 244(t)
Hyperalgesia, 238
Hyperalimentation, in neonates, 1025
Hypercalcemia, 176, 176(t), 726, 727
causes of, 203, 727(t)
electrocardiographic changes in, 368(t)
in hyperparathyroidism, management of, perioperative, 205
manifestations of, 176, 176(t), 203(t)
problems in, 1314
severe, treatment of, preoperative, 204
treatment of, 176, 726, 727
Hypercapnia, in pulmonary edema, 972
Hypercarbia, effects of, on fetus, 1103
postoperative, causes of, 81(t)
Hyperchloremia, 727
treatment of, 727
Hyperemia, zone of, in burns, 699
Hyperextension, in cervical spine instability, 467
Hyperglycemia, 727
in orthotopic liver transplantation, during neohepatic phase, 1351
treatment of, 1351
management of, 727
preoperative, in pheochromocytoma, 195
postoperative, effects of, 102
factors in, 102
treatment of, 102
Hyperinflation, in emphysema, radiographic demonstration of, 213, *215*
Hyperkalemia, 174, 175, 175(t), 725
causes of, 725(t)
critical limits of, 175
during orthotopic liver transplantation, treatment of, 1351
during renal transplantation, 1365, 1365(t)
electrocardiographic changes in, 368(t)
in end-stage renal disease, 1360, 1361
manifestations of, 174, 175, 175(t)
postoperative, effects of, 103
factors in, 103
treatment of, 103
succinylcholine-induced, in spinal cord injury, 1301, 1302
treatment of, 725
in asymptomatic patients, 175

Hypermagnesemia, 177, 177(t)
electrocardiographic changes in, 368(t)
manifestations of, 177, 177(t)
treatment of, 177
Hypermetabolic state, in thermal injuries, manifestations of, 701
Hypernatremia, 173, 173(t), 724
causes of, 724(t)
manifestations of, 173, 173(t)
treatment of, 173, 724
Hyperostosis, skeletal, idiopathic, diffuse, 463, *464*
Hyperoxia, effects of, on fetus, 1103
Hyperparathyroidism, causes of, 202(t)
definition of, 202
delayed emergence in, 164(t)
hypercalcemia in, management of, perioperative, 205
management of, perioperative, 204, 205
surgery for, complications of, 205
Hyperphosphatemia, 178, 178(t)
manifestations of, 178
treatment of, 178, 178(t)
Hyperreactivity, of airways, causes of, 955
Hyperreflexia, autonomic, 5, 1298
Hypertension, during tourniquet inflation, 1263(t)
history of, 2
in anesthetic risk, 64, 65
intracranial, benign, 157
dangers of, 771, *771*
signs of, 779
treatment of, emergency, 775, 775(t)
medication for, perioperative change in, 171
nephrology consultation in, 170, 171
on emergence, intracranial pressure control in, 780
perioperative, pharmacologic treatment of, 171(t)
postoperative, 91, 92, 92(t)
treatment of, 92
preoperative, and surgery delay, 171
pulmonary, in heart transplantation, 1328, 1329
rebound, after clonidine withdrawal, 171
treatment of, in intraoperative stroke prevention, 154, 155
Hyperthermia, 823–826
definition of, 823
differential diagnosis of, 824, 824(t)
drug reactions in, 825, 826
effects of, physiologic, 823, 824
malignant. See *Malignant hyperthermia (MH).*
mechanical factors in, 826
metabolic aberrations in, 824, 825
postoperative, 101
impact of, 101
treatment of, 101
Hyperthyroidism, assessment of, preoperative, 199
complications of, perioperative, 202
management of, 1315
perioperative, 200, 201
preoperative, 199, 199(t), 200
preoperative concerns in, 1315
signs and symptoms of, 198(t), 199, 1315, 1315(t)
Hyperthyroxinemia, euthyroid, 197
Hypertonic solutions, 720, 721
saline, 720
complications of, 720
distribution of, 720
Hypertrophic obstructive cardiomyopathy, preoperative assessment of, 138
Hyperventilation, alveolar, 807–809
causes of, 808, 808(t), 809

Hyperventilation *(Continued)*
effects of, 807, 808
central, 809
correction of, 809
definition of, 799
for abdominal surgery, 1109
for neurovascular surgery, 1294
for right ventricular failure, in heart transplantation, 1329
in intracranial pressure control, 776
preinduction, 778
prevention of, in nonobstetric surgery, in pregnant patients, 1106
Hypervolemia, in liver failure, 730
in syndrome of inappropriate antidiuretic hormone secretion, 188, 188(t)
Hypervolemic hypertensive therapy (HHT), for cerebral vasospasm, after intracranial aneurysm rupture, 1290, 1291, 1291(t)
Hypnosis, for pain, in adults, 257
Hypobaric solution, for spinal anesthesia, 517
Hypocalcemia, 175, 176, 727
causes of, 203, 727(t)
clinical features of, 203(t)
electrocardiographic changes in, 368(t)
in orthotopic liver transplantation, during anhepatic phase, 1348
during preanhepatic phase, 1347
treatment of, 1351
ionized, after cardiopulmonary bypass, 1188
manifestations of, 175, 176, 176(t)
cardiovascular, 176
central nervous system, 175, 176
postoperative, effects of, 103
factors in, 103
treatment of, 103
severe, treatment of, preoperative, 203, 204
treatment of, 727
in asymptomatic patients, 176
in symptomatic patients, 176
Hypocapnia, dilutional anemia with, 671
in cerebrovasoconstriction, 609, 610
Hypocarbia, effects of, on fetus, 1103
Hypochloremia, 727
treatment of, 726
Hypoglycemia, 727
during pediatric anesthesia, 1058, 1058(t)
in orthotopic liver transplantation, during anhepatic phase, 1348
during preanhepatic phase, 1347
in portosystemic shunting, 1130
postoperative, treatment of, 102
Hypoglycemics, oral, perioperative use of, 7
Hypokalemia, 173, 174, 174(t), 725, 726
causes of, 725(t)
critical limits of, 174
electrocardiographic changes in, 368(t)
in chronic liver disease, 1337
in elective surgery delay, 725
manifestations of, 174, 174(t)
postoperative, effects of, 103
factors in, 103
treatment of, 103
treatment of, 174, 725, 726
intravenous, 174
oral, 174
Hypomagnesemia, 177, 177(t)
electrocardiographic changes in, 368(t)
manifestations of, 177, 177(t)
treatment of, 177
Hyponatremia, 172, 172(t), 173, 724
causes of, 724(t)
factitious, vs. syndrome of inappropriate antidiuretic hormone secretion, 187, 188, 188(t)
in chronic liver disease, 1337

Hyponatremia *(Continued)*
in syndrome of inappropriate antidiuretic hormone secretion, management of, 189
manifestations of, 172, 172(t), 173
postoperative, effects of, 102, 103
factors in, 102
treatment of, 103
treatment of, 173, 724
Hypo-osmolarity, in persistent postoperative unconsciousness, 97
Hypo-osmotic fluids, administration of, in intracranial neoplasm surgery, 1308
Hypoparathyroidism, after thyroid surgery, 1316
causes of, 202(t)
definition of, 202
Hypoperfusion, cerebral, and neurologic deficit, after cardiopulmonary bypass, 327
continued, after trauma surgery, 1006
Hypophosphatemia, 177, 178, 178(t)
manifestations of, 177, 178(t)
treatment of, 178
Hypophyseal duct, neoplasm of, properties of, 1303(t)
Hypophysectomy, transsphenoidal, 1312, 1313, 1313(t)
Hypoplasia, of odontoid, 461, 462, 462(t)
Hypospadias, repair of, in children, epidural analgesia for, 268, 269
Hypotension, after aortic cross-clamp removal, 1230
after pheochromocytoma removal, 1318
control of, in cystectomy, 1243
in intraoperative myocardial ischemia, 757
during abdominal surgery, 1114, 1115, *1115*, 1115(t)
treatment of, 1114
during carotid artery surgery, electroencephalographic detection of, 401
during lower extremity joint replacement, 1249
during orthotopic liver transplantation, 1351
during pain control, in postanesthesia care unit, 76
during regional anesthesia, 537
in anaphylaxis, treatment of, 747
in shock, 663, 664
induced, for intraoperative blood loss reduction, during orthopedic surgery, 1259, *1259*
for neurovascular surgery, 1294
for otologic surgery, 1272
for parotid surgery, 1272
monitoring of, electroencephalography in, 401
intracranial, causes of, 772, 772(t)
management of, perioperative, in pheochromocytoma, 196
postoperative, 88–91
causes of, 88(t)
complications of, 88
dysrhythmias in, 90
measurement of, 88
treatment of, 90, 91
regional anesthesia and, in obstetric patient, 1092
sudden, after trauma surgery, 1006, 1006(t), 1007
supine, in pregnancy, 1003
Hypothalamic-pituitary-adrenal (HPA) axis, 189
function of, during stress, 192
steroid suppression by, susceptibility to, 192
Hypothermia, after transurethral resection of prostate, 1239
during cardiopulmonary bypass, 323, 324, 324(t)

Hypothermia (Continued)
    pediatric, 1151
    during thoracic aorta cross-clamping, 1225
    during venovenous bypass, in orthotopic
      liver transplantation, 1346, *1346*
    effects of, physiologic, 819, 819(t), 820
    fluid therapy in, 729
    for organ preservation, in orthotopic liver
      transplantation, 1338
    in anesthetized patient, development of, 817,
      818(t)
    in cerebral protection, in neurovascular sur-
      gery, 1294
    in hypothyroidism, 200
    in neonate, prevention of, 1017(t)
    in persistent postoperative unconsciousness,
      97
    in shock, 693, 694
      mechanisms of, 693, 694
    in spinal cord ischemia reduction, in thoracic
      aorta surgery, 1193
    intraoperative, 433–436
      postoperative effects of, 820–822, 821(t)
      prevention of, 433–436
      treatment of, 433–436, *436*
    pathophysiology of, 819, 819(t), 820, *820*,
      820(t)
    postoperative, 100, 101
      adverse effects of, 100, 100(t)
      causes of, 100
      prevention of, 100, 101
      shivering effects on, 100
    post-traumatic, iatrogenic, 1007, 1007(t)
    prevention of, 822, 822(t), 823
    rewarming for, and absolute hypovolemia, 89
    risk factors for, 819
    safety of, in pregnancy, 1106
    treatment of, 822, 823, 823(t)
Hypothyroidism, 1316
    airway obstruction in, 1316, 1317(t)
    assessment of, preoperative, 197
    clinical features of, 197, 198(t)
    complications of, perioperative, 201
    delayed emergence in, 164(t)
    diagnosis of, 1316
    effects of, on surgical outcome, 201
    management of, perioperative, 200
      preoperative, 197, 198
Hypotonic solutions, complications of, 729
Hypoventilation, alveolar, 800–806
    abnormal impulse conduction in, 804
    causes of, 802, 802(t), 803
    correction of, 806, *806*, 807, *807*
    effects of, 800, 801
      respiratory center depression in, 803, 804
      structural derangements in, 805, 806
      ventilatory muscle dysfunction in, 804,
        805, *805*
    definition of, 799
    on emergence, intracranial pressure control
      in, 780
    postoperative, causes of, 81(t)
      neuromuscular factors in, 84
Hypovolemia, absolute, factors in, 88, 89
    after paracentesis, 1125
    and postoperative oliguria, 95
    in syndrome of inappropriate antidiuretic
      hormone secretion, 188, 188(t)
    in trauma, inhalation anesthesia effects on,
      615
    relative, factors in, 89
Hypovolemic shock, classes of, 993, 993(t)
Hypoxemia, 782–797
    after intubation, causes of, 947, 947(t), 948
    assessment of, 786–797
    causes of, 782–785, *784*, 785(t)
    complications of, 790, *791*

Hypoxemia (Continued)
    correction of, 791, *791*, 792
      continuous positive airway pressure in,
        795
      mechanical ventilation in, 795
      oxygen therapy in, administration of, 793,
        793(t), 794, *794*, 794(t)
        adverse effects of, 792, *792*, 792(t), 793
        clinical guidelines for, 794, 795
    during anesthesia, causes of, 796
    during patient transport, monitoring of, 421,
      422
      equipment for, 425, 426
    fiberoptic bronchoscopy and, 306
    in alveolar hyperventilation, 809
    in chronic liver disease, 1336
    in facemask airway obstruction, 927
    in pulmonary edema, 972
    in shock, electroencephalographic monitoring
      of, 680
    postoperative, causes of, 77, 78, 78(t), 796
      mixed venous blood desaturation in, 80
      treatment of, 79, 80
      ventilation/perfusion mismatch in, 79
    prevention of, in apnea, 795, 796(t)
Hypoxia, cerebral, in persistent postoperative
    unconsciousness, 97
    diffusion, 796
      postoperative, 78
    during thoracic surgery, management of,
      1205, 1205(t), 1206
    effects of, on fetus, 1103
    local anesthetic overdose and, treatment of,
      635
Hypoxic drive, suppression of, and
    postoperative hypoxemia, 78
Hypoxic pulmonary vasoconstriction (HPV),
    79, 80, 1205
    in thoracoabdominal aneurysm management,
      1218, 1219

IABP. See *Intra-aortic balloon pump (IABP)*.
Ibuprofen, for pain, acute, 240(t)
    in children, 264(t)
ICP. See *Intracranial pressure (ICP)*.
ICU (intensive care unit), preoperative
    admission to, in myocardial dysfunction,
    767
ICU (intensive care unit) bed, transport of, 424,
    425
Idiopathic pain, 234
IgE, in anaphylaxis, 744, *745*
IJV. See *Internal jugular vein (IJV)*.
Ileus, after abdominal surgery, 1133
    causes of, 1133
    treatment of, 1133
    radiographic findings in, 226, *230*
Iliohypogastric blocks, in children, 268
Iliohypogastric nerves, anatomy of, 1234, *1235*
Ilioinguinal blocks, in children, 268
Ilioinguinal nerves, anatomy of, 1234, *1235*
Illicit drugs, use of, preanesthetic evaluation of,
    9
Illness, present, history of, 2
IMA (internal mammary artery), dissection of,
    1177
Imaging studies, anesthesia for, 900, *900*,
    900(t), 901, 901(t)
    risk factors in, 897–899, 898(t), 899(t)
    department for, patient transport to, 899, 900,
      900
    dipyridamole-thallium, in coronary artery
      disease evaluation, 12, 13, *13*
Imipramine, for pain, 242(t)

Immersion, in extracorporeal shock wave
    lithotripsy, physiologic effects of, 1383–
    1385, *1383–1385*, 1383(t)
Immune function, effects on, of burns, 702, 703
Immunization, for chickenpox, 863, 864
    in hepatitis prevention, 861, 861(t)
Immunoglobulin E, in anaphylactic shock, 681
Immunoglobulins, 743, 744, *744*
Immunology, 743–750
Immunosuppression, chronic, after heart
    transplantation, 1330, 1330(t)
    in orthotopic liver transplantation, 1344
    in renal transplantation, 1361, 1362
      protocols for, 1358, 1359(t)
Impact Universal ventilator, 427(t)
Impedance plethysmography (IP), in cardiac
    output measurement, 380
IMV (intermittent mandatory ventilation), 148
Inactive (indifferent) electrode, 416
Indicator-dilution, in cardiac output
    measurement, 379, 379(t)
Indocyanine green dye, in cardiac output
    measurement, 379
Indomethacin, for acute pain, 240(t)
Induction anesthesia. See *Anesthesia, induction
    of.*
Infant(s), airway management in, in
    cardiopulmonary resuscitation, 836
    closed cardiac compression in, 840, *840*
    full-term, outpatient surgery in, 1393
    hypothermia in, 819
    preterm, former, anesthetic problems in,
      1021, 1021(t)
      outpatient surgery in, 1391–1393
    "small-for-date," 1083
Infant respiratory distress syndrome (IRDS),
    1018, 1019
Infection(s), after heart transplantation, 1329,
    1330
    after trauma surgery, 1008, 1009
    arterial catheterization and, 550
    central venous catheterization and, 375
    in renal failure, 1360, 1360(t)
    pre-existing, and hyperthermia, 825
    tracheal intubation and, 456
    wound, surgical, antibiotic prophylaxis for,
      15, *16*
Infection control, in heart transplantation, 1324
    preoperative, pulmonary considerations in,
      144
Infectious waste, definition of, 115
Inferior laryngeal nerves, block of, 447
Inferior vena cava, obstruction of, nephrectomy
    and, 1242
Informed consent, for anesthesia, 1
    for vascular access, 543
Infraclavicular vein, catheterization of,
      advantages of, 546(t)
      disadvantages of, 546(t)
Infrared detectors, in temperature monitoring,
    430, *431*
Infrared spectroscopy, in anesthetic agent
    monitoring, 349(t)
Infratentorial mass lesions, abnormal
    intracranial pressure in, 776
Infusion, intravenous, for pediatric
    cardiovascular surgery, 1144
    preparation of, for pediatric cardiovascular
      surgery, 1145, 1146(t)
Infusion pumps, use of, near magnetic
    resonance imaging scanner, 915
Inguinal hernia, repair of, anesthesia for, 1134
Inguinal region, regional anesthesia of,
      complications of, 1236
      technique of, 1234–1236, *1235*, *1236*
Inhalation analgesia, in obstetric patients, 1089
Inhalation anesthesia, 606–617

Inhalation anesthesia *(Continued)*
  amount of, factors in, 608, 608(t)
  and postoperative nausea, 99
  breathing during, management of, 610–612,
    610(t), *611, 612*
  cardiac disease effects on, 1147
  circulation during, management of, 612,
    612(t), 613
  delivery of, airway management in, 922
  depth of, assessment of, 608, 608(t)
  drug interactions with, 644(t), 650, 652(t),
    654(t), 655(t)
  drugs for, cost of, 120
  effects of, on endocrine system, 614
    on fetus, 1102, 1103
    on liver, 614
    on myocardial dysfunction, 759
    on neurohumoral surgical response, 613
    on renal function, 613, 614
  elimination of, control of, 607, 608
  equilibration of, rapidity of, 607, *608*
  facemask ventilation in, 925
  for battlefield surgery, 880
  for bone marrow transplantation, 615
  for cardiovascular surgery, 1174
  for nonobstetric surgery, in pregnant patient,
    1106
  for orthotopic liver transplantation, 1344
  for outpatient surgery, 617, 1397
  for radiation therapy, 916–918, *917*
  for renal transplantation, 1364
  history of, 606, 607, 607(t)
  in asthma, 1043
    complications of, 960
  in central nervous system diseases, 608–610,
    609, 610(t)
    recovery after, 610
  in children, 1050, 1051, 1055
  in geriatric patients, 1075, 1076, *1076*
  in muscle relaxation, 615, *615*
  in obesity, 614
  in pregnancy, 616
  in puerperium, 616
  in trauma, 615, 616
  mental function changes after, persistence of,
    617
  pharmacodynamics of, 607, 608, *608*, 608(t)
  pharmacokinetics of, 607, 608, *608*, 608(t)
  prolonged, 616
  pulmonary blood flow after, 80
  selection of, factors in, 571
  uses of, 588, 589, 607
  without halogenated drug, 590
Inhibition, drug, 649
Injury Severity Score (ISS), 985
In-line traction, of cervical spine, 468
Innervation, autonomic, in coronary blood flow,
  1170
  of heart, in neonate, 1016
  of penis, 1236, *1237*
  sensory, of larynx, 1279, *1279*
Innovar, for pheochromocytoma surgery,
  1318(t)
Inotropes, action of, mechanism of, 765
  for cardiogenic shock, 761
  for perioperative myocardial dysfunction,
    765, 765(t), 766, 766(t)
    choice of, 765, 766, 766(t)
  for right ventricular infarction, 678
Inspection, in circulation monitoring, in
    anesthetized patient, 336
  in pain assessment, in adults, 238
Inspiration, mechanical, 285, 286, *287*
Inspiratory flow, generation of, 810, 811
Instrumentation, for basic monitoring, 337–339,
  338
  for spinal surgery, 1254

Insufflation, in laryngeal laser operations, 1375
Insulin, administration of, perioperative, in
    diabetes mellitus, 7, 208, 208(t)
  deficiency of, 205
Insulin tolerance tests, in Addison's disease
    diagnosis, 191
Insulinoma, 1316, 1317
Insurance, malpractice. See *Malpractice
    insurance.*
Integumentary system, in preanesthetic review
    of systems, 5
Intensive care unit (ICU), preoperative
    admission to, in myocardial dysfunction,
    767
Intensive care unit (ICU) bed, transport of, 424,
  425
Interarytenoid muscles, 448
Intercostal muscles, compromise of, in
    postoperative hypoventilation, 84
Intercostal nerve, dysfunction of, and alveolar
    hypoventilation, 804
Intercostal nerve block, 534, 535, *535*
  anatomic considerations in, 534
  drug choice for, 534
  for extracorporeal shock wave lithotripsy,
    1386, 1386(t)
  in children, 268
  needle placement for, 534, 535, *535*
  patient selection for, 534
  positioning for, 534
  potential problems with, 535
Interleukin-1, release of, in burns, 702, 702(t)
Intermediate life support, 835
Intermittent mandatory ventilation (IMV), 148
Intermittent positive-pressure ventilation
    (IPPV), during anesthesia, and hypoxemia,
    796
  in shock, 693, *693*
Internal jugular vein (IJV), catheterization of,
    500, *500*
  advantages of, 546(t)
  approach to, anterior, 551
    median, 551
    posterior, 551
  carotid artery puncture in, 551
  difficult, management of, 555, 556
  disadvantages of, 546(t)
  in heart transplantation, 1324
  precautions in, 501
  technique of, 550, 551
  structures adjacent to, 500, 501
Internal mammary artery (IMA), dissection of,
  1177
Interpleural anesthesia, complications of, 1237
  technique of, 1237
  toxicity of, 1237
Interpleural block, 535, 536, *536*
  anatomic considerations in, 535, *536*
  drug choice for, 535
  needle placement for, 536
  patient selection for, 535
  positioning for, 536
  potential problems with, 536
Interscalene block, 525–527, *527*
  anatomic considerations in, 525, 526
  drug choice for, 525
  for orthopedic surgery, 1256
  needle placement for, 526, 527, *527*
  patient selection for, 525
  positioning for, 526
  potential problems with, 527
Interspinous ligament, 459
Interstitium, pulmonary, in pulmonary edema,
  969, *970*
Intertransverse ligament, 459
Intervertebral disks, 459
  abnormalities of, epidural space in, 475, 476

Intestinal obstruction, nitrous oxide in, 1116
Intestines, motility of, after abdominal surgery,
  1133
Intoxication, alcohol, 999, 1000
  drug, 999, 1000, 1000(t)
Intra-abdominal bleeding, after trauma surgery,
  1007
Intra-abdominal pressure, increased, in reduced
    postoperative functional residual
    capacity, 79
  larynx in, 449, *449*
Intra-aortic balloon pump (IABP), for
    cardiogenic shock, 675, 676, *676*
  in myocardial ischemia, 761, *762*
  for heart failure, after cardiopulmonary
    bypass, 1184, *1184*
  radiographic findings in, 223
Intra-arterial catheterization, in cardiovascular
    surgery monitoring, 1165, *1165*
Intracranial aneurysm(s), clipping of, 1291,
  1291, 1291(t), 1292
  monitoring for, 1293
  location of, importance of, 1289, *1289*
  morbidity and mortality of, 1288
  pathogenesis of, 1288, *1288*, 1288(t)
  rupture of, 1290
    catastrophic, treatment of, 1289, *1289*
    cerebral vasospasm after, 1290, 1291,
      1291(t)
  size of, in anesthetic management, 1289,
    1289, 1290
Intracranial elastance, assessment of, 773, 774
Intracranial neoplasm(s), 1302–1309
  cerebral edema in, 1302, 1303
  growth of, 1302, *1304*, 1304(t)
  location of, 1303, 1304
  premedication in, 1306, 1306(t)
  properties of, 1302, 1302(t), 1303(t)
  size of, 1302, *1302*
  surgery of, 1304, 1305, *1305*
    anesthesia for, 1307, 1307(t)
      with pre-existing disease, 1306
    effects on, of preoperative neurologic
      function, 1305, 1306
    fluid management in, 1307–1309, 1308(t)
    monitoring in, 1306, 1306(t), 1307
  vascularity of, 1304
Intracranial pressure (ICP), 1284
  abnormal, 769–781
    causes of, 771, 772, 772(t)
    diagnosis of, 773, 775(t)
    management of, intraoperative, 775–777,
      775(t)
    control of, during anesthetic maintenance,
      778, 778(t), 779
      during emergence, 780, 780(t)
      during induction, 777, 778, 778(t)
      during patient transport, 780, 781
      in neurovascular surgery, 1293
      in traumatic head injury, 1002
      preinduction, in acute lesions, 776, 777,
        777(t)
      in chronic lesions, 777, 777(t)
  determinants of, 769–774
  effects on, of anesthesia, 774–781
    inhalation, 609, 610
  of intracranial neoplasm, 1302, *1302*
  increased, abnormal ventilation in, 814
    diagnosis of, imaging in, 1304(t)
    history of, 4
    in intracranial neoplasm surgery, 1307
    signs and symptoms of, 773, 774(t)
    with ruptured intracranial aneurysm, 1290
  measurement of, 394, *394*, 394(t), 395, 770,
    770, 771, 771(t)
  relationship of, to cerebral blood flow, 394
    to cerebral perfusion pressure, 770

Intracranial pressure (ICP) (Continued)
  status of, quick check of, 774, 775
  values for, 769, 770
Intracranial pressure-volume curve, 772, 772
Intramuscular induction, in children, 1052
Intraosseous infusion, in pediatric trauma, 1004, 1005(t), 1057, 1057
Intrathoracic pressure, increase in, larynx in, 449
Intravenous infusion, in children, for cardiovascular surgery, 1144
  for outpatient surgery, 1399, 1399(t), 1400
Intravenous regional anesthesia, in children, 1060(t), 1061
  of upper extremity, 530, 531
    drug choice for, 530
    exsanguination in, 530
    needle placement for, 530
    patient selection for, 530
    positioning for, 530
    potential problems with, 530, 531
    tourniquet inflation in, 530
Intraventricular hemorrhage (IVH), 1019, 1020
  factors predisposing to, 1019
Intubation, anatomic considerations in, 440, 441, 441
  ancillary equipment for, 315, 316
  antegrade, 937
  awake, for pharyngeal abscess, 1273
    in children, 1049, 1050
    in neonates, 1022
    problems with, 936
  bronchial, 443, 456, 948
  care after, 454
  coughing after, treatment of, 454
  difficult, 928–932
    laryngeal factors in, 448, 449
    potential for, 934–938
    with full stomach, 941, 942
    with reactive airways, 942, 942(t)
  esophageal, 456, 944, 945
    and hypoxemia, 948
    detection of, 454
  failure of, in fiberoptic bronchoscopy, 306
  fiberoptic, for otolaryngologic/maxillofacial surgery, 1280, 1281
  for abdominal surgery, 1109
  for general anesthesia, failure of, 591
  for postoperative hypoxemia, 79, 80
  hypoxemia after, causes of, 947, 947(t), 948
  in battlefield surgery, 880
  in cervical myelopathy, 1296
  in cervical radiculopathy, 1296
  in trauma, 991, 992
    craniofacial, 1278
  indications for, 938(t)
  nasal, 933, 934, 934, 935, 935(t)
    blind, 934
      awake, 936
    in spinal cord shock, 685
  nasogastric, for anesthesia induction, in orthotopic liver transplantation, 1343
  nasotracheal. See Nasotracheal intubation.
  of anesthetized patient, 938–942
    monitoring during, 336, 336
  oral cavity examination before, 440, 440
  orotracheal. See Orotracheal intubation.
  pharyngeal factors in, 441, 442
  postoperative, duration of, 87
  rapid-sequence, in spinal cord shock, 685
    risks in, 941–942
  retrograde, 937, 937
  sterile, in heart transplantation, 1325
  tracheal. See Tracheal intubation.
  transtracheal, indications for, 939, 940, 940
  ventilation/perfusion mismatch after, causes of, 948

Intubation (Continued)
  with airway neoplasia, 1274
Ionization, degree of, in local anesthetic agents, 624, 624(t)
  in intravenous anesthetic agent clearance, 599, 600
IP (impedance plethysmography), in cardiac output measurement, 380
Ipodate sodium, for hyperthyroidism, 201
IPPV (intermittent positive-pressure ventilation), during anesthesia, and hypoxemia, 796
  in shock, 693, 693
Ipratropium, 145(t)
IRDS (infant respiratory distress syndrome), 1018, 1019
Irradiance, 1372
Irradiation, diagnostic, maternal, fetal effects of, 1103, 1104
''Ischemic burden,'' 755
Ischemic cascade, 752, 753, 754
Isocarboxazid, drug interactions with, 655(t)
Isoetharine, 145(t)
  for bronchial asthma, 957(t)
Isoflurane, adverse outcome with, 70(t)
  and burst suppression, 609, 609
  and coronary steal, 1175, 1176
    in central aortic surgery, 1217
  before thoracic aorta cross-clamping, 1224
  drug interactions with, 644(t), 654(t)
  effects of, circulatory, 612(t)
    on evoked potentials, 406(t), 408(t)
    on myocardial dysfunction, 759
    physiologic, 1285(t)
  for general anesthesia, 592, 592, 593, 593(t)
  for outpatient surgery, 1397
  in geriatric patients, 1076, 1076
  in intraoperative bronchodilation, 146
  in low-pressure anesthesia machine vaporizer, concentration of, 283, 284
    misfilling of, 283–285, 285(t)
  in seizure disorders, 159
  perioperative requirements for, 657(t)
  recovery time for, 1398(t)
  selection of, factors in, 571
Isoflurophate, perioperative use of, 8
Isolation systems, in operating room, 890, 890, 891, 891
Isoniazid, drug interactions with, 645(t)
Isoproterenol, 145(t), 1182(t)
  for anaphylaxis, 748
  for bronchial asthma, 957(t), 958(t)
  for intraoperative hemodynamic stabilization, in shock, 690(t)
  for perioperative myocardial dysfunction, 766(t)
  in pediatric cardiovascular surgery, 1146(t)
  with phenylephrine, 145(t)
Isovolumic contraction, systolic pressure during, 763, 764
ISS (Injury Severity Score), 985
IVH (intraventricular hemorrhage), 1019, 1020
  factors predisposing to, 1019

Jaundice, obstructive, 1122, 1123
  abdominal muscle relaxation in, 1110, 1111
  renal failure in, 1122, 1123
Jaw, examination of, before intubation, 440
  wiring of, extubation after, 1281
Jaw thrust, for facemask airway obstruction, 926
JCAHO. See Joint Commission on Accreditation of Healthcare Organizations (JCAHO).

JCAHO Accreditation Manual for Hospitals (1992), abstract of, 49–51
Jet ventilation, in laryngeal laser operations, 1375
Joint(s), of geriatric patients, 1070
  of vertebral spine, 459
  replacement of, total. See Total joint replacement.
  septic, 1247(t)
Joint Commission on Accreditation of Healthcare Organizations (JCAHO), 32
  approach of, to quality assurance, 36–38, 37, 39
    departmental role in, 36
    freestanding review committees in, 36
    quality screening/concurrent monitoring in, 36–38, 37, 39
    retrospective review in, 36
    statistical quality control in, 36
  standards of, for quality assurance, 38–40, 40(t)
  survey of, 40, 41(t)
  ten-step process of, 38, 40(t)
Jugular bulb saturation, 398
Jugular vein, external. See External jugular vein (EJV).
  internal. See Internal jugular vein (IJV).
J-wire, threading of, difficulty in, management of, 556

Kanamycin, perioperative use of, 9(t)
Kayexalate, for hyperkalemia, 175
Kerley B lines, 216
Ketamine, drug interactions with, 652(t), 654(t)
  effects of, on evoked potentials, 406(t), 408(t)
    physiologic, 1285(t)
  for battlefield surgery, 880
  for burn surgery, 711(t)
  for cardiovascular surgery, 1174, 1175, 1175(t)
  for imaging studies, 910(t), 911(t)
  for outpatient surgery, 1396
  in children, 1056
    for intravenous induction, 1052(t)
    in premedication, 1048, 1048(t)
  in liver disease, 1344(t)
  in seizure disorders, 159
  intramuscular, for radiation therapy, 917
  intravenous, 603
  properties of, 598(t), 600(t)
Ketoacidosis, diabetic, 205, 206
Ketoconazole, drug interactions with, 647(t)
Ketoprogen, for acute pain, 240(t)
Ketorolac, for pain, acute, 240(t)
  in children, 264(t)
KIA (killed in action), 875, 877(t)
Kidney(s). See also Renal entries.
  disease of, management of, in aortic vascular surgery, 1214, 1215
    postoperative, 94, 95, 95(t)
  donor, preservation of, 1358
  dysfunction of, in chronic liver disease, 1337
  effects on, of electrical injury, 700
    of hypothermia, 820
    of orthotopic liver transplantation, during anhepatic phase, 1348
    of shock, 694
  of neonate, 1016, 1017, 1017(t)
  protection of, during renal transplantation, 1368
    intraoperative, from toxicity, 182
  response of, to acid-base imbalance, 735, 736, 736
    to contrast agent, 903

Kidney(s) (Continued)
transplantation of. See Renal transplantation.
Kidney stone, movement of, effects of, on
extracorporeal shock wave lithotripsy,
1385
Killed in action (KIA), 875, 877(t)
Kilopascals, 342
Kinins, cardiopulmonary effects of, 745
Klippel-Feil syndrome, cervical spine
anomalies in, 462, 462, 463
Knee(s), dislocation of, 1247(t)
replacement of, total, blood loss in, 1249
Korotkoff's sounds, in blood pressure
measurement, 369, 369
Korsakoff's psychosis, 165
Kyphosis, 469

Labetalol, drug interactions with, 653(t)
for perioperative hypertension, 171(t)
in pediatric cardiovascular surgery, 1146(t)
perioperative use of, pulmonary effects of,
151
Labor, analgesia for, 1085–1087, 1085(t), 1086
choice of, 1087
fetal homeostasis preservation during, 1086,
1086
pain of, aberrant, 1088, 1089, 1089(t)
anatomy and physiology of, 1087, 1087(t),
1088
premature, anesthesia and, 1102, 1104
Laboratory testing, in preanesthetic evaluation,
11, 12, 12, 12(t)
Lactated Ringer's solution, in perioperative
fluid therapy, 171
Lactic acidosis, 734, 738, 738(t), 739
causes of, 738(t)
compensation for, 739
treatment of, 739
Lactulose, for renal failure, in obstructive
jaundice, 1123
Laminectomy, 1297
Laminectomy membranes, effects of, on
postsurgical epidural blocks, 477
Laparoscopy, tracheal intubation for, 1398,
1398(t)
complications of, 1398, 1398(t)
Laparotomy, pulmonary complications after,
predictors of, 14
Laplace's law, 810, 910, 1161
application of, to aortic disease, 1213
Laryngeal cartilages, 444–446, 445
in airway obstruction, 445, 446
Laryngeal edema, tracheal intubation and, 456
Laryngeal mask airway (LMA), 301, 301
advantages of, 301
contraindications to, 301
for radiation therapy anesthesia, 917, 917
problems with, 301
Laryngeal nerve(s), inferior, blockade of, 447
recurrent, blockade of, in awake tracheal
intubation, 1280
damage to, during thyroid surgery, 1316
effects of, 1274, 1275
superior, blockade of, 446, 446, 447, 447
in awake tracheal intubation, 1279,
1280
damage to, effects of, 1274, 1275
Laryngeal tubes, 299–301, 301
use of, method of, 299–301
Laryngoscope(s), 302–305, 304
blades of, curved of, 303, 304
for tracheal intubation, 450
straight, 304
components of, 302, 303
fiberoptic, 306, 307, 307

Laryngoscope(s) (Continued)
flexible, 306
malleable, 306
rigid, Bullard, 306, 307, 307
Storz, 306
handles of, modifications of, 304, 305
in tracheal intubation, 450, 451
modifications of, 303–305
Seward, 305
Laryngoscopy, direct, failure of, 938, 939, 939
in tracheal tube placement verification,
944
fiberoptic, flexible, for potentially difficult
intubation, 937
malleable, for potentially difficult intubation, 937, 937
in children, anesthetic considerations in,
1062, 1063, 1063
Laryngospasm, 449
and facemask airway obstruction, 927
during tracheal intubation, 456
fiberoptic bronchoscopy and, 306
in intravenous induction, 590
postanesthesia, in children, 1062
Larynx, 444–450, 444–449
anatomy of, in rheumatoid arthritis, 5, 5
blood supply to, 447
evolution of, 444, 444
functions of, 444
sphincter, 448–450, 449
intubation of, difficult, 448, 449
laser surgery of, 1374–1378
safety measures in, 1377, 1378
tracheal intubation in, 1375, 1375(t), 1376,
1376(t)
alternatives to, 1375
laser-resistant wraps in, 1376, 1377,
1377(t)
muscles of, 444, 445
constricting, 448
dilating, 448, 448
intrinsic activities of, 447, 448, 448
nerve block of, indications for, 446, 446,
447, 447
nerve stimulation of, electrode placement for,
415
obstruction of, and increased postoperative
upper airways resistance, 82
of neonates, 1014, 1015
pathology of, acute, radiographic findings in,
223, 224, 225
sensory innervation of, 1279, 1279
Laser balloon angioplasty, in cardiogenic
shock, 674
Laser plume, 1372, 1373
Laser safety officer (LSO), responsibilities of,
1373, 1374
Laser surgery, genitourinary, 1243
anesthesia for, 1243
applications of, 1243
of larynx. See Larynx, laser surgery of.
Laser-resistant wraps, 1376, 1377, 1377(t)
Lasers, 1370–1379
components of, 1370, 1371, 1371
damage from, minimization of, 1373,
1373(t), 1374, 1374
thermal, 1372
definition of, 1370
fire caused by, management of, 1378, 1379,
1379(t)
for lower respiratory tract surgery, 1378
medical applications of, 1371–1374, 1371(t)–
1373(t), 1372–1374
principles of, 1370, 1371
risks associated with, 1372, 1372, 1372(t),
1373, 1373, 1373(t)
safety of, measures for, 1374, 1374

Lasers (Continued)
tissue effects of, 1371, 1372
Lasing medium, of laser, 1371, 1371
Lateral cricoarytenoid muscles, 448
Lateral decubitus position, for orthopedic
surgery, complications of, 1260, 1261
for spinal anesthesia, 517
for surgery, problems associated with, 508,
509
right, 506
Lateral extracavitary corpectomy/diskectomy,
anesthetic considerations in, 1301
Lateral femoral cutaneous nerve block, 532,
533, 533
anatomic considerations in, 533
drug choice for, 533
needle placement for, 533, 533
patient selection for, 533
positioning for, 533
"Lawnchair position," 506, 507
Lawsuit, preparation for, 57, 57(t), 58, 59(t)
medical literature review in, 58
records in, 58
Le Fort fractures, 1277, 1277
anesthetic considerations in, 1277, 1278
Leads, for electrocardiography, 361
placement of, 361, 361(t)
Left atrial catheterization, in pediatric
cardiovascular surgery, 1149
Left atrial pressure, monitoring of, in
cardiovascular surgery, 1167
Left ventricle, failure of, after cardiopulmonary
bypass, 1181, 1182, 1183(t)
free wall of, rupture of, in acute myocardial
infarction, 677
function of, assessment of, preoperative, 133,
134
methods of, 133, 134
disorder of, in noncardiac surgery outcome, 128
increased ventilatory work in, 810,
810(t)
in atherosclerosis, classification of, 1214(t)
in central aortic surgery, 1217
Left ventricular end-diastolic pressure
(LVEDP), in ischemic cascade, 753
in right ventricular dysfunction, 679
Left ventricular end-diastolic volume, in right
ventricular dysfunction, 679
Left ventricular resistance, parameters for,
691(t)
Left ventricular vent, in cardiopulmonary
bypass, 321
Leg(s). See also Lower extremity(ies).
nerve stimulation of, electrode placement for,
415
positioning of, in lateral decubitus position,
508
LES (lower esophageal sphincter), resting
pressure of, in hiatal hernia, 3
Leukocytes, polymorphonuclear, in multiple
system organ failure, 1010
Leukotrienes, cardiopulmonary effects of, 745
Levarterenol, for intraoperative hemodynamic
stabilization, in shock, 690(t)
LeVeen shunt, 1125, 1126, 1126
Levoprome, analgesic potential of, 244(t)
Levorphanol, for acute pain, 241(t)
Liability, exposure to, anesthetic record in, 20
automated anesthesia recordkeepers in, 29
types of, 59
Librium, for acute pain, 242(t)
Lidocaine, 630, 631
action of, duration of, 516
mechanism of, 846
after heart transplantation, 1327
alkalinization of, 629

Lidocaine *(Continued)*
  bupivacaine with, 630
  carbonation of, 629
  chemical structure of, 621, *621*
  for awake tracheal intubation, 1279
  for dysrhythmias, during tracheal intubation, 455
  for epidural anesthesia, 521
  for spinal anesthesia, 517
  for ventricular tachydysrhythmia, 1186(t)
  in amide metabolism, 625
  in bronchial asthma, complications of, 960
  in cardiopulmonary resuscitation, 846, 847
    complications of, 846, 847
      dosage of, 846
      indications for, 846
  in children, dosage of, 267(t)
  in liver disease, 1344(t)
  in pediatric cardiovascular surgery, 1146(t)
  intravenous, for pain, in adults, 245
  neurotoxicity of, with spinal microcatheter use, 636, 637
  perioperative use of, 6
  pharmacology of, 516(t)
  properties of, clinical, 627(t)
  toxicity of, 632, *632*, 633, *633*, 847, 847(t)
Life span, 1067, 1068
Ligaments. See also names of specific ligaments.
  of vertebral spine, 459, *460*
Ligamentum flavum, 459
Light wand, for intubation, 315, 316
LIM (line isolation monitor), 890, 891
  alarm of, sounding of, actions after, 895
Lincomycin, perioperative use of, 9(t)
Line isolation monitor (LIM), 890, 891
  alarm of, sounding of, actions after, 895
Lioresal, analgesic potential of, 244(t)
Lip, cleft, 1272, *1272*
Lipid solubility, in drug distribution, 643, 648
  of anesthetic agents, 570
    local, 623, 624(t)
Liposuction, outpatient, 1394
Liquid crystal temperature probes, 429, 430(t), *431*
Lisinopril, drug interactions with, 646(t), 655(t)
Lithium, drug interactions with, 652(t)
  effects of, on neuromuscular blockade, 651
  excretion of, diuretics in, 649
  perioperative use of, 7
Lithotomy position, for surgery, problems associated with, 509, *509*, 510
Lithotripsy, shock wave, extracorporeal. See *Extracorporeal shock wave lithotripsy (ESWL).*
Lithotripter, Dornier HM3, 1380
  grounding of, 1384
Liver. See also *Hepat-* entries.
  cancer of, orthotopic liver transplantation in, 1334
  effects on, of inhalation anesthesia, 614
    of shock, 694, 695, *695*
  in acid-base balance, 736, 737
  transplantation of, orthotopic. See *Orthotopic liver transplantation (OLT).*
Liver disease, acid-base balance in, 737
  anesthetic drugs in, 1344(t)
  chronic, conditions associated with, 1336, 1337
  classification of, 1334(t)
  delayed emergence in, 164(t)
  drug intolerance in, 1343
  end-stage, orthotopic liver transplantation in, 1333
  history of, 4
  in ester metabolism, 624
  in local anesthetic metabolism, 625

Liver disease *(Continued)*
  severity of, in prognosis, 1334, 1335
Liver failure, fluid therapy in, 730
  signs and symptoms of, 1335, 1336, 1336(t)
Liver function, changes in, in geriatric patients, 1072, 1073
  in portosystemic shunting, optimization of, 1129
  inhalation anesthesia effects on, 614
Liver resection, 1123, 1124
  blood loss in, minimization of, 1123
  problems after, 1123, 1124
  surgical risk in, 1123
  vascular exclusion in, 1123
''Liver team,'' 1340
Living-related donor harvesting, in renal transplantation, 1366–1368, *1367*
  anesthesia for, 1366, 1367
  ventilatory support for, 1367, 1368
LMA. See *Laryngeal mask airway (LMA).*
Local anesthesia, 621–637
  action of, duration of, 625, 625(t)
    improvement in, 626–629
    mechanism of, 621–625, *622, 623,* 623–625(t)
  agents for, chemical structure of, 621, *621*
    differences between, 630, 630(t), 631
    mixtures of, 629, 630
    pH adjustment of, effects of, 643
    properties of, chemical, 623, 624, 624(t)
      clinical, 627(t), 628(t)
  allergic reactions to, 635, 636, *636*, 636(t)
  applications of, clinical, 625–631, 625(t), 627(t)–629(t)
  choice of, 515, *516*, 516(t), 625, 626
  continuous infusion of, for pain control, in orthopedic surgery, 1264, 1265
  effects of, on fetus, 1103
  for pacemaker implantation, 1193
  for pain, cancer therapy–related, in children, 272
    postoperative, 246, 247, 247(t)
      dose in, 247, 247(t), 248(t)
  for stereotactic surgery, for intracranial neoplasm, 1304
  for vascular access, 544
  in autonomic nervous system blockade, 485
  in children, administration of, methods of, 268–270, *269*, 269(t)
  in transsphenoidal hypophysectomy, 1313
  intravenous injection of, inadvertent, 635, 635(t)
  metabolism of, 624, 625, 625(t)
  nerve susceptibility to, 622, 623
  peridural, administration of, monitoring of, 248–250, *251*
  pharmacology of, 516(t)
  solutions for, modifications of, 629, 630
  topical, in children, for procedural pain, 270
  toxicity of, 626, 631–637, *632–634,* 633(t), 635(t), 636(t)
    definition of, 537, 538, *538,* 538(t)
    in children, 267, 267(t)
    prevention of, 633–635, 633(t), *634,* 635(t)
    tissue, 636, 637
    treatment of, 538, 635, 635(t)
Local anesthetic bathing, in phantom limb pain prevention, 1254
Logan bow, 1272, *1272*
Longevity, 1067, 1068
Longitudinal ligaments, 459
  of cervical spine, 461, *462*
  posterior, ossification of, 463
Loop diuretics, drug interactions with, 647(t), 654(t)
Lorazepam, effectiveness of, duration of, 581
  for acute pain, 242(t)

Lorazepam *(Continued)*
  for burn surgery, 711(t)
  for imaging studies, 910(t)
  in liver disease, 1344(t)
  in premedication, 579(t), 580, *580*
  selection of, factors in, 572
Lordosis, 469
Loss of resistance technique, of epidural block needle placement, 521, 522, *522*
Low back pain, causes of, 475, *476*
Low oxygen supply pressure alarm, 277, 278, *280*
Lower esophageal sphincter (LES), resting pressure of, in hiatal hernia, *3*
Lower extremity(ies), joint replacement in, hypotension during, 1249
  nerves of, blockade of, 531–534, *531–534*
    important considerations in, 1256, 1257
    injuries of, *505*
      prevention of, surgical position in, 511(t)
Lower limb blocks, in children, 268
LSD, abuse of, diagnostic features of, 1000(t)
LSO (laser safety officer), responsibilities of, 1373, 1374
Ludwig's angina, 1273, 1273(t), 1274
  tracheotomy in, 1274
Lumbar cerebrospinal fluid catheter, in intracranial pressure measurement, 395
Lumbar microdiskectomy, anesthetic considerations in, 1300
Lumbar plexus, anatomy of, 1234, *1234*
Lumbar puncture, in geriatric patients, 1077
Lumbar radiculopathy, 1296, 1297
Lumbar spine, 471–478
  anatomy of, 471, 472, *472*
  changes in, age-related, 473
    in pregnancy, 474, *475*
  congenital anomalies of, 472, 473
  injury of, 1247(t)
  surgery of, head position in, 1299, *1299*
Lung(s), cupola of, location of, 501
  disease of, obstructive, postoperative pulmonary function tests in, 149
  expansion of, during cardiopulmonary bypass weaning, in pediatric cardiovascular surgery, 1153, *1153*
  in scoliosis, 470
  injury to, during extracorporeal shock wave lithotripsy, 1385
    thermal, 704
  mechanics of, in pulmonary edema, 972, *973*
  of neonates, 1015
  preanesthetic evaluation of, 10
  reperfusion (pump), after cardiopulmonary bypass, 1188
  surgery of, fluid volume management during, 1206
  tissue destruction in, in emphysema, radiographic demonstration of, 213, *215*
Lung resection, complications of, 147, 147(t)
  pulmonary edema after, 980
Lung volume, effects on, of pulmonary edema, 971
  maintenance of, postoperative, 146
LVEDP (left ventricular end-diastolic pressure), in ischemic cascade, 753
  in right ventricular dysfunction, 679

MAC (minimum alveolar concentration), effects on, of centrally acting antihypertensives, 656, *656*
  of anesthetic agents, 570, 571

MacIntosh curved blade, of laryngoscope, 303, *304*

Macroshock, 887, 888

Mafenide, for burn wound sepsis, 707

Magnesium, 176, 177, 177(t)
  for ventricular tachydysrhythmia, 1186(t)
  imbalance of, 727
    management of, 176

Magnesium sulfate, drug interactions with, 652(t)
  for eclamptic seizures, 158
  in preterm labor prevention, 1104

Magnet(s), effects of, on pacemakers, 894
  superconducting, hazards of, 915

Magnetic resonance imaging (MRI), 897–918
  anesthetic techniques in, 916
  contrast agents for, 914, 915, 915(t)
  effects of, 914
  equipment near, use of, 915, 916
  heat generation in, 913, 914, 914(t)
  in children, anesthetic considerations in, 1063, 1064
  indications for, 911(t)
  in intracranial pressure measurement, 395, 395(t), 780, 781
  in pain diagnosis, in adults, 239
  mechanism of, 911, 912, *915*
  risks of, 912–913, 912(t)

Major Trauma Outcome Study (MTOS), 982

Malignant hyperthermia (MH), 826–833
  acute, treatment of, 827, 828, 828(t)
  agents triggering, use of, in neuroleptic malignant syndrome, 158
  anesthetic agents in, 827, 827(t), 830
  biochemistry of, 831
  complications of, late, 828
  contracture testing in, 832
  dantrolene for, 828, 829, 829(t)
  delayed emergence in, 164(t)
  diagnosis of, 827, 827(t)
    differential, 824(t)
  genetic factors in, 831, *831*, 832, *832*
  in children, 1044–1046, 1045(t), 1046(t)
    anesthetic considerations in, 1045(t), 1046, 1046(t)
    causes of, 1045
    management of, 1046(t)
    preanesthetic assessment in, 1045, 1046
    risk factors for, 1045
  incidence of, 826, 826(t), 827
  muscle biopsy in, 833
  risk factors for, 829, 830, 830(t)
  support groups for, 832
  susceptibility to, outpatient surgery in, 1393
    prediction of, 832

Malnutrition, delayed emergence in, 164(t)

Malpractice, effects on, of technologic advances, 54
  legislation on, 33

Malpractice insurance, 60, 61
  amount of, determination of, 61
  crisis in, 53, 54
  types of, 60, 61

Mandible, abnormalities of, and difficult intubation, 930
  fractures of, 1276, 1277
    injuries associated with, 1278, 1278(t)

Manifold, of low-pressure anesthesia machine, 281, 282

Mannitol, for oliguria, 181
  for renal failure, in obstructive jaundice, 1123
  in renal function preservation, in aortic vascular surgery, 1220
  in renal transplantation, 1364

Manometer, in airway pressure monitoring, 344, 345, *347*

Manual resuscitation bag, 302, *303*

MAOIs. See *Monoamine oxidase inhibitors (MAOIs).*

MAP (mean arterial pressure), calculation of, 369
  parameters for, 691(t)

Mapleson D system, 595, *595*

Maprotiline, for pain, 242(t)

Marijuana, abuse of, diagnostic features of, 1000(t)

Marinol, analgesic potential of, 244(t)

Mask, for ventilation, during postanesthesia patient transport, 595, *595*, 595(t), 596

Mask anesthesia, in children, 1054, 1055
  indications for, 588
  with intravenous induction, 589

Mass spectroscopy, in anesthetic agent monitoring, 348, 349(t)

Masseter muscle rigidity (MMR), in malignant hyperthermia, 830, *830*, 831, 831(t)

Mast cells, in anaphylactic shock, 681, 682(t)

MAST (military antishock trousers), for shock, 666, 667
  in trauma, 994
  removal of, timing of, 1247

Mathews blade, 304

Maxillofacial surgery, 1268–1281
  airway management in, 1280, 1281, *1281*

Maximum voluntary ventilation (MVV), in thoracic surgery, 1200

MDIs (metered-dose inhalers), use of, preoperative, 144, 145(t)

Mean arterial pressure (MAP), calculation of, 369
  parameters for, 691(t)

Mean transit time, of pulmonary blood, 785

Mechanical ventilation, effects of, on fluid balance, 716
  for alveolar hyperventilation, 808
  for alveolar hypoventilation, 802, 803, 807
  for hypoxemia, 795
  for persistent pulmonary hypertension of the newborn, 1018
  in neonates, 1023, 1024
  intraoperative, 146
  postoperative, goals of, 148, 149, 149(t)
  preoperative, in pulmonary edema, 974

Mechanomyography, in neuromuscular blockade assessment, 419

Mechanoreceptors, pulmonary, in alveolar hyperventilation, 809

Meclofenamate, for acute pain, 240(t)

Meclomen, for acute pain, 240(t)

Median cubital vein, catheterization of, 498, 499

Median nerve, injury of, surgical position in, 512
  prevention of, 511(t)

Mediastinum, lesions of, 1207, *1207*

Mediators, chemical, in anaphylaxis, cardiopulmonary effects of, 744, 745
  in anaphylactic shock, 681, 682(t)
  in contrast agent reactions, 903
  of bronchospasm, in asthma, 955, 956(t)

Medical Incident Recovery Act, 33

Medical records, alteration of, 57

Medical Tracking Act of 1988, 115

Medical waste, definition of, 115

Medication(s). See also *Drug(s);* specific drugs and drug groups.
  preoperative use of, indications for, 15, 15(t), *16*, 16(t)
  review of, in preanesthetic evaluation, 5–9, 6, 7(t), *8*

Medication(s) *(Continued)*
  side effects of, vs. allergic reactions, 9

Medicine, costs of, 109–123

Medicolegal issues, 53–61
  avoidance of, 56, 57
  current status of, 54, 54(t), 55
  defense in, 57–59, 57(t), 59(t)
  scope of, 53

Medulla, function of, evaluation of, 773

Medulloblastoma, properties of, 1303(t)

Mefenamic acid, for acute pain, 240(t)

Meninges, neoplasm of, properties of, 1303(t)

Meningioma, *1304*

Meningitis, after trauma surgery, 1009
  and delayed awakening, 165
  bacterial, blunt head injury and, 1002

Mental distraction, in psychologic surgical preparation, 578

Mental function, changes in, persistence of, after inhalation anesthesia, 617
  deterioration of, in geriatric patients, causes of, 1070, 1070(t)

Meperidine, drug interactions with, 654(t), 655(t)
  for imaging studies, 911(t)
  for pain, acute, 241(t)
    in children, 264(t), 265
  for postoperative shivering, 823, 823(t)
  in liver disease, 1344(t)
  intraspinal, for acute pain, 248(t)
  intravenous, 603(t)
    patient-controlled, guidelines for, 245(t)
  properties of, 598(t), 600(t)

Mepivacaine, 631
  action of, duration of, *516*
  alkalinization of, 629
  for epidural anesthesia, 521
  pharmacology of, 516(t)
  properties of, clinical, 627(t)

MEPs (motor evoked potentials), 407, 408, *408*, 408(t)
  anesthetic agent effects on, 408, 408(t)

Mesenteric traction, and hypotension, 1115, 1115(t)

Mesocaval shunts, *1128*

Mestinon, for myasthenia gravis, 153

Metabolic acidosis, 733, 738, 738(t)
  alveolar hyperventilation with, management of, 814, 815
  causes of, 738(t)
  in orthotopic liver transplantation, during anhepatic phase, 1348, 1349
    treatment of, 1351
  respiratory acidosis with, 740, *740*
  respiratory alkalosis with, 740, *740*

Metabolic alkalosis, 739, 739(t)
  causes of, 739(t)
  compensation for, 739
  in chronic liver disease, 1337
  respiratory acidosis with, 740, *740*
  respiratory center depression in, 804
  treatment of, 739

Metabolism, changes in, after pediatric cardiopulmonary bypass, 1154, 1155
  in altered sensorium, during emergence, 98
  disorders of, in postoperative delirium, 165
  in renal failure, 1359, 1360(t)
  in septic shock, 687, *687*
  in acid-base balance, 738–740, 738(t), 739(t), *740*
  in hyperthermia, 823, 824
  in hypothermia, 819(t), 820
  in intravenous anesthetic agent clearance, 600
  increase in, after trauma surgery, 1006

Metabolism *(Continued)*
in pregnancy, 1082, 1083, 1083(t), *1084*
myocardial, during cardiopulmonary bypass, 323, 324(t)
of citrate, after liver resection, 1124
of corticosteroids, in Addison's disease, 194
of drugs, in drug interactions, 648, 649
of glucose, after liver resection, 1124
of local anesthesia, 624, 625, 625(t)
response of, to thermal injury, 701
role of, in coronary blood flow, 1170
Metacarpal veins, catheterization of, 498
Metamizol, for acute pain, 240(t)
Metaproterenol, 145(t)
for anaphylactic shock, 683(t)
for bronchial asthma, 957(t)
Metaraminol, drug interactions with, 655(t)
for intraoperative hemodynamic stabilization, in shock, 690(t)
Metastasis, intracranial, properties of, 1303(t)
Met-enkephalin, intravenous, 603(t)
Metered-dose inhalers (MDIs), use of, preoperative, 144, 145(t)
Methadone, before cardiovascular surgery, 1164(t)
for narcotic withdrawal, 867
for pain, acute, 241(t)
in children, 264(t), 265
intraspinal, 248(t)
intravenous, patient-controlled, guidelines for, 245(t)
Methemoglobin, effects of, on pulse oximetry, 354, 355
Methimazole, perioperative use of, 7
Methohexital, 602, *602*
distribution of, 602
drug interactions with, 652(t)
effects of, duration of, 602
for imaging studies, 911(t)
for intravenous induction, in children, 1052(t)
in premedication, for outpatient surgery, 1396
pediatric, 1048(t)
in seizure disorders, 159
properties of, 598(t), 600(t)
side effects of, 602
Methotrimeprazine, analgesic potential of, 242(t), 244(t)
Methoxyflurane, drug interactions with, 644(t), 654(t)
Methoxyflurane nephrotoxicity, 649
Methyldopa, drug interactions with, 654(t)
Methylene blue, effects of, on pulse oximetry, 354
Methylphenidate, analgesic potential of, 244(t)
Methylprednisolone, for traumatic cervical spine injury, 1001
high-dose, for spinal cord injury, 1302
in adrenal replacement therapy, 192(t)
Methylprednisone, for bronchial asthma, 958(t)
Methylxanthines, for bronchial asthma, 958
Metoclopramide, drug interactions with, 647(t)
for burn surgery, 711(t)
in aspiration prophylaxis, 582, 582(t), 583
complications of, 582, 583
contraindications to, 583
in children, 1049
in postoperative nausea prevention, 99
selection of, factors in, 573
Metocurine, dose of, in children, 1056(t)
Metolazone, drug interactions with, 647(t)
Metoprolol, drug interactions with, 645(t), 646(t)
Metronidazole, drug interactions with, 645(t)
Metyrapone test, in Addison's disease diagnosis, 191

Mexiletene, analgesic potential of, 244(t)
intravenous, for pain, in adults, 245
Mexitil, analgesic potential of, 244(t)
MH. See *Malignant hyperthermia (MH)*.
MI. See *Myocardial infarction (MI)*.
Microcatheter, spinal, use of, in geriatric patients, 1077
with lidocaine, 636, 637
Microdiskectomy, lumbar, anesthetic considerations in, 1300
Microprocessor-controlled oscillotonometers, in blood pressure measurement, 370, *370*, 370(t), 371
Microshock, 887, 888
Microvascular endothelium, in pulmonary edema, 969, *970*
Midazolam, before cardiovascular surgery, 1164(t)
dose of, equieffective, 658(t)
for acute pain, 242(t)
for burn surgery, 711(t)
for cardiovascular surgery, 1175(t)
for continuous sedation, in children, 270
for eclamptic seizures, 158
for imaging studies, 910(t), 911(t)
for perioperative hypertension, 171(t)
half-life of, 564, *564*
in geriatric patients, 1075, *1075*, 1075(t)
in liver disease, 1344(t)
in premedication, 579, 579(t), *580*
for outpatient surgery, 1396
in children, 580, 1048, 1048(t)
intravenous, 603, 603(t)
mortality of, causes of, 580
properties of, 598(t), 600(t)
selection of, factors in, 571, 572
transmucosal, in children, 270, 271
Midbrain, function of, evaluation of, 773
Middle ear, surgery of, 1271, *1271*
nitrous oxide for, 1271, *1271*
patient positioning for, 1271
Middle ear pressure, 1271, *1271*
Military antishock trousers (MAST), for shock, 666, 667
in trauma, 994
removal of, timing of, 1247
Military conflicts, morbidity and mortality of, analysis of, 875, 876
multitrauma in, 877, 877(t)
Military operations in urbanized terrain (MOUT), 876
Millard-Dingman retractor, 1272, *1273*
Miller blade, of laryngoscope, 303, *304*
Milrinone, for anaphylaxis, 748
Mineralocorticoids, administration of, perioperative, in Addison's disease, 193
deficiency of, in Addison's disease, treatment of, 192, 193
effects of, 189
excess of, in adrenocortical insufficiency, 1318
Minicholecystectomy, 908, 909
anesthesia for, 909
Minimum alveolar concentration (MAC), effects on, of centrally acting antihypertensives, 656, *656*
of anesthetic agents, 570, 571
"Minimum hundred criteria," in cadaveric donor harvesting, for renal transplantation, 1366
Mitral insufficiency, afterload goal for, after cardiopulmonary bypass, 1181
Mitral regurgitation, hemodynamic goals in, 1172, 1172(t), 1173
operative risks in, 1172, 1173
preoperative assessment of, 138
signs and symptoms of, 1162

Mitral stenosis, afterload goal for, after cardiopulmonary bypass, 1181
hemodynamic goals in, 1171, 1172, 1172(t)
preoperative assessment of, 138
signs and symptoms of, 1161, 1162
Mivacurium, dose of, in children, 1056(t)
in abdominal surgery, 1113
Mixed venous oximetry, 788, 788(t)
Mixed venous oxygen content, formula for, 692(t)
M-mode echocardiography, 381
MMR (masseter muscle rigidity), in malignant hyperthermia, 830, *830*, 831, 831(t)
Monitored anesthesia care, in outpatient surgery, 1400, 1401
Monitoring, after heart transplantation, 1330
basic, instrumentation for, 337–339, *338*
cardiovascular, 360–386
clinical, 333–339
application of, 333
objectives of, 333
variables in, assessment of, 333, 334, 334(t)
devices for, alarms on, activation of, 339
in anesthetic prescription, 67–69, 67(t), 69(t)
during patient transport, 421–428
effects of, on anesthetic risk, 67
electrophysiologic, in peripheral nerve injury evaluation, 162
indications for, 160, 161
fetal, 1095–1097, *1096*
in maternal trauma, 1003, 1003(t)
for general anesthesia, devices for, evaluation of, 116, 117
maintenance/repair of, 117
standards for, 116
hemodynamic, during noncardiac surgery, 135, 136, *136*
invasive, indications for, 14
in postanesthesia care unit, 73, 74
intraoperative, in ambulatory shoulder surgery, 1255
in automatic internal cardioverter-defibrillator implantation, 1195
in burns, 708, 709
in cardiovascular surgery, 1165–1169, *1166*, 1166(t)–1169(t), *1168*
pediatric, 1145, 1148–1150, 1148(t), 1149(t), *1150*
in children, 1059, 1060
in extracorporeal shock wave lithotripsy, 1384
in heart transplantation, 1323, 1324
in intracranial neoplasm surgery, 1306, 1306(t), 1307
in neurologic surgery, 1287
in neurovascular surgery, 1293
in pulmonary edema, 976, 977
in renal transplantation, 1362, 1362(t), 1363
in seizure disorders, 159–161, *160*, 160(t)
in shock, 679, 680, *680*
in spinal surgery, factors in, 1298, 1298(t), 1299
in thoracoabdominal aneurysm management, 1219
of neonates, 1025, 1026
of spinal cord function, in scoliosis, 1253, 1254
standards for, 68(t), 122, 123
invasive, in preoperative fluid deficit calculation, 722
in total joint replacement, 1249
of airway pressure, 344, 345, *347*
intraoperative, value of, 344
manometer in, 344, *347*

Monitoring (Continued)
of anesthesia machine, 294–296, 294(t)
of anesthetic agents, 348–350
potential errors in, 348–350
of carbon dioxide, 350–354, 353, 353(t)
respiratory gas drying before, 352
techiques for, 353, 353(t)
of cardiopulmonary resuscitation efficacy, 841, 842
of epidural anesthesia, in obstetric patients, 1089
of geriatric patients, 1073, 1073(t), 1074
of nervous system. See Nervous system, monitoring of.
of neuromuscular junction, 412–419
of perioperative myocardial dysfunction, 766, 767
of pregnant patient, during nonobstetric surgery, 1105
of sedation, for imaging studies, 901
of temperature, 429–436
anatomic sites for, 430–433, 431–435
probes for, 429, 430, 430, 430(t), 431
of tidal volume, 345–348, 348
end-tidal carbon dioxide in, 345, 346
setting for, alterations in, 346–348
oxygen. See Oxygen, monitoring of.
respiratory, 341–358
standards for, usefulness of, 339, 340(t)
without instruments, 334–337, 334(t), 336, 337, 337(t)
Monoamine oxidase inhibitors (MAOIs), discontinuation of, preoperative, 651, 656(t)
drug interactions with, 655(t)
use of, and hyperthermia, 825
perioperative, 7
Mononeuropathy, in pregnancy, 163
Morbidity, definition of, 63
Morphine, before cardiovascular surgery, 1164(t)
drug interactions with, 652(t)–654(t)
for pain, acute, 241(t)
in children, 264, 264(t), 265
postoperative, dose of, 247, 247(t), 248(t)
for perioperative hypertension, 171(t)
in liver disease, 1344(t)
in pediatric premedication, 1048(t)
intraspinal, 248(t)
intrathecal, after thoracic surgery, 1208
intravenous, 603(t), 604
patient-controlled, guidelines for, 245(t)
properties of, 598(t), 600(t)
selection of, factors in, 572
Morphine sulfate, for imaging studies, 911(t)
Mortality, anesthetic, risk of, 62
definition of, 63
Motor evoked potentials (MEPs), 407, 408, 408, 408(t)
anesthetic agent effects on, 408, 408(t)
MOUT (military operations in urbanized terrain), 876
Mouth, examination of, before intubation, 440, 440, 930
in temperature monitoring, 430, 431
Mouth-to-mask ventilation, in cardiopulmonary resuscitation, 837
Mouth-to-mouth ventilation, in cardiopulmonary resuscitation, 837
MRI. See Magnetic resonance imaging (MRI).
MSOF (multiple system organ failure), 1009, 1010
in burns, 702
treatment of, 1010
MTOS (Major Trauma Outcome Study), 982
MUGA (multigated angiographic) scan, in cardiac risk assessment, 133

Müller's maneuver, in heart murmur evaluation, 11(t)
Multigated angiographic (MUGA) scan, in cardiac risk assessment, 133
Multiple sclerosis, 155, 156
anesthetic considerations in, 156, 156(t)
evaluation of, preoperative, 155, 156
Multiple system organ failure (MSOF), 1009, 1010
in burns, 702
treatment of, 1010
Multitrauma, in military conflicts, 877, 877(t)
Murmur(s), evaluation of, preoperative, 135
bedside maneuvers in, 11, 11(t)
history of, 2
Muscle(s). See also names of specific muscles.
biopsy of, in malignant hyperthermia, 832
damage to, tourniquet use and, 1261, 1261(t)
respiratory, of neonates, 1015
skeletal, damage to, local anesthesia in, 637
pain in, postoperative, causes of, 104
smooth, function of, alteration of, in pregnancy, 1083(t), 1084
Muscle contracture, testing of, in malignant hyperthermia, 832
Muscle relaxants, assessment of, instrumentation for, 338, 339
drug interactions with, 658(t)
effects of, on evoked potentials, 406(t), 408(t)
on fetus, 1103
for abdominal surgery, 1110–1113, 1112, 1112(t)
for ambulatory shoulder surgery, 1255
for anesthesia induction, in renal transplantation, 1363, 1364
for battlefield surgery, 881
for facemask airway obstruction, 927
for otologic surgery, 1271, 1272
for parotid surgery, 1271, 1272
for total hip arthroplasty, 1250
in asthma, 1043
complications of, 960
in children, 1056, 1056(t)
in chronic obstructive pulmonary disease, 967
in geriatric patients, 1076
in intracranial pressure control, 776
intraoperative, 779
perioperative, 778
in myelopathy/radiculopathy, 1296
in obstetric patient, 1091, 1092
inhalation anesthesia with, 615, 615
nondepolarizing, in myasthenia gravis, 154
pharmacokinetics of, in liver disease, 1343
reversal of, inability of, and alveolar hypoventilation, 804
selection of, factors in, 573
Muscular dystrophy, 156
anesthetic considerations in, 156
Duchenne's, malignant hyperthermia in, 830
organs affected by, 156
Musculoskeletal system, changes in, in pregnancy, 1085
preanesthetic evaluation of, 5, 5
MVV (maximum voluntary ventilation), in thoracic surgery, 1200
Myasthenia gravis, 153, 154
diseases associated with, 153
evaluation of, preoperative, factors in, 153
management of, perioperative, 153, 154
postoperative, 154
Myelography, in pain diagnosis, in adults, 239
Myelopathy, 1296, 1296, 1296(t)
cervical, intubation in, 1296
positioning in, 1296
thoracic, 1296, 1297

Myocardial contusion, traumatic, assessment of, 995, 996
Myocardial depression, inhalation anesthesia and, 759
Myocardial dysfunction, 752–767, 757
alveolar hyperventilation and, 807
assessment of, 758
effects on, of inhalation anesthesia, 759
of narcotics, 759
in postoperative hypotension, 91
perioperative, monitoring of, 766, 767
treatment of, 764–767
pharmacologic, 764–766, 765(t), 766(t)
postoperative, assessment of, 763, 764, 764
quantification of, 763, 764
risk factors for, 764
preoperative patient optimization in, 767
regional anesthesia in, 759, 760
Myocardial infarction (MI), acute, complications of, mechanical, 677, 678
detection of, transesophageal echocardiography in, 382, 382, 382(t)
electrocardiographic characteristics of, 364, 365(t)
history of, 2, 2
perioperative, mortality of, 126
postoperative, 761–764
clinical presentation of, 761, 762
diagnosis of, 138
incidence of, 762
ruling out of, 762, 763, 763
timing of, 761, 762
postoperative reinfarction after, 762, 762(t)
prior, in anesthetic risk, 65
transmural, 364
vascular endothelium in, 664
Myocardial ischemia, 752–767
after cardiopulmonary bypass, and left ventricular failure, 1181, 1182, 1183(t)
and right ventricular failure, 1182
detection of, during aortic vascular surgery, 1220, 1221
electrocardiography in, 363, 363, 364, 364(t)
in coronary artery disease, 754, 755
intraoperative, 760, 760(t), 761, 761
anesthesia in, 756, 757
cardiogenic shock in, treatment of, 761
detection of, 1168, 1168(t), 1169, 1169(t)
treatment of, 760, 760(t), 761, 761
perioperative, 752–756
assessment of, 755(t)
detection of, 753, 755(t)
hemodynamic causes of, 752, 753
types of, 753, 754, 754
postoperative, factors in, 90
recognition of, 90
signs and symptoms of, 1157, 1158
silent. See Silent myocardial ischemia (SMI).
vascular endothelium in, 664, 665
Myocardium, effects on, of normovolemic anemia, 671, 671, 672
hibernating, 756
injury to, electrocardiographic characteristics of, 364, 364
metabolic requirements of, during cardiopulmonary bypass, 323, 324(t)
monitoring of, perioperative, transesophageal echocardiography in, 136
oxygen consumption by, during cardiopulmonary bypass, 323
in shock, 668–672, 669–671
oxygen supply to, demand for, 1170, 1171
during aortic vascular surgery, 1221, 1222
goals for, in coronary artery disease, 1169, 1169(t), 1170, 1170
preoperative assessment of, noninvasive, 133

Myocardium *(Continued)*
  preservation of, during thoracic aorta cross-clamping, 1224
  protection of, during cardiopulmonary bypass, 323–325, *323*, 324(t), 325(t)
  salvage of, in cardiogenic shock, 673
  stunned, 756, *756*
Myometrium, changes in, in pregnancy, 1084
Myringotomy, 1268, 1269
  in children, anesthetic considerations for, 1064
  indications for, 1268
  intravenous access for, 1268, 1269
  technique of, 1268
Myxedema coma, 198
  management of, perioperative, 200

Nail polish, effects of, on pulse oximetry, 354
Nalbuphine, for acute pain, 241(t)
  intravenous, 603(t)
    patient-controlled, guidelines for, 245(t)
Nalfon, for acute pain, 240(t)
Naloxone, drug interactions with, 654(t)
  for narcotic overdose, 164
  for spinal cord shock, 684
  in intravenous anesthetic agent reversal, 601
  in monitored anesthesia care, in outpatient surgery, 1400, 1401
  in neonatal resuscitation, 1035(t)
  in postoperative pulmonary edema, 978
  in sedation reversal, 96
  intravenous, 603(t), 604
  selection of, factors in, 573
Naltrexone, in drug abuse treatment, 867
  intravenous, 603(t)
Naproxen, for pain, acute, 240(t)
  in children, 264(t)
Narcotics, administration of, and biliary spasm, 1116, 1117
  drug interactions with, 653(t), 655(t)
  effects of, on evoked potentials, 406(t), 408(t)
    on fetus, 1103
    on myocardial dysfunction, 759
  epidural, for pain control, in postanesthesia care unit, 77
    postoperative, in geriatric patients, 1077, 1078
    in obstetric patients, 1088, 1089
  for analgesia, alternatives to, 605
  for dysrhythmias, during tracheal intubation, 455
  for orthotopic liver transplantation, 1343, 1344
  for pain, effects on, of concurrent medical condition, 237
    in postanesthesia care unit, 76
  in anesthesia induction, 604
  in asthma, 1043
  in children, 1055, 1056
  in intravenous anesthesia, 603, 603(t), 604
  in malignant hyperthermia, 827(t)
  in persistent postoperative unconsciousness, 96
  in premedication, 583
  overdose of, naloxone for, 164
  response to, in chronic renal failure, 1361
  selection of, factors in, 572, 573
  subarachnoid, for pain control, in postanesthesia care unit, 77
  use of, perioperative, pulmonary effects of, 151
    postoperative, pulmonary effects of, 146, 147

Narcotics *(Continued)*
  withdrawal from, signs and symptoms of, 867, 867(t)
Nasal airway, in cardiopulmonary resuscitation, 836
Nasal cannula, in oxygen administration, 294
Nasal decongestants, 933, 934(t)
Nasal intubation, 933, 934, *934*, *935*, 935(t)
  blind, 934
    awake, 936
  in spinal cord shock, 685
Nasoenteric tube, position of, correct, 226, *232*
Nasogastric intubation, for anesthesia induction, in orthotopic liver transplantation, 1343
Nasogastric tube, for abdominal surgery, 1117, 1118, *1118*
  emergency, rapid-sequence induction with, 1119
  in pulmonary aspiration prevention, 87
  position of, correct, 226
Nasopharynx, anatomy of, 440, 441, *441*
  in temperature monitoring, 431, 432, *432*
  of neonates, 1014
Nasotracheal intubation, 452, 453
  for anesthesia induction, in orthotopic liver transplantation, 1343
  in trauma, 992
  techniques of, 310
    blind, 453
    direct vision, 453
  tube fixation after, 454
Nausea, after outpatient surgery, treatment of, 1404, 1405(t)
  contrast agent reaction and, 902(t)
  during cesarean section, control of, 1093
  postanesthesia, in children, 1061, 1062
  postoperative, 99, 100
    prevention of, 99, 100
    risk factors for, 99
Nd:YAG (neodymium-yttrium-aluminum-garnet) laser, 1371(t)
  for genitourinary surgery, 1243
NEC (necrotizing enterocolitis), in neonates, 1028, 1029, *1029*
Neck, assessment of, before tracheal intubation, 930
  preanesthetic, 10
  injury to, airway maneuvers in, 468
    surgical positioning in, 512
  of neonate, 1015
  positioning of, in lateral decubitus position, 508
  radiography of, 223–226, *225*, *227*, *228*
  surgery of, radical, 1274, 1275
Necrotizing enterocolitis (NEC), in neonates, 1028, 1029, *1029*
Needle(s), for nerve stimulation, 415, 416
  in temperature monitoring, 429, 430, *431*
  placement of, for ankle block, 533, 534, *534*
    for axillary block, 530, *530*
    for caudal anesthesia, 523, 524, *525*
    for epidural anesthesia, 521, 522, *522*
    for femoral nerve block, 532, *532*
    for intercostal nerve block, 534, 535, *535*
    for interpleural block, 536
    for interscalene block, 526, 527, *527*
    for lateral femoral cutaneous nerve block, 533, *533*
    for regional anesthesia, intravenous, of upper extremity, 530
      nerve stimulator in, 539, 540
    for sciatic nerve block, 531, 532
    for spinal anesthesia, 517–519, *518–520*, 520
    for supraclavicular block, classic, 527, 528, *528*
      plumb-bob, 528

Negative-pressure pulmonary edema, 978, 979
Negligence, 55, 56
  comparative, 59
  definition of, 55
  in anesthetic induction, 55
  in emergence from anesthesia, 55, 56
  in postanesthesia care unit, 56
Neodymium-yttrium-aluminum-garnet (Nd:YAG) laser, 1371(t)
  for genitourinary surgery, 1243
Neohepatic phase, of orthotopic liver transplantation, 1345
  physiologic changes in, 1349–1351, *1350*
Neomycin, perioperative use of, 9(t)
Neonate(s), 1013–1035
  abdominal wall defects in, 1027, *1027*, 1028, *1028*
  airway management in, 1022, 1023
  anesthesia in, requirement for, 1013, 1014(t)
  cardiovascular system of, 1015
  congenital diaphragmatic hernia in, 1031–1033, *1032*
  esophageal atresia in, 1030, 1031, *1031*
  fluid administration in, 1024, 1025
  heat loss in, 1017, 1017(t)
  intraoperative monitoring of, 1025, 1026
  intraoperative ventilation in, 1023, 1024
  kidneys of, 1016, 1017, 1017(t)
  laboratory values in, 1017(t)
  necrotizing enterocolitis in, 1028, 1029, *1029*
  neural development in, 1013, *1014*
  pain in, perception of, 1013, 1014, *1014*
    response to, 1013, 1014
  patent ductus arteriosus in, 1029, 1030
  pre-existing medical problems in, 1017–1019
  premedication in, 1022
  preoperative fasting guidelines for, 1021, 1022
  pulmonary vascular resistance in, 1140
  pyloric stenosis in, 1026, *1026*, 1027
  respiratory system of, 1014, *1014*, 1015
  resuscitation of, 1033–1035, 1033(t), *1034*, 1035(t), 1097
    drug therapy in, 1034, 1035, 1035(t)
  tracheoesophageal fistula in, 1030, *1030*, 1031
  vascular access in, 1024
  vital signs of, 1016(t)
Neoplasm(s), airway, 1274
  intubation with, 1274
  intracranial. See *Intracranial neoplasm(s)*.
  spinal, anesthetic considerations in, 1301
Neostigmine, drug interactions with, 658(t)
  effects of, on bowel anastomosis, 1113
  in ester metabolism, 625
Nephrectomy, 1242
  anesthesia for, 1242
  complications of, 1242
  donor, positioning for, 1366, *1367*
Nephrology consultation, 170–184
  for fluid therapy, 171, 172, 172(t)
  in hypertension, 170, 171
  purpose of, 170
Nephrostomy, percutaneous, 1244
  anesthesia for, 908
  risks of, 907, 908
  technique of, 906–908, *907*
Nephrotoxicity, 182, 183
  causes of, 182
  intravenous fluids for, 182
  methoxyflurane, 649
Nephrotoxins, 182(t)
Nerve(s). See also names of specific nerves.
  compression of, in spinal disease, 1295(t)
    surgery for, 1297, *1297*
  injury to, during ambulatory shoulder surgery, 1255

Nerve(s) *(Continued)*
    in lower extremity, *505*
    in upper extremity, *505*
    intraoperative, prevention of, somatosensory evoked potentials in, 405, *405*
    regional anesthesia in, 536
    sympathetic nerve block in, 492
    tourniquet use and, 1261
    peripheral. See *Peripheral nerves.*
Nerve block(s), of larynx, indications for, 446, *446*, 447, *447*
    of lower extremity, 1256, 1257
    of spermatic cord, 1236, *1236*
    of upper extremity, 1255, 1256, *1256*
        intravenous, 1255
    peripheral, vasoconstrictor use with, 626–628
    sympathetic. See *Sympathetic nerve block(s).*
Nerve conduction, physiology of, 621, 622, *622, 623*
    velocity of, monitoring of, in seizure disorders, 160
Nerve fibers, characteristics of, 623(t)
    of autonomic nervous system, 482, *483*
Nerve stimulation, 412–419
    data from, interpretation of, 416–419
    electrode placement for, 414–416, *415*
    evoked potentials during, 417, *417*
    patterns of, assessment of, 416–419, *417, 418*, 418(t)
    supramaximal, 414, *414*
Nerve stimulator, characteristics of, 414, 414(t)
    in regional anesthesia, 539, 540
Nervous system, assessment of, in trauma, 994, 995, 995(t)
    preanesthetic, 4, 5, 11
    autonomic. See *Autonomic nervous system (ANS).*
    central. See *Central nervous system (CNS).*
    compromise of, in spinal cord shock, management of, 685
    disease of, effects of, on anesthetic management, 1286–1288, 1287(t)
        in renal failure, 1359, 1360(t)
        potassium level in, succinylcholine effects on, 156, 156(t)
        pre-existing, preoperative neurologic consultation for, 152
        progressive, in anesthetic risk, 67
    effects on, of acid-base disturbances, 741
        of Guillain-Barré syndrome, 156
        of hypothermia, 819(t), 820
        of spinal/epidural anesthesia, 163
    monitoring of, 389–409, 389(t), 390(t)
        clinical, continuous, 391, 392, 392(t)
        intraoperative, implications of, 389, 390, 390(t)
        requirements for, 390(t)
        surgical outcome with, 390
    response of, to surgery, inhalation anesthesia in, 613
    somatic, vs. autonomic nervous system, 482, 483
    sympathetic, abdominal portion of, *488*
        outflow of, dispersion/amplification of, 485
        regulation of, 483–485, *484*
Neural arch, of spine, 459
Neural canal, components of, 460
Neural development, in neonates, 1013, *1014*
Neuroaugmentation, for pain, in adults, 254, 255, 255(t)
Neurogenic pulmonary edema, 977
Neuroleptic malignant syndrome (NMS), 158
    and hyperthermia, 824(t), 825
    differential diagnosis of, 158
    incidence of, 158

Neuroleptic malignant syndrome (NMS) *(Continued)*
    malignant hyperthermia–triggering agents in, 158
    mortality of, 158
    treatment of, 158
Neuroleptics, for pain, 242(t)
Neurologic consultation, 152–168
    components of, 152, 152(t), 153
    in absence of known disease, 153
    in pre-existing disease, 152
    indications for, 152, 153(t)
    postanesthetic, 163–165, 164(t)
Neurologic examination, clinical, 390–392, 391(t)
    intraoperative, 390–392
    preoperative, 390
Neurologic function, effects on, of burns, 703
    preanesthetic evaluation of, 11
Neurologic surgery, 1283–1309
    air embolism during, 1286, 1286(t)
    anesthesia for, drug effects of, 1284, 1285, 1285(t)
        emergence from, 1287, 1288, 1309
        induction/maintenance of, 1287, 1288
    approach to, 1286–1288, 1287(t)
    fluid therapy in, 730
    homeostatic mechanisms in, 1283, 1284, *1284*
    monitoring in, 1287
    positioning for, 1286, 1286(t)
        errors in, 1286, 1286(t)
    premedication for, 1287
Neurolytic agents, for pain, in adults, 254
    in autonomic nervous system blockade, 485, 486
    spread of, during sympathetic nerve block, 492
Neuroma, injection of, for chronic pain, 254
Neuromuscular blockade, assessment of, 419
    clinical, 412, 412(t), 413, *413*, 413(t)
    drug interactions with, 657, 658, 658(t)
    effects on, of lithium, 651
    in abdominal surgery, 1111, *1112*
    in burn surgery, 709–711
    in nonimmunologic histamine release, 746
    in renal transplantation, 1364
    reversibility of, 419
    technique of, 413–416, *414*, 414(t), *415*
Neuromuscular junction, in alveolar hypoventilation, 804
    monitoring of, 412–419
Neuromuscular relaxation, for difficult intubation, 941
Neuromuscular system, disease of, in postoperative hypoventilation, 84
    electrical injury of, 700
    function of, as extubation criterion, 949
    postsynaptic, 416
    presynaptic, 416
Neuropathic pain, 234
Neuropathy, regional anesthesia in, 515
Neuropharmacology, 1283–1285, *1284*, 1285(t)
Neurophysiology, 1283–1285, *1284*, 1285(t)
Neuropraxis, prognosis in, 162
Neurosurgery. See *Neurologic surgery.*
Neurotmesis, prognosis in, 162
Neurotoxicity, of chloroprocaine, 636
    of lidocaine, with spinal microcatheter use, 636, 637
Neurovascular compromise, surgical positioning in, 504, *504*
Neurovascular surgery, 1288–1295
    anesthesia for, emergence from, 1294, 1295
        induction/maintenance of, 1293, 1293(t), 1294
    monitoring in, 1293

Neurovascular surgery *(Continued)*
    premedication for, 1292, 1293
Neutrophils, in reperfusion injury, 326
Newport E100i ventilator, 427(t)
Nialamide, drug interactions with, 655(t)
Nicomorphine, for acute pain, 241(t)
Nifedipine, analgesic potential of, 244(t)
    for perioperative hypertension, 171(t)
Nil per os (NPO) status, for outpatient surgery, 1394, 1395
    for pediatric cardiovascular surgery, 1144
    in neonates, 1021, 1022
    in pulmonary aspiration prevention, 86
    preanesthetic, duration of, 15, *16*, 17, 17(t)
Nitrates, cardiovascular effects of, 760(t)
    preoperative continuation of, 1163
    in coronary artery disease, 756
Nitric oxide, for right ventricular failure, in heart transplantation, 1329
Nitroglycerin, action of, mechanism of, 849
    before thoracic aorta cross-clamping, 1224
    drug interactions with, 646(t)
    for intraoperative myocardial ischemia, 760, *761*
    for nonobstetric surgery, in pregnant patient, 1106
    in cardiopulmonary resuscitation, 849
        complications of, 849
        dosage of, 849
        indications for, 849
    in myocardial dysfunction, in preoperative patient optimization, 767
    in pediatric cardiovascular surgery, 1146(t)
    intravenous, perioperative, value of, 136, 137
    routine use of, in cardiovascular surgery, 1171
    physiologic effects of, 1285(t)
Nitroprusside. See also *Sodium nitroprusside.*
    in pediatric cardiovascular surgery, 1146(t)
Nitrous oxide, and bowel distention, 1115, 1116, *1116*
    contraindications to, 571
    drug interactions with, 650, 654(t)
    effects of, circulatory, 612(t)
        environmental, 114
        on evoked potentials, 406(t), 408(t)
        on fetus, 1102, *1102*
        physiologic, 1285(t)
    for abdominal surgery, 1110
    for battlefield surgery, 880
    for middle ear surgery, 1271, *1271*
    for outpatient surgery, 1398
    for pediatric procedural pain, 270
    for right ventricular failure, after cardiopulmonary bypass, 1183
    in chronic obstructive pulmonary disease, 967
    in high-pressure anesthesia machine cylinder, 280, *281*
    in intestinal obstruction, 1116
    in intracranial pressure control, intraoperative, 779
    perioperative, 778
    in laryngeal laser operations, 1377
    in trauma, 615, 616
    in valvular disease, 613
    inhalation of, vascular endothelium in, 665
    perioperative requirements for, 657(t)
NMS. See *Neuroleptic malignant syndrome (NMS).*
Nociceptive pain, 234
Nocturia, in congestive heart failure, 1158
Nodes of Ranvier, local anesthesia of, 623, 623(t)
Non-A non-B hepatitis, 860
Nonchromaffin paraganglioma, anesthetic management in, 1243

Nonchromaffin paraganglioma *(Continued)*
  definition of, 1243
  preoperative treatment of, 1243
Nondepolarizing muscle relaxants,
    defasciculating dose of, 572
  drug interactions with, 645(t), 652(t), 653(t)
  for difficult intubation, 941
  in burn surgery, 710, 711
  reversal agents for, selection of, 573
Nonshivering thermogenesis, 1017
Nonsteroidal anti-inflammatory drugs
    (NSAIDs), for pain, 604
  acute, 240(t)
    in children, 264, 264(t)
      with cancer, 272
  perioperative use of, 8
Norepinephrine, 1182(t)
  for anaphylactic shock, 683(t)
  for anaphylaxis, 748
  for intraoperative hemodynamic stabilization,
      in shock, 692
  for perioperative myocardial dysfunction,
      766(t)
  for right ventricular failure, after cardiopul-
      monary bypass, 1183
  in pediatric cardiovascular surgery, 1146(t)
Nortriptyline, for pain, 242(t)
Nose, anatomy of, 440, 441, *441*
  artificial, in intraoperative hypothermia pre-
      vention, 434
  functions of, 441
NPO. See *Nil per os (NPO) status*.
NSAIDs. See *Nonsteroidal anti-inflammatory
    drugs (NSAIDs)*.
Nubain, for acute pain, 241(t)
Nuclear medicine studies, preoperative, 65, 66
Nutrition, changes in, in thermal injury, 701

O$_2$EI (oxygen extraction index), 790
Obesity, in reduced postoperative functional
    residual capacity, 79
  inhalation anesthesia in, 614
  morbid, in decreased chest wall compliance,
      814
    respiratory center depression in, 803
  preoperative pulmonary consultation in, 143
Obstetric patients, 1082–1097
  analgesia in, inhalation, 1089
  labor, 1085–1087, 1085(t), *1086*
    choice of, 1087
  anesthesia in, epidural, 1087–1089, 1087(t)–
      1089(t)
    general, 1091, 1091(t), 1092
    guidelines for, 1082(t)
    regional, 1092, 1093, *1093*
      toxic effects of, 1092
  coexisting medical/surgical problems in,
      1093–1095, *1094, 1095*
Obstructive jaundice, 1122, 1123
  effects of, on abdominal muscle relaxation,
      1110, 1111
  renal failure in, 1122, 1123
Obstructive lung disease, postoperative
    pulmonary function tests in, 149
Obstructive sleep apnea, 161
Obturator nerve, injury to, lithotomy position
    in, 510
  stimulation of, transurethral resection of
      prostate in, 1239, *1239, 1240*
Occipitoatlantoaxial articulation, *462*
Occiput, of neonate, 1015
Occurrence insurance policy, 60
Odontoid, congenital anomalies of, 461–463,
    462, 462(t)
  hypoplasia of, 461, 462, 462(t)

Odontoid *(Continued)*
  subluxation of, in rheumatoid arthritis, 464,
      465, *465*
Ohmeda 885 Field Anesthesia Machine, 878,
    878, 879, 879(t)
Ohmeda Logic 07 ventilator, 347, 427(t)
Ohm's law, 885, *886*
OKT-3, in orthotopic liver transplantation, 1344
Oligodendroglioma, properties of, 1303(t)
Oliguria, after trauma surgery, 1009, 1009(t)
  assessment of, 181
  causes of, 181, 182
    perioperative, 385, 385(t)
  definition of, 181
  differential diagnosis of, 385, 385(t)
  diuretics for, indications for, 181, 182
  in portosystemic shunting, 1130
  normovolemic, in abdominal surgery, 1120
  postoperative, 95, 95(t)
  urinary composition in, 1337(t)
OLT. See *Orthotopic liver transplantation
    (OLT)*.
Omeprazole, drug interactions with, 644(t),
    645(t)
Omnopon, for acute pain, 241(t)
Omphalocele, 1027, *1027, 1028*
Oncology, orthopedic, 1251, 1252
  procedures for, blood loss in, 1252
Oncotic pressure gradients, in colloid
    distribution, 719
Ondansetron, in postoperative nausea
    prevention, 99
Open fracture, 1247(t)
  in multiple trauma, 1246
Open heart surgery, cerebral protection during,
    barbiturates in, 328, 329
Operating room, electrical safety in, 890, *890,
    891, 891*
  occupational hazards in, 853–870
  preparation of, for trauma care, 985–990,
      987(t)
Opiates, dependence on, management of, 250–
    252
  effects of, physiologic, 1285(t)
  for postoperative pain, dose of, determination
      of, 247, 247(t), 248(t)
  intravenous, for pain, in adults, 244, 245,
      245(t)
  peridural, in respiratory depression, 248
Opioids, abuse of, diagnostic features of,
    1000(t)
  and postoperative ileus, 1133
  endogenous, release of, electrical stimulation
      for, 255
  epidural, in children, 270
  for pain, in children, 264, 264(t)
    with cancer, 272
    nonmalignant, guidelines for, 243(t)
    in adults, 240, 243(t)
  high-dose, for cardiovascular surgery, 1173,
      1175(t)
    disadvantages of, 1173, 1174, *1174*
  in abdominal surgery, 1110
  in geriatric patients, 1074, 1075
  in malignant hyperthermia, 827(t)
  in nonimmunologic histamine release, 746
  intraspinal, for acute pain, 248(t)
  intravenous, patient-controlled, guidelines
      for, 245(t)
  perioperative use of, 8, 9
  systemic, for acute pain, 241(t)
Optic nerve glioma, properties of, 1303(t)
Oral cavity, examination of, 440, *440*
Oral contraceptives, drug interactions with,
    644(t)
Oral hypoglycemics, perioperative use of, 7
Oral intubation, in spinal cord shock, 685

Oral transmucosal fentanyl citrate (OTFC), in
    children, 270
Organogenesis, anesthesia effects on, 1102
Oropharyngeal airway, in cardiopulmonary
    resuscitation, 836
Oropharynx, examination of, before intubation,
    440, *440*
Orotracheal intubation, 451, 452, *452*
  errors in, 310(t)
  failure of, 452
  in trauma, 991, 992
  techniques of, 309, 310
    curved blade, 452, *452*
    straight blade, 452
  tube fixation after, 454
Orthopedic injuries, traumatic, assessment of,
    998, 999
Orthopedic oncology, 1251, 1252
  procedures for, blood loss in, 1252
Orthopedic surgery, 1246–1265
  ambulatory, 1254, 1255
  antibiotic prophylaxis for, 1258, 1259
  blood loss during, 1259, *1259*, 1259(t), 1260
    amount of, 1260
    reduction of, 1259, 1260
  emergency, indications for, 1248
  for trauma, 1246–1248, 1247(t), *1248*
  pain control in, 1264, 1264(t), 1265, *1265*,
      1265(t)
  positioning for, 1260, 1261, *1261*
  regional anesthesia for, 1255–1258, *1256–
      1258*
    advantages of, 1257, 1258, *1258*
  tourniquets for, 1261–1263, 1261(t), 1263(t)
  urgent, indications for, 1248, *1248*
  venous thromboembolism in, 1263, 1264
    prevention of, 1263, 1264
    risk factors for, 1263
Orthotopic liver transplantation (OLT), 1333–
    1357, *1333*
  anesthesia for, equipment for, 1341
    induction of, 1342, 1343
    management of, 1343, 1344, 1344(t)
      hourly blood sampling in, 1344
  arterial pressure monitoring in, 1341, 1342
  bleeding in, 1337, 1338, 1338(t), 1339(t)
  blood/blood product availability for, 1342
  candidates for, adult, 1333, 1334
    pediatric, 1334, 1335(t)
  equipment for, 1352–1355, *1352–1355*
  immunosuppressive drugs in, 1344
  in children, 1355, 1356
  intraoperative hypotension during, 1351
  metabolic changes in, treatment of, 1351
  operating room set-up in, 1340, 1341, *1341*
  organ preservation in, 1338, 1339(t), *1340*
    solutions for, 1338, 1339(t)
  preanesthetic evaluation in, 1335–1342
    second-stage, 1340
  procedure for, length of, 1340, 1340(t)
  rapid-infusion system in, 1342, 1342(t)
  recovery after, 1356
  retransplantation after, anesthesia for, 1356
  surgical procedures after, 1356, *1356*, 1357
  surgical stages in, 1345–1351
  survival after, 1335, *1336, 1338*
  timing of, 1333
  venous access for, 1341
  venovenous bypass in, 1345, *1345*, 1346,
      1346, 1346(t)
Oscillometry, automated, in blood pressure
    measurement, 370, *370*, 370(t), 371
Osmolality, calculation of, 188
  changes in, in transurethral resection of pros-
      tate syndrome, 1240
  contrast agent effect on, 902

Osmolality *(Continued)*
plasma, calculation of, 172
in intracranial neoplasm surgery, 1308, 1308(t)
Osmotic diuresis, and postoperative polyuria, 95
vs. diabetes insipidus, 187, 187(t)
Osmotic diuretics, in pregnancy, 1106
Ossification, of posterior longitudinal ligaments, 463
Osteogenesis imperfecta, and hyperthermia, 825
Osteonecrosis, of femoral head, factors in, 1249, 1249(t), 1250
OTFC (oral transmucosal fentanyl citrate), in children, 270
Otitis media, myringotomy for, 1268, 1269
Otolaryngologic surgery, 1268–1281
airway management in, 1280, 1281, *1281*
Otologic surgery, 1271, 1272
induced hypotension in, 1272
Outcome, adverse, with general anesthesia, 70(t)
analysis of, 62–71
in quality assurance, 35, 36
analysis of, 35, 36
confounding variables in, 36
measurement of, 63, 64
patient satisfaction in, 63
peer assessment in, 63
pitfalls of, 63, 64
Outpatient surgery, 1389–1405
airway management in, 1398, 1398(t), 1399
anesthesia in, general, 1396–1398
inhalation, 617
monitored, 1400, 1401
regional, 1400
aspiration in, 1394, 1395
candidates for, unacceptable, 1390–1393
discharge criteria for, 1401, 1401(t), *1402, 1403*, 1404(t)
in children, general anesthesia for, 1397
intravenous infusions in, 1399, 1399(t), 1400
tracheal intubation for, 1398, 1399
laboratory tests for, 1390, 1391(t), 1392(t)
morbidity/mortality of, 1404, 1405
pain after, minimization of, 1404
perioperative period in, 1394, 1395
preinduction period in, 1395, 1396
procedures for, acceptable, 1393, 1394, 1394(t)
unacceptable, 1394
quality improvement programs in, 1405, 1405(t)
recovery from, 1401, 1401(t), 1402, *1402, 1403*
risk factors for, 1390(t)
screening in, 1389–1393
clinic for, 1389, 1390, *1390*
effects of, on anesthesia outcome, 1390, *1391*
purpose of, 1389
unplanned hospitalization after, 1402–1404, 1404(t)
Overhydration, and postoperative ventricular dysfunction, 89
Oxazepam, for acute pain, 242(t)
in liver disease, 1344(t)
Oximetry, dual, 790
in arterial blood gas measurement, 787
pulse. See *Pulse oximetry.*
reflectance, 354
transmission, 354
venous, mixed, 788, 788(t)
in pulmonary artery catheterization, 377, 378
Oxycodone, for acute pain, 241(t)

Oxygen, administration of, after abdominal surgery, 1132
airway management in, 921
by nasal cannula, anesthesia machine in, 294
during extubation, 454
during postanesthesia patient transport, 595, *595*, 595(t)
for shock, 666
anaphylactic, 683(t)
septic, 688
in laryngeal laser operations, 1377
in perioperative intracranial pressure control, 778
in pulmonary artery catheterization, 378, *378*, 378(t)
postoperative, 78
preoperative, in pulmonary edema, 974
to myocardium, during aortic vascular surgery, 1221, 1222
cerebral, supply/demand of, 1284
measurement of, 398–408
consumption of, by fetus, 1083
by myocardium, during cardiopulmonary bypass, 323
in shock, 668–672, *669–671*
formula for, 692(t)
in hypoxemia, 785, 785(t)
in pregnancy, *1084*
in shock, 666
content of, in arterial blood, 782–785
relationship of, to PaO_2, 782, *783*
diffusion of, blockage of, in hypoxemia, 785, 785(t)
expired, concentration of, 344
in high-pressure anesthesia machine cylinder, pressure of, 279, 280, *281*
in retinopathy of prematurity, 1020, *1020*
inspired, concentration of, 344
fraction of, PaO_2 calculation from, 342, 343, *343*
monitoring of, 343, 344
circuit valve leak in, 344
fast, 344
sensor for, diagnostic utility of, 344
misleading information from, 343, 344
regulation of, in high-pressure anesthesia machine, 277
supply of, in aortic stenosis, 1171
low, alarm for, 277, 278, *280*
to myocardium, demand for, 1170, 1171
goals for, in coronary artery disease, 1169, 1169(t), 1170, *1170*
toxicity of, 792, 793
pulmonary, postoperative, 78
transport of, in shock, 668
Oxygen challenge, in hypoxemia, 791, *792*
Oxygen dissociation curve, in hypothermia, 819(t), 820
Oxygen extraction index (O_2EI), 790
Oxygen flush valve, of high-pressure anesthesia machine, flow rate of, 280, 281
Oxygen partial pressure, alveolar-to-arterial, gradient of, 789, 790
arterial-to-alveolar, rate of, 790
indices of, 789, 790
postoperative, acceptable limits for, 77
reduction of, 77, 78, 78(t)
ratio of, to FIO_2, 790
Oxygen pressure failure safety mechanism, 278, *280*
Oxygen saturation, in pregnancy, *1084*
Oxygen therapy, for hypoxemia, 793, 793(t), 794, *794*, 794(t)
adverse effects of, 792, *792*, 792(t), 793
clinical guidelines for, 794, 795

Oxygen therapy *(Continued)*
in chronic obstructive pulmonary disease, 965
Oxygenation, cerebral, in postoperative delirium, 165
difficult, after tracheal intubation, 945–948
effects on, of abdominal surgery, 1131, 1132
of alveolar hyperventilation, 807
for anaphylaxis, 747
for laryngoscopy, in children, 1062
for persistent pulmonary hypertension of the newborn, 1018
in pulmonary edema, 972
in thoracoabdominal aneurysm management, 1218
intraoperative, for adult respiratory distress syndrome, with pulmonary edema, 976
monitoring of, 68(t)
standards for, 122
of pulmonary artery, in critical illness, 788, 788(t)
postoperative, 77–80
acceptable limits for, 77
assessment of, 77
pulmonary perfusion in, 80
tissue, in hypoxemia, 790, *791*
Oxygenator, in cardiopulmonary bypass, 321
role of, in neurologic outcome, 328
Oxygraphy, 344
with capnography, in circuit valve leak detection, 344, *346*
Oxyhemoglobin, desaturation of, intraoperative, in children, 1059, 1060
saturation of, arterial, 782–785, *783*
Oxyhemoglobin affinity, effects on, of alveolar hyperventilation, 808
of alveolar hypoventilation, 801
Oxyhemoglobin dissociation curve, 150, *150*
in congenital heart disease, 1142, *1142*
Oxymorphone, for acute pain, 241(t)
intravenous, patient-controlled, guidelines for, 245(t)
Ozone, depletion of, anesthetic agents in, 114

Pacemaker(s), 893–895, 894(t)
effects on, of magnets, 894
extracorporeal shock wave lithotripsy with, 1382
history of, 3
implantation of, anesthetic considerations in, 1193
magnetic resonance imaging with, 913
malfunction of, electrosurgical unit interference in, 894, 895, 895(t)
mechanism of, 893, 894, 894(t)
$PaCO_2$, control of, in intraoperative intracranial pressure control, 779
elevation of, in hypoxemia, oxygen therapy for, 795
relationship of, to $PETCO_2$, 351, *351*, 352
PACU. See *Postanesthesia care unit (PACU).*
PAF (platelet-activating factor), cardiopulmonary effects of, 745
Pain, acute, benzodiazepines for, 242(t)
in children, 262, 262(t)
nonopioid analgesics for, 240(t)
opioids for, intraspinal, 248(t)
systemic, 241(t)
after extracorporeal shock wave lithotripsy, 1387
after outpatient surgery, minimization of, 1404, 1405(t)
after thoracic surgery, management of, 1207, 1208, *1208*
antidepressants for, 242(t)

Pain *(Continued)*
  chronic, anesthesia for, local, 247
    regional, 254
    evaluation of, psychotherapy in, 256
    in back, anatomic factors in, 475, 476(t)
    in children, 262(t), 263
    peridural analgesia in, 250, 252(t)
  classification of, in adults, in drug therapy
    selection, 239, 240, 240(t)–242(t)
  control of, in burns, 711
    in post-anesthesia care unit, 76, 77
    postoperative, pulmonary considerations
      in, 146, 147
  during arthroscopy, causes of, 1254, 1255
  expectations for, handling of, 576, *577*
  gate control theory of, 255
  idiopathic, 234
  in adults, acute, definition of, 234
    approach to, 233, *233*, 234
    assessment of, initial, 233, *233*, 234
      laboratory studies in, 233, 234
      physical examination in, 238
    chronic, definition of, 234
    chronicity of, 234
    course of, 236
    diagnosis of, 234
      laboratory studies in, 238, 239, 239(t)
      radiography in, 238, 239, 239(t)
    duration of, 236
    history of, 234, 234(t), *235*
    intensity of, 235, *235*, 236, *236*
      individual perception of, 235, *236*
      physical signs of, 235, 236
      rating of, 235, *235*
    location of, 236
    management of, 234
      consultation for, 233–257
      peridural analgesics in, 246, *247*
      pharmacologic, 239–244, 239(t)
        concurrent medical condition in, 237
        intravenous, 244, 245, 245(t)
        monitoring in, 248–250, 248(t), *249*,
          250(t)
      techniques for, 239–250
    mechanisms of, 234, *235*
    neuroaugmentation for, 254, 255, 255(t)
    neurolytic blocks for, 254
    periodicity of, 236, *236*
    physical therapy for, 255, 256, 256(t)
    postoperative, local anesthetics for, 246,
      247, 247(t)
    psychologic/psychiatric factors in, 237,
      237(t), 238, 238(t)
      therapy for, 256, 257, 257(t)
    quality of, 236
    regional anesthesia for, 253, 254
  in altered sensorium, during emergence, 98
  in back, in pregnancy, 474
    low, causes of, 475, *476*
  in cancer, bone, 1251, 1252
  in children, 262(t), 271, 271(t), 272
    palliative management of, 272
    regional anesthesia for, 254
    steroids for, 244(t)
    treatment of, 240, *243*, 244(t), 245(t)
  in children, assessment of, 263, *263*
    preanesthetic, 263
    chronic, noncancer, 272, 273
    management of, consultation for, 261–273
    services for, 273
    measurement of, 263
    postoperative, management of, 263–265,
      264(t)
    procedural, 270, 271
      continuous sedation for, 270
      nitrous oxide for, 270
      topical local anesthesia for, 270

Pain *(Continued)*
      transmucosal drug administration for,
        270, 271
    spectrum of, 262, 262(t), 263
    undertreatment of, factors in, 261, 261(t),
      262
  in neonate, perception of, 1013, 1014, *1014*
    response to, 1013, 1014
  in orthopedic surgery, control of, 1264,
    1264(t), 1265, *1265*, 1265(t)
    postoperative, regional anesthesia for,
      1258
  in postanesthesia care unit, assessment of, 76
  in postoperative delirium, 166
  neuroleptics for, 242(t)
  neuropathic, 234
  nociceptive, 234
  nonmalignant, opioids for, guidelines for,
    243(t)
  of labor, aberrant, 1088, 1089, 1089(t)
    anatomy and physiology of, 1087, 1087(t),
      1088
    management of, 1086, 1087
  phantom limb, 1254
    causes of, 1254
    prevention of, 1254
  postanesthesia, in children, 1061
  postoperative, control of, in chronic obstruc-
    tive pulmonary disease, 967, 968
    in geriatric patients, 1077, 1078
    pathophysiology of, *246*
  psychogenic, 234
  skeletal muscle, postoperative, causes of, 104
  tourniquet. See *Tourniquet pain.*
Palate, cleft, 1272, *1273*
Palpation, in circulation monitoring, in
    anesthetized patient, 336, 337, 337(t)
  in pain assessment, in adults, 238
Pancuronium, dose of, in children, 1056(t)
  effects of, physiologic, 1285(t)
  in liver disease, 1344(t)
  in pediatric cardiovascular surgery, 1146(t)
  in renal transplantation, 1363
  selection of, factors in, 573
Pantopon, for acute pain, 241(t)
Pao$_2$, calculation of, 783, 800
    from inspired oxygen fraction, 342, 343,
      343
  postoperative, acceptable limits for, 77
    assessment of, 77
  relationship of, to arterial blood oxygen con-
    tent, 782, *783*
  to Spo$_2$, 782
PAOP. See *Pulmonary artery occlusion
    pressure (PAOP).*
PAP. See *Pulmonary artery pressure (PAP).*
Papaverine, in paraplegia prevention, after
    aortic cross-clamping, 1229
Papillary muscle, rupture of, in acute
    myocardial infarction, 678
Paracentesis, for ascites, 1124, *1124*
    delayed intravascular volume contraction
      after, 1125
Paraganglioma, nonchromaffin, anesthestic
    management in, 1243
  definition of, 1243
  preoperative treatment of, 1243
Paralysis, neuromuscular, in persistent
    postoperative unconsciousness, 96
  of vocal cords, tracheal intubation and, 456
  partial, in postoperative delirium, 166
Paraplegia, aortic cross-clamping and, 1226–
    1228
    prevention of, 1228, 1228(t), 1229
  in abdominal aortic surgery, 1229
Parasympathetic nervous system (PNS),
    postoperative activity of, factors in, 94(t)

Parasympatholysis, intraoperative, 145, 146
Parathyroid glands, diseases of, 202–205,
    202(t), 203(t)
  management of, perioperative, 204, 205
  function of, assessment of, preoperative, 202,
    203
    metabolic evaluation in, 203
  hyperplasia of, 205
  surgery of, 204, 205, 1313, 1314, *1314*
Parathyroid hormone (PTH), function of, 1313
  in calcium control, 202
  measurement of, preoperative, in parathyroid
    function assessment, 202
Parathyroidectomy, postoperative
    considerations in, 1314
Paravertebral block, 487–489, *487*, *488*
  anatomic considerations in, 487
  complications of, 487, *488*, 489
Paresthesias, regional anesthesia and, 536
Pargyline, drug interactions with, 655(t)
Parkinson's disease, 154
  anesthetic considerations in, 154
  organs affected by, 154
Paromomycin, perioperative use of, 9(t)
Parotid surgery, 1271, 1272
  induced hypotension in, 1272
Paroxysmal atrial tachycardia (PAT),
    electrocardiographic characteristics of, 366
  postoperative, 94, 94(t)
Paroxysmal nocturnal dyspnea, in congestive
    heart failure, 1158
Paroxysmal supraventricular tachycardia
    (PSVT), treatment of, emergency, 850
Partial agonists, 570
Partial-thickness burns, deep, 700
  superficial, 700
Parturition, back ache after, 478
PAT (paroxysmal atrial tachycardia),
    electrocardiographic characteristics of, 366
  postoperative, 94, 94(t)
Patent ductus arteriosus (PDA), in neonates,
    1029, 1030
Pathologic fracture, impending, stabilization of,
    1251
Patient(s), anesthetized, management of,
    monitoring in, 335–337
  conscious, management of, monitoring in,
    334, 335
    tracheal intubation in, indications for, 453,
      453(t), 454
  coverage of, in postanesthesia care unit, 73
  "do-not-resuscitate," preanesthetic evalua-
    tion of, 17
  geriatric. See *Geriatric patients.*
  obstetric. See *Obstetric patients.*
  pediatric. See *Child(ren).*
  retarded/uncooperative, dental repairs in,
    1275, 1276
  satisfaction of, in outcome measurement, 63
  surgical, positioning of. See *Position(ing), of
    surgical patient.*
Patient history, in preanesthetic evaluation, 2–5,
    3–6
  of cardiac risk, 128, 129
Patient transport, after battlefield surgery, 881
  equipment for, 424
  intracranial pressure control during, 780, 781
  intrahospital, complications of, 423
    indications for, 422, 422(t), 423
    monitoring during, 421–428
      equipment for, selection of, 425–428, *426*,
        426(t), 427(t)
    requirement for, factors in, 423
  post-transport stabilization phase of, 425
  preparation for, 423, 424
  to imaging department, 899, 900, *900*

Patient transport *(Continued)*
  to postanesthesia care unit, *594*, 595, *595*, 596
    oxygen administration during, 595, *595*, 595(t)
    ventilation during, 595, 596
  transport phase of, 424, 425
Patient-controlled analgesia (PCA), 76
  after thoracic surgery, 1207
  in children, 266, 267
  in geriatric patients, 1078
  postoperative, pulmonary considerations in, 146, 147
Patrick v Burget, 33
PCA. See *Patient-controlled analgesia (PCA)*.
Pco$_2$, changes in, effects of, 734, 735, *735*
  measurement of, 786
PCP, abuse of, diagnostic features of, 1000(t)
PDA (patent ductus arteriosus), in neonates, 1029, 1030
PEEP. See *Positive end-expiratory pressure (PEEP)*.
Peer Review Improvement Act (PRIA), 32
Peer review organizations, in quality assurance, 32, 33
  malpractice legislation effect on, 33
  role of, 32, 33
  Title 19 effect on, 33
Peer Standards Review Organization (PSRO), 32
Pelvis, fracture of, 1247(t)
  bleeding in, 1247
Pendelluft, and alveolar hypoventilation, 805
Penicillin, allergic reaction to, 9
Penile block, in children, 268
  technique of, 1236, 1237, *1237*
Penis, dorsal vein of, catheterization of, 499, 500
  innervation of, 1236, *1237*
Penlon 350 ventilator, 427(t)
Pentastarch, effects of, on coagulation, 728
Pentazocine, drug interactions with, 652(t)
  for acute pain, 241(t)
  intravenous, 603(t), 604
    patient-controlled, guidelines for, 245(t)
Pentobarbital, drug interactions with, 645(t)
  for imaging studies, 910(t), 911(t)
  in pediatric premedication, 1048(t)
Penumbra effect, 354
Percodan, for acute pain, 241(t)
Percutaneous transluminal coronary angioplasty (PTCA), in cardiogenic shock, 673, 674
  myocardial ischemia after, onset of, 1168, 1168(t)
Perfluorocarbon emulsions, in shock, 670
Perfluorochemical emulsions, 721
Perfusion, abnormal, in altered sensorium, during emergence, 98
  in conscious patients, monitoring of, 335
Perfusion pressure, during cardiopulmonary bypass, control of, 329
  for adequate cerebral blood flow, 327, *327*
  in carotid disease, 330
  low, advantages of, 327, 328(t)
  pediatric, 1151
  renal effects of, 330
Pericardial effusion, chronic, anesthetic considerations in, 1196
Pericardial tamponade, anesthetic considerations in, 1196
  signs and symptoms of, 1195, 1196
Pericardiotomy, 1195, 1196
  indications for, 1195
Pericyazine, for pain, 242(t)
Perineal relaxation, for cesarean section, 1090, 1091

Peripheral edema, fluid therapy and, 729
Peripheral nerve blocks, in children, 1060(t), 1061
  vasoconstrictor use with, 626–628
Peripheral nerves, changes in, in pregnancy, 1085
  disease of, in diabetes mellitus, 207
  injury to, detection of, somatosensory evoked potentials in, 403
    intraoperative, 161–163, 162(t)
      discovery of, actions after, 162
      during pregnancy, 162, 163
      mechanisms of, 161
      presentation of, 162, 162(t)
      prevalence of, 161
      prognosis after, 162
      therapy for, 162
    postoperative, 104
      evaluation of, 511, 512
    postpartum, 512
    surgical positioning in, 511, 511(t), 512
  of upper extremity, anatomy of, 524
  regeneration of, 162
  stimulators of, use of, in abdominal surgery, 1111, *1111*
  surgery of, electrophysiologic monitoring during, 161
Peripheral vascular disease (PVD), blood pressure differences in, 10
Peripheral venous catheterization, 498–500, *499*
  equipment for, 542, 542(t)
  in children, 500
  site for, selection of, 544, 545
  techniques of, 546, 547, *549*
    intraosseous, 499, 500, 547, *549*
    venous distention in, 546
Peritoneal lavage, diagnostic, 997
Peritoneovenous shunting, 1125, 1126, *1126*
  anesthesia administration in, 1125, 1126
  complications of, 1125, 1126, *1126*
  technique of, 1125, *1126*
Peritoneum, closure of, muscle relaxation for, inadequate, 1112, 1113
Peroneal nerve, common, injury to, lithotomy position in, 510
Perphenazine, for pain, 242(t)
Persistent pulmonary hypertension of the newborn (PPHN), 1018
PETCO$_2$, definition of, 350, 351
  monitoring of, techniques for, 353, 353(t)
  relationship of, to Paco$_2$, 351, *351*, 352
Pethidine, for acute pain, 241(t)
PFTs. See *Pulmonary function tests (PFTs)*.
pH, intracellular, definition of, 733, 734
  maintenance of, in general anesthesia, 593
  measurement of, 786
  of local anesthetics, adjustment of, 643
  relationship of, to hydrogen ion concentration, 733, 733(t)
pH stat method, of arterial blood gas analysis, 342
Phantom limb pain, 1254
  causes of, 1254
  prevention of, 1254
Pharmacodynamics, of inhalation anesthesia, 607, 608, *608*, 608(t)
Pharmacokinetics, 561–565
  of inhalation anesthesia, 607, 608, *608*, 608(t)
Pharyngeal abscess, 1273
  airway management in, 1273
Pharyngeal tracheal lumen airway (PTLA), 300
  in cardiopulmonary resuscitation, 837
Pharyngeal tubes, 299–301, *300*
  use of, method of, 299–301
Pharynx, intubation of, factors in, 441, 442

Pharynx *(Continued)*
  visualization of, before tracheal intubation, 930
Phenelzine, drug interactions with, 655(t)
  for pain, 242(t)
Phenobarbital, 159(t)
  drug interactions with, 645(t)
Phenoperidine, use of, in liver disease, 1344(t)
Phenothiazines, adverse effects of, 656(t)
  analgesic potential of, 242(t), 244(t)
  drug interactions with, 652(t)
Phenoxybenzamine, analgesic potential of, 244(t)
Phenylephrine, effects of, physiologic, 1285(t)
  for intraoperative hemodynamic stabilization, in shock, 690(t)
  for perioperative myocardial dysfunction, 766(t)
  in pediatric cardiovascular surgery, 1146(t)
  isoproterenol with, 145(t)
Phenytoin, 159(t)
  drug interactions with, 644(t), 645(t), 647(t), 652(t)
  for eclamptic seizures, 158
  perioperative use of, 7
Pheochromocytoma, 1317, 1318
  and hyperthermia, 824, 824(t)
  assessment of, preoperative, 194, 195
  clinical features of, 194
  definition of, 194
  management of, perioperative, 195, 196
    preoperative, 195, 195(t), 1317, 1318
  postoperative considerations in, 196
  removal of, anesthetic choice in, 1318, 1318(t)
    hypotension after, 1318
  screening tests for, 1317
  signs and symptoms of, 1317
Phosphate, disorders of, 727
Phosphate buffers, in acid-base balance, 736
Phosphodiesterase inhibitors, for anaphylaxis, 748
Phosphorus, 177, 178, 178(t)
  imbalance of, management of, 177
Photoplethysmography, in blood pressure measurement, 371
Phrenic nerve(s), anatomy of, 525
  blockade of, in supraclavicular block, 529
  damage to, alveolar hypoventilation in, 804
  effects of, 1275
  impairment of, in postoperative hypoventilation, 84
  location of, 500
pH-stat, 327, 328
Physical examination, in preanesthetic evaluation, 9–11, *10*, 11(t)
Physical incompatibility, of drugs, causes of, 640, 641
Physical status, ASA classification of, 127, 127(t)
Physical therapy, for pain, in adults, 255, 256, 256(t)
Physician(s), fees of, setting of, 114
  supply of, in health care cost, 114
Physician's Current Procedural Terminology, Fourth Edition, 111
Physostigmine, for anticholinergic overdose, 164
  in sedation reversal, 96
PIE (pulmonary interstitial emphysema), radiographic findings in, 216, 219, *221*
Piezoelectric crystal absorption, in anesthetic agent monitoring, 349(t)
Pilot tube, valve of, dysfunction of, 951
Pin Index Safety System (PISS), 277, *279*
''Pink puffers,'' 149

Pipeline, of high-pressure anesthesia machine, operating pressure of, 279

Piperazine, adverse effects of, 656(t)

Pipercuronium, dose of, in children, 1056(t) effects of, physiologic, 1285(t)

Piperidine, adverse effects of, 656(t)

Piroxicam, for acute pain, 240(t)

PISS (Pin Index Safety System), 277, *279*

Pituitary gland, anterior, dysfunction of, in diabetes insipidus, 187
  diseases of, 185–189, 186(t)–188(t)
  dynamic testing of, in Addison's disease diagnosis, 191
  neoplasm of, properties of, 1303(t)
  structural components of, 1312
  surgery of, 1312, *1313*

pKa, of local anesthetic agents, 624, 624(t)

Placenta, drug transport across, 566

Plasma, fresh-frozen, administration of, in orthotopic liver transplantation, 1342

Plasma osmolality (Posm), calculation of, 172
  in intracranial neoplasm surgery, 1308, 1308(t)

Plasma proteins, in drug distribution, 648

Plasmalyte A, in orthotopic liver transplantation, 1342, 1342(t)

Plasmapheresis, for myasthenia gravis, 153

Plaster splints, dangers of, 1263

Plateau waves, 770, *770*

Platelet(s), dysfunction of, after cardiopulmonary bypass, 1189
  infusion of, before aortic cross-clamp removal, 1230
  transfusion of, in splenectomy, 1122

Platelet-activating factor (PAF), cardiopulmonary effects of, 745

Plethysmography, impedance, in cardiac output measurement, 380
  in sympathetic nerve block evaluation, 486

Pleural pressure, ventilatory work in, 809, 810

Plica mediana dorsalis, 471, *472*

Plumb-bob supraclavicular block, 528, *528*

Pmv, in pulmonary edema, 970

Pneumocephalus, and delayed awakening, 165

Pneumocytes, in pulmonary edema, 969

Pneumoencephalography, technique of, 905

Pneumomediastinum, radiographic findings in, 219, *223*

Pneumonia, after trauma surgery, 1008

Pneumonitis, aspiration, 3, *3*
  during outpatient surgery, prevention of, 1395, 1395(t)

Pneumoperitoneum, radiographic findings in, 226, *231*

Pneumotachography, in tidal volume monitoring, 346

Pneumothorax, and alveolar hypoventilation, 805, 806
  during living-related donor harvesting, for renal transplantation, 1368
  needle-induced, algorithm for, *1257*
  nephrectomy and, 1242
  open, assessment of, 993
  paravertebral block and, 487, *487*
  radiographic findings in, 219, *221, 222*
  supraclavicular block and, 528
  sympathetic nerve block and, 492
  tension, after trauma surgery, 1007
    assessment of, 992, 993
    traumatic, assessment of, 995

Pneupac Model 2-R ventilator, 427(t)

PNS (parasympathetic nervous system), postoperative activity of, factors in, 94(t)

Po₂, measurement of, 786

Polio blade, 303

Polymorphonuclear leukocytes, in multiple system organ failure, 1010

Polymyxin A, perioperative use of, 9(t)

Polymyxin B, drug interactions with, 652(t)
  perioperative use of, 9(t)

Polyuria, 385, 386
  definition of, 181
  postoperative, 95, 95(t)

Polyvinyl chloride tubes, for tracheal intubation, in laryngeal laser operations, 1375(t), 1376

Pons, function of, evaluation of, 773

Ponstel, for acute pain, 240(t)

Porphyria, delayed emergence in, 164(t)
  intermittent, genetic factors in, 569

Portacaval shunts, *1127*

Portosystemic shunting, 1126–1130, *1127, 1128*, 1129(t)
  complications of, 1130
  fluid management in, 1129, 1130
  liver function in, optimization of, 1129
  postoperative outcome in, factors in, 1128, 1129(t)
  types of, 1126–1128, *1127, 1128*

Position(ing). See also names of specific positions.
  changes in, in postoperative pulmonary blood flow, 80
  for anesthesia induction, in orthotopic liver transplantation, 1343
  for axillary block, 529
  for caudal anesthesia, 523, *524*
  for donor nephrectomy, 1366, *1367*
  for epidural anesthesia, 521
  for extracorporeal shock wave lithotripsy, risks of, 1382, 1382(t), 1383
  for intercostal nerve block, 534
  for interpleural block, 536
  for interscalene block, 526
  for intracranial neoplasm surgery, 1307
  for intravenous regional anesthesia, of upper extremity, 530
  for lateral femoral cutaneous nerve block, 533
  for middle ear surgery, 1271
  for neurologic surgery, 1286, 1286(t)
    errors in, 1286, 1286(t)
  for orthopedic surgery, 1260, 1261, *1261*
  for pediatric cardiovascular surgery, 1147, 1148
  for renal transplantation, 1365
  for sciatic nerve block, 531, *531*
  for spinal anesthesia, 517
  for spinal surgery, 1299, *1299*, 1300
  for supraclavicular block, classic, 527
    plumb-bob, 528
  for vascular access, 543, 544(t)
  in cervical myelopathy, 1296
  in cervical radiculopathy, 1296
  in thoracoabdominal aneurysm management, 1219
  of surgical patient, 503–513
    complications of, 104
      incidence of, 505
    documentation of, 505, *506*
    injuries caused by, 162, 162(t), 504, 504(t), 505, 511, 511(t), 512
    sequelae of, 504, *504*
    with neck injury, 512
    with rheumatoid arthritis, 512, 513
  preoperative, in pulmonary edema, 973, 974

Positive airway pressure, effects on, of intrahospital patient transport, 422, 423
  in laryngeal laser operations, 1377

Positive end-expiratory pressure (PEEP), for hypoxia, during thoracic surgery, 1205, 1206, *1206*
  for postoperative hypoxemia, 79
  in shock, 693
  preoperative, in pulmonary edema, 974
  registration of, on breathing system pressure gauge, 288, *289*
  ventilatory work in, 810–812, *811*

Positive-pressure ventilation, urine output with, 385

Posm (plasma osmolality), calculation of, 172
  in intracranial neoplasm surgery, 1308, 1308(t)

Postanesthesia care, standards for, 73, 74(t)

Postanesthesia care unit (PACU), 73–104
  acid-base problems in, 101, 102
  administration of, 73
  admission to, 73, 74, *74*, 74(t), 75(t)
    report of, 74, 75(t)
  central nervous system function in, 95–98, 96(t), 97(t)
  complications in, 103, 104
    rate of, 73, *74*
  discharge from, criteria for, 75, 75(t), 76
    postponement of, 76
  electrocardiographic abnormalities in, 92–94, *93*, 94(t)
  glucose/electrolyte abnormalities in, 102, 103
  hypertension in, 91, 92, 92(t)
  hyperthermia in, 101
  hypotension in, 88–91, 88(t), *89*
  hypothermia in, 100, 101
  hypoxemia in, oxygen therapy for, 793, 793(t), *794*
  injuries in, 104
  laboratory tests in, 74
  monitoring in, 73, 74
  nausea and vomiting in, 99, 100
  negligence in, 56
  oxygenation in, 77–80
  pain in, assessment of, 76
    control of, 76, 77
  patient coverage in, 73
  patient transport to, *594*, 595, *595*, 596
    oxygen administration during, 595, *595*, 595(t)
    ventilation during, 595, 596
  performance evaluation in, 73
  policies and procedures of, 73
  pulmonary aspiration in, 85–87, 85(t)
    risk of, 87
  pulse oximetry in, 796, 797
  renal function assessment in, 95
  shivering in, consequences of, 821, 821(t)
    treatment of, 823, 823(t)
  ventilation in, 81–85, 81(t)–83(t), *82, 83*, 85(t)

Postanesthesia recovery, 73–104

Post–dural puncture headache, 167
  causes of, 538, 539(t)
  characteristics of, 539
  epidural blood patch for, 539
  incidence of, minimization of, 539

Posterior dural fold, in lumbar spine, 471

Posterior fossa surgery, electrophysiologic monitoring during, 161

Posterior pituitary gland, 1312

Posterior tibial nerve, in ankle block, 534

Postganglionic fibers, of sympathetic nervous system, 485

Postintubation croup, 1062

Postpartum back ache (PPB), 478

Postperfusion syndrome, 1349

Postreperfusion lung, after cardiopulmonary bypass, 1188

Post-tetanic count, in nerve stimulation, 418, 418(t)

Post-tetanic facilitation, in nerve stimulation, 418

Potassium, 173–175, 174(t), 175(t)
disorders of, 725, 725(t), 726
after pediatric cardiopulmonary bypass, 1155
in nerve conduction, 621, 622, 623
level of, in neurologic diseases, succinylcholine effects on, 156, 156(t)
low, perioperative effects of, 5, 6

Potassium titanyl phosphate laser, 1371(t)

PPB (postpartum back ache), 478

PPHN (persistent pulmonary hypertension of the newborn), 1018

PPO (preferred provider organization), 113

PR interval, alterations in, 363(t)

Prazosin, drug interactions with, 655(t)

Preanesthetic evaluation, 1–17
allergic responses in, 9
consultations in, 14, 15, 15(t)
history in, 2–5, 3–6
social, 9
in anesthetic choice, 585, 585(t)
in orthotopic liver transplantation, 1335–1342
laboratory testing in, 11, 12, 12, 12(t)
medication review in, 5–8, 6, 7(t), 8, 9(t)
nil per os (NPO) status duration in, 15, 16, 17, 17(t)
of cervical spine anomalies, 463
of "do-not-resuscitate" patient, 17
of pediatric pain, 263
physical examination in, 9–11, 10, 11(t)
preoperative medications in, 15, 15(t), 16, 16(t)
procedure for, 1, 2
purposes of, 1
special testing in, 12–14, 12(t), 13, 14(t)

Preanhepatic phase, of orthotopic liver transplantation, 1345
physiologic changes during, 1346, 1346(t), 1347

Precordial thump, in cardiopulmonary resuscitation, 841

Prednisolone, for bronchial asthma, 958(t)
in adrenal replacement therapy, 192(t)

Prednisone, complications of, 1330(t)
for bronchial asthma, 958(t)
in adrenal replacement therapy, 192(t)

Pre-eclampsia, 157, 158, 1094, 1095
delayed emergence in, 164(t)
neurologic evaluation in, 157

Preferred provider organization (PPO), 113

Preganglionic fibers, of sympathetic nervous system, 483, 484

Pregnancy, cardiopulmonary bypass in, 1106, 1107
cytomegalovirus infection in, 864
extracorporeal shock wave lithotripsy in, 1382
history of, 4
inhalation anesthesia in, 616
local anesthetic toxicity in, 634
lumbar spine changes in, 474, 475
osmotic diuretics in, 1106
physiologic changes in, 1002, 1003, 1003(t)
effects of, on anesthesia, 1100(t)
normal, 1082–1085, 1083(t), 1084
quadriplegia in, autonomic dysreflexia with, 494
surgery in, nonobstetric, 1099–1107
anesthesia for, 1099–1101, 1100(t), 1105–1107, 1105(t), 1106(t)
hyperventilation prevention in, 1106
hypothermia in, safety of, 1106

Pregnancy (Continued)
preparation for, 1104, 1105, 1105(t)
reasons for, 1099(t)
peripheral nerve injury during, 162, 163
trauma in, 1002, 1003, 1003(t)

Preinduction denitrogenation, 344, 345

Preload, control of, during thoracic aorta cross-clamping, 1226
in right ventricular failure, after cardiopulmonary bypass, 1182, 1183
goal for, after cardiopulmonary bypass, 1181
in aortic stenosis, 1171
in stroke volume, 757, 758
optimization of, in intraoperative hemodynamic stabilization, 689
quantification of, 763

Preload dependence, in end-stage heart disease, 1322

Premature ventricular contractions (PVCs), electrocardiographic characteristics of, 367
history of, 3
intraoperative, in children, 1060
postoperative, management of, 139, 139(t)
treatment of, emergency, 850

Prematurity, apnea of, 81, 82
retinopathy of, 1020, 1020, 1021
oxygen therapy in, 793

Premedication, 576–583
benzodiazepines in, 579–581, 579(t), 580
contraindications to, 578, 579(t)
drugs for, 583
for computed tomography, 910, 910(t)
for heart transplantation, 1323
for neurologic surgery, 1287
for neurovascular surgery, 1292, 1293
for orthotopic liver transplantation, 1340
for outpatient surgery, 1395, 1396
transmucosal approaches to, 1396
for renal transplantation, 1362
for spinal surgery, 1298
in bronchial asthma, 959
in children, 1046–1049, 1048(t), 1049
anticholinergic agents in, 1047
aspiration prophylaxis in, 1048, 1049, 1049
before outpatient surgery, 1395
candidates for, 1046, 1047
goals of, 1046
midazolam in, 580
sedation in, 1047, 1048, 1048(t)
in congenital heart disease, 1044
in intracranial neoplasm, 1306, 1306(t)
in neonates, 1022

Preoperative visit, 576–583
gastric content modification during, 581–583, 581, 582, 582(t)
pharmacologic evaluation in, 578, 578(t), 579

Preoxygenation, 344, 345
for general anesthesia, 586–588, 587
in apnea, in hypoxemia prevention, 795
in facemask ventilation, 925

Present illness, history of, 2

Pressure points, 504(t)
of geriatric patients, 1070

Pressure-equalizing tube, placement of, in children, 1064

Pre-use check protocols, in anesthesia machine troubleshooting, 292–294, 293(t)

PRIA (Peer Review Improvement Act), 32

Prilocaine, 631
in amide metabolism, 625
in children, dosage of, 267(t)
pharmacology of, 516(t)
properties of, clinical, 627(t)

Primidone, 159(t)

Priming, in orthotopic liver transplantation, 1342

PRO (Professional Review Organization), 32

Probe, for temperature monitoring, 429, 430, 430, 430(t), 431

Procainamide, action of, mechanism of, 847
after heart transplantation, 1327
for supraventricular tachycardia, after cardiopulmonary bypass, 1187(t)
for ventricular tachydysrhythmia, 1186(t)
in cardiopulmonary resuscitation, 847
complications of, 847
dosage of, 847
indications for, 847
in pediatric cardiovascular surgery, 1146(t)
perioperative use of, 6

Procaine, 630
action of, duration of, 516
pharmacology of, 516(t)
properties of, clinical, 628(t)

Procardia, analgesic potential of, 244(t)

Professional Review Organization (PRO), 32

Promethazine, drug interactions with, 652(t)
for imaging studies, 911(t)

Prone jackknife position, for spinal anesthesia, 517

Prone position, for caudal anesthesia, 523, 524
for surgery, problems associated with, 507, 507, 508

Propofol, drug interactions with, 653(t), 655(t), 658
effects of, on evoked potentials, 406(t), 408(t)
physiologic, 1285(t)
for imaging studies, 911(t)
for outpatient surgery, 1397, 1398, 1398(t)
in children, 1056
for intravenous induction, 1052(t)
in geriatric patients, 1075
in shock, 688
intravenous, 602, 602
properties of, 598(t), 600(t)
recovery time for, 1398(t)

Propranolol, drug interactions with, 645(t), 646(t)
use of, in liver disease, 1344(t)
perioperative, pulmonary effects of, 151

Propylthiouracil (PTU), for hyperthyroidism, 199
perioperative use of, 7

Prostaglandin E$_1$, for pediatric cardiovascular surgery, 1144, 1146(t)
for right ventricular failure, after cardiopulmonary bypass, 1183
in heart transplantation, 1328

Prostaglandins, cardiopulmonary effects of, 745
for shock, 665

Prostate, balloon dilatation of, 1237, 1238
anesthesia for, 1237, 1238
sedoanalgesia for, 1238
resection of, 1238–1240
transurethral. See *Transurethral resection of prostate (TURP)*.
surgery of, 1237–1240, 1238(t), 1239, 1239(t), 1240

Prostatectomy, open, 1238
and venous air embolism, 1238

Prosthesis, infected, removal of, blood loss in, 1249

Prosthetic heart valve, anticoagulation with, perioperative management of, 138

Protamine, after cardiopulmonary bypass, and coagulopathy, 1189
dose of, 1185–1187
pediatric, 1154
in pediatric cardiovascular surgery, 1146(t)

Protamine (*Continued*)
toxicity of, manifestations and risks of, 1187, 1188
Protein(s), metabolism of, after trauma surgery, 1006
plasma, in drug distribution, 648
ryanodine receptor, 831
serum, effects of, on serum calcium level, 1313
Protein binding, in drug distribution, 565, 648, 648(t)
of intravenous anesthetic agents, 597
of local anesthetic agents, 623, 624, 624(t), 634
Protocol, pre-use, in anesthesia machine troubleshooting, 292–294, 293(t)
Prozac, drug interactions with, 651(t)
Pseudocholinesterase, abnormal, in alveolar hypoventilation, 804
response to, genetic factors in, 569
Pseudoephedrine, drug interactions with, 655(t)
Pseudotumor cerebri, 157
PSRO (Peer Standards Review Organization), 32
PSVT (paroxysmal supraventricular tachycardia), treatment of, emergency, 850
Psychogenic pain, 234
Psychosis, Korsakoff's, 165
Psychotherapy, for pain, chronic, 256
in adults, 256, 257, 257(t)
in suicide prevention, in chronic pain, 256
PTCA (percutaneous transluminal coronary angioplasty), in cardiogenic shock, 673, 674
myocardial ischemia after, onset of, 1168, 1168(t)
PTH (parathyroid hormone), function of, 1313
in calcium control, 202
measurement of, preoperative, in parathyroid function assessment, 202
PTLA (pharyngeal tracheal lumen airway), 300
in cardiopulmonary resuscitation, 837
PTU (propylthiouracil), for hyperthyroidism, 199
perioperative use of, 7
Pudendal nerves, anatomy of, 1234
Puerperium, inhalation anesthesia in, 616
Pulmonary artery, enlargement of, in emphysema, radiographic demonstration of, 213, 216, *217*
in temperature monitoring, 431
normal anatomy of, radiographic demonstration of, 213
occlusion of, unilateral, thoracic surgery in, 1201, 1202
oxygenation of, in critical illness, 788, 788(t)
rupture of, during catheterization, factors in, 557, 557(t)
Pulmonary artery catheterization, before cardiopulmonary bypass, 1178, 1179
complications of, 377, 377(t), 557, 557(t), 558
enhancement of, 377, 378, *378*, 378(t)
equipment for, 543
in cardiovascular surgery, 1166, 1166(t), 1167(t)
pediatric, 1148(t), 1149
in heart transplantation, 1324
in myocardial ischemia detection, 1169
in aortic vascular surgery, 1221
in perioperative myocardial dysfunction monitoring, 766, 767
in renal transplantation, 1362
indications for, 14, 545, 548(t)
intraoperative, in pulmonary edema, 977
modifications of, 378, 378(t)
preoperative, in pulmonary edema, 975, 976

Pulmonary artery catheterization (*Continued*)
radiographic findings with, 223
techniques of, 557, 558
tip placement in, 376
Pulmonary artery occlusion pressure (PAOP), in perioperative myocardial ischemia assessment, 755(t)
in pulmonary edema, 972
in right ventricular dysfunction, 679
measurement of, 375, 376, 376(t)
reduction of, nitroglycerin in, 760, *761*
Pulmonary artery pressure (PAP), 375–378
in postoperative pulmonary blood flow, 80
monitoring of, in geriatric patient, 1074
indications for, 375, 376
intraoperative, 69
validity of, 376, 376(t)
waveform characteristics in, 376
Pulmonary capillary oxygen content, formula for, 692(t)
Pulmonary capillary pressure, in cardiogenic shock, 675, *675*
Pulmonary compliance, in pulmonary edema, 972, *973*
in tracheal tube placement verification, 943
reduction in, and difficult ventilation, 947
causes of, 83(t), 813
in alveolar hypoventilation, 806, *806*, 807
in facemask airway obstruction, management of, 926
intraoperative, 84
preoperative, 83, 84
treatment of, 84
ventilatory work with, 813, *813*
Pulmonary consultation, 143–151
benefits of, 143, 144
intraoperative, 145, 146
postoperative, 146–151, *147*, 147(t)–149(t), *150*
specifics of, 144, 145, 145(t)
unnecessary, 144
Pulmonary contusion, and alveolar hypoventilation, 805
traumatic, assessment of, 995
Pulmonary edema, 969–981
after battlefield surgery, 881
after cardiac surgery, 980, 981
after lung resection, 980
aortic cross-clamping in, 980
cardiogenic, radiographic findings in, 216
clinical implications of, 971, 971(t), 972, *973*
colloid therapy in, 720
differential diagnosis of, pulmonary artery catheterization in, 977
in anaphylaxis, treatment of, 747
in reduced postoperative functional residual capacity, 79
intraoperative, 976, 977
conditions associated with, 969, 970(t)
negative-pressure, 978, 979
neurogenic, 977
noncardiogenic, radiographic findings in, 216
pathogenesis of, 969, *970*
anatomic considerations in, 969, *970*
pathophysiology of, 969–971, *970*
postoperative, 978, *978*, 979, *979*, 979(t)
causes of, 978, *978*
presentation of, 969, *970*
pressure vs. permeability, 971, 971(t)
radiographic findings in, 216, *218*
re-expansion, 979
treatment of, preoperative, 973–976, 974(t), *975*
unilateral, 979, 980, *980*
Pulmonary embolism, after orthopedic surgery, with regional anesthesia, 1257, 1258
in postoperative dead space changes, 85

Pulmonary failure, acute, in shock, 695, *695*, 695(t)
Pulmonary function, as extubation criterion, 949
before intracranial neoplasm surgery, 1306
before spinal surgery, in anesthetic management, 1298
effects on, of abdominal surgery, 1130–1132, *1130*, *1131*, 1131(t)
of postoperative abdominal pain, 1131, 1131(t)
of postoperative pain control, 147
in anesthetic risk, 66
in bronchial asthma, 956, *956*, 957
in pregnant patient, during nonobstetric surgery, 1100
preanesthetic evaluation of, 13, 14, 14(t)
Pulmonary function tests (PFTs), for thoracic surgery, 1200–1202
in chronic obstructive pulmonary disease, 964, *964*, 964(t), 965
postoperative, 149, *150*
Pulmonary hypertension, in heart transplantation, 1328, 1329
Pulmonary interstitial emphysema (PIE), radiographic findings in, 216, 219, *221*
Pulmonary interstitium, in pulmonary edema, 969, *970*
Pulmonary mechanoreceptors, in alveolar hyperventilation, 809
Pulmonary system, barotrauma of, radiographic findings in, 216, 219, *221–223*
disease of, management of, in aortic vascular surgery, 1214
pre-existing, preoperative pulmonary consultation in, 143
disorders of, after cardiopulmonary bypass, 1188
fluid therapy and, 729
in chronic liver disease, 1336
in hypoxemia, 783–785, *784*, 785(t)
in shock, 692, 693, *693*
postoperative, 143, 143(t)
effects on, of immersion, for extracorporeal shock wave lithotripsy, 1384
of subarachnoid hemorrhage, 1292
postoperative pain in, 246
preanesthetic evaluation of, 3
status of, postoperative, management of, 150, *150*
Pulmonary vascular resistance (PVR), effects on, of alveolar hyperventilation, 808
of alveolar hypoventilation, 801
in congenital heart disease, 1044
in neonate, 1140
in pulmonary artery pressure monitoring, 376
in right ventricular failure, after cardiopulmonary bypass, 1183
increase in, abnormal ventilation with, control of, 814
during cardiopulmonary bypass weaning, in pediatric cardiovascular surgery, 1153, *1153*, 1153(t)
parameters for, 691(t)
Pulmonary vasculature, in pulmonary edema, radiographic demonstration of, 216, *218*
normal anatomy of, radiographic, 213
Pulse, monitoring of, in anesthetized patient, 336, 337, 337(t)
Pulse oximetry, 338, 354–356, *356*
accuracy of, 787, 787(t)
applications of, 355, 356, 787
errors in, sources of, 354, 355, *356*
in abnormal ventilation, 800
in anesthetic risk, 67
in blood gas measurement, 787, 787(t), 788
in burn surgery, 709

Pulse oximetry (Continued)
in geriatric patient, 1073
in postanesthesia care unit, 796, 797
in postoperative monitoring, 250
in shock, 679
intraoperative, in children, 1059
in neonates, 1025, 1026
principles of, 787
reliability of, 787, 788
use of, near magnetic resonance imaging
scanner, 916
Pulseless electrical activity, cardiopulmonary
resuscitation in, 851
Pump(s), centrifugal, 322, 322
in cardiopulmonary bypass, 321, 322, 322
roller, 321, 322
Pump lung, after cardiopulmonary bypass, 1188
PVCs. See Premature ventricular contractions
(PVCs).
PVD (peripheral vascular disease), blood
pressure differences in, 10
P$\bar{v}o_2$, in postoperative hypoxemia, 80
PVR. See Pulmonary vascular resistance
(PVR).
Pyloric stenosis, in neonates, 1026, 1026, 1027
Pyridostigmine, for myasthenia gravis, 153

Q waves, in myocardial infarction, 364, 365(t)
QA. See Quality assurance (QA).
QA/I (quality assessment and improvement), 36
QRS complex, 362
$\dot{Q}sp/\dot{Q}t$, calculation of, 788, 789, 789
Quadriplegia, autonomic dysreflexia with, in
pregnancy, 494
Quality assessment and improvement (QA/I),
36
Quality assurance (QA), 31–52
academic organizations in, 35
assessment in, method of, 34
ongoing, 41, 41(t), 42
automated anesthesia recordkeepers in, 28,
29
data in, aggregate, accuracy of, 34
gathering of, 34
normalized, 45
database software in, 41, 43–46, 45
selection of, 51, 52
definitions in, quality of, 34
efficiency of, 41
ground rules for, 38–40
historical considerations in, 31, 32
implementation of, 38–40
in battlefield surgery, 881, 881(t), 882
in outpatient surgery, 1405
indicators of, applicability of, 34
JCAHO approach to, 36–38, 37, 39
departmental role in, 36
freestanding review committees in, 36
quality screening/concurrent monitoring in,
36–38, 37, 39
retrospective review in, 36
statistical quality control in, 36
monthly report on, 45, 46–48
paperwork in, 35
peer review organizations in, 32, 33
process of, 35
outcome in, 35, 36
analysis of, 35, 36
confounding variables in, 36
structure in, 35
program for, characteristics of, 38
evolution of, 33, 34
pitfalls of, 33, 45
regulators of, 35
responsive action in, 45, 46–48

Quality assurance (QA) (Continued)
theoretic basis of, 35
Questionnaire, computerized, in preanesthetic
evaluation, 1, 2
"Quick connectors," 277, 279
Quincke-Babcock needle, for spinal anesthesia,
518, 518
Quinidine, after heart transplantation, 1327
drug interactions with, 646(t), 647(t), 653(t)
perioperative use of, 6
Quinine, drug interactions with, 647(t), 653(t)
Quinsy, 1273

RAAC (renin-angiotensin-aldosterone
complex), in urine output, 384
Radial artery, catheterization of, 496, 497
advantages of, 548(t)
disadvantages of, 548(t)
techiques of, 547, 548
Radial nerve, injury of, surgical position in,
512
prevention of, 511(t)
Radiant heater, in skin surface warming, 435
Radiation, coherent, 1370
medical applications of, 1371, 1371(t),
1372
production of, 1370, 1371
exposure to, damage from, mechanisms of,
898
during imaging studies, 898, 899, 899(t)
effects of, acute, 898, 899(t)
genetic, 898, 899
late, 898, 899(t)
in heat loss, 693, 694, 818, 818(t)
Radiation therapy, 897–918
anesthesia for, 916–918, 917
risks of, 916
technique of, 916
Radical head/neck surgery, 1274, 1275, 1275
Radicals, oxygen-free, in reperfusion injury,
326
Radiculopathy, 1296, 1296, 1296(t)
cervical, intubation in, 1296
positioning in, 1296
in pregnancy, 163
lumbar, 1296, 1297
thoracic, 1296, 1297
Radioallergosorbent test, in perioperative
anaphylaxis evaluation, 749, 750
Radiography, 897–918
chest. See Chest radiography.
in pain diagnosis, in adults, 239, 239(t)
of abdomen, 226, 229–232
of neck, 223–226, 225, 227, 228
Radioiodine, for hyperthyroidism, 199
Radiology, before tracheal intubation, 930
diagnostic, procedures for, 905
in trauma assessment, 995
therapeutic, nonvascular interventions in,
906–909, 906(t)
vascular interventions in, 905, 906
complications of, 906
trauma series in, 988, 988(t)
Radiology consultation, 211–232
Radionuclide angiography, before
cardiovascular surgery, 1159
gated, in coronary artery disease evaluation,
13
Radionuclide studies, preoperative, 65, 66
Raman spectroscopy, in anesthetic agent
monitoring, 348
Ranitidine, drug interactions with, 646(t)
in aspiration pneumonitis prevention, for outpatient surgery, 1395(t)
in children, 1049

Rapid-infusion system (RIS), in orthotopic liver
transplantation, 1342, 1342(t)
mechanism of, 1352, 1352, 1353, 1353
RBCs (red blood cells), administration of, in
orthotopic liver transplantation, 1342
transfusion of, in intraoperative hemodynamic stabilization, 692
RBF (renal blood flow), autoregulation of, 384
RBRV (resource-based relative-value) scale, in
health care services payment, 110–112,
112
criticism of, 111, 112
Reactive airway disease, halothane in, 611
Record, anesthetic. See Anesthetic record.
Recovery, postanesthesia, 73–104
Recruitment, alveolar, 795
Rectal induction, in children, 1052
Rectum, in temperature monitoring, 432, 433
Recurrent laryngeal nerve, blockade of, in
awake tracheal intubation, 1280
damage to, during thyroid surgery, 1316
effects of, 1274, 1275
Red blood cells (RBCs), administration of, in
orthotopic liver transplantation, 1342
transfusion of, in intraoperative hemody-
namic stabilization, 692
Red rubber tubes, for tracheal intubation, in
laryngeal laser operations, 1375(t), 1376
Re-entrant depolarization, postoperative, 93, 93
Re-entry, in dysrhythmia genesis, 365, 365
Reflectance oximetry, 354
Reflex(es), airway, loss of, in pulmonary
aspiration, 86
changes in, after heart transplantation, 1327
sympathogalvanic, during sympathetic nerve
block, 486, 487, 487
Reflex mechanism, of abdominal surgical
hypotension, 114, 115, 115
Reflex sympathetic dystrophy, pain in, in
children, 273
Regional analgesia, in children, 267–270
contraindications to, 267
pharmacology of, 267
Regional anesthesia, 514–540
advantages of, 69
cardiovascular effects of, 537
centroneuraxis blocks in, 516–524, 518–524
choice of, factors in, 515, 516, 516(t)
complications of, 536–540
contraindications to, 514, 515
effects of, on fluid balance, 715, 716
on postoperative cerebral dysfunction, in
geriatric patients, 1079, 1079
for abdominal surgery, general anesthesia
with, 1114
for extracorporeal shock wave lithotripsy,
1386, 1386(t), 1387
for orthopedic surgery, 1255–1258, 1256–
1258
advantages of, 1257, 1258, 1258
for outpatient surgery, 1400
for pacemaker implantation, 1193
for pain, after outpatient surgery, 1405(t)
in adults, 253, 254
in postanesthesia care unit, 77
for renal transplantation, 1363, 1363(t)
in autonomic dysreflexia prevention, 494
in autonomic nervous system blockade, 485
in bronchial asthma, 959, 960
in children, 1060, 1060(t), 1061, 1061
in chronic obstructive pulmonary disease,
966
in geriatric patients, 1076, 1077, 1077(t)
in hip fracture morbidity/mortality, 1257
in myocardial dysfunction, 759, 760
in obstetric patient, 1092, 1093, 1093
toxic effects of, 1092

Regional anesthesia (Continued)
  in pseudotumor cerebri, 157
  in rheumatoid arthritis, 1250, 1251
  indications for, 514, 515
  induction area for, 515
  intravenous. See Intravenous regional anesthesia.
  nerve stimulator in, 539, 540
  of inguinal region, complications of, 1236
    technique of, 1234–1236, 1235, 1236
  of lower extremity, 531–534, 531–534
  of upper extremity, 524–531, 525–530
  philosophy of, 514, 515, 515
  success of, factors in, 516
  truncal blocks in, 534–536, 535, 536
  use of, with seizure disorders, 159
Regional wall motion abnormalities (RWMAs), 1168, 1168(t)
Regurgitation, aortic, preoperative assessment of, 138
  in aortic insufficiency, 1172
  mitral. See Mitral regurgitation.
  treatment of, in pulmonary aspiration prevention, 87
Reintubation, after difficult extubation, 950
Rejection, after heart transplantation, 1330
Relaxation, in psychologic surgical preparation, 578
  neuromuscular, incomplete reversal of, 84
  of abdominal wall, 1109
  perineal, for cesarean section, 1091
  uterine, for cesarean section, 1091, 1091(t)
Renal. See also Kidney entries.
Renal blood flow (RBF), autoregulation of, 384
Renal failure, abnormalities with, 1359, 1360, 1360(t)
  after trauma surgery, 1009, 1009(t)
  anesthetic implications of, 180, 180
  causes of, in surgical patients, 181
  chronic, abnormal drug responses with, 1361, 1361(t)
    glomerular filtration rate in, 180
    history of, 4
    serum creatinine in, 180
    stages of, 179, 180, 180
  delayed emergence in, 164(t)
  drug choice in, 182, 183
  fluid therapy in, 729
  in obstructive jaundice, 1122, 1123
  postoperative, after cardiopulmonary bypass, 330
  risk factors for, perioperative, 180, 181(t)
Renal function, assessment of, in diabetes mellitus, 207
  in postanesthesia care unit, 95
  compromised, 179–182, 180, 181, 181(t), 182(t)
  in geriatric patients, 1072
  effects on, of cardiopulmonary bypass, 330
    of colloid therapy, 720
    of immersion, for extracorporeal shock wave lithotripsy, 1384
    of inhalation anesthesia, 613, 614
  preservation of, in aortic vascular surgery, 1219, 1220, 1220(t)
Renal function tests, 178, 179, 179, 180
Renal insufficiency, anesthetic implications of, 180, 180
  history of, 4
Renal transplantation, 1358–1368, 1358
  anesthesia for, immunosuppression effects on, 1361, 1362
    induction of, 1362–1364, 1362(t), 1363(t)
    maintenance of, 1364, 1365, 1365(t)
    regional, 1363, 1363(t)
  blood loss during, 1368
  cadaveric donor harvesting in, 1366, 1366(t)

Renal transplantation (Continued)
  dialysis before, 1361
  donor kidney for, preservation of, 1358
    protection of, 1368
  immunosuppression protocols in, 1358, 1359(t)
  living-related donor harvesting in, 1366–1368, 1367
  monitoring in, 1362, 1362(t), 1363
  positioning for, 1365
  postoperative care in, 1365, 1366
  premedication for, 1362
  preoperative concerns in, 1358–1362, 1360(t), 1361(t)
  revascularization in, 1364
  tissue matching for, 1358
Renal tubules, development of, in neonate, 1017
  distal, in cation exchange, 736, 736
Renin, measurement of, in Addison's disease diagnosis, 192
Renin-angiotensin-aldosterone complex (RAAC), in urine output, 384
Renoplegia, in renal function preservation, in aortic vascular surgery, 1220
Reocclusion, in cardiogenic shock, 673
Reperfusion, in cardiogenic shock, 673
Reperfusion injury, in cardiopulmonary bypass, 325, 326
Repolarization, 362
Reserpine, drug interactions with, 655(t)
Resorption atelectasis, postoperative, 78
Resource-based relative-value (RBRV) scale, in health care services payment, 110–112, 112
  criticism of, 111, 112
Respiration, disorders of, extubation in, 950
  in acromegaly, perioperative management of, 186
  in altered sensorium, during emergence, 98
  in hypothyroidism, 200
  effects on, of inhalation anesthesia, 610–612, 610(t), 611, 612
  of scoliosis, 1253
  kidney stone movement with, effects of, on extracorporeal shock wave lithotripsy, 1385
Respiratory acidosis, 733, 737, 737
  compensation for, 737, 737
  factors in, 802, 802(t), 803
  metabolic alkalosis with, 740, 740
  treatment of, 737
Respiratory alkalosis, 737, 738
  compensation for, 738
  metabolic acidosis with, 740, 740
  treatment of, 738
Respiratory center, depression of, causes of, 803, 804
  stimulation of, in alveolar hyperventilation, 808
Respiratory compromise, in anaphylactic shock, 681
Respiratory depression, and postoperative hypoxemia, 77, 78
  drug-induced, postoperative, 81
    reversal of, 81
  peridural opiates in, 248
  postanesthetic, correction of, 806
  with high-dose opioids, for cardiovascular surgery, 1173
Respiratory effort, 799
Respiratory failure, after trauma surgery, 1008
Respiratory index (RI), 790, 790(t)
Respiratory monitoring, 341–358
Respiratory quotient, formula for, 692(t)

Respiratory therapy, postoperative, indications for, 148
Respiratory tract, changes in, in pregnancy, 1084
  disorders of, Trendelenburg surgical positioning in, 510
  lower, laser surgery in, 1378
  of neonates, 1014, 1014, 1015
Restraint, for postoperative delirium, 166
Restrictive ventilatory defect (RVD), postoperative pulmonary function tests with, 149
Resuscitation, drug, for burn surgery, 709, 709(t)
  fluid, in thermal injuries, 705, 706, 706(t)
  of neonates, 1033–1035, 1033(t), 1034, 1035(t), 1097
    drug therapy in, 1034, 1035, 1035(t)
  prehospital, in shock, 666, 667
  Trendelenburg position for, 510
Retarded patients, dental repairs in, 1275, 1276
Retinopathy of prematurity (ROP), 1020, 1020, 1021
  oxygen therapy in, 793
Retractor, Millard-Dingman, 1272, 1273
Retransplantation, after orthotopic liver transplantation, anesthesia for, 1356
Retrolental fibroplasia, 1020, 1021
Retroperitoneal injuries, 1001
Revascularization, coronary, before noncardiac surgery, 134, 135
  in renal transplantation, 1364
  surgical, in cardiogenic shock, 673–675
Review of systems, in preanesthetic evaluation, 2
Revised Trauma Score, 984, 984
Rewarming, postoperative, consequences of, 821
Rheumatic fever, history of, 2
Rheumatic heart disease, in obstetric patient, 1094, 1094, 1095
Rheumatoid arthritis, 1250, 1251, 1251
  airway disorders in, 1250, 1250
  cricoarytenoid joints in, 445
  effects of, on anesthetic technique, 585(t)
    on cervical spine anatomy, 464, 465, 465
  history of, 5, 5
  regional anesthesia in, 1250, 1251
  surgical positioning in, 512, 513
  systemic involvement in, 1250
RI (respiratory index), 790, 790(t)
Richmond screw, in intracranial pressure measurement, 394, 394
Rifampin, drug interactions with, 644(t), 645(t)
Right atrial cannulation, for cardiopulmonary bypass, 1178
Right heart, function of, with left ventricular assist device, 677
Right lateral decubitus position, 506
Right upper lobe bronchus, occlusion of, and hypoxemia, 948, 948
Right ventricle, dysfunction of, acute, causes of, 679
  failure of, after cardiopulmonary bypass, causes of, 1182, 1183, 1183(t)
    in heart transplantation, 1328, 1328(t), 1329
  hypertrophy of, in emphysema, radiographic demonstration of, 216, 217
  infarction of, 678, 679, 679
    and shock, 678
    treatment of, 678, 679, 679
Right ventricular stroke work index, parameters for, 691(t)

Right-to-left shunting, in hypoxemia, 785
  increase in, and alveolar hypoventilation, 803
  physiologic, formula for, 692(t)
RIS (rapid-infusion system), in orthotopic liver
    transplantation, 1342, 1342(t)
  mechanism of, 1352, 1352, 1353, 1353
Risk, analysis of, 62–71
  anesthetic, monitoring in, 67
  factors in, perioperative, nonmodifiable, 64
    physiologic, functional, 64–67
  preoperative, assessment of, 64, 64(t)
  stratification of, 62
Ritalin, analgesic potential of, 244(t)
Robertshaw tube, 313
ROP (retinopathy of prematurity), 1020, 1020,
    1021
  oxygen therapy in, 793
Ropivacaine, 631
  properties of, clinical, 627(t)
  toxicity of, 632, 632, 633, 633
Rule of elevens, 700, 701(t)
Rule of nines, 700, 701(t)
RVD (restrictive ventilatory defect),
    postoperative pulmonary function tests
    with, 149
RWMAs (regional wall motion abnormalities),
    1168, 1168(t)
Ryanodine receptor protein, 831

Saccular aneurysm, 1211, 1212
Sacral canal, 478, 479
Sacral hiatus, 478
  in children, location of, 269, 269
Sacral spine, 478, 478, 479
  abnormalities of, 479
  anatomy of, 478, 479
Sacrum, anatomy of, surface, 523, 523
Safety, electrical, 885, 886
SAH. See Subarachnoid hemorrhage (SAH).
Salicylates, drug interactions with, 645(t)
  for acute pain, 240(t)
Saline, hypertonic, 720
    complications of, 720
    distribution of, 720
    for syndrome of inappropriate antidiuretic
        hormone secretion, 189
    in shock, 668
  intravenous, for anaphylactic shock, 683(t)
Salt, excretion of, in urine output, 385
  retention of, in urine output, 384
"Salt intolerance," 715
Saphenous nerve, in ankle block, 533
  injury to, lithotomy position in, 510
Scavenging, of anesthetic agents, 869, 870, 870
Schwannoma, acoustic, properties of, 1303(t)
Sciatic nerve, injury to, lithotomy position in,
    510
Sciatic nerve block, 531, 531, 532
  anatomic considerations in, 531
  drug choice for, 531
  needle placement for, 531, 532
  patient selection for, 531
  positioning for, 531, 531
  potential problems with, 532
Scintigraphy, thallium, in cardiac risk
    assessment, 130, 131
  preoperative, 65, 66
SCIWORA (spinal cord injury without
    radiographic abnormalities), 467, 468
Scoliosis, 469, 1252–1254, 1253
  anesthetic considerations in, 471(t)
  cause of, anesthetic implications of, 1252,
    1253
  classification of, etiologic, 469, 469(t)

Scoliosis (Continued)
  conditions associated with, 469–471, 470,
    471(t)
  correction of, anterior approach to, 1254
    indications for, 1253
  in lumbar spine, 473
  respiratory effects of, 1253
  severe, pathophysiology of, 1253, 1253
  spinal cord function in, intraoperative moni-
    toring of, 1253, 1254
Scopolamine, before cardiovascular surgery,
    1164(t)
  in postoperative nausea prevention, 99
SCPP (spinal cord perfusion pressure),
    determination of, 1192
SCr (serum creatinine), in chronic renal failure,
    180
  measurement of, indications for, 179, 180
SCS (spinal cord stimulator), for pain, in
    adults, 255, 255(t)
SCV. See Subclavian vein (SCV).
Seat belts, and traumatic abdominal injury, 998
Secobarbital, for imaging studies, 911(t)
Sedation, before cardiovascular surgery,
    considerations in, 1164, 1164(t)
  before neurovascular surgery, 1292
  before thoracic aortic surgery, 1165
  conscious, for pediatric cancer therapy–
    related pain, 272
  continuous, in children, for procedural pain,
    270
  effects of, on fetus, 1103
  for awake neurologic monitoring, 392
  for battlefield surgery, 881
  for computed tomography, 910, 910(t), 911,
    911(t)
  for imaging studies, administration of, 900,
    901
    goals of, 900, 900(t)
  for laryngoscopy, in children, 1063
  for magnetic resonance imaging, in children,
    1063, 1064
  for pediatric cardiovascular surgery, 1144
  for potentially difficult intubation, 936
  for tracheal intubation, in conscious patients,
    453
  for vascular access, 544
  in altered sensorium, during emergence, 98
  in pediatric premedication, 1047, 1048,
    1048(t)
  in persistent postoperative unconsciousness,
    96
  level of, bedside rating of, 250(t)
  postoperative, assessment of, 165(t)
  preoperative, in intracranial pressure control,
    777
Sedoanalgesia, for balloon dilatation, of
    prostate, 1238
  for extracorporeal shock wave lithotripsy,
    1386(t), 1387
  for noninvasive genitourinary surgery, 1244
Segmental wall motion abnormalities
    (SWMAs), detection of, transesophageal
    echocardiography in, 382, 382(t)
Seizure(s), 159–161
  anesthesia management in, 159
  control of, sodium thiopental in, 601
    surgery for, monitoring during, 392
  delayed emergence in, 164(t)
  evaluation of, preoperative, 159
  history of, 4
  in eclampsia, management of, 157, 158
  intracranial neoplasm and, 1305
  intraoperative monitoring of, 159–161, 160,
    160(t)
  local anesthetic overdose and, treatment of,
    635

Seizure(s) (Continued)
  treatment of, in postischemic/hypoxic brain
    injury, 166
Self-insurance, 61
Sellick maneuver, 590, 591
  in children, 1050
Sensorium, altered, during emergence,
    differential diagnosis of, 97, 97(t), 98
  treatment of, 98
Sepsis, after transurethral resection of the
    prostate, 1239
  arterial catheterization and, 550
  delayed emergence in, 164(t)
  fluid therapy in, 730
  of burn wound, 702, 707, 708
    treatment of, 707, 708
  regional anesthesia in, 515
Septic joint, 1247(t)
Septic shock, 686–688, 687
  causes of, 686, 687
  cellular mechanics of, 687, 687
  hemodynamic derangements in, 687
  management of, goals of, 687, 688
  oxygen delivery in, 688
Serax, for acute pain, 242(t)
Serum creatinine (SCr), in chronic renal failure,
    180
  measurement of, indications for, 179, 180
Service/risk profile, 36, 37
Set-point regulatory functions, changes in, in
    pregnancy, 1085
Sevoflurane, effects of, circulatory, 612(t)
  for outpatient surgery, 617, 1397
  in renal disease, 613, 614
Seward laryngoscope, 305
Shewhart, W.A., 31
Shivering, clonic, 821
  during epidural anesthesia, 818
  effects of, in febrile patients, 821, 822
    on postoperative hypothermia, 100
  postoperative, 820, 821
    consequences of, 821, 821(t)
    treatment of, 823, 823(t)
Shock, 663–695
  anaphylactic. See Anaphylactic shock.
  cardiogenic. See Cardiogenic shock.
  electric, circuit requirements for, 888, 889
    determinants of, 887, 888, 888
  fluid therapy in, 667, 668
  hematocrit in, 668
  hemodynamics of, intraoperative stabilization
    of, 689–692, 689
  hemoglobin in, 668
  hemorrhage in, evaluation of, 666, 667(t)
  hypotension in, 663, 664
  hypothermia in, 693, 694
    mechanisms of, 693, 694
  hypovolemic, classes of, 993, 993(t)
  management of, intraoperative, 688, 689
    anesthesia for, 688, 689
      induction of, 688
    pharmacologic, 665, 666
  monitoring in, 679, 680, 680
  myocardial oxygen consumption in, 668–
    672, 669–671
  organ responses to, 694, 694, 695, 695,
    695(t)
  oxygen delivery/consumption in, 666
  pulmonary dysfunction in, 692, 693, 693
  resuscitation in, prehospital, 666, 667
  right ventricular infarction and, 678
  septic. See Septic shock.
  spinal cord. See Spinal cord shock.
  vascular endothelium in, 664, 665
Shoulder(s), dislocation of, 1247(t)
  replacement of, total, blood loss in, 1249

Shoulder(s) *(Continued)*
  surgery of, ambulatory, considerations in, 1255
Shunt effect, correction of, in hypoxemia, 791, *791*
Shunt effect unit, 784
Shunt unit, 784
Shunt(ing), for thoracic aorta surgery, 1192, *1192*, 1225
  in paraplegia prevention, 1228
  in renal function preservation, in aortic vascular surgery, 1220
  intrapulmonary, physiologic, calculation of, 788, 789
  LeVeen, 1125, 1126, *1126*
  mesocaval, *1128*
  of carotid artery, electroencephalography in, 401
  peritoneovenous. See *Peritonevenous shunting.*
  portacaval, *1127*
  portosystemic. See *Portosystemic shunting.*
  right-to-left, in hypoxemia, 785
    increase in, and alveolar hypoventilation, 803
    physiologic, formula for, 692(t)
  splenorenal, *1128*
  systemic to pulmonary artery, occlusion of, during pediatric cardiopulmonary bypass, 1151
SIADH. See *Syndrome of inappropriate antidiuretic hormone (SIADH) secretion.*
Sick sinus syndrome, electrocardiographic characteristics of, 366
Sickle cell crisis, pain in, treatment of, 273
Sickling test, in congenital heart disease assessment, 1143
Siker blade, 303
Silent myocardial ischemia (SMI), 364
  and pulmonary edema, 981
  detection of, ambulatory electrocardiography in, 134
  in coronary artery disease, 754
  in geriatric patients, 1071
  morbidity and mortality of, 756(t)
  perioperative, 754, 756(t)
Silicone tubes, for tracheal intubation, in laryngeal laser operations, 1375(t), 1376
Silver nitrate, for burn wound sepsis, 708
Silver sulfadiazine, for burn wound sepsis, 707
Sims' position, for sciatic nerve block, 531, *531*
SIMV (synchronized intermittent mandatory ventilation), 148
Sinemet, in Parkinson's disease, 154
Single-twitch pattern, of nerve stimulation, 416, 417, *417*
Sinus bradycardia, electrocardiographic characteristics of, 366
  treatment of, emergency, 851
Sinus dysrhythmia, electrocardiographic characteristics of, 365, 366
Sinus node, rhythm of, in postoperative bradycardia, 94
Sinus tachycardia, electrocardiographic characteristics of, 366
  intraoperative, in children, 1060
  postoperative, 93, 94
    management of, 139
Sinusitis, 441
Sitting position, for spinal anesthesia, 517
Skeletal muscle, damage to, local anesthesia in, 637
  pain in, postoperative, causes of, 104
Skin, evaluation of, during sympathetic nerve block, 486
    preanesthetic, in children, 1041

Skin *(Continued)*
  grafting of, in burns, 708
  in temperature monitoring, 433, *434*
  injury to, lasers in, 1372
  of geriatric patients, 1070
  perfusion of, in transcutaneous blood gas measurement, 786, 787
  preparation of, for vascular access, 544
  surface of, warming of, methods of, 435, 436
Skin testing, in perioperative anaphylaxis evaluation, 750
Skull, fracture of, basilar, signs and symptoms of, 1278, 1278(t)
  neoplasm of, properties of, 1303(t)
SMI. See *Silent myocardial ischemia (SMI).*
Smokers, preoperative pulmonary consultation for, 143
Smoking, cessation of, preoperative, benefits of, 144, 145
  in chronic obstructive pulmonary disease, 966
  effects of, on aortic vascular surgery, 1214
  history of, in preanesthetic evaluation, 9
Smooth muscle, function of, alteration of, in pregnancy, 1083(t), 1084
Snow blade, 304
SNS. See *Sympathetic nervous system (SNS).*
Social history, in preanesthetic evaluation, 9
Soda lime, carbon dioxide absorption by, 287, 288(t), 356, *357*
  replacement of, 357
Sodium, 172, 172(t), 173, 173(t)
  disorders of, 723, 724, 724(t)
  in nerve conduction, 621, 622, *622*, *623*
  serum, changes in, in transurethral resection of the prostate syndrome, 1241, 1241(t)
  urinary, level of, in syndrome of inappropriate antidiuretic hormone secretion, 188
Sodium bicarbonate, action of, mechanism of, 845
  for anaphylaxis, 748
  for aortic cross-clamp removal, 1229, 1230
  for lactic acidosis, 739
  for metabolic acidosis, with alveolar hyperventilation, 814, 815
  in cardiopulmonary resuscitation, 845, 846
    administration of, route of, 846
    complications of, 846, 846(t)
    dosage of, 846
    indications for, 845
  in neonatal resuscitation, 1035(t)
  in pediatric cardiovascular surgery, 1146(t)
Sodium chloride, in perioperative fluid therapy, 171
Sodium dichloroacetate, for lactic acidosis, 739
Sodium nitroprusside, effects of, physiologic, 1285(t)
  for intraoperative myocardial ischemia, 760, 761
  for nonobstetric surgery, in pregnant patient, 1106
  for thoracic aorta surgery, 1224
    and spinal cord ischemia, 1193
Sodium pentothal, properties of, 598(t), 600(t)
Sodium thiopental, 601, 602, *602*
  distribution of, 601
  effects of, beneficial, 601
    duration of, 601
    on fetus, 1103
  in battlefield surgery, 880
  in geriatric patients, 1074
  in intraoperative intracranial pressure control, 779
  in pediatric cardiovascular surgery, 1146(t)
  in seizure control, 601
  side effects of, 601, 602

Sodium warfarin, discontinuation of, preoperative, guidelines for, 155
Soft tissue, injury to, electrical, 700
  postoperative, 103, 104
  obstruction of, in facemask airway obstruction, 926
    in increased postoperative upper airways resistance, 82
  prevertebral, radiographic findings in, 224
Solid waste, definition of, 115
Somatic nervous system, vs. autonomic nervous system, 482, 483
Somatosensory evoked potentials (SSEPs), 160
  alterations in, factors in, 406, 406(t)
  anesthetic effects on, 161, 406(t)
  definition of, 402, *403*
  in cerebral cortical function monitoring, 404, 405, *405*
  in intraoperative spinal cord function monitoring, 1253, 1254
  in thoracoabdominal aneurysm management, 1219
  monitoring of, during neurovascular surgery, 1293
  recording of, channels for, 402
    peripheral, 403
    spinal cord, 403, *403*
  use of, intraoperative, 403, 404, 404(t)
    in neurologic injury prevention, 405, *405*
Sonoclot, in coagulation disorder diagnosis, after cardiopulmonary bypass, 1190
Sore throat, tracheal intubation and, 456
Spectral array, in electroencephalography, 399, *399*
Spectroscopy, infrared, 349(t)
  mass, 348, 349(t)
  Raman, 348
Specular echos, 381
Spermatic cord, nerve block of, 1236, *1236*
Sphincter, laryngeal, 448–450, *449*
Sphincter of Oddi, contraction of, narcotic administration and, 1116, 1117
Sphygmomanometry, Doppler, 369, 370
Spina bifida, 472, 473
  epidural blockade in, 473
Spinal anesthesia, anatomic considerations in, 517, *518*
  complications of, neurologic, 163, 511
  continuous, problems with, 536, 537
  drug choice for, 517
  for abdominal surgery, 1113, 1114
  for extracorporeal shock wave lithotripsy, 1386, 1386(t)
  in children, 1060(t), 1061
  in geriatric patients, 1076, 1077, 1077(t)
  in obstetric patients, 1092, 1093
  in postoperative headache, 167
  inadvertent, during epidural anesthesia, 522, 523
  needle for, choice of, 517, 518, *518*
    placement of, 519, *519*, 520, *520*
      lumbosacral, 520, *520*
      midline, 519, *519*
      paramedian, 519, 520, *520*
  patient selection for, 517
  positions for, 517
  technique of, 516, 517
  thermoregulation during, 817, 818
Spinal angiography, risks of, 905
Spinal canal, in pregnancy, 474
Spinal cord, blood flow to, anatomy of, 1226–1228, *1227*
  autoregulation of, 1283
  during thoracic aorta cross-clamping, 1223

Spinal cord (*Continued*)
surgical blockage of, somatosensory
evoked potential monitoring in, 404
disease of, neural compression in, 1295(t)
function of, in scoliosis, intraoperative monitoring of, 1253, 1254
in thoracic spine, 468
injury to, 1301, 1302
alveolar hypoventilation and, 804
during tracheal intubation, 456
history of, 5
monitoring of, during patient transport,
428
systemic effects of, 685, 686
ischemia of, in thoracic aorta surgery, reduction of, 1193
perfusion of, control of, during thoracic aorta
cross-clamping, 1224, 1225
during descending aorta surgery, 1191,
1192
somatosensory evoked potential recording
over, 403, *403*
surgery of, 1295–1302
indications for, 1295, 1295(t), 1296
tethered, in lumbar spine, 473
Spinal cord injury without radiographic
abnormalities (SCIWORA), 467, 468
Spinal cord perfusion pressure (SCPP),
determination of, 1192
Spinal cord shock, 682–686
airway maintenance in, 685
anesthesia in, 686
induction of, 686
clinical presentation of, 684
epidemiology of, 682
management of, 685
pathophysiology of, 684, 684(t)
pharmacotherapy of, 684, 685
Spinal cord stimulator (SCS), for pain, in
adults, 255, 255(t)
Spinal fusion, epidural block in, 477, *477*
Spinal headache, in geriatric patients, 1077
Spinal microcatheter, use of, in geriatric
patients, 1077
with lidocaine, 636, 637
Spine, 458–479. See also *Vertebra(e)*.
anatomy of, vertebral, 458–460, *458–460*
cervical. See *Cervical spine*.
disease of, neural compression in, 1295(t)
embryologic development of, 458
fusion of, 1297
anesthetic considerations in, 1301
injury to, during tracheal intubation, 456
lumbar. See *Lumbar spine*.
neoplasms of, anesthetic considerations in,
1301
sacral, 478, *478*, 479
abnormalities of, 479
anatomy of, 478, 479
stabilization of, 1297
surgery of, 1295–1302
anesthesia for, 1299, 1299(t)
fluid therapy in, 1300
functional status before, importance of,
1297, 1298
indications for, 1295, 1295(t), 1296
instrumentation for, 1254
monitoring in, electrophysiologic, 161
factors in, 1298, 1298(t), 1299
somatosensory evoked potentials in,
403, 404
positioning for, 1299, *1299*, 1300
premedication in, 1298
thoracic. See *Thoracic spine*.
trauma to, anesthetic considerations in, 1301,
1302
Spinous processes, of thoracic spine, 468

Spirometry, 1200, 1201
assessment of, 1201
in bronchial asthma, 956, *956*, 957
in chronic obstructive pulmonary disease,
965
in preanesthetic evaluation, of pulmonary
function, 13, 14
in tidal volume monitoring, 345, 346
midflow measurements in, 1200, 1201
Splanchnic nerves, anatomy of, 1234
Splenectomy, 1122
platelet transfusion in, 1122
Splenorenal shunts, *1128*
Splinting, 1263
plaster, dangers of, 1263
Split function lung testing, 1201, 1202
SpO$_2$, measurement of, pulse oximetry in, 787,
787(t)
relationship of, to PaO$_2$, 782
Spondylitis, ankylosing, effects of, on cervical
spine anatomy, 465, *466*
Spondylosis, cervical, radiologic changes in,
463, 463(t)
Sprotte needle, for spinal anesthesia, 518, *518*
Squatting, in heart murmur evaluation, 11(t)
SSEPs. See *Somatosensory evoked potentials
(SSEPs)*.
ST segment, changes in, perioperative,
treatment of, 754, 755
depression of, conditions associated with,
1169(t)
displacement of, in ischemia detection, 363,
364
new-onset, 364, 364(t)
effect on, of normovolemic anemia, 671, *671*
Stadol, for acute pain, 241(t)
Standard bicarbonate, 735
Standing, in heart murmur evaluation, 11(t)
Starling equation, 719, 969–971, *970*
Stasis, zone of, in burns, 699
Status epilepticus, 167, 167(t)
treatment of, 167, 167(t)
Stein-Gates ventilator, 427(t)
Stellate ganglion, location of, 500
Stellate ganglion block, technique of, 489
Stent, placement of, in cardiogenic shock, 673,
674
Stereotactic surgery, for intracranial neoplasm,
1304, 1305, *1305*
Sternotomy, 1176
median, for automatic internal cardioverter-
defibrillator implantation, 1195
Steroids, epidural injection of, for chronic pain,
254
for pain, effects on, of concurrent medical
condition, 237
in cancer, 244(t)
for spinal cord shock, 684
hypothalamic-pituitary-adrenal axis suppression by, susceptibility to, 192, 192(t)
in intracranial pressure control, 777
replacement of, for adrenocortical insufficiency, 1318, *1319*
Stimulation, nerve. See *Nerve stimulation*.
Stomach, contents of, aspiration of, 3, *3*
full, and aspiration, 1000, 1001
difficult intubation in, 941, 942
in pregnant patient, during nonobstetric
surgery, 1100
Storz fiberoptic laryngoscope, rigid, 306
Strangulated hernia, repair of, anesthesia for,
1134
Stray capacitor, 886
Streptomycin, perioperative use of, 9(t)
Stress, hypothalamic-pituitary-adrenal axis
function during, 192
of cardiopulmonary bypass, 326, *326*

Stress (*Continued*)
of inhalation anesthesia, 613
Stress hormones, increase in, after trauma
surgery, 1006
Stress test, in cardiac risk assessment,
pharmacologic, 131, 132
preoperative, 130–132, *132*
Stretch injuries, surgical positioning in, 504,
505, *505*
"String of pearls" sign, in bowel obstruction,
226, *229*
Stroke, 154, 154(t), 155, 155(t)
cardioembolic, and delayed awakening, 165
effects of, on anesthetic technique, 585(t)
hemiparetic, succinylcholine use after, 155
perioperative, predictors of, 154, 155(t)
risk of, 154, 154(t)
prevention of, intraoperative, 155
preoperative, 154, 155
surgery after, safety of, 155
Stroke index, parameters for, 691(t)
Stroke volume, determinants of, 757, 758, *758*
parameters for, 691(t)
Stunned myocardium, 756, *756*
Stylet(s), for intubation, 315
tracheal, 451, 931, 932, *932*
for laryngotracheal anesthesia, function of,
316
liquid, in radial artery catheterization, 547,
548
Subarachnoid block, for nonobstetric surgery,
in pregnant patient, 1105
vasoconstrictor use with, 628
Subarachnoid hemorrhage (SAH), abnormal
intracranial pressure in, management of,
776
aneurysmal, classification of, 1292, 1292(t)
neurovascular surgery after, timing of, 1288
systemic effects of, 1292
Subarachnoid space, anatomy of, 460
sympathetic nerve block injection into, 492
Subclavian artery, puncture of, in
supraclavicular block, 529
Subclavian perivascular block, for orthopedic
surgery, 1256
Subclavian vein (SCV), anatomy of, on chest
radiography, 211–213
catheterization of, 501, *501*, 502
difficult, management of, 556
infraclavicular, 552, 553
lateral approach to, 553
midclavicular/medial approach to, 553
supraclavicular, 551, 552, *552*, *553*
anterior scalene/first rib approach to,
551, 552
clavicular notch approach to, 552, *553*
junctional approach to, 551, *552*, 553
technique of, 551–553, *552*, *553*
structures adjacent to, 502
Subdural bolt, in intracranial pressure
measurement, 394, *394*
Subdural hematoma, treatment of, 1005
Subdural space, anatomy of, 460
Subendocardial ischemia, perioperative, 753
Subluxation, atlantoaxial, causes of, 224, 226
radiographic findings in, 224, 226, *227*,
228
Submucosal dissection, nasal intubation and,
933, 934, *934*
Substance abuse, delayed emergence in, 164(t)
Succinylcholine, and hyperkalemia, in spinal
cord injury, 1301, 1302
contraindications to, 11
drug interactions with, 647(t), 653(t), 654(t)
effects of, on potassium level, in neurologic
diseases, 156, 156(t)

Succinylcholine *(Continued)*
  physiologic, 1285(t)
  for difficult intubation, 941
  in abdominal surgery, 1112, 1113
  in burn surgery, 710
  in children, 1056
  in pediatric cardiovascular surgery, 1146(t)
  in renal transplantation, 1363
  injection of, defasciculating drug administra-
    tion before, 591, 591(t)
  selection of, factors in, 572
  use of, after hemiparetic stroke, 155
    in liver disease, 1344(t)
Suctioning, bronchial, 443, *443*
Sufentanil, drug interactions with, 654(t)
  for cardiovascular surgery, 1175(t)
  for pain, acute, 241(t)
    in children, 265
    in liver disease, 1344(t)
  in pediatric premedication, 1048, 1048(t)
  intraspinal, 248(t)
  intravenous, patient-controlled, guidelines
    for, 245(t)
  properties of, 598(t), 600(t)
Suicide, prevention of, in chronic pain, 256
Sulindac, for acute pain, 240(t)
Superconducting magnets, potential hazards of,
  914–915
Superficial peroneal nerve, in ankle block, 533
Superficial temporal artery, catheterization of,
  498
Superior hypogastric plexus block, 489
  technique of, 490
Superior laryngeal nerve, blockade of, 446,
  446, 447, *447*
    in awake tracheal intubation, 1279, 1280
  damage to, effects of, 1274, 1275
Superior vena cava (SVC), normal anatomy of,
  on chest radiography, *212*, 213
Supine position, contoured, for surgery, 506,
  506, 507
  for surgery, problems associated with, 505–
    507, *506*, *507*
  moving from, to decubitus position, 507, 508
    to prone position, 507
Supplies, consumable, cost of, 117, 117(t)
Supraclavicular block, 527–529, *528*
  anatomic considerations in, 527
  applicability of, 529
  approach to, classic, 527, 528, *528*
    plumb-bob, 528, *528*
  drug choice for, 527
  patient selection for, 527
  potential problems with, 528, 529
Supraclavicular vein, catheterization of,
  advantages of, 546(t)
  disadvantages of, 546(t)
Supraspinous ligament, 459
Supraventricular premature impulses,
  postoperative, with aberrant conduction,
  93, *93*
Supraventricular tachycardia, history of, 3
Supraventricular tachydysrhythmias, after
  cardiopulmonary bypass, 1185, 1187(t)
Sural nerve, in ankle block, 534
Surfactant, exogenous, for infant respiratory
  distress syndrome, 1019
Surgery, battlefield. See *Battlefield surgery.*
  outpatient. See *Outpatient surgery.*
  previous, history of, 2
  psychologic preparation for, 576–578
    coping mechanisms in, 577, 578
SVC (superior vena cava), normal anatomy of,
  on chest radiography, *212*, 213
S͞vO₂, clinical significance of, 788, 788(t),
  789(t)

S͞vO₂ *(Continued)*
  monitoring of, in cardiovascular surgery,
    1167, 1167(t)
SVR. See *Systemic vascular resistance (SVR).*
Sweat tests, in sympathetic nerve block
  evaluation, 487
SWMAs (segmental wall motion
  abnormalities), detection of,
  transesophageal echocardiography in, 382,
  382
Sympathectomy, and relative hypovolemia, 89
Sympathetic nerve block(s), 485–492
  complications of, 491, 491(t)
    management of, 491, 492
  evaluation of, 486
  in children, 268
  indications for, 485, 485(t)
  lumbar, 489, *490*
  preparation for, 486
  radiologic assistance during, 490, 491
  regional, intravenous, 489
  technique of, 489, 490, *490*
  types of, 489(t)
Sympathetic nervous system (SNS), abdominal
  portion of, *488*
  activity of, postoperative, and relative hypo-
    volemia, 89
    factors in, 94(t)
  dysfunction of, in spinal cord injury, 1301
  effects on, of alveolar hypoventilation, 801
  in postoperative hypertension, 91, 92, 92(t)
  outflow of, dispersion/amplification of, 485
  regulation of, 483–485, *484*
Sympathogalvanic reflex, during sympathetic
  nerve block, 486, 487, *487*
Sympathomimetics, drug interactions with,
  654(t), 655(t)
  for intraoperative hemodynamic stabilization,
    in shock, 690, 690(t)
  in postoperative pulmonary blood flow, 80
Synapses, of autonomic nervous system, 482
Synchronized intermittent mandatory
  ventilation (SIMV), 148
Syncope, in aortic stenosis, 1161
Syndrome of inappropriate antidiuretic
  hormone (SIADH) secretion, 187–189,
  187(t), 1309
  causes of, 188
  diagnosis of, 187, 188, 188(t)
  management of, 188, 189
Systemic to pulmonary artery shunt, occlusion
  of, during pediatric cardiopulmonary
  bypass, 1151
Systemic vascular resistance (SVR), decrease
  in, postoperative, effects of, 90, 91
  during nonpulsatile cardiopulmonary bypass,
    330
  effects on, of alveolar hyperventilation, 807,
    808
    of immersion, for extracorporeal shock
      wave lithotripsy, 1383
  in aortic insufficiency, 1172
  in congenital heart disease, 1044
  parameters for, 691(t)
Systolic pressure, rate of, during isovolumic
  contraction, 763, 764

T wave, changes in, in ischemia, 363, *363*
T₃ (triiodothyronine), 196, 196(t)
T₄ (thyroxine), perioperative use of, 7
  ratio of, to thyroid-stimulating hormone, 197
  synthetic, for hypothyroidism, 197, 198
Tachycardia, and postoperative hypotension, 91
  atrial, paroxysmal, postoperative, 94, 94(t)

Tachycardia *(Continued)*
  control of, preoperative, in pheochromocy-
    toma, 195, 195(t)
  sinus. See *Sinus tachycardia.*
  supraventricular, history of, 3
  ventricular. See *Ventricular tachycardia.*
Tail coverage insurance, 60
Talwin, for acute pain, 241(t)
TBSA (total body surface area), in burns, 699–
  701, *701*
TCD (transcranial Doppler) ultrasonography,
  clinical applications of, 396–398
  in cerebral blood flow measurement, 396–
    398, *396*, *397*
TEE. See *Transesophageal echocardiography
  (TEE).*
Teeth. See also entries beginning *Dent-.*
  examination of, before intubation, 440
TEF (tracheoesophageal fistula), in neonate,
  1030, *1030*, 1031
TEG (thromboelastography), in coagulation
  disorder diagnosis, after cardiopulmonary
  bypass, 1190
  in orthotopic liver transplantation, 1353–
    1355, *1354*, *1355*
Temperature, ambient, compensation for, low-
  pressure anesthesia machine vaporizer in,
  282
  assessment of, instrumentation for, 338
  barometric, compensation for, low-pressure
    anesthesia machine vaporizer in, 282
  control of, in spinal cord shock, 686
  core, measurement of, 433, *435*
  effects on, of orthotopic liver transplantation,
    during anhepatic phase, 1348
    during preanhepatic phase, 1347
  fluctuations in, 817–832
    intraoperative, in children, 1060
  intraoperative, standards for, 123
  maximum, in malignant hyperthermia, 827,
    827(t)
  monitoring of, 429–436
    anatomic sites for, 430–433, *431–435*
    during sympathetic nerve block, 486
    in burn surgery, 709, 710
    in cardiovascular surgery, 1167, 1168,
      1168
    in geriatric patient, 1073
    in pediatric cardiovascular surgery, 1149,
      1150
    intraoperative, standards for, 68(t)
    probes for, 429, 430, *430*, 430(t), *431*
  of geriatric patients, 1070
  room, regulation of, in intraoperative hypo-
    thermia prevention, 433, 434
Temporal artery, catheterization of, advantages
  of, 548(t)
  disadvantages of, 548(t)
  superficial, catheterization of, 498
Temporomandibular joint (TMJ), injury of,
  effects of, 1278
Tenoxicam, for acute pain, 240(t)
TENS (transcutaneous electrical nerve
  stimulation), for pain, in adults, 254, 255
Tensilon, in myasthenia gravis, 154
Tension pneumothorax, after trauma surgery,
  1007
  assessment of, 992, 993
  traumatic, assessment of, 995
Ten-Twenty Electrode System, in
  electroencephalography, 398, 399, *399*
Teratogenicity, of anesthesia, 1102, 1102(t)
Terbutaline, 145(t)
  for bronchial asthma, 958(t)
Tetanic nerve stimulation, 418
Tetany, alveolar hyperventilation and, 807

Tetracaine, 631
 action of, duration of, *516*
 for spinal anesthesia, 517
 in children, dosage of, 267(t)
 pharmacology of, 516(t)
 properties of, clinical, 628(t)
Tetracycline, drug interactions with, 654(t)
 perioperative use of, 9(t)
Tetrahydrocannabinol, analgesic potential of,
 244(t)
Texas Health Policy Task Force Study, 54, 55
Thallium scintigraphy, in cardiac risk
 assessment, 130, 131
 preoperative, 65, 66
Thallium-201 perfusion scan, before
 cardiovascular surgery, 1158, 1159
Theophylline, drug interactions with, 644–
 646(t), 652(t), 653(t)
 for contrast agent reactions, 904
 preoperative blood level of, measurement of,
 150
 use of, intraoperative, 146
 with halothane, 150
Thermal injuries, 699–711
 and pulmonary injury, 704
 anesthesia for, 708–711
 classification of, 700, 701, *701*, 701(t)
 compartment syndromes in, assessment of,
 706, 707
 pathology of, 699, 700
 pathophysiology of, 701–704
 therapy of, definitive, 705–708
 initial, 704, 705
Thermistors, in temperature monitoring, 429
Thermocouples, in temperature monitoring, 429
Thermodilution, in cardiac output measurement,
 379, 379(t)
Thermogenesis, nonshivering, 1017
Thermography, in pain diagnosis, in adults, 239
Thermoregulation, after trauma surgery, 1006
 during anesthesia, 817, 818, *818*, 818(t)
 during emergence, 821, 821(t)
Theta rhythm, in electroencephalography, 400,
 400
Thiamylal, drug interactions with, 652(t)
Thiazide diuretics, drug interactions with,
 647(t)
 perioperative use of, 5, *6*
Thionamides, for hyperthyroidism, 201
Thiopental, contraindications to, 571
 drug interactions with, 652(t)
 for imaging studies, 910(t), 911(t)
 for intravenous induction, in children,
 1052(t)
 half-life of, 564, *564*
 in liver disease, 1344(t)
 in pediatric premedication, 1048(t)
 perioperative requirements for, 657(t)
 recovery time for, 1398(t)
Thioridazine, for pain, 242(t)
Thioxanthine, adverse effects of, 656(t)
 for pain, 242(t)
Third space losses, 716
 in abdominal surgery, 1119
 in renal transplantation, 1365
 intraoperative, in children, 1058
 postoperative, and absolute hypovolemia, 88
 replacement of, 723
Thoracic aorta, cross-clamping of,
 hemodynamic goals in, 1224
 precautions in, 1223–1225
 disease of, 1162, *1162*
 hemodynamic goals in, 1173, 1173(t)
 rupture of, 1162
 surgery of, anesthesia for, 1190–1193, *1192*
 sedation before, 1165
 shunting in, 1192, *1192*

Thoracic duct, location of, 501
Thoracic myelopathy, 1296, 1297
Thoracic radiculopathy, 1296, 1297
Thoracic spine, 468–471
 anatomy of, 468, 469
 curvature of, abnormal, 469, 469(t), *470*
 injury of, 1247(t)
 instability of, 471
 surgery of, head position in, 1299, *1299*
Thoracic surgery, 1200–1208
 anesthesia for, management of, 1202–1206,
 1202(t), *1203*, *1204*, 1205(t), *1206*
 complications of, pulmonary, classification
 of, 148(t)
 elective, delay of, pulmonary considerations
 in, 147, *147*
 functional residual capacity after, 79
 hypoxia during, management of, 1205,
 1205(t), *1206*
 pain after, management of, 1207, 1208, *1208*
 pulmonary consultation before, 143
 pulmonary function testing for, 1200–1202
 risk of, chronic obstructive pulmonary disease in, 966, 966(t)
Thoracoabdominal aneurysm, management of,
 1218, 1219
 repair of, 1216
Thoracolumbar spine, injury to, mechanisms of,
 471
Thoracotomy, anterior, for automatic internal
 cardioverter-defibrillator implantation,
 1195
 complications of, pulmonary, 147, 147(t)
Thorax, injuries of, traumatic, abdominal
 injuries with, 1005
 radiography of, 211–223
Three breath rule, 588
Throat, sore, tracheal intubation and, 456
Thrombocytopenia, after cardiopulmonary
 bypass, 1189
Thromboelastography (TEG), in coagulation
 disorder diagnosis, after cardiopulmonary
 bypass, 1190
 in orthotopic liver transplantation, 1353–
 1355, *1354*, *1355*
Thromboembolism, in persistent postoperative
 unconsciousness, 97
 pulmonary, after orthopedic surgery, with
 regional anesthesia, 1257, 1258
 venous, after orthopedic surgery, 1263, 1264
 prevention of, 1263, 1264
 risk factors for, 1263
Thrombolysis, in cardiogenic shock, 673, 674
 beta-blocker use after, 674
Thrombosis, arterial catheterization and, 549,
 550
 deep vein, after transurethral resection of the
 prostate, 1239, 1240
 venous, perioperative, antibiotic prophylaxis
 for, 15, 16(t)
 risk groups for, 16(t)
Thrombus, formation of, vascular endothelium
 in, 664
Thyroarytenoid muscles, external, 448
 internal, 448
Thyroid, desiccated, for hypothyroidism, 198
Thyroid arteries, location of, 500, 501
Thyroid cartilage, 444, *445*
 attachments of, 444, *445*
Thyroid gland, diseases of, 196–202, 196(t),
 198(t), 199(t)
 clinical features of, 198(t)
 history of, 4
 medication for, perioperative use of, 7
 dysfunction of, diagnosis of, 196, 196(t), 197
 in nonthyroidal illness, 197
 function of, testing of, 1314, 1315, 1315(t)

Thyroid gland *(Continued)*
 surgery of, 1314–1316
 recurrent laryngeal nerve damage during,
 1316
Thyroid hormone, administration of,
 perioperative, in hypothyroidism, 200
 biosynthesis of, 1314, *1315*
 level of, changes in, in nonthyroidal illness,
 197
 normalization of, for hyperthyroidism, 199,
 199(t)
 synthesis of, blockade of, 199
Thyroid storm, 199
 and hyperthermia, 824, 824(t)
 manifestations of, 1315, 1315(t)
Thyroiditis, Hashimoto's, 197
Thyroid-stimulating hormone (TSH), level of,
 changes in, in nonthyroidal illness, 197
 ratio of, to thyroxine, 197
Thyrotoxic crisis, 199
Thyrotoxicosis, cardiovascular effects of, 1315,
 1316
 treatment of, 1316(t)
Thyrotropin-releasing hormone (TRH), 196,
 196(t)
Thyroxine (T$_4$), perioperative use of, 7
 ratio of, to thyroid-stimulating hormone, 197
 synthetic, for hypothyroidism, 197, 198
L-Thyroxine, for hypothyroidism, 197, 201
Ticlid, in intraoperative stroke prevention, 155
Ticlopidine, in intraoperative stroke prevention,
 155
Tidal volume, monitoring of, 345–348, *348*
 end-tidal carbon dioxide in, 345, 346
 settings for, alterations in, 346–348
Tilt test, in dialysis patient, 183
Timolol, cardiovascular response to, 8, *8*
Tissue damage, MRI-induced, 913
Tissue elastance, in intracranial neoplasm, 1308
Tissue perfusion, restoration of, in trauma, 994
TMJ (temporomandibular joint), injury of,
 effects of, 1278
TNF (tumor necrosis factor), release of, in
 burns, 702, 702(t)
Tocainide, analgesic potential of, 244(t)
Tocolysis, prophylactic, during anesthesia,
 1104
Toe, in temperature monitoring, 433
Tolectin, for acute pain, 240(t)
Tolmetin, for acute pain, 240(t)
Tongue, displacement of, and difficult
 intubation, 930
 of neonates, 1014
Tonocard, analgesic potential of, 244(t)
Tonometry, arterial, in blood pressure
 measurement, 371
"Tonsil position," 1270, *1270*
Tonsillectomy, in children, 1064
 outpatient, 1393, 1394
Topical anesthesia, for awake tracheal
 intubation, 453, 1279
 to nose, 441
Toradol, for acute pain, 240(t)
Total body surface area (TBSA), in burns, 699–
 701, *701*
Total hip arthroplasty, blood loss in, 1249
 muscle relaxation during, 1250
Total joint replacement, 1248–1250, 1249(t)
 blood loss in, 1249, 1249(t)
 fluid requirements in, 1248, 1249
 in lower extremity, hypotension during, 1249
 invasive monitoring in, 1249
 without cement, 1250
Total knee replacement, blood loss in, 1249
Total shoulder replacement, blood loss in, 1249
Tourniquet(s), deflation of, intraoperative, 1262

Tourniquet(s) *(Continued)*
  physiologic effects of, 1263
  for arthroscopy, 1255
  for orthopedic surgery, 1261–1263, 1261(t),
    1263(t)
  inflation of, bleeding distal to, 1262
    for intravenous regional anesthesia, of
      upper extremity, 530
    hypertension during, 1263(t)
  inflation/release scheme for, 1262
  pressure of, optimal, 1262
  use of, complications of, 1261, 1261(t)
Tourniquet pain, causes of, 1262, 1263
  characteristics of, 1262, 1263(t)
  definition of, 1262, 1263, 1263(t)
  regional anesthesia in, 1258
Trace gas, exposure to, 868–870
  effects of, 868, 869
  sources of, 869, 869(t)
Trachea, anatomy of, 442, *442*, 443, *443*
  cross-sectional area of, in difficult intubation,
    932
  injuries of, traumatic, assessment of, 997
  of neonates, 1015
Tracheal extubation, in bronchial asthma, 960
  in spinal cord shock, 686
  intracranial pressure control during, 780
  postoperative, criteria for, 149(t)
  risks of, 310(t)
Tracheal intubation, 450–456
  advantages of, 450
  and soft tissue injury, 104
  atlanto-occipital gap effect on, 464
  awake, 1279, *1279*, 1280
    laryngeal nerve block in, recurrent, 1280
      superior, 1279, 1280
    patient preparation for, 1279
    translaryngeal analgesia for, 1280
  complications of, 455, *455*, 455(t), 456
  difficult, 442
    difficult ventilation/oxygenation after,
      945–948, 945(t)
    potential for, 936–938, *937*
  endoscopy with, 930, 931
  equipment for, 450, *450*, 451, *451*
  failure of, 456
    causes of, 928, *929*
    consequences of, 928
  for assisted ventilation, 450
  for laparoscopy, 1398, 1398(t)
    complications of, 1398, 1398(t)
  for refractory facemask airway obstruction,
    928
  in burn surgery, 711
  in cardiopulmonary resuscitation, 837
  in children, 1052
    for outpatient surgery, 1398, 1399
  in conscious patients, indications for, 453,
    453(t), 454
  in inhalation anesthesia, 589
  in laryngeal laser operations, 1375, 1375(t),
    1376, 1376(t)
    alternatives to, 1375
    laser-resistant wraps in, 1376, 1377,
      1377(t)
  in neonatal resuscitation, 1034
  in thermal injuries, 705
  in traumatic cervical spine injury, 1001
  indications for, 450
  physical examination in, 930
  purposes of, 928
  radiologic assessment before, 930
  risks of, 310(t)
  technical errors in, 931, 931(t)
  techniques of, 451–453, *452*
Tracheal tube(s), 450, 451
  construction of, 451

Tracheal tube(s) *(Continued)*
  diameter of, selection of, 932, 932(t)
  in ventilatory work, 811
  laser-resistant, 1377, 1377(t)
  malpositioning of, in alveolar hypoventila-
    tion, 802
  placement of, 942–944
    verification of, 942–944, 943(t)
  special purpose, 451
Tracheal tug, in anesthetized patient, 335, 336
Tracheitis, tracheal intubation and, 456
Tracheobronchial rupture, double-lumen tube
  in, 315
Tracheobronchial tree, anatomy of, *1203*
Tracheoesophageal fistula (TEF), in neonate,
  1030, *1030*, 1031
Tracheotomy, complications of, 317
  elective, for potentially difficult intubation,
    937, 938
  emergency, 940–941, 992
  for airway maintenance, 316, 317
  for pharyngeal abscess, 1273
  for proximal airways obstruction, 82
  in Ludwig's angina, 1274
  in thermal injuries, 705
  indications for, 1281
  tubes for, 317
Traction, in-line, of cervical spine, 468
  mesenteric, and hypotension, 1115, 1115(t)
Train-of-four pattern, of nerve stimulation, 417,
  417, 418
TRAM (transport remote acquisition monitor),
  424, *425*
Tranquilizers, in battlefield surgery, 881
  in chronic renal failure, 1361
  in malignant hyperthermia, 827(t)
Transcranial Doppler (TCD) ultrasonography,
  clinical applications of, 396–398
  in cerebral blood flow measurement, 396–
    398, *396*, *397*
Transcutaneous electrical nerve stimulation
  (TENS), for pain, in adults, 254, 255
Transducer(s), fluid-coupled, fidelity of, 372,
  372
  in blood pressure measurement, 371,
    371(t), 372
  in intracranial pressure measurement, 394,
    394, 395
Transesophageal echocardiography (TEE),
  clinical uses of, 380, 382, *382*, 382(t), 383
  future applications of, 383
  in aortic disease diagnosis, 1212, 1213(t)
  in burn surgery, 709
  in cardiac output measurement, 380, 381,
    381
  in myocardial ischemia detection, in aortic
    vascular surgery, 1220, 1221
    intraoperative, 755(t), 1169
  methodology of, 380
  perioperative, in myocardial monitoring, 136,
    767
  problems in, 383
  vs. electrocardiography, 382
Transfusion, of blood. See *Blood transfusion.*
  of platelets, in splenectomy, 1122
  of red blood cells, in intraoperative hemody-
    namic stabilization, 692
Transhepatic procedures, 908
Translaryngeal analgesia, for awake tracheal
  intubation, 1280
Translaryngeal jet ventilation, 1280, *1281*
Transmission oximetry, 354
Transmural ischemia, perioperative, 754, *754*
Transplantation, of bone marrow, inhalation
  anesthesia in, 615
  of heart. See *Heart transplantation.*
  of kidneys. See *Renal transplantation.*

Transplantation *(Continued)*
  of liver, orthotopic. See *Orthotopic liver
    transplantation (OLT).*
Transport remote acquisition monitor (TRAM),
  424, *425*
Transsphenoidal hypophysectomy, 1312, 1313,
  1313(t)
Transtracheal catheter ventilation, in
  cardiopulmonary resuscitation, 838–840,
  839
Transurethral resection of prostate (TURP),
  1238–1240
  anesthesia for, 1238
  coexisting disease with, 1238(t)
  complications of, 1238–1240, *1239*, 1239(t),
    1240
  fluid therapy in, 729, 730
Transurethral resection of prostate (TURP)
    syndrome, 730, 1240–1242
  causes of, 1240
  definition of, 1240
  diagnosis of, 1241, *1241*, 1241(t)
  treatment of, 1241, 1242
Tranylcypromine, drug interactions with, 655(t)
Trauma, 982–1010
  assessment of, history in, 990, 991, 991(t)
    initial, 990–999, 991(t), 995(t), *996–998*
    primary survey in, 990–995
    secondary survey in, 995–999
  categorization of, 982
  costs of, 983
  craniofacial. See *Craniofacial trauma.*
  emergency department preparation in, 985–
    990
  epidemiology of, 982–984, 983(t)
  fiberoptic bronchoscopy and, 306
  hypothermia in, 819
  in children, 1003–1005, 1004(t), 1005(t)
  in pregnancy, 1002, 1003, 1003(t)
  inhalation anesthesia in, 615, 616
  injuries in, severity of, assessment of, 984,
    984(t), 985
  multiple, 1005, 1006
    open fracture in, 1246
  operating room preparation in, 985–990
  orthopedic, 1246–1248, 1247(t), *1248*
  postoperative complications in, 1006–1010,
    1006(t), 1007(t), 1009(t)
  resuscitation in, strategy for, 990–999,
    993(t)–995(t)
  rural, 983
  significance of, 982, 983, 983(t)
  system for, expediting of, 988–990, 988(t),
    989
  to head, intracranial pressure control after,
    776, 777, 777(t)
  urban, 983
Trauma alert, 985
  operating room response to, 987
Trauma system, definition of, 983
Trauma team, members of, 985–987, 987(t)
Trazodone, drug interactions with, 651(t)
  for pain, 242(t)
Trendelenburg position, for surgery, problems
  associated with, 510
TRH (thyrotropin-releasing hormone), 196,
  196(t)
Triage, in battlefield surgery, 882
  in trauma care, 985, *986*
Triamcinolone, for bronchial asthma, 958(t)
Triazolam, for acute pain, 242(t)
  selection of, factors in, 572
Tricyclic antidepressants, drug interactions
  with, 650, 651
  for pain, effects on, of concurrent medical
    condition, 237
  use of, and hyperthermia, 826

Tricyclic antidepressants (Continued)
   perioperative, 7
Trifluoperazine, for pain, 242(t)
Triiodothyronine (T₃), 196, 196(t)
Trilisate, for acute pain, 240(t)
Trimethaphan, drug interactions with, 652(t)
   effects of, physiologic, 1285(t)
   for nonobstetric surgery, in pregnant patient, 1106
Trimethoprim-sulfamethoxazole, drug interactions with, 645(t)
Trimipramine, for pain, 242(t)
Tri-Service Anesthesia apparatus, 879, 879, 880
Tris(hydroxymethyl)aminomethane buffer, for lactic acidosis, 739
TRISS score, 985
Truncal blocks, 534–536, 535, 536
TSH (thyroid-stimulating hormone), level of, changes in, in nonthyroidal illness, 197
   ratio of, to thyroxine, 197
Tube(s). See also names of specific types of tubes.
   for tracheotomy, 317
   management of, during patient transport, 424
Tube changer, 316, 952
Tuberculosis, 865
Tubocurarine, dose of, in children, 1056(t)
Tumor(s). See also specific sites of tumors.
   in abnormal intracranial pressure, 772, 773
   of brain. See Intracranial neoplasm(s).
Tumor necrosis factor (TNF), release of, in burns, 702, 702(t)
Tuohy needle, for epidural anesthesia, 521, 521
TURP. See Transurethral resection of prostate (TURP).
TURP syndrome. See Transurethral resection of prostate (TURP) syndrome.
Two-dimensional echocardiography, 381
Tympanic membrane, in temperature monitoring, 431, 432

Ulnar nerve, injury of, surgical position in, 512
   prevention of, 511(t)
   stimulation of, electrode placement for, 414, 415, 415
Ultrasonography, continuous-wave, in cardiac output measurement, 380
   Doppler, pulsed-wave, in cardiac output measurement, 380
   transcranial, clinical applications of, 396–398
      in cerebral blood flow measurement, 396–398, 396, 397
Umbilical bridge, 1117, 1118
Umbilical catheterization, in neonate, 1024
Unconsciousness, persistent, differential diagnosis of, 96, 96(t)
United States, health care system in, cost containment in, 112–114
Universal precautions, in human immunodeficiency virus infection prevention, 856, 856(t)
Upper extremity(ies), intravenous regional anesthesia of. See Intravenous regional anesthesia, of upper extremity.
   nerves of, injuries of, 505
      peripheral, anatomy of, 524
Upper extremity nerve blocks, 524–531, 525–530, 1255, 1256, 1256
   anatomic considerations in, 524, 525
   intravenous, 1255
Upper respiratory infection (URI), in children, 1041, 1042
Urban warfare, 876
Urea, synthesis of, in acid-base balance, 737

Urea nitrogen, 178
Uremia, abnormal drug responses with, 1361, 1361(t)
   anesthetic implications of, 183, 184
   signs and symptoms of, 1360(t)
   water/electrolyte imbalance in, 183, 183(t)
Uremic syndrome, 182, 183
Urethroscopy, 1244
URI (upper respiratory infection), in children, 1041, 1042
Uric acid, measurement of, in syndrome of inappropriate antidiuretic hormone secretion, 188
Urinalysis, preoperative, indications for, 178
Urinary tract infection (UTI), after trauma surgery, 1008
   extracorporeal shock wave lithotripsy with, 1382
   history of, 4
Urine, composition of, in oliguria, 1337(t)
   monitoring of, in thoracoabdominal aneurysm management, 1219
   volume of, 178
Urine output, 384–386
   factors in, 384, 384, 384(t), 385
   in preoperative fluid deficit calculation, 722
   monitoring of, guidelines for, 180, 181, 181(t), 182(t)
      in burn surgery, 709
      in cardiovascular surgery, 1167
      in geriatric patient, 1074
Use-dependent block, in local anesthesia, 622, 623
Uteroplacental perfusion, anesthesia effects on, 1101, 1101(t)
Uterus, relaxation of, for cesarean section, 1091, 1091(t)
   vasoconstriction of, in pregnant patient, anesthesia effects on, 1101
UTI (urinary tract infection), after trauma surgery, 1008
   extracorporeal shock wave lithotripsy with, 1382
   history of, 4

v wave, 373
VADs (ventricular assist devices), for heart failure, after cardiopulmonary bypass, 1184, 1184(t), 1185
   in cardiogenic shock, 676, 677
   left, right heart function with, 677
Vagal block, of larynx, 446
Vagus nerve, location of, 500
Valium, for acute pain, 242(t)
Valproic acid, 159(t)
   drug interactions with, 645(t)
Valsalva's maneuver, in heart murmur evaluation, 11(t)
Valve(s), cardiac, abnormalities of, and postoperative hypotension, 90
   function of, assessment of, after cardiopulmonary bypass, 1185
      transesophageal echocardiography in, 383
   flow control, of low-pressure anesthesia machine, 281
   inspiratory, leak in, in capnography, 354, 355
   unidirectional, of breathing system, incompetency of, 286, 287
Valvular heart disease, history of, 2
   inhalation anesthesia in, 613
   perioperative management of, 137, 137(t), 138
   signs and symptoms of, 1161, 1162
Valvuloplasty, mitral, balloon, 138

Vancomycin, drug interactions with, 652(t)
   in bacterial endocarditis prophylaxis, 15(t)
Vaporizer(s), draw-over, in battlefield surgery, 879, 879
   of low-pressure anesthesia machine, accuracy of, at very low fresh gas flow rates, 283, 284
      in ambient temperature compensation, 282
      in barometric temperature compensation, 282
      in fluctuating back pressure compensation, 282, 283
      misfilling of, effects of, 283–285, 285(t)
      variable-bypass, 282, 283
   VerniTrol, in battlefield surgery, 878, 879, 879
Variable-bypass vaporizer, of low-pressure anesthesia machine, 282, 283
Varicella-zoster virus (VZV), epidemiology of, 862
   incidence of, 862
VAS (visual analogue scale), in pain rating, 235, 235
   use of, after thoracic surgery, 1208, 1208
Vascular access, 542–558
   analgesia/anesthesia/sedation for, 544
   equipment for, 542, 542(t), 543, 543(t)
   for myringotomy, 1268, 1269
   in burns, 708
   in children, 1056, 1057, 1057
   in neonates, 1024
   in pediatric trauma, 1004
   informed consent for, 543
   positioning for, 543, 544(t)
   preparation for, 543, 544, 544(t)
      skin, 544
Vascular bed, evaluation of, during sympathetic nerve block, 486
Vascular endothelium, in shock, 664, 665
Vascular exclusion, in liver resection, 1123
Vascular surgery, cardiac risk factors in, assessment of, 132, 133
   noncardiac, cardiac risk with, 126, 126(t)
   pain after, local anesthetics for, 247
Vascular system, anatomy of, 496–502
Vascular trauma, sympathetic nerve block and, 492
Vascularity, of intracranial neoplasm, 1304
Vasoactive drugs, for cardiopulmonary bypass weaning, in pediatric cardiovascular surgery, 1152
   for intraoperative hemodynamic stabilization, in shock, 689–691, 690, 690–692(t)
   in autonomic dysreflexia prevention, 494
Vasoconstriction, cerebral, alveolar hyperventilation and, 807
   for intraoperative blood loss, in burns, 708
   in cardiopulmonary resuscitation, 849, 850
   local anesthesia with, effects of, 626
      toxicity of, prevention of, 634, 635
   pulmonary, hypoxic, 1205
      ablation of, during anesthesia, 796
      in thoracoabdominal aneurysm management, 1218, 1219
   topical, in nasal intubation, 933, 934(t)
   urine output with, 384
   uterine, in pregnant patient, anesthesia effects on, 1101
Vasodilation, production of, local anesthetic agents in, 624, 624(t)
   urine output with, 385
Vasogenic edema, 1302
Vasopressin, deficiency of, in diabetes insipidus, 186
   response to, vs. diabetes insipidus, 187, 187(t)

Vasopressin *(Continued)*
  secretion of, ectopic, surgical treatment of,
    191
Vasopressors, for postoperative hypotension, 91
Vasospasm, cerebral, after intracranial
    aneurysm rupture, 1290, 1291, 1291(t)
  detection of, transcranial Doppler ultraso-
    nography in, 397, *397*
  preoperative treatment of, effects of, on
    anesthetic management, 1291
Vd. See *Volume of distribution (Vd)*.
Vecuronium, dose of, in children, 1056(t)
  effects of, physiologic, 1285(t)
  for abdominal surgery, 1113
  for burn surgery, 711(t)
  for renal transplantation, 1363
  in liver disease, 1344(t)
  selection of, factors in, 573
Vein(s). See also names of specific veins.
  normal anatomy of, on chest radiography,
    211–213, *214*
Vena cava, inferior, obstruction of,
    nephrectomy and, 1242
Venous access, for orthotopic liver
    transplantation, 1341
Venous air embolism, open prostatectomy and,
    1238
Venous cannula, in cardiopulmonary bypass,
    320
Venous catheterization, 544, 545, 545(t)
  site for, selection of, 544, 545, 546(t), 547(t)
Venous drainage, during pediatric
    cardiopulmonary bypass, 1151
Venous plexus, epidural, in pregnancy, 474,
    475
Venous return, 320
  impedance to, postoperative, and relative hy-
    povolemia, 89
Venous thrombosis, in orthopedic surgery,
    1263, 1264
  prevention of, 1263, 1264
  risk factors for, 1263
  in pregnant patient, during nonobstetric sur-
    gery, 1100
  perioperative, antibiotic prophylaxis for, 15,
    16(t)
  risk groups for, 16(t)
Venovenous bypass (VVB), in orthotopic liver
    transplantation, 1345, *1345*, 1346, *1346*,
    1346(t)
  effects on, of anhepatic phase, 1347, 1348
Ventilation, abnormal, 799–815
  signs and symptoms of, 800
    therapy for, 814, 815
  acid-base balance in, 734, *734*, 735, *735*,
    737, *737*, 738, 741
  alveolar, improvement in, larynx in, 449
  assessment of, in trauma, 992, 993
    instrumentation for, 338
  assisted, tracheal intubation for, 450
  bag-valve, 301, 302, *303*
  changes in, in pregnancy, 1083, 1084, *1084*
  control of, for postischemic/hypoxic brain
      injury, 166
    mechanisms of, 81
  dead space, in hypoxemia, 784
  difficult, after tracheal intubation, 945–948,
      945(t)
  disorders of, in hypoxemia, 783, 784, *784*
  during patient transport, equipment for, 426–
      428, 426(t), 427(t)
  effects on, of aging, 1071, 1072, 1072(t)
    of inhalation anesthesia, 610
  facemask. See *Facemask ventilation*.
  failure of, acute, after abdominal surgery,
      1132
    cardiogenic, correction of, 806

Ventilation *(Continued)*
  for anaphylaxis, 747
  for general anesthesia, failure of, 591
  for laryngoscopy, in children, 1062, *1063*
  for rapid-sequence induction, in emergency
      abdominal surgery, 1118
  in anesthetized patient, monitoring of, 335,
      336, *336*
  in battlefield surgery, 881
  in cardiopulmonary resuscitation, methods
      of, 837
  in conscious patients, monitoring of, 334,
      335
  in neonatal resuscitation, 1034
  in pulmonary edema, 972
  inappropriate, consequences of, 295
    management of, 295, 296
  intraoperative, for adult respiratory distress
      syndrome, with pulmonary edema, 976
    in neonates, 1023, 1024
      monitoring of, 68(t)
      standards for, 122, 123
  jet, translaryngeal, 1280, *1281*
  mandatory, intermittent, 148
    synchronized, 148
  manual, during one-lung anesthesia, 1206
    in inhalation anesthesia, 588, 589
  mechanical. See *Mechanical ventilation*.
  monitoring of, variables in, 334(t)
  muscles of, dysfunction of, and alveolar
      hypoventilation, 804, 805, *805*
    work of, increased, 809
  one-lung, considerations in, 1204, 1205
    in thoracoabdominal aneurysm manage-
      ment, 1218, 1218(t)
    inhalation anesthesia in, 612, *612*
  positive-pressure, urine output in, 385
  postoperative, 81–85, 81(t)–83(t), *82*, *83*,
      85(t)
    assessment of, 84
    failure of, increased carbon dioxide pro-
      duction in, 85
    reduction in, factors in, 81, 81(t), 82
  support of, during postanesthesia patient
      transport, 595, 596
    devices for, 595, *595*
    in burn surgery, 710
    in living-related donor harvesting, for
      renal transplantation, 1367, 1368
    in mediastinal lesions, 1207, *1207*
Ventilation/perfusion index, 790
Ventilation-perfusion mismatch, after
    abdominal surgery, 1131, 1132
  after intubation, causes of, 948–949
  carbon dioxide monitoring in, 351, 352
  in general anesthesia, 593, 594
  in geriatric patients, 1072
  in hypoxemia, 784, *784*
    postoperative, 79
  in scoliosis, 470
  with double-lumen tube use, 314, 315(t)
Ventilation/perfusion scanning, 1201
Ventilator(s), alarm of, activation of, during
    nasogastric intubation, 1117
  anesthesia, 276–297
  disorders of, in alveolar hypoventilation, 802,
      802(t), 803
  Dräger, 347
  for patient transport, 426, 426(t), 427, 427(t)
  malfunction of, in alveolar hyperventilation,
      808
  of anesthesia machine, hose of, elimination
      of, 296
  Ohmeda, 347, 427(t)
  use of, near magnetic resonance imaging
      scanner, 915

Ventilatory work, 799, 800, *800*, 800(t), 809–
    814
  airway obstruction in, 812, *812*, 813
  assessment of, 799
  carbon dioxide production in, 814
  causes of, 810–812, *811*
  clinical correlates of, 799, 800
  effects of, 809, 810, *810*, 810(t)
  increased dead space in, 814
  respiratory effort in, 799
  respiratory mechanics in, 800, 800(t)
Ventral hernia, repair of, anesthesia for, 1133
Ventricle(s), compliance of, in pulmonary
    artery pressure monitoring, 376, 376(t)
  dysfunction of, postoperative, factors in, 89,
      90
  function of, anesthetic effects on, assessment
      of, transesophageal echocardiography
      in, 383, 383(t)
    determination of, cardiac catheterization
      in, 1160
    in intraoperative hemodynamic stabiliza-
      tion, 689
  hypertrophy of, in aortic stenosis, 1161
  left. See *Left ventricle*.
  right. See *Right ventricle*.
Ventricular assist devices (VADs), for heart
    failure, after cardiopulmonary bypass,
    1184, 1184(t), 1185
  in cardiogenic shock, 676, 677
  left, right heart function with, 677
Ventricular asystole, treatment of, emergency,
    850, 851
Ventricular catheter, in intracranial pressure
    measurement, 394, *394*
Ventricular defibrillation, in cardiopulmonary
    resuscitation, 841–843, *843*
Ventricular depolarization, 362
Ventricular dysrhythmias, after
    cardiopulmonary bypass, 1185, 1186(t)
  electrocardiography in, 367
Ventricular fibrillation, during pediatric
    cardiopulmonary bypass, 1151
  electrocardiographic characteristics of, 367
  fine, treatment of, epinephrine in, 844, 845
  postoperative, 94
  treatment of, emergency, 841–843, *843*, 850
Ventricular premature contractions (VPCs),
    origination of, 92, 93, *93*
Ventricular septal rupture, in acute myocardial
    infarction, 677, 678
Ventricular tachycardia, electrocardiographic
    characteristics of, 367
  postoperative, 94
  treatment of, emergency, 843, *844*, 850
Ventriculography, nuclide, gated, in cardiac
    risk assessment, 133
  technique of, 905
VEPs (visual evoked potentials), 407
Verapamil, after heart transplantation, 1327
  drug interactions with, 645(t), 646(t), 652(t),
      655(t)
  for supraventricular tachycardia, after cardio-
      pulmonary bypass, 1187(t)
VerniTrol vaporizer, in battlefield surgery, 878,
    879, *879*
Versed, for acute pain, 242(t)
Vertebra(e), anatomy of, 458–460, *458–460*
  joints of, 459
  ligaments of, 459, *460*
  of lower cervical spine, 461
Vertebral arteries, anatomy of, 525
  location of, 500, 501
Vertebral body, 458, 459, *459*
Vertebral column. See *Spine*.
Vertebrectomy, 1297
Vicodin, for acute pain, 241(t)

Vincristine, for bone cancer, 1252
Viomycin, perioperative use of, 9(t)
Vision, disturbances of, in diabetes mellitus, 207
Vistaril, analgesic potential of, 244(t)
Visual analogue scale (VAS), in pain rating, 235, *235*
    use of, after thoracic surgery, 1208, *1208*
Visual evoked potentials (VEPs), 407
Vital signs, assessment of, frequency of, 339
    preanesthetic, 9, 10, *10*
    in children, 1038, 1039(t)
    in neonates, 1016(t)
    in pediatric trauma, 1004, 1004(t)
    in preoperative fluid deficit calculation, 722
Vitamin D, in calcium control, 202
Vocal cords, intubation of, failure of, 931, 932, *932*
    paralysis of, tracheal intubation and, 456
Voiding, necessity of, for outpatient discharge, 1401
Volume of distribution (Vd), changes in, effects of, on fat-soluble drugs, 565, *565*
        on water-soluble drugs, 565, *565*
    effects on, of protein binding, 565
    factors in, 643
    of intravenous anesthetic agents, 597, 597(t), 598
Vomiting, after outpatient surgery, treatment of, 1404, 1405(t)
    contrast agent reaction in, 902(t)
    control of, for cesarean section, 1093
    cricoid pressure release in, 1119
    in facemask airway obstruction, management of, 926
    postanesthesia, in children, 1061, 1062
    postoperative, 99, 100
        risk factors for, 99
    preoperative assessment for, 1404(t)
    treatment of, in pulmonary aspiration prevention, 87

Vomitus, aspiration of, during outpatient surgery, 1395
VPCs (ventricular premature contractions), origination of, 92, 93, *93*
V̇/Q̇ index (VQI), 790
VVB (venovenous bypass), in orthotopic liver transplantation, 1345, *1345*, 1346, *1346*, 1346(t)
    effects on, of anhepatic phase, 1347, 1348
VZV (varicella-zoster virus), epidemiology of, 862
    incidence of, 862

Wake-up test, 390, 391, 1253
    complications of, 391
    technique of, 391, 391(t)
    validity of, 391
Wall motion, abnormal, in preoperative cardiac risk assessment, 132, 133
Warfarin, drug interactions with, 644(t)–646(t)
    perioperative use of, 8
Wartime surgery, 874, 875
    advances made by, 874, 875
Waste, hospital. See *Hospital waste.*
    infectious, definition of, 115
    medical, definition of, 115
    solid, definition of, 115
Water, body, balance of, 715, *715*
    distribution of, 714, *714*
    imbalance of, in uremia, 183, 183(t)
Water solubility, in drug distribution, 643, 648
Water vapor, in anesthetic agent monitoring, 348, 349
WBC (white blood cell) count, in congenital heart disease assessment, 1142, 1143
Weaning, from cardiopulmonary bypass, 1179–1181, *1180*
    after heart transplantation, 1327–1329, 1328(t), 1329(t)

Weaning *(Continued)*
    after pediatric cardiovascular surgery, 1152, *1152*, 1152(t), 1153
    postoperative, criteria for, 149(t)
        from ventilatory support, in chronic obstructive pulmonary disease, 967
Weight, loss of, preoperative, benefits of, 144, 145
    normal, in children, 1038, 1039(t)
    preanesthetic evaluation of, 9
Wernicke's disease, 165
Western blot, in human immunodeficiency virus infection diagnosis, 855
Wheezing, intraoperative, causes of, 960(t)
    treatment of, 967, 967(t)
Whitacre needle, for spinal anesthesia, 518, *518*
White blood cell (WBC) count, in congenital heart disease assessment, 1142, 1143
White tube, 313
Whitehead blade, 304
Whitlow, herpetic, 862
Wisconsin solution, 1338, 1339(t)
Witness, expert, anesthesiologist as, 59, 60
    qualifications of, 60, 60(t)
Wound(s), burn, sepsis of, 707, 708
        treatment of, 707, 708
    surgical, infection of, antibiotic prophylaxis for, 15, *16*
    wartime, mortality of, 881(t)

x descent, 373
Xenon, radioactive, in cerebral blood flow measurement, 395, *395*

y descent, 374

Zone of coagulation, in burns, 699
Zone of hyperemia, in burns, 699
Zone of stasis, in burns, 699